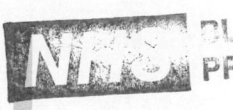
# Clinical Anesthesia Practice

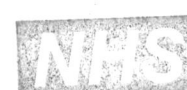

# Clinical Anesthesia Practice

## 2ND Edition

**Robert R. Kirby, M.D.**
Professor of Anesthesiology
University of Florida College of Medicine
Chief, Anesthesiology
North Florida/South Georgia Veterans Health System
Malcom Randall Veterans Affairs Medical Center
Gainesville, Florida

**Nikolaus Gravenstein, M.D.**
Jerome H. Modell Professor and Chairman
Department of Anesthesiology, and
Professor of Neurosurgery
University of Florida College of Medicine
Gainesville, Florida

**Emilio B. Lobato, M.D.**
Associate Professor of Anesthesiology
University of Florida College of Medicine
Assistant Chief of Anesthesiology
North Florida/South Georgia Veterans Health System
Malcom Randall Veterans Affairs Medical Center
Shands Hospital at the University of Florida
Gainesville, Florida

**Joachim S. Gravenstein, M.D., Dr.h.c.**
Graduate Research Professor Emeritus
Department of Anesthesiology
University of Florida College of Medicine
Gainesville, Florida

**W.B. SAUNDERS COMPANY**
*A Harcourt Health Sciences Company*
Philadelphia London New York St. Louis Sydney Toronto

**W.B. SAUNDERS COMPANY**
*A Harcourt Health Sciences Company*

The Curtis Center
Independence Square West
Philadelphia, Pennsylvania 19106

**Library of Congress Cataloging-in-Publication Data**

Clinical anesthesia practice/Robert R. Kirby . . . [et al.].—2nd ed.

p. ; cm.

Includes bibliographical references and index.

ISBN 0–7216–8566–8

1. Anesthesiology.    I. Kirby, Robert R.
   [DNLM: 1. Anesthesia. WO 200 C6412 2002]

RD81.C584 2002    617.9′6—dc21                    2001020604

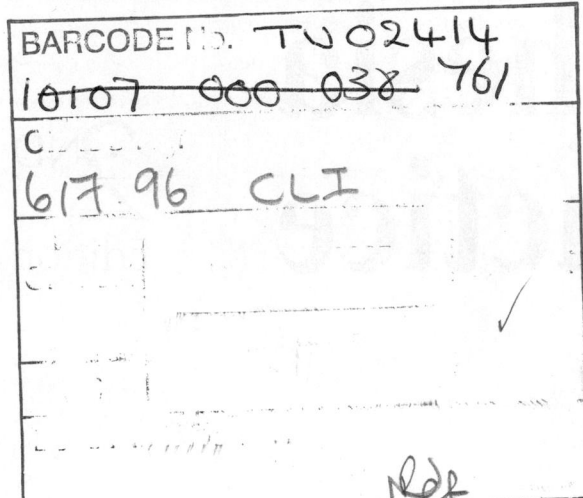

*Acquisitions Editor:*  Allan Ross
*Senior Developmental Editor:*  Ann Ruzycka
*Manuscript Editor:*  Amy L. Cannon
*Production Manager:*  Guy Barber
*Senior Illustration Specialist:*  Walt Verbitski

CLINICAL ANESTHESIA PRACTICE                                ISBN 0–7216–8566–8

Printed in the United States of America.

Last digit is the print number:     9   8   7   6   5   4   3   2   1

*Haven M. Perkins, M.D., was the first resident in Anesthesiology at the University of Florida College of Medicine. He received his training under J. S. Gravenstein, M.D., one of the editors of this edition. "Perk" had already been trained as a general surgeon and a thoracic and cardiovascular surgeon before he embarked on his new career in the fledgling anesthesiology department in Gainesville. He never left, as a result of which he participated in more than 30 years' training of anesthesiology residents. For many years, he "ran the VA," and he was single-handedly responsible for making anesthesiology the most popular rotation through the mid-1990s. Every woman was "daughter" to him. Some felt he used this term because he wasn't too good with names. We think it was simply a reflection of his fatherly approach (he never forgot the men's names).*

*Perk was a skilled clinician and a great teacher. Whenever you got into trouble, you always felt better when he walked into the room. He was a rarity in that he was liked and respected by the surgeons, and we never saw him engaged in an argument with them. He simply looked at them, perhaps with a slight frown, and the problem was resolved. In June 2000, he died, but his legacy continues here and in all the far-flung places where the residents he trained now practice. He is missed, but his memory will always be cherished.*

ROBERT R. KIRBY, M.D.

# Contributors

**Patricia L. Abbitt, M.D.**
Professor of Radiology, Department of Radiology, University of Florida College of Medicine, Gainesville, Florida
*Radiology Consultation*

**John G. Augoustides, M.D.**
Assistant Professor of Anesthesia, University of Pennsylvania School of Medicine; Staff, Department of Anesthesia, University of Pennsylvania Health System, Philadelphia, Pennsylvania
*Surgery of the Descending Thoracic Aorta*

**R. Dennis Bastron, M.D.**
Professor of Anesthesiology and Professor and Head, Department of Humanities in Medicine, Texas A&M University System Health Sciences Center, Texas A&M College of Medicine; Senior Staff Anesthesiologist, Scott and White Memorial Hospital and Clinic, Temple, Texas
*Nephrology Consultation*

**Jerry J. Berger, M.D.**
Associate Professor of Anesthesiology, Department of Anesthesiology, University of Florida College of Medicine; Director, Acute Pain Service, Shands Hospital at the University of Florida, Gainesville, Florida
*Genitourinary Surgery*

**David R. Bevan, M.D., M.A., M.B., M.R.C.P., F.R.C.P.C., F.R.C.A.**
Professor, Department of Anesthesia, University of Toronto; Anesthesiologist-in-Chief, University Health Network and Mount Sinai Hospital, Toronto, Ontario, Canada
*Clinical Applications of Acid-Base Chemistry and Physiology*

**Mark L. Blas, M.D.**
Assistant Professor of Anesthesiology, Department of Anesthesiology, University of Florida College of Medicine; Staff Anesthesiologist, North Florida/South Georgia Veterans Health System, Malcom Randall Veterans Affairs Medical Center, Gainesville, Florida
*Heart and Lung Transplantation*

**Monica Botero, M.D.**
Assistant Professor of Anesthesiology, Department of Anesthesiology, University of Florida College of Medicine; Staff Anesthesiologist, North Florida/South Georgia Veterans Health System, Malcom Randall Veterans Affairs Medical Center, Gainesville, Florida
*Anesthesia for Adult Cardiovascular Surgery*

**David L. Brown, M.D.**
Professor of Anesthesia, Department of Anesthesia, University of Iowa; Professor and Head, Department of Anesthesia, University of Iowa Health Care, Iowa City, Iowa
*Risk and Outcome Analysis: Myths and Truths; Regional Anesthesia*

**Brian A. Broznick, C.T.P.C.**
President/CEO, Center for Organ Recovery and Education, Pittsburgh, Pennsylvania
*Overview of Organ Transplantation*

**Scott J. Bullard, M.D.**
Staff Anesthesiologist, Trinity Anesthesia Associates, Trinity Hospital, Minot, North Dakota
*Hypoxemia; Abnormal Ventilation*

**Roy D. Cane, M.D.**
Professor and Vice Chair, Department of Anesthesiology, Northwestern University Medical School, Chicago, Illinois
*Hypoxemia; Abnormal Ventilation*

**Lawrence J. Caruso, M.D.**
Assistant Professor of Anesthesiology, Department of Anesthesiology, University of Florida College of Medicine, Gainesville, Florida
*Fluids, Electrolytes, Blood, and Blood Substitutes*

**John Casto, M.D.**
Clinical Instructor, Department of Anesthesiology, West Virginia University Hospital School of Medicine; Clinical Instructor, Department of Anesthesiology, West Virginia University Hospital, Morgantown, West Virginia
*Anesthesia for Mass Casualty and Disaster Situations*

## Donald Caton, M.D.

Professor of Anesthesiology, Department of Anesthesiology; Professor of Obstetrics and Gynecology, Department of Obstetrics and Gynecology, University of Florida College of Medicine, Gainesville, Florida

*The Obstetric Patient*

## Jesse L. Chai, M.D.

Department of Radiology, Brigham and Women's Hospital, Boston, Massachusetts

*Radiology Consultation*

## David P. Ciceri, M.D.

Assistant Professor of Anesthesiology; Chief, Division of Critical Care, Department of Anesthesiology; Co-Director, Surgical Intensive Care Unit, Scott and White Memorial Hospital, Temple, Texas

*Nephrology Consultation*

## Jerry A. Cohen, M.D.

Associate Professor of Anesthesiology, Department of Anesthesiology, University of Florida College of Medicine; Chief, Liver Transplant Anesthesia, Shands Hospital at the University of Florida, Gainesville, Florida

*Quality Assurance in Anesthesiology*

## E. Stuart Cornett, M.D.

Chief Resident, West Virginia University School of Medicine, Morgantown, West Virginia

*Anesthesia for Mass Casualty and Disaster Situations*

## Meredith J. Craigie, M.B.B.S., F.A.N.Z.C.A.

Senior Consultant, Department of Paediatric Anaesthesia, Women's and Children's Hospital, North Adelaide, Australia

*Pain Management Consultation in Pediatric Patients*

## Edward T. Crosby, M.D.

Professor, University of Ottawa; Consultant, Department of Anesthesiology, Ottawa Hospital—General Campus, Ottawa, Ontario, Canada

*The Spine*

## Joseph M. Darby, M.D.

Associate Professor of Critical Care Medicine, University of Pittsburgh School of Medicine; Medical Director of Trauma and ICU, UPMC Presbyterian University Hospital, Pittsburgh, Pennsylvania

*Overview of Organ Transplantation*

## Laurie K. Davies, M.D.

Associate Professor of Anesthesiology, Department of Anesthesiology, University of Florida College of Medicine; Chief, Pediatric Cardiothoracic Anesthesia, Shands Hospital at the University of Florida, Gainesville, Florida

*Anesthesia for Pediatric Cardiovascular Surgery*

## Donn H. Dennis, M.D.

Associate Professor of Anesthesiology and Pharmacology and Experimental Therapeutics, University of Florida College of Medicine, Gainesville, Florida

*Laparoscopic Procedures*

## Cheryl L. Dixon, M.D.

Staff Anesthesiologist, Anesthesia Consultants, P.A., Jacksonville, Florida

*Pain Management Consultation in Adult Patients*

## Eddy N. Duncan, M.D.

Staff Anesthesiologist, Biloxi Regional Medical Center, Biloxi, Mississippi

*Pain Management Consultation in Adult Patients*

## Thomas J. Ebert, M.D., Ph.D.

Professor of Anesthesiology and Adjunct Professor of Physiology, Medical College of Wisconsin; Staff Anesthesiologist, Veterans Affairs Medical Center, Milwaukee, Wisconsin

*Autonomic Nervous System and Sympathetic Blockade*

## Roderic G. Eckenhoff, M.D.

Austin Lamont Professor of Anesthesia, University of Pennsylvania; Director of Research, Department of Anesthesia, Hospital of the University of Pennsylvania, Philadelphia, Pennsylvania

*Basic Pharmacologic Applications in Anesthesia*

## James Eckhart, A.B., J.D.

Practicing Lawyer and Partner, Kubicki Draper P.A., Miami; Chief Defense Counsel, Anesthesiologists' Professional Assurance Company, Coral Gables, Florida

*Medicolegal Issues and Concerns*

## Jay S. Ellis, M.D.

Clinical Associate Professor, University of Texas Health Science Center at San Antonio, San Antonio; Chief Military Consultant for Anesthesiology to the Air Force Surgeon General, Wilford Hall Medical Center, Lackland AFB, Texas

*Local Anesthetics*

## F. Kayser Enneking, M.D.

Associate Professor of Anesthesiology, Department of Anesthesiology, University of Florida College of Medicine; Medical Director, Florida Surgical Center, Gainesville, Florida

*Anesthesia for Orthopedic Surgery*

## Tammy Y. Euliano, M.D.

Assistant Professor of Anesthesiology, Department of Anesthesiology, University of Florida College of Medicine; Chief, Obstetric Anesthesia, Shands Hospital at the University of Florida, Gainesville, Florida

*The Obstetric Patient*

## Jeffrey M. Feldman, M.D., M.S.E.

Adjunct Associate Professor of Anesthesiology, MCP/Hahnemann School of Medicine, Philadelphia, Pennsylvania; Anesthesiologist, Virtua Memorial Hospital, Mount Holly, New Jersey; Consulting Medical Director, Draeger Medical Incorporated, Telford, Pennsylvania

*The Anesthetic Record*

## Lynne Ferrari, M.D.

Associate Professor, Anesthesiology, Harvard Medical School; Medical Director, Perioperative Services, The Children's Hospital, Boston, Massachusetts

*Otolaryngologic and Maxillofacial Surgery*

## Michael A. Frölich, M.D., D.E.A.A.

Assistant Professor of Anesthesiology, Department of Anesthesiology, University of Florida College of Medicine; Chief, Division of Obstetric Anesthesiology, Shands Hospital at the University of Florida, Gainesville, Florida

*Nonobstetric Surgery in the Pregnant Patient*

## Andrea Gabrielli, M.D.

Assistant Professor of Anesthesiology, Department of Anesthesiology, University of Florida College of Medicine; Medical Director, Hyperbaric Chamber, Shands Hospital at the University of Florida, Gainesville, Florida

*Management of the Difficult Airway*

## Phillip Gaukroger, M.B.B.S., F.A.N.Z.C.A.

Clinical Lecturer, University of Adelaide; Senior Consultant, Paediatric Anaesthesia, Women's and Children's Hospital, North Adelaide, Australia

*Pain Management Consultation in Pediatric Patients*

## Gordon L. Gibby, M.D.

Associate Professor of Anesthesiology, Department of Anesthesiology, University of Florida College of Medicine, Gainesville, Florida

*Radiologic Procedures, Computed Tomography Scans, Magnetic Resonance Imaging, and Radiation Therapy*

## Hugh C. Gilbert, M.D.

Associate Professor, Department of Anesthesiology, Northwestern University, Chicago; Senior Attending Physician, Evanston/Northwestern Health Care, Evanston Hospital, Evanston, Illinois

*Cardiovascular Monitoring*

## Julian M. Goldman, M.D.

Associate Professor of Anesthesiology, University of Colorado School of Medicine, Denver, Colorado; Vice President of Medical Affairs, Masimo Corporation, Irvine, California

*Respiratory Monitoring*

## Michael L. Good, M.D.

Professor of Anesthesiology, Department of Anesthesiology, University of Florida College of Medicine; Chief of Staff, North Florida/South Georgia Veterans Health System, Malcom Randall Veterans Affairs Medical Center, Gainesville, Florida

*The Anesthesia Machine, Anesthesia Ventilator, Breathing Circuit, and Scavenging System*

## Salvatore R. Goodwin, M.D.

Chairman, Department of Anesthesiology and Critical Care, Nemours Children's Clinic, Jacksonville, Florida

*Drug Interactions*

## Alexander W. Gotta, M.D.

Professor Emeritus of Anesthesiology, State University of New York, Downstate Medical Center, Brooklyn, New York

*Otolaryngologic and Maxillofacial Surgery*

## Christopher M. Grande, M.D., M.P.H.

Executive Director, International Trauma Anesthesia and Critical Care Society, Baltimore, Maryland; Lecturer in Anesthesiology, Harvard Medical School and Staff Anesthesiologist, Department of Anesthesiology, Perioperative and Pain Medicine, Brigham and Women's Hospital, Boston, Massachusetts; Professor, Department of Anesthesiology, Jon C. Moore Trauma Center, Robert C. Byrd Health Sciences Center, West Virginia University School of Medicine, Morgantown, West Virginia; Professor and Special Consultant for Trauma, Department of Anesthesiology, Erie County Medical Center, SUNY Buffalo School of Medicine, Buffalo, New York

*Anesthesia for Mass Casualty and Disaster Situations*

## Dietrich Gravenstein, M.D.

Assistant Professor of Anesthesiology, Department of Anesthesiology, University of Florida College of Medicine, Gainesville, Florida

*Respiratory Monitoring*

## Joachim S. Gravenstein, M.D., Dr.h.c.

Graduate Research Professor Emeritus, Department of Anesthesiology, University of Florida College of Medicine, Gainesville, Florida

*Critical Incident Management; Introduction to Monitoring: Clinical Monitoring; General Anesthesia: Induction, Maintenance, and Emergence*

## Nikolaus Gravenstein, M.D.

Jerome H. Modell Professor and Chairman, Department of Anesthesiology, and Professor of Neurosurgery, University of Florida College of Medicine, Gainesville, Florida

*Vascular Access; Positioning the Surgical Patient*

## Sergio Gregoretti, M.D.

Professor of Anesthesiology, Department of Anesthesiology, University of Alabama at Birmingham, Birmingham, Alabama

*Abdominal Surgery*

## Ake Grenvik, M.D., Ph.D.

Distinguished Service Professor of Critical Care Medicine, University of Pittsburgh School of Medicine, Pittsburgh, Pennsylvania
*Overview of Organ Transplantation*

## Gregory M. Gullahorn, M.D.

Clinical Instructor, Anesthesiology and Critical Care Medicine, Naval Medical Center and University of California at San Diego; Staff Anesthesiologist, Scripps Clinic and Research Foundation, Green Hospital, La Jolla, California
*Monitoring During Patient Transport*

## Maximilian W. B. Hartmannsgruber, M.D., F.C.C.M.

Assistant Professor of Anesthesiology, Yale University School of Medicine, New Haven, Connecticut
*Thermal Injuries: Pathophysiology and Anesthetic Considerations*

## Stephen O. Heard, M.D.

Professor of Anesthesiology and Surgery, University of Massachusetts Medical School; Executive Vice-Chair and Co-Director, Surgical Intensive Care Units, University of Massachusetts Memorial Medical Center, Worcester, Massachusetts
*Preanesthetic Evaluation*

## Jan C. Horrow, M.D.

Clinical Professor, Anesthesiology, MCP-Hahnemann University, Philadelphia; Medical Director, Clinical Research, Astrazeneca LP, Wayne, Pennsylvania
*Electrical Safety*

## Christopher F. James, M.D.

Assistant Professor of Anesthesiology, Mayo Graduate School, Jacksonville; Courtesy Visiting Associate Professor of Anesthesiology, University of Florida, Gainesville; Director, Obstetric Anesthesia, Mayo St. Luke's Hospital and Mayo Clinic, Jacksonville, Florida
*Nonobstetric Surgery in the Pregnant Patient*

## Gregory M. Janelle, M.D.

Assistant Professor of Anesthesiology, Director of Perioperative Echocardiography, Department of Anesthesiology, University of Florida College of Medicine, Gainesville, Florida
*Anesthesia for Adult Cardiovascular Surgery*

## Ilkka Kalli, M.B.A., M.D., Ph.D.

Associate Professor of Anesthesiology, Department of Anesthesiology, University of Florida College of Medicine, Gainesville, Florida; Senior Staff Anesthesiologist, Department of Anesthesiology and Intensive Care Medicine, Helsinki University Central Hospital; Medical Advisor, Datex-Ohmeda Division, Instrumentarium Corporation, Helsinki, Finland
*Neuromuscular Block Monitoring*

## Robert E. Kettler, M.D.

Associate Professor of Anesthesiology, Medical College of Wisconsin; Associate Professor of Anesthesiology, Froedtert Memorial Lutheran Hospital–East, Milwaukee, Wisconsin
*Autonomic Nervous System and Sympathetic Blockade*

## Robert R. Kirby, M.D.

Professor of Anesthesiology, University of Florida College of Medicine; Chief, Anesthesiology, North Florida/South Georgia Veterans Health System, Malcom Randall Veterans Affairs Medical Center, Gainesville, Florida
*Medicolegal Issues and Concerns; General Anesthesia: Induction, Maintenance, and Emergence; Fluids, Electrolytes, Blood, and Blood Substitutes; Cardiopulmonary Resuscitation*

## Samsun Lampotang, Ph.D.

Associate Professor of Anesthesiology, Department of Anesthesiology; Affiliate Associate Professor of Mechanical Engineering and Affiliate Associate Professor of Electrical and Computer Engineering, University of Florida College of Medicine, Gainesville, Florida
*The Anesthesia Machine, Anesthesia Ventilator, Breathing Circuit, and Scavenging System*

## Paul Langevin, M.D.

Associate Professor of Anesthesiology, Yale University School of Medicine; Attending Staff in Anesthesiology and Critical Care, VA Connecticut Health Care System, West Haven, Connecticut
*Pulmonary Consultation; Occupational Hazards in the Operating Room*

## A. Joseph Layon, M.D.

Professor of Anesthesiology, Surgery, and Medicine, University of Florida College of Medicine; Medical Director, Gainesville Fire Rescue Service, Gainesville, Florida
*Thermal Injuries: Pathophysiology and Anesthetic Considerations; Occupational Hazards in the Operating Room; Management of the Difficult Airway*

## Thomas W. Lebert II, M.D.

Staff Anesthesiologist, St. Joseph's Hospital; Managing Partner, Physician Specialists in Anesthesia, P.C., Atlanta, Georgia
*Nonobstetric Surgery in the Pregnant Patient*

## Jerrold H. Levy, M.D.

Professor of Anesthesiology, Emory University School of Medicine; Director, Cardiothoracic Anesthesiology, Emory Healthcare, Atlanta, Georgia
*Allergy and Immunology*

## Monte Lichtiger, M.D.

Director and Chairman, Claims Management, Anesthesiologists' Professional Assurance Company, Coral Gables, Florida
*Medicolegal Issues and Concerns*

## Richard Lilly, Jr., B.A., M.D.

Professor and Chairman, Department of Anesthesiology, University of Connecticut School of Medicine, Farmington; Director of Anesthesiology, Hartford Hospital, Hartford, Connecticut

*Temperature Management and Aberrations*

## Marian C. Limacher, M.D.

Professor of Medicine, Division of Cardiovascular Medicine, University of Florida College of Medicine, Gainesville, Florida

*Cardiology Consultation*

## Emilio B. Lobato, M.D.

Associate Professor of Anesthesiology, University of Florida College of Medicine; Assistant Chief of Anesthesiology, North Florida/South Georgia Veterans Health System, Malcom Randall Veterans Affairs Medical Center; Director, Cardiac Anesthesia, Shands Hospital at the University of Florida, Gainesville, Florida

*Vascular Access; Anesthesia for Adult Cardiovascular Surgery; Heart and Lung Transplantation*

## Martin J. London, M.D.

Professor of Clinical Anesthesia, University of California, San Francisco; Attending Anesthesiologist, San Francisco Veterans Affairs Medical Center, San Francisco, California

*Myocardial Ischemia and Dysfunction*

## Salvatore LoPalo, C.R.N.A., M.S., M.A.

Associate in Anesthesiology, Department of Anesthesiology, University of Florida College of Medicine; Administrative Officer, Anesthesiology Service, North Florida/South Georgia Veterans Health System, Malcom Randall Veterans Affairs Medical Center, Gainesville, Florida

*Occupational Hazards in the Operating Room*

## Anne C. P. Lui, M.Sc., M.D., F.R.C.P.C.

Assistant Professor, University of Ottawa; Active Attending Staff, The Ottawa Hospitals, Civic Campus, Ottawa, Ontario, Canada

*The Spine*

## Michael E. Mahla, M.D.

Professor of Anesthesiology and Neurosurgery, University of Florida College of Medicine, Gainesville, Florida

*Monitoring the Nervous System; Neurologic Surgery*

## Timothy W. Martin, M.D., M.B.A.

Associate Professor of Anesthesiology, University of Arkansas for Medical Sciences; Chief, Division of Pediatric Anesthesia, Arkansas Children's Hospital, Little Rock, Arkansas

*The Neonate; The Pediatric Patient*

## James B. Matthews III, J.D.

Partner, Matthews & Steel, Atlanta, Georgia

*Medicolegal Issues and Concerns*

## Roger S. Mecca, M.D.

Chairman, Department of Anesthesiology, and Executive Director, Surgical Services, Danbury Hospital, Danbury, Connecticut

*Postanesthesia Recovery*

## Richard J. Melker, M.D., Ph.D.

Professor of Anesthesiology, Pediatrics, and Biomedical Engineering, University of Florida College of Medicine, Gainesville, Florida

*Airway Devices and Their Application; Cardiopulmonary Resuscitation*

## Luis G. Michelsen, M.D.

Associate Professor, Department of Anesthesiology, Division of Cardiothoracic Anesthesia and Critical Care, Emory University School of Medicine, Atlanta, Georgia

*Cardiopulmonary Bypass*

## Terri G. Monk, M.D.

Professor of Anesthesiology, Department of Anesthesiology, University of Florida College of Medicine, Gainesville, Florida

*Outpatient Anesthesia*

## Sreenivasa S. Moorthy, M.B.B.S., M.D.

Professor of Anesthesia, Indiana University Medical Center; Chief, Anesthesia Department, Roudebush Veterans Affairs Medical Center, Indianapolis, Indiana

*Anesthesia for Patients With Bronchial Asthma or Chronic Obstructive Lung Disease*

## Robert C. Morell, M.D.

Associate Professor of Anesthesiology and Medical Director, Preoperative Assessment Center, Wake Forest University School of Medicine, Winston-Salem, North Carolina

*Positioning the Surgical Patient*

## Timothy E. Morey, M.D.

Assistant Professor of Anesthesiology, University of Florida College of Medicine, Gainesville, Florida

*Laparoscopic Procedures*

## Thomas C. Mort, M.D.

Clinical Associate of Anesthesiology and Associate Director, Surgical Intensive Care Unit, Hartford Hospital; Associate Professor of Surgery, University of Connecticut School of Medicine, Hartford, Connecticut

*Temperature Management and Aberrations*

## David W. Mozingo, M.D.

Associate Professor of Surgery and Anesthesiology, University of Florida College of Medicine; Director, Shands Burn Center at the University of Florida, Gainesville, Florida

*Thermal Injuries: Pathophysiology and Anesthetic Considerations*

## Antoni M. Nejman, M.D.

Assistant Professor of Anesthesia, University of Miami School of Medicine; Director, Cardiac Surgical Intensive Care, Jackson Memorial Hospital, Miami Beach, Florida
*Muscle Relaxants; Sedation and Analgesia*

## Scott H. Norwood, M.D.

Clinical Associate Professor, University of Texas Health Science Center–Houston; Director, Trauma Services, East Texas Medical Center, Tyler, Texas
*Trauma and Shock*

## Azriel Perel, M.D.

Professor and Chairman, Department of Anesthesiology and Intensive Care, Sheba Medical Center, Tel Aviv University, Tel-Hashomer, Israel
*Pulmonary Edema*

## Carl E. Ravin, M.D.

Professor and Chairman, Department of Radiology, Duke University Medical Center, Durham, North Carolina
*Radiology Consultation*

## Richard J. Rogers, M.D., Ph.D.

Assistant Professor of Anesthesiology, Department of Anesthesiology, University of Florida College of Medicine; Associate Medical Director, Florida Surgical Center, Gainesville, Florida
*Intravenous Anesthetic Agents*

## Kathryn Rouine-Rapp, M.D.

Associate Professor of Clinical Anesthesia, Department of Anesthesia, University of California School of Medicine, San Francisco, California
*Myocardial Ischemia and Dysfunction*

## Ray Roy, Ph.D., M.D.

Professor and Chair, Department of Anesthesiology, Wake Forest University School of Medicine, Winston-Salem, North Carolina
*The Geriatric Patient*

## William R. Runciman, M.D.

Professor and Head, Departments of Anaesthesia and Intensive Care, Royal Adelaide Hospital, Adelaide, Australia
*Critical Incident Management*

## Mark T. Scarborough, M.D.

Associate Professor, Department of Orthopedic Surgery and Rehabilitation, University of Florida College of Medicine, Gainesville, Florida
*Anesthesia for Orthopedic Surgery*

## Eran Segal, M.D.

Director, General Intensive Care Unit, Department of Anesthesiology and Intensive Care, Sheba Medical Center, Sackler School of Medicine, Tel Aviv, Israel
*Pulmonary Edema*

## Michael Seropian, M.D., F.R.C.P.C.

Assistant Professor of Anesthesiology and Pediatrics, Doernbecher Children's Hospital, Oregon Health Sciences University, Portland, Oregon
*Inhalation Agents*

## Avner Sidi, M.D.

Associate Professor of Anesthesiology, University of Florida College of Medicine, Gainesville, Florida; Associate Professor, Tel Aviv University, Tel Aviv, Israel; Vice Chairman and Head of PACU, Anesthesiology Department, The Chaim Sheba Medical Center, Tel-Hashomer, Israel
*Orthotopic Liver Transplantation; Renal Transplantation*

## Ian Smith, B.Sc., M.B.B.S., F.R.C.A., M.D.

Senior Lecturer in Anaesthesia, Keele University, Staffordshire, United Kingdom; Consultant Anaesthetist, North Staffordshire Hospital, Stoke-on-Trent, United Kingdom
*Outpatient Anesthesia*

## Dale E. Solomon, M.D.

Staff Anesthesiologist, San Antonio Area Hospitals, San Antonio, Texas
*Neurologic Consultation*

## Diane Solomon, M.D.

Associate Professor of Neurology, University of Texas Health Science Center at San Antonio, San Antonio; Chief of Neurology, South Texas VA Hospital System, Kerrville, Texas
*Neurologic Consultation*

## Jennifer E. Souders, M.D.

Assistant Professor, Department of Anesthesiology, University of Washington and Veterans Medical Center, Puget Sound Health Care System, Seattle, Washington
*Respiratory Monitoring*

## Donald S. Stevens, M.D.

Assistant Professor of Anesthesiology, University of Massachusetts Medical School, Worcester; Medical Director, Center for Pain Management, Marlborough Hospital, Marlborough, Massachusetts
*Preanesthetic Evaluation*

## Wendell C. Stevens, M.D.

Professor Emeritus of Anesthesiology, Oregon Health Sciences University; Volunteer, Clinical Faculty, Department of Anesthesiology, Oregon Health Sciences University Hospital; Anesthesiology Staff, Veterans Administration Medical Center, Portland, Oregon
*Inhalation Agents*

## Joanne M. Stoner, M.D.

Staff Anesthesiologist, Kosair Children's Hospital; Clinical Assistant Professor, Department of Anesthesiology, University of Louisville, Louisville, Kentucky
*The Neonate; The Pediatric Patient*

**Susan Stuart, R.N.**

Center for Organ Recovery and Education, Pittsburgh, Pennsylvania
*Overview of Organ Transplantation*

**Cheri A. Sulek, M.D.**

Associate Professor of Anesthesiology, Department of Anesthesiology, University of Florida College of Medicine; Staff Anesthesiologist, North Florida/South Georgia Veterans Health System, Malcom Randall Veterans Affairs Medical Center, Gainesville, Florida
*Intracranial Pressure*

**Colleen A. Sullivan, M.B., Ch.B.**

Retired Clinical Professor of Anesthesiology, State University of New York, Downstate Medical Center, Brooklyn, New York
*Otolaryngologic and Maxillofacial Surgery*

**Jerry J. Tomasovic, M.D.**

Clinical Professor of Pediatrics, University of Texas Health Science Center at San Antonio; Pediatric Neurologist, Texas Association of Pediatric Neurology, Texas Neurosciences Institute, San Antonio, Texas
*Neurologic Consultation*

**Felipe Urdaneta, M.D.**

Assistant Professor of Anesthesiology, Department of Anesthesiology, University of Florida College of Medicine, Gainesville, Florida
*Vascular Access*

**Van L. Vallina, M.D.**

Trauma Surgeon, East Texas Medical Center, Tyler, Texas
*Trauma and Shock*

**Leroy D. Vandam, Ph.B., M.D., M.A. (Hon.)**

Professor of Anesthesia Emeritus, Harvard Medical School; Chairman of Anaesthesia Emeritus, Brigham and Women's Hospital, Boston, Massachusetts
*Clinically Relevant Airway Anatomy*

**Mark Veerman, Pharm.D.**

Clinical Associate Professor, University of Florida College of Pharmacy; Department of Pharmacy, Shands Hospital at the University of Florida, Gainesville, Florida
*Drug Interactions*

**Jeffrey S. Vender, M.D., F.C.C.M.**

Professor and Associate Chairman, Department of Anesthesiology, Northwestern University Medical School, Chicago; Chairman, Department of Anesthesiology, and Director, Critical Care Services, Evanston Northwestern Healthcare, Evanston, Illinois
*Cardiovascular Monitoring*

**Walter W. Virkus, M.D.**

Assistant Professor, Department of Orthopedic Surgery, Rush Medical College, Chicago, Illinois
*Anesthesia for Orthopedic Surgery*

**Lisette Volckmar, B.A., M.D.**

Former Instructor, Hospital of the University of Pennsylvania, Philadelphia, Pennsylvania; Staff Attending, Vanguard Anesthesia Associates
*Basic Pharmacologic Applications in Anesthesia*

**Stuart J. Weiss, Ph.D., M.D.**

Associate Professor of Anesthesia, Department of Anesthesia, University of Pennsylvania School of Medicine; Director of Intraoperative Echocardiographic Services, Hospital of the University of Pennsylvania, Philadelphia, Pennsylvania
*Surgery of the Descending Thoracic Aorta*

**Sno E. White, M.D.**

Clinical Assistant Professor of Anesthesiology, Department of Anesthesiology, University of Florida College of Medicine, Gainesville, Florida
*The Preoperative Visit and Premedication*

**William C. Wilson, M.D., M.A.**

Associate Clinical Professor, Anesthesiology and Critical Care Medicine, University of California at San Diego Medical Center, San Diego, California
*Anesthetic Considerations for Thoracic Surgery*

**Susan Stuart, R.N.**

**Cheri A. Sulek, M.D.**

**Colleen A. Sullivan, M.E., Ch.B.**

**Jerry F. Tomasovic, M.D.**

**Felipe Urdaneta, M.D.**

**Van L. Valdez, M.D.**

**Leroy C. Vandam, Ph.D., M.D., M.A. (Hon)**

**Mark Wetzman, Pharm.D.**

**Jeffrey S. Vender, M.D., F.C.C.M.**

**Walter W. Virkus, M.D.**

**Lisette Whitehead, B.A., M.D.**

**Stuart I. Weiss, Ph.D., M.D.**

**Scott Willis, M.D.**

**William C. Wilson, M.D., M.A.**

# Preface

In 1994, when the first edition of this textbook was published, we wrote in the preface, "Why . . . in the face of apparent plenty [of anesthesiology texts], should this textbook have been conceived, let alone published?" In 2001, the same question is still relevant because even more reference sources are available now than was the case 7 years ago. Originally, we felt a book that focused on the clinically relevant aspects of anesthesiology practice could be of value to the resident-in-training and to the practitioner faced with an unusual case, the fine points of which might not be immediately apparent. The format was "question and answer," much like case discussion conferences that are so popular in training programs. No pretense was made that this approach was encyclopedic; rather, it was pragmatic, with pearls being slipped into the discussion from time to time by the authors, who were chosen as much for their clinical expertise as for their academic prowess.

Since 1994 we continually have assessed whether we accomplished our goal. Based upon some of the published reviews that examined our efforts, the answer appeared to be "yes"—at least in part. Discussions with some of our most vociferous critics (our in-training residents) seemed to substantiate this viewpoint. And yet it was clear to us that some rather significant shortcomings were present. One example: Although we had a rather extensive chapter on the monitoring and assessment of neuromuscular blockade, we did not have a chapter on neuromuscular blocking agents. That oversight has been corrected in this edition. A very discerning critic reported that, "On the down side there is no intensive care section . . . and some of the diagrams and photographs are poorly reproduced. . . ." In the planning stages, we had debated the pros and cons of devoting a section of the book to critical care medicine because one of us (RRK) has devoted the majority of his career to this subspecialty area; the American Board of Anesthesiology requires training in this area; and a certificate of added qualification is awarded to those anesthesiologists who successfully complete fellowship training in critical care and pass an examination. In the end, we felt that the amount of critical care subject material that could be presented in a volume of limited size would be insufficient for these purposes. We still feel that way and, therefore, have not added a section to the second edition.

In most respects, we have adhered to the concepts and formatting of the first edition. The question and answer style seems to be very popular in focusing study, and the emphasis on clinical aspects of everyday problems has been well received. One glaring oversight in the first edition was the use of "an incredible potpourri of measurement units that would torment anyone trying to prepare for examination. For example, one author, when discussing gas pressures talks about pounds per square inch, millimeters of mercury, and centimeters of water almost without drawing breath." The fault, of course, did not reside with the author, but with us, the editors, for not rectifying the situation before the chapter appeared in print. A major effort has been expended to bring some order out of the chaos. In trying to "keep up with the times," we have deleted a few chapters that perhaps are not as relevant as they seemed in the early 1990s, and we have added a few that represent significant departures from the traditional practice of anesthesiology.

As was true with the first edition, this one is not encyclopedic, but we believe it is useful clinically, and we hope it is relevant to the evolving and ever-changing scope of our specialty. Only the discerning reader will be able to judge whether we have been successful. Dr. Julius Comroe once wrote that he welcomed suggestions for additional material for a new edition of a previous textbook, as long as the suggestion contained a recommendation for the deletion of an equal amount! We echo his sentiments.

As has so often been the case, our thanks (grudgingly) are extended to Lew Reines, former President and CEO of The W.B. Saunders Company. Somehow, he always managed to persuade us to take on yet another authoring-editing-publishing task, despite our strong avowal not to do so. Thanks also to Allan Ross, one of Lew's right-hand men, who spearheaded this effort. Hope Olivo, who has been the true power behind the successful completion of our previous publishing efforts, deserves special accolades. Without her, none of this ever would happen!

ROBERT R. KIRBY, M.D.
NIKOLAUS GRAVENSTEIN, M.D.
EMILIO B. LOBATO, M.D.
JOACHIM S. GRAVENSTEIN, M.D.

# Preface to the First Edition

In the 1960s, when one of us (RRK) received his training, the number of anesthesiology textbooks was limited. Authors such as Wylie, Churchill-Davidson, Dripps, Eckenhoff, Vandam, Adriani, Cullen, Moore, Lee, and Collins were well known to practicing anesthesiologists and residents alike. By the early 1980s, when NG was in training, an explosion in anesthesia publishing was already underway. New names—Miller, Stoelting, Gregory, Orkin, Cooperman, Cousins, Blitt, Martin, Shnider, Barash, Benumof, Kaplan, and others too numerous to mention—became as well known as their predecessors. Their books were comprehensive, informative, and, in many cases, encyclopedic. More texts already were available than most practitioners could hope to read and assimilate in a lifetime.

Why then, in the face of apparent plenty, should this textbook have been conceived, yet alone published? We are convinced that an approach to clinical anesthesia that differs in several ways from that presented in available texts can be of practical use. Specifically, our goal has been to incorporate the clinical practice of anesthesia, equivalent to two volumes, under a single cover. To do so, we have divided the text roughly as follows. The first nine sections (54 chapters) deal with fundamental concepts with which everyone who practices or is learning about anesthesia should be familiar. The subject matter is generic in the sense that the information is applicable to almost any case. Rather than to make these discussions all-encompassing, we asked the contributors to focus their discussions on what they consider to be the *clinically relevant* and, to the reader, *clinically applicable* features of the particular concepts being considered.

In order to provide up-to-date, expert treatments with a fresh outlook, we chose many contributors who have published or lectured on their topics but have not written on the same topics in one of the major anesthesiology texts. This arrangement allows the reader to obtain a different perspective in areas where opinions and approaches are divergent; conversely, it may confirm that an approach to a case is standard when it mirrors information that is available in other writings.

The 10th section (comprising 26 chapters) arises out of our observation that, when preparing for a type of case we have not done recently (or may never have done before), we are often frustrated by having to piece together the relevant facts from numerous sources. For that reason, we asked the contributors to include the relevant anatomy, physiology, pharmacology, and surgical procedure/anesthetic interactions in their approach to clinical management. Specifically, they were requested to organize their discussions as if they were describing their approach to a colleague who had not dealt with a particular problem for some time. In all cases, they were requested to provide "tips" or "pearls" that they have found useful in their practice and that are of practical use even if they are not validated scientifically.

We also requested that contributors don their soothsayer caps whenever possible and project what future major advances or changes appear likely in their specialties and subspecialties. The reader exposed to such prognostication may thus be stimulated to peruse a scientific article on a subject with no apparent current clinical relevance, but which he or she recognizes as having the potential to become a "hot" topic in the next few years.

We attempted to render each of the chapters similar one to another with respect to style but without altering the flavor of each individual author's contributions. Usually, a reference text is perused to answer a question. Therefore, we have introduced each major topic with a question, and this question is followed by the information that provides the answer. The discerning reader will note duplication of some subject matter and even of a few illustrations in some chapters. This approach was deliberate on our part and is based on our annoyance when we must break our trains-of-thought while reading intently and are referred to another part of a book for a figure, table, or related discussion. Although we have not resolved this problem completely, we have tried to make chapters stand on their own merit as much as possible.

Our sincere thanks go to Lew Reines, President and Chief Executive Officer of W.B. Saunders Company, who finally convinced us (we think!) that this effort was worthwhile. The editors also commend the work of the copy editor, Frank Messina, who achieved the miraculous with late entries and revisions and whose gracious cooperation was indispensable in maintaining the high standards set forth for this book. Finally, the editors thank Hope Olivo, our assistant editor, who, as so often in the past, made it all possible!

We wish to dedicate this textbook to T. W. Andersen, M.D., Professor of Anesthesiology, who has been a mentor, teacher, friend, and role model for faculty and residents alike at the University of Florida for over 30 years.

ROBERT R. KIRBY, M.D.
NIKOLAUS GRAVENSTEIN, M.D.

# Contents

# Toward a Safer Practice

CHAPTER

## 1

# Preanesthetic Evaluation

Stephen O. Heard

Donald S. Stevens

First impressions often have lasting effects. The preanesthetic evaluation is likely to be the first time a patient interacts with a member of the anesthesia department. Although the evaluation encounter usually is brief, it is important. This chapter examines the first encounter between a patient and the anesthesiologist and gives practical suggestions to the anesthesiologist about how to improve the skills needed to perform the preanesthetic evaluation.

## PURPOSES

### What Are the Purposes of the Preoperative Evaluation?

The preoperative evaluation is important for three reasons[1]: meeting the patient, delineating the problem, and obtaining informed consent.

## Meeting the Patient

First, the anesthesiologist is able to meet the patient. Although busy clinicians may downplay this interaction, many studies have shown that the preoperative interview is effective in reducing a patient's anxiety.[2–4] In light of current practice, it is assumed (but unclear) that this effect continues from the time the patient is evaluated by a member of an anesthesia department to when he or she is provided intraoperative care by another member of the department.

## Delineating the Problem

Second, the anesthesiologist is able to delineate the current problem through the medical history, physical examination, and laboratory studies. Coexisting problems are also determined and evaluated.

## Obtaining Informed Consent

Third, the anesthesiologist is able to obtain the patient's informed consent for anesthesia procedures.[1]

# PROCEDURES

## How Is Information Obtained?

Much of the preoperative evaluation can be done by reviewing the patient's medical record. However, examining, counseling, and reassuring the patient are still essential aspects of the preoperative assessment.

## Communicating Information

Changes in medical and surgical practice that have occurred over the past several decades have revolutionized the method by which the preoperative evaluation is completed. Large numbers of patients now have surgery in the ambulatory setting or are admitted to the hospital on the day of surgery instead of the night before. One consequence of this practice is that the anesthesiologist sometimes must interview and examine the patient in the preoperative holding area. A significant proportion of hospitals and medical centers has established preoperative evaluation clinics whereby the evaluation and work-up of patients are directed by the anesthesiologist.[5] Although this practice may be efficient, reduce the time and cost of preoperative evaluations, and shorten the length of stay, the anesthesiologist who evaluated the patient preoperatively is often not the one who will administer the anesthesia. Care must be taken to ensure good communication between the preoperative clinic and operating room personnel to avoid delays or cancellation of procedures.

## Computerized Questionnaires

Ideally, a personal interview is part of the initial preoperative evaluation. Several computerized questionnaires have been developed to assist in obtaining the medical history of the patient. Although one might expect patient responses to such questionnaires to be incomplete, one study has indicated that they are as accurate and helpful in obtaining the medical history as the interview.[6] It is important to emphasize that the purpose of these questionnaires is not to replace the personal interview but to assist the physician in obtaining the history and to suggest what laboratory tests should be ordered. Using these questionnaires can make the personal interview much more efficient.

# PATIENT HISTORY

## What Can Be Learned From the History of the Present Illness?

Knowledge of the current surgical problem is crucial. The anesthetic management depends on the type of surgery to be performed. The disease state being treated may also have implications for anesthetic management or may suggest other underlying medical conditions. For example, pneumoencephalus after skull fracture is a contraindication to the use of nitrous oxide. A craniotomy in the sitting position for a posterior fossa tumor places the patient at risk for venous air emboli. The possibility of emboli prompts consideration of preoperative echocardiography to assess for patent foramen ovale, insertion of a central venous catheter, use of precordial Doppler ultrasound, and particularly careful monitoring of end-tidal carbon dioxide. A parathyroidectomy for hypercalcemia should alert the anesthesiologist to the possibility of an undiagnosed multiple endocrine neoplasia syndrome.

The specifics regarding any organ system involvement by a primary process in a patient undergoing surgical treatment should be strongly considered.

## Why Are the Previous Surgical and Anesthetic Histories Important?

Previous surgery may affect the anesthetic plan. For instance, the patient with limited neck motion after a cervical fusion may be managed differently than a patient with a normal airway. Also, presence of an arteriovenous dialysis fistula would contraindicate placement of an intravenous catheter or blood pressure (BP) cuff on the involved extremity.

## Adverse Drug Reactions

Important information is obtained from prior anesthetic experience. Previous adverse reactions to particular anesthetic agents would presumably preclude their use for the impending anesthetic procedure. In particular, the interviewer should determine whether the patient has ever had a prolonged episode of paralysis following succinylcholine administration or whether the patient (or a family member) has ever been thought to have malignant hyperthermia.

## Questions to Ask

Information about adverse drug reactions can be obtained easily by asking the patient such questions as, "Have you had any operations before?" "What kind of anesthesia did you have?" "Did you have any problems with the anesthesia?" Unexpectedly specific answers, such as "I'm allergic to Anectine [succinylcholine chloride]," have been obtained by such questioning. Most commonly, nausea and vomiting are reported as problems. If these types of side effects are almost always present postoperatively, then use of a technique aimed at limiting these complications (eg, a regional or propofol-based anesthetic and early antiemetic therapy) might be helpful.

## What Can Be Learned From the Medical History?

Obtain as complete a medical history as possible before anesthetizing the patient. Many different approaches can be used, but regardless of which one is chosen, the anesthesiologist should be sure that all relevant information is obtained. Our approach is based on a review of systems, as follows.

### Cardiovascular System

Questions concerning the cardiovascular system should focus on determining the existence of a history of hypertension, valvular or ischemic heart disease, and peripheral vascular insufficiency. Presence of arrhythmias as well as a pacemaker also needs to be determined.

### Hypertension

If the patient has a history of hypertension, the anesthesiologist should inquire about the duration of the disease and the length and adequacy of treatment. Patients with untreated or inadequately treated hypertension may have a greater risk of perioperative hemodynamic fluctuations, resulting in increased morbidity.[7–10] It is also helpful to ask what the patient's normal BP is and what the lowest routine check BP was because the spot check during the preoperative visit will typically be higher than usual and thus would suggest different intraoperative goals.

### Valvular Disease

The patient should be questioned about his or her history of rheumatic fever or heart murmurs, especially if a history of syncope is elicited. Syncope is associated with mitral valve prolapse, hypertrophic cardiomyopathy, and severe aortic stenosis.

### Coronary Artery Disease

Patients of appropriate age should be asked if they have a history of angina, myocardial infarction (MI), or congestive heart failure (CHF). The risk of perioperative morbidity and mortality associated with surgery in patients who have suffered an MI <6 months before surgery (*recent MI*) appears to be lower today than that reported in the 1960s and 1970s.[11–14] The risk of morbidity and mortality for those patients with an MI ≥6 months before surgery (*remote MI*) is also lower today compared with data from those earlier studies. However, there are not enough data in the more recent studies to demonstrate whether there are differences in morbidity and mortality between those patients with a recent MI and those with a remote MI who are undergoing noncardiac surgery (Fig. 1–1).[15] Thus, a recent MI still dictates that elective surgery be delayed or, if surgery is urgent, that invasive hemodynamic monitoring be contemplated during and after the procedure.

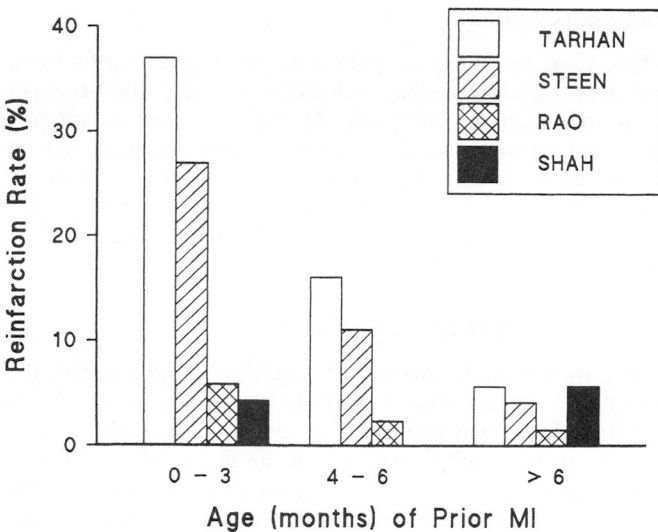

**FIGURE 1–1.** Reinfarction rates from several studies in patients who have had prior myocardial infarction (MI). (Adapted from McCulloch HA, Sprague DH. Myths in vascular anesthesia. *Probl Anesthesiol.* 1991;5:453–467.)

Angina of new onset or a change in a previous anginal pattern should be a warning that the patient be evaluated more thoroughly before surgery. In many cases, a cardiologist should assist with this evaluation.

### Symptomatic Arrhythmias

Symptomatic arrhythmias can also be important aspects of a patient's history. Palpitations often indicate premature ventricular contractions that may require treatment before elective surgery. A history of a rapid heartbeat can indicate paroxysmal supraventricular tachycardia, which may arise during surgery. Several types of arrhythmias are associated with increased perioperative cardiac risk: a rhythm other than sinus, premature atrial contractions, and 5 or more premature ventricular contractions per minute.[16]

### Pacemakers

Inquiries as to the presence, type, and location of a pacemaker should be made, as well as the date and results of the most recent evaluation and underlying rhythm. Because electrocautery can interfere with pacemaker function, reprogramming the pacemaker to an asynchronous mode before surgery may be indicated. Presence of a pacemaker also suggests the use of bipolar cautery, where feasible. Moreover, the older practice of using a magnet to convert a demand pacemaker to an asynchronous pacemaker[17] may not work well with newer pacing devices and is discouraged.[18] Reports of patients whose pacemakers have been reprogrammed to unwanted rates by the use of a magnet are found in the literature.[19,20] Use of the appropriate type of pacemaker interrogation and reprogramming devices, with the assistance of a cardiologist, is the safest course.[18]

Identifying the pacemaker's location allows intraoperative placement of the electrocautery grounding pad in a location where the current flow from the electrocautery at the surgical site is least likely to pass through or near the pacemaker.

## Pulmonary System

Questions related to the pulmonary system should focus on a history of emphysema, bronchitis, asthma, recent upper respiratory tract infection (URTI), productive or nonproductive cough, or sinusitis. The patient's exercise capacity should be elicited by asking such questions as, "Can you climb up one flight of stairs?" and "Are you out of breath at the top?" Remember that dyspnea may also be the presenting symptom for cardiovascular problems.

### Chronic Obstructive Lung Disease

In patients with chronic obstructive lung disease, the amount of sputum that is expectorated per day should be determined. A change in the amount or color of the sputum from its usual quality may indicate an acute URTI. Elective surgery in the presence of a current or recent URTI is controversial.[21–24] Proceeding with general anesthesia and elective surgery must be weighed against the potential complications associated with such infections (eg, laryngospasm, hypoxemia).

### Miscellaneous Conditions

The anesthesiologist should remember that a nonproductive cough may be the sole manifestation of asthma or silent regurgitation and aspiration of stomach contents.[25,26] Nasotracheal intubation may be contraindicated in patients with a history of sinusitis or nasal polyposis.

## Gastrointestinal System

### Aspiration of Gastric Contents

One of the most feared anesthetic complications is pulmonary aspiration of gastric contents. The anesthesiologist must determine whether the patient is at risk for developing aspiration pneumonitis if regurgitation and aspiration occur during anesthesia and surgery. Pain, recent injury, insufficient duration of fasting, diabetes mellitus, obesity, pregnancy, and use of narcotics, β-adrenergic agents, and anticholinergic agents can delay gastric emptying or alter lower esophageal sphincter tone, thus theoretically increasing the risk of aspiration.[27–29] A hiatal hernia is believed to increase the risk for aspiration, but reflux symptoms (eg, acid taste), rather than the hiatal hernia itself, probably better identify the patient at risk and suggest the patient most likely to benefit from antacid prophylaxis (Fig. 1–2).[30]

### Liver Disease

A history of blood transfusions, hepatitis, hematemesis, or hematochezia should also be elicited. When indicated, questions concerning chronic liver disease (eg, cirrhosis and hypoalbuminemia) need to be asked because the pharmacokinetics and pharmacodynamics of various drugs often will be altered in such disease. Coagulation studies may also be abnormal in patients with altered liver function.

## Genitourinary System

### Renal Insufficiency

Renal insufficiency may be a manifestation of diseases of organ systems other than the genitourinary (GU) system. Thus,

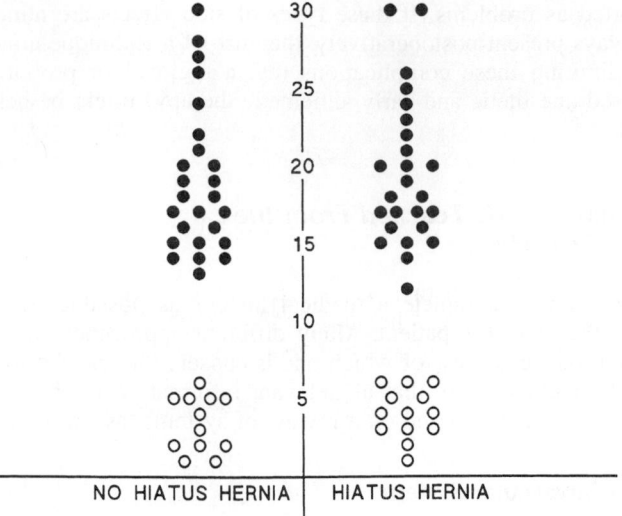

**FIGURE 1–2.** Resting lower esophageal sphincter (LES) pressure (in millimeters of mercury) in patients with or without a hiatal hernia and with (open circles) or without (filled circles) the symptoms of reflux. LES pressures were higher in patients without symptoms of reflux irrespective of the presence of a hiatal hernia. (Reprinted from Cohen S, Harris LD. Does hiatus hernia affect competence of the gastroesophageal sphincter? *N Engl J Med.* 1971;284:1053, by permission of the *New England Journal of Medicine.*)

the patient with diabetes mellitus, connective tissue disease, hypertension, or peripheral vascular disease (PVD) should be carefully questioned about signs and symptoms of renal insufficiency. In patients with chronic renal failure, the anesthesiologist should be sure to establish the time of the patient's last dialysis because significant changes in blood volume and serum potassium level may occur before and after dialysis.

### Urinary Tract Infection

Inquiries into recent or chronic urinary tract infections should also be made. This is particularly relevant in cases in which the GU tract will be instrumented intraoperatively.

### Pregnancy

In women of childbearing age, the possibility of pregnancy should be considered, and appropriate inquiries should be made.

## Endocrine System

### Diabetes Mellitus

All patients should be asked whether they have diabetes mellitus. Diabetic patients are at risk for silent myocardial ischemia, autonomic neuropathy, and gastroparesis. Attention should be carefully focused on the cardiovascular system as well as on other end-organ systems. Direct laryngoscopy and intubation also appears to be more difficult in this patient population.[31,32]

### Adrenal Suppression and Corticosteroids

In those patients with diseases in which corticosteroid use is common (eg, asthma, ulcerative colitis, or rheumatoid arthritis), the anesthesiologist should inquire as to the dose and the time of last use of corticosteroids. The incidence of adrenal suppression is not predictable and depends on the potency and frequency of steroid dose and on the length of steroid therapy. Suppression can occur with cumulative doses of prednisone <0.4 g and can last for as long as 1 year following cessation of steroid therapy (Fig. 1–3).[33]

### Thyroid Disease

In patients with thyroid disease, the adequacy of thyroid hormone replacement therapy (for hypothyroidism) or antithyroidal treatment (for hyperthyroidism) should be established. Although recent retrospective data suggest that elective anesthesia and surgery can be performed on patients with stable hypothyroidism,[34,35] delay of elective operations is prudent to allow for adequate thyroid hormone replacement.[36]

### Miscellaneous

Other endocrine disease, such as primary hyperparathyroidism, may suggest the existence of an underlying multiple endocrine neoplasia syndrome. Further evaluation may be needed to rule out endocrine abnormalities, such as pheochromocytoma or medullary carcinoma of the thyroid gland.

## Neurologic System

The anesthesiologist should ask the patient whether he or she has a history of central or peripheral nervous system problems. These queries are particularly germane if a regional anesthetic technique is contemplated.

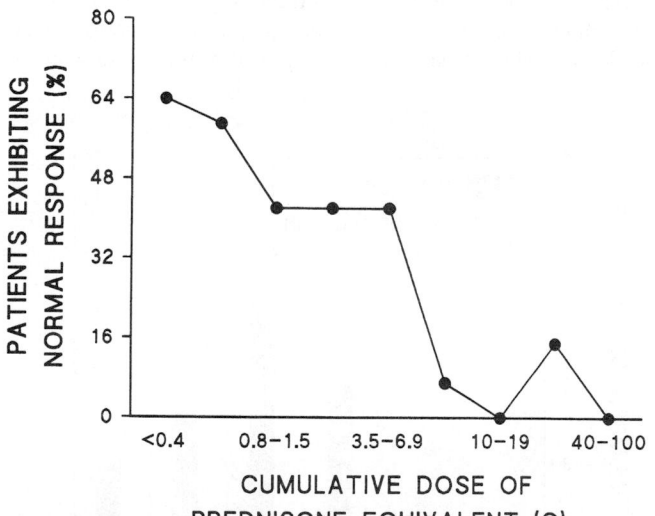

**FIGURE 1–3.** Relationship between the cumulative dose of glucocorticoid and the adrenal response to exogenous corticotropin-releasing hormone. A normal response was a 1.5-fold increase in the plasma cortisol level to at least a level of 276 nmol/L or a peak cortisol level of 552 nmol/L. A *blunted response* was a plasma cortisol level between 83 and 276 nmol/L after corticotropin-releasing hormone administration or an increase of <1.5 times the basal level if the basal level was >179 nmol/L. *No response* was defined as basal and stimulated cortisol levels of <83 nmol/L. (Adapted from information appearing in Schlaghecke R, Kornely E, Santen RT, et al. The effect of long-term glucocorticoid therapy on pituitary-adrenal responses to exogenous corticotropin-releasing hormone. *N Engl J Med.* 1992;326:226, by permission of the *New England Journal of Medicine.*)

### Intracranial Pressure

If the patient has an intracranial lesion, symptoms of intracranial hypertension should be sought. Pituitary lesions may cause endocrine abnormalities that must be carefully managed in the perioperative period. A history of recent transient ischemic attack, with signs and symptoms of <24 hours' duration; reversible ischemic neurologic deficits, with signs and symptoms of <72 hours' duration; or cerebrovascular accidents ("completed strokes") suggests that careful neurologic evaluation be undertaken before proceeding with surgery.

### Seizures

The anesthesiologist should ask the patient about a history of seizures, particularly their type, frequency, last occurrence, as well as what type, if any, of anticonvulsants the patient is receiving.

### Spinal Cord Injuries

In patients with spinal cord injury, the level of the neurologic deficit must be determined. Episodes of autonomic hyperreflexia can occur with cutaneous stimulation or distention of a hollow viscus with deficits above T7.[37] Recent spinal cord lesions preclude the use of succinylcholine because of the potential for massive release of intracellular potassium caused by the proliferation of extrajunctional acetylcholine receptors on which succinylcholine also acts.[38]

## Musculoskeletal System

A history of rheumatoid arthritis may indicate several problems that need to be evaluated.[39] Airway management can be more difficult owing to altered laryngeal anatomy (Fig. 1–4) and decreased range of joint motion (spine and temporomandibular joint). Cervical spine instability may also exist at the atlantoaxial joint, requiring that special precautions be taken during intubation. The use of routine preoperative cervical radiographs to diagnose cervical spine instability is controversial; some recommend routine screening,[40] whereas others conclude that preoperative cervical films are not needed in the asymptomatic patient.[41] Because of the reduced range of motion in arthritic joints, positioning the patient can be difficult after anesthetic induction.[42]

The presence of a muscular disorder, such as a muscular dystrophy, should also be ascertained. Specific anesthetic agents, such as succinylcholine, are contraindicated in patients with such a disorder.

## Integumentary System

Recent burns contraindicate the use of depolarizing muscle relaxants because of the danger of hyperkalemia.[38] If emergent surgery is required, careful airway evaluation and assessment of the adequacy of fluid resuscitation also are essential.[43]

## Hematologic System

Asking about previous bleeding problems and about the need for blood transfusions almost always identifies the patient who may develop perioperative hemorrhage.[44] In addition, if the preoperative assessment is performed sufficiently

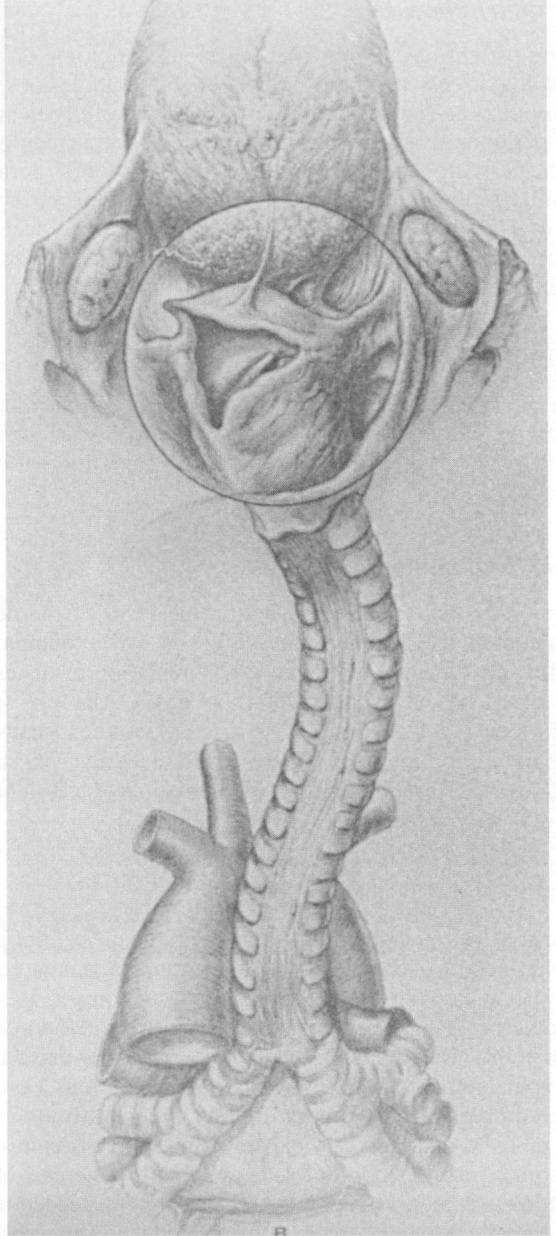

**FIGURE 1–4.** The effect of severe erosive polyarticular arthritis on the anatomy of the larynx and trachea. The larynx is rotated, deviated, and tilted forward; the trachea becomes redundant. (From Keenan MA, Stiles CM, Kaufman RL. Acquired laryngeal deviation associated with cervical spine disease in erosive polyarticular arthritis. *Anesthesiology.* 1983;58:441.)

early, the anesthesiologist can identify a patient who is suitable for preoperative autologous blood donation. Use of recombinant erythropoietin also can increase the efficiency of preoperative autologous blood donation (Fig. 1–5).[45]

## MEDICATIONS

### What Medications Should Be Continued or Stopped Before Surgery?

#### Antihypertensives

In general, antihypertensive agents other than diuretics should be continued up to the time of surgery. Many studies

have documented the adverse hemodynamic effects of discontinuing β-adrenergic blockers or clonidine in the perioperative period.[46,47] Indeed, recent data suggest that perioperative administration of atenolol for 7 days to patients with or at risk for coronary artery disease (CAD) reduces postoperative myocardial ischemia and may decrease the risk of postoperative death.[48,49]

#### Diuretics

Use of diuretics is usually stopped before surgery. Patients taking thiazides frequently have hypokalemia regardless of potassium supplementation or the use of potassium-sparing agents.[50] Serum potassium concentrations <3.5 mEq/L occur in 15% of patients, and concentrations <3.0 mEq/L occur in 10%.

The perioperative consequences of a low serum potassium level are being refined. Data from the 1980s suggested that complications secondary to hypokalemia were not as severe as once was believed (Fig. 1–6).[50,51] However, a more recent study evaluating hypokalemia in cardiac surgery patients indicated that preoperative potassium levels below 3.5 mEq/L are associated with increased perioperative arrhythmias and the need for cardiopulmonary resuscitation.[52]

#### Digitalis Glycosides

Digoxin use should be continued in the perioperative period. It is efficacious in patients with CHF in New York Heart Association classifications III or IV.[53] However, more recent data suggest that its utility in atrial fibrillation is limited.[54,55]

#### Antianginal Medication

Use of all medications used to treat angina pectoris, including nitrates, calcium channel blockers, and β-adrenergic receptor blockers should be continued up to the time of surgery.[47,56]

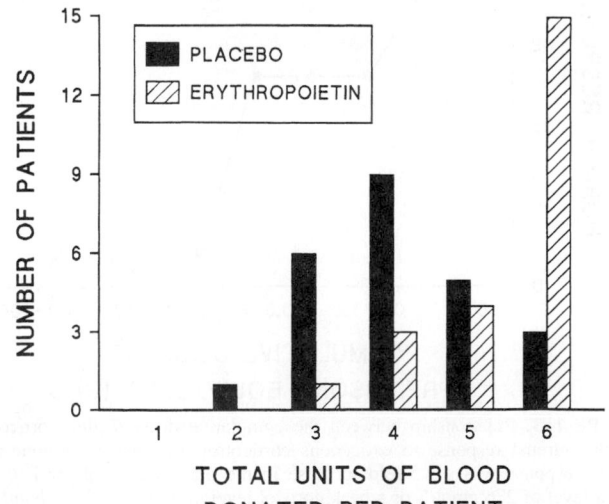

**FIGURE 1–5.** Efficiency of preoperative autologous blood donation in patients receiving erythropoietin compared with those given a placebo. Erythropoietin-treated patients were able to donate significantly more units of blood than were placebo-treated patients. (Adapted from Goodnough LT, Rudnick S, Price TH, et al. Increased preoperative collection of autologous blood with recombinant human erythropoietin therapy. *N Engl J Med.* 1989;321:1163, by permission of the *New England Journal of Medicine.*)

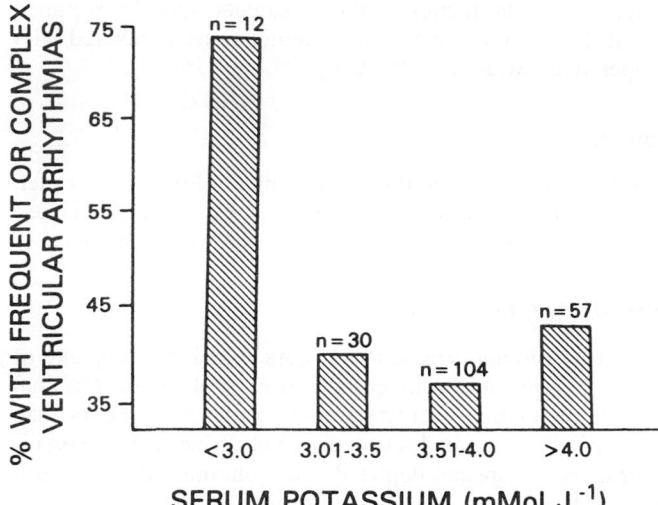

**FIGURE 1–6.** Incidence of frequent or complex ventricular arrhythmias as a function of serum potassium levels in hypertensive men taking thiazide diuretics. Those patients with a serum potassium level of $\leq 3$ mmol/L had a significantly higher incidence of arrhythmias compared to those with patients with potassium levels $>3$ mmol/L. (Redrawn from Siegel D, Hulley SB, Black DM, et al. Diuretics, serum and intracellular electrolyte levels, and ventricular arrhythmias in hypertensive men. *JAMA.* 1992;267:1083–1089. Copyright 1992, American Medical Association.)

If taken orally, they should be given at their usual dosing interval. If required, they can be given during surgery as well.

### Antiarrhythmic Agents

Depending on their original indication, antiarrhythmic medications should be continued in the perioperative period. However, several of these drugs can have significant side effects relevant to anesthesia. The administration of quinidine to patients with stable digoxin blood levels causes a decrease in the clearance of digoxin and may result in toxicity.[57] Both quinidine and procainamide can cause prolonged QT syndrome.

Disopyramide is a myocardial depressant and may increase the cardiac depression observed with volatile anesthetics. Amiodarone has been associated with altered thyroid function, particularly thyrotoxicosis, and with hypersensitivity pneumonitis.[58]

Intravenous lidocaine is a commonly used antiarrhythmic agent. Remember that this drug decreases the minimum alveolar concentration for volatile anesthetic agents and has been used as an adjunct to intravenous anesthetic techniques in the past.

### Bronchodilators

Inhaled $\beta_2$-agonists are central in the management of patients with reactive airway disease. These medications should be continued up to (and through) surgery. Inhaled anticholinergics and corticosteroids should also be continued.

The role of aminophylline in the management of the patient with bronchospastic disease is controversial. Although aminophylline is an effective bronchodilator, it does not add significantly to the bronchodilating effects of inhaled $\beta$-adrenergic or anticholinergic agents.[59] In addition to inhibiting phosphodiesterase, aminophylline causes the release of norepinephrine.

However, aminophylline does have anti-inflammatory properties and can decrease the requirements for inhaled steroids.[60]

Because halothane sensitizes the myocardium to circulating catecholamines, the combined use of aminophylline and halothane may result in ventricular arrhythmias.[61] In addition, toxic serum concentrations of aminophylline may occur in the perioperative period due to alterations in drug metabolism by the liver that have been induced by changes in the parenteral nutritional content.[62]

Our practice is to give aminophylline only if a patient is receiving a stable dose preoperatively. Otherwise, we avoid aminophylline and instead use nebulized bronchodilators and corticosteroids for reactive airway disease. If a patient uses nebulized medications routinely, we administer them 30 to 60 minutes preoperatively.

Cromolyn sodium has no bronchodilating properties but inhibits mast cell degranulation and is useful for prophylaxis.[60]

There are several leukotriene receptor antagonists and inhibitors of leukotriene synthesis that are now available for clinical use. Some (zileuton and zafirlukast) can increase serum concentrations of warfarin and other medications.[60]

### Insulin and Oral Hypoglycemic Agents

#### Insulin

The optimal management of blood glucose levels in the diabetic patient remains controversial; "tight" and "loose" control regimens have been proposed.[63] Those who favor tight control argue that better management of the perioperative blood glucose level results in decreased postoperative morbidity, including fewer wound infections and enhanced wound healing.[64]

Those who favor loose control believe that sound data supporting the notion that tight control reduces perioperative morbidity are lacking, the resources needed for tight control are too expensive, and that without these resources, the danger of hypoglycemia is significant.[65]

We favor loose control. If the patient has adult-onset insulin-dependent diabetes mellitus, one half to two thirds of the usual dose of insulin is administered on the morning of surgery after an intravenous infusion of a dextrose-containing crystalloid solution has been started.[63] Capillary glucose monitoring at the time of intravenous catheter placement is recommended perioperatively to dictate additional subcutaneous or intravenous doses of insulin.

#### Oral Hypoglycemic Agents

Oral hypoglycemic agents should not be administered on the day of surgery, particularly those agents with a long duration of action, such as chlorpropamide, glipizide, and glyburide. They bind ionically to serum albumin and may be displaced from their binding sites by drugs used in the perioperative period.[66] Asymptomatic hypoglycemia can occur in the somnolent postoperative patient who has been taking long-acting oral hypoglycemic drugs.

### Corticosteroids

The patient who is taking corticosteroids or adrenocorticotropic hormone should receive appropriate perioperative corticosteroid replacement (Table 1–1). For the patient who is

**TABLE 1–1.** Perioperative Glucocorticoid Coverage for Patients Based on Degree of Stress

| Degree of Stress | Dosage | | |
|---|---|---|---|
| | Preoperative | Intraoperative* | Postoperative |
| Minor | Usual AM | 25 mg | Usual PM |
| Moderate | Usual AM | 50 mg | 20 mg hydrocortisone every 8 h for 1 to 2 d |
| Major | Usual AM | 50 mg | 50 mg hydrocortisone every 8 h for 2 to 3 d |

*Hydrocortisone or glucocorticoid equivalent.
From Narr BJ. Preanesthetic evaluation. In: Murray MJ, Cousin DB, Pearl RG, et al, eds. *Critical Care Medicine: Perioperative Management.* Philadelphia, Pa: Lippincott-Raven; 1997:11–18.

taking a corticosteroid with a potency of >300 mg of hydrocortisone per day, hydrocortisone is not substituted for the perioperative steroid treatment; the routine dose of steroid can be administered. For example, if a patient is taking 3 mg of dexamethasone every 6 hours, this daily dose meets the stress dose requirements of surgery. The patient will be protected from adrenal insufficiency if this drug and dosing regimen is continued perioperatively.

## Thyroid Medication

Because of its long half-life (7 days), thyroxine does not have to be given on the day of surgery. Antithyroid medications include methimazole and propylthiouracil. These agents should be administered on the morning of surgery.

## Anticonvulsant Medications

The use of anticonvulsant medications should be continued up to the time of surgery. Many anticonvulsants induce the hepatic microsomal enzyme system and may cause alterations of the pharmacokinetics of other perioperative medications, particularly barbiturates and nondepolarizing muscle relaxants.

However, recent treatment with anticonvulsants may *not* have the desired effect. The prophylactic value of phenytoin in reducing the incidence of seizures in patients who have suffered closed head injuries is only effective during the first week of therapy; thus, the anesthesiologist still should be wary of seizures perioperatively despite prophylactic preventive therapy.[67]

## Antipsychotics and Antidepressants

Antipsychotics and antidepressants are usually administered up to the time of the surgical procedure. However, several special situations deserve consideration.

### Monoamine Oxidase Inhibitors

Monoamine oxidase inhibitors are generally discontinued 2 weeks before surgery. They have been implicated in a number of adverse reactions in the perioperative period, including hyperthermia, especially in association with meperidine administration, cardiac arrhythmias, and death. There have been several reports of patients taking monoamine oxidase inhibitors who had uneventful anesthetic procedures. The risk of administering anesthetics to these patients must be weighed against the possible psychiatric complications associated with preoperative cessation of the drug.[68,69]

### Lithium

Lithium carbonate, used in the treatment of bipolar disorder, can potentiate the effect of muscle relaxants, may decrease anesthetic requirements, and can alter free water clearance.

### Tricyclic Antidepressants

The tricyclic antidepressants (TCAs) block the reuptake of norepinephrine and, with chronic use, deplete the terminal nerve stores of this neurotransmitter. Patients on TCAs may manifest an exaggerated response to ephedrine if their norepinephrine stores are not depleted and a diminished response if they are. It is easiest to simply substitute phenylephrine as the vasopressor of choice in patients taking TCAs. Although animal studies suggest an interaction of TCAs with pancuronium and halothane, resulting in the development of fatal ventricular arrhythmias, there are no published clinical reports suggesting such an interaction in human beings.

## Anti-Inflammatory Drugs

Anti-inflammatory agents affect coagulation owing to their effect on platelets. Aspirin irreversibly acetylates the platelet enzyme cyclooxygenase-1 (COX-1, a constitutive enzyme), resulting in decreased platelet aggregation for the life of the platelet (7-10 days).[70] Other nonsteroidal anti-inflammatory drugs (NSAIDs) appear to inhibit the same enzyme but do so reversibly, with effects lasting at most 2 days after a single NSAID dose.[71] More recent data suggest that hemorrhagic complications associated with spinal or epidural anesthesia are not increased when preoperative antiplatelet medications are administered.[72] A class of investigational anti-inflammatory drugs, the cyclooxygenase-2 (COX-2) inhibitors, is now available. COX-2 is an enzyme that is induced by the cytokines, various growth factors, and endotoxin and is found at sites of inflammation. Thus, selective COX-2 inhibitors may reduce inflammation without causing other side effects such as renal insufficiency, gastrointestinal bleeding, and inhibition of platelet aggregation.[73] The 2 COX-2 inhibitors approved for use in the United States are rofecoxib and celecoxib.

Although discontinuation of aspirin 7 days and NSAIDs 48 hours before neuraxial blockade was recommended in the past, a consensus statement from the American Society of Regional Anesthesia indicated this is no longer necessary if other forms of anticoagulation are not used.[74]

## Anticoagulants

In general, use of anticoagulants should be discontinued before a surgical procedure. In some cases, their effects may require reversal before surgery can proceed. If the patient is receiving warfarin and surgery is urgent, fresh frozen plasma should be given for quick reversal of the anticoagulant effect. Remember that this effect is transient, and additional units of fresh frozen plasma may be required as the coagulation factors are metabolized. If surgery is elective, an oral dose of 5 to 10 mg of phytonadione (vitamin $K_1$) should cause the prothrombin time to normalize within 24 hours, although longer periods may be needed for maximum effect.[75] Use of vitamin $K_1$, however, makes subsequent oral re-anticoagulation following surgery more difficult.

If a heparin infusion is used, it may be stopped 3 to 4 hours before surgery, allowing sufficient time for the return of normal coagulation. If reversal is urgently needed, protamine sulfate can be used.

Special mention must be made of low molecular weight heparin (LMWH). Case reports and series have documented a higher than normal risk of neuraxial bleeding when LMWH is used in conjunction with a neuraxial anesthetic or analgesic regimen. For those patients who are receiving low-dose LMWH (eg, 0.5 mg/kg enoxaparin), the needle should be placed at least 10 to 12 hours after the last dose. High-dose therapy (1 mg/kg) dictates needle placement 24 hours beyond the last dose.[76]

### Antineoplastic Agents

Cancer patients should be asked about the chemotherapeutic agents used in their treatment. The anesthesiologist should determine what agents were given and how long ago they were administered. In addition, an assessment of bone marrow recovery should be made.

### *Doxorubicin*

Specific problems also exist apart from bone marrow suppression. Adverse effects of doxorubicin on the heart have been well described.[77] The anesthesiologist needs to determine the total dose given to the patient. If the administration is recent, a myocardial inflammation also occurs transiently. Although myocardial damage can be detected by subendocardial biopsies after cumulative doses of 250 mg/m$^2$, clinically significant CHF is rare with doses <500 mg/m$^2$.[77] Concurrent administration of cyclophosphamide and doxorubicin increases the risk of cardiac toxicity. If the patient reports symptoms suggestive of CHF, an assessment of cardiac function (echocardiogram) should be undertaken preoperatively.

### *Bleomycin*

Bleomycin can cause interstitial pulmonary fibrosis and may sensitize the lungs to damage from inspired oxygen concentrations >28%.[78] If there is a history of bleomycin use, particularly if the dose is >500 mg, it is wise to limit the perioperative inspired oxygen concentration to <30% while carefully monitoring the patient's arterial hemoglobin oxygen saturation using pulse oximetry. Administration of corticosteroids preoperatively may help prevent perioperative respiratory failure in patients with a history of bleomycin treatment.[79]

### Antiglaucoma Agents

Use of antiglaucoma agents is routinely continued in the perioperative period. Two important medications in this class are the cholinesterase inhibitors: echothiophate and isoflurophate. They irreversibly inhibit plasma cholinesterase, which prolongs the duration of action of succinylcholine.[80]

Systemic absorption of ophthalmic medication may also occur in those patients who use ophthalmic β-blockers (eg, timolol). The cardiovascular reserve to stress may be blunted in such patients.[81]

### Antibiotics

Many antibiotics, particularly the aminoglycosides, potentiate neuromuscular blockade. This effect can present difficulties in the reversal of neuromuscular relaxation at the end of surgery or in the presence of a respiratory acidosis. A partial list is presented in Table 1–2.[82]

### Opioids and Benzodiazepines

Opioids and benzodiazepines are sometimes withheld after midnight the night before surgery. However, this course of action leaves a patient's preoperative pain untreated or may precipitate panic attacks or withdrawal symptoms. These drugs should be continued until the time of surgery. If the use of oral medications is deemed unwise, parenteral therapy can be instituted instead.

## ALLERGIC RESPONSES

### *What Specific Information Is Important?*

#### Allergic Responses Versus Side Effects

Any allergies to medications must be documented, and the exact nature of the allergic responses should be determined and included in the record. This documentation is important because patients may confuse side effects with allergic responses. For example, codeine may cause nausea (a side effect) or a pruritic rash (an allergic response), but either may be interpreted as an allergy by the patient. Also, tachycardia due to epinephrine mixed with lidocaine given for dental procedures may lead the patient to say that he or she is allergic to local anesthetics.

#### True Allergies

A 10% to 15% rate of allergic cross-reaction exists between penicillins and cephalosporins. In patients with a history of immediate hypersensitivity reaction to penicillin (eg, anaphy-

**TABLE 1–2.** Interaction Among Antibiotics, Muscle Relaxants, Neostigmine, and Calcium*

| Antibiotic | DTc | Succinylcholine | Neostigmine | Calcium |
|---|---|---|---|---|
| Neomycin | Yes | Yes | Usually | Usually |
| Streptomycin | Yes | Yes | Usually | Usually |
| Gentamicin | Yes | † | Sometimes | Usually |
| Kanamycin | Yes | Yes | Sometimes | Sometimes |
| Paromomycin | Yes | † | Yes | Yes |
| Viomycin | Yes | † | Yes | Yes |
| Polymyxin A | Yes | † | No | No |
| Polymyxin B | Yes | Yes | No‡ | No |
| Colistin | Yes | Yes | No | Sometimes |
| Tetracycline | Yes | No | Partially | Partially |
| Lincomycin | Yes | † | Partially | Partially |
| Clindamycin | Yes | † | Partially | Partially |

*Increase in neuromuscular block from antibiotic.
†Not studied.
‡Block is augmented by neostigmine.
dTc, d-tubocurarine-like drugs, which include other nondepolarizing muscle relaxants.
From Savarese JJ, Miller RD, Lien CA, et al. Pharmacology of muscle relaxants and their antagonists. In: Miller RD, ed. *Anesthesia.* 4th ed. New York, NY: Churchill Livingstone; 1994:417–487.

lactic shock, angioedema, and hives), a cephalosporin should not be used as a substitute antibiotic. Cephalosporins may be used if a history of a delayed type of allergic reaction to penicillins *only* is elicited.

Allergies to iodine-containing compounds preclude the use of agents that contain iodine (eg, metocurine). If intravenous radiographic contrast agents are absolutely required, pretreatment with corticosteroids and antihistamines can be used to decrease or eliminate the allergic response.[83]

### Anesthetic Agents

True allergy to anesthetic agents is extremely rare. Allergy to ester-based local anesthetic agents may actually be an allergy to *p*-aminobenzoic acid, a metabolite of that group of compounds. Allergies to the amide local anesthetics have been reported but are even more rare than those observed with ester anesthetics. Intradermal challenge testing for true allergy to local anesthetics can be done before elective surgery or elective nerve block through consultation with an allergist.[84] Similar testing can also be used for other medications.

### Latex Allergy

Since the mid-1980s, awareness of allergies to latex has emerged. Exposure of a sensitized individual to latex can result in urticaria, allergic rhinoconjunctivitis, asthma, or anaphylaxis.[85] Patients who appear to be at increased risk for latex allergy include those who require chronic and repeated instrumentation of the GU tract, receive barium enemas through a latex balloon tip, have multiple drug allergies, and have occupational exposure to latex (including health care personnel).[86] As part of their preoperative evaluation, all patients should be asked about a possible latex allergy. Appropriate precautions can then be undertaken in the perioperative period.

## SOCIAL HISTORY

### Why Is the Social History Important?

#### Smoking and Alcohol

Questions concerning tobacco and alcohol use need to be asked, including those addressing the amount and duration of consumption. Cigarette smoke has many adverse effects, including alteration of mucus secretion and clearance and decrease of small airway caliber. It also may alter the immune response. The chronic smoker should be encouraged to abstain from smoking for at least 2 months before the operation.[87] Stopping smoking for even <24 hours may produce benefits in cardiovascular physiology[88] but will not affect postoperative pulmonary complications.[89]

#### Illicit Drug Use

Inquiries into illicit or recreational drug use or behavior that would place a patient into a high-risk group for infection with HIV also need to be made. Once drug use is identified (whether it is prescribed or illicit), strategies for the prevention or treatment of withdrawal syndromes in the perioperative period can be formulated.

The patient who is suffering from a withdrawal syndrome should not undergo anesthesia and surgery unless the surgery is urgent. Also, an increased requirement for opioids should be expected both intraoperatively and postoperatively in patients who have a preoperative history of medicinal opioid use or opioid abuse.

Questions concerning anabolic steroid use should be asked of athletes because these drugs can have significant side effects on the liver, primarily cholestatic hepatitis.[90]

## PHYSICAL EXAMINATION

### What Should Be Checked?

#### General Assessment

A quick general assessment of the patient frequently provides important information. For example, cyanosis may be observed; if it is present, a careful examination of the cardiovascular and pulmonary systems should be performed. A pulse oximeter-determined baseline arterial oxygen saturation value confirms or refutes the clinical impression of cyanosis. The chronically ill-appearing patient with anasarca has an altered volume of distribution for most of the drugs that are used in the perioperative period.

#### Vital Signs

Vital signs, including weight (in kilograms), should be documented. In patients with PVD, BP is measured in both arms. Up to 21% of such patients present with a pressure disparity of >20 mm Hg between the 2 extremities that is presumably due to atherosclerosis (Fig. 1–7).[91] Such differences in pressure require a change in the location of a radial artery catheter because the arm with the higher BP reflects the central arterial pressure more accurately.

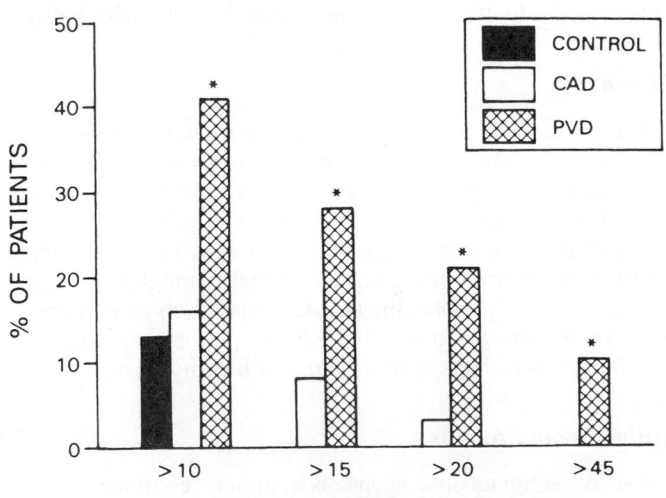

**FIGURE 1–7.** Systolic blood pressure differences between the right and left arm in 3 groups of patients: control patients without atherosclerotic disease, patients with coronary artery disease (CAD), and patients with peripheral vascular disease (PVD). There is a significantly greater number of patients with PVD who have systolic pressure differences between the 2 arms compared with the other 2 groups. (Adapted from Frank SM, Norris EJ, Christopherson R, et al. Right- and left-arm discrepancies in vascular surgery patients. *Anesthesiology.* 1991;75:457.)

If available, a preoperative baseline measure of hemoglobin saturation ($Sp_{O_2}$) is also of value because it not only identifies a respiratory abnormality but also establishes a realistic goal for postoperative saturation before the patient is discharged from the postanesthesia recovery area. The need for supplemental oxygen is also assessed. In many institutions, $Sp_{O_2}$ has become the fifth vital sign, with pain score being the sixth.

## Airway

An accurate assessment of the airway must be made and includes examination of cervical spine mobility, temporomandibular joint function, and dentition. Problems with orotracheal intubation may be expected in those patients who are unable to open their mouths >4 cm; whose distance from the thyroid notch to the mandible is <3 fingerbreadths; who have a high, arched palate; who demonstrate decreased cervical spine mobility; or who have an oropharyngeal (Mallampati) class of III or IV (Fig. 1–8).[92,93]

These tests have come under criticism. Individually, they lack specificity and have a low positive predictive value for difficult intubations.[94] Accuracy will improve if the airway is evaluated while the patient is sitting, the head is in full extension, the tongue is protruded, the patient is making vocal sounds, and the distance is measured from the thyroid cartilage to just inferior to the mentum.[95] A multivariate risk index (Table 1–3) appears to be more accurate than the oropharyngeal classification.[96] A simplified airway risk index of ≥4 exceeds the specificity of a Mallampati class III for predicting laryngoscopic views of grades III and IV. The use of an acoustic reflection device may also prove to be of value in predicting difficult intubations.[97]

## Dentition

Examination of the teeth is important as well. The presence of chipped or otherwise damaged teeth should be noted on

**TABLE 1–3.** Multivariate Predictors of Difficulty With Tracheal Intubation

| Variable | Simplified Airway Risk Index Weighting* |
|---|---|
| *Mouth Opening* | |
| ≥4 cm | 0 |
| <4 cm | 1 |
| *Thyromental Distance* | |
| >6.5 cm | 0 |
| 6.0-6.5 cm | 1 |
| <6.0 cm | 2 |
| *Mallampati Class* | |
| I | 0 |
| II | 1 |
| III | 2 |
| *Neck Movement* | |
| >90° | 0 |
| 80-90° | 1 |
| <80° | 2 |
| *Ability to Protrude the Lower Jaw* | |
| Yes | 0 |
| No | 1 |
| *Body Weight* | |
| <90 kg | 0 |
| 90-110 kg | 1 |
| >110 kg | 2 |
| *History of Difficult Intubation* | |
| None | 0 |
| Questionable | 1 |
| Definite | 2 |

*The risk index score represents the sum of the individual risk factor weightings (eg, a patient with Mallampati class II who is unable to protrude the lower jaw, weighs >110 kg, and has a questionable history of difficult intubation would be assigned a simplified airway risk score of 5. (From el-Ganzouri AR, McCarthy RJ, Tuman KJ, et al. Preoperative airway assessment: predictive value of a multivariate risk index. *Anesth Analg.* 1996;82:1200.)

the medical record. Teeth that are in imminent danger of falling out should be pulled before the administration of anesthesia to avoid aspiration. This procedure, of course, must be done with the patient's consent.

## Neck

Examination of the neck should be performed in addition to the airway examination just described. A carotid bruit indicates the presence of PVD and may be an indication for further evaluation but does not necessarily reflect an increased risk for a perioperative stroke.[98] Palpation of the thyroid gland can also be performed quickly and easily.

## Lungs

Auscultation of the lungs may reveal evidence of disease in otherwise asymptomatic individuals and may indicate that further evaluation is needed. Bronchospasm in an asthmatic patient who has been cleared for surgery indicates that the patient has not been prepared optimally. Similarly, evidence of rales or wheezing in a patient with a history of CHF may be suggestive of subclinical CHF. Diaphragmatic excursion should be checked if an interscalene block is planned because ipsilateral phrenic nerve paralysis occurs regularly with this technique.[99]

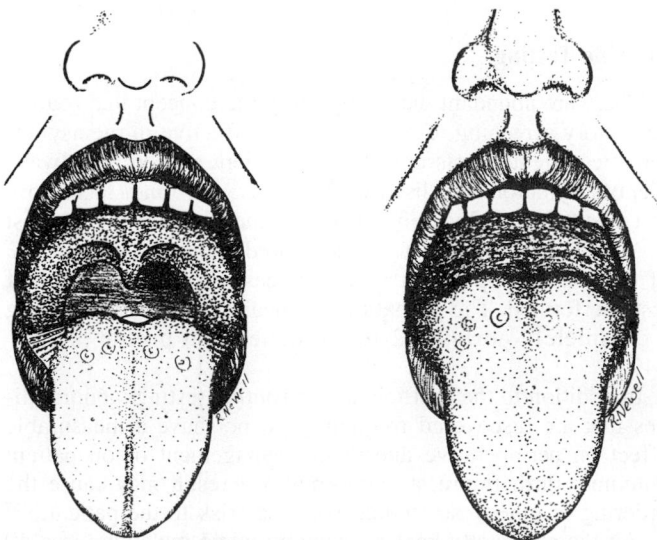

**FIGURE 1–8.** Examples of Mallampati *(left)* class I (faucial pillars; soft palate and uvula are visible) and *(right)* class III (no pharyngeal structures are seen) airways. Difficulty may be encountered when intubating the patient with the class III airway. (From Mallampati SR, Gugino LD, Gatt SP, et al. A clinical sign to predict difficult tracheal intubation: a prospective study. *Can Anaesth Soc J.* 1985;32:429.)

**TABLE 1–4.** Useful Bedside Maneuvers to Determine the Type of Cardiac Murmur

| Type of Murmur | Müller Maneuver | Valsalva Maneuver | Squatting | Standing | Amyl Nitrate |
|---|---|---|---|---|---|
| Right-sided heart murmurs | ↑ | | Should ↑ | | ↑ |
| Hypertrophic cardiomyopathy | ↓ | ↑ | ↓ | ↑ | ↑ |
| Aortic stenosis | | ↓ | Should ↑ | ↓ | ↑ |
| Mitral regurgitation | | | Should ↑ | ↓ | ↓ |
| Mitral valve prolapse | ± | ± | | ↑ | ± |
| Aortic insufficiency | | | ↑ | | ↓ |
| Pulmonic stenosis | | | | ↓ | ↑ |
| Tricuspid regurgitation | | | | ↓ | ↑ |
| Pulmonic regurgitation | | | | | ↑ |

Reproduced with permission from Rothman A, Goldberger AL. Aids to cardiac auscultation. *Ann Intern Med.* 1983;99:346.

## Heart

Examination of the heart should include an assessment of the heart rate and rhythm (regular, irregular, presence of extrasystolic beats) and determination of whether murmurs, extra heart sounds (eg, a third heart sound), or jugular venous distention are present. Determination of the type of murmur may be assisted by the use of amyl nitrate and several bedside maneuvers (Table 1–4).[100, 101]

## Extremities and Back

The extremities and back should also be examined. If use of a regional anesthetic is contemplated, examination of the injection site is important to identify that it is clear of lesions and that the appropriate landmarks are present to determine the feasibility of the technique.

A modification of the Allen test (Table 1–5)[102] is usually performed to provide some assessment of the adequacy of ulnar collateral flow if cannulation of the radial artery is considered. However, the utility of this test in patients without PVD has been called into question.[103] Because this test does not cost anything and has no risk associated with it, and because the results may alter choice of the cannulation site, it is difficult to convincingly argue against its use.

## Neurologic Function

If a regional anesthetic technique is planned, the anesthesiologist should document the neurologic function in the area to be anesthetized. Likewise, if the patient is to be operated on in an unusual position, the anesthesiologist should determine the neurologic function of areas that could be affected by the position. A corollary to this approach is to have the patient assume the anticipated intraoperative position to determine whether it is easily tolerated.

## Preexisting Deficits

Documentation of preexisting neurologic deficits is important, especially considering that 15% of closed malpractice claims made against anesthesiologists involved peripheral nerve injury after anesthesia.[104] If a neurologic deficit is present, succinylcholine may be contraindicated owing to increased muscle membrane chemosensitivity and resultant hyperkalemia.[38]

# LABORATORY TESTING

## What Tests Are Appropriate?

Extensive information has been published since the 1990s regarding routine preoperative blood tests. The most important screening "test" to detect disease processes is still a thorough history and physical examination.

## Routine Testing

There are abundant data supporting the concept that routine laboratory screening tests are not cost-effective in the asymptomatic patient.[1] Tests are often inefficient and do not always identify symptomatic disease.[105] Because a *normal* laboratory test result is usually defined as the mean value for the test ± 2 SD, an *abnormal* test result predictably appears in 5% of the healthy population[106] and increases with the number of tests performed. The probability of healthy individuals having a completely normal 12-test biochemical profile is only 54%.[106]

In addition to the inefficiency of routine testing, abnormalities that are discovered frequently do not have a measurable effect on perioperative anesthetic management or on patient outcome; furthermore, an abnormal test result may cause the ordering of other tests, which increases risk to the patient.[1,107]

For the apparently healthy, asymptomatic male who is <40 years of age and who is undergoing surgery with minimal expected blood loss, no preoperative blood testing is necessary.[1,107] Those patients with underlying disease as detected by history and physical examination should undergo preoperative testing.[1,107,108]

**TABLE 1–5.** Modified Allen Test

Both radial and ulnar arteries are compressed
The patient clenches and unclenches the fist repeatedly until the palm develops pallor
One of the arteries is released
The amount of time required for blushing of the palm is noted
The procedure is repeated for the other artery
Normal palmar blushing should be evident within 7 s
An equivocal test is 8-14 s
An abnormal test is present if it takes 15 s or longer for the palm to blush
A pulse oximeter may also be helpful to determine the time to return of flow

From Seneff M. Arterial line placement and care. In: Irwin RS, Cerra FB, Rippe JM, eds. *Intensive Care Medicine.* 4th ed. Philadelphia, Pa: Lippincott-Raven; 1999:36–46.

## Electrocardiogram

The utility of routine electrocardiograms (ECGs) is also questionable. Abnormal ECG findings are common in surgical patients, and the prevalence of these findings increases with age.[109] Abnormal findings usually do not alter perioperative medical management.[109,110] The significance of the abnormalities depends in part on the prevalence of the disease state. In young, healthy patients, Q waves or ST-T wave changes usually are not due to ischemic heart disease.[109]

The probability of detecting cardiac disease based on the admission ECG and not during the taking of the patient history or physical examination is low irrespective of age, but it increases in patients >44 years of age or in those who also have a history of a cardiac abnormality.[109]

Although there is no consensus when a routine preoperative ECG should be obtained,[109] it is reasonable to request one for patients older than 40 to 50 years of age, particularly if a history of cardiac disease is suggested.[106,108–110]

## Previous Tests

If a patient has normal complete blood cell count; sodium, potassium, and creatinine levels; prothrombin time; and partial thromboplastin times within 1 year before surgery, the likelihood that a current preoperative value is abnormal is <0.5%,[111] whereas up to 20% of preoperative tests results will be abnormal if a previous test result is also abnormal.[111]

Despite specific criteria for preoperative tests, more recent data suggest that a large number of unnecessary tests are still ordered and that indicated testing is often not performed.[112] Implementation of hospital preoperative testing guidelines can decrease unnecessary testing by approximately 30%.[113] Table 1–6 presents proposed guidelines for the minimal amount of preoperative testing for a number of disease categories.[108]

# SPECIAL TESTING

## When Should Additional Testing Be Performed?

### Coronary Artery Disease

Each year, approximately 7 to 8 million noncardiac surgical patients are at risk for cardiac morbidity and mortality.[114] A significant number of these patients have undetected CAD. Preoperative identification of this high-risk group is not only important but also necessary to identify the severity, stability, and prior treatment of the disease.[115] The American College of Cardiology and American Heart Association convened a task force that developed a Bayesian approach to delineate which patients should be candidates for further preoperative testing. Clinical markers of risk, the functional capacity of the patient, and the risk of specific surgical procedures were blended to develop algorithms (Fig. 1–9A–C) to assist clinicians in assessing the patient with CAD.

### Noninvasive Testing

A number of noninvasive tests are available to assist in the evaluation of the patient with known or suspected CAD.

**Dipyridamole-Thallium or Adenosine-Thallium Imaging.** Dipyridamole and adenosine are potent coronary artery vasodilators and divert coronary blood flow from areas with fixed arterial lesions. Thallous chloride Tl 201 is taken up by normal myocytes and is detected by scintigraphy. The thallium is administered after the vasodilator has been infused. Areas of the myocardium that do not take up thallium during and after dipyridamole or adenosine-induced vasodilation are considered areas of infarct. Areas of the myocardium that do not take up thallium during vasodilation but do so afterward (reperfusion defect) are considered at risk for ischemia and infarction (Fig. 1–10).

This type of imaging is also helpful in detecting significant CAD in high-risk patients who cannot be tested using other methods (eg, patients with PVD who cannot perform treadmill testing). If the reperfusion defect is sufficiently severe, the patient may be referred for coronary angiography and possible angioplasty or revascularization instead of undergoing the scheduled elective procedure. This strategy has come into question; retrospective reviews and decision analyses have suggested that invasive cardiac evaluation and selective coronary revascularization are not justified for the majority of patients, including those with extensive CAD.[116,117] However, the knowledge that a particular patient is at high risk for perioperative ischemia or infarction is still highly useful information because monitoring or anesthetic techniques and postoperative care strategy (eg, β-blockade) might change. Published negative predictive values exceed 95%, whereas the positive predictive values range from 5% to 25%.[118]

**Other Tests.** Echocardiographic observation of new or worsening wall motion abnormalities during an infusion of dobutamine is helpful in detecting CAD. A normal dobutamine stress echocardiogram has a negative predictive value of 93% to 100%, whereas the presence of a new or worsening wall motion abnormality is of value in risk prediction in patients with clinical markers of CAD but not in patients without risk factors.[118] Preoperative ischemia detected by Holter monitoring may identify vascular surgery patients at risk for perioperative cardiac events.[119] Echocardiography and gated radionuclide angiography can be useful ancillary tests in those patients with a history of cardiac dysfunction because such tests can also assess the degree and location of cardiac wall motion abnormalities.

## Pulmonary Function

### Spirometry

For those patients undergoing nonthoracic surgery, few studies exist that validate the clinical usefulness of routine pulmonary function testing in the preoperative period.[120,121] Spirometry is no better than a careful history and physical examination in predicting postoperative pulmonary complications following upper abdominal surgery.[122,123] In addition, no single abnormal finding on standard pulmonary function testing contraindicates surgery. Patients with a forced expiratory volume in 1 second ($FEV_1$) as low as 0.45 L have tolerated surgery.[123]

Several easily obtained clinical parameters are predictive of postoperative pulmonary complications (Table 1–7).[124] For those patients in whom a pneumonectomy is contemplated, more extensive testing that includes split pulmonary function testing, exercise studies, and right-sided heart catheterization with pulmonary artery (PA) pressure measurements is generally indicated.[122–124]

**TABLE 1–6.** Suggested Minimal Preoperative Test Requirements

| Preoperative Diagnosis | ECG | CXR | Hct/Hb | CBC | Electrolytes | BUN/Creatinine | Glucose | Coagulation | LFT | Medication Levels | Ca++ |
|---|---|---|---|---|---|---|---|---|---|---|---|
| ***Cardiac Disease*** | | | | | | | | | | | |
| History of myocardial infarction | X | | | | ± | | | | | | |
| Stable angina | X | | | | ± | | | | | | |
| Congestive heart failure | X | ± | | | | | | | | | |
| Hypertension | X | ± | | | X* | ± | | | | X† | |
| Chronic atrial fibrillation | X | | | | | X | | | | | |
| Peripheral vascular disease | X | | | | | | | | | | |
| ***Valvular Heart Disease*** | X | ± | | | | | | | | | |
| ***Pulmonary Disease*** | | | | | | | | | | | |
| Emphysema | X | ± | | | | | | | | X‡ | |
| Asthma | | | | | | | | | | | |
| Chronic bronchitis | X | ± | | X | | | | | | | |
| ***Diabetes*** | X | ± | | | ± | X | X | | | | |
| ***Hepatic Disease*** | | | | | | | | | | | |
| Infectious hepatitis | | | | | | | | X | X | | |
| Alcohol/drug induced | | | | | | | | X | X | | |
| Tumor infiltration | | | | | | | | X | X | | |
| ***Renal Disease*** | | | X | | X | X | | | | | |
| ***Hematological Disorders*** | | | | X | | | | | | | |
| ***Coagulopathies*** | | | | X | | | | X | | | |
| ***Central Nervous System Disorders*** | | | | | | | | | | | |
| Stroke | X | | | X | X | | X | | | | |
| Seizures | X | | | X | X | | X | | | X | |
| Tumor | X | | | X | | | | | | | |
| Vascular/aneurysms | X | | X | X | | | | | | | |
| ***Malignancy*** | | | X | X | X | | | | | | X |
| ***Hyperthyroidism*** | X | | X | | X | | | | | | |
| ***Hypothyroidism*** | X | | X | | X | | | | | | |
| ***Cushing Syndrome*** | | | | X | X | | X | | | | |
| ***Addison Disease*** | | | | X | X | | X | | | | |
| ***Hyperparathyroidism*** | X | | X | | | X | | | | | X |
| ***Hypoparathyroidism*** | X | | | | | | | | | | X |
| ***Morbid Obesity*** | X | ± | | X | X | X | X | | | | |
| ***Malabsorption/Poor Nutrition*** | | | | X | | | | ± | | | |
| ***Select Drug Therapies*** | | | | | | | | | | | |
| Digoxin (digitalis) | X | | | | ± | | | | | X | |
| Anticoagulants | | | X | | | | | X | | | |
| Dilantin | | | | | | X | | | | X | |
| Phenobarbital | | | | | | | | | | X | |
| Diuretics | | | | | X | X | X | | | | |
| Steroids | | | | X | | | X | | | | |
| Chemotherapy | | | | X | | | | | | | |
| Aspirin/nonsteroidal anti-inflammatory drug | | | | | | | | | | | |
| Theophylline | | | | | | | | | | X | |

*Patients on diuretics.
†Patients on digoxin.
‡Patients on theophylline.
X, obtained; ±, consider; BUN, serum urea nitrogen; Ca++, calcium; CBC, complete blood cell count; CXR, chest radiograph; ECG, electrocardiogram; Hct/Hb, hematocrit/hemoglobin; LFT, liver function test.
From Fischer SP. Cost-effective preoperative evaluation and testing. *Chest.* 1999;115:98S.

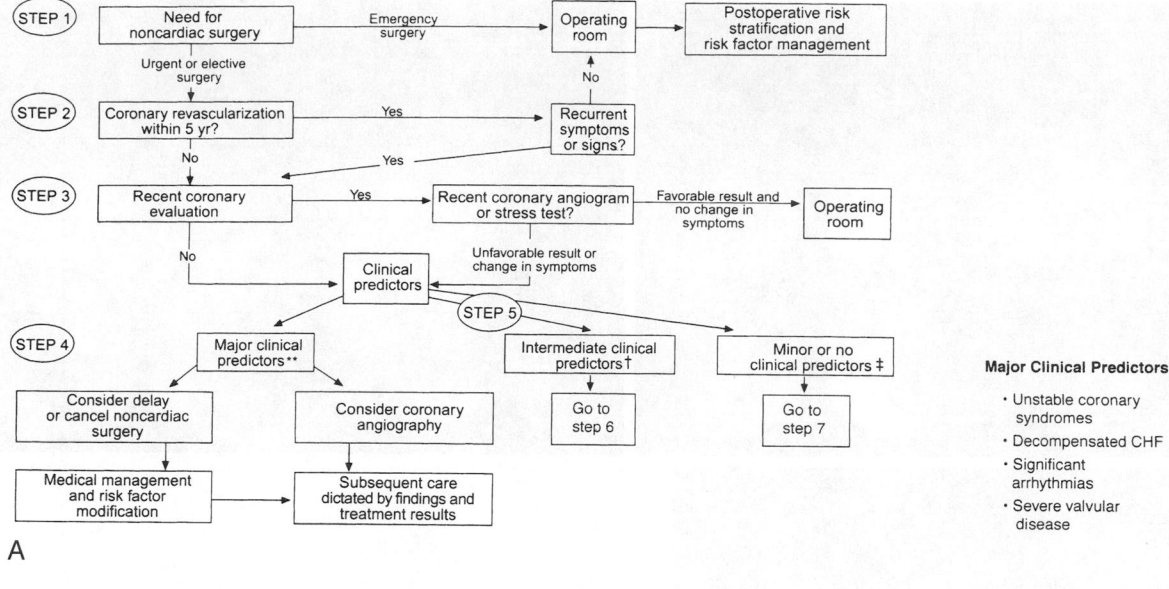

**Major Clinical Predictors \*\***

· Unstable coronary syndromes
· Decompensated CHF
· Significant arrhythmias
· Severe valvular disease

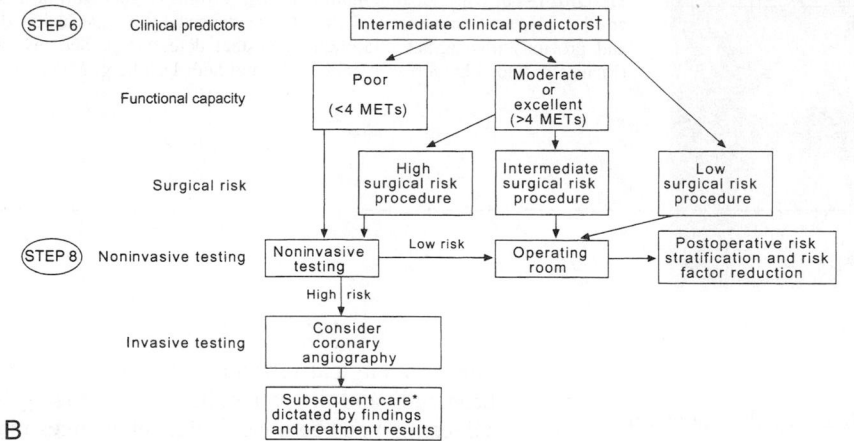

**Intermediate Clinical Predictors †**

· Mild angina pectoris
· Prior MI
· Compensated or prior CHF
· Diabetes mellitus

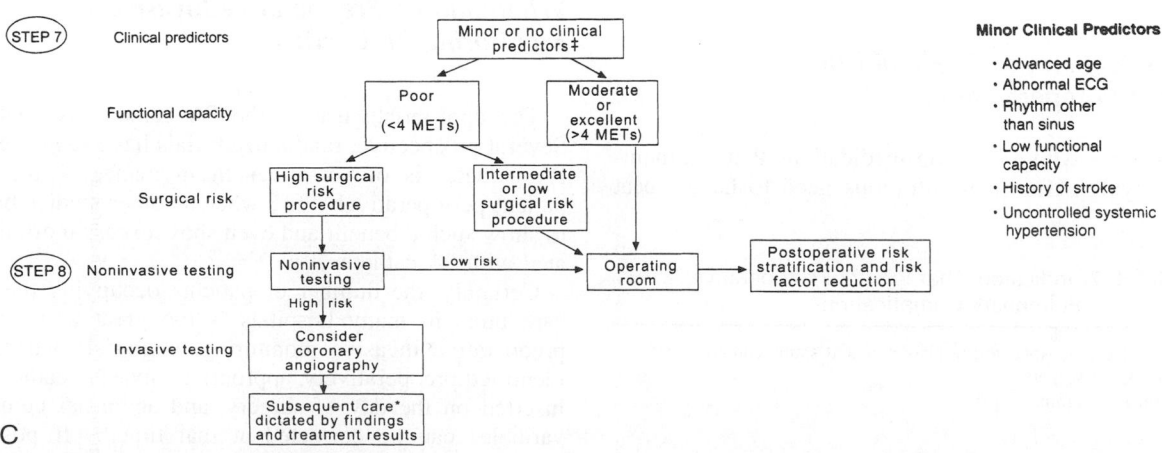

**Minor Clinical Predictors ‡**

· Advanced age
· Abnormal ECG
· Rhythm other than sinus
· Low functional capacity
· History of stroke
· Uncontrolled systemic hypertension

**FIGURE 1–9.** *A–C,* Stepwise approach to preoperative cardiac assessment. Subsequent care may include cancellation or delay of surgery, coronary revascularization followed by noncardiac surgery, or intensified care. In step 6, an example of poor functional capacity (<4 METs) is light work around the house (dusting, dishes) and an example of moderate or excellent functional capacity (>4 METs) is climbing a flight of stairs. MET, metabolic equivalent. (From Guidelines for perioperative cardiovascular evaluation for noncardiac surgery. Report of the American College of Cardiology/American Heart Association Task Force on Practice Guidelines. *Circulation.* 1996;93:1278–1317.)

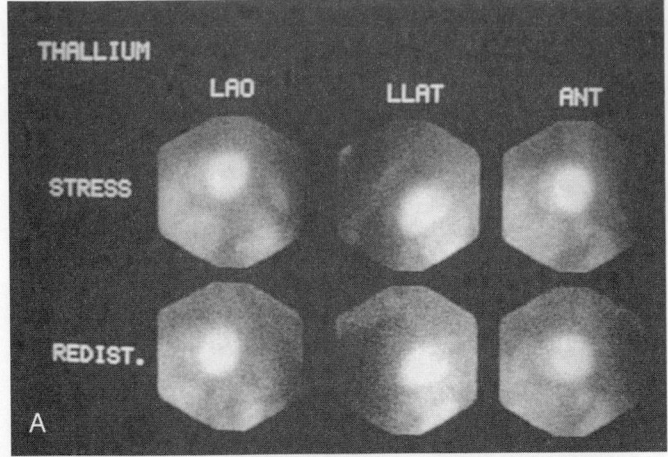

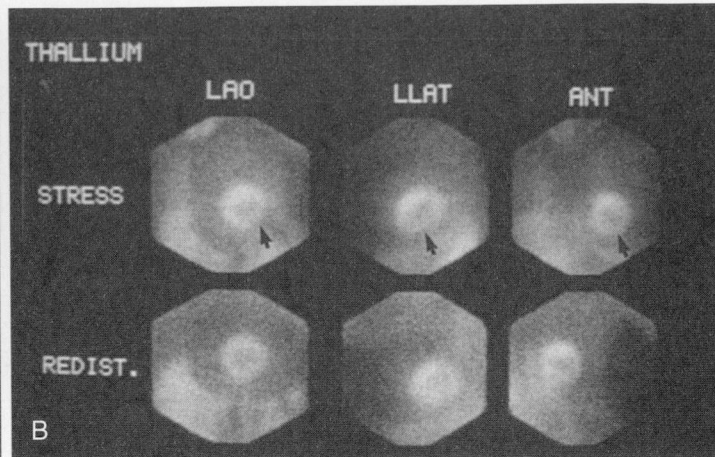

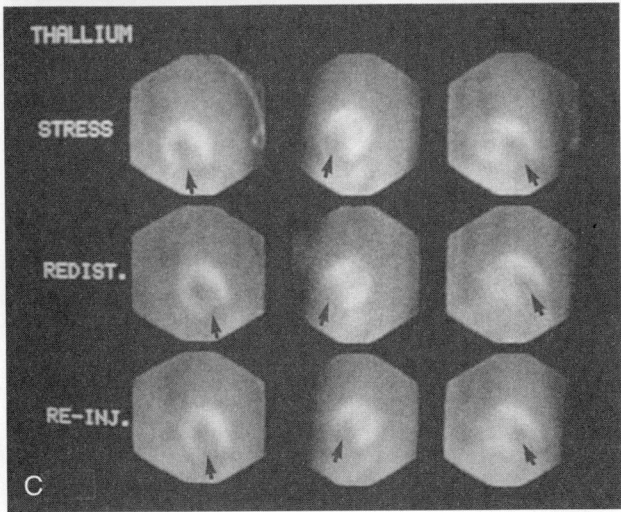

**FIGURE 1–10.** Dipyridamole-thallium images from patients with normal coronary arteries (*A*), coronary artery disease (as evidenced by a reperfusion defect [*B*]), and previous myocardial infarction (persistent defect [*C*]). See text for details. (Images provided by Jeffrey Leppo, MD, and Seth Dahlberg, MD.)

## Arterial Blood Gas Analysis

In addition to a careful clinical evaluation, the most important and easily obtained test relating to pulmonary function is the arterial blood gas measurement.[123] In the absence of neuromuscular disease or drug-induced alveolar hypoventilation, an arterial carbon dioxide tension ($Pa_{CO_2}$) >45 mm Hg reliably predicts pulmonary complications.[121]

## Which Medication Levels Should Be Determined Preoperatively?

Not all patients who are taking medications that are monitored by assaying serum concentrations need to have repeat

**TABLE 1–7.** Indicators That Predict Postoperative Pulmonary Complications

American Society of Anesthesiologists physical status category >II
Upper abdominal surgery
Residual intra-abdominal sepsis
Age >59 y
Obesity
Preoperative stay >4 d
Colorectal or gastroduodenal surgery
Cardiac surgery with pleurotomy
Preoperative $Pa_{CO_2}$ >45

assays before a surgical procedure. If a medication has been taken chronically and the patient has been clinically stable, no additional testing need be done.[125] Recent changes in dosing or in the clinical condition make determination of the serum concentration of the medication in question prudent.

## When Should Preoperative Invasive Monitoring Be Used?

The appropriate use of the PA catheter is controversial. Several prospective, randomized trials have suggested that the PA catheter is of some benefit in managing the high-risk patient perioperatively,[126,127] whereas other studies have failed to show such a benefit and even show excess mortality associated with PA catheter use.[128,129]

Certainly, the number of patients occupying the intensive care units in many hospitals is too great to allow routine preoperative invasive monitoring. High-risk patients can be identified preoperatively, appropriate invasive catheters can be inserted on the day of surgery, and abnormal hemodynamic variables can be corrected at that time.[127] If postoperative surgical intensive care is anticipated, arrangements should be made preoperatively. Surgery should not begin on patients requiring such care until a bed is available in the surgical intensive care unit.

## CONSULTATIONS

### When Is Preoperative Consultation Appropriate?

After the history and physical examination are completed and the laboratory data have been reviewed, additional testing or treatment may be indicated. Assistance from other medical specialists is appropriate to help better prepare the patient for surgery or to perform additional diagnostic tests.

When requesting the services of a consultant, the anesthesiologist should ask a specific question rather than request preoperative clearance. Without specific direction, the consultant, who may lack an understanding of intraoperative practice, often suggests methods of intraoperative monitoring, medication use, or anesthetic techniques that are inappropriate or condescending.[130]

A growing number of medical centers have developed preoperative anesthesia consultation clinics where anesthesiologists direct the evaluation of patients deemed at high risk for anesthesia and surgery.[5,131] The interviewing anesthesiologist should contact the consultant directly by telephone to discuss the specifics of the situation and to expedite the consultation. This approach helps to prevent delays in elective surgical cases.

### How Is the Risk of Anesthesia Estimated?

The overall risk of death from anesthesia in several reports ranges from 0.01% to 0.0005%.[132] This range is for primary anesthetic mortality only and not for anesthetic-associated deaths from iatrogenic causes. A preoperative grading system that evaluates patients according to their general state of health and the severity of their underlying diseases was first published by Saklad.[133] This system was later revised into the American Society of Anesthesiologists (ASA) Physical Status Scale (Table 1–8).[134]

Although interobserver variations in score assignment and vagueness in the definitions have been noted,[135] several studies showed the ASA physical status scale to be a good predictor of noncardiac deaths when it is applied to total operative mortality.[136,137] The scale is much less sensitive when it is used as a means to predict anesthesia-related deaths.[138]

**TABLE 1–8.** American Society of Anesthesiologists Physical Status Scale

| Category | Description |
|---|---|
| I | Normal, healthy patient |
| II | Mild systemic disease; no functional limitation |
| III | Severe systemic disease; definite functional limitation |
| IV | Severe systemic disease that is a constant threat to life |
| V | Moribund patient who is unlikely to survive 24 h with or without operation |
| VI | Patient declared brain-dead whose organs are being removed for donation |
| E | Emergency operation |

## PREOPERATIVE MEDICATIONS

### What Medications Should Be Given Preoperatively?

As discussed previously, the most important medications should be continued on the day of surgery. Other specific medication needs are discussed next.

#### Antibiotics

If the patient is at risk for the development of infective endocarditis, appropriate antibiotic prophylaxis should be instituted. Table 1–9 provides the most recent American Heart Association guidelines for perioperative endocarditis prophylaxis.[139]

Many patients receive preoperative prophylactic antibiotics to reduce the incidence of wound or prosthetic device-related infections. Such antibiotics must be given no earlier than 2 hours before incision; otherwise, their effectiveness is reduced (Fig. 1–11).[140]

#### Aspiration Prophylaxis

Those patients at risk for vomiting and aspiration of gastric contents should receive prophylaxis with nonparticulate antacids or histamine$_2$ blockers with or without metoclopramide.[141] Proton pump inhibitors such as omeprazole are also effective in keeping gastric pH above 2.5.[142] Routine use of these agents is not recommended in patients at low risk for pulmonary aspiration.[143]

#### Prophylaxis for Venous Thrombosis

Some patients are at high risk for the development of venous thrombosis in the perioperative period (Table 1–10).

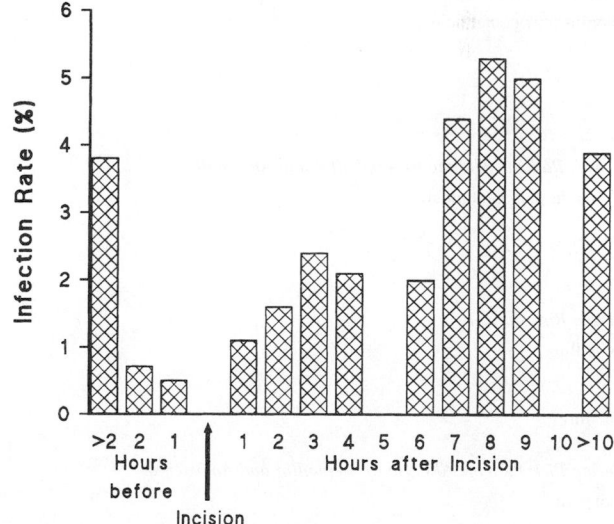

**FIGURE 1–11.** Surgical wound infection rates as a function of the time of initial perioperative antibiotic dose. There is a significant trend toward higher infection rates for each hour that antibiotic administration was delayed following surgical incision. (Reprinted from Classen DC, Evans RS, Pestotnik SL, et al. The timing of prophylactic administration of antibiotics and the risk of surgical-wound infection. *N Engl J Med.* 1992;326:281, by permission of the *New England Journal of Medicine.*)

**TABLE 1–9.** Bacterial Endocarditis Prophylaxis

**Cardiac Conditions for Which Prophylaxis Is Recommended**

*High-Risk Category*

Prosthetic cardiac valves, including bioprosthetic and homograft valves
Previous bacterial endocarditis
Complex cyanotic congenital heart disease (eg, single ventricle states, transposition of the great arteries, tetralogy of Fallot)
Surgically constructed systemic pulmonary shunts or conduits

*Moderate-Risk Category*

Most other congenital cardiac malformations
Acquired valvular dysfunction (eg, rheumatic heart disease)
Hypertrophic cardiomyopathy
Mitral valve prolapse with valvular regurgitation or thickened leaflets

**Surgical Procedures for Which Prophylaxis Is Recommended**

*Dental Procedures*

Those known to induce gingival or mucosal bleeding

*Respiratory Tract*

Tonsillectomy or adenoidectomy
Surgical operations that involve respiratory mucosa
Bronchoscopy with a rigid bronchoscope

*Gastrointestinal Tract*

Sclerotherapy for esophageal varices
Esophageal stricture dilation
Endoscopic retrograde cholangiography with biliary obstruction
Biliary tract surgery
Surgical operations that involve intestinal mucosa

*Genitourinary Tract*

Prostatic surgery
Cystoscopy
Urethral dilation

**Standard Prophylactic Regimen for Patients at Risk**

| *Drug* | *Dosing Regimen*\*† |
|---|---|
| *Standard General Prophylaxis* | |
| Amoxicillin | *Adults:* 2.0 g orally 1 h before procedure<br>*Children:* 50 mg/kg orally 1 h before procedure |
| *Allergic to Penicillin* | |
| Clindamycin | *Adults:* 600 mg orally 1 h before procedure<br>*Children:* 20 mg/kg orally 1 h before procedure |
| *or*<br>Cephalexin‡ or cefadroxil‡ | *Adults:* 2.0 g orally 1 h before procedure<br>*Children:* 50 mg/kg orally 1 h before procedure |
| *or*<br>Azithromycin or clarithromycin | *Adults:* 500 mg orally 1 h before procedure<br>*Children:* 15 mg/kg orally 1 h before procedure |
| *Patients Unable to Take Oral Medications* | |
| Ampicillin | *Adults:* 2.0 g IM or IV within 30 min before procedure<br>*Children:* 50 mg/kg IM or IV within 30 min before procedure |
| *Patients Allergic to Penicillin and Unable to Take Oral Medications* | |
| Clindamycin | *Adults:* 600 mg IV within 30 min before procedure<br>*Children:* 20 mg/kg IV within 30 min before procedure |
| *or*<br>Cefazolin‡ | *Adults:* 1.0 g IM or IV within 30 min before procedure<br>*Children:* 25 mg/kg IM or IV within 30 min before procedure |
| *High-Risk Patients* | |
| Ampicillin plus gentamicin | *Adults:* ampicillin 2.0 g IM or IV plus gentamicin 1.5 mg/kg (not to exceed 120 mg) within 30 min of starting procedure; 6 h later, ampicillin 1 g IM/IV or amoxicillin 1 g orally<br>*Children:* ampicillin 50 mg/kg IM or IV (not to exceed 2.0 g) plus gentamicin 1.5 mg/kg within 30 min of starting procedure; 6 h later, ampicillin 25 mg/kg IM/IV or amoxicillin 25 mg/kg orally |
| *High-Risk Patients Allergic to Ampicillin and Amoxicillin* | |
| Vancomycin plus gentamicin | *Adults:* vancomycin 1.0 g IV over 1–2 h plus gentamicin 1.5 mg/kg IV/IM (not to exceed 120 mg); complete injection/infusion within 30 min of starting procedure<br>*Children:* vancomycin 20 mg/kg IV over 1–2 h plus gentamicin 1.5 mg/kg IV/IM; complete injection/infusion within 30 min of starting procedure |
| *Moderate-Risk Patients* | |
| Amoxicillin | *Adults:* amoxicillin 2.0 g orally 1 h before procedure<br>*Children:* amoxicillin 50 mg/kg orally 1 h before procedure |
| *or*<br>Ampicillin | *Adults:* ampicillin 2.0 g IM/IV within 30 min of starting procedure<br>*Children:* ampicillin 50 mg/kg IM/IV within 30 min of starting procedure |
| *Moderate-Risk Patients Allergic to Ampicillin and Amoxicillin* | |
| Vancomycin | *Adults:* vancomycin 1.0 g IV over 1–2 h; complete infusion within 30 min of starting procedure<br>*Children:* vancomycin 20 mg/kg IV over 1–2 h; complete infusion within 30 min of starting procedure |

\*Total children's dose should not exceed adult dose.
†No second dose of vancomycin or gentamicin is recommended.
‡Cephalosporins should not be used in individuals with immediate-type hypersensitivity reaction (urticaria, angioedema, or anaphylaxis) to penicillins.
IM, intramuscular; IV, intravenous.
Modified from Dajani AS, Taubert KA, Wilson W, et al. Prevention of bacterial endocarditis. Recommendations by the American Heart Association. *JAMA.* 1997;277:1794–1801. Copyright 1997, American Medical Association.

**TABLE 1–10.** Risk Levels for Venous Thromboembolism

|  | Low | Moderate | High | Highest |
|---|---|---|---|---|
| Calf vein thrombosis | 2% | 10%–20% | 20%–40% | 40%–80% |
| Proximal vein thrombosis | 0.4% | 2%–4% | 4%–8% | 10%–20% |
| Clinical pulmonary embolism | 0.2% | 1%–2% | 2%–4% | 4%–10% |
| Fatal pulmonary embolism | 0.002% | 0.1%–0.4% | 0.4%–1.0% | 1%–5% |
| Successful preventive strategies | No specific measures | LDUH (q12h), LMWH, IPC, and ES | LDUH (q8h), LMWH and IPC | LMWH, oral anticoagulants, IPC (+ LDUH or LMWH), and ADH |

Low, Patients <40 y with no clinical risk factors undergoing uncomplicated minor surgery.

Moderate, Patients 40–60 y with no additional risk factors undergoing any surgery (major or minor), patients <40 y with no additional risk factors undergoing major surgery, or patients with risk factors undergoing minor surgery.

High, Patients >60 y without additional risk factors undergoing major surgery, patients 40–60 y who have additional risk factors undergoing major surgery, or patients with myocardial infarction, and medical patients with risk factors.

Highest, Patients >40 y with prior venous thromboembolism, with malignant disease, or in a hypercoagulable state undergoing major surgery, patients with elective major lower extremity orthopedic surgery, hip fracture, stroke, multiple trauma, or spinal cord injury.

ADH, adjusted dose heparin; ES, elastic compression stockings; IPC, intermittent pneumatic compression devices; LDUH, low dose unfractionated heparin; LMWH, low molecular weight heparin.

Modified from Clagett GP, Anderson FA Jr, Geerts W, et al. Prevention of venous thromboembolism. *Chest.* 1998;114:531S–560S.

Prophylactic measures should be used. Various methods include the use of low-dose heparin, LMWH, heparinoids, intermittent calf compression, warfarin (particularly after total hip replacement), or dextran.[144] Regrettably, studies indicate methods to prevent venous thromboembolism are underutilized.[145]

## "NIL PER OS" STATUS

### How Long Should a Patient Not Be Allowed to Take Anything by Mouth?

The duration of preoperative fasting has come under scrutiny since the late 1980s. The stomach empties clear liquids in 1 to 2 hours but takes >3 hours to clear solids.[146] Studies indicate that in both children and adults (ASA I or II), gastric volume and pH are unchanged after ingestion of 2 to 3 mL/kg of clear liquids (eg, tea, coffee, fruit juice without pulp, and water) 2 to 3 hours before the scheduled start of surgery compared with those of the gastric contents of patients who fasted for >6 hours (Fig. 1–12).[147–150] Practice guidelines have recently been published by the ASA and the summary recommendations are presented in Table 1–11.[143]

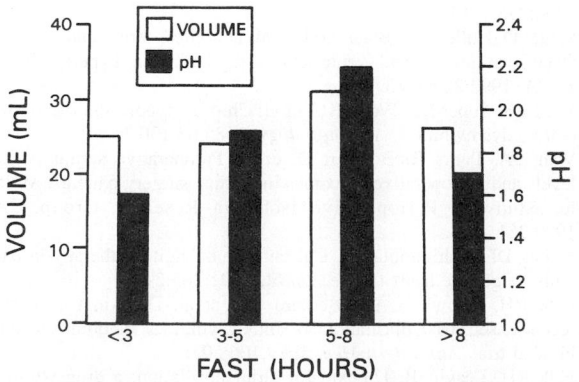

**FIGURE 1–12.** Gastric volume and pH as a function of preoperative duration of fast for liquids. There are no significant differences among groups. (Data from Scarr M, Maltby JR, Jani K, et al. Volume and acidity of residual gastric fluid after oral fluid ingestion before elective ambulatory surgery. *Can Med Assoc J.* 1989;141:1151.)

### How Should the "Do-Not-Resuscitate" Patient Be Treated?

Approximately 15% of patients with do-not-resuscitate orders undergo a surgical procedure.[151] These patients present a special problem to the anesthesiologist: should the do-not-resuscitate orders be suspended during anesthesia and surgery?

Because the administration of anesthesia involves the use of potent cardiovascular depressants and often requires some degree of resuscitation (whether it be with fluids, inotropes, or vasopressors), some anesthesiologists recommend that do-not-resuscitate orders be suspended in the perioperative period.[151–154] In the preoperative evaluation, the patient's do-not-resuscitate status should be clarified. If the goals of surgery and anesthesia are consistent with that clarification and if the patient and health care team agree, the operation can proceed. Appropriate resuscitative and supportive measures can then be undertaken should hemodynamic instability or arrest occur in the perioperative period as a result of the anesthesia or surgery.

**TABLE 1–11.** Suggested Fasting Guidelines for Elective Surgical Patients

| Ingested Material | Minimum Fasting Period* (h) |
|---|---|
| Clear liquids† | 2 |
| Breast milk | 4 |
| Infant formula | 6 |
| Nonhuman milk‡ | 6 |
| Light meal§ | 6 |

These recommendations apply to healthy patients who are undergoing elective procedures. They are not intended for women in labor. Following the guidelines does not guarantee complete gastric emptying.

*The fasting periods noted above apply to all ages.

†Examples of clear liquids include water, fruit juices without pulp, carbonated beverages, clear tea, and black coffee.

‡Since nonhuman milk is similar to solids in gastric emptying time, the amount ingested must be considered when determining an appropriate fasting period.

§A light meal typically consists of toast and clear liquids. Meals that include fried or fatty foods or meat may prolong gastric emptying time. Both the amount and type of foods ingested must be considered when determining an appropriate fasting period.

From Practice guidelines for preoperative fasting and the use of pharmacologic agents to reduce the risk of pulmonary aspiration: application to healthy patients undergoing elective procedures. A report by the American Society of Anesthesiologists Task Force on Preoperative Fasting. *Anesthesiology.* 1999;90:899.

If the cause of the arrest is the patient's underlying condition or is believed to be irreversible, resuscitative efforts do not have to be instituted.[152] The most important point that needs to be emphasized is that good preoperative communication and agreement must be present among physicians, the patient, and the members of the patient's family.[152]

## References

1. Roizen MF. Preoperative evaluation. In: Miller RD, ed. *Anesthesia*. New York, NY: Churchill Livingstone; 1994:827.
2. Egbert LD, Battit GE. The value of the preoperative visit by the anesthetist. *JAMA*. 1963;185:553.
3. Egbert LD. Preoperative anxiety: the adult patient. *Int Anesthesiol Clin*. 1986;24:17.
4. Leigh JM, Walker J, Janaganathan P. Effect of preoperative anaesthetic visit on anxiety. *BMJ*. 1977;2:987.
5. Pollard JB, Zboray AL, Mazze RI. Economic benefits attributed to opening a preoperative evaluation clinic for outpatients. *Anesth Analg*. 1996;83:407.
6. Lutner RE, Roizen MF, Stocking CB, et al. The automated interview versus the personal interview. Do patient responses to preoperative health questions differ? *Anesthesiology*. 1991;75:394.
7. Prys-Roberts C, Meloche R, Foëx P. Studies of anaesthesia in relation to hypertension, I: cardiovascular responses of treated and untreated patients. *Br J Anaesth*. 1971;43:122.
8. Goldman L, Caldera DL. Risks of general anesthesia and elective operation in the hypertensive patient. *Anesthesiology*. 1979;50:285.
9. Bedford RF, Feinstein B. Hospital admission blood pressure: a predictor for hypertension following endotracheal intubation. *Anesth Analg*. 1980;59:367.
10. Asiddao CB, Donegan JH, Whitesell RC, et al. Factors associated with perioperative complications during carotid endarterectomy. *Anesth Analg*. 1982;61:631.
11. Tarhan S, Moffitt EA, Taylor WF, et al. Myocardial infarction after general anesthesia. *JAMA*. 1972;220:1451.
12. Steen PA, Tinker JH, Tarhan S. Myocardial reinfarction after anesthesia and surgery. *JAMA*. 1978;239:2566.
13. Rao TL, Jacobs KH, El-Etr AA. Reinfarction following anesthesia in patients with myocardial infarction. *Anesthesiology*. 1983;59:499.
14. Shah KB, Kleinman BS, Sami H, et al. Reevaluation of perioperative myocardial infarction in patients with prior myocardial infarction undergoing noncardiac operations. *Anesth Analg*. 1990;71:231.
15. McCulloch HA, Sprague DH. Myths in vascular anesthesia. *Probl Anesthesiol*. 1991;5:453.
16. Goldman L, Caldera DL, Nussbaum SR, et al. Multifactorial index of cardiac risk in noncardiac surgical procedures. *N Engl J Med*. 1977;297:845.
17. Simon AB. Perioperative management of the pacemaker patient. *Anesthesiology*. 1977;46:127.
18. Bourke ME. The patient with a pacemaker or related device. *Can J Anaesth*. 1996;43:R24.
19. Domino KB, Smith TC. Electrocautery-induced reprogramming of a pacemaker using a precordial magnet. *Anesth Analg*. 1983;62:609.
20. Shapiro WA, Roizen MF, Singleton MA, et al. Intraoperative pacemaker complications. *Anesthesiology*. 1985;63:319.
21. Cohen MM, Cameron CB. Should you cancel the operation when a child has an upper respiratory tract infection? *Anesth Analg*. 1991;72:282.
22. DeSoto H, Patel RI, Soliman IE, et al. Changes in oxygen saturation following general anesthesia in children with upper respiratory infection signs and symptoms undergoing otolaryngological procedures. *Anesthesiology*. 1988;68:276.
23. Tait AR, Reynolds PI, Gutstein HB. Factors that influence an anesthesiologist's decision to cancel elective surgery for the child with an upper respiratory tract infection. *J Clin Anesth*. 1995;7:491.
24. Steward DJ. Assessment of pediatric patients for general anesthesia: the child with an upper respiratory infection and the ex-premature infant. *Semin Pediatr Surg*. 1999;8:13.
25. Irwin RS, Corrao WM, Pratter MR. Chronic persistent cough in the adult: the spectrum and frequency of causes and successful outcome of specific therapy. *Am Rev Respir Dis*. 1981;123:413.
26. Corrao WM, Braman SS, Irwin RS. Chronic cough as the sole presenting manifestation of bronchial asthma. *N Engl J Med*. 1979;300:633.
27. Olsson GL, Hallen B, Hambraeus-Jonzon K. Aspiration during anaesthesia: a computer-aided study of 185,358 anaesthetics. *Acta Anaesthesiol Scand*. 1986;30:84.
28. Knieriem K, Stehling L. Aspiration pneumonitis. *Semin Anesth*. 1990;9:54.
29. Mittal RK, Balaban DH. The esophagogastric junction. *N Engl J Med*. 1997;336:924.
30. Cohen S, Harris LD. Does hiatus hernia affect competence of the gastroesophageal sphincter? *N Engl J Med*. 1971;284:1053.
31. Hogan K, Rusy D, Springman SR. Difficult laryngoscopy and diabetes mellitus. *Anesth Analg*. 1988;67:1162.
32. Warner ME, Contreras MG, Warner MA, et al. Diabetes mellitus and difficult laryngoscopy in renal and pancreatic transplant patients. *Anesth Analg*. 1998;86:516.
33. Schlaghecke R, Kornely E, Santen RT, et al. The effect of long-term glucocorticoid therapy on pituitary-adrenal responses to exogenous corticotropin-releasing hormone. *N Engl J Med*. 1992;326:226.
34. Drucker DJ, Burrow GN. Cardiovascular surgery in the hypothyroid patient. *Arch Intern Med*. 1985;145:1585.
35. Weinberg AD, Brennan MD, Gorman CA, et al. Outcome of anesthesia and surgery in hypothyroid patients. *Arch Intern Med*. 1983;143:893.
36. Litt L, Roizen MF. Anesthetic and surgical risk in hypothyroidism [letter]. *Arch Intern Med*. 1984;144:657,660.
37. Schonwald G, Fish KJ, Perkash I. Cardiovascular complications during anesthesia in chronic spinal cord injured patients. *Anesthesiology*. 1981;55:550.
38. Gronert GA, Theye RA. Pathophysiology of hyperkalemia induced by succinylcholine. *Anesthesiology*. 1975;43:89.
39. Keenan MA, Stiles CM, Kaufman RL. Acquired laryngeal deviation associated with cervical spine disease in erosive polyarticular arthritis. Use of the fiberoptic bronchoscope in rheumatoid disease. *Anesthesiology*. 1983;58:441.
40. Kwek TK, Lew TW, Thoo FL. The role of preoperative cervical spine x-rays in rheumatoid arthritis. *Anaesth Intensive Care*. 1998;26:636.
41. Campbell RS, Wou P, Watt I. A continuing role for preoperative cervical spine radiography in rheumatoid arthritis? *Clin Radiol*. 1995;50:157.
42. Popitz MD. Anesthetic implications of chronic disease of the cervical spine. *Anesth Analg*. 1997;84:672.
43. Vassalo SA, Martyn JAJ. Pathophysiology and anesthetic management of burn injury. *Semin Anesth*. 1989;8:275.
44. Rapaport SI. Preoperative hemostatic evaluation: which tests, if any? *Blood*. 1983;61:229.
45. Goodnough LT, Rudnick S, Price TH, et al. Increased preoperative collection of autologous blood with recombinant human erythropoietin therapy. *N Engl J Med*. 1989;321:1163.
46. Kaplan JA, Dunbar RW, Bland JW, et al. Propranolol and cardiac surgery: a problem for the anesthesiologist? *Anesth Analg*. 1975;54:571.
47. Goldman L. Noncardiac surgery in patients receiving propranolol. Case reports and recommended approach. *Arch Intern Med*. 1981;141:193.
48. Wallace A, Layug B, Tateo I, et al. Prophylactic atenolol reduces postoperative myocardial ischemia. McSPI Research Group. *Anesthesiology*. 1998;88:7.
49. Mangano DT, Layug EL, Wallace A, et al. Effect of atenolol on mortality and cardiovascular morbidity after noncardiac surgery. Multicenter Study of Perioperative Ischemia Research Group [published erratum appears in *N Engl J Med*. 1997;336:1039]. *N Engl J Med*. 1996;335:1713.
50. Siegel D, Hulley SB, Black DM, et al. Diuretics, serum and intracellular electrolyte levels, and ventricular arrhythmias in hypertensive men. *JAMA*. 1992;267:1083.
51. Vitez TS, Soper LE, Wong KC, et al. Chronic hypokalemia and intraoperative dysrhythmias. *Anesthesiology*. 1985;63:130.
52. Wahr JA, Parks R, Boisvert D, et al. Preoperative serum potassium levels and perioperative outcomes in cardiac surgery patients. Multicenter Study of Perioperative Ischemia Research Group. *JAMA*. 1999;281:2203.
53. Kulick DL, Rahimtoola SH. Current role of digitalis therapy in patients with congestive heart failure. *JAMA*. 1991;265:2995.
54. Falk RH, Knowlton AA, Bernard SA, et al. Digoxin for converting recent-onset atrial fibrillation to sinus rhythm. A randomized, double-blinded trial. *Ann Intern Med*. 1987;106:503.
55. Falk RH, Leavitt JI. Digoxin for atrial fibrillation: a drug whose time has gone? *Ann Intern Med*. 1991;114:573.
56. Böttiger BW, Fleischer F. Medical therapy for coronary heart disease. Perioperative relevance. *Anaesthesist*. 1994;43:699.
57. Grace AA, Camm AJ. Quinidine. *N Engl J Med*. 1998;338:35.
58. Hilleman D, Miller MA, Parker R, et al. Optimal management of

amiodarone therapy: efficacy and side effects. *Pharmacotherapy.* 1998;18:138S.

59. Moan MJ, Fanta CH. Bronchodilator therapy in the management of acute asthma. *Compr Ther.* 1995;21:421.

60. Drugs for asthma. *Med Lett Drugs Ther.* 1999;41:5.

61. Roizen MF, Stevens WC. Multiform ventricular tachycardia due to the interaction of aminophylline and halothane. *Anesth Analg.* 1978;57:738.

62. Pantuck EJ, Pantuck CB, Weissman C, et al. Effects of parenteral nutritional regimens on oxidative drug metabolism. *Anesthesiology.* 1984;60:534.

63. Schwartz JJ, Rosenbaum SH, Graf GJ. Anesthesia and the endocrine system. In: Barash PG, Cullen BF, Stoelting RK, eds. *Clinical Anesthesia.* Philadelphia, Pa: Lippincott-Raven; 1996:1055.

64. Palumbo PJ. Blood glucose control during surgery [editorial]. *Anesthesiology.* 1981;55:94.

65. Roizen MF. Is tight perioperative control of diabetes warranted? *Anesthesiology.* 1982;56:242.

66. Stoelting RK. *Pharmacology and Physiology in Anesthetic Practice.* Philadelphia, Pa: Lippincott-Raven; 1999:427.

67. Temkin NR, Dikmen SS, Wilensky AJ, et al. A randomized, double-blind study of phenytoin for the prevention of post-traumatic seizures. *N Engl J Med.* 1990;323:497.

68. Smith MS, Muir H, Hall R. Perioperative management of drug therapy, clinical considerations. *Drugs.* 1996;51:238.

69. Abdi S, Fishman SM, Messner E. Acute exacerbation of depression after discontinuation of monoamine oxidase inhibitor prior to cardiac surgery. *Anesth Analg.* 1996;83:656.

70. Macdonald R. Aspirin and extradural blocks. *Br J Anaesth.* 1991;66:1.

71. Cronberg S, Wallmark E, Söderberg I. Effect on platelet aggregation of oral administration of 10 non-steroidal analgesics to humans. *Scand J Haematol.* 1984;33:155.

72. Horlocker TT, Wedel DJ, Schroeder DR, et al. Preoperative antiplatelet therapy does not increase the risk of spinal hematoma associated with regional anesthesia. *Anesth Analg.* 1995;80:303.

73. Rofecoxib for osteoarthritis and pain. *Med Lett Drugs Ther.* 1999;41:59.

74. Urmey WF, Rowlingson J. Do antiplatelet agents contribute to the development of perioperative spinal hematoma? *Reg Anesth Pain Med.* 1998;23:146.

75. Majerus PW, Broze GJ, Miletich JP, et al. Anticoagulant, thrombolytic, and antiplatelet drugs. In: Hardman JG, Limbird LE, eds. *Goodman and Gilman's The Pharmacological Basis of Therapeutics.* New York, NY: McGraw-Hill; 1996:1341.

76. Horlocker TT, Wedel DJ. Neuraxial block and low-molecular-weight heparin: balancing perioperative analgesia and thromboprophylaxis. *Reg Anesth Pain Med.* 1998;23:164.

77. Chabner BA, Allegra CJ, Curt GA, et al. Antineoplastic agents. In: Hardman JG, Limbird LE, eds. *Goodman and Gilman's The Pharmacological Basis of Therapeutics.* New York, NY: McGraw-Hill; 1996:1233.

78. Waid-Jones MI, Coursin DB. Perioperative considerations for patients treated with bleomycin. *Chest.* 1991;99:993.

79. Ingrassia TS 3d, Ryu JH, Trastek VF, et al. Oxygen-exacerbated bleomycin pulmonary toxicity. *Mayo Clin Proc.* 1991;66:173.

80. Cavallaro RJ, Krumperman LW, Kugler F. Effect of echothiophate therapy on the metabolism of succinylcholine in man. *Anesth Analg.* 1968;47:570.

81. Leier CV, Baker ND, Weber PA. Cardiovascular effects of ophthalmic timolol. *Ann Intern Med.* 1986;104:197.

82. Savarese JJ, Miller RD, Lien CA, et al. Pharmacology of muscle relaxants and their antagonists. In: Miller RD, ed. *Anesthesia.* New York, NY: Churchill Livingstone; 1994:417.

83. Lasser EC, Berry CC, Talner LB, et al. Pretreatment with corticosteroids to alleviate reactions to intravenous contrast material. *N Engl J Med.* 1987;317:845.

84. Levy JH. *Anaphylactic Reactions in Anesthesia and Intensive Care.* Boston, Mass: Butterworths-Heinemann; 1992.

85. Sussman GL, Beezhold DH. Allergy to latex rubber. *Ann Intern Med.* 1995;122:43.

86. Hancock DL. Latex allergy: prevention and treatment. *Anesth Rev.* 1994;21:154.

87. Warner MA, Offord KP, Warner ME, et al. Role of preoperative cessation of smoking and other factors in postoperative pulmonary complications: a blinded prospective study of coronary artery bypass patients. *Mayo Clin Proc.* 1989;64:609.

88. Pearce AC, Jones RM. Smoking and anesthesia: preoperative abstinence and perioperative morbidity. *Anesthesiology.* 1984;61:576.

89. Bluman LG, Mosca L, Newman N, et al. Preoperative smoking habits and postoperative pulmonary complications. *Chest.* 1998;113:883.

90. Wilson JD. Androgens. In: Hardman JG, Limbird LE, eds. *Goodman and Gilman's The Pharmacological Basis of Therapeutics.* New York, NY: McGraw-Hill; 1996:1441.

91. Frank SM, Norris EJ, Christopherson R, et al. Right- and left-arm blood pressure discrepancies in vascular surgery patients. *Anesthesiology.* 1991;75:457.

92. Stone DJ, Gal TJ. Airway management. In: Miller RD, ed. *Anesthesia.* Vol 2. New York, NY: Churchill Livinstone; 1994:1403.

93. Mallampati SR, Gatt SP, Gugino LD, et al. A clinical sign to predict difficult tracheal intubation: a prospective study. *Can Anaesth Soc J.* 1985;32:429.

94. Tse JC, Rimm EB, Hussain A. Predicting difficult endotracheal intubation in surgical patients scheduled for general anesthesia: a prospective blind study. *Anesth Analg.* 1995;81:254.

95. Lewis M, Keramati S, Benumof JL, et al. What is the best way to determine oropharyngeal classification and mandibular space length to predict difficult laryngoscopy? *Anesthesiology.* 1994;81:69.

96. el-Ganzouri AR, McCarthy RJ, Tuman KJ, et al. Preoperative airway assessment: predictive value of a multivariate risk index. *Anesth Analg.* 1996;82:1197.

97. Eckmann DM, Glassenberg R, Gavriely N. Acoustic reflectometry and endotracheal intubation. *Anesth Analg.* 1996;83:1084.

98. Ropper AH, Wechsler LR, Wilson LS. Carotid bruit and the risk of stroke in elective surgery. *N Engl J Med.* 1982;307:1388.

99. Urmey WF, Talts KH, Sharrock NE. One hundred percent incidence of hemidiaphragmatic paresis associated with interscalene brachial plexus anesthesia as diagnosed by ultrasonography. *Anesth Analg.* 1991;72:498.

100. Etchells E, Bell C, Robb K. Does this patient have an abnormal systolic murmur? *JAMA.* 1997;277:564.

101. Rothman A, Goldberger AL. Aids to cardiac auscultation. *Ann Intern Med.* 1983;99:346.

102. Seneff M. Arterial line placement and care. In: Irwin RS, Cerra FB, Rippe JM, eds. *Intensive Care Medicine.* 4th ed. Philadelphia, Pa: Lippincott-Raven; 1999:36.

103. Slogoff S, Keats AS, Arlund C. On the safety of radial artery cannulation. *Anesthesiology.* 1983;59:42.

104. Kroll DA, Caplan RA, Posner K, et al. Nerve injury associated with anesthesia. *Anesthesiology.* 1990;73:202.

105. Pauker SG, Kopelman RI. Trapped by an incidental finding. *N Engl J Med.* 1992;326:40.

106. Cebul RD, Beck JR. Biochemical profiles. Applications in ambulatory screening and preadmission testing of adults. *Ann Intern Med.* 1987;106:403.

107. Narr BJ, Hansen TR, Warner MA. Preoperative laboratory screening in healthy Mayo patients: cost-effective elimination of tests and unchanged outcomes. *Mayo Clin Proc.* 1991;66:155.

108. Fischer SP. Cost-effective preoperative evaluation and testing. *Chest.* 1999;115:96S.

109. Goldberger AL, O'Konski M. Utility of the routine electrocardiogram before surgery and on general hospital admission. Critical review and new guidelines. *Ann Intern Med.* 1986;105:552.

110. Turnbull JM, Buck C. The value of preoperative screening investigations in otherwise healthy individuals. *Arch Intern Med.* 1987;147:1101.

111. Macpherson DS, Snow R, Lofgren RP. Preoperative screening: value of previous tests. *Ann Intern Med.* 1990;113:969.

112. Blery C, Charpak Y, Szatan M, et al. Evaluation of a protocol for selective ordering of preoperative tests. *Lancet.* 1986;1:139.

113. Mancuso CA. Impact of new guidelines on physicians' ordering of preoperative tests. *J Gen Intern Med.* 1999;14:166.

114. Mangano DT. Perioperative cardiac morbidity. *Anesthesiology.* 1990;72:153.

115. Eagle KA, Brundage BH, Chaitman BR, et al. Guidelines for perioperative cardiovascular evaluation for noncardiac surgery. Report of the American College of Cardiology/American Heart Association Task Force on Practice Guidelines. Committee on Perioperative Cardiovascular Evaluation for Noncardiac Surgery. *Circulation.* 1996;93:1278.

116. Mason JJ, Owens DK, Harris RA, et al. The role of coronary angiography and coronary revascularization before noncardiac vascular surgery. *JAMA.* 1995;273:1919.

117. Massie MT, Rohrer MJ, Leppo JA, et al. Is coronary angiography necessary for vascular surgery patients who have positive results of dipyridamole thallium scans? *J Vasc Surg.* 1997;25:975; discussion 982.

118. Hollenberg SM. Preoperative cardiac risk assessment. *Chest.* 1999;115:51S.

119. Raby KE, Goldman L, Creager MA, et al. Correlation between preoperative ischemia and major cardiac events after peripheral vascular surgery. *N Engl J Med.* 1989;321:1296.

120. American College of Physicians. Preoperative pulmonary function testing. *Ann Intern Med.* 1990;112:793.

121. Smetana GW. Preoperative pulmonary evaluation. *N Engl J Med.* 1999;340:937.

122. Gass GD, Olsen GN. Preoperative pulmonary function testing to predict postoperative morbidity and mortality. *Chest.* 1986;89:127.

123. Zibrak JD, O'Donnell CR, Marton K. Indications for pulmonary function testing. *Ann Intern Med.* 1990;112:763.

124. Hall JC, Tarala RA, Hall JL, et al. A multivariate analysis of the risk of pulmonary complications after laparotomy. *Chest.* 1991;99:923.

125. Troupin AS. Diagnostic decision. The measurement of anticonvulsant agent levels. *Ann Intern Med.* 1984;100:854.

126. Boyd O, Grounds RM, Bennett ED. A randomized clinical trial of the effect of deliberate perioperative increase of oxygen delivery on mortality in high-risk surgical patients. *JAMA.* 1993;270:2699.

127. Berlauk JF, Abrams JH, Gilmour IJ, et al. Preoperative optimization of cardiovascular hemodynamics improves outcome in peripheral vascular surgery. A prospective, randomized clinical trial. *Ann Surg.* 1991;214:289; discussion 298.

128. Tuman KJ, McCarthy RJ, Spiess BD, et al. Effect of pulmonary artery catheterization on outcome in patients undergoing coronary artery surgery. *Anesthesiology.* 1989;70:199.

129. Valentine RJ, Duke ML, Inman MH, et al. Effectiveness of pulmonary artery catheters in aortic surgery: a randomized trial. *J Vasc Surg.* 1998;27:203; discussion 211.

130. Choi JJ. An anesthesiologist's philosophy on "medical clearance" for surgical patients. *Arch Intern Med.* 1987;147:2090.

131. Berger JJ. The patient for outpatient surgery, part I: preoperative evaluation. *Probl Anesth.* 1991;5:613.

132. Ross AF, Tinker JH. Anesthesia risk. In: Miller RD, ed. *Anesthesia.* New York, NY: Churchill Livingstone; 1994:791.

133. Saklad M. Grading of patients for surgical procedures. *Anesthesiology.* 1941;2:281.

134. American Society of Anesthesiologists. New classification of physical status. *Anesthesiology.* 1963;24:111.

135. Reiling RB, Christou NV. Nonemergency surgery, I: initial evaluation and preoperative planning. In: Wilmore DW, Brennan MF, Harken AH, eds. *Care of the Surgical Patient. Perioperative Management and Techniques.* Vol 1. Sect 5. New York, NY: Scientific American; 1997:1.

136. Goldman L. Cardiac risks and complications of noncardiac surgery. *Ann Intern Med.* 1983;98:504.

137. Freeman WK, Gibbons RJ, Shub C. Preoperative assessment of cardiac patients undergoing noncardiac surgical procedures. *Mayo Clin Proc.* 1989;64:1105.

138. Ross AF, Tinker JH. Risk and anesthesia. In: Breslow MJ, Miller CF, Rogers MC, eds. *Perioperative Management.* St Louis, Mo: CV Mosby; 1990:13.

139. Dajani AS, Taubert KA, Wilson W, et al. Prevention of bacterial endocarditis. Recommendations by the American Heart Association. *JAMA.* 1997;277:1794.

140. Classen DC, Evans RS, Pestotnik SL, et al. The timing of prophylactic administration of antibiotics and the risk of surgical-wound infection. *N Engl J Med.* 1992;326:281.

141. Davies JM, Davison JS, Nimmo WS, et al. The stomach: factors of importance to the anaesthetist. *Can J Anaesth.* 1990;37:896.

142. Moore J, Flynn RJ, Sampaio M, et al. Effect of single-dose omeprazole on intragastric acidity and volume during obstetric anaesthesia. *Anaesthesia.* 1989;44:559.

143. Practice guidelines for preoperative fasting and the use of pharmacologic agents to reduce the risk of pulmonary aspiration: application to healthy patients undergoing elective procedures: a report by the American Society of Anesthesiologist Task Force on Preoperative Fasting. *Anesthesiology.* 1999;90:896.

144. Clagett GP, Anderson FAJ, Geerts W, et al. Prevention of venous thromboembolism. *Chest.* 1998;114:531S.

145. Anderson FAJ, Wheeler HB, Goldberg RJ, et al. Physician practices in the prevention of venous thromboembolism. *Ann Intern Med.* 1991;115:591.

146. Minami H, McCallum RW. The physiology and pathophysiology of gastric emptying in humans. *Gastroenterology.* 1984;86:1592.

147. Crawford M, Lerman J, Christensen S, et al. Effects of duration of fasting on gastric fluid pH and volume in healthy children. *Anesth Analg.* 1990;71:400.

148. Shevde K, Trivedi N. Effects of clear liquids on gastric volume and pH in healthy volunteers. *Anesth Analg.* 1991;72:528.

149. Hutchinson A, Maltby JR, Reid CR. Gastric fluid volume and pH in elective inpatients, part I: coffee or orange juice versus overnight fast. *Can J Anaesth.* 1988;35:12.

150. Scarr M, Maltby JR, Jani K, et al. Volume and acidity of residual gastric fluid after oral fluid ingestion before elective ambulatory surgery. *Can Med Assoc J.* 1989;141:1151.

151. Truog RD. Do-not-resuscitate orders during anesthesia and surgery. *Anesthesiology.* 1991;74:606.

152. Cohen CB, Cohen PJ. Do-not-resuscitate orders in the operating room. *N Engl J Med.* 1991;325:1879.

153. Couper C. DNR in the OR. *JAMA.* 1992;267:1465; discussion 1466.

154. Franklin C, Rothenberg DM. DNR in the OR. *JAMA.* 1992;267:1465; discussion 1466.

# 2

# The Anesthetic Record

Jeffrey M. Feldman

The year is 1894, and E. A. Codman, a surgical house officer at the Massachusetts General Hospital, is about to create the first anesthesia record.[1] Listen, if you will, to the quiet of the surgical suite. The anesthetist drops ether while the surgeon busies himself with the surgical procedure at hand, the silence broken only by the occasional clang of a metal instrument and some quiet conversation. Picture Codman, with pen in hand, scribbling heart and respiratory rates every 5 minutes (Fig. 2–1).

Today, most anesthesiologists are still scribbling heart and respiratory rates as part of the anesthesia record, although the rhythm of the operating room is anything but quiet, with monitors beeping, lights blinking, pagers buzzing, phones ringing, and a host of operating room sounds in the background. Even though the amount of information documented in the record has certainly increased, what has changed most dramatically is the significance of the anesthesia record for those who provide anesthesia. Little did Codman know that what began as an academic exercise would become a fundamental—and controversial—part of anesthesia practice.

One of the first skills taught to trainees in anesthesia is how to create an anesthetic record. Trainees learn that preparation of a quality anesthesia record requires careful attention to detail. The record should be legible, complete, and accurate. After an appreciation is gained of the many functions of the record, the diligent clinician endeavors to create a useful document.

Underlying the meticulous creation of the record is concern about liability exposure. Given the rather aggressive medicolegal climate in the United States, such concern is reasonable and appropriate. No doubt, the ultimate form of the record is influenced by the manner in which each individual who has contributed to its preparation reacts to liability potential. Some anesthesiologists feel that the most detailed, high-quality record possible is the best defense. Others may not include details of every physiologic change, arguing that fluctuations in vital signs typical during anesthesia may be misinterpreted as potentially harmful by a lay reviewer.

These emotions and concerns about the record have led to a great deal of controversy regarding how the anesthesia record should be kept. The demands on the clinician in the operating room have made quality handwritten recordkeeping increasingly difficult. Technology to perform automated recordkeeping is progressing and offers the potential to improve the recordkeeping process but has met with limited acceptance.

The intent of this chapter is to explore the issues important to quality recordkeeping and the suitability of both handwritten and automated anesthesia records to that task.

## PURPOSES OF THE RECORD

The purpose of the first anesthesia record is subject to debate.[1] Cushing has written that a wager between Codman and himself concerning who was the best "etherizer" was the

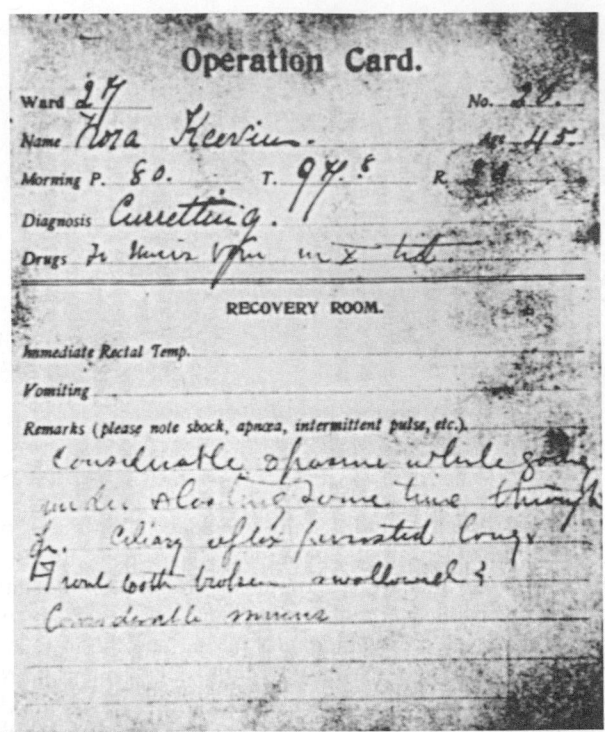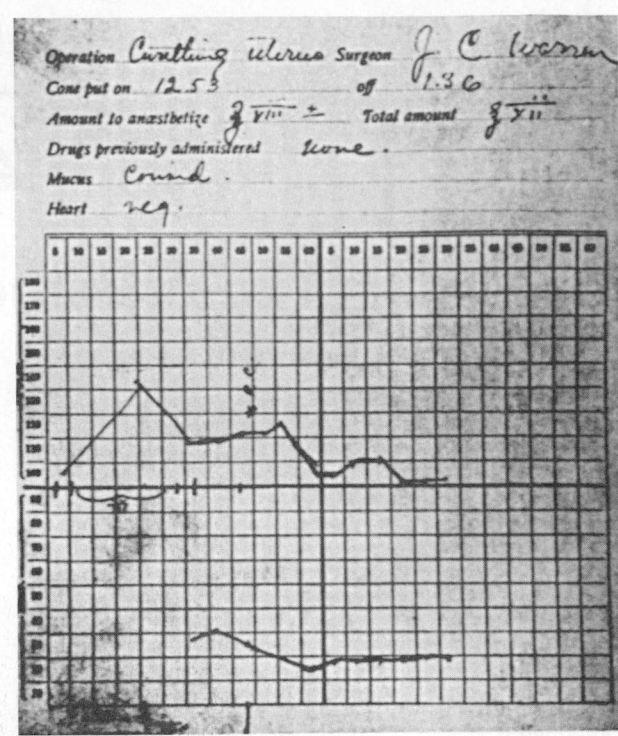

**FIGURE 2–1.** An early anesthesia record created by Codman. (From Beecher HK. The first anesthesia records. *Surg Gynecol Obstet.* 1940;71:689–693. By permission of *Surgery, Gynecology, & Obstetrics.*)

motivation for the first anesthesia records. Codman, noting Cushing's flair for the dramatic, explained that F. B. Harrington, Codman's chief when he was a house officer, suggested that anesthesia records be kept to document the anesthetic course. It is certain, however, that there were probably few individuals other than Dr Codman and his colleagues who took an interest in their content.

Current handwritten records are subjected to much more intense scrutiny. Not only is the primary anesthetist interested in the content of the record but also other physicians and nurses, the anesthesiologists who will care for the patient in the future, administrators, accountants, peer review organizations, researchers, and attorneys who may require access to it[2] (Table 2–1). Although the modern anesthesia record serves many masters and contains more information than did the first record, the basic approach to recordkeeping has changed little.

## How Is It Used?

A study of the patient record conducted by the Institute of Medicine of the National Academy of Sciences highlights its many different uses. Four categories of use were identified: direct patient care, administration and management, reimbursement, and research (Table 2–2). These uses are considered primary if they are associated with the provision of patient care (ie, with the provision, management, or reimbursement of care services) and secondary if they do not influence the encounter between provider and patient directly but rather influence the environment in which care is provided.[3] To emphasize issues important to anesthesia practice, the following uses of the anesthesia record are considered: patient care, administration (including reimbursement), research and education, and medicolegal purposes.

### Patient Care

As an instrument for patient care, the anesthesia record serves both intraoperative and postoperative functions. For the intraoperative anesthesia care provider, the anesthesia record functions as both a logbook and a clinical management tool.[4]

### Logbook

The clinician uses the anesthesia record as a logbook to record information about the patient that should be readily

**TABLE 2–1.** Individual Users of the Record

| Patient Care Delivery (Providers) | Patient Care Management and Support |
|---|---|
| Chaplains | Administrators |
| Dental hygienists | Financial managers and accountants |
| Dentists | Quality assurance managers |
| Laboratory technologists | Records professionals |
| Nurses | Risk managers |
| Occupational therapists | Unit clerks |
| Optometrists | Utilization review managers |
| Pharmacists | **Patient Care Reimbursement** |
| Physical therapists | |
| Physicians | Benefit managers |
| Physician assistants | Insurers (federal, state, and private) |
| Podiatrists | **Other** |
| Psychologists | |
| Radiology technologists | Accreditors |
| Respiratory therapists | Government policymakers and legislators |
| Social workers | Lawyers |
| **Patient Care Delivery (Consumers)** | Health care researchers and clinical investigators |
| Patients | Health sciences journalists and editors |
| Families | |

Reprinted with permission from Dick RS, Steen EB, eds. *The Computer-Based Patient Record: An Essential Technology for Health Care.* Copyright 1991 by the National Academy of Sciences. Courtesy of the National Academy Press, Washington, DC.

**TABLE 2–2.** Primary Uses of Patient Records

| Patient Care Delivery (Patient) | Patient Care Management |
|---|---|
| Document services received | Document case mix in institutions and |
| Constitute proof of identity | practice |
| Self-manage care | Analyze severity of illness |
| Verify billing | Formulate practice guidelines |
| **Patient Care Delivery** | Manage risk |
| **(Provider)** | Characterize the use of services |
| Foster continuity of care (ie, | Provide the basis for utilization review |
| serve as a communication tool) | Perform quality assurance tests |
| Describe diseases and causes | **Patient Care Support** |
| (ie, support diagnostic work) | Allocate resources |
| Support decision-making about | Analyze trends and develop forecasts |
| diagnosis and treatment of | Assess workload |
| patients | Communicate between departments |
| Assess and manage risk for | **Billing and Reimbursement** |
| individual patients | |
| Facilitate care in accordance with | Document services for payments |
| clinical practice guidelines | Bill for services |
| Document patient risk factors | Submit insurance claims |
| Assess and document patient | Adjudicate insurance claims |
| expectations and patient | Determine disabilities (eg, workmen's |
| satisfaction | compensation) |
| Generate care plans | Manage costs |
| Determine preventive advice or | Report costs |
| health maintenance infomation | Perform actuarial analysis |
| Remind clinicians (eg, screens, | |
| age-related reminders) | |
| Support nursing care | |
| Document services provided (eg, | |
| drugs, therapies) | |

Reprinted with permission from Dick RS, Steen EB, eds. *The Computer-Based Patient Record: An Essential Technology for Health Care.* Copyright 1991 by the National Academy of Sciences. Courtesy of the National Academy Press, Washington, DC.

available. For example, preoperative data, patient medications, patient weight, allergies, and perhaps a succinct list of medical problems are included. This information is typically transcribed from the medical record into the record or preoperative evaluation note because it otherwise may not be easily found when needed. It provides a useful summary for other anesthetists who become involved with the patient.

Documentation of the anesthetic care is the most obvious role of the record as a logbook. This documentation should include location of the operating room, time of the operation, identification numbers for the anesthesia machine, notes on airway management and other procedures, list of the drugs and fluids administered, and record of vital signs. All practicing clinicians are familiar with this aspect of the record and with the difficulty maintaining a quality contemporaneous record when occupied with patient care.

### Clinical Management Tool

As the record evolves, a trend plot is created that may indicate a change that is not apparent from observing individual values on the monitor. When multiple parameters are plotted together, the relationship between these parameters (eg, heart rate and blood pressure) can indicate subtle but important physiologic changes (eg, progressive hypovolemia). The relationship between drug doses and physiologic response demonstrates the dose-response relationship for the individual patient. For the clinician who assumes responsibility for anesthesia care from another individual, the carefully constructed record can be invaluable for developing and continuing an appropriate anesthetic plan.

Postoperative users include the physicians and nurses who care for the patient in the postanesthesia care unit (PACU), on the postoperative surgical ward, or in the intensive care unit. These physicians and nurses consult the anesthesia record for information about intraoperative blood loss, fluids and drugs administered, and overall physiologic stability. The other postoperative beneficiaries of a quality record are the anesthesiologists and anesthetists who consult the record when preparing to administer a subsequent anesthetic to the same patient.

### Administration

Whereas the primary purpose of the record traditionally has been to facilitate the management of patient care, the growth of managed health care has increased the importance of the administrative functions. The administrative uses of the record have become fundamental to the successful delivery of health care. Several aspects of the administrative use of the record are identifiable:

1. The individuals responsible for the administration of the department must make decisions about such aspects as the quality of care, outcome of patients, implications of practice patterns, and use of manpower. The information in the anesthesia record constitutes the documentation necessary for making and supporting these decisions.
2. Hospital administrators also rely on the information in the anesthesia record to make decisions regarding use of pharmaceuticals, equipment, and supplies. As anesthesia practices expand to the office environment, these administrative functions typically assumed by the facility can become the responsibility of the anesthesia providers. Careful tracking of these costs through recordkeeping are essential to a successful practice.
3. Reimbursement for anesthesia services has become an increasingly complex undertaking given the number of third-party payers and the regulations applied to reimbursement for anesthesia services. The anesthesia record is the primary document that confirms the billing information. Auditors seek to confirm entries on the anesthesia record by comparing them with information in other documentation, such as nurse's notes and the surgeon's dictation. All documents must be in agreement if questions about billing practices are to be avoided.
4. Quality assurance and peer review auditors examine the anesthesia record to fulfill their responsibilities. Accreditation agencies require ongoing quality assurance programs and carefully audit records for this information. As managed care becomes more prevalent, quality assurance activities that document the complication rate may be used as a means to compare the services rendered by different providers and to provide guidance for awarding contracts and determining reimbursement.

### Research and Education

Educational activities are served whenever a record is reviewed with the goal of improving care. Conferences that focus on discussion of a difficult case use the record as the primary documentation of events. Research activities are also facilitated by an accurate record. Despite the limitations of retrospective chart review, a careful review of records can help to identify undesirable practice patterns.

## Medicolegal Purposes

As any practicing anesthesiologist knows, the importance of the anesthesia record as a medicolegal document cannot be understated. During anesthesia-related legal proceedings, the anesthesia record undergoes intense scrutiny. Verbal testimony regarding the quality of care has little credibility if the anesthesia record does not corroborate the testimony. The attorney for a plaintiff often asserts, "If it isn't charted, it didn't happen."

Because most clinicians are consumed with patient care activities during anesthetic induction, emergence, and emergencies, little information is recorded on the anesthesia record during these times. However, during these periods, physiologic changes are typically most dramatic, and the greatest potential for serious problems exists.

## What Constitutes a Meaningful Record?

The anesthesia record serves many users, but the responsibility for creating the record lies only with the anesthesia provider. How can the individual clinician develop a record that serves the purposes of all its potential users? What information should be included? How should the information be organized and presented?

A meaningful record should be a complete rendition of events that anyone can review to understand what has transpired. Furthermore, sufficient detail should be included to identify the cause or causes of significant intraoperative and postoperative events. This description of the meaningful record is easier to state than it is to achieve in practice. The clinician may not always appreciate the wide range of information of interest to all potential users of the record. The most diligent clinician may simply not have enough time (or space) while caring for the patient during surgery to include all the pertinent data. Finally, the record may not present information in a manner conducive to interpretation. Both the information content and the manner in which the information is presented are important aspects of a meaningful record.

## What Information Should the Record Contain?

The American Society of Anesthesiologists (ASA) has developed a sample anesthetic record as a model for clinicians (Fig. 2–2). This record is intended to be modified by the user for the needs of his or her practice and exemplifies both the range of information that should be included and the difficulty in portraying this information in a usable format. One glance at this record and one is immediately struck by the density of the print. The appearance is due to the need to represent an extensive amount of information on an 8½- × 11-inch piece of paper. The limitations of this format notwithstanding, when this record is completed faithfully, much useful information is recorded.

## Equipment Checks and Airway Management

The ASA record incorporates details that are applicable to every anesthetic procedure: confirmation that equipment is checked, details of the monitors used, a record of the catheters inserted, airway management notes, and emergence (PACU) transfer notes. Of these details, confirmation that equipment is checked should be indicated clearly to avoid citation by accreditation auditors. Notes on management of the airway should be explicit and legible, especially when airway management is not straightforward. No patient should be resubjected to the risks of an airway problem simply because the previous occurrence was poorly documented.

## Data Sufficient to Re-Create the Anesthetic Course

The ASA format perpetuates the habit of recording vital signs at 5-minute intervals, which, although rooted in tradition, serves the purposes of the recordkeeper more than the record. Important physiologic changes are in no way related to a 5-minute interval. Some physiologic changes require intervention much more rapidly than every 5 minutes. Therefore, a 5-minute interval for vital sign recording does not reflect true physiologic variation. When the patient is stable, recording vital signs every 5 minutes is perhaps too frequent. When an important event occurs, however, accurate recordkeeping is essential; yet, the current format does not allow sufficient resolution or space for a meaningful reflection of what transpired.

Much information indicated in the ASA record is not applicable to most anesthetic procedures. Large spaces are dedicated to obstetric and regional anesthesia notes, even though these are used in the minority of anesthetic procedures. The obstetric anesthesia note space accommodates triplet delivery, which occurs rarely even with the increasing application of in vitro fertilization. Space for blood gas analysis results and for central venous pressure and pulmonary artery occlusion pressure measurements is also unlikely to be used in most anesthetic procedures. Although the ASA record was not intended to be used in its entirety, many record forms include space for information that is rarely recorded at the expense of room to record other information more legibly and completely.

## POSTANESTHESIA DOCUMENTATION

### What Is Important?

Postanesthesia documentation is required at the time of discharge from the recovery room and 1 day or more after the anesthetic procedure, particularly if a complication occurs. With the increase in same-day surgery, documentation of discharge readiness has become an important issue. Whenever a patient is allowed to leave the PACU, some assessment of physiologic stability should be documented.

For the patient returning home, documentation should include not only that the patient is awake but also that he or she is able to take fluid by mouth, ambulate, and, in most centers, void. Although the inpatient need not ambulate, physiologic stability and some assessment of pain control should be documented. Furthermore, if a problem occurred in the PACU, the treatment rendered and the effectiveness of that treatment should be documented.

The postanesthesia documentation that occurs after discharge from the PACU should indicate that a postoperative visit occurred and should identify problems that relate to the

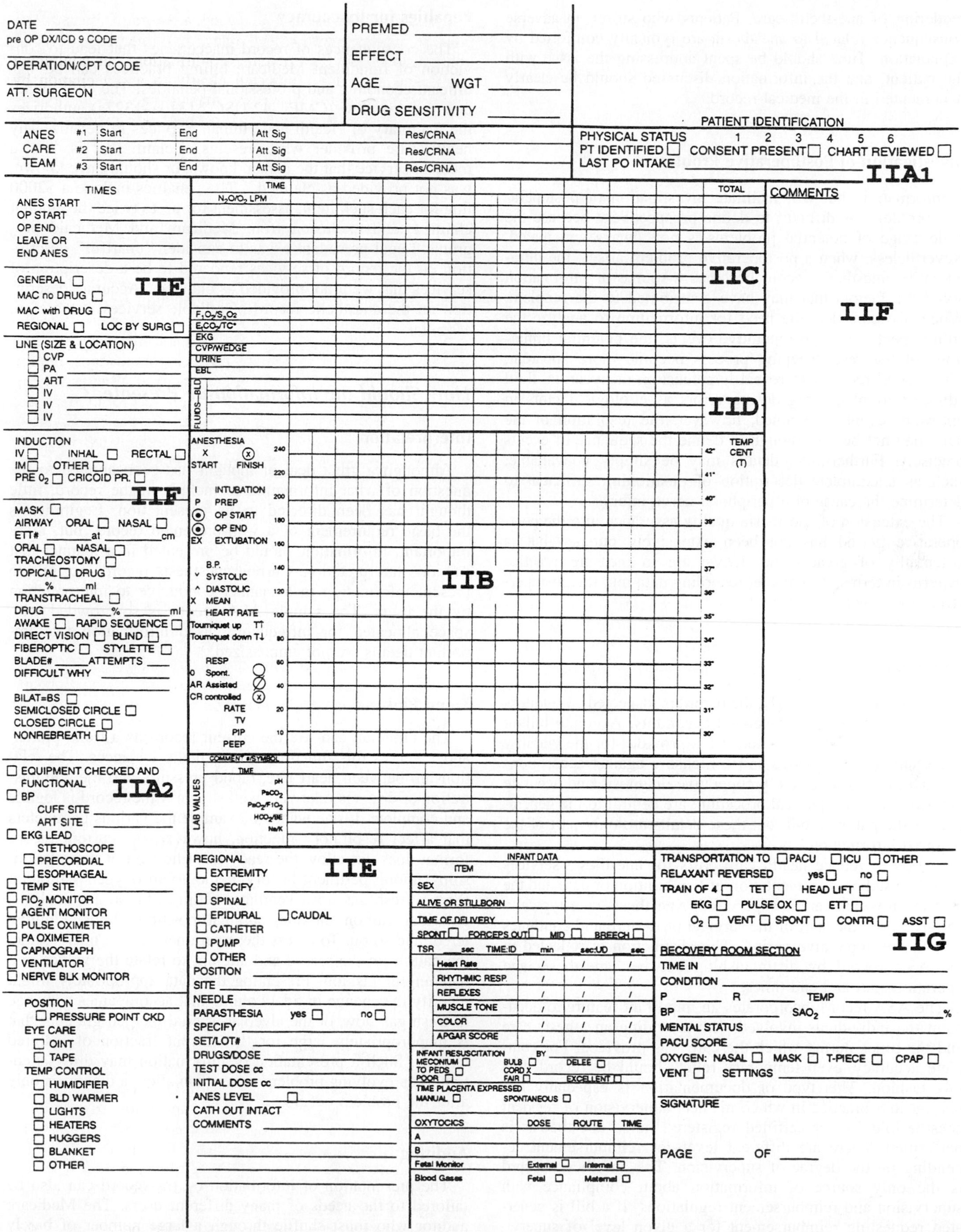

DATE _____
pre OP DX/ICD 9 CODE _____

OPERATION/CPT CODE _____

ATT. SURGEON _____

PREMED _____
EFFECT _____
AGE _____ WGT _____
DRUG SENSITIVITY _____

PATIENT IDENTIFICATION

| ANES | #1 | Start | End | Att Sig | | Res/CRNA |
| CARE | #2 | Start | End | Att Sig | | Res/CRNA |
| TEAM | #3 | Start | End | Att Sig | | Res/CRNA |

PHYSICAL STATUS 1 2 3 4 5 6
PT IDENTIFIED ☐ CONSENT PRESENT ☐ CHART REVIEWED ☐
LAST PO INTAKE _____ **IIA1**

TIMES
ANES START _____
OP START _____
OP END _____
LEAVE OR _____
END ANES _____

TIME
N₂O/O₂ LPM

TOTAL COMMENTS

GENERAL ☐ **IIE**
MAC no DRUG ☐
MAC with DRUG ☐
REGIONAL ☐ LOC BY SURG ☐

F₁O₂/SₐO₂
E₁CO₂/TC°
EKG
CVP/WEDGE
URINE
EBL
FLUIDS—BLD

**IIC**
**IIF**
**IID**

INDUCTION
IV ☐ INHAL ☐ RECTAL ☐
IM ☐ OTHER ☐ _____
PRE O₂ ☐ CRICOID PR. ☐ **IIF**

MASK ☐
AIRWAY ORAL ☐ NASAL ☐
ETT# ___ at ___ cm
ORAL ☐ NASAL ☐
TRACHEOSTOMY ☐
TOPICAL ☐ DRUG _____
___% ___ml
TRANSTRACHEAL ☐
DRUG ___% ___ml
AWAKE ☐ RAPID SEQUENCE ☐
DIRECT VISION ☐ BLIND ☐
FIBEROPTIC ☐ STYLETTE ☐
BLADE# ___ ATTEMPTS ___
DIFFICULT WHY _____

BILAT=BS ☐
SEMICLOSED CIRCLE ☐
CLOSED CIRCLE ☐
NONREBREATH ☐

ANESTHESIA
X (x) 240
START FINISH
I INTUBATION
P PREP 200
⊙ OP START
⊙ OP END
EX EXTUBATION 160
B.P.
ˇ SYSTOLIC 140
^ DIASTOLIC 120
X MEAN
• HEART RATE 100
Tourniquet up T↑
Tourniquet down T↓ 80
RESP 60
O Spont.
AR Assisted 40
CR controlled
RATE 20
TV
PIP 10
PEEP

**IIB**

TEMP CENT (T)
42° 41° 40° 39° 38° 37° 36° 35° 34° 33° 32° 31° 30°

☐ EQUIPMENT CHECKED AND FUNCTIONAL **IIA2**
☐ BP
CUFF SITE _____
ART SITE _____
☐ EKG LEAD
STETHOSCOPE
☐ PRECORDIAL
☐ ESOPHAGEAL
☐ TEMP SITE
☐ FIO₂ MONITOR
☐ AGENT MONITOR
☐ PULSE OXIMETER
☐ PA OXIMETER
☐ CAPNOGRAPH
☐ VENTILATOR
☐ NERVE BLK MONITOR

COMMENT #/SYMBOL
TIME
pH
PaCO₂
PaO₂/F1O₂
HCO₂/BE
Na/K
LAB VALUES

POSITION
☐ PRESSURE POINT CKD
EYE CARE
☐ OINT
☐ TAPE
TEMP CONTROL
☐ HUMIDIFIER
☐ BLD WARMER
☐ LIGHTS
☐ HEATERS
☐ HUGGERS
☐ BLANKET
☐ OTHER _____

REGIONAL **IIE**
☐ EXTREMITY
SPECIFY _____
☐ SPINAL
☐ EPIDURAL ☐ CAUDAL
☐ CATHETER
☐ PUMP
☐ OTHER _____
POSITION _____
SITE _____
NEEDLE _____
PARASTHESIA yes ☐ no ☐
SPECIFY _____
SET/LOT# _____
DRUGS/DOSE _____
TEST DOSE cc _____
INITIAL DOSE cc _____
ANES LEVEL _____
CATH OUT INTACT
COMMENTS _____

INFANT DATA
| ITEM | | | |
| SEX | | | |
| ALIVE OR STILLBORN | | | |
| TIME OF DELIVERY | | | |
SPONT ☐ FORCEPS OUT ☐ MID ☐ BREECH ☐
TSR ___ sec TIME:ID ___ min ___ sec:UD ___ sec
| Heart Rate | / | / | / |
| RHYTHMIC RESP. | / | / | / |
| REFLEXES | / | / | / |
| MUSCLE TONE | / | / | / |
| COLOR | / | / | / |
| APGAR SCORE | / | / | / |
INFANT RESUSCITATION BY
MECONIUM ☐ BULB ☐ DELEE ☐
TO PEDS ☐ CORD X
POOR ☐ FAIR ☐ EXCELLENT ☐
TIME PLACENTA EXPRESSED
MANUAL ☐ SPONTANEOUS ☐
| OXYTOCICS | DOSE | ROUTE | TIME |
| A | | | |
| B | | | |
Fetal Monitor External ☐ Internal ☐
Blood Gases Fetal ☐ Maternal ☐

TRANSPORTATION TO ☐ PACU ☐ ICU ☐ OTHER
RELAXANT REVERSED yes ☐ no ☐
TRAIN OF 4 ☐ TET ☐ HEAD LIFT ☐
EKG ☐ PULSE OX ☐ ETT ☐
O₂ ☐ VENT ☐ SPONT ☐ CONTR ☐ ASST ☐
**IIG**
RECOVERY ROOM SECTION
TIME IN _____
CONDITION _____
P ___ R ___ TEMP ___
BP ___ SAO₂ ___%
MENTAL STATUS _____
PACU SCORE _____
OXYGEN: NASAL ☐ MASK ☐ T-PIECE ☐ CPAP ☐
VENT ☐ SETTINGS _____
SIGNATURE _____
PAGE ___ OF ___

**FIGURE 2–2.** Sample anesthetic record proposed by the American Society of Anesthesiologists. (From American Society of Anesthesiologists, Park Ridge, Ill.)

rendering of anesthetic care. Patients who suffer an adverse consequence related to anesthesia are typically comforted by explanation. Time should be spent addressing the issue with the patient, and the information discussed should be clearly documented in the medical record.

## Investigation of Postoperative Problems

Information that will facilitate investigation of postoperative problems is difficult to define prospectively because the wide range of potential problems is not always anticipated. Nevertheless, when a postoperative problem arises, the intraoperative anesthetic record becomes a source of information about the factors that may have contributed to the problem. When one considers the need for information to analyze the entire spectrum of postoperative events, the potential limitations of the recordkeeping process become more apparent. The current record can reveal hypotension, tachycardia, fluid administration, or drug dosing errors as etiologic factors in untoward events. As noted, however, the resolution of the data may not be fine enough to define the sequence of events precisely. Furthermore, details may be simply unavailable, such as a complete description of positioning sufficient to determine the cause of a peripheral nerve injury.

The extension of anesthesia quality assurance into the postoperative period has not been extensively pursued but is potentially of great value. If we are to measure practice patterns in terms of outcome, recording data into the postoperative period will be essential.

## Billing Data

As mentioned previously, the record is inspected by auditors to verify that bills are generated accurately. Accurate billing practice is a vital function because it provides for the viability of the anesthesia practice and can ensure against accusations of fraud. Inclusion of the preoperative diagnosis and accurate description of the surgical procedure are central to the generation of the patient's bill, but these details are only part of the required information.

Efforts to reduce health care costs for anesthesia services have focused on documentation of the duration of care and the manner in which care is supervised. Anesthesia care typically begins before the start of the surgical procedure and continues into the postoperative period. This distinction is reflected in the ASA record by distinguishing between anesthesia and operation start and end times.

The ASA record incorporates an important feature to document the individuals involved with providing anesthesia care and the times during which the care was provided. For complete accuracy, even temporary relief should be recorded in this fashion. This type of documentation is especially important in a practice in which medical supervision of resident anesthesiologists or certified registered nurse anesthetists is performed. There are different levels of reimbursement depending on the degree of supervision. The anesthesia record is the only source of information about compliance with supervision and reimbursement regulations. If a bill is generated requesting reimbursement for a given level of supervision, the records completed at that time should indicate the same level of supervision as indicated in the bill.

## Penalties for Inaccuracy

The consequences of record inaccuracies that lead to conviction of fraudulent Medicare billing practices can be significant economic and professional penalties. The civil monetary penalties law (CMPL 42 USC §1320a–1327a) authorizes the Secretary of Health and Human Services to penalize any health care provider who presents a claim that is "for a medical service that the person knows, or should have known, was not provided as claimed." The penalties include a $2000 fine for each such item, assessment for up to twice the amount claimed, and exclusion from Medicare and Medicaid programs. Legal precedent exists to consider "unartful" description on the record of services rendered to be a description of services that were not provided as claimed.[5] Accurate description on the anesthetic record of billable services is therefore essential.

## How Should the Information Be Presented?

### Interpretation

Although a great deal of thought has been applied to the question of what information to include in the record, little thought has been directed to its presentation. Legibility is the basic requirement of a well-presented record, but, more important, information should be presented in a manner that supports interpretation. Current anesthesia records do little to present information in a manner conducive to interpretation by the users. The sample ASA record is so crowded with space allocated for infrequently used information that important details are not emphasized.

### Trend Plotting

The clinician can use the current record as a trend plotter, and it serves this function well in many instances. The relationship between heart rate, blood pressure, and the administration of drugs is relatively well shown if the record is legible and complete. If one wants to examine the various parameters that affect respiratory function, however, the current record format does not allow the ready identification of the relationships among pertinent history, hemoglobin oxygen saturation ($SpO_2$), fresh gas flow, ventilator settings, blood gas analysis, end-tidal carbon dioxide, surgical position, fluids administered, and so on. To assess these parameters, one must extract the data from the record and attempt to relate the values in a meaningful fashion. Presenting the data appropriately might identify the change in tidal volume that accompanies a change in fresh gas flow, or the alveolar-arterial oxygen gradient that is inappropriately large for the current fraction of inspired oxygen. Such a presentation of information may draw attention to an evolving problem rather than allow a diagnosis only after the problem occurs.

### Auditing

The presentation of information on the record can also be tailored to the needs of many different users. The Medicare auditor who must shuffle through a large number of barely legible, poorly organized records is more likely to find fault simply owing to an inability to locate appropriate information.

If the important information is clearly displayed, it becomes more difficult to find fault where none exists.

The ASA-proposed record is one example of the type of information and detail necessary to develop a meaningful record. The conventional format has important limitations, however, especially with regard to the manner in which information is presented. As the number of the record's users and uses increases, their needs cannot be ignored. We must divorce ourselves from conventional notions about the anesthesia record and consider new methods of recordkeeping that better serve the needs of anesthesiologists and others who use it. We must examine not only the form and content of the record but also the ability of the handwritten record to satisfy recordkeeping needs now and in the future.

## CREATING THE RECORD

The foregoing discussion created a perspective on the essential elements of a quality anesthetic record. Although the record traditionally has been created by hand, technology for creating it automatically is proliferating. Given the importance of the record, the means by which it is created merits close inspection. Clearly, the handwritten record may not be an adequate document. Unfortunately, automated anesthesia recordkeepers (AARKs) may not be the indispensable tools their proponents would have us believe.

### What Are the Handwritten Record's Strengths?

The handwritten anesthesia record has many strengths. It is portable, can be used at the bedside, and is easily integrated into the crowded anesthesia workspace. All clinicians possess the skills to create a record. *Soft data*, such as the subjective descriptions of managing an airway or performing a procedure, are easily recorded.[6] These are obvious strengths and the primary reasons that the use of the handwritten anesthesia record has become entrenched in clinical practice.

The handwritten record must satisfy other requirements in which its strengths are not as obvious. The clinician must have the time available to create the record. The record must also be accurate, complete, and legible. The process of recordkeeping must not interfere with patient care.

The literature contains numerous studies that compare handwritten recordkeeping to AARKs. A critical review of these studies highlights the strengths and limitations of each method of recordkeeping.

### How Much Time Is Spent Recordkeeping?

Time demands in the operating room are significant. The clinician must not only manage the patient and facilitate the surgical procedure but also communicate with the laboratory, manage infusion pumps, insert monitoring devices, and troubleshoot equipment. Therefore, the time required to maintain the record has increased significantly and often exceeds the time available for contemporaneous handwritten entry.

### AARK Versus Handwritten Recordkeeping

The time spent in recordkeeping during coronary artery bypass[7] and general surgical procedures[8] has been studied by means of videotape examination of these procedures. Meijler compared the studies by equating the tasks studied and by plotting the results on the same graph[9] (Fig. 2–3). The task of logging data on the chart consumed 6% of the anesthesiologists' time during general surgery and 12% of their time during coronary artery bypass surgery.

Proponents of automated recordkeeping contend that with

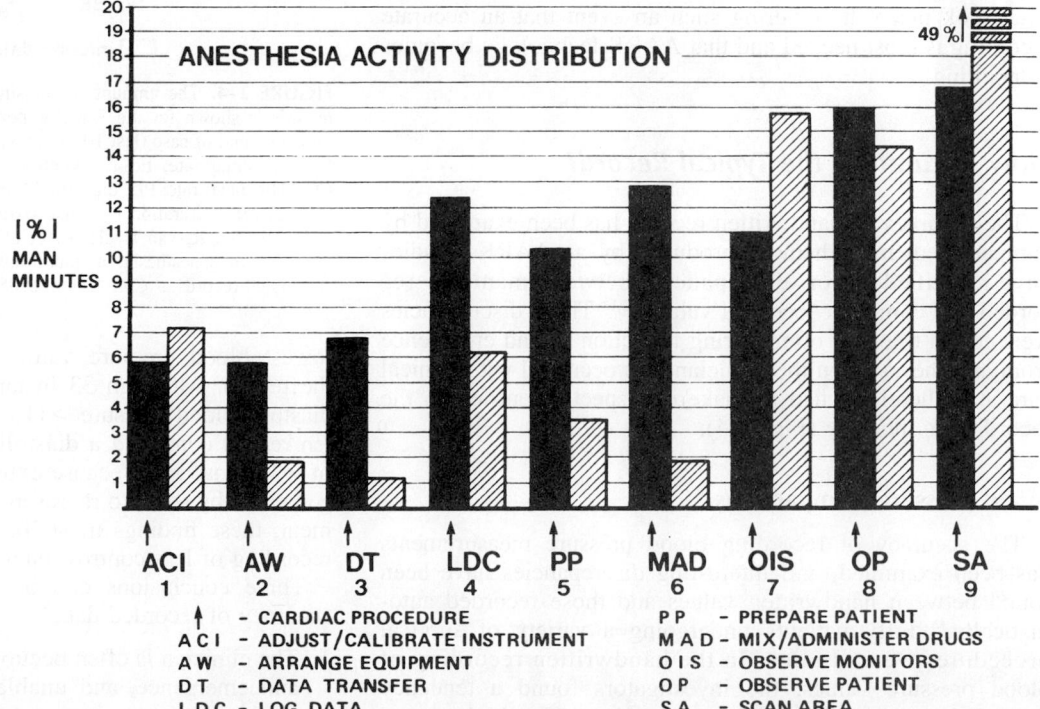

**FIGURE 2–3.** The only available quantitative information on anesthesia workload is presented in the figure. The time spent on 9 subtasks in percentage of work-minutes is plotted for cardiac surgical procedures (*solid columns*) and general procedures (*slashed columns*). (From Meijler AP. *Automation in Anesthesia: A Relief? A Systematic Approach to Computers in Patient Monitoring.* New York, NY: Springer-Verlag; 1987:23.)

ANESTHESIA ACTIVITY DISTRIBUTION

[%] MAN MINUTES

49 %

| ACI | AW | DT | LDC | PP | MAD | OIS | OP | SA |
| 1 | 2 | 3 | 4 | 5 | 6 | 7 | 8 | 9 |

↑ – CARDIAC PROCEDURE
A C I – ADJUST/CALIBRATE INSTRUMENT
A W – ARRANGE EQUIPMENT
D T – DATA TRANSFER
LDC – LOG DATA

P P – PREPARE PATIENT
M A D – MIX/ADMINISTER DRUGS
O I S – OBSERVE MONITORS
O P – OBSERVE PATIENT
S A – SCAN AREA

its application, the anesthetist could spend less time keeping a record and, therefore, have additional time to manage the anesthetic procedure. For this contention to be true, less time should be required to keep a record using an AARK than is needed for handwritten recordkeeping. Because an AARK records monitored data automatically, the user should be spared the time usually required to transcribe data from the monitors. Time savings may be offset, however, by the increased time spent entering notations into the AARK. This task may be more awkward than handwritten notation.

Task-analysis studies have compared the time spent recordkeeping when using a manual chart and an AARK in an effort to determine the true impact of the recordkeeping tool on the time spent recordkeeping. Task-analysis studies have been performed in both the cardiac surgery setting[10] and in varied anesthetic procedures.[11] Both studies found that the total time spent recordkeeping with either method was between 10% and 15% of the time spent in all activities. The automated recordkeeping took somewhat less time in both studies than manual recordkeeping, although the difference was small. Because the AARK technology records monitored data automatically, the difficulty entering annotations into the automated system seemed to offset the time saving of automated recording. Perhaps future improvements in technology, such as handwriting or voice recognition, will reduce the effect of this disadvantage of the AARK technology.

Although the overall percentage of available time devoted to recordkeeping during anesthesia is of interest, it does not reflect those situations in which 100% of the anesthetist's attention is directed to the patient and, thus, no time for recordkeeping is available. An AARK is capable of recording monitored information with a resolution that reflects true physiologic change. Reflecting this detail in recordkeeping is not possible for a human being, particularly when intensive patient care demands exist. Every practitioner has experienced the frustration that occurs after management of a serious adverse event in the operating room when it is virtually impossible to create an accurate and complete rendition of what took place. It is during such an event that an accurate recording is most needed and that AARK technology becomes compelling.

## How Accurate Is the Typical Record?

The accuracy of handwritten records has been examined by comparing them with those produced by an AARK. Studies have identified major discrepancies between manually recorded and computer-recorded values.[12,13] These discrepancies were found to occur often during induction of and emergence from anesthesia when the clinician was occupied with clinical care and, therefore, had to make retrospective entries on the record from memory (Fig. 2–4).

### Blood Pressure Comparisons

The accuracy of recording blood pressure measurements has been examined, and interesting discrepancies have been found between handwritten values and those recorded automatically.[14] Fifty patients undergoing a variety of surgical procedures were studied. In the handwritten recording of blood pressure values, the investigators found a tendency toward the elimination of extreme values. The highest and

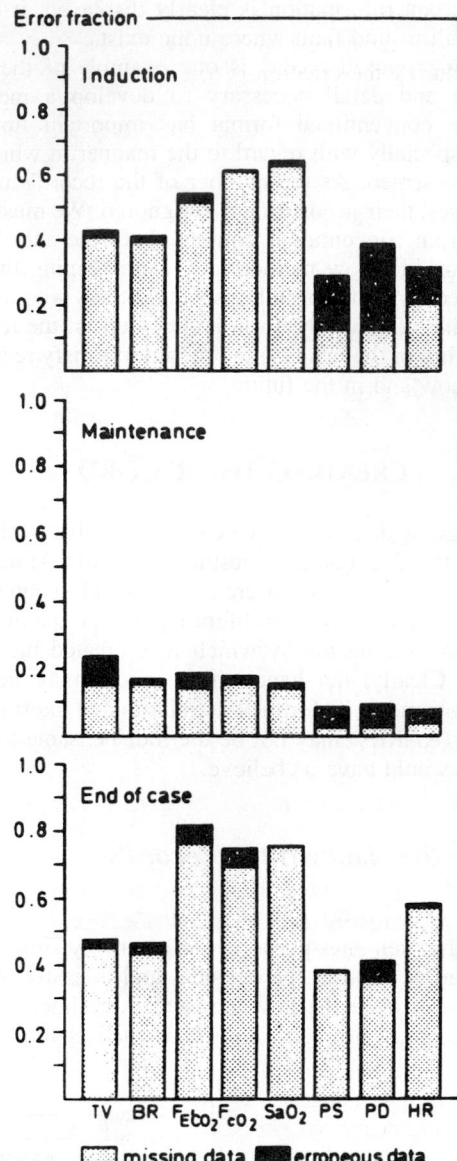

**FIGURE 2–4.** The amount of missing and erroneous data on handwritten records is shown for the 3 major periods of anesthesia: induction (first 15 minutes), end of case (last 10 minutes), and maintenance (period in between). BR, breathing rate; $F_{CO_2}$, oxygen fraction in the circuit; $FET_{CO_2}$, end-tidal $CO_2$; HR, heart rate; PD, diastolic blood pressure; PS, systolic blood pressure; $Sa_{O_2}$, oxygen saturation by pulse oximetry; TV, tidal volume. (From Lerou JGC, Dirksen R, van Daele M, et al. Automated charting of physiological variables in anaesthesia: a quantitative comparison of handwritten versus automated records. *J Clin Monit.* 1988;4:37–47.)

lowest blood pressure values measured did not appear on the record. Although 33 instances of automatically recorded diastolic blood pressure >110 mm Hg occurred, no handwritten record contained a diastolic blood pressure measurement of >110 mm Hg. Because extremes in blood pressure may be construed by some to represent suboptimal anesthetic management, these findings most likely represent a bias toward the recording of less controversial values.

Three conclusions can be drawn from these studies on accuracy of recorded data:

1. The clinician is often occupied, especially during induction and emergence, and unable to make timely notations on the record.

2. Entries made from memory are often inaccurate.
3. A bias, whether it be conscious or unconscious, is likely present during the creation of the handwritten record.

## AARK Artifacts

The handwritten record may be inaccurate for a number of reasons, but the automated record may also be flawed. An AARK records exactly what is displayed on the monitor, whether or not it is artifactual.[15,16] Two studies of the incidence of artifact recorded by AARKs demonstrated that a small percentage of data (between 0.1% and 6%, depending on the parameter of interest) is artifactual.[15,16] Of perhaps greater interest, however, is that both studies demonstrated that the incidence of artifact decreased as AARK technology matured. This may be related to advances in monitoring technology, AARK technology, or both.

Artifactual data usually appear on the record as markedly different from the other values recorded. As such, artifact is unlikely to be regarded as a manifestation of poor anesthetic management.

## How Complete Is the Record?

AARKs seem to create a more accurate rendition of monitored parameters than does the clinician. Can the AARK facilitate the creation of a more complete record as well?

### Entry Frequency

An anesthetic record can be incomplete because data are not entered at the desired resolution. For most handwritten records, data are recorded every 5 minutes for the most frequently recorded information and every 15 minutes for other parameters, such as $SpO_2$. As noted earlier, this frequency, although well accepted, is not indicative of important physiologic changes. Significant heart rate and blood pressure alterations can occur within seconds. This interval is not practical for a human data recorder, but AARKs with modern computer technology can acquire data well within the frequency of physiologic changes. One approach to avoid storing large amounts of normal data would be to program the automated record to eliminate high-resolution normal data but to retain a high resolution during periods of interest.

The printed record generated by an AARK typically displays data at the intervals customary on handwritten records. AARK systems that record data to magnetic disk actually do so more frequently than is printed on the handwritten record. If these *magnetic records* are retained, events can be reviewed in much greater detail than that provided by either the printed or handwritten records.

### Messages, Checklists, and Automated Prompts

AARKs can also be programmed to determine whether the information entered onto the record is complete. Messages, checklists, or automated prompts can be programmed into an AARK as reminders to the user to be sure that essential items are included. For example, before the record is considered complete, the AARK can check to ensure that billing information or any other required details are complete. It can then prompt the user for additional information as it is needed.

## Is the Record Legible?

The light-hearted comment often made to someone with illegible handwriting that he or she would make a good physician has an unfortunate ring of truth. In fact, many health care professionals either have poor handwriting or the legibility of their handwriting deteriorates when they attempt to record rapidly changing events. Figure 2–5A shows examples of a typical automated record, and Figure 2–5B shows a representative handwritten record. The automated record is clearly the more legible of the two.

Why is legibility important? Obviously, an illegible record fails to serve the function for which it was created, that is, the documentation of the course of an anesthetic procedure. Furthermore, an illegible anesthetic record may have serious medicolegal implications. A jury may interpret a sloppy record as an indication of a sloppy approach to patient care. If important data are missing from the record, it may prove difficult to alter the jury's interpretation.

## Do AARKs Interfere With Vigilance?

One purported advantage of the handwritten record is that the physical act of entering data on the record makes the clinician aware of physiologic trends. Does the clinician using an AARK suffer a decrement in vigilance by having monitored data charted automatically? Investigators have used different strategies to determine the impact of an AARK on vigilance.

One approach used has been to document the clinician's awareness of the most recent vital signs. For this study, investigators randomly entered the operating room and both record the most current monitor data and ask the anesthetist to recall the same data without looking at the monitors. The investigators studied two groups of users: one using AARK technology and the other keeping records manually. The difference between the recalled and the actual data was used as an indicator of vigilance, using predefined clinically relevant error limits for the difference. Using this vigilance measure, there was no impact on vigilance by either recordkeeping technique.[11]

The impact of recordkeeping on vigilance has also been investigated using a defined vigilance task. In one case, the investigators added a number to the display on a physiologic monitor and asked the resident anesthetist to indicate when the number had changed from 5 to 10. The response time to a random change in this number was recorded under two different conditions for each resident: during manual recordkeeping by the anesthetist and when the complete record was kept by an assistant without any input from the anesthetist. There was no difference in response to the vigilance task under each set of conditions, indicating that the act of recordkeeping may not be required to maintain vigilance.[17] In a similar study, a vigilance task was created using a red light mounted adjacent to the patient monitor. Resident anesthetists were randomly assigned to use manual recordkeeping or AARK technology. The response time to noting that the light had been turned on was recorded. No difference in response time (*vigilance latency*) was noted between the two recordkeeping methods.[10]

The evidence to date suggests that maintaining vigilance does not depend on the manner in which the anesthetic record

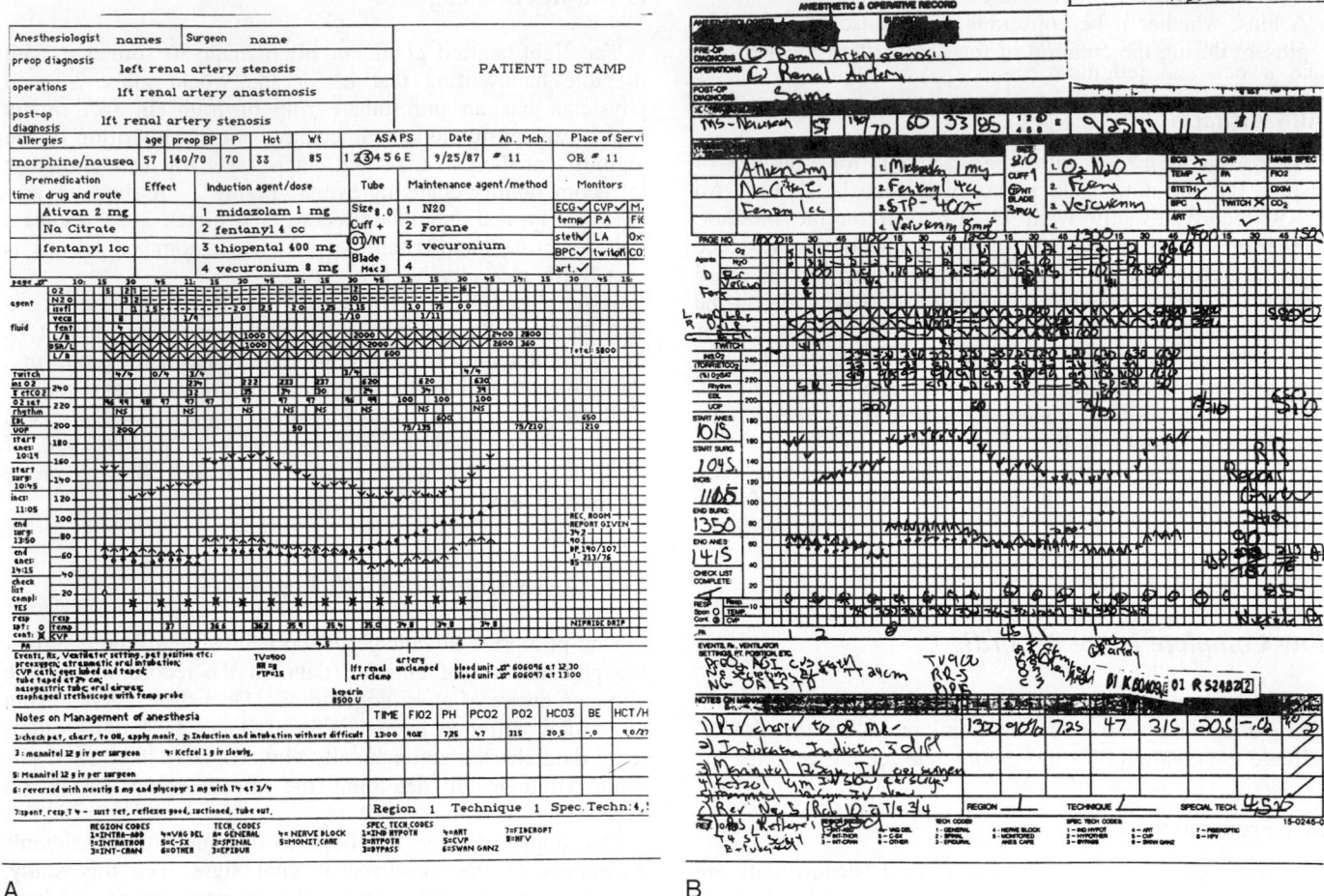

A

B

**FIGURE 2–5.** *A*, Representative automated anesthetic record. *B*, The same record shown as it would be handwritten. (From Gravenstein JS. The uses of the anesthesia record. *J Clin Monit.* 1989;5:251–255.)

is kept. It is difficult to answer this question definitively because both defining and studying vigilance are somewhat elusive. Ideally, one would like to study the response time to true clinical events that require a rapid response and the impact on patient outcome of those types of events when using each recordkeeping approach. The patient numbers that would be required to have a scientifically valid sample are prohibitive, as is the challenge to collecting the data. The existing data do, however, offer some comfort that the introduction of AARK technology is unlikely to have a major negative impact on either vigilance or patient outcome.

## THE AUTOMATED ANESTHESIA RECORD

### *Unnecessary Technology or an Indispensable Tool?*

We have seen that the AARK offers many advantages over the handwritten record. The true utility of the AARK is a topic of heated debate, and the technology has yet to be embraced by more than a small percentage of clinicians. AARK proponents assert that this technology provides a higher-quality and more complete, accurate, and legible record than handwritten recording. Detractors of AARKs believe that

reduced vigilance is a problem and that recording of artifactual data may open the possibility of medicolegal exposure. How can these opposing views be resolved? Will AARK technology ultimately fade away, or will it become an integral part of the anesthesia workplace?

To gain acceptance into routine clinical practice, a new device must satisfy one or more of the following criteria[18]:

- Improve patient care
- Reduce physician workload
- Decrease cost
- Be medicolegally compelling
- Perform one or more important tasks that would otherwise not be done

Does AARK technology satisfy any of these criteria?

### *Can an AARK Improve Patient Care?*

No data are available to document that AARKs improve patient care. Further, a study is unlikely to collect such data, given the low incidence of patient injury due to anesthesia and the multitude of factors that potentially contribute to such injury. AARKs may improve care by increasing the amount of time available to observe the patient, or they may be detrimental by reducing the awareness of monitored data. Given the paucity of objective information, each user must make a personal judgment about the potential impact on patient care. In any event, AARKs are unlikely to gain acceptance based on the criteria of improved patient care.

## Do AARKs Reduce the Physician's Workload?

Clearly, AARKs reduce the work associated with entering physiologic data on the record because these data are recorded automatically. The clinician using an AARK, however, is not freed from all recordkeeping activities because demographic, procedural, and drug information must still be entered manually. Current AARK technology does not provide a method for entering information that can be more conveniently entered by hand.

Of the data entry devices that have been tried, including bar code readers,[19] voice recognition systems,[20] and touch screens,[21] none has replaced the keyboard. Great strides have been made in both voice recognition technology and handwritten input. Both of these technologies have great promise; however, many clinicians do not have typing skills, and manual annotation remains awkward. Prerecorded annotations can reduce the amount of manual entry required but do not eliminate it entirely. The workload advantages of the AARK are apparent during those situations when all attention must be directed to the patient; however, such situations likely do not occur frequently enough to drive acceptance of the technology.

## Is an AARK Cost-Effective?

As the cost of medical care continues to escalate, the cost of any new technology is increasingly a factor in its acceptance. At first glance, it appears that AARKs are excessively expensive, and this is likely a major factor in their rather slow acceptance. The only costs associated with the handwritten record are those incurred by printing forms and buying pens. The cost of one AARK (which can function only in one location) approaches the cost of an integrated physiologic monitor. The question of whether an AARK can pay for itself remains to be answered, but careful analysis can provide some insight into this issue.

### The Cost of Anesthesia Practice

The cost of anesthesia practice (practice overhead) includes personnel costs as well as the costs of drugs, supplies, and equipment. Different practice patterns can lead to a different cost basis for the same case. Induction agents, muscle relaxants, and anesthetic vapors all have different costs, and the selection of individual agents can alter the expense significantly. More costly choices do not amount to a large expense for an individual case but become significant when multiplied by the thousands of cases performed annually in most institutions. To understand whether costs are appropriate, the use of more costly drugs and supplies with potential advantages must be analyzed with an eye toward determining whether these advantages are realized. The clinical information included in the record, such as ASA status, case type, and duration, must

be combined with the drug use information to understand the value of the choices made and dollars spent. Can AARK technology help to address this aspect of practice costs?

A sustained reduction in pharmaceutical costs of $30 000 per month over 3 years using the data available from an AARK system has been reported.[22] This group used the data available from an AARK system to determine the actual number of vials or ampules of drug used for each procedure. This information was combined with pharmacy inventory data to generate costs for 22 commonly used drugs, which were updated monthly and presented to the department. Unit costs of these drugs were updated every 6 months, and anesthesia providers were encouraged to use less costly drugs whenever feasible. Use of a specific drug was reviewed every 2 to 3 months along with the pertinent literature on that agent. Any cases identified through the quality assurance review of anesthetic records as undesirable outcomes were examined to determine the role, if any, of drug choice.

Savings were calculated by comparison to a 3-month reference period before the start of the cost-saving initiative. Although savings related to better choices of drugs typically have a one-time effect on the bottom line, the authors indicated that availability of an AARK system allowed for these cost savings to be continually tracked and sustained over time. Other reports corroborated that an ongoing process is needed if the savings are to be sustained over time,[23] and an AARK or other suitable information tool can facilitate that process.

There is additional experience using an AARK system to drive a value-based analysis of costs for drugs and supplies as they relate to the duration and complexity of individual cases.[24] Investigators used the ASA Relative Value Scale as a means to find the cost per unit rather than the cost per case for drugs and supplies. They concluded that adjusting the cost basis in this fashion facilitates comparison of costs among providers as well as institutions and serves as a reliable benchmark because it accommodates the complexity of differences among cases. This approach was not reported as a method to save dollars directly but rather as a reliable auditing tool to understand the reasons for drug costs. Such a tool can be invaluable for determining appropriate budgets and distinguishing between potential opportunities for cost reduction and areas in which attempts to reduce costs are not likely to be productive.

### Billing and Collection

Because the AARK is used to record information necessary for billing purposes, it may help to improve collections, although it is certainly possible to have an efficient billing and collection system without this technology. The requirements for proper billing continue to increase in complexity, in part because of the number of different payers and the varied payment models that have evolved. The US Health Care Finance Administration, which administers Medicare and Medicaid payments, follows a traditional fee-for-service model and continues to modify the rules for anesthesia billing. These rules, particularly with regard to the level of supervision in the anesthesia care team model, necessitate careful documentation to generate a proper bill and to prove that billing practices are proper when faced with an audit.

At the other end of the payment model spectrum, some payers are offering a fixed fee per insured patient per month to a health care system for hospital-based services. Maintaining financial viability in the face of this type of payment structure can be challenging. If the type and complexity of services to patients exceed projections, financial losses are a certainty. Tracking utilization carefully is essential to understanding and documenting the actual financial risk incurred as well as to negotiating successfully with the various parties involved.

There is no question that any modern billing system is completely dependent on information technology. For the most part, these systems use information that is entered manually from data collected in the operating room. As a bedside data collection tool, AARKs are an ideal link for the billing system. As the AARK systems are integrated with billing systems, clerical processing of billing information can be reduced or eliminated. As a result, bills should be generated more quickly and with fewer errors. If done correctly, the overhead associated with the billing process should be reduced, not to mention the ability to document proper billing practices. Although the cost savings of this process remain to be documented, the Workgroup for Electronic Data Interchange of the US Department of Health and Human Services estimates that automating the flow of information between insurers and health care providers could reduce health care costs in the range of $4 to $10 billion.[25]

## Quality Assurance

AARKs can also facilitate tasks that now consume both clerical and physician time in an anesthesia practice. Quality assurance analysis is required of all anesthesia practices and is increasingly scrutinized by hospital-accrediting agencies. A busy anesthesia practice generates a large amount of quality assurance information that must be processed and analyzed. The AARK stores a large amount of the information that is necessary to support quality assurance. That information can be transferred automatically to quality assurance software to generate the appropriate reports, thus reducing clerical and physician time devoted to updating quality assurance records. In addition, because the AARK data are more complete and accurate than those obtained from the handwritten record, quality assurance should be better when the data have been collected using an AARK.

Although no one to date has evaluated the overall cost-effectiveness of AARKs, some potential major advantages can translate into significant cost savings and offset the cost of the devices. As AARK technology matures, its costs may decrease, and AARKs will evolve into sophisticated data management systems that improve the quality and efficiency of not only recordkeeping but also billing and quality assurance.

## Does an AARK Increase or Decrease Liability Exposure?

When viewed from a medicolegal perspective, AARK technology is highly controversial. It is striking, however, that professionals who defend physicians overwhelmingly support the use of automated records. The consensus of these individuals is that the poor or incomplete anesthesia record is the greatest obstacle to successful defense against a malpractice claim.[26] Crawford Morris, an attorney experienced in de-

fending physicians in malpractice litigation, wrote the following about AARKs:

*With the use of such devices, each side is going to lose some malpractice cases it might have won with poorly decipherable records, and vice versa, but on balance, the presentation of actual facts should not only promote justice but also lead to more reasonable settlements.*[27]

To date, no malpractice claims have been won or lost because of the use of an AARK. As their application proliferates, malpractice litigation ultimately involves data collected by AARKs. The role of the AARK in litigation will almost certainly have a major impact on acceptance of the technology.

## Can an AARK Facilitate New Tasks?

AARKs have the potential to perform information management functions that are not currently possible. This potential will ultimately drive their acceptance. An increasing demand is being placed on the anesthesia record for information. Following is the foremost recommendation of an Institute of Medicine study on the computer-based patient record:

*Health care professionals and organizations should adopt the computer-based patient record (CPR) as the standard for medical and all other records related to patient care.*[28]

The basis for this recommendation is the recognition that the computer-based patient record, of which the AARK is one element, will facilitate access to information in ways that are not possible with current approaches to recordkeeping.

## Access to Medical Records

Merely obtaining an old medical record can be a frustratingly slow process, whereas the pressure to care for more patients in less time is increasing. Patients are often poor historians and do not relate significant past complications that could be readily gleaned from their old charts if they were available. The AARK offers the potential to archive patient records and make them immediately accessible when needed.

## Research Activities

Any number of research activities can be supported if accurate information is entered into the record. Retrospective chart reviews can provide useful information but are hampered by the difficulty involved in locating information and by the inconsistency of information entered onto the record.

In the future, studies will be facilitated by AARK technology. Data that are collected in the operating room will be more easily categorized and analyzed. Studies involving more than one institution will be feasible because data formats will be standardized and readily exchangeable. The ability to combine data between institutions is especially appealing to study anesthesia morbidity and mortality, which requires large groups of patients to obtain statistically meaningful results.

## Should You Adopt AARK Technology for Your Practice?

Although AARK technology has not been widely adopted to date, there are a number of departments that have both succeeded and failed in their efforts to replace the handwritten record with this technology. The lessons learned in this process are instructive for those considering the adoption of this technology.

One department implemented AARK technology by installing the units on a surprise basis with little advance discussion among members of the department. Recordkeeping devices were installed in all noncardiac operating rooms, and utilization reached 90% of possible cases. Despite this widespread use, the members of the department were never enthusiastic about the technology, and it was ultimately rejected. The reasons for failure were reported to be the lack of involvement of anesthesia department members and hospital administrators in the decision to adopt the technology as well as a lack of a workable training mechanism for the residents, who were the primary users.[29]

A successful implementation of the identical AARK technology has also been reported. In this case, success was attributed to unequivocal support for the technology by both hospital and departmental leadership. Support by hospital administration guaranteed initial and continued funding. Another key component to the success was establishing a successful training program that included members of the user group, such as faculty, residents, and nurse anesthetists, who could serve as a resource for members of their peer group. This approach to training helped to ensure that enthusiasm among the users would develop and sustain use of the technology.[30]

A definitive discussion of whether to adopt AARK technology in favor of the handwritten record is beyond the scope of this chapter. Indeed, the answer to this question is complicated. The technology remains expensive, and ultimately the culture must change such that the users become enthusiastic about this new method of recordkeeping. For this to occur, training must be considered, but, ultimately, the technology must bring value to clinical practice. Institutions already committed to widespread use of information technology have been among the first to take this step. As the AARK systems evolve from recordkeepers to full-fledged information systems and the information needs of anesthesia practice become compelling, widespread adoption will likely be inevitable.

## CONCLUSIONS

The anesthetic record is the final arbiter of the manner in which patient care is rendered. The record no longer exists solely for the benefit of its creator. As viewed by other users, it is a reflection of the person caring for the patient. To create an effective record, anesthetists must think of the manner in which they would like each user of the records to view the care they provide.

It is becoming increasingly difficult to satisfy all the demands now being placed on the handwritten anesthetic record. In addition, a clear mandate is emerging to move to computer-based patient records. For the anesthesia community to satisfy this mandate, AARK technology needs to be closely examined. AARKs have the potential to improve patient care in a multitude of ways. Not only can information be presented in a fashion that aids clinical decision-making but also the accessibility and quality of data will be improved.

Outcomes research, which requires extensive data collection procedures, often by many institutions, will be enhanced through the definition of uniform information formats. Costs will be contained through improved efficiency and better data for accounting procedures. If we continue to think of the AARK only as an alternative means to reproduce the existing anesthesia record, acceptance will remain slow and the rewards limited. We must think beyond existing concepts of what the record presently is to what it might become if we use the technologies available.

## References

1. Beecher HK. The first anesthesia records. *Surg Gynecol Obstet.* 1940;71:689.
2. Gravenstein JS. The uses of the anesthesia record. *J Clin Monit.* 1989;5:256.
3. The computer-based patient record: meeting health care needs. In: Dick RS, Steen EB, eds. *The Computer-Based Patient Record: An Essential Technology for Health Care.* Washington, DC: National Academy Press; 1991:34.
4. Gravenstein JS. The automated anesthesia record. *Int J Clin Monit Comput.* 1986;3:131.
5. *Anesthesiologists Affiliated v Sullivan,* 941 F2d 678 (8th Cir 1991).
6. Introduction. In: Dick RS, Steen EB, eds. *The Computer-Based Patient Record: An Essential Technology for Health Care.* Washington, DC: National Academy Press; 1991:14.
7. Kennedy PJ, Feingold A, Wiener EL, et al. Analysis of tasks and human factors in anesthesia for coronary artery bypass. *Anesth Analg.* 1976;55:374.
8. Boquet G, Bushman JA, Davenport HT. The anaesthetic machine, a study of function and design. *Br J Anaesth.* 1980;52:61.
9. Meijler AP. *Automation in Anesthesia: A Relief? A Systematic Approach to Computers in Patient Monitoring.* New York, NY: Springer-Verlag; 1987:23.
10. Weinger MB, Herndon OW, Gaba DM. The effect of electronic recordkeeping and transesophageal echocardiography on task distribution, workload and vigilance during cardiac anesthesia. *Anesthesiology.* 1997;87:144.
11. Allard J, Dzwonczyk DY, Yablok D, et al. Effect of automatic record keeping on vigilance and record keeping time. *Br J Anaesth.* 1995;74:619.
12. Zollinger RM, Kreul JF, Schneider AJL. Man-made versus computer-generated anesthesia records. *J Surg Res.* 1977;22:419.
13. Lerou JGC, Dirksen R, van Daele M, et al. Automated charting of physiological variables in anesthesia: a quantitative comparison of automated versus handwritten anesthesia records. *J Clin Monit.* 1988;4:37.
14. Cook RI, McDonald JD, Nunziata E. Differences between handwritten and automatic blood pressure records. *Anesthesiology.* 1989;71:385.
15. Edsall DW. Analysis and frequency of artifacts generated by anesthesia information management systems. *Anesthesiology.* 1990;73:A481.
16. Stanley TE, Smith LR, White WD, et al. Incidence of vital sign artifact in automated anesthesia records. *Anesthesiology.* 1990;73:A483.
17. Loeb RG. Manual record keeping is not necessary for anesthesia vigilance. *J Clin Monit.* 1995;11:9.
18. Gravenstein N, Feldman JM. Anesthesia records and automation. *Semin Anesth.* 1989;8:119.
19. Block FE, Burton LW, Rafal MD, et al. Two computer-based anesthetic monitors: the DUKE automatic monitoring equipment (DAME) system and the microdame. *J Clin Monit.* 1985;1:30.
20. Brien RA, Smith NT, Quinn ML, et al. The accuracy of voice recognition in the operating room. *Anesthesiology.* 1988;69:A331.
21. Klocke H, Inform D, Trispel S, et al. An anesthesia information system for monitoring and recordkeeping during surgical anesthesia. *J Clin Monit.* 1986;2:246.
22. McNitt JD, Bode ET, Nelson RE. Long-term pharmaceutical cost reduction using a data management system. *Anesth Analg.* 1998;87:837.

23. Johnstone RE, Jozefczyk KG. Cost of anesthetic drugs: experiences with a cost education trial. *Anesth Analg.* 1994;78:766.

24. Dexter F, Lubarsky DA, Gilbert BC, et al. A method to compare costs of drugs and supplies among anesthesia providers. *Anesthesiology.* 1998;88:1350.

25. McIlrath S. Panel wants most paper claims to go the way of the dinosaur. *Am Med News.* August 10, 1992:1.

26. Gibbs RF. The present and future medicolegal importance of recordkeeping in anesthesia and intensive care: the case for automation. *J Clin Monit.* 1989;5:251.

27. Morris C. Legal aspects of monitoring. In: Gravenstein JS, Newbower RS, Ream AK, et al, eds. *The Automated Anesthesia Record and Alarm Systems.* Boston, Mass: Butterworth Scientific; 1987:270.

28. Dick RS, Steen EB, eds. Summary. In: *The Computer-Based Patient Record: An Essential Technology for Healthcare.* Washington, DC: National Academy Press; 1991:6.

29. Block FE, Reynolds KM, McDonald JS. The Diatek Arkive "organizer" patient information system: experience at a university hospital. *J Clin Monit.* 1998;14:89.

30. Coleman RL, Stanley T, Gilbert WC, et al. The implementation and acceptance of an intra-operative anesthesia information management system. *J Clin Monit.* 1997;13:121.

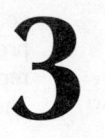

# Quality Assurance in Anesthesiology

Jerry A. Cohen

*Those who fail to remember the past are condemned to repeat it.*

GEORGE SANTAYANA

## THE DEVELOPMENT OF BASIC PRINCIPLES

In the broad sense, quality management (QM), which includes quality improvement, increases the likelihood that medical intervention will improve patient outcome and reduces the probability that it will precipitate a bad outcome.[1] When QM works effectively, it provides a systematic mechanism by which problems are detected and corrected, efficiency is improved, and care is rendered in a manner convenient for patients and health care providers. When it fails, usually from superficiality or disuse, the history of practice problems is repeated. Quality assurance (QA) and its basis is riddled with acronyms; refer to Table 3–1 for an alphabetized list.

In October 1988, at the American Society of Anesthesiologists (ASA) Workshop on Quality Assurance held at the annual meeting in San Francisco,[2] the question was asked, "How many people are here because they are interested in passing the Joint Commission on Accreditation of Healthcare Organizations (JCAHO) audit, and how many people are here because they would like to learn more about how to evaluate and improve quality?" About 99% of the attendees indicated that their major motivation was passing the JCAHO audit, and only 1% were interested in using QA techniques to improve their practice. Just 3 years later, in June 1991, at another ASA workshop for QA and risk management, the same question was asked.[3] This time the answers were reversed; 99% of the attendees indicated that they wanted to improve the quality of their practice and reduce their perceived quality problems, and only 1% were primarily concerned about passing the next JCAHO audit.

Interest in quality improvement as a management tool has continued to be a major topic in the literature of corporate management, in the popular press, and in medicine. Provision of the best possible quality of care is now perceived as more efficient, more economical, more profitable, and less of a liability than the alternative. In addition, JCAHO has made performance improvement a key element in accreditation,[4] in

**TABLE 3–1.** Acronyms Used in Quality Assurance

| | |
|---|---|
| AMH | *Accreditation Manual for Hospitals* |
| APO | Adverse patient outcomes |
| ASA | American Society of Anesthesiologists |
| CAMH | *Comprehensive Accreditation Manual for Hospitals* |
| COBRA | Comprehensive Omnibus Budget Reconciliation Act |
| CQI | Continuous quality improvement |
| DRG | Diagnosis-related group |
| HCFA | Healthcare Financing Administration |
| HCQIA | Healthcare Quality Improvement Act |
| JCAHO | Joint Commission on Accreditation of Healthcare Organizations |
| MADOM | *Manual for Anesthesia Department Organization and Management* |
| PARR | Postanesthesia recovery room |
| PPS | Prospective payment system |
| PRIA | Peer Review Improvement Act |
| PRO | Professional review organization |
| PSRO | Peer standards review organization |
| QA | Quality assurance |
| QI | Quality improvement |
| QA/I | Quality assurance/improvement |
| QM | Quality management |
| TEFRA | Tax, Equity, and Fiscal Responsibility Act |

a very real sense unifying many of the goals of accreditation and QM.

## HISTORICAL CONSIDERATIONS

### *How Did the "Quality" Concept Enter Medical Practice?*

#### The Agricultural Experience

Major concepts of statistical quality control were derived to a great extent from agriculture. Contributors such as E. A. Fisher, who applied the science of mathematical statistics to agricultural problems, eventually developed statistical methods by which complex interactions could be analyzed. Two individuals who contributed greatly to the concept of analysis of variance were W. Edwards Deming and W. A. Shewhart. Their understanding of the relationship of inherent variation in processes, control limits, and outcome subsequently led to the notion that complex undertakings, such as medical performance and outcome, can also be expected to perform within limits determined by the underlying structure and process of medical practice.[5]

Although Deming's original writings were highly technical and difficult to read, even when they were intended for the public, the methodology used and its impact on the rise of Japanese industry were captured in an accessible, well-written book by Mary Walton, *The Deming Management Method*.[6] Today, we use Deming's principles of statistical quality control to improve practices that work and to eliminate those that do not. At the same time, we attempt to improve the efficiency and economy of medical practice.

A condensed historical timeline of QM developments is provided in Table 3–2.

### *What Was the Stimulus for Early Quality Assurance Development?*

Because of the poor quality of American hospitals at the beginning of the 20th century, a major effort to improve the

standards of care developed. The Flexner Report,[7] Codman Survey,[8] and early work by the American College of Surgeons coalesced into the Hospital Standardization Program. This program eventually became highly effective. In the initial report of 1917, 87% of the hospitals surveyed failed the audit; later, only 6% of hospitals failed a much more rigorous audit.

Because the program had expanded and required more resources than the American College of Surgeons could provide, the Joint Commission on Accreditation of Hospitals (JCAH) was established in 1951. This commission was composed of the American Hospital Association, the American Medical Association, the American Dental Association, the American College of Physicians, and the American College of Surgeons.

From its beginning to the present, hospital accreditation has dwelt largely on the area of quality and the observance of quality standards. Seventy-eight percent of the average JCAHO audit and >60% of the contingencies have dealt with QA in recent years. Although the current JCAHO audit is, in theory, voluntary, successful passage is required for Medicare reimbursement. This fact alone has made JCAHO the most influential purveyor of QA concepts in American medicine.

Clearly, when Codman made his well-known speech in 1914 and stated that hospitals should look critically at their outcomes and strong and weak points, contrast their results with other hospitals, base physician credentials on demonstrated ability, and be forthcoming about bad outcomes as a lever for increasing resources, he was nearly three fourths of a century early in his pronouncements. His key concepts, although extremely well developed and the impetus for the current hospital survey system, were left to twist idly in the wind and had to be rediscovered later by people such as Avedis Donabedian,[9] and even later, systematically applied to health care by George Labovitz through his company, Organizational Dynamics, Inc.[10]

**TABLE 3–2.** Timeline of Quality Management Developments

| Year | Development |
|---|---|
| 1914 | Codman's speech about analyzing outcome as a basis for improvement and mission planning |
| 1917 | Hospital Standardization Program, an outgrowth of the Flexner Report, the Codman Survey, and the American College of Surgeons |
| 1951 | JCAH formed |
| 1965 | Social Security Act establishes Medicare; deems JCAH the accrediting body for Medicare |
| 1972 | PSRO legislation |
| 1982 | TEFRA law establishes the Peer Review Improvement Act, replaces PSRO with PRO |
| 1983 | DRGs become part of the Social Security Act; prospective payment system established |
| 1985 | COBRA—mandates quality review and discharge planning |
| 1986 | HCQIA—mandates Federal QA data bank |
| 1988 | *Wall Street Journal* reports dozens of JCAHO accredited hospitals fail state inspection |
| 1992 | JCAHO announces Agenda for Change with notion of CQI |
| 1993 | Organizational Dynamics, Inc. introduces CQI for physicians and the FADE process |

COBRA, Comprehensive Omnibus Budget Reconciliation Act; CQI, continuous quality improvement; DRGs, diagnosis-related groups; FADE, *f*ocus on and characterize problems and determine the desired state that should be achieved, *a*nalyze the data that form a compelling basis for *d*eveloping and executing and evaluating solutions; HCQIA, Health Care Quality Improvement Act; JCAH, Joint Commission on Accreditation of Hospitals; JCAHO, Joint Commission on Accreditation of Healthcare Organizations; PRO, professional review organization; PSRO, peer standards review organization; QA, quality assurance; TEFRA, Tax, Equity, and Fiscal Responsibility Act.

Despite the increasing role of JCAHO in improving medical practice, its seal of approval has come under fire. On October 12, 1988, the *Wall Street Journal* published a chilling article including a list of dozens of JCAHO-accredited hospitals that had failed state inspections between 1986 and 1988.[11]

As a result of this and other pressures, JCAHO responded with the *Agenda for Change,*[12] which introduced practice parameters as part of the concept that standards of practice could improve outcome. JCAHO also outlined a system for ongoing quality analysis and assessment and by 1992 had begun to foster the notion of continuous quality improvement (CQI).[13] The immense task of bringing a standardized approach to QM was the central preoccupation of JCAHO in the 1990s. The Indicator Monitoring System, ORYX, and other performance improvement initiatives, based to a large extent on the theories of Labovitz,[10] have found their way into the *Comprehensive Accreditation Manual for Hospitals.*[4]

## PEER REVIEW ORGANIZATIONS

### What Were the Legislative Initiatives?

To a great extent, the battle between cost and quality has been spearheaded by a series of legislative initiatives. The Social Security Act of 1965 established Medicare and with it the requirement for JCAH accreditation. Utilization review soon followed in the Social Security Act of 1967. To review the quality and appropriateness of care and to establish some form of ongoing review, the Peer Standards Review Organization (PSRO) was enacted into law in 1972. A decade of profound disinterest in the PSRO followed because physicians saw it more as an intrusion than a help.

Subsequently, as part of the Tax, Equity, and Fiscal Responsibility Act in 1982, the Peer Review Improvement Act was passed, which replaced the PSRO with the Professional Review Organization (PRO). Some critics commented that the PRO was merely the PSRO without standards. The next year, 1983, saw the implementation of diagnosis-related groups as part of the Social Security Act. This act mandated the prospective payment system and had almost no QA measures. The deficit soon was remedied by the Comprehensive Omnibus Budget Reconciliation Act of 1985, in which QA and discharge planning were mandated.

The flurry of legislative activity culminated in 1986 in the Health Care Quality Improvement Act, which mandated a federal databank for reporting QA issues. The items to be reported included any restriction of privileges for >30 days, liability settlements, professional society restrictions, and restrictions of a practitioner's medical license.

### What Is the Role of the Peer Review Organization?

Mark Holoweiko, writing in *Medical Economics,*[14] quoted William Roper, then head of the Health Care Financing Administration (HCFA) and later Deputy Assistant to the President for Domestic Policy: "The time has come for the federal government to become intricately involved in the writing of medical-practice standards." Roper anticipated that the PRO would be the government's agent in this effort. Although this statement did not mark the beginning of the federal government's interest in controlling the quality of care for which it paid, it was a major cannonball delivered across the bow of organized medicine. It represents the continuing contest between the cost and quality of care, characterized by the PRO's third contract cycle.

The PRO was largely responsible for administrating HCFA's quality intervention plan, which included sanctions for quality deficiencies. The legitimacy of quality review provided by the PRO rested to a large extent on the validity of the governmental assumption that health care providers will render poor care because of the combination of financial incentives and disincentives introduced by the prospective payment system.

The adversarial nature of the PRO with respect to medical practice included its punitive measures, bureaucratic orientation, negative rather than positive incentives, and overconcentration on case outliers, all of which have been a continuing annoyance to physicians. This irksome set of characteristics was not helped by the lack of demonstrated effect on outcome. Consequently, the National Academy of Sciences Institute of Medicine recommended that Congress totally redesign the PRO to oversee Medicare quality in a manner to reflect realistic and meaningful standards and to improve outcome.[15] Since the fourth scope of work, the PRO has taken a serious interest in quality improvement. It has undertaken a number of studies of care pathways, based on nationally accepted standards.

### What Is the Impact of Malpractice Legislation and Tort Law?

The courts have established some general guidelines regarding the relationship of hospitals to the physicians to whom they extend privileges.[16,17] In these corporate negligence cases, the responsibility of hospitals to guarantee the extension of clinical privileges only to physicians who are well qualified was established as a matter of law.

### How Does Title 19 Protect Peer Reviewers?

Defects in the law of the state of Oregon, demonstrated in the continuing case of *Patrick v Burget,*[18] were instrumental in the genesis of protective federal legislation. In this suit, brought by a physician who was deprived of his right to practice by the peer review committee of his hospital, the committee was held liable under the antitrust laws for improper restraint of trade. Further, confidential documents involving the review process were exposed to public scrutiny.

This frightening precedent was promptly dealt with on the federal level. The Health Care Quality Improvement Act extended protection via Title 19 of the Social Security Act to peer reviewers. Under the provisions of this act, peer reviewers who act on a reasonable belief that they are improving the quality of care, who make a reasonable effort to obtain the appropriate and relevant facts in the case, who provide appropriate notice to physicians being reviewed, who give them an opportunity to rebut the charges, and who base their decisions on the facts of the case are immune to prosecution or suit under the Federal Antitrust Laws.

The act further protects the peer review and QA documents from exposure in medical malpractice cases and specifically provides for up to 6 months of imprisonment, a $1000 fine, or both, for individuals who expose these documents improperly through any publication, distribution, or factual description outside the peer review process.

Regardless of legislative initiatives, the real solution to liability and exposure is the observance of scrupulously fair procedures for peer review, including written criteria for review that are made part of the hospital bylaws.

## CURRENT QUALITY ASSURANCE

### What Are Its Common Problems?

The difficulties in developing a productive QA program are numerous. The QA infrastructure sometimes develops in a manner that is overly complex and inefficient. The database produced by that system may not be sufficiently robust or accurate to describe the quality of each service's activities in a meaningful fashion. As such, it cannot form the foundation for significant action. Several internal and external problems reduce the productivity of a QA program.

### Evolution Through Reaction to JCAHO

QA evolved as a reaction to JCAHO demands, which have been advanced in a manner that has often lacked detail and consistency. Although JCAHO has been our greatest stimulus to develop quality assessment and improvement techniques, its leadership has straddled the fence on the specifics of implementation, causing great confusion to those attempting to comply. Its pilot studies on quality indicators revealed a simplistic approach that contrasts markedly with the detailed pilot study of severe morbidity and mortality performed by the Battelle Human Affairs Research Center and the ASA.[19] JCAHO methodology was characterized by the development of a few indicators of severe morbidity and mortality that pertain to a small minority of patients. They poorly reflect the overall quality of the hospital and the concerns of most patients.[20] A robust, meaningful database probably is not much more expensive than the abbreviated one advocated by JCAHO, which chose a simple system to make it more palatable.

Herein lies one of the principal paradigms for failure in QA: adoption of an overly simple system in order to obtain acceptance. This approach fails because it does not produce meaningful assessment and action in a predictable fashion. It fails in particular institutions because many hours are spent by the medical staff to produce reports (the necessary paperwork), but little real improvement in quality is derived from the effort. This produces frustration and cynicism. Recently, JCAHO has become more responsive to the criticism that its accreditation process should become less pejorative and more useful as a tool for improvement. ORYX and the Indicator Monitoring System, as well as increasing emphasis on CQI, are evidence of changes in JCAHO's direction.

### Gathering of Data

The indicators used by the medical staff to reflect quality of care may be gathered in a manner that produces statistical inaccuracy. The QA staff can help individual specialties by

analyzing the medical record post hoc to determine the occurrence of indicators such as those listed in Table 3–3. Because data are gathered not only by nonphysicians who are unfamiliar with the patients but also long after the problem occurred, they are often incomplete. Data are more accurate when they are gathered as closely as possible to the event that is to be monitored. This is enhanced by making the gathering of

**TABLE 3–3.** Quality Assurance Report Form

**Airway**

**Difficult intubation, unexpected** (visualization problem, >2 attempts, special technique, reintubation, surgical airway, emergency use of succinylcholine)

**Obstruction** requiring intervention (more than airway insertion, jaw thrust, or positive pressure)

**Trauma** requiring treatment or explanation to patient (damage to teeth, uvula, vocal cords, oral mucosa)

**Cardiovascular**

**Cardiac arrest**

**Death**

**Ischemia or Rule Out Myocardial Infarction** requiring escalation of care (more than transient ST changes)

**Hemodynamic instability** requiring intervention (>2 doses of ephedrine in 1 h, unplanned vasopressor, depressor, or antiarrhythmic infusion; unplanned fluid bolus >2 L

**Miscellaneous**

**Cancellation of operation**

**Delay of operation** (incomplete work-up, patient medically unprepared, equipment problem)

**Emergency call button pushed**

**Nausea and vomiting** causing a delay in discharge or requiring treatment

**Pain problem** causing a delay in discharge

**Parenteral line problem** leading to escalation of care (vascular obstruction, hemothorax, pneumothorax, exploration of site)

**Other problem** not on form requiring escalation of care or causing morbidity

**Respiratory**

**Desaturation** (<92%) requiring >2 L nasal $O_2$

**Decreased compliance** requiring treatment (bronchodilators, chest tube, bronchoscopy)

**Ventilatory insufficiency** requiring support or antagonism of sedative drugs (includes aspiration, apnea, $CO_2$ retention)

**Neurologic**

**CNS injury or mental status change** unrelated to surgical procedure (stroke, lateralizing weakness)

**Nerve injury**

**Prolonged sedation**—unintubated patient not oriented >2 h postoperatively

**Regional or Pain Block**

**Complication** (wet tap, toxicity, high spinal, persistent paresthesia)

**Duration** delaying discharge

**Surgical block inadequate**—general endotracheal anesthesia required

**Pain block inadequate** requiring replacement or analgesia by other route

**Discharge**

**>3 h in postanesthesia care unit (PACU)**

**>2 h in PACU**

**Delay in transfer** from PACU (intensive care unit, ward, transportation not ready)

**Prolonged observation** due to protocol (tonsillectomy and adenoidectomy, malignant hyperthermia)

**Unplanned**

For each problem, describe the cause, treatment, and outcome below:

data an integral part of the recordkeeping routine. Electronic medical record systems have the potential to make data gathering a highly accurate and relatively painless process.

## Applicability of Indicators

The indicators used to reflect quality may apply to a minority of patients. Because most systems are driven by regulators, we tend to direct our efforts toward assessment of the worst possible problems. In fact, few patients suffer the extremes in poor quality of care, but many have minor and frequent problems that are annoying, prolong their hospital stay, and reduce profitability.

## Method of Assessment

The way in which recognized problems in care are assessed may prevent systematic action. Assessments should be clear and forthright. Labeling problems as *expected, unexpected,* and *possibly outside the standards of care* does not express the true preventability or severity of the problems being addressed. These categories do not even exist along the same continuum and, at best, are ambiguous and perhaps disingenuous.

The tendency of hospitals to adopt obscure assessment categories derives in part from legal concerns that labels, such as *preventable/nonpreventable,* treated *properly/improperly,* and leading to *short-term/permanent damage,* or escalation of care could have adverse tort claim effects. Because federal statutes limit the discovery of QA data, however, this specter has not materialized.

To be useful, any assessment system should reflect the medical, ethical, and legal severity of the problems observed. We must differentiate between trivial problems and those that lead to escalation of care, severe morbidity, or even death. The system should account for the preventability of the event. (Is it unrelated to our process, or is it something we can improve?) Finally, it should form the basis for effective action.

## Accuracy of Aggregate Data

Methodology may be inadequate to obtain consistently accurate aggregate data that serve to inform practitioners and the hospital administration of the quality of care. Many institutions use a mixture of normalized data (the frequency of events per patient at risk or per other meaningful cohort grouping) and nonnormalized data (total number of events without reference to a denominator). Also, when the data are gathered by nonphysician QA workers rather than concurrently with patient care, the number of problems detected may represent only a fraction of the total. Therefore, the data that are obtained cannot serve as a barometer of the current status, nor can they be the basis for meaningful improvement. A well-structured, robust system is less expensive to operate and more productive in terms of improving quality of care, public image, and profitability.

To be useful, data should include relevant measurements of how well the structure, process (including practice parameters generally accepted as leading to good outcome), and outcome of current medical practices are functioning (ie, how often a good or bad outcome occurs per patient at risk). Compilation of statistics that are not related to risk or cost of care are largely noncontributory and wasteful of resources.

Much of the information needed for computing frequency statistics is available in existing hospital databases, especially those that form the cohort denominators. Rekeying of these data is wasteful. The relevant data should be centralized as much as possible and distributed in a common electronic form for QA review and use. This method provides a cost-effective uniform standard for calculating frequency statistics.

## Quality of Definitions

Quality and the purpose of QA may be poorly defined. A well-understood concept of what constitutes quality should lead to the development of meaningful indicators based on the scope of care, including all services and therapeutic modalities, their desired outcome, and their associated risks. Problem and outcome indicators must be designed by the individual specialties in terms meaningful to their practice. Some of these indicators may require long-term follow-up (eg, neurologic dysfunction, efficacy of pain therapies, or headache secondary to lumbar puncture).

A 2-tiered system of quality assessment bookkeeping—one for JCAHO and one that we report in our specialty journals or talk about in the lounge—must be eliminated by devising a scientifically meaningful database and using it to guide change. This approach should have a positive impact on the economics of care and could lead to sustained demonstrable improvements in outcome.

## Academic Organization and Care Path Models

Academic institutions often have an organizational structure that parallels that of the affiliated medical school, which time and tradition have made virtually unchangeable. Although several layers of this system could be eliminated, most academic hospitals choose to retain the departmental organizational skeleton. The strengths of departmental organization and current technology can be used in these institutions to help facilitate individual departmental QA programs. Departments should retain the role of developing meaningful quality indicators and providing the QA system with realistic definitions of quality.

The department-oriented quality program tends to insulate each medical department from the others and further insulates nursing and operations groups from each other and from the medical staff. The care path model differs significantly from the traditional departmental model. In the care path model, data are collected from each patient as the patient proceeds along the continuum from admission to discharge. The indicators of care are selected to monitor the effectiveness and efficiency of care along the path. Complications are just one problem that affects the path by creating a longer path to the desired outcome. This model requires that care path teams, such as for stroke, chronic pain, solid organ transplantation, or ischemic cardiac disease, replace departments as the central quality monitoring unit. Each team is composed of physicians, nurses, and operations personnel who are involved in activities related to the path. This tends to eliminate departmental silos and breaks down traditional barriers to improvement.

## Role of Hospital Quality Improvement Departments

The hospital QA service can provide basic support for the medical staff to collect data for problems related to individual patients. Physicians have more confidence in data they collect as a matter of course than in distantly post hoc data gathered by others.

Existing data can be provided in electronically usable form. Hospital computer resources can help to customize existing software, resulting in uniformity, standardization, and a marked reduction in personnel requirements. The departmental QA officer can then review only the outliers of quality instead of screening chart after chart. Time saved allows for review of the big picture and formulation of meaningful action.

### Regulators

Some problems in dealing with our regulators are not of our making. To resolve these problems, we must continue to work with them to establish firmly what the ground rules are, although we must not make them the centerpiece of our QA program. Although the specifics in the JCAHO accreditation manual[4] and the ASA *Manual for Anesthesia Department Organization and Management* (MADOM)[21] are not exquisitely detailed, their intent is clear. JCAHO wants physicians to develop a system for monitoring quality that has some meaning with respect to outcome.

## What Is the Theoretic Basis of Medical Quality Assurance?

Some of the concepts of industrial QA were translated into medical terms by Donabedian.[9,22] The overall goal of his unified quality assessment theory was to advance simple but powerful principles that would expose the sources of variation in medical management, then to reduce them by making the outcomes of care more predictable.

To achieve this goal, the quality assessment process is divided into 3 functionally related categories: structure, process, and outcome. A quality indicator may fall into one or more of these divisions. Donabedian postulated that the structures and processes of medical care cause the observed outcomes.

### Structure

Quality indicators that are primarily structural are derived from the institutional elements that support care. These include elements relating to the physical plant, including the anesthetic gas delivery system, the anesthesia machine and its components, disposable equipment, the logistic means by which items are supplied to the anesthesiologist, and the patient-monitoring systems. Also included are the means of deploying personnel, established operating room safety procedures, and well-accepted management algorithms, such as basic cardiac life support or the Harvard anesthesia practice standards[23,24] and those of the ASA.[21]

### Process

Process elements are derived from the generally accepted techniques, methodologies, and judgment processes that contribute to patient care. These include the indications for anesthetics, blood components, drugs, invasive monitoring, and pain management.

### Outcome

Changes in structure and process are generally systematic and should lead to improvement in outcome by reducing the frequency of problem events related to these elements. To be useful, structure and process review requires specific criteria defining the problem area to be improved, the goals of improvement stated in terms of enhanced outcome and performance, and a description of the changes in process that are to be used to effect the improvement. If the problems, goals, or methodologies are poorly defined, improvement is unlikely.

Similarly, if the structural and process elements of practice are not reviewed continuously over time, improvement may be ephemeral. For example, if a QA program detected a large number of hypotensive episodes attributable to rapid vancomycin infusions (ie, red man syndrome),[25] improving the structures and processes involved should lead to improved outcome. This goal might be accomplished by pretreating patients with an antihistamine, by using only infusion pumps to deliver the drug over a 1-hour period, or by infusing the drug even more slowly over an 8-hour period before surgery.

Such changes in the structure and process of vancomycin administration should reduce the number of reactions related to rapid administration virtually to zero. In this case, the goal, the methods to achieve that goal, and the resulting outcome are clear and achievable. Continued monitoring of the problem ensures that the improvement is sustained.

### Problems of Analysis

Outcome cannot be improved directly, except by time travelers and other miracle workers; rather, it improves as a consequence of improved structure or process or a change in the overall severity of patients' illness. Review of outcome is useful principally to determine the consequences that the structure and process elements have on care. Outcome elements include mortality and morbidity rates, overuse or underuse of blood products and monitoring techniques, cost of care, length of stay, and patient satisfaction. To the extent that outcome reflects the impact that antecedent structures and processes have on care, it is a useful measurement, but it should not be used alone as a quality indicator. It can serve best as a gross confirmation of the success or failure of changes to improve defined endpoints of care.

### Confounding Variables

Outcome assessment is limited by several factors. In medicine, unlike industry, many uncontrollable variables in patients' physiology and behavior conspire to limit the effectiveness of the health care system. Hence, poor outcome does not always indicate substandard care.[26]

The relationship of process and structure to outcome may be obscured by confounding offsetting variables. Outcome can best be understood in relationship to the severity of preexisting illness, but even MedisGroups admission severity groups fail to give unbiased estimates of outcome.[27] This limitation severely reduces our ability to compare the standard expected outcome, weighted for severity of illness, with the actual outcome. It also compromises efforts by JCAHO and the PROs to set simple normative standards for outcome.

Adverse outcomes may be delayed, thereby obscuring problems in care. Such is the case with hepatitis or HIV. The effect of knowing the severity of outcome biases the review of process.[28] Reviewers regularly judge care to be substandard when they are told that permanent injury or death occurred.

Overzealous reliance on outcome assessment may lead to the temptation to manipulate the case mix inappropriately. Both individuals and institutions may improve their outcome statistics by reducing the number of high-risk admissions.[29] For all of these reasons, changes in outcome resulting from system-wide changes in process and structure are useful measurements of the effectiveness of change. However, outcome is not, in itself, an independent indicator of quality.

## What Is the Approach to Quality Management of JCAHO?

More than any other body, JCAHO has the greatest single influence on medical QA because of its roots and its quasi-regulatory status. JCAHO sets forth its theory and regulations in the annual *Accreditation Manual for Hospitals* (AMH).

Building on the concepts of structure, process, and outcome, JCAHO has transformed QA from an almost useless bureaucratic waste of paper into a reasonably scientific approach to quality assessment and improvement (QA*/I). Some of this transformation, as noted previously, occurred in response to external criticism.[11]

### Statistical Quality Control

In developing the concept of QA/I, JCAHO borrowed heavily from the theories of statistical quality control, especially those of Deming[5] and Labovitz.[10] It has at times developed its methodology before its theory, such as when it mandated the development of indicators of care before clearly explaining their basis in the service and risk profile (Fig. 3–1). On balance, the history of QA, under the aegis of JCAHO, has

---

*QA variably refers to quality assessment or quality assurance. Used by JCAHO, it normally refers to quality assurance. A more modern term that merges both concepts is *quality management* (QM).

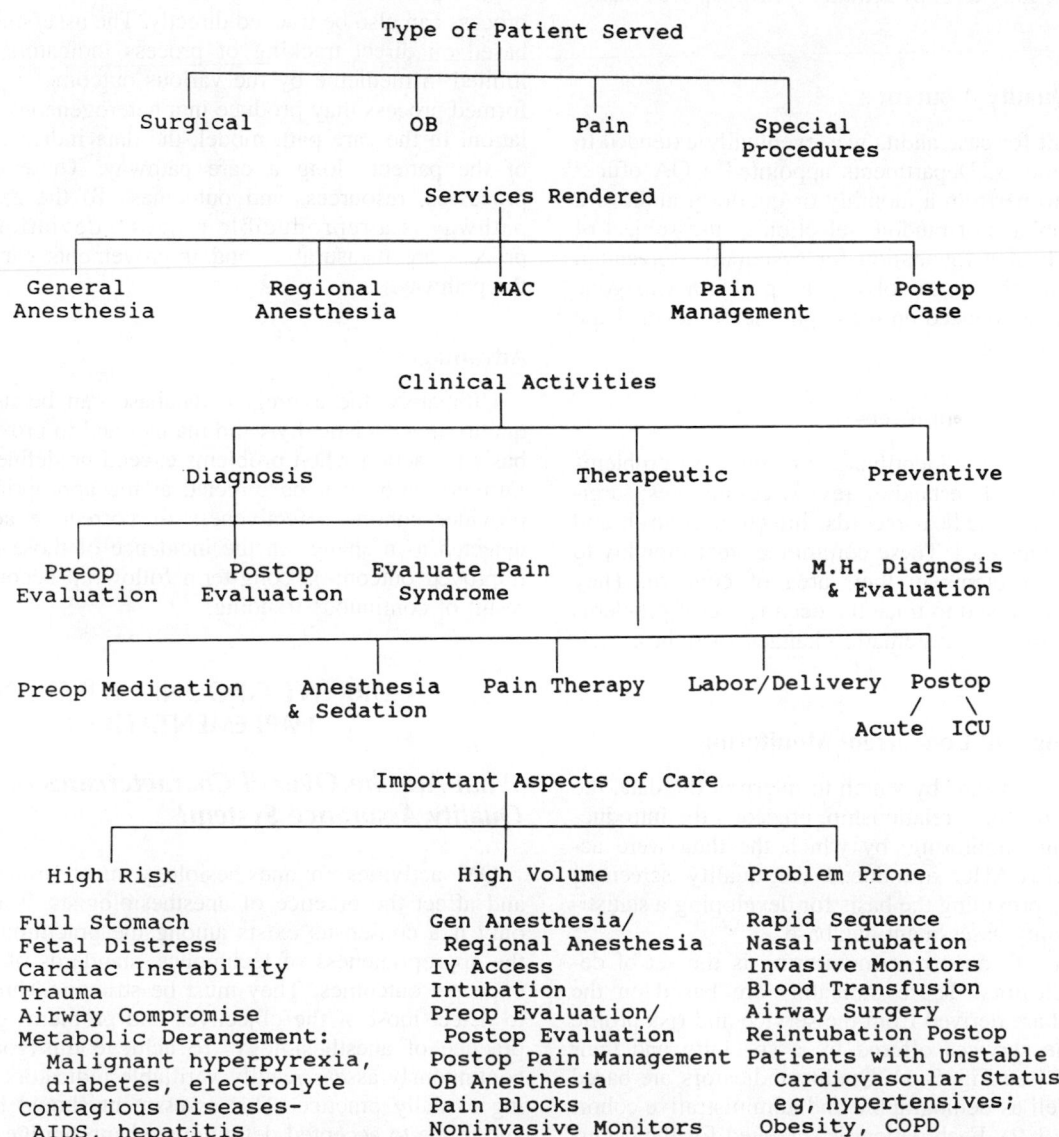

**FIGURE 3–1.** Risk service profile. (From Cohen JA. Quality assurance and risk management. In: Gravenstein N, ed. *Manual of Complications in Anesthesia.* Philadelphia, Pa: JB Lippincott; 1991:1–44.)

been a gradual evolution from procedure and diagnosis spot checks to the use of aggregate data gathered concurrently with patient care, divided into relevant cohort groupings, and stated in terms of frequency of occurrence.

## Retrospective Review

In the 1970s and early 1980s, JCAHO promoted retrospective review in the form of the problem-oriented medical audit, also espoused by Brown.[30] Essential elements of quality assessment were promulgated: identification of the problem, determination that it was a real problem affecting outcome, investigation of its exact cause (structure and process), and implementation of corrective action.

Without the concept of a logical set of indicators and an aggregate database, the case audit method did not evaluate medical practice comprehensively. It depended on the episodic identification of problems from various sources (eg, incident reports, mortality and morbidity conferences), but without prioritization in terms of the source or the level of the problem. The audits were conducted often enough to please JCAHO; however, long-term systematic follow-up was inadequate.

## Departmental Quality Assurance

The requirement for case audits was eventually extended to individual departments. Departments appointed a QA officer who was tasked to perform a monthly or quarterly audit of a problem. The problems of random selection of the subject of the audit, the lack of a foundation for systematic screening, and the assumption that once solved, the problem was gone forever were now reproduced on the departmental level. Time was wasted; little changed.

## Freestanding Review Committees

The need for systematic identification of ongoing problems eventually gave rise to freestanding review committees: surgical tissue, blood use, medical records, infection control, and pharmacy and therapeutics. These committees met monthly to evaluate specific problems in their area of concern. They began to compile data and to trace the occurrence of problems with the goal of making systematic changes to reduce their frequency.

## Quality Screening and Concurrent Monitoring

Paradoxically, the means by which to interpret the data, the structure-process-outcome relationship, preceded the introduction of concurrent monitoring, by which the data were acquired. In 1984, JCAHO introduced the quality screening concept,[31] thereby providing the basis for developing a statistically credible quality assessment database.

The foundation of concurrent monitoring is the set of defined quality indicators. These indicators are based on the scope of care and are derived from the service and risk profile that describes the services offered by a specialty and their associated risks[32] (see Fig. 3–1). Quality indicators are based on the risks as well as demographic and administrative cohort groupings[32] (Fig. 3–2). Each patient is screened for the occurrence of the defined indicators according to predefined criteria.[33]

Quality indicators are usually adverse patient outcomes, but they may also be positive occurrences. Generic indicators include cohort groupings such as anesthetic type or ASA physical status. The criteria (eg, acceptable upper and lower limits of blood pressure) are used to determine the occurrence of an indicator. Other criteria are used to determine the severity, preventability, and cause of the observed indicator.

Data for each patient are combined to form an aggregate database that can be tabulated to show the difference in problems between corresponding cohort groupings. Because all patients are screened, the incidence of adverse patient outcomes or other indicators can be trended. If the data are entered into a computerized database, a powerful, statistically valid description of the quality indicators of a department results.

## Limitations

The usefulness of this database is limited only by the definition of the criteria on which it is founded and by the fact that it is largely outcome driven. If standards of practice or resource and efficiency goals are used to develop indicators, process can also be tracked directly. The assessment of quality based on direct tracking of process indicators, however, is limited in medicine by the various outcomes a properly performed process may produce in a heterogeneous patient population. In the care path model, the data indicate the progress of the patient along a care pathway. These data refer to processes, resources, and outcomes. To the extent that the pathway is a reproducible process, deviations from that process are measurable, and improvements can be made to the pathway.

## Advantages

Ultimately, the aggregate database can be used to assess quality in a statistically valid manner and to provide a rational basis for action when problems exceed predefined thresholds. Further, action can be directed at the appropriate patient or provider cohort. Effectiveness of corrective action can be detected as a change in the incidence of those problems (ie, improved outcome). Long-term follow-up becomes a natural result of continuous trending.

# CURRENT GROUND RULES AND IMPLEMENTATION

## What Are the Overall Characteristics of a Quality Assurance System?

QM activities in anesthesiology must primarily evaluate and affect the practice of anesthesiologists. They can do so only if a consensus exists among the practitioners regarding the appropriateness of techniques, standards of practice, and expected outcomes. They must be structured broadly enough to detect most of the objectives and problems generic to the practice of anesthesiology. To achieve this goal, QM must continuously assess readily verifiable indicators of care relating to daily practice. This assessment should be reasonable and relate to accepted definitions of appropriate practice. The assessment of the frequency of problems, their degree of preventability and appropriateness of treatment, and their dis-

CLINICAL QUALITY ASSURANCE <u>PEER REVIEW</u> AUDIT
(Return form with anesthesia record to OR desk.
Do not make copies.  Do not attach to patient record.)

Date _____
OR# _____
Operation _____
ASA Class _____

Pre op:  [ ] Complete
         [ ] Completed in OR (e.g., labs)
         [ ] Incomplete (explain below)
         [ ] Made by another anesthetist
         [ ] Plan changed (explain below)

Anesthetic [ ] General    [ ] Regional    [ ] MAC
Anesthesiologist _____
Surgeon _____
Recovery Room Nurse _____

Anesthesiology Resident _____
Surgery Resident _____
Discharge:[ ] ONR  [ ] ICU  [ ] Ward  [ ] Home

[ ] NO UNTOWARD EVENTS                    [ ] UNTOWARD EVENTS (check below)

OR RR        **Airway**
__ __  Chipped tooth/loosened tooth
__ __  Stridor, Laryngospasm, Obstruction
__ __  Failed rapid sequence induction
__ __  Nose bleed or other trauma of airway
__ __  Inability to intubate by route
          originally planned
__ __  Esophageal intubation
__ __  Lip trauma
__ __  Accidental extubation

             **CV**
__ __  Death
__ __  Cardiac arrest
__ __  Significant Hypertension (sustained
          >30% above preop systolic)
__ __  Significant Hypotension (sustained
          <30% below preop diastolic)
__ __  Significant Bradycardia (30% below
          preop or that associated with
          hypotension)
__ __  Significant Tachycardia (30% above
          preop or that associated with
          hypertension)
__ __  Myocardial ischemia/MI suspected
__ __  Congestive heart failure/pulmonary edema
__ __  Dysrhythmia associated with one or
          more of above

        **Discharge planning**
__  Unplanned outpatient admission
__  Unplanned transfer to ICU
__  Unplanned return to OR
__  Unscheduled ONR
__  > 3 hr. stay in RR
__  Delayed waiting for M.D. to evaluate
__  Delayed waiting for X-ray
__  Delayed waiting for Room
__  Delayed for medical reasons
__  Other delay (explain below)

OR RR        **Respiratory**
__ __  Post op ventilatory assistance
          (unplanned)
__ __  Significant Hypoxemia/hypercapnia
__ __  Pneumothorax
__ __  Inappropriate bronchial
          intubation
__ __  Aspiration-respiratory
          distress syndrome
__ __  Reintubation (other than accidental
          extubation)
__ __  Bronchospasm

        **Miscellaneous**
__ __  Other (describe below)
__ __  Hyperpyrexia >38 C
__ __  Hypothermia <34 C (uninduced)
__ __  Wrong medication/dose given
          (describe below)
__ __  Drug reaction (allergic/adverse)
__ __  Intravascular line problem
__ __  Delayed or erroneous lab report/other
__ __  Nausea and vomiting
__ __  Equipment failure (explain below)
__ __  Pain medication delayed/inadequate

     **Regional (including pain therapy)**
__ __  Pain unresponsive to block
__ __  Failed block, inadequate block
__ __  Toxic reaction
__ __  Excessive block (high spinal)
__ __  Wet tap (epidural)

        **Neurological**
__ __  Prolonged neuromuscular block
__ __  Prolonged sedation
__ __  Peripheral nerve injury
__ __  Stroke
__ __  Recall
__ __  Seizure
__ __  Other damage (explain below)

For each of the above, describe briefly on back:

Event location    [ ] OR        [ ] RR

A)  Cause of Event
B)  Treatment of Event
C)  Result of Treatment

**FIGURE 3–2.** Example of a quality assurance report form. (From Cohen JA. Quality assurance and risk management. In: Gravenstein N, ed. *Manual of Complications in Anesthesia.* Philadelphia, Pa: JB Lippincott; 1991:1–44.)

tribution among cohorts (eg, patient, provider, location) should lead to actions that improve outcome. Improved outcome should be evident from subsequent QA data.

### Industrial Quality Control Methodology

Most of the objectives of QA/I in medicine parallel those in industrial quality control. The industrial model of statistical quality control discussed previously is largely applicable.[5] In industry, variation is an expected part of all processes. It results from the way in which the system is defined and taught and how and what support equipment is used. Individual performance is limited by variation engendered primarily by the system, by chance, and to a lesser extent by individuals, especially if they are well trained. As long as individual performance is within defined acceptable standards, outcome remains within predictable limits (ie, the system is in control). Improved outcome depends on continuous small improvements in the structure and process of the system.

## Quality Monitoring

Quality monitoring focuses on indicators of outcome that relate to the practice of anesthesia. Standards should be adopted with the goal of improving predictability of outcome by reducing the variability in performance. When performance variation goes beyond acceptable limits, improvement first should be sought through systematic changes in the process of anesthesia rather than through disciplinary actions directed at the practitioners. To do so, performance limits must be stated in terms of thresholds for acceptable outcome. This process is often definable by the frequency of adverse outcomes. Action to change the system is taken if the frequency of adverse outcomes exceeds agreed-on threshold levels.

## Meaningful Data

Meaningful action must be based on a statistically valid assessment of the aggregate database. It requires analysis of the differences between expected and actual outcome, subdivided into cohort groups (eg, providers, anesthetic techniques, physical status, locations, discharge destinations, acute postoperative monitoring). The cause of the observed disparities must be identified in terms of structure and process components that can be changed. Provider behavior is modified only if it remains outside of performance limits. The modified process or standards should produce a reduction in preventable problems detected by the QA program. The monitoring-analysis-change cycle is continual and should result in steady improvement.

## *What Are the Essential Standards of JCAHO?*

The principles promulgated by JCAHO for focusing on priority issues have been outlined in the last several AMHs. A specific person, usually the departmental chairman, is responsible for monitoring and evaluation of quality.

The QA process is based on an understanding of the scope of care and of those important aspects from which specific quality indicators are developed. Action is taken when established thresholds are exceeded to correct the systematically identified problems. The quality indicator data-gathering process is ongoing and is used to assess the effectiveness of changes. All providers are regularly informed of the findings and actions of the QA program.

JCAHO incorporated vast amounts of QA theory into its accreditation manual. Almost one third of the 1999 MADOM,[21] published by the ASA, deals with QM and JCAHO regulations. Although the regulations change somewhat from year to year, this is an excellent source of additional detailed information. The elements of structure, process, and outcome described by Donabedian,[9] the notion of performance limits and quality improvement described by Deming,[5,6] and the concepts of how to focus on quality issues and improve process elaborated by Labovitz[10] have led to a gradual refinement of JCAHO theories regarding QA and the rules by which those theories are to be implemented.

The term *quality assurance* has become a liability to JCAHO, which changed it to *quality assessment* and added *quality improvement.* Interestingly, *quality assessment* was a term in use more than a decade ago by the JCAH and does have the advantage of being value neutral. The QA concept became infused with the notion that it is a method for removing the "bad apples" from medicine, with the dubious expectation that medical practice will, therefore, improve. The term *quality management* is more useful in representing the goals of this discipline: the use of systematic data to effect strategic improvements in health care delivery that leads to more efficient, more effective care at a lower cost by eliminating error and improving process. As such, it is not a tool for passing a JCAHO survey so much as a strategic planning tool used to increase the probability of institutional survival. Although JCAHO cannot abandon its role as a regulator, it is becoming more collaborative as a QM consultant.

## New Directions

Beginning with the 1992 AMH,[13] JCAHO initiated a major effort to encourage the application of the principle of CQI, a part of the *Agenda for Change.*[12] The concept of indicators of care and a database derived from the services and risks presented to patients by various services, methods of monitoring, and trending remain largely the same.

Most important in the JCAHO AMH, there has been a steady decrease after 1992 in the total number of standards and a transfer of some of the standards previously under surgery and anesthesia to the medical staff and performance improvement sections. Standards affecting anesthesia include the general staff standards for review of surgical and other invasive procedures and blood or blood product use. Standards for sedation by nonanesthesiologists have been brought into close alignment with the standards for anesthesia. Current standards, objectives, and intents are well documented in the ASA MADOM.[34,35] Because standards change over time, the latest edition of the MADOM and AMH should be consulted for the most current authoritative opinion.

Emphasis on continuous improvement rather than on solving isolated nonsystemic problems continues to evolve but appears to be more a philosophic reorientation than a change in methodology. JCAHO is now emphasizing the problems resulting from the overall process of care and service rather than the performance of individual physicians. The purpose is to provide a means by which CQI is possible even when problems are not clearly above threshold levels. Rather than being purely department based, contemporary quality review requires cross-departmental attention to problems that involve patients whose care depends on many different hospital services.

Trending of individual performance is expected to demonstrate quality problems resulting more from flaws in the existing systems rather than individual flaws. Evaluation of individual performance will remain a secondary objective.

## JCAHO SURVEY

## *What Preparations Should Be Made?*

The JCAHO survey is voluntary and is paid for by the institution under review. Although passing the JCAHO survey is desirable and prestigious and certifies the institution for Medicare reimbursement, it is not essential, and the survey does not replace state-mandated audits. Some hospitals choose not to endure the rigors of a JCAHO audit to qualify for Medicare, opting instead for a direct audit by HCFA. The latter organization does not charge for the audit, and the process is somewhat simpler.

Passing the JCAHO survey requires a thorough understanding of the principles applied to the institution or department under review. In addition, a familiarity with the current regulations applicable to medical staff and entire perioperative pathways is essential. A summary of the current JCAHO standards can be found in the ASA's MADOM.[34] The numbering of these standards changes somewhat from year to year, but the principles are fairly consistent.

Review the general principle outlined in the AMH[13] and the ASA MADOM.[21] This should include the last several editions because surveyors also have trouble remembering all of the changes and tend to have a fairly "holographic" view of standards formed over a period of years. The following should serve as a general guide to JCAHO's belief system:

1. Procedures that require review are most importantly those that are routinely performed, have high risk, or are suspected or known to be prone to problems. This is an old concept, now applied specifically to invasive procedures. This type of review is to be made in a systematic manner and is geared toward improving the performance of individuals who are having problems.

2. Specific areas of evaluation of patient care with respect to invasive procedures include (a) selection of the appropriate procedure, (b) preparation of patients for the procedure, (c) performance of the procedure and monitoring of patients during the procedure, and (d) postprocedure care.

3. Drug use evaluation is aimed at an ongoing criteria-based process designed to improve the effectiveness of drug use. Included are (a) evaluation of the appropriateness of medications prescribed, (b) appropriate preparation and dispensing of medication, (c) appropriate administration, and (d) monitoring of medication effects.

4. Similarly, review of blood and blood component administration is mandated to make sure that (a) appropriate blood components are ordered, (b) their distribution and dispensing are appropriate, (c) they are given in an appropriate manner, and (d) the effects of blood and blood component administration are appropriately monitored. Specific criteria for the administration of blood are conspicuously absent. Review is limited to components that are used in high volume, pose a substantial risk, and are known or thought to be potentially problematic. As is the JCAHO tradition, specifics are absent.

5. Quality is now defined as that which increases the probability of a desired outcome. Emphasis is now more patient based than physician or service based. The overall thrust of this change is to try to deal with the multiple interrelated problems within an institution instead of attributing them to individual physicians. To implement these changes, JCAHO now requires that administrative organizational leaders undergo specific education in quality improvement.

6. Monitoring quality of care includes the identification of the important aspects of care. The most important aspects of care are considered to be those that occur frequently and affect large numbers of patients who are hospitalized where care is not properly provided or is provided when not properly indicated. In-depth evaluation of particular care problems is indicated when important single events or a pattern of problems exists. This requirement is not a departure from previous JCAHO guidelines; new is the encouragement to initiate improvement or changes in policy to improve overall performance.

7. Organized anesthesia services are directed by a physician member of the medical staff with appropriate clinical and administrative experience. This individual makes recommendations regarding clinical privileges of all licensed independent practitioners and personally provides, or provides through his or her designees, the formulation of mechanisms and material to help provide uniform quality of anesthesia services throughout the hospital. These mechanisms include means to ensure that anesthesia services are consistent with patients' needs and the current standards of practice, the type and amount of physical resources necessary for administering anesthesia and providing resuscitative measures, and approaches to monitoring and evaluating effectively the quality of anesthesia care provided by individuals in *any* department, including ambulatory, dental, emergency, obstetric, and psychiatric care, special care, and special procedures units within a hospital.

8. Guidelines must be developed to include those for administering general anesthesia with an anesthesia machine, the use of safety devices including but not limited to oxygen analyzers, pressure and disconnect alarms, product identification number index safety systems, gas-scavenging systems, and oxygen pressure interlock systems. It also appears that the chief of anesthesia services is responsible for not only policies related to the giving of anesthetics by an anesthesiologist but also the administration of anesthesia in other departments as well as the hospital's cardiopulmonary resuscitation program.

9. A preanesthetic evaluation is mandated for every patient for whom anesthesia is contemplated (note the language). It includes gathering sufficient information to formulate an anesthetic plan intelligently. Objective diagnostic data, an interview with the patient, and a discussion of the patient's medical, anesthetic, and drug history, as well as a review of his or her physical status, are required. It also includes a determination that the patient is an appropriate candidate for the anesthetic planned. Before the induction of anesthesia, this determination must be made by a licensed independent practitioner with appropriate clinical privileges. Immediately before the induction of anesthesia, patients must be reevaluated and equipment, drugs, and gas supplies checked. Patients must be appropriately monitored during anesthesia. Documentation is required for monitoring data; the dosage of all drugs and agents used; the type and amounts of fluids administered, including blood and blood products; the technique or techniques used; unusual events during the anesthetic period; and the status of patients at the conclusion of anesthesia, including vital signs and other information relevant to the continued care of the patient by the postoperative recovery staff.

10. A patient's postoperative status is evaluated on admission to and discharge from the postanesthesia recovery room. Documentation includes vital signs and level of con-

sciousness, intravenous fluid and drugs administered, unusual events or postoperative complications, and the management of those events. Discharge from the postanesthesia recovery room is the responsibility of a licensed independent practitioner with appropriate clinical privileges. If this person is not physically present, his or her name must be recorded in the patient's medical record along with the relevant criteria applied to determine the readiness for discharge. These criteria must have been previously approved by the medical staff.

11. Patients with the same health status and condition must receive comparable levels of quality of surgery and anesthesia care throughout the hospital. This section addresses the need for uniformity between different areas of the hospital, in particular the need for the standards in ambulatory surgery to be identical to those for inpatient surgery and the need to provide outpatients with a means of obtaining assistance in the event of postoperative complications. The standards specifically mandate that patients who receive other than local anesthesia on an ambulatory basis be accompanied at discharge by a designated individual who is responsible for the patient.

In summary, JCAHO will be looking for evidence of performance improvement at the time of the survey. The classic JCAHO 10-step process is outlined in Table 3–4. Surveyors will expect to find a system that evaluates the critical issues of quality based on a systematic data-gathering process that makes successful attempts to correct identified problems. The hospital's chief of staff and QM director are generally no longer available at the time of the departmental interview. In fact, much of the departmental review may come from the department's QA reports and from on-site conversations and observations in the operating room by the surveyor.

### The Survey Process

A survey team spends 3 to 5 days in the hospital. This team has at least one physician member. After an opening conference with the hospital executive administration and a review of the hospital rules, regulations, medical staff bylaws, and departmental quality reports, the surveyors conduct a leadership interview. Here, the surveyors make sure that hospital leadership is conversant with the QM structure, issues that are exposed by quality surveillance, and the progress of efforts made to improve quality and correct problems. They may review the activities of the hospital's CQI teams. Surveyors

**TABLE 3–4.** The Classic Joint Commission on Accreditation of Healthcare Organizations Ten-Step Process

1. Assign responsibility for monitoring and evaluation.
2. Delineate scope of care provided.
3. Identify important aspects of care.
4. Identify clinical care indicators.
5. Establish thresholds that trigger evaluation.
6. Monitor each indicator by collecting ongoing data.
7. Evaluate care when thresholds are reached.
8. Take actions to correct identified problems.
9. Assess effectiveness of actions:
   Improved outcome
   Decreased incidence of problems
   Increased productivity
10. Communicate results.

then visit all patient care areas and speak directly with members of the health care team, including physicians, nurses, and service personnel. A complete tour of the operating rooms, preoperative areas, and postoperative recovery areas is made. At the end of the survey, the surveyors meet again with the hospital leadership to discuss their findings and issue a preliminary report. This process is summarized in the *Comprehensive Accreditation Manual for Hospitals*[4] and in the ASA's MADOM.[35]

The JCAHO survey differs from those conducted by HCFA or the PRO. The JCAHO audit surveys the quality process but does not specifically look at outcome, whereas the PRO and HCFA audits are more intensely focused on outcome. JCAHO audits are voluntary, but HCFA (Medicare) audit is required if JCAHO accreditation is not obtained.

## FUNDAMENTAL CHALLENGES IN REDESIGNING QUALITY MANAGEMENT AS A STRATEGIC PLANNING TOOL FOR THIS CENTURY

### What Are the Problems That Departments and Health Care Organizations Face in Using Quality Management as a Strategic Tool for Success?

#### Lack of Common Perspectives and Sense of Mission

A lack of common perspectives and sense of mission can defeat any attempt to use QM as a strategic planning tool. Yet it is exactly this tool that would save many health care institutions in an increasingly competitive environment. Various divisions (medical, nursing, and operations staff) tend to regard quality from their own unique perspectives. Operations tends to concentrate on the structural elements, nursing on processes, and medical staff on outcomes, especially as applied to adverse outcomes. In this last respect, the physicians resemble the risk management approach to quality assessment. Consequently, each of these divisions tends to evaluate quality in ways that they cannot share easily.

#### Lack of a Unifying Comprehensive Theory of Relevant Quality Assessment

Among many medical departments, indicators of care are often a patchwork of relatively unrelated "dysquality" indicators resulting, in part, from attempts to please JCAHO with insufficient attention to institutional needs. Some organizations have developed indicators that measure a variety of things that can go wrong over a wide range of severity (eg, from nausea to death), with major variations in impact on outcome, arranged in no particular priority, acquired by means of questionable accuracy. This may be a small exaggeration, but not by much. On an enterprise-wide level, it is essential to report systematically measures of desired outcome and how frequently they are achieved (eg, vascular graft patency, organ transplant survival, and improved survival after tissue plasminogen activator or angioplasty). Many of us are beset by systems that do not help us to plan, strategically, on systematically acquired data. To manage quality successfully, a health care organization needs a comprehensive theory on how they will be using QM, what role it will play in the advancement of their enterprise, and how to administer it.

## Lack of Unified Infrastructure

The infrastructure of QM (what actually is done from day to day in terms of data gathering and analysis) needs to be unified conceptually across the enterprise so that the basic concepts are the same in medicine, nursing, pharmacy, nutritional services, site maintenance, risk management, credentialing, and so forth. Some of the major challenges to making QM a strategic planning tool are listed in Table 3–5. Although each area has a different component of the overall mission and different data to evaluate its success in meeting its mission components, the methodology should be essentially the same. Many of the quality data are poorly integrated across health care organizations. Quality-related activities, such as credentialing, incident reporting, QA/I, risk management, medical records, and surgical review, proceed as parallel activities without being well integrated. Each surveillance entity appreciates only its "part of the elephant."

Consequently, the overall incidence of various problems, the appropriate denominators with which to calculate frequency, and the incidence of various problems are not known accurately. Clearly, an integrated measurement system with a master repository of data is needed. Each of the above entities, for example, should draw on a common set of data. To do this they all have to identify the same event in the same manner, through a common data system, using the same nomenclature. This requires a global system for measuring and distributing quality data.

## The Positive Effects of Continuous Quality Improvement

When an organization's staff accepts a single, uniform, institution-wide quality improvement model that defines how to identify problems and analyze their root causes, and then develops and executes a plan for improvement based on that model, it has adopted the essential concepts required for successful CQI. These concepts are delineated in Table 3–6.

A single, unified methodology is also likely to be much less expensive and easier to support than a series of uncoordinated, nonuniform efforts. Uniformity also facilitates problem solving by having different groups work through a single care pathway. In making successful quality improvements, organizations transcend the boundaries of divisions and act in a coherent cross-functional manner.

**TABLE 3–5.** Challenges to Making Quality Management a Strategic Planning Tool

| |
| --- |
| Lack of common view of structure, process, and outcome among staff |
| Inadequate commitment to QM to make critical decisions |
| No decision support system to gather meaningful data |
| Mistaking quality management and regulatory missions |
| Relying only on "dysquality" (adverse outcome) measurements |
| Indirect measurement using charge-surrogates |
| Failure to understand the critical waypoints on the care pathway |
| Not measuring the critical waypoints on the care pathway |
| No concept of how to form teams that use common QI principles |

QI, quality improvement; QM, quality management.

**TABLE 3–6.** Summary of Ground Rules for Continuous Quality Improvement

| |
| --- |
| Establish a concept of mission—starting with service/risk profile as it relates to internal and external customers. |
| Adopt standards where they exist to: |
|    Reduce variability—reduce performance limits |
|    Emphasize systems change rather than people change |
|    Promote systems testing rather than people testing |
| Define thresholds for outcome (performance limits): |
|    Define the current expected outcome. |
|    Define limits of variation (unacceptable outcome). |
|    Caveat—undesirable outcome indicates a problem with structure, process, or provider, but not which one. |
| Monitor indicators of outcome that relate to clinical process. |
| Analyze differences between expected and actual outcome for: |
|    Providers |
|    Structure elements |
|    Locations |
|    Techniques |
| Relate differences observed to their root causes: |
|    Eliminate useless processes—eg, fetal monitoring |
|    Promote useful ones—eg, oximetry |
| Modify the process and establish new standards: |
|    Emphasize process change: do not "round up the usual suspects" |
|    Modify behavior only if consistently outside of performance limits |
| Redefine thresholds; repeat monitoring-analysis-change process. |

## What Are the Keys to Overcoming the Challenges?

1. Define the data that indicate performance by creating a structured database. Some of these data will relate to outcomes of care, length of stay and turnover (in the hospital, intensive care unit, operating room, PACU, pain clinic, registration department, preoperative clinic); consistency and proficiency with which staff members perform; how often staff have to treat complications and perform other types of rework; and patient satisfaction. Some of the data may relate to regulatory requirements not obviously connected to the perceived institutional mission. The data, as a whole, should demonstrate how the institution compares with its competitors in a way that convinces its customers that it is the best place for health care or, conversely, pinpoints problem areas.
2. Review the *value* of all data currently gathered. Data cost money; justify the effort of gathering it. Make sure that the data fulfill a clear need or stop measuring them.
3. Find ways to gather the needed data that are part of patient care and routine business whenever possible. Make maximal use of existing information, such as clinical outcome measurements currently tabulated by departments to measure performance, but avoid simply throwing data into the mix because they are easy to find; unneeded data also have a price.
4. Ensure that measurements are made in a way that compels benchmarking internally and externally.
5. Consciously encourage insightful analysis of the data and pithy reporting. Allow various divisions to gather whatever data they wish, but make sure that they report only those measurements that support the quality decision-making process.

## Ten Steps to Success With Quality Teams

Teams need a blueprint or agenda that delineates the entire process from the point of problem detection (opportunity to

# Conscious Sedation CQI Team

| Focus: Problem Statement | Analyze: Data Collection for Causes |
|---|---|
| **Problem Statement:** As part of the JCAHO survey, it was determined that the medical record did not uniformly document that the patient was a suitable candidate for conscious sedation as determined by the physician. Attempts to correct this by modifying existing policy demonstrated inconsistent preoperative evaluation, intraprocedure monitoring and postprocedure care practices.<br><br>**Impact:** Conscious Sedation could potentially have been given to a patient who was not an appropriate candidate for it or in a manner that did not account for that patient's needs, thereby increasing the risk of an adverse event.<br><br>**Desired State:** Preanesthetic evaluation of the patient is completed and documented in the medical record prior to administration of Conscious Sedation so that it is given only to patients in whom it is appropriate and in a manner that takes each patient's needs into account. Intraprocedure monitoring and postprocedure recovery standards are uniform and safe throughout the institution. The staff participating in sedation understands its principles and requirements and is capable of basic life support. Documentation of sedation is uniform and complete.<br><br>A | 1. Prior institutional activities were evaluated with respect to the desired state. The following initial needs were identified: a) Reviewing the current sedation policy with respect to any evolving internal and external need; b) Formulating changes in that policy to be approved by the Executive Committee; c) Educating the Nursing and Medical Staff; and d) Management of the policy, *ie*, authority with regard to the policy in order to achieve departmental and divisional alignment with the policy.<br>2. A four-month audit of charts was performed to reassess compliance with the existing sedation policy. Records of patients from GI, ER, Cardiac Cath Lab, Pediatric Renal, and Pediatric Pulmonary were reviewed. Pre-, intra-, and postop documentation was uniformly appropriate in ER, GI, and Cardiac Cath lab, the latter of which was not reviewed by JCAHO.<br>3. The Medical Departmental Chairs were sent a request for evaluation of compliance with the current policy by evaluating the charts of patients to whom their members gave sedation, and to assess how the current policy should be revised to allow better compliance in the future. Some departments do not use sedation; compliance with policy varied from 57% to 80% in the others.<br>4. The team extensively interviewed a cross-section of the nursing and medical staffs. These interviews made it clear that there were problems with the definition of sedation and the application of current policy that varied from area to area. The presence of variation in practice represented a potential accreditation, quality of care, and risk management hazard. The applicability of the current policy to the ICU and pediatric patients was especially problematic. Central to this issue was the need for a clear definition of sedation/analgesia in contradistinction to usage of sedative drugs in a manner that has little potential for causing loss of airway or cardiac reflexes.<br>5. The team found that there was also a clear resource constriction that impacts the ability of areas that understand how to apply the policy, but are not able to consistently do so. In particular, their ability to properly monitor patients in transport and in preprocedure holding areas is compromised by a lack of transport monitoring equipment, sufficient properly trained personnel, and physical space dedicated to pre- and postprocedure care for patients undergoing sedation. This was acutely felt in Radiology, Radiation Oncology, and the Bone Marrow Transplant Unit, where sedated patients may be at risk when in transport or in hallways awaiting procedures. |

| Develop: Solutions & Recommendations | Execute: Implementing Solutions | Evaluate: Track Solutions, Hold the Gain |
|---|---|---|
| 1. For all of these reasons, the Committee has therefore reviewed the policy, with the assistance of the Department of Pediatrics, to eliminate ambiguities and make the policy more generally applicable to all patients in order to eliminate multiple standards of care.<br>2. The Committee worked with the outpatient clinics to make policies in these two areas identical so that practices would be uniform.<br>3. Information tools regarding requirements for patient selection and for documenting administration of sedating agents were developed and/or amended. In particular, a basic pre-anesthesia form was developed to ensure that the medical database was complete for patients receiving Conscious Sedation.<br>4. Specific areas utilizing Conscious Sedation were instructed in development of specific assessment and monitoring forms to document processes unique to their services based on the basic requirements for pre anesthesia assessment.<br>5. Requirements for credentials in sedation were revised to specify BLS training as a means of standardizing staff capabilities.<br>6. A quality monitoring process was developed.<br>7. A plan for disseminating information was developed to educate the Medical Staff.<br><br>B | 1. Final draft of the policy.<br>2. Numerous letters to house staff and medical staff as well as a presentation at the annual medical staff meeting.<br>3. Credentialling process in place and functioning.<br>4. Continued monitoring of medical records for problems.<br>5. Designation of team members as persons available to answer questions about sedation during all weekday business hours.<br>6. Continued development of a site change to allow centralization of pre- and post-procedure care.<br>7. Discussion of the practicality of a sedation "flying team" to provide sedation in areas that only need it occasionally.<br>8. Acquisition of literature and posters on sedation provided by the Anesthesia Patient Safety Foundation. | 1. Monthly reviews of compliance have been performed using the HIRM staff. These reviews are reported to the HIRM and Sedation Committees.<br>2. A continuing quality review process is being developed by MCEC to track problems and variances in sedation performance. These findings will be reported regularly to QEC.<br>3. Targeted educational activities will be launched as problem areas are identified.<br>4. Continued credentialling will be governed by performance measures as tracked by the quality measurement process.<br>5. The CQI process will be used to improve the hospital infrastructure as needed to maintain a safe environment for sedation. |

**FIGURE 3–3.** Example of the FADE system for quality improvement teams and improving the quality of documentation for conscious sedation.

improve) to the action that improves it. To do this in practical terms, they must:

1. Clearly define the mission of QM in the context of the mission of the enterprise.
2. Determine the broad categories of data that support measuring how well they are meeting that mission and use it to formulate a defined database.
3. Critically assess the data they have gathered and what they are missing.
4. Design a process for justifying what data are gathered and use it to delete unneeded data and acquire new data.
5. Assign the individual data to a category in the defined database.
6. Determine the best method, place, time, and frequency to gather each datum. This may involve assignments to various departments or divisions.
7. Determine how best to aggregate and display the data for analysis.
8. Determine where and by whom the various data should be analyzed. This will vary, depending on the data.
9. Define the endpoints of analysis and who will be responsible for recommending action.
10. Develop a plan for educating the organization's staff about the new QM system. This includes rewriting the quality plan, policies, and procedures.

A systematic way that quality teams focus on problems and arrive at solutions was described by Organizational Dynamics, Inc.[10] The FADE system provides a blueprint for helping these teams:

**F** Focus on and characterize problems and determine the desired state that should be achieved
**A** Analyze the data that form a compelling basis for improvement
**D** Develop solutions
**E** Execute and evaluate solutions

An example of using this process to resolve problems with documentation and adherence to proper standards for conscious sedation is shown in Figure 3–3.

## QUALITY ASSURANCE IN ANESTHESIA PRACTICE

### How Can It Work Efficiently?

The principles discussed in this chapter are more easily implemented in anesthesiology than in many other areas of medicine. Anesthesiologists tend to view their activities as a pathway, with a discrete beginning and end, along which are a series of reproducible processes and outcomes. The importance of physical and organizational structure is clear. The data-driven nature of anesthesiology, coupled with an organized way of recording those data, facilitates the maintenance of an aggregate database. The highly focused scope of care and well-defined expectations easily translate into standards of practice and an accepted set of quality indicators. In a way, QM programs in anesthesiology are prototypical of what is likely to develop in other areas of medicine as their activities become more precisely defined.

### Ongoing Measurement

At the foundation of improvement is an ongoing measurement of the state of affairs. A summary of the steps used in our institution is outlined in Table 3–7. Quality indicators should be collected on all patients and combined to form an aggregate database. This can be done most easily by attaching an indicator form to the anesthesia record (see Fig. 3–2). The form can be completed by the anesthesia provider during the case and passed on to the postanesthesia care unit staff for their additions. A short summary of the cause, treatment, and result of treatment facilitates the assessment of problem cases without the need to perform a detailed chart review. The finished forms should be deposited in a central location for collection. Other forms can facilitate postoperative follow-up (Fig. 3–4).

### Computerized Data Entry

After being checked for completeness, the information can be entered into a computerized database (example provided in Fig. 3–5). Although this process is not absolutely necessary, cross-tabulation of data, division of data into cohort groupings, and frequency calculations can be automated with the appropriate software. Hand calculation is not only time-consuming but also requires marked constriction of the data analysis to be affordable. By contrast, software is consistently

**TABLE 3–7.** Guide to Data Collection and Entry

1. Use a QA report form such as that in Figure 3–2 to document basic demographic data and adverse events.
2. Make sure that the providers know how to fill out the form and that they understand how to fill out the description of events section. These descriptions enable the QA review officer to assess and code events without reviewing each medical record.
3. Attach the QA report form to the anesthesia record or billing form so that the providers do not have to look for it separately. This maximizes ease of compliance.
4. Provide a single central location for the QA forms. Keeping them with the billing form or the department's copy of the anesthesia record works well. If you collect the operative data, you need to designate a location for postoperative evaluation forms.
5. Make sure that a QA form is filled out for each case. Cross-check the QA forms against the operating room log daily and make sure that missing data are obtained promptly.
6. Enter the data into the database or import data from another source, such as the billing database.
7. Code incomplete entries. Use the database to summarize incomplete QA reports to track incomplete forms. Recode incomplete to complete when the record is corrected (completed).
8. Separate the QA forms without adverse events from the others. Give the forms with events to the QA officer for assessment (coding and narrative summary) of each of the events. The QA officer should number and code each event, indicate if further audit is necessary, and write a brief narrative summary. For efficiency, you may restrict the narratives to the records with at least one code-2 event.
9. Collect the coded forms and enter the assessment codes and narrative comments on the database. Code the audits as pending (P) on the database. This allows you to use the database to produce the summary of audited cases. Use this report to help you when ordering medical records for auditing.
10. Submit the medical records for further audit to the QA officer when available and type in the case review audit reports.
11. Transcribe the case review audits and enter any resulting changes in the database. Change the audit code from pending (P) to audited (A).
12. Use the database software to generate the reports.

QA, quality assessment.

DEPARTMENT OF ANESTHESIOLOGY  NAME:

FORM TYPE 1
**POST-OP ANESTHESIA EVALUATION**  MEDICAL RECORD NUMBER:

Postoperative Diagnosis:  Post op day: **#**

| Operation: surgery: | Anesthetic: [G] [R] [M] | Anesthesiologist: | Resident: | Date of |

Postoperative Notes:

| | Y | N | | COMMENTS |
|---|---|---|---|---|
| Sore Throat | | | | |
| Drug Reaction | | | | |
| Nausea/Vomiting | | | | |
| Muscle Pain | | | | |
| Respiratory Distress | | | | |
| Nerve Injury | | | | |
| Stroke | | | | |
| Headache | | | | |
| Recall | | | | |
| CV Instability | | | | |
| Cardiac Arrest | | | | |
| M. I. | | | | |
| Death | | | | |
| Organ Failure | | | | |
| Escalation of Care | | | | |
| Other | | | | |

RECOMMENDATIONS:

Physicians signature:

Date:_____ Time:_____

**FIGURE 3–4.** Example of a postoperative report form.

accurate, does not receive a salary, takes no coffee breaks, and has no personal agenda.

The computerized database can import data from other computer databases; trend volume and quality indicators by month or provider; trend adverse event indicators by month; filter and sort the data; display reports graphically or print tabular reports; and provide various summary reports, including adverse event assessments and recommendations. It can calculate indicators for the entire patient population, those with events, or the percentage of patients with events. Such software is commercially available and ranges considerably in price.

### Desirable Characteristics of Computerized Systems

Although a database system can simplify the handling of even large amounts of data, it requires organization, beginning with a logical series of menus that guide you in using the system. A well-organized top-level menu should branch no more than 2 or 3 times before reaching an essential function. All of the basic functions of the system should be accessible from the main menu. Use of the functions is guided by a series of online instructions and tables. Validity checks can detect mistakes immediately and prompt appropriate correc-

**\*\*VIEWING Qa-9192 TABLE, WITH 5039 RECORDS (1 NEW) - 6030KB ON DISK\*\***

| F1=Help | F2=End Mode | F3=Top F4=Bottom | F7=Form/TableF9=Edit | F10=Edit Menu |
|---|---|---|---|---|
| Del=-Rec | F5, Del=-Let | **QUALITY ASSURANCE - DATA FORM** | | Rec # 5039 |

**FIGURE 3–5.** Example of information that can be entered into a computerized database. This should include basic demographics, case-specific and event-specific data, and a characterization of events and actions taken.

**Patient ln:** Monroe        **fn:** Marla        **Number:** 38-20-36        Date: 1/20.92
**Age:** 3 (P, N, I, T, 1-9)

**O.R.:** 14        **Operation:** Total knee arthroplasty

**ASA** Class: 2        **Anesthetic:** G   (G, R, M, P)        **Discharge:** WARD   (HOME, WARD, ICU)

**Anesthesiologist:** 025        **Resident/Anesthetist:** 115        **PARU Nurse:** 000
**Surgeon/Other:** 000        **Resident/Assistant:** 000

**Pre op:** C   (C, COR, I)        **By:** A   (A, 0)        **Database:** C   (C, I)

**Event** 1: D. 3h        **Assess** 1: 2        **Severity** 1: A        **Location** 1: RR        **Audit:**
(Code) 2: N. Sed        (Code 2: 2        (Code 2: A        (OR, RR, 2: RR        (A, P)
3:        1-3) 3:        A-E) 3:        PO) 3:

| **Summary of Problem:** | **Action/Recommendation:** |
|---|---|
| Lock out on PCA set to 5 min, leading to excessive sedation in this 40 kg patient | Inservice training on proper setting of lock out on PCA pumps scheduled |

tions. Such a system should provide an easy-to-use but robust capacity to enter data, manage data files, alter look-up tables, add users, maintain security, sort the database, and generate and review past reports graphically or on paper.

### Responsive Action

The trended data form the basis for actions taken to reduce the observed incidence of problems. Other data contribute to the decision to take action, such as the evaluation of sentinel events or referrals from other departments or the hospital QA committee or other quality-monitoring committees, such as pharmacy, blood use, or infection control. The relevant findings should be reviewed quarterly and summarized in a report or minutes (Fig. 3–6). Effective actions should produce a decrease in the observed problem indicators.

### How Important Are Normalized Data?

Use of normalized data to compute QA statistics is essential for valid inferences. The probability that the analysis of QA data will lead to actions that improve the quality of care is critically dependent on the quality of the data. Conclusions may be erroneous if the problems and cohort groupings of the patients with adverse events (numerator) are evaluated without respect to the total population at risk. When problems in the numerator are divided by the total population in the corresponding denominator, however, the relative distribution of the data, and hence the conclusions, may change. The relationship of the incidence of adverse events to total number of adverse events within cohorts is often poor.[36]

Use of nonnormalized data to point to the source of problems among providers is inaccurate because of the wide disparities in caseload. The distribution of totals grossly distorts the apparent relative occurrence of common events. Providers who have a heavy caseload often have a higher total number but much lower incidence of adverse events than those who provide fewer anesthetics.

The apparent increase in gross problem rates associated with increasing ASA physical status ranking among patients undergoing regional anesthesia is apparent only from the incidence statistics, not from the enumeration of totals. The influence of physical status on the gross adverse event rate is similarly obscured by evaluating the numerator alone. Thus, the numerators of care (total numbers of events) must always be analyzed in relationship to the denominators of care that provide the context in which these events occur. Otherwise, meaningless statistics may lead to spurious efforts to improve quality.

### What Are the Pitfalls in a Nutshell?

The major pitfall in any QA program is inconsistent reporting of data. Until data are derived directly from the electronic medical record from monitoring systems,[37] provider-generated reports will still be essential. To avoid resistance engendered by the additional time needed to fill out a quality audit, a succinct check-off form should be used. Demographic data can be imported from existing databases to avoid unnecessarily encumbering anesthetists.

To avoid inaccuracies caused by fear of self-reporting, providers must participate in the development of the QM program, including the standards of practice, indicators, and ground rules for assessment of data. Confidentiality of data must be absolute. Appropriate resources, such as a personal computer and a part-time clerk, must be provided.

At least one department member must take charge of the system and be willing to spend 1 to 2 hours a week evaluating the data and occasionally reviewing cases that represent severe problems. Finally, meaningful improvements in the structure and process of practice must result in improved outcome, or the entire QA system will degenerate into a meaningless pantomime.

REPORTING PERIOD: *month, year*
DEPARTMENT: *Anesthesiology*

# Minutes
## Quality Assurance Committee
### *DEPARTMENT OF ANESTHESIOLOGY*

**Meeting Date:**

**Meeting Called to Order at:**

**Meeting Place:**

**Those who were** required to be **present** and were (listed alphabetically):

**Those who were** required to be present but were **absent** (listed alphabetically):

<u>Old Business</u>:

<u>Follow up on referrals/issues from the following</u>:

<u>Medical Staff Monitors (concurrent generic monitors)</u>:

<u>Blood Utilization (transfusion practice)</u>:

<u>Medical Records</u>:

<u>Surgical Case Review</u>:

<u>Unscheduled Ambulatory Admissions</u>:

<u>Pharmacy and Therapeutics</u>:

<u>Infection Control</u>:

<u>Other referrals</u>:

<u>Other</u>:

**FIGURE 3–6.** Example of format for taking minutes of the quality assurance committee.

New Business:

Medical Staff Monitors and referrals for the month of:

1. Volume: Total cases __.  See also Volume Indicator Reports

2. Quality Review:

    a.   General Summary:

        1) General Review/Analysis - See also Analysis of Adverse Events Report

        2) Generic trends by month and provider - See also Adverse Event by Month Reports

    b.   Case Reviews - internal and external referrals (next pages)

Utilization Review Referrals:

Blood Utilization (transfusion practice):

Medical Records:

Surgical Case Review:

Unscheduled Ambulatory Admissions:

Pharmacy and Therapeutics:

Infection Control:

Other referrals:

Other:

**Meeting adjourned at:**

_____      _____
Chairman, Quality Assurance Committee    Chairman, Department of
    Department of Anesthesiology          Anesthesiology

**FIGURE 3–6** *Continued*

## References

1. Cohen JA. Quality assurance initiatives. *Probl Anesth*. 1991;5:277.
2. American Society of Anesthesiologists. *Workshop on Quality Assurance, San Francisco*. Park Ridge, Ill: American Society of Anesthesiologists; 1988.
3. American Society of Anesthesiologists. *Workshop on Quality Assurance, Milwaukee*. Park Ridge, Ill: American Society of Anesthesiologists; 1991.
4. Joint Commission on Accreditation of Healthcare Organizations. *Comprehensive Accreditation Manual for Hospitals*. Chicago, Ill: Joint Commission on Accreditation of Healthcare Organizations; January 1998–August 1999.
5. Deming W. *Out of the Crisis*. Cambridge, Mass: Institute for Advanced Engineering Studies; 1986:484.
6. Walton M. *The Deming Management Method*. Chicago, Ill: Putnam; 1986.
7. Anonymous. What is the safest anesthetic? *JAMA*. 1887;8:520.
8. Codman EA. *A Study in Hospital Efficiency*. Boston, Mass: Thomas Todd; 1918.
9. Donabedian A. The quality of medical care: methods for assessing and monitoring the quality of care for research and quality assurance programs. *Science*. 1978;200:856.
10. Organizational Dynamics, Inc. *CQI for Physicians—Facilitator Manual*. Burlington, Mass: Organizational Dynamics, Inc; 1993.
11. Bogdanich W. Small comfort: prized by hospitals, accreditation hides perils patients face. *Wall Street Journal*. October 12, 1988;212(12):A1, A12.
12. Task forces lay groundwork for new survey process. In: Joint Commission on Accreditation of Healthcare Organizations. *Agenda for Change Update*. Vol 1. No 1. Chicago, Ill: Joint Commission on Accreditation of Healthcare Organizations; 1987:1.
13. Joint Commission on Accreditation of Healthcare Organizations. *Accreditation Manual for Hospitals*. Chicago, Ill: Joint Commission on Accreditation of Healthcare Organizations; 1992.
14. Holoweiko M. What cookbook medicine will mean for you. *Med Econom*. 1989;66:118.
15. Lohr KN. Institute of Medicine (IOM) study urges a major shift in QA strategy. *QA Rev*. 1990;2:1.
16. *Darling v Charleston Community Memorial Hospital*, 33 Ill2d 326, 211 NE2d 253 (1965).
17. *Johnson v Misericordia Community Hospital*, 99 Wis2d 708, 301 NW2d 156 (1981).
18. *Patrick v Burget*, 800 F2d (9th Cir 1986).
19. Battelle Human Affairs Research Center. *Study Coordinators Manual—ASA/CDC Anesthesia Mortality and Morbidity Study*. Washington, DC: Battelle; 1988.
20. Eichhorn JW. Quality assurance in anesthesiology. In: *International Anesthesia Research Society 1989 Review Course Lectures*. International Research Society; Cleveland, Ohio: March 1989:36–42.
21. Apfelbaum JL, Zerwas JM, eds. *Manual for Anesthesia Department Organization and Management*. Park Ridge, Ill: American Society of Anesthesiologists; 1999.
22. Donabedian A. Evaluating the quality of medical care. *Milbank Mem Fund Q*. 1966;44:166.
23. Eichhorn JH, Cooper JB, Cullen DJ, et al. Anesthesia practice standards at Harvard: a review. *J Clin Anesth*. 1988;1:55.
24. Eichhorn JH, Cooper JB, Cullen DJ. Standards for patient monitoring during anesthesia at the Harvard medical school. *JAMA*. 1986;256:1017.
25. Polk RE, Healy DP, Schwartz LB, et al. Vancomycin and the redman syndrome: pharmacodynamics of histamine release. *J Infect Dis*. 1988;157:502.
26. Schroeder SA, Kabcenall AI. Do bad outcomes mean substandard care? [editorial]. *JAMA*. 1991;265:1995.
27. Blumberg MS. Biased estimates of expected acute myocardial infarction mortality using MedisGroups admission severity groups. *JAMA*. 1991;265:2965.
28. Caplan RA, Posner KL, Cheney FW. Effect of outcome on physician judgements of appropriateness of care. *JAMA*. 1991;265:1957.
29. Ferrante J. What can medical sociologists say about clinical outcome measurements? *Am J Publ Health*. 1978;77:1155.
30. Brown E. Quality assurance in anesthesiology: the problem-oriented audit. *Anesth Analg*. 1984;63:611.
31. Joint Commission on Accreditation of Healthcare Organizations. *Accreditation Manual for Hospitals*. Chicago, Ill: Joint Commission on Accreditation of Healthcare Organizations; 1984.
32. Cohen JA. Quality assurance and risk management. In: Gravenstein N, ed. *Manual of Complications in Anesthesia*. Philadelphia, Pa: JB Lippincott; 1991:1.
33. Roberts JS, Walczak RM. Toward effective quality assurance: the evolution and current status of the JCAH standard. *QRB Qual Rev Bull*. 1984;8:11.
34. Cohen JA, ed. *JCAHO Standards, Intents, and Examples of Anesthesia Care in ASA MADOM*. Park Ridge, Ill: American Society of Anesthesiologists; 1999:77.
35. Cohen JA, Phillip BK. *How to Prepare for a Joint Commission Survey in MADOM*. Park Ridge, Ill: American Society of Anesthesiologists; 1999:77.
36. Cohen JA. Normalizing data improves quality assurance inference. *Anesthesiology*. 1992;77:A1099.
37. Edsall DW. Quality assessment with a computerized anesthesia information management system (AIMS). *Qual Rev Q*. June 1991:182.

CHAPTER

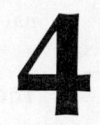

4

# Medicolegal Issues and Concerns

Monte Lichtiger
James Eckhart
James B. Matthews III
Robert R. Kirby

# PART I

# THE DEFENSE PERSPECTIVE

Monte Lichtiger
James Eckhart

## INTRODUCTION

### What Is the Scope of the Medicolegal Problem?

Since the 1950s, the incidence of personal injury suits against physicians has increased tremendously. General practice physicians in the 1940s and 1950s lacked the scientific armamentarium and the technologic advances that we have today. However, they made up for this deficiency with the rapport they developed with their patients. These patients knew their physicians well, thought of them as benefactors of society, and realized that they had limitations.

### The Impact of Specialization

With increasing emphasis on specialization, medical science advanced so rapidly that an individual could not keep abreast of all the advances in the many specialties and subspecialties. However, physicians could truly cure or effectively treat many of the ailments that people were prone to develop. New devices capable of diagnosing diseases in their early stages were introduced. Better therapeutic modalities were commonplace. Indeed, life expectancy itself increased rapidly, and the geriatric age group became an increasingly large percentage of the total population.

Patients now came to their physicians with great expectations. They saw these physicians as all-knowing individuals who could take care of almost all of their illnesses. Excellent results were not merely desired, they were expected. Should problems occur someone must, presumably, be at fault. Consequently, physicians were sued not only for negligence but also for the unexpected, poor result.

### Interpersonal Relationships

The age of specialization brought great medical advances, but often lost was the personal relationship patients had with their physicians. The greater abilities of physicians to cure disease led to their spending less time with patients to provide emotional support. Patients had difficulties relating to their physicians, and physicians were thought of as impersonal. Therefore, patients had no qualms about suing them if they were unhappy with the results of their therapy.

### Public Perception

Compounding this state of affairs was the fact that the old country physician, who was paid with poultry and produce, no longer existed. Physicians were not viewed as benefactors of humankind. To the contrary, they had an exceptionally high income and were perceived as individuals earning their fortune from the ills of humanity. This image was, of course, aided by the increased cost of this better medical care and the fact that many physicians adorned themselves with the external accoutrements of success.

### The Effect of Malpractice Insurance

Patients also became aware of the fact that physicians carried professional liability insurance. Consequently, should they have any positive feelings toward the physician against whom they wished to bring suit, they could rationalize these feelings with the knowledge that it was the insurance carrier, not the physician, who would compensate them. "It's just business, not personal."

### The Contribution of Plaintiff Attorneys

The change in medical science, the change in attitudes of physicians in developing rapport with their patients, the increase in the cost of health care, and the knowledge of the existence of malpractice insurance led to what has been called the *malpractice crisis*. To be complete, another factor must be mentioned—the increased number of attorneys in this country, some of whom viewed physicians with their malpractice insurance as legitimate targets, with little regard as to whether negligence had occurred. If a poor result was associated with a sympathy factor that would sway a jury, they were eager to institute a suit.

## THE MALPRACTICE INSURANCE CRISIS

### How Did It Arise?

In many cases, the previously mentioned circumstances led juries with little medical or economic knowledge to award millions of dollars to the "victims" of medical malpractice. This upward spiral in awards eventually led to escalating insurance premiums, as well as to the financial failure of many insurance carriers in a number of states, and became what physicians refer to as the *malpractice insurance crisis*.

### How Did Anesthesiologists Fare?

Anesthesiologists, in particular, were singled out as high-risk physicians. They spent most of their time in high-risk environments (ie, the operating room, the emergency room, the intensive care unit). They also had little time (or inclination) to develop rapport with their patients. In fact, patients rarely knew their anesthesiologist. He or she simply was that physician who put them to sleep. They had little or no knowledge of what this physician had to do while they were anesthetized. Indeed, many patients felt that after the anesthesiologists gave them an injection to put them to sleep, they left the operating room.

This patient perception, coupled with the lack of rapport between the patient and the anesthesiologist, contributed to the malpractice problem in anesthesiology. Malpractice insurance premiums rose precipitously as insurance carriers had large verdicts returned against anesthesiologists. The incidence of anesthetic problems was low, but their severity was extremely high.[1] Hypoxia or anoxia led to brain damage. Medication and technical errors when performing central nervous system blocks led to paralysis.

## CURRENT STATUS

### Is the Situation Getting Worse?

The previously referred to medical advances, of course, also took place in anesthesiology. Since 1990, we have witnessed the advent of new monitoring techniques and seen the expansion of our pharmacologic armamentarium. These new drugs and monitors enhance patients' safety and can prevent poor results. In essence, the techniques of the physiology laboratory have been brought into the operating room. Not uncommonly, patients are monitored with central venous, arterial, and pulmonary artery catheters to determine a number of directly measured variables and various calculated derivatives (Table 4–1).

The American Society of Anesthesiologists has also published rather specific standards regarding intraoperative and perioperative monitoring.[2] The most notable inclusions are the routine use of pulse oximetry in the operating and recovery rooms and identification of carbon dioxide in the expired gas of any patient in whom an endotracheal tube is inserted.

### What Is the Impact of Technologic Advances on Malpractice Actions?

Technologic advances in anesthesiology have improved patients' safety and seem to have decreased the number of

**TABLE 4–1.** American Society of Anesthesiologists' Statement on Invasive Monitoring in Anesthesiology

A major contribution to the current practice of medicine is made by the galaxy of monitoring equipment and techniques developed in the past 2 decades. They have had a vital role in improving our ability to prevent, recognize, and treat many conditions that previously contributed to morbidity and mortality.

These techniques, particularly those involving insertion of central venous pressure (CVP) monitoring lines, intra-arterial catheters (A-lines), and Swan-Ganz catheters (PA lines), all carry with their application some varying degree of risk to a patient. This statement attempts to minimize such risk by outlining our position on the provision of such procedures in the delivery of anesthesia care by anesthesia care team personnel.

*The decision to use invasive monitoring is a medical judgment and should therefore be made only by a qualified physician.*

*Invasive monitoring techniques should be prescribed by a physician. Depending on its risk, each should be applied only by a competent and trained physician or under the personal and immediate medical direction of such a competent and responsible physician.*

Training and credentialing of nonphysician members of the anesthesia care team who may perform invasive monitoring techniques should be approved at the local medical staff level by the anesthesia department and the active medical staff.

Some of the invasive monitoring tasks, namely the insertion of CVP lines placed via the upper extremity and of arterial lines (A-lines), may be delegated to properly trained and credentialed members of an anesthesia care team. Performance, however, should be under the immediate and personal medical direction of the leader of the team, preferably an anesthesiologist.

Insertion of pulmonary artery catheters is a relatively hazardous procedure and should only be done by a properly trained physician.

Excerpted from the American Society of Anesthesiologists' Statement on Invasive Monitoring in Anesthesiology, 1984, of the American Society of Anesthesiologists. A copy of the full text can be obtained from ASA, 520 North Northwest Highway, Park Ridge, IL 60068–2573.

anesthetic mishaps,[3] although this point is debated.[4] These results should decrease our medicolegal problems, and our experience is that this is, in fact, the case. One of the major problems leading to large judgments against anesthesiologists was brain damage secondary to unrecognized esophageal intubation.[5] This problem arises less frequently now, but it has not disappeared.[6] However, it has been replaced in part by brain damage secondary to the inability to establish an airway. Thus, better monitoring permits us to diagnose the misplaced tube if the monitor is on and the alarms are enabled, but it does not secure the airway for us. The bottom line, however, is that early diagnosis frequently leads to correction. Therefore, it is probable that, overall, anesthetic complications related to the airway are declining.

### With These Technological Advances, Are There Any Remaining Areas of Concern?

The answer to this question is an emphatic *yes*. An anesthesiologist must accept the limits of his or her competence. In our experience, a substantial number of malpractice claims occur when physicians exceed the boundaries of their competence and practice in areas in which they are not proficient; some even dabble at the fringes of accepted anesthetic practice. One problem area that is currently emerging is the practice of pain management. Plaintiffs are increasingly using the argument that anesthesiologists are providing services that are beyond the scope of their specialty. Is the implantation of spinal stimulators part of anesthetic practice? What training has the anesthesiologist had that qualifies him or her to perform this procedure?

A physician must show that he or she is qualified by education, training, and experience to perform a procedure. If an anesthesiologist takes a weekend course in spinal stimulator implantation, does that qualify him or her to return to practice and begin implanting these devices in patients? Should an adverse incident occur, neurosurgeons might be happy to testify against the anesthesiologist, feeling that such procedures more properly are in the realm of neurosurgery. They may also feel that their livelihood is being threatened. No doubt "turf battles" and economic self-interest motivate physicians to testify against their colleagues.

This scenario plays directly into the hands of the plaintiff attorney. Instead of anesthesiologists defending their actions based on standard of care, causation, and informed consent, they must now also defend these actions as being within the specialty of anesthesiology. Anesthesiologists must remain mindful of those territorial areas that overlap other medical disciplines and must be prepared to show their qualifications and justifications for what was done.

### Are Anesthetic Medicolegal Problems Decreasing?

A decrease in anesthetic problems should reduce anesthetic medicolegal problems, which in turn should be reflected by reduced premiums for malpractice insurance. If this sequence is correct, we can conclude that medicolegal problems for anesthesiologists, indeed, are declining. From 1990 to 2000, these premiums decreased about 40% for anesthesiologists. We even witnessed a reclassification of anesthesiologists by many insurance carriers from insurance rate or risk classification 5 to 3 on a scale of 1 to 7. Category 1 represents the benchmark, for example, a physician not engaged in invasive procedures. Within 10 years we moved from among the highest insurance risk groups to among the lowest.

It is doubtful that this trend will continue. With the increase in the number of pain centers in the United States and the number of physicians treating pain syndromes, an increase in the frequency of anesthesia claims is now seen in this field. This observation could compel insurance carriers to increase premiums for those anesthesiologists practicing pain medicine.

## The Texas Health Policy Task Force Study

The improvement in anesthetic risk classification may reflect overall improvement in the malpractice situation in general. Plaintiff attorneys and defendant physicians and hospitals have traditionally been adversarial in and out of the courtroom. Inflammatory rhetoric has obscured the facts concerning how serious the problem of malpractice is and how much it costs.

One published study was funded jointly by the Texas Hospital Association, Texas Medical Association, and Texas Trial Lawyers' Association.[7] Apart from the uniqueness reflected by the cooperation of these often contentious groups, the findings were remarkable and included the following:

1. Few claimants receive multimillion-dollar payments.
2. Overall caps tend to shift rather than reduce overall costs.
3. Few cases are resolved by jury judgments.
4. Noneconomic damages do not appear to be a major factor in payments to claimants.

Of perhaps more interest to physicians was the finding that the economic impact of medical malpractice to total health care expenditures in Texas was 0.62% (~$260 million). This figure was close to national findings of 0.74% reported to Congress in March 1992 by the Congressional Budget Office.[8] Presumably, these findings are applicable to anesthesiologists. Although these dollar amounts are significant, they are less than generally had been assumed.

## NEGLIGENCE

### *Where Do Problems of Negligence Arise?*

#### Anesthetic Induction

Years ago, we would answer this question by stating that most of our problems occurred during anesthetic induction, although this perception was disputed as early as 1976.[9] Many problems were related to improper intubation (ie, esophageal intubation). As was already stated, undiagnosed endotracheal tube misplacement now is less common. However, the esophagus and mainstem bronchus still are intubated on occasion, the problem is not detected, and injury or death may result. Esophageal perforation or tearing still occurs. We also have alluded to the fact that the inability to establish or maintain an airway is a significant cause of hypoxic damage.[9,10] Despite our better monitoring techniques, we still have major problems associated with induction and airway maintenance, even when regional techniques are used.

#### Negligence

Legally, *negligence* is the failure to use reasonable care, that is, the level of care, skill, and treatment that, in light of all relevant circumstances, is recognized as acceptable and appropriate by reasonably careful physicians in the same field. The term *ordinary care* is sometimes substituted.

Is the inability to intubate a patient negligence? Many expert witnesses are willing to state under oath that it is. However, a responsible and honest expert witness will admit that some patients have anatomy that misleads an anesthesiologist; they appear to have a feasible airway yet are difficult or impossible to intubate by the conventional approach. A physician is negligent only if he or she does not have and use a plan (eg, algorithm) to manage these patients. In the case of an esophageal intubation, most expert witnesses would concede that placement of the tube in the esophagus is not negligent, per se; however, failure to recognize that esophageal intubation has occurred is negligent. Every anesthesiology department should have such a plan that is consistent with the equipment and expertise available to it. For example, fiberoptic intubation techniques should not be included in a department's scheme if a fiberoptic bronchoscope is unavailable.

Also, members of a department must be familiar with that department's policies and procedures. If, for example, the policies and procedures state that patients in whom muscle relaxants are used must be monitored with a nerve stimulator, then this policy must be followed; to do otherwise constitutes negligence. Because policies and procedures vary from department to department and are periodically updated, it is important to familiarize yourself with them.

Aspiration of gastric contents may also occur during induction (and emergence), especially in a patient with a full stomach. This problem is a known complication of anesthesia, but lawsuits for death or brain damage secondary to aspiration continue to appear. Anesthesiologists must document all the steps taken to prevent this complication. Their best defense rests with demonstrating awareness of the potential problem and a complete record showing that their management was aimed at avoiding it (eg, antacid prophylaxis and induction with cricoid pressure).

The largest awards for negligence against anesthesiologists have been for incidents resulting in brain damage. Most of these are related to hypoxic or anoxic encephalopathy secondary to failure to establish an airway. Attempts to intubate a patient with a difficult airway can be traumatic. Bleeding with possible blood aspiration, avulsion of laryngeal cartilages, vocal cord damage, and perforation of the trachea, esophagus, or pyriform sinuses may result. The latter problems may lead to pneumothorax, pneumomediastinum, and subcutaneous emphysema. Although problems can arise at any time during an anesthetic,[9] the most damaging ones do so during induction.

#### Emergence

Emergence from anesthesia can be fraught with problems. Again, the most severe cases relate to death and brain damage. One of the most important incidents leading to severe problems is premature extubation of the trachea, for example, in a patient with Ludwig's angina. If the patient was intubated successfully, an anesthesiologist may be comfortable with extubation once the patient awakens and is able to follow commands. All too often, however, delayed respiratory obstruction occurs, after which the patient may be more difficult to intubate than before surgery. The ensuing hypoxia may lead to death or brain damage.

Other respiratory problems that may occur during emergence include aspiration pneumonitis, laryngeal spasm, and noncardiogenic pulmonary edema. The latter problem may be related to airway obstruction and negative-pressure pulmonary edema,[11] aspiration of gastric contents, and central nervous system hypoxia. The results of a traumatic intubation may not be noted until after the patient has emerged from anesthesia and has been extubated. Documentation in the record that a patient is able to follow simple commands and has no evidence of residual neuromuscular blockade is strong evidence that a conservative approach was taken regarding timing of extubation. It also decreases the impact of a negligence accusation.

## How Do Postanesthesia Care Unit Problems Impact Anesthesiologists?

An anesthesiologist's responsibility for care does not end with a patient's arrival in the postanesthesia care unit (PACU). Indeed, in most institutions, the PACU is under the direction of the anesthesiology department. Many legal precedents hold anesthesiologists responsible for the caliber of care rendered by a hospital's PACU employees. If a patient in a PACU suffers an adverse outcome as a result of a nurse's negligence, the anesthesiologist often is named in the suit. If not named as a defendant because he or she left the patient in the PACU in an unsafe condition (eg, still anesthetized so that airway obstruction was possible), the anesthesiologist is often designated as the physician who has the responsibility for care given by the nurse. Minimum documentation in the record should include the following:

- Record of acceptable vital signs
- Note of a formal transfer of patient care responsibility from the anesthesiologist to the PACU nurse
- A PACU recovery score document that the transfer of responsibility took place, was organized, and was appropriate

Since the late 1990s, we have witnessed an increased number of cases of severe outcome in the PACU. As intraoperative monitoring has improved, we have noted fewer cases of hypoxic brain damage in the operating room and more in the PACU. This observation has prompted insurance carriers to require improved PACU monitoring as a condition for coverage. We can hope that better PACU monitoring (eg, pulse oximetry) will decrease morbidity and mortality in this area.

If an emergency occurs in the PACU, ideally an anesthesiologist should respond. However, if all the anesthesiologists are busy with patients in the operating rooms, a plan must be available to the PACU nurses so that they know who to call for the emergency.[2] The plan may include coverage of an operating room case by a Certified Registered Nurse Anesthetist to free up an anesthesiologist for the PACU. Alternatively, an intensivist, an emergency room physician, or an emergency team in the institution must be designated so that help is available in the PACU. Whatever plan is formulated must be designed to provide expedient and appropriate care.

Such a plan, if accepted at the institution, ameliorates an anesthesiologist's liability for any alleged negligence in the PACU. The specifics of the plan differ from hospital to hospital. However, it must be a workable approach to emergencies occurring in the PACU, and it must be accepted by all parties involved.

## FUTURE PROBLEMS

### How Can They Be Avoided?

#### Vigilance

Vigilance is one of the most important characteristics that anesthesiologists can bring to bear. (Is the antonym *negligence?*) Close monitoring with an awareness of the pitfalls of monitoring devices is essential. However, with the increased importance that monitoring has assumed in our practices, we must remember to pay close attention to our patients. Not uncommonly, cases arise in which too much attention was given to the monitors and too little to the patient.

As an example, a patient suffered a cardiac arrest with resultant brain damage secondary to an obstructed endotracheal tube, even though a pulse oximeter was in use. The physician, who was alerted to the problem by the oximeter's alarm, spent a great deal of time readjusting the oximeter probe and monitor while his patient was hypoxic. We must first assume that the monitor is correct and check the patient.[4] The monitors should be checked only after we have satisfied ourselves that the patient is all right. Do not shoot the messenger.

#### Patient Rapport

Good patient rapport is another important aspect of care that must be pursued to avoid future problems. Lawsuits are easier to initiate against someone with whom one does not have a positive relationship. Conversely, a patient may be reluctant to pursue legal action against a physician who has taken a great deal of time to explain the anticipated procedures, who has answered questions, and who has generally attempted to make the upcoming surgery and anesthesia as comfortable as possible. This concept was espoused by an anesthesiologist who wrote a letter to the editor encouraging other anesthesiologists to ensure that our role in patient care is properly presented to the media. He felt that to do so would enhance our stature with the public:

*One thing we learned after the expenditure of huge sums of money on public relations consultants was the fact that "we have met the enemy, and they is us." Failure to carry out meaningful preoperative and postoperative interviews with patients was determined to be a glaring deficit shared by a majority of anesthesiologists.*[12]

We must spend some time with our patients and show that we are both informed and caring individuals. Physicians are human, and human beings sometimes make mistakes. It is surprising how forgiving patients can be if we demonstrate humanity when dealing with them.

## The Hospital Record and Anesthesia

We must also have thorough records and record events appropriately:

- Write legibly and use ink when charting.
- Make all entries promptly and use only acceptable abbreviations.
- Date, time, and sign each entry. On the anesthesia record, timing and dating are routine, but anesthesiologists often are less compulsive in this regard when writing preoperative notes.
- Cosign, with date and time, the anesthesia preoperative evaluation if it was performed by another member of your department. This measure confirms in the record that you are informed about the patient before caring for him or her.
- Cross out all errors in charting with a single line, and initial and date these corrections.

To a jury, a sloppy record designates a sloppy physician.

As an example, a certified registered nurse anesthetist (CRNA) had written the following statement in the Comments section of her anesthesia record, allegedly at the conclusion of the case: "Suctioned, SV (spontaneous ventilation), extubated, to RR." Before any of these documented events, however, the patient sustained a cardiac arrest; he died 2 weeks later. The CRNA, at some point, wrote over the above entry, stating instead that the supervising anesthesiologist was paged to the operating room. She then testified, in video deposition, that no overwrite occurred; it only *appeared* that her original note was present. A court order resulted in the production of 5 of her other anesthesia records in which the identical "original note" statement also was present. The jury was not impressed when this point and several others related to inaccurate recordkeeping were demonstrated at trial. They awarded the decedent's family $3.6 million.

The anesthetic record should tell a complete story of what occurred in the operating room. The plaintiff always argues that if it was not charted, it was not done; thus, details regarding positioning changes and any notable occurrences are important to record. The record is a medicolegal document that can, if complete, represent the anesthesiologist as well as an attorney, if not better. Finally, the medical record is not an editorial forum, and one must resist making editorial comments in it about a patient's care by yourself or others.

## ADVERSE EVENTS

### What Should Be Done If an Adverse Event Occurs?

An adverse event should be reported promptly to your insurance carrier and risk manager. This process is not only important for your ultimate defense but also may be required so that your insurance policy covers any potential expenses that arise out of the adverse event. It also alerts your carrier to hidden cases and allows them to review and collect facts, settle, assume hospital bills, or prepare a defense. You should also write down your own recollection of the events involved while they are fresh in your mind. Keep this narrative in a safe place where you can retrieve it in the future. Some plaintiff attorneys may wait to file suit in the hope that the defendant will have forgotten many of the facts of the case.

Remember to preserve any evidence that relates to the problem, including equipment that may have malfunctioned and medications.[13,14] This action may be a great help to you and may also protect other patients in your institution.

### How Should You Interact With the Patient and Family?

Maintain good rapport with the patient and the patient's family. You must present yourself as a concerned physician. As stated previously, people can be very forgiving if they are treated with care and regard. Explain the problem in terms that they can understand. A logical explanation of the complication may help the patient and family accept the outcome.

### What Should Not Be Done?

Above all, do not attempt to cover up the incident either in the medical records or in talking to the patient. When this action is discovered, as it almost always is, you will be confronted by an angry patient and his or her attorney. Hiding a problem can also result in punitive charges being brought against you. An award for punitive damages usually is not covered by your insurance carrier.

### Alteration of Records

Some physicians have tried to conceal their liability by altering medical records. To do so is unethical and dishonest. This approach should never even be considered. Handwriting experts may be called on to examine these records and are almost always able to detect these changes. When they testify at trial, you will lose all credibility.

Examination of medical records has become scientific. An expert in this field is able to discern if the record was altered some time after it was initially entered. One of the ways in which this determination is made is by ink analysis. Ink manufacturers change certain fluorescent components in their inks on a yearly basis at the direction of the Internal Revenue Service to enable them to detect recent changes in records made by taxpayers. Chromatographic studies can also be performed on the ink in the records. A needle is used to punch out a sample from the chart, and the ink is separated from the paper by a solvent. Chromatographic studies on this dissolved ink can then establish the manufacturer of the ink as well as the year it was made.

Other examinations routinely used include infrared reflectance and infrared luminescence photography, which demonstrate differences in writing instruments. Precision typewriter grids are also available and can show where additions have been made when the records are reinserted into the typewriter.

One of the most interesting new instruments, designed to detect interlineation and substitution of pages, is an electrostatic detection apparatus, which makes a permanent record of indentations appearing on the surface of a sheet of paper. One can actually read the writing that was present before the changes were made. These are just some of the modern technology methods that are now available to detect record changes.

If an addition or alteration is made, it should be as with

any other record change (ie, a single line through the deleted comment with your initials and date in such a way that the original comment is still legible). For late additions, identify them as such, time, date, and sign. In general, however, little is gained by late entries or deletions, even when they are made according to the appropriate protocol.

## Contact With the Plaintiff's Attorney

You should avoid all contact with the plaintiff's attorney. Do not discuss the case with anyone except your attorney or a representative of your insurance company. Be careful not to make any derogatory remarks or loose comments about patients or colleagues. Be in control at all times while speaking about the adverse incident. Furthermore, do not mention anything about a report you may have written, either for yourself or your insurance company. And remember, do not admit liability that has yet to be determined.

## DEFENSE

### How Does One Prepare?

Assuming you obtained informed consent and have not done anything to cover up the incident, you are now ready to prepare for your defense. Some steps can be taken to assist in your defense before reporting the incident to your carrier and before an attorney is assigned to represent you. These steps are often the key to a successful outcome of your case, whether you are appearing before an institutional review panel, a state regulatory body, or a jury (Table 4–2).

### Copies of Pertinent Records

Obtain complete copies of all pertinent hospital records as quickly as possible. By obtaining your copies early, you protect yourself from the hospital's locking up the chart, which could prevent you from reviewing these records. By copying the records soon after the incident, you obtain excellent evidence to demonstrate late entries, changes, or attempts to alter the records by others involved in the case. Remember that even minor changes or attempts at altering the records can destroy the credibility of the person making them. Should another physician or nurse make such alterations, your defense is solidified.

Prepare a legible verbatim copy of your records and a narrative summary of events. Aside from the embarrassment of not being able to read your own chart entries, a thought or idea that was in your mind at the time of the incident is often lost because a word or phrase cannot be read. At times, the

**TABLE 4–2.** How to Prepare for a Possible Lawsuit

Obtain complete copies of all records.
Make written verbatim copies of records.
Do not discuss the case or make written reports unless such activities are protected from later discovery.
If served with suit papers, do not discuss anything with the patient, family, or opposing attorney.
Obtain supporting medical literature and read it.
Be active in your defense.

emergent nature of an incident precludes a contemporaneous entry in the medical records.

Certainly, even the most compulsive physician will not be able to chart everything as accurately as desired. However, by preparing a summary immediately after the incident (no matter how time-consuming or unpleasant), events can be kept in perspective for questions that will almost certainly arise. Furthermore, this summary allows you to detail what actually occurred better than the chart entries alone. The combination of the two can greatly assist you in whatever defense is ultimately presented.

### Discussion of the Case

Do not discuss the incident with anyone who may be on the other side. Resist the temptation to discuss the case with the other physicians or personnel involved. Any such discussions that are not in the context of a quality assurance or attorney-client discussion, especially if written, are discoverable and can become evidence against you. Decline to meet with the hospital's risk manager unless you are certain that your conversation is legally protected from discovery. You must also be aware of the fact that the hospital may become your adversary in court.

Never talk to the patient, the patient's family, or the patient's attorney once you have been served with suit papers or a preliminary presuit screening notice. Whatever you say (or write) at that point can and will be used against you. It will not change their decision to proceed with the suit.

### Review of Medical Literature

Obtain medical literature that supports your diagnosis and treatment. If possible, do so early while the facts of the case are still fresh in your mind. Such action will help in your defense later when your insurance carrier and your attorney become involved. It will also assist you by suggesting potential expert witnesses for your defense.

This supporting literature gives you a psychologic advantage, as well. It demonstrates to your attorney and your insurance carrier that what you did is an accepted practice. It helps to educate your attorney and helps him or her plan for your defense. This approach provides everyone involved in your defense with a positive outlook. It certainly is preferable to just telling your defense team that you followed an accepted practice. Without supporting medical literature, they may be skeptical about your actions until an expert is retained to verify your position. This action also demonstrates your concern and interest in assisting with the defense.

### How Active Should Your Participation Be?

Become actively involved in your defense. All defense attorneys appreciate a client who is willing to spend the time to become involved in the defense of a claim. Anesthesiologists too often assume that their attorney will take care of everything. They fail to spend the necessary time to educate the attorney about the medical issues of a case. This educational process helps the anesthesiologist and lawyer gain confidence in each other and creates a sense of teamwork. The members of this team can feel comfortable enough to discuss the weaknesses of the case and to analyze them rationally when preparing the defense. The anesthesiologist will also feel more secure in questioning his or her lawyer about how things are proceeding and what can be expected in the future.

Proper preparation is the key to a successful defense. It includes explaining the following:

1. The facts and circumstances
2. How the medical literature supports your actions
3. Any deviations from accepted standards

Do not assume that the case will go away and do not avoid addressing any mistakes you made (no matter how painful). If you fail to do so during your preparation, you will be even more uncomfortable explaining your actions at a deposition or a hearing; by then it may be too late.

A major problem in every case is finding a good expert. This is an area in which you can truly provide assistance. As the medical practitioner, you will know the leading physicians in the area of anesthesia involved in your case. Your input will continue to build confidence between you and your attorney.

Once you have taken a position on the record under oath, it is almost impossible to change without losing credibility. Ask your counsel to discuss all the ramifications of the case with you so that you are fully prepared and have no surprises when you give your testimony. Follow the advice of your attorney and ask questions about the legal sequence of events if you do not understand what is going to happen. This action helps to eliminate the fear and uncertainty surrounding litigation. Remember that you know more medicine than the plaintiff's attorney. You really have the upper hand if you use your head and stay in control. A good defense counsel will be able to prepare you for your deposition and for any trick questions you may be asked.

## What Do the Plaintiff and Defense Look for in a Record?

States differ in terms of what information is admissible and what is discoverable at the time of trial. Generally speaking, physicians should recognize that a good attorney, whether plaintiff or defendant, will look at the documents summarized in Table 4–3. Once these records are obtained, the attorney

**TABLE 4–3.** Documents of Particular Interest to Plaintiff Attorneys

Complete set of hospital records, including those from the emergency room, postanesthesia care unit, intensive care unit, and labor and delivery areas, including obstetric and other logs, as well as an autopsy report (if available). (Nurses' notes are heavily scrutinized because they are often much more detailed than those of physicians.)

Complete sets of records from all physicians who provided treatment.

Health care provider certificates or applications for state licensure and hospital staff privileges

Corporate information on your professional group

Medical staff bylaws and the rules and regulations of the departments involved in the case

Incident reports if discoverable in your state

Pharmacy drug log

Medical bills

will ascertain the defendant's education, training, and qualifications.

The extent of independent recollection of events in the case must be learned during the discovery period to prevent sudden "convenient" recall testimony at the time of trial. The records will be scrutinized to develop a sequence of events that will be covered in detail during the testimony of all involved parties. Everything from the first visit or contact through history, physical examination, diagnostic tests, and findings and the medical significance of all of these items will be covered.

Conversations with the plaintiff will also be explored, as will the treatment given and any communication with other physicians and medical personnel involved in the plaintiff's care. The anesthetic given and the thought processes behind your decisions will also be considered. Alternative methods of care will be discussed, including your reasons for adopting or rejecting them. Any possible conflicts in the records and testimony will be explored thoroughly.

### Evidence of Finger Pointing

In particular, the opposing attorney will look for inconsistencies and finger pointing. Again, the hospital record should not be used for airing grievances or editorializing; however, this practice sometimes occurs despite all instructions to avoid it. The defendant anesthesiologist should be aware of other physicians' notes that suggest his or her culpability. The defendant should also look for any nursing notes that are incomplete or that conflict with his or her notes or recollection of the facts. The anesthesiologist must pay particular attention to notes made in the PACU.

Attorneys will also examine the original records to determine if anything has been rewritten or changed. Of course, a record that is too neat also arouses suspicion. Remember that almost without exception, every negligence case changes in theory as the case develops and discovery proceeds. This fact of life results from the witnesses' interpretation of the records and testimony, which often depends on what is in their own best interest.

### Are There Cases in Which Everything Goes Smoothly?

It is rare to see a case in which everything goes beautifully. Even the most defensible cases have weak points. For example, the medical facts can be supportive, there can be excellent expert witnesses, and the defendant physician can be a terrific witness. Yet the anesthesia record can have a gap in charting, or sympathy can be a factor that a plaintiff attorney will exploit. The following 2 cases represent the extremes of "good" and "bad" defense cases.

#### CASE HISTORY 1

One of the better cases that we defended involved a 44-year-old woman with chronic back pain. She gave a history of multiple back surgeries as well as the implantation of a spinal stimulator. When our anesthesiologist saw the patient, she was taking pain medications chronically. A morphine patient-controlled analgesia (PCA) infusion was started. However, the patient complained that she was not getting good pain relief. The surgeon then ordered sedatives to help the patient sleep. The PCA recording showed that the patient stopped using the PCA shortly after receiving the sedatives. The nurses documented good respiration up until 6:30 the next morning. At 7:30 AM, the patient was found dead and resuscitation was unsuccessful. A drawer full of prescription medications was found at the patient's bedside.

An autopsy summarized the patient's problems as atherosclerosis, pulmonary emphysema, and diverticulitis. The cause of death was occlusive atherosclerotic cardiovascular disease. A drug screen revealed a postmortem blood opiate level (free and bound opiate) of 0.46 µg/mL. The plaintiff's expert anesthesiology witness stated that the patient died of an "excessive amount of narcotic." The witness felt that the anesthesiologist (our insured) ordered too much morphine because he thought that the patient had developed tolerance. However, the witness opined that the PCA device may also have malfunctioned, and even more drug could have been administered than was ordered.

When the medical examiner who performed the autopsy was deposed, he never deviated from his opinion that the patient died as a result of her atherosclerosis. He acknowledged that the inventory of medications delivered with her body included Halcion (triazolam), Soma (carisoprodol), Xanax (alprazolam), and Talwin (pentazocine lactate). However, the toxicology results did not show a large quantity of any medication in her system. He also ruled out an overdose of morphine as a cause of her death. He stated that a morphine overdose usually leaves foam in the mouth or the endotracheal tube. He further pointed out that the patient's death was sudden.

The plaintiff's anesthesia expert felt that the blood level of morphine found at autopsy was consistent with an overdose. He stated that patients with coronary atherosclerosis could still die from an overdose of morphine. However, he did not know what the ratio of free morphine to total morphine was, and he could not explain the fact that the patient's respiratory rate was within the normal range >4 hours after her last dose of morphine. To explain this discrepancy, he just said that the nurses' charting of the vital signs was obviously wrong.

A professor of pharmacology at the University of Florida felt that the claim had absolutely no merit. He was ready and willing to help us at trial. The associate dean of the college of pharmacy at a major university was also willing to testify. He also explained the high postmortem blood level of morphine found in this patient by a phenomenon known as *rebound distribution*. Essentially, drugs within the body tissues move back into the bloodstream after death. This fact makes postmortem blood analysis inaccurate.

A forensic pathologist explained the relationship between free and total morphine when death is caused by an overdose of morphine. He stated that the ratio of free to total morphine in the bloodstream is ≥50% in individuals dying of morphine overdose. He pointed out that said ratio was only 16% in our patient.

The case did go to trial, and our physician was an excellent witness on his own behalf. He came across as a competent and caring physician. In answering questions, he talked directly to the jury. He explained why this patient was a candidate for PCA morphine. He explained that the dosage of morphine administered was not high and that she did not die of a morphine overdose.

In his closing argument to the jury, the plaintiff's attorney asked for $1 450 000. He suggested an apportionment of 80% responsibility for the hospital and 20% for our anesthesiologist. The jury returned a verdict in favor of our physician. However, they found for the plaintiffs and against the hospital in the total sum of $175 000.

## CASE HISTORY 2

This case involved a 54-year-old woman with a many-year history of lumbar spine problems. She previously had a herniated disk, which was treated with a chymopapain injection. She had some pain relief, but she continued to have pain that became progressively more severe. She was then admitted for a lumbar laminec-

tomy, posterior fusion with bone grafting, and spinal instrumentation.

Anesthesia was induced with propofol and maintained with nitrous oxide, oxygen, and narcotic. Intubation was accomplished easily and muscle relaxation was maintained. The patient's systolic blood pressure was kept in the 80 to 90 mm Hg range to facilitate the surgical procedure and minimize blood loss. Metoprolol tartrate (Lopressor) and hydralazine HCl (Apresoline) were used to maintain this blood pressure.

The patient was extubated after more than 9 hours of anesthesia and brought to the PACU. The PACU score was recorded as 3 on the patient's admission to that unit. She was pale and unresponsive, although she did open her eyes once. Her oxygen saturation decreased, and an airway was inserted. There was no response to insertion of the airway. A little later, posturing was noted. Repeated doses of naloxone were administered. No change was noted in the patient's condition; she remained unresponsive to all types of stimulation and demonstrated decerebrate posturing when transferred to a special care unit. A neurology consultant felt that brainstem injury was likely, and a computed tomography scan was ordered. It showed massive cerebral infarctions and possible uncal herniation. The patient's family was informed of the poor prognosis and requested a "Do not resuscitate" order. The patient remained comatose with decerebrate posturing until her death. The family refused an autopsy.

The claim against the anesthesiologist as alleged by the plaintiff's experts was divided into 2 portions:

1. An unnecessary state of deliberate hypotension was induced by administering a combination of potent drugs.
2. The anesthesiologist failed to appropriately monitor the condition of the patient thereafter.

According to these experts, the patient became dangerously hypotensive during her surgery. They claimed that this hypotension caused a lack of perfusion to the brain, which resulted in massive cerebral infarction.

The defense expert felt that there were weaknesses in the case, but based on the chart, he did not think that the anesthesiologist did anything wrong. However, he did point out that the patient's usual blood pressures were in the 140 to 150 mm Hg range, not the level that was recorded in the operating room. He also pointed out that the mean arterial blood pressures were in the mid–50 mm Hg during surgery. The insured felt that the patient's injury was secondary to an embolic event. He asked that we obtain both a neurologist and a neuroradiologist to review the films.

When our neurologist reviewed the computed tomography scan, he felt that it looked more like a hypoxic injury than an embolic event but said that he would defer to a neuroradiologist. Unfortunately, the neuroradiologist also felt that the brain injury was secondary to hypoxia. Upon hearing this, our insured asked us to find another neuroradiologist to look at the films. A second (and later a third) neuroradiologist again read the scan as demonstrating hypoxic injury.

Our attorneys then received repeated requests from our insured to allow him to submit a written summary of the case to our experts. They explained that they could not do so, because that summary would then be discoverable. He then wanted to speak to the experts to explain the case. It became obvious that he could not accept the experts' opinions (on both sides) that placed some blame on him regarding the outcome.

Because our insured's deposition was being scheduled, we now had great concerns as to how he would handle his own deposition. Physicians must listen to their lawyers' instructions as to how to handle certain issues when they are being deposed. Unfortunately, some physicians are not "controllable" no matter how much time their attorney spends with them to prepare for the deposition. A good witness is better than good facts.

Our physician did not handle himself well at his deposition. He started answering the plaintiff attorney's questions even before they were completed. In essence, we had a defendant who was in denial and who was not a good witness.

The plaintiff's case was in fact becoming stronger. That side had good experts in anesthesiology, neurology, and neuroradiology. The decedent's family members were excellent, sympathetic witnesses. It was time to think about settlement. The damages in the case were estimated to be >$2 million. This was greater than the limits of the insured's policy; the insured's assets had to be protected. After negotiations, the anesthesiologist's liability was settled for $850 000.

## TYPES OF LIABILITY

### How Do They Differ?

#### Individual Liability

Most states have statutes or case decisions defining or interpreting what is meant by this aspect of fault determination. If you are the only one sued, individual liability is apparent. The problem occurs when many parties are potentially responsible.

#### Joint and Several Liability

Under the doctrine of joint and several liability, a plaintiff who recovers a judgment against only 1 defendant can recover against that defendant or any other defendants for any reason he or she chooses. Consequently, a defendant found to be only 1% at fault may pay the entire judgment, allowing another more responsible defendant to escape payment entirely. Clearly, this distribution of blame is inequitable.

#### Comparative Negligence

Most state jurisdictions now have elected to use a comparative negligence system, in which the percentage of fault is equated with the percentage of liability. However, as with most things in law, the manner in which this doctrine is applied to defendants varies. Some states have adopted the principle of pro rata contribution among defendants, in which one's percentage of fault is one's percentage of the judgment recoverable. Other states have a sliding scale of fault. One example of this system is a state in which a defendant found to be ≥20% at fault would be in a situation in which joint and several liability was applicable. However, if his or her percentage of fault was determined to be <20%, pro rata contribution would apply. Anesthesiologists must be aware of the laws in their states to understand how the theory of joint and several liability impacts their practices.

## THE ANESTHESIOLOGIST AS AN EXPERT WITNESS

### What Is the Desired Role?

The role of expert witnesses in a medical malpractice case is crucial in determining the case outcome. Expert witnesses provide testimony about whether a breach in the standard of care occurred and whether that breach was the proximate cause of the injury sustained. The suggestion has been made that an expert witness should render an honest opinion based on scientific principles and facts. The American Society of Anesthesiologists suggests that at a minimum, expert witnesses should be qualified for their role and should follow a clear and consistent set of ethical guidelines (Table 4–4). In theory, either side, plaintiff or defendant, should be able to use the testimony regardless of who retained the expert.

Unfortunately, in the real world, this idealistic approach is rarely the case. Perhaps it should not be. A completely bland recitation of facts and principles by an uninspired witness is unlikely to be comprehensible and may well be soporific. Both the plaintiff and defendant want an expert who testifies enthusiastically and favorably for their side yet is believable. This need has led to shopping for experts to provide the desired testimony. Certainly, the proliferation of expert witness services and brokering agencies attests to this situation. Also, some itinerant medical testifiers constantly solicit attorneys, thus demeaning both the legal and medical professions.

### How Is Accountability Determined?

Irresponsible medical experts (so-called hired guns) can testify to anything they wish. They may be devious, partisan,

**TABLE 4–4.** American Society of Anesthesiologists' Guidelines for Expert Witness Qualifications and Testimony

The integrity of the civil litigation process in the United States depends in part on the honest, unbiased testimony of expert witnesses. Such testimony serves to clarify and explain technical concepts and to articulate professional standards of care. The American Society of Anesthesiologists supports the concept that such expert testimony by anesthesiologists should be readily available, objective, and unbiased. To limit uninformed and possibly misleading testimony, experts should be qualified for their role and should follow a clear and consistent set of ethical guidelines.

**Expert Witness Qualifications**

1. The physician (expert witness) should have a current valid and unrestricted state license to practice medicine.
2. The physician should be board certified in anesthesiology or hold an equivalent specialist qualification as recognized by the American Board of Anesthesiology.
3. The physician should be familiar with the clinical practice of anesthesiology at the time of the occurrence and should have been actively involved in clinical practice at the time of the event.

**Guidelines for Expert Testimony**

1. The physician's review of the medical facts should be thorough and impartial and should not exclude any relevant information to create a view favoring either the plaintiff or the defendant. The ultimate test for accuracy and impartiality is willingness to prepare testimony that could be presented unchanged for use by either the plaintiff or defendant.
2. The physician's testimony should reflect an evaluation of performance in light of generally accepted standards, neither condemning performance that clearly falls within generally accepted practice standards nor endorsing or condoning performance that clearly falls outside accepted medical practice.
3. The physician should make a clear distinction between medical malpractice and adverse outcomes not necessarily related to negligent practice.
4. The physician should make every effort to assess the relationship of the alleged substandard practice to the patient's outcome. Deviation from a practice standard is not always causally related to a poor outcome.
5. Fees for expert testimony should relate to the time spent and in no circumstances should be contingent on outcome of the claim.
6. The physician should be willing to submit such testimony for peer review.

Excerpted from the American Society of Anesthesiologists' Guidelines for Expert Witness Qualifications and Testimony, 1990, of the American Society of Anesthesiologists. A copy of the full text can be obtained from ASA, 520 North Northwest Highway, Park Ridge, IL 60068–2573.

and uninformed physicians who can present to a jury outrageous testimony that is completely unfounded and without merit. In our present system, they usually need not fear accountability for their testimony. Without such accountability, hired guns can provide their often ludicrous opinions for many years. The only problem they may encounter is a well-prepared attorney on the other side who is aware of this expert's prior testimony. The hired gun can then be exposed during cross-examination.

## What Are the Qualifications of an Expert Witness?

Part of the reason for this problem relates to the lack of precise qualifications that an expert witness should possess before being allowed to testify. The various state legislatures have been reluctant to define such qualifications. Consequently, individual courts have wide latitude in allowing testimony from expert witnesses. In fact, most courts permit almost any type of medical testimony to be presented, as long as it helps the jury to understand the evidence or to determine a fact in question. The response to an opposing attorney's objections is that the weight to be given to the testimony is for the jury to decide.

Without a medical expert, usually a plaintiff will not do well. Few medical malpractice cases can be successfully tried without a medical expert. Fortunately, the defense bar has started some clearinghouse organizations to gather information on these hired gun experts. This information results in a more effective cross-examination, enabling attorneys to eliminate many of these physicians who constantly testify in a manner adverse to the medical profession.

## What Is Being Done by Professional Medical Organizations?

Similar efforts are now taking place in some medical specialty organizations. The American Medical Association and numerous medical specialty organizations are in the process of creating guidelines for expert witnesses' qualifications. They are also seeking ways of providing some means of accountability for their testimony. Until this goal is accomplished, true medical experts should be objective, render honest and scientifically valid opinions, and present what the standard of care was at the time of the occurrence, not what it is today if standards have changed. They should also recognize the wide range of acceptable medical approaches when presenting their expert opinions. To do otherwise is irresponsible and is a disservice to the medical profession.

## MALPRACTICE INSURANCE

### What Types Are Available?

Space does not allow an exhaustive discussion of the many types of insurance policies available. However, two basic types of insurance can be purchased by physicians.

### Occurrence

The first type of malpractice insurance is the traditional *occurrence policy* (almost nonexistent nowadays), which insures for damage that occurs during the policy period, regardless of when the claim is made. The occurrence determines whether or not coverage is applicable.

### Claims-Made

The more common form of insurance is the *claims-made* policy. Generally speaking, this policy covers only those claims made during the policy period. Unfortunately, there are many variations of claims-made policies. Each particular policy should be carefully read before you purchase the insurance to ensure that you are receiving the coverage you desire. Some, for example, may require both the occurrence and the claim to take place during the policy period. Others may require that both the claim and report of the occurrence be made during the policy period. In other words, some claims-made policies are more limited than others in the coverage they provide.

Some companies, however, cover the insured anesthesiologist forever on any case for which an incident report was filed with the company during the policy period. In essence, this policy becomes an occurrence policy for those claims for which an incident report was filed during the policy period.

### Tail Coverage

To further protect yourself when insured with a claims-made policy, it is advisable to purchase extended reported or *tail coverage*. Then, if you have not reported a potential claim to your prior carrier to activate coverage, your tail coverage should provide coverage with your current carrier.

### Self-Insurance

*Self-insurance* is another alternative to the traditional insurance company policies. Two general forms of self-insurance are available. The first requires the individual to join a group or association of licensed individuals in the same profession, who then establish a trust fund to provide coverage. This type of insurance is strictly regulated by statutes in the states where it is allowed.

The second form is self-insurance in the literal sense, with the individual physician meeting the financial responsibility required by state statutes. In general, some type of bond is purchased from a licensed surety, or an escrow account is established with the required money. Of course, if a judgment is rendered in excess of the amount of the bond or escrow account required, the physician can be personally liable. This fact should be considered before choosing any self-insurance program. Furthermore, if involved in one of these programs, physicians obviously should take the necessary steps to try to make themselves judgment proof.

### Going Bare

Finally, physicians may elect to practice while uninsured ("going bare"). In this case, they are banking on the injured party looking to others for his or her damages. This is an extremely risky position to take because of the personal asset exposure plus the need to pay for legal defense, which can be costly.

### How Much Malpractice Insurance Should One Have?

The answer to this question varies from one locale to another.[15] For those physicians practicing in states having a state insurance fund to protect them, they need only secure the limits required by that state. Other physicians must decide on coverage with which they are comfortable. Frequently, hospital attorneys or risk managers may be in a position to suggest appropriate insurance limits based on their experience with jury verdicts in that community. We recognize that finances may dictate the amount of coverage that an individual physician can purchase. Notwithstanding that fact, limits of $1 million are almost always sufficient to resolve a case and to protect the assets of the individual physician.

Finally, protect yourself by checking the details of your insurance policy. Understand the insurance carrier's rules for obtaining coverage, such as what incidents to report, the policy period, limits of coverage, and exclusions. Should you have questions, contact your agent, and, if necessary, ask for a written explanation. Every practitioner should read and understand his or her policy.

# PART II
# THE PLAINTIFF PERSPECTIVE

James B. Matthews III

## INTRODUCTION

### Why Do Patients Consult Lawyers?

Contrary to the belief held by many physicians, most patients do not visit attorneys because of greed. Money is not the primary goal. In my experience, most prospective plaintiffs believe, for a variety of reasons, that something was done wrong. Perhaps the patient underwent a routine shoulder arthroscopy and suffered severe brain damage. The family wants an explanation for this unexpected outcome. Not satisfied with the explanation provided by the orthopedic surgeon or the anesthesiologist, the family contacts an attorney.

Another reason that medical malpractice attorneys are contacted by patients or their families following a bad outcome or complication is because a nurse or another physician has suggested that an attorney be consulted. At least half of my clients contact lawyers for this reason. Usually, a subsequent treating physician or a nurse has been critical of the medical care that was provided.

A patient also may contact a lawyer following a bad result because the physician refused to speak with the patient about the problem or acted rudely, defensively, or indifferently when discussing the outcome. People who normally look with distaste upon the legal profession feel that they have no place else to turn when they perceive that the physician is uncaring.

Medical malpractice cases usually are filed by lawyers who specialize in such cases. These lawyers are not always the first ones contacted by the patient or his or her family. Most often, the patient has contacted another lawyer, who recognizes that medical negligence cases are not within his or her area of expertise. This lawyer will then contact a lawyer who has been known to successfully handle such cases. A review of the cases in my law firm showed that 65% of our medical negligence clients were referred by other lawyers; 25% were referred by physicians.

### What Does the Plaintiff Attorney Do Next?

After being contacted about a potential case, usually the first thing that the attorney does is meet with the patient or, if the patient has died, with the family.

During this initial meeting, the experienced malpractice attorney will ask the patient what he or she thinks was done wrong. Usually, questions have been left unanswered by the treating physician or other medical personnel. The lawyer must be acutely aware that poor communication or a simple misunderstanding does not equal negligence on the part of the physician. Although the reason for seeking legal consultation may be the personality of the physician, the malpractice attorney is primarily interested in the medical care. He or she will hear the plaintiff's version of all relevant facts. At the same time, he or she will be evaluating the plaintiff's appearance, character, and credibility and will attempt to find out whether any factors attributable to the patient contributed to the bad outcome. The malpractice attorney recognizes that potential plaintiffs are sometimes eager to blame the physician but reluctant to admit that their own conduct may have played a role. For example, the patient who aspirated in the PACU may claim to have forgotten to tell the anesthesiologist that he had eaten eggs and bacon 3 hours before surgery, despite being asked.

The attorney also will be on the lookout for whiners and those who have done their own medical research and now believe they are experts on the medical care at issue. The attorney will also be careful when considering a case that has already been turned down by another attorney. Before going further, the attorney should contact the other attorney to find out the reasons for the rejection of the case.

Assuming that the prospective plaintiff's case seems to have merit, at least on the surface, the attorney will have the client sign authorizations allowing him or her to obtain the client's medical records.

Finally, the attorney must elicit information about the extent of the client's injury and its current and future implications. Unless these damages are significant, it usually will not be economically feasible for the attorney to pursue an investigation into the case. Medical malpractice attorneys are paid on a contingent fee basis, not by the hour. The attorney's fee depends upon the amount recovered in the lawsuit. The attorney who repeatedly takes cases with relatively minor injuries will quickly find that his or her medical negligence practice is not profitable.

A responsible plaintiff's lawyer (they do exist) does not want to file cases that lack merit against anyone, including physicians. Attorneys are ethically obligated to file lawsuits only if they truly believe that they can prove that the defendant's negligence led to a person's injuries. Another reason that experienced medical malpractice lawyers do not want to file nonmeritorious cases is that, given their contingent fee agreement with the client, they will not be paid unless the case is financially successful. Attorneys invest thousands of hours and hundreds of thousands of dollars to pursue malpractice cases. They do not want to make this investment and lose. The best way for the attorney to guard against such a loss is to be careful to accept only cases of true medical negligence.

## What Must the Plaintiff Prove?

The medical malpractice lawyer must always keep in mind the elements that a plaintiff must prove in order to prevail. A malpractice case is a type of civil litigation. It is not a criminal case. The physician will not be found *guilty* or *not guilty*. Unlike a criminal case, there is no requirement of proof beyond a reasonable doubt. Each of the elements of the plaintiff's case must be proved by evidence, which, if placed on a "scale of justice," would tilt the scale in favor of the plaintiff by a *preponderance of the evidence:*

1. The plaintiff must prove that the defendant physician owed a duty to the plaintiff. In cases in which the physician is a treating physician (eg, the anesthesiologist in charge), this duty arises out of the physician-patient relationship.
2. The plaintiff must prove that the physician was negligent. As was mentioned earlier, in medical malpractice cases, negligence is defined as conduct that falls below the standard of care as practiced by physicians generally under the same or similar circumstances. To establish the standards of care, the plaintiff's attorney will need to retain so-called expert witnesses.
3. Finally, the plaintiff must prove that the physician's violation of the standard of care caused the injury that was sustained. Lawyers refer to this element as *proof of causation.* This proof must be made by what is known as a *reasonable degree of medical certainty* or a *reasonable degree of medical probability.* In most jurisdictions, these terms mean that it is more likely than not that the plaintiff's injury resulted from the alleged negligence of the physician.

## What Documents Should Be Obtained?

If the plaintiff's attorney chooses to proceed with the investigation of a potential medical malpractice case, it is essential that he or she obtain all medical records and medical bills. Other documents will be relevant at a later time, but they cannot always be obtained during this investigatory stage before the lawsuit is filed. These documents include pharmacy logs, hospital policies and procedures, and contracts between the hospital and the anesthesia group.

The medical chart is usually the single most important part of a medical negligence case. An inaccurate or incomplete medical chart can make or break the plaintiff's case. When the rationale for a medical decision is absent from the chart or when the chart is silent regarding crucial acts, the plaintiff's case is strengthened. Communication is important in the practice of medicine, and much of the communication between medical providers is done in a patient's chart. If the chart is illegible or incomplete, the jury is more likely to believe that the medical care was also sloppy.

*The chart should never be altered.* This dictum, which was emphasized earlier, cannot be stated too strongly. Most states

have laws making the alteration of medical records a crime. Cases of doubtful liability have been won by plaintiffs who discovered an alteration in the medical records. If a physician or other health care provider alters the medical records and is caught, he or she will lose the case. *The physician should never believe that he or she will not be caught.* Experienced malpractice attorneys always ask to see the *original* hospital chart. They are adept at finding areas in which alterations might occur. If chart alteration is discovered, it will become the focus of the plaintiff's case at trial. The physician will lose the most important trial battle—credibility.

The plaintiff's attorney will compare the medical record with the medical bill. The chart may show that a particular drug was not given. If the medical bill shows a charge for this drug, the accuracy of the chart is called into question.

## Medical Research

The experienced medical malpractice plaintiff attorney will not simply interview the client, gather and review medical records, and then decide whether to accept the case. He or she must first know or teach himself or herself about the pertinent area of medicine. There should be an exhaustive literature search that covers medical textbooks and journals. After this process of self-education is complete, the attorney should, once again, review the medical records, using this new information to re-evaluate the case. Having a working knowledge of the medical aspects of the case will also make it much easier to converse with potential expert witnesses.

Some attorneys employ nurses or physicians as part of their staff whose job is to review the records, identify issues, and locate relevant medical literature. Other attorneys will ask a physician who is a friend or acquaintance to review the records. This physician may or may not be a specialist in the specific area of medicine that is involved in the case. Usually, however, this physician can identify the issues and let the attorney know when a case is obviously without merit.

## Consulting Experts

After interviewing the plaintiff, receiving and reviewing the medical records, gaining a basic understanding of the subject matter of the case from the medical literature, and then re-evaluating the case, the attorney's next step is to have the records reviewed by physicians who are willing and able to objectively evaluate the medical care and treatment received by the patient.

Even after determining that the patient's claim seems to have merit, a good medical malpractice attorney still will not file a lawsuit until he or she has retained a qualified and well-respected physician in the particular specialty involved to give yet another evaluation of the case. So-called hired guns or prostitutes who make a living giving questionable testimony against physicians should never be used. When an attorney is having a case reviewed by a physician, he or she is relying heavily on the physician's opinion. When a hired gun manipulates the standard of care and causes an unknowing plaintiff's attorney to incorrectly believe that he or she has a meritorious claim, a great disservice is done, not only to the medical profession but also to the legal system.

Most experienced malpractice attorneys do not use this type of expert. It is really not that difficult to find qualified, reputable physician-experts who will objectively review cases and give unbiased opinions. My practice starts by contacting physicians who are obviously at the top of their specialty. Their names can be found in the medical literature and by speaking with other physicians. When we contact these true experts, we ask if they will agree to review a case objectively without knowing whether the attorney who is requesting the review represents the patient or the defendant physician. Some are too busy. Others simply do not want to be involved in a medicolegal matter. Most, however, welcome this opportunity for peer review.

This true expert may not agree to testify for the plaintiff despite his or her belief that medical negligence did occur. Even if the expert does not agree to testify, he or she can be a valuable consultant to the plaintiff's attorney. Most importantly, armed with an objective opinion by an unbiased expert, the plaintiff attorney can justify the time and expense involved in the pursuit of a medical negligence case.

## AFTER THE LAWSUIT IS FILED

I have had several cases in which a physician, having been served with the lawsuit, contacts the patient or the patient's family in an attempt to clear up the misunderstanding. The misunderstanding never has been cleared up, and the plaintiff's case usually has been enhanced as a result of this conversation.

I have also had cases in which the physician contacted me. In these instances, the physician feels that it is necessary to explain actions or omissions. These phone calls always have worked to the physician's detriment.

## THE DEFENSE LAWYER

Most physicians have liability insurance. As a consequence, the insurance company will refer the case to a lawyer who specializes in the defense of medical malpractice cases. Often, much of the work on the case is then delegated to a less experienced associate. This situation can be confusing for the physician, who did not choose the lawyer. The goal of the insurer is not necessarily the goal of the physician. The insurer wants to save money. The physician may want to preserve his or her reputation by quietly settling or by insisting on a trial. The physician's insurance company may not really care about the physician's state of mind or his or her desire to end the case against him or her. This can be true, even if the insurance company is owned by physicians or a medical association and writes medical malpractice insurance only.

Medical malpractice defense lawyers and physicians are busy people. I can usually tell when busy schedules have interfered with the preparation of the physician's case. Usually, it is the physician who has failed to properly prepare with the defense counsel. The physician should not simply "let the lawyer handle it." He or she must be involved in the case, however distasteful it is. The physician should attempt to educate his or her attorney about the relevant medical issues and supply him or her with pertinent medical literature. The physician should be blunt and honest and should not tell the lawyer what he or she thinks the lawyer wants to hear; he or she should tell the truth, regardless of its impact on the case. Occasionally, a defense attorney will encourage the

physician to embellish or stretch the truth. The physician should resist this temptation. If caught by a skilled plaintiff attorney, the physician's credibility will be undermined, and the effect can be devastating at trial.

## THE PHYSICIAN'S DEPOSITION

The deposition of the defendant physician is usually the most important part of the discovery in the medical malpractice case. It is the plaintiff attorney's opportunity to see what kind of witness the defendant will make at trial. The skilled plaintiff attorney will be looking for an emotional element that can increase the chances of success in the case and enhance its value. The most compelling factor that the plaintiff's attorney is looking for is one that can destroy the physician's defense. This factor is indifference on the part of the defendant physician. The plaintiff's attorney knows that, at trial, if the jury perceives that the physician does not care, the plaintiff will win the case.

The physician's attitude may be reflected in the way that he or she dresses. He or she should be well dressed and should appear professional and conservative. I was involved in one case in which the defendant anesthesiologist arrived at his deposition dressed in blue jeans and a Hell's Angels T-shirt. On one hand, my client, the husband of the deceased patient, was boiling mad but managed to retain his composure. On the other hand, I was delighted with the physician's appearance and with his cavalier attitude during the deposition.

Certain emotions do not go over well in litigation. The defendant physician who becomes agitated, argumentative, indifferent, or defensive during deposition will damage his or her case. Probably the biggest mistake that I see physicians make during medical malpractice litigation is their failure to thoroughly prepare for their deposition. This can be the fault of the defense lawyer as much as the physician.

Physicians also make a big mistake during their deposition when they fail to admit the obvious. For example, during the deposition of a defendant anesthesiologist, the physician testified under oath that he never used a peripheral nerve stimulator during or after arthroscopic shoulder surgery, that he did not know anyone else who did so, and that it was not required by written hospital policy. The physician apparently forgot that he had done a shoulder arthroscopy case involving the same patient 12 months earlier in which he had used a peripheral nerve stimulator. In addition, his nurse anesthetist testified that the physician always used a peripheral nerve stimulator during arthroscopic shoulder surgery. Later in the case, the physician's partners all testified that they used a nerve stimulator during arthroscopic shoulder surgery. To top it off, the hospital's written policy stated that a peripheral nerve stimulator should *always* be used during arthroscopic shoulder surgery, and the policy had been authored 4 years earlier by the defendant physician when he was the chair of the hospital's department of anesthesiology. In reality, failure to use the nerve stimulator probably had little to do with the lawsuit. However, once the physician would not admit an obvious, albeit relatively minor mistake, the nerve stimulator (and the physician's credibility) became a key part of the case.

Another mistake that I see in depositions is made by physicians who sometimes insist on relying on their memory without referring to the medical records. If the physician's memory of something that occurred 4 years earlier differs from the written record, a skilled plaintiff's attorney will seize the discrepancy in an attempt to discredit the physician's credibility.

## CONCLUSION

In the final analysis, a medical malpractice attorney should not file a lawsuit unless he or she is convinced that a strong case of substandard medical care can be made and that the substandard care directly caused the patient's injury or death. Other factors, such as the personalities and attitudes of the parties, have some bearing on the ongoing evaluation of a medical negligence case. The focus, however, should be the medical care.

## References

1. Brunner EA. Analysis of anesthetic mishaps. The National Association of Insurance Commissioners' closed claim study. *Int Anesthesiol Clin.* 1984;22:17.
2. Standards for basic anesthetic monitoring. In: American Society of Anesthesiologists. *Directory of Members.* Chicago, Ill: American Society of Anesthesiologists; 2001:493.
3. Eichhorn JH. Prevention of intraoperative anesthesia accidents and related injury through safety monitoring. *Anesthesiology.* 1989;70:572.
4. Orkin FK. Practice standards. The Midas touch or the emperor's new clothes? *Anesthesiology.* 1989;70:567.
5. Caplan RA, Posner KL, Ward RJ, et al. Adverse respiratory events in anesthesia: a closed claims analysis. *Anesthesiology.* 1990;72:828.
6. Caplan RA. The closed claims project: looking back, looking forward. *ASA Newslett.* 1999;63:7.
7. Tonn and Associates. *Medical and Hospital Professional Liability: A Report Prepared for the Texas Health Policy Task Force.* July 1992.
8. Rerschauer R. *Congressional Budget Office Testimony, Ways and Means.* Washington, DC: US House of Representatives; March 4, 1992.
9. Taylor G, Larson CP Jr, Prestwich R. Unexpected cardiac arrest during anesthesia and surgery. An environmental study. *JAMA.* 1976;236:2758.
10. Cheney FW, Posner KL, Caplan RA. Adverse respiratory events infrequently leading to malpractice suits. A closed claims analysis. *Anesthesiology.* 1991;75:932.
11. Sulek C, Kirby RR. The recurring problem of negative-pressure pulmonary edema. *Curr Rev Clin Anesth.* 1998;18:241.
12. Cheney F. [Letter to the editor]. *ASA Newslett.* 1990;54:4.
13. Spooner RB, Kirby RR. Equipment-related anesthetic incidents. *Int Anesthesiol Clin.* 1984;22:133.
14. Cooper JB, Cullen DJ, Eichhorn JH, et al. Administrative guidelines for response to an adverse anesthesia event. The Risk Management Committee of the Harvard Medical School Department of Anaesthesia. *J Clin Anesth.* 1993;5:79.
15. Cheney FW. How much professional liability coverage is enough? Lessons from the ASA closed claims project. *ASA Newslett.* 1999;63:19.

# 5

# Risk and Outcome Analysis: Myths and Truths

## David L. Brown

Since the introduction of effective inhalational anesthetics in the mid-1800s, the term *anesthetic risk* has often been used interchangeably with *anesthetic mortality*. Perhaps this fundamental confusion in conceptualizing anesthetic risks has to do with a somewhat unique aspect of anesthesia. Intraoperative anesthesia care, except in rare circumstances, is not therapeutic. The best we can hope for as anesthesiologists is that patients emerge from the anesthetic in no worse physiologic state than when anesthesia was induced.

The problem has become accentuated since the 1950s with the ever-increasing narrow focus on specialization and subspecialization in medical practice. This factor allows patients to receive care predicated on the latest advances in a specialty; however, it often prevents a single physician from being in a position to weigh comprehensively all risk and benefit decisions. Because it is easier to understand *perioperative death* than the more elusive anesthetic risk, many take the less rigorous approach and accept death due to anesthesia as the essence of anesthetic risk.

## RISK STRATIFICATION

### What Is the Risk of Anesthetic Mortality?

It has been suggested that the overall risk of anesthetic-related mortality is about 1 death per 10 000 anesthetic procedures. Nevertheless, this easy-to-conceptualize incidence blurs many subtleties. For instance, the collaborative confidential inquiry into perioperative death (CEPOD) conducted in England in the mid-1980s showed that unequivocal anesthetic mortality occurred at a rate of 1 in about 185 000 anesthetics.[1] Natof, in a survey of ambulatory surgical centers spanning 1975 to 1980, reported a rate of anesthetic mortality of 1 in about 450 000 anesthetics.[2] Eichhorn and colleagues evaluated anesthetic-related deaths and severe central nervous system injury in patients classified as American Society of Anesthesiologists (ASA) physical status I and II in the Harvard-affiliated hospitals during the years 1976 to 1988. They found a rate of anesthetic death or significant central nervous system injury of 1 per 112 000 anesthetics.[3]

## What Do These Data Mean?

For ASA *status I or II,* patients undergoing non–life-threatening surgery, it is likely that the incidence of anesthetic mortality is on the favorable side of 1 per 100 000 anesthetics. In higher-risk patients, those with more physiologic dysfunction or those undergoing life-threatening procedures, the anesthetic-related mortality rate is likely higher. The difficulty in these more critically ill patients is that the specific cause of death is often blurred between a patient's disease, the surgical procedure, and the anesthetic care. Because anesthetic mortality in healthy patients occurs so infrequently, it is important to begin to understand and define the more frequently occurring nonmortal anesthetic complications.

## How Should We Define and Assess Anesthetic Complications?

One of the difficulties in understanding anesthetic complications is the confusion that exists between complications and physiologic side effects related to anesthetics. The most evident example of this confusion has to do with blood pressure decreases related to anesthetic drugs. The literature is replete with references to hypotension as a complication of various anesthetic techniques; nevertheless, many of these are likely simply physiologic responses to vasodilation accompanying both general and regional anesthetics.

This imprecision in language should be a principal focus of ongoing anesthesia outcome analyses. I believe the term *complication* should be reserved for those situations in which a morbidity measure reaches a predetermined threshold of severity. This approach certainly makes outcome analyses more complex; however, over time, it also increases the precision of our language and deepens our understanding of anesthetic complications.

## OUTCOME MEASUREMENT

## Are Morbidity and Mortality Suitable Indicators?

Morbidity and mortality are certainly the most useful measures of anesthetic outcome. The difficulty arises in agreeing on their definitions. For example, should a death occurring 7 days after operation be considered an anesthetic mortality, but one occurring 8 days after an anesthetic be excluded? This question has practical implications because critical care medicine increasingly prolongs the lives of the most at-risk and critically ill patients.

## How Should Mortality Be Defined?

Mortality is a suitable measure of outcome, and the focus of our research should be to agree on suitable time-linked mortality measures. Moving the time limit for mortality toward operation improves its specificity but clearly decreases its sensitivity.

## How Is Morbidity Defined?

The question of morbidity as an appropriate measure of outcome is even more complex because most morbid events do not have a uniformly agreed-upon definition (as does mortality). It is in this area of anesthetic outcome analysis that imprecision in language most often confuses morbidity and side effects.

To measure anesthetic morbidity accurately, the morbid event should require either additional therapy, prolongation of the patient's hospitalization, or a patient's dissatisfaction. If 1 of these 3 requirements is fulfilled before determining that morbidity occurred, practical precision in our outcome language will be increased.

Despite this belief, circumstances exist in which intermediate variables, such as myocardial ischemia, may be practical measures of anesthetic outcome. Slogoff and Keats showed that an intermediate variable (myocardial ischemia) is linked to the development of perioperative myocardial infarctions (MIs).[4] Other intermediate variables, such as patient temperature, can be linked to adverse outcomes and may be appropriately included in outcome analysis after that link is established.[5]

## When and by Whom Should Anesthetic Outcome Be Measured?

The measurement of anesthetic outcome is inevitably time linked. The length of outcome observation is necessarily shorter for outpatients than for critically ill inpatients. Once again, the length of time needs to be determined by multiple factors, including the magnitude and urgency of the operation, the patient's age, ASA physical status assessment, and others appropriate for given surgical and anesthetic techniques.

## Is Peer Assessment Appropriate?

Another aspect of outcome measurement that needs to be considered when undertaking outcome studies is the reliability of peer assessments of anesthetic outcome. Goldman showed that in peer assessment, physicians' agreement regarding the quality of care is only slightly better than the level expected by chance.[6] Likewise, Caplan and colleagues have shown that knowledge of the severity of outcome of an injury related to anesthetic care influences a reviewer's judgment of the appropriateness of that care.[7] These studies highlight that retrospective outcome analyses can be significantly influenced by reviewer bias, and they suggest that reviewers of medicolegal situations are likely influenced by the severity of outcome when determining the appropriateness of care.

## Can the Process Be Improved?

An extension of this observation is that to accumulate data in an objective fashion, the data collection should be "unhooked" from individuals providing clinical anesthetic care. Cohen and associates took this approach in their study of anesthetic outcome in Winnipeg.[8] Their study design template is likely an effective method of data collection; however, it is more expensive for an independent observer to categorize morbidity and mortality in anesthetic practice than is self-reporting by practitioners.

## What Is the Role of Patient Satisfaction?

Another aspect of outcome analysis receiving increasing attention is the linking of patient satisfaction with anesthetic care and outcome measurements. In this age of consumerism, not surprisingly, quality anesthetic practice may be tied to patients' satisfaction with the care provided. Today, there are few data to substantiate this concept as a valid measure of anesthetic outcome or quality anesthetic practice, but it will likely and appropriately be studied as a measure of outcome in the near future.

## How Is the Statistical Problem of Rare Events Addressed?

Anesthetic care has become increasingly safe through the years, a positive development. When events occur infrequently, however, statistical analysis is problematic.

### Pitfalls

Statistical analysis is the means by which the effects of random variation are estimated. When we use inferential statistics to formulate conclusions about a larger group from a selected number of individuals (a sample), we take risks. As an example, during a multiinstitutional English report involving 108 878 patients and 2391 deaths, the author stated:

*Although we examined more than 100,000 operations, the numbers were still too small to allow analysis of the risk of the preoperative conditions for specific operations or even separately for males and females.*[9]

### Data Dredging

As computerization of clinical databases has become commonplace, one of the statistical problems in outcome studies is the use of multiple comparisons. As investigators attempt to generate hypotheses from many of these databases, the problem of data dredging can occur. That is, any time they compare 20 outcome measures from the database, one of the observations of $P < .05$ is likely to be erroneous because the commonly accepted statistical handling of a type I error sets the alpha at 1 per 20 observations (or 0.05).

To highlight the issues involved in studying rare events, consider that in the 1970s, the estimated cost to study general anesthetic agents and outcome in a multiinstitutional prospective evaluation of 17 000 patients was >$1 million.[9]

### Default Mode of Anesthetic Prescription

The final difficulty in understanding anesthetic risk and outcome is the implicit bias that technique comparisons use a general anesthetic as the benchmark of measure. Most anesthesiologists' default mode of anesthetic prescription is general anesthesia.

As previously outlined, when morbid or mortal events occur infrequently, it is difficult and expensive to document an improvement in outcome related to anesthetic technique, especially in this era of relative anesthetic safety. We should be willing to state, in order to be scientifically honest, that in particular patient situations, neither general nor regional anesthesia has been shown to be safer (J.B. Forrest, personal communication, 1986). Detailed risk-benefit analysis demands that we be honest in this regard, both for our patients and for our legal colleagues, who frequently become involved in patient care after adverse outcomes.

## PREOPERATIVE RISK ASSESSMENT

Because anesthetic care is not therapeutic, the focus of most of our preoperative risk management efforts has been to ensure that patients are physiologically optimized when they arrive in the operating room.

## Which Perioperative Risk Factors Are Not Modifiable?

Anesthesiologists know that perioperative risk variables fall into two broad classes. Some, such as a patient's age, intended operation, urgency of operation, personnel experience, and the institution in which the procedure is to be performed, are impossible (or nearly so) to change preoperatively. Conversely, a number of patient variables (organ system physiologic function) may be amenable to optimization before operation. These issues are next addressed sequentially.

## What Is the Impact of Advanced Age?

The most striking example in this category is a patient's age. Most clinicians assume that as patients age, perioperative and mortality risks increase. Many investigations suggest, however, that age is primarily a marker of an increasing number of concurrent diseases or physiologic derangements.[10] The CEPOD study showed that about 80% of perioperative deaths occurred in patients >65 years of age.

An additional relationship of age to perioperative risks is the life expectancy remaining for elderly patients undergoing operation. Decisions to operate or not to operate are often affected by a misunderstanding of the extent of life remaining for 85- to 90-year-old patients[11] (Table 5-1). Many more years are predicted actuarially for elderly patients than physicians weighing risk-benefit decisions realize.

## What Are the Effects of the Personnel and Institution?

Other nonmodifiable risk factors are the personnel and institution involved. Slogoff and Keats showed that the incidence of myocardial ischemia accompanying coronary artery bypass grafting procedures may vary depending on the indi-

**TABLE 5–1.** Geriatric Life Expectancy

| Current Age (y) | Estimated Years of Life Remaining | |
| --- | --- | --- |
| | *Men* | *Women* |
| 65 | 14 | 18 |
| 67 | 12 | 16 |
| 70 | 11 | 14 |
| 75 | 9 | 11 |
| 80 | 7 | 9 |
| 85 | 5 | 7 |

Modified from Eiseman B. *What Are My Chances?* Philadelphia, Pa: WB Saunders; 1980:15.

vidual delivering the anesthetic.[4] This concept has been strengthened by data from Merry and colleagues, who also showed that specific anesthesiologists affect perioperative outcome.[12] Although the concept is speculative, specific surgical colleagues probably can also be linked to changes in perioperative outcome.

After a decision has been made to operate, the institution in which the operation is to be performed most often is not alterable. For specific operations, a frequency-dependent minimum exists, below which perioperative outcomes are less desirable.[13] Additionally, for what are thought to be similar types of institutions, such as academic centers performing coronary artery bypass grafting procedures, even in age- and disease-matched patients, a 21-fold variation in perioperative mortality can result.[14]

## When Is the Type of Surgery a Factor?

Other factors that affect perioperative risk relate to the surgical procedure itself. Superficial operations, such as repair of fractures of the extremities, are associated with a lower risk for adverse outcomes than are intrathoracic, major intraabdominal, or intracranial procedures.[15,16]

An additional feature having a major influence over adverse perioperative outcome is the elective or emergent nature of the operation. Although elective and emergent procedures may never be the same for a similar operation, emergent conditions increase the risk for adverse outcome by a factor of 3-fold to 6-fold.[17–19]

## FUNCTIONAL PHYSIOLOGIC RISK FACTORS

### Which Cardiovascular Functions Are Important?

#### Hypertension

Treatment of even mild hypertension prolongs life.[20] Between 10% and 50% of an anesthesiologist's patients, depending on the type of practice, may have hypertension. Thus, this risk factor must be analyzed. Some studies suggest that mild to moderate hypertension is not associated with adverse perioperative outcome.

Improved vasoactive drugs have led some investigators to believe that uncontrolled hypertension should not postpone a scheduled surgical procedure.[21] This study of about 1000 patients with hypertension must be placed in perspective. The patients all received a general anesthetic. Whether their data can be applied to patients receiving regional anesthesia must remain speculative. Additionally, only a limited number of patients with severe hypertension were included in the investigation, making a type II (false negative) statistical error possible.

#### Coronary Artery Disease

Patients with coronary artery disease are widely variable, ranging from those experiencing only angina to others with documented MI. Prior MI has a time-linked relationship to adverse perioperative myocardial events. The link of angina to adverse outcomes is less clear.[22]

Anesthesiologists have interpreted Rao and colleagues' data to suggest that the well-established truism that surgical procedures should be postponed for 6 months after an MI when possible may no longer be valid.[23] Nevertheless, a preponderance of evidence, even in Rao's study, shows that performing a surgical procedure within 6 months of prior MI significantly increases the perioperative risk for subsequent myocardial events.[22]

Why recent MI markedly increases surgical risk is not clear, nor is the reason that an interval of 6 months affords risk reduction. One may speculate that this interval is necessary for healing or for scarring of the myocardium to mature. Likewise, this time may be necessary for the development of sufficient collateral circulation to protect areas of myocardium at risk in the perimeter around prior infarcts.

#### Congestive Heart Failure

Congestive heart failure (CHF) is associated with significant morbidity and mortality in the perioperative period. In Goldman's study, patients who were >40 years of age and who developed CHF had a 57% incidence of perioperative mortality.[24] The best preoperative predictors of postoperative heart failure are jugular venous distention and third heart sounds or a prior history of CHF.[25] Important valvular heart disease, particularly aortic stenosis, has also been reported to cause new or worsening heart failure in 20% of those so affected.[23]

Complicating analyses of the impact of CHF on adverse perioperative outcomes are the different and often clinically imprecise criteria used to diagnose the condition. Postoperative myocardial reinfarction occurs at a higher rate in patients with preoperative CHF.[25] Mangano and colleagues found that a history of CHF was a univariant predictor of adverse postoperative cardiac outcome.[26]

### Is an Admission Electrocardiogram Useful?

An admission electrocardiogram (ECG) is usually obtained for patients older than some predetermined age, which varies by institution. The usefulness of this practice continues to be debated. Moorman and colleagues[27] evaluated ECGs in 1410 general medical patients and found that the admission ECG provided new information in only 1% of patients with no cardiac problems suggested by history or physical examination. In patients suspected of having cardiac problems, admission ECGs provided additional information in 6.9% of cases.[27]

## Indications

Some have suggested that Moorman's findings indicate that a preoperative ECG is unnecessary in patients with no evidence of cardiac disease. In this study, however, 75% of the 1410 admission ECGs were abnormal. Because these patients were scheduled for surgery, it remains speculative whether obtaining a preoperative ECG would allow alteration of anesthetic management to lower the risk for adverse cardiac outcomes.

Despite the scarcity of outcome data, a preoperative ECG to evaluate cardiovascular risk factors probably is reasonable in men aged 40 years or older; in patients with hypertension, peripheral vascular disease, or diabetes; in patients at risk for electrolyte abnormalities; in patients undergoing intrathoracic, intraperitoneal, aortic, major neurologic, or emergency surgery; and in patients with a history of physical findings suggestive of heart disease, including arrhythmias.

## Other Tests

Technologic advances in noninvasive cardiac function assessment provide a number of options in preoperative cardiac assessment. The difficulties anesthesiologists experience in understanding the optimal use of these tests include the fact that traditional lower-cost tests are not discarded as new (and expensive) noninvasive tests become practical. The most important risk management decision for anesthesiologists, I believe, is to voice concerns to our cardiologist colleagues. By the time an individual patient is evaluated, a multitude of tests have often already been performed. A practical discussion may better focus the preoperative evaluation.

### Echocardiography

Patients often undergo an echocardiographic study before their surgical procedure; this study is an excellent means to assess valvular and overall ventricular functions. A significantly decreased ejection fraction, in the 25% to 35% range, likely identifies a high-risk group.[28] Remember, however, that preoperative ejection fraction measurements assess only function. A normal ejection fraction does not exclude the presence of significant coronary artery disease.[29]

### Radionuclide Studies

A patient who has a history suggestive of myocardial ischemia and who has not undergone a thallium radionuclide–type study is unusual today. Thallium acts like potassium and follows myocardial perfusion. In a normal patient, an image of homogeneous myocardial perfusion results. A scar in the myocardium, similar to that found after an MI, is identified as a cold spot.

To understand the use of thallium imaging, one must be familiar with stress thallium scans. Exercise or dipyridamole is used to produce coronary vasodilation during a thallium scan. An immediate image is obtained, followed by another after a 2- to 3-hour delay. If homogeneous perfusion is shown on the initial and delayed scans, the study is interpreted as normal. If a defect is noted on the initial scan and is not observed on the delayed scan, a diagnosis of viable myocardium at risk is made. If the initial scan shows a defect that persists to the delayed scan, a fixed defect, such as MI, is diagnosed.

Boucher and colleagues in 1985 published a widely discussed study suggesting that preoperative dipyridamole-thallium imaging could predict adverse cardiac outcomes in patients undergoing peripheral vascular surgery.[30] Several permutations of this work have been developed since that time. Overall thallium redistribution does indicate a high incidence of adverse cardiac outcomes; however, a normal dipyridamole-thallium scan does not ensure an uneventful postoperative course.[31]

### Exercise Studies

Further confounding the appropriate use of nuclear medicine studies are reports by Gerson and coworkers[32,33] in which bicycle exercise testing was a better predictor of perioperative pulmonary, cardiac, and combined cardiopulmonary complications than were nuclear medicine studies. An inability to perform 2 minutes of supine bicycle exercise sufficient to raise the heart rate above 99 beats per minute was the best predictor of adverse cardiac events in patients undergoing elective noncardiac surgery. Elderly patients who were able to perform this bicycle exercise had a 5-fold to 6-fold reduction in major perioperative pulmonary, cardiac, and combined cardiopulmonary complications.

## How Important Are Pulmonary Risk Factors?

The ASA closed-claims project showed that at least one third of all claims against anesthesiologists are related to respiratory events.[34] European data also suggest that most adverse outcomes are related to cardiopulmonary complications after operation.[15] The difficulty for a clinical anesthesiologist is highlighted by the data presented by Caplan and colleagues showing that even patients with normal lung function may experience postoperative pulmonary complications.[34]

In patients with abnormal pulmonary function, no single test accurately predicts postoperative complications.

### Operative Site

The incidence of postoperative pulmonary complications increases if the operative site involves the upper abdomen and diaphragm.[35] Provision of adequate analgesia is one means of limiting the adverse effects of such operations. Despite using adequate analgesia, however, Ford and associates showed that after these procedures, a shift from abdominal to rib cage breathing still occurs.[36] These data suggest that either direct diaphragmatic irritation or initiation of a neural reflex becomes established and inhibits diaphragmatic function.

### Chronic Obstructive Lung Disease

Another well-established perioperative risk factor for pulmonary complications is chronic obstructive lung disease. Because postoperative pulmonary changes are primarily restrictive in character, a patient with underlying chronic obstructive lung disease may be especially compromised. A number of studies indicated that a combination of pulmonary function tests, such as forced vital capacity, forced expiratory volume in one second ($FEV_1$), and maximal voluntary ventilation, are the best predictors of postoperative respiratory dysfunction.[37–40]

A discussion with our pulmonary colleagues about the ideal method of evaluating patients with significantly compromised pulmonary function should occur in advance of the need for such evaluations. Despite increased risk, patients with an $FEV_1$ as low as 0.45 L may survive the perioperative period.[40]

## Asthma

Asthmatic patients, or those with reversible airflow obstruction, also are at increased perioperative risk. Common dictum suggests that avoidance of a general anesthetic and tracheal tube minimizes asthmatic exacerbations.[41] Shnider and Papper studied 687 asthmatic patients in a group of >55 000 patients (1.2% prevalence of asthma) requiring anesthesia.[42] In those asthmatic patients whose wheezing was quiescent preoperatively, 6.5% wheezed intraoperatively (40% on induction and 60% during anesthetic maintenance). Increasing age increased the incidence of exacerbation. Contrary to traditional teaching, patients undergoing regional anesthesia had the same incidence of intraoperative wheezing as nonintubated patients receiving general anesthesia.

Gold and Helrich reviewed the perioperative course of about 200 asthmatic patients and documented that the site of surgical procedure is an important predictor in the asthma exacerbation equation.[43] They found that the highest incidence of pulmonary complications occurred during upper abdominal procedures.

To minimize risks, anesthesiologists should ensure that asthmatic patients are in their optimal condition, and an anesthetic approach tailored for the specific patient should be developed. Postoperative analgesia requirements should be considered before formulating an intraoperative anesthetic plan.

## Routine Chest Radiographs

The question of obtaining a routine chest radiograph before surgical procedures has been better defined over time. Roizen suggested that the risks of chest radiography probably exceed its benefits if a patient does not have symptoms and is <60 years of age.[44] He emphasized that this assumption is predicated on maximizing the benefit to society in general rather than to individual patients.

## *What Is the Impact of Neurologic Dysfunction?*

Preoperative neurologic dysfunction often influences anesthetic selection. Little information suggests, however, that well-conducted general or regional anesthesia significantly alters the incidence of adverse neurologic outcome. Preoperative concern about patients with cerebrovascular disease has been prevalent for years. I believe that the primary benefit of identifying cerebrovascular disease preoperatively is that it highlights a patient's risk for adverse cardiovascular outcome, such as MI.[45]

## Blood Pressure Control

A generally accepted dictum is that blood pressure in patients with cerebrovascular disease needs to be maintained at a higher level perioperatively than in patients without a history of cerebrovascular disease. Data gathered from patients who were resuscitated after cardiac arrest and who died from 1 day to several weeks later suggest, however, that the risk for precipitating brain infarcts by lowering blood pressure is not much greater in atherosclerotic than in nonatherosclerotic patients.[46]

## Carotid Bruits

Between 4% and 5% of patients >45 years of age have asymptomatic carotid bruits.[47] When patients who are >55 years of age and who are undergoing elective surgery are considered, the incidence increases to 14%.[48] The presence of a carotid bruit suggests that a patient has a higher risk for atherosclerosis involving other blood vessels. MI occurs 2.5 times more commonly in patients with asymptomatic bruits than in age-matched controls.[47]

## Progressive Neurologic Disease

Neurologic dysfunction often affects anesthetic prescription for patients with progressive neurologic diseases. In many cases, anesthesiologists alter their usual prescription of a regional anesthetic in favor of a general anesthetic for fear that the regional technique might be implicated in further deterioration of neurologic function. No data show that a well-conducted regional anesthetic places patients with conditions such as diabetes mellitus or other peripheral neuropathies at higher risk than a well-conducted general anesthetic. Nevertheless, a thorough discussion with a patient is indicated before the surgical procedure if one believes a regional anesthetic has advantages.

# ANESTHETIC PRESCRIPTION

## *What Is the Proper Role of Monitoring?*

One of the first decisions required when considering anesthetic prescription is what monitoring devices to use. Risk management in this area has been affected by the ASA's basic intraoperative monitoring standards, the latest revision of which became effective in January 1999 (see Appendix, Chapter 18).

Since anesthesiologists began monitoring patients with a finger on the pulse many years ago, new monitoring devices have been resisted by many. One early report suggesting that ECG was useful as an intraoperative monitor documented an 80% incidence of arrhythmias during surgical procedures.[49] A reviewer questioned whether this high incidence was clinically significant and whether the advances in operating room monitoring were justified. He stated, "It seems to me that the question is not whether irregularities occur or what causes them particularly, but whether the patient gets through the operation."[49]

This same tone has been taken by many anesthesiologists as additions have been made to what is considered basic intraoperative monitoring (Table 5–2).

## *Does Monitoring Reduce Anesthetic Risk?*

One of the difficulties in assessing whether added monitoring decreases the risks of operation is that most devices have

**TABLE 5–2.** Basic Intraoperative Monitors, Circa 1994

| | |
|---|---|
| Automated blood pressure | Precordial and esophageal stethoscope |
| Electrocardiograph | Circuit oxygen analyzer |
| Pulse oximeter | Airway pressure (high or low) |
| Capnometer | Temperature probe |

been included in the monitoring schema before randomized studies documenting their usefulness. One of the most discussed recent additions is pulse oximetry as a continuous monitor during administration of all anesthetics. No randomized prospective study documents its value, and in fact, one large prospective study of 20 802 patients could not show that pulse oximetry affected early postanesthesia outcome.[50] Eichhorn, however, presented retrospective data suggesting a lowered incidence of perioperative complications since its introduction.[3]

The ASA closed-claims database has been analyzed to determine whether negative outcomes could have been prevented by the proper use of additional monitoring devices. More than 1000 cases were reviewed, and >30% of the negative outcomes were believed to have been preventable by the application of additional monitors, chiefly pulse oximetry plus capnometry.[51] When Caplan and colleagues looked at the ASA closed-claims database and assessed adverse outcomes related to respiratory events, they stated that 72% of the adverse outcomes could have been prevented by better monitoring.[34]

## Does Monitoring Introduce Additional Problems?

A report by Kestin and colleagues highlighted one of the increasing difficulties of intraoperative monitoring.[52] In a pediatric population, they assessed the significance of auditory alarms that sounded during routine anesthetics. Seventy-five percent of all auditory alarms did not originate from changes in the physiologic variables for which the monitor was designed, and only 3% presented any patient risk.[52] Although many industrial suppliers are addressing this issue, nonintegrated and nonhierarchic alarms remain one of the unsolved problems of risk management in patient monitoring.

## When Is Patient Risk Increased?

When anesthesiologists become concerned about higher levels of risk in surgical patients, they often escalate the monitoring schema to include invasive hemodynamic devices. Many believe this continuous assessment of arterial or pulmonary arterial blood pressure creates a margin of safety. Some operations, such as cardiac surgery, carotid endarterectomy, and aortic aneurysm repair, would be *difficult* to conduct without continuous invasive monitors. Nevertheless, few data suggest that invasive hemodynamic monitors have *lowered* perioperative risks.

Additional advantages of direct over noninvasive blood pressure monitoring include reduced intraoperative workload, immediate detection of the hemodynamic effects of cardiac arrhythmias or surgical manipulation of vascular structures, and better assessment of lower blood pressures.[53]

## Direct Arterial Pressure Monitoring

In any risk-benefit analysis, the benefits of a technique (monitor) must be weighed against the risks of the device itself. One of the factors encouraging widespread use of direct systemic arterial blood pressure monitoring is the minimal risk attendant to its use. Superficial skin infections occur in about 4% of patients,[54,55] and radial artery occlusion may occur in up to 40% of patients.[56,57] Nevertheless, compromise of hand or digits is rare and does not appear to result in the absence of concurrent vasopressor therapy, multiple particulate emboli from the heart, or prolonged periods of low cardiac output.

## Central Venous and Pulmonary Artery Pressure Monitoring

Central pressure monitoring, including central venous pressure (CVP) and pulmonary artery pressure (PAP) monitoring, has increased since the 1970s, partly because of its widespread application in cardiovascular surgical patients. Once again, randomized trials do not document its effectiveness. It seems unlikely that such trials will ever be performed effectively.

### Complications

Unlike direct systemic arterial blood pressure monitoring, the risks associated with both CVP and PAP monitoring must be seriously considered in risk-benefit analyses. Carotid artery puncture, infection, thrombosis of central veins, and pulmonary artery rupture (including death) occur with these techniques. Despite these problems, the pulmonary artery catheter has made available tremendous amounts of information to anesthesiologists, allowing classification of many perioperative disease states into understandable terms and treatment regimens.

### Application

The prescription of invasive central monitoring for an individual patient must be predicated on many of the factors already discussed. Shoemaker and colleagues proposed that the use of a pulmonary artery catheter to direct "supraphysiologic cardiovascular function" lowered perioperative deaths in high-risk general surgical patients.[58] This thesis, however, has not been corroborated by any well-designed, randomized clinical studies. The final choice about using pulmonary artery and central venous catheters needs to be based on the anesthesiologist's institution and practice style. I believe that CVP monitoring alone to direct hemodynamic therapy is misguided in many situations. The risks of adverse outcomes are lower with CVP catheters than with PAP catheters; however, useful hemodynamic information is less frequently obtained from the former devices. An increasingly acceptable alternative to both CVP and PAP monitoring is the use of transesophageal echocardiography.

## Anesthesia Awareness Monitoring

Processed electroencephalography has evolved through many forms since the 1980s.[59] The current most popular version of processed electroencephalographic monitoring is the Bispectral Index (BIS; Aspect Medical Systems, Natick,

Mass). The BIS value is claimed to minimize awareness by being a surrogate for anesthetic depth.[60] At present, no randomized, blinded trials confirm this claim, although the device has many enthusiastic proponents. I believe we need to await additional studies before widely embracing this monitor.

## What Advantages Accrue to Regional Anesthesia?

Advantages of regional anesthesia over general anesthesia are difficult to confirm in most circumstances. In certain clinical situations, however, regional techniques are clearly advantageous. A decreased incidence of deep vein thrombosis follows neuraxial blocks during hip repair and prostatectomy.[61] Fewer episodes of CHF occur during low spinal anesthesia.[62] Organ function also appears better preserved, and decreased morbidity and possibly reduced mortality are noted in critically ill patients for whom prolonged epidural analgesia is used in the intensive care unit.[63,64]

A long-quoted criticism of regional anesthesia is that it takes too long, an accurate assessment if such techniques are infrequently used.[65] Because many anesthesia trainees have limited access to comprehensive regional anesthesia experience, the development of efficient regional anesthesia skills may be difficult.[66] Conversely, if regional anesthesia is conducted in a comprehensive manner using induction rooms and appropriate levels of sedation, skilled anesthesiologists can keep turnover time to a minimum and provide efficient anesthetic care.

## Postoperative Analgesia

If a stand-alone regional anesthetic is used before surgical incision or as part of a general anesthetic technique, postoperative pain may be lessened for a period of time even after the local anesthetic effect has resolved. Tverskoy and colleagues showed that regional anesthesia during herniorrhaphy is associated with less postoperative pain than are general anesthesia and routine opioids for postoperative analgesia in similar patients.[67] My belief is that the advantages of regional anesthesia, in most circumstances, are related to prolonged postoperative analgesia and regional anesthesia techniques moving toward peripheral blocks.[68] This effect may be amplified further by the immune dysfunction associated with opioids.[69]

## What Advantages Accrue to General Anesthesia?

A recurring theme during preoperative discussion with many surgical patients is their desire to be asleep. If anesthesiologists interpret this to mean a patient wishes a general anesthetic, appropriate prescription can be difficult. From the times of Crile[70] and Lundy,[71] it has been clear that most patients prefer to be amnestic for their operative experience. With the addition of anesthetic agents such as midazolam, propofol, and fentanyl and its congeners, amnesia for the operative experience does not preclude a regional anesthetic. Conversely, as noted earlier, in only a few situations is it clear that regional anesthesia has advantages over general anesthesia. Therefore, administration of a general anesthetic for almost any operative procedure may be easily justified.

## Which Considerations Are Important?

General anesthetic techniques can be provided with quite different methods. Primarily inhalational anesthesia, using the lungs as the route of anesthetic uptake, or higher-dose opioid techniques, using intravenous administration, can be applied with equal facility. When higher-dose opioid techniques are used, however, that consideration must include the need for postoperative mechanical ventilation. This is less common in the era of focus on decreased hospital stay.

### Familiarity

Despite the concept that one should administer that general anesthetic technique with which one has had the most experience, recent data from the multiinstitutional general anesthetic study by Forrest and colleagues show that statistically different incidences of adverse outcomes depend on the general anesthetic technique chosen[16] (Table 5–3). Thus, hypertension is more common with fentanyl, ventricular arrhythmias are more common with halothane, and tachycardia is more common when isoflurane is used as a primary anesthetic agent.[16]

### Data Interpretation

Additional information about differences in general anesthetic prescription comes from a contrary interpretation of the data of Yeager and colleagues.[63] They showed that prolonged epidural analgesia in high-risk patients lowered their risk of morbidity and mortality, compared with patients receiving a moderate- to high-dose fentanyl general anesthetic. The striking differences perhaps would not have been as large if the patients receiving general anesthesia had received a lower dose of opioid or an inhalational-based anesthetic.

As a result of the moderate- to high-dose opioid technique chosen in the general anesthetic group, patients required on average >80 hours of tracheal intubation and mechanical ventilation, compared with about 7 hours for patients having regional anesthesia. Perhaps what really was shown in this study was that prolonged postoperative mechanical ventilation is not as risk free as many anesthesiologists believed. This alternative interpretation must remain speculative because it was not designed as part of the original study.

Additional data highlight the differences between general anesthetic techniques. Anand and Hickey found that infants anesthetized for the repair of complex congenital heart lesions had lower perioperative mortality when administered a high-dose sufentanil anesthetic that was continued into the postoperative period, compared with a similar group receiving a

**TABLE 5–3.** Severe Adverse Anesthetic Outcome in General Anesthesia

| Anesthetic | Percentage of Patients With Adverse Outcome | | |
| --- | --- | --- | --- |
| | *Tachycardia* | *Hypertension* | *Ventricular Arrhythmia* |
| Halothane | 0.7 | 0.5 | 8.6* |
| Isoflurane | 1.5* | 0.8 | 0.8 |
| Fentanyl | 1.0 | 2.4* | 1.3 |

*Significantly different from other anesthetics.
From Forrest JB, Rehder K, Cahalan MK, et al. Multicenter study of general anesthesia, III: predictors of severe perioperative adverse outcomes. *Anesthesiology.* 1992;76:3.

traditional halothane technique.[72] This study is sound in design and, coupled with data from Forrest and colleagues,[16] suggests that anesthesiologists using primarily general anesthetic techniques must be willing to alter their anesthetic prescription to specific patient requirements.

## POSTOPERATIVE ANALGESIA

Interest in postoperative analgesia care for surgical patients has humanitarian as well as practical implications. The benefit of anesthesia is that patients are able to undergo a surgical procedure without the mortal pain that accompanied surgical care before the 1840s.

Although most anesthesiologists are supportive of the advances made in postoperative analgesia, some suggest that acute postoperative pain services are not in their best interests. This concept smacks of those mid-1840s days when some physicians criticized the introduction of effective general anesthetics.[73] Because anesthesia practice is based on the basic concept of pain relief, it seems important that anesthesiologists continue to advance patient care in that area.

### What Are the Advantages?

On the practical side, increasing evidence suggests that the nervous system and its pain recognition components are not the hard-wired structures that many of us learned in medical school. Rather, prevention of pain through the use of more effective regional analgesic or parenteral techniques may affect the degree of pain a patient experiences at a time remote from the anesthetic and analgesic intervention.[74]

Yeager and coworkers[63] and Tuman and colleagues[64] demonstrated that epidural analgesia carried into the postoperative period of high-risk surgical patients can reduce the mortality and morbidity associated with these surgical procedures. Tverskoy and colleagues found that a common surgical procedure, inguinal herniorrhaphy, is associated with less postoperative pain if a regional anesthetic technique is used as part of the anesthesia.[67]

### What Are the Risks?

If analgesia were prescribed and carried out without any associated increased morbidity, this discussion would be moot. Almost all analgesia, however, is associated with small but measurable risks[75] (Table 5–4). Epidural opioid analgesia provides excellent analgesia for major intraabdominal proce-

dures,[63,64] but it may lead to respiratory depression. Should this potential problem prevent anesthesiologists from prescribing the technique? Probably not. The often forgotten part of the risk-benefit equation is that respiratory depression accompanies routine parenteral opioid analgesia.[76–78]

An additional risk that has developed with the use of neuraxial analgesia is neuraxial bleeding when neuraxial anesthesia or analgesia is carried out in patients receiving low molecular weight heparin. It is clear that the larger doses of low molecular weight heparin used in the United States have created an increased risk compared with patients receiving the same techniques in many European countries[79] (Table 5–5).

**TABLE 5–5.** Recommendations for Patients Receiving Low Molecular Weight Heparin and Neuraxial Anesthesia

1. Monitoring of Factor-Xa level is not recommended. The Factor-Xa level is not predictive of the risk for bleeding and is, therefore, not helpful in the management of patients undergoing neuraxial blocks.
2. Antiplatelet or oral anticoagulant medications administered in combination with LMWH may increase the risk for spinal hematoma. Concomitant administration of medications affecting hemostasis, such as antiplatelet drugs, standard heparin, or dextran, represents an additional risk for hemorrhagic complications perioperatively, including spinal hematoma. Education of the entire patient care team is necessary to avoid potentiation of the anticoagulant effects.
3. Presence of blood during needle and catheter placement does not necessitate postponement of surgery. However, initiation of LMWH therapy in this setting should be delayed for 24 h postoperatively. Traumatic needle or catheter placement may signify an increased risk for spinal hematoma, and it is recommended that this consideration be discussed with the surgeon.
4. Patients taking preoperative LMWH can be assumed to have altered coagulation. A single-dose spinal anesthetic may be the safest neuraxial technique in patients receiving preoperative LMWH. In these patients, needle placement should occur at least 10 to 12 h after the LMWH, whereas patients receiving higher doses of LMWH (eg, enoxaparin 1 mg/kg twice daily) will require longer delays (24 h). Neuraxial techniques should be avoided in patients administered a dose of LMWH 2 h preoperatively (general surgery patients) because needle placement would occur during peak anticoagulant activity.
5. Patients with postoperative initiation of LMWH thromboprophylaxis may safely undergo single-dose and continuous catheter techniques. The first dose of LMWH should be administered no earlier than 24 h postoperatively and only in the presence of adequate hemostasis. In addition, it is recommended that indwelling catheters be removed before initiation of LMWH thromboprophylaxis. If a continuous technique is selected, the epidural catheter may be left indwelling overnight and removed the following day, with the first dose of LMWH administered 2 h after catheter removal.
6. The decision to implement LMWH thromboprophylaxis in the presence of an indwelling catheter must be made with care. Extreme vigilance of the patient's neurologic status is warranted. An opioid or dilute local anesthetic solution is recommended in these patients to allow frequent monitoring of neurologic function. If epidural analgesia is anticipated to continue for more than 24 h, LMWH administration may be delayed (in selected cases) or an alternate method of thromboprophylaxis may be selected (eg, external pneumatic compression), based on the risk profile for the individual patient. These decisions should be made preoperatively to allow optimal management of both postoperative analgesia and thromboprophylaxis.
7. For any LMWH prophylaxis regimen, the timing of catheter removal is of paramount importance. Catheter removal should be delayed for at least 10 to 12 hours after a dose of LMWH. A true normalization of the patient's coagulation status could be achieved if the evening dose of LMWH was not given and the catheter was removed the following morning (24 h after the last dose). Again, subsequent dosing should not occur for at least 2 h after catheter removal.

LMWH, low molecular weight heparin.

**TABLE 5–4.** Major Risks Associated With Analgesia Techniques

| Analgesia Technique | Complication | Incidence |
|---|---|---|
| Peridural opioid | Severe respiratory depression | 1:500 to 1:100[75, 77] |
| Parenteral opioid (intravenous, subcutaneous, intramuscular) | Respiratory depression | 1:100[78] |
| Intercostal nerve block | Symptomatic pneumothorax | 1:1100[79] |

## What Are the Costs?

Yeager and colleagues included data about physician and hospital costs associated with random assignment to traditional or epidural analgesia techniques.[63] Although their study was small, including only 53 patients, the costs associated with epidural analgesia were significantly less overall than those associated with traditional analgesia.

Because physicians and hospital administrators are most comfortable in thinking of medical costs in an unbundled fashion, many fail to recognize that money spent for analgesia may, in the long run, save money during the period of an entire hospitalization. If techniques allow patients to return to their jobs sooner because of improved analgesia, further decreases in incremental costs may accrue.

## References

1. The lessons of CEPOD [editorial]. *Br J Anaesth.* 1988;60:753.
2. Natof HE. Complications. In: Wetchler BV, ed. *Anesthesia for Ambulatory Surgery.* Philadelphia, Pa: JB Lippincott; 1985:349.
3. Eichhorn JH. Prevention of intraoperative anesthesia accidents and related severe injury through safety monitoring. *Anesthesiology.* 1989;70:572.
4. Slogoff S, Keats AS. Does perioperative myocardial ischemia lead to postoperative myocardial infarction? *Anesthesiology.* 1985;62:107.
5. Frank SM, Fleisher LA, Breslow MJ, et al. Perioperative maintenance of normothermia reduces the incidence of morbid cardiac events. *JAMA.* 1997;277:1127
6. Goldman RL. The reliability of peer assessments of quality of care. *JAMA.* 1992;267:958.
7. Caplan RA, Posner KL, Cheney FW. Effect of outcome on physician judgments of appropriateness of care. *JAMA.* 1991;265:1957.
8. Cohen MM, Duncan PG, Pope WDB, et al. A survey of 112,000 anaesthetics at one teaching hospital (1975–83). *Can Anaesth Soc J.* 1986;33:22.
9. Fowkes FGR, Lunn JN, Farrow SC, et al. Epidemiology in anaesthesia, III: mortality risk in patients with coexisting physical disease. *Br J Anaesth.* 1982;54:819.
10. Cohen MM, Duncan PG, Tate RB. Does anaesthesia contribute to operative mortality? *JAMA.* 1988;260:2859.
11. Eiseman B. *What Are My Chances?* Philadelphia, Pa: WB Saunders; 1980.
12. Merry AF, Ramage MC, Whitlock RML, et al. First-time coronary artery bypass grafting: the anaesthetist as a risk factor. *Br J Anaesth.* 1992;68:6.
13. Luft HS, Bunker JP, Einthoven AC. Should operations be regionalized? The empirical relation between surgical volume and mortality. *N Engl J Med.* 1979;301:1364.
14. Kennedy JW, Kaiser GC, Fischer LD, et al. Clinical and angiographic predictors of operative mortality from the collaborative study in coronary artery surgery (CASS). *Circulation.* 1981;63:793.
15. Pedersen T, Eliasen K, Henriksen E. A prospective study of risk factors and cardiopulmonary complications associated with anaesthesia and surgery: risk indicators of cardiopulmonary morbidity. *Acta Anaesthesiol Scand.* 1990;34:144.
16. Forrest JB, Rehder K, Cahalan MK, et al. Multicenter study of general anesthesia, III: predictors of severe perioperative adverse outcomes. *Anesthesiology.* 1992;76:3.
17. Practice standards: the Midas touch or the emperor's new clothes? [editorial]. *Anesthesiology.* 1989;70:567
18. Tiret L, Desmonts JM, Hatton F, et al. Complications associated with anaesthesia: a prospective survey in France. *Can Anaesth Soc J.* 1986;33:336
19. Tiret L, Hatton F, Desmonts JM, et al. Prediction of outcome anaesthesia in patients over 40 years: a multifactorial risk index. *Stat Med.* 1988;7:947.
20. The Hypertension Detection and Follow-Up Program. The effect of treatment on mortality in "mild" hypertension: results of the hypertension detection and follow-up program. *N Engl J Med.* 1982;307:976.
21. Goldman L, Caldera DL. Risks of general anesthesia and elective operation in the hypertensive patient. *Anesthesiology.* 1979;50:285.
22. Ross AF, Tinker JH. Cardiovascular disease. In: Brown DL, ed. *Risk and Outcome in Anesthesia.* Philadelphia, Pa: JB Lippincott; 1992:39–76.
23. Rao TLK, Jacobs KH, El-Etr AA. Reinfarction following anesthesia in patients with myocardial infarction. *Anesthesiology.* 1983;59:499.
24. Goldman L, Caldera DL, Southwick FS, et al. Cardiac risk factors and complications in noncardiac surgery. *Medicine.* 1978;57:357.
25. Goldman L. Cardiac risks and complications of noncardiac surgery. *Ann Surg.* 1983;198:780.
26. Mangano DT, Browner WS, Hollenberger M, et al. Association of perioperative myocardial ischemia with cardiac morbidity and mortality in men undergoing noncardiac surgery. *N Engl J Med.* 1990;323:1781.
27. Moorman JR, Hlatky MA, Eddy DM, et al. The yield of the routine admission electrocardiogram: a study in a general medical service. *Ann Intern Med.* 1985;103:590.
28. Pasternack PF, Imparato AM, Bear G, et al. The value of radionuclide angiography as a predictor of perioperative myocardial infarction in patients undergoing abdominal aortic aneurysm resection. *J Vasc Surg.* 1984;1:320.
29. Moraski RE, Russell RO, Smith M, et al. Left ventricular function in patients with and without myocardial infarction and one, two, or three vessel coronary artery disease. *Am J Cardiol.* 1975;35:1.
30. Boucher CA, Brewster DC, Darling RC, et al. Determination of cardiac risk by dipyridamole-thallium imaging before peripheral vascular surgery. *N Engl J Med.* 1985;312:389.
31. Eagle KA, Boucher CA. Cardiac risk of noncardiac surgery. *N Engl J Med.* 1989;321:1300.
32. Gerson MC, Hurst JM, Hertzberg VS, et al. Cardiac prognosis in noncardiac geriatric surgery. *Ann Intern Med.* 1985;103:832.
33. Gerson MC, Hurst JM, Hertzberg VS, et al. Prediction of cardiac and pulmonary complications related to elective abdominal and noncardiac thoracic surgery in geriatric patients. *Am J Med.* 1990;88:101.
34. Caplan RA, Posner KL, Ward RJ, et al. Adverse respiratory events in anesthesia: a closed claims analysis. *Anesthesiology.* 1990;72:828.
35. Meneely GR, Ferguson JL. Pulmonary evaluation and risk in patient preparation for anesthesia and surgery. *JAMA.* 1961;175:1074.
36. Ford GT, Whitelaw WA, Rosenal TW, et al. Diaphragm function after upper abdominal surgery in humans. *Am Rev Respir Dis.* 1983;127:431.
37. Latimer RC, Dickman M, Day WC, et al. Ventilatory patterns and pulmonary complications after upper abdominal surgery determined by preoperative and postoperative computerized spirometry and blood gas analysis. *Am J Surg.* 1971;122:622.
38. Gracey DR, Divertie MB, Didier EP. Preoperative pulmonary preparation of patients with chronic obstructive pulmonary disease. *Chest.* 1979;76:123.
39. William CD, Brenowitz JB. Prohibitive lung function and major surgical procedures. *Am J Surg.* 1976;132:763.
40. Milledge JS, Nunn FJ. Criteria for fitness for anesthesia in patients with chronic obstructive lung disease. *BMJ.* 1975;3:670.
41. Kingston HGG, Hirschman CA. Perioperative management of the patient with asthma. *Anesth Analg.* 1984;63:844.
42. Shnider SM, Papper EM. Anesthesia for the asthmatic patient. *Anesthesiology.* 1961;22:886.
43. Gold MI, Helrich M. A study of complications related to anesthesia in asthmatic patients. *Anesth Analg.* 1963;42:283.
44. Roizen MF. Preoperative evaluation. In: Miller RD, ed. *Anesthesia.* New York, NY: Churchill Livingstone; 1990:753.
45. Dexter DD, Whisnant JP, Connolly DC, et al. The association of stroke and coronary heart disease: a population study. *Mayo Clin Proc.* 1987;62:1077.
46. Torvik A, Skullerud K. How often are brain infarcts caused by hypotensive episodes? *Stroke.* 1976;7:255.
47. Wolf PA, Kannel WB, Sorlie P, et al. Asymptomatic carotid bruit and risk of stroke: the Framingham study. *JAMA.* 1981;245:1442.
48. Ropper AH, Wechsler LR, Wilson LS. Carotid bruit and the risk of stroke in elective surgery. *N Engl J Med.* 1982;307:1388.
49. Kurtz CM, Bennett JH, Shapiro HH. Electrocardiographic studies during surgical anesthesia. *JAMA.* 1936;106:434.
50. Moller JT, Pedersen T, Rasmussen L, et al. Randomized evaluation of pulse oximetry in 20,802 patients (I and II). *Anesthesiology.* 1993;78:436, 445.
51. Tinker JH, Dull DL, Caplan RA, et al. Role of monitoring devices in prevention of anesthetic mishaps: a closed claims analysis. *Anesthesiology.* 1989;71:541.
52. Kestin IG, Miller BR, Lockhart CH. Auditory alarms during anesthesia monitoring. *Anesthesiology.* 1988;69:106.
53. Wagner DL. Hemodynamic monitoring. In: Brown DL, ed. *Risk and Outcome in Anesthesia.* 2nd ed. Philadelphia, Pa: JB Lippincott; 1992:283–312.
54. Pinilla JC, Ross DF, Martin T, et al. Study of the incidence of intravascu-

lar catheter infection and associated septicemia in critically ill patients. *Crit Care Med.* 1983;11:21.

55. Gardner RM, Schwartz R, Wong HC. Percutaneous indwelling radial artery catheters for monitoring cardiovascular function: prospective study of the risk of thrombosis and infection. *N Engl J Med.* 1974;290:1227.

56. Slogoff S, Keats AS, Arlund C. On the safety of radial artery cannulation. *Anesthesiology.* 1983;59:42.

57. Bedford RF, Wollman H. Complications of percutaneous radial artery cannulation: an objective prospective study in man. *Anesthesiology.* 1973;38:228.

58. Shoemaker WC, Appel PL, Kram HB, et al. Prospective trial of supranormal values of survivors as therapeutic goals in high-risk surgical patients. *Chest.* 1988;94:1176.

59. Rampil IJ. A primer for EEG signal processing in anesthesia. *Anesthesiology.* 1998;89:980.

60. Todd MM. EEGs, EEG processing, and the bispectral index [editorial]. *Anesthesiology.* 1998;89:815.

61. Brown DL. Anesthetic choice. In: Brown DL, ed. *Risk and Outcome in Anesthesia.* Philadelphia, Pa: JB Lippincott; 1992:193–234.

62. Greene NM. *Physiology of Spinal Anesthesia.* Baltimore, Md: Williams & Wilkins, 1981:93.

63. Yeager MP, Glass DD, Neff RK, et al. Epidural anesthesia and analgesia in high-risk surgical patients. *Anesthesiology.* 1987;66:729.

64. Tuman KJ, McCarthy RJ, March RJ, et al. Effects of epidural anesthesia and analgesia on coagulation and outcome after major vascular surgery. *Anesth Analg.* 1991;73:696.

65. Bonica JJ. Regional anesthesia in private practice. *Anesthesiology.* 1960;21:554.

66. Bridenbaugh LD. Are anesthesia resident programs failing regional anesthesia? *Reg Anesth.* 1982;7:26.

67. Tverskoy M, Cozacov C, Ayache M, et al. Postoperative pain after inguinal herniorrhaphy with different types of anesthesia. *Anesth Analg.* 1990;70:29.

68. Horlocker TT. Peripheral nerve blocks: regional anesthesia for the new millennium [editorial]. *Reg Anesth Pain Med.* 1998;23:237.

69. Yeager MP, Colacchio TA, Yu CT, et al. Morphine inhibits spontaneous and cytokine-enhanced natural killer cell cytotoxicity in volunteers. *Anesthesiology.* 1995;83:500.

70. Crile GW. Nitrous oxide anaesthesia and a note on anociassociation, a new principle in operative surgery. *Surg Gynecol Obstet.* 1911;13:170.

71. Lundy JS. Balanced anesthesia. *Minn Med.* 1926;9:399.

72. Anand KJS, Hickey PR. Halothane-morphine compared with high-dose sufentanil for anesthesia and postoperative analgesia in neonatal cardiac surgery. *N Engl J Med.* 1992;326:1.

73. Brown DL. Anesthesia risk: a historical perspective. In: Brown DL, ed. *Risk and Outcome in Anesthesia.* Philadelphia, Pa: JB Lippincott; 1992:1–35.

74. Dickenson AH, Sullivan AF. Subcutaneous formalin-induced activity of the dorsal horn neurons in the rat: differential response to an intrathecal opiate administered pre or post formalin. *Pain.* 1987;30:349.

75. Moore DC, Bridenbaugh LD. Intercostal nerve block in 4,333 patients. *Anesth Analg.* 1962;41:1.

76. Ready LB, Loper KA, Nessly M, et al. Postoperative epidural morphine is safe on surgical wards. *Anesthesiology.* 1991;75:452.

77. Rawal N, Arner S, Gustafsson LL, et al. Present state of extradural and intrathecal opioid analgesia in Sweden. *Br J Anaesth.* 1987;59:791.

78. Miller RR, Greenblatt DG, eds. *Drug Effects in Hospitalized Patients: Experiences of the Boston Collaborative Drug Surveillance Program, 1966–75.* New York, NY: John Wiley & Sons; 1976.

79. Horlocker TT, Wedel DJ. Neuraxial block and low-molecular-weight heparin: balancing perioperative analgesia and thromboprophylaxis. *Reg Anesth Pain Med.* 1998;23(6 Suppl 2):164.

CHAPTER

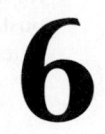

# 6

# Postanesthesia Recovery

Roger S. Mecca

*What Is the Significance of Oliguria?*

*What Should Be Done If Oliguria Persists?*

## CENTRAL NERVOUS SYSTEM FUNCTION

*What Causes Prolonged Unconsciousness After Anesthesia?*

*What Should Be Done If the Cause Is Indeterminate?*

*Why Does Altered Sensorium Occur After Anesthesia?*

*What Therapy Is Appropriate?*

## POSTOPERATIVE NAUSEA AND VOMITING

*What Is the Impact?*

*What Are the Risk Factors?*

*How Are Postoperative Nausea and Vomiting Prevented and Treated?*

## POSTOPERATIVE HYPOTHERMIA

*Why Does Hypothermia Develop?*

*What Are the Adverse Effects?*

*Why Is Shivering Detrimental?*

*How Is Hypothermia Attenuated or Prevented?*

## POSTOPERATIVE HYPERTHERMIA

*What Is the Impact?*

*How Is Hyperthermia Treated?*

## POSTOPERATIVE ACID-BASE PROBLEMS

*Why Does Respiratory Acidemia Occur?*

*Why Does Metabolic Acidemia Occur?*

*Why Does Respiratory Alkalemia Occur?*

*Why Does Metabolic Alkalemia Occur?*

## POSTOPERATIVE GLUCOSE AND ELECTROLYTE ABNORMALITIES

*Why Does Hyperglycemia Occur?*

*Why Does Hypoglycemia Occur?*

*Why Does Hyponatremia Occur?*

*Why Does Hypokalemia Occur?*

*Why Does Hyperkalemia Occur?*

*Are Calcium and Magnesium Important?*

## MISCELLANEOUS POSTOPERATIVE COMPLICATIONS

*What Are the Causes of Corneal Injury?*

*Why Does Soft Tissue Trauma Occur?*

*When Is Trauma to the Airways a Problem?*

*What Neurologic Injuries May Be Seen After Regional Anesthesia?*

*What Factors Predispose to Peripheral Nerve Injury?*

*What Visual Disturbances May Occur?*

*What Problems Are Associated With Positioning?*

*How Do Injuries Occur in the Postanesthesia Care Unit?*

*What Are the Causes of Postoperative Skeletal Muscle Pain?*

A contemporary postanesthesia care unit (PACU) provides an optimal postoperative recovery for each patient, with minimal risk, inconvenience, and expense. It also offers an organized clinical environment that enhances a practitioner's ability to perform individualized, problem-oriented assessment and care. Facility design, staffing, and equipment requirements for a modern PACU are reviewed elsewhere.[1] Standards for postanesthesia care developed by the American Society of Anesthesiologists are listed in Table 6–1.

## GENERAL CONCERNS

The administrative structure of a PACU affects the quality of clinical care, the medical liability exposure of staff and facility, and the environmental safety of physicians and PACU nurses. Clear lines of authority avoid confusion about which physician is responsible when clinical decisions are necessary. Collaborative management between a medical director and the PACU manager facilitates oversight of clinical services, promotes performance improvement, and ensures compliance with clinical and regulatory policies.

The PACU should be administratively positioned as a component of a larger surgical service governed by an interdisciplinary group of professionals. This arrangement fosters continuity of care and minimizes interface problems with the operating room (OR), the ambulatory discharge area, and the inpatient floor. The most important linkage is with the intraoperative anesthesiology service. In a study of 37 000 patients, 22.1% suffered a minor anesthesia-related event or complication that prolonged PACU stay and consumed PACU resources.[2] Coordination among services can reduce the incidence and effects of such events.[3]

### *What Are the Minimal Administrative Considerations?*

#### Patient Coverage

Policies governing patient coverage by PACU nurses must define staffing competencies, a method of assigning patients, and minimal staff-to-patient ratios. Assign each patient a primary PACU nurse on admission. Generally, a PACU nurse should not be responsible for more than 2 patients. At times, patient acuity or age makes one-to-one coverage appropriate. In other circumstances, lower acuity patients, such as those awaiting transfer, may safely be covered at lower staff-to-patient ratios. Ensure that a sufficient number of trained PACU nurses are always available to provide each patient with immediate, focused care without jeopardizing the care of others. Create a clear, well-understood procedure for mobilizing the anesthesiologist responsible for each patient's recovery. Finally, the PACU must have a procedure that ensures the availability of another physician capable of managing postoperative complications if the anesthesiologist is temporarily unavailable.

#### Performance Evaluation

Aggressive staff development, performance evaluation, and interdisciplinary medical education help ensure that PACU nurses have sufficient skill and judgment to recognize evolving problems regarding airway management, pulmonary function, and cardiovascular dynamics. The ability to interact with demanding patients under trying circumstances with a positive and supportive demeanor is an essential skill. Friendliness of surgical services staff fosters a pleasant and safe care environment and is a key determinant of patient satisfaction.[4]

**TABLE 6–1.** Standards for Postanesthesia Care

These standards apply to postanesthesia care in all locations. These standards may be exceeded based on the judgment of the responsible anesthesiologist. They are intended to encourage quality patient care, but cannot guarantee a specific patient outcome. They are subject to revision from time to time as warranted by the evolution of technology and practice. Under extenuating circumstances, the responsible anesthesiologist may waive the requirements marked with an asterisk (*); it is recommended that when this is done, it should be so stated (including the reasons) in a note in the patient's medical record.

**Standard I**

*All patients who have received general anesthesia, regional anesthesia, or monitored anesthesia care shall receive appropriate postanesthesia management.*†

1. A postanesthesia care unit (PACU) or an area that provides equivalent postanesthesia care shall be available to receive patients after anesthesia care. All patients who receive anesthesia care shall be admitted to the PACU or its equivalent, except by specific order of the anesthesiologist responsible for the patient's care.
2. The medical aspects of care in the PACU shall be governed by policies and procedures that have been reviewed and approved by the Department of Anesthesiology.
3. The design, equipment, and staffing of the PACU shall meet requirements of the facility's accrediting and licensing bodies.

**Standard II**

*A patient transported to the PACU shall be accompanied by a member of the anesthesia care team who is knowledgeable about the patient's condition. The patient shall be continually evaluated and treated during transport with monitoring and support appropriate to the patient's condition.*

**Standard III**

*Upon arrival in the PACU, the patient shall be reevaluated and verbal report provided to the responsible PACU nurse by a member of the anesthesia care team who accompanies the patient.*

1. The patient's status on arrival in the PACU shall be documented.
2. Information concerning the preoperative condition and the surgical and anesthetic course shall be transmitted to the PACU nurse.
3. The member of the Anesthesia Care Team shall remain in the PACU until the PACU nurse accepts responsibility for the nursing care of the patient.

**Standard IV**

*The patient's condition shall be evaluated continually in the PACU.*

1. The patient shall be observed and monitored by methods appropriate to the patient's medical condition. Particular attention should be given to monitoring oxygenation, ventilation, circulation, and temperature. During recovery from all anesthetics, a quantitative method of assessing oxygenation, such as pulse oximetry, shall be employed in the initial phase of recovery.* This is not intended for application during the recovery of the obstetrical patient in whom regional anesthesia was used for labor and vaginal delivery.
2. An accurate written report of the PACU period shall be maintained. Use of an appropriate PACU scoring system is encouraged for each patient on admission, at appropriate intervals before discharge and at the time of discharge.
3. General medical supervision and coordination of patient care in the PACU should be the responsibility of an anesthesiologist.
4. There shall be a policy to ensure the availability in the facility of a physician capable of managing complications and providing cardiopulmonary resuscitation for patients in the PACU.

**Standard V**

*A physician is responsible for the discharge of the patient from the PACU.*

1. When discharge criteria are used, they must be approved by the Department of Anesthesiology and the medical staff. They may vary depending on whether the patient is discharged to a hospital room, to the intensive care unit, to a short-stay unit or home.
2. In the absence of the physician responsible for the discharge, the PACU nurse shall determine that the patient meets the discharge criteria. The name of the physician accepting responsibility for discharge shall be noted on the record.

---

*Under extenuating circumstances, the responsible anesthesiologist may waive the requirements marked with an asterisk (*). Approved by House of Delegates on October 12, 1988 and last amended on October 19, 1994.

†Refer to *Standards of Post Anesthesia Nursing Practice, 2000.* Cherry Hill, NJ: The American Society of PeriAnesthesia Nurses; 2000: 1–85, for issues of nursing care.
From *2001 ASA Directory of Members.* Park Ridge, Ill: American Society of Anesthesiologists; 2001:494–495.

---

Topics relevant to postanesthesia care should be incorporated into continuing medical education programs of anesthesiologists, surgeons, and other physicians performing invasive procedures. Peer review proceedings of the corresponding medical staff departments must address clinical management of patients in the PACU.

## Policies and Procedures

A comprehensive PACU policy and procedure manual ensures that clinical care and administrative performance are optimum. Policies must also address medical ethics (eg, informed consent, patient confidentiality, do-not-resuscitate status), environmental safety for patients and staff, regulatory compliance, and cost. Avoid creating unrealistic policies that cannot be followed. The inevitable lack of compliance interferes with accreditation and makes appropriate clinical activity appear to fall below an unachievable local standard. Review policies yearly to keep pace with changing standards and new modalities. Interdisciplinary quality improvement and risk management minimize liability and ensure that care in the PACU remains safe, appropriate, and current.

## Patient Safety

The PACU environment must be safe for both patients and staff. Staffing arrangements have to provide appropriate coverage and skill mix to deal with unforeseen crises at any time. Ideally, all nurses should have PACU certification. Staffing should always meet appropriate standards.[5] If non-PACU trained staff are deployed, it is the medical director's role to ensure that they are supervised and that a sufficient number of certified personnel is always available.

The PACU staff acts as a patient's advocate during periods of diminished competence. Each patient's privacy and dignity need to be preserved, and the patient's rights to informed consent for additional procedures and to compliance with advance directives must be safeguarded.[6] For both medical safety and liability reasons, PACU leaders have to examine the potential for patients to be assaulted during recovery.

Strictly regulate access to the PACU and appropriately monitor staff activity. Review the advisability of cross-gender care, especially during periods when staff are relatively unobserved.

## Staff Safety

Also make the environment safe for professionals. Strict compliance with policies governing disposal of "sharps" and infection control is essential. Staff must observe procedures that protect against blood-borne pathogens, tuberculosis, or methicillin-resistant staphylococci.[7] Make sure that suitable masks, gloves, and eye protection are always available, including fitted personal respirators if appropriate. Keep vaccinations of PACU staff current, including that for hepatitis B. Adequate help should be available so that an individual does not risk personal injury from lifting and positioning patients, or when dealing with emergence reactions. Assess PACU air turnover to ensure that the staff is not exposed to high levels of trace anesthetic gases. Routine monitoring of trace gas levels is unnecessary.[8]

## *Does Every Patient Need to Go Through the Postanesthesia Care Unit?*

The postoperative care that a patient requires varies with underlying illness, the duration and complexity of anesthesia and surgery, and the risk for postoperative complications. As anesthetic and surgical techniques have improved, minimal physiologic impairment after surgery has allowed many patients to bypass the PACU and to recover safely in a less intense setting. The patient avoids the inconvenience, stress, and expense of a PACU admission; reunites with family sooner; and recovers more comfortably in a recliner with music, television, food, and other amenities not usually available in a PACU. Bypassing the PACU allows the facility to dedicate scarce, expensive PACU resources to patients who benefit the most.

## Fast-Track Recovery

After straightforward surgical procedures performed using local anesthetic infiltration, digital blocks, or field blocks with moderate sedation, patients can be transferred directly from the OR to a discharge area. Selected patients who meet PACU discharge criteria in the OR at the end of a general or major regional anesthetic procedure may also bypass the PACU.[9] Anesthetic techniques using short-acting agents and bispectral index monitoring facilitate rapid emergence with minimal side effects.[10] Bypassing the PACU does not eliminate the need to deal with pain and postoperative nausea and vomiting (PONV).[11] Failure to provide adequate analgesia and control of emesis derails even the most organized fast-track discharge program. Whenever there is concern about a patient's ability to recover safely in a lower intensity setting, admit to a full-service PACU.

## Customized Postanesthesia Care

In an era of resource limitations, one objective is to provide exactly the level of postanesthesia support and monitoring each patient needs within staffing and facility constraints. Customizing postanesthesia care can be accomplished by creating two or more discrete PACUs or by offering different levels of monitoring and coverage in one comprehensive unit. Every surgical service must establish triage criteria, monitoring requirements, and staffing levels that acknowledge the techniques and skills of the medical staff and the needs of the patient population being served. Ensure that creative recovery protocols meet regional regulatory requirements and national standards.

A full-service PACU will always be necessary for acute postoperative management, given the incidence of complications after anesthesia and surgery. Figure 6–1, from a prospective study of 18 000 PACU patients, illustrates the frequency of adverse postoperative events.[12] As the population ages and complication rates climb in the face of dwindling resources,[13] maintaining appropriate PACU capacity will be increasingly essential.

## Cost-Effectiveness of Postanesthesia Care

There is growing interest in reducing the cost of the PACU portion of surgical care. Besides eliminating admission to the

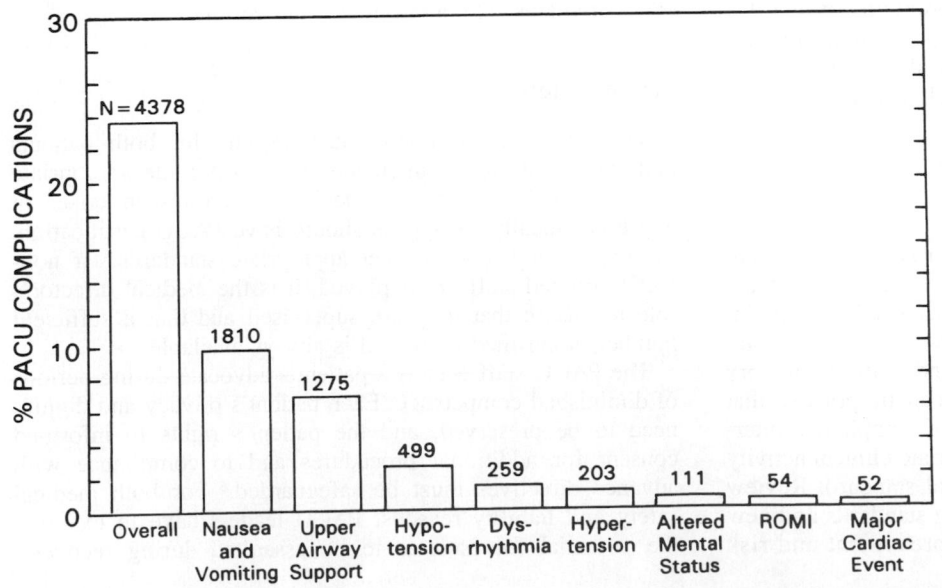

**FIGURE 6–1.** Major PACU complications by percentage of occurrence and number of patients (*above the bars*) experiencing each complication. Nausea and vomiting were the most frequently observed PACU complications, occurring in 1810 patients (9.8%). PACU, postanesthesia care unit; ROMI, rule out myocardial infarction. (From Hines R, Barash PG, Watrous G, et al. Complications occurring in the postanesthesia care unit: a survey. *Anesth Analg.* 1992;74:503.)

PACU altogether, focus falls on expensive medications (eg, antiemetics and sedatives) and on the duration of stay in the PACU. Actual medication expenditures are small per patient and usually justifiable in terms of shortening length of stay or improving patient outcome and satisfaction. Innovative care could shorten length of stay in the PACU and discharge unit, but the actual impact is frequently reduced by transportation delays, surgeon discharge delays, persistence of pain or nausea, or waiting for space.[14,15] Also, beware of cost-saving measures in other areas that increase the cost of PACU care. For example, if switching to cheaper, longer acting muscle relaxants significantly increases length of stay and complication rates in the PACU, the organization realizes no net savings.[16]

### The Illusion of Cost Savings

There is a difference between creating an opportunity for cost savings and actually reducing the PACU cost per case. Nurse staffing is the largest component of variable direct costs in the PACU.[17] Shortening PACU length of stay or innovative scheduling of cases creates an opportunity for savings that is realized only if the number of paid nursing hours is reduced or if more patients are serviced using the same nursing hours. Often, hard-won opportunities for savings are consumed by ineffective scheduling, staff subterfuge, or investment of excess nursing hours in low-yield clerical or maintenance tasks. This may result in patient care being pushed toward the margin of safety for a negligible payback in savings. Objectively assess the real yield from cost reduction in the PACU.

## What Are the Initial Steps on Admission?

### Assessment and Monitoring

When a patient is admitted to a PACU, record the heart rate, systemic blood pressure (BP), and ventilatory rate initially, at least every 5 minutes for the first 15 minutes, and at least every 15 minutes thereafter. Document an axillary or oral temperature at least on admission and discharge and more frequently if appropriate. Rectal, tympanic, or esophageal determination may be more accurate when core temperature assessment is important.

Document the level of consciousness, airway patency, character of ventilation, and skin color. Every patient is continuously monitored using pulse oximetry and single-lead continuous electrocardiography (ECG). Continuous capnographic monitoring is not essential unless a patient requires mechanical ventilation or is at risk for compromised ventilation. Output from arterial, central venous, and pulmonary artery (PA) catheters is transduced and recorded.

### Transfer to the Postanesthesia Care Unit Staff

Before anesthesiology personnel transfer responsibility for a patient's care, the PACU staff should be given ample time to ascertain admission vital signs and to record a succinct clinical report (Table 6–2). If a postoperative complication arises, this information will facilitate rapid evaluation and intervention by a physician who may be unfamiliar with the patient. A standardized format printed on the PACU record is useful.

**TABLE 6–2.** Postanesthesia Care Unit Admission Report

**Pertinent History**
   Significant medical illnesses
   Pertinent previous surgery
   Chronic medications (last dose)
   Medication allergies and sensitivities
**Preoperative Status**
   Premedication and preoperative meds NPO status
   Acute conditions (ischemia, dehydration)
   Traumatic injuries
**Intraoperative Factors**
   Surgical procedure
   Surgeon and anesthesiologist
   Estimated blood loss and replacement
   Urine output
   Type of anesthetic and specific agents
   Other medications (steroids, diuretics, antibiotics)
   Amount and time of narcotic administration
   Intraoperative vital sign ranges
   Amount and type of intravenous fluids
   Intraoperative laboratory findings
   Relaxant and reversal status
   Unexpected surgical and anesthetic events
**Status on Admission to PACU***
   Heart rate and rhythm
   Size and location of intravenous catheters
   Systemic pressure
   Function and readings, invasive monitors
   Airway patency and ventilatory adequacy
   Endotracheal tube position
   Level of consciousness
   Anesthetic equipment (epidural catheters)
   Intravascular volume status
   Overall assessment of status
**Postoperative Instructions**
   Acceptable vital sign ranges
   Therapeutic goals and end points
   Acceptable urine output and blood loss
   Orders for therapeutic interventions
   Anticipated cardiovascular problems
   Surgical instructions (positioning, wound care)
   Anticipated airway and ventilatory status
**Location of the Responsible Anesthesiologist**
   Diagnostic tests to be secured

*Determined and documented in conjunction with PACU staff.
NPO, nil per os (nothing by mouth); PACU, postanesthesia care unit.

Review orders for required laboratory evaluations or therapeutic interventions and clearly identify the responsible anesthesiologist. Complete a final check of intravenous catheters, endotracheal or chest tubes, and monitoring devices. Never leave a patient with PACU personnel if there is uncertainty about airway patency, ventilation, or hemodynamic stability. If complications arise, comprehensive reporting, careful and legible documentation, and consistent transfer practices decrease clinical risks and reduce liability exposure.

### Routine Laboratory Tests

Avoid routine postoperative laboratory testing. Rather, order tests such as hematocrit and electrolyte determinations, arterial blood gas (ABG) measurements, ECG, and chest radiography individually based on each patient's requirements. Avoiding unnecessary testing is one reliable way to decrease the actual cost per case of PACU care.

## When Is a Patient Ready to Leave the Postanesthesia Care Unit?

The decision to release a patient from a PACU is based on both objective and subjective criteria. Scoring systems that quantify physical status and facilitate assessment[18-21] do not replace an individual evaluation.

## Physiologic Assessment

Generally, the systemic BP and heart rate should be relatively constant for at least 30 minutes before transfer from the PACU. Make sure that airway protective reflexes are sufficiently recovered to prevent aspiration and that pulse oximetry verifies that the patient will maintain oxygenation on the discharge fraction of inspired oxygen ($FIO_2$). Also ensure that pulmonary function is adequate to overcome potential minor deterioration in ventilation or oxygenation. Before discharge, patients should be alert enough to evaluate their physical condition, communicate perceived problems, and summon assistance if necessary. Complete rewarming is not necessary, but resolution of shivering and discomfort is. Check that intravascular volume and peripheral perfusion are adequate, and assess the need to void. Evaluate potential adverse surgical sequelae or complications from preexisting conditions like coronary artery disease (CAD), diabetes, or bronchospastic disease.

## Late Interventions

Assess the peak impact of late therapeutic interventions before discharge. After discontinuing supplemental oxygen ($O_2$), observe for 15 minutes to detect unexpected hypoxemia with room air ventilation. Patients should be observed for at least 15 minutes for cardiovascular or ventilatory side effects of administered medications (eg, narcotics and sedatives, antihypertensives, calcium channel or β-adrenergic blockers, antidysrhythmics). Observation is also necessary after reinforcement of regional analgesic techniques.

## Postponement of Discharge

In an ideal setting, every patient should be discharged from the PACU by an anesthesiologist who uses consistent criteria to evaluate the anesthetic, the PACU course, and the patient's condition (Table 6-3). If patients are transferred from the PACU based on a discharge scoring system, have a knowledgeable physician clear the patient's condition before discharge from the facility or within a few hours of admission to a patient floor.

Consider the patient's destination, especially for an ambulatory patient who will be leaving the medical facility. Remember, the intensity and scope of care decrease significantly when a patient is discharged to anywhere but a special care unit. If doubt remains about a patient's viability outside the PACU, either postpone the discharge or transfer the patient to a specialized unit for extended care and monitoring.

## PAIN CONTROL

### What Is an Acceptable Approach to Postoperative Pain Management?

Control of postoperative pain is a high priority for both anesthesiologists and patients.[22] The clinical endpoint for postoperative analgesic therapy is relief of surgical pain without undesired side effects.

**TABLE 6-3.** Criteria for Discharge From a Postanesthesia Care Unit*

**General**
Oriented to time, place, and surgical procedure
Follows simple instructions
Adequate strength and mobility for minimal self-sufficiency
Suitable control of nausea and vomiting
Appropriate appearance without cyanosis or splotches
Control of acute surgical complications (bleeding, edema, diminished pulses)
Status is appropriate for destination
Ambulate without dizziness, hypotension, or support (ambulatory patients)
Ability to drink or eat if deemed appropriate (ambulatory patients)

**Airway Maintenance**
Adequate level of consciousness
Protective reflexes (swallow, gag) intact
Absence of stridor, retraction, or other signs of obstruction
Assistance not needed for airway support

**Ventilation and Oxygenation**
Spontaneous ventilatory rate >10, <30
Forced vital capacity about twice tidal volume
Adequate ability to cough and clear secretions
Qualitatively acceptable work of breathing

**Systemic Blood Pressure, Heart Rate and Rhythm**
Within ±20% resting preoperative value
Relatively constant for at least 30 min
Acceptable intravascular volume status
Resolution or clearance of any new arrhythmia
Suspicion of myocardial ischemia clarified

**Renal Function**
Urine output >30 mL/h (catheterized patients)
Appropriate color and appearance of urine, notation of hematuria
Follow-up orders if spontaneous voiding has not occurred

**Metabolic, Laboratory Values**
Acceptable hematocrit for hydration, blood loss and potential blood loss
Appropriate blood glucose and electrolyte status
Chest radiograph, electrocardiogram, and other tests reviewed

**Analgesia**
Ability to localize and identify intensity of surgical pain
Adequate analgesia 15–20 min since last narcotic
Appropriate orders for analgesics at destination

*Clinical judgment should supersede guidelines because every patient will not meet these criteria. If any doubt exists about a patient's viability beyond the PACU, discharge should be delayed.

Create an analgesic continuum for each patient that matches the "discomfort curve" for the procedure. In a study of postoperative pain in 10 008 ambulatory patients, 5.3% related severe pain in the PACU, but only 1.7% reported severe pain in the discharge area. Surprisingly, 5.3% related severe pain again 24 hours after surgery[23] (Fig. 6-2). Careful planning of analgesic requirements and medication transitions can provide seamless pain control for all patients.

### How Should the Intensity and Severity of Pain Be Assessed?

#### Intensity

The intensity of pain after a given surgical procedure is affected by surgical skill, anesthetic technique, and the individual patient's pain tolerance. Postoperative pain is neither uniform nor homogeneous. The intensity and nature of pain differ between movement and rest.[24] Postoperative pain is often perceived as being relatively intense for the first 2 or 3 postoperative days despite analgesic regimens. The correlation

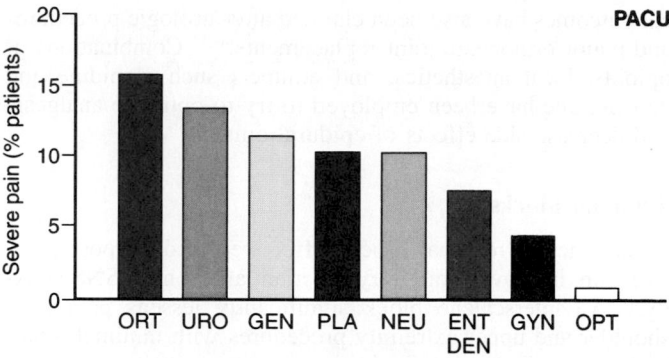

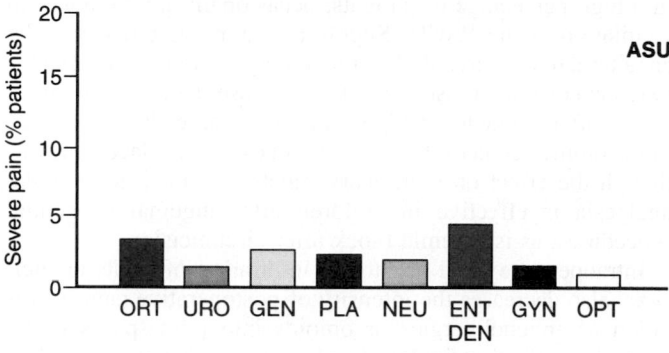

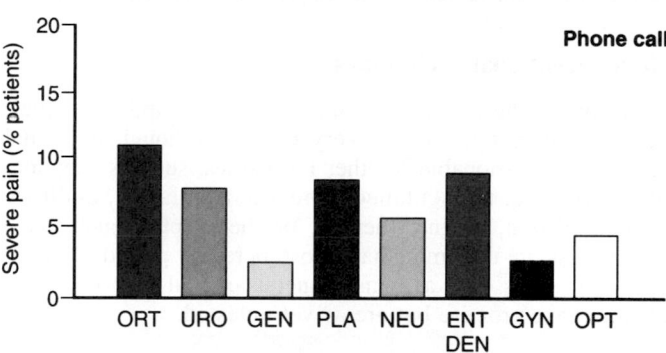

**FIGURE 6–2.** Percentage of patients with severe pain in the PACU, in the ASU, and during a 24-hour postanesthesia telephone call. ASU, ambulatory surgery unit; DEN, dental; ENT, ear, nose, and throat; GEN, general surgery; GYN, gynecologic; NEU, neurosurgical; OPT, ophthalmologic; ORT, orthopedic; PACU, postanesthesia care unit; PLA plastic; URO, urologic. (From Chung F, Ritchie E, Su J. Postoperative pain in ambulatory surgery. *Anesth Analg.* 1997;85:808.)

between cognitive perception of postoperative pain and sympathetic nervous system (SNS) response is unpredictable because of cultural, psychological, and cardiovascular variations among patients. Some patients exhibit hypertension, tachycardia, and ectopic cardiac complexes on the ECG with minimal complaint of discomfort. Others perceive severe pain without evidence of unusual autonomic nervous system tone.

Inadequate postoperative analgesia is a major source of preoperative fear and of postoperative dissatisfaction for surgical patients.[25] In the PACU, well-meaning practitioners frequently misjudge an individual patient's degree of postoperative pain. Inexperienced nurses tend to overestimate the amount of discomfort, whereas the experienced tend to underestimate.[26] Either error generates a level of analgesia that does not match the patient's needs. Patients are sometimes undermedicated to avoid potential side effects of high-dose

narcotics. The individual with the incision is usually the most proficient at assessing postoperative pain. The analgesic regimen is successful when the patient agrees that it is.

## Appropriateness of Pain

Before medicating a patient, make sure the nature and degree of pain are consistent with the operative procedure and anesthetic technique. This helps to avoid inadvertently masking signs of an evolving surgical complication or unrelated condition.

Remember that central nervous system (CNS) manifestations of hypoxemia, respiratory acidemia, or cerebral hypoperfusion often mimic signs of postoperative pain, especially after general anesthesia. Administration of parenteral analgesic or sedative medication can acutely exacerbate hypoventilation or hypotension, leading to cardiorespiratory collapse. Careful assessment of arousal and orientation, as well as systemic perfusion pressure and minute ventilation, usually identifies these patients.

## Fear and Anxiety

Fear, anxiety, or agitation often accentuates a patient's reaction to pain during emergence from anesthesia. Titration of intravenous diazepam or midazolam decreases these psychogenic components, although benzodiazepines can delay discharge somewhat and may paradoxically increase opioid requirements through central actions on γ-aminobutyric acid receptors.

Be sure to differentiate between analgesic and sedative requirements. Opiates are ineffective sedatives, whereas benzodiazepines and other sedatives do not provide significant analgesia. Choice of the wrong type of medication only increases unnecessary side effects. A calm and reassuring manner shown by the anesthesiologist and PACU personnel can be as important as sedative medication.

## Hypotension Following Pain Relief

Relief of pain or removal of offensive stimuli decreases SNS activity and level of arousal. This is generally positive because it controls postoperative hypertension, tachycardia, and agitation. Decreased venous adrenergic tone or narcotic-induced histamine release, however, can cause venous dilation, reduced cardiac output, and hypotension. Hypovolemic patients who rely on high levels of SNS activity to support their cardiovascular status are at especially high risk. Any normotensive or hypotensive patient with signs and symptoms of severe postoperative pain is likely hypovolemic, especially if tachycardia is present. A decreased level of arousal secondary to analgesia may interfere with airway patency or increase the risk for aspiration should regurgitation or vomiting occur.

## Narcotics

Surgical pain can be effectively treated with intermittent intravenous opiate administration using long-acting agents such as morphine.[27] Shorter acting narcotics such as fentanyl may be more appropriate in ambulatory settings,[28] but shorter duration of action can leave patients with inadequate analgesia after discharge.[29] Large doses of narcotics may be required by patients with high levels of preoperative pain or with tolerance from chronic opioid or alcohol use.[30] The endpoint is safe relief of pain, not a dosage threshold.

Intravenous narcotic titration achieves a safe, appropriate level of analgesia with minimal risk for respiratory or cardiovascular depression. Onset time and peak effects are most predictable with intravenous administration. Intravenous opiate loading is important for the transition to patient-controlled analgesia (PCA), a widely used postoperative modality. Make sure that the physician responsible for regulating postoperative PCA is familiar with the patient's intraoperative and PACU narcotic tally.

## Alternate Routes of Opioid Administration

Intramuscular administration of analgesics is less desirable because onset is delayed, uptake is unpredictable in hypothermic patients, and larger doses are required. Also, a high percentage of intramuscular injections are actually subcutaneous, leading to even poorer predictability. Selected children may benefit from rectal or nasal analgesics. Oral and transdermal routes are relatively ineffective during immediate postoperative recovery.

## Nonnarcotic Analgesics

Nonnarcotic analgesics generally cannot replace narcotics for PACU applications unless surgical pain is minimal. Supplementation of narcotic analgesia with agents like ibuprofen, acetaminophen, ketamine, or clonidine, however, reduces narcotic requirements and side effects.[31–34] Ketorolac is an effective analgesic and antiinflammatory agent, although its antiplatelet properties may increase the risk for postoperative hemorrhage in some patients.[35,36] The addition of ketorolac may decrease ischemic events in patients with CAD through both analgesia and antiplatelet actions.[37] N-methyl-D-aspartate antagonists such as dextromethorphan are claimed beneficial for inflammatory components of pain.[38] Be aware that hypotension can occur after administration or adjuncts. Elimination of offending stimuli through repositioning, extubation of the trachea, or removal of a urinary catheter also helps decrease postoperative discomfort.

## *What Alternative Techniques Are Useful?*

### Epidural and Subarachnoid Narcotics

Epidural or subarachnoid narcotics can yield prolonged postoperative analgesia in selected patients.[39–41] Both immediate and delayed ventilatory depression, however, can occur secondary to vascular uptake and rostral cerebrospinal fluid (CSF) spread; thus, careful ventilatory monitoring is important.[39,42,43] Nausea and pruritus are bothersome side effects. Nausea usually resolves with administration of antiemetics, whereas pruritus often responds to naloxone infusion. Ondansetron has been proposed to treat pruritus as well as opiate-induced nausea.[44] The addition of local anesthetics to epidural narcotic regimens augments postoperative analgesia but adds the risk for motor blockade or subarachnoid injection.

Epidural techniques are particularly useful after major abdominal or thoracic surgery and to facilitate weaning patients with morbid obesity or severe chronic obstructive lung disease (COLD) from mechanical ventilation. Improvements in surgi-

cal outcomes have also been claimed after urologic procedures and major orthopedic joint replacements.[45,46] Combinations of opioids, local anesthetics, and adjuncts such as clonidine and neostigmine have been employed to try to optimize analgesia and decrease side effects of epidural opiates.[40]

### Regional Blocks

Long-acting regional blocks effectively reduce postoperative pain, improve ventilatory function, and control SNS activity.[43] An interscalene block significantly lessens pain after shoulder and upper extremity procedures with minimal motor impairment. Ipsilateral diaphragmatic paresis, however, occurs in a high percentage of patients, occasionally interfering with ventilation in the PACU. Suprascapular nerve block may be an alternative to avoid this potentially serious side effect.[47] Percutaneous intercostal blocks decrease analgesic requirements after thoracic or high abdominal procedures, such as thoracotomy, cholecystectomy, or chest tube placement, although the effect on pulmonary function is unclear.[48] Caudal analgesia is effective in children after inguinal or genital procedures, as is a penile block after circumcision.

Intraoperative local anesthetic infiltration of joints or incisions also decreases the intensity of postoperative pain. Instillation of anticholinergics or opioids into joint spaces is described as effective for low-level postoperative analgesia.[49]

### Nonconventional Techniques

Positive auditory input during surgery may influence analgesic requirements and recovery course, although its actual efficacy is questionable.[50] Other modalities, such as acupuncture, hypnosis, transcutaneous nerve stimulation, auditory overstimulation, magnet therapy, or therapeutic touch, have limited use in the immediate postoperative period. Cutting edge modalities, such as transcutaneous cranial electrical stimulation, have promise but are as yet untested.[51]

### Summary

When PCA, prolonged epidural analgesia, sustained regional analgesia, or multimodal analgesia is used for postoperative pain control, planning the therapy and assessing the risks are essential. Initiate the analgesic regimen at the induction of surgical anesthesia and continue it throughout the anesthetic procedure and the PACU course. If an extended modality fails, exercise caution before switching to a second therapy in order to minimize the complexity of management and the risk for complications after transfer from the PACU.

## POSTOPERATIVE PULMONARY FUNCTION

Mechanical, hemodynamic, and pharmacologic factors related to surgery and anesthesia profoundly affect postoperative pulmonary function.[52] Predicting which patients are at risk for which complications is difficult. Preexisting conditions, such as obesity, heavy smoking, sleep apnea, severe asthma, and COLD, increase the risk for postoperative ventilatory events.[53] Preoperative pulmonary function testing has limited predictive value for postoperative complications,[42,54] perhaps with the exception of bronchospasm in smokers.[55]

## *How Is Postoperative Oxygenation Assessed?*

Systemic arterial partial pressure of oxygen ($PaO_2$) is a reliable index of $O_2$ transfer from alveolar gas to pulmonary venous blood. Arterial hemoglobin $O_2$ saturation measured by pulse oximetry ($SpO_2$) indicates adequacy of arterial oxygenation but yields little information on alveolar-arterial gradients.[56] Accuracy of pulse oximetry is also affected by changes in hemoglobin capacity (eg, carboxyhemoglobin, methemoglobin) and by patient motion.[57] Mixed venous $O_2$ content, venous hemoglobin saturation, and arterial pH are useful as indicators of peripheral $O_2$ delivery and consumption.

Even though $PaO_2$ may be adequate, arterial perfusion pressure, cardiac output, or distribution of systemic blood flow may not be sufficient to maintain tissue oxygenation. Tissue ischemia can also occur with normal $PaO_2$ secondary to anemia, hemoglobin dissociation abnormalities, peripheral shunting, and poisoning with carbon monoxide (CO) or cyanide.

Pulse oximetry monitoring is essential throughout the PACU stay and especially after discontinuation of supplemental $O_2$. Neither careful clinical observation nor assessment of cognitive function reliably detects hypoxemia in PACU patients.[58,59]

## Acceptable Limits

In the PACU, an acceptable lower limit for $PaO_2$ at a given $FIO_2$ must be estimated for each patient. This estimate may be based on the preoperative $SpO_2$. Reduction of $PaO_2$ to <60 mm Hg causes significant arterial hemoglobin desaturation, although tissue $O_2$ delivery can still be adequate. Increasing the $PaO_2$ to >100 mm Hg offers little benefit because hemoglobin saturation is only minimally increased and the volume of additional $O_2$ dissolved in serum is negligible. Maintaining the $PaO_2$ between 80 and 100 mm Hg (saturation >93%-95%) ensures adequate arterial oxygen content with minimal intervention.

Higher $PaO_2$ levels have a beneficial effect in patients with CO poisoning or severe anemia. During routine postoperative mechanical ventilation, if the $PaO_2$ exceeds 80 mm Hg ($SpO_2$ >93%) with a 0.4 $FIO_2$ and 5 cm $H_2O$ positive end-expiratory pressure (PEEP) or continuous positive airway pressure (CPAP), patients usually sustain adequate oxygenation after tracheal extubation.

## *What Postoperative Factors Cause a Decreased Alveolar Oxygen Partial Pressure?*

Many factors reduce arterial hemoglobin saturation with $O_2$ after surgery (Table 6–4).

## Respiratory Depression and Apnea

If uptake of $O_2$ from the alveoli exceeds delivery by fresh gas ventilation, the alveolar partial pressure of oxygen ($PAO_2$) and the $PaO_2$ both fall. Moderate hypoventilation as seen with respiratory center depression from opioid administration usually causes hypercarbia before hypoxemia, especially when

**TABLE 6–4.** Causes of Hypoxemia in the Postanesthesia Care Unit

**Ventilation-Perfusion Mismatch: Distribution of Ventilation**
   Atelectasis secondary to reduced functional residual capacity
   Hydrostatic pulmonary edema and increased lung water
   Postobstructive pulmonary edema
   Mucus plugging and airway obstruction
   Mainstem intubation and lobar bronchus occlusion
   Aspiration
**Ventilation-Perfusion Mismatch: Distribution of Perfusion**
   Variations in pulmonary artery pressure
   Gravitational effects secondary to positioning
   Pulmonary arteriolar dilation from drugs, sepsis, cirrhosis
   Decreased hypoxic pulmonary vasoconstriction
   Varying airway pressure
**Reduced $PaO_2$**
   Severe hypoventilation
   Decreased hypoxic ventilatory drive
   Airway obstruction
**Reduced Mixed Venous $PO_2$**
   Accentuates impact of ventilation-perfusion mismatch

patients are given supplemental oxygen. Reduced $PaO_2$ and arterial $O_2$ desaturation are also caused by periodic apnea. Cessation of fresh gas delivery during total apnea causes a rapid reduction of the $PaO_2$ and severe hypoxemia. The rate of $PaO_2$ decline varies with age, body habitus, degree of underlying illness, and initial $PaO_2$[60] (Fig. 6–3). If obesity or surgical factors reduce the functional residual capacity (FRC), the decreased volume of $O_2$ available in the lungs accelerates the development of hypoxemia.

## Suppression of Hypoxic Drive

Normally, the carotid bodies increase in ventilation in response to a fall in the $PaO_2$. PACU patients are at greater risk for hypoxemia caused by hypoventilation because opiates, sedatives, and residual anesthetics suppress this hypoxic respiratory drive. A portion of the hypoxic drive is mediated by cholinergic pathways; thus, residual neuromuscular paralysis may also suppress its effectiveness.[61] Although rare in postoperative patients, hypoventilation due to supplemental $O_2$ in patients with severe COLD is also caused by hypoxic drive suppression.

## Airway Obstruction

Partial upper airway obstruction or an increase in small airway resistance usually does not reduce ventilation enough to affect $PaO_2$, especially if supplemental $O_2$ is being administered. Complete airway obstruction by soft tissues or laryngospasm leads to rapid depletion of alveolar $O_2$, as does a severe increase in airway resistance that prevents effective ventilation. The rate of $PaO_2$ decline during severe hypoventilation is patient dependent but rapid.[60]

## Diffusion Hypoxia

At the end of a general anesthetic, outpouring of relatively insoluble nitrous oxide into the alveoli can displace alveolar gas. The $PAO_2$ can fall to dangerous levels if a patient is hypoventilating or breathing ambient air. Administration of 100% $O_2$ to dilute the alveolar nitrous oxide maintains $PAO_2$ and minimizes risk for hypoxemia. This problem usually oc-

## TIME TO HEMOGLOBIN DESATURATION WITH INITIAL F$_{AO_2}$ = 0.87

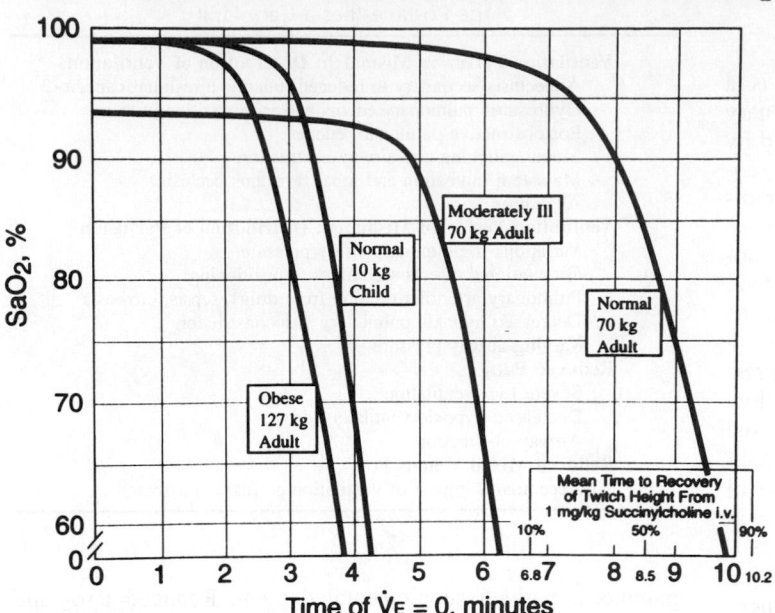

**FIGURE 6–3.** Rate of SpO$_2$ decline versus duration of apnea in various types of patients. FAO$_2$, fraction of alveolar O$_2$; SaO$_2$, oxygen saturation, arterial; V̇E, expired volume per unit time. (From Benumof JL, Dagg R, Benumof R. Critical hemoglobin desaturation will occur before return to an unparalyzed state following 1 mg/kg intravenous succinylcholine. *Anesthesiology.* 1997;87:979.)

curs in the OR but may present in the PACU if a patient is hypoventilating on admission.

### How Does Maldistribution of Ventilation Cause Ventilation-Perfusion Mismatch and Postoperative Hypoxemia?

Ventilation-perfusion (V̇/Q̇) mismatch resulting from loss of volume in dependent lung areas commonly causes hypoxemia in the PACU. Reduction of the FRC decreases radial traction on small airways, promoting airway collapse and atelectasis.[62] Hypoventilation of dependent lung is particularly damaging because gravity directs pulmonary blood flow to these poorly ventilated areas.[63] V̇/Q̇ mismatching can progressively deteriorate for 36 hours after surgery.

### What Factors Reduce the Functional Residual Capacity?

#### Age and Chronic Lung Disease

Older patients and those with COLD are at increased risk for reduced FRC after surgery because they already have lower airway traction and some airway closure at end expiration.

#### Obesity and Increased Intraabdominal Pressure

Obesity or increased intraabdominal pressure decreases lung volume by limiting diaphragmatic excursion and lung expansion. Low pulmonary compliance, caused by increased lung water, atelectasis, pleural effusions, or restrictive disorders, also promotes loss of lung volume. During upper abdominal surgery, peritoneal distention, retraction, packing, and external abdominal compression by leaning surgical assistants also contribute.[64] The prone, lithotomy, and Trendelenburg positions are disadvantageous in obese patients.

### Thoracic Operations

Reduction of FRC and V̇/Q̇ mismatching frequently occur during thoracic surgery, especially with one-lung anesthesia.[65] Direct surgical compression, the weight of unsupported mediastinum, and displacement of the paralyzed dependent diaphragm into the chest cavity reduce dependent lung volume. Gravity and lymphatic obstruction lead to accumulation of interstitial fluid, which accentuates V̇/Q̇ mismatching and causes a "down lung syndrome," which appears as unilateral pulmonary edema on a chest radiograph. Increased blood flow through the dependent lung worsens intrapulmonary shunting, especially when volatile anesthetic agents interfere with hypoxic pulmonary vasoconstriction (HPV).

### Pulmonary Edema

Acute postoperative pulmonary edema caused by overhydration, ventricular dysfunction, or increased capillary permeability interferes with V̇/Q̇ matching and also with O$_2$ diffusion. Edema and loss of lung volume also occur after strong inspiratory efforts against an obstructed airway (negative pressure pulmonary edema).[66]

### Miscellaneous Causes of Decreased Lung Volume

Pneumothorax, hemothorax, pulmonary contusion, and intrapulmonary hemorrhage all alter V̇/Q̇ matching and promote hypoxemia. Mucus plugging or severe bronchospasm promotes hypoventilation of distal air spaces, as does obstruction of larger airways by mainstem bronchial intubation, foreign body aspiration, or external compression. Partial right mainstem intubation and right upper lobe collapse are a frequently overlooked cause of postoperative hypoxemia.

### What Treatment Is Indicated for Maldistribution of Ventilation?

Conservative measures to restore lung volume in the PACU often produce improvement in arterial oxygenation. Deep ventilation, vigorous cough, and chest physiotherapy mobilize secretions, increase FRC, and acclimate a patient to incisional discomfort associated with deep inspiration. Incentive spirometry is helpful to maintain FRC. Intermittent positive pressure breathing techniques are probably less effective, but CPAP is a valuable adjunct that may be applied with a mask or nasal prongs. If possible, obese patients should recover in a semisitting position to reduce the pressure of abdominal contents against the diaphragm.

### Analgesia

Pain with deep inspiration encourages rapid, shallow breathing, which provides adequate minute ventilation but fails to restore and maintain lung volume. Adequate analgesia is vital, especially after upper abdominal or thoracic surgery. Continuous regional analgesia is helpful in weaning patients with limited pulmonary reserve from ventilatory support.[42]

### Continuous Positive Airway Pressure or Positive End-Expiratory Pressure

CPAP is effective for restoring and maintaining FRC. It can be delivered at low levels by face or nasal mask for several hours to maintain the $PaO_2$ until the loss of lung volume resolves. Lack of patient acceptance or persistent arterial hypoxemia, however, may necessitate tracheal intubation for delivery of CPAP. Usually, 5 to 10 cm $H_2O$ of CPAP or PEEP supports $PaO_2$ without causing hypotension or increased intracranial pressure. Positive pressure ventilation should be added only if the arterial partial pressure of carbon dioxide ($PaCO_2$), the arterial pH, and the work of breathing indicate ventilatory insufficiency.

If the $PaO_2$ does not improve with 5 to 10 cm $H_2O$ of positive pressure, the cause of hypoxemia should be reevaluated. Higher positive pressure is seldom effective unless serious pulmonary pathology, such as acute respiratory distress syndrome (ARDS), is present. Pressures >10 to 15 cm $H_2O$ cause cardiovascular compromise and an increased incidence of barotrauma.[67] High airway pressure may worsen $\dot{V}/\dot{Q}$ matching by increasing vascular resistance in compliant lung, thereby diverting blood flow to poorly ventilated areas.

### Intubation

In general, intubated patients should exhale against some positive pressure. Tracheal intubation eliminates so-called physiologic PEEP, which probably helps to maintain lung volume during spontaneous ventilation. Exposing an intubated patient to ambient pressure can lead to gradual reduction of the FRC and arterial hypoxemia. Young, slender patients can tolerate short periods of ambient pressure and are able to restore the FRC easily after extubation. The routine use of PEEP or CPAP in such healthy patients is probably not indicated.

### Is Postoperative Oxygenation Affected by Pulmonary Perfusion?

The distribution of pulmonary blood flow is determined by PA and venous pressures and by arteriolar and capillary resistance. These factors are affected by airway pressure, gravity, lung volume, and cardiovascular dynamics. Blood flow distribution is also modulated by HPV, which diverts flow away from poorly ventilated air spaces with low $PaO_2$.[68] In postoperative patients, inappropriate distribution of pulmonary perfusion interferes with $\dot{V}/\dot{Q}$ matching and causes hypoxemia.

### Changes in Pulmonary Artery Pressure

In the PACU, increased adrenergic tone caused by pain, hypoxemia, or acidemia can increase cardiac output and pulmonary vascular resistance, thus elevating PA pressure. High PA pressure can increase blood flow to nondependent lung areas, through the bronchial circulation, and through pulmonary arteriovenous anastomoses, thereby interfering with $\dot{V}/\dot{Q}$ matching.

A reduction of PA pressure can also interfere with $\dot{V}/\dot{Q}$ matching. If perfusion to the upper parenchyma is compromised by decreased PA pressure while low compliance and atelectasis in dependent lung redistributes fresh ventilation to upper parenchyma, regional $\dot{V}/\dot{Q}$ mismatch results. A low PA pressure also reduces the differences in flow resistance among areas of the vascular bed, impairing the effectiveness of HPV. HPV varies with PA pressure in a bimodal fashion.

### Position Changes

Position affects oxygenation if gravity augments blood flow to areas with reduced ventilation. Placing a patient with a unilateral ventilatory deficiency such as pneumonia or a mainstem intubation lateral with the poorly ventilated lung dependent can seriously reduce $PaO_2$; placing the poorly ventilated lung in a nondependent position can improve arterial oxygenation. Placing a diseased lung in a nondependent position, however, increases the risk for drainage of purulent or obstructing material to the unaffected, dependent lung.

### Changes in Airway Pressure and Lung Volume

Pulmonary blood flow distribution is also affected by airway pressure. Positive pressure lung inflation may increase resistance in both intra-alveolar and extra-alveolar vessels, whereas spontaneous negative pressure inspiration probably decreases extra-alveolar vascular resistance. A decrease in capillary transmural pressure gradients caused by reduction of dependent lung volume may increase vascular resistance and improve $\dot{V}/\dot{Q}$ matching by diverting blood away from poorly ventilated areas. Redistribution of flow to nondependent lung, however, could worsen matching. Clinically, the net impact of lung volume changes on distribution of pulmonary perfusion is difficult to predict.

### Drug and Humoral Effects

Inhalation anesthetics or sympathomimetic drugs that alter pulmonary vascular pressures also affect $\dot{V}/\dot{Q}$ matching. Nitrous oxide and ketamine cause direct pulmonary vascular constriction, whereas nitroglycerin, phentolamine, and sodium nitroprusside cause pulmonary vasodilation. Inhalation anesthetics and vasodilators impair HPV, contributing to an increased alveolar-arterial $O_2$ gradient during general anesthesia. The effects of anesthetics on HPV persist well into the recovery period.

Antihypertensives and β-mimetic drugs probably interfere with $\dot{V}/\dot{Q}$ matching and oxygenation. Circulating humoral substances related to inadequate hepatic metabolism appear to cause poor $\dot{V}/\dot{Q}$ matching and hypoxemia in patients with cirrhosis of the liver. Endotoxin impairs HPV, contributing to hypoxemia in patients with systemic sepsis.

### Therapy

$\dot{V}/\dot{Q}$ abnormalities are more easily resolved by improving the distribution of ventilation than by manipulating pulmonary blood flow. Maintenance of a relatively normal PA pressure probably optimizes the perfusion component of $\dot{V}/\dot{Q}$ matching. Avoiding the placement of severely underventilated lung regions in a dependent position improves oxygenation. Weaning from β-mimetic or vasodilatory medications may also improve $Pa_{O_2}$, but the therapeutic benefits of the medications usually require that they be continued.

## Does Desaturation of Mixed Venous Blood Contribute to Arterial Hypoxemia?

The mixed venous partial pressure of $O_2$ ($P\bar{v}_{O_2}$) varies with cardiac output, arterial $O_2$ content, tissue $O_2$ extraction, and the proportional contributions of different tissue beds to mixed venous blood. If $Pa_{O_2}$ decreases or global tissue extraction increases, the $P\bar{v}_{O_2}$ falls. Shivering and hypermetabolism lower $P\bar{v}_{O_2}$ primarily by increasing tissue $O_2$ consumption.

A low $P\bar{v}_{O_2}$ amplifies the impact of $\dot{V}/\dot{Q}$ mismatch on $Pa_{O_2}$ because blood with lower $P\bar{v}_{O_2}$ flowing through poorly ventilated lung causes a larger proportional reduction of $Pa_{O_2}$ after equilibration in pulmonary veins. Reduced $P\bar{v}_{O_2}$ also increases the extraction of $O_2$ from alveoli, accelerating the decline in $PA_{O_2}$ if hypoventilation or airway obstruction reduces fresh gas delivery to the alveoli. The impact of low $P\bar{v}_{O_2}$ can be attenuated with supplemental $O_2$.

## Is Oxygen-Carrying Capacity an Important Factor in Postoperative Oxygenation?

### Anemia

Preoperative anemia and intraoperative hemorrhage determine how low a patient's red blood cell mass and oxygen-carrying capacity fall after surgery. Reduction of hematocrit caused by dilution has less impact on oxygen-carrying capacity. The hematocrit at which oxygen delivery becomes insufficient to match tissue needs is highly patient dependent and varies with cardiac reserve, oxygen consumption, hemoglobin dissociation, $Pa_{O_2}$, blood flow distribution, and other factors. For each patient, there is a minimal hematocrit below which tissues are forced to use inefficient anaerobic metabolism, generating a lactic acidemia. Patients with vascular disease are at increased risk for vital organ ischemia as hematocrit falls.

### Carbon Monoxide Poisoning

Hemoglobin reversibly binds CO with 200 times the affinity of oxygen. Resulting carboxyhemoglobin prevents the binding of oxygen and impedes the dissociation of oxygen molecules from unaffected oxyhemoglobin. During general anesthesia,

patients can be exposed to CO generated by a reaction between inhalation anesthetics and dry $CO_2$-absorbing agents, such as soda lime and Baralyme. Overall incidence of CO exposure is estimated as 0.26%, but risk is nearly doubled to 0.46% for first cases of the day and to a frightening 2.9% for first cases performed in peripheral anesthetizing locations.[69,70]

Hypoxia related to CO poisoning is insidious and difficult to recognize. Symptoms of low to moderate CO exposure include irritability, altered visual and motor skills, headache, nausea, and vomiting. All these nonspecific symptoms are frequently exhibited by patients in the PACU. In contrast to desaturated hemoglobin, carboxyhemoglobin seldom causes cyanosis. Pulse oximeters read carboxyhemoglobin as oxyhemoglobin; hence, $Sp_{O_2}$ is falsely high. The $Pa_{O_2}$ can be high on ABG analysis even though little oxygen is being carried to the periphery. In short, a PACU patient can be severely hypoxic and still appear well oxygenated by routine indices. A laboratory co-oximeter differentiates between carboxyhemoglobin and oxyhemoglobin values.

## Should Oxygen Be Administered Postoperatively?

The risk for postoperative hypoxemia leads some practitioners to administer supplemental $O_2$ prophylactically to all patients during initial recovery, including those given regional anesthetics. The rationale is that oxygen is a benign, low-cost drug that is beneficial to a large number of patients. Other clinicians choose to administer $O_2$ only to patients at high risk for hypoxemia or as necessary based on $Sp_{O_2}$ readings.[71,72] The rationale for avoiding oxygen in patients who will not clearly benefit is the cost associated with the therapy, the patient's dislike of wearing oxygen apparatus, and the minimal risk from hyperoxia and oxygen equipment. Hypoventilating patients may also be more easily identified as the $Sp_{O_2}$ decreases.

### Value of Supplemental Oxygen

There is no correct answer. The value of supplemental oxygen in some patients is clear. Increasing $O_2$ content in the FRC delays the onset of serious hypoxemia caused by airway obstruction or hypoventilation,[73] so that oxygen has a prophylactic value. Supplemental $O_2$ often improves hypoxemia caused by $\dot{V}/\dot{Q}$ mismatching, although the impact of a given $FI_{O_2}$ is variable. A patient's actual $FI_{O_2}$ is difficult to predict with use of face masks, tents, or nasal prongs because ambient air is entrained during inspiration.[74] Hypoxemia caused by true shunting is often not improved by supplemental $O_2$ because shunted blood is not exposed to increased $FI_{O_2}$, whereas blood passing ventilated alveoli is already fully saturated. Hypoxemia caused by low $\dot{V}/\dot{Q}$ units improves because high $FI_{O_2}$ augments $O_2$ delivery to marginally ventilated air spaces.

If anemia or carboxyhemoglobinemia has reduced the oxygen-carrying capacity, supplemental oxygen helps maximize the saturation of available hemoglobin. Increased $Pa_{O_2}$ also displaces CO from hemoglobin, although this effect is relatively minor with the low $FI_{O_2}$ levels usually administered in the PACU. Administration of 100% oxygen markedly accelerates the elimination of CO. In severe cases, hyperbaric oxygen therapy may be indicated.

It is difficult to predict which patients will become hypoxemic in the PACU or when the hypoxemia will occur. Obese patients, those with lung disease, children with perioperative upper respiratory infections or adenotonsillar hypertrophy, patients recovering from upper abdominal or thoracic surgical procedures, and patients with preoperative hypoxemia are probably at increased risk.[75–77] The incidence of hypoxemia in postoperative patients is high. In one recent study of PACU patients placed on room air, 30% of children <1 year old, 20% of children 1 to 3 years old, 14% of children 3 to 14 years old, and 7.8% of adults had hemoglobin saturations fall below 90%, with many in each group falling below 85%[78] (Fig. 6–4). Hypoxemia frequently occurs after regional anesthesia[43,44]; however, administration of supplemental $O_2$ in the PACU does not guarantee that hypoxemia will not develop.[79]

### Risks of Oxygen: Resorption Atelectasis and Pulmonary Oxygen Toxicity

Risk of oxygen administration is minimal. Some drying of nasal or oral mucosa may occur at higher flow rates, and placing a rigid oxygen mask near the eyes likely increases the incidence of corneal abrasion during emergence.

At an $FIO_2$ >0.8, replacement of inert nitrogen with $O_2$

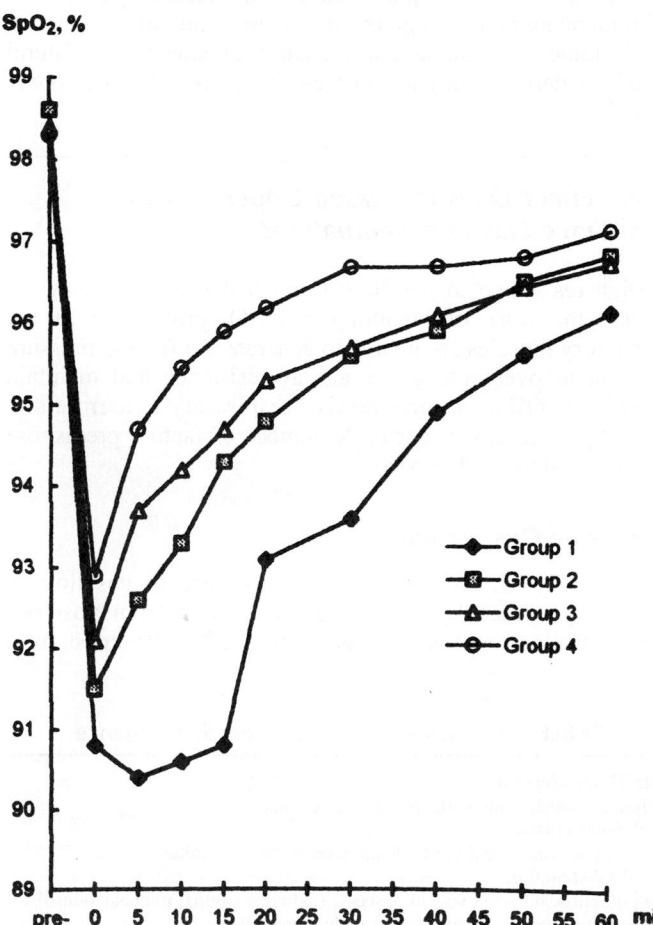

**SpO2, %**

**FIGURE 6–4.** $SpO_2$ versus time during the first hour in the postanesthesia care unit in various patients spontaneously ventilating on room air after general anesthesia (group 1, ages 0-1 year; group 2, 1-3 years; group 3, 3-14 years; group 4, 14-58 years). $SpO_2$, oxygen saturation as measured by pulse oximetry. (From Xue FS, Huang YG, Tong SY, et al. A comparative study of early postoperative hypoxemia in infants, children, and adults undergoing elective plastic surgery. *Anesth Analg.* 1996;83:709.)

in poorly ventilated alveoli may cause resorption atelectasis because oxygen is extracted from alveoli faster than it is replenished. Inspiration of 100% $O_2$ for 24 to 36 hours may generate early pulmonary $O_2$ toxicity, which can progress to alveolar epithelial degeneration and capillary leak pulmonary edema.[80] Severe hyperoxia can also precipitate grand mal seizures. Risk of $O_2$ toxicity is increased in patients undergoing hyperbaric $O_2$ therapy but is unchanged after bleomycin therapy.

Neither resorption atelectasis nor oxygen toxicity is of concern to most PACU patients. Nevertheless, $PaO_2$ should be maintained below 150 to 175 mm Hg, given adequate arterial saturation. The routine use of humidified $O_2$ yields little additional benefit unless tracheal intubation or tracheotomy inhibits natural humidification.

## POSTOPERATIVE VENTILATION

Effective alveolar ventilation delivers fresh gas to perfused alveoli and washes out a sufficient volume of $CO_2$ to match peripheral $CO_2$ production. Ventilation of dead space (ie, airways and nonperfused alveoli) does not participate in gas exchange. $PaCO_2$ rises if the amount of $CO_2$ excreted through ventilation falls below the amount of $CO_2$ produced per unit time.

### What Are the Physiologic Control Mechanisms?

Ventilation is regulated primarily by medullary center receptors that are sensitive to pericellular pH in CSF. When hypercarbia causes CSF acidosis, neural output increases the ventilatory rate and tidal volume, augmenting minute ventilation and reducing $PaCO_2$. Consequent resolution of CSF acidosis creates a negative feedback loop that keeps $PaCO_2$ relatively constant.

Minute ventilation also responds to peripheral chemoreceptors that guard against hypoxemia secondary to hypoventilation by monitoring carotid $PaO_2$. Respiratory rate, depth, and pattern may be further modulated by neural elements such as chest wall mechanoreceptors, parenchymal stretch receptors, and J-receptors. Subconscious and conscious cortical input can override these physiologic regulating mechanisms.[81]

### What Factors Reduce Ventilatory Drive?

Many factors increase $PaCO_2$ during the immediate postoperative period (Table 6–5).

### Drug-Induced Respiratory Depression

Residual effects of intravenous opioids or inhalational anesthetics blunt the ventilatory sensitivity to both hypercarbia and hypoxemia.[82,83] Sedatives depress ventilation through direct depression of ventilatory drives, synergistic actions with opiates or anesthetics, and blunting of the conscious will to ventilate.[84,85] Analgesic medications given in the PACU exert an additive depressant effect. The time, amount, and route of all respiratory depressant medications given to patients must

**TABLE 6–5.** Causes of Postoperative Hypoventilation and Hypercarbia

**Decreased Ventilatory Drive**
 Depression of pH drive by anesthetics, narcotics, or sedatives
 Suppression of hypoxic drive
 Abrupt withdrawal of noxious stimuli
 Sedation with decreased volitional will to ventilate
 Emergence of chronic drive problems (sleep apnea)
 Chronic $CO_2$ retention
 Intracranial pathology
**Increased Work of Breathing**
 Increased upper or small airway resistance
 Decreased lung compliance
 Decreased chest cavity compliance
 Increased intra-abdominal pressure and gastric distention
**Decreased Mechanical Capacity**
 Ventilatory muscle fatigue
 Neuromuscular paralysis
 Splinting against a painful incision
 Phrenic nerve paresis or anesthesia
 Chronic obstructive changes
 Recurrence of chronic neuromuscular weakness
**Increased Dead Space**
 Pulmonary air or thromboembolism
 Airway expansion secondary to continuous positive pressure
 Gas trapping secondary to airway resistance and high ventilation rates
 Acute respiratory distress syndrome with microvascular destruction
**Increased $CO_2$ Production**
 Reversal of neuromuscular relaxant and warming
 Increased work of breathing
 Shivering
 Fever and sepsis
 Hyperalimentation
 Malignant hyperthermia

be clearly documented. Mild respiratory acidemia is expected in postoperative patients. A cautious balance must be struck to establish a safe degree of postoperative ventilatory depression with an acceptable level of discomfort or anxiety.[86]

Patients suffering from abnormal $CO_2$ and pH responses associated with morbid obesity, chronic upper airway obstruction, chronic $CO_2$ retention, or sleep apnea disorders exhibit blunted $CO_2$ responses and are often sensitive to respiratory depressants. They are at increased risk for inadequate postoperative ventilation, especially if their hypoxic drive is suppressed by medications.[87]

Hypoventilation secondary to depressed ventilatory drive is often difficult to diagnose. Serious hypoventilation often begins insidiously during transfer to the PACU.[77] Intravenous narcotics administered toward the end of surgery can exert a peak ventilatory depressant effect in the PACU. Certain neuroleptic or opiate anesthetic techniques may generate delayed respiratory depression.[88] Medullary centers that regulate autonomic activity are also depressed; thus, usual SNS responses to acidemia and hypoxemia (eg, agitation, tachycardia, and hypertension) are blunted. $SpO_2$ is often maintained as $PaCO_2$ rises, especially in patients receiving supplemental oxygen. Patients may communicate lucidly and even complain of severe pain while suffering significant opioid-induced hypoventilation.[89] A high index of suspicion helps identify patients with depressed ventilatory drive.

## Reversal of Respiratory Depression

Careful titration of intravenous naloxone reverses respiratory depression from opioids without affecting analgesia. In-

travenous flumazenil counteracts depression from benzodiazepines.[90,91] Neither naloxone nor flumazenil effectively restores hypoxic drive in a sedated PACU patient.

## Decreased Level of Arousal

In addition to residual sedation, abrupt diminution of a noxious stimulus (eg, extubation of the trachea or administration of a postoperative regional analgesic block) reduces excitation that counteracts medication-induced respiratory depression. Hypoventilation or airway obstruction may result.

## Apnea of Prematurity

After anesthesia, the risk for apnea in preterm infants varies with postconceptional age[92] and preoperative hematocrit.[93] The type of anesthetic administered may influence the incidence of postoperative apnea and bradycardia. All preterm infants <60 weeks total age (gestational and postnatal) should be monitored for at least 12 hours after surgery and perhaps admitted overnight.[94]

## Neurologic Impairment

Hypoventilation or apnea can be the presenting symptom of intracranial hemorrhage or edema, especially after posterior fossa craniotomy. Damage to the carotid bodies after bilateral carotid endarterectomy sometimes ablates peripheral hypoxic drive.[95]

## *What Effect Does Increased Upper Airway Resistance Have on Ventilation?*

High resistance to gas flow through the upper airway increases the work of breathing and $CO_2$ production. If the inspiratory muscles are unable to generate a sufficient pressure gradient to overcome upper airway resistance and maintain alveolar ventilation, progressive respiratory acidemia and acute hypoxemia can occur. A number of factors predispose to this problem (Table 6–6).

## Soft Tissue Obstruction

In the PACU, increased airway resistance to gas flow is commonly caused by pharyngeal obstruction from posterior tongue displacement or soft tissue collapse.[96,97] Weakness from

**TABLE 6–6.** Causes of Increased Airway Resistance

**Soft Tissue Necrosis**
 Tongue, tonsils, adenoids, hematoma, edema
**Laryngeal Obstruction**
 Laryngospasm, vocal cord edema, foreign body, vomitus
**Fixed Obstruction**
 Epiglottitis, retropharyngeal abscess, Ludwig's angina, tracheal stenosis, extrinsic compression, kinked endotracheal tube
**Bronchospasm**
 Suctioning, aspiration, tracheal intubation, allergic reactions, pulmonary embolization
**Airway Edema**
 Asthma, smoking
**Loss of Radial Traction**
 Chronic obstructive lung disease

residual neuromuscular relaxation[98] or myasthenia gravis[99] is sometimes contributory but seldom significantly compromises airway patency.

Immediate relief of airway obstruction is essential. Simple maneuvers, such as jaw lift, mandible elevation, lateral positioning, or placement of an oropharyngeal or nasopharyngeal airway, usually relieve pharyngeal obstruction. Improving the level of consciousness is useful.

Edema worsens postoperative airway obstruction by soft tissues, especially after carotid endarterectomy, thyroid surgery, or other procedures on the neck.[100] Nebulized vasoconstrictors may help to a limited degree, but systemic steroids have little effect. Patients with C1 esterase inhibitor deficiency can develop severe, refractory angioneurotic edema after even slight surgical trauma to the upper airway.[101]

Pathologic conditions, such as epiglottitis, pharyngeal abscess, or tumor encroachment on the airway, generate acute, profound obstruction to airflow. Any extrinsic upper airway compression from an expanding neck hematoma or dressing should be relieved.

### Laryngeal and Tracheal Obstruction

Edema of the vocal cords, glottis, or tracheal mucosa sometimes reduces upper airway caliber after extubation of the trachea, bronchoscopy, or airway surgery.[102] This problem is common in children. Complete obstruction from edema at this level is rare, and airway compromise can often be ameliorated with nebulized racemic epinephrine inhaled in $O_2$. Again, systemic steroid administration appears to have little effect.

Laryngospasm triggered by extubation[103] or minor airway stimulation frequently causes significant airway obstruction in recovering patients as laryngeal constrictor muscles acutely occlude the tracheal inlet and severely reduce airflow. The incidence of laryngospasm is increased after upper airway surgery, in children with upper respiratory infections,[104] in smokers,[105] in patients with irritable airway conditions, and in children chronically exposed to secondhand smoke.[106,107]

Assuming that an airway is clear of vomitus or foreign bodies, most episodes of laryngospasm resolve spontaneously or with application of gentle positive pressure in the oropharynx using 100% $O_2$. For prolonged laryngospasm, a small dose of succinylcholine (eg, 0.1 mg/kg) yields sufficient relaxation to restore airway patency. Use of larger dosages increases the risk for hypoxemia if supplemental ventilation is not supplied.[60]

More distal large airway obstruction from extrinsic compression or tracheal stenosis is unusual.

### Emergency Treatment

Occasionally, standard airway maneuvers fail, and tracheal intubation is indicated to restore airway patency. Emergency intubation in this setting is risky[108] because patients may be hypoxemic or hypercarbic after a period of airway obstruction. Every attempt should be made to oxygenate and ventilate the patient before intubation. The most experienced operator should use the fastest, highest yield approach to secure the airway. If obstruction is caused by soft tissue pathology or edema, even minor trauma from instrumenting the airway can create an irreversible obstruction. Use of sedatives or muscle relaxants to facilitate intubation can worsen obstruction by compromising the patient's volitional efforts to maintain the airway and by eliminating spontaneous ventilation.

If tracheal intubation or face mask ventilation proves impossible, one is faced with a life-threatening emergency. Keep equipment and personnel necessary for emergency cricothyroidotomy or tracheotomy readily available. Cricothyroidotomy using a 14-gauge intravenous catheter attached to a high-pressure $O_2$ source permits oxygenation and marginal ventilation until the airway can be secured (Figs. 6–5 and 6–6). This subject is covered in more detail in Chapter 53.

## What Is the Impact of Distal Airway Resistance on Postoperative Ventilation?

High resistance to gas flow through small airways increases the work of breathing and the time required for exhalation. Consequent trapping of end-expiratory gas leads to increased dead space ventilation and progressive hypercarbia, especially as work of breathing increases $CO_2$ production. Both inspiratory and expiratory muscles fatigue from sustaining high pressure gradients required to overcome airway resistance. If resistance does not improve, ventilatory failure leads to severe hypercarbia and hypoxemia (see Table 6–6).

### Pathophysiology

Simply put, resistance to gas flow varies inversely with the fourth power of airway radius during laminar airflow, so that reduction of the airway cross-sectional area significantly increases airway resistance. Pharyngeal or tracheal stimulation

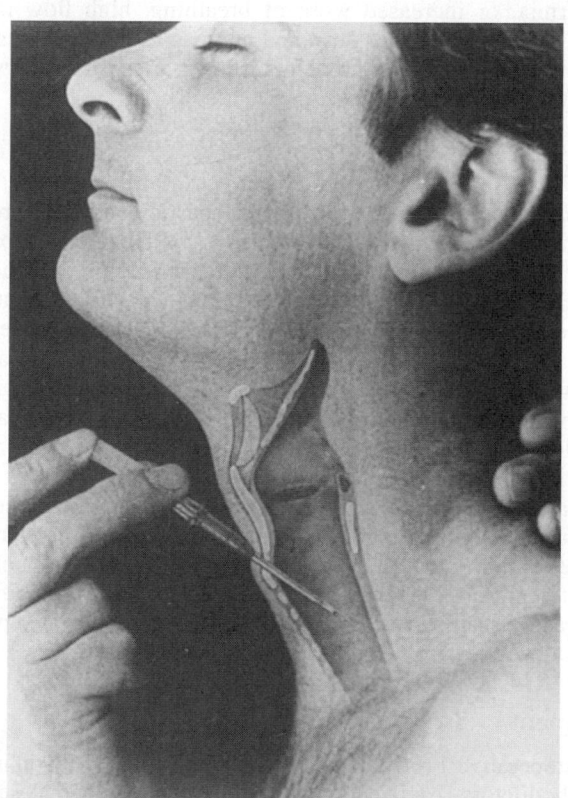

**FIGURE 6–5.** Cricothyroidotomy using large-bore (12- to 14-gauge) intravenous catheter. (From Benumof JF. *Clinical Procedures in Anesthesia and Intensive Care.* Philadelphia, Pa: JB Lippincott; 1992:199.)

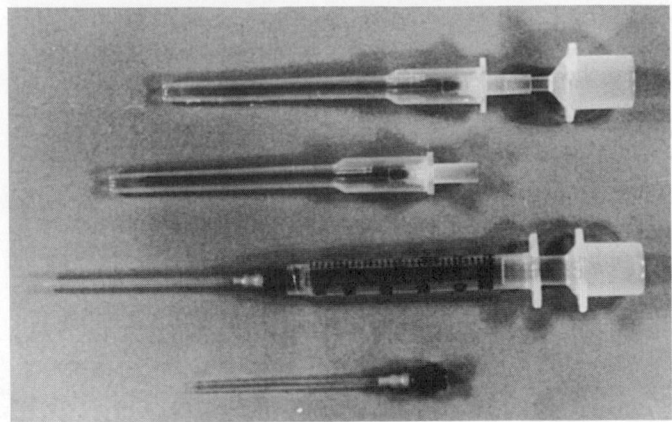

**FIGURE 6–6.** Devices for attaching a cricothyroidotomy catheter to a positive pressure source for ventilation. An adapter from a 3.0-mm-ID pediatric tracheal tube fits directly into the Luer lock on the catheter. An adapter from a 7.0-mm-ID endotracheal tube fits into the barrel of a 3-mL syringe, which in turn engages the Luer lock on the catheter. ID, inside diameter.

from secretions, suctioning, aspiration, or intubation elicits reflex constriction of bronchial smooth muscle, especially as the bronchodilatory effects of inhalation anesthetics wane. Histamine release caused by medication or allergic reactions can also cause bronchospasm.

Decreased airway caliber is worsened by airway wall edema in patients with chronic reactive airway disease. Reduction of radial airway traction secondary to decreased lung volume also decreases airway cross-sectional area in patients with COLD, obesity, excess lung water, or hypoexpansion.

If ventilatory requirements are increased by shivering, hyperthermia, or increased work of breathing, high flow rates cause chaotic turbulent flow and increased flow resistance. (Flow resistance during turbulent airflow varies inversely with the fifth power of the radius.)

### Diagnosis

Smokers and patients with bronchospastic conditions are at risk for bronchospasm after surgery.[109,110] Preoperative spirometric evidence of increased airway resistance predicts postoperative bronchospasm.[55] A forced vital capacity expiration often exposes high airway resistance in spontaneously ventilating patients. Resistance is higher during expiration because positive intrathoracic pressure compresses intermediate diameter airways. Increased airway resistance does not always cause audible turbulent airflow (wheezing) because ventilation may be so restricted that no sound is produced.

Signs of increased small airway resistance mimic those of decreased pulmonary compliance. Spontaneously breathing patients exhibit increased work of breathing, accessory muscle recruitment, and labored ventilation with either condition, whereas mechanically ventilated patients exhibit elevated peak inspiratory pressure.

### Treatment of Bronchospasm

Postoperative bronchospasm usually resolves with inhaled bronchodilators. Alert patients often respond to their baseline regimen of albuterol, pirbuterol, or salmeterol inhalers. Isoetharine or metaproterenol nebulized in $O_2$ is also effective. Intramuscular or sublingual terbutaline can be added. Patients

whose bronchospasm is resistant to $\beta_2$-sympathomimetic medications may respond to an anticholinergic medication such as atropine or ipratropium. An aminophylline loading dose and maintenance infusion or epinephrine infusion can be used if ventilation is still compromised. Treatment of bronchospasm should always include an attempt to eliminate the offending laryngeal or tracheal stimulus.

Increased small airway resistance caused by mechanical factors such as loss of lung volume or pulmonary edema is usually refractory to bronchodilators. Incentive spirometry or deep tidal ventilation can restore lung volume and increases external radial traction on small airways, thereby decreasing flow resistance. If high airway resistance is caused by increased lung water, reduction of left ventricular filling pressures is beneficial. An acute exacerbation of chronic bronchospasm may appear resistant to bronchodilators because prolonged contraction of airway smooth muscle causes venous and lymphatic obstruction in airway walls. Airway wall edema and interstitial fluid accumulation persist even after smooth muscle relaxation occurs.

### *How Does Reduction of Pulmonary Compliance Interfere With Ventilation?*

Factors that reduce pulmonary compliance, the change in lung and chest wall volume per unit change in transthoracic pressure, increase work of breathing (Table 6–7). Low compliance causes ventilatory muscle fatigue, which leads to increased work of breathing, hypoventilation, and respiratory acidemia. Low compliance also causes decreased lung volume, which leads to $\dot{V}/\dot{Q}$ mismatching and hypoxemia.[111]

### Preoperative Factors

Postoperative pulmonary compliance depends in part on preoperative status. Obesity reduces compliance, especially if adipose tissues compress the thoracic cage in the supine or lateral positions.[112] Increased intraabdominal pressure due to obesity, pregnancy, tumor, ascites, or bowel obstruction impedes diaphragmatic excursion, reduces FRC, and promotes airway closure and atelectasis. Reexpansion of atelectatic parenchyma and airways requires extra energy expenditure.

Pulmonary contusion, consolidation, or hemorrhage interferes with lung expansion and accentuates the work of breathing. Restrictive lung diseases, musculoskeletal abnormalities, intrathoracic tumors or aneurysms, and massive cardiomegaly also reduce compliance. Increased pulmonary fluid and blood

**TABLE 6–7.** Causes of Reduced Pulmonary Compliance

**Preoperative**
Obesity
Increased intra-abdominal pressure (pregnancy, ascites, tumor, bowel obstruction)
Pulmonary parenchymal problems (contusion, tumors, edema, restrictive diseases)
**Intraoperative**
Mainstem intubation
Abdominal manipulations
Hemothorax, pneumothorax
Unusual positions (lateral decubitus, prone without chest rolls)
Restrictive dressings

volume secondary to hydrostatic or high-permeability pulmonary edema increase the weight and inertia of the lungs, whereas accumulation of fluid in air spaces interferes with the modulation of surface tension by pulmonary surfactant.

### Intraoperative Factors

Intraoperative factors that promote atelectasis and reduce compliance include gastric or bowel distention, intraabdominal manipulation, intraperitoneal fluid accumulation, mainstem tracheal intubation, excessive airway suctioning, and hemothorax or pneumothorax. Mediastinal compression and interstitial fluid accumulation lower compliance in the dependent lung after prolonged lateral positioning during thoracic surgery. Tight chest or abdominal dressings also contribute.

### Treatment

In the PACU, allowing patients to recover in a semisitting (60° inclination) rather than supine or full sitting position improves diaphragmatic excursion and decreases work of breathing. Deep breathing, chest physiotherapy, incentive spirometry, PEEP, and CPAP are useful to restore inflation. Remember that in patients with COLD, positive airway pressure can overdistend the highly compliant lungs past the equilibrium point of the chest cavity, paradoxically increasing the muscular effort required to breathe.

## What Neuromuscular Problems Interfere With Ventilation?

### Inadequate Muscle Relaxant Reversal

Incomplete reversal of neuromuscular relaxation is a serious potential cause of postoperative hypoventilation. Residual paralysis impairs cough, reduces the ability to overcome increase airway resistance, and compromises airway patency and protection.[113,114] Use of shorter acting agents or combinations of agents may decrease the incidence of residual paralysis but does not eliminate the problem.[115]

Marginal reversal of paralysis is insidious. It is easier to identify an agitated, uncoordinated patient with severe airway obstruction than a somnolent patient with marginal neuromuscular function who exhibits only mild stridor. Respiratory acidemia or regurgitation and aspiration may occur well after admission to the PACU, when observation is less intense.

### Neuromuscular Abnormalities

Administration of muscle relaxants to patients with neuromuscular deficiencies such as myasthenia gravis, Eaton-Lambert syndrome, periodic paralysis, or muscular dystrophies often results in prolonged paralysis. These patients may suffer postoperative ventilatory insufficiency, even when relaxants are omitted as well, and therefore deserve especially careful observation and monitoring.[99]

Neuromuscular relaxation can be inadvertently potentiated by antibiotics, furosemide, phenytoin, and propranolol as well as by hypocalcemia or hypermagnesemia.[116,117] Patients with atypical pseudocholinesterase have a dramatic increase in the duration of succinylcholine-induced paralysis.

### Diaphragmatic and Intercostal Muscle Function Compromise

Strength and coordination of diaphragmatic contraction are probably compromised in certain postoperative patients, reducing their ability to deal with decreased compliance or increased ventilatory demands.[118] Residual thoracic spinal or epidural blockade impedes external intercostal muscle function and can reduce ventilatory ability, especially in patients with COLD. Morphine may also compromise intercostal function, further compounding ventilatory inadequacy.

### Phrenic Nerve Impairment

Phrenic nerve impairment due to trauma, thoracic or neck surgery, or interscalene anesthesia immobilizes the ipsilateral hemidiaphragm.[119] Use of more dilute local anesthetic solutions for interscalene blocks may reduce the incidence of ventilatory impairment without compromising analgesia.[120] Although adequate ventilation can usually be maintained with one hemidiaphragm and marginal ventilation with only the external intercostal muscles, increased work of breathing or ventilatory demands may precipitate ventilatory failure.[121] Patients with Guillain-Barré syndrome, cervical spinal cord trauma, or severe kyphosis or scoliosis are at risk for postoperative ventilatory insufficiency.[122]

### Flail Chest

Paradoxic inspiratory chest wall collapse secondary to flail chest impedes thoracic cavity expansion so that ventilatory failure occurs. Loss of compliance from an underlying pulmonary contusion undoubtedly is of greater significance with respect to ventilatory impairment than is the flail.

## How Is the "Mechanical" Ability to Ventilate Assessed?

Simple bedside tests help assess the mechanical ability to ventilate. A forced vital capacity of >10 to 12 mL/kg and inspiratory pressure more negative than $-25$ cm $H_2O$ usually indicate adequate ventilatory muscle strength, although many patients with chronic lung diseases cannot meet these criteria preoperatively. The ability to sustain head elevation for longer than 5 seconds in a supine position likely ensures ability to sustain ventilation but probably does not predict recovery of airway protective reflexes.[123] Conventional tactile train-of-four assessment accurately assesses ability to ventilate but often fails to identify levels of paralysis that interfere with protective reflexes.[124] Hand grip, pedal flexion, and other maneuvers are less reliable indicators.

### Clinical Appearance

Patients who are hypoventilating secondary to mechanical difficulty exhibit obvious clinical signs. Upper airway obstruction causes stridor, rocking motions of the epigastrium, recruitment of accessory muscles, and limited chest wall excursion. Increased small airway resistance causes wheezing, labored ventilation, and prolonged expiration. Residual paralysis generates characteristic uncoordinated, flopping motions, difficulty swallowing, and marked agitation. Low compliance causes rapid, shallow ventilation, recruitment of accessory muscles, and labored inspiration. In addition, patients often exhibit agitation and air hunger with each of these problems.

Occasionally, a patient exhibits signs of postoperative ventilatory insufficiency when minute ventilation is actually adequate. Splinting inspiration against a painful incision can present as a rapid, shallow breathing pattern characteristic of inadequate ventilation. Incisional pain, however, seldom causes respiratory acidemia, and the labored ventilatory pattern usually disappears with analgesia. Prolonged ventilation with small tidal volumes caused by thoracic restriction or reduced compliance often leads to dyspnea, labored breathing, and accessory muscle recruitment despite appropriate minute ventilation. This problem also occurs during *mechanical* ventilation with low inspired volumes. Providing patients with a large, satisfying lung expansion decreases afferent input from pulmonary stretch receptors and relieves these symptoms. Hyperventilation to compensate for metabolic acidemia may generate tachypnea and labored ventilation that mimics mechanical difficulty. When assessing potential ventilatory insufficiency, always evaluate the $Pa_{CO_2}$ and pH.

## How Does Increased Dead Space Interfere With Ventilation?

Ventilation of air spaces that are not perfused (ie, dead space ventilation) does not contribute to $CO_2$ excretion, whereas ventilation of alveoli with high $\dot{V}/\dot{Q}$ is less effective in removing $CO_2$. If dead space volume increases while tidal volume remains constant, the fraction of each inspiration wasted in dead space; that is, the dead space-to-tidal volume ratio ($V_{DS}/V_T$) increases. A decreased tidal volume also increases $V_{DS}/V_T$.

High dead space necessitates a proportionally larger increase in minute ventilation to meet increased ventilatory demands. Patients with a high $V_{DS}/V_T$ are therefore at greater risk for postoperative ventilatory failure. A $V_{DS}/V_T$ between 0.55 and 0.60 (normal, 0.30) usually necessitates mechanical assistance to maintain adequate ventilation and $CO_2$ excretion. A ratio >0.60 to 0.65 often precludes adequate ventilation with conventional positive pressure ventilation. High-frequency ventilation may facilitate $CO_2$ removal at higher $V_{DS}/V_T$.

### Changes in Dead Space

A number of factors affect dead space after surgery (Table 6–8).

**TABLE 6–8.** Factors Causing Changes in Dead Space

**Decrease**
  Tracheal intubation, tracheostomy, high-frequency ventilation
**Increase**
  Circuit valve reversal
  Prolonged inspiratory-to-expiratory ratios, mechanical ventilation
  Positive end-expiratory pressure and continuous positive airway pressure
  Increased airways resistance (eg, gas trapping)
  Embolic phenomena (air, fat, thrombus)
  Shock, pulmonary hypotension
  Acute respiratory distress syndrome

### Mechanical Factors That Increase Dead Space

Tracheal intubation or tracheotomy reduces upper airway dead space by about 75%. Valve reversal in ventilator circuits or incorrect connection of expiratory tubing could promote rebreathing of exhaled gas rich in $CO_2$. PEEP or CPAP marginally increases anatomic dead space by expanding airway volume, especially if pulmonary compliance is high. Interruption of expiration by a subsequent inspiration forces spent alveolar gas back into exchanging air spaces, mimicking an increase in dead space. This gas trapping and $CO_2$ retention occurs when high airway resistance lengthens the time required for complete exhalation. During mechanical ventilation, the same problem occurs if prolonged inspiratory-to-expiratory time ratios or excessive ventilatory rates are used.

### Embolic Phenomena

Pulmonary embolization with air, thrombus, cellular debris, or foreign matter interferes with perfusion of ventilated alveoli and increases physiologic dead space.[125] The impact of high $\dot{V}/\dot{Q}$ on $CO_2$ excretion is often masked by increased minute ventilation mediated by reflex responses to emboli or ventilatory response to hypercarbia. Trending the gradient of end-expiratory partial pressure of carbon dioxide ($P_{ET}CO_2$) to $Pa_{CO_2}$ is useful to detect embolization.

### Other Causes

Pulmonary hypotension increases $V_{DS}/V_T$ by reducing perfusion to well-ventilated nondependent alveoli.[126] If a pathologic process destroys pulmonary microvasculature, an irreversible increase in dead space occurs. ARDS related to sepsis, massive transfusion, trauma, or hypoxemia progressively increases $V_{DS}/V_T$.

## When Does Increased Carbon Dioxide Production Lead to Postoperative Ventilatory Failure?

$CO_2$ production varies directly with metabolic rate, body temperature, and substrate availability. General anesthesia reduces $CO_2$ production up to 40% as hypothermia lowers metabolic activity and neuromuscular relaxation reduces baseline muscle tone. Postoperative warming restores metabolic rate, $O_2$ consumption, and $CO_2$ production toward normal.

### Causes

Shivering, increased work of breathing, SNS activity, and carbohydrate metabolism during hyperalimentation could accelerate $CO_2$ production after surgery. Even small increases in postoperative $CO_2$ production can precipitate respiratory acidemia if ventilatory reserve is compromised. Malignant hyperthermia dramatically increases $CO_2$ production, rapidly exceeding normal ventilatory capacity and causing severe respiratory acidemia.

### Treatment

Control of $CO_2$ production in the PACU usually involves control of shivering using warming lights, blankets, forced warm air systems, or fluid warmers. A variety of medications have been studied to treat shivering (see later), and in rare cases, neuromuscular relaxation can be used. In the PACU, the need to control $CO_2$ production by adjusting hyperalimentation or treating malignant hyperthermia is rare.

If dead space in a mechanically ventilated patient is so high that mechanical ventilation can no longer control the $Paco_2$, paralysis and deliberate hypothermia may reduce $CO_2$ production and improve acid-base status.

## PULMONARY ASPIRATION SYNDROME

Morbidity from pulmonary aspiration in the perioperative period varies with the type and volume of aspirate.

Aspiration of acidic gastric contents is most feared, although other aspiration syndromes occur (Table 6–9).

## *What Other Types of Aspiration Occur?*

### Clear Oral Secretions

Aspiration of oral secretions during face mask ventilation, extubation of the trachea, or emergence from anesthesia is common and usually insignificant. Usually, transient cough or laryngospasm is the only sequela. Repeated aspiration of large volumes may promote small airway obstruction or infection.

### Blood

Blood aspiration secondary to trauma, epistaxis, or surgical bleeding in the airway is cleared from air spaces by mucociliary transport or by resorption and phagocytosis. The impact on pulmonary function is generally minimal, although the radiographic presentation can be dramatic. Secondary infection may occur, especially if bits of tissue or purulent matter are also aspirated. Massive blood aspiration interferes with gas exchange and may cause pulmonary hemochromatosis. Residual fibrinous deposits also increase morbidity.

### Solid Foreign Matter

Aspiration of solid foreign matter, such as food, teeth, pieces of dental appliances, or small objects, causes persistent cough and diffuse reflex bronchospasm. Obstruction of the trachea or mainstem bronchi causes acute, life-threatening impairment of ventilation and oxygenation. Localized complications of obstruction in smaller airways, such as distal atelectasis and infection, are treatable with antibiotics and conservative pulmonary care once the obstructing matter is expelled or removed through bronchoscopy.

**TABLE 6–9.** Aspiration Syndromes

Acid
Clear oral (saliva)
Blood
Solid foreign matter (eg, food, coins, buttons, teeth)

## *What Problems Result From Aspiration of Acidic Gastric Contents?*

Aspiration of acidic gastric contents causes bronchospasm, hypoxemia, and atelectasis. Subsequent chemical pneumonitis leads to airway epithelial degeneration, interstitial and alveolar edema, and air space hemorrhage. A fulminating ARDS with high-permeability pulmonary edema, $\dot{V}/\dot{Q}$ mismatch, and marked reduction in compliance often follows.[127] Destruction of pneumocytes reduces surfactant activity, whereas damage to the pulmonary microvasculature increases pulmonary vascular resistance and $V_{DS}/V_T$. If the patient survives, later sequelae include accumulation of fibrinous deposits, hyaline membrane formation, and emphysematous changes caused by parenchymal destruction.

### Severity

Severity and degree of resolution probably depend on the volume and pH of the aspirate. Morbidity sharply increases when the pH is $<2.0$ to 2.5. Aspiration of fluid with higher pH is somewhat less damaging but still interferes with surfactant activity and disrupts pulmonary function.[128] Morbidity also increases as the volume of aspirate increases.

Pneumonitis is more severe if partially digested food is aspirated as well. Food particles obstruct small airways and promote secondary bacterial infection. Aspirated vegetable matter causes a chronic granulomatous reaction resembling that caused by miliary tuberculosis.[129]

## *What Factors Increase the Risk for Aspiration?*

### Loss of Protective Airway Reflexes

The risk for aspiration is particularly high if protective airway reflexes, such as cough, swallowing, gagging, and laryngospasm, are suppressed by depressant medications such as inhalation anesthetics, barbiturates, and opiates.[130] Impairment of protective reflexes by residual neuromuscular paralysis is common and may not be obvious. Patients can sustain spontaneous ventilation, pass a head-lift test, and have a tactile train-of-four ratio $>0.7$ but still exhibit impaired airway reflexes and esophageal constrictor function secondary to residual paralysis.[123,124] The train-of-four ratio may need to exceed 0.9 before resolution of clinically evident neuromuscular block is achieved.[131] Risk for aspiration may also be increased if reversal is omitted after paralysis with short-acting relaxants.[132]

Trauma or anesthesia of the airway or of the laryngeal and pharyngeal muscle innervation seriously compromises airway reflexes. The effects of intraoperative interventions to reduce airway irritability such as topical local anesthetics or laryngeal nerve blocks can persist well into the PACU stay, decreasing a patient's airway protection.

### Vomiting, Gastric Contents, and the Gastroesophageal Junction

Postoperative vomiting is still a significant problem. Whenever gastric contents enter the pharynx, the risk for aspiration increases. Risk also increases if patients requiring emergency surgery have large volumes of intragastric food and fluid. Many factors interfere with gastric emptying, including bowel obstruction, pain, anxiety, narcotics, salt depletion, and peristaltic abnormalities.

Pregnancy and morbid obesity result in increased gastric volume and hyperacidity. An associated mechanical displacement of the gastroesophageal junction interferes with sphincter integrity. Abnormalities that affect gastroesophageal tone or swallowing (eg, achalasia, hiatal hernia, esophageal diverticula or tumors, and amyotrophic lateral sclerosis) also increase the risk for regurgitation and aspiration.

### Level of Consciousness

The deeper the level of residual anesthesia a patient exhibits on admission to the PACU, the greater the risk for aspiration. This results not only from blunting of airway reflexes but also from the lack of volitional ability to handle oral contents. Diminishing a patient's level of arousal with additional sedative or analgesic medications in the PACU increases the risk for aspiration. Finally, hypotension, hypoxemia, or acidemia raises the risk for aspiration by causing both obtundation and emesis.

### Anatomic Distortion

Soft tissue trauma interferes with afferent sensory input from the airway and with swallowing and other motor aspects of airway protective reflexes. Mandibular fixation impedes expulsion of vomitus, blood, or secretions from the mouth. Instruments necessary to release the fixation apparatus should be available in the PACU.

## What Steps Should Be Taken to Prevent Aspiration?

### Nil Per Os Status

Prevention of aspiration is critical because therapy is limited. Traditionally, anesthesiologists maintained a nil per os (NPO) status for at least 8 to 12 hours before induction of anesthesia. Analysis of outcomes after revision of preoperative fasting guidelines has demonstrated the safety of shorter NPO periods for clear liquids and for feedings in young children.[133–135] The effectiveness of NPO status for generating an "empty" stomach before elective surgery is questionable anyway.[136] Nevertheless, vigilance for potential regurgitation and aspiration is prudent for any patient with a history of recent ingestion.

### Antiemetics

Risk for aspiration is a consideration when deciding whether antiemetic prophylaxis is appropriate. If vomiting occurs in the PACU, weigh the risk for side effects from antiemetic treatment against the risk for aspiration for each individual patient. Cost should not be part of this analysis. Make every effort to avoid PONV in patients who are at high risk for aspiration (eg, mandibular fixation, decreased level of consciousness, impaired swallowing).

### Nonparticulate Antacids

Nonparticulate antacids, such as sodium citrate, increase the pH of gastric fluid without excessively increasing volume. Particulate antacids should be avoided because subsequent aspiration of these medications causes chronic granulomatous reactions.

### Histamine Blockers and Metoclopramide

Histamine $H_2$ blockers, such as cimetidine and ranitidine, increase the pH and decrease the production of gastric fluid, whereas metoclopramide improves gastroesophageal sphincter tone and accelerates gastric emptying.[137]

### Nasogastric Suction

Gastric contents should be emptied as much as possible after anesthetic induction, although nasogastric suction is often ineffective to remove particulate matter. Presence of a nasogastric tube during emergence helps relieve gastric distention from trapped gas but interferes with gastroesophageal sphincter integrity and sometimes promotes retching.

### Positioning

Trendelenburg positioning may promote regurgitation, but it also aids in clearing vomitus once regurgitation has occurred. Head elevation should be avoided if airway reflexes are marginal because establishing a gravitational gradient from pharynx to lungs promotes aspiration.

## How Long Should Patients Remain Intubated?

Patients at high risk for aspiration should remain intubated until restoration of airway reflexes is complete. Endotracheal intubation does not preclude aspiration.[138] Appropriate pharyngeal suctioning reduces the incidence of silent aspiration past a nonsealing cuff. Tracheal tube cuff deflation increases risk for aspiration because the rigid tube prevents laryngeal closure.

Before extubation, completely suction the pharynx. Cuff deflation and extubation should be performed at end inspiration with positive airway pressure to promote vigorous expulsion of material trapped below the vocal cords but above the inflated cuff. After extubation, airway reflexes can be temporarily impaired, and patients should be carefully monitored.

## What Should Be Done If Vomiting or Regurgitation Occurs?

### Airway Management

If gastric secretions appear in the pharynx, rotate the head into a lateral position and suction the pharynx. Use great care when clearing the airway of a patient with a cervical spine injury.

Tracheal intubation may be indicated if airway reflexes are compromised. If intubation is performed, suction the trachea through the tube before instituting positive pressure ventilation. This action avoids spreading aspirated material into distal airways. Instilling saline or alkalizing solutions into the tracheal tube is contraindicated. Determining tracheal aspirate pH is of no value because buffering is almost immediate. Assessment of pH in a pharyngeal aspirate is more reliable but of little practical value.

### Assessment and Intervention for Possible Aspiration

If aspiration is suspected, monitor the patient carefully for 24 to 48 hours. If the likelihood of significant aspiration is small and if hypoxemia, wheezing, cough, or radiographic abnormalities do not appear within 4 to 6 hours, outpatients can be discharged. Inform the responsible physician about the possibility of aspiration. The patient and family must receive clear instructions to monitor for fever, cough, malaise, chest discomfort, or other symptoms of pneumonitis. Instruct them to call the facility or their physician about any problems. A follow-up telephone call to the patient is essential.

In cases with a high likelihood of serious aspiration, the patient should remain in the facility for a sufficient period to assess the problem. Serial temperature checks, differential white blood cell counts, ABG determinations, and pulmonary function testing are helpful. Infiltrates can appear on repeated chest radiographs anytime within 24 to 36 hours, and hypoxemia may evolve insidiously as lung pathology progresses. Chest physiotherapy and incentive spirometry may help minimize atelectasis and $\dot{V}/\dot{Q}$ mismatching. Medications for preexisting chronic pulmonary conditions such as asthma should be reinstituted.

### *What Should Be Done When Aspiration Is Documented?*

If aspiration causes hypoxemia, increased airway resistance, or pulmonary edema, institution of mechanical ventilation with supplemental $O_2$ and PEEP or CPAP is often necessary. Therapy is similar to that used for ARDS. High-permeability pulmonary edema should not be treated with diuretics unless high ventricular filling pressures are present. Hypovolemia caused by fluid loss into the lungs may necessitate aggressive fluid resuscitation.

Steroids do not yield improvement in long-term outcome after aspiration. Prophylactic antibiotic administration promotes colonization by resistant organisms. If bacterial infection appears, institute specific antibiotic therapy based on sputum culture results. If culture results are equivocal, broad-spectrum antibiotics should cover gram-negative rods and anaerobes, including *Bacteroides fragilis.*[139]

### POSTOPERATIVE HYPOTENSION

Hypotension in the immediate postoperative period is a common problem (Table 6–10). Systemic hypotension can lead to hypoperfusion of vital organs. Inadequate $O_2$ delivery causes tissue hypoxia, inefficient aerobic metabolism, and lactic acid accumulation. In response to decreases in intravascular pressure and acidemia, the SNS increases heart rate and

**TABLE 6–10.** Causes of Postoperative Hypotension

**Spurious**
 Inappropriately small blood pressure cuff
 Improperly zeroed arterial catheter
 Damped arterial catheter trace
**Absolute Hypovolemia**
 Inadequate replacement of preoperative deficits, third space losses, and intraoperative blood loss
 Occult or continued hemorrhage in postanesthesia care unit
 Increased venous capacity with rewarming
**Relative Hypovolemia**
 Sympathectomy secondary to regional anesthetics
 Decreased α-adrenergic venous tone
 Direct venodilation by medications (furosemide, morphine, nitrates)
 Venodilation secondary to α-adrenergic blockade (droperidol, chlorpromazine)
 Venodilation secondary to histamine release (barbiturates, relaxants, morphine)
 Allergic or anaphylactoid reactions, anaphylaxis
 Decreased venous return (caval compression, high airway pressure, tension pneumothorax)
 Interference with ventricular filling (pericardial tamponade)
**Ventricular Dysfunction**
 Acute ischemic myocardiopathy
 Overhydration, ventricular dilation, and nonischemic failure
 Reduced endogenous sympathetic nervous system activity
 β-Receptor or calcium channel blockade
 Severe acidemia or alkalemia
 Decreased ionized calcium, acute steroid deficiency
 Acute valvular dysfunction, air embolism, thromboembolism
**Arrhythmia**
 Bradycardia (sinus or heart block) with decreased cardiac output
 Tachyarrhythmia with decreased ventricular filling
 Tachycardia with underlying valvular lesions
 Life-threatening ventricular tachycardia, fibrillation, or asystole
**Decreased Systemic Vascular Resistance**
 Sympathectomy from major regional anesthetics
 Direct arterial dilating medications (hydralazine, nitroprusside)
 α-Adrenergic blockade (droperidol, chlorpromazine)
 Decreased endogenous sympathetic nervous system tone
 Blunted baroreceptor function, intracranial pathology
 Severe hypoxemia or acidemia
 Arteriolar dilation secondary to sepsis, blood components
 Acute steroid deficiency

contractility, systemic vascular resistance (SVR), and venous tone.

The SNS also diverts perfusion to the brain, heart, and kidneys, where autoregulatory arteriolar dilation helps to preserve blood flow. When hypotension causes symptoms of hypoperfusion to these vital systems (eg, nausea, disorientation, loss of consciousness, angina, or oliguria), the body's compensatory reserve already has been expended.

### *What Are the Complications of Hypotension?*

Complications of hypotension include myocardial, cerebral, and renal ischemia or infarction. Viability of the spinal cord or bowel can be jeopardized, and the risk for deep vein thrombosis may be increased by low venous flow velocities. Decreased hepatic $O_2$ delivery may trigger alternate pathways for drug metabolism and lead to hepatic damage from the accumulation of toxic metabolites.

The minimal acceptable systemic BP is higher in patients with chronic hypertension, arteriosclerotic disease, fixed stenotic vascular lesions, increased intracranial pressure, or conditions that interfere with autoregulation.

### Is the Measurement Valid?

Ensuring the accuracy of a low BP reading avoids the risk for iatrogenic hypertension from inappropriate treatment. Inappropriately large cuffs yield artificially low values. BP cuff width should equal about two thirds of arm circumference.

If an arterial catheter transducer system is improperly zeroed or damped by air bubbles or catheter obstruction, readings can be erroneously low. Arterial constriction can reduce radial or even brachial intraarterial readings below the central pressure in hypothermic patients or in those receiving α-adrenergic receptor agonist medications.

### What Is Absolute Hypovolemia?

Absolute hypovolemia implies that the total intravascular volume is insufficient to support ventricular filling and cardiac output. SNS responses mediated by baroreceptor reflexes usually can maintain systemic pressure despite a 15% to 20% loss of intravascular volume. Greater deficits overcome the SNS compensation, and systemic BP falls.

#### Inadequate Blood and Fluid Replacement

Postoperative hypovolemia is frequently caused by inadequate replacement of preoperative fluid deficits, evaporative losses during surgery, and blood loss. In the PACU, hypovolemia is exacerbated by additional hemorrhage, insensible fluid loss, and exudation of fluid into tissues. Blood loss from intramuscular hemorrhage after trauma or orthopedic procedures, diffuse oozing related to acute coagulopathy, or retroperitoneal bleeding can be difficult to recognize. Third space losses continue for 24 to 48 hours and can lead to profound hypovolemia through the accumulation of ascites, pulmonary edema, or anasarca.

#### Hypothermia and Rewarming

On admission to the PACU, arterial and venous constriction caused by hypothermia often masks absolute hypovolemia. When a hypothermic patient rewarms, venous capacitance increases, afterload decreases, and hypovolemia causes hypotension.[140] Whenever a patient is admitted with a low core body temperature, PACU staff should suspect that hypovolemia may acutely reduce systemic BP during rewarming. This problem is an excellent rationale for maintaining body temperature during surgery.

### What Is Relative Hypovolemia?

Relative hypovolemia implies that an otherwise normal intravascular volume is inadequate to maintain BP.

#### Decreased Sympathetic Nervous System Activity

Increased venous capacitance due to chemical sympathectomy after spinal or epidural anesthesia reduces ventricular

filling pressures and prevents venoconstriction in response to hemorrhage or position changes.

After general anesthesia, vasovagal responses, extubation of the trachea, or relief of pain can suddenly reduce SNS activity and increase venous capacity. Medications with α-adrenergic receptor–blocking properties, such as droperidol and chlorpromazine, increase venous capacity, as do those that dilate veins, such as nitrates or furosemide.

#### Histamine Release

After allergic responses or administration of medications such as barbiturates or morphine, histamine release may cause significant venous pooling. Blood products or low molecular weight dextrans sometimes cause venous dilation, which probably is secondary to histamine release.

#### Impedance to Venous Return

Factors that impede venous return to the right atrium cause relative hypovolemia. These include compression of thoracic veins by positive pressure ventilation or tension pneumothorax, and inferior vena caval compression by a gravid uterus or increased intraabdominal pressure. Acute pericardial tamponade also impedes ventricular filling.

### How Is Intravascular Volume Status Assessed?

On admission to the PACU, review each patient's preoperative fluid status, estimated blood loss, and intraoperative fluid loss and replacement. Also, complete a qualitative assessment of current intravascular volume and hemostasis. The variation of systolic BP on an arterial catheter or pulse oximeter waveform (Fig. 6–7) during ventilation provides a qualitative warning of reduced intravascular volume.[141,142] Generating a sustained increase in mean arterial pressure by lifting the patient's legs to increase venous return could also reveal hypovolemia in selected cases.

Urine output is a potentially misleading index of intravascular volume because surgery and anesthesia interfere with renal concentrating ability. Also, unrecognized hyperglycemia promotes glycosuria and osmotic diuresis, which overcomes the kidney's ability to retain fluid.

If intravascular volume status is uncertain, insertion of a central venous or PA catheter helps assess right or left ventricular filling pressures. Esophageal Doppler or echocardiographic monitoring can also be helpful to determine ventricular filling.

### Is Ventricular Dysfunction Present?

Hypotension from ventricular dysfunction is relatively uncommon in postoperative patients. This problem usually occurs in patients who have impaired baseline ventricular contractility and who require elevated left ventricular end-diastolic pressure (LVEDP) and intense SNS activity to maintain cardiac output.

#### Overhydration and Ventricular Dilation

In patients with impaired ventricular contractility, overhydration causes ventricular dilation, decreased cardiac output,

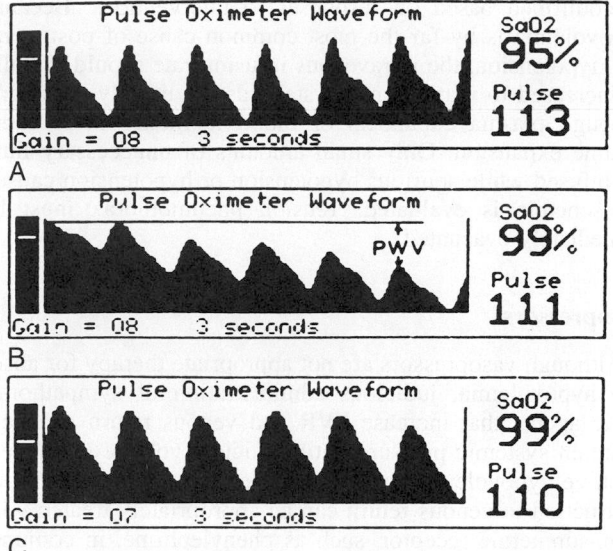

**FIGURE 6–7.** Pulse oximeter waveform representation. *A*, When the patient arrived in the operating room, CVP was 8 mm Hg. Little variation was seen in the waveform with positive pressure ventilation. *B*, After third space translocation and blood loss, CVP was 4 to 5 mm Hg. The pulse waveform varied with respiration. The method for measuring PWV is shown. *C*, After fluid resuscitation, CVP was 8 mm Hg. The pulse waveform no longer shows significant variation with respiration. CVP, central venous pressure; PWV, pulse waveform variation. (From Partridge BL. Use of pulse oximetry as a noninvasive indicator of intravascular volume status. *J Clin Monit.* 1987;3:263, with kind permission from Kluwer Academic Publishers.)

hydrostatic pulmonary edema, and hypotension. Excessive intravascular volume may initially be concealed in patients recovering from spinal or epidural anesthesia because sympathectomy dramatically increases venous capacity. When SNS blockade resolves, a characteristically high level of SNS outflow causes venoconstriction and an acute increase of central vascular volume.

Massive pulmonary thromboembolism or air embolism impedes right ventricular outflow and often presents with systemic hypotension.

### Drug and Metabolic Effects

Patients with severe ventricular dysfunction who rely on maximal SNS activity may exhibit hypotension after administration of β-adrenergic receptor blocking drugs or analgesics. During postoperative regional blocks, intravascular injection of local anesthetic or uptake from highly vascular tissues may cause severe myocardial depression. Residual alveolar partial pressures of inhalation anesthetics marginally reduce ventricular contractility and decrease SNS outflow, limiting cardiac output to a small degree.

Severe acidemia reduces ventricular performance by interfering with endogenous or exogenous catecholamine–receptor interaction and by directly depressing SNS outflow. Severe alkalemia has similar effects. Ventricular contractility may be marginally compromised by decreased ionized calcium from acute alkalemia, dilution, or chelation by banked blood preservatives.

### Is Myocardial Ischemia Present?

Hypotension and tachycardia may precipitate postoperative myocardial ischemia or infarction in patients with CAD.[143]

Inadequate aortic diastolic BP reduces myocardial perfusion pressure. Tachycardia in response to hypotension, pain, acidemia, anxiety, or medications reduces time available for coronary perfusion during diastole. Myocardial $O_2$ consumption goes up if demand for cardiac output is increased during shivering or if ventricular wall tension is increased by high SVR or overhydration. Hypoxemia, anemia or carboxyhemoglobinemia can generate myocardial ischemia despite adequate coronary perfusion. The lowest tolerable hematocrit is highly individualized to each patient but is generally higher in patients with vascular disease.[144]

### Recognition

Postoperative ischemia is often difficult to recognize, and risk for early morbidity is still high. Among patients with coronary disease, risk is higher with a history of smoking, congestive heart failure, or hypertension.[145,146] Risk is significant after both general and regional anesthetics and higher after emergency surgery.[147]

Most episodes of postoperative angina are silent.[148] Analgesia from residual anesthetics or narcotics treats anginal as well as incisional pain. Chest pain may also be attributed to discomfort from upper abdominal incisions, esophageal reflux, vomiting, or gastric distention.

Routine ECG monitoring is relatively nonspecific for evaluation of ischemic changes but remains the standard in most PACUs. Lead V5 has a higher yield. The value of ST segment depression as a predictor of outcome has been questioned.[37] A high incidence of benign postoperative dysrhythmias makes identification of ischemia-induced dysrhythmias difficult.

Hypotension secondary to ischemic ventricular dysfunction is a late, serious sign that warns of rapid progression to irreversible infarction. Close evaluation of hemodynamic responses to fluid challenge, ST segment and T wave morphology on 12-lead ECG, and assessment of cardiovascular dynamics may uncover ischemia before hypotension occurs. Careful control of precipitating factors and timely therapy are important to decrease morbidity.

### What Is the Effect of Decreased Systemic Vascular Resistance?

Decreased SVR is an important cause of postoperative hypotension associated with regional anesthesia, vasoactive blood components, and rewarming, although venous dilation also plays a role. Severe systemic acidemia (pHa ≤6.8) reduces SVR by a direct vasodilatory effect and by interfering with catecholamine interactions with α-adrenergic receptors. Hydralazine and nitroprusside reduce SVR by dilating muscular arterioles, whereas α-adrenergic receptor and ganglionic blocking drugs interfere with peripheral SNS activity.

Hypotension during systemic sepsis is often related to a low SVR caused by endotoxin, although myocardial depression is superimposed in end stages. Decreased SVR can also be caused by blunted baroreceptor function[95] or by intracranial pathology. SVR falls during acute postoperative steroid deficiency when exogenous steroids have suppressed the pituitary-adrenal axis. Hypotension is usually preceded by lethargy, fever, or nausea and accompanied by hyperkalemia, hyponatremia, and hypoglycemia. Response to supplemental steroids is often dramatic.

### What Arrhythmias Reduce Blood Pressure?

Postoperative hypotension caused by a cardiac dysrhythmia is more common in patients with a history of myocardial disease or rhythm disturbance. Slow sinus or nodal bradycardia simply decreases cardiac output and BP, as does a slow ventricular rhythm associated with complete heart block. Loss of atrial contribution to filling during atrial fibrillation can reduce cardiac output in patients with noncompliant ventricles.

Paroxysmal atrial tachycardia (PAT), atrial fibrillation or flutter, and fast ventricular tachycardias that generate ventricular rates of >140 to 150 beats per minute often do not provide adequate diastolic intervals for ventricular filling. Stroke volume, cardiac output, and systemic BP all decrease. Needless to say, ventricular fibrillation, asystole, or electromechanical dissociation causes lethal reduction in cardiac output.

### Why Are Valvular Abnormalities Particularly Dangerous?

PACU patients often exhibit high levels of SNS activity, which can precipitate hypotension in patients with valvular abnormalities. Tachycardia in a patient with mitral stenosis interferes with left ventricular filling, increases left atrial pressure, and decreases cardiac output and systemic pressure. With mitral regurgitation, high SVR increases the regurgitant fraction and compromises cardiac output. Postoperative tachycardia in a patient with aortic stenosis reduces systolic ejection time and increases LVEDP, promoting decreased cardiac output and ventricular dilation. Increased contractility or heart rate causes similar problems in patients with hypertrophic subaortic stenosis.

### What Treatment Is Indicated?

A 20% to 30% reduction of systolic BP below chronic preoperative levels is usually an indication for therapy, as is the appearance of symptoms referable to vital organ hypoperfusion. If a high risk for hypotensive complications is present, acceptable limits for pressure and heart rate should be defined when the patient is admitted to the PACU.

Before treatment is initiated, the pressure determination should be quickly validated. Cardiac rate and rhythm, breath sounds, and $O_2$ saturation should be checked immediately. Depending on the circumstances, a 12-lead ECG, an ABG sample, or a chest radiograph may be ordered. Every hypotensive patient should receive supplemental $O_2$.

Infusions that can cause vasodilation should be discontinued, and recent drug administration should be noted. Simple maneuvers, such as lateral uterine displacement in pregnant patients or supine positioning and elevating the legs of patients with orthostatic changes, should be used if appropriate. It is still controversial whether Trendelenburg positioning actually augments venous return.

For severe, acute hypotension, palpation of carotid or femoral pulses and auscultation of heart sounds are useful qualitative indicators of central BP. Cardiopulmonary resuscitation must be instituted immediately if pulses are absent.

#### Initial Therapy

Therapy should be directed toward the specific problem responsible for reducing systemic BP. The etiology should be confirmed based on responses to interventions. Because hypovolemia is by far the most common cause of postoperative hypotension, the intravenous infusion rate should initially be increased to maximum. Crystalloids are usually sufficient, although plasma expanders or blood facilitates more rapid volume expansion. Only small amounts of unnecessary fluid are infused while spurious hypotension or hypotension caused by ischemia is evaluated. Tension pneumothorax must be immediately evacuated.

#### Vasopressors

Although vasopressors are not appropriate therapy for absolute hypovolemia, judicious administration of sympathomimetic agents that increase SVR and venous return can help maintain systemic pressure until sufficient volume is infused. Relative hypovolemia caused by increased venous capacity or obstruction to venous return can be appropriately treated with an α-adrenergic receptor, such as phenylephrine, in conjunction with fluid therapy. Ephedrine is less desirable because an increase in heart rate and contractility is usually unnecessary. Its ready availability, however, makes it a popular choice.

#### Treatment of Myocardial Dysfunction

If 300 to 500 mL of fluid does not improve BP, myocardial dysfunction should be considered a possible cause of hypotension. When hypotension is caused by myocardial ischemia, resolution of ischemia usually restores baseline myocardial function. Therapy of acute ischemia is dependent on the circumstances. In the presence of significant hypotension, support of aortic diastolic pressure with an α-adrenergic receptor agonist such as phenylephrine and reduction of LVEDP with nitroglycerin help maximize the coronary artery perfusion pressure. Control of heart rate with analgesics, sedatives, and especially β-adrenergic receptor blockers is essential.[149–151]

If dysfunction is not related to ischemia, drugs that augment contractility, such as ephedrine, dopamine, dobutamine, or amrinone, in conjunction with carefully titrated systemic vasodilators, often restore cardiac output and systemic pressure.

Because therapy for ischemia can acutely worsen hypotension cause by hypovolemia, decreased SVR, or nonischemic ventricular dysfunction, it is critical that the diagnosis of ischemia be accurate. Suspicion that hypotension is caused by ventricular dysfunction is an indication for echocardiography or PA catheterization to measure cardiac output and left ventricular filling.

#### Treatment of Arrhythmias

Hypotension from PAT often responds to alteration of cardiac conduction rates by vagal maneuvers or medications, whereas digitalization or calcium channel blockade reduces the ventricular rate during atrial fibrillation. Low-energy (50 J) direct current cardioversion can be used if hypotension due to a tachydysrhythmia is life-threatening.

Hypotension secondary to sinus bradycardia unrelated to hypoxemia almost always resolves after administration of atropine, glycopyrrolate, or ephedrine. Refractory bradycardia caused by sinus node disease or complete heart block often requires intravenous administration of epinephrine or isoproterenol, or cardiac pacing.

## Treatment of Decreased Systemic Vascular Resistance

Low SVR with high cardiac output sometimes can be resolved with phenylephrine, although norepinephrine infusion may be required with advanced sepsis or catecholamine depletion.

## POSTOPERATIVE HYPERTENSION

Moderate elevation of systemic BP is acceptable in the PACU, but significant hypertension increases morbidity and should be aggressively evaluated and treated.[53] Hypertension increases hemorrhage and third space losses after surgery. Disruption of major vascular suture lines can also occur. Ventricular dilation or myocardial fiber stretch secondary to high LVEDP can cause cardiac arrhythmias, whereas an increase in wall tension may precipitate myocardial ischemia. Hypertension also exacerbates increased intracranial pressure, cerebral edema, intracranial hemorrhage, and elevated intraocular pressure.

If a BP cuff is inappropriately small, it yields erroneously high readings. This is a particular problem in the evaluation of obese patients. An improperly zeroed or calibrated transducer or an excessive amount of resonance and electronic "overshoot" can lead to overestimation of systolic pressure with an arterial catheter.

### What Is the Role of Sympathetic Nervous System Activity?

Hypertension due to increased SNS activity after surgery reflects either an appropriate response to noxious stimuli or an adverse physiologic condition (Table 6–11).

### Increased α-Adrenergic Stimulation

Enhanced α-adrenergic receptor stimulation causes arteriolar and venous constriction, increasing SVR and venous return respectively. Increased $\beta_1$-adrenergic receptor stimulation increases heart rate and ventricular contractility. After surgery, patients with preexisting hypertension often exhibit noncompliant arteriosclerotic vasculature and elevated peripheral vascular tone mediated by the renin-angiotensin system. Baroreceptor control of heart rate is also impaired,[152] especially after administration of anticholinergic medications during reversal of neuromuscular relaxants.[153] Each of these factors causes exaggerated BP responses to stimuli in the PACU.

Abnormally high SNS activity can occur as a baseline condition or can be caused by exogenous sympathomimetics or, rarely, by monoamine oxidase inhibition or pheochromocytoma.

### Other Precipitating Factors

Intravascular volume expansion from infusions during surgery increases cardiac output and BP despite compensatory decreases in SVR and heart rate, especially in hypothermic, vasoconstricted patients. After carotid endarterectomy, abnormal baroreceptor sensitivity can produce significant hypertension.[154] Central SNS regulation of BP can be disrupted by cerebrovascular accidents, hypoxic encephalopathy, increased intracranial pressure, or osmotic changes, causing severe hypertension.

### How Should Hypertension Be Treated?

Treatment of postoperative hypertension is usually indicated when systolic or diastolic pressure exceeds 120% to 130% of resting pressure or when signs of complications, such as headache, bleeding, visual changes, angina, or ST segment depression, occur.

Patients with increased intracranial pressure, open eye injury, mitral regurgitation, or intracardiac shunts are at increased risk for morbidity and should be treated more aggressively. To avoid hypoperfusion of vital organs in patients with chronic hypertensive disease, pressure should not be reduced below preoperative baseline levels.

### Therapy

Elimination of increased SNS activity by administering analgesics for pain or sedatives for anxiety, correcting acidemia or hypoxemia, or decompressing the urinary bladder often suffices. Intravenous labetalol,[155] esmolol,[156] or nicardipine[157] in small incremental doses is useful for short-term pressure control, as is a combination of intravenous hydralazine and propranolol. Clonidine is useful for both augmenting postoperative analgesia and BP control.[152] Clonidine may also blunt the postoperative SNS response to stimuli.[158] Potent intravenous vasodilators, such as sodium nitroprusside and nitroglycerin, should be reserved for severe or refractory hypertension.

## POSTOPERATIVE ELECTROCARDIOGRAPHIC ABNORMALITIES

Often, after anesthesia, morphology or rhythm changes are seen on the ECG that suggest abnormal myocardial physiology and yet are unrelated to clinical signs or symptoms of

**TABLE 6–11.** Factors That Increase Postoperative Sympathetic Activity

| | | |
|---|---|---|
| Increased sympathetic activity | Noxious stimuli | Surgical pain, discomfort, anxiety, full bladder, tracheal intubation, carinal stimulation |
| | Adverse physiologic conditions | Hypercarbia or acidemia, hypoxemia, hypotension, hypoglycemia, congestive heart failure, myocardial ischemia, increased intracranial pressure, atelectasis, pulmonary embolism |
| | Medications | Vasopressors, bronchodilators, antihypertensives, anesthetics |
| Decreased parasympathetic activity | Parasympatholytic medications | Atropine, glycopyrrolate, pancuronium, gallamine |

actual pathology.[159] These findings are probably caused by a combination of autonomic nervous system imbalance, electrophysiologic effects of inhalation anesthetics, electrolyte imbalance, and hypothermia.[160,161]

Transient alterations in axis, intraventricular conduction, P wave and T wave morphology, and ST segments almost always resolve spontaneously within 3 to 6 hours. Repeat ECG recording and perhaps CK-MB enzyme determinations are appropriate in higher risk patients if ECG changes are strongly indicative of myocardial ischemia.

Ventricular arrhythmias that exist preoperatively usually reappear in the PACU, often with somewhat decreased frequency. Presence of a preoperative dysrhythmia is not usually predictive of postoperative outcome.[162]

### What Is the Significance of Premature Complexes?

#### Atrial

An aberrant impulse from the atrium, atrioventricular (AV) node, or upper bundle of His generates an atrial premature contraction (APC) with an early but otherwise normal QRS complex. In postoperative patients, APCs usually reflect increased SNS activity and seldom lead to hemodynamic compromise. Control of SNS activity (pain management, sedation) is usually sufficient to eliminate APCs.

#### Ventricular

Most abnormal QRS complexes seen on PACU monitors represent aberrantly conducted supraventricular complexes or reentrant arrhythmias. Differentiation from actual ventricular ectopy is important because reentry and aberrant conduction seldom reflect cardiac pathology or require treatment. Frequent ventricular ectopy may also be benign, particularly if it was evident preoperatively. Frequent multifocal ventricular ectopy, however, sometimes reflects a serious underlying abnormality that could degenerate into a more threatening dysrhythmia.

#### Ectopic Ventricular Depolarizations

A spontaneous depolarization that originates in ventricular conducting tissue generates a ventricular premature complex (VPC) with a wide, bizarre QRS complex. Not all peculiar QRS complexes are VPCs. True VPCs usually occur at varying intervals from previously normal QRS complexes because they are random ventricular events. Also, the interval between previous and subsequent normal QRS complexes is usually twice the normal interval (compensatory pause).

Spontaneous ventricular depolarization is associated with excess SNS activity, which accelerates spontaneous ventricular depolarization rates or fosters the emergence of parasystolic foci. Treatment involves eliminating the cause of increased SNS activity or administration of β-adrenergic receptor–blocking medications to reduce ventricular depolarization rates. Ventricular depolarization is also associated with excess parasympathetic nervous system (PNS) activity. When the PNS reduces the rate of supraventricular pacemakers, ventricular escape beats emerge. Treatment using vagolytic or sympathomimetic medications accelerates supraventricular pacemaker rates.

Myocardial fiber stretch, digitalis toxicity, electrolyte disturbances, and mechanical stimulation from central catheters cause ectopic ventricular depolarization. Catheter-induced arrhythmias are best treated by withdrawing the catheter from the ventricle or atrium.

Ventricular depolarizations that do not respond to control of SNS tone or other conservative measures may indicate that myocardial ischemia is causing nonphysiologic impulse generation in the ventricle. In addition to resolving ischemia, administration of intravenous antidysrhythmic agents, such as lidocaine, bretylium, or procainamide, can be useful to control ischemic ventricular automaticity.

#### Supraventricular Premature Impulses With Aberrant Conduction

If a premature atrial depolarization enters the ventricular conduction system before complete recovery of excitability, asynchronous ventricular depolarization generates wide, high-amplitude ECG complexes similar to PVCs. These aberrantly conducted supraventricular impulses often resemble normal QRS complexes in general shape and are sometimes preceded by a P wave that may be different from the normal P waves. The interval between a previous and subsequent normal QRS is usually less than twice the normal interval (noncompensatory pause).

Supraventricular impulses with aberrant conduction are common during recovery from anesthesia and are generally benign. Increased SNS activity is the usual cause, but delayed recovery of conducting tissues caused by chronic disease, general anesthetics, or electrolyte abnormalities also favors aberrant conduction. If the frequency compromises cardiac output, control of SNS activity usually restores regular rhythm.

#### Reentrant Depolarization

If a sinus impulse is delayed in a ventricular conduction pathway long enough to encounter tissue that has recovered excitability, the impulse causes a second, reentrant depolarization that spreads throughout the heart. Reentrant depolarizations resemble PVCs because they generate wide, high amplitude complexes with full compensatory pauses. However, reentrant depolarizations are uniform in configuration, follow the preceding normal complex by a constant interval (fixed coupling), and often appear in a bigeminal pattern.

In postoperative patients, reentry is often related to increased SNS activity, especially after halothane anesthesia. Control of SNS tone and elimination of factors that cause conduction delay or nonuniform recovery of excitability usually suppress reentry dysrhythmias.

### When Is Tachycardia Significant?

#### Sinus Tachycardia

Sinus tachycardia, the most common dysrhythmia encountered in the PACU, reflects increased SNS activity and is usually harmless. It seldom interferes with ventricular filling but can reduce cardiac output in patients with stenotic valvular lesions. During tachycardia, decreased diastolic filling time can precipitate acute myocardial ischemia in patients with

CAD. Sinus tachycardia also exacerbates postoperative hypertension.

Because increased SNS activity can be caused by serious conditions such as acidemia, hypoxemia, or malignant hyperthermia, it is important to identify and treat the underlying cause. Intravenous fluids to counteract hypovolemia, analgesics to treat postoperative pain, or sedatives to calm anxiety usually help resolve tachycardia. Relief of bladder distention by catheterization often slows the sinus rate. When tachycardia presents a medical risk and the underlying cause is beyond control, β-adrenergic receptor blockade is useful. Digoxin is ineffective unless ventricular failure is the underlying cause.

## Atrial Fibrillation and Atrial Flutter

Untreated atrial fibrillation (AF) can generate ventricular rates in excess of 150 beats per minute and may appear as a nearly regular supraventricular tachycardia on ECG. Patients recovering from thoracic surgical procedures exhibit a higher incidence of postoperative atrial fibrillation, as do patients with mitral valvular disease or pulmonary embolism.[163]

Treatment involves decreasing the number of impulses that can traverse the AV node per minute by administering digoxin or calcium channel blockers. β-Adrenergic receptor blockade may also slow rate and promote conversion. Direct current cardioversion is indicated in urgent circumstances.

Atrial flutter is rare in postoperative patients. It usually presents with a rapid, regular ventricular rate at some fraction of the atrial rate. Decreasing the ventricular rate and regulating atrial electrical activity are the major goals of therapy.

## Paroxysmal Atrial Tachycardia

PAT is usually caused by circus reentry in conduction tissue, although a small percentage of cases result from discrete, rapidly firing groups of atrial pacemaker cells. The excessive ventricular rate sometimes interferes with ventricular filling and reduces cardiac output.

Treatment of PAT involves slowing cardiac conduction velocity to interrupt reentrant synchrony. This allows a dominant pacemaker to recapture the heart at a slower rate. Depression of conduction by residual anesthetic levels may contribute to the relative rarity of PAT in the PACU setting. Increasing PNS influence on the heart (Table 6–12) resolves PAT. Digoxin or calcium-channel blockers can also be useful. PAT caused by a rapidly firing atrial pacemaker may slow with β-adrenergic receptor blockade.

## Ventricular Tachycardia and Fibrillation

Postoperative ventricular tachycardia or fibrillation usually reflects severe myocardial ischemia, systemic acidemia, or hypoxemia. Controlled ventilation and oxygenation, management of systemic pH, cardiopulmonary resuscitation, and cardioversion are mainstays of therapy.

## *When Is Postoperative Bradycardia Significant?*

### Sinus Bradycardia

A decrease in SNS activity or an increase in PNS activity slows spontaneous depolarization in supraventricular pace-

**TABLE 6–12.** Factors That Increase Postoperative Parasympathetic Influence

| Increased Parasympathetic Activity | Decreased Sympathetic Activity |
|---|---|
| *Vagal Reflexes* <br> Carotid sinus massage, gagging, Valsalva maneuver, rectal examination, increased ocular pressure, bladder distention, pharyngeal stimulation | *Sympathectomy* <br> T1–4 spinal or epidural sympathectomy; decreased stimulus (analgesia, tracheal extubation); emptying bladder; severe acidemia or hypoxemia |
| *Parasympathomimetic Medications* <br> Cholinesterase inhibitors (neostigmine, edrophonium); α-adrenergic medications (phenylephrine, norepinephrine); narcotics (morphine, fentanyl); succinylcholine | *Sympatholytic Medications* <br> β-Blockers (propranolol, esmolol); narcotics, sedatives, general anesthetics; ganglionic blockers, local anesthetics |

makers, leading to sinus bradycardia. The sinus rate also falls with sick sinus syndrome, sinus nodal ischemia, or severe hypoxemia. Hypotension usually does not result until the rate falls below 40 to 45 beats per minute. In postoperative patients, sinus bradycardia frequently occurs with sudden increases in PNS activity (ie, vasovagal episodes). As management of epidural analgesia has become more prevalent in the PACU, sinus bradycardia related to onset of sympathectomy is also seen more frequently.

Sinus bradycardia is benign unless it causes hypotension or an unacceptable number of ventricular escape beats. In the PACU, therapy involves restoration of SNS tone. Excess PNS activity usually responds to muscarinic blocking drugs, such as atropine or glycopyrrolate, whereas decreased SNS activity is usually resolved with a β-mimetic drug such as ephedrine. Frequency of bradycardia after spinal anesthesia may be reduced by placing the patient in a semisitting position.[164] If bradycardia reflects acute hypoxemia, immediate restoration of oxygenation is essential.

### Nodal Rhythm

The sinus node sometimes appears more sensitive to increased PNS influence than other pacemakers. Autonomic imbalance can promote emergence of a "nodal" pacemaker in the lower AV node or bundle of His. A nodal rhythm can also emerge if sinus node impulses are prevented from reaching the ventricle by sinus nodal exit block or AV nodal block.

In the PACU, nodal rhythm occurs in patients with underlying conduction disease, in those recovering from regional anesthetic with high levels, after inhalation anesthesia, and during periods of increased PNS tone. If the ventricular rate is sufficient to maintain cardiac output and BP, nodal rhythm does not require treatment. Lack of coordinated atrial contraction, however, can decrease cardiac output by 10% to 15%, especially in patients with noncompliant ventricles. If hypotension occurs, atropine or β-mimetic medications may restore the sinus node as the dominant pacemaker, although sometimes they only increase the nodal rate. BP support may be necessary until spontaneous resolution occurs.

### Idioventricular Bradycardia

Idioventricular bradycardia almost always reflects a serious condition such as third-degree heart block, myocardial ischemia, severe hypoxemia, or profound acidemia. A slow idio-ventricular rhythm seldom generates an adequate BP. Epineph-rine, isoproterenol, or cardiac pacing is effective to accelerate ventricular rate. Vagolytic medications do not increase the depolarization rates of ventricular pacemakers. If acute third-degree AV nodal block is secondary to digitalis toxicity or ischemia, however, atropine sometimes improves AV nodal conduction and allows supraventricular impulses to reach the ventricles.[165]

## POSTOPERATIVE RENAL PROBLEMS

### How Is Renal Function Assessed?

#### Ability to Void

Urinary output helps assess postoperative renal and cardiac status. In the PACU, the frequency, amount, and general nature of urinary output should be documented for all patients. Those with indwelling catheters should have urine output recorded hourly, whereas patients without catheters should be encouraged to void before discharge.

Opiates and parasympathomimetic side effects of regional anesthetics accentuate urinary sphincter tone and lead to difficulty with micturition.[166] Urinary retention is common after inguinal and genital surgery and frequently delays discharge.[167] If a patient cannot spontaneously void, monitoring after discharge from the PACU is necessary to avoid urinary retention. It is reasonable to discharge inpatients to a surgical floor and selected ambulatory surgical patients from the facility before they void.[168] Ambulatory patients should be given a specific time interval in which to void (eg, 10-12 hours after discharge). If retention persists beyond that interval, instruct the patient to contact a health care facility. Higher than average return rates after urologic procedures are partially related to urinary retention.[169]

Before discharge, the degree of bladder distention should be assessed. Patients with high urinary bladder volumes may require catheterization to relieve distention. Neither patients nor staff are particularly accurate at assessing bladder volumes by sensation or physical examination, respectively.[170] A portable ultrasonic bladder scanner is useful to determine bladder volume.

#### Urine Characteristics as Indices of Renal Function

Assessment of postoperative urine output as the sole index of renal function can be misleading because osmotic diuresis or the effects of surgery and anesthesia interfere with renal regulatory mechanisms. Urine color is a poor predictor of renal concentrating ability but can suggest pyuria, hematuria, or myoglobinuria.

A urine sodium concentration far below serum concentration indicates renal tubular viability, as does a urine potassium concentration above serum concentration. Urine osmolarity better reflects tubular function than does specific gravity. An osmolarity of >450 mOsm/L implies intact tubular concentrating ability.

Acidification or alkalization of urine requires intact tubular function so that urine pH reflects tubular viability. Electrolyte osmolarity and pH values close to those in serum can be normal or may signify acute tubular necrosis.

Although more comprehensive tests, such as creatinine clearance or fractional excretion of sodium, are better indicators of renal function, they are more applicable to post-PACU follow-up than to short-term PACU care.

### What Is the Significance of Polyuria?

A number of conditions cause postoperative polyuria (Table 6–13). Profuse urine output usually reflects the excretion of generous intraoperative fluid administration. Sustained polyuria (>4-5 mL/kg/h) that compromises intravascular volume and systemic BP, however, sometimes reflects abnormal regulation of free water clearance. Polyuria also can be caused by persistent effects of intraoperatively administered diuretics. High-output renal failure should also be considered.

#### Osmotic Diuresis

Osmotic diuresis secondary to hyperglycemia and glycosuria can generate massive urine output, especially if glucose-containing crystalloid solutions are used to replace urinary losses. Once urine and serum glucose determinations reveal the problem, glucose restriction is the only therapy required for this self-limited process. Clearance of intraoperatively administered mannitol can also cause postoperative osmotic diuresis.

#### Diabetes Insipidus

Polyuria caused by diabetes insipidus can occur after intracranial surgery, pituitary ablation, or head trauma. Increased intracranial pressure or inadvertent omission of preoperative vasopressin also interferes with free water reabsorption. Comparison of electrolytes and osmolarity between urine and serum is diagnostic, and the administration of vasopressin is therapeutic.

#### Nephrotoxicity From Inhalation Anesthetics

Inorganic fluoride released during metabolism of inhalational anesthetics can cause a transient reduction in renal concentrating ability. High levels of inorganic fluoride lead to nephrotoxicity and renal tubular necrosis. Older inhalation anesthetics, such as enflurane, released relatively small amounts of fluoride, causing a transient decrease in maximal tubular concentrating ability after prolonged anesthesia.

Interaction between sevoflurane and carbon dioxide absorbents (soda lime and Baralyme) generates a vinyl ether compound designated Compound A. The amount of Compound A produced varies directly with sevoflurane concentration and with the degree of absorbent dryness, and inversely with flow rate.[171] In human beings, defluoridation of Compound A by cytochrome P450 yields an increase in free inorganic fluoride.

**TABLE 6–13.** Causes of Postoperative Polyuria

---

Liberal intraoperative fluid administration
Diuretics
High output renal failure
Osmotic diuresis (glucose, mannitol)
Diabetes insipidus (central or nephrogenic)

---

**TABLE 6–14.** Causes of Postoperative Oliguria

Inadequate intraoperative fluid administration
Hypotension
Elevated antidiuretic hormone secretion (pain, anxiety, stress)
Hyponatremia
Acute renal insufficiency (acute tubular necrosis)
Ureteral ligation
Catheter occlusion
Renal vascular occlusion
Narcotic administration
Residual effects of spinal, epidural, caudal anesthesia

Compound A is lethal to rats in high concentrations and nephrotoxic in lower concentrations.

Although transient increases in protein excretion and decreases in concentrating ability may occur, use of sevoflurane for prolonged general anesthesia has little serious impact on renal function.[172] Given the relationship between Compound A and dry $CO_2$ absorbents, PACU staff should be aware that polyuria or proteinuria may be related to Compound A exposure in patients who received sevoflurane during first cases or cases performed in peripheral anesthetizing locations.

## What Is the Significance of Oliguria?

Urine volume of <0.5 mL/kg/h usually reflects an appropriate kidney response to hypovolemia but can be caused by elevated antidiuretic hormone levels, systemic hypotension, or abnormal renal function (Table 6–14). Always evaluate oliguria, especially after procedures involving aortic cross-clamping, possible ureteral ligature, severe hypotension, or massive transfusion.

Check urinary catheter patency because obstruction by blood clots or debris mimics oliguria, as does positioning that forces the catheter tip above the urine level in the bladder. For patients without urinary catheters, assessment of bladder fullness by ultrasonic scan helps to differentiate between urinary retention and oliguria.

### Hypovolemia

To assess whether oliguria represents a response to hypovolemia, give a 300- to 500-mL intravenous crystalloid bolus after urine samples for electrolyte and osmolarity testing are obtained. If output does not improve, a larger fluid bolus or a diagnostic trial of 5 mg of furosemide is appropriate. Furosemide increases urine output if oliguria is caused by increased tubular reabsorption.

Hypoperfusion due to systemic hypotension can reduce urine output. The systemic BP that provides minimally adequate renal perfusion varies, depending on the usual preoperative pressure.

## What Should Be Done If Oliguria Persists?

If oliguria persists despite adequate hydration, perfusion pressure, and a small furosemide challenge, the possibility of ureteral obstruction, acute tubular necrosis, renal artery or vein occlusion, or inappropriate antidiuretic hormone secretion must be evaluated. Intravenous pyelography, angiography, or radioisotope imaging helps to clarify current renal status, whereas PA catheterization or echocardiography can determine the adequacy of cardiovascular function. Osmotic or loop diuretics and low-dose dopamine or dobutamine are probably useful to attenuate renal damage. Perioperative administration of desmopressin usually has minimal effect on postoperative urinary output.

# CENTRAL NERVOUS SYSTEM FUNCTION

## What Causes Prolonged Unconsciousness After Anesthesia?

Ninety percent of patients regain consciousness within 15 minutes of admission to the PACU. Unconsciousness that persists beyond 15 minutes can be considered prolonged.[173] When evaluating prolonged unconsciousness after anesthesia, review the level of preoperative responsiveness to exclude chronic mental dysfunction and drug or alcohol intoxication (Table 6–15). Also note all depressant medications administered before and during surgery.

During physical examination, pupillary size and responses

**TABLE 6–15.** Differential Diagnosis of Persistent Unconsciousness

| **Routine Causes** | |
| --- | --- |
| Residual depression from general anesthetics | Usually resolves within 60–90 min |
| Excessive narcotic administration | Identify and treat with naloxone titration |
| Long-acting sedative premedication | Either medical drugs or substance abuse; if benzodiazepines, treat with flumazenil |
| Preoperative exhaustion | Causes deep sleep; arousable with stimulus |
| Preoperative decreased level of consciousness | Intoxication, chronic low level of arousal |
| **Global Physiologic Disorders** | |
| Profound residual neuromuscular paralysis | Precluded if any motor responses noted |
| Systemic hypotension | Severe if hypoperfusion causes unconsciousness |
| Profound hypoxemia | Airway obstruction, hypoventilation |
| Marked hypercarbia or $CO_2$ narcosis | High $CO_2$ as sedative; often with hypoxemia |
| Severe hypoglycemia | Suspicion indicates 50% dextrose trial |
| Hypothermia | Below 30°C, unusual cause or deep sedation |
| Severe hyperglycemia or hyperosmolarity | Unusual, treated with insulin and potassium |
| Hyponatremia or hypoosmolality | Treated with furosemide to waste free water |
| **Central Nervous System Dysfunction** | |
| Seizure activity | Seizure or postictal phase decreased responses |
| Intraoperative cerebral anoxia | Hypotension, disconnection, arrhythmia |
| Unrecognized subarachnoid injection of regional anesthesia | Can occur with general-regional techniques |
| Undiagnosed preoperative high intracranial pressure or subdural hematoma | Multitrauma with unrecognized head injury |
| Cerebral embolism | Fibrillation, air embolism, invasive catheters |
| Stroke or increased intracranial pressure | Mostly after carotid, cardiac, neurosurgery |

are unreliable diagnostic indices because many drugs affect pupillary signs. The rate and character of spontaneous breathing help assess adequacy of ventilation and, to a lesser extent, oxygenation, whereas systemic BP and heart rate shed light on adequacy of cerebral perfusion and the prevailing level of autonomic tone. A firm tactile stimulus is often more effective than verbal stimulation to elicit arousal, perhaps because it recruits the reticular activating system.

## Inhalation Anesthetics

Residual sedation from intraoperative medications frequently causes somnolence in the PACU. Inhalation anesthetics are more likely to prolong unconsciousness after long surgical procedures, especially in obese patients. If high inspired concentrations of such agents are continued through the end of surgery to facilitate deep extubation, patients often appear unresponsive early in the PACU course.

## Narcotics

Intraoperatively administered narcotics or sedatives generally cause dose-related sedation. Perioperative administration of long-acting sedatives, such as lorazepam, scopolamine, pentobarbital, hydroxyzine, or promethazine, significantly prolongs emergence. Ventilatory rate and depth are reasonable indicators of the degree of central depression caused by opioids.

If unconsciousness persists beyond 60 to 90 minutes, low-dose intravenous naloxone in 40-μg increments every 2 minutes will reverse the sedative and respiratory depressant effects of intraoperative opioids without precipitating dangerous reversal of analgesia. A maximal dose of 200 to 400 μg should increase ventilatory rate and arousal unless a patient has been massively overdosed with opioids.

## Sedative Drugs

Flumazenil, a competitive benzodiazepine antagonist, is useful to identify and reverse sedation from benzodiazepines,[174] although residual sedative effects of the benzodiazepines may recur after the drug's 1-hour duration of action. Intravenous physostigmine, 1.25 mg, may nonspecifically counteract sedation from residual inhalation anesthetics, anticholinergics, tricyclic antidepressants, and other sedatives.[175] Lack of response to adequate doses of naloxone, flumazenil, or physostigmine does not categorically preclude unrecognized preoperative or intraoperative overdose with sedative medications as a possible cause.

## Neuromuscular Paralysis

Profound residual neuromuscular paralysis can mimic unconsciousness and should be considered in patients with unrecognized neuromuscular disease, phase II blockade caused by excessive succinylcholine administration, or pseudocholinesterase deficiency. It is unlikely, however, that a conscious patient admitted to the PACU would be weakened to a point that paralysis would mimic complete unconsciousness. Any purposeful motion, spontaneous ventilation, reflex activity, or other evidence of neuromuscular function eliminates residual paralysis as an explanation for prolonged unresponsiveness.

## Metabolic Abnormalities

Unconsciousness from hypoglycemia is a medical emergency that requires immediate treatment. If hypoglycemia is suspected, an immediate empiric trial of intravenous 50% dextrose should be administered while serum glucose determination is pending.

Hypoosmolarity secondary to acute hyponatremia can affect consciousness; thus, serum electrolyte concentrations and osmolarity should be checked. A serum sodium concentration of <125 mEq/L is cause for concern, as is a serum osmolarity of <260 mOsm/L. Glucose and electrolyte determinations also reveal whether severe hyperglycemia or hypernatremia is causing acute hyperosmolar coma.

ABG analysis assesses whether unrecognized hypoxemia or marked hypercarbia with $CO_2$ narcosis is contributing to unconsciousness. Severe hypoxemia is unlikely with continuous pulse oximetry monitoring; however, there is a small but real possibility of coma caused by cerebral hypoxia secondary to CO poisoning. Trauma patients could be exposed to CO before emergency surgery, or patients receiving general anesthesia could be exposed through the interaction between inhalation anesthetics and $CO_2$ absorbents.

## Less Common Etiologies

Preoperative exhaustion sometimes delays emergence from an anesthetic, especially if sleep patterns are interrupted in children undergoing emergency surgery at night. Caffeine withdrawal is an uncommon cause that may contribute in patients who are heavy caffeine users (eg, >10 cups per day). Intravenous caffeine promptly reverses this rare cause of delayed emergence.

Hypothermia with core temperatures of <33°C impairs consciousness and accentuates the depressant effects of some medications. Fixed pupillary dilation, areflexia, and coma can occur at core temperatures of <30°C.

On rare occasion, a patient will feign unresponsiveness or suffer a hysterical reaction that presents as unconsciousness.[176]

## What Should Be Done If the Cause Is Indeterminate?

A thorough, carefully documented neurologic evaluation in consultation with a neurologist should be carried out if the cause of unconsciousness is still unclear.

### Central Nervous System Pathology

Subclinical seizures secondary to delirium tremens or an underlying seizure disorder can present as unresponsiveness in the PACU, as can CNS depression due to intravenous local anesthetic toxicity or inadvertent subarachnoid injections during analgesic blocks.[177] Unrecognized intraoperative cerebral hypoxia secondary to severe hypotension, dysrhythmias, or hypoxemia must be considered. Trauma victims should be evaluated for covert head trauma or increased intracranial pressure. Increased intracranial pressure due to bleeding or edema also causes unconsciousness after intracranial surgery. Even in the absence of pathology, patients are sometimes slow to emerge after long intracranial procedures.[178]

Cerebral embolism is another possible problem after vascular surgery or after the insertion of internal jugular, subclavian, or intraarterial catheters. A history of atrial fibrillation, carotid disease, or hypercoagulability increases the risk for thromboembolism.[179] Air embolism through a right-to-left intracardiac shunt and intracerebral hemorrhage secondary to hypertension also cause postoperative coma.

Cerebrovascular accidents are rare in lower risk patients and usually occur later in the postoperative course.[180]

## Why Does Altered Sensorium Occur After Anesthesia?

Inappropriate mental reactions ranging from lethargy and confusion to extreme disorientation and physical combativeness occur in the PACU (Table 6–16), especially during early emergence. These emergence reactions are disturbing to staff and other patients. Emergence reactions carry substantial risk for injury, including contusion or fracture due to contact with equipment or bed side rails, corneal abrasion due to dislodged $O_2$ apparatus, and sprains due to violent struggling. Combative, thrashing patients jeopardize suture lines, vascular grafts, and orthopedic fixation. They also dislodge drains, tracheal tubes, or vascular catheters. High SNS activity in agitated patients causes tachycardia and hypertension, with the potential for serious medical complications. The risk for injury to the PACU staff struggling to contain a combative patient is also significant.

### TABLE 6–16. Differential Diagnosis of Altered Sensorium During Emergence

| General Causes | Effects |
| --- | --- |
| Disorientation during emergence | Poor integration of sensory input, 10 min |
| Postoperative surgical pain | Treatment with analgesia if pain is clearly from procedure |
| Nonsurgical discomfort | Full bladder, nausea, gastric distention, positioning |
| Postoperative anxiety or fear | Separation from parents, emotional diagnoses, death |
| Inability to move, poor positioning | Escalating combativeness against restraint |
| Individual variation | Affected by intelligence, culture, gender, retardation |
| Unrecognized preoperative intoxication | Marked combativeness, disorientation |
| Scopolamine, ketamine, or etomidate | Occasional postoperative dysphoria |
| Atropine or meperidine | Rare anticholinergic-induced postoperative delirium |
| **Serious Underlying Abnormalities** | |
| Pulmonary dysfunction | Increased work of breathing, poor expansion, vascular distention |
| Hypoxemia | Clouding of sensorium, disorientation, mild agitation |
| Hypercarbia or acidemia | Marked agitation, disorientation, dyspnea, tachypnea |
| Hypotension | Cerebral hypoperfusion, confusion, nausea, somnolence |
| Hypoglycemia | Agitation, confusion, disorientation, sympathetic nervous system activity |
| Hyponatremia or hypoosmolality | Confusion, visual disturbances, seizures |
| Residual paralysis | Terrified, flopping motions mimic agitation |

## Patients at Risk

Although difficult to predict, extreme emergence reactions are more prevalent in children and young adults, especially after inhalation anesthesia with sevoflurane and desflurane.[181] Parental separation increases anxiety in young children. Elderly patients may recover cognitive function more slowly.[182,183]

Psychological, ethnic, and cultural differences have some role,[184,185] especially if a language barrier interferes with reassurance by the PACU staff. Oral fixation or tracheal intubation interferes with communication and generates frustration or fear. Preoperative psychological status often complicates the emergence of individuals with mental retardation, clinically evident psychiatric disorders, organic brain dysfunction, or hostile affect. The incidence of stormy emergence is probably higher after procedures that are associated with unusual anxiety or emotion, such as breast or testicular biopsies. Recall of intraoperative events may generate severe panic and anxiety during emergence.[186]

## Failure to Process Sensory Input

For a short period during emergence from general anesthesia, the ability to process and react to sensory input is impaired. Lack of integration may present as gradually clearing somnolence, disorientation, and sluggish mental responsiveness or as wide emotional swings with uncontrollable weeping. An occasional patient exhibits escalating combativeness against positioning and restraint.

## Sedatives and Psychiatric Drugs

Preoperative administration of long-acting sedatives or psychogenic medications clouds the sensorium and causes disorientation in the PACU. Preoperative alcohol or drug abuse often generates bizarre emergence behavior secondary to either residual intoxication or withdrawal.[187]

Disorientation, paranoia, and combativeness after parenteral scopolamine administration can be treated with intravenous physostigmine. Prolonged preoperative meperidine therapy or atropine premedication can also cause anticholinergic-induced postoperative delirium.[188,189] Etomidate induction may be associated with increased postoperative restlessness.[190] Postoperative dysphoria and hallucination secondary to acute ketamine reactions are rare but real. Droperidol occasionally generates acute dysphoria and agitation during recovery.

## Pain and Discomfort

Pain or discomfort amplifies confusion, agitation, and aggressive behavior during emergence; hence, adequate postoperative analgesia is essential early in the PACU course.[191] Urinary bladder or gastric distention generates marked discomfort and agitation in emerging patients. Tracheal or nasogastric tubes, urinary catheters, infiltrated vascular catheters, tight dressings, and painful phlebotomy are also troublesome.

Unusual sources of pain, such as corneal abrasion, entrapment of sensitive body parts, or small pieces of equipment left beneath a patient, are occasionally responsible. Nausea and dizziness are distressing, as is severe pruritus caused by medication reactions.

## Position and Restraint

Obese patients and those with gastroesophageal reflux or pulmonary congestion sometimes struggle vigorously to move from a supine into a semisitting position. Emerging patients often fight vigorously against physical restraint until the restraint is relaxed. Partial neuromuscular paralysis causes severe agitation during emergence, even if ventilation is adequate. Residual paralysis elicits violent, uncoordinated motion that may be mistaken for disorientation or combativeness.

## Respiratory Dysfunction

Confusion, delirium, or combativeness after anesthesia sometimes indicates serious respiratory dysfunction. Hypoxemia causes disorientation, clouded mentation, or agitation that is similar to that caused by pain. Respiratory acidemia also elicits profound agitation, although if hypercarbia is caused by respiratory center suppression, the visible responses may be reduced by coincident depression of other higher CNS functions. Hypercarbia without acidemia is usually asymptomatic unless $CO_2$ narcosis causes somnolence and disorientation. Acute respiratory alkalemia during hyperventilation causes dizziness, anxiety, and confusion.

Increased work of breathing from high airway resistance or partial upper airway obstruction causes marked agitation, as does the inability to cough or clear secretions. Pulmonary vascular engorgement or early interstitial pulmonary edema yields symptoms of chest fullness and air hunger well before airway flooding occurs.

Restriction of inspiratory volume by tight dressings, gastric distention, splinting, and inappropriately low tidal volume settings during mechanical ventilation cause vague manifestations similar to air hunger. This phenomenon is probably mediated by stretch receptors that monitor lung volume. Agitation caused by problems with the mechanics of ventilation can be profound, even though ventilation and oxygenation are adequate.

## Abnormal Perfusion

Lactic acidemia caused by poor peripheral perfusion results in anxiety and disorientation. Cerebral hypoperfusion is associated with lethargy, disorientation, agitation, or combativeness. Sedatives or analgesics administered to quell anxiety or pain may lead to cardiopulmonary collapse.

## Metabolic Changes

Metabolic abnormalities can interfere with lucidity. Acute hyponatremia and hypoosmolarity after transurethral prostatic resection markedly cloud the sensorium, although glycine toxicity may also play a part.[192] Cerebral fluid shifts that affect mentation can occur after dialysis, acute repletion of severe dehydration, or massive fluid infusion. Moderate hypoglycemia results in significant agitation or diminished responsiveness, whereas acute hyperglycemia due to excess glucose infusion or insufficient insulin can reduce consciousness.

Hypothermic patients exhibit reduced cognitive performance during emergence.

## Primary Neurologic Problems

A primary neurologic problem must be considered once reversible causes of delirium or agitation are eliminated. Seizure activity in patients with epilepsy, head trauma, chronic alcohol abuse, or cocaine intoxication can mimic agitation and combativeness and can generate disorientation and somnolence during the postictal phase.[187] Patients with cerebral embolism, hemorrhage, or infarct sometimes present with disorientation, inability to vocalize, or a reduced level of consciousness.[193]

### What Therapy Is Appropriate?

There is no effective prophylaxis against altered mental status in the PACU, and therapy is generally supportive. In children, use of preoperative sedatives does not appear to decrease the incidence of emergence delirium.[194] Most emergence reactions disappear as residual anesthesia resolves, although unpleasant sequelae can persist.[194,195] Reassuring a patient that he or she is doing well is invaluable, especially if the patient's and surgeon's name are frequently used and the time and location are emphasized. Allowing a patient to determine his own position is also helpful.

Of course, adequate analgesia is essential. A small amount of sedative is sometimes useful to reduce fear or anxiety. Before treatment, identify whether a patient is reacting to pain or to anxiety. Narcotics are relatively poor sedatives, whereas benzodiazepines or barbiturates are ineffective analgesics.

Use physical restraint only when a patient's physical safety is in jeopardy. Altered mental status caused by a physiologic abnormality, such as hypoxemia, acidemia, hypoglycemia, or hypotension, should be treated by resolving the underlying problem.

## POSTOPERATIVE NAUSEA AND VOMITING

PONV remains a significant problem during recovery. Avoidance of PONV is considered a major priority by both physicians and patients alike.[22]

### What Is the Impact?

The incidence of PONV varies widely with age, surgical procedure, and anesthetic technique. Incidence in the PACU is lower than incidence over 24 to 48 hours because emesis frequently occurs after discharge from the PACU.[196] Delayed emesis may be related to timing of oral intake or to waning effects of perioperative antiemetics. PONV often delays PACU discharge or necessitates admission of ambulatory patients, reducing efficiency and satisfaction of patients and surgeons.

Vomiting is unpleasant for patients and staff and poses genuine medical risks. Aspiration of gastric contents is a major risk, especially if airway reflexes are marginal or postoperative oral fixation interferes with airway clearance. Increased intra-abdominal pressure during vomiting jeopardizes abdominal or inguinal closures, whereas increased central venous pressure may increase morbidity after ocular, tympanic, or intracranial procedures. The SNS responses to vomiting and to pain from movement elevate the heart rate and BP, increasing the risk for myocardial ischemia and dysrhythmias.

Gagging and retching may also elicit a parasympathetic response with bradycardia and hypotension.

## What Are the Risk Factors?

### Demographic Factors

Many demographic factors appear to increase the risk for PONV or to predict its emergence. One large prospective study of 17 638 ambulatory patients[196] found an increased risk in younger patients, with likelihood of PONV decreasing 13% per decade of age. Women had a 3 times higher incidence than men. Risk for emesis was increased with general anesthesia and varied directly with duration of general anesthesia. Ear, nose, and throat and dental procedures had a high incidence (14.3%), followed by orthopedic shoulder procedures and plastic procedures. A history of preoperative emesis or motion sickness has some predictive value. Undergoing a general anesthetic near menses increases the incidence of vomiting in women,[197] perhaps related to an increase in circulating $E_2$ estrogen levels. The risk for PONV is also high after procedures involving extraocular muscles[198] or middle ear manipulation, peritoneal or intestinal irritation, and testicular traction.[199] Smokers have a significantly lower risk for PONV than nonsmokers.[196,200]

### Contributing Factors

The pathophysiology of PONV is complex and multifactorial. Risk for PONV is likely increased by starvation, gastric irritation, the effect of anesthetics on chemotactic centers, autonomic imbalance, and postoperative pain.[196] Swallowed blood or tissue promotes PONV, as does accumulation of gas in the stomach. General anesthesia generates more immediate postoperative vomiting than does regional, although vomiting frequently occurs when parenteral narcotics are required as the regional block resolves.

### Anesthetic Agents

Although controversy will undoubtedly continue, it seems clear from recent meta-analyses that exclusion of nitrous oxide from an anesthetic reduces the incidence of postoperative vomiting.[201,202] The incidence of PONV does not appear to differ significantly among the potent inhalation anesthetics, although sevoflurane may generate a marginally higher incidence.

Barbiturate induction appears less offensive than ketamine or etomidate; propofol induction may have the lowest incidence. Narcotic analgesics probably increase PONV when compared with "pure" inhalational or propofol infusion techniques, especially in ambulatory surgical patients.[196]

Nonnarcotic analgesics, such as ketorolac, in conjunction with small doses of narcotics, may reduce the severity of emesis. It is unclear whether neostigmine administered during reversal of neuromuscular relaxants or physostigmine given to counteract sedation also increases the incidence of PONV. Anticholinergics used for reversal of paralysis may also affect incidence.[203]

## How Are Postoperative Nausea and Vomiting Prevented and Treated?

Several interventions help to prevent PONV. Adequate postoperative analgesia is important, as is limiting postoperative vestibular stimulation by minimizing brisk head motion. Avoiding gastric distention by evacuation of stomach contents with an orogastric tube is of questionable value. Maintaining adequate hydration appears to reduce the incidence of PONV,[204] but initiation of postoperative drinking is frequently a triggering event. It is sometimes appropriate to discharge children or high-risk patients before they take oral fluids.[205] Whether this decreases the incidence of vomiting or merely delays its onset is unclear.

It is important to remember that nausea and vomiting are also signs of serious underlying physiologic abnormalities. Before instituting treatment, it is important to evaluate for hypotension, increased intracranial pressure, hypoxemia, hypoglycemia, or gastric bleeding.

### Antiemetic Therapy

A staggering number of studies have attempted to elucidate which medications are most effective for the prophylaxis and treatment of PONV, with respect to both efficacy and cost-effectiveness. Although universal consensus has yet to be reached, three medications emerge as mainstay antiemetics for PONV: droperidol, ondansetron, and metoclopramide.[198,206] Among the three, droperidol and ondansetron are probably equal in effectiveness and patient satisfaction,[207] whereas metoclopramide holds a weak third place.[208] Given the different loci of action for these antiemetics, combination therapy may generate better results by treating two or more precipitating factors simultaneously.[209,210]

### Droperidol

The potent antiemetic effect of intravenous droperidol is clear, and it has remained a cornerstone of therapy. Intravenous droperidol decreases the incidence and severity of PONV, although its efficacy varies among procedures and individual patients. A total dose of 1 to 2 µg/kg (0.625 mg to 1.25 mg in adults) appears optimally effective and seldom causes excessive sedation.[207]

For patients who have already received prophylaxis, intravenous droperidol effectively treats breakthrough nausea in the PACU. Although resulting sedation may delay discharge, the delay secondary to untreated PONV is usually greater. The α-adrenergic receptor–blocking properties of droperidol can precipitate hypotension in hypovolemic patients. Transient restlessness or sedation and rare extrapyramidal side effects are usually inconsequential.[208,211]

### Ondansetron and Other 5-Hydroxytryptamine Antagonists

Ondansetron, a serotonin receptor blocker, is a useful antiemetic to treat PONV. Optimal intravenous dosage in adults appears to be 4 mg. Administration near the end of surgery or on admission to the PACU appears most effective.[212] Ondansetron may be particularly useful for PONV caused by blood or other substances that stimulate the enterochromaffin cells of the gastric lining.[213] Ondansetron has notably few side effects, although headache can be troublesome,[208] and a small percentage of patients exhibit a transient elevation of liver enzymes after its intravenous administration.[214] Although the drug is costly, the potential yield from avoiding unnecessary admission, shortening PACU length of stay, and improving patient satisfaction is well worth its expense.

Granisetron, tropisetron, dolasetron, and the newer ramosetron have all been studied.[215–217] Although each has demonstrable antiemetic properties compared with placebo, none yet surpasses ondansetron for efficacy and cost-effectiveness.

### Metoclopramide

Intravenous metoclopramide, alone or with droperidol, decreases the incidence of PONV. Whether metoclopramide merely reduces gastric volume or has an additional central antiemetic action is unclear. Rarely, it causes dysphoria.

### Less Effective Antiemetic Medications

Propofol has short-term antiemetic properties that make it an appealing agent for induction and maintenance of anesthesia, especially in patients at high risk for PONV[218]; however, it does not compare with droperidol or ondansetron as a first-line antiemetic agent.[198] Dexamethasone has an antiemetic effect, particularly when employed during upper airway procedures such as adenotonsillectomy.[219] Whether its effect is secondary to its antiinflammatory properties or to a direct antiemetic action is unclear.[220]

Although cimetidine and ranitidine (Zantac) decrease gastric acidity and ranitidine improves gastric emptying, neither has significant efficacy for the treatment of PONV. Dimenhydrinate and thiethylperazine also appear less effective. Intravenous scopolamine causes unacceptable psychogenic reactions when used as an antiemetic. Low efficacy and a tendency to cause visual disturbances make transdermal scopolamine a poor substitute for other agents.[221] Ephedrine may be effective for PONV related to ambulation or motion, but its efficacy is unclear.[222] The antiemetic effect of midazolam in children may be related to the relationship between crying or agitation and nausea.

### Alternative Therapies

Acupuncture stimulation and acupressure have been shown to reduce the incidence of postoperative vomiting.[223] These modalities are not commonly used and would need to be clearly superior to antiemetic medications before they gained wide acceptance.

## POSTOPERATIVE HYPOTHERMIA

Although intraoperative temperature maintenance is prevalent, many patients still exhibit hypothermia after surgery. The level at which the body actively begins to regulate temperature (ie, the thermoregulatory threshold) is decreased by about 2.5°C during general anesthesia.[224]

### Why Does Hypothermia Develop?

During surgery, heat is lost through evaporation during skin preparation, by airway humidification of dry gases, and through radiation and convection from the skin and surgical wound. A reduction in core temperature is accelerated by low ambient temperatures and cold intravenous fluids.[224]

The ability to maintain body temperature is compromised even after temperature reaches the reset thermoregulatory threshold. Paralysis and anesthesia impair shivering, and nonshivering thermogenesis is relatively ineffective in adults. Peripheral thermoregulatory vasoconstriction decreases heat loss but is less effective in anesthetized patients.

Heat loss is about the same during general and regional anesthesia, but rewarming is slower after regional anesthetics because residual vasodilation and paralysis interfere with heat generation and retention. Infants are at increased risk because their body mass is relatively low compared with surface area. Cachectic, traumatized, and burned patients are prone to more serious temperature reduction.

### What Are the Adverse Effects?

Adverse effects are many and varied (Table 6–17). Hypothermia increases postoperative morbidity because it increases SNS activity, elevates peripheral vascular resistance, and decreases venous capacitance.[225] Risk for adverse cardiac events, such as myocardial ischemia, is increased.[226] The temperature corrected alveolar-arterial gradient for oxygen becomes larger.[227] Hypoperfusion of peripheral tissues promotes hypoxia and metabolic acidemia, jeopardizing the viability of marginal tissue grafts. Increased avidity of hemoglobin for $O_2$ further compromises oxygenation in hypothermic tissues. Visceral sequestration of platelets, decreased platelet function, and reduced activity of clotting factors may cause mild coagulopathy. Patients become moderately hyperglycemic. Cellular immune responses are compromised,[228] and postoperative infection rates rise.[229]

The minimal alveolar concentration of inhalation anesthetics decreases 5% to 7% per 1°C reduction in core temperature, accentuating sedation from residual alveolar partial pressures. Decreased biotransformation and reduced perfusion may increase the duration of sedation and neuromuscular relaxation.

Severe hypothermia interferes with cardiac rhythm generation and impulse conduction, lengthening PR, QRS, or QT intervals and generating J waves on ECG. The risk for dysrhythmia after mechanical stimulation of the myocardium is increased, and spontaneous ventricular fibrillation can occur at temperatures of <28°C.

Hypothermia also complicates care rendered in the PACU. Thermoregulatory vasoconstriction interferes with the reliabil-

**TABLE 6–17.** Adverse Effects of Hypothermia

Increased systemic vascular resistance
Decreased venous capacitance
Hypoperfusion
Increased hemoglobin affinity
Decreased metabolic biotransformation
Increased sedation
Hyperglycemia
Platelet sequestration
Decreased renal function
Cardiac dysrhythmias
Shivering

ity of pulse oximetry, intraarterial pressure monitoring, and peripheral nerve stimulation. Hypothermic patients remain in the PACU an average of 90 minutes longer than normothermic patients and 40 minutes longer if complete rewarming is excluded as a discharge criterion.[230]

## Why Is Shivering Detrimental?

During emergence from general anesthesia, hypothalamic regulation steps up metabolic activity and generates shivering to increase endogenous heat production.[231] The intensity of postoperative shivering is sometimes accentuated by inhalation anesthetic–related tremor, which manifests both clonic and tonic components. The former may be triggered by hypothermia but appears related to decreased cortical influence on spinal cord reflexes.

Postoperative shivering increases the risk for incidental trauma and makes routine PACU care more difficult. Shivering increases $O_2$ consumption and $CO_2$ production by up to 800%. The associated increase in cardiac output and minute ventilation may precipitate myocardial ischemia or ventilatory failure in patients with CAD or limited ventilatory reserve.[226,232]

### Treatment

Morphine, meperidine, sufentanil, propofol, droperidol, physostigmine, clonidine, butorphanol, nalbuphine, chlorpromazine, methylphenidate, and magnesium all have been advocated to suppress shivering.[233–235] Withholding the reversal of neuromuscular relaxants in intubated, ventilated, sedated patients attenuates shivering but increases rewarming time. Additional relaxant administration in the PACU to eliminate shivering in patients with limited cardiac reserve is an option but is usually not indicated.

For most PACU patients, shivering during resolution of mild to moderate hypothermia is uncomfortable but self-limited and inconsequential. It needs no treatment other than reassurance and warming.

## How Is Hypothermia Attenuated or Prevented?

During surgery, covering exposed body and head surfaces and warming of ambient air, intravenous fluids, and irrigating solutions are useful to counteract temperature loss. Surface or radiant warmers and heated humidification of inspired gases also help.

All hypothermic patients should receive supplemental $O_2$ in the PACU. Reduction of core temperature is <2 to 3°C in most patients; thus, spontaneous rewarming during recovery is usually sufficient, although moderate shivering often occurs. Patients undergoing prolonged major surgical procedures with significant fluid replacement can suffer more profound hypothermia. Core temperature of <35°C is an indication for assisted rewarming using heating blankets, reflective coverings, radiant lighting, or forced air. As body temperature rises, hypotension caused by increasing venous capacitance can occur.

## POSTOPERATIVE HYPERTHERMIA

### What Is the Impact?

Fever is less common than hypothermia in the PACU. Self-limited hyperthermia is occasionally caused by close draping or aggressive heat preservation in the OR. Postoperative fever from atelectasis or respiratory infection secondary to lost lung volume or retained secretions occurs more often after PACU discharge. Unrecognized intraoperative aspiration sometimes presents with fever in the PACU. Exacerbation of infection during tonsillectomy or appendectomy, abscess drainage, and urinary tract manipulation are other frequent causes. Emergence of preexisting influenza, sinusitis, otitis, or upper respiratory infection may also generate fever.

Increased body temperature is a presenting sign of a drug or transfusion reaction. Muscarinic blocking agents like atropine interfere with cutaneous cooling and can contribute to postoperative fever. Increased temperature occurs during malignant hyperthermia, but other signs, such as tachycardia, rigidity, acidemia, and hypercarbia, generally precede it. Rare causes of hypermetabolism, such as thyroid storm, must also be considered.

### How Is Hyperthermia Treated?

Therapy for fever is generally supportive. Chest physiotherapy, incentive spirometry, and administration of antipyretics are usually sufficient. If a drug or transfusion reaction is suspected, the offending medication or blood product should be withheld. The physician responsible for long-term care should be notified to observe for a more serious problem.

## POSTOPERATIVE ACID-BASE PROBLEMS

### Why Does Respiratory Acidemia Occur?

Respiratory acidemia frequently occurs in the PACU because inhalation anesthetics, opioids, and sedative medications promote hypoventilation. Hypercarbia and acidemia are usually mild in awake, spontaneously breathing patients. Residual neuromuscular paralysis, increased airway resistance, or decreased pulmonary compliance, however, can impede ventilation and generate progressive respiratory acidemia despite appropriate CNS drive to breathe. Elevated $CO_2$ production caused by shivering, fever, hyperalimentation, or malignant hyperthermia amplifies the problem, as does increased dead space.

### Effects

Respiratory acidemia causes agitation, confusion, dyspnea, and tachypnea as well as hypertension, tachycardia, and dysrhythmias due to increased SNS activity. When caused by CNS depression, SNS activity is less intense because central autonomic responses are also depressed. Cerebral blood flow increases and intracranial pressure rises in patients with head injury, intracranial tumor, or cerebral edema.[236] In patients with CAD, myocardial blood flow is also increased in proportion to increased cardiac index.[237] At low pH, heart rate and BP decrease precipitously.

## Treatment

Compensation is limited for acute respiratory acidemia because the kidneys require many hours to conserve enough bicarbonate. Therapy involves correction of the imbalance between effective alveolar ventilation and $CO_2$ production. Reversal of narcotics or neuromuscular relaxants, relief of airway obstruction, or improvement of ventilatory mechanics may suffice. If $CO_2$ elimination cannot be maintained with spontaneous ventilation, tracheal intubation and mechanical ventilation are required. Reducing $CO_2$ production by controlling fever, shivering, and work of breathing may be helpful, but extreme measures such as core cooling or paralysis are seldom appropriate.

## Why Does Metabolic Acidemia Occur?

Postoperative metabolic acidemia sometimes reflects ketoacidosis in severely diabetic patients. Elevated serum glucose levels and urinary or blood ketones are diagnostic. Patients suffering from renal failure, renal tubular acidosis, or small bowel drainage often exhibit preoperative metabolic acidemia. Overdose with phenformin, aspirin, or methanol rarely causes postoperative metabolic acidemia. Excessive saline infusion during surgery can cause a self-limited, moderate hyperchloremic acidemia in the PACU.[238] Substitution of lactated Ringer's solution helps resolve this problem.

After ketoacidosis or a known metabolic problem is excluded, postoperative metabolic acidemia almost always reflects lactic acid accumulation secondary to insufficient delivery or use of $O_2$ in tissues. Peripheral hypoperfusion is often caused by low cardiac output due to hypovolemia, sympathectomy, or cardiac failure. Intense arteriolar constriction due to hypothermia reduces tissue perfusion, as does inappropriate distribution of peripheral blood flow.

Hypoxemia from pulmonary dysfunction, decreased oxygen-carrying capacity from anemia or carbon monoxide poisoning, and hemoglobin dissociation abnormalities can all contribute to lactic acidemia after surgery.

## Effects

Signs of metabolic acidemia are similar to those of respiratory acidemia. The sympathetic response to acute metabolic acidemia is usually somewhat less than that to respiratory acidemia because hydrogen and bicarbonate ions cross the blood-brain barrier with more difficulty than $CO_2$.

## Treatment

A spontaneously ventilating patient should generate a respiratory compensation to offset metabolic acidemia, but anesthetic agents and narcotics can suppress the ventilatory response. Therapy should resolve the condition causing accumulation of metabolic acid. Fluids and intravenous insulin, potassium, and glucose are used to treat ketoacidosis. After cardiac output and systemic BP are improved, mild lactic acidemia resolves spontaneously through acid metabolism and renal excretion of hydrogen ions. Rewarming also improves perfusion. Intravenous sodium bicarbonate or a suitable substitute helps restore pH toward normal when acidemia is severe or progressive despite other therapy.

## Why Does Respiratory Alkalemia Occur?

Pain or anxiety during emergence commonly causes spontaneous hyperventilation and acute respiratory alkalemia. Pain from clumsy blood sampling sometimes generates a spurious alkalemia on ABG. Pathologic causes of spontaneous hyperventilation include cerebrovascular accident, sepsis, or paradoxical CNS acidosis.

Excessive mechanical ventilation frequently causes postoperative respiratory alkalemia, especially when hypothermia or paralysis has reduced $CO_2$ production.

## Effects

In PACU patients, acute respiratory alkalemia causes confusion or dizziness, atrial dysrhythmias, and mild cardiac conduction abnormalities. Alkalemia decreases cerebral blood flow and may lead to hypoperfusion and cerebral ischemia in patients with cerebrovascular disease. Avidity of hemoglobin for oxygen is increased; thus, peripheral unloading of oxygen is reduced. More severe alkalemia precipitates muscle fasciculation or tetany resulting from reduction of serum ionized calcium. High pH levels directly depress cardiovascular and CNS function and interfere with catecholamine receptor function.

## Treatment

Large renal time constants for bicarbonate excretion limit metabolic compensation for acute respiratory alkalemia. Correction of respiratory alkalemia necessitates reduction of effective alveolar ventilation, usually through the administration of analgesics and sedatives to control pain and anxiety. Rebreathing of exhaled $CO_2$ or addition of $CO_2$ to inspired gases is seldom useful in the PACU.

## Why Does Metabolic Alkalemia Occur?

New-onset metabolic alkalemia is unusual during the immediate recovery period. Preoperative vomiting, gastric suctioning, dehydration, or potassium wasting may generate a known alkalemia that persists through surgery. Metabolism of excess sodium lactate or citrate in blood products usually requires 24 hours to generate significant bicarbonate, but excessive bicarbonate administration causes postoperative metabolic alkalemia.

## Treatment

Retention of $CO_2$ to compensate for metabolic alkalemia is rapid but limited because hypoventilation causes hypoxemia at some point. Hydration and correction of hypochloremia and hypokalemia are important for the kidneys to retain hydrogen and to excrete bicarbonate. Hydrochloric acid infusion through a central venous catheter is seldom necessary but is effective to treat severe, life-threatening metabolic alkalemia. Acetazolamide is useful if hypochloremia has been corrected.

# POSTOPERATIVE GLUCOSE AND ELECTROLYTE ABNORMALITIES

## Why Does Hyperglycemia Occur?

Glucose infusions and stress response commonly elevate serum glucose levels in patients recovering from surgery, but hyperglycemia may also indicate severe insulin deficiency and evolving ketoacidosis in diabetic patients.

### Effects and Treatment

Short duration, moderate hyperglycemia (200-300 mg/dL) probably has little adverse effect and usually resolves spontaneously. Higher glucose levels cause glycosuria and osmotic diuresis and reduce the accuracy of serum electrolyte determinations. Severe hyperglycemia increases serum osmolarity and generates cerebral disequilibrium and hyperosmolar coma.

Treatment of severe hyperglycemia includes titration of intravenous regular insulin by small incremental bolus or continuous infusion. Potassium replacement and monitoring of serial blood glucose levels are essential.

## Why Does Hypoglycemia Occur?

Hypoglycemia in the PACU can be caused by endogenous insulin secretion or by inadvertent or excessive insulin administration. Sedation or excessive SNS activity may mask signs and symptoms of hypoglycemia during recovery. Serious postoperative hypoglycemia is rare and easily treated by intravenous administration of 50% dextrose followed by glucose infusion.

## Why Does Hyponatremia Occur?

Postoperative hyponatremia occurs if excess free water is infused or absorbed during surgery. Uptake of sodium-free irrigating solution during hysteroscopy or through prostatic venous sinuses during transurethral prostatic resection are classic examples.[192] The effects of glycine or its metabolite, ammonia, can exacerbate the signs. Inappropriate secretion of antidiuretic hormone, prolonged labor induction with oxytocin, and respiratory uptake of nebulized water droplets can also result in free water retention.

Excess intraoperative administration of isotonic saline can expand extracellular volume and lead to excretion of large amounts of hypertonic urine, causing iatrogenic hyponatremia through desalination.[239]

### Effects and Treatment

Symptoms of moderate hyponatremia include nausea, agitation, disorientation, and visual disturbances. More severe dilution causes unconsciousness, decreased effectiveness of airway reflexes, and grand mal seizures.

Therapy of acute hyponatremia incorporates water restriction in mild cases and infusion of normal saline with intravenous furosemide in moderate to severe cases. Infusion of hypertonic saline with careful monitoring of serum sodium concentration and osmolarity is effective in particularly severe instances. Care should be taken to avoid volume overload and desalination.

## Why Does Hypokalemia Occur?

A potassium deficit caused by chronic diuretic administration, prolonged nasogastric suctioning, or vomiting usually underlies postoperative hypokalemia. Dilution, urinary and hemorrhagic losses, and insulin therapy often exacerbate potassium deficits. A shift of potassium into cells during β-adrenergic receptor therapy or acute respiratory alkalemia acutely exacerbates hypokalemia in the PACU.

### Effects and Treatment

Postoperative hypokalemia is usually inconsequential but occasionally can generate serious dysrhythmia, especially in patients taking digitalis preparations. Hypokalemic patients should be closely observed during infusion of calcium, insulin, or β-mimetic medications and during periods of increased SNS activity.

Addition of supplemental potassium to routine intravenous fluids usually restores an acceptable serum concentration, but infusion of concentrated solutions through a central catheter may be necessary. Correction of serum concentration does not imply repletion of the total body deficit.

## Why Does Hyperkalemia Occur?

Postoperative hyperkalemia can result from excessive potassium administration, chronic renal failure, or malignant hyperthermia. Acute acidemia exacerbates postoperative hyperkalemia by shifting potassium from cells to the serum. Succinylcholine may increase serum potassium to dangerous levels in patients with burns or old neurologic injuries. Potassium levels may also rise during reperfusion of severely ischemic tissue.

### Effects and Treatment

The major complication of hyperkalemia is cardiac dysrhythmia culminating in cardiac arrest at levels of >7.5 to 8 mEq/dL. Intravenous insulin and glucose acutely lower the serum potassium level, whereas intravenous calcium transiently counters myocardial effects. Whenever an unusually high serum potassium level appears with no apparent cause, suspect spurious hyperkalemia caused by a hemolyzed specimen or sampling near an intravenous infusion containing potassium or banked blood.

## Are Calcium and Magnesium Important?

Hypocalcemia is rarely a problem in the PACU. Massive fluid replacement or underlying parathyroid disease reduces total body calcium, although symptomatic hypocalcemia seldom occurs. A rare patient will manifest hypocalcemia after parathyroid excision. Transfusion of blood containing chelating agents also rarely causes symptomatic hypocalcemia. Magnesium plays a key role in neuromuscular function after surgery,[117] and in maintenance of cardiac rhythm and conduction.[240]

### Effects and Treatment

Hypocalcemia secondary to surgical parathyroidectomy usually takes several hours to cause clinical symptoms but can present with acute laryngospasm within 3 hours. Further reduction of the critical ionized fraction by metabolic or respiratory alkalemia may cause myocardial conduction and contractility abnormalities, decreased vascular tone, or tetany. Administration of calcium to hypocalcemic patients improves cardiovascular dynamics and response to intravenous fluids. Calcium salts are no longer recommended during cardiopulmonary resuscitation unless hypocalcemia is known to be present.

# MISCELLANEOUS POSTOPERATIVE COMPLICATIONS

Anesthetized or emerging patients can suffer incidental trauma from equipment, positioning, and nonsurgical manipulations.

## What Are the Causes of Corneal Injury?

Corneal abrasion is the most common eye injury related to surgery,[241] although conjunctivitis and chemical injuries from exposure to irritating solutions are also seen. Corneal injury due to drying or inadvertent eye contact during airway manipulation occurs more frequently in elderly patients, after long cases, with lateral positioning, and after head and neck surgery.[242] The injury causes pain, photophobia, tearing, and decreased visual acuity. Fluorescein staining is useful for diagnosis, and treatment with artificial tears and eye closure is primarily symptomatic. Abrasions usually heal spontaneously within 72 hours, but severe injury can lead to cataract formation and impaired vision.

## Why Does Soft Tissue Trauma Occur?

Oral soft tissue trauma frequently results from laryngoscopy, indwelling airways, or biting. Lip, tongue, or gum abrasions require only an ice pack for treatment, but penetrating injuries caused by entrapment of tissue between the teeth and laryngoscope blade or airway may benefit from topical antibiotic application.

Upper airway edema or hematoma due to traumatic or difficult tracheal intubation must be considered before extubation. Nebulized racemic epinephrine may reduce stridor and edema. A dental consultation should be obtained if teeth or dental appliances are loosened or broken, and the patient should be monitored for signs of foreign body aspiration.[243]

## When Is Trauma to the Airways a Problem?

Tracheal intubation causes sore throat and hoarseness in 20% to 50% of patients. Symptoms vary with the degree of trauma during laryngoscopy or oropharyngeal suctioning, the duration of tracheal intubation, and the type of tube.[244] Sore throat from expansion of cuff volume with nitrous oxide can be attenuated by inflating the cuff with a sample of the anesthetic mixture. Mucosal irritation often presents as unquenchable dryness in the mouth and throat. Lubrication of tubes with anesthetic ointments probably does not help and may cause additional irritation to the tracheal mucosa. Sore throat can also be caused by breathing dry gases or by trauma resulting from oral airways and suctioning.

In children, the severity of postextubation laryngeal edema or tracheitis depends on age, intubation trauma, duration of intubation, and degree of movement with the tracheal tube in place. Cool mist therapy is usually sufficient, although racemic epinephrine often helps to relieve the signs of upper airway obstruction.

Other traumatic complications of laryngoscopy and intubation include desquamation of mucosa, vocal cord avulsion, airway wall ulceration, tracheal perforation, and hypoglossal, lingual, or recurrent laryngeal nerve damage.[245]

## What Neurologic Injuries May Be Seen After Regional Anesthesia?

### Postdural Puncture Headache

Despite progress with spinal needle design, postdural puncture headache still occurs and often manifests first in the PACU. Headache is more frequent after difficult subarachnoid anesthetics with multiple attempts[246] and after dural puncture during attempted epidural placement. Subarachnoid air bubbles from loss of resistance testing may contribute to headache after attempted epidural anesthesia.[247] In the PACU, treatment of headache is supportive with hydration, analgesics, and positioning, although in clear cases, early epidural blood patch may be appropriate.

### Needle Injury

Risk for mechanical nerve injury during placement of regional anesthetics is small but real.[248,249] In the PACU, patients may complain of residual paresthesia, dysesthesia, or focal numbness related to trauma from regional anesthesia placement. These symptoms are almost always transient. In one large study, 6.3% of 4767 patients having spinal anesthesia suffered paresthesia during placement, but only 0.126% had persisting symptoms.[250] Treatment should include analgesics, reassurance, and notification of the primary physician for follow-up. Close observation is necessary to ensure that neurologic symptoms do not predict a more serious complication.

### Chemical Injury

During recovery from spinal anesthesia, some patients exhibit buttock pain, lower extremity discomfort, and other signs of sacral neurologic irritation. This finding is more common after spinal anesthesia with 5% lidocaine, in obese patients, and after procedures in lithotomy position.[251] Symptoms are usually transient and are treated supportively.

Rarely, a patient exhibits severe headache and meningeal signs secondary to chemical meningitis after injection of a spinal anesthetic solution that is contaminated or that is outside an acceptable pH range.

## What Factors Predispose to Peripheral Nerve Injury?

Peripheral nerve compression against hard surfaces during general or regional anesthesia sometimes causes permanent sensory and motor deficits, as do stretch injuries resulting from inadvertent hyperextension of an extremity.[248] Whenever pressure-related bruising or skin breakdown is noted, underlying nerve damage must be considered. Unfortunately, many postoperative neuropathies occur without an identifiable cause. This is particularly true of ulnar neuropathy, which may be related to preexisting subclinical impairment,[252] subtle positioning problems,[253] or increased sensitivity of the ulnar nerve to ischemia.[254] Any complaint of pain, numbness, or weakness during PACU evaluation should be evaluated and documented. Notification of the physician responsible for long-term care is essential to ensure follow-up.

## What Visual Disturbances May Occur?

Visual acuity is often transiently impaired during emergence. Autonomic side effects of medications impair accommodation, and residual ocular lubricant clouds vision. Occlusion of retinal perfusion by ocular compression can generate postoperative visual disturbances ranging from loss of acuity to permanent blindness.[255] Ischemic optic atrophy can also occur without evidence of external compression of the globes.[256] Risk is especially high after prolonged prone procedures and in patients with vascular disease and anemia. PACU staff should be alert for complaints of visual impairment and should perform a cursory check of vision in patients at high risk for ischemic optic atrophy.

## What Problems Are Associated With Positioning?

Ischemia and necrosis of soft tissue can occur during long surgical procedures, especially if pressure points are not properly padded. Entrapment of breasts, genitalia, ears, and skin folds may cause necrosis, especially in the lateral or prone positions. Scalp pressure may cause localized alopecia. Regional ischemia secondary to arterial inflow occlusion is possible, although rare. Joint or muscle hyperextension can cause postoperative pain, stiffness, backache, and even joint instability.

## How Do Injuries Occur in the Postanesthesia Care Unit?

Incidental injury also occurs in the PACU, especially with thrashing during emergence. Bruising resulting from contact with stretcher rails, damage to dental appliances from biting on rigid airways, and corneal injury caused by rigid disposable face masks are relatively common. Dislocation or infiltration of vascular catheters can lead to hematoma formation or extravasation of caustic medications. Discovery of a complication in the PACU requires careful documentation, notification of primary physicians, consultation of appropriate specialists, and assiduous follow-up.

## What Are the Causes of Postoperative Skeletal Muscle Pain?

Postoperative muscle pain undoubtedly is caused by various intraoperative factors. Prolonged immobility and excessive muscle stretch during positioning often contribute to stiffness and aching after surgery. Symptoms referable to joint hyperextension also lead to postoperative complaints or soreness.

Fasciculation during depolarizing blockade with succinylcholine has been implicated as a cause of postoperative myalgia.[257] Acute myalgia occurs less frequently after administration of other relaxants; it also occurs in patients receiving no relaxant whatsoever. Delayed-onset muscle fatigue that appears days after surgery usually resolves spontaneously.

### References

1. DeFranco M. Planning the physical structure of the PACU. In: Frost EAM, ed. *Post Anesthesia Care Unit.* St Louis, Mo: CV Mosby; 1990:187.
2. Bothner U, Georgieff M, Schwilk B. The impact of minor perioperative anesthesia related incidents, events and complications on postanesthetic care unit utilization. *Anesth Analg.* 1999;89:507.
3. Waddle JP, Evers AS, Piccirillo JF. Postanesthesia care unit length of stay: quantifying and assessing dependent factors. *Anesth Analg.* 1998;87:628.
4. Tarazi E, Philip B. Friendliness of OR staff is top determinant of patient satisfaction with outpatient surgery. *Am J Anesthesiol.* 1998;4:154.
5. Sullivan E, Mamaril M, Bauer J, et al. *Standard of Peri-Anesthesia Nursing Practice.* Thorofare, NJ: American Society of Post-Anesthesia Nurses; 1998.
6. Clemency MV, Thompson NJ. Do not resuscitate orders in the perioperative period: patient perspectives. *Anesth Analg.* 1997;84:859.
7. Tait AR. Occupational transmission of tuberculosis: implications for anesthesiologists. *Anesth Analg.* 1997;5:444.
8. McGregor DG, Senjem DH, Mazze RI. Trace nitrous oxide levels in the postanesthesia care unit. *Anesth Analg.* 1999;89:472.
9. Dexter F, Macario A, Manberg PJ, et al. Computer simulation to determine how rapid anesthetic recovery protocols to decrease time for emergence or increase the phase I postanesthetic care unit bypass rate affect staffing of an ambulatory surgery center. *Anesth Analg.* 1999;88:1053.
10. Gan TJ, Glass TS, Windsor A, et al. Bispectral index monitoring allows faster emergence and improved recovery from propofol, alfentanil, and nitrous oxide anesthesia. *Anesthesiology.* 1997;87:808.
11. Song D, Joshi G, White PF. Fast track eligibility after ambulatory anesthesia: a comparison of desflurane, sevoflurane, and propofol. *Anesth Analg.* 1998;86:267.
12. Hines R, Barash PG, Watrous G, et al. Complications occurring in the postanesthesia care unit: a survey. *Anesth Analg.* 1992;74:503.
13. Kolpfenstein CE, Herrmann FR, Michel JP, et al. The influence of an aging surgical population on the anesthesia workload: a ten year survey. *Anesth Analg.* 1998;86:1165.
14. Chung F: Recovery pattern and home readiness after ambulatory surgery. *Anesth Analg.* 1995;80:896.
15. Pavlin DJ, Rapp SE, Polissar NL, et al. Factors affecting discharge time in adult outpatients. *Anesth Analg.* 1998;87:816.
16. Ballantyne JC, Chang Y. The impact of choice of muscle relaxant on postoperative recovery time: a retrospective study. *Anesth Analg.* 1997;85:476.
17. Dexter F, Tinker JH. Analysis of strategies to decrease post anesthesia care unit costs. *Anesthesiology.* 1995;82:94.
18. Aldrete JA, Kroulik D. A postanesthetic recovery score. *Anesth Analg.* 1970;49:924.
19. Aldrete JA. The post-anesthesia recovery score revisited. *J Clin Anesth.* 1995;7:89.
20. White PF, Song D. New criteria for fast tracking after outpatient anesthesia: a comparison with the modified Aldrete's scoring system. *Anesth Analg.* 1999;88:1069.
21. Chung F, Chen VW, Ong D. A post-anesthetic discharge scoring system for home readiness after ambulatory surgery. *J Clin Anesth.* 1995;7:500.
22. Macario A, Weinger M, Truong P, et al. Which clinical anesthesia outcomes are both common and important to avoid? The perspective of a panel of expert anesthesiologists. *Anesth Analg.* 1999;88:1085.
23. Chung F, Ritchie E, Su J. Postoperative pain in ambulatory surgery. *Anesth Analg.* 1997;85:808.
24. Lynch EP, Lazor MA, Gellis J, et al. Patient experience of pain after elective non cardiac surgery. *Anesth Analg.* 1997;85:117.
25. Rawal N. 10 Years of acute pain services: achievements and challenges. *Reg Anesth Pain Med.* 1999;24:68.

26. Rundshagen I, Schnabel K, Standl T, et al. Patients' vs. nurses' assessments of postoperative pain and anxiety during patient or nurse controlled analgesia. *Br J Anaesth.* 1999;82:374.

27. Sear JW. Recent advances and developments in the clinical use of IV opioids during the perioperative period. *Br J Anaesth.* 1998;81:38.

28. Peng PWH, Sandler AN. A review of the use of fentanyl analgesia in the management of acute pain in adults. *Anesthesiology.* 1999;90:576.

29. Claxton AR, McGuire G, Chung F, et al. Evaluation of morphine versus fentanyl for postoperative analgesia after ambulatory surgical procedures. *Anesth Analg.* 1997;84:509.

30. Slappendel R, Weber EWG, Bugter MLT, et al. The intensity of preoperative pain is directly correlated with the amount of morphine needed for postoperative analgesia. *Anesth Analg.* 1999;88:146.

31. Plummer JL, Owen H, Ilsley AH, et al. Sustained release ibuprofen as an adjunct to morphine patient controlled analgesia. *Anesth Analg.* 1996;83:92.

32. Korpela R, Korvenoja P, Meretoja OA. Morphine sparing effect of acetaminophen in pediatric day case surgery. *Anesthesiology.* 1999;91:442.

33. Schug SA, Sidebotham DA, McGuinnety M, et al. Acetaminophen as an adjunct to morphine by patient controlled analgesia in the management of acute postoperative pain. *Anesth Analg.* 1998;87:368.

34. Suzuki M, Tsuedo K, Lansing P, et al. Small dose ketamine enhances morphine induced analgesia after outpatient surgery. *Anesth Analg.* 1999;89:98.

35. Strom BL, Berlin JA, Kinman JL, et al. Parenteral ketorolac and risk of gastrointestinal and operative site bleeding: a post-marketing surveillance study. *JAMA.* 1996;275:376.

36. Reuben SS, Connelly NR, Lurie S, et al. Dose-response of ketorolac as an adjunct to morphine patient controlled analgesia in patients after spinal fusion surgery. *Anesth Analg.* 1998;87:98.

37. Beattie WS, Warriner CB, Etches R, et al. The addition of continuous intravenous infusion of ketorolac to a patient controlled analgetic morphine regime reduced postoperative myocardial ischemia in patients undergoing elective total hip or knee arthroplasty. *Anesth Analg.* 1997;84:715.

38. Henderson DJ, Withington BS, Wilson JA, et al. Perioperative dextromethorphan reduces postoperative pain after hysterectomy. *Anesth Analg.* 1999;89:399.

39. Gwirtz KH, Young JV, Byers RS, et al. The safety and efficacy of intrathecal opioid analgesia for acute postoperative pain: seven years experience with 5969 surgical patients at Indiana University Hospital. *Anesth Analg.* 1999;88:599.

40. DeLeon-Casasola OA. Postoperative epidural opioid analgesia. *Anesth Analg.* 1996;83:867.

41. Ballantyne JC, Carr DB, DeFerranti S, et al. The comparative effects of postoperative analgesic therapies on pulmonary outcome: cumulative meta-analyses of randomized, controlled trials. *Anesth Analg.* 1998;86:598.

42. Boylan JF, Katz J, Kavanagh BP, et al. Epidural bupivacaine-morphine analgesia versus patient controlled analgesia following abdominal aortic surgery. *Anesthesiology.* 1998;89:585.

43. Motamed C, Spencer A, Farhat F, et al. Postoperative hypoxaemia: continuous extradural infusion of bupivacaine and morphine vs patient controlled analgesia with intravenous morphine. *Br J Anaesth.* 1998;80:742.

44. Capdevila X, Barthelet Y, Biboulet P, et al. Effects of perioperative analgesic technique on the surgical outcome and duration of rehabilitation after major knee surgery. *Anesthesiology.* 1999;91:8.

45. Borgeat A, Stirnemann HR: Ondansetron is effective to treat spinal or epidural morphine-induced pruritus. *Anesthesiology.* 1999;90:432.

46. Allen HW, Liu SS, Ware PD, et al. Peripheral nerve blocks improve analgesia after total knee replacement surgery. *Anesth Analg.* 1998;87:93.

47. Ritchie ED, Tong D, Chung F, et al. Suprascapular nerve block for postoperative pain relief in arthroscopic shoulder surgery: a new modality. *Anesth Analg.* 1997;84:1306.

48. Ross WB, Tweedle JH, Leong YP, et al. Intercostal blockade and pulmonary function after cholecystectomy. *Surgery.* 1989;105:166.

49. Yang LC, Chen LM, Wang CJ, et al. Postoperative analgesia by intra-articular neostigmine in patients undergoing knee arthroscopy. *Anesthesiology.* 1998;88:334.

50. Van der Laan WH, van Leeuwen BL, Sebel PS, et al. Therapeutic suggestion has no effect on postoperative morphine requirements. *Anesth Analg.* 1996;82:148.

51. Mignon A, Laudenbach V, Guischard F, et al. Transcutaneous cranial electrical stimulatiuon (Limoge's currents) decrease early buprenorphine analgesic requirements after abdominal surgery. *Anesth Analg.* 1996;83:771.

52. Rose DK, Cohen MM, Wigglesworth DF, et al. Critical respiratory events in the postanesthesia care unit: patient, surgical and anesthetic factors. *Anesthesiology.* 1994;81:410.

53. Chung F, Mezei G, Tong D: Pre-existing medical conditions as predictors of adverse events in day case surgery. *Br J Anaesth.* 1999;83:262.

54. Lawrence VA, Dhanda R, Hilsenbeck SG, et al. Risk of pulmonary complications after elective abdominal surgery. *Chest.* 1996;110:774.

55. Warner DO, Warner MA, Offord KP, et al. Airway obstruction and perioperative complications in smokers undergoing abdominal surgery. *Anesthesiology.* 1999;90:372.

56. Moller JT, Johannessen NW, Espersen K, et al. Randomized evaluation of pulse oximetry in 20,802 patients: preoperative events and postoperative complications. *Anesthesiology.* 1993;78:445.

57. Barker SJ, Shah MK. Effects of motion of the performance of pulse oximeters in volunteers. *Anesthesiology.* 1996;85:774.

58. Russell GB, Graybeal JM. Persistent occurrence of postoperative arterial oxygen desaturations despite oxygen therapy. *Anesthesiology.* 1990;73:A540.

59. Kimovec MA, Grutsch JF, Napcil JA. Incidence of postoperative hypoxemia prior to recovery room discharge. *Anesthesiology.* 1989; 71:A373.

60. Benumof JL, Dagg R, Benumof R. Critical hemoglobin desaturation will occur before return to an unparalyzed state following 1 mg/kg intravenous succinylcholine. *Anesthesiology.* 1997;87:979.

61. Erikson LI. The effects of residual neuromuscular blockade and volatile anesthetics on the control of ventilation. *Anesth Analg.* 1999;89:243.

62. Rothen HU, Sporre B, Engberg G, et al. Airway closure, atelectasis and gas exchange during anaesthesia. *Br J Anaesth.* 1998;81:681.

63. Pelosi P, Croci M, Ravagnan I, et al. The effects of body mass on lung volumes, respiratory mechanics, and gas exchange during general anesthesia. *Anesth Analg.* 1998;87:654.

64. Karayiannakis AJ, Makki GG, Mantzioka A, et al. Postoperative pulmonary function after laparoscopic and open cholecystectomy. *Br J Anaesth.* 1996;77:448.

65. Weisman C. Pulmonary function after cardiac and thoracic surgery. *Anesth Analg.* 1999;88:1272.

66. Jackson FN, Rowland V, Corssen G: Laryngospasm induced pulmonary edema. *Chest.* 1980;78:819.

67. Haake R, Schlichtig R, Ulstad DR, et al. Barotrauma: pathophysiology, risk factors, and prevention. *Chest.* 1987;91:608.

68. Hambraeus-Jonzon K, Bindslev L, Mellgard Aj, et al. Hypoxic pulmonary vasoconstriction in human lungs: a stimulus response study. *Anesthesiology.* 1997;86:308.

69. Baxter PJ, Garton K, Kharasch ED. Mechanistic aspects of carbon monoxide formation from volatile anesthetics. *Anesthesiology.* 1998;89:929.

70. Woehick HJ, Dunning M, Connolly LA. Reduction in the incidence of carbon monoxide exposures in humans undergoing general anesthesia. *Anesthesiology.* 1997;87:228.

71. Fu ES, Neymour R, Downs JB. Routine supplemental oxygen is not necessary during post-anesthesia recovery. *Anesth Analg.* 1999;88:S39.

72. DeBenedeto RJ, Craves SA, Gravenstein N, et al. Pulse oximetry monitoring can change routine oxygen supplementation practices in the postanesthesia care unit. *Anesth Analg.* 1994;78:365.

73. Stone JG, Cozine KA, Wald A. Nocturnal oxygenation during patient controlled analgesia. *Anesth Analg.* 1999;89:104.

74. Gibson RL, Comer PB, Beckman RW. Actual tracheal oxygen concentrations with commonly used oxygen equipment. *Anesthesiology.* 1976;44:71.

75. Isono S, Sha M, Suzukawa M, et al. Preoperative nocturnal desaturations as a risk factor for late postoperative nocturnal desaturations. *Br J Anaesth.* 1998;80:602.

76. Xue FS, Li BW, Zhang GS, et al. The influence of surgical sites on early postoperative hypoxemia in adults undergoing elective surgery. *Anesth Analg.* 1999;88:213.

77. Kataria BK, Harnik EV, Mitchard R, et al. Postoperative arterial oxygen saturation in the pediatric population during transportation. *Anesth Analg.* 1988;67:280.

78. Xue FS, Huang YG, Tong SY, et al. A comparative study of early postoperative hypoxemia in infants, children, and adults undergoing elective plastic surgery. *Anesth Analg.* 1996;83:709.

79. Moller JT, Wittrup M, Johansen SH. Hypoxemia in the postanesthesia care unit: an observer study. *Anesthesiology.* 1990;73:890.

80. Klein J. Normobaric pulmonary oxygen toxicity. *Anesth Analg.* 1990;70:195.

81. Shea SA, Walter J, Pelley K, et al. The effect of visual and auditory stimuli upon resting ventilation in man. *Respir Physiol.* 1987;68:345.

82. Jordan C. Assessment of the effects of drugs on respiration. *Br J Anaesth.* 1982;54:763.

83. Dahan A, Sarton E, Teppema I, et al. Sex related differences in the influence of morphine on ventilatory control in humans. *Anesthesiology.* 1998;88:903.

84. Bailey PL, Pace NL, Ashburn MA. Frequent hypoxemia and sedation with midazolam and fentanyl. *Anesthesiology.* 1990;73:826.

85. Etches RC. Respiratory depression associated with patient controlled analgesia: a review of eight cases. *Can J Anaesth.* 1994;41:125.

86. Borgbjerg FM, Nielsen K, Franks J. Experimental pain stimulates respiration and attenuates morphine induced respiratory depression: a controlled study in human volunteers. *Pain.* 1996;64:123.

87. Strauss SG, Lynn AM, Bratton SL, et al. Ventilatory response to $CO_2$ in children with obstructive sleep apnea from adenotonsillar hypertrophy. *Anesth Analg.* 1999;89:328.

88. Krane BD, Kreutz JM, Johnson DL, et al. Alfentanil and delayed respiratory depression: case studies and review. *Anesth Analg.* 1990;70:557.

89. Wheatley RG, Shephard D. Jackson IJB, et al. Hypoxaemia and pain relief after upper abdominal surgery: comparison of IM and patient controlled analgesia in the postoperative patient. *Br J Anaesth.* 1992;69:558.

90. Gross JB, Weller RS, Conard P, et al. Flumazenil antagonism of midazolam-induced ventilatory depression. *Anesthesiology.* 1991;75:179.

91. Gross JB, Blouin RT, Zandsberg S, et al. Effect of flumazenil on ventilatory drive during sedation with midazolam and alfentanil. *Anesthesiology.* 1996;85:713.

92. Kurth CD, Spitzer AR, Broennle AM, et al. Postoperative apnea in preterm infants. *Anesthesiology.* 1987;66:483.

93. Welborn LG, Hannallah RS, Luban NL, et al. Anemia and postoperative apnea in former preterm infants. *Anesthesiology.* 1991;74:1003.

94. Welborn LG, Rice LJ, Hannallah RS, et al. Postoperative apnea in former preterm infants: prospective comparison of spinal and general anesthetics. *Anesthesiology.* 1990;72:838.

95. Wade JG, Larson CP Jr, Hickey RF. Effect of carotid endarterectomy on carotid chemoreceptor and baroreceptor function in man. *N Engl J Med.* 1977;282:823.

96. Drummond GB. Comparison of sedation with midazolam and ketamine: effects on airway muscle activity. *Br J Anaesth.* 1996;76:663.

97. Mathru M, Esch O, Lang J, et al. Magnetic resonance imaging of the upper airway. *Anesthesiology.* 1996;84:273.

98. D'Honneur G, Lofaso F, Drummond GB, et al. Susceptibiity to upper airway obstruction during partial neuromuscular block. *Anesthesiology.* 1998;88:371.

99. Putnam MT, Wise RA. Myasthenia gravis and upper airway obstruction. *Chest.* 1996;109:400.

100. Carmichael FJ, Mcguire GP, Wong DT, et al. Computed tomographic analysis of airway dimensions after carotid endarterectomy. *Anesth Analg.* 1996;83:12.

101. Jansen NF, Weiler JM. C1 esterase inhibitor deficiency, airway compromise, and anesthesia. *Anesth Analg.* 1998;87:480.

102. Ho LI, Harn HJ, Lien TC, et al. Postextubation laryngeal edema in adults: risk factor evaluation and prevention by hydrocortisone. *Intensive Care Med.* 1996;22:933.

103. Asai T, Koga K, Vaughan RS: Respiratory complications associated with tracheal intubation and extubation. *Br J Anaesth.* 1998;80:767.

104. Schreiner MS, O'Hara I, Markakis DA, et al. Do children who experience laryngospasm have an increased risk of upper respiratory tract infection? *Anesthesiology.* 1996;85:475.

105. Schwilk B, Bothner U, Schraag S, et al. Perioperative respiratory events in smokers and nonsmokers undergoing general anesthesia. *Acta Anaesthesiol Scand.* 1997;41:348.

106. Lakshmipathy N, Bokesch PM, Cowan DE, et al. Environmental tobacco smoke: a risk factor for pediatric laryngospasm. *Anesth Analg.* 1996;82:724.

107. Skolnick ET, Vomvolakis MA, Buck KA, et al. Exposure to environmental tobacco smoke and the risk of adverse respiratory events in children receiving general anesthesia. *Anesthesiology.* 1998;88:1144.

108. Mort TC. Unplanned tracheal extubation outside the operating room: a quality improvement audit of hemodynamic and tracheal airway complications associated with emergency tracheal reintubation. *Anesth Analg.* 1998;86:1171.

109. Kablain CS, Yarnold PR, Grammer LC. Low complication rate of corticosteroid-treated asthmatics undergoing surgical procedures. *Arch Intern Med.* 1995;155:1379.

110. Warner DO, Warner MA, Barnes RD, et al. Perioperative respiratory complications in patients with asthma. *Anesthesiology.* 1996;85:460.

111. NHLBI Workshop summary. Respiratory muscle fatigue: report of the Respiratory Muscle Fatigue Workshop Group. *Am Rev Respir Dis.* 1990;142:474.

112. Joris JL, Hinque VL, Laurent PE, et al. Pulmonary function and pain after gastroplasty performed via laparotomy or laparoscopy in morbidly obese patients. *Br J Anaesth.* 1998;80:133.

113. Berg H, Viby-Mogensen J, Roed J, et al. Residual neuromuscular block is a risk factor for postoperative pulmonary complications: a prospective, randomized, and blinded study of postoperative pulmonary complications after atracurium, vecuronium, and pancuronium. *Acta Anaesthesiol Scand.* 1997;41:1095.

114. Freund PR, Bowdle TA, Posner KL, et al. Cost effective reduction of neuromuscular blocking drug expenditures. *Anesthesiology.* 1997;87:1044.

115. Bevan DR, Kahwaji R, Arsermino JM, et al. Residual block after mivacurium with or without edrophonium reversal in adults and children. *Anesthesiology.* 1996;84:362.

116. Spacek A, Nick LS, Neiger FX, et al. Augmentation of the rocuronium-induced neuromuscular block by the acutely administered phenytoin. *Anesthesiology.* 1999;90:1551.

117. Fuchs-Buder T, Wilder-Smith OH, Borgeat A, et al. Interaction of magnesium sulfate with vecuronium induced neuromuscular block. *Br J Anaesth.* 1995;74:405.

118. Sharma RR, Axelsson H, Oberg A, et al. Diaphragmatic activity after laparoscopic cholecystectomy. *Anesthesiology.* 1999;91:406.

119. Casati A, Fanelli G, Cedrati V, et al. Pulmonary function changes after interscalene brachial plexus anesthesia with 0.5% and 0.75% ropivacaine: a double blind comparison with 2% mepivacaine. *Anesth Analg.* 1999;88:587.

120. Al-Kaisy AA, Chan VWS, Perlas A. Respiratory effects of low dose bupivacaine interscalene block. *Br J Anaesth.* 1999;82:217.

121. Loh L, Hughes JMB, Newson Davis J. The regional distribution of ventilation and perfusion in paralysis of the diaphragm. *Am Rev Respir Dis.* 1979;119:121.

122. Troyer AD, Heilporn A. Respiratory mechanics in quadriplegia: the respiratory function of the intercostal muscles. *Am Rev Respir Dis.* 1980;122:591.

123. Kopman AF, Yee PS, Neuman GG. Relationship of the train-of-four fade ratio to clinical signs and symptoms of residual paralysis in awake volunteers. *Anesthesiology.* 1997;86:765.

124. Kopman AF, Ng J, Zank LM, et al. Residual postoperative paralysis: pancuronium versus mivacurium, does it matter? *Anesthesiology.* 1996;85:1253.

125. Parmet JL, Horrow JC, Berman AT, et al. The incidence of large venous emboli during total knee arthroplasty without pneumatic tourniquet use. *Anesth Analg.* 1998;87:439.

126. Khambatta HJ, Stone JG, Matteo RS. Effect of sodium nitroprusside induced hypotension on pulmonary deadspace. *Br J Anaesth.* 1982;54:1197.

127. Mathay MA, Rosen GD. Acid aspiration induced lung injury: new insights and therapeutic options. *Am J Respir Crit Care Med.* 1996;154:277.

128. Schwartz DJ, Wynne JW, Gibbs CP. The pulmonary consequences of aspiration of gastric contents at pH values greater than 2.5. *Am Rev Respir Dis.* 1980;121:119.

129. Vidyarthi SC. Diffuse miliary granulomatosis of the lungs due to aspirated vegetable cells. *Arch Pathol.* 1967;83:215.

130. Laxmaiah M, Colliver JA, Marrero TC, et al. Assessment of age related acid aspiration risk factors in pediatric, adult, and geriatric patients. *Anesth Analg.* 1985;64:11.

131. Eriksson LI, Sundman E, Olsson R, et al. Functional assessment of the pharynx at rest and during swallowing in partially paralyzed humans: simultaneous videomanometry and mechanomyography of awake human volunteers. *Anesthesiology.* 1997;78:1035.

132. Tramer MR, Fuchs-Buder T. Omitting antagonism of neuromuscular block: effect on postoperative nausea and vomiting and risk of residual paralysis. A systematic review. *Br J Anaesth.* 1999;82:379.

133. American Society of Anesthesiologists Task Force on Preoperative Fasting. Practice guidelines for preoperative fasting and the use of pharmacologic agents to reduce the risk of pulmonary aspiration: application to healthy patients undergoing elective procedures. *Anesthesiology.* 1999;90:896.

134. Warner MA, Warner ME, Warner DO, et al. Perioperative pulmonary aspiration in infants and children. *Anesthesiology.* 1999;90:66.

135. Splinter WM, Schreiner MS. Preoperative fasting in children. *Anesth Analg*. 1999;89:80.

136. Harter RL, Kelly WB, Kramer MG, et al. A comparison of the volume and pH of gastric contents of obese and lean surgical patients. *Anesth Analg*. 1998;86:147.

137. Solanki DR, Suresh M, Ethridge HC. The effects of intravenous cimetidine and metoclopramide on gastric volume and pH. *Anesth Analg*. 1984;63:599.

138. Petring OU, Adelhoj B, Jensen BN, et al. Prevention of silent aspiration due to leaks around cuffs of endotracheal tubes. *Anesth Analg*. 1986;65:777.

139. Bartlett JG, Gorbach SL, Finegold S. The bacteriology of aspiration pneumonia. *Am J Med*. 1974;56:202.

140. Ivanov J, Weisel RD, Mickelborough LL, et al. Rewarming hypovolemia after aortocoronary bypass surgery. *Crit Care Med*. 1984;12:1049.

141. Partridge BL. Use of pulse oximetry as a noninvasive indicator of intravascular volume status. *J Clin Monit*. 1987;3:263.

142. Rooke GA, Schwid HA, Shapira Y. The effect of graded hemorrhage and intravascular volume replacement on systolic pressure variation in humans during mechanical and spontaneous ventilation. *Anesth Analg*. 1995;78:46.

143. Mangano DT. Perioperative cardiac morbidity. *Anesthesiology*. 1990;72:153.

144. Wahr JR. Myocardial ischaemia in anaemic patients. *Br J Anaesth*. 1998;81(suppl 1):10.

145. Eagle KA, for the CASS Investigators and University of Michigan Heart Care Program. Cardiac risk of noncardiac surgery: influence of coronary disease and type of surgery in 3368 operations. *Circulation*. 1997;96:1882.

146. Howell SJ, Sear JW, Sear YM, et al. Risk factors for cardiovascular death within 30 days after anaesthesia and urgent or emergency surgery: a nested, case controlled study. *Br J Anaesth*. 1999;82:679.

147. Bois S, Couture P, Boudreault D, et al. Epidural analgesia and intravenous patient controlled analgesia result in similar rates of postoperative myocardial ischemia after aortic surgery. *Anesth Analg*. 1997;85:1233.

148. Badner NH, Knill RL, Brown JE, et al. Myocardial infarction after noncardiac surgery. *Anesthesiology*. 1998;88:572.

149. Mangano DT, Layug EL, Wallace A, et al., for the Multicenter Study of Perioperative Ischemia Research Group. Effect of atenolol on mortality and cardiovascular morbidity after non cardiac surgery. *N Engl J Med*. 1996;335:1713.

150. Raby KE, Brull SK, Timimi F, et al. The effect of heart rate control on myocardial ischemia among high risk patients after vascular surgery. *Anesth Analg*. 1999;88:477.

151. Wallace A, Layug B, Tateo I, et al. Prophylactic atenolol reduces postoperative myocardial ischemia. *Anesthesiology*. 1998;88:7.

152. Parlow JL, Begou G, Sagnard P, et al. Cardiac baroreflex during the postoperative period in patients with hypertension: the effect of clonidine. *Anesthesiology*. 1999;90:681.

153. Van Vlymen JM, Parlow JL. The effects of reversal of neuromuscular blockade on autonomic control in the perioperative period. *Anesth Analg*. 1997;84:148.

154. Satiani B, Vasko JS, Zarins CK. Hypertension following carotid endarterectomy. *Arch Surg*. 1982;1117:1073.

155. Leslie JB, Kalayjian RW, Sirgo MA, et al. Intravenous labetalol for treatment of postoperative hypertension. *Anesthesiology*. 1987;67:413.

156. Kataria BK, Bubois MY, Gadde PL, et al. Evaluation of intravenous esmolol for treatment of postoperative hypertension. *Anesth Analg*. 1990;70:S192.

157. IV Nicardipine Safety Group. Efficacy and safety of intravenous nicardipine in the control of postoperative hypertension. *Chest*. 1991;99:393.

158. Dorman T, Clarkson K, Rosenfeld BA, et al. Effects of clonidine on prolonged postoperative sympathetic response. *Crit Care Med*. 1997;25:1147.

159. Breslow MJ, Miller CF, Parker SD, et al. Changes in T-wave morphology following anesthesia and surgery: a common recovery room phenomenon. *Anesthesiology*. 1986;64:398.

160. Atlee JL, Bosnjak ZJ. Mechanisms for cardiac dysrhythmias during anesthesia. *Anesthesiology*. 1990;72:347.

161. Amar D, Fleisher M, Pantuck CB, et al. Persistent alterations of the autonomic nervous system after noncardiac surgery. *Anesthesiology*. 1998;89:30.

162. Mahla E, Rotman B, Rehak P, et al. Perioperative ventricular dysrhythmias in patients with structural heart disease undergoing noncardiac surgery. *Anesth Analg*. 1998;86:16.

163. Amar D, Roistacher N, Burt M, et al. Clinical and echocardiographic correlates of symptomatic tachydysrhythmias after non cardiac thoracic surgery. *Chest*. 1995;108:349.

164. Ponhold H, Vicenzi MN. Incidence of bradycardia during recovery from spinal anaesthesia: influence of patient position. *Br J Anaesth*. 1998;81:723.

165. Gauss A, Hubner C, Radermacher P, et al. Perioperative risk of bradyarrhythmias in patients with asymptomatic chronic bifascicular block or left bundle branch block: does an additional first degree atrioventricular block make any difference? *Anesthesiology*. 1998;88:679.

166. Kamphius ET, Ionescu TI, Kuipers PWG, et al. Recovery of storage and emptying functions of the urinary bladder after spinal anesthesia with lidocaine and with bupivacaine in men. *Anesthesiology*. 1998;88:31.

167. Pavlin DJ, Rapp SE, Polissar NL, et al. Factors affecting discharge time in adult outpatients. *Anesth Analg*. 1998;87:816.

168. Marshall SI, Chung F. Discharge criteria and complications after ambulatory surgery. *Anesth Analg*. 1999;88:508.

169. Twersky R, Fishman D, Homel P. What happens after discharge? Return hospital visits after ambulatory surgery. *Anesth Analg*. 1997;84:319.

170. Pavlin DJ, Pavlin EG, Gunn HC, et al. Voiding in patients managed with or without ultrasound monitoring of bladder volume after outpatient surgery. *Anesth Analg*. 1999;89:90.

171. Fang ZX, Kandel L, Laster MJ, et al. Factors affecting production of compound A from the interaction of sevoflurane with baralyme and soda lime. *Anesth Analg*. 1996;82:775.

172. Higuchi H, Sumita S, Wada H, et al. Effects of sevoflurane and isoflurane on renal function and on possible markers of nephrotoxicity. *Anesthesiology*. 1999;89:307.

173. Zelcer J, Wells DG. Anaesthetic-related recovery room complications. *Anaesth Intensive Care*. 1996;15:168.

174. Ghoneim MM, Dembo JB, Block RI. Time course of antagonism of sedative and amnesic effects of diazepam by flumazenil. *Anesthesiology*. 1989;70:899.

175. Bourke DL, Rosenberg M, Allen PD. Physostigmine: effectiveness as an antagonist of respiratory depression and psychomotor effects caused by morphine or diazepam. *Anesthesiology*. 1984;1:523.

176. Adams AP, Goroszeniuk T. Hysteria: a cause of failure to recover after anaesthesia. *Anaesthesia*. 1991;46:932.

177. Douglass JH, Ross JD, Bruce DL. Delayed awakening due to lidocaine overdose. *J Clin Anesth*. 1989;2:126.

178. Schubert A, Mascha EJ, Bloomfield EL, et al. Effect of cranial surgery and brain tumor size on emergence from anesthesia. *Anesthesiology*. 1996;85:513.

179. Gutierrez IZ, Barone DL, Makula PA, et al. The risk of perioperative stroke in patients with asymptomatic carotid bruits undergoing peripheral vascular surgery. *Am Surg*. 1987;53:487.

180. Larsen SF, Zaric D, Boysen G. Postoperative cerebrovascular accidents in general surgery. *Acta Anaesthesiol Scand*. 1988;32:698.

181. Welborn LG, Hannallah RS, Norden JM, et al. Comparision of emergence and recovery characteristics of sevoflurane, desflurane, and halothane in pediatric ambulatory patients. *Anesth Analg*. 1996;83:917.

182. Dodds C, Allison J. Postoperative cognitive deficit in the elderly surgical patient. *Br J Anaesth*. 1998;81:449.

183. Williams-Russo P, Urquhart BL, Sharrock NE, et al. Postoperative delirium: predictors and prognosis in elderly orthopedics patients. *J Am Geriatr Soc*. 1992;40:759.

184. Jamison RN, Parris WC, Maxson WS. Psychological factors influencing recovery from outpatient surgery. *Behav Res Ther*. 1987;25:31.

185. Taenzer P, Melzack R, Jeans ME. Influence of psychological factors in postoperative pain, mood, and analgesic requirements. *Pain*. 1986;24:331.

186. Schwender D, Kunze-Kronawitter H, Dietrich P, et al. Conscious awareness during general anaesthesia: patients' perceptions, emotions, cognition and reactions. *Br J Anaesth*. 1998;80:133.

187. Spies CD, Rommelspacher H: Alcohol withdrawal in the surgical patient: prevention and treatment. *Anesth Analg*. 1999;88:946.

188. Hammon K, Demartino BK. Postoperative delirium secondary to atropine premedication. *Anesth Prog*. 1985;32:107.

189. Eisenrath SJ, Goldman B, Douglas J, et al. Meperidine induced delirium. *Am J Psychiatry*. 1987;144:1062.

190. Heath PJ, Kennedy DJ, Ogg TW, et al. Which intravenous induction agent for day surgery? A comparison of propofol, thiopentone, methohexitone, and etomidate. *Anaesthesia*. 1988;43:365.

191. Lynch EP, Lazor MA, Gellis JE, et al. The impact of postoperative pain on the development of postoperative delirium. *Analgesia*. 1998;86:781.

192. Gravenstein D. Transurethral resection of the prostate: a review of the pathophysiology and management. *Anesth Analg.* 1997;84:438.

193. Oliver SB, Cucchiara RF, Warner MA, et al. Unexpected focal neurologic deficit on emergence from anesthesia: a report of three cases. *Anesthesiology.* 1987;67:823.

194. Kain ZN, Mayes LC, Wang SM, et al. Postoperative behavioral outcomes in children: effects of sedative premedication. *Anesthesiology.* 1999;90:758.

195. Suresh D. Nightmares and recovery from anesthesia. *Anesth Analg.* 1991;72:404.

196. Sinclair DR, Chung F, Mezei G. Can postoperative nausea and vomiting be predicted? *Anesthesiology.* 1999;91:109.

197. Beattie WS, Lindblad T, Buckley DN, et al. Menstruation increases the risk of nausea and vomiting after laparoscopy: a prospective, randomized study. *Anesthesiology.* 1993;78:272.

198. Tramer M, Moore A, McQuay H. Prevention of vomiting after paediatric strabismus surgery: a systematic review using the numbers needed to treat method. *Br J Anaesth.* 1995;75:556.

199. Palazzo MG, Strunin L. Anesthesia and emesis, I: etiology. *Can Anaesth Soc J.* 1984;31:178.

200. Duncan PG, Cohen MM, Tweed WA, et al. The Canadian four centre study of anaesthetic outcomes, III: are anaesthetic complications predictable in day surgical practice? *Can J Anaesth.* 1992;39:440.

201. Divatia JV, Vaidya MS, Badwe RA, et al. Omission of nitrous oxide during anesthesia reduces the incidence of postoperative nausea and vomiting: a meta-analysis. *Anesthesiology.* 1996;85:1055.

202. Hartung J. Twenty four of twenty seven studies show a greater incidence of emesis associated with nitrous oxide than with alternative anesthetics. *Anesth Analg.* 1996;83:114.

203. Chibber AK, Lustik SJ, Thakur R, et al. Effects of anticholinergics on postoperative vomiting, recovery, and hospital stay in children undergoing tonsillectomy with or without adenoidectomy. *Anesthesiology.* 1999;90:697.

204. Yogendran S, Kumar B, Cheng D, et al. A prospective, randomized double blinded study of the effect of intravenous fluid therapy on adverse outcomes from outpatient surgery. *Anesth Analg.* 1995;80:682.

205. Fengling J, Norris A, Chung F, et al. Should adult patients drink fluids before discharge from ambulatory surgery? *Anesth Analg.* 1998;87:306.

206. Tramer MR, Walder B. Efficacy and adverse effects of prophylactic antiemetics during patient controlled analgesia therapy: a quantitative systematic review. *Anesth Analg.* 1999;88:1354.

207. Fortney JT, Gan TJ, Graczyk S, et al. A comparison of the efficacy, safety, and patient satisfaction of ondansetron versus droperidol as antiemetics for elective outpatient surgical procedures. *Anesth Analg.* 1998;86:731.

208. Domino KB, Anderson EA, Polissar NL, et al. Comparative efficacy and safety of ondansetron, droperidol, and metoclopramide for preventing postoperative nausea and vomiting: a meta analysis. *Anesth Analg.* 1999;88:1370.

209. Steinbrook RA, Freiberger D, Gosness JL, et al. Prophylactic antiemetics for laparoscopic cholecystectomy: ondansetron versus droperidol plus metoclopramide. *Anesth Analg.* 1996;83:1081.

210. McKenzie R, Lim NT, Riley TJ, et al. Droperidol/ondansetron combination controls nausea and vomiting after tubal banding. *Anesth Analg.* 1996;83:1218.

211. Melnick BM. Extrapyramidal reactions to low-dose droperidol. *Anesthesiology.* 1988;69:424.

212. Tang J, Wang B, White P, et al. The effect of timing of ondansetron administration on its efficacy, cost effectiveness, and cost benefit as a prophylactic antiemetic in the ambulatory setting. *Anesth Analg.* 1998;86:274.

213. Hamid SK, Selby IR, Sikich N, et al. Vomiting after adenotonsillectomy in children: a comparison of ondansetron, dimenhydrinate, and placebo. *Anesth Analg.* 1999;86:496.

214. Tramer MR, Reynolds JM, Moore A, et al. Efficacy, dose-response, and safety of ondansetron in prevention of postoperative nausea and vomiting: a quantitative, systematic review of randomized, placebo controlled trials. *Anesthesiology.* 1997;87:1277.

215. Fujii Y, Saitoh Y, Tanaka H, et al. Comparison of ramosetron and granisetron for prevention of postoperative nausea and vomiting after gynecologic surgery. *Anesth Analg.* 1999;89:476.

216. Chan MT, Chui PT, Ho WS, et al. Single dose tropisetron for preventing postoperative nausea and vomiting after breast surgery. *Anesth Analg.* 1998;87:931.

217. Kovac AL, Scuderi PE, Boerner TR, et al. Treatment of postoperative nausea and vomiting with single intravenous doses of dolasetron mesylate: a multicenter trial. *Anesth Analg.* 1997;85:546.

218. Gan TJ, Glass PSA, Howell ST, et al. Determination of plasma concentrations of propofol associated with 50% reduction in postoperative nausea. *Anesthesiology.* 1997;87:779.

219. Pappas ALS, Sukhani R, Hotaling AJ, et al. The effect of preoperative dexamethasone on the immediate and delayed postoperative morbidity in children undergoing adenotonsillectomy. *Anesth Analg.* 1998;87:57.

220. Wang JJ, Shung TH, Lee SC, et al. The prophylactic effect of dexamethasone on postoperative nausea and vomiting in women undergoing thyroidectomy: a comparison of droperidol with saline. *Anesth Analg.* 1999;89:200.

221. Tigerstedt I, Salmela L, Aromaa U. Double-blind comparison of transdermal scopolamine, droperidol, and placebo against postoperative nausea and vomiting. *Acta Anesthesiol Scand.* 1988;32:454.

222. Rothenberg DM, Parnass SM, Litwack K, et al. Efficacy of ephedrine in the prevention of postoperative nausea and vomiting. *Anesth Analg.* 1991;72:58.

223. Lee A, Done ML. The use of non-pharmacologic techniques to prevent postoperative nausea and vomiting: a meta analysis. *Anesth Analg.* 1999;88:1362.

224. Sessler DI. Perioperative hypothermia. *N Engl J Med.* 1997;336:1730.

225. Frank SM, Higgins MS, Fleisher LA, et al. The adrenergic, respiratory, and cardiovascular effects of core cooling in humans. *Am J Physiol.* 1997;272:R557.

226. Frank SM, Fleisher LA, Breslow MJ, et al. Perioperative maintenance of normothermia reduces the incidence of morbid cardiac events: a randomized clinical trial. *JAMA.* 1997;277:1127.

227. Hansen D, Syben R, Vargas O, et al. The alveolar arterial difference in oxygen tension increases with temperature corrected determination during moderate hypothermia. *Anesth Analg.* 1999;88:538.

228. Beilin B, Shavit Y, Razumovsky J, et al. Effects of mild perioperative hypothermia on cellular immune responses *Anesthesiology.* 1998;89:1133.

229. Kurz A, Sessler DI, Lenhardt R, et al. Perioperative normothermia to reduce the incidence of the surgical would infection and shorten hospitalization. *N Engl J Med.* 1996;334:1209.

230. Lenhardt R, Marker E, Goll V, et al. Mild intraoperative hypothermia prolongs post anesthetic recovery. *Anesthesiology.* 1997;87:1318.

231. Horn EP, Sessler DI, Standl T, et al. Non-thermoregulatory shivering in patients recovering from isoflurane or desflurane anesthesia. *Anesthesiology.* 1998;89:878.

232. MacIntyre PE, Pavin EG, Dwersteg JF. Effect of meperidine on oxygen consumption, carbon dioxide production, and respiratory gas exchange in post anesthesia shivering. *Anesth Analg.* 1987;66:751.

233. Horn EP, Standl T, Sessler DI, et al. Physostigmine prevents postanesthetic shivering as does meperidine or clonidine. *Anesthesiology.* 1998;88:108.

234. Kurz A, Ikeda T, Sessler DI, et al. Meperidine decreases the shivering threshold twice as much as the vasoconstriction threshold. *Anesthesiology.* 1997;86:1046.

235. Wang JJ, Ho ST, Lee SC, et al. A comparison among nalbuphine, meperidine, and placebo for treating postanesthetic shivering. *Anesth Analg.* 1999;88:686.

236. Brian JE. Carbon dioxide and the cerebral circulation. *Anesthesiology.* 1998;88:1365.

237. ABG Kazmaier S, Weyland A, Buhre W, et al. Effects of respiratory alkalosis and acidosis on myocardial blood flow and metabolism in patients with coronary artery disease. *Anesthesiology.* 1998;89:831.

238. Scheingraber S, Rehm M, Sehmisch C, et al. Rapid saline infusion produces hyperchloremic acidosis in patients undergoing gynecologic surgery. *Anesthesiology.* 1999;90:1265.

239. Steele A, Gowrishankar M, Abrahamson S, et al. Postoperative hyponatremia despite near-isotonic saline infusion: a phenomenon of desalination. *Ann Intern Med.* 1997;126:20.

240. Gomez MN. Magnesium and cardiovascular disease. *Anesthesiology.* 1998;89:222.

241. Gild WM, Posner KI, Caplan RA, et al. Eye injuries associated with anesthesia: a closed claims analysis. *Anesthesiology.* 1992;76:204.

242. Roth SR, Thisted RA, Erickson JP, et al. Eye injuries after nonocular surgery: a study of 60,965 anesthetics from 1988–1992. *Anesthesiology.* 1996;85:1020.

243. Warner ME, Benenfeld SM, Warner MA, et al. Peri-anesthetic dental

injuries: frequency, outcomes and risk factors. *Anesthesiology.* 1999;90:1302.

244. Stout DM, Bishop MJ, Dwersteg JF, et al. Correlation of endotracheal tube size with sore throat and hoarseness following general anesthesia. *Anesthesiology.* 1987;67:419.

245. Keane WM, Denneny JC, Rowe LD, et al. Complications of intubation. *Ann Otol Rhinol Laryngol.* 1982;91:584.

246. Seeberger MD, Kaufmann M, Staender S, et al. Repeated dural punctures increase the incidence of post dural puncture headache. *Anesth Analg.* 1996;82:302.

247. Aida S, Taga K, Yamakura T, et al. Headache after attempted epidural block. *Anesthesiology.* 1998;88:76.

248. Cheney FW, Domino KB, Caplan RA, et al. Nerve injury associated with anesthesia: a closed claims analysis. *Anesthesiology.* 1999;90:1062.

249. Auroy Y, Narchi P, Messiah A, et al. Serious complications related to regional anesthesia: results of a prospective survey in France. *Anesthesiology.* 1997;87:479.

250. Horlocker TT, McGregor DG, Matsushige DK, et al. A retrospective review of 4767 consecutive spinal anesthetics: central nervous system complications. *Anesth Analg.* 1997;84:578.

251. Hodgson PS, Neal JM, Pollock JE, et al. The neurotoxicity of drugs given intrathecally (spinal). *Anesth Analg.* 1999;88:797.

252. Warner MA, Warner DO, Matsumoto JY, et al. Ulnar neuropathy in surgical patients. *Anesthesiology.* 1999;90:54.

253. Prielipp RC, Morell RC, Walker FO, et al. Ulnar nerve pressure: influence of arm position and relationship to somatosensory evoked potentials. *Anesthesiology.* 1999;91:345.

254. Swenson JD, Hutchinson DT, Bromberg M, et al. Rapid onset of ulnar nerve dysfunction during transient occlusion of the brachial artery. *Anesth Analg.* 1998;87:677.

255. Myers MA, Hamilton SR, Bogosian AJ. Visual loss as a complication of spine surgery: a review of 37 cases. *Spine.* 1997;22:1325.

256. Williams EL, Hart WM, Templehoff R. Postoperative ischemic optic neuropathy. *Anesth Analg.* 1995;80:1018.

257. Pace NL. Prevention of succinylcholine myalgias: a meta analysis. *Anesth Analg.* 1990;70:477.

CHAPTER

# 7

# Critical Incident Management

William R. Runciman

Joachim S. Gravenstein

## HUMAN ERROR

*How Can We Prevent or Avoid Critical Incidents?*

*What Problems Can Arise During a Crisis?*

## CRITICAL INCIDENTS

*How Is a Critical Incident Defined?*

*What Factors Are Associated With Critical Incidents?*

*How Can We Detect Dangerous Trends, Whether Brought About by Human Error or as a Consequence of Developments Beyond Our Control?*

## EMERGENCY MANAGEMENT

*In Case of Trouble, How Can We Best Initiate Appropriate Therapy?*

No single precaution, no isolated effort, and no clever apparatus can guarantee safe anesthesia. Countless pitfalls await the clinician. Human errors set the stage for critical incidents that can mushroom into crises. We need to be aware of these incidents in order to prevent or avoid them. Only when we know how to detect the first indications of an adverse trend can we hope to avert a crisis. However, should a crisis develop, we must be prepared to coordinate the efforts of a team because no practitioner can hope to manage a full-blown crisis single-handedly.

## HUMAN ERROR

### How Can We Prevent or Avoid Critical Incidents?

The extensive literature and distressing experiences show that most crises, excluding natural disasters, are brought about by human error. This is true for accidents in atomic power plants, aviation, shipping, road traffic, and medicine.[1] Although we bemoan the frequency of such human errors, we can take heart in the fact that many can be prevented by (1) being well informed (through education, experience, and good data management), (2) being technically capable (by good

training, experience, and dexterity), and (3) using up-to-date equipment.

Modern anesthesia machines, for example, are equipped with numerous features that would be superfluous were it not for our propensity to commit errors from time to time. For example, the pin index system on compressed gas cylinders makes it difficult (but not impossible) to attach a nitrous oxide cylinder to an oxygen yoke. The oxygen proportioning system that ensures the delivery of no less than 25% oxygen makes it difficult (but not impossible) to administer a less than safe concentration of oxygen. The color-coding and labeling of drug vials and syringes help to avoid (but does not eliminate) the administration of the wrong drug. These and many other safety features would not be necessary were we infallible. However, being imperfect, we cannot justify working with equipment that lacks available safety features.

### What Problems Can Arise During a Crisis?

Under the category of human error, we must also consider common problems that arise once a crisis has developed. Even experienced clinicians may commit errors in an emergency, particularly when challenged not only by the patient's problems but also by other responsibilities in the operating room. A clinician may be in denial, ignoring the signals that indicate the emergency or underestimating the seriousness of the problem. This can delay the switch from the "business as usual" to the "emergency" mode with a consequent and dangerous holdup in treatment.

Pressures during an emergency may set the stage for slip-ups (eg, *syringe swap,* in which the clinician picks up the wrong syringe because it is near the appropriate one). Other clinicians may gamble on the statistics of likelihood, ignoring data that point to a rare situation. All too often, clinicians disregard mounting evidence that the adopted diagnosis is wrong and that the difficulties lie elsewhere—a common human failure known as *confirmation bias.* Others, overwhelmed by diagnostic possibilities, vacillate and thus treat nothing with decisiveness.

## CRITICAL INCIDENTS

### How Is a Critical Incident Defined?

In 1978 and 1984, Cooper and coworkers published their classic studies of critical incidents.[2,3] They defined a *critical incident* as a human error or equipment failure that could have led (if not discovered or corrected in time) or did lead to an undesirable outcome, ranging from a prolonged hospital stay (or increased stay in a recovery room or an intensive care unit) to death. Table 7–1 shows the most frequent critical incidents and illustrates the diverse pedigree, ranging from judgmental errors (eg, overdoses) to slip-ups.

### What Factors Are Associated With Critical Incidents?

Cooper's team also listed factors associated with critical incidents (Table 7–2), factors we should recognize and avoid.[3] Some of these factors reflect situations that must be anticipated in teaching institutions; many factors, however, will arise in any anesthesia setting. Observe that the classic study by Cooper and colleagues[3] is now many years old. New studies may show a different ranking of problems. More recently, Australian investigators published an extensive study of critical incidents. In general, their findings buttress the observations by Cooper and his team even though the Australian colleagues used a different definition of a *critical incident,* namely any unintended event that reduced or could have reduced the safety margin for the patient.[4]

**TABLE 7–1.** Most Frequent Critical Incidents

| Incident Description | No. of Incidents |
| --- | --- |
| Breathing circuit disconnection during mechanical ventilation | 57 |
| Syringe swap | 50 |
| Gas flow control error | 41 |
| Loss of gas supply | 32 |
| Intravenous tubing disconnection | 24 |
| Vaporizer off unintentionally | 22 |
| Drug ampule swap | 21 |
| Drug overdose (syringe, judgmental) | 20 |
| Drug overdose (vaporizer, technical) | 20 |
| Breathing circuit leak | 19 |
| Unintended extubation | 18 |
| Misplaced endotracheal tube | 18 |
| Breathing circuit misconnection | 18 |
| Inadequate fluid replacement | 15 |
| Premature extubation | 15 |
| Ventilator malfunction | 15 |
| Misuse of blood pressure monitor | 15 |
| Breathing circuit control technical error | 15 |
| Wrong choice of airway management technique | 13 |
| Laryngoscope malfunction | 12 |
| Wrong intravenous tubing used | 12 |
| Hypoventilation (human error only) | 11 |
| Drug overdose (vaporizer, judgmental) | 9 |
| Drug overdose (syringe, technical) | 9 |
| Wrong choice of drug | 7 |
| **Total** | **508** |

From Cooper JB, Newbower RS, Kitz RJ. An analysis of major errors and equipment failures in anesthesia management: considerations for prevention and detection. *Anesthesiology.* 1984;60:34–42.

**TABLE 7–2.** Factors Associated With Critical Incidents

| Associated Factor | No. of Incidents |
| --- | --- |
| Failure to check | 223 |
| First experience with situation | 208 |
| Inadequate total experience | 201 |
| Inattention to carelessness | 166 |
| Haste encouraged by situation | 131 |
| Unfamiliarity with equipment or device | 126 |
| Visual restriction | 83 |
| Inadequate familiarity with anesthetic technique | 79 |
| Other distracting simultaneous anesthesia activities | 71 |
| Teaching in progress | 60 |
| Excessive dependence on other personnel | 60 |
| Unfamiliarity with surgical procedure | 59 |
| Lack of sleep and/or fatigue | 55 |
| Insufficient supervision | 52 |
| Failure to follow personal routine | 41 |
| Inadequate supervision | 34 |
| Conflicting equipment design | 34 |
| Unfamiliarity with drug | 32 |
| Failure to follow institutional practice | 31 |

From Cooper JB, Newbower RS, Kitz RJ. An analysis of major errors and equipment failures in anesthesia management: considerations for prevention and detection. *Anesthesiology.* 1984;60:34–42.

### How Can We Detect Dangerous Trends, Whether Brought About by Human Error or as a Consequence of Developments Beyond Our Control?

#### Algorithms

Whether stressed by a developing crisis or lulled into apathy by a boring routine, it is useful to follow a methodical plan to detect dangerous trends. For this purpose, Runciman and colleagues[5] urged the adoption of 2 algorithms (Tables 7–3 and 7–4). The algorithms were based on hundreds of observed critical events and offer an ordered review of the majority of findings that could reveal impending problems.[5] In many critical incidents, adherence to these algorithms would have expedited the detection of the trend and thus the treatment of the problem.

The algorithms use the mnemonic acronym *COVER ABCD* and *A SWIFT CHECK. COVER* deals with issues arising from the gas supply, anesthesia machine, breathing circuit, ventilator, and endotracheal tube. A review of cases from the Australian study[4] suggested that COVER would have been helpful in virtually all relevant cases and that a solution would have been obtained in <60 seconds:

**C** Circulation and color
**O** Oxygen delivery, oximeter, and oxygen analyzer
**V** Ventilation and vaporizer
**E** Endotracheal tube and eliminate machine
**R** Review monitors and equipment

The anesthetist should observe the patient and scan equipment at least every 5 minutes, with the check running from *C* to *O* to *V* to *E* to *R*. The information should be viewed in the context of the data gathered in the last one or several checks. Following is a list of which areas are checked with each letter:

**C** Assess pulse, blood pressure (peripheral arterial and, when available, pulmonary artery, central venous), electrocardiogram, and peripheral circulation.

**TABLE 7–3.** Crisis Management Algorithm: Memorize and Practice*

| | | |
|---|---|---|
| **C** | Circulation | Establish adequacy of peripheral circulation (rate, rhythm, and character of pulse). If pulseless (3%), start CPR, get help, and complete COVER as soon as possible. |
| | Color | Note saturation; look for central cyanosis. Use pulse oximetry if possible. Test probe on own finger if necessary while proceeding with the next steps. |
| **O** | Oxygen | Check rotameter settings, ensure inspired mixture is not hypoxic. Adjust inspired oxygen concentration to 100%, and note that only the oxygen flowmeter is operating (2%). |
| | Oxygen analyzer | Check that the oxygen analyzer shows a rising oxygen concentration distal to the common gas outlet (0.2%). |
| **V** | Ventilate | Ventilate the lungs by hand to assess circuit integrity, airway patency, compliance, and air entry by feel, observation, and auscultation; inspect capnograph trace (20%). Note settings and levels of agents. |
| | Vaporizer | Check all vaporizer filler and drainage ports, seatings and connections for liquid or gas leaks during pressurization of the system; consider the possibility of the wrong agent being in the vaporizer (4%). |
| **E** | Endotracheal tube | Check the endotracheal tube; ensure it is patent with no leaks, kinks, or obstructions. Check capnograph for tracheal placement and oximeter for possible endobronchial intubation. If necessary, adjust tube, deflate cuff, pass a catheter, or remove and replace (14%). |
| | Elimination | Eliminate the anesthetic machine and ventilate with self-inflating bag with 100% $O_2$ (from alternative source if necessary). Retain gas monitor sampling port but be aware of possible gas sampling or gas monitor problems (15%). Remove the filter in the breathing circuit if there is any chance that it is or may become blocked with secretions, blood, vomitus, or pulmonary edema fluid. Also, see *K* in Table 7–4. |
| **R** | Review monitors | Review all monitors in use. All monitors should have been correctly placed, checked, and calibrated (eg, oximeter, capnograph, ECG, BP, circuit pressure, neuromuscular monitoring electrodes) (4%). |
| | Review equipment | Review all other equipment in contact with or relevant to the patient (eg, diathermy, humidifiers, heating blankets, endoscopes, probes, prostheses, retractors) (2%). |
| **A** | Airway | Check patency of the nonintubated airway. Consider laryngospasm (6%), presence of foreign body (1%), or aspiration/regurgitation (5%) (total, 12%). |
| **B** | Breathing | Assess pattern, adequacy, and distribution of ventilation. Consider, examine, and auscultate for hypoventilation (2%), bronchospasm (2%), pulmonary edema, lobar collapse, and pneumothorax or hemothorax (1%) (total, 5%). |
| **C** | Circulation | Evaluate peripheral perfusion, pulse, blood pressure, ECG, and filling pressures (where possible) and any possible obstruction to venous return, raised intrathoracic pressure (eg, inadvertent PEEP), direct interference to (eg, stimulation by central line), or tamponade of the heart. Note any trends on patient records. Bradycardia/arrhythmia (5%), tachycardia/arrhythmia (2%), hypotension (5%), hypertension (1%), ischemia (1%) (total, 14%). |
| **D** | Drugs | Review intended, and consider possible unintended, drug or substance administration. Consider whether the problem may be due to an unexpected drug effect, failure of administration (eg, kinked cannula, extravasation), or wrong dose, route, or manner of administration of an intended or wrong drug. Review all possible routes of drug administration (total, 3%). |

*For use on patients breathing gas from an anesthetic machine: COVER ABCD with tracheal tube; AB COVER ABCD with mask.

BP, blood pressure; CPR, cardiopulmonary resuscitation; ECG, electrocardiogram; PEEP, positive end-expiratory pressure.

Data from Runciman WB, Webb RK, Klepper ID, et al. The Australian Incident Monitoring Study. Crisis management—validation of an algorithm by analysis of 2000 incident reports. *Anaesth Intensive Care.* 1993;21:579–592.

**O** Review the settings of flowmeters for oxygen and other gases; check the reading of the oxygen analyzer and pulse oximeter.

**V** Listen to the lungs; if a ventilator is in use, check peak inspiratory pressure. Always check tidal volume, respiratory rate, and capnogram. Changes in $CO_2$ production (hyperthermia) or delivery (circulatory failure or embolism) can be seen best when the ventilator setting has not been changed and end-tidal $CO_2$ trends are rising or falling. Such changes are common (20%[4]) and may be obscured with manual (or spontaneous) ventilation. Occasionally, clinicians accustomed to relying on the ventilator will forget to switch back to mechanical ventilation after testing the feel of the bag. The vaporizer setting (Is it still appropriate for the patient?) and function (leaks, level) need to be checked; an analyzer for gaseous anesthetics makes it easy. The analyzer may also (depending on the type) discover and indicate the rare event of the vaporizer having been filled with the wrong agent.

**E** The endotracheal tube deserves frequent checking. With changes in position, it can slip into a mainstem bronchus or out of the larynx; it can kink; and, in children and particularly infants, it can become obstructed with secretions. If nitrous oxide is present, deflate the cuff every 20 minutes because the gas causes the cuff to swell. When refilling the cuff, allow a leak when the desired peak inspiratory pressure is exceeded by about 5 cm $H_2O$. If a problem remains obscure, eliminate possible problems arising from the anesthetic machine or breathing circuit by disconnecting at the endotracheal tube and ventilating with a self-inflating bag. Use an independent source of oxygen while ensuring that anesthesia is maintained with an intravenous agent.

**R** Review all monitors and confirm that they have been properly calibrated. In 4% of incidents in the Australian study,[4] the critical incidents involved monitors, and in 2%, they were related to other equipment (cauterizers, humidifiers, warming blankets, endoscopes, probes, prostheses, retractors, and others).

For a complete explanation of ABCD, see Table 7–3.

A SWIFT CHECK starts with four important A's:

1. **Awareness.** The extensive use of narcotics (which may not blot out memory) and muscle relaxants has increased the occurrence of awareness during general anesthesia (depriving the patient of the ability to communicate awareness).

2. **Air embolism.** Air embolism is a common complication in patients sitting up for neurosurgical procedures. It can

**TABLE 7–4.** A SWIFT CHECK*

| | Condition | Comments |
|---|---|---|
| **A** | Air embolus | Hypotension, hypocarbia |
| | Anaphylaxis | Hypotension/bronchospasm/urticaria |
| | Air in pleura | Pneumothorax, any unexpected circulatory or respiratory deterioration |
| | Awareness | Dilution of anesthetic gases, resistant patient, failure to deliver |
| **S** | Surgeon/situation | Vagal stimulation, caval compression, bleeding, direct myocardial stimulation |
| | Sepsis | Hypotension, desaturation, acidosis, hyperdynamic circulation, ARDS, rigors |
| **W** | Wound | Trauma, bleeding, tamponade, pneumothorax, problems due to retractors |
| | Water intoxication | Electrolyte disturbance, fluid overload |
| **I** | Infarct | Myocardial conduction ST or rhythm problem, hypotension, or cardiac output |
| | Insufflation | Vagal tone, reduced venous return, pulmonary or paradoxical arterial gas embolism |
| **F** | "Fat" syndrome | Desaturation and/or hypotension, especially after induction and in the lithotomy position (with obesity or distended abdomen); profuse bronchial secretions† |
| | Full bladder | Marked hemodynamic changes and/or sympathetic stimulation |
| **T** | Trauma | Spinal injury, undiagnosed subdural or extradural hematoma, bronchial or diaphragmatic injury, ruptured viscus, concealed hemorrhage, myocardial contusion |
| | Tourniquet down | Local anesthetic toxicity, unseen bleeding, failed block |
| **C** | Catheter/IV cannula | Leaks, blocks, failure to deliver, wrong drug or label, wrong connection/site, trauma |
| | Chest drain problems | Tube not in or out, clamped, kinked, blocked, wrongly connected |
| | Cement | Hemodynamic change with methylmethacrylate |
| **H** | Hyper-/Hypothermia | Tachycardia and hypercarbia/poor perfusion, ECG changes |
| | Hypoglycemia | Inappropriate or inadvertent insulin administration preoperatively, fasting and β-blockers, hepatic compromise and β-blockers |
| **E** | Embolus | Fat, thrombus, amniotic fluid; hypotension, hypocarbia, hypoxia, ECG changes |
| | Endocrine | Hyperthyroid or hypothyroid/adrenal medullar or cortex/pituitary/diabetes/5-hydroxytryptamine |
| **C** | Check | Right patient, right operation, right surgeon, correct side, correct body part |
| | Check | Case notes and old notes for preoperative status, diseases, drugs, and conditions |
| **K** | K+ | Potassium and any other electrolyte abnormality (hyper or hypo), ECG changes |
| | Keep | Patient "asleep" (eg, with diazepam, ketamine) until a new anesthetic machine can be obtained |

**Note:** 99.9% of incidents should be identified by the end of this acronym. If the problem has not been solved, direct the available resources to its solution. Get skilled and experienced help. Work from first principles. Think laterally.

*COVER ABCD covers 95% of incidents, 3% of which are cardiac arrests. A SWIFT CHECK handles the remaining 5%. This list should be immediately available in the operating room. Conditions listed under *A* make up 4% of problems (~1% each). The remainder (A SWIFT CHECK) either contribute to cardiac arrests (eg, vagal stimulation, bleeding, infarct) or make up most of the rest of 1% of incidents.

†>90% of causes of desaturation are corrected by COVER ABCD; this category represents most of the remainder.

ARDS, acute respiratory distress syndrome.

Data from Runciman WB, Webb RK, Klepper ID, et al. The Australian Incident Monitoring Study. Crisis management—validation of an algorithm by analysis of 2000 incident reports. *Anaesth Intensive Care.* 1993;21:579–592.

occur whenever the operative site is above the level of the right atrium or whenever the central venous pressure drops low enough to admit air, for example, during a gasp or negative inspiratory pressure. Air embolism has been reported in patients lying prone for back surgery, lying on their sides for hip surgery, and lying on their backs for breast surgery. Air can enter when infusion tubing, drip sets, and warming coils have not been properly flushed and purged of air. Tumor, clot (common in knee arthroplasty), and bone cement can also lead to pulmonary embolism with hypoxemia and hypotension, which may present difficult diagnostic puzzles.

3. **Air in pleura (pneumothorax).** An undiagnosed bleb can burst with little provocation, or a broken rib can puncture the lung. We might injure the lung during insertion of a central venous or pulmonary artery catheter or by exerting excessive airway pressure.

4. **Anaphylaxis.** For reasons not well understood, latex allergy has become so common that the American Society of Anesthesiologists published a booklet describing it.[6] This allergy is particularly worrisome because it may develop without an obvious relationship to the induction of anesthesia or to the beginning of the procedure. In addition to the well known anaphylactic reactions to antibiotics

and radiopaque dyes, heparin, muscle relaxants (including, although rare, succinylcholine), and thiopental can trigger anaphylactic reactions that may be fatal if not recognized and treated expeditiously.

A SWIFT CHECK (see Table 7–4) may trigger a helpful association if the problem still remains obscure. Caplan and colleagues[7] concluded from their study of closed claims related to gas delivery equipment that more than half of the adverse outcomes could have been prevented by the use of pulse oximetry and capnography, monitoring techniques that have been adopted in many countries as minimal standards.

### Clinical Factors

However, even when the difficulties do not arise from the gas delivery system, capnography and pulse oximetry will signal problems whether brought about by malignant hyperthermia, myocardial infarction, cardiac tamponade, or pneumothorax (Table 7–5). Gaba and colleagues[8] listed numerous clinical emergencies that can lead to death and enumerated the findings that are likely to be observed. Table 7–5 illustrates how many different situations may lead to changes in blood

**TABLE 7–5.** Changes in Vital Signs Are Nonspecific

| Problem | BP | HR | SpO$_2$ | ETCO$_2$ | PIP | Breath Sounds |
|---|---|---|---|---|---|---|
| Breathing system obstruction | Up | Up | Down | Down | Up | Abnormal |
| Transfusion reaction | Down | Up | Down | Down | Up | Abnormal |
| Anaphylaxis | Down | Up | Down | Down | Up | Abnormal |
| Pulmonary edema | Down | Up | Down | Down | Up | Abnormal |
| Aspiration | | Up | Down | Down | Up | Abnormal |
| Asthma | | Up | Down | Down | Up | Abnormal |
| Myocardial infarction | Down | Up | Down | Down | | Abnormal with edema |
| Cardiac tamponade | Down | Up | Down | Down | | Normal |
| Pulmonary embolism | Down | Up | Down | Down | | Normal |
| Hemorrhage | Down | Up | | Down | | Normal |
| Esophageal intubation | Up | Up | Down | Absent | Up | Abnormal |
| Light anesthesia | Up | Up | | | | Normal |
| Malignant hyperthermia | | Up | Down | Up | | Normal |
| Disconnect | Up | Up | Down | Absent | Down | Abnormal |
| Endobronchial intubation | | Up | Down | Down | Up | Abnormal |
| Pneumothorax | Down | Up | Down | Down | Up | Abnormal |
| Addison crisis | Down | Up | | Down | | Normal |

BP, blood pressure; ETCO$_2$, end-tidal carbon dioxide; HR, heart rate; PIP, peak inspiratory pressure.

pressure, heart rate, oxygen saturation, end-tidal CO$_2$ values, peak inspiratory pressure, and breath sounds.

Some of the empty spaces in Table 7–5 will begin to show abnormal values or directions; others will reverse direction when a problem fully develops or persists. For example, severe hypoxemia is associated with bradycardia; malignant hyperthermia will eventually cause hypotension; the asthmatic patient can develop hypertension and only later hypotension; light anesthesia is not invariably associated with tachycardia and hypertension; and a myocardial infarction is not always accompanied by tachycardia. Nevertheless, Table 7–5 demonstrates the diagnostic challenges the clinician faces when things begin to go wrong.

Table 7–5 also shows that the often neglected peak inspiratory pressure deserves to be monitored. This pressure and end-tidal CO$_2$ values may be obscured when the clinician gets the feel of the bag and manually hyperventilates instead of watching tidal volume and peak inspiratory pressure in a patient requiring mechanical ventilation of the lungs. Yet, changes (or no changes) in peak inspiratory pressure can help rule in or out several diagnoses. Exhaled carbon dioxide points to specific problems when it is absent (disconnection) and when it rises (with fever and in malignant hyperthermia). Auscultation is still valuable and will often be abnormal and diagnostic.

With rare exception, vital signs will signal trouble; however, more often than not, they do not pinpoint the diagnosis. Usually, the diagnosis can be made only when vital signs, clinical signs, the patient's history, and the surgical procedure are taken into consideration. For some conditions, special monitors such as transesophageal echocardiography, pulmonary artery catheter, electroencephalogram, or transcranial Doppler may greatly aid in eliminating some diagnoses, thus narrowing the choices. However, in the majority of cases, these special tools are not in use.

We often find it difficult to draw a line between acceptably reduced blood pressure and dangerously low blood pressure. For example, young adults may have daytime pressures of 120/80 mm Hg, but during physiologic sleep in the wee hours of the night their pressures can drop to 80/50 mm Hg. The resting pressures of older adults do not decrease by as large a percentage. Other vital signs also have a wide physiologic range. Unfortunately, we do not know whether physiologic extremes that are well tolerated are equally well suffered when induced by anesthetic or surgical interventions.

## Alarms

Modern anesthesia equipment and monitors are equipped with numerous alarms. Ideally, the alarms should reset themselves whenever the clinical context so indicates. For example, a low CO$_2$ alarm during intubation is not only annoying, it is not helpful. Current alarm technology has not reached a level of sophistication that would obviate that category of false alarms. Yet, even the sometimes annoying, and often false, alarms should be suffered because, in general, alarms serve a valuable function. Before induction of anesthesia, alarms should be set to match the patient's status and the expected range of values. For example, it makes little sense to set the alarm for a threshold of inspired oxygen concentration at 21% if the patient is to receive 50% oxygen in air or nitrous oxide. In case of trouble with the delivery of oxygen, the alarm would sound much later than the onset of the problem. Similarly, the blood pressure and heart rate alarms should be set at levels appropriate for the patient. Conversely, be aware of what variables your anesthesia equipment does *not* protect with an alarm. For example, on many older anesthesia machines, only an aneroid pressure gauge displays airway pressures. We have no monitors or alarms for intravenous fluids given by drip or intravenous drugs injected by hand. No infusion pump knows what it is infusing, but many will alarm when they fail to deliver what they were set to infuse. It is easy to make medication errors with respect to type of drug, dose, or route of administration.

## EMERGENCY MANAGEMENT

### In Case of Trouble, How Can We Best Initiate Appropriate Therapy?

In the event of a cardiac arrest, follow the guidelines described in Chapter 47. It is useful to practice crisis management with all members of the surgical team, as advocated by

Gaba and associates.[8] Following are four basic rules that apply to the management of any crisis, be it a cardiac arrest or any other acute, life-threatening problem:

1. Call for help and do so early. Time and again we are reminded that the successful management of most crises requires more than a lone anesthetist. In the ongoing British study, National Confidential Enquiry Into Perioperative Deaths, the point is made that "Anaesthetists must have appropriately skilled and dedicated non-medical assistants."[9] This is true for most complex cases and especially true for a crisis.
2. Immediately inform the surgeon, radiologist, or whoever performs the procedure for which you are giving anesthesia of the crisis. This is important not only because continuation of the procedure may add new problems but also because the surgeon may be responsible for the problem (eg, a retractor on the vena cava or the heart). A joint decision must be made by the anesthesiologist and surgeon whether and how quickly an ongoing operation must be abandoned.
3. Establish a team and identify the team leader. More often than not, the anesthetist will assume that role. Without a firm command structure, individual well-intentioned efforts may work against each other or be redundant, leaving other tasks undone or unattended. Remember that some efforts require the full attention of a single person. For example, when treating malignant hyperthermia, the preparation of dantrolene will fully occupy one member of the team. The anesthesiologist must delegate that type of responsibility in order to be free to guide the overall resuscitation efforts.
4. Appoint one individual, usually a nurse or technician, to be the sole recorder of all events: vital signs, drugs, fluids, and resuscitation efforts. The time of these events and who

did what should be documented. After the crisis, the team should meet for an analysis of what was done. It is vital that the details of such a meeting (when, where, who was present) be clearly documented. Additional information about the patient's history and preceding events and activities that might not have been obvious during the event now need to be recorded. The longer this important step is delayed, the less accurate will be the analysis. The effort should result in a comprehensive account of the crisis and its management. The report can be the basis for evaluating what was done and what might be done better. It will be a most useful document should a claim be brought against the team or one of its members.

### References

1. Kohn LT, Corrigan JM, Donaldson MS. *To Err Is Human. Building a Safer Health System.* Washington, DC: National Academy Press; 2000.
2. Cooper JB, Newbower RS, Long CD, et al. Preventable anesthesia mishaps: a study of human factors. *Anesthesiology.* 1978;49:399.
3. Cooper JB, Newbower RS, Kitz RJ. An analysis of major errors and equipment failures in anesthesia management: considerations for prevention and detection. *Anesthesiology.* 1984;60:34.
4. Webb RK, Currie M, Morgan CA, et al. The Australian Incident Monitoring Study: an analysis of 2000 incident reports. *Anaesth Intensive Care.* 1993;21:520.
5. Runciman WB, Webb RK, Klepper ID, et al. The Australian Incident Monitoring Study. Crisis management—validation of an algorithm by analysis of 2000 incident reports. *Anaesth Intensive Care.* 1993;21:579.
6. American Society of Anesthesiologists. *Natural Rubber Latex Allergy.* Park Ridge, Ill: American Society of Anesthesiologists; 1999.
7. Caplan RA, Vistica MF, Posner KL, et al. Adverse anesthetic outcomes arising from gas delivery equipment: a closed claims analysis. *Anesthesiology.* 1997;87:741.
8. Gaba DM, Fish KJ, Howard SK. *Crisis Management in Anesthesiology.* New York, NY: Churchill Livingstone; 1994.
9. Summary of the 1993/94 Report. Available at: http://ncepod.org.uk/csumms93.htm. Accessed October 23, 2000.

# Preoperative Consultations

CHAPTER

## 8

# Cardiology Consultation

Marian C. Limacher

## RISK FACTORS FOR CARDIAC EVENTS

*What Are the Risks?*

*How Is the Level of Cardiac Risk Evaluated?*

*What Can Be Done to Modify Risk?*

## THE ROLE OF THE CARDIOLOGIST

The goal of a cardiac evaluation before surgery should not be *clearance* because there is no accepted understanding of what that term means nor how such a decision is derived. Rather, cardiac consultation before surgery should evaluate the patient's current cardiac status, estimate the risk of cardiac problems developing in the perioperative period, and offer recommendations to manage the observed conditions. In fact, identifying and managing long-term cardiac risk factors before surgery are likely to be more important than modifying them in the immediate perioperative period.

The primary reason for assessing the cardiac risks of a specific patient undergoing a given procedure is that the likelihood of a cardiac event is directly related to the burden of underlying cardiovascular disease. Although it has been suggested that the purpose of the preoperative cardiology assessment should be to answer the question, "Can this patient reasonably have noncardiac surgery?"[1] most authors and recommendations focus on the assessment of underlying cardiac disease in regard to its immediate and long-term management.[2–4] In order to optimize perioperative patient assessment and management, collaboration among surgeon, anesthesiologist, and consulting physician is required. Each brings expertise and perspective that can be most effectively used when collegial communication is established within a team framework.

Several reports have documented discrepancies in the reasons for consultation and the ultimate function of the consultation itself. Some problems surrounding consultations follow[5–8]:

- Reason for the consultation may not be specified.
- Consultants' recommendations are commonly ignored.
- Recommendations themselves may not provide any real management instructions.

The importance of communication (or lack thereof) among team members was highlighted in a report about the intended purpose and perceived utility of preoperative cardiology consultations.[8] In a survey of anesthesiologists, surgeons, and cardiologists, they reached consensus about several important purposes of a cardiology consultation:

- Treating an inadequately treated cardiac condition before surgery
- Providing data to use in anesthesia management
- Diagnosing the medical condition before surgery

However, there were discrepancies regarding the importance of the following points:

- Suggesting intraoperative monitoring (anesthesiologists and surgeons said such recommendations were much less important than did cardiologists)
- Suggesting intraoperative treatment modalities when not requested
- Advising the safest type of anesthesia (anesthesiologists responded that this was unimportant)

The majority of anesthesiologists reported they "seldom or never" felt obligated to follow a cardiologist's recommendations, and only 16.6% reported they "frequently or always" felt obligated to follow recommendations. There was also disagreement regarding which physician (surgeon, anesthesiologist, primary physician, or consultant) was responsible for making sure the patient's condition was medically optimal before surgery and which physician had the ultimate authority to determine that an elective case could proceed. The most common deficiencies of cardiologists, as reported by anesthesiologists, were failing to give specific facts, failing to write legibly, attempting to dictate type of anesthesia, and giving suggestions outside the realm of individual competence.[8]

The authors also provided a chart review of 55 completed surgeries with consultations. The authors found that 58% of the surgeries did not have a specific reason for the consultation documented in the chart. The consultations were highly variable in content: 32.7% contained no recommendation (many contained the phrase "cleared for surgery"); 16% gave advice for placing a pulmonary artery catheter; 7% recommended continuing current medications. More than 90% of the consultations reviewed were for patients with known medical problems already being treated; 89% of the procedures planned were in categories classified as low or intermediate risk; and few specific recommendations were made. Therefore, it is likely that many of the cardiology preoperative consultations conducted were unnecessary.[8]

This chapter provides a review of the factors that have been identified as contributing to risk for cardiac events in noncardiac surgical procedures, describes important features of the approach to evaluating risk, suggests which interventions may reduce the risk of a perioperative cardiac event, and concludes with guidelines for when a cardiology consultation should be requested and what it should contain. The reader is referred to the comprehensive American College of Cardiology (ACC)/American Heart Association (AHA) Guidelines for Perioperative Cardiovascular Evaluation for Noncardiac Surgery for additional background.[3]

## RISK FACTORS FOR CARDIAC EVENTS

### What Are the Risks?

The triggers for acute myocardial ischemia are complex and may differ in individual patients. Simple imbalance between supply and demand not only can be induced by the stress of procedures in patients with fixed coronary artery atherosclerosis but also can be altered by drug and technique interventions. The more common and concerning culprit for unstable syndromes and myocardial infarction (MI) is plaque rupture with thrombosis. Because we have yet to be able to identify who is at greatest risk for this cascade of events and have even less understanding of the factors leading to coronary endothelial dysfunction, the ability to identify and intervene with surgical procedures to prevent complications from coronary artery disease (CAD) currently relies on an understanding of risk factors identified from careful analyses of reported surgical cases.

The risk of a patient experiencing a perioperative cardiovascular event is influenced by the underlying presence and severity of cardiac disease as well as by the type of surgery itself. Among the most striking factors predicting an adverse cardiac event is recent MI. Early reports indicated a rate of reinfarction or cardiac death of >30% when noncardiac surgery was performed within the first 3 months following MI, 15% at 4 to 6 months, and approximately 5% after 6 months. Subsequent studies reported a much lower risk but included selected patients who had undergone overall risk assessment and intensive intraoperative and postoperative monitoring and management.[9,10] Another reported series of consecutive pa-

tients undergoing urgent or emergent vascular surgery in the 1980s within 6 weeks of MI revealed that cardiac risks were still high[11] (Fig. 8–1).

The risk of a particular surgery for a given patient has at least two components. First, the type of patient typically undergoing a particular procedure may be at greater risk for a cardiac event than patients in the general population, as in the case of a patient with severe peripheral vascular disease (PVD). As demonstrated by many studies, patients with PVD invariably have underlying CAD, and many are diabetic.[12] Therefore, the patient himself or herself is at increased risk for a cardiac event. Second, the hemodynamic stress associated with the specific surgical procedure may impart cardiac risk. Operations that predictably cause increases, decreases, or wide variations in heart rate, blood pressure (BP), intravascular volume, clotting tendencies, oxygenation, and neurohumoral activation are associated with greater cardiac risks. For major emergency surgery, many of these factors are activated, and in most series, emergency surgery, per se, emerges as an important risk factor for cardiovascular complications.

However, many of the factors that would be likely to increase the risk for an acute cardiac event appear to be well controlled during modern anesthesia.[13] Although some agents may provoke myocardial ischemia to a greater degree than others,[14,15] most studies have been unable to demonstrate differences in cardiac outcomes related to the choice of primary anesthetic agent or with different routes of administration (eg, epidural versus general).[16–18] Therefore, the choice of anesthetic agent and route of administration is always best left to the judgment of the anesthesiologist. Any recommendation by the cardiology consultant regarding his or her choice of one anesthetic mode or agent over another should not be considered.

As defined by the ACC/AHA Task Force, procedures in which the combined perioperative MI and death rate are ≥5% constitute high-risk procedures.[3] Emergency major operations and aortic and peripheral vascular surgery fall into this category (Table 8–1). Intermediate risk surgical procedures generally have cardiac-mortality risks <5%. Low-risk surgical procedures have reported cardiac-mortality risks <1%. Notably, the ACC/AHA Task Force does not recommend further cardiac testing or evaluation for patients undergoing these low-

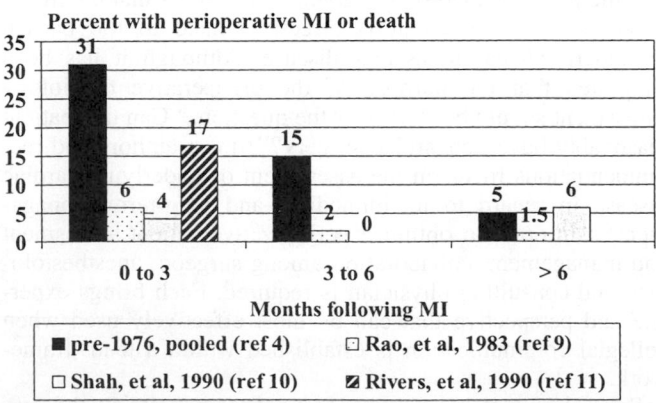

**FIGURE 8–1.** Rates of reinfarction or cardiac death with noncardiac surgery performed 0 to 3 months, 3 to 6 months, or >6 months after myocardial infarction. (Modified from Rivers SP, Scher LA, Gupta SK, et al. Safety of peripheral vascular surgery after recent acute myocardial infarction. *J Vasc Surg.* 1990;11:70.)

**TABLE 8–1.** Classification of Cardiac Risk for Noncardiac Surgical Procedures

*High:* **Risk of Cardiovascular Event or Death ≥5%**
Emergency major operations, particularly in the elderly
Aortic and other major vascular
Peripheral vascular
Anticipated prolonged surgical procedures associated with large fluid shifts and/or blood loss
*Intermediate:* **Risk of Cardiovascular Event or Death <5%**
Carotid endarterectomy
Head and neck
Interperitoneal and intrathoracic
Orthopedic
Prostate
*Low:* **Risk of Cardiovascular Event or Death <1%**
*(Cardiac evaluation not recommended)*
Endoscopic procedures
Superficial procedures
Cataract
Breast

From Eagle KA, Brundage BH, Chaitman BR, et al. Guidelines for perioperative cardiovascular evaluation for noncardiac surgery. Report of the American College of Cardiology/American Heart Association Task Force on Practice Guidelines (Committee on Perioperative Cardiovascular Evaluation for Noncardiac Surgery). *Circulation.* 1996;93:1278.

risk procedures if no history or examination factors warrant additional evaluation.[3]

## How Is the Level of Cardiac Risk Evaluated?

### Preoperative Evaluation

Virtually all patients undergoing a surgical procedure requiring regional or general anesthetic agents will have a preoperative assessment by the anesthesia team. The general assessment, including symptoms, exercise tolerance, prior medical diagnoses (including cardiac), medications, tests, and interventions, and a physical examination will be performed in the preoperative setting. It is important to remember that many patients will have been under the care of a primary care physician or cardiologist and may have had an assessment before the initial surgical referral. Obtaining results of previous pertinent evaluations, tests, hospitalizations, and medications is an important step in the patient evaluation.

It is likewise important to consider that some of the patients who seek attention for a surgical procedure will not have had adequate cardiovascular assessment for many years, if ever. Thus, the preoperative evaluation affords an opportunity to obtain an overall assessment of cardiac risk and permits planning for needed follow-up for ongoing long-term health beyond the scope of the planned surgical procedure.

### Cardiovascular History

In obtaining the history, several key features are crucial in order to assess cardiac risk. Patients should be specifically asked about diagnoses such as angina, MI, congestive heart failure (CHF), heart murmur, and symptomatic dysrhythmia. In addition, the presence and treatment of risk factors should be documented, including high cholesterol levels, diabetes and glycemic control, hypertension, family history of premature CAD, and cigarette smoking. The patient's functional capacity can be briefly estimated by asking several questions about

usual physical activity (Table 8–2). The metabolic equivalent (MET) level is particularly important to determine because both perioperative and long-term cardiac risk are increased in patients unable to achieve a level of energy expenditure of at least 4 METs.[3]

### Physical Examination

The physical examination focusing on cardiovascular findings should include careful ascertainment of vital signs, height and weight, and particular attention to pulses and BP in each arm. Attention should be paid to the carotid pulse contour, presence of bruits, jugular venous pressure and waves, auscultation of the lungs and heart, and palpation of the precordium. The presence of a murmur should direct further assessment by echocardiography if not already obtained. Additionally, the need for antibiotic prophylaxis can be determined.[19] Other important assessments are abdominal auscultation and palpation and examination of the extremities for edema and pulses.

Cardiac testing and treatments generally have the same indications as in the nonsurgical setting. The risks and long-term benefits must be considered for each procedure or intervention; the task is not only to "get the patient through" the proposed surgical procedure but also to alleviate symptoms, improve quality of life, or increase longevity. "No test should be performed unless it is likely to influence patient treatment."[3]

### Clinical Predictors

The original preoperative risk assessment tools used clinical assessments. The earliest system of preoperative assessment was developed by the American Society of Anesthesiologists and standardized by Dripps.[20] In this system, a normal, healthy patient is assigned Class 1; a patient with mild systemic disease is Class 2; a patient with severe systemic disease that limits activity but is not incapacitating is Class 3; a patient

**TABLE 8–2.** Estimated Energy Requirements for Common Activities

| 1 MET | Can you take care of yourself? |
|---|---|
| | Can you eat, dress, or use the toilet? |
| | Can you walk indoors around the house? |
| | Can you walk a block or two on level ground at 2-3 mph? |
| | Can you do light housework, such as dusting or washing dishes? |
| 4 METs | Can you climb a flight of stairs or walk up a hill? |
| | Can you walk on level ground at 4 mph? |
| | Can you run a short distance? |
| | Can you do heavy housework, such as scrubbing floors or lifting or moving heavy furniture? |
| | Do you participate in moderate recreational activities, such as golf, bowling, dancing, doubles tennis, or throwing a baseball or football? |
| >10 METs | Do you participate in strenuous sports, such as swimming, singles tennis, football, basketball, or skiing? |

MET, metabolic equivalent.
Data from Eagle KA, Brundage BH, Chaitman BR, et al. Guidelines for perioperative cardiovascular evaluation for noncardiac surgery. Report of the American College of Cardiology/American Heart Association Task Force on Practice Guidelines (Committee on Perioperative Cardiovascular Evaluation for Noncardiac Surgery). *Circulation.* 1996;93:1278; Hlatky MA, Boineau RE, Higginbotham MB, et al. A brief self-administered questionnaire to determine functional capacity (the Duke Activity Status Index). *Am J Cardiol.* 1989;64:651; and Fletcher GF, Balady G, Froelicher VF, et al. Exercise standards: a statement for healthcare professionals from the American Heart Association. *Circulation.* 1995;91:580.

**TABLE 8–3.** Goldman's Multifactorial Cardiac Risk Index

| | | |
|---|---|---|
| History | Myocardial infarction within 6 months | 10 |
| | Age >70 y | 5 |
| Physical examination | S3 gallop or jugular venous distension | 11 |
| | Important aortic stenosis | 3 |
| Electrocardiogram | Rhythm other than sinus or sinus plus APBs on last preoperative electrocardiogram | 7 |
| | >5 premature ventricular beats per minute at any time preoperatively | 7 |
| Poor general medical status (any of these) | Pao$_2$ <60 mm Hg; Paco$_2$ >50 mm Hg; K$^+$ <3.0 mEq/L; HCO$_3^-$ <20 mmol/L; BUN 50 mg/dL; creatinine >3 mg/dL; abnormal SGOT; signs of chronic liver disease; patient bedridden from noncardiac causes | 3 |
| Intraperitoneal, intrathoracic, or aortic surgery | | 3 |
| Emergency operation | | 4 |
| | **Total** | **53** |

APB, atrial premature beat; BUN, serum urea nitrogen; SGOT, aspartate aminotransferase.

Reprinted from Goldman L, Caldera D, Nussbaum SR, et al. Multifactorial index of cardiac risk in non-cardiac surgical procedures. *N Engl J Med.* 1977;197:848 by permission of the *New England Journal of Medicine.*

**TABLE 8–5.** Detsky's Multifactorial Index

| | | |
|---|---|---|
| Coronary artery disease | MI within 6 months | 10 |
| | MI >6 months ago | 5 |
| | Canadian Cardiovascular Society Angina | |
| | Class III | 10 |
| | Class IV | 20 |
| Alveolar pulmonary edema | Within 1 week | 10 |
| | Ever | 5 |
| Valvular disease | Suspected critical aortic stenosis | 20 |
| | Rhythm other than sinus or sinus + APBs on the last perioperative ECG; >5 premature ventricular contractions at any time prior to surgery | 5 |
| Poor general medical status | Pao$_2$ <60 mm Hg; Paco$_2$ >50 mm Hg; K +, 3.0 mEq/L; HCO$_3^-$ <20 mEq/L; BUN >50 mg/dL; creatinine >3 mg/dL; abnormal SGOT; signs of chronic liver disease; patient bedridden from noncardiac cause | 5 |
| Age >70 y | | 5 |
| Emergency operation | | 10 |

APB, atrial premature beat; BUN, serum urea nitrogen; SGOT, aspartate aminotransferase.

Data from Detsky AS, Abramo HB, McLaughlin JR, et al. Predicting cardiac complications in patients undergoing non-cardiac surgery. *J Gen Intern Med.* 1986;1:213.

with incapacitating systemic disease that is a constant threat to life is Class 4; and a moribund patient not expected to survive 24 hours with or without surgery is Class 5. Increasing mortality was shown to be associated with higher classes.[18]

Goldman and colleagues developed a multifactorial cardiac risk index (Table 8–3) emphasizing clinical history, physical examination, and specific laboratory measures.[21] Numeric points are assigned to various components of the risk index, and risk of complications have been shown to be related to higher point totals[21] (Table 8–4). Other modifications have been proposed by Detsky and associates[22] (Tables 8–5 and 8–6) and Larsen and coworkers (Table 8–7).[23] The clinical risk indices have been shown to effectively determine the level of cardiac risk for patients undergoing noncardiac surgery, but these indices have limited positive predictive value[24] (Fig. 8–2).

A classification of clinical markers of perioperative cardiovascular risk has been developed by the ACC/AHA Task Force[3] (Table 8–8). According to this classification, major predictors of cardiovascular risk include the following:

- Active or unstable cardiac disease, which would impart increased risk for morbidity and mortality even without concomitant noncardiac surgery
- Recent MI (<30 days)
- Unstable angina
- Severe angina

- Decompensated CHF
- High-grade atrioventricular heart block
- Symptomatic arrhythmias in the presence of underlying heart disease
- Supraventricular arrhythmias with uncontrolled ventricular response
- Severe valvular disease (particularly aortic stenosis)[3]

In the study by Ashton and coworkers, CAD resulted in a relative risk of 10.5 for perioperative MI following major noncardiac surgery.[25]

According to the ACC/AHA Task Force's classification of clinical markers of perioperative cardiovascular risk, intermediate predictors of increased cardiovascular risk include the following[3]:

- Mild angina pectoris
- Prior MI (>3-6 months)
- Compensated or prior diagnosis of CHF
- Diabetes mellitus

Risk predictors of minor importance include the following[3]:

- Advanced age (>70 years)
- Abnormal electrocardiogram

**TABLE 8–4.** Prediction of Perioperative Cardiac Complications by Points in the Goldman Index

| | Point Total | Cardiac Deaths (%) | Other Life-Threatening Complications* (%) |
|---|---|---|---|
| Class I | 0–5 | 0.2 | 0.7 |
| Class II | 6–12 | 2.0 | 5.0 |
| Class III | 13–25 | 2.0 | 11.0 |
| Class IV | ≥26 | 56 | 22.0 |

*Nonfatal myocardial infarction, congestive heart failure, and ventricular tachycardia.
Reprinted from Goldman L, Caldera D, Nussbaum SR, et al. Multifactorial index of cardiac risk in non-cardiac surgical procedures. *N Engl J Med.* 1977;197:848 by permission of the *New England Journal of Medicine.*

**TABLE 8–6.** Likelihood Ratios of Perioperative Cardiac Complications* (Using Detsky's Point Scale)

| Class (Points) | Major Surgery | Minor Surgery | All Surgery |
|---|---|---|---|
| I (0–15) | 0.42 | 0.39 | 0.43 |
| II (15–30) | 3.58 | 2.75 | 3.38 |
| III (> 30) | 14.93 | 12.20 | 10.60 |

*Defined as myocardial infarction pulmonary edema, ventricular tachycardia or fibrillation, new or worsening congestive heart failure, and coronary insufficiency.
From Detsky AS, Abrams HB, McLaughlin JR, et al. Predicting cardiac complications in patients undergoing non-cardiac surgery. *J Gen Intern Med.* 1986;1:217.

**TABLE 8–7.** Larsen Risk Scale

|  | Points |
|---|---|
| ***Congestive Heart Failure*** | |
| Persistent pulmonary congestion | 12 |
| Previous pulmonary edema | 8 |
| Neither, but previous heart failure | 4 |
| ***Ischemic Heart Disease*** | |
| Myocardial infarction within 3 months | 11 |
| Older infarction or angina | 3 |
| ***Diabetes Mellitus*** | ***3*** |
| Serum creatinine >0.13 mmol/L | 2 |
| Emergency operation | 3 |
| ***Major Surgical Procedure*** | |
| Aortic surgery | 5 |
| Other intraperitoneal/pleural operation | 3 |

Data from Matthay RA. Chronic airway diseases. In: Wyngaarden JB, Smith LH Jr, Bennett JC, eds. *Cecil Textbook of Medicine.* Vol 1. 19th ed. Philadelphia, Pa: WB Saunders; 1992:386.

- Nonsinus rhythm
- Poor functional capacity (<4 METs)
- History of stroke
- Uncontrolled hypertension

## Additional Testing

### Electrocardiogram

In healthy populations, routine 12-lead electrocardiograms (ECGs) provide little information for medical decisions.[26] Resting ECG abnormalities are common and increase with advanced age, hypertension, underlying cardiac disease, and unknown factors. In a large epidemiologic study of men and women between ages 18 and 65 years, 55% of ECG tracings were normal, but 20% of women and 9% of men had ST depression.[27] In a hypertensive population, left ventricular (LV) hypertrophy was found in 21.3% of men and 14.6% of women, with 41% having normal ECGs.[28]

Among patients admitted to a general hospital, routine preoperative ECGs revealed findings considered abnormal in 7.4% of patients over age 40 and in only 4.5% under age 40. When ECGs were evaluated in the setting of an abnormal physical finding or history of cardiac diagnosis, 31% were abnormal.[29] Another study of routine preoperative ECGs demonstrated that abnormalities were more common with increasing age and with Class 2 or higher American Society of Anesthesiologists Physical Status Classification. Of 877 patients, 45% had abnormal ECGs.[30] Among ambulatory surgery patients, routine ECGs commonly (42.7%) were abnormal, but only 1.6% of patients experienced an adverse cardiac event with low-risk surgery.[31]

Abnormalities on routine resting ECGs that are associated with increased cardiac events include nonsinus rhythm, bundle branch block, Q wave infarctions, ST segment shifts, and left axis deviation.[32–35] Unfortunately, there is no evidence that discovering these abnormalities alters management or outcome with elective noncardiac surgery. Despite these observations, ECGs are universally performed before planned surgery. Future investigations might define the cost-benefit ratio for the preoperative ECG and perhaps refine the indications for ordering. It is likely that the ECG will remain a part of the complete preoperative work-up because the practice is so ingrained. The preoperative team should be cautioned that clinically low-risk patients are unlikely to have any ECG abnormalities and patients at higher risk may have more abnormalities but that further evaluation and intervention will usually be guided by other factors.

### Echocardiography

Transthoracic echocardiography is a common noninvasive technique used to assess cardiac structure and function. As-

**TABLE 8–8.** Clinical Predictors of Increased Perioperative Risk for Cardiovascular Events (Myocardial Infarction, Congestive Heart Failure, Death)

**Major**
Unstable coronary syndromes
  Recent myocardial infarction (7–30 d) with evidence of important ischemic risk by clinical symptoms or noninvasive study
  Unstable or severe angina (Canadian Class III or IV), including "stable" angina in sedentary patients
Decompensated congestive heart failure
Significant arrhythmias
  High-grade atrioventricular (A-V) block
  Symptomatic ventricular arrhythmias in the presence of underlying heart disease
  Supraventricular arrhythmias with uncontrolled ventricular rate
Severe valvular disease
  Aortic stenosis
  Severe aortic or mitral insufficiency with compromised ventricular function
**Intermediate**
Mild angina pectoris (Canadian Class I or II)
Prior myocardial infarction by history or pathological Q waves (confirmed by wall motion study if no other documentation)
Compensated or prior congestive heart failure
Diabetes mellitus
**Minor**
Advanced age (>70 y)
Abnormal ECG (left ventricular hypertrophy, left bundle branch block, ST-T abnormalities)
Rhythm other than sinus (eg, atrial fibrillation)
Low functional capacity (eg, inability to climb one flight of stairs with a bag of groceries)
History of stroke
Uncontrolled hypertension

A-V, atrioventricular; ECG, electrocardiogram.
Data from Pasteur W. Active lobar collapse of the lung after abdominal operations: a contribution to the study of post-operative lung complications. *Lancet.* 1910;2:1080.

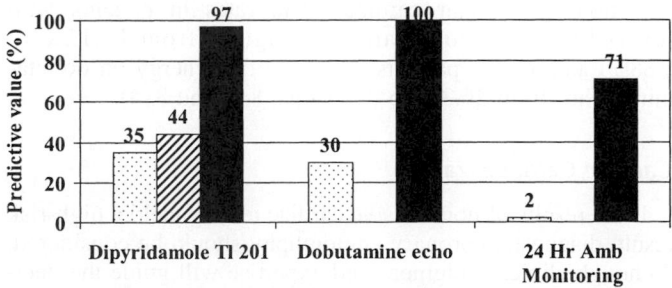

**FIGURE 8–2.** Positive and negative predictive value for *serious postoperative cardiac events* (defined as death, myocardial infarction, pulmonary edema, or unstable angina) in patients undergoing dipyridamole–thallium 201, dobutamine echocardiography, or 24-hour ambulatory monitoring before planned vascular surgery. (Reprinted from *Clinical Cardiology* 1995, Vol 18:447 with permission from Clinical Cardiology Publishing Company, Inc.)

□ + Pred value (reversible defect)  ▨ + Pred value (severe defect)
■ Negative Predictive Value

sessment of LV ejection fraction has been reported to be valuable in determining perioperative complications, with a resting ejection fraction <35% discriminating risk. Reduced LV function, however, is primarily predictive of postoperative CHF, not MI or ischemia.[36] Most studies of LV function as a screening technique for preoperative assessment have been conducted using radionuclide angiography.[37–43] Resting LV function, however, has not been found to be consistently predictive of perioperative ischemic events. Accordingly, determination of resting LV function has been designated a *Class III Indication* (ie, a condition for which there is evidence or general agreement that the procedure is not necessary) by the ACC/AHA Task Force of Practice Guidelines Committee on Perioperative Cardiovascular Evaluation for Noncardiac Surgery.[3]

Despite these reports and despite the recommendations of the ACC/AHA Task Force, transthoracic echocardiography is frequently performed as a preoperative assessment of LV function. One study reported that an LV ejection fraction of <50% has a sensitivity of 78% and a specificity of 81% for predicting cardiac morbidity in the perioperative state. The positive predictive value of an abnormal ejection fraction was only 20%, with a negative predictive value of 97%.[44]

Another study prospectively performed transthoracic echocardiograms on 368 male patients before elective noncardiac surgery. Lower ejection fraction was correlated with combined cardiac events (MI, cardiac death, unstable angina, CHF, and ventricular tachycardia); however, the echocardiographic measurements did not add any significant information to known clinical risk factors when each individual adverse event was analyzed. The sensitivity and positive predictive values for echocardiographic measurements remained quite low for predicting cardiac events (sensitivity, 28%-31%; predictive value, 0.06 for ischemic events, 0.4 for all cardiac events.)[45]

Assessment of resting ejection fraction provides accurate information about baseline global and regional function, but it offers no information about function under stress, which is more likely to detect myocardium at risk for an ischemic event. In view of the existing evidence, resting echocardiography, in the absence of suspected valvular disease or suspected but undiagnosed LV dysfunction, cannot be recommended for routine use.

### Exercise Capacity

Functional capacity has been shown to be one of the most important factors for predicting perioperative cardiac risk.[4] Exercise ECG (treadmill testing) can be used to quantitate functional capacity. An early study by Cutler and colleagues demonstrated that vascular surgery patients at highest risk were those who were able to achieve <75% of the predicted maximal heart rate and who had ST segment changes.[46] Maximal predicted heart rate is estimated by the following formula:

$$220 - \text{Patient's Age}$$

Conversely, the ability to achieve >75% or 85% predicted heart rate is associated with substantially lower risk.[45,47] Two other studies of patients over age 65 undergoing major abdominal or thoracic noncardiac surgery demonstrated that the ability to reach a heart rate of at least 100 beats per minute with supine bicycle exercise was a better predictor of cardiac complications than findings on the exercise ECG or radionu-

clide ejection fraction.[48,49] Because patients with good exercise tolerance or good performance on an exercise test are at reduced risk, no further cardiac evaluation is needed after following the decision steps outlined by the ACC/AHA Task Force[3] (Table 8–9). Functional capacity can be readily estimated by asking about common daily activities, as outlined in Table 8–2.[3,4,50,51]

### Pharmacologic Stress Testing

Unfortunately, many patients are unable to exercise because of conditions frequently causing referral for the proposed surgical intervention (eg, orthopedic problems, severe PVD). In these patients, the assessment of functional capacity is more difficult. Symptoms of angina cannot be used as an indirect assessment of functional capacity because inactivity may not result in reproducible exertional symptoms. In these patients, a variety of pharmacologic stress tests have been developed and used.

It is important to realize the proper role of other types of cardiac testing, however. Several studies have emphasized that additional testing adds little to the clinical risk assessment for patients within the lowest or highest risk categories, but that there is incremental value to applying a careful testing strategy to those assessed to have an intermediate level of risk.[52,53] Although primarily tested on the high-risk patient population undergoing vascular surgery, many studies have demonstrated that preoperative thallium testing can stratify cardiac risk.[54–58]

Shaw and associates prepared a meta-analysis of the 15 published reports using dipyridamole thallium 201 or dobutamine echocardiography for perioperative cardiac risk stratification before vascular surgery.[59] All 15 studies were consecutive series and most were not blinded (although 3 of 5 echocardiographic studies and 4 of 10 nuclear studies did have blinded interpretation of the imaging modality). Possibly as a result of nonblinding, 6% of patients in the nuclear reports and 2.8% of echocardiographic study patients had their vascular surgery canceled. Preoperative coronary angiography was performed in 20% of nuclear patients and 11.7% of echocardiographic patients, with 5% and 6.4% of patients undergoing preoperative revascularization, respectively. The negative predictive value for a normal dipyridamole study was 3.16% and 0.37% for a normal dobutamine echocardiographic study.[59] In those who underwent revascularization before vascular surgery because of abnormal test results, there was a reduction in vascular cardiac event rates in patients with reversible defects on thallium imaging (from 18.12% to 5.88%) and among patients with new dyssynergy on dobutamine echo (from 26.3% to 0)[59] (Figs. 8–3 and 8–4).

### Cardiac Catheterization

If the results of noninvasive cardiac testing yield a high-risk result, diagnostic coronary angiography should be considered. Although clinical judgment and expertise will guide the decision regarding need for catheterization, a published consensus recommended that catheterization be performed if (1) BP falls >10 mm Hg during exercise with associated ischemic changes on ECG; (2) stress myocardial perfusion scan reversibility is demonstrated in 50% or more of single-photon emission computed tomographic slices, and (3) stress echocardiographic ischemia is detected in >5 LV wall segments (using a 16-segment model), in ≥2 coronary artery zones, or in 4 seg-

**TABLE 8–9.** Stepwise Approach to Preoperative Evaluation of the Cardiac Patient for Noncardiac Surgery

**Step 1. Is the Operation an Emergency?**
Yes   Proceed directly with surgery.
No    Go to Step 2.

**Step 2. Has the Patient Had Coronary Revascularization Within 5 Years?**
Yes   Does the patient have signs or symptoms of recurrent disease?
  Yes   Go to Step 3.
  No    Proceed with surgery.
No    Go to Step 3.

**Step 3. Has the Patient Had a Coronary Evaluation Within the Past 2 Years?**
Yes   Are symptoms stable or unchanged?
  Yes   Proceed with surgery.
  No    Go to Step 4.
No    Go to Step 4.

**Step 4. Does the Patient Have Any Major Clinical Predictors of Risk (unstable coronary syndrome, decompensated CHF, hemodynamically significant arrhythmias, severe valvular disease)?**
Yes   Perform specific evaluation based on clinical findings (catheterization echocardiograms, intensive medical management, intervention based on accepted indications).
No    Go to Step 5.

**Step 5. Does the Patient Have Any Intermediate Clinical Predictors (mild angina, prior MI, compensated or prior CHF, diabetes)?**
Yes   Go to Step 6.
No    Go to Step 7.

**Step 6. Does the Patient Have a Functional Capacity >4 METs?**
Yes   Is the planned surgery a high risk procedure (aortic surgery, peripheral vascular surgery, prolonged procedure with large fluid shifts and/or blood loss involving the abdomen, thorax, or head and neck)?
  Yes   Go to Step 8.
  No    Proceed with surgery.
No    Go to Step 8.

**Step 7. Does the Patient Have Minor (age >70, abnormal ECG, nonsinus rhythm, low functional capacity, prior stroke, uncontrolled hypertension) or No Clinical Predictors?**
Yes   Does the patient have a functional capacity >4 METs?
  Yes   Proceed with surgery.
  No    Is the planned surgery high risk?
    Yes   Go to Step 8.
    No    Proceed with surgery.
No    Proceed with surgery.

**Step 8. Perform Noninvasive Testing (exercise ECG, pharmacologic myocardial perfusion scan, dobutamine echocardiogram).**
***High-Risk Result?***
*High-Risk Exercise ECG*
+ Findings at <4 METs or HR <100 or <70% predicted maximal HR. (Horizontal or downsloping ST depression >0.1 mV; ST-elevation >0.1 mV in noninfarct lead; 5 or more leads with ST shifts >0.1 mV; ST changes persist >3 min after exercise; typical angina during test.)
*High-Risk Thallium/Perfusion Scan*
Large or multiple redistribution areas.
*High-Risk Dobutamine Echocardiogram*
New cardiography or worsening wall motion abnormality.
    Yes   Consider catheterization.
    No    Proceed with surgery.
***Intermediate-Risk Result?***
Use clinical judgement about catheterization or medical management.
***Low or Normal Result?***
Proceed with surgery.

CHF, congestive heart failure; ECG, electrocardiogram; HR, heart risk; MET, metabolic equivalent; MI, myocardial infarction.
Data from Pasteur W. Active lobar collapse of the lung after abdominal operations: a contribution to the study of post-operative lung complications. *Lancet.* 1910;2:1080.

ments perfused by the left anterior descending artery.[60] Other findings on testing were met with discrepant or uncertain decisions for catheterization.[60]

Mason and colleagues evaluated the question of whether perioperative coronary angiography and revascularization improves short-term outcomes in patients undergoing noncardiac vascular surgery. They found, using decision analysis methods, that having preoperative coronary angiography would result in lower mortality rates if vascular surgery was canceled in patients with nonrevascularizable CAD or with high-risk procedures with a high cardiac complication rate.[61] The ACC/AHA Task Force offers indications for coronary angiography in the preoperative evaluation[3] (Table 8–10). Catheterization should only be performed when clinical indications suggest the patient will have important coronary artery abnormalities (as determined by the established assessment criteria listed); when the patient is a candidate (and is willing) to undergo coronary revascularization if the findings at catheterization

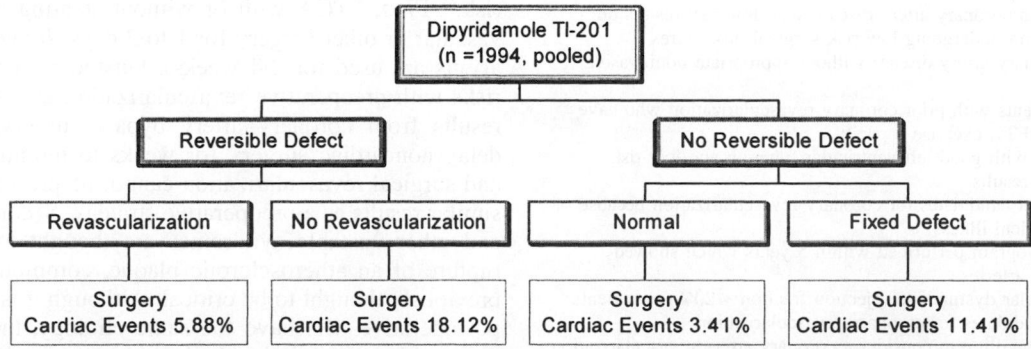

**FIGURE 8–3.** Cardiac event rates after risk stratification by dipyridamole–thallium 201 testing in 1994 patients from 10 studies. If a reversible defect was detected, patients who had coronary revascularization before noncardiac vascular surgery had a three-fold reduction in cardiac events. (Modified. Reprinted with permission from the American College of Cardiology, *Journal of the American College of Cardiology,* 1996, Vol 27:787.)

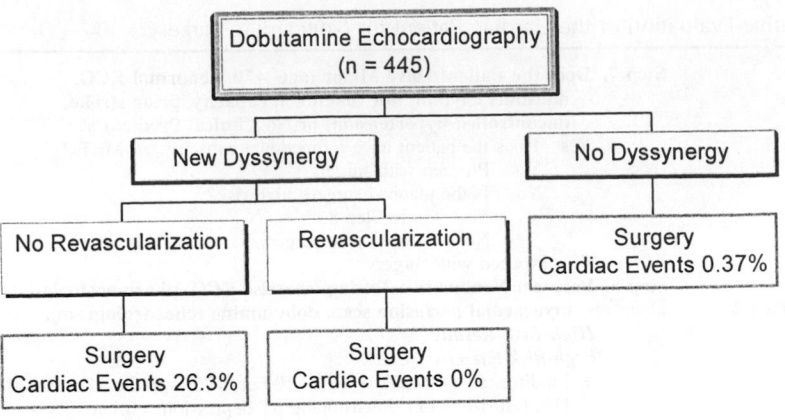

**FIGURE 8–4.** Cardiac event rates after preoperative dobutamine stress testing in 445 patients from five studies. If new wall motion abnormalities (new dyssynergy) was detected and coronary revascularization was undertaken, no perioperative cardiac events occurred with vascular surgical procedures. (Modified. Reprinted with permission from the American College of Cardiology, *Journal of the American College of Cardiology,* 1996, Vol 27:787.)

warrant intervention; and when the findings will affect management.

## What Can Be Done to Modify Risk?

### Coronary Interventions

One of the major themes of the report by the ACC/AHA Task Force of Practice Guidelines Committee on Perioperative Cardiovascular Evaluation for Noncardiac Surgery in 1996 was that *intervention is rarely necessary to lower the risk of surgery.*[3] There is limited information on the safety and effi-

**TABLE 8–10.** Indications for Perioperative Coronary Angiography

**Class I (conditions for which there is evidence for or general agreement that a procedure be performed or a treatment is of benefit)**
Patients with suspected or proven coronary artery disease
  High-risk results during noninvasive testing (see Table 8–9.)
  Angina pectoris unresponsive to adequate medical therapy
  Patients with unstable angina
  Nondiagnostic or equivocal results from noninvasive testing in a patient with high clinical risk undergoing a high-risk surgical procedure.
**Class II (conditions for which there is a divergence of evidence or opinion about performing the procedure)**
  Intermediate-risk results during noninvasive testing
  Nondiagnostic or equivocal noninvasive test in a clinically lower risk patient undergoing a high-risk surgical procedure
  Urgent noncardiac surgery in a patient convalescing from an acute myocardial infarction
  Perioperative myocardial infarction
**Class III (conditions for which there is evidence and/or general agreement that the procedure is not necessary)**
  Patients with known coronary artery disease with low-risk results on noninvasive testing undergoing low-risk surgical procedures
  Screening for coronary artery disease without appropriate noninvasive testing
  Asymptomatic patients with prior coronary revascularization who have excellent ($\geq 7$ METs) exercise capacity
  Mild stable angina with good left ventricular function and low-risk noninvasive test results
  Patients who are not candidates for coronary revascularization because of concomitant medical illness
  Prior coronary angiogram performed within 5 years which showed normal coronary arteries
  Severe left ventricular dysfunction (ejection fraction <20%) in patients felt not to be candidates for coronary revascularization
  Patients who are unwilling to consider a coronary artery revascularization procedure

MET, metabolic equivalent.

cacy of coronary revascularization procedures performed before noncardiac surgery.

### Percutaneous Transluminal Coronary Angioplasty

In a 50-patient case series, percutaneous transluminal coronary angioplasty (PTCA) was performed in patients with abnormal noninvasive tests. Five patients required urgent coronary artery bypass surgery after angioplasty. The perioperative MI rate following vascular surgery that was performed an average of 9 days after angioplasty was 5.6% and the mortality rate was 1.9%.[62]

Elmore and associates compared preoperative angioplasty with coronary bypass surgery in patients with abdominal aortic aneurysms. In this retrospective analysis, only 100 of 2452 patients underwent coronary revascularization before aortic surgery. Most patients were at high risk with symptomatic coronary disease. The majority underwent coronary artery bypass surgery (86%) and 14% underwent angioplasty. The revascularized patients had no mortality with aortic surgery, although the angioplasty group more commonly had late cardiac complications.[63] Another retrospective study examined 148 patients who underwent angioplasty before major noncardiac surgery (ie, abdominal, vascular, or orthopedic). Fewer deaths and cardiac complications occurred in the revascularized patients.[64] These studies were done before the era of intracoronary stent implantation and are limited by their lack of randomized treatment assignment.

Goldman pointed out several caveats to the current practice of preoperative cardiac testing and risk stratification that may lead to the practice of preoperative revascularization to reduce risk.[65] First, PTCA with or without stenting may only delay vascular or other surgery for 1 to 2 days (longer if antiplatelet agents are used for 2-4 weeks), but the reductions in cardiac risks with preoperative revascularization are largely based on results from coronary artery bypass surgery, which would delay noncardiac surgery for weeks to months. Thus, PTCA and surgical revascularization cannot be presumed to produce similar results as a preoperative strategy. Second, Q wave MIs and other unstable syndromes are thought to be caused by rupture of an atherosclerotic plaque, commonly at a site not previously thought to be critical. Although it is not certain that postoperative MIs have the same etiology, the abnormalities detected by preoperative testing may not be the correct markers for events related to unstable coronary syndromes. Thus, the value of performing procedures to reduce risk of a high-risk procedure may not be the optimal strategy, and the development of further recommendations must await the results of randomized testing and other studies.[65]

### Coronary Artery Bypass Surgery

Coronary artery bypass surgery has also been performed in high-risk patients before planned noncardiac surgery. In the Coronary Artery Surgery Study (CASS) registry, the mortality rate for noncardiac surgery was 0.9% in patients who had undergone prior coronary artery bypass graft (CABG) and 2.4% in patients who had not. However, the mortality rate with the CABG procedure was 1.4%, resulting in a combined mortality that was not different from patients undergoing noncardiac surgery without prior revascularization.[34]

The European Coronary Surgery Study Group examined the results of patients with PVD within the large randomized study assigned to coronary bypass surgery or medical management. The long-term (8-year) survival for patients with PVD who underwent coronary bypass surgery was 85%, compared with 57% for those receiving medical management.[66] An analysis of the CASS registry patients, who underwent coronary angiography before noncardiac surgery, revealed that patients undergoing *high-risk surgical procedures* (defined as major abdominal, vascular, thoracic, or head and neck operations) had higher rates of perioperative MI or death if treated medically than if they had undergone coronary artery bypass surgery. However, the study was conducted between 1974 and 1979 with nonrandomized treatment assignment.[67] Differences in patient characteristics between the two treatment groups cannot be excluded.

Despite the potential benefit for surgical coronary revascularization, it is also important to recognize that coronary artery bypass surgery is a riskier procedure in patients with PVD than in those without it.[68] A report documented that PVD patients undergoing CABG had similar mortality to those without vascular disease but a 3.6-fold increase in major morbidity (MI, pneumonia, reintubation, prolonged ventilator support, mediastinitis, postoperative bleeding requiring reoperation, cardiac arrest requiring cardiopulmonary resuscitation, cerebral vascular accident, heart block requiring permanent pacing, colonic ischemia, pancreatitis, cholecystitis, and sepsis).[69]

When and whether patients should be referred for preoperative coronary revascularization before planned major noncardiac (usually vascular) surgery cannot be answered with certainty. A randomized clinical trial has been recommended because of the enormous costs involved with staged strategies.[70] There is currently one randomized study underway, the Veterans Affairs Cooperative Study on Coronary Artery Revascularization Prior to Peripheral Vascular Surgery (CARP).[71] This study randomized patients with revascularizable lesions to receive coronary revascularization (either percutaneous or operative) before planned vascular surgery or to proceed directly to vascular surgery. Enrollment began in 1998 and 3.5 years of follow-up are planned. Until the results of randomized studies are known, the indications for coronary revascularization are essentially unchanged from those recommended for patients who are not planning noncardiac surgery.[72,73]

Examples of patients in whom CABG is considered to be indicated include those with acceptable coronary revascularization risk and suitable viable myocardium with left main stenosis, 3-vessel coronary disease with LV dysfunction, 2-vessel coronary disease involving severe obstruction of the proximal left anterior descending artery, and intractable coronary ischemia despite maximal medical therapy. These indications emphasize that revascularization is indicated for improvement of long-term outcome and not to improve the cardiac risks for pending noncardiac surgery.

The timing of noncardiac surgery following indicated PTCA is not clear. Early surgery (within several days) may increase cardiac risk because of increased early risks of closure and thrombosis. However, delay for several months may increase the likelihood of restenosis. One approach would be to delay noncardiac surgery for several days to reduce the risks of plaque instability.[3]

### Medical Interventions

Perioperative treatment of the surgical patient for known or presumed coronary disease has been attempted with a number of agents. For the most part, these studies have been small clinical trials with hemodynamic or ischemic endpoints. An early report demonstrated a reduction in frequency of ST-segment depression on ECG monitoring using oral β blockers 2 hours preoperatively in patients with mild hypertension. Of the 89 patients on β blockers, only 2 were found to have ST changes, compared with 11 of 39 (28%) receiving control medication.[74] Pasternack and associates reported that oral metoprolol given immediately before surgery and followed by intravenous drug resulted in less intraoperative ischemia and lower rates of MI after vascular surgery.[75,76]

Mangano and coworkers conducted a prospective, randomized, double-blind, placebo-controlled trial of atenolol in patients undergoing noncardiac surgery. Cardiac events (MI, unstable angina, need for coronary artery bypass surgery, and CHF), as well as overall survival, were significantly better at 6 months, 1 year, and 2 years after surgery[77] (Figs. 8–5 and 8–6). The majority of the improvement (15% increase in absolute rate of event-free survival) not only was found within the first 6 to 8 months after surgery but also persisted for at least 2 years.[77] These effects cannot be attributed solely to the perioperative use of atenolol alone. Patients in the atenolol group tended to remain on β blockers and receive angiotensin-converting enzyme inhibitors compared with those in the placebo group, who were more likely to receive calcium channel blockers.[78]

Thus, preoperative and perioperative β blockers are safe and have long-term benefit in patients undergoing major noncardiac surgery, likely for the same reasons β blockers are beneficial in patients with MI. Whether all patients undergoing surgery should receive β blockers is not known, but patients with known coronary disease or at high risk for coronary disease should remain on β blockers if they are already prescribed, including intravenous β blockers during and immediately following surgery. Patients at risk for CAD should receive β blockers as described by Mangano and associates.[77]

The use of nitroglycerin as a prophylactic agent for patients at risk for or with ischemic coronary disease has been demonstrated in one study to reduce intraoperative myocardial ischemia.[79] However, other studies have not shown benefit.[80–82] The lack of effect of nitroglycerin may be due to competing vasodilating effects of the nitroglycerin and anesthetic agents. Patients with active signs of myocardial ischemia who are not hypertensive should use nitroglycerin.[3] Other uses may be

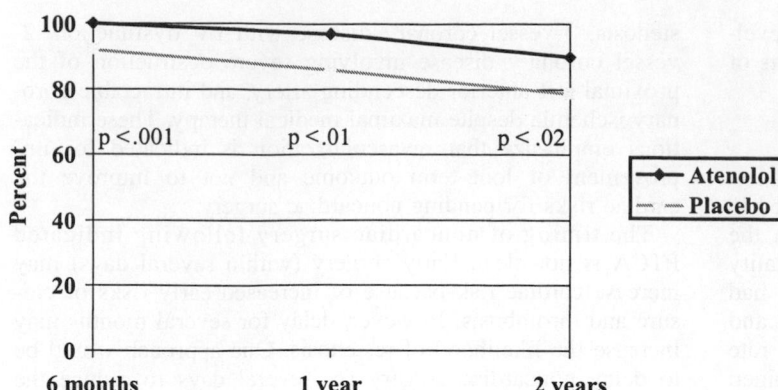

**FIGURE 8–5.** Overall survival rates from 6 months to 2 years for patients receiving atenolol immediately preceding noncardiac surgery and continued through the hospital stay. (Data from Mangano DT, Layug EL, Wallace A, et al. Effect of atenolol on mortality and cardiovascular morbidity after noncardiac surgery. *N Engl J Med.* 1996;335:1713.)

individualized, and the potential for hypotension, particularly in the presence of hypovolemia, must be carefully evaluated.[3] Few other medical interventions to reduce perioperative myocardial ischemia have been tested.

## Use of Invasive Monitoring

### Pulmonary Artery Catheterization

Only one study has tested the value of aggressive preoperative hemodynamic assessment and management utilizing pulmonary artery catheterization. Berlauk and coworkers conducted a randomized trial of patients undergoing peripheral vascular reconstruction.[83] Using a detailed algorithm, patients who achieved optimal hemodynamic endpoints (ie, pulmonary capillary wedge pressure between 8 and 15 mm Hg, cardiac index $\geq 2.8$ L/min/m², and systemic vascular resistance $<1100$ dynes/s/cm⁵) had fewer intraoperative events and fewer cardiac complications, although there was no difference in MI or nonarrhythmogenic cardiac death.[83] Intensive preoperative preparation and perioperative management may benefit some high-risk patients, particularly those with heart failure and hemodynamic instability, but such management cannot be recommended routinely.[3]

### Transesophageal Echocardiography

The use of intraoperative transesophageal echocardiography (TEE) has become commonplace, particularly for cardiac procedures and in high-risk cardiac patients undergoing noncardiac surgery. Prospective evaluation of intraoperative TEE has found little incremental value compared with other risk assessment methods.[84] However, others reported that approximately 15% of patients may have management changes determined by TEE, particularly in older patients ($>66$ years).[85] TEE is also thought to be important for monitoring and managing patients undergoing cardiac surgery.[86]

It is important that those who perform TEE undergo appropriate training. Guidelines for performing studies have been published.[87] In the absence of large scale outcome studies and cost-effectiveness data, the true value of TEE in evaluating and managing patients undergoing noncardiac surgery cannot yet be determined.

## THE ROLE OF THE CARDIOLOGIST

The strategy for cardiac risk assessment in the preoperative patient (see Table 8–9) may be implemented by the referring physician, surgeon, anesthesiologist, or cardiologist. One method would be for the operative team physicians to follow the outlined steps until an abnormal or high-risk result is identified, after which the cardiologist could be consulted. Alternatively, particularly for patients with known major clinical risks (see Table 8–8) or high risk findings on any previous testing, a cardiologist could be consulted before embarking on the stepped approach in Table 8–9. If all parties agreed to systematically follow the stepwise preoperative evaluation, much of the variability in approach to the presurgical patient would be eliminated.

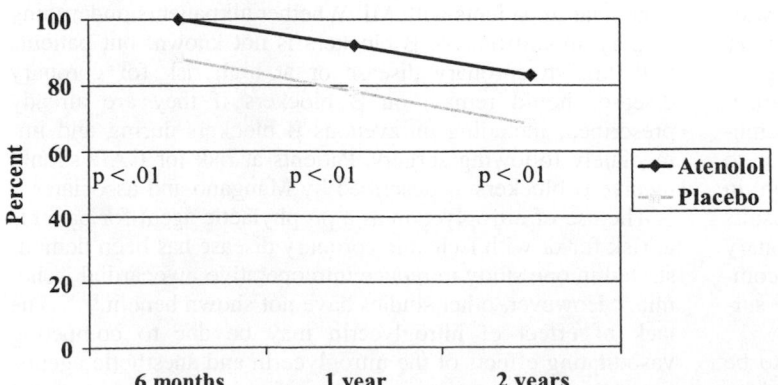

**FIGURE 8–6.** Survival without cardiac events (myocardial infarction, unstable angina, need for coronary artery bypass surgery, congestive heart failure) from 6 months to 2 years for patients receiving atenolol immediately preceding noncardiac surgery and continued through the hospital stay. (Data from Mangano DT, Layug EL, Wallace A, et al. Effect of atenolol on mortality and cardiovascular morbidity after noncardiac surgery. *N Engl J Med.* 1996;335:1713.)

## References

1. Bodenheimer MM. Noncardiac surgery in the cardiac patient: what is the question? *Ann Intern Med.* 1996;124:763.
2. Fleisher LA, Eagle KA. Screening for cardiac disease in patients having noncardiac surgery. *Ann Intern Med.* 1996;124:767.
3. Eagle KA, Brundage BH, Chaitman BR, et al. Guidelines for perioperative cardiovascular evaluation for noncardiac surgery. Report of the American College of Cardiology/American Heart Association Task Force on Practice Guidelines (Committee on Perioperative Cardiovascular Evaluation for Noncardiac Surgery). *Circulation.* 1996;93:1278.
4. Goldman L. Cardiac risk in noncardiac surgery: an update. *Anesth Analg.* 1995;80:810.
5. Kleinman B, Czinn E, Shah K, et al. The value to the anesthesia-surgical care team of the preoperative cardiac consultation. *J Cardiothorac Anesth.* 1989;3:670.
6. Rudd P, Siegler M, Byyny RL. Preoperative diabetic consultations: a plea for improved training. *J Med Educ.* 1978;53:590.
7. Mackenzie TB, Popkin MK, Callies AL, et al. The effectiveness of cardiology consultation: concordance with diagnostic and drug recommendations. *Chest.* 1981;79:16.
8. Katz RI, Barnhart JM, Ho G, et al. A survey on the intended purposes and perceived utility of preoperative cardiology consultations. *Anesth Analg.* 1998;87:830.
9. Rao TLK, Jacobs KH, El-Etr AA. Reinfarction following anesthesia in patients with myocardial infarction. *Anesthesiology.* 1983;59:499.
10. Shah KB, Kleinman BS, Sami H, et al. Reevaluation of perioperative myocardial infarction in patients with prior myocardial infarction undergoing noncardiac operations. *Anesth Analg.* 1990;71:231.
11. Rivers SP, Scher LA, Gupta SK, et al. Safety of peripheral vascular surgery after recent acute myocardial infarction. *J Vasc Surg.* 1990;11:70.
12. Hertzer NR, Beven EG, Young JR, et al. Coronary artery disease in peripheral vascular patients: a classification of 1000 coronary angiograms and results of surgical management. *Ann Surg.* 1984;199:223.
13. Reiz S. Perioperative management of the cardiac patient undergoing noncardiac surgery. New anaesthesia techniques: is there a real benefit for the cardiac high-risk patient? *Acta Anaesthesiol Scand Suppl.* 1997;111:17.
14. Helman JD, Leung JM, Bellows WH, et al. The risk of myocardial ischemia in patients receiving desflurane versus sufentanil anesthesia for coronary artery bypass graft surgery. *Anesthesiology.* 1992;77:47.
15. Hohner P, Backman C, Diamond G, et al. Anaesthesia for abdominal aortic surgery in patients with coronary artery disease, part II: effects of nitrous oxide on systemic and coronary haemodynamics, regional ventricular function and incidence of myocardial ischaemia. *Acta Anaesthesiol Scand.* 1994;38:793.
16. Slogoff S, Keats AS, Dear WE. Steal-prone coronary anatomy and myocardial ischemia associated with four primary anesthetic agents in humans. *Anesth Analg.* 1991;72:22.
17. Forrest JB, Cahalan MK, Rehder K. Multicenter study of general anesthesia, II: results. *Anesthesiology.* 1990;72:262.
18. Baron J-F, Bertand M, Barre E, et al. Combined epidural and general anesthesia versus general anesthesia for abdominal aortic surgery. *Anesthesiology.* 1991;75:611.
19. Dajani AS, Bisno AL, Chung KJ, et al. Prevention of bacterial endocarditis: recommendations by the American Heart Association. *JAMA.* 1990;264:2920.
20. American Society of Anesthesiologists. New classification of physical status. *Anesthesiology.* 1963;24:111.
21. Goldman L, Caldera D, Nussbaum SR, et al. Multifactorial index of cardiac risk in non-cardiac surgical procedures. *N Engl J Med.* 1977;197:845.
22. Detsky AS, Abrams HB, McLaughlin JR, et al. Predicting cardiac complications in patients undergoing non-cardiac surgery. *J Gen Intern Med.* 1986;1:217.
23. Larsen SF, Olesen KH, Jacobsen E, et al. Prediction of cardiac risk in non-cardiac surgery. *Eur Heart J.* 1987;8:179.
24. Younis LT, Miller DD, Chaitman BR. Preoperative strategies to assess cardiac risk before noncardiac surgery. *Clin Cardiol.* 1995;18:447.
25. Ashton C, Peterson N, Wray N, et al. The incidence of perioperative myocardial infarction in men undergoing noncardiac surgery. *Ann Intern Med.* 1993;118:504.
26. Nissan R, Encarnacion M. Clinical value of the electrocardiogram in ambulatory care. *J Fam Pract.* 1987;24:361.
27. Jonsson B, Astrand I. Electrocardiographic findings in men and women aged 18-65. *Scand J Soc Med.* 1977;5:41.
28. Zamboni S, Ambrosio BG, Bertoldero G, et al. Electrocardiograms in hypertensive subjects from a population random sample: basic characteristics and correlations with some biological variables. *G Ital Cardiol.* 1985;15:375.
29. Sommerville TE, Murray WB. Information from routine preoperative chest radiography and electrocardiography. *S Afr Med J.* 1992;81:190.
30. McCleane GJ, McCoy E. Routine preoperative electrocardiography. *Br J Clin Pract.* 1990;44:92.
31. Gold BS, Young ML, Kinman JL, et al. The utility of preoperative electrocardiograms in the ambulatory surgical patient. *Arch Intern Med.* 1992;152:301.
32. Cooperman M, Pflug B, Martin EW Jr, et al. Cardiovascular risk factors in patients with peripheral vascular disease. *Surgery.* 1978;84:505.
33. Goldman L, Caldera DL, Southwick FS, et al. Cardiac risk factors and complications in non-cardiac surgery. *Medicine.* 1978;57:357.
34. Foster ED, Davis KB, Carpenter JA, et al. Risk of noncardiac operation in patients with defined coronary disease: the Coronary Artery Surgery Study (CASS) registry experience. *Ann Thorac Surg.* 1986;41:42.
35. Rettke SR, Shub C, Naessena JM, et al. Significance of mildly elevated creatine kinase (myocardial band) activity after elective abdominal aortic aneurysmectomy. *J Cardiothorac Vasc Anesth.* 1991;5:425.
36. Baron JF, Mundler O, Bertrand M, et al. Dipyridamole-thallium scintigraphy and gated radionuclide angiography to assess cardiac risk before abdominal aortic surgery. *N Engl J Med.* 1994;330:663.
37. Fletcher JP, Antico VR, Gruenewald S, et al. Risk of aortic aneurysm surgery as assessed by preoperative gated heart pool scan. *Br J Surg.* 1989;76:26.
38. Pederson T, Kelbaek H, Munck O. Cardiopulmonary complications in high-risk surgical patients: the value of preoperative radionuclide cardiography. *Acta Anaesthesiol Scand.* 1990;34:183.
39. Lazor L, Russell JC, DaSilva J, et al. Use of the multiple uptake gated acquisition scan for the preoperative assessment of cardiac risk. *Surg Gynecol Obstet.* 1988;167:234.
40. Pasternack PF, Imparato AM, Bear G, et al. The value of radionuclide angiography as a predictor of perioperative myocardial infarction in patients undergoing abdominal aortic aneurysm resection. *J Vasc Surg.* 1984;1:320.
41. Mosley JG, Clarke JM, Ell PJ, et al. Assessment of myocardial function before aortic surgery by radionuclide angiocardiography. *Br J Surg.* 1985;72:886.
42. Kazmers A, Cerqueira MD, Zierler RE. The role of preoperative radionuclide ejection fraction in direct abdominal aortic aneurysm repair. *J Vasc Surg.* 1988;8:128.
43. Fiser WP, Thompson BW, Thompson AR, et al. Nuclear cardiac ejection fraction and cardiac index in abdominal aortic surgery. *Surgery.* 1983;94:736.
44. Ouriel K, Green RM, DeWeese JA, et al. Outpatient echocardiography as a predictor of perioperative cardiac morbidity after peripheral vascular surgical procedures. *J Vasc Surg.* 1995;22:671.
45. Halm EA, Browner WS, Tubau JF, et al. Echocardiography for assessing cardiac risk in patients having noncardiac surgery. *Ann Intern Med.* 1996;125:433.
46. Cutler BS, Wheeler HT, Paraskos JA, et al. Applicability and interpretation of electrocardiographic stress testing in patients with peripheral vascular disease. *Am J Surg.* 1981;141:501.
47. McPhail N, Calvin JE, Shariatmadar A, et al. The use of preoperative exercise testing to predict cardiac complications after arterial reconstruction. *J Vasc Surg.* 1988;7:60.
48. Gerson MC, Hurst JM, Hertzberg VS, et al. Cardiac prognosis with noncardiac geriatric surgery. *Ann Intern Med.* 1985;103:832.
49. Gerson MC, Hurst JM, Hertzberg VS, et al. Prediction of cardiac and pulmonary complications related to elective abdominal and noncardiac thoracic surgery in geriatric patients. *Am J Med.* 1990;88:101.
50. Hlatky MA, Boineau RE, Higginbotham MB, et al. A brief self-administered questionnaire to determine functional capacity (the Duke Activity Status Index). *Am J Cardiol.* 1989;64:651.
51. Fletcher GF, Balady G, Froelicher VF, et al. Exercise standards: a statement for healthcare professionals from the American Heart Association. *Circulation.* 1995;91:580.
52. Eagle KA, Coley CM, Newell JB, et al. Combining clinical and thallium data optimizes preoperative assessment of cardiac risk before major vascular surgery. *Ann Intern Med.* 1989;110:159.
53. L'Italien GJ, Paul SD, Hendel RC, et al. Development and validation of a Bayesian model for perioperative cardiac risk assessment in a cohort of 1,081 vascular surgical candidates. *J Am Coll Cardiol.* 1996;27:779.
54. Raby K, Goldman L, Granger M, et al. Correlation between preoperative ischemia and major cardiac events after peripheral vascular surgery. *N Engl J Med.* 1989;321:1296.

55. Lette J, Waters D, Cerino M, et al. Preoperative coronary artery disease risk stratification based on dipyridamole imaging and a simple three-step, three-segment model for patients undergoing noncardiac vascular surgery or major general surgery. *Am J Cardiol.* 1992;69:1553.

56. Bry JD, Belkin M, O'Donnell TF Jr, et al. An assessment of the positive predictive value and cost-effectiveness of dipyridamole myocardial scintigraphy in patients undergoing vascular surgery. *J Vasc Surg.* 1994;19:112.

57. McFalls EO, Doliszny KM, Grund F, et al. Angina and persistent exercise thallium defects: independent risk factors in elective vascular surgery. *J Am Coll Cardiol.* 1993;21:1348.

58. Brown KA, Rowen M. Extent of jeopardized viable myocardium determined by myocardial perfusion imaging best predicts perioperative cardiac events in patients undergoing noncardiac surgery. *J Am Coll Cardiol.* 1993;21:325.

59. Shaw LJ, Eagle KA, Gersh BJ, et al. Meta-analysis of intravenous dipyridamole–thallium-201 imaging (1985 to 1994) and dobutamine echocardiography (1991 to 1994) for risk stratification before vascular surgery. *J Am Coll Cardiol.* 1996;27:787.

60. Cohen MC, Eagle KA. Expert opinion regarding indications for coronary angiography before noncardiac surgery. *Am Heart J.* 1997;134:321.

61. Mason JJ, Owens DK, Harris RA, et al. The role of coronary angiography and coronary revascularization before noncardiac vascular surgery. *JAMA.* 1995;273:1919.

62. Huber KC, Evans MA, Bresnahan JF, et al. Outcome of noncardiac operations in patients with severe coronary artery disease successfully treated preoperatively with coronary angioplasty. *Mayo Clin Proc.* 1992;67:15.

63. Elmore JR, Hallett JW Jr, Gibbons RJ, et al. Myocardial revascularization before abdominal aortic aneurysmorrhaphy: effect of coronary angioplasty. *Mayo Clin Proc.* 1993;68:637.

64. Allen JR, Helling TS, Hartzler GO. Operative procedures not involving the heart after percutaneous transluminal coronary angioplasty. *Surg Gynecol Obstet.* 1991;173:285.

65. Goldman L. Cardiac risk for vascular surgery [editorial comment]. *J Am Coll Cardiol.* 1996;27:799.

66. European Coronary Surgery Study Group. Long-term results of prospective randomized study of coronary artery bypass surgery in stable angina pectoris. *Lancet.* 1982;2:1173.

67. Eagle KA, Rihal CS, Mickel MC, et al. Cardiac risk of noncardiac surgery: influence of coronary disease and type of surgery in 3368 operations. *Circulation.* 1997;96:1882.

68. Birkmeyer JD, O'Connor GT, Quinton HB, et al. The effect of peripheral vascular disease on in-hospital mortality rates with coronary artery bypass surgery. *J Vasc Surg.* 1995;21:445.

69. Mesh CL, Cmolik BL, Van Heekeren DW, et al. Coronary bypass in vascular patients: a relatively high-risk procedure. *Ann Vasc Surg.* 1997;11:612.

70. Domanski M, Ellis S, Eagle K. Does preoperative coronary revascularization before noncardiac surgery reduce the risk of coronary events in patients with known coronary artery disease? *Am J Cardiol.* 1995;75:829.

71. McFalls EO, Ward HB, Krupski WS, et al. Prophylactic coronary artery revascularization for elective vascular surgery: study design. Veterans Affairs Cooperative Study Group on Coronary Artery Revascularization Prophylaxis for Elective Vascular Surgery. *Control Clin Trials.* 1999;20:297.

72. Guidelines and indications for coronary artery bypass graft surgery: a report of the American College of Cardiology/American Heart Association Task Force on Assessment of Diagnostic and Therapeutic Cardiovascular Procedures (Subcommittee on Coronary Artery Bypass Graft Surgery). *J Am Coll Cardiol.* 1991;17:543.

73. Guidelines for percutaneous transluminal coronary angioplasty: a report of the American College of Cardiology/American Heart Association Task Force on Assessment of Diagnostic and Therapeutic Cardiovascular Procedures (Committee on Percutaneous Transluminal Coronary Angioplasty). *J Am Coll Cardiol.* 1993;22:233.

74. Stone JG, Foex P, Sear JW, et al. Myocardial ischemia in untreated hypertensive patients: effect of a single small oral dose of a beta-adrenergic blocking agent. *Anesthesiology.* 1988;68:495.

75. Pasternack PF, Grossi EA, Bauman FG, et al. Beta blockade to decrease silent myocardial ischemia during peripheral vascular surgery. *Am J Surg.* 1989;158:113.

76. Pasternack PF, Imparato AM, Baumann FG, et al. The hemodynamics of beta-blockade in patients undergoing abdominal aortic aneurysm repair. *Circulation.* 1987;76(3pt2):III1.

77. Mangano DT, Layug EL, Wallace A, et al. Effect of atenolol on mortality and cardiovascular morbidity after noncardiac surgery. *N Engl J Med.* 1996;335:1713.

78. Eagle KA, Froelich JB. Reducing cardiovascular risk in patients undergoing noncardiac surgery [editorial]. *N Engl J Med.* 1996;335:1761.

79. Coriat P, Daloz M, Bousseau D, et al. Prevention of intraoperative myocardial ischemia during noncardiac surgery with intravenous nitroglycerin. *Anesthesiology.* 1984;61:193.

80. Dodds TM, Stone JG, Coromilas J, et al. Prophylactic nitroglycerin infusion during noncardiac surgery does not reduce perioperative ischemia. *Anesth Analg.* 1993;76:705.

81. Gallagher JD, Moore RA, Jose AB, et al. Prophylactic nitroglycerin infusions during coronary artery bypass surgery. *Anesthesiology.* 1986;64:785.

82. Thomson IR, Mutch WA, Culligan JD. Failure of intravenous nitroglycerin to prevent intraoperative myocardial ischemia during fentanyl-pancuronium anesthesia. *Anesthesiology.* 1984;61:385.

83. Berlauk JF, Abrams JH, Gilmour IJ, et al. Preoperative optimization of cardiovascular hemodynamics improves outcome in peripheral vascular surgery: a prospective, randomized clinical trial. *Ann Surg.* 1991;214:289.

84. Eisenberg MJ, London MJ, Leung JM, et al. Monitoring for myocardial ischemia during noncardiac surgery. A technology assessment of transesophageal echocardiography and 12-lead electrocardiography. The Study of Perioperative Ischemia Research Group. *JAMA.* 1992;268:210.

85. Suriani RJ, Neustein S, Shore-Lesserson L, et al. Intraoperative transesophageal echocardiography during noncardiac surgery. *J Cardiothorac Vasc Anesth.* 1998;12:274.

86. Mishra M, Chauhan R, Sharma KK, et al. Real-time intraoperative transesophageal echocardiography—how useful? Experience of 5,016 cases. *J Cardiothorac Vasc Anesth.* 1998;12:625.

87. Shanewise JS, Cheung AT, Aronson S, et al. ASE/SCA guidelines for performing a comprehensive intraoperative multiplane transesophageal echocardiography examination: recommendations of the American Society of Echocardiography Council for Intraoperative Echocardiography and the Society of Cardiovascular Anesthesiologists Task Force for Certification in Perioperative Transesophageal Echocardiography. *Anesth Analg.* 1999;89:870.

# Pulmonary Consultation

Paul B. Langevin

Pulmonary complications are the most frequently reported causes of morbidity and mortality after surgery,[1,2] especially after procedures involving the abdomen and thorax.[3,4] When possible, identification of patients at risk—to allow appropriate interventions that limit that risk—is imperative before surgical intervention. In cases in which the history and physical examination indicate a respiratory condition that may alter the risk of the planned surgery or the perioperative management, a pulmonary consultation may be indicated if any of the following three criteria are true:

1. The diagnosis is still not clear to the anesthesiologist after a thorough history and physical examination.
2. The severity of the disorder is not adequately evaluated.
3. The patient's pulmonary status is not optimized.

Beyond these measures, preoperative consultation with a pulmonologist may provide a helpful perspective on which to base recommendations for postoperative management.

Finally, there are some patients who are at risk for pulmonary complications because of factors unrelated to the respiratory system (eg, cardiac disease, debilitation, immunosuppression, malnutrition). Although these patients occasionally benefit from pulmonary consultation, help with management of the underlying condition frequently is of greater value.

What constitutes a postoperative pulmonary complication is not clearly defined, a fact that may explain the range of reported complication rates.[5] Its ambiguity notwithstanding,[6] the incidence of postoperative pulmonary complications has been reported to reach 75% in some patient populations.[7,8] Prolonged mechanical ventilation, pneumonia, atelectasis, chest radiograph changes, and respiratory failure are the most commonly reported postoperative pulmonary complications. In some studies, the lengths of stay in the intensive care unit (ICU) and in the hospital in general have been suggested as factors in the genesis of pulmonary problems, including nosocomial infections. Clearly, the causes of postoperative pulmonary complications are multifactorial.[6] The risk of postoperative pulmonary complications is increased by age extremes,[9] smoking,[10–13] preexisting lung disease,[11,12,14] type of surgery,[2,15] anesthesia duration,[13,16] and the patient's poor general health.[9] In patients exhibiting one or more of these risk factors, pulmonary consultation may be of particular benefit in doing the following:

1. Evaluating whether current therapy is adequate or prescribing more aggressive intervention when necessary

2. Suggesting prophylaxis against predictable postoperative events
3. Better estimating the pulmonary risks and benefits and the probable outcome of the planned surgical procedure

Patients with preexisting lung disease are at considerable risk; the greater the number of risk factors, the more likely a complication is to occur.[17] However, the normal consequences of a surgical intervention may compromise patients who do not suffer from underlying lung disease but nevertheless have limited reserve.[18,19] Identification of patients who may be at risk for postoperative pulmonary complications is relatively simple compared with the considerably more complex task of modifying that risk. Not performing the planned procedure may be an option in extreme cases, but beyond this option, few data indicate which interventions, if any, are the most beneficial. The consultant's recommendation not to perform an operation implies that he or she understands the consequences both of the planned intervention and its cancellation.

## PREOPERATIVE CONSIDERATIONS

### What Are Pulmonary Function Tests?

Pulmonary function tests (PFTs) are noninvasive tools that characterize respiratory function by doing the following:

1. Measuring a variety of lung volumes
2. Examining respiratory mechanics
3. Evaluating gas exchange

These tests only assess function, not etiology; thus, PFTs rarely help the physician make a specific diagnosis. Furthermore, patients who do not admit to symptoms that limit their activity, even after careful history and physical examination, are unlikely to benefit from PFTs (Fig. 9–1). Rather, PFTs derive their value from confirming a presumptive diagnosis, documenting the progress of a disease, and evaluating any therapeutic intervention. Together with analysis of arterial blood gas (ABG) values, PFTs may be the least expensive method of evaluating patients with suspected lung disease[20] and may be particularly useful when patients present with a mixed disorder (eg, chronic obstructive lung disease [COLD] and restrictive lung disease [RLD]).

Spirometry, a component of PFTs, is a noninvasive test that can be used to examine static lung volumes and dynamic gas flows (respiratory mechanics). Static volumes can be combined in various ways to give defined capacities (Fig. 9–2). The volume of air moving past the lips can be measured over time (Fig. 9–3), and flow can be evaluated against volume to give rise to a flow-volume loop (Fig. 9–4). Patients can be asked to perform specific maneuvers, such as inhaling maximally and exhaling as fast as possible, and the volume of gas that can be forcibly exhaled in a given amount of time, such as 1 second ($FEV_1$), can be determined. Clearly, these measurements are dependent on the patient's effort in performing them; a low value that suggests poor functional capacity may only reflect suboptimal effort. In an attempt to overcome this bias, effort-independent measurements (eg, forced expiratory flow, midexpiratory phase [$FEF_{25\%-75\%}$]) can also be made.

Based on these measurements, lung diseases may be classi-

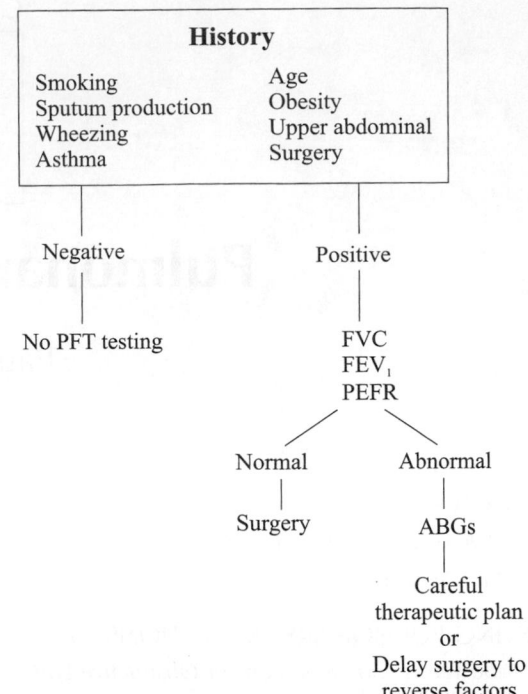

**FIGURE 9–1.** A systematic approach to the evaluation of patients undergoing operations. ABG, arterial blood gas; $FEV_1$, forced expiratory volume in 1 second; FVC, forced vital capacity; PEFR, peak expiratory flow rate; PFT, pulmonary-function test. (From Celli BR. What is the value of preoperative pulmonary function testing? *Med Clin North Am.* 1993;77:309–325.)

fied as obstructive or restrictive (Table 9–1). Although the majority of patients suffer from obstructive disease, restrictive diseases encompass a greater diversity of disorders.[21]

### Obstructive Lung Diseases

Obstructive diseases are characterized by abnormally slow alveolar emptying (Fig. 9–5). This aberrancy results in air trapping (incomplete expiration before the next breath) and increased static volumes (eg, residual volume [RV], total lung volume) and capacities (eg, functional residual capacity [FRC]). Obstructive diseases also reduce the $FEV_1$; although the total amount of gas that can be exhaled, the *vital capacity* (VC), tends to be preserved, it takes longer to exhale the volume. Hence, the $FEV_1$- forced vital capacity (FVC) ratio is reduced in obstructive disorders, and depression of this ratio is considered the hallmark of obstructive lung disease.

Obstructive ventilatory disorders may have a reversible component. Asthma, to a large extent, is a reversible disorder in which periods of quiescence are punctuated by acute episodes of distress. These episodes are largely treatable, and the obstruction to airflow (bronchospasm) can be relieved by appropriate therapy. COLD tends to be irreversible in that the underlying injury is structural, permanent, and minimally amenable to therapy. In reality, most patients manifest both a reversible and irreversible component.

### Restrictive Lung Disorders

Restrictive disorders result from an inability of the alveoli to fill properly. Although emptying may also be impaired, this problem results from abnormal recoil of the tissue rather than

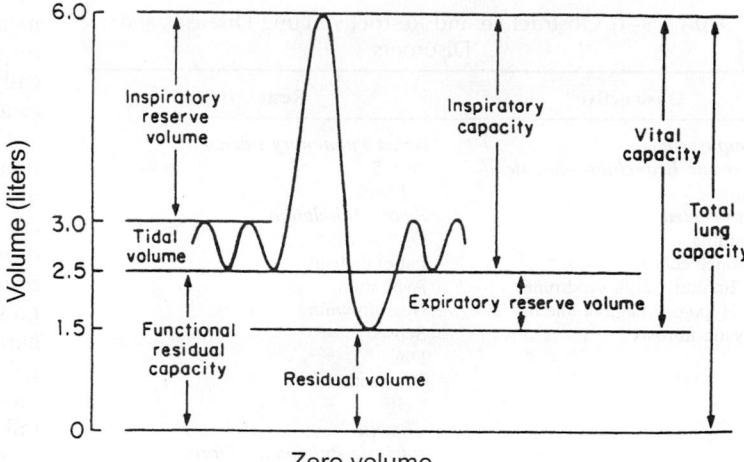

**FIGURE 9–2.** Lung volumes and lung capacities. (From Yao FSF. Asthma-chronic obstructive pulmonary disease (COPD). In: Yao FSF, Artusio JF Jr, eds. *Anesthesiology: Problem Oriented Patient Management.* 3rd ed. Philadelphia, Pa: JB Lippincott; 1993:6.)

from narrowing of the airways. Resultant lung volumes are small, and air trapping is atypical. Restrictive disorders are *intrinsic* when the disease process involves the lung parenchyma and *extrinsic* when expansion of the alveoli is impeded by external compression (see Table 9–1). In restrictive diseases, lung volumes and capacities are reduced (see Fig. 9–5); although the $FEV_1$ is decreased as well, this decrease is in direct proportion to reductions in the FVC, thus preserving the $FEV_1$-FVC ratio.

It should be clear that PFT values are not pathognomonic of any specific disease. Rather, they can suggest a differential diagnosis of disorders that impair pulmonary function in similar ways (obstructive versus restrictive). Although these tests have been overused in the past with little benefit to the patient, in certain cases, they may be of great use in assessing the risk for postoperative pulmonary complications (Table 9–2). For example, PFTs may be nearly indispensable in evaluating whether a patient is a suitable surgical candidate for a proposed pulmonary resection.

## How Can the Data Be Applied?

### Pulmonary Resection

Pulmonary resection requires preoperative confirmation that the remaining lung tissue will be adequate to support the patient's respiratory needs postoperatively. This determination usually is made by performing PFTs, including the $FEV_1$ and a ventilation-perfusion ($\dot{V}/\dot{Q}$) scan, to measure the fraction of the total lung perfusion in the area of proposed resection ($FQ_{resection}$). These values are then multiplied ($FEV_1 \times 1$ $FQ_{resection}$) to estimate the postoperative $FEV_1$. If the $FEV_1$ after operation is estimated to exceed 30% of what it should be for a patient of that height, gender, and age ($\approx 800$ mL for most adults), resection may be considered.

It should be realized that this is a long range estimate of the function that the patient is expected to regain after recovering from the surgical insult; such recovery may require several months. Therefore, when a resection is performed in which the patient's postoperative $FEV_1$ approaches 30% of predicted, it may be necessary to support ventilation for some

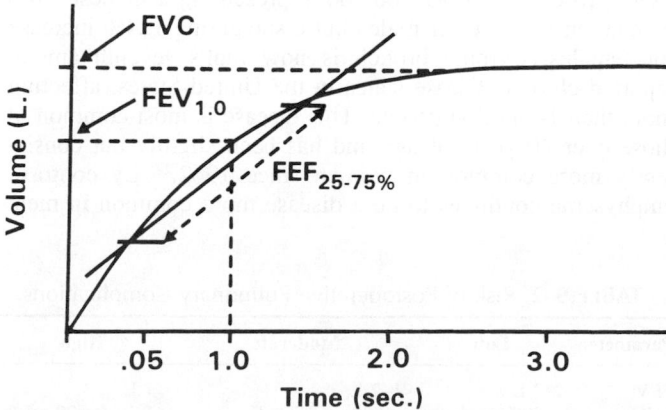

**FIGURE 9–3.** Normal spirogram with the relevant components illustrated. FEF, forced expiratory flow; $FEV_1$, forced expiratory volume in 1 second; FVC, forced vital capacity. (From Boysen PG. Preoperative assessment of the patient undergoing noncardiac thoracic surgery. In: Mangano DT, ed. *Preoperative Cardiac Assessment.* Society of Cardiovascular Anesthesiologists Monograph. NLM 8917861. Philadelphia, PA: JB Lippincott; 1990:127.)

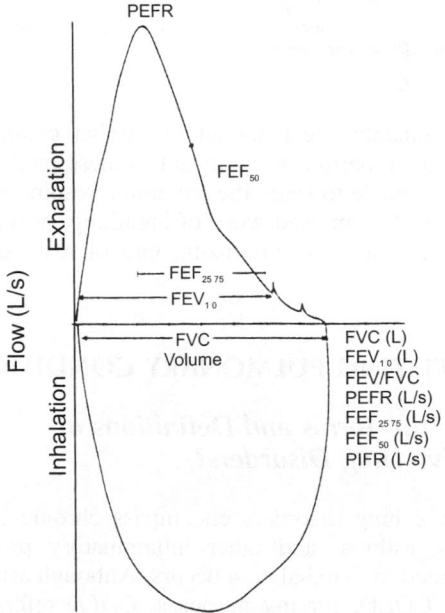

**FIGURE 9–4.** A forced vital capacity (FVC) is obtained using a flow-versus-volume loop. The forced expiratory volume at 1 second ($FEV_1$), FVC, peak expiratory flow rate (PEFR), forced expiratory flow between 25% and 75% of vital capacity ($FEF_{25-75}$), and forced expiratory flow at 50% of vital capacity ($FEF_{50}$) can also be calculated. PIFR, peak inspiratory flow rate. (From Boysen PG. Evaluation of the patient with pulmonary disease. In: Rogers MC, Tinker JH, Covino BG, eds. *Principles and Practice of Anesthesiology.* St Louis, Mo: Mosby–Year Book; 1993:232–241.)

**TABLE 9–1.** Obstructive and Restrictive Lung Diseases and Disorders

| Obstructive | Restrictive |
|---|---|
| *Emphysema* | *Acute Pulmonary Edema* |
| *Chronic Bronchitis—Simple* | ARDS |
| Simple | Shock |
| *Obstructed* | *Smoke Inhalation* |
| Asthma | O₂ toxicity |
| Bronchiectasis | Fat embolism |
|   Immotile cilia syndrome | Aspiration |
|   Hypogammaglobulinemia | Near-drowning |
| Cystic fibrosis | Sepsis |
| | DIC |
| | Pancreatitis |
| | CHF |
| | *Chronic* |
| | *Intrinsic Pulmonary Fibrosis* |
| | Sarcoidosis |
| | Eosinophilic granuloma (histiocytosis) |
| | Hypersensitive pneumonitis |
| | Pulmonary alveolar proteinosis |
| | *Lymphangiomyomatosis* |
| | Extrinsic |
| |   Pleura and mediastinum |
| |     Effusion |
| |     Mediastinal mass |
| |     Pneumothorax |
| |     Pneumomediastinum |
| |   Neuromuscular disease |
| |     Guillain-Barré syndrome |
| |     Myasthenia gravis |
| |     Eaton-Lambert syndrome |
| |     Muscular dystrophies |
| |     Spinal cord transection |
| |     Flat chest |
| |   Ankylosing spondylitis |
| |   Kyphoscoliosis |
| |   Pectus |
| |   Obesity |
| |   Ascites |

ARDS, acute respiratory distress syndrome; CHF, congestive heart failure; DIC, disseminated intravascular coagulation.

time. Unfortunately, the potential for further compromise in the postoperative period is significant in these patients. Every effort must be made to spare the remaining respiratory reserve by decreasing the imposed work of breathing, providing adequate pain control, and minimizing loss of respiratory muscle strength.

## PREEXISTING PULMONARY CONDITIONS

### What Are the Terms and Definitions of Obstructive Lung Disorders?

Obstructive lung disorders encompass chronic bronchitis, emphysema, asthma, and other inflammatory processes in which obstruction to exhalation occurs. Although asthma often is listed as COLD, for my purposes, *COLD* refers to long-standing, continuous obstruction to airflow in emphysema, chronic bronchitis, or both. *Asthma,* as was mentioned previously, has periods of normalcy punctuated by acute exacerbations of obstruction.

*Emphysema* is characterized by the progressive and permanent destruction of alveolar septa that results in the enlarge-

ment of the terminal air spaces, including the alveoli and respiratory bronchioles. Emphysema, therefore, is a pathologically definable entity. In contrast, chronic bronchitis may refer to a wider range of disorders.

*Chronic bronchitis* is defined by excessive mucus production resulting in a cough with expectoration for at least 3 months during 2 consecutive years. This condition may be associated with a constant obstruction to airflow (*obstructive bronchitis*). If it is not, the condition represents *simple chronic bronchitis.* Few patients with simple chronic bronchitis progress to *chronic obstruction.* The latter condition results from narrowing of the small airways (<2 mm diameter) due to goblet cell hyperplasia (elevated Reid index), intraluminal mucus plugging, bronchial smooth-muscle hypertrophy, and inflammation and edema of the mucosa and submucosa.

Superimposed on this anatomic narrowing of the airways may be a physiologic, bronchospastic element as well. When this condition is present, the patient is said to have *chronic asthmatic bronchitis.* The bronchospastic component of this condition results from reactivity of the bronchial smooth muscle; it is variably relieved by bronchodilator therapy.

In summary, COLD includes a spectrum of lung disorders, ranging from emphysema at one extreme to chronic asthmatic bronchitis at the other. All of them share a characteristic slowing of expiratory airflow. The site of injury in emphysema is the alveolus and respiratory bronchiole, although the pathologic changes of chronic bronchitis occur in the conducting bronchioles. Although the predominant injury determines the primary presentation of the patient, most patients with COLD manifest a mixed picture, having some components from both ends of the spectrum (Table 9–3).

### How Is Chronic Obstructive Lung Disease Characterized?

#### Prevalence and Diagnosis

The prevalence of COLD increased by 60% between 1982 and 1994, affecting more than 16 million Americans. Although COLD encompasses a number of disorders, emphysema and chronic bronchitis account for the overwhelming majority. Between 1979 and 1995, the mortality rate for COLD rose to 25.6 per 100 000, representing a modest 3.6% population increase for males but a staggering 124% increase for females. Chronic bronchitis now ranks seventh among reported chronic disease states in the United States, affecting more than 14 million people. This disease is most common in those over 40 years of age and has been slightly but consistently more common in women since 1962.[22] By contrast, emphysema continues to be a disease more common in men,

**TABLE 9–2.** Risk of Postoperative Pulmonary Complications

| Parameter | Low | Moderate | High |
|---|---|---|---|
| FEV₁ | >2 L | 1–2 L | <1 L |
| FVC | >50% predicted | <50% predicted | <1.5 L or 20 mL/kg |
| FEV₁/FVC | >70% predicted | >35%, <50% predicted | <35% predicted |
| FEF₂₅₋₇₅ | >50% | <50% predicted | |

FEF₂₅₋₇₅, forced expiratory flow between 25% and 75% of vital capacity; FEV₁, forced expiratory volume in 1 second; FVC, forced vital capacity.

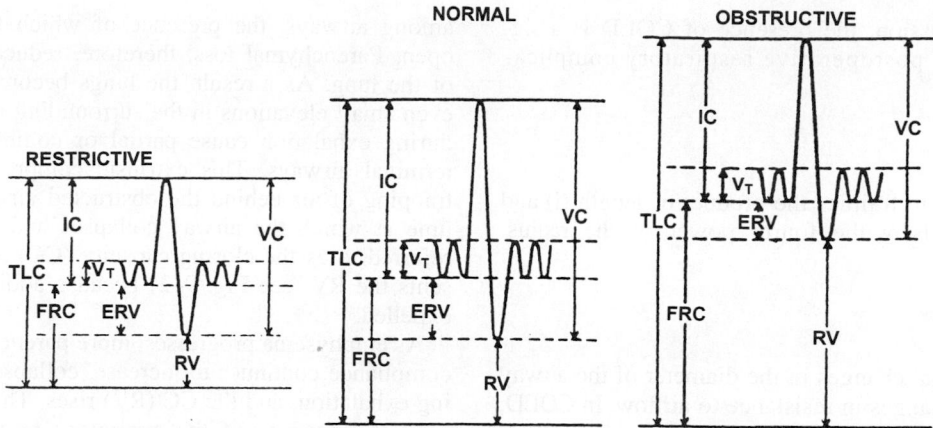

**FIGURE 9–5.** In the presence of restrictive lung disease, VC, RV, FRC, and TLC are decreased. In the presence of obstructive lung disease, the VC is normal to decreased, the RV and FRC are increased, the TLC is normal to increased, and the RV-TLC ratio is increased. ERV, expiratory reserve volume; FRC, functional residual capacity; IC, inspiratory capacity; RV, residual capacity; TLC, total lung capacity; VC, vital capacity; $V_T$, tidal volume. (Data from Stoelting RK, Dierdorf SF. Restrictive lung disease. In: Stoelting RK, Dierdorf SF, eds. *Anesthesia and Co-Existing Disease.* 3rd ed. New York, NY: Churchill Livingstone; 1993:160; and Stoelting RK, Dierdorf SF. Chronic obstructive pulmonary disease. In: Stoelting RK, Dierdorf SF, eds. *Anesthesia and Co-Existing Disease.* 3rd ed. New York, NY: Churchill Livingstone; 1993:139.)

affecting about 1.9 million people.[22] Because adolescent girls are smoking at nearly three times the rate of their male cohorts, the overall predominance of COLD can be expected to transition from males to females in about 30 years.[23]

All forms of chronic bronchitis are related to smoking.

However, for reasons that remain obscure, <20% of smokers develop significant obstruction to airflow.[23] The diagnosis of COLD is one of exclusion, and it is made after infections of the upper respiratory tract, allergic responses, and parenchymal or endobronchial diseases have been ruled out. More

**TABLE 9–3.** Chronic Obstructive Lung Disease: Salient Features

|  | Predominantly Emphysema | Predominantly Bronchitis |
|---|---|---|
| Age at time of diagnosis (y) | 60± | 50± |
| Dyspnea | Fever; insidious | Mild, often with chest infection |
| Cough | After dyspnea starts | Before dyspnea starts |
| Sputum | Scanty, mucoid | Copious, purulent |
| Bronchial infections | Less frequent | More frequent |
| Respiratory insufficiency episodes | Often terminal | Repeated |
| Weight loss | Often marked | Usually slight or absent |
| Chest examinations | Quiet chest (except slight wheeze at end expiration), marked hyperinflation | Noisy chest, slight hyperinflation |
| Chest film | "Hyperinflation" ± bullous changes, small heart | Increased bronchovascular markings at bases, large heart |
| Physiologic tests |  |  |
|   Total lung capacity | Increased | Normal or slightly decreased |
|   Residual volume | Markedly increased | Moderately increased |
|   Lung compliance, static | Increased | Near normal |
|   Lung compliance, dynamic | Normal or slightly low | Very low |
|   Lung recoil | Markedly reduced | Variable |
|   Inspiratory resistance | Normal | Increased |
|   Chronic $Paco_2$ (mm Hg) | 35–40 | 50–60 |
|   Chronic $Pao_2$ (mm Hg) | 65–75 | 45–60 |
|   Hematocrit (%) | 35–45 | 50–55 |
|   Pulmonary hypertension |  |  |
|     Rest | None to mild | Moderate to severe |
|     Exercise | Moderate | Worsens |
|   Cor pulmonale | Rare, except terminally | Common |
|   Elastic recoil | Severely damaged | Normal |
|   Resistance | Normal to slight increase | High |
|   Diffusing capacity | Decreased | Normal to slight decrease |
|   Cardiac output | Often low | Usually near normal |

Data from Honig EG, Ingram RH Jr. Chronic bronchitis, emphysema, and airways obstruction. In: Fauci AS, Martin JB, Braunwald E, et al, eds. *Harrison's Principles of Internal Medicine.* Vol 2. 14th ed. New York, NY: McGraw Hill; 1998 and Matthay RA. Chronic airways disease. In: Wyngaarden JB, Smith LH Jr, Bennett JC, eds. *Cecil Textbook of Medicine.* Vol 1. 19th ed. Philadelphia, Pa: WB Saunders; 1992:386.

germane to this discussion, the presence of COLD is a significant predictor of postoperative respiratory complications.[24,25]

## Pathophysiology

Resistance is equal to 8 times the product of length (l) and viscosity ($\eta$), divided by the fourth power of the radius, multiplied by pi ($\pi$):

$$R = 8l\eta/\pi r^4$$

Hence, even minimal changes in the diameter of the airway produce significant changes in resistance to airflow. In COLD, airflow is impeded during expiration by one or more of three factors that narrow the airways:

1. Thickening of the wall
2. Decline in the elastic recoil of the lung
3. Collapse of the airway

Hypertrophy and contraction of the bronchial smooth muscle thicken the airway wall at the expense of the lumen. Loss of lung parenchyma, in particular the alveolar septa, compromises the geometry of the small airways that normally are stented open by the presence of this tissue. Increased compliance of the remaining lung tissue makes it much easier to compress the airways when the intrapleural pressure is increased during normal exhalation. In addition, any accumulation of mucus narrows the airway further, thereby increasing the resistance and impeding airflow even more.

### Chronic Bronchitis

In response to bronchial irritation in chronic bronchitis, mucus production is stimulated and ciliary clearance depressed. As a result, copious amounts of mucus are deposited in the airways, reducing the diameter and the airflow. In addition, the function of the alveolar macrophage is compromised, resulting in lower resistance to pulmonary infection, higher numbers of bacteria in the sputum, and greater inflammation and edema. Hence in chronic bronchitis, the airways are mechanically narrowed due to smooth-muscle hypertrophy, inflammation, edema, goblet cell hyperplasia, increased mucus secretion, and decreased mucus clearance. Much of this process is irreversible. The indolent mechanical decrease in patency may be punctuated by episodes of increased irritability of the bronchial smooth muscle that exacerbate the obstruction. These episodes may or may not be related to bacterial or viral infection. Patients with chronic bronchitis frequently suffer from elements of cardiac disease, including arrhythmia (eg, atrial fibrillation), pulmonary hypertension, and cor pulmonale. Acute infections, bronchospasm, and cardiac complications represent reversible components of the disease that may be treatable.

### Emphysema

Unlike chronic bronchitis, in which the conducting airways are narrowed due to pathologic changes intrinsic to them, in emphysema, the airways are narrowed due to extrinsic compression resulting from the destruction of alveolar septa. The loss of lung parenchyma eliminates the tethering effect among airways, the presence of which tends to hold them open. Parenchymal loss, therefore, reduces the elastic recoil of the lung. As a result, the lungs become so compliant that even small elevations in the surrounding intrapleural pressure during exhalation cause partial or complete collapse of the terminal airways. This extrinsic compression results in the trapping of air behind the obstructed airways. The lung volume at which the airway collapses and obstructs airflow is referred to as the closing capacity (CC) and, in effect, represents the RV (see Fig. 9–2) because additional air cannot be expelled.

As emphysema progresses, more parenchyma are destroyed, compliance continues to increase, collapse occurs earlier during exhalation, and the CC (RV) rises. The increase in the RV is at the expense of the expiratory reserve volume (ERV). With more advanced disease, the CC approaches the FRC. That is, the patient cannot forcibly exhale more air because the airways are completely collapsed at that lung volume. At this point, the ERV is zero, the patient can only exhale to the FRC, and the RV, CC, and FRC are equal. Progression of the disorder increases the RV, CC, and FRC still further. Any additional increase in compliance results in air trapping, and the lungs become hyperinflated with a consequent increase in the RV and FRC.

With further progression, the CC and FRC continue to rise, and tidal volume breathing must occur at higher lung volumes. The result is a profound increase in the work of breathing because breathing occurs at an elevated FRC and a less favorable position on the pulmonary compliance curve. Because the airways are so easily collapsed, increases in intrapleural pressure that are required for effective coughing become difficult, thus limiting the patient's ability to clear secretions and severely impeding bronchopulmonary toilet. When coupled with increased mucus production, secretions collect in the airways, increasing their resistance still further and promoting bacterial growth. The end result is a predisposition of the patient to pneumonia.

## Staging and Severity of Disease

No standardized staging system for COLD exists.[26,27] However, the $FEV_1$ correlates directly with morbidity and mortality. Based on this relationship, the American Thoracic Society established criteria for three stages of disease:

**Stage I.** $FEV_1$ >50% of predicted flow, and the disease minimally affects the patient's life. Most patients with COLD have stage I disease.

**Stage II.** $FEV_1$ = 35% to 49% of predicted flow. A minority of patients are involved at this stage, but it has a significant impact on the quality of life.

**Stage III.** $FEV_1$ <35% of predicted flow, and the disease is associated with severely limited reserve and severe symptoms.[28]

In terms of perioperative pulmonary complications, patients with stage I disease have risks similar to patients without COLD and should not require special interventions.[29] Patients with stage II and stage III disease, however, should benefit greatly from aggressive perioperative pulmonary management, as evidenced by improved outcome and a reduced cost of care.[11,15,30,31]

## What Measures Can Be Taken to Optimize Pulmonary Function in Patients With Chronic Obstructive Lung Disease?

### Cessation of Smoking

First and foremost, *smoking must stop*, and exposure to known irritants should be limited as much as possible. COLD is a progressive disease with an annual decline in the $FEV_1$ that accelerates over time. The most desirable therapeutic interventions are those that not only relieve obstruction but also reverse the disease or at least slow the rate of loss of pulmonary function. The Lung Health Study, a 5-year evaluation of more than 6000 patients, demonstrated that although bronchodilators relieved obstruction, only cessation of smoking altered the disease process.[32] A more detailed discussion of the detrimental effects of tobacco use may be found in the section, "Why Does Smoking Play a Pivotal Role in the Development of COLD?" that follows later in the chapter. Patients anticipating surgery are best served by an 8-week hiatus from smoking before the procedure.[31]

Because emphysema results from a loss of tissue, the bronchospastic component of the disease is typically less prominent than in chronic bronchitis. Unfortunately, from the standpoint of perioperative optimization, on one hand, the reversible component of the disease may be considerably less in those with emphysema compared with patients with chronic bronchitis. On the other hand, patients with emphysema are less likely to develop bronchospasm intraoperatively or to require postponement of surgery in order to optimize their physical status. As was stated previously, however, most patients present with elements of both emphysema and chronic bronchitis. To the extent that any component of the disease is reversible, it should be treated preoperatively.

### Oxygen Therapy

Oxygen ($O_2$) is the most potent pulmonary vasodilator known, with the possible exception of nitric oxide. Pulmonary vasodilation reduces pulmonary vascular resistance and, therefore, right ventricular afterload. Thus, the administration of $O_2$ to patients with a $PaO_2$ <55 mm Hg improves right ventricular failure, alleviates cor pulmonale, increases exercise tolerance, and improves survival (Fig. 9–6).[33,34] Additionally, nocturnal hypoxemia may be prevented by the administration of supplemental $O_2$ during sleep, thereby preventing cardiac arrhythmias that occur during nocturnal arterial desaturation. This finding may explain why delivery of supplemental $O_2$ for longer periods derives additional benefit in these patients. Because $O_2$ selectively dilates the vasculature in ventilated areas of the lung, $\dot{V}/\dot{Q}$ matching will improve, enhancing arterial oxygenation. Indications for $O_2$ therapy are listed in Table 9–4.

### Bronchodilator Therapy

#### β₂-Agonists

β₂-Agonists increase the concentration of cyclic adenosine monophosphate (cAMP) in the airway smooth muscle, resulting in relaxation. These agents are capable of producing a 20%[35] to 47%[36] rise in the $FEV_1$ in patients suffering from COLD. β₂-Agonists currently available may be aerosolized, oral, or parenteral. Aerosolized agents are delivered by a

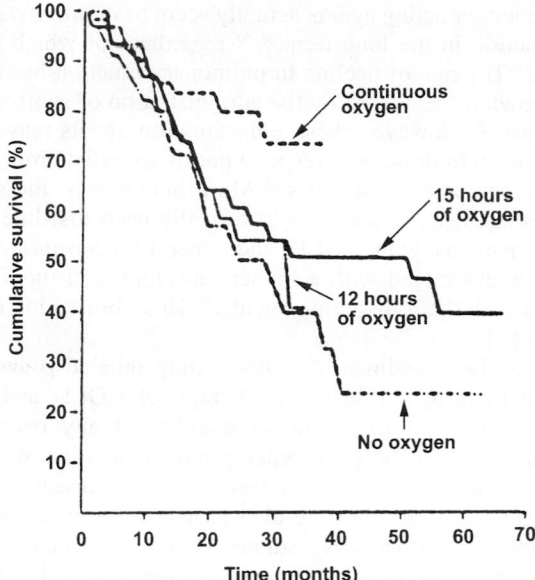

**FIGURE 9–6.** Use of oxygen and survival in patients with chronic obstructive pulmonary disease receiving continuous oxygen, no oxygen, or 12 and 15 hours of oxygen. (From Bertka KR, Wunderink RG. Outpatient management of COPD. *Am Fam Phys.* 1988;37:265–280.)

nebulizer or metered-dose inhaler (MDI). Although controversy surrounds discussions of which delivery mode is better,[37–42] aerosolized administration is the most common delivery method and offers several advantages, including direct delivery to the target organ, less systemic effect, and lower required dose.[43] Unfortunately, many patients use their inhalers incorrectly,[44] making oral agents (ie, bambuterol) a reasonable, although inadequately studied, alternative. Nonetheless, oral administration of β₂-agonists is not benign,[45] and, although the systemic effects of these drugs may be limited and tolerable, they should be used only in patients who are unable to use inhalers.

Aerosolized agents may be of long or short duration. Recent data suggest that the longer acting aerosols (formoterol, salmeterol) may be more effective than those of shorter duration (eg, albuterol),[46] but this point remains debatable.[47] Neverthe-

**TABLE 9–4.** Indications for Long-Term Oxygen Therapy

**Absolute**
$PaO_2$ ≤55 mm Hg or $SaO_2$ ≤88%
**In Presence of Cor Pulmonale**
$PaO_2$ 55–59 mm Hg or $SaO_2$ ≥89%
ECG evidence of P pulmonale, hematocrit >55%, congestive heart failure
**Only in Specific Situations**
$PaO_2$ ≥60 mm Hg or $SaO_2$ ≥90%
With lung disease and other clinical needs, such as sleep apnea with nocturnal desaturation not corrected by CPAP
If the patient meets criteria at rest, $O_2$ should also be prescribed during sleep and exercise and appropriately titrated.
If the patient is normoxemic at rest but desaturates during exercise or sleep ($PaO_2$ ≤55 mm Hg), $O_2$ should be prescribed for these indications. Also consider nasal CPAP or BiPAP.

BiPAP, bilevel positive airway pressure; CPAP, continuous positive airway pressure; ECG, electrocardiogram; $O_2$, oxygen.
From American Thoracic Society, 1995, Medical Section of the American Lung Association: standards for the diagnosis and care of patients with chronic obstructive pulmonary disease. *American Journal of Respiratory and Critical Care Medicine*, Vol 152:S77–S120. Official Journal of the American Thoracic Society. © American Lung Association.

less, the longer acting agents actually seem to improve respiratory function in the long term,[48–50] regardless of which agent is used.[51] The rate of decline in pulmonary function has never been shown to be altered by the administration of short-acting $\beta_2$-agonists.[23] However, these long duration agents may offer benefits even to those who respond poorly to initial bronchodilator therapy with $\beta_2$-agonists.[52] More importantly, the short-acting $\beta$-agonists, which have historically been first-line therapy for patients with COLD and other bronchospastic diseases, are associated with a higher morbidity and mortality[30] not seen with the long-acting agents.[28] This observation needs further study.

Despite these findings, the short-acting inhaled $\beta$-agonists continue to have a role in the therapy of COLD and may be useful in maximizing the elimination of any reversible component of bronchospasm when prompt resolution of symptoms is needed, as in acute exacerbations of the disease. Acute improvement in airflow may also promote the expectoration of secretions. Retrospective studies have shown that the use of preoperative, short-acting bronchodilators is correlated with a decreased incidence of postoperative pulmonary complications[11]; prospective studies reveal a similar decline in postoperative pneumonia in patients treated preoperatively with bronchodilators and steroids.[2,19] Although it is likely that longer acting agents will prove equally effective, no data currently substantiate this possibility. It will be enlightening to see if the long- and short-acting $\beta$-agonists offer comparable reductions in perioperative complications when they are standardized for similar $FEV_1$.

The maximal dose of a $\beta$-agonist that should be administered, especially in an acute disease exacerbation, is unclear. Mestitz and colleagues showed that the response to terbutaline was still increasing, even after a cumulative dose of 40 mg had been administered.[53] Such doses, however, are associated with intolerable side effects including tremor, palpitation, and dysrhythmia. Hyperkalemia can develop secondary to the sympathomimetic stimulation of renin secretion. Recommended doses of the $\beta$-agonists are given in Table 9–5.

## Anticholinergic Agents

Like the $\beta_2$-agonists, anticholinergic agents are available as parenteral (eg, atropine, glycopyrrolate) or aerosolized (eg, ipratropium bromide) preparations. Parasympathetic stimulation of the airways results in the release of neuronal acetylcholine, stimulating the muscarinic (M3) receptor on the surface of the smooth-muscle cell. Stimulation of this receptor on the bronchial smooth muscle activates guanylate cyclase, which increases the cytoplasmic concentration of cyclic guanosine monophosphate, causing the cell to contract. Stimulation of the M3 receptor on the submucosal glands increases their secretions.[54]

Anticholinergic agents block the M3 receptors on both the submucosal glands and the smooth-muscle cells in the airway wall, thereby reducing secretion[55] and contraction. The viscosity of secretions is also reduced.[56] In contrast to its effects on patients with asthma, ipratropium bromide is more effective than the $\beta$-agonists in severe COLD. In severe COLD, parasympathetic tone is one of the few reversible features. Furthermore, ipratropium bromide does not inhibit mucociliary clearance as do atropine and glycopyrrolate.[57] M3-specific antagonists (hexahydrosiladifenidol and 4-deoxyadenosine monophosphate) are under development and may alleviate many of the adverse effects (eg, dry mouth, tachycardia) associated with anticholinergics.

Ipratropium can be delivered by aerosol and produces a maximum response with 0.4 to 0.6 mg doses.[58] Anticholinergic agents, in combination with the $\beta_2$-agonists, seem to yield greater benefit than either agent alone.[59] Whether these agents are additive or synergistic is unclear. Their combined efficacy in COLD seems rather less than it is in asthma[60] or simple bronchitis.[61,62] Many physicians combine anticholinergics and $\beta_2$-agonists in the treatment of patients with COLD. This approach may provide added benefit and does not seem to have any undesirable effects. Use of these agents with steroids is discussed later, in the section, "What Is the Role for Steroids in Chronic Obstructive Lung Disease?"

**TABLE 9–5.** Sympathomimetic Bronchodilator Dosages

| Bronchodilator | MDI Dose | MDI Puffs | Standard Doses of Inhalent Solutions* | Equivalent MDI Puffs From Inhalent Dose* |
|---|---|---|---|---|
| Epinephrine (Adrenalin, Primatene Mist, and others) | 0.16–0.15 mg | 2–4 every 4–6 h | 0.25–0.5 mL (1.25–11 mg) | 5–70 |
| Isoproterenol (Isuprel, Medihaler-Iso) | 0.08–0.13 mg | 2–4 every 4–6 h | 0.25–0.5 mL (1.25–2.5 mg) | 10–30 |
| Isoetharine (Bronkometer, Bronkosol, Arm-A-Med, and so on) | 0.34 mg | 1–2 every 4 h | 0.25–1 mL (2.5–10 mg)† or 1.25–5 mL (2.5–5 mg)† | 7–30 |
| Metaproterenol (Alupent) | 0.65 | 1–2 every 3–4 h | 0.2–0.3 mL (10–15 mg)† or 2–5 mL (10 mg)† or 2–5 mL (15 mg)† | 15–23 |
| Terbutaline (Brethaire, Brethine)‡ | 0.20 mg | 2 every 4–6 h | 0.25–0.5 mL (0.25–0.5 mg) | — |
| Albuterol (Proventil, Ventolin) | 0.09 mg | 1–2 every 4–6 h | 0.5 mL (2.5 mg)† or 3.0 mL (2.5 mg)† | 27 |
| Pirbuterol (Maxair) | 0.20 mg | 1–2 every 4–6 h | — | — |
| Bitolterol (Tornalate) | 0.37 mg | 2 every 4–8 h | 0.25–1 mL (0.5–2 mg) | 1–5 |
| Salmeterol (Serevent) | 0.02 mg | 2 every 12 h | — | — |

*Unit dose is standard dose recommended for adults. Amount is usually available in 0.25–2.5 mL, and percentage delivered to lungs depends on both nebulizer and breathing technique used.
†Dosage depends on brand.
‡Marketed for subcutaneous use.
MDI, metered-dose inhaler.
From American Thoracic Society, 1995, Medical Section of the American Lung Association: standards for the diagnosis and care of patients with chronic obstructive pulmonary disease. *American Journal of Respiratory and Critical Care Medicine*, Vol 152:S99. Official Journal of the American Thoracic Society. © American Lung Association.

## How Do Infections Affect Pulmonary Function?

COLD patients suffer from frequent chest infections, which further decrease their lung function for up to 90 days.[63] Acute respiratory infections are known to increase reactivity of the airways and increase mucus secretion. Infection-induced inflammation, coupled with airways and alveolar edema, adds resistance and further increases the diffusion barrier for $O_2$. Hence, treatment of respiratory infections should be early and aggressive, particularly in those who require surgical intervention and may be at increased risk of respiratory failure.[64]

## How Are Respiratory Infections Treated?

Presence of a noneosinophilic, purulent sputum suggests an infection in patients with a history of COLD and should be treated with a 7 to 10 day course of tetracycline, ampicillin, or double strength trimethoprim-sulfamethoxazole.[8] Failure of the sputum to clear is more frequently the result of poor airway drainage than an inappropriate choice of antibiotic but should warrant a sputum culture and sensitivity test, nonetheless. Although half of all hospital-acquired pneumonias occur in surgical patients,[2] preoperative antibiotics should be reserved for patients with COLD, purulent sputum, and a productive cough. The primary bacterial infections found in these patients include *Haemophilus influenzae, Streptococcus pneumoniae,* and typical oropharyngeal flora.

Yearly vaccination for influenza and vaccination against pneumococcus every 6 years seems prudent, even if benefit remains unproven.[65] Amantadine and zanamivir (Relenza) should be started in unvaccinated patients within the first 24 to 48 hours of an acute influenza infection, if possible.

## What Is the Role for Steroids in Chronic Obstructive Lung Disease?

Steroids may be beneficial in the treatment of COLD,[66] and some evidence suggests their use retards the decline in $FEV_1$.[67] However, these findings await confirmation from studies that have specifically included patients with asthma and asthmatic bronchitis.[68,69]

### Administration

Steroids may be administered systemically or with an MDI. Inhaled steroids are effective in the treatment of acute exacerbations. They spare the adrenal axis, thereby avoiding many of the complications of systemic steroids in older patients with diabetes, cataracts, and osteoporosis. Inhaled steroids also avoid the risk of systemic secondary infection but do predispose patients to oral thrush. When systemic steroids are required, they should be started at least 12 hours before surgery, although methylprednisolone (125 mg) may have an appreciable effect in 6 hours. When implemented, systemic steroids should be administered in high doses[70] only for the briefest time possible and then stopped, tapering if necessary.

### Phosphodiesterase Inhibitors

Although theophylline has long been used in the treatment of patients suffering from COLD, its relative potency has been questioned; it is unclear if the drug affords more bronchodilating effects than the β-agonists alone.[23] Nevertheless, some data suggest that combination therapy with theophylline and the β-agonists may be markedly better than either agent alone in treating patients with irreversible disease.[71]

Theophylline alleviates morning dyspnea, perhaps by reducing the overnight decline in the $FEV_1$.[72] Furthermore, theophylline improves collateral ventilation, increases mucociliary clearance, stimulates central respiratory drive, strengthens respiratory muscles, and may reduce airway inflammation.[73] The phosphodiesterase inhibitors (PDEIs) also elevate cardiac output. These potentially beneficial effects notwithstanding, the weak bronchodilating properties of these drugs, in conjunction with their narrow therapeutic index and pernicious side effects, suggest their use be reserved for those with continued bronchospasm after other interventions have been maximized. Finally, theophylline may be of benefit in patients suffering from respiratory fatigue during ventilator weaning protocols; this effect is likely attributable to the drug's effect on the respiratory musculature.[74]

## How Is Pulmonary Toilet Improved?

Humidification of inspired gas may help to prevent drying of secretions, although nebulized water or saline has not been shown to be effective in promoting expectoration. Oral expectorants, including guaifenesin and saturated solutions of sodium iodide, are without documented benefit and may actually be harmful. Iodinated glycerol may relieve coughing and chest discomfort but fails to improve the $FEV_1$ or reduce symptoms of dyspnea.[75] Although *N*-acetylcysteine loosens inspissated mucus plugs, perhaps improving the clearance of secretions, the drug can actually induce bronchospasm and has not been shown to improve the $FEV_1$.[76] I use *N*-acetylcysteine in a mixture with albuterol. Chest physical therapy and postural drainage are of limited usefulness except in those with seriously impaired cough.

### $\alpha_1$-Antitrypsin Therapy

$\alpha_1$-Antitrypsin (AAT) is indicated in patients with documented phenotypic proteinase inhibitor ($Pi^{null}$ or $Pi^Z$) AAT deficiency.[77] The drug is typically administered weekly but may be equally effective if given less frequently.[78]

## How Does Asthma Compare With Other Obstructive Ventilatory Disorders?

In the past, our understanding of asthma centered on the bronchospastic component of the disorder, and our therapy was directed at relieving contraction of the bronchial smooth muscle. Since the early 1990s, we have come to understand that asthma is an inflammatory disorder, with bronchospasm being only a small part of the process. Yet the bronchospastic element remains the focus of most clinicians because the drugs currently available for the treatment of asthma are largely bronchodilators (corticosteroids being a notable exception). Clinicians other than pulmonologists must begin to understand the pathogenesis and pathophysiology of asthma because the next generation of drugs available for the treatment of the disease are sure to be directed against specific mediators of the inflammatory process.

## Characteristics

*Asthma* is a disorder characterized by hyperresponsiveness of the tracheobronchial tree to a variety of stimuli, which leads to narrowing of the airways, increased resistance to airflow, and increased work of breathing.[79] It is distinguished from COLD in several ways:

1. Resolution of airway obstruction occurs between attacks (ie, the disorder is reversible).
2. Total lung capacity and RV, although increased during an attack, resolve between attacks.
3. ABG analysis in asthma patients is notable for hypoxemia and hypocapnia until the patient becomes fatigued, whereas in patients with chronic bronchitis, ABG analysis demonstrates a normal, if not increased, $PaCO_2$.

## Demographics

Asthma may develop at any age but usually presents early in life. Approximately 80% of patients develop symptoms before age 40 and more than half before age 10. Asthma remains the most common chronic disease of children. Boys are affected twice as often as girls, but the prevalence of the disease is gender-equal by age 30. The disease affects 4% to 5% of the US population, accounting for nearly 17 million patients. Approximately 5600 people die of asthma complications each year in the United States. This figure represents a 25% increase in the mortality rate between 1979 and 1995. The Centers for Disease Control and Prevention further reported that the prevalence of asthma in the US population is clearly increasing, perhaps related to environmental factors.[80]

## Pathogenesis and Pathophysiology

Asthma has been classified as allergic, idiosyncratic, or mixed. *Allergic asthma* tends to develop earlier in life than the idiosyncratic form and is frequently associated with other manifestations of immune hyperresponsiveness including urticaria, rhinitis, eczema, and elevated IgE levels. Conversely, *idiosyncratic* and *mixed* disorders develop later in life in patients who lack a personal or family history of allergy. In reality, the etiology of asthma remains unknown and probably represents a group of distinct disorders, all of which share similar, if not common, final pathways.

A number of conditions exist in asthmatic patients that narrow the airways and increase airflow resistance, including epithelial hyperplasia, accumulation of secretions in the lumen of the airway, edema in the airway wall, and bronchiole smooth-muscle contraction. A variety of stimuli invoke inflammatory processes that result in the release of mediators capable of precipitating this tetrad. Among these mediators is histamine, which is released from the increased numbers of mast cells present in the bronchioles of people with asthma. Histamine produces smooth-muscle contraction through direct stimulation of the bronchiolar histamine receptor type I ($H_1$), increases capillary permeability, and causes dilation of the pulmonary vascular bed. Histamine also increases the release of kallikreins by mast cells. Kallikreins are enzymes that cause production of bradykinin and related compounds from their precursors in the circulation. Unfortunately, there are no kallikrein inhibitors or antagonists yet available.

The airways of people with asthma are populated with plasma cells and lymphocytes.[81–83] Lymphocytes of the $TH_2$ phenotype respond to antigens in the "allergic repertoire" of the individual by releasing cytokines, including interleukin 3 (IL-3), IL-4, and IL-5.[84,85] IL-3 and IL-5 are chemotactic for eosinophils. Presumably, plasma cells produce antigen-specific immunoglobulin E (IgE), which binds to IgE-specific receptor sites on the surface of mast cells and eosinophils.[86] This molecule primes the mast cells, eosinophils, and alveolar macrophages, all of which contain enzymes essential for the production of the leukotrienes (LTs) that are derived from arachidonic acid present in the cell membrane (Fig. 9–7).[87] Specifically, LTC4 and LTB4 are derived from arachidonic acid by reactions catalyzed by 5-lipoxygenase, LTC4 synthetase, and 5-lipoxygenase–activating protein. Once produced, LTC4 is secreted by these cells and converted extracellularly to LTD4 and LTE4, previously referred to as the *slow-reacting substances of anaphylaxis* (see Fig. 9–7).

These leukotrienes are intense contractile agonists that increase vascular permeability, produce edema, stimulate mucus secretion, and inhibit its removal.[88–90] LTC4 and LTD4 are 3000 times more potent than histamine in stimulating contraction of the bronchial smooth muscle. Acetylcholine released from the intrapulmonary efferent distribution of the vagus nerve stimulates the bronchial smooth muscle directly via the M3 subtype muscarinic receptor, which can amplify the inflammatory response.[91–93] This finding explains the utility of atropine and its analogues (eg, ipratropium bromide) in relieving smooth-muscle constriction. Substance P, neurokinin A, and neurokinin B are peptides of similar structure called *tachykinins*. These compounds are released from the afferent

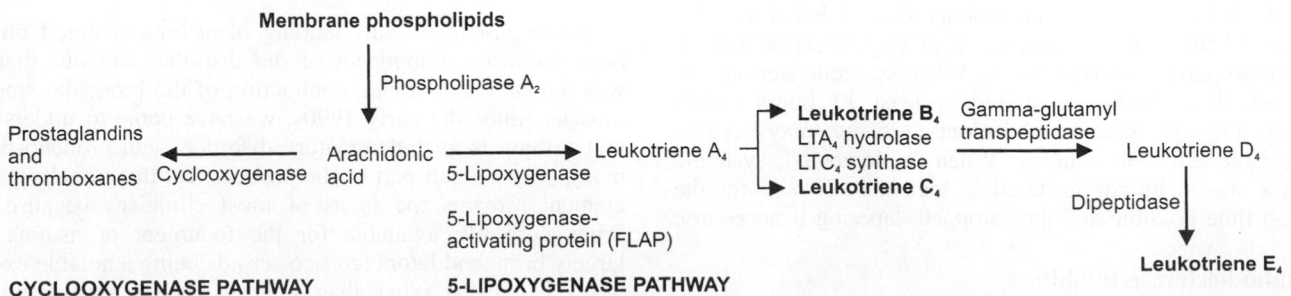

**FIGURE 9–7.** Inflammatory mediators in asthma. (Reprinted, with permission, from *Postgrad Med* 1998;103(3):63. © 1998, The McGraw-Hill Companies.)

limb of the pulmonary innervation into the walls of the airways where they stimulate agonist-specific, receptor-mediated, smooth-muscle constriction and mucus secretion. As yet, no inhibitors of the leukotrienes, the enzymes that produced them, or the tachykinins are commercially available.

Hyperplasia of the mast cells and the bronchial epithelium, infiltration by neutrophils and CD4[+] lymphocytes, hypertrophy of the glandular mucosa, dilation of the vasculature, and, less often, actual thickening of the basement membrane all contribute to the inflammatory process in asthma and narrow the airway. In addition, eosinophils infiltrate the tissue where they elaborate major basic protein and eosinophilic cationic protein that can denude the epithelium, forming creola bodies in the airway lumen as the epithelium is sloughed.[81,82,94–97] Denudation of the airways may stimulate neural afferents, further intensifying the inflammatory response[93] (Figs. 9–8 and 9–9).

The intensity of these inflammatory reactions in asthmatic patients greatly exceeds that for similar stimuli in nonasthmatic patients.[98] This response is mediated by histamine and bradykinin, as well as a multitude of leukotrienes and prostaglandins, and seems to be present, albeit to a lesser extent, in the first degree relatives of asthmatic patients.[99,100] Airway reactivity increases with continued or repetitive exposure to the inciting antigen and may resolve, often completely, when exposure is terminated.[101–103]

Diverse stimuli cause elaboration of the mediators discussed and, undoubtedly, others (eg, platelet-activating factor). These mediators result in sustained contraction of the bronchial smooth muscle, increased secretion of mucus, impaired mucociliary transport, vascular engorgement, and edema. Typically, the airways become narrowed as they become more edematous, highly vascularized, and hypercellular.

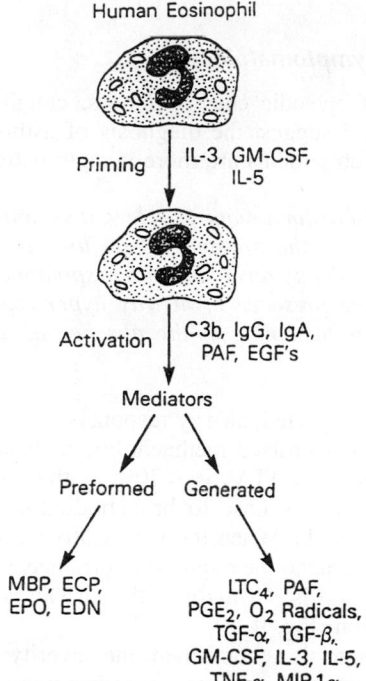

**FIGURE 9–9.** Eosinophil priming and activating stimuli and resultant mediators of inflammation. C3b, complement protein 3B; ECP, eosinophil cationic protein; EDN, eosinophil-derived neurotoxin; EGF, epidermal growth factor; EPO, eosinophil perioxidase; GM-CSF, granulocyte-macrophage colony-stimulating factor; Ig, immunoglobulin; IL, interleukin; LTC$_4$, leukotriene C$_4$; MBP, major basic protein; O$_2$, oxygen; PAF, platelet-activating factor; PGE$_2$, prostaglandin E$_2$; TGF, transforming growth factor; TNF-$\alpha$, tumor necrosis factor-$\alpha$; MIP-1$\alpha$, macrophage inflammatory peptide-1$\alpha$. (From Goldstein RA. Asthma. *Ann Intern Med.* 1994;121:703.)

Airway inflammation and the immune processes associated with it may result from exposure to pollutants or allergens, especially from viral infections of the upper respiratory tract. Ozone[104] and nitrogen dioxide,[105] which are found in polluted air, increase airway reactivity, but sulfur dioxide does not.[106] Viral infections of the upper respiratory tract can precipitate severe symptoms, and airways remain hyperreactive for weeks.[107] Asthmatic patients demonstrate increases in airway resistance in the minutes following exposure to immunologically active substances,[103,104,108–110] which may continue for protracted periods.[110] Nonantigenic stimuli presumably trigger a similar cascade of responses; even the nocturnal circadian increases in airway tone increase from the typical 10% for healthy patients to as much as 50% in asthmatic patients. These nocturnal changes are directly proportional to the severity of disease and correlate with the nocturnal dyspnea common in people with asthma.[111–113]

In summary, in patients with asthma, an aggressive inflammatory response is mounted to infection, allergens, environmental and occupational pollutants, drugs, exercise, and emotional stress. The result is narrowing of the airways, increased work of breathing, and hypoxia due to profound mismatch. Their daytime symptoms may appear minimal, but if a history of difficult evenings is not solicited, the patient may proceed to the operating suite under the care of an anesthesiologist who is unaware that the disease is out of control. Asthma is episodic and, thus, the temporary lack of symptoms should not impart a sense of security to those performing the anesthetic.

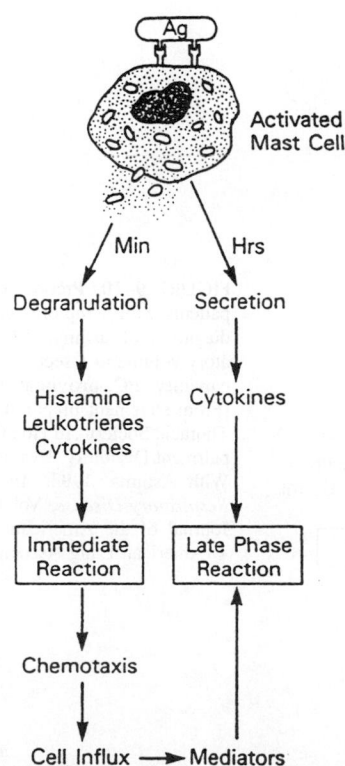

**FIGURE 9–8.** Mast cell–dependent immediate and late-phase reactions. Ag, antigen. (From Goldstein RA. Asthma. *Ann Intern Med.* 1994;121:702.)

## Evaluation

### History and Symptomatology

A history of episodic chest tightness, cough, dyspnea, or wheezing should suggest the diagnosis of asthma, especially in cases in which patients are more symptomatic at night.

*The diagnosis of asthma requires relevant symptoms (currently or by history) and the presence of airflow limitation that is partially or completely reversible either spontaneously or after treatment, or the presence of airway hyperresponsiveness to methacholine or histamine in the absence of airflow limitation.*[114]

If asthma is suspected, airway responsiveness must be evaluated using a standardized methacholine or histamine inhalation test,[115] unless the $FEV_1$ is <70% of the predicted value, in which case the response to bronchodilator should be assessed (see Fig. 9–1). When the provocative concentration of histamine or methacholine required to produce a 20% decrease in the $FEV_1$ ($PC_{20}$) is <8 mg/mL, the airway is hyperresponsive by definition (Fig. 9–10) .

Once the diagnosis is confirmed, the severity of the disease must be assessed when patients are symptomatic (Table 9–6). Between exacerbations, however, the history elicited by the anesthesiologist should include determination of the type of asthma (eg, intrinsic, extrinsic, exercise-induced, or allergen-induced), severity, duration, and any known stimuli that may worsen the condition of the patient. The intensity and the frequency of attacks, as well as the therapy required to treat them, may be quite telling. Sensitivity of the patient to sulfites (≈25% of asthmatic patients) or susceptibility to acute attacks

with weather changes (exposure to cold dry air is actually used to diagnose the condition) can forewarn the anesthesiologist to avoid certain interventions (Table 9–7) and to consider techniques that reduce the potential for iatrogenic causes of an attack (eg, warm humidified circuit).

### The Asthma Attack

Symptomatic patients present with tachypnea, hyperinflation, prolonged expiration, and a polyphonic wheeze. Tachypnea results from stimulation of intrapulmonary neurons that increase the gain of the oscillatory feedback to respiratory centers in the central nervous system. The presence of wheezing does not confirm the diagnosis of an asthmatic attack, but its absence in a symptomatic patient with asthma suggests a profound obstruction and minimal airflow that represent a medical emergency.

**TABLE 9–6.** Severity of Expiratory Airflow Obstruction

|  | FEV (% Predicted) | $FEF_{25\%-75\%}$ (% Predicted) | $Pao_2$* (mm Hg) | $Paco_2$* (mm Hg) |
|---|---|---|---|---|
| Mild (asymptomatic) | 65–80 | 60–75 | >60 | <40 |
| Moderate | 50–64 | 45–59 | >60 | <45 |
| Marked | 35–49 | 30–44 | <60 | >50 |
| Severe (status asthmaticus) | <35 | <30 | <60 | >50 |

*Values are estimates.
$FEF_{25\%-75\%}$, forced expiratory flow, midexpiratory phase; FEV, forced expiratory volume.
From Bronchial asthma. In: Stoelting RK, Dierdorf SF, eds. *Anesthesia and Co-Existing Disease.* 3rd ed. New York, NY: Churchill Livingstone; 1993:151.

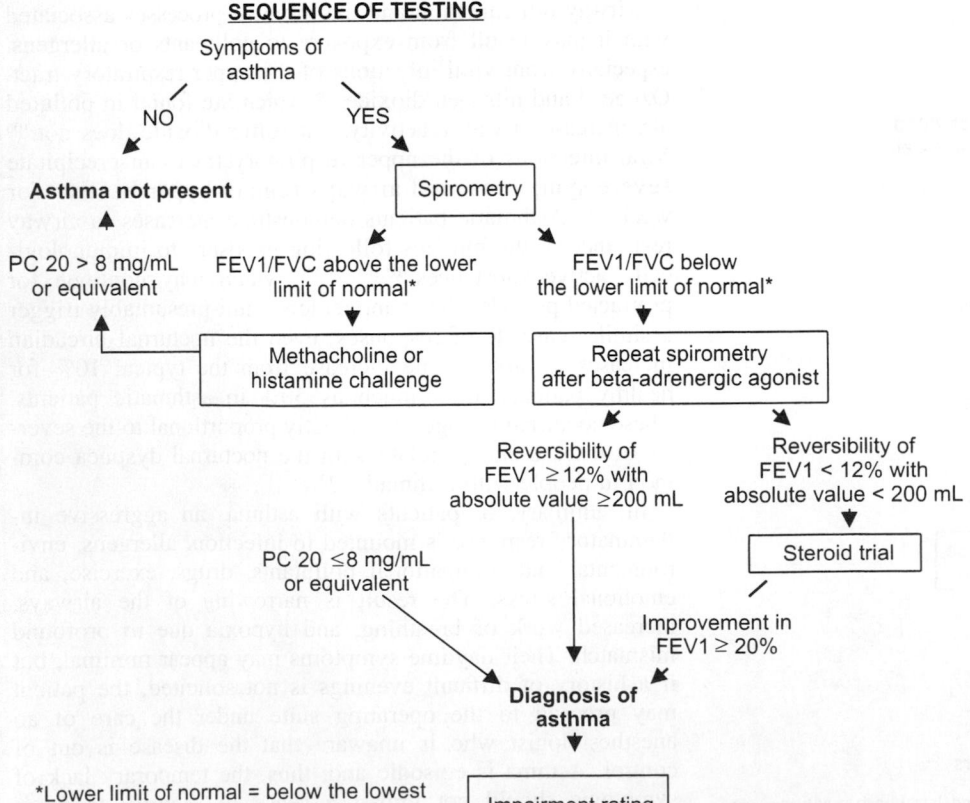

**SEQUENCE OF TESTING**

FIGURE 9–10. Preoperative evaluation of patients with symptoms consistent with the diagnosis of asthma. $FEV_1$, forced expiratory volume in 1 second; FVC, forced vital capacity; PC, provocative concentration. (From statement prepared by the American Thoracic Society Ad Hoc Committee on Impairment/Disability Evaluation in Subjects With Asthma, 1993, *American Review of Respiratory Disease,* Vol 147:1057. Official Journal of the American Thoracic Society. © American Lung Association.

**TABLE 9–7.** Representative Drugs Containing Sulfites

| Drug | Company |
|------|---------|
| Norepinephrine | Levophed |
| EpiPen (epinephrine) | Dey |
| Lidocaine 0.5% | Astra |
| Phenylephrine injection | Baxter |
| Bupivacaine MPF with epinephrine | AstraZeneca |
| Lidocaine MPF with epinephrine | AstraZeneca |
| Epinephrine in Tubex | Wyeth-Ayerst |
| Epinephrine injection | Elkins-Sinn |
| Lidocaine hydrochloride with epinephrine injection | Elkins-Sinn |

Courtesy of the Drug Information Services at the University of Florida, Gainesville, Florida.

Rhonchi suggest that secretions are pooled in the airways. Use of the accessory muscles during inspiration typifies the difficulty with exhalation and air trapping, forcing the patient to breathe at an increased FRC; this is consistent with the hyperresonance noted by percussion. Tachycardia is typically present, even in the absence of methylxanthines or β-agonists. It commonly is associated with a pulsus paradoxus, the magnitude of which correlates with the degree of obstruction. Conversely, the degree of dyspnea is frequently unrelated to the severity of obstruction and better correlates with the acuteness of the attack. Patients suffering from attacks caused by nonsteroidal anti-inflammatory agents or tartrazine dyes often present with intense congestion of the conjunctiva and nasal mucosa.

A chest radiograph is not indicated for asymptomatic patients and is probably unnecessary for those with mild to moderate complaints who have no findings other than wheezing. In severe cases, the chest radiograph is frequently normal, save for signs of hyperinflation (eg, depressed diaphragms, radiolucent lung fields, increased distance between ribs), but it should be obtained to rule out complications of severe attacks, including pneumomediastinum, pneumothorax, or infection. An electrocardiogram usually is unnecessary, typically demonstrating sinus tachycardia. It may reveal generous P waves (P pulmonale), right axis deviation, or right bundle branch block. These findings may be absent; when present, they are transient and resolve with amelioration of the attack. Sputum may be copious or absent, serous or thick, and colored (yellow to green) or clear; it may contain Charcot-Leyden crystals, Curschmann spirals, and, frequently, eosinophils but must be evaluated by gram stain to be of any value.

### Making the Diagnosis

PFTs are essential for diagnosis. The diagnosis of asthma is made when the $FEV_1$-FVC ratio is below the fifth percentile of the normal population, and when the $FEV_1$ improves by at least 12% (200 mL) from baseline after the administration of bronchodilators (which confirms significant reversibility) in the context of a consistent history and physical examination. Alternatively, a 20% improvement in airflow following institution of steroids may confirm the diagnosis when the response to bronchodilators is <12%.[114] It is important to note that also in asthma, flow rates are reduced and airway resistance is increased throughout the vital capacity because obstruction occurs in all levels of the airways, which may help distinguish it from COLD. During attacks, peak expiratory flow rates (PEFRs) are simple, rapid, and easily obtained at the bedside.

The PEFR correlates with the degree of obstruction and therefore the severity of the attack. Maximal midexpiratory flow rate and $FEV_1$ are also decreased during attacks and also correlate with PEFR. As an attack subsides, flow rates and resistances initially normalize at high vital capacities because airway changes resolve in the large airways before doing so in the small airways. Serial evaluation of FEF is useful in determining when an elective procedure should be performed because the expiratory flow at the end of the vital capacity will remain depressed until the attack has completely resolved. Because asthma is a disease of the airways, static measurements reveal few changes, although total lung capacity and RV will increase during an attack and normalize when the attack subsides.

### Therapy

The treatment of asthma may include receptor-specific agonists, receptor-specific antagonists, PDEIs, glucocorticoids, and anti-inflammatory agents such as disodium cromoglycate. When the airway is particularly reactive, the response to bronchodilators is greater, and the therapy required to control symptoms is increased.[110] However, these agents definitely do not lessen reactivity of the airways.[116–119] Bronchodilators increase the intracellular cAMP concentration, resulting in smooth-muscle relaxation,[120] increased ciliary transport,[121] decreased vascular permeability,[122] and inhibition of the release of acetylcholine from airway parasympathetic neurons.[123]

### β-Agonists

The β-agonists may be administered by nebulizer, MDI, or in oral or parenteral form (subcutaneous, intramuscular, or intravenous). Although many of these drugs are $β_2$ selective, those that are cannot be given parenterally. Up to 50% of patients do not use inhalers correctly.[124–126] Unfortunately, all of the parenteral agents are associated with significant systemic effects including tremor, palpitations, and tachycardia. These effects are dose-dependent and, although tremor is clearly attributable to direct stimulation of the $β_2$ receptor on the neuron, palpitations and tachycardia may result from the $β_1$ activity of these drugs or in response to the $β_2$ mediated vasodilation.[127]

Electrolyte changes are typically small but do occur at higher doses.[124–126] At least one case of diabetic ketoacidosis has been reported.[128] Patients with exercise-induced or extrinsic symptoms can use an MDI immediately before exposure to the offending agent with excellent results and few side effects. Those who suffer only a few attacks per year may also benefit from the occasional use of these medications. In the past, patients with moderate to severe asthma have been admonished to use their inhaler every 6 to 8 hours, regularly. However, longer acting agents with a duration of action up to 12 hours that can be delivered by an MDI have proven useful in the relief of nocturnal dyspnea and may offer some advantage.[129] A bronchospastic response to the use of these MDI drugs probably results from preservatives but is quite rare.[130] Concern has been voiced about an increased incidence of death with $β_2$-agonists. Originally studied in New Zealand,[131] it is unclear whether this relationship holds true for all β-agonists[132] or solely for fenoterol.[133]

Preoperative use of the β-agonists in patients who require surgery is prudent. The side effects from single dose administration of a β₂ selective agent are minimal and may inhibit the bronchospastic response to the intense stimulation of an endotracheal tube (ETT), should one prove necessary. These drugs may be delivered with an MDI by giving two puffs with 5 minutes between them. This sequence allows the second puff to reach deeper into the airways after the first puff dilates the more proximal airways. Patients should exhale to RV and then actuate the inhaler as they begin to inspire to total lung capacity, holding their breath at full inflation for 5 seconds. Actuation of the MDI at the beginning of inspiration ensures that the medication is contained in the deeply inhaled gas, although holding the breath allows droplets of the aerosol to deposit in the deepest regions of the airways.

A spacer can be added for patients who cannot coordinate these activities. Those individuals with symptoms, audible wheezing, or moderate disease may benefit more from nebulized delivery of the β-agonists; the addition of a second drug or an oral agent may be considered. Parenteral administration is associated with significant side effects and should be reserved for attacks and those with severe disease. Whether continued use of β₂-agonists can render the patient tachyphylactic to these agents is unclear.

### Anticholinergics

Ipratropium bromide is a cholinergic antagonist that can be delivered by an MDI or a nebulizer. As a quaternary salt, it lacks the central nervous system side effects associated with atropine but remains a potent bronchodilator. Its primary mechanism of action is to block the release of acetylcholine from the neurons innervating the tracheobronchial tree.[57] The drug is ineffective against the response to antigens[134] and does not inhibit reactivity of the airways.[135] The combination of β-agonists and anticholinergics may be more effective than either drug alone, although their combined use extends the duration of action.[136] In some patients, the combination of these agents has proven useful and may reduce the incidence of acute attacks. Given that their peak effect is not reached for 30 to 60 minutes, it remains doubtful that an acute episode of bronchospasm will be relieved by ipratropium without the concomitant use of a β-agonist.

### Steroids

Patients who remain symptomatic despite combination therapy with bronchodilators frequently benefit from a course of steroids. Oral prednisone (40-60 mg/d) tapered over 7 to 14 days is useful for outpatients. Severe bronchospasm that is not immediately life threatening may be treated with intravenous hydrocortisone (2 mg/kg followed by 0.5 mg/kg/h). Objective benefit (improved PEFR) usually is noted in about 12 hours. Life-threatening bronchospasm following the introduction of an ETT should be treated with 125 mg of methylprednisolone every 6 hours. Four to 6 hours may be required before appreciable improvement occurs.

These drugs have profound systemic effects, and the prescription of steroids has been traditionally eschewed except as a last resort. Introduction of inhaled steroids has radically changed this concept; many now say that given the inflammatory nature of the disease and the limited systemic effects of their use, aerosolized steroids should be first-line therapy.

Inhaled steroids lower airway activity and can reduce or replace oral steroids.[137,138] The main side effects of inhaled steroids at the recommended dose are oral thrush and dysphonia, which may be minimized with the use of a spacer.[139] The effect of the inhaled steroids is dose-dependent; improved effect has been reported with twice the recommended dose.[140–142] Unfortunately, as the dose increases, so does systemic absorption and untoward side effects including bone resorption,[143] depressed growth in children,[144] steroid purpura,[145] cataracts,[146] and suppression of the adrenal axis.[147,148] Preoperative treatment with steroids delivered by an MDI has few, if any, deleterious effects and may be of great benefit in patients prone to bronchospasm.

The mechanisms of action of steroids in the treatment of asthma remain uncertain. However, these drugs are known to reduce the number of inflammatory cells and inhibit the action of the enzyme phospholipase A₂, which catalyzes the formation of arachidonic acid.[149,150] Interestingly, steroids do not seem to inhibit mast cell degranulation,[151] although airway reactivity does decline with continued use.[152,153] Steroids are not bronchodilators; whether they potentiate the activity of the β-agonists remains open to debate.[154–156] The inhaled formulations are less effective in the presence of severe obstruction, probably due to ineffective delivery.[157]

### Phosphodiesterase Inhibitors

The methylxanthines (aminophylline and theophylline) are type I PDEIs that have been shown to relax bronchial smooth muscle but do not increase the intracellular concentration of cyclic adenosine monophosphate at therapeutic concentrations. Furthermore, other PDEIs that do increase the cAMP concentration are not bronchodilators, leaving open to question the exact nature of their mechanism of action. Alternatively, the PDEIs do inhibit adenosine stimulation of secretion by mast cells, increase mucociliary transport and diaphragmatic contractility, and stimulate the respiratory centers in the medulla.[158,159] Whether methylxanthines are synergistic with β-agonists is unclear,[160] although the drugs do alleviate symptoms in patients with chronic asthma[161] and reduce their need for corticosteroids.[162] With only about one fourth the bronchodilating effect of the β-agonist, aminophylline lacks significant benefit in the treatment of acute asthmatic attacks[163] and has no appreciable effect on the hyperresponsiveness of the airways.[164]

Note that theophylline is the active compound, and aminophylline (the intravenous preparation) contains 85% theophylline by weight. Therefore, intravenous aminophylline should be given at 1.2 times the desired dose of theophylline. A loading dose (5-6 mg/kg) followed by a continuous infusion, 0.2 to 0.5 mg/kg/h, can be given to patients who develop acute bronchospasm. Loading doses should be avoided in patients already taking oral theophylline, and doses should be reduced in the elderly and in patients with congestive heart failure or liver disease.

Clearance of theophylline is decreased during acute febrile episodes. Cimetidine, erythromycin, allopurinol, and propranolol slow theophylline metabolism; doses should be reduced accordingly. Conversely, patients who smoke or are treated with phenobarbital or phenytoin (Dilantin) will require higher doses to achieve the desired serum concentrations.[158] The bronchodilating effect of the drug is directly proportional to the log of the serum concentration between 3 and 25 μg/mL. Bronchodilation is slightly below 10 μg/mL, and toxicity rapidly increases as doses exceed 25 μg/mL. Hence, the therapeutic range has been arbitrarily established at 10 to 20 µg/mL, although some patients will exhibit excellent control at lower levels although others will require higher serum concentrations. Signs of toxicity include nervousness, nausea, vomiting, abdominal pain, headache, seizures, and cardiac dysrhythmias. Drug levels should be monitored because seizure and dysrhythmia can present without more benign symptoms of toxicity preceding them.

### Antihistamines

Given that histamine is one of the central mediators of the airway inflammatory response mounted in asthmatic patients, and given its ability to increase vasodilation and vascular permeability and induce bronchospasm, blockade of the histamine receptor should alleviate these effects. Before the development of specific $H_1$ blocking agents, the lack of response to the antihistamines was attributed to a lack of specificity for the receptor of interest. Unfortunately, new $H_1$-specific antihistamines (eg, terfenadine, astemizole, azelastine, and citerizine) offer little advantage and exhibit weak bronchodilating effects.[165,166] Even ketotifen, a specific $H_1$ antagonist that also inhibits mast cell degranulation, has proven to be a trivial addition to the more conventional therapy discussed previously.[167,168]

### Leukotriene Antagonists

Several leukotriene antagonists have failed to demonstrate real promise, although many of these compounds are still undergoing clinical trials.[169] However, zileuton (Zyflo) is a 5-lipoxygenase inhibitor that inhibits production of the leukotrienes. It is a bronchodilator and may prove to be of some benefit if used consistently.[170]

### Anesthesia Intervention Outside the Operating Room

The anesthesiologist may be called to assist in the management of asthmatic patients in the emergency room or ICU. When the PEFR or $FEV_1$ decline to 40% and fail to improve despite continuously inhaled $\beta_2$-agonists, anticholinergics, aminophylline, and steroids, hospital admission is indicated. The actual definition of status asthmaticus is as follows:

*a particularly severe asthmatic attack, usually requiring hospitalization, that does not respond adequately to ordinary therapeutic measures.[171]*

These patients should be admitted to an environment where they can be monitored for the development of pneumothorax, pneumomediastinum, and respiratory failure. Supplemental $O_2$ should be administered, and refractory hypoxia or hypercapnia should be treated with intubation performed in a manner that will not further exacerbate the bronchospasm.

### Pregnant Asthmatic Patients

Anesthesiologists may also be consulted by obstetricians caring for pregnant women with asthma. Symptoms may improve or worsen during pregnancy, and treatment should be similar to that in nonpregnant patients, except that terbutaline should be avoided if delivery is desirable. Anticholinergics

should be administered with the knowledge that fetal tachycardia and delayed onset of fetal bradycardia may result, and mucolytics should be avoided. Tetracycline can be used to treat many atypical respiratory infections that can be associated with asthmatic attacks but should be avoided in pregnancy.

## Why Does Smoking Play a Pivotal Role in the Development of Chronic Obstructive Lung Disease?

Smoking accounts for >80% of the risk of developing COLD, yet for unknown reasons, only 15% of smokers develop clinically significant disease.[172,173] Cigarette smoking accounts for nearly 400 000 preventable deaths each year (about one sixth the mortality) in the US population. Cigarette use is more closely linked with health risks than pipe smoking, cigar smoking, or chewing tobacco because cigarette smokers inhale. Tobacco smoke is a mixture of particulate matter (tar), nicotine, water vapor, and other gases including carbon monoxide, sulfur dioxide, and nitric oxide. Substances contained in cigarette smoke number in the thousands, and many are ciliotoxic. Although tar is the primary carcinogen, many of the gases are absorbed and exert systemic effects. The risks of cigarette smoking are varied (Table 9–8) and correlate with the number of cigarettes smoked, depth of inhalation, duration of the habit, and age at which it began.

Comorbid factors include hypertension, hypercholesterolemia, and asbestos exposure, all of which are synergistic rather than additive. Smokers who do not have comorbid factors still have twice the risk of coronary artery disease found in age-matched nonsmokers. Ninety percent of patients with peripheral vascular disease (including cerebrovascular disease) smoke, and the incidence of aortic disease (atherosclerosis and aneurysm) is high. The $FEV_1$ normally declines by approximately 30 mL/y, but this decline is accelerated by cigarette smoking.[174] Cessation, even after a long history of

---

**TABLE 9–8.** Increased Risks for Cigarette Smokers

**Cardiovascular Disease**
Coronary artery disease
Peripheral vascular disease
Aortic aneurysm
Stroke
**Carcinoma**
Lung
Larynx, oral cavity, esophagus
Bladder, kidney
Pancreas
**Lung Disorders**
Carcinoma (as noted above)
Chronic bronchitis with airflow obstruction
Emphysema
**Complications of Pregnancy**
Infants—small for gestational age, higher perinatal mortality
Maternal complications—placenta previa, abruptio placentae
**Gastrointestinal Complications**
Peptic ulcer
Esophageal reflux
**Other**
Altered drug metabolism

From Burns DM. Tobacco and health. In: Wyngaarden JB, Smith LH Jr, Bennett JC, eds. *Cecil Textbook of Medicine.* Vol 1. 19th ed. Philadelphia, Pa: WB Saunders; 1992:34.

smoking, returns the patient to the normal curve but does not afford recovery of lost function (Fig. 9–11).

## Lung Cancer

Lung cancer claims more lives than any other type of malignancy in both men and women. Whereas cigarette smoking was a predominantly male habit before the 1930s, young women are now smoking at a greater rate than young men. Smoking causes all four known types of lung cancer: large cell, small cell, squamous cell, and adenocarcinoma; >80% of patients with lung cancer smoke. In addition, cigarette smoking increases the incidence of laryngeal and pharyngeal cancer, as well as cancer of the oral cavity, particularly in those who consume alcohol. Many of the substances contained in tobacco smoke are complete carcinogens that can be absorbed, predisposing patients to cancer of the bladder, pancreas, stomach, kidney, and cervix.

## Surgical Risks

In the surgical population, continued smoking is known to be associated with increased pulmonary complications postoperatively.[175] Cessation of smoking for >8 weeks decreases pulmonary morbidity. Presumably, mucociliary function improves over the 8 weeks after smoking is stopped, promoting pulmonary clearance of secretions. This observation also explains why pulmonary complications actually increase if smoking is halted for <2 weeks preoperatively.[10] Those who smoke heavily have more pulmonary complications than light smokers. Furthermore, carboxyhemoglobin levels are higher in heavy smokers, who should be treated with $O_2$-enriched air preoperatively in an effort to displace hemoglobin-bound carbon monoxide. The fraction of inspired $O_2$ ($FIO_2$) will, of course, be inversely proportional to the duration of therapy required (Table 9–9). Cessation of smoking alone may alleviate respiratory symptoms and improve function. If symptoms persist despite cessation of these activities, medical management is indicated.

**TABLE 9–9.** Carbon Monoxide Hemoglobin Equilibrium at a Barometric Pressure of 1 atm

| Parts per Million CO Inhaled | Carboxyhemoglobin Saturation (%) | | |
|---|---|---|---|
| | *15% O₂* | *18% O₂* | *21% O₂* |
| 1 | 0.62 | 0.46 | 0.38 |
| 3 | 1.12 | 0.83 | 0.69 |
| 5 | 1.61 | 1.19 | 0.99 |
| 7 | 2.09 | 1.55 | 1.30 |
| 8.7 | 2.50 | 1.85 | 1.55 |
| 10 | 2.81 | 2.08 | 1.75 |
| 25 | 6.25 | 4.68 | 3.94 |
| 30 | 7.34 | 5.51 | 4.65 |
| 35 | 8.41 | 6.33 | 5.34 |
| 50 | 11.47 | 8.71 | 7.38 |
| 70 | 15.24 | 11.69 | 9.96 |
| 90 | 18.71 | 14.49 | 12.40 |
| 100 | 20.34 | 15.83 | 13.57 |
| 300 | 43.14 | 35.84 | 31.81 |
| 500 | 55.80 | 48.17 | 43.69 |
| 700 | 63.85 | 56.53 | 52.05 |
| 900 | 69.43 | 62.58 | 58.25 |
| 1000 | 71.62 | 65.01 | 60.78 |
| 3000 | 88.36 | 84.82 | 82.30 |
| 5000 | 92.69 | 90.33 | 88.58 |
| 7000 | 94.69 | 92.91 | 91.58 |
| 9000 | 95.83 | 94.42 | 93.33 |
| 10 000 | 96.24 | 94.96 | 93.96 |
| 30 000 | 98.76 | 98.32 | 97.94 |
| 50 000 | 99.28 | 99.02 | 98.78 |
| 70 000 | 99.50 | 99.32 | 99.15 |
| 90 000 | 99.63 | 99.49 | 99.35 |

With permission, from the *Annual Review of Pharmacology and Toxicology*, Volume 15 © 1975 by Annual Reviews www.AnnualReviews.org.

## What Factors Characterize Restrictive Lung Disease?

*Obstructive* lung diseases are characterized by an increased total lung capacity and decreased expiratory flow rates, whereas *restrictive* disease represents a group of disorders in which total lung capacity and compliance are reduced and the expiratory flow rate is relatively normal (Fig. 9–12). Restrictive diseases may be intrinsic or extrinsic to the lung and acute or chronic in onset. RLD that develops acutely results

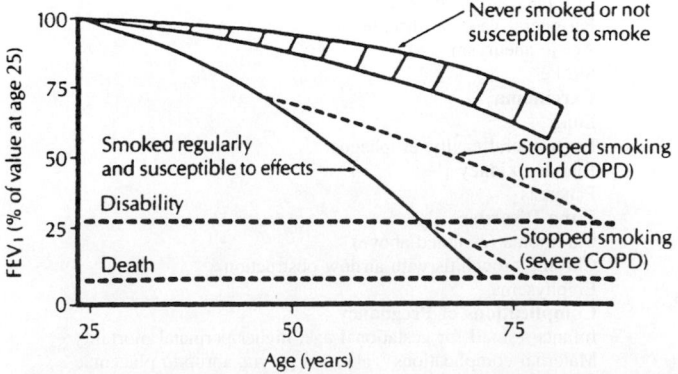

**FIGURE 9–11.** Smoking and its effects on the decline of lung function. The upper curve shows the normal age-related decline in lung function in nonsmokers. The lower curves show the accelerated loss of lung function in smokers. Dotted line shows that the decline in $FEV_1$ (forced expiratory volume in 1.0 second) is slowed if smoking is stopped. The patient who is already disabled at the time of smoking cessation may still die of respiratory disease. (From Bertka KR, Wunderink RG. Outpatient management and COPD. *Am Fam Phys.* 1988;37:265–280.)

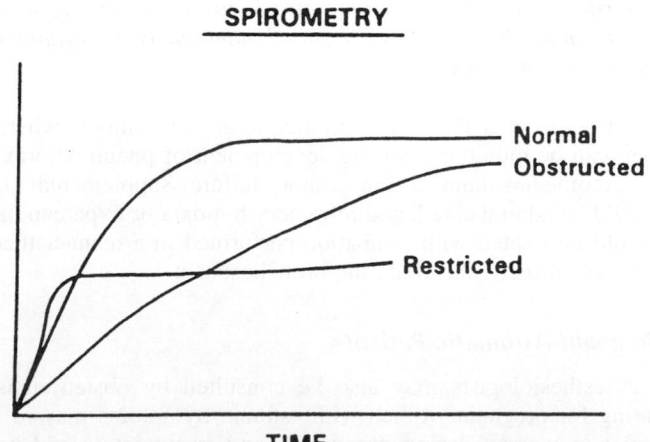

**FIGURE 9–12.** Comparison of spirometry in normal, obstructed and restricted patients.

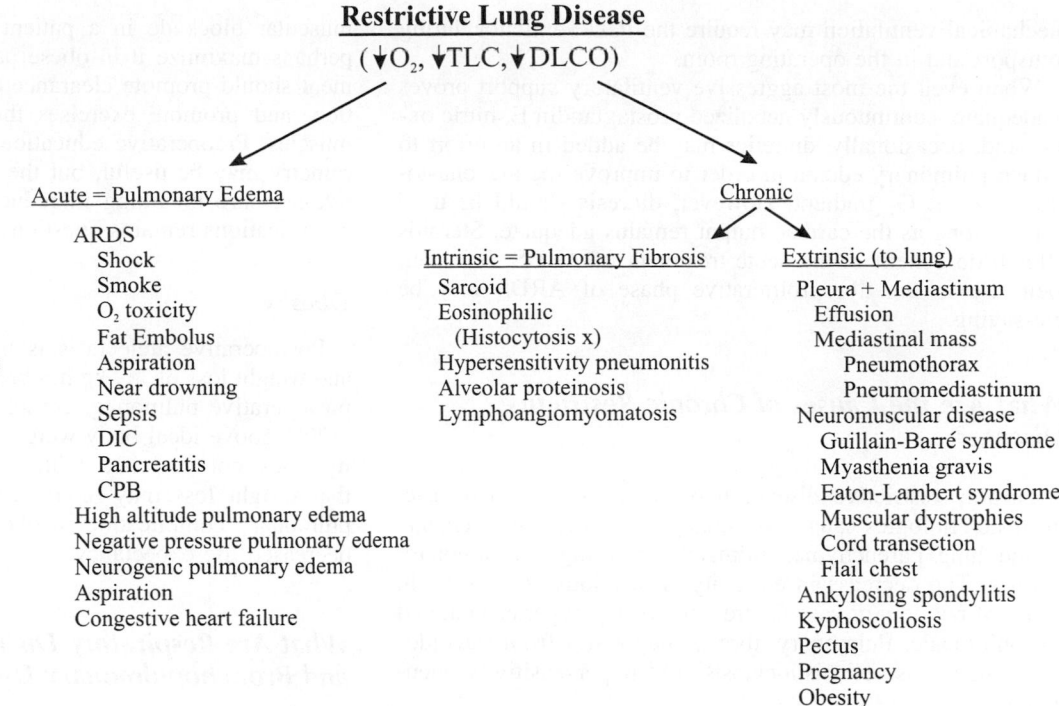

**Restrictive Lung Disease**
($\downarrow O_2$, $\downarrow TLC$, $\downarrow DLCO$)

Acute = Pulmonary Edema

ARDS
  Shock
  Smoke
  $O_2$ toxicity
  Fat Embolus
  Aspiration
  Near drowning
  Sepsis
  DIC
  Pancreatitis
  CPB
High altitude pulmonary edema
Negative pressure pulmonary edema
Neurogenic pulmonary edema
Aspiration
Congestive heart failure

Chronic

Intrinsic = Pulmonary Fibrosis
  Sarcoid
  Eosinophilic
    (Histocytosis x)
  Hypersensitivity pneumonitis
  Alveolar proteinosis
  Lymphoangiomyomatosis

Extrinsic (to lung)
  Pleura + Mediastinum
    Effusion
    Mediastinal mass
      Pneumothorax
      Pneumomediastinum
  Neuromuscular disease
    Guillain-Barré syndrome
    Myasthenia gravis
    Eaton-Lambert syndrome
    Muscular dystrophies
    Cord transection
    Flail chest
  Ankylosing spondylitis
  Kyphoscoliosis
  Pectus
  Pregnancy
  Obesity
  Ascites

**FIGURE 9–13.** Restrictive lung disease.

from the accumulation of fluid in the interstitium of the lungs, causing them to become stiff and noncompliant. As such, it constitutes the early stage of pulmonary edema, which is a component of adult respiratory distress syndrome (ARDS). Fluid may accumulate as a result of increased permeability of the pulmonary capillaries (noncardiogenic) or due to an increase in the capillary hydrostatic pressure (cardiogenic). In either case, *acute* restrictive disease is always intrinsic to the lung.

RLD may also be chronic and insidious in nature, in which case it can result from slowly evolving changes in the elastic elements of the lung (*intrinsic*) or from disorders that do not involve the lungs, per se, but nevertheless compromise their function by limiting their capacity and producing a measurable decrease in compliance (*extrinsic*) (Fig. 9–13).

Whether the disorder causing the restriction is intrinsic or extrinsic, chronic or acute, the work of breathing is increased, and patients become dyspneic in an effort to expand their lungs in the face of decreased compliance. Patients with obstructive lung disease tend to breathe deeply with rapid inspiration. Expiration is prolonged, providing additional time for exhalation to compensate for the decrease in expiratory flow rate. By contrast, patients with restrictive disease breathe rapidly and shallowly to limit the work of breathing. The $PaCO_2$ may actually be decreased; the diffusing capacity of lung for carbon monoxide (DLCO) frequently is decreased in restrictive disorders.

## What Are the Causes of Acute Restrictive Disease?

### Acute Respiratory Distress Syndrome

#### Signs and Symptoms

ARDS is characterized by noncardiogenic pulmonary edema, decreased pulmonary compliance, decreased FRC, and hypoxemia that results from intrapulmonary shunt. Patients developing this syndrome appear dyspneic, tachypneic, and tachycardic. Chest radiographs reveal bilateral pulmonary infiltrates with a ground glass appearance that may progress to complete opacification.

As the disease progresses, compliance deteriorates and pulmonary artery pressure rises, even as the pulmonary artery occlusion pressure remains normal or decreases. Increasing supplemental $O_2$ may be inadequate compensation for the severe hypoxia that develops due to increasing intrapulmonary shunt, necessitating greater ventilatory support. Pneumonia is coexistent with ARDS in 50% of cases.[176] More than 50% of patients with ARDS die,[177] typically from multisystem organ failure. Until recently, advances in positive pressure-ventilation and pulmonary care, although supportive, failed to alter the mortality rate. Newer techniques employing low tidal volumes and pressures may reverse this finding.[178] The syndrome may develop from any etiology that results in injury to the pulmonary capillary endothelium, including hypotension, pancreatitis, sepsis, toxic inhalation, toxic ingestion, near drowning, and aspiration.

### Treatment

The goal of therapy in ARDS is to maintain a $PaO_2$ >60 mm Hg ($O_2$ saturation as measured by pulse oximetry [$SpO_2$] ≥90%). Treatment should be accomplished with the lowest inspired concentration of $O_2$ possible, using the least ventilatory support tolerable. In most cases, pulmonary compliance is sufficiently compromised that positive end-expiratory pressure (PEEP) will be required, and higher $O_2$ concentrations are needed to maintain the $PaO_2$ ≥60 mm Hg. Patients in this condition are critically dependent on mechanical ventilation and may deteriorate rapidly when they are transported outside the ICU. Adequate ventilation in the operating room may not be possible with the anesthesia machine ventilator. Continued mechanical ventilation may require the ICU ventilator during transport and in the operating room.

When even the most aggressive ventilatory support proves inadequate, continuously nebulized prostaglandin E, nitric oxide, and, occasionally, diuretics may be added in an effort to reduce pulmonary edema in order to improve the alveolar-to-arterial (A-a) $O_2$ gradient. However, diuresis should be used only as long as the cardiac output remains adequate. Steroids offer little benefit in the acute treatment of ARDS; however, their use in the fibroproliferative phase of ARDS may be life-saving.

## What Are the Causes of Chronic Restrictive Disease?

Chronic restrictive disease may be intrinsic or extrinsic. Intrinsic etiologies cause slow changes in the elastic elements of the lung parenchyma, ultimately resulting in pulmonary fibrosis. The decrease in elasticity is insidious and results in a loss of pulmonary vasculature, pulmonary hypertension, and cor pulmonale. Pulmonary fibrosis may result from sarcoidosis, Langerhans cell histiocytosis, and hypersensitivity pneumonitis.

Indolent extrinsic disorders include a host of etiologies that prevent the lung from expanding due to their effects on the thoracic cage. Thoracic deformity as a result of trauma (flail chest), congenital defects, or kyphoscoliosis of the spine prevent the typical bucket-handle motion (up and out) of the chest wall, thus altering the mechanics of breathing and limiting inflation. Cough, necessary to clear secretions adequately, is frequently impaired as well, resulting in recurrent pneumonia and potentially leading to an obstructive component.

Neuromuscular disorders such as the muscular dystrophies, myasthenia gravis, Eaton-Lambert syndrome, and spinal cord injury compromise the function of respiratory muscles, thereby limiting vital capacity and the ability to cough. Injury to the phrenic nerve from malignant disease, from aortic aneurysm, or after thoracic surgery may be unilateral or bilateral. Of interest, paralysis of one hemidiaphragm is usually an asymptomatic finding on chest radiograph. Space occupying lesions, such as a large pleural effusion, mesothelioma, or a mediastinal mass, can prevent normal lung expansion. Pleural fibrosis due to hemothorax, empyema, or pleurodesis typically leads to a minor restrictive defect. Although many of these conditions are insidious in their onset, they tend to be progressive, ultimately leading to respiratory insufficiency, pulmonary hypertension, and cor pulmonale.

### Preoperative Care

Preoperative evaluation of patients with known or suspected RLD should include PFTs if the patient is symptomatic, especially if activity is limited. Flow-volume loops, peak flow, total lung capacity, RV, and vital capacity should be determined and ABG analyzed. Many of these measurements are effort-dependent; nevertheless, a vital capacity of <15 mL/kg (normal = 70 mL/kg) or an elevated $PaCO_2$ correlate with an increased risk of postoperative pulmonary complications.

Once the presence and severity of the disorder have been confirmed, a serious attempt to diagnose the etiology of the disease should be made. Anesthetic management may depend on this determination. For example, one would limit neuro-

muscular blockade in a patient with myasthenia gravis but perhaps maximize it in obese patients. Preoperative management should promote clearance of secretions, eradicate infection, and promote exercises that strengthen the respiratory muscles. Preoperative education in the use of incentive spirometry may be useful, but the efficacy of intermittent positive-pressure breathing in reducing postoperative pulmonary complications remains questionable.

### Obesity

Postoperative atelectasis is increased in obese patients,[179] and weight loss of >9 kg has been correlated with a decline in postoperative pulmonary complications in patients remaining >20% above ideal body weight.[180] However, surgical mortality does not correlate with obesity.[181] These data suggest that weight loss may reduce the incidence of postoperative pulmonary complication in obese patients known to have a decreased life expectancy.

## What Are Respiratory Distress Syndrome and Bronchopulmonary Dysplasia?

### Respiratory Distress Syndrome

Respiratory distress syndrome (RDS), historically known also as *hyaline membrane disease* (HMD), is a neonatal form of RLD and is similar to ARDS. Before the 26th week of gestation, the developing lung tissue lacks the type II alveolar pneumocytes required to secrete a complex mixture of phospholipids, which is called *surfactant*. These compounds reduce the surface tension of the alveoli and dramatically increase lung compliance. Type II pneumocytes are numerous at 35 weeks, but infants who are born prematurely are deficient in surfactant. Inadequate amounts of surfactant cause *RDS* (HMD). This condition is characterized by elevated surface tension, decreased lung compliance, and alveolar collapse. A significant shunt fraction leads to hypoxemia and metabolic acidosis.

RDS accounts for more than half of all neonatal deaths in premature babies. Infants with RDS may require mechanical ventilation with high $FIO_2$, high airway pressures, and PEEP. Synthetic surfactant and high frequency ventilation often reduce the level of support required and the associated complications. In neonatal level 3 centers, significant improvement in outcome of low birthweight is clearly demonstrated. Premature infants requiring ventilatory support who received a 42-day course of dexamethasone (0.5 mg/kg) recovered pulmonary function more rapidly and were weaned from the ventilator significantly faster than patients receiving more limited steroids or none at all.[182]

### Bronchopulmonary Dysplasia

Bronchopulmonary dysplasia (BPD) represents the chronic sequela of RDS and the consequent need for supplemental $O_2$ and ventilatory support. Signs of BPD are present within 24 hours in >10% of infants requiring $O_2$ for the treatment of RDS. Generally speaking, the more serious the RDS, the more support is required, and the more likely that BPD will develop.

The airways of children with BPD are hyperresponsive and demonstrate an increased resistance. The lungs are less compliant, and mismatch is present. These changes, as in ARDS, result in greater shunt (increased A-a $O_2$ partial pressure gradient), more dead space ventilation (increased gradient between end-tidal $CO_2$ and $PaCO_2$), tachypnea, and a 25% increase in $O_2$ consumption. Children with a history of RDS can be assumed to have some degree of BPD, the severity of which will be correlated with the intensity of the therapy required to treat the RDS. They manifest stiff lungs and intraoperatively will need a high $FIO_2$ and mechanical ventilation. The severe bronchospastic component of the disease suggests that a deep surgical plane of anesthesia be obtained before instrumenting the airway.

Pulmonary dysfunction will be greatest in the first year following the onset of RDS; children surviving this year have a good prognosis. BPD can often be improved by the administration of steroids, which can be given by aerosol or systemically. Nebulized and parenteral delivery is equally effective; however, aerosolized preparations reduce many of the detrimental effects of parenteral administration such as increased caloric consumption and decreased growth.[183]

## What Issues Are Important Concerning Infectious Disease and Control?

### Pneumonia

Over 4.5 million people in the United States contract pneumonia each year; it remains the sixth leading cause of death in this country. Three hundred thousand of these patients acquire the infection while hospitalized. Obviously, elective operations should be deferred until the infection resolves, but emergent cases and procedures that are required in intubated, critically ill patients will need to be performed in the operating room under less favorable conditions.

*Pneumonia* is an infection of the lung parenchyma characterized by poor oxygenation of the arterial blood because of intrapulmonary shunt and increased A-a gradient. These changes result from the accumulation of fluid in the alveoli and interstitium of the lung.

### Lobar

Lobar pneumonia is an acute febrile illness that results from infection of the lung with *S. pneumoniae*. It may involve one or more lobes of the lungs. In addition to fever, symptoms include dyspnea, tachypnea, pain on the side of the infection, and expectoration of bloody sputum.

Initially, the affected tissue is congested but soon becomes red and solid (*red hepatization*) as blood and exudative fluid fill the alveoli (*consolidation*). It is during this time that hypoxia develops, with patients becoming symptomatic when the $O_2$ saturation reaches 85% or less. Hypoxia stimulates tachypnea. Breathing is shallow, as is typical of restrictive disorders, possibly as a result of pain. A heightened sensitivity of the vagal afferents innervating the alveoli through the Hering-Breuer reflex also may explain the respiratory pattern.[184,185] Tidal volume may fall to $\leq 3$ mL/kg, but minute ventilation is increased, and the carbon dioxide content declines by an average of 15%. The arterial pH remains normal to slightly elevated, indicative of a partially compensated respiratory alkalosis.[186]

About 1 to 2 weeks later, if the patient survives, the blood

and exudate are degraded and reabsorbed (*gray hepatization*). At this point, the blood vessels in the affected region are obliterated, and the blood flow is redirected to better ventilated areas. Consequently, oxygenation improves, and the alkalosis resolves.

### Bronchopneumonia

Bronchopneumonia is characterized by an even higher degree of desaturation than lobar pneumonia and is associated with hypercapnia and a compensated respiratory acidosis, rather than hypocapnia and a respiratory alkalosis. The carbon dioxide content in the arterial blood may reach 80 mL/dL. In lobar pneumonia, consolidated areas of the lung are poorly ventilated but they are aerated. As a result, carbon dioxide continues to diffuse from the blood into the alveolar space, and the increased minute ventilation eliminates the gas. In bronchopneumonia, alveoli are completely cut off from any ventilation due to plugging of the airways with mucus and exudative fluid. The amount of absolute shunt exceeds the increase in alveolar ventilation, and carbon dioxide accumulates.

Pneumonia may progress to septicemia, and systemic $O_2$ delivery is challenged by perfusion with blood that has a low $O_2$ content. The widened A-a gradient can be treated with supplemental $O_2$, but shunt cannot be overcome by simply increasing the $FIO_2$. Increasing the $FIO_2$ >70% may actually increase the amount of shunt[187]; therefore, respiratory support must be optimized in an effort to improve $O_2$ delivery.[187] Toward this end, pulmonary toilet is paramount, and bronchodilators should be used in an effort to ventilate all alveoli that are perfused. Antibiotic therapy directed at the culpable organisms should be aggressive to eradicate the infection.

Mechanical ventilation should be optimized for a minute ventilation that yields a normal pH; a tidal volume and rate that do not produce excessive airway pressures; a $FIO_2$ that provides a $PaO_2$ >60 mm Hg; and PEEP that increases the $PaO_2$ without reducing cardiac output. Finally, because the A-a gradient is directly proportional to interstitial pulmonary edema, fluids should be minimized to the extent that will allow preservation of cardiac output in an effort to reduce the hydrostatic pressure in the pulmonary capillaries.

## INTRAOPERATIVE CONSIDERATIONS

### How Should Anesthetic Management Be Tailored?

Patients with significant lung disease should be diagnosed preoperatively and the severity of their disease documented. The anesthesiologist then may tailor the anesthetic to the patient. For example, one might want to choose a neuraxial block for a patient with severe asthma who requires an abdominal procedure in an effort to avoid complications associated with intubating the trachea. Alternatively, the same procedure might be better performed under a general anesthetic in a patient with severe COLD who may not tolerate any loss of respiratory muscle function. In the latter case, postoperative pain management becomes critical, and the need to extubate the patient should be obvious. A complete discussion of the anesthetic considerations associated with specific disorders can be found in this text (see Chapters 54 and 64) and elsewhere.[188,189]

### How Does Intubation Predispose to Infection?

The pathogenesis of pneumonia in patients who remain intubated may result from aspiration of bacteria colonizing the oropharynx and proximal gastrointestinal (GI) tract. A review of 16 independent studies suggests that decontamination of the GI tract in intubated patients lowers the incidence of nosocomial pneumonia and tracheobronchitis.[190] However, at least one study of >120 intubated patients showed that the GI tract was not the source of tracheobronchial tree colonization and revealed that no cases of ventilator-associated pneumonia were attributable to organisms that came from the GI tract.[191] Aspiration of colonized secretions may be the pathogenic mechanism involved in the development of postoperative pneumonias, although the incidence of pneumonia is also increased in patients who remain bedridden and those with nasogastric intubation.[192–194]

Intubated patients are not ambulatory, postural drainage is reduced, atelectasis is frequent, and cough is impossible in the presence of an ETT, all of which facilitate colonization of bacteria and their accumulation in secretions that pool in the distal airways. These factors may predispose to pneumonia. Besides the infectious disease concerns associated with the presence of an ETT, the cost and intensity of care required for patients who remain intubated should prompt extubation whenever appropriate and possible.

### What Surgical Issues Are Pertinent to Postoperative Pulmonary Complications?

The incidence of postoperative pulmonary complications is inversely proportional to the distance of the surgical site from the diaphragm.[29,195,196] Pulmonary complications following surgery include pneumonia, pneumonitis, atelectasis, mucus plugging, lobar collapse, and pulmonary embolus. These complications are associated with prolonged hospital stay and increased morbidity and mortality; the incidence may reach 50% in some patient populations.

Although the development of any of these complications may be multifactorial, decreases in lung volumes caused by alterations in respiratory mechanics are central to all, except possibly pulmonary embolus. All patients are at risk for postoperative respiratory complications following upper abdominal and thoracic surgery.[6,194–196] In patients with more than stage I disease, mortality may reach 5% and morbidity may exceed 80%,[197] primarily because ventilation becomes dependent on the accessory muscles of respiration instead of the diaphragm.[194] This finding is not attributable to pain, but it may explain why deep breathing, incentive spirometry, or intermittent positive-pressure breathing fails to completely eliminate postoperative pulmonary complications.

The pulmonary consequences of surgery are attributable to both surgery and anesthesia.[193,195] Complications for upper abdominal procedures are so prevalent in patients with stage II and stage III disease that elective surgery should be avoided whenever possible.[197] When surgery must be performed, lapa-

roscopic alternatives should be considered[198] and the anesthetic tailored to the patient.[30,194]

### Functional Residual Capacity

Decreases in lung volumes—specifically, the FVC and FRC—result from changes in chest wall mechanics and impaired function of the respiratory muscles. Recumbency compromises the FRC by as much as 28% in the supine position and even more in the Trendelenburg position.[199] The induction of anesthesia and muscle paralysis may reduce the FRC an additional 18%,[200,201] and peritonitis, ascites, pleural effusion, or obesity further compromises it.

The FRC is critical for proper pulmonary function. Pulmonary compliance is maximized and the work of breathing minimized at this volume. Because compliance decreases at lung volumes below the normal FRC, the tendency for atelectasis is increased. Adequacy of FRC ensures adequate oxygenation between ventilations by minimizing alveolar collapse and shunt. The FRC is reduced following lower abdominal, upper abdominal, and thoracic surgery by 15%, 30%, and 35%, respectively,[202–204] and may remain so for up to 6 months.[205,206]

### Closing Volume

Decreases in FRC are compounded by increases in the closing volume (CV). CV is the volume of gas in the lungs when the distal airways in the primarily dependent regions of the lungs are compressed. Such compression prevents expiration. The FRC normally is 40% of the lung capacity, and the CV is about 20%.[207,208] Typically, expiration continues from all alveoli (including dependent alveoli) down to the FRC. At FRC, all airways are still patent and do not begin to close unless forced exhalation reduces the lung volume below this level.

If at any time CV exceeds FRC, the airways collapse at CV, trap gas distally, and produce an increase in the end-expiratory volume that is above normal FRC. This condition produces relative hyperinflation at end expiration, decreases compliance, and increases work of breathing for the same tidal volume breath. Furthermore, air trapping due to premature airway closure impairs gas exchange, thereby promoting absorption atelectasis, $\dot{V}/\dot{Q}$ mismatch, and shunt. In addition, closure of the airways impedes normal drainage of secretions, increasing the potential for pneumonitis. Conditions that increase CV include age (CV = FRC in the supine position at age 40 and in the standing position at age 65), smoking, bronchospasm, airway secretions, fluid overload, anesthesia, and surgery.[209–211]

## POSTOPERATIVE ISSUES

### What Procedures Are Prone to Postoperative Pulmonary Complications?

#### Abdominal

Nearly one third of patients undergoing abdominal procedures develop postoperative pulmonary complications. Factors that reduce FRC are responsible, including abdominal muscle dysfunction, ascites, the supine position, and diaphragmatic dysfunction.[192] Transdiaphragmatic pressure is reduced by 70% one day after surgery and does not return to normal for at least one week.[212] Upper abdominal procedures have a 1.5 times greater adverse impact on respiratory function than do lower abdominal procedures.[192] The incidence of pulmonary complications may reach 70% in patients requiring operations in the upper abdomen[8,11,25,29] compared with only 4% for urologic procedures.[213]

Spirometry is a poor predictor of postoperative pulmonary complications in the general surgical population.[214] The patient's preoperative condition, history of smoking, obstructive disease, obesity, chronic bronchitis,[2,192,215] and possibly age[9] seem to be the most important predictors. As was noted previously, colonizing bacteria in the stomach and placement of a nasogastric tube also are correlated with an increased incidence of pneumonia.[192,193]

Major abdominal vascular surgery is associated with mechanical ventilation for at least 24 hours in 24% of patients with moderate to severe COLD.[216] Prolonged ventilation was significantly more frequent in patients with major blood loss who were cigarette smokers and had preoperative hypoxemia.

## Esophagectomy

Twenty-five percent to 50% of patients undergoing esophagectomy sustain postoperative pulmonary complications.[217] The likelihood that pulmonary compromise will develop is increased by age, preexisting COLD, decreased respiratory reserve, poor nutrition, low spirometric indices, and impaired diffusing capacity.[218] The potential for pulmonary complications is increased further by the amount of mediastinal dissection, blood loss, placement and location of a reconstructed organ in the chest cavity (substernal worse than posterior mediastinal), and development of a pleural effusion.[219] The type of incision also affects pulmonary compromise postoperatively (isolated left thoracotomy > Ivor-Lewis technique [right thoracotomy and laparotomy] > transhiatal approach that avoids thoracotomy in favor of abdominal and cervical incisions).[220,221] Injury to the recurrent laryngeal nerve impairs cough generation and further increases the probability of respiratory complications and continued ventilatory support postoperatively.[222]

Given the high incidence of pulmonary complications and possible mortality associated with this intervention, a complete preoperative evaluation of the surgical candidate's pulmonary function is warranted and should be used to determine exactly how the resection will be performed.

## Thoracotomy

Approximately 85% of patients undergoing a lung mass resection have COLD. Thirty percent will sustain severe pulmonary dysfunction preoperatively.[223] The resection of lung tissue and changes in chest wall mechanics jointly contribute to the development of postoperative pulmonary complications. Vital capacity may be decreased by 30% after simple thoracotomy and remain depressed for up to 6 months. Resection of functional lung tissue, on the other hand, permanently reduces lung function by as much as 50% in pneumonectomy. Estimates of permanent loss of functional reserve correlate with the amount of normal tissue resected: wedge, 0 to 10% loss; segmentectomy, 5% to 10% loss; and lobectomy, 10% to 20% loss.[197]

PFTs can be used to predict which patients are at the highest risk and thus require more specific evaluation such as $\dot{V}/\dot{Q}$ scintigraphy or exercise testing. If postoperative $FEV_1$ postoperatively is expected to be ≥40% of the normal value based on the patient's age, height, and gender, surgery should proceed. Alternatively, if the patient's maximal $O_2$ consumption ($\dot{V}O_2$) is between 10 and 15 mL/kg/min, postoperative pulmonary complications are likely; if the $\dot{V}O_2$ is <10 mL/kg/min, death is probable.[224]

Which patients are at greatest risk for a pulmonary complication can be assessed reasonably well. Clinical assessment of the pulmonary reserve, such as the stair climbing effort or the 6-minute walk distance, are more valuable than is preoperative spirometry.[223] Measurements of gas exchange and $O_2$ consumption, although markedly better than spirometry and less dependent on patient effort than tests designed to assess pulmonary reserve, are no panacea. The most reliable factors are patient age and predicted postoperative $D_{LCO}$.[225]

Every effort should be made to optimize cardiorespiratory function preoperatively. Patients should be instructed in the proper use of incentive spirometry. The surgical approach should be the least traumatic possible (ie, muscle sparing incisions to reduce pain and preserve strength). Thoracoscopic procedures are promising in this regard. Patients should be extubated early, if possible, to avoid ETT complications and to enable effective cough and clearance of secretions.

When patients cannot be extubated safely, continuous positive airway pressure to support the FRC and pressure support ventilation to minimize the imposed work of breathing seem to be preferable. Postoperative pain must be optimally controlled in an effort to promote spontaneous ventilation, to maximize the FRC, and to minimize atelectasis and the work of breathing, all of which reduce the need for extended intubation and ventilatory support. In those patients who require prolonged intubation, pulmonary toilet should be aggressive.

## Cardiac Surgery

Pulmonary complications occur in up to 40% of cardiac cases[226] and include prolonged ventilatory support, pneumonitis, bronchospasm, atelectasis, and lobar collapse. Preoperative spirometry is a poor predictor of postoperative pulmonary function after cardiac surgery, yet COLD remains the most common cause of pulmonary dysfunction in patients presenting for cardiac surgery.[29]

The incidence is highest in patients undergoing cardiopulmonary bypass, who sustain insult not only from the invasion of the chest wall but also from the effects of the inflammatory mediators released during extracorporeal circulation. Changes in the mechanics of the chest wall result in a decrease in FRC that remains decreased by 20% at the time of discharge and does not return to normal for nearly 3 months.[227,228]

Elderly patients tolerate the respiratory stress of cardiac surgery less well than younger patients. Advanced age and the mammary artery dissection independently contribute to the decrease in FRC following cardiac surgery.[227,228] Injury to the phrenic nerve is increased from 5% to 30%, and left lower lobe collapse increases from 30% to 80% when iced slush is used to cool the myocardium.[229] The A-a $O_2$ partial pressure gradient is increased 150% following extracorporeal circulation due to an increase in shunt from 3% to 30%.

Increase in shunt develops within the first 24 hours after bypass. Presumably it also results from the release of inflammatory mediators generated by interaction between blood and the bypass circuit. However, this possibility has not been established. The lesion, whatever its cause, does not resolve for nearly 6 weeks.[230] Minimally invasive procedures ("off-pump coronary artery bypass graft") avoid cardiopulmonary bypass entirely. Whether the postoperative pulmonary problems also will be eliminated remains to be seen. Following cardiac procedures, COLD patients should be managed with a combination of inhaled $\beta_2$-agonists and inhaled anticholinergic agents.[231,232]

## References

1. Bartlett R, Bremman ML, Gazzaniga AB, et al. Studies on the pathogenesis and prevention of postoperative pulmonary complications. *Surg Gynecol Obstet*. 1973;137:925.
2. Garibaldi RA, Britt MR, Coleman ML, et al. Risk factors for postoperative pneumonia. *Am J Med*. 1981;70:677.
3. Pasteur W. Active lobar collapse of the lung after abdominal operations: a contribution to the study of post-operative lung complications. *Lancet*. 1910;2:1080.
4. Busch E, Verazin G, Antkowiak JG, et al. Pulmonary complications in patients undergoing thoracotomy for lung carcinoma. *Chest*. 1994;105:760.
5. Celli BR. What is the value of preoperative pulmonary function? Validity, indication, and benefits. *Med Clin North Am*. 1993;7:309.
6. Zibrak JD, O'Donnell CR. Indication for preoperative pulmonary function testing. *Clin Chest Med*. 1993;14:227.
7. Kroehke K, Lawrence VA, Theroux JF, et al. Operative risk in patients with severe obstructive pulmonary disease. *Arch Intern Med*. 1993;152:967.
8. Stein M, Cassara EL. Preoperative pulmonary evaluation and therapy for surgery patients. *JAMA*. 1970;211:787.
9. Mohr DN. Estimation of surgical risk in the elderly: a correlative review. *J Am Geriatr Soc*. 1983;31:99.
10. Warner MA, Divertie MB, Tinker JH. Preoperative cessation of smoking and pulmonary complications in coronary artery bypass patients. *Anesthesiology*. 1984;60:380.
11. Gracey DR, Divertie MB, Didier EP. Preoperative pulmonary preparation of patients with chronic obstructive pulmonary disease. *Chest*. 1979;76:123.
12. Tarhan S, Mottitt E, Sessler AD, et al. The risk of anesthesia and surgery in patients with chronic bronchitis and chronic obstructive pulmonary disease. *Surgery*. 1973;74:720.
13. Wong DH, Weber EC, Schell MJ, et al. Factors associated with postoperative complications in patients with severe chronic obstructive pulmonary disease. *Anesth Analg*. 1995;80:276.
14. Carr HD, Stevens PM, Adamiya R. Preoperative pulmonary function and complications after cardiovascular surgery. *Chest*. 1979;80:276.
15. Celli BR, Rodriguez K, Snider GL. A controlled trial of intermittent positive pressure breathing, incentive spirometry and deep breathing exercises in preventing pulmonary complications after abdominal surgery. *Am J Respir Dis*. 1984;130:12.
16. Yeager MP, Glass DD, Neff RK, et al. Epidural anesthesia and analgesia in high-risk surgical patients. *Anesthesiology*. 1987;66:729.
17. Mitchell CK, Smoger SH, Pfeifer MP, et al. Multivariate analysis of factors associated with postoperative pulmonary complications following general elective surgery. *Arch Surg*. 1998;133:194.
18. Prys-Roberts C, Nunn JF, Dobson RH, et al. Radiologically undetectable pulmonary collapse in the supine position. *Lancet*. 1967;2:399.
19. Berson W, Adriani J. "Silent" regurgitation and aspiration during anesthesia. *Anesthesiology*. 1954;15:644.
20. Tisi GM. Preoperative evaluation of pulmonary function, validity, indications, and benefits. *Am Rev Respir Dis*. 1979;119:293.
21. Kipp VJ, Arora SK, Boysen PG. Pulmonary consultation. In: Murray MJ, Coursin DB, Pearl RC, et al, eds. *Critical Care Medicine Perioperative Management*. Philadelphia, Pa: Lippincott-Raven; 1997:400.
22. Adams PF, Marano MA. Current estimates from the National Health Interview Survey, 1994. National Center for Health Statistics. *Vital Health Stat*. 1994;10:193.
23. Matthay RA. Chronic airway diseases. In: Wyngaarden JB, Smith LH Jr, Bennett JC, eds. *Cecil Textbook of Medicine*. Vol 1. 19th ed. Philadelphia, Pa: WB Saunders; 1992:386.
24. Carr DT. Education of patients about lung cancer. *Chest*. 1979;76:122.
25. Wightman JA. A prospective study of the incidence of postoperative pulmonary complications. *Br J Surg*. 1968;55:85.
26. Sweer L, Zwillich CW. Dyspnea in the patient with chronic pulmonary disease: etiology and management. *Clin Chest Med*. 1990;11:417.
27. Mahler DA, Weinberg DH, Wills CK, et al. The measurement of dyspnea. Contents, interobserver agreement, and physiologic correlates of two new clinical indexes. *Chest*. 1984;85:751.
28. American Thoracic Society. Lung function testing: selection of reference values and interpretative strategies. *Am Respir Dis*. 1991;144:1202.
29. Kroenke K, Lawrence VA, Theroux JF, et al. Postoperative complications after thoracic and major abdominal surgery in patients with and without obstructive lung disease. *Chest*. 1993;104:1445.
30. Hall JC, Tarala R, Harris J, et al. Incentive spirometry versus routine chest physiotherapy for prevention of pulmonary complications after abdominal surgery. *Lancet*. 1991;337:953.
31. Warner MA, Offord KP, Warner ME, et al. Role of preoperative cessation of smoking and other factors in postoperative pulmonary complications: a blinded prospective study of coronary artery bypass patients. *Mayo Clin Proc*. 1989;64:609.
32. Anthonisen NR, Connett JE, Kiley JP, et al. Effects of smoking intervention and the use of an inhaled anticholinergic bronchodilator on the rate of decline of $FEV_1$. The Lung Health Study. *JAMA*. 1994;272:1497.
33. Morrison D, Skwarski KM, MacNee W. The adequacy of oxygenation in patients with hypoxic chronic obstructive pulmonary disease treated with long-term domiciliary oxygen. *Respir Med*. 1997;91:287.
34. Gorecka D, Gorzelak K, Sliwinski B, et al. Effect of long-term oxygen therapy on survival in patients with chronic pulmonary disease with moderate hypoxaemia. *Thorax*. 1997;52:674.
35. O'Driscoll BR, Taylor RJ, Horsley MG, et al. Nebulized salbutamol with and without ipratropium bromide in acute airflow obstruction. *Lancet*. 1989;1:1418.
36. Rebuck AS, Chapman KR, Abboud R, et al. Nebulized anticholinergic and sympathomimetic treatment of asthma and chronic obstructive airways. *Am J Med*. 1987;82:59.
37. Madsen EB, Bundgaard A, Hidinger KG. Cumulative dose-response study comparing terbutaline pressurized aerosol administered via a pear shaped spacer and terbutaline in a nebulized solution. *Eur J Clin Pharmacol*. 1982;23:27.
38. Harber P, SooHoo K, Tashkin DP. Is the $MVV:FEV_1$ ratio useful for assessing spirometry validity? *Chest*. 1985;88:52.
39. Morley TF, Marozsan E, Zappasodi SJ, et al. Comparison of beta-adrenergic agents delivered by nebulizer versus metered dose inhaler with InspirEase in hospitalized asthmatic patients. *Chest*. 1988;94:1205.
40. Turner JR, Corkery KJ, Eckman D, et al. Equivalence of continuous flow nebulizer and metered-dose inhaler with reservoir bag for treatment of acute airflow obstruction. *Chest*. 1988;93:476.
41. Berenberg MJ, Baigelman W, Cupples LA, et al. Comparison of metered-dose inhaler attached to an Aerochamber with an updraft nebulizer for the administration of metaproterenol in hospitalized patients. *J Asthma*. 1985;22:87.
42. Jasper AC, Mohsenifar Z, Kahan S, et al. Cost-benefit comparison of aerosol bronchodilator delivery methods in hospitalized patients. *Chest*. 1987;91:614.
43. Roche N, Chinet T, Huchon G. Ambulatory inhalation therapy in obstructive lung disease. *Respiration*. 1997;64:121.
44. van der Palen J, Klein JJ, Kerkhoff AH, et al. Evaluation of the effectiveness of four different inhalers in patients with chronic obstructive pulmonary disease. *Thorax*. 1995;50:1183.
45. Cazzola M, Calderaro F, Califano C, et al. Oral bambuterol compared to inhaled salmeterol in patients with partially reversible chronic obstructive pulmonary disease. *Eur J Clin Pharmacol*. 1999;54:829.
46. Cazzola M, Santangelo G, Piccolo A, et al. Effect of salmeterol and formoterol in patients with chronic obstructive pulmonary disease. *Pulm Pharmacol*. 1994;7:103.
47. Cazzola M, Spina D, Matera MG. The use of bronchodilators in stable chronic obstructive pulmonary disease. *Pulm Pharmacol Ther*. 1997;10:129.
48. Schultze-Werninghause G. Multi-center 1-year trial on formoterol, a new long-acting beta 2-agonist, in chronic obstructive airway disease. *Lung*. 1990;168(suppl):83.
49. Thomson NC, Angus R, Quebe-Fehling E, et al. Efficacy and tolerability of formoterol in elderly patients with reversible obstructive airway disease. *Respir Med*. 1998;92:562.
50. Maesen FP. Eformoterol versus salbutamol in patients with ROAD. *Br J Clin Pract Symp Suppl*. 1995;81:8.
51. Vervloet D, Ekstrom T, Pel R, et al. A 6-month comparison between

formoterol and salmeterol in patients with reversible obstructive airways disease. *Respir Med.* 1998;92:836.

52. Cazzola M, Vinciguerra A, DiPenna F, et al. Early reversibility to salbutamol does not always predict bronchodilation after salmeterol in stable chronic obstructive pulmonary disease. *Respir Med.* 1998;92:1012.

53. Mestitz H, Copland JM, McDonald CF. Comparison of outpatient nebulized dose inhaler terbutaline in chronic airflow obstruction. *Chest.* 1989;96:1237.

54. Subtypes of Muscarinic Receptors V. Proceedings of the 5th International Symposium, Newport Beach, California, October 22-24, 1992. *Life Sci.* 1993;52:405.

55. Ghafouri MA, Patil KD, Kass I. Sputum changes associated with the use of ipratropium bromide. *Chest.* 1984;86:387.

56. Chapman KR. The role of anticholinergic bronchodilators in adult asthma and chronic obstructive pulmonary disease. *Lung.* 1990;168(suppl):295.

57. Gross NJ. Ipratropium bromide. *N Engl J Med.* 1988;319:486.

58. Gross NJ, Petty TL, Friedman M, et al. Dose response to ipratropium as a nebulized solution in patients with chronic obstructive pulmonary disease. A three-chapter study. *Am Rev Respir Dis.* 1989;139:1188.

59. O'Driscoll BR, Kay EA, Taylor RJ, et al. A long-term prospective assessment of home nebulizer treatment. *Respir Med.* 1992;86:317.

60. Tonnesen F, Laursen LC, Evald T, et al. Bronchodilating effect of terbutaline powder in acute severe bronchial obstruction. *Chest.* 1994;105:697.

61. Brown IG, Chan CS, Kelly CA, et al. Assessment of the clinical usefulness of nebulized ipratropium bromide in patients with chronic airflow limitation. *Thorax.* 1984;39:272.

62. Gross NJ, Skorodin MS. Anticholinergic, antimuscarinic bronchodilators. *Am Rev Respir Dis.* 1984;129:856.

63. Fletcher T, Peto R, Tinker C, et al. *The Natural History of Chronic Obstructive Lung Disease in Working Men in London.* New York, NY: Oxford University Press; 1976.

64. Ferguson GT, Cherniack RM. Management of chronic obstructive pulmonary disease. *N Engl J Med.* 1993;328:1017.

65. Spika JS, Fedson DS, Facklam RR. Pneumococcal vaccination. Controversies and opportunities. *Infect Dis Clin North Am.* 1990;4:11.

66. Oh SH, Patterson R. Surgery in corticosteroid-dependent asthmatics. *J Allergy Clin Immunol.* 1974;53:345.

67. Benhamou D, Girault C, Faure C, et al. Nasal mask ventilation in acute respiratory failure. Experience in elderly patients. *Chest.* 1992;102:912.

68. Dompeling E, van Schack CP, van Grunsven PM, et al. Slowing the deterioration of asthma and chronic obstructive pulmonary disease observed during bronchodilator therapy by adding inhaled corticosteroids. A 4-year prospective study. *Ann Intern Med.* 1993;118:770.

69. van Schayck CP, Dompeling E, van Herwaarden CL, et al. Bronchodilator treatment in moderate asthma or chronic bronchitis: continuous or on demand? A randomized controlled study. *BMJ.* 1991;303:1426.

70. Muir JF, Godard PH, Verhaert, et al. Seventy-two hour comparison of methylprednisolone suleptanate and methylprednisolone sodium succinate in patients with acute asthma. *Br J Clin Pract.* 1996;50:440.

71. Thomas P, Pugsley JA, Steward JH. Theophylline and salbutamol improve pulmonary function in patients with irreversible chronic obstructive pulmonary disease. *Chest.* 1992;101:160.

72. Martin RJ, Pak J. Overnight theophylline concentrations and effects on sleep and lung function in chronic obstructive pulmonary disease. *Am Rev Respir Dis.* 1992;145:540.

73. Ziment I. Pharmacologic therapy of obstructive airway disease. *Clin Chest Med.* 1990;11:461.

74. Murciano D, Auclair MH, Pariente R, et al. A randomized, controlled trial of theophylline in patients with severe chronic obstructive pulmonary disease. *N Engl J Med.* 1989;320:1521.

75. Petty TL. The National Mucolytic Study. Results of a randomized, double-blind, placebo-controlled study of iodinated glycerol in chronic obstructive bronchitis. *Chest.* 1990;97:75.

76. Boman G, Backer U, Larsson S, et al. Oral acetylcysteine reduces exacerbation rate in chronic bronchitis: report of a trial organized by the Swedish Society for Pulmonary Disease. *Eur J Respir Dis.* 1983;64:405.

77. Wewers MD, Casolaro MA, Sellers SE, et al. Replacement therapy for alpha 1-antitrypsin deficiency associated with emphysema. *N Engl J Med.* 1987;316:1055.

78. Hubbard RC, Sellers S, Czerski D, et al. Biochemical efficacy and safety of monthly augmentation of therapy for alpha 1-antitrypsin deficiency. *JAMA.* 1988;260:1259.

79. McFadden ER Jr. Asthma. In: Fauci AS, Braunwald E, Isselbacher KJ,

et al, eds. *Harrison's Principles of Internal Medicine.* 14th ed. New York, NY: McGraw Hill; 1998:1419.

80. American Lung Association. The asthma survey: asthma fact sheet. Available at: http://www.lungusa.org/asthma/merck_fact.html. Accessed November 13, 2000.

81. Lozewicz S, Gomez E, Ferguson H, et al. Inflammatory cells in the airways in mild asthma. *BMJ.* 1988;297:1515.

82. Beasley R, Roche WR, Roberts JA, et al. Cellular events in the bronchi in mild asthma and after bronchial provocation. *Am Rev Respir Dis.* 1989;139:806.

83. Jeffery PK, Wardlaw AJ, Nelson FC, et al. Bronchial biopsies in asthma. An ultrastructural, quantitative study and correlation with hyperactivity. *Am Rev Respir Dis.* 1989;140:1745.

84. Soloperto M, Mattoso VL, Fasoli A, et al. A bronchial epithelial cell-derived factor in asthma that promotes eosinophil activation and survival as GM-CSF. *Am J Physiol.* 1991;260(6pt1):L530.

85. Sedgwick JB, Calhoun WJ, Gleich GJ, et al. Immediate and late airway response of allergic rhinitis patients to segmental antigen challenge. Characterization of eosinophil and mast cell mediators. *Am Rev Respir Dis.* 1991;144:1274.

86. Busse WW, Calhoune WF, Sedgwick JD. Mechanism of airway inflammation in asthma. *Am Rev Respir Dis.* 1993;147(6pt2):s20.

87. Keenan JM. Asthma management. The case for aiming at control rather than merely relief. *Postgrad Med.* 1998;103:53.

88. Wasserman SI. Mediators of immediate hypersensitivity. *J Allergy Clin Immunol.* 1983;72:101.

89. Kaliner M. Asthma and mast cell activation. *J Allergy Clin Immunol.* 1989;83(2pt2):510.

90. Drazen JM, Austen KF. Leukotrienes and airway responses. *Am Rev Respir Dis.* 1987;136:985.

91. Djukanovic R, Roche WR, Wilson JW, et al. Mucosal inflammation in asthma. *Am Rev Respir Dis.* 1990;142:434.

92. Leff AR, Hamann KJ, Wegner CD. Inflammation and cell-cell interactions in airway hyperresponsiveness. *Am J Physiol.* 1991; 260(4pt1):L260.

93. Barnes PJ. Neuropeptides and asthma. *Am Rev Respir Dis.* 1991;143 (3pt2):s28.

94. Laitinen LA, Heino M, Laitinen A, et al. Damage of the airway epithelium and bronchial reactivity in patients with asthma. *Am Rev Respir Dis.* 1985;131:599.

95. Bousquet J, Chanez P, Lacoste JY, et al. Eosinophilic inflammation in asthma. *N Engl J Med.* 1990;323:1033.

96. Wardlaw AJ, Dunnette S, Gleich GJ, et al. Eosinophils and mast cells in bronchoalveolar lavage in subjects with mild asthma. Relationship to bronchial hyperreactivity. *Am Rev Respir Dis.* 1988;137:62.

97. Adelroth E, Rosenhall L, Johansson SA, et al. Inflammatory cells and eosinophilic activity in asthmatics investigated by bronchoalveolar lavage. The effects of antiasthmatic treatment with budesonide or terbutaline. *Am Rev Respir Dis.* 1990;142:91.

98. National Asthma Education Program Expert Panel Report. *Guidelines for the Diagnosis and Management of Asthma.* Washington, DC: US Department of Health and Human Services; 1991:35. Report No. 01:3042.

99. Konig P, Godfrey S. Prevalence of exercise-induced bronchial lability in families of children with asthma. *Arch Dis Child.* 1973;48:513.

100. Deal EC Jr, McGadden ER Jr, Ingram RH Jr, et al. Airway responsiveness to cold air and hyperpnea in normal subjects and in those with hay fever and asthma. *Am Rev Respir Dis.* 1980;121:621.

101. Boulet LP, Cartier A, Thomson NC, et al. Asthma and increases in nonallergic bronchial responsiveness from seasonal pollen exposure. *J Allergy Clin Immunol.* 1983;71:399.

102. Cartier A, Thomson NC, Frith PA, et al. Allergen-induced increase in bronchial responsiveness to histamine: relationship to the late asthmatic response and change in airway caliber. *J Allergy Clin Immunol.* 1982;70:170.

103. Platts-Mills TA, Tovey ER, Mitchell EB, et al. Reduction of bronchial hyperreactivity during prolonged allergen avoidance. *Lancet.* 1982;2:675.

104. Holtzman MJ, Cunningham JH, Sheller JR, et al. Effect of ozone on bronchial reactivity in atopic and nonatopic subjects. *Am Rev Respir Dis.* 1979;120:1059.

105. Orehek J, Massari JP, Gayrad P, et al. Effect of short-term, low-level nitrogen dioxide exposure on bronchial sensitivity of asthmatic patients. *J Clin Invest.* 1976;57:301.

106. Sheppard D, Epstein J, Bethel RA, et al. Tolerance of sulfur dioxide-induced bronchoconstriction in subjects with asthma. *Environ Res.* 1983;30:412.

107. Empey DW, Laitinen LA, Jacobs L, et al. Mechanisms of bronchial hyperreactivity in normal subjects after upper respiratory tract infection. *Am Rev Respir Dis.* 1976;113:131.

108. Mussaffi H, Springer C, Godfrey S. Increased bronchial responsiveness to exercise and histamine after allergen challenge in children and asthma. *J Allergy Clin Immunol.* 1986;77(1pt1):48.

109. Thorpe JE, Steinberg D, Bernstein IL, et al. Bronchial reactivity increases soon after the immediate response in dual-responding asthmatic subjects. *Chest.* 1987;91:21.

110. Hargreave FE, Ryan G, Thomson NC, et al. Bronchial responsiveness to histamine or methacholine in asthma: measurement and clinical significance. *J Allergy Clin Immunol.* 1981;68:347.

111. Smolensky MH, Barnes PJ, Reinberg A, et al. Chronobiology and asthma, I: day-night differences in bronchial patency and dyspnea and circadian rhythm dependencies. *J Asthma.* 1986;23:321.

112. Hetzel MR, Clark TJ. Comparison of normal and asthmatic circadian rhythms in peak expiratory flow rate. *Thorax.* 1980;35:732.

113. Turner-Warwick M. Epidemiology of nocturnal asthma. *Am J Med.* 1988;85(1B):6.

114. American Thoracic Society. Guidelines for the evaluation of impairment/disability in patients with asthma. Medical Section of the American Lung Association. *Am Rev Respir Dis.* 1993;147:1056.

115. Juniper EF, Cockcroft DW, Hargreave FE. Histamine and methacholine inhalation tests: tidal breathing method. Laboratory procedure and standardization. *Canadian Thoracic Society Statement.* Lund, Sweden: AB Draco; 1991.

116. Cockcroft DW, Murdock KY. Comparative effects of inhaled salbutamol, sodium cromoglycate, and beclomethasone dipropionate on allergen-induced early asthmatic responses, late asthmatic responses, and increased bronchial responsiveness to histamine. *J Allergy Clin Immunol.* 1987;79:734.

117. Kraan J, Koeter GH, v d Mark TW, et al. Changes in bronchial hyperreactivity induced by 4 weeks of treatment with antiasthmatic drugs in patients with allergic asthma: a comparison between budesonide and terbutaline. *J Allergy Clin Immunol.* 1985;76:628.

118. Kerrebijn KF, van Essen-Zandvliet EE, Neijens HJ. Effect of long-term treatment with inhaled corticosteroids and beta-agonists on the bronchial responsiveness in children with asthma. *J Allergy Clin Immunol.* 1987;79:653.

119. Haahtela T, Jarvinen M, Kava T, et al. Comparison of a beta 2-agonist, terbutaline, with an inhaled corticosteroid, budesonide, in newly detected asthma. *N Engl J Med.* 1991;325:388.

120. Stiles GL, Caron MG, Lefkowitz RJ. Beta-adrenergic receptors: biochemical mechanisms of physiological regulation. *Physiol Rev.* 1984;64:661.

121. Santa Cruz R, Landa J, Hirsch J, et al. Tracheal mucous velocity in normal man and patients with obstructive lung disease: effects of terbutaline. *Am Rev Respir Dis.* 1974;109:458.

122. Basran GS, Paul W, Morley J, et al. Adrenoceptor-agonist inhibition of the histamine-induced cutaneous response in man. *Br J Dermatol.* 1982;107(suppl 23):140.

123. Rhoden KJ, Meldrum LA, Barnes PJ. Inhibition of cholinergic neurotransmission in human airways by beta 2-adrenoceptors. *J Appl Physiol.* 1988;65:700.

124. Leitch AG, Clancy LJ, Costello JF, et al. Effect of intravenous infusion of salbutamol on ventilatory response to carbon dioxide and hypoxia and on heart rate and plasma potassium in normal men. *BMJ.* 1976;1(6006):365.

125. Kallenbach J, Joffe BI, Zwi S, et al. Metabolic and cardiovascular effects of salbutamol in atopic subjects with and without asthma. *Scand J Respir Dis.* 1979;60:44.

126. Nogrady SG, Hartley JP, Seaton A. Metabolic effects of intravenous salbutamol in the course of acute severe asthma. *Thorax.* 1977;32:559.

127. McFadden ER Jr. Beta 2 receptor agonist: metabolism and pharmacology. *J Allergy Clin Immunol.* 1981;68:91.

128. Leslie D. Generalized allergic reaction to monocomponent insulin. *BMJ.* 1977;145:28.

129. Derom EY, Pauwels RA, Van der Straeten ME. The effect of inhaled salmeterol on methacholine responsiveness in subjects with asthma up to 12 hours. *J Allergy Clin Immunol.* 1992;89:811.

130. Nicklas RA. Current issues on asthma drugs: impact on clinical trial methodology. *J Asthma.* 1992;29:69.

131. Crane J, Pearce N, Flatt A, et al. Prescribed fenoterol and death from asthma in New Zealand, 1981-83: case-control study. *Lancet.* 1989;1:917.

132. Spitzer WO, Suissa S, Ernst P, et al. The use of beta-agonists and the risk of death and near death from asthma. *N Engl J Med.* 1992;326:501.

133. CSM Working Party. β-agonist use in asthma. Current Problems in Pharmacovigilance. 1992;33.

134. Cockcroft DW, Ruffin RE, Hargreave FE. Effect of Sch 1000 in allergen-induced asthma. *Clin Allergy.* 1978;8:361.

135. Howarth PH, Durham SR, Lee TH, et al. Influence of albuterol, cromolyn sodium and ipratropium bromide on the airway and circulating mediator responses to allergen bronchial provocation in asthma. *Am Rev Respir Dis.* 1985;132:986.

136. Shenfield GM. Combination bronchodilator therapy. *Drugs.* 1982;24:414.

137. Rafferty P, Tucker LG, Fergusson RJ, et al. Comparison of budesonide and beclomethasone dipropionate in patients with severe chronic asthma: assessment of relative prednisolone-sparing effects. *Br J Dis Chest.* 1985;79:244.

138. American Academy of Allergy and Immunology Study Group. Treatment of mild to moderate asthma: comparison of aerosolized beclomethasone and oral theophylline. *Am Acad Resp Dis.* 1991;143:A265.

139. Toogood JH, Jennings B, Greenway RW, et al. Candidiasis and dysphonia complicating beclomethasone treatment of asthma. *J Allergy Clin Immunol.* 1980;65:145.

140. Toogood JH. High-dose inhaled steroid therapy for asthma. *J Allergy Clin Immunol.* 1989;83(2pt2):528.

141. Salmeron S, Guerin JC, Godard P, et al. High dose of inhaled corticosteroids in unstable chronic asthma. A multicenter, double-blind, placebo-controlled study. *Am Rev Respir Dis.* 1989;140:167.

142. Malo JL, Cartier A, Merland N, et al. Four-times-a-day dosing frequency is better than a twice-a-day regimen in subjects requiring a high-dose inhaled steroid budesonide, to control moderate to severe asthma. *Am Rev Respir Dis.* 1989;140:624.

143. Pouw EM, Prummel MF, Oosting H, et al. Beclomethasone inhalation decreases serum osteocalcin concentrations. *BMJ.* 1991;302:677.

144. Wolthers OD, Pedersen S. Growth of asthmatic children during treatment with budesonide: a double blind trial. *BMJ.* 1991;303(6795):163.

145. Capewell S, Reynolds S, Shuttleworth D, et al. Purpura and dermal thinning associated with high dose inhaled corticosteroids. *BMJ.* 1990;300(6739):1548.

146. Kewley GD. Possible association between beclomethasone diproprionate aerosol and cataracts. *Aust Paediatr J.* 1980;16:117.

147. Smith MJ, Hodson ME. Effects of long-term inhaled high dose beclomethasone dipropionate on adrenal function. *Thorax.* 1983;38:676.

148. Law CM, Marchant JL, Honour JW, et al. Nocturnal adrenal suppression in asthmatic children taking inhaled beclomethasone dipropionate. *Lancet.* 1986;1(8487):942.

149. Baigelman W, Chodosh S, Pizzuto D, et al. Sputum and blood eosinophils during corticosteroid treatment of acute exacerbations of asthma. *Am J Med.* 1983;75:929.

150. Flower RJ. Eleventh Gaddum memorial lecture. Lipocortin and the mechanism of action of the glucocorticoids. *Br J Pharmacol.* 1988;94:987.

151. Djukanovic R, Wilson JW, Britten KM, et al. Effect of an inhaled corticosteroid on airway inflammation and symptoms in asthma. *Am Rev Respir Dis.* 1992;145:669.

152. Vathenen AS, Knox AJ, Wisniewski A, et al. Time course of change in bronchial reactivity with an inhaled corticosteroid in asthma. *Am Rev Respir Dis.* 1991;143:1317.

153. Kraan J, Koeter GH, van der Mark TW, et al. Dosage and time effects of inhaled budesonide on bronchial hyperreactivity. *Am Rev Respir Dis.* 1988;137:44.

154. Ellul-Micallef R, Fenech FF. Intravenous prednisolone in chronic bronchial asthma. *Thorax.* 1975;30:312.

155. McFadden ER Jr, Kiser R, deGroot WJ, et al. A controlled study of the effects of single doses of hydrocortisone on the resolution of acute attacks of asthma. *Am J Med.* 1976;60:52.

156. Molema J, Lammers JW, van Herwaarden CL, et al. Effects of inhaled beclomethasone dipropionate on beta 2-receptor function in the airways and adrenal responsiveness in bronchial asthma. *Eur J Clin Pharmacol.* 1988;34:577.

157. Brogden RN, Pinder RM, Sawyer PR, et al. Beclomethasone dipropionate inhaler: a review of its pharmacology, therapeutic value and adverse effects, I: asthma. *Drugs.* 1975;10:166.

158. Hendeles L, Weinberger M. Theophylline. A "state of the art" review. *Pharmacotherapy.* 1983;3:2.

159. Persson CG. Overview of effect of theophylline. *J Allergy Clin Immunol.* 1986;78(4pt2):780.

160. Svedmyr K. Beta 2-adrenoceptor stimulants and theophylline in asthma therapy. *Eur J Respir Dis Suppl.* 1981;116:1.

161. Weinberger M, Hendeles L. Experience with theophylline for the management of chronic asthma. *Eur J Respir Dis Suppl.* 1980;109:120.

162. Nassif EG, Weinberger M, Thompson R, et al. The value of maintenance theophylline in steroid-dependant asthma. *N Engl J Med.* 1981;304:71.

163. Rossing TH, Fanta CH, Goldstein DH, et al. Emergency therapy of asthma: comparison of the acute effects of parenteral and inhaled sympathomimetics and infused aminophylline. *Am Rev Respir Dis.* 1980;122:365.

164. Dutoit JL, Salome CM, Woolcock AJ. Inhaled corticosteroids reduce the severity of bronchial hyperresponsiveness in asthma but oral theophylline does not. *Am Rev Respir Dis.* 1987;136:1174.

165. Holgate ST, Finnerty JP. Antihistamines in asthma. *J Allergy Clin Immunol.* 1989;83(2pt2):537.

166. Rafferty P, Holgate ST. Histamine and its antagonists in asthma. *J Allergy Clin Immunol.* 1989;84:144.

167. Tinkleman DG, Webb CS, Vanderpool GE, et al. The use of ketotifen in the prophylaxis of seasonal allergic asthma. *Ann Allergy.* 1986;5:213.

168. Loftus BG, Price JF. Long-term, placebo-controlled trial of ketotifen in the management of preschool children with asthma. *J Allergy Clin Immunol.* 1987;79:350.

169. Busse WW, Gaddy JN. The role of leukotriene antagonists and inhibitors in the treatment of airway disease. *Am Rev Respir Dis.* 1991;143(5pt2):S103.

170. Israel E, Fischer AR, Rosenberg MA, et al. The pivotal role of 5-lipoxygenase products in the reaction of aspirin-sensitive asthmatics to aspirin. *Am Rev Respir Dis.* 1993;148(6pt1):1447.

171. *Dorland's Pocket Medical Dictionary.* 24th ed. Philadelphia, Pa: WB Saunders; 1989.

172. US Surgeon General. *The Health Consequence of Smoking: Chronic Obstructive Lung Disease.* Washington, DC: US Department of Health and Human Services; 1984. DHHA Publication No. 84-50205.

173. Sherrill DL, Lebowitz MD, Burrows B. Epidemiology of chronic obstructive pulmonary disease. *Clin Chest Med.* 1990;11:375.

175. Dockery DW, Speizer FE, Ferris BG Jr, et al. Cumulative and reversible effects of lifetime smoking on simple tests of lung function in adults. *Am Rev Respir Dis.* 1988;137:286.

176. Pearce AC, Jones RM. Smoking and anesthesia: preoperative abstinence and perioperative morbidity. *Anesthesiology.* 1984;61:576.

177. DeCamp MM, Demling RH. Posttraumatic multisystem organ failure. *JAMA.* 1988;260:530.

178. The Acute Respiratory Distress Syndrome Network. Ventilation with lower tidal volumes as compared with traditional tidal volumes for acute lung injury and the acute respiratory distress syndrome. *N Engl J Med.* 2000;342:1301.

179. Meduri GU, Headley AS, Golden E, et al. Effect of prolonged methylprednisolone therapy in unresolving acute respiratory distress syndrome: a randomized controlled trial. *JAMA.* 1998;280:159.

180. Latimer RG, Dickman M, Day WC, et al. Ventilatory patterns and pulmonary complications after upper abdominal surgery determined by preoperative and postoperative computerized spirometry and blood gas analysis. *Am J Surg.* 1971;122:622.

181. Gould AB. Effect of obesity on respiratory complications following general anesthesia. *Anesth Analg.* 1962;41:448.

182. Mohr DN, Jett JR. Preoperative evaluation of pulmonary risk factors. *J Gen Intern Med.* 1988;3:277.

183. Cummings JJ, D'Eugenio DB, Gross SJ. A controlled trial of dexamethasone in preterm infants at high risk for bronchopulmonary dysplasia. *N Engl J Med.* 1989;320:1505.

184. Cloutier MM. Nebulized steroid therapy in bronchopulmonary dysplasia. *Pediatr Pulmonol.* 1993;15:111.

185. Dunn JS. The effects of multiple embolism of pulmonary arterioles. *QJM.* 1920;13:129.

186. Binger CA, Moore RL. Changes in carbon dioxide tension and hydrogen ion concentration of the blood following multiple pulmonary embolism. *J Exp Med.* 1927;45:633.

187. Meakins J, Davies HW. Observations on the gases in human arterial and venous blood. *J Pathol Bacteriol.* 1920;23:451.

188. Suter PM, Fairley B, Isenberg MD. Optimum end-expiratory airway pressure in patients with acute pulmonary failure. *N Engl J Med.* 1975;292:284.

189. Stoelting RK, Dierdorf SF. *Anesthesia and Co-Existing Disease.* 3rd ed. New York, NY: Churchill Livingstone; 1993.

190. Gol MK, Karahan M, Ulus AT, et al. Bloodstream, respiratory, and deep surgical wound infections after open heart surgery. *J Card Surg.* 1998;13:252.

191. Kollef MH. The roles of selective digestive tract decontamination on

mortality and respiratory tract infections. A meta-analysis. *Chest.* 1994;105:1101.

192. Cardenosa Cendrero JA, Sole-Violan J, Bordes Benitez A, et al. Role of different routes of tracheal colonization in the development of pneumonia in patients receiving mechanical ventilation. *Chest.* 1999;116:462.

193. Mitchell C, Garrahy P, Peake P. Postoperative respiratory morbidity: identification and risk factors. *Aust N Z J Surg.* 1982;52:203.

194. Ephgrave KS, Kleiman-Wexler R, Pfaller M, et al. Postoperative pneumonia: a prospective study of risk factors and morbidity. *Surgery.* 1993;114:815.

195. Ford GT, Rosenal TW, Clergue F, et al. Respiratory physiology in upper abdominal surgery. *Clin Chest Med.* 1993;14:237.

196. Celli BR. Perioperative respiratory care of the patient undergoing upper abdominal surgery. *Clin Chest Med.* 1993;14:253.

197. Merli GJ, Weitz HH. Approaching the surgical patient. Role of the medical consultant. *Clin Chest Med.* 1993;14:205.

198. American Thoracic Society. Standards for the diagnosis and care of patients with chronic obstructive pulmonary disease. American Thoracic Society. *Am J Respir Crit Care Med.* 1995;152(5pt2):s77.

199. MacFayden BV Jr, Wolfe BM, McKernan JB. Laparoscopic management of the acute abdomen, appendix, and small and large bowel. *Surg Clin North Am.* 1992;72:1169.

200. Juno J, Marsh HM, Knopp TJ, et al. Closing capacity in awake and anesthetized-paralyzed man. *J Appl Physiol.* 1978;44:238.

201. Bergman NA, Tien YK. Contribution of the closure of pulmonary units to impaired oxygenation during anesthesia. *Anesthesiology.* 1983;59:395.

202. Gilmour I, Burnham M, Craig DB. Closing capacity measurement during general anesthesia. *Anesthesiology.* 1976;45:477.

203. Ali J, Weisal RD, Layug AB, et al. Consequences of postoperative alterations in respiratory mechanics. *Am J Surg.* 1974;128:376.

204. Meyers JR, Lembeck L, O'Kane H, et al. Changes in functional residual capacity of the lung after operation. *Arch Surg.* 1975;110:576.

205. Vaughan RW, Wise L. Choice of abdominal operative incision in the obese patient: a study using blood gas measurements. *Ann Surg.* 1975;181:829.

206. Craig DB. Postoperative recovery of pulmonary function. *Anesth Analg.* 1981;60:46.

207. Bastin R, Moraine JJ, Bardocsky G, et al. Incentive spirometry performance. A reliable indicator of pulmonary function in the early postoperative period after lobectomy? *Chest.* 1997;111:559.

208. Buist AS. New test to assess lung function. The single-breath nitrogen test. *N Engl J Med.* 1975;293:438.

209. Closing volume. *Lancet.* 1972;2(7783):908.

210. Muravchick S. Anesthesia for the elderly. In: Miller RD, ed. *Anesthesia.* 3rd ed. New York, NY: Churchill Livingstone; 1990:1969.

211. Rehder K, Marsh HM, Rodarte JR, et al. Airway obstruction. *Anesthesiology.* 1977;47:40.

212. Alexander JI, Spence AA, Parikh RK, et al. The role of airway closure in postoperative hypoxaemia. *Br J Anaesth.* 1973;45:34.

213. Simonneau G, Vivien A, Sartene R, et al. Diaphragm dysfunction induced by upper abdominal surgery: role of postoperative pain. *Am Rev Respir Dis.* 1983;128:899.

214. Pedersen T, Viby-Mogensen J, Ringsted C. Anaesthetic practice and postoperative pulmonary complications. *Acta Anaesthesiol Scand.* 1992;36:812.

215. Lawrence VA, Page CP, Harris GD. Preoperative spirometry before abdominal operations. A critical appraisal of its predictive value. *Arch Intern Med.* 1989;149:280.

216. Dilworth JP, White RJ. Postoperative chest infection after upper abdominal surgery: an important problem for smokers. *Respir Med.* 1992;86:205.

217. Jayr C, Matthay MA, Goldstone J, et al. Preoperative and intraoperative factors associated with prolonged mechanical ventilation. A study in patients following major abdominal vascular surgery. *Chest.* 1993;103:1231.

218. Law SY, Folk M, Wong J. Risk analysis in resection of squamous cell carcinoma of the esophagus. *World J Surg.* 1994;18:339.

219. Hennessey TPJ. Respiratory complications in oesophageal surgery. In: Peracchia A, Rosati R, Bonavina L, eds. *Recent Advances in Diseases of the Esophagus.* Milan, Italy: Monduzzi Editore; 1996:537.

220. Ferguson MK, Martin TR, Reeder LB. Determinants of pulmonary complications following esophagectomy. In: Peracchia A, Rosati R, Bonavina L, eds. *Recent Advances in Diseases of the Esophagus.* Milan, Italy: Monduzzi Editore; 1996:527.

221. Stark SP, Romberg MS, Pierce GE, et al. Transhiatal versus transthoracic esophagectomy for adenocarcinoma of the distal esophagus and cardia. *Am J Surg.* 1996;172:478.

222. Ferguson MK, Martin TR, Reeder LB, et al. Mortality after esophagectomy: risk factor analysis. *World J Surg.* 1997;21:599.

223. Bartels H, Stein HJ, Siewert JR. Early extubation vs prolonged ventilation after esophagectomy: a randomised prospective study. In: Peracchia A, Rosati R, Bonavina L, eds. *Recent Advances in Diseases of the Esophagus.* Milan, Italy: Monduzzi Editore; 1996:537.

224. Marshall MC, Olsen GN. The physiologic evaluation of the lung resection candidate. *Clin Chest Med.* 1993;14:305.

225. Olsen GN. The evolving role of exercise testing prior to lung resection. *Chest.* 1989;95:218.

226. Ferguson MK, Reeder LB, Mick R. Optimizing selection of patients for major lung resection. *J Thorac Cardiovasc Surg.* 1995;109:275.

227. Hammermeister KE, Burchfiel C, Johnson R, et al. Identification of patients at greatest risk for developing major complications at cardiac surgery. *Circulation.* 1990;82(5 suppl):IV380.

228. Shapira N, Zabatino SM, Ahmed S, et al. Determinants of pulmonary function in patients undergoing coronary bypass operations. *Ann Thorac Surg.* 1990;50:268.

229. Berrizbeitia LD, Tessler S, Jacobwitz IJ, et al. Effect of sternotomy and coronary bypass surgery on postoperative pulmonary mechanics. Comparison of internal mammary and saphenous vein bypass grafts. *Chest.* 1989;96:873.

230. Efthimiou J, Butler J, Woodham C, et al. Diaphragm paralysis following cardiac surgery: role of phrenic nerve cold injury. *Ann Thorac Surg.* 1991;52:1005.

231. Taggart DP, el-Fiky M, Carter R, et al. Respiratory dysfunction after uncomplicated cardiopulmonary bypass. *Ann Thorac Surg.* 1993; 56:1123.

232. Matthay MA, Wiener-Kronish JP. Respiratory management after cardiac surgery. *Chest.* 1989;95:424.

CHAPTER

# 10

# Neurologic Consultation

Diane Solomon
Dale E. Solomon
Jerry J. Tomasovic

*How Does Nerve Injury Present?*

*What Should Be Done After a Potential Nerve Injury Is Discovered?*

*What Is the Prognosis?*

*What Therapy Is Available?*

*What Nerve Injuries Are Common in Pregnancy?*

## NEUROLOGIC COMPLICATIONS AFTER SPINAL OR EPIDURAL ANESTHESIA

*Why Do They Occur?*

## POSTANESTHETIC NEUROLOGIC EXAMINATION

*When Should the Anesthesiologist Become Concerned About Delayed Awakening?*

*How Should Evaluation Proceed?*

## POSTOPERATIVE DELIRIUM

*What Are the Causes?*

## POSTISCHEMIC/HYPOXIC BRAIN INJURY

*What Can Be Done?*

*Can Outcome Be Predicted After Cardiac Arrest?*

*How Is Brain Death Diagnosed?*

## POSTOPERATIVE HEADACHE

*What Diagnostic Work-Up Is Reasonable?*

## CONCLUSION

Patients with neurologic disease present unique challenges to anesthesiologists in the perioperative period. Many neurologic diseases are rare and are even more rarely encountered in the operating room, yet they have associated manifestations that require specific knowledge for optimal perioperative management. A neurologist as consultant can provide assistance in the perioperative period by doing the following:

1. Preoperatively identifying and optimizing medical management of neurologic disorders
2. Providing advice about perioperative management of patients with specific neurologic diseases
3. Performing intraoperative electrophysiologic assessments
4. Diagnosing and treating postoperative sequelae and complications

The intent of this chapter is to provide answers to questions that anesthesiologists might commonly ask a neurologist and to share with neurologists the unique challenges that an anesthesiologist encounters while caring for patients with neurologic disease.

## THE PERIOPERATIVE NEUROLOGIC CONSULTATION

### What Are the Components of an Effective Consultation?

An effective neurologic consultation (Table 10–1) begins with a clear communication of the questions the consultant

**TABLE 10–1.** Effective Consultation Requirements

Direct contact between the consulting and consultant physicians
Limited number of recommendations
Emphasis on high-priority recommendations
Specification of drug, dosage, route, and duration
Continued follow-up and repeated offering of recommendations

needs to address. When the question is ill defined or nebulous, the resultant assessment and recommendations are also likely to be vague. Even when the cause of the problem is unknown, a directed question can be formulated. For example, "Does this patient have a reversible neurologic condition?" is a better consult request than "Please see postoperative patient in coma."

Next, the degree of urgency must be adequately communicated to the consultant. Thus, a patient in status epilepticus represents a more urgent problem than does a work-up of a perioperative nerve injury.

The consultant then gathers data (history, physical examination, diagnostic tests) to formulate an opinion. Ideally, data gathering and interpretation of findings by the consultant are performed independently to remove the bias of previous examinations and assessments. A neurologist's skill in taking detailed histories and performing expert neurologic examinations is extremely important at this point.

Finally, the consultant communicates his or her assessment and recommendations to the physician requesting the consult. This communication should be brief, specific to the question, diplomatic, and timely. The recommendations should include contingency plans for courses that the disease process is likely to take as well as subsequent tests that might be needed during the perioperative period. Follow-up by the consultant can ensure that potential new problems are adequately addressed.[1]

The spectrum of circumstances for which a neurologic consultation might be requested is summarized in Table 10–2.

### What Should a Routine Preoperative Neurologic Evaluation Comprise?

#### Preexisting Disease

First, the presence of known preexisting disease should be well documented, with particular attention to the disease duration, current manifestations, drug therapy, physical examination findings, and laboratory data that substantiate the diagnosis. Whenever inconsistencies are noted between the current findings and the presumed diagnosis, further investigation is needed. In addition, careful testing of disabilities immediately before surgery allows more accurate postanesthetic assessment of neurologic dysfunction.

#### Absence of Known Disease

##### History

For patients without known neurologic diseases, a screening history and physical examination detect most neurologic diseases that have important anesthetic consequences. Every patient should be specifically questioned about a history of headache, loss of consciousness, weakness, and focal neurologic symptoms such as transient monocular blindness, diplopia, numbness, and dysphagia.

**Preoperative Diagnosis of Neurologic Signs or Symptoms**

Headache
Spells
Transient or chronic focal symptoms
Weakness
Movement disorder
Altered mental status

**Preoperative Assessment of Chronic Disease**

Poorly controlled seizures
Myasthenia gravis
Pseudotumor cerebri
Parkinson's disease
Multiple sclerosis
Muscular dystrophy
Symptomatic carotid disease

**Intraoperative Monitoring of Neurologic Function**

Electroencephalography or evoked responses for cerebral ischemia
Somatosensory evoked responses for spine surgery
Brainstem auditory evoked responses for posterior fossa surgery
Electromyography and nerve conduction velocity for cranial or peripheral nerve monitoring

**Postoperative Complications**

Failure to awaken, coma
Delirium, encephalopathy
New focal neurologic sign or nerve injury
Headache
Seizure
Brain death determination

---

Headache may denote tumor or other mass lesions, increased intracranial pressure (ICP), hydrocephalus, intracranial aneurysm, or arteriovenous malformation.

Loss of consciousness, described as fainting or blackouts, may indicate cardiovascular disease or a seizure disorder. Weakness, when diffuse, may suggest the presence of neuromuscular diseases (eg, muscular dystrophy [MD], myasthenia gravis, or a polyneuropathy), endocrine disorders, or metabolic disorders. Unilateral episodes of weakness are most often associated with stroke, transient ischemic attack (TIA), or spinal root disease.

Finally, focal neurologic symptoms may be due to various central and peripheral neurologic diseases and may indicate that further neurologic evaluation is necessary.

### Physical Findings

Patients with identified and unstable disease or new symptoms or who are undergoing procedures that place them at risk for postoperative neurologic dysfunction should undergo more in-depth evaluation, perhaps by a neurologist.

## MYASTHENIA GRAVIS

### What Factors Are Important in Preoperative Evaluation?

Myasthenia gravis is caused by autoantibodies against nicotinic acetylcholine receptors in the neuromuscular junction, resulting in weakness and easy fatigability.[2] All muscles can be affected, but those of most concern to an anesthesiologist are the pharyngeal/laryngeal muscles protecting the airway

and the muscles of respiration. These muscles must be assessed by testing the gag reflex, the ability to handle secretions, and the force of cough. Most patients should undergo pulmonary function studies to help anticipate the need for postoperative ventilatory assistance. Predictors of the need for postoperative mechanical ventilation include a duration of the disease >6 years, a history of chronic respiratory disease, pyridostigmine dose >750 mg/day, and vital capacity <2.9 L.[3] More recently, multivariate discriminant analysis has identified the forced vital capacity, midmaximal expiratory flow, forced expiratory flow (midexpiratory phase), and the patient's gender as variables that predict the need for postoperative ventilatory support.[4]

### Drug Therapy

Accurate documentation of baseline strength is important. If a patient is weak, drug therapy should be maximized before elective surgery. Anticholinesterase drugs are used to prevent metabolism of acetylcholine at the neuromuscular junction. The most frequently used is pyridostigmine (Mestinon) at doses averaging 60 mg orally every 4 to 6 hours. If the disease is not controlled with pyridostigmine, steroids are usually added. However, approximately 8% of cases of myasthenia gravis transiently worsen when steroid therapy is initiated.

Immunosuppressive agents are used in severe myasthenia or if the response to steroids is inadequate. A full response to steroids or chemotherapeutic agents may take weeks to months. Plasmapheresis may provide the most rapid improvement in poorly controlled cases. When pheresis was provided 1 to 4 times at 2 to 13 days before thymectomy in patients with severe myasthenia, the need for postoperative mechanical ventilation, time to extubation, and length of stay in the intensive care unit all decreased.[5]

### Associated Diseases

A search for frequently associated diseases, including thyroid disease, rheumatoid arthritis, systemic lupus erythematosus, and pernicious anemia, should be made.

### How Is the Patient Managed Perioperatively?

Preoperative sedation is titrated carefully because narcotics and benzodiazepines can affect respiratory and neuromuscular function. Most antibiotics except penicillins and cephalosporins can exacerbate weakness. Preoperative anticholinesterase medications are continued until the day of surgery. Patients treated with steroids should receive perioperative coverage.

Awake intubation or rapid sequence induction with cricoid pressure is used in patients with bulbar involvement. Use of succinylcholine is avoided because patients are resistant to it, it has the potential for phase II blockade, and its action is prolonged because of anticholinesterase therapy. In most cases, tracheal intubation can be performed without pharmacologically induced muscle relaxation, often with deep inhalation anesthesia alone.[6–8]

Drugs (eg, magnesium, local anesthetics, cardiac antidysrhythmics) and other factors (hypothermia, respiratory acidosis) that can potentiate nondepolarizing muscle relaxants should be avoided. Patients may be extremely sensitive to nondepolarizing muscle relaxants. When further muscle relaxation is needed, small doses of nondepolarizing relaxants can be titrated with monitoring of neuromuscular blockade. Atracurium appears to be the relaxant of choice.[9] Rocuronium at one fourth the usual dose has been used successfully.[10]

Reversal of nondepolarizing muscle relaxants is performed in a titrated fashion with 1 to 2 mg of neostigmine every 5 minutes to avoid anticholinergic overdose, resultant cholinergic crisis, and an increase in weakness.

## What Are the Postoperative Concerns?

If a patient is unable to resume oral pyridostigmine, it can be given intravenously at approximately one-thirtieth of the oral dose.[11] In the past, a Tensilon test frequently was performed in the postoperative period to distinguish cholinergic toxicity from worsening primary myasthenic weakness. Edrophonium (Tensilon) is a short-acting and rapid acting anticholinesterase that improves weakness in myasthenic patients except in cases of excessive anticholinesterase medication. In the latter circumstance, the cholinergic effect of edrophonium causes increased weakness.

Because most neurologists no longer use large doses of pyridostigmine and anesthesiologists limit their use of cholinergic drugs, cholinergic crisis is now uncommon as a cause of worsening weakness. Unless large doses of neostigmine are given as a muscle relaxant reversal, the Tensilon test is usually unnecessary. If patients are difficult to wean after restarting anticholinesterase therapy, plasmapheresis is begun. Protocols vary, but most begin with a whole volume plasma exchange each day for 2 to 3 days, followed by alternate-day exchanges, depending on the clinical response. Postoperative pain control can be problematic. For postoperative analgesia, intrathecal morphine has been reported to cause less diminution of pulmonary function than intravenous morphine.[12]

## PARKINSON'S DISEASE

## Which Organ Systems Can Be Affected?

Depletion of dopamine in the striatonigral pathways of the basal ganglia causes the neurologic manifestations of Parkinson's disease: tremor, rigidity, bradykinesia, and impairment of postural and righting reflexes. Autonomic dysfunction results in orthostatic hypotension, impaired thermoregulation, and labile hemodynamics during anesthesia. There is a tendency toward dementia, delirium, and psychosis.[13]

Pharyngeal/laryngeal muscle dysfunction may place patients with Parkinson's disease at an increased risk for aspiration. In addition, difficulty in eating and swallowing may affect the blood volume and nutritional status. Restrictive pulmonary disease results from rigidity and bradykinesia of the respiratory muscles and spinal kyphosis. Preoperative pulmonary function studies, arterial blood gas analysis, and pulmonary teaching are often recommended.

## What Are the Medical Treatments?

Early Parkinson's disease may require no treatment. Selegiline hydrochloride is a monoamine oxidase B (MAOB) inhibitor, often begun early in the course of the disease because of a probable neuroprotective effect. It achieves benefit by reducing oxidative stress.[14] It is metabolized to amphetamine derivatives and also has a minor symptomatic treatment role. Anticholinergics may relieve the pill-rolling rest tremor typical of Parkinson's disease, and amantadine is an antiviral agent that improves bradykinesia and rigidity.[15] Both tend to be used to greatest benefit earlier in the course of the disease. Cognitive side effects can be significant, particularly in the elderly and in combination with other medications.

Carbidopa-levodopa (Sinemet) is the most effective and most frequently used drug to treat Parkinson's disease.[16] Bradykinesia, rigidity, and rest tremors improve with levodopa. Side effects include nausea, dyskinesias, and hallucinations, especially when levodopa is combined with other antiparkinsonian medications. It can sensitize the myocardium to arrhythmias and cause hypotension.[17,18] A long-acting form of carbidopa-levodopa is available and is helpful for patients with end-of-dose motor fluctuations or those requiring frequent dosing.

Dopamine agonists are traditionally used as adjunctive treatment to levodopa when wearing-off fluctuations develop. More recently, dopamine agonists have been used as primary monotherapy in Parkinson's disease. This approach has the advantage of delaying the use of levodopa and onset of the dyskinesias that ultimately occur with its use. The dopamine agonists include bromocriptine, pergolide, ropinirole, and pramipexole.[19]

Catechol-$O$-methyltransferase (COMT) and dopa decarboxylase are the enzymes that metabolize levodopa. Entacapone extends the effects of carbidopa-levodopa by blocking COMT.[20,21] Prolonging levodopa reduces or prevents end-of-dose wearing-off. Dyskinesias, diarrhea, and orange discoloration of the urine can occur. MAO inhibitors should not be used with entacapone. The exception is selegiline, which has been shown to be safe at doses ≤10 mg/day. Potentiation may occur if other drugs metabolized by COMT, such as isoproterenol, epinephrine, norepinephrine, dopamine, dobutamine, methyldopa, apomorphine, isoetharine, and bitolterol, are used with entacapone.[22]

## What Are the Surgical Treatments?

For patients with advanced Parkinson's disease who become resistant to medical therapy, three surgical approaches are used: ablative surgery, deep brain stimulation, and restorative therapy.

### Ablative Surgery

Ablative surgery of the globus pallidus reduces tremor, rigidity, bradykinesia, and the dyskinesias induced by levodopa.[23] The benefit occurs contralateral to the side on which the precise lesion is made. Thalamotomy reduces only tremor of the limbs on the opposite side.[24] Risk of intracerebral hemorrhage is 2% to 4%.[25] If ablative surgery is performed bilaterally, there is a risk of worsening of speech and cognitive function.

### Deep Brain Stimulation

Deep brain stimulation is a relatively nondestructive way to block the activity of the target brain tissue. High-frequency stimulating electrodes are placed in the nucleus ventralis intermedius of the thalamus, the internal segment of the globus pallidus, or the subthalamic nucleus.[26-30] At this time, only deep brain stimulation of the thalamus is approved by the US Food and Drug Administration (FDA). Stimulation parameters are adjustable, and bilateral stimulation does not cause cognitive problems.[31]

## Restorative Therapies

Restorative therapies refer to the experimental transplantation of fetal cells and growth factor infusion. The goal is to replace the lost dopaminergic brain cells or promote survival of these cells.[32] So far, none of the restorative therapies under investigation appears to offer as much consistent improvement in parkinsonian symptoms as lesion surgery or deep brain stimulation.

## *What Are the Anesthetic Considerations?*

Carbidopa-levodopa and other antiparkinsonian medications should be given preoperatively with a sip of water. When the pharyngeal/laryngeal musculature is affected, rapid sequence induction with cricoid pressure is used. Moderated doses of cardiodepressant anesthetics are used because of altered homeostatic adrenergic responses to hypotension. Succinylcholine was reported in one case to cause hyperkalemia.[33] Normal responses to nondepolarizing muscle relaxants have been reported.[34]

Antidopaminergic drugs such as metoclopramide, droperidol, and chlorpromazine should be avoided. Selegiline should not be used with the narcotic meperidine because of the possibility of a severe adverse reaction of agitation, stupor, muscle rigidity, and hyperthermia.[35] An acute dystonic reaction after alfentanil in a patient with untreated Parkinson's disease has been reported.[36]

Regional anesthetic techniques can be used, but positioning may be difficult. Patients should be awake, and special attention should be given to verification of intact or at least baseline pharyngeal/laryngeal reflexes and adequate pulmonary function before extubation.

Withdrawal of carbidopa-levodopa in the postoperative period can cause severe exacerbation of symptoms. Therapy should be restarted as soon as possible to prevent irreversible rigidity and bradykinesia. In patients who are unable to take medications orally or by gastric tube, parenterally administered anticholinergic drugs such as trihexyphenidyl, benztropine, or diphenhydramine can be administered.

Other postoperative care is centered on pulmonary toilet and prevention of thromboses and, most important, early physical therapy and ambulation. Postoperative delirium is not uncommon and may be due to preexisting dysfunction, intravenous anticholinergics, or medication withdrawal.[37]

Ablative procedures and deep brain stimulation are almost always carried out under local anesthesia. The use of intravenous low-dose narcotics for pain and glycopyrrolate to prevent bradycardia is part of the anesthetic conduct, as well as patient monitoring for blood pressure (BP), heart rate, electrocardiogram (ECG), and pulse oximetry.

**TABLE 10–3.** Perioperative Stroke Risk

| Surgery | Incidence (%) | Range (%) |
|---|---|---|
| General | 0.2 | 0.1–0.4 |
| Peripheral vascular | 1.5 | 1–2 |
| Cardiac | 4 | 1–6 |
| Carotid artery | 4 | 1–8 |

Data from Lee T, Goldman L. Role of the consultant. In: Breslow M, Miller C, Rogers M, eds. *Perioperative Management.* St Louis, Mo: CV Mosby; 1990:49, and Landercasper J, Merz BJ, Cogbill TH, et al. Perioperative stroke risk in 173 consecutive patients with a past history of stroke. *Arch Surg.* 1990;125:986.

# STROKE

## *What Is the Risk?*

Perioperative stroke risk depends on the type of surgery. Cumulative data indicate that stroke incidence ranges from as low as 0.2% for patients undergoing general surgery to 4% in patients having cardiac or carotid surgery (Table 10–3). If patients with a history of cerebrovascular disease are excluded, the risk of stroke in adults undergoing general surgery decreases by more than half. Additional risk predictors include peripheral vascular disease, hypertension, atrial fibrillation, and possibly age >70 years[38,39] (Table 10–4).

## *What Preventive Strategies May Be Used?*

### Preoperative

Treatment of coronary artery disease, atrial fibrillation, and hypertension should be optimized before surgery. New atrial fibrillation should be converted to normal sinus rhythm, if possible, or the ventricular rate should be well controlled in chronic atrial fibrillation. Guidelines have been generated by an expert consensus panel[40] recommending that most patients with atrial fibrillation be treated with oral anticoagulation (target international normalized ratio [INR] 2.0-3.0).[41] Chronic anticoagulation is currently the widely endorsed therapy for all patients with atrial fibrillation who are >75 years (approximately half of patients with atrial fibrillation) and a large fraction of younger patients with atrial fibrillation with risk factors who can safely receive warfarin. Risk factors (in addition to age >75 years) are hypertension, prior stroke or TIA, and poor left ventricular function.[42]

Asymptomatic carotid stenosis probably does not warrant carotid endarterectomy (CEA) based on recent evidence.[43] Approximately half the strokes that occur in the territory of an asymptomatic carotid artery are not caused by large artery

**TABLE 10–4.** Predictors of Perioperative Stroke

| Predictor | Relative Risk |
|---|---|
| Prior stroke/transient ischemic attack | 20 |
| Peripheral vascular surgery | 8 |
| Atrial fibrillation | 4 |
| Advanced age | ? |

Data from Larsen SF, Zaric D, Boysen G. Postoperative cerebrovascular accidents in general surgery. *Acta Anaesthesiol Scand.* 1988;32:698, and Hart RG, Easton JD. Management of cervical bruits and carotid stenosis in preoperative patients. *Stroke.* 1983;14:290.

occlusion but are cardioembolic or of small vessel disease origin. The low risk of large artery stroke in asymptomatic patients (in contrast to symptomatic patients) does not justify the risk of carotid surgery. Preoperative management should focus on identifying and treating other stroke risk factors in these patients.

The cause of past strokes and TIAs should be determined. This work-up includes a computed tomographic (CT) scan of the brain to rule out intracerebral hemorrhage or subdural hematoma; carotid screening with carotid ultrasonography/Doppler; and cardiac monitoring with echocardiography, if a patient has a history of coronary artery disease, valvular heart disease, or cardiac dysrhythmias. In patients with known atrial fibrillation or those considered at high risk for emboli of cardiac origin (large left atrial size, stroke in posterior cerebral artery territory), a transesophageal echocardiogram should be considered if a transthoracic echocardiogram is nonrevealing.[44] Unlike transesophageal echocardiography, transthoracic echocardiography does not easily visualize the left atrium, and clots often are missed.

Preventive therapy is directed by the stroke's cause. If carotid ultrasonography or Doppler identifies stenosis of ≥70% on the symptomatic side of the stroke or TIA, angiography anticipating CEA should be done before elective surgery.[45] Noncardioembolic strokes without significant carotid disease are primarily treated with antiplatelet agents. Aspirin, extended-release dipyridamole-aspirin combination, clopidogrel, and ticlopidine have been shown significantly to reduce stroke.[46] Ticlopidine is associated with a 1% risk of neutropenia and requires biweekly complete blood cell counts (CBCs) with differentiation for at least 3 months.[47]

If a cardiac thrombus is identified, sodium warfarin is usually given for a minimum of 3 months and then as indicated by repeat echocardiogram. Patients with atrial fibrillation and stroke should be treated with lifelong warfarin.

### Intraoperative

Intraoperative stroke prevention involves BP control and optimal oxygen transport. Most strokes occur postoperatively and are not a result of intraoperative hypotension even in the presence of carotid occlusive disease.[48] An exception to this observation is that intraoperative hypotension may have a role in stroke during aortic surgery. These patients have a high likelihood of carotid disease, and transient acute hypotension is common at the time of vessel clamp release, thus increasing the risk of stroke.[38]

It is commonly recommended that mean perfusion pressure be maintained at >50 mm Hg in patients with significant occlusive carotid disease. However, no controlled, prospective studies address this issue. A transcranial Doppler study showed that when mean arterial pressure was kept >60 mm Hg, blood flow velocity was maintained despite severe unilateral stenosis.[49] However, Brusino and colleagues[50] found no difference in cerebral blood flow in a patient with >80% bilateral carotid stenosis at mean arterial pressures of 35 and 85 mm Hg. Cerebral autoregulation appears to remain intact over a wide range of pressures despite old age and severe cerebrovascular disease if a vasoconstrictor is used to increase the mean arterial pressure and thereby the cerebral perfusion pressure.

## What Is the Acute Treatment of Perioperative Stroke?

If stroke occurs, emergent CT is indicated to rule out intracerebral hemorrhage. Vital signs are initially followed every 15 minutes and the head is elevated 30°. Important laboratory values include glucose, chemistry, CBC, INR, and partial thromboplastin time. ECG or cardiac monitoring is appropriate, and a chest radiograph is obtained to identify neurogenic pulmonary edema and aspiration pneumonia. Euvolemia is the goal. Because 5% dextrose and water is hypoosmolar, it should be avoided. No food or liquid is given orally until the risk for aspiration has been assessed. Anticonvulsants are not begun prophylactically, but they are given for observed seizures or subclinical seizures identified by electroencephalography (EEG) in the comatose patient.[51]

### Hypertension

Relative hypotension (eg, BP 100/60 mm Hg), normally well tolerated by the brain with intact autoregulation, causes the ischemic penumbra to progress to infarction. Therefore, physicians should avoid overzealous treatment of mild to moderate hypertension in the days immediately after ischemic stroke (for up to 6 weeks).[52]

Perfusion pressure plays a substantial role in the development of ischemia and infarction. The threshold below which it is unsafe to lower mean arterial pressure in the setting of acute stroke is unknown and is likely related to the baseline "set point" of an individual patient. Multiple reports of symptomatic deterioration with lowering BP in the acute phase of stroke have led to the general acceptance of not treating routine hypertension in acute ischemic stroke. For patients who are not candidates for therapy with tissue plasminogen activator (TPA), a thrombolytic agent that dissolves clots, it is recommended that BP not be treated unless the diastolic pressure is >120 and the systolic >220 mm Hg. Treating at a lower BP threshold may be necessary if there is associated myocardial ischemia or dissecting aortic aneurysm. A hyperperfusion syndrome with brain hemorrhage and swelling is a known complication of untreated hypertension after revascularization procedures such as CEA and may occur with TPA.[53] Treatment of elevated BP in patients with acute ischemic stroke receiving TPA is more aggressive than that recommended for patients with ischemic stroke in general.[54]

Agents that are easily titrated and predictable should be used to avoid uncontrolled, prolonged hypotension. Intravenous labetalol is often used, except in patients with asthma, acute congestive heart failure, or atrioventricular conduction block. Intravenous enalapril is a slow onset alternative, and nitroprusside is easily titratable. Sublingual nifedipine is avoided because of its association with precipitous drops in BP and the inability carefully to titrate the appropriate dose. When the diastolic BP is >120 mm Hg or the systolic BP is >220 mm Hg, decreasing these values by 15% in the first 24 hours is an appropriate goal for many patients.[55]

### Oxygenation in Acute Stroke

A pulse oximeter is used to monitor oxygen saturation in patients with acute stroke, with the $Pao_2$ kept at >95%. Cheyne-Stokes respiration has been thought typically to accompany bilateral or deep brain damage. However, it occurs in over half of all patients with stroke, in both unilateral supratentorial and infratentorial lesions. This nonspecific breathing pattern is associated with relative decreases in oxygen saturation that may harm tissue in the ischemic penumbra, and supplemental oxygen may be beneficial.[56]

Sleep apnea occurs with high frequency in patients in the acute phase of stroke and should be considered in patients with habitual snoring, decreased oxygen saturation, or severe stroke.[57]

### Glucose Management

Hyperglycemia is believed to harm tissue in the ischemic penumbra by promoting lactic acidosis. Clinical standards dictate keeping the glucose <150 to 180 mg/dL. Conversely, hypoglycemia can be associated with focal neurologic deficits such as aphasia or hemiparesis and mental status changes.

### Antithrombotic and Antiplatelet Therapy

TPA can be given only after a CT scan documents absence of hemorrhage. The window of opportunity appears to be limited to 3 hours.[58, 59] Although 12% of patients return to normal function with TPA, 6% have intracerebral hemorrhage as a result of TPA. TPA is usually not an option in perioperative stroke because of the risk of hemorrhage at the surgical site. Major surgery within 14 days and arterial puncture within 7 days are stated exclusions.[58] The exclusion of arterial puncture within 7 days applies to a noncompressible site; for example, TPA with compression could be considered in a patient sustaining stroke during cardiac catheterization.

Early aspirin use (within 1 to 2 days) reduces early recurrent stroke or death for 1 patient with stroke per 100 treated. Approximately 1 patient in 200 experiences serious non–central nervous system bleeding due to aspirin.[60,61] Intracranial hemorrhage is excluded by CT and the risk of incisional bleeding is assessed before beginning an antiplatelet agent.

The value of heparin for acute ischemic stroke continues to be debated. Low-dose subcutaneous heparin is useful (and safe) for prevention of deep venous thrombosis in nonambulatory patients, but higher doses had no benefit for short-term neurologic outcomes in patients with stroke.[60] Whether heparin is effective in aborting progressive ischemic stroke (more frequent with vertebrobasilar ischemia) is unproved; anecdotal experience suggests benefit. Low molecular weight heparins (LMWHs) and heparinoids theoretically have advantages over unfractionated heparin because of better bioavailability and perhaps less bleeding. A large trial with an LMWH showed no overall benefit for mortality or disability.[62] A heparinoid agent given within 24 hours of acute stroke also showed no benefit at 3 months.[63]

Pending further data, heparin probably should not be given routinely to patients with acute ischemic stroke, except for deep venous thrombosis prophylaxis. Use for progressing ischemic stroke is reasonable but of unproven benefit.[64] In the setting of a cardiac thrombus, acute anticoagulation carries the risk of hemorrhagic transformation of the infarct. If possible, anticoagulation is delayed for 3 to 10 days depending on the size of the infarct (larger infarcts warrant a longer delay).[65]

### When Are Antiplatelet Agents and Anticoagulants Stopped Before Surgery?

Guidelines for discontinuing aspirin depend on the vascularity of the surgical site and the judgment of the surgeon. For most operations, aspirin is stopped 5 to 10 days before surgery and restarted 48 to 72 hours after surgery. Aspirin usually is not stopped before CEA and is continued immediately afterward.[45] One study suggests expeditious resumption of aspirin therapy is especially important to prevent myocardial infarction in patients post-CEA.[66] The other antiplatelet agents are similar to aspirin in terms of their effect on bleeding time, and similar guidelines are appropriate.

Guidelines for stopping anticoagulants before surgery depend on the risk for thrombotic complications. If the elective surgical patient is at relatively low risk, it may be reasonable to stop the warfarin with an anticipated decline in the INR of perhaps 1 unit/day. If the patient needs surgery unexpectedly and the INR is only modestly elevated (<6), low doses of vitamin K (1-2.5 mg orally) should be given and may return the INR to the therapeutic range without inducing the level of refractoriness seen with larger does of vitamin K. More serious presentations may warrant larger doses of vitamin K, fresh frozen plasma, or factor concentrates.[67]

For patients at high risk for thromboembolism, it may be necessary to convert to heparin anticoagulation before surgery, interrupt the heparin as required for the procedure, and re-anticoagulate after surgery, first with heparin, then with warfarin. This process may require several days of hospitalization. Alternatives for patients at less risk include stopping warfarin 4 to 5 days before surgery, replacing it with low-dose (5000 U subcutaneously) heparin or LMWH before surgery, then resuming with warfarin after surgery. For some gynecologic and orthopedic surgeries, it may be safe to lower the warfarin dose and operate at an INR of 1.3 to 1.5. (An INR of 1.3 to 1.5 is not protective against stroke but allows a more rapid transition to a therapeutic INR after surgery.) The warfarin dose can be lowered 4 to 5 days before surgery and supplemented with low-dose heparin after surgery.[68]

In the patient who requires dental surgery or extraction, a 4.8% solution of tranexamic acid may be used as a mouthwash. The use of 10 mL 4 times a day for 7 days has been shown to prevent serious bleeding in patients undergoing dental surgery maintained on full-dose warfarin therapy. ε-Aminocaproic acid mouthwash also has been used successfully.[69]

## When Is It Safe to Operate After a Stroke?

By convention, anesthesia and surgery are delayed 4 to 6 weeks after acute stroke. This practice is based on our knowledge of loss of autoregulation in the ischemic penumbra surrounding the infarct. Neuronal perfusion is directly related to systemic BP when autoregulation is absent. This relationship puts the susceptible periinfarct tissue at high risk for irreversible damage from relatively mild hypotension.

## How Long Should Succinylcholine Be Avoided After a Hemiparetic Stroke?

Unless a compelling reason necessitates the use of succinylcholine, it should probably be avoided for the remainder of the patient's life if there is stroke-associated paresis. However, a hyperkalemic response to succinylcholine has not been reported >6 months after stroke.[70]

## MULTIPLE SCLEROSIS

### *What Elements Are Necessary in the Preoperative Evaluation?*

#### Clinical Findings

White matter degeneration in the brain of patients with multiple sclerosis can cause diverse clinical findings. Sensory, motor, autonomic, optic, and integrative pathways all may be affected. Respiratory function may be affected by demyelinating lesions of the cervical spinal cord or medullary respiratory centers.[71] Pulmonary function studies and arterial blood gas analysis should be obtained to evaluate the respiratory reserve. Pharyngeal/laryngeal muscle dysfunction places some patients at increased risk for aspiration of gastric contents. Patients with paraplegia or quadriplegia may be prone to autonomic hyperreflexia. Symptoms or signs of this syndrome should be sought.

#### Medications

Some medications used to treat associated spasticity have anesthetic implications.[70] Propantheline can potentiate nondepolarizing neuromuscular relaxants, delay gastric emptying, and cause autonomic blockade. Baclofen and dantrolene may potentiate nondepolarizing muscle relaxants. A more recently approved medication for spasticity, tizanidine, is a short-acting, centrally active $\alpha$-adrenergic receptor agonist. It is thought to reduce spasticity by increasing presynaptic inhibition of motor neurons. The sedative and hypotensive effects of anesthetic drugs are exaggerated in patients taking tizanidine.[72] Diazepam potentiates the sedative effects of anesthetic drugs. Carbamazepine increases resistance to nondepolarizing muscle relaxants.

A history of recent (within 1 year) steroid therapy should be elicited. Exacerbations are sometimes treated with steroids, and stress coverage for surgery often is necessary. Chemotherapeutic agents may cause bone marrow suppression.

### *What Are the Anesthetic Considerations?*

Spinal and epidural anesthesia have been reported to cause exacerbations of the disease but may be used when other patient factors argue against general anesthesia.[73,74] Intrathecal local anesthetics are thought to be neurotoxic to demyelinated axons in the spinal cord, making low-concentration epidural anesthesia preferable.[75] When general anesthesia is chosen, rapid sequence induction is indicated if pharyngeal/laryngeal muscle involvement is present. Invasive hemodynamic monitoring is warranted in the presence of autonomic insufficiency.[76] The volatile anesthetics have not been shown to exacerbate multiple sclerosis.[77,78]

Succinylcholine may cause significant potassium release with multiple sclerosis (Table 10–5). Close monitoring of neuromuscular function is needed when nondepolarizing muscle relaxants are used because they may have an exaggerated or prolonged effect. Hyperthermia should be avoided because exacerbation of multiple sclerosis weakness can occur as a consequence of fever.[79] Patients with multiple sclerosis comprise one of the few noncardiac surgical groups in which active cooling is indicated. The disease may be worsened

**TABLE 10–5.** Neurologic Diseases in Which Succinylcholine May Cause an Exaggerated Potassium Release

| Neurologic Disease | Period of Vulnerability |
|---|---|
| Anterior horn disease (amyotrophic lateral sclerosis) | Not reported |
| Encephalitis | Not reported |
| Head injury | Not reported |
| Hemiplegia (stroke) | 7 d–6 mo |
| Multiple sclerosis | Not reported |
| Muscle denervation | 3 wk–3 mo |
| Muscular dystrophy* | Always |
| Myotonia* | Always |
| Paraplegia (traumatic) | 3 wk–3 mo |
| Parkinson disease | ? If any |
| Subarachnoid hemorrhage | Not reported |
| Tetanus | Not reported |

*Increased susceptibility to succinylcholine–induced malignant hyperthermia.
Modified from Azar I. The response of patients with neuromuscular disorders to muscle relaxants: a review. *Anesthesiology.* 1984;61:173.

simply by the stress of anesthesia and surgery, and patients should be told this before surgery.

## MUSCULAR DYSTROPHY

### *Which Organ Systems Are Affected?*

Of most interest to anesthesiologists is that MD may affect the muscles of the pharynx and glottis, respiratory system, and cardiovascular system. Delayed gastric emptying, difficulty with swallowing, and inability to handle secretions place patients at risk for perioperative aspiration. In addition, glottic muscle weakness may restrict expiratory airflow.

Respiratory muscle dysfunction often manifests as tachypnea, smaller tidal volumes, and paradoxical breathing with use of accessory muscles of respiration. Many times, baseline respiratory function appears normal, but reserve is severely limited. In addition, the ventilatory response to hypercapnia and hypoxemia may be depressed.

Myocardial function can be severely compromised in myotonic dystrophy, Duchenne MD, Becker MD, limb-girdle dystrophy, and fascioscapulohumeral MD.[80] Cardiac conduction abnormalities are common. Preoperative testing, including ECG and some measure of myocardial contractility (echocardiogram or multigated angiogram), should be performed.

### *What Are the Anesthetic Considerations?*

In patients with Duchenne and Becker MD, rhabdomyolysis may develop after administration of succinylcholine or exposure to volatile inhalation agents.[81] They should be treated as if they are susceptible to malignant hyperthermia. Cardiac arrest has been reported even with total intravenous anesthesia.[82] During surgery, patients with MD most often require assisted or controlled ventilation to compensate for the negative effects of anesthetics on muscle function and ventilatory response to elevated $PaCO_2$. ECG and frequent BP monitoring are important to assess the effect of anesthesia on cardiac function. When cardiac reserve is compromised before surgery, invasive hemodynamic monitoring is indicated. Patients with Duchenne MD are more sensitive to nondepolarizing muscle relaxants.[83] Postoperatively, the trachea is extubated when patients are awake and baseline motor function has returned, and when weaning criteria are met (ie, peak negative pressure at least −20 to −30 cm $H_2O$ and vital capacity at least 15 mL/kg with acceptable arterial blood gas values and pH).

## DYSTONIA

### What Is It?

Dystonias are sustained contractions of muscles that result in abnormal twisting or posturing. They may be sustained, intermittent and focal, or generalized, and they are classified by the patient's age at onset, the distribution of the muscles affected, and etiology. Most adult-onset dystonias are idiopathic or primary, excluding drug reactions. Secondary dystonias involve other areas of the central nervous system in addition to the basal ganglia, so that the clinical manifestations are not limited to a disorder of movement. Several hereditary neurometabolic and degenerative neurologic disorders may cause dystonia secondarily.

### Wilson Disease

Wilson disease is an autosomal recessive disorder with progressive lenticular degeneration and liver cirrhosis that is associated with prominent dystonic posturing. It is caused by a defect of copper metabolism and decreased ceruloplasmin synthesis (the serum enzyme that binds copper). The improvement after treatment with penicillamine is sometimes dramatic.[84] Dystonia may also result from anoxic brain injury, heavy metal toxicity, encephalitis, and focal cerebral disease, including stroke, head trauma, multiple sclerosis, and brain tumors.[85]

### Focal Dystonias

The focal dystonias common in adulthood include blepharospasm (forced, involuntary eye closure), oromandibular dystonia (face, jaw, or tongue), cervical dystonia or torticollis (neck), writer's cramp (action-induced dystonic contraction of hand muscles), and spasmodic dysphonia. Blepharospasm begins with increased blinking and often progresses to a debilitating disorder of functional blindness. The onset is in the fifth to sixth decades. A patient who presents with dystonia in one area may acquire dystonia in other craniocervical areas over time.[86]

### What Is the Treatment?

#### Medical

Torticollis or cervical dystonia is the most common form of focal dystonia presenting for treatment. The scalene, sternocleidomastoid, and trapezius muscles are most often affected. Patients with this condition may have neck rotation, flexion or extension, head tilt, lateral shift, or a combination of these.[87,88] Patients with a twisted neck should be evaluated for secondary, structural abnormalities. If there are any findings on history or examination suggestive of an orthopedic cause (atlantoaxial dislocation, cervical fracture, degenerative disk disease, osteomyelitis, or Klippel-Feil syndrome), magnetic resonance imaging (MRI) of the cervical spine should be performed.[89]

Most patients with focal dystonia are now treated with local injections of botulinum toxin. From 70% to 92% obtain relief of abnormal postures with injections repeated every 3 to 6 months. Side effects may include excessive weakness in the injected or adjacent muscles, but this can usually be avoided with proper selection of muscles for injection and by reducing the dose. Resistance develops in some patients and appears to be linked to the development of antibodies.[90–93] Physical therapy has limited benefit in mildly affected patients. Pharmacotherapeutic agents that may be useful in small doses early in therapy include anticholinergics, baclofen, and benzodiazepines.

#### Surgical

In medically intractable cases of dystonia, surgical procedures may be beneficial. For torticollis, denervation of the anterior roots of the upper cervical nerves and sometimes the spinal accessory nerve can provide relief.[94,95] Similarly, blepharospasm is sometimes treated with orbital myectomy when botulinum therapy has been unsuccessful. Fixed lesions, such as infarction of the basal ganglia or posttraumatic lesions, are associated with hemidystonia and have the best surgical response to thalamotomy.[96] Thalamotomy is performed using local anesthesia so that the patient can give feedback in assessing the effect of electrical stimulation and lesion placement on the dystonia.

### What Are the Anesthetic Considerations?

Few published accounts exist of anesthetic management of patients with dystonia or torticollis. Surgical release or application of halo devices may be undertaken in patients with torticollis.[97] Airway considerations are paramount because prolonged contraction causes facial asymmetry and fixation of the head, jaw, and cervical spine even in the presence of complete pharmacologic neuromuscular blockade.

Based on clinical judgment, many patients require awake tracheal intubation before induction of general anesthesia. Alternatively, maintenance of spontaneous ventilation during induction of anesthesia or placement of a laryngeal mask airway seems appropriate. When kyphoscoliosis is present, the patient should be evaluated for restrictive lung disease and appropriate precautions taken to ensure adequate pulmonary function in the postoperative period. There appears to be no contraindication to succinylcholine because the muscle is normal; in fact, overstimulation of neuromuscular receptors is occurring.[98,99]

Severe dystonic reactions and opisthotonos can occur during and after the administration of general anesthesia. This usually, but not always, occurs after antidopaminergic drugs have been given.[100,101]

## GUILLAIN-BARRÉ SYNDROME

### How Is the Nervous System Affected?

Guillain-Barré syndrome presents most often after an otherwise inconsequential viral infection but has been reported in postoperative patients without evidence of antecedent viral infection.[80] It consists of a symmetric ascending weakness evolving over several days and caused by demyelination of peripheral nerves.

In half of these cases, cranial nerve involvement compromises respiratory and bulbar function. Sensory deficits can occur. Autonomic dysfunction is common, resulting in hemodynamic instability. Nerve conduction studies reveal slowed conduction velocities early and denervation potentials late in the course of the disease. Other polyneuropathies may mimic the disease.

## What Are the Anesthetic Implications?

With regard to muscle weakness, attention to airway management and respiratory support is similar to that with MD. Succinylcholine may cause massive potassium release in chronically denervated muscles (see Table 10–5). Depending on the stage of the disease, patients may have decreased or increased sensitivity to nondepolarizing muscle relaxants.[102] Close hemodynamic monitoring, including continuous ECG and intra-arterial BP monitoring, is indicated because of the instability of the cardiovascular system with resultant lability of heart rate and BP. Central venous or pulmonary artery catheter monitoring may be useful to ensure euvolemia because with autonomic insufficiency, heart rate and BP are unreliable indicators of the volume status.

# HUNTINGTON'S DISEASE

## What Are the Anesthetic Considerations?

Huntington's disease is a genetically transmitted condition associated with neuronal destruction in the caudate nucleus and putamen. Patients manifest progressive chorea, dementia, and depression. They may have prolonged sedation with normal doses of induction drugs. Also, prolonged paralysis with succinylcholine has been suggested, although it has not been confirmed in other reports.[103] Anticholinergic drugs may exacerbate the choreiform movements.[104] Because of involvement of the pharyngeal musculature, an increased risk of aspiration may be present in the perioperative period.[105]

Haloperidol, a butyrophenone, is most commonly used to treat the choreiform movements. The $\alpha$-adrenergic blocking properties of this agent may potentiate hypotension during induction or maintenance of anesthesia, whereas the sedative properties potentiate the hypnotic and respiratory depressant effects of anesthetic drugs.

# PSEUDOTUMOR CEREBRI

## What Is It?

Pseudotumor cerebri (also called *idiopathic* or *benign intracranial hypertension*) is a syndrome that causes elevated ICP without an intracranial mass. It occurs 4 to 8 times more frequently in women than in men[106] and is associated with headache, papilledema, visual disturbances, and cranial nerve dysfunction (usually of cranial nerve VI).[107] The etiology is most often idiopathic but can include abnormalities of cerebral

venous drainage, cerebrospinal fluid (CSF) secretion/outflow, or endocrine, metabolic, and immunologic diseases. The lumbar CSF pressure is elevated to >200 mm $H_2O$. Lumbar CSF drainage is often beneficial in treating symptoms of headache but should be done only after a mass lesion has been ruled out with contrast CT scanning or MRI.[108] Hydrocephalus is not present; in fact, the ventricles are normal or small.

## How Is Anesthesia Managed?

### Preoperative Management

Careful preoperative documentation of the current visual abnormalities is important to assess postoperative dysfunction adequately. Patients undergoing spinal or epidural anesthesia may benefit from a CT scan of the head to rule out impending herniation syndromes. When the condition has been stable for months or years, anesthesia and surgery can proceed. However, recent deterioration in visual acuity or cranial nerve function necessitates further assessment and therapy before surgery. Perioperative steroid coverage is required for patients who have recently been treated with steroids.

### Regional Anesthesia

Spinal anesthesia is safe in most cases and even has been advocated because CSF drainage, which constitutes part of the normal therapy for this condition, may be instituted immediately before injection of the spinal anesthetic in many patients.[109,110] Epidural anesthesia is a less desirable choice because injection of fluid into the epidural space increases the ICP.

### General Anesthesia

When general anesthesia is necessary, drugs and techniques that actually decrease or prevent increases in ICP are used. Abnormal responses to muscle relaxants have not been reported, nor do these patients appear more sensitive to sedative-hypnotics. Because most patients with pseudotumor cerebri are obese, standard techniques for induction, emergence, and extubation of obese patients should be instituted.

# NEUROLEPTIC MALIGNANT SYNDROME

## What Is It?

Neuroleptic malignant syndrome (NMS) is an idiosyncratic reaction that occurs in one of two pharmacologic settings:

1. NMS occurs after withdrawal of dopaminergic agonists used for treatment of parkinsonism.[111]
2. NMS occurs after administration of drugs that cause central dopaminergic blockade of the striatum. These drugs include agents used in the perioperative period (chlorpromazine, droperidol, metoclopramide, prochlorperazine), neuroleptics used primarily in psychiatry (butyrophenones, phenothiazines, and thioxanthenes), and many other drugs.

NMS most often occurs when these drugs are administered at dosages within the therapeutic range.[112] It is seen in approximately 1 in 100 to 1 in 1000 patients treated with neuroleptic medications.[113] Because other drugs besides neuroleptics can cause the illness, the name *drug-induced central hyperthermic syndrome* has been proposed, a term that identifies the pathophysiologic process and distinguishes the disease from malignant hyperthermia.[114]

Because dopamine is an integral neurotransmitter both in thermoregulatory neural pathways of the hypothalamus and in striatal motor projections, interference with dopaminergic activity can lead to impairment of temperature regulation and drug-induced parkinsonism. Fever results from altered thermoregulation in the face of increased thermogenesis due to exaggerated muscle activity, such as tremor or rigidity. Thus, NMS should be suspected in the proper pharmacologic setting when parkinsonism or other movement disorders, such as dystonia, are associated with fever. Autonomic instability, altered mental status, and an elevated creatine kinase may be present.[113] Metabolic changes in peripheral skeletal muscle have also been implicated in the pathogenesis of the disease.[115]

The rigidity of NMS is commonly the "lead pipe" type, but akinesia, dyskinesia, waxy flexibility, and cogwheeling have been reported. Involvement of the chest wall may impair ventilation. Dysautonomia may present as pallor, diaphoresis, tachycardia, cardiac arrhythmias, and BP swings. Nearly all patients have mental status changes, including confusion, delirium, agitation, or frank coma. No laboratory studies are diagnostic. The creatine kinase is usually elevated because of unrelenting muscle contraction. There may be lactic acidosis superimposed on respiratory acidosis. Death is usually due to respiratory insufficiency or aspiration pneumonia.[116]

## What Is the Differential Diagnosis?

Fever and movement disorder may also be seen in a variety of other clinical situations (Table 10–6). Encephalitis and meningitis may have a similar presentation, as may idiopathic or drug-induced parkinsonism with ongoing infection, heat stroke, malignant hyperthermia, and alcohol or benzodiazepine withdrawal.

Lethal catatonia, a psychiatric disorder resulting in continuous, uncontrollable motor activity and hyperthermia, is often included in the differential diagnosis. Central anticholinergic syndrome may cause fever and abnormal motor responses, and physostigmine should be therapeutic in this condition.

**TABLE 10–6.** Differential Diagnosis of Neuroleptic Malignant Syndrome

---

Alcohol withdrawal
Brain tumors
Cerebrovascular infarct or hemorrhage
Drugs (salicylates, dopamine inhibitors and antagonists,
    stimulants, psychedelics, monoamine oxidase inhibitors,
    anesthetics, anticholinergics)
Encephalitis/encephalomyelitis
Heat stroke
Lethal catatonia
Metabolic abnormalities
Parkinsonism with infection
Pheochromocytoma
Seizures
Systemic lupus erythematosus
Thyroid storm

---

MAO inhibitors taken in conjunction with meperidine, tricyclic antidepressants, or selective serotonin reuptake inhibitors can cause an NMS-like syndrome termed *serotonin syndrome*.[117]

## What Is the Treatment?

The initial treatment of NMS is supportive. Neuroleptic medication is stopped. Adequate oxygenation and ventilation are ensured if necessary, with tracheal intubation, mechanical ventilation, and muscle paralysis. Nondepolarizing muscle relaxants provide paralysis in NMS. Hyperpyrexia is treated with cooling blankets, cool water baths, and antipyretics. Cardiovascular stability is achieved with fluid and vasopressors in hypotensive patients and with vasodilators or β-adrenergic blocking agents when severe hypertension is present. Dantrolene can improve muscle rigidity and aid in lowering fever, but an improvement in mortality rates has not been consistently demonstrated.[118] The dopamine agonists, carbidopa-levodopa, amantadine, and bromocriptine can shorten the duration of the illness and probably lower mortality rates.[112] A stepped approach to drug therapy based on the degree of temperature elevation has been proposed.[118] When myoglobinuria is present, vigorous fluid therapy and alkalinization of the urine are necessary to prevent renal failure.

Since 1980, the overall mortality rate of NMS has declined from 30% to 10% or less.[112,119] Excess mortality occurs when NMS is associated with myoglobinemia and renal failure.

## What Are the Anesthetic Considerations?

Patients with a history of NMS may present for surgery. It is probably safe to rechallenge patients with antidopaminergic drugs if their use is thought necessary, but a period of at least 2 weeks should have passed since recovery from the acute episode.[111,112]

### Safety of Malignant Hyperthermia–Inducing Agents

Succinylcholine has been used many times in patients with NMS, although a case of succinylcholine-induced hyperkalemia has been reported.[120] Nondepolarizing muscle relaxants are safe to use. Patients with a history of NMS have been repeatedly anesthetized with volatile anesthetics, emphasizing the basic pathophysiologic difference between NMS and malignant hyperthermia.

## KNOWN SEIZURE DISORDERS

## What Is Important in the Preoperative Evaluation?

In patients who have a known seizure disorder and are being treated with anticonvulsants, the type of seizures and their frequency, drug therapy, and serum drug concentrations should be known. For patients whose seizure disorder is well controlled or who experience only absence (petit mal) seizures, surgery can proceed without adjustment of their usual anticonvulsant regimen. Patients who have experienced an increasing frequency of seizures or who have frequent, generalized tonic-clonic seizures should be evaluated for potential causes of exacerbation of seizures.

Common contributors include medication noncompliance, alcohol, and illness. Electrolyte, creatinine, and albumin determinations; a CBC with differential; and urinalysis are performed. If the anticonvulsant level is subtherapeutic, the patient is given a loading dose of the applicable agent.

## How Are Anticonvulsants Handled Perioperatively?

Table 10–7 lists the available anticonvulsants. Since 1993, the FDA has approved 7 completely new anticonvulsants as well as new formulations of 5 established anticonvulsants.[121] Established therapeutic levels for those anticonvulsants are listed in Table 10–8. Most patients maintain acceptable blood levels of drug by taking the usual oral dose of medication with sips of water during the *nil per os* (NPO) preoperative period. For patients who remain in NPO status postoperatively, the oral medications can be given by nasogastric tube; alternatively, a change to intravenous phenytoin or phenobarbital can be made.

When poor oral absorption can be anticipated in elective surgery, a switch to phenytoin or sodium valproate several weeks before surgery allows attainment of steady-state levels

**TABLE 10–7.** Anticonvulsant Medications

| Drug | Usual Daily Dosage (Adults) | Common Side Effects |
|---|---|---|
| Carbamazepine | 800-1600 mg | Somnolence, dizziness, diplopia, ataxia, nausea, vomiting, rash, hyponatremia |
| Ethosuximide | 750-1500 mg | Sleep disturbance, drowsiness, hyperactivity, nausea, vomiting |
| Felbamate | 2400-3600 mg | Insomnia, dizziness, headache, ataxia, nausea, vomiting, anorexia, weight loss |
| Gabapentin | 1800-3600 mg | Fatigue, dizziness, ataxia, somnolence |
| Lamotrigine | 300-500 mg | Rash, dizziness, ataxia, headache, somnolence, nausea, rhinitis, diplopia, blurred vision |
| Levetiracetam | 1000-3000 mg | Somnolence, asthenia, agitation, anxiety, depression, psychosis |
| Oxcarbazepine | 1200-2400 mg | Somnolence, dizziness, diplopia, ataxia, nausea, vomiting, rash, hyponatremia |
| Phenobarbital | 1-4 mg/kg | Sedation, lethargy, behavioral changes, hyperactivity, ataxia, nausea, rash, tolerance, dependence |
| Phenytoin | 300-400 mg | Rash, ataxia |
| Primidone | 500-1000 mg | Sedation, lethargy, behavioral changes, hyperactivity, ataxia, nausea, rash, tolerance, dependence |
| Tiagabine | 32-56 mg | Fatigue, dizziness, somnolence, nervousness, asthenia, headache, tremor, nausea |
| Topiramate | 200-400 mg | Abnormal thinking, impaired concentration, fatigue, dizziness, ataxia, somnolence, nausea, agitation, nystagmus, headache, speech disorder, paresthesia, tremor, agitaton, amnesia, depression, diplopia |
| Valproate | 1000-3000 mg | Tremor, alopecia, weight gain, nausea, vomiting, easy bruising |

**TABLE 10–8.** Established* Therapeutic Levels of Anticonvulsants

| Drug | Therapeutic Level (μg/mL) |
|---|---|
| Carbamazepine | 4-12 |
| Ethosuximide | 40-100 |
| Felbamate | 32-137 |
| Gabapentin | 2-3 |
| Phenobarbital | 15-40 |
| Phenytoin | 10-20 |
| Primidone | 5-12 |
| Valproate | 50-100 |

*Therapeutic levels have not been established for the newer anticonvulsants: lamotrigine, levetiracetam, oxcarbazepine, tiagabine, topiramate.

and avoidance of an intravenous or intramuscular loading dose. Extended-release formulations of carbamazepine provide reliable serum drug levels with twice-daily dosing regimens, possibly an advantage during the perioperative period. Oxcarbazepine, chemically similar to carbamazepine, has a longer half-life than the regular formulation of carbamazepine and provides effective twice-daily dosing.[122]

Valproic acid given rectally to children has good absorption.[123] A preceding cleansing enema is required for predictable absorption. Rectal absorption of carbamazepine is unreliable. A rectal gel form of diazepam also is available.

## How Is Anesthesia Managed?

### Regional Anesthesia

Although toxic doses of local anesthetics can cause seizures, no evidence shows that the serum concentrations associated with routine epidural or brachial plexus anesthesia are unsafe in patients with a seizure disorder. Nevertheless, when regional anesthesia is chosen, it is prudent, when possible, to use spinal anesthesia, with its much lower local anesthetic dose.

### General Anesthesia

Many of the intravenous and inhaled anesthetics in common use can enhance or suppress seizure activity, depending on the dose administered and the clinical situation. Ketamine (especially when combined with theophylline) and methohexital have been reported to be epileptogenic in patients with a seizure disorder.[124]

Enflurane, at high doses (2.5%) with hyperventilation ($PaCO_2$ ≤25 mm Hg), produces EEG evidence of seizure activity.[125,126] Avoidance of enflurane use is recommended, as is maintenance of normocarbia in the perioperative period. Halothane may be metabolized to a greater extent because of the upregulation of hepatic microsomal enzymes, resulting in a potentially increased incidence of hepatotoxicity.[124] Isoflurane is a potent anticonvulsant.[127] Postoperative seizures have been reported with sevoflurane, but desflurane appears to lack seizure-inducing activity.[128,129]

Etomidate precipitates seizures in epileptic patients[130] and in 20% of nonepileptic patients during open heart surgery.[131] Propofol may induce seizure activity in patients with preexisting central nervous system disease, with increases in spike activity at sedative doses but suppression of activity at high doses.[132–134]

**TABLE 10–9.** Treatment of Generalized Tonic-Clonic Status Epilepticus

**Immediate Intervention (First 10 min)**

1. Support circulation.
2. Support respiration; most, if not all, patients should be intubated.
3. Draw blood for anticonvulsant levels, glucose, electrolytes, complete blood count, calcium.
4. Measure arterial blood gas values.
5. Administer 50 mL of 50% glucose IV.
6. Administer 100 mg thiamine IM.

**Intermediate Intervention (Second 10 min)**

1. Diazepam, 10 mg (lorazepam 4 mg) at 2-4 mg/min until seizure stops or to a total of 30 mg (lorazepam 12 mg). For children, diazepam 0.1 mg/kg, up to 0.3 mg/kg, is given over 5 to 30 min.
2. Slow infusion (<50 mg/min) of phenytoin to a total of 20 mg/kg. (Fosphenytoin may be given at 150 phenytoin equivalents/min as a safe substitute for phenytoin. If status continues after 20 mg/kg, give additional phenytoin or fosphenytoin at 5 mg/kg increments to a maximum dose of 30 mg/kg.)
3. Perform general and neurologic examination with attention to evidence of primary or secondary trauma, pupils, fundi, extremity movements, pathologic reflexes.

**Further Intervention (Next 40-60 min If Seizures Persist)**

1. Phenobarbital IV at 50 mg/min to a total of 20 mg/kg. Intubation and ventilation are required.
2. Thiopental drip (1 g/500 mL) *or* general anesthesia with pentobarbital, midazolam, or propofol to obtain electroencephalographic burst suppression. Intubation, ventilation, and vasopressors are required.

IM, intramuscular; IV, intravenous.

**TABLE 10–10.** Electroencephalographic Waveform: Characteristics and Interpretation

| Rhythm | Frequency (Hz) | State of Arousal |
| --- | --- | --- |
| Delta | 0-4 | Coma, hypoxia/ischemia, deep anesthesia |
| Theta | 4-8 | Sleep, surgical anesthesia |
| Alpha | 8-13 | Relaxed, eyes closed, light anesthesia |
| Beta | 13-30 | Awake, alert, low-dose barbiturate |

Awareness of the sedative side effects of this group of drugs and their effect on hepatic metabolism and protein binding of concurrently administered drugs is important. In addition, chronic phenytoin and carbamazepine therapy have been associated with resistance to nondepolarizing neuromuscular relaxants.

## What Is the Definition and Treatment of Status Epilepticus?

When seizures are so frequent that recovery of function does not occur between them, status epilepticus is present. Immediate and aggressive treatment is necessary to prevent permanent neurologic damage associated with this entity. Table 10–9 presents a protocol for treatment.[135]

## INTRAOPERATIVE MONITORING

## What Is Available?

### Electroencephalography

The EEG measures the summation of spontaneous brain electrical activity immediately adjacent to recording electrodes placed on the scalp or on brain tissue itself. The raw EEG can record voltage changes with time over a large percentage of the brain using a 16-channel montage. By noting the frequency of the resultant electrical waveform (in hertz) and its amplitude and symmetry, inferences can be made about the degree of activation and metabolic state of the underlying brain (Table 10–10). For example, increasing frequency of the waveform is associated with seizure activity and with use of low-dose barbiturates and ketamine. Low-frequency, high-amplitude waveforms are associated with narcotic anesthesia and deeper levels of inhalational anesthesia. Low-frequency, low-amplitude activity may occur with hypoxia, ischemia, and higher-dose barbiturates. Finally, an isoelectric EEG is found with brain death, severe hypothermia, profound hypoperfusion, barbiturate-induced coma, and twice minimal alveolar concentration (2 × MAC) levels of isoflurane.

Computer processing of the raw EEG transforms the data into power (amplitude squared) versus frequency and can display the data in a graphically simplistic manner. For example, the compressed spectral array monitor plots power versus frequency over time in a three-dimensional plot, often with a display of the spectral edge frequency—that is, the frequency below which 97% of the power is occurring (Fig. 10–1). Processed EEG monitors are primarily used to detect global cerebral ischemia and miss episodes of focal ischemia that can be detected by a 16-channel raw EEG.

### Evoked Potentials

Evoked potentials (often also referred to as *evoked responses*) measure the electrical response in the central nervous

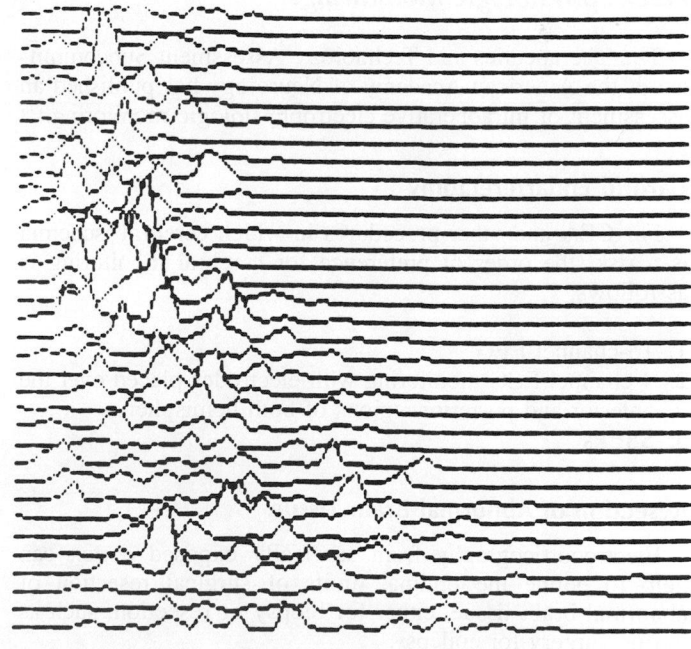

**FIGURE 10–1.** Compressed spectral array plotting of power and frequency against time. This frequency domain display allows easy recognition of frequency concentration shifts over long periods. However, the large amplitude of some traces can obscure activity in others. (From Kirby RR. Monitoring of neurologic function. In: Civetta JM, Taylor RW, Kirby RR, eds. *Critical Care*. Philadelphia, Pa: JB Lippincott; 1988:353.)

system to a stimulus applied to a more peripheral nerve. The clinical use of evoked potentials requires that (1) an intact neural pathway be accessible for stimulation distally and monitoring proximally, and (2) this neural pathway be anatomically proximate or physiologically similar to the neural elements at risk during surgery. By signal averaging and electronic filtering, the low-amplitude evoked potentials can be recorded and analyzed for their latency (time from stimulation to generation of an electrical signal) and amplitude. In addition, near field (close to the recording electrode, eg, the cerebral cortex) and far field (recording deeper transmission through deeper brain structures, eg, brainstem) potentials can be recorded.

Current evoked potential modalities include (1) somatosensory evoked potentials (SSEPs), elicited by stimulating a peripheral nerve in the arm or leg and recording the nerve impulse at the scalp, over the spine, at an interspinous ligament, or in an epidural space; (2) brainstem auditory evoked potentials (BAEPs), in which cranial nerve VIII is stimulated with an audible click and recording of the generated potentials in the brainstem occurs over the posterior scalp; and (3) visual evoked potentials, in which cranial nerve II is stimulated with flashes of light and potentials are recorded over the anterior cranial fossa.

### Electromyography and Nerve Conduction Velocity

In addition, electromyography (EMG) and nerve conduction velocity monitoring can be used by surgeons to assess the integrity of motor and cranial nerve pathways during dissection of proximate tissue.

## What Are the Indications for Electrophysiologic Monitoring?

The Therapeutics and Technology Assessment Subcommittee of the American Academy of Neurology has published an assessment of intraoperative electrophysiologic monitoring.[136]

### Carotid Endarterectomy

For CEA and other procedures in which cerebral ischemia is a risk, the order of preference for cerebral monitoring is as follows:

1. 16-channel EEG
2. 4-channel EEG monitoring with electrodes placed over the anterior and posterior regions of both hemispheres
3. SSEPs

### Resection of Abnormal Brain Tissue

Electrocorticography from surgically exposed cortex can help to define the optimal limits of surgical resection of abnormal brain tissue, either for biopsy or resection, such as during surgery for epilepsy.

### Posterior Fossa Surgery

During posterior fossa surgery, BAEPs and facial nerve (VII) monitoring by nerve stimulation with EMG are indicated to identify cranial nerve impairment caused by compression, retraction, or ischemia.

### Spine Surgery

Somatosensory evoked potential monitoring is indicated during orthopedic spine surgery, especially scoliosis surgery and neurosurgical spinal cord surgery, and when the thoracic aorta is cross-clamped.[137,138]

### Peripheral Nerve Grafting/Dissection

Electromyography and nerve conduction velocity measurements are indicated for identifying peripheral nerves that are damaged and need grafting, for identifying nerve pathways and monitoring their function during surgical dissection, and for monitoring nerve function during intraoperative procedures (traction, compression, limb positioning) that may damage nerves.

The Therapeutics and Technology Assessment Subcommittee cautions that intraoperative monitors not be used in clinical situations where the risk of nervous system damage is low. When the risk is high, electrophysiologic monitoring is probably safe and efficacious.

In addition to these published recommendations, many anesthesiologists are using the EEG and SSEPs to monitor depth of anesthesia, to ensure adequate brain and spinal cord perfusion during induced hypotension, and to achieve an isoelectric EEG pattern when the brain is at risk for ischemic events.

## What Are the Anesthetic Effects on Evoked Potential Monitoring?

Most intravenous and inhalational anesthetics affect the SSEPs to a variable and inconsistent degree, with cortical SSEPs recorded from the scalp affected more than subcortical SSEPs or BAEPs. Barbiturates cause a small increase in the latency and decrease the amplitude but do not abolish the SSEPs even when the cortical EEG is isoelectric. The volatile anesthetics and nitrous oxide have the greatest effect on cortical SSEPs by increasing the latency and decreasing the amplitude of the recorded potential.[139] Opiates tend to decrease the amplitude and increase the latency of recorded potentials, but clinically useful SSEPs can be obtained even with high-dose narcotic anesthesia. Etomidate, ketamine, and propofol may actually potentiate SSEPs.[140]

The most common technique for maintenance of anesthesia during SSEP monitoring uses narcotics, usually fentanyl, supplemented with 60% nitrous oxide or 1% isoflurane. General anesthesia appears to have little effect on either peripheral (eg, cervical SSEPs) or short-latency auditory evoked potentials.[141]

The most important anesthetic factors in producing an easily interpretable recording are that the depth of anesthesia be maintained at a stable level during baseline and subsequent monitoring and that the person interpreting the evoked potentials be made aware when clinical circumstances dictate a change in the anesthetic technique. Other physiologic variables must be maintained constant, such as body temperature, acid-base status, hematocrit, and BP.[142]

## PERIPHERAL NERVE INJURY

### How Common Is It?

Historical data indicate that nerve injury occurs in approximately 0.1% of anesthetized patients.[143] Surgery for myocardial revascularization carries an incidence of nerve injury of 2.6% to 13%.[144–146] Surgical positions other than level supine probably increase the risk of nerve injuries.[147] Muscle relaxants, which allow abnormal stretching of limbs, have been implicated as a risk factor for nerve injury.[148] Ulnar nerve injury is not uncommon even after spinal anesthesia or monitored anesthesia care,[149] and may not be a preventable complication.[150]

### What Are the Mechanisms?

Nerves may be injured by various mechanisms. Ischemia due to mechanical pressure can be caused by external compression, traction, or stretching. Other causes include interruption of blood flow or inadequate oxygen supply due to vascular disease, anemia, or hypotension. Direct trauma may result from surgical misadventure, needle trauma, and intraneural injection.

The incidence of nerve injury is increased when paresthesias are sought during performance of a nerve block.[151] It may be less when the level of the black needle is parallel to the direction of the nerve fibers and when a long-tapered rather than short-tapered needle encounters a nerve.[152,153] Neurotoxicity due to high perineural concentrations of local anesthetics can occur. Lidocaine has been implicated as being neurotoxic in the subarachnoid space, especially when high concentrations settle in a small portion of the subarachnoid space, or when stretching of nerve fibers occurs, as with the lithotomy position.[154] Various chemical compounds (ie, local anesthetics at high concentration, antibiotics, electrolyte solutions, and bactericidal and chemotherapy agents), when injected into the subarachnoid space or around peripheral nerves, are potentially toxic.

### Which Nerves Are Most Likely to Be Injured?

The database of the American Society of Anesthesiologists Closed Claim Study reports that the second most common cause of claims (16%) is nerve injury. Ulnar nerve injuries were the most common (28% of total nerve injuries), followed by brachial plexus (20%), lumbosacral nerve root (16%), and spinal cord (13%), then sciatic, median, radial, femoral, and other nerves.[155] Overall, nerve injuries were equally divided between men and women, although a 3:1 male predominance was noted in ulnar nerve injury, similar to the 5:1 predominance cited in another study.[156]

### How Does Nerve Injury Present?

Analysis of ulnar nerve injuries showed that 21% presented immediately postoperatively. The remainder were first detected as long as a month after surgery. The presenting symptoms may include paresthesia, dysesthesia, weakness, clumsiness, or pain in the affected nerve distribution. Many nerve injuries may be subtle or not appreciated by a patient, such as Horner syndrome (after cervical sympathetic chain injury) or a unilateral phrenic nerve palsy. A postanesthetic nerve assessment directed by the intraoperative position has been advocated.[156] Table 10–11 lists nerves at particular risk with different intraoperative positions.

### What Should Be Done After a Potential Nerve Injury Is Discovered?

First, reversible causes of nerve dysfunction should be sought and rectified. This process may include release of orthopedic casts and traction devices, correction of anemia, or surgical decompression of nerves compressed by edema, hematoma, or surgical devices.

### History and Physical Findings

A detailed history and neurologic examination most often reveal which nerves are affected and why. First, the nature of the nerve deficit (sensory, motor, both; unilateral, bilateral) should be determined. Next, whether the suspected lesion can be explained on an anatomic basis (peripheral nerve, nerve root, or spinal cord lesion) or on a physiologic basis—for example, residual local anesthetic or neuromuscular blockade, electrolyte abnormality, or coexisting nerve-muscle disease—should be established. Finally, whether surgical trespass or positioning could have caused the lesion is determined.[157,158] Examples include lithotomy position (affecting the peroneal nerve) and inguinal exploration (affecting the femoral nerve). When a spinal or epidural hematoma is suspected, immediate myelography, CT, or MRI is indicated.

### Electrophysiologic Studies

Electrophysiologic measurements may help to localize the nerve lesion and determine whether loss of axonal continuity has occurred. EMG signs of muscle denervation (fibrillation potentials and positive sharp waves) do not become evident until 2 to 3 weeks after the nerve injury; even then they are not 100% sensitive or specific for axonal loss. This is a critically important feature because an EMG in the immediate postoperative period can implicate the presence of a preexisting pathologic process. Therefore, it can serve as a baseline

**TABLE 10–11.** Relationship Between Positioning and Potential Nerve Injury

| Position | Nerves at Risk |
|---|---|
| Supine | Ulnar, suprascapular |
| Fracture table (vertical perineal post) | Obturator, pudendal, common peroneal |
| Lithotomy | Obturator, peroneal, femoral, saphenous |
| Sitting | Ulnar, sciatic, cervical spinal cord |
| Trendelenburg (shoulder braces) | Brachial plexus, long thoracic |
| Lateral decubitus | Brachial plexus, peroneal, cervical sympathetic chain, facial nerve |
| Prone | Brachial plexus, ulnar, lateral femoral cutaneous, facial, optic |

for later studies when pathologic changes attributable to the perioperative period should become evident. Nerve conduction studies can localize the area along the course of the nerve that has become injured. Later, motor and sensory evoked responses may indicate when regeneration is occurring.[159]

## What Is the Prognosis?

The prognosis depends on the mechanism of injury. Neurapraxia is an injury in which a portion of the nerve fibers becomes demyelinated but the continuity of the nerve and the endoneural sheath is preserved. Remyelination allows recovery of function in 6 to 8 weeks.

Axonotmesis occurs when complete disruption of axons takes place within an intact epineural and perineural sheath. In this type of lesion, recovery depends on regeneration of neurons in endoneural tubes. Spontaneous recovery can occur, with a favorable prognosis after months to years. A rule of thumb is that the nerve regenerates at a rate of 1 mm/day. Thus, a proximal injury requires longer to recover than a distal one.

Neurotmesis is complete transection of the axon and myelin sheath. With the fascicular anatomy disrupted, connective tissue proliferation and scarring occur in the nerve, preventing spontaneous generation down the nerve tract. These injuries are sometimes amenable to surgical repair.[160]

## What Therapy Is Available?

Little can be done to aid nerve regeneration after traumatic nerve injuries. If nerve transection has occurred, reapproximation of the nerve ends may allow some regeneration to occur. A clean laceration caused by a slip of the scalpel in the operating room should be immediately repaired. If the injury is less well demarcated, nerve repair should be delayed 3 to 6 weeks. Determination must be made in the immediate postoperative period that the nerve dysfunction is not due to extrinsic compression that can be relieved surgically.

Control of metabolic factors, such as diabetes and uremia, and nutritional supplementation in patients with hypovitaminosis caused by alcoholism or nutritional diseases may speed recovery. Antiinflammatory medications may lessen the extent of the injury. Carbamazepine and phenytoin have been used to treat painful dysesthesia. Finally, sympathectomy may be needed to treat causalgia.[160,161]

## What Nerve Injuries Are Common in Pregnancy?

Neurologic complications are common in parturients who do not receive an anesthetic, occurring perhaps in 1 of 3000 deliveries.[162,163] Thus, polyneuropathies and mononeuropathies should be identified in the preanesthetic period so that anesthetic procedures can be eliminated in the differential diagnosis of a neuropathy that is discovered postpartum.

Many mononeuropathies that in nonpregnant patients would be attributed to the anesthetic or positioning can be caused by pregnancy and childbirth. For example, brachial plexus and lateral femoral cutaneous nerve injury can be caused by weight gain and changes in spinal curvature. A median neuropathy at the wrist is common.[164] Peripartum ulnar neuropathy has been described.

Vaginal delivery may injure the femoral nerve, the obturator nerve, and the lumbosacral plexus.[165] Surgical procedures, vaginal instruments, and stirrups can injure the femoral nerve, lumbosacral trunk, and peroneal nerves, respectively. The weight of a term fetus and the effects of pregnancy can injure the sciatic nerve and cause radiculopathies. Radiculopathies may present at any time in the peripartum period with severe weakness. Bladder dysfunction is not uncommon after delivery. Backache occurs in approximately 40% of parturients not receiving an epidural anesthetic.[166]

In evaluating parturients for postanesthetic nerve injury, the clinician should remember that repeated injection of long-acting local anesthetics (as with labor analgesia) can produce a long-lasting effect. The partition coefficient of the anesthetic, in effect, concentrates the drug in the neural tissue.[167,168] Duration and difficulty of labor, use of instruments and retractors, and local anesthetics injected by the obstetrician are also important in determining the etiology of nerve lesions.

## NEUROLOGIC COMPLICATIONS AFTER SPINAL OR EPIDURAL ANESTHESIA

### Why Do They Occur?

Although nerve lesions associated with spinal or epidural anesthesia are exceedingly rare and probably occur no more frequently than with general anesthesia, permanent nerve damage can occur.[169,170] Lumbosacral nerve injury has been reported and seems to be associated with paresthesia or pain on advancing the needle or during injection. Needle trauma to the spinal cord is unreported in the literature.[171] The toxic effects of local anesthetics, their preservatives, or both have been thought to cause neural deficits,[172,173] cauda equina syndrome,[174] and backache.[175] Meningitis—bacterial or aseptic—can result from subarachnoid or epidural injection.[176–180] Several case reports describe spinal epidural abscesses after needle instrumentation.[181,182]

Epidural hematomas can occur regardless of whether a patient is undergoing anticoagulation.[183] Unintentional injection of toxic substances into the subarachnoid space may cause adhesive arachnoiditis; a technique has been described for "washing out" toxic substances.[184] Dural puncture can cause headache and has been associated with postoperative hearing loss and cranial nerve abnormalities.[185,186]

Spinal anesthesia has been implicated in exacerbation of multiple sclerosis. Back pain occurs with a frequency of a few percent after spinal or epidural anesthesia but may be just as frequent after general anesthesia. Preservative-free 2-chloroprocaine has been implicated as a cause of back pain.[175] Finally, paraplegia has occurred after epidural anesthesia without the presence of abscess or hematoma. Arterial hypotension and body positioning were thought to have contributed to spinal cord ischemia.[187]

## POSTANESTHETIC NEUROLOGIC EXAMINATION

Many physical findings that are considered pathologic in healthy patients are commonly found in patients emerging from anesthesia. It is not unusual to find sustained ankle clonus, muscle spasticity, an up-going plantar response (positive Babinski sign), and nonreactive pupils as long as 40 minutes after anesthesia.[188,189] However, all abnormal findings should be symmetric, and a new unilateral finding of weakness, pathologic reflexes, or cranial nerve dysfunction requires immediate investigation.

A patient with a prior stroke or other intracranial process occasionally manifests lateralizing neurologic signs on awakening from general anesthesia. If the signs resolve within 30 minutes, they may be attributed to *differential awakening*.[189] This entity is distinct from a procedure-related neurologic deficit, which recovers more slowly, if at all. Theories that explain the phenomenon of differential awakening speculate that injured tissue is more sensitive to low concentrations of anesthetic; that injured tissue is less well perfused, and therefore requires a longer time for drug elimination; or that compensatory pathways that evolve during recovery of the injured tissue function only when the patient is in the completely awake state.[190]

## When Should the Anesthesiologist Become Concerned About Delayed Awakening?

### Drug Effects

Impaired cerebral functioning in the postoperative period is a normal consequence of the pharmacologically induced anesthetic state. Lingering effects of anesthetic drugs are expected to depress mental function for a variable time after the end of surgery. In addition, antiemetics, analgesics, and the psychological response to pain may alter the postoperative mental status.

Clearly, most cerebral dysfunction is due to the effects of administered drugs. For example, after anesthesia with isoflurane, cerebral dysfunction can persist for days.[191] This effect may be due to the prolonged half-life of inhaled anesthetics in brain tissue.[192] Natural sleep patterns are disturbed for several days after surgery.[193] Even small antiemetic doses of droperidol can cause prolonged sedation in patients after ambulatory surgery.[194]

The concept that most postoperative cerebral dysfunction is drug induced is reinforced by the knowledge that although prolonged postanesthetic sedation is frequently encountered, new neurologic events occur with an incidence of <1 in 2500 general anesthetics.[195]

No guidelines state at what point postoperative sedation has become prolonged, and clinical experience remains the most important factor in deciding when emergence has become excessively delayed. Expectations of emergence from anesthesia are strongly influenced by the type, route, and total dose of administered drug and must take into account patient characteristics that influence the pharmacodynamics and pharmacokinetics of those drugs. Even in patients who are susceptible to prolonged sedation, awakening should be expected to occur by 60 to 90 minutes after arrival in the postanesthesia care unit.[196] When emergence from anesthesia seems abnormal or prolonged compared with the clinician's expectations, further neurologic evaluation should be carried out.

## How Should Evaluation Proceed?

When emergence from anesthesia has taken longer than expected, a systematic work-up is required. The differential diagnosis is not unlike that of any patient with coma or excessive somnolence, and diagnosis should first rule out reversible conditions that can cause permanent neurologic injury. Afterward, less threatening yet common causes of prolonged sedation or coma are sought based on the patient's medical history, drug history, and perioperative course. Finally, less common etiologies are considered.

Most important, the airway, ventilation, and circulation are assessed and supported if necessary. Adequate blood oxygenation, ventilation, and perfusion are verified by arterial blood gas analysis, BP measurement, and determination of hematocrit. Hypoglycemia is ruled out by serum glucose measurement. The presence of ongoing seizure activity is carefully sought, by EEG examination if necessary, because status epilepticus can cause permanent dysfunction if untreated.

Intracranial pathologic processes, which may require immediate intervention, include subarachnoid or intracerebral hemorrhage, tumor edema, or cerebral ischemia after cerebrovascular surgery. In most cases, neurosurgical emergencies present with lateralizing neurologic signs such as asymmetric motor activity, reflexes, or pupillary findings. Cyanide toxicity should be considered in patients who have received sodium nitroprusside.

After these problems are addressed, a careful search of the medical record, a more complete neurologic examination, and further laboratory studies are carried out in a search for the most likely cause of neurologic dysfunction.

The medical record must be examined for preexisting medical conditions that predispose to metabolic abnormalities. Table 10–12 lists medical conditions that may delay emergence from anesthesia. Laboratory studies are carried out according to the likelihood of causative factors based on the medical

**TABLE 10–12.** Conditions That May Delay Emergence

| Condition | Associated Problems |
|---|---|
| Diabetes mellitus | Hypoglycemia, ketoacidosis, nonketotic hyperosmolar coma, hyponatremia, stroke |
| Hepatic disease | Hepatic encephalopathy, altered drug pharmacokinetics, hypoglycemia, intracranial hemorrhage, cerebral edema, acidosis |
| Renal failure | Uremia, acidosis, hyponatremia, hypocalcemia, hypermagnesemia, hypoglycemia, cerebral edema, altered drug pharmacokinetics, postdialysis syndrome |
| Hypothyroidism | Hypothermia, increased sensitivity to anesthetics, hyponatremia, hypoglycemia |
| Hyperparathyroidism | Hypercalcemia |
| Seizure disorder | Ongoing seizure activity, postictal state, toxic anticonvulsant levels |
| Alcoholism | Acute ethanol intoxication, Wernicke encephalopathy, Korsakoff psychosis, subdural hematoma, hypoglycemia |
| Adrenal insufficiency | Altered pharmacodynamics and pharmacokinetics, hyponatremia, hypoglycemia |
| Malignant hyperthermia | Acidosis, hypoxemia, electrolyte abnormalities |
| Sepsis | Impaired cerebral metabolism, anemia, hypotension, acidosis |
| Fat embolism | Impaired cerebral metabolism |
| Porphyria | Altered porphyrin metabolism |
| Preeclampsia, eclampsia | Hypermagnesemia, seizure, cerebral edema, intracranial hemorrhage, venous sinus thrombosis |
| Substance abuse | Drug interactions, acute intoxication |
| Cancer | Hypercalcemia, hyponatremia, brain tumor edema |
| Malnutrition | Altered pharmacokinetics, hypoglycemia |

history. The medication list is carefully searched for drugs with sedative side effects such as clonidine, methyldopa, lithium, lidocaine, and antihistamines. Anesthetic and other perioperative drugs are surveyed to ascertain that they were given in an amount appropriate for the patient.

Narcotics, benzodiazepines, inhaled anesthetics, anticholinergics, droperidol, and muscle relaxants may cause failure to arouse. Narcotic overdose tends to be indicated by slow, deep respirations and miotic pupils, whereas patients with residual volatile anesthetic usually have faster, shallow respirations and pupils that are not small. Patients who are unarousable because of muscle paralysis demonstrate minimal to no response to electrical nerve stimulation.

## Drug Overdose

When drug overdose is either relative (eg, patient sensitivity or synergistic drug interaction) or absolute (eg, administration error or unanticipated short procedure), specific antagonists should be administered to rule out neurologic injury. Naloxone, administered intravenously in titrated doses of 20 to 40 μg, reverses the sedation and respiratory depression of narcotics without causing severe pain, hypertension, and tachycardia. Flumazenil given in 0.2-mg increments promptly reverses benzodiazepine-induced sedation. It should be used cautiously in patients receiving continuous benzodiazepine or tricyclic antidepressant therapy. Physostigmine, 1 to 2 mg intravenously, can reverse the sedation of anticholinergic drugs, droperidol, and inhaled anesthetics. Finally, neostigmine or edrophonium is used to reverse neuromuscular blockade.

## Surgical Procedures

Certain surgical procedures are commonly associated with neurologic dysfunction. After transurethral resection of the prostate, hyponatremia is a common cause of mental dysfunction, and glycine absorption can cause blindness. Stroke is more common after carotid and open heart surgery than after general surgery. Hypocalcemia is relatively more common after thyroid or parathyroid surgery. Vasospasm may cause coma after surgery for cerebral aneurysm when subarachnoid hemorrhage has occurred. The anesthesia record is carefully surveyed for evidence of hypotension/hypoxemia, which may be causing postischemic/hypoxic encephalopathy. Hypothermia may cause coma, in addition to potentiating anesthetic drugs and muscle relaxant effect.

Assessment should carefully rule out lateralizing signs in motor function and reflexes or pupillary findings that indicate focal cerebral lesions. When these are suspected, immediate cranial imaging is necessary.

## Rare Events

Finally, rare events must be considered. Cardioembolic stroke may occur in patients with cardiac dysrhythmias or congestive heart failure. Echocardiography may detect intracardiac thrombi. Paradoxical air embolism through a patent foramen ovale can occur after procedures in which the surgical incision is higher than the central venous pressure level, and paradoxical $CO_2$ embolism after abdominal $CO_2$ insufflation has been reported. Embolic events should evidence lateralizing signs on neurologic examination but do not necessarily show immediate changes with cranial imaging techniques.

Pneumocephalus can occur after neurosurgical procedures that drain CSF. Unrecognized seizure activity during the intraoperative period may cause a postictal state that manifests as difficulty in arousal. Preoperative illicit drug use should be considered. If a spinal or epidural anesthetic was administered, total spinal anesthesia may have occurred.

Finally, meningitis and encephalitis should be ruled out by lumbar puncture in patients with fever and depressed mental function, especially in the presence of a stiff neck and when other causes of cerebral dysfunction have been eliminated. Table 10–13 presents an algorithm for assessing patients with postoperative coma.

# POSTOPERATIVE DELIRIUM

## *What Are the Causes?*

Some patterns of emergence from anesthesia are clearly abnormal. Delirium—a confusional state involving altered sensorium that is often associated with agitation, restlessness, and combativeness—is probably the most common abnormal postanesthetic condition. As with delayed emergence, various external factors influenced by psychological and physiologic patient characteristics can cause postoperative delirium.

## Differential Diagnosis

The differential diagnosis of postoperative delirium includes many of the causative factors for encephalopathy in the general population. In addition, many of the conditions, which in a more severe form cause coma or delayed emergence, in a less severe form present as delirium.

## Cerebral Oxygenation

Of greatest importance is the quick ruling out of disturbances in cerebral oxygen delivery and utilization, pulmonary ventilation, and arterial circulation. Thus, the initial evaluation includes the determination of arterial blood gases and oxyhemoglobin saturation, hematocrit, BP, and blood glucose levels.

**TABLE 10–13.** Assessment of Postoperative Coma, Sedation, Delirium

**Immediately**

1. Ensure adequate airway, oxygenation, ventilation: verify with arterial blood gas analysis.
2. Ensure adequate cerebral perfusion and energy utilization: check blood pressure, glucose; rule out seizures and cyanide toxicity.
3. Check for lateralizing signs that may indicate an intracranial mass lesion and impending herniation.

**Further Testing (Directed by History and Neurologic Examination)**
*Medical/Surgical Problem? Drug Effect? New Neurologic Deficit?*

- History: Electrolytes, blood urea nitrogen, magnesium, calcium, ammonia, thyroid function, alcohol level, temperature
- CT scan or MRI, angiogram, electroencephalogram
- Specific reversal agents: naloxone, flumazenil, physostigmine
- Check serum level: lidocaine, phenobarbital, phenytoin, magnesium
- Check neuromuscular function with nerve stimulator
- Lumbar puncture, evoked potentials

CT, computed tomography; MRI, magnetic resonance imaging.

A partially obstructed airway or ventilator dyssynchrony can cause severe agitation.

## New or Preexisting Medical Problems

After airway, breathing, and circulation problems are ruled out, other diagnoses are entertained. Preexisting medical or psychiatric conditions, new neurologic conditions, drug side effects, intraoperative complications, and metabolic and endocrine abnormalities are sought. Table 10–9 lists medical conditions that can result in coma; however, delirium may also be the initial presentation.

Glucose-containing solutions administered to malnourished, alcoholic patients can result in Wernicke disease and Korsakoff psychosis. Patients with organic brain syndromes, mental retardation, personality disorders, and psychiatric illness are more prone to postoperative delirium or agitation. Patients at the extremes of age have a higher incidence of stormy emergence and postoperative delirium. Those with acute psychosis may appear to have delirium.

## Metabolic and Endocrine Factors

Metabolic and endocrine factors may be causative, including electrolyte abnormalities, uremia, hepatic dysfunction, hypothyroidism and hyperthyroidism, and adrenal disease. Also, sepsis, fat embolism, encephalitis, meningitis, malignant hyperthermia, and NMS may result in delirium.

## Brain Injury

Brain injury after ischemic/hypoxic events may also present as encephalopathy. Neurologic examination should be especially tuned to lateralizing signs indicating the presence of stroke, hemorrhage, or other intracranial mass lesion.

## Drugs

Delirium is most commonly caused by the side effects or sequelae of preoperatively or intraoperatively administered drugs. Commonly implicated drugs are ketamine, atropine, scopolamine, droperidol, lidocaine, and cimetidine. Probably every drug administered by anesthesiologists, including antibiotics, has been blamed for causing delirium.

## Pain

Some patients react to severe pain with restlessness, agitation, and confusion. Occult causes of discomfort may be present, such as tight surgical dressings, bladder or gastric distention, intravenous infiltration, and nausea.

## Restraint/Partial Paralysis

Physical restraint in some patients may cause extreme agitation that can present as delirium. Finally, patients who are partially paralyzed may be restless and unable to speak as they attempt to breathe. Fortunately, in most cases, delirium is due simply to a loss of higher integrative functions because of residual anesthesia and resolves as the anesthetic state abates.

# POSTISCHEMIC/HYPOXIC BRAIN INJURY

## What Can Be Done?

### General Measures

In most cases, patients with this type of brain injury—for example, that caused by cardiac arrest, arterial hypoxemia, or both—should receive primarily supportive care. Strict attention to hemodynamics and maintenance of at least normal and perhaps supranormal BPs may ensure perfusion of areas of brain at risk during the postinjury phase.[197,198] Vasopressors may be needed to maintain BP after euvolemia is attained with dextrose-free intravenous fluids. Cerebral metabolism should be minimized when possible. Induced hypothermia has been advocated; certainly, hyperthermia is to be avoided.[199] Small doses of intravenous chlorpromazine (Thorazine), 1 to 2 mg, to inhibit normal temperature regulation may be helpful in this regard as long as hypotension is avoided.

### Seizures

Evidence of seizure activity should be quickly abated with sodium thiopental, phenytoin, or a benzodiazepine titrated as needed. Sedative drugs, however, alter the results of prognostic neurologic examinations.

### Pharmacologic Agents

Various pharmacologic agents, including steroids,[200] barbiturates,[201] and calcium channel blockers,[202,203] have been administered to comatose survivors of cardiac arrest without evidence of benefit in clinical trials. The 30° head-up position may help maintain cerebral perfusion pressure by enhancing jugular venous drainage.

### Ventilatory Support

Controlled ventilation is maintained for several hours or until normal pulmonary function and adequate mental status are ensured. The use of hyperventilation is controversial.[204] Straining, bucking on the ventilator, and excessive muscle activity are controlled with muscle relaxants if needed.

### Miscellaneous Support

Severe hyperglycemia is avoided, the hematocrit is kept in the 30% range, and the serum osmolality is kept between normal and 320 mOsm/L. ICP is not normally elevated after global brain ischemia, but imaging or physical examination evidence of elevated ICP warrants ICP monitoring. When ICP is found to be elevated, normal protocols involving hyperventilation, osmotic/loop diuretics, barbiturates, and hypothermia can be followed.

In the future, other therapies, including free radical scavengers and blockers of excitatory neuroreceptors,[205,206] other regulators of humorally mediated responses,[207] induced hypertension, hypothermic cardiopulmonary bypass,[208] or selective brain cooling[209] may be used.

## Can Outcome Be Predicted After Cardiac Arrest?

A multitude of patient characteristics at the time of cardiac arrest influence the eventual outcome. These factors include age, concurrent drug therapy, hematocrit, serum glucose level, body temperature, reperfusion pattern, acid-base status, serum osmolality, and premorbid conditions of the brain. Levy and colleagues observed physical signs that predicted the eventual level of recovery after 1 year[210] (Table 10–14). For example, patients who on initial examination (within 6 hours of injury) had intact pupillary reflexes, flexor or extensor motor responses, and at least roving conjugate eye movements went on to independent function most of the time. SSEPs have been shown to have high sensitivity and specificity for predicting outcome after anoxic/ischemic coma.[211,212] Unfortunately, no clinical or laboratory test is 100% predictive of eventual neurologic outcome.[213,214]

### How Is Brain Death Diagnosed?

The diagnosis of brain death is made when signs of brain activity are absent and the patient is comatose in the absence of drug intoxication, hypothermia, or reversible metabolic, electrolyte, or endocrine disturbances.[215] Spontaneous respiratory activity does not occur despite elevations in $PaCO_2$ of >50 to 60 mm Hg and evidence that peripheral neuromuscular function is intact. Electrical nerve stimulation or the presence of spinal reflexes demonstrates that apnea is not due to chemical paralysis.

Absence of brainstem reflexes, including the pupillary response to light, the corneal reflex, and the vestibuloocular reflex (ice-water calorics), must be demonstrated. Spinal reflexes to somatic stimulation may be present, but cranial nerve responses and decorticate/decerebrate posturing are absent. EEG, cerebral angiography, and positron emission tomography can verify the diagnosis of brain death but are not essential.[216]

## POSTOPERATIVE HEADACHE

### What Diagnostic Work-Up Is Reasonable?

Headache is a frequent complaint in the general population and has a reported incidence of 13% to 80% after general anesthesia.[217,218] Bromide, a byproduct of halothane metabolism, can cause headache in up to 60% of patients anesthetized with halothane.[219] However, one survey of >18 000 patients admitted to the postanesthesia care unit did not list headache as a complication.[220] Thus, patients complaining of headache deserve further evaluation (Table 10–15).

**TABLE 10–14.** Predicting Outcome After Cardiac Arrest

| Time | Good Prognosis | Poor Prognosis |
|---|---|---|
| Initial examination | Roving conjugate (or better) eye movements | Absent pupillary reflexes |
| | Extensor or flexor motor response | No motor response |
| 3 days | Orienting eye movements, withdrawal or purposeful motor responses | Extensor or flexor motor response |
| 1 week | Obeys commands | Spontaneous eye opening only |

From Levy DE, Caronna J, Singer B, et al. Predicting outcome from hypoxic-ischemic coma. *JAMA.* 1985;253:1420. Copyright 1985, American Medical Association.

**TABLE 10–15.** Differential Diagnosis of Postanesthetic Headache

Mass lesion
  Tumor, aneurysm
  Hematoma, arteriovenous malformation
Increased intracranial pressure
  Cerebral edema, venous sinus thrombosis
  Hydrocephalus
  Malignant hypertension
Cerebrovascular insufficiency
Hypercapnia
Meningitis/encephalitis
Pneumocephalus
Postdural puncture
Posttraumatic (concussion, closed head injury)
Preeclampsia
Hypoglycemia
Referred pain
  Sinusitis
  Degenerative spine disease
  Carotid dissection
  Increased intraocular pressure
Migraine headache
Cluster headache
Tension headache
Caffeine withdrawal
Anemia/polycythemia
Vasodilator: nitroglycerin, nitroprusside
Vasoconstrictor: phenylephrine

### History

The preanesthetic case history should be reviewed to determine whether a long-standing syndrome is present (eg, migraine or cluster headaches) and whether risk factors are present for conditions that might cause headache. For example, patients with coagulopathy would be at higher risk for a subdural hematoma, hypertensive patients for intracerebral bleeds, patients with collagen vascular diseases for vasculitic headaches, and febrile patients for meningitis.

Coffee drinkers who abstain from caffeine intake on the day of surgery may be at increased risk for withdrawal headache.[217] The medication record should be reviewed because vasodilators, such as nitroglycerin, can also cause headache.

### Examination

Malignant hypertension should be ruled out by BP determination. A careful neurologic and funduscopic examination should be performed to rule out the presence of mass lesions and elevated ICP. Laboratory studies should include hematocrit, white blood cell count, and blood glucose determination. When a mass lesion is suspected, CT scanning of the head is indicated.

### Spinal Anesthesia

Patients who had spinal anesthesia are at risk for postdural puncture headache. This problem occurs more frequently in young women and pregnant patients, when larger cutting-tipped needles are used, when the needle bevel is oriented perpendicular to the spine, and perhaps when the needle passes through povidone-iodine solution.[221]

A postdural puncture headache begins within 12 to 48 hours after dural puncture or when a patient first assumes an upright position. The headache is most often described as being frontal, radiating toward the occiput, dull or throbbing, and almost invariably relieved by a horizontal body position. Visual and auditory disturbances are common, and nausea and vomiting are a frequent accompaniment. Cranial nerve abnormalities, especially diplopia (VI) and hearing loss (VIII), may be encountered.

If a headache that resembles a postdural puncture headache does not respond to conservative measures such as hydration or administration of analgesics or caffeine, or if it continues after epidural blood patch, further diagnostic endeavors must be undertaken. Postpartum patients present additional diagnostic dilemmas because the incidence of postpartum headache without anesthesia has been estimated at 30% to 40%[222] and because these patients are at risk for unusual causes of headaches such as venous sinus thrombosis, cerebral edema due to hypertensive disease of pregnancy,[223] subarachnoid hemorrhage, pituitary tumors, and cerebral choriocarcinoma.[224]

## CONCLUSION

Working together, anesthesiologists and neurologists can effect optimal perioperative care of patients with chronic or acute neurologic disease. Neurologists have specific and detailed knowledge about the diagnosis, pathophysiology, and therapy of unique disease processes, whereas the knowledge and skills of anesthesiologists are required to support patients through various pharmacologic, hemodynamic, and respiratory challenges.

## *References*

1. Lee T, Goldman L. Role of the consultant. In: Breslow M, Miller C, Rogers M, eds. *Perioperative Management.* St Louis, Mo: CV Mosby; 1990:49.
2. Baraka A. Anaesthesia and myasthenia gravis. *Can J Anaesth.* 1992;39:476.
3. Leventhal S, Orkin F, Hirsh R. Prediction of the need for postoperative mechanical ventilation in myasthenia gravis. *Anesthesiology.* 1980;53:26.
4. Naguib M, elDawlatly AA, Ashour M, et al. Multivariate determinants of the need for postoperative ventilation in myasthenia gravis. *Can J Anaesth.* 1996;43:1006.
5. d'Empaire G, Hoaglin D, Perlo V, et al. Effect of prethymectomy plasma exchange on postoperative respiratory function in myasthenia gravis. *J Thorac Cardiovasc Surg.* 1985;89:592.
6. Kiran U, Choudhury M, Saxena N, et al. Sevoflurane as a sole anaesthetic for thymectomy in myasthenia gravis. *Acta Anaesthesiol Scand.* 2000;44:351.
7. Tortosa JA, Hernandez-Palazon J. Anaesthesia for laparoscopic cholecystectomy in myasthenia gravis: a non–muscle relaxant technique [letter]. *Anaesthesia.* 1997;52:807.
8. Lorimer M, Hall R. Remifentanil and propofol total intravenous anaesthesia for thymectomy in myasthenia gravis. *Anaesth Intensive Care.* 1998;26:210.
9. Brown T, Gebert R, Meretoja O, et al. Myasthenia gravis in children and its anaesthetic complications. *Anaesth Intensive Care.* 1990;18:466.
10. Sanfilippo M, Fierro G, Cavalletti MV, et al. Rocuronium in two myasthenic patients undergoing thymectomy. *Acta Anaesthesiol Scand.* 1997;41:1365.
11. Merli G, Bell R. Preoperative management of the surgical patient with neurologic disease. *Med Clin North Am.* 1987;71:511.
12. Nilsson E, Perttunen K, Kalso E. Intrathecal morphine for post-sternotomy pain in patients with myasthenia gravis: effects on respiratory function. *Acta Anaesthesiol Scand.* 1997;41:549.
13. Adams RD, Victor M. Parkinson's disease. In: *Principles of Neurology.* 6th ed. New York, NY: McGraw-Hill; 1997:1067.
14. LeWitt PA. Deprenyl's effect at slowing progression of parkinsonian disability: the DATATOP Study. The Parkinson Study Group. *Acta Neurol Scand Suppl.* 1991;136:79.
15. Parkes JD, Baxter RC, Marsden CD, et al. Comparative trial of benzhexol, amantadine, and levodopa in the treatment of Parkinson's disease. *J Neurol Neurosurg Psychiatry.* 1974;37:422.
16. Lees AJ. Levodopa: the gold standard in the management of Parkinson's disease. In: Poewe W, Lees AJ, eds. *Twenty Years of Madopar: New Avenues.* New York, NY: Editiones Roche; 1994:55.
17. Young RR. The differential diagnosis of Parkinson's disease. *Int J Neurol.* 1977;120:210.
18. Severn AM. Parkinsonism and the anaesthetist. *Br J Anaesth.* 1988;61:761.
19. Inzelberg R, Carasso RL, Schechtman E, et al. A comparison of dopamine agonists and catechol-o-methytransferase inhibitors in Parkinson's disease. *Clin Neuropharmacol.* 2000; 23:262.
20. Ruottinen HM, Rinne UK. A double-blind pharmacokinetic and clinical dose-response study of entacapone as an adjuvant to levodopa therapy in advanced Parkinson's disease. *Clin Neuropharmacol.* 1996;19:283.
21. Ruottinen HM, Rinne UK. Entacapone prolongs levodopa response in a one month double blind study in parkinsonian patients with levodopa related fluctuations. *J Neurol Neurosurg Psychiatry.* 1996;60:36.
22. Lyytinen J, Kaakkola S, Ahtila S, et al. Simultaneous MAO-B and COMT inhibition in L-dopa-treated patients with Parkinson's disease. *Mov Disord.* 1997;12:497.
23. Lang AE, Lozano AM, Montgomery E, et al. Posteroventral medial pallidotomy in advanced Parkinson's disease. *N Engl J Med.* 1997;337:1036.
24. Koller WC, Pahwa R, Lyons KE, et al. Surgical treatment of Parkinson's disease. *J Neurol Sci.* 1999:167:1.
25. Starr PA, Vitek JL, Bakay RA. Ablative surgery and deep brain stimulation for Parkinson's disease. *Neurosurgery.* 1998;43:989.
26. Benabid AL, Pollak P, Gao DM, et al. Chronic electrical stimulation of the ventralis intermedius nucleus of the thalamus as a treatment of movement disorders. *J Neurosurg.* 1996;84:203.
27. Koller W, Pahwa R, Busenbark K, et al. High-frequency unilateral thalamic stimulation in the treatment of essential and parkinsonian tremor. *Ann Neurol.* 1997;42:292.
28. Kumar R, Lozano A, Montgomery E, et al. Pallidotomy and deep brain stimulation of the pallidum and subthalamic nucleus in advanced Parkinson's disease. *Mov Disord.* 1998;13(suppl 1):73.
29. Kumar R, Lazano AM, Kim YJ, et al. Double-blind evaluation of the effects of subthalamic nucleus (STN) deep brain stimulation (DBS) in advanced Parkinson's disease. *Neurology.* 1998;51:850.
30. Limousin P, Krack P, Pollak P, et al. Electrical stimulation of the subthalamic nucleus in advanced Parkinson's disease. *N Engl J Med.* 1998;339:1105.
31. Kumar R, Lazano AM, Sime E, et al. Comparative effects of unilateral and bilateral subthalamic nucleus deep brain stimulation. *Neurology.* 1999;53:561.
32. Clarkson ED, Freed CR. Development of fetal neural transplantation as a treatment for Parkinson's disease. *Life Sci.* 1999;65:2427.
33. Gravlee GP. Succinylcholine-induced hyperkalemia in a patient with Parkinson's disease. *Anesth Analg.* 1980;59:444.
34. Nuizzi DA, et al. The lack of effect of succinylcholine on serum potassium in patients with Parkinson's disease. *Anesthesiology.* 1989;71:322.
35. Zornberg GL, Bodkin JA, Cohen BM. Severe adverse interaction between pethidine and selegiline [letter]. *Lancet.* 1991;337:246.
36. Nietz B. Acute dystonia after alfentanil in untreated Parkinson's disease. *Anesth Analg.* 1991;72:557.
37. Golden WE, Lavender RC, Metzer WS. Acute postoperative confusion and hallucinations in Parkinson's disease. *Ann Intern Med.* 1989;111:218.
38. Hart RG, Hindman B. Mechanisms of perioperative cerebral infarction. *Stroke.* 1982;13:766.
39. Larsen SF, Zaric D, Boysen G. Postoperative cerebrovascular accidents in general surgery. *Acta Anaesthesiol Scand.* 1988;32:698.
40. Laupacis A, Albers G, Dalen J, et al. Antithrombotic therapy in atrial fibrillation. *Chest.* 1998;114(suppl 5):579.
41. Hart RG. Intensity of anticoagulation to prevent stroke in patients with atrial fibrillation [letter]. *Ann Intern Med.* 1998;128:408.
42. Hart RG, Halperin JL. Atrial fibrillation and thromboembolism: a decade of progress in stroke prevention. *Ann Intern Med.* 1999;131:688.
43. Inzitari D, Eliasziw M, Gates P, et al. The causes and risk of stroke in patients with asymptomatic internal-carotid-artery stenosis. *N Engl J Med.* 2000;342:1693.
44. Manning WJ, Douglas PS. Transesophageal echocardiography and atrial fibrillation: added value or expensive toy? *Ann Intern Med.* 1998;128:685.

45. North American Symptomatic Carotid Endarterectomy Trial Collaborators. Beneficial effect of carotid endarterectomy in symptomatic patients with high-grade carotid stenosis. *N Engl J Med.* 1991;325:445.

46. Albers GW, Tijssen JG. Antiplatelet therapy: new foundations for optimal treatment decisions. *Neurology.* 1999;53(7 suppl 4):S25.

47. Hass WK, Easton JD, Adams HP Jr, et al. Ticlopidine Aspirin Stroke Study Group: a randomized trial comparing ticlopidine hydrochloride with aspirin for the prevention of stroke in high-risk patients. *N Engl J Med.* 1989;321:501.

48. Limburg M, Wijdicks EF, Li H. Ischemic stroke after surgical procedures: clinical features, neuroimaging, and risk factors. *Neurology.* 1998;50:895.

49. Von Reutern GM, Hetzel A, Bernbaum D, et al. Transcranial Doppler ultrasonography during cardiopulmonary bypass in patients with severe carotid stenosis or occlusion. *Stroke.* 1988;19:674.

50. Brusino FG, Reves JG, Smith LR, et al. The effect of age on cerebral blood flow during hypothermic cardiopulmonary bypass. *J Thorac Cardiovasc Surg.* 1989;97:541.

51. McDowell FH, Brott TG, Goldstein M, et al. Stroke the first six hours. *J Stroke Cerebrovasc Dis.* 1993;3:133.

52. Britton M, Faire UD, Helmers C. Hazards of therapy for excessive hypertension in acute stroke. *Acta Med Scand.* 1980;207:253.

53. Lisk DR, Grotta JC, Lamki LM, et al. Should hypertension be treated after acute stroke? A randomized controlled trial using single photon emission computed tomography. *Arch Neurol.* 1993;50:855.

54. Bath FJ, Bath PMW. What is the correct management of blood pressure in acute stroke? The Blood Pressure in Acute Stroke Collaboration. *Cerebrovasc Dis.* 1997;7:205.

55. Adams HP, Brott TG, Furlan AJ, et al. Guidelines for thrombolytic therapy for acute stroke: a supplement to the guidelines for the management of patients with acute ischemic stroke. A statement for healthcare professionals from a special writing group of the Stroke Council, American Heart Association. *Circulation.* 1996;94:1167.

56. Nachtmann A, Siebler M, Rose G, et al. Cheyne-Stokes respiration in ischemic stroke. *Neurology.* 1995;45:820.

57. Bassetti C, Aldrich MS, Chervin RD, et al. Sleep apnea in patients with transient ischemic attack and stroke: a prospective study of 59 patients. *Neurology.* 1996;46:1167.

58. NINDS rt-PA Stroke Study Group. Tissue plasminogen activator for acute ischemic stroke. *N Engl J Med.* 1995;333:1581.

59. Barber PA, Zhang J, Demchuk AM, et al: Why are stroke patients excluded from TPA therapy? An analysis of patient eligibility. *Neurology.* 2001;56:1015.

60. International Stroke Trial Collaborative Group. The International Stroke Trial (IST): a randomised trial of aspirin, subcutaneous heparin, both, or neither among 19,435 patients with acute ischaemic stroke. *Lancet.* 1997;349:1569.

61. Chinese Acute Stroke Trial Collaborative Group. Chinese Acute Stroke Trial. *Lancet.* 1997;349:1641.

62. Hommel M, for the FISS bis Investigators Group. Fraxiparine in ischemic stroke study (FISS bis). *Cerebrovasc Dis.* 1998;8(suppl 4):63.

63. The Publications Committee for the Trial of ORG 10172 in Acute Stroke Treatment (TOAST) Investigators. Low molecular weight heparinoid, ORG 10172 (danaparoid), and outcome after acute ischemic stroke: a randomized controlled trial. *JAMA.* 1998;279:1265.

64. Hart RG, Benavente O, Lalonde DR, et al. What's new in stroke? update 1998. *Tex Med.* 1998;94(5):44.

65. Hornig CR, Bauer T, Simon C, et al. Hemorrhagic transformation in cardioembolic cerebral infarction. *Stroke.* 1993;24:465.

66. Mayo Asymptomatic Carotid Endarterectomy Study Group. Results of a randomized controlled trial of carotid endarterectomy for asymptomatic carotid stenosis. *Mayo Clin Proc.* 1992;67:513.

67. Kearon C, Hirsh J. Management of anticoagulation before and after elective surgery. *N Engl J Med.* 1997;336:1506.

68. Hirsh J, Dalen JE, Anderson DR, et al. Oral anticoagulants: mechanism of action, clinical effectiveness, and optimal therapeutic range. *Chest.* 1998;114:445S.

69. Soute JC, Oliver A, ZuaZuJausoro I, et al. Oral surgery in anticoagulated patients without reducing the dose of oral anticoagulant: a prospective randomized study. *J Oral Maxillofac Surg.* 1996;54:27.

70. Kearse L. Neurologic disorders and spinal cord injuries. In: Cheng EY, Kay J, eds. *Manual of Anesthesia and the Medically Compromised Patient.* Philadelphia, Pa: JB Lippincott; 990:317.

71. Smeltzer SC, Skurnick JH, Troiano R, et al. Respiratory function in multiple sclerosis: utility of clinical assessment of respiratory muscle function. *Chest.* 1992;101:479.

72. Ueno K, Miyai K, Mitsuzane K. Phenytoin-tizanidine interaction [letter]. *DICP.* 1991;25:1273.

73. Warren T, Datta S, Ostheimer G. Lumbar epidural anesthesia in a patient with multiple sclerosis. *Anesth Analg.* 1982;61:1022.

74. Bader AM, Hunt Co, Datta A, et al. Anesthesia for the obstetric patient with multiple sclerosis. *J Clin Anesth.* 1988;1:21.

75. Alderson JD. Intrathecal diamorphine and multiple sclerosis. *Anaesthesia.* 1990;45:1084.

76. Jones RM, Healy T. Anaesthesia and demyelinating disease. *Anaesthesia.* 1980;35:879.

77. Jones RM, Healy T. Anesthesia for the obstetric patient with multiple sclerosis. *J Clin Anesth.* 1988;1:21.

78. Kohno K, Uchida H, Yamamoto N, et al. Sevoflurane anesthesia in a patient with multiple sclerosis. *Masui.* 1994;43:1229.

79. Guthrie TC, Nelson DA. Influence of temperature changes on multiple sclerosis: critical review of mechanisms and research potential. *J Neurol Sci.* 1995;129:1.

80. Borel C. Neuromuscular disease. In: Breslow M, Miller C, Rogers M, eds. *Perioperative Management.* St Louis, Mo: CV Mosby; 1990:417.

81. Goresky GV, Cox RG. Inhalation anesthetics and Duchenne's muscular dystrophy [editorial]. *Can J Anaesth.* 1999;46:564.

82. Irwin MG, Henderson M. Cardiac arrest during major spinal scoliosis surgery in a patient with Duchenne's muscular dystrophy undergoing intravenous anaesthesia. *Anaesth Intensive Care.* 1995;23:626.

83. Ririe DG, Shapiro F, Sethna NF. The response of patients with Duchenne's muscular dystrophy to neuromuscular blockade with vecuronium. *Anesthesiology.* 1998;88:351.

84. Starosta-Rubinstein S, Youg AAAB, Kluin K, et al. Clinical assessment of 31 patients with Wilson's disease. *Arch Neurol.* 1987;44:365.

85. Marsden DC. Investigation of dystonia. *Adv Neurol.* 1988;50:35.

86. Patrinely JP, Anderson RL. Essential blepharospasm: a review. *Geriatr Ophthalmol.* 1986;2:27.

87. Chan J, Brin MF, Fahn S. Idiopathic cervical dystonia: clinical characteristics. *Mov Disord.* 1991;6:119.

88. Jankovic J, Leder S, Warner D, et al. Cervical dystonia: clinical findings and associated movement disorders. *Neurology.* 1991;41:1088.

89. Brin MF. Torticollis (cervical dystonia). In: Johnson RT, Griffin JW, eds. *Current Therapy in Neurologic Disease.* 4th ed. St Louis, Mo: Mosby-Year Book; 1993:266.

90. National Institutes of Health Consensus Development Conference Statement. Clinical use of botulinum toxin. *Arch Neurol.* 1991;48:1294.

91. Munchau A, Bhatia KP. Uses of botulinum toxin injection in medicine today. *BMJ.* 2000;320:161.

92. Dutton JJ. Botulinum-A toxin in the treatment of craniocervical muscle spasms: short- and long-term, local and systemic effects. *Surv Ophthalmol.* 1996;41:51.

93. Jankovic J. Medical therapy and botulinum toxin in dystonia. *Adv Neurol.* 1998;78:169.

94. Bertrand C, Molina-Negro P, Bouvier G, et al. Observations and analysis of results in 131 cases of spasmodic torticollis after selective denervation. *Appl Neurophysiol.* 1987;50:319.

95. Bertrand C, Molina Negro P, Martinez SN. Technical aspects of selective denervation for spasmodic torticollis. *Appl Neurophysiol.* 1982;45:326.

96. Andrew J, Fowler CJ, Arrison MJ. Stereotaxic thalamotomy in 55 cases of dystonia. *Brain.* 1983;106:981.

97. Oh I, Nowacek CJ. Surgical release of congenital torticollis in adults. *Clin Orthop.* 1978;131:141.

98. Walajahi FH, Karasic LH. Anesthetic management of a patient with dystonia musculorum deformans. *Anesth Analg.* 1984;63:616.

99. Davis NL, David R. Anesthetic management of a patient with dystonia musculorum deformans. *Anesthesiology.* 1975;42:630.

100. Dehring DJ, Gupta B, Peruzzi WT. Postoperative opisthotonus and torticollis after fentanyl, enflurane and nitrous oxide. *Can J Anaesth.* 1991;38:919.

101. Stemp LI, Taswell C. Spastic torticollis during general anesthesia: case report and review of receptor mechanisms. *Anesthesiology.* 1991;75:365.

102. Fiacchino F, Gemma M, Bricchi M, et al. Hypo- and hypersensitivity to vecuronium in a patient with Guillain-Barré syndrome. *Anesth Analg.* 1994;78:187.

103. Browne MG, Cross R. Huntington's chorea. *Br J Anaesth.* 1981;53:136.

104. Stewart JT. Huntington's disease. *Am Fam Physician.* 1988;37:105.

105. Cangemi CF, Miller RJ. Huntington's disease: review and anesthetic case management. *Anesth Prog.* 1998;45:150.

106. Duncan FJ, Corbett J, Wall M. The incidence of pseudotumor cerebri. *Arch Neurol.* 1988;45:875.

107. Baker RS, Bauman RJ, Buncic JR. Idiopathic intracranial hypertension (pseudotumor cerebri) in pediatric patients. *Pediatr Neurol.* 1989;5:5.

108. Corbett JJ, Mehta M. Cerebrospinal fluid pressure in normal obese subjects and patients with pseudotumor cerebri. *Neurology.* 1983;33:1386.

109. Paruchuri SR, Lawlor M, Kleinhomer K, et al. Risk of cerebellar tonsillar herniation after diagnostic lumbar puncture in pseudotumor cerebri [letter]. *Anesth Analg.* 1993;77:403.

110. Abouleish E, Ali V, Tang R. Benign intracranial hypertension and anesthesia for cesarean section. *Anesthesiology.* 1985;63:705.

111. Granner MA, Wooten GF. Neuroleptic malignant syndrome or parkinsonism hyperpyrexia syndrome. *Semin Neurol.* 1991;11:228.

112. Caroff SN, Mann SC. Neuroleptic malignant syndrome. *Med Clin North Am.* 1993;77:185.

113. Heiman-Patterson TD. Neuroleptic malignant syndrome and malignant hyperthermia: important issues for the medical consultant. *Med Clin North Am.* 1993;77:477.

114. Heyland D, Sauve M. Neuroleptic malignant syndrome without the use of neuroleptics. *CMAJ.* 1991;145:817.

115. Dickey W. The neuroleptic malignant syndrome. *Prog Neurobiol.* 1991;36:425.

116. Schneider SML. Neuroleptic malignant syndrome: controversies in treatment. *Am J Emerg Med.* 1991;9:360.

117. Keltner N, Harris CP. Serotonin syndrome: a case of fatal SSRI/MAOI interaction. *Perspect Psychiatr Care.* 1995;33:33.

118. Gratz SS, Levinson DF, Simpson GM. The treatment and management of neuroleptic malignant syndrome. *Prog Neuropsychopharmacol Biol Psychiatry.* 1992;16:425.

119. Lev R, Clark RF. Neuroleptic malignant syndrome presenting without fever: case report and review of the literature. *J Emerg Med.* 1994;12:49.

120. George A, Wood C. Succinylcholine-induced hyperkalemia complicating the neuroleptic malignant syndrome. *Ann Intern Med.* 1987;106:172.

121. Cramer JA, Fisher R, Ben-Menachem E, et al. New antiepileptic drugs: comparison of key clinical trials. *Epilepsia.* 1999;40:500.

122. Tecoma ES. Oxcarbazepine. *Epilepsia.* 1999;40(suppl 5):S37.

123. Woody R, Grollady E, Fiedorek S. Rectal anticonvulsants in seizure patients undergoing gastrointestinal surgery. *J Pediatr Surg.* 1989;24:474.

124. Modica PA, Tempelhoff R, White PF. Part 1: pro- and anticonvulsant effects of anesthetics. *Anesth Analg.* 1990;70:433.

125. Lebowitz MH, Blitt CD, Dillon JB. Enflurane-induced central nervous system excitation and its relation to carbon dioxide tension. *Anesth Analg.* 1972;51:355.

126. Burchiel KJ, Stockard JJ, Calverley RK, et al. Relationship of pre and postanesthetic EEG abnormalities to enflurane-induced seizure activity. *Anesth Analg.* 1977;56:509.

127. Modica PA, Tempelhoff R, White PF. Part 2: pro- and anticonvulsant effects of anesthetics. *Anesth Analg.* 1990;70:303.

128. Rampil IJ, Lockhart SH, Eger EI, et al. The electroencephalographic effects of desflurane in humans. *Anesthesiology.* 1991;74:434.

129. Komatsu H, Taie S, Endo S, et al. Electrical seizure during sevoflurane anesthesia in two pediatric patients with epilepsy. *Anesthesiology.* 1994;81:1535.

130. Ebrahim ZY, DeBoer GE, Luders H, et al. Effect of etomidate on the electroencephalogram of patients with epilepsy. *Anesth Anal.* 1986;65:1004.

131. Krieger W, Copperman J, Laxer KD. Seizures with etomidate anesthesia. *Anesth Analg.* 1985;64:1226.

132. Cochran D, Price W, Gwinnutt CL. Unilateral convulsion after induction of anaesthesia with propofol. *Br J Anaesth.* 1996;74:26.

133. Ebrahim ZY, Schubert AS, Van Ness P, et al. The effect of propofol on the electroencephalogram of patients with epilepsy. *Anesth Analg.* 1994;78:275.

134. Smith M, Smith SJ, Scott CA, et al. Activation of the electrocorticogram by propofol during surgery for epilepsy. *Br J Anaesth.* 1996;76:499.

135. Manners JM, Wills A. Post-operative convulsions: a review based on a case report. *Anaesthesia.* 1971;26:66.

136. Therapeutics and Technology Assessment Subcommittee of the American Academy of Neurology. Assessment: intraoperative neurophysiology. *Neurology.* 1990;40:1644.

137. McTaggart Cowan RA. Somatosensory evoked potentials during spinal surgery. *Can J Anaesth.* 1998;45:460.

138. Nuwer MR. Spinal cord monitoring. *Muscle Nerve.* 1999;22:1620.

139. Sloan TB. Anesthetic effects on electrophysiologic recordings. *J Clin Neurophysiol.* 1998;15:217.

140. Goodrich JT. Electrophysiologic measurements: intraoperative evoked potential monitoring. *Anesthesiol Clin North Am.* 1987;5:477.

141. Gugino V, Chabot R. Somatosensory evoked potentials. *Int Anesthesiol Clin.* 1990;28:154.

142. Levine R. Short-latency auditory evoked potentials: intraoperative applications. *Int Anesthesiol Clin.* 1990;28:147.

143. Thompson GE, Lui A. Perioperative nerve injury. In: Benumof JL, Saidman LJ, eds. *Anesthesia and Perioperative Complications.* St Louis, Mo: Mosby-Year Book; 1992:160.

144. Lederman R, Breuer A, Hanson M, et al. Peripheral nervous system complications of coronary artery bypass graft surgery. *Ann Neurol.* 1982;12:297.

145. Keates J, Innocenti D, Ross D. Mononeuritis multiplex, a complication of open-heart surgery. *J Thorac Cardiovasc Surg.* 1975;69:820.

146. Merchant RN, Brown WF, Watson BV. Peripheral nerve injuries in cardiac anesthesia. *Can J Anaesth.* 1990;37:5152.

147. McAlpine FS, Seckel BR. The peripheral nervous system. In: Martin JT, ed. *Positioning in Anesthesia and Surgery.* 2nd ed. Philadelphia, Pa: WB Saunders; 1987:303.

148. Parks B. Postoperative peripheral neuropathies. *Surgery.* 1973;74:348.

149. Warner MA, Warner ME, Martin JT. Ulnar neuropathy: incidence, outcome, and risk factors in sedated or anesthetized patients. *Anesthesiology.* 1994;81:1332.

150. Stoelting RK. Postoperative ulnar nerve palsy: is it a preventable complication? *Anesth Analg.* 1993;81:1332.

151. Selander D, Edshage S, Wolff T. Paresthesiae or no parasthesiae? Nerve lesions after axillary blocks. *Acta Anaesthesiol Scand.* 1979;23:27.

152. Rice ASC, McMahon SB. Peripheral nerve injury caused by injection needles used in regional anesthesia: influence of bevel configuration, studies in a rat model. *Br J Anaesth.* 1992;69:433.

153. Selander D, Brattsand R, Lundborg G, et al. Local anesthetics: importance of mode of application, concentration and adrenaline for the appearance of nerve lesions. *Acta Anaesthesiol Scand.* 1979;23:127.

154. Pollock JE, Neal JM, Stephenson CA, et al. Prospective study of the incidence of transient radicular irritation in patients undergoing spinal anesthesia. *Anesthesiology.* 1996;84:1361.

155. Cheney FW, Domino KB, Caplan RA, et al. Nerve injury associated with anesthesia: a closed claims analysis. *Anesthesiology.* 1999;90:1062.

156. Cameron M, Stewart O. Ulnar nerve injury associated with anesthesia. *Can Anaesth Soc J.* 1975;22:253.

157. Aldrete J. Recovery room assessment. In: Martin J, ed. *Positioning in Anesthesia and Surgery.* Philadelphia, Pa: WB Saunders; 1987:329.

158. Chadwick HS, Ross BK. Causes and consequences of maternal-fetal perianesthetic complications. In: Benumof JL, Saidman LJ, eds. *Anesthesia and Perioperative Complications.* St Louis, Mo: Mosby-Year Book; 1992:520.

159. Dawson DM, Krarup C. Perioperative nerve lesions. *Arch Neurol.* 1989;46:1355.

160. Ducker T. Management of peripheral nerve injuries. In: Salcman E, ed. *Neurologic Emergencies Recognition and Management.* 2nd ed. New York, NY: Raven Press; 1990:221.

161. Massey EW, Cefalo RC. Managing the carpal tunnel syndrome of pregnancy. *Contemp Obstet Gynecol.* 1977;9:39.

162. Massey EW. Mononeuropathies in pregnancy. *Semin Neurol.* 1988;8:193.

163. Hill EC. Maternal obstetric paralysis. *Am J Obstet Gynecol.* 1962;83:1452.

164. Berry PR, Wallis WE. Venepuncture nerve injuries. *Lancet.* 1977;1:1236.

165. Adelman J, Goldberg G, Puckett J. Postpartum bilateral femoral neuropathy. *Obstet Gynecol.* 1973;42:845.

166. Grove LH. Backache, headache and bladder dysfunction after delivery. *Br J Anaesth.* 1973;45:147.

167. Pathy G, Rosen M. Prolonged block with recovery after extradural analgesia for labour. *Br J Anaesth.* 1975;47:520.

168. Cuerdan C, Buley R, Downing JW. Delayed recovery after epidural analgesia for labour. *Anaesthesia.* 1977;32:773.

169. Kane R. Neurologic deficits following epidural or spinal anesthesia. *Anesth Analg.* 1981;60:150.

170. Vandam L, Dripps R. A long-term follow-up of 10,098 spinal anesthetics. *Surgery.* 1955;38:463.

171. Murphy TM, O'Keeffe D. Complications of spinal, epidural and caudal anesthesia. In: Benumof JL, Saidman LJ, eds. *Anesthesia and Perioperative Complications.* St Louis, Mo: Mosby-Year Book; 1992:38.

172. Wang BC, Hillman DE, Spielholz NI, et al. Chronic neurological deficits and Nesacaine-CE: an effect of the anesthetic, 2-chloroprocaine, or the antioxidant, sodium bisulfite? *Anesth Analg.* 1984;63:445.

173. Reisner L, Hochman B, Plumer M. Persistent neurologic deficit and adhesive arachnoiditis following intrathecal 2-chloroprocaine injection. *Anesth Analg.* 1980;59:452.

174. Rigler M, Drasner R, Krejcie T, et al. Cauda equina syndrome after continuous spinal anesthesia. *Anesth Analg.* 191;72:275.

175. Fibuch E, Opper S. Back pain following epidurally administered Nesacaine-MPF. *Anesth Analg.* 1989;69:113.

176. Ready LB, Helfer D. Bacterial meningitis in parturients after epidural anesthesia. *Anesthesiology.* 1989;71:988.

177. Goldman WW, Sanford JP. An "epidemic" of chemical meningitis. *Am J Med.* 1960;29:94.

178. Berga S, Trierweiler MW. Bacterial meningitis following epidural anesthesia for vaginal delivery: a case report. *Obstet Gynecol.* 1989;74:437.

179. McHale S, Clark MM. Meningitis after spinal anaesthesia. *Anaesthesia.* 1990;45:987.

180. DiGiovanni AJ, Galbert MW, Phillips JN. "Chemical meningitis" tied to cleaning fluid bacteria. *JAMA.* 1970;214:2129.

181. Goucke CR, Graziotti P. Extradural abscess following local anaesthetic and steroid injection for chronic low back pain. *Br J Anaesth.* 1990;65:427.

182. Baker A, Ojemann R, Swartz M, et al. Spinal epidural abscess. *N Engl J Med.* 1975;293:463.

183. Owens E, Kasten G, Hessel E. Spinal subarachnoid hematoma after lumbar puncture and heparinization: a case report, review of the literature and discussion of anesthetic implications. *Anesth Analg.* 1986;65:1201.

184. Tartiere J, Gerard JL, Peny J, et al. Acute treatment after accidental intrathecal injection of hypertonic contrast media. *Anesthesiology.* 1989;71:169.

185. Fog J, Wang L, Sundberg A, et al. Hearing loss after spinal anesthesia is related to needle size. *Anesth Analg.* 1990;70:517.

186. Robles R. Cranial nerve paralysis after spinal anesthesia. *Northwest Med.* 1968;67:845.

187. Bromage P. "Paraplegia following epidural analgesia": a misnomer. *Anaesthesia.* 1976;31:947.

188. Rosenberg H, Clofine R, Bialik O. Neurologic changes during awakening from anesthesia. *Anesthesiology.* 1981;54:125.

189. Cucchiara RF. Differential awakening [letter]. *Anesth Analg.* 1992;75:467.

190. McCulloch PR, Milne B. Neurological phenomena during emergence from enflurane or isoflurane anesthesia. *Can J Anaesth.* 1990;37:739.

191. Davison L, Steinhelber J, Eger E, et al. Psychological effects of halothane and isoflurane anesthesia. *Anesthesiology.* 1975;43:313.

192. Mills P, Sessler D, Moseley M, et al. An in vivo $^{19}$F nuclear magnetic resonance study of isoflurane elimination from the rabbit brain. *Anesthesiology.* 1987;67:169.

193. Knill R, Moote C, Skinner M, et al. Anesthesia with abdominal surgery leads to intense REM sleep during the first postoperative week. *Anesthesiology.* 1990;73:52.

194. Melnick B, Sawyer R, Karambelkar D, et al. Delayed side effects of droperidol after ambulatory general anesthesia. *Anesth Analg.* 1989;69:748.

195. Crosby G. Impaired central nervous system function. In: Benumof JL, Saidman LJ, eds. *Anesthesia and Perioperative Complications.* St Louis, Mo: Mosby-Year Book; 1992:356.

196. Mecca RS. Complications during recovery. *Int Anesthesiol Clin.* 1991;29:37.

197. Safar P. Cerebral resuscitation after cardiac arrest: a review. *Circulation.* 1986;74(suppl 4):IV-138.

198. Sterz F, Leonov Y, Safar P, et al. Hypertension with or without hemodilution after cardiac arrest in dogs. *Stroke.* 1990;21:1178.

199. Sterz F, Safar P, Tisherman S, et al. Mild hypothermic cardiopulmonary resuscitation improves outcome after prolonged cardiac arrest in dogs. *Crit Care Med.* 1991;19:379.

200. Jastremski M, Sutton-Tyrrell K, Vaagenes P, et al. Glucocorticoid treatment does not improve neurological recovery following cardiac arrest. *JAMA.* 1989;262:3427.

201. Brain Resuscitation Clinical Trial I Study Group. A randomized clinical study of thiopental loading in comatose survivors of cardiac arrest. *N Engl J Med.* 1986;314:397.

202. Brain Resuscitation Clinical Trial II Study Group. A randomized clinical study of a calcium-entry blocker (lidoflazine) in the treatment of comatose survivors of cardiac arrest. *N Engl J Med.* 1991;324:1225.

203. Roine R, Kaste M, Kinnunen A, et al. Nimodipine after resuscitation from out of hospital ventricular fibrillation. *JAMA.* 1990;264:3171.

204. Loughhead MG. Brain resuscitation and protection. *Med J Aust.* 1988;148:458.

205. Bocher, A Zornow MH. Lamotrigine inhibits extracellular glutamate accumulation during transient global cerebral ischemia in rats. *Anesthesiology.* 1997;86:459.

206. Safar P. Resuscitation from clinical death: pathophysiologic limits and therapeutic potentials. *Crit Care Med.* 1988;16:923.

207. Farbiszeroshi R, Chwiecko M, Ustymowicz J. The 21 aminosteroid U-743899 protects the antioxidant enzymes in ischemia (reperfusion-induced rat brain damage). *Eur J Pharmacol.* 1994;270:263.

208. Safar P. Cerebral resuscitation after cardiac arrest: research initiatives and future directions. *Ann Emerg Med.* 1993;22:324.

209. Safar P, Klain M, Tisherman S. Selective brain cooling after cardiac arrest. *Crit Care Med.* 1996;24:911.

210. Levy DE, Caronna J, Singer B, et al. Predicting outcome from hypoxic-ischemic coma. *JAMA.* 1985;253:1420.

211. Zandbergen EG, de Haan RJ, Stoutenbeek CP, et al. Systematic review of early prediction of poor outcome in anoxic-ischaemic coma. *Lancet.* 1998;352:1808.

212. Chen R, Bolton CF, Young B. Prediction of outcome in patients with anoxic coma: a clinical and electrophysiologic study. *Crit Care Med.* 1996;24:672.

213. Reinmuth O, Vagnes P, Abramson N, et al. Predicting outcome after resuscitation from clinical death. *Crit Care Med.* 1988;16:1043.

214. Berek K, Jeschow M, Aichner F. The prognostication of cerebral hypoxia after out-of-hospital cardiac arrest in adults. *Eur Neurol.* 1997;37:135.

215. The Quality Standards Subcommittee of the American Academy of Neurology. Practice parameters for determining brain death in adults. The Quality Standards Subcommittee of the American Academy of Neurology. *Neurology.* 1995;45:1012.

216. Critchley E. *Neurological Emergencies.* Philadelphia, Pa: WB Saunders; 1988:88.

217. Fennelly M, Galletly DC, Purdie GI. Is caffeine withdrawal the mechanism of postoperative headache? *Anesth Analg.* 1991;72:449.

218. Cosh PH. Headache after general anesthesia. *Anaesthesia.* 1988;43:889.

219. Tyrrell M, Feldman S. Headache following halothane anesthesia. *Br J Anaesth.* 1968;40:99.

220. Hines R, Barash P, Watrous G, et al. Complications occurring in the postanesthesia care unit. *Anesth Analg.* 1992;74:503.

221. Gurmarnik S. Skin preparation and spinal headache. *Anaesthesia.* 1988;43:1057.

222. Stein G, Morton J, Marsh A, et al. Headaches after childbirth. *Acta Neurol Scand.* 1984;69:74.

223. Reik L. Headaches in pregnancy. *Semin Neurol.* 1988;8:187.

224. Fox M, Harms R, Davis D. Selected neurologic complications of pregnancy. *Mayo Clin Proc.* 1990;65:1595.

**11**

# Nephrology Consultation

### R. Dennis Bastron
### David P. Ciceri

## PURPOSE OF THE CONSULTATION
*What Questions Should Be Addressed?*

## HYPERTENSION
*How Is the Efficacy of Antihypertensive Therapy Assessed?*
*What Are Allowable Blood Pressure Limits?*
*When Should Surgery Be Delayed?*
*Is Perioperative Medication Change Indicated?*
*Is Clonidine a Problem?*

## FLUID THERAPY
*How Are Intravenous Fluids Chosen?*
*What Fluids Are Useful?*
*Is Dextrose a Problem?*
*When Can Dextrose Be Administered?*
*What Is the Role of Sodium?*
*What Is the Significance of Hyponatremia?*
*What Is the Significance of Hypernatremia?*

## POTASSIUM
*What Is the Significance of Hypokalemia?*
*What Is the Significance of Hyperkalemia?*

## CALCIUM
*What Is the Significance of Hypocalcemia?*
*What Is the Significance of Hypercalcemia?*

## MAGNESIUM
*How Is Magnesium Imbalance Managed?*
*What Is the Significance of Hypomagnesemia?*
*What Is the Significance of Hypermagnesemia?*

## PHOSPHORUS
*How Is Phosphorus Imbalance Managed?*
*What Is the Significance of Hypophosphatemia?*
*What Is the Significance of Hyperphosphatemia?*

## RENAL FUNCTION TESTS
*When Is Urinalysis Useful?*
*Of What Significance Is the Urine Volume?*
*What Does Serum Urea Nitrogen Indicate?*
*When Is Serum Creatinine Measurement Useful?*

## COMPROMISED RENAL FUNCTION
*Are the Changes Acute or Chronic?*
*What Are the Hallmarks of Chronic Failure?*
*When Should Urine Output Be Monitored?*
*What Are Oliguria and Polyuria?*
*Why Is Oliguria Present?*
*Is Sophisticated Testing Necessary?*

## RENAL TOXICITY
*What Are the Causative Factors?*
*How Are the Kidneys Protected?*
*What Intravenous Fluids Are Best?*
*How Does Renal Failure Affect Drug Choice and Dosage?*

## DIALYSIS PATIENTS
*Why Is Timing Important?*
*Is a Tilt Test Advisable?*
*What Blood Studies Are Important?*
*How Should Arteriovenous Fistulas or Other Dialysis Sites Be Managed?*
*Why Is the Postoperative Period Critical?*
*What Are the Anesthetic Implications?*

Identification of an electrolyte abnormality often results in a nephrology consult. A range outside of which a laboratory value signifies severe electrolyte imbalance is somewhat meaningless because each patient responds differently to electrolyte changes. For example, a patient with slowly developing hyponatremia may be symptom free with a serum sodium level of 120 mEq/L, whereas another patient with acute hyponatremia may have major symptoms at a serum sodium level of 130 mEq/L. In this chapter, *severe electrolyte imbalance* is defined as a disorder that causes signs or symptoms or is outside of the range that a patient's current physicians feel confident about treating.

Similarly, chronic renal disease is characterized by slow, irreversible, progressive loss of nephrons and is accompanied by compensatory changes in the remaining nephrons. Patients pass through several stages before they develop uremia and require dialysis. Each stage has anesthetic implications, but a preoperative nephrology consultation is usually not necessary until the patient requires dialysis. In contrast, patients with acute renal failure (ARF) should have a nephrologist involved in their care as soon as practical.

## PURPOSE OF THE CONSULTATION

### What Questions Should Be Addressed?

A nephrology consultation should answer these questions:

1. What is the patient's diagnosis and pathophysiology?
2. Is the patient in optimal condition for anesthesia and surgery?
3. If not, what must be done to make the patient's condition optimum?

This information is valuable to help plan the timing of nonemergency surgery. Specifically, a nephrologist can help with perioperative fluid management, antihypertensive therapy, selection and dosage of certain drugs, and dialysis if necessary. A consultation is superfluous when a patient's problems do not lie outside the confidence zone of the treating physicians, when the consultation indicates something that is already known (eg, "monitor the patient and keep the patient well oxygenated"), or when the advice is outside the consultant's area of expertise (eg, "general anesthesia is contraindicated").

## HYPERTENSION

About 10% of Americans are hypertensive, and nearly 12 million develop renal disease annually.[1] The size of the patient population that is anesthetized determines the frequency of nephrology consultations that are requested, but this number is probably small.

### How Is the Efficacy of Antihypertensive Therapy Assessed?

In the mid-1980s, patients were admitted to the hospital one or two days before surgery, and several recorded blood pressure (BP) measurements were usually available to evaluate control of a patient's hypertension. Today, the odds are that your first contact with a patient will be in the preoperative holding area, and perhaps one BP measurement will be recorded in the chart. It may be recorded in several places by different people, but it is uncanny how the numbers are the same. This BP value probably was measured just as the patient had been told that the risks of surgery and anesthesia may include death, coma, and permanent neurologic damage. It

often is higher than usual, and it is on this insufficient information that a judgment must be made about whether the antihypertensive therapy is adequate.

### What Are Allowable Blood Pressure Limits?

If the BP is <160 mm Hg systolic and <90 mm Hg diastolic, there probably is no problem. If it is 190/100 mm Hg, the anesthetist should be concerned but can medicate the patient to see whether decreasing anxiety or pain decreases the BP. If the diastolic BP exceeds 110 mm Hg, it is not controlled by the current therapy.[2]

To assess the effectiveness of treatment, the patient's usual BP (many hypertensive patients know this value) must be known. Whether the patient is adequately treated, has a rare pathologic process (thyrotoxicosis, pheochromocytoma), or has some temporary and reversible cause of hypertension (severe pain, distended bladder) must then be determined. Also of concern is the possibility of a drug reaction (eg, phenylephrine eye or nose drops), withdrawal (eg, missed morning dose), or interaction (eg, meperidine and monoamine oxidase inhibitor).

### When Should Surgery Be Delayed?

Surgery normally should not be delayed for a patient whose diastolic pressure is <110 mm Hg. When the diastolic pressure exceeds 110 mm Hg, several determinations should be made while you try therapeutic maneuvers. These include catheterization of the bladder or administration of sedatives, tranquilizers, narcotics, vasodilators, β-blockers, or calcium channel blockers (Table 11–1). After the pressure decreases to a tolerable range (and it almost always does), proceed with anesthesia. Careful BP control intraoperatively and, perhaps more importantly, postoperatively is essential.[3–5] When the inevitable peaks and valleys of BP occur, react appropriately but do not overreact.

Delay surgery only in the following rare circumstances:

- The diastolic BP cannot be controlled (ie, it is >110 mm Hg).
- You suspect thyrotoxicosis or pheochromocytoma.
- The patient has myocardial ischemia or congestive heart failure.
- Signs and symptoms of previously undiagnosed end-organ failure (renal, central nervous system [CNS]) are present.

### Is Perioperative Medication Change Indicated?

Changing a patient's medication in the perioperative period may cause an unsteady state that can be more of a problem than if the medication were not changed. The medication schedule usually should be maintained right up to the time of surgery. Any doses scheduled after the nil per os (NPO) period can safely be taken with a sip of water. If the patient is taking a diuretic for BP control rather than for congestive heart failure, the morning dose on the day of surgery can be omitted.

**TABLE 11–1.** Useful Drugs for Treating Perioperative Hypertension

| Drug | Dose | Route | Action |
|------|------|-------|--------|
| Hydralazine | 5 mg every 5 min | Intravenous | Direct vasodilator |
| Labetalol | 5–20 mg | Intravenous | α- or β-blocker |
| Nifedipine | 10 mg | Sublingual | Calcium channel blocker |
| Diazepam | 2–10 mg | Intravenous | Tranquilizer |
| Midazolam | 1–2 mg | Intravenous | Tranquilizer |
| Fentanyl | 50–100 μg | Intravenous | Narcotic |
| Morphine | 2–10 mg | Intravenous | Narcotic |

### Is Clonidine a Problem?

Rebound hypertension may occur after withdrawal of clonidine. It is more common at doses >0.6 mg daily and can be treated with direct vasodilators (especially α-methyldopa, which is also centrally active), adrenergic antagonists, or calcium channel blockers. When the parenteral clonidine preparations used in Europe becomes available in the United States, this issue will become moot. Until then, clonidine patches can be used to replace the oral clonidine. Because these patches require a 2- to 3-day absorption period, one approach is to apply a clonidine patch on the morning of day 1 and give the usual oral dose. Then, on day 2, the BP is checked. If it is elevated, half the usual oral dose is given; if not, the dose remains unchanged. On day 3, the BP is checked again to verify that the patch is effective.

## FLUID THERAPY

### How Are Intravenous Fluids Chosen?

This discussion is limited to routine surgery and does not address the colloid and crystalloid debate or blood component replacement for patients in shock (see Chapter 40). Surgical patients need salt.[6,7] The practice of giving 5% dextrose in water (D₅W) as the only intravenous fluid for intraoperative and postoperative patients has been abandoned. The questions of importance are which salt solution to use and whether the solution should contain dextrose.

### What Fluids Are Useful?

The most common salt solutions available in surgical suites are 0.9% sodium chloride (NS) and lactated Ringer's solution (LR).[8,9] The use of LR is generally safe despite theoretic considerations about the presence of lactate.[10] On the other hand, NS is a perfectly acceptable solution for intraoperative use as well, despite the excess chloride.[11] With few exceptions—primarily patients with severe electrolyte imbalance—it does not make a difference whether NS or LR is used. Sometimes, the best solution is whatever is warm.

### Is Dextrose a Problem?

The dextrose question is a little more complicated (Table 11–2). Historically, intravenous glucose was administered to surgical patients for several reasons. Glucose protected the liver from the toxic effects of chloroform. In the era when salt was not given to patients in the perioperative period, D₅W was the primary alternative. Moreover, with long preoperative fasting periods, physicians feared that some patients would become symptomatically hypoglycemic.

In the early days of surgical treatment of morbid obesity, many deaths were caused by embolic phenomena. These were thought to be a result of elevated levels of free fatty acids, which are suppressed by administering dextrose.

Maternal administration of dextrose during labor has been shown to cause severe hypoglycemia in the newborn. Administration of intravenous glucose can increase the damage caused by experimentally induced brain ischemia. Moreover, many patients who receive >1 L of 5% dextrose in LR develop significant hyperglycemia. On the basis of this information, many anesthesiologists have abandoned the use of dextrose-containing solutions in the operating room.

### When Can Dextrose Be Administered?

Opponents of dextrose solutions intraoperatively take the approach that no one really needs glucose, that it is harmful in a parturient, and that it may be harmful in certain patients, including those undergoing cardiac surgery, carotid artery surgery, and neurosurgery and those suffering cardiac arrest.

Some patients who are maintained NPO for long periods before surgery, who are malnourished, or who are morbidly obese may receive some benefit from dextrose. Certainly, a diabetic patient who has received insulin should have some dextrose if the NPO period is prolonged.

### What Is the Role of Sodium?

Sodium is the major solute in extracellular fluid and is the major determinant of extracellular fluid volume and osmol-

**TABLE 11–2.** To Sweeten or Not to Sweeten, That Is the Question

| No Sugar | Consider Sugar |
|----------|----------------|
| Parturient | Diabetic patient who received insulin |
| Global central nervous system ischemia related to Neurosurgery Spinal column surgery Carotid artery surgery Cardiopulmonary bypass | Prolonged fast |
| Diabetic patient with elevated blood sugar | Starvation Morbid obesity |

**TABLE 11–3.** Signs and Symptoms of Hyponatremia

| | |
|---|---|
| Anorexia | Nausea |
| Confusion | Vomiting |
| Disorientation | Stupor |
| Apathy | Seizures |
| Headache | Deep tendon reflexes |
| Muscle cramps | Coma |
| Lethargy | |

ality.[10] Glucose and urea contribute lesser amounts to osmolality. Sodium concentration (140 ± 5 mEq/L), osmolality (287 ± 7 mOsm/kg), and extracellular fluid volume, especially the circulating blood volume, are regulated closely by the body. Plasma osmolality (Posm) can be estimated as follows:

$$Posm = 2[Na^+] \text{ Glucose} + (mg/dL)/18 + \text{Serum Urea Nitrogen (mg/dL)}$$

A measured osmolality >9 mOsm/kg from that calculated indicates the presence of exogenous molecules such as mannitol or radiographic dyes. Alterations in sodium concentration result when a disproportionate change in either sodium or water occurs. These changes may be associated with normal or abnormal physiologic mechanisms, normal or abnormal osmolality, and normal or abnormal total body water. To evaluate patients with sodium imbalance, the general fluid status (volume, osmolality) as well as the renal response (urine volume, osmolality, and sodium excretion) should be known. A carefully taken history and a physical examination reveal the cause of sodium imbalance in most patients.

## What Is the Significance of Hyponatremia?

Hyponatremia can be caused by water intoxication, rarely because of polydipsia. More often, it is caused by decreased glomerular filtration rate (GFR), decreased obligatory solute excretion, or chemical interference with the diluting mechanism, especially by thiazide diuretics. It may be encountered with stress, decreased thyroid or adrenal function, diuretic administration, or the syndrome of inappropriate release of antidiuretic hormone.[12]

### Manifestations

Serum sodium concentration and signs or symptoms are often poorly correlated. Patients are more likely to develop symptoms with rapid or extreme changes. The signs and symptoms of hyponatremia (Table 11–3) usually begin with anorexia, confusion, headaches, and muscle cramps, progressing to nausea, vomiting, and personality changes and finally to convulsions, coma, and death. Acute symptomatic hyponatremia is associated with significant morbidity and mortality. Chronic symptomatic hyponatremia has a lower mortality rate, and chronic asymptomatic hyponatremia is associated with a low mortality rate. Nevertheless, relatively low levels of hyponatremia, especially in young women, may result in death or permanent neurologic sequelae.

### Treatment

A good rule of thumb is to treat rapidly if hyponatremia occurred rapidly and to treat slowly if it evolved slowly. It is important to treat any associated abnormality in intravascular volume. Asymptomatic reaction to mild hyponatremia is treated by restricting water intake to <1 L/d. Excess fluid can be calculated as follows:

$$\text{Water Excess (kg)} = \text{Weight (kg)} \times 0.6 \times 140 - [Na^+]/140$$

**Example:** A 70-kg patient has a serum sodium concentration of 126 mEq/L.

$$\begin{aligned} \text{Water Excess} &= [70 \times 0.6] \times 140 - 126/140 \\ &= 42 \times 0.1 \\ &= 4.2 \text{ kg (L)} \end{aligned}$$

Patients with acute neurologic symptoms are treated more aggressively.

$$\text{Sodium Deficit (mEq)} = \text{Weight (kg)} \times 0.6 \times (140 - [Na^+])$$

A useful rule of thumb is that an infusion of 1 mEq/kg of sodium per hour raises the serum sodium level 2 to 3 mEq/L. Another method for rapid correction of symptomatic hyponatremia is to administer furosemide (1 mg/kg), measure the hourly sodium excretion, and replace it with 3% sodium chloride (sodium concentration of 513 mEq/L). The goal is to increase serum sodium concentration 1 to 2 mEq/L/h. Stop aggressive treatment when relief of symptoms occurs and a sodium level between 120 and 130 mEq/L is achieved. More rapid correction or overcorrection may cause fluid overload or potentially fatal CNS complications (ie, central pontine myelinolysis). Intravenous sodium bicarbonate, 2 mL/kg over several minutes, increases serum sodium by about 6 mEq/L in infants and small children.

## What Is the Significance of Hypernatremia?

Hypernatremia is rarely caused by excessive sodium intake (eg, saltwater near-drowning, accidental substitution of salt for sugar in infant formula, problems during hypertonic saline abortions). More often, the cause is limited access to water or inability to ingest water to replace renal or extrarenal water loss (diabetes insipidus [central or nephrogenic], osmotic diuresis, excessive sweating, diarrhea). A carefully taken history is helpful in diagnosing the cause of hypernatremia.

### Manifestations

Acutely increased serum osmolality initially causes intracellular dehydration of the brain, with restlessness, lethargy, and headache. This complex may progress to confusion, seizures, coma, and death (Table 11–4). The brain responds to this dehydration by forming intracellular solutes (idiogenic os-

**TABLE 11–4.** Signs and Symptoms of Hypernatremia

| | |
|---|---|
| Restlessness | Deep tendon reflexes |
| Lethargy | Seizures |
| Headache | Muscle tone |
| Disorientation | Stupor |
| Confusion | Coma |

moles) with partial restoration of intracellular volume. This process begins within 4 to 6 hours and takes several days to reach equilibrium. The presence of idiogenic osmoles in chronic hypernatremia makes rapid correction dangerous because of a resulting predisposition to cerebral edema.

### Treatment

Calculate total water deficit by the following formula:

$$\text{Water Deficit (kg)} = (\text{Weight [kg]} \times 0.6) \times (Na^+ - 140)/140$$

The treatment of hypernatremia is to control shock, if present, with crystalloids or colloids to stabilize the cardiovascular system. Treat accompanying acidosis with sodium bicarbonate only if the pH is <7.20. Replace the calculated fluid deficit slowly with hypotonic fluid (0.25 or 0.5 NS). The goal is to decrease plasma osmolality by no more than 2 mOsm/kg/h. Measure plasma sodium and osmolality every 2 hours.

While treating either hyponatremia or hypernatremia, always remember to consider and treat the underlying disease.

## POTASSIUM

Potassium is the second most abundant cation within the body and the major intracellular cation. The intracellular concentration of potassium is about 150 mEq/L. About 2% of total body potassium is extracellular, with a concentration of 3.5 to 4.5 mEq/L.[12,13]

### What Is the Significance of Hypokalemia?

Hypokalemia can occur without a change in total body content when extracellular potassium moves to the intracellular space (internal shift). Shifts of potassium into cells occur with metabolic or respiratory alkalosis, endogenous or exogenous catecholamines (especially β-adrenergic receptor agonists), and elevated insulin levels. Alkalosis predictably decreases serum potassium concentrations about 0.5 mEq/L for each 0.1 increase in pH (10 mm Hg decrease in arterial partial pressure of carbon dioxide [$Pa_{CO_2}$]).

Inadequate intake of potassium as a cause of hypokalemia is relatively unusual because the kidneys can decrease obligatory potassium losses to about 10 to 30 mEq/d. It may occur in starvation and anorexia nervosa as well as in elderly and alcoholic patients. Excessive potassium loss usually causes the hypokalemia. These losses may be through the skin (excessive sweating), gastrointestinal tract (vomiting, diarrhea), or kidneys (diuretics, hyperaldosteronism).[13]

### Manifestations

Because the ratio of intracellular to extracellular potassium determines cell membrane potential, most of the signs and symptoms of hypokalemia are related to cells that depolarize (Table 11–5). With moderate hypokalemia, patients may develop muscle weakness, cramps, fatigue, and decreased gastrointestinal motility with constipation or ileus. More severe hypokalemia (usually <2.5 mEq/L) may cause paralysis (including respiratory), rhabdomyolysis, and decreased vascular

**TABLE 11–5.** Signs and Symptoms of Hypokalemia

Digitalis toxicity
Electrocardiogram changes (flattened T waves, depressed ST segments, prolonged PR interval, U waves)
Muscle weakness
Constipation
Ileus
Orthostatic hypertension
Vasodilation
Rhabdomyolysis
Arrhythmias
Paralysis

resistance. Electrocardiographic (ECG) changes include flattening of the T waves and depressed ST segments; susceptibility to atrial and ventricular arrhythmias is increased, especially in the presence of digitalis.

### Critical Limits

The old rule of canceling surgery for patients with potassium levels of <3 or even <3.5 mEq/L is not valid. Surgery should not be canceled for symptom-free, chronically moderately hypokalemic, nondigitalized patients without ECG changes. Most patients with potassium levels of <2.7 mEq/L have ECG changes. Hypokalemia in patients taking digitalis and patients with ischemic heart disease or cardiomyopathy is of greater concern because these patients may be more susceptible to arrhythmias.

When anesthetizing a hypokalemic patient, maneuvers such as hyperventilation and administration of sodium bicarbonate, glucose, insulin, or catecholamines should be avoided because they further decrease the serum potassium level. Techniques or drugs associated with a higher incidence of arrhythmias (eg, halothane, atropine) should also not be used. Hypokalemia is worsened by dopamine or epinephrine administration and lowers the threshold for epinephrine-induced arrhythmias. Hypokalemia may increase the effectiveness of nondepolarizing muscle relaxants and may increase the requirement for reversal agents for the neuromuscular blocking drugs.

### Treatment

The primary treatment of asymptomatic hypokalemia is to address the cause. Each 1 mEq/L decrease in serum potassium concentration approximates a 200 to 400 mEq total body deficit.

### Oral

The deficit should be replaced slowly, preferably by mouth, over several days while monitoring both serum levels and urinary excretion. Rapid intravenous replacement may be hazardous because of rapid changes in the intracellular-to-extracellular ratio and, therefore, the cell membrane potential.

### Intravenous

Treat symptomatic hypokalemia with intravenous potassium using ECG monitoring. The maximal recommended rate of replacement is 0.5 to 0.7 mEq/kg/h given in a maximal concentration of 80 to 120 mEq/L. Hyperkalemia is possible with rapid intravenous potassium administration, especially in insulin-dependent diabetic patients and patients receiving nonselective β-blockers.

## What Is the Significance of Hyperkalemia?

Shifts of potassium from intracellular to extracellular fluid or an increase in total body potassium from excessive load or diminished excretion of potassium can cause hyperkalemia.[11] Significant internal shifts (ie, intracellular to extracellular) can be caused by respiratory or metabolic acidosis. Acute hyperosmolality of extracellular fluid (eg, hyperglycemia, mannitol, radiocontrast media) increases serum potassium by 0.3 to 0.5 mEq/L for each 10 mOsm/kg increase in plasma osmolality. Anesthesiologists are familiar with the rise in plasma potassium after succinylcholine administration and associated with malignant hyperthermia. Deficiencies in insulin (diabetes), catecholamines (eg, with β-blockers), and aldosterone decrease cellular potassium uptake. When these deficiencies occur in combination (severe diabetes) and in the presence of an increased potassium load (eg, vigorous exercise in a patient taking β-blockers) or decreased excretory ability (ARF or chronic renal failure, use of potassium-sparing diuretics), clinically significant and even fatal hyperkalemia can occur.

Increased potassium loads result from exogenous or endogenous sources. Exogenous potassium loads are usually iatrogenic, in the form of potassium salts administered orally or intravenously for potassium replacement, or incidentally (eg, large doses of potassium penicillin). Endogenous sources include cell lysis, trauma, rhabdomyolysis, hypercatabolic states (eg, malignant hyperthermia), and hemolysis (eg, gastrointestinal tract hemorrhage, resolution of massive hematomas). Excessive loads are rarely a problem without diminished cellular uptake or renal excretion of potassium.

Severely decreased GFR, hypoaldosteronism, angiotensin-converting enzyme inhibitors, and aldosterone-blocking agents (eg, spironolactone, triamterene amiloride) cause decreased renal potassium excretion.

### Manifestations

Signs and symptoms of hyperkalemia are usually absent or insignificant with plasma levels of <6 mEq/L and are frequent and severe with levels of >8 mEq/L (Table 11–6). ECG changes begin with peaked T waves and prolongation of the PR interval, progressing to disappearance of P waves, widening of the QRS complex to a sine wave configuration, and finally ventricular fibrillation or asystolic cardiac arrest. These ECG abnormalities are accentuated by concomitant hyponatremia, hypocalcemia, and acidosis. Vasodilation and hypotension may occur, along with paresthesias, weakness, and eventually paralysis of extremity and respiratory muscles.

### Critical Limits

The adage about canceling elective surgery if the potassium level exceeds 5.5 mEq/L needs reevaluation. The most common cause of hyperkalemia in surgical patients is chronic renal failure. Many patients with chronic renal failure tolerate high levels of potassium without signs or symptoms. Consider dialysis of patients who often exceed this level several times a week.

In the patient with chronic hyperkalemia, we proceed with anesthesia when there is a moderate elevation of serum potassium and there are no ECG changes. Elective surgery should be delayed if the process is acute, if the cause is unknown, or if the patient has heart disease (especially conduction defects) that may predispose to dysrhythmias. Finally, if a patient has diabetes, is taking β-blockers, or has symptoms suggestive of hyperkalemia (including ECG changes), delay is also recommended.

When anesthesia is conducted in a hyperkalemic patient, certain drugs (eg, succinylcholine) and techniques that lead to acidosis (eg, hypoventilation) are avoided, intravenous glucose is infused, and hyperventilation is used.

### Treatment

#### Asymptomatic

In patients with asymptomatic hyperkalemia, the cause of the hyperkalemia is treated or corrected. These patients are managed by decreasing oral potassium intake, administering loop diuretics to increase potassium excretion, and, if indicated, using ion exchange resin (sodium polystyrene sulfonate [Kayexalate]) or dialysis. The dose of sodium polystyrene sulfonate is 15 to 30 g in 20% sorbitol orally or 50 g rectally; this regimen removes 0.5 to 1 mEq of potassium per gram of resin.

#### Symptomatic

Muscle weakness or ECG changes in any patient constitutes a medical emergency. Treatment must counteract the membrane effects of hyperkalemia (calcium) to cause internal shifts of potassium into cells (bicarbonate, glucose, insulin). These regimens have a relatively rapid onset (within minutes) and short duration (15-60 minutes).

Administration of calcium (1-2 g of calcium chloride or 30-60 mL of calcium gluconate) should be assessed with constant ECG monitoring and stopped when the abnormal ECG changes reverse. Calcium is used with caution in patients taking digitalis to avoid toxicity. It must never be mixed with bicarbonate or it precipitates.

Insulin (with or without dextrose), sodium bicarbonate, hyperventilation, and inhaled $\beta_2$-adrenergic receptor agonists cause internal shifts of potassium.[14] These modalities have a somewhat slower onset and longer duration of action. Because none actually lowers total body potassium, begin ion exchange therapy or dialysis as soon as practical.

**TABLE 11–6.** Signs and Symptoms of Hyperkalemia

Electrocardiogram changes (peaked T waves, prolonged PR intervals, bradycardia, absent P waves, widened QRS complex, sine wave pattern)
Paresthesias
Arrhythmias
Vasodilation
Hypotension
Paralysis

## CALCIUM

Bone contains >99% of the total body calcium; about 0.6% is intracellular, and 0.1% is in the extracellular fluid. Most intracellular calcium is in various membrane structures. The free, ionized intracellular calcium is 100 to 200 nmol/L. Ionized calcium serves many second messenger functions and regulates several enzyme systems.[15]

Extracellular calcium exists in 3 phases:

1. Ionized (about 50%)
2. Complexed to various anions (about 10%)
3. Bound to plasma proteins, mostly albumin (40%)

Ionized calcium is physiologically active and should be measured to guide therapy. Many laboratories still measure total calcium. Changes in ionized and total calcium are frequently not proportionate. As examples, hypoalbuminemia decreases total extracellular calcium without affecting ionized calcium; alkalosis increases protein binding and decreases ionized calcium without changing total calcium concentration; and hyponatremia also increases protein binding but to a lesser extent. Normal levels of total serum calcium are 8.5 to 10.5 mg/dL (2.0-2.5 mEq/L).

## What Is the Significance of Hypocalcemia?

Hypocalcemia is present when the ionized calcium is <1 mmol/L or 4 mg/dL. Hypocalcemia can occur because of increased sequestration of calcium (hyperphosphatemia, chelation with citrate of ethylenediaminetetraacetic acid, acute pancreatitis, rhabdomyolysis, bone deposition from osteoblastic metastases, or severe osteitis fibrosa cystica). Significant hypocalcemia due to citrate intoxication associated with blood transfusion is extremely rare and is transient when it does occur. Other causes include hypoparathyroidism, hypomagnesemia, vitamin D deficiency, phenytoin, sepsis, and mithramycin.

### Manifestations

The symptoms of hypocalcemia are primarily neuromuscular and cardiovascular (Table 11–7).

### Central Nervous System

CNS symptoms begin with lethargy and depression and may progress to psychosis, dementia, and seizures. Neuromuscular excitability begins with paresthesias and hyperreflexia. A positive *Chvostek sign* (facial twitching when the facial nerve is tapped) and *Trousseau sign* (carpal spasm after 3 minutes of arm ischemia) may occur. With progression, patients develop muscle cramps and finally tetany and laryngeal stridor.

**TABLE 11–7.** Signs and Symptoms of Hypocalcemia

| | |
|---|---|
| Paresthesias | Bone pain |
| Muscle cramps | Depression |
| Chvostek sign | Dementia |
| Trousseau sign | Tetany |
| Lethargy | Hypotension |
| Seizures | Arrhythmias* |
| Fractures | |

*Especially heart block and ventricular fibrillation.

### Cardiovascular System

Cardiovascular signs and symptoms include prolonged QT interval, heart block, hypotension, heart failure, and ventricular fibrillation. The response to digitalis is decreased. All of these symptoms may be exacerbated by concurrent hypomagnesemia, alkalosis, or hyperkalemia.

### Treatment

### Asymptomatic

Hypocalcemia should be treated to avoid progression to potentially fatal symptoms. If a patient does not have symptoms, give oral calcium, vitamin D supplements, and perhaps a thiazide diuretic to reduce urinary calcium loss. Treat hyperphosphatemia, if present, before calcium is supplemented. Calcium supplementation should proceed cautiously in patients taking digitalis to avoid digitalis toxicity.

### Symptomatic

Treat patients with severe, symptomatic hypocalcemia or an ionized calcium of <3.2 mg/dL (0.8 mmol/L) urgently with an initial bolus of intravenous calcium followed by an infusion. Monitor replacement by frequent determinations of ionized calcium. Administer calcium in a dose just sufficient to reverse the symptoms and normalize the plasma concentration. Begin oral calcium and vitamin D supplements as soon as possible.

The intravenous preparations are calcium gluconate 10% and calcium chloride 10%. Calcium gluconate produces less venous irritation. A bolus dose of 10 to 30 mL over 10 to 15 minutes is followed by an infusion of 10 to 15 mg of calcium per kilogram of body weight in 1 L of $D_5W$ over 4 to 6 hours. Each 10 mL of calcium gluconate contains 93 mg (4.7 mEq) of calcium. Calcium chloride (273 mg, 14 mEq/10 mL) is given through a central venous catheter in the same doses (about one third the volume) as calcium gluconate.

## What Is the Significance of Hypercalcemia?

Hypercalcemia occurs when calcium enters the extracellular fluid faster than regulatory hormones (parathyroid hormone and vitamin D) or renal excretory mechanisms can respond or when disorders of the hormones are present. More than one mechanism is usually involved. Increased intestinal absorption, increased bone release, and decreased renal excretion usually occur together in significant hypercalcemia. The most common causes of hypercalcemia are hyperparathyroidism, vitamin D intoxication, certain malignancies, chronic renal failure, milk-alkali syndrome, and iatrogenic causes.

### Manifestations

Signs and symptoms (Table 11–8) include depression, lethargy, confusion, coma, muscle weakness, and decreased deep tendon reflexes. Hypertension is common, and dysrhythmias and digitalis toxicity may occur. ECG changes include shortening of the QT interval. Gastrointestinal symptoms include nausea, vomiting, and constipation. Metastatic calcification may cause pruritus, band keratopathy, and conjunctivitis.

**TABLE 11–8.** Signs and Symptoms of Hypercalcemia

| | |
|---|---|
| Nausea | Depression |
| Vomiting | Hypertension |
| Decreased deep tendon reflexes | Digitalis toxicity |
| Shortened QT interval | Peptic ulcer |
| Constipation | Arrhythmias |
| Lethargy | Coma |
| Muscle weakness | |

## Treatment

Most cases of hypercalcemia should be treated. Treatment of the causative disorder usually suffices in symptom-free patients. The main treatment of acute symptomatic hypercalcemia is a brisk saline diuresis (5-10 L/d) induced by rapid administration of intravenous saline. This approach must proceed cautiously in patients with significant heart disease.

After the diuresis is established, it can be enhanced by the administration of furosemide, 20 to 40 mg given intravenously every 2 to 3 hours. Urinary losses of sodium, potassium, and magnesium should be measured and replaced. Hemodialysis may be necessary in patients with a low GFR. Other therapies (eg, biphosphonate, mithramycin) are appropriate in certain patients with hypercalcemia but would require consultation.

## MAGNESIUM

### How Is Magnesium Imbalance Managed?

Like calcium, magnesium is primarily an intracellular ion, only 1% to 2% being extracellular. Of the extracellular magnesium, about 60% is free, 15% is complexed to anions, and 25% is protein bound. Magnesium is an essential cofactor in >300 enzymatic reactions.

### What Is the Significance of Hypomagnesemia?

Normal plasma magnesium concentrations are between 1.7 and 2.7 mg/dL (1.4-2.3 mEq/L). Internal shifts are rarely a cause of hypomagnesemia. The most common causes are decreased intestinal absorption (starvation, alcoholism, malabsorption, diarrhea) and increased renal excretion (diuresis). Urine excretion is usually appropriately low (<10 mg/dL) when the cause is intestinal and is higher (>10 mg/dL) when the cause is renal.

### Manifestations

Hypomagnesemia is common in postoperative patients in an intensive care unit. It may be accompanied by hypocalcemia and hypokalemia, which exacerbate the signs and symptoms. Symptoms similar to those of hypokalemia include apathy, nausea, positive Chvostek's and Trousseau's signs, muscle spasticity, increased deep tendon reflexes, tetany, and seizures. Ventricular dysrhythmias may occur, especially in patients taking digitalis (Table 11–9). Hypomagnesemia may hamper treatment of hypokalemia because it interferes with establishing the normal transcellular gradient for potassium and often must be corrected to correct the potassium deficit.

**TABLE 11–9.** Signs and Symptoms of Hypomagnesemia

| | |
|---|---|
| Increased deep tendon reflexes | Nausea |
| Chvostek sign | Apathy |
| Trousseau sign | Tetany |
| Muscle spasticity | Arrhythmias |

## Treatment

Patients with seizures, tetany, or dysrhythmias should receive 100 to 200 mg (8-16 mEq) of magnesium intravenously over 10 to 15 minutes. With less severe symptoms, the infusion can proceed intravenously at a rate of 12 mg/kg/d. Deep tendon reflexes should be checked frequently and the infusion stopped if they decrease. Asymptomatic hypomagnesemia is treated with oral supplementation.

### What Is the Significance of Hypermagnesemia?

Hypermagnesemia is almost always iatrogenic (from treatment of preeclampsia) or due to uncontrolled magnesium intake (in antacids, cathartics) in patients with severe reductions in GFR.

### Manifestations

Signs and symptoms (Table 11–10) include lethargy, confusion, nausea, hypotension, muscle weakness, decreased deep tendon reflexes, arrhythmias, respiratory paralysis, and coma. Hypermagnesemia increases the effectiveness of both depolarizing and nondepolarizing neuromuscular blocking agents.

### Treatment

Mild, asymptomatic hypermagnesemia does not need treatment other than to limit magnesium intake. If the plasma magnesium level is >10 mg/dL or if the patient has developed symptoms, administer calcium intravenously to provide 15 mg/kg over a 4-hour period. If renal function permits, establish a diuresis by volume expansion and loop diuretics. Otherwise, dialysis may be necessary.

## PHOSPHORUS

### How Is Phosphorus Imbalance Managed?

Only about 0.03% of total body phosphorus is in plasma; the remainder exists in bone (85%) and cells (14%). Intracellular phosphorus is critically important in most cell functions. Plasma inorganic phosphate is primarily dibasic ($HPO_4^{-2}$) and monobasic phosphate ($H_2PO_4^-$). Changes in albumin concentration do not influence plasma phosphorus levels.

**TABLE 11–10.** Signs and Symptoms of Hypermagnesemia

| | |
|---|---|
| Muscle weakness | Confusion |
| Decreased deep tendon reflexes | Hypotension |
| Nausea | Coma |
| Lethargy | Arrhythmias |

**TABLE 11–11.** Signs and Symptoms of Hypophosphatemia

| | |
|---|---|
| Paresthesias | Seizures |
| Muscle weakness | Hemolysis |
| Confusion | Rhabdomyolysis |
| Irritability | Decreased cardiac output |
| Stupor | Coma |

Normal plasma inorganic phosphorus concentrations are 2.5 to 4.5 mg/dL in adults and 3.5 to 6.0 mg/dL in children. Significant internal redistribution occurs with respiratory alkalosis but not metabolic alkalosis or glucose or insulin administration. Hypophosphatemia secondary to respiratory alkalosis is asymptomatic.

## What Is the Significance of Hypophosphatemia?

Hypophosphatemia can result from decreased absorption (starvation, alcoholism, phosphate binders, vitamin D deficiency) and from excessive renal loss (hyperparathyroidism, carbonic anhydrase inhibitors).

### Manifestations

Symptoms of hypophosphatemia are largely attributable to decreased intracellular adenosine triphosphate and impaired oxygen delivery secondary to decreased red blood cell 2,3-diphosphoglycerate (Table 11–11). These include irritability, confusion, stupor, coma, seizures, paresthesias, muscle weakness, hemolysis, rhabdomyolysis, and decreased cardiac output. There is poor correlation between plasma and total body phosphorus. Symptoms usually do not occur until the total body deficit exceeds 10 g.

### Treatment

Hypophosphatemia is treated by increasing oral phosphorus intake. If the plasma phosphorus is <1.5 mg/dL or if a patient has symptoms, give intravenous phosphorus, 2.0 to 7.5 mg/kg, 3 to 4 times daily until the plasma concentration exceeds 2.0 mg/dL (Table 11–12). Do not give parenteral phosphorus in the presence of hypocalcemia. Give phosphorus cautiously if the GFR is reduced. Metastatic calcification can occur if the phosphorus and calcium product exceeds 60.

**TABLE 11–12.** Electrolyte Solutions Useful in Treating Electrolyte Imbalance*

3% NaCl: 513 mEq/L Na$^+$
Calcium gluconate: 10% = 93 mg (4.7 mEq) Ca$^{2+}$/10 mL
Calcium chloride: 10% = 273 mg (14 mEq) Ca$^{2+}$/10 mL
Magnesium sulfate
    50% = 50 mg (4 mEq) Mg$^{2+}$/mL
    25% = 25 mg (2 mEq) Mg$^{2+}$/mL
    10% = 10 mg (1 mEq) Mg$^{2+}$/mL
Sodium phosphate = 93 mg PO$_4^-$/mL (4 mEq/mL Na$^+$)
Potassium phosphate = 93 mg PO$_4^-$/mL (4 mEq/mL K$^+$)

*See text for doses and indications.

## What Is the Significance of Hyperphosphatemia?

Hyperphosphatemia may result from internal shifts (hemolysis, rhabdomyolysis, tumor lysis), excessive exogenous load (phosphorus-containing antacids, enemas, laxatives), or diminished excretion (decreased GFR). Renal dysfunction is almost always a factor.

### Manifestations

Symptoms are generally attributed to secondary changes in calcium concentration and ectopic tissue deposition with calcium. A phosphorus and calcium concentration product of ≥60 must be treated aggressively.

### Treatment

In the presence of adequate renal function, the treatment consists of volume expansion to increase the GFR. Once accomplished, a carbonic anhydrase inhibitor (acetazolamide) is administered. The alternative is hemodialysis. Less severe or asymptomatic hyperphosphatemia is treated by decreasing phosphorus intake and the cautious use of phosphorus binders such as oral antacids containing aluminum, magnesium, or calcium (Table 11–13; see Table 11–12).

## RENAL FUNCTION TESTS

Clinically available methods for evaluating renal function include urinalysis and measurement of urine output, BUN, serum creatinine (Scr), and rarely, creatinine clearance (C$_{cr}$).[16] All have significant limitations that should be considered when interpreting results.

### When Is Urinalysis Useful?

Urinalysis is one of the most common laboratory tests ordered for preoperative patients. It is more useful to establish a diagnosis of urinary tract disease than to evaluate renal function. The presence of protein, sugar, and abnormal sediment tells little about kidney function. In most cases, urine concentration and pH cannot be interpreted meaningfully. Extremely concentrated or dilute urine (specific gravity 1.025 or ≤1.005) indicates that the renal concentrating or diluting mechanisms are functioning. These values may also give an idea of the patient's fluid status at the time the specimen was collected.

### Of What Significance Is the Urine Volume?

Urine volume is a nonspecific indicator of renal function because many factors influence urine output, including protein and fluid intake, nonrenal fluid loss, stress, pain, drugs, and cardiovascular status. Therefore, a great deal must be known about a patient to judge the appropriateness of the urine output. Normal urine output is in the range of 0.7 to 1.5 mL/kg/h. Under unusual circumstances, it may be lower or higher. Despite the limitations of urine output as a measure of renal

**TABLE 11–13.** Summary of Signs and Symptoms of Electrolyte Imbalance

| Sign or Symptom | ↓ Na⁺ | ↑ Na⁺ | ↓ K⁺ | ↑ K⁺ | ↓ Ca²⁺ | ↑ Ca²⁺ | ↓ Mg²⁺ | ↑ Mg²⁺ | ↓ PO₄⁻³ |
|---|---|---|---|---|---|---|---|---|---|
| Lethargy | + | + | | | + | + | | + | |
| Coma | + | + | | | | + | | + | + |
| Seizures | + | | | | + | | + | | + |
| ↑ Deep tendon reflexes | | + | | | + | | + | | |
| ↓ Deep tendon reflexes | + | | | | | + | | + | |
| Muscle weakness | | | + | + | | + | | | + |
| Positive (+) Trousseau sign | | | | | + | | + | | |
| Positive (+) Chvostek sign | | | | | + | | + | | |
| Electrocardiogram changes | | | + | + | + | + | + | + | |
| Rhabdomyolysis | | | + | | | | | | + |

function, it is the most routinely available if not the best test in the operating room.

### What Does Serum Urea Nitrogen Indicate?

Urea nitrogen is an end product of hepatic protein metabolism. Ingestion of large amounts of protein, catabolic states, anabolic steroids, and blood in the gut all increase urea nitrogen production. Urea nitrogen is freely filterable by the kidneys and is both secreted and reabsorbed by the tubules. The amount reabsorbed increases as urine flow decreases. If all factors are constant, an inverse relationship between GFR and BUN exists (Fig. 11–1). Oliguria, hypercatabolism, and blood in the gut may increase the BUN without a decrease in GFR.

With complete cessation of glomerular filtration, the BUN rises about 10 to 20 mg/dL/d. After massive trauma, sepsis, or other problems associated with hypercatabolic states, the BUN may rise as much as 100 mg/dL/d. Elevation of the BUN-to-Scr ratio, which is normally 10:1, may mean that extracellular fluid depletion is causing the azotemia. Severe liver disease, decreased protein intake, and extracellular volume expansion decrease the BUN.

### When Is Serum Creatinine Measurement Useful?

The Scr level is also inversely proportional to GFR (see Fig. 11–1). Creatinine is produced by muscle, and its rates of production and release are related to the muscle mass. Creatinine is freely filtered by the glomeruli; little is secreted or reabsorbed by the tubules. The equation Scr × GFR is a constant. If GFR is halved, Scr doubles. This relationship holds only when a steady state exists.

If GFR ceases, the Scr rises about 0.5 to 1.0 mg/dL/d (Fig. 11–2). This increase may be much greater with severe trauma or rhabdomyolysis. Because creatinine production is related to muscle mass, loss of muscle tissue with renal failure may result in a deceptively low Scr level. Neither BUN nor Scr values accurately reflect acute changes in GFR.

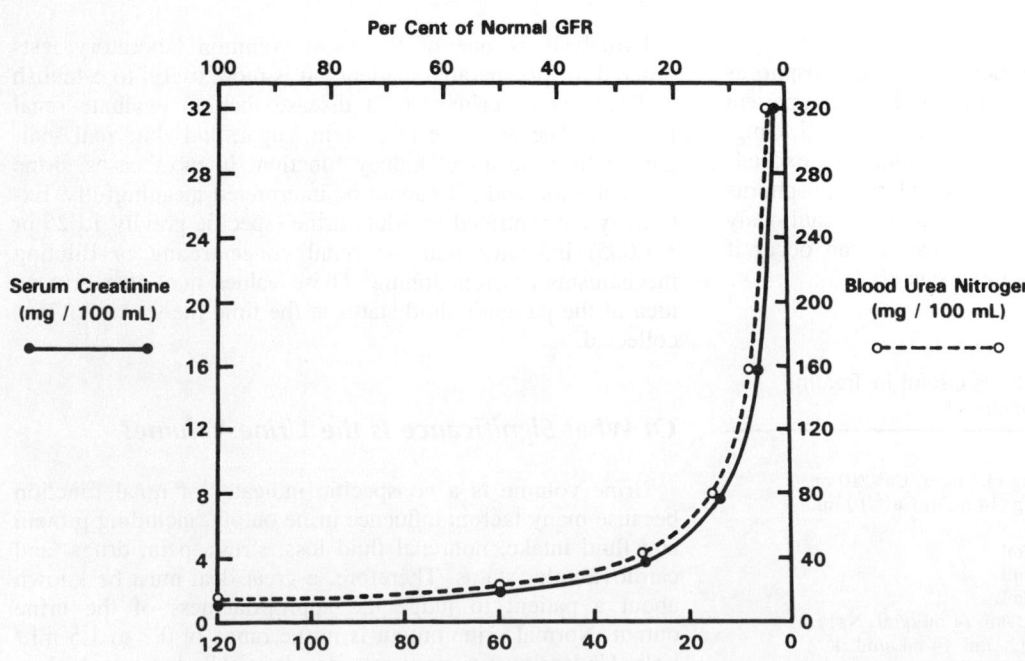

**Per Cent of Normal GFR**

**Serum Creatinine (mg / 100 mL)**

**Blood Urea Nitrogen (mg / 100 mL)**

**GFR (mL / min)**

**FIGURE 11–1.** Theoretical relationship among blood urea nitrogen (BUN), serum creatinine (Scr), and glomerular filtration rate (GFR). (From Kassirer JP. Clinical evaluation of kidney function: glomerular function. *N Engl J Med.* 1971; 285:385, by permission of the *New England Journal of Medicine.*)

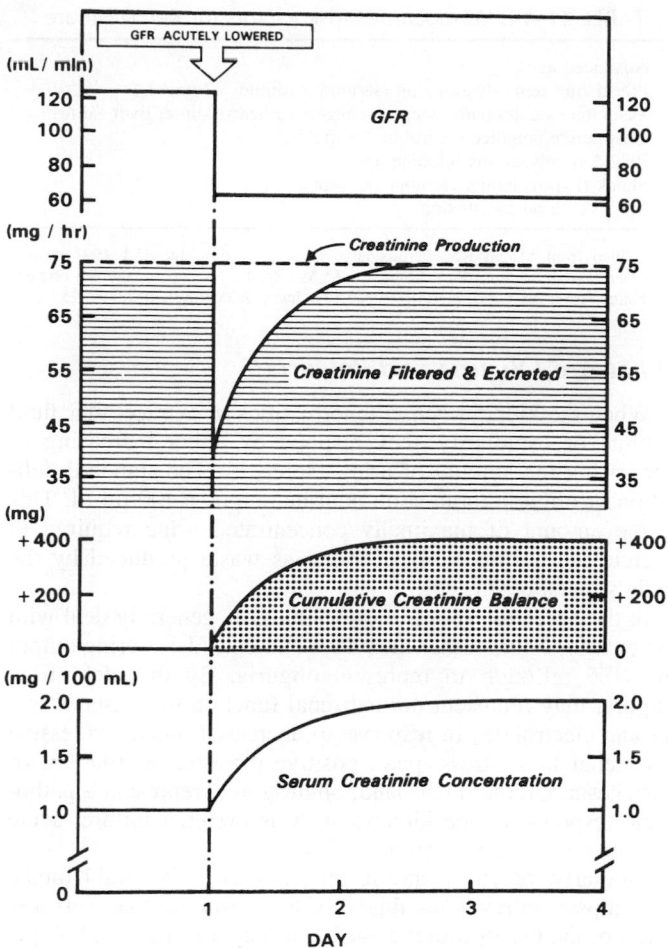

**FIGURE 11–2.** Effects of an acute decrease in glomerular filtration rate (GFR) on creatinine balance, excretion, and serum concentration. (From Kassirer JP. Clinical evaluation of kidney function. *N Engl J Med.* 1971;285:385, by permission of the *New England Journal of Medicine.*)

A more accurate method for determining GFR uses $C_{cr}$, which can be calculated as follows:

$$C_{cr} = U_{cr} \times V/P_{Cr}$$

where $U_{cr}$ is the urine creatinine concentration, V is urine volume during a given period of time, and $P_{Cr}$ is the plasma creatinine concentration sampled during the urine collection period.

This test is fraught with collection errors and is rarely available (or appropriate) in the acute situation usually found in the operating room. It is, however, useful in patients with chronic renal dysfunction and in some patients in the intensive care unit. Like Scr determination, $C_{cr}$ is not an accurate estimate of GFR unless a steady state exists.

## COMPROMISED RENAL FUNCTION

The kidneys are the primary organs for maintaining homeostasis of the internal milieu. This function is accomplished by glomerular filtration and by tubular secretion and absorption. When the ability to maintain homeostasis is interfered with by physiologic, pathologic, or pharmacologic means, renal dysfunction exists. Changes can be gradual (eg, aging, chronic

renal disease) or abrupt (eg, renal artery thrombosis, diuretics, acute tubular necrosis).

### Are the Changes Acute or Chronic?

When we think of compromised renal function, we are usually concerned with ARF or chronic renal failure. ARF can be oliguric (urine output <400 mL/d) or nonoliguric (urine output >400 mL/d). Inadequately treated functional renal failure may eventuate in acute tubular necrosis.[17]

### What Are the Hallmarks of Chronic Failure?

Patients with chronic renal failure may pass through several stages (Fig. 11–3).

#### Decreased Renal Reserve

Until about 60% of nephron mass is lost, patients are in a stage of decreased renal reserve. They generally have no signs or symptoms of renal dysfunction and present no special problems for the anesthesiologist.

#### Early Renal Insufficiency

Subsequently, patients enter the stage of renal insufficiency and may develop mild degrees of azotemia, anemia, and acidosis; decreased concentrating ability; and nocturia. Any decrease in effective circulating blood volume in these patients can cause devastating further deterioration of renal function. Implications of even a small decrease in GFR are illustrated in Figure 11–4. The main anesthetic implications of renal insufficiency are, therefore, careful attention to fluid replacement and renal perfusion. With this in mind, these patients can surely undergo major surgery.

#### Advanced Renal Insufficiency

As renal disease evolves, azotemia, anemia, and acidosis become more severe. Isosthenuria, polyuria, nocturia, hyperchloremia, hyperphosphatemia, hyponatremia, and hypocal-

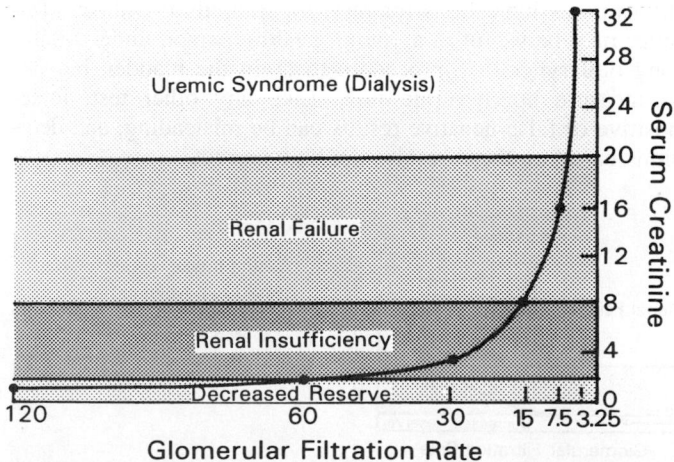

**FIGURE 11–3.** Changes in glomerular filtration rate and serum creatinine in chronic renal failure. (Modified from Bastron RD. Chronic renal failure, clinical implications. In: *Current Reviews in Clinical Anesthesia, 1982.* Lesson 8. Vol 3. Miami, Fla: Current Reviews in Clinical Anesthesia; 1982:60.)

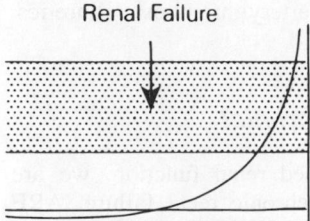

**FIGURE 11–4.** The patient with renal failure requires strict attention to fluid balance and aseptic technique. (Modified from Bastron RD. Chronic renal failure, clinical implications. In: *Current Reviews in Clinical Anesthesia, 1982.* Lesson 8. Vol 3. Miami, Fla: Current Reviews in Clinical Anesthesia; 1982:63.)

cemia are common. Infection is a constant threat. The major anesthetic problems in patients with renal failure are drug elimination, fluid balance, and sepsis (Fig. 11–5).

## Decompensation

With further progression, decompensation occurs. Uremia and all the manifestations of renal disease become overt. Significant anesthesia implications of uremia are discussed later in this chapter.

## When Should Urine Output Be Monitored?

No hard and fast rules are available to determine when to measure urine output. Certain perioperative risk factors (Table 11–14), high-risk procedures (Table 11–15), and nephrotoxins (Table 11–16) are associated with higher incidences of ARF.

Some factors, such as shock, massive blood transfusion, aortic cross-clamping, hemolysis, rhabdomyolysis, and major trauma, are strong indications for monitoring urine output. Others are relative indicators for such monitoring. As an example, measurement of urine output in a patient with preexisting renal dysfunction undergoing major bowel surgery is advisable but is unnecessary during less extensive surgery, such as hernia repair, cataract extraction, or median nerve decompression. This decision is clinical, and common sense serves as a guide.

Note that indications for monitoring urine output are not the same as indications for inserting a urethral catheter. The latter may be useful in a young, healthy person undergoing a long otolaryngologic procedure to drain the bladder, but not to measure hourly urine flow. Like any other test, false-positive or false-negative results can be misleading, and decisions based on those results can be incorrect.

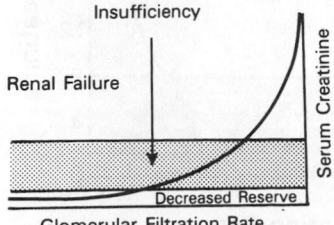

**FIGURE 11–5.** The primary concern in renal insufficiency is meticulous fluid replacement. (Modified from Bastron RD. Chronic renal failure, clinical implications. In: *Current Reviews in Clinical Anesthesia, 1982.* Lesson 8. Vol 3. Miami, Fla: Current Reviews in Clinical Anesthesia; 1982:63.)

**TABLE 11–14.** Perioperative Risk Factors for Renal Failure

Advanced age
Preexisting renal dysfunction (serum creatinine >2 mg/dL)
Vasomotor nephropathy (sepsis, congestive heart failure, liver failure)
Obstructive jaundice (bilirubin >8 mg/dL)
Rhabdomyolysis, myoglobinemia
Shock (hypovolemic, cardiogenic, septic)
Massive blood transfusion

Modified from Sladen RN. Perioperative renal protection. In: *ASA 1991 Annual Refresher Course Lectures.* Park Ridge, Ill: ASA; 1991:1–7. A copy of the full text can be obtained from ASA, 520 North Northwest Highway, Park Ridge, IL 60068-2573.

## What Are Oliguria and Polyuria?

When the kidneys sense abnormalities in extracellular fluid volume or osmolarity, they respond by either increasing or decreasing the amount of urine excreted.[18] The standard definition of oliguria in an adult is urine output <400 mL/d. This is the amount of maximally concentrated urine required to excrete the normal daily nitrogenous waste produced by the body's metabolism.

In the operating room, anesthesiologists generally deal with patients for hours rather than days and consider a urine output of <0.5 mL/kg/h to represent oliguria. By this definition, oliguria may represent normal renal function to conserve water and electrolytes in response to decreased intake, excessive extrarenal loss, stress, pain, positive pressure ventilation, or anesthesia. On the other hand, oliguria may represent a pathologic response of the kidneys such as prerenal failure, acute tubular necrosis, or postrenal failure.

Similarly, polyuria may result from excessive fluid intake (polydipsia, intravenous fluids), a high osmotic load (glycosuria), or the use of diuretic agents. It may also be a pathologic response to central or renal diabetes insipidus, severe hypokalemia, or high-output renal failure. The diagnosis can be made on the basis of a carefully taken history, physical examination, and laboratory tests.

## Why Is Oliguria Present?

The cause of normally occurring oliguria (long-term NPO status, stress, pain, or anesthesia) is usually apparent. The main problem is oliguria in patients with the previously mentioned risk factors. High-risk patients with oliguria should be evaluated systematically to exclude or prevent ARF. One such approach is discussed next.

### Likely Causes

The main causes of renal failure in surgical patients follow:

1. Prerenal (hypovolemia, pump failure)
2. Intrinsic acute tubular necrosis (vascular, toxic)
3. Postrenal (obstruction, extravasation)

### Assessment

The first step in the evaluation of oliguric patients is to be certain that urine being formed can flow to the collection

**TABLE 11–15.** High-Risk Procedures

Cardiac surgery
Aortic cross-clamp
Biliary tract surgery (sepsis, obstructive jaundice)
Complicated obstetrics
Major trauma

**TABLE 11–16.** Nephrotoxins

| Endogenous nephrotoxins | Myoglobin |
| --- | --- |
| | Hemoglobin |
| | Conjugated bilirubin |
| | Uric acid |
| Exogenous nephrotoxins | Volatile anesthetic agents with fluoride metabolites; antibiotic agents (aminoglycosides, amphotericin B); immunosuppressives (cyclosporine, *cis*-platinum); contrast dyes (especially in dehydrated, elderly, hypertensive, diabetic patients); low-molecular-weight dextrans |

Modified from Sladen RN. Perioperative renal protection. In: *ASA 1991 Annual Refresher Course Lectures.* Park Ridge, Ill: ASA; 1991:1–7. A copy of the full text can be obtained from ASA, 520 North Northwest Highway, Park Ridge, IL 60068-2573.

receptacle. Insert a urethral catheter or irrigate a catheter that is already in place. Be sure that all collection tubing is properly connected and patent. Male patients with pelvic trauma should have an injection urethrogram before insertion of a urethral catheter. Anuria is a hallmark of postrenal failure, although oliguria or intermittent anuria is more common.

The second and most important step is to be certain that perfusion is optimum. Correction of preload (effective circulating blood volume); cardiac rate, rhythm, and contractility; and afterload (peripheral vascular resistance) is critical.[19] The approach may be as simple as a fluid challenge or may entail the use of the most sophisticated cardiac monitoring devices and the infusion of potent drugs, depending on the clinical situation. Remember that many critically ill patients need to be hyperdynamic—that is, they require a higher than normal filling pressure and cardiac index.

### Indications for Diuretics

Most of the time, these steps are sufficient to evaluate and treat oliguric patients. If the cause of oliguria is prerenal, it should be reversed by providing optimal perfusion. If a patient remains oliguric despite optimal perfusion, diuretics may be helpful.[20]

Mannitol, 12.5 to 25 g, or furosemide, 1 to 2 mg, can be administered intravenously. Mannitol increases blood volume and should be used with caution in patients with heart disease. If a low dose of furosemide is not effective, a second dose of up to 1 mg/kg may be given. If oliguria persists, assume that the patient has acute tubular necrosis. If urine output increases, carefully monitor and maintain the patient's volume and electrolyte status. Consider a nephrology consultation for any patient who requires this latter step.

Diuretics may be indicated in well-hydrated patients in several circumstances.[21] These include cardiopulmonary bypass, aortic cross-clamp, or kidney transplantation. They may be requested by a urologist to increase urine flow (eg, to make the ureteral orifices easier to identify during cystoscopy) or by a neurosurgeon or ophthalmologist to decrease intracranial or intraocular pressure, respectively. The only contraindication to diuretics is volume depletion, which may be aggravated by the diuretic administration.

Occasionally, a lung-versus-kidney or heart-versus-kidney situation is encountered with respect to therapy. With careful monitoring of renal, pulmonary, and cardiac function, this dilemma should not occur often. When it does, erring in favor of the kidneys is recommended. Numerous interventions are available for congestive heart failure but none for acute tubular necrosis. Pulmonologists and cardiologists do not always agree with this approach. When it is necessary to choose among these vital organs, the decision is made on a case-by-case basis.

### Is Sophisticated Testing Necessary?

The fractional excretion of sodium, the renal failure index, and other urinary indices for differentiating prerenal failure from acute tubular necrosis are of limited clinical value for an anesthesiologist. We have never seen them used in the operating room and only rarely in the intensive care unit when an aggressive approach to oliguria, such as outlined earlier, is used. If you believe these indices to be necessary, a nephrology consultation is required. If you anticipate using any of them, be sure to collect the urine and plasma samples for analysis before giving any diuretic agents.

## RENAL TOXICITY

### What Are the Causative Factors?

A wide variety of compounds, including heavy metals, organic solvents, analgesics, antibiotics, radiocontrast dyes, and anesthetics, can be nephrotoxic. Of most interest to anesthesiologists are antibiotics, radiocontrast dyes, and anesthetics. The prototypical nephrotoxic antibiotic is gentamicin. Gentamicin nephrotoxicity can be limited by measuring peak and trough levels, keeping them below toxic levels, and monitoring Scr values for signs of decreased renal function. This speaks in favor of giving gentamicin in the operating room by slow infusion rather than as a bolus.

Nephrotoxicity due to radiocontrast dyes can be minimized by avoiding dehydration. Prolonged use of enflurane can produce sufficient free inorganic fluoride to damage kidneys. Enflurane should probably not be used in patients with existing renal dysfunction.

### How Are the Kidneys Protected?

Duration of insult is probably the most important factor causing renal dysfunction during and after high-risk procedures. Anesthesiologists have little or no control over a procedure's duration. The best one can do is to ensure adequate cardiac output and circulating blood volume to minimize vasoconstriction and to maximize renal perfusion.

Hypotension associated with vasoconstriction (low cardiac output or circulating blood volume) is associated with a higher incidence of postoperative dysfunction than is hypotension caused by vasodilators. Use monitoring techniques appropriate for the patient, surgeon, and surgical procedure.

### What Intravenous Fluids Are Best?

Intraoperative fluid therapy is aimed at replacing fluids lost by normal body functions that are not replaced during the NPO period as well as blood and third space losses caused by the surgical procedure. The main concern is to maintain adequate circulating blood volume and extracellular fluid volume. This goal is best achieved with salt solutions, either isotonic NS or nearly isotonic LR.

The main argument against balanced salt solutions such as LR is that they contain potassium, and patients with renal failure may be hyperkalemic. Realistically, the 4 mEq/L of potassium in the balanced salt solutions does no harm. NS may be selected for use if a patient is significantly hyperkalemic or will be receiving large volumes of banked blood that will provide a large potassium load. Otherwise, it makes no difference which fluid is chosen.

### How Does Renal Failure Affect Drug Choice and Dosage?

Patients with uremic syndrome may have unusual responses to drugs for several reasons.[20,21] Protein binding is abnormal, and drugs, such as sodium thiopental, that are highly protein bound may cause exaggerated or prolonged effects. Pseudocholinesterase levels may be diminished but rarely enough to cause clinically significant prolongation of succinylcholine-induced blockade (and presumably that of mivacurium).

Electrolyte imbalance, especially hypokalemia and hypermagnesemia, may potentiate the neuromuscular blocking agents. Drugs, such as gallamine, that are totally dependent on renal excretion, should be used with caution if at all. Other drugs depend on renal excretion of active metabolites (eg, meperidine). Most drugs that are partially dependent on renal excretion require smaller than usual doses or longer intervals between doses.

#### Preoperative Blood Levels

Renal dysfunction per se is not an indication to measure any drug level. The usual indication for monitoring drug levels is to confirm a clinical impression that drug levels are subtherapeutic, therapeutic, or toxic. This same indication should be used for patients with renal failure.

### DIALYSIS PATIENTS

In addition to the usual concerns for any preoperative patient, the main consideration for preoperative patients on dialysis is to assess the adequacy of dialysis. Dialysis replaces the kidneys to maintain homeostasis of the internal milieu as well as possible. It should correct water and electrolyte imbalance (Table 11–17) as well as several other abnormalities associated with the uremic syndrome.

### Why Is Timing Important?

Determine the time of the last dialysis, which ideally should be within 24 hours. Serum electrolytes measured the day of surgery should be within normal limits if dialysis is adequate. Verifying the absence of hypertension and comparison of predialysis and postdialysis weight are the best clinical methods for determining the status of the water balance. Patients usually know their dry weight and the amount of fluctuation in weight that they experience with each dialysis cycle.

Nephrologists often remove more water than usual in preoperative patients to allow the anesthesiologist to give more intravenous salt solutions during the procedure.

**TABLE 11–17.** Water and Electrolyte Imbalance in Uremia

| ↑ Intake | ↓ Intake, extrarenal loss |
|---|---|
| Hypervolemia | Hypovolemia |
| Peripheral edema | Hypotension |
| Pulmonary edema | Shock |
| Ejection murmurs | ↑ $H^+$, $PO_4^{-3}$, $Mg^{2+}$, $K^+$ |
| Hypertension | ↓ $Na^+$, $Ca^{2+}$ |
| Encephalopathy | |

Modified from Bastron RD. Chronic renal failure, clinical implications. In: *Current Reviews in Clinical Anesthesia.* Lesson 8. Vol 3. Miami, Fla: Current Reviews in Clinical Anesthesia; 1982.

### Is a Tilt Test Advisable?

Although theoretically attractive, a tilt test to determine adequacy of autonomic nervous system function is not necessary. A patient's response to anesthesia and blood loss is determined primarily by the effective circulating blood volume and is treated accordingly, regardless of the results of a tilt test.

### What Blood Studies Are Important?

Be aware of the degree of anemia and how well it is tolerated. If a patient is inadequately dialyzed or has just recently been dialyzed, check for clotting abnormalities. Inadequately dialyzed patients may have abnormal platelet function; the best test for this situation is determination of bleeding time. Recently dialyzed patients may still be heparinized or may develop rebound heparinization (Table 11–18), which can be excluded by an activated clotting time. Because most of these patients have received multiple transfusions, they should be considered at increased risk for hepatitis or HIV infection.

If a patient is confused or nauseated and has been dialyzed in the immediate preoperative period, the disequilibrium syndrome may be to blame. This condition results from cerebral edema subsequent to a decrease in plasma osmolality relative to cerebral osmolality. It requires up to 24 hours to resolve. Such patients should be treated as though they had increased intracranial pressure if postponement of the procedure is not an option.

### How Should Arteriovenous Fistulas or Other Dialysis Sites Be Managed?

Dialysis sites are the lifeline of these patients and must be protected carefully. Do not measure BP or start intravenous infusions on the arm with an arteriovenous fistula; carefully protect the fistula from external pressure, kinking, or obstruc-

**TABLE 11–18.** Abnormalities Caused by Dialysis

Rebound heparinization
Disequilibrium syndrome
Encephalopathy
Hepatitis, human immunodeficiency virus
Ascites, pericardial effusion
Hypersplenism

Modified from Bastron RD. Chronic renal failure, clinical implications. In: *Current Reviews in Clinical Anesthesia.* Lesson 8. Vol 3. Miami, Fla: Current Reviews in Clinical Anesthesia; 1982.

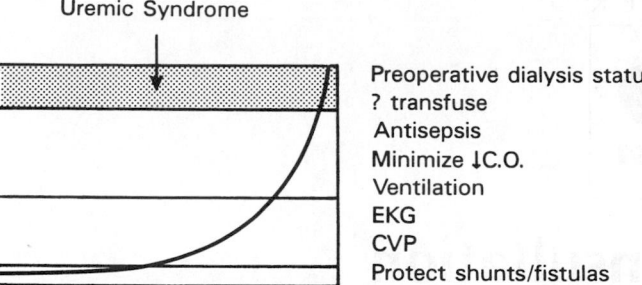

Uremic Syndrome

Preoperative dialysis status
? transfuse
Antisepsis
Minimize ↓C.O.
Ventilation
EKG
CVP
Protect shunts/fistulas

**FIGURE 11–6.** Anesthetic implications of uremia and dialysis. (Modified from Bastron RD. Chronic renal failure, clinical implications. In: *Current Reviews in Clinical Anesthesia, 1982*. Lesson 8. Vol 3. Miami, Fla: Current Reviews in Clinical Anesthesia; 1982:63.)

tion due to arm flexion; and when feasible, do not place intravenous infusion catheters in veins that may be needed later for arteriovenous fistulas. Document on the anesthesia record that the fistula was protected and functioning.

## Why Is the Postoperative Period Critical?

Postoperatively, these patients may develop a hypercoagulable state. This problem may explain why arteriovenous fistulas clot at this time. Therefore, fistulas must be carefully protected in the postoperative period as well. The lumen of temporary dialysis catheters may be filled with a solution containing 10 000 U of heparin per milliliter. If one of these must be used for intravenous access, aspirate to clear it of heparin before injecting anything through the catheter.

## What Are the Anesthetic Implications?

The importance of preoperative dialysis cannot be overemphasized (Fig. 11–6). Adequate dialysis corrects the problems caused by fluid and electrolyte imbalance. Evaluate and treat anemia according to your hospital's current guidelines. Compensation for severe anemia involves increased cardiac output, which reduces available cardiac reserve, and increased red blood cell 2,3-diphosphoglycerate, which shifts the oxygen dissociation curve to the right (more favorable for tissue oxygenation). Therefore, avoid or minimize reductions in cardiac output and increases in pH during anesthesia. Blood gas partition coefficients may be reduced by as much as 20% in patients with severe anemia, affecting induction and recovery times from inhaled anesthetics.

Monitor the ECG with particular attention to electrolyte-related changes. Poorly prepared patients may have hyperkalemic metabolic acidosis with compensatory hyperventilation. Failure to maintain hyperventilation may result in more severe acidosis and a catastrophic rise in serum potassium levels.

Immunosuppressive drugs used in transplant recipients potentiate a natural susceptibility to infections. Therefore, special attention to aseptic technique is important when performing any invasive procedure. Hepatitis is endemic in the dialyzed population, and appropriate precautions including vaccination should be followed.

All types of anesthetic techniques and agents have been used successfully in dialyzed patients and transplant recipients. No single agent or technique is always appropriate.[22–24] A choice is made on the basis of the principles discussed, the patient's psychological and physiologic state, and the requirements of the surgical procedure.

### References

1. Roberts SL, Tinker JH. Cardiovascular disease. In: Brown DL, ed. *Risk and Outcome in Anesthesia*. Philadelphia, Pa: JB Lippincott; 1988:34.
2. Brown DL, Thompson GE. Anesthetic choice. In: Brown DL, ed. *Risk and Outcome in Anesthesia*. Philadelphia, Pa: JB Lippincott; 1988:166.
3. Prys-Roberts C. Anesthetic management of the hypertensive patient. *Acta Anaesthesiol Belg.* 1988;39(suppl 2):9.
4. Miller ED Jr. Anesthesia and the hypertensive patient. *IARS 1987 Review Course Lectures*. Cleveland, Ohio: International Anesthesia Research Society; 1987:6.
5. Miller ED Jr. Perioperative hypertension: an overview. ASA 42nd Annual Refresher Course Lectures and Clinical Update Program. Park Ridge, Ill: American Society of Anesthesiologists; 1991. No. 331.
6. Berry FA. *Anesthetic Management of Difficult and Routine Pediatric Patients*. 2nd ed. New York, NY: Churchill Livingstone; 1990:89.
7. Cheung AT, Chernow B. Perioperative electrolyte disorders. In: Benumof JL, Saidman JL, eds. *Anesthesia and Perioperative Complications*. St Louis, Mo: Mosby–Year Book; 1992:466.
8. Gravenstein JS. Fluid and electrolytes and acid-base balance. In: Gravenstein N, ed. *Manual of Complications During Anesthesia*. Philadelphia, Pa: JB Lippincott; 1991:353.
9. Cogan MG. *Fluid and Electrolytes: Physiology and Pathophysiology*. Norwalk, Conn: Appleton & Lange; 1991.
10. Williams EL, Hildebrand KL, McCormick SA, et al. The effect of intravenous lactated Ringer's solution versus 0.9% sodium chloride solution on serum osmolality in human volunteers. *Anesth Analg*. 1999;88:99.
11. Scheingraber S, Rehm M, Sehmisch C, et al. Rapid saline infusion produces hyperchloremic acidosis in patients undergoing gynecologic survey. *Anesthesiology*. 1999;90:1265.
12. Kokko JP, Tannel RL. *Fluids and Electrolytes*. 2nd ed. Philadelphia, Pa: WB Saunders; 1990.
13. Solomon RJ, Katz JD. Disturbances of potassium homeostasis. In: Stoelting RK, Barash PG, Gallagher TJ, eds. *Advances in Anesthesia*. Vol 3. Chicago, Ill: Year Book Medical Publishers; 1986:169.
14. Allan M, Dunlay R, Copkney C. Nebulized albuterol for acute hyperkalemia in patients on hemodialysis. *Ann Intern Med*. 1989;110:426.
15. Prielipp R, Zaloga GP. Calcium action and general anesthesia. In: Stoelting RK, Barash PG, Gallagher TJ, eds. *Advances in Anesthesia*. Vol 8. St Louis, Mo: Mosby–Year Book; 1991:241.
16. Kaufman BS, Contreras J. Preanesthetic assessment of the patient with renal disease. *Anesthesiol Clin North Am*. 1990;8:677.
17. Takala J, Ruokonen E, Kari A. Acute renal failure. *Anesthesiol Clin North Am*. 1988;6:173.
18. Prough DS. Oliguria: significance and management. *IARS 1987 Review Course Lectures*. Cleveland, Ohio: International Anesthesia Research Society; 1987:112.
19. Prough DS, Zaloga G. Hypovolemia and renal dysfunction. In: Benumof JL, Saidman LJ, eds. *Anesthesia and Perioperative Complications*. St Louis, Mo: Mosby–Year Book; 1992:434.
20. Sladen RN. Perioperative renal protection. *ASA 42nd Annual Refresher Course Lectures and Clinical Update Program*. Park Ridge, Ill: American Society of Anesthesiologists; 1991, No. 255.
21. Prough DS. Perioperative management of acute renal failure. In: Stoelting RK, Barash PG, Gallagher TJ, eds. *Advances in Anesthesia*. Vol 5. Chicago, Ill: Year Book Medical Publishers; 1988:192.
22. Barr L, Miller ED Jr. Preserving renal function. *Anesthesiol Rep*. 1989;1:290.
23. Gelman S. Preserving renal function during surgery. *IARS 1991 Review Course Lectures*. Cleveland, Ohio: International Anesthesia Research Society; 1992:88.
24. Borland LM, Cook DR. Anesthesia for organ transplantation. In: Stoelting RK, Barash PG, Gallagher TJ, eds. *Advances in Anesthesia*. Vol 3. Chicago, Ill: Year Book Medical Publishers; 1986:12.

CHAPTER

# 12

# Radiology Consultation

Patricia L. Abbitt

Jesse L. Chai

Carl E. Ravin

## THE THORAX

*What Factors Affect Chest Film Assessment?*

*What Is the Normal Anatomy on the Chest Radiograph?*

*What Are the Radiographic Findings in Emphysema?*

*What Are the Radiographic Findings of Pulmonary Edema?*

*What Are the Radiographic Findings of Pulmonary Barotrauma?*

*What Are the Common Radiographic Findings in Catheter and Tube Placement?*

## THE NECK

*What Are the Radiographic Findings of Acute Laryngeal Pathology?*

*What Are the Radiographic Findings of Atlantoaxial Subluxation?*

## THE ABDOMEN

*What Are the Radiographic Manifestations of Bowel Obstruction?*

*What Are the Radiographic Findings of Pneumoperitoneum?*

*What Is the Correct Gastric or Enteric Tube Position?*

The purpose of this chapter is to demonstrate normal plain film anatomy of the thorax, neck, and abdomen and to illustrate pathologic processes in these regions that are of clinical concern to an anesthesiologist.

## THE THORAX

### What Factors Affect Chest Film Assessment?

Initial review of a chest radiograph should include assessment of the radiographic technique, the patient's position, and the lung volumes. Understanding the factors that vary from film to film enables an observer to discriminate more easily among technical variation, true pathology, and normal anatomy.

### Positioning of Film

Most preoperative chest films are taken with a patient standing at a 6-foot focal film distance (from the radiographic tube to the radiographic film) and are exposed at full inspiration. Almost all normal radiographic measurements of structures in the thorax are defined only for the standard erect posteroanterior (PA) chest film.

However, most films of critically ill patients, such as those in intensive care units, are performed in an anteroposterior (AP) projection with a patient supine and a focal film distance of 40 to 48 inches. This difference in technique results in significant magnification of many intrathoracic structures, particularly those located more anteriorly in the chest, such as the heart. In addition, the change in position from erect to supine often results in increased venous volume, causing additional enlargement of venous structures.

### Patient Position

Interpreting films of critically ill patients may be difficult. Rotation of the patient's body can confound findings. Not infrequently, a patient is imaged in a semierect position, which is particularly confusing because the patient's actual position can vary from almost supine to almost erect. Lung volumes are often low. Assessing the patient's position (generally indicated on the film by the technologist) is especially important when looking for pneumothoraces or pleural fluid because air and fluid move freely in the pleural space in the absence of adhesions.

Thus, a pneumothorax would be visible in the apex of the chest of a patient in the erect position. In a patient in the supine position, a pneumothorax would be anterior and medial and would be difficult or impossible to see on a single AP view of the chest. Fluid would be posterior and basal with a patient in the erect position, and posterior and medial with a patient supine. In some cases, fluid actually is better seen in a lateral view if a patient must remain supine.

### Radiographic Techniques

Moreover, radiographic technique can vary greatly, depending on the experience of the technologist. For the most part, any judgment regarding edema, pulmonary vascularity, and heart size should be made cautiously on low lung volume films. In addition, edema can appear worse on light, underexposed films or appear improved with larger lung volumes on dark, overexposed films. A dark film should always be viewed over a bright light in addition to the standard view box.

## What Is the Normal Anatomy on the Chest Radiograph?

Chest radiography is invaluable in assessing placement of endotracheal tubes (ETTs), central venous and pulmonary artery catheters, monitoring devices, and pacemakers. Understanding normal anatomy helps to identify the location of these devices.

Figure 12–1 demonstrates the normal anatomy of a PA and lateral chest radiograph.[1–3]

### Central Venous Structures of Interest

The subclavian vein is the continuation of the axillary vein and courses along the inner surface of the clavicle. It joins the internal jugular vein to form the brachiocephalic vein behind the sternoclavicular joint. The left brachiocephalic vein courses obliquely downward and to the right; the right brachiocephalic vein passes directly downward behind the manubrium. The union of the brachiocephalic veins forms the superior vena cava (SVC), which then enters the right atrium. The right atrium forms the right-sided border of the normal cardiac silhouette on a frontal chest film. A normal-sized right ventricle is not seen on a frontal chest radiograph.

At about the level of T4, the azygos vein arches forward over the right mainstem bronchus to empty into the back wall of the SVC (Fig. 12–2). Enlargement of the azygos vein is seen in disease states that result in elevated right heart end-diastolic pressures, tricuspid insufficiency, or increased venous return such as right-sided heart failure or inferior vena cava obstruction. An azygos vein diameter <10 mm as seen en face on a standard PA chest radiograph is considered normal. A measurement >10 mm is considered pathologic except in pregnant women.[4]

### Cardiomediastinal Silhouette

The left border of the cardiomediastinal silhouette is formed (superiorly to inferiorly) by the left subclavian artery, the aortic arch, the pleural reflection from the aorta onto the main pulmonary artery, the left border of the main pulmonary artery, the left atrial appendage, and the left ventricle.

On the lateral view, the right ventricle is the most anterior border-forming structure of the heart and normally abuts the sternum; it generally occupies no more than one third of the distance from the anterior costophrenic angle to the sternomanubrial joint.

The left ventricle is the chamber that most frequently enlarges in adults and tends to enlarge more posteriorly than laterally. An often-cited sign of left ventricular enlargement is the Hoffmann-Rigler sign (Fig. 12–3).

### Heart Size

The normal heart size on a standard PA chest radiograph ranges from 11.5 to 15.5 cm. The widely used *50% rule* for describing the upper limits of normal for the cardiothoracic ratio should be used with caution because at least 10% of normal patients exceed this ratio. In addition, patients with small hearts that subsequently enlarge pathologically sometimes do not approach this 50% ratio.[5]

### Airway and Pulmonary Arteries

On the frontal view, the trachea divides at the carina into the right and left mainstem bronchi at approximately the level of T5. On the lateral view, the trachea ends in a rounded radiolucent structure that represents the distal left mainstem and left upper lobe bronchus (see Fig. 12–1C). Above the left mainstem bronchus, another rounded lucent structure representing the right upper lobe bronchus can occasionally be seen. The left pulmonary artery arches over the left mainstem bronchus. Projected anterior to the left mainstem bronchus is the right pulmonary artery.

### Pulmonary Vasculature

Appreciation of normal pulmonary vascularity is best learned through experience. The normal pulmonary vasculature radiates from the hilum and branches toward the periphery of the lung. On a normal erect chest radiograph, the upper lung vessels are smaller and less numerous than those in the lower lung fields because of differences in blood flow related to hydrostatic pressure differences. The differences between the upper and lower lobe vessels tend to disappear on a supine chest radiograph as the hydrostatic pressure differences between the upper and lower lungs are eliminated.

## What Are the Radiographic Findings in Emphysema?

The role of chest radiography in diagnosing emphysema has been the subject of contentious debate. Most radiologists are uncomfortable with the term *chronic obstructive pulmonary disease* because it describes function (or malfunction) and is therefore a clinical diagnosis. *Emphysema,* on the other hand, is defined structurally as enlargement of air spaces distal to the terminal respiratory bronchiole accompanied by destruction of the alveolar walls.[6] Although some experts believe that emphysema is a pathologic rather than a radiologic diagnosis, we are comfortable with the diagnosis of emphysema because radiographs reflect structure. However, in general, when the disease is evident radiographically, clinical and physiologic clues to the diagnosis are also evident, and the disease is often advanced.

### Hyperinflation

Various criteria have been proposed for diagnosing emphysema radiographically. Those relating to hyperinflation appear to be the most reproducible and reliable, whereas those reflecting tissue destruction are subject to more intraobserver and interobserver variation.

Signs of hyperinflation include the following:

1. Depression and flattening of the hemidiaphragms, with blunting of the costophrenic angles on the PA or lateral

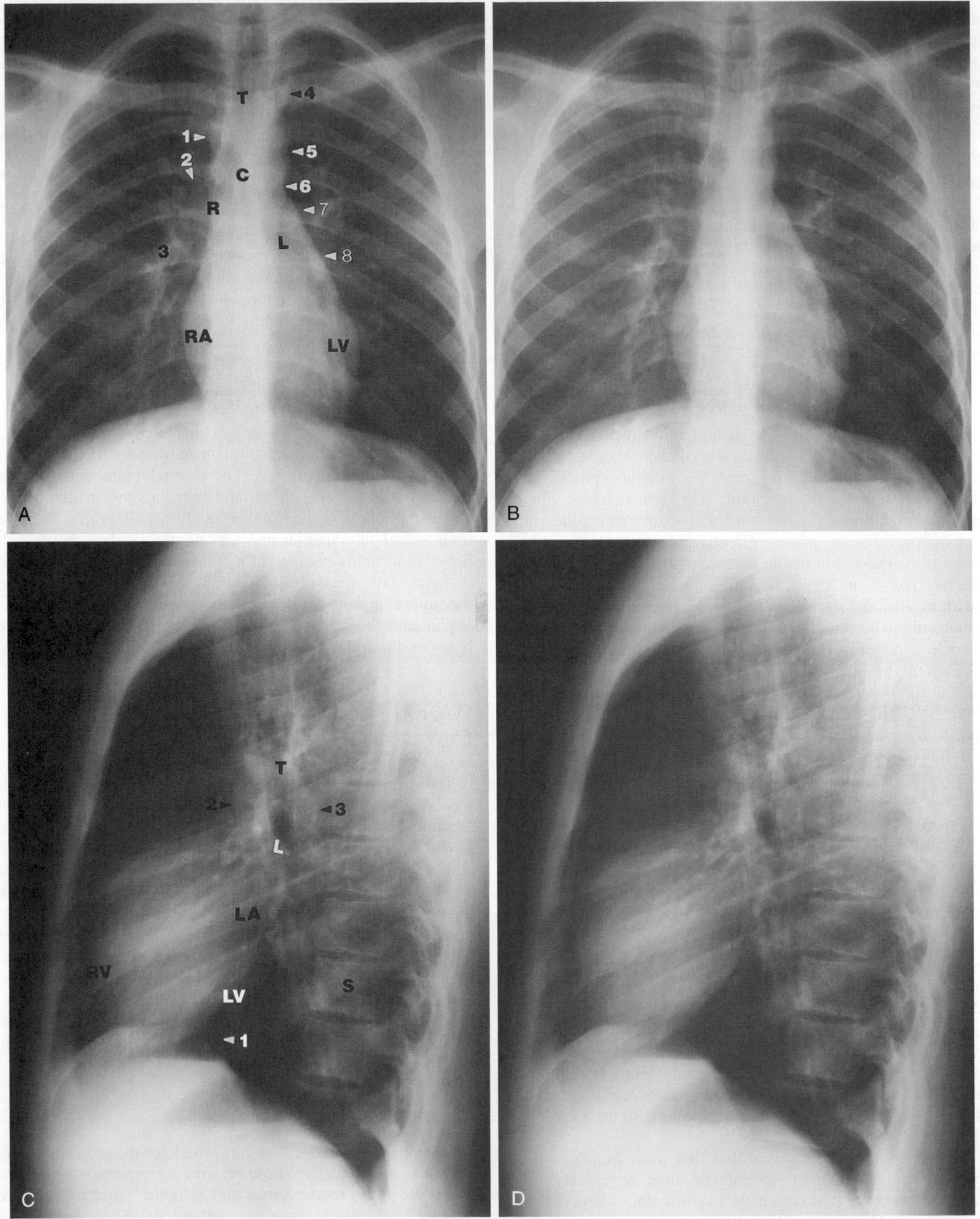

**FIGURE 12–1.** Normal chest film. *A,* PA view: 1, superior vena cava; 2, azygos vein; 3, right interlobar pulmonary artery; 4, left subclavian artery; 5, aortic arch; 6, pleural reflection from aorta onto main pulmonary artery; 7, main pulmonary artery; 8, left atrial appendage. *B,* Same PA view without labels. *C,* Lateral view. The right upper lobe bronchus is not visualized on this film: 1, inferior vena cava; 2, right pulmonary artery; 3, left pulmonary artery. *D,* Same lateral view without labels. C, carina; L, left mainstem bronchus; LA, left atrium; LV, left ventricle; PA, posteroanterior; R, right mainstem bronchus; RA, right atrium; RV, right ventricle; S, spine; T, trachea.

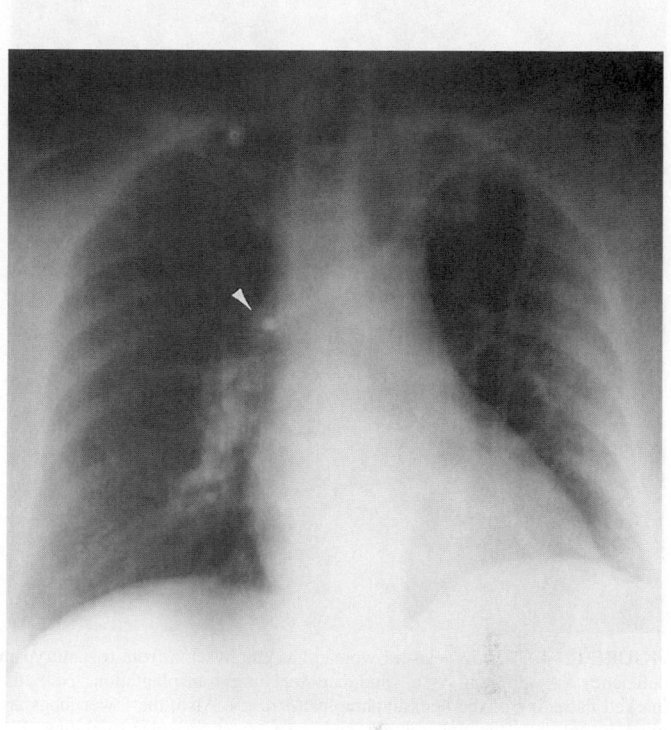

**FIGURE 12–2.** The course of the azygos vein is more clearly delineated on this film because of inadvertent placement of a catheter into the azygos vein. This left subclavian catheter traverses the left brachiocephalic vein and the superior vena cava and then courses posteriorly into the azygos vein. The distal 5 cm of the catheter is in the azygos vein (*arrowhead*). (Courtesy of James Chen, MD.)

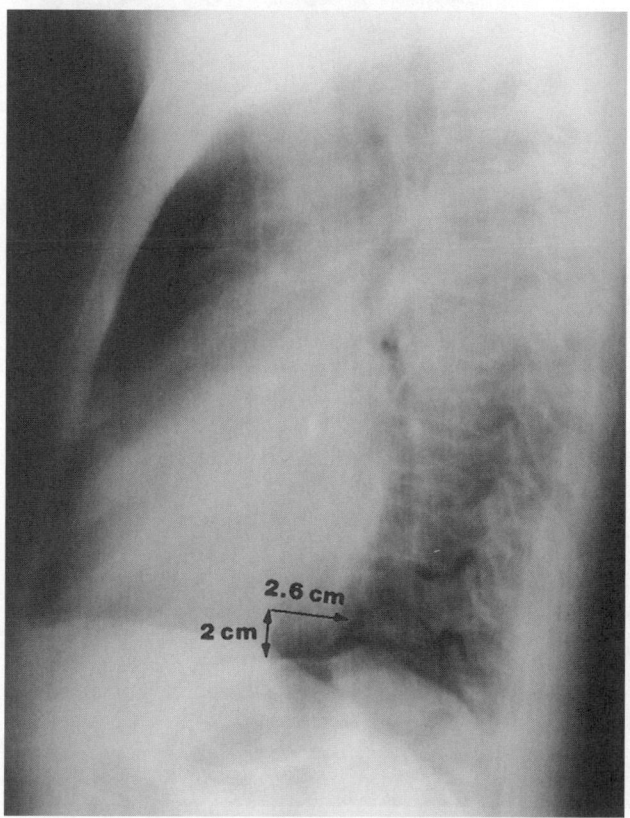

**FIGURE 12–3.** Hoffmann-Rigler sign. On the lateral view, a measurement of >1.7 cm at a point 2 cm cephalad from the crossing of the inferior vena cava with the left ventricle indicates left ventricular enlargement. The measurement should be made on a plane parallel to the endplates of the vertebral bodies of the spine. This sign is not specific in the presence of a pectus excavatum deformity and right ventricular hypertrophy because both of these processes tend to displace the left ventricle posteriorly even in the absence of left ventricular enlargement. Also, a true lateral film is required for utilization of this sign because the left ventricle can be positioned more posteriorly on a rotated film. This 42-year-old man has marked left ventricular enlargement secondary to mitral valvular insufficiency. The measurement of 2.6 cm greatly exceeds the upper limits of normal.

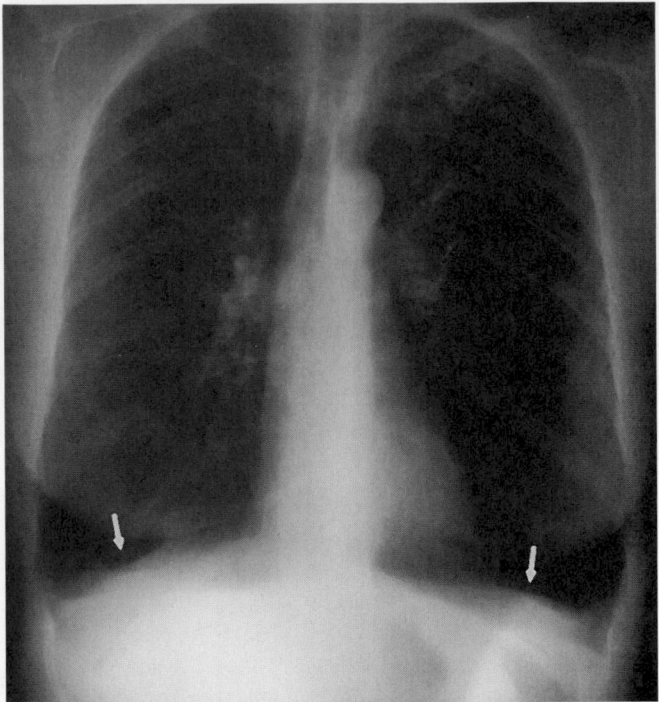

**FIGURE 12–4.** This 52-year-old woman has emphysema from $\alpha_1$-antitrypsin deficiency ($A_1AD$) and is a candidate for lung transplantation. Note the marked flattening of the hemidiaphragms (*arrows*). Also, the lower lungs are more lucent than the upper lungs and have fewer vascular markings. The emphysematous changes in $A_1AD$ are typically more prominent in the bases of the lungs.

view. The contour of the hemidiaphragms is more important than the actual level. If the highest level of a hemidiaphragm is <1.5 cm above a line drawn from the costophrenic angle to the vertebrophrenic junction, the diaphragm can be regarded as flat (Fig. 12–4).
2. Increased retrosternal space on the lateral view. Radiolucency measuring 2.5 cm or more from the sternum to the most anterior margin of the ascending aorta is considered abnormal.[7,8]

### Tissue Destruction

Discerning tissue destruction can be difficult. Alterations of the normal branching pattern of pulmonary vascularity with displacement of vessels around areas of pulmonary destruction constitute a reliable radiographic sign. Increased lucency within the lungs corresponds to abnormal enlargement of air spaces associated with alveolar destruction. The lucencies may be focal or diffuse. Focal lucencies may reflect bullae, which are thin-walled air-filled spaces >1 cm (Fig. 12–5). They appear radiographically as well-demarcated avascular spaces. Blebs, another finding in emphysema, are collections of air within the layers of the visceral pleura that are not generally as large as bullae.[9]

### Pulmonary Artery Enlargement

Complications of emphysema or any other long-standing pulmonary disease include pulmonary arterial hypertension. A

characteristic finding is enlargement of the central pulmonary arteries (Fig. 12–6). Increase in diameter of the right descending (*interlobar*) pulmonary artery (>16 mm in men and >15 mm in women) has been shown to correlate well with the diagnosis of pulmonary arterial hypertension.[10]

### Right Ventricular Hypertrophy

Long-standing pulmonary arterial hypertension can lead to right ventricular hypertrophy or cor pulmonale (Fig. 12–7). Roentgenologically, right ventricular hypertrophy may be difficult to detect, especially in emphysematous patients with generous lung volumes. Comparison with prior films is helpful to determine interval increase in size of the right ventricle.

### *What Are the Radiographic Findings of Pulmonary Edema?*

When pulmonary capillary pressure is markedly increased or when the permeability of the capillary wall is increased above normal, excess fluid tends to accumulate in the interstitial space. This can be seen on the chest film by increased interstitial markings, interstitial thickening, and vascular structures that appear indistinct. When the quantity of fluid in-

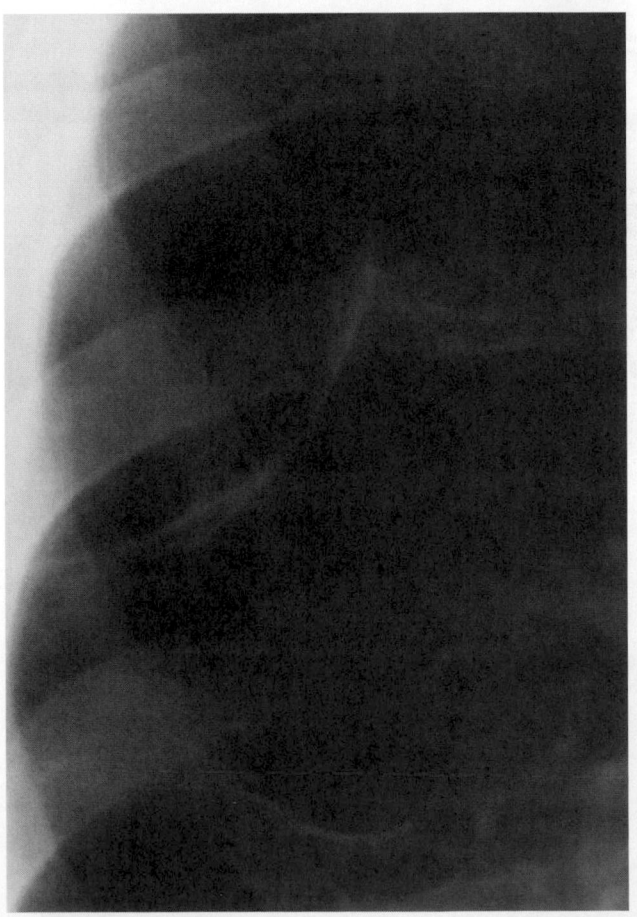

**FIGURE 12–5.** Bullae are seen radiographically as thin curvilinear lines demarcating avascular spaces.

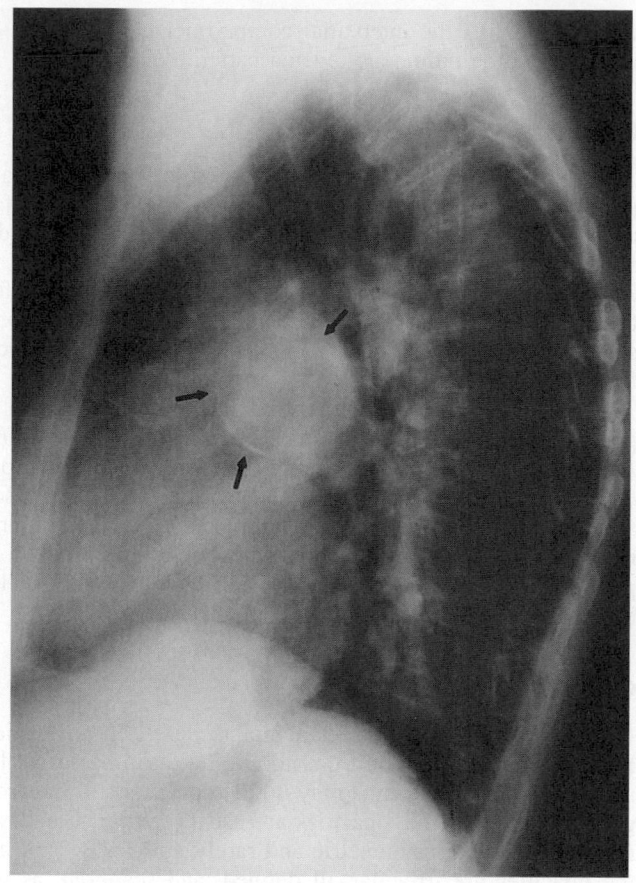

**FIGURE 12–6.** This 67-year-old woman has long-standing pulmonary arterial hypertension from an atrial septal defect. On the lateral view, the right pulmonary artery (*arrows*) is markedly enlarged and calcified. (Courtesy of Edward Patz, MD.)

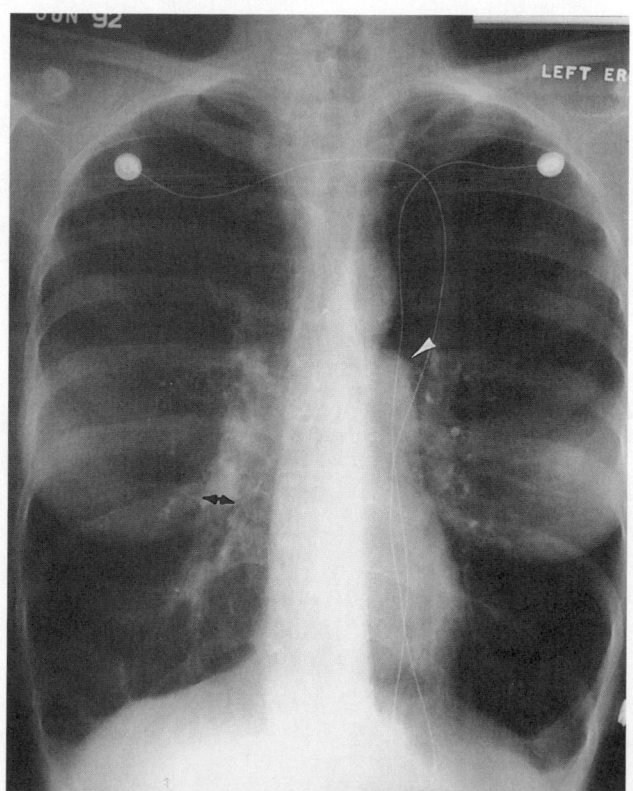

**FIGURE 12–7.** This 43-year-old woman has severe emphysema, pulmonary arterial hypertension, and cor pulmonale. Note the marked flattening of the hemidiaphragms. The main pulmonary artery (*white arrowhead*) is enlarged, the right interlobar pulmonary artery (*double-headed arrow*) measures 17 mm, and the right ventricle is enlarged.

creases and fills the interstitial compartment, fluid floods the alveoli, and the pulmonary edema pattern develops.

## Pulmonary Vasculature

Pulmonary edema most commonly results from elevated pulmonary venous pressure secondary to left-sided heart failure. Detecting early interstitial edema can be difficult and is subject to considerable interobserver variability. One of the earliest radiographic signs is loss of the normal sharp definition of the pulmonary vessels. With increasing venous pressure, vasoconstriction occurs in the lower lungs, and blood flow is redistributed from the lower to the upper lungs.

Later, septal lines secondary to interstitial fluid may be present. The most common form, often referred to as *Kerley B lines,* are short (<2 cm), straight, thin lines oriented perpendicular to the pleural surface, and they are most clearly seen along the lateral border of the lower lungs or in the retrosternal region (Fig. 12–8). Peribronchial thickening may occur in the perihilar regions. Subpleural edema, which is manifested as thickened interlobar fissures, may also be noted.[11]

## Cardiogenic Pulmonary Edema

Interstitial edema precedes alveolar edema. In any patient, however, the progression from normal fluid to interstitial fluid to overt pulmonary edema may not be documented. In cardiogenic alveolar edema, opacities are usually bilateral and symmetric but can be asymmetric and rarely unilateral. Typically, the opacities are irregular, ill defined, and scattered, as well as more confluent in the medial third of the lungs. The "butterfly" or "bat wing" pattern describes a distribution of alveolar edema in a bilateral perihilar configuration. This pattern was initially described in and is more common with uremia, but the pattern may also be seen in congestive heart failure.[12,13]

## Congestive Heart Failure

In congestive heart failure, the heart is usually enlarged, and pleural effusions are generally present. The left ventricle is the chamber that most commonly enlarges (Fig. 12–9). A normal heart size associated with cardiogenic edema is noted in acute myocardial infarctions or dysrhythmias (Fig. 12–10). Resolution of the edema generally begins peripherally and ends medially. The radiographic findings may lag behind the clinical findings but generally clear rapidly once therapy is instituted.

## Noncardiogenic Pulmonary Edema

The pulmonary findings of noncardiogenic pulmonary edema resemble those of cardiogenic edema. However, heart size is generally normal. Common causes include acute increase in intracranial pressure, inhalation of noxious substances, anaphylaxis, drug reactions, and sepsis.

## Adult Respiratory Distress Syndrome

The pulmonary edema of adult respiratory distress syndrome is generally associated with altered permeability of the

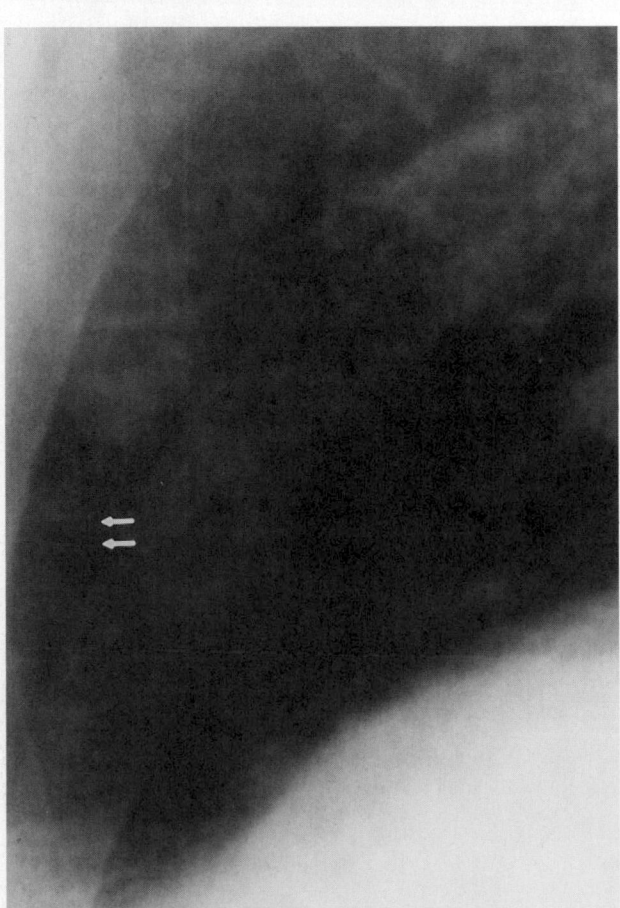

**FIGURE 12–8.** Septal lines (*arrows*) are best seen along the lateral borders of the lower lungs (as in this case) and in the retrosternal space.

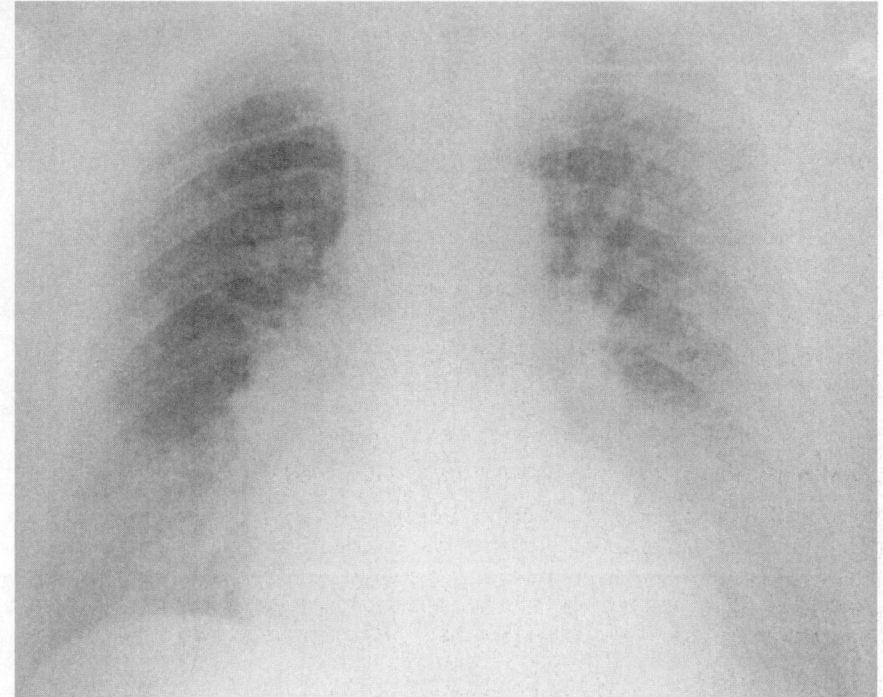

**FIGURE 12–9.** This 34-year-old woman developed postpartum congestive heart failure. Interstitial edema is demonstrated by interstitial thickening and septal lines.

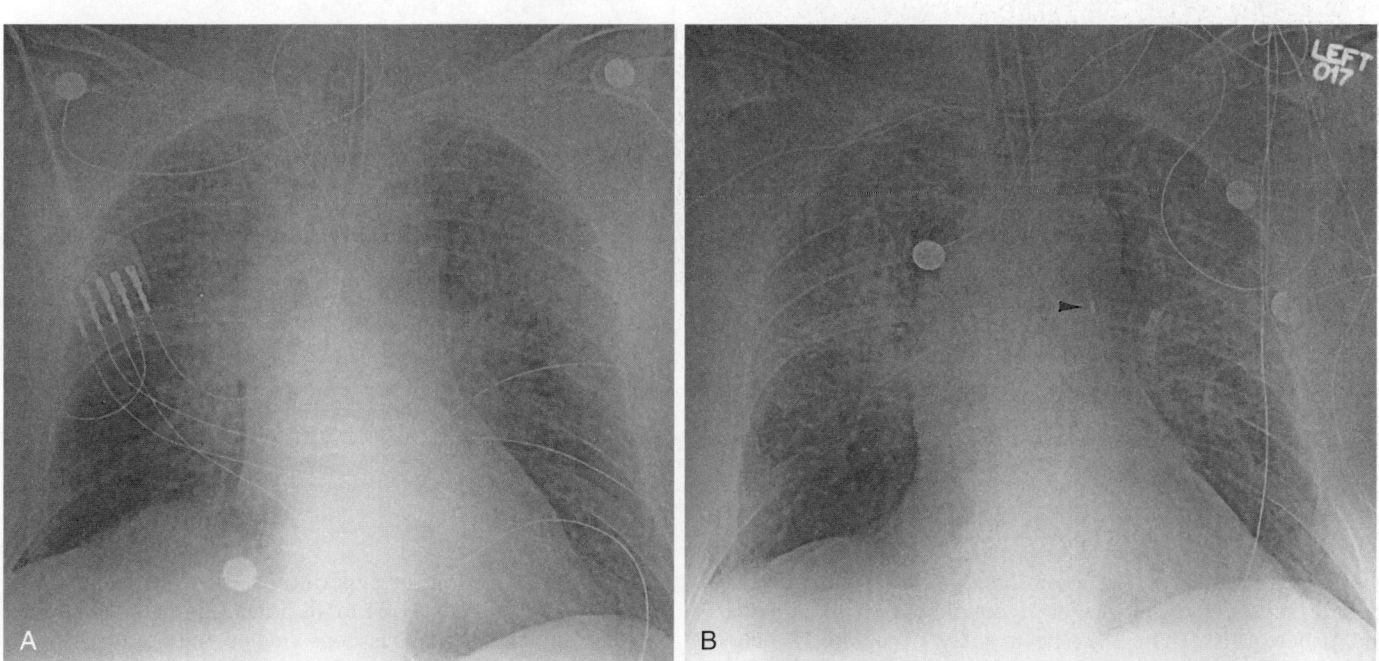

**FIGURE 12–10.** This 74-year-old man suffered an acute myocardial infarction. *A,* Initial chest radiograph reveals bilateral hazy perihilar opacities consistent with cardiogenic pulmonary edema. The heart size is normal; this can be seen in the setting of acute myocardial infarction. The endotracheal tube is in satisfactory position. *B,* The bilateral perihilar opacities are improved after diuretic therapy and placement of an intra-aortic balloon pump *(arrowhead).* There has been interval placement of a pulmonary artery catheter via a femoral vein.

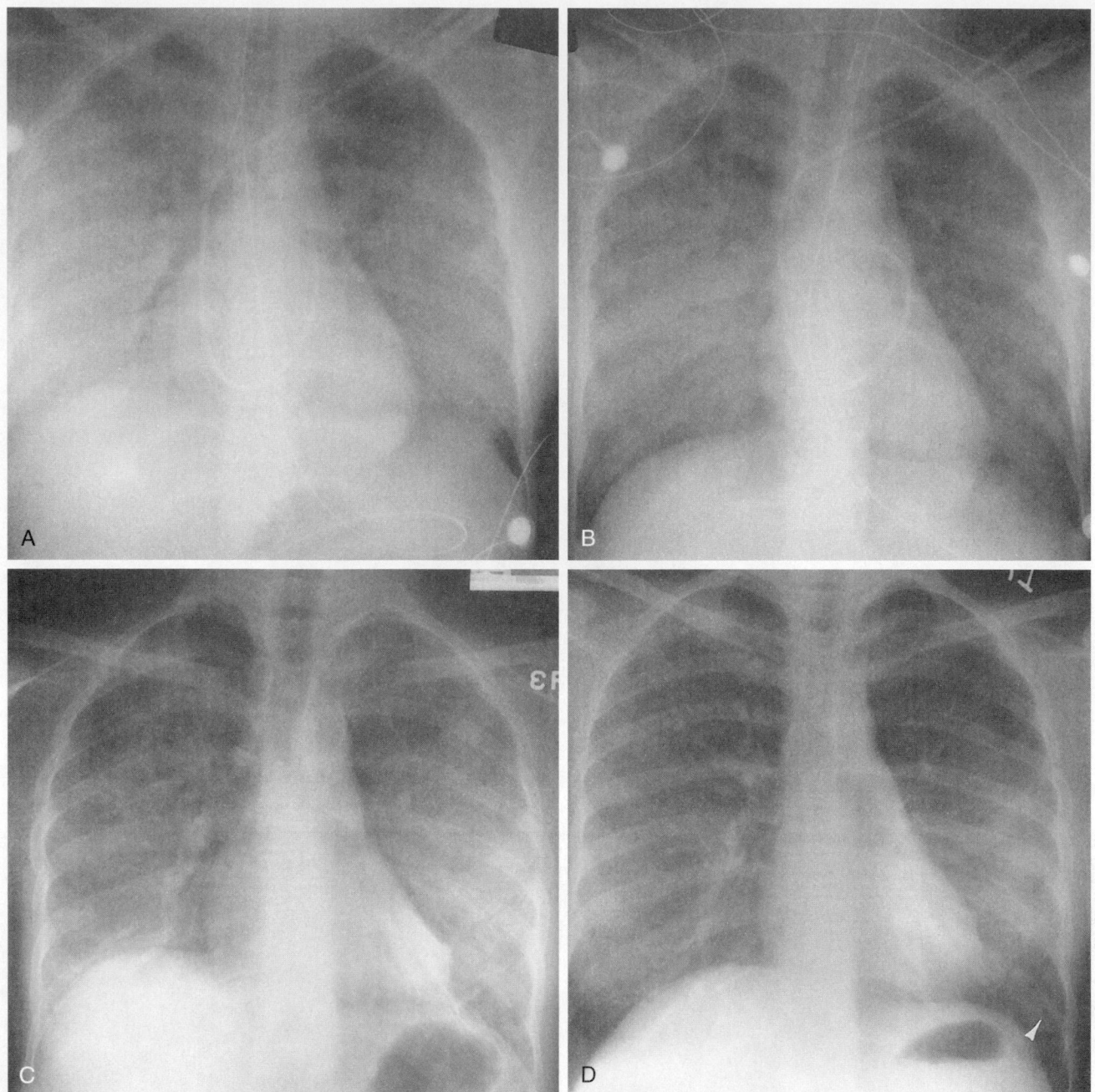

**FIGURE 12–11.** This 16-year-old girl was brought comatose and hypotensive into the emergency room following an overdose of ethchlorvynol (Placidyl). The patient subsequently developed adult respiratory distress syndrome. *A,* Chest radiograph taken 4 hours after admission reveals bilateral dense alveolar opacities. The endotracheal tube is in satisfactory position with the tip 2 cm above the carina. The Swan-Ganz catheter terminates in the right ventricular outflow tract and needs to be advanced. *B,* Chest radiograph taken 2 days later demonstrates slight interval clearing of the alveolar opacities. The endotracheal tube tip is now 2 cm above the thoracic inlet, and the Swan-Ganz catheter tip is now in the proximal right pulmonary artery. *C,* Three weeks later, interstitial opacities remain. *D,* Chest radiograph taken 3 months later reveals resolution of the opacities except for minimal scarring (*arrowhead*) at the left lung base.

pulmonary capillaries. The most common precipitating events include sepsis, hypotensive or hypovolemic shock, trauma, and pancreatitis. There may be a delay of up to 12 hours between the clinical onset of respiratory failure and radiographic abnormality.

At 12 to 24 hours, patchy irregular opacities appear bilaterally and resemble those of cardiogenic edema. However, cardiomegaly, pleural effusions, and cephalization of the pulmonary vessels are generally absent unless these abnormalities were preexistent.

If pleural effusions are present, an underlying infection,

pulmonary infarction, or superimposed cardiogenic failure should be considered. At 24 to 48 hours, the patchy opacities coalesce into homogeneous consolidated regions. By 5 to 7 days, the consolidation often becomes inhomogeneous, suggesting improved aeration.

As aeration improves with treatment, a coarse reticular pattern is seen and corresponds pathologically to fibrin deposition on the alveolar walls. The radiographic findings may revert to normal in 2 to 3 weeks (Fig. 12–11) or may progress to pulmonary fibrosis.[11,14,15]

Mechanical ventilation improves lung expansion and consequently often improves the radiographic picture of diffuse pulmonary parenchymal disease even if clinical findings do not suggest improvement. Conversely, when mechanical support is discontinued, radiographic findings associated with hypoaerated lungs may falsely suggest worsening of the parenchymal process despite an improving clinical picture.[16]

## What Are the Radiographic Findings of Pulmonary Barotrauma?

### Pulmonary Interstitial Emphysema

When intra-alveolar pressure rises and an alveolus ruptures, air dissects along the bronchovascular bundle. The condition of air in the interstitium is termed *pulmonary interstitial emphysema*. When positive pressure ventilation is a cause of this complication, the spaces around the bronchi and vessels become filled with air. Radiographically, these dilated structures resemble tortuous bubbles, 2 to 3 mm in diameter, which radiate outward from the hilum (Fig. 12–12). Inspiratory and expiratory films demonstrate that these structures do not decompress. With continued positive pressure ventilation, these structures dilate even more and can enlarge into large cysts.

Pulmonary interstitial edema is more commonly encountered in children than adults and usually resolves when positive pressure ventilation is stopped.[17] If the air decompresses by bursting through the visceral pleura into the pleural space, pneumothorax results. If the air decompresses into the mediastinum, pneumomediastinum results. Generally, when interstitial air is noted, every attempt to minimize progression should be made, usually by attempting to decrease ventilator pressures.

### Pneumothorax

The radiographic diagnosis of pneumothorax is established when the visceral pleural line is visualized. In an erect patient, air in the pleural space normally rises to the apex of the hemithorax and causes local compression of the lung (Fig. 12–13). In a supine patient, air rises to the most superior portion of the hemithorax, which, in this position, is located near the hemidiaphragm in the anteromedial and subpulmonic recesses. A deep costophrenic sulcus may be seen, and the upper quadrant of the abdomen may be relatively lucent (Fig. 12–14).[18,19]

If a pneumothorax is suspected clinically but not demonstrated radiographically, a lateral decubitus view often establishes the diagnosis because the pleural line is more easily seen along the lateral chest wall, where there are fewer confounding shadows. An expiratory film may also be used. Computed tomography scanning will reveal smaller pneumothoraces than those detectable on plain films.

*Tension pneumothorax* is a clinical diagnosis, not a radiologic one. Shift of the mediastinum toward the contralateral side does not necessarily indicate increased pressure from the pneumothorax.[11] A pneumothorax that develops in a mechanically ventilated patient is likely to become a tension pneumothorax if not treated appropriately.

### Pneumomediastinum

Pneumomediastinum is manifested radiographically as lateral displacement of the mediastinal pleural line or as linear vertically oriented collections of air in the mediastinum. The line is usually more evident on the left, and a longitudinal

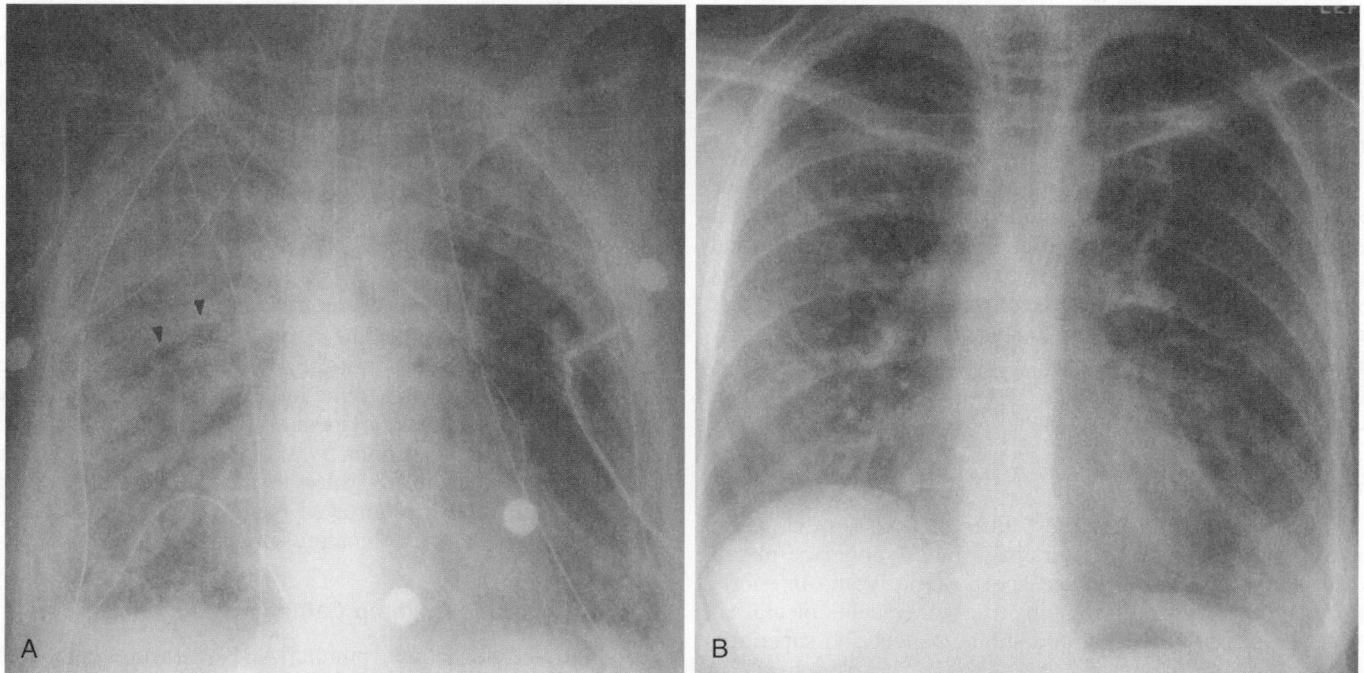

**FIGURE 12–12.** This 19-year-old woman had a prolonged course in an intensive care unit secondary to meningococcemia and adult respiratory distress syndrome. *A*, Multiple tortuous radiolucencies (*arrowheads*) represent air within the bronchovascular sheaths, a finding of pulmonary interstitial emphysema. *B*, Three months later, coarse interstitial opacities reflect pulmonary fibrosis, a complication of adult respiratory distress syndrome and oxygen toxicity.

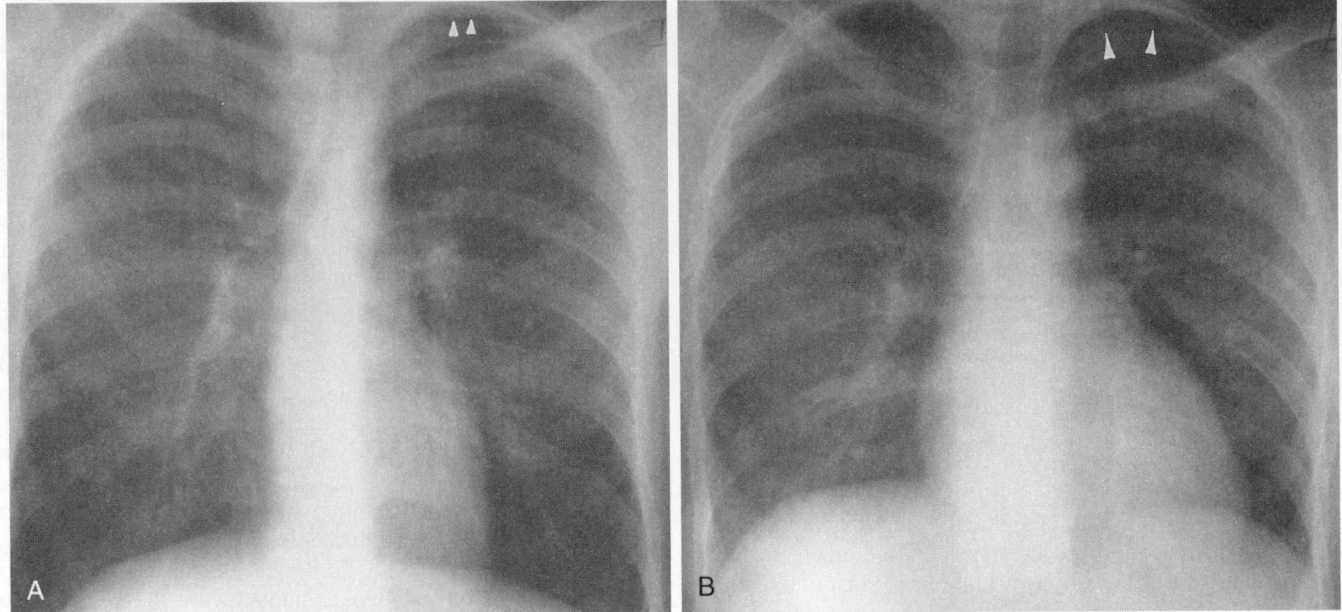

**FIGURE 12–13.** *A,* On this upright inspiratory film, a left apical pneumothorax is demonstrated by visualization of the visceral pleural line *(arrowheads).* *B,* The visceral pleural line *(arrowheads)* is more easily seen on the expiratory film.

line can be seen paralleling the heart and sometimes the aorta (Fig. 12–15).

Pneumothorax is a common complication of pneumomediastinum and results from rupture of the mediastinal pleura. Air in the mediastinal space can extend into the soft tissues of the neck and into the retroperitoneum.

The presence of subcutaneous emphysema on a radiograph may be one of the first signs of barotrauma, and the development of a pneumothorax or pneumomediastinum should be suspected if subcutaneous air is observed.

## What Are the Common Radiographic Findings in Catheter and Tube Placement?

### Endotracheal Tubes

Most ETTs are marked by a radiodense stripe that extends to the tip. The tip of a single-lumen ETT is ideally placed in the region of the thoracic inlet and should be no more distal than 2 cm from the carina.[20] Intubating a mainstem bronchus results in atelectasis or collapse of the contralateral lung and may result in barotrauma of the portion of the lung that is selectively aerated. In contrast, a proximal intubation predisposes to inadvertent extubation and laryngeal or tracheal stenosis. (The vocal cords are located at the level of ≈C5-6.)

### Chest Tubes

The correct position for chest tubes depends on the reason for placement. Pleural fluid drainage tubes should be placed posteriorly for a supine patient and posteriorly and inferiorly for an ambulatory patient. A tube used to evacuate pleural air should be placed anteriorly in a supine patient and superiorly in an ambulatory patient.

### Central Venous Catheters

Because as many as one third of central venous catheters are initially malpositioned, placement should be checked ra-

diographically. The distal tip of the catheter should be located in the SVC, proximal to but not in the right atrium. Extension into the right atrium or beyond predisposes to perforation of the heart by the catheter tip.[21] Extension into the region of the tricuspid valve can cause valvular insufficiency as well as ectopy.

Overinsertion of the catheter into the right ventricle also predisposes to ectopy and perforation of the heart.[22] The ideal catheter tip position zone is proximal to the right atrium within the SVC above the pericardial reflection, with the catheter tip parallel to the SVC (Fig. 12–16). In addition, to minimize the chance of SVC perforation, the catheter tip should not have an impingement angle with the SVC of >40°.[22] Because of the close anatomic relationship between the subclavian vein and the underlying lung, pneumothorax is a complication that occurs following subclavian line placement and should also be ruled out.

### Pulmonary Artery Catheters

Pulmonary artery catheters are typically radiodense. The tip should be placed in either the right or left pulmonary artery or in a main descending branch. The catheter tip should be no more than 2 cm lateral to the hilum; otherwise, pulmonary infarction or perforation may result.

Central venous and pulmonary artery catheters may knot or break, with subsequent migration of the free fragment. Such fragments can often be retrieved using interventional radiographic techniques, thus obviating surgery.

### Intra-Aortic Balloon Pump Catheters

An intra-aortic balloon pump (IABP) measures about 26 cm in length and has a radiodense marker at the tip, which is inserted proximally. The proximal end of the IABP should be placed just distal to the aortic arch so that the left subclavian artery or left common carotid artery is not occluded. Distally, the balloon should be above the origins of the renal and celiac

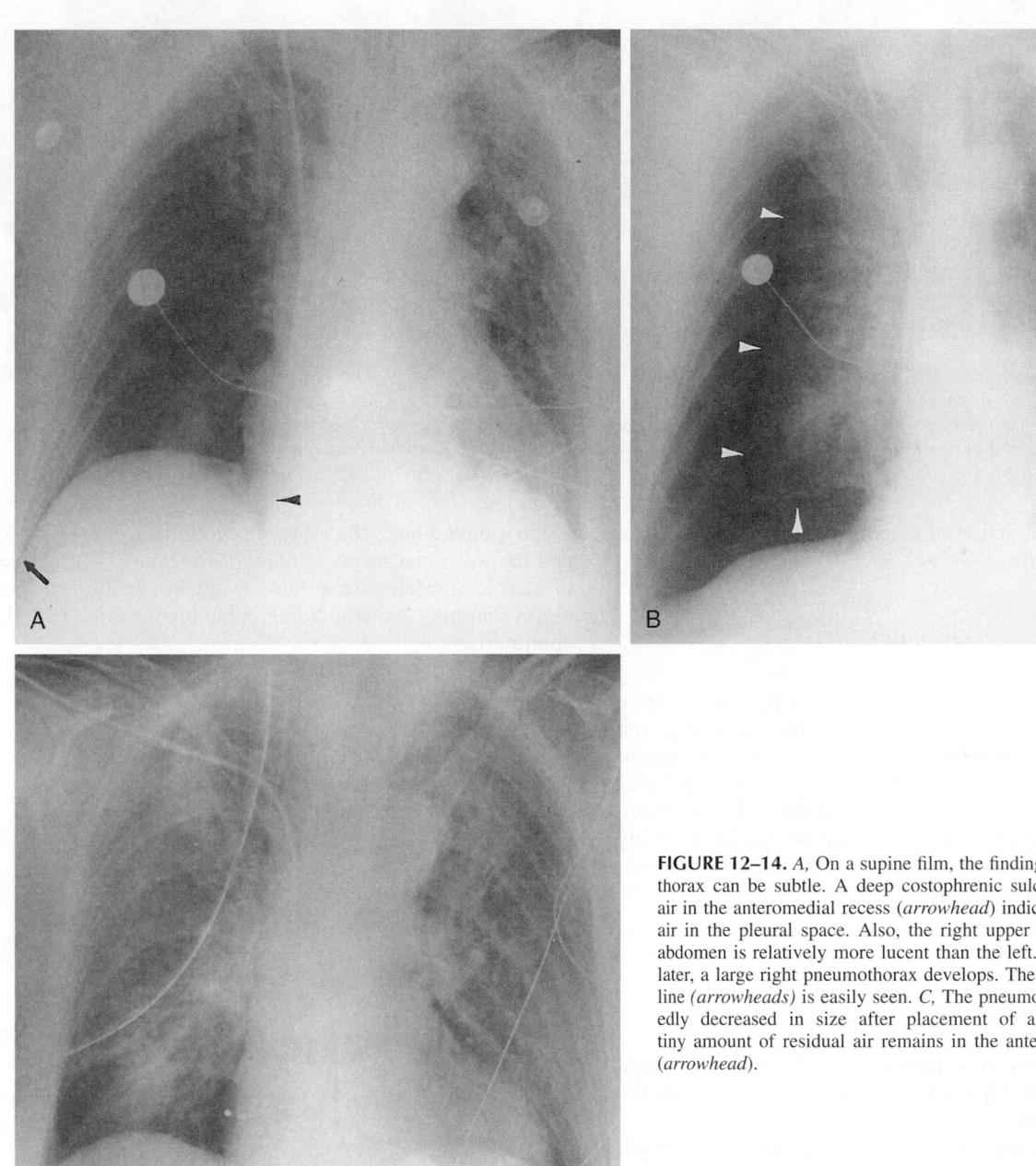

**FIGURE 12–14.** *A,* On a supine film, the findings of a pneumothorax can be subtle. A deep costophrenic sulcus *(arrow)* and air in the anteromedial recess *(arrowhead)* indicate that there is air in the pleural space. Also, the right upper quadrant of the abdomen is relatively more lucent than the left. *B,* Three hours later, a large right pneumothorax develops. The visceral pleural line *(arrowheads)* is easily seen. *C,* The pneumothorax is markedly decreased in size after placement of a chest tube. A tiny amount of residual air remains in the anteromedial recess *(arrowhead).*

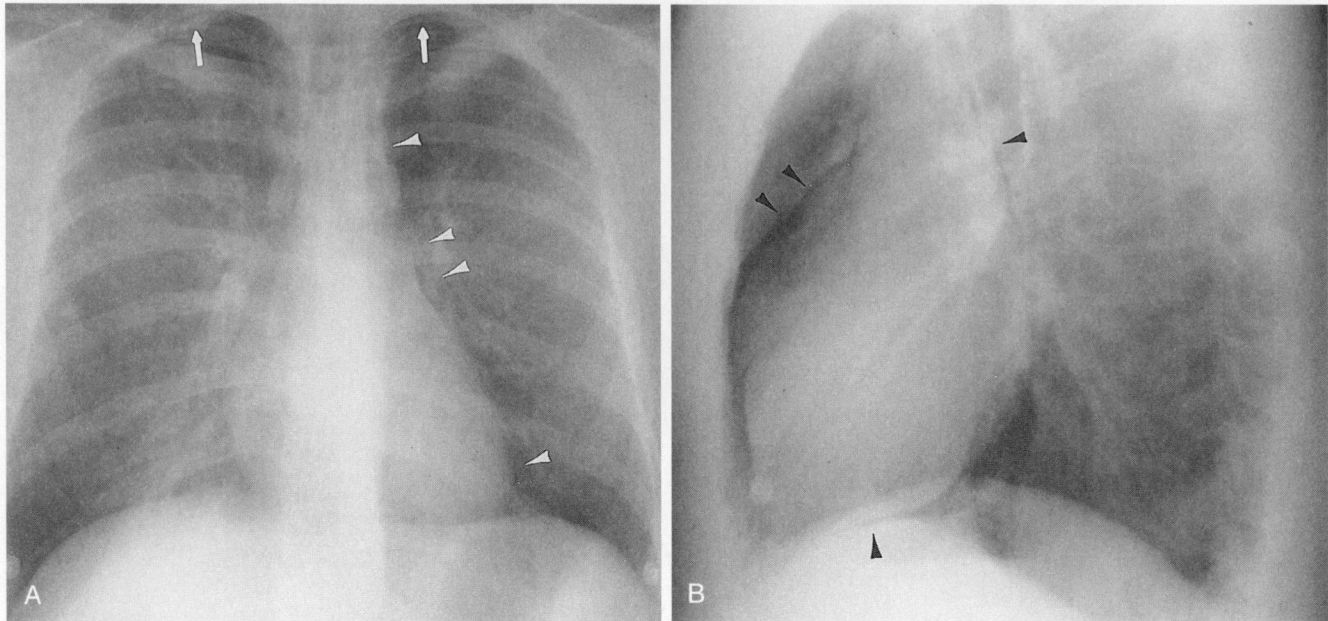

**FIGURE 12–15.** This 20-year-old man developed chest pain following cocaine use. *A,* Pneumomediastinum is demonstrated by visualization of a line (*arrowheads*) paralleling the heart and aortic arch. Small biapical pneumothoraces (*arrows*) are present. Subcutaneous air is seen as streaky radiolucencies projecting over the upper mediastinum. *B,* Air in the mediastinal space (*arrowheads*) is easily seen on the lateral film.

arteries to avoid obstruction of these arteries when the balloon inflates during diastole.[21]

## THE NECK

Regardless of etiology, diseases of the upper airway often lead to obstruction. Any insult to the larynx and trachea can result in airway compromise that may require the urgent attention of an anesthesiologist. Children are especially susceptible because of the smaller caliber of their airways. Frontal and lateral radiographs of the neck are useful for detecting pathologic processes. The lateral view demonstrates the majority of abnormalities.

### What Are the Radiographic Findings of Acute Laryngeal Pathology?

The anatomy of the soft tissues of the larynx in a normal adult is illustrated in Figure 12–17. The anatomy is similar in children older than 3 years.

The vallecular recess is an air-containing structure between the base of the tongue and the epiglottis. The epiglottis has a smooth anterior surface and a pointed superior tip. The aryepiglottic folds arise from the tip of the epiglottis and continue posteriorly and inferiorly to end in the arytenoid area.

### Epiglottitis

Swelling of the epiglottis or aryepiglottic folds can be life-threatening. The most common cause is epiglottitis, which occurs in all age groups but more commonly in children. Epiglottitis is manifested radiographically as enlargement of the epiglottis so that it becomes a thumblike mass rather than

a thin, pointed one. The aryepiglottic folds become thickened, and the vallecular recess is obliterated (Fig. 12–18). Ingestion of caustic substances may also result in swelling of the epiglottis and may create a radiographic picture similar to that in epiglottitis.[21]

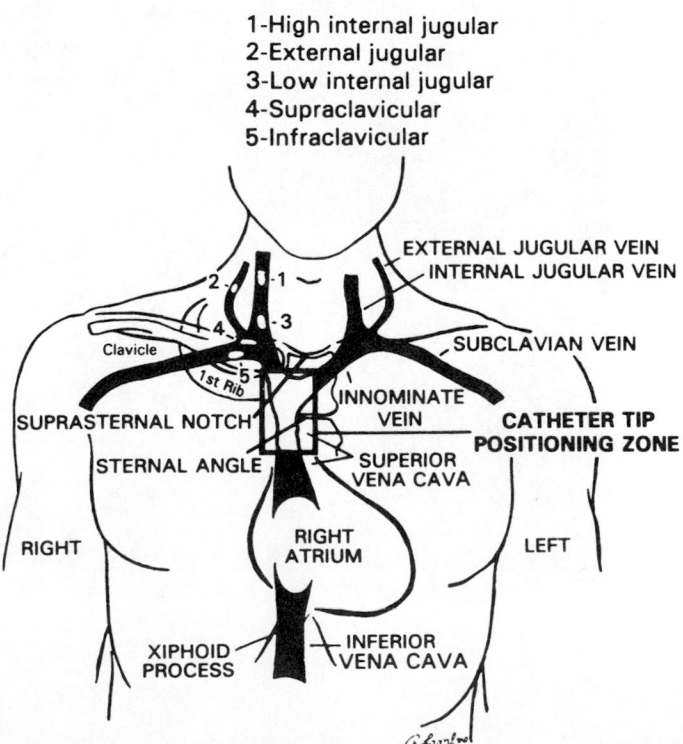

1-High internal jugular
2-External jugular
3-Low internal jugular
4-Supraclavicular
5-Infraclavicular

**FIGURE 12–16.** Central venous access sites and catheter tip positioning zone. (From Triple Lumen Central Venous Catheter [package insert]. Bloomington, Ind: Cook Critical Care, a division of Cook, Inc; 1986.)

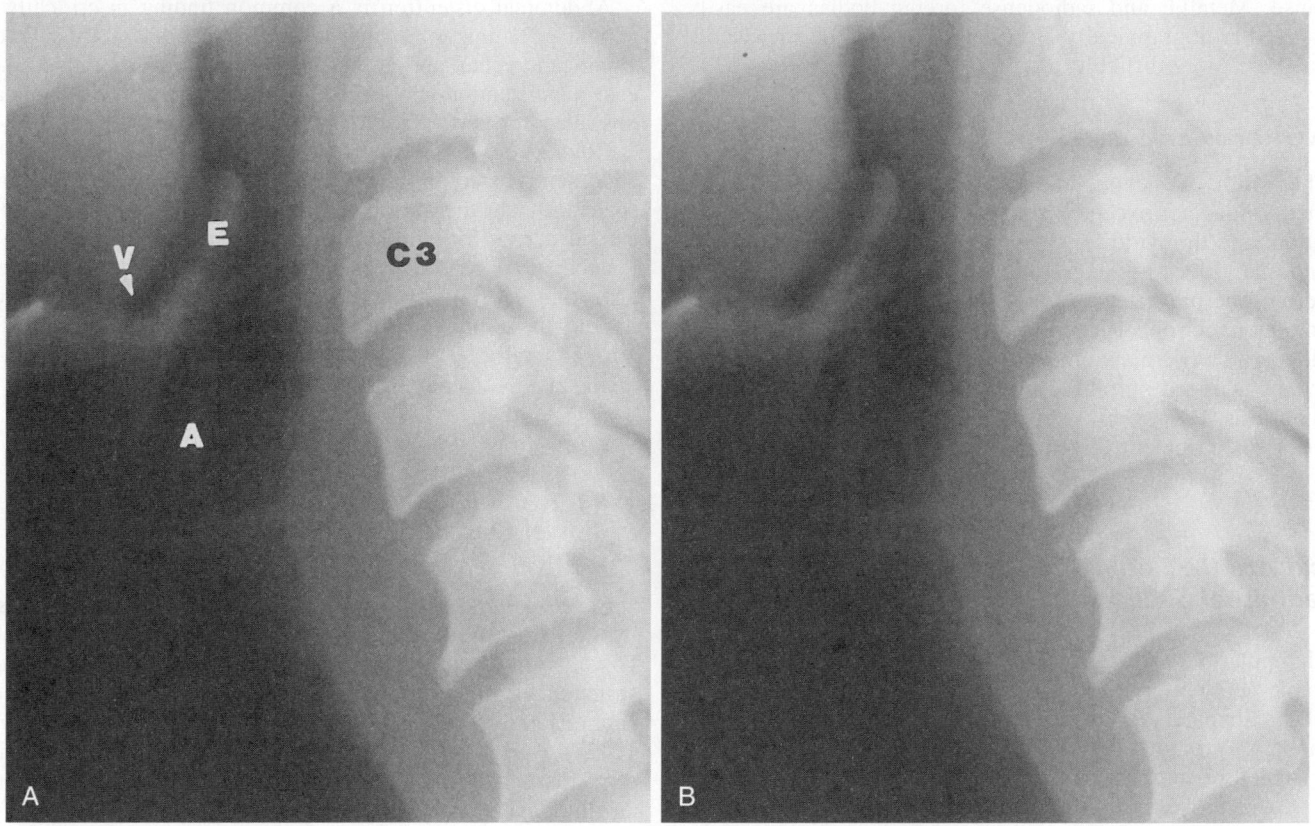

**FIGURE 12–17.** *A,* The normal soft tissues of the neck in an adult. The prevertebral soft tissues are normal anterior to the C3 vertebral body. *B,* Same lateral view of the neck without labels. A, aryepiglottic folds; E, epiglottis; V, vallecular recess.

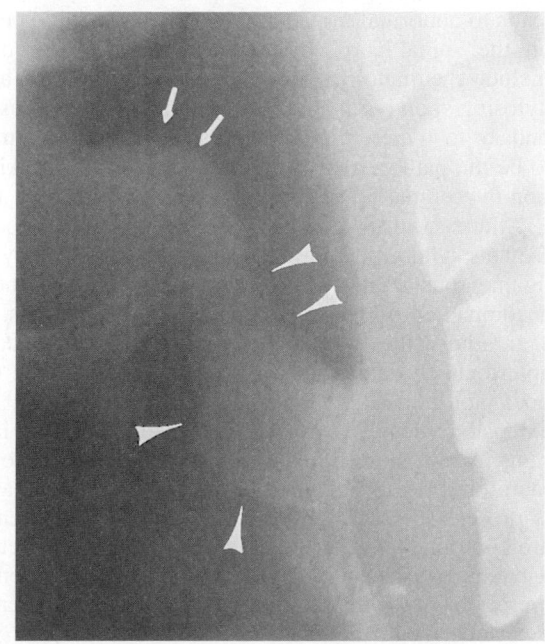

**FIGURE 12–18.** Epiglottitis in an adult. The epiglottis (*arrows*) is enlarged and blunted, and the aryepiglottic folds (*arrowheads*) are markedly thickened. The vallecular recess is obliterated. (Courtesy of Phyllis Kornguth, MD.)

## Foreign Bodies

Aspiration of a foreign body can also lead to airway compromise. Metallic and radiodense foreign bodies are easily visualized radiographically. Substances such as plastic, wood, or food are more difficult to detect.

## Prevertebral Soft Tissues

The width of the prevertebral soft tissues anterior to C3 normally does not exceed 4 to 5 mm with the neck in neutral position, and the width of the retrotracheal tissues anterior to C6 normally does not exceed 22 mm in adults and 14 mm in children. The prevertebral soft tissues enlarge in the presence of infection (retropharyngeal abscess), trauma, neoplasia, and angioneurotic edema. Sometimes, pockets of radiolucent air may be visualized on plain films in patients with retropharyngeal abscess. Prevertebral soft tissue swelling associated with anterior displacement and narrowing of the airway suggests airway compromise.

## What Are the Radiographic Findings of Atlantoaxial Subluxation?

Manipulation of the head and neck in the presence of an unstable cervical spine can lead to injury to the spinal cord, resulting in paralysis or death. Most cervical spine injuries secondary to trauma are known or suspected by the anesthesiologist before intubation. Atlantoaxial subluxation, however, can be overlooked. High-risk patients should be screened so that they can be appropriately managed in the operating room.

## Causes

The transverse atlantal ligament holds the dens adjacent to the anterior arch of C1. Disruption or laxity of this ligament leads to abnormal movement of C1 on C2, which can impinge on the spinal cord. Inflammatory causes are common and include rheumatoid arthritis, juvenile rheumatoid arthritis, ankylosing spondylitis, and pharyngitis. Ligamentous laxity secondary to hyperemia from adjacent inflammation is thought to be the pathogenesis. The incidence of atlantoaxial subluxation in rheumatoid patients is estimated to be 20% to 25%.[23–25]

Atlantoaxial instability is also encountered in patients with Down's syndrome and is presumed to be secondary to inherent ligamentous laxity. Traumatic causes are rare and are often accompanied by fractures of the odontoid process.

In adults, the distance between the posterior surface of the anterior arch of the atlas and the anterior surface of the dens does not normally exceed 2.5 mm on neutral, flexion, or extension views. The normal distance in children is 3.5 to 4.5 mm. When these measurements are exceeded on carefully monitored flexion and extension series, atlantoaxial instability is present (Figs. 12–19 and 12–20). Flexion-extension views are contraindicated when a dens fracture is suspected or when a patient is insensitive to pain. Flexion and extension views are performed when an alert cooperative patient can carefully flex and extend the neck, usually bound by pain with movement. An inebriated or sedated patient will not be asked to do flexion or extension views.

# THE ABDOMEN

Abdominal distention is a common finding in critically ill patients. Radiographic monitoring is necessary to rule out significant acute abdominal pathology. For the most part, gaseous distention is not disconcerting unless bowel loops are obstructed or perforation has occurred.

Colonic gas is normally located in the periphery of the abdomen. The colon has haustral markings that are irregularly spaced, indent the surface of the colon, and do not typically extend across the whole lumen. Gas in the small bowel is located more centrally in the abdomen. Small bowel loops have thin, closely spaced lines that extend across the whole lumen; these lines represent the valvulae conniventes. The normal small bowel loop is generally no more than 3 cm in diameter.

## What Are the Radiographic Manifestations of Bowel Obstruction?

Seventy-five percent of small bowel obstructions are caused by adhesions. Other causes include hernia, gallstone ileus, volvulus, intussusception, and neoplasm. In small bowel obstruction, air-filled or fluid-filled small bowel loops are dilated, and relatively little gas or stool is seen in the colon (Fig. 12–21). Upright or decubitus films may demonstrate a "string of pearls" sign (Fig. 12–22), which represents multiple small air-fluid levels in the small bowel.

In large bowel obstruction, the colon is dilated to the level of obstruction (Fig. 12–23). The sigmoid, cecum, and transverse colon are affected, in decreasing order of frequency. The small bowel may or may not be dilated, depending on the competency of the ileocecal valve. Carcinomas account for the majority of colonic obstructions. Diverticulitis and volvulus are frequently encountered but are less common causes of colonic obstruction.

## Ileus

*Adynamic ileus* is characterized by generalized dilation of the stomach, small bowel, and colon without an underlying mechanical obstruction. *Colonic ileus* refers to generalized dilation of the colon without obstruction. Ileus is a common finding following surgery and trauma and is also associated with sepsis, electrolyte imbalances, and drugs such as narcotics. Differentiating between a low colonic obstruction and ileus can be difficult. Prone or left lateral decubitus views may rule out a low colonic obstruction by demonstrating air rising into the rectum (Fig. 12–24).[26]

A subclassification of colonic ileus is cecal ileus, in which the cecum is dilated out of proportion to the remainder of the colon. The major risk of cecal ileus is perforation, especially when the cecum is mobile and rotates anteromedially. Risk of perforation correlates more with the duration of dilation than with actual cecal size. Aggressive decompression measures should be considered when the cecum is dilated >10 cm for more than 2 to 3 days.[27]

*Text continued on page 229*

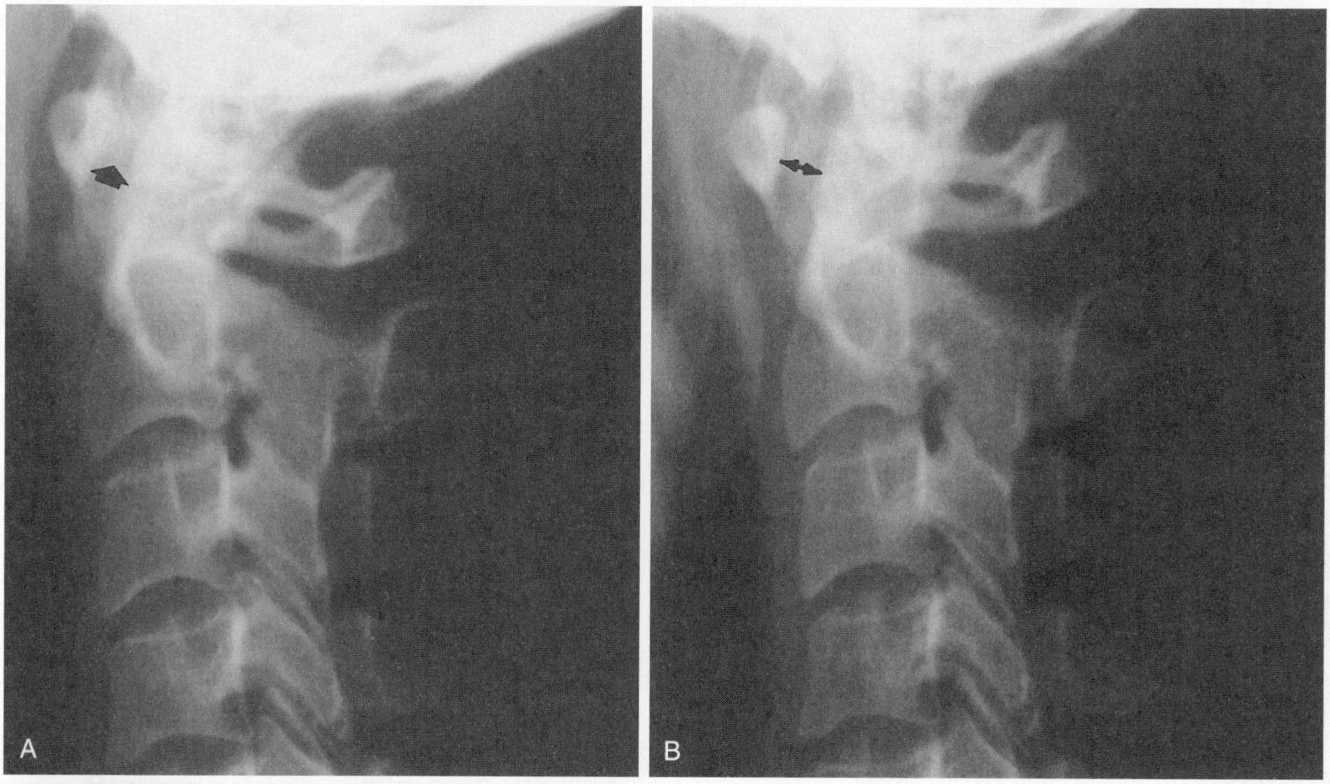

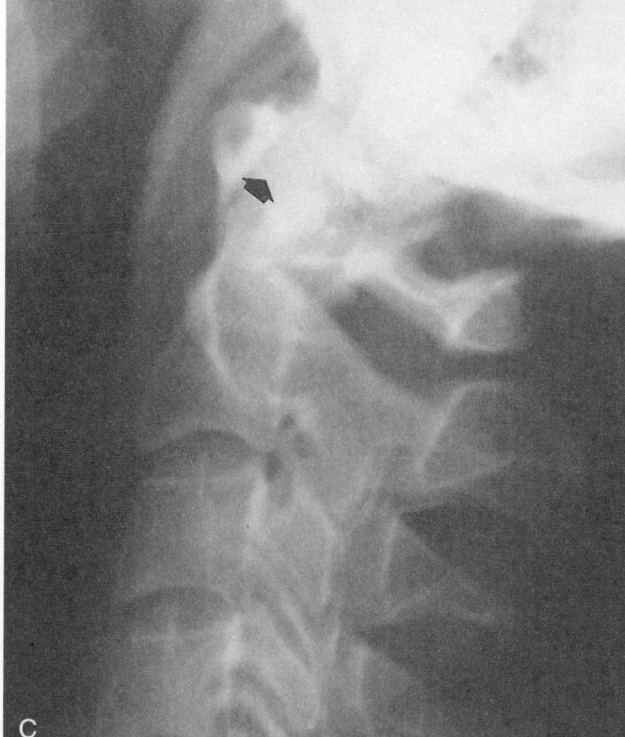

**FIGURE 12–19.** This 42-year-old man has rheumatoid arthritis and atlantoaxial instability. *A,* Lateral view of the cervical spine in neutral position reveals that the predental space (*arrow*) measures 6 mm. *B,* A limited flexion view demonstrates the interval (*double-headed arrow*) increasing to 7 mm. *C,* The predental space (*arrow*) decreases to 5 mm on the extension view.

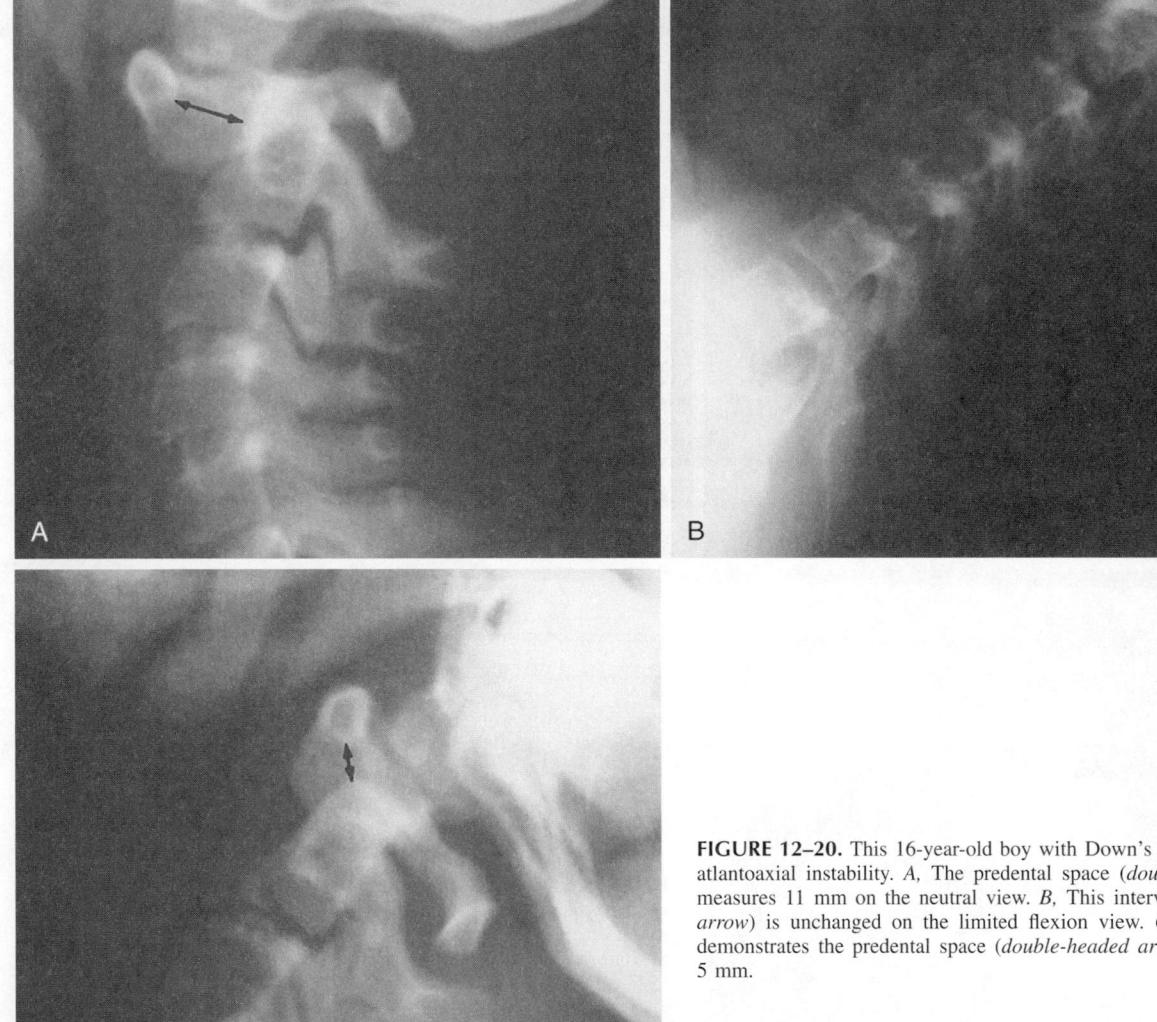

**FIGURE 12–20.** This 16-year-old boy with Down's syndrome also has atlantoaxial instability. *A,* The predental space (*double-headed arrow*) measures 11 mm on the neutral view. *B,* This interval (*double-headed arrow*) is unchanged on the limited flexion view. *C,* Extension view demonstrates the predental space (*double-headed arrow*) decreasing to 5 mm.

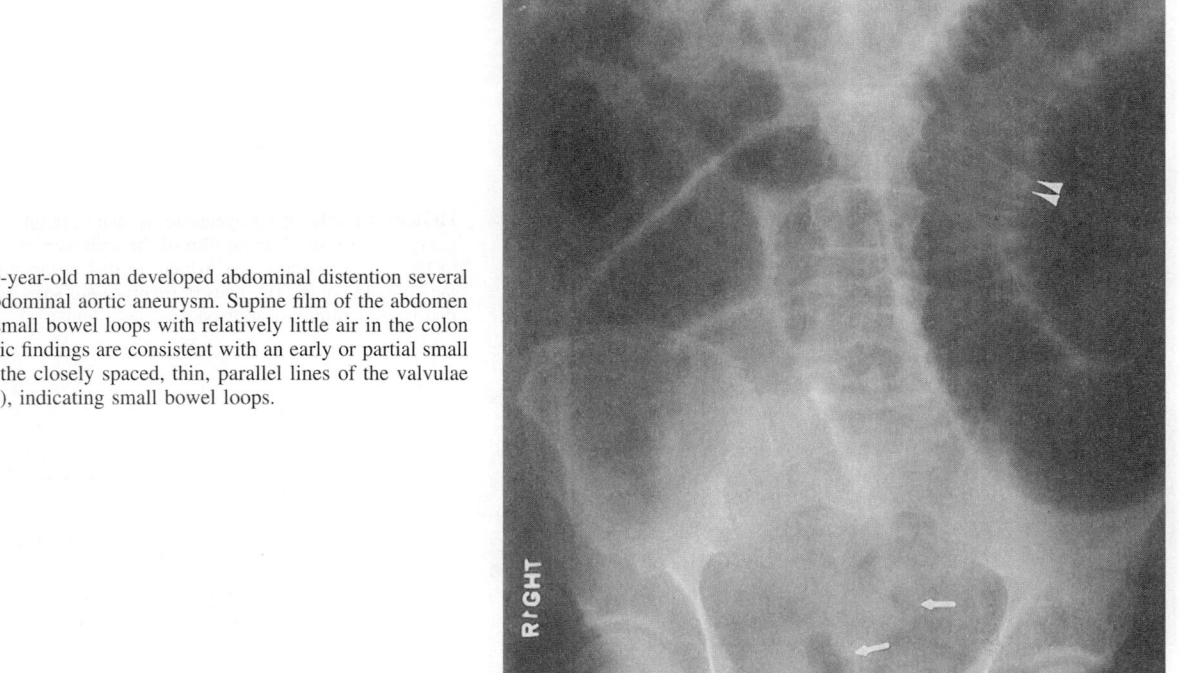

**FIGURE 12–21.** This 60-year-old man developed abdominal distention several days after repair of an abdominal aortic aneurysm. Supine film of the abdomen reveals multiple dilated small bowel loops with relatively little air in the colon (*arrows*). The radiographic findings are consistent with an early or partial small bowel obstruction. Note the closely spaced, thin, parallel lines of the valvulae conniventes (*arrowheads*), indicating small bowel loops.

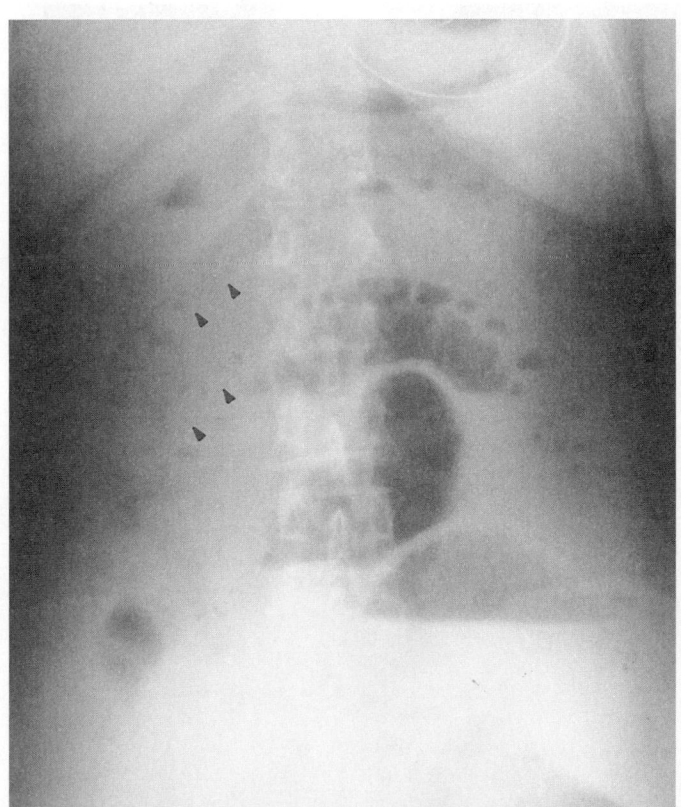

**FIGURE 12–22.** Upright abdominal film of a 62-year-old woman demonstrates the "string of pearls" sign (*arrowheads*) of small bowel obstruction. (Courtesy of Reed P. Rice, MD.)

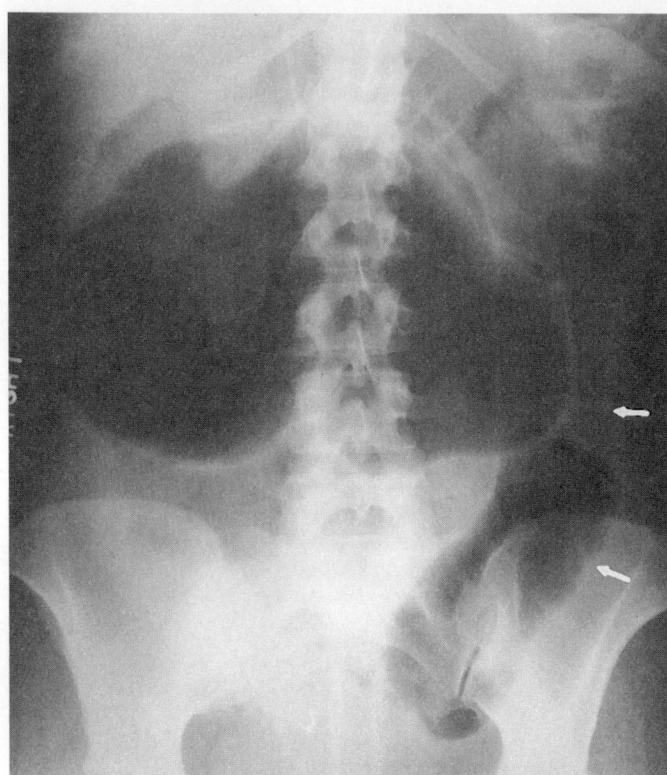

**FIGURE 12–23.** This 31-year-old woman developed colonic obstruction from serosal metastases. Supine film of the abdomen reveals dilated colonic loops to the level of obstruction, which, in this instance, is the distal segment of the sigmoid colon. The haustra (*arrows*) are seen as irregularly spaced lines that in general do not traverse the entire lumen.

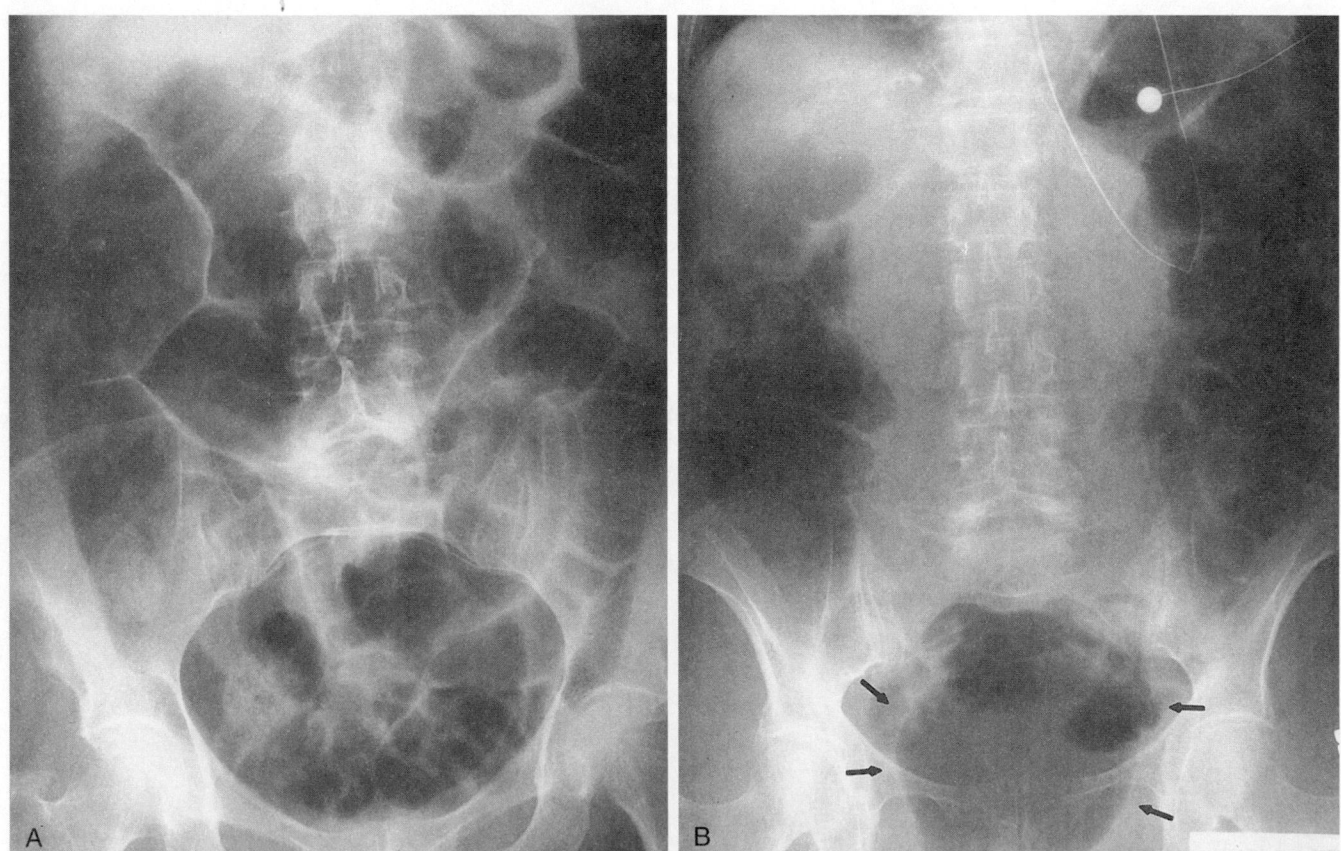

**FIGURE 12–24.** This 60-year-old woman presented with abdominal distention. *A*, Supine film of the abdomen reveals air in dilated colonic and small bowel loops. These findings do not distinguish between adynamic ileus and large bowel obstruction with an incompetent ileocecal valve. *B*, Prone film demonstrates air rising into the rectum (*arrows*), a finding seen in adynamic ileus. (Courtesy of Reed P. Rice, MD.)

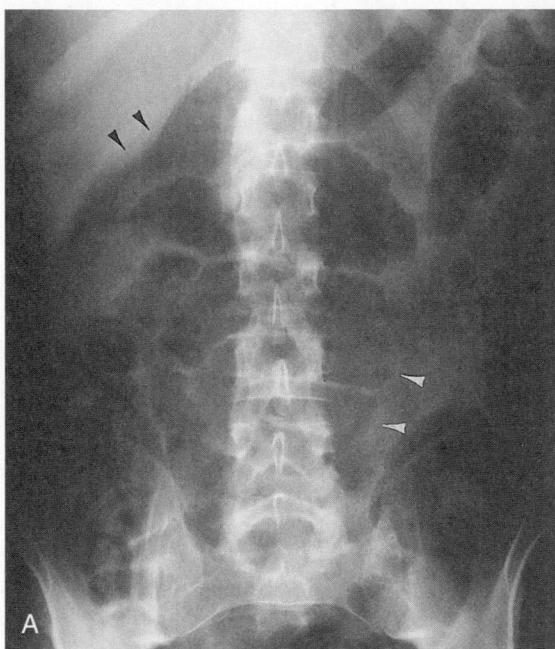

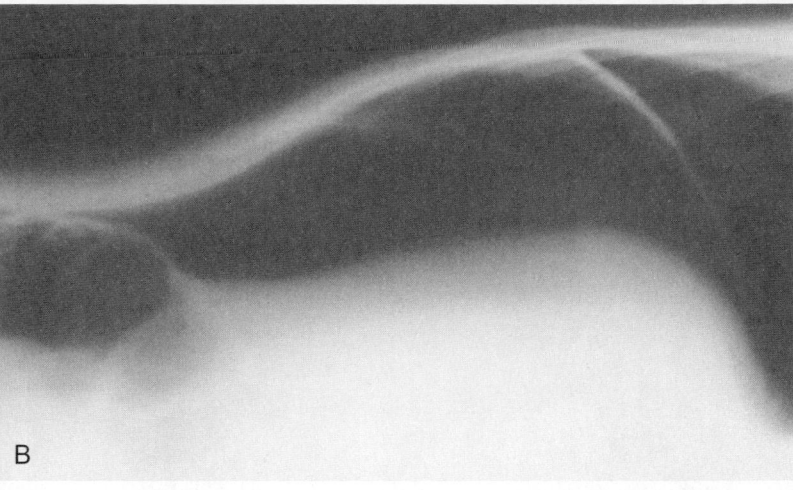

**FIGURE 12–25.** This 22-year-old man presented with abdominal pain. *A,* Supine film of the abdomen reveals a large amount of extraluminal subhepatic air (*black arrowheads*) and air outlining the bowel walls (*white arrowheads*). *B,* Left lateral decubitus film confirms the findings of pneumoperitoneum. (Courtesy of Reed P. Rice, MD.)

## What Are the Radiographic Findings of Pneumoperitoneum?

A plain film of the abdomen is performed with a patient supine, and the radiographic findings of pneumoperitoneum on a supine film can be quite subtle. Radiographic findings (Figs. 12–25 and 12–26) include the following:

1. Outlining of the bowel wall by air inside and outside the lumen (Rigler sign)
2. Outlining of the falciform ligament by air
3. Lucency in the right upper quadrant, indicating air anterior to the liver
4. Subhepatic air
5. Triangular extraluminal lucencies between bowel loops

When pneumoperitoneum is suspected but not readily detected on a supine abdominal film, a left lateral decubitus or an upright film often simplifies diagnosis.[26,28] Pneumoperitoneum is an expected finding in patients who have recently undergone abdominal surgery or who are on peritoneal dialysis.

## What Is the Correct Gastric or Enteric Tube Position?

### Nasogastric

Nasogastric tubes are used to relieve gastric distention. Most nasogastric tubes have radiopaque linear markers that are continuous except in the region of the side port. The side port should be located in the stomach and specifically should not be positioned in the distal esophagus. Positioning of a

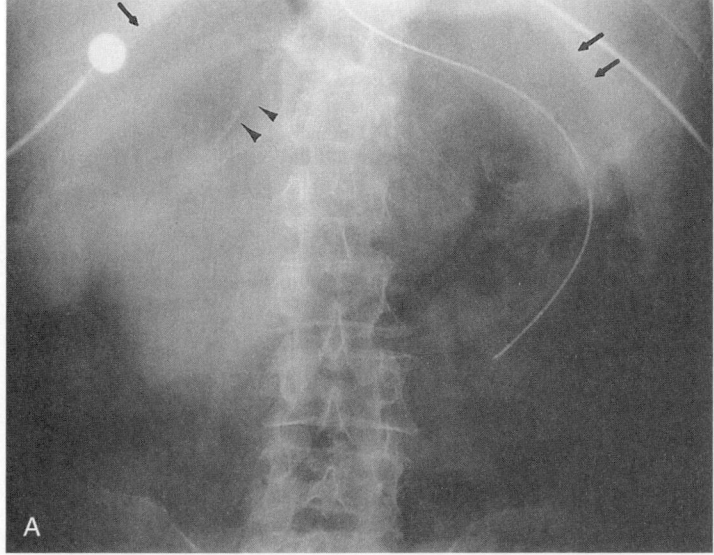

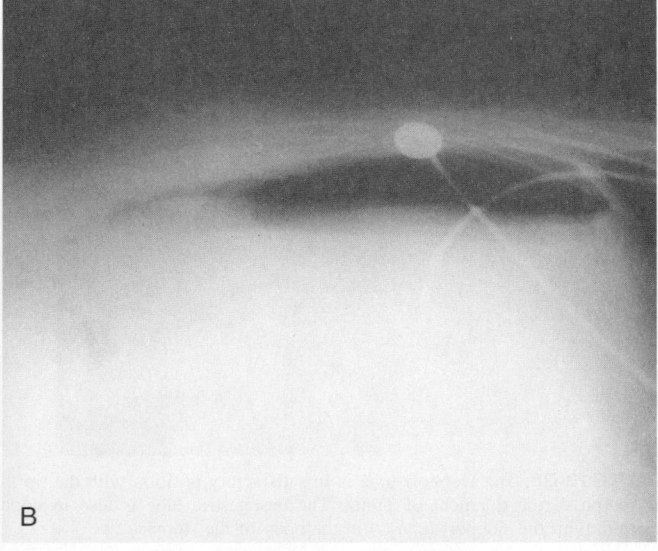

**FIGURE 12–26.** *A,* Pneumoperitoneum on this supine film is demonstrated by the outlining of the falciform ligament (*arrowheads*) by air and relative radiolucency (*arrows*) in the upper abdomen. *B,* Left lateral decubitus view reveals air rising superior to the liver.

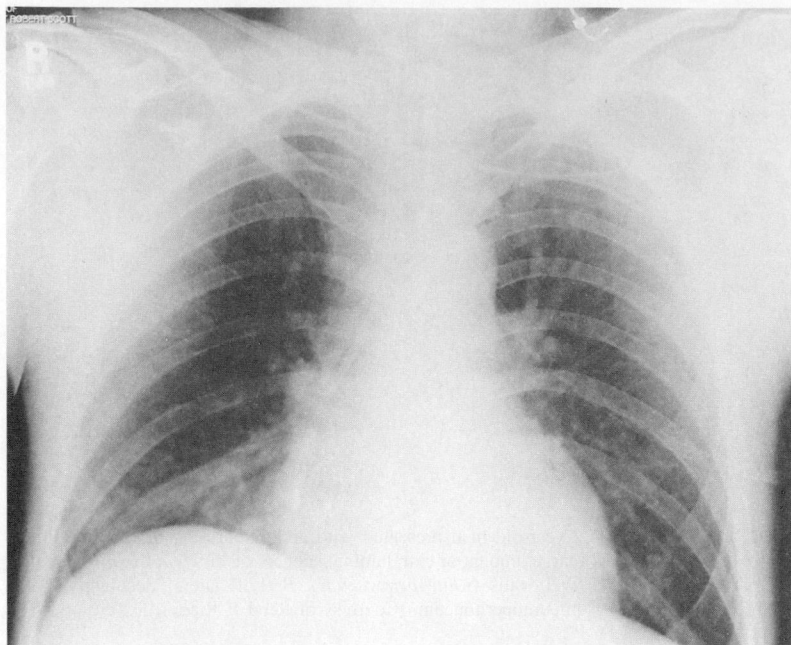

**FIGURE 12–27.** The nasogastric tube appears to have cannulated the right mainstem bronchus.

side port in the distal esophagus or at the gastroesophageal junction predisposes to aspiration. A nasogastric tube can also be inadvertently placed in a mainstem bronchus or can be coiled in a hiatal hernia.

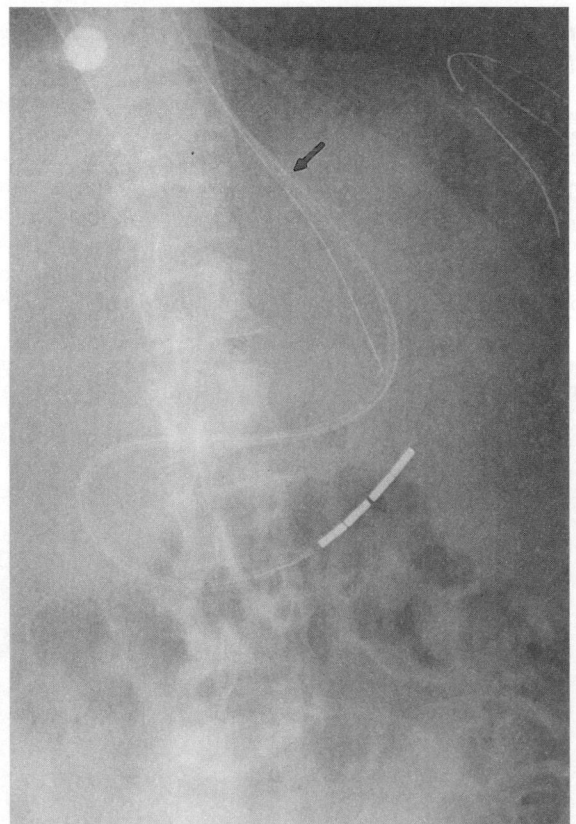

**FIGURE 12–28.** The Dobhoff tube is in satisfactory position with the tip in the region of the ligament of Treitz. The nasogastric tube is also in good position, with the sideport (*arrow*) in the body of the stomach.

## Nasoenteric

The course of nasoenteric tubes is more difficult to visualize radiographically; most have radiodense tips. The position of a nasoenteric feeding tube should be checked radiographically before starting tube feedings.

Complications from these tubes are related to malpositioning and include mainstem bronchus intubation (Fig. 12–27), pneumothorax, and perforation of a mediastinal structure. Many clinicians place these tubes fluoroscopically to avoid these complications. The tip should be located in the third or fourth portion of the duodenum to avoid aspiration of tube feedings (Fig. 12–28). However, no study has confirmed that intragastric feeding is less safe in the absence of gastroesophageal reflux, gastroparesis, or gastric outlet obstruction.[29]

## References

1. Godwin JD, Chen JTT. Thoracic venous anatomy. *AJR Am J Roentgenol.* 1986;147:674.
2. Ravin CE. Introduction to chest radiography. In: Putman CE, Ravin CE, eds. *Textbook of Diagnostic Imaging.* Philadelphia, Pa: WB Saunders; 1988:413.
3. Heitzman ER. *The Mediastinum: Radiologic Correlations With Anatomy and Pathology.* 2nd ed. Berlin, Germany: Springer Verlag; 1988.
4. Felson B. *Chest Roentgenology.* Philadelphia, Pa: WB Saunders; 1973.
5. Simon G. *Principle of Chest X-Ray Diagnosis.* 3rd ed. London, United Kingdom: Butterworth; 1971.
6. American Thoracic Society. Chronic bronchitis, asthma, and pulmonary emphysema: statement by the committee on diagnostic standards for nontuberculous respiratory disease. *Am Rev Respir Dis.* 1962;85:762.
7. Pratt PC. Role of conventional chest radiography in diagnosis and exclusion of emphysema. *Am J Med.* 1987;82:998.
8. Pratt PC. Radiographic appearance of the chest in emphysema. *Invest Radiol.* 1987;22:927.
9. Heitzman ER. *The Lung: Radiologic Pathologic Correlations.* St Louis, Mo: CV Mosby; 1984.
10. Chang CH. The normal roentgenographic measurement of the right descending pulmonary artery in 1,085 cases. *AJR Am J Roentgenol.* 1962;87:929.
11. Pare JA, Fraser RG. *Synopsis of Diseases of the Chest.* Philadelphia, Pa: WB Saunders; 1983.

12. Nessa CG, Rigler LG. The roentgenological manifestations of pulmonary edema. *Radiology.* 1941;37:35.

13. Hodson CJ. Pulmonary oedema and the "bat's wing" shadow. *J Fac Radiol.* 1950;1:176.

14. Joffe N. Roentgenologic findings in post-shock and postoperative pulmonary insufficiency. *Radiology.* 1970;94:369.

15. Ostendorf P, Birzle H, Vogel W, et al. Pulmonary radiographic abnormalities in shock. *Radiology.* 1975;115:257.

16. Johnson TH, Altman AR, McCaffree RD. Radiologic considerations in the adult respiratory distress syndrome treated with positive and expiratory pressure (PEEP). *Clin Chest Med.* 1982;3:89.

17. Swischuk LE. Respiratory system. In: Swischuk LE, ed. *Imaging of the Newborn, Infant, and Young Child.* 3rd ed. Baltimore, Md: Williams & Wilkins; 1989:1.

18. Rhea JT, van Sonnenberg E, McLoud TC. Basilar pneumothorax in the supine adult. *Radiology.* 1979;133:593.

19. Tocino IM, Miller MH, Fairfax WR. Distribution of pneumothorax in the supine and semirecumbent critically ill adult. *AJR Am J Roentgenol.* 1985;144:901.

20. Goodman LR, Putman CE. *Critical Care Imaging.* Philadelphia, Pa: WB Saunders; 1992.

21. Ellis L, Vogel S, Copeland E. Central venous catheter vascular erosions. Diagnosis and clinical course. *Ann Surg.* 1989;209:475.

22. Blackshear RH, Gravenstein N. Critical angle of incidence for delayed vessel perforation by central venous catheter: a study of in vivo data [abstract]. *Ann Emerg Med.* 1992;21:659.

23. Conlon PW, Isdale IC, Rose BS. Rheumatoid arthritis of the cervical spine: an analysis of 333 cases. *Ann Rheum Dis.* 1966;25:120.

24. Resnick D, Niwayama G. *Diagnosis of Bone and Joint Disorders.* 2nd ed. Philadelphia, Pa: WB Saunders; 1988.

25. Mathews JA. Atlanto-axial subluxation in rheumatoid arthritis. *Ann Rheum Dis.* 1969;28:260.

26. Rice RP. The plain film of the abdomen. In: Tavaras JM, Ferrucci JT, eds. *Radiology: Diagnosis-Imaging-Intervention.* Vol 4. Philadelphia, Pa: JB Lippincott; 1990:1.

27. Johnson CD, Rice RP, Kelvin FM, et al. The radiologic evaluation of gross cecal distension: emphasis on cecal ileus. *AJR Am J Roentgenol.* 1985;145:1211.

28. Laufer B. The left lateral view in the plain film assessment of abdominal distention. *Radiology.* 1976;119:265.

29. Gutierrez ED, Balfe DM. Fluoroscopically guided nasoenteric feeding tube placement: results of a 1-year study. *Radiology.* 1991;178:759.

# 13

# Pain Management Consultation in Adult Patients

Eddy N. Duncan

Cheryl L. Dixon

The role of the anesthesiologist as a pain management consultant is changing rapidly. Pain management has evolved into a legitimate subspecialty and is no longer a "black art." Our understanding of the anatomic and physiologic mechanisms of pain is expanding almost daily. As basic scientists discover more and more pieces to the pain puzzle, our pharmacologic and therapeutic options expand as well. The goal of this chapter is to delineate a clinical approach to the adult patient that elicits the correct pain diagnosis and allows full consideration and implementation of all therapeutic options.

## THE ADULT PAIN MANAGEMENT CONSULTATION

### What Is the Best Approach?

On the first day of the "pain rotation," an anesthesiology resident must experience the same feelings of inadequacy that medical students feel as they try to complete their first history and physical examination, differential diagnosis, and treatment plan. The principles of medical diagnosis are applicable to the pain patient, regardless of the nature and duration of the problem.

#### Initial Assessment

Portenoy outlined an approach to pain diagnosis in patients with cancer that can be modified to apply to the evaluation and assessment of all patients with pain[1] (Fig. 13–1). With this problem-solving strategy in mind, even the beginning

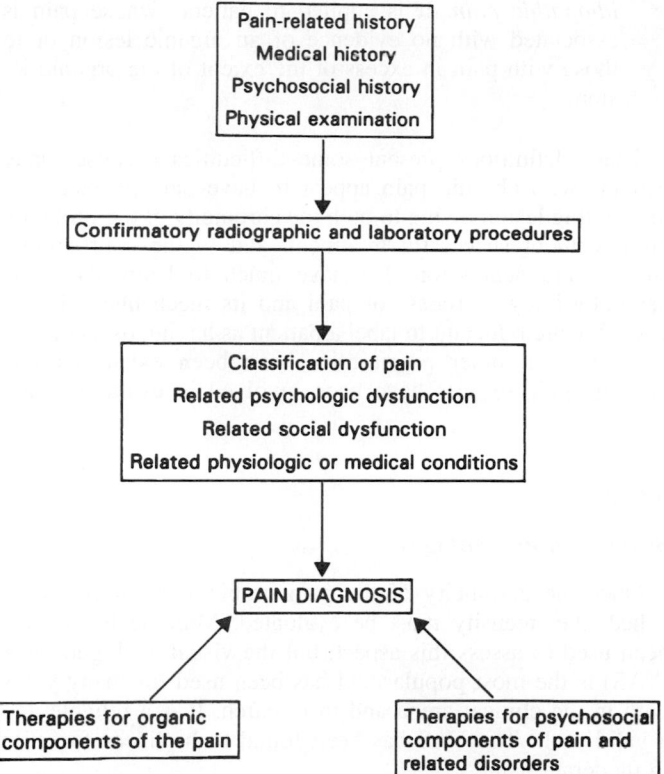

**FIGURE 13–1.** The pain diagnosis incorporates the multifactorial nature of pain and its associated symptoms and signs and is a guide to targeting interventions appropriately and efficiently. See text for the various classifications of pain. (From Portenoy RK. Diagnosis of cancer pain syndromes. In: Field H, ed. *Pain Syndromes in Neurologic Practices.* New York, NY: Butterworth; 1990:240.)

pain management consultant can be successful both in diagnosing and treating pain.

Several basic components to the evaluation process must be thoroughly examined (Table 13–1). The consultant must assess key elements of a pain-related history; understand the impact that psychologic, psychiatric, and social factors have on the problem; and know when to ask for further evaluation. This approach is basic to all pain consultations, aids in the classification of pain, and expedites the eventual diagnosis. A basic medical history is imperative to pain diagnosis, therapeutic strategy, and prediction of outcome. A generalized physical examination and detailed examination of the targeted area should also be performed.

## Laboratory Assessment

Based on the information obtained, the consultant next uses laboratory testing to aid in the differential diagnosis. The most

**TABLE 13–1.** Key Points in Obtaining a Thorough Pain History

Definition of the pain problem (acute, chronic, or cancer related; nociceptive or neuropathic)
Course of the pain problem from the onset
Characteristics of the pain intensity (quality, duration, periodicity, location, and distribution)
Exacerbating factors
Associated factors (stress, depression, sleep disturbances)
Current therapeutic modalities
Results of all diagnostic and therapeutic procedures

common tests (selectively applied based on the previously obtained information) include spine radiography, computed tomography (CT), magnetic resonance imaging (MRI), myelography, electromyography, nerve conduction studies, bone scanning, and determination of complete blood count, erythrocyte sedimentation rate, and vitamin $B_{12}$ and folate levels.

## Diagnosis

Once this information is gathered, the pain and associated medical and psychosocial conditions can be classified and a pain diagnosis established. Not until this problem-solving approach has been performed thoroughly can the patient be adequately treated with an expected good outcome. The methodology used distinguishes a "block" clinic from a "pain" clinic. Therapeutic options specific to the classification of pain as well as to the individual patient can then be recommended.

## Treatment

Treatment options to be discussed in greater detail later include pharmacologic approaches by all routes (oral to neuraxial); regional anesthetic techniques (single injection to neurolytic blockade); neuroaugmentation, including transcutaneous electrical nerve stimulation (TENS) and spinal cord stimulation; and psychiatric and psychologic therapy.

Patients experiencing pain with an expected short duration and a limited etiology (eg, postoperative pain in young, healthy adults) usually require only a simple therapeutic modality. Patients with pain of long duration and no chance of medical recovery (eg, that associated with metastatic prostate cancer) require the most attention and inventive strategies. Regardless of a patient's location in this spectrum, the pain management consultant can offer something that is of help, often with tremendous success and to the patient's delight.

## *What Are the Key Historical Elements?*

Before discussing a pain problem with a patient, the anesthesiologist should have an understanding of the definitions of pain because treatment options vary accordingly. The Subcommittee on Taxonomy of the International Association for the Study of Pain has published definitions to be used by all those working in the field of pain management. The universally accepted definition of pain is "an unpleasant sensory and emotional experience associated with actual or potential tissue damage, or described in terms of such damage."[2]

## Chronicity

Bonica took this definition one step further by differentiating acute from chronic pain.[3] This modifier is vitally important because the etiology, pathophysiology, symptomatology, diagnosis, and therapy of both are potentially different.

### *Acute Pain*

*Acute pain,* as defined by Bonica, "is a complex constellation of unpleasant sensory, perceptual, and emotional experiences and certain autonomic, psychologic, emotional, and behavioral responses."[3] Patients with acute pain do not have a psychopathologic process as a primary cause of their problem. Their pain is self-limiting in nature and usually resolves within days to weeks.

### Chronic Pain

*Chronic pain* is "pain that persists a month beyond the usual course of an acute disease or a reasonable time for an injury to heal, or that is associated with a chronic pathologic process that causes continuous pain, or the pain recurs at intervals for months or years."[3] It may well have an associated psychopathologic process, either as a cause or result, and may be associated with an irreversible pathophysiologic process if not recognized and treated in a timely fashion. Chronic pain may be caused by cancer, in which case additional pathophysiologic factors are introduced and variations in treatment modalities are used.

The term *chronic, benign pain* describes nonmalignant pain; nothing is benign about chronic pain, which can be devastating to both patients and associates. Bonica[3] recommended that the term *chronic pain* be reserved for nonmalignant pain and that *cancer pain* be used for those pain problems related to a malignant process. Finally, adding to the complexity of the problem is the well-known fact that patients with malignancies can have acute and chronic pain.

### Mechanisms

Another way to define pain uses a mechanistic approach that removes the emotional aspect of pain and suffering but is helpful in determining the best medical approach to the underlying problem. Portenoy proposed three general mechanisms of chronic pain that might be helpful in classification: nociceptive, neuropathic, and psychogenic pain[4] (Fig. 13–2).

**Nociceptive pain.** This is pain that occurs under normal conditions and is related to ongoing activation of nociceptive pathways of somatic or visceral origin.

**Neuropathic pain.** This type of pain is related to the pathologic effects of an injury to a nerve, a nerve plexus, or the central nervous system (CNS).

**Psychogenic pain.** Historically, psychogenic pain was termed *idiopathic pain.* It is applied to patients whose pain is associated with no evidence of an organic lesion or to those with pain in excess of the extent of the organic lesion.

These definitions present some difficulties because many patients with chronic pain appear to have pain in excess of the inciting lesion owing to both the chronicity of the problem, often without successful treatment, and to the confounding anxiety and depression. We have much to learn about the pathophysiologic process of pain and its mechanisms in the CNS. We are reluctant to label a patient as having psychogenic pain until all other possibilities have been exhausted and multiple pain experts have been involved in evaluation and treatment.

### Intensity

#### Scales and Percentages

Once the chronicity of the pain problem has been established, the intensity must be evaluated. Multiple tools have been used to assess this aspect, but the visual analogue scale (VAS) is the most popular and has been used for many years both in the clinical arena and in research. It is a reliable and a valid tool.[5] The VAS has been found to be linear for mild to moderate pain.[6]

In the traditional use of the VAS, the patient is shown a 10-cm line with endpoint descriptors of "no pain" on the left and "worst pain imaginable" on the right. The patient is then asked to place a mark at the position that represents his or her current level of pain[7] (Fig. 13–3). Some patients find it easier to use if the numeric scale is already present on the line; others are able only to use words to describe their pain level (see Fig. 13–3).

Another method of evaluation that is useful in elderly patients involves the use of percentages. Many such patients can tell the clinician what percentage of pain they experience out of 100%, or what percentage decrease in pain they achieve in response to treatment, but have tremendous difficulty in using a 0-to-10 scale. The key is to find the method of

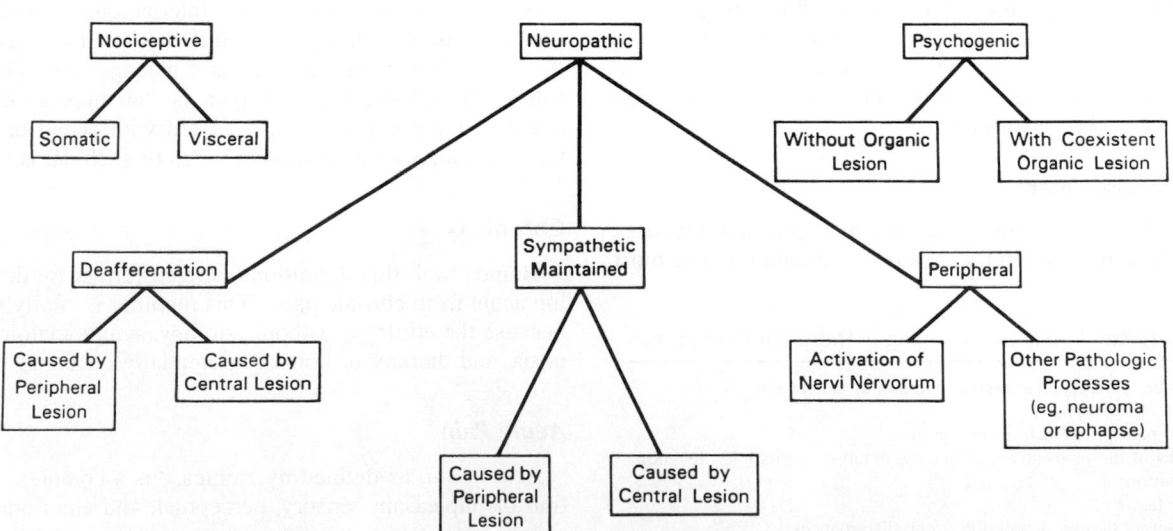

**FIGURE 13–2.** Proposed taxonomy of chronic pain based on presumed pathophysiologic distinctions. (From Portenoy RK. Mechanisms of clinical pain, observations and speculations. *Neurol Clin.* 1989;7:207.)

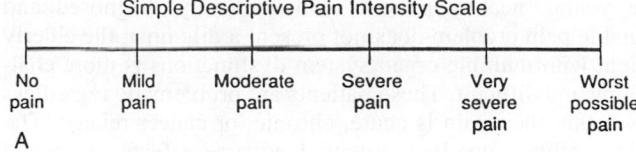

Simple Descriptive Pain Intensity Scale

| No pain | Mild pain | Moderate pain | Severe pain | Very severe pain | Worst possible pain |

A

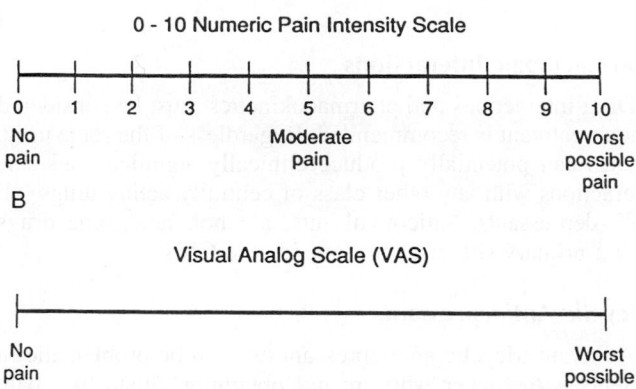

0 - 10 Numeric Pain Intensity Scale

| 0 No pain | 1 | 2 | 3 | 4 | 5 Moderate pain | 6 | 7 | 8 | 9 | 10 Worst possible pain |

B

Visual Analog Scale (VAS)

| No pain | | Worst possible pain |

C

**FIGURE 13–3.** Examples of pain intensity and pain distress scales. *A,* Descriptive pain intensity scale. *B,* Numeric pain intensity scale (0-10). *C,* Visual analogue scale (modified from source). (From Acute Pain Management Guideline Panel, US Department of Health and Human Services. *Acute Pain Management: Operative or Medical Procedures and Trauma.* Clinical Practice Guideline. Rockville, Md: Agency for Health Care Policy and Research, Public Health Service; 1992:116. Publication AHCPR 92-0032.)

pain assessment that works for each patient and then use it consistently.

### Individual Perception

One major point that must be understood when pain is assessed is the belief that the most reliable indicator of pain is the patient's reporting.[8] Loeser developed a model of the components of pain that well illustrates this point[9] (Fig. 13–4). It incorporates the physiologic processing of pain (nociception); the perceptions (pain) and emotional responses to the pain (suffering); and the only assessable part (pain behavior). The anesthesiologist must constantly remind himself or herself that pain behavior—that is, what the patient does or does not say or do—is the *only* measurable component. In so doing, any temptation to second guess this evaluation process is quickly discarded.

### Physical Signs

The pain management novice is tempted to rely on objective measures such as heart rate, blood pressure, and facial expressions when assessing pain or pain management techniques. Although these signs should be included in the evaluation process, they are not as reliable as the patient's self-report, especially in the setting of chronic pain, where the neuroendocrine stress response tends to be blunted.[10]

An example familiar to anesthesiologists is the patient in the postanesthesia care unit who sleeps intermittently yet complains of pain when awake. This scenario is easy to understand when the intraoperative drug history is reviewed. As long as centrally acting drugs influence the patient's level of consciousness, he or she may legitimately feel pain when

awake yet intermittently fall asleep until the blood level of the sedative/hypnotic/analgesic combination deteriorates. Withholding appropriate pain medications at that point delays not only a satisfactory degree of pain management but also the postanesthesia care unit discharge.

### Quality

The quality of pain can be a clue to its etiology. Examples of differentiating pain descriptors include cutaneous (sharp, pricking, burning, throbbing, stabbing); deep somatic (dull, aching, diffuse); visceral (vague, poorly localized, diffuse dull, aching); and sympathetic (burning, aching, throbbing).

Similarities between deep somatic (ie, in muscles, tendons, joints, and bones) and visceral pain have been noted. The characteristics are similar, but significant differences involve the pain pathways and the embryologic origin of the structures involved. Although sensory innervation involves A delta and C fibers, those fibers traveling from the viscera run in association with the sympathetic fibers. Also, the structures involved in deep somatic pain are of mesodermal origin, whereas those of the viscera are of endodermic origin.

### Duration and Periodicity

The duration and periodicity of pain are also characteristics that are helpful in a differential diagnosis. Lewis described many well-known pains using a time-intensity curve that incorporates the length of time between episodes, the way pain starts, and the rate of rise, frequency, and rate of decline of the curve[11] (Fig. 13–5). Questions to elicit this information address whether the pain is intermittent or continuous, or pulsatile or wavelike. The relationship in time to injuries, changes in weather, stressful life events, and medical problems can all be helpful as well.

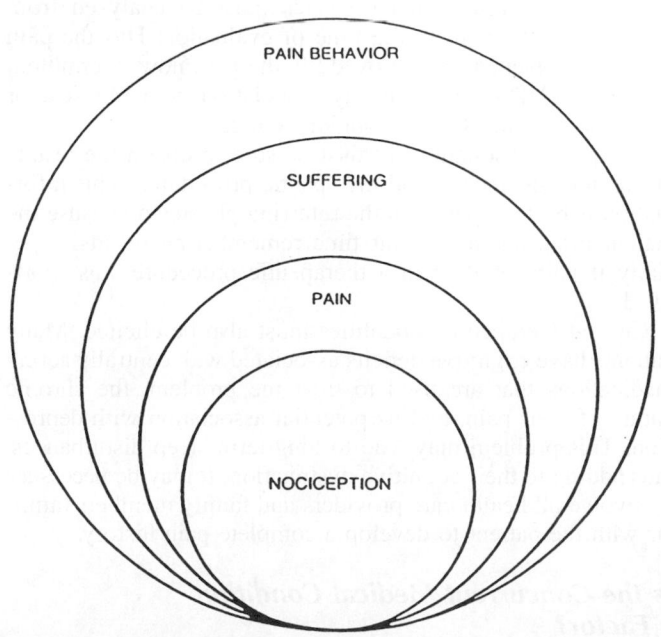

**FIGURE 13–4.** A multifaceted model of the components of pain. (From Loeser JD. Concepts of pain. In: Staton-Hicks M, Boas R, eds. *Chronic Low Back Pain.* New York, NY: Raven Press; 1982:146.)

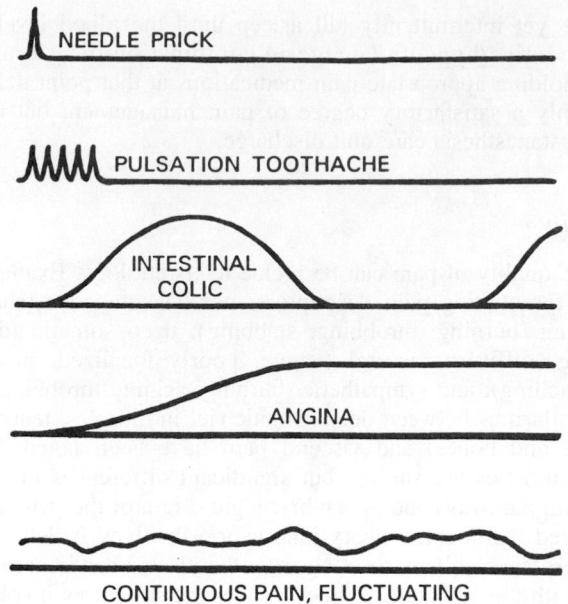

**FIGURE 13–5.** Diagram illustrating time-intensity curves of various well-known pains, namely, needle prick, pulsating toothache, intestinal colic, angina, and continuous fluctuating pain. (From Lewis T. *Pain.* New York, NY: MacMillan; 1942:173.)

### Location

The location of pain also is a key to its diagnosis. This fact must be tempered with the realization that only cutaneous pain is well localized. Deep somatic pain and visceral pain may be difficult to locate because of the amount of referred pain involved. Furthermore, sympathetically mediated pain does not follow classic dermatome distributions.

### Course

It is important to determine exacerbating factors and relieving maneuvers, particularly if the pain is chronic or cancer related. For all pain problems except the most acute, the previously discussed characteristics must be analyzed from the onset of the pain to the time of evaluation. Has the pain intensity worsened or improved? Is the pain now intermittent or constant? Does it have any association with physical or emotional stress? Has the location changed?

The pain consultant also must be sure to obtain the results of previous diagnostic and therapeutic procedures. This information is best sought from the referring physician because the patient often has a difficult time remembering results, especially if pain relief from a therapeutic procedure was short-lived.

Current therapeutic modalities must also be elicited. Many patients have cognitive deficits associated with centrally acting medications that are used to treat the problem, the chronic nature of their pain, and its potential association with depression. This problem may lead to long-term sleep disturbances, thus adding to their cognitive dysfunction. It may be necessary to involve all health care providers and family members familiar with the patient to develop a complete pain history.

### Is the Concurrent Medical Condition a Factor?

The next step in the development of a pain diagnosis involves obtaining a separate medical history (see Fig. 13–1).

The young, healthy patient with an easily diagnosed and treatable pain problem does not present a dilemma; the elderly patient with multiple organ system dysfunctions is more challenging and difficult. These patients are problematic regardless of whether their pain is acute, chronic, or cancer related. The major problem involves potential adverse effects associated with both pharmacologic and nonpharmacologic treatment options.

### Pharmacologic Interactions

Drug interactions and pharmacokinetics must be considered when treatment is recommended. Regardless of the route used, opiates can potentially produce clinically significant adverse interactions with any other class of centrally acting drugs (all CNS depressants, anticonvulsants, alcohol, and some drugs with a primary site of action outside the CNS).

#### Tricyclic Antidepressants

Adjuvant tricyclic antidepressant use can be problematic in patients with cancer who are not obtaining satisfactory pain relief with opiates alone. Even a low dose of amitriptyline can cause delirium and major management problems.[12] This drug interaction may take hours to days to resolve once the source of the problem has been identified owing to the long half-life of the tricyclic antidepressant. Obviously, dose titration is crucial in these and similar patients and requires close observation and gradual increase in the antidepressant dose while all other drug doses are maintained at a stable level.

Tricyclic antidepressants are metabolized by the cytochrome $P_{450}$ enzyme system. Any medication that inhibits that system can increase tricyclic antidepressant plasma levels, sometimes dramatically, leading to toxicity. Many medications can impede the $P_{450}$ system; most likely pertinent to the pain management specialist are the selective serotonin reuptake inhibitor antidepressants (fluoxetine, paroxetine, sertraline). Care must be taken if the concurrent administration of these two classes of medications is desired; a reduction in dosage of one or both medications may be necessary to avoid tricyclic toxicity.[13]

#### Tramadol

The centrally acting analgesic tramadol (Ultram) has become a popular pain medication in the United States. Unfortunately, tramadol can have significant interactions with other medications frequently used in pain management. Tramadol lowers the seizure threshold, and seizures have been reported in patients taking tramadol within the recommended dosage range. The seizure risk is increased in patients who concomitantly use both tramadol and any other medication that also lowers the seizure threshold. Many medications, including serotonin reuptake inhibitors, tricyclic antidepressants, and neuroleptics, lower the seizure threshold. The risk of seizures in patients taking tramadol may also be increased in patients with a history of epilepsy or head trauma. Naloxone administration in the setting of tramadol overdose may increase the seizure risk.[14] Caution should be used in the administration of tramadol in these settings.

#### Steroids

Treatment for several types of low back pain involves the placement of steroids in the epidural space. Although the depot form is used, gradual uptake occurs with the potential for systemic effects. A common problem in patients with diabetes mellitus is an increase in the insulin or oral hypoglycemic requirements and the need for stricter diet control. Thus, a plan for close monitoring of blood glucose must be in place before administration of depot steroid to a diabetic patient.

Steroids administered by any route may cause serious gastrointestinal bleeding problems in patients who are taking aspirin or nonsteroidal antiinflammatory drugs. Both of these drug therapies may be overlooked by the patient during the medical and drug history unless questions are specifically asked.

## Pharmacokinetic Alterations

The pharmacokinetics of medications used in the treatment of pain may be altered by hepatic, renal, or cardiac disease. Cirrhosis and liver failure can result in decreases in drug clearance, decreases in enzymatic biotransformation, and a greater potential for drug sensitivity and toxicity. The reduction in plasma proteins results in a greater delivery of larger amounts of free drug to target organs.[15]

Renal dysfunction can lead to an increase in plasma drug levels or in their active metabolites because of decreased clearance or uremia-induced hypoalbuminemia.[16]

Cardiac dysfunction, particularly congestive heart failure, results in decreased blood flow to both the liver and the kidneys, further impairing hepatic clearance, biotransformation, and renal elimination.[17] Obviously, prescribing medications to patients in pain with major systemic disease, those taking other medications, or both, must be done with great caution, reductions in dose, and close communication with the patient's primary physician.

## Nonpharmacologic Interactions

Nonpharmacologic treatment options might also be problematic in patients with significant medical problems. Such patients most likely have difficulty participating in active exercise programs that are often imperative in the recovery process of a myofascial pain problem. The primary physician can help to determine the acceptable level of physical activity.

## What Is the Impact of Psychologic or Psychiatric Dysfunction?

Psychologic and psychiatric factors may play important roles in the perception and response to pain. Pain becomes a problem once it can no longer be ignored. At this point, the emotional or affective aspects of the pain become increasingly important[18] (Table 13–2).

The Minnesota Multiphasic Personality Inventory reveals that patients with chronic pain have higher scores in hysteria, depression, and hypochondriasis.[19] Such patients have a reduction in their scores once their pain is treated successfully.[20]

## Emotional Disorders

Emotional disorders often predispose to increased susceptibility or decreased tolerance for pain. Such problems include major depression, dysthymia, somatization, conversion disor-

**TABLE 13–2.** Psychologic Effects of Pain

| | |
|---|---|
| Depressed mood | Reduced libido |
| Sleep disturbance | Irritable |
| Somatic preoccupation | Anxiety |
| Reduced activity | |

From Pelz M, Mersky H. A description of the psychological effects of chronic painful lesions. *Pain.* 1982;14:293.

ders, hypochondriasis, and psychogenic pain.[21] Depression impairs the patient's ability to cope with the pain, whereas somatization disorder and hypochondriasis result in a persistent search for the etiology of the pain problem, often involving invasive tests and surgery. Obviously, when such a problem might exist, a screening evaluation by a trained psychiatrist is needed.

## Environmental Factors

Environmental factors influence a patient's response to pain. The consequences of a person's pain behavior are at the heart of this relationship. Behavior may be rewarded or punished, depending on environmental factors. The learning model of pain holds that reinforcement of pain behavior sustains it even in the absence of the noxious somatic stimulus that initially elicited the pain.[22]

The issue of disability payments is a common problem seen in patients with chronic pain. Financial compensation for pain and injury is a positive reinforcer to continue the pain and to stay away from work. Inactivity is another commonly seen problem. Initially, avoiding activity lessens the pain; eventually, the inability to be active is reinforced by the avoidance of unpleasant tasks or the attention of family members, or both. Physicians often contribute to this problem in their attempts to identify the organic cause of the pain without evaluating the other possible psychosocial etiologies.

Preliminary questions that need be asked to screen for these features are listed in Table 13–3.

## How Should the Physical Examination Be Approached?

The physical examination is crucial to the differential pain diagnosis. It includes a general examination as well as a

**TABLE 13–3.** Screening Questions to Detect Psychologic, Psychiatric, Emotional, and Environmental Problems

Have you felt sad, blue, depressed, hopeless, down in the dumps lately?
Have you noticed a decrease in your appetite or weight loss?
Are you able to sleep at night?
Have you lost interest in your usual pleasurable activities?
Have you noticed a loss of energy or the onset of fatigue?
Are you able to concentrate in your usual fashion?
Have you had recurrent thoughts of death or suicide?
Have you at any time had psychiatric or psychological treatment for any condition?
Has anyone in your family been diagnosed with a psychiatric problem?
Do others consider you a sickly person?
If your present pain condition was caused on or by your job, do you feel that your employer has treated you fairly?
Have you received compensation for your injury?
Are you bringing suit because of your pain?
Do you expect to sue or are you thinking about suing?
When you are in pain, what does your spouse do?

thorough evaluation of the painful region. Height, weight, blood pressure, heart rate, respiratory rate, and temperature are essential as screening data. A complete cardiopulmonary examination is also mandatory, as is a screening neurologic examination that includes assessment of cranial nerve function, spinal nerve function (sensory and motor), coordination, and cerebral function. The anesthesiologist should explain to the patient that this initial examination process is for screening purposes to assure the physician that nothing is missed. Otherwise, a patient will be confused and possibly resentful when the initial examination involves nonpainful areas. Examination of the most painful area should be performed last so as not to interfere with the rest of the process.

## The Painful Area

### Inspection

Inspection gives further evidence that is needed to make the correct pain diagnosis. When pain is secondary to chronic reflex sympathetic dystrophy, the skin in the involved area is mottled, often sweaty, and sustains hair loss; ridging of the nails is common. Patients with myofascial pain may exhibit observable muscle asymmetry in the area of muscle spasm, or they may experience limited range of motion. Denervation hypersensitivity can be observed in skin supplied by damaged nerve roots when cool air provokes the pilomotor reflex.[23] This response may be short-lived, occurring at the time of undressing and possibly resolving shortly thereafter, but it can be reproduced by stroking or scratching the affected area.

### Palpation

Palpation adds more information on which to base the pain diagnosis. In myofascial pain, tender muscle areas are palpable as nodules or bands; palpation reproduces the patient's pain. The patient may jump or withdraw when relatively light pressure is applied to these tender areas. The muscle itself may even twitch under the palpating finger (jump sign), further supporting the diagnosis.[24]

In some neuropathic pain problems, sensation is diminished in the dermatomal distribution of the affected nerve or nerves, whereas the surrounding areas may reveal hyperesthesia, dysesthesia, allodynia, or hyperalgesia. These findings are elicited by gently stroking the contralateral mirror-image region first, followed by the affected area. If the affected area is more sensitive than the normal region, the patient is said to have hyperesthesia; dysesthesia is an unpleasant sensation, and allodynia is pain elicited by a nonpainful stimulus.[2] Also seen with neuropathic pain is an increased response to a painful stimulus that is termed *hyperalgesia*.[2] It can be elicited by pinprick testing that compares normal and painful areas. Palpation over a neuroma, also classified as neuropathic by some, reproduces the sharp, shooting pain that is the patient's major complaint.

### What Laboratory or Radiographic Data Are Necessary to Make a Pain Diagnosis?

Although pain management experts rely heavily on physical examination, they also find specific tests to be of value[25] (Table 13–4). Usually, patients coming to a chronic pain clinic

**TABLE 13–4.** Useful Laboratory and Radiographic Tests in Pain Evaluation

| | |
| --- | --- |
| Plain radiography | Laboratory tests (other than blood tests) |
| Computed tomography scan | Complete blood cell count |
| Electromyography | Thermography |
| Contrast radiography | Electroencephalography |
| Nuclear medicine | Electrocardiography |

From Rudy TE, Turk DC, Brena SF. Differential utility of medical procedures in the assessment of chronic pain patients. *Pain.* 1988;34:167.

or center have had these studies performed in the recent past. The pain management consultant must interpret these tests appropriately and know when to order further tests.

## Radiographic Studies

Radiographic studies are useful in evaluation of a number of musculoskeletal pain problems, including arthritis, bone tumors (primary and metastatic), and fractures. The physician must always remember to correlate the radiologic study with the clinical picture because there are numerous documented cases of pathologic findings on radiologic examinations of asymptomatic patients.[26]

### Computed Tomography Scans

CT scans are commonly used to evaluate the spine. The spinal cord and any extrinsic defects in the canal may be visualized, as can facet joint disease and spinal stenosis. The CT scan is noninvasive and thus preferable to myelography, which carries potential significant risks.

### Myelography

Myelography is helpful to determine whether a patient has a surgically correctable disease and, if so, to localize the lesion before surgery. Over 90% of lumbar herniated disks are diagnosed by CT scanning alone; the myelogram is reserved for those cases in which CT scanning fails to find an abnormality.[27] The myelogram is unsurpassed in its ability to define spinal cord and nerve root anatomy, but carries the risks of an invasive procedure and postdural puncture headache.

### Magnetic Resonance Imaging

MRI is noninvasive and visualizes the spinal anatomy in much the same way as contrast myelography, but without the associated risks. The MRI is superior for the evaluation of intervertebral disk disease and is the examination of choice for many spinal conditions.

## Electromyography

Electromyography is useful in the diagnosis of nerve trauma, plexopathies or nerve root lesions, diffuse polyneuropathies, and primary muscle diseases.

## Screening Laboratory Studies

The causes of painful neuropathies are extensive; laboratory screening studies may include determination of complete blood counts, erythrocyte sedimentation rate, and muscle enzyme levels; serum protein electrophoresis; immunoglobulin measurement; lupus erythematosus cell preparation; antinuclear antibodies; glucose tolerance testing; vitamin $B_{12}$, folate, and niacin determination; and serologic assay for syphilis.

## Thermography

Thermography has been used to diagnose many pain syndromes. However, because the test measures surface temperature, it yields positive results in many situations and cannot necessarily be used as a specific diagnostic tool. It may be useful in the following situations: soft tissue injury, nerve root compression or irritation, bone and joint disorders, myofascial pain syndromes, neurovascular compression, sprains, infections, and sympathetically mediated pain.

## MANAGEMENT TECHNIQUES

Once the history, physical examination data, and laboratory results have been obtained and a pain diagnosis determined, a treatment plan is generated. Treatment should provide the most benefit with the least side effects. Unfortunately, the diagnosis is not always readily apparent on the first visit, and the patient may require several trials, a combination of treatments, or both. Combination therapy often minimizes side effects and maximizes pain relief by blocking pain pathways at multiple sites in the peripheral nervous system and CNS.

## *What Is the Basis of Pharmacologic Approaches?*

Table 13–5 lists the major classes of drugs that are available for consideration. Some are not indicated for every patient. A long-acting opiate such as morphine sulfate is not the drug of choice in a patient with postoperative pain in whom the problem is expected to be short-lived. Similarly, a short-acting drug that must be administered in multiple doses each day is less than desirable for the management of a long-term, chronic pain problem.

## Classification of Pain and Associated Drug Therapy

Drug therapies are often selected in accordance with the classification of pain the patient is experiencing. Primary drugs used for acute pain include nonopiate and opiate analgesics and occasionally a benzodiazepine[28] (Tables 13–6 to 13–8). Patients with chronic pain present a different therapeutic dilemma because of the chronicity of the disease and the

**TABLE 13–5.** Major Drug Classifications Used in Pain Management

| | |
|---|---|
| Nonopiate analgesics | Corticosteroids |
| Opiate analgesics | Analeptics |
| Local anesthetics | Neuroleptics |
| Antidepressants | Antihistamines |
| Anticonvulsants | Benzodiazepines |
| Muscle relaxants | Miscellaneous (eg, baclofen, clonidine) |
| Sympatholytics | |

potential for psychologic involvement. With these facts in mind, the most common drug therapies include use of nonopiate analgesics, antidepressants, oral local anesthetics (eg, mexiletine), anticonvulsants, neuroleptics, sympatholytics, and miscellaneous drugs such as baclofen[29] (Tables 13–9 and 13–10).

One principle to follow in the prescription of pain medication to chronic pain patients is to avoid the long-term use of medications known to produce tolerance and physical dependence until all other options have undergone adequate trials (including a multidisciplinary inpatient program, when appropriate). Occasionally, such medications may be necessary in the beginning (eg, use of a muscle relaxant such as cyclobenzaprine for myofascial pain). The pain consultant should be certain to prescribe a short course of any such medication and to follow these patients closely until they no longer require medications to control their problem.

## *Opioids and Nonmalignant Pain*

A growing body of literature concerns opioid therapy for the treatment of chronic (nonmalignant) pain. Significant controversy surrounds this issue.[30–32] Discussion issues include analgesic efficacy, tolerance, goals, risk of adverse pharmacologic outcomes, toxicity, side effects, drug dependence, and drug addiction.[30] Many experts believe that a subset of patients with chronic pain obtains improved pain relief without significant toxicity or addiction. The practitioner should be aware of the recommendations for opioid therapy[30] (Table 13–11). The physician should also keep in mind that regulation of controlled substance prescription by physicians is primarily at the state level, with laws varying from state to state.

## *Cancer Pain*

Patients with cancer pain present a different set of problems owing to the nature of the disease and the impact it has on the patient and the family.[33–35] Such patients can experience a combination of acute and chronic pain and often have a limited life expectancy. Therefore, they have even more medication needs as well as some unique problems specific to their group.

The World Health Organization (WHO) has developed a three-step analgesic ladder that is applicable to all patients with cancer pain both in developed and undeveloped countries[33] (Fig. 13–6). In addition, use of corticosteroids, analeptics, neuroleptics, antihistamines, and miscellaneous drugs such as antiemetics and anticonstipation agents must be considered early[35] (Tables 13–12 to 13–15).

## *Known Efficacy*

Appropriate pharmacotherapy may be chosen based on drug groups that are known to be efficacious in the treatment of a specific pain syndrome or problem. The simplest mechanistic approach, after determining if the pain is acute, chronic, or cancer related, is to classify the pain as nociceptive or neuropathic.

Physicians of all specialties know the utility of nonopiate and mild opiate analgesics for the treatment of nociceptive pain related to injury, particularly musculoskeletal injuries. However, once the problem outlives the usual course of healing, such therapies often cease to be effective. At this point,

**TABLE 13–6.** Nonopioid Analgesics for the Treatment of Acute Pain

| Agent | Adult Dose (mg PO) | Interval (h) | Maximum Daily Dose (mg) | Comments |
|---|---|---|---|---|
| **Salicylates** | | | | |
| Aspirin | 500–1000 | 4–6 | 6000 | 1. Gastrointestinal upset and bleeding<br>2. Irreversible decrease in platelet aggregation |
| Diflunisal (Dolobid)* | 1000 initial<br>500 subsequent | 8–12 | 1500 | No antiplatelet effect at lower doses |
| Choline magnesium trisalicylate (Trilisate) | 1000–1500 | 12 | 4000 | No antiplatelet effect |
| Acetaminophen | 500–1000 | 4–6 | 4000 | Hepatotoxic with sustained high doses |
| **NSAIDs** | | | | |
| Ibuprofen | 200–400 | 4–6 | 3200 | **NSAIDs**<br>1. Reversible decrease in platelet aggregation<br>2. Can produce gastrointestinal effects<br>3. Can cause renal insufficiency<br>4. Can cause central nervous system impairment |
| Naproxen* | 500 initial, 250 subsequent | 12 | 1250 | |
| Fenoprofen (Nalfon) | 300–600 | 6–8 | 3000 | |
| Celecox (cyclooxygenase inhibitor) | 100–200 | 24 | 200 | |
| Rofecoxib (cyclooxygenase inhibitor) | 12.5–50 | 24 | 50 | |
| Indomethacin* | 25 | 8–12 | 150 | |
| Sulindac (Clinoril) | 150–200 | 12 | 400 | |
| Mefenamic acid (Ponstel) | 500 initial, 250 subsequent | 6 | 1000 | Do not use longer than 7 d |
| Meclofenamate (Meclomen) | 50 | 6 | 400 | |
| Tolmetin (Tolectin) | 400 | 8 | 2000 | |
| Piroxicam (Feldene)* | 10 | 12 | 30 | |
| Ketoprogen* | 50 | 6–8 | 300 | |
| Diclofenac* | 50–100 | 6–12 | 200 | |
| Ketorolac (Toradol)* | PO 10 | 6 | 40 | Do not use longer than 5 d |
| | IV 30 | 6 | 120 | |
| Tenoxicam† | 20 | 24 | 20 | |
| Celebrex | | | | |

*Injectable form is available in some countries.
†IM or IV route only.
IM, intramuscular; IV, intravenous; NSAIDs, nonsteroidal antiinflammatory drugs; PO, oral.
From Task Force on Acute Pain. Ready BH, Edwards WT, eds. *Management of Acute Pain: A Practical Guide.* Seattle, Wash: IASP Publications; 1992:11–21.

**TABLE 13–7.** Systemic Opioids for the Treatment of Acute Pain

| Drug | Route of Administration (mg/kg) | Front Load*† (mg/kg) | Maintenance Dose‡ (mg/kg) | Frequency§ (h) |
|------|--------------------------------|---------------------|--------------------------|----------------|
| *Agonist* | | | | |
| Codeine | PO | 1.5 | 0.75 | 3–4 |
| | SC, IM | 1.0 | 0.5 | 3–4 |
| Hydrocodone (Vicodin)‖ | PO | 0.15 | 0.07–0.15 | 4–6 |
| Oxycodone (Percodan) | PO | 0.15 | 0.07–0.15 | 3–4 |
| Morphine | PO | 0.5–1.0 | 0.5–1.0 | 4 |
| | Slow-release | 1.0 | 1.0–2.0 | 12 |
| | PO¶ | 1.0 | 1.0–2.0 | 12 |
| | SC, IM | 0.15 | 0.1–0.2 | 3–4 |
| | IV | 0.15 | 0.01–0.04 per h | PRN, continuous |
| Meperidine (Pethidine) | PO | 2.5–3.5 | 1.5–3.0 | 3–4 |
| | SCI, IM | 1.5–2.0 | 1.0–1.5 | 3–4 |
| | IV | 1.5–2.0 | 0.3–0.6 per h | Continuous |
| Omnopon (Pantopon) | SC, IM | 0.3 | 0.1–0.2 | 4 |
| Hydromorphone (Dilaudid) | PO | 0.04–0.08 | 0.04–0.08 | 3 |
| | SC, IM | 0.02–0.04 | 0.03–0.06 | 3 |
| | IV | 0.02 | 0.01 per h | Continuous |
| Nicomorphine†† | SC, IM | 0.15 | 0.1–0.2 | 3–4 |
| | IV | 0.15 | 0.01–0.04 per h | Continuous |
| Diamorphine†† (Heroin) | SC, IM | 0.03–0.07 | 0.01–0.04 | 2 |
| | IV | 0.03–0.07 | 0.01–0.04 per h | 2 |
| Oxymorphone | SC, IM | 0.15 | 0.1–0.2 | 3–4 |
| Methadone | PO | 0.2–0.4 | 0.1–0.4 | **, ‡‡ |
| | SC, IM | 0.14 | 0.1–0.2§§ | **, ‡‡ |
| | IV | 0.15 | | |
| Levorphanol | PO | 0.02–0.04 | 0.02–0.04 | **, ‡‡ |
| | SC, IM | 0.02 | 0.01§§ | **, ‡‡ |
| | IV | 0.02 | | |
| Fentanyl | IV | 0.0008–0.0016 | 0.0003–0.0016 per h | Continuous |
| | Transdermal | | | |
| Sufentanil | IV | 0.001–0.0003 | Not established | — |
| Alfentanil‖ ‖ | IV | 0.03–0.05 | 0.06–0.09 per h | Continuous |
| *Mixed Agonist-Antagonists* | | | | |
| Pentazocine¶¶ (Talwin) | PO | 1.5–2.5 | 1.0–1.5 | 6 |
| | SC, IM | 1.0 | 0.7–1.0 | 6 |
| | IV | 1.0 | 0.7–1.0 per h | 6 |
| Nalbuphine (Nubain) | SC, IM | 0.05–0.01 | 0.05–0.1 | 3–4 |
| | IV | 0.05–0.01 | 0.05–0.1 per h | 3–4 |
| Butorphanol¶¶ (Stadol) | SC, IM | 0.03 | 0.02–0.04 | 3 |
| | IV Intranasal | 0.03 | 0.02–0.04 | 3 |
| *Partial Agonist* | | | | |
| Buprenorphine (Buprenex) | Sublingual | 0.006 | 0.004 | 6–8 |
| | SC, IM | 0.004 | 0.002 | 6 |
| | IV | 0.004 | 0.002 per h | 6 |

*IV front-loading dose should be titrated slowly to reduce risk of overdose.
†Except in pediatric patients, body weight is not an accurate predictor of effective opioid dose. Titration to desired effect for each patient is necessary.
‡If pain breakthrough occurs before administration of scheduled maintenance dose, give one additional maintenance dose and continue schedule.
§Maintenance dose is usually approximately one half the effective loading dose.
‖Available only in combination with aspirin or acetaminophen in the United States.
¶Nearest dosage increment must be chosen; if tablets are broken, immediate release can occur.
**Metabolic normeperidine accumulates; central nervous system stimulation can lead to seizures; higher doses or prolonged infusions are not recommended.
††Not available in the United States.
‡‡Watch for accumulation, especially after 48 h of administration.
§§Long duration of action renders drug unsuitable for continuous infusion.
‖ ‖Short duration of action makes IV infusion the only practical route of administration.
¶¶Can precipitate withdrawal in opioid-dependent patients.
IM, intramuscular; IV, intravenous; PO, oral; SC, subcutaneous.
From Task Force on Acute Pain. Ready BH, Edwards WT, eds. *Management of Acute Pain: A Practical Guide.* Seattle, Wash: IASP Publications; 1992:11–21.

**TABLE 13–8.** Benzodiazepines as Adjuncts in the Treatment of Acute Pain

| | Half-Life of Drug or Metabolites (h) | Route | Adult Dose (mg) | Interval (h) | Comments |
|---|---|---|---|---|---|
| Diazepam (Valium) | 30–60 | PO | 2–10 | 6 | 1. Injection is painful |
| | | IV | 2–5 | 3–4 | 2. Long-acting active metabolite |
| Chlordiazepoxide (Librium) | 5–15 | PO | 10–25 | 8–12 | |
| | | IM, IV | 5–25 | 6–8 | |
| Flurazepam (Dalmane) | 50–100 | PO | 10–30 | 12–24 | Hypnotic |
| Lorazepam (Ativan) | 10–20 | PO | 0.5–3 | 6–12 | May accumulate in elderly patients |
| | | | 0.5–2 | 6–12 | |
| Oxazepam (Serax) | 5–10 | PO | 10–20 | 6–8 | |
| Triazolam (Halcion) | 1.3–3 | PO | 0.125–0.5 | 8–12 | Hypnotic |
| Midazolam (Versed) | 1.2–12 | IM | 1–3 | 2–4 | 1. Amnesia is pronounced |
| | | IV | 0.5–2 | 0.3–3 | 2. Well suited to IV infusion (0.5–5 mg/h) |

IM, intramuscular; IV, intravenous; PO, oral.
From Task Force on Acute Pain. Ready BH, Edwards WT, eds. *Management of Acute Pain: A Practical Guide.* Seattle, Wash: IASP Publications; 1992:11–21.


**TABLE 13–9.** Dosages and Effects of Antidepressants Used in Pain Management

| | | | | Adverse and Side Effects | |
|---|---|---|---|---|---|
| Drug | Initial Dosage* | Maintenance Dosage* | Efficacy in Depression | *Orthostatic Hypotension* | *Sedation* |
| **Heterocyclics** | | | | | |
| Tricyclics | 10–300 | 10–150 | + + + + | + + | + + + |
| Amitriptyline | | | | | |
| Clomipramine | 20–200 | 20–150 | + + + + | + + | + + |
| Desipramine | 75–300 | 75–100 | + + + + | + + | − |
| Doxepin | 30–300 | 30–200 | + + + + | + + | + + + + |
| Imipramine | 20–300 | 20–150 | + + + + | + + + | + |
| Nortriptyline | 50–150 | 50–150 | + + + + | + | + |
| Trimipramine | 50–225 | 75–150 | + + + + | + + | + + + |
| Maprotiline | 75–300 | 75–125 | + + + + | + | + + |
| Trazodone | 50–600 | 100–300 | + + +? | + + | + + + |
| **Monoamine Oxidase Inhibitor** | | | | | |
| Phenelzine | 45–90 | 45–75 | + + | + + + | − |

Antidepressant dose reflects material from the clinical literature cited in this chapter and the author's personal experience.
+ + + +, marked; + + +, moderate; + +, mild; +, minimal; −, absent; ?, questionable (data inadequate). Only values in vertical columns should be compared.
From Monks R. Psychotropic drugs. In: Bonica JJ, ed. *The Management of Pain.* Philadelphia, Pa: Lea & Febiger; 1990:1676.


**TABLE 13–10.** Dosages and Side Effects of Neuroleptics Used for Pain Management

| | | | Side and Adverse Effects | |
|---|---|---|---|---|
| Drug | Initial Dosage* (mg/d PO) | Maintenance Dosage† (mg/d PO) | Anticholinergic | *Autonomic (Hypotension)* |
| **Phenothiazines** | | | | |
| Chlorpromazine | 75–500 | 25–150 | + + + | + + + |
| Fluphenazine | 1–10 | 1–3 | + | + |
| Methotrimeprazine | 5–100 | 15–50 | + + + | + + + |
| Pericyazine | 5–200 | 5–100 | + + + | + + + |
| Perphenazine | 8–64 | 4–16 | + + | + + |
| Thioridazine | 10–200 | 25–75 | + + + | + + + |
| Trifluoperazine | 3–20 | 3–10 | + | + |
| **Thioxanthenes** | | | | |
| Chlorprothixene | 50–200 | 50–150 | + + + | + + + |
| Flupenthixol | 0.5–2 | 0.5–1 | + | − |
| **Miscellaneous** | | | | |
| Haloperidol | 0.5–15 | 0.5–10 | + | + |

*Neuroleptic doses reflect data from the clinical material cited in this chapter and from the author's personal experience.
†Modified from Baldessarini RJ. Drugs and the treatment of psychiatric disorders. In: Goodman L, Gilman AG, eds. *The Pharmacological Basis of Therapeutics.* 7th ed. New York, NY: Macmillan; 1985.
PO, oral; + + +, moderate; + +, mild; +, minimal; −, absent. Only values in vertical columns should be compared.
From Monks R. Psychotropic drugs. In: Bonica JJ, ed. *The Management of Pain.* Philadelphia, Pa: Lea & Febiger; 1990:1676–1689.

**TABLE 13–11.** Proposed Guidelines in the Management of Opioid Maintenance Therapy for Nonmalignant Pain

1. Should be considered only after all other reasonable attempts at analgesia have failed.
2. A history of substance abuse should be viewed as a relative contraindication.
3. A single practitioner should take primary responsibility for treatment.
4. Patients should give informed consent before the start of therapy; points to be covered include recognition of the low risk of psychological dependence as an outcome, potential for cognitive impairment with the drug alone and in combination with sedative/hypnotics, and understanding by female patients that children born when the mother is on opioid maintenance therapy will likely be physically dependent at birth.
5. After drug selection, doses should be given on an around-the-clock basis; several weeks should be agreed upon as the period of initial dose titration, and although improvement in function should be continually stressed, all should agree to at least partial analgesia as the appropriate goal of therapy.
6. Failure to achieve at least a partial analgesia at relatively low initial doses in the nontolerant patient raises questions about the potential treatability of the pain syndrome with opioids.
7. Emphasis should be given to attempts to capitalize on improved analgesia by gains in physical and social function.
8. In addition to the daily dose determined initially, patients should be permitted to escalate dose transiently on days of increased pain; two methods are acceptable: (1) prescription of an additional 4 to 6 "rescue doses" to be taken as needed during the month; and (2) instruction that 1 or 2 extra doses may be taken on any day, but they must be followed by an equal reduction of dose on subsequent days.
9. Most patients should be seen and drugs prescribed at least monthly. Patients should be assessed for the efficacy of treatment, adverse drug effects, and the appearance of either misuse or abuse of the drugs during each visit. The results of the assessment should be clearly documented in the medical record.
10. Exacerbations of pain not effectively treated by transient, small increases in dose are best managed in the hospital, where dose escalation, if appropriate, can be observed closely, and return to baseline doses can be accomplished in a controlled environment.
11. Evidence of drug hoarding, acquisition of drugs from other physicians, uncontrolled dose escalation, or other aberrant behaviors should be followed by tapering and discontinuation of opioid maintenance therapy.

Reprinted by permission of Elsevier Science Publishing Co, Inc, from Chronic opioid therapy in non-malignant pain, by RK Portenoy, *Journal of Pain and Symptom Management*, Vol 5(Suppl):546. Copyright 1990 by the US Cancer Pain Relief Committee.

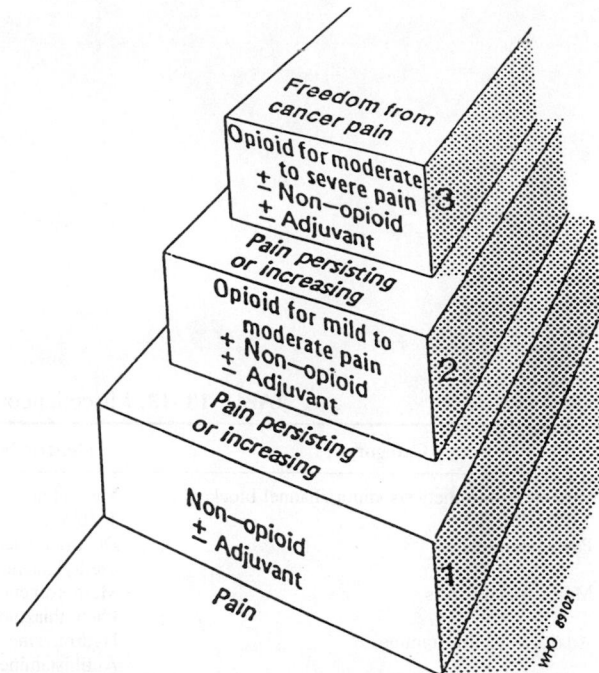

**FIGURE 13–6.** The World Health Organization three-step analgesic ladder. (Reproduced, by permission, from *Cancer Pain Relief and Palliative Care. Report of a WHO Expert Committee. Geneva, Switzerland: World Health Organization; 1990:9. WHO Technical Report Series No. 804.)*

antidepressants that are efficacious in both nociceptive and neuropathic pain problems should be considered.[36]

For neuropathic pain problems not controllable with antidepressants, oral local anesthetics, sympatholytics, anticonvulsants, neuroleptics, and baclofen use should be considered.[37–42] The order in which the drugs are chosen is based on the degree of pain, the potential for side effects, and the known efficacy of the drug for a particular pain syndrome. The consultant must have a thorough understanding of the pharmacology of the chosen drug and of the pathophysiology and proven treatment modalities for each pain problem before instituting a treatment plan.

## When Is the Intravenous Route Appropriate?

### Opiates

Although intravenous opiates have long been used for acute pain problems, only recently have anesthesiologists successfully managed acute pain with inventive, invasive techniques. Intravenous opiate delivery, whether by intermittent bolus, continuous infusion, or a combination of the two, is appropriate for any patient experiencing acute pain that is uncontrollable with oral opiates or other analgesics or who is unable to take medications by mouth[28] (Table 13–16; see also Table 13–7). Included are postoperative patients, patients with cancer pain with an acute exacerbation, obstetric patients, patients with burns, intensive care unit patients, and patients with chronic pain in the acute phase of their disease (eg, those with cardiac pain, herpes zoster, or sickle cell crisis).

Regardless of whether the pain problem is acute, chronic, or cancer related, the oral route should be used as soon as possible. Conversion from parenteral to oral opiates should take into consideration the previous 24-hour needs that produced adequate analgesia as well as the length of time opiate therapy has been required[43] (Table 13–17). If such therapy is for a single dose, then a 1:6 intramuscular-to-oral ratio is used; if the patient requires opiate therapy for some time, a 1:2 to a 1:3 ratio is more appropriate.[44]

### Lidocaine and Mexiletine

Intravenous lidocaine is used successfully for many neuropathic pain problems.[45] Although this approach was reported

**TABLE 13–12.** Steroid Therapy for Cancer Pain

| Dose | Dexamethasone | Pain |
|---|---|---|
| Low | 2–4 mg PO bid or tid | Soft tissue infiltration |
| Moderate | 4–8 mg PO bid or tid | Nerve compression, visceral distention, lymphedema |
| High | 4–12 mg PO tid or qid | Increased intracranial pressure |

PO, oral.
From Patt RB, Szalados JE, Wu CL. Pharmacotherapeutic guidelines. In: Patt RB, ed. *Cancer Pain.* Philadelphia, Pa: JP Lippincott; 1993:574.

**TABLE 13–13.** Miscellaneous Drugs With Analgesic Potential

| Category | Generic Name | Trade Name | Dose Range | Comments |
|---|---|---|---|---|
| Oral local anesthetics/sodium channel blockers | Mexiletine | Mexitil | 600–1200 mg/d | 1 |
| | Tocainide | Tonocard | 400–600 mg tid | 2 |
| Psychostimulants | Dextroamphetamine | Dexedrine | 5–15 mg q 6–12 h | 3 |
| | Methylphenidate | Ritalin | 5–30 mg bid | 3 |
| Major tranquilizers | Methotrimeprazine | Levoprome | 10–50 mg q 4–8 h | 4 |
| | Phenothiazines | — | — | 5 |
| Anxiolytic/antihistamines | Hydroxyzine | Vistaril, Atarax | 50–100 mg q 4–6 h | 6 |
| | Antihistamines | | | 7 |
| | Benzodiazepines | | | 8 |
| Miscellaneous | Baclofen | Lioresal | 20–80 mg/d | 9 |
| | Nifedipine | Procardia | 10–120 mg/d | 10 |
| | Phenoxybenzamine | Dibenzyline | 10–120 mg/d | 11 |
| | Clonidine | Catapres | 0.2–24 mg/d | 12 |
| | Tetrahydrocannibinol | Marinol | 2.5–25 mg/d | 13 |

**Comments**

1. Frequently considered for management of neuropathic pain in patients who have failed trials of antidepressants, anticonvulsants, or both. Potential adverse effects include cardiac dysrhythmia, confusion, dysarthria, nystagmus, tremor, nausea, vomiting, and constipation.
2. Considered as a third-line drug for neuropathic pain for patients who have failed trials of antidepressants, anticonvulsants, and mexiletine. Side effect profile similar to but more severe than that of mexiletine. In addition, administration has been associated with rare incidences of pneumonitis, hepatitis, and immunologic, allergic, and psychotic reactions.
3. Primary indication is as a psychostimulant to enhance alertness in patients with opioid-induced sedation. Analgesic effect has been demonstrated with some reliability, although pain per se is not a primary indication. Although not indicated as an analgesic, its analgesic effect, together with its rapid antidepressant activity, are beneficial side effects.
4. Phenothiazine. Available only in parenteral (intramuscular) form, although there is anecdotal support for safe intravenous use. Equianalgesic with morphine (15 mg methotrimeprazine = 10 mg morphine sulfate). Use is associated with sedation, making it a good choice in anxious patients with advanced illness who have not responded to more conventional analgesics or who are unable to take opioids. Potent antiemetic. Use may be associated with the appearance of extrapyramidal signs (see text for details).
5. With the exception of methotrimeprazine, generally regarded as not possessing intrinsic analgesic activity, although sedative and antiemetic properties make these agents useful in the treatment of agitation, nausea, and vomiting.
6. Antihistamine. Only drug of this class with demonstrated analgesic activity. Often coadministered with an opioid for acute pain and anxiety. Intramuscular injection may be painful. Not recommended in the management of chronic cancer pain.
7. With the exception of hydroxyzine, generally regarded as not possessing intrinsic analgesic activity, although sedative and antipruritic actions may be useful.
8. Direct analgesic/coanalgesic activities have not been demonstrated. Well-established role in treatment of insomnia and anxiety. May have an indirect role in managing pain when complaints are presumed to stem in large part from anxiety or sleep deprivation. Should not be used as a substitute for analgesics.
9. Antispasmodic agent (($\gamma$)-aminobutyric acid analogue). Has not been studied in patients with cancer but may be useful as an adjunctive pharmacologic agent in the treatment of neuropathic pain.
10. Calcium channel blocker. Has not been studied in patients with cancer pain. Anecdotal support for use as a systemic vasodilator in the presence of sympathetically maintained pain. Common adverse effects include orthostatic hypotension, headache, and peripheral edema.
11. $\alpha$-Adrenergic antagonist. Has not been studied in patients with cancer pain. Anecdotal support for use as a systemic vasodilator in the presence of sympathetically maintained pain. Common adverse effects include orthostatic hypotension, headache, and peripheral edema.
12. Centrally acting antihypertensive. Has not been studied in cancer pain. Indications for use still unclear. Analgesic by intraspinal routes; available as transdermal patch; used as an adjunct in the management of opioid and nicotine withdrawal.
13. Cannabinoid/psychotropic. Capacity to relieve pain is controversial. Use is associated with psychomimetic effects that many patients find undesirable. Indication is mainly as an antiemetic and, more recently, an appetite stimulant.

From Patt RB, Szalados JE, Wu CL. Pharmacotherapeutic guidelines. In: Patt RB, ed. *Cancer Pain.* Philadelphia, Pa: JB Lippincott; 1993:574.

**TABLE 13–14.** Recommended Prophylactic Antiemetics

| | |
|---|---|
| Prochlorperazine (Compazine), 5 mg PO every 4 h (range: 5 mg every 6 h to 20 mg every 4 h) | |
| If the above is too sedating or ineffective: | Haloperidol (Haldol), 0.5 mg PO every 8 h (range: 0.5 mg every 12 h to 1.0 mg every 4 h) |
| If sedation is desired in an agitated, nauseated patient: | Chlorpromazine (Thorazine), 10 mg PO every 4 h (range: 10 mg every 6 h to 25 mg every 4 h) |
| If gastric outlet obstruction is a problem, switch to or add to above: | Metoclopramide (Reglan), 10 mg PO every 8 h (range: 10 mg every 8 h to 20 mg every 6 h) |

PO, oral.

From Patt RB, Szalados JE, Wu CL. Pharmacotherapeutic guidelines. In: Patt RB, ed. *Cancer Pain*. Philadelphia, Pa: JB Lippincott; 1993:574.

previously,[46–48] renewed interest developed with the introduction of mexiletine, an oral analogue to parenteral local anesthetics.[49]

The first studies of this approach involved diabetic patients with neuropathy.[50] After a 1 mg/kg lidocaine bolus given over 2 to 3 minutes, an infusion was instituted with 4 mg/kg over 30 minutes. A significant number of these patients experienced improvement in pain that lasted days to weeks. A follow-up study showed the utility of mexiletine in long-term treatment when the intravenous therapeutic result was short-lived.[51] Subsequently, this therapy has been found to be useful in patients with burn pain,[52] postherpetic neuralgia,[53] and neuropathic pain in a variety of other syndromes.[49]

Because mexiletine takes several days to have an effect, acute pain may be treated with intravenous lidocaine initially; if this drug is effective, mexiletine is started at 5 to 10 mg/kg/d in divided doses.[51]

The most common side effects of mexiletine use are nausea,

**TABLE 13–15.** Bowel Preparation Protocol

Begin with a stool softener and gentle laxative
  Diocytil sodium sulfosuccinate, 100 mg, plus casanthranol, 30 mg (Peri-Colace), 1 capsule PO tid (range: 1 capsule qd to 2 capsules tid)
  Docusate calcium, 60 mg, plus Danthron, 50 mg (Doxidan), 1 capsule bid (range: 1 capsule qd to 2 capsules tid)
  Docusate sodium, 50 mg, plus senna, 187 mg (Senokot S), 1 tablet PO tid (range: 1 tablet qd to 4 tablets tid)
If no bowel movement in any 48-h period, add one of the following:
  Senna (Senokot), 187 mg, 2 to 3 tablets PO hs (range: 2 tablets hs to 4 tablets tid)
  Bisacodyl (Dulcolax), 10–15 mg PO hs (range: 5 mg hs to 15 mg tid)
  Milk of magnesia, 30–60 mL PO hs (range: once to twice per day)
  Haley's M-O, 30–60 mL PO hs (range: qd to bid)
  Lactulose (Chronulac: 10 g/15 mL), 30–45 mL PO hs (range: 15–60 mL hs *or* bid)
If no bowel movement by 72 h, perform rectal examination to rule out impaction
  If not impacted, try one of the following: bisacodyl (Dulcolax) suppository, 10 mg, magnesium citrate, 8 oz PO, senna extract (X-Prep liquid), 2.5 oz PO, mineral oil, 30–60 mL PO, Fleet enema
  If implacted
    Manually disimpact if stool is soft enough (consider pretreatment of patient with analgesic or tranquilizer)
    Soften with glycerin suppository or olive oil retention enema, then disimpact manually
    Follow-up with enema or enemas of choice (eg, tap water, soap suds) until clear and then increase intensity of daily bowel preparation

hs, bedtime; PO, oral.

From Patt RB, Szalados JE, Wu CL. Pharmacotherapeutic guidelines. In: Patt RB, ed. *Cancer Pain*. Philadelphia, Pa: JB Lippincott; 1993:574.

**TABLE 13–16.** Guidelines for Patient-Controlled Intravenous Opioid Administration*

| Drug (Concentration) | Size of Bolus (mg) | Lockout Interval (min) |
|---|---|---|
| Morphine (1 mg/mL) | 0.5–2.5 | 5–10 |
| Meperidine (10 mg/mL) | 5–25 | 5–10 |
| Hydromorphone (0.2 mg/mL) | 0.05–0.25 | 5–10 |
| Methadone (1 mg/mL) | 0.5–2.5 | 8–20 |
| Oxymorphone (0.25 mg/mL) | 0.2–0.4 | 8–10 |
| Fentanyl (0.01 mg/mL) | 0.010–0.020 | 3–10 |
| Sufentanil (0.002 mg/mL) | 0.002–0.005 | 3–10 |
| Nalbuphine (1 mg/mL) | 1–5 | 5–15 |
| Buprenorphine (0.03 mg/mL) | 0.03–0.1 | 8–20 |

*Individual patient requirements vary widely. Small doses should be used initially for elderly or very sick patients.

From Task Force on Acute Pain. Ready BH, Edwards WT, eds. *Management of Acute Pain: A Practical Guide*. Seattle, Wash: IASP Publications; 1992:11–21.

tremor, and dizziness; therefore, dose titration is imperative in patients with a predisposition to any of these side effects. The gastrointestinal side effects can be minimized if the medication is taken with food.

## What Is the Value of Peridural Analgesics in Acute Pain?

As mentioned previously, the type of pain experienced is a primary determinant of the appropriateness of therapy. Peridural opiates have different indications in acute, chronic, and cancer-related pain.

Most literature has focused on the use of peridural opiates in the acute pain setting. Bonica summarized the clinical responses to acute pain in relationship to each level affected in the CNS[54] (Fig. 13–7).

### Pulmonary Changes

The pulmonary system is the most affected and most important organ system in relation to potential postoperative complications. After upper abdominal surgery, atelectasis, pneumonia, and arterial hypoxemia develop in up to 70% of patients.[55] These complications are related to reductions in vital capacity, functional residual capacity, tidal volume, and the forced expiratory volume in 1 second. The ability to cough and clear secretions is reduced, as is chest wall compli-

**TABLE 13–17.** Oral-to-Parenteral Dose Ratios and Equianalgesic Doses for Various Opioids (Reference Dose: 10 mg Morphine Intramuscularly to Treat Severe Pain)

| Drug | Oral Dose | Oral-to-Parenteral Dose Ratio | Parenteral Dose |
|---|---|---|---|
| Morphine | | | |
|   Single dose | 60 mg | 6:1 | 10 mg |
|   Repeated dose | 30 mg | 3:1 | 10 mg |
| Hydromorphone | 8 mg | 5:1 | 1.6 mg |
| Methadone | 20 mg | 2:1 | 10 mg |
| Levorphanol | 2 mg | 1:1 (approximate) | 2 mg |
| Meperidine | 300 mg | 4:1 | 75 mg |
| Codeine | 200 mg | 1.5:1 | 130 mg |

From Hill CS. Oral opioid analgesics. Patt RB, ed. In: *Cancer Pain*. Philadelphia, Pa: JB Lippincott; 1993:137.

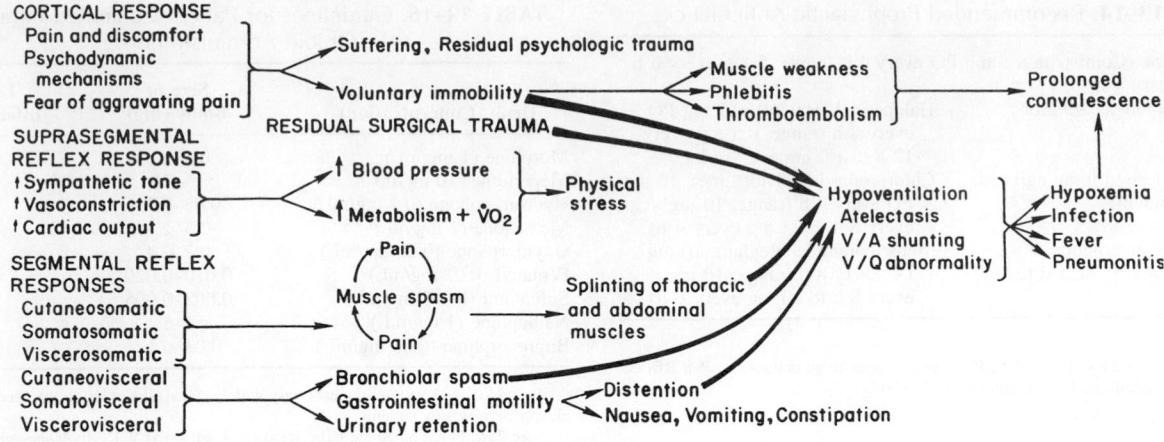

**FIGURE 13–7.** Schematic depiction of the pathophysiology of postoperative pain. (From Bonica JJ. Postoperative pain. In: Bonica JJ, ed. *The Management of Pain*. 2nd ed. Philadelphia, Pa: Lea & Febiger; 1990:466.)

ance.[55–57] The changes in respiratory mechanics are greatest after thoracic and upper abdominal procedures and least after extraabdominal and nonthoracic procedures.[56,58,59] Even pain from peripheral surgical procedures, such as major orthopedic surgery, can produce pulmonary dysfunction.[60]

### Cardiovascular Function

The cardiovascular system is also affected. Pain activates the sympathetic nervous system and the neuroendocrine system, producing multiple responses that affect myocardial oxygen supply and demand. The addition of these stress responses to a patient with known cardiovascular disease increases the potential for ischemia and cardiac failure.[61,62] In addition, pain affects the development of deep venous thrombosis by way of platelet-fibrinogen activation and impairs a patient's ability to ambulate, with resulting decreased venous flow.[63–65]

### Gastrointestinal Problems

The gastrointestinal system becomes problematic with the development of postoperative ileus, which is thought to occur in response to spinal reflexes triggered by pain and the stress of the surgical procedure.[66,67] If these expected postoperative responses to surgery and pain are superimposed on preexisting cardiopulmonary illness or morbid obesity, the outcome is questionable without good pain control.

### Outcome Studies

Studies have been completed in an attempt to determine whether peridural analgesia can alter the impact that acute pain has on the pathophysiologic changes discussed earlier. The neuroendocrine response is decreased to a greater extent when pain is adequately controlled with epidural opiates than when it is managed with intravenous opiates alone.[68–71] Epidural morphine also improves postoperative immune function and nitrogen balance.[72] Postoperative epidural opiate analgesia is said to improve pulmonary function and reduce morbidity compared with patient-controlled analgesia with morphine.[73]

A decreased incidence in pulmonary complications follows upper abdominal[72,74,75] or thoracic[57,76,77] procedures when postoperative epidural analgesia is used. These same observations apply to patients with morbid obesity. Epidural morphine compared with intramuscular morphine in obese patients results in less sedation, earlier ambulation, return of bowel function, and fewer pulmonary complications.[75]

Epidural or intrathecal opiates given for postoperative pain management may improve cardiac outcome.[78–80] Finally, epidural analgesia may reduce morbidity and mortality in high-risk patients.[81]

### What Is the Effect of Added Local Anesthetics?

The combination of peridurally administered local anesthetics and opiates more completely blunts the neuroendocrine response than the use of opiates alone[64,68,70,82] and relieves pain better than the use of local anesthetics alone.[83] However, no difference in postoperative pulmonary morbidity or mortality results. Local anesthetics administered through site-specific epidural catheters significantly decrease hospital stays after major abdominal or hip operations compared with intramuscularly administered morphine.[84,85]

### Vascular Surgery

Both morbidity and mortality after major vascular surgery may be improved with intraoperative epidural anesthesia followed by postoperative epidural analgesia. Postoperative epidural analgesia may be more important than intraoperative epidural anesthesia in reducing cardiac morbidity, whereas the reverse is probably true in reducing graft thrombosis in lower extremity vascular surgery.[80] More confirmatory research is needed in this area before firm conclusions can be drawn.

### Hip Arthroplasties

Epidural anesthesia followed by use of epidural local anesthetics for postoperative pain relief can reduce the incidence of lower extremity thrombosis and pulmonary embolism in patients undergoing total hip arthroplasties.[65] Local anesthetics perhaps increase fibrinolytic activity and inhibit platelet aggregation.[86,87] Similar results have been demonstrated in patients undergoing total knee arthroplasty.[80]

## Gastrointestinal Motility

Several studies show an improvement in postoperative gastrointestinal motility with peridural local anesthesia or analgesia that is not seen with epidural opiate administration.[88] In fact, both epidural and parenteral use of opiates delay return of bowel function, although this effect is more pronounced with parenteral administration.[75,89-91] The use of bupivacaine for postoperative epidural analgesia with or without epidural morphine resulted in a significant improvement in gastrointestinal motility after colectomy.[92] A significant reduction in hospital stay follows use of epidural opiates or local anesthetics for perioperative pain relief.[84,92-94]

## Chronic Pain Syndromes

In addition to blunting the responses to acute pain, local anesthetics administered by multiple routes may prevent chronic pain syndromes related to surgical procedures. The best examples include prevention of acute and chronic pain associated with iliac crest bone donor sites by local anesthetic infusions through iliac crest catheters,[95] and of phantom limb pain with peridural local anesthetics and opiates.[96,97] This idea of "preemptive analgesia" dates back to the early 1900s. The postoperative mortality rate was thought to be significantly reduced if the transmission of the response to the surgical procedure (pain or stress) could be blocked before the incision.[98] More recent studies have supported this observation; patients require significantly less postoperative analgesia when local anesthetic blockade is provided before the surgical incision.[99-101]

Factors to consider when deciding whether peridural opiates, local anesthetics, or both, might be beneficial to the acute pain patient are summarized in Table 13–18.

## How Is the Dose of Peridural Opiates and Local Anesthetics Determined?

### Opiates

Most clinicians initially used morphine as the drug of choice for peridural postoperative pain management. Table 13–19 is an excellent guide for determining the dose of epidural morphine, taking into consideration the patient's age, site of the surgical incision, and site of the epidural catheter.[28] Morphine is now commonly administered successfully by

**TABLE 13–18.** Situations in Which Peridural Opiates, Local Anesthetics, or Both Might Be Beneficial

**Surgical Considerations**

Thoracoabdominal procedures, major vascular procedures, major orthopedic procedures, urologic procedures, cesarean sections
Increased risk associated with ileus, risk of the development of chronic pain

**Medical Considerations**

Cardiovascular diseases, pulmonary disease, obesity, multisystem disease, high-risk patients, elderly

**Patient-Related Factors**

History of a good past experience with epidural analgesia, desire for health care professionals to manage their pain control
No patient preference but the procedure or the underlying medical problem suggests benefit of epidural analgesia
Desire for regional anesthesia

**TABLE 13–19.** Initial Dose (mg) of Epidural Morphine for Incisional Pain*

| | | Thoracic Surgery | |
| Patient Age (y) | Nonthoracic Surgery (Lumbar or Caudal Catheter) | *Thoracic Catheter* | *Lumbar Catheter* |
| --- | --- | --- | --- |
| 15–44 | 4 | 4 | 5 |
| 45–65 | 3 | 3 | 4 |
| 66–75 | 2 | 2 | 3 |
| 76+ | 1 | 1 | 2 |

*These doses should be considered only as guidelines. They are based on the use of undiluted 0.1% preservative-free morphine. Safe and effective doses for individual patients may vary considerably.

From Task Force on Acute Pain. Ready BH, Edwards WT, eds. *Management of Acute Pain: A Practical Guide.* Seattle, Wash: IASP Publications; 1992:11–21.

constant infusions in an attempt to minimize the periods of pain experienced with intermittent bolus injections[102] (Table 13–20). Again, the dose is based on the site of incision and, to a lesser extent, on the site of catheter insertion. Table 13–21 summarizes the dosing intervals of all the commonly used opiates for both intrathecal and epidural administration.[28]

### Local Anesthetics

Many practitioners add local anesthetics in analgesic doses to gain their previously described benefits and to minimize the side effects of opiates. Bupivacaine at concentrations of 0.0625% to 0.25% is frequently used; alternatively, ropivacaine at 0.1% to 0.2% is gaining popularity.[103,104] Patient-controlled epidural analgesia has become increasingly popular. One technique is outlined in Table 13–22.[105] Following these guidelines, a self-administered dose of morphine can reach 1.2 mg/h in addition to the superimposed background infusion of 0.4 mg/h. This total is a significant dose for an elderly patient or one with any degree of opiate sensitivity. A lower dose or a longer lockout interval may be appropriate in such patients.

## Why and How Should Patients Be Monitored?

Problems that require special monitoring include sedation and respiratory depression. Sedation may result from the direct

**TABLE 13–20.** Recommended Epidural Morphine Doses for Various Surgical Procedures

| | Doses | |
| Operation | *(mg/h)* | *(mL/h)* |
| --- | --- | --- |
| Total hip arthroplasty | 0.2–0.5 | 2–5 |
| Prostatectomy | 0.3–0.8 | 3–8 |
| Total abdominal hysterectomy* | 0.4–1.0 | 4–10 |
| Colectomy | 0.4–1.0 | 4–10 |
| Hepatic resection | 0.5–1.0 | 5–10 |
| Cholecystectomy | 0.6–1.0 | 6–10 |
| Total knee arthroplasty | 0.5–1.5 | 5–15 |
| Thoracotomy | | |
|    Lumbar | 0.8–1.5 | 8–15 |
|    Thoracic | 0.3–0.6 | 3–6 |

*Rates given are for lumbar catheters unless otherwise specified.

From Benson JP. Organization of a postoperative pain service. In: Miller RD, ed. *Anesthesia Update no. 6, Supplement to Anesthesia.* 3rd ed. New York, NY: Churchill Livingstone; 1992:137–153.

**TABLE 13–21.** Intraspinal Opioids for the Treatment of Acute Pain

| Drug | Single Dose* (mg) | Infusion Rate† (mg/h) | Onset (min) | Duration of Single Dose‡ (h) |
|---|---|---|---|---|
| *Epidural* | | | | |
| Morphine | 1–6 | 0.1–1.0 | 30 | 6–24 |
| Meperidine | 20–150 | 5–20 | 5 | 4–8 |
| Methadone | 1–10 | 0.3–0.5 | 10 | 6–10 |
| Hydromorphone | 1–2 | 0.1–0.2 | 15 | 10–16 |
| Fentanyl | 0.025–0.1 | 0.025–0.10 | 5 | 2–4 |
| Sufentanil | 0.01–0.06 | 0.01–0.05 | 5 | 2–4 |
| Alfentanil | 0.5–1 | 0.2 | 15 | 1–3 |
| *Subarachnoid* | | | | |
| Morphine | 0.1–0.3 | | 15 | 8–24* |
| Fentanyl | 0.005–0.025 | | 5 | 3–6 |

*Low doses may be effective when administered to the elderly or when injected in the cervical or thoracic region.

†If combining with a local anesthetic, consider using 0.0625% bupivacaine.

‡Duration of analgesia varies widely; higher doses produce longer duration.

From Task Force on Acute Pain. Ready BH, Edwards WT, eds. *Management of Acute Pain: A Practical Guide.* Seattle, Wash: IASP Publications; 1992:11–21.

central effects of the opiate secondary to the hypercarbia associated with opiate-induced respiratory depression or from the additive effects of other adjuvant medications. It should be thought of as a sign of respiratory depression until proven otherwise.

## Respiratory Depression

Peridural opiate-related respiratory depression occurs in two phases.

### Early

Early respiratory depression is caused by systemic absorption of the opiate through the epidural veins. This effect may be of more concern with the use of potent lipophilic agents, such as fentanyl and sufentanil, and occurs within the first 1 to 2 hours after administration. The degree of respiratory depression is similar to that seen with an equivalent dose of parenterally administered opiate.[106]

### Late

The late phase of respiratory depression occurs primarily with hydrophilic opiates, such as morphine, that tend to accumulate in the cerebrospinal fluid and spread rostrally to the

**TABLE 13–22.** Usual Parameters Used for Epidural Infusion Patient-Controlled Analgesia (Plain Preservative-Free Morphine 0.2 mg/mL or With Additional 0.1% to 0.125% Bupivacaine)

| Parameter | Amount |
|---|---|
| Load | 2–3 mg of morphine |
| Infusion | 0.4 mg/h |
| Patient-controlled dose | 0.2 mg |
| Lockout | 10 min |

From Walmsley PNH. Patient-controlled epidural analgesia. In: Sinatra RS, Hord AH, Ginsberg B, et al, eds. *Acute Pain: Mechanisms and Management.* St Louis, Mo: Mosby–Year Book; 1992:312–325.

brainstem respiratory centers. This problem is noted between 8 and 12 hours after the opiate administration.[107]

## Nursing Care

The best monitor to ensure patient safety is a well-trained, vigilant nurse. One of the contraindications to peridural opiate analgesia is inadequate nursing education.[108] Standard orders must accompany the institution of peridural opiate therapy and should include the monitoring procedures that are expected to occur. Figure 13–8 is an example of the epidural order form used at the Shands Hospital at the University of Florida in Gainesville.

## Techniques

Standard monitoring procedures include frequent checks of respiratory rate and the level of sedation[109] (Table 13–23). Ready suggested the use of a respiratory monitor for patients with the following risk factors: age ≥50 years; American Society of Anesthesiologists physical status 3, 4, or 5; thoracic or upper abdominal incisions; surgical procedures lasting >4 hours; concomitant use of long-acting anesthetics, opiates, or other CNS depressants either before or during surgery; and epidural morphine dose of ≥6 mg or intrathecal morphine dose of ≥0.5 mg.[110] High-risk patients should be monitored more extensively in intensive care units or in intermediate care units where the nurse-to-patient ratio is greater than on a medical-surgical floor.

### Peridural Local Anesthetics

In patients receiving local anesthetics through an epidural catheter, hypotension may develop related to the sympathetic blockade, extensive sensory blockade, and muscle weakness if an excessive dose or inappropriately placed catheter is used. Vital signs should be taken according to protocol as ordered, but in the case of local anesthetics, additional orthostatic blood pressure checks may be necessary as well. Nursing assessment should also include testing for sensation and strength in the lower extremities before ambulation and with each routine pain assessment. This level of nursing assessment, coupled with that of the pain consultant (Fig. 13–9), minimizes the attendant risks.

### Pulse Oximetry

Pulse oximetry is an alternative monitoring technique on the ward that best identifies respiratory depression if a patient is not receiving supplemental oxygen. Periodic end-tidal carbon dioxide checks are also useful in the high-risk patient. The risk of respiratory depression from peridural opiate therapy is 0.2% to 0.4%.[109,111] Pulse oximetry is less sensitive than respiratory rate in detecting respiratory depression, and its use may be unwarranted if a nurse monitors the respiratory rate every 1 to 2 hours.[112]

## When Should Patients With Cancer Receive Peridural Analgesia?

### Indications

Most physicians who work with patients with cancer pain believe that 80% of their patients' pain can be controlled with

ADDRESSOGRAPH:

**PHYSICIAN'S ORDERS
SHANDS at the
UNIVERSITY OF FLORIDA**

*Generic equivalent permitted unless this square
initialed by physician.* ➡️

| DATE/TIME | EPIDURAL / INTRATHECAL NARCOTIC          DOCTOR'S ORDERS | |
|---|---|---|
| | 1) | This patient is receiving epidural/intrathecal narcotics. Notify APS on arrival. Label head of bed, front of chart, infusion bag. (Beeper #393-5300) | |
| | 2) | Epidural/intrathecal bolus of duramorph _____ mg @ _____ AM/PM. | |
| | 3) | Epidural infusion of:  a)  Morphine Sulfate 50 micrograms/ml with Bupivacaine 1/16%. | |
| | (Circle One)  b)  Morphine Sulfate 50 micrograms/ml with Bupivacaine 0.1%. | |
| | c)  Hydromorphone 20 ug/ml. + Bupivacaine 1/16%. | |
| | d)  Hydromorphone 20 ug/ml. + Bupivacaine 0.1%. | |
| | e)  Other | |
| | 4) | Basal infusion at _____ ml/hr, PCEA dose _____ ml, Delay _____ min, 1 hr max _____ ml, Bolus _____ ml. | |
| | 5) | **NO ADDITIONAL NARCOTICS, SEDATIVES OR ANTIEMETICS WITHOUT CLEARANCE FROM APS.** | |
| | 6) | Continuous Pulse oximetry with low saturation alarm set at 90% until d/c'd by APS. | |
| | 7) | Monitor and record respiratory rate, level of consciousness, and $SpO_2$ q2hr until d/c'd by APS. | |
| | 8) | Maintain venous access until routine monitoring resumed. | |
| | 9) | Assess and record pain score (VAS) and side effects q 2 hr **while awake.** | |
| | 10) | If patient is receiving epidural bupivacaine: | |
| | 1)  Take and record B/P lying and sitting prior to ambulation. | |
| | 2)  Assess sensation changes and motor strength BLE prior to getting patient OOB. | |
| | 3)  Notify APS for decreased sensation or decreased motor strength lower extremities, or orthostatic B/P change. | |
| | 4)  Initial ambulation with assistance only. | |
| | 11) | Lower extremity neuro checks for sensation and hip flexion as well as inquiry about back pain Q 4h. | |
| | Call APS for change in exam or symptoms. | |
| | 12) | **Managing side effects:** | |
| | a)  **Itching:**   Naloxone (400 mcg/ml): | |
| | **Adult:** 40 mcg (0.1 ml) IV, then place remainder of vial in >500 cc maintenance IV fluids, | |
| | run @ maintenance rate up to 1 liter.    **Call APS if ineffective.** | |
| | **Child:** 1-2 mcg/kg bolus, then 0.5-1.0 mcg/kg/hr. prn.    **Call APS if ineffective.** | |
| | b)  **Nausea:  Adult:** Droperidol 0.625 mg (1/4 ml) IV x 2, may repeat every 8 hr. prn. | |
| | **If ineffective, give ondansetron 4mg IV x 2 prn.** | |
| | **Child:** Droperidol 0.31 mg (1/8 ml) IV x 2.  **If ineffective, give ondansetron 2mg IV x 2 prn.** | |
| | c)  **Urinary retention > 8°** : Notify APS. | |
| | d)  **Respiratory: Adult:** RR < 12/min. **Child:** school age RR <16, preschool RR <20, or $SpO_2$ | |
| | consistently <90%. Notify APS. | |
| | e)  **Resp. rate: Adult:** <8/min,  **Child:** school age RR <12, preschool RR <16 or pt. unresponsive: | |
| | 1. Turn off epidural infusion. | |
| | 2. Give naloxone (400 mcg/ml): **Adult** - 100 mcg (1/4 ml) IV  **Child:** 10.0 mcg/kg, | |
| | repeat until responsive or RR >12/min. in adults, > 16 in school age child, > 20 in preschool child. | |
| | 3. Notify APS, STAT. (Beeper #393-5300) | |
| | f)  **Sedation:** Notify APS for patient who does not arouse to normal verbal stimulation. | |
| | 13) | Naloxone 0.4 mg/cc **attached** to epidural pump with syringe and needle **if patient travels off unit.** | |
| | Call APS for pulse oximeter orders **if patient must travel off unit.** | |
| | 14) | **NOTIFY APS BEFORE GIVING LOVENOX / FRAGMIN / IV HEPARIN / COUMADIN** | |

REV. 4/00

CHART COPY

**FIGURE 13–8.** Physician order sheet. (Courtesy of Shands Hospital at the University of Florida, Gainesville, Fla.)

**TABLE 13–23.** Example of Bedside Sedation Scale

| Sedation | Description |
|---|---|
| 0 (None) | Alert |
| 1 (Mild) | Occasionally drowsy; easy to arouse |
| 2 (Moderate) | Frequently drowsy; easy to arouse |
| 3 (Severe) | Somnolent; difficult to arouse |
| S (Sleeping) | Normal sleep; easy to arouse |

From Ready LB, Loper KA, Nessly M, et al. Postoperative epidural morphine is safe on surgical wards. *Anesthesiology.* 1991;75:452.

oral analgesics, following the WHO three-step program.[113] However, 60% to 80% of terminally ill patients with cancer still have significant pain.[114] Patients most likely to benefit from invasive delivery systems for analgesic therapy include those receiving around-the-clock strong opiates in adequate doses but without adequate pain relief; those with intolerable side effects from systemic opiates; and those without a tumor in the epidural space or thecal sac.[115]

A therapeutic trial of peridural opiate therapy, usually with morphine, is used to ensure that the patient will experience adequate pain relief. The dose to be used for the trial is based on the patient's previous 24-hour morphine requirement.

### Changeover to Peridural Administration

A conversion schema[116] should include the 24-hour oral morphine requirement change to parenteral morphine (see Table 13–17), the 24-hour nonmorphine requirement change to parenteral morphine, and administration of one half of this calculated dose (owing to incomplete cross-tolerance). The epidural morphine dose is equal to the 24-hour parenteral morphine dose divided by 10; the intrathecal morphine dose is equal to the epidural dose divided by 10.

Concern about opiate withdrawal during the changeover to the peridural route of administration is justified. Withdrawal can be avoided if the initial 24-hour opiate dose reduction is no more than 50% and if further reductions are limited to 20% of the original need per day. A positive response to this therapeutic trial is found when the patient reports a 50% reduction in pain, a 50% reduction in the 24-hour opiate requirement, or both.[116]

### Delivery System

Once a positive therapeutic trial has been established, the appropriate delivery system must be chosen. A commonly held practice is to use an entirely implantable system for any patient with a life expectancy >3 months; patients with an anticipated life expectancy <3 months are candidates for a tunneled epidural catheter with an external pump for continuous infusion or use of intermittent injections[116] (Fig. 13–10).

Other issues to be considered include patient preference, home support available to the patient, physician preference, cost, drug or dose requirements, and location and type of pain. The issues of surgical complications (bleeding, infection, pump pocket seroma, cerebrospinal fluid leaks, and postspinal headache), mechanical complications, and pharmacologic management through the chosen delivery system must be well considered ahead of time. The patient and his or her family members should be aware of the potential problems and solutions.

## When Should Patients With Chronic Pain Receive Peridural Analgesia?

Considerable controversy surrounds peridural opioids in this patient population. Concerns about stable opiate use and efficacy, addiction, tolerance, and dependence, whether founded or not, are widespread. These patients normally do not have a limited life expectancy. Patients with chronic pain can be helped with this therapy. Successful case reports describe implantable infusion systems.[111] The reversible nature of the procedure, even though it initially involves surgical implantation at a significant cost, makes it more desirable and less risky than irreversible neuroablative procedures.

The patient selection criteria proposed by Krames are reasonable, taking into account that the long-term effects of intraspinal infusional therapy are unknown[116] (Table 13–24). These criteria state that the patient with chronic pain should have tried all nonopiate and opiate medications as well as all the other pain management treatment modalities before the institution of neuraxial opiate therapy.[117]

## CONTROVERSIES

### How Should Patients With Opiate Dependence Be Managed?

Opiate dependence must be evaluated for its cause, which may be any of the following:

1. The appropriate use of opiates without psychologic dependence or drug-seeking behavior, as in patients with cancer
2. The appropriate use of opiates, with psychosocial and physiologic reinforcers, as in patients with chronic pain
3. Drug tolerance, physical dependence, and psychologic dependence from the use of illegal drugs or alcohol
4. The potential for psychologic dependence, but current lack of tolerance or dependence, as in the recovering alcoholic or substance abuser[112]

### General Principles

Several general principles of management deserve attention. The expected result of the operation and the reason for preoperative opiate use will determine the therapeutic plan for postoperative pain management.[118] If the preoperative pain problem is expected to be cured by the surgical procedure, the opiates can be quickly and easily weaned after surgery. But if the reason for the use of preoperative opiates will not be eliminated, the need will continue. This is not the time to begin an opiate taper. In fact, every effort should be made to

**TABLE 13–24.** Selection Criteria for Opioid Infusional Therapy for Patients With Non–Cancer-Related Pain

Therapy of last resort
Baseline neurologic examination
Psychological report unequivocally stating nonfunctional pain state

Reprinted by permission of Elsevier Science Publishing Co, Inc, from Intrathecal infusional therapies for intractable pain: patient management guidelines, by Krames ES. *Journal of Pain and Symptom Management,* Vol 8:36. Copyright 1993 by the US Cancer Pain Relief Committee.

**SHANDS HOSPITAL**
at the University of Florida
Gainesville, Florida  32610

**History**

**Physical Examination**

**Progress Notes**

Patient Name:                          MR#:

---

### Anesthesiology Pain Service

Date:                      Time:                      POD:                      Catheter Day:

Patient report:

Pain location:                                              VAS: rest _____ move _____ /10

Side effects:  *Sedation _____   **Nausea _____   Pruritus _____   Urinary retention _____

Current therapy:

SaO2: _____ RA ___ O2 ___ Tx: _____ L/min      RR: _____ /min    Incentive spirometer _____ cc

O2 saturation trend last 8 hrs.: _____

B/P: _____ Tmax: _____ Wt.: _____ kg

Motor exam:                                              Sensory exam:

Site:  L _____ T _____ :  Clean/dry _____      Other: _____

Assessment:

Plan:

☐ Continue current therapy.

☐ Change analgesics as follows:

☐ Treat side effects as follows:

☐ Discontinue therapy today. Further analgesic orders per primary service.

/APS

**0 = none    1 = no tx required    2 = tx with relief    3 = tx without relief

*Sedation:    0 = None    1 = arouses to voice    2 = requires physical stimulation

            3 = Unarousable    5 = Normal sleep

Rev 9 92                                                                                PS3079099215C

**FIGURE 13–9.** University of Florida daily assessment form. (Courtesy of Shands Hospital at the University of Florida, Gainesville, Fla.)

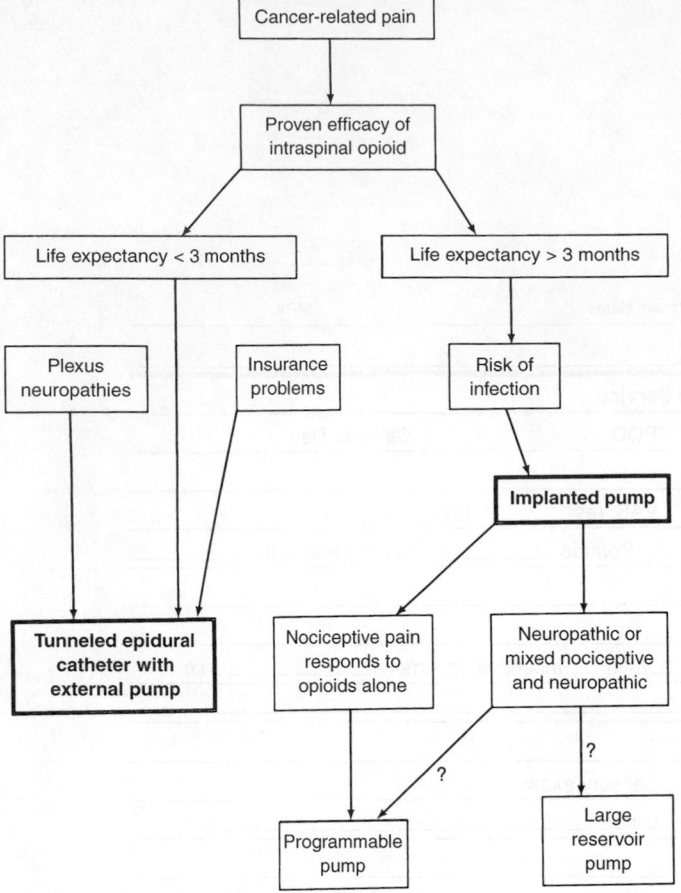

**FIGURE 13–10.** Algorithm for choosing the appropriate peridural opiate delivery system in patients with cancer pain. (Reprinted by permission of Elsevier Science Publishing Co, Inc, from Intrathecal infusional therapies for intractable pain: patient management guidelines, by ES Krames, *Journal of Pain and Symptom Management,* Vol 8:36. Copyright 1993 by the US Cancer Pain Relief Committee.)

control postoperative pain. Confidence in the patient-physician relationship will increase, thus allowing the potential for successful dependency treatment once the acute pain problem has resolved. The patient and all involved health care providers should be well informed as to the plan for both short- and long-term management.

## Specific Methods

Specific management includes all of the techniques discussed previously. Some caveats include a preferred avoidance of opiate use in recovering addicts and the fear of loss of control by others. Intravenous patient-controlled analgesia is useful in the second group of patients because it does not carry the risk of renewed or worsening dependence.[119] In addition, this technique prevents withdrawal as long as opiate agonist-antagonists are not used. Epidural opiate analgesia is useful in the opiate-tolerant patient without psychologic dependence as long as an equivalent dose is prescribed to avoid withdrawal. The dose of epidural opiate is selected based on the previous opiate use, as follows:

1. Convert the average daily preoperative opiate use to its intravenous morphine equivalent.

2. Divide this dose by 24 to obtain the hourly intravenous morphine equivalent.
3. Divide by 4 to obtain the hourly epidural morphine equivalent.[118]

## Psychologic Dependence

Patients with psychologic opiate dependence do not do well with epidural opiate analgesia because they do not experience the central effect they normally obtain. They demand much higher doses than the physician feels comfortable prescribing and do better with an equivalent dose of intravenous opiate. Local anesthetics administered by peripherally placed catheters or epidural catheters are useful to reduce postoperative pain and opiate needs. The opiate dose equivalent to that used before surgery should be prescribed by way of intravenous patient-controlled analgesia to prevent opiate withdrawal.

### Benzodiazepines

Benzodiazepines are useful in allaying anxiety but should be avoided in opiate-dependent patients who are naive to this class of drugs.[118] They must be used in larger doses than normal in those patients who are also dependent on them. Most other adjuvant drugs do not have a role in the treatment of acute pain.

### Specific Abuse Behavior

Specific abuse behavior should be recognized and dealt with firmly and consistently by all health care providers. Limits must be set to avoid ongoing and excessive negotiations regarding drug use for pain management. Other consultants should be used early in difficult cases. Psychologists, psychiatrists, substance abuse experts, and neurologists can be most helpful.

## Who Is at Risk for a Peridural Hematoma?

### Patients Receiving Subcutaneous Standard Heparin

During subcutaneous (mini-dose) prophylaxis, there is no contraindication to the use of neuraxial techniques. The risk of neuraxial bleeding may be reduced by delaying the heparin injection until after the block, and may be increased in debilitated patients or after prolonged therapy.[120]

### Patients Receiving Low Molecular Weight Heparin

The decision to perform a neuraxial block on a patient receiving perioperative low molecular weight heparin (LMWH) must be made on an individual basis by weighing the risk of spinal hematoma with the benefits of regional anesthesia for a specific patient. The American Society of Regional Anesthesia has issued the following recommendations to minimize the risk of spinal hematoma[120]:

1. Monitoring of laboratory results (ie, antifactor Xa level) is not predictive of bleeding and therefore not recommended.

2. Antiplatelet or oral anticoagulant medication administered in combination with LMWH may increase the risk of spinal hematoma.

3. The presence of blood during needle and catheter placement does not necessitate postponement of surgery. However, initiation of LMWH therapy in this setting should be delayed for 24 hours after surgery.

4. Patients on preoperative LMWH can be assumed to have altered coagulation; a single-dose spinal anesthetic may be the safest neuraxial technique in this setting, with needle placement at least 10 to 12 hours after the last LMWH dose.

5. The first dose of LMWH should be administered no sooner than 24 hours after surgery, and indwelling catheters should be removed before this dosing.

6. The decision to implement LMWH therapy in the presence of an indwelling catheter must be made with care, and extreme vigilance must be used in monitoring the patient's neurologic status.

7. Catheter removal should be delayed for at least 10 to 12 hours after an LMWH dose. Subsequent dosing should not occur for at least 2 hours after catheter removal.

### Patients Who Are Anticoagulated During and After Surgery

The literature is somewhat more thorough concerning the issue of epidural catheter placement in patients who are to receive anticoagulation intraoperatively, postoperatively, or both. Odoom and Sih reported no side effects related to hemorrhage or hematoma in 950 patients receiving preoperative oral anticoagulants and intraoperative intraarterial heparin infusions at a rate of 250 to 300 μg/min.[121] They placed epidural catheters after induction of general anesthesia and left them in place for 48 hours.

Baron and coworkers also reported no untoward neurologic events attributable to an epidural hematoma in 912 patients. Patients in this group were anticoagulated transiently with heparin, 75 U/kg; this elevated their activated partial thromboplastin time to 100 seconds or more.[122]

Rao and El-Etr prospectively reviewed the results of 3164 patients who received epidural anesthesia and 847 patients who received spinal anesthesia for vascular surgery.[123] The patients were given 500 units of heparin every 3 minutes during surgery to maintain an activated clotting time level twice baseline. The catheters were removed 24 hours after surgery just before the next dose of heparin. The only untoward events were complaints of postoperative paresthesias (4 patients with epidural anesthesia, 1 patient with spinal anesthesia) that resolved spontaneously, and of low back pain (9 patients with epidural anesthesia, 6 patients with spinal anesthesia) that resolved with analgesia therapy.

As expected, case reports describe epidural and subdural hematomas with anticoagulation, with and without regional anesthesia.[124–126] Recommendations based on the preceding information follow[126]:

1. Avoid lumbar puncture in a patient who is receiving anticoagulants or who has known coagulopathy or significant thrombocytopenia, except in extraordinary circumstances.

2. Discuss the risks and benefits of regional anesthesia with a patient and document the discussion if this approach is chosen in the face of anticoagulation.

3. Use an atraumatic midline approach to the peridural space.

4. Monitor anticoagulation activity and minimize heparin doses.

5. Use short-acting local anesthetics intraoperatively to allow immediate assessment of motor and sensory function.

6. Remove catheters when the heparin levels are low, as determined by appropriate laboratory studies.

7. Continue to monitor the patient's neurologic status closely during the hospital stay and at the follow-up visit.

8. Evaluate the spine radiologically if prolonged, severe low back pain occurs with or without neurologic signs, local tenderness, fever, or leukocytosis.

The choice of analgesics should minimize the degree of sensory and motor block to ensure complete assessment of the neurologic status.[120]

## REGIONAL ANESTHETIC TECHNIQUES

Regional anesthesia and pain management represent different areas of anesthetic practice; however, considerable overlap between these two areas occurs. Most important is knowing *when* to apply the regional techniques in pain management. Such techniques are used diagnostically, prognostically, prophylactically, and therapeutically. With the exception of peridural analgesia, no concise recommendations for regional anesthetic techniques exist in pain management. Nevertheless, some principles that help with everyday decision making can be followed[127]:

1. Use data from the history, physical, laboratory, and radiologic examinations to determine both the classification and the location of the pain problem.

2. Use the least invasive and lowest-risk procedure possible (eg, administer a trigger-point injection first when trying to differentiate between low back pain of myofascial origin and nerve root irritation).

3. Use diagnostic nerve blocks *only* when alternative therapy that will then be as successful and as long lasting is available. (Note: short-term pain relief is almost always possible with some type of regional anesthetic technique, but this relief may give the patient with chronic benign pain a false sense of hope, and the patient may be devastated once the block wears off.)

4. Know the literature with regard to the etiology of the pain problem you are attempting to treat and familiarize yourself with the treatments that have been most successful in the past. A wealth of knowledge that dates back many decades is still valid in this subspecialty. Your patients deserve the benefit of both the historical and current literature when deciding on the best course of action.

5. Combine other modalities of pain management, such as physical or psychologic therapy, to gain the best result possible. Rarely does nerve block alone cure a pain problem of a magnitude that prompts a patient to seek the help of a pain management expert.

A more extensive set of principles is available for review if these techniques are to become a part of pain management practice.[128]

## What Techniques Are Applicable?

### Continuous Catheter Infusions for Acute Pain

Repeated injections into nerves or nerve plexuses are less than desirable from the standpoint of patient comfort and manpower requirements. Placement of a catheter into the nerve sheath or plexus sheath permits a continuous infusion, thus eliminating those problems. Catheters have been used, among other locations, in the wound, in nerve sheaths after amputation, in the brachial plexus, and in the sciatic nerve sheath.[129–132] Lower extremity catheters are indicated when only one extremity is involved or when a patient's medical status dictates a minimum of hemodynamic change.

### Cancer Pain

Once oral analgesics no longer control the pain, cause intolerable side effects, or both, and once the pain is well localized, well characterized, somatic or visceral in origin, and does not comprise a component of a pain syndrome characterized by multifocal aches and pains, regional techniques may be considered.[133] They should always be used prognostically before neurolytic or ablative procedures to predict efficacy and to allow the patient to experience the expected loss of sensation.

Specific somatic blocks, trigger-point injections, and sympathetic nerve blocks are also useful in the treatment of cancer pain related to reflex sympathetic dystrophy, some neuropathic conditions, and acute and chronic herpes zoster.[134] Last, regional techniques can be used as an alternative to opioid analgesics in crisis management due to intractable pain. This approach allows the reversal of tolerance that would otherwise occur, especially as the tumor process progresses.

### Chronic Pain

The patient with chronic benign pain can also benefit from regional anesthetic techniques in some of the same situations as the patient with cancer pain.

#### Epidural Steroid Injection

Epidural steroid injections are a popular treatment modality for many spine-related pain conditions. They appear to be most efficacious in conditions of nerve root irritation; their efficacy in spinal stenosis is controversial, and they are rarely effective in spondylosis and functional low back pain.[135]

The following are guidelines for epidural steroid injections:

1. Place the patient in the lateral decubitus position with the affected side down because the steroid becomes hyperbaric when it is mixed with saline or local anesthetic.
2. Once the epidural space is located, mix the steroid with 2 to 4 mL of saline or local anesthetic. The patient may experience transient radicular pain with the injection.
3. Clear the steroid from the needle before its removal from the epidural space.
4. Keep the patient in position with the affected side down for at least 10 minutes to ensure that the steroid has had time to bathe the affected nerve root.
5. If local anesthetic has been used, test for correct placement of the drug by having the patient perform a straight leg

test; performance should be improved compared with that of the preinjection period.
6. Warn the patient that the local anesthetic effect (if used) wears off in a number of hours and that the full steroid effect may not be apparent for 5 to 6 days.

#### Neuroma Injection

Another commonly used technique involves the injection of local anesthetics and steroids into the area of a neuroma. Nerves can be trapped in scar tissue after surgery or other injury and can be treated effectively in this manner. Corticosteroids suppress spontaneous ectopic discharges from entrapped nerves, stabilizing the nerve membrane for 2 weeks or longer.[136] The injection of a combination of local anesthetic and depot corticosteroid is useful in the treatment of myofascial pain with trigger points, arthritic joint pain, and facet joint pain.[137–140]

## NEUROLYTIC BLOCKS

### When and How Are They Used?

A neurolytic block involves the application of a chemical agent onto or into a nerve, the epidural space, the subdural space, or the subarachnoid space to destroy the axon or the cell bodies of somatic nerves, sympathetic nerves, or both. The agents most frequently used are phenol, alcohol, or glycerol. Although many clinicians perform neurolytic blocks for chronic benign pain, the risk of a severe neuralgia during nerve regeneration has led experts in the field of pain management to state that "with few special exceptions, neurolytic block of somatic spinal nerves should not be done in patients with nonmalignant chronic pain."[141] On the other hand, if a series of prognostic blocks with local anesthetic relieves cancer pain in a patient with limited life expectancy, the neurolytic block is indicated. The increasing popularity of neuraxial analgesia has supplanted neurolytic blocks to some extent because of the effectiveness and safety of neuraxial techniques. The principles of neurolytic block application, combined with the general principles of regional anesthetic techniques used for pain management, are as follows[141]:

1. Only physicians with extensive experience, skill, and knowledge of the procedures and the management of chronic pain should perform neurolytic blocks.
2. Neurolytic blocks should be used in conjunction with all other appropriate pain management techniques because they do not necessarily relieve all pain and eventually lose effectiveness.
3. Careful patient selection should be combined with the least invasive technique that has the least side effects and the best potential for pain relief.
4. The patient and the patient's family must be informed regarding the details of the procedure, the expected outcome, and the potential side effects and complications.
5. The neurolytic block should be preceded by two or three diagnostic or prognostic blocks with local anesthetic.
6. Assessment of the results of the block necessitates close observation by the physician, nurses, and the patient's family members and must take into consideration the many

factors that can influence a patient's report of pain relief or lack thereof.

7. Pain relief in a patient previously requiring large doses of opiate analgesics carries the risk of causing respiratory depression (as the respiratory stimulus is removed) and withdrawal symptoms (if the opiate is stopped too quickly).

# NEUROAUGMENTATION

## How Does a Transcutaneous Electrical Nerve Stimulator Work?

Two basic mechanisms may explain the effective pain relief found with TENS and spinal cord stimulation. However, the true mechanism of pain relief with these modalities remains uncertain.

### Gate Control

The first mechanism involves an understanding of the gate control theory of pain, which was first described by Melzack and Wall in 1965.[142] A delta and C fibers are responsible for the transmission of pain to the spinal cord. Once they synapse on interneurons in the substantia gelatinosa, the "gate" is opened, reducing presynaptic inhibition and allowing the painful stimulus to continue up the central neuraxis.

When transmission from large-diameter, myelinated A fibers occurs (carrying sensations of light touch and pressure), the gate closes, facilitating presynaptic inhibition of the gelatinosa cells and blocking the flow of painful information. Neurostimulation is thought to involve stimulation of the large-diameter A fibers, thus blocking the transmission of pain through the C fibers to the brain.

### Release of Endogenous Opioids

Electrical stimulation also may release endogenous opioid-like substances that act at the opiate receptors in the CNS to mediate the pain response. β-Endorphin levels are elevated in the plasma[143] and in the cerebrospinal fluid[144] regardless of which mode of stimulation is used. However, other investigators have found no difference in endorphin levels before, during, or after TENS therapy.[145]

## Who Is a Candidate for a Transcutaneous Electrical Nerve Stimulator Unit?

### Acute Pain

Most research evaluating the effectiveness of a TENS has been done in the area of acute pain. Ordog found TENS to be useful for sprains, lacerations, fractures, hematomas, and contusions and as effective as acetaminophen with codeine.[146] It is also useful for postoperative pain, dental pain, and the pain of labor and delivery.[147–149]

### Chronic Pain

TENS is reported to be effective in the treatment of chronic low back pain, peripheral neuropathies, postherpetic neuralgia, reflex sympathetic dystrophy, phantom limb pain, arthritis, and pain associated with malignancies.[150–154] Although a decline in use occurs with time, Johnson and associates reported that 58% of patients surveyed found that the efficacy remained unchanged with long-term use (mean duration, 4 years).[155] As can be seen from the preceding list of indications, most of the successfully treated pain problems are of neuropathic origin. Those of nociceptive origin are less likely to respond to TENS.[156]

## When Is a Spinal Cord Stimulator Considered?

The classic indication for spinal cord stimulation is neuropathic pain of an extremity that has failed pharmacologic, surgical, physical, and psychologic therapies. Spinal cord stimulation has been successfully used in postlaminectomy syndrome, arachnoiditis, intercostal neuralgia, complex regional pain syndrome, peripheral neuropathy, phantom limb pain, radiculopathy, peripheral pain associated with ischemic vascular disease, and postherpetic neuralgia.[157,158] This therapy has been in use since the late 1970s, with reported variable responses. Initial enthusiasm after the first trials in the 1970s subsided over time when long-term relief was not always as good as anticipated. This finding possibly was a result of "uncritical overuse" of this reversible and extremely safe surgical treatment.[155]

In the 1970s, the introduction of percutaneous dorsal column stimulators (DCSs) also met with the same level of enthusiasm owing to their ease of insertion and decreased invasiveness. Similarly, however, the number of late failures caused significant reevaluation of the use and indications for the DCS and spinal cord stimulator. A review of >500 patients treated with DCSs up to 1978 showed a long-term satisfactory outcome rate of between 30% and 40%.[159] The incidence of successful results after 4 years was only 26%.[159] With the percutaneous approach, the short-term success rate reportedly is ≤80%; the long-term success rate is ≤50%.[160] A list of indications is presented in Table 13–25.[161]

# PHYSICAL THERAPY

Rehabilitation and physical therapy have been used for the treatment of acute injuries for many years and with great success. Problems develop when patients have pain that is out of proportion to their injury and that prevents completion of therapy to aid recovery. In many cases, physical therapists can decrease acute, subacute, and chronic pain problems. Patients with cancer pain also should have the benefit of physical therapy during all phases of their disease, including the terminal stage, when the risk of pain is highest.

Three goals of physical therapy used specifically for pain control are described by Yeh and colleagues[162]:

1. Determination of the most effective means of decreasing pain
2. Correction of the identified dysfunction or dysfunctions
3. Restoration of a patient's confidence in his or her ability to move and to enjoy physical activity by reducing the fear of further injury or pain

**TABLE 13–25.** Neurogenic, Neuropathic, Deafferentiation, and Other Pain Syndromes Likely to Respond to Dorsal Column Stimulators

**Peripheral Nerve and Root Lesions**

Posttraumatic neuropathy:
  Trauma due to injuries, surgery, entrapment, or incisional scar
  Causalgia and reflex sympathetic dystrophy
  Postamputation pain (stump and phantom)
  Coccygodynia
Diabetic neuropathy
Plexus lesions induced by trauma, malignancy, and radiation*
Rhizopathy
  Postherpetic neuralgia
  Cervical syndrome
  Low back pain (particularly radicular pain due to arachnoiditis and
    epidural fibrosis)

**Spinal Cord Lesions**

Postcordotomy dysesthesia
Multiple sclerosis
Paraplegia (radicular pain at level of lesion and pain below level of lesion
  with preservation of sensibility)

**Peripheral Vascular Disease**

*Plexus avulsion pain is not likely to respond to dorsal column stimulation.
From Meyerson BA. Electrical stimulation of the spinal cord and brain. In: Bonica JJ, ed. *The Management of Pain*. Philadelphia, Pa: Lea & Febiger; 1990:1862–1877.

## When Should Physical Therapy Be Prescribed?

### Therapeutic Exercise

In acute pain states, active exercise may be contraindicated owing to the potential for further injury or problems with healing. The advice of an orthopedist or a physiatrist should be sought in this circumstance. In the healing phase, passive range-of-motion exercises are indicated to maintain muscle and joint mobility.

Once healing has occurred and chronic pain is the main problem, the patient must be encouraged to increase activity, first with the aid of analgesics and injections when appropriate. Eventually, with improved pain control, there is minimal or no need for any other management technique. When a specific chronic pain problem such as reflex sympathetic dystrophy or radicular pain is treated, physical therapy may be prescribed immediately after a regional anesthetic technique if one is used initially.

The goals of physical therapy in cancer pain initially are the same as for acute and chronic pain. In advanced stages,

**TABLE 13–26.** Therapeutic Heating Modalities

| Primary Mode of Heat Transfer | Modality | Depth |
|---|---|---|
| Conduction | Hot packs | Superficial heat |
| | Paraffin bath | Superficial heat |
| Convection | Hydrotherapy | Superficial heat |
| | Fluidotherapy | Superficial heat |
| Conversion | Infrared | Superficial heat |
| | Shortwaves | Deep heat |
| | Microwaves | Deep heat |
| | Ultrasound | Deep heat |

From Lee MHM, Itoh M, Yang G-FW, et al. Physical therapy and rehabilitation medicine. In: Bonica JJ, ed. *The Management of Pain*. 2nd ed. Philadelphia, Pa: Lea & Febiger; 1990:1769–1788.

the specific needs of the cancer patient population come into play, including respiratory management to allow free and effective breathing, encouragement of independence in daily living (eg, the ability to transfer from bed to wheelchair), and relaxation therapy (both peripheral and general).[162,163]

### Other Options

Besides therapeutic exercise, the physical therapist has many other options for pain management. Techniques to consider include thermotherapy[164] (Table 13–26), cryotherapy (cold packs, vapo-coolant sprays), electrotherapy (iontophoresis, TENS), and passive mechanotherapies (massage, manipulation, traction). Because these interventions are applied without *active* patient participation, some experts question their utility in the treatment of chronic pain. Although the final goal is independent, pain-free activity without analgesics, the initial treatment phase is a time for building trust between the patient and health care provider. Few patients will be successful if they are asked to begin a vigorous exercise program that involves a painful extremity without the application of analgesic techniques.

## PSYCHOLOGIC THERAPY

### When Should a Psychologist or Psychiatrist Become Involved?

After thorough evaluation and assessment of psychosocial dysfunction, the appropriate psychologic intervention can be applied. Psychiatrists and psychologists are trained in many of the techniques used. Choosing the appropriate specialist is based on that person's level of interest and expertise in the interventional therapy requested.

### Suicide Precautions

It is crucial to have access to psychiatrists who are willing to evaluate and treat severely depressed patients who are suicidal. The psychologist often uncovers the suicidal intention during the initial assessment. The psychiatrist is then consulted to confirm the diagnosis and admit the patient to the psychiatric unit, if needed. This task can be emotional and difficult, not only for the patient but also for his or her family and health care providers. All involved must understand that the decision for psychiatric admission is made with the patient's best interest in mind and to allow further therapy to help alleviate depression and pain.

### Chronic Pain Evaluation

Aside from this rare but important need for psychiatric support, a psychiatrist or a psychologist can and should evaluate all patients with chronic pain as part of the multidisciplinary approach to chronic pain management. The interventions used are adjuvants to the medical treatments discussed earlier. The objective of such therapy is to change the perception of pain by altering the meaning of the pain experience or the affect associated with it, by changing the pain behavior and expression, or both. Many times, an accurate medical diagnosis and treatment plan fails without this additional psychologic

**TABLE 13–27.** Major Types of Cognitive-Behavioral Therapies for Pain

**Cognitive Restructuring**

Patients are taught to monitor and evaluate negative thoughts and to generate more accurate and adaptive cognitions. *Example:* A patient with chronic pain who responds to increased pain by thinking, "I can't take this anymore" is taught to examine such thoughts and develop more accurate and adaptive ones; for example, "Is it really true that I can't deal with this? No. It may be difficult, but I've done it before and can do it again."

**Coping Skills Training**

Patients are provided a rationale for the use of techniques and then taught various skills for managing pain stress.

*Relaxation*

*Example:* Physical or mental relaxation methods

*Imagery*

*Example:* Imagining pleasant scenes

*Coping Self-Statements*

*Examples:* "Relax." "I can cope." "Focus on what you have to do."

From Turner JA, Romano JM. Cognitive-behavioral therapy. In: Bonica JJ, ed. *The Management of Pain.* 2nd ed. Philadelphia, PA: Lea & Febiger; 1990:1711–1721.

treatment. Family members or loved ones also must be incorporated into the treatment plan to ensure a successful therapeutic trial. Patients with acute pain also can benefit from many of these same therapies, particularly if a history of chronic pain is present. The additional psychologic problems associated with death and dying experienced by patients with cancer pain can be tempered by many of the same techniques.

## What Are Appropriate Cognitive and Behavioral Interventions?

No psychologic technique is appropriate for all patients with pain. Each situation requires careful evaluation, possibly over many return visits, to determine the best approach. Several techniques are potentially useful, including cognitive-behavioral therapy, biofeedback therapy, hypnosis, and psychotherapy.

### Cognitive-Behavioral Therapy

The idea behind the application of cognitive-behavioral treatment strategies[165] (Table 13–27) is that a patient can learn to change the negative impact of pain, thus decreasing suffering and pain behavior (see Fig. 13–4) and increasing control over the pain. These techniques have been found to be useful in a variety of pain problems.

### Biofeedback

Biofeedback is a different approach that uses an electronic device to detect and amplify biologic responses and convert them into information that patients can use to change their response to the pain. This technique has been found to be successful in the treatment of tension or migraine headaches, myofascial pain, and temporomandibular joint syndrome.

### Hypnosis

Hypnosis has been successful in reducing or eliminating a variety of clinical pain problems, including acute and chronic pain syndromes.

### Psychotherapy

Last, psychotherapy is defined as any form of treatment for mental illness, behavioral maladaptation, and other problems assumed to be of an emotional nature. The therapist deliberately establishes a professional relationship with a patient for the purpose of modifying, removing, or retarding existing symptoms, attenuating or reversing disturbed patterns of behavior, and promoting positive personality growth and development.[166] This type of therapy must be chosen carefully and is appropriate when[167]:

1. Much or all of the problem seems to follow from a psychologic disorder without a major physical contribution.
2. Emotional changes have developed in response to suffering related to a prolonged and severe illness without evidence of premorbid predisposition to psychologic illness.
3. The aim of treatment is to change subjective distress related to relationships, conflicts, and the sense of self.

The major types of psychotherapy used in the treatment of patients with chronic pain include supportive, dynamic, family, and group therapies.

### References

1. Portenoy RK. Diagnosis of cancer pain syndromes. In: Field H, ed. *Pain Syndromes in Neurologic Practices.* New York, NY: Butterworth; 1990:237.
2. Mersky H, ed. Classification of chronic pain: description of chronic pain syndromes and definition of pain terms. *Pain.* 1986;S1(suppl 3):217.
3. Bonica JJ. Definitions and taxonomy of pain. In: Bonica JJ, ed. *The Management of Pain.* Philadelphia, Pa: Lea & Febiger; 1990:18.
4. Portenoy RK. Mechanisms of clinical pain, observations and speculations. *Neurol Clin.* 1989;7:205.
5. Revill SI, Robinson JO, Rosen M, et al. The reliability of a linear analogue for evaluating pain. *Anaesthesia.* 1976;31:1991.
6. Myles PS, Troedel S, Boquest M, et al. The pain visual analog scale: is it linear or nonlinear? *Anesth Analg.* 1999;89:1517.
7. Acute Pain Management Guideline Panel, US Department of Health and Human Services. *Acute Pain Management: Operative or Medical Procedures and Trauma.* Clinical Practice Guideline. Rockville, Md: Agency for Health Care Policy and Research, Public Health Service; 1992:116. Publication AHCPR 92-0032.
8. National Institutes of Health Consensus Panel. The integrated approach to the management of pain. *J Pain Symptom Manage.* 1987;2:35.
9. Loeser JD. Concepts of pain. In: Staton-Hicks M, Boas R, eds. *Chronic Low Back Pain.* New York, NY: Raven Press; 1982:145.
10. Beyer JE, McGrath PJ, Berde CN. Discordance between self-report and behavior pain measures in children age 3-7 years after surgery. *J Pain Symptom Manage.* 1990;5:350.
11. Lewis T. *Pain.* New York, NY: MacMillan; 1942:173.
12. Bruera E, Ripamonti C. Adjuvants to opioid analgesics. In: Pratt RB, ed. *Cancer Pain.* Philadelphia, Pa: JB Lippincott; 1993:143.
13. Amitryptyline. *Physicians' Desk Reference.* 53rd ed. Montvale, NJ: Medical Economics; 1999:3418.
14. Tramedal. *Physicians' Desk Reference.* 53rd ed. Montvale, NJ: Medical Economics; 1999:2255.
15. Stoelting RK. Pharmacokinetics and pharmacodynamics of injected and inhaled drugs. In: Stoelting RK, ed. *Pharmacology and Physiology in Anesthetic Practice.* Philadelphia, Pa: JB Lippincott; 1987:2.
16. Reidenberg MM. Effect of disease states on plasma protein binding of drugs. *Med Clin North Am.* 1974;58:1103.
17. Hudson RJ. Basic principles of pharmacology. In: Barash PG, Cullen BF, Stoelting RK, eds. *Clinical Anesthesia.* Philadelphia, Pa: JB Lippincott; 1989:137.
18. Pelz M, Merskey H. A description of the psychological effects of chronic painful lesions. *Pain.* 1982;14:293.
19. Sternbach RA, Wolf SR, Murphy RW, et al. Traits of pain patients: the low-back "loser." *Psychosomatics.* 1973;14:226.
20. Sternbach RA, Timmermans G. Personality changes associated with reduction of pain. *Pain.* 1975;1:177.

21. Fields HL. The psychology of pain. In: Fields HL, ed. *Pain*. New York, NY: McGraw-Hill; 1987:171.

22. Fordyce WE. The acquisition of operant pain. In: Fordyce WE, ed. *Behavioral Methods for Chronic Pain and Illness*. St Louis, Mo: Mosby; 1976:41.

23. Gunn CC, Milbrandt E. Early and subtle signs of low back pain. *Spine*. 1978;3:267.

24. Travell J. Myofascial trigger points: clinical view. *Adv Pain Res Ther*. 1976;1:919.

25. Rudy TE, Turk DC, Brena SF. Differential utility of medical procedures in the assessment of chronic pain patients. *Pain*. 1988;34:167.

26. Frymoyer JW. Back pain and sciatica. *N Engl J Med*. 1988;318:291.

27. Schipper J, Kardaun JWPF, Braakman R, et al. Lumbar disk herniation: diagnosis with CT or myelography? *Radiology*. 1987;165:227.

28. Task Force on Acute Pain. *Management of Acute Pain: A Practical Guide*. Seattle, Wash: IASP Publications; 1992:11.

29. Monks R. Psychotropic drugs. In: Bonica JJ, ed. *The Management of Pain*. 2nd ed. Philadelphia, Pa: Lea & Febiger; 1990:1676.

30. Portenoy RK. Chronic opioid therapy in non-malignant pain. *J Pain Symptom Manage*. 1990;5(suppl):S46.

31. Fishbain DA, Rosomoff HL, Rosomoff RS. Review article: drug abuse, dependence, and addiction in chronic pain patients. *Clin J Pain*. 1992;8:77.

32. Portenoy RK, Foley KM. Chronic use of opioid analgesics in nonmalignant pain: report of 38 cases. *Pain*. 1986;25:171.

33. World Health Organization. *Cancer Pain Relief and Palliative Care*. Geneva, Switzerland: World Health Organization; 1990:9. WHO Technical Report Series 804.

34. Levy MH. Pain management in advanced cancer. *Semin Oncol*. 1985;12:394.

35. Patt RB, Szalados JE, Wu CL. Pharmacotherapeutic guidelines. In: Patt RB, ed. *Cancer Pain*. Philadelphia, Pa: JB Lippincott; 1993:574.

36. Onghena P, Van Houdenhove B. Antidepressant-induced analgesia in chronic nonmalignant pain: a meta-analysis of 39 placebo-controlled studies. *Pain*. 1992;49:205.

37. Tanelian DL, Brosse WG. Neuropathic pain can be relieved by drugs that are use-dependent sodium channel blockers: lidocaine, carbamazepine, and mexiletine. *Anesthesiology*. 1991;74:949.

38. Davis KD, Treede RD, Raja SN, et al. Topical application of clonidine relieves hyperalgesia in patients with sympathetically maintained pain. *Pain*. 1991;47:309.

39. Raskin NH, Levinson SA, Hoffman PM, et al. Post-sympathectomy neuralgia: amelioration with diphenylhydantoin and carbamazepine. *Am J Surg*. 1974;128:75.

40. Kocher R. Use of psychotropic drugs for the treatment of chronic severe pain. *Adv Pain Res Ther*. 1976;1:579.

41. Fromm GH, Terrence CF, Chattha AS. Baclofen in the treatment of trigeminal neuralgia: double-blind study and long-term follow-up. *Ann Neurol*. 1984;15:240.

42. Ghostine SY, Comair YG, Turner DM, et al. Phenoxybenzamine in the treatment of causalgia. *J Neurosurg*. 1984;60:1263.

43. Hill CS. Oral opioid analgesics. In: Patt RB, ed. *Cancer Pain*. Philadelphia, Pa: JB Lippincott; 1993:137.

44. Patt RB, Szalados JE, Wu CL. Pharmacotherapeutic guidelines. In: Patt RB, ed. *Cancer Pain*. Philadelphia, Pa: JB Lippincott; 1993:565.

45. Marchettini P, Lacerenza M, Marangoni C, et al. Lidocaine test in neuralgia. *Pain*. 1992;48:377.

46. Graubard DJ, Robertazzi RW, Peterson MC. One year's experience with intravenous procaine. *Anesth Analg*. 1948;27:222.

47. Boas RA, Covino BG, Shahnarian A. Analgesic responses to IV lignocaine. *Br J Anaesth*. 1982;54:501.

48. Edwards WT, Habib F, Burney RG, et al. Intravenous lidocaine in the management of various chronic pain states: a review of 211 cases. *Reg Anesth*. January-March 1983;1.

49. Glazer S, Portenoy RK. Review article: systemic local anesthetics in pain control. *J Pain Symptom Manage*. 1991;6:30.

50. Kastrup J, Peterson P, Dejgard R, et al. Intravenous lidocaine infusion: a new treatment of chronic painful diabetic neuropathy? *Pain*. 1987;28:69.

51. Dejgard A, Peterson P, Kastrup J. Mexiletine for treatment of chronic painful diabetic neuropathy. *Lancet*. 1988;1:9.

52. Jönsson A, Cassuto J, Hanson B. Inhibition of burn pain by intravenous lignocaine infusion. *Lancet*. 1991;338:151.

53. Dixon CL, Berger JJ. Intravenous lidocaine in the treatment of postherpetic neuralgia [abstract]. *Reg Anesth*. 1992;17(suppl):61.

54. Bonica JJ. Postoperative pain. In: Bonica JJ, ed. *The Management of Pain*. 2nd ed. Philadelphia, Pa: Lea & Febiger; 1990:466.

55. Brown DL, Carpenter RL. Perioperative analgesia: a review of risks and benefits. *J Cardiothorac Anesth*. 1990;4:363.

56. Ali J, Weisel RD, Layug AB, et al. Consequences of postoperative alterations in respiratory mechanics. *Am J Surg*. 1974;128:376.

57. Buckley DN, MacIntosh J, Beattie WS. Epidural analgesia prevents loss of lung volume [abstract]. *Anesthesiology*. 1990;73(suppl):A764.

58. Craig DG. Postoperative recovery of pulmonary function. *Anesth Analg*. 1981;60:46.

59. Mankikian B, Cantineau JP, Bertrand M, et al. Improvement of diaphragmatic function by a thoracic extradural block after upper abdominal surgery. *Anesthesiology*. 1988;68:379.

60. Modig J. Respiration and circulation after total hip replacement surgery: a comparison between parenteral analgesics and continuous lumbar epidural block. *Acta Anaesthesiol Scand*. 1976;20:225.

61. Christopherson R, Rock P, Parker S, et al. Tachycardia occurs more frequently postoperatively than intraoperatively in patients at risk for perioperative myocardial ischemia. *Anesthesiology*. 1989;71:A950.

62. Ellis JE, Busse JR, Foss JF, et al. Postoperative management of myocardial ischemia. *Anesth Clin*. 1991;9:609.

63. Breslow MJ. Neuroendocrine responses to surgery. In: Breslow MJ, Miller CF, Rogers MC, eds. *Perioperative Management*. St Louis, Mo: Mosby–Year Book; 1990:180.

64. Cousins MJ. Acute pain and the injury response: immediate and prolonged effects. *Reg Anesth*. 1989;16:162.

65. Modig J, Borg T, Karlström G, et al. Thrombo-embolism after total hip replacement: role of epidural and general anesthesia. *Anesth Analg*. 1983;62:174.

66. Bing HI. Viscerocutaneous and cutaneovisceral thoracic reflexes. *Acta Med Scand*. 1936;89:57.

67. Nimmo WS. Effect of anaesthesia on gastric motility and emptying. *Br J Anaesth*. 1984;56:29.

68. Philbin DM, Rosow CE, Schneider RC, et al. Fentanyl and sufentanil anesthesia revisited: how much is enough? *Anesthesiology*. 1990;73:5.

69. Suchner U, Rothkopf MM. Metabolic effects of the neuroendocrine stress response. *Anesth Clin North Am*. 1988;6:1.

70. Ruthberg H, Hakanson E, Anderberg B, et al. Effect of extradural administration of morphine or bupivacaine on the endocrine response to upper abdominal surgery. *Anaesthesia*. 1985;40:748.

71. Traynor C, Paterson JL, Ward ID, et al. Effects of extradural analgesia and vagal blockade on the metabolic and endocrine response to upper abdominal surgery. *Br J Anaesth*. 1982;54:319.

72. Kehlet H. Modification of responses to surgery by neural blockade: clinical implications. In: Cousins MJ, Bridenbaugh PO, eds. *Neural Blockade in Clinical Anesthesia and Management in Pain*. 2nd ed. Philadelphia, Pa: JB Lippincott; 1988:145.

73. Bell SD. The correlation between pulmonary function and resting and dynamic pain scores in post-aortic surgery patients. *Anesth Analg*. 1991;72:S18.

74. Hendolin H, Lahtinen J, Lärsimies E, et al. The effect of thoracic epidural analgesia on respiratory function after cholecystectomy. *Acta Anaesthesiol Scand*. 1987;31:645.

75. Rawal N, Sjöstrand U, Christoffersson E, et al. Comparison of intramuscular and epidural morphine for postoperative analgesia in the grossly obese: influence of postoperative ambulation and pulmonary function. *Anesth Analg*. 1984;63:583.

76. Hasenbos M, van Egmond J, Gielen M, et al. Post-operative analgesia by high thoracic epidural versus intramuscular nicomorphine after thoracotomy, part III: the effect of pre- and post-operative analgesia on morbidity. *Acta Anaesthesiol Scand*. 1987;31:645.

77. Shulman M, Sandler AN, Bradley JW, et al. Post-thoracotomy pain and pulmonary function following epidural and systemic morphine. *Anesthesiology*. 1984;61:569.

78. El-Baz N, Goldin M. Continuous epidural infusion of morphine for pain relief after cardiac operations. *J Thorac Cardiovasc Surg*. 1987;93:878.

79. Vanstrum GS, Bjornson KM, Ilko R. Postoperative effects of intrathecal morphine in coronary artery bypass surgery. *Anesth Analg*. 1988;67:261.

80. Moore JM, Liu SS. How acute pain management affects outcome. *Tech Reg Anesth Pain Manage*. 1997;1:64.

81. Yeager MP, Glass DD, Neff RK, et al. Epidural anesthesia and analgesia in high risk surgical patients. *Anesthesiology*. 1987;66:729.

82. Waskinck J, Hurford W, Gelb C, et al. Epidural opioid analgesia does not alter the neuro-endocrine response to thoracotomy. *Anesth Analg*. 1990;70:S422.

83. Scott NB, Mogensen T, Bigler D, et al. Continuous thoracic extradural 0.5% bupivacaine with or without morphine: effect on quality of blockade, lung function and surgical stress response. *Br J Anaesth*. 1989;62:252.

84. Bonnet F, Blery C, Zatan M, et al. Effect of epidural morphine on postoperative pulmonary function. *Acta Anaesthesiol Scand.* 1984;28:147.

85. Pflug AE, Murphy TM, Butler SH, et al. The effects of postoperative peridural analgesia on pulmonary therapy and pulmonary complications. *Anesthesiology.* 1974;41:8.

86. Borg T, Modig J. Potential antithrombotic effect of local anesthetics due to their inhibition of platelet aggregation. *Acta Anaesthesiol Scand.* 1985;29:739.

87. Modig J, Borg T, Bagge L, et al. Role of epidural and of general anesthesia in fibrinolysis and coagulation after total hip replacement. *Br J Anaesth.* 1983;55:625.

88. Ahn H, Bronge A, Johansson K, et al. Effect of continuous postoperative epidural analgesia on intestinal motility. *Br J Surg.* 1988;75:1176.

89. England DW, Davis JJ, Timmins AE, et al. Gastric emptying: a study to compare the effects of intrathecal morphine and i.m. papaveretum analgesia. *Br J Anaesth.* 1987;59:1403.

90. Scheinin B, Asantila R, Orko R. The effect of bupivacaine and morphine on pain and bowel function after colonic surgery. *Acta Anaesthesiol Scand.* 1987;31:161.

91. Grass JA, Sakina NT. Epidural anesthesia and analgesia results in shorter hospital stay after total abdominal hysterectomy [abstract]. *Reg Anesth.* 1992;17(suppl):77.

92. Liu SS, Carpenter RL, Mackey DC, et al. Effects of perioperative analgesic technique on rate of recovery after colon surgery. *Anesthesiology.* 1995;83:757.

93. Bellamy CD, McDonnell FJ, Colclough GW. Postoperative epidural pain management results in shorter hospital stay than IV PCA morphine: a comparison in anterior cruciate ligament repair [abstract]. *Anesthesiology.* 1989;71(suppl):A685.

94. Dixon CL, Sefton W, Gravenstein N. Epidural analgesia after donor nephrectomy decreases duration of hospitalization [abstract]. *Reg Anesth.* 1992;17(suppl):75.

95. Brull SJ, Lieponis JV, Murphy MJ, et al. Acute and long-term benefits of iliac crest donor site perfusion with local anesthetics. *Anesth Analg.* 1992;74:145.

96. Jacobson L, Chabal C. Prolonged relief of acute post-amputation phantom limb pain with intrathecal fentanyl and epidural morphine. *Anesthesiology.* 1989;71:984.

97. Bach S, Noreng MF, Tjellden NU. Phantom limb pain in amputees during the first 12 months following limb amputation, after preoperative lumbar epidural blockade. *Pain.* 1988;33:297.

98. Crile GW, Lower WE. *Anoci-association.* Philadelphia, Pa: WB Saunders; 1914.

99. Tverskoy M, Cozacov C, Ayache M, et al. Postoperative pain after inguinal herniorrhaphy with different types of anesthesia. *Anesth Analg.* 1990;70:29.

100. McQuay HJ, Carroll D, Moore RA. Postoperative orthopedic pain: the effect of opiate premedication and local anesthetic blocks. *Pain.* 1988;33:291.

101. Jebeles JA, Reilly JS, Gutierrez JF, et al. The effect of pre-incisional infiltration of tonsils with bupivacaine on the pain following tonsillectomy under general anesthesia. *Pain.* 1991;47:305.

102. Benson JP. Organization of a postoperative pain service. In: Miller RD, ed. *Anesthesia Update No. 6: Supplement to Anesthesia.* 3rd ed. New York, NY: Churchill Livingstone; 1992:137.

103. Kampe S, Weigand C, Kaufman J, et al. Postoperative analgesia with no motor block by continuous epidural infusion of ropivacaine 0.1% and sufentanil after total hip replacement. *Anesth Analg.* 1999;89:395.

104. Scott DA, Blake D, Buckland M, et al. A comparison of epidural ropivacaine infusion alone and in combination with 1, 2, and 4 microg/ml fentanyl for seventy-two hours of postoperative analgesia after major abdominal surgery. *Anesth Analg.* 1999;88:857.

105. Walmsley PNH. Patient-controlled epidural analgesia. In: Sinatra RS, Hord AH, Ginsberg B, et al, eds. *Acute Pain: Mechanisms and Management.* St Louis, Mo: Mosby–Year Book; 1992:312.

106. Sinatra RS. Pharmacokinetics and pharmacodynamics of spinal opioids. In: Sinatra RS, Hord AH, Ginsberg B, et al, eds. *Acute Pain: Mechanisms & Management.* St Louis, Mo: Mosby–Year Book; 1992:102.

107. Kafer ER, Brown JT, Scott DD, et al. Biphasic depression of ventilatory responses to $CO_2$ following epidural morphine. *Anesthesiology.* 1983;58:418.

108. Ready LB, Oden R, Chadwick HS, et al. Development of an anesthesiology-based postoperative pain management service. *Anesthesiology.* 1988;68:100.

109. Ready LB, Loper KA, Nessly M, et al. Postoperative epidural morphine is safe on surgical wards. *Anesthesiology.* 1991;75:452.

110. Ready LB. Regional analgesia with intraspinal opioids. In: Bonica JJ, ed. *The Management of Pain.* 2nd ed. Philadelphia, Pa: Lea & Febiger; 1990:1967.

111. Rawal N, Arner S, Gustafsson LL, et al. Present state of extradural and intrathecal opioid analgesia in Sweden. *Br J Anaesth.* 1987;59:791.

112. Stevens RA, de Leon-Casasola O. What have we learned about acute postoperative epidural pain management since 1988? *Tech Reg Anesth Pain Manage.* 1997;1:59.

113. Ventafridda V, Tamburini M, Caraceni A, et al. A validation study of the WHO method for cancer pain relief. *Cancer.* 1987;59:851.

114. Foley KM. Treatment of cancer pain. *N Engl J Med.* 1985;313:84.

115. Krames ES, Gershow J, Glassberg A, et al. Continuous infusion of spinally administered narcotics for the relief of pain due to malignant disorders. *Cancer.* 1985;56:696.

116. Krames ES. Intrathecal infusional therapies for intractable pain: patient management guidelines. *J Pain Symptom Manage.* 1993;8:36.

117. Plummer JL, Cherry DA, Cousins MJ, et al. Long-term spinal administration of morphine in cancer and non-cancer pain: a retrospective study. *Pain.* 1991;44:215.

118. Hord AH. Postoperative analgesia in the opioid-dependent patient. In: Sinatra RS, Hord AH, Ginsberg B, et al, eds. *Acute Pain: Mechanisms and Management.* St Louis, Mo: Mosby–Year Book; 1992:390.

119. Stacey BR, Brody MC, Burke DF. Patients with a substance abuse history can effectively use PCA [abstract]. *Anesthesiology.* 1990;73(suppl):A759.

120. Enneking FK, Benzon H. Oral anticoagulants and regional anesthesia: a perspective. *Reg Anesth Pain Manage.* 1998;23(suppl 2):140.

121. Odoom JA, Sih IL. Epidural analgesia and anticoagulant therapy. *Anaesthesia.* 1983;38:254.

122. Baron HC, LaRaja RD, Rossi G, et al. Continuous epidural analgesia in the heparinized vascular surgical patient: a retrospective review of 912 patients. *J Vasc Surg.* 1987;6:144.

123. Rao TLK, El-Etr AA. Anticoagulation following placement of epidural and subarachnoid catheters: an evaluation of neurologic sequelae. *Anesthesiology.* 1981;55:618.

124. Owens EL, Kasten GW, Hessel EA. Spinal subarachnoid hematoma: a case report, review of the literature, and discussion of anesthetic implications. *Anesth Analg.* 1986;65:1201.

125. Helperin SW, Cohen DD. Hematoma following epidural anesthesia: report of a case. *Anesthesiology.* 1971;35:641.

126. DeAngelis J. Hazards of subdural and epidural anesthesia during anticoagulant therapy: a case report and review. *Anesth Analg.* 1972;51:676.

127. Dixon, CL. Preoperative assessment for regional anesthesia. *Probl Anesth.* 1991;5:591.

128. Bonica JJ, Buckley FP. Regional analgesia with local anesthetics. In: Bonica JJ, ed. *The Management of Pain.* 2nd ed. Philadelphia, Pa: Lea & Febiger; 1990:1883.

129. Levack SP, Holmes JD, Robertson JS. Abdominal wound perfusion for the relief of postoperative pain. *Br J Anaesth.* 1986;58:615.

130. Malawer MM, Buck R, Khurana JS, et al. Postoperative infusional continuous regional analgesia. *Clin Orthop.* 1991;266:227.

131. Rosenblatt R, Pepitone-Rockwell R, McKillop RJ. Continuous axillary analgesia for traumatic hand injury. *Anesthesiology.* 1979;51:565.

132. Smith BD. Continuous sciatic nerve block. *Anaesthesia.* 1984;39:155.

133. Patt RB, Jain S. Therapeutic decision-making for invasive procedures. In: Patt RB, ed. *Cancer Pain.* Philadelphia, Pa: JB Lippincott; 1992:275.

134. Ferrer-Brechner T. Anesthetic techniques for the management of cancer pain. *Cancer.* 1989;63:2343.

135. Honorio TB. Epidural steroids. In: Raj PP, ed. *Pain Medicine: A Comprehensive Review.* St. Louis, Mo: Mosby; 1996:261.

136. Devor M, Govrin-Lippimann R, Raber P. Corticosteroids suppress ectopic neural discharge originating in experimental neuromas. *Pain.* 1985;22:127.

137. Simons DG. Myofascial pain syndromes of head, neck and low back. *Pain Res Clin Manage.* 1988;3:186.

138. Pybus PK. Control of pain and stiffness in osteoarthritis of the hand. *S Afr Med J.* 1981;59:514.

139. Dory MA. Arthrography of the cervical facet joints. *Radiology.* 1983;148:379.

140. Wedel DJ, Wilson PR. Cervical facet arthrography. *Reg Anesth.* 1985;10:7.

141. Bonica JJ, Buckley FP, Moricca G, et al. Neurolytic blockade and hypophysectomy. In: Bonica JJ, ed. *The Management of Pain.* 2nd ed. Philadelphia, Pa: Lea & Febiger; 1990:1980.

142. Melzack R, Wall PD. Pain mechanisms: a new theory. *Science.* 1965;150:971.

143. Hughes GS, Lichstein PR. Response of plasma beta-endorphins to TENS in healthy subjects. *Phys Ther.* 1984;64:1062.
144. Facchinetti F, Sforza G. Central and peripheral beta-endorphin response to TENS. *NIDA Res Monogr.* 1986;75:555.
145. O'Brien WJ, Rutan FM. Effect of TENS on human blood beta-endorphin levels. *Phys Ther.* 1984;64:1367.
146. Ordog GJ. TENS vs oral analgesic: a randomized double-blind controlled study in acute traumatic pain. *J Emerg Med.* 1987;5:6.
147. Schomberg FL, Carter-Baker SA. Transcutaneous electrical nerve stimulation for postlaparotomy pain. *Phys Ther.* 1983;63:188.
148. Solomon FA, Vierstein MC. Reduction of postoperative pain and narcotic use by TENS. *Surgery.* 1980;87:142.
149. Warfield CA. Physical therapy for pain relief. *Hosp Pract.* 1984;19:84E.
150. Gersh MR, Wolf SL. Applications of transcutaneous electrical stimulation in the management of patients with pain. *Phys Ther.* 1985;65:314.
151. Melzack R. TENS for low back pain: a comparison of TENS with massage for pain and range of motion. *Phys Ther.* 1983;63:489.
152. Carabelli RA, Kellerman WC. Phantom limb pain: relief by application of TENS to contralateral extremity. *Arch Phys Med Rehabil.* 1985;66:466.
153. Robaina FJ, Rodriguez JL. TENS and spinal cord stimulation for pain relief in reflex sympathetic dystrophy. *Stereotact Funct Neurosurg.* 1989;52:53.
154. Wolf SL, Gersh MR. Examination of electrode placements and stimulating parameters in treating chronic pain with conventional TENS. *Pain.* 1981;11:37.
155. Johnson MI, Ashton CH, Thompson JW. An in-depth study of long-term users of transcutaneous electrical nerve stimulation (TENS): implications for clinical use of TENS. *Pain.* 1991;44:221.
156. Meyerson BA. Electrostimulation procedures: effects, presumed rationale, and possible mechanisms. *Adv Pain Res Ther.* 1983;5:495.

157. Leak WD, Ansel AE. Neural stimulation: Spinal cord and peripheral nerve stimulation. In: Raj PP, ed. *Pain Medicine: A Comprehensive Review.* St. Louis, Mo: Mosby; 1996:328.
158. Hua SE, Levy RM. Epidural spinal cord stimulation for chronic pain control. In: Benzon HT, Raja SN, Borsook D, et al, eds. *Essentials of Pain Medicine and Regional Anesthesia.* New York, NY: Churchill Livingstone; 1999:112.
159. Sedan R, Lazorthes Y. La neurostimulation electrique therapeutique. *Neurochirurgia.* 1978;24(suppl 1):1.
160. Urban BJ, Nashold BS. Percutaneous epidural stimulation of the spinal cord for relief of pain. *Neurosurgery.* 1978;48:323.
161. Meyerson BA. Electrical stimulation of the spinal cord and brain. In: Bonica JJ, ed. *The Management of Pain.* 2nd ed. Philadelphia, Pa: Lea & Febiger; 1990:1862.
162. Yeh C, Gonyea MB, Lemke J, et al. Physical therapy: evaluation and treatment of chronic pain. In: Aronoff GM, ed. *Evaluation and Treatment of Chronic Pain.* Baltimore, Md: Urban & Schwarzenberg; 1985:251.
163. Marcant D, Rapien C-H. Role of the physiotherapist in palliative care. *J Pain Symptom Manage.* 1993;8:68.
164. Lee MHM, Itoh M, Yang G-FW, et al. Physical therapy and rehabilitation medicine. In: Bonica JJ, ed. *The Management of Pain.* 2nd ed. Philadelphia, Pa: Lea & Febiger; 1990:1769.
165. Turner JA, Romano JM. Cognitive-behavioral therapy. In: Bonica JJ, ed. *The Management of Pain.* 2nd ed. Philadelphia, Pa: Lea & Febiger; 1990:1711.
166. *OHIP Schedule of Benefits.* Ontario, Canada: Ministry of Health, Physician's Services; 1984.
167. Tunks ER, Merskey H. Psychotherapy in the management of chronic pain. In: Bonica JJ, ed. *The Management of Pain.* 2nd ed. Philadelphia, Pa: Lea & Febiger; 1990:1751.

# Pain Management Consultation in Pediatric Patients

Phillip B. Gaukroger

Meredith J. Craigie

The past few decades have seen an escalation of interest in the management of all forms of pain in children. In the early 1980s, Mather and Mackie studied the incidence of postoperative pain in 170 children.[1] They found that children had severe pain, analgesia was often not ordered, and there was a marked reluctance to administer narcotic analgesics. In many cases, the doses of medication were too small and too infrequent. Children expressed a fear of intramuscular injections and preferred to put up with pain.

A review of the literature at the time reveals that there was little known about pediatric pain relief. The pharmacology of analgesics in children was largely unknown and methods of administration and doses of analgesics were merely scaled-down adult regimens. Myths were common. Special pediatric needs were not appreciated.

Considerable developments have since occurred. Increased knowledge and the development of techniques to suit the unique needs of children have done much to reduce needless suffering of pain.

## PEDIATRIC PAIN MANAGEMENT

### *What Myths Have Been Dispelled?*

#### Commonly Accepted Myths

Table 14–1 summarizes the reasons for past ignorance about pediatric pain. Clearly, many myths were promulgated for

**TABLE 14–1.** Reasons for Undertreatment of Pediatric Pain

| | |
|---|---|
| Myths | Children don't feel pain<br>Children don't remember pain<br>Children will become addicted to narcotics |
| Attitudes | Pain is character-building<br>It is not a painful operation<br>Children are powerless |
| Research difficulties | Measuring pediatric pain<br>Technical (eg, blood sampling in small children)<br>Ethical |
| Poor education | Medical<br>Nursing<br>Allied health professionals<br>Child and parent |
| Poor clinical application | Unsuitable methods (eg, intramuscular injections)<br>Drugs not approved for children<br>Poor prescribing practices<br>Acute pain management poorly developed in adult practice |
| Economic | Difficult to demonstrate cost-effectiveness of pain management in children |

years and tended to be handed down as gospel. Several deserve special comment.

The myth that children and infants do not feel pain has probably arisen from arguments that myelination of nerves is incomplete at birth. The immaturity of nervous tissue, however, has not affected pain perception.

In 1987, Anand and Hickey demonstrated that infants who underwent surgery with little or no analgesia mounted a significant stress response as measured by the release of catecholamines, growth hormone, glucagon, and corticosteroids and the suppression of insulin release.[2] This work dispelled the myth that neonates do not feel pain, and subsequent studies showed that outcome can be improved by the provision of adequate anesthesia and analgesia.[3–6]

The myth that children do not remember pain is often used as an argument for infants undergoing neonatal circumcision without anesthesia. However, behavioral changes persist in infants who have undergone surgery without pain relief or who undergo many painful procedures in neonatal intensive care units.[7, 8] Furthermore, addiction has never been documented to be a problem in the management of acute pain.[9]

### Research and Education Issues

Pediatric pain research has been difficult. Assessment and measurement of pain in such a wide range of ages and developmental stages are clearly more difficult than in adults. Technical problems such as collection of adequate quantities of blood for pharmacokinetic studies exist. Ethical issues such as consent are more complex in children.

Education about pain management was absent from past syllabuses and texts. Pain relief tended not to be discussed in the past, but it is clear now that both children and parents benefit from knowledge about pain relief methods.

Clinical issues are relevant. Methods of drug delivery designed specifically for children were uncommon until recently. Many drugs are restricted or not specifically approved for use in children.

### Financial Incentives

A strong financial impetus has encouraged improved chronic pain management in adults. The costs of third-party claims, Workers' Compensation injuries, and sickness benefits are considerable. Arguments for the cost-effectiveness of pediatric pain management are more difficult to advance; rather, improvements in pediatric pain management are based on humanitarian and ethical issues.[10]

## SPECTRUM OF PEDIATRIC PAIN

### What Types of Pain Do Children Experience?

Clear differences are demonstrated in the spectrum of pain experienced by children and adults (Table 14–2). Because of these differences, many adult pain relief therapies and experiences may not be appropriate in pediatrics.

### Acute Pain in Children

Acute pain is the most common pain experienced by children. In adults, chronic noncancer and cancer pain is common. Postoperative pain management is of obvious importance to pediatric anesthesiologists and is an area in which the benefits of improved pain management are readily seen.

Procedural pain causes considerably more distress in children, especially if recurrent procedures are required. The difficulty in explaining the benefits of blood tests, lumbar punctures, and intravenous insertions to small children is obvious. Burns and trauma present major pain management problems and may require ongoing pain therapy for weeks to months.

### Cancer Pain

Pediatric cancers are uncommon, constituting only 1% of all malignancies. Hematologic malignancies predominate and have much higher cure rates than do adult cancers. Therapy is thus much more aggressive, and therapy-related pain is more common in children. This is in contrast to adult cancer pain, which usually occurs during the terminal phase of the illness and is most commonly due to tumor spread.

**TABLE 14–2.** Spectrum of Pediatric and Adult Pain

| Pediatric | Adult |
|---|---|
| ***Acute Pain—Common*** | |
| Postoperative | Postoperative |
| Procedural | Trauma |
| Trauma | Burns |
| Burns | |
| ***Cancer Pain*** | |
| Therapy-related pain predominates | Tumor-related pain predominates |
| ***Chronic Noncancer Pain*** | |
| Juvenile chronic arthritis | Low back pain |
| Headache | Cervical pain |
| Recurrent abdominal pain | Postherpetic neuralgia |
| Sickle cell disease | Phantom limb pain |
| Hemophilia | Workers' Compensation injuries |
| Sympathetically maintained pain | Sympathetically maintained pain |
| Progressively debilitating diseases | Neuralgias |
| Miscellaneous | Miscellaneous |

## Noncancer Pain

Chronic noncancer pain is relatively common in both adults and children but is much less likely to be debilitating in children. As seen in Table 14–2, the diseases causing chronic pain in children are vastly different from those in adults.

## ASSESSMENT AND MEASUREMENT OF PAIN IN CHILDREN

Poor assessment of pain in children was a major factor inhibiting early research. Considerable effort has been expended in the development of suitable pain measurement and assessment tools.[11–13] Although numerous methods are now available, none is universally accepted and none is truly applicable to all age groups.[14]

### *What Methods Are Clinically Useful?*

In clinical practice, routine recording of pain as a nursing observation is becoming standard practice and is to be encouraged because it increases awareness, allows more rational decisions to be made about therapy, and gives a more accurate picture of how the patient has progressed. Simple verbal rating scales for pain and side effects such as sedation, nausea, and vomiting are easy to understand and have been a useful first step toward more accurate recording and interpretation of these important observations.[15,16] However, for the purposes of research, validated methods are required.

### Self-Reporting

Because pain is a subjective phenomenon, self-report methods such as the 10-cm visual analogue scale (VAS) have become universally accepted for use by adults. The use of a VAS in children is limited by the child's cognitive development. The standard 10-cm VAS can be used reliably by most children as young as 6 to 7 years.

Most children >3 years can communicate that they feel pain or hurt. Self-report measures can be applied, but methods that are easily understood by a child are more likely to be successful.[13] The use of happy and sad faces is the most common modification to the VAS[13,16] (Fig. 14–1). It is important to make the child aware that the faces communicate their feelings about pain and not other emotions.

### Behavioral Methods

Behavioral methods are necessary for measurement of pain in smaller children and infants. Behavioral changes associated with pain can be classified as simple motor responses, crying, facial expressions, and other, more complex patterns. The major limitations of behavioral methods are that some have been designed to measure responses to a specific procedure (eg, heel lance) and some can be applied only to a limited age group.[12,17]

### Physiologic Measures

Physiologic variables such as pulse rate and blood pressure, transcutaneous oxygenation, palmar sweating, and hormonal levels change with painful experiences; however, no physiologic responses directly reflect a child's perception of pain.[11,18]

## POSTOPERATIVE PAIN MANAGEMENT

Postoperative pain is the most common type treated by pediatric anesthesiologists. It is also an area that is undergoing considerable improvement, with the introduction of newer techniques.

### *What Are the General Considerations?*

It is preferable to prevent pain rather than treat it.[19] With respect to postoperative pain, a child is better managed if he or she arrives in the recovery room comfortable from a loading dose of opioid or local anesthetic. If children are allowed to wake up in severe pain, more opioid will be required to settle them down. Opioids given in the recovery room should be titrated intravenously for rapid onset of effect.

The concept of preemptive analgesia has found some popularity in recent years.[20] It involves administering analgesia before the onset of pain, thus preventing "wind-up" in the pain receptors. Proponents believe that postoperative analgesic requirements will be less than if analgesia is administered at the end of surgery. Although this concept has considerable merit and is the way most anesthesiologists practice, it is difficult to demonstrate additional benefits.

### Preanesthetic Assessment

The anesthesiologist needs to plan postoperative analgesia during the preoperative visit. Not only do the child, parent, and ward staff benefit from this knowledge but also the anesthesiologist can plan for rational use of analgesic drugs. If opioid analgesics are to be used, we encourage anesthesiologists to use the same opioid during surgery as will be prescribed after surgery.

### Psychological Needs

The psychological needs of children must be considered. Parental presence and comforting help most children experiencing pain; therefore, it is common and appropriate to permit parents to be with their children during the postanesthesia recovery period.

Children benefit from an honest explanation of how much pain they are likely to experience and how it will be relieved. They are then able to prepare themselves psychologically and clinically appear to cope with painful surgery much better. Many school-aged children wish to know more about postop-

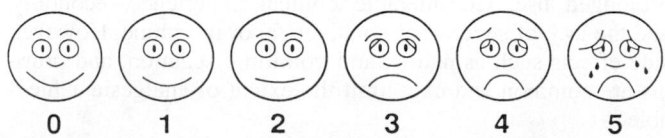

**FIGURE 14–1.** Face 0, very happy, has no hurt; face 1, still happy, but not quite as happy as "0"; face 2, not very happy or sad, kind of "in between," hurts just a little bit; face 3, sad, hurts a little more; face 4, even sadder and hurts a whole lot; face 5, very, very sad, hurts as bad as it can be. (Courtesy of Perdue Frederick Co, Norwalk, Conn.)

erative pain and prefer an honest explanation of how much pain they are likely to experience.

## Staff Education

Education and support for ward nursing and medical staffs are essential to implement new techniques and improve the way other techniques are managed.[21, 22] The greatest benefits in postoperative pain management are achieved in the general wards rather than the high-care areas; hence, the general wards should not be ignored when new techniques are introduced. Commonly used drugs are illustrated in Table 14–3.

## How Should Acetaminophen Be Used?

Acetaminophen is a useful analgesic and antipyretic drug that is well tolerated by children. It is most often used for minor procedures, for outpatient surgery, and to supplement regional blockade. The principal questions are "How much should I give?" and "When should I give it?"

Manufacturers' recommendations of 12.5 mg/kg are inadequate for analgesia. For postoperative pain, doses of 15 to 20 mg/kg every 4 hours and rectal doses of 20 to 30 mg/kg every 6 hours are required.[23, 24] A commonly suggested maximum daily dose is 100 mg/kg/day. Hepatic toxicity is uncommon in children and has not been reported with this dose. However, doses should be reduced or an alternative drug used in the child who is febrile, dehydrated, or malnourished.[25, 26]

Oral doses take approximately 30 minutes and rectal doses approximately 60 minutes for effect. Thus, premedication with 20 mg/kg of acetaminophen orally, 30 to 60 minutes before the operation, is sensible, especially for ear-nose-throat, ophthalmologic, dental, and minor general surgical procedures. A commonly used alternative is to give 40 mg/kg rectally immediately after induction of anesthesia. Both methods are preferable to attempting to administer acetaminophen after surgery in the recovery room or on return to the ward.

**TABLE 14–3.** Pediatric Analgesic Dosage Guidelines

| Drug | Prescription | Comments |
|---|---|---|
| **Simple Analgesics** | | |
| Acetaminophen | 15-20 mg/kg PO q 4 h | Minor procedures with local |
| | 20-30 mg/kg PR q 6 h | anesthetic infiltration |
| NSAIDs | | Nonsedating; inhibit platelet function |
| Naproxen | 5-7 mg/kg q 12 h | Available in syrup, tablets, suppositories |
| Ibuprofen | 4-8 mg/kg q 6 h | Syrup, tablets, over-the-counter |
| **Opioid Analgesics** | | |
| Codeine | 0.5-1 mg/kg q 4 h | Partial agonist |
| Morphine | See text | Most commonly used |
| Meperidine | See text | Not for prolonged use (normeperidine toxicity) |
| Methadone | 0.2 mg/kg IV bolus | Intraoperative single dose |
| | 0.2 mg/kg PO q 12 h | Oral starting dose for prolonged pain |
| Fentanyl | 1-3 μg/kg/h infusion | Short-acting drug |

IV, intravenous; NSAIDs, nonsteroidal antiinflammatory drugs; PO, orally; PR, rectally.

## What Is the Value of Nonsteroidal Antiinflammatory Drugs?

The use of nonsteroidal antiinflammatory drugs (NSAIDs) remains controversial in pediatric anesthetic practice. Aspirin fell from favor in pediatric practice when its potential association with Reye syndrome was described.[27] For this reason, and because of the well-documented side effects of gastric irritation and platelet dysfunction, aspirin is not used for pediatric postoperative pain management.

Other NSAIDs, such as ibuprofen, diclofenac, and naproxen, are available in pediatric formulations and are commonly used for children in many countries. These drugs provide equal or better analgesia than acetaminophen, do not sedate, and do not predispose to as much nausea and vomiting as opioids. However, they have more serious side effects than acetaminophen. Problems of platelet dysfunction, gastric irritation, renal failure, and potential precipitation of asthma prevent their more widespread use. In most institutions, NSAIDs are not administered routinely but are considered when opioid side effects become troublesome. Because NSAIDs are also antipyretic, if concern about masking a fever is an issue, an opioid analgesic is preferred.

The parenteral NSAID, ketorolac,[28] is still being evaluated, but it may overcome some of the logistical problems of trying to administer NSAIDs orally or rectally to children in the perioperative period. Manufacturers' recommendations in some countries prevent its use in children <16 years of age. An initial dose of 1 mg/kg intramuscularly or intravenously is commonly used, followed by 0.5 mg/kg every 12 hours.[29]

## When Are Opioids Indicated?

Where pain is not likely to be ameliorated by simple analgesics or local anesthesia, opioid analgesics remain the drugs of choice. Healthy children ≥3 months of age absorb, metabolize, and excrete opioids similarly to healthy young adults. Studies by Hertzka and colleagues suggest that children >6 months have no more respiratory depression than adults.[30] Premature and term newborns, on the other hand, have reduced clearance of most opioids[31, 32] and possibly increased blood-brain barrier permeability. These factors, combined with their immature responses to hypoxia and hypercarbia, render them more susceptible to the respiratory depressant effects of opioids.[33]

### Morphine

Morphine remains the opioid of choice for postoperative pain, although fentanyl, oxycodone, codeine, and sufentanil are common alternatives. Meperidine is falling from favor because of its potential to cause convulsions, particularly with prolonged use. Considerable clinical experience, economy, and the lack of superior alternatives favor morphine. However, side effects such as nausea and vomiting, sedation, and pruritus are common and may limit the extent of analgesia achievable.[34]

### Fentanyl and Sufentanil

Fentanyl and sufentanil are more lipid-soluble drugs that, because of rapid redistribution, have a relatively short duration of action. They cause little histamine release, an attribute that is especially useful in patients with opioid-induced pruritus or rash. Disadvantages include skeletal muscle rigidity at higher doses. For postoperative pain, they are best administered as continuous infusions because of their short duration of effect.

## Methadone

Methadone has been considered for postoperative pain but has a long half-life of approximately 19 hours, making it slightly difficult to titrate. However, a loading dose of 0.1 to 0.2 mg/kg at the start of anesthesia may provide postoperative analgesia for most of the first day.[35] If overdose occurs, the side effects also will be long lasting. Most anesthesiologists prefer a more titratable drug for postoperative analgesia.

Methadone can be a useful alternative to morphine in situations of prolonged opioid requirement such as severe burns or palliative care.[36]

## Codeine

Codeine is a partial-agonist opioid still in common use for pediatric analgesia. Clinically, it appears to have fewer side effects than the full-agonist drugs, but it also appears to have an analgesic ceiling effect. It is commonly used when postoperative pain is not severe and sedation is to be avoided, as in neurosurgery. It is frequently used as an adjunct to acetaminophen. One in every 10 to 20 patients lacks the ability to metabolize codeine to its active metabolite, morphine. In these patients, it is presumed ineffective.

## Other Drugs

Other opioids are available, but none offers any significant advantage over those discussed earlier. Drugs commonly used for postoperative pain have not changed in recent years. For pediatric patients, the method of administration is more important than the choice of drug; the greatest advances in pediatric postoperative pain management have been made in this area.

## TECHNIQUES OF ANALGESIC ADMINISTRATION

A bewildering array of methods of administering opioids to children has been devised, including oral, rectal, intravenous, subcutaneous, oral transmucosal, nasal transmucosal, transdermal, and inhalational routes.[37] How does the clinician sift through this array to decide what is the most appropriate method for pediatric patients?

Considerations include the advantages and disadvantages of each method (Table 14–4), the age and cognitive development of the child, and the interest of staff in considering the use of alternative methods.

### Is the Intramuscular Route Outmoded?

Intramuscular opioid administration was the mainstay of analgesia for decades in both adults and children. However, such injections should never be used routinely in children.

**TABLE 14–4.** Methods of Opioid Delivery in Children

| Method | Advantages | Disadvantages |
|---|---|---|
| Oral | Simple<br>Acceptable to children | Difficult if child vomiting<br>Variable effect and speed of onset |
| Rectal | Simple<br>Effective in vomiting child<br>No special equipment needed | May be disliked by child<br>May be socially unacceptable |
| Intramuscular | No special equipment needed | Children hate injections<br>Variable effect<br>Encourages pain cycle |
| Intravenous | | |
| Boluses | Avoids painful injections<br>Quick onset | Frequent doses required<br>Time-consuming method |
| Infusion | Continuous analgesia<br>Avoids injections | Needs close observation<br>Incident pain difficult to control |
| Patient-controlled analgesia | Patient in control<br>Allows for variability<br>High patient satisfaction<br>Safety<br>Reduced nursing staff workload | Expensive equipment<br>Requires staff training |
| Subcutaneous | Relatively simple<br>Continuous analgesia<br>Needle site discomfort | Variability in response<br>Slow onset |
| Epidural | Good-quality analgesia<br>Often less sedation | Invasive technique<br>Urinary retention more common<br>Pruritus more common |
| Transmucosal | Simple administration<br>Bypasses first-pass metabolism<br>Avoids needles | Taste may be deterrent<br>Needs cooperation |
| Transdermal | Simple<br>Acceptable to children | Slow onset, slow offset<br>Incident pain difficult to control |

The most common fear children have of hospitals is needles. Children are quick to discover that the expression of pain after surgery is frequently followed by an intramuscular injection. The child then denies pain to avoid further injections. In children requiring frequent hospitalization, this fear becomes a major management problem. Clearly, pain-free methods of administering analgesics are essential.

Intravenous and oral routes of administration are the most useful current methods. Various options are available for intravenous opioids. Most pediatric institutions offer three methods of administration: intermittent intravenous boluses as necessary, continuous infusions, and patient-controlled analgesia (PCA).

### How Should Intermittent Intravenous Boluses Be Used?

This technique involves the injection of boluses of morphine 0.05 to 0.1 mg/kg or meperidine 0.5 mg/kg directly into the side port of the intravenous infusion device over a 5-minute period. Alternatively, these doses can be infused over 20 minutes through a burette.

This technique is advantageous because it is painless, and

intravenous boluses work more quickly than intramuscular or subcutaneous injections. However, it should be used only after minor procedures, when the administration of opioids is unlikely to be needed after the first postoperative day, or in situations where the clinician is unsure whether opioids will be required at all.

The disadvantages of intravenous boluses are that in smaller children, small increments of the drug have to be calculated and drawn up, which can incur calculation and administration errors. Also, if pain is more severe, doses have to be given at 1- to 2-hour intervals, which is time consuming for ward nurses. In this situation, a continuous intravenous infusion or PCA is more suitable.

### How Are Intravenous Infusions Administered?

This method was described in children in the early 1980s[38, 39] and was a considerable advance over intramuscular administration. The argument for continuous administration is that it provides smooth, consistent analgesia by maintaining a constant blood level of the drug. Intravenous infusions have become one of the most commonly accepted methods of pediatric postoperative pain relief.

Infusions are most commonly used when moderate or severe pain is expected, usually in preschool children and those unsuitable for PCA. Infusions are, in effect, scheduled rather than administered on an as-needed basis. Hence, they require closer observation to allow titration, lest drug accumulation and attendant side effects occur.

Syringe pumps are commonly used for intravenous infusions. A simple regimen is to add 0.5 mg/kg of morphine to a 50-mL syringe and dilute to 50 mL with normal saline. The infusion is then run at 0 to 4 mL/hour (ie, 0-40 µg/kg/hour of morphine). Most institutions encourage ward nurses to use their discretion in varying this infusion rate within the prescribed limits. We allow our ward nurses to administer bolus doses of 30 µg/kg at their discretion to control incident pain or quickly relieve high levels of pain. If pain is not controlled with up to 3 bolus doses over 2 hours, review by a physician is required.

### Background Versus Incident Pain

Achieving constant blood levels of opioids is desirable, but it is not the only factor to be considered in achieving good analgesia. Postoperative pain is not constant. We must consider control of both background pain (pain that occurs when the patient lies still in bed) and incident pain (pain on movement or with procedures such as physiotherapy and removing drains, dressings). Background pain is well managed with intravenous infusions; incident pain is more difficult to control and requires bolus dose administration, preferably before the activity.

### How Do Infants Differ?

Infants <3 months of age can accumulate morphine.[32] Therefore, in this group, we use a modified regimen using the same concentration of morphine but with a reduced infusion rate of 0 to 2 mL/hour (0-20 µg/kg/hour). Most infusions are

run at 10 µg/kg/hour. These infants require closer observation than that usually available on most general wards. Apnea monitoring, continuous pulse oximetry, and a high level of nursing care are highly desirable.

Morphine infusions can also be delivered through a typical intravenous set and burette run through an infusion pump. In this situation, 0.5 mg/kg morphine (or 5 mg/kg meperidine) is added to 500 mL of normal saline or 5% dextrose in water ($D_5W$) and run as a continuous infusion at up to 40 mL/hour. The burette should contain ≤1 hour's infusion to prevent the contents of the bag being inadvertently emptied into the patient.

### Is Patient-Controlled Analgesia Useful?

PCA has become the standard of care for acute pain management with opioids. Its use in children was described in the late 1980s.[40, 41] Initial fears regarding the ability of children to administer their own pain relief were unfounded; the technique has been used in children as young as 4 years but is most commonly reserved for children >6 years of age.[42, 43]

The fundamental difference between PCA and staff-administered techniques is the issue of control. The psychological benefits of "control" in children and adolescents, in particular, should not be underestimated. The commonly recognized benefits are individualization of the patient's opioid requirement, better control of incident pain, high patient and parental satisfaction, and safety.

There are some practical differences that need to be considered when PCA is prescribed in children.

### Management

Many hospitals prefer not to set a lower age limit but offer PCA to all children who can understand the simple concept of pressing a button when they hurt.[44] The child is asked to explain in his or her own words what the machine is for, so that the clinician is satisfied that the child comprehends. With this precaution taken, most children ≥7 years of age have no trouble with PCA.

PCA is also better managed if the parents are able to reinforce this concept before and after surgery. However, parents are *not* allowed to press the button because to do so removes the fundamental safeguard with PCA—that is, that the patient has to be awake and able to press a button to receive morphine.

All children benefit from the explanation that analgesics do not completely take the pain away but merely bring it down to a level that is well tolerated. The setting of honest and realistic goals is important.

### Prescribing

The settings need to vary with the size of the child; therefore, most regimens are related to body weight. Common settings for morphine follow:

- Bolus dose: 15 to 20 µg/kg
- Lockout interval: 5 minutes
- Background infusion (if used): 4 to 10 µg/kg/hour

A concentration of 10 to 20 μg/mL is commonly used in the PCA syringe. Care must be taken with most systems to ensure that the bolus dose size remains above 0.5 mL.[45]

## Background Infusion

The use of a background infusion remains controversial in adult practice but may have some advantages in children.[46, 47] The advantages include better pain control and a better sleep pattern, but the disadvantages are that the inherent safety of PCA may be compromised and nausea, vomiting, and sedation may be more common. For this reason, background infusions are usually reserved for children who have undergone major surgery, who are on long-term PCA therapy, or who are deemed unable to use PCA. The background infusion is usually discontinued after 1 to 2 days.

Long-term PCA for children with prolonged acute pain episodes such as those with burns, cancer, and sickle cell disease is a promising technique.[43, 48, 49] Giving these children control of their pain medication over longer periods is of psychological as well as pharmacologic benefit.

## REGIONAL BLOCKADE

The swing toward greater use of regional analgesia in children has been well justified. The advantages and disadvantages are listed in Table 14-5. The benefits of most importance clinically are the ability of local anesthetics to produce complete analgesia without sedation, without opioid side effects, and with a quicker recovery. However, because of dislike of needles and reduced cooperation in smaller children, regional blockade is rarely the sole anesthetic technique; it is more often used to provide intraoperative and postoperative analgesia.[50-53]

### When Is It Contraindicated?

Absolute contraindications are similar to those for adults. The presence of infection near the site of the block, coagulopathy, and the lack of consent are obvious contraindications. Relative contraindications include ongoing degenerative axonal disease, meningomyelocele, or uncorrected hypovolemia with central neuraxis blocks, and the possibility of compartment syndromes in patients with plaster casts. In these situations, the benefits need to be considered against the disadvantages and discussed with the parents and surgeon before deciding to proceed with the block.[54, 55]

### How Does Local Anesthetic Pharmacology Differ in Children?

Differences in children relate mainly to neonates and infants. Older children handle local anesthetics in a manner similar to young adults. Esters such as tetracaine are metabolized by plasma cholinesterase, and infants <6 months of age have reduced levels of this enzyme.[56] However, no evidence suggests that this difference is of clinical importance.

With amides, plasma protein binding and hepatic clearance need to be considered. Neonates may be at increased risk of

**TABLE 14-5.** Regional Analgesia in Children

| Advantages | Disadvantages |
| --- | --- |
| Total pain reflief is possible | Technical expertise required |
| No sedation | Usually requires general anesthesia |
| Quick recovery | Risk of local anesthetic toxicity |
| Control of muscle spasm, bladder spasm, and the like | May mask pressure necrosis or compartment syndrome |
| | Technical problems with catheter techniques |
| Usually fever side effects | Other side effects (eg, motor block, urinary retention) |

local anesthetic toxicity because of reduced levels of albumin and α$_1$-acid glycoproteins[57] that allow higher levels of free drug in the plasma. Immature hepatic enzyme systems compound this problem by also increasing free drug levels. These observations are clearly important for bupivacaine, which is highly plasma protein bound. Ropivacaine is of less concern because it has a much more favorable cardiotoxic profile than bupivacaine, although it is similarly highly protein bound.[58] On the other hand, the greater volume of distribution in neonates may confer some protection against local anesthetic toxicity.

### Is Local Anesthetic Toxicity a Problem?

Cardiovascular and central nervous system toxicity from local anesthetics was thought to be uncommon in children.[51] However, general anesthesia masks signs of central nervous system toxicity, so it is difficult to assess. A number of reported cases of bupivacaine toxicity have encouraged a review of risk factors for seizures from local anesthetic use in children.[59]

Suggested maximum doses of local anesthetics are listed in Table 14-6. Plasma bupivacaine levels after caudal blockade with 3 mg/kg bupivacaine have been reported to be within safe limits[60] and may be lower than those in adults. These recommendations assume that the local anesthetic has not been injected intravenously or intraarterially, in which case toxic effects occur at much lower doses.

### What Are the Common Local Anesthetic Techniques?

Many procedures performed on children are suitable for the application of regional techniques. Benefits are seen particu-

**TABLE 14-6.** Suggested Maximum Local Anesthetic Doses in Children

| Anesthetic | Dosage |
| --- | --- |
| Lidocaine | 7 mg/kg |
| Lidocaine with epinephrine | 10 mg/kg |
| Prilocaine | 8 mg/kg (not in neonates) |
| Bupivacaine | 3 mg/kg |
| Bupivacaine with epinephrine | 5 mg/kg |
| Etidocaine | 4 mg/kg |
| Tetracaine | 2 mg/kg |
| Ropivacaine | Maximum not available |

larly in children undergoing outpatient surgery, where rapid return to normal function is important.

## Infiltration

This is the simplest and one of the most reliable applications of local anesthesia. Wound infiltration of up to 3 mg/kg (1.2 mL/kg) of plain 0.25% bupivacaine at the end of minor general surgical and plastic surgical procedures prevents a child from waking up in significant pain. This approach is particularly suitable in neonates and infants undergoing inguinal herniorrhaphy or pyloromyotomy.

Other forms of analgesia (eg, acetaminophen) may be required after the local anesthetic effect dissipates. Counsel the parents about what dose to administer to the child after leaving the hospital and about timing it so that the drug effect is present before the local anesthetic wears off.

## Lower Limb Blocks

Femoral nerve blocks are commonly used in children presenting with femoral shaft fractures. They not only provide analgesia for the application of traction but prevent painful muscle spasm. Continuous femoral blockade through a 19-gauge epidural catheter may prolong the benefits of this technique. Combined blockade of the femoral nerve and lateral cutaneous nerve of the thigh may be useful in providing analgesia for skin graft donor sites.[61, 62]

Sciatic nerve blockade has been used for procedures on the foot in children, and posterior, anterior, and lateral approaches have been described.[63-65] Other nerve blocks around the knee are sometimes useful.[66] The main limitation to peripheral blocks is the concern, particularly by orthopedic surgeons, that compartment syndromes and pressure necrosis will not be recognized in patients with plaster casts. Many anesthesiologists do not have sufficient technical expertise to perform certain blocks reliably, in which case some other form of analgesia is used. Again, we need to recognize the need for alternative analgesia when the block wears off.

## Brachial Plexus Blocks

Brachial plexus blockade is easily performed in children using the commonly described approaches for adults. These blocks are uncommon, however, because of the need for general anesthesia or heavy sedation to perform the blocks, thus negating some of their advantages.

## Penile Blocks

Penile blocks are often used as an alternative to caudal analgesia after circumcision[67, 68] because they are easy to perform. In the hands of many pediatric anesthesiologists, caudal blockade is more reliable.

## Ilioinguinal and Iliohypogastric Blocks

Ilioinguinal and iliohypogastric nerve blocks[69] can be simply inserted during inguinal surgery either under direct vision by the surgeon or percutaneously by the anesthesiologist. Wound infiltration is usually performed as well to cover the skin incision. The femoral nerve occasionally is blocked, in which case the child is unable to ambulate until the block recedes.

## Intercostal Block

Intercostal nerve blocks may be used to supplement analgesia after thoracotomy and in patients with rib fractures. Interpleural analgesia has been described in children[70] but has limited application because unilateral subcostal incisions are uncommon in pediatric surgery.

## Sympathetic Block

Sympathetic blockade may be indicated in children with peripheral ischemia after accidental intraarterial injections or for the treatment of sympathetically maintained pain. Stellate ganglion block[71] and lumbar sympathetic block can be performed in children using techniques similar to those used in adults. Neurolytic blockade is rarely performed in children.

If prolonged sympathetic blockade is required, continuous catheter administration of bupivacaine can be used for lumbar sympathetic blockade, and axillary catheter or interpleural administration of bupivacaine can be used for upper limb sympathetic blockade. Surgical sympathectomy may be indicated if a good response is obtained after the block. Details of the performance of these blocks can be found in several reviews.[50, 51, 72, 73]

## *What Is the Role for Epidural Techniques?*

Epidural techniques have been used widely in adults and are gaining general acceptance in children.[74] No method of providing epidural analgesia is universally accepted. Options for the anesthesiologist are to decide whether to use a single-shot or continuous technique, whether the caudal or lumbar approach is appropriate, and which drug or drug combination should be used.[75, 76]

## Indications

The type of surgery is the major determinant of whether an epidural technique is suitable. Table 14–7 provides suggested guidelines for the applicability. Urologic surgery is particularly suitable.

## Circumcision

Children undergoing circumcision under general anesthesia are usually given 0.5 mL/kg of 0.25% bupivacaine or 0.2% ropivacaine into the caudal space. Intraoperative and postoperative analgesia usually lasts 4 to 6 hours.[77, 78] The child awakens clear headed and with no pain and can usually eat and drink more quickly than after opioid analgesia. A single-shot technique is used because these children are treated as outpatients. As with infiltration techniques, parents should be advised concerning appropriate analgesia (eg, acetaminophen, 15-20 mg/kg orally every 4 hours) after the caudal block wears off.

## Hypospadias Repair

Hypospadias repair can be particularly distressing to children of all ages, especially those who return for repeat proce-

**TABLE 14–7.** Indications for Epidural Analgesia in Children

| Method of Administration | Procedure |
| --- | --- |
| Single shot caudal | Circumcision |
| | Rectal prolapse |
| | Imperforate anus procedures |
| | Hypospadias |
| | Lower limb procedures |
| | Inguinal surgery (hernia, hydrocele, orchidopexy) |
| Continuous caudal catheter | Hypospadias |
| | Epispadias |
| | Perineal surgery for ambiguous genitalia |
| Continuous lumbar epidural | Lower abdominal urologic procedure |
| | Pyeloplasty |
| | Abdominal tumor surgery |
| | Spinal surgery |
| Continuous thoracic epidural | Thoracotomy |
| | Major upper abdominal surgery |
| | Chest trauma (less common in children) |

**Comments**

Lumbar and thoracic catheters may be placed by caudal route.
Continuous methods are used when children already have a urinary catheter.
Single-shot caudals need to be followed by other suitable analgesic techniques.
Single-shot caudals are mostly bupivacaine or ropivacaine alone.
Continuous techniques are mostly low-dose bupivacaine/fentanyl mixtures.
Single-shot and intermittent epidural morphine are used in some centers.

dures or second-stage repairs. In the past, it was common practice to administer single-shot caudal epidural blocks to these children, and they would subsequently be managed with intermittent acetaminophen or intravenous opioids. In our experience, the use of continuous epidural infusions through caudal epidural catheters has been successful.

## Lower Abdominal Surgery

Lower abdominal operations such as ureteral reimplantation, other bladder operations, and flank operations such as pyeloplasty are also suitable for continuous epidural techniques. These children all have urinary catheters inserted as part of their surgery, thus removing the worry of urinary retention as a complication. Reduction of bladder spasm is often cited as an advantage over systemically administered opioids. Catheters for these procedures are usually placed by a lumbar approach, although in children it is easy to feed epidural catheters up to the lumbar or even thoracic level from the caudal canal.[78–80]

## Differences in Children

Caudal catheters are easily placed because the sacral hiatus is easily accessible in children[79, 80] (Fig. 14–2). Catheters placed through an 18- or 19-gauge Tuohy or Crawford needle are fed several centimeters into the epidural space. Those supplied with 18-gauge sets are less likely to kink, block, or cause syringe pump occlusion.

The most difficult part of the procedure is to provide a comfortable, secure dressing. Transparent plastic adhesive dressings and Hypafix (Smith & Nephew) achieve this better than traditional tapes and prevent soiling of the site. Syringe pumps are the most accurate way of infusing the smaller volumes of drugs required in children.

## Management of Continuous Epidural Mixtures

An epidural mixture can easily be prepared by adding 20 mL of 0.25% bupivacaine, 2 mL (100 μg) fentanyl, and 28 mL of saline to a 50-mL syringe. The final concentration is bupivacaine 0.1% (1 mg/mL) and fentanyl 2 μg/mL. Many other combinations are possible, but it is important that the mixture be balanced between local anesthetic and opioid effects. The low concentration of bupivacaine has the advantage of not causing leg weakness, which may be otherwise distressing for children and limit early mobilization. Ropivacaine 0.1% is a suitable alternative to bupivacaine.[78]

Low-dose epidural mixtures can provide complete pain relief after procedures such as hypospadias repair and almost complete relief after lower abdominal urologic procedures. Required infusion rates vary with the type of procedure and the site of the catheter. In general, for lower abdominal surgery (and also thoracic surgery), the aforementioned mixture can be infused at rates of up to 0.2 mL/kg/hour. For a continuous sacral block, 0.1 mL/kg/hour usually provides excellent analgesia.

Although continuous epidural analgesia can provide pain relief for orthopedic procedures and other abdominal operations, the frequent need for urinary catheterization militates against its general use and favors, instead, well-administered systemic opioids.

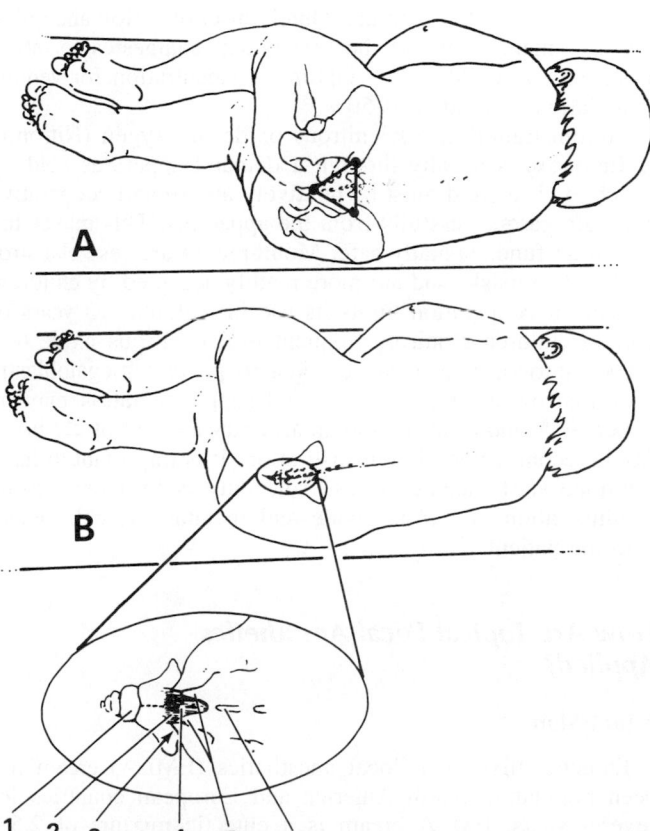

**FIGURE 14–2.** Localization of the sacral hiatus in children. *A,* Landmarks: the equilateral triangle. *B,* The sacrococcygeal membrane. 1, Coccyx; 2, sacrococcygeal membrane; 3, sacrococcygeal joint; 4, site of puncture; 5, sacral cornua; 6, spinous process of L5. (Reproduced with permission from Dalens BJ, ed. *Pediatric Regional Anesthesia.* Boca Raton, Fla: CRC Press; 1990:361. Copyright CRC Press, Boca Raton, Fla.)

## Epidural Opioids as Sole Agents

Epidural opioids are less commonly used as sole agents in children. Epidural morphine in a single dose of approximately 0.05 mg/kg provides analgesia lasting 10 to 12 hours.[81–83] Delayed respiratory depression is uncommon in children, but it has been described[84] and necessitates a higher degree of respiratory monitoring. Side effects such as nausea, vomiting, urinary retention, and pruritus may be troublesome.

For these reasons, many anesthesiologists prefer to use more lipophilic agents such as fentanyl by infusion or PCA.[76] If used alone, epidural opioids in children provide no apparent additional benefits over well-administered systemic opioids.

## PROCEDURAL PAIN IN CHILDREN

Procedural pain is a common problem in pediatric hospitals and presents major difficulties in management. Painful dressing changes, suturing, intravenous cannulation, phlebotomy, lumbar punctures, and bone marrow aspirations strike fear into many children and constitute some of the main reasons why children may be afraid of hospitals. Various options are available to reduce these fears.

### When Is Nitrous Oxide Useful?

The analgesic effects of nitrous oxide have been well known since the 19th century. Quick onset of action and quick recovery make it one of the best potent analgesics for short procedures in children.[37, 85] Optimal concentration for venous cannulation in children is 50%.[86]

Administration of 50% nitrous oxide in oxygen (Nitronox or Entonox) is usually through a demand apparatus held by the child. The child must be relatively awake and cooperative to obtain gas successfully from the apparatus. This makes the technique fundamentally safe. Mouthpieces are less claustrophobic than masks and are more readily accepted by children.

Lack of cooperation limits its use in children <5 years of age. In children requiring frequent use of nitrous oxide (eg, cancer, burns), care must be taken to prevent megaloblastic bone marrow changes. Folinic acid supplementation may be of benefit,[87] and restriction to an arbitrary amount of ≤1 hour/day is recommended in our institution. It is important to have a trained staff member whose sole duty is to supervise the administration of nitrous oxide and maintain verbal contact with the patient.

### How Are Topical Local Anesthetics Applied?

#### Intact Skin

Eutectic mixture of local anesthetics (EMLA) cream has been popular in North America and European countries for several years. EMLA cream is a eutectic mixture of 2.5% lidocaine and 2.5% prilocaine that penetrates the relatively impermeable barrier provided by skin. Most experience has been with venous cannulation,[88–90] but EMLA is also useful before lumbar puncture, for superficial skin procedures, and for other needle procedures, such as accessing implanted access ports.

An EMLA cream is applied under an occlusive dressing and needs to be on the skin for at least 1 hour before the procedure. Methemoglobinemia can result from the prilocaine component when used in small infants,[91] but the mixture is considered safe in infants >3 months of age.[92]

### Wound Analgesia and Suturing

EMLA cream is not recommended for use in wounds and on broken skin. To overcome this problem and to provide analgesia for wound suturing, a topical anesthetic solution containing tetracaine 0.5%, epinephrine (adrenaline) 1:2000, and cocaine 11.8% (TAC) has been developed.[93–95]

This solution is instilled into the wound and then onto a gauze on the wound for 10 to 20 minutes. When it is removed, painless suturing is possible, although supplementary lidocaine infiltration is occasionally required. Because TAC solution is a potent vasoconstrictor, it should not be used in areas supplied by an end artery. Clinical signs of cocaine toxicity are rare.[96]

### Is Intravenous Sedation an Option?

The use of short-acting analgesics and sedatives (commonly fentanyl and midazolam) for short, painful procedures, usually in pediatric oncology patients, is referred to as *intravenous sedation*. The report of the Consensus Conference on the Management of Pain in Childhood Cancer[97] provided suitable guidelines for the management of procedural pain in these children.

#### Fentanyl

Fentanyl, 1 to 2 μg/kg intravenously, can be given concurrently for analgesia. Intravenous sedation must be undertaken in a room with appropriate resuscitation facilities and should be administered by well-trained medical staff. Continuous monitoring with pulse oximetry is essential.

#### Midazolam

Midazolam is useful not only for its anxiolysis but also for amnesia. Children who are sleepy from midazolam rarely have any recall of painful procedures. This drug is especially useful for children who undergo frequent burn or oncology procedures. Midazolam is titrated to effect intravenously with 0.05-mg/kg increment, or given orally 0.5 to 1 mg/kg 15 to 30 minutes before the procedure.

### Is Transmucosal Drug Administration of Value?

Both fentanyl and midazolam are highly lipid-soluble drugs that are well absorbed across the oral mucosa, making them suitable for transmucosal premedication before procedures or the induction of anesthesia. The benefits of transmucosal administration are rapid onset and absence of first-pass metabolism.

### Fentanyl

Oral transmucosal fentanyl citrate has been evaluated both as an anesthetic premedicant[98–100] and as an analgesic before painful procedures.[101] It is presented in the form of a lollipop that is sucked (not eaten) 10 to 30 minutes before the painful procedure. Nausea, vomiting, and facial pruritus can occur.

### Midazolam

Transmucosal application of intravenous midazolam has been described by both intranasal and sublingual routes.[102] Not surprisingly, most children find the transnasal route unacceptable; it offers no advantage over the oral route. The commonly used dose is 0.2 mg/kg.

## Are Nonpharmacologic Techniques Useful?

Children are excellent subjects for behavioral techniques, especially patients with cancer or burns.[103–105] Hypnotherapy and other strategies such as distraction and relaxation should be considered as part of the overall management of procedural pain and should complement pharmacologic management.

## ANALGESIA FOR BURNS

Pain management in children with burns presents considerable difficulties because of the need to perform frequent, painful procedures and the often lengthy rehabilitation. These problems are compounded by the devastating cosmetic and social effects of a burn injury, not only on the child but also on the family.

Pain results from the initial injury, daily or twice-daily dressing changes, surgical débridement, and skin grafting procedures. Several weeks or, in severe cases, several months may elapse before skin coverage is complete. These children frequently benefit from hypnosis and the entire spectrum of behavioral methods in combination with pharmacologic techniques.[102, 103]

## What Pharmacologic Techniques Are Useful?

Most children with >10% burn surface area require intravenous access. In this situation, most children are managed initially with an intravenous morphine infusion or PCA. PCA has been described in children with burns for periods of up to 131 days.[43] In this series of 11 children, PCA was started at the time of first débridement, usually 7 to 10 days after the burn. A perceived benefit of PCA was that the children were given control over their pain, a positive psychological effect. There was considerable variability in morphine requirements. Tolerance developed in 3 children, but it was easily managed by increasing doses. All children weaned themselves from opioids when skin closure was complete and painful procedures were no longer required.

Various techniques are available to ameliorate the pain of dressing changes. If intravenous access is available, titration with midazolam and fentanyl (see "Procedural Pain in Children," earlier) is commonly used. If not, inhalational analgesia

**TABLE 14–8.** Differences Between Pediatric and Adult Cancers

|  | Children | Adults |
|---|---|---|
| Incidence | Uncommon (1%) | Common (99%) |
| Tumors | Many hematologic | Mostly solid tumors |
| Outcome | Mostly curable | Mostly incurable |
| Treatment | Very aggressive | Less aggressive |
| Pain problems | Therapy-related pain common | Tumor-related pain common |
| Palliative care | Usually short (weeks) | Often months/years |
| Bony metastases | Uncommon | More common |
| Managed by | Oncology team | Variety of specialties |

with nitrous oxide is a useful patient-controlled method for school-aged children. A protocol must, however, be at hand to avoid bone marrow toxicity. Oral premedication with midazolam, 0.5 to 1.0 mg/kg, has a reliable amnesic and anxiolytic effect and is used in conjunction with oral morphine, 0.5 mg/kg. These therapies should be used from the outset instead of waiting for pain management difficulties to develop.

Longer-term analgesia may also be achieved with oral slow-release morphine preparations or oral methadone.[36] Additional analgesia may still be required to ease the acute pain of dressing changes.

## CANCER PAIN

Pain is common in children with cancer,[106] and the importance of adequately managing it cannot be overestimated.

## How Does Pediatric Cancer Pain Differ?

Fundamental differences must be considered in the types of cancer pain experienced by children (Table 14–8). For this reason, extrapolation of adult cancer pain management practices to pediatric patients is difficult.

Pediatric cancers are relatively uncommon. Only 1% of cancers occur in children. Many general practitioners have no experience with pediatric cancer, the treatment of which is largely confined to larger pediatric institutions. Types of cancers experienced by children are listed in Table 14–9. Almost half of pediatric malignancies are hematologic; carcinomas are rare. Bony metastasis—the most common cause of adult cancer pain—is rare in children.

Survival rates from pediatric cancers are increasing because of improvements in aggressive chemotherapy, radiation therapy, and surgery. However, such therapy causes many pain management problems. Bone marrow aspirations, lumbar punctures, intravenous therapy, and surgery are frequent, and

**TABLE 14–9.** Incidences of Pediatric Malignancies

| | |
|---|---|
| Leukemias | 30% |
| Cerebral tumors | 18% |
| Lymphoma | 13% |
| Neuroblastoma | 11% |
| Wilms tumor | 10% |
| Bone tumors | 5% |
| Miscellaneous | 13% |

painful complications such as oral mucositis and infections may develop. Therapy-related pain, therefore, predominates in children.

Pediatric palliative care is a slowly evolving specialty because most communities have too few cases. Most children and their parents prefer palliative care to be provided in the home environment, where children are happy with their surroundings and usually have parents and siblings to provide care.

## How Is Therapy-Related Pain Managed?

A variety of options are available. Placement of long-term central venous catheters reduces problems of intravenous access and phlebotomy; and simplifies the administration of intravenous sedation or general anesthesia.

### General Anesthesia

Bone marrow biopsies and lumbar punctures remain a major pain management problem. In some countries, general anesthesia is routinely used. The procedures are painless, and intravenous therapy or phlebotomy can also be performed while the child is anesthetized. Although some children dislike general anesthesia, it is close to the ideal for most.

### Intravenous Sedation

In hospitals where general anesthesia is not feasible, intravenous sedation, often with midazolam and fentanyl, is used. Nitrous oxide is a suitable alternative. These methods are considerably more reliable and acceptable to these children than intramuscular opioid analgesia.

### Opioids and Local Anesthetics

Oral mucositis is a painful ulceration of the upper alimentary tract frequently encountered after bone marrow transplantation. Patients usually are unable to swallow and often experience extreme discomfort. Systemic opioids (often using PCA), topical local anesthetics, and mouthwashes are the mainstay of providing comfort.

### Behavioral Intervention

In addition to the pharmacologic approaches, behavioral and psychological interventions are important, especially in children whose treatments may take several years. Hypnosis, distraction, and relaxation are commonly used in children.

## How Is Pediatric Palliative Care Pain Managed?

Making the decision to administer palliative care is stressful for children, parents, hospital, and community staff. The decision to discontinue treatment is often made after considerable time and effort with aggressive therapies, and it is difficult for parents to accept that their child's disease is not curable.

The likelihood of pain depends on the type of neoplasia. Leukemias usually produce generalized bone pain during the terminal stages. Medulloblastomas may spread caudally from the posterior fossa and cause spinal pain. Bone tumors may cause pain from local spread or metastases. Neuroblastomas often cause abdominal and chest pain because of tumor spread and may give rise to neuropathic pain from nerve compression.

An analgesic ladder similar to the one proposed by the World Health Organization is worthwhile, but many of the medications used are different in children. Therapy must be individualized to the needs of each child.[107-109]

### Acetaminophen and Codeine

Mild pain is often treated with simple analgesics such as intermittent acetaminophen and codeine. Syrup, tablet, or rectal formulations are used according to the child's preference.

### Nonsteroidal Antiinflammatory Drugs

The NSAIDs are a useful next step, especially if bone pain is present. The platelet dysfunction caused by NSAIDs can occasionally lead to problems such as nosebleeds in children who are thrombocytopenic, but the benefits in terms of quality of pain relief often outweigh this disadvantage in the palliative care situation. Drugs such as naproxen need to be administered twice daily and are available in tablet, syrup, and suppository formulations.

### Opioids

Opioids are often required in combination with NSAIDs, and longer-acting preparations are useful for most children with cancer pain. Slow-release morphine tablets or sachets, methadone syrup, and oxycodone slow-release tablets or suppositories are three commonly used drugs, the choice depending on which route of administration is suitable for the individual child. Vomiting may prevent the reliable use of the oral route, necessitating rectal administration.

Intravenous and subcutaneous infusions[110] are often not required until the child is no longer ambulatory. Epidural opioids,[111] with or without local anesthetics, are rarely required for children when other routes are used in an appropriate manner. Many children acquire progressive tolerance to opioids and require escalating doses. Side effects such as nausea, constipation, and pruritus need to be anticipated and treated before they become severe. If drowsiness and reduced ambulation are not major considerations, midazolam, administered orally, rectally, or parenterally, is a useful drug to reduce distress.

### Other Drugs

Other adjuvants may be required. Nortriptyline syrup or amitriptyline tablets may help to promote sleep and are particularly useful if neuropathic pain is present. Carbamazepine or phenytoin is usually also required for neuropathic pain; plasma levels should approximate the lower end of the anticonvulsant range.

## CHRONIC NONCANCER PAIN

The spectrum of chronic, noncancer pain problems in children is vastly different from that in adults (see Table 14–2).

Although many of these problems are common in children (headaches occur in 75%), they are rarely debilitating. Most are managed by pediatricians, pediatric neurologists, rheumatologists, psychiatrists, and psychologists and rarely require the services of a pediatric anesthesiologist. However, as with adult pain management, a multidisciplinary approach is useful for difficult chronic pain problems.

## What Treatments Are Required?

### Headache

Headache is common in children and adolescents, and efforts are initially focused on ruling out serious causes. Tension headaches and migraines are most common and, if mild, are treated conservatively with rest, simple over-the-counter analgesics (see Table 14–3), physical measures such as massage, and psychological strategies such as relaxation and biofeedback training.[112, 113] More difficult cases may require more aggressive drug therapy in addition to these measures.

### Abdominal Pain

Recurrent abdominal pain is another relatively common pediatric problem (15% of schoolchildren); to find a clear-cut organic cause for this problem is uncommon.[113] If recurrent abdominal pain is troublesome, these children are most often referred to a pediatrician, pediatric gastroenterologist, or pediatric surgeon for investigation and treatment.

### Complex Regional Pain Syndromes

Complex regional pain syndromes have been poorly recognized in children until recently. Female adolescents are more likely to have the syndrome (female-to-male ratio ≈6:1).[114] No uniform method of management is available, although a combination of physical therapies, psychological assessment and therapy, and sympathetic blockade may offer the best combination for more difficult cases.[115, 116] A comprehensive treatment approach based on experience at The Children's Hospital in Boston was outlined by Berde and colleagues.[112]

Sickle cell crisis causes episodic pain because of occlusion of small blood vessels and distal infarction. Painful episodes may be mild and respond to simple analgesics such as codeine, acetaminophen, or ibuprofen. When pain is severe, parenteral opioids may be required. They should not be withheld because of fear of addiction. The harmful effects of uncontrolled pain outweigh this fear in most cases. PCA is useful because children and adolescents react positively to being able to control this aspect of their care.[117, 118]

## PAIN MANAGEMENT SERVICES FOR CHILDREN

Pediatric pain management services are becoming common in major institutions.[119] There has been a considerable increase in the number of hospitals providing pediatric pain management facilities, particularly in North America. This trend is likely to continue, although cost constraints in many countries have inhibited such growth.

## How Are Anesthesiology Departments Involved?

Many anesthesiology departments, particularly in specialty pediatric hospitals, provide acute pain management services for children and respond to requests for PCA and epidural techniques. The question of expanding this "informal" therapy to include services for pediatric cancer pain, palliative care, burns, procedural pain, and the wide range of chronic noncancer pain in children must be answered by individual departments.

An acute pain management service[120–122] is the most common first option because it requires fewer resources than does a full multidisciplinary pain management service. The pain management problems encountered are relevant to anesthetic practice. Good working relationships with surgical colleagues and nursing staff are essential for the smooth running of such a service.

### Extended Acute Pain Management

My experience has been in providing an extended acute pain management service that is involved with cancer pain, burns, and procedural pain, all of which are experienced on the hospital campus. A small amount of community palliative care work is provided.

The anesthesiologist's involvement in all areas is to facilitate and coordinate pain management methods within the hospital and to provide hospital protocols, prescription guidelines, education, and maintenance of pain management equipment. Individual surgeons are encouraged to participate in managing the common techniques, including PCA, although prescribing, machine programming, and overall supervision of such techniques remain with anesthetic personnel. There is no outpatient service.

Chronic pain problems continue to be managed by appropriate pediatric specialties and, if severe, may be referred to adult pain management services. Pediatric pain services must always be individualized to suit the clinical workload of a particular institution, and we must respect the opinions and needs of clinicians in the anesthesiology department and the other clinical services.

### Comprehensive Multidisciplinary Pain Management

The third option is to provide maximum care in the form of a comprehensive multidisciplinary pain management service.[123] This service requires input from specialists in anesthesia, pediatric surgery, orthopedics, neurosurgery, pediatric medicine, psychiatry, psychology, nursing, social work, pharmacology, and rheumatology who have a dedicated interest in pediatric pain management. Several key individuals should coordinate the service to receive patients from an extensive referral base. Although this approach is ideal for major pediatric referral centers, cost constraints and the recruitment of sufficiently interested people are commonly encountered difficulties.

Many comprehensive clinics (ie, oncology and burns) already have weekly multidisciplinary group meetings to discuss patient management problems. This group usually consists of physicians, ward nurses, ward play leader, hospital school teacher, community nurse representative, clinical psychologist, social worker, and sometimes research staff. The addition of an acute pain management specialist such as an anesthesiologist is valuable.

## Pain Interest Groups

Another simple option is to set up a pain interest group. These groups have regular meetings to discuss pain management problems in an institution and assist in coordinating the way pain is managed. They can offer advice and opinions concerning individual cases. Such a group requires interested people from anesthesiology, surgery, medicine, psychiatry, nursing, social work, and allied specialties and should be open to anyone in the hospital who is interested.

## *References*

1. Mather L, Mackie J. The incidence of postoperative pain in children. *Pain.* 1983;15:271.
2. Anand KJS, Hickey PR. Pain and its effects in the human neonate and fetus. *N Engl J Med.* 1987;317:1321.
3. Anand KJS, Sippell WG, Aynsley-Green A. Randomised trial of fentanyl anaesthesia in preterm babies undergoing surgery: effects on the stress response. *Lancet.* 1987;1:243.
4. Anand KJS, Sippell WG, Schofield NM, et al. Does halothane anaesthesia decrease the metabolic and endocrine stress responses of newborn infants undergoing operation? *BMJ.* 1988;296:668.
5. Anand KJS, Hickey PR. Halothane-morphine compared with high-dose sufentanil for anesthesia and postoperative analgesia in neonatal cardiac surgery. *N Engl J Med.* 1992;326:1.
6. Wolf AR, Doyle E, Thomas E. Modifying infant stress responses to major surgery: spinal vs extradural vs opioid analgesia. *Paediatr Anaesth.* 1998;8:305.
7. Marshall RE, Stratton WC, Moore JA, et al. Circumcision: effects on newborn behavior. *Infant Behav Dev.* 1980;3:1.
8. Taddio A, Goldbach M, Ipp M, et al. Effect of neonatal circumcision on pain responses during vaccination in boys. *Lancet.* 1995;345:291.
9. Porter J, Jick H. Addiction rare in patients treated with narcotics [letter]. *N Engl J Med.* 1980;302:123.
10. Walco GA, Cassidy RC, Schechter NL. Pain, hurt and harm: the ethics of pain control in infants and children. *N Engl J Med.* 1994;331:541.
11. Sweet S, McGrath PA. Physiological measures of pain. In: Finley GA, McGrath PJ, eds. *Measurement of Pain in Infants and Children.* Seattle, Wash: IASP Press; 1998:59.
12. McGrath PA. Behavioral measures of pain. In: Finley GA, McGrath PJ, eds. *Measurement of Pain in Infants and Children.* Seattle, Wash: IASP Press; 1998:83.
13. Champion GD, Goodenough B, von Baeyer CL, et al. Measurement of pain by self-report. In: Finley GA, McGrath PJ, eds. *Measurement of Pain in Infants and Children.* Seattle, Wash: IASP Press; 1998:123.
14. Hester NO, Foster RL, Jordan-Marsh M, et al. Putting pain measurement into clinical practice. In: Finley GA, McGrath PJ, eds. *Measurement of Pain in Infants and Children.* Seattle, Wash: IASP Press; 1998:179.
15. Gaukroger PB. Paediatric analgesia—which drug? which dose? *Drugs.* 1991;41:52.
16. Bieri D, Reeve RA, Champion GD, et al. The Faces Pain Scale for the self-assessment of the severity of pain experienced in children: development, initial validation, and preliminary investigation for ratio scale properties. *Pain.* 1990;41:139.
17. Craig KD. The facial display of pain. In: Finley GA, McGrath PJ, eds. *Measurement of Pain in Infants and Children.* Seattle, Wash: IASP Press; 1998:103.
18. McGrath PA. An assessment of children's pain: a review of behavioral, physiological and direct scaling techniques. *Pain.* 1987;31:147.
19. Cousins MJ. Prevention of postoperative pain. In: Bond MR, Charlton JE, Woolf CJ, eds. *Proceedings of the VIth World Congress on Pain.* New York, NY: Elsevier; 1991:41.
20. Berry FA. Preemptive analgesia for postoperative pain [editorial]. *Paediatr Anaesth.* 1998;8:187.
21. Goddard JM, Pickup SE. Postoperative pain in children. *Anaesthesia.* 1996;51:588.
22. Coleman SA, Booker-Milburn J. Audit of postoperative pain control: influence of a dedicated acute pain nurse. *Anaesthesia.* 1996;51:1093.
23. Korpela R, Korvenoja P, Meretoja OA. Morphine-sparing effect of acetaminophen in pediatric day-case surgery. *Anesthesiology.* 1999;91:442.
24. Anderson B, Kanagasundarum S, Woollard G. Analgesic efficacy of paracetamol in children using tonsillectomy as a pain model. *Anaesth Intensive Care.* 1996;24:669.
25. Anderson BJ. What we don't know about paracetamol in children [review]. *Paediatr Anaesth.* 1998;8:451.
26. Morton NS, Arana A. Paracetamol-induced fulminant hepatic failure in a child after 5 days of therapeutic doses [case report]. *Paediatr Anaesth.* 1999;9:463.
27. Barrett MJ, Hurwitz ES, Schonberger LB, et al. Changing epidemiology of Reye's syndrome in the United States. *Pediatrics.* 1986;77:598.
28. Maunuksela E-L, Olkkola KT, Kokki H. Pharmacokinetics of intravenous ketorolac and its efficacy in relieving postoperative pain in children [abstract]. *J Pain Symptom Manage.* 1991;6:143.
29. Splinter WM, Reid CW, Roberts DJ, et al. Reducing pain after inguinal hernia repair in children. *Anesthesiology.* 1997;87:542.
30. Hertzka RE, Gauntlett IS, Fisher DM, et al. Fentanyl-induced respiratory depression: effects of age. *Anesthesiology.* 1989;70:213.
31. Koren G, Butt W, Chinyanga H, et al. Postoperative morphine infusion in newborn infants: assessment of disposition characteristics and safety. *J Pediatr.* 1985;107:963.
32. Kart T, Christup LL, Rasmussen M. Recommended use of morphine in neonates, infants and children based on a literature review, part 1: pharmacokinetics [review]. *Paediatr Anaesth.* 1997;7:5.
33. Kart T, Christup LL, Rasmussen M. Recommended use of morphine in neonates, infants and children based on a literature review, part 2: clinical use [review]. *Paediatr Anaesth.* 1997;7:93.
34. Esmail Z, Montgomery C, Court C, et al. Efficacy and complications of morphine infusions in postoperative paediatric patients. *Paediatr Anaesth.* 1999;9:321.
35. Berde CB, Beyer JE, Bournaki M-C, et al. Comparison of morphine and methadone for prevention of postoperative pain in 3- to 7-year-old children. *J Pediatr.* 1991;119:136.
36. Williams PI, Sarginson RE, Ratcliffe JM. Use of methadone in the morphine-tolerant burned paediatric patient. *Br J Anaesth.* 1998;80:92.
37. Gaukroger PB. Novel techniques of analgesic delivery. In: Schechter N, Berde CB, Yaster M, eds. *Pain Management in Children and Adolescents.* Baltimore, Md: Williams & Wilkins; 1992:195.
38. Bray RJ. Postoperative analgesia provided by morphine infusion in children. *Anaesthesia.* 1983;38:1075.
39. Dilworth NM, MacKellar A. Pain relief for the pediatric surgical patient. *J Pediatr Surg.* 1987;22:264.
40. Rodgers BM, Webb CJ, Stergios D, et al. Patient-controlled analgesia in pediatric surgery. *J Pediatr Surg.* 1988;23:259.
41. Gaukroger PB, Tomkins DP, Van der Walt JH. Patient-controlled analgesia in children. *Anaesth Intensive Care.* 1989;17:264.
42. Gaukroger PB. Patient-controlled analgesia in children. In: Schechter N, Berde CB, Yaster M, eds. *Pain Management in Children and Adolescents.* Baltimore, Md: Williams & Wilkins; 1992:203.
43. Gaukroger PB, Chapman MJ, Davey RB. Pain control in paediatric burns: the use of patient-controlled analgesia (PCA). *Burns.* 1991;17:396.
44. Gaukroger PB, Tomkins DP, van der Walt JH. Letter to the editor. *J Pediatr Surg.* 1988;23:1227.
45. Patient-controlled analgesic infusion pumps. *Health Devices.* 1988;17:137.
46. Berde CB, Lehn BM, Yee JD, et al. Patient-controlled analgesia in children and adolescents: a randomised, prospective comparison with intramuscular administration of morphine for postoperative analgesia. *J Pediatr.* 1991;118:460.
47. Doyle E, Harper I, Morton NS. Patient controlled analgesia with low dose background infusions after lower abdominal surgery in children. *Br J Anaesth.* 1993;71:818.
48. Mowbray MJ, Gaukroger PB. The use of long-term patient-controlled analgesia in children. *Anaesthesia.* 1990;45:941.
49. Shapiro B, Cohen D, Howe C. Use of patient-controlled analgesia for patients with sickle cell disease [abstract]. *J Pain Symptom Manage.* 1991;6:176.
50. Brown TCK, Schulte-Steinberg O. Neural blockade for pediatric surgery. In: Cousins MJ, Bridenbaugh PO, eds. *Neural Blockade in Clinical Anesthesia and Management of Pain.* 2nd ed. Philadelphia, Pa: JB Lippincott; 1988:669.
51. Arthur DS, McNicol LR. Local anaesthetic techniques in paediatric surgery. *Br J Anaesth.* 1986;58:760.
52. Dalens B. Regional anesthesia in children. *Anesth Analg.* 1989;68:654.

53. Yaster M, Maxwell LG. Pediatric regional anesthesia. *Anesthesiology.* 1989;70:324.
54. Berde C. Regional anesthesia in children—what have we learned [editorial]? *Anesth Analg.* 1996;83:897.
55. Strafford MA, Wilder RT, Berde CB. The risk of infection from epidural analgesia in children: a review of 1620 cases. *Anesth Analg.* 1995;80:234.
56. Zsigmond EK, Downs JR. Plasma cholinesterase activity in newborns and infants. *Can Anaesth Soc J.* 1971;18:278.
57. Wood M, Wood AJJ. Changes in plasma drug binding and alpha-1 acid glycoprotein in mother and newborn infant. *Clin Pharmacol Ther.* 1979;19:426.
58. McClure JH. Ropivacaine [review]. *Br J Anaesth.* 1996;76:300.
59. Berde CB. Convulsions associated with pediatric regional anesthesia. *Anesth Analg.* 1992;75:164.
60. Eyres RL, Bishop W, Oppenheim RC, et al. Plasma bupivacaine concentrations in children during caudal epidural anaesthesia. *Anaesth Intensive Care.* 1983;11:20.
61. McNicol LR. Lower limb blocks for children: lateral cutaneous and femoral nerve blocks for postoperative pain relief in paediatric practice. *Anaesthesia.* 1986;41:27.
62. Brown TCK, Dickens DRV. A new approach to lateral cutaneous nerve of thigh block. *Anaesth Intensive Care.* 1986;14:126.
63. Dalens B, Tanguy A, Vanneuville G. Sciatic nerve blocks in children: comparison of the posterior, anterior, and lateral approaches in 180 pediatric patients. *Anesth Analg.* 1990;70:131.
64. McNicol LR. Sciatic nerve block for children: sciatic nerve block by the anterior approach for postoperative pain relief. *Anaesthesia.* 1985;40:410.
65. Guardini R, Waldron BA, Wallace WA. Sciatic nerve block: a new lateral approach. *Acta Anaesthesiol Scand.* 1985;29:515.
66. Kempthorne PM, Brown TCK. Nerve blocks around the knee in children. *Anaesth Intensive Care.* 1984;12:14.
67. Bacon AK. An alternative block for post circumcision analgesia. *Anaesth Intensive Care.* 1977;5:63.
68. Serour F, Cohen A, Mandelberg A, et al. Dorsal penile nerve block in children undergoing circumcision in a day-care surgery. *Can J Anaesth.* 1996;8:954.
69. Casey WF, Rice LJ, Hannallah RS, et al. A comparison between bupivacaine instillation versus ilioinguinal/iliohypogastric nerve block for postoperative analgesia following inguinal herniorrhaphy in children. *Anesthesiology.* 1990;72:637.
70. McIlvaine WB, Chang JHT, Jones M. The effective use of intrapleural bupivacaine for analgesia after thoracic and subcostal incisions in children. *J Pediatr Surg.* 1988;23:1184.
71. Parris WC, Reddy BC, White HW, et al. Stellate ganglion blocks in pediatric patients. *Anesth Analg.* 1991;72:552.
72. Dalens B, ed. *Pediatric Regional Anesthesia.* Boca Raton, Fla: CRC Press; 1991.
73. Saint-Maurice C, Schulte-Steinberg O. *Regional Anesthesia in Children.* Norwalk, Conn: Appleton & Lange/Mediglobe; 1990.
74. Rowney DA, Doyle E. Epidural and subarachnoid blockade in children [review]. *Anaesthesia.* 1998;53:980.
75. Lin Y-C, Sentivany-Collins SK, Peterson KL, et al. Outcomes after single-injection caudal epidural versus continuous infusion epidural via caudal route approach for postoperative analgesia in infants and children undergoing patent ductus arteriosus ligation. *Paediatr Anaesth.* 1999;9:139.
76. Caudle DL, Freid EB, Bailey AG, et al. Epidural fentanyl infusion with patient-controlled epidural analgesia for postoperative analgesia in children. *J Pediatr Surg.* 1993;28:554.
77. Ivani G, Mereto N, Lampugnani E, et al. Ropivacaine in paediatric surgery: preliminary results. *Paediatr Anaesth.* 1998;8:127.
78. Da Conceicao MJ, Coelho L, Khalil M. Ropivacaine 0.25% compared with bupivacaine 0.25% by the caudal route. *Paediatr Anaesth.* 1999;9:229.
79. Bosenberg AT, Bland BAR, Schulte-Steinberg O, et al. Thoracic epidural anaesthesia via caudal route in infants. *Anesthesiology.* 1988;69:265.
80. Rasch DK, Webster DE, Pollard TG, et al. Lumbar and thoracic epidural analgesia via the caudal approach for postoperative pain relief in infants and children. *Can J Anaesth.* 1990;37:359.
81. Tyler DC, Krane EJ. Epidural opioids in children. *J Pediatr Surg.* 1989;24:469.
82. Krane EJ, Jacobson LE, Tyler DC. Caudal epidural morphine in children: A comparison of three doses [abstract]. *Anesthesiology.* 1988;69:A763.
83. Glenski JA, Warner MA, Dawson B, et al. Postoperative use of epidurally administered morphine in children and adolescents. *Mayo Clin Proc.* 1984;59:530.
84. Krane EJ. Delayed respiratory depression in a child after caudal epidural morphine. *Anesth Analg.* 1988;67:79.
85. Miser AW, Ayesh D, Broda E, et al. Use of a patient-controlled device for nitrous oxide administration to control procedure-related pain in children and young adults with cancer. *Clin J Pain.* 1988;4:5.
86. Henderson JM, Spence DG, Komocar LM, et al. Administration of nitrous oxide to pediatric patients provides analgesia for venous cannulation. *Anesthesiology.* 1990;72:269.
87. Amos RJ, Amess JAL, Nancekievill DG, et al. Prevention of nitrous oxide-induced megaloblastic changes in bone marrow using folinic acid. *Br J Anaesth.* 1984;56:103.
88. Maunuksela E-L, Korpela R. Double-blind evaluation of a lignocaine-prilocaine cream (EMLA) in children. *Br J Anaesth.* 1986;58:1242.
89. Hallen B, Olsson GL, Uppfeldt A. Pain-free venipuncture: effect of timing of application of local anaesthetic cream. *Anaesthesia.* 1984;39:969.
90. Hallen B, Uppfeldt A. Does lidocaine-prilocaine cream permit pain free insertion of IV catheters in children? *Anesthesiology.* 1982;57:340.
91. Frayling IM, Addison GM, Chattergee K, et al. Methaemoglobinaemia in children treated with prilocaine-lignocaine cream. *BMJ.* 1990;301:153.
92. Selbst SM. Managing pain in the pediatric emergency department. *Pediatr Emerg Care.* 1989;5:56.
93. Pryor GJ, Kilpatrick WR, Opp AR. Local anesthesia in minor lacerations: topical TAC versus lidocaine infiltration. *Ann Emerg Med.* 1980;9:568.
94. Bonadio WA. TAC: a review. *Pediatr Emerg Care.* 1989;5:128.
95. Bonadio WA, Wagner V. Efficacy of tetracaine-adrenaline-cocaine topical anesthetic without tetracaine for facial laceration repair in children. *Pediatrics.* 1990;86:856.
96. Fitzmaurice LS, Wasserman GS, Knapp JF, et al. TAC use and absorption of cocaine in a pediatric emergency department. *Ann Emerg Med.* 1990;19:515.
97. Zeltzer LK, Altman A, Cohen D, et al. Report of the Subcommittee on the Management of Pain Associated With Procedures in Children With Cancer. *Pediatrics.* 1990;86:826.
98. Nelson PS, Streisand JB, Mulder SM, et al. Comparison of oral transmucosal fentanyl citrate and an oral solution of meperidine, diazepam, and atropine for premedication in children. *Anesthesiology.* 1989;70:616.
99. Streisand JB, Stanley TH, Hague B, et al. Oral transmucosal fentanyl citrate premedication in children. *Anesth Analg.* 1989;69:28.
100. Ashburn MA, Streisand JB, Tarver S, et al. Oral transmucosal fentanyl citrate for premedication in pediatric outpatients. *Can J Anaesth.* 1990;37:857.
101. Schechter NL, Weisman SJ, Rosenblum M, et al. Oral transmucosal fentanyl citrate for pediatric procedures: a randomised clinical trial. *J Pain Symptom Manage.* 1991;6:178.
102. Karl HW, Larach MG, Ruffle JM. Transmucosal midazolam for preinduction of anesthesia in pediatric patients: comparison of intranasal and sublingual routes [abstract]. *Anesthesiology.* 1991;75:A922.
103. Zeltzer LK, Jay SM, Fisher DM. Management of pain associated with pediatric procedures. *Pediatr Clin North Am.* 1989;36:941.
104. Osgood PF, Szyfelbein SK. Management of burn pain in children. *Pediatr Clin North Am.* 1989;36:1001.
105. Maron M, Bush JP. Burn injury and treatment pain. In: Bush JP, Harkins SW, eds. *Children in Pain: Clinical and Research Issues From a Developmental Perspective.* New York, NY: Springer-Verlag; 1991:275.
106. Miser AW, Dothage JA, Wesley RA, et al. The prevalence of pain in a pediatric and young adult cancer population. *Pain.* 1987;29:73.
107. Dangel T. Chronic pain management in children, part I: cancer and phantom limb pain. *Paediatr Anaesth.* 1998;8:5.
108. Berde C, Ablin A, Glazer J, et al. Report of the Subcommittee on Disease-Related Pain in Childhood Cancer. *Pediatrics.* 1990;86:818.
109. Miser AW, Miser JS. The treatment of cancer pain in children. *Pediatr Clin North Am.* 1989;36:979.
110. Miser AW, Moore L, Greene R, et al. Prospective study of continuous intravenous and subcutaneous morphine infusions for therapy-related or cancer-related pain in children and young adults with cancer. *Clin J Pain.* 1986;2:101.
111. Collins JJ, Brier HE, Sethna NF, et al. Regional anesthesia for pain associated with terminal pediatric malignancy. *Pain.* 1996;65:63.
112. Berde CB, Anand KJS, Sethna NF. Pediatric pain management. In: Gregory GA, ed. *Pediatric Anesthesia.* 2nd ed. New York, NY: Churchill Livingstone; 1989:679.

113. McGrath PA. *Pain in Children: Nature, Assessment and Treatment.* New York, NY: The Guilford Press; 1990:251.

114. Wilder RT, Berde CB, Wolohan M, et al. Reflex sympathetic dystrophy in children: clinical characteristics and follow-up of 70 patients. *J Bone Joint Surg Am.* 1992;74:910.

115. Walker SM, Cousins MJ. Complex regional pain syndromes, including "reflex sympathetic dystrophy" and "causalgia" [review]. *Anaesth Intensive Care.* 1997;25:113.

116. Dangel T. Chronic pain management in children, part II: reflex sympathetic dystrophy. *Paediatr Anaesth.* 1998;8:105.

117. Shapiro BS. The management of pain in sickle cell disease. *Pediatr Clin North Am.* 1989;36:1029.

118. Shapiro B, Cohen D, Howe C. Use of patient-controlled analgesia for patients with sickle cell disease [abstract]. *J Pain Symptom Manage.* 1991;6:176.

119. Berde CB, Sethna NF, Masek B, et al. Pediatric pain clinics: recommendations for their development. *Pediatrician.* 1989;16:94.

120. Ready LB, Oden R, Chadwick HS, et al. Development of an anesthesiology-based postoperative pain management service. *Anesthesiology.* 1988;68:100.

121. Ready LB. Acute pain services: an academic asset. *Clin J Pain.* 1989;5(suppl 1):S28.

122. Gaukroger PB. An acute pain management service for children. *Pain.* 1990 (suppl 5):S6.

123. Berde CB, Lacouture PG, Masek BJ, et al. Initial experience with a pediatric pain treatment service. *Pain.* 1987 (suppl 4):S99.

# Tools of the Trade and Their Applications

# The Anesthesia Machine, Anesthesia Ventilator, Breathing Circuit, and Scavenging System

Samsun Lampotang

Michael L. Good

## TROUBLESHOOTING THE GAS DELIVERY SYSTEM

*What Needs to Be Checked?*

*How Well Are Systems Checked?*

*Are Pre-Use Check Protocols Useful?*

*Why Do Pre-Use Check Protocols Fail?*

*What Is the Revised Food and Drug Administration Pre-Use Check Protocol?*

*How Has the Revised Food and Drug Administration Pre-Use Check Performed?*

## MONITORING THE ANESTHESIA MACHINE

*How Do Anesthesia Gas Machines Injure Patients?*

*What Are the Consequences of Inspiring a Hypoxic Gas?*

*Must All Anesthesia Gas Delivery Systems Provide Supplemental Oxygen?*

*What Malfunctions Cause Respiration of Hypoxic Gas?*

*Can the Anesthesia Machine Provide Oxygen Through a Nasal Cannula?*

*What Are the Consequences of an Inappropriate Anesthetic Dose?*

*What Malfunctions Cause an Inappropriate Anesthetic Dose?*

*What Are the Consequences of Inadequate Ventilation?*

*What Should Be Done if a Machine Malfunction Is Suspected?*

## STANDARDS AND CHANGES IN ANESTHESIA MACHINE DESIGN

*What Are They?*

## RECENTLY INTRODUCED ANESTHESIA MACHINES

*What Are the Major Differences?*

*Why Pressure Controlled Ventilation?*

*What Are the Disadvantages of Pressure Controlled Ventilation*

## FUTURE DEVELOPMENTS

*What Changes Are Anticipated?*

*When Is an Anesthesia Machine Obsolete?*

For many years, the Jackson design (circa 1915),[1] embodied by the Ohmeda (Madison, Wis) Modulus series and the North American Dräger (NAD) (Telford, Pa) Narkomed series of anesthesia machines has been the main conceptual design used in most anesthesia machines in North America. In recent years, new machines, such as the Datex-Ohmeda (Madison, Wis) anesthesia delivery unit (ADU) and the Dräger Julian (Telford, Pa), which differ substantially from the Jackson design (eg, operation controlled by microprocessors, electronic flow control, integrated monitoring), have been approved for use in North America.

The eloquent simplicity of early anesthesia systems, such as the Morton inhaler, demanded few technical skills but great clinical acumen from the anesthesiologist. Today, oxygen ($O_2$) and anesthetic gases are precisely metered, mixed, measured, and delivered into the lungs of the patient. The patient's pulmonary ventilation is assessed with a spirometer and capnograph and is automatically delivered by a mechanical ventilator.

The drawback of this enhanced precision in gas delivery and pulmonary ventilation is a proportional increase in the complexity of anesthesia gas delivery systems. Contemporary anesthesia machines contain hundreds of functionally distinct components and have dozens of controls that need to be adjusted, numerous gauges and displays that must be watched, and a multitude of possible failure modes.

## BASIC CONCEPTS

The anesthesia gas delivery system has three primary functions:

1. To provide $O_2$
2. To blend and deliver an anesthetic gas mixture
3. To support ventilation of the patient's lungs

### *What Are the Four Component Subsystems?*

A better understanding of the anesthesia gas machine is achieved by functionally dividing it into four component subsystems (Fig. 15–1). Pipeline and cylinder gas supplies (usually $O_2$ and nitrous oxide, and sometimes helium and xenon) are connected to the *high-pressure system.* Concealed within the anesthesia machine, the high-pressure system connects to the *low-pressure system,* in which an $O_2$ and anesthetic gas mixture (often called the *fresh gas mixture*) is blended according to the control settings. The fresh gas mixture passes through the fresh gas hose into the *breathing system,* which includes the mechanical ventilator. The *scavenging system* collects excess gas from the breathing system and delivers it to the waste gas evacuation system.

### Monitoring Instruments

Note that this classification scheme does not include monitoring instruments (eg, $O_2$ analyzer, capnograph, and pulse oximeter) as a component subsystem of the anesthesia machine. Although they play an important role in monitoring anesthesia machine performance,[2] monitors may or may not

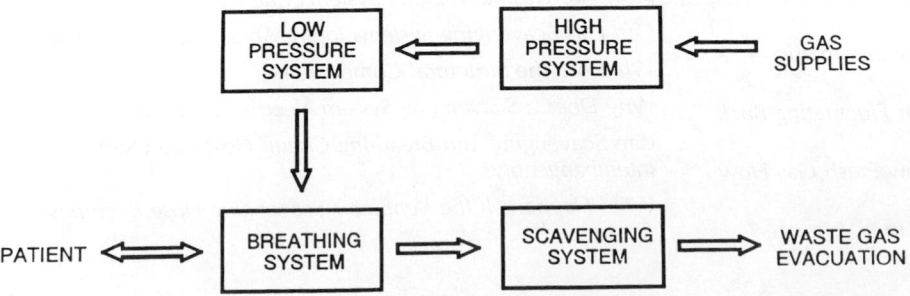

**FIGURE 15–1.** Gas flow through the four component subsystems of an anesthesia machine.

**TABLE 15–1.** Structures and Safety Features in the High-Pressure System

**Structures**
Pipeline gas inlets and check valves
Cylinder gas inlets and check valves
Cylinder hanger yokes
Cylinder pressure regulator
Gas supply pressure gauges
$O_2$ (ventilator) power outlet
$O_2$ flush valve
Second-stage $O_2$ pressure regulator
**Safety Features**
Diameter index safety system
Pin index safety system
Low $O_2$ supply pressure alarm
$O_2$ pressure failure safety mechanism (fail-safe system)

be built-in features of an anesthesia gas delivery system. Descriptive and technical aspects of monitoring instruments, as well as their vital role in monitoring a patient's physiologic status, are discussed in separate chapters of this textbook.

# HIGH-PRESSURE SYSTEM

## *What Are the Structural Components?*

### Gas Sources

The structures and safety features of the high-pressure system are listed in Table 15–1 and illustrated graphically in Figure 15–2. The pipeline gas inlets (see Fig. 15–2.1) provide connection sites for high-pressure gas hoses (see Fig. 15–2.2) that are connected to the hospital's pipeline gas supply (see Fig. 15–2.3). Hanger yokes enable us to attach cylinders of compressed gas to the anesthesia machine. When a gas cylin-

der is connected to the yoke and the stem valve on the cylinder is opened, gas can flow through the cylinder gas inlet (see Fig. 15–2.4) into the anesthesia machine. Check valves (see Fig. 15–2.5) are located on the machine side of both the pipeline and the cylinder inlets and prevent gas from leaking retrograde through the back of the anesthesia machine. On machines that accommodate more than one cylinder of each gas, the cylinder inlet check valves also prevent gas from a cylinder with higher pressure from transfilling a second cylinder with lower pressure.

### Pressure Regulation

Pressure gauges (see Fig. 15–2.6), which are typically located on the front or side of the anesthesia machine, indicate the gas pressure in the hospital pipeline and cylinders. The pressure in a cylinder of medical gas is related to the volume of compressed gas in the cylinder and to the physical characteristics of the contained gas—specifically, to whether the gas enters the liquid phase when compressed at room temperature.

Regardless of the pressure in the cylinder, which may be as high as 2200 pounds/square inch gauge (psig) ($x$ psig = $\left[\frac{x}{14.7}\right]$ + 1 atmosphere; 2200 psig = 151 atm), the cylinder pressure regulator (see Fig. 15–2.7) reduces pressure to about 45 psig (4 atm), which is below the 50- to 55-psig (4.4-4.74 atm) operating pressure of the hospital pipeline gas supply. This pressure differential (pipeline gas at 50 psig [4.4 atm]; cylinder gas at 45 psig [4 atm]) allows the pipeline gas to be used preferentially if the anesthesia machine is connected to the hospital pipeline gas supply and if a reserve gas cylinder is simultaneously (and inadvertently) left open.

### *Oxygen*

The $O_2$ portion of the high-pressure system also includes an $O_2$ power outlet (see Fig. 15–2.8), which is typically

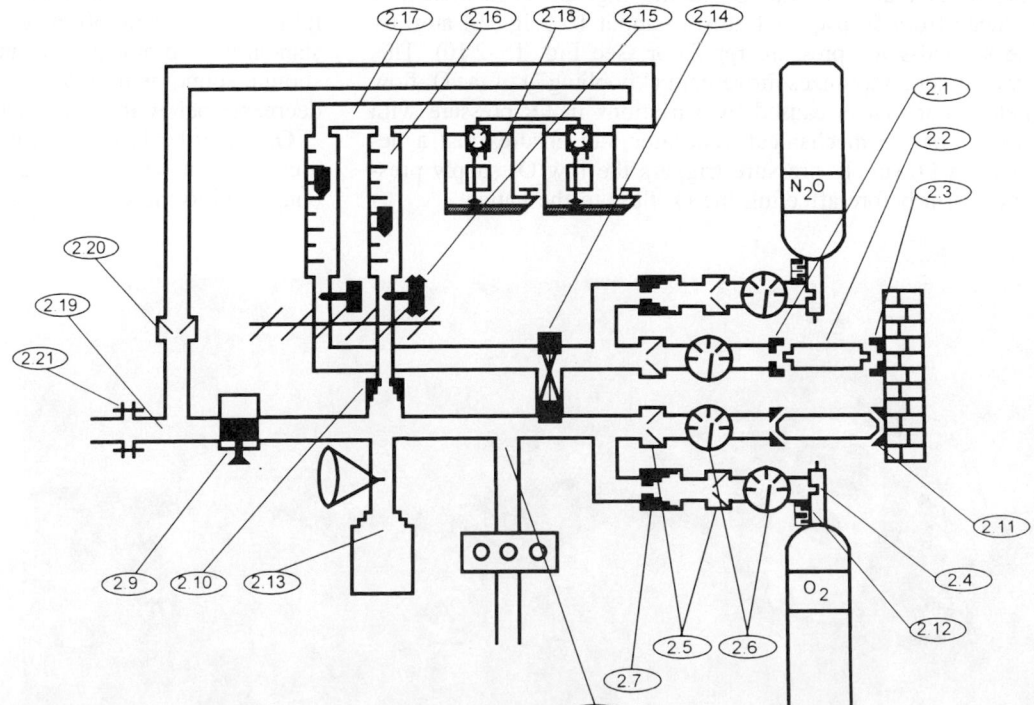

**FIGURE 15–2.** Simplified schematic diagram of an anesthesia machine (see text for details).

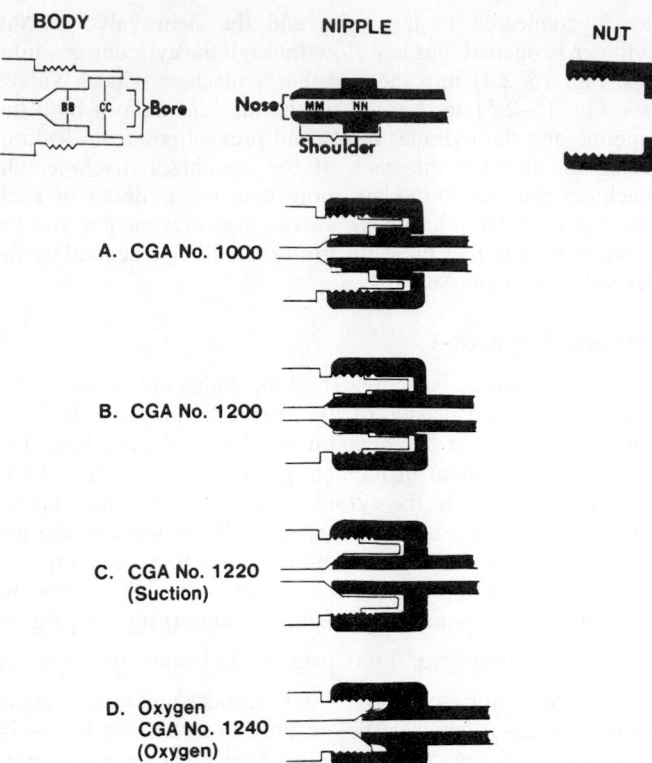

**FIGURE 15–3.** Diameter Index Safety System (1000 Series). With increasing compressed gas association (CGA) number, the small shoulder of the nipple becomes larger and the large diameter becomes smaller. Noninterchangeability of connections is ensured because either MM will be too large for BB or NN will be too large for CC if assembly of a nonmating body and nipple is attempted. (From Dorsch JA, Dorsch SE. *Understanding Anesthesia Equipment.* 2nd ed. Baltimore, Md: Williams & Wilkins; 1984:25.)

connected to a pneumatically driven mechanical ventilator, and the $O_2$ flush valve (see Fig. 15–2.9). On Datex-Ohmeda anesthesia machines, the $O_2$ in the high-pressure system is reduced from 50 psig (4.4 atm) to about 16 psig (2.1 atm) by the second-stage pressure regulator (see Fig. 15–2.10). This arrangement minimizes movement ("bobbing") of the $O_2$ flow meter float that is caused by variations in $O_2$ pressure with cycling of the mechanical ventilator and ensures that a decreasing $O_2$ supply pressure triggers the low $O_2$ supply pressure alarm before affecting the $O_2$ flow to the patient.

## Safety Features

A number of safety features are built into the high-pressure system. All are designed to prevent the anesthesia machine from delivering hypoxic gas.

### Diameter Index Safety System Connections

The Diameter Index Safety System (DISS; see Fig. 15–2.11) is designed to prevent the misconnection of a gas supply hose to the wrong pipeline gas inlet (eg, nitrous oxide [$N_2O$] supply hose connected to the $O_2$ pipeline inlet). The DISS standard specifies nut, nipple, and thread combinations (Fig. 15–3) that preclude such incorrect interconnections.

### Quick Connectors

Many hospital pipeline systems use so-called quick connectors (Fig. 15–4) that allow faster connection of gas supply hoses to the pipeline outlets than do the DISS connectors, which are more tedious to screw on and off. The quick connector systems are also specifically designed to prevent misconnections.

### Pin Index Safety System Connections

Analogous to the DISS is the Pin Index Safety System (PISS; see Fig. 15–2.12), which uses unique pin and receptacle combinations (Fig. 15–5) on cylinder hanger yokes to prevent the misconnection of a gas cylinder to the wrong cylinder inlet. The PISS system can be inappropriately defeated by pulling out the pins or by placing extra washers between the hanger yoke and the cylinder stem.

### Low Oxygen Supply Pressure Alarm

The low $O_2$ supply pressure alarm (see Fig. 15–2.13) is designed to warn the anesthesiologist when the $O_2$ pressure falls below about 30 psig (3 atm). Machine performance standards recommend that an alarm that cannot be disabled should sound within 5 seconds if the $O_2$ supply pressure decreases below the manufacturer-specified threshold level.[3]

One anesthesia machine manufacturer implements this device mechanically by using a pressure reservoir and a reed connected to the $O_2$ high-pressure line (Fig. 15–6). When the

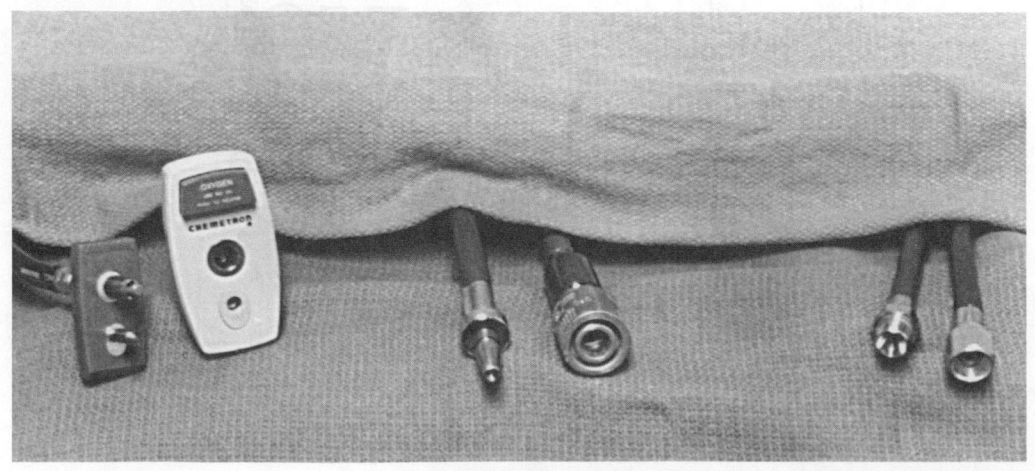

**FIGURE 15–4.** Examples of quick connectors, which, like Diameter Index Safety System connectors, prevent misconnections of high-pressure gas hoses. The quick coupler and the attached hose should be color-coded for the specific gas.

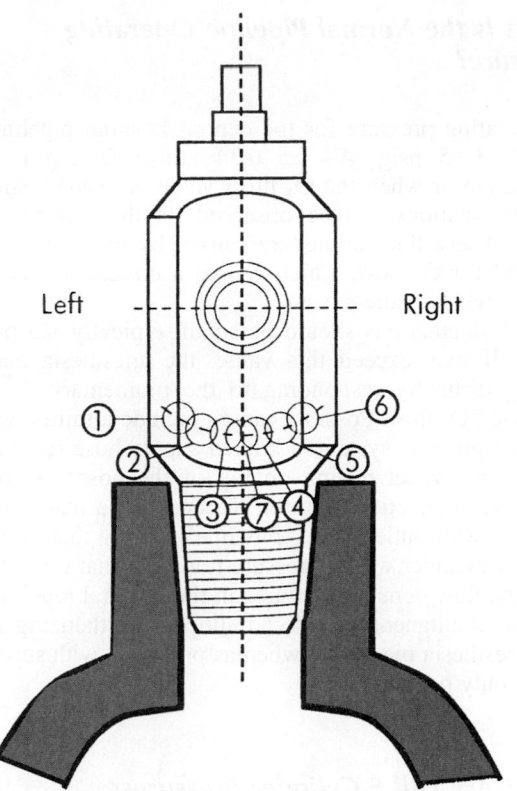

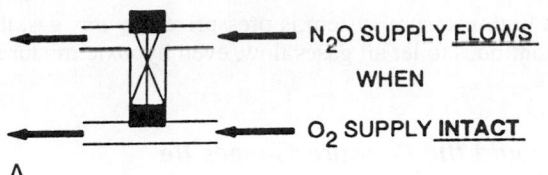

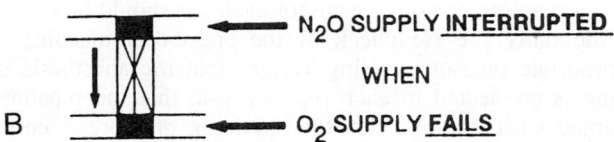

**FIGURE 15–7.** Oxygen pressure failure safety mechanism (fail-safe). *A,* When the oxygen system is pressurized, the fail-safe mechanism allows nitrous oxide to flow through the anesthesia machine. *B,* If the oxygen supply pressure decreases below the manufacturer's preset threshold (eg, 25 psig), the fail-safe mechanism shifts to interrupt the flow of nitrous oxide, either completely or in proportion to the decrease in oxygen pressure. (From Good ML, Cooper JB. Monitoring the anesthesia machine. In: Saidman LJ, Smith NT, eds. *Monitoring in Anesthesia.* 3rd ed. Boston, Mass: Butterworth-Heinemann; 1993:381.)

**FIGURE 15–5.** Pin Index Safety System pin location. Perspective shown looking at the placement of holes in the tank. Pins are placed precisely complementary in the tank yoke. Two pins are used to identify each type of gas. (From Eichhorn JH, Ehrenwerth J. Medical gases: storage and supply. In: Ehrenwerth J, Eisenkraft JB, eds. *Anesthesia Equipment: Principles and Applications.* St Louis, Mo: Mosby–Year Book; 1993:9.)

anesthesia machine is first connected to a high-pressure $O_2$ source (pipeline or cylinder) and is turned on, gas flows from the high-pressure line into the pressure reservoir, causing the reed to sound an alarm.

This feature explains why the low $O_2$ supply pressure alarm is activated when the anesthesia machine is first turned on. When the pressure in the reservoir equilibrates with the high-pressure $O_2$ line, gas stops flowing across the reed, and the alarm is silent. If the $O_2$ supply pressure decreases below a preset threshold, usually 30 psig (3 atm), gas begins to flow

from the pressure reservoir into the $O_2$ high-pressure line, once again causing the alarm to sound.

### Oxygen Pressure Failure Safety Mechanisms

Perhaps the most inappropriately named safety feature of the high-pressure system is the $O_2$ pressure failure safety mechanism (see Fig. 15–2.14). This device is often referred to only as the *fail-safe,* implying that it eliminates the possibility of the anesthesia machine delivering hypoxic gas. The $O_2$ pressure failure safety mechanism arrests (Ohmeda machines) or proportionally reduces (NAD machines) the flow of non-$O_2$ gases when the pressure in the $O_2$ pipeline decreases to $\leq 25$ psig (2.7 atm) (Fig. 15–7).

Continued flow of $N_2O$, helium, or other non-$O_2$ gases in the absence of $O_2$ quickly causes the gas mixture inspired by the patient to become hypoxic. Note, however, that if the $O_2$ pipeline or cylinder is pressurized with a gas other than $O_2$ (eg, argon), the fail-safe does not activate. As long as the $O_2$

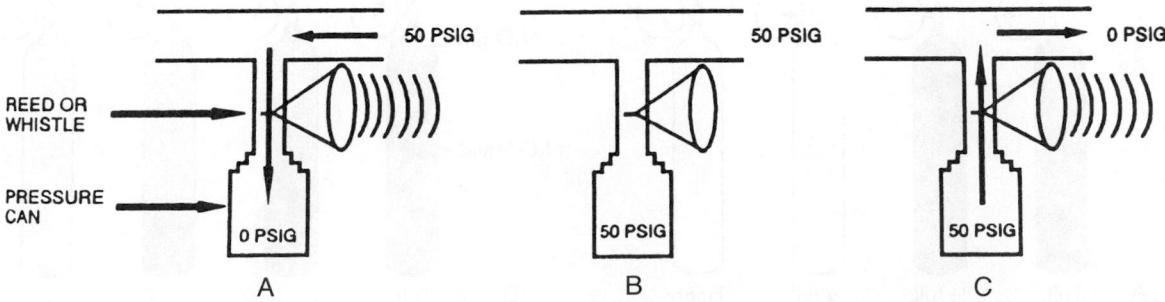

**FIGURE 15–6.** Low oxygen supply pressure alarm. *A,* When the anesthesia machine is connected to the oxygen supply and is turned on, oxygen at about 50 psig rushes by a reed or whistle as it passes into the pressure can. *B,* When oxygen pressure remains above a manufacturer's preset threshold (eg, 30 psig), the can remains pressurized, and the reed or whistle is silent. *C,* If the oxygen supply pressure drops below the manufacturer's preset threshold, gas rushes from the pressure can into the depressurized oxygen supply and causes the reed or whistle to sound the low oxygen supply pressure alarm. (From Good ML, Cooper JB. Monitoring the anesthesia machine. In: Saidman LJ, Smith NT, eds. *Monitoring in Anesthesia.* 3rd ed. Boston, Mass: Butterworth-Heinemann; 1993:381.)

line in the high-pressure system is pressurized by *any* gas, the fail-safe continues to let all gases flow, even hypoxic mixtures.

## When Should the Pressure Gauges Be Checked?

### Pipeline

The pipeline pressure gauge for each gas should be included in the daily pre-use check of the anesthesia machine. An appropriate pressure reading verifies that the anesthesia machine is connected to each pipeline gas, that the pipeline is charged with gas, and that the operating pressure is correct. Each gauge should be checked periodically during the anesthetic procedure to verify that the correct pressure is maintained. Occasionally, pipeline pressure is lost or may change dramatically (eg, decrease to 25 psig [2.7 atm]). Unexpected and confusing changes in machine performance (eg, switching from pipeline to cylinder gas source) may result if the anesthesiologist is unaware of the change in the gas supply pressure.

### Cylinder

To obtain an accurate cylinder pressure reading, the gauge must read zero before the cylinder is opened. If the cylinder pressure gauge does not read zero, depressurize by disconnecting the pipeline supply and pressing the $O_2$ flush button until the gauge reads zero. If depressurization of the cylinder gauge is impractical, the pressure reading on opening the cylinder can be trusted only if the new reading is higher than the original nonzero reading. Pressure in the $O_2$ cylinders should be checked each day as part of the pre-use machine check. Pressure in other gas cylinders ($N_2O$, air, helium) needs to be checked only according to periodic maintenance schedules, depending on local usage and practice. After checking the pressure in the gas cylinders, be sure to close the stem valve to prevent undesired leakage or inadvertent use of the cylinder gas.

## What Is the Normal Pipeline Operating Pressure?

Operating pressure for the central hospital pipeline should be 50 ± 5 psig (4.4 ± 0.34 atm).[4] During mechanical ventilation or when the $O_2$ flush valve is opened, small pressure fluctuations can be observed on the pipeline pressure gauge. These fluctuations are caused by the momentary high demand for $O_2$ flow, which causes a corresponding decrease in the high-pressure system.

Such fluctuations should be small, typically <5 psig (0.34 atm).[4] If they exceed this value, the anesthesia machine is having difficulty responding to the momentary demand for increased $O_2$ flow. Possible causes include a failure within the hospital pipeline system, a kinked supply hose (eg, caused by a machine wheel resting on top of the hose), an otherwise defective connection between the anesthesia machine and the pipeline wall outlet, or a "pipeline" supply that is actually a large H-cylinder with a pressure regulator that cannot keep up with the flow demand. Failures in the hospital pipeline system should simultaneously affect multiple anesthetizing locations and anesthesia machines, whereas problems with supply hoses affect only one site.

## What Are Full E-Cylinder Pressures?

### Oxygen

A full E-cylinder contains 660 L of $O_2$ and has a pressure of at least 1900 psig (131 atm).[5] Oxygen remains in the gaseous phase when compressed at room temperature. Thus, the amount of gas remaining in an E-cylinder is directly proportional to its pressure (Fig. 15–8A). In other words, the volume of $O_2$ remaining in the cylinder is equal to the cylinder pressure (psig) multiplied by 660 L, and divided by 1900 psig (131 atm). At 950 psig (66 atm), 330 L of $O_2$ remains compressed in the cylinder, and at 475 psig (33 atm), 165 L of $O_2$ remains.

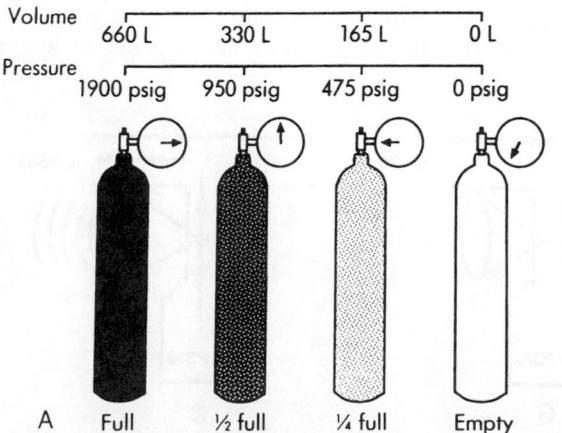

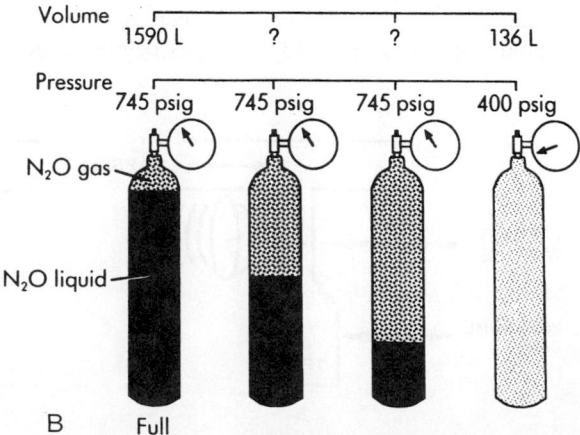

**FIGURE 15–8.** *A,* Oxygen remains a gas under high pressure. The pressure falls linearly as the gas flows from the cylinder; thus, in contrast to nitrous oxide, the oxygen pressure remaining always reflects the amount of gas remaining in the cylinder. *B,* At ambient temperature (20°C), nitrous oxide liquefies under high pressure, and the pressure of the gas above the liquid remains constant *independently* of how much liquid remains in the cylinder. Only when all the liquid has evaporated does the pressure start to fall; as the residual gas flows from the cylinder, the pressure falls rapidly. (From Eichhorn JH, Ehrenwerth J. Medical gases: storage and supply. In: Ehrenwerth J, Eisenkraft JB, eds. *Anesthesia Equipment: Principles and Applications.* St Louis, Mo: Mosby–Year Book; 1993:5.)

## Nitrous Oxide

A full E-cylinder of $N_2O$ contains 1600 L and has a pressure of approximately 750 psig (52 atm). Nitrous oxide enters the liquid phase when it is compressed at room temperature. As long as any of the $N_2O$ in the E-cylinder is in the liquid phase, the pressure remains 750 psig (52 atm) (see Fig. 15–8B). When the volume of $N_2O$ remaining in the cylinder reaches about 255 L (one sixth of its initial value), all of the $N_2O$ in the cylinder is in the gaseous phase.[6] From this point on, pressure correlates directly with the volume remaining, just as with $O_2$. Thus, an $N_2O$ E-cylinder with a pressure of 750 psig (52 atm) may contain as little as 255 L or as much as 1600 L of gaseous $N_2O$. Only by weighing the cylinder and also knowing the weight of the empty cylinder can one ascertain the exact amount of gas remaining. At a pressure of 375 psig (26.5 atm), 128 L of $N_2O$ remains within the cylinder; at 187 psig (13.7 atm), 64 L remains.

## Practical Applications

These relationships are used to determine how long an anesthesia machine can function on the reserve E-cylinder gas supplies. For example, suppose general anesthesia is needed in a remote site that is not supplied with pipeline gas. An E-cylinder of $O_2$ has a pressure of 1000 psig (69 atm), and an E-cylinder of $N_2O$ has a pressure of 745 psig (52 atm). Assuming fresh gas flows of 5 L/min each for $O_2$ and $N_2O$, how long can anesthesia be provided? Using the previously described relationships, 1000 psig corresponds to 347 L of $O_2$, which will last longer than 1 hour at a flow rate of 5 L/min. At a pressure of 745 psig (52 atm), the $N_2O$ E-cylinder contains any value between 255 and 1600 L, which, in a worst case scenario, provides a 5 L/min flow for 51 minutes.

For spontaneous respiration or manual positive pressure ventilation administered with the breathing bag, these calculations are sufficient. If an $O_2$-powered mechanical ventilator is used, however, you must also account for the extra usage. Oxygen usage by mechanical ventilators varies widely, ranging from 5 to 28 L/min. This additional usage is at least equal to the patient's minute ventilation.[7] Thus, if minute ventilation is 5 L, total $O_2$ usage per minute is at least 10 L. Because only 347 L of $O_2$ is left in the E-cylinder, anesthesia and mechanical ventilation with the $O_2$-powered ventilator can be provided for just over 30 minutes.

When using E-cylinders as the sole gas source, it is practical to obtain an anesthesia machine that has two $O_2$ hanger yokes and inlet ports. This setup allows one $O_2$ cylinder to be used while the other is being exchanged.

## What Is the Flow Rate When the Oxygen Flush Valve Is Pressed?

Note that the $O_2$ flush valve provides a direct connection between $O_2$ at 50 psig (4.4 atm) in the high-pressure system and the breathing system, which is in continuity with the patient's lungs (see Fig. 15–2.9). When the $O_2$ flush valve is depressed, the breathing system is flooded with 35 to 75 L/min of $O_2$.

If the adjustable pressure-limiting (APL, or *pop-off*) valve is partially or completely closed during spontaneous ventila-

tion, or if the pressure relief (spill) valve in the mechanical ventilator is closed during mechanical inspiration, this high flow may cause pressure to increase rapidly in the breathing system, potentially leading to cardiovascular compromise and pulmonary barotrauma.

To help guard against this complication, push the $O_2$ flush valve in short, intermittent bursts while observing the patient's chest or the airway pressure gauge. Never hold the flush valve open during the inspiratory phase of mechanical ventilation.[8] Alternatively, turn the ventilator off before pressing the flush button, but remember to turn the ventilator back on afterward.

## How Can a Hypoxic Gas Mixture Be Delivered With a Fail-Safe Mechanism?

The fail-safe designation is misleading because it implies that the anesthesia machine cannot deliver a hypoxic gas mixture. Unfortunately, the device protects against only the continued flow of $N_2O$ or other non-$O_2$ gas (eg, helium) after a loss of $O_2$ supply pressure. As was already discussed, if a non-$O_2$ pressurized gas source is attached inadvertently to the $O_2$ source, the fail-safe will be defeated.

Several other mechanisms can also cause a hypoxic gas mixture, including a contaminated $O_2$ pipeline or cylinder supply, inadequate $O_2$ flow, hypoxic $N_2O$–$O_2$ fresh gas flows, and leaks in the low-pressure system.[9] Although devices such as the fail-safe decrease the likelihood of hypoxic gas delivery, they do not eliminate it. Anesthesiologists must use calibrated $O_2$ analyzers with an audible alarm to ensure that a rare, but often lethal, hypoxic inspired gas mixture is rapidly detected.

## LOW-PRESSURE SYSTEM

## What Are the Structural Components?

### Flow Control Valves

The components and safety features in the low-pressure system are listed in Table 15–2 and illustrated graphically in Figure 15–2. The high-pressure system is separated from the low-pressure system by the flow control valves (see Fig. 15–2.15). As gas passes through the small orifice of the flow control valve, its pressure drops substantially. The flow control valves are simple but relatively precise variable-orifice needle valves. The anesthetic gas mixture is blended by turning the flow control valves to adjust the flow of $O_2$, $N_2O$, air, or

**TABLE 15–2.** Structures and Safety Features in the Low-Pressure System

| |
|---|
| **Structures** |
|    Flow control valves |
|    Flow meters (flow tubes) |
|    Manifold |
|    Calibrated vaporizers |
|    Common gas outlet check valve |
|    Common gas outlet |
| **Safety Features** |
|    Touch-indexed (fluted) $O_2$ flow control knob |
|    Hypoxic guard (link or proportioned) |
|    Minimal $O_2$ flow |
|    Vaporizer interlock–exclusion system |

other gases (eg, helium) that may be installed in a particular anesthesia machine.

### Flow Meters

As gas emerges from the flow control valve, it passes immediately into a flow meter (see Fig. 15–2.16). (Many anesthesiologists incorrectly state that they "adjust the flow meter." Technically speaking, one adjusts the flow control *valve* and observes the resulting flow on the flow *meter*.) Most anesthesia machines use a float or bobbin within a tapered, calibrated flow tube to measure the flow of gas emerging from the flow control valve. The greater the flow, the higher the float is lifted in the flow tube. Floats and flow tubes are calibrated as a pair for a specific gas. Use a flow meter only with the gas for which it was calibrated; if either the float or the tube is damaged, both must be replaced, or gas flow will be measured incorrectly.

### Manifold

Anesthesia machines usually have at least two, often three, and sometimes four or more separate gas sources, each with its own flow control valve and flow meter. Because the purpose of the low-pressure system is to blend a gas mixture, the gas emerging from each flow meter must be joined together; this junction takes place in the manifold (see Fig. 15–2.17) of the low-pressure system.

### Calibrated Vaporizers

As the gas mixture emerges from the flow meters and travels through the low-pressure system manifold, it may detour through one of the calibrated vaporizers (see Fig. 15–2.18) attached to the manifold. Contemporary anesthesia vaporizers are usually of the variable bypass type and are temperature compensated. The volatile anesthetic desflurane has a high vapor pressure and boils at 22.8°C, requiring a special Tec 6 desflurane vaporizer (Ohmeda, Madison, Wis).

### Common Gas Outlet

The low-pressure system arbitrarily ends with the common gas outlet (see Fig. 15–2.19). Some Ohmeda anesthesia machines position a common gas outlet check valve (see Fig. 15–2.20) just proximal to the outlet. The check valve is designed to prevent retrograde flow from the flush valve or breathing system into the low-pressure system. Newer anesthesia machines use special antidisconnect connectors (see Fig. 15–2.21) to help prevent accidental disconnection of the fresh gas hose from the common gas outlet.

### *Is the Arrangement of the Gas Flow Meters Important?*

Yes, the arrangement of the gas flow meters is important. The $O_2$ flow meter should connect to the manifold at the point closest to the common gas outlet.[10] This arrangement is safest if a leak occurs in one of the flow tubes or in the manifold. For example, let us assume that a 2-gas anesthesia machine with $N_2O$ and $O_2$, each flowing at 1 L/min, has a 1.5-L/min leak in one of the flow tubes (Fig. 15–9). If the $O_2$ flow meter is positioned farther from the common gas outlet than the $N_2O$ flow meter (see Fig. 15–9A and B), about 1 L/min of $O_2$ and 0.5 L/min of $N_2O$ escape through the leak; 0.5 L/min of pure $N_2O$ flows through the common gas outlet to the patient; and a hypoxic gas mixture rapidly develops in the breathing system.

Consider the same situation, but switch the order of the $O_2$ and $N_2O$ flow meters such that the $O_2$ flow meter is closest to the common gas outlet (see Fig. 15–9C and D). In this configuration, 1 L/min of $N_2O$ and 0.5 L/min of $O_2$ escape through the leak in the manifold, whereas 0.5 L/min of $O_2$ flows to the common gas outlet. Although the patient does not receive the intended 50:50 $N_2O$–$O_2$ gas mixture, the inspired gas is not hypoxic.

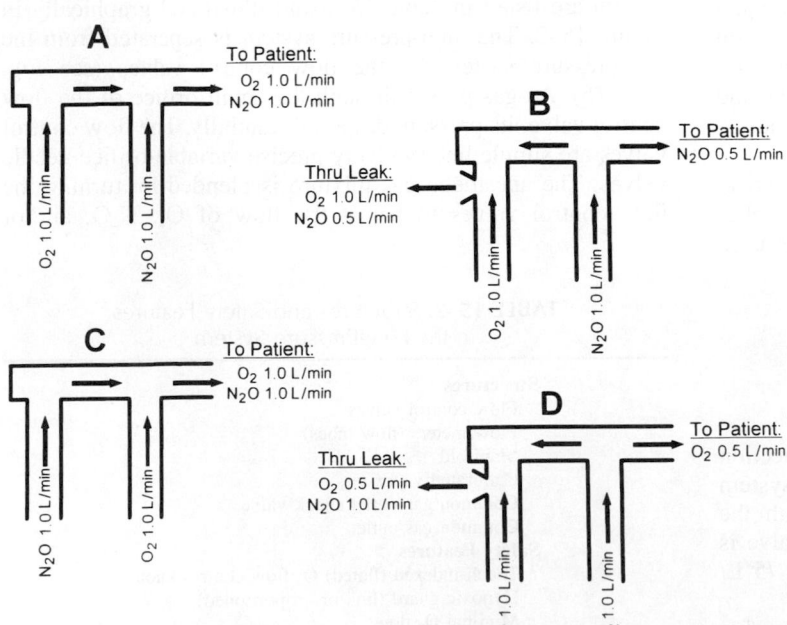

**A**

To Patient:
$O_2$ 1.0 L/min
$N_2O$ 1.0 L/min

Thru Leak:
$O_2$ 1.0 L/min
$N_2O$ 0.5 L/min

$O_2$ 1.0 L/min    $N_2O$ 1.0 L/min

**B**

To Patient:
$N_2O$ 0.5 L/min

$O_2$ 1.0 L/min    $N_2O$ 1.0 L/min

**C**

To Patient:
$O_2$ 1.0 L/min
$N_2O$ 1.0 L/min

Thru Leak:
$O_2$ 0.5 L/min
$N_2O$ 1.0 L/min

$N_2O$ 1.0 L/min    $O_2$ 1.0 L/min

**D**

To Patient:
$O_2$ 0.5 L/min

$N_2O$ 1.0 L/min    $O_2$ 1.0 L/min

**FIGURE 15–9.** Optimal arrangement of flow meters in low pressure system (see text for explanation).

## How Do Variable-Bypass Vaporizers Meter Anesthetic Vapor?

The functional components of a variable-bypass vaporizer (Fig. 15–10) include the gas inlet (see Fig. 15–10.1), bypass channel, vaporizing chamber (see Fig. 15–10.5), concentration control (see Fig. 15–10.2), temperature compensator (see Fig. 15–10.3 and 15–10.6), fluctuating back pressure compensator (see Fig. 15–10.4), bypass control valve (see Fig. 15–10.8), and gas outlet (see Fig. 15–10.7). When the concentration control is in the off position, the inlet and outlet port valves close, isolating the vaporizer from the fresh gas flow. When the concentration control is turned on, the vaporizer inlet and outlet port valves open, and the fresh gas mixture flows into the vaporizer.

From this point, the fresh gas flow is divided; most flows through the bypass channel and the remainder through the vaporizing chamber. The portion that travels along each route depends on the concentration control setting and on the temperature compensator. As the concentration control setting increases, the proportion of gas directed into the vaporizing chamber increases (see Fig. 15–10.10). Gas passing through the chamber becomes fully saturated with anesthetic vapor; as it emerges, it rejoins the gas passing through the bypass channel and exits through the vaporizer outlet port.

## Do Contemporary Vaporizers Compensate for Ambient Temperature?

Contemporary anesthetic vaporizers are temperature compensated. The temperature-compensating mechanism includes a sensing component (see Fig. 15–10.6) and a valve (see Fig. 15–10.3). As the liquid anesthetic cools, the temperature-compensating valve directs more gas into the vaporizing chamber, and vice versa. Thus, the vaporizer automatically compensates for changes in the vaporization of liquid anesthetic at different temperatures.

## Do Contemporary Vaporizers Compensate for Barometric Pressure?

Although the volumetric concentration (ie, volume/volume percent) of the anesthetic vapor emerging from a vaporizer is dependent on barometric pressure, compensation for changes in barometric pressure do not occur within contemporary vaporizers. Remember that the partial pressure (ie, millimeters of mercury) and not the concentration (ie, percentage) of anesthetic agent correlates with depth of anesthesia. Thus, although a vaporizer set to deliver 1% isoflurane at sea level delivers about 2% when the barometric pressure is decreased to 380 mm Hg, the gas mixture has an isoflurane partial pressure of about 7 mm Hg—the same as it would at sea level. Anesthetic potency is unchanged.

If the barometric pressure were increased to 1520 mm Hg, the 1% vaporizer setting actually would deliver 0.5%. Again, however, the partial pressure of isoflurane is 7 mm Hg. Thus, even though the vaporizer does not possess a formal barometric pressure compensator, and although changes in barometric pressure alter the volumetric concentration of the anesthetic output, the applicable physical principles of anesthetic vaporization enable the vaporizer to perform in a satisfactory manner.

## Do Contemporary Vaporizers Compensate for Fluctuating Back Pressure?

Intermittently fluctuating pressure in the breathing system, such as that generated by positive pressure ventilation or by intermittent pressing and releasing of the $O_2$ flush valve, causes fluctuating back pressure to be transmitted into the low-pressure system. Earlier vaporizer designs were susceptible to this pumping effect.[11, 12] When breathing system pressure was increased sufficiently, the pressure and, therefore, the volume of gas in both the vaporizing chamber and the bypass channel also increased. When the pressure was released, gas in the vaporizing chamber was able to flow retrograde into the bypass channel as it decompressed. The result of this pumping effect was an increased concentration of anesthetic delivered. New anesthetic vaporizers (Tec 4, Tec 5 [Ohmeda machines] and Dräger Vapor 19.1 [NAD machine]) incorporate mechanisms that decrease the size of the vaporizing chamber relative to the bypass channel and increase the volume of the inflow channel. Accordingly, vapor-saturated gas cannot make its way back into the bypass channel, and thus the pumping effect is prevented.

## Are Contemporary Vaporizers Accurate at Low Fresh Gas Flow Rates?

Some clinicians erroneously claim that vaporizer output is inaccurate at low fresh gas flow rates. During low-flow anesthesia, when only a small volume of fresh gas is added to the breathing circuit, the patient rebreathes much of his or her exhaled gas, which markedly changes the composition of the fresh gas. Constant flow performance data clearly demonstrate that anesthetic vaporizers are accurate, even when the fresh gas flow is only 500 mL/min (Fig. 15–11).

## What Happens If the Wrong Agent Is Added to a Vaporizer?

The concentration of anesthetic that emerges from the vaporizer depends on the vaporization characteristics of the

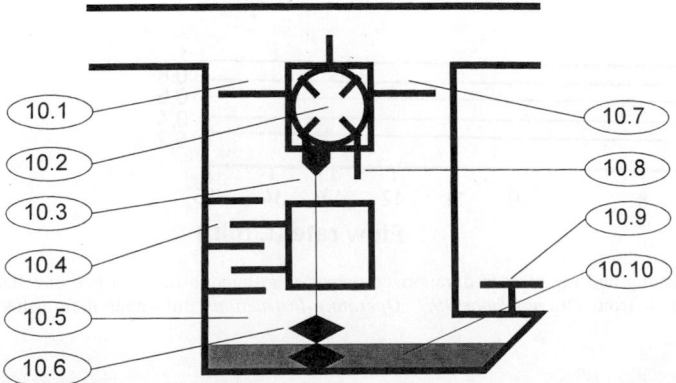

**FIGURE 15–10.** Cutaway view of a variable bypass, temperature compensated vaporizer (see text for explanation).

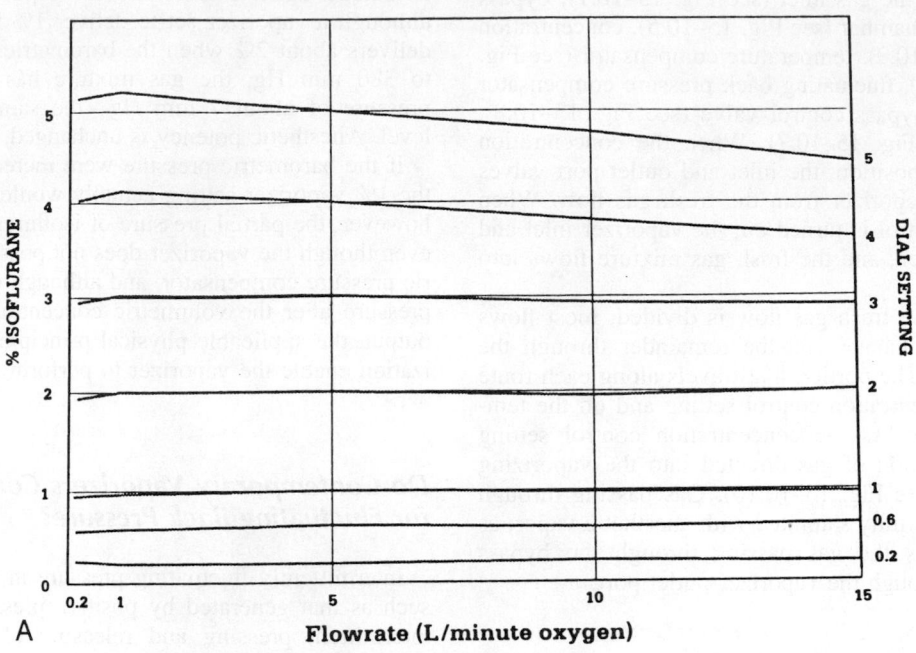

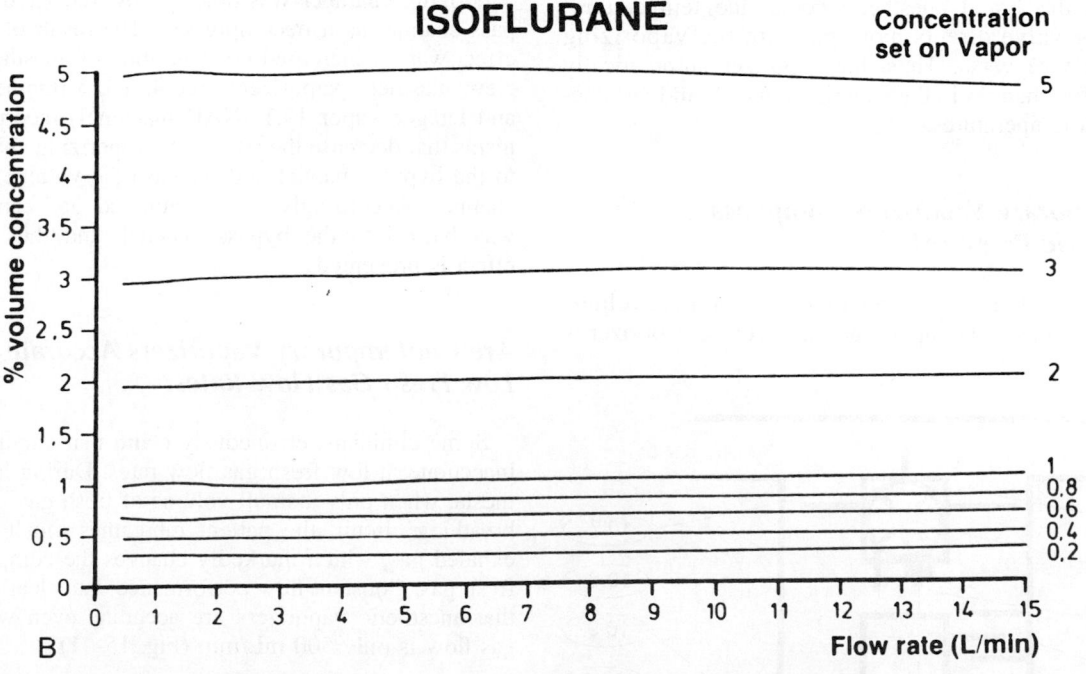

**FIGURE 15–11.** Performance graphs comparing the vaporizer control ("dial") setting and the measured vaporized output as a function of fresh gas flow. (*A* from *Tec 5 Operation and Maintenance Manual*. Madison, Wis: Ohmeda; 1989. *B* from *Dräger-Vapor 19.1, Operating Instructions*. Information furnished courtesy of Drägerwerk AG of Lübeck, Germany.)

**TABLE 15–3.** Structures and Safety Features in the Breathing System

**Structures**
Fresh gas hose
Fresh gas inlet
Inspiratory unidirectional valve
Expiratory unidirectional valve
Breathing hoses
Y-piece
Adjustable pressure-limiting or pop-off valve
$CO_2$ absorber housing
$CO_2$ absorbent canister
"Airway" (breathing system) pressure gauge
Return tube
Breathing bag
Bag/ventilator selector switch
Ventilator drive gas tube
Ventilator hose
Mechanical ventilator control unit
Ventilator bellows
Ventilator pressure relief ("spill") valve
**Safety Features**
Antidisconnect fresh gas hose connectors
Antidisconnect pressure sampling line connections
Ventilator low airway pressure alarm
Ventilator pressure-limiting adjustment knob
Ventilator pressure relief valve

agent. Isoflurane and halothane have nearly identical vaporization constants; thus, the concentration of anesthetic emerging from the vaporizer should be similar even if misfilling occurs. Halothane, however, is more potent than isoflurane. Therefore, the patient receives a relative overdose when an isoflurane vaporizer is filled with halothane. In general, the difference in anesthetic potency (ie, the minimum alveolar concentration) is of greater significance than differences in vapor pressure.

## BREATHING SYSTEM

### What Are the Structural Components?

Structures and safety features in the breathing system are listed in Table 15–3 and illustrated in Figure 15–12. The anesthetic gas mixture blended in the low-pressure system is delivered through the fresh gas hose (see Fig. 15–12.1), which connects to the breathing system at the fresh gas inlet (see Fig. 15–12.2) on the carbon dioxide ($CO_2$)-absorbent canister (see Fig. 15–12.3).

The circle anesthesia breathing system includes the inspiratory (see Fig. 15–12.4) and expiratory (see Fig. 15–12.5) unidirectional valves, breathing hoses (see Fig. 15–12.6), and Y-piece (see Fig. 15–12.7). Located on the $CO_2$-absorbent canister are the APL or pop-off valve (see Fig. 15–12.8); "airway" or, more precisely, breathing system pressure gauge (see Fig. 15–12.9); return tube (see Fig. 15–12.10); breathing bag (see Fig. 15–12.11); and the bag/ventilator selector switch (see Fig. 15–12.12).

Also included are the mechanical ventilator and associated components, specifically the ventilator hose (see Fig. 15–12.13), mechanical ventilator control unit (see Fig. 15–12.14), drive gas tube, ventilator bellows (see Fig. 15–12.15), and ventilator pressure relief (*spill*) valve (see Fig. 15–12.16). Note that if the bellows is not mounted directly on the ventilator control unit, a longer, nonstandard, wire-reinforced drive gas tube is required.

### Safety Features

Although many equipment related injuries are caused by problems in the breathing system, relatively few safety features are found in this portion of the anesthesia machine. Newer anesthesia machines have antidisconnect fresh gas hose connectors on both the machine and circuit side of the fresh gas hose rather than the older push-fit–type connectors. Also, contemporary anesthesia ventilators include a ventilator low airway pressure alarm that is designed to warn the clinician in the event of a partial or complete disconnection. Generally, mechanical inspiration is aborted if the airway pressure exceeds the high-pressure limit.

### When Is Carbon Dioxide Removed From the Respiratory Gas?

Despite its deceiving simplicity, tracing the flow of gas through a circle anesthesia breathing system is more difficult

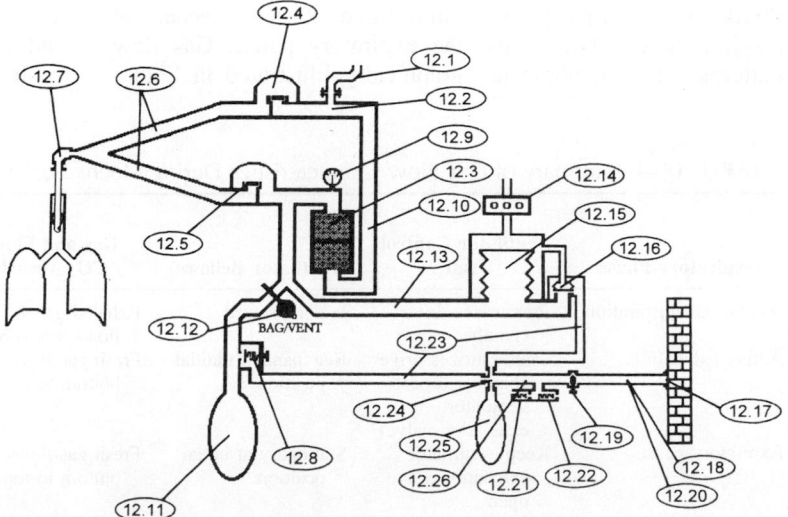

**FIGURE 15–12.** Simplified schematic diagram of the breathing and scavenging systems (see text for explanation).

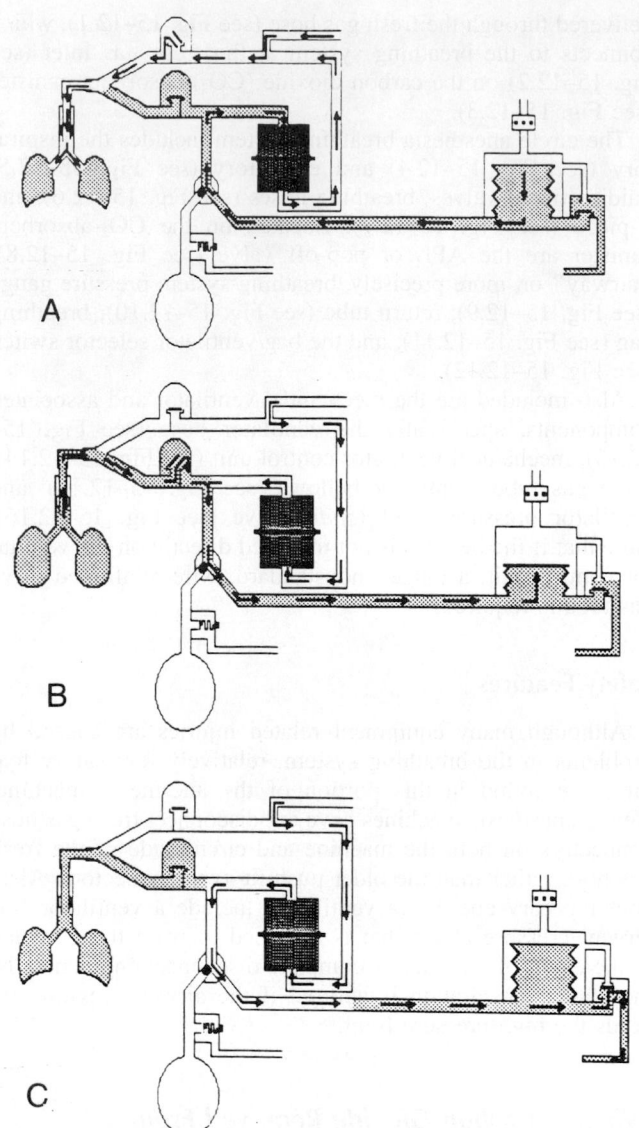

**FIGURE 15–13.** Gas flow through the circle anesthesia breathing system during the three phases of mechanical ventilation. *A*, Mechanical inspiration. *B*, Expiration. *C*, Expiratory pause. (See text for explanation.)

15–13, summarized in Table 15–4, and described in detail in the following sections. For an animation of the flow of gases in a circle breathing circuit, see the Internet site, http://www.anest.ufl.edu/vam.[13]

### Mechanical Inspiration

The control unit of the mechanical ventilator can be thought of as a timer and flow controller. When it initiates a mechanical breath, a high flow of drive gas (usually $O_2$ or an $O_2$-air mixture from the $O_2$ high-pressure system and entrained air) passes into the outer drive chamber of the mechanical ventilator (see Fig. 15–13A). The duration of this high-flow state (*mechanical inspiration*) and the flow rate of gas delivered to the outer chamber are determined by the tidal volume and inspiratory flow or inspiratory-to-expiratory ratio and respiratory rate settings on the control unit.

Pressurization within the drive chamber compresses the bellows and "pushes" gas, under positive pressure, into the ventilator hose and the breathing circuit. Pressure against the machine side of the expiratory unidirectional valve causes it to close, preventing gas from entering the expiratory limb of the circuit. Thus, the gas moves down through the $CO_2$-absorber and up the return tube that is concealed within. At the top of the $CO_2$ absorber, the positive pressure breath from the ventilator is augmented by the continuously flowing fresh gas mixture. The combined gas volume moves through the inspiratory unidirectional valve, down the inspiratory limb, through the Y-piece and endotracheal tube, and into the patient's lungs.

The drive gas delivered by the ventilator control unit during mechanical inspiration also pressurizes the upper side of the ventilator pressure relief valve, closing off access to the scavenging system and momentarily turning the circle breathing system into a closed breathing circuit for the duration of mechanical inspiration. Pressing the $O_2$ flush button during mechanical inspiration introduces 35 to 75 L/min of $O_2$ into a closed system and poses the risk for barotrauma. This is the rationale for the earlier recommendation of never activating the $O_2$ flush button during mechanical inspiration on an anesthesia machine of traditional design.

### Exhalation

The exhalation phase of the respiratory cycle commences as soon as the ventilator control unit ends the inspiratory phase and depressurizes the outer drive chamber of the mechanical ventilator by opening the ventilator exhalation valve that re-

than it appears. To understand this gas flow better, one can divide the respiratory cycle into three phases: mechanical inspiration, exhalation, and the expiratory pause. Gas flow patterns for each phase are graphically illustrated in Figure

**TABLE 15–4.** Summary of Gas Flow Characteristics During Mechanical Ventilation Through a Circle Anesthesia Breathing System

| Respiratory Phase | Ventilator Control Unit | Ventilator Bellows | Gas and Flow in $CO_2$ Absorber | Flow in Return Tube | Fresh Gas Flow | Ventilator Pressure Relief Valve |
|---|---|---|---|---|---|---|
| Mechanical inspiration | Pressurizes drive chamber | Is compressed | Exhaled gas with $CO_2$ flows top to bottom | Bottom to top | Toward inspiratory limb | Closed |
| Active exhalation | Depressurizes drive chamber (opens ventilator exhalation valve) | Reexpands to initial position | Fresh gas flows bottom to top | Top to bottom | Into return tube and absorbent canister | Closed |
| Expiratory pause | Keeps ventilator exhalation valve open | Stationary at initial position | Fresh gas flows bottom to top | Top to bottom | Into return tube and absorbent canister | Open |

leases the drive gas to atmosphere. Elastic recoil of the patient's lungs pushes gas through the airway and Y-piece and into the expiratory limb.

As the exhaled gas passes into the absorber, it is joined by the continuously flowing fresh gas mixture (see Fig. 15–13B). When the inspiratory unidirectional valve closes at the beginning of exhalation, the fresh gas flow can no longer continue its course into the patient; instead, the path of least resistance is now retrograde, down the return tube, and back through the $CO_2$ absorber, where it joins the exhaled gas from the patient's lungs. This gas mixture (exhaled and fresh gas) then passes through the bag/ventilator selector switch and ventilator hose and into the ventilator bellows, which reexpands to its initial position.

When the ventilator bellows reaches the top of its housing, pressure momentarily begins to increase in the breathing system, as evidenced by the momentary swelling of the bellows. As soon as the pressure reaches about 3 cm $H_2O$, however, the ventilator pressure relief valve opens to allow the remaining exhaled gas to enter the waste gas scavenging system. The ventilator pressure relief valve present in standing bellows ventilators is responsible for the "intrinsic" positive end-expiratory pressure (PEEP) of 2 to 3 cm $H_2O$ associated with standing bellows ventilators in the North American market.

The ventilator relief valve consists mainly of a weighted diaphragm. The weight keeps the diaphragm closed when there is no pressure buildup in the bellows, ensuring that the bellows is first completely refilled before excess gas is allowed to flow to the scavenging system. When the pressure inside the bellows acting on the underside of the diaphragm is sufficient to overcome the weight, the ventilator relief valve opens.

## Expiratory Pause

The time between the end of exhalation and the start of the next mechanical inspiration is designated as the *expiratory pause*. No gas movement occurs in or out of the patient's lungs nor in the inspiratory and expiratory limbs of the breathing system. However, fresh gas continues to flow into the absorbent canister (see Fig. 15–13C). The path of least resistance for this gas is also down the return tube, retrograde through the $CO_2$-absorbent canister, through the bag/ventilator selector switch and ventilator hose, into the ventilator bellows, and out the ventilator pressure relief valve. The fresh gas flow during this phase begins to purge the $CO_2$-containing gas from the ventilator hose and ventilator bellows. The degree to which purging occurs is dependent on the fresh gas flow rate and on the duration of the expiratory pause. Thus, at high fresh gas flow rates (eg, >12 L/min), the circle system can be used as a nonrebreathing system, and it allows adequate ventilation, even without $CO_2$ absorbent.

## What Is the Effect of a Torn Ventilator Bellows?

An intact bellows separates the circuit gas from the ventilator drive gas, which is $O_2$ (factory setting) in Ohmeda machines and an air-$O_2$ mixture in NAD Narkomed machines. With modern anesthesia ventilators such as the Ohmeda 7800, a torn bellows will not cause hyperventilation. In most cases, a bellows tear does not necessarily mean that the drive gas will enter the circuit and raise the fraction of inspired oxygen ($FIO_2$) or lighten anesthesia, except at high tidal volumes and low fresh gas flows. A bellows tear will, however, allow circuit gas to bypass the scavenging system and exhaust directly into the ambient air through the ventilator exhalation valve, causing room contamination.[14] An animation of the flow of gas during a bellows tear can be found at a website developed and maintained by the University of Florida Department of Anesthesiology.[13]

Note that certain ventilators, such as the Ohmeda 7800 ventilator and Datex-Ohmeda ADU, can use either medical air or oxygen as the drive gas. One of the rationales often put forward for using oxygen as the drive gas is that if there is a bellows tear, ingress of drive gas into the breathing circuit will result in an increase of $FIO_2$ rather than a potentially hypoxic mixture, should the drive gas be, for example, nitrogen. Recent studies indicate that, although this may have been true with much older ventilators, with modern ventilators such as the Ohmeda 7800, there is no clinical effect on $FIO_2$ with a bellows tear.[14] Furthermore, it can be argued that with the widespread availability of oxygen monitoring in North America, a bellows tear in a medical air-driven bellows will be detected by the $FIO_2$ monitor.

Another reason advanced for the use of oxygen as the drive gas in ventilators is that dried, filtered air is more expensive than $O_2$. This explanation appears counterintuitive if one considers that the manufacture of $O_2$ requires compression, purification, cooling, and compression to liquefy air, followed by fractional distillation to separate $O_2$ from nitrogen and argon. In addition, transport of the liquid $O_2$ (LOX) in special tankers and the rental of an insulated, on-site LOX tank also add cost, compared with in-hospital air compressors, filters, and desiccators. On the other hand, the capital cost of the compressors and affiliated equipment, depreciation, and routine maintenance need to be added to the cost of producing compressed air. A further argument could be made that, for hospitals with existing air compressors with spare capacity, switching to medical air as the drive gas represents an additional usage that does not cause an incremental increase in capital cost. A benefit of using air as the drive gas is that there is no longer a need to switch to manual ventilation when the reserve $O_2$ E-cylinder is in use to maximize its life.

## What Is the Effect of an Incompetent Unidirectional Valve?

The flow of gas during the three phases of respiration can be reexamined in the case of an incompetent inspiratory valve and an incompetent expiratory valve.

### Inspiratory Valve

With an incompetent, stuck-open inspiratory valve, mechanical inspiration proceeds normally because the inspiratory valve is supposed to be open at this time. During exhalation, however, the inspiratory valve fails to close, and part of the exhaled gas enters the inspiratory limb. If the volume of the exhaled gas entering the inspiratory limb exceeds the volume of the inspiratory hose, the excess gas passes down the return tube, enters the absorbent canister, and $CO_2$ is removed. During the expiratory pause, fresh gas flows retrograde through the return tube, flushing the $CO_2$-containing gas into the $CO_2$ absorber.

With the next mechanical inspiration, previously exhaled gas in the inspiratory limb is pushed back into the patient's lungs, causing $CO_2$ rebreathing. Because the volume of most standard breathing hoses is 300 to 600 mL, and because the tidal volume for adults exceeds the volume of the breathing hose, some fresh gas eventually reaches the patient's lungs, resulting in a minimal inspired $CO_2$ level of 0 mm Hg. Thus, an incompetent inspiratory valve causes partial rebreathing, the amount of which is determined primarily by the volume of the inspiratory hose relative to the tidal volume. The shape of the capnogram will reveal the problem, showing a sloping decline in $CO_2$ level from the end-tidal $CO_2$ value to 0 mm Hg, instead of the normal sharp drop.

## Expiratory Valve

When the expiratory valve is stuck open, exhalation proceeds normally because the expiratory valve is supposed to be open at this time. During mechanical inspiration, however, the expiratory valve fails to close. A portion of the inspiratory gas from the ventilator bellows is thus directed to the patient through the expiratory limb, and rebreathing of $CO_2$ results. In this case, the abnormal reservoir for $CO_2$ includes not only the expiratory limb but also the gas in the ventilator hose and ventilator bellows (2 L or more). Thus, an incompetent expiratory valve causes significantly more $CO_2$ rebreathing than does an incompetent inspiratory valve.

## What Is the Compliance of the Breathing Hoses?

The compliance of anesthesia breathing hoses varies greatly, depending on the type and manufacturer (Table 15–5). Most anesthesiologists use the term *compliance* to include collectively the distensibility of the breathing hose and volume of gas that can be compressed within it. This information is important to determine the volume of gas trapped in the

breathing system that does not reach the patient's lungs. It is calculated as the plateau inspiratory pressure (Pplat) minus PEEP (if applied), multiplied by the breathing circuit compliance. If Pplat is 23 cm $H_2O$, intrinsic PEEP is 3 cm $H_2O$, and the circuit compliance is 7 mL/cm $H_2O$, the volume of gas compressed within the hoses during mechanical inspiration is 140 mL. For an adult with an 800-mL tidal volume, this loss is not clinically significant. For a small child with a 300-mL tidal volume, however, it represents almost a 50% decrease.

Gas compressed within and distending the breathing hoses during mechanical inspiration does not enter the patient's lungs. During exhalation, the breathing hoses decompress, and the trapped gas exits with gas from the patient's lungs through the expiratory hose. Thus, a spirometer located on the expiratory limb includes both gas components (patient-ventilated and compressed gas) and may mislead the anesthesiologist into thinking that the patient's tidal volume is appropriate when it actually is low. The compliance of a breathing circuit can be estimated by occluding the Y-piece, pressurizing the circuit by cycling the ventilator, and observing the exhaled volume measured by a spirometer adjacent to the expiratory valve. The compliance (expressed as mL/cm $H_2O$) is determined from the exhaled volume and the measured circuit pressure minus the PEEP level, or the 3 cm $H_2O$ of intrinsic PEEP.

## How Is Carbon Dioxide Removed From the Respiratory Gas?

### Chemical Absorbent

During inspiration, the gas from the previous exhalation is directed through the $CO_2$-absorbent canister that contains a chemical $CO_2$ absorbent. Such absorbents, most commonly soda lime or Baralyme, chemically remove $CO_2$ from the gas. The chemical reactions require water and produce heat (Table 15–6).

### Dye Indicator

The $CO_2$ absorbent includes a dye indicator designed to turn the normally white absorbent to a purple color when it is

**TABLE 15–5.** Compression Volume Versus Pressure*

| | Peak Inflation Pressure (cm $H_2O$) | | | | |
|---|---|---|---|---|---|
| Circuit | *10* | *20* | *30* | *40* | *50* |
| *Mapleson D Circuits* | | | | | |
| Bain† | 20 | 60 | 100 | 120 | 167 |
| Piggyback† | 27 | 67 | 127 | 147 | 180 |
| Our own† | 27 | 53 | 94 | 120 | 160 |
| *Circle Circuits* | | | | | |
| Adult rubber | 127 | 240 | 353 | 487 | 600 |
| Adult rubber† | 147 | 267 | 380 | 547 | 687 |
| Adult plastic | 74 | 147 | 220 | 294 | 347 |
| Adult plastic† | 100 | 187 | 274 | 360 | 447 |
| Adult wire | 53 | 127 | 187 | 240 | 294 |
| Adult wire† | 74 | 147 | 220 | 280 | 353 |
| Pediatric rubber | 53 | 107 | 167 | 207 | 260 |
| Pediatric rubber† | 67 | 133 | 200 | 267 | 320 |
| Pediatric plastic | 53 | 113 | 174 | 233 | 267 |
| Pediatric plastic† | 67 | 140 | 200 | 274 | 333 |

*This table presents the mean volume of compressed oxygen (in milliliters) of 6 determinations at each peak inflation pressure (in centimeters of water).
†Study was carried out with a heated humidifier (see text for details).
From Coté CJ, Petkau AJ, Ryan JF, et al. Wasted ventilation measured in vitro with eight anesthetic circuits with and without inline humidification. *Anesthesiology.* 1983;59:442.

**TABLE 15–6.** Chemical Reactions of Carbon Dioxide With Soda-Lime (Top) and Baralyme (Bottom)

$$CO_2 + H_2O \rightleftarrows H_2CO_3$$
$$H_2O + 2NaOH \ (KOH) \rightleftarrows Na_2CO_3 \ (K_2CO_3) + heat$$
$$Na_2CO_3 \ (K_2CO_3) + Ca \ (OH)_2 \rightleftarrows CaCO_3 + 2NaOH \ (KOH)$$
$$Ba \ (OH)_2 + 8H_2O + CO_2 \rightleftarrows BaCO_3 + 9H_2O + heat$$
$$9H_2O + 9CO_2 \rightleftarrows 9H_2CO_3$$
$$9H_2CO_3 + 9Ca \ (OH_2) \rightleftarrows 9CaCO_3 + 18H_2O + heat$$

exhausted and no longer capable of removing $CO_2$. Normally, the dye indicator performs as it should. However, the color change is not permanent and may fade over time. Fluorescent lights also adversely affect absorbent performance.[15] Capnography serves as an additional and perhaps more reliable means to detect exhausted $CO_2$ absorbent, which is indicated by an elevated inspiratory baseline.

In certain instances, referred to as *tunneling,* respiratory gas may channel through the inner core of the absorbent-filled canister and exhaust this portion. The outer rim of absorbent remains white, concealing the purple, exhausted absorbent core. In this situation, the dye indicator change is not visible to the anesthesiologist; however, the capnograph detects the problem.

### Carbon Monoxide Poisoning

Excessively dry $CO_2$ absorbent will react with volatile anesthetics to create carbon monoxide. The first clinical manifestations of this phenomenon occurred mostly on Monday mornings, thus the term *Monday morning syndrome* associated with this hazard. If a machine is left with the $O_2$ flow meter running over the weekend, the $CO_2$ absorbent will dry out and will be more likely to generate carbon monoxide on exposure to volatile anesthetics. The general recommendation is to discard the $CO_2$ absorbent if it is suspected that it has dried out from exposure to a continuous flow of dry gas. $CO_2$ absorbents containing calcium hydroxide instead of sodium or potassium hydroxide have been shown to minimize the formation of carbon monoxide and compound A after exposure to sevoflurane, desflurane, isoflurane, and enflurane.[16]

### *What Is Compound A?*

Compound A is fluoromethyl-2,2-difluoro-1-(trifluoromethyl)vinyl ether, a product of degradation of sevoflurane when the agent is given during low-flow anesthesia. Although nephrotoxic to rats, it has not been shown to reach nephrotoxic levels in clinical practice.[17]

### *Why Does Positive End-Expiratory Pressure Not Register on the Breathing Pressure Gauge?*

The airway pressure gauge (which, as noted before, is more correctly called the *breathing system pressure gauge*) is typically positioned within the $CO_2$-absorbent canister on older machines (see Fig. 15–12.9). In this position, it is a long distance from the patient's airway and separated from it by

the inspiratory and expiratory unidirectional valves. When PEEP is added to the breathing circuit, typically through the placement of a valve on the expiratory port of the absorbent canister, the end-expiratory pressure is maintained on the patient side of the unidirectional valves but is not transmitted into the absorbent canister. Thus, the pressure gauge indicates only peak inspiratory pressure and returns to zero during exhalation.

On newer anesthesia machines, the gauge remains on the absorbent canister, but the pressure sensor is tunneled through the canister to measure the pressure on the patient side of the unidirectional valve (Fig. 15–14). In this position, it is closer to the patient's airway, more accurately reflects the pressure there, and registers PEEP.

### *What Is the Difference Between an Upright and a Hanging Bellows?*

An ascending (upright) bellows ascends during exhalation and descends during inspiration. A descending (hanging) bellows descends during exhalation and ascends during inspiration. Hence, the terms *ascending* and *descending* refer to the motion of the bellows during exhalation. The important difference between the two is that the ascending bellows requires that the patient's exhaled gas fill it, whereas the descending bellows refills on its own because gravity pulls it back to its initial position. In the event of a disconnection within the breathing system, the descending bellows ventilator continues to refill and to cycle. By contrast, the ascending bellows ventilator collapses, triggering the ventilator's low airway pressure alarm and alerting the anesthesiologist that a problem exists (Fig. 15–15).

Most anesthesia ventilators used on human patients in North America at present have upright bellows. In contrast, hanging bellows are commonly used in Europe. With the widespread availability of monitoring, a disconnection with a hanging bellows ventilator will be readily detected by the monitoring equipment (low airway pressure, low $CO_2$ waveform). Actually, an anesthesia machine incorporating a hanging bellows (Julian, Dräger Medical Inc.) has been approved for sale in the United States by the US Food and Drug Administration (FDA). The safety features of the Julian that mitigate the risks associated with the hanging bellows are listed subsequently.

The bellows is lighter than a traditional hanging bellows so that gravity generates a smaller suction effect through a disconnection. A small flow resistance is deliberately added to impede the exhaust of drive gas out of the bellows compartment during exhalation. The value of the flow resistance is designed to offset the reduced weight of the bellows. As a result, the bellows may fall on its own during a disconnection but will do so slowly so that the effect of a disconnection or leak on bellows motion will be quite noticeable. The bellows is designed to require exhaled gas to descend. A high fresh gas flow may conceivably cause the bellows to fall, but much of the fresh gas would also exit the circuit through the disconnection, and the rate of descent is reduced to some extent relative to an airtight breathing circuit. In addition, an optical sensor at the base of the bellows compartment detects when the bellows has reached the bottom and will set off an alarm if that does not occur. Finally, the machine is designed with integrated pressure and $CO_2$ monitoring, which was not the case in machines of the past with a descending bellows.

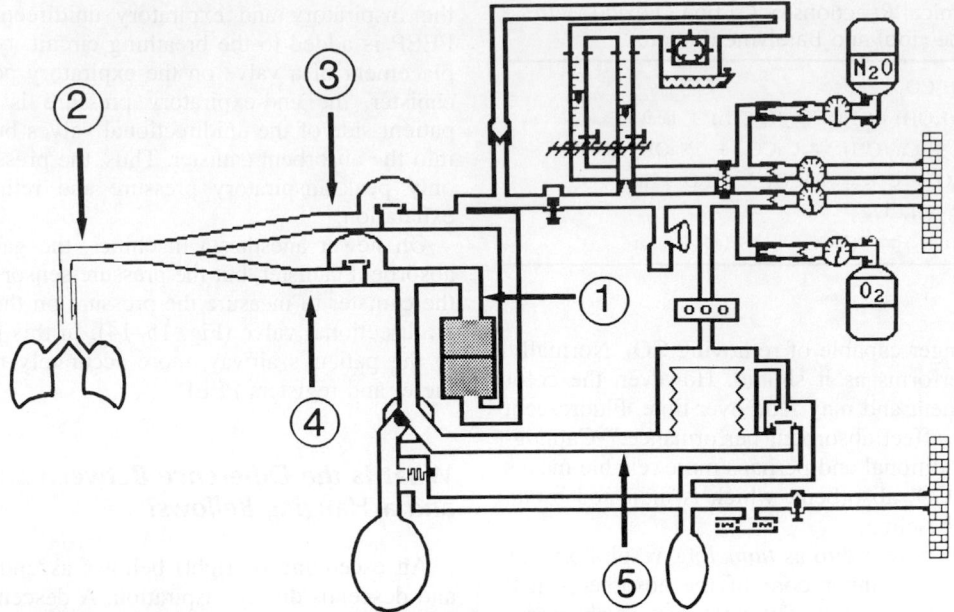

**FIGURE 15–14.** Breathing system pressure sensor sites. *1,* In older breathing systems, pressure is sensed within the absorber canister. Positive end-expiratory pressure (PEEP), which is constrained to the patient side of the unidirectional valves, does not register when breathing system pressure is sensed in this location. *2,* If breathing system pressure is measured close to the patient's airway, it more accurately reflects pressure in the patient's lungs. However, pressure sensors that are connected at this site tend to promote displacement of endotracheal tubes, are sometimes bulky, and increase the number of potential disconnection sites. *3 & 4,* Breathing system pressure sensors placed on the patient side of unidirectional valves correctly register PEEP when present. Site 4 is preferred to site 3 because at site 3, pressure fluctuations are registered (and prevent low-pressure alarms from sounding) with a disconnection if a partial obstruction occurs between the pressure sensor and the patient's airway. *5,* Breathing system pressure should never be measured in the ventilator portion of the breathing system. Again, breathing system pressure fluctuations may register even though a complete disconnection has occurred further downstream. (Modified from Good ML, Cooper JB. Monitoring the anesthesia machine. In: Saidman LJ, Smith NT, eds. *Monitoring in Anesthesia.* 3rd ed. Boston, Mass: Butterworth-Heinemann; 1993:387.)

## WASTE GAS SCAVENGING SYSTEMS

### Why Do We Need Scavenging Systems?

Concerns have been voiced about the mutagenicity, carcinogenicity, organ toxicity, and adverse reproductive effects of inhaled anesthetics. A recent American Society of Anesthesiologists (ASA) publication[18] developed by the ASA Task Force on Trace Anesthetic Gases found that "studies have not shown an association between trace levels of waste anesthetic gases found in *scavenged* anesthetizing locations and adverse health effects to personnel." The publication recommended

scavenging of waste anesthetic gases at all anesthetizing locations, noting that with scavenging and appropriate work practices, trace levels of anesthetic gases are within the exposure limits recommended by regulatory agencies.

### How Are Gas Scavenging Systems Classified?

Gas scavenging systems are classified (Table 15–7) as active or passive and as valved ("closed") or valveless ("open"). A vacuum source (see Fig. 15–12.17), vacuum hose

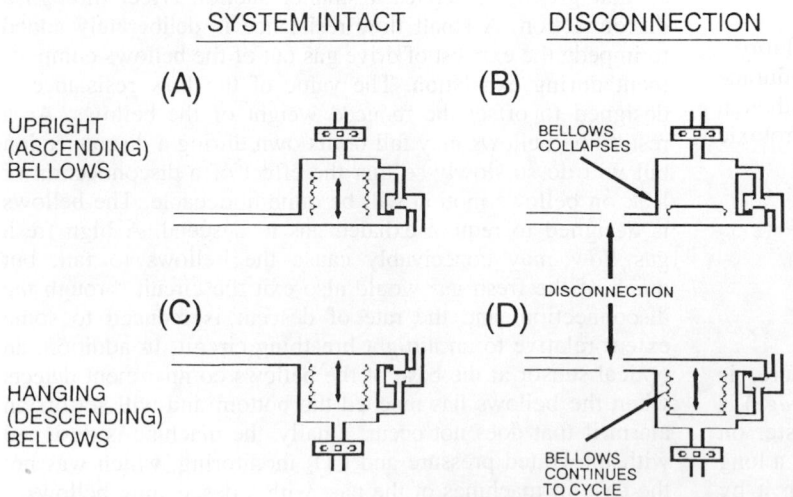

| SYSTEM INTACT | DISCONNECTION |
|---|---|

UPRIGHT (ASCENDING) BELLOWS — (A)

(B) BELLOWS COLLAPSES

DISCONNECTION

HANGING (DESCENDING) BELLOWS — (C)

(D) BELLOWS CONTINUES TO CYCLE

**FIGURE 15–15.** Comparison of an upright (ascending) and hanging (descending) bellows mechanical ventilator during disconnection. The upright bellows ventilator cycles normally when the breathing system is intact (*A*) but collapses during disconnection (*B*) because the patient's exhaled gas no longer lifts the bellows back to its initial position. The hanging bellows ventilator cycles normally when the breathing system is intact (*C*); it continues to cycle up and down despite a disconnection (*D*) because the bellows is pulled by gravity to its initial position. (From Good ML, Cooper JB. Monitoring the anesthesia machine. In: Saidman LJ, Smith NT, eds. *Monitoring in Anesthesia.* 3rd ed. Boston, Mass: Butterworth-Heinemann; 1993:386.)

**TABLE 15–7.** Classification of Gas Scavenging Systems

| Manufacturer | Model | Active | Passive | Valved* | Valveless† |
|---|---|---|---|---|---|
| Ohmeda (Madison, Wis) | Waste gas scavenging interface valve | X‡ | X‡ | X | |
| North American Dräger (Telford, Pa) | Scavenger interface for air conditioning systems | | X | X | |
| | Scavenger interface for suction systems | X | | X | |
| | Open reservoir scavenger | X | | | X |

*Also referred to as *closed.*
†Also referred to as *open.*
‡This scavenging system can be used in either an active or a passive configuration.

(see Fig. 15–12.18), and vacuum control (see Fig. 15–12.19) distinguish an active scavenging system, whereas a waste gas evacuation hose (see Fig. 15–12.20) replaces these components in a passive scavenging system.

The negative pressure (vacuum) source of the active scavenging system, usually a component of the hospital pipeline system, actively pulls the excess gas from the anesthesia machine, transports it through the hospital gas disposal system, and typically releases it from the roof. Passive scavenging systems do not require the vacuum source; instead, they rely on a slight positive pressure to push the waste gas out through the waste gas evacuation hose and into the gas disposal system.

## Can Gas Scavenging Systems Injure Anesthetized Patients?

If excessive positive or negative pressure develops in the scavenging system, it can be transmitted back through the breathing system to the patient's lungs. To minimize the likelihood of these events, both active and passive scavenging systems include a positive pressure relief mechanism (see Fig. 15–12.21) to vent undesired positive pressure. Note that there is no alarm to inform the user that circuit gas is being insidiously spewed into ambient air. Active scavenging systems also include a negative pressure relief mechanism (see Fig. 15–12.22) to dissipate undesired negative pressure. Some systems use gravity-driven or spring-loaded valves for the positive and negative pressure relief mechanisms. Other systems accomplish the same objectives without valves. These safety features do not protect the patient if the scavenging hoses are obstructed between the breathing circuit and the safety valve, as might occur with improper connections or kinking of hoses.

**TABLE 15–8.** Structures and Safety Features of the Gas Scavenging System

**Structures**
- Collecting hoses (19-mm yellow connectors for older machines; 30-mm magenta connectors for newer machines)
- Inlet ports
- Reservoir
- Manifold
- Vacuum port and control (active)
- Exhaust port and evacuation hose (passive)

**Safety Features**
- 19-mm or 30-mm connectors
- Positive pressure relief mechanism
- Negative pressure relief mechanism

## What Are the Structural Components?

The structures and safety features of the waste gas scavenging system are listed in Table 15–8 and illustrated in Figure 15–12. Excess anesthetic gas must be collected from the APL and ventilator pressure relief valves (see Fig. 15–12.8 and 15–12.16). A scavenging system collecting hose (see Fig. 15–12.23) connects each of these to the scavenging system intake ports (see Fig. 15–12.24). The scavenging system may have just one intake port that must be divided to allow both collecting hoses to be connected. If more than two intake ports are present, those not in use should be capped off to ensure proper function of the scavenging system.

The vacuum control (see Fig. 15–12.19) typically is an adjustable needle valve that controls the flow rate of gas from the scavenging system into the hospital gas disposal system. A gas reservoir (see Fig. 15–12.25) is also required to buffer the intermittent outflow of waste gases from the breathing circuit. The vacuum hose, vacuum control, intake ports, and reservoir bag are joined together by the scavenging system manifold (see Fig. 15–12.26), which is also called the scavenging system *interface* because it interfaces the anesthesia machine and the hospital gas disposal system. The passive scavenging system has a waste gas evacuation hose (see Fig. 15–12.20). This hose connects the scavenging manifold with the environment into which the waste gas will be delivered (eg, a nonrecirculating air conditioning intake duct or an open window).

## Why Does a Scavenging System Need a Gas Reservoir?

The flow rate of gas from the breathing system into the scavenging system can be calculated as the total fresh gas flow into the breathing system minus the rate of $O_2$ consumption and other gas uptake by the patient (eg, $N_2O$ during induction) plus the rate of $CO_2$ production and other gas elimination by the patient into the breathing system (eg, $N_2O$ during emergence) minus leaks (including gas sampled by the gas analyzer). During maintenance anesthesia, with minimal gas uptake or elimination, the total flow of gas into the scavenging system is about the same as the total fresh gas flow rate. Unfortunately, knowledge of the total flow of gas into the scavenging system is of little use clinically because gas does not flow into the scavenging system at a continuous rate but rather in discrete "boluses."

### Positive Pressure Ventilation

Table 15–4 and Figure 15–13 demonstrate that when the patient's lungs are mechanically ventilated, gas enters the scavenging system through the ventilator pressure relief valve only during late exhalation and the expiratory pause after the ventilator bellows has returned to its full position. When the anesthesiologist delivers positive pressure breaths manually with the breathing bag, gas enters the scavenging system when the breathing system pressure exceeds the opening pressure of the APL valve.

## Spontaneous Breathing

Because spontaneous breathing is often assisted with manual ventilation, the selector knob is usually set in the manual position. However, a patient can also be breathing spontaneously with the selector knob set to the ventilator position, although in this configuration, it is impractical to assist the patient's respiration. When the patient breathes spontaneously, gas enters the scavenging system through the APL valve (pressure relief valve) only during late expiration and the expiratory pause after the breathing bag (bellows) is fully distended.

## Reservoir Function

Regardless of the mode of ventilation, gas delivery to the scavenging manifold is discontinuous and can be high when the $O_2$ flush is activated. Gas flow out of the scavenging system, however, is continuous and constant. Therefore, the gas reservoir—typically, a bag or canister—is needed to provide buffering between the discontinuous flow into and continuous flow out of the scavenging system. Without a reservoir (see Fig. 15–12.25), excessively high vacuum would be required to capture all the waste gas; more likely, inadequate vacuum levels would result in spillage of waste anesthetic gas into the operating room environment.

## Vacuum Control

From the preceding discussion, one deduces that if the volume of the gas reservoir is adequate, the vacuum flow rate should be set slightly greater than the total fresh gas flow rate. In clinical practice, however, this precise an adjustment is difficult. With one open reservoir system, the flow induced by the vacuum is adjusted using a flow meter.[19] For systems that use a reservoir bag, the vacuum level is adjusted until the reservoir bag is neither fully collapsed nor fully distended.

Recall, however, that each time the rate of fresh gas flow into the breathing system changes, the rate of gas flow out of the breathing system and into the scavenging system also changes. The rate of fresh gas flow changes many times during a typical anesthetic procedure because high flow rates of $O_2$ (eg, 6-12 L/min) are provided during denitrogenation and mask ventilation before intubation; high flows (eg, 5 L/min) of $O_2$ and $N_2O$ or air occur during the rapid uptake phases; low or very low flows (eg, 0.5-2 L/min) are provided during maintenance anesthesia; periodic increases to higher flow (3-5 L/min) are used to quickly increase or decrease the concentration of volatile agent in the breathing system; and a return to high flows (eg, 5 L/min) occurs just before emergence to hasten elimination of anesthetic gases from the breathing system. To prevent the reservoir bag from overdistending or collapsing, each change in fresh gas flow would need to be accompanied by a concomitant change in the vacuum control knob.

### Practical Considerations

Because this approach is not clinically practical, we must choose the "lesser of two evils": (1) having the reservoir bag fully distended and venting anesthetic gas into the room, with a risk for excessively high airway pressures if the positive pressure relief mechanism fails; or (2) allowing the reservoir bag to be fully collapsed and air-conditioned room air to be entrained, with the risk for subatmospheric pressures if the negative pressure relief mechanism fails.

In our opinion, the fully collapsed bag is a more attractive option. During pre-use check of the anesthesia machine, we follow the advice of a colleague: we completely close the vacuum control knob (clockwise) and then open it one-half turn counterclockwise (personal communication, Dr. David G. Bjoraker, 1991). This technique results in a collapsed reservoir bag at low fresh gas flow rates and in a partially distended reservoir bag at high flow rates. The one-half turn may have to be adjusted in each practitioner's institution, depending on the strength of the vacuum.

## Can Scavenging and Breathing Circuit Hoses Be Used Interchangeably?

Scavenging and breathing system hoses are similar in appearance. For safety reasons, however, scavenging collecting hoses are fitted with 19-mm (30-mm on newer machines) connectors and breathing hoses with 22-mm connectors. The 19-mm (30-mm) connectors are often color-coded with yellow (magenta on newer machines) tape or molded from yellow (magenta) plastic to distinguish them clearly from breathing hoses, which have black or clear plastic connectors.

Misconnection of scavenging hoses so that exhalation is blocked has the disastrous consequence of barotrauma.

## What Happens If the Ventilator Scavenging Hose Becomes Obstructed?

Obstruction of either gas collecting hose is dangerous because it prevents gas from exiting the breathing system. Because fresh gas continues to flow in, breathing system and airway pressures increase dramatically and rapidly, leading to barotrauma. Typical clinical findings include subcutaneous emphysema of neck and face, pneumothorax, pneumomediastinum, pneumoperitoneum, and possibly dissection of air into the mesentery with air surrounding the intestines. Tension pneumothorax and cardiovascular collapse lead to death unless the syndrome is discovered and treated in time.

During manual positive pressure ventilation, the anesthesiologist usually recognizes that a problem exists because the breathing bag "gets stiff" and continues to distend even though the APL valve is fully opened. With mechanical ventilation, however, this important clinical sign is not available because the bag is not held in the hand. A distended ventilator bellows, abnormal ventilator sounds, or elevated airway pressures may be the first clues. Ideally, the airway pressure is monitored close to the endotracheal tube. As an additional safety feature to protect the patient against excessive airway pressure, inflate the cuff of the endotracheal tube so that it can function as a safety valve. That is, enable the cuff to leak when the desired peak airway pressure is exceeded by a few centimeters of water pressure.

Precautions to prevent injury include keeping scavenging hoses as short as possible so that they are not run over and obstructed by the wheels of the anesthesia machine. Never use adhesive tape to mate a 22-mm breathing hose connector incorrectly to a 19-mm mount. The tape can work itself free and obstruct the lumen of the collecting hose, and this obstruction will not be visible. This particular failure mode has been eliminated with the newer 30-mm connector. Patency of the scavenging collecting hoses should be assessed during the pre-use check of the anesthesia machine.

## TROUBLESHOOTING THE GAS DELIVERY SYSTEM

Anesthesiologists must apply their technical knowledge of the anesthesia machine by (1) conducting a pre-use check each day before first use, (2) monitoring the performance of the machine during an anesthetic procedure, and (3) troubleshooting the machine to identify and correct malfunctions when they occur.

### What Needs to Be Checked?

Equipment malfunction is an infrequent but recurrent cause of critical incidents. Numerous case reports describing injuries and "near misses" resulting from equipment malfunction fill the anesthesia literature. Nearly every component of the anesthesia gas delivery system has been implicated. In one large study of untoward outcomes in anesthesia, injury from equipment malfunction (including breathing system disconnection) accounted for about 14% of all critical incidents.[20]

Patients are usually not directly injured by an equipment failure. Instead, the equipment malfunction compounds and worsens an evolving crisis in which the primary causative factor is a human error.[21] In large surveys of critical anesthesia incidents, "failure to check" is one of the most frequently cited "associated factors."[22]

### A Critical Example

Suppose that a syringe of succinylcholine is mislabeled as fentanyl. During monitored anesthesia care, the patient receives 100 μg (2 mL) of "fentanyl," promptly "has a seizure," and becomes apneic. Anticipating a spontaneously breathing patient, the anesthesiologist failed to check the anesthesia machine before beginning the anesthetic procedure. Now, a malfunctioning bag/ventilator selector switch prevents the patient from receiving positive pressure ventilation by either the breathing bag or the mechanical ventilator. The backup self-inflating resuscitation bag is missing from the anesthesia cart. The patient suffers several minutes of hypoxemia before a Mapleson circuit and E-cylinder of $O_2$ are brought to the operating room, assembled, connected, and used to restore ventilation. The primary problem was human error, namely the mislabeling of a syringe. However, the patient would have done well if the anesthesia machine and the backup ventilation equipment had been present and properly checked before the case began.

### How Well Are Systems Checked?

Can anesthesia practitioners properly check an anesthesia gas machine? In the early 1980s, Buffington and coworkers studied the ability of anesthesia personnel to detect anesthesia machine malfunctions.[22] Anesthesia machines were preconfigured with five machine faults:

1. Removal of inspiratory and expiratory unidirectional check valves
2. Removal of the PISS, which allowed interchange of $N_2O$ and $O_2$ reserve E-cylinders
3. Malfunction of the fail-safe mechanism
4. Interchange of $O_2$ and cyclopropane flow tubes
5. Misfilling of the halothane vaporizer with methoxyflurane

Anesthesiologists were asked to examine the anesthesia machines and determine what was wrong. On average, only 2.2 of the five faults were identified. No faults were detected by 7.3% of participants, and only 3.4% detected all five faults. Participants with >10 years of clinical anesthesia practice identified more faults (2.46) than did those with less experience (2.04). No correlation was found between professional background (physician, nurse, technician, dentist, designer, manufacturer, or service personnel) and the number of faults detected.

### Are Pre-Use Check Protocols Useful?

Because "failure to check" can set the stage for a critical incident, manufacturers of anesthesia machines, the ASA, the Anesthesia Patient Safety Foundation (APSF), and the FDA support the use of pre-use check protocols to help anesthesia practitioners ensure that their anesthesia machine is properly functioning and fit for patient use. The FDA designed a generic protocol, entitled *Anesthesia Apparatus Checkout Recommendations,* that was first published in 1986[23] and has since been widely disseminated.[24, 25]

The effectiveness of the FDA protocol was subsequently evaluated in the early 1990s.[26] Residents in training and private practitioners attending continuing medical education meetings were challenged to identify one set of four machine faults using their own check methods, and then a different set of four machine faults using the FDA protocol. The specific machine faults included a malfunctioning $O_2$-to-$N_2O$ ratio protection system, malfunctioning fail-safe mechanism, malfunctioning $O_2$ analyzer, leak in the low-pressure system, leak in the mechanical ventilator, leak in the vaporizer, incompetent unidirectional valve, and a leak in the high-pressure system.

Participants detected an average of only 1.03 of four faults (25.8%) using their own check methods and only 1.20 of four faults (29.9%) using the FDA check protocol. Only the malfunctioning $O_2$-to-$N_2O$ ratio protection system was detected more frequently using the FDA check protocol than the participants' own methods. The investigators concluded that the "mere introduction of the FDA checklist did not improve the ability of anesthesiologists to detect anesthesia machine faults."[26]

### Why Do Pre-Use Check Protocols Fail?

Two important considerations help us to understand why detailed pre-use check protocols by themselves fail to improve the ability to detect anesthesia machine malfunctions.

### Understanding

The written protocol provides specific instruction for completing the pre-use check, but it does not help one to understand the anesthesia machine.

### Length of the Pre-Use Check List

A factor contributing to poor acceptance and understanding of the pre-use machine check is its length. Older protocols included 70 or more individual tasks and took 10 minutes or more to complete. They included checking machine components that fail infrequently and that do not immediately jeopardize the patient when they do fail. Newer anesthesia machines like the Datex-Ohmeda AS/3 ADU incorporate semiautomated pre-use checks that reduce the time required for a check by the user. In the ADU, a complete system check lasts about 3 to 4 minutes, during which time the user can perform other tasks. In an emergency, the user can bypass the automated pre-use check. The system checks gas supply pressures, $N_2O$ delivery, hypoxic mixture prevention, agent delivery, automatic and manual ventilation, and circuit leaks.

## What Is the Revised Food and Drug Administration Pre-Use Check Protocol?

Table 15–9 shows the revised pre-use check protocol. It emphasizes components that fail frequently or that can quickly and severely jeopardize the safety of the anesthetized patient. Other components are relegated to periodic maintenance.

For example, the $O_2$ supply pressure fail-safe mechanism is a durable mechanical device that rarely fails. Even if it does fail, it does not injure the anesthetized patient except with a simultaneous loss of the $O_2$ supply pressure. Even in this worst case scenario, the low $O_2$ supply pressure alarm on the anesthesia machine, the low $O_2$ supply pressure alarm on the mechanical ventilator, the $O_2$ analyzer, and eventually the pulse oximeter alarm should warn of a developing hypoxic gas mixture in sufficient time for corrective action to be taken.

## How Has the Revised Food and Drug Administration Pre-Use Check Performed?

The revised FDA pre-use check protocol can be completed in 5 minutes or less. A study of 22 subjects indicated that the revised FDA checklist was not more effective than the user's own methods in detecting faults. Using their own methods, 54.5% of anesthesia providers did not discover >50% of an initial set of four faults. Using the revised FDA checklist, 40.9% of the same users did not detect >50% of a different set of four faults. There was no statistical difference ($P$ = .479) in fault detection scores.[27]

In another study involving 29 anesthesiology residents, 69% of faults were detected with the revised FDA pre-use check. After instructional review, 86% of faults were detected by the same group of subjects. The authors noted that they did not achieve the high detection rate they sought, even with instructional review and intensive teaching.[28]

Its recommendation is generally not applicable to newer machines like the Dräger Julian, Datex-Ohmeda Aestiva, and Siemens KION (Siemens-Elema AB, Solna, Sweden). Gener-

ally, the manufacturer provides a recommended checklist in the user's manual that should be adapted by each institution to fit local clinical practice.

## MONITORING THE ANESTHESIA MACHINE

### How Do Anesthesia Gas Machines Injure Patients?

The primary purposes of an anesthesia gas machine are listed:

1. To provide $O_2$
2. To blend an anesthetic gas mixture
3. To facilitate spontaneous, assisted, or controlled ventilation of the patient's lungs

Accordingly, anesthesia gas machines injure patients when they do the following:

1. Cause the patient to respire a hypoxic gas mixture
2. Deliver an incorrect anesthetic dose
3. Inappropriately ventilate the patient's lungs

### What Are the Consequences of Inspiring a Hypoxic Gas?

Inspiring a hypoxic gas mixture (one that contains <21% $O_2$) rapidly causes oxyhemoglobin desaturation. In general, irreversible hypoxic injury of the central nervous system is thought to begin after about 4 minutes of arterial desaturation. Surprisingly, no or only small changes in hemodynamic variables are initially observed even when arterial hypoxemia is severe, a strong argument in favor of pulse oximetry!

### Must All Anesthesia Gas Delivery Systems Provide Supplemental Oxygen?

Anesthesia gases can be delivered to the patient's lungs using room air, without supplemental $O_2$. For example, a drawover vaporizer system,[29] which is often used for providing anesthesia in a military environment, in developing countries, and in other locations without compressed $O_2$ supplies, can deliver anesthesia gases to the patient using room air. All but the healthiest of patients, however, require supplemental $O_2$ administration to maintain arterial $O_2$ saturation during mechanical ventilation.[30] Thus, to be of use in contemporary civilian anesthesia practice, the anesthesia machine must provide $O_2$ and a control system to meter its release into the inspired gas mixture.

### What Malfunctions Cause Respiration of Hypoxic Gas?

Malfunctions that allow the anesthesia machine to deliver a hypoxic gas mixture are shown in Table 15–10. The entire list of problems may or may not be applicable to a specific

**TABLE 15–9.** Anesthesia Apparatus Checkout Recommendations (1993)

This checkout or a reasonable equivalent should be conducted before administration of anesthesia. These recommendations are only valid for an anesthesia system that conforms to current and relevant standards and includes an ascending bellows ventilator and at least the following monitors: capnograph, pulse oximeter, oxygen analyzer, respiratory volume monitor (spirometer), and breathing system pressure monitor with high- and low-pressure alarms. *This is a guideline that users are encouraged to modify to accommodate differences in equipment design and variations in local clinical practice. Such local modifications should have appropriate peer review.* Users should refer to the operator's manual for the manufacturer's specific procedures and precautions, especially the manufacturer's low-pressure leak test (step 5).

**Emergency Ventilation Equipment**
*1. Verify that backup ventilation equipment is available and functioning.

**High-Pressure System**
*2. Check $O_2$ cylinder supply.
    a. Open $O_2$ cylinder and verify that it is at least half full (about 1000 psi).
    b. Close cylinder.
*3. Check central pipeline supplies.
    a. Check that hoses are connected and that pipeline gauges read about 50 psi.

**Low-Pressure System**
*4. Check initial status of low-pressure system.
    a. Close flow control valves and turn vaporizers off.
    b. Check fill level and tighten vaporizers' filler caps.
*5. Perform leak check of machine low-pressure system.
    a. Verify that the machine's master switch and flow control valves are off.
    b. Attach "suction bulb" to common (fresh) gas outlet.
    c. Squeeze bulb repeatedly until fully collapsed.
    d. Verify that bulb stays *fully* collapsed for at least 10 seconds.
    e. Open one vaporizer at a time and repeat steps *c* and *d* above.
    f. Remove suction bulb and reconnect fresh gas hose.
*6. Turn on machine's master switch and all other necessary electrical equipment.
*7. Test flow meters.
    a. Adjust flow of all gases through their full range, checking for smooth operation of floats and undamaged flow tubes.
    b. Attempt to create a hypoxic $O_2$–$N_2O$ mixture and verify correct changes in flow and alarm operation.

**Scavenging System**
*8. Adjust and check scavenging system.
    a. Ensure proper connections between the scavenging system and both the APL (pop-off) valve and the ventilator relief valve.
    b. Adjust waste gas vacuum (if possible).
    c. Fully open APL valve and occlude Y-piece.
    d. With minimal $O_2$ flow, allow scavenging reservoir bag to collapse completely, and verify that absorber pressure gauge reads about zero.
    e. With the $O_2$ flush activated, allow the scavenger reservoir bag to distend fully, and then verify that absorber pressure gauge reads <10 cm $H_2O$.

**Breathing System**
*9. Calibrate $O_2$ monitor.
    a. Ensure that monitor reads 21% in room air.
    b. Verify that low $O_2$ alarm is enabled and functioning.
    c. Reinstall sensor in circuit and flush breathing system with $O_2$.
    d. Verify that monitor now reads >90%.
10. Check initial status of breathing system.
    a. Set selector switch to bag mode.
    b. Check that breathing circuit is complete, undamaged, and unobstructed.
    c. Verify that $CO_2$ absorbent is adequate.
    d. Install breathing circuit accessory equipment (eg, humidifier, positive end-expiratory pressure valve) to be used during the case.
11. Perform leak check of the breathing system.
    a. Set all gas flows to zero (or minimum).
    b. Close APL (pop-off) valve and occlude Y-piece.
    c. Pressurize breathing system to about 30 cm $H_2O$ with $O_2$ flush.
    d. Ensure that pressure remains fixed for at least 10 seconds.
    e. Open APL (pop-off) valve and ensure that pressure decreases.

**Manual and Automatic Ventilation Systems**
12. Test ventilation systems and unidirectional valves.
    a. Place a second breathing bag on Y-piece.
    b. Set appropriate ventilator parameters for next patient.
    c. Switch to automatic ventilation (ventilator) mode.
    d. Turn ventilator on and fill bellows and breathing bag with $O_2$ flush.
    e. Set $O_2$ flow to minimum, other gas flows to zero.
    f. Verify that during inspiration, bellows delivers appropriate tidal volume and that during expiration, bellows fills completely.
    g. Set fresh gas flow to about 5 L/min.
    h. Verify that the ventilator bellows and simulated lungs fill *and empty appropriately* without sustained pressure at end expiration.
    i. *Check for proper action of unidirectional valves.*
    j. Exercise breathing circuit accessories to ensure proper function.
    k. Turn ventilator off and switch to manual ventilation (bag/APL) mode.
    l. Ventilate manually and ensure inflation and deflation of artificial lungs and appropriate feel of system resistance and compliance.
    m. Remove second breathing bag from Y-piece.

**Monitors**
13. Check, calibrate, or set alarm limits of all monitors (capnometer, pulse oximeter, oxygen analyzer, respiratory volume monitor (spirometer), pressure monitor with high and low airway pressure alarms).

**Final Position**
14. Check final status of machine; make sure that:
    a. Vaporizers are off.
    b. APL valve is open.
    c. Selector switch is moved to bag mode.
    d. All flow meters read zero (or minimum).
    e. Patient suction level is adequate.
    f. Breathing system is ready to use.

*If an anesthesia provider uses the same machine in successive cases, these steps need not be repeated or may be abbreviated after the initial checkout.
APL, adjustable pressure-limiting

**TABLE 15–10.** Malfunctions That Result in Hypoxic Gas

| | |
|---|---|
| Obstructed fresh gas hose | Leak in the low-pressure system |
| Hypoxic fresh gas flow ratios | Loss of $O_2$ supply pressure |
| Inaccurate flow meters | Contaminated $O_2$ supply |
| Inadequate $O_2$ flow | |

make and model of anesthesia machine. However, if the $O_2$ pipeline or cylinder provides a gas other than $O_2$, the anesthesia machine will deliver hypoxic gas. This type of malfunction, whether due to a pipeline cross-over or a direct misfilling, can be detected only with a functioning $O_2$ analyzer. Leaks in the low-pressure system of the anesthesia machine may also cause a hypoxic gas mixture if $O_2$ is preferentially lost through the leak (see Fig. 15–9).

An inadequate flow rate of $O_2$ may also lead to a hypoxic gas mixture. Consider fresh gas flow rates of 300 mL/min for both $O_2$ and $N_2O$. The $O_2$ concentration emerging from the fresh gas hose is 50%. A typical adult patient, however, consumes about 250 mL of $O_2$ each minute. Thus, the net delivery of $O_2$ to the breathing system is 50 mL/min, whereas that of $N_2O$ (assuming minimal uptake or elimination) is 300 mL/min. Over time, the $O_2$ concentration approaches 16%, eventually causing oxyhemoglobin desaturation.

## Can the Anesthesia Machine Provide Oxygen Through a Nasal Cannula?

Because supplemental $O_2$ is often administered to nonintubated, spontaneously breathing patients through a nasal cannula during regional or monitored anesthesia care, an attractive feature of some anesthesia machines is a separate flow control and flow meter for metering $O_2$.

Without this secondary system, the anesthesiologist who desires to administer $O_2$ through a nasal cannula must attach that cannula to the common gas outlet on the anesthesia machine or connect it to the Y-piece of the breathing system. The first option requires temporary disassembly of the machine. In the event of complications requiring emergent transition to general anesthesia, the nasal cannula must be disconnected from the common gas outlet and the fresh gas hose reconnected.

The second option is fraught with several problems. First, because the resistance of the nasal cannula tubing is high, a significant amount of pressure is required to push $O_2$ flow through it; therefore, if the APL valve is not fully closed, an indeterminate amount of $O_2$ escapes into the scavenging system and is not delivered to the patient. Even if the pop-off valve is closed, because of the relative compliance of the breathing system and breathing bag, a limited (usually about 3 L/min) and indeterminate amount of $O_2$ is delivered through the nasal cannula.

## What Are the Consequences of an Inappropriate Anesthetic Dose?

Anesthetic overdose or underdose may injure the patient. An underdose may lead to awareness and recall and, in some patients, to sympathetic stimulation that results in tachycardia and hypertension. Depending on the underlying medical prob-

lems, this sympathetic stimulation may have adverse sequelae (eg, myocardial ischemia). An anesthetic overdose results in hypotension, may cause bradycardia, and, if severe enough, eventually leads to cardiovascular collapse.[31]

## What Malfunctions Cause an Inappropriate Anesthetic Dose?

Anesthetic underdose and overdose are most often related to titration errors by the anesthesiologist. However, faults within the machine may also cause problems. A leak in the low-pressure system allows anesthetic gas to escape into the operating room and not be delivered to the breathing system. A vaporizer that is filled with the wrong anesthetic agent may also cause an anesthetic underdose or overdose, depending on the specific type of vaporizer and the anesthetic with which it is filled. Spillage of liquid anesthetic into the breathing system may also cause an inadvertent overdose.

## What Are the Consequences of Inadequate Ventilation?

Inadequate ventilation leads initially to hypercapnia and eventually to hypoxemia. Hypercapnia increases pulmonary vascular resistance and causes changes in acid-base regulation, serum potassium concentration, cerebral blood flow, and sympathetic stimulation, whereas prolonged hypoxemia leads to irreversible central nervous system damage.

## What Should Be Done If a Machine Malfunction Is Suspected?

The course of action taken when an anesthesia machine malfunction is discovered or suspected depends on the specific clinical circumstances. The anesthesiologist should have a systematic, organized, and rehearsed plan for responding to equipment malfunction. However, the cardinal principle should be that the patient takes priority over debugging of the machine. Effective use of resources at the anesthesia provider's disposal is also crucial, for example, requesting the help of an anesthesia technician so that the anesthesia provider can focus on patient care. The management of crises calls for the establishment of leadership and clear communication, and effective use of resources is emphasized. For a discussion, see Chapter 7.

### Hypoxic Gas Mixture

If the $O_2$ analyzer indicates a hypoxic gas mixture, we recommend immediate disconnection of the patient from the anesthesia machine. If the patient is not breathing spontaneously, ventilation can be supported using a self-inflating resuscitation bag. A Mapleson breathing circuit is not an ideal backup ventilation system unless it is accompanied by a separate E-cylinder of $O_2$ and a pressure regulator. An independent $O_2$ pressure source is necessary with the Mapleson circuit; if the anesthesia machine is suspected of delivering hypoxic gas, one does not want to connect it to the Mapleson circuit. Conversely, the self-inflating resuscitation bag can be used with or without an $O_2$ supply.

## Inappropriate Anesthetic Dose

### Underdose

If an anesthetic underdose is suspected, the concentration on the vaporizer is increased in an attempt to deliver additional anesthetic. At some point, the concentration set on the vaporizer will seem inappropriately high; at this time, a vaporizer or machine malfunction will be suspected.

The liquid fill level on the vaporizer should be checked to ensure that the vaporizer is filled with liquid anesthetic. Also, check the filler cap (see Fig. 15–10.9) and drain port to ensure that they are closed tightly. Small leaks in this portion of the anesthesia machine can result in the loss of all or nearly all of the anesthetic vapor. If these maneuvers do not improve the situation, use another vaporizer or intravenous anesthetics. Appropriate service personnel should be contacted to verify vaporizer performance and to check the contents of the vaporizer.

### Overdose

If an anesthetic overdose is suspected, first turn off the vaporizer and turn on high fresh gas flows to wash the volatile agent from the breathing system. If an overdose continues to be suspected, smell the gas emerging from the fresh gas hose; minimal volatile odor should be present with the vaporizer turned off. Finally, disconnect the patient from the machine to guarantee that a volatile anesthetic agent is not being inhaled.

### Anesthetic Agent Analysis

The clinical utility of an anesthetic agent monitor is readily apparent when one considers machine malfunctions that cause these problems. Without such a monitor, the anesthesiologist must make decisions with incomplete data; differentiation of patient variation and errors in titration from anesthesia equipment malfunction is difficult and sometimes impossible. Anesthetic agent analyzers eliminate this uncertainty.

## Inadequate Ventilation

If inadequate ventilation is suspected, or if data from the spirometer and capnograph indicate such a condition, the cause must be sought. Leaks are suggested by low inspiratory pressure, whereas high inspiratory pressure suggests obstruction. When searching for the location of a breathing system leak, we divide the anesthesia machine into three components:

1. The ventilator
2. The breathing system
3. The endotracheal tube and patient

### Ventilator

Ventilator-associated problems are easily eliminated by switching to the breathing bag and manually inflating the patient's lungs. If the leak disappears, its location is pinpointed to the ventilator portion of the breathing system.

### Breathing System

If the leak persists, disconnect the patient from the breathing system, occlude the Y-piece, close the APL valve, and perform the standard positive pressure leak check of the breathing system. If it fails to hold 30 cm $H_2O$ pressure for 10 seconds, the site of the leak is in the breathing system.

### Endotracheal Tube

If the breathing system is leak free, the leak most likely involves the endotracheal tube cuff or a misplaced endotracheal tube. A leak around the endotracheal tube cuff is easily confirmed by placing a stethoscope over the larynx and auscultating during sustained application of positive pressure in the breathing system; if a leak is present, a rush of gas can be heard.

## STANDARDS AND CHANGES IN ANESTHESIA MACHINE DESIGN

### What Are They?

Anesthesia gas delivery systems are durable and dependable pieces of equipment. Historically, anesthesia machine manufacturers followed the guidelines of the American National Standards Institute, which published standards for anesthesia machines in the Z-79 document.[32] Subsequently, for legal and other reasons, the American Society for Testing and Materials (ASTM) took over. Anesthesiologists play a prominent role in the ASTM committee that develops the anesthesia machine standards. Voluntary anesthesia machine performance guidelines published in the ASTM F1161 document[33] have now been superseded by ASTM F1850-98.[3] The major philosophical difference between F1850-98 and F1161 is that the newer standards are performance based (specifying *what* it must do rather than specifying *how* it must be done). Because conformance to the ASTM standards helps the FDA approval process, a multitude of new anesthesia machine designs have appeared on the North American market recently, as a result of the new ASTM standards.

### Integration of Monitoring Instruments

Notable recent changes include the integration of monitoring instruments into the anesthesia machine. This feature ensures that the monitoring instruments are turned on with the anesthesia machine (an F1161 requirement for the $O_2$ analyzer). Such integration also enables all data, on both patient and machine, to be available on a common database, which lends itself to automated anesthesia recordkeeping.

### Elimination of the Ventilator Hose

Elimination of the ventilator hose represents an attractive design improvement because critical incident studies indicated that ventilator hose disconnection was a frequent problem. This configuration prevents disconnection of the ventilator hose from either its canister attachment or its attachment to the ventilator bellows because no ventilator hose is present to disconnect.

### Isolation of the Adjustable Pressure-Limiting Valve

Isolation of the APL valve from the breathing system during mechanical ventilation is another important improvement. In this position, even if the valve is inadvertently left open during mechanical ventilation, the entire ventilator breath will be delivered to the patient; no gases will leak out of the open APL valve.

### Measurement of Breathing System Pressure

Finally, newer anesthesia machines measure the breathing system pressure on the patient side of the inspiratory unidirectional valve. This previously discussed design improvement allows the airway pressure gauge, which is still physically located on the absorbent canister, to identify and measure PEEP.

## RECENTLY INTRODUCED ANESTHESIA MACHINES

### What Are the Major Differences?

Major significant differences in new anesthesia machines are the addition of pressure control ventilation and tighter integration of the ventilator and monitoring equipment into the anesthesia machine to generate a comprehensive anesthesia workstation.

### Pressure Control Ventilation

Pressure control ventilation (PCV) is a time-cycled mode of positive pressure ventilation that is different from traditional volume-controlled, pressure-limited, time-cycled ventilation (VCV). During PCV, respiratory rate and inspiratory-to-expiratory ratio are selected, just like in VCV, resulting in a given inspiratory time. Instead of picking a set tidal volume, however, a target pressure is titrated by the user, generally based on observed chest rise. Later on, the set pressure level can be adjusted based on end-tidal $CO_2$ concentration, just like in VCV.

In some anesthesia ventilators that offer PCV, such as the Datex-Ohmeda ADU, the rise time of pressure from the PEEP level (if used) to the target pressure can also be selected by the user as a percentage of the total inspiratory time (Ti). The Datex-Ohmeda ADU offers a selection of fast (10% of Ti), medium (50% of Ti), and slow (90% of Ti) pressure rise times.

### Why Pressure Controlled Ventilation?

PCV is particularly indicated for pediatric patients because the uncuffed endotracheal tubes used with these patients introduce a leak of unknown size that may also vary during a case. Therefore, during VCV, the user cannot compensate for the leak, a priori, by simply adding the leaked volume to the set tidal volume. The premise behind PCV is that during a no-flow condition, as may occur at the end of PCV, airway pressure, P, is dictated solely by compliance, C, and the volume, V, delivered to the lungs:

$$P = V/C$$

If insufficient volume has been delivered, pressure will be lower than the target pressure. Assuming an infinite flow

delivery capability from the ventilator, flow will increase, feeding both the lungs and the leak until airway pressure matches the target pressure. PCV, compared with VCV, also provides a safety feature in the case of a mainstem (endobronchial) intubation, which coincidentally appears to be more common in children. The reduced (by about half) compliance of the intubated lung side results in the pressure target being reached, with half of the volume preventing overinflation of the intubated lung side, as would occur with VCV.

### What Are the Disadvantages of Pressure Controlled Ventilation?

Because of the shape of the pressure curve during inspiration with PCV, the mean airway pressure over time is higher than with VCV, leading to higher intrathoracic pressures that adversely affect cardiac output. The ability to ramp the pressure slowly (eg, the 90% Ti pressure rise on the ADU), instead of generating an abrupt step input in pressure, decreases mean airway pressure and may reduce the adverse effect of PCV on cardiac output.

For a detailed listing of the features in the more recently introduced anesthesia machines, the reader is referred to the Emergency Care Research Institute (ECRI) publication *Healthcare Product Comparison System: Anesthesia Units.*[34]

## FUTURE DEVELOPMENTS

### What Changes Are Anticipated?

Europe has been at the forefront of many of the recent technical innovations regarding anesthesia machines. For example, most of the new anesthesia machines being introduced to the US market come from Europe, where designers have had a much freer hand in the past. To get a preview of what the future holds, it helps to look at current developments in Europe.

Xenon, an inert gas obtained from distillation of air, is touted to be a desirable (but expensive) anesthetic. With the availability of microprocessor-controlled anesthesia machines that automatically perform closed-circuit anesthesia, xenon anesthesia becomes a practical possibility.

Intravenous anesthesia is gaining ground, especially with the advent of target-controlled infusion that provides the practicality of a minimum alveolar concentration equivalent for intravenous anesthesia.

In the future, also look for more options to appear, perhaps including features to facilitate closed-circuit anesthesia by feedback control.

Tighter integration of the ventilator within the anesthesia machine will also enable more safety features, such as automatic abortion of mechanical inspiration if the $O_2$ flush is concurrently pressed, a current barotrauma hazard in older ventilators. Some machines, such as the Datex-Ohmeda Aestiva, already possess this safety feature. Better integration of the ventilator will also allow more user-friendly operation. For example, in the Aestiva anesthesia machine, a single action (flipping the ventilation mode selector knob) is required to switch from manual to mechanical ventilation, compared with up to three separate actions (flip selector knob, close

APL valve, flip ventilator on/off switch) for an older machine like the Ohmeda Modulus I.

One could argue that the full potential of the widespread availability of monitoring has not yet been realized. As older machines and their legacy are phased out, and monitoring becomes ubiquitous, manufacturers will be able to promote novel and more efficient designs. We expect to see machine designs (eg, the Dräger Julian) as well as changes in procedures and practices (eg, use of medical air as the ventilator drive gas) that will exploit the ready availability of monitoring while challenging current dogma, such as "hanging bellows are unsafe" and "use $O_2$ as the drive gas."

## When Is an Anesthesia Machine Obsolete?

Exactly when an anesthesia gas machine becomes obsolete is difficult to determine. Intuition suggests that the design and safety features of contemporary anesthesia machines should decrease the incidence of patient injuries attributable to equipment malfunction and that older anesthesia machines without these features should no longer be used. However, solid scientific data addressing this issue are lacking. The suggestion has been advanced that more harm than good may result when a practitioner with years of experience who uses a particular "outdated" anesthesia gas machine is forced to replace it with a new, "safer" anesthesia machine with which he or she is much less familiar.

Yet, certain types of equipment-related patient injuries appear to be recurrent problems. For example, the copper kettle and Vernitrol vaporizers frequently caused anesthetic overdoses in the past. They are no longer commercially available, and service contracts for them are no longer available; thus, in effect, they have been declared obsolete.

After a panel discussion at the 1989 annual meeting, the ASA Committee on Equipment and Standards proposed the following *Policy for Assessing Obsolescence,* which was subsequently approved by the ASA Board of Directors[35]:

*The age of an anesthesia machine has not been demonstrated to be a factor in anesthetic mishaps. An anesthesia gas machine, however, which no longer functions as designed and is not modified to meet acceptable levels of performance and monitoring should not be used.*

*Each anesthesia department should establish a protocol to assure that all anesthesia staff members are qualified in the operation of each type of gas machine, ventilator, and monitor in use.*

The APSF Committee on Technology addressed obsolescence as it relates to anesthesia equipment,[35] noting that "age alone does not create obsolescence . . . neither does the failure to continue in widespread use." Modularity is viewed as an attractive feature that prevents obsolescence because "failure of a module does not render the entire system obsolete."

Specific definitions of obsolescence are provided with regard to maintenance (eg, cost required to keep device working is too great), reliability (eg, the device is not as fail-safe as newer devices), ergonomics (eg, avoidable injuries occur owing to user errors), and function (eg, higher morbidity than with newer alternatives) of anesthesia equipment.

*1. Time alone does not adequately characterize changes in function.*

*2. Failure with wear can be reversed with repair or replacement. A time threshold removes the option of repair.*

*3. Innovation does not occur at a constant rate. A time threshold can therefore trigger unnecessary replacement or delay necessary replacement.*

*4. A time threshold increases the probability of inadequate maintenance of older equipment (i.e., older equipment is not serviced if it is expected to be replaced by newer equipment).*

*5. A time threshold implies economic stability for manufacturers, even if they do not innovate, and thus reduces the incentive to innovate.*

*6. A time threshold causes economic expense for users, whether or not it is required for patient safety.*

In the end, every practitioner must decide whether his or her anesthesia machine or any other piece of anesthesia equipment is obsolete. As should be evident from the aforementioned ASA and APSF documents, functionality and safety features, not age, are the characteristics on which this determination should be based. Anesthesia machine standards, such as ASTM F1161 and ASTM F1850-98, and ASA Practice Guidelines, as well as texts such as this edition, are designed to help each practitioner make an educated decision.

## References

1. Jackson DE. Anesthesia equipment from 1914 to 1954 and experiments leading to its development. *Anesthesiology.* 1955;16:953.
2. Good ML, Cooper JB. Monitoring the anesthesia machine. In: Saidman LJ, Smith NT, eds. *Monitoring in Anesthesia.* Boston, Mass: Butterworth-Heinemann; 1993.
3. *Standard Specification for Particular Requirements for Anesthesia Workstations and Their Components*: West Conshohocken, Pa: American Society for Testing and Materials; August 1998: F 1850.
4. *Health Care Facilities: NFPA 99.* Quincy, Mass: National Fire Protection Association; 1990:59.
5. *Characteristics and Safe Handling of Medical Gases.* Publication P-2. 7th ed. Arlington, Va: Compressed Gas Association; 1989.
6. Eisenkraft JB. The anesthesia delivery system: part one. *Progr Anesth.* 1989;3:1.
7. Raessler KL, Kretzman WE, Gravenstein N. Oxygen consumption by anesthesia ventilators. *Anesthesiology.* 1988;69:A271.
8. Andrews JJ. Inhaled anesthetic delivery systems. In: Miller RD, ed. *Anesthesia.* 5th ed. New York, NY: Churchill Livingstone; 2000:174.
9. Good ML, Paulus DA. Equipment. In: Gravenstein N, ed. *Complications During Anesthesia.* Philadelphia, Pa: JB Lippincott; 1991.
10. Eger EI, Hylton RR, Irwin RH, Guadagni N. Anesthetic flow meter sequence: a cause for hypoxia. *Anesthesiology.* 1963;24:396.
11. Hill DW, Lowe HJ. Comparison of concentration of halothane in closed and semiclosed circuits during controlled ventilation. *Anesthesiology.* 1962;23:291.
12. Hill DW. The design and calibration of vaporizers for volatile anaesthetic agents. *Br J Anaesth.* 1968;40:648.
13. Lampotang S, Dobbins W, Good ML, et al. Interactive Teaching Software: Interactive, Web-Based, Educational Simulation of an Anesthesia Machine. Available at: http://www.anest.ufl.edu/vam. Accessed November 6, 2000.
14. Lampotang S, Chen BX, Good ML. Ventilator performance without a bellows: an explanation [abstract]. *Anesthesiology.* 1996;85:3A:A443.
15. Andrews JJ, Johnston RV, Bee DE, et al. Photodeactivation of ethyl violet: a potential hazard of Sodasorb. *Anesthesiology.* 1990;72:59.
16. Murray JM, Renfrew CW, Bedi A, et al. A new carbon dioxide absorbent for use in anesthetic breathing systems. *Anesthesiology.* 1999;91:1342.
17. Kharasch ED, Jubert C. Compound A uptake and metabolism to mercapturic acids and 3,3,3-trifluoro-2-fluoromethoxypropanoic acid during low-flow sevoflurane anesthesia: biomarkers for exposure, risk assessment, and interspecies comparison. *Anesthesiology.* 1999;91:1267.
18. American Society of Anesthesiologists. *Waste Anesthetic Gases: Information for Management in Anesthetizing Areas and the Postanesthesia Care*

*Unit (PACU)*. Available at: http://www.asahq.org/ProfInfo/wasteanes-gases.html. Accessed November 6, 2000.

19. *North American Dräger Operator Instruction Manual: Open Reservoir Scavenger*. Telford, Pa: North American Dräger; 1986.

20. Cooper JB, Newbower RS, Kitz RJ. An analysis of major errors and equipment failures in anesthesia management: considerations for prevention and detection. *Anesthesiology*. 1984;60:34.

21. Gaba DM, Maxwell M, DeAnda A. Anesthetic mishaps: breaking the chain of accident evolution. *Anesthesiology*. 1987;66:670.

22. Buffington CW, Ramanathan S, Turndorf H. Detection of anesthesia machine faults. *Anesth Analg*. 1984;63:79.

23. Food and Drug Administration. *Anesthesia Apparatus Checkout Recommendations*. Rockville, Md: Federal Register; February 1987.

24. Carstensen P. FDA issues pre-use checkout. *Anesth Patient Safety Found Newslett*. 1986;1:13.

25. *American Society of Anesthesiologists Newsletter*. Park Ridge, Ill: American Society of Anesthesiologists; October 1986:5.

26. March MG, Crowley JJ. An evaluation of anesthesiologist's present checkout methods and the validity of the FDA checklist. *Anesthesiology*. 1991;75:724.

27. Manley R, Cuddeford JD. An assessment of the effectiveness of the revised FDA checklist. *J Am Assoc Nurse Anesthetists*. 1996;64:277

28. Olympio MA, Goldstein MM, Mathes DD. Instructional review improves performance of anesthesia checkout procedures. *Anesth Analg*. 1996;83:618.

29. Mackie A. Drawover anaesthetic systems. *Anaesthesia*. 1987;42:299.

30. Borland CW, Herbert P, Pereira NH, et al. Evaluation of a new range of air drawover vaporizers: the PAC series-laboratory and field studies. *Anaesthesia*. 1983;38:852.

31. Keenan RL, Boyan CP. Cardiac arrest due to anesthesia: a study of incidence and causes. *JAMA*. 1985;253:2373.

32. *Minimum Performance and Safety Requirements for Components and Systems of Continuous Flow Anesthesia Machines for Human Use: ANSI Z79.8-1979*. New York, NY: American National Standards Institute; 1979.

33. *Standard Specification for Minimum Performance and Safety Requirements for Components and Systems of Anesthesia Gas Machines: F1161-88*. Philadelphia, Pa: American Society for Testing and Materials; 1989.

34. ECRI. *Healthcare Product Comparison System: Anesthesia Units*. August 1999. Available at: http://www.ecri.org/documents/Anesthesia_Units.pdf. Accessed November 6, 2000.

35. Lees DE. Older anesthesia equipment target of study, panel: ASA policy recommended. In: Eichhorn JH, ed. *Anesthesia Patient Safety: A Modern History; The Formative Years, 1986–1993*. Pittsburgh, PA: Anesthesia Patient Safety Foundation; 1993:143.

CHAPTER

# 16

# Airway Devices and Their Application

Richard J. Melker

Establishment of a patent airway is essential to the practice of anesthesiology. Indeed, anesthesiologists must be procedural experts for high-quality airway management. To this end, familiarity with airway equipment is mandatory. Airway devices can be divided into two broad categories: (1) those that are essential and must be available, regardless of the anesthetic technique (face masks, oral and nasal airways, laryngoscopes, and endotracheal tubes [ETTs]); and (2) those that are ancillary or adjunctive and used to facilitate airway control as dictated by the patient's peculiar anatomic characteristics, pathologic problem, or the surgical procedure (fiberoptic bronchoscopes [FOBs], lightwands, specialized or modified laryngoscopes, tube changers, and other related devices).

In the operating room (OR), airway management may be performed simply with basic devices for oxygen ($O_2$) delivery such as a nasal cannula or face mask. Complete airway control is achieved by tracheal intubation and manual or mechanical ventilation. During emergencies, cricothyroidotomy or tracheotomy may be used. Various resources are used to facilitate airway access, successful airway control, and adequate ventilation and oxygenation. This chapter addresses the different types of airway devices and their indications, contraindications, complications, techniques of utilization, maintenance, and care.

## ORAL AND NASAL AIRWAYS

### What Are Their Clinical Applications?

During anesthetic induction or emergence, patients often manifest signs and symptoms of airway obstruction. The most common cause is the tongue falling back into the oropharynx. Displacement of the mandible anteriorly and backward head tilt (Jackson position) usually relieves the obstruction. Failure to correct the problem necessitates the use of an oral or nasal airway, which provides an artificial passage to airflow by separating the tongue from the posterior pharyngeal wall.[1,2]

An oral airway is preferred to a nasal airway during induction owing to its ease of insertion and lesser likelihood of causing trauma and bleeding. During emergence, a nasal airway is much better tolerated because it reduces gagging, vomiting, and laryngeal spasm. An oral airway may also be inserted after orotracheal intubation to prevent the patient from biting the ETT. The oral airway facilitates insertion of an esophageal stethoscope and nasogastric tube and allows suctioning of the mouth and oropharynx as necessary.

A nasal tube may be particularly useful in patients who have masseter spasm or trismus. If the nares are partially blocked, or if pharyngeal obstruction is only partially relieved by a nasal airway, an oral airway is preferable; however, it should be avoided in conscious or uncooperative patients. Nasal airways are contraindicated in the presence of coagulopathy, basal skull fracture, and nasopharyngeal infection or anatomic deformity.

### How Are They Inserted?

#### Oral

Oral airways are metallic, black rubber, or, most commonly, plastic devices in the shape of an "S" or semicircular curve. They are available in various sizes, ranging from those suitable for neonates to those for adults. An appropriate size holds the tongue in the normal anatomic position and follows its natural curvature. Adult sizes range from 80 to 100 mm (also labeled as numbers 3, 4, and 5). Sizes for children range from 50 to 70 mm (numbers 0, 1, and 2). Smaller airways also are available for premature and newborn infants.

Most commonly used are the S-shaped Guedel and Berman airways (Fig. 16–1). The Guedel design has a large flange, a reinforced bite area, and a large tubular lumen for increased air exchange and insertion of a suction catheter. A specially designed metal airway (Patil-Syracuse endoscopic airway) is available for use during fiberoptic tracheal intubation. This device has a central groove to hold the endoscope in the midline. A slit is provided distally to direct it into the larynx. Lateral channels are also provided for suctioning.

The Williams airway intubator (round hole airway) is cylindric on its proximal half and open on the distal half of the lingual surface (see Fig. 16–1). It serves as an oropharyngeal airway, a means of intubating the trachea, and a guide for fiberoptic laryngoscope placement.

Insertion of an oral airway is enhanced with a tongue blade that depresses the tongue and moves it laterally. The oral airway is inserted by turning the curved side up, then by advancing it toward the posterior end of the tongue while rotating it 90° downward into the position of function. Alter-

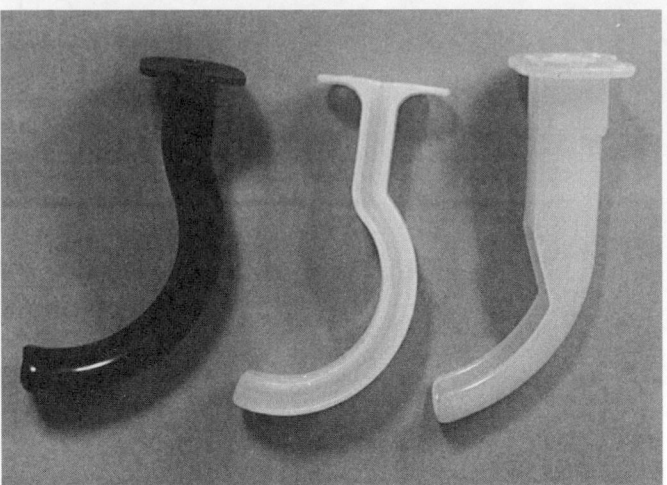

**FIGURE 16–1.** The Guedel oral airway (left) is commonly made of black rubber and is provided with a tubular lumen that facilitates airway exchange and insertion of suction catheters. The Berman oral airway (center) is a plastic device similar in shape to the Guedel airway but is not provided with an air channel. The Williams airway intubator (right) is made of plastic and is cylindric on its proximal half and open on the distal half of the tongue surface. It has a central opening to allow passage of fiberoptic airway devices, endotracheal tubes, and suction catheters.

natively, it may be inserted upside down and rotated 180° into the proper position.

### Problems

Problems associated with oral airway insertion are uncommon. The gag reflex may be elicited in conscious or lightly anesthetized patients, as may coughing, vomiting, laryngospasm, and bronchospasm. Therefore, they should be used only in unconscious, well-anesthetized, or comatose patients. Improper placement may push the tongue against the pharynx and aggravate airway obstruction. Malposition also can traumatize the teeth, tongue, and pharynx. Placement should be checked periodically, especially in long procedures.

If the patient's mouth cannot be pried open, and if time permits, a useful approach is to insert two tongue blades, one on top of the other, between the molars and then to place additional tongue blades between them until an adequate mouth opening is achieved.

#### Nasal

A nasal airway is a soft rubber or pliable plastic, uncuffed tube approximately 15 cm in length. It is useful for short-term airway management and is inserted through the naris into the posterior pharynx. It is better tolerated in conscious patients, in those with sensitive gag reflexes, or in instances when the oral route is inaccessible because of oral or lower facial trauma. Measurement of the tube size is based on its outer diameter and circumference and expressed in French sizes 28 to 30 for women and 32 to 34 for men. Smaller nasal airways for pediatric patients are also available. Most commonly used are the straight red rubber Rusch airway, the neoprene rubber Bardex airway, and the soft, pliable plastic modified Saklad nasal airway (Fig. 16–2). A binasal airway can also be used and is provided with an adaptor that may be connected to the anesthesia machine.

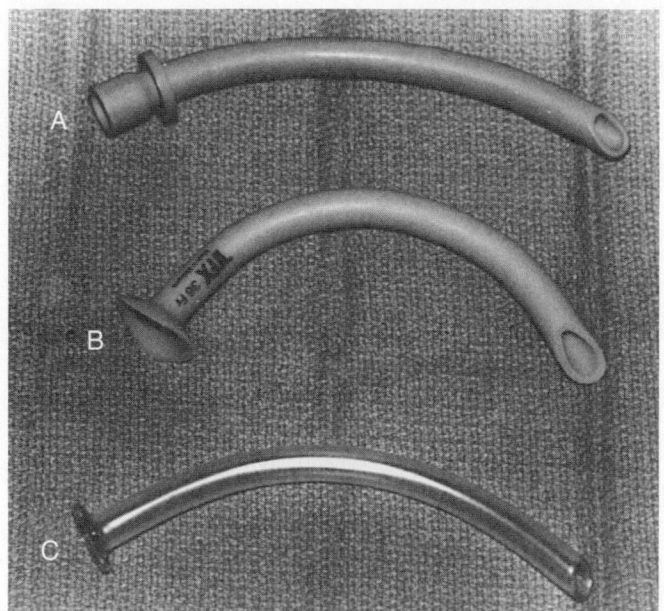

**FIGURE 16–2.** Nasal airways. *A,* The Rusch nasal airway is a soft red rubber device with a firm, adjustable flange at the nasal end and a bevel at the pharyngeal end. *B,* The Bardex airway is a soft rubber nasal airway with a large flange at the nasal end and a bevel at the pharyngeal end. *C,* The modified Saklad-type nasal airway is made of plastic and has a small flange at the nasal end and a blunted bevel at the pharyngeal end.

Several important points should be remembered during insertion. First, the more patent naris should be selected. In patients with septal deviation, the airway should be inserted in the side with the smaller external orifice because the ipsilateral nasal chamber is usually larger. Second, the nasal tube should be adequately lubricated with lidocaine jelly to facilitate insertion. A local vasoconstrictor like phenylephrine or 4% cocaine should be applied before insertion to minimize bleeding. Third, the length of the nasal tube to be inserted can roughly be estimated by measuring the distance from the nasal tip to the external auditory meatus. The tip of the nasal airway should be directed perpendicular to the face, not toward the cribriform plate. Insertion should be done smoothly and slowly; any resistance requires that the tube be gently rotated until no obstruction is felt. The tip of the airway should be at a point just above the epiglottis.

### Problems

Complications associated with nasal airway insertion include epistaxis and nasopharyngeal trauma. Aspiration into the lower airway may occur. A large safety pin inserted off center at the top prevents this problem. A nasal airway should not be used in any patient with suspected or proven basilar skull fracture; otherwise, it may be passed into the cranium.

## ESOPHAGEAL, PHARYNGEAL, AND LARYNGEAL TUBES

### How Are They Used?

Other devices for maintenance of a patent airway are available, but their role in the OR is undefined. They are confined mainly to emergency situations and out-of-hospital resuscitation and include the esophageal obturator airway (EOA), the pharyngeal tracheal lumen airway (PTLA), and the esophageal tracheal Combitube (ETC). Conversely, the binasal pharyngeal airway (BNPA) and laryngeal mask airway (LMA) have been used with variable success in the OR.

### Esophageal Obturator Airway

The EOA is a plastic tube 34 cm long with a balloon at its distal end designed to be inflated in the esophagus[3] (Fig. 16–3). Sixteen holes, 3 mm in diameter, are present in the upper third of the tube and allow for the passage of air during ventilation. The EOA is attached to a self-sealing face mask and is inserted into the esophagus at a level just distal to the carina. Insertion does not require visualization and is facilitated by grasping the mandible between the thumb and the index finger and lifting it forward while the tube is inserted into the esophagus with the other hand. The balloon is inflated with 30 mL of air once the tube is in place, and the mask is fitted to the face. Air is blown into the tube through the small holes in the upper part of the tube into the airways. Inflation of the balloon prevents gas passage into the stomach.

Unfortunately, no convincing evidence of EOA effectiveness exists for clinical situations in which it has been used, (eg, during cardiopulmonary resuscitation in prehospital cardiac arrest).[4–6] Complications, some of which are fatal, include esophageal rupture, inadvertent tracheal intubation and occlusion, massive gastric distention, vomiting, and aspiration.[7–9]

### Pharyngeal Tracheal Lumen Airway

The PTLA is a modification of the EOA. This device consists of two tubes: an ETT and a shorter tube that is designed to terminate in the hypopharynx.[10] A large, 150- to 200-mL cuff is attached proximal to the port of the pharyngeal tube; inflation prevents oral and nasal secretions from entering the airway and prevents oral escape of air delivered via the pharyngeal tube.[11] A smaller, 30-mL distal cuff is attached to the ETT.

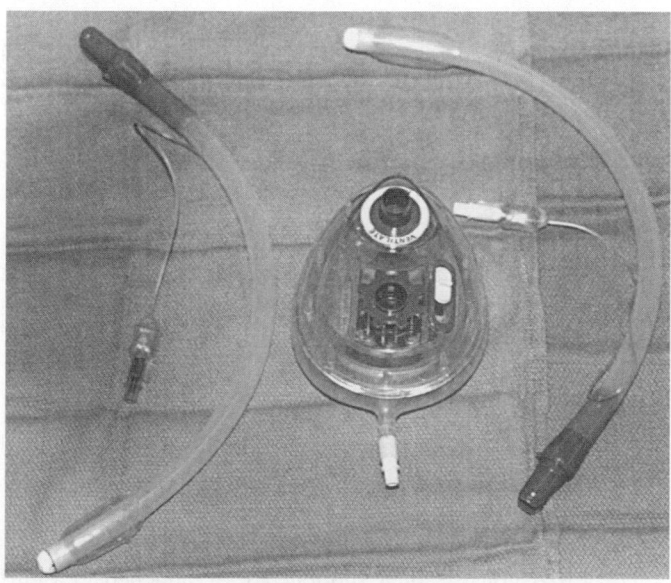

**FIGURE 16–3.** The esophageal obturator airway.

The PTLA also is inserted blindly, allowing placement of the ETT component into the trachea or esophagus. Once the airway is in position, air is injected into the balloon port, inflating both the oropharyngeal and ETT cuffs. Air is then blown into the pharyngeal tube. If lung inflation occurs, a resuscitator bag is attached to the tube, and ventilation is continued. If lung inflation does not occur when the pharyngeal tube is ventilated, the ETT is in the trachea. The resuscitator bag is then attached to the ETT and ventilation initiated, following which the pharyngeal balloon is deflated. Unlike the EOA, the face mask is not required to maintain an effective seal.

### Esophageal Tracheal Combitube

The ETC is a variant of the PTLA. Its proximal cuff is smaller than that of the PTLA and is placed between the base of the tongue and the hard palate.[12] It is inserted in the same manner as the PTLA. Ventilation is similar to that of the EOA except for the absence of a face mask.

#### Advantages

Considerable data have been generated on the use of the ETC in the prehospital, emergency department, and intensive care unit (ICU) settings. Few comparative, controlled studies have been performed, especially in the OR setting. Studies of anesthesia practice patterns in the United States show that training in the use of the ETC is sporadic.[13,14]

#### Problems

Although the ETC has been suggested to be of particular value in patients with suspected cervical spine injury, one study showed that blind insertion was impossible in 66% of patients placed in a rigid cervical collar before induction of the anesthesia.[15] Several publications have documented complications from the use of the ETC, including esophageal lacerations.[16,17] In a comparative study of the ETC with the LMA and ETT, the ETC had a significantly higher rate of complications, especially hematomas.[18]

In light of the documented complications with this device and number of other adjunct devices available, recommendation for the use of the ETC in anesthesia cannot be justified. Further, use of the device is complicated and, unless it is used on a regular basis, it is doubtful that a practitioner will remember how to use the device correctly under the stress of an emergency situation.

### Binasal Pharyngeal Airway

The BNPA is made up of 2 soft nasopharyngeal tubes connected to a suitable 15-mm male adaptor[19] (Fig. 16–4). It is inserted in both nares in a manner similar to that for a single nasal airway. This airway has been successfully used to ventilate patients in the OR.[20] Gastric dilation is unlikely because excess air escapes through the mouth. The BNPA is contraindicated in patients with full stomachs and specifically recommended only during difficult intubation when skilled personnel or more sophisticated equipment are not available.

### Laryngeal Mask Airway

The LMA consists of a shortened ETT attached to a cuff of a shallow face mask[20] (Fig. 16–5). It conforms to the shape

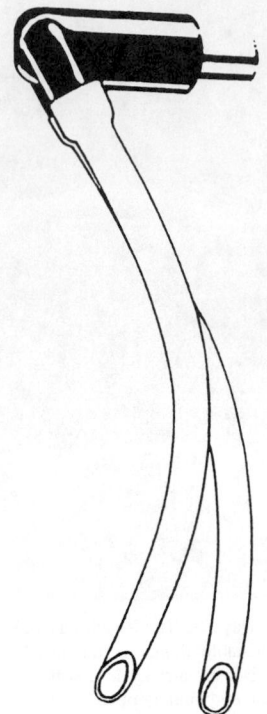

**FIGURE 16–4.** Binasal pharyngeal airway.

of the laryngeal inlet and can be inserted without direct visualization. The tube is inserted facing backward and is rotated 180° as it is passed downward into the larynx. Inflation of the cuff holds the device in place over the larynx, and the position of the mask is adjusted if a good seal is not obtained. This device does not require a laryngoscope for insertion. It is expensive but can be autoclaved and is reusable. It is widely used in the United Kingdom for airway management during general anesthesia[21] and has gained considerable popularity in the United States. The LMA is available in various sizes (sizes 1, 2, 2½, 3, 4, and 5) for neonates, infants, children, and adults.

In 1997, a new version of the LMA, the intubating LMA (ILMA), was introduced.[22] The advantage of this version is that it is designed to be used not only as an airway adjunct but also as a guide for endotracheal intubation. Several design changes were made to improve the device and facilitate endotracheal intubation.

The ILMA consists of a short, curved stainless steel tube with attached cuff and guiding handle. The rigid structure facilitates one-handed placement. The internal diameter (ID) of the device has been increased to allow passage of an 8-mm ID ETT, and the ILMA can be removed after ETT insertion. In addition, an epiglottis elevating bar has been added to ensure that the epiglottis does not obstruct the intubation attempt.

The initial study in 100 patients showed a 93% success rate at intubation after placement of the ILMA. Subsequent studies, including a study performed in 110 patients, have documented an extremely high rate of successful intubation after placement of the device.[23]

#### Advantages

Smith and White found the LMA to be associated with fewer episodes of desaturation, less difficulty in maintenance

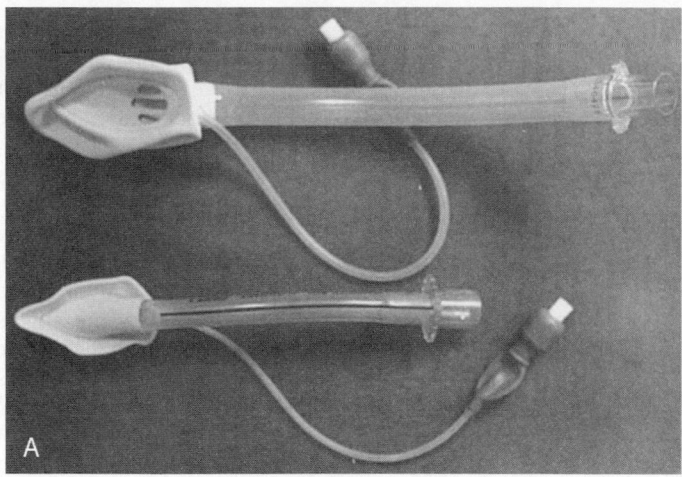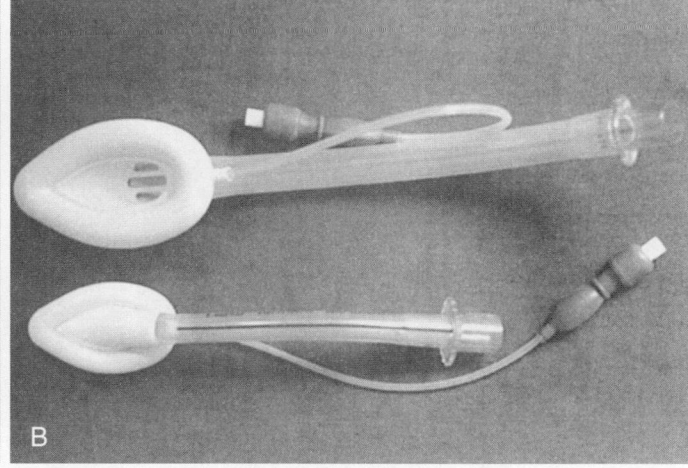

**FIGURE 16–5.** The laryngeal mask airway (LMA). *A,* A correctly deflated LMA that forms a smooth, flat wedge-shaped structure, allowing easy passage around the back of the tongue and behind the epiglottis. *B,* Properly inflating an LMA with the correct volume of air allows proper positioning of the device and provides a seal around the laryngeal aperture.

of a patent airway, and decreased arm and hand fatigue compared with a conventional face mask.[24] It can serve as an emergency airway during difficult intubation or when ventilation is not possible with a standard face mask and bag.[25–27] It can also serve as an airway conduit for an intubating tracheal stylet or FOB, through which an ETT may be passed when airway management or intubation is difficult.[28–30] Fiberoptic diagnostic visualization of the airway and fiberoptic laser ablation of tracheobronchial tree tumors are facilitated, as is management of patients with facial burns and those who need multiple anesthetics in a short time.[30–33] Finally, it may be useful in patients with unstable cervical spines because its insertion does not require neck manipulation.[34]

Introduction of the ILMA has further strengthened the position of this device as a major adjunct for patients who cannot be intubated by direct laryngoscopic visualization. Two studies have demonstrated the ILMA to be superior to the LMA during manual in-line neck stabilization.[35,36]

### Problems

The most common problems during insertion are failure to achieve correct placement as a result of inadequate anesthesia or inadequate relaxation; failure to negotiate the 90° turn from the posterior pharynx to the hypopharynx; and the selection of the wrong LMA size.[28] The device is difficult to insert in patients with small mouths, large tongues or tonsils, or a posteriorly displaced pharynx. The esophagus may be exposed to positive pressure, resulting in gastric dilation and regurgitation. Failed insertion occurs in as many as 5% of attempts. Cricoid pressure may have to be released for proper placement of the ILMA and subsequent advancement of an ETT.[37]

### Contraindications

The LMA is contraindicated in patients with a pharyngeal or laryngeal pathologic process, in patients who are at risk of regurgitation or aspiration or who have blood present in the upper airway, or cases in which >25 cm H₂O peak inflation pressure is required to ventilate the lungs. It is relatively contraindicated for situations in which tracheal intubation cannot be performed immediately, such as in a patient in the prone position or when the operating table is away from the anesthesiologist's field.[38]

### Cuffed Oropharyngeal Airway

The cuffed oropharyngeal airway (COPA) is a recently introduced device to add to the adjunct armamentarium of the anesthesiologist. It is clearly marketed as a competitor to the LMA. Greenberg and Toung first reported on its use in 1992.[39] Numerous studies have evaluated it and compared it with the LMA.[40–43]

The COPA is essentially a Geudel airway with a large cuff attached. The cuff is designed to produce an airtight seal with the pharynx, retract the base of the tongue, elevate the epiglottis, and provide a patent airway. The cuff is inflated from a pilot balloon. It is available in four sizes and can be held in place by an elastic strap (Fig. 16–6).

In a randomized trial in 453 patients undergoing routine procedures, the devices were found to be equivalent in terms of ease of placement, physiologic alterations, and overall clinical problems associated with use. The LMA was associated with a higher first attempt success rate and less manipulation. The COPA was associated with less sore throat and blood on the device at time of removal.[42] A study comparing

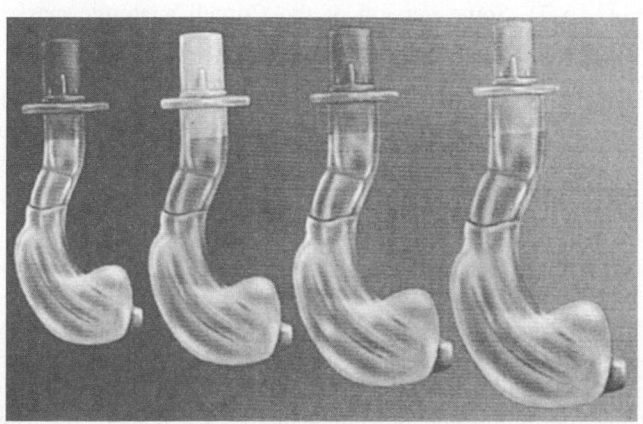

**FIGURE 16–6.** The cuffed oropharyngeal airway.

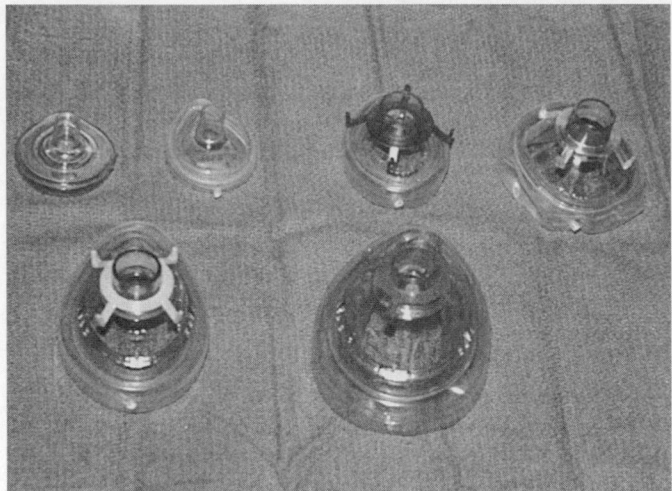

**FIGURE 16–7.** The most commonly used face mask is made of clear, colorless plastic with a soft, pliable rim. It is available in various sizes for children and adults.

the pressor response of the COPA with that of the LMA showed smaller cardiovascular changes with the COPA.[44]

Problems and complications reported with the COPA are similar to those found with the LMA. As with the LMA, the design continues to evolve and further studies comparing the two devices can be anticipated in the hopes of elucidating if one has an advantage over the other in certain difficult airway scenarios.

## FACE MASK AND BAG VALVE VENTILATION

Before tracheal intubation, and sometimes throughout surgery, oxygenation is achieved by ventilating the patient through a face mask. Available face masks are made of black rubber or colorless, clear plastic. An ideal face mask should be large enough to fit snugly over the patient's mouth and nose. It should have a soft, pliable rim to create an effective seal with the cheeks. A clear mask is preferred because it provides direct visualization of the mouth, lips, and nose, as well as emesis or secretions. An airtight seal is necessary to allow adequate ventilation and avoids escape of the anesthetic agent during induction.

Various mask sizes are available for children and adults (Fig. 16–7). Some version of the Cornell anatomic mask is most commonly used in adults, whereas the Rendell-Baker-Soucek mask is commonly used in children because it is relatively flat, conforms well to a child's face, and has minimal dead space. The Patil-Syracuse endoscope face mask may be used during fiberoptic tracheal intubation. It has a port for the bronchoscope and permits ETT insertion.

### How Should a Face Mask Be Applied?

Face mask placement can be achieved by single-handed or double-handed technique. With the former method, the anesthesiologist fits the mask snugly on the patient's face, using the thumb and the index finger in a pincer grip while displacing the mandible upward and lifting the chin with the

other three fingers. The middle finger is placed on the anterior mandible, the ring finger is midway between the mandibular angle and the chin, and the little finger rests on the angle of the jaw. Pressure on the soft tissues should be avoided because it can raise the base of the tongue and cause airway obstruction. It is also uncomfortable and sometimes painful to the awake patient.

On occasion, ventilation may be inadequate or airway obstruction may be unrelieved with the single-handed technique. If an oral or nasopharyngeal airway does not relieve the obstruction, the mask can be held by both hands. The fingers are placed as with the single-handed technique but on both sides of the face. The chin is lifted, and the mandible is pulled upward. An assistant is necessary to provide manual ventilation if the patient is not breathing spontaneously.

### What Problems May Occur?

Problems associated with mask ventilation include inability to ventilate, pressure damage to soft tissues and the eyes, gastric distention, and pulmonary aspiration of gastric contents. If a tight mask strap is left in place over the facial nerve for a prolonged period, a facial nerve palsy may result. Cricoid pressure (Sellick maneuver) may be applied during prolonged mask ventilation to avoid regurgitation of gastric contents. Decompressing the stomach with a nasogastric tube may reduce gastric distention but does not guarantee an empty stomach.

### Is a Manual Resuscitator Bag Necessary in the Operating Room?

Although mask ventilation is readily achieved by connecting the face mask to the anesthesia machine circuit, in the rare instance of machine or breathing circuit failure, a manual resuscitator bag is mandatory. A manual bag also may be necessary or desirable during transport to the postanesthesia care unit or ICU. Various designs are available, but a self-inflating, manual resuscitation bag is preferable because it allows ventilation even if the $O_2$ supply is cut off (Fig. 16–8).

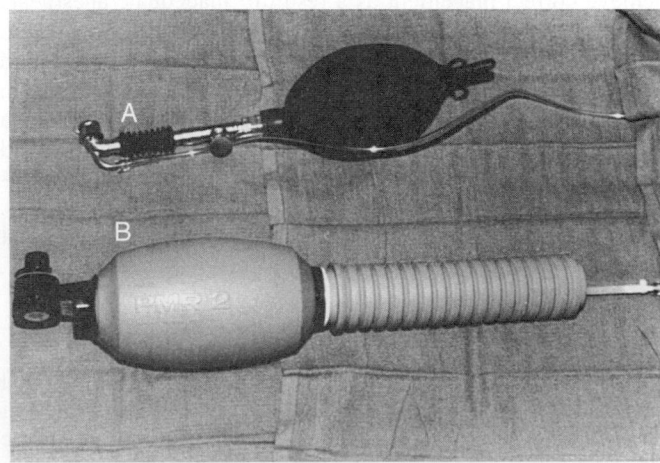

**FIGURE 16–8.** Commonly available manual resuscitation bags. *A,* The Mapleson bag is not self-inflating and requires a continuous oxygen source for proper functioning. *B,* A self-inflating manual resuscitator allows ventilation even if the oxygen supply is cut off.

The standard parts should include a delivery port with a 15-mm inside diameter and a 22-mm outside diameter that can be connected to an ETT or to a face mask. The self-inflating system must allow delivery of an $O_2$-rich mixture. It should have a valve that allows both spontaneous and controlled positive-pressure ventilation. A positive end-expiratory pressure valve can also be incorporated. Pediatric manual resuscitation bags are usually provided with a 25- to 30-cm $H_2O$ pop-off valve to avoid excessive positive airway pressure. Because the bag is usually reusable and is dismantled during cleaning, proper functioning and, especially, appropriate valve component reassembly must be ensured before any attempt to use it is made.

# LARYNGOSCOPES

## What Are the Components?

### Handles

The basic rigid laryngoscope incorporates a handle that allows attachment of various blade types. The power source is provided by batteries (C cells for adult handles and AA cells for pediatric handles). The handle surface is roughened to allow a better grip. The top has a crossbar to which the blade adapter locks. When the blade is snapped into the position of use, current flows between electrical contacts at its base and the handle, and the bulb is illuminated. To ensure proper contact, the electrical contacts should be clean. The blade should be detached from the handle or folded when it is not in use. Failure of the bulb to illuminate indicates low battery power, bulb failure, improper blade positioning, or use of a wrong blade (eg, the handle for fiberoptic blades cannot be used for standard blades with replaceable light bulbs because the contact points differ). The light source of a standard rigid laryngoscope is the light bulb; the light source for the fiberoptic bundle is in the handle.

### Blades

The laryngoscope blade has four main parts: the light source, the flange, the spatula, and the blade tip. The light source allows illumination and visualization of the airway, whereas the flange helps to guide the ETT. The spatula provides the means to compress and manipulate the tongue and soft tissue while the blade tip presses on the vallecula (curved blade) or supports the epiglottis (straight blade) for vocal cord exposure.

## How Are Blades Shaped?

### Curved

The MacIntosh (MAC) curved blade is designed to elevate the epiglottis when its tip is pressed into the vallecula. It provides increased space during intubation, reduces trauma to the teeth and epiglottis, and purportedly is associated with a reduced incidence of laryngospasm because it does not touch the lower surface of the epiglottis. The MAC 1 (87 mm in length) is used for infants, whereas the MAC 2 (108 mm in length) is used for children. The MAC 3 (130 mm in length)

is most frequently used in adults, although a MAC 4 (158 mm in length) can be useful in large adults. The curved blade has a ridge that prevents the tongue from intruding into the path of vision. However, the ridge may also provide a fulcrum for leverage against the upper teeth when improper techniques are used. The light source is located one third of the blade length from the tip.

### Straight

Straight blades commonly have a straight tip (the Jackson-Wisconsin blade) or a curved tip (the Miller blade). The blade is designed to be placed directly behind the epiglottis, which is then elevated directly to expose the vocal cords. It is the preferred blade for small children and is advantageous when the mouth opening is small or when the larynx is "anterior." It also has a left-sided ridge that protects the visual pathway from obstruction by the tongue. Its light source is located just behind the blade tip on the right side of the Miller blade and on the left side of the Jackson-Wisconsin blade.

The Miller blade is the most popular of the straight blades and is available in various sizes, depending on patient age. The Miller 0 is intended for premature infants and newborns, the Miller 1 for infants and toddlers, the Miller 2 for older children and average adults, and the Miller 3 for large adults. A Miller 4 is also available. Jackson-Wisconsin blades come in three sizes. A modification of this blade, the Wisconsin-Hippe blade, is especially designed for infants (9 months-2 years of age). Figure 16–9 shows the two most commonly used laryngoscope blades.

## What Modifications Are Available?

### Curved Blades

#### Siker

This blade allows visualization of an anterior larynx through a stainless steel, mirrored surface that reflects an inverted image of the cords.[45] This feature makes the blade difficult to use without practice, especially if the patient has a small mouth.[45,46]

#### Huffman

A prism clipped to the base of the blade allows the user to see the blade's tip without inversion of the image.[29,46,47] It is useful during difficult intubation when the larynx cannot be readily visualized with standard blades.

#### Bizarri-Guiffrida

This is a modified MAC blade with the left ridge removed and a light bulb placed in the blade's midportion.[48] It allows easy insertion in a patient with a small oral opening, a short, thick neck, or an extremely anterior larynx.

#### Fink

The Fink blade is a modified curved blade with the left ridge reduced in size at the hook, a wider spatula, and an increased curvature at the tip. Unlike in the Bizarri-Guiffrida blade, the light source is closer to the tip.

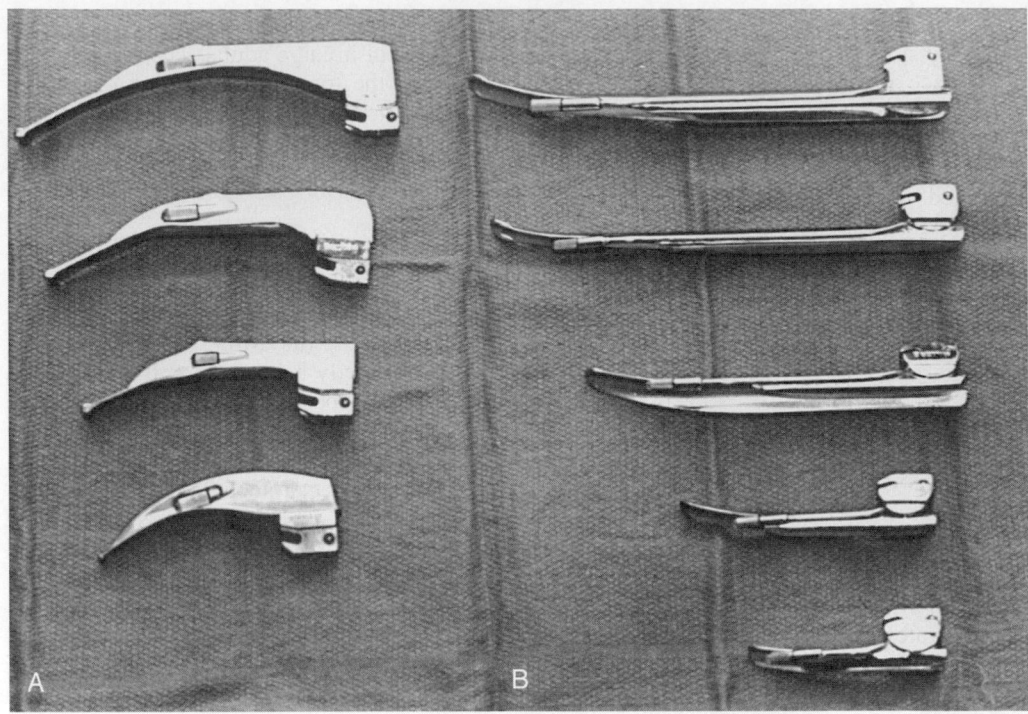

**FIGURE 16–9.** Laryngoscope blades. *A*, Curved (Macintosh) blades. *B*, Straight (Miller) blades.

## Polio

The angle formed by the blade and the handle is more obtuse[49–51] (Fig. 16–10), allowing easier insertion into the mouth. It is useful in patients with increased anteroposterior chest wall diameter that impedes handle rotation and blade insertion.

## Blechman

The Blechman blade has an angled tip to elevate the glottis further in a patient with a short neck. Viewing is enhanced by removal of part of the flange near the lock of the blade.

## Straight Blades

### Guedel

The angle between the handle and the blade is 72° instead of 90°. The light bulb is located just behind the slightly curved tip.

### Flagg

This blade has a C-shaped flange. An angle of 90° is formed between the blade and handle, and the light bulb is located just behind the tip.

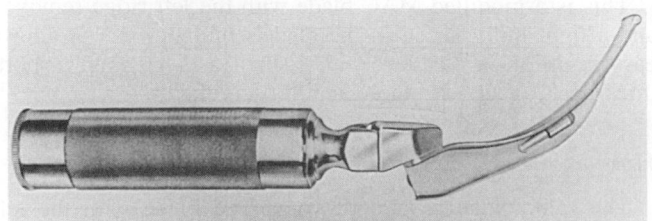

**FIGURE 16–10.** The Polio laryngoscope. (From Dorsch JA, Dorsch SE. *Understanding Anesthesia Equipment.* Baltimore: Williams & Wilkins; 1975:236.)

## Whitehead

This blade has a smaller left-sided ridge. It allows easy insertion in a patient with a small mouth opening and reduces pressure against the upper teeth.

## Bennett

A reduced left-sided ridge (as with the Whitehead blade) is present, and the angle formed between the handle and the blade is 72° when in a position of function (as with the Guedel blade).

## Snow

This blade has a reduced left-sided flange and a raised tip.

## Eversole

The C-shaped ridge is reduced over the distal half of the blade.

## Bellhouse

The Bellhouse blade is modified by a forward angulation of 115° at the midpoint.[52] The spatula has vertical and horizontal components that are significantly lower than in the MAC blade. The light bulb is located near the tip. Alternatively, a prism can be added for a better view of the larynx.

## Bainton

The Bainton blade is a tubular straight blade that can displace tissues circumferentially, permitting rapid viewing of the larynx when the pharyngeal space is limited. A tube 7 cm in length is present in the distal portion, and an intraluminal light source is protected from tissues that might otherwise cover and obstruct it.

### Mathews

This blade is designed for difficult nasopharyngeal intubation. It has a unique petalloid configuration that allows the tip of the ETT to be guided between the vocal cords. Its peculiar shape also allows better visualization of the hypopharynx and the supraglottic area.

## Handles

### Stunted Handle

This handle has a reduced height to facilitate blade insertion. It is particularly useful in patients with increased anteroposterior chest wall diameter, in pregnant patients, in patients with large breasts, or in morbidly obese patients whose body habitus causes the standard handle to press on the chest wall during insertion. The stunted handle has largely replaced the Polio blade in this respect.

### Howland Adapter Handle

The handle is modified to allow changes in the angle between the handle and the blade.[46,53] It decreases the angle that the blade makes with the horizontal axis of the patient and brings the handle forward, thus improving exposure. It may, however, be more difficult to use in patients with increased anteroposterior chest wall diameter.

### Seward Laryngoscope

This modified laryngoscope has a narrow handle and a small, straight blade. It facilitates intubation of neonates and infants by improving access into the mouth and exposure of the larynx.

Other modifications incorporate adjustable double-angle or multiple-angle adapters that are useful in a patient with a receding mandible, anterior larynx, protruding teeth, bullneck, facial fractures, and decreased jaw mobility.[54-56]

## BRONCHOSCOPES

Bronchoscopic devices allow direct visualization of the airway and can be used as a means to pass an ETT. They permit verification of tube position and evaluation of the airway in patients with diffuse parenchymal lung disease, atelectasis, hemoptysis, and blunt chest trauma. Aspirates and tissue samples can be obtained for microbiologic, cytologic, or chemical analysis, and foreign bodies, excessive secretions, and blood clots can be removed from the airway.[57] Effective use of a bronchoscope requires skill and experience and should not be relegated to the novice.

### What Types Are Available?

Available types include diagnostic (Negus and Storz), rigid intubating (Magill), rigid Venturi (Sanders injector), and flexible FOBs.[58]

### Diagnostic Bronchoscopes

Diagnostic bronchoscopes are rigid instruments inserted through the mouth to examine the trachea and the major bronchi. They allow extraction of foreign bodies and endobronchial resection of granulomatous tissue after prolonged or traumatic intubation. They can be fitted with a fiberoptic light source. The Storz bronchoscope can be used to ventilate a patient, using either the Sanders injector or through connection to a standard breathing circuit.

### Rigid Intubating Bronchoscope

The rigid Venturi bronchoscope has a jet ventilator attachment.[59] It allows continuous ventilation and extends bronchoscopy time. However, the fraction of inspired $O_2$ available to the patient at the distal end of the bronchoscope is unpredictable as a result of air entrainment by the $O_2$ jet. Lung ventilation may be inadequate, especially if airway resistance is increased.

### Flexible Fiberoptic Bronchoscope

The flexible FOB is inserted through the nose or mouth and allows direct visualization up to the fifth bronchial branching. It is frequently used for preoperative assessment and management of a potentially difficult airway; as a conduit for the ETT during intubation; to verify correct single-lumen or double-lumen tracheal tube position; and to facilitate intubation in awake patients and bronchial toilet.[60-64] Considerable training and continued use are required, especially if it is to be used in difficult airway situations. It is associated with few complications, allows excellent exposure of the tracheobronchial tree, and does not require general anesthesia during induction.

## What Should an Anesthesiologist Know About Fiberoptic Bronchoscopes?

### Components

The standard flexible FOB has three basic components: the light source, the elongated flexible portion, and the handle with the control section. The elongated flexible portion is marked in centimeters throughout most of its length and is provided with a distal bending section. The upward or downward movement of the tip can be controlled by manipulating the knob on the handle.

A channel or side port at the control section is provided, allowing $O_2$, local anesthetic, and irrigation fluid administration; attachment to a vacuum source permits the suctioning of secretions. It also provides access for a guidewire over which an ETT can be passed. A wire basket can be placed for the removal of foreign bodies from the airway, and a biopsy forceps or cytologic brush can be used to sample tissue for cytopathologic studies.

The handle has an adjustable proximal eyepiece and a control knob for upward and downward manipulation of the distal end. Pediatric and adult-sized bronchoscopes are available. A 4.5-mm ETT is the smallest tube that passes over current commercially available FOBs. A teaching head may be fitted over the control section to allow others to see the airway as the operator manipulates the instrument. If the bronchoscope is inserted orally in an awake patient, a specially designed hollow oral airway (oral airway intubator) should be used to protect the instrument against damage from patient biting.[65,66]

## Maintenance

The FOB is an expensive and delicate instrument. To ensure that it survives and functions properly, appropriate handling and storage are mandatory. Before use, a clear, water-soluble lubricant should be applied to the elongated flexible portion of the ETT.[46,53] Propylene glycol-containing ointments should be avoided because they may damage the covering. An antifogging substance can be applied to the lens.

The distal end should be dipped in warm water for 30 seconds to minimize fogging, and suction should be applied to extricate any secretion remaining in the instrument. Unnecessary bending of the flexible portion should be avoided to prevent breaking the fiberoptic bundles. Fracture or break of individual fibers results in small black dots in the field of view.

After use, the distal end of the scope should be dipped in soap and water and suction applied to remove any secretions. Sterilization may be done by soaking the flexible portion in a 30% ethanol solution or by gas sterilization. An anesthesia technician should be familiar with the care and cleaning of the instrument according to the individual manufacturer's specific recommendations.

## Potential Problems

### Hypoxemia

A number of complications are associated with the FOB, which has an overall complication rate of 6.5% to 8.1% and an associated mortality rate of 0.01% to 0.04%.[67–70] Minor complications include bleeding, nausea, vomiting, vasovagal reaction, and fever. The patient may become hypoxic owing to prolonged suctioning, endotracheal instillation of lidocaine or irrigant, or respiratory depression secondary to sedative use. Hypoxemia-induced catecholamine release can predispose a patient to myocardial ischemia, cardiac dysrhythmia, hypotension, and, in rare instances, cardiac arrest. The incidence of bronchoscopy-induced hypoxemia is decreased by delivery of 100% $O_2$ by a face mask with either a bronchoscope adapter or with a suction port throughout the procedure; by shortening the bronchoscopy time; by suctioning secretions intermittently for 10 seconds at a time or less; and by carefully titrating sedatives.

### Laryngospasm/Bronchospasm

Laryngospasm or bronchospasm is seen in 0.1% to 0.4% of patients. It is more common in patients with reactive airway disease. Bronchodilator therapy before the procedure reduces the incidence of this problem.

### Trauma

Damage to laryngeal, tracheal, and bronchial mucosa may occur; pneumothorax rarely has been observed. Epistaxis and severe hemorrhage may occur during nasal insertion of the bronchoscope. Other reported problems include allergic reaction to the premedications or local anesthetic, aphonia, pneu-

monia, mechanical trauma, subglottic edema, and upper airway obstruction on passage of the bronchoscope through an area of tracheal stenosis.

### Failure to Intubate

Failure to thread the ETT over the bronchoscope after it has been inserted into the trachea is occasionally encountered.[71] The point of obstruction during oral bronchoscopy is commonly caused by the catching of the bevel at the distal end of the ETT by the right arytenoid cartilage, thus hindering smooth advancement into the trachea. Rotation of the ETT's radiopaque stripe to the patient's right places the Murphy tip under and slightly anterior to the epiglottis and corrects the problem. Similarly, during nasal fiberoptic intubation, obstruction may result owing to catching of the Murphy tip on the epiglottis. Rotation of the ETT (positioning the stripe to the patient's left, which places the tip posteriorly) usually facilitates passage.

### Miscellaneous Considerations

Certain conditions are associated with increased risks of complications. Bronchoscopy should not be performed when an experienced bronchoscopist is not available or when a patient is uncooperative. Patients with an unstable cardiac history, bleeding diathesis, untreated asthma, chronic obstructive lung disease, active untreated tuberculosis, advanced malignancy, persistent hypoxemia with supplemental $O_2$, and persistent hyperbaric pulmonary hypertension are poor candidates.

## FIBEROPTIC LARYNGOSCOPES

## What Types Are Available?

Newer devices with fiber-guided light paths for airway visualization and illumination are available.[53] They include flexible, malleable, and specialized rigid types.

### Flexible Fiberoptic Laryngoscope

The flexible fiberoptic laryngoscope is similar to the bronchoscope. It is useful for oral and nasal intubation and has a laryngoscopic handle, an optic bundle, and a port for suctioning or administration of $O_2$, local anesthetics, and irrigants. Its light source may be supplied by portable batteries in the handle; alternatively, a separate, high-intensity source may provide light through a fiberoptic cable. The eyepiece is adjustable, and a control knob can be manipulated to move the tip of the bundle upward or downward.

### Rigid Storz Fiberoptic Laryngoscope

The rigid Storz laryngoscope is similar to a rigid bronchoscope and has excellent optical characteristics. The rigid stylet has a narrow diameter, which allows the ETT to be placed over it. Because of its rigidity, patient conformation to the configuration of the laryngoscope through neck extension may be necessary. It is, therefore, contraindicated in patients with suspected cervical injury. A fiberoptic cable attached to a high-intensity source provides illumination.

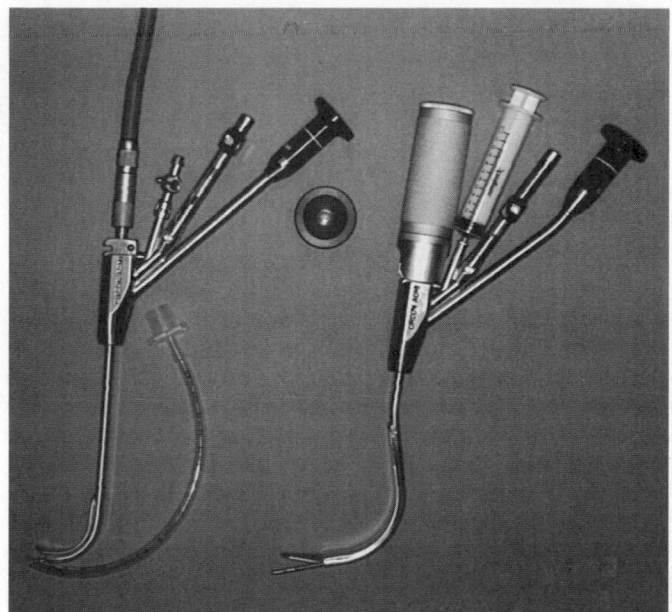

**FIGURE 16–11.** The Bullard laryngoscope. The pediatric Bullard laryngoscope *(left)* has a fiberoptic cable attachment. Note that the blade is smaller and that a pediatric endotracheal tube is held in place by a grasping forceps at the Murphy eye. The adult Bullard laryngoscope *(right)* is shown with a laryngoscope handle as the light source. The smaller working part has a syringe attachment to show the site to administer drugs, oxygen, or emergent solutions. The larger working part is used for insertion of the intubation forceps or a dedicated stylet. (From Bjoraker DG. The Bullard intubating laryngoscope. *Anesthesiol Rev.* 1990;17:64.)

## Rigid Bullard Fiberoptic Laryngoscope

The Bullard laryngoscope is used primarily for indirect oral laryngoscopy.[72–76] Because of its shape and low blade profile, it requires minimal manipulation of the head and neck. It is useful in patients with abnormal or difficult airways and is available in adult and pediatric sizes (Fig. 16–11).

Components include a handle, a blade that angulates 90° from the handle, and a halogen bulb that is powered by two C cells or by a light post that accepts a fiberoptic cable from a light source. It has a fixed-focus eyepiece with an optional snap-on diopter corrector. A teaching attachment provides an additional eyepiece.

Two working ports are between the handle and the viewing arm. The smaller one has a female Luer lock and may be used to administer $O_2$, local anesthetics, or irrigant solution, or to suction. A larger working port is used for insertion of an intubation forceps or a dedicated stylet. This port can be plugged by a rubber stopper if the smaller port is being used for suctioning or the administration of drugs or $O_2$. The pediatric Bullard laryngoscope is provided with a shorter blade and is recommended for use in patients up to 10 years of age.[73]

### Insertion

The instrument may be inserted orally in a manner similar to that used for an oral airway. Several techniques of tracheal intubation have been described.[69] A dedicated grasping forceps can be inserted through a channel in the scope to hold the ETT in place at the Murphy eye. The scope and the ETT are then inserted together into the oropharynx. Once the larynx is

identified, the ETT is advanced by applying pressure on the thumb lever at the proximal end of the forceps. Additional pressure on the lever releases the ETT, which is then inserted to its proper depth in the trachea.

The instrument also functions as a regular laryngoscope. A dedicated stylet may be attached at the same site as the forceps, thus maintaining the tube closely applied to the underside of the blade. The entire apparatus is introduced into the pharynx. Once the larynx is visualized, the tube is advanced into its proper position using the right hand. It allows minimal displacement of the tongue or epiglottis for visualization of the vocal cords, making awake intubation more comfortable than conventional laryngoscopy. It is safe for patients with an unstable neck and avoids the complications associated with nasal intubation.

### Problems

Problems encountered with this instrument include inadvertent laceration of the ETT cuff by the forceps teeth during insertion and failure to intubate adults with longer necks owing to inadequate blade length. Complications associated with standard oral laryngoscopy may also be encountered.

The instrument is expensive. Maintenance and cleaning require proper training. It has several potential mechanical problems, and considerable training and familiarization are required before it can be used, especially in patients with difficult airways.

## What Are the New Fiberoptic Imaging Devices?

A plethora of new imaging devices have been introduced since the mid-1990s. They generally fall into two categories: imaging ETTs and imaging stylets (ISs). Table 16–1 summarizes some of these new products.

### Imaging Endotracheal Tube

The visualized ETT incorporates imaging and illumination fibers in the wall of an ETT, as well as an air flow lumen that can be used to rinse the lens. The device is designed primarily for use in the ICU, where tube position and tracheobronchial secretions are of continuing concern. The image is viewed on a monitor and allows continuous evaluation of airway status distal to the end of the tube.

In a study of 20 OR patients, and subsequently 20 ICU

**TABLE 16–1.** Commercial Optical Stylet Systems

| System | Fiber | Pixels | Flex | View | Hold |
|---|---|---|---|---|---|
| Bonfils | Glass | 12K | Rigid | Eyepiece | Dagger |
| Fiberview | Glass | 10K | Malleable | Eyepiece | Dagger |
| Nanoscope | Plastic | 7K | Malleable | Monitor | Pen |
| PSS-6 | Glass | ? | Malleable | Eyepiece | Dagger |
| Shikani | Glass | 30K | Malleable | Eyepiece/monitor | Pistol |
| StyletScope | Plastic | 3K | Rigid except for tip | Eyepiece/monitor | Pen |
| VETT | Glass | 10K | Malleable | Monitor | Pen |
| VOIS | Glass | 10K | Malleable | Monitor | Pen |

VETT, visualized endotracheal tube; VOIS, video-optical intubation stylet.

patients, the device was found to be easy to use, allowing verification of tube position and decision making on when to suction the airway.[77] In one instance, the lens could not be cleaned of dried secretions.

## Imaging Stylet Systems

IS systems have been available since the 1970s, when American Optical introduced a malleable stylet with imaging and illumination fibers for direct visualization through an eyepiece. Apparently the device was not embraced owing to a price of $4000.

More recently, several stylet-based imaging devices have been introduced, some rigid, others malleable; some using glass optical fiber, others plastic; and some using an eyepiece for viewing and others a monitor. The chief advantages of these devices over conventional laryngoscopy are that the image is from the distal end of the ETT and that the device, when loaded into an ETT, can often be used without a laryngoscope.

### Shikani Seeing Stylet

The Shikani device is similar to the original American Optical system and can be used with either an eyepiece or with a video monitor. It contains both illumination and imaging glass fibers and is malleable. The fiberoptic bundle contains 30 000 fibers and provides a high-quality image.

**Advantages.** When used with a video system, this device has several advantages over conventional laryngoscopic intubation. First, it allows visualization at the distal tip of the ETT and can be used with or without a laryngoscope. A study in 120 patients demonstrated the ease of use and value of this device.[78] It has several advantages over the conventional FOB, primarily because it requires no change in psychomotor skill to use the fiberoptic version, and thus there is essentially no learning curve compared with the FOB.

**Disadvantages.** The version with an eyepiece uses a pistol grip and requires the endoscopist to place his or her face directly above the patient, making the device far more difficult to use.

### Imaging Stylet

The IS is similar to the video version of the Shikani Seeing Stylet but has the advantage of using plastic optical fiber (Fig. 16–12). This greatly reduces the cost of the device, allows greater bending of the stylet without breaking fibers, and allows the potential for a disposable device.

In a study performed at our institution comparing a prototype IS with FOB and direct laryngoscopy (27, 29, and 25 patients, respectively), I found that even when IS was used by novices with no prior training with the device, there was a lower incidence of sore throat compared with direct laryngoscopy.[79]

### Video-Optical Intubation Stylet

The video-optical intubation stylet is actually several versions of an IS. In one version, it is used in conjunction with a Schroeder stylet, whereas in others it is similar to the video version of the Shikani and to the IS. Studies indicate similar advantages compared with standard laryngoscopy.[80,81]

### StyletScope

This device is similar to those described previously. It incorporates a plastic imaging fiber, is rigid except for a movable tip, and can be used with an eyepiece or video system. Several studies again testify to the advantages of these simple imaging systems compared with direct laryngoscopy and FOB.[82,83]

### The Emerging Role of Stylet-Based Imaging Systems

It is clear from the studies cited in the preceding sections that stylet-based imaging systems provide significant advantages over direct laryngoscopy and FOB in certain situations, particularly unanticipated difficult airways. It is clear that there will be further evolution of these systems and that, in time, they may reduce the reliance on direct laryngoscopy and thus avoid its many complications. One report predicts that video imaging systems will become the norm in anesthesia practice.[84]

## SINGLE-LUMEN ENDOTRACHEAL TUBES

### How Are They Constructed?

#### Materials

ETT design has progressed hand-in-hand with the development of anesthesia. Current ETTs are made of polyvinyl

## Imaging Stylet

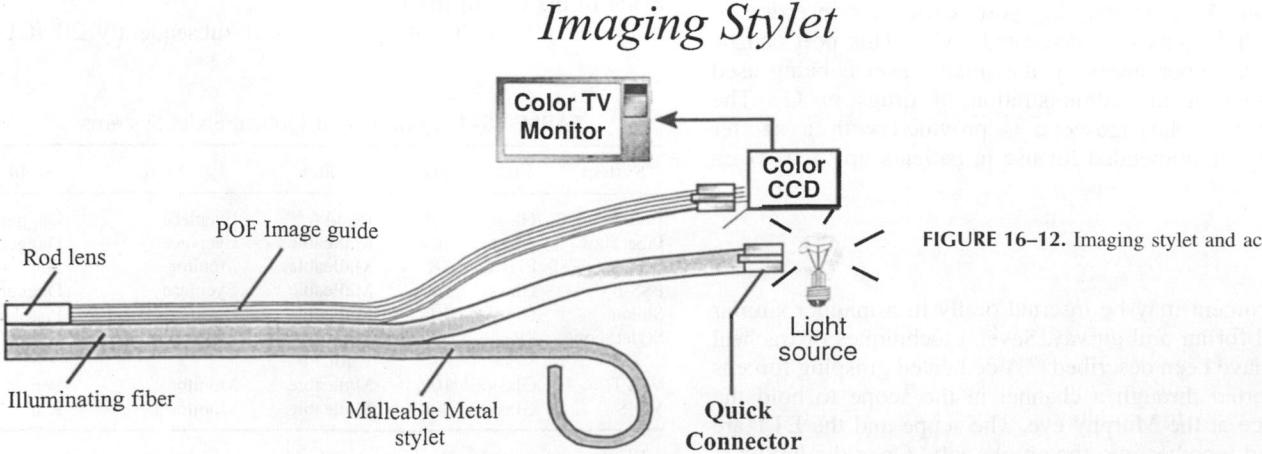

**FIGURE 16–12.** Imaging stylet and accessories.

chloride, medical grade silicone rubber, nylon, or Teflon.[85] Polyvinyl chloride is most commonly used. In its pure form, polyvinyl chloride is brittle, hard, inflexible, and translucent, and it degrades easily when exposed to heat. Chemicals are added during the manufacturing process to increase its flexibility (plasticizers) and stability (stabilizers).

Medical grade silicone rubbers are opaque and flexible. They bend easily, a quality that sometimes interferes with insertion unless a stylet is used.

Nylon tubes are rigid, lightweight, and reusable. Their chemical composition is variable, but they are nontoxic to tissues and can be sterilized by autoclaving. Teflon tubes are hard, rigid, reusable plastic tubes that can be boiled, steam autoclaved, or chemically sterilized.

Because of the many chemicals used in the manufacture of ETTs, extensive testing has been done to ensure patient safety. Most tubes are stamped "I.T." (Implant Tested) or "Z-79" (Z-79 Committee of the American National Standards Institute) to indicate that they have been tissue tested and are free of toxicity or irritant properties.

## Components

Standard ETTs have several important parts:

1. The *bevel* is the distal, stented end of the tube.
2. The *cuff* is the inflatable sleeve around the distal end of the ETT that is inflated to provide an effective seal between the tube and the trachea.
3. The *machine* or proximal portion projects from the patient and is attached to the breathing circuit by a 15-mm adaptor.
4. The *pilot balloon* connects to the cuff and gives some indication of the cuff inflation pressure—in such instances, pressure is controlled through a pressure-regulating valve incorporated in the pilot balloon.
5. The *inflating pilot tube* connects the pilot balloon to the cuff.
6. The *Murphy eye* is a side port near the distal end of the tube that allows ventilation when the main port is occluded by secretions, blood clot, or tracheal wall. Not all ETTs have a Murphy eye.

## Calibration and Dimensions

ETTs are calibrated in internal and external diameter (millimeters) as well as in length (centimeters). Oral and nasal tubes have a radius of curvature of 14 cm ± 10%. The bevel angle of oral and nasal tubes is 45° and 30°, respectively, in relation to their long axis, except for smaller nasal tubes (<6-mm ID), which have a bevel angle similar to that of the oral tube. The bevel opening faces left in oral tubes; nasal tube bevels face in either direction.

The cuff length is usually 2 to 4 cm, and the maximum length of the cemented end is 1.0 cm. The distance between the cemented end of the cuff and the tip of the ETT is usually <13 mm except in tubes with an ID ≤4.5 mm, in which the distance is 5 to 6 mm. Cuff sizes vary with tube size.

Pediatric ETTs have single and double black marks located 2 and 3 cm from the tip of the tube, respectively. ETTs are also provided with a stripe of radiopaque material along the wall to facilitate confirmation of tube position. Uncuffed tubes usually are used for children younger than 6 years of age.

Because the smallest portion of the pediatric airway is at the level of the cricoid cartilage, which is circumferential, an appropriately selected uncuffed tube provides an adequate seal.

### Special Modifications

Single-lumen tubes are most commonly used and can be inserted orally or nasally. They may be cuffed or uncuffed and vary in size from 2.5 to 11.0 mm ID. Preformed or Ring-Adair-Elwyn tubes are also available in oral and nasal forms. The portions that emerge from the nose or mouth are angulated to direct their proximal path away from the surgical field. They are useful in oromaxillofacial surgery.

Armored, anode, or wire-reinforced tubes have a spiral metal wire or nylon filament embedded in their wall that provides resistance to kinking or collapse. Their flexibility necessitates the use of a stylet during insertion. Owing to their flexibility and kink resistance, they may also be inserted through a tracheotomy or laryngectomy stoma and fastened to the skin.

The guidable tube (Endotrol) has a built-in tip control system and is useful for blind nasal or difficult oral intubation. A ring or trigger at the machine (proximal) end of the tube is provided with a thread that runs through a channel in the inner curvature of the tube wall up to its distal end. Traction on the ring decreases the radius of the tube's distal end, causing the curvature to increase and facilitating its guidance into the larynx.

Other single-lumen tubes are designed specifically for laser surgery.[86] Double-cuffed, silicone-coated metal tubes decrease the risk of fire associated with airway laser use but are expensive. Protected ETTs (wrapped with metallic tapes) also reduce the fire hazard. When properly wrapped with metallic tape or copper foil, red rubber tubes are more flame resistant than are polyvinyl chloride, stainless steel Laser-Flex, and other commercially available laser-resistant tubes; however, the cuff still remains unprotected.

## *How Are Tube Size and Length Chosen?*

### Adults

Oral intubation usually requires an 8.0- to 9.0-mm-ID ETT for men and a 7.0- to 8.0-mm-ID tube for women. Tubes that are 1 mm smaller are used for nasal intubation. The tube's length from the alveolar ridge to the tip is usually 20 to 22 cm for women and 22 to 24 cm for men. For nasotracheal intubation, 2 to 3 cm is added to the length from the naris to the tube tip.

### Children

For children, the ID of the ETT is selected on the basis of age and size (Table 16–2). A tracheal tube one size above and below the calculated size should be immediately available to allow proper selection after visualization of the glottic opening. The following formulas can be used to calculate uncuffed tube sizes for children 6 years of age or younger:

$$\text{Size (mm ID)} = 4 + \frac{\text{Age (y)}}{4}$$

**TABLE 16–2.** Recommended Sizes for Pediatric Endotracheal Tubes

| Age of Patient | Internal Diameter of Tube (mm)* |
|---|---|
| Newborn | 3.0 |
| 6 mo | 3.5 |
| 18 mo | 4.0 |
| 3 y | 4.5 |
| 5 y | 5.0 |
| 6 y | 5.5 |
| 8 y | 6.0 |
| 12 y | 6.5 |
| 16 y | 7.0 |

*One size larger or one size smaller should be allowed for individual intra-age variations.

Modified from Florete OG. Airway management. In: Civetta JM, Taylor RW, Kirby RR, eds. *Critical Care.* 2nd ed. Philadelphia, Pa: JB Lippincott; 1991:1427.

Alternatively, this formula can be used:

$$\text{Size (mm ID)} = \frac{16 \text{ to } 18 + \text{Age (y)}}{4}$$

An ideally sized tube allows a leak at 20 to 25 cm $H_2O$ of airway pressure. If the leak occurs at $\leq 10$ cm $H_2O$, the tube should be replaced with the next larger size (eg, from 4.0 to 4.5).

The depth to which the tube should be inserted may also be calculated using a formula based on the child's age:

$$\text{Oral Tube Length (cm)} = \frac{12 + \text{Age (y)}}{2}$$

$$\text{Nasal Tube Length (cm)} = \frac{15 + \text{Age (y)}}{2}$$

These values estimate the distance of the tracheal tube from the alveolar ridge or naris to the tip positioned in the midtrachea.

## Why Is the Correct Size Important?

### Cuff Inflation

Appropriate ETT size and length are important, especially in children. Too large a tube may cause laryngotracheal trauma or failure to intubate. A higher incidence of postoperative sore throat, laryngeal damage, and tracheal stenosis also occurs when a tube that is too large is used. An inappropriately small tube may result in gas leakage, especially if it is uncuffed; conversely, with a cuffed tube, the cuff may have to be excessively inflated to maintain a seal, thereby creating a high-pressure cuff.

### Resistance

Work of breathing and airway resistance vary inversely with tube size. For a 1-mm decrease in the ID of the ETT, the work of breathing increases by 34% to 154%, and the airway resistance increases by 25% to 100%.[87] This factor also emphasizes the importance of not using a tube that is too small.

### Positioning

In adults, the correct position of the tracheal tube tip is approximately 5 cm above the carina. Neck extension moves the tip an average of 1.9 cm away from the carina toward the pharynx, whereas flexion moves it toward the carina. Lateral rotation moves the tube 0.7 cm away from the carina.[88] In children, the length of the trachea varies with age. The vocal cord-to-carina distance in newborns is approximately 4 cm.

Because the tube tip moves with head movement, the best approach is to verify position by auscultation with the neck flexed and extended after intubation to identify a tube that is positioned too deeply (potential mainstem intubation) or not deeply enough (potential extubation).

## How Is Intubation Performed?

### Orotracheal

Orotracheal intubation is most commonly used because it permits direct airway visualization. It is fast and easy to perform in awake, sedated, or fully anesthetized and paralyzed patients. Awake intubation requires patient cooperation. It may be advantageous because airway reflexes are maintained with minimal depression of the cardiovascular, respiratory, and nervous systems. However, gagging and vomiting may be induced. General anesthesia ensures patient "cooperation," removes language barriers, provides amnesia, and promotes muscle relaxation. However, airway reflexes are lost, inability to intubate may occur, and adverse drug reactions, although rare, may result.

### Initial Steps

Administration of 100% $O_2$ for at least 1 minute (preferably 3-5 minutes) before intubation promotes denitrogenation, corrects underlying hypoxemia, and provides a buffer against development of hypoxia. The patient's head is placed in the sniffing position, aligning the axial plane of the mouth, pharynx, and trachea. A pillow or blanket elevates the head 10 cm above the shoulders and helps to align the pharyngeal and laryngeal axes.

### Positioning

The anesthesiologist stands behind the patient, with the bed height adjusted so that the patient's head is at the level of the xiphoid. He or she holds the laryngoscope with the left hand so that the blade is below the hypothenar eminence. The right hand tilts the patient's head back, automatically opening the patient's mouth. Occasionally, the right hand may be placed inside the patient's mouth to open the jaw using the crossed-finger or scissors maneuver, which depresses the lower teeth with the thumb and raises the upper teeth with the index finger.

### Blade Insertion

The laryngoscope blade is inserted at the right side of the mouth along the groove between the tongue and alveolar ridge; the tongue is swept to the left side by the flange of the blade as it is gently and deliberately advanced. A key concept to ensure optimal visualization is not to allow any part of the

**TABLE 16–3.** Common Errors During Intubation

| Step | Error | Correction |
|------|-------|------------|
| Position | Axes not aligned | Put patient in "sniffing" position |
| Mouth opening | Mouth not wide open | Tilt back head or open mouth using crossed-finger technique |
| Blade insertion | Wrong size or wrong blade | Change blade |
| | Blade not inserted on right side of tongue | Withdraw blade and reinsert on the right side |
| Vocal cord exposure | Leverage rather than traction | Keep wrist rigid and pull handle upward and apply traction |
| Tube introduction | Obscuring line of vision of tube | Reinsert tube along right side of mouth lateral to path of blade |
| | Failure to maintain natural curve of tube | Use a stylet |
| | Angulation of trachea due to excessive traction | Release traction |
| Tube position | Endobronchial intubation/esophageal intubation | Auscultate for breath sounds; check chest radiograph |
| | Inadvertent extubation | Secure and tape tube in place |

Adapted with permission in 2001, from Salem MR, Mathrabhutham M, Bennett EJ. Difficult intubation. *N Engl J Med.* 1976;295:879. Copyright © 1976 Massachusetts Medical Society. All rights reserved.

tongue to appear on the right side of the blade. A curved blade follows the base of the tongue anterior to the epiglottis, with the tip in the vallecula. Gentle upward traction on the vallecula opens the epiglottis and exposes the vocal cords. A straight blade tip is used to lift the epiglottis. Once the blade is inserted, the handle is pulled forward; in this way, wrist flexion is avoided. This movement allows elevation of the tongue and visualization of the vocal cords. It also avoids injury to the teeth and maintains the larynx within sight.

### Tube Insertion

Once the vocal cords are seen, the ETT is inserted at the right side of the mouth just lateral to the laryngoscope. An assistant may retract the right corner of the mouth to facilitate tube insertion. The tube is gently advanced between the vocal cords. A stylet may be used to guide the ETT into the larynx, but it should be removed as soon as the tube tip passes the cords. The tube is advanced 2 to 4 cm beyond the glottic opening in a child and several centimeters beyond disappearance of the cuff from view in an adult. The laryngoscope blade is then removed, and the proximal end of the tube is attached to the breathing circuit.

### Cuff Inflation

The tube cuff is inflated with sufficient air to create a seal while positive-pressure breaths are delivered. Chest movement is observed. Bilateral auscultation of the chest in the axillary area and over the epigastrium helps to confirm tube position.

Table 16–3 lists the common errors that occur during intubation and the means to correct them.[89]

### Nasotracheal

Although most patients are intubated orally, certain clinical situations require nasotracheal intubation. Patients with an unstable cervical spine who are conscious, those with a fractured mandible, neck abnormalities, temporomandibular problems, or oropharyngeal infection, and those scheduled for oral or facial surgery may be candidates for nasotracheal intubation.

This technique is more difficult to perform, takes longer, and is more traumatic than oral intubation and often causes epistaxis. It may be performed blindly or under direct visualization with conventional laryngoscopy or FOB. Nasotracheal intubation is avoided in patients with basal skull fractures or a bleeding diathesis, those receiving anticoagulant therapy, those with nasal obstruction or nasal fractures, or those at risk for bacteremia (ie, patients with heart prosthesis or valvular disease). Details are provided in Chapter 53.

### Problems/Considerations

Problems may occur any time during intubation, after placement, during extubation, and after extubation[89] (Table 16–4).

### What Problems Are Associated With Cuff Inflation?

ETTs for adults and children >6 to 8 years of age are provided with inflatable cuffs at the distal end. The cuff serves

**TABLE 16–4.** Risks of Tracheal Intubation/Extubation

| Time | Tissue Injury | Mechanical Problems | Other |
|------|---------------|---------------------|-------|
| Tube placement | Corneal abrasion; nasal polyp dislodgment; bruise/laceration of lips/tongue; tooth extraction; retropharyngeal perforation; vocal cord tear; cervical spine subluxation or fracture; hemorrhage; turbinate bone avulsion | Esophageal/endobronchial intubation; delay in cardiopulmonary resuscitation | Dysrhythmia; pulmonary aspiration; hypertension; hypotension |
| Tube in place | Tear/abrasion of larynx, trachea, bronchi | Airway obstruction; migration of tube; ignition of tube during laser surgery | Bacterial infection (secondary); pulmonary aspiration; paranasal sinusitis; problems related to mechanical ventilation (eg, pulmonary barotrauma) |
| Extubation | Damage to vocal cords (failure to deflate cuff) | Difficult extubation; airway obstruction from blood; foreign bodies, dentures, or throat packs | Pulmonary aspiration; laryngeal edema; laryngospasm; tracheomalacia |

Modified from Florete OG. Airway management. In: Civetta JM, Taylor RW, Kirby RR, eds. *Cricital Care.* 2nd ed. Philadelphia, Pa: JB Lippincott; 1991:1427.

two purposes. It creates a seal against the underlying tracheal mucosa, reducing the likelihood of aspiration of pharyngeal or gastric contents. It also helps prevent air leakage, thereby facilitating positive-pressure ventilation.

Many misconceptions exist about the physiology of ETT cuff design. For most OR patients, this is of little import because most have relatively normal lung compliance and airway resistance and can be ventilated at low inflation pressures. However, an occasional patient requires high inflation pressures because of underlying disease or injury. In these instances, meticulous attention to cuff inflation pressure is important to prevent iatrogenic tracheal injury.

Computed tomographic studies demonstrate that <35% of patients have the C-shaped trachea configuration shown in textbooks. Figure 16–13 shows the range of tracheal shapes and their frequency.[90] These findings are quite different from those reported from autopsy studies. Of course, in reality there is a continuum of tracheal shapes, and any classification is arbitrary. Because inflated cuffs have a circular cross section, it is easy to recognize why fully inflated cuffs would inadequately seal various tracheal shapes. The six tracheal shapes have been classified into low intracuff pressure tracheas and high intracuff pressure tracheas based on the intracuff pressure required for a circular-shaped cuff to seal the trachea adequately.[91] This study also showed that tracheal shape can vary widely, even in the same subject, depending on the distance from the vocal cords (Fig. 16–14).

A magnetic resonance imaging study demonstrated that the greatest changes in cross-sectional area of the trachea during airway maneuvers occur just above the thoracic inlet, the location where most ETTs are placed.[92] What is still unknown is what normal tracheal compliance is or how it changes with advancing age. It has been shown by computed tomography that cross-sectional shape is virtually circular in young children and changes with age.[93,94] It is also known that the tracheal rings may calcify, particularly in elderly patients. It can be inferred from these data that tracheal rings change from circular and extremely compliant to other, less compliant shapes with age, in some cases becoming rigid with calcification. Why the rings take various shapes is unknown, but perhaps the distance between the rings spanned by the mem-

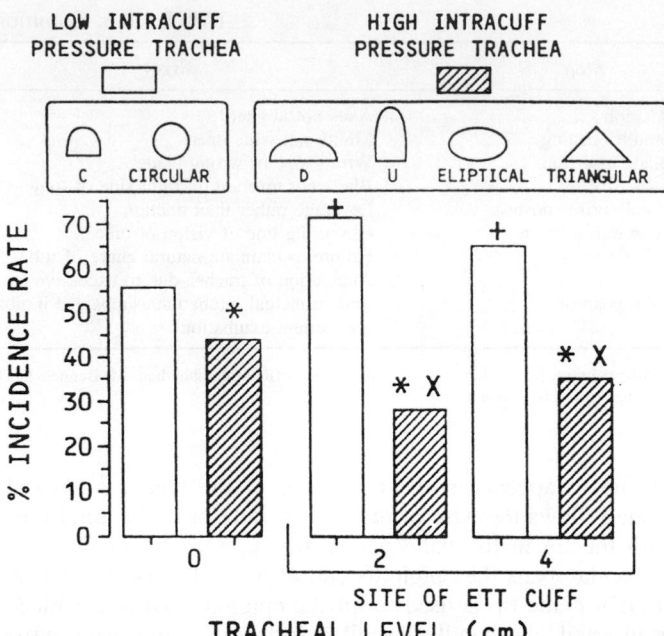

**FIGURE 16–14.** The six tracheal shapes (see Fig. 16–13) are classified into low-pressure tracheas and high-pressure tracheas based on the intracuff pressure required for a circular-shaped cuff to seal the trachea adequately.

branous portion of the trachea helps determine shape. These observations explain why high-pressure, low-volume cuffs are more likely to cause injury even with normal compliance and airway resistance.

### High-Pressure, Low-Volume Cuffs

Early ETT cuffs were usually made of latex and were noncompliant and spherical, and thus had a small area of contact with the tracheal wall. If the trachea is a shape other than circular and is fairly rigid, it is possible to seal only the cuff either by distorting the trachea to conform to the shape of the cuff or by distorting the cuff to assume the shape of the trachea, as illustrated in Figure 16–15.[95,96] This would require extremely high intracuff pressures. In either case, there would be areas of contact between the cuff and tracheal wall where the cuff-to-tracheal wall pressure greatly exceeded the capillary perfusion pressure of the mucosa (25-35 mm Hg), leading to ischemia, which, if persistent, leads to tracheal necrosis, stricture, or fistula formation. These injuries were usually more severe over the tracheal rings and wall than in the posterior membranous trachea.[96–98] These cuffs would also often expand asymmetrically, deforming the trachea and eventually producing tracheal dilation. The latex composition probably also played a part in mucosal injury.

### High-Volume, Low-Pressure Cuffs

High-volume, low-pressure cuffs were the solution to the aforementioned problems because they adapt to the shape of the trachea as long as the inflation pressures are low. Further, they are much longer (sausage shaped), allowing more surface area for a seal, and are made of less-damaging material (polyvinyl chloride). The lower cuff-to-tracheal wall pressure results in less mucosal injury,[99–101] but pressure of even 25 mm Hg can cause partial obstruction to mucosal perfusion.[102–105]

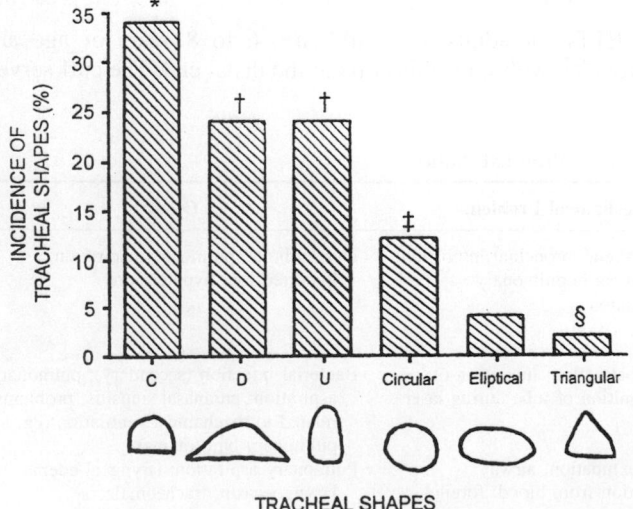

**FIGURE 16–13.** Tracheal cross-sectional shapes and their incidence in humans.

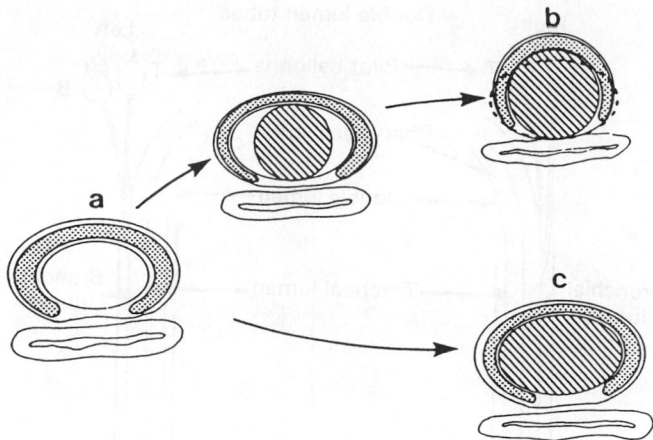

**FIGURE 16–15.** Mechanism of tracheal injury by high-pressure cuff inflation. A high-pressure cuff produces a narrow, spherical structure with a small area of tracheal contact. It expands the trachea until the normal C-shape of the tracheal form is lost and the trachea assumes the cuff's shape. Pressure on the tracheal wall exceeds capillary perfusion pressure, resulting in mucosal ischemia, inflammation, hemorrhage, and ulceration. This ultimately leads to tracheal dilation, granuloma formation, tracheomalacia, tracheal stenosis, and, in some instances, erosion into the innominate artery. (From Cooper JD, Grillo HC. The evolution of tracheal injury due to ventilatory assistance through cuffed tubes: a pathologic study. *Ann Surg.* 1969;169:334.)

Even at a low cuff-to-tracheal wall pressure, cuffs cause tracheal injury, probably because of the movement of the tube in the trachea during ventilation and the polyvinyl chloride, which can adhere to tracheal epithelium. This results in denuded cilia and often loss of the epithelial layer.[102–107] Figure 16–16 shows a comparison of the pressure-volume curves of high-pressure and low-pressure cuffs before and after placement in the trachea, clearly illustrating the significant difference in intracuff pressure necessary to effect a seal.

## Cuff Size

Although modern ETTs are classified as low-pressure and high-volume, not all behave the same way under different

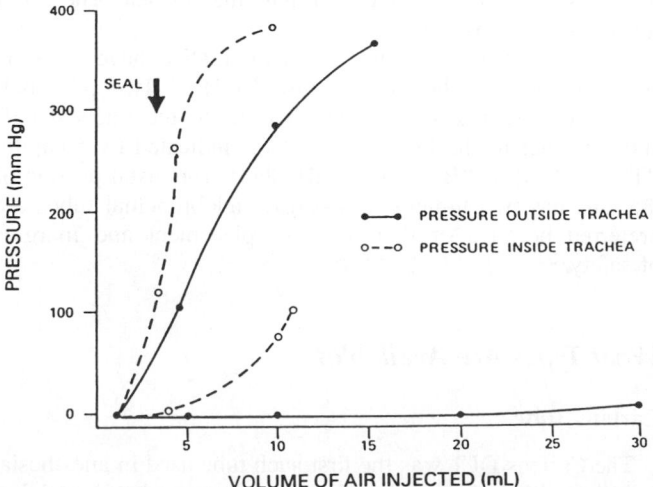

**FIGURE 16–16.** Difference in volume and pressure curves of low-pressure and high-pressure endotracheal tube cuffs. *Solid* and *dotted lines* show the volume and pressure curves of low-pressure and high-pressure cuffs, respectively. (From Dunn CR, Dunn DL, Moser KH. Determinants of tracheal injury by cuffed tracheostomy tubes. *Chest.* 1974;65:128.)

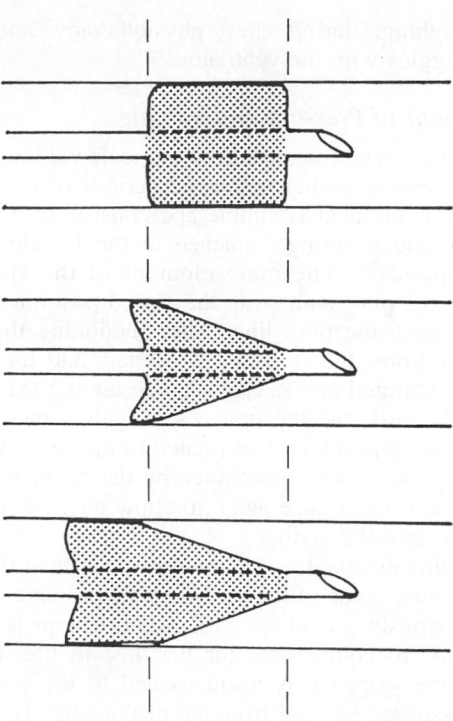

**FIGURE 16–17.** Effect of increased peak airway pressure on an endotracheal tube cuff's shape (see text for explanation). (From Guyton DC. Endotracheal and tracheotomy tube cuff design: influence on tracheal damage. *Crit Care Updates.* 1990;1:1.)

clinical settings.[108] Cuffs of nearly identical diameter (IDs 1.5 times that of the trachea) but of different lengths provide an equal and adequate tracheal seal at peak inflation pressures <25 mm Hg. When lung compliance is reduced and peak inflation pressure is increased to 80 cm $H_2O$, shorter cuffs need an inflation pressure of nearly 50 mm Hg compared with an inflation pressure of only 30 mm Hg in longer ones. The difference in performance is attributed to the length of their tracheal contact. The distal ends of both cuffs collapse when the peak airway pressure is increased, whereas the proximal end bulges outward, changing the cuff shape from cylindric to conical[108] (Fig. 16–17).

## Inflation Volume and Pressure

As lung compliance decreases or airway resistance increases, the volume of gas placed in the cuff must be increased to maintain a seal. This results in distortion of either the cuff or the tracheal shape. At some point, the maximum "tracheal stretch" is reached, with severe damage ensuing. At this point, a low-pressure cuff becomes a high-pressure cuff as cuff-to-tracheal wall pressure increases above acceptable limits.[108] During general anesthesia with nitrous oxide, intracuff pressure increases because of nitrous oxide diffusion into the cuff.[109–111] This can be prevented by inflating the cuff with gas from the breathing circuit rather than with air.[112,113]

After prolonged intubation, cuff pressures have been observed to decrease with time, although the magnitude of decrease and time were not correlated.[114] This reduction is believed to be due to diffusion of gas and to slow movement (creeping) of plastic in the cuff. Intermittent increases occur during positive-pressure ventilation if the airway pressure exceeds that in the cuff. Transient large increases are seen during coughing, during chest physiotherapy, and when a patient struggles with the ventilator.[115]

### Measurement of Pressure and Volume

Measurement and monitoring of intracuff volume and pressure are necessary during prolonged periods of tracheal intubation. The equipment is simple and consists of a sphygmomanometer and a syringe attached to the female port of a 3-way stopcock.[85] The male element of the stopcock is attached to the pilot balloon in the closed position to prevent air escape from the pilot line. After suctioning the pharynx free of secretions, the stopcock is opened, and the entire air volume is aspirated and measured. The air is then reinjected back into the cuff, and the stopcock is again turned to the off position. The stopcock is then rotated to the second orifice to allow cuff pressure to be measured by the sphygmomanometer. It is then rotated once again to allow air from the cuff to be aspirated into the syringe.

The volume obtained at this point is lower than the original volume because some of the air filling the pressure-measuring system previously was in the cuff. Additional air is reinjected into the cuff to compensate for that lost to the manometer tube, and the stopcock is again rotated to the position that allows pressure to be read from the manometer. This pressure is higher than the initial reading and is the true intracuff pressure, compensated for the volume of air in the manometer.

### Minimal-Leak Cuff Inflation

To minimize the possibility of an excessively high intracuff pressure, the minimal-leak inflation technique is increasingly preferred. The cuff is inflated during positive-pressure ventilation until total occlusion occurs between the cuff and the tracheal wall. Air is then gradually aspirated until a minimal air leak is heard at peak inspiratory pressure. The tidal volume is then adjusted to compensate for the minimal loss through the leak in this system. This approach minimizes tracheal damage at low to moderate peak inflation pressure but not when high ventilatory pressure is necessary.

### No-Leak Cuff Inflation

In some clinical situations, the minimal-leak technique may not be helpful, and total occlusion is desirable, particularly for patients who aspirate repeatedly, have poor lung compliance, or require high levels of positive end-expiratory pressure to maintain adequate ventilation and oxygenation. In these instances, a no-leak technique with minimal occluding volume is used to inflate the cuff. This approach requires around-the-clock frequent monitoring of intracuff pressure and volume.

To ensure that minimum pressure and volume are used, the cuff is inflated and deflated in a manner similar to that for the minimal-leak technique. Once a minimal leak is observed, an additional volume of air is slowly injected until no leak is appreciated. This process is periodically repeated. This technique of cuff pressure inflation is prevalent in the OR to avoid contamination of the room with anesthetic gases.

## DOUBLE-LUMEN ENDOTRACHEAL TUBES

### What Is Their Role?

Double-lumen tubes (DLTs) are primarily used for one-lung ventilation.[116] These devices functionally consist of two tubes

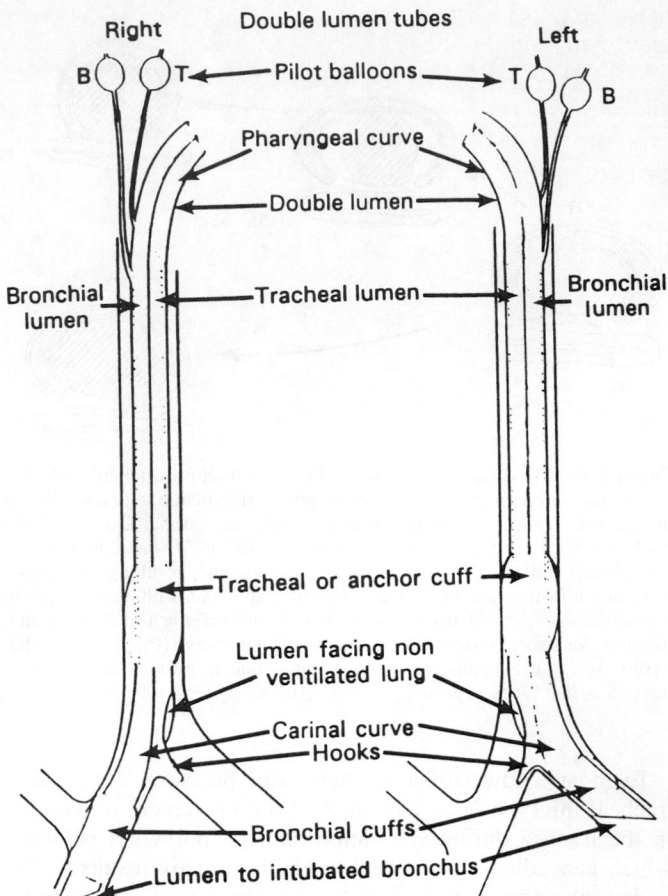

**FIGURE 16–18.** Parts of right- and left-sided double-lumen tubes. (From Vaughan RS. Endobronchial intubation. In: Latto IP, Rosen M, eds. *Difficulties in Tracheal Intubation.* London, United Kingdom: Bailliere Tindall; 1983:158.)

attached together, side by side, with one side longer than the other and with the tip curved to the longer side. They are available with a left- or right-sided orientation. The former allows placement of the left catheter into the left mainstem bronchus and the right catheter into the trachea. The latter functions in opposite fashion.

Regardless of the type or manufacturer, DLTs have common characteristics, as shown in Figure 16–18.[117] Two pilot balloons are provided, one of which leads to the tracheal cuff and the other to the bronchial cuff (as indicated by a capital "T" [trachea] or "B" [bronchial] label). The distal portion of the tube has two lumens. Left-sided endobronchial tubes are preferred because of their ease of placement and margins of safety.

### What Types Are Available?

#### Carlens Tube

The Carlens DLT was the first such tube used in anesthesia. It is left sided and made of soft rubber or plastic and has tracheal and bronchial cuffs, two pilot balloons, and a carinal hook to facilitate tube placement and avoid distal tube movement. Occasionally, the carinal hook may be amputated during or after intubation, which may make intubation difficult. It may also cause laryngeal trauma, tube malposition, or physical interference during surgery.[118] Four sizes are available: 35, 37, 39, and 41 French (with IDs of 5.0, 5.5, 6.0, and 6.5 mm, respectively).

## White Tube

The White tube is essentially a right-sided Carlens tube.[119] It has a slotted cuff on its right side, thus permitting right upper lobe ventilation.

## Bryce Smith Tube

The Bryce Smith tube has right-sided and left-sided versions. It lacks a carinal hook, and the right-sided version has a slotted cuff that promotes right upper lobe ventilation.

## Robertshaw Tube

The Robertshaw tube has an enlarged lumen to decrease resistance to airflow and facilitate suctioning of secretions.[120] The original version was made of reusable red rubber, but this has been replaced by a modern version made of disposable, clear, nontoxic, tissue-implantable plastic.[121] It does not have a carinal hook; this facilitates tube insertion and permits ligation of a mainstem bronchus close to the carina for pneumonectomy.[122] Left-sided or right-sided tubes are available. The right-sided version has a slotted tip in the endobronchial cuff, permitting right upper lobe ventilation. The left-sided model has a beveled bronchial lumen with restricted bronchial cuff inflation on the medial side. This design reduces interference with right lung ventilation.

Tube sizes are 28, 35, 37, 39, and 41 French (with IDs for each lumen of 4.5, 5.0, 5.5, 6.0, 6.5 mm, respectively). Only a left-sided tube is available in the 28-French size. Both cuffs are low pressure and high volume. The bronchial cuff is bright blue, allowing easy recognition during FOB. The tube also has a black radiopaque line at the end of both lumens that is used as a radiographic marker. Malleable stylets and nonadhering suction catheters are usually provided in the package of the disposable Robertshaw tube.

## What Are the Indications?

For thoracotomies requiring ventilation of the left lung and collapse of the right, a left-sided DLT should be used. For left thoracotomies, either a left-sided or right-sided tube may be used. If a right-sided tube is selected, the ventilation slot in the endobronchial cuff should be closely opposed to the right upper lobe orifice to permit unobstructed right upper lobe ventilation. The best way to achieve this precise positioning of the ventilation slot is to position it using the flexible FOB. Otherwise, because of wide anatomic variation in the exact position of the right upper lobe opening and in the length of the right mainstem bronchus, the slot of the endobronchial cuff may not be in proper position, resulting in the risk of inadequate right upper lobe ventilation. This problem accounts for the popularity of the left-sided tube even during left lung surgery.[123,124] If the left mainstem bronchus needs to be clamped, the DLT can be pulled back into the trachea and used as a single-lumen tracheal tube to ventilate the right lung.

## What Are the Contraindications?

The presence of strictures, tumors, tracheobronchial disruption, extraluminal compression of the airway (eg, aortic arch aneurysm), or any lesion along the double tube's pathway contraindicates DLT use. Such tubes are relatively contraindicated in patients with full stomachs or at high risk of aspiration; critically ill patients with a single-lumen ETT in place who cannot tolerate even a short period of removal from mechanical ventilation; and instances in which it is difficult or impossible to perform conventional, direct vision intubation.[116] Tenting of the left mainstem bronchus with a takeoff angulation from the trachea of ≥90° may make insertion of the left endobronchial tube extremely difficult and hazards left mainstem bronchus injury.

## How Are They Inserted?

Insertion of the DLT may be performed using conventional laryngoscopy or FOB. If conventional laryngoscopy is selected, a MAC blade is preferable because it approximates the tube's curvature. Once the vocal cords are visualized, the tube is inserted into the mouth with the concave side up; it is then rotated 90°. As the tube tip passes the larynx, the stylet is removed, and the tube is rotated 90° back to the original position to advance the bronchial portion into the appropriate bronchus. Turning the head and neck to the opposite side may facilitate insertion. Advancement continues until the proximal end of the double-lumen binder mold is near or at the level of the teeth, or when mild resistance to further advancement is encountered, indicating that the tube tip is positioned endobronchially. The tracheal and bronchial cuffs are then inflated. In general, <3 mL of air is required to inflate the bronchial cuff.

## Verification of Placement

Bilateral ventilation is checked by delivering several positive-pressure breaths, auscultating breath sounds, and observing the chest. If only one side of the chest moves and unilateral breath sounds are appreciated, both lumens may have entered a single mainstem bronchus. The cuffs should be deflated and the tube withdrawn 1 to 2 cm at a time. The cuffs are reinflated, the chest is observed for movement, and the lungs are auscultated until bilateral chest movement is seen and breath sounds are heard equally in both lung fields.

If the tube is in its proper place, clamping of one connecting tube results in disappearance of breath sounds on the ipsilateral side. Only the contralateral side of the chest rises and falls with ventilation, giving it a rocking boat motion. Tube condensation is observed only on exhalation from the ventilated side. The ventilated lung should feel reasonably compliant and easy to ventilate.

Breath sounds should be equally appreciated at the basal, medial, and apical portions. If right-sided apical breath sounds are not audible, the upper lobe on that side may not be ventilated. Pulling the tube back 1 cm at a time until apical breath sounds are heard corrects the problem. If the lumen cap is opened proximal to the clamp, no air leakage should be noted to indicate adequate seal by the bronchial cuff. Once the clamp is removed and the lumen cap is replaced, bilateral breath sounds and chest movement should be observed. Further confirmation of tube placement must be done by chest radiography or fiberoptic visualization.

## Malpositioning

If the patient is moved and repositioned, tube position should again be reconfirmed; head flexion may advance the tracheal tube into the mainstem bronchus or cut off right upper lobe ventilation. Head extension may cause the bronchial cuff to move out of the mainstem bronchus.[125,126]

Three major malpositions of the DLT have been described after blind insertion[126] (Fig. 16–19). They can be ascertained by chest auscultation combined with unilateral clamping and by endobronchial cuff inflation-deflation. When the left cuff is inflated and the left lumen is clamped, ventilation occurs only through the right lumen. In all three malpositions, this maneuver results in blockage of the right lumen, and breath sounds are either absent or diminished. When the left cuff is deflated, breath sounds are heard only on the left if the tube is too far into the left bronchus; bilateral breath sounds are heard if the tube is out too far in the trachea; and only right breath sounds are appreciated if the tube is too far into the right bronchus.

If the patient has preexisting lung disease, breath sounds may not be a good indicator of proper tube positioning, and FOB should be used to confirm position. The tube may be only slightly malpositioned and thus is difficult to diagnose. Also, surgical manipulation, head movement, or patient turning during the procedure may change the position of the tube. In all cases, ready access to and use of FOB is considered by many to be essential to avoid complications of malpositioning.

## Fiberoptic Bronchoscopic Examination

The blind method of DLT insertion is associated with a high rate of failure and malposition (25%-48%), even when clinical signs indicate proper tube position.[127,128] FOB is associated with a more accurate placement.[123,128–130] Some argue, however, that routine use of FOB to position a DLT is unnecessary, expensive, and time consuming and discourages the use of such tubes.[131,132] Furthermore, movement of the tube is likely to occur several times during surgery as a result of the patient's positioning, surgical procedure, or head movement, making the use of FOB impractical.

Nevertheless, most anesthesiologists use an FOB to confirm tube position. It may be passed through the tracheal lumen to check the position of both the bronchial cuff and the tracheal lumen opening relative to the mainstem bronchus that leads to the other lung. Insertion of the instrument into the tracheal lumen should provide a clear view of the carina, the ETT going into the appropriate bronchus, and the upper surface of the blue bronchial balloon visible just below the carina. FOB readily detects gross malposition and excessive bronchial cuff inflation pressure that results in cuff herniation, carinal deviation, and excessive left lumen constriction. In addition, it localizes the right upper lobe ventilation slot of the right-sided DLT and its relation to the right upper lobe orifice.

A pediatric FOB is preferred for insertion and confirmation of tube position because it can pass down the lumens of all commercially available DLTs. Once the tube is in the trachea, positive-pressure ventilation may be continued during bronchoscopy by inserting the bronchoscope through a self-sealing diaphragm in the elbow connector to the bronchial lumen.

## What Are the Potential Complications?

### Ventilation-Perfusion Mismatch

Several complications of DLTs have been reported. The most common is arterial hypoxemia after induction and insertion of the tube.[133] Arterial desaturation may result from obstruction of the right upper lobe bronchus or increased shunt secondary to ventilation-perfusion mismatch during one-lung ventilation. It may also result from excessive intraalveolar pressure when the tidal volume delivered to one lung remains the same as it was originally for both lungs. To minimize this

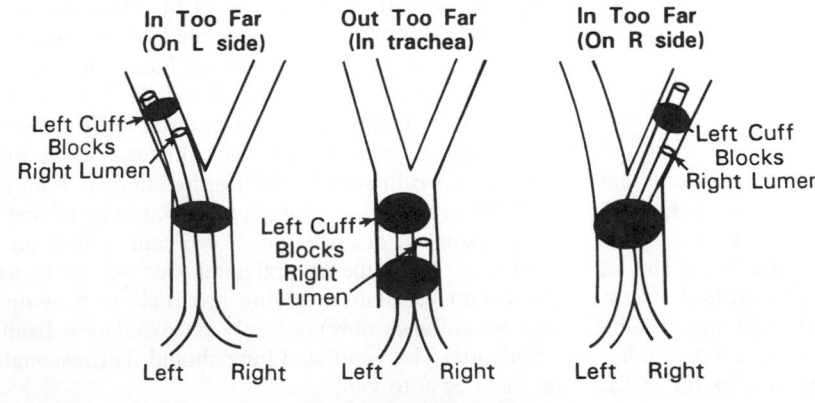

| Procedure | Breath Sounds Heard | | |
|---|---|---|---|
| Clamp Right Lumen Both Cuffs Inflated | Left | Left and Right | Right |
| Clamp Left Lumen Both Cuffs Inflated | None or Very ⬇⬇ | None or Very ⬇⬇ | None or Very ⬇⬇ |
| Clamp Left Lumen Deflate Left Cuff | Left | Left and Right | Right |

**FIGURE 16–19.** Different types of double-lumen tube malpositioning. (From Benumof JL. Anesthesia for thoracic surgery. In: *IARS 1988 Review Course Lectures.* Baltimore, Md: Williams & Wilkins; 1988:120.)

**TABLE 16–5.** Approaches to Independent Lung Ventilation in Lateral Decubitis Position

| "Dependent" Lung | "Up" Lung |
|---|---|
| 1. Ventilate | 1. Provide CPAP (5-10 cm $H_2O$; apneic oxygenation) |
| 2. Ventilate | 2. Provide constant CPAP, apneic oxygenation, periodic ventilation |
| 3. Ventilate with CPAP (5-10 cm $H_2O$) | 3. Do not ventilate |
| 4. Provide high-frequency ventilation | 4. Ventilate with or without CPAP |

CPAP, continuous positive airway pressure.

problem, the fraction of inspired $O_2$ may be increased to 1.0, the tidal volume appropriately reduced, and the respiratory rate increased to maintain the same minute ventilation.

Use of volatile anesthetics that increase the shunt through pulmonary vasodilation may have to be discontinued and intravenous agents substituted. If hypoxemia persists, one of the approaches listed in Table 16–5 is suggested. Persistent hypoxemia is unusual if the ventilated lung receives a fraction of inspired $O_2$ of 1.0 and the nonventilated lung is inflated with $O_2$ and 5 cm positive end-expiratory pressure.

## Tube Malposition

The most common cause of malposition is selection of a tube that is inappropriately long, allowing its placement too far into the bronchus.[133,134] Malposition may result in airway obstruction, atelectasis, inability to isolate and collapse the lung, and $O_2$ desaturation. If the DLT is too large, it may be difficult to position into the appropriate bronchus. Proper tube selection and FOB obviate this problem.

## Tracheobronchial Rupture

A dreaded complication of DLT insertion is tracheobronchial rupture.[135–137] Risk factors include insertion by inexperienced operators, use of intubating stylets, multiple vigorous attempts at intubation, presence of tracheobronchial abnormalities, overdistention of the tracheal or bronchial cuff, and advanced patient age.[138–141] Diagnosis can be difficult, and clinical signs such as hemorrhage, cyanosis, subcutaneous emphysema, pneumothorax, or compliance changes may be absent or slow to develop.

To prevent this problem, the bronchial cuff should not be inflated with >2 to 3 mL of air and should be deflated before the patient is moved. The integrity of the intubated bronchus can be checked with the bronchial cuff deflated at the time of testing of the resected bronchus for air leak.

## Miscellaneous Problems

Other reported complications include traumatic laryngitis,[118] cardiac arrest due to pulmonary outflow tract obstruction,[112] and suture of a pulmonary vessel to the DLT.[142,143] Trauma during extubation may also occur and includes slight bleeding and ecchymosis of mucous membranes, arytenoid dislocation, laryngeal and vocal cord damage, and accidental tooth extraction.

## ANCILLARY EQUIPMENT

Several ancillary devices facilitate intubation. These include specialized forceps, flexible lumen finders, tube changers, laryngotracheal anesthesia kits, malleable stylets, lighted stylets, and lightwands.

### *How Is the Intubating Forceps Used?*

The forceps is used during direct laryngoscopy to direct the tip of the ETT into the glottic inlet. The Magill forceps has a handle angle relative to its length of approximately 50°. The Rovenstein forceps has a 90° handle angulation and a deeper tip with which to grasp the ETT. The Aillon forceps is provided with a spring-loaded handle and is used to grasp and bend the ETT's tip to align it with the laryngeal axis. The forceps is usually held in the right hand and is used to grasp the ETT distally above the point of attachment of the cuff. The tube is advanced by an assistant while the operator directs it to the glottic opening with the aid of the forceps.[144,145]

### *Is a Stylet Helpful?*

A stylet is an elongated, malleable introducer made from a variety of materials, including copper wire, coat hanger wire, brass rods, flexible stainless steel, or disposable plastic rods.[146–148] When inserted into an ETT, it permits customizing of the tube's shape to facilitate intubation. The stylet is lubricated and passed into the ETT, and the distal end is bent gradually in a J or "hockey stick" shape. The tube is inserted with the curvature directed toward the coronal plane (glottic opening).

A stylet should not protrude through the Murphy eye or the tip of the ETT, nor should it be used to force entry into the trachea. Instead, its tip should lie at least 2 cm from the tube's end to avoid trauma and possible perforation of the larynx, trachea, or esophagus. Its proximal end should be bent over the rim of the 15-mm adaptor to avoid accidental advancement beyond the tube tip during intubation. It should be withdrawn once the tube is seen to pass the vocal cords.

Because most intubations can be performed rapidly and safely without a stylet, I do not recommend that a stylet be used routinely; it should be reserved for rapid sequence induction or emergency intubation, when a difficult airway is anticipated, or if an armored tube is used. Although a stylet is used primarily for oral intubation, it may be used for nasotracheal intubation.[146] Reported complications of stylet use include bleeding, hematoma formation, submucosal dissection, tracheobronchial rupture, esophageal perforation, pneumomediastinum, and pneumothorax.

### *What Is a Lightwand?*

A flexible, battery operated stylet (lightwand) with a smooth tip and a bulb at its distal end for illumination is available.[149–154] The lightwand is lubricated and placed inside the ETT, and the distal end is preformed to the anticipated path of entry to the glottic opening. The stylet is inserted orally and transilluminates the neck when it passes through the vocal cords. A bright, cherry red glow is appreciated at the region of the cricothyroid membrane, indicating proper positioning of the stylet. If the stylet is somewhere else, the light is noted laterally or not at all. The transillumination is most easily observed in a dark room. Once the characteristic glow is noted, the tube is passed over the lightwand into the trachea.

### Insertion

This technique of insertion does not require direct laryngoscopy and can be performed safely in adults and children.[152–154] It has been used for routine and difficult intubation in awake as well as in anesthetized patients. Its greatest value is in patients whose glottic opening cannot be completely visualized by direct laryngoscopy. Minimal movement of the neck is required; thus, it may also be useful in patients with suspected neck injury.

### Potential Problems

Blood and secretions in the oropharynx do not interfere with use of the lightwand, as they might with direct laryngoscopy or fiberoptic intubation. The lightwand cannot be used in children <5 years of age or in those requiring an ETT <5.5 mm ID because of the bulb size. Problems associated with its use are uncommon and include hoarseness, postoperative sore throat, and cricoarytenoid subluxation. Complications associated with the use of the lightwand are similar to those occasionally seen with a malleable stylet.

### What Is a Flexible Lumen Finder?

Another modification of the stylet is a flexible lumen finder and intubation guide.[155] It has a proximal control handle, trigger, inner rod, and notched outer tube that allows the operator's right hand to maneuver the distal tip with the proximal trigger. The smooth, flexible tip can be directed anteriorly, posteriorly, or laterally. The distal 5 cm should be well lubricated before the ETT is inserted through it. Direct laryngoscopy is performed, and the stylet tip is maneuvered toward the glottic inlet. Once the distal tip of the finder enters the trachea, the tracheal tube is advanced, and the lumen finder is removed.

### How Does the Laryngotracheal Anesthesia "Stylet" Function?

Although a laryngotracheal anesthesia kit usually is used to spray topical anesthesia into the larynx and trachea, it may also function as a stylet. The distal end is inserted into the Murphy eye of the ETT. After direct laryngoscopy, the tip is directed into the rima glottidis.[156] The ETT is then advanced over the elongated portion. The tube often hangs up on the laryngeal inlet when it is advanced over the stylet. This problem is usually resolved by rotating the ETT 90° to 180°.

### What Is a Tube Changer?

A tube changer is a hollow or solid elongated plastic tube that can be used to exchange a malfunctioning ETT or as an introducer during initial intubation in a patient with a difficult airway. To change the tube, the tube changer is first lubricated and inserted into the trachea through the in situ ETT, which is then pulled out while the position of the tube changer is maintained. A new ETT is then inserted over the tube changer into proper position. The tube changer is withdrawn, and the tube is secured.

Hollow tube changers can be connected to a high-pressure $O_2$ source, and oxygenation can be achieved with either $O_2$ insufflation or ventilation using a Sanders injector. Suction catheters may function as tube changers but are a less-secure option because they are too flexible and often of insufficient length. Complications associated with tube changer manipulation are similar to those encountered with stylets. An additional reported complication is bronchial rupture caused by a tube changer that has advanced beyond the carina.

## ALTERNATIVE MANAGEMENT TECHNIQUES

The incidence of failed tracheal intubation ranges from 5 to 35 per 10 000 patients.[157–160] Inability to mask-ventilate and intubate patients ranges from 0.01 to 2.0 per 10 000 patients.[161,162] Failure to oxygenate and ventilate patients is responsible for 50% to 75% of cardiac arrests during general anesthesia.[162–164] Hence, alternative methods of securing the airway must be available. These include needle cricothyroidotomy with transtracheal jet ventilation,[165–168] percutaneous cricothyroidotomy,[169–173] surgical cricothyroidotomy or tracheotomy,[174–176] and retrograde tracheal intubation. Percutaneous cricothyroidotomy is easier and safer than emergency tracheotomy.[174–178]

### When Is Retrograde Catheter Placement Useful?

Retrograde tracheal intubation is indicated when translaryngeal intubation fails and the glottic inlet is not totally obstructed.[179–187] The procedure can be done in an awake, sedated, or anesthetized patient, and the ETT can be passed orally or nasally. It involves puncture of the cricothyroid membrane with a hollow needle, followed by passage of a wire or small catheter through the membrane and upward into the pharynx. The posterior pharynx is visualized, and the catheter is grasped with a forceps and directed toward the mouth or nose. It is then used as a guide to insert the ETT into the airway. Once the ETT is seen to pass through the cords, the catheter is gently removed, and the tube is secured in place. Clinical signs as previously described should be observed for proper tube placement.

Although its success rate is high, the technique is time consuming and sometimes difficult to perform. It is not popular among anesthesiologists and serves only as a last resort when other, easier methods, such as fiberoptic intubation or percutaneous cricothyroidotomy, fail to secure the airway. Complications include inability to secure the airway, minor bleeding at the puncture site or nose, hematoma formation, and barotrauma. Potential complications observed during percutaneous cricothyroidotomy and standard translaryngeal intubation may occur.

## *When Is Tracheotomy Performed?*

Emergency tracheotomy should be performed only by a trained surgeon. Indications include rare instances of laryngeal trauma and emergency airway control in infants.[185] Elective tracheotomy is indicated for relief of upper airway obstruction, to improve suctioning, to reduce work of breathing, to improve airway access for prolonged mechanical ventilation, to assist in weaning mechanically ventilated patients with marginal pulmonary function, to reduce dead space, and to relieve patient discomfort. It generally should not be done in patients with fresh sternotomies because of the danger of the spread of infection from the stoma to the surgical site. It also should be avoided in most cases of emergency airway access because of a high morbidity and mortality rate.[186,187] Emergent tracheotomy has a reported complication rate of as high as 42%; the mortality rate is 2% to 5% even in elective cases.[186,188–191]

## Tube Types

"Standard" tubes consist of an inner and outer cannula, an obturator, a flange, and a cuff. The inner cannula has a 15-mm universal adapter that can be connected to a self-inflating bag or to the anesthesia machine breathing circuit. The cannula is made of metal or plastic and is shorter, wider, and less curved than a standard ETT. Only implant-tested tubes should be used, and a low-pressure, high-volume cuff is preferable. A tracheotomy button is available to maintain a tracheostomy stoma after decannulation when there are doubts about whether a patient can chronically maintain a patent airway without the tracheotomy tube. A fenestrated tracheotomy tube allows breathing through the upper respiratory tract, permitting phonation and humidification of the inspired gas.

## Early Complications

Early complications include pneumothorax, subcutaneous emphysema, bleeding, aspiration, and aerophagia. The most important and potentially lethal complication is tube displacement after initial insertion. Blind attempts to reinsert the tube may cause tracheal compression and upper airway obstruction. If the tube is displaced and the path to the trachea is not clear, translaryngeal intubation should be attempted to secure the airway. If necessary, a pediatric laryngoscope can be used to visualize the trachea directly through the stoma, and careful cannulation can be performed with a small, cuffless ETT. Once the patient is stable, the tracheotomy tube can be reinserted.

## Late Complications

Late complications include lower respiratory tract infection, which is observed in >50% of patients,[191] stricture, tracheal stenosis, erosion of the brachiocephalic artery with tracheobrachiocephalic fistula formation, and tracheal hemorrhage.[191] Tracheal necrosis and tracheoesophageal fistula may be caused by excessive intracuff pressure or by a poorly fitting tracheotomy tube.[192] Other chronic problems include swallowing dysfunction, tube obstruction, aspiration, stomal infection, and unsightly scar formation.

## References

1. Applebaum EL, Bruce DL. A short history of tracheal intubation. In: Applebaum EL, Bruce DL, eds. *Tracheal Intubation.* Philadelphia, Pa: WB Saunders; 1976:1.
2. Welch GW, Rippe JW. Airway management and endotracheal intubation. In: Rippe JM, Irwin RS, Alpert JS, et al, eds. *Intensive Care Medicine.* Boston, Mass: Little, Brown & Co; 1985:1.
3. Smith JP, Bodai BI, Seifkin A, et al. The esophageal obturator airway: a review. *JAMA.* 1983;250:1081.
4. Meislin HW. The esophageal obturator airway: a study of respiratory effectiveness. *Ann Emerg Med.* 1980;9:54.
5. Schofferman J, Oill P, Lewis AD. The esophageal obturator airway: a clinical evaluation. *Chest.* 1984;69:63.
6. Smith JP, Bodai BI, Aubourg R, et al. A field evaluation of the esophageal obturator airway. *J Trauma.* 1983;23:317.
7. Harrison EE, Ward HJ, Bleman RW. Esophageal perforation following use of the esophageal obturator airway. *Ann Emerg Med.* 1980;9:21.
8. Jancey W, Wear SR, Kamajian G. Unrecognized tracheal intubation: a complication of the esophageal obturator airway. *Ann Emerg Med.* 1980;9:18.
9. Key GK. Use of the esophageal obturator airway with a report of an unusual complication. *Postgrad Med.* 1980;67:189.
10. Niemann JT, Rosborough JP, Myers R, et al. The pharyngeo-tracheal lumen airway: preliminary investigation of a new adjunct. *Ann Emerg Med.* 1984;13:591.
11. Bartlett RL, Martin SD. The pharyngeo-tracheal lumen airway: an assessment of airway control in the setting of upper airway hemorrhage. *Ann Emerg Med.* 1987;16:343.
12. Frass M, Frenzer R, Zdrahl F, et al. The esophageal tracheal Combitube: preliminary results with a new airway for CPR. *Ann Emerg Med.* 1987;16:768.
13. Koppel JN, Reed AP. Formal instruction in difficult airway management: a survey of anesthesiology residency programs. *Anesthesiology.* 1995;83:1343.
14. Rosenblatt WH, Wagner PH, Ovassapian A, et al. Practice patterns in managing the difficult airway by anesthesiologists in the United States. *Anesth Analg.* 1998;87:155.
15. Mercer MH, Gabbott DA. Insertion of the Combitube airway with the cervical spine immobilised in a rigid cervical collar. *Anaesthesia.* 1998;53:971.
16. Mercer MH, Gabbott DA. The influence of neck position on ventilation using the Combitube airway. *Anaesthesia.* 1998;53:146.
17. Vezina D, Lessard MR, Bussieres J, et al. Complications associated with the use of the esophageal-tracheal Combitube. *Can J Anaesth.* 1998;45:76.
18. Oczenski W, Krenn H, Dahaba AA, et al. Complications following the use of the Combitube, tracheal tube and laryngeal mask airway. *Anaesthesia.* 1999;54:1161.
19. Elam JO, Titel JH, Feingold A, et al. Simplified airway management during anaesthesia or resuscitation: a binasal pharyngeal system. *Anesth Analg.* 1969;48:407.
20. Brain AIJ. The laryngeal mask: a new concept in airway management. *Br J Anaesth.* 1983;55:801.
21. Leach AB, Alexander CA. The laryngeal mask: an overview. *Eur J Anaesthesiol Suppl.* 1991;4:19.
22. Kapila A, Addy EV, Verghese C, Brain AI. The intubating laryngeal mask airway: an initial assessment of performance. *Br J Anaesth.* 1997;79:710.
23. Agro F, Brimacombe J, Carassiti M, et al. The intubating laryngeal mask: clinical appraisal of ventilation and blind tracheal intubation in 110 patients. *Anaesthesia.* 1998;53:1084.
24. Smith I, White PF. Use of the laryngeal mask airway as an alternative to a face mask during outpatient arthroscopy. *Anesthesiology.* 1992;77:850.
25. Brain AIJ. The laryngeal mask: a new concept in airway management. *Br J Anaesth.* 1983;55:801.
26. Calder I, Ordman AJ, Jackowski A, et al. The brain laryngeal mask airway: an alternative to emergency tracheal intubation [case report]. *Anaesthesia.* 1990;45:137.
27. Riley RH, Swan HD. Value of the laryngeal mask during thoracotomy [letter]. *Anesthesiology.* 1992;77:1051.
28. Benumof JL. Laryngeal mask airway: indications and contraindications. *Anesthesiology.* 1992;77:843.
29. Benumof JL. Management of the difficult airway: with special emphasis on the awake tracheal intubation. *Anesthesiology.* 1991;75:1087.
30. Brimacombe J. The laryngeal mask airway and flexible bronchoscopy [letter]. *Thorax.* 1991;46:591.
31. Walker RWM, Murrel D. Yet another use for the laryngeal mask airway. *Anaesthesia.* 1991;46:591.
32. Tanigawa K, Inoue Y, Iwata S. Protection of recurrent laryngeal nerve during neck surgery: a new combination of neutracer, laryngeal mask

airway, and fiberoptic bronchoscope [letter]. *Anesthesiology.* 1991;74:918.

33. Grebenik CR, Ferguson C, White A. The laryngeal mask airway in pediatric radiotherapy. *Anesthesiology.* 1990;72:474.

34. Logan AS. Use of the laryngeal mask in a patient with an unstable fracture on the cervical spine [letter]. *Anesthesia.* 1991;46:987.

35. Asai T, Wagle AU, Stacey M. Placement of the intubating laryngeal mask is easier than the laryngeal mask during manual in-line neck stabilization. *Br J Anaesth.* 1999;82:712.

36. Asai T, Murao K, Tsutsumi T, et al. Ease of tracheal intubation through the intubating laryngeal mask during manual in-line head and neck stabilization. *Anaesthesia.* 2000;55:82.

37. Harry RM, Nolan JP. The use of cricoid pressure with the intubating laryngeal mask. *Anaesthesia.* 1999;54:656.

38. Fisher JS, Ananthanarayan C, Edelist G. Role of the laryngeal mask in airway management. *Can J Anaesth.* 1992;39:1.

39. Greenberg RS, Toung T. The cuffed oro-pharyngeal airway: a pilot study. *Anesthesiology.* 1992;77:A558.

40. Brimacombe JR, Brimacombe JC, Berry AM, et al. A comparison of the laryngeal mask airway and cuffed oropharyngeal airway in anesthetized adult patients. *Anesth Analg.* 1998;87:147.

41. Hsu YW, Pan MH, Huang CJ, et al. Comparison of the cuffed oropharyngeal airway and laryngeal mask airway in spontaneous breathing anesthesia. *Acta Anaesthesiol Sin.* 1998;36:187.

42. Greenberg RS, Brimacombe J, Berry A, et al. A randomized controlled trial comparing the cuffed oropharyngeal airway and the laryngeal mask airway in spontaneously breathing anesthetized adults. *Anesthesiology.* 1998;88:970.

43. Voyagis GS, Dimitriou VK, Kyriakis KP. Comparative evaluation of the prolonged use of the cuffed oropharyngeal airway and the laryngeal mask airway in spontaneously breathing anaesthetized patients. *Eur J Anaesthesiol.* 1999;16:371.

44. Casati A, Cappelleri G, Fanelli G, et al. The pressor response after laryngeal mask or cuffed oropharyngeal airway insertion. *Acta Anaesthesiol Scand.* 1999;43:1053.

45. Siker ES. A mirror laryngoscope. *Anesthesiology.* 1956;17:38.

46. Finucane BT, Santora A. Difficult intubation. In: *Principles of Airway Management.* Philadelphia, Pa: FA Davis; 1988.

47. Huffman JP, Elam JO. Prisms and fiberoptics for laryngoscopy. *Anesth Analg.* 1971;50:64.

48. Dorsch JA, Dorsch SE, eds. *Understanding Anesthesia Equipment.* Baltimore, Md: Williams & Wilkins; 1975.

49. Huffman JP. The development of optical prism instruments to view and study the human larynx. *J Am Assoc Nurse Anesth.* 1970;38:197.

50. Weeks DB. A new use for an old blade. *Anesthesiology.* 1974;40:200.

51. Kessell J. A laryngoscope for obstetrical use. *Anaesth Intensive Care.* 1977;5:265.

52. Bellhouse CP. An angulated laryngoscope for routine and difficult tracheal intubation. *Anesthesiology.* 1988;69:126.

53. Roberts JT. *Fundamentals of Tracheal Intubation.* New York, NY: Grune & Stratton; 1983.

54. Patil VU, Stehling LC, Zander HL. An adjustable laryngoscope handle for difficult intubation. *Anesthesiology.* 1984;60:609.

55. Dhara SS, Cheong TW. An adjustable multiple angle laryngoscope adaptor. *Anaesth Intensive Care.* 1991;19:243.

56. Nunn G. A new laryngoscope. *Anaesthesia.* 1987;42:877.

57. Corwin RW, Irwin RS. Bronchoscopy. In: Rippe JM, Irwin RS, Alpert JS, et al, eds. *Intensive Care Medicine.* Boston, Mass: Little, Brown & Co; 1985:73.

58. Vaughan RS. Endobronchial intubation. In: Latto IP, Rosen M, eds. *Difficulties in Tracheal Intubation.* London, United Kingdom: Bailliere Tindall; 1983:162.

59. Sanders R. Two ventilating attachments for bronchoscopes. *Del Med J.* 1968;39:170.

60. Landa JF. Indications for bronchoscopy. *Chest.* 1978;73(suppl):686.

61. Sackner MA. State of the art: bronchofiberoscopy. *Annu Rev Respir Dis.* 1975;111:62.

62. Udaya BS, Prakash MD, Stubbs SE. Bronchoscopy: indications and technique. *Semin Respir Med.* 1981;3:17.

63. Fulkerson WJ. Current concepts: fiberoptic bronchoscopy. *N Engl J Med.* 1984;311:511.

64. Dellinger DP. Fiberoptic bronchoscopy in adult airway management. *Crit Care Med.* 1990;18:882.

65. Williams RT, Maltabey JR. Airway intubator. *Anesth Analg.* 1982;61:309.

66. Hogan K, Harpier MH, Pollard BJ. Use of a pharyngeal guide to aid intubation with the fiberoptic laryngoscope. *Anaesth Intensive Care.* 1984;12:18.

67. Pereira W Jr, Kounet DM, Snider GL. A prospective cooperative study of complications following flexible fiberoptic bronchoscopy. *Chest.* 1978;73:813.

68. Suratt PM, Smiddy JF, Gruber B. Deaths and complications associated with fiberoptic bronchoscopy. *Chest.* 1976;69:747.

69. Credle WF, Smiddy JF, Elliott RC. Complications of fiberoptic bronchoscopy. *Am Rev Respir Dis.* 1974;109:67.

70. Simpson FB, Arnold AG, Purvis A, et al. Postal survey of bronchoscopic practice by physicians in the United Kingdom. *Thorax.* 1986;41:311.

71. Katsnelson T, Frost EA, Farcon E, et al. When the endotracheal tube will not pass over flexible fiberoptic bronchoscope. *Anesthesiology.* 1992;76:151.

72. Saunders PR, Geisecke AH. Clinical assessment of the adult Bullard laryngoscope. *Can Anaesth Soc J.* 1989;36:S118.

73. Bjoraker DG. The Bullard intubating laryngoscopes. *Anesthesiol Rev.* 1990;17:64.

74. Gorback MS. Management of the challenging airway with the Bullard laryngoscope. *J Clin Anaesth.* 1991;3:473.

75. Borland LM, Caselbrant M. The Bullard laryngoscope: a new indirect oral laryngoscope (pediatric version). *Anesth Analg.* 1990;70:105.

76. Dyson A, Harris J, Bhatia K. Rapidity and accuracy of tracheal intubation in a mannequin: comparison of the fiberoptic with the Bullard laryngoscope. *Br J Anaesth.* 1990;65:268.

77. Frass M, Kofler J, Thalhammer F, et al. Clinical evaluation of a new endotracheal tube. *Anesthesiology.* 1997;87:1262.

78. Shikani AH. New "seeing" stylet-scope and method for the management of the difficult airway. *Otolaryngol Head Neck Surg.* 1999;120:113.

79. Gravenstein D, Melker RJ, Lampotang S. Clinical assessment of a plastic optical fiber stylet for human tracheal intubation. *Anesthesiology.* 1999;91:648.

80. Wiess M. Management of difficult tracheal intubation with a video-optically modified Schroeder intubation stylet. *Anesth Analg.* 1997;85:1181.

81. Weiss M. Video-intuboscopy: a new aid to routine and difficult tracheal intubation. *Br J Anaesth.* 1998;80:525.

82. Kitamura T, Yamada Y, Du HL, et al. An efficient technique for tracheal intubation using the StyletScope alone. *Anesthesiology.* 2000;92:1210.

83. Kitamura T, Yamada Y, Du HL, et al. Efficiency of a new fiberoptic stylet scope in tracheal intubation. *Anesthesiology.* 1999;91:1628.

84. Vlessides M. Video intubation in the 21st century. *Anesthesiol News Special Rep.* 1999;25:97.

85. Caldwell SL, Sullivan KN. Artificial airways. In: Burton GG, Hodgin JF, eds. *Respiratory Care. A Guide to Clinical Practice.* Philadelphia, Pa: JB Lippincott; 1984:493.

86. Sosis MB. What is the safest endotracheal tube for Nd-YAG laser surgery? A comparative study. *Anesth Analg.* 1989;69:802.

87. Bolder PM, Healey TEJ, Bolder AR. The extra work of breathing through adult endotracheal tubes. *Anesth Analg.* 1986;65:853.

88. Conrardy PA, Goodman LR, Lainge F, et al. Alteration of endotracheal tube position: flexion and extension of the neck. *Crit Care Med.* 1976;4:8.

89. Florete OG Jr: Airway management. In: Civetta JM, Taylor RW, Kirby RR, eds. *Critical Care.* Philadelphia, Pa: JB Lippincott; 1992:1419.

90. Williams LA, Banner MJ, Melker RJ. Tracheal shapes: implications for endotracheal tube cuff design. *Anesthesiology.* 1995;83:A262.

91. Fontes ML, Setaro J, Matthew JP, et al. *Anesthesiology.* 1997;87:A208.

92. Schmalfuss IM, Mancuso AA, Melker RJ, et al. Magnetic resonance imaging (MRI) of the upper trachea during quiet respiration and Valsalva maneuver. In: ASNR and ASHNR Annual Meeting Syllabus. Atlanta, Ga: April 3–8, 2000. Page 170.

93. Griscom NT, Wohl ME, Fenton T. Dimensions of the trachea to age 6 years related to height. *Pediatr Pulmonol.* 1989;6:186.

94. Griscom NT, Wohl ME. Dimensions of the growing trachea related to body height: length, anteroposterior and transverse diameters, cross-sectional area, and volume in subjects younger than 20 years of age. *Am Rev Respir Dis.* 1985;131:840.

95. Cooper JD, Grillo HC. Analysis of problems related to cuffs on endotracheal tubes. *Chest.* 1972;62:24S.

96. Cooper JD, Grillo HC. The evolution of tracheal injury due to ventilatory assistance through cuffed tubes: a pathologic study. *Ann Surg.* 1969;169:334.

97. Cooper JD, Grillo HC. Experimental production and prevention of injury due to cuffed tracheal tubes. *Surg Gynecol Obstet.* 1969;129:1235.

98. Grillo HC, Cooper JD, Geffin B, et al. A low pressure cuff for tracheostomy tubes to minimize tracheal injury. *J Thorac Cardiovasc Surg.* 1971;62:898.

99. Ching NP, Nealon TB Jr. Clinical experience with new low-pressure, high-volume tracheostomy cuffs: importance of limiting intracuff pressure. *N Y State J Med.* 1974;74:2379.

100. Dobrin P, Canfield T. Cuffed endotracheal tubes: mucosal pressure and tracheal wall blood flow. *Am J Surg.* 1977;133:562.

101. Leigh JM, Maynard JP. Pressure on the tracheal mucosa from cuffed tubes. *BMJ.* 1979;1:1173.

102. Nordin U. The trachea and cuff-induced tracheal injury. *Acta Otolaryngol Suppl (Stockh).* 1977;345:1.

103. Bjorkund S, Ekedahl C, Hansson PG, et al. Experimental tracheal wall injury. *Acta Otolaryngol (Stockh).* 1973;75:387.

104. Dobrin P, Canfield T. Cuff endotracheal tubes: mucosal pressures and tracheal wall blood flow. *Am J Surg.* 1972;133:562.

105. Nordin U, Lindholm CE, Wolfgast M. Blood flow in the rabbit tracheal mucosa under normal conditions and under the influence of tracheal intubation. *Acta Anaesthesiol Scand.* 1977;21:8.

106. Klainer AS, Turndorf H, Wen-Hsien WV, et al. Surface alterations due to endotracheal intubation. *Am J Med.* 1975;58:674.

107. Dunn CR, Dunn DL, Moser KM. Determinants of tracheal injury by cuffed tracheostomy tubes. *Chest.* 1974;65:128.

108. Guyton DC. Endotracheal and tracheotomy tube cuff design: influence on tracheal damage. *Crit Care Updates.* 1990;1:1.

109. Stanley TH, Kawamura R, Graves C. Effects of nitrous oxide on volume and pressure of endotracheal tube cuffs. *Anesthesiology.* 1974;41:256.

110. Stanley TH. Effects of anesthetic gases on endotracheal tube cuff gas volumes. *Anesth Analg.* 1974;53:480.

111. Stanley TH. Nitrous oxide and pressures and volumes of high and low pressure endotracheal tube cuffs in intubated patients. *Anesthesiology.* 1975;42:637.

112. Stanley TH, Liu WS. Tracheostomy and endotracheal tube cuff volume and pressure changes during thoracic operations. *Ann Thorac Surg.* 1975;20:144.

113. Ravenas B, Lindholm CE. Pressure and volume changes in tracheal tube cuffs during anesthesia. *Acta Anaesthesiol Scand.* 1976;20:321.

114. Jacobsen L, Greenbaum R. A study of intracuff pressure measurements, trends and behaviour in patients during prolonged periods of tracheal intubation. *Br J Anaesth.* 1981;53:97.

115. Mackenzie CF, Klose S, Browne DRG. A study of inflatable cuffs on endotracheal tubes. *Br J Anaesth.* 1976;48:105.

116. Benumof JL. *Anesthesia for Thoracic Surgery.* Philadelphia, Pa: WB Saunders; 1987.

117. Vaughan RS. Endobronchial intubation. In: Latto IP, Rosen M, eds. *Difficulties in Tracheal Intubation.* London, United Kingdom: Bailliere Tindall; 1983:156.

118. Newman RW, Finer GE, Downs JE. Routine use of the Carlens double-lumen endobronchial catheter: an experimental and clinical study. *J Thorac Cardiovasc Surg.* 1961;42:326.

119. White G. A new double lumen tube. *Br J Anaesth.* 1960;32:232.

120. Robertshaw F. Low resistance, double-lumen endobronchial tubes. *Br J Anaesth.* 1962;34:576.

121. Clapham MC, Vaughan RS. Bronchial intubation: a comparison between polyvinyl chloride and red rubber double lumen tubes. *Anaesthesia.* 1985;40:1111.

122. Zeitlin GL, Short DH, Ryder GH. An assessment of the Robertshaw double-lumen tube. *Br J Anaesth.* 1965;57:858.

123. Benumof JL, Partridge BL, Salvatierra C, et al. Margin of safety in positioning double-lumen endotracheal tubes. *Anesthesiology.* 1987;67:729.

124. Black AMS, Harrison GA. Difficulties with positioning Robertshaw double lumen tubes. *Anaesth Intensive Care.* 1975;3:299.

125. Saito S, Dohi S, Naito H. Alteration of double-lumen endobronchial tube position by flexion and extension of the neck. *Anesthesiology.* 1985;62:696.

126. Benumof JL. Anesthesia for thoracic surgery. In: *1988 Review Course Lectures.* International Anesthesia Research Society. Baltimore, Md: Williams & Wilkins; 1988:120.

127. Read NC, Friday CD, Eason CN. Prospective study of the Robertshaw endobronchial catheter in thoracic surgery. *Ann Thorac Surg.* 1977;24:156.

128. Smith GB, Hirsch NP, Ehrenwerth J. Sight and sound: can double-lumen endotracheal tubes be placed accurately without fiberoptic bronchoscopy? *Anesth Analg.* 1986;65:S1.

129. Ovassapian A, Braunschweig R, Joshi CW. Endobronchial intubation using a flexible fiberoptic bronchoscope. *Anesthesiology.* 1983;59:501.

130. Shinnick JP, Freedman AP. Bronchofiberscopic placement of a double-lumen endotracheal tube. *Crit Care Med.* 1982;10:544.

131. Burk WJ. Should a fiberoptic bronchoscope be routinely used to position a double-lumen tube? *Anesthesiology.* 1988;68:826.

132. Grum D, Porembka D. Misconceptions regarding double tubes and bronchoscopy. *Anesthesiology.* 1988;68:826.

133. Wilson RS. Endobronchial intubation. In: Kaplan JA, ed. *Thoracic Anesthesia.* New York, NY: Churchill Livingstone; 1983:389.

134. Brodsky JB, Shulman MS, Mark JB. Malposition of left-sided double lumen endobronchial tubes. *Anesthesiology.* 1985;62:667.

135. Wagner DL, Gammage GW, Wong ML. Tracheal rupture following the insertion of a disposable double lumen endotracheal tube. *Anesthesiology.* 1985;63:698.

136. Heiser M, Steinberg JJ, MacVaugh H III, et al. Bronchial rupture, a complication of use of the Robertshaw double-lumen tube. *Anesthesiology.* 1979;51:88.

137. Foster JNG, Lau OJ, Alimo EB. Ruptured bronchus following endobronchial intubation. *Br J Anaesth.* 1983;55:687.

138. Hood RM, Sloan HE. Injuries of the trachea and major bronchi. *J Thorac Cardiovasc Surg.* 1959;18:458.

139. Tornvall SS, Jackson KH, Oyanedel ET. Tracheal rupture: complication of cuffed endotracheal tube. *Chest.* 1971;69:237.

140. Blanc FV, Trembal NAG. Complications of tracheal intubation: a new classification and a review of the literature. *Anesth Analg.* 1976;53:202.

141. Thompson DS, Reed RC. Rupture of the trachea following endotracheal intubation. *JAMA.* 1968;204:995.

142. Wells DG, Zelcer J, Podolakin W, et al. Cardiac arrest from pulmonary outflow tract obstruction due to a double lumen tube. *Anesthesiology.* 1987;66:422.

143. Dryden GE. Circulatory collapse after pneumonectomy (an unusual complication from the use of a Carlens catheter): a case report. *Anesth Analg.* 1977;56:451.

144. Bearman AJ. Device for nasotracheal intubation. *Anesthesiology.* 1962;23:130.

145. Munson ES, Cullen SC. Endotracheal intubation in a patient with ankylosing spondylitis of the cervical spine. *Anesthesiology.* 1965;26:365.

146. Cass NM, James NR, Lines V. Difficult direct laryngoscopy complicating intubation for anaesthesia. *BMJ.* 1956;ii:488.

147. Bowen RA. An introducer for difficult intubation. *Anaesthesia.* 1967;22:150.

148. Brechner VL. Unusual problems in the management of airways: flexion extension mobility of the cervical vertebrae. *Anesth Analg Curr Res.* 1968;47:362.

149. Ducrow M. Throwing light on blind intubation. *Anaesthesia.* 1978;33:827.

150. Elis DG, Jackymec A, Kaplan RE, et al. Guided orotracheal intubation in the operating room using a lighted stylet: a comparison with direct laryngoscopic technique. *Anesthesiology.* 1986;64:823.

151. Weis FR, Hatton MN. Intubation by the use of the light wand: experience in 253 patients. *J Oral Maxillofac Surg.* 1989;47:577.

152. Rayburn RL. Light wand intubation [letter]. *Anaesthesia.* 1979;34:677.

153. Holzman RS, Nargozian CD, Florence B. Lightwand intubation in children with abnormal airways. *Anesthesiology.* 1988;69:784.

154. Fox DJ, Matson MD. Management of the difficult pediatric airway in an austere environment using the lightwand. *J Clin Anesth.* 1990;2:123.

155. Rao TLK, Mathru M, Gorski DW, et al. Experience with a new intubation guide for difficult tracheal intubation. *Crit Care Med.* 1982;10:882.

156. Rosenberg MB. Use of the LTA kit as a guide for endotracheal intubation. *Anesth Analg.* 1977;56:287.

157. Samsoon GLT, Young JRB. Difficult tracheal intubation: a retrospective study. *Anaesthesia.* 1987;42:487.

158. Lyons G. Failed intubation. *Anaesthesia.* 1985;40:759.

159. Cormack RS, Lehane J. Difficult tracheal intubation in obstetrics. *Anaesthesia.* 1984;39:1105.

160. Glassenburg R, Vaisrub N, Albright G. The incidence of failed intubation in obstetrics: is there an irreducible minimum? [abstract]. *Anesthesiology.* 1990;73:A1061.

161. Tunstall ME. Failed intubation in the parturient [editorial]. *Can J Anaesth.* 1989;36:611.

162. Keenan RL, Boyan CP. Cardiac arrest due to anesthesia. *JAMA.* 1985;253:2373.

163. Holland R. Anesthesia-related mortality in Australia. *Int Anesthesiol Clin.* 1984;22:61.

164. Tiret L, Desmonts JM, Hatton F, et al. Complications associated with anaesthesia: a prospective survey in France. *Can Anaesth Soc J.* 1986;33:336.

165. Benumof JL, Scheller MS. The importance of transtracheal jet ventilation in the management of the difficult airway. *Anesthesiology.* 1989;71:769.

166. Griggs WM, Worthley LIG, Gillegan GE, et al. A simple percutaneous tracheostomy technique. *Surg Gynecol Obstet.* 1990;170:543.

167. Toye FJ, Weinstein JD. Clinical experience with percutaneous tracheostomy and cricothyroidotomy in 100 patients. *J Trauma.* 1988;26:1034.

168. Wain JC, Wilson DJ, Mathisen DJ. Clinical experience with mini-tracheostomy. *Ann Thorac Surg.* 1990;49:881.

169. Walls RM. Cricothyroidotomy. *Emerg Med Clin North Am.* 1988;6:725.

170. Mace SE. Cricothyrotomy. *J Emerg Med.* 1988;6:309.

171. Roven AN, Clapham MC. Cricothyroidotomy. *Ear Nose Throat J.* 1983;62:68.

172. Corke C, Cranswick P. A Seldinger technique for mini-tracheostomy insertion. *Anaesth Intensive Care.* 1988;16:206.

173. Melker RJ, Banner MJ. Work imposed by breathing through cricothyrotomy tube. Paper presented at: 6th World Congress on Emergency and Disaster Medicine; September 6–18, 1989; Hong Kong.

174. Boyd AD, Romita MC, Conlan AA, et al. A clinical evaluation of cricothyrotomy. *Surg Gynecol Obstet.* 1979;149:365.

175. Essess BA, Jafek BW. Cricothyroidotomy: a decade of experience in Denver. *Ann Otol Rhinol Laryngol.* 1987;96:519.

176. O'Connor JV, Reddy K, Ergin MA, et al. Cricothyroidotomy for prolonged ventilatory support after cardiac operations. *Ann Thorac Surg.* 1988;39:353.

177. Sise MJ, Shaelford SR, Cruickshank JC, et al. Cricothyroidotomy for long term tracheal access. *Ann Surg.* 1984;200:13.

178. Kress TD, Balasbramanian S. Cricothyroidotomy. *Ann Emerg Med.* 1982;11:197.

179. Waters DJ. Guided blind endotracheal intubation. *Anaesthesia.* 1963;18:158.

180. Powell WF, Ozdil T. A translaryngeal guide for tracheal intubation. *Anesth Analg.* 1967;46:231.

181. Bourke D, Levesque PR. Modification of retrograde guide for endotracheal intubation. *Anesth Analg.* 1974;53:1013.

182. Harmaer M, Vaughan RS. Guided blind oral intubation. *Anaesthesia.* 1980;35:921.

183. Robert KW. New use for Swan-Ganz introducer wire. *Anesth Analg.* 1981;60:67.

184. Borland LM, Swan DM, Leff S. Difficult pediatric intubation: a new approach to the retrograde technique. *Anesthesiology.* 1981;55:577.

185. Piotrowskii JJ, Moore EE. Emergency department tracheostomy. *Emerg Med Clin North Am.* 1988;6:737.

186. Heffner JE, Miller KS, Sahn SA. Tracheostomy in the intensive care unit, part I: indications, technique, and management. *Chest.* 1986;90:269.

187. Heffner JE, Sahn SA. The technique of tracheostomy and cricothyroidotomy. *J Crit Care Illness.* 1987;2:79.

188. Meade JW. Tracheotomy: its complications and their management. *N Engl J Med.* 1961;264:587.

189. Heffner JE, Miller KS, Sahn SA. Tracheostomy in the ICU, part 2: complications. *Chest.* 1986;90:430.

190. Selecky PA. Tracheostomy: a review of present-day indications, complications, and care. *Heart Lung.* 1974;3:272.

191. Cross AS, Roup B. Role of respiratory assistance devices on endemic nosocomial pneumonia. *Am J Med.* 1981;70:681.

192. Thomas AN. The diagnosis and treatment of tracheoesophageal fistula caused by cuffed tracheal tubes. *J Thorac Cardiovasc Surg.* 1973;65:612.

CHAPTER

17

# Cardiopulmonary Bypass

## Luis G. Michelsen

DISCONTINUATION OF CARDIOPULMONARY BYPASS

*Is Cardiopulmonary Bypass Just Stopped Abruptly at the End of the Procedure?*

*When and How Can Cardiopulmonary Bypass Be Discontinued?*

Initial attempts at performing cardiac surgery without any support were severely limited by the problems of hemorrhage, air entrainment, and poor exposure. The use of cross circulation by Lillehei in 1954,[1] although successful in some cases, meant that the operation was risky not only to the patient but also to the person who served as circulatory support. A major factor in the advancement of cardiac surgery was the development of cardiopulmonary bypass (CPB) by Gibbon and colleagues.[2] Through the use of plastic tubing, a reservoir, a pump, and an oxygenator, the blood could be routed away from the heart and lungs, giving the surgeon the time and the ability to see inside the heart. Although the underlying principles and mechanics of CPB are essentially unchanged, significant developments have been achieved in the materials used. In addition, there is now a greater understanding of the complex cellular changes produced when all of the blood volume comes in contact with artificial tubing and filters. This chapter focuses on the practical aspects and implications of CPB.

## CARDIOPULMONARY BYPASS: CONCEPT AND INDICATIONS

The basic concept is to divert the circulation from the heart and lungs into a machine that performs the main functions of those organs. Blood is drained from the right venous system, typically the right atrium or venae cavae, and returned to the aorta. Plastic tubing is used to drain venous blood into a reservoir. Drainage occurs by gravity; this explains why the CPB machine is placed at a lower height than the patient. The reservoir allows mixing of the blood, removal of bubbles, and addition of fluids or drugs. The temperature of the blood can also be increased or decreased through a heat exchanger located next to the venous reservoir. Oxygenation of the blood is accomplished through an oxygenator. The oxygenator also allows the removal of carbon dioxide ($CO_2$) and the exchange of vaporized anesthetic gases. The blood is then returned under pressure (pumped) through plastic tubing back to the patient.

### What Are the Main Forms of Bypass and How Are They Used?

Total or "full" CPB requires complete isolation of the venous return by cannulating each vena cava separately and placing tourniquets around them. This complete isolation is useful when the chambers of the heart are opened during the operation because otherwise air could enter into the circuit. Just as important, blood in the field would make it difficult for the surgeon to see inside the heart. Cardiac valve surgery and repair of intracardiac defects are usually done with total CPB.

Partial CPB occurs when some of the blood flows through the heart and lungs and another portion flows through the machine. This situation is present at the initiation of total CPB and during its discontinuation. For many cardiac surgeries, a single cannula that drains the right atrium and inferior vena cava (IVC) is used. Although, technically, some of the blood may be able to go into the right ventricle, the surgery can be done without problem, provided that the venous drainage is adequate and that the right chambers are not opened surgically. Coronary artery and aortic surgery are usually done in this way.

Blood can be diverted from the left atrium to the aorta, bypassing only the left ventricle. Because the blood in the left atrium has already gone through the lungs, oxygenation is not necessary. This form of bypass is known as *left-heart bypass* and is used mainly to support the circulation during thoracic aortic surgery. Diversion of the blood from the right atrium to the pulmonary artery (PA) (*right-heart bypass*) is used much less commonly, mainly in some pediatric cardiac surgeries.

During liver transplantation surgery, marked hemodynamic changes occur during occlusion and reopening of the IVC and portal vein.[3] Venovenous bypass can be used in this situation, routing blood from the IVC and portal vein to a tributary of the superior vena cava (SVC) such as the axillary or subclavian vein.[4]

### Is Bypass Used Only for Surgery on the Heart?

CPB or one of its forms of circulatory support can also be used in several other situations (Table 17–1):

1. Surgery on major vessels such as the aorta and venae cavae
2. Surgeries in which oxygenation by the lungs is compromised (bilateral lung transplantation and some tracheobronchial surgeries)
3. Surgeries in which the circulation needs to be stopped (resection of giant intracranial aneurysms, removal of major arteriovenous malformations)
4. When circulatory support is needed (venovenous bypass for liver transplantation, circulatory support during high-risk angioplasty)

**TABLE 17–1.** Indications for Cardiopulmonary Bypass

| |
|---|
| **Cardiac Surgery** |
|     Coronary arteries |
|     Cardiac valves |
|     Repair of cardiac defects |
|     Aortic surgery |
| **Pulmonary Surgery** |
|     Lung transplantation |
|     Complete tracheobronchial interruption |
| **Neurosurgery** |
|     Giant intracranial aneurysms |
|     Large arteriovenous malformations |
| **Other Surgeries** |
|     Inferior vena cava surgery |
|     Liver transplantation |
|     Large mediastinal masses |
|     Trauma |
| **Other Procedures** |
|     High-risk angioplasty |
|     Treatment of hypothermia |

## COMPONENTS AND MECHANICS OF CARDIOPULMONARY BYPASS

### *What Are the Different Parts of Cardiopulmonary Bypass and How Do They Work?*

#### Venous Cannulas

The CPB circuit starts with the venous cannulas. These are large plastic tubes that, as previously noted, are placed through incisions into the right atrium or venae cavae. The cannulas are designed to facilitate blood return and usually have multiple orifices near the tip. Their wall may have a wire reinforcement to prevent kinking. Venous cannulas that have a single set of orifices near the tip are known as *single stage cannulas.* Dual stage cannulas have a first set of orifices near the tip (first stage) that drain the blood from the IVC. A second set of orifices (second stage) is located several centimeters from the tip, and the diameter of the cannula increases at this point (Fig. 17–1). The second stage drains the blood pooled in the right atrium from drainage of the SVC and the coronary sinus. A dual stage cannula is placed through the right atrium, but its tip is directed into the IVC.

#### Venous Tubing

The venous cannulas are connected to transparent plastic tubing that drains the blood to the CPB machine. The venous tubing has a large diameter to facilitate flow. Its walls do not have to be thick because this is a low pressure system. The venous blood that is drained to the machine is known as the *venous return.* The venous return depends mainly on gravity, the patient's intravascular volume, and the position of and resistance from the venous cannula and tubing.

Important points to remember about venous tubing include the following:

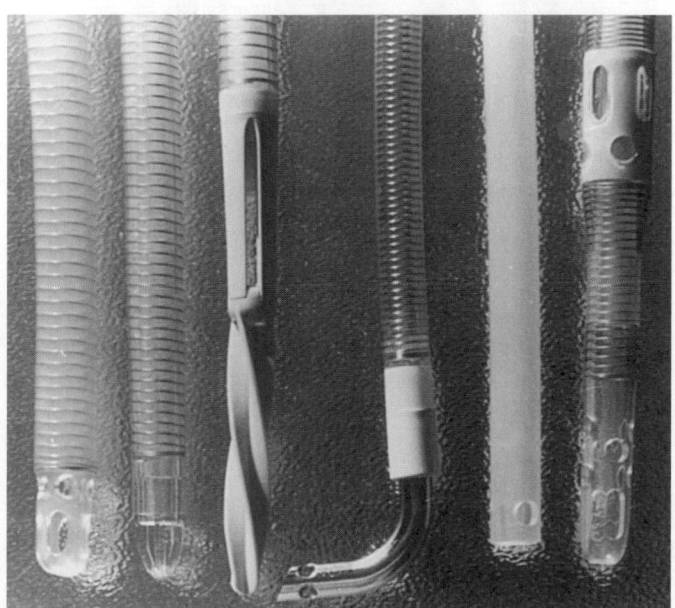

**FIGURE 17–1.** Different venous cannulas. *Far right* is a dual-stage cannula, whereas the others are single stage. Note that most have a wire reinforcement in the wall to prevent kinking.

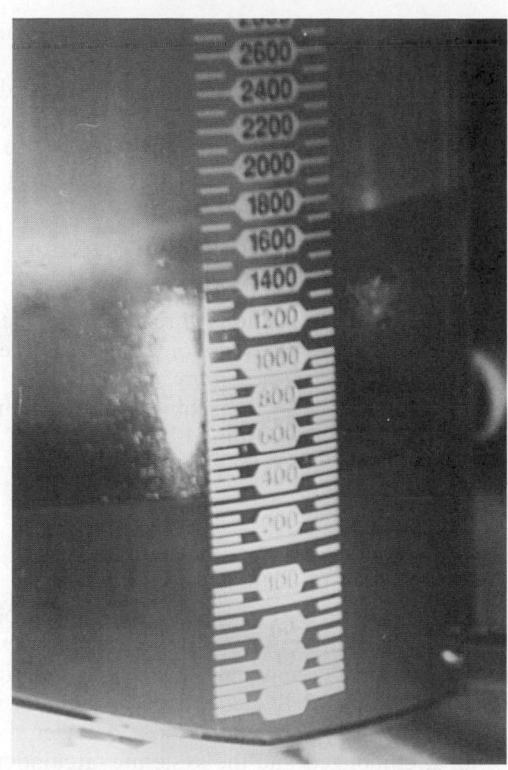

**FIGURE 17–2.** Venous reservoir and volume scale. Note the cone shape at the bottom of the reservoir and the change in the scale at that level to indicate smaller volumes better.

- Because of the thin wall, the venous tubing can be kinked easily. If there is a decrease in the venous return to the pump, check that the tubing is not kinked.
- The height of the operating table can affect the venous drainage into the pump. If venous return needs to be increased, ask the surgeon if the operating table can be elevated.
- When significant amounts of air are entrained, a large bubble may obstruct the gravity drainage of the venous tubing. This is known as an *air lock.* If this happens, be prepared to assist the perfusionist by manipulating the venous tubing so that the air pocket advances and drains into the venous reservoir.

#### Venous Reservoir

The venous blood is collected in a plastic transparent container known as the *venous reservoir.* The venous reservoir serves as a mixing chamber where additional fluids and drugs can be added as well as a place for removal of air bubbles and for mixing drainage from other reservoirs. It also gives the perfusionist an idea of the volume available to be returned to the patient at any given time. The reservoir has a scale in milliliters and is cone shaped at its bottom to give the perfusionist a better appreciation of when it is becoming empty (Fig. 17–2). A low volume in this reservoir should alert the perfusionist that it will soon be empty and that air can accidentally be pumped into the arterial circulation.

Important points to remember follow:

- Because of the shape of the venous reservoir, there may appear to be an acceptable volume even though it is almost empty. Make sure to look at the scale to determine the volume available.

- Some pumps are equipped with optical sensors to detect a low volume in the venous reservoir as well as air detectors that interrupt the pump if air enters the arterial line. However, the best monitor overall is an alert perfusionist. Avoid unnecessarily distracting the perfusionist.

### Cardiotomy Reservoir

Blood that the surgeon suctions directly from the heart, pericardium, and pleural spaces is sometimes returned to a separate container called a *cardiotomy reservoir*. The advantage of a separate cardiotomy reservoir is additional filtering and defoaming of the suctioned blood.

### Oxygenator

There are two basic types of oxygenators available: bubble and membrane oxygenators. In bubble oxygenators, a thin column of blood is directly exposed to multiple bubbles of oxygen. Small bubbles are efficient for oxygenation, whereas larger ones improve $CO_2$ removal. The fraction of inspired oxygen ($FIO_2$) in the gas delivered to the oxygenator is kept close to 1.0 because oxygen bubbles pose a lower risk than bubbles of air if embolized into the systemic circulation. This type of system is relatively simple and inexpensive but has several disadvantages. The bubbles have to be removed from the blood in a defoaming chamber, where the foam floats to the top and the blood is removed from the bottom. Incomplete removal of the bubbles results in gas embolism. Because the $FIO_2$ is kept fixed, both oxygenation and removal of $CO_2$ depend on gas flow and cannot be controlled independently.[5] The direct contact of the bubbles with blood results in hemolysis and denaturing of plasma proteins.[6] This problem, as well as gaseous embolism, intensifies with longer durations of CPB and limits the length of time that a bubble oxygenator can be used safely.

In membrane oxygenators, an artificial membrane is interposed between blood and gas. Polypropylene is the most common material used for this purpose, although silicone membranes are also available. Oxygenation and $CO_2$ removal can be controlled independently in a membrane oxygenator; altering the $FIO_2$ controls oxygenation, and $CO_2$ removal is affected by the gas flow rate (also called *sweep rate*).[5] Membrane oxygenators have a much higher resistance to blood flow because the blood has to go through multiple small channels. For this reason, membrane oxygenators are usually placed after the pump.

### Heat Exchanger

The heat exchanger can be in different places but is often located in the venous reservoir/oxygenator assembly. A heat exchanger is necessary because the blood circulating outside the body is exposed to the room air temperature and cools. The heat exchanger allows the blood to be cooled down further, if desired, or to be rewarmed. The exchanger typically consists of tubes or coils through which water of the desired temperature circulates. The blood outside the coils is cooled or warmed depending on the water temperature. Heat exchangers are efficient, particularly for cooling. Rewarming is a slower process because the temperature difference between

the water bath and the blood is kept low. Excessive gradients ($>8°$-$10°C$) between the water bath and the blood should be avoided because they can result in formation of gas bubbles in the blood as well as denaturing of proteins. For the same reason, the bath temperature should not go higher than $42°C$.

### Pump

The most common type of pump used is the positive displacement or roller pump. In this type of pump, the plastic tubing containing the blood is compressed between a roller and the curved walls that surround the roller (Fig. 17–3). The flow depends on the internal diameter of the tubing, the amount of compression, and the number of revolutions of the roller. The degree of compression can be manually adjusted during the setup of the pump and is important because excessive compression results in injury to the blood cells and damage to the tubing, whereas inadequate compression leads to inefficient pumping.

Typically, the roller pump located at the left of the CPB machine is the main roller pump, and it returns the blood under pressure to the body. Additional roller pumps are used for suction and delivery of cardioplegia (Fig. 17–4). The amount of blood being pumped by the main roller is displayed at the pump console in liters per minute and is equivalent to the cardiac output; it indicates how much blood is circulating in the body. Roller pumps are able to pump against a great resistance, and an abrupt kinking of the arterial line can result in excessive pressure and disruption of the circuit. The pressure at which blood is being pumped is therefore routinely measured. This pressure is not equal to the arterial pressure of the patient because of resistance in the return circuit. The

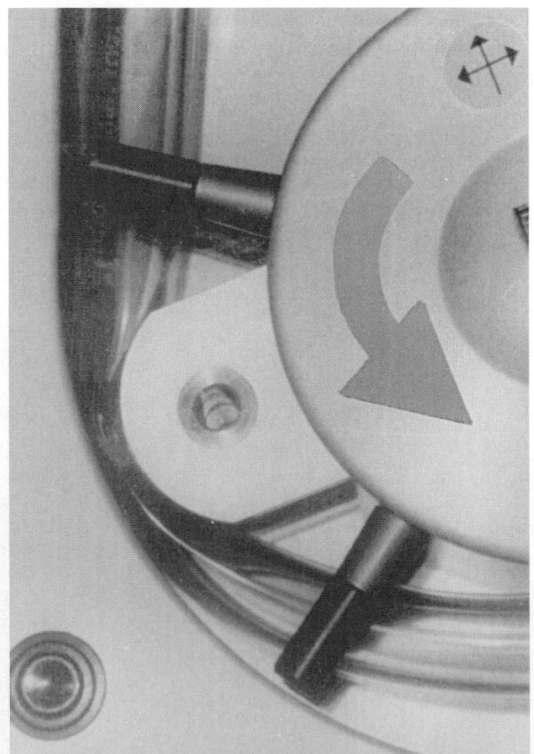

**FIGURE 17–3.** Close-up view of a positive displacement or roller pump, which turns (*arrow*) and compresses the plastic tubing, displacing the fluid inside.

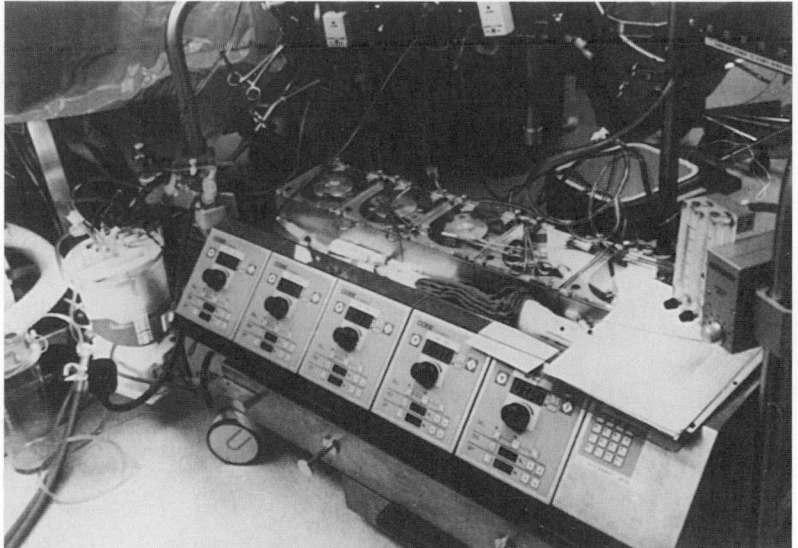

**FIGURE 17–4.** A cardiopulmonary bypass machine setup during cardiac surgery. The roller pump located at the left is the main roller pump returning blood to the patient and replacing the heart. The other roller pumps are used for suctioning and delivery of cardioplegia.

importance of this pressure is discussed later in the section, Monitoring During Cardiopulmonary Bypass.

The roller pump delivers blood at a constant rate. Some roller pumps can be set to deliver the blood in a pulsatile manner, during which they alternate rapid and slower rotation. This form of pumping increases the shear stress and is not often used.

Another type of pump is the centrifugal or vortex pump. In this pump, a cone-shaped plastic housing contains smaller cones attached to a base with a circular magnet. Rotation of the magnet makes the smaller cones rotate within the housing. Blood enters through the top of the cone and is expelled by centrifugal force through an outlet at the base (Fig. 17–5). Centrifugal pumps are affected by the pressure downstream and therefore are less likely to result in disruption of the circuit if the pressure increases abruptly because of a kink or

a clamp. However, blood flow decreases to the patient if the afterload increases. An advantage of centrifugal pumps is that they do not pump large volumes of air because this stops the functioning of the pump. However, smaller amounts of air can be accidentally pumped.[7] Centrifugal pumps are often used in left-heart bypass during thoracoabdominal aortic surgery, as well as during venovenous bypass for liver transplantation.

Remember the following:

- If the roller pump returning blood to the patient fails, one of the roller pumps used for suction may be used to replace it.
- Most roller pumps give a display of their output in liters per minute. However, older pumps may display only the number of revolutions per minute. In this case, it is necessary to know the volume displaced per revolution to obtain the total volume given per minute.

### Filters

An arterial filter is commonly used between the pump and the patient. This filter prevents the embolization of particles larger than 20 to 40 µm, depending on the filter used. Particles arise not only from the patient but also from pieces of tubing and plastic connectors. As particles become trapped in the filter, resistance to blood flow through it can markedly increase. To permit changing the filter without having to stop the circulation, a parallel circuit is located next to it (Fig. 17–6).

### Arterial Cannula

The arterial cannula returns the oxygenated blood to the patient. For CPB, the most common site of cannulation is the ascending aorta. However, because the arterial tree does not have valves, cannulation is possible in other arterial vessels, such as the femoral artery. In such a case, the blood flows in a reverse or retrograde fashion all the way to the ascending aorta.

To avoid creating a large orifice at the site of aortic cannulation, arterial cannulas usually are narrower at their tip. The disadvantage to this is increased resistance to flow and a

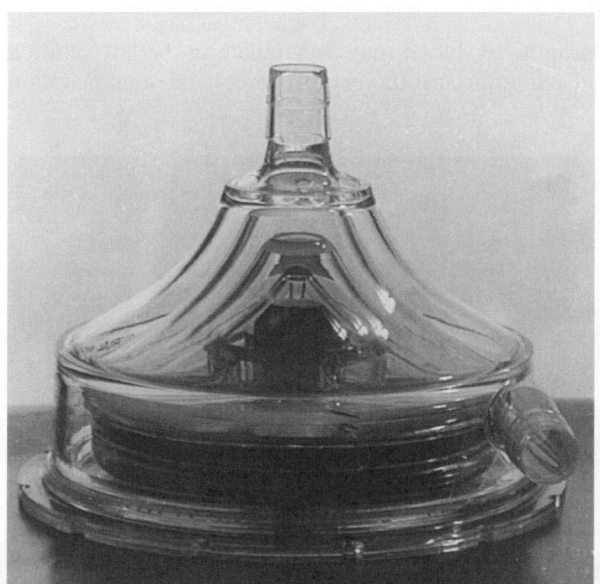

**FIGURE 17–5.** A centrifugal pump housing with its inner cones. Rotation of the magnet in the base moves the inner cones and creates a vortex, which takes blood from the top of the cone and expels it through the outlet port at the base.

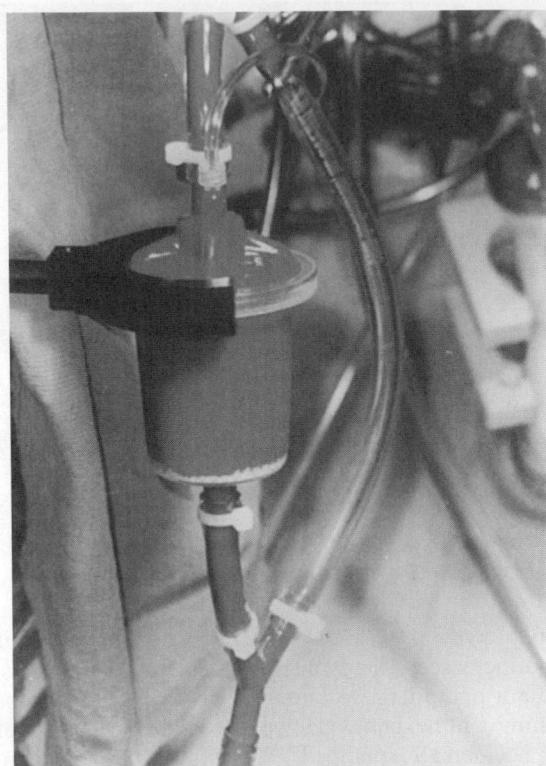

**FIGURE 17–6.** Arterial filter. Note the circuit (with a clamp) parallel to the filter. This permits the filter to be bypassed if it becomes obstructed.

pressure gradient across this narrowing. For a given patient, the surgeon tries to select the arterial cannula that will give the best balance between tip size and resistance to flow. Figure 17–7 illustrates some of the arterial cannulas available.

Significant complications can arise from cannulation of the aorta. Aortic tears and bleeding can occur during both placement and removal of the cannula. Atheromas present in the wall at the site of cannulation or directly in the path of the returning jet of blood can result in distal arterial embolism and organ damage such as stroke.[8] Although the surgeon occasionally may be able to feel an atheroma by palpating the wall, epiaortic echocardiography is much more reliable at identifying such a problem and should be used whenever there is any suspicion or likelihood that the patient may have atheromatous disease of the ascending aorta. Air bubbles need to be completely removed, and the arterial cannula and tubing should be checked before infusing any volume through the cannula into the patient. Failure to do so results in arterial embolism with potential end-organ damage.

A much-feared complication is acute dissection of the aorta because it carries a high mortality rate. Aortic dissection can occur during cannulation or any point thereafter. A bluish discoloration of the aortic wall may be noted on the surgical field, although it may not be visible if it affects the posterior portion or if scarring from previous surgery covers the aortic wall.[9] Most often, the perfusionist notes that the pressure in the arterial line is high because of increased resistance to flow across the arterial cannula and that venous return diminishes while the systemic blood pressure (BP) decreases.[10] Transesophageal or epiaortic echocardiography can help establish the diagnosis.[11] The treatment consists of cannulation of the true arterial lumen, inducing profound hypothermia and repairing or replacing the ascending aorta.

Several points to remember about arterial cannulas follow:

- At the time of placement or removal of the arterial cannula, it is desirable to decrease the BP so that there is less tension on the aortic wall. The systolic BP is decreased to a target range of 90 to 100 mm Hg, although the number selected should take into consideration the patient's coexisting diseases.
- Significant bleeding can occur at the time of placement or removal of the arterial cannula. Be prepared to infuse volume rapidly at such times. Once the cannula is in place and secured, fluid from the pump can be infused through it.
- When the arterial cannula has been placed and connected to the plastic tubing, test it by infusing a small amount of volume (50 mL) through it. If correctly placed, there should not be excessive resistance or increased line pressure, and no changes should be observed in the aortic wall.
- The jet of blood flow delivered to the aorta through the cannula can be directed to a single arterial branch such as the innominate artery. This results in excessive blood flow to this area and insufficient flow to others. Such a problem should be suspected if edema, rhinorrhea, or marked blanching of one side of the face occurs.[12–14]

## Cardioplegia Circuit

The basic function of the cardioplegia is to prevent the heart from beating while the surgeon operates on it. Cardioplegia also delivers oxygen and removes products of metabolism. A separate circuit is used to administer the cardioplegia. This inflow consists of the cardioplegia solution, which may be mixed and diluted with oxygenated blood from the pump. Cooling is achieved by passing the solution through a coil immersed in cold water or ice. The solution is then infused to the patient while pressure and flow are monitored. The implications of cardioplegia and myocardial protection are discussed later in the section, Myocardial Protection and Cardioplegia.

## Vent

During CPB, blood may accumulate in the left ventricle as a result of aortic insufficiency, cardioplegia administration, or

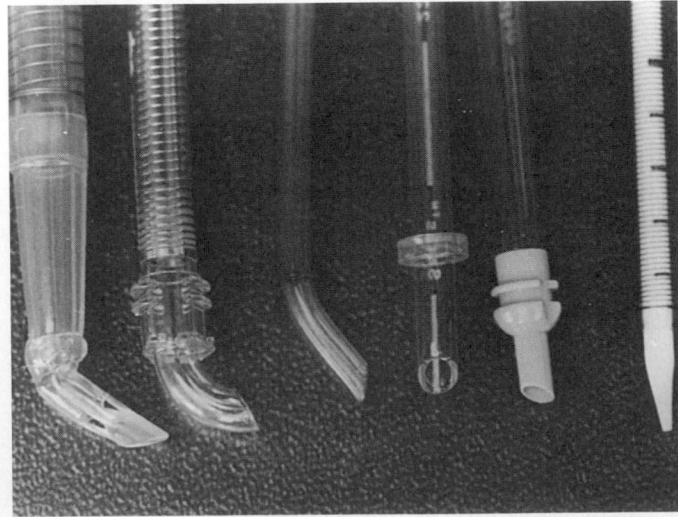

**FIGURE 17–7.** Different arterial cannulas. Note narrowed tips.

some blood going through the pulmonary circuit. As the blood accumulates, it distends the ventricle and, by increasing the intraventricular pressure, decreases perfusion to the myocardium. To treat this problem, a catheter or vent is placed—usually through a pulmonary vein—into the left atrium or ventricle. The blood suctioned through the vent is returned to the CPB machine. A vent can be placed in the PA, but if the mitral valve remains competent, blood may still accumulate in the left ventricle as a result of aortic insufficiency. Finally, a vent also is often placed in the aortic root to aspirate the cardioplegia administered through the coronary sinus and to remove air.

### What Is Port Access Cardiopulmonary Bypass?

With the development of minimally invasive techniques to reduce postoperative morbidity and length of stay, alternative cannulas and techniques have been developed. In a procedure evolved from laparoscopic surgical techniques, ports or small incisions are made in the chest to perform cardiac surgery. CPB is achieved using standard circuits but specialized cannulas[15] (Fig. 17–8). Arterial cannulation is done through a cannula in the femoral artery. Venous cannulation requires a long cannula placed through a femoral vein and advanced, under echocardiographic or fluoroscopic guidance, to the junction of the IVC and right atrium. Because of the length and size of the cannula, venous return may be inadequate and is often enhanced by using low-grade suction.

Occlusion of the aorta and administration of cardioplegia is done using a specialized catheter placed through the femoral artery. An inflatable balloon at its end positioned just above the coronary arteries allows occlusion of the aorta. This catheter is called the *endoaortic clamp,* and through its lumen cardioplegia can be delivered or blood can be vented. The endoaortic clamp is placed using transesophageal echocardiography or fluoroscopy. Its position needs to be monitored because migration toward the heart results in aortic insufficiency, whereas distal migration may result in obstruction of vessels of the aortic arch and cerebral hypoperfusion.[16] Cardioplegia can also be administered in the coronary sinus using a catheter

placed through an internal jugular vein. The catheter is positioned in the coronary sinus using the same imaging guidance already noted. Finally, the heart can also be vented by advancing a catheter through an internal jugular vein into the PA.

Complications related to the placement and use of each of these specialized cannulas can occur.[17] There is controversy over the advantages of port access surgery, and only a small proportion of all cardiac surgeries is done with this technique.

## ANTICOAGULATION AND REVERSAL

### Why Is Anticoagulation Necessary for Cardiopulmonary Bypass?

Anticoagulation is needed because contact of the blood with the plastic surfaces and filters in the pump would otherwise lead to diffuse coagulation and death. Anticoagulation needs to be maintained at all times while the patient is on CPB.

### What Is Given for Anticoagulation and How Much?

Heparin is the drug of choice because it acts quickly, is effective, and its action can be reversed. Doses of heparin between 300 and 400 U/kg are most commonly used. Heparin produces anticoagulation in just a few minutes and is administered intravenously before the surgeon is ready to place the cannulas for CPB.

### How Does One Know That the Patient Is Anticoagulated?

For patients undergoing CPB, coagulation is monitored in the operating room using the activated clotting time (ACT). This simple test measures in seconds the time it takes for blood to clot once it is placed in a glass tube that has an activator. The activators used most commonly are celite and

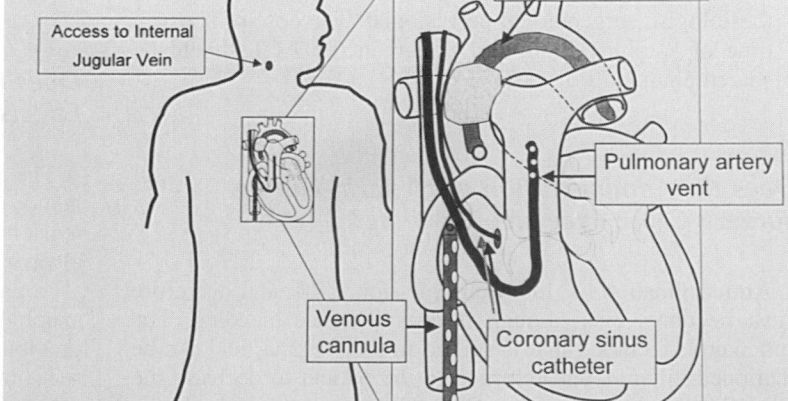

**FIGURE 17–8.** The catheters used for port-access cardiac surgery and their positions in relation to the heart.

kaolin. In this test, blood from a patient normally clots in approximately 120 seconds (range, 100-140). For CPB, the goal is to increase the ACT to >400 seconds.

The anticoagulating effect of heparin depends on the levels of circulating antithrombin III (AT III). Patients with low levels of AT III may not show as much prolongation of the ACT as expected and are labeled *heparin resistant.* This situation is seen in patients who have been on heparin infusions for several days and, if necessary, can be treated by administering AT III.

The half-life of heparin is approximately 90 minutes. Taking this into consideration as well as the ACT, heparin should be redosed if needed to maintain anticoagulation.

### Does It Matter Which Kind of Heparin Is Used to Anticoagulate the Patient?

Commercially available heparin is obtained from cow lungs (beef heparin) or pork intestines (porcine heparin). Although there may be some small variability in the response to a specific type of heparin, and some claims have been made indicating that problems such as heparin-induced thrombocytopenia are less common in patients who receive porcine heparin,[18] either type can be used for anticoagulation. The concentration for the two kinds of heparin is different and therefore dosing should always be based on the content and not on volume.

Several points should be noted about using heparin:

- Aspirate from the central line before giving the heparin to ensure that there is blood return. However, do not assume that the patient is anticoagulated because heparin was administered. It is necessary to confirm the effect by measuring the ACT because a catheter may not be where expected or the incorrect drug may be injected.
- Clot formation requires enzymatic activity, and this activity is markedly decreased with hypothermia. The ACT may not reliably indicate the effect of heparin during hypothermia because it will be prolonged even if the patient has low levels of heparin.
- The metabolism of heparin is also affected by temperature. With rewarming, heparin is metabolized faster and the ACTs should be done more often at this time.
- It is critical to maintain communication between the anesthesiologist, surgeon, and perfusionist. The dose of heparin, time of administration, and effect on the ACT should be shared among all of them.

### Does the Administration of Heparin During Surgery Cause Excessive Bleeding?

Anticoagulation is indispensable for CPB and therefore must be done, even though it does increase bleeding. The anticoagulated blood that is spilled in the surgical field can be suctioned, filtered, and returned to the patient to decrease the need for blood transfusions. Once CPB is terminated and the cannulas are removed, anticoagulation is no longer desirable and heparin is reversed.

### What Can Be Done to Decrease Bleeding During Cardiac Surgery?

Bleeding during cardiac surgery is influenced by many factors, such as the surgical technique and results, duration of bypass, platelet count, body size, fibrinolysis, and preexisting coagulopathy. Careful attention to and treatment of those factors that can be modified can be helpful. Aprotinin is a serine protease inhibitor that inhibits fibrinolysis. Prophylactic administration of aprotinin can reduce bleeding, particularly in high-risk patients.[19-22] Other antifibrinolytics such as tranexamic and aminocaproic acids have also been used. Although most studies have not found them as effective as aprotinin, their substantially lower cost makes them a viable alternative.[23] Normovolemic hemodilution with autologous intraoperative donation and postbypass retransfusion is also used to avoid exposing some of the patient's platelets to the deleterious effects of CPB.

Note the following about aprotinin:

- Aprotinin is derived from cow lung and can lead to the development of antibodies. Reexposure to aprotinin, particularly within 6 months, can lead to an anaphylactic reaction.[24] Give a small test dose before giving a load of the drug; in high-risk cases, do not give it until CPB can be rapidly initiated in case of cardiovascular collapse.
- Aprotinin can cause prolongation of the ACT when celite is used as the reagent. Kaolin ACT tubes should be used when aprotinin is administered, so that the ACT reflects more closely the effect of heparin and not that of aprotinin.[25]

### How Are the Effects of Heparin Reversed?

Protamine, a basic protein derived from salmon sperm, antagonizes the effect of heparin. Every milligram of protamine neutralizes approximately 1 mg of heparin (1 mg of heparin is equivalent to 100 U). The dose of protamine given can be based on direct measurement of circulating heparin or, more commonly, on how much heparin is estimated to still be circulating considering the initial dose, time of administration, and half-life of the drug. Once administered, the neutralizing effect of protamine occurs quickly, and the ACT can be measured after 5 minutes to determine if it has returned to normal.

### Does Protamine Have Any Important Side Effects?

The administration of protamine can result in significant hemodynamic changes. Bolus administration results in hypotension in virtually all patients, and thus protamine should always be given as a slow infusion.

In previously sensitized patients, protamine can result in an anaphylactic reaction. Patients who have received protamine previously for cardiac or vascular surgery are at increased risk. Protamine is also present in NPH insulin, and diabetic patients who have used this type of insulin have a greater risk of a reaction (although the overall incidence remains <1% for this group as a whole).[26] However, even patients who have never been previously exposed to protamine can have an anaphylactoid reaction to it.[27] Hypotension, pulmonary hypertension, capillary leak, and pulmonary edema can all occur.

Protamine given alone is a weak anticoagulant and because of this, excessive doses of protamine should be avoided. Anticoagulation due to excessive protamine should be suspected when additional doses of protamine given to treat a mildly elevated ACT result in further increases in the ACT.

Protamine rapidly binds to the circulating heparin. However, heparin that is bound to tissues may reappear in the circulation once the heparin level in blood decreases. This later reappearance of heparin is called *heparin rebound.* There is controversy over how significant this problem is. Even if it does occur, heparin rebound can be treated with small (30-50 mg) doses of additional protamine.

There are several points to remember about protamine:

- Accidentally administering protamine during CPB is likely to be lethal to the patient. Develop safety habits to avoid a drug error, such as not drawing protamine until it is needed, clearly labeling the syringe, and storing it in a different place than heparin.
- Protamine is strongly basic and causes precipitation when it comes into contact with many drugs. Avoid mixing protamine with other drugs.
- Once protamine is administered, the blood from the surgical field should not be suctioned into the CPB machine because clots can form in the oxygenator. To avoid this, always notify the perfusionist when protamine is started.
- If significant hypotension develops during protamine administration, slow down the infusion or stop it until the problem is corrected. A severe reaction to protamine may require reheparinization and return to CPB.
- Clotting of a coronary artery graft can be mistaken for a protamine reaction because the symptoms are similar (hypotension, increased PA pressure), and it occurs when anticoagulation is reversed. Identifying changes in the electrocardiogram (ECG) or echocardiogram that indicate regional ischemia as well as palpating clot in the graft can help determine the true problem.

## MONITORING DURING CARDIOPULMONARY BYPASS

### How Is the Patient Monitored During Cardiopulmonary Bypass?

Monitoring during CPB involves a continuation of the monitoring used during surgery, as well as additional monitoring used exclusively for CPB.

### Blood Pressure

Continuous measurement of the BP with an arterial catheter is necessary for several reasons. The BP can change suddenly, which makes continuous display necessary. During CPB, the BP is usually not pulsatile and, therefore, techniques used to measure the BP under normal conditions, such as a sphygmomanometer or Doppler ultrasonography, are not useful during CPB.

The place where the arterial catheter is inserted can affect the pressure measured. Under normal conditions, the pressure measured in a place relatively distant from the heart, such as the radial artery, is not different from the central aortic pressure: the systolic pressure is slightly higher and the mean is almost identical.

However, during CPB, several factors may change this relationship. Vasodilation of the capillary bed during bypass, decrease in the diameter of the radial artery, and measurement downstream can all work together to produce a much lower radial artery than central aortic pressure.[28,29] Although such a discrepancy often is not appreciated until weaning from CPB is attempted, this phenomenon can occur soon after the initiation of bypass and should be considered whenever a patient has unexplained hypotension during bypass.[30] The surgeon can directly measure the pressure in the aorta with a small needle to determine the central aortic pressure. Gradients of 30 to 50 mm Hg are not unusual. If a large gradient is found, a catheter can be placed in the femoral artery, which usually correlates better with the central aortic pressure (Fig. 17–9). The radial-to-aortic pressure discrepancy usually improves some time (30 minutes to several hours) after discontinuing CPB.[31]

### Electrocardiogram

In addition to showing the changes in the ST segment and T waves seen with ischemia, the ECG is useful for following the effects of hyperkalemic arrest from the cardioplegia as well as evaluating rhythm disturbances once the cross-clamp is removed. Electrical artifacts may interfere with the ECG during CPB; this issue is discussed in the section, Myocardial Protection and Cardioplegia (Fig. 17–10).

### Pump Pressure

The blood returning to the patient from the pump has to overcome the resistance of the tubing and the smaller diameter of the aortic cannula compared with the aortic lumen. The difference between the pressure at which the blood is pumped and the pressure it has in the patient's body is known as the

FIGURE 17–9. Difference in blood pressure between radial and femoral artery catheters at the end of cardiopulmonary bypass. In this case, there is a difference of 85 mm Hg for systolic and 46 mm Hg for mean pressure.

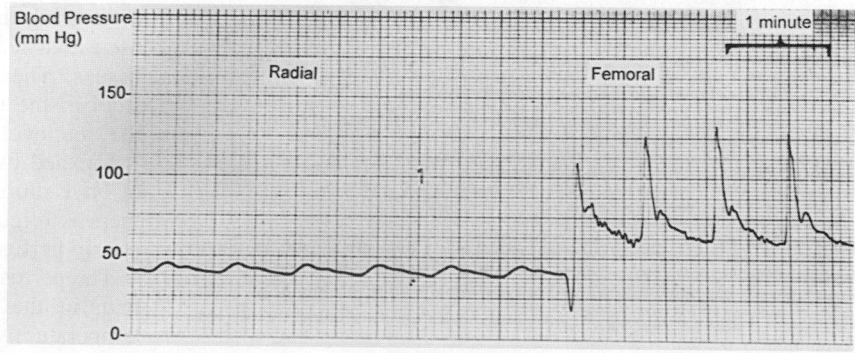

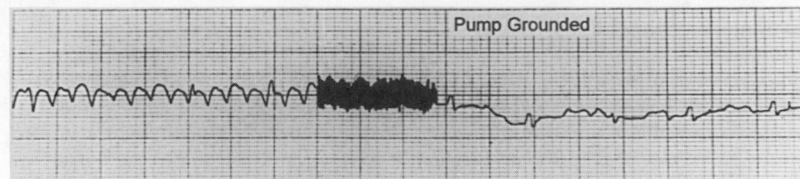

*pump gradient.* This gradient depends on the size of the cannula, tubing, temperature, hematocrit, and flow. Usually it is in the 100- to 200-mm Hg range. Gradients >250 mm Hg, particularly with decreased flow, suggest an obstruction. This can occur in the pump (ie, arterial filter) or in the patient (aortic dissection), and should be treated accordingly.

## Central Venous Pressure

Because of the drainage of blood by gravity into the venous reservoir, the central venous pressure during CPB should be close to zero or even a negative number. Measuring this pressure during CPB is important because its elevation (>10 mm Hg) may be an indicator of poor venous drainage through the cannulas, resulting in venous obstruction. Elevated venous pressure from venous obstruction results in a lower perfusion pressure for the organs affected, as well as edema and congestion. In addition, because of poor venous return, the perfusionist is often forced to add fluids into the venous reservoir, resulting in hemodilution and more edema.

## Pulmonary Artery Pressure

When the patient has a PA catheter in place, the pressure measured should be low during CPB because of the lack of blood flow in the pulmonary circulation. However, accumulation of blood in the left ventricle and left atrium from conditions such as aortic insufficiency can lead to increased PA pressures. It is important to notify the surgeon if this occurs. Placing a drain or vent should relieve the increased pressure; this is usually done through a pulmonary vein. Failure to treat this problem can cause decreased myocardial perfusion and pulmonary edema (Fig. 17–11).

With initiation of CPB, the heart decreases in size and,

because of this change, the PA catheter may migrate distally. In addition, the PA catheter becomes stiffer with lower body temperatures. These two factors may result in perforation of the PA by the catheter tip. This can be avoided by withdrawing the catheter a few centimeters when CPB is initiated.

## Oxygen Saturation

During pulsatile circulation, the peripheral oxygen saturation can be measured with a pulse oximeter. During CPB, the pulse oximeter usually does not give a reading because of the lack of pulsatility. Instead, oxygen saturation is measured at the venous inflow to obtain a mixed venous oxygen saturation ($S\bar{v}O_2$) and is used as an indicator of global perfusion. The perfusionist tries to maintain the $S\bar{v}O_2$ above 60%. Lower numbers may be due to inadequate pump flow, low hematocrit, increased consumption, or other problems.

The oxygen saturation is also measured in the arterial line and indicates if the oxygenator is saturating the blood with oxygen. With adequate oxygenation, the arterial saturation is typically 98% to 100%.

## Temperature

During CPB, the patient is cooled or rewarmed by having the blood circulate through the heat exchanger. Changing the temperature of the blood does not result in a uniform temperature change throughout the body. Well-perfused organs tend to follow the temperature of the water bath, whereas poorly perfused ones lag behind. During bypass, the temperature should be monitored at different places to determine if the desired level of cooling or rewarming has been achieved. Although none of the temperature monitoring sites indicates the true brain temperature,[32] the nasopharyngeal temperature is a reasonable alternative and should be monitored routinely. Excessive rewarming is particularly dangerous for the brain because it increases brain oxygen consumption and worsens the effect of decreased perfusion. This temperature should not be allowed to exceed 37.5°C. The PA and esophageal temperatures reflect the central core temperature before CPB, but during bypass, they can be markedly affected by the temperature of fluids used for mediastinal irrigation or cooling of the heart. This should be taken into consideration when monitoring these values. The rectal or bladder temperature is used as a reflection of the slower warming, poorly perfused tissues. These sites can also have pitfalls; the presence of stool in the rectum acts as an insulator and does not reflect the true level of cooling or warming. The bladder temperature is affected by the amount of urine produced. In the presence of brisk diuresis, it mirrors the blood temperature, whereas if there is oliguria, the bladder temperature is closer to that of poorly perfused organs.[33]

The perfusionist also monitors the temperature of the water bath in the heat exchanger as well as the venous blood temperature. As mentioned earlier, a temperature difference

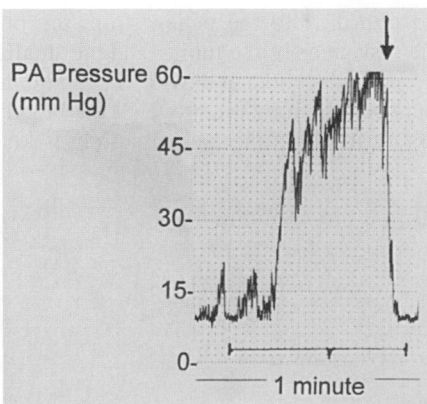

**FIGURE 17–11.** Elevated pulmonary artery (PA) pressure during cardiopulmonary bypass as a result of left ventricular distention produced by aortic insufficiency. The PA pressure elevation resolved with placement of a vent *(arrow)* in a pulmonary vein. If untreated, such condition could rapidly lead to pulmonary edema.

>8°C between the water bath and the blood during rewarming can result in bubbles coming out of solution and gas embolism.

## Pump Flow

The amount of blood being returned to the patient per minute is the pump flow or output and is equivalent to the cardiac output measurement. This number is displayed continuously, and correlating it with the $S\bar{v}O_2$ helps determine if the blood supply matches the demand.

## Other Pump Monitors

Because one of the greatest hazards of CPB is the accidental pumping of air into the arterial circulation, a bubble detector is commonly used. For this same reason, a blood level detector is installed in the venous reservoir, informing the perfusionist when dangerously low levels are reached. Continuous blood gas monitoring is sometimes used, although blood more commonly is sampled for determination of arterial gases at 20- to 60-minute intervals, depending on the conditions. A gas analyzer similar to that used in the anesthesia machine can also be used to determine the content of the gas delivered to the oxygenator (usually oxygen, although $CO_2$ and inhaled anesthetics may be added). The pressure at which the cardioplegia is delivered as well as the flow and volume are routinely measured.

## Other Patient Monitors

As mentioned in the section, Anticoagulation and Reversal, the ACT is followed to ensure that anticoagulation is reached and maintained. In addition, heparin levels can be determined using specialized cartridges.

Renal function is monitored by measuring urine output. The large amounts of fluids added to prime the pump as well as mannitol should lead to increased diuresis. However, the lack of pulsatile perfusion and hypothermia decreases urine production. Overall, urine output is usually >0.5 mL/kg/h during periods of normothermia. Higher urine outputs may be desirable when large volumes of fluid and potassium are given through the cardioplegia solution. Loop diuretics such as furosemide are used in these cases to increase urine output.

Perfusion and function of the brain may be monitored by using the electroencephalogram, the bispectral index (a processed electroencephalogram), cerebral oxymetry, or, in special cases, measurement of the jugular venous saturation.

## MYOCARDIAL PROTECTION AND CARDIOPLEGIA

### What Is Cardioplegia and Why Is It Used?

CBP allows the circulation to be sustained while surgery is performed on the heart. However, even when empty, the heart will continue to beat. Blood flowing through the coronary arteries and returning through the coronary sinus and thebesian veins may limit the surgeon's view. To provide a bloodless and immobile heart, cardioplegia is given into the coronary circulation. The word *cardioplegia* is derived from *cardio* (heart) and *plegia* (paralysis) and gives a good indication of its purpose. Administration of a solution high in potassium to the heart results in diastolic arrest. Cooling the heart decreases its metabolic activity and oxygen consumption, but by stopping the electrical activity, an even more dramatic reduction in myocardial oxygen consumption is produced[34] (Fig. 17–12). However, the cardioplegia solution does more than stop the electromechanical activity of the heart. It delivers oxygen and nutrients, removes byproducts of metabolism, cools or rewarms the heart, and acts as a buffer.

### What Are the Ingredients of Cardioplegia?

Cardioplegia can be blood based or crystalloid based. Blood-based cardioplegia takes oxygenated blood and dilutes it further with fluids. One part of fluid is added to 4 parts of blood (4:1 dilution), resulting in a hematocrit of 16% to 18%. Such a low hematocrit is used because cardioplegia is given at a low temperature (4°-12°C). At such temperatures, the viscosity of blood increases significantly; higher hematocrits result in sludging and poor perfusion. In addition, the metabolic requirements of the cardiac muscle decrease markedly, and only small amounts of oxygen are needed.

This principle of low oxygen consumption with hypothermia is what allows crystalloid cardioplegia to meet the needs of cold myocardium. Oxygen is bubbled in the crystalloid and dissolves into it. The tissues take the dissolved oxygen; in a cold and electrically silent heart, this provides the amount of oxygen needed.

The specific composition of cardioplegia depends on the preferences of the surgeon; many different combinations exist, but some general principles apply. Electrical arrest is produced by high concentrations of potassium (15-30 mEq/L). Once electrical activity has stopped, lower amounts of potassium are used in retrograde cardioplegia because larger volumes

**FIGURE 17–12.** Effect of hypothermia and electrical activity on myocardial metabolism. $M\dot{V}O_2$, myocardial oxygen consumption. (From Buckberg GD, Brazier JR, Nelson RL, et al. Studies of the effect of hypothermia on regional myocardial blood flow and metabolism during cardiopulmonary bypass, I: the adequately perfused beating, fibrillating and arrested heart. *J Thorac Cardiovasc Surg.* 1977;73:87.)

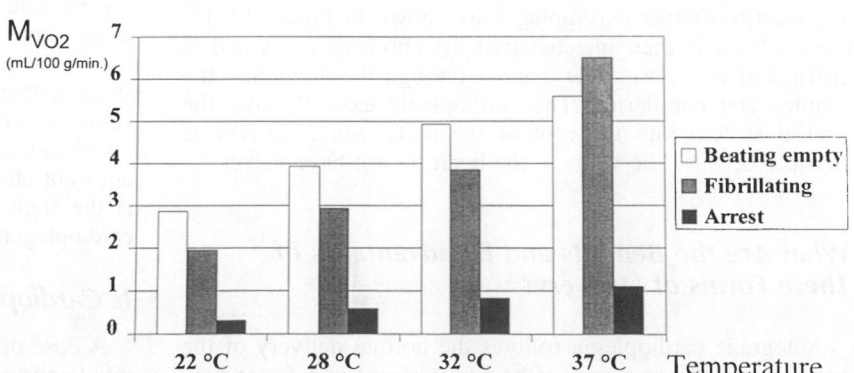

result in marked systemic hyperkalemia. Myocardial cells need calcium to contract, so it might be expected that its presence would not be necessary in cardioplegia. However, if calcium is not added to the cardioplegia, ischemic contracture of the heart can occur during reperfusion (a condition also known as *stone heart*), and thus calcium is added in small doses. The osmolarity of the solution is regulated by the addition of albumin or mannitol. Mannitol also can potentially serve as a free radical scavenger. Glucose is used as a metabolic substrate and, in some cases, simple amino acids such as aspartate or glutamate are added for the same purpose.

## How Is Cardioplegia Given?

There are two main routes to deliver cardioplegia. With *antegrade* cardioplegia, the solution follows the usual path of the circulation: from arteries to arterioles to capillaries, draining out through the venous system. *Retrograde* cardioplegia implies that the solution is infused in an opposite direction to the usual path of the circulation: from veins to capillaries to arteries.

### Antegrade Cardioplegia

The first step is application of a cross-clamp to the ascending aorta, above the coronary arteries, to isolate the coronary circulation. The cardioplegia solution is then injected into the root of the aorta, from which it distributes through the coronary arteries. An initial dose is given based on the size and muscle mass of the heart. This volume typically ranges from 0.5 to 1.5 L for an adult patient. Additional doses are given every 20 to 30 minutes for as long as cardiac arrest is needed.

Another possibility is injection of the cardioplegia directly into the ostia of the coronary arteries. This is done in cases where the aorta is opened, such as aortic valve surgery. A special tip is used to ensure an adequate seal without damaging the coronary arteries.

Cardioplegia can also be injected into the grafts that are sewn to the coronary arteries. Measuring the flow of cardioplegia down a graft gives the surgeon an idea of the quality of the anastomosis and of the circulation beyond it.

### Retrograde Cardioplegia

With *retrograde* cardioplegia, a catheter is placed in the coronary sinus, which normally drains the venous blood from the heart into the right atrium. Some of the specialized catheters used to deliver cardioplegia are shown in Figure 17–13. Cardioplegia is then injected into the coronary sinus and is distributed in a retrograde manner through the veins into the venules and capillaries. The cardioplegia exits through the arterial system into the root of the aorta. Such delivery is possible because the veins in the heart do not have valves.

## What Are the Benefits and Disadvantages of These Forms of Delivery?

Antegrade cardioplegia follows the normal delivery of the circulation and can therefore be administered at a faster flow

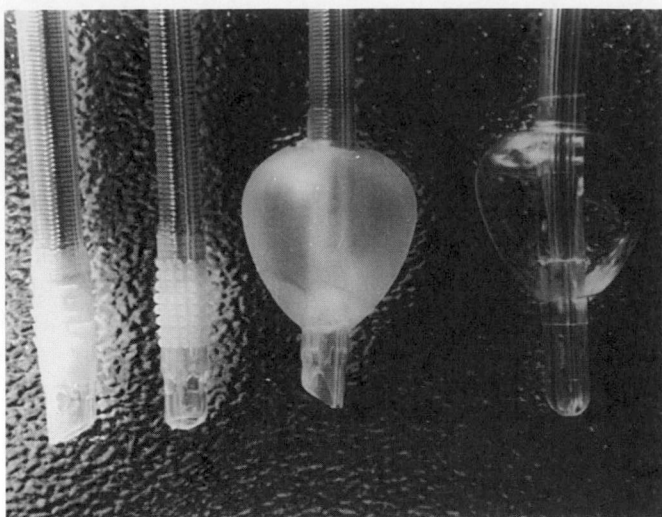

**FIGURE 17–13.** Catheters used for retrograde delivery of cardioplegia through the coronary sinus. Some have an inflatable balloon to prevent the cardioplegia from leaking back into the right atrium.

rate and pressure. However, atherosclerosis and obstructions in the coronary arteries limit or completely impede delivery of cardioplegia to areas of the heart that may be at precisely the highest risk of ischemia. Introduction of air bubbles into the coronary circulation is also possible and undesirable. Injection in the aortic root requires the aortic valve to be competent; otherwise the cardioplegia fills the left ventricle instead of distributing down the coronaries. Administration directly into the coronary ostia is done only when the aortic root is opened. The surgery must be interrupted while the cardioplegia is delivered, and thus injury to the coronary ostia is possible. Delivery through a graft reaches only the area of myocardium supplied by that vessel, and care must be taken not to embolize air or atheromatous material disturbed while sewing the graft.

Retrograde cardioplegia requires placing a specialized cannula in the coronary sinus. Placement of this cannula is not always easy and, on occasion, injury and perforations to the coronary sinus may occur. The venous system does not normally carry blood under elevated pressure and doing so may lead to myocardial edema. To prevent this, the pressure in the coronary sinus is monitored and not allowed to increase over 40 to 50 mm Hg. Because the volume has to be injected slowly, it is administered continuously or over longer periods. Venting of the aortic root is also necessary to allow the fluid to exit. An advantage of retrograde cardioplegia is that the venous system does not develop atheromas that obstruct delivery and can, therefore, distribute the cardioplegia solution to areas where the arterial system is totally obstructed. However, not all the arterial supply of the heart drains into the coronary sinus system. Part of the venous drainage is through thebesian veins directly into the right ventricle as well as through arteriovenous sinusoids. Therefore, retrograde cardioplegia does not effectively protect all of the heart. At particular risk is the right ventricle, which receives small amounts of the cardioplegia administered retrograde.

## Is Cardioplegia Always Given Cold?

A dose of cardioplegia may be given at or near normothermic temperatures. This is often done at the end of the cardiac arrest, allowing the temperature of the muscle to return toward normal before contraction starts.

## Does Cardioplegia Always Work?

Properly administered cardioplegia should result in cardiac arrest. However, if there is uneven distribution, segments of the heart may continue to have electrical activity (usually fibrillation). It is important to monitor the ECG in search of such a condition so that additional cardioplegia can be given. Uneven or inadequate administration of cardioplegia can also occur if there is aortic insufficiency, if the aortic clamp is improperly applied, if there is marked ventricular hypertrophy, or if the coronary sinus retrograde cardioplegia catheter is improperly positioned. Certain congenital anomalies (persistent left SVC and unroofed coronary sinus) can also prevent retrograde cardioplegia from distributing evenly.

## How Does the Heart Start Beating Again?

Once the aortic clamp is removed, the blood washes away the cardioplegia. In a number of cases, this is enough for spontaneous regular electrical activity to start. In other instances, the heart fibrillates and electrical cardioversion is necessary. On other occasions, marked bradycardia or even asystole occurs, requiring temporary pacing.

Things to remember during and after cardioplegia follow:

- Antegrade cardioplegia should cause electrical silence. Monitor the ECG and inform the surgeon if electrical activity is present. Some slow electrical activity may continue during retrograde cardioplegia because of the lower potassium concentrations often used.
- The ECG can be affected by electrical interference from the pump, particularly static electricity generated by friction with the plastic tubing. If the heart appears immobile but electrical activity is seen on the ECG, ask the perfusionist to ground the pump before deciding if ventricular fibrillation is present (see Fig. 17–10).
- Monitor the systemic glucose and levels of potassium during cardioplegia administration. Although some elevation is expected, inform the surgeon if the systemic potassium level exceeds 7.0 mEq/L and be prepared to treat hyperglycemia if the glucose levels exceed 150 to 180 mg/dL.
- As a bolus of cardioplegia is returned to the circulation, hypotension is often observed. This may be caused by hypertonic solutions resulting in vasodilation or from release of vasodilators such as adenosine from the coronary endothelium. Be prepared to treat hypotension when cardioplegia is given rapidly.

## ANESTHESIA DURING CARDIOPULMONARY BYPASS

### How Are Patients Kept Anesthetized During Cardiopulmonary Bypass?

Although mainly oxygen and $CO_2$ are exchanged through the oxygenator, other gases such as anesthetic vapors may be added or removed. An anesthetic vaporizer placed before the inflow of the oxygenator allows continued administration of inhaled anesthetic during CPB.

Anesthesia may also be maintained during CPB with the use of intravenous agents. Opioids such as fentanyl combined with benzodiazepines or hypnotics such as propofol can be used.

When using muscle relaxants, the anesthesiologist must balance the advantage of avoiding patient movement with the difficulty of determining if the patient is adequately anesthetized once paralysis is present. During CPB, tachycardia is no longer a manifestation of light anesthesia because of the use of cardioplegia. The vasodilation that often occurs with CPB counteracts the hypertension of light anesthesia. In addition, the anesthesiologist can erroneously assume that the hypotension is due to excessive anesthesia and incorrectly reduce the amount of anesthetic given. Hypothermia can abolish diaphoresis and hyperthermia can cause it, making this sign unreliable as a manifestation of light anesthesia. As a compromise, lower doses of muscle relaxants can be used so that patient movement is still detected. Monitoring with a nerve stimulator allows precise titration so that 1 to 2 twitches are present.

Given the limitations in determining depth of anesthesia during CPB, the bispectral index can be a useful tool in this situation. It must be kept in mind that opioids, even in high doses, do not produce amnesia and that supplemental hypnotics are needed. The bispectral index can be affected by changes in temperature, BP, and flow to the brain, as well as by artifacts such as those resulting from muscular activity, pacemakers, and electrical interference.

During periods of partial CPB such as during initiation or weaning, part of the blood flow goes through the lungs and part through the bypass circuit. In such situations, if inhaled anesthetic is administered at only one place such as the CPB machine, the remaining flow behaves as a shunt and dilutes the final concentration of anesthetic. To administer a steady concentration of inhaled anesthetic during such conditions (parallel circulation), the vaporizers in the anesthesia and CPB machines must be open at the same concentration.

Inhaled anesthetics are myocardial depressants in varying degrees and can also affect the vascular tone. Because of these properties, the anesthesiologist may elect to discontinue their use at certain times, particularly if there is difficulty in weaning from CPB. Intravenous anesthetics should be administered when this is done to prevent the patient from awakening. This point needs to be emphasized because it can be forgotten in the midst of treating hemodynamic instability.

Remember the following about anesthesia during CPB:

- Just as metabolism decreases with hypothermia, it increases during rewarming. Consider the need for redosing drugs such as heparin and anesthetics when rewarming is initiated.
- The plastic of some oxygenators and venous reservoirs may crack or even shatter if liquid anesthetic is spilled on it. The anesthetic vaporizer should be kept away from the oxygenator and should be filled before starting CPB. If refilling of the vaporizer is needed during CPB, hold a towel underneath to catch any spilled fluid.
- The initiation and discontinuation of CPB can be associated with hemodynamic instability. In such conditions, marked reduction or even discontinuation of the inhaled anesthetic

may be necessary. Be prepared to administer intravenous drugs at those times to prevent intraoperative awareness.

## PHYSIOLOGY OF CARDIOPULMONARY BYPASS

### What Happens to the Blood Pressure and Flow During Cardiopulmonary Bypass?

As blood is diverted from the heart to the CPB machine, the pulse pressure decreases and the arterial tracing becomes a flat line with minimal or no pulsatile variation (Fig. 17–14). The initiation of CPB is characterized by a decrease in the mean arterial pressure. This is the result of a decrease in the systemic vascular resistance, which in turn is the product of several factors. The plastic tubing, venous reservoir, and oxygenator are primed with fluids. This volume is approximately 1.5 to 2 L, although the exact volume depends on the type of oxygenator and tubing used. When this fluid enters in the circulation, it results in abrupt hemodilution and a marked reduction in the viscosity of blood. The reduction in viscosity accounts for most of the reduction in systemic vascular resistance, although other factors implied are the absence of pulsatile pressure and the brief circulation of fluid that does not carry oxygen, resulting in reflex vasodilation.[35]

The CPB machine is able to pump as high as the dials are set. However, there are tradeoffs. The mechanical pumping results in trauma to the cells present in the blood. Therefore, the higher the pump flows, the greater trauma and destruction

of red blood cells and platelets. During CPB, it is necessary to balance the desired pump flow and pressure with the desire to avoid trauma to the blood cells. In addition, the morbidity of CPB is related to the amount of arterial embolism produced. Embolism has many sources (air, fat, plastic, atheroma) and occurs despite the use of filters. The higher the pump flow, the higher the embolic load to the patient. Although there is disagreement regarding the optimal pump flow, in general, flow rates of 2.0 to 2.4 L/min/m² are used at normothermia. As the patient is cooled, oxygen consumption decreases, and lower flows can be used.

### What Is the Normal Blood Pressure During Cardiopulmonary Bypass?

There is controversy over what is an acceptable BP during CPB, with studies showing conflicting results.[36–40] A recent study from one institution found a decrease in cardiac and neurologic morbidity in a selected group of patients if the mean arterial BP was kept between 80 to 100 mm Hg (or at least was attempted to be kept at such a level) rather than at 50 to 60 mm Hg.[41,42] However, the number of patients studied is not large enough to resolve the controversy, and important questions about differences between the two groups have been raised.[43,44]

Cerebral blood flow, as well as flow to many other organs, is autoregulated. That is, the organ regulates the vascular tone of the vessels supplying it, so that even if the pressure changes (within a certain range), the blood flow remains unaltered. The lower limit of 50 mm Hg is used because of studies indicating that this is the lower limit of pressure at which cerebral autoregulation is maintained.[45–47] This lower limit of cerebral autoregulation is further decreased during hypothermic CPB.[45,48] In addition, the widespread use of high perfusion pressures can result in potential increases in the embolic load and of bleeding in the surgical field.[44] From a practical standpoint, a range of 50 to 90 mm Hg is used at most centers.

When evaluating the pressure during CPB, it is important to address several questions:

1. Where is the pressure being measured, and is it accurate? As discussed previously, measurement in a peripheral artery may not be an accurate reflection of the central pressure.
2. What is the temperature? Because of decreased metabolism with hypothermia, lower perfusion pressures may be better tolerated at low temperatures.
3. What is the hematocrit? The hematocrit as well as the temperature affects the viscosity, and viscosity in turn affects the pressure obtained for a given flow.
4. What concomitant disease does the patient have? Patients with chronic hypertension shift their autoregulation curve and are likely to require higher perfusion pressures. Patients with severe atherosclerosis, diabetes, and intravascular obstructions may require higher pressures as well.

Note the following points about the administration of medication during CPB:

- Before treating the BP during CPB, always make sure that the transducers are appropriately zeroed and that there is

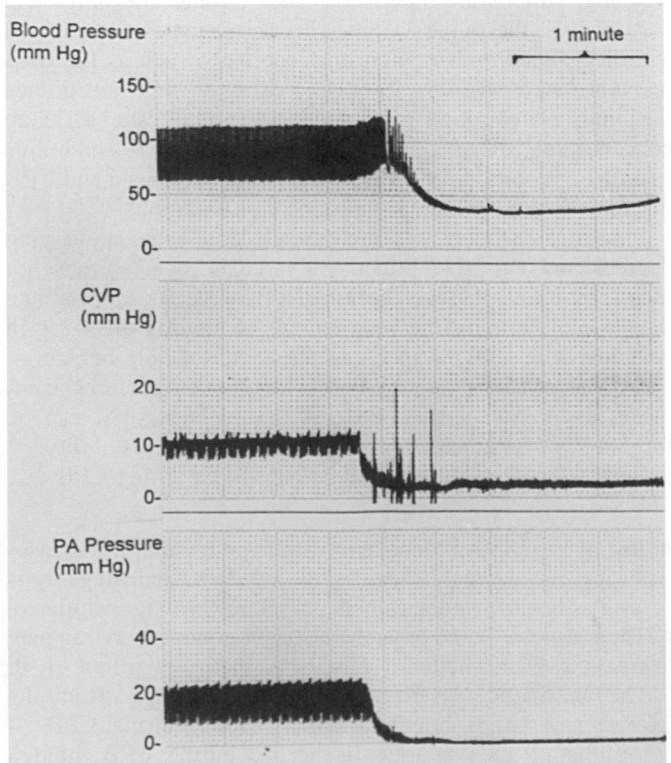

**FIGURE 17–14.** Effect of initiating cardiopulmonary bypass (CPB) on the hemodynamic tracings. Notice the disappearance of pulsatility with full CPB as well as profound reduction in the central venous pressure (CVP) and pulmonary artery (PA) pressure.

no unintended administration of vasodilators or vasoconstrictors.

- During CPB, vasoactive drugs should be administered at the pump to ensure adequate delivery. Do not administer drugs in the right ventricle or PA because these areas are being bypassed from the main blood flow.
- The administration of cardioplegia and the reinfusion of blood accumulated in the pleural cavities are often associated with vasodilation and hypotension. Be prepared to treat the BP at those times (Fig. 17–15).
- Marked hypotension or hypertension may be a sign of a severe problem such as cannula malposition and aortic dissection. Take this into consideration before treating the BP with vasoactive medications.

## What Happens to the Body Temperature During Cardiopulmonary Bypass?

The fluids use to prime the pump are at room temperature. In the absence of active rewarming, CPB results in cooling of the patient. The amount of cooling depends on the temperature of the fluids in the pump. In the heat exchanger, the blood circulates through coils immersed in a water bath. By changing the temperature of the water bath, the blood can be cooled or warmed as desired. Complex cases may require the use of profound hypothermia, although hypothermia is often induced even for simple cases.

## Is Hypothermia Undesirable During Cardiopulmonary Bypass?

Some of the most severe consequences of hypothermia, such as decreased myocardial contractility and ventricular fibrillation, do not affect the blood flow to the patient because the pump maintains the circulation. Hypothermia can indeed have other undesirable side effects, such as decreased platelet function, increased blood viscosity, vasoconstriction, and hyperglycemia. However, the benefits of decreased metabolism, reduced oxygen consumption (allowing lower pump flows and reduced trauma to the red cells), and reduction in the excitotoxic cascade (decreasing the effect of cerebral ischemia) outweigh the detrimental effects.[49] The degree of hypothermia

necessary to obtain beneficial effects is often mild (32°-35°C), a value often obtained by allowing the temperature to drift.[50,51] In contrast, active efforts to maintain the patient's warmth through CPB have been associated with an increased incidence of neurologic injury.[52,53]

Remember the following about rewarming following hypothermia during CPB:

- Cooling occurs rapidly, but the speed of rewarming is limited by the need to keep a temperature gradient of <8°C between the water bath and the blood.[54] Rewarming should start ahead of time so that the patient does not have to be on CPB longer than necessary.
- The surgeon usually estimates when it is time to start rewarming. However, while concentrating on the surgery, he or she may forget. If this seems to be the case, ask the surgeon if rewarming should start.
- Redistribution of heat from the core to the periphery occurs after CPB. To avoid a rapid loss of heat, ensure that the patient has rewarmed uniformly before discontinuing CPB.

## Why Do Patients Have Greater Generalized Edema After Cardiac Surgery Than After Other Surgeries?

The circulation of blood through the plastic surfaces and filters used in CPB results in a massive activation of complement.[55] In addition, endotoxins are released, and these in turn stimulate the production of cytokines by macrophages.[56] The inflammatory response increases with the duration of CPB and is responsible for multiple pathologic changes, including injury to capillary membranes, leakage of fluid into extravascular compartments (third space), alterations in cellular immunity, pulmonary dysfunction, renal insufficiency, and alterations in hemostasis.[57] Hemodilution and changes in oncotic pressure may also contribute to the development of edema.

## Can This Inflammatory Response Be Prevented?

Corticosteroids are administered before surgery to decrease the inflammatory response. Although some studies report de-

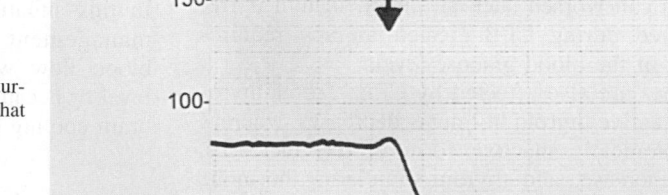

**FIGURE 17–15.** Decrease in the systemic blood pressure during cardiopulmonary bypass after infusing blood *(arrow)* that had extravasated into the pleural cavity.

creases in complement levels and other markers of inflammation, changes in outcome are more difficult to prove.[58–60] Because steroids can have detrimental effects, such as immunosuppression and hyperglycemia, the potential benefits must be balanced with known risks before a decision is made to administer them. Nonsteroidal anti-inflammatory drugs can also decrease some of the markers of inflammation, but because they interfere with platelet function, their use is also controversial.

Significant efforts have been spent trying to develop plastic surfaces that do not cause a widespread inflammatory response. Perhaps the best example is the use of heparin-bonded circuits, which were initially developed to decrease or abolish the need for anticoagulation. Heparin-bonded tubing and heparin-coated oxygenators can reduce complement activation and the inflammatory response, although it is controversial whether this reduction is clinically significant for most patients and justifies the additional cost.[61–64]

Other attempts to prevent the inflammatory response include the use of aprotinin, milrinone, and different antibiotics. Although there is evidence to indicate that each of these therapies can have some effect on the inflammatory response, multiple factors influence the body's response, and therefore their primary effects rather than reduction of inflammation dictate when to use them.[55,65–68]

## Is Cardiopulmonary Bypass Stressful?

Despite the administration of anesthesia, CPB results in a significant stress response. The plasma levels of catecholamines rise, presumably as a response to the changes that characterize CPB: hemodilution, nonpulsatile flow, hypothermia, and activation of complement.[69,70] The levels of catecholamines remain high because hypothermia slows their breakdown, and bypassing the heart and lungs circumvents important organs for their metabolism.[10] Levels of other hormones, such as cortisol and vasopressin, also increase during bypass.

## Are There Other Endocrine Changes With Cardiopulmonary Bypass?

Hyperglycemia is often encountered during CPB. This is the result of increased catecholamine levels producing increased glycogenolysis and decreased insulin response to hyperglycemia with hypothermia. In addition, insulin may bind to the plastic tubing in the CPB circuit, and the kidneys tend to reabsorb large amounts of filtered glucose.[71] Because neurologic injury can always potentially occur with cardiac surgery, and hyperglycemia can worsen such an injury, insulin is frequently administered during CPB.[72] Such therapy requires careful monitoring of the blood glucose levels.

Thyroid hormones are also affected by CPB. Triiodothyronine ($T_3$), the most active thyroid hormone, decreases, whereas reverse $T_3$ (a biologically inactive form of $T_3$) increases. Thyroxine levels increase, and thyroid-stimulating hormone levels fall.[73] Replacement of thyroid hormone during bypass has been attempted, with mixed results. It is not recommended as a routine treatment but can be considered in patients who are difficult to wean from CPB because of decreased cardiac output.[74,75]

## What Are Alpha-Stat and pH-Stat Acid-Base Management?

As hypothermia is induced during CPB, the solubility of $CO_2$ and oxygen increases, resulting in a lower $PCO_2$ and an increase in pH. When analyzing the blood gases during hypothermia, there are two different ways to look at the results: alpha-stat and pH-stat.

### Alpha-Stat

When blood gases are measured, the machine warms the sample to 37°C. Alpha-stat management aims to keep the results of the warmed sample at a $PCO_2$ of approximately 40 mm Hg and a pH of 7.40. The basis for this is that histidine (important in maintaining the intracellular charge state) maintains a constant alpha ratio of dissociated and undissociated forms despite the change in temperature, therefore maintaining neutrality within the cell.[76]

### pH-Stat

In contrast, in pH-stat management, a nomogram is used to convert the result obtained by the machine to that expected at the patient's actual temperature—a process known as *temperature correction.*

## How Is Temperature Correction Actually Done?

From the practical point of view, alpha-stat implies managing the blood gases as in normothermia, ignoring the patient's actual temperature. In contrast, with pH-stat the blood gas is found to be increasingly alkalotic with hypothermia, and $CO_2$ gas is added to the circuit to correct this finding.

## How Does This Affect the Patient?

Adding $CO_2$ to the patient results in cerebral vasodilation. This was thought initially to be beneficial and was advocated as a way of improving neurologic outcome.[77] However, most studies have found that pH-stat management resulted in unchanged or even worse neurologic outcomes.[78–80] Because many of the adverse neurologic outcomes in cardiac surgery are the result of embolism, increasing the cerebral blood flow may result in an increase in the embolic load. In addition, vasodilation may produce a shunting of blood from areas that need the perfusion to others that do not.[78,81]

In neonates and children, where deep hypothermia and circulatory arrest are not uncommon, BP and flow can be low. In this situation, some of the studies indicate that pH-stat management may be beneficial, perhaps because cerebral blood flow would otherwise fall below the autoregulation level or because cerebral vasodilation results in more uniform brain cooling during the induction of hypothermia.[82–84]

## How Much Fluid Should Be Given on Bypass?

Normally during surgery, fluids are administered based on estimated losses or measurement of filling pressures. However,

CPB creates a unique situation. The filling pressures are low or even negative and do not reflect the volume status of the patient. Fluid losses are difficult to estimate because of the amount of blood and fluid present in the extracorporeal and cardioplegia circuits. Therefore, fluid is added so that a minimum operating level is maintained in the venous reservoir. If the venous reservoir is filled up, fluid can be removed through diuresis or ultrafiltration.

## At What Level Should the Hematocrit Be During Cardiopulmonary Bypass?

The priming fluid used to fill the CPB tubing and reservoir results in hemodilution during CPB. A lower hematocrit during CPB is acceptable because hypothermia decreases oxygen consumption and blood flow is maintained by the pump. Equally important, hypothermia results in increased blood viscosity. Without hemodilution, the elevated viscosity would result in an increased resistance to circulation once the temperature decreased.

There is disagreement about how low the hematocrit can be maintained without compromising organ function.[85] Studies in animals suggest that at normothermia, a hematocrit of 18% or more is needed to maintain cerebral oxygen supply, with lower values tolerated as the temperature decreases. However, patients often have coexisting disease,[86] which raises concerns about profound anemia resulting in inadequate oxygen delivery, thus causing complications.[87,88] As a general (although somewhat arbitrary) guideline for adult patients, the hematocrit during normothermia is usually kept >20% at normothermia and >16% during hypothermia.

The following should be remembered when considering at what level the hematocrit should remain during CPB:

- The administration of a vasodilator during CPB can result in blood being pooled in the peripheral circulation and lead to a rapid decrease in the volume of the venous reservoir. Always notify the perfusionist when giving a drug with vasodilating properties, including inodilators such as amrinone and milrinone, so that dangerously low volumes in the pump are avoided.
- Before deciding to transfuse a patient based on the hematocrit, check the volume in the venous reservoir and ask the surgeons to suction the blood from the mediastinum and pleural cavities. If the volume available in the reservoir is >600 to 700 mL, the hematocrit can be increased through diuresis or hemofiltration.

## LUNGS AND CARDIOPULMONARY BYPASS

## What Should Be Done With the Lungs During Cardiopulmonary Bypass?

During partial CPB, blood still flows through the lungs, and ventilation should be continued to avoid having this portion of blood behave as a shunt. Once full CPB has been obtained, blood flow through the lungs is minimal, and ventilation is no longer necessary. There is some debate about whether the lungs should be completely deflated or if it is better to have low levels (5 cm $H_2O$) of continuous positive airway pressure (CPAP). Most studies suggest that gas exchange deteriorates after CPB regardless of the modality used, although CPAP may be slightly better overall.[89–91]

## Why Does Lung Function Deteriorate After Cardiopulmonary Bypass?

A number of factors have been suggested as contributing to this phenomenon, including fluid extravasation, complement activation, and leukocyte sequestration in the lungs. However, the most important causes appear to be residual atelectasis and cardiogenic pulmonary edema.[92,93]

## CENTRAL NERVOUS SYSTEM AND CARDIOPULMONARY BYPASS

## What Problems Can Occur in the Central Nervous System With Cardiopulmonary Bypass?

It is difficult to separate the problems caused by CPB, per se, from those events that are closely associated with it, such as arterial cannulation and cardiac surgery, and therefore they are all grouped together. Stroke is one of the most feared complications, occurring in 2% to 3% of patients undergoing coronary artery bypass grafting and increasing in incidence with combined procedures.[94,95] Surprisingly, the incidence is not necessarily higher with valve surgery despite the fact that cardiac chambers are opened and air is entrained—this has been attributed to procedures of shorter duration.[96] Much more common is the occurrence of neuropsychological dysfunction, which is detected with specialized examinations[97] and is manifested as changes in concentration, motor dexterity, and psychomotor speed. The incidence varies from 20% to 79%.[98] The etiology of central nervous system changes is multifactorial and includes macroembolism and microembolism, hypoperfusion, reperfusion injury, inflammation, edema, and thrombosis.[99,100]

## Can These Problems Be Decreased or Prevented?

A number of factors, including age, type of procedure, and preexisting disease, cannot be modified. Reduction of central nervous system complications has focused on detection of specific sites of aortic atherosclerosis using echocardiography and modification of the cannulation site, decreasing the manipulation and clamping of the aorta, shortening the duration of CPB, evaluating for carotid disease, use of improved oxygenators and filters, and use of retrograde cerebral perfusion in selected cases.[101–105] As mentioned previously, hypothermia, even of only 2°C or 3°C below normal, offers substantial protection.[50,51] The use of barbiturates, propofol (to induce burst suppression), and steroids remains controversial because of conflicting results.[106–109]

**TABLE 17–2.** Prevention of Renal Insufficiency in
Cardiac Surgery

**Improve Cardiac Output**
Treat heart failure
Control hypertension
**Avoid Nephrotoxic Drugs**
Aminoglycosides
Nonsteroidal anti-inflammatory drugs
Angiotensin-converting enzyme inhibitors
Contrast agents
**Control Hyperglycemia**
Insulin infusion
**Decrease CPB Time**
Simpler surgery
Off CPB surgery (coronary artery bypass grafting)*
**Fluids**
Monitor and maintain preload
**Medications**
Dopamine (low doses)*
Fenoldopam (low doses)*
Mannitol (osmotic diuresis)
Furosemide
New drugs (ularitide)†

*Controversial therapy.
†Experimental therapy.
CPB, cardiopulmonary bypass.

## RENAL FUNCTION AND CARDIOPULMONARY BYPASS

### What Changes in Renal Function Can Cardiopulmonary Bypass Cause?

During CPB, renal vascular resistance increases while renal blood flow and glomerular filtration decrease, probably because of the increase in catecholamines, lack of pulsatility, activation of complement, inflammation, embolism, and hemolysis.[69,110] Most patients tolerate these changes and recover. However, if preexisting renal function is impaired (preexisting renal insufficiency, advanced age, heart failure, type 1 diabetes mellitus), the risk of renal failure increases significantly.[111] Other important risk factors for renal dysfunction after cardiac surgery include prolonged CPB (>3 hours) and a low cardiac output state.[111–113] The overall incidence of renal dysfunction (serum creatinine >2.0 mg/dL) in patients undergoing coronary artery bypass grafting is approximately 8%.[111]

### What Can Be Done to Prevent Renal Dysfunction During Cardiac Surgery?

Some of the most important considerations are outlined in Table 17–2. A low cardiac output is a significant risk factor for renal insufficiency and is actively treated in the hope of decreasing the incidence of this complication. A number of drugs used perioperatively can worsen renal function and should be avoided (see Table 17–2). Although diabetes is likely a marker of vascular disease, preoperative hyperglycemia is associated with a significant increase in renal insufficiency.[111] The use of low doses of dopamine ("renal dose") is controversial, as is the use of more specific dopaminergic agonists.[114,115] However, the mortality rate of patients in whom renal failure develops after cardiac surgery exceeds 50%—a

powerful incentive to intervene.[111,112,116] Ularitide, also known as urodilatin, is an atrial natriuretic peptide that appears to be useful in preliminary studies for the treatment of oliguric renal failure after cardiac surgery.[117–119]

Note the following about preventing renal dysfunction during cardiac surgery:

- Overdistention of the left ventricle during CPB can rapidly result in pulmonary edema. Notify the surgeon of any mean PA pressure >20 mm Hg during full CPB, so that appropriate venting can be done (see Fig. 17–11).
- Just as hypothermia decreases the incidence on neurologic injury, hyperthermia markedly increases it. Monitor the nasopharyngeal temperature and avoid excessive rewarming of the patient (temperature >37.5°C).
- Large volumes of fluid and potassium are given by retrograde cardioplegia. Follow the amount of cardioplegia given and be prepared to administer diuretics to prevent excessive hemodilution and hyperkalemia.

## OTHER CONSIDERATIONS

### What Happens If the Electrical Power Fails During Cardiopulmonary Bypass?

If electrical power to the roller pump ceases because of a power outage or electrical malfunction, circulation stops. Every hospital should have a backup power supply that provides electrical power to critical areas such as the operating room during an outage. In addition, many CPB machines are connected to an uninterrupted power supply, which is essentially a battery that provides electrical power until the main power is restored. Finally, the main roller pump can be manually powered by using a hand crank. The anesthesiologist should ensure that this hand crank is always available and be prepared to help the perfusionist in such an event (Fig. 17–16).

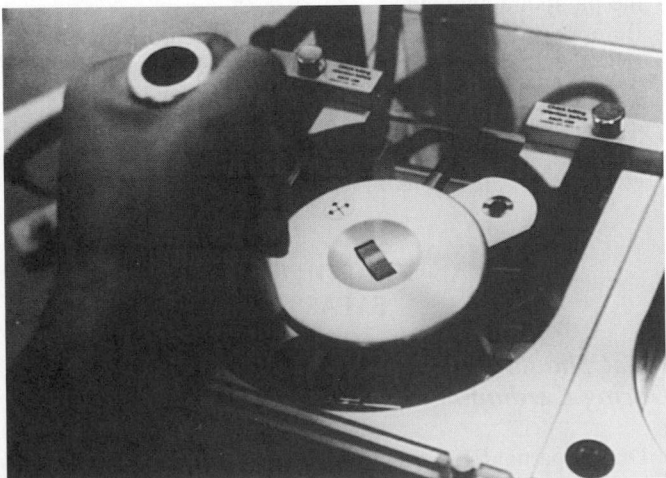

**FIGURE 17–16.** Hand crank used manually to power the main roller pump. Because the output display also is lost with power failure, the roller is turned, taking into account the blood level in the reservoir and S$\bar{v}$O$_2$ (if the S$\bar{v}$O$_2$ monitor battery is operational).

**TABLE 17–3.** Conditions Needed Before Attempting to Wean From Cardiopulmonary Bypass

**Surgical Conditions**
  All chambers closed
  Sutures checked for leaks
  Air removed from chambers
  Vent suction stopped
  Caval tourniquets released
**Metabolic Conditions**
  Normothermia
  Acid-base balanced
  Electrolyte abnormalities (potassium, calcium) corrected
  Hematocrit acceptable*
  Anticoagulation maintained
  $S\bar{v}O_2$ >50%
**Anesthetic Conditions**
  Anesthesia during transition period maintained*
**Equipment Conditions**
  Monitors on transducers rezeroed
  Table flat and level
**Medications**
  Emergency drugs ready
  Check what is and what is not infusing
**Cardiac Conditions**
  Heart rate 75-100 bpm*
  Rhythm
    Sinus rhythm ideal
    Alternatives: atrial pacing, atrioventricular pacing, ventricular pacing
  Afterload in range (mean arterial pressure >50, <100 mm Hg at full flow)
**Pulmonary Conditions**
  Ventilatory circuit connnected
  Secretions suctioned
  Lungs reexpanded, oxygen on

*Determined by the patient's condition.

## DISCONTINUATION OF CARDIOPULMONARY BYPASS

### Is Cardiopulmonary Bypass Just Stopped Abruptly at the End of the Procedure?

Separation from CPB is a process that requires several steps and adequate preparation. It is not an emergency, and time should be allowed to discontinue the pump support gradually.

The process of discontinuing CPB is called *weaning*, reflecting that it is normally done in steps rather than abruptly.

### When and How Can Cardiopulmonary Bypass Be Discontinued?

Certain conditions must be met before weaning is attempted and are listed in Table 17–3. It is important to keep these requirements in mind at all times because interruptions during the weaning process are not uncommon.[120] It is easy to become focused on cardiac performance and forget, for example, that ventilation has stopped. Another important point is that clear communication between the anesthesiologist, the surgeon, and the perfusionist should be maintained, with one person directing the weaning process.

The process of discontinuing CPB involves resuming the functions taken over by the bypass machine: ventilation and pumping. Ventilation is restarted with the appropriate tidal volume and rate. Given the potential for hemodynamic instability and the importance of oxygen delivery, 100% oxygen is administered.

The volume available in the venous reservoir, the pump flow, and $S\bar{v}O_2$ are monitored closely during the weaning process. The circulatory support is decreased by partially clamping the venous return tubing, allowing the heart to start filling with blood. As the heart begins to contribute to the circulation, the pump flow is decreased. This process is continued until the heart is adequately filled (as estimated by the filling pressures and appearance of the heart) and the BP is acceptable with low pump flows. At this point, the pump is stopped and the patient is assessed, making sure that oxygenation, ventilation, and circulation are appropriate. If the heart appears to be distending during the weaning process or the BP is not acceptable, weaning should be halted and the problem corrected. Poor ventricular function, prolonged cardiac ischemic time, and technical difficulties with the surgery are all good reasons to proceed cautiously. The cannulas should not be removed until it is clear that the patient is stable.

Remember the following when considering discontinuing CPB:

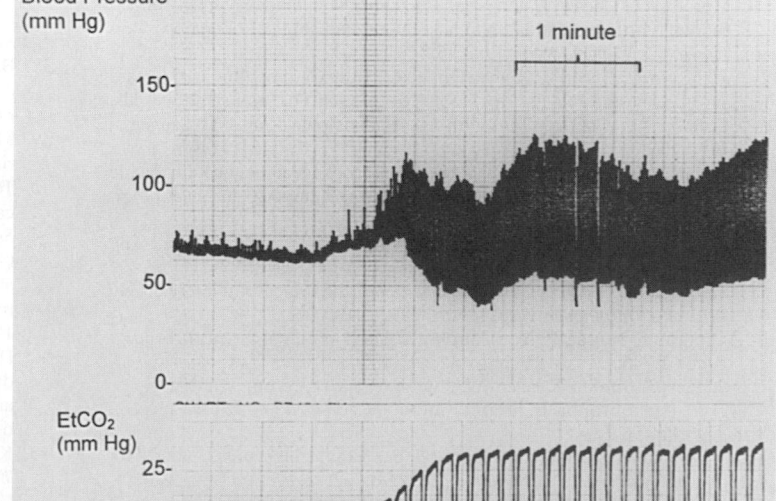

**FIGURE 17–17.** Arterial tracing and end-tidal $CO_2$ ($P_{ETCO_2}$) curves during weaning from cardiopulmonary bypass. The $P_{ETCO_2}$ curve can be used as a gross indicator of cardiac output during weaning.

- Observe the surgical field when reexpanding the lungs. Even with the pleurae intact, it is often possible to determine if both lungs are inflating. Also make sure that the lungs do not overexpand and distort an internal mammary artery graft or compress the heart.

- Once weaning from CPB is attempted, a flat PA tracing when the patient has a pulsatile arterial tracing suggests that the PA catheter is in a wedged position. The PA catheter should be withdrawn until a PA tracing is obtained.

- As cardiac output and blood flow increase, the exhaled $CO_2$ increases toward normal values (Fig. 17–17). Failure of the exhaled $CO_2$ curve to rise may be an early indication of poor cardiac output, although problems such as endotracheal tube displacement or a kinked sampling line should also be considered.

- Even though maneuvers to remove air from the heart are done before weaning, air removal is only partial until substantial blood is flowing through the pulmonary circulation. Be prepared for air removal during weaning and halt weaning if abrupt ST segment elevation suggestive of coronary air embolism is noted on the ECG.

## References

1. Lillehei C. Controlled cross circulation for direct-vision intracardiac surgery: correction of ventricular septal defects, atrioventricularis communis and tetralogy of Fallot. *Postgrad Med.* 1955;17:388.

2. Gibbon JJ, Dobell A, Voigt G, et al. The closure of interventricular septal defects in dogs during open cardiotomy with the maintenance of cardio-respiratory functions by a pump oxygenator. *J Thorac Surg.* 1954;28:235.

3. Shaw B, Martin D, Marquez J, et al. Venous bypass in clinical liver transplantation. *Ann Surg.* 1984;200:524.

4. Griffith B, Byers W, Hardesty R, et al. Venovenous bypass without systemic anticoagulation for transplantation of the human liver. *Surg Gynecol Obstet.* 1985;160:270.

5. Pearson D. Bubble and membrane oxygenators. *Semin Thorac Cardiovasc Surg.* 1990;2:213.

6. van Oeveren W, Kazatchkine M, Descamps-Latscha B, et al. Deleterious effects of cardiopulmonary bypass: a prospective study of bubble versus membrane oxygenation. *J Thorac Cardiovasc Surg.* 1985;89:888.

7. Stammers A. Extracorporeal devices and related technologies. In: Kaplan JA, Reich DL, Konstadt SN, eds. *Cardiac Anesthesia.* Vol 1. 4th ed. Philadelphia, Pa: WB Saunders; 1999:1017.

8. Katz E, Tunick P, Rusinek H, et al. Protruding aortic atheromas predict stroke in elderly patients undergoing cardiopulmonary bypass: experience with intraoperative transesophageal echocardiography. *J Am Coll Cardiol.* 1992;20:70.

9. Murphy D, Craver J, Jones E. Recognition and management of ascending aortic dissection complicating cardiac surgical operations. *Ann Thorac Cardiovasc Surg.* 1983;85:247.

10. Mangano CM, Hill L, Cartwright CR, et al. Cardiopulmonary bypass and the anesthesiologist. In: Kaplan JA, Reich DL, Konstadt SN, eds. *Cardiac Anesthesia.* Vol 1. 4th ed. Philadelphia, Pa: WB Saunders; 1999:1061.

11. Troianos C, Savino J, Weiss R. Transesophageal echocardiographic diagnosis of aortic dissection during cardiac surgery. *Anesthesiology.* 1991;75:149.

12. Ross W, Lake C, Wellons H. Cardiopulmonary bypass complicated by inadvertent carotid cannulation. *Anesthesiology.* 1981;54:85.

13. Sudhaman D. Accidental hyperperfusion of the left carotid artery during CPB. *J Cardiothorac Vasc Anesth.* 1991;5:100.

14. Chapin J, Nance P, Yarbrough J. Facial paleness. *Anesth Analg.* 1982;61:745.

15. Stevens J, Burdon T, Peters W, et al. Port-access coronary artery bypass grafting: a proposed surgical method. *J Thorac Cardiovasc Surg.* 1996;111:567.

16. Siegel L, St Goar F, Stevens J, et al. Monitoring considerations for port-access surgery. *Circulation.* 1997;96:562.

17. Fann J, Pompili M, Stevens J, et al. Port-access cardiac operations with cardioplegic arrest. *Ann Thorac Surg.* 1997;63:S35.

18. Warkentin T, Kelton J. Heparin and platelets. *Hematol Oncol Clin North Am.* 1990;4:243.

19. Levy J, Pifarre R, Schaff H, et al. A multicenter, double-blind, placebo-controlled trial of aprotinin for reducing blood loss and the requirements for donor-blood transfusion in patients undergoing repeat coronary artery bypass grafting. *Circulation.* 1995;92:2236.

20. Lemmer JJ, Stanford W, Bonney S, et al. Aprotinin for coronary bypass operations: efficacy, safety and influence on early saphenous vein graft patency. A multicenter, randomized, double-blind, placebo controlled study. *J Thorac Cardiovasc Surg.* 1994;107:543.

21. Dietrich W, Barankay A, Hahnel C, et al. High-dose aprotinin in cardiac surgery: three years' experience in 1,784 patients. *J Cardiothorac Vasc Anesth.* 1992;6:324.

22. Royston D. High-dose aprotinin therapy: a review of the first five years' experience. *J Cardiothorac Vasc Anesth.* 1992;6:76.

23. Manucci P. Drug therapy: hemostatic drugs. *N Engl J Med.* 1998;339:245.

24. Dietrich W, Spathe P, Ebell A, et al. Prevalence of anaphylactic reactions to aprotinin: analysis of two hundred forty-eight reexposures to aprotinin in heart operations. *J Thorac Cardiovasc Surg.* 1997;113:194.

25. Feindt P, Seyfert U, Volkmer I, et al. Celite and kaolin produce differing activated clotting times during cardiopulmonary bypass under aprotinin therapy. *J Thoracic Cardiovasc Surg.* 1994;42:218.

26. Levy J, Schwieger I, Zaidan J. Evaluation of patients at risk for protamine reactions. *J Thorac Cardiovasc Surg.* 1989;98:200.

27. Horrow J. Protamine allergy. *J Cardiothorac Vasc Anesth.* 1988;2:225.

28. Bazaral M, Welch M, Golding L, et al. Comparison of brachial and radial arterial pressure monitoring in patients undergoing coronary artery bypass surgery. *Anesthesiology.* 1990;73:38.

29. Baba T, Goto T, Yoshitake A, et al. Radial artery diameter decreases with increased femoral to radial arterial pressure gradient during cardiopulmonary bypass. *Anesth Analg.* 1997;85:252.

30. Rich G, Lubanski R, McLoughlin T. Differences between aortic and radial artery pressure associated with cardiopulmonary bypass. *Anesthesiology.* 1992;77:63.

31. Pauca A, Wallenhaupt S, Kon N. Reliability of the radial arterial pressure during anesthesia: is wrist compression a possible diagnostic test? *Chest.* 1994;105:69.

32. Stone JG, Young WL, Smith CR, et al. Do standard monitoring sites reflect true brain temperature when profound hypothermia is rapidly induced and reversed? *Anesthesiology.* 1995;82:344.

33. Horrow JC, Rosenberg H. Does urinary catheter temperature reflect core temperature during cardiac surgery? *Anesthesiology.* 1988;69:986.

34. Buckberg G, Brazier J, Nelson R, et al. Studies of the effect of hypothermia on regional myocardial blood flow and metabolism during cardiopulmonary bypass, I: the adequately perfused beating, fibrillating and arrested heart. *J Thorac Cardiovasc Surg.* 1977;73:87.

35. Gordon R, Ravin M, Rawitscher R, et al. Changes in arterial pressure, viscosity and resistance during cardiopulmonary bypass. *J Thorac Cardiovasc Surg.* 1975;69:552.

36. Slogoff S, Girgis K, Keats A. Etiologic factors in neuropsychiatric complications associated with cardiopulmonary bypass. *Anesth Analg.* 1982;61:903.

37. Slogoff S, Reul G, Keats A, et al. Role of perfusion pressure and flow in major organ dysfunction after cardiopulmonary bypass. *Ann Thorac Surg.* 1990;50:911.

38. Bashein G, Townes B, Nessly M, et al. A randomized study of carbon dioxide management during hypothermic cardiopulmonary bypass. *Anesthesiology.* 1990;72:7.

39. McKann G, Goldsborough M, Borowicz L Jr, et al. Predictors of stroke risk in coronary artery bypass patients. *Ann Thorac Surg.* 1997;63:516.

40. Townes B, Bashein G, Hornbein T, et al. Neurobehavioral outcomes in cardiac operations: a prospective controlled study. *J Thorac Cardiovasc Surg.* 1989;98:774.

41. Gold J, Charlson M, Williams-Russo P, et al. Improvement of outcomes after coronary artery bypass: a randomized trial comparing intraoperative high versus low mean arterial pressure. *J Thorac Cardiovasc Surg.* 1995;110:1302.

42. Hartman G, Yao F, Bruefach M, et al. Severity of aortic atheromatous disease diagnosed by transesophageal echocardiography predicts stroke and other outcomes associated with coronary artery surgery: a prospective study. *Anesthesiology.* 1996;83:701.

43. Keats A, Slogoff S. Perfusion pressure and coronary bypass [letter]. *J Thorac Cardiovasc Surg.* 1996;112:204.

44. Cartwright CR, Mangano CM. Con: during cardiopulmonary bypass for elective coronary artery bypass grafting, perfusion pressure should not

routinely be greater than 70 mm Hg. *J Cardiothorac Vasc Anesth.* 1998;12:361.

45. Murkin J, Farrar J, Tweed WA, et al. Cerebral autoregulation and flow/metabolism coupling during cardiopulmonary bypass: the influence of $PaCO_2$. *Anesth Analg.* 1987;66:825.

46. Aladj L, Croughwell N, Smith L, et al. Cerebral blood flow autoregulation is preserved during cardiopulmonary bypass in isoflurane-anesthetized patients. *Anesth Analg.* 1991;76:48.

47. Schell R, Kern FH, Greeley WJ, et al. Cerebral blood flow and metabolism during cardiopulmonary bypass. *Anesth Analg.* 1993;76:849.

48. Shaw P, Bates D, Cartilidge N, et al. Long-term intellectual dysfunction following coronary artery bypass graft surgery: a six-month followup study. *QJM.* 1987;62:259.

49. Williams W, Davtyan H, Drazanova M. Hypothermia, cardiac surgery and cardiopulmonary bypass. In: Mora C, ed. *Cardiopulmonary Bypass: Principles and Techniques of Extracorporeal Circulation.* Vol 1. New York, NY: Springer-Verlag; 1995:40.

50. Wong B, McLean R, Naylor C, et al. Central nervous system dysfunction following warm and hypothermic cardiopulmonary bypass. *Lancet.* 1992;339:1383.

51. Cook D. Changing temperature management for cardiopulmonary bypass. *Anesth Analg.* 1999;88:1254.

52. Martin T, Craver J, Gott J, et al. Prospective, randomized trial of retrograde warm-blood cardioplegia: myocardial benefit and neurologic threat. *Ann Thorac Surg.* 1994;57:298.

53. Mora C, Henson M, Weintraub W, et al. The effect of temperature management during cardiopulmonary bypass on neurologic and neuropsychologic outcomes in patients undergoing coronary revascularization. *J Thorac Cardiovasc Surg.* 1996;112:514.

54. Rajek A, Lenhardt R, Sessler D, et al. Tissue heat content and distribution during and after cardiopulmonary bypass at 17°C. *Anesth Analg.* 1999;88:1220.

55. Wan S, LeClerc J, Vincent J. Inflammatory response to cardiopulmonary bypass: mechanisms involved and possible therapeutic strategies. *Chest.* 1997;112:676.

56. Nilsson L, Kulander L, Sven-Olov N, et al. Endotoxins in cardiopulmonary bypass. *J Thorac Cardiovasc Surg.* 1990;100:770.

57. Hall R, Smith M, Rocker G. The systemic inflammatory response to CPB. *Anesth Analg.* 1997;85:766.

58. Engelman R, Rousou J, Flack JE 3rd, et al. Influence of steroids on complement and cytokine generation after cardiopulmonary bypass. *Ann Thorac Surg.* 1995;60:801.

59. Hill G, Alonso A, Thiele G, et al. Glucocorticoids blunt neutrophil CD11b surface glycoprotein upregulation during cardiopulmonary bypass. *Anesth Analg.* 1995;79:23.

60. Chaney M, Nikolov P, Blakeman B, et al. Hemodynamic effects of methylprednisolone in patients undergoing cardiac operation and early extubation. *Ann Thorac Surg.* 1999;67:1006.

61. Ranucci M, Massucco A, Pessotto R, et al. Heparin-coated circuits for high-risk patients: a multicenter, prospective, randomized trial. *Ann Thorac Surg.* 1999;67:994.

62. Gu Y, Oeveren W, Akkerman C, et al. Heparin-coated circuits reduce the inflammatory response to cardiopulmonary bypass. *Ann Thorac Surg.* 1993;55:917.

63. Videm V, Svennig J, Fosse E, et al. Reduced complement activation with heparin-coated oxygenator and tubings in coronary bypass operations. *J Thorac Cardiovasc Surg.* 1992;103:806.

64. Boroweic J, Thelin S, Bagge L, et al. Heparin-coated circuits reduce activation of granulocytes during cardiopulmonary bypass. *J Thorac Cardiovasc Surg.* 1992;104:642.

65. Hill G, Pohorecki R, Alonso A, et al. Aprotinin reduces interleukin-8 production and lung neutrophil accumulation after cardiopulmonary bypass. *Anesth Analg.* 1996;83:696.

66. Mollhoff T, Loick H, Van Aken H, et al. Milrinone modulates endotoxemia, systemic inflammation, and subsequent acute phase response after cardiopulmonary bypass (CPB). *Anesthesiology.* 1999;90:72.

67. Bauernschmitt R, Lange R, Mehmanesh H, et al. Immunomodulatory effects of perioperative antibiotic therapy in patients undergoing cardiopulmonary bypass. *Cardiovasc Eng.* 1999;4:3.

68. Picone A, Lutz C, Finck C, et al. Multiple sequential insults cause postpump syndrome. *Ann Thorac Surg.* 1999;67:978.

69. Reeves J, Karp R, Buttner E, et al. Neuronal and adrenomedullary catecholamine release in response to cardiopulmonary bypass in man. *Circulation.* 1982;66:49.

70. Philbin D, Levine F, Kono K. Attenuation of the stress response to cardiopulmonary bypass by the addition of pulsatile flow. *Circulation.* 1981;64:808.

71. Brade H, Cheema-Dhadli S, Mazer CD, et al. Hyperglycemia during normothermic cardiopulmonary bypass: the role of the kidney. *Ann Thorac Surg.* 1998;65:1588.

72. Lanier W. Glucose management during cardiopulmonary bypass: cardiovascular and neurologic implications. *Anesth Analg.* 1991;72:423.

73. Reinhardt W, Mocker V, Jockenhovel F, et al. Influence of coronary artery bypass surgery on thyroid hormone parameters. *Horm Res.* 1997;47:1.

74. Broderick TJ, Wechsler AS. Triiodothyronine in cardiac surgery. *Thyroid.* 1997;7:133.

75. Bennett-Guerrero E, Jimenez JL, White WD, et al. Cardiovascular effects of intravenous triiodothyronine in patients undergoing coronary artery bypass graft surgery: a randomized, double-blind, placebo-controlled trial. Duke T3 Study Group [see comments]. *JAMA.* 1996;275:687.

76. Reeves R. An imidazole alphastat hypothesis for vertebrate acid-base regulation: tissue carbon dioxide content and body temperature in bullfrogs. *Respir Physiol.* 1972;14:219.

77. Wollman H, Stephan G, Clement A, et al. Cerebral blood flow in man during extracorporeal circulation. *J Thorac Cardiovasc Surg.* 1966;52:558.

78. Henriksen L. Brain luxury perfusion during cardiopulmonary bypass in humans: a study of the cerebral blood flow response to changes in $CO_2$, $O_2$ and blood pressure. *J Cereb Blood Flow Metab.* 1986;6:366.

79. Prough D, Stump D, Roy R, et al. Response of cerebral blood flow to changes in carbon dioxide tension during hypothermic cardiopulmonary bypass. *Anesthesiology.* 1986;64:576.

80. Murkin J, Martzke J, Buchanan A, et al. A randomized study of the influence of perfusion technique and pH management strategy in 316 patients undergoing coronary artery bypass surgery. *J Thorac Cardiovasc Surg.* 1995;110:349.

81. Engelhardt W, Dierks T, Pause M, et al. Early cerebral functional outcome after coronary artery bypass surgery using different acid-base management during hypothermic cardiopulmonary bypass. *Acta Anaesthesiol Scand.* 1996;40:457.

82. Pua HL, Bissonnette B. Cerebral physiology in paediatric cardiopulmonary bypass. *Can J Anaesth.* 1998;45:960.

83. Kurth C, O'Rourke M, O'Hara I. Comparison of pH-stat and alpha-stat cardiopulmonary bypass on cerebral oxygenation and blood flow in relation to hypothermic circulatory arrest in piglets. *Anesthesiology.* 1998;89:110.

84. Hindman B. Choice of alpha-stat or pH-stat management and neurologic outcomes after cardiac surgery. *Anesthesiology.* 1998;89:5.

85. Gruber EM, Jonas RA, Newburger JW, et al. The effect of hematocrit on cerebral blood flow velocity in neonates and infants undergoing deep hypothermic cardiopulmonary bypass. *Anesth Analg.* 1999;89:322.

86. Cook DJ, Orszulak TA, Daly RC. Minimum hematocrit at differing cardiopulmonary bypass temperatures in dogs. *Circulation.* 1998;98(19 suppl):II170.

87. Busch T, Sirbu H, Aleksic I, et al. Anterior ischemic optic neuropathy: a complication after extracorporal circulation. *Ann Thorac Cardiovasc Surg.* 1998;4:354.

88. Shapira OM, Kimmel WA, Lindsey PS, et al. Anterior ischemic optic neuropathy after open heart operations. *Ann Thorac Surg.* 1996;61:660.

89. Magnusson L, Zemgulis V, Wicky S, et al. Effect of CPAP during cardiopulmonary bypass on postoperative lung function: an experimental study. *Acta Anaesthesiol Scand.* 1998;42:1133.

90. Gilbert TB, Barnas GM, Sequeira AJ. Impact of pleurotomy, continuous positive airway pressure, and fluid balance during cardiopulmonary bypass on lung mechanics and oxygenation. *J Cardiothorac Vasc Anesth.* 1996;10:844.

91. Cogliati AA, Menichetti A, Tritapepe L, et al. Effects of three techniques of lung management on pulmonary function during cardiopulmonary bypass. *Acta Anaesthesiol Belg.* 1996;47:73.

92. Rady M, Ryan T, Starr N. Early onset of acute pulmonary dysfunction after cardiovascular surgery: risk factors and clinical outcome. *Crit Care Med.* 1997;25:1831.

93. Weissman C. Pulmonary function after cardiac and thoracic surgery. *Anesth Analg.* 1999;88:1272.

94. Roach G, Kanchuger M, Mangano CM, et al. Adverse cerebral outcomes after coronary bypass surgery. *N Engl J Med.* 1996;335:1857.

95. Wolman RL, Nussmeier NA, Aggarwal A, et al. Cerebral injury after cardiac surgery: identification of a group at extraordinary risk. Multicenter Study of Perioperative Ischemia Research Group (McSPI) and the Ischemia Research Education Foundation (IREF) Investigators. *Stroke.* 1999;30:514.

96. Ahlgren E, Aren C. Cerebral complications after coronary artery bypass

and heart valve surgery: risk factors and onset of symptoms. *J Cardiothorac Vasc Anesth.* 1998;12:270.

97. Rolfson DB, McElhaney JE, Rockwood K, et al. Incidence and risk factors for delirium and other adverse outcomes in older adults after coronary artery bypass graft surgery. *Can J Cardiol.* 1999;15:771.

98. Martzke J, Murkin J, Buchanan A. A prospective survey of cognitive function following coronary artery bypass (CAB). *J Clin Exp Neuropsychol.* 1991;14:A60.

99. Libman RB, Wirkowski E, Neystat M, et al. Stroke associated with cardiac surgery: determinants, timing, and stroke subtypes. *Arch Neurol.* 1997;54:83.

100. Brooker RF, Brown WR, Moody DM, et al. Cardiotomy suction: a major source of brain lipid emboli during cardiopulmonary bypass. *Ann Thorac Surg.* 1998;65:1651.

101. Bar-El Y, Goor D. Clamping of the atherosclerotic ascending aorta during coronary artery bypass operations: its cost in strokes. *J Thorac Cardiovasc Surg.* 1992;104:469.

102. Taggart DP, Bhattacharya K, Meston N, et al. Serum S-100 protein concentration after cardiac surgery: a randomized trial of arterial line filtration. *Eur J Cardiothorac Surg.* 1997;11:645.

103. Hogue CW Jr, Murphy SF, Schechtman KB, et al. Risk factors for early or delayed stroke after cardiac surgery. *Circulation.* 1999;100:642.

104. Davila-Roman VG, Phillips KJ, Daily BB, et al. Intraoperative transesophageal echocardiography and epiaortic ultrasound for assessment of atherosclerosis of the thoracic aorta. *J Am Coll Cardiol.* 1996;28:942.

105. Rokkas CK, Kouchoukos NT. Surgical management of the severely atherosclerotic ascending aorta during cardiac operations. *Semin Thorac Cardiovasc Surg.* 1998;10:240.

106. Nussmeier N, Arlund C, Slogoff S. Neuropsychiatric complications after cardiopulmonary bypass: cerebral protection by a barbiturate. *Anesthesiology.* 1986;64:165.

107. Zaidan J, Klochany A, Martin W, et al. Effect of thiopental on neurologic outcome following coronary artery bypass grafting. *Anesthesiology.* 1991;74:406.

108. Roach G, Newman M, Murkin J, et al. Ineffectiveness of burst suppression therapy in mitigating perioperative cerebrovascular dysfunction. *Anesthesiology.* 1999;90:1255.

109. Pascoe EA, Hudson RJ, Anderson BA, et al. High-dose thiopentone for open-chamber cardiac surgery: a retrospective review. *Can J Anaesth.* 1996;43:575.

110. Mori A, Watanabe K, Onoe M. Regional blood flow in the liver, pancreas and kidney during cardiopulmonary bypass. *Arch Surg.* 1988;124:458.

111. Mangano CM, Diamondstone L, Ramsay J, et al. Renal dysfunction after myocardial revascularization: risk factors, adverse outcomes, and hospital resource utilization. *Ann Intern Med.* 1998;128:194.

112. Llopart T, Lombardi R, Forselledo M, et al. Acute renal failure in open heart surgery. *Ren Fail.* 1997;19:319.

113. Chertow GM, Lazarus JM, Christiansen CL, et al. Preoperative renal risk stratification. *Circulation.* 1997;95:878.

114. Carcoana OV, Hines RL. Is renal dose dopamine protective or therapeutic? Yes. *Crit Care Clin.* 1996;12:677.

115. Singer I, Ebstein M. Potential of dopamine A-1 agonists in the management of acute renal failure. *Am J Kidney Dis.* 1998;31:743.

116. Chertow GM, Levy EM, Hammermeister KE, et al. Independent association between acute renal failure and mortality following cardiac surgery. *Am J Med.* 1998;104:343.

117. Meyer M, Wiebe K, Wahlers T, et al. Urodilatin (INN:ularitide) as a new drug for the therapy of acute renal failure following cardiac surgery. *Clin Exp Pharmacol Physiol.* 1997;24:374.

118. Valsson F, Ricksten SE, Hedner T, et al. Effects of atrial natriuretic peptide on acute renal impairment in patients with heart failure after cardiac surgery. *Intensive Care Med.* 1996;22:230.

119. Meyer M, Uberbacher HJ, Bohm E, et al. Ularitide: from renal natriuretic peptide to clinical trials. *Curr Opin Nephrol Hypertens.* 1996;5:364.

120. Michelsen L, Shanewise J. Discontinuation of cardiopulmonary bypass. In: Mora C, ed. *Cardiopulmonary Bypass: Principles and Techniques of Extracorporeal Circulation.* Vol 1. New York, NY: Springer-Verlag; 1995:281.

# Monitors and Their Applications

CHAPTER

## 18

# Introduction to Monitoring: Clinical Monitoring

### Joachim S. Gravenstein

## HISTORICAL CONSIDERATIONS

### Why Monitor Without Instruments?

Anesthesiology pioneers monitored ventilation, circulation, and skin color without the help of instruments. Then, one by one, monitoring instruments appeared, but often they were adopted only years after they had become available. Sphygmomanometers and thermometers only enhanced the qualitative clinical judgment by adding quantitative assessments; others captured data that escaped the human senses, such as the electrocardiogram (ECG), electroencephalogram, and analyses of physiologic gases.

In many parts of the world, thousands of anesthetics are still administered daily without the help of modern anesthesia machines, ventilators, and monitoring instruments. Every expert in the field, however accustomed to advanced instrumentation, should be able to do as well as those forced to work without the help of modern tools. The requisite clinical skills must be practiced. Skills to care for a patient in the most primitive of circumstances may be required in an emergency in which no instruments are available.

Even with all currently used instruments, clinical skills still make the difference in outcome for some patients. Two examples illustrate this. In the first example, a pneumothorax develops in a patient, perhaps spontaneously, without provocation. No currently used instrument routinely available in the operating room can make the diagnosis, but inspection, palpation, and auscultation will. In the second example, inspection of face and eyes shows venous congestion in case of obstruction of veins draining the head. No current, routinely used instrument can make that diagnosis.

## UNDERLYING CONCEPTS

### What Are the Principal Objectives Served by Monitoring? (Is There a Sixth Sense in Monitoring?)

Experienced clinicians appear to have an intuition or sixth sense for perceiving trouble. They may identify a problem well before it becomes obvious. That sixth sense deserves continual cultivation. This sense is not limited to the changes in vital signs of the patient but extends to the entire clinical process, whether a surgical operation or a diagnostic procedure under anesthesia. We pick up important information, often difficult to put into words, by watching the body language of the operator and the way in which the surgical team cooperates, by assessing the available resources, and by judging the expertise brought to bear. The skills to evaluate these clues are not taught in training programs. There is, however, no doubt that with experience, clinicians develop a sixth sense that helps in detecting and possibly deflecting problems before they cause harm to the patient.

## What Is the Monitoring Routine?

Today, as was the case a century and a half ago, all monitoring starts with inspection, auscultation, and palpation—that is, with the clinical assessment of the patient. This routine continues to come first because many clinical signs are subtle, and as yet no instruments exist that can detect them.

### Titration

We titrate the effects of anesthetic and adjuvant drugs, such as a muscle relaxant, or adjust the ventilator to a desired end-tidal carbon dioxide tension. If patients' responses to drugs were predictable, we could dose all medications in milligrams per kilogram per unit time, and titration would not be necessary.

### Safety

We look for unexpected perturbations of vital functions before a patient suffers harm—for example, from hypotension when the surgeon compresses the vena cava or from hypotension and hypoxia when a pneumothorax affects circulation and ventilation.

### Equipment Function

We monitor equipment function because malfunction can cause injury—for example, from an occluded scavenger system or when a gas other than oxygen ($O_2$) comes through the oxygen flow meter.

## In What Order Should We Sample Monitored Data?

Monitoring can be pursued according to a geographic or a conceptual approach. Both have proponents.

### Geographic Approach

The geographic approach calls for scanning of all variables in a predetermined sequence, such as starting with a patient's left hand, which might carry a pulse oximeter probe; working up the arm and checking the intravenous site; auscultating across the chest for breath and heart sounds; progressing to the other arm to measure blood pressure (BP); and moving

**TABLE 18–1.** Monitoring Variables*

| Ventilation | Circulation |
| --- | --- |
| Gas supply | Patient's color (perfusion) |
| Gas flow rates | Skin (pale, vasoconstricted) |
| Inspired gas concentrations | Mucous membranes/wound |
|   Oxygen | Appearance of skin (moist/dry) |
|   Carbon dioxide (system | Heart sounds |
|     OK?) | Arterial pressure |
|   Anesthetic vapors | Venous pressure |
| Peak inspiratory pressures |   Neck veins |
| End-expiratory pressures |   Other veins |
| Bellows or bag excursions | Electrocardiogram (rate and rhythm) |
| Tidal volume | Pulse oximeter saturation (plethysmogram) |
| Respiratory rate | Capnogram (pulmonary circulation) |
| Expired gas concentrations | Urine output |
| Patient's color | Cerebral perfusion |
| Chest excursion |   Conscious → orientation |
| Patterns of breathing |   Unconscious |
| Breath sounds |   Pupils |
| Pulse oximeter saturation | Electroencephalogram, evoked potentials |

*Grouped according to the conceptual approach and combining clinical observation and use of instruments.

down to the wrist of the right hand to the nerve stimulator. An alternative geographic sequence calls for scanning the instruments from one side to the other, regardless of their physiologic relationship.

### Conceptual Approach

The conceptual approach, in contradistinction, calls for assessment of variables according to physiologic systems. The practitioner may start with ventilation, which in most patients under general anesthesia includes the system that brings gases to the patient, and then move to the circulation (Table 18–1). Other systems can be added, including neuromuscular integrity (the feel of the bag or the peak inspiratory pressure, how relaxed the muscles are in the surgical field, and the response to nerve stimulation) or metabolic variables such as control of blood sugar or regulation of electrolytes and pH.

The conceptual system has intellectual appeal because a clinician thinks in terms of concepts and systems rather than individual variables. Ideally, the geographic and the conceptual system should merge—that is, monitoring instruments should be arranged according to concepts rather than by dint of their size and their ability to fit in this or that empty hole on the anesthesia machine. The following discussion adopts the conceptual approach.

## BASIC MONITORING WITHOUT INSTRUMENTS (OTHER THAN A STETHOSCOPE)

First we address the basics: monitoring without instruments, which is essential and continuous yet is the least expensive of all monitoring approaches. According to the *Oxford English Dictionary*, both *continual* and *continuous* have been used to mean "incessant, perpetual, without intermission." However, the word *continual* is sometimes used to describe actions that are repeated with brief intermissions. The American Society of Anesthesiologists has embraced the latter definition of *continual* (see Appendix), and reserves the word *continuous* for actions without interruption.

## How Should Conscious Patients Be Monitored?

If patients are awake; oriented to person, time, and place; and can answer questions, their brains are adequately perfused and oxygenated and cerebral metabolism is within acceptable limits. Talking with conscious patients is the best monitor. It reassures patients and represents good clinical practice. As long as the brain receives adequate blood and $O_2$, we may assume that other organs are adequately perfused and that BP is satisfactory. Remember, however, that in anemic patients, the heart with its high $O_2$ extraction may be at greater risk than the brain. Myocardial oxygenation may be impaired secondary to low perfusion or low arterial $O_2$ content, particularly in patients with heart disease. Maintain contact with the patient to assess cerebral function, but do not forget the heart. Good care of the conscious patient includes frequently touching the patient to feel the pulse, mop a brow, or adjust a pillow, drape, or blanket. Patients are justifiably anxious. Concern shown by the clinician and the human touch go a long way toward lessening anxiety.

## Ventilation

If the patient is dozing or sleeping, make sure that ventilation remains adequate. Remember that even in light-skinned patients, cyanosis is a late and unreliable sign of deoxygenation.[1] Table 18–2 includes data from an old study that is still valid. Of course, pulse oximetry can be enormously helpful in the early detection of respiratory problems *provided* the patient is not breathing more $O_2$ than found in room air. When $O_2$ is given, the patient's respiration may be depressed, $PaCO_2$ may rise, yet the pulse oximeter may continue to report good oxygenation. Under those circumstances, respiratory depression can be missed for some time. In particular, when giving $O_2$, monitor the breathing pattern.

### Pattern of Breathing

During normal sleep, healthy people breathe so quietly that inspiration and expiration are barely discernible. Any deviation from a peaceful, regular, and smooth pattern of breathing must raise questions. Such deviations typically occur in a progression, from the most subtle signs in patients minimally affected by disease or weakness to grossly obvious manifestations of severe respiratory impairment. The signs of breathing discussed in the following sections are ranked from subtle to obvious. The anesthesiologist should make it a habit to check for abnormal signs. If none is detected, so much the better. Attempts to bring modern monitoring instruments and methods of analysis to bear on this meet a number of hurdles, among them the fact that the introduction of spirometry, as benign as it is, does change the pattern of breathing.[2]

**Respiratory Rate.** You may have to listen to breath sounds, for example in the jugular notch, or put your hand on the patient's epigastrium to count respirations. Fewer than 12 breaths per minute in an adult should raise questions. With central depression of ventilation brought about by narcotics, the breathing pattern may be unremarkable, but a slow respiratory rate often shows the effects of narcosis. However, a slow respiratory rate (ie, <8 breaths per minute) is not an absolute indication of respiratory depression and often is inadequate for assessment. The lowering of a respiratory rate from 16 to 20 breaths per minute to 10 to 14 breaths per minute may be a more important indication of impending respiratory depression than is a specific, low respiratory rate.[3]

**Abdominal Motion.** With quiet ventilation in a healthy subject, abdominal motion is barely noticeable. In distressed patients, the abdomen may rise during inspiration. During expiration, the muscles of the abdomen may tighten. That pattern is typically observed in patients with obstructive pulmonary disease. Because of obstruction and the loss of elastic recoil of the lungs, these patients must exhale actively using accessory muscles of respiration.

It is easy to imagine what happens when such a patient's abdominal muscles are paralyzed, such as during spinal or epidural anesthesia. Active expiration is impossible, and a patient is unable to exhale fully. The functional residual capacity is likely to increase. A desperate situation can arise in asthmatic patients, in whom a high epidural or spinal anesthetic blocks not only the abdominal muscles but the sympathetics without inhibiting the vagus innervation, resulting in greater vulnerability to bronchial constriction.

**Chest Motion.** Healthy patients, breathing quietly, show little motion of the chest. During inspiration, the chest may rise slightly and symmetrically. Tightening of the intercostal muscles during inspiration cannot be seen. However, when the intercostal muscles are paralyzed and a patient is inhaling forcefully, the intercostal spaces may retract, together with the jugular area just above the sternum. This is most noticeable in children and cachectic patients. In thin, spontaneously breathing patients, intercostal retraction is helpful in identifying the level of a spinal or epidural block.

In spontaneously breathing patients who have upper airway obstruction or are weakened by neuromuscular disease, the chest may show a paradoxical motion, the so-called rocking of the boat. The upper anterior chest sinks instead of rising during inspiration, while the abdomen rises.

**Breath Sounds.** That we can and will listen to the breath sounds goes without saying. These sounds should be of equal quality on the left and right. In children, breath sounds are easy to hear, regardless of where the stethoscope is applied. In adults, the loudest sounds are heard over the trachea in the suprasternal notch, where air passes by with great velocity during each breath. There, we can also hear if a patient swallows, gags, or retches and if, once he or she is intubated and mechanically ventilated, the cuff on the endotracheal tube leaks. The patient's chest should be auscultated in front and laterally on both sides. In the recumbent patient, beginning pulmonary edema may be heard better in the posterior axillary line than anteriorly. We care for many patients with a history

**TABLE 18–2.** Percentage of Observers Who Detected Cyanosis in White Men

| $PaO_2$ | No Cyanosis | Slight Cyanosis | Definite Cyanosis |
|---|---|---|---|
| 100–96 | 68 | 26 | 6 |
| 95–91 | 43 | 40 | 17 |
| 90–86 | 32 | 37 | 31 |
| 85–81 | 14 | 37 | 49 |
| 80–76 | 10 | 40 | 50 |
| 75–71 | 3 | 22 | 75 |

From Comroe JH Jr, Botelho S. The unreliability of cyanosis in the recognition of arterial anoxemia. *Am J Med Sci.* 1947;214:1.

of wheezing. Make sure wheezing does not worsen after the administration of drugs such as antibiotics or narcotics or other drugs that may release histamine.

## Circulation

### Perfusion

I like to inspect a patient's palpebral conjunctiva. My impression is that it turns pale early in hypovolemia and anemia and that it is less likely to be blanched by vasoconstriction than are the nail beds. Check it before starting anesthesia and whenever questions about hypovolemia or anemia arise.

### Cardiac Function

Auscultation of breath and heart sounds with a precordial stethoscope is routine in some centers and, unfortunately, is being abandoned in others. No other instrument ties the clinician to his or her patient, costs less, is less likely to fail, and offers breath-by-breath and beat-by-beat data better than the precordial stethoscope.

The first heart sound is produced by vibration of the taut atrioventricular valves, the second by vibration of the semilunar valves. In addition, vibrations of the ventricular wall and, for the second sound, the walls of the aorta and pulmonary artery contribute to the heart sounds. Thus, whenever the contractile force of the heart decreases and BP falls, the vibrations diminish and the heart sounds become muffled.

Of course, in addition to characterizing the heart sounds, auscultation gives continuous information about heart rate and, to a degree, rhythm. Explore where the heart sounds are heard best. Sometimes, in obese and emphysematous patients, the suprasternal notch also transmits heart sounds more clearly than does the precordium.

## How Should Anesthetized Patients Be Monitored?

### Ventilation

Is a patient getting $O_2$? If the pulse oximeter oxygen saturation ($SpO_2$) drops or the patient turns blue, it makes little sense to start fretting over ventilation, shunts, alveolar dead space, and the like when the problem all along is the supply of $O_2$. Therefore, first make sure that $O_2$ is available to the patient. Your checklist (you could be modern and call it an *algorithm*) should be as follows:

$O_2$ Flow Meter $\rightarrow$ Inspired $O_2$ Concentration $\rightarrow$ Ventilation

That inspection should require <10 seconds; then proceed.

### Inspection and Palpation: The Tracheal Tug

During normal ventilation in healthy people, the larynx does not move. With beginning emphysema and in patients with muscle weakness, mild respiratory obstruction, or processes that interfere with normal gas exchange, such as pneumonia, the larynx moves down a little with every inspiration. If the reader is young and healthy, he or she should now put a hand over his or her larynx and observe the lack of motion with normal ventilation. Now take a rapid, gasping deep breath and feel how the larynx moves down during inspiration; that is a tracheal tug.

Check your patient before starting anesthesia. If no tracheal tug is felt, the patient should not have one after recovery from anesthesia. If one develops, search for an explanation. The most common causes are muscle relaxant "hangover," with weakening of the respiratory muscles; partial obstruction of the upper airway; and atelectasis. Patients with lung disease exhibit a postoperative tracheal tug with little provocation. They are the very patients likely to have respiratory complications.

Tracheal tugs can be so subtle that the clinician cannot discern them by inspection, particularly in obese patients with a short neck. Put your hand over the larynx or place three fingers along the larynx and trachea and feel for the tug. Do this before starting anesthesia and again before leaving a patient in the postanesthesia care unit.

The more severe the problem with ventilation, the more pronounced is the tracheal tug. First, only the larynx moves a few millimeters, then, with graver respiratory problems, even the floor of the mouth tightens with every inspiration. With severe respiratory distress, the nares may flare and the mouth may open with every inspiratory gasp. The extreme form is seen in agonal breathing.

## Tube Position

### Check the Chest

Listen over the anterior chest and in the axillary line before induction of anesthesia to obtain baseline impressions. After intubation, do two things:

1. Listen for breath sounds over the left and right chest, in front, and in the axillary lines. Remember that it is not always easy to determine whether the endotracheal tube has slipped into a mainstem bronchus. The tip may have been located just over the carina; on flexion of the patient's head, it may have descended into a bronchus, most often, but not invariably, to the right.
2. Feel for the endotracheal tube cuff. It should be palpable just under the larynx in the jugular notch. I gently increase and decrease the volume in the cuff by pushing and releasing the plunger of the inflating syringe while I palpate the trachea between larynx and jugular notch. In most adult patients, the position of the cuff can be confirmed: if you can feel it, the tip of the tube cannot be in a mainstem bronchus, *but it can be in the esophagus.*[4] Some clinicians press on the trachea and feel for the transmitted pulsation in the partially compressed pilot balloon; others squeeze the pilot balloon and feel over the trachea.

Fastening the tube to the skin over the maxilla (rather than the cheek) prevents it from being pushed in all the way or coming out altogether. The lip and the skin over the cheek are quite loose and can give the tube enough slack to get where it is not supposed to go—namely, into a mainstem bronchus or, particularly in infants, out of the larynx.

### Check the Trachea

The breath sounds heard over the trachea are loud and serve well to monitor breathing (and the absence of a discon-

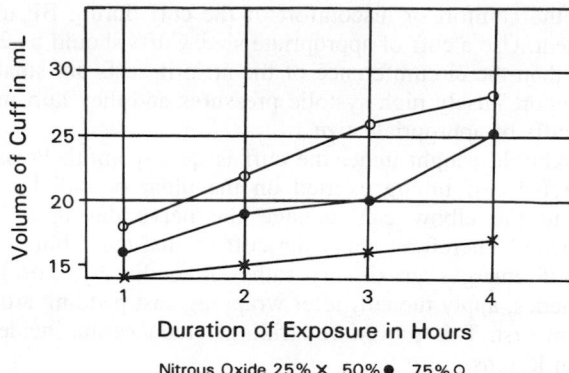

**FIGURE 18–1.** Volume of 10-mL cuff of a 34-French latex rubber endotracheal tube exposed to nitrous oxide. (From Stanley TH, Kawamura R, Graves C. Effects of nitrous oxide on volume and pressure of endotracheal tube cuffs. *Anesthesiology.* 1974;41:256.)

nection), particularly during mechanical ventilation. It is also useful to listen there while applying a little positive inspiratory pressure to discover leaks around the endotracheal tube. Optimally, the inflated cuff should form a safety valve: with the desired peak inspiratory pressure exceeded by only a few millimeters of mercury, the cuff *should* leak. This can prevent barotrauma and can be lifesaving if a malfunction of the system prevents exhalation. Usually, the cuff is overinflated, exerting >25 mm Hg pressure on the mucous membrane of the trachea. Particularly in hypotensive patients, such pressure jeopardizes perfusion of the fine ciliary epithelium.

Because the cuff swells during nitrous oxide ($N_2O$) anesthesia (Fig. 18–1), I recommend deflating it approximately every half hour until a leak can be heard and then inflating it just enough to make the leak disappear. An alternative is to fill the cuff with $N_2O$ and $O_2$ from the breathing circuit, which eliminates the gradient of $N_2O$ pressure across the membrane of the cuff. The gas can easily be obtained from the gas sampling port at the elbow connector.

### Check the Breathing Hose

Some surgical procedures preclude application of the stethoscope to the chest or the suprasternal notch. Remember that you can clearly hear breath sounds after putting the stethoscope over the expiratory hose of the breathing circuit or the endotracheal tube. Indeed, you can listen to breath sounds by putting the expiratory hose to your ear. Try it. Breath sounds over the breathing tubes tend to be harsher in mechanically ventilated patients than in those breathing spontaneously.

### Circulation

Our principal concern is perfusion of the vital organs—the brain and heart. If a patient is anesthetized, the adequacy of cerebral circulation is difficult to judge. The following are a few clinical signs that can prove useful.

### Inspection

A patient's mucous membranes should be pink in areas well above the heart. Remember that blood pools in dependent areas, which appear to be pink. They blanch with pressure

and then refill, even in severe hypotension, although perhaps not as briskly as normal.

Also look at the eyes. I recommend taping patients' eyes *only* when there is danger of damaging them. At all other times, we should not deprive ourselves of the advantage of checking pupil size; they should be constricted when all is well, and the palpebral conjunctiva should be well perfused and pink.

Look at the veins. In the areas hydrostatically below the right atrium, the veins should be dilated if blood volume is adequate and if the patient's sympathetic system is not working overtime. Use a patient's hand veins for a quick and rough estimate of right atrial pressure. Lift the hand until it is at the same height as the right atrium. Then raise it until the veins collapse and measure how much above the right atrium the hand veins collapsed. Of course, during this maneuver there should be no constriction to blood flow between hand and heart, that is, there should be no BP cuff and the arm should be abducted approximately 45°.

The same maneuver can be performed by using a simple U-tube concept: open a stopcock of the intravenous infusion tubing to air, hold the open stopcock at heart level, and slowly lift it, watching where the meniscus of water begins to recede into the tubing. You can also put tubing on the stopcock and watch the water level (Fig. 18–2). The smaller the intravenous catheter, the more time it takes for the system to equalize its pressure.

### Palpation

**Pulse.** Feel the pulse. Before the introduction of the precordial or esophageal stethoscope, it was customary to hold a

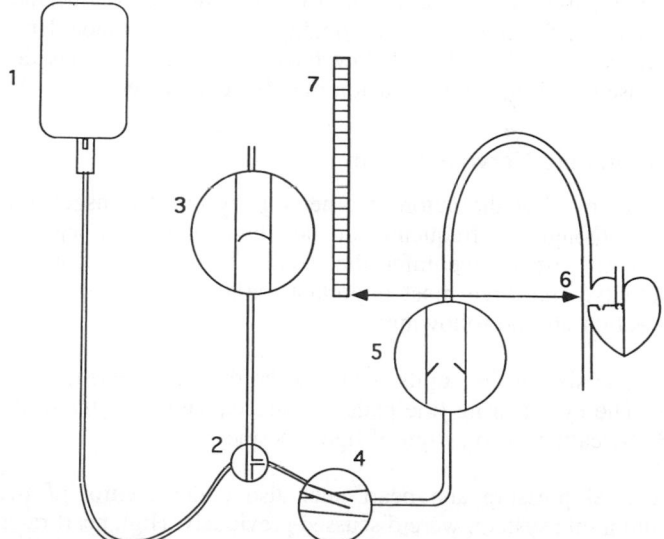

**FIGURE 18–2.** A simple, clinical estimation of central venous pressure (CVP): 1, intravenous solution bag; 2, 3-way stopcock connecting vein to open-ended tubing; 3, meniscus of fluid in open-ended tubing; 4, catheter or needle in peripheral vein; 5, valve in vein; 6, superior vena cava; 7, measuring stick. When estimating CVP, fill the open-ended tubing with intravenous fluid and hold the end of the tubing well above the level of the right atrium. Turn the stopcock to allow fluid to drain into the vein. The fluid stops flowing when the pressure in the system and the CVP equalize. Because there are valves in peripheral veins, it is important to let the fluid drain into the vein rather than wait for blood to return from the vein into the tubing. Watch for respiratory fluctuations if the patient's lungs are being mechanically ventilated. This is a good sign indicating that the venous passage is not obstructed. Instead of attaching the tubing to watch the meniscus, the open stopcock can simply be lifted until a meniscus forms.

finger over the external maxillary, temporal, or preauricular artery. I do not recommend keeping a finger on the carotid artery because compression of that vessel may not be tolerated well by patients with easily compromised carotid blood flow.

Heart rate can reveal a great deal. Tachycardia does not invariably signal hypovolemia, and hypovolemia is not invariably accompanied by tachycardia. Nevertheless, hemorrhage must be ruled out when the heart rate accelerates.

A simple rule of thumb calls for feeling the radial artery pulse. If it is palpable, the pressure is presumably acceptable (perhaps ≥90 mm Hg systolic); if it is absent, feel for the carotid artery pulse. If it is palpable but the radial pulse is not, the pressure may be approximately 60 mm Hg systolic.

**Capillary Refill.** Momentarily blanch the skin or a nail bed to look for capillary refill. It should occur promptly, in no more than approximately 1 second. Raise the patient's hand or pick the point highest above the heart when checking capillary refill. This test provides only rough estimates. But surely, if the capillaries of a finger held well above the heart refill quickly after blanching, perfusion must be at least adequate to push blood into the finger. Remember, capillary refill is a useless test when performed on a finger that is held below the level of the heart. There, gravity refills even in the absence of measurable arterial pressure.

### Auscultation

Listening to the heart sounds in an anesthetized patient is more important than in an awake patient, whose adequacy of cerebral perfusion you can monitor by nothing more than a conversation. Listen for muffled heart sounds and for dysrhythmias.

If a patient had a carotid bruit before induction of anesthesia, listen for the bruit. The quality of its sound should not change. If it does, blood flow through the stricture has decreased, and cerebral perfusion may be jeopardized.

### Autonomic Nervous System

We monitor the autonomic nervous system by inspection, even though we frequently do not think of it as a separate system; instead, we infer the depth of anesthesia from its activity. The three most important variables assessed by inspection are the following:

1. The size of the pupils (worry when they are dilated)
2. The eyes tearing (the patient is inadequately anesthetized)
3. Sweating (also a sign of light anesthesia).

Arterial pressure and heart rate, also under control of the autonomic system, were discussed previously. High heart rates and systolic pressure are taken as evidence of light anesthesia. A rare patient becomes bradycardic and hypotensive in response to pain.

## BASIC MONITORING INSTRUMENTATION

### What Should Be Done First?

#### Blood Pressure Cuff Application

As a general principle, establish baseline data before starting anesthesia. These data include arterial BP. Ask patients about the comfort or discomfort of the cuff during BP measurement. Use a cuff of appropriate size. Cuffs should be 20% wider than the circumference of the arm; if cuffs are smaller, they report falsely high systolic pressures and they hurt more than cuffs of appropriate size.

A skinfold caught under the cuff is quite painful. Pressure of the BP cuff tubing exerted on the ulnar or radial nerve close to the elbow can damage the nerve during a long anesthetic.[5] Therefore, apply the cuff so that the tubing from the cuff emerges proximally rather than distally. For long anesthetics, apply the cuff after wrapping cast padding around the arm first. This procedure strikingly reduces the incidence of skin lesions.

Traditionally, the cuff is applied to the upper arm, leaving the elbow joint free for access to the brachial artery, where the stethoscope is applied. With the oscillometric technique, the cuff can also be wrapped around the forearm or the leg. The forearm is suitable if that extremity is needed for venous cannulation, which can then be obtained proximally. If the cuff is applied to the leg, place it just above the ankle, where it hurts less than higher up and is remote from the otherwise vulnerable superficial peroneal nerve. Avoid the thigh whenever possible.

Wherever you apply the cuff, be sure that it is at the same level as the heart—as is true for the upper arm in a resting patient.

### Blood Pressure Variation

Normally, small differences in systolic and diastolic pressure are noted, depending on where the pressure is measured, even if the sites of cuff application are all at the same (heart) level. Check the pressure in both arms (and legs) if there is the least suspicion that the patient may have vascular abnormalities or diseases that would lead to unequal arm (or leg) pressures. Systolic pressure tends to be higher in the lower than in the upper extremity. Mean pressure must decrease with the distance from the heart because it is related to the flow of blood down a pressure gradient. If systolic pressure is higher in the lower extremity than in the aorta, it must mean that the pressure waveform changes so that the mean pressure can be lower in the face of a higher systolic pressure. The preinduction BP should be close to the values recorded before surgery, possibly a little higher if the patient is anxious. If not, check for an explanation (mechanical, eg, a cuff too small for the patient; or changes that require your attention before inducing anesthesia).

### Pulse Oximetry

Record the $SpO_2$ while the patient is breathing room air. Again, make sure the probe is comfortable. Some probes can be pushed too far onto the finger or taped too tightly and can cause sloughing of the fingertip.

### Electrocardiographic Monitoring

Run an ECG strip before inducing anesthesia. Obtain at least a $V_5$ tracing in adults to record whether this patient had dysrhythmias, flipped T waves, or ST segment depression. Even with a 3-lead ECG, a useful, if modified, lead $V_5$ tracing can be obtained (Fig. 18–3).

Once anesthesia is under way, proceed system by system,

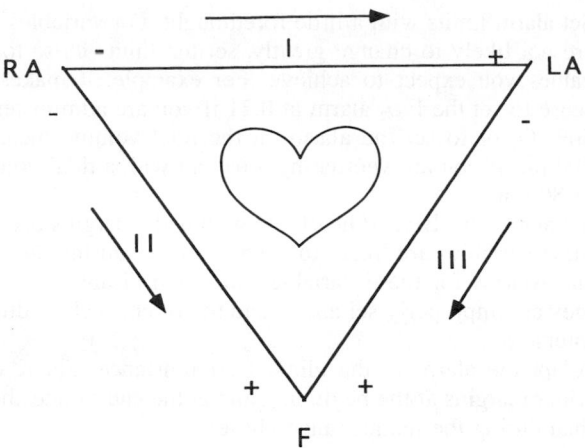

**FIGURE 18–3.** The traditional Einthoven triangle shows the classic limb leads. Remember that the exploring electrode is always positive. For a modified $VC_5$, place the F (left leg) over the anterior axillary line in the fifth intercostal space, move the right arm electrode close to the manubrium, and run lead II.

using all electronically or mechanically monitored variables *in addition* to the clinical assessment without instruments.

### How Is Ventilation Assessed?

Start with the supply of $O_2$; check the pressure gauge, flow meters, and fraction of inspired $O_2$ ($FIO_2$); proceed to check gas exchange with tidal volume and end-tidal carbon dioxide ($PETCO_2$; ~35 mm Hg, or 4%). Also make sure that end-tidal $O_2$ concentration (if available) is reasonable, that is, 3% to 6% (~40 mm Hg) below the inspired $O_2$ concentration once the patient has reached steady state.

There should be no $CO_2$ in the inspired gas. If there is, your instrument may be sluggish (damped waveform) or noisy (artifact), or there is rebreathing of $CO_2$. If the inspired $PCO_2$ is <4 mm Hg, the patient will not be harmed, but your system deserves an examination to explain the observation.

Capnography has now assumed an important place in monitoring for safety. The two completely preventable causes of major disasters in anesthesia can be detected by capnography: esophageal intubation and disconnection (see Chapter 19). Check $SpO_2$. Remember the advantages of observing the patient, as described earlier.

### How Is Circulation Assessed?

Start assessing the circulation by measuring BP. It might decrease with injection of intravenous induction agents, increase with intubation, and settle down to steady, slightly reduced values during anesthesia maintenance. If you use an automated noninvasive method for BP measurement—for example, an oscillometric device—let it cycle once a minute during induction but do not forget to reset it to a lower cycling frequency (ie, once every 3-5 minutes) for the balance of the anesthetic. Even at that frequency, petechial hemorrhages develop in many patients under the cuff, usually longitudinal, where folds of the cuff press into the skin or where skinfolds are compressed by the cuff.

Remember also that our blood vessels are alive and reac-

tive. It is quite possible to have constricted vessels (and low pressures) in the periphery (eg, radial and digital arteries) and high pressures in the aorta. Monitor lead $V_5$ (best for detecting ST segment depression) and lead II (best for P wave monitoring), if you can look at two leads at once.

Remember the advantages of observing a patient, as described earlier. In addition to listening to the precordial stethoscope, insert an esophageal stethoscope if a patient is intubated. Advance it to optimize the auscultation of heart sounds.

### How Is Temperature Assessed?

Feel a patient's forehead, even though you cannot determine his or her temperature to the exact degree. If a patient feels hot or cold but a temperature probe reports differently, use another probe or check the temperature the old-fashioned way, with a system used by nurses (electronic or mercury). Put the probe under the tongue or in the axilla. It will not give you a continuous reading, but it will tell whether you need to worry about your patient.

During general anesthesia, temperature is most conveniently measured in the esophagus, even though numerous other sites are available: the nose, the rectum, the forehead (with a strip that changes color and numbers), the tympanic membrane or the ear canal, the bladder or the pulmonary artery, and finally the axilla. Any of these sites is preferable to not measuring temperature at all. All have their drawbacks.

For routine monitoring, you need not worry about accuracy or about how closely the temperature you measure reflects core temperature. You need to know whether your patient is running a fever or is becoming too cold. In either case, you need to act (see Chapter 48).

### How Is Muscle Relaxation Assessed?

Once a patient is paralyzed, it becomes difficult to gauge the degree of relaxation by means other than a nerve stimulator, affectionately known as a *twitch monitor.* Apply the electrodes close to the wrist over the ulnar nerve so that their current stimulates nerve rather than muscle. The nerve stimulator delivers a direct current; however, if you put the electrodes close together (ie, 2 cm apart), you need not worry about which is the anode and which is the cathode. If not, the negative electrode should be distal and over the nerve. Optimally, you should increase the stimulating current until you obtain a maximum response, then set the stimulator to 10% above that maximum value. However, do not do that until a patient is asleep, because the current is painful.

#### Practical Applications

Many nerve stimulators offer the option of delivering single shocks, single shocks repeated every second, train-of-four shocks, train-of-four shocks repeated every 10 seconds, or tetany. There is a science to nerve stimulation and the interpretation of the responses (see Chapter 22). A simple clinical approach calls for turning on the stimulator as soon as the anesthetic is induced, selecting the optimal power setting, and setting it to single stimuli to be repeated every second while the first dose of the muscle-relaxing drug takes effect. Once the response to stimulation is absent, intubation is appropriate, provided the patient is adequately anesthetized. After that, switch to train-of-four stimulation or some other method with which you are comfortable and periodically assess the degree of relaxation.

## How Often Should Vital Signs Be Checked?

Ideally, patients should be monitored continuously. Although we can and should inspect without interruption and listen to the precordial or esophageal stethoscope continuously, many variables cannot be monitored without interruption. A simple formula lets clinicians determine the minimal monitoring intervals[5]:

$$TT_{max} = delta_{max}/slope_{max}$$

where $TT_{max}$ is the maximum interval between determinations, $delta_{max}$ is the maximum difference the clinician is willing to ascribe to acceptable physiologic variability, and $slope_{max}$ is the maximum rate of change the clinician foresees for this variable in this particular patient.

For example, $delta_{max}$ for BP might be set at 50 mm Hg, meaning that a change of that magnitude would require attention. BP $slope_{max}$ might be set as a 50 mm Hg change in 60 seconds. One postulates that short of a cardiac arrest, the pressure is not likely to change faster than that. The monitoring interval, therefore, would be set at once a minute, as suggested during induction of anesthesia. With invasive monitoring, of course, continuous readings are available. For the average anesthetic, we might assume 50 mm Hg for $delta_{max}$ and set a $slope_{max}$ of 180 seconds, which would give a monitoring interval for BP of 3 minutes.

## How Should Alarms on Monitoring Devices Be Set?

Today, many monitors have automatic alarms that are useless or harmful if not properly used. Do not treat them nonchalantly. Numerous disasters and lost lawsuits have resulted when anesthesiologists have disabled or turned off an alarm and forgotten to turn it back on or ignored it.

Important points follow:

1. Use the alarms. *Do not disable them.* If you must disable them, do so temporarily; make a positive identification of the alarm and its origin, take the necessary action, and turn it back on as soon as possible.

2. Set alarm limits with a little forethought. For variables that are not likely to change greatly, set the limits close to the values you expect to achieve. For example, it makes no sense to set the $FIO_2$ alarm at 0.21 if you are administering 50% $O_2$ or to set the alarm on the tidal volume meter at 300 mL if you are ventilating a patient with a tidal volume of 800 mL.

3. Set alarms for BP and heart rate with wide margins because these variables are likely to change greatly during anesthesia. Alarms for these variables are often disabled because they are improperly set and sound too often, such as during intubation.

4. Adapt the alarm to the clinical circumstance. Set it with wider margins at the beginning and at the end of anesthesia than during the maintenance phase.

## Are Monitoring Standards Useful?

Many countries have adopted minimal monitoring standards. The World Federation of Anesthesia Societies in 1992 adopted an international version, showing different levels appropriate to the resources of individual countries.[6] The 1998 Standards published by the American Society of Anesthesiologists are presented in the Appendix at the end of this chapter.

Many questions must be raised about standards. Are they helpful? The answer depends not only on how they affect outcome (not known) but on how they affect the practice of the specialty (also not known). Can we drop standards that require expensive systems? Should instruments that are now available or likely to become available be incorporated into existing standards? Would practice standards (or guidelines), rather than or in addition to equipment standards, be useful? Anesthesiology has made a dramatic step in adopting a first set of standards and guidelines, which are being updated. The clock will not be turned back.

### References

1. Comroe JH Jr, Botelho S. The unreliability of cyanosis in the recognition of arterial anoxemia. *Am J Med Sci.* 1947;214:1.
2. Ayoub J, Cohendy R, Dauzat M, et al. Non-invasive quantification of diaphragm kinetics using m-mode sonography measurement technique. *Can J Anaesth.* 1997;44:739.
3. Bailey PL. Opioid-induced respiratory depression. *Curr Rev Clin Anesth.* 1997;17:191.
4. Stirt JA. Endotracheal tube misplacement. *Anaesth Intensive Care.* 1982;10:274.
5. Gravenstein JS, DeVries A, Beneken JEW. Sampling intervals for clinical monitoring of variables during anesthesia. *J Clin Monit.* 1989;5:17
6. The International Task Force on Anaesthesia Safety. International standards for a safe practice of anaesthesia. [Adopted by the World Federation of Societies of Anaesthesiologists 13 June 1992]. *Eur J Anaesthesiol.* 1993;10(S7):12.

# Appendix

## STANDARDS FOR BASIC ANESTHETIC MONITORING

(Approved by House of Delegates on October 21, 1986, and last amended on October 21, 1998)

These standards apply to all anesthesia care, although in emergency circumstances, appropriate life support measures take precedence. These standards may be exceeded at any time based on the judgment of the responsible anesthesiologist. They are intended to encourage high-quality patient care, but observing them cannot guarantee any specific patient outcome. They are subject to revision from time to time, as warranted by the evolution of technology and practice. They apply to all general anesthetics, regional anesthetics and monitored anesthesia care. This set of standards addresses only the issue of basic anesthetic monitoring, which is one component of anesthesia care. In certain rare or unusual circumstances, (1) some of these methods of monitoring may be clinically impractical and (2) appropriate use of the described methods may fail to detect untoward clinical developments. Brief interruptions of continual* monitoring may be unavoidable. *Under extenuating circumstances, the responsible anesthesiologist may waive the requirements marked with a dagger* (†). It is recommended that when this is done, it should be so stated (including the reasons) in a note in the patient's medical record. These standards are not intended for application to the care of the obstetric patient in labor or in the conduct of pain management.

### STANDARD I

Qualified anesthesia personnel shall be present in the room throughout the conduct of all general anesthetics, regional anesthetics, and monitored anesthesia care.

## Objective

Because of the rapid changes in a patient's status during anesthesia, qualified anesthesia personnel shall be continuously present to monitor the patient and provide anesthesia care. In the event there is a direct known hazard, eg, radiation, to the anesthesia personnel which might require intermittent remote observation of the patient, some provision for monitoring the patient must be made. In the event that an emergency requires the temporary absence of the person primarily responsible for the anesthetic, the best judgment of the anesthesiologist will be exercised in comparing the emergency with the anesthetized patient's condition and in the selection of the person left responsible for the anesthetic during the temporary absence.

Appendix excerpted from *ASA Directory of Members 2001* of the American Society of Anesthesiologists. A copy of the full text can be obtained from ASA, 520 North Northwest Highway, Park Ridge, IL 60068-2573.

*Note that *continual* is defined as "repeated regularly and frequently in steady rapid succession," whereas *continuous* means "prolonged without any interruption at any time."

### STANDARD II

During all anesthetics, the patient's oxygenation, ventilation, circulation, and temperature shall be continually evaluated.

## Oxygenation

### Objective
To ensure adequate oxygen concentration in the inspired gas and the blood during all anesthetics.

### Methods
1. Inspired gas: During every administration of general anesthesia using an anesthesia machine, the concentration of oxygen in the patient's breathing system shall be measured by an oxygen analyzer with a low oxygen concentration limit alarm in use.†
2. Blood oxygenation: During all anesthetics, a quantitative method of assessing oxygenation such as pulse oximetry shall be employed.† Adequate illumination and exposure of the patient are necessary to assess color.†

## Ventilation

### Objective
To ensure adequate ventilation of the patient during all anesthetics.

### Methods
1. Every patient receiving general anesthesia shall have the adequacy of ventilation continually evaluated. Qualitative clinical signs such as chest excursion, observation of the reservoir breathing bag, and auscultation of breath sounds are useful. Continual monitoring for the presence of expired carbon dioxide shall be performed unless invalidated by the nature of the patient, procedure, or equipment. Quantitative monitoring of the volume of expired gas is strongly encouraged.†
2. When an endotracheal tube or laryngeal mask is inserted, its correct positioning must be verified by clinical assessment and by identification of carbon dioxide in the expired gas. Continual end-tidal carbon dioxide analysis, in use from the time of endotracheal tube/laryngeal mask placement until extubation/removal or initiating transfer to a postoperative care location, shall be performed using a quantitative method such as capnography, capnometry, or mass spectroscopy.†
3. When ventilation is controlled by a mechanical ventilator, there shall be in continuous use a device that is capable of detecting disconnection of components of the breathing system. The device must give an audible signal when its alarm threshold is exceeded.
4. During regional anesthesia and monitored anesthesia care, the adequacy of ventilation shall be evaluated, at least, by continual observation of qualitative clinical signs.

## Circulation

### Objective

To ensure the adequacy of the patient's circulatory function during all anesthetics.

### Methods

1. Every patient receiving anesthesia shall have the electrocardiogram continuously displayed from the beginning of anesthesia until preparing to leave the anesthetizing location.†
2. Every patient receiving anesthesia shall have arterial blood pressure and heart rate determined and evaluated at least every 5 minutes.†
3. Every patient receiving general anesthesia shall have, in addition to the above, circulatory function continually evaluated by at least one of the following: palpation of a pulse, auscultation of heart sounds, monitoring of a tracing of intra-arterial pressure, ultrasound peripheral pulse monitoring, or pulse plethysmography or oximetry.

## Body Temperature

### Objective

To aid in the maintenance of appropriate body temperature during all anesthetics.

### Methods

Every patient receiving anesthesia shall have temperature monitored when clinically significant changes in body temperature are intended, anticipated, or suspected.

CHAPTER

# 19

# Respiratory Monitoring

Dietrich Gravenstein

Julian M. Goldman

Jennifer E. Souders

Modern practitioners rely on traditional physical examination skills and numerous new and technically complex devices to monitor the patient's respiratory status. A thorough understanding of the strengths and limitations of each of our monitor and equipment options is essential to maximize our diagnostic ability and intelligently guide our therapeutic intervention.

## INDIRECT ASSESSMENT OF RESPIRATION AND OXYGENATION

### Are Clinical Skills Still Necessary?

Modern electronic instruments have added valuable capabilities to our monitoring efforts. Yet, even the most sophisticated monitor cannot replace the vigilant clinician. On the one hand, modern instruments do not cover a number of signals of great importance to the clinician, in particular the quality of breath sounds and the motion of the chest or larynx with respiration. On the other hand, artifacts or failures of modern equipment can be disastrous if not recognized by the alert clinician as such.

The redundant assessment of heart rate by electrocardiography (ECG), automated sphygmomanometry, and pulse oximetry can compensate for the failure of one or the other instrument. When monitoring ventilation and respiration, a variety of signals can point to trouble. These include old-fashioned physical examination, oximetry (inspired and expired and pulse oximetry), monitoring the adequacy of ventilation, and finally looking at the brain and heart with the help of different sensors.

### What Can Physical Examination Reveal?

We should look at our instruments as complementing a good physical examination. First, one must observe that the endotracheal tube (ETT) has really slipped through the glottic opening and then confirm, by capnometry, the continuous presence of exhaled $CO_2$. During the management of a patient in cardiac arrest, ventilating the lungs may not generate a capnogram. The clinician will have to rely on auscultation, observing chest expansion and deflation, and condensation within an ETT to rule out airway obstruction, esophageal intubation, or disconnection of the circuit.[1]

At times, the physical examination may be misleading. For example, cyanosis is recognized as a condition usually reflecting tissue ischemia. The human eye first perceives the blue tint in skin or mucosa when 5 g/dL blood or more of deoxygenated hemoglobin (Hgb) is present.[2,3] Thus, when an anemic patient with 10 g Hgb/dL blood becomes cyanotic, it suggests that the patient has desaturated to <50%, whereas a polycythemic patient with 20 g Hgb/dL blood who becomes cyanotic could have a saturation of 75%. Therefore, although the existence of cyanosis is always of concern, it is a vastly more serious finding in anemic patients.

### Are Organ-Specific Monitors of Oxygenation Available?

Severe anemia and inadequate tissue perfusion or oxygenation will damage the brain or heart. The ECG, echocardiograph, and the electroencephalograph (EEG) will show changes when these organs suffer a critical lack of oxygen. Cerebral oximetry generates more direct evidence of brain oxygenation.

### Electrocardiography and Transesophageal Echocardiography

Ischemia in the heart often manifests as ST segment depression or T wave inversion. The 5-lead intraoperative ECG, monitoring leads II and $V_5$ simultaneously, is capable of detecting 80% of ischemic events that would manifest as ST segment changes.[4] The advent of transesophageal echocardiography has allowed continuous intraoperative imaging of the heart. The skilled clinician can observe the effects of ischemia as wall segments become hypokinetic or dyskinetic even before ECG changes are evident.[5,6]

### Cerebral Assessment of Oxygenation

#### Electroencephalography

Continuous EEG has been successfully employed as a clinical monitor for cerebral ischemia during carotid endarterectomy and cardiopulmonary bypass procedures, among others. The association of reduced EEG activity and irregular slowing with cerebral ischemia when observed during steady-state anesthesia is well established.[7,8]

#### Near Infrared Light-Based Measurement

Cerebral oximetry, as performed by the INVOS 3100 (Somanetics Corp, Troy, Mich), employs near infrared (NIR) spectroscopy to interrogate regional brain oxygenation ($rSo_2$). Its use as a clinical monitor has been described in numerous reports.[9-11] The brain is interrogated by introducing NIR light that traverses skin, bone, and brain and measuring what is scattered back to several sensor sites. Because the light must traverse skin, which is perfused by blood delivered by the external carotid artery, the relative contribution of extracranial blood to the signal has been questioned. The question of the influence of extracranial blood flow is yet to be answered. Some investigators have found extracranial blood flow to be of no significant influence,[12] whereas others disagree.[13,14]

Reflection spectrophotometry is a second noninvasive method for interrogating the oxygenation status of the brain. This method, as found in the NIRO 500 (Hamamatsu Photonics Corp, Osaka, Japan), uses four wavelengths of NIR light that are transmitted through the scalp, skull, and brain and are reflected back to one sensor. A monitor then calculates the changes in the reduction/oxidation ratio of cytochrome a, $a_3$.[15,16] This method, although not as widely utilized as the INVOS cerebral oximeter, also has been demonstrated to track hypoperfusion and hypoxemia.[17] It may even permit detection of small changes in cerebral oxygenation during induction of general anesthesia[18] but, because this method follows intracellular oxygenation, it may not be very sensitive or accurate at detecting subcritical changes in cerebral oxygenation.

In summary, ECG and transesophageal echocardiography monitor the oxygen-dependent function of the heart. When changes in their signals are detected, the differential diagnosis must include deficient delivery of oxygen. EEG, although sensitive to changes in depth of anesthesia, will also reliably respond to ischemia once anesthetic depth has reached steady state. The ultimate clinical use of the NIR brain oxygenation monitors remains to be established.

## PULSE OXIMETRY

### What Does a Pulse Oximeter Really Measure?

Pulse oximetry computes arterial $O_2$ saturation by using variations in the absorption of light in the red and infrared (IR) wavelengths caused by the pulsation of arterial blood.[19] Arterial $O_2$ saturation determined by a pulse oximeter is designated as $SpO_2$ (Fig. 19–1). Increased arterial blood flow during systole expands tissue beds by delivering additional blood with each pulse and absorbing a little more light. By working only with the pulsatile signal, the pulse oximeter can ignore light absorption by nonpulsatile elements in the light transmission pathway (eg, tissue, bone, pigmented skin, and nonpulsatile venous and arterial blood).[20] The technology just described is called *transmission oximetry* and uses light at wavelengths of 660 nm (visible red light, primarily absorbed by reduced hemoglobin) and 910 or 940 nm (invisible IR light, primarily absorbed by oxyhemoglobin). A newer technology exploits *reflectance oximetry*, which monitors $SpO_2$ by measuring light reflected from perfused tissues. This approach is advantageous for monitoring sites that cannot be transilluminated (eg, the pulmonary artery).

### What Is the Difference Between Functional and Fractional Saturation?

Oximeters display either functional or fractional $SpO_2$. Functional saturation is defined as the oxyhemoglobin concentration, divided by the concentrations of oxyhemoglobin and deoxyhemoglobin combined, multiplied by 100. These two hemoglobin species participate in oxygen transport. Fractional saturation also recognizes the species of hemoglobin not participating in oxygen transport. A fractional saturation calculation includes concentrations of methemoglobin and carboxyhemoglobin in the denominator of the equation. In pulse oximetry, these species are not measured, and the instrument makers assign them an average value. Thus, oximeters displaying functional saturation will report slightly higher saturations than oximeters displaying fractional saturation. This difference has not been shown to be of clinical importance. Refer to the manufacturer's manual to determine whether the instrument reports functional saturation:

$$SpO_2 = \frac{HbO_2}{HbO_2 + Hb}$$

or fractional saturation:

$$SpO_2 = \frac{HbO_2}{HbO_2 + Hb + metHb + COHb + Others}$$

### What Are Potential Sources of Error?

Performance limitations of pulse oximetry intraoperatively are well documented. In a study of more than 9000 computerized anesthesia records, loss of the pulse oximetry signal for at least 10 minutes occurred in over 9% of cases.[21] In a study of 10 000 anesthetics, it was shown that failure to monitor $SpO_2$ occurs more commonly in sicker patients (7.2% of American Society of Anesthesiologists physical status IV patients).[22]

#### Nail Polish

Both nail polish and synthetic nails occasionally interfere with pulse oximetry. Obviously, opaque nail polish diminishes the intensity of transmitted light and may result in decreased signal strength.[23] Nail polish that incorporates a blue pigment can cause a similar artifactual lowering of the reported $SpO_2$ value. One can either ask the patient to remove nail polish on one finger or place the probe sideways to transilluminate through the lateral aspect of the finger or select another probe site, all reasonable options for a patient with an expensive manicure who is undergoing outpatient surgery. Alternatively, you can check the baseline $SpO_2$ using the polished nail and determine if the pulse oximeter gives a valid reading and proceed accordingly.

#### Insufficient Signal Strength

If the emitter-detector is improperly aligned or placed so that the part of the light beam misses perfused tissue, the

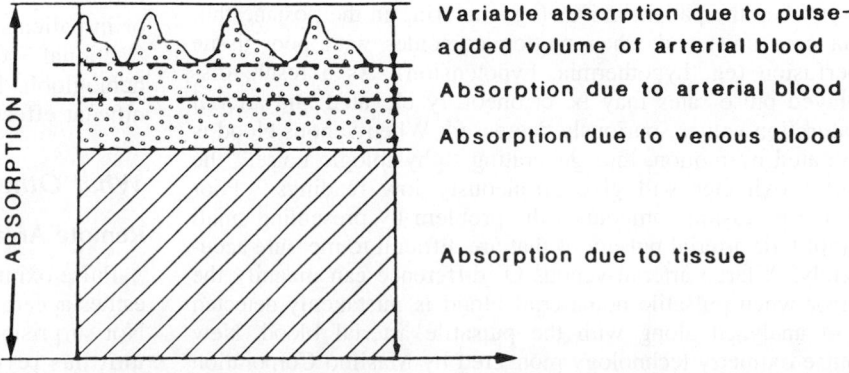

**FIGURE 19–1.** Tissue composite showing dynamic and static components that affect light absorption during pulse oximetry. (Adapted from *Ohmeda 3700, Pulse Oximeter Users Manual.* Madison, Wis: Ohmeda; 1989:22. Provided by Ohmeda, Inc, The BOC Group.)

Variable absorption due to pulse-added volume of arterial blood

Absorption due to arterial blood

Absorption due to venous blood

Absorption due to tissue

ABSORPTION

TIME

instrument will typically report no signal at all of a falsely low saturation. A falsely low saturation is obviously the more bothersome problem and is thought to result from incorporation of venous pulsations, thus contaminating what is presumed to be a purely arterial signal. Patients who are warm and peripherally vasodilated are most prone to show this phenomenon, termed the *penumbra effect*.[24] Placing the sensing site more proximal (ie, over larger arterial or capillary vessels) resolves the problem. Incorrect emitter-detector alignment will also magnify motion artifacts.

Patients who are vasoconstricted from cold, shock, vasculitis, or drugs and who have reduced blood flow through the fingertips also present difficulties.[25] In such circumstances, the amplitude of the arterial optical plethysmogram can decrease to less than 1% (100% assumed to be the standard of optimally peripheral perfusion) and may be difficult to detect and measure. Unless the reduced flow stems from occlusive disease of the digital arteries, the problem can be remedied by warming the hand or increasing local blood flow by performing a digital nerve block with an epinephrine-free local anesthetic or the application of topical nitroglycerin.[26] Newer pulse oximetry technologies can more reliably measure arterial pulsations of small amplitude.[27]

Other causes of low perfusion, such as arterial compression or hypotension, or nothing more than an elevated arm, can similarly diminish the signal that the pulse oximeter needs to detect; in fact, the pulse oximeter probe can be positioned specifically to aid in detecting arterial pulsations.

## Noisy Signals

Noisy signals are commonly caused by ambient light (especially IR warming lights), motion, and stray electromagnetic energy from the electrosurgical unit Stealth Station Camera (Medtronics, Broomfield, Colo) or magnetic resonance imaging (MRI). Excessive ambient light overwhelms the photodetection circuit and makes it more difficult to detect the desired red and IR signals. Electrosurgical units and ambient light can cause either falsely high or falsely low saturations and heart rates. The entry of ambient light may be reduced with a close-fitting probe and may be blocked with an opaque probe cover. Some new sensor designs incorporate electromagnetic shielding in the sensor and sensor cable and reduce the entry of ambient light. MRI interferes with pulse oximetry (and vice versa) and can cause abrupt changes in $SpO_2$ with the start of imaging.

Accurate pulse oximetry measurement is particularly difficult when the patient moves (eg, shivering in the postanesthesia care unit) and when motion coincides with poor tissue perfusion (eg, hypothermia, hypotension). As a result, displayed pulse rates may be erroneously elevated and arterial saturation values spuriously decreased. When venous blood is agitated by motion, thus generating "physiologic noise," the pulse oximeter will give erroneously low readings.[28] Poor tissue perfusion compounds the problem by presenting small amplitude arterial pulsations that are difficult to measure accurately. A large arterial-venous $O_2$ difference can magnify the error when pulsatile nonarterial blood is mistakenly detected and analyzed along with the pulsatile arterial blood. New pulse oximetry technology pioneered by Masimo Corporation (Irvine, Calif) uses adaptive filters to obtain motion resistant pulse oximetry. It also offers improved performance in low perfusion states. This signal processing approach can remove motion-induced noise from the oximetry signal when the noise frequency differs from arterial pulsation frequency. As a result of adaptive filtering, digital signal processor-based noise filters, and electromagnetic shielding, new pulse oximetry technology boasts improved clinical "up time" and resistance to conditions that produce false alarms.[29] Historically, the techniques required to reduce false alarms have resulted in decreased sensitivity to detecting hypoxemic episodes.[30] In contrast, despite the reduction in false alarms with new pulse oximetry technology, sensitivity to the detection of true hypoxemic episodes is not diminished—it is enhanced.[31-33]

Motion of the probe may cause the data to be incorrect or missing altogether. The readings may increase or decrease to a default $SpO_2$ value of 82% to 85%, which implies a red-to-IR light transmission ratio of 1 (corresponding to an $SpO_2$ of 82%-85%). In comparison to clip-on probes, the adhesive probes designed for single-patient use (and hence more expensive) usually provide more reliable readings during motion and less tissue compression, thereby not exacerbating the problems existing when tissue perfusion is low. Extensive effort has been put into the successful development of probes that are less sensitive to motion, including coupling of the ECG signal to the oximeter and novel signal extraction technology.[33]

An additional source of error arises when a large dicrotic notch is detected as a separate heartbeat, causing the displayed pulse rate to be twice the actual pulse rate.[26]

## Dyes and Abnormal Hemoglobins

Dyes and abnormal hemoglobins, other sources of pulse oximetry errors, deserve mention. Methylene blue, indocyanine green, and indigo carmine cause transient, apparent desaturation when administered intravenously. Methylene blue has the most profound and complex effects on $SpO_2$. It both produces and clears methemoglobin, causes a transient increase in cardiac output followed by cardiac depression, and has an absorbance peak at 668 nm that interferes with the oximeter's detection of red absorbance and thus falsely indicates desaturation.[20]

Methemoglobin can cause falsely high or low $SpO_2$ readings, depending on the relative amounts of oxyhemoglobin and reduced hemoglobin. However, as the methemoglobin level increases, the $SpO_2$ decreases to 80% to 85% and then remains constant.

Pulse oximeters read carboxyhemoglobin as approximately 90% saturated oxyhemoglobin. Therefore, carboxyhemoglobin can falsely present elevated $SpO_2$ readings in heavy smokers or in patients with carbon monoxide poisoning if their actual, fractional $SaO_2$ levels are low in the face of elevated carboxyhemoglobin levels. Fetal hemoglobin has no clinically significant effect on pulse oximetry.[34]

## What Other Applications Are Useful?

### Remote Areas/Transport

Pulse oximetry has become a standard of care in the postanesthesia care unit that parallels that in the operating room. Not surprisingly, its introduction into the postanesthesia care unit has revealed a high incidence of postanesthetic hypoxemia.[35] Peripheral vasoconstriction and motion increases the failure rate of conventional pulse oximetry in this setting.[36] In areas where parenteral sedation is given (eg, dental offices, angiography suites, endoscopy units, office-based anesthesia), pulse oximetry should be the monitoring standard as well.

We use pulse oximetry to monitor critically ill (and especially ventilator-dependent) patients during transport to and from the intensive care unit. Poor perfusion and movement artifact may reduce its reliability in this group of patients.

## Circulatory Assessment

The plethysmographic display of the pulse oximeter has been proposed as a means of monitoring the circulation. Although clinicians have used this display to estimate intravascular volume status, the technique has limited clinical applicability.[37] On the one hand, many pulse oximeters feature an automated scaling of the plethysmographic display to compensate for alterations in amplitude. For instance, changes in saturation change plethysmographic amplitude. Some newer pulse oximeters display a perfusion index that is related to plethysmogram amplitude and may overcome limitations of current instruments in steady-state conditions but should be cautiously interpreted because this signal is affected by hemoglobin concentration and transilluminated blood volume, which may vary and does not measure flow. On the other hand, the finger plethysmogram may change dramatically, owing to changes in regional rather than systemic blood flow. This is particularly true in the awake patient, in whom a startling noise may cause a marked decrease in the amplitude of the plethysmogram. In the lightly anesthetized patient, a noxious surgical stimulus can produce the same change in amplitude.

Pulse oximetry also has been used to assess the palmar collateral circulation before arterial cannulation. However, its ability to detect even minute pulsations (ie, <10% of the normal blood flow) can be deceptive because such pulsations may be present in the absence of adequate collateral flow.[38–40]

## Blood Pressure

The disappearance of the plethysmographic waveform during slow inflation of the blood pressure (BP) cuff can provide an estimate of systolic BP.[41] We have found this to be an effective technique for measuring BP in pediatric patients undergoing general anesthesia. Note that this technique of BP determination is best observed during *inflation*. Systolic pressure corresponds to the *loss* of the plethysmographic signal. During deflation of the cuff, reacquisition of the pulse signal is sufficiently slow that this endpoint predictably underestimates systolic pressure.

## Monitoring Inspired Oxygen Concentration

Monitoring the fraction of inspired oxygen ($FIO_2$) delivered to a patient has been advocated as an intraoperative monitoring standard by the American Society of Anesthesiologists since 1986. The $O_2$ monitor, when it incorporates an activated low-concentration alarm, provides an easy and inexpensive way to alert the clinician.

When oxygen concentration is measured by a relatively slowly responding sensor placed in the inspiratory limb of the circle breathing circuit, it indicates the concentration but not the volume of oxygen the *circuit is delivering* to the patient. In other words, we may be delivering an adequate concentration of oxygen, but it is a volume that fails to meet the

patient's oxygen requirement. Only if the fresh gas flow (FGF) is so high as to prevent rebreathing of exhaled gas will the oxygen analyzer (placed in the inspiratory hose) reflect the concentration of oxygen in the FGF. Of course, it does not give any indication of the expired $O_2$ concentration. If the expired concentration falls below 16% or 17%, the patient's oxygen demand may not be met. Pulse oximetry can confirm an underlying oxygen deficit. In short, although we want to know the concentration of oxygen delivered to the patient, we cannot limit our curiosity to what this monitoring technology offers.

### Sensor Position

Because the sensor is typically placed in the inspiratory limb of the breathing circuit near the inspiratory valve, it cannot measure a change in $O_2$ concentration resulting from air entrainment in the circuit at a site distal to it. Therefore, a spontaneously breathing patient could be inspiring room air around a deflated ETT cuff or through a partially disconnected or leaking circuit that would escape detection by an $O_2$ sensor in the inspiratory limb.

## *How Can the Oxygen Sensor Mislead Us?*

### Calibration

$O_2$ analyzers can produce incorrect values as a result of faulty initial calibration. Therefore, we recommend that the analyzer be calibrated at least once daily, usually during the initial anesthesia machine check, and that it be calibrated with room air as opposed to 100% $O_2$ to maximize its accuracy in the low concentration range and to facilitate the detection of a hazardously low concentration. In addition to faulty calibration, some of the commonly used older polarographic or galvanic $O_2$ sensors have been reported to be sensitive to nitrous oxide ($N_2O$), particularly as the battery power for the sensor fails.[42]

Once the analyzer is calibrated, the alarm limits should be set a little below the oxygen concentration to be delivered. For example, if the clinician plans to give 50% oxygen, the alarm limit should be set at 40% or 45% oxygen. To set it at 21% would delay the detection of a problem that had caused the oxygen concentration to drop from 50% to 21%.

## *Can the Oxygen Sensor's Diagnostic Utility Be Improved?*

One method is to place the sensor in the expiratory limb, which facilitates the detection of leaks or disconnections. However, moisture condensation on the sensor can damage it and render it useless.[43] Moving the location of the $O_2$ sensor is not even an option in many newer anesthesia machines, because they have incorporated their $O_2$ analyzers into the $CO_2$ absorber canister. Perhaps for reasons of durability and reducing liability, manufacturers want to prove that their machines *deliver* a sufficient $O_2$ concentration, although we would prefer to know that a patient *receives* $O_2$ sufficient to meet the patient's requirements. Hence, enthusiasm has surrounded the development and use of "fast" airway $O_2$ sensors that actually create an $O_2$ waveform or oxygram, showing inspired and expired oxygen concentrations.

### What Is Fast Oxygen Monitoring?

*Fast O$_2$ monitoring* refers to the use of rapidly responding (eg, 0%-95% in 150 ms) O$_2$ analyzers that measure inspired and expired O$_2$ at the mouth or ETT.[44] Current technologies capable of fast O$_2$ analysis include mass spectroscopy, Raman spectroscopy, and paramagnetic O$_2$ analysis. (Mass spectroscopy and Raman spectroscopy are described further in the section, Agent Monitoring.)

### Paramagnetic Sensors

Paramagnetic O$_2$ sensors take advantage of the fact that O$_2$ is one of only a few molecules that has two electrons in unpaired orbits, allowing it to exhibit a magnetic property. The paramagnetic sensor uses an alternating magnetic field to generate a pressure in the presence of O$_2$ molecules. The difference in pressure between a reference cell and a sample cell is proportional to the difference in O$_2$ partial pressures. When used with a sufficiently small sample cell, the paramagnetic sensor provides a fast response time that gives breath-by-breath measurements of inspired and expired oxygen.[45]

### Oxygraphy

*Oxygraphy,* which is the continuous waveform display of these breath-by-breath O$_2$ time-concentration waveform measurements, may detect ventilatory abnormalities such as circuit disconnections and leaks in a fashion similar to that for capnography (the CO$_2$ time-concentration waveform).

### Oxygen Delivery and Uptake

The difference between the inspired and expired O$_2$ concentrations ($\Delta$O$_2$) can be measured. This value provides a noninvasive estimate of the relationship between alveolar O$_2$ delivery (a function of F$_{IO_2}$ and alveolar ventilation) and alveolar O$_2$ uptake (primarily affected by pulmonary blood flow and mixed venous O$_2$). Hence, inadequate O$_2$ delivery for a given O$_2$ consumption can be detected. An increase in the $\Delta$O$_2$ has been demonstrated to be a more sensitive indicator of alveolar hypoventilation than a change in SpO$_2$.[46]

### Denitrogenation

Another useful application of oxygraphy involves examining the decrease in $\Delta$O$_2$ as a patient breathes 100% O$_2$. With FGF set high enough (at least minute volume) to prevent rebreathing of exhaled gas, the progress of denitrogenation can be monitored. As demonstrated in Figure 19–2, the decrease in alveolar nitrogen (N$_2$) concentration is accompanied by a complementary increase in the alveolar O$_2$ concentration. Figure 19–2 illustrates that alveolar N$_2$ can be rapidly exchanged for O$_2$ in a healthy patient who takes big (approaching vital capacity) breaths. In contrast, during quiet breathing, N$_2$ wash-

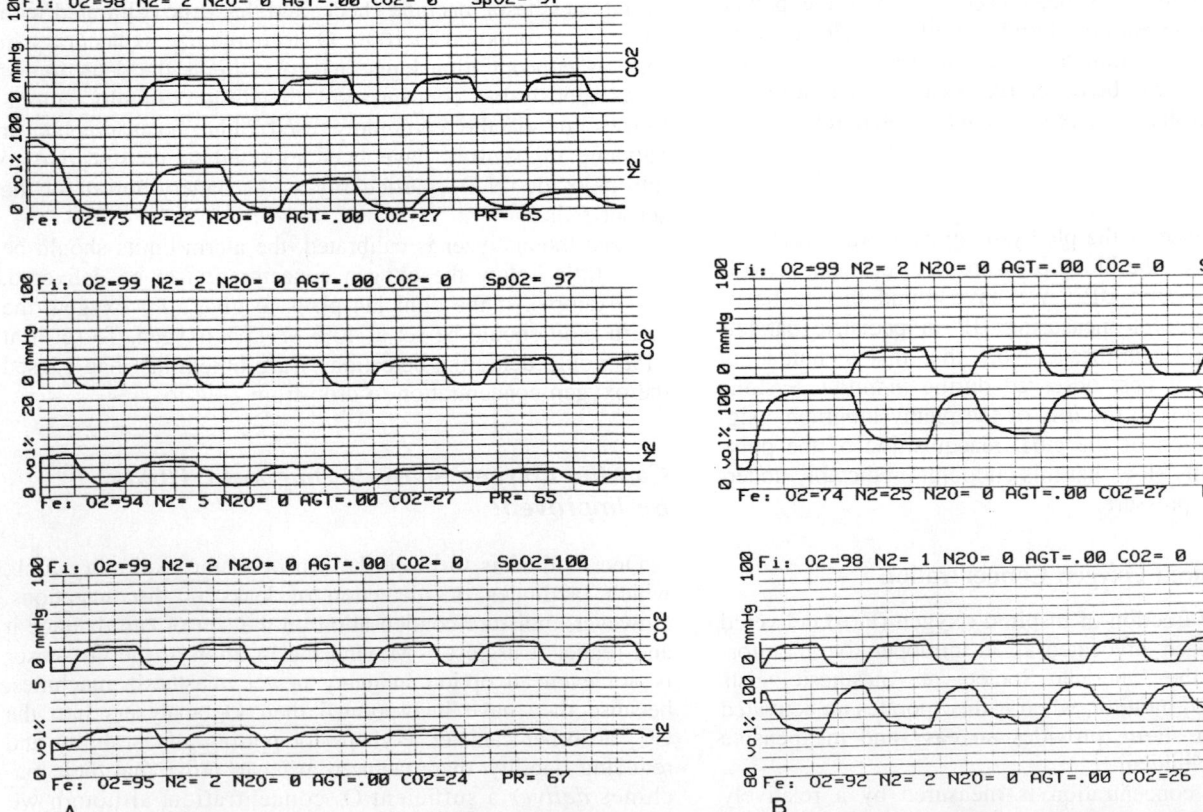

**FIGURE 19–2.** *A,* Preinduction denitrogenation (commonly called *preoxygenation*). Breathing pure O$_2$ exchanges N$_2$ for O$_2$ in the patient's pulmonary functional residual capacity. The capnogram and N$_2$ curve from this patient breathing O$_2$ by face mask illustrate the rapid decline in expired N$_2$ concentration. Nitrogen washout in this healthy adult patient is almost complete after four large breaths. (Note that the N$_2$ scale is different on each printout. Gas analyzed by Datex-Ohmeda Rascal II Raman spectroscopic analyzer.) *B,* Preinduction denitrogenation oxygram. Simultaneous oxygram and capnogram from same patient and under same conditions as in *A.* The end-tidal O$_2$ concentration rises as N$_2$ washout occurs. (Note that the O$_2$ scale is different on each printout.)

out requires between 2 and 3.5 minutes in a healthy patient and 10 to 12 minutes in a patient with emphysema.[47]

### Detection of Circuit Valve Leaks

We have compared the efficacy of oxygraphy with that of capnography for the detection of circle-circuit valve leaks and spontaneous respiratory efforts during mechanical ventilation. In our experiments, performed with a mechanical lung and mass spectrometer, oxygraphy was not as useful as capnography for detecting an expiratory valve leak (Fig. 19–3).

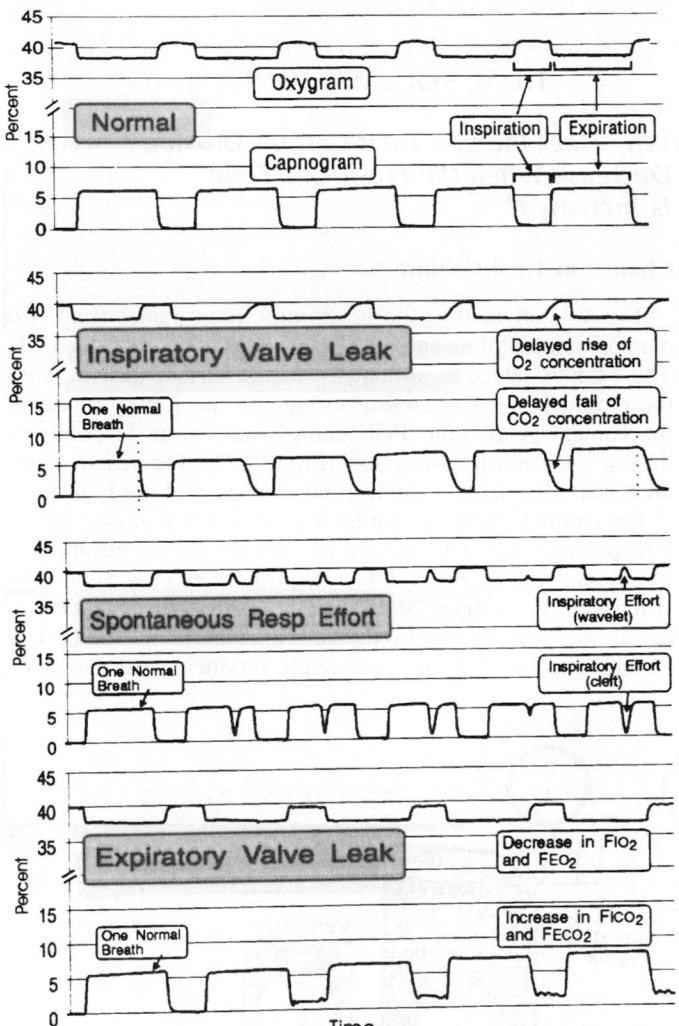

**FIGURE 19–3.** Oxygrams and capnograms with valve defects. Comparison of the capnogram and oxygram during ventilation by a mechanical lung with a volume-cycled ventilator and an adult circle breathing circuit. Inspiratory and expiratory valve leaks were produced by elevating the valve disks. Spontaneous inspiratory efforts during expiration (cleft) were produced by manually expanding the lung bellows during expiration. In all examples, the oxygram is similar to a capnogram that is flipped over vertically. Abnormalities that produce clear morphologic changes are apparent on both gas concentration tracings. However, the expiratory gas rebreathing that results from an expiratory valve leak primarily changes the concentration, and not the morphology, of the waveforms. Thus, the slow decrease in inspired and expired $O_2$ concentrations is the only evidence of the defect. Although concentration changes are also the only abnormalities evident on the capnogram, the baseline change is more obvious because the capnogram rises above its normally zero baseline. In contrast, the oxygram's baseline normally varies with inspired $O_2$ concentration. The *vertical dotted lines* on the inspiratory valve leak tracing indicate the beginning of inspiration. (See Figure 19–9 for a complete explanation of this valve defect.)

## AIRWAY PRESSURE MONITORING

### What Is the Value of Intraoperative Measurement?

Continuous intraoperative airway pressure monitoring offers many benefits, particularly when high-pressure and low-pressure alarms and a graphic pressure-time display are used. The likelihood of barotrauma can be reduced by adjusting the ventilator's tidal volume (VT) and inspiratory flow rate to optimize peak and mean airway pressures. In addition, some newer anesthesia ventilators can be set to terminate inspiration at a predetermined "safe" peak airway pressure. A loss of pressure, as occurs with a disconnection, can be similarly detected. Compliance changes, including those caused by ETT obstruction, bronchospasm, or pneumothorax, will cause changes in the peak airway pressure. Finally, an airway pressure monitor allows a rough evaluation of a patient's respiratory mechanics before extubation through measurement of the negative inspiratory and positive expiratory pressures.

### Does a Manometer in the Breathing Circuit Accurately Measure Intratracheal and Circuit Pressure?

Not always. It overestimates intratracheal pressure during mechanical ventilation and underestimates it during spontaneous breathing. The error is a function of inspiratory flow and ETT size (Fig. 19–4). The pressure difference across a small pediatric ETT can easily exceed 20 cm $H_2O$. When knowledge of the precise intratracheal pressure is important, application of an end-inspiratory hold or plateau (ie, a period of no flow, therefore no resistance) allows the circuit and intratracheal pressures to equilibrate.

The simulator tracings (Fig. 19–5) illustrate the relationship

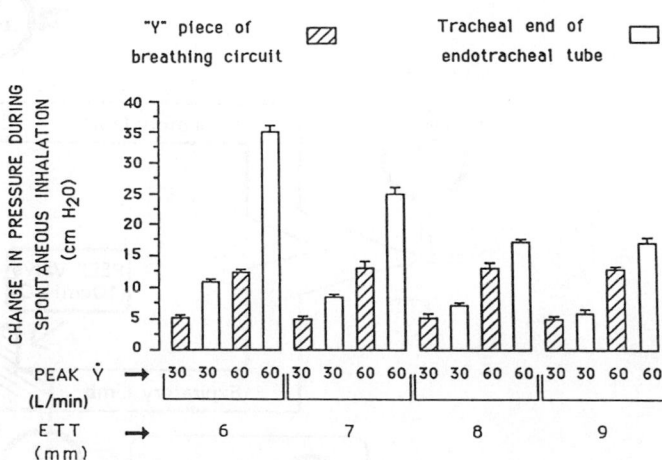

**FIGURE 19–4.** Comparison of pressure changes measured at the Y-piece of the breathing circuit tubing and at the tracheal (or carinal) end of the endotracheal tube during spontaneous inhalation at different peak sinusoidal inspiratory flow rate demands (V) with four different tube sizes (6.0, 7.0, 8.0, and 9.0). Note that the narrower the internal diameter of the tube and the greater the peak inspiratory flow rate demand, the greater the discrepancy between pressures measured at the Y-piece and at the tracheal end of the tube. Measuring pressure at the Y-piece results in significant underestimations of pressure changes, especially when the endotracheal tube has a small internal diameter and the peak inspiratory flow rate demand is high.

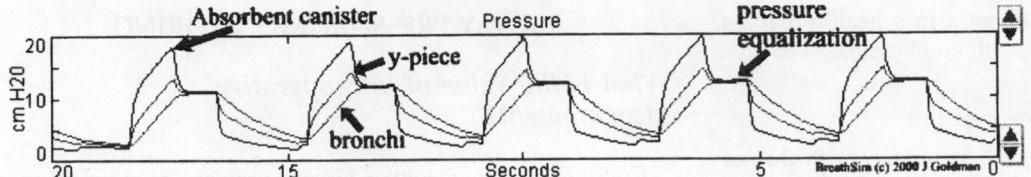

of alveolar pressure, Y-piece pressure, and $CO_2$ absorbent canister pressure throughout the respiratory cycle. Note the pressure gradient produced as the inspiratory gas flows through various breathing system components. As a result of resistance to gas flow, the pressure upstream ($CO_2$ absorbent canister) is higher than at the Y-piece, which is higher than bronchial pressure. The brief end-inspiratory pause produces a period of zero flow, which allows the pressure at the three sites to equilibrate. One could also place a pressure sensor at the tracheal tip of the ETT to obtain a measure of true airway pressure.

### Sensor Location

The location of the pressure sensor may also influence accuracy. Positioning the pressure sensor within the $CO_2$ absorber canister, as is the case in older anesthesia machines, produces an incorrect positive end-expiratory pressure (PEEP) measurement due to isolation of the sensor by the inspiratory valve (Fig. 19–6). PEEP devices usually are added between the expiratory limb and the expiratory valve. Therefore, the PEEP-induced circuit pressure increase occurs only in that portion of the circuit bounded by the inspiratory valve and the PEEP valve. To detect PEEP, the measurement must take place anywhere in the patient segment of the circuit between the two valves. The old Ohio Anesthesia Absorber incorporated a pressure gauge in the canister. Although this measured

intracanister pressure, it did not measure pressure produced with a typical PEEP valve. It would detect inadvertent PEEP produced by other factors, such as a scavenger valve defect. (See Chapter 15 for additional discussion.)

## TIDAL VOLUME MONITORING

### Why Does the End-Tidal Carbon Dioxide Decrease When the Fresh Gas Flow Is Increased?

#### Change in Tidal Volume

The $V_T$ delivered to the breathing circuit comes from two parallel sources: the ventilator bellows excursion and the FGF. The FGF is added continuously to the circuit gas; because the circuit pop-off is closed during the inspiratory phase of mechanical ventilation, FGF contributes to the inspired $V_T$ during mechanical inspiration (Fig. 19–7). The resultant increase is a function of the inspiratory time and the FGF.

For example, with a ventilator-delivered $V_T$ of 600 mL at a respiratory rate of 10 breaths per minute and an inspiratory-to-expiratory (I:E) ratio of 1:2, inspiratory time is 2 seconds. If the FGF is 6 L/min, 200 mL will be added to each 600-mL breath that is delivered by the ventilator bellows. The patient actually receives 800 mL per breath, producing a discrepancy

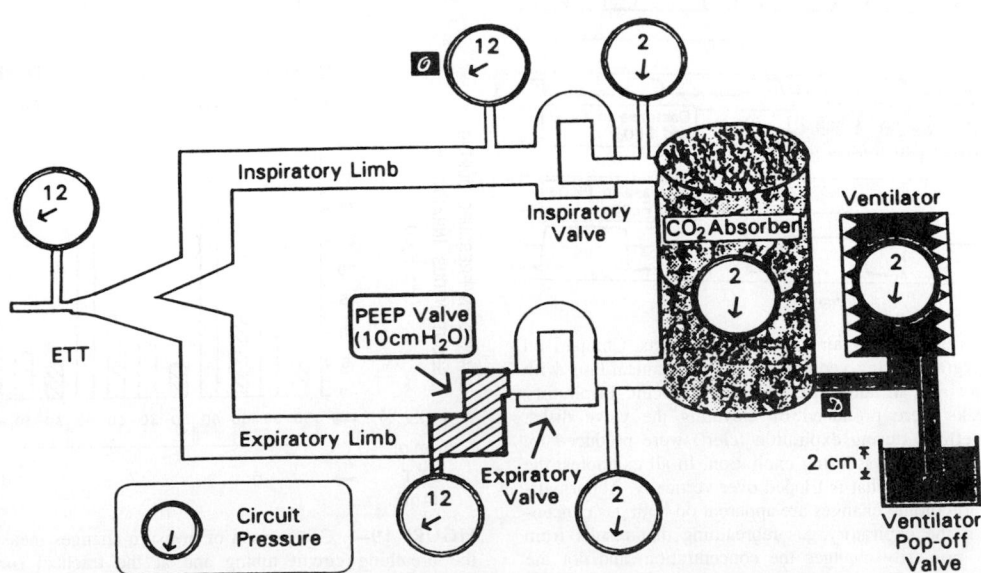

**FIGURE 19–6.** Breathing circuit pressure distribution. Schematic diagram of circle breathing circuit (during expiration) with a PEEP valve added to the expiratory limb. Ventilator bellows, which rise on expiration, incorporate a low pressure pop-off valve to maintain positive pressure within the bellows during expiration (depicted here by a water column valve). Note that with the PEEP valve placed at the expiratory valve, the pressures on the circuit side are different from those on the canister side of the inspiratory and expiratory valves. Currently, both North American Dräger (Telford, Pa) and Datex-Ohmeda (Madison, Wis) supply anesthesia machines that incorporate adjustable PEEP valves into the absorber head in locations that differ from those shown on this figure (and from each other). The Datex-Ohmeda machine measures circuit pressure at O in the figure, and the Dräger machine incorporates the PEEP valve and measures circuit pressure at D. Both machines correctly measure circuit pressure on the patient side of the PEEP valves. (See text for discussion.)

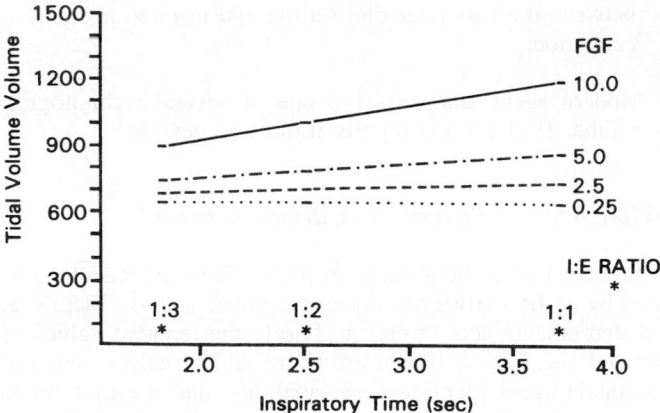

**FIGURE 19–7.** The effect of the ratio of inspiratory time to expiratory time (I:E) and fresh gas flow on the delivered $V_T$ as determined with a test lung. The ventilator was set for a $V_T$ of 600 mL by observing the bellows excursion at 8 breaths per minute. I:E was 1:3, 1:2, and 1:1 at the corresponding inspiratory times, indicated by *asterisks.* Data are means ± SD. (From Gravenstein N, Banner MJ. Tidal volume changes due to the interaction of anesthesia machine and anesthesia ventilator. *J Clin Monit.* 1987;3:187.)

between the set $V_T$ (noted on the ventilator control panel or the ventilator bellows excursion) and the measured $V_T$.

If the FGF is decreased to 2 L/min, only 66 mL is added to each 600-mL breath. The effect of changes in FGF on delivered $V_T$ may be particularly important for children immediately after induction of general anesthesia when FGF is reduced from a very high to a lower value and just before emergence when a low FGF is increased to a higher one. An analogous effect on $V_T$ occurs when the I:E ratio is reduced (ie, the longer the inspiratory [I] time, the larger the $V_T$).

The design of new anesthesia machine ventilators eliminates or reduces the effect of FGF on $V_T$ during mechanical ventilation.

## Spirometer Design

Several factors influence the discrepancy between the set and delivered $V_T$ measured by an in-circuit spirometer. Different spirometer designs are affected by various breathing circuit conditions and flow patterns.

### Turbine

A *rotating mechanical* (turbine) spirometer's accuracy may be reduced at low flow rates because of the inertia of the turbine element. If moisture condenses on the turbine, its mass may increase so that low gas flows do not initiate turbine rotation, falsely indicating absence of gas flow.

### Pneumotachograph

A pneumotachograph calculates flow by measuring the pressure drop across a flow resistor (eg, fine mesh screen) located in the circuit. The resultant pressure drop is a function of the flow. The Datex-Ohmeda Capnomac Ultima (Datex Ohmeda, Madison, Wis) uses a unique implementation of pneumotachography to measure flow at the ETT and produce flow-volume and pressure-volume loops. Correct interpretation of the flow-induced pressure drop depends on careful calibration of the pneumotachograph with a specific ETT size.

A change in placement of the pneumotachograph (eg, from the proximal side to the distal side of an elbow connector) also may necessitate recalibration. Gas composition changes during an anesthetic procedure are analyzed by the Ultima, which automatically compensates the pneumotachograph's calibration to maintain accuracy in the presence of gas density changes. A pneumotachograph offers the benefits of potentially high accuracy, but it may incorrectly measure circuit flow if not used with careful attention to detail.

## Does Changing the Tidal Volume on the Ventilator Cause a Corresponding Change of the Patient's Tidal Volume?

### Circuit Compression and Expansion

Anesthesia ventilators with bellows compress the bellows with $O_2$ to drive circuit gas into a patient's lungs. The set $V_T$ is the volume that would be delivered by the ventilator into a chamber at ambient pressure. However, for the volume to be delivered into a patient's lungs and the anesthesia circuit, it must be pressurized; this pressure increase compresses some gas within the ventilator bellows, ventilator hose, $CO_2$ absorber, and breathing circuit. The actual volume delivered to a patient's lungs reflects the set $V_T$ minus the resultant volume of gas compressed during inspiration. Additional $V_T$ loss occurs as a result of expansion of the breathing circuit tubing. The longer and more compliant the breathing circuit, the greater is the loss of volume delivered to the patient.

Subtle differences between the methods of operation of the Datex-Ohmeda (Datex-Ohmeda, Madison, Wis) and North American Dräger (Telford, Pa) anesthesia machine ventilators influence the effect of pulmonary compliance on apparent delivered volume.

### Datex-Ohmeda Ventilator

The Datex-Ohmeda ventilator bellows always fills to its capacity (~1600 mL). It then partially empties when a volume of gas equal to the set $V_T$ is introduced into the bellows housing, compresses the bellows, and forces circuit gas into the patient. Because the bellows is emptying against the resistance imposed by an increasing circuit pressure, the driving gas introduced around the bellows will be compressed, resulting in a smaller bellows volume change (as indicated by a reduction in bellows excursion) than would be expected. In other words, the bellows may descend only to the 650-mL mark on the bellows housing despite a $V_T$ setting at 800 mL. If the exhaled $V_T$ is measured after a return to ambient pressure, the volume will reexpand to a value close to the set $V_T$. In contrast, the patient's lung volume increases only by a volume equal to the compressed breath (650 mL in this example). This effect can be partially offset by increasing the set $V_T$ until the bellows descends the desired amount.

The newer Datex-Ohmeda 7900-series ventilator uses inspiratory and expiratory limb sensors to adjust bellows excursions and deliver the set $V_T$ volume. When FGF is changed, the system will compensate for the altered contribution of FGF to $V_T$ by adjusting bellows excursion over approximately 6 to 12 breaths.

### Dräger Ventilator

The classic Dräger ventilator uses an adjustable stop to limit bellows capacity. Ventilator inspiratory flow is adjusted to ensure complete emptying of the bellows. If the bellows' capacity is adjusted to 800 mL, this volume, measured at ambient pressure, is delivered. However, it is variably compressed during inspiration, depending on the peak inspiratory pressure. The reduction in actual lung volume change that results from $V_T$ compression is similar to that which occurs with the Datex-Ohmeda ventilator. However, with the Dräger ventilator, there is no objective indication of this volume compression. The new horizontal piston Dräger ventilator uses sophisticated volume compensation techniques more accurately to deliver the set $V_T$ over a large range of $V_T$.

### Summary

The design of the ventilator may also affect $V_T$ delivery. Additional circuit volume increases circuit compliance. With a set $V_T$ of 600 mL, the residual volume of the Datex-Ohmeda bellows is 1 L more than the classic Dräger bellows. Hence, a larger total volume is present in the Datex-Ohmeda system than in the Dräger system, even if the patient circuit, soda lime canister, and ventilator hose volumes are the same.

The breathing circuit spirometer measures only that *gas that flows by it in the expiratory limb* (gas exhaled by a patient and gas that distends the circuit or is compressed within it during inspiration). It does not include the portion of the $V_T$ that is sequestered in the ventilator, ventilator hose, and soda lime canister. Only when the FGF is sufficient to make up this lost volume will the set and measured exhaled $V_T$ values match.

Hence (in the older systems):

$$V_T \text{ Delivered to Patient} = \text{Bellows Excursion} + FGF \times T_I - \text{Gas Lost to Compression and Circuit Compliance}$$

where FGF = mL/s and $T_I$ = inspiratory time (seconds).

## AGENT MONITORING

### What Is the Value of Monitoring Anesthetic Concentration?

There are numerous benefits to monitoring anesthetic concentration:

1. Allows detection of an overdose due to human error or malfunction of the vaporizer.
2. Enables precision timing of reaching MAC-awake and achievement of a desired or target end-tidal concentration.[48,49]
3. Can detect the wrong vapor brought about by a vaporizer filled with the wrong agent. Only agent-specific monitors offer this advantage.
4. Allows observation of inhalation kinetics.
5. Provides assurance that the desired concentration is actually delivered, particularly when low flows cause equilibrium to be reached slowly and produce a large discrepancy

between the vaporizer dial setting and inspired agent concentration.

Modern agent analyzers use one of several technologies. See Table 19–1 for a comparison of these devices.

### What Are the Potential Sources of Error?

Ethanol has an IR absorption peak within the wavelengths used by an IR analyzer to detect anesthetic agents. Therefore, exhaled ethanol acts to elevate falsely the reported values of exhaled anesthetics. If you are using an IR analyzer without automatic agent identification capability, and the monitor is set to read enflurane or isoflurane, ethanol vapor will have minimal effects. In contrast, if halothane is selected, ethanol can artifactually increase the halothane reading by 3.5 times the blood alcohol percent concentration. We can apply this phenomenon to our clinical practice by selecting halothane during preoxygenation to detect potential interference by ethanol. This effect could also be anticipated in the presence of other organic hydrocarbons that have similar IR absorption (ketones, methanol, or isopropyl alcohol).[50]

### "Unusual" Gases

Ethanol, which could constitute only a small fraction of the gas mixture, would affect the mass spectrometer minimally. However, other unusual gases may have a more profound effect. The mass spectrometer reports each detected gas as a fraction of all the detectable gases. Because those used in anesthesiology usually do not detect nonanesthetic gases, their presence is ignored. Thus, the mass spectrometer may report falsely elevated levels of anesthetic agents in the presence of nondetectable gases such as helium or other organic hydrocarbons.

If we administer 20% helium, the isoflurane concentration is read according to its fraction in the remaining 80% of the respiratory gas that the mass spectrometer "sees"; a 1% dial setting on the vaporizer is associated with a 1.25% reading on the mass spectrometer. (Explained another way, if a patient inspires a mixture of helium 33%, $O_2$ 33%, and $N_2$ 33%, a clinical mass spectrometer that is not designed to detect helium would report concentrations of $O_2$ 50% and $N_2$ 50%.) If a metered-dose inhaler is used during mass spectroscopy, the propellant, a chlorofluorocarbon like the volatile agents, artifactually increases the reported anesthetic concentration.

In contrast to mass spectroscopy, Raman spectroscopy reports the measured concentration of each detectable gas present. Thus, the Raman spectrometer should continue to provide accurate values for anesthetics even in the presence of unidentifiable gases.

### Water Vapor

All agent analyzers are affected by water vapor. IR analyzers are subject to interference by water vapor, particularly in the $CO_2$ absorption wavelengths. A wet sample cell causes an increase in the baseline and end-tidal values.

Mass spectrometers and Raman analyzers are subject to mechanical failure as a result of water condensate in the sample cell. In addition, mass spectrometers yield errors in measurement if the analyzed gas is not dried for the same

**TABLE 19–1.** Comparison of Methods Used for Anesthetic Agent Analysis*

| Technology | Principle of Operation | Benefits | Weaknesses | Notes |
|---|---|---|---|---|
| IR spectroscopy | Anesthetic agents absorb certain IR wavelengths. Concentration is determined by the absorption difference between the sample cell (which contains the gas to be analyzed) and reference cell (a sealed cell containing a known gas concentration). | Newer analyzers with automated agent detection (*agent ID*) identify agent in vaporizer and obviate manual agent selection.[47] | In many analyzers, the user must select the specific agent to be analyzed. Mistakenly selecting the wrong agent results in an inaccurate value. This test cannot detect $O_2$, $N_2$, argon, or other nonpolar molecules. | Older monitors are being replaced by IR monitors that can identify specific anesthetic agents automatically. |
| Piezoelectric crystal adsorption | Measurement is performed by 2 quartz crystals: 1 is coated with a synthetic oil that adsorbs agents, the other serves as a reference. Adsorption of agent molecules (or water) on the crystal's surface decreases the crystal's vibrational frequency as a function of agent concentration. | Although the agent must be selected, the displayed error due to incorrect agent selection (with halothane, enflurane, and isoflurane) is minimal. (Error with desflurane may be higher.) Calibration requirements are needed infrequently. | Agent to be measured must be selected manually. Test cannot be used for measurement of $CO_2$ or other respiratory gases. | Developed in 1982 but not in widespread use. |
| Raman spectroscopy | Raman scattering describes the phenomenon in which sample gas illuminated by light (usually a laser beam) reemits a small portion of the light at a different wavelength. Analysis of the resultant Raman spectrum identifies and quantifies the sampled gases. | Test reports the measured concentration of each gas detected (in contrast to mass spectroscopy). Therefore, the presence of undetectable gases does not influence the measured concentration of the identified gases. All gases are measured. | Like mass spectroscopy, frequent calibration is required. Laser light source has a limited life span. | Improvements in solid-state laser technology may permit further miniaturization. |
| Mass spectroscopy | Sampled gases are ionized, and the resultant particles are deflected by a magnetic field in a vacuum chamber. The particles are separated by their mass-charge ratios. Each gas produces particles with an identifiable pattern of mass-charge ratios. | There is a potentially long delay time if long sample tubing is used in a multiplexed (shared) installation. | It reports each detected gas as a fraction of all detected gases. Therefore, it gives incorrect results if an undetected gas (eg, helium) dilutes the other gases. | Single-user monitors are becoming available but remain expensive. |

*In order of increasing list price of a representative monitor of each technology.
IR, infrared.

reasons that they yield errors when nonstandard gases are present. Raman spectrometers have a separate scattering peak for water that is far removed from the peaks for other respiratory gases.

Piezoelectric crystal adsorption monitors are sensitive to water molecules deposited on the measuring crystal's surface. The water is misidentified as an anesthetic agent and produces an artifactual increase in agent concentration.

### *Eliminating Water From Sampling Lines*

To have dry gas for analysis, many agent monitors use in line hydrophobic filters and frequently combine them with Nafion tubing. Nafion is a copolymer of tetrafluoroethylene and a fluorosulfonyl monomer that selectively adsorbs water without affecting the other respiratory gases present in the sample. After water vapor is adsorbed to the inner surface of Nafion tubing, it passes through the wall and evaporates.

Because Nafion is ineffective in eliminating water droplets, it is most efficacious when used at the airway where the water is still vaporized, rather than near the analyzer at which point it has condensed. The unique properties of Nafion also allow selective removal of alcohols, ketones, and some ethers, thus decreasing interference from these compounds.

Simpler solutions include positioning the sampling site such that it is in a nondependent position. If an artificial nose is used, it is placed between the patient and sampling site, thereby eliminating most of the water vapor before it reaches the sample line.

### Calibration, Leaks, Machine Faults

Three other reasons for apparent gas analysis errors should be considered if the displayed concentrations seem inaccurate:

1. The gas monitor requires calibration.
2. The gas monitor is not sampling what you think it is (the sampling catheter may have a leak).
3. The anesthesia machine is not delivering the gas mixture that you think it is.

### *Calibration*

Begin your evaluation with two simple tests: (1) let the monitor sample room air, then (2) exhale into the sampling catheter. Room air provides known concentrations of $CO_2$ (0%), $O_2$ (21%), and $N_2$ (79%) (these commonly quoted estimates ignore the presence of argon and trace concentrations of $CO_2$). If these values are not displayed, the monitor requires calibration (or perhaps servicing). If room air is measured correctly, your exhaled gas provides $CO_2$ at 33 to 38 mm Hg. If room air values were correct but your exhaled gas showed abnormal values, try repeating the test with a new gas-sampling catheter. The monitor may be aspirating room air through a discontinuity in the sampling catheter, resulting in dilution of the respiratory gas sample.

### Inappropriate Gas Delivery

If the monitor passes these tests, it should be performing adequately for clinical purposes. If sampling from the anesthesia machine now shows unexpected readings, consider the possibility that the anesthesia machine is delivering an incorrect gas mixture. For example, a vaporizer may require calibration or the $FIO_2$ may be decreased because $N_2$ is accumulating in the circuit during a low-flow or closed-circuit anesthetic.

### Sampling Line Leak

Inspection of the capnogram (the respiratory $CO_2$ concentration-time tracing) may provide a clue about the equipment problem. Figure 19–8 shows $CO_2$ and $N_2$ waveforms collected during and after correction of small and large gas monitor sampling catheter leaks. In the top printout, a small sampling catheter leak produced a small rise in the terminal portion of the capnogram's alveolar plateau.

The capnogram abnormality associated with a sampling line leak is subtle and may not arouse suspicion by itself. However, the concentration of $N_2$ and its waveform are also abnormal. Because the patient was breathing a mixture of $O_2$, $N_2O$, and

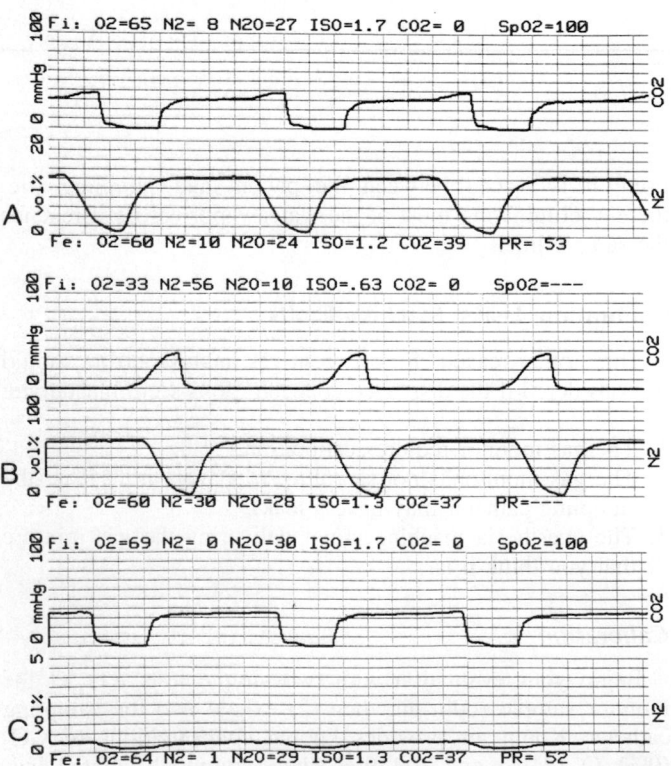

**FIGURE 19–8.** Large, small, and corrected respiratory gas monitor sampling catheter leak. $N_2$ and $CO_2$ concentration-time curves aspirated from a circle-circuit Y-piece during intermittent positive-pressure ventilation of an anesthetized adult patient. *A,* Small leak in gas monitor sampling catheter. *B,* Large sampling catheter leak. *C,* Leak eliminated. Note that the $N_2$ scale is different on each printout. (See text for discussion.)

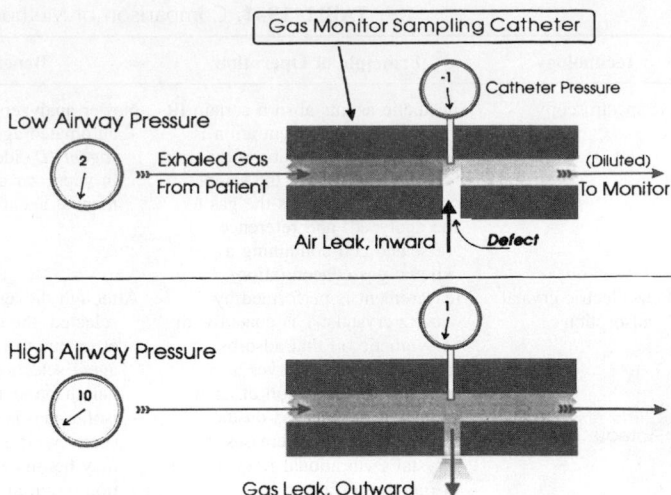

**FIGURE 19–9.** The monitor continuously aspirates sample gas; this generates a negative pressure (compared with ambient pressure), which entrains room air into the gas sample. When circuit pressure rises (during intermittent positive pressure ventilation), the sample catheter pressure rises (and usually becomes greater than ambient pressure). Room air is no longer entrained, and the gas sample may be accurately measured (although the capnogram is distorted). (Figure 19–8 shows resultant $CO_2$ and $N_2$ waveforms.)

isoflurane, we should not detect more than a small amount of (residual) $N_2$. Inspection of the $N_2$ waveform (see Fig. 19–8A) reveals that the $N_2$ concentration varied from 1% to 12% during the respiratory cycle and that its concentration decreased as the capnogram's alveolar plateau suddenly increased.

Figure 19–9 is a schematic representation of a segment of gas-sampling catheter. During the early part of expiration, the gas monitor samples respiratory gas that has been diluted by the aspiration of room air through a leak in the sampling catheter. When the ventilator cycles and pressurizes the breathing circuit and gas-sampling catheter, room air entrainment stops and an undiluted sample is aspirated by the gas monitor. The point of pressurization of the breathing circuit is evident on the $N_2$ tracing; note that $N_2$ concentration falls toward zero as room air entrainment stops.

### Circuit Leaks and Air Embolization

Analysis of the sampling catheter leak underscores the value of a monitor that can detect $N_2$. The same principle—that of observing an unexpectedly high concentration of $N_2$—applies to detecting breathing circuit discontinuities that entrain room air. Similarly, entrainment of air into the venous system (venous air embolization), with subsequent elimination of atmospheric $N_2$ by the lungs, can be detected by noting a sudden if very small increase in concentration of expired $N_2$.[51]

## CARBON DIOXIDE MONITORING

### What Is Meant by End-Tidal Carbon Dioxide?

The $PETCO_2$ is the partial pressure of exhaled $CO_2$ obtained at the end of a tidal breath. It is measured by selecting the

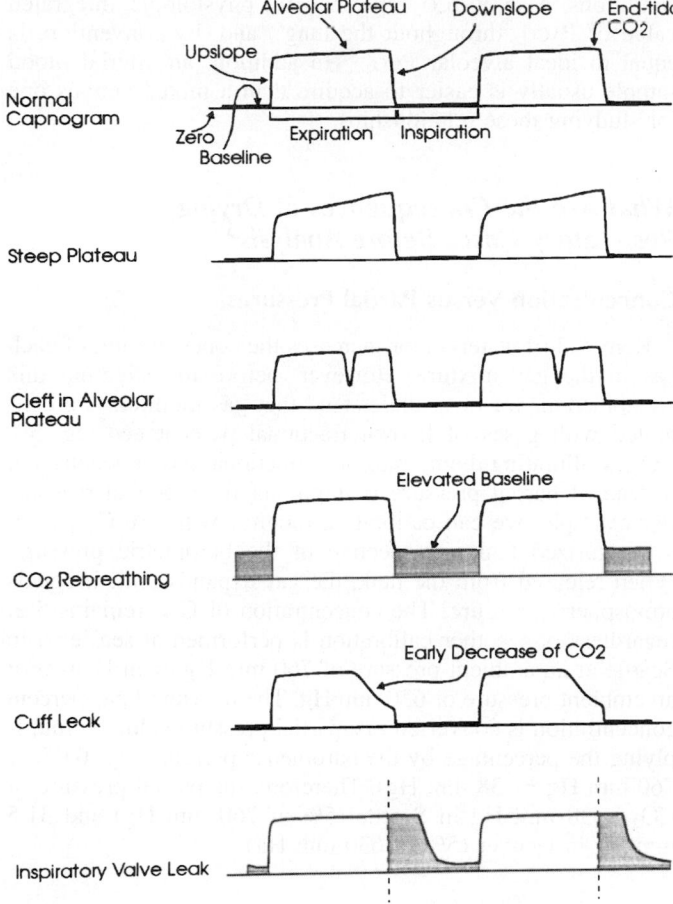

**FIGURE 19–10.** Typical capnograms. Note that baseline, upslope, and alveolar plateau correspond approximately to phase I, phase II, and phase III, respectively, of the classic physiologic description of a single breath analysis of $CO_2$.[59] These capnograms may be seen with a circle breathing circuit and mechanically ventilated patient. *Shaded areas* indicate duration and concentration of rebreathed $CO_2$. *Dotted lines* of inspiratory valve leak tracing indicate the point at which inspiration began and at which point the capnogram should be returning to baseline. (This phenomenon is explained in detail in Figure 19–13.)

highest concentration of $CO_2$ achieved in a single breath and is usually indicated by the terminal portion of the alveolar plateau of the capnogram (Fig. 19–10). Respiratory $CO_2$ concentration may be measured by a capnometer, which displays only the $CO_2$ concentration (peak or instantaneous), or by a capnograph, which displays the $CO_2$ concentration-time waveform.

The key principle underlying the significance of $PETCO_2$ is that it is an end-tidal gas sample composed primarily of alveolar gas. The concentration of $CO_2$ in alveolar gas is, in turn, used to estimate $PaCO_2$ noninvasively. When $PETCO_2$ differs from $PaCO_2$, we can glean clinically relevant information from the $P(a - ET)CO_2$ difference.

Of course, the process really is not that straightforward. Because of the complex nature of pulmonary gas exchange and the effects of mixing expired gas and ventilatory gas at the sampling site, confirmation that alveolar gas is being sampled may be difficult to ascertain. Therefore, a *capnometer,* which only indicates the $CO_2$ concentration (eg, with a bar graph or digital display) but does not have a graphic display, may lead to errors in measuring and interpreting the $PETCO_2$. Even when using a capnograph, we must be suspi-

cious that a $PETCO_2$ value that was not measured at the terminal portion of a capnogram with a normal alveolar plateau may substantially underestimate the $PaCO_2$.

As an example, the capnogram with the steep plateau in Figure 19–10 could have been measured from a patient with severe obstructive lung disease. The steep plateau may indicate that expiration was not complete before the ventilator produced the next inspiration and returned the capnogram to baseline. Had expiration been permitted to continue, the capnogram would have continued to rise and may have finally measured a sample of undiluted alveolar gas. It is also possible that the $PETCO_2$ measured with a steep alveolar plateau is greater than $PaCO_2$, but this finding is unusual.

Another example of a potential difficulty in determining alveolar $CO_2$ occurs when capnography is applied to nonintubated patients. Expiratory gas can be sampled by modifying nasal cannulas or by inserting a sampling catheter in the naris, among other methods. A reliable alveolar sample that reflects $PaCO_2$ may be obtained, but only from a capnogram with a normal alveolar plateau and only if the ventilation-perfusion ratio of the patient is normal.[52,53]

## What Is the Relationship Between $PETCO_2$ and $PaCO_2$?

$PETCO_2$ may be greater than, equal to, or less than the $PaCO_2$. This variable relationship is influenced by the sampling technique, equipment, and a patient's (patho)physiology (Fig. 19–11). In healthy patients, the $P(a - ET)CO_2$ difference is about 5 mm Hg, but it varies during the course of an anesthetic.[54,55]

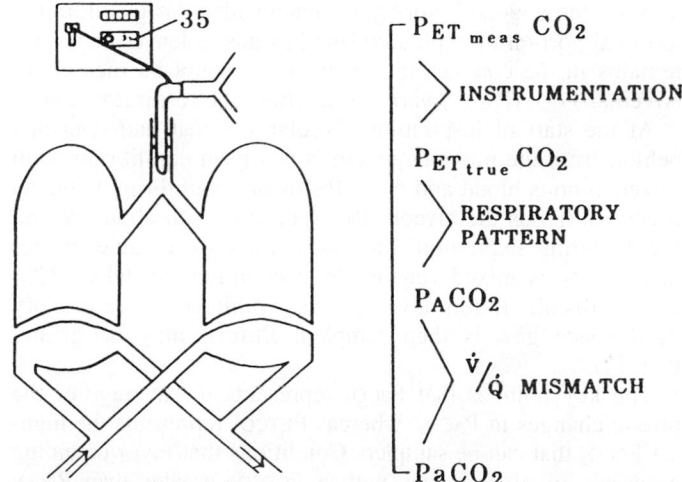

**FIGURE 19–11.** The difference between $PaCO_2$ and $PETCO_2$ can be divided into three components. The first component is the difference between $PaCO_2$ and $PACO_2$. Ventilation-perfusion mismatching causes this component of the $PaO_2$-$PETCO_2$ difference to increase. The second component is the difference between $PaCO_2$ and true $PETCO_2$ ($PET_{true}CO_2$). Respiratory patterns that do not deliver mixed alveolar gas to the upper airway (eg, rapid shallow breathing) increase this component of the $PaCO_2$-$PETCO_2$ difference. The third component is the difference between $PET_{true}CO_2$ and measured $PETCO_2$ ($PET_{meas}CO_2$). This component of the $PaCO_2$-$PETCO_2$ difference increases in the presence of problems related to instrumentation (eg, miscalibrated $CO_2$ analyzer, sampling line leak). (From Good ML. Capnography: uses, interpretation, and pitfalls. In: *Refresher Courses in Anesthesiology.* Vol 18. Park Ridge, Ill: American Society of Anesthesiologists; 1990:185.)

To consider the relationship between $P_{ETCO_2}$ and $Pa_{CO_2}$, we must first consider the factors that impede acquisition of an alveolar gas sample. Obstruction to expiratory gas flow, as in asthma or with a partially occluded ETT, produces an artifactually low $P_{ETCO_2}$ because a true end-exhaled sample is not obtained. Sampling from a loose-fitting or large dead space face mask causes dilution of the alveolar sample with fresh gas. The presence of a leak in the sampling catheter permits aspiration of room air by the gas monitor, again producing an artifactually low $P_{ETCO_2}$.

In patients with severe pulmonary ventilation-perfusion $(\dot{V}/\dot{Q})$ abnormalities, such as may be induced by pulmonary hypotension or a pulmonary embolus, alveoli with little or no pulmonary blood flow (high $\dot{V}/\dot{Q}$) contribute their gas (which has not acquired $CO_2$) to gas from normally perfused alveoli. If these groups of alveoli empty in parallel, the average exhaled $CO_2$ is lower than the concentration in the normally perfused alveoli, and $P_{ETCO_2}$ is lower than "true" alveolar $CO_2$. The resulting alveolar dead space (and dead space ventilation) decreases $P_{ETCO_2}$ without necessarily producing an abnormal alveolar plateau.[56] Conversely, patients in whom part of the pulmonary arterial blood flow fails to perfuse ventilated alveoli will dump venous blood into the arterialized blood leaving the lung. Such a shunt will also result in a larger than normal difference between end-tidal and arterial $CO_2$ concentration without affecting the shape of the capnogram.

## If Conditions Are Perfect, Will $P_{ETCO_2}$ Equal $Pa_{CO_2}$?

Although clinicians expect $P_{ETCO_2}$ to be close to $Pa_{CO_2}$, here is a different question: what does the $P_{ETCO_2}$ value actually represent? In the ideal setting (assuming normal physiology), the end-expiratory gas contains alveolar gas from the terminal portion of expiration (the last gas to leave the alveoli remains in the conducting airways and cannot be measured). Alveolar $P_{CO_2}$ ($PA_{CO_2}$) varies throughout the respiratory cycle.

At the start of inspiration, alveolar gas that had remained behind from the previous breath is nearly in equilibrium with mixed venous blood and has a $PA_{CO_2}$ of about 44 mm Hg. As fresh gas floods the alveoli, $PA_{CO_2}$ decreases to about 39 mm Hg.[54] During expiration, the $PA_{CO_2}$ rises to a value greater than $Pa_{CO_2}$ as mixed venous blood continues to deliver $CO_2$ to the alveoli. If this alveolar gas, undiluted by respiratory dead space gas, is then sampled, $P_{ETCO_2}$ may be greater than $Pa_{CO_2}$.

The key point is that $Pa_{CO_2}$ represents the average of the phasic changes in $PA_{CO_2}$, whereas $P_{ETCO_2}$ represents the highest $PA_{CO_2}$ that can be sampled. Conditions that favor obtaining a sample of alveolar gas with a $P_{ETCO_2}$ greater than $Pa_{CO_2}$ include healthy lungs, minimal alveolar dead space, low respiratory rate, and large $V_T$.[57] These conditions promote equilibration of end-expiratory gas with mixed venous gas.

## Why Is the Relationship Between $P_{ETCO_2}$ and $Pa_{CO_2}$ Emphasized?

This relationship is emphasized for several reasons. The parameter that we wish to know is $Pa_{CO_2}$; effort is thus placed on assessing its relationship to $P_{ETCO_2}$ under varying clinical conditions. Also, $P_{ETCO_2}$ represents the physiologic, integrated value of $Pa_{CO_2}$ throughout the lung[56] and, by convention, is equal to ideal alveolar $P_{CO_2}$.[54] In addition, an arterial blood sample usually is easier to acquire than a mixed venous one for studying these relationships.

## What Are the Consequences of Drying Respiratory Gases Before Analysis?

### Concentration Versus Partial Pressures

Removal of water vapor increases the concentration of each gas in the gas mixture. However, before investigating this phenomenon, we must understand that gas monitors are calibrated with gases of known fractional percentages (eg, 5% $CO_2$). Calibrating the monitor to a fractional gas concentration instead of partial pressure is important for practical reasons. For example, we can calibrate a monitor with 5% $CO_2$ from a pressurized tank, irrespective of the barometric pressure. When released from the tank, the gas expands until it equals atmospheric pressure. The concentration of $CO_2$ remains 5%, regardless of whether calibration is performed at sea level in Seattle at an ambient pressure of 760 mm Hg or in Denver at an ambient pressure of 630 mm Hg. The measured gas percent concentration is converted to a partial pressure value by multiplying the percentage by the barometric pressure (eg, $0.05 \times$ 760 mm Hg = 38 mm Hg). Therefore, the partial pressure of $CO_2$ is 38 mm Hg in Seattle (5% of 760 mm Hg) and 31.5 mm Hg in Denver (5% of 630 mm Hg).

### Practical Implications

The implication of calibrating a monitor with dry gas and then measuring water vapor-saturated exhaled gas is that if the $P_{ETCO_2}$ is 38 mm Hg, the equivalent fraction of $CO_2$ in saturated alveolar gas is 5% (38 mm Hg/760 mm Hg). Because we know that saturated water vapor exerts a constant partial pressure of 47 mm Hg at body temperature, we can also calculate the concentration of water vapor: 47 mm Hg/760 mm Hg = 6.2%.

Let us assume that $O_2$ is the only other gas present and that its concentration is 88.8% (675 mm Hg/760 mm Hg). If water vapor were removed from the alveolar gas sample, the remaining $O_2$ and $CO_2$ would increase in concentration but their relative proportions would remain unchanged. Therefore, the new concentration of $CO_2$ would be its old concentration (5%) divided by the fractional sum of $CO_2$ and $O_2$, or 5%/(0.05 + 0.888) = 5.3%. Similarly, the new concentration of $O_2$ would be 94.6%.

A more common and mathematically equivalent way of calculating the expected concentration change that results from removal of water vapor is to divide the partial pressure by (760 − 47) mm Hg. For example, the new concentration of $CO_2$ would be 38 mm Hg/(760 − 47) mm Hg = 5.3%.

### Open and Closed Systems

If we had sealed these gases in a box (closed system) before removing the water vapor, the number of molecules of $CO_2$ and $O_2$ could not change and, by definition, the partial pressures of the $CO_2$ and $O_2$ would be unchanged despite an increase in the concentration of each gas. However, drying of the gas sample is occurring within the monitor or Nafion gas-sampling line, which is an open system, so that additional gas can replace the water vapor as it is removed. Therefore, the number of molecules of $CO_2$ and $O_2$ increases in proportion to the increase in concentration of these gases as water vapor is removed. The new partial pressures of these gases can be calculated by multiplying the new concentrations by 760 mm Hg. From our previous example, the new $P_{CO_2}$ is 5.3% of 760 mm Hg, or $0.053 \times 760$ mm Hg = 40.3 mm Hg.

## Summary

The gas monitor analyzes the dried (or a gas with the assumed low relative humidity of the ambient air) sample gas and measures 5.3% $CO_2$. If the monitor displays a gas concentration as a partial pressure, it may calculate 5.3% of 760 mm Hg and report $P_{ETCO_2}$ as 40.5 mm Hg, or it may adjust the partial pressure value to reflect saturated alveolar conditions by calculating 5.3% of $(760 - 47)$ mm Hg and report $P_{ETCO_2}$ as 38 mm Hg.

Respiratory physiology nomenclature conventions recommend displaying the fractional percentage unchanged (eg, 5.3% $CO_2$) while displaying the partial pressure ($P_{ETCO_2}$) adjusted to saturated conditions.[58] Unfortunately, not all monitors correct their partial pressure measurement to water vapor-saturated conditions, and whether a specific monitor is displaying dry or water vapor-saturated gas partial pressure is not readily apparent.

Another confounding problem is that only partial drying of the gas sample may occur before analysis. An interesting consequence of this artifactual increase in $P_{ETCO_2}$ is a reduction in the apparent difference between $Pa_{CO_2}$ and $P_{ETCO_2}$.

## What Is the Difference Between Mainstream and Sidestream Capnographs?

A mainstream analyzer uses a cuvette attached to the ETT to measure $CO_2$. The IR optics are located in the cuvette itself, so that analysis of the gas sample is rapid. In contrast, a sidestream analyzer must aspirate the gas sample through a sampling catheter. Therefore, the sidestream analyzer imposes an additional delay in sampling and modest slurring of the waveform due to the transit of the gas sample in the sampling catheter[59] and large water traps that function like capacitors or by low aspiration sampling rates employed to conserve respiratory gas. The fidelity of the capnogram can be affected by the sampling location and technique. Loss of fidelity will complicate capnogram morphology analysis and may yield erroneous peak and trough $CO_2$ values, especially in neonates ventilated at high respiratory rates.

The advantage of the mainstream analyzer is the high fidelity of the resultant capnograms. Disadvantages include the cost and fragility of some brands of cuvettes. In addition, the cuvette adds apparatus dead space to the breathing circuit, is relatively heavy, and is awkward and bulky.

We prefer sidestream analyzers because the lightweight and inexpensive disposable sampling catheter permits flexibility in selecting a gas-sampling location. Also, many modern sidestream analyzers incorporate oxygen and agent analyzers, offering much more information than traditional capnographs. One disadvantage of sidestream analyzers is their need to aspirate sufficient gas (about 200 mL/min) from the breathing

circuit. This necessitates special consideration during low-flow or closed-circuit anesthesia for pediatric applications where the removed volume becomes a significant fraction of the minute volume. The aspirated volume can be returned to the breathing circuit.

A new sidestream technology (Microstream, Oridion Medical Inc, Jerusalem, Israel; www.oridion.com) uses laser-based IR technology and a small sample cell (15 µL) to permit high-fidelity $CO_2$ analysis with low sample aspiration rates (50 mL/min).[60]

## Chemical Detectors

A third technology for $P_{ETCO_2}$ monitoring is the chemical detector. The chemical reaction $CO_2 + CO_3^- + H_2O \rightleftarrows 2HCO_3^-$ drives a pH reaction to one of six color zones. These devices are disposable and semi-quantitative, add 38 mL of apparatus dead space, and are not recommended for more than 10 minutes' use. This technology should be considered a backup rather than a primary technique in the operating room (Table 19–2). However, it is useful in remote locations to confirm ETT placement and the effectiveness of cardiopulmonary resuscitation.

## What Can Be Learned by Examining Capnogram Morphology?

We can learn much about patients and equipment by examining a capnogram. Figure 19–9 shows capnogram nomenclature and several classic capnogram abnormalities that may be observed with a circle breathing circuit attached to a mechanically ventilated patient. The normal capnogram is labeled to explain the various parts of the waveform. Note that the baseline of the capnogram should be zero; if it is not, the patient is inhaling $CO_2$. Be aware, however, that in children with rapid respiratory rates a sidestream analyzer may slur the capnogram, falsely showing $CO_2$ during inspiration. The following are examples of conditions that could produce the capnograms illustrated in Figure 19–10.

### Steep Plateau

An upward sloping plateau will be seen in a patient with bronchoconstriction or during ventilation at a slow respiratory rate and large $V_T$. Typically, a patient with bronchospasm will have a peak $P_{ETCO_2}$ at end of expiration markedly lower

**TABLE 19–2.** Comparison of Chemical and Electronic Detectors

| Characteristic | Chemical Devices | Sidestream Electronic Devices | Mainstream Electronic Devices |
|---|---|---|---|
| Breath-by-breath | + | + | + |
| Increased dead space | + + | − | ± |
| Quantitative | − | + | + |
| Long-term use | − | + | + |
| Requires calibration gas | − | + | − |
| Respiratory rate | − | + | + |
| Alarm | − | + | + |
| Diagnose hypercapnia | − | + | + |
| Power requirement | − | + | + |

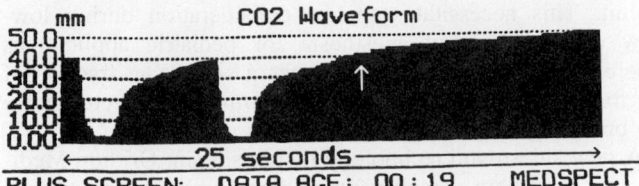

**FIGURE 19–12.** Steep alveolar plateau. In this adult patient with severe obstructive pulmonary disease, the apparent $P_{ETCO_2}$ on the capnogram misrepresents alveolar $P_{CO_2}$. The first capnogram demonstrates an abnormally steep alveolar plateau. It appears that $P_{ETCO_2}$ is 39 mm Hg. When expiration was permitted to continue uninterrupted for about 18 seconds, expired $CO_2$ concentration increased to 50 mm Hg as alveolar $CO_2$ finally reached the endotracheal tube sampling site. Arterial $P_{CO_2}$ was 55 mm Hg. (The *vertical white arrow* indicates the point at which inspiration would have begun had mechanical ventilation not been interrupted.)

than the $Pa_{CO_2}$. This difference is due, in part, to prolonged expiration that does not have enough time to run its full course so that an adequate alveolar gas sample is not obtained before initiation of the next inspiration. Therefore, as illustrated in Figure 19–12, we can improve the estimation of $Pa_{CO_2}$ in these patients by permitting expiration to continue for 10 to 20 seconds and noting the peak $CO_2$ concentration.

### Alveolar Plateau Cleft

A cleft in the alveolar plateau results from $CO_2$-free gas passing from the inspiratory limb and back toward the patient (and $CO_2$ sampling site) during expiration. This transient reversal of gas flow briefly decreases the concentration of $CO_2$ until expiration recommences. The cleft sometimes results from the sudden release of a surgeon's elbow pressure from a patient's chest. It often heralds a patient's recovery of neuromuscular function and the return of (weak) spontaneous respirations. In a normally functioning circle breathing circuit, the regular repetitive appearance of a cleft is a sensitive indicator of spontaneous inspiratory efforts. Such efforts deserve our attention: is the patient's $Pa_{CO_2}$ high because of relative hypoventilation or is the patient "light," making respiratory efforts in response to painful stimuli?

### Elevated Baseline

$CO_2$ appearing during inspiration indicates either an exhausted $CO_2$ absorber or an incompetent expiratory valve, leading to bidirectional flow in the expiratory limb of the breathing circuit. In either case, during inspiration, $CO_2$-laden expired gas mixes with fresh gas from the inspiratory limb and is inspired with it. If the expiratory valve is absent, no recognizable undulations may occur in the capnogram.

### Early Decrease of Carbon Dioxide

A leaking ETT cuff may permit the escape of ventilating gas past the cuff and into the upper airway during inspiration and expiration.

### Inspiratory Valve Leak

A leaking inspiratory valve causes an abnormally prolonged downslope brought about by admixing exhaled $CO_2$ to the

fresh gas delivered in the inspiratory hose (Fig. 19–13). In patients with fast respiratory rates, the slope may not reach baseline.

## What Lies on the Horizon for Carbon Dioxide Monitoring in the Operating Room?

As the transition of care from the operating room to the intensive care unit continues to blur, one intensive care unit monitor may soon appear in the operating room. A recent addition to the family of noninvasive respiratory monitors (CO$_2$SMO Plus!, Novametrix Medical Systems, Wallingford, Conn) measures and trends alveolar minute ventilation and $CO_2$ elimination and calculates physiologic dead space (Fig. 19–14). It simultaneously monitors the volume-based expirogram and $CO_2$ concentrations rather than only the traditional time-based capnogram.[61] We may also see the use of artificial intelligence-based capnogram analysis systems to facilitate the diagnosis of intraoperative ventilatory problems.[62] Preliminary investigations of the monitor suggest it may have a role in critical care settings to assist with management and weaning of mechanically ventilated patients.[63,64] Continuous calculations of the dead space can detect the development of dead space ventilation and thus contribute to the early detection of a pulmonary embolus.[65,66] Efforts are also currently underway to develop a monitor of continuous oxygen consumption (D. Corsali, Novametrix, oral communication, October 1999).

### Intraoperative Spirometry

Normally, exhaled $V_T$ is not actually measured as a volume. Rather, it is calculated by integrating expiratory flow with respect to time. When analyzed more carefully, inspiratory and expiratory flow data may convey valuable information about the patient's ventilation.

## What Is the Pressure-Volume Loop?

The pressure-volume loop, often called the *dynamic compliance loop,* plots inspiratory and expiratory volume on the abscissa against pressure on the ordinate. Figure 19–15 shows compliance curves. In the spontaneously breathing person, the loop will tightly straddle the zero-pressure line because the pressure changes measured at the mouth will be low, indeed, a little negative during inspiration, a little positive during expiration. Figure 19–15A shows a dynamic compliance loop of a person breathing through an anesthesia circle. The loop shows the effects of resistance, which makes it necessary for the patient to generate enough pressure to overcome the resistance offered by the breathing system and its valves.

With mechanical ventilation, the entire loop moves to the right of the zero-pressure line (see Fig. 19–15B) because during inspiration, the ventilator generates pressure that, at first slowly, inflates the lungs, whereas during expiration, deflation of the lungs is retarded by the system. The resulting loop depicts the *hysteresis* (Greek for deficiency), the volume of which represents the work required to overcome the tissue resistance of lungs and thorax. Figure 19–15C shows two loops—one obtained with reduced compliance when the right main stem bronchus had been intubated, and one obtained

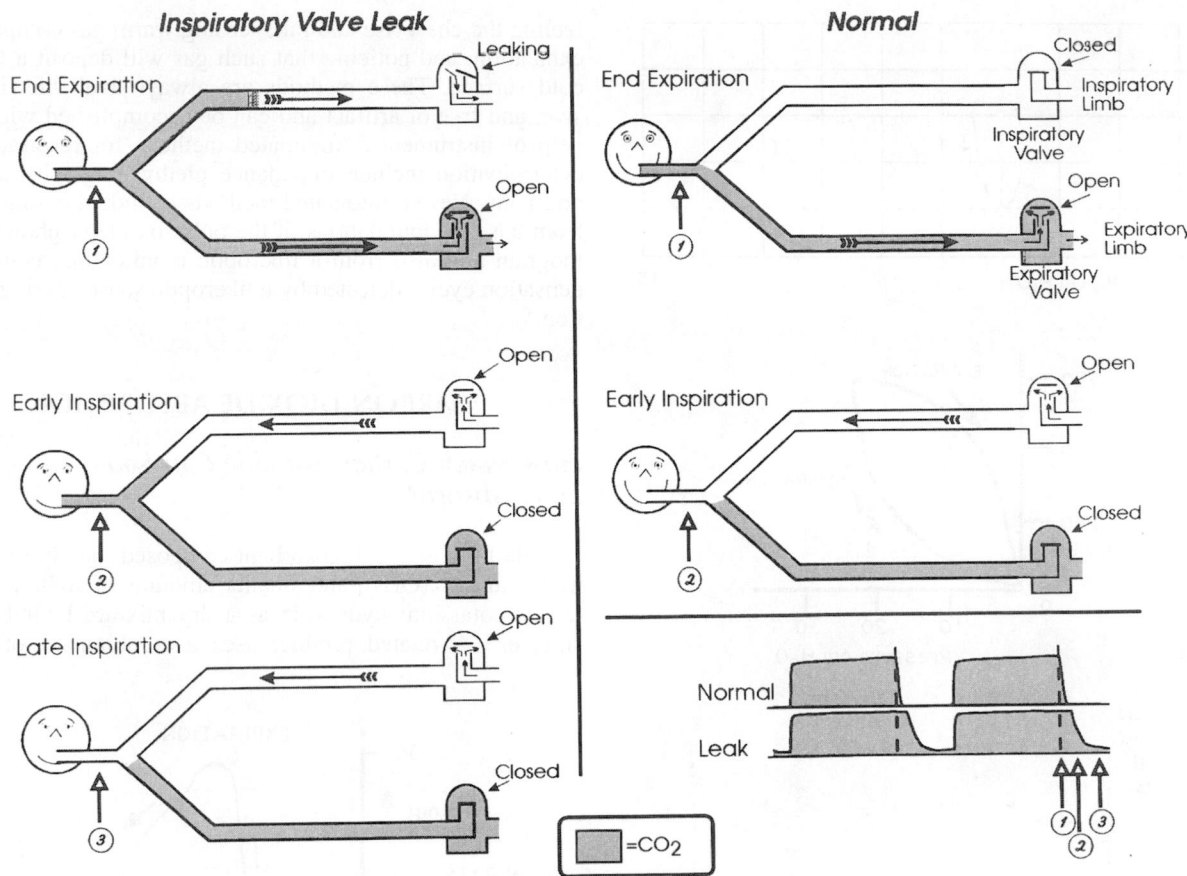

**FIGURE 19–13.** Pattern of gas flow with a leaking inspiratory valve. Diagram of $CO_2$ flow in a circle breathing circuit with a leaking inspiratory valve and under normal conditions. Normally during expiration, $CO_2$-laden expiratory gas flows only through the expiratory limb and is measured by the capnograph (1). Then, as inspiration begins, fresh gas (devoid of $CO_2$) flows through the inspiratory limb and is sampled by the capnograph (2). This results in the rapid downslope of the capnogram during inspiration. If the inspiratory valve leaks and permits bidirectional gas flow, expired gas will flow through both the expiratory and inspiratory limbs of the circuit during expiration. Then, as inspiration begins, the capnogram will demonstrate the continued presence of $CO_2$ at the endotracheal tube (2). As inspiration progresses, the inspired limb $CO_2$ may completely wash into the patient or a residual amount may still remain at the end of inspiration (3). The gradual washout of $CO_2$ from the inspiratory limb produces a capnogram with a prolonged plateau and an abnormal downslope. The severity of $CO_2$ rebreathing depends on the amount of reverse flow in the inspiratory limb. The capnogram may return to baseline during inspiration if the tidal volume is large relative to the volume of gas that flows backward into the inspiratory limb.

after pulling the ETT back into the trachea. Observe that the loops do not come back to baseline because the breathing system, with its valves and the standing bellows, causes a little positive pressure to remain after exhalation. With PEEP,

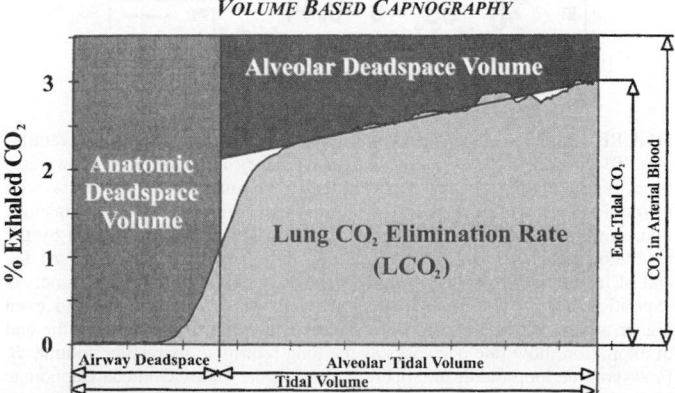

**FIGURE 19–14.** Single breath $CO_2$ elimination method. The percentage of exhaled $CO_2$ is plotted against tidal volume.

the loop will move farther away from the zero line, showing the imposed pressure at end expiration.

### What Is the Flow-Volume Loop?

The flow-volume loop plots inspiratory and expiratory flow rate (in liters per minute) on the ordinate and cumulative volume (inspired and expired) on the abscissa. The breath begins at 0 flow and 0 volume on the right side of the graph, as shown in Figure 19–16A. Observe that a downward deflection represents inspiration. Ideally, during inspiration, flow rate becomes steady as volume increases during inspiration powered by the ventilator. Because the ventilator drives inspiration, the flow-volume loop becomes more interesting during expiration when resistance to exhalation affects the rate at which gas is expelled from the lungs (see Fig. 19–16B).

It will also expose breathing system leaks when caused by escape of respiratory gases distal to the flow measuring site.

### Did They Teach About These Curves During Pulmonary Medicine Rotation?

Probably not. The spirometry curves that are typically analyzed to assess pulmonary function and identify airway ob-

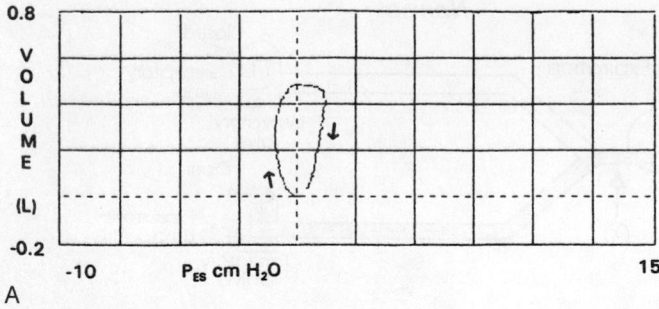

A

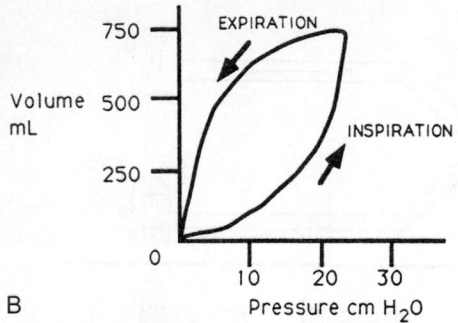

B

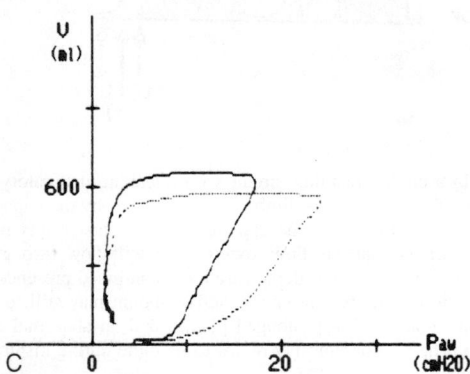

C

FIGURE 19–15. *A,* Compliance loop during spontaneous ventilation while breathing into an anesthesia circle breathing system. With inspiration, the pressure falls *(to the left)* while volume rises. *B,* An idealized volume-pressure (dynamic compliance) loop during mechanical ventilation. *C,* Compliance loop with intubation of a mainstem bronchus. The loop with *dotted lines* represents one-lung ventilation. The compliance loop improves (lower pressure—larger volume) with retraction of the tip of the endotracheal tube into the trachea. (From Gravenstein JS, Paulus DA, Hayes TJ. *Gas Monitoring in Clinical Practice.* 2nd ed. Boston, Mass: Butterworth-Heinemann; 1995:78.)

struction are based on tests conducted on spontaneously breathing, compliant patients. As a result of the confounding elements introduced by a patient's ability and cooperation, these are *effort dependent* and *effort independent* tests. In contrast, the anesthetized patient's inspiratory flow pattern will be determined primarily by the ventilator's inspiratory flow characteristics, whereas the expiratory flow pattern is always effort independent. There can be no effort-based peak expiratory flow measurement. Nevertheless, intraoperative spirometry can provide valuable information, as shown in Figures 19–15 and 19–16.

### What Is New in Breath Rate Detection?

Nothing can displace the old-fashioned way of counting respiration by listening to the breath sounds and watching and

feeling the chest rise and fall, sensing warm gas escape during exhalation, and noticing that such gas will deposit a fog on a cold surface. These methods are always available, inexpensive, and free of artifact and can be accomplished without the help of instruments. Automated methods for respiratory rate determination include impedance plethysmography and capnography. Newer automated methods include deriving the rate from baseline undulations of the pulse oximeter photoplethysmogram and also from a fiberoptic monitor that counts condensation cycles detected by a fiberoptic sensor during exhalation.[67]

## CARBON DIOXIDE ABSORPTION

### How Much Carbon Dioxide Can Soda Lime Absorb?

Soda lime is a $CO_2$ absorbent composed mainly of calcium hydroxide $[Ca(OH)_2]$ and smaller amounts of sodium hydroxide or potassium hydroxide as a dry mixture bound to inert silicate.[68] A related product uses a combination of barium

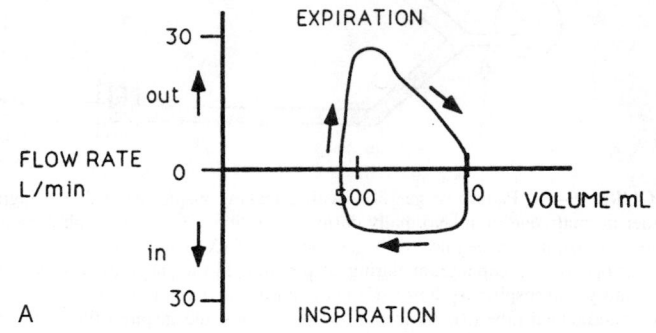

A

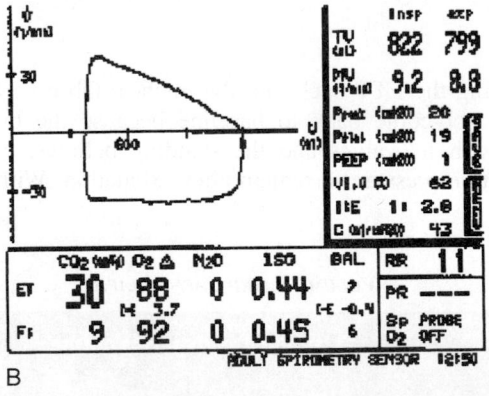

B

FIGURE 19–16. *A,* Idealized flow-volume loop during mechanical ventilation. To generate a flow-volume loop, inspiratory and expiratory flow rates (L/min) are plotted against the cumulative volume. The loop starts with inspiration (zero volume, zero flow) at the right of the abscissa. With inspiration, flow rate that increased *(plotted downward)* rapidly is sustained by the ventilator, which increases the inspired volume *(plotted to the left).* At the end of inspiration, flow rate drops to zero and volume remains the same. As expiration begins, flow rate increases rapidly (up to 30 L/min—and even higher with coughing) as the elastic forces of the lungs expel gas. At the end of expiration, flow rate decreases as the lung returns to its resting volume. *B,* Flow-volume loop (adult intraoperative) using the Datex-Ohmeda Capnomac Ultima. (*A* from Gravenstein JS, Paulus DA, Hayes TJ. *Gas Monitoring in Clinical Practice.* 2nd ed. Boston, Mass: Butterworth-Heinemann; 1995:77. *B* courtesy of Datex Ohmeda, Madison, Wis.)

hydroxide (as an octahydrate compound) and sodium hydroxide as the absorbent (Baralyme). Barium hydroxide is heavier than calcium hydroxide. Therefore, under ideal conditions, 100 g of soda lime absorbs 23 L of $CO_2$, whereas 100 g of barium hydroxide absorbs only 18 L.

During closed-circuit anesthesia, when all $CO_2$ produced by a patient must be absorbed, the amount of time to exhaustion of the $CO_2$ absorber can be calculated if you know its absorbing capacity. In a properly packed canister, 100 g of soda lime should absorb a minimum of 15 L of $CO_2$ before the exiting gas exceeds 1% $CO_2$. The average to maximum production of $CO_2$ in healthy adult males under general anesthesia is between 12 and 18 L per hour. Therefore, about 100 g of fresh soda lime is required to absorb all of the $CO_2$ produced during each hour of general anesthesia; for added safety, the usual estimate is 1 kg of soda lime for every 8 hours of use.

Because the average $CO_2$ absorber holds two soda lime containers, each of 1- to 1.5-kg capacity, a total of 16 hours of $CO_2$-absorbing capacity should be possible with a new canister of soda lime. In semi-closed anesthesia systems, a portion of the $CO_2$ is vented to the scavenging system; hence the $CO_2$ absorbent lasts longer. The higher the FGF, the longer the absorbent lasts (Fig. 19–17).

Calcium hydroxide is consumed during the process of $CO_2$ absorption, which proceeds in three steps as follows:

1. $2CO_2 + 2H_2O \rightarrow 2H_2CO_3$
2. $2H_2CO_3 + 2NaOH + 2KOH \rightarrow Na_2CO_3 + K_2CO_3 + 4H_2O$
3. $Na_2CO_3 + K_2CO_3 + 2Ca(OH)_2 \rightarrow 2CaCO_3 + 2NaOH + 2KOH$

## What Factors Govern the Efficiency of Absorption?

The efficiency of $CO_2$ absorption can be influenced by the physical characteristics of the carbon dioxide absorber and how it is packed into the canister.

### Shape

Soda lime granules have irregular shapes to increase the surface area for $CO_2$ absorption.

### Size

Limitation of granule size to 4 to 8 mesh optimizes the surface area without increasing the resistance to breathing. (*Mesh* is a measure designating screen size as the number of openings per linear inch.)

### Hardness

Granules must have a specific minimum hardness to minimize the formation of caustic dust particles that might be inhaled.

### Packing

Granules must be firmly packed to prevent *channeling*, which is the formation of vertical pathways with low resistance to gas flow. Channeled gases contact only a small portion of the absorbent granules, thus allowing $CO_2$-containing gas to pass through the absorber canister and be rebreathed.

## When Is the Soda Lime Nearly Exhausted?

To facilitate recognition of soda lime's loss of $CO_2$-absorbing capacity, manufacturers incorporate an indicator dye in the granules. This indicator, ethyl violet, has a critical pH of 10.3. As calcium hydroxide is consumed and the pH in the canister falls, the indicator dye turns purple. The color change becomes more prominent as the absorbing capacity is progressively exhausted.

The manufacturer of Sodasorb (W. R. Grace & Co, Dewey and Almy Chemical Division, Atlanta, Ga) recommends that the upper canister be replaced when the majority of visible granules just begin to show a change in color. The lower canister, which is generally spared by the $CO_2$-containing gas flow, is then switched to the upper location. Another option is to compare the temperature of the two canisters by touching them with the back of your hand. The reaction sequence described is exothermic. When the lower canister is warmer, the upper canister is depleted.

North American Dräger and Datex-Ohmeda recommend changing soda lime when any visible color change is present. We cannot find any evidence to support this wasteful ap-

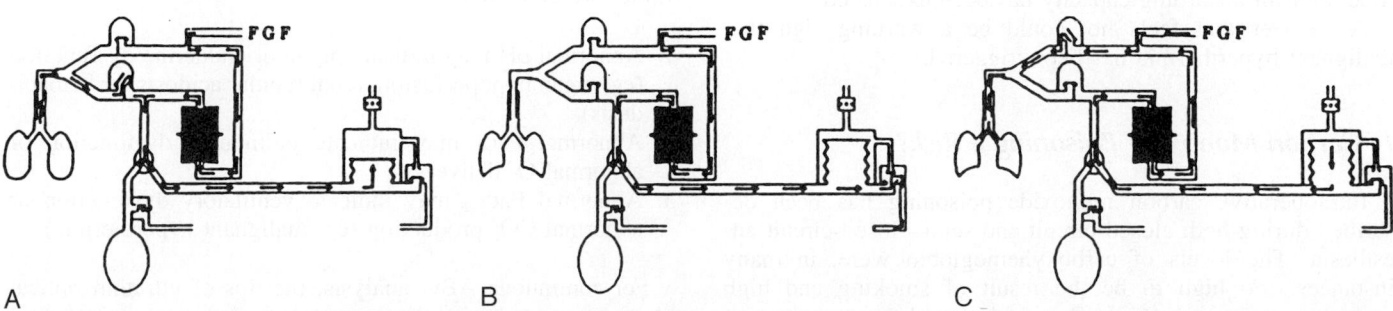

**FIGURE 19–17.** Mechanism by which the rate of fresh gas flow affects the $CO_2$ absorbent. $CO_2$-containing gases are represented by the *blacked-in portions* of the circuit. *A,* $CO_2$-containing gases from the patient pass through the ventilator hose into the ventilator bellows during exhalation. *B,* $CO_2$-containing gases pass through the ventilator hose, into the ventilator bellows, and out of the spill valve during the respiratory pause. *C,* Gases flow retrograde through the absorbent during inspiration. (From Öhrn M, Gravenstein N, Good ML. Duration of carbon dioxide absorption by soda lime at low rates of fresh gas flow. *J Clin Anesth.* 1991;3:104. Reproduced by permission of Butterworth-Heinemann.)

proach. Our practice is to remove the upper canister and replace it with the lower as soon as a color change is noted in the lower canister (proof that $CO_2$ is passing through the upper canister).

## Is a Carbon Dioxide Absorber Without Purple Discoloration Fresh?

Maybe not. The indicator dye helps only when the anesthesia machine is in use. If the machine has been allowed to stand idle for more than 30 minutes without exposure to $CO_2$, the soda lime may regenerate a small amount of absorptive capacity, increasing the pH sufficiently to cause the indicator to revert to a colorless state. In this instance, the absence of a color change belies the presence of nearly exhausted absorbent with limited remaining capacity. It is thus evident that white Sodasorb always has absorptive capacity, but its whiteness is not a quantitative indication. Sodasorb that is purple, however, is always at or very near the point of clinical—not chemical—exhaustion.

Fluorescent light can generate ethyl violet, which may mask the exhaustion of the carbon dioxide absorber. In addition, ethyl violet decays with time after a container of soda lime has been opened, even if it is stored in the dark.[69]

Finally, unknown to you, your absorbent may be of a type that lacks an indicator, in which case the color change that you are expecting will never occur. Without capnography, you would not know that the patient is rebreathing $CO_2$ until abnormal vital signs aroused your suspicion and prompted you to perform an arterial blood gas (ABG) analysis. If $CO_2$ rebreathing is documented by the appearance of inspired $CO_2$ on the capnogram, exhausted $CO_2$ absorbent can be differentiated from an incompetent expiratory valve by increasing the FGF to exceed the minute ventilation. This process converts the circle system into a nonrebreathing circuit and should return the capnogram to normal if the $CO_2$ absorbent is exhausted.

## Why Is the Soda Lime Canister Warm?

The chemical reaction of $CO_2$ with a strong base is exothermic; therefore, a warm canister signals active $CO_2$ absorption. The temperature is not proportional to the remaining absorptive capacity and may not decrease as the absorber is nearing exhaustion. The canister may remain warm for considerable time after all absorbing capacity has been exhausted.

A canister that feels hot could be a warning sign that malignant hyperthermia has been triggered.

## Is Carbon Monoxide Poisoning a Risk?

Intraoperative carbon monoxide poisoning has been described during both closed-circuit and semi–closed-circuit anesthesia. The levels of carboxyhemoglobin were, in many instances, too high to be the result of smoking and high enough to cause poisoning. One study noted that the cases of unexplained poisoning tended to be the first anesthetic cases on Monday mornings. Apparently, this was because of the prolonged contact of fluorinated anesthetics with the dry absorbent–generated carbon monoxide.[70]

Many now flush the absorber with fresh gas after prolonged idle periods. The small number of reported cases of carbon monoxide contamination should not discourage the use of a $CO_2$ absorbent.

A new $CO_2$ absorbent, Superia (Molecular Products Ltd, Essex, England; www.molecularproducts.co.uk and www. lowflow.net) does not contain added sodium, potassium, or barium hydroxides and therefore is noncorrosive and generates minimal amounts of carbon monoxide and Compound A. Clinically acceptable $CO_2$ absorption characteristics were obtained by advanced physical processing of the absorbent material.

# DIRECT MONITORING OF RESPIRATION AND OXYGENATION

## Arterial Blood Gas Analysis

Despite advances in new, sophisticated, noninvasive monitoring techniques, the analysis of ABG partial pressures and pH remains essential for a thorough evaluation of respiratory and overall physiologic function in anesthetized patients.

## Why Are the Measurements Important?

### Verify the Normal

Certain physiologic parameters must be within a narrow range for homeostasis. In fact, *we treat these numbers* (normally we treat the patient) for the following reasons:

1. Arterial pH is corrected to ensure an optimal milieu for the functioning of enzymes and drugs.
2. $PaO_2$ is normalized to permit cellular aerobic metabolism.
3. $PaCO_2$ is regulated to maintain normal organ perfusion because of its pervasive interaction via the sympathetic nervous system and as a therapeutic intervention (eg, control of intracranial hypertension).

### Identify the Abnormal

In addition to the previously cited reasons, ABG analysis is used to indicate the presence of abnormal physiologic states. Once identified, diagnosis and treatment of the underlying problem can proceed, so that the pathology and not just the values are corrected:

1. Abnormal pH may indicate organ or endocrine dysfunction (eg, organ hypoperfusion, renal tubular acidosis, or ketoacidosis).
2. Abnormal $PaO_2$ may indicate pulmonary dysfunction or abnormal $O_2$ delivery.
3. Abnormal $PaCO_2$ may indicate ventilatory dysfunction or abnormal $CO_2$ production (eg, malignant hyperthermia).

For continuous ABG analysis, the tips of ultrathin optical fibers are coated with fluorescent dyes that alter their optical properties as the concentrations of specific interactive substances change.[71,72] Agilent Technologies (Böblingen, Germany) markets a monitor that incorporates electrochemical pH and $PaCO_2$ in addition to fiberoptic $PaO_2$ elements on a thin, flexible sensor array that may be inserted into a 20-gauge arterial catheter and maintained in situ for several days.

## What Is Measured and What Is Calculated?

Clinical blood gas machines use three electrodes: one each for $PaCO_2$, $PaO_2$, and pH. These variables are directly measured and may be temperature corrected before display (more about temperature correction later). In contrast, bicarbonate ($HCO_3^-$), base excess, and percentage saturation of hemoglobin by $O_2$ ($SaO_2$) are calculated from the directly measured variables. ($SaO_2$ can be directly measured with a spectrophotometric automatic hemoglobin analyzer, or co-oximeter.)

### Units of Measurement

The newest measurement system, Système Internationale (SI), is in use in many countries but has not yet achieved popularity in the United States. These values are based on meter-kilogram-second units and do not include gravity-based units such as millimeters of mercury. The kilopascal (kPa) is the appropriate SI unit for the description of clinical pressure measurement. One kilopascal is equal to 7.50 mm Hg or 10.2 cm $H_2O$. Although kilopascals were introduced a number of years ago, their acceptance as the clinical unit of measure of fluid pressures has been delayed for reasons described by Nunn as "an entirely specious attachment to the mercury or water manometer."[73]

## How Quickly Must a Blood Sample Be Analyzed?

Most clinicians accept the observation that if a sample is stored in a plastic syringe at room temperature, no significant abnormalities will be induced by waiting up to 20 minutes before analysis.[74] Exceptions to this rule are blood samples from patients who are polycythemic or who have leukocytosis and a higher total metabolic rate of the white blood cells. However, some investigators recommend a more conservative time limit of 10 minutes if the sample is not stored on crushed ice (ie, at 0°C).[75] Regardless of philosophy, no harm results from analyzing it even sooner or, conversely, putting it on ice if there is uncertainty about how much time will elapse before analysis. Note that when whole blood samples for ABG analysis are stored on crushed ice, glass syringes may confer more stability than plastic syringes.[76]

It is important to be careful to avoid producing foam when aspirating arterial blood and to eliminate all air bubbles. Residual air in the sample syringe will begin to equilibrate with the blood sample and alter the $PaO_2$ and $PaCO_2$ within 2 minutes.[77]

## Should the Arterial Blood Gas Analysis Be Performed at a Standard Temperature of 37°C Even When the Patient's Temperature Is Lower or Higher?

Blood gas analyzers are warmed and perform their measurements with the blood sample brought to exactly 37°C. This is useful because we are familiar with physiologic principles at a normal body temperature. When the temperature drops, more gas goes into the solution. However, the pH rises by about 0.015°C because hemoglobin binds more hydrogen ions when cooled. Obviously, the opposite happens in hyperthermia. It is possible to determine or calculate the pH, bicarbonate, and partial pressures of gases at whatever the patient's temperature. However, we do not find this helpful because we do not have ready reference to what "normal" values at abnormal body temperature should be. Further discussion can be found in the medical literature.[78,79]

## If the Fraction of Inspired Oxygen Is Known, How Can the Predicted $PaO_2$ Be Calculated?

Several methods predict what the $PaO_2$ should be when a given $FIO_2$ is breathed. For a normal adult breathing room air at sea level, the $PaO_2$ can be estimated by the following equations[76]:

$$PaO_2 \text{ in mm Hg} = 102 - \frac{Age}{3}$$

$$PaO_2 \text{ in kPa} = 13.6 - 0.044 \,(Age)$$

If a patient with lung disease breathes supplemental $O_2$, an accurate estimate of $PaO_2$ can be obtained by measuring the $FIO_2$, calculating the pulmonary shunt fraction, and using the isoshunt diagram to diagram plots of $FIO_2$ against $PaO_2$ for a range of calculated shunt values[80] (Fig. 19–18).

In contrast to estimating $PaO_2$, calculating the $PAO_2$ is considerably simpler, as long as we do not require great accuracy. For *clinical* purposes, the following form of the alveolar air equation can be used:

$$PAO_2 = PIO_2 - \frac{PaCO_2}{R}$$

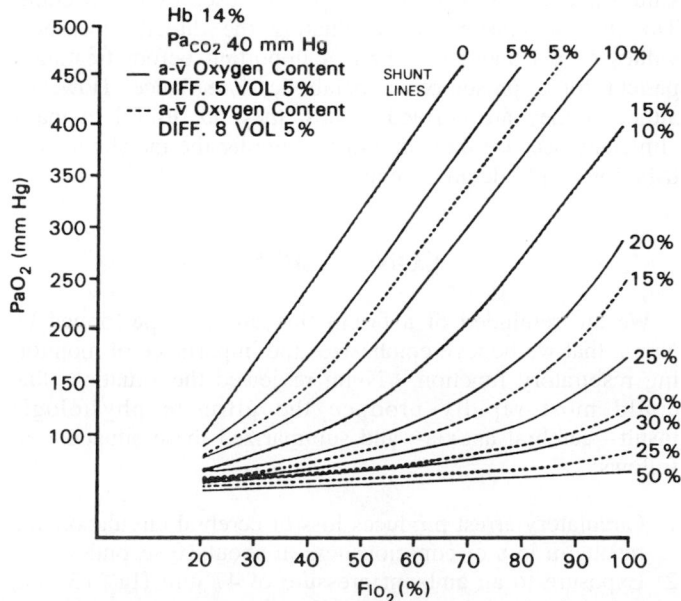

**FIGURE 19–18.** Theoretic relationships between $PaO_2$ and $FIO_2$ for different values of shunt at two different values of arterial/mixed venous $O_2$ content difference. Note that the curves are displaced but that their pattern is unaltered. (From Benatar SR, Hewlett AM, Nunn JF. The use of iso-shunt lines for control of oxygen therapy. *Br J Anaesth.* 1973;45:713.)

where R is the respiratory exchange ratio (equal to pulmonary $CO_2$ elimination/$O_2$ consumption) and $P_{IO_2}$ is the inspired partial pressure of $O_2$.

This equation is appropriate for a calculation performed intraoperatively when a simple and easy estimate of the alveolar-arterial oxygen difference (P[A − a]$O_2$) is necessary and less accuracy is acceptable. This form of the alveolar air equation does not account for differences in the volume of inspired and expired gas due to the respiratory exchange ratio or to the exchange of inert gases.[73] Despite these shortcomings, this estimate of the $P_{AO_2}$ can be used to evaluate a patient's pulmonary function (as reflected by the P[A − a]$O_2$ difference); even patients with normal lungs have a difference of about 15 mm Hg (2 kPa).

## How Are Respiratory and Metabolic Disturbances Differentiated?

A systematic approach to ABG interpretation simplifies intraoperative diagnosis and treatment of acid-base derangements that inevitably arise during anesthesia. We suggest first examining the pH value to determine whether acidemia or alkalemia is present. This initial assessment is followed by evaluation of the $P_{aCO_2}$, which is elevated in the presence of respiratory acidosis and decreased in the presence of respiratory alkalosis. Finally, the values for bicarbonate and base excess are examined; a low bicarbonate and negative base excess indicate a metabolic acidosis, whereas an elevated bicarbonate and base excess are associated with metabolic alkalosis. Obviously, different combinations of acid-base derangements can be present simultaneously and can infrequently produce an overall normal pH (see Chapter 41 for additional discussion).

An important fact to consider when interpreting ABGs is that the values for both bicarbonate and base excess are calculated by the blood gas analyzer; hence, they are derived values that vary based on the algorithm used by the machine. This is one reason why evaluating the directly measured values of pH and $P_{aCO_2}$ first is important before treating a patient for a presumptive metabolic disturbance. However, although they are derived values, they are useful to many clinicians because they simplify assigning the metabolic contribution of pH derangements.

## CONCLUSION

We are reminded of a fascinating analysis, performed by Nunn, that we believe emphasizes the importance of monitoring respiratory function.[73] Nunn reviewed the situations that could most rapidly produce the ultimate physiologic insult—cerebral anoxia—and summarized these situations as follows:

1. Circulatory arrest produces loss of cerebral circulation and results in loss of consciousness in about 10 seconds.
2. Exposure to an ambient pressure of 47 mm Hg (6.3 kPa) causes body fluids to boil. Water vapor replaces alveolar gas, and consciousness is lost in one circulation time (~15 seconds).
3. Hyperventilation with pure $N_2$ washes out alveolar $O_2$ and produces cerebral anoxia in about 30 seconds.

4. Inhalation of pure $N_2O$ produces loss of consciousness more slowly than inhalation of $N_2$ (unspecified time). The difference in speed of action occurs because $N_2O$ is more soluble than $N_2$, so that removal of $N_2O$ from the lungs by pulmonary blood flow decreases the rate of rise of alveolar $N_2O$, and hence the resultant fall in $P_{AO_2}$ is slowed.
5. Apnea ultimately leads to loss of consciousness, but the time to development of cerebral anoxia is dependent on the rate of $O_2$ consumption and alveolar $O_2$ stores. Loss of consciousness could occur within 90 seconds of apnea (after breathing room air).

Respiratory monitoring permits immediate detection of four of these five causes of cerebral anoxia; an altimeter detects the remaining cause. Although these scenarios represent the extremes of untoward events, they do underscore the value of such respiratory monitoring.

## Acknowledgments

We express our gratitude to our colleagues for their thoughtful comments: Robert W. Phelps, MD, PhD; Paul S. Nelson, MD; Lyle E. Kirson, DDS; and Robert J. Kopotic, MSN, RRT.

## References

1. Birmingham PK, Cheney FW, Ward RJ. Esophageal intubation: a review of intubation techniques. *Anesth Analg*. 1986;65:886.
2. Lundsgaard C, Van Slyke DD. Cyanosis. *Medicine*. 1923;2:1.
3. Braunwald E. Hypoxia, polycythemia, and cyanosis. In: Isselbacher KJ, Braunwald E, Wilson JD, et al, eds. *Harrison's Principles Of Internal Medicine*. 3rd ed. New York, NY: McGraw-Hill; 1994:178–183.
4. London MJ, Hollenberg M, Wong MG, et al. Intraoperative myocardial ischemia: localization by continuous 12-lead electrocardiography. *Anesthesiology*. 1988;69:232.
5. Clements FM, deBruijn NP. Perioperative evaluation of regional wall motion by transesophageal two-dimensional echocardiography. *Anesth Analg*. 1987;66:249.
6. Smith JS, Cahalan MK, Benefiel DJ, et al. Intraoperative detection of myocardial ischemia in high-risk patients: electrocardiography versus two-dimensional transesophageal echocardiography. *Circulation*. 1985;72:1015.
7. Sharbrough FW, Messick JM, Sundt TM. Correlation of continuous electroencephalograms with cerebral blood flow measurements during carotid endarterectomy. *Stroke*. 1973;4:674.
8. Messick JM, Casement B, Sharbrough FW, et al. Correlation of regional cerebral blood flow (rCBF) with EEG changes during isoflurane anesthesia for carotid endarterectomy: critical rCBF. *Anesthesiology*. 1987;66:344.
9. Ganzel BL, Edmonds HL, Pank JR, et al. Neurophysiologic monitoring to assure delivery of retrograde cerebral perfusion. *J Thorac Cardiovasc Surg*. 1997;113:748.
10. Dujovny M, Slavin KV, Luer MS, et al. Transcranial cerebral oximetry and carotid cavernous fistula occlusion. *Acta Neurochir*. 1995;133:83.
11. Pollard V, Prough DS, DeMelo AE, et al. Validation in volunteers of a near-infrared spectroscope for monitoring brain oxygenation in vivo. *Anesth Analg*. 1996;82:269.
12. Samra SK, Stanley JC, Zelenock GB, et al. An assessment of contributions made by extracranial tissues during cerebral oximetry. *J Neurosurg Anesth*. 1999;11:1.
13. Kytta J, Ohman J, Paivi T, et al. Extracranial contribution to cerebral oximetry in brain dead patients: a report of six cases. *J Neurosurg Anesth*. 1999;11:252.
14. Germon TJ, Evans PD, Barnett NJ, et al. Cerebral near infrared spectroscopy: emitter-detector separation must be increased. *Br J Anaesth*. 1999;82:831.
15. Jobsis FF, Keizer JH, LaManna JC, et al. Reflectance spectrophotometry of cytochrome a, a$_3$ in vivo. *J Appl Physiol*. 1977;43:858.
16. Grubhofer G, Tonninger W, Keznickl P, et al. A comparison of the monitors INVOS 3100 and NIRO 500 in detecting changes in cerebral oxygenation. *Acta Anaesth Scand*. 1999;43:470.
17. Yamada S, Brauer F, Knierim D, et al. Safety limits of controlled hypotension in humans. *Acta Neurochir Suppl (Wien)*. 1988;42:14.

18. Lovell AT, Owen-Reece H, Elwell CE, et al. Continuous measurement of cerebral oxygenation by near infrared spectroscopy during induction of anesthesia. *Anesth Analg.* 1999;88:554.

19. Severinghaus JW, Honda Y. History of blood gas analysis, VII: pulse oximetry. *J Clin Monit.* 1987;3:135.

20. Kelleher JF. Pulse oximetry. *J Clin Monit.* 1989;5:37.

21. Reich DL, Timcenko A, Bodian CA, et al. Predictors of pulse oximetry data failure. *Anesthesiology.* 1996;84:859.

22. Moller JT, Pedersen T, Rasmussen LS, et al. Randomized evaluation of pulse oximetry in 20,802 patients, I: design, demography, pulse oximetry failure rate, and overall complication rate. *Anesthesiology.* 1993;78:436.

23. Coté CJ, Goldstein EA, Fuchsman WH, et al. The effect of nail polish on pulse oximetry. *Anesth Analg.* 1988;67:683.

24. Kelleher JF, Ruff RH. The penumbra effect: vasomotion-dependent pulse oximeter artifact due to probe malposition. *Anesthesiology.* 1989;71:787.

25. Reed HL, Pepper S, Armstrong D, et al. Oxygen saturation of brachial venous blood correlates with fingertip temperatures between 11 and 39 degrees C. *Aviat Space Environ Med.* 1989;60:1068.

26. Severinghaus JW, Kelleher JF. Recent developments in pulse oximetry. *Anesthesiology.* 1992;76:1018.

27. Barker SJ, Novak S, Morgan S. The performance of three pulse oximeters during low perfusion in volunteers. *Anesthesiology.* 1997;87:A409.

28. Hay WW. Pulse oximetry: as good as it gets? *J Perinatol.* 2000;20:181.

29. Malviya S, Reynolds PI, Voepel-Lewis T, et al. False alarms and sensitivity of conventional pulse oximetry versus the Masimo SET technology in the pediatric postanesthesia care unit. *Anesth Analg.* 2000;90:1336.

30. Witucki PJ, Bell SJ. Comparison of three new technology pulse oximeters during recovery from extreme exercise in adult males. *Crit Care Med.* 1999;27:A87(224).

31. Tremper KK. Pulse oximetry's final frontier. *Crit Care Med.* 2000;28:1584.

32. Bohnhorst B, Peter CS, Poets CF. Pulse oximeters' reliability in detecting hypoxemia and bradycardia: comparison between a conventional and two new generation oximeters. *Crit Care Med.* 2000;28:1565.

33. Barker SJ, Shah NK. The effects of motion on the performance of pulse oximeters in volunteers (revised publication). *Anesthesiology.* 1997;86:101.

34. Pologe JA, Raley DM. Effects of fetal hemoglobin on pulse oximetry. *J Perinatol.* 1987;7:324.

35. Canet J, Ricos M, Vidal F. Early postoperative arterial desaturation: determining factors and response to oxygen therapy. *Anesth Analg.* 1989;69:207.

36. Dumas C, Wahr J, Tremper KK. Clinical evaluation of a prototype motion artifact resistant pulse oximeter in the recovery room. *Anesth Analg.* 1996;83:269.

37. Partridge BL. Use of pulse oximetry as a noninvasive indicator of intravascular volume status. *J Clin Monit.* 1987;3:263.

38. Lawson D, Norley I, Korbon G, et al. Blood flow limits and pulse oximeter signal detection. *Anesthesiology.* 1987;67:599.

39. Cheng EY, Lauer KK, Stommel KA, et al. Evaluation of the palmar circulation by pulse oximetry. *J Clin Monit.* 1989;5:1.

40. Glavin RJ, Jones HM. Assessing collateral circulation in the hand—four methods compared. *Anaesthesia.* 1989;44:594.

41. Wallace CT, Baker JD III, Alpert CC, et al. Comparison of blood pressure measurement by Doppler and by pulse oximetry techniques. *Anesth Analg.* 1987;66:1018.

42. Piernan S, Roizen MF, Severinghaus JW. Oxygen analyzer dangerous—senses nitrous oxide as battery fails. *Anesthesiology.* 1979;50:146.

43. Westenskow DR, Jordan WS, Jordan R, et al. Evaluation of oxygen monitors for use during anesthesia. *Anesth Analg.* 1981;60:53.

44. Linko K, Paloheimo M. Inspiratory end-tidal oxygen content difference: a sensitive indicator of hypoventilation. *Crit Care Med.* 1989;17:345.

45. Merilainen PT. A differential paramagnetic sensor for breath-by-breath oximetry. *J Clin Monit.* 1990;6:65.

46. Linko K, Paloheimo M. Monitoring of the inspired and end-tidal oxygen, carbon dioxide, and nitrous oxide concentrations: clinical applications during anesthesia and recovery. *J Clin Monit.* 1989;5:149.

47. Boothby WM, Lundin G, Helmholz HF Jr. Gaseous nitrogen elimination test to determine pulmonary efficiency. *Proc Soc Exp Biol Med.* 1948;67:558.

48. Gaumann DM, Mustaki JP, Tassonyi E. MAC-awake of isoflurane, enflurane and halothane evaluated by slow and fast alveolar washout. *Br J Anaesth.* 1992;68:81.

49. Stoelting RK, Longnecker DE, Eger E II. Minimum alveolar concentrations in man on awakening from methoxyflurane, halothane, ether and fluroxene anesthesia: MAC awake. *Anesthesiology.* 1970;33:5.

50. Guyton DC, Gravenstein N. Infrared analysis of volatile anesthetics: impact of monitor agent setting, volatile mixtures, and alcohol. *J Clin Monit.* 1990;6:203.

51. Matjasko J, Petrozza P, Mackenzie CF. Sensitivity of end-tidal nitrogen in venous air embolism detection in dogs. *Anesthesiology.* 1985;63:418.

52. Bowe EA, Boysen PG, Broome JA, et al. Accurate determination of end-tidal carbon dioxide during administration of oxygen by nasal cannulae. *J Clin Monit.* 1989;5:105.

53. McNulty SE, Roy J, Torjman M, et al. Relationship between arterial carbon dioxide and end-tidal carbon dioxide when a nasal sampling port is used. *J Clin Monit.* 1990;6:93.

54. Nunn JF, Hill DW. Respiratory dead space and arterial to end-tidal $CO_2$ tension difference in anesthetized man. *J Appl Physiol.* 1960;15:383.

55. Raemer DB, Francis D, Philip JH, et al. Variation in $P_{CO_2}$ between arterial blood and peak expired gas during anesthesia. *Anesth Analg.* 1983;62:1065.

56. Fletcher R, Jonson B, Cumming G, et al. The concept of deadspace with special reference to the single breath test for carbon dioxide. *Br J Anaesth.* 1981;53:77.

57. Bhavani Shankar K, Maseley H, Vemula V, et al. Physiological dead space during general anaesthesia for caesarean section. *Can J Anaesth.* 1987;34:373.

58. Severinghaus JW. Water vapor calibration errors in some capnometers: respiratory conventions misunderstood by manufacturers? *Anesthesiology.* 1989;70:996.

59. Gravenstein JS, Paulus DA, Hayes TJ. *Capnography in Clinical Practice.* Stoneham, Mass: Butterworths; 1989.

60. Colman Y, Krauss BK. Microstream capnography technology: a new approach to an old problem. *J Clin Monit Comput.* 1999;15:403.

61. Arnold JH, Thompson JE, Arnold LW. Single breath $CO_2$ analysis: description and validation of a method. *Crit Care Med.* 1996;24:96.

62. Goldman JM. Considerations for developing a clinical capnogram monitoring system. *Biomed Sci Instrum.* 1998;34:197.

63. Sungur M, Banner MJ, Gabrielli A, et al. Lung carbon dioxide elimination rate ($L_{CO_2}$) correlates with physiologic deadspace volume during mechanical ventilatory support. *Crit Care Med.* 1999;27:A91.

64. Hubble CL, Gentile MA, Tripp DS, et al. Dead space to tidal volume ratio predicts successful extubation in infants and children. *Crit Care Med.* 2000;28:2034.

65. Anderson JT, Owings JT, Goodnight JE. Bedside noninvasive detection of acute pulmonary embolism in critically ill surgical patients. *Arch Surg.* 1999;134:869.

66. Patel MM, Rayburn DB, Browning JA, et al. Neural network analysis of the volumetric capnogram to detect pulmonary embolism. *Chest.* 1999;116:1325.

67. Larsson C, Staun P. Evaluation of a new fibre-optical monitor for respiratory rate monitoring. *J Clin Monit.* 1999;15:295.

68. *The Sodasorb Manual of Carbon Dioxide Absorption.* Atlanta, Ga: WR Grace & Co, Dewey and Almy Chemical Division; 1962.

69. Andrews JJ, Johnston RV Jr, Bee DE, et al. Photodeactivation of ethyl violet: a potential hazard of Sodasorb. *Anesthesiology.* 1990;72:59.

70. Moon RE, Ingram C, Brunner EA, et al. Spontaneous generation of carbon monoxide within anesthetic circuits [abstract]. *Anesthesiology.* 1991;75:A873.

71. Shapiro BA. In-vivo monitoring of arterial blood gases and pH. *Respir Care.* 1992;37:165.

72. Greenblott G, Barker SJ, Tremper KK, et al. Detection of venous air embolism by continuous intraarterial oxygen monitoring. *J Clin Monit.* 1990;6:53.

73. Nunn JF. *Applied Respiratory Physiology.* 3rd ed. Boston, Mass: Butterworths; 1987.

74. Nanji AA, Whitlow KJ. Is it necessary to transport arterial blood samples on ice for pH and gas analysis? *Can Anaesth Soc J.* 1984;31:568.

75. Lenfant C, Aucutt C. Oxygen uptake and change in carbon dioxide tension in human blood stored at 37°C. *J Appl Physiol.* 1965;20:503.

76. Mahoney JJ, Harvey JA, Wong RJ, et al. Changes in oxygen measurements when whole blood is stored in iced plastic or glass syringes. *Clin Chem.* 1991;37:1244.

77. Biswas CK, Ramos JM, Agroyannis B, et al. Blood gas analysis: effect of air bubbles in syringe and delay in estimation. *BMJ.* 1982;284:923.

78. Ream RK, Reitz BA, Silverberg G. Temperature correction of $P_{CO_2}$ and pH in estimating acid-base status. *Anesthesiology.* 1982;56:41.

79. Nattie EE. The alphastat hypothesis in respiratory control and acid-base balance. *J Appl Physiol.* 1990;69:1201.

80. Benatar SR, Hewlett AM, Nunn JF. The use of iso-shunt lines for control of oxygen therapy. *Br J Anaesth.* 1973;45:713.

# 20

# Cardiovascular Monitoring

Hugh C. Gilbert

Jeffrey S. Vender

## THE ELECTROCARDIOGRAM

## ARTERIAL BLOOD PRESSURE

## CENTRAL VENOUS PRESSURE

## PULMONARY ARTERY PRESSURE

## CARDIAC OUTPUT

## TRANSESOPHAGEAL ECHOCARDIOGRAPHY

## URINE OUTPUT

Cardiovascular monitoring remains an essential component of anesthesia care. Today, cardiovascular monitoring encompasses a variety of instrumentation and sophisticated technology that extends the capability of anesthesiologists to monitor the effects of anesthetics and surgery beyond the basic senses. This chapter examines key elements and specific techniques that are useful in monitoring the adequacy of cardiac and circulatory function during anesthesia care.

## THE ELECTROCARDIOGRAM

The electrocardiogram (ECG) was the first electronic monitor to be employed intraoperatively.[1] Described principally as a means of detecting intraoperative arrhythmias, the continuous display of the ECG has been and remains an important component of routine intraoperative monitoring.[2] ECG is inexpensive and simple to use and provides clinicians with continuous information that has proved to be of diagnostic and prognostic value.

## What Is the Value of Monitoring the Electrocardiogram During Anesthesia?

ECG monitoring is necessary to identify arrhythmias that occur during anesthesia care. Disturbances in cardiac rhythm often occur in sick patients and may be associated with the administration of anesthesia.[3] Although most intraoperative arrhythmias are of no clinical consequence, there is always the potential for the development of an arrhythmia that becomes clinically significant and requires the alteration of the anesthetic management plan, the addition of specific drug therapy, or even cardioversion. Table 20–1 lists intraoperative factors that may be associated with the development of arrhythmias. Patients with preexisting heart disease are more prone to developing arrhythmias in the perioperative period.[4]

Because intraoperative arrhythmias occur frequently, it is necessary for anesthesiologists to become skillful in monitoring and interpreting ECG changes. The prevalence of coronary artery disease has focused attention on the potential for using ECG criteria for the diagnosis and treatment of intraoperative ischemia and infarction.[5]

## What Does the Electrocardiogram Represent?

The ECG provides a graphic record of the alterations in electrical potentials that result from the continuous transfer of ions across membranes in the electrically active cells of the heart over time. Although the electrical gradients that result from the depolarization and repolarization potentials of the atrium and ventricle are small, recording impulse formation and conduction is easily performed.

A multitude of electrode arrays and instrumentation are available. Intraoperatively, interest is focused on alterations of atrial depolarization, atrioventricular (AV) conduction, ventricular depolarization, and ventricular repolarization.

### Factors That Determine Electrocardiographic Deflections

When bipolar electrodes are used, a current vector in the direction of the positive electrode results in an upward deflection. A downward deflection occurs when the current flow is reversed. If an electrode pair is perpendicular to the current flow, no deflection occurs. If the electrode pair is parallel to the current flow, the resulting recording has a maximal deflection.

An infinite number of bipolar electrode pairs are possible.

**TABLE 20–1.** Factors That May Contribute to Intraoperative Dysrhythmias

| Factor | Mechanism |
| --- | --- |
| Inhalational anesthetic agents | Reentry, sensitization |
| Hyperventilation | Hypokalemia, alkalosis |
| Electrolyte imbalance | Reentry, automaticity |
| Endotracheal intubation | Autonomic activation |
| Preexisting cardiac disease | Myocardial ischemia; conduction defects |
| Catheter guidewire insertions | Irritation of myocardium |
| Drug interaction | Sensitization |
| Retractor pushing into heart | Irritation of myocardium |

Twelve standardized lead positions are recognized. The electrical signals obtained from surface electrodes require amplification in order to be displayed. Modern ECG monitors facilitate the processing of these signals, permitting real time analysis of events of interest.

## What Leads Are Used Intraoperatively?

Intraoperative electrocardiography is based on information obtained from placing either three or five surface leads. Three leads placed on both arms and the left leg can be used to monitor the standard limb leads (I, II, III) or any modified bipolar lead. A fourth lead, the right leg lead, is necessary to establish a reference ground for the augmented leads (augmented voltage, unipolar right arm lead [aVR], left arm lead [aVL], unipolar left leg lead [aVF]). Many microprocessor-based intraoperative monitors require application of the right leg lead (green lead) to reduce interference and to permit arrhythmia processing.

### Color Coding

Color coding the standard leads permits quick identification of the proper electrode pairs. In the United States, the color coding listed here is followed:

**White lead** is applied to the right arm.
**Green lead** is applied to the right leg.
**Black lead** is placed on the left arm.
**Red lead** is applied to the left leg.
**Brown chest lead** is used to monitor unipolar V leads.

An easy mnemonic to remember limb lead placement considers the patient a driver of a car. The left leg operates the brake (red), the right leg operates the gas (green), the driver's left arm gets suntanned (black), while the right arm remains pale (white).

By convention, lead I detects the potential difference from the right arm to the left arm, lead II detects the potential difference from the right arm to the left leg, and lead III detects the potential difference from the left arm to the left leg.

### Augmented and Precordial Leads

The augmented leads (aVR, aVL, and aVF) use a zero potential indifferent electrode by connecting three limb leads to 5000-$\Omega$ resistors. This indifferent central terminal serves as a common negative electrode. The positive, exploring electrode can be switched from the right arm, left arm, or left leg, representing the positive electrodes for the aVR, aVL, and aVF leads, respectively. The precordial leads ($V_1$-$V_6$) constitute the unipolar leads recorded during a standard 12-lead ECG.

### 5-Lead Cable Systems

A 5-electrode cable enables display of a precordial lead by placing an electrode on each extremity and the remaining electrode (brown lead) over the precordium. During anesthesia, this unipolar lead is usually placed along the anterior axillary line in the fifth intercostal space ($V_5$). A 5-lead cable

**TABLE 20–2.** Electrocardiogram Electrode Placement Options for Three-Lead Cables

| Limb Leads | White | Black | Red | Switch | Benefit |
|---|---|---|---|---|---|
| Lead I | Right arm (−) | Left arm (+) | Ground | Lead I | Lateral ischemia |
| Lead II | Right arm (−) | Ground | Left leg (+) | Lead II | Dysrhythmias, inferior ischemia |
| Lead III | Ground | Left arm (−) | Left leg (+) | Lead III | Inferior ischemia |
| *Modified Bipolar Leads—Infinite Varieties* | | | | | |
| MV$_5$ | Right arm (−) | V$_5$ (+) | Ground | Lead I | Anterior ischemia |
| CS$_5$ | Subclavicular (−) | V$_5$ (+) | Ground | Lead I | As above |
| CB$_5$ | Scapula (−) | V$_5$ (+) | Ground | Lead I | Like true V$_5$ |
| MCL$_1$ | Ground | Subclavicular (−) | V$_1$ (+) | Lead III | Dysrhythmias |

(+), positive electrode; (−), negative electrode; B, back; C or CL, central; M, modified; S, subclavicular; V$_5$, precordial positions.
From Griffin RM, Kaplan JA. Bipolar leads for use with three electrodes. In: Thys DM, Kaplan JA, eds. *The ECG in Anesthesia and Critical Care.* New York, NY: Churchill Livingstone; 1987:20.

permits the intraoperative monitoring of 6 of the 12 standard leads (I through aVF) as well as a precordial lead of choice. When monitoring a precordial unipolar lead, all of the limb leads serve as the indifferent central terminal (negative).

### 3-Lead Cable Systems

Table 20–2 depicts commonly used lead placements for intraoperative monitoring when using a 3-lead cable ECG system. If the shoulders, precordium, and left leg are available for electrode placement, using the MV$_5$ array (white is right arm; black is V$_5$ precordial position; red is left leg) permits monitoring of a modified V$_5$ lead when the selector switch is turned to "lead I" and the standard lead II when the selector is turned to "lead II." Monitoring the modified V$_5$ and lead II offers excellent capability of detecting ischemia of the inferior and anterior myocardium as well as arrhythmias.

## What Are the Characteristics of the Electrocardiogram That Interest Anesthesiologists?

The quality of intraoperative ECG waveforms is dependent on the following six electrical linkages:

Heart→Skin→Electrode→Lead→Cable→ECG Amplifier→Display

### Atrial Depolarization

Atrial depolarization is evident by the development of the P wave (Fig. 20–1). The size and shape of the P wave depend on the vector relationship between atrial depolarization and the monitoring lead displayed. In normal sinus rhythm, the P wave is upright in I and II and is inverted in aVR. After the depolarization of both atria, a delay in the conduction of the depolarization potential (PR interval) is associated with the ejection of blood into the ventricles.

### Ventricular Depolarization

After conduction through the AV node, the electrical impulse is transmitted through the bundle of His to the left and right bundle branches, Purkinje fibers, and both ventricles. Like its atrial counterpart, the size and projection of the depolarization vector of the ventricles vary depending on the spatial relationship of the monitoring lead and the propagation of ventricular depolarization.

The ventricular depolarization ECG wave is termed the *QRS complex* (see Fig. 20–1). Numerous variations can be observed. By definition, the first positive deflection is called an *R wave*. R waves can be preceded or trailed by negative deflections termed *Q waves* and *S waves*, respectively. Secondary positive deflections are labeled *R$^1$*.

### Ventricular Repolarization

Unlike depolarization, which is propagated throughout the heart from cell to cell, repolarization is an energy-dependent process that occurs at a specific rate in each myocardial cell. Although the summation of repolarization is manifest on the ECG by the T wave, its orientation during monitoring is complex and also includes the preceding ST segment and occasionally a following U wave. With a limb lead, V$_5$, or MV$_5$, the ST segment is normally isoelectric, and the T wave vector is usually positive.

### Signal Fidelity

Any decrease in fidelity or artifact interferes with the user's ability to identify abnormalities. Table 20–3 lists patient and equipment factors that can degrade the fidelity of the ECG monitored display.

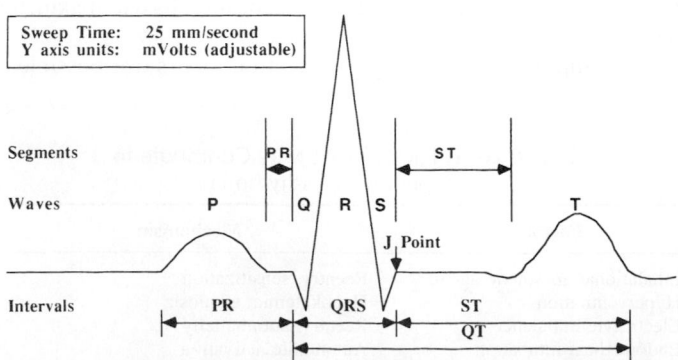

**FIGURE 20–1.** The electrocardiogram waves and intervals. (From Horan E. Electrocardiography and vectorcardiography in heart disease. In: Braunwald E, ed. *Heart Disease: A Textbook of Cardiovascular Medicine.* Philadelphia, Pa: WB Saunders; 1980.)

**TABLE 20–3.** Trouble-Shooting Electrocardiogram

### Summary of Causes

#### Patient Factors

Electrodes over muscles
Loose electrodes
Hairy skin
High skin resistance
Excessive shivering

#### Equipment Factors

"Dried-out" electrodes
Corroded connectors
Ungrounded equipment
Lead wire strain
Broken connection
Interference from adjacent electrical cables

### Corrective Action

Prepare skin
Reapply electrodes
Replace cable connections
Remove faulty equipment
Reposition cables

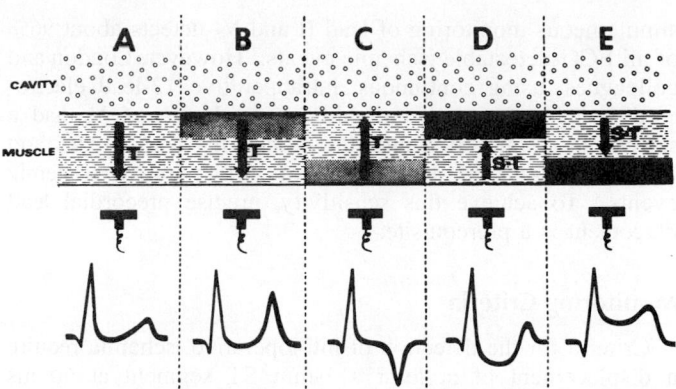

**FIGURE 20–2.** The T-wave vector during ischemia and injury recorded from an epicardial electrode. *A,* normal; *B,* subendocardial ischemia; *C,* subepicardial ischemia; *D,* subendocardial infarction; *E,* subepicardial infarction. (From Schamroth L. *The ECG of Coronary Artery Disease.* Oxford, United Kingdom: Blackwell; 1984.)

## Information Derived From Monitoring the Electrocardiogram

Monitoring the ECG is mandated in all patients undergoing anesthesia care. In healthy patients, the ECG helps assess heart rate and rhythm disturbances. In patients with cardiovascular diseases, intraoperative ECG monitoring provides data that are helpful in assessing ischemia, acute infarctions, dysrhythmias, electrolyte imbalances, and chamber enlargement. Table 20–4 lists conditions often associated with alteration in the ECG waves and intervals.

A strip chart ECG recording is valuable for evaluating the size, shape, and character of the ECG waves and determining ST and T wave changes. Comparisons between preoperative ECG tracings and baseline intraoperative and subsequent recordings can assist in defining the importance and course of intraoperative changes.

## How Does the Electrocardiogram Help Identify Intraoperative Ischemia?

During periods of coronary insufficiency, repolarization of ischemic myocardial cells is delayed, and electrical events in the region of ischemia manifest as changes in the ST segment and the T wave. Although ECG changes during ischemia, injury, and infarction are specific when recorded from epicardial electrodes, detection from surface electrodes may be confusing because of technical aspects of electrode placement and the frequency response of the recording system employed. Instrumentation and practice standards for ECG monitoring in special care units have been formulated.[6]

## Classic Changes

This section summarizes the classic changes associated with ischemia using an epicardial electrode. During periods of subendocardial ischemia, there is an unopposed increase in the repolarization vector that results in tall, upright T waves. If the ischemia becomes transmural, the direction of repolarization travels from the endocardium to the epicardium, producing an inverted T wave. Figure 20–2 demonstrates the ST and T wave changes observed when recording from the region of ischemia. Ischemic changes are best observed in leads that are parallel to the T wave vector.

ST and T wave changes often result from conduction defects, left ventricular hypertrophy, electrolyte disorders, and drug effects. Data from exercise stress testing suggest that

**TABLE 20–4.** Alterations of Electrocardiographic Waves and Intervals

| Alteration | ECG Abnormality | Associated Conditions and Potential Causes |
| --- | --- | --- |
| Shortened PR interval | <200 ms | Preexcitation: Wolff-Parkinson-White, junctional rhythm |
| Prolonged PR interval | 1st-degree block | Normal athletes, vagotonia, digitalis |
| | 2nd-degree block | Vagotonia, heart disease, new MI |
| Atrioventricular block | 3rd-degree block | Inferior wall MI |
| Q waves | Q waves | MI: idiopathic hypertrophic subaortic stenosis |
| QRS complex | Left bundle branch block | MI, IHD |
| | Right bundle branch block | MI, IHD |
| QT interval (corrected for heart rate) | Prolonged | IHD, hypocalcemia |
| | | Hypomagnesemia |
| | Shortened | Hypercalcemia |
| ST segment | Depression | IHD, LVH conduction defects, digitalis |
| | Elevation | Myocardial injury, MI, LVH |
| T wave | Tall peaked | Hyperkalemia, IHD |
| | Inverted | MI, ventricular hypertrophy, etc. |
| U wave | Present | Hypokalemia, hypercalcemia, thyrotoxicosis |
| | Inverted | LVH, IHD, intracranial hemorrhage |

ECG, electrocardiogram; IHD, ischemic heart disease; LVH, left ventricular hypertrophy; MI, myocardial infarction.

simultaneous monitoring of lead II and $V_5$ detects about 96% of all ECG-detectable ischemic events.[7] However, London and colleagues, using continuous, intraoperative 12-lead electrocardiography, found that monitoring leads II and $V_5$ had a sensitivity of only 80% and that monitoring leads II, $V_4$, and $V_5$ is necessary to detect 96% of intraoperative ischemic events.[8] To achieve this sensitivity, precise precordial lead placement is a prerequisite.

## Monitoring Criteria

Criteria for the detection of intraoperative ischemia require a displacement of at least a 1-mm ST segment at 60 ms after the J point and was adopted from the American Heart Association criteria for detecting ischemia during exercise. A more inclusive set of criteria has been used by London and colleagues[8] for determining the incidence of intraoperative myocardial ischemia using continuous 12-lead electrocardiography, as follows:

1. New ST depression of >1 mm (0.1 mV) in a horizontal or downsloping ST segment measured 60 ms after the J point
2. ST segment depression >1.5 mm in a slowly upsloping ST segment
3. ST segment elevation >1.5 mm from baseline in a non–Q wave lead
4. ST segment elevation >1 mm if associated with a simultaneous ST elevation of >1.5 mm in another ECG lead

ST segment changes that occurred during dysrhythmias do not always indicate ischemia. Displacement that meets inclusion criteria must be interpreted cautiously when observed in populations that are not at risk for myocardial ischemia or when observed on ECG monitoring systems in which the characteristics of electronic filtering are unknown.[9]

## New-Onset ST Segment Displacement

Studies in patients undergoing coronary artery bypass grafting or major vascular surgery have demonstrated a high incidence of new-onset ST segment displacement.[10, 11] When new-onset ST segment displacement occurs in high risk patients, intraoperative myocardial ischemia should be suspected, even if the ECG changes are not accompanied by hypertension and tachycardia.

## Silent Ischemia

Silent ischemia occurs in patients with asymptomatic coronary artery disease as well as in patients recovering from myocardial infarction (MI).[12] Most of these events are unrelated to major alterations in heart rate or blood pressure (BP).[13] Although ECG monitoring is not as sensitive as wall motion monitoring by means of echocardiography in assessing intraoperative ischemia, its ubiquity makes it the most accessible and universal intraoperative monitor for ischemia.

## ST Segment Analysis

Little information is available regarding the diagnostic precision of clinicians in assessing intraoperative ECG ST segment changes. London and colleagues suggested that by using a clinical display and 3-lead or 5-lead cables, a sensitivity of

75% may be expected.[8] Intraoperative ST segment evaluation lends itself to computer analysis, and several reports suggest that this technology enhances both sensitivity and specificity.[14]

Automated detection enhances intraoperative precision in detecting ischemia. Modern trending devices detect 80% to 100% of ECG-detectable ischemic events.[15,16] The ST segment is measured as the vertical difference between the T-P isoelectric point (reference) and the ST point (60-80 ms after the J point). Interrogation points can be manually set on many monitors to enhance precision. ST segment measurements are stored in memory with graphic programs for display on the monitor screen. Alarm limits can be set to warn when ischemia develops. Representative samples of the average digitized signals are often displayed for comparison with the ECG sweep. Conduction disturbances, T wave inversion, and tachycardia can limit the precision of automated ST segment monitoring.

## What Are the Characteristics of Myocardial Injury and Infarction?

### Injury

Early ischemia results in a current of injury, which accounts for ST and T wave changes. If conditions causing subendocardial injury currents are reversed, the ST segment changes resolve. If the area of ischemia increases to include the epicardium, an endocardial-to-epicardial injury current is established. The result is ST-T wave elevation in leads facing the current vector and ST-T wave depression in opposite leads.[17] Figure 20–3 illustrates ST-T wave changes involving the anterior, inferior, and posterior walls monitored from an epicardial electrode. If conditions responsible for injury currents are not reversed, MI results.

### Infarction

Myocardium that has undergone *transmural* necrosis is no longer electrically active, and depolarization cannot occur. Q

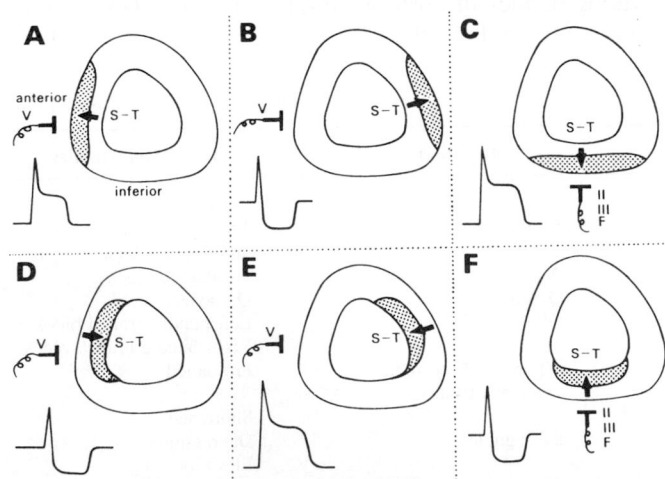

**FIGURE 20–3.** Injury patterns. *A–C,* The theoretic electrocardiogram observed during epicardial injury of the anterior, posterior, and inferior walls. *D–F,* Subendocardial injury of corresponding areas of myocardium. (From Schamroth L. *The ECG of Coronary Artery Disease.* Oxford, United Kingdom: Blackwell; 1984.)

**TABLE 20–5.** Electrocardiographic Evidence for Q-Wave Infarctions

| Left Ventricular Infarctions | |
|---|---|
| Anteroseptal | Abnormal Q: $V_1$, $V_2$, $V_3$ |
| Anterior | Abnormal Q: $V_2$, $V_3$, $V_4$ |
| Anterolateral | Abnormal Q: $V_2$, $V_3$, $V_4$ |
| Inferior | Abnormal Q: II, III, aVF |
| Posterior | Abnormal wide R wave: $V_1$ and $V_2$ |
| **Right Ventricular Infarctions** | Abnormal Q: II, III, aVF, ST segment elevation in right precordial leads: ($V_{3R-6R}$) |

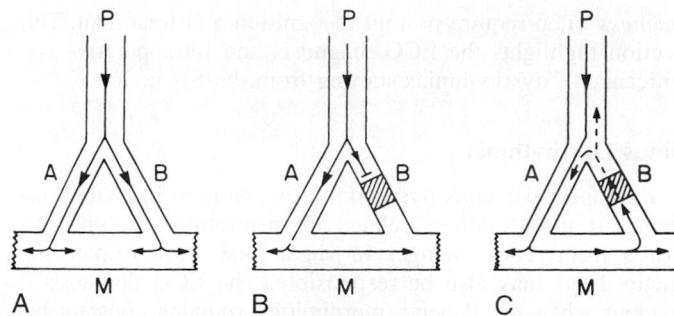

**FIGURE 20–4.** Reentry arrhythmia genesis. *A,* Normal conduction. *B,* Area of impaired conduction. *C,* Reentry activation of B after its recovery. M, myocardium; P, P wave. (From Chou Te-C. *Electrocardiography in Clinical Practice.* Philadelphia, Pa: WB Saunders; 1991.)

waves are recorded from leads facing the infarct. Abnormal Q waves (Q wave >0.04 s) are the classic finding after transmural necrosis. Unfortunately, localization of infarction by ECG patterns of necrosis is imprecise, particularly when conduction disturbances exist. The pathologic correlation between transmural infarction and the presence of Q waves is often incomplete. Table 20–5 lists ECG findings that are expected after MIs associated with Q waves. Non–Q wave infarction is also a well-recognized clinical entity.

## How Do Dysrhythmias Originate?

For simplicity, dysrhythmias are described as resulting from abnormalities of impulse formation, impulse conduction, or combinations thereof. Electrophysiologic studies have identified four phases to describe the transmembrane potential changes in electrically active cells of the heart. If the resting potential of these cells is reduced or intracellular $K^+$ or $Ca^{2+}$ ion currents are appreciably altered, abnormal automaticity or irritability often results.

Spontaneous diastolic depolarization (phase 4 of the action potential) usually occurs in the sinoatrial (SA) node. In a normal heart, automaticity (spontaneous diastolic depolarization) is a characteristic of the heart's conducting system. Ectopic beats or abnormal rhythms can be expected if the SA node is suppressed, if the conduction pathways are altered, or if the automaticity of other cardiac cells of the conduction system is enhanced.

### Dysrhythmia Genesis

The genesis and propagation of dysrhythmias are often complex. Dominant pacemaker function may shift from the SA node to subsidiary pacemakers. Local cellular changes occurring in the atria, AV node, or ventricles may induce abnormal spontaneous diastolic depolarization, which, if conducted, produces an ectopic beat. The refractory period for myocardial fibers is long. Therefore, a normal or ectopic impulse must remain active somewhere in the heart in order to reexcite a portion of the heart.

### Reentry

Reentry, precipitated by slow conduction and unidirectional conduction block, explains the genesis of many dysrhythmias. Figure 20–4 depicts the genesis of a ventricular dysrhythmia by reentry, resulting from slow conduction and a unidirectional conduction block in the Purkinje fibers. This mechanism

has been implicated in the genesis of lethal dysrhythmias accompanying MI.[18]

### Automaticity

All currently administered potent inhalational agents affect automaticity.[19] The effects are complex, involving the entire conduction cascade, and may influence impulse formation and conduction. Drug effects, sympathetic stimulation, electrolyte imbalance, and metabolic factors often contribute to the genesis of intraoperative dysrhythmias. Cardiac and antidysrhythmic drugs potentially alter the membrane permeability of ions responsible for normal conduction. Confounding variables such as digitalis, hyperkalemia, and preexisting heart block often make it difficult to define the etiologic events contributing to the genesis of an intraoperative dysrhythmia. Table 20–6 lists many of the dysrhythmias that may occur during anesthesia care.

## What Are the Characteristics of Atrial Dysrhythmias?

Although the mechanism for the genesis of intraoperative dysrhythmias is always important, *hemodynamic conse-*

**TABLE 20–6.** Intraoperative Dysrhythmias

| Mechanism | Location | Electrocardiogram Finding |
|---|---|---|
| Enhanced automaticity | SA node | Sinus tachycardia |
| Sympathetic stimulation | Atria,* AV node | Supraventricular tachycardia |
| Drugs, electrolyte disturbances | Atria* | PAC |
| Metabolic diseases, hyperthermia | Ventricle* | PVC |
| Reduced automaticity | SA node | Bradycardia, PAC |
| Parasympathetic stimulation | Atria* | Bradycardia, junctional rhythm |
| Drugs, electrolyte disturbances | Atria,* His, AV node, ventricle | Bradycardia or tachycardia, junctional rhythm, PVCs |
| Reentry | Atria* | Atrial flutter, fibrillation |
| Diseases | Purkinje fibers | Ventricular tachycardia |
| Electrolyte disturbances | Ventricle* | Ventricular tachycardia, ventricular fibrillation |

*Indicates cardiac tissues that normally do not demonstrate spontaneous diastolic depolarization.

AV, atrioventricular; PAC, premature atrial contraction; PVC, premature ventricular contraction; SA, sinoatrial.

*quences* often require prompt recognition and treatment. This section highlights the ECG diagnosis and intraoperative significance of dysrhythmias starting from the SA node.

## Sinus Dysrhythmia

Intraoperative sinus dysrhythmia is common in healthy patients. It most often is related to inspiration and probably arises from reflex changes in vagal tone. Parasympathomimetic drugs may also be responsible. The ECG diagnosis is evident when the P wave morphology remains constant but the PR interval varies, usually at slow sinus rates. Sinus dysrhythmia occurs frequently in children.

## Sinus Bradycardia

In adults, sinus bradycardia is defined as a heart rate of >60 beats per minute (BPM). The intraoperative ECG has a normal P wave and normal PR interval. Sinus bradycardia may be prevalent in healthy athletic adults and in patients taking β-blockers or calcium channel blockers. Hypothyroidism or hypothermia can also depress SA function. Sinus bradycardia is commonly associated with acute MI.[20] It may occur intraoperatively as a vagal response to traction of the mesentery, as a result of the stretching of extraocular muscles in children, or after the second intravenous administration of succinylcholine. New-onset bradycardia associated with hypotension, ventricular dysrhythmia, or signs of diminished perfusion require prompt evaluation and treatment.

## Sinus Tachycardia

In adults, a sinus heart rate of >100 BPM defines sinus tachycardia. The ECG monitor displays normal P waves, but the PR interval may shorten. ST segment depression is occasionally associated with fast rates, and the QT interval is shortened. Differentiation of pure sinus tachycardia from other supraventricular tachycardias is often difficult when the heart rate is >150 BPM. Finding P waves cements the diagnosis and may require changing monitor leads (eg, from $V_5$ to II). Sinus tachycardia can occur under various clinical situations. The underlying disorder (eg, hypovolemia, hypoxemia, hyperthermia, sympathetic response, pain, drug effects) warrants treatment depending on the etiology. Patients with ischemic heart disease and tachycardia are at risk for ischemia if myocardial oxygen demand exceeds supply. Tachycardia predisposes to this because it disproportionally reduces the time in diastole, which is when most myocardial perfusion occurs.

## Sick Sinus Syndrome

The ECG characteristics of sick sinus syndrome are bradycardia, sinus arrest, bradycardia, or tachycardia. The etiology appears to be multifactorial.[21] Patients with sick sinus syndrome have a diminished response to intravenous atropine.[22] The condition is often observed in patients with ischemic cardiomyopathies or hypertensive heart disease. Intraoperative treatment may require β-agonists or pacing.

## Paroxysmal Atrial Tachycardia

Paroxysmal atrial tachycardia (PAT) is an uncommon intraoperative dysrhythmia that is often initiated and sustained by reentrant or ectopic atrial foci (see Fig. 20–4). In healthy patients, PAT is usually short lived and has no significant hemodynamic effects. Atrial rates of 100 to 250 BPM are followed by normal-appearing QRS complexes. Secondary ST segment and T wave changes may suggest ischemia. P waves may be difficult to identify. Digitalis toxicity is a common cause of PAT with associated heart block. Sustained PAT (unlike paroxysmal supraventricular tachycardia) usually indicates organic heart disease. Under anesthesia, PAT may predispose to severe hemodynamic deterioration.[23]

## Atrial Flutter

Atrial flutter results from circus movement. Saw-tooth flutter (F) waves of constant timing and morphology distinguish atrial flutter (240-350 BPM) from atrial fibrillation (AF), which has fibrillatory (f) waves of irregular timing and morphology at rates of >350 BPM. ST segment tracking during atrial flutter is difficult. Most patients with atrial flutter have organic heart disease. Other causes include pulmonary disease, hyperthyroidism, and pericarditis.

## Atrial Fibrillation

As with atrial flutter, atrial fibrillation results from an induced circus movement. However, the chaotic depolarizations in the atria are conducted through the AV junction at random intervals. In AF, P waves are absent, and the atrial rate is rapid (350-700 BPM). The RR intervals are typically irregular. Fibrillatory waves are often identifiable in right precordial leads. The most common causes include coronary artery disease, valvular heart disease, hypertensive heart disease, congestive heart failure (CHF), chronic obstructive lung disease, and pulmonary embolism.

## What Are the Characteristics of Atrioventricular Dysrhythmias?

The AV junction retards conduction from the atria to the ventricles. AV junction cells are capable of spontaneous phase 4 depolarization. Under anesthesia, the AV junction may become the dominant pacemaker if SA node automaticity is slowed or fails. The ECG monitor usually displays a rate of 40 to 60 BPM and a normal-appearing Q wave. P waves may precede, coincide with, or follow the QRS complex, depending on the location of the junctional pacemaker and the relative velocity of conduction to the atria and ventricles. Intraoperative junctional rhythms are commonly associated with decreases in BP.[24]

If the SA node or the atria lose their automaticity, the AV junction normally assumes pacemaker function. Reentrant and automatic junctional mechanisms have been described to occur at the AV junction. Premature junctional beats or junctional tachycardias may occur under anesthesia. The effect of potent inhalational agents on AV nodal function remains obscure. Enhancement of impulse formation occasionally occurs in the AV node, producing accelerated AV junctional rhythms.

## What Are the Characteristics of Atrioventricular Block?

Independent atrial and ventricular rates define AV dissociation. It is always a secondary phenomenon that develops from other disturbances in cardiac rhythm, such as heart block, default of the primary pacemaker with escape of a subsidiary pacemaker, or usurpation by a faster pacemaker.[25]

## Complete Block

Serious reductions in cardiac output (CO) often result when AV conduction is blocked. If a complete disruption occurs, the atria beat at the rate set by the SA node, and the ventricular rate is determined by a slower pacemaker situated in the AV node, in the bundle of His, or within the ventricular muscle. During complete disruption (third-degree AV block), the ECG displays P and QRS-T waves that may have normal morphology but are asynchronous. New-onset third-degree block often requires drug therapy or pacing.

## Incomplete Block

Incomplete disruptions of AV conduction may also be of clinical importance. Disruption can occur after acute MI. Gradually increasing PR intervals, followed by nonconducted P waves (Wenckebach phenomenon), is the ECG hallmark of a Mobitz type I block. Mobitz I block usually results from an abnormality of the AV node, and Mobitz II blocks usually occur in the bundle of His or the bundle branches. First-degree AV block (PR interval >0.20 s) is common and usually does not influence anesthesia management.

## What Are the Characteristics of Ventricular Dysrhythmias?

### Premature Ventricular Contractions

Premature ventricular contractions (PVCs) alter the sequence of coordinated ventricular contraction. The QRS complex is abnormal and prolonged; ST-T wave changes are expected because ventricular repolarization is also abnormal. P waves are not associated with PVCs, but retrograde depolarization or blocked sinus beats may add confusing appearances to the complexes. Premature atrial contractions (PACs) with aberrant ventricular conduction may mimic the wide and bizarre QRS complexes that result from ventricular ectopy. They may or may not reset the sinus rhythm and are not hemodynamically significant.

PVCs are commonly observed with preexisting cardiac disease. They may be observed in healthy patients during periods associated with sympathetic stimulation. New-onset PVCs may be ominous signs of impending life-threatening dysrhythmias, MI, ongoing myocardial ischemia, digitalis toxicity with hypokalemia, or hypoxemia due to any cause. Therefore, the occurrence of PVCs during anesthesia requires prompt identification of any clinical aberrations that may be corrected.

Intraoperative PVCs are significant when they are frequent (>6 per minute), are multifocal, occur early in the normal cardiac cycle (R on T), or occur after recent MI. Continuation of PVCs may lead to the development of ventricular tachycardia (VT) or ventricular fibrillation (VF).

### Ventricular Tachycardia

Intraoperative VT is not commonly observed other than in cardiac surgery. It occurs when three or more PVCs occur in a row.[26] The conduction pattern is aberrant, and AV dissociation is frequently present. The rhythm is usually regular, with a heart rate of 100 to 250 BPM. Recognition of VT is important because the acute onset of VT is often hemodynamically significant, may be life-threatening, and requires immediate treatment.

### Ventricular Fibrillation

Ventricular fibrillation is characterized by rapid, disorganized depolarization of the ventricles. The ECG displays irregular complexes. Discrete QRS-T waves are not present. During VF, cardiovascular collapse is expected because VF does not permit effective ventricular ejection. The causes of intraoperative VF include ongoing hypoxia, severe myocardial ischemia, electric shock, hyperkalemia, hypothermia, and malignant hyperpyrexia.

## What Electrocardiographic Changes Occur With Electrolyte Disturbances?

Intraoperative electrolyte disturbances, especially significant changes in potassium and calcium, are often heralded by changes in the ECG. Unfortunately, the electrocardiographic changes associated with electrolyte disturbances are often nonspecific. Classically, hyperkalemia is associated with tall peaked T waves and hypokalemia as well as hypocalcemia with flattened T waves.

# ARTERIAL BLOOD PRESSURE

Estimates of the arterial BP (ABP) predominantly depend on the generation and propagation of the arterial pressure wave. Measurement of ABP remains an essential element of anesthesia care.

## What Are the Characteristics of the Arterial Pressure Waveform?

Immediately after ventricular ejection, a fluid wave begins in the central aorta and propagates throughout the arterial tree. As the peripheral vasculature divides, the contour, size, and character of the arterial pressure wave vary. Factors contributing to the propagation and character of the pressure pulse include the energy content imparted by ventricular systole (1-600 W), contour transformation by the vascular tree, and reflective waves produced at the periphery (Table 20–7).

### Wave Reflection and Propagation

Wave reflection and propagation vary with physiologic and pathologic conditions. In most species, the systolic pressure

**TABLE 20–7.** Factors Influencing the Characteristics of the Arterial Pressure Wave

Dynamics of pulsatile flow
Acceleration and deceleration of blood
Elasticity of the large conducting arteries
Modulated impedance to flow (systemic vascular resistance)

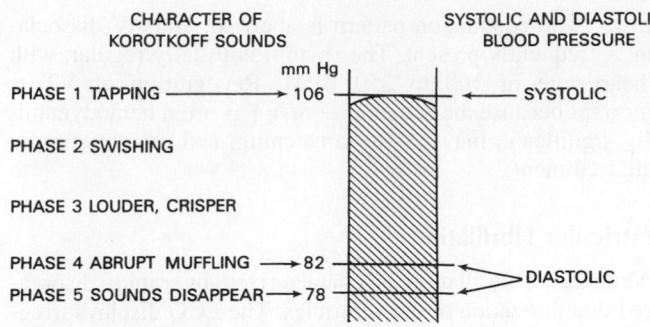

CHARACTER OF KOROTKOFF SOUNDS

SYSTOLIC AND DIASTOLIC BLOOD PRESSURE

mm Hg

PHASE 1 TAPPING → 106 ← SYSTOLIC

PHASE 2 SWISHING

PHASE 3 LOUDER, CRISPER

PHASE 4 ABRUPT MUFFLING → 82

PHASE 5 SOUNDS DISAPPEAR → 78

DIASTOLIC

**FIGURE 20–5.** Graphic representation of the relationship of the Korotkoff sounds to blood pressure measurement. (From Stobo JD, ed. *The Principles and Practice of Medicine.* 23rd ed. Norwalk, Conn: Appleton & Lange; 1984.)

component of the arterial pulse wave is augmented as the wave passes from the central aorta into the peripheral vessels. Similarly, the diastolic component is lowered. Peripheral wave artifacts can exceed central aortic pressure measurements by 20% to 30%. Figure 20–5 demonstrates the changes in size and shape of the pressure wave observed at various sites.[27] Occlusive vascular disease, dynamically changing peripheral vascular resistance, and the physical constraints of the measuring system often influence the pulse contour.

## How Is Blood Pressure Measured Noninvasively?

### Manual (Nonautomated) Techniques

Palpatory or auscultatory measurements are the traditional methods employed to monitor BP. Inflation of a BP cuff above systolic pressure flattens the underlying regional artery. With gradual deflation, the pressure at which arterial flow resumes can be determined if the encircling cuff is attached to a calibrated manometer.

The endpoint for arterial flow can be determined using several methods. Palpation of a distal pulse during slow deflation of a BP cuff provides a reasonable estimate of systolic BP (SBP). Today, palpatory techniques are a valuable backup when primary monitoring techniques fail or require verification. Sophisticated modifications are possible when pulse oximeter finger probes, indwelling arterial catheters, or Doppler ultrasound (US) transducers are used to determine the point at which distal arterial flow resumes.

### *Auscultation of Korotkoff Sounds*

Auscultation of Korotkoff sounds permits estimation of SBP and diastolic BP (DBP). Mean arterial pressure (MAP) can be calculated using an estimating equation:

$$MAP = \text{Diastolic Pressure} + \tfrac{1}{3} (\text{Systolic} - \text{Diastolic}) \text{ Pressure}$$

Korotkoff sounds result from turbulent flow within an artery in response to the mechanical deformation from the BP cuff (see Fig. 20–5). SBP is signaled by the appearance of the first Korotkoff sound. Disappearance of the sounds or a change to a muffled tone signals the DBP. The detection of sound

changes is subjective and prone to errors based on deficiencies in sound transmission or poor hearing. Cuff deflation rates also influence accuracy. Quick deflations (>3 mm Hg/s) underestimate BP and may be unreliable during conditions of low flow.[28]

Nonautomated BP measurements are reasonably accurate when aneroid gauges are within calibration, the encircling cuff is appropriately positioned, the initial inflation is greater than the true systolic pressure, and Korotkoff sounds or arterial pulse wave are properly identified.

The accuracy of a BP estimate is, to a great extent, dependent on the proper use of the encircling BP cuff. Too small a cuff, in particular, results in BP estimates that are high. A larger than necessary cuff does not significantly affect accuracy as long as the pressure of the cuff is transmitted to the underlying artery and compresses it.[29] The optimal width of a BP cuff is 40% of the circumference of the arm.[30]

### *Doppler Sphygmomanometry*

Doppler sphygmomanometry detects the audible Doppler shift after the restoration of distal blood flow on deflation of a BP cuff. Studies have shown excellent correlation with direct arterial measurements.[31] This method is popular to confirm SBP in low flow states.

### Automated Devices

Since 1976, microprocessor-controlled oscillotonometers (MCOs) have largely replaced auscultatory and palpatory techniques for routine intraoperative BP monitoring. Advantages of these devices are listed in Table 20–8. Oscillometry measures mean BP by sensing the point of maximal fluctuations produced while a BP cuff is deflated.

### *Methodology*

Modern MCOs measure systolic, diastolic, and mean pressures by sampling oscillations in the cuff and determining parameter identification points (PIPs) for each respective measurement.[32] A generic MCO senses cuff pressure with a transducer, and the output is digitized for processing. After the cuff is inflated by an air pump, pressure is held constant while oscillations are sampled. If no oscillations are detected, the cuff pressure is greater than ABP; the computer then opens a deflation valve for sampling at the next lower level. MCOs assign the systolic pressure to the point of appearance of pressure oscillations in the cuff; MAP is the pressure at which maximal oscillations occur; and diastolic pressure is the point of maximal oscillatory decline.

Artifact-rejection algorithms are implemented by the step-

**TABLE 20–8.** Benefits of Microprocessor-Controlled Oscillotonometers

Hands-free operation
Programmable time cycle
Adaptable to all age groups
Measures mean, systolic, and diastolic pressures
Functions on all extremities
Programmable alarms
Integration within monitoring systems
Documented accuracy in wide range of patients

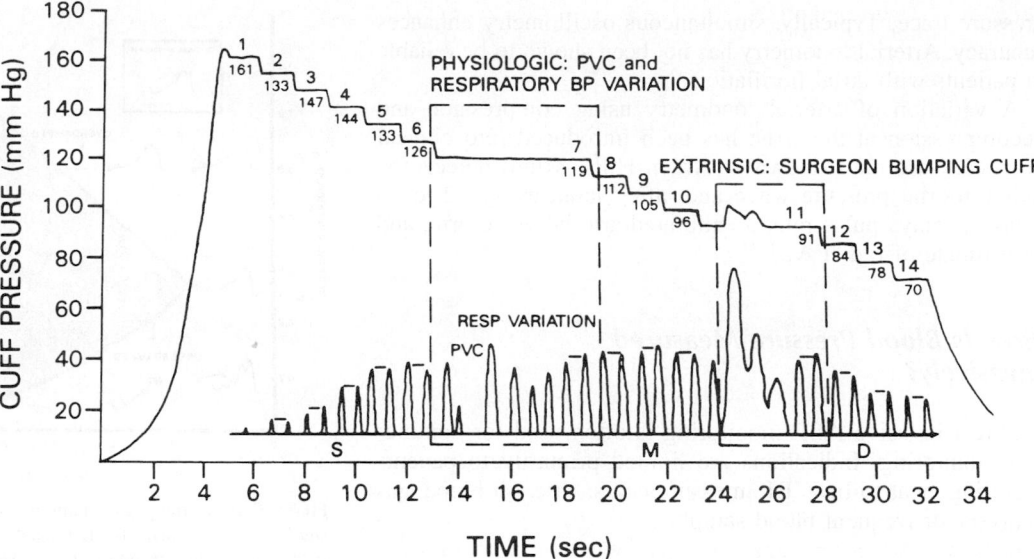

**FIGURE 20–6.** Diagram of microprocessor-controlled oscillotonometer operation. In this illustration, motion artifact, premature ventricular contraction, and respiratory artifacts are demonstrated. BP, blood pressure; PVC, pressure volume curve; Resp, respiratory. (From Ramsey M. Blood pressure monitoring: automated oscillometric devices. *J Clin Monit.* 1991;7:56.)

wise deflation–PIPs cycle. MCOs compare the amplitude of oscillation pairs and numerically display their estimates. This technique requires that a patient be relatively still. A dysrhythmia such as AF, in which the amplitude of successive pulses varies widely, renders accurate measurements problematic. Figure 20–6 graphically depicts the responses of an MCO in operation. During this inflation cycle, respiratory variation, a PVC, and cuff movement are demonstrated.

### Accuracy

Automated oscillometry correlates well with direct intra-arterial measurement of mean BP and DBP.[33] Underestimation of SBP may occur, with mean errors reported from −6.9 to −8.6 mm Hg, compared with direct radial artery pressures.[34] The Association for the Advancement of Medical Instrumentation recommends that MCOs have a mean error of <5 mm Hg compared with a centrally placed arterial catheter.[35]

Oscillometry requires the careful evaluation of several cardiac cycles at each increment of deflation in order to smooth out pronounced respiratory variations or motion artifacts. Cuff movement or erratic pulse transmission influences accuracy. Difficulties can be expected when shock or hypotension reduces the ability to sense wave oscillations. Shivering produces motion artifacts that degrade MCO performance. The time necessary to display the measured MAP and the estimates of systolic and diastolic pressures vary, depending on the proprietary software that integrates the inflation-deflation cycle and the analysis of the amplitude of oscillations. Many MCOs offer end-users a STAT mode, in which the inflation-deflation cycle is shortened. In the STAT mode, accuracy is compromised, but new data are made available up to 3 times per minute.

### Benefits and Risks

MCOs have simplified the task of obtaining accurate intra-operative BP measurements. Improper cuff deflation has the potential to promote venous congestion. Placement of an automated BP cuff on the same extremity in which venous access has been established influences the rate of fluid administration and can impair drug administration. This problem is particularly annoying during a rapid-sequence induction. The potential for direct compression of superficial peripheral nerves is minimized by careful cuff application.[36]

### Photoplethysmography

Peñaz developed a method for BP monitoring that holds the size of the digital arteries of a finger constant and alters the pressure within a finger cuff.[37] The Finapres device uses infrared light and detects oscillations within the finger cuff. These oscillations correspond to the arterial pressure trace.

Clinical trials in healthy patients undergoing routine surgical procedures suggest that digital photoplethysmography correlates with direct ABP measurements. Arterial spasm after cardiopulmonary bypass or the administration of phenylephrine affected the reliability of early prototypes.[38] The device is also susceptible to hydrostatic errors resulting from changing the position of the transducer-servo mechanism. Finapres methodology is still attractive and continues to be supported.[39,40]

### Arterial Tonometry

Satisfactory estimates of the BP waveform and measurement of systolic, mean, and diastolic pressures can be obtained using arterial tonometry. Arterial tonometry incorporates an array of piezoelectric pressure transducers placed on the wrist over the radial artery. The transducer assembly contains an air chamber that places sufficient pressure on the skin to flatten the wall of the artery, at which time the intraarterial BP is transmitted through the subcutaneous tissues and is sensed at the skin.

The accuracy of arterial tonometry requires tension exerted on the artery to be perpendicular to the sensor. Clinical tonometry monitors incorporate a computer analysis of the multiple sensors to determine which transducer elements faithfully monitor the flattened arterial wall. Clinical studies demonstrate a close correlation between arterial tonometry and intraarterial BP.[41] Arterial tonometry provides end-users with a real time continuous waveform representation of the arterial pressure trace. Typically, simultaneous oscillometry enhances accuracy. Arterial tonometry has not been shown to be reliable in patients with atrial fibrillation.[42]

A variation of arterial tonometry using compression and decompression at the wrist has been introduced into clinical practice. Vasotrac (Medwave, Arden Hills, Minn) detects the radial arterial pressure wave and, after about every 12 to 15 beats, displays pulse rate, a calibrated arterial waveform, and an estimate of radial ABP.[43]

## How Is Blood Pressure Measured Invasively?

Direct invasive ABP monitoring is often used for continuous monitoring. Indications are limited primarily to patients requiring beat-to-beat BP measurements, arterial blood gas analysis, or frequent blood sampling.

## Components

All intravascular pressure measurements require placement of a catheter into a vessel and attachment to a rigid fluid-filled tubing. The tubing links the pressure wave to a transducer that converts pressure (force per unit area) into an electrical signal that is amplified and filtered electronically. This processed electrical signal is displayed as the monitored pressure tracing.

Cardiovascular pressure waves have unique shapes that are often characterized as complex periodic sine waves. High-fidelity recordings and analysis of the arterial pressure tracing (Fourier series of power spectrum analysis) indicate that the arterial pressure wave contains frequencies from 1 to 30 Hz (1 Hz = 60 cycles/s). Most of the frequency components are <10 Hz.

The behavior of transducers, fluid couplings, signal amplification, and display can be described by a second-order differential equation in which the mass, elasticity, and resistance of the transducing system are related to input. Solution of the equation predicts the transduced arterial pressure trace and characterizes the system's performance. Table 20–9 lists the properties of a fluid-coupled transducing system.

## Fidelity

The fidelity of any fluid-coupled transducing system is constrained by two properties: damping ($\zeta$) and natural frequency (Fo) (Fig. 20–7). Optimizing $\zeta$ and Fo permits the to-and-fro movement of the coupling fluid and transducer to reproduce faithfully the range of frequencies contained in the pressure wave (the system's bandwidth).

**TABLE 20–9.** Properties of Fluid-Coupled Transducing Systems

| Feature | Definition |
|---|---|
| Frequency response | How faithfully the display of pressure equals the input pressure wave. Ideally, fluid-coupled pressure transducing systems have a flat frequency response up to 20 Hz. |
| Natural frequency | The frequency at which the system resonates |
| Fo or resonant frequency | When input frequencies approach Fo, amplifications and distortion of output result. |

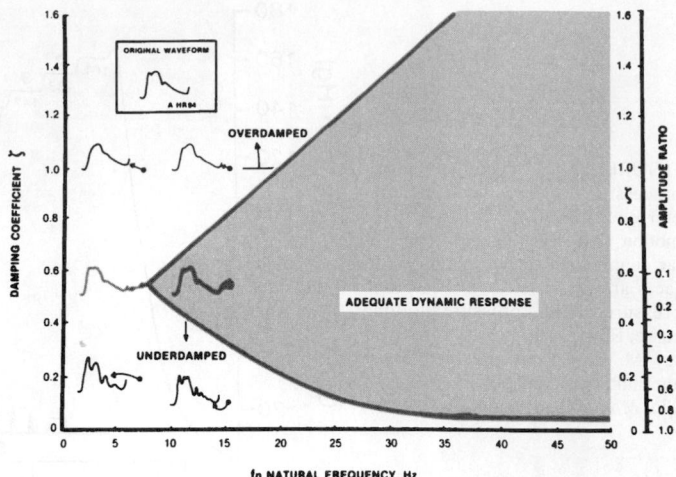

**FIGURE 20–7.** Ranges of damping coefficients and natural frequencies. The *shaded area* represents the regions of best fidelity. (From Gardner RM. Blood pressure: dynamic response needs. *Anesthesiology.* 1981;54:227.)

### Natural Frequency

Fo describes the tendency for the measuring system to resonate. Conventional disposable transducers, coupled with 60 inches of pressure tubing, have an Fo of about 20 to 40 Hz. Should the Fo approach the frequencies found in the arterial pressure wave (<10 Hz), estimates of the SBP increase because the fluid-filled coupling system resonates.

### Damping Coefficient

The damping coefficient describes the tendency for fluid in the measuring system to extinguish motion. Damping lowers the effective bandwidth. If the system is underdamped ($\zeta = 0.2$), the effective bandwidth is reduced by about two thirds of the Fo. Figure 20–7 demonstrates the effect of damping on the character of an arterial pressure trace. Fidelity is optimized when catheters and tubing are stiff, the mass of the fluid is small, the number of stopcocks is limited, and the connecting tubing is as short as possible. Small air bubbles lower the Fo of catheter-transducer systems.[44,45] Larger bubbles dampen the pulse pressure wave.

In clinical practice, underdamped catheter-transducer systems tend to overestimate systolic pressure by 15 to 30 mm Hg and amplify artifact (catheter whip). Overdamping reduces the fidelity of the system, underestimates the systolic pressure, and overestimates the diastolic pressure. The MAP value is most resistant to inadequate frequency response or damping characteristics.

### Clinical Applications

Damping and Fo can be estimated when a strip-chart recorder is available. After cannulation and zeroing, a rapid high-pressure flush is initiated while the system's output is recorded. Fluid-coupled transducer systems show a square wave followed by oscillations during the fast flush. Natural frequency is estimated by dividing the paper speed by the distance measured between two consecutive oscillations. Damping is estimated by the ratio of the amplitude of the first and second oscillations. Figure 20–8 demonstrates the calculation of Fo and $\zeta$ using the fast flush test.

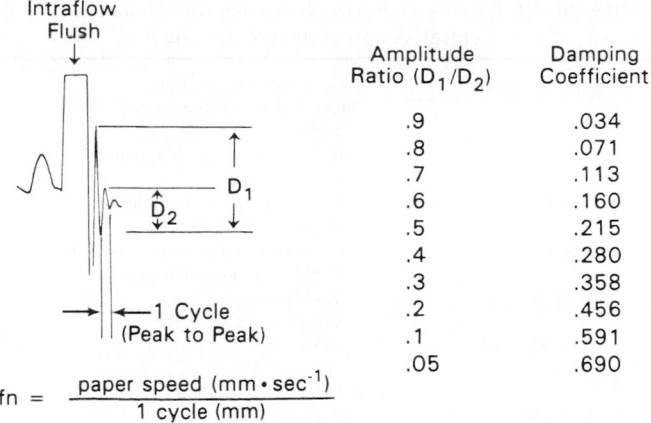

$$fn = \frac{\text{paper speed (mm} \cdot \text{sec}^{-1})}{1 \text{ cycle (mm)}}$$

| Amplitude Ratio ($D_1/D_2$) | Damping Coefficient |
|---|---|
| .9 | .034 |
| .8 | .071 |
| .7 | .113 |
| .6 | .160 |
| .5 | .215 |
| .4 | .280 |
| .3 | .358 |
| .2 | .456 |
| .1 | .591 |
| .05 | .690 |

**FIGURE 20–8.** Example of the fast flush test methodology for determining damping and natural frequency. (From Bedford RF, Shah NK. Blood pressure monitoring: invasive and noninvasive. In: Blitt CD, Hines RL, eds. *Monitoring in Anesthesia and Critical Care Medicine*. New York, NY: Churchill Livingstone; 1994:93.)

If a pen recorder is not present, observation of the display during a fast flush test identifies systems that oscillate. Systems with damping coefficients of 0.4 to 0.6 perform ideally (they are optimally damped). For the most part, transducer systems used in clinical anesthesia are underdamped ($\zeta$ = 0.2-0.36). Monitor manufacturers filter the transducer signal to remove the higher harmonic frequencies carried in the electrical signal. The accuracy and reliability of disposable pressure transducers, coupled with modern pressure monitors, has been reviewed by Gardner.[46]

## Arterial Cannulation

The radial artery is most commonly used for ABP monitoring. Alternative cannulation sites are listed in Table 20–10. Site selection should be based on ease of access and the adequacy of collateral circulation.

### Complications and Their Prevention

Abnormal radial artery blood flow after the removal of arterial catheters occurs frequently. Studies suggest that blood flow normalizes in 3 to 70 days.[47,48] Radial artery thrombosis can be minimized by using nontapered 20- to 22-gauge catheters constructed of Teflon and reducing the duration of arterial cannulation.[49] Using a catheter smaller than 20 gauge when the wrist circumference is <15 cm may also decrease the risk for thrombosis. The potential for thromboembolism may be diminished by compressing the proximal and distal artery while aspirating the cannula during removal.[50]

### Risk for Infection

Peripheral arterial catheters and catheter monitoring systems can become infected. Current guidelines suggest that in adults, replacement of peripheral arterial catheters and disposables should be performed no more frequently than every 4 days. In high-grade bacteremia, catheters should be replaced 24 to 48 hours after the start of appropriate antimicrobial therapy.[51]

Ischemia following radial artery cannulation resulting from thrombosis, proximal or distal embolization, and prolonged shock has been described.[52] Contributing factors include severe atherosclerosis, diabetes mellitus, low CO, intense peripheral vasoconstriction, or use of vasoconstrictors. Ischemia, hemorrhage, thrombosis, embolism, cerebral air embolism, aneurysm formation, and arteriovenous fistula formation have occurred as the result of arterial cannulation, arterial blood sampling, or pressure flushing.

Continuous flush devices are incorporated into disposable transducer kits and infuse fluid at 3 to 6 mL/h. In neonates, the infusion volume may contribute to fluid overload. Continuous flush devices have little effect on the BP measurement. However, pressurized flush devices may serve as a source of air embolism. Removing air from the pressure bag, stopcocks, and tubing minimizes the potential for air embolism and reduces damping.

## CENTRAL VENOUS PRESSURE

### Where Are Catheters Placed?

Central venous pressure (CVP) cannulas are important portals for intraoperative vascular access. Table 20–11 lists clinical indications for intraoperative CVP cannula placement. The right internal jugular vein is the preferred site of cannulation by anesthesiologists because it is accessible from the head of the operating table, has a relatively predictable anatomy, is usually the larger jugular vein, and is associated with a high success rate in both adults and children.[53]

Left-sided internal jugular cannulation can also be used but should be considered a second choice. It is less desirable because of the potential for damage of the thoracic duct, puncture of the apex of the left lung, and difficulty in maneuvering and positioning catheters through the left jugular–left subclavian junction. The potential for accidental puncture of the left carotid artery and embolization to a more commonly dominant left cerebral hemisphere is often cited as an additional reason to avoid this site.

Alternatively, right and left external jugular and subclavian

**TABLE 20–10.** Arterial Cannulation Sites

| Radial | Preferred site for routine cannulation |
|---|---|
| Ulnar | Ulnar nerve adjacent; primary source of hand blood flow |
| Axillary | Insertion site at junction of pectoralis major and deltoid muscle; specialized catheter kit available |
| Femoral | Easy access in low-flow state; longer catheters preferred; preferred access for intraaortic balloon; potential for local and retroperitoneal hemorrhage |
| Dorsalis pedis | Small vessel; adequate collateral flow needs verification |

From Gilbert HC, Vender JS. Monitoring the anesthetized patient. In: Barash PG, Cullen BF, eds. *Clinical Anesthesia*. 2nd ed. Philadelphia, Pa: JB Lippincott; 1992:748.

**TABLE 20–11.** Indications for Intraoperative Central Venous Cannulation

Vascular access: rapid infusion of fluids; parenteral alimentation; central drug infusion
Monitoring central venous pressure
Access portal: pulmonary artery catheterization; transvenous pacemaker
Therapeutic uses: treatment of venous air embolism

veins can be used. A J-tipped guidewire increases the success of central catheter placement through the external jugular veins. The success and safety of central venous cannulation requires knowledge of regional anatomy and attention to detail (see Chapter 27).

## What Are the Normal Pressure Waveforms?

CVP monitoring measures and displays a waveform that resembles the right atrial pressure (RAP). Conditions affecting RAP are reflected by changes in the CVP. The normal CVP waveform is depicted in Figure 20–9.

### a Wave

The a wave reflects the pressure change associated with atrial contraction following the P wave of the ECG. It occurs at the end of ventricular diastole and provides the "atrial kick" that primes the right ventricle.

### c Wave

As the right atrium relaxes, the right ventricle contracts. The resulting upward motion of the tricuspid valve is reflected by a transient increase in pressure—the c wave. Because it occurs in early systole (ventricular), it follows the QRS complex.

### x Descent

As ventricular systole continues, the relaxed right atrium is pulled down. This motion is reflected by a decrease in RAP that is termed the *x descent*.

### v Wave

The last positive wave, the v wave, results when venous filling of the atrium occurs (atrial diastole).

### y Descent

The y descent is ascribed to the opening of the tricuspid valve, which rapidly empties blood from the right atrium into the right ventricle.[54]

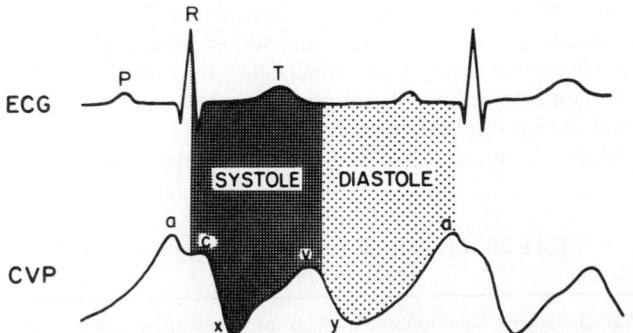

**FIGURE 20–9.** The relationship of normal central venous pressure (CVP) waves to ventricular systole and diastole. ECG, electrocardiogram. (From Mark JB. Central venous pressure monitoring: clinical insights beyond the numbers. *J Cardiothorac Vasc Anesth.* 1991;5:163.)

**TABLE 20–12.** Factors That May Influence the Character of the Central Venous Pressure Tracing

| | |
|---|---|
| Cardiac factors | Heart rate and rhythm |
| | Conduction disturbances |
| | Tricuspid valve function |
| | Right ventricular compliance |
| | Cor pulmonale |
| Intrathoracic pressure | Pneumothorax or hemothorax |
| | Mechanical ventilation |
| Blood volume | Changes in intravascular volume |
| | Rapid fluid administration |
| Drug therapy | Vasodilators |
| | Vasopressors |
| Pulmonary emboli | Blood |
| | Fat |
| | Air |
| Artifacts | Catheter kinks |
| | Catheter obstruction |

## What Data Obtained From Central Venous Pressure Monitoring Are of Interest to Anesthesiologists?

Many factors influence the character of the CVP tracing and often have diagnostic significance (Table 20–12). Table 20–13 lists features of interest to anesthesiologists. Prominent v waves in the CVP tracing are suggestive of right ventricular papillary muscle ischemia and tricuspid regurgitation. The CVP waveform in patients with diminished right ventricular compliance often demonstrates elevated pressures with prominent a and v waves that create an M or W configuration.[55]

CVP monitoring is helpful in the diagnosis and treatment of pericardial tamponade. As the CVP tracing becomes monophasic, the y descent is lost. Equalization of CVP, right ventricular and pulmonary artery (PA) diastolic pressures, and PA occlusion pressure (PAOP) is characteristic of hemodynamically significant pericardial constriction and tamponade.[56] With adequate drainage, a dramatic drop in filling pressures, restoration of SBP, and normalization of the CVP waveform should occur.

## What Conditions Warrant Central Venous Catheter Placement?

Central venous access is indicated in patients with hypovolemia, multiple trauma, or shock and whenever surgical proce-

**TABLE 20–13.** Clinical Significance of Central Venous Pressure Morphology

| Changes in Morphology | Common Clinical Conditions |
|---|---|
| Fusion of a and c waves | Sinus tachycardia |
| Absent a waves | Atrial fibrillation |
| Large a waves | Impaired atrial emptying |
| | Tricuspid stenosis |
| | Right ventricular hypertrophy |
| | Acute lung injury |
| | Chronic obstructive pulmonary disease |
| | Pulmonary hypertension |
| Giant v waves | Tricuspid regurgitation |
| Large a, v waves; prominent x, y descent | Constrictive pericarditis |
| Rapid x descent and blunted y descent | Pericardial tamponade |

**TABLE 20–14.** Mean Central Venous Pressure Numbers: Guide to Fluid Resuscitation?

| Clinical Situations | Ventilation | Range of Values (cm H₂O) |
|---|---|---|
| Healthy patients | Spontaneous | −2 to +6 |
| | Mechanical | +4 to +12 |
| Surgical patients (mild hypovolemia) | Spontaneous | −4 to +2 |
| | Mechanical | 0 to +3 |
| Critically ill patients (severe hypovolemia) | Spontaneous | −6 to 0 |
| | Mechanical | −4 to +1 |
| Fluid resuscitation | Mechanical | +10 to +15 |

dures may be associated with large fluid shifts. For patients in shock, a subclavian approach may be preferred because the subclavian vein has a constant size regardless of intravascular volume status. In contrast, the caliber and ease of cannulation of the jugular vein are completely pressure dependent. Monitoring is often indicated in cardiac procedures (CVP or CVP port of a PA catheter) and in patients with preexisting cardiovascular disease.

Table 20–14 focuses attention on the difficulty in interpreting the clinical relevance of mean CVP numbers.

Changes in the numbers during anesthesia care are often helpful in monitoring fluid resuscitation and assessing the need for a PA catheter. At higher CVP values, however, intraoperative fluid management is best guided by advancing intraoperative monitoring. Options include floating a PA catheter or performing transesophageal echocardiography (TEE).

## What Are the Complications?

Potentially serious complications have been described for virtually every vascular access location. Table 20–15 lists complications of CVP placement that are common to all central venous access sites.

## Carotid Puncture

Carotid puncture is a common problem during internal jugular vein cannulation. Ensuring that venous cannulation has occurred before placing large-bore sheaths reduces the potential for cannulation of the internal carotid artery. Use of either ultrasound imaging or a hand-held Doppler probe reduces the likelihood of carotid puncture. Measuring the pres-

**TABLE 20–15.** Complications Common to All Central Venous Cannula Placement Techniques

Accidental arterial puncture
   Hematoma
   False aneurysm
   Arteriovenous fistula formation
Dysrhythmias
Perforation of vein
Injury to surrounding structures
Clot and fibrinous sleeve formation
Thrombosis
Catheter-related infections
Guidewire embolus
Bleeding

sure within a small gauged pilot catheter or observing the falling height of a column of blood in an elevated extension tube connected to the needle before inserting a large-bore sheath minimizes unintentional carotid cannulation.

### Dysrhythmias

Dysrhythmias are most commonly associated with mechanical irritation of the myocardium by the guidewire. The guidewire is normally at least twice as long as the catheter; limiting its insertion distance to <15 cm avoids most dysrhythmias. Prevention of improper catheter position-related injuries is predicated on review of the follow-up chest radiograph to identify that the catheter tip is within the superior vena cava, not the right atrium, and relatively parallel to it. The appearance of tenting of the superior vena cava or coiling of the catheter at the tip may portend delayed perforation.[57]

### Miscellaneous Insertion Problems

Additional complications inherent to internal jugular and subclavian access include pneumothorax from puncture of pleura or lung, arterial puncture leading to hemothorax or hemomediastinum, puncture of the lymphatic ducts leading to chylothorax or chylomediastinum, pleural effusion, and brachial plexus injury. Isolated case reports underscore the potential for serious complications, including death from exsanguination.

### Infection

Central venous catheters are identified as significant sources of nosocomial infections and sepsis. Catheter contamination may occur during insertion (poor technique), as a result of colonization from a distant infected site (hematogenous spread), or as a consequence of skin contamination at the insertion site. Maximal barrier precautions are recommended even when catheters are placed in the operating room.

The practice of using transparent polyurethane dressings has been associated with an increased risk for bacterial colonization.[58] Introducers and catheters should remain in place for as short an interval as clinically practical. Recent data suggest reduced colonization and infection with the introduction of antibiotic-coated catheters. Prevention of catheter-related infections requires knowledge of and adherence to institutional guidelines for dressing and tubing changes.

## PULMONARY ARTERY PRESSURE

Flow-directed balloon flotation PA catheters continue to be important tools for the quantitative assessment of cardiopulmonary function. PA catheters augment CVP monitoring, which often provides unreliable estimates of left ventricular filling pressures. This disparity is particularly true of patients who are elderly or have preexisting cardiopulmonary disease.[59]

PA catheters have engendered significant controversy as to their clinical value.[60,61] We acknowledge that a long-standing debate exists and is relevant to the clinical application of PA catheter use. Observational data and case-matching studies have attempted to examine the value of PA catheter monitoring in a variety of acute care settings. The current data fall short of answering the question of value because of many confounding variables. Rational use of more expensive, invasive monitoring tools such as PA catheters requires a disciplined logic to identify where clinical application will provide the greatest benefit and to ensure that end-user knowledge and experience is adequate.[62,63]

### What Are the Indications?

PA pressure monitoring was originally used to aid in the management of complicated MI.[64] Indications continue to be broadly defined. If one views the PA catheter as a physiologic monitor, insertion should be guided by the need for information to diagnose and treat the underlying condition. PA catheter monitoring provides anesthesiologists the unique opportunity to assess intracardiac pressures, thermodilution CO, mixed venous oxygenation, oxygen transport and delivery, and derived hemodynamic indices (Table 20–16). This information can often help to define clinical problems, monitor the progression of hemodynamic dysfunctions, and guide the adequacy of and response to therapy.[63] Although technologic factors often influence the accuracy and precision of PA pressure monitoring, proponents believe that treatment decisions are often enhanced even though the issue of enhanced outcomes is much less certain.[60,65]

### Clinical Applications

The measurement of intracardiac pressures is helpful to assess left ventricular preload, pulmonary hypertension, and cardiac or noncardiac causes of pulmonary edema. Analysis of the CVP and PA port pressure waveforms provides diagnostic insights regarding the functional characteristics of rapid and reproducible ($\pm 10\%$) measurements of thermodilution CO. CO measurements are helpful to assess cardiac function, calculate oxygen delivery ($\dot{D}O_2$), and evaluate alterations in cardiac performance. Mixed venous blood samples (or measurement of $O_2$ saturation by reflectance oximetry) are necessary to calculate intrapulmonary and intracardiac shunts.

### Hemodynamic Assessment

Hemodynamic management is often predicated on the manipulation of preload, afterload, and contractility. Several of the derived indices of hemodynamic function necessitate CO

**TABLE 20–16.** Derived Hemodynamic Variables

| Name | Abbreviation | Calculation |
|------|--------------|-------------|
| Cardiac index | CI | CO/body surface area |
| Systemic vascular resistance | SVR | (MAP − CVP/CO) × 80 |
| Pulmonary vascular resistance | PVR | (MPAP − PWP/CO) × 80 |
| Stroke index | SI | CI/heart rate |
| Left ventricular stroke work index | LVSWI | SI × (MAP − PWP) × 0.0136 |
| Right ventricular stroke work index | RVSWI | SI × (MAP − CVP) × 0.0136 |

CO, cardiac output; CVP, central venous pressure; MAP, mean arterial pressure; MPAP, mean pulmonary artery pressure; PWP, pulmonary wedge pressure.
From Gilbert HC, Vender JS. Monitoring the anesthetized patient. In: Barash PG, Cullen BF, eds. *Clinical Anesthesia.* 2nd ed. Philadelphia, Pa: JB Lippincott; 1992:752.

measurement. Table 20–16 lists derived hemodynamic variables that generally require PA catheter insertion. The PA catheter is used to measure the PAOP. PAOP is used to assess left ventricular preload and, by inference, left ventricular end-diastolic volume (LVEDV) by reflecting changes in left ventricular end-diastolic pressure (LVEDP).

The clinical value of the PAOP is based on the assumption that an open conduit from the catheter tip to the left ventricle results when the PA catheter is in the wedged position. During end-diastole, cessation of forward blood flow occurs, and a static fluid column is presumed to exist from the left ventricle to the PA catheter tip. Ideally, changes in LVEDP are reflected by all proximal pressures (ie, PA end-diastolic pressure, PAOP, pulmonary venous pressure, and left atrial pressure). Technically, the PAOP is not always the same as the true pulmonary capillary pressure.[66]

### What Factors Affect Data Validity?

#### Pulmonary Vascular Resistance

Normally, pulmonary vascular resistance (PVR) and the impedance to pulmonary blood flow are minimal. Any significant increase in PVR alters the relationship between PAOP and PA end-diastolic pressure. Acute or chronic parenchymal pulmonary disease, pulmonary emboli, alveolar hypoxia, acidosis, hypoxemia, and many inflammatory mediators or vasoactive drugs may increase PVR. Tachycardia shortens ventricular diastole, reducing distal runoff of pulmonary blood flow and increasing PVR.[67] During these conditions, the PA end-diastolic pressure cannot be assumed to reflect distal diastolic pressures, including the PAOP.

#### Pulmonary Artery Catheter Tip Placement

Accurate measurement of PAOP can also be affected by the position of the catheter tip in the PA and by changes in intrathoracic pressure. Gravity-dependent differences in the alveolar, PA , and venous pressures are well known. West and colleagues describe three zones that define these interrelationships.[68] Only in zone III do pulmonary arterial and venous pressures consistently exceed alveolar pressure. Therefore, only zone III locations meet the requirement for uninterrupted blood flow and continuous communication with distal intracardiac pressures.[69] Increase in alveolar pressure, decrease in perfusion (eg, hypovolemia, hypotension, reduced CO), or changes in posture may convert areas of zone III to either zone I or II. Accurate measurement necessitates a PA catheter tip to be placed in zone III. Because PA catheters are flow directed, they usually advance to areas of highest blood flow. A lateral chest radiograph to ascertain that the catheter tip is below the level of the left atrium can confirm proper catheter position. Factors that influence the accuracy and validity of the PAOP are listed in Table 20–17.

#### Waveform Characteristics

When the PA balloon is inflated and the catheter tip is in the wedged or occluded location, the pressure tracing looks like the CVP or atrial trace. It has been assumed that in normal circumstances, the PAOP is a good reflection of pulmonary capillary pressure. It is now believed that many fac-

**TABLE 20–17.** Factors Affecting the Accuracy of Pulmonary Artery Occlusion Pressure Measurements

| Factor | Potential Effect |
|---|---|
| Increases in pulmonary vascular resistance (eg, acidosis, alveolar hypoxia, hypoxemia, chronic pulmonary disease) | PAD > PAOP |
| Increases in airway pressure (eg, PEEP therapy, reactive airway diseases) | PAOP > LAP |
| Mitral stenosis | LAP > LVEDP |
| Left atrial myxoma | |
| Abnormal ventricular compliance | LVEDP > LVEDV |

LAP, left atrial pressure; LVEDP, left ventricular end-diastolic pressure; LVEDV, left ventricular end-diastolic volume; PAD, pulmonary artery diastolic pressure; PAOP, pulmonary artery occlusion pressure; PEEP, positive end-expiratory pressure.

tors have disparate influences on pulmonary arterial and venous resistance, thereby limiting the clinical significance of changes in PAOP. PA v waves are present at the end of ventricular systole when the left atrium is maximally filled. The size of the v wave is most often associated with changes in left atrial compliance rather than regurgitant volume.

Decreases in left ventricular compliance, aortic regurgitation, and premature closure of the mitral valve may reverse the normal pressure gradient so that the LVEDP is greater than the left atrial pressure.[70,71] Therefore, accuracy of the measured pulmonary pressures and their correlation with LVEDP do not always ensure a valid reflection of left ventricular preload.

## Ventricular Compliance

The relationship between LVEDP and LVEDV is not linear. Changes in ventricular compliance result from inherent alterations in ventricular stiffness.[72] Ventricular compliance is a dynamic factor that can be influenced by many physiologic and pathologic variables. Factors that affect ventricular compliance are shown in Table 20–18. Appropriate use of PA catheters necessitates an appreciation and understanding of these pitfalls and limitations.[73]

## *What Do the Numbers Mean?*

The preceding discussion emphasized many factors that affect the *character* of the PA tracing as well as the absolute

**TABLE 20–18.** Factors That Influence Ventricular Compliance

**Decreased Left Ventricular Compliance**

Myocardial ischemia
Restrictive myopathies
Right-to-left intraventricular shunts
Aortic stenosis
Cardiac tamponade
Myocardial fibrosis
Inotropic drugs
Chronic hypertension

**Increased Ventricular Compliance**

Vasodilator therapy
Mitral regurgitation
Congestive myopathies
Aortic regurgitation

From Gilbert HC, Vender JS. Monitoring the anesthetized patient. In: Barash PG, Cullen BF, eds. *Clinical Anesthesia*. 2nd ed. Philadelphia, Pa: JB Lippincott; 1992:755.

numbers. PA catheters, by virtue of their multiple ports, provide simultaneous measurements of CVP and PAOP. These numbers, along with information obtained from thermodilution CO measurements, enhance assessment of fluid status and cardiac performance. However, use of the numbers is sometimes difficult.

Consider the example of a failing left ventricle versus new-onset left ventricular ischemia. In both situations, the LVEDP may have the same absolute value. However, the intraventricular volumes are likely to be different because the conditions may be associated with dissimilar changes in ventricular compliance. To assume that abnormal values by themselves mandate specific therapeutic interventions is unwise.

Recognition of artifacts, understanding of clinical circumstances in which PA catheter data may be misleading or difficult to obtain, and knowledge of the interaction of pathophysiologic states and diseases common to surgical patients define the cognitive skill of clinicians who use these catheters to their patient's advantage.

For many years, anesthesiologists have debated the worth of PA monitoring, particularly with respect to its value as a sensitive indicator of new-onset ischemia.[74] Many cardiac anesthesiologists do not routinely insert PA catheters. Patients with poor left ventricular function (ejection fraction <0.4), documented left ventricular wall motion abnormality, recent MI, significant angina, or documented left main (or left main equivalent) stenosis are often considered candidates for PA monitoring. This is not to suggest that PA catheter monitoring is superior to other monitoring options, such as TEE. Monitoring patients with cardiac impairments requires a knowledgeable anesthesia care team to minimize complications and to maximize the clinical value.[75]

## *What Are the Complications?*

PA catheters are associated with numerous complications.[76] Factors that appear to reduce complications include experience, appropriate supervision, and attention to details. One large study suggests a low incidence of morbidity and mortality,[77] but isolated case reports indicate that PA catheters have significant comorbidity and comortality. Most complications can be categorized into three groups:

1. Insertion risks
2. Catheter passage risks (advancement and removal)
3. Risks associated with use (maintenance)

### Insertion

Insertion risks are identical to those described for CVP cannulation.

### Advancement and Removal

Complications of advancement and removal are related to problems associated with cardiac performance or structure. Dysrhythmias are the most common complication of catheter passage.[78] Right bundle branch block and even complete heart block have been reported. If complete heart block is a concern, as in patients who have a preexisting left bundle branch block and in whom a superimposed right bundle branch block would

**TABLE 20–19.** Complications of Pulmonary Artery Catheter Passage

| |
|---|
| Dysrhythmias |
| Knotting |
| Valvular damage |
| Perforation of the atrium, ventricle, or pulmonary artery |
| Heart block |
| Kinking or coiling |

From Gilbert HC, Vender JS. Monitoring the anesthetized patient. In: Barash PG, Cullen BF, eds. *Clinical Anesthesia.* 2nd ed. Philadelphia, Pa: JB Lippincott; 1992:755.

result in complete heart block, a catheter with pacing capabilities should be considered.

Table 20–19 lists some of the complications that have been associated with catheter advancement and removal. Difficult insertions can be anticipated in patients who have right ventricular enlargement, low-flow states, or tricuspid valvular disease. In these situations, patient positioning (head up, right side down),[79] deep breathing, or fluoroscopic guidance may be necessary.

### Maintenance

Numerous complications have been associated with the continued use of PA catheters[80] (Table 20–20). The most dramatic and potentially catastrophic complication is PA perforation and hemorrhage.[81,82] Predisposing risk factors include hypothermia, pulmonary hypertension, advanced age, female gender, and poor technique. Perforations and subsequent hemorrhage can be avoided by restricting overwedging through rigorous monitoring of the PA tracing during gradual balloon inflation, continuously monitoring the PA pressure tracing to recognize spontaneous wedging, and minimizing the number of balloon inflations. Serious pulmonary hemorrhage from PA perforation is associated with hemoptysis and has a high incidence of mortality.

Catheter-related infections (sepsis or endocarditis) are well-recognized causes of morbidity that can be minimized when infection control protocols are implemented.[83] Because the benefit of long-term PA catheter monitoring is controversial, removal should be considered at the earliest appropriate opportunity based on clinical need and benefit.

### *How Is Pulmonary Artery Catheter Use Enhanced?*

Several modifications enhance PA catheter monitoring capabilities. The first significant improvement was the incorporation of a thermistor at the tip, enabling CO measurement by

**TABLE 20–20.** Complications of Pulmonary Artery Catheter Maintenance

| |
|---|
| Thrombosis |
| Pulmonary artery rupture |
| Sepsis |
| Endocarditis |
| Balloon rupture |
| Pulmonary infarction |
| Thrombocytopenia |
| Dysrhythmias |

thermodilution. Other features include intracardiac pacing, mixed venous oximetry, right ventricular ejection fraction (RVEF), and continuous CO monitoring.

### Mixed Venous Oximetry

Advances in fiberoptic technology led to the development of PA catheters that can continuously monitor mixed venous $O_2$ saturation ($S\bar{v}O_2$). The accuracy of these in vivo measurements has been confirmed by comparison studies with co-oximetry. Continuous $S\bar{v}O_2$ monitoring provides a minute-to-minute reflection of total tissue $O_2$ balance, which defines the relationship between $\dot{D}O_2$ and $O_2$ consumption ($\dot{V}O_2$).

### Oxygen Delivery, Demand, and Consumption

Understanding the value of continuous $S\bar{v}O_2$ monitoring necessitates a review of the factors influencing $O_2$ demand, $\dot{D}O_2$, and $\dot{V}O_2$. Oxygen demand cannot be measured directly. It represents the global oxygen requirement to maintain normal aerobic metabolism. However, the balance between $\dot{D}O_2$ and $\dot{V}O_2$ can be quantified.

The key measurements necessary for evaluating oxygen delivery and transport are CO, arterial oxygen saturation, and hemoglobin concentration. $\dot{V}O_2$ can also be measured directly by several methods. In this discussion, the indirect Fick method is underscored because it requires the use of a thermodilution CO catheter. $\dot{D}O_2$ (mL/min) equals $CaO_2$ (mL/L) times CO (L/min). $CaO_2$ can be estimated by multiplying hemoglobin concentration by the volume of oxygen that is transported by hemoglobin (1.34 times the saturation of the hemoglobin). Dissolved oxygen can also be calculated (0.003 × $PaO_2$) and is often added for completeness. $\dot{D}O_2$ can be approximated by measuring the CO and multiplying by the hemoglobin concentration times 13.8. The constant 13.8 represents the volume of $O_2$ carried by hemoglobin (g/L). This equation does not include the dissolved $O_2$ content, which in most cases is insignificant. $\dot{V}O_2$ is determined by the difference between arterial and venous $O_2$ content times CO. It is the numerator in the Fick equation. The relationships among $S\bar{v}O_2$, $\dot{V}O_2$, and CO is demonstrated in the following equation:

$$S\bar{v}O_2 = SaO_2 - \dot{V}O_2/(Hemoglobin \times 13.8) \times CO$$

where $SaO_2$ represents the percentage of $O_2$ saturation of arterial hemoglobin.

### Clinical Implications

Increases in $O_2$ extraction are reflected by a decrease in $S\bar{v}O_2$. At critical $\dot{D}O_2$ levels, the $S\bar{v}O_2$ plateaus because the $\dot{V}O_2$ is at maximal levels.[84] When the $S\bar{v}O_2$ is <30%, tissue $O_2$ balance is compromised, and anaerobic metabolism ensues. $S\bar{v}O_2$ is determined by the previously mentioned variables and, therefore, is not exclusively a reflection of changes in CO.

Figure 20–10 demonstrates the $S\bar{v}O_2$ recording of a patient recovering from cardiac surgery. In this example, a decrease in $S\bar{v}O_2$ was observed despite marked increases in CO, suggesting an imbalance between $\dot{D}O_2$ and $\dot{V}O_2$. A reduction in $\dot{V}O_2$ (reduced shivering) restored the balance between $\dot{V}O_2$ and $\dot{D}O_2$, reflected by a step-up of the $S\bar{v}O_2$ despite a decrease in CO.

Mixed venous oximetry is a powerful tool for both diagnos-

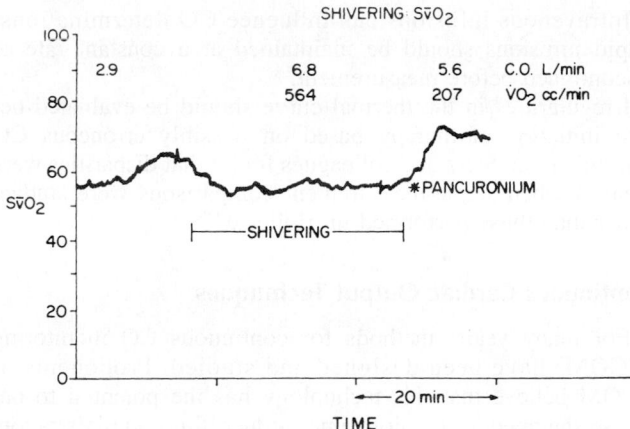

**FIGURE 20–10.** Effects of increased $\dot{V}O_2$ (shivering) on the balance of oxygen delivery ($\dot{D}O_2$) and $O_2$ consumption ($\dot{V}O_2$) as reflected by changes in mixed venous $O_2$ saturation ($S\bar{v}O_2$).

tic and therapeutic assessments of critically ill patients. The combination of continuous $SaO_2$ and $S\bar{v}O_2$ monitoring (dual oximetry) provides continuous information regarding the cardiopulmonary effects of positive end-expiratory pressure.[85] Coupling dual oximetry with estimates of carbon dioxide production can provide alternative estimates of CO.[86]

As with all monitoring, technologic and physiologic limitations affect clinical utility. Although low $S\bar{v}O_2$ often is considered ominous, a normal or high $S\bar{v}O_2$ does not always indicate adequate tissue $O_2$ balance. $S\bar{v}O_2$ is a global measurement. Table 20–21 lists some of the pathophysiologic conditions that may be associated with normal or high $S\bar{v}O_2$. Although there are no controlled studies examining the impact of $S\bar{v}O_2$ monitoring on outcome, intraoperative $S\bar{v}O_2$ monitoring is commonly recommended for complex cardiac and vascular surgery as well as for patients with multiorgan system disease.

### Other Modifications

Table 20–22 lists other adaptations that have been engineered into flow-directed PA catheters. Monitoring of RVEF requires a rapid-response thermistor for quantification of the beat-to-beat variations in PA temperature. Ejection fraction estimates are reasonably accurate so long as regurgitant flow or cardiac dysrhythmias are not present.[87] Knowledge of right ventricular volume could be useful in patients with acute lung injury or cardiac tamponade, or during positive-pressure ventilation. Urban and associates have demonstrated acute decreases in RVEF and increases in PA pressures during complex hip arthroplasties.[88] The value of and appropriate

**TABLE 20–21.** Clinical Conditions Associated With Normal or High Venous Oxygen Saturation

| |
|---|
| Sepsis |
| Peripheral shunts |
| Left-to-right intracardiac shunts |
| Arteriovenous fistulas |
| Paget's disease |
| Cirrhosis |
| Cyanide toxicity |
| Unintentional wedging of $S\bar{v}O_2$ pulmonary artery catheter |

$S\bar{v}O_2$, Mixed venous oxygen saturation.

**TABLE 20–22.** Pulmonary Artery Catheter Modifications

| Modification | Utility |
|---|---|
| Pacing wires and leads | Atrial and ventricular pacing |
| | Electrocardiogram dysrhythmia diagnosis |
| Ventricular ports | Placement of Chandler's wire |
| | Ventricular pacing |
| Infusion port | Central drug infusion |
| Fast thermistors | Right ventricular ejection fraction measurements |
| Heating filaments | Continuous thermal cardiac output monitoring |
| Fiberoptic transmission | Monitoring of oxygen saturation |

clinical situations for monitoring RVEF during anesthesia care have not been fully explored.

## CARDIAC OUTPUT

CO and hemodynamic variables derived from estimates of BP and flow are important indices of myocardial performance and the circulatory system. Estimates of CO, although not a routine measurement during anesthesia, are of great importance when managing critically ill patients or patients with documented or newly acquired cardiac dysfunction.[89]

### How Is Cardiac Output Measured Invasively?

The earliest technique for CO measurement was proposed by Adolph Fick in 1870. Fick found that the size of a fluid stream can be calculated by instilling an indicator into the stream and measuring the concentration difference over time between the inflow and outflow. Traditionally, $O_2$ has been used as the indicator substance, and CO is determined by measuring the $\dot{V}O_2$ and dividing it by the arterial-venous $O_2$ content difference.

Invasive and novel noninvasive methodology based on adaptations of Fick's principle are available for clinical use. The direct Fick CO measurement technique is the standard by which other methods are judged. Implicit in its use is the assumption that a steady state exists with respect to $O_2$ saturation, $\dot{V}O_2$, and CO during the period of data collection. Values are inaccurate if cardiac, pulmonary, or hepatic shunts are present.[90] The traditional Fick CO determination has been replaced by the thermodilution technique that was introduced into clinical practice in 1971.[91] However, indicator dilution methodology that formerly used indocyanine dye, or more recently lithium dilution, is again receiving attention as an alternative to more invasive methods.

### Indicator Dilution Techniques

#### Indocyanine Green Dye

Indicator dilution determinations of CO are based on a concept proposed by Stewart and tested by Hamilton and colleagues.[92] A known amount of indicator is injected into a CVP catheter, arterial blood is withdrawn at a constant rate, and a concentration-time curve is quantified. Computers calculate the average concentration over time. In adults, 50 mL of blood is withdrawn during each calculation. In children, 4 to

5 mL can be used without sacrificing accuracy.[93] After each determination, the blood can be returned to the patient.

### Thermodilution

Thermodilution CO determination (TDCO) is the most widely used adaptation of the indicator dilution principle. This technique was first described by Fegler in 1954.[94] Today, 5% dextrose or 0.9% saline is injected into the central venous port of a thermodilution PA catheter. A thermistor at the catheter tip records the decrease in temperature as blood, cooled by the injectate, passes through the PA. Computers contend with the complexity of the thermodilution CO equation, which, although similar to that for dye dilution, includes the following factors: specific heat and gravity of blood and indicator, volume of the injectate, catheter size, and area of the blood temperature curve.

**Accuracy.** Unlike dye dilution, the small amount of injected indicator in TDCO does not recirculate. Comparison studies suggest that either room-temperature or iced injectate can be used with equal accuracy for clinical measurements of TDCO when a 10-mL injectate volume is used.[95] Iced injectate produces more accurate results in children and adults when a 5 mL injectate is used. Properly performed, TDCO correlates well with both direct Fick and dye dilution determinations.[96,97] Triplicate determinations may be averaged to increase precision. Differences in values of 12% to 15% are not of clinical significance. Factors that influence the accuracy and precision of TDCO determinations are listed in Table 20–23.

**Sources of Error.** Observation of the thermal curve is helpful in assessing the accuracy of TDCO determinations. Low-amplitude curves result when CO is high or injectate volume is too small, the temperature differential between injectate and the patient is small, or the thermistor is improperly positioned.[98] Tricuspid or pulmonic regurgitation and intracardiac shunts may produce recirculation errors.[98] A diminished height of the concentration-time (thermodilution) curve can also occur from incomplete filling of the syringe, from loss of injectate through leaks, or from a thrombus insulating the PA thermistor. Each of these conditions results in a falsely high CO measurement.

**TABLE 20–23.** Accuracy and Precision of Thermodilution Measurements

**Theoretic Concerns**

Steady state of cardiac output during measurement sequence
Steady-state blood volume

**Sources of Errors**

Intracardiac shunts
Computational error due to programming mismatch
Thermistor drift and thermal noise
Variable rate of injectate administration
Coadministration of cool intravenous fluids
Respiratory cycle variation

**Factors That Enhance Accuracy and Precision**

Measure at peak inspiration or end expiration
Injectate rate of 2–4 s
Constant, precise injectate volume
Delay repetition of injections for 60–90 s
Accurate injectate temperature
Observation of the temperature decay curve
Average of three measurements

Intravenous infusions can influence CO determinations. Rapid infusions should be maintained at a constant rate or discontinued before measurement.[98]

Irregularities in the thermal curve should be evaluated before initiation of therapy based on possibly erroneous CO determination. Stetz and colleagues found that disparities were greatest when single-measurement comparisons were studied rather than those performed in triplicate.[99]

### Continuous Cardiac Output Techniques

For many years, methods for continuous CO monitoring (CCOM) have been designed and studied. Proponents of CCOM believe that this technology has the potential to decrease therapeutic decision time, reduce fluid administration, and reduce infection risks. CCOM is less labor intensive than traditional thermodilution.

### Invasive Techniques

Thermal convection principles permit an adaptation of the PA catheter that places a heating filament proximal to the thermistor. Heat from the filament is used as the indicator.[100] Several variations of this concept are available. Studies evaluating the accuracy, precision, and physiologic benefits continue to define areas in which this technology can assist in clinical decision making.[101]

The safety of the heating filament has been established as long as the temperature is kept <44°C and the power input is <15 W.[102] Continuous CO monitoring may provide logistical advantages.[103,104] Questions regarding the accuracy and response times continue to be reported.[105] Thermal methods for continuous CO monitoring require thermal stability. Errors due to temperature fluctuations can limit the usefulness of filament convection methods.

## How Is Cardiac Output Measured Noninvasively?

The quest for technically simple, noninvasive methods to estimate CO has a long history. Several methods are available for clinical use.

### Impedance Plethysmography

Impedance plethysmography (IP) is based on measurement of the pulsatile change in resistance during the cardiac cycle. Four electrodes are applied to the neck and thorax. Impedance measurements are made in two pairs while a continuous small electric current is applied across the thorax. The maximal rate of impedance change during systole (max $dZ/dT$) is proportional to the stroke volume and the ventricular ejection time.[106]

CO monitors based on IP are commercially available. Electrode placement is an important source of error.[107] Impedance signal processing is susceptible to motion artifacts and requires a stable ECG. Chest deformities and the thoracic fluid content can influence accuracy.[108] Although IP has not gained wide use, the technique offers clinicians a quick method for determining CO with minimal risk to patients.[109] Difficulties in signal acquisition and processing (eg, during electrocautery) have limited the acceptance of IP as a monitoring modality.

## Continuous or Pulsed-Wave Doppler Ultrasonography

Continuous or pulsed-wave Doppler US can measure the velocity of blood in the ascending aorta. CO is calculated by multiplying the time-weighted average velocity of blood flow by an estimate of aortic cross-sectional area. Aortic area can either be measured or predicted from a nomogram based on the patient's height, weight, age, and gender.

The accuracy and precision of Doppler-derived CO estimates are dependent on the reliability of the estimate of aortic diameter and the alignment of the Doppler probe to the blood flow jet in the aorta. Velocity measurements are most accurate when the Doppler beam and flow are parallel. When done from an esophageal location, a correction factor is used to estimate total CO from the velocity measurements obtained from interrogation of the descending thoracic aorta.

Modern transesophageal probes and instrumentation are promising techniques for monitoring CO *noninvasively and continuously* in critical care settings. The close proximity of the esophagus to the descending aorta provides end-users with an excellent opportunity to obtain stable measurements for longer periods of time. Substantial evidence has emerged suggesting that the esophageal Doppler technology is a reasonable clinical tool.[110] Like most technologies, programmed training enhances precision.[111,112] Esophageal Doppler technology is appealing for use in infants and young children.[113]

Transesophageal Doppler instruments appear to have robust performance and are simple to employ.[114] The flow time corrected for heart rate has been suggested as a reasonable estimate of preload, and the peak flow velocity can estimate changes in myocardial contractility.[115]

## Pulse Contour Analysis

Arterial pulse contour analysis (PCCO) represents another novel, minimally invasive method for estimating CO. This requires using a special arterial thermodilution catheter in patients who also have a central venous catheter. PCCO represents a minimally invasive system that calculates stroke volume from the contour of the arterial pressure curve. The PCCO system (Pulsion Medical Systems, Munich, Germany) calculates stroke volume using the Wesseling algorithm.[116] PCCO requires calibration using a thermodilution methodology whereby injectate is administered in a central venous portal, and the thermal dilution curve is obtained at a peripheral artery (femoral or axillary). Clinical testing in cardiac surgical patients comparing PCCO to intermittent thermodilution and impedance CO estimates suggests that PCCO offers clinicians a minimally invasive approach. Its accuracy requires recalibration if significant changes in peripheral vascular resistance occur.[117]

## Partial Carbon Dioxide Rebreathing Technique

For many years, it has been known that under steady-state conditions, the classic Fick equation can be reformulated by substituting $\dot{V}CO_2/R$ for $\dot{V}O_2$, where R equals the respiratory quotient (0.8). Manipulations of Fick's concepts using $CO_2$ as the indicator provide a useful method for estimating CO nearly continuously (every 3 minutes) and noninvasively. Modified Fick $CO_2$ methodology assumes that the hemoglobin and R remain constant during the measurement cycle. If these conditions are met, one can estimate CO by measuring $\dot{V}CO_2$, $SaO_2$, and end-tidal $CO_2$ ($ETCO_2$).[118,119]

NICO (Novametrix Medical Systems, Wallingford, Conn) provides clinicians with a respiratory sensor monitoring system that estimates pulmonary blood flow by further adaptation of the modified $CO_2$ Fick concept termed *partial $CO_2$ rebreathing*. This system estimates pulmonary blood flow from changes in $\dot{V}CO_2$ and estimated arterial $CO_2$ resulting from a sudden, brief, controlled change in dead space. If one assumes a steady state before, during, and immediately after rebreathing, it is possible to determine CO by monitoring the exhaled volume and tracking a high-fidelity trace of the exhaled concentration of $CO_2$ and oxygen saturation as measured by pulse oximetry ($SpO_2$). The NICO computer calculates an estimate for Q using the modified $CO_2$ Fick equation. After the rebreathing maneuver, the first estimate is subtracted from the value obtained after 30 seconds of rebreathing, where Q is estimated from the change in $\dot{V}CO_2$, and the change in $PaCO_2$ is estimated from the change in $ETCO_2$. The resulting equation for pulmonary capillary blood flow (PCBF) is as follows:

$$PCBF = \Delta \dot{V}CO_2 / S\Delta ETCO_2$$

where S is the slope of the $CO_2$ dissociation curve.

Partial rebreathing is noninvasive, near continuous, and derived from familiar monitoring technology. The reliability of the partial rebreathing methodology has been reported.[118] The system assumes a stable arterial–to–$ETCO_2$ gradient and estimates the intracardiac shunt to get from pulmonary capillary blood flow to total CO from the Nunn nomogram.[118]

## TRANSESOPHAGEAL ECHOCARDIOGRAPHY

TEE adds a new dimension to intraoperative monitoring because it creates beat-to-beat cardiac imaging (structure and function) with the capability of measuring intracardiac, pulmonary, and aortic blood flow. This approach offers information that complements data obtained from surface ECGs, invasive hemodynamic monitoring, and clinical signs. In experienced hands, TEE provides important information about the onset of myocardial ischemia, valvular competency, blood flow during diastole and systole, estimates of chamber volumes, quantification of CO, and estimates of regional myocardial function.

### What Are the Clinical Applications?

Despite the potential for esophageal damage (especially in the patient with dysphagia or stricture) or irritation, TEE has an excellent record of safety with few reports of complications. As anesthesiologists learn to use TEE, its application for intraoperative clinical decision making expands to include estimation of preload and measurement of stroke volume,[120] tracking of changes in left ventricular filling during noncardiac surgery,[121] assessment of intraoperative inotropy after cardiopulmonary bypass, and determination of the incidence and location of intracardiac air or other embolic material. Enhancements in instrumentation and computer software have improved the quality of images. Unfortunately, the equipment is expensive and user unfriendly. The learning curve for clinical interpretation requires considerable hands-on training. A perioperative certification examination developed by the National Board of Echocardiography is offered to anesthesiologists who wish to demonstrate expertise in TEE.

## How Does Transesophageal Echocardiography Work?

### Methodology

Modern intraoperative TEE uses Doppler-shifted US to penetrate intracardiac structures. The TEE processes reflected sound waves using complex instrumentation to depict graphically the size and shape of the heart chambers during filling and ejection. Direction of blood flow across valves, intracardiac chambers, proximal coronary and pulmonary arteries, and pulmonary veins can be determined. Valvular motion can be depicted, and the presence or absence of intracardiac masses or septal defects can be defined.

Sound is transmitted through matter (water, tissue) as ripples (sine waves) that are depicted when the amplitude of the sound energy is plotted against time. When sound waves enter a homogeneous medium, the velocity of the wave is constant and equals the product of the cycle length and frequency: $V = f(\lambda)$.

The ability of US to discern structures depends on the distance between the structures, the interface between the objects of interest, the frequency of the probing wave, and attenuation of this frequency by intervening tissues.

### Transesophageal Versus Transthoracic Techniques

Modern TEE uses high-frequency US (2.5-7.5 MHz) to probe the heart through the thin-walled esophagus. Although the US beams are weakened as they penetrate tissues, the beating heart is ideal for US probing because strong reflections, termed *specular echos,* are produced at the blood-tissue interfaces. TEE is more sensitive than transthoracic techniques because penetration of the chest wall is avoided, the lungs do not interfere with imaging, and higher frequencies may be used.

## What Are the Types of Echocardiograms?

The display produced by US probing is called an *echocardiogram.* Transesophageal equipment can produce echocardiograms using various formats (Fig. 20–11). A complete intraoperative TEE evaluation includes 2-dimensional (2-D) imaging and Doppler flow studies. Other specialized TEE interrogations have also been developed for intraoperative use. These investigational TEE procedures often require sophisticated computerization and are beyond the scope of this discussion.

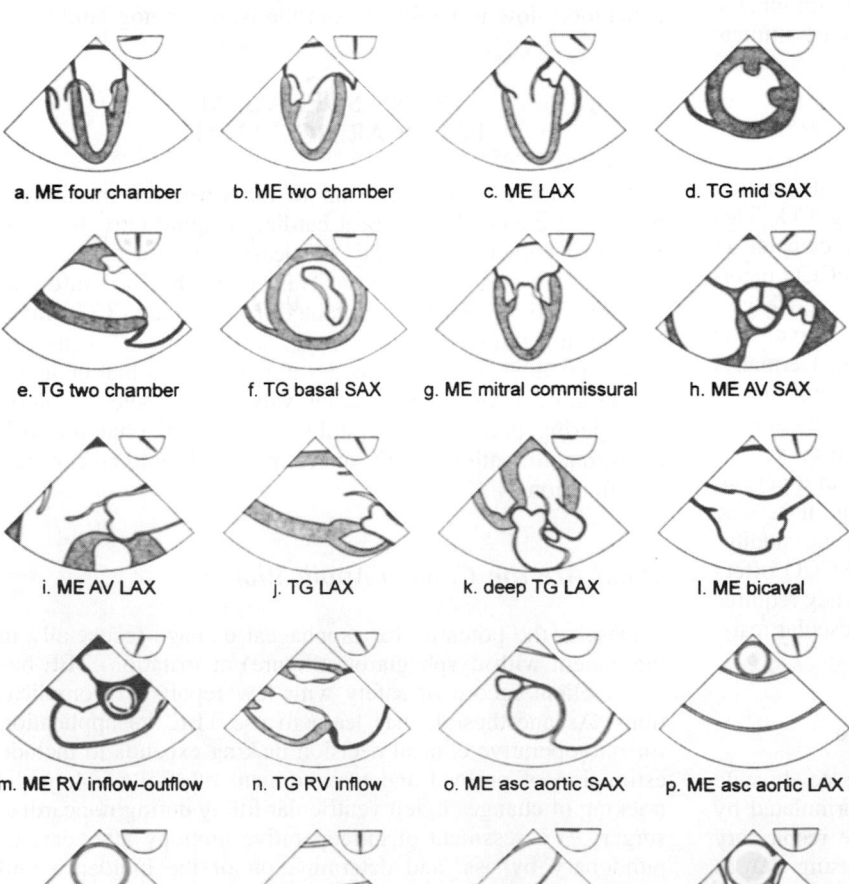

a. ME four chamber  b. ME two chamber  c. ME LAX  d. TG mid SAX

e. TG two chamber  f. TG basal SAX  g. ME mitral commissural  h. ME AV SAX

i. ME AV LAX  j. TG LAX  k. deep TG LAX  l. ME bicaval

m. ME RV inflow-outflow  n. TG RV inflow  o. ME asc aortic SAX  p. ME asc aortic LAX

q. desc aortic SAX  r. desc aortic LAX  s. UE aortic arch LAX  t. UE aortic arch SAX

**FIGURE 20–11.** Cross-sectional views of a comprehensive transesophageal echocardiography (TEE) examination using a multiplane TEE probe. asc, ascending; AV, aortic valve; desc, descending; LAX, long axis; ME, midesophageal; RV, right ventricle; SAX, short axis; TG, transgastric; UE, upper esophagus. (From Shanewise JS, Cheung AT, Aronson S, et al. ASE/SCA guidelines for performing a comprehensive intraoperative multiplane transesophageal echocardiography examination. *Anesth Analg.* 1999;89:870.)

## M-Mode Studies

M-mode echocardiograms (time-motion displays) are produced when a US beam is aimed at oscillating cardiac structures, and the reflected beam is displayed as wavy lines (due to oscillations of intervening heart tissues). Distance away from the transducer is displayed on the vertical axis, and time is displayed on the horizontal axis. Intraoperative M-mode echocardiograms are valuable because M-mode transducers can track rapidly moving structures such as valve leaflets.

## 2-Dimensional

2-D echocardiograms result when the TEE collects a series of B-mode (brightness mode) scans and aligns them in their appropriate anatomic orientation. Four approaches have been engineered to acquire the B-mode scan lines that create 2-D echocardiograms. Many crystals or a rapidly moving single crystal creates multiple views of cardiac structures that can be graphically reconstructed and collated into a 2-D image. Multiplane probes permit stepwise TEE interrogations by fine mechanical or electronic rotation of the scanning plane to 180°. Figure 20–11 depicts the 20 cross-sectional views recommended for a comprehensive TEE examination.[122]

Multiplane 2-D echocardiograms display cardiac structures with amazing clarity. The imaging process is minimally invasive, and no adverse effects of TEE US have been reported. 2-D scans depend on the reflected waves that are perpendicular to the US beam. Three-dimensional (3-D) reconstructions of TEE images are also feasible.[123] Esophageal probes (modified gastroscopes) can be positioned to optimize the spatial resolution of the scans. Figure 20–12 depicts the positioning of the TEE esophageal probe during a TEE examination. At each level, structures of interest are present, and the operator

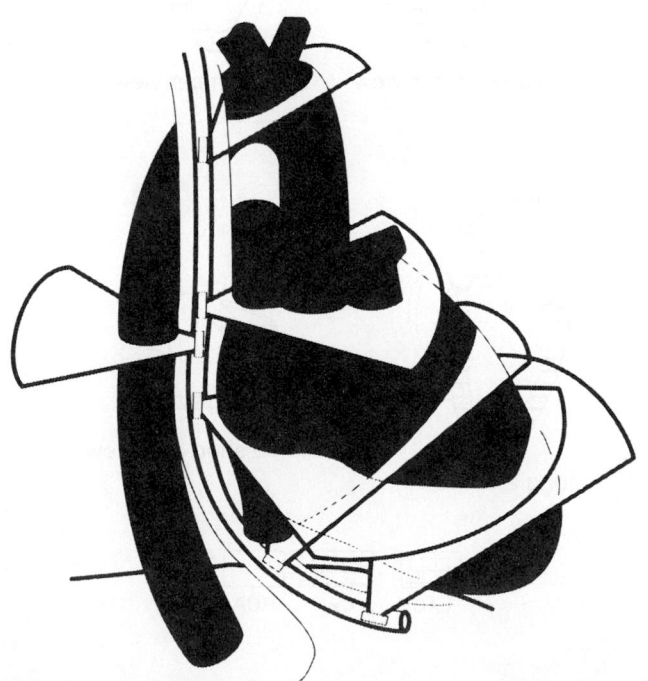

**FIGURE 20–12.** Graphic depiction of the positioning of a transesophageal echocardiography (TEE) probe during a comprehensive TEE examination. (Redrawn from Sutherland GR, Roelandt JPTC. Transesophageal echocardiography. In: *Clinical Practice*. London, United Kingdom: Gower Medical Publishing; 1991.)

must be skilled in orienting the esophageal probe to produce the best images.[124]

## Doppler Flow

Color imaging is based on the principle of Doppler-shifted US and uses sophisticated processing of the reflected echo waves to estimate flow characteristics. Because the velocity of the wave (pulsed or continuous) through the tissues is nearly constant, the distance between interfacing tissues can be determined by timing the reflected wave at the probe site. The shift of the frequency and amplitude of the reflected waves can be processed to provide color flow enhancement. Flow in the direction of the transducer is depicted as red and that away from the transducer is shown in blue. Increasing velocity in either direction is depicted by increases in the intensity of color shading.

These studies are useful to verify cardiac anatomy, identify intracardiac shunts, assess valvular regurgitation or stenosis, and evaluate myocardial perfusion.[125] Contrast echocardiograms are made by enhancing the echo characteristic of blood using saline "microbubbles." Alternatively, echo-dense contrast materials can be used to assess coronary blood flow.

Pulsed Doppler studies provide quantitative estimates of flow as long as the sampling frequency is higher than the velocities measured. If the Doppler shift exceeds half the sampling rate (Nyquist limit), the direction of flow is ambiguously presented as a signal of the highest velocity in the opposite direction (aliasing). Aliasing can be used to define areas of increased flow. Pulsed Doppler flow studies are range gated and susceptible to aliasing when blood is examined at high velocities.

Continuous wave Doppler permits measurement of high-flow velocities but lacks range resolution. Pulsed-wave Doppler permits measurement of blood flow at a specific location but cannot discriminate high flows without aliasing. Color flow Doppler imaging uses pulsed Doppler information and encodes mean velocities with 16 to 32 shades of colors. Color flow processing reduces the frame refresh rate, density of scan lines, frequency of resolution, and depth of simultaneous 2-D scanning.[126] Intraoperative color flow studies have been found to be sensitive indicators of mitral regurgitation.[127]

## *What Are the Clinical Uses?*

### Intraoperative Monitoring

Before the design of practical TEE probes, anesthesiologists, cardiologists, and cardiac surgeons depended on transthoracic and epicardial echocardiography for intraoperative cardiac and aortic imaging. These techniques, although helpful, were cumbersome to perform and had limited resolution.

Intraoperative TEE, unlike other cardiovascular monitors, provides almost real time beat-to-beat information about valvular function and cardiac filling and ejection. The clinical interpretation of wall motion abnormalities is a sensitive method to assess intraoperative ischemia. Table 20–24 lists the grading criteria used to quantify wall motion abnormalities. In the future, electronic processing of echocardiographic signals may assist clinicians in monitoring myocardial performance automatically. TEE monitoring during cardiac surgery has flourished. The role of TEE as an intraoperative monitor in noncardiac surgery and critical care is also expanding.

**TABLE 20–24.** Qualitative Grading of Wall Motion Abnormalities

| Grade | Wall Motion | Radial Shortening and Thickening |
|---|---|---|
| 1 | Normal | >30% |
| 2 | Mild hypokinesis | 10%–30% |
| 3 | Severe hypokinesis | <10% |
| 4 | Akinesia | None |
| 5 | Dyskinesia | Paradoxical bulging out and thinning |

Modified from Cahalan MK. Transesophageal echocardiography: should I be using it? In: *ASA Annual Refresher Course Series.* Vol 48. Park Ridge, Ill: American Society of Anesthesiology; 1997.

## Detection of Myocardial Infarction

For many years, graded reductions in myocardial perfusion pressure have been known to be associated with quantifiable alterations in wall motion.[128] During cardiac catheterization, cardiologists grade regional wall motion by assessing systolic ventriculographic patterns. Similarly, TEE images can be used to detect segmental wall motion abnormalities (SWMA). 2-D imaging and cineangiography show excellent correlation.[129] Acute intraoperative myocardial ischemia can be assessed by evaluating SWMA and wall thickening. By convention, 16 TEE segments describe left ventricular wall motion. Intraoperative SWMA analysis requires three short-axis views—basal, midpapillary, and apical—to assess intraoperative myocardial ischemia. The basal and midpapillary views are each divided into six segments. The apical view yields four additional segments[130] (Fig. 20–13A).

An experienced echocardiographer can provide sensitive and specific assessment of the location and extent of intraoperative ischemia. Figure 20–13B illustrates the relationship between myocardial blood supply and regional segments as observed by TEE. Intraoperative SWMA changes can be qualitatively graded, and their location may have significance with respect to specific vessel distribution. Similarly, TEE quantification of left ventricular end-diastolic volume and end-diastolic area correlates well with other accepted methods, suggesting that intraoperative TEE can serve as a sensitive, minimally invasive, intraoperative volume monitor.[131]

## Comparison With Electrocardiographic Monitoring

Monitoring for SWMA has been found to be more sensitive than intraoperative ST segment ECG monitoring for early detection of intraoperative ischemia.[132] Leung and colleagues evaluated the prognostic value of intraoperative TEE and compared SWMA with two-channel ECG monitoring.[133] TEE was more sensitive than ECG and was particularly useful in detecting ischemic changes occurring in the posterior or lateral quadrants of the left ventricle.

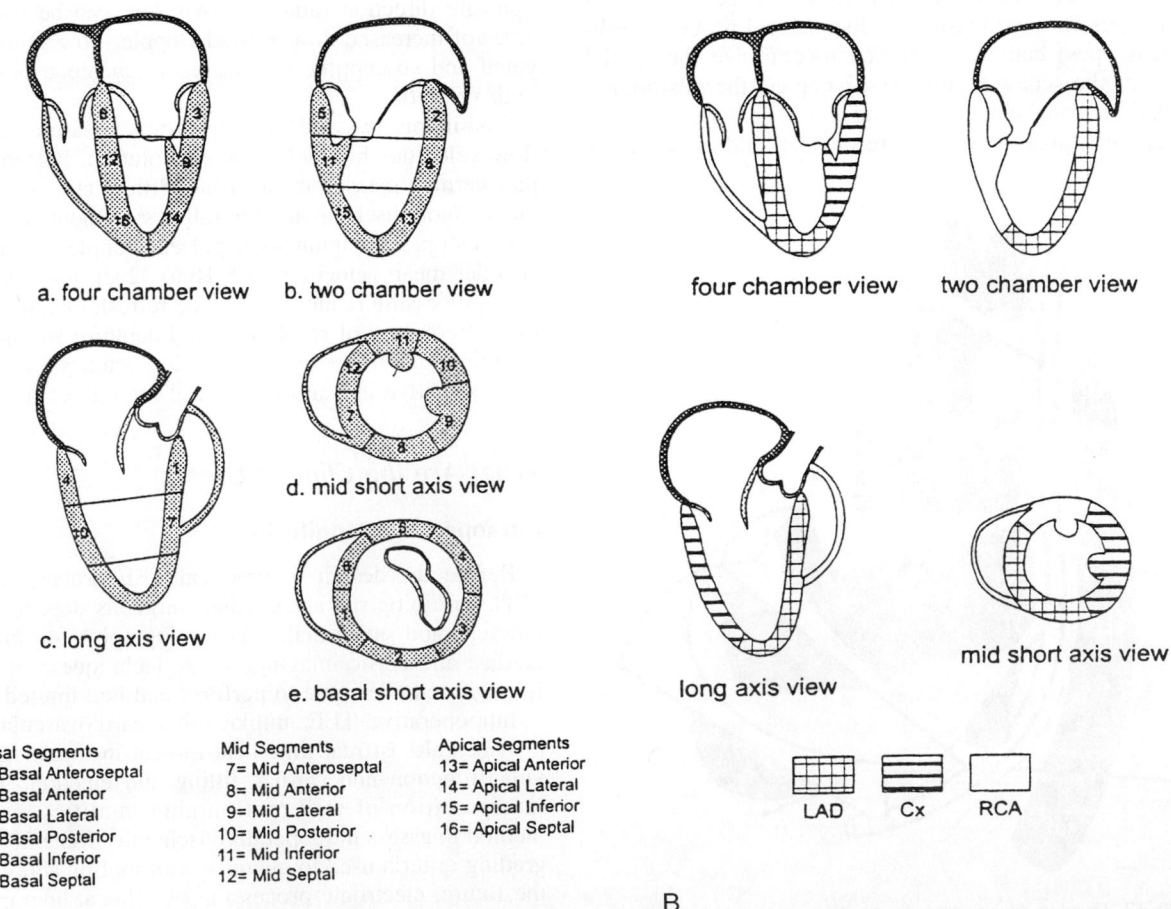

a. four chamber view    b. two chamber view

c. long axis view    d. mid short axis view

e. basal short axis view

four chamber view    two chamber view

long axis view    mid short axis view

**Basal Segments**
1= Basal Anteroseptal
2= Basal Anterior
3= Basal Lateral
4= Basal Posterior
5= Basal Inferior
6= Basal Septal

**Mid Segments**
7= Mid Anteroseptal
8= Mid Anterior
9= Mid Lateral
10= Mid Posterior
11= Mid Inferior
12= Mid Septal

**Apical Segments**
13= Apical Anterior
14= Apical Lateral
15= Apical Inferior
16= Apical Septal

LAD    Cx    RCA

A    B

**FIGURE 20–13.** *A,* Graphic depiction of the 16-segment model of the left ventricle used to assess wall motion abnormalities. *B,* Graphic depiction of typical regional perfusion by the major coronary arteries. Cx, circumflex; LAD, left anterior descending; RCA, right coronary artery. (From Shanewise JS, Cheung AT, Aronson S, et al. ASE/SCA guidelines for performing a comprehensive intraoperative multiplane transesophageal echocardiography examination. *Anesth Analg.* 1999;89:870.)

No other pathologic process has been found to produce acute SWMA to the same degree as myocardial ischemia that results from the acute disruption of myocardial blood flow. Conversely, correction of myocardial blood flow reverses SWMA associated with coronary insufficiency.[134]

## Assessment of Ventricular Dysfunction

Low-output syndromes may occur with right ventricular dysfunction, left ventricular dysfunction, and biventricular dysfunction. TEE is acknowledged as an important diagnostic tool in discriminating biventricular dysfunction.[135] TEE is helpful in identifying causes of severe intraoperative hypotension. No other intraoperative monitoring modality is capable of quickly differentiating hemodynamic derangements associated with tumors, valve dysfunction, pseudomasses, thrombi, vegetations, or air.

## Future Applications

Pioneering TEE studies have confirmed its sensitivity as a qualitative monitor of ischemia. For the technique to become popular as an intraoperative monitor, it must be determined that SWMA can be detected with confidence in all patients at risk for myocardial ischemia by practicing anesthesiologists. Current methodology cannot be considered a standard monitor until all practicing anesthesiologists learn to identify wall motion abnormalities. Today, TEE supplements but does not replace ECG monitoring. To that end, biplane probes, split-screen displays, and enhanced computer graphics may facilitate intraoperative interpretation of SWMA. Quantitative computer analysis of SWMA is undergoing investigation. In some centers, TEE intraoperative images can be electronically transmitted to off-site echocardiographers for consultation.

## Analysis of Valvular Function

TEE has advantages over precordial echocardiographic imaging techniques in assessing the structure and function of the cardiac valves. Higher quality images are provided without compromising the sterility of the surgical field. Analysis of mitral regurgitation is often dramatic when color flow studies are performed. Color flow mapping is helpful in ascertaining diastolic and systolic flow within the atria, across the valves, and in the pulmonary veins.

The clinical performance of prosthetic heart valves and complicating factors such as perforation of leaflets and intracardiac fistulas can be evaluated before and after surgical correction. With increasing degrees of mitral regurgitation, antegrade systolic flow in the pulmonary veins becomes abnormal. Experienced echocardiographers can also help cardiac surgeons identify potential problems that may occur during rewarming and before cessation of cardiopulmonary bypass.

## Effects of Anesthesia

Several investigations have focused attention on the use of echocardiography to assess the effect of anesthesia on ventricular function. Narcotic techniques appear to have little effect on ventricular function. Potent inhalational agents vary in their effects. Clinical assessment of myocardial performance using echocardiographic indices requires careful consideration of loading conditions, heart rate, and differences in blood-gas and tissue-blood partition coefficients of potent inhalational agents.

## Additional Applications

### Aortic Dissection

TEE is a valuable tool for assessing aortic dissections. Comparison studies have demonstrated equivalent sensitivity and specificity with angiography and computed tomographic scanning.[136] Intraoperative monitoring permits assessment of aortic valve function, estimation of luminal thrombus, delineation of aortic size and the extent of dissection, presence of pericardial fluid, involvement of the coronary ostia with subsequent myocardial ischemia, and quantification of flow in the false lumen.

### Detection of Atheromas

Cerebral vascular accidents after open heart surgery are a leading cause of morbidity and mortality. An epiaortic echoprobe is more sensitive in delineating atheromas than direct palpation by surgeons.[137] Intraoperative US scanning of the ascending aorta to guide aortic cannulation site choice may reduce the frequency of stroke related to atheromatous embolization associated with cardiac surgery.[138,139]

### Embolic Events

TEE is of great value in monitoring for intraoperative embolic events. Unlike conventional monitoring for air embolus, TEE offers capabilities to monitor and diagnose systemic as well as venous embolic events. TEE has been demonstrated to be particularly sensitive in detecting venous air embolism. Although the sensitivity of TEE to check for residual intracardiac air after heart surgery is well established, its utility has been questioned.[140]

### Congenital Lesions

Miniaturized TEE probes permit the monitoring of shunts, regurgitant, and obstructive lesions in infants as small as 3 kg.[141,142] Intraoperative TEE has been advocated for assessing the surgical repair of a wide spectrum of congenital lesions. TEE probe insertion in small infants can be associated with hemodynamic dysfunction or elevated airway pressures.[143]

## Final Issues

Although wide applications for intraoperative TEE monitoring are possible, its availability is limited because of its expense and complexity. The use of TEE as a diagnostic tool for defining cardiac morphology is well established. Its role as an integral intraoperative monitor is well established. Intraoperative TEE data often influence the conduct of anesthesia care.

Despite the potential for esophageal injury, continued observation has not revealed increased risks for esophageal damage. Pharyngeal and especially esophageal injury during placement, as well as laryngeal trauma after prolonged TEE, have been described. The size of TEE probes (6-11 mm) makes esophageal passage difficult in some patients. It is useful to consider placement under partial, direct laryngoscopic, pharyngeal exposure to facilitate easy and atraumatic probe placement in the anesthetized patient.

A complete history of esophageal problems should be taken from all patients for whom TEE is planned. Esophageal tumor or stricture contraindicates TEE evaluation. Esophageal varices have been cited as a contraindication as well, but TEE use during liver transplantation is common and without reported sequelae. Thus, esophageal varices probably should not preclude TEE monitoring if the benefits of TEE placement outweigh the risks.

## URINE OUTPUT

The production of urine and its composition offer anesthesiologists insights into the adequacy of the circulation and intraoperative renal function. The kidneys, more than any other organ, have a central role in the regulation of blood volume, extracellular fluid volume, osmolality of body fluids, concentration of ions, acidity, and excretion of drugs and metabolic byproducts. Thus, their function is a reflection of overall cardiovascular performance and stability. For this reason, monitoring the quality and quantity of urine output is included in this chapter. The indications for bladder catheterization are listed in Table 20–25.

### What Factors Determine Urine Output?

Urine homeostasis results from two variables—glomerular filtration and tubular reabsorption. Additionally, unwanted substances can be cleared by tubular secretion. In healthy kidneys, the glomerular filtration rate (GFR) is autoregulated by pressure inside the glomerular capillaries and outside Bowman capsule and by the colloid oncotic pressure (COP).

### Autoregulation of Glomerular Filtration and Renal Blood Flow

The mechanisms for autoregulation of glomerular filtration and renal blood flow (RBF) are complex. When the GFR falls, the concentration of sodium at the macula densa decreases. The reduction of sodium and chloride ions at the macula densa initiates two responses: the afferent arterioles dilate, and the juxtaglomerular cells release renin, causing the formation of angiotensin II. Angiotensin II induces efferent arterioles to constrict, favoring the reabsorption of water and electrolytes by reducing peritubular pressure and increasing

**TABLE 20–25.** Indications for Bladder Catheterization and Monitoring of Urine Output

---

Procedures with an anticipated duration >4 h
All pelvic surgical procedures (potential damage to ureters)
When large blood losses are anticipated
When excessive fluid replacement is anticipated
During deliberate hypotensive anesthesia
When diuretics are to be administered
All major vascular procedures requiring aortic cross-clamp
Most intracranial neurosurgical procedures
All procedures using cardiopulmonary bypass
All procedures performed after major trauma or burns
When monitoring hourly urine output is deemed helpful

---

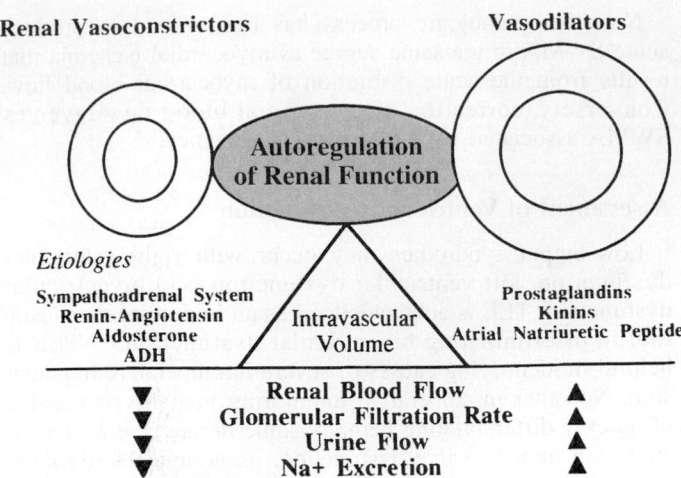

**FIGURE 20–14.** Graphic illustration of the complexity of factors that influence renal function during anesthesia care. ADH, antidiuretic hormone.

the COP of the peritubular capillaries. Feedback mechanisms that enhance tubular reabsorption of water and salt reduce the quantity of urine production.

Healthy kidneys autoregulate RBF and GFR as long as the MAP is sustained between 80 and 180 mm Hg.[144] The precise mechanism for autoregulation is not fully understood. Apart from autoregulation, renal function is controlled by the interaction of complex neurohumoral systems that are influenced by trauma, surgical stress, and drug therapy to various degrees (Fig. 20–14).

### What Factors Promote Vasoconstriction and Salt Retention?

Each day, 160 to 180 L of water is filtered by the kidneys. This ultrafiltrate of plasma contains 300 mOsm of solute per liter. Nephrologists define *oliguria* as a reduction of urine output to <0.3 mL/kg/h. Anesthesiologists become concerned when intraoperative urine output falls to <0.5 to 1 mL/kg/h. Studies suggest that the effects of anesthetic agents and techniques on renal function are mediated by extrarenal circulatory changes rather than by direct action on kidney function.[145] Surgical wounds often promote the stimulation of systems that foster vasoconstriction and salt retention.

### Catecholamines

The release of norepinephrine from autonomic nerve fibers and stimulation of the adrenal medulla diminish GFR and RBF. Slight α-adrenergic stimulation is not associated with significant changes and causes more efferent than afferent arteriolar constriction, and thus may actually increase urine production. However, high-level α-adrenergic stimulation promotes afferent arteriolar vasoconstriction, decreasing RBF and GFR. β-Adrenergic stimulation is associated with the release of renin from the juxtamedullary apparatus. Therefore, increases in adrenergic tone associated with intraoperative events may promote vasoconstriction and sodium retention.

### Renin-Angiotensin-Aldosterone Complex

The renin-angiotensin-aldosterone complex is important in regulating GFR, vasoconstriction, and salt homeostasis. Renin release is controlled by several factors. Baroreceptors in the renal afferent arterioles are primary modulators of the renin-angiotensin-aldosterone complex. β-Adrenergic receptors in the vicinity of the juxtaglomerular cells also influence the release of renin. In addition to its vascular and renal effects, angiotensin II activation promotes the secretion of aldosterone from the zona glomerulosa of the adrenal cortex. Aldosterone increases sodium and water absorption from the distal convoluted tubules.

## Antidiuretic Hormone

Antidiuretic hormone (ADH) secretion is normally stimulated by changes in osmolality, blood volume, and BP; however, it is also influenced by surgical stimulation. Inappropriate ADH secretion after major surgery may result in fluid retention, hypoosmolality, and hyponatremia.[146]

## Positive Pressure Ventilation

Positive pressure ventilation, with or without positive end-expiratory pressure, often diminishes urine production. This effect results from a contraction of the central circulation (decreased venous return) that concomitantly reduces RBF. Sympathetic, ADH, and renin-angiotensin modulations are the responses that maintain central arterial circulation. For a more extensive review of the effects of positive pressure ventilation on renal function and the enigmatic associated hormonal interactions, refer to the reports by Berry,[147] Sladen and colleagues,[148] and Hemmer and associates.[149]

## What Factors Promote Vasodilation and Salt Excretion?

A protective role has been defined for the production of intrarenal prostaglandins.[150] During periods of hypotension or ischemia or after catecholamine or angiotensin II stimulation, local prostaglandin production is increased. Prostaglandins produce renal vasodilation, maintain intrarenal hemodynamics, and block sodium reabsorption within the distal convoluted tubules. Renal prostaglandins modulate renin secretion.[151] Intrarenal kinins also have prominent roles in producing vasodilation and enhancing the actions of prostaglandins.[152]

A series of peptides that have been extracted from atrial tissues promote natriuresis and interact with the renin-aldosterone axis.[153] If hypotension and hypovolemia ensue during anesthesia, release of renin and atrial natriuretic hormone is triggered. Atrial natriuretic hormone inhibits the release of renin, blocks angiotensin-induced vasoconstriction, and blocks aldosterone release, thereby promoting vasodilation and salt-losing urine production.

## Why Does Oliguria Occur?

Oliguria is common postoperatively. Intraoperative oliguria is usually associated with decreases in circulating blood volume because of inadequate fluid replacement or hidden fluid losses. If severe and persistent hypotension occurs, the potential for oliguric renal failure must be considered in the early postoperative period.

**TABLE 20–26.** Evaluation of Perioperative Oliguria

| Test | Prerenal | Renal |
|---|---|---|
| Urinary Na⁺ (mEq/L) | <20 | >40 |
| Urine osmolarity (mOsm/L) | >500 | <350 |
| Urine/plasma osmolarity ratio | >1.3 | <1.1 |
| Urine/plasma urea ratio | >8 | <3 |
| Urine/plasma creatinine ratio | >40 | <20 |
| Fractional excretion of Na⁺ (%) | <1 | >2 |

Modified from Bauman LA, Prough DS. Acute perioperative renal dysfunction. In: Vender JS, Spies BD, eds. *Post Anesthesia Care*. Philadelphia, Pa: WB Saunders; 1992:147.

## Differential Diagnosis

Urinary diagnostic tests are helpful to distinguish the cause of acute oliguria. Laboratory evaluation of renal function is based on examination of the urine formed elements and blood and urine chemistry studies. Creatinine, urea, and sodium in plasma and urine are central to differentiating prerenal and renal causes of oliguria. Urinalysis may help to differentiate renal from tubular obstruction by assessing the presence or absence of granular casts, epithelial cells, or urine histiocytes.

Table 20–26 lists laboratory values that help to distinguish prerenal and renal oliguria. Urine osmolarity and urine sodium values are readily available intraoperatively. Urea, creatinine, and the fractional excretion of sodium can be measured in the early postoperative period. Potential causes of postoperative oliguria are multifactorial (Table 20–27).

## Why Does Polyuria Occur?

A number of physiologic and pathologic processes may result in an increase in urine production. If the kidneys' ability

**TABLE 20–27.** Causes of Perioperative Oliguria

| Postrenal etiologies | Catheter obstruction | Kink |
|---|---|---|
| | Ureteral obstruction | Calculi |
| | | Benign prostatic hypertrophy |
| | | Surgical accidents |
| | Extravasation of urine | Catheter disconnection |
| | | Rupture of bladder |
| | | Ureteral disruption |
| Prerenal etiologies | Hypovolemia | Hypotension |
| | | Hemorrhage |
| | | Fluid sequestration |
| | | Diuretic dependence |
| | Cardiovascular failure | Sepsis |
| | | Myocardial ischemia |
| | | Left heart failure |
| | Vascular obstructions | Renal artery (thrombosis or embolus) |
| | | Renal vein (thrombosis) |
| Renal etiologies | Intravascular hemolysis | Transfusion reactions |
| | | Eclampsia |
| | | Immune complexes |
| | Rhabdomyolysis | Malignant hyperpyrexia |
| | | Trauma |
| | | Muscle disease |
| | Nephrotoxins | Drug reactions |
| | | Immune complexes |

Modified from Dooley JR, Mazze RI. Oliguria. In: Orkin FR, Cooperman LH, eds. *Complications in Anesthesia*. Philadelphia, Pa: JB Lippincott; 1983:406.

to concentrate or dilute is impaired, urine production can be affected. Intraoperative polyuria requires evaluation.

## Fluid Drug Therapy

If hypotonic fluids are administered preoperatively, one should anticipate decreased ADH secretion in response to decreases in serum osmolarity. Glucose-containing fluids often produce an osmotic diuresis because the glucose load may exceed the renal threshold for reabsorption. Reducing glucose administration to <100 g during surgery diminishes the incidence of glucose-mediated, intraoperative polyuria.

## Diuretics

Perioperative diuretic therapy may also account for increased urine production. Diuretics are often administered to neurosurgical or ophthalmologic patients. Mannitol is an important component of cardiopulmonary bypass primes and cardioplegia solutions.

## Diabetes Insipidus

The potential for surgically induced diabetes insipidus should be entertained after neurosurgical procedures near the supraopticohypophyseal axis. In most instances, adequate stores of ADH are present to maintain water conservation for 12 hours.

## Anesthetic Agents

Most anesthetic agents and techniques lower GFR and RBF, so that urine output is diminished compared with the awake state.[154] These effects are related to changes in renal hemodynamics and are readily reversible.

A syndrome of polyuric renal failure, characterized by loss of concentrating ability and progressive azotemia, sometimes occurs after the administration of methoxyflurane. Studies of rats[155] and human beings[156] show that inorganic fluoride (Fi) is responsible for this reversible renal tubular dysfunction. Fi is a metabolite of methoxyflurane, enflurane, and sevoflurane.[157] Isoflurane and halothane produce negligible amounts of Fi. In most instances, the threshold for Fi-induced polyuric renal failure approaches 100 to 150 $\mu$mol/L. Toxicity may be enhanced by the concomitant administration of aminoglycosides or by prolonged anesthetic exposure in patients with previous renal dysfunction.

## References

1. Kuntz CM, Bennett JH, Shapiro H. Electrocardiographic studies during surgical anesthesia. *JAMA.* 1936;106:434.
2. American Society of Anesthesiologists. *Standards for Basic Intraoperative Monitoring: Approved October 21, 1986.* Park Ridge, Ill: American Society of Anesthesiologists; 1998.
3. Katz RL, Bigger JT. Cardiac arrhythmias during anesthesia and operation. *Anesthesiology.* 1970;33:193.
4. Mahla E, Rotman B, Rehak P, et al. Perioperative ventricular dysrhythmias in patients with structural heart disease undergoing noncardiac surgery. *Anesth Analg.* 1998;86:16.
5. Mangano DT. Peri-operative cardiac morbidity. *Anesthesiology.* 1990;72:153.
6. Mirvis DM, Berson AS, Goldberger AL, et al. Instrumentation and practice standards for electrocardiographic monitoring in special care units. *Circulation.* 1989;79:464.
7. Blackburn H, Katigbak R. What electrocardiographic leads to take after exercise? *Am Heart J.* 1964;67:184.
8. London MJ, Hollenberg M, Wong MG, et al. Intraoperative myocardial ischemia: localization by continuous 12-lead electrocardiography. *Anesthesiology.* 1988;69:232.
9. Palmer CM, Norris MC, Giudici MC, et al. Incidence of electrocardiographic changes during cesarean delivery under regional anesthesia. *Anesth Analg.* 1990;70:36.
10. Slogoff S, Keats AS. Does perioperative myocardial ischemia lead to postoperative myocardial infarction? *Anesthesiology.* 1985;62:107.
11. Slogoff S, Keats AS, Davod Y, et al. Incidence of perioperative myocardial ischemia detected by different electrocardiographic systems. *Anesthesiology.* 1990;73:1074.
12. Epstein SE, Quyyumi AA, Bonow RD. Current concepts: myocardial ischemia—silent or symptomatic? *N Engl J Med.* 1988;318:1038.
13. Kotter GS, Bernstein JS, Kotrly KJ, et al. ECG changes detect coronary artery bypass graft occlusion without hemodynamic instability. *Anesth Analg.* 1984;63:1133.
14. Kotrly KJ, Kotter GVS, Mortara D, et al. Intraoperative detection of myocardial ischemia with an ST segment trend monitoring system. *Anesth Analg.* 1984;63:343.
15. Ellis JE, Shah MN, Briller JE, et al. A comparison of methods for the detection of myocardial ischemia during noncardiac surgery: automated ST-segment analysis systems, electrocardiography and transesophageal echocardiography. *Anesth Analg.* 1992;75:764.
16. Wajon P, Lindsay G. Detection of postoperative myocardial ischemia by bedside ST-segment analysis in coronary artery bypass graft patients. *J Cardiothorac Vasc Anesth.* 1998;12:620.
17. Gunnar RM, Pietras RJ, Blackaller J, et al. Correlation of vectorcardiographic criteria for myocardial infarction with autopsy findings. *Circulation.* 1967;35:158.
18. Wit AL, Bigger JT Jr. Possible electrophysiological mechanisms for lethal arrhythmias accompanying myocardial ischemia and infarction. *Circulation.* 1975;52(6 suppl):III96.
19. Basnijak ZJ, Kampine JP. Effects of halothane, enflurane, and isoflurane on the SA node. *Anesthesiology.* 1983;58:314.
20. Meltzer LE, Kitchell JB. The incidence of arrhythmias associated with acute myocardial infarction. *Prog Cardiovasc Dis.* 1966;9:50.
21. Rubeinstein JJ, Schulman CL, Yurchak PM, et al. Clinical spectrum of the sick sinus syndrome. *Circulation.* 1972;46:5.
22. Rosen KM, Loeb HS, Sinno MZ, et al. Cardiac conduction in patients with symptomatic sinus node disease. *Circulation.* 1971;43:836.
23. Sprague DH, Mandel SD. Paroxysmal supraventricular tachycardia during anesthesia. *Anesthesiology.* 1977;46:75.
24. Haldemann G, Schoer H. Haemodynamic effect of transient atrioventricular dissociation in general anesthesia. *Br J Anaesth.* 1972;44:159.
25. Chou TE-C. *Electrocardiography in Clinical Practice.* Philadelphia, Pa: WB Saunders; 1991.
26. Kastor JA, Horowitz LN, Harken AH, et al. Clinical electrophysiology of ventricular tachycardia. *N Engl J Med.* 1981;304:1004.
27. MacDonald DA. *Blood Flow in Arteries.* London, United Kingdom: Edward Arnold; 1974.
28. Cohn JN. Blood pressure measurement in shock. *JAMA.* 1967;199:118.
29. Simpson JA, Jamieson G, Dickhaus DW, et al. Effect of site of cuff bladder on accuracy of measurement of indirect blood pressure. *Am Heart J.* 1965;70:206.
30. Geddes LA. *The Direct and Indirect Measurement of Blood Pressure.* Chicago, Ill: Year Book Medical Publishers; 1970.
31. Stegall HF, Kardon MB, Kemmerer WT. Indirect measurement of arterial blood pressure by Doppler ultrasonic sphygmomanometry. *J Appl Physiol.* 1968;25:793.
32. Ramsey M. Blood pressure monitoring: automated oscillometric devices. *J Clin Monit.* 1991;7:56.
33. Hynson JM, Sessler DI, Moayeri A, et al. Thermoregulatory and anesthetic-induced alterations in the differences among femoral, radial and oscillometric blood pressures. *Anesthesiology.* 1994;81:1411.
34. Ramsey M. Noninvasive automatic determination of mean arterial blood pressure. *Med Biol Eng Comput.* 1979;17:11.
35. Instrumentation (AAMI). *Proposed Standard for Electronic or Automated Sphygmomanometers.* Arlington, Va: Association for the Advancement of Medical Instrumentation; 1992.
36. Sy WP. Ulnar nerve palsy possibly related to use of automatically cycled blood pressure cuff. *Anesth Analg.* 1981;60:687.
37. Peñaz J. Photoelectric measurement of blood pressure volume and flow in the finger. *Digest, 10th International Conference of Medical Biological Engineers.* 1973:104.

38. Kurki T, Smith NT, Head N, et al. Noninvasive continuous blood pressure measurement from the finger: optimal measurement conditions and factors affecting reliability. *J Clin Monit.* 1987;3:6.

39. Langewouters GJ, Settels JJ, Roelandt R, et al. Why use Finapres or Portapres rather than intra-arterial or intermittent non-invasive techniques of blood pressure measurement? *J Med Eng Technol.* 1998;22:37.

40. Silke B, McAuley D. Accuracy and precision of blood pressure determination with the Finapres: an overview using re-sampling statistics. *J Hum Hypertens.* 1998;12:403.

41. Siegel LC, Brock-Utne JG, Brodsky JB. Comparison of arterial tonometry with radial artery catheter measurements of blood pressure in anesthetized patients. *Anesthesiology.* 1994;81:578.

42. Searle NR, Perrault J, Ste-Marie H, et al. Assessment of arterial tonometer (N-CAT) for the continuous blood pressure measurement in rapid atrial fibrillation. *Can J Anaesth.* 1993;40:388.

43. Belini K, Ozaki M, Hynson J, et al. A new noninvasive method to measure blood pressure. *Anesthesiology.* 1999;91:686.

44. Gardner RM. Blood pressure-dynamic response needs. *Anesthesiology.* 1981;54:227.

45. Hipkins SF, Rutten AJ, Runciman WB. Experimental analysis of catheter-manometer systems in vitro and in vivo. *Anesthesiology.* 1989;71:893.

46. Gardner RM. Accuracy and reliability of disposable pressure transducers coupled with modern pressure monitors. *Crit Care Med.* 1996;24:879.

47. Slogoff S, Keats AS, Arlund C. On the safety of radial artery cannulation. *Anesthesiology.* 1980;59:42.

48. Bedford RF, Wollman H. Complications of percutaneous radial artery cannulation: an objective prospective study in man. *Anesthesiology.* 1973;38:232.

49. Davis FM, Steward JM. Radial artery cannulation. *Br J Anaesth.* 1980;52:674.

50. Bedford RF. Removal of radial artery thrombi following percutaneous cannulation for monitoring. *Anesthesiology.* 1977;46:430.

51. Pearson ML. Guideline of prevention of intravascular device-related infections. *Am J Infect Control.* 1996;24:262.

52. Vender JS, Watts RD. Differential diagnosis of hand ischemia in the presence of an arterial cannula. *Anesth Analg.* 1982;61:465.

53. Sanford TJ. Internal jugular vein cannulation versus subclavian cannulation: an anesthesiologist's view: the right internal jugular vein. *J Clin Monit.* 1985;1:58.

54. Mark JB. Central venous pressure monitoring: clinical insights beyond the numbers. *J Cardiothorac Vasc Anesth.* 1991;5:163.

55. Trager MA, Feinberg BI, Kaplan JA. Right ventricular ischemia diagnosed by an esophageal electrocardiogram and right atrial pressure tracing. *J Cardiothorac Anesth.* 1987;1:123.

56. Sharkey SW. Beyond the wedge: clinical physiology and the Swan-Ganz catheter. *Am J Med.* 1987;83:111.

57. Tocino IM, Watanube A. Impending catheter perforation of superior vena cava: radiographic recognition. *Am J Roentgenol.* 1986;146:487.

58. Hoffman KK, Weber DJ, Gregory P, et al. Transparent polyurethane film as an intravenous catheter dressing. *JAMA.* 1992;276:2072.

59. Samii K, Counseiller C, Viars P. Central venous pressure and pulmonary wedge pressure. *Arch Surg.* 1976;111:1122.

60. Connors AF, Speroff T, Dawson NV, et al. The effectiveness of right heart catheterization in the initial care of critically ill patients. *JAMA.* 1996;276:889.

61. Dalen JE, Bone RC. Is it time to pull the pulmonary artery catheter? *JAMA.* 1996;276:916.

62. Tumen KJ, Roizen MF. Outcome assessment and pulmonary artery catheterization: why does the debate continue? *Anesth Analg.* 1997;84:1.

63. Vender JS. Pulmonary artery catheter monitoring. *Anesth Clin North Am.* 1988;6:743.

64. Swan HJC, Ganz W, Forrester JS, et al. Catheterization of the heart in man with the use of flow-directed balloon-tipped catheters. *N Engl J Med.* 1970;283:447.

65. Vender JS. Resolved: a pulmonary artery catheter should be used in the management of the critically ill patient. *J Cardiothorac Vasc Anesth.* 1998;12(2 suppl 1):9.

66. Collee GG, Lynch KE, Hill RD, et al. Bedside measurement of pulmonary capillary pressure in patients with acute respiratory failure. *Anesthesiology.* 1987;66:614.

67. Tumen KJ, Carroll GC, Ivankovich AD. Pitfalls of interpretations of pulmonary artery catheter data. *J Cardiovasc Anesth.* 1989;3:625.

68. West JB, Dollery CT, Naimark A. Distribution of blood flow in isolated lung: relation to vascular and alveolar pressures. *J Appl Physiol.* 1984;19:713.

69. Marini JJ. Obtaining meaningful data from the Swan-Ganz catheter. *Crit Care Clin.* 1988;2:572.

70. Carlile PV. Pitfalls in the interpretation of hemodynamic data. *Prog Crit Care Med.* 1985;2:69.

71. Jardin F, Farcot JC, Boisante L, et al. Influence of positive end-expiratory pressure on left ventricular performance. *N Engl J Med.* 1981;305:387.

72. Weber KT, Janiold JS, Shroff S, et al. Contractile mechanics and interaction of the right and left ventricles. *Am J Cardiol.* 1981;47:686.

73. Marini JJ. Hemodynamic monitoring with the pulmonary artery catheter. *Crit Care Clin.* 1986;2:551.

74. Kaplan JA, Wells PH. Early diagnosis of myocardial ischemia using the pulmonary arterial catheter. *Anesth Analg.* 1981;60:792.

75. Iberti TJ, Fischer EP, Leibowitz AB, et al. A multicenter study of physician's knowledge of the pulmonary artery catheter. Pulmonary Artery Study Group. *JAMA.* 1990;264:2928.

76. Puri VK, Carlson RW, Bander JT, et al. Complications of vascular catheterization in the critically ill. *Crit Care Med.* 1980;8:495.

77. Shah KB, Rao TLK, Laughlin S, et al. A review of pulmonary artery catheterization in 6,245 patients. *Anesthesiology.* 1984;61:27.

78. Voukydis PC, Cohen SI. Catheter-induced arrhythmias. *Am Heart J.* 1974;88:588.

79. Keusch DJ, Winters S, Thys DM. The patient's position influences the incidence of dysrhythmias during pulmonary artery catheterization. *Anesthesiology.* 1989;70:582.

80. Kelso LA. Complications associated with pulmonary artery catheterization. *New Horizons.* 1997;5:259.

81. Mullerworth MH, Angelopoulos P, Couyant MA, et al. Recognition and management of catheter-induced pulmonary artery rupture. *Ann Thorac Surg.* 1998;66:1242.

82. Klafta JM, Olson JP. Emergent lung separation for management of pulmonary artery rupture. *Anesthesiology.* 1997;87:1248.

83. Yunis N, Crausman RS. Sepsis and the pulmonary artery catheter. *Medicine and Health Rhode Island.* 1997;80:413.

84. Mohsinifar Z, Goldbach P, Tachkin DP, et al. Relationship between $O_2$ delivery and $O_2$ consumption in the adult respiratory distress syndrome. *Chest.* 1983;84:267.

85. Räsänen J, Downs JB, DeHaven B. Titration of continuous positive airway pressure by real-time dual oximetry. *Chest.* 1987;92:853.

86. Brandi LS, Bertolini R, Pieri M, et al. Comparison between cardiac output measured by thermodilution technique and calculated by $O_2$ and modified $CO_2$ Fick methods using a new metabolic monitor. *Intensive Care Med.* 1997;23:908.

87. Dhainaut JF, Brunet F, Monsallier JF, et al. Bedside evaluation of right ventricular performance using a rapid computerized thermodilution method. *Crit Care Med.* 1987;15:148.

88. Urban MK, Sheppard R, Gordon MA, et al. Right ventricular function during revision total hip surgery. *Anesth Analg.* 1996;82:1225.

89. Singer M. Cardiac output in 1998. *Heart.* 1998;79:425.

90. Taylar SH, Silke B. Is the measurement of cardiac output useful in clinical practice? *Br J Anaesth.* 1988;60:90s.

91. Ganz W, Donoso R, Marcus HS, et al. A new technique for measurement of cardiac output by thermodilution in man. *Am J Cardiol.* 1971;27:392.

92. Hamilton WF, Moore JW, Kinsman JM, et al. Studies on the circulation. IV. Further analysis of the injection method and of changes in hemodynamics under physiologic and pathologic condition. *Am J Physiol.* 1932;99:534.

93. Truccone NJ, Spontnitz HM, Gersony WM, et al. Cardiac output in infants and children after open-heart surgery. *J Thorac Cardiovasc Surg.* 1976;71:410.

94. Fegler G. Measurement of cardiac output in anesthetized animals by thermodilution method. *Q J Exp Physiol.* 1954;39:153.

95. Shellock FG, Riedinger MS, Bateman TM, et al. Thermodilution cardiac output determination in hypothermic postcardiac surgery patients: room vs. iced temperature injectate. *Crit Care Med.* 1983;11:668.

96. Fischer AP, Benis AM, Jurado RA, et al. Analysis of errors in measurement of cardiac output by simultaneous dye and thermal dilution in cardiothoracic surgical patients. *Cardiovasc Res.* 1978;12:190.

97. Levitt JM, Replogle RL. Thermodilution cardiac output: a critical analysis and review of the literature. *J Surg Res.* 1979;27:392.

98. Wetzel RC, Latson TW. Major errors in thermodilution cardiac output measurement during rapid volume infusion. *Anesthesiology.* 1985;62:684.

99. Stetz CW, Miller RG, Kelly CE, et al. Reliability of the thermodilution method in the determination of cardiac output in clinical practice. *Am Rev Respir Dis.* 1982;126:1002.

100. Yelderman M. Continuous measurement of cardiac output with the use of stochastic system identification techniques. *J Clin Monit.* 1990;6:322.

101. Lefrant J-Y, Bruelle P, Ripart J, et al. Cardiac output measured in critically ill patients: comparison of continuous and conventional thermodilution techniques. *Can J Anaesth.* 1995;42:972.

102. Yelderman M, Quinn M, McKown R. Thermal safety of a filamented pulmonary artery catheter. *J Clin Monit.* 1992;8:147.

103. Greim CA, Roewer N, Thiel H, et al. Continuous cardiac output monitoring during adult liver transplantation: thermal filament technique versus bolus thermodilution. *Anesth Analg.* 1977;85:483.

104. Burchell SA, Yu M, Takiguchi SA, et al. Evaluation of a continuous cardiac output and mixed venous oxygen saturation catheter in critically ill surgical patients. *Crit Care Med.* 1977;25:388.

105. Boldt J, Menges T, Wollbruck M, et al. Is continuous cardiac output measurement using thermodilution reliable in the critically ill patient? *Crit Care Med.* 1994;22:1913.

106. Kubicek WG, Karnegis JN, Patterson RP, et al. Development and evaluation of an impedance cardiac output system. *Aerosp Med.* 1966;37:1208.

107. Bernstein DP. A new stroke volume equation for thoracic electrical bioimpedance: theory and rationale. *Crit Care Med.* 1986;14:902.

108. Wong DH, Tremper KK, Stemmer EA, et al. Noninvasive cardiac output: simultaneous comparison of two different methods with thermodilution. *Anesthesiology.* 1990;72:784.

109. Weiss S, Calloway E, Cairo J, et al. Comparison of cardiac output measurements by thermodilution and thoracic electrical bioimpedance in critically ill versus non-critically ill patients. *Am J Emerg Med.* 1995;13:626.

110. Singer M. Esophageal Doppler monitoring of aortic blood flow: beat by beat cardiac output monitoring. *Int Anesth Clin.* 1993;31:99.

111. Siegel LC, Pearl RG. Noninvasive cardiac output measurement: troubled technologies and troubled studies. *Anesth Analg.* 1992;74:790.

112. Lefrant JH, Bruelle P, Aya AG, et al. Training is required to improve the reliability of esophageal Doppler to measure cardiac output in critically ill patients. *Intensive Care Med.* 1998;24:347.

113. Gueugniaud PY, Muchada R, Moussa M, et al. Continuous oesophageal aortic blood flow echo-Doppler measurement during general anaesthesia in infants. *Can J Anaesth.* 1997;44:745.

114. Valtier B, Cholley BP, Belot JF, et al. Noninvasive monitoring of cardiac output in critically ill patients using transesophageal Doppler. *Am J Respir Crit Care Med.* 1998;158:77.

115. Marik PE. Pulmonary artery catheterization and esophageal Doppler monitoring in the ICU. *Chest.* 1999;116:1085.

116. Wesseling KH, de Wit B, Weber JAP, et al. A simple device for the continuous measurement of cardiac output. *Adv Cardiovasc Physiol.* 1983;5:16.

117. Rodig C, Prasser C, Keyl C, et al. Continuous cardiac output measurement: pulse contour analysis vs thermodilution technique in cardiac surgical patients. *Br J Anaesth.* 1999;82:525.

118. Jaffe MB. Partial $CO_2$ rebreathing cardiac output: operating principles of the NICO system. *J Clin Monit.* 1999;15:387.

119. Mahutte CK, Jaffe MB, Chen PA, et al. $O_2$ Fick and modified $CO_2$ monitoring by the Fick cardiac outputs. *Crit Care Med.* 1994;22:86.

120. Martin RW, Bashein G. Measurement of stroke volume with three-dimensional transesophageal ultrasonic scanning: comparison with thermodilution measurement. *Anesthesiology.* 1989;70:470.

121. Roizen MF, Beaupre PN, Alpert RA, et al. Monitoring with two-dimensional transesophageal echocardiography: comparison of myocardial function in patients undergoing supraceliac, suprarenal-infrarenal or infrarenal aortic occlusion. *J Vasc Surg.* 1984;1:300.

122. Shanewise JS, Cheung AT, Aronson S, et al. ASE/SCA guidelines for performing a comprehensive intraoperative multiplan transesophageal echocardiography examination: recommendations of the American Society of Echocardiography Council for intraoperative echocardiography and the Society of Cardiovascular Anesthesiologists Task Force for Certification in Perioperative Transesophageal Echocardiography. *Anesth Analg.* 1999;89:870.

123. Nanda NC, Pinheiro L, Sanyal R, et al. Multiplane transesophageal echocardiographic imaging and three-dimensional reconstruction: a preliminary study. *Echocardiography.* 1992;9:667.

124. Powis RL, Powis W. *A Thinker's Guide to Ultrasonic Imaging.* Baltimore, Md: Urban & Schwarzenberg; 1984.

125. Lang RM, Feinstein SB, Feldman T, et al. Contrast echocardiography for evaluation of myocardial perfusion: effects of coronary angioplasty. *J Am Coll Cardiol.* 1986;8:232.

126. Kisso J, Adams DB, Belkin RN. Doppler color flow imaging. New York, NY: Churchill Livingstone; 1988.

127. Czer LSC, Maurer G, Bolger AF, et al. Intraoperative evaluation of mitral regurgitation by Doppler color flow mapping. *Circulation.* 1987;76(suppl 3):III.

128. Forrester JS, Wyatt HL, Paluz PL, et al. Functional significance of regional ischemic contraction abnormalities. *Circulation.* 1976;54:64.

129. Kisslo J, Robertson D, Gilbert B, et al. A comparison of real-time, two-dimensional echocardiography and cineangiography in detecting left ventricular asynergy. *Circulation.* 1977;55:134.

130. Schiller NB, Shah PM, Crawford M, et al. Recommendation for quantitation of the left ventricle by two-dimensional echocardiography. American Society of Echocardiography Committee on Standards, Subcommittee of Quantitation of Two-Dimensional Echocardiograms. *J Am Soc Echocardiogr.* 1989;2:358.

131. Horpole DH, Clements FM, Quill T, et al. Right and left ventricular performance during and after abdominal aortic aneurysm repair. *Ann Surg.* 1989;209:356.

132. Smith JS, Cahalan MK, Benefiel DJ, et al. Intraoperative detection of myocardial ischemia in high risk patients: electrocardiography versus two-dimensional transesophageal echocardiography. *Circulation.* 1985;72:1015.

133. Leung JM, O'Kelly B, Browner WS, et al. Prognostic importance of postbypass regional wall motion abnormalities in patients undergoing coronary artery bypass graft surgery. *Anesthesiology.* 1989;71:16.

134. Koolen JJ, Visser CA, Van Wezel WB, et al. Influence of coronary artery bypass surgery on regional left ventricular wall motion: an intraoperative two-dimensional transesophageal echocardiography study. *J Cardiothorac Anesth.* 1987;1:276.

135. Davuka-Rinab VGM, Waggoner AD, Hokins WE, et al. Right ventricular dysfunction in low output syndrome after cardiac operations: assessment by transesophageal echocardiography. *Ann Thorac Surg.* 1996;62:319.

136. Erbel R, Engberding R, Daniel W, et al. Echocardiography in diagnosis of aortic dissection. *Lancet.* 1989;1:457.

137. Ohteki H, Itoh T, Matsuaki M, et al. Intraoperative ultrasonic imaging of the ascending aorta in ischemic heart disease. *Ann Thorac Surg.* 1990;50:539.

138. Kouchoukos NT, Wareing TH, Daily BB, et al. Management of the severely atherosclerotic aorta during cardiac operations. *J Card Surg.* 1994;9:490.

139. Wareing, Davila-Roman VG, Barzilai B, et al. Management of the severely atherosclerotic ascending aorta during cardiac operations: a strategy for detection and treatment. *J Thorac Cardiovasc Surg.* 1992;102:453.2

140. Topol EJ, Humphrey LS, Borkon AM, et al. Value of intraoperative left ventricular microbubbles detected by transesophageal two-dimensional echocardiography in predicting neurologic outcome after cardiac operations. *Am J Cardiol.* 1985;56:773.

141. Ritter SB. Transesophageal real-time echocardiography in infants and children with congenital heart disease. *J Am Coll Cardiol.* 1991;18:1991.

142. Muhiudeen IA, Roberson DA, Silverman NH, et al. Intraoperative echocardiography for evaluation of congenital heart defects in infants and children. *Anesthesiology.* 1992;76:165.

143. Gilbert TB, Panico FG, McGill WA, et al. Bronchial obstruction by transesophageal echocardiography probe in a pediatric patient. *Anesth Analg.* 1992;76:1172.

144. Shipley RE, Study RS. Changes in renal blood flow, extraction of insulin, glomerular filtration rate, tissue pressure and urine flow with acute alterations of renal artery pressure. *Am J Physiol.* 1951;197:676.

145. Sladen RN. Effect of anesthesia and surgery on renal function. *Crit Care Clin.* 1987;3:373.

146. Bartter FC, Schwartz WB. The syndrome of inappropriate secretion of antidiuretic hormone. *Am J Med.* 1967;42:790.

147. Berry A. Respiratory support and renal function. *Anesthesiology.* 1981;55:655.

148. Sladen A, Laver MB, Pontoppidan H. Pulmonary complications and water retention in prolonged mechanical ventilation. *N Engl J Med.* 1968;279:448.

149. Hemmer M, Viguerat CE, Suter PM, et al. Urinary antidiuretic hormone excretion during mechanical ventilation and weaning in man. *Anesthesiology.* 1980;52:399.

150. Anggard E, Oliw E. Formation and metabolism of prostaglandins in the kidney. *Kidney Int.* 1981;19:771.

151. Gerber JG, Olsen RD, Nies AS. Interrelationship between prostaglandins and renin release. *Kidney Int.* 1981;19:816.

152. Nasjletti A, Malik KU. Renal kinin-prostaglandin relationship: implications for renal function. *Kidney Int.* 1981;19:860.

153. Laragh JH. Atrial natriuretic hormone, the renin-aldosterone axis, and blood pressure-electrolyte homeostasis. *N Engl J Med.* 1985;313:1330.

154. Priano LLO. Effects of anesthetic agents on renal function. In: Barash PG, ed. *Refresher Courses in Anesthesiology.* Vol 13. Philadelphia, Pa: JB Lippincott; 1985:143.

155. Cousins MJ, Mazze RI, Kosek JC. The etiology of methoxyflurane nephrotoxicity. *J Pharmacol Exp Ther.* 1974;190:523.

156. Cousins MJ, Mazze RI. Methoxyflurane nephrotoxicity: a study of dose response in man. *JAMA.* 1973;225:1611.

157. Kharasch ED. Biotransformation of sevoflurane. *Anesth Analg.* 1995;81(6 suppl):S27.

# 21

# Monitoring the Nervous System

## Michael E. Mahla

The central and peripheral nervous systems (CNS; PNS) can be readily examined in an awake patient to determine whether they are functioning normally. This examination may consist of a neurologic physical examination and laboratory tests such as an electroencephalogram (EEG), a magnetic resonance imaging (MRI) study, or both. Abnormalities of the CNS (eg, aneurysms, tumors), its supporting structures (eg, spondylitic myelopathy, scoliosis), or its blood supply (eg, carotid artery arteriosclerosis, thoracoabdominal aortic or intracranial aneurysms) may require surgery for correction. When surgery is required, the patient must be prevented from experiencing the pain associated with operation.

Some operations may be performed under local or regional anesthesia with the patient awake. The parts of the patient's nervous system not anesthetized may then be examined while surgery is being performed. However, local or regional anesthesia is inadequate for many operations, and general anesthe-

**TABLE 21–1.** Monitors of the Nervous System

**Monitors of Blood Flow**

Blood pressure
Intracranial pressure
Jugular venous $Po_2$
Radioactive ($^{133}Xe$) washout
Transcranial Doppler blood flow velocity
Cerebral oximetry
Near-infrared spectroscopy (NIRS)

**Monitors of Function**

Discontinuous: wake-up test

*Neurologic Examination*

Continuous: local or regional technique

**Electroencephalogram**

Scalp recordings (unprocessed, processed)
Direct cortical recordings

**Evoked Potentials**

*Somatosensory*

Cortical: scalp recordings; cortical recordings
Subcortical: surface recordings; direct recordings
Peripheral: surface recordings; direct nerve recordings

*Auditory*

Brainstem (BAEPs)
Middle latency cortical (MLAEPs)

*Visual (VEPs)*

Cortical
Direct nerve recordings

*Motor (MEPs)*

Electrical or magnetic cortical stimulation
Electrical or magnetic spinal cord stimulation

*Electromyography*

Peripheral muscle recordings
Facial nerve monitoring: active and passive
Other cranial nerve monitoring

**TABLE 21–2.** Surgical Procedures in Which Electrophysiologic Monitoring Is Used Successfully

| Operation | Monitor |
|---|---|
| Carotid endarterectomy | Awake patient, EEG, SSEP, TCD, rCBF, cerebral oximetry |
| Thoracoabdominal aneurysm repair, coarctation of aorta repair | SSEP, MEP |
| Posterior spinal fusion, anterior cervical fusion, vertebral body resection | SSEP, MEP, wake-up test |
| Intracranial aneurysm clipping | SSEP, VEP, BAEP, EEG, TCD, rCBF |
| Resection of intracranial or spinal cord tumor | SSEP, BAEP, VEP, EEG, EMG, MEP |
| Selective dorsal rhizotomy | EMG, SSEP |
| Induced hypotension (during many different operations) | EEG, SSEP, BAEP |
| Microvascular decompression of cranial nerve V or VII | BAEP, EMG |

BAEP, brainstem auditory evoked potential; EEG, electroencephalogram; EMG, electromyogram; MEP, motor evoked potential; rCBF, regional cerebral blood flow (using $^{133}Xe$); SSEP, somatosensory evoked potential; TCD, transcranial Doppler; VEP, visual evoked potential.

---

sia must be used. When general anesthesia is used, the nervous system can no longer be assessed by neurologic examination unless the patient is awakened during the operation. Over the past several decades, clinicians have begun to use tests previously used only in the diagnostic laboratory as continuous intraoperative monitors for various portions of the CNS and PNS.

Nervous system monitors may be divided into those that assess nervous system blood flow and those that assess nervous system function (Table 21–1). This chapter provides an overview and clinical examples of how different diagnostic tests have been adapted for such monitoring during surgery. Common surgical procedures in which such monitors have been found useful are presented in Table 21–2.

## IMPLICATIONS FOR INTRAOPERATIVE MANAGEMENT

For a monitor of the nervous system to have maximum utility, it must meet the requirements set forth in Table 21–3. Monitors measure function only at the time they are being used. No monitor in the operating room (OR) has been shown to change or reliably predict outcome. The electrocardiogram (ECG) used in the OR can detect only a small fraction of the number of instances of myocardial ischemia that occurs during surgery, even if it is watched continuously (and it is not).

Certainly, patients with intraoperative ischemia detected by ECG have a higher likelihood of perioperative myocardial infarction (MI), but ECG detection of intraoperative ischemia does not reliably predict MI, nor does its absence guarantee that MI will not occur postoperatively.

No studies demonstrate that monitoring of the ECG during surgery reduces the likelihood of perioperative MI or even of ischemia, yet intraoperative ECG monitoring is a standard of care. Most clinicians who routinely use neurologic monitoring have become convinced of its utility, not because scientific studies have demonstrated its usefulness but rather because cases in which major changes in therapy guided by monitoring have resulted in good outcome. These clinicians would be totally unwilling at this point in time to participate in prospective studies designed to test the utility of neurologic monitoring, just as many anesthesiologists would be uncomfortable with testing the utility of pulse oximetry, capnometry, and blood pressure (BP) monitoring.

## How Well Do Monitors of Neurologic Function Predict Outcome?

Numerous retrospective studies have addressed this question. Most used either EEG, somatosensory evoked potentials (SSEPs), or brainstem auditory evoked potentials (BAEPs)

**TABLE 21–3.** Requirements for a Nervous System Monitor

The monitor must reflect the function of the part of the nervous system at risk from either surgery or compromise of blood supply.
The operator must understand the anatomic pathways assessed by the monitor and the pathophysiologic mechanisms of injury that might occur during surgery.
The monitor should be used continuously, if possible, particularly during periods of risk.
The number of other factors affecting the monitor must be kept to a minimum.
Strict quality control must be observed to avoid technical problems with recordings.

as monitors of neurologic function, and their results were impressive. In a series of >1000 patients undergoing carotid endarterectomy at the Mayo Clinic, no patient awakened with a new neurologic deficit that was not detected by EEG.[1] Monitoring of evoked potentials has a similar accuracy record for scoliosis surgery.[2–7] However, a few cases have been reported in which neurologic monitoring was used and bad neurologic outcome occurred, even though there were no changes in the monitored parameters (ie, false-negative results).[8,9] Indeed, it would be extremely surprising if such cases were not reported. However, in a large, multicenter survey, the total reported false-negative rate was only 0.063%, or roughly 6 in 10 000 patients.[10]

Even if all of the individually reported false-negative results were valid (most were not), the number of such events is exceedingly small compared with the total number of patients monitored.[11] Many of these results were generated by an inappropriate use of the monitor. For example, the monitored pathway did not correspond to the part of the nervous system at risk from the operation, or inadequate quality control resulted in technical problems with the recordings. However, some of the reports of unacceptable outcomes have improved our understanding of how well the function of the monitored pathway predicts the function of adjacent areas of the brain and spinal cord. As a result, we are better able to define the monitor's limitations.[9,12]

Cases in which a perceived or real failure of a monitor occurred must be kept in perspective. When used carefully and appropriately, intraoperative neurologic monitoring appears to be useful for the early detection of a change in the monitored function and for the initiation of therapeutic interventions to prevent permanent neurologic injury.

## THE CLINICAL NEUROLOGIC EXAMINATION

### Why Is Preoperative Assessment Important?

If the clinical neurologic examination is to be used as a monitor of function during surgery (or after emergence from anesthesia), the clinician must know the level of baseline function. A patient who cannot perform a task preoperatively cannot be expected to perform this task during surgery or postoperatively. For example, if a wake-up test is planned during scoliosis surgery, one should ensure that the necessary commands (eg, "move your toes," and "squeeze my hand") can be followed preoperatively. A patient with a preexisting motor weakness from a stroke often does not function at baseline level immediately following carotid endarterectomy. On the contrary, preexisting neurologic deficits may be transiently aggravated by general anesthesia. A patient with a preoperative mild residual left hemiparesis, for example, may experience a more dense motor weakness for a few hours postoperatively.

### How Can the Examination Be Used Intraoperatively?

#### The Wake-Up Test

The neurologic examination may be used intraoperatively either intermittently (the wake-up test) or continuously (during local or regional anesthesia). The wake-up test is used to test neurologic function following a reversible surgical manipulation that has the potential to cause neurologic damage. Nothing is gained by awakening a patient to assess neurologic function if nothing can be done to correct a problem that is detected.

The wake-up test can be used safely only when movement will not cause damage. As an example, waking a patient following clipping of an aneurysm to assess function is extremely hazardous. Movement of a patient secured in a pin head holder may cause cervical spine injury as well as severe scalp lacerations. In addition, coughing, straining, and hypertension associated with wake up may cause cerebral swelling. The test is most commonly used following distraction of the spinal column during surgery for correction of kyphoscoliosis.

#### Techniques

Table 21–4 shows one of the many effective techniques for applying the wake-up test. The hypnotic (but not the analgesic) component of the anesthetic is reversed for a brief period, and the patient is asked to follow simple commands with both the upper extremities (not at risk from surgery) and the lower extremities (at risk from surgery). The patient must follow a command voluntarily. Interruption of the blood supply to the corticospinal tracts in the thoracic spinal cord results in complete failure of voluntary lower extremity movement. Reflex movement in response to pain, however, will still be intact as long as blood supply to the lumbar cord is intact and the patient is not experiencing "spinal shock." Thus, grasping the leg and applying a painful stimulus may evoke movement of the leg via spinal reflex and is not an appropriate method of applying the wake-up test.

#### Validity

The wake-up test has been considered for many years to be the gold standard for assessment of spinal cord function during

---

**TABLE 21–4.** How May the Wake-Up Test Be Performed?

**Before Surgery**

Document the level of preoperative neurologic function. Can the patient understand and perform the necessary commands?

Discuss the test to prepare the patient psychologically and to reduce intraoperative panic.

**Anesthetic Technique**

Narcotic infusion with potent inhalation agent; ± nitrous oxide, partial neuromuscular blockade

**Before Wake Up**

Document at least 2 of 4 twitches with blockade monitor, and partially reverse relaxant if needed (not usually necessary).

**Wake Up**

1. Discontinue administration of potent inhalation agent and nitrous oxide.
2. Continue narcotic infusion.
3. Begin calling patient by name until he or she responds.
4. Ask the patient to squeeze your hand and then to let go. Asking the patient to let go differentiates a voluntary response from a spinal reflex grasp.
5. After the patient voluntarily follows an upper extremity command, ask the patient to move toes and feet. For completeness, strength in each leg should be compared with that in the arms. Having the patient move the leg in response to pain is not a valid wake-up test. Movement following painful stimulus is a reflex and tests only lumbar cord function.
6. Sensation to a pinprick may be tested in a similar fashion, beginning with the upper extremities and continuing with the lower extremities.

scoliosis surgery. However, its sensitivity is open to question. The test is applied only intermittently. Long periods occur in which nervous system function is unknown. Thus, the effects of induced hypotension, which potentially places spinal cord function at risk, particularly when distraction is applied to the spinal column, is not assessed except during the test performance.

The appropriate time or times to apply the wake-up test are not clear. Both the spinal cord and brain have gray and white matter. Gray matter has a higher metabolic need for oxygen ($O_2$) and stops functioning within seconds after a complete interruption in blood supply. White matter, which consumes much less $O_2$, may continue to function for many minutes after a complete interruption. Partial interruption of blood supply to white matter may take much longer (even hours) to manifest loss of function. Thus, a wake-up test applied immediately after spinal column distraction may fail to detect loss of blood flow to white matter pathways in the midthoracic spinal cord (the area at highest risk for ischemia) and cannot reliably detect partial loss of blood flow that may later become critical.

In summary, the wake-up test can evaluate both motor and sensory function at the time it is applied. It cannot assess function at other times during the procedure. Despite these shortcomings, results of the wake-up test seem to correlate well with neurologic outcome (only a few reported cases and in one case in my personal experience did a patient demonstrate a neurologic deficit postoperatively that was not detected by an intraoperative wake-up test).[13,14] With increasing experience with electrophysiologic monitoring of the spinal cord (both sensory and motor), the wake-up test is being omitted entirely in many centers, unless electrophysiologic changes occur that do not make sense clinically or monitoring is not possible because of preexisting nervous system pathology (eg, cerebral palsy) or anesthetic-related problems.[7]

### Potential Complications

The wake-up test is potentially dangerous because the patient may become agitated and dislodge monitoring, life-support, and surgical instrumentation. Ideally, the test is applied in conjunction with other less dangerous and more continuous forms of neurologic function monitoring. In this way, it can be used as a confirmatory test when the results of other monitoring are uninterpretable or when such monitoring suggests a potential problem that, for example, occurs at an unexpected time or does not make sense clinically.

### Ankle Clonus Test

A modification of the wake-up test that does not require patient cooperation has been proposed and tested in a single study. This test is based on the observation that in the early recovery phase from general anesthesia, sustained ankle clonus is normally easy to elicit. The reason for this is thought to be continued loss of cortical inhibitory function in the early phases of recovery from anesthesia. In the face of spinal cord damage from scoliosis surgery, the reflex arc that produces clonus is interrupted, and clonus cannot be elicited. In a study of 1121 patients, all six patients who subsequently developed a neurologic deficit failed to demonstrate clonus when anesthesia was lightened. There were only three false-positive results in the series (three patients who failed to demonstrate

**TABLE 21–5.** Some Procedures During Which the Clinical Neurologic Examination Has Been Applied, and Anesthetic Techniques That May Be Used in Them

| Procedure | Anesthetic Technique or Techniques |
| --- | --- |
| Carotid endarterectomy | Local infiltration, cervical plexus block, interscalene block, ± sedation |
| Electrocorticography and resection of seizure focus | Local infiltration, multiple nerve blocks, ± sedation |
| Resection of brain tumor from eloquent area of the cortex | Local infiltration, multiple nerve blocks, ± sedation |
| Non-neurologic surgery on patient with head or neck injury following trauma or otherwise unstable central nervous system function | Local infiltration, nerve blocks, epidural or spinal anesthesia, ± sedation |

clonus who were neurologically normal).[15] It is unclear how this test could be applied in the patient with preexisting neurologic dysfunction. If results of this study can be duplicated, this test may have clinical value when neurologic monitoring is not available. This test would seem to have lower risk than the formal wake-up test.

### Continuous Clinical Monitoring

Table 21–5 lists operations in which local or regional anesthesia has been used successfully for continuous clinical CNS assessment. The level of sedation and airway accessibility are two special considerations during these operations (Table 21–6).

Continuous assessment of the awake patient is extremely useful in any situation in which unstable CNS function may occur. Patients under local or regional anesthesia who have an unstable neck (eg, those with rheumatoid arthritis or cervical myelopathy secondary to degenerative arthritis) may be positioned while they are awake, and neurologic examination can be conducted during surgery. A patient with compromised blood supply to the head (severe carotid stenosis) may be assessed continuously to make certain that his or her cerebral perfusion is adequate to supply the brain's needs. Neurologic function may be monitored similarly in carotid surgery during application of a carotid cross-clamp.

**TABLE 21–6.** Special Considerations for Monitoring of the Central Nervous System in the Awake Patient

**Sedation**

Overuse of sedation makes this type of monitoring useless.

***Recommended Drugs***

*Narcotics*

Fentanyl, sufentanil, alfentanil, remifentanil

*Hypnotics*

Propofol, midazolam,* droperidol

*Amnestics*

Midazolam*

**Airway**

If the surgery itself limits airway access carefully consider risk-benefit ratio for sedation.

*Avoid use during electrocorticography for location of seizure focus, as this drug or any in its class may depress any seizure activity.

The clinical neurologic examination also is particularly useful during non-CNS surgery following trauma that produces a closed head injury or cervical spine injury. If regional or local anesthesia is feasible and not contraindicated for other reasons (eg, the presence of coagulopathy, lack of cooperation, or combativeness on the part of the patient), continuous awake neurologic assessment enables the anesthesiologist to detect neurologic deterioration associated with cerebral edema or delayed intracranial hematoma formation, particularly if intracranial pressure (ICP) monitoring is not available.

In the case of a neck injury and an unstable cervical spine, the neurologic examination can be followed closely during and following positioning for surgery to ensure that the position has not compromised spinal cord function.

## Surgery to Control Seizures

Patients have surgery to control seizures because medical treatment has proved unsuccessful or has produced significant side effects. The location of the seizure focus may be determined by several methods, including preoperative EEG scalp recording, continuous EEG monitoring, recording from depth EEG electrodes or subdural grid electrodes placed in the OR, and intraoperative direct cortical EEG mapping.

If the location of the focus involves brain tissue that controls important neurologic function such as speech or motor activity, resection might produce an unacceptable neurologic injury. In the awake patient, the function of the area of the brain that is the source of the seizure activity may be tested. An electric current is applied directly to the applicable portion of the cortex. This current causes the patient to experience sensation or movement of a particular portion of the body or temporarily results in the cessation of function of that area of the brain. If application of the electric current to an area of active epileptic activity causes the patient to stop talking until the current is removed, resection of that area of the cortex will likely produce postoperative aphasia. The surgeon can then assess the cost-benefit ratio of resection. Newer, rapidly reversible intravenous anesthetics, such as propofol and remifentanil, combined with bispectral index monitoring (BIS) (author's experience) have made this type of monitoring procedure much more feasible and pleasant for the patient.[16,17] The level of consciousness may be controlled so precisely that the patient may be deeply sedated for the unpleasant portions of the procedure (opening and closing) and wide awake during the critical times of the operation.

### Candidates

Patients who undergo awake monitoring for either neurologic or non-neurologic surgery must be chosen carefully. Those who are anxious or who cannot understand what is happening may require so much sedation to tolerate the procedure that an adequate clinical examination cannot be carried out.

When the planned surgical procedure is conducted near to or on the head and neck and limits access to the airway, patients frequently feel claustrophobic. Special care with positioning and surgical draping is needed to provide an open space around the face, to allow free breathing, and to permit the patient to maintain visual contact with the surroundings. If neurologic deterioration that results in compromised ventilation occurs, quick access to the airway is necessary. This factor must be considered when determining the advisability of awake CNS monitoring.

### Sedation and Analgesia

Awake neurologic monitoring may be difficult during lengthy procedures. A 3-hour limit is probably expedient. Patients often become uncomfortable after lying in the same position for a prolonged period; they may require analgesics and sedation to tolerate the procedure. At some point, such therapy may decrease the sensitivity and specificity of the neurologic examination to detect injury.

Some investigators recommend propofol infusion for "unconscious sedation" during longer procedures that require only limited patient cooperation. For example, during craniotomy for electrocorticography and cortical mapping, the patient may be maintained with propofol during the relatively painful opening portion of the operation.[16–18] Propofol may then be discontinued, and the patient returns rapidly to baseline neurologic function for the testing period.

This technique has three drawbacks. First, neurologic monitoring is no longer continuous; therefore, it is not helpful during operations such as carotid endarterectomy in which continuous CNS assessment is desirable. Second, oversedation with loss of airway patency and aspiration may occur, although use of BIS monitoring may help avoid that complication. Third, some drug effect will persist into the testing period, and the results of neurologic testing, particularly during EEG monitoring, will be affected.[19] The use of propofol for sedation, however, seems to minimize that problem.[17]

## CEREBRAL BLOOD FLOW MONITORING DURING GENERAL ANESTHESIA

During general anesthesia, the clinical neurologic examination, except during the wake-up test, cannot be performed for obvious reasons. Thus, complete functional monitoring is impossible. However, two other techniques can be readily performed: cerebral blood flow (CBF) monitoring (direct and indirect) and partial functional monitoring (EEG, SSEP and BAEP, motor evoked potentials [MEPs], and electromyography [EMG]).

### Why Is Cerebral Blood Flow Monitoring Important?

The brain has a high metabolic $O_2$ requirement. When blood flow falls below a level sufficient to meet the cerebral metabolic requirements for $O_2$ ($CMRO_2$), cerebral function fails before cellular integrity is lost (resulting in permanent damage). Thus, if CBF is restored in a timely fashion, function is also restored without permanent damage. If CBF falls further, insufficient $O_2$ is available to supply energy for cell maintenance and brain cells die. Flow may be monitored indirectly, directly, or by measuring the balance between cerebral $O_2$ supply and demand (Table 21–7).

### How Is Indirect Assessment Performed?

The most commonly monitored parameter that gives information about the adequacy of the blood supply to the brain is

**TABLE 21–7.** Brain and Spinal Cord Blood Flow Monitors

| Monitor Type | Method of Assessment | Location of Blood Flow |
|---|---|---|
| Monitors that measure blood flow indirectly | Blood pressure | B, SC |
| | Intracranial pressure | B, SC |
| Monitors that measure blood flow directly | Radioactive $^{133}$Xe washout | B |
| | Transcranial Doppler blood flow velocity | B |
| | Cerebral oximetry | B |
| Monitor that measures balance between O$_2$ supply and demand directly | Jugular venous pO$_2$ | B |
| | Cerebral oximetry | B |
| Monitors that measure balance between supply and demand functionally | EEG | B |
| | SSEPs | B, SC |
| | MEPs | B, SC |

B, brain; EEG, electroencephalogram; MEP, motor evoked potential; SC, spinal cord; SSEP, somatosensory evoked potential.

**TABLE 21–8.** Some Conditions in Which Autoregulation May Fail

Head trauma
Subarachnoid hemorrhage
Brain tumor
Hypoxemia
Hypercarbia
High concentration of volatile anesthetic

---

BP. Normally, the relationship between BP and CBF is described by the cerebral autoregulation curve (Fig. 21–1). *Cerebral perfusion pressure* (CPP) is defined as the mean arterial pressure (MAP) minus the ICP or central venous pressure (CVP), whichever is higher:

$$CPP = MAP - ICP \text{ (or CVP)}$$

CBF is normal and constant over perfusion pressures that range from 50 to 150 mm Hg (see Fig. 21–1). If cerebral autoregulation is intact and ICP is known and constant, BP may be used to indirectly monitor the adequacy of CBF. BP that maintains CPP between 50 mm Hg and 150 mm Hg provides adequate CBF in normal patients.

### What Are the Limitations?

The most important limitation to BP monitoring of CBF is uncertainty regarding the limits of cerebral autoregulation and whether autoregulation is intact in the individual patient. Patients with poorly controlled hypertension generally have higher limits for cerebral autoregulation. This effect is reflected by a rightward shift of the curve in Figure 21–1. These limits return to normal with control of BP.[20,21] The actual limits for autoregulation in an individual patient are not known unless CBF is actually measured.

Autoregulation is impaired in many patients with intracranial pathology; in such patients, knowledge of CBF may be critically important (Table 21–8). The actual relationship between BP and blood flow in these patients is unknown without some measurement of CBF or cerebral function. BPs

within the normal range may be inadequate to maintain sufficient CBF. Anesthetic drugs may also impair cerebral autoregulation and change the relationship between BP and CBF, even when autoregulation is intact.

Finally, knowledge of cerebral perfusion pressure is only part of the story. The brains of anesthetized patients have a significantly lower requirement for O$_2$ and may be able to tolerate significantly lower perfusion pressures. I have seen many examples in which BPs significantly lower than baseline have *not* produced any changes in monitored neurologic function.

### Decreased Cerebral Perfusion Pressure

If CPP decreases to <50 mm Hg, cerebral and spinal cord blood flow decrease linearly with BP. The BP at which CBF becomes inadequate depends on the mechanism of BP reduction and, again, cannot be known for certain without some measurement of cerebral function (level of consciousness, EEG, or evoked potentials). I have observed unexpectedly normal evoked potentials during aneurysm clipping performed with sustained, severe sodium nitroprusside-induced hypotension (MAP = 30 mm Hg). CBF was maintained at acceptable levels despite the low perfusion pressure because of the cerebral vasodilating effects of nitroprusside.

### Increased Cerebral Perfusion Pressure

In normotensive patients with increases in CPP to >150 mm Hg, blood flow varies directly with BP. As CBF increases, cerebral edema, intracranial hemorrhage, or both, become more likely. Until either of these events occurs, function remains normal.

### Clinical Implications

BP is not a sensitive monitor of CBF when CPP is outside the limits of autoregulation. The likelihood of blood flow abnormalities that will produce functional damage to the brain probably increases with the duration and magnitude of CPP variance from the autoregulatory limits.

The discussion thus far has ignored changes in ICP. Many patients have a constant, normal ICP during surgery; changes in CBF are related to changes in BP alone. However, ICP may be variable in patients with different types of CNS pathology. Unless ICP is measured, CPP is unknown.

### Summary

Because BP measurement is noninvasive and easy to perform, it is the most frequently used monitor of CBF. In normal patients (ICP = ≈10 mm Hg), BP relates directly to CPP

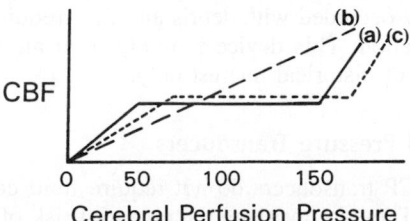

**FIGURE 21–1.** Relationship between cerebral blood flow and cerebral perfusion pressure. a, Normal; b, failure of autoregulation; c, hypertensive patient.

and is a reasonably good indicator of CBF. In patients with intracranial pathology or with altered autoregulation secondary to hypertension or drug administration, BP, at best, crudely estimates CBF and may be misleading. Generally, BP should be kept within the awake range throughout which function is documented. If it must be adjusted outside this range for surgical or medical reasons, some form of functional monitoring is needed.

### How Does Intracranial Pressure Relate to Cerebral Blood Flow?

The relationship between ICP and CBF in normal patients is also described by the cerebral autoregulation curve (see Fig. 21–1). If BP is constant, as ICP rises, CPP falls. Changes in blood flow will not occur until the limits for autoregulation are exceeded. However, in patients with impaired autoregulation (see Table 21–8 and Fig. 21–1*B*), CBF, as noted previously, varies directly with CPP (ie, the curve is "straightened"). In these patients, as ICP rises, CBF falls, unless BP increases by the same amount.

ICP commonly refers to supratentorial pressure measured in the subarachnoid space on the surface of the brain—subdural, epidural, or intraventricular—and is usually thought of as relatively constant in different areas of the brain. However, ICP reflects complex interactions within the craniospinal system, and pressure may be quite different in the various intracranial and intraspinal compartments.

### How Is Intracranial Pressure Measured?

ICP can be measured using any of the techniques shown in Table 21–9.

### Ventricular Catheter

Fluid-coupled ICP measurement is perhaps the least controversial method when it is performed with a ventricular catheter (Fig. 21–2). A small burr hole is made in the head, and a needle is passed through the dura and the substance of the brain into the lateral ventricle. A catheter is passed through the needle, and the needle is removed. The catheter is connected to a fluid-filled system and attached to a pressure transducer that is zeroed at the level of the foramen of Monro, which corresponds roughly to the surface landmarks of the nasion, the inion, or the external auditory meatus. *Note: This transducer system should not be attached to a flush system of any sort. If it is, infusion of fluid into the ventricle will occur, resulting in potentially disastrous elevations in ICP. Because*

**TABLE 21–9.** Methods of Intracranial Pressure Assessment

Lumbar cerebrospinal fluid pressure
Fluid-coupled transducer systems
    Ventriculostomy
    Subdural bolt (the Richmond screw)
Implanted intracranial transducer
    Optical methods
    Pressure transducer
Neuroradiologic studies

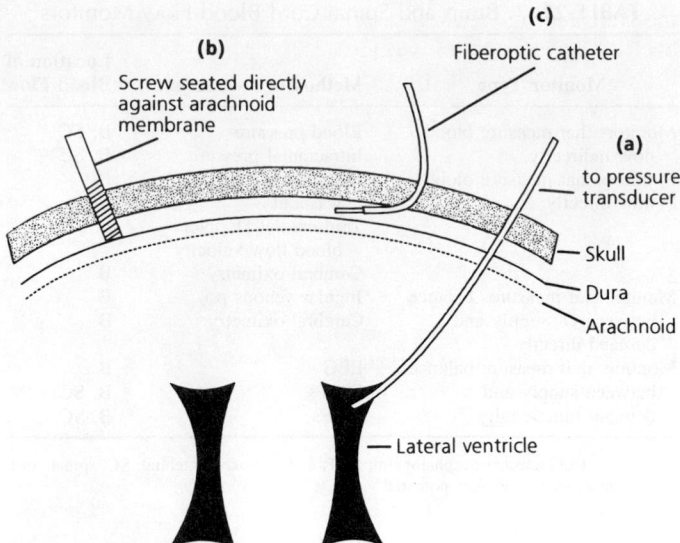

**FIGURE 21–2.** Schematics of intracranial pressure monitors. a, Ventriculostomy; b, Richmond screw; c, fiberoptic intracranial pressure transducer.

*this system does not involve blood, the catheter is unlikely to become occluded, and flush systems are not needed.*

A ventricular catheter is felt by many to provide the most accurate monitor of ICP. A major advantage of this system is that it can be both diagnostic and therapeutic because cerebrospinal fluid (CSF) may be removed during treatment for elevated ICP. Complications associated with insertion and use include an approximately 1% risk of bleeding[22] and an infection rate as high as 6.3% if the device is left in place for more than a few days.

### Subdural Bolt

The second fluid-coupled ICP measurement device is the subdural bolt or Richmond screw (see Fig. 21–2). A small incision is made in the scalp, and a small twist drill hole is made in the skull. The dura is opened, and a hollow bolt is screwed through the skull so that the open end protrudes 1 to 2 mm below the inner table and rests directly against the brain surface. The hole in the skull is sealed. The hollow bolt is filled with fluid and connected through fluid-filled tubing to a pressure transducer. Again, no flush device should be attached. The transducer is zeroed at the level of the foramen of Monro.

The Richmond screw reportedly gives readings that are lower than those for simultaneously recorded intraventricular pressure. Some feel that this discrepancy is caused by the leaking of fluid around the bolt. A major disadvantage of this system when compared with the ventriculostomy catheter is that the bolt cannot be used therapeutically to aspirate CSF. It is also easily occluded with debris and thus requires frequent, careful irrigation. This device is rarely used anymore and is now largely of historical interest only.

### Intracranial Pressure Transducers

Several ICP transducers do not require fluid coupling (see Fig. 21–2). They do not share the potential risk of inadvertent attachment of heparin flush to the transducer. The level at which these transducers are zeroed is not important because the transducers themselves are intracranial. The major drawback of these systems, again, is their inability to be used therapeutically for CSF withdrawal. The sensing catheters also are quite expensive and are not designed for multiple patient use.

### Lumbar Cerebrospinal Fluid Catheters

Lumbar CSF pressure may be measured easily by inserting a small, fluid-filled catheter designed for epidural use into the subarachnoid space through a Tuohy needle. This catheter is attached to a transducer again without a flushing device. Lumbar CSF pressure correlates well with ICP, provided that the transducer is zeroed at the level of the foramen of Monro and that the lumbar CSF space communicates with the lateral ventricles.

Any blockage of CSF circulation may prevent this communication. Hence, lumbar CSF pressure may be substantially lower than supratentorial ICP. Such a blockage makes insertion of a lumbar catheter dangerous as well; leakage of CSF from the lumbar space increases the pressure gradient between the supratentorial and lumbar compartments and may cause downward herniation of the intracranial contents.

### Scanning Techniques

Computed tomography (CT) and MRI scans of the head can give information about increased ICP. However, both studies are intermittent and their results can be misleading, thus they should not be considered as monitors. Evidence of increased ICP on CT or MRI scans is by no means quantitative and does not substitute for pressure measurements (Table 21–10).

**TABLE 21–10.** Computed Tomography and Magnetic Resonance Imaging Indicators of Elevated Intracranial Pressure

Shift of structures
Small or absent ventricles
Loss of cortical folds
Loss of cerebrospinal fluid in prepontine
   and mesencephalic cisterns
Cerebral edema (white matter)
Tumor with hydrocephalus
Tumor $\geq 3$ cm with edema

## DIRECT MEASUREMENT OF CEREBRAL BLOOD FLOW

### How Is Regional Blood Flow Assessed?

Direct measurements of regional CBF are not commonly used. The only practical intraoperative measurement involves injection of a radioactive isotope of xenon into the carotid artery, followed by measurement of the radioactivity washout with a gamma detector placed over a specific area of the brain (Fig. 21–3). This method cannot measure CBF over other areas of the brain and cannot distinguish flow at different depths (gray and white matter). Rather, regional CBF measurements reflect average gray-white matter flow. The technique is not continuous; therefore, during most of the operation, CBF is unknown. Indirect measurements, in contradistinction, can be used continuously. Despite its shortcomings, this method has been used in combination with other continuous monitoring methods, particularly during carotid endarterectomy surgery.[1]

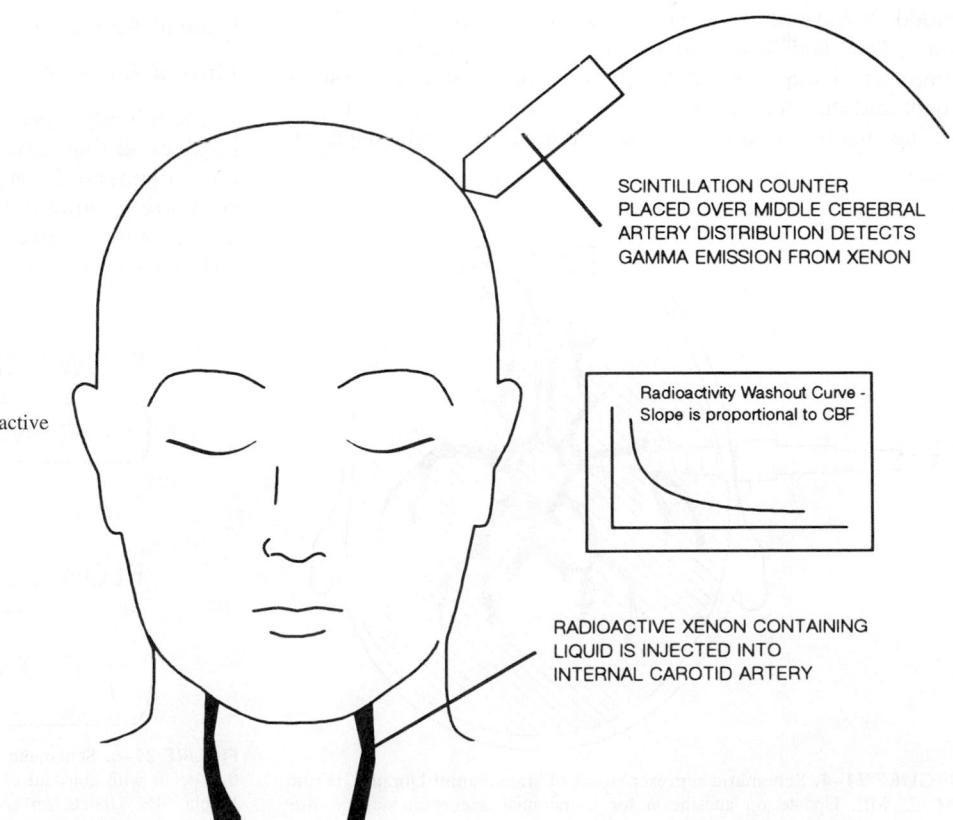

SCINTILLATION COUNTER
PLACED OVER MIDDLE CEREBRAL
ARTERY DISTRIBUTION DETECTS
GAMMA EMISSION FROM XENON

Radioactivity Washout Curve -
Slope is proportional to CBF

RADIOACTIVE XENON CONTAINING
LIQUID IS INJECTED INTO
INTERNAL CAROTID ARTERY

**FIGURE 21–3.** Schematic representation of radioactive xenon cerebral blood flow measurement.

## *How Is Transcranial Doppler Ultrasound Used?*

An easy-to-apply, direct, continuous, and noninvasive monitor of CBF employs transcranial Doppler (TCD) ultrasound (US). It has found increasing application as a monitor in the OR and intensive care unit (ICU).

### Methodology

US waves are used to measure the velocity of blood flow in the basal arteries of the brain. These waves are transmitted through the relatively thin temporal bone (Fig. 21–4). When they contact moving red blood cells, they are reflected at a changed frequency through the brain and skull back to a detector. The change in frequency as blood cells move toward or away from the US transmitter and detector is an example of Doppler-shifted US that is related to the velocity and direction of flow. Velocity increases during systole and decreases during diastole; blood in the center of the lumen moves faster than does that near the vessel wall, producing a spectrum of flow velocities. This spectrum resembles the shape of the waveform produced by an intra-arterial pressure transducer (Fig. 21–5).

TCD flow velocity measurements are most commonly and easily made in the middle cerebral and internal carotid arteries but are also possible in other vessels, including the anterior cerebral, anterior communicating, posterior cerebral, posterior communicating, and basilar arteries.

### Flow Velocity and Cerebral Blood Flow Relationships

Two assumptions must be made in order for TCD-measured blood flow velocity to have a direct relationship with CBF. First, flow and flow velocity are directly related only if the diameter of the artery at the point of flow velocity measurement and the measurement angle of the Doppler probe (angle of insonation) remain constant (Fig. 21–6). The angle of

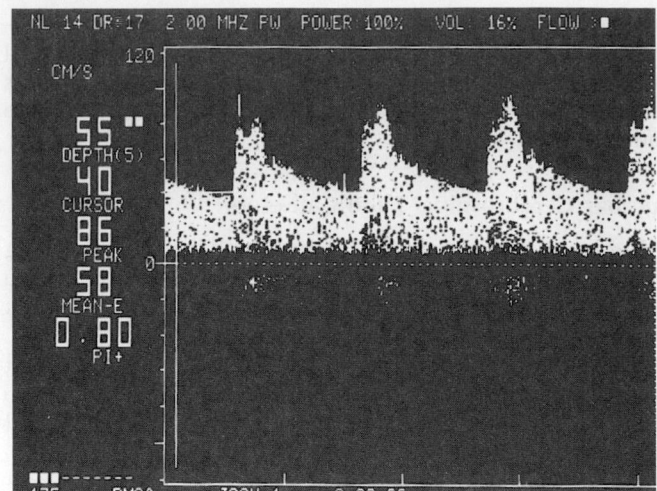

**FIGURE 21–5.** Typical transcranial Doppler waveform showing middle cerebral artery blood flow velocity spectrum.

insonation may be kept constant by rigidly mounting the TCD probe on the patient's head with a headset. Second, the blood flow in the basal arteries of the brain must be directly related to cortical CBF.

Neither of these assumptions has been proven. TCD technology has not been adequately validated in a large series of intraoperative cases against established monitors of CBF, such as the EEG, or against direct cortical CBF measurements, although evidence is accumulating that in some clinical circumstances, TCD may be used effectively to at least follow trends in cerebral blood flow, if not cerebral blood flow itself.[23–26]

### Clinical Applications

#### *Carotid Endarterectomy*

The initially reported, major intraoperative use of TCD US involves testing CBF adequacy while the carotid artery is cross-clamped during carotid endarterectomy. Studies that compare gamma detector-measured CBF with TCD US-derived middle cerebral artery flow have not shown a particularly strong correlation.[27] In addition, the period of carotid

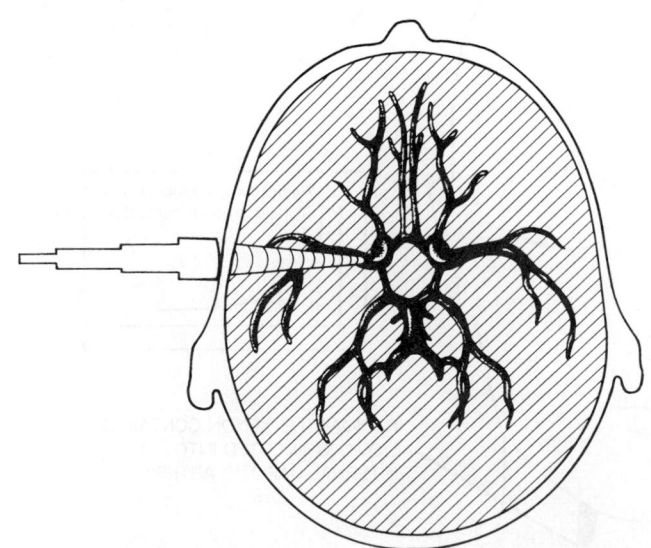

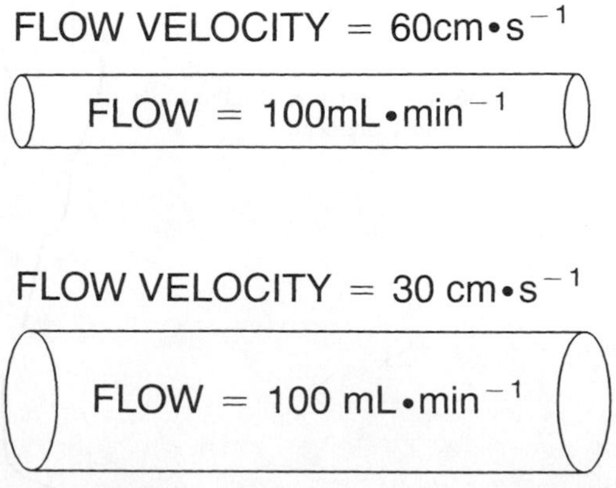

**FIGURE 21–4.** Schematic representation of transcranial Doppler. (From Mahla ME. Update on anesthesia for intracranial aneurysm surgery. *Adv Anesth.* 1993;10:103.)

$$\text{FLOW VELOCITY} = 60 \text{cm} \cdot \text{s}^{-1}$$

$$\text{FLOW} = 100 \text{mL} \cdot \text{min}^{-1}$$

$$\text{FLOW VELOCITY} = 30 \text{ cm} \cdot \text{s}^{-1}$$

$$\text{FLOW} = 100 \text{ mL} \cdot \text{min}^{-1}$$

**FIGURE 21–6.** Schematic representation of changes in blood flow velocity that occur with constant blood flow and a change in artery diameter. (From Mahla ME. Update on anesthesia for intracranial aneurysm surgery. *Adv Anesth.* 1993;10:103.)

cross-clamping is only a small portion of the time that the patient with carotid disease is at risk for ischemia; most strokes occur at other times during or after surgery. Few data are available about the nature and degree of acceptable TCD changes during the remainder of the operation. There is even controversy about the degree of acceptable change in cerebral blood flow velocity during clamping, although most studies will cite a reduction of between 50% and 80% as significant. Studies have also appeared that question the relevance of an even higher percentage reduction in blood flow velocity.[28–30] In one study that compared TCD blood flow velocity measurements with EEG and SSEP monitoring, the authors concluded that using the 70% decrease criterion for shunting will lead to unnecessary shunting in some patients (ie, some patients with this degree of decreased flow velocity showed *no* changes in SSEP or EEG).[28]

Use of TCD to detect emboli during carotid surgery, however, appears to be much more promising. Although it would seem that using TCD for this purpose would be labor-intensive (observation and counting of emboli), manufacturers are rapidly developing automated algorithms for detection and quantification of emboli that approach the accuracy of the human eye and ear.[31] One study demonstrated that simply the use of TCD monitoring during carotid surgery could train surgeons to change their techniques in a fashion that reduces the incidence and severity of intraoperative embolization.[32] The immediate auditory feedback to the surgeons provides ideal immediate feedback for learning. This observation is particularly important because several studies have suggested that a high postendarterectomy intraoperative emboli load predicts postoperative stroke, cerebral ischemia, or even carotid thrombosis.[33–36]

TCD also appears to have value in detecting patients at risk for postoperative hyperperfusion with resultant cerebral edema and hemorrhage. Significant preoperative carotid stenosis can result in significant downstream vasodilation with loss of autoregulation. Restoration of blood inflow in these patients can result in cerebral hyperemia, hemorrhage, and stroke. TCD can easily detect patients with persistently high postoperative blood flow velocities, allow for more aggressive reduction of BP in these patients, and perhaps even produce a reduction in the incidence of intracranial hemorrhage.[37–39]

Normal variations in blood flow velocities during surgery in patients without cerebrovascular disease appear to be large[40] and there is no agreement on the acceptable degree or duration of intraoperative changes, or, for that matter, on the significance of intraoperative changes. Thus, in the early 21st century, TCD US cannot be recommended as the optimal sole monitor of CBF during carotid surgery. The awake patient and EEG and SSEP monitoring appear to be more sensitive and specific monitors. TCD US technology likely has a supplementary role to other monitoring, particularly when it is used for detection of emboli before, during, and following endarterectomy.[41]

### Cardiopulmonary Bypass

These measurements also have been made during cardiopulmonary bypass to assess CBF[42] and to detect emboli.[43] Based on a limited number of studies involving a small number of patients, correlation between CBF and TCD US measurements is not particularly good[44–46] and appears to be influenced by whether the management of arterial carbon dioxide partial

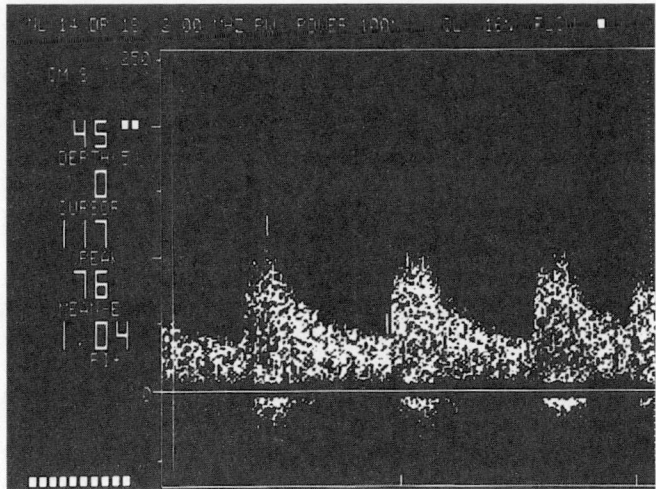

**FIGURE 21–7.** Typical transcranial Doppler waveform in a patient before the development of cerebral vasospasm following subarachnoid hemorrhage.

pressure ($PaCO_2$) is based on temperature-corrected (poor correlation) or uncorrected blood gas measurements. Emboli are readily detected, but studies to determine whether the incidence and severity of TCD US-detected emboli correlate with neurologic outcome do *not* suggest a particularly good correlation.[47,48]

### Detection of Vasospasm

Measurements of CBF with TCD have also had considerable application in the ICU. There was considerable early enthusiasm for the use of TCD in detection and documentation of the severity of vasospasm following subarachnoid hemorrhage.[49,50] As the diameter of the arterial lumen decreases with vasospasm, the velocity of blood flowing through the narrowed vessel must increase if flow is to be maintained (Figs. 21–7 and 21–8). Early detection would allow prophylactic treatment and close monitoring. In addition, preoperative evidence of vasospasm in asymptomatic patients with subarachnoid hemorrhage could alert the anesthesiologist to the patient

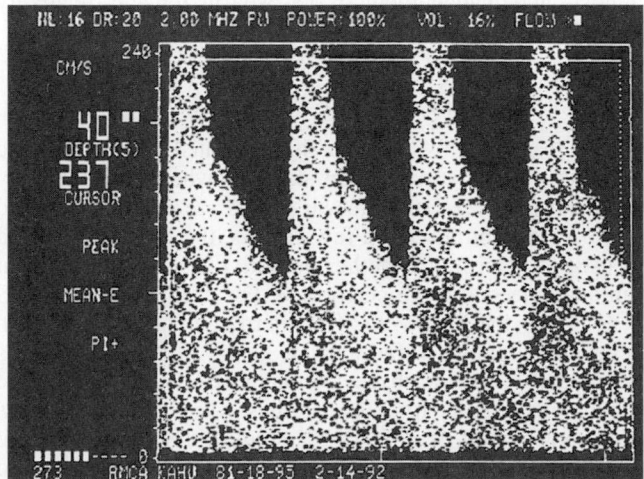

**FIGURE 21–8.** Typical transcranial Doppler waveform in a patient after the development of cerebral vasospasm following subarachnoid hemorrhage. Note greatly increased flow velocity compared with that in Figure 21–7.

who may be at greater risk for ischemia during hypotension, if hypotension is needed for aneurysm clipping. More experience with TCD and several subsequent studies have shown that the interpretation, particularly of single TCD studies without a longer term trend, is not so simple.

First of all, autoregulation is frequently impaired following subarachnoid hemorrhage. Use of hypervolemic hypertensive therapeutic regimens in these patients would thus be expected to have a significant effect on TCD measured blood flow velocities. In one study, 10 of 19 patients showed a significant rise in blood flow velocities that directly paralleled increases in MAP. In seven of these patients, the blood flow velocity increased sufficiently to change the interpretation of the grade of vasospasm.[51] Thus, the induced hypertension itself can actually make the disease process appear to worsen.

Second, insonation of cerebral blood vessels is somewhat of an art and requires considerable operator skill. By no means is the entire cerebral circulation examined by this method. It is quite possible for even a skilled operator to be unable to examine large segments of both the proximal and distal major cerebral vessels in an individual patient. One recent study showed that single positron emission CT was able to detect delayed ischemia where TCD showed no problem.[52]

Third, many patients with significantly elevated blood flow velocities never show any evidence of delayed ischemic deficit.[53,54] One study suggested that patients with elevated flow velocities without neurologic deficit may actually be experiencing hyperemia.[54] Hypertensive, hypervolemic therapy in these patients could actually be harmful and produce significant cerebral edema or even hemorrhage.

Fourth, preexisting hypertension with resultant chronic cerebrovascular changes may also alter the sensitivity and specificity of TCD diagnosis of vasospasm. In these patients, even moderately increased flow velocities that would not normally cause concern may be significant.[55] A recent study reflects a growing consensus among physicians caring for patients with subarachnoid hemorrhage.[56] Only low (<120 cm/s) or very high (>200 cm/s) flow velocities reliably predicted the absence or presence of clinically significant angiographic vasospasm. Intermediate velocities were not reliable for use in either diagnosis or in following treatment of vasospasm. The initial enthusiasm for this diagnostic tool has cooled somewhat, and the appropriate role for TCD in the diagnosis and management of vasospasm remains relatively poorly defined.

### Confirmation of Brain Death

In the early 1990s, studies demonstrated a characteristic blood flow velocity pattern in patients who were clinically brain dead (Fig. 21–9).[57] Measurements are easily performed at the bedside. Initially, in a few centers, the TCD US method was used to determine whether definitive studies to document brain death needed to be performed. For example, if TCD US did not show the flow velocity pattern characteristic of brain death, angiographic or radioactive xenon blood flow studies were unlikely to show absent cortical CBF. Transport of these critically ill patients for CBF studies was thus unnecessary. On the other hand, if a TCD US study did show the pattern characteristic of brain death (see Fig. 21–9), the patient could be transported for definitive blood flow studies without further delay or expenditure of resources. Further studies documenting the sensitivity and specificity have, for the most part,

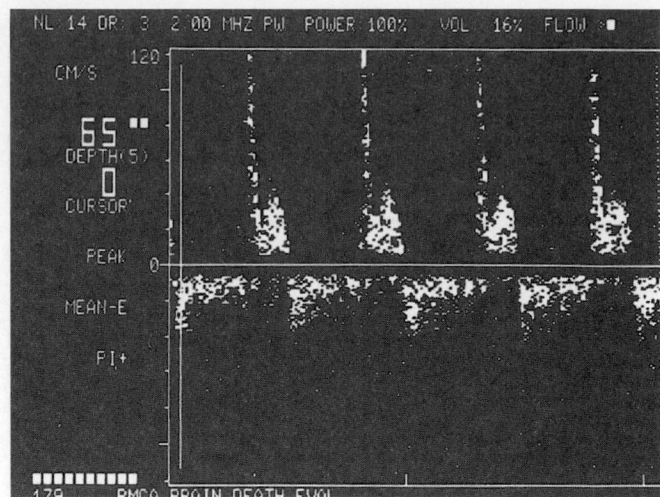

**FIGURE 21–9.** Transcranial Doppler waveform in a patient with intracranial circulatory arrest. Note reversal of blood flow direction during diastole.

demonstrated that the TCD is a sensitive and reliable tool for the diagnosis of intracranial circulatory arrest. Recently, a Task Force of the World Federation of Neurology concluded:

*Extra- and intracranial Doppler sonography is a useful confirmatory test to establish irreversibility of cerebral circulatory arrest as an optional part of a brain death protocol.*[58]

They concluded that TCD was especially valuable when drugs rendered the use of EEG unreliable. Two cautionary studies have appeared, however. One suggested that, especially in children, it is unclear how long the pattern of circulatory arrest needs to be present before it can be considered irreversible. Two patients were reported who demonstrated diastolic flow reversal who, with subsequent rapid intervention, survived in one case with normal function and in the other case with significant impairment.[59] The other study examined 15 patients with a *clinical* diagnosis of brain death. The results of EEG, TCD, Xe[133] washout cerebral blood flow studies, and cerebral angiography were compared.[60] These authors found that angiography and Xe[133] measurements were the most reliable tests, and that both TCD and EEG had false-positive and false-negative findings. All studies showed that in a significant number of patients, no waveforms at all could be recorded.

### Summary

In the early 21st century, the appropriate and optimal use of this monitoring device is still not clear. Most promising uses appear to be detection (and potentially treatment) of emboli during carotid vascular surgery, diagnosis and treatment of cerebral vasospasm, and diagnosis of intracranial circulatory arrest. One area of interesting research where the device shows some promise is in the diagnosis and management of elevated ICP, but it is still too early to say whether the device will find use in this area.

Technically satisfactory recordings cannot be obtained in some patients (particularly elderly women), thus rendering TCD US diagnosis or monitoring useless. When recordings can be made, TCD US is attractive because it is a continuous method and easy to use. It clearly is of benefit in the laboratory evaluation of patients with cerebrovascular disease and is finding use as a monitor during cerebrovascular surgery.

## BALANCE OF CEREBRAL OXYGEN SUPPLY AND DEMAND: JUGULAR BULB SATURATION

Cerebral $O_2$ demand (requirement) varies with changing CNS conditions. Reduction of brain temperature by 5°C may reduce $O_2$ needs by $\geq 35\%$. CBF may be adequate for cerebral function and cellular integrity at 32°C but inadequate at 37°C. Cerebral $O_2$ delivery varies with CBF and $O_2$ content. Cerebral function is determined by the *balance* between cerebral $O_2$ demand and supply. Thus, numerical values of CBF, taken alone, do not guarantee either preservation or loss of function; they must be interpreted with regard to $O_2$ demand and supply.

Clinically applicable direct measurements of $O_2$ demand are not available at this time. The EEG can be used to assess $O_2$ demand indirectly. Generation of spontaneous electrical activity uses roughly 50% of the total $O_2$ consumed by the brain. As a corollary, if drugs are given to totally suppress spontaneous electrical activity, the $O_2$ demand will be reduced by about 50%.

### How Is Jugular Bulb Saturation Used?

Measurements that reflect the balance between $O_2$ supply and demand, however, can be made directly or by measuring the $O_2$ saturation in the jugular venous blood ($S\bar{v}O_2$) returning from the brain. A catheter is advanced retrograde under fluoroscopic guidance in the jugular vein until its tip lies in the jugular bulb. Blood can then be aspirated and saturation measured. When cerebral $O_2$ delivery falls (as a result of decreased blood $O_2$ content, decreased CBF, or both), cerebral $O_2$ extraction increases. This change results in decreased $S\bar{v}O_2$ of venous blood returning from the brain. Measurement also can be made continuously using a small fiberoptic catheter similar to that used to measure mixed venous $O_2$ saturation in the pulmonary artery. Catheters are currently being designed and tested that are manufactured specifically for this use.[61]

Jugular $S\bar{v}O_2$ monitoring has been used primarily in head trauma patients who require control of increased ICP with hyperventilation or barbiturates, or both.[62] Hyperventilation decreases CBF; too much can produce cerebral ischemia. Several clinical series have described knowledge of jugular $S\bar{v}O_2$ as helpful in detecting excessive hyperventilation.[62–65] Although hyperventilation was found to lower ICP, the accompanying decrease in CBF caused $O_2$ delivery to fall below demand. These data suggested that another technique to control ICP (eg, barbiturate coma, ventriculostomy, or CSF drainage) might be safer.

Several problems occur with this technique. Blood in a single jugular bulb comes from sources on both sides of the brain (70% ipsilateral, 30% contralateral). This measurement technique evaluates the *global* balance between cerebral $O_2$ supply and demand. Inadequate CBF to a small area of cortex may be masked by blood that has a higher $S\bar{v}O_2$ from areas of adequately perfused brain in either hemisphere.[66–68] One study nicely demonstrated a marked regional heterogeneity in venous $O_2$ saturation.[69] Thus, a high saturation can be falsely reassuring. More importantly, placement of a catheter in the

jugular vein may block jugular outflow or cause thrombosis after prolonged use. Even unilateral placement sometimes impedes jugular outflow sufficiently to raise ICP in patients with decreased intracranial compliance. These problems have prevented widespread use of such monitoring, although judging from the case reports and reviews available in the literature, interest in and use of this type of monitoring is continuing to increase.

Intraoperative monitoring of jugular venous $O_2$ saturation has found much more limited use and cannot yet be recommended for routine use in any procedure that risks cerebral ischemia. Research continues with monitoring of jugular venous oxygen saturation ($J\bar{v}O_2$) during cerebrovascular surgery, cardiopulmonary bypass, and even induced hypotension in the elderly.[70–74]

## CEREBRAL OXYGEN SUPPLY-DEMAND BALANCE: THE ELECTROENCEPHALOGRAM

When $O_2$ delivery falls below a level sufficient to meet the $CMRO_2$, function fails. Because function is disrupted before cellular integrity is lost, monitors of function provide early warning of inadequate $O_2$ supply and provide opportunity to correct this problem before irreversible damage occurs. Such monitors can be used to guide therapy when CNS $O_2$ supply may be compromised during surgery and to detect surgically induced structural damage that produces changes in function.

The function of some motor and sensory pathways, as well as the spontaneous electrical activity of the cerebral cortex, is easily monitored during general anesthesia. These pathways and spontaneous electrical activity of the cerebral cortex reflect only a portion of the entire nervous system. Changes in one monitored parameter may *imply* damage to other nearby areas of the nervous system; however, damage to unmonitored portions of the nervous system may occur without detection. Thus, when areas of the nervous system that cannot be monitored are at risk during surgery, false-negative monitoring patterns should be expected.

### What Is the Electroencephalogram?

The EEG recorded from the scalp is a summation of excitatory and inhibitory postsynaptic potentials produced in the pyramidal layer of the cerebral cortex. These electrical signals range in amplitude from $<10$ $\mu V$ to around 100 $\mu V$.

### Recording

As with recording of the ECG, EEG electrodes are placed in a standardized fashion so that tracings from one person may be compared either with later tracings from the same person or with those of others. The International Ten-Twenty Electrode System[75] (Fig. 21–10) places EEG electrodes or electrodes for recording evoked potentials over specific areas of the cerebral cortex and is based on measurements made between pairs of specific sites on the patient's head. Each recording point is designated with a letter and a number and can often be associated with underlying CNS structures; for example, $C_3$, $C_z$, and $C_4$ are all associated with the motor cortex. By convention, recording electrodes placed over the

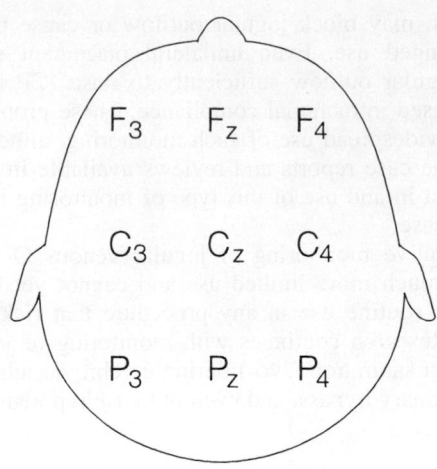

SCHEMATIC OF THE 10-20 SYSTEM

**FIGURE 21–10.** Schematic representation of the Ten-Twenty System of electrode placement.

right hemisphere are even-numbered, and those placed over the left hemisphere are odd-numbered. Midline electrodes are designated by a "z."

These electrodes are connected in pairs to an amplification system and their recordings are displayed, just as with the ECG, as a plot of voltage versus time. Each EEG channel represents the electrical activity of one electrode pair. The recording of multiple EEG channels simultaneously on paper at speeds of up to 3 cm/s creates a large amount of online data; a technician or neurologist must monitor the EEG output constantly for maximum utility.

## Alternative Displays

Reduction in the number of channels or simplification and suitable formatting of data enable personnel, such as anesthesiologists, who also have other intraoperative tasks, to use the EEG for intraoperative monitoring. The display can be simplified through signal processing techniques,[76] which include power spectrum analysis, frequency analysis, filtering,

and rectification. Data are displayed in time-compressed formats such as compressed spectral array and density spectral array (Fig. 21–11). Of extreme importance, however, is the retention of access to the real-time, unprocessed EEG. Except for gross artifact rejection by voltage criteria, these simplified monitors do not yet have the ability to distinguish brain activity from other biologic signals (eg, ECG) or noise. Noise is processed as if it were electrical brain activity.

### Number of Leads for Meaningful Data

The largest clinical series that examined the usefulness of EEG monitoring during carotid surgery used 16 channels of acquired data for analysis.[1] Although no carefully performed studies have compared lesser numbers of channels systematically to the 16-channel unprocessed recordings, limited data suggest that fewer numbers of channels may be useful. One study compared 2-channel, computer-processed EEGs interpreted by an inexperienced observer with 16-channel hard copy EEGs monitored by a trained technician and a neurologist. The inexperienced observer was able to identify 75% of the significant EEG changes seen on the 16-channel EEG.[77] This study suggests that even 2-channel EEGs (one channel examining each cerebral hemisphere) are useful for monitoring a carotid endarterectomy. One channel on each hemisphere helps to differentiate EEG changes that are caused by global factors (eg, anesthetic drugs) from those changes that are caused by more regional factors (eg, carotid cross-clamping).

## What Is the Significance of Electroencephalogram Frequency and Amplitude?

For pattern recognition in the EEG, the complex waveforms are described in terms of frequency (cycles per second = Hertz) and amplitude (voltage). Four basic EEG rhythms or frequency patterns are analyzed (Fig. 21–12): delta (0-4 Hz); theta (4-8 Hz); alpha (8-13 Hz); and beta (>13 Hz).

Delta rhythm occurs during deep sleep and deep anesthesia and in many pathologic states such as ischemia, drug overdose, and severe metabolic derangements. Theta rhythm is

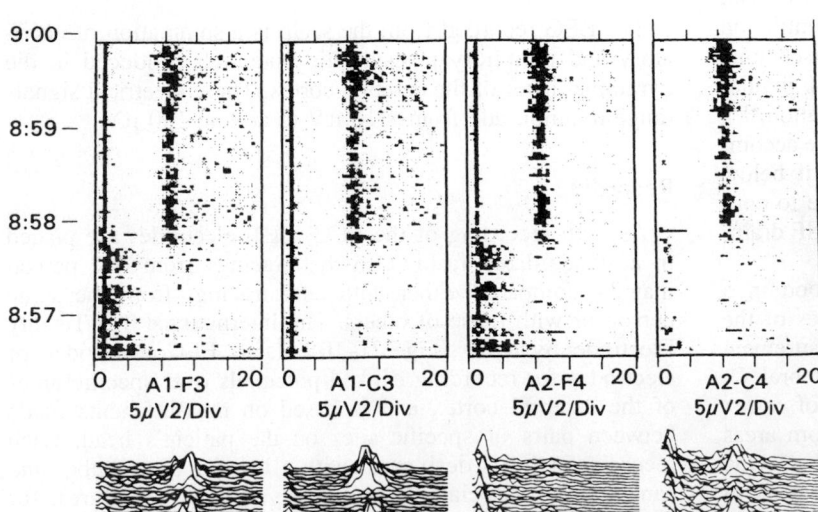

**FIGURE 21–11.** Processed electroencephalogram. The two most common types of electroencephalographic processing are density spectral array (*top*) and compressed spectral array (*bottom*).

## EEG FREQUENCY PATTERNS

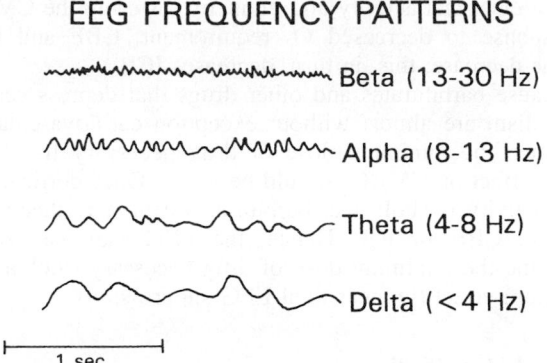

Beta (13-30 Hz)

Alpha (8-13 Hz)

Theta (4-8 Hz)

Delta (<4 Hz)

1 sec

**FIGURE 21–12.** Electroencephalogram frequency patterns in order of declining frequency.

commonly seen during general anesthesia and may occur during the same pathologic states in which delta rhythm is seen. Alpha rhythm can be recorded, mainly over the occipital region, in an alert, relaxed patient whose eyes are closed. During lighter surgical planes of anesthesia, this 8- to 13-Hz activity can be recorded over much of the cortex but especially in the anterior leads.

Beta rhythm accompanies mental concentration or may be induced with low doses of many sedative and hypnotic drugs such as barbiturates or benzodiazepines. Deep anesthesia, ischemia, or other pathologic states abolish both alpha and beta frequencies, after which slower frequencies predominate.

Changes in EEG amplitude normally result from synchronization or desynchronization of cortical electrical activity. Larger EEG amplitude is seen during sleep or surgical anesthesia. However, deep levels of anesthesia cause a loss in EEG amplitude, secondary to direct depression of cortical neuronal activity. Awakening usually produces a decrease in amplitude and the appearance of higher frequency patterns such as beta rhythm. An extremely strong stimulus under anesthesia may cause the appearance of an alerting pattern that consists of high-voltage delta and theta frequency patterns.

### How Is the Electroencephalogram Useful to the Anesthesiologist?

#### Relationship to Brain Function

EEG activity—that is, cortical electrical activity—requires roughly 50% of the total $O_2$ consumed by the brain; the remaining 50% is needed to maintain cellular integrity. When $O_2$ delivery is compromised by either hypoxemia or decreased blood supply, $O_2$ that ordinarily would be used to produce electrical activity is instead diverted to maintain cellular integrity. Depression of EEG activity thus reflects decreased $O_2$ delivery.

#### Practical Considerations

The first step in using an unfamiliar monitor is to define it in terms of a monitor that is familiar. ECG is routinely used by anesthesiologists who have learned the various normal and abnormal ECG patterns that may occur during surgical operations. For example, ST segment depression immediately causes concern about myocardial ischemia. Interpretation of

CNS monitoring also involves pattern recognition. Slowing of the EEG (Fig. 21–13) may be associated with cerebral ischemia. Interventions based on recognition of these patterns may be made in much the same fashion in which interventions are made after recognition of ECG changes.

The most important intraoperative use for the EEG is to monitor $O_2$ supply and demand balance in the cerebral cortex. In a large series of patients undergoing carotid endarterectomy at the Mayo Clinic,[1] the EEG was compared with regional CBF using the $^{133}$Xe washout method. This study validated the EEG as an indicator of the adequacy of regional CBF.

Normal CBF in gray and white matter averages 50 mL/100 g/min. With most anesthetic techniques, the EEG begins to become abnormal when CBF falls to 20 mL/100 g/min. However, the threshold for EEG changes appears to be much lower (8-10 mL/100 g/min) when isoflurane or sevoflurane are used.[78,79] Cellular survival is not threatened until CBF falls to 12 mL/100 g/min (lower with isoflurane and sevoflurane). Thus, a margin of safety is present between the time at which the EEG becomes abnormal and that at which cellular damage begins to occur. Severe anemia and decreases in $O_2$ saturation also decrease $O_2$ delivery. The EEG activity becomes abnormal once increased blood flow cannot compensate for decreased arterial $O_2$ content.

### Why Is the Electroencephalogram Useful During Carotid Surgery?

#### Determination of Inadequate Oxygen Delivery

Serious intraoperative reduction in cerebral $O_2$ supply may result from surgical factors (eg, carotid cross-clamping) that are usually beyond the anesthesiologist's control and from factors that the anesthesiologist can correct. Reduction in CBF produced by hyperventilation, hypotension, or temporary occlusion of major blood vessels sometimes is corrected by reducing ventilation, by restoring normal BP, or, in the case of temporary vessel occlusion, by increasing BP above normal. Because the EEG correlates with CBF adequacy, it serves as a monitor of the effectiveness of therapy instituted to correct ischemia.

Ideally, EEG use is continuous; yet, it has been described most frequently as a spot check to determine the need for shunt placement after carotid cross-clamping in anesthetized patients. However, this short-term use detects only a small

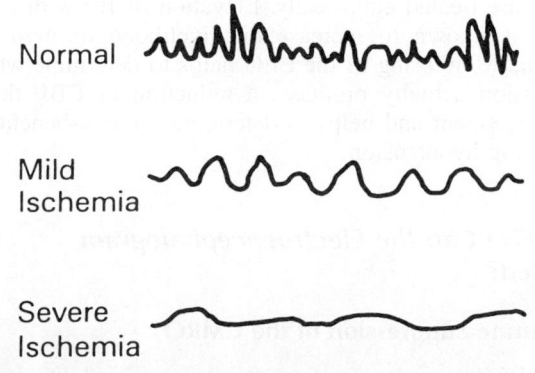

Normal

Mild
Ischemia

Severe
Ischemia

**FIGURE 21–13.** Schematic of electroencephalogram changes during ischemia.

portion of the neurologic injuries that can occur during and after carotid surgery. Critical carotid luminal narrowing risks cerebral hypoperfusion during hypotension or positioning. These problems will be missed if the EEG is not monitored continuously.

## Shunt Placement

If monitoring of the EEG could be proved scientifically to reduce the incidence of stroke, the question introducing this section would require no discussion. Data demonstrating this ability, however, do not exist. What information is available is less than satisfactory. In a large series of patients undergoing carotid endarterectomy with selective shunting who were monitored with 16-channel unprocessed EEG, no patient awakened with a new neurologic deficit that was not predicted by EEG.[1] Transient, correctable EEG changes were not associated with stroke, but persistent changes were shown to be related to stroke.

Based on laboratory data, the ischemic tolerance of neural tissue is directly related to both the severity of CBF reduction and the duration of the insult.[80] Because the EEG detects reductions in CBF that would not otherwise be apparent in unmonitored patients and thus permits intervention that may correct the problem (usually placement of a shunt), EEG monitoring should be useful in reducing the incidence of stroke when selective shunting is used.

More difficult to prove is that EEG monitoring is useful when all patients are shunted during carotid clamping. Such monitoring has detected correctable shunt malfunction, and investigators have described hypotension-related EEG changes in patients with critical stenoses and poor collateral circulation.[81,82]

Finally, three recent studies strongly suggest that shunting of patients without evidence of decreased cerebral perfusion actually increases the incidence of stroke. One of these, a multicenter study of 1495 carotid endarterectomies monitored with TCD showed a >6-fold increase in stroke rate when patients were shunted without evidence of cerebral ischemia.[83] Two recent studies involving EEG also demonstrated a significant reduction in stroke rate when EEG was used for selective shunting as compared with routine shunting of patients whenever the carotid artery was cross-clamped (0.5% versus 4% in one study and 0.3% versus 2.2% in the other).[84,85]

## Hypotension

Without EEG monitoring, BP decreases that occur during surgery are treated empirically. Elevation of BP with a vasopressor is known to increase the likelihood of myocardial ischemia. Monitoring of the EEG helps to determine whether hypotension actually produces a reduction in CBF that requires treatment and helps to determine the risk-benefit ratio for treating hypotension.

## How Else Can the Electroencephalogram Be Used?

### Barbiturate Suppression of the CMRO$_2$

The EEG may be used to monitor cerebral O$_2$ demand. Barbiturates administered to lower ICP do so by depressing

cortical electrical activity and, thus, by lowering the CMRO$_2$. In response to decreased O$_2$ requirement, CBF and blood volume decrease; this, in turn, decreases ICP.

Because barbiturates and other drugs that depress cerebral metabolism are almost without exception cardiovascular depressants, the minimum dose of drug necessary for the intended effect on CMRO$_2$ should be given. Once cortical electrical activity is abolished, barbiturates cannot further reduce CMRO$_2$, CBF, or ICP. Hence, the EEG may be used to determine the minimum dose of drug necessary to obtain the maximum effect (ie, near total EEG suppression).

### Induced Hypotension

Monitoring cerebral cortical function during induced hypotension or cardiopulmonary bypass is a logical extension of EEG use in carotid surgery. Carefully controlled studies appearing in the literature describe the use of EEG for these purposes, but the monitoring methods and EEG changes used to guide therapy vary widely from institution to institution, and little standardization of intraoperative techniques exists. A recent randomized study of 16 patients used significant induced hypotension (MAP = 50 mm Hg) and hemodilution (hematocrit = 20%) to reduce blood loss during major orthopedic surgery.[86] The control group (n = 6) was maintained within 20% of baseline BP without hemodilution. The safety of hypotension was monitored with EEG, Jvo$_2$, and mixed venous O$_2$ saturation. In the study group, the total transfusion requirement was 1440 mL, of which only 225 mL was homologous blood. In the control group, the total transfusion requirement was 2650 mL, all of which was homologous blood. Only one patient in the study group and all patients in the control group required ICU admission for treatment of moderate-severe tissue edema and metabolic acidosis. There were no cerebral complications in either group. Although this is a small study, the data suggest that significant hypotension, even in the elderly, may be induced safely with appropriate CNS monitoring. Much more work in this area is needed before this approach can be recommended.

## What Effects Do Anesthetic Drugs Have on the Electroencephalogram?

Low doses of potent inhalation agents with nitrous oxide produce an active EEG with alpha and beta frequencies present. Steady-state anesthesia, regardless of the agent used, usually produces a stable EEG pattern. Be aware that deep anesthesia and ischemia produce similar EEG changes. In both cases, fast activity is replaced by slower, larger EEG waveforms. As anesthesia is further deepened or as ischemia worsens, additional slowing occurs, and the EEG amplitude decreases and ultimately becomes flat (isoelectric).

Boluses of anesthetic drugs may produce large EEG changes that are indistinguishable from those seen during ischemia; such changes in the anesthetic regimen should be avoided during surgery, especially at times when ischemia is a risk. Unfortunately, most strokes during carotid vascular surgery do not occur during the period surrounding cross-clamping. Thus, stable anesthetic technique throughout surgery is critical, despite the fact that carotid vascular surgery is commonly associated with wide swings in BP. In addition, monitoring of areas that are not at risk for ischemia during surgery may help to distinguish anesthetic effect, which should be global, from surgically induced decreases in blood flow, which may be regional only.

## Can Anesthetic Depth Be Determined From the Electroencephalogram?

Until recently, the answer to that question would be probably not. Multiple studies using various types of EEG processing—including relative power, spectral edge frequency, median power frequency, and others—have been performed to see whether EEG can predict movement on skin incision or even awareness or recall. Although some of the processed parameters showed some promise, none of them attained the degree of reliability that would assure the practicing anesthesiologist that his or her patient was adequately anesthetized during a given surgical stimulus or procedure.[87-93]

In the mid-1990s, Aspect Medical Systems of Newton, Massachusetts, completed extensive testing of a new method of processing information contained in the EEG and designed a monitor of the hypnotic effect of anesthetic drugs. They called this monitored parameter the Bispectral Index.[94,95] Instead of analyzing linear parameters of the EEG signal, this technology used a technique developed for other non-EEG waveform analyses called *bispectral analysis*. This method searches for relationships among different frequencies that constitute a given complex waveform, such as the EEG. Simply put, in the awake state, the brain has many complex functions that must occur simultaneously. The resulting EEG waveforms correlating to these functions are complex and do not appear—even to sophisticated computer programs—to have recognizable relationships among the many different frequencies present. As the patient becomes more sedated (depth of hypnosis increases), many of the independent functions stop, and relationships begin to appear among the many different EEG frequencies.

The BIS is a dimensionless number that is related to the degree of frequency interdependencies present at a given time. The lower the number, the more relationship there is among the EEG frequencies present. Over the years, the algorithm has been adjusted and validated based on data obtained from thousands of patients undergoing anesthesia with many different types of drugs.[96] Table 21–11 shows the significance of the range of BIS values commonly seen.

Potential uses for this device are great, and scientific studies in all of these areas are beginning to appear. Theoretically, BIS could be used to titrate the anesthetic so precisely that many outpatients could entirely bypass the recovery room.[97-99] Operations in which key parts require patient cooperation but

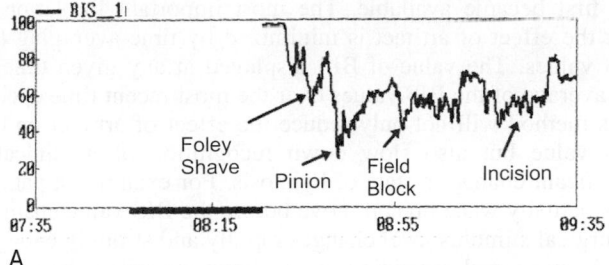

A

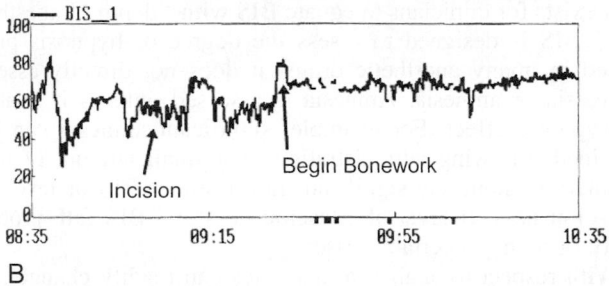

B

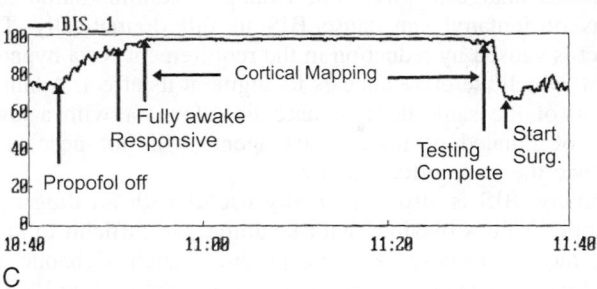

C

**FIGURE 21–14.** Bispectral Index (Aspect Medical Systems, Newton, Mass) during awake craniotomy for functional mapping of the speech area before resection of a seizure focus. Patient was not intubated and breathed spontaneously throughout. *A,* Propofol dosage was adjusted to produce deeper levels of sedation for performance of painful procedures such as Foley placement, pinion placement, performance of field block, and initial incision and bone work. *B,* Once painful portions were completed, propofol level was decreased to keep the patient just barely unconscious until the surgeon was ready for testing. *C,* Discontinuation of propofol resulted in rapid return of normal consciousness and a fully cooperative patient. After testing was complete, the propofol was reinstituted to allow the patient to be comfortable during brain resection and closure.

otherwise are better performed with the patient asleep or deeply sedated may benefit from BIS monitoring. Awake craniotomies for functional mapping of the brain before surgery to eliminate a seizure focus have been performed using this technique,[100] and an example from a case at the University of Florida is shown in Figure 21–14.

Clinicians at the University of Florida and elsewhere have observed that drug dosages, especially during monitored anesthesia care and total intravenous anesthetics, may be significantly reduced, leading to rapid emergence times. Although no studies have shown that the actual incidence of awareness under anesthesia has decreased with the use of this monitor, this should theoretically be possible. Finally, BIS shows promise for monitoring the depth of sedation in the ICU environment.[101-103]

The monitor still does have some limitations, mainly with respect to artifact recognition and rejection, but significant improvements have been made in this area since BIS monitor-

**TABLE 21–11.** The Bispectral Index

| Value of Bispectral Index | Clinical State of the Patient |
|---|---|
| 90–100 | Awake, verbalizing spontaneously, amnesia is uncommon |
| 80–90 | Drowsy but easily arousable, amnesia is prominent |
| 70–80 | Frequently asleep, arousable with strong stimulus, amnesia is very prominent |
| <70 | Unconscious |
| <40 | Deep coma |

ing first became available. The most important limitation is that the effect of artifact is minimized by time-averaging the BIS values. The value of BIS displayed at any given time is the average of the BIS values over the most recent time epoch. This method will not only reduce the effect of artifact on the BIS value but also slow down recognition of a clinically significant change in state of hypnosis. For example, a patient may actually wake up and move before the BIS value changes if surgical stimulus level changes rapidly and strongly enough.

I have several remaining reservations regarding the use of BIS for assessing the depth of the hypnotic state. The temptation exists for clinicians to equate BIS with "depth of anesthesia." BIS is designed to assess the degree of hypnosis produced by many anesthetic drugs; it does not directly assess analgesia or amnesia. Amnesia is assessed only as it relates to hypnotic effect. For example, significant amnesia can be obtained following administration of a small amount of midazolam without any significant fall in either BIS or level of consciousness. If level of consciousness and BIS fall, probability of amnesia certainly rises.

With respect to analgesia, narcotics can readily change the BIS value, but they do so indirectly, and BIS is not designed to assess analgesic level. For example, administration of a bolus of fentanyl can cause BIS to fall dramatically. This effect is caused by reduction in the requirement for a hypnotic agent, which therefore appears to augment its effect. Administration of the same dose of narcotic, alone or with a lower dose of inhaled or intravenous agent, will not necessarily produce the same effect on BIS.

Finally, BIS is also not equally useful with all drugs. For example, values obtained with ketamine are difficult to interpret, largely because ketamine produces such a chaotic and different EEG pattern from any other anesthetic drug.[104,105]

Other EEG analysis techniques, as well as the middle latency auditory evoked response, also show promise for assessing some aspects of anesthetic depth. No other techniques or devices have achieved the level of simplicity or scientific validation as the BIS at this point in time. Because of the high level of interest in this approach to monitoring, other devices are in various stages of development so that anesthesiologists will have choices in this area as they currently do with other monitoring technologies.

### What Information Is Not Provided by Electroencephalogram Monitoring?

EEG monitoring provides information about the overall electrical functioning of the cerebral cortex but not much information about the subcortical brain, spinal cord, or cranial and peripheral nerves. The functioning of CNS sensory or motor pathways that may be at risk during surgical procedures is monitored using SSEPs and MEPs.

### CEREBRAL OXYGEN SUPPLY AND DEMAND: EVOKED POTENTIALS

The EEG records *spontaneous* electrical activity produced by the CNS. Sensory evoked potentials (SEPs) consist of CNS electrical activity that is evoked by sensory stimuli (electrical, auditory, or visual). SEPs are of three types: (1) peripheral or cranial nerve, (2) subcortical, and (3) cortical.

### From Where Are Evoked Potentials Recorded?

Evoked potentials (EPs) from peripheral nerves that are generated by propagated action potentials usually are recorded directly over the nerve or plexus and are large. Subcortical EPs are produced by synaptic activity generated in subcortical groups of nerve cells and action potentials traveling on connecting nerve pathways. They cannot usually be recorded near the cells or pathways that produce the EPs and therefore have small amplitude. Instead, they are recorded over the spinal cord and brainstem.

Cortical EPs, as with the EEG, are produced by the summation of postsynaptic potentials in the pyramidal layer of the cerebral cortex and also have a small amplitude. These EPs are recorded over the cerebral cortex. The amplitude of spontaneous background EEG activity is generally much larger than that of either subcortical or cortical EPs and easily obscures these smaller signals. This problem is solved through the application of filtering and signal-averaging techniques.

### How Do Evoked Potentials Appear, and How Are They Described?

EPs are described in terms of latency and amplitude (Fig. 21–15). *Latency* is the time measured from the application of the stimulus to the point of maximum amplitude of the EP. Some types of EPs have more than one peak. Latency measured between EP peaks (*interpeak latency*) is often important clinically. *Amplitude* is defined as the voltage difference between two peaks of opposite polarity or between an EP peak and a reference level that represents zero potential.

### What Are Somatosensory Evoked Potentials?

SSEPs monitor the function of the somesthetic sensory system that extends throughout the PNS and CNS. Thus, peripheral nerve, spinal cord, and subcortical and cortical structures in the brain may be monitored. The somesthetic system carries sensory information, including that concerning vibration, proprioception, and light touch. An SSEP is generated when repetitive electrical stimuli are applied to a peripheral nerve, and many single responses are averaged to record the evoked response. Responses may be recorded over the

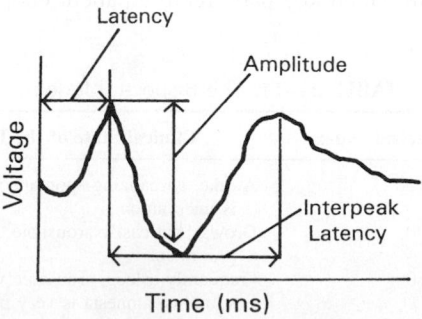

**FIGURE 21–15.** Evoked potentials are described in terms of time after stimulus (latency) and size (amplitude).

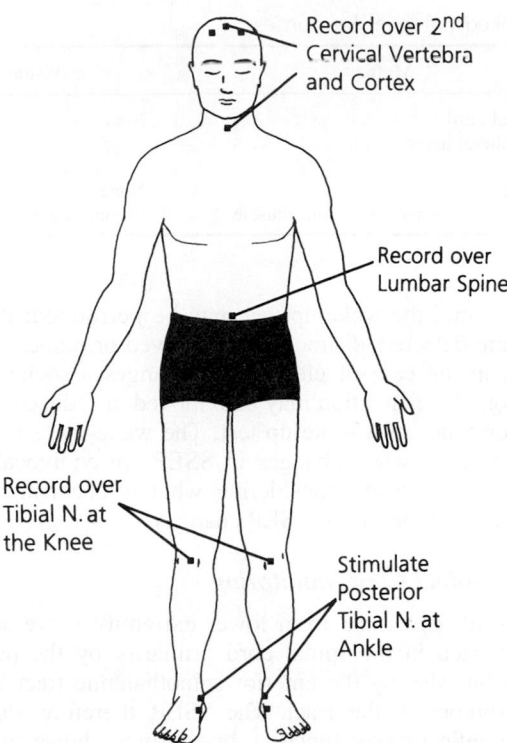

**FIGURE 21–16.** Schematic representation of spinal cord monitoring showing sites of recording electrode placement. (Note that some of the electrodes that are placed posteriorly are shown on the anterior view.)

peripheral nerve, nerve plexus, spinal cord, brainstem, and cerebral cortex (Fig. 21–16). Recording sites are related directly to the somesthetic pathway. As with the EEG, cortical recording electrode locations are based on the International Ten-Twenty System of electrode placement.

### Recording Channels

The number of recording channels varies with the type of case being monitored. In an ideal situation, recordings should be made over each peripheral nerve being stimulated, the spinal cord rostral to the nerve's entry, the second cervical vertebra, and the opposite cerebral cortex. In addition, if possible, a portion of the somatosensory system not at risk from surgery should also be monitored to help differentiate surgically related changes from the previously mentioned changes in SSEPs produced by global factors such as anesthetic drugs. Thus, during a right carotid endarterectomy, cortical responses to both left and right median nerve stimulation should be recorded. During surgery for correction of thoraco-lumbar scoliosis, responses from both posterior tibial nerves, as well as from at least one median nerve, are desirable. Generally, these requirements translate into at least four channels of data.

### Usefulness of Peripheral and Spinal Cord Recordings

#### Adequacy of Stimulus

The most important use of peripheral nerve recordings is to make certain that a stimulus is actually reaching the CNS. If the SSEP disappears during a surgical procedure, one must ensure that the cause is not failure to stimulate adequately. A peripheral nerve response rules out this technical failure.

### Peripheral Nerve Injuries

Recordings over the peripheral nerves and plexuses also have been useful during surgical explorations of peripheral nerve injuries and may help to direct the most appropriate treatment of these lesions (ie, lesion resection and nerve grafting versus leaving the nerve intact with lysis of scar and adhesions).[106,107] If SSEPs can be recorded on both sides of a peripheral nerve lesion, neurolysis usually suffices to improve function. If proximal recording cannot be obtained, resection of the lesion and nerve grafting is needed.

### Technical Failure and Choice of Anesthetic

Recordings over the spinal cord also ensure against technical failure. In addition, they monitor spinal cord function below the level of electrode placement. In the case of operations on the spinal cord or on the spinal column, if recordings over the spinal cord rostral to the operative site can be made, cortical recordings become less important. Recordings made over the spinal cord are much less sensitive to the effects of anesthetic drugs than are recordings made over the cortex (Fig. 21–17). Reliance on spinal recordings allows the anesthesiologist much greater freedom in drug choice. Spinal recordings, however, give little information about cortical function and show only that a stimulus has reached the CNS.

### Significant Changes

Because factors other than surgery may alter the SSEP signal, the clinician must be able to decide when a change is significant and requires treatment. On the basis of many clinical series (not studies) and of studies addressing the effects of different anesthetic agents on the SSEP (Table 21–12), many experts quote a 50% decrease in amplitude or a 10% increase in latency as the degree of change that should provoke concern. Amplitude changes are considered the more

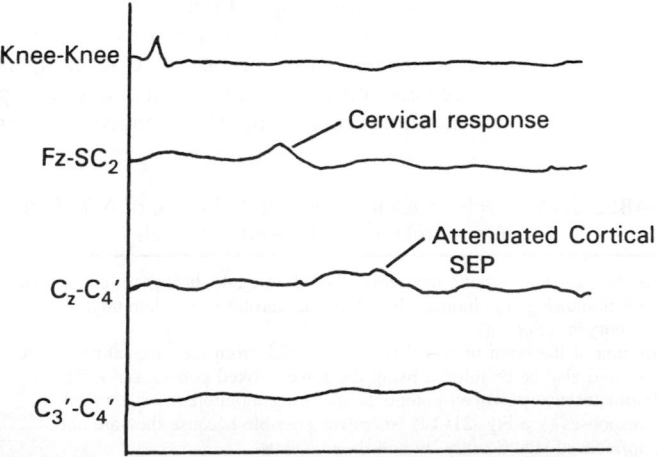

**FIGURE 21–17.** Cervical somatosensory evoked potential responses are not affected by high concentrations of potent inhalation agents.

**TABLE 21–12.** Anesthetic Susceptibility of Evoked Potential Responses

| | Somatosensory | Auditory | Motor | Visual |
|---|---|---|---|---|
| Resistant | Peripheral nerve<br>Lumbar/thoracic potentials<br>Subcortical potential at $C_2$ | Brainstem | Spinal cord<br>Peripheral nerve | None |
| Moderate | Primary cortical response | Middle latency responses | None | None |
| Severe | Long latency responses | Long latency responses | All responses recorded from muscle | Primary cortical response |

important factor in most cases, but in actuality, serious SSEP changes will generally show significant changes in both latency and amplitude.

In an environment where factors known to influence the SSEP (eg, anesthetic drugs, temperature, or $Paco_2$) cannot be controlled, these guidelines may be appropriate. If tight control of these factors can be maintained (Table 21–13), any amount of event-related change in the SSEP should be considered significant. In the absence of any observable event occurring around the time of an SSEP change, the aforementioned latency and amplitude criteria should be used to help decide when a change needs to be investigated urgently.

## How Are Somatosensory Evoked Potentials Used Intraoperatively?

### Spinal Operations

Spinal cord monitoring is the most widely applied intraoperative use of SSEPs, particularly during spinal instrumentation for the treatment of kyphoscoliosis. It has been used to a lesser extent during other operations on the spinal cord and its supporting structures, such as resection of spinal cord tumors or vascular malformations, diskectomies, and stabilization procedures for trauma or degenerative disease.

The incidence of postoperative paraplegia following posterior spinal fusion for scoliosis ranges from approximately 1% to 10%, depending on the type of instrumentation used. The highest incidence occurs when sublaminar wires are used, as with the Luque fusion. Before intraoperative SSEPs came into common use, the wake-up test was used to assess lower extremity motor function intraoperatively. This test has the advantage of being simple and inexpensive. However, as was discussed previously, it has numerous disadvantages. Also, it is only an intermittent monitor of spinal cord function.

In contrast, SSEP monitoring may be performed continuously, and trauma associated with intraoperative wake up is avoided. In most centers, clinicians now omit the wake-up test if SSEPs are monitored and remain unchanged. If clear

**TABLE 21–13.** Techniques to Minimize Influence of Anesthetics on Interpretation of Evoked Potentials

No changes in anesthetic technique should be made during critical periods of monitoring (eg, induced hypotension, carotid cross-clamping, aneurysm clipping).

An area of the brain or spinal cord not at risk from the surgical procedure should also be monitored using the same evoked potential modality.

If somatosensory evoked potentials are being monitored, use cervical responses (see Fig. 21–17) whenever possible because they are not influenced significantly by anesthetic agents.

If cervical responses cannot be recorded or if evoked potentials susceptible to anesthetics must be monitored, use favorable anesthetic techniques.

changes occur, the wake-up test may be performed; if motor deficits are detected, distraction is removed or reduced. Alternatively, in the case of clear SSEP changes associated with distraction, the distraction may be removed or reduced without the performance of a wake-up test. The wake-up test is more commonly used when changes in SSEP are equivocal or do not make sense when considering what is occurring during surgery at the time of the SSEP changes.

### Anterior Spinal Cord Monitoring

The SSEP generated from lower extremity nerve stimulation is carried in the spinal cord primarily by the posterior columns but also by the anterior spinothalamic tract and the ventral spinocerebellar tract. The SSEP, therefore, does not primarily reflect motor function. Interestingly, however, SSEP monitoring during posterior spinal fusion has correlated well with postoperative sensory and motor neurologic outcome.[2–5,7] In some previously discussed case reports, however, SSEPs did not change during surgery, and the patients awakened with motor deficits (false-negative results).[8,9]

Few case reports or case series have appeared in the literature since the early 1990s specifically addressing this issue. A few of these are, however, of note. Colleagues at the University of Toronto, where a well-established monitoring program exists, report a 1.1% false-negative rate during unspecified "spinal surgery" (3 of 272 patients with suitable baseline tracings).[108] Another series involving only anterior thoracic vertebrectomies reported a false-negative rate of 9%.[109] These cases are extremely rare, and I have never observed a case during a spinal column surgical procedure where there were no significant SSEP changes, and the patient awakened with any evidence of spinal cord damage. I have, however, observed failure of the SSEP to detect individual nerve root damage in the cauda equina, which is not surprising because the SSEP really only monitors the nerve roots involved with the nerve being stimulated. Many of the false-negative cases are controversial. When I have consulted on outside cases, all of the cases reviewed arose from poor quality baseline tracings. In many of the cases I reviewed, there were actually no reproducible responses present, even at baseline. Even if all the reported data are correct, the reported false-negative rate is still 1%, or likely much less, a frequency not approached by any other intraoperative monitor. MEPs may be useful in overcoming this limitation of SSEPs.

Occasionally, technically satisfactory waveforms cannot be obtained. In this case, the wake-up test must be used, if feasible, to monitor spinal cord function.

### Operations That Jeopardize Spinal Cord Blood Flow

SSEPs have been used to monitor spinal cord function during operations on the thoracic aorta (aneurysm or coarctation correction) with variable results. A normal SSEP at the conclusion of the operation clearly does not guarantee normal postoperative motor function. The most important factor in predicting ultimate outcome with SSEP monitoring is the duration of time over which the SSEP is lost during aortic cross-clamping.[110-115] Restoration of a normal SSEP after aortic cross-clamping release does not ensure a good outcome if the SSEP was lost for >14 minutes during cross-clamping. Loss of SSEPs for <14 minutes, with subsequent return to normal, is associated with good outcome during coarctation repair.[110]

Changes in the SSEP during surgery may be corrected by a trial of clamp reposition, shunting, induced hypertension, spinal fluid drainage, or intercostal reimplantation in an attempt to reestablish adequate spinal cord blood flow. Well-documented reports indicate that if normal SSEPs are continuously monitored and remain unchanged throughout surgery, major new neurologic deficits will not occur.

## Are Somatosensory Evoked Potentials Useful for Monitoring Cerebral Cortical Function?

Cortical structures can also be monitored by SSEPs. Inadequate perfusion of the somatosensory cortex eliminates the cortical but not the subcortical components. The reduction in CBF necessary to suppress the SSEP appears slightly greater than that needed to suppress the EEG; thus, SSEPs may not be as sensitive as the EEG.[116] Such monitoring is successful during procedures that may compromise blood flow, including carotid endarterectomy, cerebral aneurysm clipping (Fig. 21–18), induced hypotension before aneurysm clipping, and arteriovenous malformation resection.

Correlation of SSEP recordings with neurologic outcome is strong, particularly when the middle and anterior cerebral circulations are involved. Irreversible loss of the SSEP nearly

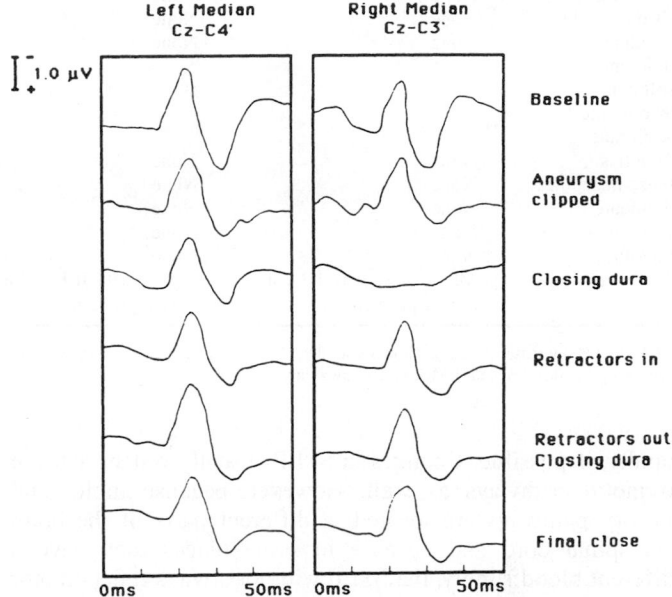

**Sequential Median Nerve SEP**

**Left MCA Aneurysm Surgery**

**FIGURE 21–19.** Somatosensory evoked potential change caused by kinking of the middle cerebral artery after removal of frontal and temporal lobe retraction following the placement of an aneurysm clip. (From Mahla ME. Update on anesthesia for intracranial aneurysm surgery. *Adv Anesth.* 1993;10:113.)

always predicts postoperative sensory and motor deficits. Preservation of cortical SSEPs is associated with an unchanged neurologic examination in the vast majority of patients.[117-121] False-negative monitoring patterns usually occur during neurovascular procedures that involve the basilar and posterior cerebral circulations. Large portions of the brainstem may become ischemic or suffer infarction with no effect on the somatosensory pathway or the SSEP.[122]

## Are Somatosensory Evoked Potentials Helpful in Preventing Neurologic Injury?

As with other monitors, no carefully controlled studies prove that SSEP monitoring improves outcome following neurologic surgery. The absence of such outcome studies, however, should not prevent clinicians from using this monitoring modality. It has an excellent overall correlation with neurologic outcome. Feedback to the surgeon is rapid; this, in turn, enables rapid intervention—either surgical or anesthetic—to prevent permanent neurologic deficit. In Figure 21–19, note that the cortical SSEP disappeared following middle cerebral artery aneurysm clipping after removal of retraction from the frontal and temporal lobes. The brain then shifted, causing the clip to kink the middle cerebral artery. Retractors were again placed, and the clip position was adjusted so that no further problems occurred. Prompt feedback prevented a major neurologic injury.

Provided that other factors affecting SSEPs are kept constant, increases in latency and decreases in amplitude are ominous signs; surgical causes should be sought and corrected

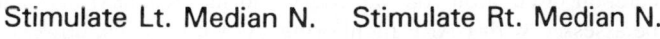

**Stimulate Lt. Median N.    Stimulate Rt. Median N.**

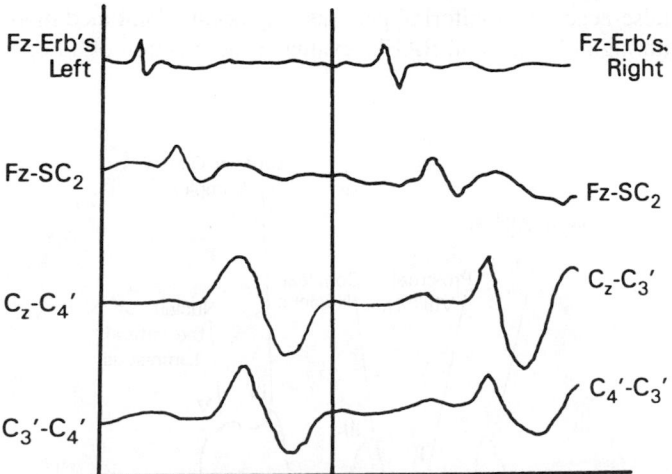

**FIGURE 21–18.** Changes in the cortical somatosensory evoked potential ipsilateral to the aneurysm is likely caused by the surgery. Bilateral changes are likely caused by anesthesia. Monitoring a part of the central nervous system not at risk for surgical manipulation allows this differentiation. In this figure, both hemispheres are monitored by sequential stimulation of the median nerve.

**TABLE 21–14.** Effects of Anesthetics on Somatosensory Evoked Potentials[123–130]

| Anesthetic Drug | Effect on Peripheral Nerve Potential | Effect on Subcortical Potential | Effect on Cortical Potential Latency | Effect on Cortical Potential Amplitude |
|---|---|---|---|---|
| Barbiturates | None | None | 1 to 2+ D | 1 to 3− D |
| Nitrous oxide | None | None | 1+ | 1 to 2− D |
| Halothane | None | None | 1 to 4+ D | 1 to 4− D |
| Enflurane | | | | |
| Isoflurane | | | | |
| Sevoflurane | | | | |
| Desflurane | | | | |
| Narcotics | None | None | ± | ± |
| Benzodiazepines | None | None | 1+ | 1 to 2− |
| Etomidate | None | None | 1+ | 2 to 4+ D |
| Ketamine | None | None | 1+ | 1 to 2+ |
| Propofol | None | None | 1+ to 2+ D | 1 to 2− D |
| Muscle relaxants | May clarify if EMG noise is a problem | May clarify if EMG noise is a problem | None; may clarify if EMG noise is present | None; may clarify if EMG noise is present |

1+, >10% increase; 2+, >20% increase; 3+, >50% increase; 4+, ≥100% increase; 1−, >10% decrease; 2−, >20% decrease; 3−, >50% decrease; 4−, incompatible with monitoring; D, dose-related; EMG, electromyogram.

rapidly, if possible. Changes in SSEPs usually reflect damage to motor pathways as well. However, because motor and sensory pathways are located in different parts of the brain and spinal cord and because in some places they have a different blood supply, the SSEP will not always reflect motor function. Such monitoring is most effective when a large area of brain or spinal cord or its blood supply is threatened during surgery.

## What Factors Other Than Surgical Damage Change the Somatosensory Evoked Potentials?

Intraoperative depression of SSEPs can be caused by decreased body temperature, cold irrigation to the surgical field, hypoxemia, variations in $Paco_2$, and anesthetic agents. Of these, changes in anesthetic drug dose are the most significant (Table 21–14).[123–133] Most of these factors can be kept constant during SSEP monitoring.

## What Do Brainstem Auditory Evoked Potentials Monitor?

The BAEP is a monitor of auditory system function, which begins with the eighth cranial nerve and extends up through the medulla and pons to the temporal lobe.[134–136] BAEPs are the subcortical components of the auditory evoked response and monitor function of the eighth cranial nerve and brainstem auditory pathway up through the nucleus of the lateral lemniscus (Fig. 21–20). The stimulus is a loud, repetitive click delivered to the patient by small ear inserts placed in the external auditory canal. Because recording electrodes cannot be placed close to the brainstem, the BAEP is recorded from the scalp quite far from the generating structures. It is thus small, and as many as 2000 repetitions may be required to produce a good averaged response.

## Use During Surgery

Intraoperative monitoring of BAEPs has been used most frequently for monitoring eighth nerve and brainstem function

during surgical procedures in the posterior fossa. This monitoring has been used successfully by surgeons attempting to preserve hearing during resection of acoustic neuromas.[137–142] Preservation of an unchanged BAEP is associated with functional hearing postoperatively. Loss of all components of the BAEP predicts deafness. Recently, electrocochleography and recording of the compound nerve action potential directly from the eighth cranial nerve seems to have improved the sensitivity and specificity of monitoring during resection of acoustic neuromas.

During microvascular decompression of the fifth or seventh cranial nerve in the posterior fossa (the Jannetta procedure), retractor placement may damage the eighth nerve and cause postoperative deafness (Fig. 21–21). Detection of ischemia of the eighth nerve allows retractors to be repositioned before irreversible damage occurs. Monitoring BAEPs has made possible a reduction of the incidence of deafness associated with the Jannetta procedure.[143–146]

Brainstem function during surgery involving the posterior cerebral circulation (basilar artery and its branches) also can be assessed with BAEP monitoring. As with SSEPs, however, false-negative monitoring patterns may occur. Combined monitoring of SSEPs and BAEPs evaluates the function of a larger

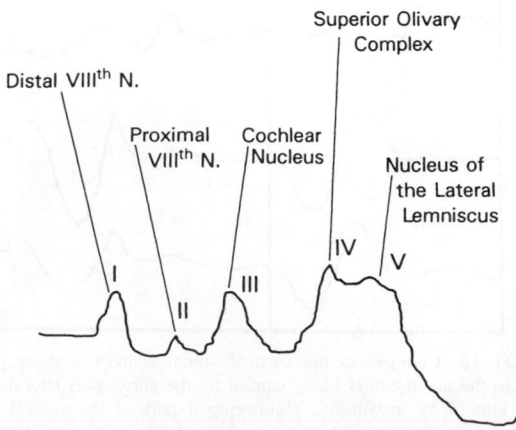

**FIGURE 21–20.** Brainstem auditory evoked potential. The generator of each wave is shown.

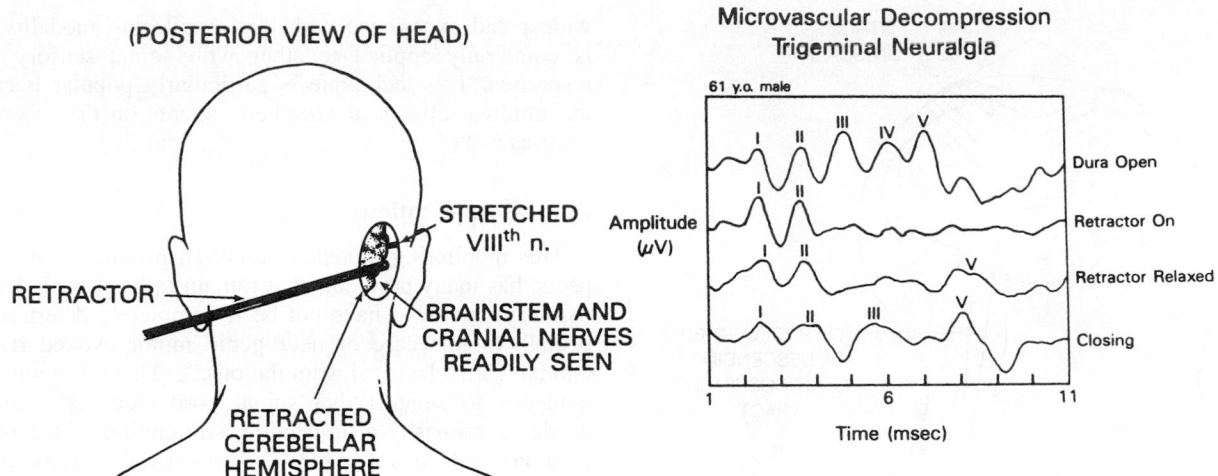

**FIGURE 21–21.** Cerebellar retraction during the Jannetta procedure stretches the eighth nerve.

portion of the brainstem and may be more useful than isolated monitoring of either EP during vascular surgery in this region.

### Factors Other Than Surgical Damage That Change the Brainstem Auditory Evoked Potentials

Resistance to nonsurgical factors, such as hypothermia and anesthetic drugs, is greater with BAEPs than with other EPs. They may be recorded successfully during any anesthetic technique. In contrast with SSEP monitoring, changes in anesthetic technique (Table 21–15) are unlikely to produce a change in the BAEP waveform that will be mistaken for a surgically induced change.

### What Do Visual Evoked Potentials Monitor?

Visual evoked potentials (VEPs) reflect the function of the visual pathway, which extends from the optic nerve through

**TABLE 21–15.** Effects of Anesthetics on Brainstem Auditory Evoked Potentials[123,134–136]

| Anesthetic Drug | Effect on I-V Interpeak Latency | Effect on Amplitude of Wave V | Clinical Significance* |
|---|---|---|---|
| Barbiturates | Increases | Decreases | None |
| Nitrous oxide | Minimal | Minimal | None |
| Halothane | Increases | Decreases | Minimal |
| Enflurane | | | |
| Isoflurane | | | |
| Sevoflurane† | | | |
| Desflurane† | | | |
| Narcotics | None | None | None |
| Benzodiazepines | Minimal | Minimal | Minimal |
| Etomidate | Minimal | Minimal | None |
| Ketamine | | | |
| Propofol | | | |
| Muscle relaxants (all types) | None | None | None |

*Clinical significance is based on criteria for significant changes at the University of Florida.

†Little scientific data are available, but no evidence exists to suggest that these agents would behave differently from other potent inhaled agents.

the chiasm to the visual cortex. The VEP is generated primarily by the visual cortex. Intraoperatively, the stimulus is usually applied by goggles that deliver a repetitive bright flash through closed eyelids. Contact lenses containing light-emitting diodes also have been applied directly to the cornea. This arrangement takes up less space and is less likely to interfere with surgical exposure; also, when contact lenses are used, a closed eyelid does not interfere with delivery of the stimulus as it does when goggles are used. Recordings are from scalp electrodes placed over the calcarine cortex.

### Use During Surgery

VEPs are not widely used during surgery. They have been used for visual function monitoring in operations near the optic nerve and chiasm (most commonly during pituitary surgery). They can also be monitored during resection of intracranial tumors such as meningiomas that involve or compress the optic nerve.

Correlation between changes in VEPs and outcome has not been evaluated in a large series of patients. Which VEP changes during manipulation of the optic nerve and chiasm are normal and which are ominous have not been identified. The major reasons for this lack of data are difficulties with stimulus application and the exquisite sensitivity of the VEP to anesthetic agents. Some investigators believe that VEPs are too variable intraoperatively to be of any clinical use.[147–150]

### What Are Motor Evoked Potentials?

MEP monitoring was developed specifically to assess the function of motor pathways; thus, it overcomes one of the major limitations of SSEP monitoring. Many variants exist. The most common involves placement of stimulating electrodes on the scalp over the motor cortex; an electrical current is passed through the motor cortex transcranially to provide stimulation. Magnetic stimulation of the motor cortex also has been used. A powerful magnetic stimulator is placed on the scalp over the motor cortex. Brief repetitive applications of a strong magnetic field induce current in the motor cortex and produce an MEP. Both methods also probably activate surrounding cortical structures as well as subcortical white matter pathways (sensory and motor) (Fig. 21–22).

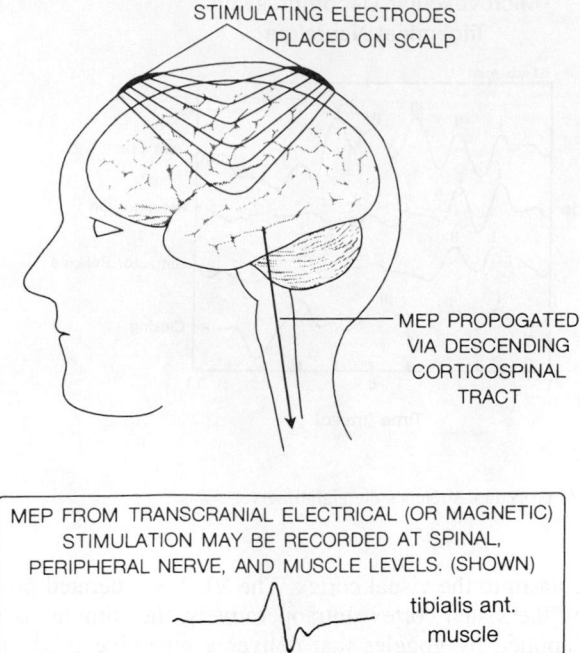

STIMULATING ELECTRODES
PLACED ON SCALP

MEP PROPOGATED
VIA DESCENDING
CORTICOSPINAL
TRACT

MEP FROM TRANSCRANIAL ELECTRICAL (OR MAGNETIC)
STIMULATION MAY BE RECORDED AT SPINAL,
PERIPHERAL NERVE, AND MUSCLE LEVELS. (SHOWN)

tibialis ant.
muscle

**FIGURE 21–22.** Schematic representation of transcranial motor evoked potential for magnetic stimulation. Electrodes are replaced by a magnetic coil that is positioned over the motor strip.

Propagation of the stimulus is blocked by synapses in all of the ascending (*sensory*) pathways, but the stimulus is propagated easily via descending pathways. The evoked responses may be recorded over the spinal cord, the peripheral nerve, and the involved muscle (EMG) (see Fig. 21–22). To enhance the MEP, these responses may be averaged in the same manner as for SEPs; however, averaging often is unnecessary.

Early studies with both electrical and magnetic stimulation involved application of a single stimulus pulse followed by recording of the descending responses. Anesthetic effects on these recordings were profound and prohibited the use of virtually all traditional anesthetic techniques. Anesthetic techniques producing the most reliable results involved total intravenous anesthesia, most commonly with a combination of an etomidate and narcotic infusion with carefully titrated muscle relaxation. Muscle relaxation was needed to prevent gross patient movements but had to be carefully controlled to preserve and record electrical response (EMG) from muscle.[151,152] More recent use of trains of stimuli, either magnetic or electrical, has allowed additional use of more traditional anesthetic techniques. Before this, the reluctance of many anesthesiologists to use accommodating anesthetic techniques prevented widespread successful applications of either of these techniques. However, with application of newer stimulation techniques and more traditional anesthetics, use of transcranial stimulation techniques are likely to become more widespread.[153–155] Transcranial stimulation has not yet been approved by the US Food and Drug Administration, although considerable experience exists that would suggest that these techniques are safe for use.

A third method to produce the MEP involves electrical stimulation of the spinal cord above the area at risk during surgery. Responses are recorded over the peripheral nerve (neurogenic motor evoked potentials) and muscle. There is widespread experience with this monitoring modality, and it is commonly applied together with somatosensory evoked responses. This technique is particularly popular because of the minimal effects of anesthetic agents on the recorded responses.[7,156–161]

## Clinical Applications

This monitoring modality, although promising in some aspects, has many problems that remain to be solved. The exact pathways involved have not been completely determined, especially in the case of neurogenic motor evoked responses (spinal cord electrical stimulation).[162] There is considerable evidence to suggest that spinal cord electrical stimulation produces primarily a descending stimulation of the posterior columns and an antidromically conducted sensory response recorded over peripheral nerves. Except in the case of spinal cord electrical stimulation, intraoperative experience remains relatively limited but is growing fast. Multiple reports suggest that transcranial MEP monitoring during surgery on the spine or its blood supply may be useful,[163–169] but the level of experience with this monitoring technique does not begin to approach that with somatosensory evoked responses. Recent data suggest that MEPs may be no more effective in predicting motor function following major aortic surgery than are SSEPs.[170] Responses recorded over the lumbar cord are insensitive indicators of motor function following aortic cross-clamping in several animal models.[171,172]

## Anesthetic Effects

Anesthetic agent effects are surprisingly profound, particularly on EMG recordings of the MEP produced by either transcranial electrical or magnetic stimulation (Table 21–16).[173–178] Recordings produced by stimulation of the spinal cord are less sensitive to anesthetic agents. However, as noted above, use of trains of stimuli can overcome the effects of anesthesia and allow the use of generally up to 1 MAC of inhaled anesthetic agent along with opiates. Nitrous oxide up to 50% can be successfully used but becomes problematic when potent inhaled agents are added.[153,179–182] Transcranial magnetic stimulation techniques appear more sensitive to the effects of anesthesia than those involving electrical stimulation.[180]

**TABLE 21–16.** Effects of Anesthetics on Motor Evoked Potentials: Transcranial Magnetic and Electrical

| Anesthetic Drug | Muscle Potential |
|---|---|
| Barbiturate | P |
| Nitrous oxide | P (D) |
| Halothane | P |
| Enflurane | |
| Isoflurane | |
| Narcotics | A |
| Benzodiazepines | P |
| Ketamine | A |
| Etomidate | A |
| Propofol | ?P* |
| Muscle relaxant | A† |

*Conflicting data in literature.
†Provided that one to two twitches are maintained.
A, acceptable; D, dose dependent; P, prohibitive in clinically used concentrations <1 minimum alveolar concentration.

## Safety

Limited data are available regarding the short-term or long-term safety of magnetic or electrical transcranial stimulation of the cortex, and there is currently no convincing evidence that either technique produces short- or long-term harm. Neither stimulation method, however, is approved for use in human beings; at this time, transcranial MEP monitoring should be considered promising. Some centers are now using this form of monitoring without patient consent, whereas others still consider the technique to be experimental and require approved protocols and informed consent.

## FACIAL NERVE MONITORING

### Why Is It Important?

Some operations in the posterior fossa, particularly those involving resection of acoustic neuromas and the base of the skull, may result in damage to the facial nerve (cranial nerve VII). Postoperative weakness or paralysis of the facial nerve produces serious morbidity. First, eye closure may be incomplete, producing corneal drying and damage; second, muscles of facial expression can fail to function, with resulting serious disfigurement.

### How Can It Be Monitored During Surgery?

#### Direct Observation

The simplest method involves direct observation of the face while the surgeon uses a nerve stimulator to locate the facial nerve in the surgical field. This method is limited for several reasons. First, the facial nerve is not assessed except when the surgeon attempts to locate it with a nerve stimulator. Serious damage that will not be detected can occur at other times during surgery (eg, during exposure of an acoustic tumor over which the facial nerve has been stretched). Second, the face may not be readily visible for direct observation. For example, during procedures conducted in the three-quarter prone position—commonly used for posterior fossa explorations—the face cannot be seen unless the clinician crawls under the table and shines a light on it.

#### Electromyography

For facial nerve monitoring, EMG recording needles are placed in the orbicularis oculi and orbicularis oris muscles (Fig. 21–23). To locate the facial nerve, a repetitive electrical stimulus is applied, and EMG activity is recorded from these muscles (Fig. 21–24). The EMG response is displayed on a screen and converted to an audio signal that gives immediate, direct feedback to the surgeon.

#### Passive Monitoring

The facial nerve may also be passively monitored. Whenever surgical manipulation involves touching of or retraction on the facial nerve, spontaneous electrical activity increases, and the audio signal, which sounds like static on a radio, immediately alerts the surgeon to the proximity of the nerve.

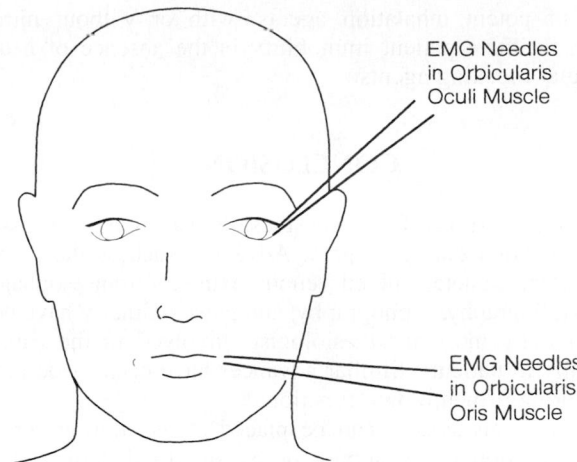

**FIGURE 21–23.** Schematic representation of facial nerve monitor.

EMG Needles in Orbicularis Oculi Muscle

EMG Needles in Orbicularis Oris Muscle

### Summary

These techniques are much more reliable than mere observation for facial twitching. Facial nerve monitoring leads to improved facial nerve function following acoustic tumor removal.[183–186] The EMG is also safer than facial observation because it is a continuous monitor, and the anesthesiologist does not have to disturb the arrangement of equipment, personnel, or drapes to see the patient's face. Motor cranial nerves III, IV, VI, X, XI, and XII also can be monitored in a similar fashion to detect surgical trauma in the posterior fossa.

### Can Neuromuscular Blocking Agents Be Used?

For EMG monitoring to be successful, the patient cannot be completely paralyzed. One study demonstrated that partial paralysis (twitch height 50% of control) is compatible with successful location of the facial nerve.[187] Another study suggested that even total peripheral blockade is compatible with successful recordings following facial nerve stimulation.[188] Whether such paralysis affects the sensitivity of passive facial nerve monitoring is unclear. Many experts involved in seventh nerve monitoring, including myself, still recommend complete avoidance of neuromuscular blockade during the time at which the facial nerve is considered at risk. Higher concentra-

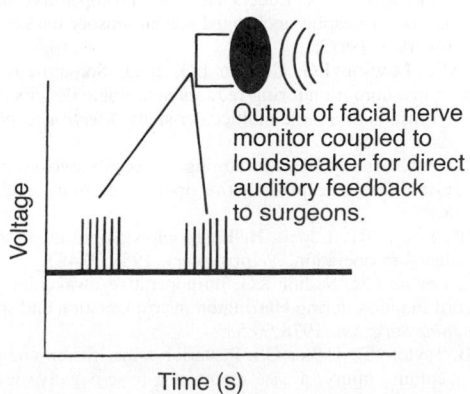

Voltage

Output of facial nerve monitor coupled to loudspeaker for direct auditory feedback to surgeons.

Time (s)

**FIGURE 21–24.** Active monitoring of the facial nerve.

tions of potent inhalation agents, with or without nitrous oxide, facilitate patient immobility in the absence of neuromuscular blocking agents.

## CONCLUSION

A large portion of the anesthesiologist's job is to assess organ function during surgery. Advances such as the pulmonary artery catheter, mixed venous oximetry, transesophageal echocardiography, capnography, and pulse oximetry have been mastered by most anesthesiologists involved in the care of critically ill patients. Similar advances have been made in the monitoring of neurologic function.

The nervous system can be placed at risk during surgery by a reduction in $O_2$ supply or by structural damage from positioning or surgical manipulation. Monitoring gives information about blood flow or neurologic function that would not otherwise be available. The surgeon can alter the procedure, and the anesthesiologist may intervene to increase BP, change patient position, increase the amount of inspired $O_2$, or administer drugs to decrease $O_2$ demand, thus restoring blood flow or CNS function to normal levels. Anesthesiologists should embrace CNS monitoring as a part of their practice when they provide perioperative care for patients at risk for neurologic damage.

## References

1. Sundt TM Jr, Sharbrough FW, Piepgras DG, et al. Correlation of cerebral blood flow and electroencephalographic changes during carotid endarterectomy: with results of surgery and hemodynamics of cerebral ischemia. *Mayo Clin Proc.* 1981;56:533.
2. Nash CL, Lorig RA, Schatzinger LA, et al. Spinal cord monitoring during operative treatment of the spine. *Clin Orthop.* 1977;126:100.
3. Dinner DS, Lüders H, Lesser RP, et al. Intraoperative spinal somatosensory evoked potential monitoring. *J Neurosurg.* 1986;65:807.
4. York DH, Chabot RJ, Gaines RW. Response variability of somatosensory evoked potentials during scoliosis surgery. *Spine.* 1987;12:864.
5. Bieber E, Tolo V, Uematsu S. Spinal cord monitoring during posterior spinal instrumentation and fusion. *Clin Orthop.* 1988;229:121.
6. Grundy BL, Nash CL, Brown RH. Arterial pressure manipulation alters spinal cord function during correction of scoliosis. *Anesthesiology.* 1981;54:249.
7. Padberg AM, Wilson-Holden TJ, Lenke LG, et al. Somatosensory- and motor-evoked potential monitoring without a wake-up test during idiopathic scoliosis surgery. An accepted standard of care. *Spine.* 1998;23:1392.
8. Ginsburg HH, Shetter AG, Raudzens PA. Postoperative paraplegia with preserved intraoperative somatosensory evoked potentials: a case report. *J Neurosurg.* 1985;63:296.
9. Lesser RP, Raudzens PA, Lüders H, et al. Postoperative neurological deficits may occur despite unchanged somatosensory evoked potentials. *Ann Neurol.* 1986;19:22.
10. Nuwer MR, Dawson EG, Carlson LG, et al. Somatosensory evoked potential spinal cord monitoring reduces neurologic deficits after scoliosis surgery: results of a large multicenter study. *Electroencephalogr Clin Neurophysiol.* 1995;96:6.
11. Friedman WA, Grundy BL. Monitoring of sensory evoked potentials is highly reliable and helpful in the operating room. *J Clin Monit.* 1987;3:38.
12. Little JR, Lesser RP, Lüders H. Electrophysiologic monitoring during basilar aneurysm operation. *Neurosurgery.* 1987;20:421.
13. Hall JE, Levine CR, Sudhir KG. Intraoperative awakening to monitor spinal cord function during Harrington instrumentation and spine fusion. *J Bone Joint Surg Am.* 1978;60:533.
14. Ben DB, Taylor PD, Haller GS. Posterior spinal fusion complicated by posterior column injury: a case report of a false-negative wake-up test. *Spine.* 1987;12:540.
15. Hoppenfeld S, Gross A, Andrews C, et al. The ankle clonus test for

assessment of the integrity of the spinal cord during operations for scoliosis. *J Bone Joint Surg Am.* 1997;79:208.
16. Herrick IA, Craen RA, Gelb AW, et al. Propofol sedation during awake craniotomy for seizures: patient-controlled administration versus neurolept analgesia. *Anesth Analg.* 1997;84:1285.
17. Herrick IA, Craen RA, Gelb AW, et al. Propofol sedation during awake craniotomy for seizures: electrocorticographic and epileptogenic effects. *Anesth Analg.* 1997;84:1280.
18. Silbergeld DL, Mueller WM, Colley PS, et al. Use of propofol (Diprivan) for awake craniotomies: technical note. *Surg Neurol.* 1992;38:271.
19. Oei-Lim VL, Kalkman CJ, Bouvy-Berends EC, et al. A comparison of the effects of propofol and nitrous oxide on the electroencephalogram in epileptic patients during conscious sedation for dental procedures. *Anesth Analg.* 1992;75:708.
20. Hoffman WE, Miletich DJ, Albrecht RF. The influence of antihypertensive therapy on cerebral autoregulation in aged hypertensive rats. *Stroke.* 1982;13:701.
21. Paulson OB, Strandgaard S, Edvinsson LTI. Cerebral autoregulation. *Cerebrovasc Brain Metab Rev.* 1990;2:161.
22. Sundbarg G, Nordstrom CH, Soderstrom S. Complications due to prolonged ventricular fluid pressure recording. *Br J Neurosurg.* 1988;4:485.
23. ter Minassian A, Melon E, Leguerinel C, et al. Changes in cerebral blood flow during $PaCO_2$ variations in patients with severe closed head injury: comparison between the Fick and transcranial Doppler methods. *J Neurosurg.* 1998;88:996.
24. Fukushima U, Sasaki S, Okano S, et al. The comparison between the cerebral blood flow directly measures and cerebral flow velocity in the middle and basilar cerebral arteries measured by transcranial Doppler ultrasonography. *J Vet Med Sci.* 1999;61:1293.
25. Muller M, Reiche W, Langenscheidt P, et al. Ischemia after carotid endarterectomy: comparison between transcranial Doppler sonography and diffusion-weighted MR imaging. *Am J Neuroradiol.* 2000;21:47.
26. Els T, Daffertshofer M, Schroeck H, et al. Comparison of transcranial Doppler flow velocity and cerebral blood flow during focal ischemia in rabbits. *Ultrasound Med Biol.* 1999;25:933.
27. Halsey JH, McDowell HA, Gelmon S, et al. Blood velocity in the middle cerebral artery and regional cerebral blood flow during carotid endarterectomy. *Stroke.* 1989;20:53.
28. Lacroix H, Beyene G, Van Hemelrijck J, et al. Is transcranial Doppler useful in the detection of internal carotid artery cross-clamp intolerance? *Cardiovasc Surg.* 1999;7:203.
29. Arnold M, Sturzenegger M, Schaffler L, et al. Continuous intraoperative monitoring of middle cerebral artery blood flow velocities and electroencephalography during carotid endarterectomy. A comparison of the two methods to detect cerebral ischemia. *Stroke.* 1997;28:1345.
30. Cao P, Giordano G, Zannetti S, et al. Transcranial Doppler monitoring during carotid endarterectomy: is it appropriate for selecting patients in need of a shunt? *J Vasc Surg.* 1997;26:973.
31. Cullinane M, Reid G, Dittrich R, et al. Evaluation of new on-line automated embolic signal detection algorithm, including comparison with panel of international experts. *Stroke.* 2000;31:1335.
32. Smith JL, Evans DH, Gaunt ME, et al. Experience with transcranial Doppler monitoring reduces the incidence of particulate embolization during carotid endarterectomy. *Br J Surg.* 1998;85:56.
33. Gaunt ME. Transcranial Doppler: preventing stroke during carotid endarterectomy. *Ann R Coll Surg Engl.* 1998;80:377.
34. Lennard N, Smith J, Dumville J, et al. Prevention of postoperative thrombotic stroke after carotid endarterectomy: the role of transcranial Doppler ultrasound. *J Vasc Surg.* 1997;26:579.
35. Spencer MP. Transcranial Doppler monitoring and causes of stroke from carotid endarterectomy. *Stroke.* 1997;28:685.
36. Levi CR, O'Malley HM, Fell G, et al. Transcranial Doppler detected cerebral microembolism following carotid endarterectomy. High microembolic signal loads predict postoperative cerebral ischaemia. *Brain.* 1997;120(pt4):621.
37. Dalman JE, Beenakkers IC, Moll FL, et al. Transcranial Doppler monitoring during carotid endarterectomy helps to identify patients at risk of postoperative hyperperfusion. *Eur J Vasc Endovasc Surg.* 1999;18:222.
38. Pascazio L, Regina G, Perilli F, et al. Investigation on cerebral hemodynamics in patients with carotid disease receiving carotid endarterectomy. *Clin Hemorheol Microcirc.* 1999;21:395.
39. Gossetti B, Martinelli O, Guerrichio R, et al. Transcranial Doppler in 178 patients before, during, and after carotid endarterectomy. *J Neuroimaging.* 1977;7:213.
40. Pashayan AG, Mahla ME. Unpublished data.
41. Spencer MP, Thomas GI, Nicholls SC, Sauvage LR. Detection of middle

cerebral artery emboli during carotid endarterectomy using transcranial Doppler ultrasonography. *Stroke.* 1990;21:415.

42. van der Linden J, Wessler O, Tyden H, et al. Transcranial Doppler versus thermodilution measurements of cerebral blood flow during cardiac surgery. *J Cardiothorac Anesth.* 1989;3:68.

43. van der Linden J, Casimir-Ahn H. When do cerebral emboli occur during open heart operations? A transcranial Doppler study. *Ann Thorac Surg.* 1991;51:237.

44. Grocott HP, Amory DW, Lowry E, et al. Transcranial Doppler blood flow velocity versus 133Xe clearance cerebral blood flow during mild hypothermic cardiopulmonary bypass. *J Clin Monit Comput.* 1998;14:35.

45. Nuttall GA, Cook DJ, Fulgham JR, et al. The relationship between cerebral blood flow and transcranial Doppler blood flow velocity during hypothermic cardiopulmonary bypass in adults. *Anesth Analg.* 1996;82:1146.

46. Weyland A, Stephan H, Kazmaier S, et al. Flow velocity measurements as an index of cerebral blood flow. Validity of transcranial Doppler sonographic monitoring during cardiac surgery. *Anesthesiology.* 1994;81:1401.

47. Jacobs A, Neveling M, Horst M, et al. Alterations of neuropsychological function and cerebral glucose metabolism after cardiac surgery are not related only to intraoperative microembolic events. *Stroke.* 1998;29:660.

48. Braekken SK, Russell D, Brucher R, et al. Cerebral microembolic signals during cardiopulmonary bypass surgery. Frequency, time of occurrence, and association with patient and surgical characteristics. *Stroke.* 1997;28:1988.

49. Sloan MA, Haley EC Jr, Kassell NF, et al. Sensitivity and specificity of transcranial Doppler ultrasonography in the diagnosis of vasospasm following subarachnoid hemorrhage. *Neurology.* 1989;39:1514.

50. Grosset DG, Straiton J, du Trevou M, et al. Prediction of symptomatic vasospasm after subarachnoid hemorrhage by rapidly increasing transcranial Doppler velocity and cerebral blood flow changes. *Stroke.* 1992;23:674.

51. Manno EM, Gress DR, Schwamm LH, et al. Effects of induced hypertension on transcranial Doppler ultrasound velocities in patients after subarachnoid hemorrhage. *Stroke.* 1998;29:422.

52. Lewis DH, Newell DW, Winn HR. Delayed ischemia due to cerebral vasospasm occult to transcranial Doppler. An important role for cerebral perfusion SPECT. *Clin Nucl Med.* 1997;22:238.

53. Ekelund A, Saveland H, Romner B, et al. Is transcranial Doppler sonography useful in detecting late cerebral ischaemia after aneurysmal subarachnoid hemorrhage? *Br J Neurosurg.* 1996;10:19.

54. Meixensberger J, Hamelbeck B, Dings J, et al. Critical increase of blood flow velocities after subarachnoid hemorrhage: vasospasm versus hyperaemia. *Zentralbl Neurochir.* 1996;57:70.

55. Ekelund A, Saveland H, Romner B, et al. Transcranial Doppler ultrasound in hypertensive versus normotensive patients after aneurysmal subarachnoid hemorrhage. *Stroke.* 1995;26:2071.

56. Vora YY, Suarez-Almazor M, Steinke DE, et al. Role of transcranial Doppler monitoring in the diagnosis of cerebral vasospasm after subarachnoid hemorrhage. *Neurosurgery.* 1999;44:1237.

57. Petty GW, Mohr JP, Pedley TA, et al. The role of transcranial Doppler in confirming brain death. *Neurology.* 1990;40:300.

58. Ducrocq X, Hassler W, Moritake K, et al. Consensus opinion on diagnosis of cerebral circulatory arrest using Doppler-sonography: Task Force Group on cerebral death of the Neurosonology Research Group of the World Federation of Neurology. *J Neurol Sci.* 1998;159:145.

59. Chiu NC, Shen EY, Lee BS. Reversal of diastolic cerebral blood flow in infants without brain death. *Pediatr Neurol.* 1994;11:337.

60. Paolin A, Manuali A, Di Paola F, et al. Reliability in diagnosis of brain death. *Intensive Care Med.* 1995;21:657.

61. Howard L, Gopinath SP, Uzura M, et al. Evaluation of a new fiberoptic catheter for monitoring jugular venous oxygen saturation. *Neurosurgery.* 1999;44:1280.

62. Sheinberg M, Kanter MJ, Robertson CS, et al. Continuous monitoring of jugular venous oxygen saturation in head-injured patients. *J Neurosurg.* 1992;76:212.

63. Feldman Z, Robertson CS. Monitoring of cerebral hemodynamics with jugular bulb catheters. *Crit Care Clin.* 1997;13:51.

64. Matz PG, Pitts L. Monitoring in traumatic brain injury. *Clin Neurosurg.* 1997;44:267.

65. Robertson CS, Gopinath SP, Goodman JC, et al. Sjvo2 monitoring in head-injured patients. *J Neurotrauma.* 1995;12:891.

66. Metz C, Holzschuh M, Bein T, et al. Monitoring of cerebral oxygen metabolism in the jugular bulb: reliability of unilateral measurements in severe head injury. *J Cereb Blood Flow Metab.* 1998;18:332.

67. Gupta AK, Hutchinson PJ, Al-Rawi P, et al. Measuring brain tissue oxygenation compared with jugular venous oxygen saturation for monitoring cerebral oxygenation after traumatic brain injury. *Anesth Analg.* 1999;88:549.

68. Gopinath SP, Valadka AB, Uzura M, et al. Comparison of jugular venous oxygen saturation and brain tissue Po2 as monitors of cerebral ischemia after head injury. *Crit Care Med.* 1999;27:2337.

69. Komiyama M, Kan M, Shigemoto T, et al. Marked regional heterogeneity in venous oxygen saturation in severe head injury studied by superselective intracranial venous sampling: case report. *Neurosurgery.* 1999;45:1469.

70. ter Minassian A, Poirier N, Pierrot M, et al. Correlation between cerebral oxygen saturation measured by near-infrared spectroscopy and jugular oxygen saturation in patients with severe closed head injury. *Anesthesiology.* 1999;91:985.

71. Kadoi Y, Kawahara F, Fujita N. [Malfunctioning of cerebral function monitors in three cases of carotid endarterectomy]. *Masui.* 2000;49:40.

72. Souter MJ, Andrews PJ, Alston RP. Propofol does not ameliorate cerebral venous oxyhemoglobin desaturation during hypothermic cardiopulmonary bypass. *Anesth Analg.* 1998;86:926.

73. Grubbofer G, Lassnigg AM, Schneider B, et al. Jugular venous bulb oxygen saturation depends on blood pressure during cardiopulmonary bypass. *Ann Thorac Surg.* 1998;65:653.

74. Jansen GF, van Praagh BH, Kedaria MB, et al. Jugular bulb oxygen saturation during propofol and isoflurane/nitrous oxide anesthesia in patients undergoing brain tumor surgery. *Anesth Analg.* 1999;89:358.

75. Jasper HH. The ten-twenty electrode system of the International Federation. *Electroencephalogr Clin Neurophysiol.* 1958;10:371.

76. Rampil IJ. A primer for EEG signal processing in anesthesia. *Anesthesiology.* 1998;89:980.

77. Spackman TN, Faust RJ, Cucchiara RF, et al. A comparison of aperiodic analysis of the EEG with standard EEG and cerebral blood flow for the detection of ischemia. *Anesthesiology.* 1987;66:229.

78. Messick JM Jr, Casement B, Sharbrough FW, et al. Correlation of regional cerebral blood flow (rCBF) with EEG changes during isoflurane anesthesia for carotid endarterectomy: critical rCBF. *Anesthesiology.* 1987;66:344.

79. Grady RE, Weglinski MR, Sharbrough FW, et al. Correlation of regional cerebral blood flow with ischemic electroencephalographic changes during sevoflurane-nitrous oxide anesthesia for carotid endarterectomy. *Anesthesiology.* 1998;88:892.

80. Sundt TM Jr, Michenfelder JD. Focal transient ischemia in the squirrel monkey: effect on brain adenosine triphosphate and lactate levels with electrocorticographic and pathologic correlation. *Circ Res.* 1972;30:703.

81. Silbert BS, Koumoundouros E, Davies MJ, et al. Comparison of the processed electroencephalogram and awake neurologic assessment during carotid endarterectomy. *Anaesth Intensive Care.* 1989;17:298.

82. Whittemore AD, Kauffman JL, Kohler TR, et al. Routine electroencephalographic (EEG) monitoring during carotid endarterectomy. *Ann Surg.* 1983;193:707.

83. Halsey JH Jr. Risks and benefits of shunting in carotid endarterectomy. The international transcranial Doppler collaborators. *Stroke.* 1992;23:1583.

84. Salvian AJ, Taylor DC, Hsiang YN, et al. Selective shunting with EEG monitoring is safer than routine shunting for carotid endarterectomy. *Cardiovasc Surg.* 1997;5:481.

85. Plestis KA, Loubser P, Mizrahi EM, et al. Continuous electroencephalographic monitoring and selective shunting reduces neurologic morbidity rates in carotid endarterectomy. *J Vasc Surg.* 1997;25:620.

86. Shapira Y, Gurman G, Artru AA, et al. Combined hemodilution and hypotension monitored with jugular bulb oxygen saturation, EEG, and ECG decreases transfusion volume and length of ICU stay for major orthopedic surgery. *J Clin Anesth.* 1997;9:643.

87. Dwyer RC, Rampil IJ, Eger EI II, et al. The electroencephalogram does not predict depth of isoflurane anesthesia. *Anesthesiology.* 1994;81:403.

88. Schwender D, Daunderer M, Mulzer S, et al. Spectral edge frequency of the electroencephalogram to monitor "depth" of anaesthesia with isoflurane or propofol. *Br J Anaesth.* 1996;77:179.

89. Rampil IJ, Laster MJ. No correlation between quantitative electroencephalographic measurements and movement response to noxious stimuli during isoflurane anesthesia in rats. *Anesthesiology.* 1992;77:920.

90. Rampil IJ, Matteo RS. Changes in EEG spectral edge frequency correlate with the hemodynamic response to laryngoscopy and intubation. *Anesthesiology.* 1987;67:139.

91. Sidi A, Halimi P, Cotev S. Estimating anesthetic depth by electroencephalography during anesthetic induction and intubation inpatients undergoing cardiac surgery. *J Clin Anesth.* 1990;2:101.

92. Gurman GM. Assessment of depth of general anesthesia. Observations on processed EEG and spectral edge frequency. *Int J Clin Monit Comput.* 1994;11:185.

93. Drummond JC, Brann CA, Perkins DE, et al. A comparison of median frequency, spectral edge frequency, a frequency band power ratio, total power, and dominance shift in the determination of depth of anesthesia. *Acta Anaesthesiol Scand.* 1991;35:693.

94. Sigl JC, Chamoun NG. An introduction to bispectral analysis for the electroencephalogram. *J Clin Monit.* 1994;10:392.

95. Billard V, Gambus PL, Chamoun N, et al. A comparison of spectral edge, delta power, and bispectral index as EEG measures of alfentanil, propofol, and midazolam drug effect. *Clin Pharmacol Ther.* 1997;61:45.

96. Sebel PS, Lang E, Rampil IJ, et al. A multicenter study of bispectral electroencephalogram analysis for monitoring anesthetic effects. *Anesth Analg.* 1997;84:891.

97. Song D, van Vlymen J, White PF. Is the bispectral index useful in predicting fast-track eligibility after ambulatory anesthesia with propofol and desflurane? *Anesth Analg.* 1998;87:1245.

98. Dexter F, Macario A, Manberg PJ, et al. Computer simulation to determine how rapid anesthetic recovery protocols to decrease the time for emergence or increase the phase I postanesthesia care unit bypass rate affect staffing of an ambulatory surgery center. *Anesth Analg.* 1999;88:1053.

99. Gan TJ, Glass PS, Windsor A, et al. Bispectral index monitoring allows faster emergence and improved recovery from propofol, alfentanil, and nitrous oxide anesthesia. BIS Utility Study Group. *Anesthesiology.* 1997;87:808.

100. Hans P, Bonhomme V, Born JD, et al. Target-controlled infusion of propofol and remifentanil combined with bispectral index monitoring for awake craniotomy. *Anaesthesia.* 2000;55:255.

101. Shapiro BA. Bispectral index: better information for sedation in the intensive care unit? *Crit Care Med.* 1999;27:1663.

102. Simmons LE, Riker RR, Prato BS, et al. Assessing sedation during intensive care unit mechanical ventilation with the Bispectral Index and the Sedation-Agitation Scale. *Crit Care Med.* 1999;27:1499.

103. De Deyne C, Struys M, Decruyenaere J, et al. Use of continuous bispectral EEG monitoring to assess depth of sedation in ICU patients. *Intensive Care Med.* 1998;24:1294.

104. Hirota K, Kubota T, Ishihara H, et al. The effects of nitrous oxide and ketamine on the bispectral index and 95% spectral edge frequency during propofol-fentanyl anaesthesia. *Eur J Anaesthesiol.* 1999;16:779.

105. Friedberg BL. The effect of a dissociative dose of ketamine on the bispectral index (BIS) during propofol hypnosis. *J Clin Anesth.* 1999;11:4.

106. Landi A, Copeland SA, Wynn-Parry CB, et al. The role of somatosensory evoked potentials and nerve conduction studies in the surgical management of brachial plexus injuries. *J Bone Joint Surg.* 1980;4:492.

107. Oberle JW, Antoniadis G, Rath SA, et al. Value of nerve action potentials in the surgical management of traumatic nerve lesions. *Neurosurgery.* 1997;41:1337.

108. Manninen PH. Monitoring evoked potentials during spinal surgery in one institution. *Can J Anaesth.* 1998;45(5pt1):450.

109. Deutsch H, Arginteanu M, Manhart K, et al. Somatosensory evoked potential monitoring in anterior thoracic vertebrectomy. *J Neurosurg.* 2000;92(2 suppl):155.

110. Kaplan BJ, Friedman WA, Alexander JA, Hampson SR. Somatosensory evoked potential monitoring of spinal cord ischemia during aortic operations. *Neurosurgery.* 1986;19:82.

111. Crawford ES, Mizrahi EM, Hess KR, et al. The impact of distal aortic perfusion and somatosensory evoked potential monitoring on prevention of paraplegia after aortic aneurysm operation. *J Thorac Cardiovasc Surg.* 1988;95:357.

112. Maeda S, Miyamoto T, Murata H, et al. Prevention of spinal cord ischemia by monitoring spinal cord perfusion pressure and somatosensory evoked potentials. *J Cardiovasc Surg.* 1989;30:565.

113. Laschinger JC, Cunningham JN, Cooper MM, et al. Monitoring of somatosensory evoked potentials during surgical procedures on the thoracoabdominal aorta, I: relationship of aortic cross-clamp duration, changes in somatosensory evoked potentials, and incidence of neurologic dysfunction. *J Thorac Cardiovasc Surg.* 1987;94:260.

114. Cunningham JN, Laschinger JC, Spencer FC. Monitoring of somatosensory evoked potentials during surgical procedures on the thoracoabdominal aorta, IV: clinical observations and results. *J Thorac Cardiovasc Surg.* 1987;94:275.

115. Faberowski LW, Black S, Trankina MF, et al. Somatosensory-evoked potentials during aortic coarctation repair. *J Cardiothorac Vasc Anesth.* 1999;13:538.

116. Branston NM, Symon L, Crockard HA, et al. Relationship between the cortical evoked potential and local cortical blood flow following acute middle cerebral artery occlusion in the baboon. *Exp Neurol.* 1974;45:195.

117. Friedman WA, Chadwick GM, Verhoeven FJS, et al. Monitoring of somatosensory evoked potentials during surgery for middle cerebral artery aneurysms. *Neurosurgery.* 1991;29:83.

118. Schramm J, Koht A, Schmidt G, et al. Surgical and electrophysiologic observations during clipping of 134 aneurysms with evoked potential monitoring. *Neurosurgery.* 1990;26:61.

119. Mooij JJA, Buchthal A, Belopavlovic M. Somatosensory evoked potential monitoring of temporary middle cerebral artery occlusion during aneurysm operation. *Neurosurgery.* 1987;21:492.

120. Lopez JR, Chang SD, Steinberg GK. The use of electrophysiologic monitoring in the intraoperative management of intracranial aneurysms. *J Neurol Neurosurg Psychiatry.* 1997;66:189.

121. Sako K, Nakai H, Kawata Y, et al. Temporary arterial occlusion during anterior communicating or anterior cerebral artery aneurysm operation under tibial nerve somatosensory evoked potential monitoring. *Surg Neurol.* 1998;49:316.

122. Little JR, Lesser RP, Lüders H. Electrophysiological monitoring during basilar aneurysm operation. *Neurosurgery.* 1987;20:421.

123. Sebel PS, Ingram DA, Flynn PJ, et al. Evoked potentials during isoflurane anaesthesia. *Br J Anaesth.* 1986;58:580.

124. Drummond JC, Todd MM, U HS. The effect of high dose sodium thiopental on brainstem auditory and median nerve somatosensory evoked responses in humans. *Anesthesiology.* 1985;63:249.

125. McPherson RW, Sell B, Traystman RJ. Effects of thiopental, fentanyl and etomidate on upper extremity somatosensory evoked potentials in humans. *Anesthesiology.* 1986;62:626.

126. McPherson RW, Mahla ME, Johnson R, et al. Effects of enflurane, isoflurane and nitrous oxide on somatosensory evoked potentials during fentanyl anesthesia. *Anesthesiology.* 1985;62:626.

127. Schubert A, Drummond JC, Peterson DO, et al. The effect of high-dose fentanyl on human median nerve somatosensory-evoked responses. *Can J Anaesth.* 1987;34:35.

128. Sloan TB, Ronai AK, Toleikis JR, et al. Improvement of intraoperative somatosensory evoked potentials by etomidate. *Anesth Analg.* 1988;67:582.

129. Koht A, Schütz W, Schmidt G, et al. Effects of etomidate, midazolam, and thiopental on median nerve somatosensory evoked potentials and the additive effects of fentanyl and nitrous oxide. *Anesth Analg.* 1988;67:435.

130. Maurette P, Simeon F, Castagnera L, et al. Propofol anaesthesia alters somatosensory evoked cortical potentials. *Anaesthesia.* 1988;43(suppl):44.

131. Schindler E, Thiel A, Muller M, et al. Changes in somatosensory evoked potentials after sevoflurane and isoflurane. A randomized phase II study. *Anaesthesist.* 1996;45(suppl 1):S52.

132. Bernard JM, Pereon Y, Fayet G, et al. Effects of isoflurane and desflurane on neurogenic motor- and somatosensory-evoked potential monitoring for scoliosis surgery. *Anesthesiology.* 1996;85:1013.

133. Schindler E, Muller M, Zickmann B, et al. Modulation of somatosensory evoked potentials under various concentrations of desflurane with and without nitrous oxide. *J Neurosurg Anesthesiol.* 1998;10:218.

134. Drummond JC, Todd MM, Schubert A, et al. Effect of the acute administration of high dose pentobarbital on human brainstem auditory and median nerve somatosensory evoked responses. *Neurosurgery.* 1987;20:830.

135. DuBois MY, Sato S, Chassy J, et al. Effects of enflurane on brainstem auditory evoked responses in humans. *Anesth Analg.* 1982;61:898.

136. Manninen PH, Lam AM, Nicholas JF. The effects of isoflurane and isoflurane-nitrous oxide anesthesia on brainstem auditory evoked potentials in humans. *Anesth Analg.* 1985;64:43.

137. Watanabe E, Schramm J, Strauss C, et al. Neurophysiologic monitoring in posterior fossa surgery, II: BAEP-waves I and V and preservation of hearing. *Acta Neurochir (Wien).* 1989;98:118.

138. Moller AR. Monitoring auditory function during operations to remove acoustic tumors. *Am J Otol.* 1996;17:452.

139. Battista RA, Wiet RJ, Paauwe L. Evaluation of three intraoperative auditory monitoring techniques in acoustic neuroma surgery. *Am J Otol.* 2000;21:244.

140. Colletti V, Fiorino FG, Carner M, et al. Mechanisms of auditory impairment during acoustic neuroma surgery. *Otolaryngol Head Neck Surg.* 1997;117:596.

141. Roberson JB Jr, Jackson LE, McAuley JR. Acoustic neuroma surgery:

absent auditory brainstem response does not contraindicate attempted hearing preservation. *Laryngoscope*. 1999;109:904.

142. Matthies C, Samii M. Management of vestibular schwannomas (acoustic neuromas): the value of neurophysiology for intraoperative monitoring of auditory function in 200 cases. *Neurosurgery*. 1997;40:459.

143. Moeller AR, Moeller MB. Does intraoperative monitoring of auditory evoked potentials reduce incidence of hearing loss as a complication of microvascular decompression of cranial nerves? *Neurosurgery*. 1989;24:257.

144. Rizvi SS, Goyal RN, Calder HB. Hearing preservation in microvascular decompression for trigeminal neuralgia. *Laryngoscope*. 1999;109:591.

145. Hatayama T, Moller AR. Correlation between latency and amplitude of peak V in the brainstem auditory evoked potentials: intraoperative recordings in microvascular decompression operations. *Acta Neurochir (Wien)*. 1998;140:681.

146. Acevedo JC, Sindou M, Fischer C, et al. Microvascular decompression for the treatment of hemifacial spasm. Retrospective study of a consecutive series of 75 operated patients—electrophysiologic and anatomical surgical analysis. *Stereotact Func Neurosurg*. 1997;68(1-4pt1):260.

147. Raudzens PA. Intraoperative monitoring of evoked potentials. *Ann N Y Acad Sci*. 1982;388:308.

148. Grundy BL. Monitoring of sensory evoked potentials during neurosurgical operations: methods and applications. *Neurosurgery*. 1982;11:556.

149. Chacko AG, Babu KS, Chandy MJ. Value of visual evoked potential monitoring during trans-sphenoidal pituitary surgery. *Br J Neurosurg*. 1996;10:275.

150. Jones NS. Visual evoked potentials in endoscopic and anterior skull base surgery: a review. *J Laryngol Otol*. 1997;111:513.

151. Taniguchi M, Nadstawek J, Langenbach U, et al. Effects of four intravenous anesthetic agents on motor evoked potentials elicited by magnetic transcranial stimulation. *Neurosurgery*. 1993;33:407.

152. Yang LH, Lin SM, Lee WY, et al. Intraoperative transcranial electrical motor evoked potential monitoring during spinal surgery under intravenous ketamine or etomidate anesthesia. *Acta Neurochir (Wien)*. 1994;127:191.

153. Ubags LH, Kalkman CJ, Been HD. Influence of isoflurane on myogenic motor evoked potentials to single and multiple transcranial stimuli during nitrous oxide/opioid anesthesia. *Neurosurgery*. 1998;43:90.

154. Jones SJ, Harrison R, Koh KF, et al. Motor evoked potential monitoring during spinal surgery: responses of distal limb muscles to transcranial cortical stimulation with pulse trains. *Electroencephalogr Clin Neurophysiol*. 1996;100:375.

155. Chen R, Gerloff C, Classen J, et al. Safety of different inter-train intervals for repetitive transcranial magnetic stimulation and recommendations for safe ranges of stimulation parameters. *Electroencephalogr Clin Neurophysiol*. 1997;105:415.

156. Bernard JM, Pereon Y, Fayet G, et al. Effects of isoflurane and desflurane on neurogenic motor- and somatosensory-evoked potential monitoring for scoliosis surgery. *Anesthesiology*. 1996;85:1013.

157. Darden BV II, Hatley MK, Owen JH. Neurogenic motor evoked-potential monitoring in anterior cervical surgery. *J Spinal Disord*. 1996;9:485.

158. Owen JH, Bridwell KH, Grubb R, et al. The clinical application of neurogenic motor evoked potentials to monitor spinal cord function during surgery. *Spine*. 1991;16(8 suppl):S385.

159. Owen JH, Jenny AB, Naito M, et al. Effects of spinal cord lesioning on somatosensory and neurogenic-motor evoked potentials. *Spine*. 1989;14:673.

160. Owen JH, Laschinger J, Bridwell K, et al. Sensitivity and specificity of somatosensory and neurogenic-motor evoked potentials in animals and humans. *Spine*. 1988;13:1111.

161. Pereon Y, Bernard JM, Fayet G, et al. Usefulness of neurogenic motor evoked potentials for spinal cord monitoring: findings in 112 consecutive patients undergoing surgery for spinal deformity. *Electroencephalogr Clin Neurophysiol*. 1998;108:17.

162. Rose RD. Removing the antidromically driven sensory component from cervically evoked motor potentials. *Med Hypotheses*. 1998;50:147.

163. Edmonds HL Jr, Paloheimo MP, Backman MH, et al. Transcranial magnetic motor evoked potentials for functional monitoring of motor pathways during scoliosis surgery. *Spine*. 1989;14:683.

164. Owen JH, Bridwell KH, Grubb R, et al. The clinical application of neurogenic motor evoked potentials to monitor spinal cord function during surgery. *Spine*. 1991;16(8 suppl):S385.

165. Macri S, de Monte A, Greggi T, et al. Intraoperative spinal cord monitoring in orthopaedics. *Spinal Cord*. 2000;38:133.

166. Lubitz SE, Keith RW, Crawrod AH. Intraoperative experience with neuromotor evoked potentials. A review of 60 consecutive cases. *Spine*. 1999;24:2030.

167. Mochida K, Komori H, Okawa A, et al. Evaluation of motor function during thoracic and thoracolumbar spinal surgery based on motor-evoked potentials using train spinal stimulation. *Spine*. 1997;22:1385.

168. Nagle KJ, Emerson RG, Adams DC, et al. Intraoperative monitoring of motor evoked potentials: a review of 116 cases. *Neurology*. 1996;47:999.

169. Lang EW, Beutler AS, Chesnut RM, et al. Myogenic motor-evoked potential monitoring using partial neuromuscular blockade in surgery of the spine. *Spine*. 1996;21:1676.

170. Sueda T, Okada K, Watari M, et al. Evaluation of motor- and sensory-evoked potentials for spinal cord monitoring during thoracoabdominal aortic aneurysm surgery. *Jpn J Thorac Cardiovasc Surg*. 2000;48:60.

171. Elmore JR, Gloviczki P, Harper CM, et al. Spinal cord injury in experimental thoracic aortic occlusion: investigation of combined methods of protection. *J Vasc Surg*. 1992;15:789.

172. Elmore JR, Gloviczki P, Harper CM, et al. Failure of motor evoked potentials to predict neurologic outcome in experimental thoracic aortic occlusion. *J Vasc Surg*. 1991;14:131.

173. Zentner J, Albrecht T, Heuser D. Influence of halothane, enflurane, and isoflurane on motor evoked potentials. *Neurosurgery*. 1992;31:298.

174. Jellinek D, Platt M, Jewkes D, et al. Effects of nitrous oxide on motor evoked potentials under total anesthesia with intravenously administered propofol. *Neurosurgery*. 1991;29:558.

175. Ghaly RF, Stone JL, Levy WJ, et al. The effect of etomidate on motor evoked potentials induced by transcranial magnetic stimulation in the monkey. *Neurosurgery*. 1990;27:936.

176. Zentner J, Kiss I, Ebner A. Influence of anesthetics—nitrous oxide in particular—on electromyographic response evoked by transcranial electrical stimulation of the cortex. *Neurosurgery*. 1989;24:253.

177. Kalkman CJ, Drummond JC, Ribberink AA, et al. Effects of propofol, etomidate, midazolam, and fentanyl on motor evoked responses to transcranial electrical or magnetic stimulation in humans. *Anesthesiology*. 1992;76:502.

178. Kalkman CJ, Drummond JC, Kennelly NA, et al. Intraoperative monitoring of tibialis anterior muscle motor evoked responses to transcranial electrical stimulation during partial neuromuscular blockade. *Anesth Analg*. 1992;75:584.

179. Thees C, Scheufler KM, Nadstawek J, et al. Influence of fentanyl, alfentanil, and sufentanil on motor evoked potentials. *J Neurosurg Anesthesiol*. 1999;11:112.

180. Ubags LH, Kalkman CJ, Been HD, et al. A comparison of myogenic motor evoked responses to electrical and magnetic transcranial stimulation during nitrous oxide/opioid anesthesia. *Anesth Analg*. 1999;88:568.

181. Pechstein U, Nadstawek J, Zentner J, et al. Isoflurane plus nitrous oxide versus propofol for recording of motor evoked potentials after high frequency repetitive electrical stimulation. *Electroencephalogr Clin Neurophysiol*. 1998;108:175.

182. Zentner J, Thees C, Pechstein U, et al. Influence of nitrous oxide on motor-evoked potentials. *Spine*. 1997;22:1002.

183. Harner SG, Daube JR, Ebersold MJ, et al. Improved preservation of facial nerve function with use of electrical monitoring during removal of acoustic neuromas. *Mayo Clin Proc*. 1987;62:92.

184. Fenton JE, Chin RY, Shirazi A, et al. Prediction of postoperative facial nerve function in acoustic neuroma surgery. *Clin Otolaryngol*. 1999;24:483.

185. Kartush JM. Intra-operative monitoring in acoustic neuroma surgery. *Neurol Res*. 1998;20:593.

186. Grey PL, Moffat DA, Palmer CR, et al. Factors which influence the facial nerve outcome in vestibular schwannoma surgery. *Clin Otolaryngol*. 1996;21:409.

187. Lennon RL, Hosking MP, Daube JR, et al. Effect of partial neuromuscular blockade on intraoperative electromyography in patients undergoing resection of acoustic neuromas. *Anesth Analg*. 1992;75:729.

188. Brauer M, Knuettgen D, Quester R, et al. Electromyographic facial nerve monitoring during resection for acoustic neurinoma under moderate to profound levels of peripheral neuromuscular blockade. *Eur J Anaesthesiol*. 1996;13:612.

# 22

# Neuromuscular Block Monitoring

## Ilkka S. Kalli

Neuromuscular blocking agents (NBAs) were brought into clinical practice over 50 years ago as adjuvants to inhalation anesthesia and to facilitate surgery. Initially, after a few years, they were abandoned as unsafe; these drugs paralyze voluntary muscles and hence also weaken spontaneous breathing. Later, when intubation and control of ventilation were developed, use of NBAs became a safe routine in anesthesia. However, their history was repeated in the postanesthesia care unit (PACU), where residual neuromuscular block may increase the patient's risk.[1,2]

Modern NBAs have an excellent toxicity profile, and their site of action at the neuromuscular junction is quite specific. Barring allergic reactions, an overdose does not lead to toxic manifestations. Yet, an overdose does delay the return of neuromuscular integrity and increases the need for antagonists. Therefore, it is important to monitor the degree of blockade. Nerve stimulators, when used appropriately, allow optimal dosing according to patients' needs and ensure well-timed and safe recovery. In today's managed care, the anesthetist may also face new requirements or constraints. Selection of drugs based on their cost is one consideration, as is the requirement of "fast tracking" or early discharge of the patient.[3–5] Use of the nerve stimulator to optimize drug administration can be of significant help to the anesthetist who must balance different obligations.

## POSTOPERATIVE RESIDUAL NEUROMUSCULAR BLOCKADE

### What Is Its Significance?

Improper timing of administration or too large a dose of NBA may cause postoperative residual block. When the long-acting NBAs are used, the postoperative incidence of residual block can exceed 40%.[1] The newer, intermediate-acting drugs may have a better safety record.[6] Detection of postoperative residual block is important because it may increase respiratory complications[7,8] and the risk of aspiration.[9]

Attempts to judge recovery from the effects of NBAs based on clinical criteria and without the aid of a peripheral nerve stimulator may result in failure to appreciate significant residual neuromuscular blockade.[6] Significant amounts of NBA may still be in the body, but without any clinical symptoms due to neuromuscular block (Table 22–1). Beside NBAs, inhalation agents and analgesics contribute to respiratory depression in postoperative recovery. Their central actions are not easy to distinguish from the suspected effects of NBAs solely on the basis of clinical signs.

## ASSESSMENT OF BLOCK

### What Is the Value of Clinical Signs?

Assessment of neuromuscular block by clinical signs is based on a group of traditional tests that assess muscle force and ventilation[3] (Table 22–2). Typically, head lift sustained for 5 seconds is regarded as a standard clinical assessment of adequate recovery from neuromuscular blockade.[9] Clinical signs, however, cannot replace use of the nerve stimulator

**TABLE 22–1.** Receptor Occupancy and Assessment of Neuromuscular Function

| Method of Assessment | NBA Occupation of Receptors (%)* | Limitations of the Method |
|---|---|---|
| Tidal volume | 75-80 | Insensitive, altered significantly by anesthetic agents |
| Twitch height by nerve stimulator | 75-80 | Insensitive, uncomfortable |
| Tetanic stimulation by nerve stimulator (30 Hz) | 75-80 | Insensitive, uncomfortable |
| Vital capacity | 75-80 | Insensitive, patient cooperation required |
| TOF by nerve stimulator | 75-80 | TOF ratio must be >50% to be visible |
| Tetanic stimulation | 50 | Painful |
| Head lift or hand grip | 33 | Patient cooperation required |

*Percentage of receptors occupied by NBA before appearance of clinical signs.
NBA, neuromuscular blocking agent; TOF, train-of-four.

because assessment in anesthetized patients can be misleading. Tests performed in the PACU usually require patient cooperation. Pediatric patients rarely offer cooperation during emergence from anesthesia. Leg lift and loud cry have been suggested as clinical parameters for their neuromuscular recovery.[10] Many tests try to verify the patient's adequate spontaneous breathing, but this must be assessed with caution. Lingering anesthetic or analgesic effects, despite apparent adequate ventilation and normal tidal volume, can still impair airway reflexes. Numerous investigators have compared recovery assessed by clinical signs with that by the evoked nerve stimulation method (Fig. 22–1). Such studies increase our understanding of the value and limitations of clinical observations.

### How Should Nerve Stimulators Be Used?

The nerve stimulator delivers a pattern of short square-wave pulses to the nerve at short intervals, usually every 10 to 20 seconds. A square-wave, direct current impulse of 0.1 to 0.3 milliseconds' duration is required and is provided by most commercial nerve stimulators. Longer stimulus impulse duration may cause repetitive firing of the nerve with an unpredictable response.

The evoked muscle response (a twitch) is then evaluated by observing the evoked muscle contractions, such as thumb adduction. Visual or tactile observation enables the clinician to detect the type of the block and to make *subjective*, semi-quantitative estimates of its magnitude. The more advanced, *objective* method, which uses a measurement sensor attached to the muscle, allows the degree of block to be more precisely quantified.

### Why Should the Stimulus Be Supramaximal?

Each muscle fiber contracts according to an all-or-none principle. A supramaximal stimulus ensures that all muscle fibers contract simultaneously, maintaining a stable response during surgery (Fig. 22–2). After induction of anesthesia, but before neuromuscular block, that stimulus current which elic-

its maximal contraction of the muscle is determined. This process involves increasing the stimulus output from the nerve stimulator and noting the current required to reach maximal contraction. The thumb response is maximal when it does not increase in spite of a further increase in the stimulus current.[11]

For improved stability, the current is then increased from that level by 10% to 20% (*supramaximal stimulus*). Calibration to the supramaximal current should be performed for each case, instead of simply using the maximum output of the stimulator. Too high a stimulus current can interfere with assessment of response and cause direct contractions of arm muscles. Automated neuromuscular monitors usually find the supramaximal stimulus automatically, and then calibrate and store the initial responses in memory.

### Should the Skin Be Prepared, and What Type of Electrodes Should Be Used?

The resistance between the skin and the electrode may change over time. It is therefore important that the current

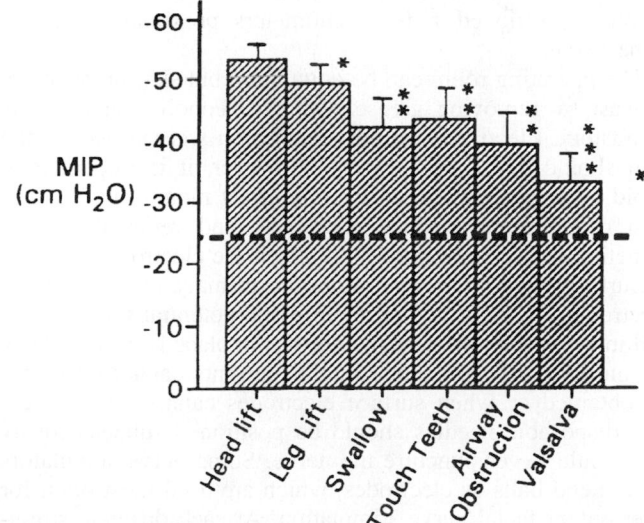

**FIGURE 22–1.** Levels of neuromuscular blockade with *d*-tubocurarine in awake volunteers indicated by maximum inspiratory pressure (MIP ± standard error of the mean), below which the indicated clinical maneuvers could not be accomplished. Head lift was the most sensitive indicator of neuromuscular blockade with *d*-tubocurarine. No maneuvers indicating airway protection could be accomplished by any of the subjects at an MIP of $-25$ cm $H_2O$. The asterisks indicate statistical significance compared with that level of MIP (*$P < .01$; **$P < .2$; ***$P < .05$). (From Pavlin EG, Holle RH, Schoene RB. Recovery of airway protection compared with ventilation in humans after paralysis with curare. *Anesthesiology.* 1989;70:383.)

**TABLE 22–2.** Classic Clinical Signs of Recovery From Neuromuscular Block

| | | |
|---|---|---|
| Head lift (5 s) | Swallow | Vital capacity |
| Eye opening | Grip strength | Maximal inspiratory pressure |
| Tongue protrusion | Tidal volume | Leg lift (pediatric patients) |

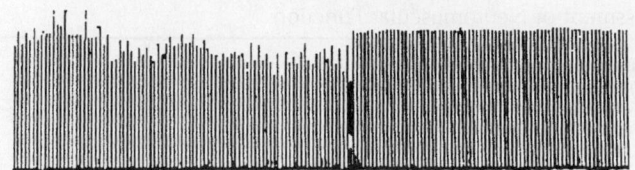

**FIGURE 22–2.** Submaximal versus supramaximal stimulation. The left half of the stimulus response recording demonstrates the variability with submaximal nerve stimulation, whereas the right half represents the stable response to supramaximal stimuli.

level, once set, remain steady throughout the operation. Commercial nerve stimulators must deliver constant current output in spite of changes in skin resistance. Typically, the skin impedance may vary between 1 and 5 k$\Omega$, and with surface electrodes, the required stimulus current usually varies between 20 and 60 mA. Current requirements with needle electrodes are small, often <10 mA. For routine clinical practice, electrocardiogram-type surface electrodes are usually best, provided that they are fresh. They should be attached cautiously, avoiding leakage of the electrode jelly, which can form a conductive bridge that short circuits the two electrodes. The small diameter of the stimulation electrodes ensures that the stimulus current flows to the underlying nerve and not to the surrounding tissues.

### The Stimulator Has Leads Marked + and −; Does It Matter?

Positioning of the stimulus electrodes has an impact on the evoked response.[12–14] Usually, the two nerve stimulator leads have been marked for polarity as positive or negative. The negative stimulus electrode should be positioned on the ulnar nerve, 2 cm proximal to the skin crease of the wrist. Requirements for the positive stimulus electrode are less rigid; it is often positioned a few centimeters proximal along the same nerve.

The operating room can be quite busy, but skin preparation, at least by removing grease with an alcoholic detergent, is mandatory. Electrodes do not attach on a wet surface, so the skin should be allowed to dry. However, it is important to avoid cooling, which may severely affect monitoring.[15] Abrasion of skin may reduce resistance, and removal of hair sometimes may be necessary to attach the electrodes.

Surface electrodes are always the primary choice. Needle electrodes are invasive and there is the potential for infection and injury if the arm with the needles in place is moved. They are an option if sufficient stimulus currents cannot otherwise be obtained or when surface electrodes cannot be attached. The disposable needles should be positioned subcutaneously but should never puncture the nerve. Some nerve stimulators have metal balls as electrodes, which are used most often for intermittent facial nerve stimulation. At each different stimulus, the position may change, making comparison between consecutive stimuli difficult. However, the count of train-of-four (TOF) responses can easily be calculated.

### Where Should the Electrodes Be Applied?

The ulnar nerve at the wrist is by far the most common site for monitoring neuromuscular block (Fig. 22–3). The ulnar

nerve originates in the C8 to T1 levels of the spinal cord. It descends medial to the axillary artery to the middle of the arm. From there, it angles dorsally and laterally to pass behind the medial epicondyle of the humerus, then down the ulnar side of the forearm to the hand. At the wrist, the ulnar nerve lies on the radial side of the flexor carpi radialis tendon.

Of the four thenar muscles, the deep branch of the ulnar nerve innervates the adductor pollicis and the deep branch of the flexor pollicis brevis. The median nerve innervates the other muscles of the thumb (abductor brevis, opponens, and the superficial part of flexor pollicis).

The ulnar nerve innervates all hypothenar muscles (opponens, palmaris brevis, abductor, and flexor brevis). The lumbrical muscles are innervated either by the median nerve (usually I and II) or by the ulnar nerve (III and IV). There are four dorsal and three palmar interosseal muscles, which are innervated by the deep branch of the ulnar nerve.

Measurement of the evoked muscle response is usually based on adduction of the thumb. The anesthetist should observe movement only of the thumb. Assessing the block by movement of fingers 2 through 4 of the hand is misleading. Such movement can be caused by direct muscle stimulation, particularly if the stimulus electrodes are attached over the arm muscles proximal to the wrist.

### Which Other Sites Are Available If the Hand Cannot Be Used?

Because of the type of surgery, the ulnar nerve cannot always be used, but there are other sites available. Based on

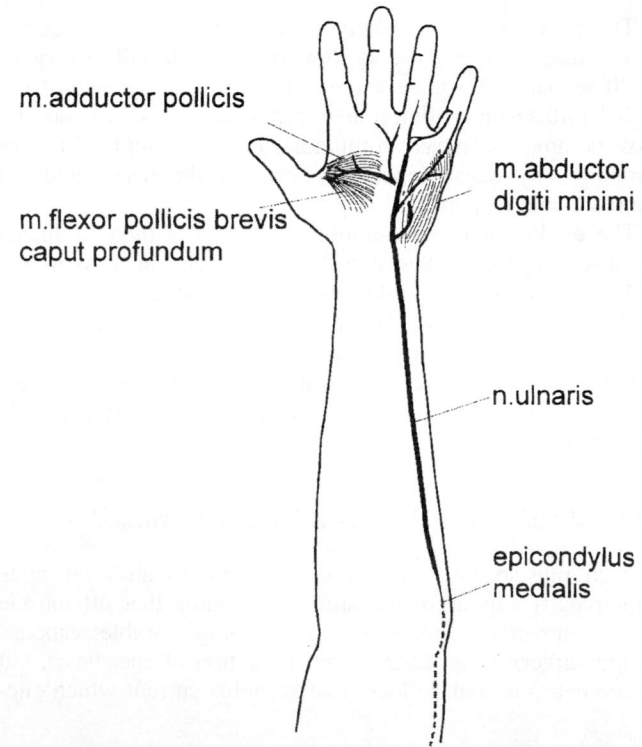

**FIGURE 22–3.** Ulnar nerve-innervated hand muscles suitable for monitoring of neuromuscular block. Stimulation of the nerve evokes contraction of the adductor pollicis muscle, which results in thumb adduction. Hence, the thumb is the recommended site for assessment of the mechanical twitch response. Other ulnar nerve-innervated hand muscles include the hypothenar (m. abductor digiti minimi) and the first dorsal interosseous (near the adductor pollicis, but on the dorsal side of the hand).

histologic structure and muscle fiber composition, the slow- and fast-contracting muscles of the body have different sensitivities to NBAs. Hence, the evoked responses from different sites cannot be directly compared. The degree of innervation, blood flow, and temperature of the monitored muscle also may affect the evoked response.

Because it is one of the rapidly contracting muscles, the adductor pollicis at the hand is relatively sensitive to NBAs. Compared with the diaphragm, neuromuscular block at the hand has a slower onset and recovery, making the hand a safe site for assessment of residual blockade. In general, if the adductor pollicis response has recovered sufficiently, recovery in the diaphragm is even better.[16,17] The onset of neuromuscular block in the larynx is more rapid than in the adductor pollicis, which may be helpful for the timing of intubation[18] (Fig. 22–4). These differences explain why the diaphragm may still contract when the hand is already fully paralyzed. Hence, hiccupping or coughing during deep levels of block does not indicate a lack of neuromuscular blockade. Incidentally, near the end of expiration on the capnogram, minor inspiratory deflections can sometimes be seen. Diaphragmatic contraction can cause such "curare clefts." Before administering more drug, the anesthesiologist should check whether the patient is normocapnic or the level of anesthesia is adequate.

### Is the Facial Nerve Suitable for Monitoring?

The temporal branch of the facial nerve is easily accessible for application of nerve stimulation electrodes during anesthesia[19] (Fig. 22–5). The evoked responses can be assessed at the orbicularis oculi muscle. Typically, facial muscles recover from paralysis more rapidly than the skeletal muscles of the extremities. Hence, their response resembles that of the diaphragm and larynx, and patients may be judged ready for intubation earlier than according to the response at the hand.[20]

### Can the Leg Be Used for Monitoring?

Monitoring at the leg can be an alternative if the hand cannot be used.[21] In general, the results are clinically relevant,

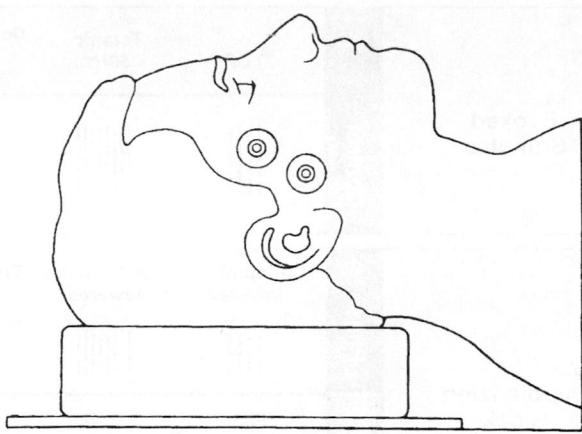

**FIGURE 22–5.** Positioning of stimulating electrodes over the facial nerve. The electrode nearest the eye is negative. (Modified from Caffrey RR, Warren ML, Becker KE Jr. Neuromuscular blockade monitoring comparing the orbicularis oculi and adductor pollicis muscles. *Anesthesiology.* 1986;65:96.)

in spite of some reported differences from the adductor pollicis response.[22,23] Stimulation of the common peroneal nerve around the head of the fibula results in ankle flexion. Stimulation of the posterior tibial nerve in its course behind the medial malleolus causes contractions of the flexor hallucis brevis muscle with plantar flexion.

## CLINICAL APPLICATIONS

### What Patterns of Stimulation Are Best?

In the beginning, single-twitch (ST) and tetanic stimulation were used. The use of TOF stimulation was first suggested by Ali and coworkers in 1970[24] to standardize assessment of fade after repeated stimuli. Today, TOF monitoring represents the standard of care, allowing for adjustment of surgical levels of block simply by observing the evoked muscle contractions. In addition, recording of the TOF response with a sensor attached to the muscle enables measurement of residual block. Double-burst stimulation (DBS), the newest stimulus technique, has been claimed to detect small amounts of residual block even without recording devices. Figure 22–6 shows characteristic stimulus responses during depolarizing and nondepolarizing neuromuscular block.

### Tetanic Stimulation

Tetanic nerve stimulation uses relatively high-frequency currents of 50 to 100 Hz. In normal conditions of neuromuscular transmission, the 50-Hz stimulus for 5 seconds usually results in a sustained contraction. In contrast, the nondepolarizing NBAs cause a typical fade, and the tetanic response is not sustained. During the pure depolarizing block induced by succinylcholine, the tetanic response is sustained. However, fade occurs once a phase II block develops, which can happen with repeated or large bolus doses or with continuous infusion.

Tetanic stimulation can be used only during anesthesia because a muscle contraction is painful. At the end of anesthesia, some practitioners like to elicit a 50-Hz tetanic contraction, which is thought to detect a residual block. It has been questioned, however, whether such an observation really is

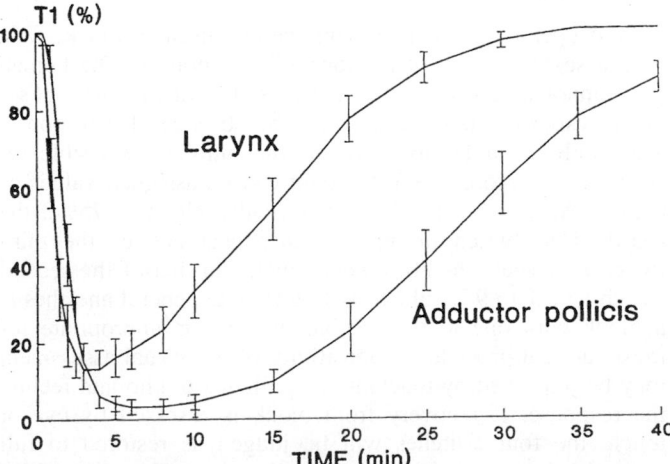

**FIGURE 22–4.** After a single dose of vecuronium (0.07 mg/kg), both onset of and recovery from the neuromuscular blockade occur more rapidly in the larynx than in the thumb (adductor pollicis). (From Donati F, Plaud B, Bevan DR. Vecuronium neuromuscular blockade at the adductor muscle of the larynx and at the adductor pollicis. *Anesthesiology.* 1991;74:833.)

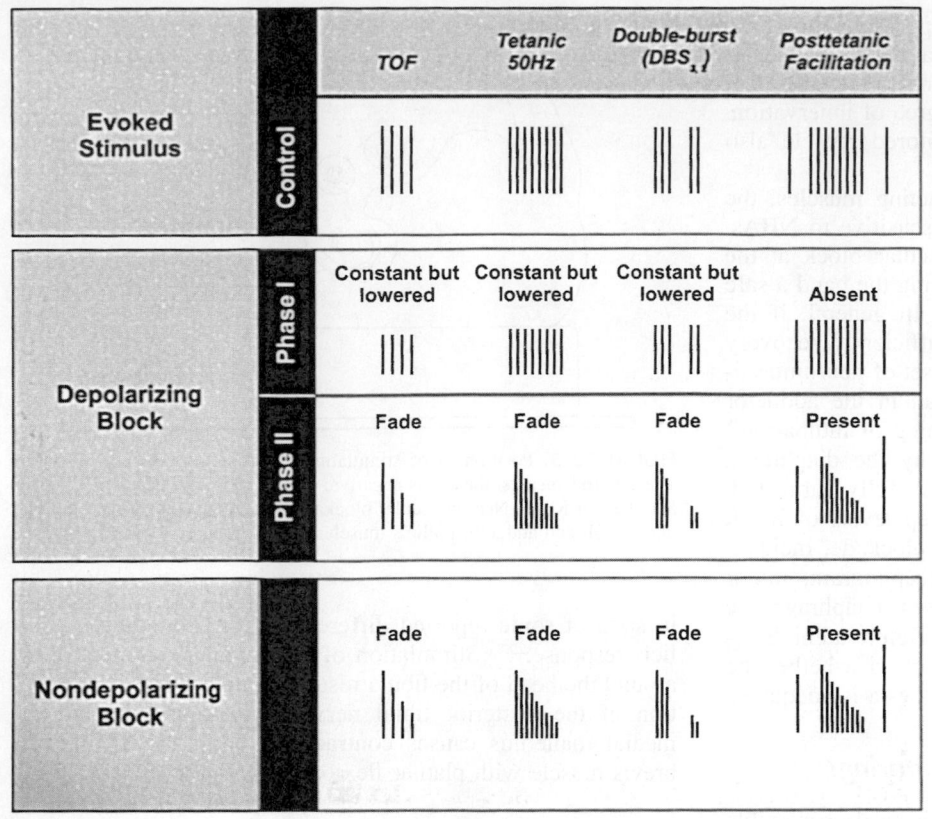

**FIGURE 22–6.** Supramaximal nerve stimulation responses during depolarizing and nondepolarizing block.

reliable.[25] Stimulus at higher frequency (100 Hz) has been claimed to work better. That claim, too, is controversial; even without NBAs, some patients show fading with such high-frequency stimulation. A few patients recall tetanic stimulation as an annoying way to wake up from anesthesia. In short, tetanic stimulation does not offer information that the TOF does not provide more reliably.

## Single Twitch

In the ST stimulation mode, a single supramaximal electrical stimulus pulse of 0.2 to 0.3 millisecond is applied to a motor nerve. ST can be repeated every 1 to 10 seconds (ie, at a frequency of 1-0.1 Hz). Today, ST has rather limited application, but it can be used to time the onset of neuromuscular block in preparation for tracheal intubation. At the onset of neuromuscular block, the observable decline in the ST response occurs when approximately 75% to 80% of receptors are blocked. However, all responses disappear when 90% to 95% of the receptors are blocked, which means that the window of clinical utility is narrow. For all practical purposes, TOF stimulation gives the same information and more.

## Train-of-Four

In TOF stimulation, four supramaximal electrical stimuli are generated at 0.5-second intervals (ie, at a frequency of 2 Hz). TOF can be used for monitoring throughout the procedure, from induction to recovery and extubation.[24,26] With repeated nerve stimulation, fade occurs, which is the progressive decrease in the evoked response as repetitive stimulation depletes the acetylcholine available in the prejunctional nerve

ending. The practical rule of thumb is that a stimulus pattern should not be repeated more often than every 10 to 12 seconds. If the rate is faster, consecutive stimuli may interfere with each other, altering the response at the level of the neuromuscular junction.

Fade always occurs with nondepolarizing NBAs. In contrast, fade is not seen with depolarizing phase I block. In the latter case, the four TOF responses decline evenly after a dose of succinylcholine. However, fade appears after a high dose, with the development of phase II depolarizing block.

## Train-of-Four Count

In deepening nondepolarizing neuromuscular block, fade progresses with each of the four TOF responses. The human eye cannot assess the small changes that distinguish subsequent responses, but it can detect the absence of a response. That ability enables us to report the number of visible responses. Therefore, the TOF count can be assigned values of 0 to 4. At deep levels of neuromuscular block (~75%), the fourth TOF twitch disappears. Disappearance of the third twitch represents the 80% block level, and that of the second twitch a 90% to 95% block. With adequate general anesthesia, a block with one to two visible twitches is appropriate for most surgical procedures. Sensitivity of the visual assessment may be improved by touching the patient's thumb and feeling the response. If recovery from block is assessed by eye or touch, the four twitches will be judged as restored to full strength while the level of block still is deep. Hence, the TOF count is suitable for judging levels of surgical neuromuscular blockade, but measurement of residual neuromuscular block at recovery requires the use of specific sensors.[27]

## Posttetanic Count

A tetanic stimulus, if given during a partial nondepolarizing block, increases the evoked response to the following STs. This phenomenon is called *posttetanic potentiation* or *facilitation* (PTF), and it can be useful in the estimation of deep neuromuscular blockade.[28] Without any responses to TOF or ST stimulation, it is difficult to measure the time elapsed before the drug level in the effector site drops sufficiently to allow these responses to reappear. In such situations, a posttetanic count (PTC) can be used to get an estimate.[29,30] To that end, tetanic 50-Hz stimulation is applied for 5 seconds (thought to mobilize acetylcholine at the nerve endings and set up the possibility of PTF). After a 3-second pause, continuous ST stimulation at 1 Hz is started. If responses after the PTF are detected, their number is counted. The larger the PTC (ie, the number of detected responses), the sooner the first TOF response will return. The PTC should not be obtained more often than every 6 minutes to avoid fatiguing the system.[31] A PTC of 10 or more indicates that the first TOF response will develop in a matter of minutes. If the block is excessive, and no evoked responses are seen, the PTC test fails to give any estimate; however, the anesthesiologist must first check the monitoring system to rule out a technical reason for lack of response (eg, loose connection, weak battery, dry electrode).

With deep levels of neuromuscular blockade, antagonists should never be given; their administration must wait until the block starts to recover. Usually it is appropriate to initiate reversal with neostigmine when one to two TOF responses are detected. This rule works especially well with drugs of intermediate duration because neostigmine then has enough time to reach its peak effect.

## Double-Burst Stimulation

DBS originally was thought to increase the likelihood of a correct tactile or visual assessment of a residual block.[32,33] DBS consists of two stimuli separated by 750 milliseconds, each consisting of 50-Hz tetanic bursts. Two modifications have been tested. In the DBS-3.3 mode, both of the short bursts comprise three tetanic pulses. In the DBS-3.2 mode, three pulses are followed by a burst of two. In either case, DBS elicits fade during nondepolarizing block because the two pulses are clearly separated.

Compared with the TOF monitor, which measures the response with a sensor, DBS cannot achieve the same accuracy during recovery.[34] However, when monitoring intense neuromuscular block, with no responses visible, the DBS response may reappear earlier than the TOF response. Hence, DBS may be an alternative to PTC measurement.[35]

## *What Objective Methods Are Available to Quantify the Response to Nerve Stimulation?*

Objective measurement of the evoked response allows increased accuracy compared with subjective assessment by the human observer. To quantify the evoked response, a measurement sensor must be attached to the target muscle. In particular, this makes the quantification of residual neuromuscular block possible. Many commercial devices allow automated monitoring of neuromuscular block at repeated intervals. Most also trigger an alarm if the level of block unexpectedly changes from that desired. Trends and graphic display of the response can give a more comprehensive picture of neuromuscular management. It may even be feasible to transfer that information to the automated anesthesia record.

Automated monitors of neuromuscular block usually can estimate the supramaximal current, and they also store the preblock TOF response as a reference value for later calculations. Most use TOF stimulation, basing the objective quantification of the response on one or more of the following variables:

- The ratio (T1%) of the first TOF response to the preblock reference is calculated and then used to assess the ST response. At the onset of blockade, T1% reflects fast changes; during surgical levels of blockade, when the first twitch usually remains visible, this ratio can be helpful in the administration of drugs. Estimates of residual block are based only on the TOF ratio calculations, however; neither T1% nor ST can provide that information.

- The TOF count, which was explained earlier, needs to be assessed every few minutes throughout the case. However, this repetitive task is easy to automate by using a simple piezoelectric sensor. Whether the clinician uses TOF count or T1% is a matter of personal preference. Both give the same information. However, T1% is often used for research, whereas the TOF count is less technical and may be better suited for clinical work.

- The TOF ratio is calculated by dividing the fourth response by the first response. For example, when all the responses are of the same size (eg, as occurs during succinylcholine phase I block with no fade), the TOF ratio is 1.0. The significant benefit of TOF ratio measurement is that there is no need for a reference value, which makes the estimation rather reliable. Hence, it is the most important single value to quantify residual neuromuscular blockade. Indeed, the human observer cannot estimate residual curarization reliably by eye or touch alone. In the past, TOF ratios of approximately 0.7 were regarded as acceptable, but that may not be enough. More recent studies have elucidated the risk factors associated with residual blockade and recommend better restoration of muscle strength. Hence, more complete recovery with TOF ratios in the range of 0.8 to 0.9 should be the goal.[3,8]

## Mechanomyography

The first sensors to measure the strength of muscle contraction, such as a rubber balloon fixed in the palm, were nonspecific and of limited accuracy. Improved accuracy was obtained by mechanomyography (MMG), a technique that measures the force of contraction of the muscle with a force displacement transducer. The devices are not small, and the hand must be fixed on an arm board.[36] Typically, evoked ulnar nerve stimulus responses are measured at the preloaded thumb. It is not easy to adjust the direction and position of the transducer, so an isometric adductor pollicis contraction is obtained. Because MMG has been used mostly for research, it has become the gold standard for neuromuscular monitoring research. Characteristic of the MMG TOF response is that in the beginning of monitoring, the response tends to increase gradually. Hence, the initial setup and stabilization of monitoring can be a time-consuming and distracting effort.

## Evoked Electromyography

After supramaximal nerve stimulation, the evoked compound muscle action potential (CMAP; evoked electromyography [EMG]) can be measured on the muscle. This response can be used for quantification of neuromuscular blockade. The contraction is always preceded by an electrical muscle action potential. Hence, the CMAP should not be equated with the motion of the thumb or MMG.[37,38] The CMAP response on the monitored muscle comprises the sum of single-fiber action potentials. That compound response is typically biphasic and of short duration (usually <20 milliseconds). Using modern electronics, the CMAP is easy to measure. The integrated area under the CMAP response curve is most often used for quantification. Deepening neuromuscular block results in a diminishing CMAP response amplitude and area.[39,40]

## *Electrode Positioning*

A total of five surface electrodes are needed for CMAP monitoring. The ulnar nerve (or some other site) is stimulated as usual with two electrodes. The CMAP response is recorded by two measurement electrodes, which must be positioned precisely to monitor the correct muscle. For successful monitoring, fresh electrocardiogram-type surface electrodes must be used. The electrode jelly must not be dry, but neither should it leak to the outside of the electrode. Insertion of a needle into a contracting muscle to measure its response is neither recommended nor necessary. The fifth electrode serves as the neutral reference, usually placed at the wrist distal to stimulus electrodes. Figure 22–7 shows the positioning of the surface electrodes for evoked EMG monitoring.

The active measurement electrode is placed on the muscle belly of either the adductor pollicis or the abductor digiti minimi (hypothenar) muscle. A third alternative, the first dorsal interosseous muscle, may be the best choice for clinical practice. This location is easy to identify, and the dorsum of the hand remains dry even with nonpremedicated patients. The site on the dorsal side of the hand is relatively insensitive to hand movement. Because the thumb need not be free in interosseous monitoring, keeping the patient's hand clenched in a fist may further stabilize monitoring. For adequate CMAP responses, the passive recording electrode needs to be positioned outside any active muscle (Fig. 22–8); my recommendation is to use the nearest finger.

Once the electrodes have been properly attached, the response remains fairly steady. However, gross movements, like repositioning of the upper extremity or moving the patient to the prone position, may change the previous reference value because of the altered position of the thumb in relation to the electrode. The drawback of EMG monitoring is its downward baseline drift, which occurs typically during the first 30 minutes of monitoring.[41] Cooling of the hand or a change in electrode impedance has been thought to be responsible, but more studies are needed. These effects usually alter the T1% response; after a complete recovery, it may reach a level of only approximately 80% of the preblock reference value. By definition, the TOF ratio is independent of the reference, and

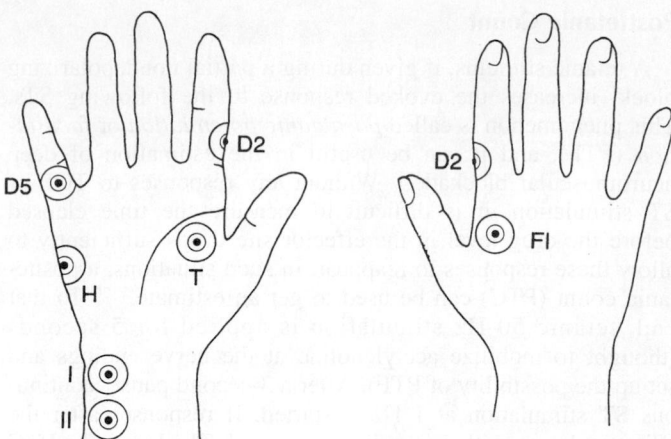

**FIGURE 22–7.** Stimulus and recording electrode positions for evoked electromyographic monitoring. The negative (I) and positive (II) stimulating electrodes are attached over the ulnar nerve at the wrist. For recording the response, it is important to position the active electrode on the muscle motor point. The indifferent electrode needs to be outside the active muscle; hence, the nearest finger is a good choice. The 3 ulnar nerve-innervated muscles for the active electrode position are the adductor pollicis (thenar; T), abductor digiti minimi (hypothenar; H), or the first dorsal interosseous (FI). D2 and D5 indicate the indifferent electrodes on the second or fifth finger. Hence, 1 of the 3 pairs of recording electrodes (T-D2, FI-D2, or H-D5) can be used. (Modified from Kalli I. Effect of surface electrode position on the compound action potential evoked by ulnar nerve stimulation during isoflurane anaesthesia. *Br J Anaesth.* 1990;65:495. © The Board of Management and Trustees of the *British Journal of Anaesthesia.* Reproduced by permission of Oxford University Press/*British Journal of Anaesthesia.*)

hence the measurement of residual block is not affected (Fig. 22–9). Graphic trends clearly illustrate changes in neuromuscular blockade. Evoked EMG monitoring became popular in the early 1980s, when the first commercial devices were launched on the market. Compared with MMG, it offers a less tedious alternative for objective monitoring of neuromuscular blockade. It has become a widely used research tool that also can be adapted to clinical routine (Fig. 22–10), but many

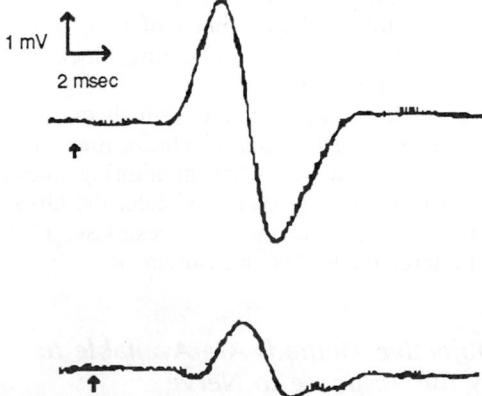

1 mV

2 msec

**FIGURE 22–8.** The high-amplitude, biphasic evoked electromyographic response (*top*), which was obtained before the onset of neuromuscular block, indicates correct positioning of the recording electrode on the adductor pollicis muscle. The multiphasic, low-amplitude response (*bottom*) demonstrates the effect of false electrode positioning on the response curve. (Modified from Kalli I. *Monitoring of Neuromuscular Blockade by Electromyography, With Special Reference to Clinical Application in Anaesthetized Infants and Children* [dissertation]. Helsinki, Finland: Helsinki University; 1991:30.)

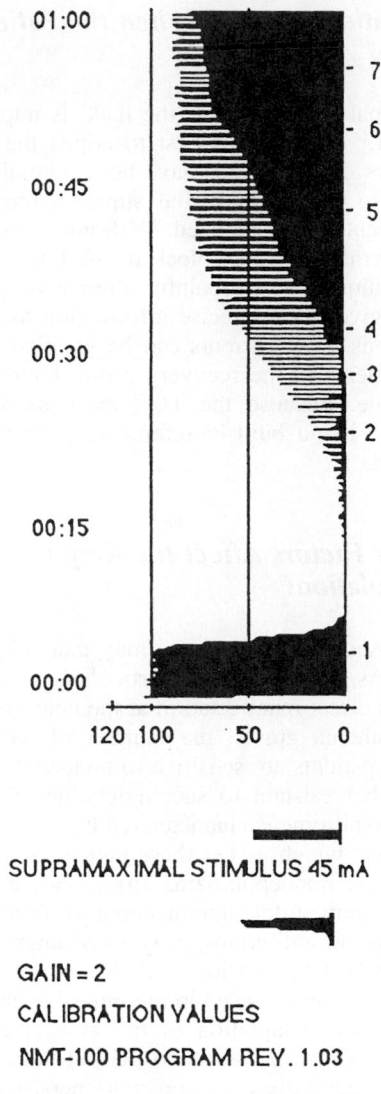

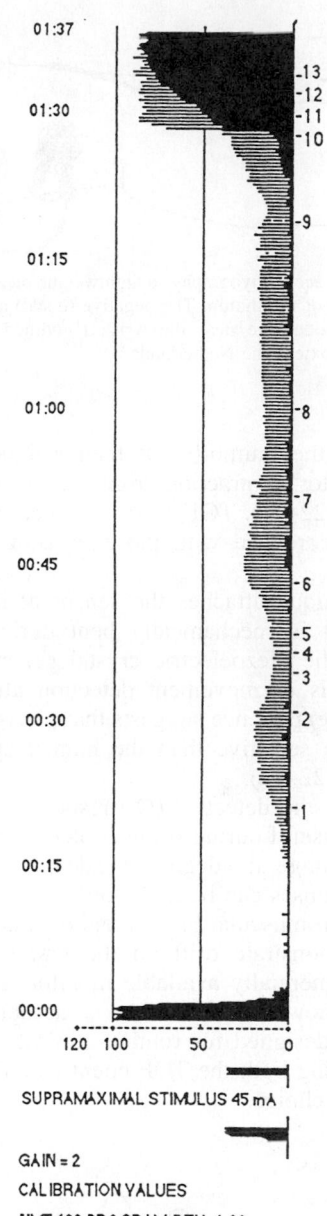

**FIGURE 22–9.** Evoked electromyographic recording showing the effect of 0.05 mg/kg vecuronium administered to the adult patient anesthetized for herniotomy. The first (T1) and the fourth (T4) response of each train-of-four (TOF) are converted into bars. During restoration of neuromuscular transmission, T1 often fails to reach the level of the preblock control. The TOF ratio, which is the measure of adequate clinical recovery, is obtained by dividing T4 by T1; hence, it is independent of any control value. (From Kalli I. *Monitoring of Neuromuscular Blockade by Electromyography, With Special Reference to Clinical Application in Anaesthetized Infants and Children* [dissertation]. Helsinki, Finland: Helsinki University; 1991:27.)

regard the need to position five electrodes as a constraint to its widespread use.

## Are Piezoelectric Sensors a Clinical Alternative?

Piezoelectric movement or acceleration transducers, which can simply be taped or fixed to the thumb, may be a lightweight alternative for routine anesthesia and intensive care. Accelomyography is a variant of the piezoelectric sensor technique in which a small, light transducer is usually attached

**FIGURE 22–10.** Evoked electromyographic recording closely demonstrating changes when the atracurium infusion is adjusted manually to achieve a steady state during intravenous general anesthesia. Event numbers to the right of the recording refer to the following clinical comments. (1) Spontaneous recovery of neuromuscular blockade after administration of the bolus dose (atracurium 0.4 mg/kg) has begun. Atracurium infusion is initiated at the rate of 0.6 mg/kg/h. (2) The initial infusion rate turns the spontaneous recovery to deepening blockade. (3-4) Infusion stopped. (5) Spontaneous recovery of neuromuscular blockade again detected. (6) New infusion rate of 0.5 mg/kg/h. (7) Neuromuscular blockade deepens and the infusion rate is decreased to 0.4 mg/kg/h. (8) Slightly deepening neuromuscular blockade. Consequently, the infusion rate is decreased to 0.35 mg/kg/h, resulting in a steady state. (9) Infusion stopped. Short drop in T1 level is caused by a minor bolus dose when the syringe is loosened. (10) Partial spontaneous recovery is enhanced by edrophonium with atropine, resulting in the complete recovery of T1 and T4. (11-13) Again, the completely recovered T1 level does not reach the preoperative control level, but the fully recovered train-of-four ratio of 1.0 indicates complete clinical recovery. (From Kalli I. *Monitoring of Neuromuscular Blockade by Electromyography, With Special Reference to Clinical Application in Anaesthetized Infants and Children* [dissertation]. Helsinki, Finland: Helsinki University; 1991:17.)

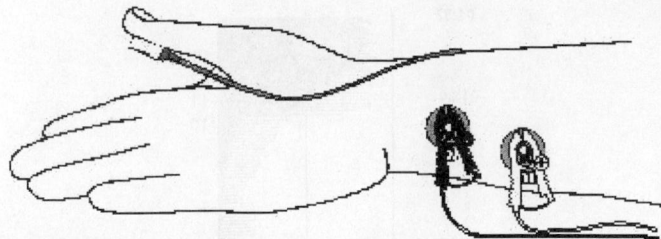

**FIGURE 22–11.** In accelomyography, a lightweight piezoelectric sensor is attached near the tip of the thumb. The negative (distal) and positive (proximal) stimulus electrodes are near the wrist. (Modified from material by Organon Teknika, Boxtel, The Netherlands.)

near the tip of the thumb.[42,43] It then estimates the degree of thumb adductor contraction from the acceleration of the movement (Fig. 22–11). TOF ratios obtained by accelomyography are in accordance with those measured by MMG or evoked EMG.

Another technique attaches the sensor at the base of the thumb, where it is mechanically bent during movement.[44] When twisted, the piezoelectric crystal generates a voltage, creating the basis of movement detection after ulnar nerve stimulation. My experience suggests that piezoelectric sensors are clearly more sensitive than the human eye in detecting movement (Fig. 22–12).

Calculation of the detected TOF responses gives the TOF count, which is useful during surgical block. From the proportional voltage change, the degree of fade between the first and fourth TOF responses can be measured.

Typically, neuromuscular block monitors that use piezoelectric sensors demonstrate drift on the first twitch response. Hence, the commercially available monitors in this category usually do not show the T1% value, an acceptable solution if the devices are designed for routine clinical use and not for research. Providing both the TOF count and TOF ratio offers the clinician the choice.

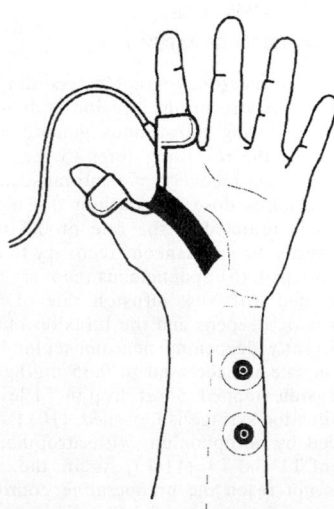

**FIGURE 22–12.** A piezoelectric movement transducer is placed between the thumb and the index finger and secured by a piece of tape. Optimized for clinical work, it detects the number of counts during surgical block but can also measure the postoperative recovery of the train-of-four ratio. (Modified from material by Datex-Ohmeda, Helsinki, Finland.)

## Can Stimulation Be Used When the Patient Is Awake?

Supramaximal stimulation of the hand is unpleasant to an awake subject.[14] Hence, it is best to adjust the current only after analgesics or anesthetics have been administered. There is no reason to use anything but supramaximal stimulation when the patient is anesthetized.[11,12] Sometimes, when there is doubt concerning residual block in the PACU, use of submaximal stimulus as a less painful alternative has been suggested[17]; this gives more precise information than assessment by clinical signs. Low currents can be justified because with spot measurements in the recovery room, long-term stability is not an issue. Because the TOF ratio, as a measure of residual block, has a built-in reference, preinduction values are not needed.

## What Other Factors Affect the Response to Nerve Stimulation?

Some diseases and medications may markedly modify the effect of NBAs. Monitoring is particularly important if the disease has its direct manifestation at the neuromuscular junction. In myasthenia gravis, the number of receptors is decreased. Such patients are sensitive to nondepolarizing NBAs, but they can be resistant to succinylcholine. Eaton-Lambert (myasthenic) syndrome is characterized by a decreased release of acetylcholine, which makes these patients sensitive to both depolarizing and nondepolarizing drugs. Some medications, such as magnesium sulfate administered to obstetric patients[45] or aminoglycoside antibiotics, may have unexpected effects on neuromuscular transmission.

NBAs are increasingly used in the intensive care unit (ICU) to improve patient adaptation to the mechanical ventilator. Mounting evidence shows that ICU patients treated with NBAs for days[4,46,47] may demonstrate persistent weakness, leading to delayed weaning and prolonged hospital stay. Although not always a routine procedure in the ICU, intermittent monitoring using a nerve stimulator should always be considered. Assessment of block only by observing patient movement may be misleading; such movement may demonstrate pain, but deepening the neuromuscular block is no cure for that. Indeed, adequate analgesia and sedation are crucial for patients undergoing neuromuscular block.

## References

1. Viby-Mogensen J, Jorgensen BC, Ording H. Residual curarization in the recovery room. *Anesthesiology.* 1979;50:539.
2. Miller RD. How should residual neuromuscular blockade be detected? [editorial] [see comments]. *Anesthesiology.* 1989;70:79.
3. Kopman AF, Yee PS, Neuman GG. Relationship of the train-of-four fade ratio to clinical signs and symptoms of residual paralysis in awake volunteers [see comments]. *Anesthesiology.* 1997;86:765.
4. Zarowitz BJ, Rudis MI, Lai K, et al. Retrospective pharmacoeconomic evaluation of dosing vecuronium by peripheral nerve stimulation versus standard clinical assessment in critically ill patients. *Pharmacotherapy.* 1997;17:327.
5. Lubarsky DA, Glass PS, Ginsberg B, et al. The successful implementation of pharmaceutical practice guidelines: analysis of associated outcomes and cost savings. SWiPE Group. Systematic Withdrawal of Perioperative Expenses [see comments]. *Anesthesiology.* 1997;86:1145.
6. Bevan DR, Smith CE, Donati F. Postoperative neuromuscular blockade:

a comparison between atracurium, vecuronium, and pancuronium. *Anesthesiology.* 1988;69:272.

7. Eriksson LI, Sato M, Severinghaus JW. Effect of a vecuronium-induced partial neuromuscular block on hypoxic ventilatory response. *Anesthesiology.* 1993;78:693.

8. Berg H, Roed J, Viby-Mogensen J, et al. Residual neuromuscular block is a risk factor for postoperative pulmonary complications: a prospective, randomised, and blinded study of postoperative pulmonary complications after atracurium, vecuronium and pancuronium. *Acta Anaesthesiol Scand.* 1997;41:1095.

9. Pavlin EG, Holle RH, Schoene RB. Recovery of airway protection compared with ventilation in humans after paralysis with curare [see comments]. *Anesthesiology.* 1989;70:381.

10. Mason LJ, Betts EK. Leg lift and maximum inspiratory force, clinical signs of neuromuscular blockade reversal in neonates and infants. *Anesthesiology.* 1980;52:441.

11. Kopman AF, Lawson D. Milliamperage requirements for supramaximal stimulation of the ulnar nerve with surface electrodes. *Anesthesiology.* 1984;61:83.

12. Berger JJ, Gravenstein JS, Munson ES. Electrode polarity and peripheral nerve stimulation. *Anesthesiology.* 1982;56:402.

13. Rosenberg H, Greenhow DE. Peripheral nerve stimulator performance: the influence of output polarity and electrode placement. *Can Anaesth Soc J.* 1978;25:424.

14. Brull SJ, Silverman DG. Pulse width, stimulus intensity, electrode placement, and polarity during assessment of neuromuscular block [see comments] [published erratum appears in *Anesthesiology.* 1996;84:1014]. *Anesthesiology.* 1995;83:702.

15. Heier T, Caldwell JE, Eriksson LI, et al. The effect of hypothermia on adductor pollicis twitch tension during continuous infusion of vecuronium in isoflurane-anesthetized humans. *Anesth Analg.* 1994;78:312.

16. Pansard JL, Chauvin M, Lebrault C, et al. Effect of an intubating dose of succinylcholine and atracurium on the diaphragm and the adductor pollicis muscle in humans. *Anesthesiology.* 1987;67:326.

17. Brull SJ, Ehrenwerth J, Connelly NR, et al. Assessment of residual curarization using low-current stimulation. *Can J Anaesth.* 1991;38:164.

18. Donati F, Meistelman C, Plaud B. Vecuronium neuromuscular blockade at the adductor muscles of the larynx and adductor pollicis. *Anesthesiology.* 1991;74:833.

19. Caffrey RR, Warren ML, Becker KE Jr. Neuromuscular blockade monitoring comparing the orbicularis oculi and adductor pollicis muscles. *Anesthesiology.* 1986;65:95.

20. Donati F, Meistelman C, Plaud B. Vecuronium neuromuscular blockade at the diaphragm, the orbicularis oculi, and adductor pollicis muscles. *Anesthesiology.* 1990;73:870.

21. Leslie K, Iatrou CC, Jones K, et al. Common peroneal nerve stimulation for neuromuscular monitoring: evaluation in awake volunteers and anesthetized patients. *Anesth Analg.* 1999;88:197.

22. Beemer GH. Monitoring neuromuscular blockade with calf stimulators. *Anaesth Intensive Care.* 1987;15:375.

23. Saitoh Y, Koitabashi Y, Makita K, et al. Train-of-four and double burst stimulation fade at the great toe and thumb. *Can J Anaesth.* 1997;44:390.

24. Ali HH, Utting JE, Gray C. Stimulus frequency in the detection of neuromuscular block in humans. *Br J Anaesth.* 1970;42:967.

25. Dupuis JY, Martin R, Tessonnier JM, et al. Clinical assessment of the muscular response to tetanic nerve stimulation. *Can J Anaesth.* 1990;37:397.

26. Ali HH, Savarese JJ, Lebowitz PW, et al. Twitch, tetanus and train-of-four as indices of recovery from nondepolarizing neuromuscular blockade. *Anesthesiology.* 1981;54:294.

27. Viby-Mogensen J, Jensen NH, Engbaek J, et al. Tactile and visual evaluation of the response to train-of-four nerve stimulation. *Anesthesiology.* 1985;63:440.

28. Ali HH, Savarese JJ. Monitoring of neuromuscular function. *Anesthesiology.* 1976;45:216.

29. Muchhal KK, Viby-Mogensen J, Fernando PU, et al. Evaluation of intense neuromuscular blockade caused by vecuronium using posttetanic count (PTC). *Anesthesiology.* 1987;66:846.

30. Viby-Mogensen J, Howardy-Hansen P, Chraemmer-Jorgensen B, et al. Posttetanic count (PTC): a new method of evaluating an intense nondepolarizing neuromuscular blockade. *Anesthesiology.* 1981;55:458.

31. Howardy-Hansen P, Viby-Mogensen J, Gottschau A, et al. Tactile evaluation of the posttetanic count (PTC). *Anesthesiology.* 1984;60:372.

32. Engbaek J, Ostergaard D, Viby-Mogensen J. Double burst stimulation (DBS): a new pattern of nerve stimulation to identify residual neuromuscular block [see comments]. *Br J Anaesth.* 1989;62:274.

33. Drenck NE, Ueda N, Olsen NV, et al. Manual evaluation of residual curarization using double burst stimulation: a comparison with train-of-four. *Anesthesiology.* 1989;70:578.

34. Fruergaard K, Viby-Mogensen J, Berg H, et al. Tactile evaluation of the response to double burst stimulation decreases, but does not eliminate, the problem of postoperative residual paralysis. *Acta Anaesthesiol Scand.* 1998;42:1168.

35. Kirkegaard Nielsen H, May O. Double burst stimulation for monitoring profound neuromuscular blockade: a comparison with posttetanic count and train of four. *Acta Anaesthesiol Belg.* 1992;43:253.

36. Epstein RA, Epstein RM. The electromyogram and the mechanical response of indirectly stimulated muscle in anesthetized man following curarization. *Anesthesiology.* 1973;38:212.

37. Kopman AF. The relationship of evoked electromyographic and mechanical responses following atracurium in humans. *Anesthesiology.* 1985;63:208.

38. Engbaek J, Ostergaard D, Viby-Mogensen J, et al. Clinical recovery and train-of-four ratio measured mechanically and electromyographically following atracurium. *Anesthesiology.* 1989;71:391.

39. Engbaek J, Skovgaard LT, Fries B, et al. Monitoring of neuromuscular transmission by electromyography (II): evoked compound EMG area, amplitude and duration compared to mechanical twitch recording during onset and recovery of pancuronium-induced blockade in the cat. *Acta Anaesthesiol Scand.* 1993;37:788.

40. Kalli I. Effect of isometric thumb preload on the evoked compound muscle action potential. *Br J Anaesth.* 1993;70:92.

41. Meretoja OA, Theroux M. Can final EMG baseline be used as a reference to calculate neuromuscular recovery? *Acta Anaesthesiol Scand.* 1997;41:492.

42. Jensen E, Viby-Mogensen J, Bang U. The Accelograph: a new neuromuscular transmission monitor. *Acta Anaesthesiol Scand.* 1988;32:49.

43. Saitoh Y, Fujii Y, Ueki M, et al. Accelographic and mechanical posttetanic count and train-of-four ratio assessed at the great toe. *Eur J Anaesthesiol.* 1998;15:649.

44. Kern SE, Johnson JO, Westenskow DR, et al. An effectiveness study of a new piezoelectric sensor for train-of-four measurement [see comments]. *Anesth Analg.* 1994;78:978.

45. Kwan WF, Lee C, Chen BJ. A noninvasive method in the differential diagnosis of vecuronium-induced and magnesium-induced protracted neuromuscular block in a severely preeclamptic patient. *J Clin Anesth.* 1996;8:392.

46. Rudis MI, Sikora CA, Angus E, et al. A prospective, randomized, controlled evaluation of peripheral nerve stimulation versus standard clinical dosing of neuromuscular blocking agents in critically ill patients [see comments]. *Crit Care Med.* 1997;25:575.

47. Frankel H, Jeng J, Tilly E, et al. The impact of implementation of neuromuscular blockade monitoring standards in a surgical intensive care unit. *Am Surg.* 1996;62:503.

# 23

# Monitoring During Patient Transport

Gregory M. Gullahorn

BASIC CONSIDERATIONS
*Why Monitor?*
*What Does Intrahospital Transport Entail?*

A RATIONAL APPROACH
*What Factors Determine Monitoring Requirements?*
*How Is a Patient Prepared for Transport?*
*How Is the Transport Phase Managed?*
*What Problems Occur in the Posttransport Stabilization Phase?*

SELECTION OF MONITORS
*What Factors Should Be Considered?*

Anesthesiologists use a vast array of monitors to assess the physiologic status of patients as well as the functional status of the anesthesia machine, ventilator, and other life support equipment. Such monitoring is applied not only in the operating room (OR) and intensive care unit (ICU) but also in the postanesthesia care unit (PACU) and emergency department, where anesthesiologists may routinely be involved in patients' care. We feel uncomfortable managing critically ill or anesthetized patients without monitoring in such settings; yet, what parameters should be monitored while transporting patients between these locations or to other diagnostic and therapeutic areas in the hospital is less clear. A number of questions must be addressed.

## BASIC CONSIDERATIONS

### *Why Monitor?*

Patients who have serious illnesses or injuries or who are anesthetized may have altered organ system function and abnormal responses to stress.[1,2] We use our senses—and monitors as an extension of these senses—to identify trends or problems that require intervention and then to assess the effects of therapy. Monitors that check functions on which our treatment may have an impact are clearly the most efficacious (ie, pulse oximeters to evaluate the adequacy of oxygenation in anesthetized or sedated patients, or those with compromised respiratory status, and electrocardiography [ECG] in patients at risk for cardiac dysrhythmias).

In the OR and the ICU, these monitors are well established (see also Chapters 20-22, 48). In all settings, simple inspection is the most basic and least invasive form of monitoring. Precordial or esophageal stethoscopes, pulse oximetry, ECG, blood pressure (BP) (invasive or noninvasive) measurement, inspired gas monitoring, and capnography now represent standards of care in the OR. Temperature monitoring and assessment of neuromuscular activity are indicated by a patient's status and the surgery. During general anesthesia with controlled ventilation, spirometry is strongly recommended, and continuous use of a disconnect detection system is required.[3]

Anesthesiologists would be hesitant to administer a full induction dose of sodium thiopental to a pale, diaphoretic trauma victim and would pause before performing laryngoscopy and intubation on a patient with an intracranial aneurysm without measuring BP. At the end of surgery, however, less concern may be directed to a patient who is making a quick trip from the OR to the PACU or the ICU. In this era of managed care, we may be pushed not to delay transfer if a transport monitor is not readily available, with the justification that the time frame will be short. Realistically, however, is the potential for fluctuations in BP, changes in heart rate or rhythm, problems with oxygenation or unplanned extubation any less during this transport process, and are these considerations less important because of the hopefully limited time frame?

Hypoxemia is common during emergence from anesthesia. Similarly, patients who are intubated and ventilated may be at risk for hypocapnia and hemodynamic changes during transport. Patients who are critically ill or who have undergone major surgical procedures may experience hypotension, hypertension, or cardiac dysrhythmias.

### Cardiovascular Changes

Using a complex mobile monitoring system, Taylor and colleagues found life-threatening dysrhythmias in 22 of 50 cardiac patients during intrahospital transport, with some dysrhythmias in fully 80% of patients.[4] Insel and colleagues examined cardiovascular changes occurring during transport from the OR to the ICU after major general or vascular surgery, carotid endarterectomy, or coronary artery bypass. In the first three groups, significant increases in BP, pulse, and initial lability were noted. In the major vascular/general surgery group, 20% of patients required vigorous fluid resuscitation for hypotension on arrival in the ICU, and 36% required either nitroglycerin or sodium nitroprusside for control of hypertension.[5] In a more recent study of cost and complications during in-hospital transport, Hurst and coworkers identified at least one significant physiologic change in 66% of transported patients, lasting a minimum of 5 minutes.[6] Changes in heart rate or blood pressure were the most common.

## Hypoxemia

Hypoxemia may also be common. Tyler and associates reported a 35% incidence of decreased oxyhemoglobin saturation (SaO$_2$) to <90% during the transport of adults from the OR to the PACU; 12% fell to <85%.[7] Healthy pediatric patients appear to be equally at risk. Kataria and coworkers found that even with 3 minutes of 100% O$_2$ administration after surgery, a significant age-related reduction in SaO$_2$ occurred during a 120- to 180-second transfer to the PACU. The mean SaO$_2$ was 88% in children <6 months of age.[8]

Tomkins and colleagues examined children with American Society of Anesthesiologists physical status I or II and found that 24% had an SaO$_2$ <90% during the first 10 minutes after anesthesia. Clinical signs such as cyanosis or upper airway obstruction correlated poorly with measured hypoxemia.[9] "Modest" desaturation was also demonstrated in adult patients during transfer from an anesthesia induction room to the OR. Despite an average transfer time of only 51 seconds, 21 of 25 patients had a decline in SaO$_2$. In 2 patients, a decrease to 90% occurred. All patients were either apneic or breathing room air.[10]

Hensley and colleagues, in a study of patients being prepared for cardiac surgery, found that after a standard premedication with morphine and scopolamine, 60% had an arterial oxygen saturation measured by pulse oximetry (SpO$_2$) of <90%. All patients were awake or judged to be easily arousable, and almost half actually required additional sedation during placement of invasive monitors.[11]

Although the risk of hypoxemia in most postsurgical patients during a brief transfer from the OR to the PACU is minimized by routine administration of supplemental O$_2$, the potential for mishaps probably increases with prolonged transit times en route to an ICU and in patients with preexisting or new-onset pulmonary disease. In these patients, it may be necessary to verify the adequacy of treatment by monitoring SpO$_2$.

## *What Does Intrahospital Transport Entail?*

Many experienced anesthesiologists correctly assume that the potential for clinically significant problems during transfer from the OR is fairly remote except in specific population groups; the challenge is to identify those at risk. The possibility of adverse events may be just as pronounced in other types of intrahospital transport. Venkataraman and Orr defined four common scenarios for intrahospital transport[12] (Table 23–1).

## Conceptual Differences

Vigilance is the cornerstone of anesthesiology and is vital in all transport scenarios. However, differences do exist. When

**TABLE 23–1.** Common Intrahospital Transport Scenarios

**Movement From Critical Care Areas**
OR TO PACU
OR to ward
ICU ward
**One-way Transfer to Critical Care Areas**
ED to OR or ICU
Ward to OR or ICU
**Round-Trip Transport Between Critical Care and Noncritical Care Areas**
ICU to radiology and back
ICU to cardiac catheterization laboratory and back
**Transfer Between Critical Care Areas**
ICU to OR
OR to ICU or PACU
ED to OR or ICU

ED, emergency department; ICU, intensive care unit; OR, operating room; PACU, postanesthesia care unit.

patients leave a critical care setting, their physiologic status should be stable, with continued normalization expected. They no longer need as intensive monitoring as they had in the OR or ICU. Major risks involve airway problems or changing level of consciousness.

Patients being taken to a critical care area, however, present different problems. Examples include trauma victims transported to the OR after initial resuscitation in the emergency room or septic patients who have deteriorated on the ward and are now being transferred to the ICU. In these settings, the baseline requirements for monitoring are increasing as the potential for significant physiologic changes grows.

## Secondary Insults

In head-injured patients, *secondary insults* such as hypoxia, hypotension, and intracranial hypertension clearly worsen outcome.[13] Andrews and colleagues found secondary insults during transport in 47% of patients being transferred from the emergency department. Eighty percent of these patients sustain secondary injuries within 4 hours of their transfer.[14] Significantly, Gentlemen and Jennet reported airway compromise in 43 of 164 head-injured patients on arrival at a neurosurgical unit; 15% to 22% of patients were hypoxic.[13] Patients who sustained a secondary insult were much more likely to end up dead, vegetative, or severely disabled compared with those who did not (76% versus 44%). Better monitoring of these patients might have a profound impact on outcome if problems leading to secondary injury can be identified and corrected.

## Critical Care Transport

Modern critical care units provide extensive monitoring of physiologic functions and multiple life support modalities. The ICU concentrates equipment and personnel who are experienced in managing severely ill or injured patients, as well as the complications they may experience. For those of us involved in critical care, transporting patients from the ICU to other parts of the hospital and back is sure to evoke anxiety. Any anesthesiologist may be called on to assist in this process, however. The provision of sedation or anesthetic support for unstable or combative patients who must undergo computed tomographic (CT) scans, angiography, other invasive radiologic procedures, magnetic resonance imaging, or even radiation therapy is increasingly common.

## Transport of Anesthetized Patients

Movement of critically ill or anesthetized patients to and from these ancillary areas presents special logistical and clinical challenges; the decision to proceed with such moves must carefully weigh the potential benefits of the planned procedure or test against the potential for misadventure. In Hurst and colleagues' study of 100 surgery and trauma patients transported from the ICU for diagnostic studies, 66% had significant physiologic changes lasting >5 minutes, and in 1992 resulted in an average patient charge of $612, with an actual cost to the hospital of $452. Of the diagnostic studies, 61% resulted in no change in management. Angiography or abdominal CT scan studies were most likely to effect a change in management, whereas head CT scans were the least.[6] Venkataraman and Orr divide adverse events during transport into physiologic changes and equipment mishaps.[12] Small changes in heart rate or BP may be of no consequence, whereas unplanned extubation or the loss of intravenous access in a patient requiring multiple pressors for hemodynamic support can be lethal. The potential exists for changes or problems to occur in virtually all organ systems (Table 23–2). Clearly, early detection of such changes is critically important for definitive intervention.

## Mortality

In the 1970s, Waddell reported a 5-month study of both critically ill ICU patients and postoperative patients who had undergone at least one intrahospital transport. Among the critically ill patients, one per month sustained cardiac arrest or died of causes attributed to the transport process.[15]

A review of interhospital transport of critically ill pediatric patients by Kanter and associates, in 1992, showed an excess morbidity rate of 9.6% attributed to the transport process alone, compared with control ICU patients who did not undergo transport.[16]

## Mechanically Ventilated Patients

Many patients in an ICU require ventilatory support and are prone to transport complications related to inadvertent changes in tidal volume, minute ventilation, continuous positive airway pressure (CPAP), or ventilatory mode. These changes may adversely affect the cardiovascular system, intracranial pressure (ICP), or cerebral perfusion pressure. Patients with pulmonary hypertension, and especially those with right-to-left intracardiac shunts, may be particularly sensitive to changes in $Paco_2$ and ventilation.

Braman and colleagues prospectively studied changes in arterial blood gas partial pressures and hemodynamic parameters in 36 ventilator-dependent patients who required procedures outside the ICU.[17] Two groups were examined: the first was ventilated manually during transport and the second by a portable, volume-limited ventilator (with settings matched to the bedside ventilator). Several patients in both groups had significant (>10 mm Hg) changes in $Paco_2$ and pH, as well as hypotension; however, the incidence was considerably greater in the manually ventilated group (75% versus 44%), and new cardiac dysrhythmias developed in 2 patients. Hypotension and dysrhythmias were strongly correlated with blood gas deterioration.

Gervais and associates found that both manual ventilation

**TABLE 23–2.** Potential Complications During Transport

| Physiologic | Technical |
| --- | --- |
| ***Respiratory*** | |
| Hypoxemia/desaturtion | Airway obstruction/loss of unprotected airway |
| Hypercapnia/respiratory acidosis | Unplanned extubation |
| Hypocapnia/respiratory alkalosis | Endotracheal tube obstruction |
| Tachypnea/bradypnea | Inability to match bedside ventilator mode/parameters |
| Bronchospasm | Lack of central oxygen lines at diagnostic/procedure locations |
| Aspiration | |
| Pneumothorax | Loss of oxygen supply |
| Increased airway pressures and hemodynamic compromise | Chest tube loss or malfunction |
| ***Cardiovascular*** | |
| Hypotension/hypertension | Electrocardiograph lead disconnect/artifact |
| Hypervolemia/fluid overload | |
| Hypovolemia/bleeding | Invasive arterial or venous catheter loss/disconnect |
| Congestive heart failure/pulmonary edema | Vasoactive drug infusion disconnect/loss/bolus |
| Ischemia/infarction | Monitor failure |
| Arrhythmias/cardiac arrest | Pacemaker malfunction |
| Decreased cardiac output | IABP malfunction |
| Shock/inadequate tissue perfusion | Inability to fit IABP in elevator |
| Compromise of anastomoses/grafts/bypasses | Transducer artifact/malfunction |
| ***Neurologic*** | |
| Increased intracranial pressure | Change in position |
| Decreased cerebral perfusion pressure | Inability to maintain spine stabilization/traction |
| Inadequate cerebral blood flow | Inability to maintain adequate head-up positioning |
| Excessive cerebral blood flow/blood volume | Inadequate/excessive sedation or analgesia |
| Seizures | Intracranial pressure monitor loss or malfunction |
| Cerebral edema | |
| Cerebral hemorrhage | Ventriculostomy loss |
| Stroke | Loss of electrophysiologic or electroencephalographic monitoring |
| Herniation | |
| ***Other*** | |
| Metabolic acidosis/alkalosis | Tangled/mislabeled infusion and monitoring catheters |
| Hyperglycemia/hypoglycemia | Pulled surgical drain/catheter |
| Hypothermia/hyperthermia | Pulled nasogastric or feeding tube |
| Oliguria/diabetes insipidus | Pulled Foley catheter |
| | Difficulty with temperature control |
| | Malfunction of compression stockings |
| | Missed medications/therapies |
| | Infusion pump battery loss |
| | Bed malfunction |
| | Elevator malfunction |

IABP, intraaortic balloon pump.

without volume monitoring and portable mechanical ventilation with preset but unmonitored volumes resulted in significant decreases in $Paco_2$ and increases in pH.[18] These changes were not noted when tidal volume was controlled using a spirometer during manual ventilation.

Palmon and colleagues examined the efficacy of end-tidal $CO_2$ ($Petco_2$) monitoring in controlling $Paco_2$ during hand ventilation for transport.[19] Three groups were studied: (1) a no-monitor, (2) a monitor-blind, and (3) a monitored group. Ventilation was performed by experienced anesthesia residents during transports lasting an average of 5 to 6 minutes. Although there were no differences in pretransport and posttransport $Paco_2$ levels among groups, there was significantly more individual variability in the no-monitor and monitor-blind groups. Ten patients in the no-monitor and monitor-blind groups had a >10 mm Hg difference in baseline and posttransport $P_{ETCO_2}$, whereas no patient in the monitored group had a difference >7 mm Hg.[19]

Tobias and associates studied the effects of manual ventilation during transportation on $P_{ETCO_2}$ in children who were being hyperventilated to a $Paco_2$ of 25 to 30 mm Hg for control of ICP.[20] Patients ranged in age from 7 months to 14 years. Despite attempting to match ventilation, unintentional excessive hyperventilation occurred >62% of the time. Twenty-three percent of measurements showed a $P_{ETCO_2}$ <20 mm Hg, and $P_{ETCO_2}$ values were between 25 and 30 mm Hg only 31% of the time.[20] Excessive hyperventilation may have the unintended consequence of increasing regional areas of cerebral ischemia, particularly in patients with cerebral vasospasm.

### Adverse Effects of Positive Airway Pressure

Changes in airway pressure may have profound impact on venous return, BP, and intracranial elastance. Unrecognized changes in $Po_2$, $Pco_2$, pH, and BP are potentially deleterious for patients with coronary or cerebrovascular disease, congenital heart disease, pulmonary hypertension, and especially head injuries. Such patients are of particular concern because they are likely to undergo multiple transports to CT or magnetic resonance imaging scanning facilities, the OR, or the angiography suite.

In Gentleman and Jennet's review, more than one third of deaths in patients referred to a neurosurgical unit had avoidable contributing factors.[13] Andrews and coworkers' series showed that during transport of head-injured patients from the ICU, pretransfer insults (eg, episodes of hypotension, hypoxia, or intracranial hypertension) were predictive of increased ICP during transport and the likelihood of further insults during the first 4 hours after return to the ICU.[14] This observation supports the admonition that adequate resuscitation and stabilization are vital before transport.

Bekar and colleagues looked at changes in severely head-injured patients who were transported for follow-up CT scans.[21] All patients were intubated and mechanically hyperventilated to $Paco_2$ of 27 to 30 mm Hg. They were sedated with propofol and fentanyl by infusion and also received vecuronium for neuromuscular blockade by infusion. In addition to standard monitors, all patients had a ventriculostomy and a fiberoptic ICP monitor. During transportation, patients were manually ventilated. Sixty percent of patients had an increase in ICP, with an average increase of 27%. The highest values were during the CT scan itself, when patients were prone. A mean decrease in $Paco_2$ of 16% was noted during manual ventilation.[21]

### Complications

Smith and colleagues reviewed 125 intrahospital transports from the ICU to identify factors related to mishaps.[22] The latter were defined as events having a detrimental effect on a patient's stability (eg, monitor failure, intravenous catheter infiltration or disconnect, vasoactive drug infusion disconnect, ventilator disconnects, extubation, invasive monitor- or line-related mishaps). More than one third of transports involved at least one mishap, and 11% involved multiple events. On return to the ICU, 24% of patients were judged to be less stable.

### Intensive Care Unit to Computed Tomography Scanner

Several interesting factors were apparent in this series. Mishaps were more common during transport to the CT scanner than to any other location, especially when a delay occurred at the destination. Transfer of a patient from the bed to the scanner and physical isolation during scanning were believed to be significant contributors. Overall, 75% of mishaps occurred at the study site. Surprisingly, no correlation was noted between the number of catheters and monitors and the likelihood of mishaps, nor was an increased incidence of mishaps noted during emergent transports, perhaps reflecting increased vigilance in these settings.

### Critical Care to Critical Care

When a patient is transferred between critical care areas (from the OR to ICU or from the ICU to OR), isolation in remote areas of the hospital with limited resources is unlikely. Nevertheless, issues involving the transport process are still relevant. Just as Insel and associates showed significant hemodynamic changes in adults during transfer from the OR to the ICU,[5] Venkataraman and Orr demonstrated major cardiorespiratory changes in children going from the OR to the ICU, many of whom required interventions such as ventilator changes or vasoactive infusions to stabilize.[12] Petre and co-workers noted that patients with complex cardiothoracic problems may leave the OR with multiple inotropic or vasoactive infusions, invasive monitors, and at times pacemakers and intraaortic balloon pumps, all requiring monitoring and adjustment during the transport process.[23] They found that patients frequently arrived in the ICU in unstable condition.

I frequently am asked to maintain tight control of moderate induced hypotension in awake patients immediately after complex neurovascular or cardiovascular procedures during emergence from anesthesia, transport to the ICU, and transfer to the critical care team. This approach is vital after resection of high-flow arteriovenous malformations to prevent hemorrhage and edema and requires close and constant monitoring. The same potential for physiologic deterioration certainly is present when patients are transferred from the ICU to the OR; in this setting, the added factor of an emergent situation is often present. Even when patients remain stationary in the ICU, critical illness by its nature causes physiologic changes. Hurst and colleagues, in their study of cost and complications during in-hospital transport, found that 60% of control patients who remained in the ICU had significant physiologic changes during a time equivalent to a transport.[6]

## A RATIONAL APPROACH

### What Factors Determine Monitoring Requirements?

Cost-benefit relationships have been demonstrated with monitors and monitoring.[1,2] The costs may be economic (related to the equipment), physical (iatrogenic injury to the patient), or a combination of the two (increased time or personnel requirements). Benefits are related to improved patient care, reduced complications, shorter ICU or hospital stays, and, it is hoped, better outcomes.

## Risk Analysis

Risks and costs increase with progression from simple clinical observation, to noninvasive equipment-assisted monitoring, to invasive monitors; clearly, not all monitors are needed for all patients. A decision about what monitors should be used during transport must be based on an individual patient's physiologic status and the stress imposed by injury, disease process, surgery, anesthesia, and medications. These needs are modified by the length and type of transport. General guidelines can be developed for the previously mentioned scenarios described by Venkataraman and Orr.[12]

Patients should be stabilized as much as possible before any movement.[12-15,17,22,24,25] In healthy patients after elective surgery, a regular heart rate and rhythm, adequate airway with regular respirations, and acceptable BP before transfer usually are all that is required.

## How Is a Patient Prepared for Transport?

In critically ill patients, transport should be broken down into the *preparatory phase, transport phase,* and *posttransport stabilization.*[12] The first phase should start with the carefully weighed decision to transport made by the primary members of the critical care, trauma, or surgical team (including the anesthesiologist). Once this decision is made, adequate and appropriate personnel should be gathered, and a careful systems review of the patient should be made to determine if any further interventions can optimize stabilization of the patient.

If a patient is receiving vasoactive infusions, he or she should be in a steady state, not in a continuous state of flux.[24] In patients with shock due to trauma, volume resuscitation should be well underway or complete before movement, and all necessary vascular catheters should be in place. If BP cannot be stabilized, surgical exploration and control of bleeding must take precedence over *any* further diagnostic procedures.[13,14]

A ventriculostomy catheter can be placed in the OR in hypotensive trauma victims with severe head injury during other surgical exploration, and an air ventriculogram used to lateralize a mass lesion if the ICP is increased. Control of the airway and some level of adequate oxygenation and ventilation should be achieved. In a neurologically injured or impaired patient (or any patient with a depressed level of consciousness) who is not intubated, careful consideration should be given to securing the airway electively before transport.

Burn patients, those with significant smoke inhalation, and patients with facial, neck, or chest trauma may also be at risk for airway compromise. Intubation in a controlled setting may be appropriate before any prolonged transport or diagnostic procedure.

In 1993, a joint task force consisting of members from the American College of Critical Care Medicine, Society of Critical Care Medicine, and American Association of Critical Care Nurses developed and published guidelines for intrahospital and interhospital transport of the critically ill.[26] These mandate that all patient care units shall have written transport policies addressing coordination and communication, personnel, equipment, and monitoring.

## Coordination and Communication

Before transport/transfer of a critically ill patient, discussion should take place from physician to physician and nurse to nurse regarding the patient's condition and treatment plan, if care is to be transferred. Coordination with security personnel and personnel at ancillary locations is essential to ensure that there are no unforeseen delays en route and that the receiving location is ready to accept the patient. Elevators may be reserved for patient transport at a designated time, or a key operator can accompany the team. Confirmation that the receiving location is ready to accept the patient *and* immediately begin the procedure or test is mandatory. If the responsible physician is not accompanying the patient, he or she should be informed of the transport and that an acute event may occur outside of the ICU. Finally, the rationale for the transport, as well as the patient's condition during transport, should be documented in the chart.[26]

## Personnel

The appropriate number and type of personnel to accompany a patient vary according to individual needs and physiologic status. At a minimum, two people must accompany the patient, one of whom is the patient's critical care nurse or a designated and specially trained critical care transport nurse.[26] Nursing care is vital to patient care in the ICU and is mandatory during transport to ensure that vasoactive infusions are adjusted, medications administered, and accurate records maintained. When a patient is unstable or is at risk for airway problems, a physician who is familiar with the patient and skilled in managing tracheal intubation and other potential complications should be present.[24,25,27] A respiratory therapist or perfusionist may be required for specific problems.

Stearley described the development of the STAT Nurse Program at the University of Missouri.[28] One specially trained ICU transport nurse is available each shift to assist with patient transport/transfers. They also respond to "codes," assist with postoperative admission, help troubleshoot monitors and systems, and provide assistance with intravenous insertion throughout the hospital. He reported a reduced complication rate during transport compared with other published studies (15.5% overall versus ≤75%) and a significant cost savings to the hospital. The STAT nurse not only provided appropriate care for the transported patient but also eased the burden on patient care for those remaining in the ICU. Stearley calculated that each STAT nurse position provided an impact equivalent to 1.84 regular ICU nurse full-time equivalents.[28]

## Equipment and Supply Needs

A routine set of equipment for any critical care transport should include a cardiac monitor/defibrillator and basic airway management supplies, including a self-inflating resuscitation bag and mask, airways, a laryngoscope with appropriate blades, and appropriate-size endotracheal tubes. An adequate oxygen supply must allow a 30-minute reserve, in addition to anticipated needs for full support during the period outside of the ICU. The consequences of a depleted oxygen supply are devastating and inexcusable.[24,26]

In addition to basic resuscitation drugs, such as epinephrine, atropine, and lidocaine, any scheduled or anticipated medications should accompany the patient (eg, antibiotics, sedatives, muscle relaxants), and guidelines should be written for their use if the physician is not present. Medications administered by infusion should be maintained by battery-operated volumetric pumps. Finally, adequate intravenous fluids should be brought along to allow for ongoing maintenance requirements, as well as crystalloids, colloids, or blood products as indicated for resuscitation.

Parameters to be monitored during transport must be transferred to portable monitors. Dedicated transport beds with built-in monitors may seem attractive; however, the risk of dislodging catheters and an endotracheal tube or of inducing changes in ICP with a patient's movement suggests that patients should be transported in their ICU beds whenever possible. Self-contained critical care transport carts may be attached or detached quickly from the ICU bed. These are set up with appropriate monitors, compressed gas cylinders, transport or ICU ventilators, infusion pumps, and battery power sources.[29–32] During monitor transfer, brief periods of blackout for the parameters being transferred often are needed to permit rezeroing of transducers.

### The Transport Remote Acquisition Monitor System

The transport team must be familiar with the operation and function of the additional equipment. One concept that has been developed to ease this problem is the transport remote acquisition monitor (TRAM) system. The TRAM is designed around a self-contained data acquisition and processing module, to which ECG leads, invasive or noninvasive pressure transducers, pulse oximeter probes, temperature probes, and other monitoring modalities may be attached. This module may be plugged into a permanent (fixed) OR or bedside monitor; before disconnection from the primary monitor, it is linked to the portable TRAM liquid crystal display screen. When a patient is moved, the module is simply removed from the fixed monitor and "follows" the patient without the need to detach any of the monitoring lines.[33]

An alternative approach to avoid gaps is to duplicate monitoring between the bedside and transport systems. This process involves placing a separate set of ECG pads and leads for the transport monitor if cardiac rhythm is a concern, and measuring BP noninvasively while invasive lines are transferred. Several of the new ICU and OR monitors allow the transfer of modules for individual monitoring parameters between bedside and transport monitors or at least have compatible cable connections. The real utility of these systems is evident when multiple invasive monitors are to be followed or a patient must be transported to an intermediate location (eg, CT scan or angiography) en route between the OR and ICU.

### Management of Tubing

Not only must monitoring be transferred in preparation for transport but also care must be taken to ensure that the various infusion tubing and cables are organized and identifiable. Patient safety necessitates that lines and infusions not be confused, yet we are all aware of the unseen hand of entropy and the apparently spontaneous chaotic "spaghetti" that may develop. An inadvertent fluid bolus through infusion tubing filled with a vasoactive medication obviously can have serious consequences. Our approach has been to try to simplify things as much as possible. At least one "free" route for intravenous administration should be maintained in all patients, but other access ports may be flushed and capped off if they are not required during transport. If possible, all infusions should be placed through a single, separate port. Bundling of lines and

cables, along with adequate labeling, may be helpful. Velcro straps or even the corrugated plastic tubing from a breathing circuit can also be very helpful for managing multiple tubing.

### The Intensive Care Unit Bed

The Cleveland Clinic has developed an elegant system to increase safety and efficiency during transfer of patients undergoing cardiothoracic surgery. Their concept centers around the ICU bed as the primary transport device with which they interface other equipment (Fig. 23–1). Monitoring is based on the TRAM system in the OR, during transport, and in the ICU. At the head of the bed is a bracket designed to hold all the patient-monitoring transducers and the TRAM display. The TRAM module is placed in a receptacle under the bed. An infusion rack is used for all intravenous infusion fluids and medications and incorporates intravenous hooks, an adjustable intravenous pole, and volumetric pumps. This rack is suspended from an overhead mount in the OR, then attached to the side of the ICU bed for transport, and then once again suspended from a ceiling mount in the ICU. Thus, the

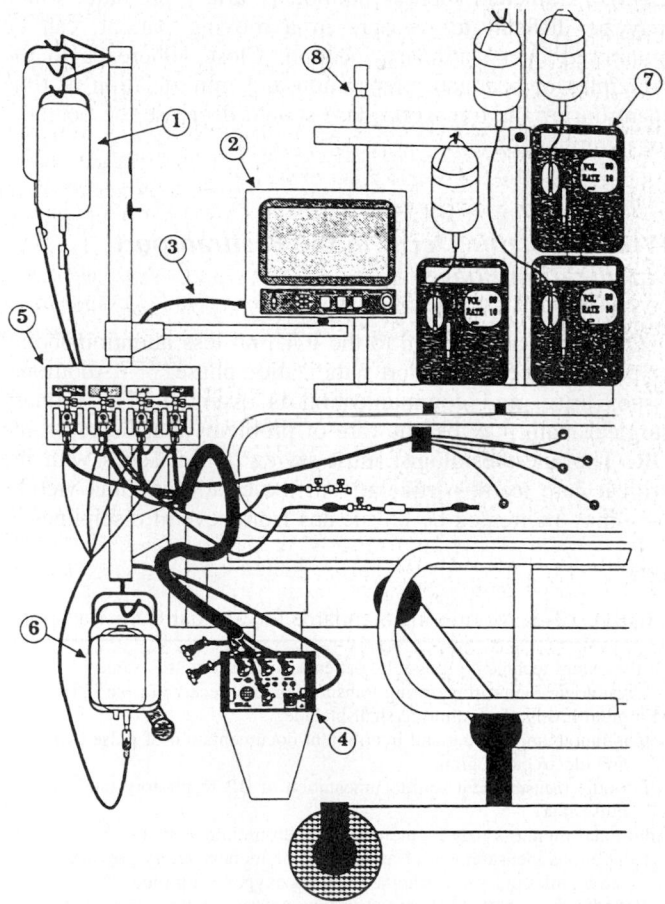

**FIGURE 23–1.** Integrated transport system. Support pole at head (1) holds pressure transducer mount (5) and pressurized flush solution (6) as well as hooks for intravenous solutions. The transport remote acquisition monitor (TRAM) display screen (2) is mounted on the pole by a moveable side arm and is connected to the TRAM module (4) by an electrical cord (3). The infusion bracket (8) is mounted on the side of the bed, and can support multiple intravenous solutions and up to 6 infusion pumps (7). (From Hendren W, Higgins T. Immediate postoperative care of the cardiac surgical patient. *Semin Thorac Cardiovasc Surg.* 1991;3:6.)

monitoring system and infusion/medication systems follow the patient as a unit.

Although the hardware for this system in 1988 cost more than $1000 per bed, it was believed to be cost-effective because of an estimated 50% time savings in the transport process and increased ability of transport personnel to focus on a patient rather than on movement of equipment.[23,34] Even if this particular system is too complex for some institutions, the concept of maintaining uninterrupted monitoring and moving infusions as a unit is worth noting.

### How Is the Transport Phase Managed?

During the transport phase, the goal is to provide the same level of care as the patient had in the OR or ICU: (1) maintain stability of the patient through monitoring, (2) continue the present ongoing management, and (3) avoid iatrogenic mishaps.[12] Every attempt should be made to return monitoring and care to the ICU level during the diagnostic or therapeutic procedure. This point is emphasized by the combined task force on the transfer of critically ill patients, in addition to guidelines setting minimum monitoring standards[26] (Table 23–3). Parameters such as pulmonary artery pressure, which may be difficult to measure in a moving patient, can be monitored in a stationary location. Close adherence to the principles of adequate preparation and minimization of time spent during the transport phase should decrease the potential for complications.

### What Problems Occur in the Posttransport Stabilization Phase?

On arrival at or return to the ICU, no less attention should be paid to the posttransport stabilization phase.[5,13,22] Additional issues arise, and communication is essential. The primary surgical team may be unaware of problems that began in the OR. The anesthesiologist must review these issues with the critical care team, particularly in the case of trauma victims who may be treated by physicians from several disciplines.[27]

---

**TABLE 23–3.** Monitoring Standards for Critical Care Transport

To the extent technically possible, patients must receive the same physiologic monitoring during transport as they receive in the ICU.
Minimum levels of monitoring shall include:
  Continuous monitoring and intermittent documentation of pulse oximetry and electrocardiogram
  Periodic measurement and documentation of BP, respiratory rate, and pulse rate
Additional monitors may be indicated based on clinical status:
  Continuous measurement of arterial BP, pulmonary artery pressure, intracranial pressure, or mixed venous oxygen saturation
  Periodic measurement of central venous pressure, pulmonary artery occlusion pressure or cardiac output
  Capnography
Intubated patients should have airway pressure monitored.
  Transport ventilators must have disconnect and high-pressure alarms
  Ventilators must be able to match the minute ventilation, fraction of inspired oxygen, and positive end-expiratory pressure the patient is receiving in the ICU

---

BP, blood pressure; ICU, intensive care unit.

## SELECTION OF MONITORS

### What Factors Should Be Considered?

Monitoring procedures may individualized, depending on the transport scenario and the individual patient's physiology. Observation alone can provide information on respiratory pattern, signs of obstruction, skin color, and gross tissue perfusion. Through touch and auscultation, we add measures of cardiac rate and rhythm, ventilation, and some approximation of BP. Simple communication and interaction can often yield a fairly good measure of level of consciousness and gross neurologic functioning.

The feasibility and ease of monitoring additional parameters during transport and in remote locations have been increased dramatically by the evolution of small, lightweight, battery-operated devices. A variety of models are available, from several manufacturers. Many of these have the capability to monitor ECG, noninvasive BP, one or two invasive pressures, $SpO_2$, temperature, and $PETCO_2$ (Fig. 23–2).

### Hypoxemia

The evidence for hypoxemia after general anesthesia in all age groups is now quite convincing; thus, the routine use of supplemental $O_2$ during transport to the PACU is justifiable. When underlying pulmonary disease or the nature of the surgical procedure suggests that a patient may not be able to maintain adequate oxygenation with simple face mask or blow-by $O_2$, observation, including pulse oximetry, should take place in the OR using the transport mode of supplemental $O_2$. The practitioner can assess the rate and depth of respirations by feeling exhalations on the palm of the hand while helping to support the airway (Fig. 23–3). The precordial stethoscope permits simultaneous monitoring of heart rate and rhythm (as well as tone) and breath sounds, with the patient on his or her side and the occiput cushioned. In this position, soft tissues are pulled forward and away from the airway, decreasing obstruction and allowing secretions (or emesis, should it occur) to drain out of the corner of the mouth.[1]

### Cardiopulmonary Assessment

Additional monitors may be desirable in individual patients, even during the brief transfer to the PACU, but observation and a stethoscope usually suffice. If a patient was anesthetized in a location other than the OR and a longer transfer is required, a pulse oximeter is advisable. ECG monitoring and automated noninvasive BP monitoring are desirable if a potential exists for volume shifts or bleeding during transport. Such occurrences may be noted after invasive radiologic or angiographic procedures. Various lightweight, battery-operated transport monitors follow these parameters and also allow vascular pressures to be transduced.

During transfer from the ICU or PACU to the ward, clinical observation should form the basis of monitoring. Unless a patient is moved to a stepdown unit or a telemetry ward, ECG and BP measurement are not required. If a patient has been receiving supplemental $O_2$, however, and may continue to need it on the ward, $O_2$ should be administered during transport.

Critically ill patients, and those undergoing invasive hemo-

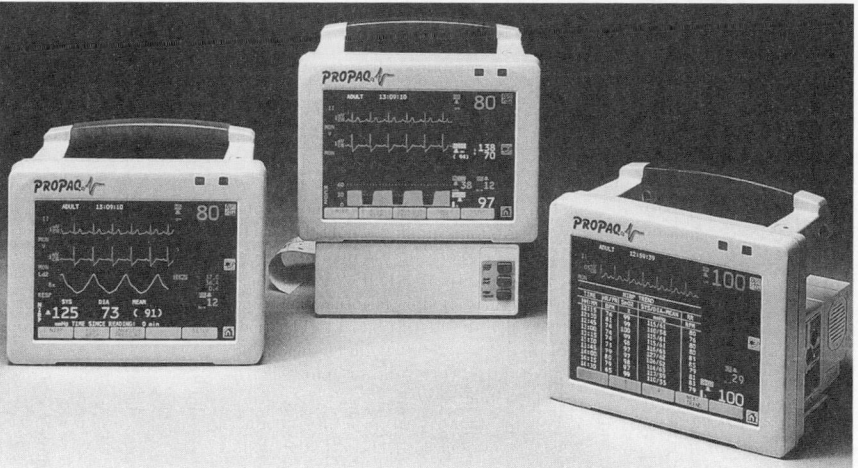

**FIGURE 23–2.** Three Propaq CS portable monitors. Each is a battery-operated monitor for fixed or transport use, capable of monitoring the electrocardiogram, pulse oximeter arterial oxygen saturation, noninvasive blood pressure, invasive pressures, and mainstream or sidestream end-tidal $CO_2$. Weight, 7.6 lb. (Courtesy of Welch Allyn Protocol, Beaverton, Ore.)

dynamic or ICP monitoring, should continue to have those parameters monitored during transport.

## Ventilator-Dependent Patients

Ventilator-dependent patients are clearly at risk for deterioration during critical care transport. How ventilation should be accomplished and what additional monitors should be used are pertinent questions during transport. Gervais and colleagues showed that manual ventilation with spirometry measurement prevents alterations in arterial blood gas and hemodynamic changes that accompany unmonitored manual ventilation or use of a transport ventilator.[18] Weg and Haas found that stable hemodynamic and respiratory status for most patients could be maintained by a trained respiratory therapist using manual ventilation matched to the inspired $O_2$ and minute ventilation of the bedside ventilator.[35] Other investigators have reported similar findings, although a tendency toward hyperventilation with bag inflation compared with that using a transport ventilator is noteworthy[36] (Table 23–4). My experience suggests that most ventilator-dependent patients can be satisfactorily managed for brief transfers using a Mapleson D circuit with a gauge attached to monitor airway pressures. This combination allows some control over positive end-expiratory pressure (PEEP) and prevents overdistension and barotrauma.[24]

### Choice of Ventilator

Critically ill patients may require high levels of CPAP or complex ventilatory modes such as pressure control ventilation with inverse inspiration-to-expiration ratios to maintain oxygenation. In these patients, manual ventilation is likely to be ineffective, and a transport ventilator must be used. Branson and McGough conducted an extensive review of transport ventilators, and their characteristics are summarized in Table 23–5.[36] Unfortunately, the modes of an ICU ventilator (intermittent mandatory ventilation, pressure support ventilation, CPAP/PEEP, pressure control ventilation, and so on) may be different or impossible to match with these devices. The safest approach whenever possible in such cases may be to use the ICU ventilator for transport and, if necessary, for any surgical procedure in the OR.[24] The ventilator may be moved independently, with compressed gas tanks as part of a transport cart or, in some cases, on the patient's bed.[31] One interesting new series of ventilators developed by Bird Products Corporation (Palm Springs, Calif) uses a turbine instead of compressed gas to power mechanical ventilation. One model, the AVSIII

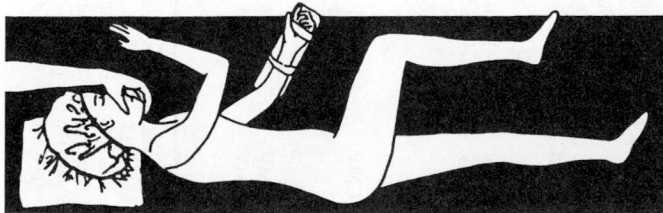

**FIGURE 23–3.** The optimal position of an unconscious patient during transport from the operating room to the postanesthesia care unit. The patient is placed on his or her side. If the patient had been in a lateral position during the operation, he or she is positioned with the side with the incision down. Straighten the lower leg and flex the upper leg 90° at hip and knee. This provides stability to the hip. Bring both arms and hands forward to stabilize the shoulder girdle. Support the head by placing a pillow or folded blanket under the occiput so that the face is turned slightly downward; this causes the jaw and tongue to fall forward, preventing obstruction while allowing saliva, gastric juice, or vomitus to drain from the mouth rather than pool in the hypopharynx. (From Gravenstein J, Paulus D. *Monitoring Practice in Clinical Anesthesia.* Philadelphia, Pa: JB Lippincott; 1982:33.)

**TABLE 23–4.** Comparing Self-Inflating Bag and Transport Ventilator

|  | Conventional Ventilation Before Transport | Self-Inflating Bag Used During Transport | Transport Ventilator Used During Transport |
|---|---|---|---|
| pHa | 7.39 ± 0.3 | 7.51 ± 0.2* | 7.40 ± 0.3 |
| $Paco_2$ (mm Hg) | 39 ± 4 | 30 ± 3* | 39 ± 3 |
| $Pao_2$ (mm Hg) | 116 ± 17 | 109 ± 24 | 117 ± 20 |
| Heart rate (beats per minute) | 106 ± 23 | 115 ± 19 | 109 ± 25 |
| Systolic pressure (mm Hg) | 130 ± 36 | 112 ± 24 | 136 ± 31 |
| Diastolic pressure (mm Hg) | 86 ± 12 | 73 ± 10 | 81 ± 20 |

Average transport time = 9 ± 3 minutes during manual ventilation with a self-inflating bag; 8 ± 3 minutes during ventilation with a transport ventilator.
*$P < .05$ compared with conventional ventilation.
pHa, arterial pH.
From Branson RD, McGough EK. Transport ventilators. *Probl Crit Care.* 1990;4:261.

**TABLE 23–5.** Ventilatory and Monitoring Characteristics of Transport Ventilators

| Ventilator | Cycling Variables | Modes | Rate (Breaths per Minute) | Tidal Volume (mL) | Minute Volume (L/min)* | I:E Ratio (Minimum) | Peak Flow Rate (L/min) | FiO$_2$ | PEEP (cm H$_2$O)† | Alarms | Monitoring | Demand-Flow Valve | Manual Breath |
|---|---|---|---|---|---|---|---|---|---|---|---|---|---|
| Hamilton Max | Time | IMV, CMV | 2–30 | 50–1500 | 45.0 | 1:1 | 90 | 1.0 | No | Low inlet pressure and low battery (audible and visual) High airway pressure (audible) | Airway pressure | Yes | Yes |
| Biomed IC2A | Time | CMV, IMV, CPAP | 1–66 | 130–2500 | 37.5 | 4:1 | 75 | 1.0 | 0–25 | None | Airway pressure | No‡ | Yes |
| Healthdyne 105 | Time | IMV, CPAP, CMV | 1–150 | 10–4000 | 20.0 | 4:1 | 60 | 0.21–1.0 | 0–20 | Audible/visual; low/high pressure, low inlet pressure, system interrupt, insufficient expiratory time, reverse I:E, power loss, disconnect | Airway pressure | No, continuous flow only | Yes |
| Impact Universal | Time | CMV | 14, 20, 30 child; 12, 18 adult | 10–1250 | 22.5 | 1:2 | 90 | 1.0 | No | Visual low battery; audible high pressure | None | No | Yes |
| Life Support Products Auto Vent 2000 | Time | IMV, CMV | 8–20 | 400–1200 | 24.0 | 1:1 | 48 | 1.0 | No | High pressure audible | None | Yes | No |
| Life Support Products Auto Vent 3000 | Time | IMV, CMV | 9–27 child; 8–20 adult | 200–600 child; 400–1200 adult | 24.0 adult; 16.0 child | 1:1 | 48 | 1.0 | No | High pressure audible | None | Yes | No |
| Newport E100I | Time or pressure | IMV, CMV, A/C, CPAP | 1–80 | 100–3600 | 36.0 | 1:1 | 72 | 0.21–1.0 | 0–25 | Visual/audible high/low pressure, inspiration time too long | Airway pressure | No, continuous flow only | Yes |
| Ohmeda Logic 07 | Time | CMV | 10–40 | 100–2000 | 20.0 | 1:2 | 65 | 0.5 or 1.0 | No | High pressure audible | Airway pressure | No | No |
| Penlon 350 | Time | CMV | 10–85 | 10–300 neonate/child; 50–2000 adult | 0.1–9.0 neonate/child; 1.0–3.0 adult | 2:1 | 60 | 1.0 | No | High pressure audible | Airway pressure | No | No |
| Pneupac Model 2-R | Time | CMV1 | 1, 12, 13, 14, 16, 19, and 21 | 340–1450 | 16.0 | 1:1.5 | 40 | 0.45 or 1.0 | No | High pressure audible | None | No | No |
| Stein-Gates | Time | CMV | 1–150 | 30–3000 | 20.0 | 2:1 | 45 | 1.0 | No | None | None | No | No |
| Bird Space Technologies Mini-TXP | Time | CMV | 4–15 | 50–2500 | 30.0 | 1:2 | 120 | 0.45–0.8 | No | None | None | No | Yes |

A/C, assist/control; CMV, controlled mechanical ventilation; CPAP, continuous positive airway pressure; FiO$_2$, fraction of inspired oxygen; IMV, intermittent mandatory ventilation; I:E, inspiration-to-expiration; PEEP, positive end-expiratory pressure.

*Maximum available minute volume with an I:E of 1:1.

†PEEP can be provided in all ventilators with an external PEEP valve.

‡During spontaneous inhalation, the ventilator cycles "on," but the exhalation valve remains depressurized to allow venting of gas to the atmosphere. Depending on the inspiratory flow rate and time settings, gas flow rate for a specific duration of time is available for spontaneous breathing. The system does not function as a demand-flow valve.

From Branson RD, McCough EK. Transport ventilators. *Probl Crit Care.* 1990; 4:264.

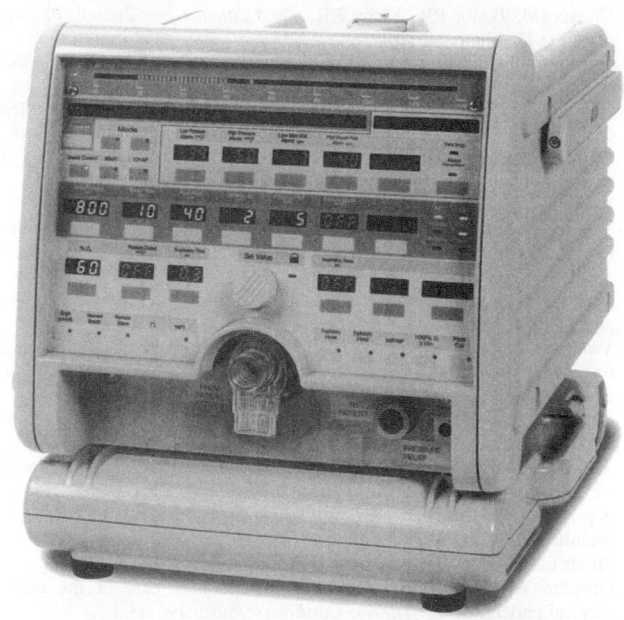

**FIGURE 23–4.** Bird AVSIII Ventilator. This self-contained, turbine-powered ventilator is capable of operating without a compressed gas source. It offers a full range of ventilatory modalities, and is mobile with a battery pack. Weight, <15.5 kg; dimensions, 13 × 14.5 × 11 in. (Courtesy of Bird Products Corp, Palm Springs, Calif.)

(Fig. 23–4), is capable of a full range of ventilatory modes, including controlled ventilation, assist/control, synchronized intermittent mandatory ventilation, pressure support ventilation, pressure control ventilation, inverse inspiratory-expiratory ratio, volume-assured pressure support—as well as combinations—yet weighs only 15.5 kg and measures approximately 1 cubic foot. Such ventilators combine complex support in the ICU with the flexibility of moving with the patient during transport, avoiding the potential complications associated with changing ventilatory modes or to manual ventilation.

In addition to pulse oximetry, ventilated patients should have airway pressure monitored during transport. A spirometer is helpful to ensure adequate and consistent tidal volumes. At the minimum, a colorimetric $CO_2$ detector should be available. Critically ill patients, especially those with reduced intracranial elastance or pulmonary hypertension, should have continuous end-tidal $CO_2$ monitoring.[19–21,31,37] Capnography should be considered during the transport of intubated pediatric patients.[20]

## Head-Injured Patients

Patients with a neurologic injury present special challenges. Clinical examination remains the best monitor of neurologic status, both during transport and in the ICU. Unfortunately, the need to pursue diagnostic studies in an uncooperative patient or perform surgical procedures may necessitate sedation or other medications that can obscure neurologic findings. Sedation and intubation in a relatively controlled setting, before transport to the CT scanner or other areas of the hospital, is often advisable. Short-acting sedatives, especially propofol and perhaps remifentanil, are useful, allowing rapid emergence so that patients may be clinically assessed at the end of the transport or procedure.

Patients with severe head injuries or other causes of in-

creased ICP are likely to have ICP monitors in place. They are intubated and are likely to be hyperventilated and in a 20° to 30° head-up position. Newer modalities include somatosensory evoked potential monitoring and jugular bulb oximetry. These patients are at high risk for secondary insults, yet are also quite likely to require transport for radiologic studies or to the OR.

Although jugular bulb oximetry and evoked potential monitoring are unnecessary during transport, oxygenation, BP, and end-tidal $CO_2$ should be maintained as constant as possible. The head-up position should be continued. Because ICP changes are common during transport, ICP monitoring should be continued. This assessment is easily accomplished with the newer fiberoptic devices but may require careful attention to transducer height and monitor function if a ventriculostomy catheter or Richmond bolt is being used.

## Spinal Cord–Injured Patients

Spinal cord–injured patients present special logistical concerns related to the traction and stabilization devices that may be used. Any movement or transport should be performed in consultation with a member of the neurosurgical team. Airway protection in spinal cord injury must also take into consideration the potential for progressive ventilatory muscle insufficiency. Although this problem is unlikely to occur rapidly, it must be addressed before any prolonged transport.

## Hemodynamically Unstable Patients

Optimal preparation is crucial to the safe transport of hemodynamically unstable patients. Resuscitation fluids should be available with blood (if appropriate), together with a plentiful supply of any infusions or medications. Consideration should be given to having at least one individual available for the sole purpose of fluid or blood administration and to ensure that the nurse or other designated individual has uninterrupted access to vasoactive infusions.

## *References*

1. Gravenstein J, Paulus D. *Monitoring Practice in Clinical Anesthesia.* Philadelphia, Pa: JB Lippincott; 1982.
2. Blitt C. A philosophy of monitoring. In: Blitt C, ed. *Monitoring in Anesthesia and Critical Care Medicine.* New York, NY: Churchill Livingstone; 1985:1.
3. American Society of Anesthesiologists. *Standards for Basic Anesthesia Monitoring.* Approved by the House of Delegates October 21, 1986 and last amended October 21, 1998. Park Ridge, Ill: American Society of Anesthesiologists Directory; 2001:493.
4. Taylor J, Landers C, Cholay J, et al. Monitoring high-risk cardiac patients during transportation. *Lancet.* 1970;2:1205.
5. Insel J, Weissman C, Kemper M, et al. Cardiovascular changes during transport of critically ill and postoperative patients. *Crit Care Med.* 1986;14:539.
6. Hurst J, Davis K, Johnson D, et al. Cost and complications during in-hospital transport of critically ill patients: a prospective cohort study. *J Trauma.* 1992;33:582.
7. Tyler I, Tatisara B, Winter P, et al. Continuous monitoring of arterial oxygen saturation with pulse oximetry during transfer to the recovery room. *Anesth Analg.* 1985;64:1108.
8. Kataria B, Harnik E, Mitchard R, et al. Postoperative arterial oxygen saturation in the pediatric population during transportation. *Anesth Analg.* 1988;67:280.
9. Tomkins D, Gaukroger P, Bentley M. Hypoxia in children following general anesthesia. *Anaesth Intensive Care.* 1988;16:177.
10. Riley R, Davis N, Finucane K, et al. Arterial oxygen saturation in

anaesthetised patients during transfer from induction room to operating room. *Anaesth Intensive Care.* 1988;16:182.

11. Hensley F, Dodson D, Martin D, et al. Oxygen saturation during placement of invasive monitoring in the premedicated, unanesthetized cardiac patient. *Anesthesiology.* 1986;65:A22

12. Venkataraman S, Orr R. Intrahospital transport of critically ill patients. *Crit Care Clin.* 1992;8:525.

13. Gentleman D, Jennet B. Audit of transfer of unconscious head-injured patients to a neurosurgical unit. *Lancet.* 1990;335:330.

14. Andrews P, Piper I, Dearded N, et al. Secondary insults during intrahospital transport of head-injured patients. *Lancet.* 1990;335:327.

15. Waddell G. Movement of critically ill patients within hospital. *BMJ.* 1975;2:417.

16. Kanter R, Boeing N, Hannan W, et al. Excess morbidity associated with interhospital transport. *Pediatrics.* 1992;90:893.

17. Braman S, Dunn S, Amico C, et al. Complications of intrahospital transport in critically ill patients. *Ann Intern Med.* 1987;107:469.

18. Gervais H, Eberle B, Konietzke D, et al. Comparison of blood gases of ventilated patients during transport. *Crit Care Med.* 1987;15:761.

19. Palmon S, Liu M, Moore L, et al. Capnography facilitates tight control of ventilation during transport. *Crit Care Med.* 1996;24:608.

20. Tobias J, Lynch A, Garrett J. Alterations of end-tidal carbon dioxide during the intrahospital transport of children. *Pediatr Emerg Care.* 1996;12:249.

21. Bekar A, Ipekoglu Z, Türeyen K, et al. Secondary insults during intrahospital transport of neurosurgical intensive care patients. *Neurosurg Rev.* 1998;21:98.

22. Smith I, Fleming S, Cernaianu A. Mishaps during transport from the intensive care unit. *Crit Care Med.* 1990;18:278.

23. Petre J, Bazaral M, Estafanous F. Patient transport: an organized method with direct clinical benefits. *Biomed Instrum Technol.* 1989;23:100.

24. Melker R, Gallagher TJ. Transport of the critically ill/injured patient. In: Civetta JM, Taylor RW, Kirby RR, eds. *Critical Care.* 2nd ed. Philadelphia, Pa: JB Lippincott; 1992:1797.

25. Fromm R, Dellinger R. Transport of critically ill patients. *J Intensive Care Med.* 1992;7:223.

26. Guidelines Committee of the American College of Critical Care Medicine; Society of Critical Care Medicine and American Association of Critical Care Nurses Transfer Guidelines Task Force. Guidelines for the transfer of critically ill patients. *Crit Care Med.* 1993;21:931.

27. Watson C, Norfleet E. Anesthesia for trauma. *Crit Care Clin.* 1986;2:717.

28. Stearley H. Patients' outcomes: intrahospital transportation and monitoring of critically ill patients by a specially trained ICU nursing staff. *Am J Crit Care.* 1998;7:282.

29. Kondo K, Herman S, O'Reilly P, et al. Transport system for critically ill patients. *Crit Care Med.* 1985;13:1081.

30. Vandermeersch E, Muller E, Mulier J, et al. A new mobile artificial respiration and monitoring system for transporting critically ill (emergency) patients. *Anasth Intensivther Notfallmed.* 1988;23:276.

31. Link J, Krause H, Wagner W, et al. Intrahospital transport of critically ill patients. *Crit Care Med.* 1990;18:1427.

32. Schirmer U, Heinrich H, Siebeneich H, et al. Safe intraclinical transfer of intensive care patients: a concept to avoid monitoring and treatment gaps. *Anasthesiol Intensivmed Notfallmed Schmerzther.* 1991;26:112.

33. Weinfurt P. TRAM: a new concept in transport monitoring. *Int J Clin Monit Comput.* 1987;4:149.

34. Hendren W, Higgins T. Immediate postoperative care of the cardiac surgical patient. *Semin Thorac Cardiovasc Surg.* 1991;3:3.

35. Weg J, Haas C. Safe intrahospital transport of critically ill ventilator-dependent patients. *Chest.* 1989;96:631.

36. Branson RD, McGough EK. Transport ventilators. *Probl Crit Care.* 1990;4:254.

37. End-tidal carbon dioxide measurement in emergency medicine and patient transport. *Health Devices.* 1991;20:35.

# Clinically Relevant Anatomy

CHAPTER

## 24

# Clinically Relevant Airway Anatomy

Leroy D. Vandam

PHYLOGENETIC CONSIDERATIONS
*What Are the Effects of the Erect Position?*

TOPICAL ANATOMY OF THE AIRWAY
*How Should the Oral Cavity Be Examined?*
*What Anatomic Considerations Are Important for Intubation?*
*What Pharyngeal Factors Are Important for Intubation?*

THE TRACHEA
*What Anatomic Considerations Are Important?*

THE LARYNX
*What Are Its Functions?*
*What Are the Laryngeal Cartilages?*
*When Is a Nerve Block of the Larynx Performed?*
*What Should Be Known About Laryngeal Blood Supply?*
*What Are the Intrinsic Muscle Actions?*
*Why Is Intubation Sometimes Difficult?*
*What Are the Sphincter Functions of the Larynx?*

TRACHEAL INTUBATION
*What Are the Advantages?*
*What Equipment Should Be Available?*
*Which Techniques Are Preferred?*
*When Is Tracheal Intubation Performed in the Conscious Patient?*
*Why Does Coughing Occur, and How Is It Treated?*
*What Factors Affect Tube Movement?*
*How Is Esophageal Intubation Detected?*
*How Is Extubation Performed?*
*Why Is Extubation Sometimes Difficult?*

*What Precautions Are Necessary?*
*What Are the Complications of Tracheal Intubation?*

Perhaps it is superfluous to state that maintenance of the airway is one of two essentials of anesthetic management, the other being circulatory homeostasis. In support of this tenet are those reports originating from closed-claim analyses of medicolegal actions in which respiratory events involving hypoxia formed the single largest class of adverse anesthetic events, occurring in 762 of 2046 cases.[1] Relatively infrequent were airway trauma, pneumothorax, subcutaneous emphysema, aspiration of gastric contents into the lungs, barotrauma, and bronchospasm.

In the conscious state, exchange of oxygen ($O_2$) and carbon dioxide ($CO_2$) in the lungs is vital to survival. During anesthesia, any difficulty that might have existed beforehand is surely magnified by sedatives, central depressant effects of general anesthetics, neuromuscular blocking agents, the supine position with relaxation of the jaw, or any of the many unusual body positions required for surgical procedures. Despite these findings, and 150 years after the introduction of anesthesia, airway management continues to bedevil anesthesiologists, as demonstrated by a spate of articles, symposia, and monographs on the subject. Perhaps the prevalence of this ever-increasing technology in anesthesia has influenced clinicians to no longer be the observant physicians they once were.

In their respective fields, medical specialists, particularly radiologists and surgeons, are obliged to be experts in anatomy on which they base their diagnoses and need for operations. Nevertheless, I am unaware of any sustained effort on the part of anesthesiologists to return to the dissecting room to learn the essentials of how the airway is related to the maneuvers they perform. Because recall of details once learned in medical school is hardly possible, we must rely instead on textbook illustrations, radiographs, or observations made during operation—hardly substitutes for the 3-dimensional views, relationship of structures, and tissue textures of the anatomy we should have in mind.

## PHYLOGENETIC CONSIDERATIONS

Problems with the airway are of evolutionary origin, dating back to primordial times when $O_2$ transport became necessary for survival: the development of gills in fish, the emergence of aquatic creatures from the sea, the development of the extremities for locomotion, and, finally, bipedalism.[2] These phylogenetic matters are emphasized in the subsequent discussion on laryngeal anatomy.

### What Are the Effects of the Erect Position?

Anthropologists have advanced several theories for the change from four-footed to two-footed locomotion: the need to use one pair of extremities for foraging, for climbing, for defense, or for traveling distances in search of food while carrying the young in the arms.[3]

Despite these advantages that distinguish anthropoids from other mammalian species, the erect position has its tradeoffs.[4] The cranium became set at a right angle to the vertebral column, thus detouring and adding resistance to airflow in respiration; the eyes became centered for vision, with loss of part of the lateral visual fields; and the more mobile cervical spine became susceptible to degenerative changes with aging as well as the liability of injury and trauma to the spinal cord. Further, the use of only two extremities in locomotion and running and the inability to gallop have placed obligate two-footed species at a disadvantage with the felines, hounds, and horses in the matter of speed.

## TOPICAL ANATOMY OF THE AIRWAY

Since the introduction of artificial airways to improve gas exchange—initially, simple oropharyngeal or nasopharyngeal devices and tracheotomy in an emergency and, later, tracheal intubation—the need to examine the existing features of the airway beforehand has been emphasized. Most misadventures can be avoided by this appraisal alone. With the patient's head at a right angle to the spine, some of the probable difficulties encountered in airway establishment are noticeable (Table 24–1). Nevertheless, despite attempts to predict difficulty in airway placement, one occasionally encounters unforeseen problems and must be ready for any contingency.

**TABLE 24–1.** Examination of the Airway: Clues to Problems

Inability to open the mouth widely
Temporomandibular joint problems: pain, masseter spasm, trismus
Protruding upper incisors
Agnathia
Nasal obstruction: old fractures, posterior choanal atresia
Hypertrophied tonsils and adenoids
Ankylosis of the cervical spine; dislocation, fractures
Short, thick, muscular neck; "turkey" neck; scarring from burns
Congenital malformations
Endocrine disease; acromegaly, goiter, exophthalmos

### How Should the Oral Cavity Be Examined?

Kaban[5] described the manner in which the airway should be examined before induction of anesthesia. In addition to other obligatory elements of the physical examination, this approach impresses patients with the seriousness of the anesthetic experience.

#### Face and Jaw

One should inspect the structure of the face and jaws with regard to mask fit during induction. A large protruding nose, a receding jaw, a wide mouth, or a heavy beard can hinder a tight mask fit required for assisted ventilation and oxygenation. As clues to temporomandibular joint dysfunction and the accompanying pain that often presents as neuralgia or headache postoperatively, one should look for hypomobility or the possibility of dislocation of the jaw during intubation by listening for clicking sounds as well as by elicitation of pain.

#### Mouth and Oropharynx

The mucous membranes of the mouth and tongue and their coloration may offer clues to underlying disease: anemia, leukoplakia, or early epidermoid carcinoma. The soft palate and uvula should be observed as a patient says "ah" to exclude cranial nerve dysfunction and deviation of the tongue (Fig. 24–1), and the tongue should be examined to determine whether it is excessively large as it is protruded.

With use of a wooden tongue depressor, the oropharynx is examined for any pathologic changes in the faucial pillars and tonsils while watching for secretions from the salivary ducts.

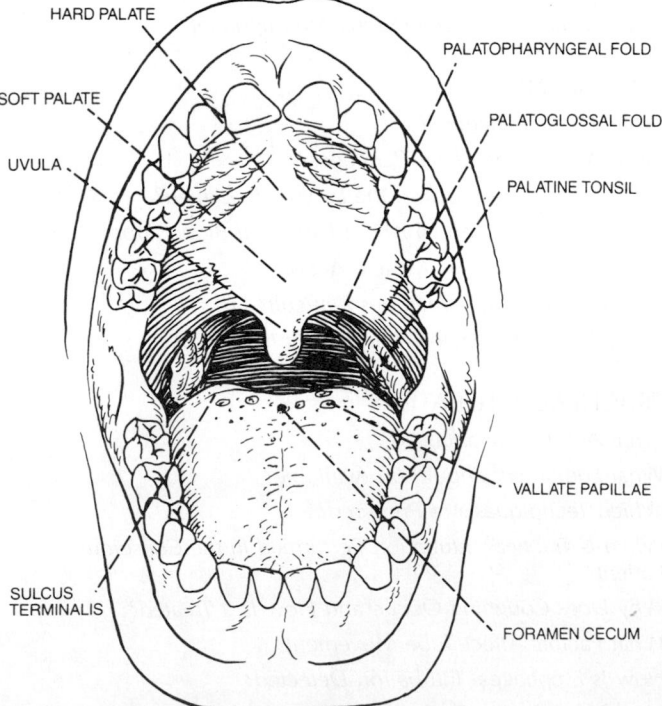

**FIGURE 24–1.** The open mouth showing the base of the tongue, uvula, and faucial pillars. (From Snell RS, Katz J. *Clinical Anatomy for Anesthesiologists.* Norwalk, Conn: Appleton & Lange; 1988. Reproduced with permission of The McGraw-Hill Companies.)

For example, clear saliva should issue from the parotid duct adjacent to the second molar maxillary teeth. Pharyngeal anatomy is particularly relevant when placing a laryngeal mask airway.

### Teeth and Dental Appliances

Observe tooth structure and examine for the presence of periodontal infection, caries, looseness, and the general state of dental hygiene as well as for edentia and prostheses. Although removable bridgework should be taken out before induction of anesthesia, a mask fit is more easily obtained if complete dental plates are retained. The risk here is the possible loss of dentures if they are removed and misplaced during the course of anesthesia. Any detected abnormalities should be noted in the patient's chart along with informing the patient that injury may occur during anesthesia. Before intubation, when there is concern, the teeth can be protected against damage by means of a malleable mold.

## What Anatomic Considerations Are Important for Intubation?

The airway extends from the nostrils to the pulmonary alveoli, but for intubation purposes only, the distance to the tracheal bifurcation is pertinent. Proctor[6] defined the *upper airway* as consisting of the area of airflow between nasal passages and larynx, the former from the nostrils to the posterior termination of the nasal septum; the nasopharynx from the end of the septum to the lower border of the soft palate; and the pharynx from the soft palate to the larynx. Under some circumstances, the mouth is also included as part of the airway.

### Nose and Nasopharynx

The nasal passage is a double airway with a complex shape. The nasopharynx is the region where closure can separate the nasal passage from the pharynx; the pharynx is an airway common to both nasal and oronasal breathing and, along with the larynx, more or less forms a bottleneck.

The tip of the nose with its nostrils is fairly mobile and prone to necrosis of the skin if a tracheal tube is allowed to exert pressure. This mobile area of the nose consists of several hyaline cartilages, which articulate with the nasal bones laterally and the maxillary and frontal bones superiorly (Fig. 24–2). Cartilages can be injured or even fractured as a result of rough treatment. The nares, or external choanae, are larger in diameter than the posterior choanae, which lead to the nasopharynx. Both dilation and stabilization of the nares are afforded by the dilator nares muscles. Dilation of the nostrils can be seen during respiratory distress (*air hunger*) in human beings and is commonly seen in animals running at high speed.

### Functions

As stated by Courtiss and colleagues,[7] the nose offers several basic functions: air conditioner, air cleaner, airway, olfaction, phonation, and reflex responder. Flow of air is both laminar and turbulent, with the main flow passing through the

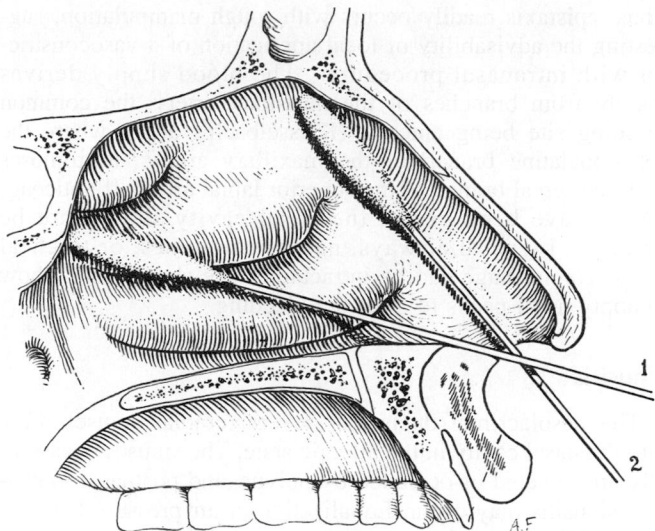

**FIGURE 24–2.** The lateral wall of the nasal cavity showing the vestibule-like entry, the turbinates, the hard and soft palates, and the adjacent sinuses. The swabs (1 and 2) illustrate how topical anesthesia may be applied to the mucous membranes. Notice the space below the inferior turbinate, where there is more room for the passage of air. (From Labat G. *Regional Anesthesia: Its Technical and Clinical Application*. 2nd ed. Philadelphia, Pa: WB Saunders; 1928.)

middle meatus; that flow, in turn, is influenced by mucus, ciliary action, and vasoconstriction or vasodilation.

**Warming and Humidification.** During inspiration, air is warmed nearly to body temperature before reaching the larynx, a conditioning process requiring 75 to 100 calories of energy expenditure per day. About 90% humidification is achieved before air reaches the lungs, consuming about 1 L/d of water.

**Air Cleansing.** Air cleansing, an essential protective measure, includes impingement of gross particles suspended in air, with the larger particles caught in the vibrissae of the nostrils and electrostatic changes causing adhesion of others. The cilia of the upper airway, with their covering mobile blanket of mucus, constantly propel foreign particles toward the exterior, and coughing is the main means by which larger foreign bodies are expelled.

**Airway.** In adults, the nasal airway is about 10 to 14 cm in length, divided into two parts by the septum and convoluted by the scroll-like structure of the turbinate cartilages (superior, middle, and inferior conchae attached to the lateral wall) (see Fig. 24–2). The entrance to the nose forms a funnel-shaped vestibule. The entry initially points upward, so that the nostrils should be lifted to form a straight passage when inserting a nasal airway. Beyond the vestibule, the passage becomes horizontal but slopes backward, widens at the nasopharynx, and then makes a 90° curve downward toward the larynx.

The roof of the nose is formed by the olfactory plate. For some obscure reason, anosmia has been reported as a complication of general anesthesia. In the supine position, the nasal cavity slopes downward, and the greater space for airway placement lies below the inferior turbinate (see Fig. 24–2).

### Epistaxis

Because of the air-conditioning function of the nasal passages, the mucous membranes are highly vascular and erectile.

Thus, epistaxis readily occurs with rough manipulation, suggesting the advisability of local application of a vasoconstrictor with intranasal procedures. The blood supply derives mainly from branches of the maxillary artery, the common bleeding site being anterior (Kiesselbach's area), where the sphenopalatine branch of the maxillary artery anastomoses with the septal branch of the superior labial artery. If anticoagulants have been given, the nasal cavity should not be breached by nasal airways, nasogastric tubes, or tracheal tubes. Hemorrhage can be intractable; one should know how to apply nasal packs to stem the bleeding.

## Sinusitis

The nasolacrimal ducts and several cranial sinuses drain into the nasal cavity in the allergic state. The sinuses occasionally are infected or occluded by polyps, and postnasal intubation sinusitis may occur. Equalization of air pressure between the middle ear and pharynx is provided by the eustachian tubes, which can be obstructed by a nasotracheal tube.

## Topical Anesthesia

The nose inside and out is innervated by the superior, medial, and inferior branches of the trigeminal nerve. Terminal nerve endings are superficial in the mucosa, rendering them easily susceptible to topical anesthesia. Rhinoplasty and other surgical procedures performed on the nose are readily accomplished under regional anesthesia. Injection at the exiting foramina of the infratrochlear and external nasal extensions of the maxillary divisions of the trigeminal nerves is easily accomplished.

## What Pharyngeal Factors Are Important for Intubation?

The shape of the pharynx resembles a flattened cylinder, constantly changing contour by constriction or relaxation of the pharyngeal muscles and positioning of the soft palate, uvula, and tongue (see Fig. 24–1). During examination, the tongue can be drawn forward to widen the oropharyngeal cavity in order to visualize the structures more clearly and to apply topical anesthesia. This capability is particularly important during placement of a laryngeal mask airway. Although direct laryngoscopy has become a lost art among most physicians,[8] the anesthesiologist, using head and laryngeal mirrors with reflected light, should be proficient in examining the larynx to detect pathologic changes and to observe movement of the vocal cords.

## Potential Difficulties in Intubation

As a simple means of detecting possible difficulty in tracheal intubation, Mallampati and colleagues[9] showed that the size of the tongue at its base is a major factor (see Fig. 24–1). If the base of the tongue when protruded is sufficiently large and the faucial pillars and uvula are concealed during laryngoscopy, the larynx will be overshadowed and its visualization made difficult. In a prospective study, the degree of obscuration by the tongue of faucial pillars and uvula was graded and matched with subsequent ability to expose the glottis fully (see Chapter 1, Fig. 1–8). Grades I and II were compatible with adequate exposure, and grades III and IV were predictive of inadequate exposure, findings of statistical significance.

Another means of predicting difficult intubation is by using ultrasound scanning, a noninvasive means of visualizing the vocal cords and larynx.

## Anticipated Problems

Proctor[6] stated that the pharynx and larynx compose, in essence, a bottleneck of the airway. This dictum is most evident in neonates and younger children, in whom the presence of infection, mucosal swelling, inspissated secretions, enlarged adenoids and tonsils, and various degrees of choanal atresia can virtually obstruct the airway. The consequent increase in airway resistance may set off a vicious circle, with development of negative pressure causing the tongue and epiglottis to fall backward into the air passages; emergency treatment (laryngeal intubation and, occasionally, tracheotomy) may be required.

In adults, severe infection can also lead to airway difficulty in the presence of epiglottitis. Further, sleep apnea can cause major physiologic changes. The cause of sleep apnea has not been established, but many studies implicate a discordant action of the glossal and pharyngeal muscles.

## THE TRACHEA

## What Anatomic Considerations Are Important?

The trachea, about 15 cm in length in adults, extends from the cricoid cartilage of the larynx to the bronchial bifurcation, about at the level of the fifth thoracic vertebra and the manubrium sterni (Fig. 24–3). Hyaline cartilaginous rings, about 3 to 5 of which are palpable in the neck, encircle the trachea, maintaining its patency. Tracheotomy or tracheostomy is preferably performed below the level of the first cartilage to avoid development of chondritis in the cricoid ring.

The cartilages are incomplete posteriorly, joined by fibroelastic tissue and highly reactive smooth muscle, Reisseisen muscle (Fig. 24–4), under the same autonomic innervation as the gut. Thus, the trachea dilates during inspiration and narrows during expiration, almost completely closing during cough to enhance development of positive intrathoracic pressure. The epithelial lining is composed of stratified ciliated columnar epithelium and mucus-secreting goblet cells (Fig. 24–5) under ciliary action. The mucus covering propels microparticles in an oral direction.

## Mainstem Intubation

Because the right lung consists of 3 lobes, the right mainstem bronchus is larger in diameter than the left, diverging from the trachea at a lesser angle to the midline (see Fig. 24–3). Consequently, foreign bodies preferentially lodge there, and inadvertent bronchial intubation usually occurs on that side. In children, this difference is less pronounced, and thus right-sided lodging of foreign bodies is less frequent. Further, the bronchus to the right upper lobe arises a mere 2 cm below the bifurcation, whereas the left upper lobe bronchus originates about 5 cm below the bifurcation. As a result, inflation of the cuff on an ordinary or double-lumen tracheal

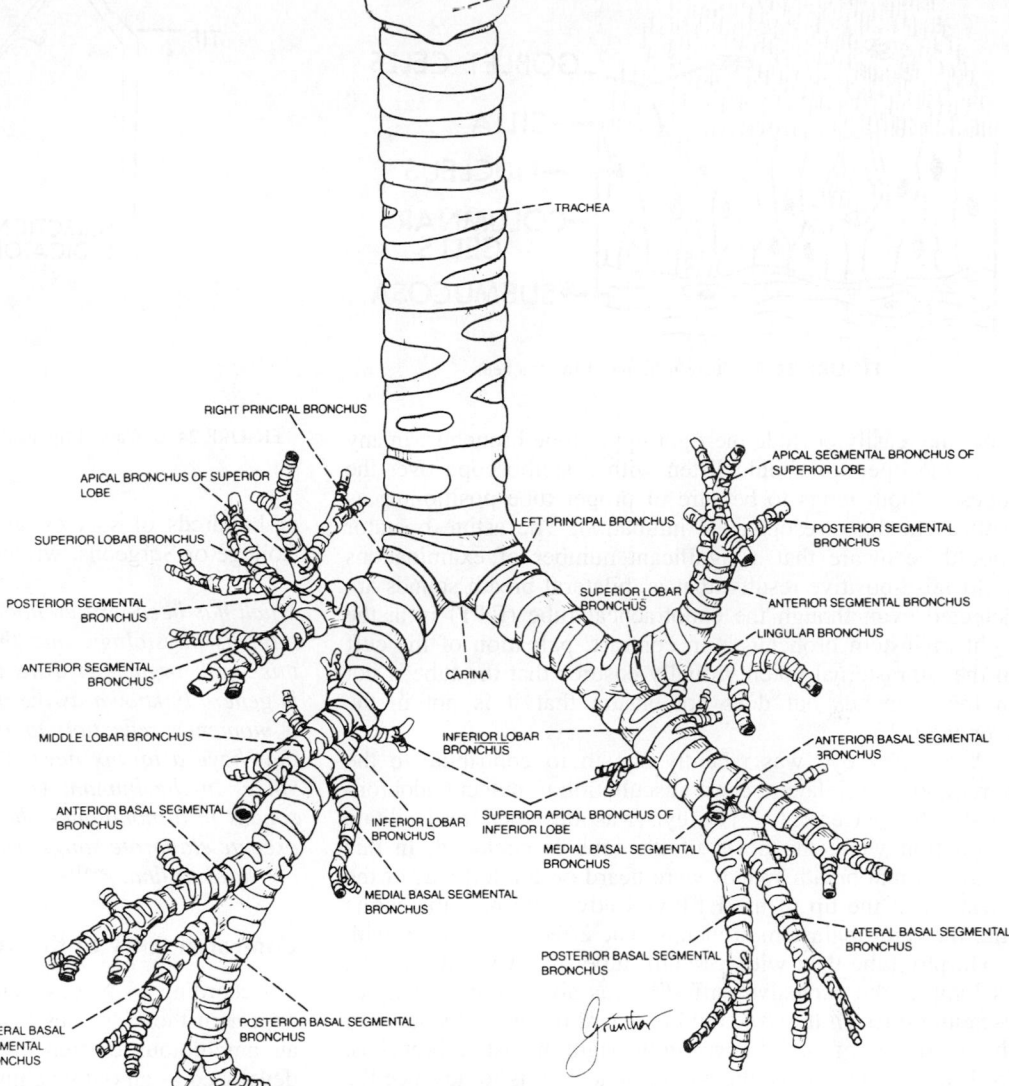

**FIGURE 24–3.** The trachea and its bifurcation. Notice the lesser angle at which the right mainstem bronchus derives from the trachea as well as the high exit of the bronchus of the upper lobe. Conversely, observe the greater angle of departure of the left mainstem bronchus and the relatively lower exits of the bronchus to the upper lobe. (From Snell RS, Karz J. *Clinical Anatomy for Anesthesiologists.* Norwalk, Conn: Appleton & Lange; 1988. Reproduced with permission of The McGraw-Hill Companies.)

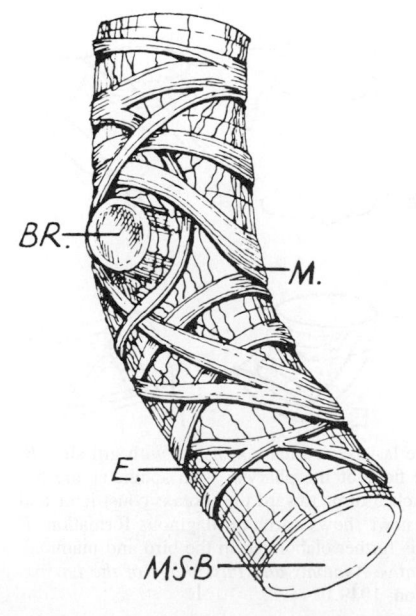

**FIGURE 24–4.** Smooth muscle (M) and elastic fibers (E) of the trachea at a place where a branch (BR) departs from the mainstem bronchus (MSB) of the lung. By contracting and relaxing, the smooth muscle (Reisseisen) with its spiral arrangement can cause marked changes in both length and caliber of the trachea and bronchi. (From Vandam LD. The functional anatomy of the lung. *Anesthesiology.* 1952;13:130.)

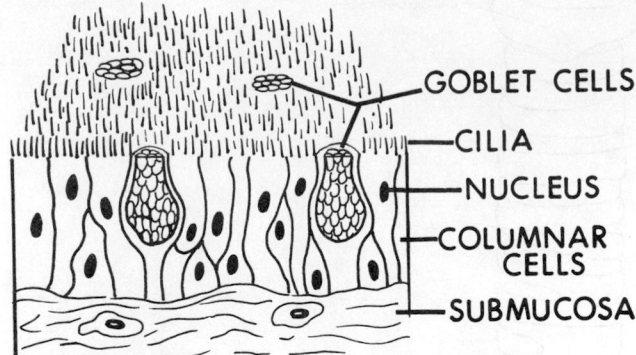

FIGURE 24–5. Mucosal lining of the trachea.

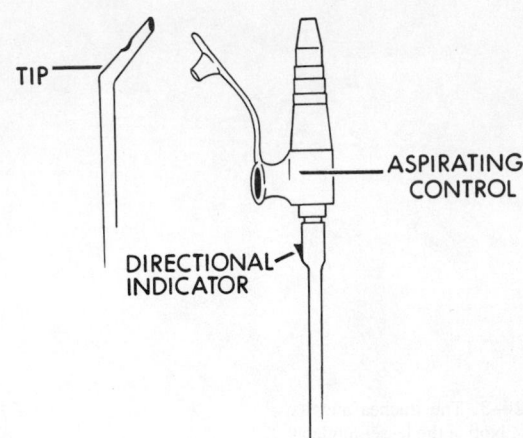

FIGURE 24–6. Curved-tip suctioning catheter with directional indicator.

tube may easily occlude the right upper lobe bronchus. In any case, the operator should listen with a stethoscope over the lobes of both lungs to be sure of proper tube positioning as well as to detect esophageal intubation. The astute operator should be aware that a significant number of examinations yield false-positive results; that is, bilateral breath sounds are detected even though the endotracheal tube (ETT) is in the right mainstem bronchus.[10] In contrast, palpation of the cuff in the suprasternal notch virtually ensures that the tube is not in the bronchus but does not ensure that it is not in the esophagus.[11]

A Murphy eye was recently shown to contribute to the unreliability of bilateral chest auscultation to detect endobronchial tube placement.[12] The eye was designed to facilitate ventilation when the bevel of the tube is occluded. In this study, normal breath sounds were heard on the left side of the chest when the tip of the ETT was advanced past the carina into the right mainstem bronchus. The effect was greater with a Murphy tube than with a Magill tube (no eye). Apparently, as long as the occlusive cuff still was above the carina, gas escaping through the eye could be heard on the left side, even though the tip of the ETT was in the right mainstem bronchus. In difficult intubations, the natural tendency is to advance the ETT farther than is necessary, thereby predisposing to bronchial placement; this work suggests that standard auscultation may not detect the error.

### Bronchial Suctioning

Because of the difference in the angles of the right and left mainstem bronchi, Kubota and associates[13] found that catheters used for suctioning of secretions or treatment of atelectasis entered the right bronchus in about 85% of insertions and the left bronchus in about 11%, coiling up in the upper airway in the remaining 4%. To circumvent this haphazard approach to selective bronchial suctioning, Kubota's group developed a curved-tip catheter with a guide mark at the proximal end to indicate the direction of the curve in its rotation (Fig. 24–6). With this method, they achieved a success rate ranging from 80% to 97% for left bronchial catheterization. Later, and with equal success, they used a J-shaped catheter tip to aspirate the upper lobe bronchi on either side.

## THE LARYNX

### *What Are Its Functions?*

#### Phonation

Negus,[2] an eminent British laryngologist who studied the comparative anatomy of the larynx by dissecting the larynges

of hundreds of species stored in the museum of the Royal College of Surgeons, wrote the following:

*Much has been written about the larynx, its anatomical structure, its physiology, and the diseases that affect it. And yet, this small organ performs its work enshrouded in mystery. It is generally known as the organ of voice, and yet it takes but a moment's reflection to observe that thousands of species that have a larynx never (or practically never) make use of voice. In the human, voice is a poor thing—the individual speaks in a monotone—the range is limited—few are able to execute elaborate songs. Those can sing through a wide range are hard to find.*[2(p444)]

### Control of Entry to the Respiratory Tract

According to Negus,[2] elements of a larynx first began to appear in those species that emerged from the sea to take up an amphibious existence (Fig. 24–7). When the lung buds developed as an outpouching of the foregut, a sphincter mechanism was required to prevent inundation of the lungs on reentry to the aqueous milieu. As a consequence, it is worth noting that the pharmacologic reactions of tracheal smooth

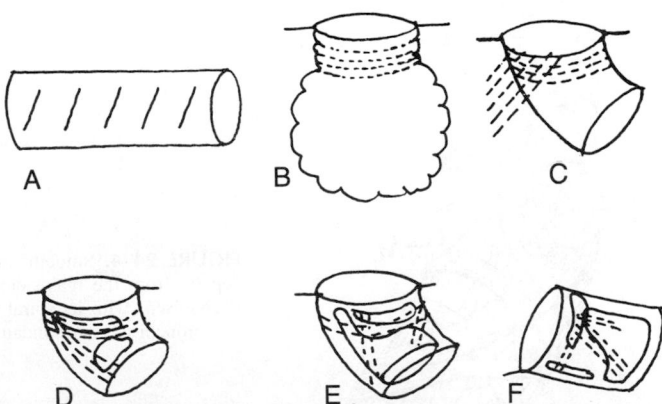

FIGURE 24–7. Evolution of the larynx. *A,* Pharynx of fish with gill slits. *B,* Pulmonary outgrowth from the floor of the pharynx with sphincter mechanism. *C,* In the mudfish, the trachea turns toward the thorax; constrictor and dilator fibers are seen. *D,* The newt shows early cartilaginous formation. *E* and *F,* Cartilaginous formation is further elaborated in the bird and mammal. (From Negus VE. *The Comparative Anatomy and Physiology of the Larynx.* New York, NY: Grune & Stratton; 1949.)

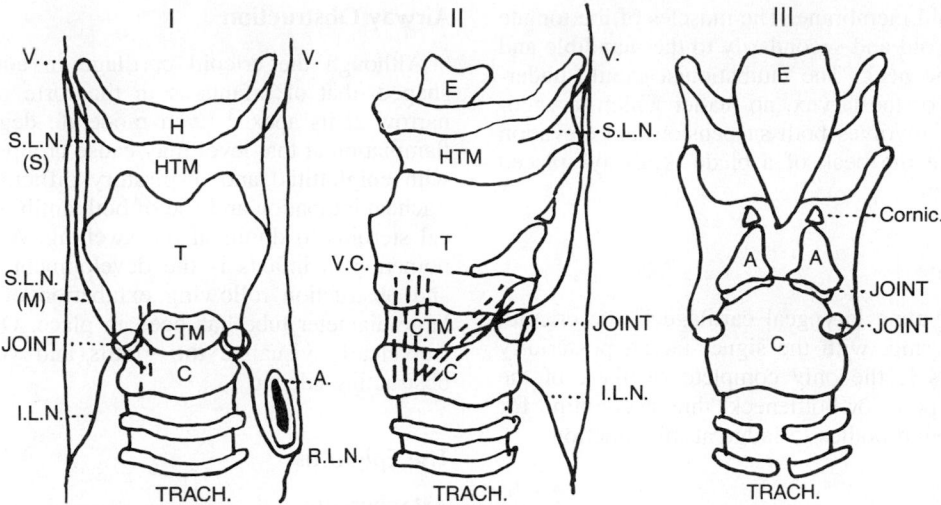

**FIGURE 24–8.** The cartilages of the larynx and the nerve supply in anterior (I), lateral (II), and posterior (III) views. The thyroid (T), cricoid (C), and arytenoid (A) cartilages are the essential elements. Epiglottis (E), corniculate cartilages (Cornic), and cuneiform cartilages (not shown) are of little functional importance. Note the presence of synovial membrane-lined joints between arytenoid and cricoid cartilages and between cricoid and thyroid cartilages. These joints permit movement, owing to action of the intrinsic muscles in the former case and to contraction of the cricothyroid muscle (*dotted lines*) in the latter. The hyoid bone (H), the hypothyroid membrane (HTM), and the cricothyroid membrane (CTM) are important landmarks both for regional anesthesia and for resuscitation. The vagus (V) exits from the superior laryngeal nerve (SLN) and provides sensory function (S) to the upper portion of the larynx and motor function (M) to the only intrinsic muscle, the cricothyroid muscle. Contraction of the latter rotates the cricoid cartilage and tenses the vocal cords. The inferior laryngeal nerves (ILNs) are also mixed nerves, providing sensory function to the lower larynx and motor function to all of the intrinsic muscles. (From Vandam LD. Functional anatomy of the larynx. *Wkly Anesth Update.* 1977;1:2.)

muscle present in mammals are the same as those of the intestinal tract, based presumably on their similar autonomic innervation.

A primitive sphincter is present at the aditus to the lungs in the lungfish (Kamongo of East Africa), then elaborated in the evolutionary ascent through amphibians, avians, and mammals. Thus, from the human standpoint, even though voice appears to be the dominant function, the larynx must be viewed as a valvular mechanism controlling entrance to the respiratory tract.

Valves of any kind, whether physiologic (in living creatures) or elements of machinery (anesthetic apparatus), consist of a housing within which the moving parts perform their function. The human larynx is described here in that context.

## What Are the Laryngeal Cartilages?

Because of their subcutaneous location in the anterior triangles of the neck, most of the structures of the larynx are easily palpable and serve as topographic landmarks for performance of such maneuvers as tracheal intubation, regional anesthesia, and resuscitation, such as in cricothyroidotomy or tracheostomy. In preparation for tracheal intubation, these structures should be examined beforehand.

## The Thyroid Cartilage

Nine cartilages comprise the larynx (Fig. 24–8), of which the largest is the hyaline thyroid cartilage, so called because it is shaped like a shield. The broad laminae of this cartilage meet anteriorly at an acute angle to form a prominence (Adam's apple) in men that is less acute in women. Masculinizing tumors in women cause male-type morphologic changes as well as deepening of the voice.

### Attachments

The broad plates of the cartilage serve as attachments for the sternothyroid, sternohyoid, cricothyroid, and strap muscles in the neck (Fig. 24–9), which serve to tether the larynx during such functions as swallowing, sneezing, vomiting, and coughing. Innervation of these muscles comes from the ansa hypoglossi, with elements contributed by the hypoglossal nerves and branches of the cervical plexus, thus suggesting the interactive complexity of laryngeal function.

Superiorly, the thyroid cartilage is attached to the hyoid

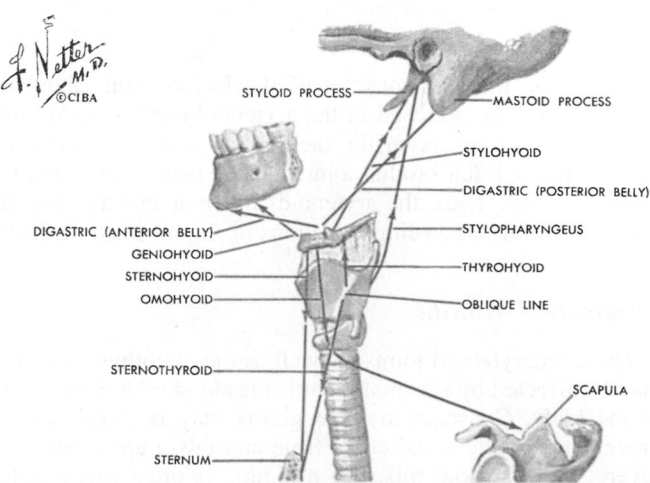

**FIGURE 24–9.** The extrinsic muscles of the larynx and their action. Notice the direction of action of these muscles and their attachment to the hyoid bone, sternum, mandible, mastoid and styloid processes of the temporal bone, scapula, and thyroid cartilage. During a variety of physiologic functions (eg, voice production, swallowing, coughing, sneezing, use of the shoulder girdle), these muscles act jointly to tether the larynx. (From Saunders WH. The larynx. *Clin Symp.* 1964;16:75.)

bone by the thyrohyoid membrane. The muscles of the tongue are attached to the hyoid and secondarily to the mandible and other structures of the neck. The intubationist should understand that intubation of the larynx, no matter which laryngoscopic blade is used, involves both suspension and elevation of the larynx because the beak of a blade is always placed beneath the hyoid bone.

## The Cricoid Cartilage

A second, large hyaline laryngeal cartilage is the cricoid, shaped like a signet ring, with the signet facing posteriorly (see Fig. 24–8). This is the only complete cartilage of the airway, a narrowing point or bottleneck, thus accounting for the propensity of foreign bodies to lodge at this junction.

### Attachments

As part of the larynx, the cricoid is attached to the thyroid cartilage by the cricothyroid membrane, which is immediately subcutaneous, easily palpated, and readily incised in the midline for large needle insertion or incision during resuscitation.

Invagination of the membrane contributes to formation of the true and false vocal cords internally. Further, the cricoid lies at the level of the sixth cervical vertebra (C6), serving as a landmark for a stellate ganglion nerve block, whereby the injecting needle strikes the prominent Chassaignac tubercle of the C6. The cricoid cartilage also articulates with the thyroid cartilage bilaterally by way of diarthrodial joints, permitting a rocking motion of the former in an anteroposterior direction under the action of the external cricothyroid muscles. This motion serves to tense the vocal cords.

## The Arytenoid Cartilages

The remaining cartilages of functional significance are the paired arytenoids (ladle-shaped), which sit atop the signet portion of the cricoid posteriorly.

### Attachments

All of the intrinsic muscles of the larynx, both abductor and adductor, are attached to the arytenoid cartilages. Motion of these cartilages is again facilitated by the presence of synovium-lined diarthrodial joints located between the cricoid and arytenoids. Thus, the arytenoids move anteriorly, posteriorly, or laterally according to actions of the intrinsic muscles.

### Rheumatoid Arthritis

The cricoarytenoid joints, as well as the cricothyroid joints, may be affected by rheumatoid arthritis along with other joints in the body. Consequently, the glottis may be narrowed as movements of the vocal cords (true and false) are limited. In severely arthritic patients, this affliction is often revealed by a high-pitched, weak voice concomitant with a fixed lordotic cervical spine and ankylosis of the temporomandibular joints. Tracheal intubation thus becomes difficult, and a tracheal tube of smaller diameter should be selected, particularly for nasotracheal intubation, which may be the approach of choice in the presence of an arthritic spine.

## Airway Obstruction

Although the cricoid cartilage in adults is cylindrically shaped, that of infants is in the form of an inverted cone, narrow at its apex.[14] Even moderate degrees of mucosal inflammation at that level may cause croup (often in association with epiglottitis) and respiratory difficulty, calling for early tracheal intubation and use of both antibiotics and adrenocortical steroids to diminish the swelling. A second related phenomenon in infants is the development of subglottic edema and obstruction following extubation of the trachea after a large-diameter tube has been in place. On laryngoscopy, one can clearly visualize the glottis and vocal cords with the obstructing edema.

## The Epiglottis

### Attachments

The remainder of the laryngeal cartilages are of little functional significance, and they are mostly vestigial elements (see Fig. 24–8). The largest of this group is the fibrocartilaginous epiglottis (petiole or petal), the stem of which is attached to the interior of the thyroid cartilage above the false cords. On the oropharyngeal side, it is attached to the base of the tongue by the hyoepiglottic ligament, a vestige of a muscle in lower species that apposed the epiglottis to the uvula and soft palate.

### Function

In running animals and infants, the epiglottis is elongated so that its approximation to the palate effectively separates the nasopharyngeal and oropharyngeal cavities. This arrangement permits a running, predatory animal with its long snout to maintain a streamlined airway to the glottis and trachea while retaining access of air to the olfactory plate for scenting prey.

Occasionally, in human beings, inflammation can result in epiglottitis and edema,[15] which may obstruct the airway. Contrary to popular opinion, the epiglottis does not serve, as does a cover on a box, to close the glottis. Rather, during swallowing and in other functions in which the airway must close, the larynx is apposed to the base of the tongue by action of the extralaryngeal muscles.[16]

From the standpoint of topical anesthesia, the oral surface of the epiglottis receives its innervation from the glossopharyngeal nerve and the laryngeal surface from the sensory division of the superior laryngeal branch of the vagus.

## The Corniculate and Cuneiform Cartilages

The paired corniculates (horn-shaped) and the cuneiforms (wedge-shaped) are mainly of evolutionary interest (see Fig. 24–8). The corniculates can be seen as translucent structures during laryngoscopy or can be palpated in anatomic specimens as horn-shaped objects at the tips of the arytenoids, where they once functioned as attachments or davits for the cricopharyngeal sphincter muscles.

### Functions

In lower species and in the developmental stages of human beings, the wedge-shaped cuneiform cartilages are present in the aryepiglottic folds, perhaps adding to their stiffness (as in a starched collar) and width and possibly protecting the glottis against aspiration of liquids and foreign bodies. Because human fetuses and infants recapitulate phylogeny, these paired cartilages and the aryepiglottic folds, as well as the epiglottis, are quite prominent and are to be reckoned with during laryngoscopy.[13]

## When Is a Nerve Block of the Larynx Performed?

Before discussion of the actions of the intrinsic muscles of the larynx, a description of their innervation is necessary. Topical anesthesia of the airway is easily accomplished because of the submucosal location of sensory nerve endings. The larynx, in its entirety—both sensory and motor—is supplied by the vagus nerve, although elements of the glossopharyngeal nerve may be present by means of the 10th nerve nucleus in the hindbrain (see Fig. 24–8).

### Vagal Block

The vagi enter and exit from the skull together with the glossopharyngeal and spinal accessory nerves and jugular veins. As practiced by Mushin,[17] nerve block of the vagi at the jugular foramina provided superb conditions for tracheal intubation in awake patients, although the accompanying glossopharyngeal and spinal accessory paralysis led to respiratory obstruction.

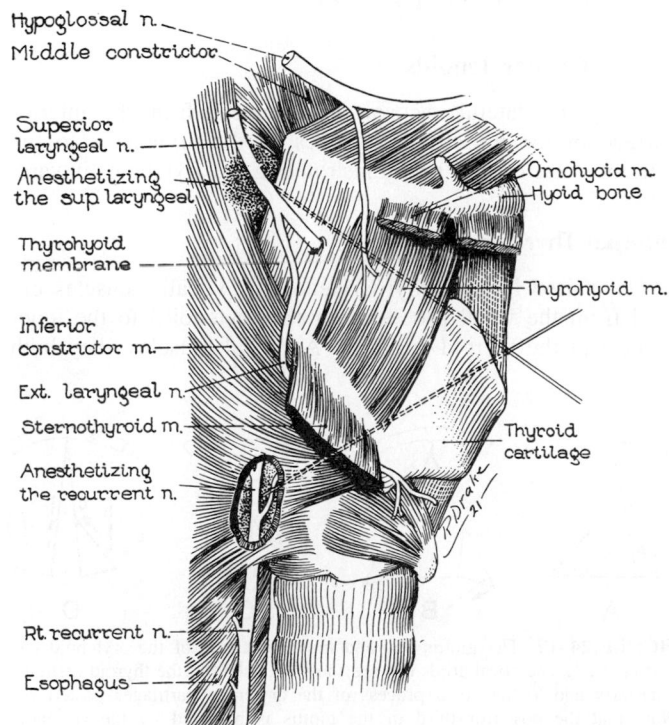

**FIGURE 24–10.** Nerve supply to the larynx from the vagus nerve. Notice the internal branch (sensory) of the superior laryngeal nerve as it pierces the thyrohyoid membrane and the external branch (motor), the external laryngeal nerve, which supplies the cricothyroid muscle. Also shown is the recurrent branch of the vagus as it ascends toward the larynx. *Dotted lines* show the needle pathway for injection of the superior and inferior laryngeal nerves through the thyroid notch. (From Labat G. *Regional Anesthesia: Its Technical and Clinical Application.* 2nd ed. Philadelphia, Pa: WB Saunders; 1928:143.)

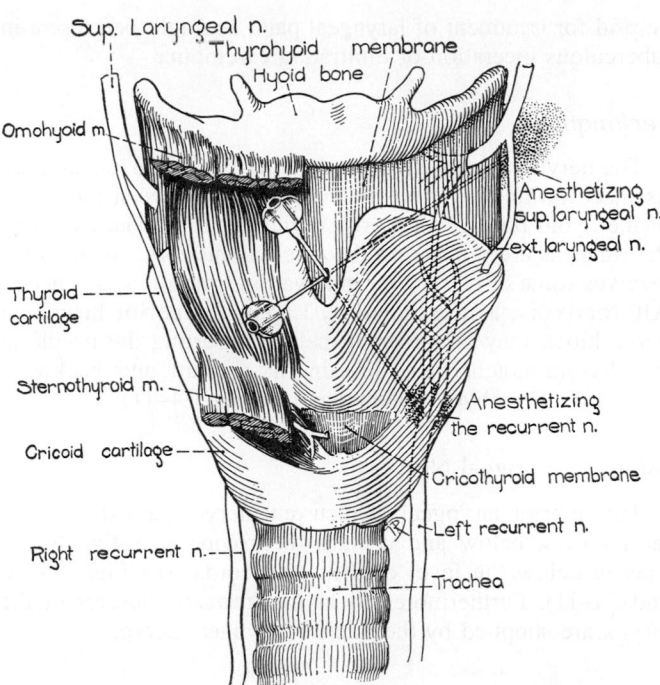

**FIGURE 24–11.** Approach to local anesthetic injection of the superior laryngeal nerve. (From Labat G. *Regional Anesthesia: Its Technical and Clinical Application.* 2nd ed. Philadelphia, Pa: WB Saunders; 1928:143.)

When vocal cord paralysis is found in any patient, in addition to the more common causes, the anesthesiologist should consider the possible presence of a brainstem lesion and examine for accompanying paralysis of the glossopharyngeal and spinal accessory nerves.

### Superior Laryngeal Nerves

One branch of the vagus, the mixed motor and sensory superior laryngeal nerve, leaves the parent nerve at the site of the nodose ganglion at the base of the skull. (A ganglion always implies the presence of sensory neuronal bodies.) An internal branch pierces the hyothyroid membrane to provide sensation to the larynx and part of the pharynx (glossopharyngeal plexus) above the level of the vocal cords (Figs. 24–10 and 24–11).

The motor branch of the superior laryngeal nerve supplies the only extrinsic muscle of the larynx, the cricothyroid (see Figs. 24–8, 24–10, and 24–11). Because of both vertical and diagonal fiber direction and because of the cricothyroid joint, contraction of the cricothyroid muscles causes a rocking motion of the cricoid in the sagittal plane, thus tensing the vocal cords. This action occurs because the arytenoids move with the cricoid, and the internal thyroarytenoid muscle or musculus vocalis is stretched.

### Effects of Nerve Block

Nerve block of the superior laryngeal nerve at its entry to the hyothyroid membrane, along with performance of pharyngeal and transtracheal topical anesthesia, provides excellent conditions for tracheal intubation in awake patients. Sensory anesthesia of the larynx and trachea is obtained, and the vocal cords are relaxed. Superior laryngeal nerve block is also helpful for treatment of laryngeal pain, as might be present in tuberculous ulceration of infiltrating carcinoma.

### Technique

The nerve is anesthetized by fanning out of the needle after its insertion anterior to a fingertip placed between the cornu of the hyoid bone and superior cornu of the thyroid cartilage. Paresthesias are referred to the external auditory canal, which receives some of its sensory innervation from the vagus nerve. Alternatively, as described by Labat,[18] superior laryngeal nerve block may be accomplished by inserting the needle at the thyroid notch, then directing it upward and backward toward the thyrohyoid membrane (see Fig. 24–11).

### Inferior Laryngeal Nerves

The inferior laryngeal or recurrent nerves pass toward the larynx from below and upward to provide sensation to the trachea below the level of the vocal cords (see Figs. 24–10 and 24–11). Furthermore, all of the intrinsic muscles of the larynx are supplied by the inferior laryngeal nerve.

### Anatomic Relationships

On the left, the inferior laryngeal nerve is truly recurrent as it encircles the arch of the aorta close to the ligamentum arteriosum (the obliterated ductus arteriosus). Thus, the left or recurrent nerve is more subject to injury not only during thyroidectomy but also during ligation of a patent ductus arteriosus. Injury can also be due to pressure from an expanding aortic aneurysm but is rarely caused by atrial enlargement in mitral stenosis.

### Technique

The inferior nerve can be anesthetized close to the inferior cornu of the thyroid. Anesthetization of the superior and inferior nerves along with superficial cervical plexus block permit performance of laryngectomy solely under regional anesthesia.

## What Should Be Known About Laryngeal Blood Supply?

The blood supply to the larynx derives from the inferior laryngeal branch of the thyrocervical trunk of the first portion of the subclavian artery and the superior laryngeal artery (the first branch of the external carotid). Because the inferior laryngeal artery lies close to the recurrent laryngeal nerve, injury to the nerve may occur in attempts to control bleeding during thyroidectomy, the most common cause of vocal cord paralysis. Because the nerves may already have divided into their branches at that point, vocal cord paralysis may be partial or complete, depending on the number of branches injured and, incidentally, accounting for the variable positions of the cords found in paralysis.

## What Are the Intrinsic Muscle Actions?

As noted, all of the intrinsic muscles of the larynx are supplied by the recurrent laryngeal nerves, and they may be grouped according to dilator (abductor) or constrictor (adductor) action. The muscles extend between the muscular processes of the arytenoid cartilages at one end to the cricoid or thyroid cartilage at the other. In evolutionary development, the constrictors dominate because only one set of dilators is present. Figure 24–12 gives a view of the glottis as seen at laryngoscopy. One can see how the muscles act during adduction or abduction of either the true or false vocal cords (ventricular bands).

### Laryngeal Dilators

The posterior, paired cricoarytenoid muscles connect the posterior aspects of the vocal processes of the arytenoids to the broad, posterior plate of the cricothyroid cartilage, thus rotating the arytenoids laterally to abduct the cords. These are the only dilator muscles. Consequently, when the cords are found in adduction after nerve injury, paralysis is usually presumed to be the cause (posticus paralysis) (Fig. 24–13; see Fig. 24–12).

### Laryngeal Constrictors

Several muscles form a complete sphincter for the larynx (see Figs. 24–12 and 24–13).

### Interarytenoids

The interarytenoids, transverse and oblique, bring the arytenoids together. The transverse elements ascend in the aryepiglottic folds as the aryepiglottic muscles.

### Lateral Cricoarytenoids

The paired lateral cricoarytenoids extend from the anterior surface of the muscular processes of the arytenoids to the interior of the cricoid ring, thus rotating the arytenoids inward.

### Internal Thyroarytenoids

The paired internal thyroarytenoid or vocalis muscles extend from the vocal processes of the arytenoids to the inner surface of the thyroid cartilage. As vocal muscles, they both

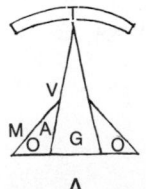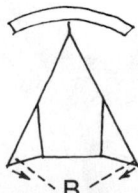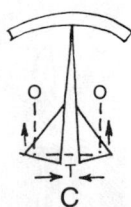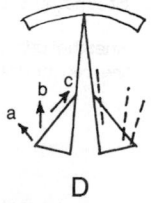

**FIGURE 24–12.** The glottis (G) and movement (M) of the arytenoid (A) cartilages. *A,* The vocal cords (V) are shown attached to the thyroid cartilage anteriorly and to the vocal process of the arytenoid cartilages posteriorly. Note that the posterior third of the glottis is bounded by the arytenoid cartilages, covered with squamous epithelium. *B,* The action of the posterior cricoarytenoid muscles is shown, attached to the posterior face of the arytenoid cartilages, thus opening the glottis. *C,* The glottis is nearly closed, owing to the action of the transverse interarytenoid (T) and oblique interarytenoid (O) muscles. *D,* The remainder of the adductors are shown, indicating action of the lateral cricoarytenoid muscles (a), action of the external thyroarytenoid muscles (b), and action of the internal thyroarytenoid or vocalis muscles (c). (From Vandam LD. Functional anatomy of the larynx. *Wkly Anesth Update.* 1977;1:95.)

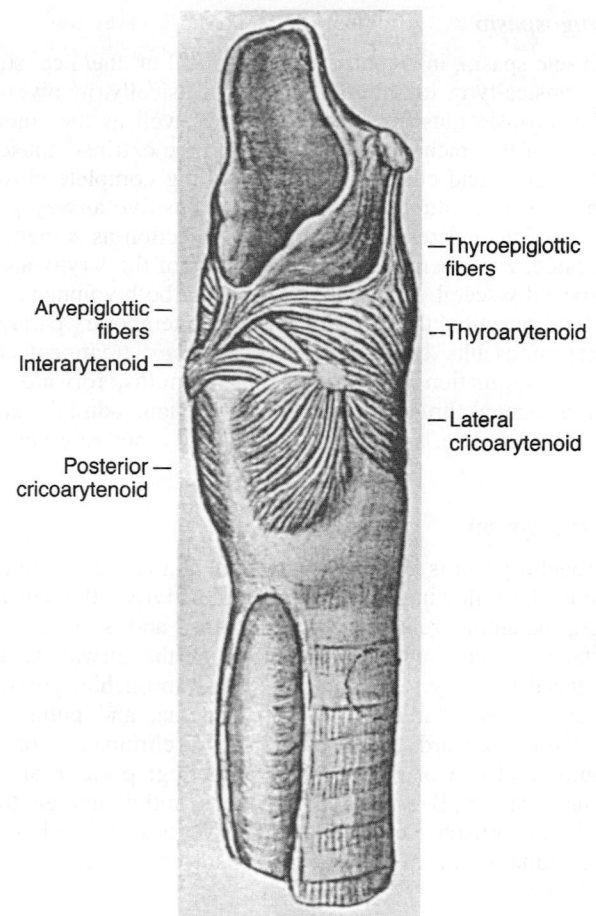

**FIGURE 24–13.** The dilator muscles of the larynx (posterior cricoarytenoid) and the components of the sphincteric group. Note how the latter form a complete sphincter around the larynx. Note also the height of the larynx from the cricoid cartilage below to the tip of the epiglottis above. (From Negus VE. *The Comparative Anatomy and Physiology of the Larynx.* New York, NY: Grune & Stratton; 1949.)

close the glottis and tense the cords (as do the extrinsic cricothyroid muscles). The vocal cords are covered by stratified squamous epithelium, the source of epidermoid carcinoma. Vocal cord polyps are more likely to develop at the posterior third of the glottis, where a tracheal tube might lie against the underlying vocal processes of the arytenoids. Movement of the larynx in light planes of anesthesia (swallowing, cough) may abrade the epithelium. During healing of the ulceration, fibrous organization results in polyp formation with continued cord movement. Postintubation polyp formation, not a rare complication, is suggested by chronic hoarseness. An unusual complication of prolonged intubation, in addition to tracheal erosion and stenosis, is arytenoid cartilage dislocation.

### External Thyroarytenoids

The paired external thyroarytenoid muscles extend from the vocal processes of the arytenoids at a higher level to the interior of the thyroid cartilage, thus forming the ventricular bands (see Figs. 24–12 and 24–13). An evagination of the larynx between the true and false cords forms the laryngeal ventricles and Morgagni vestigial saccules.

## Why Is Intubation Sometimes Difficult?

Anesthetists should realize that the larynx is of considerable depth, extending from the level of the C3 to the C6 (Fig. 24–14). In difficult intubations, the problem is not so much that the larynx is "too anterior," as often stated (it is always anterior in the neck), but that it is relatively high in a short, thick-necked patient. Visualization of the glottis is difficult because of the correspondingly more acute angle between the oropharynx and pharynx, hence the need for a tracheal tube stylet, curved blade, or fiberoptic laryngoscope.

## What Are the Sphincter Functions of the Larynx?

In addition to its function in vocalization, the larynx also serves as a true valve of the respiratory tract.

### Increase in Intrathoracic Pressure

To increase intrathoracic pressure, as in the Valsalva maneuver and during coughing or sneezing, the larynx must close before thoracic pressure can be raised.

### Increase in Intraabdominal Pressure

Similarly, to increase intraabdominal pressure, the diaphragm must be stabilized by laryngeal closure before the abdominal muscles can contract effectively as during urination, defecation, or bearing down in labor (Fig. 24–15). Further, when the upper extremities are used for lifting or for "chinning" on a bar, the shoulder girdle muscles attached to

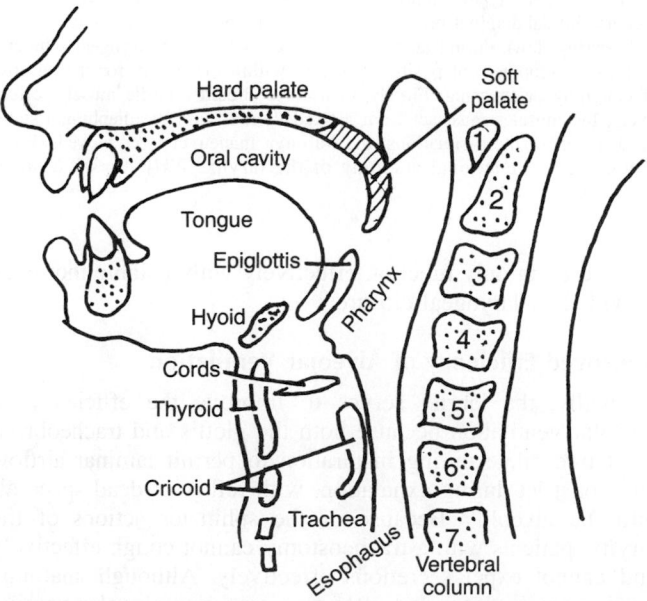

**FIGURE 24–14.** Sagittal section through the upper airway. Note that the larynx, from the tip of the epiglottis to the cricoid cartilage below, corresponds to a span of four cervical vertebrae (C3 through C6). If intubation is difficult, it is not because the larynx lies anteriorly (it always does) but because it is relatively high on the cervical column in the short-necked person. The angle between oral cavity and pharynx is acute and is not easily negotiated on intubation. (From Vandam LD. Functional anatomy of the larynx. *Wkly Anesth Update.* 1977;1:95.)

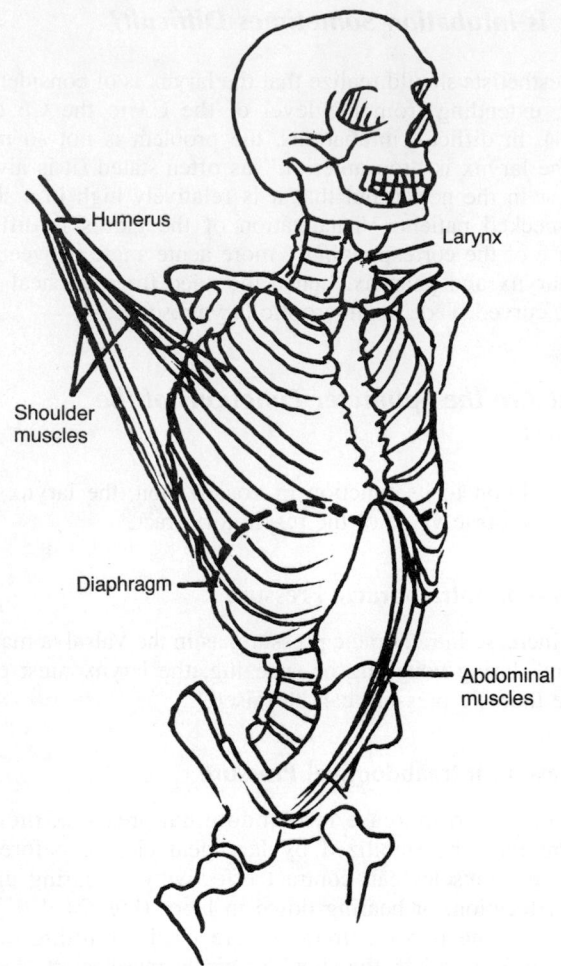

**FIGURE 24–15.** Sphincter mechanism of the larynx. Closure of the larynx stabilizes the volume of air within the thorax and fixes the diaphragm *(dotted line)*. This permits the abdominal muscles to contract effectively and to increase intraabdominal pressure for such functions as urination, defecation, and bearing down during labor. Similarly, closure of the laryngeal sphincter permits development of positive pressure within the thorax for the purpose of coughing or sneezing. Finally, to use the shoulder girdle muscles effectively, the muscles must act from a fixed thorax, with the diaphragm stabilized. In all of these situations, the Valsalva maneuver is employed. (From Vandam LD. Functional anatomy of the larynx. *Wkly Anesth Update.* 1977;1:95.)

the chest can only function effectively with a stable thorax as provided by laryngeal closure.

### Improved Efficiency of Alveolar Ventilation

Finally, the larynx serves to improve the efficiency of alveolar ventilation because both the glottis and tracheobronchial tree dilate during inspiration to permit laminar airflow and constrict during exhalation, with reflux of dead space air into the alveoli.[19] Because of the sphincter actions of the larynx, patients with a tracheostomy cannot cough effectively and cannot expel secretions effectively. Although anatomic dead space is decreased after tracheostomy, alveolar ventilation is not as efficient: respiratory rate increases, and a minor degree of respiratory alkalosis develops.

### Reflex Airway Closure

Laryngospasm and bronchospasm are manifestations of the reflex defensive system of the lungs.

#### Laryngospasm

Muscle spasm, in response to mechanical or chemical stimuli intrinsically or to painful stimuli extrinsically, involves all of the intrinsic muscles of the larynx as well as the smooth muscles of the tracheobronchial tree and the extrinsic muscles of the larynx and chest wall. The resulting complete closure of the airway is stubbornly resistive to positive airway pressure and does not respond to atropine injection as sometimes advocated. However, because the muscles of the larynx are of the special visceral variety, thus permitting both voluntary and involuntary action, they readily respond to temporary paralysis by neuromuscular blocking agents. Standard treatment consists of elimination of the offending stimulus, forward and upward manual thrusts of the jaw, intravenous administration of succinylcholine, and $O_2$ given by positive pressure ventilation.

#### Bronchospasm

Bronchospasm is a complex phenomenon caused by one or more of the following: parasympathetic activity, allergens and drugs, histamine release, prostaglandins, and slow-reacting substance of anaphylaxis. Narrowing of the airway is also influenced by body temperature, extrinsic bronchial pressure, congestive heart failure, pulmonary edema, and pulmonary embolism. Standard therapy consists of elimination of the stimulus and one or more of the following: positive airway pressure with $O_2$, β-sympathetic agonists, anticholinergic therapy, hydrocortisone, occasionally intravenous aminophylline, and elimination of any chest wall spasm with a neuromuscular blocker.

## TRACHEAL INTUBATION

### What Are the Advantages?

Patency of the airway is reasonably ensured for several reasons. Secretions can be removed from the tracheobronchial tree with relative ease. Positive pressure can be applied to the airway without distention of the stomach; a patient can be placed in any position during operation, with less chance of compromising the airway; and the anesthetist can be seated at a distance from the patient while still maintaining control of respiration.

### Assisted Ventilation

Intubation is necessary to assist ventilation in patients with ventilatory insufficiency and to protect the lungs when laryngeal reflexes are compromised. Tracheal intubation is mandatory in patients at high risk for aspiration of gastric contents and in operations such as thoracotomy when positive pressure ventilation is paramount.

Intubation is also indicated in the prone, sitting, lateral, or Trendelenburg position, in which maintenance of an airway by mask and application of positive pressure ventilation would be unreliable. It is also necessary in operations on patients with an already compromised airway.[20]

### What Equipment Should Be Available?

#### Laryngoscope

To expose the glottis, a laryngoscope is used. The instrument is made of metal and consists of a handle, a blade, and

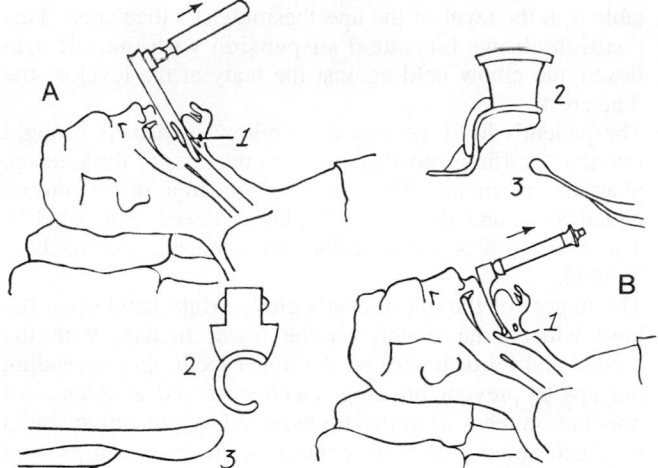

**FIGURE 24–16.** Upward lift of laryngoscopy at 45° angle to expose the glottis. *A,* Straight blade beneath the (1) epiglottis. 2, End view of the straight blade with semicircular construction to keep tongue to the left. 3, Tip of the straight blade to lift the hyoid bone when placed beneath the epiglottis. *B,* Curved blade proximal to the (1) glottis. 2, End view of the curved blade with right-angle construction to keep the tongue to the left; the flange lifts the tongue. (From Dripps RD, Eckenhoff JE, Vandam LD. *Introduction to Anesthesia: The Principles of Safe Practice.* 1st ed. Philadelphia, Pa: WB Saunders; 1957.)

light source. The handle contains batteries that provide current for the light bulb fitted into the tip of the blade, the latter with a hook-on attachment to the handle. In cross section, the C-shaped blade displaces the tongue to the left, away from the path of vision, and space is maintained on the right for passage of a tracheal tube (Fig. 24–16).

## Blades

Laryngoscope blades come in two principal types, curved and straight, varying in size for use in infants, children, or adults. Many varieties of both curved and straight blades have been designed to facilitate passage of a tracheal tube; however, an accomplished anesthesiologist can manage with two or three blades at most. Disposable blades are available to avoid transmission of infectious disease. A flexible fiberoptic bronchoscope is used for intubation under difficult conditions (for a more detailed discussion, see Chapter 16).

## Tracheal Tubes

Most tracheal tubes are disposable and consist of clear, pliable polyvinylchloride with little tendency to kink. They are sterilized with ethylene oxide by the manufacturer and thoroughly vented before use. At body temperature, the tubes mold to the contour of the upper airway and present a smooth interior for easy passage of suction catheters or a flexible bronchoscope.

### Construction

Tracheal tubes are of measured length, marked in 0.5-cm increments according to diameter, with inflatable cuffs optional above 5 mm, and with a Magill or a Murphy tip. The latter has an opening opposite the bevel. They are usually longer than necessary when received from the manufacturer and benefit from shortening to lessen the possibility of bron-

chial intubation or to prevent kinking at the nose or mouth. After the proximal end of the tube is cut, the connector should be firmly reinserted.

### Cuffs

Built-in cuffs are used in adults and older children; when inflated, the cuff ensures a closed system, permitting easy control of ventilation and minimizing the possibility of aspiration of vomitus or blood. Cuffs may be of the high-pressure or low-pressure variety, depending on the volume of air required for inflation. When inflated, a high-pressure cuff is short; thus, a small surface is in contact with the tracheal wall and a high internal cuff pressure is required to seal the trachea. Low-pressure cuffs offer both a larger volume and diameter plus a broad contact with the tracheal wall.

When a cuff is overinflated, regardless of type (high-pressure, low-volume; or low-volume, high-pressure), excessive pressure on the tracheal wall may cause mucosal ischemia; therefore, the cuff is inflated with only enough air to obtain a seal. Esophageal temperature probes and nasogastric tubes may readily pass into the trachea beside a low-pressure cuff. Cuffed tracheal tubes usually incorporate a pilot balloon with a self-sealing valve at the inflation site. Moreover, the cuffs are permeable to nitrous oxide and, over time, increase in volume and pressure[21]; thus, during a prolonged anesthetic, the volume should be readjusted to prevent excessive pressure.

### Special Purpose Tracheal Tubes

A number of special purpose tracheal tubes are available, as follows:

- Armored or anode tubes are reinforced with coiled wire to prevent occlusion from external pressure or kinking. Noncollapsible tubes are useful in patients with a tracheostomy and in operations performed with a patient in the sitting or face-down position with the head sharply flexed. Magill forceps or a stylet is needed for insertion.
- Preformed tubes have molded angles placed at the point of emergence from the mouth or nose; the molded curve minimizes kinking and obstruction.
- Pediatric tubes are small, <5 mm in diameter, and generally without a cuff.
- Laser-shield tubes (various types) have been made of silicone impregnated with metal particles covering the main shaft and cuff to withstand laser-induced heat and ignition. Nitrous oxide should not be used during anesthesia, and the cuff should be inflated with sterile saline.
- Double-lumen tubes are used for selective ventilation of the lungs or airway protection.

See Chapter 16 for additional discussion of special-purpose tracheal tubes.

### Accessory Intubating Instruments

#### Stylets

A stylet made of malleable metal or plastic is inserted in a tracheal tube to improve the curvature and add stiffness to it. The stylet is lubricated to aid in its withdrawal and should not protrude beyond the tip.

### Intubating Forceps

Magill intubating forceps are used to assist in passage of flaccid or regular tracheal tubes, to aid in passage of a nasogastric tube, or to insert pharyngeal packing. Damage to the cuff may occur if handled with forceps.

## Which Techniques Are Preferred?

The mode of intubation is predicated not only on the site of operation but also on the projected need for postoperative ventilation.

### Orotracheal Intubation

Before induction of anesthesia, all necessary equipment should be tested and readied for use. A tube of appropriate diameter and length should be selected: in women, 7.5 mm inside diameter; in men, 8 to 9 mm inside diameter. The tube should be cut to size before intubation and examined for patency, and the cuff should be inflated to detect air leak. The adapter placed in the proximal end should fit snugly, lying at the level of the teeth; otherwise, its projection may lead to kinking. The tube is kept in its clean wrapper and not handled until ready for insertion.

After preoxygenation and induction of anesthesia, relaxation is usually achieved with a neuromuscular blocker, and the lungs are oxygenated by positive pressure ventilation before attempted intubation. In teaching, an instructor should set a limit of 45 seconds for placement of the tube; in failed intubation, a second period of ventilation with $O_2$ should follow.

### Comparison of Straight- and Curved-Blade Techniques

Theoretically, the advantages of the curved blade relate to the sensory innervation of the laryngeal or inferior surface of the epiglottis, where sensation is derived from the superior laryngeal branch of the vagus. Stimulation by a straight blade placed beneath the epiglottis is believed to predispose more to laryngospasm and cough. The pharyngeal or superior surface is innervated by the glossopharyngeal nerve, stimulation of which is less likely to cause spasm. Further, the curved blade allows more room for passage of the trachea between the teeth than does a straight blade. Occasionally, however, exposure of the glottis is not as good as that obtained with the straight blade, and a stylet may be required to improve the curvature of the tube.

When a patient's mouth cannot be opened widely, as when the teeth protrude or are in poor condition or in stout-necked patients, a curved blade is more useful. If the glottis is not easily exposed, depression of the cricoid cartilage (Sellick maneuver)[22] by an assistant may help, although suspension of the larynx is impeded. This maneuver is commonly used to prevent regurgitation of stomach contents during induction of anesthesia.

### Curved-Blade Technique

The maneuvers are as follow:

• The height of the operating table is adjusted so that the table is at the level of the anesthesiologist's iliac crest. This position allows laryngeal suspension with the left arm flexed and elbow held against the body at the level of the iliac crest.

• The patient's head, resting on a pillow or pad, is brought into the "sniffing" position to align the axes of the trachea, pharynx, and mouth. The head is extended at the atlantooccipital joint, and the cervical spine is flexed (Fig. 24–17). This position was first described by Bannister and Macbeth in 1944.[23]

• The fingers of the anesthetist's gloved right hand open the jaws widely, the thumb on the lower molars, with the second and third fingers on the upper teeth, thus spreading the lips to prevent bruising. Gentleness and avoidance of pressure on teeth or gums are essential. A protective shield or plastic mold placed over the upper incisors can prevent damage.

• Held in the left hand, the moistened or lubricated laryngoscope blade is introduced at the right side of the mouth and advanced in the midline, displacing the tongue to the left. The epiglottis is then seen at the base of the tongue, the tip of the blade fitting into the vallecula (see Fig. 24–16). The wrist is held rigid to avoid using the upper teeth as a fulcrum for the laryngoscope blade. A forward and upward lift of the laryngoscope and blade stretches the hypoepiglottic ligament, thus folding the epiglottis upward and further exposing the glottis. As a result, the larynx is suspended on the tip of the blade by means of the hyoid bone.

• The tracheal tube, with cuff deflated and concavity directed anterolaterally, is passed to the right of the laryngoscope through the glottis into the trachea until the cuff passes 2 to 3 cm beyond the vocal cords.

The glottis occasionally is not fully visible, but intubation is possible when only the arytenoid cartilages and posterior commissure are seen. A curved stylet helps to direct the tube anteriorly.

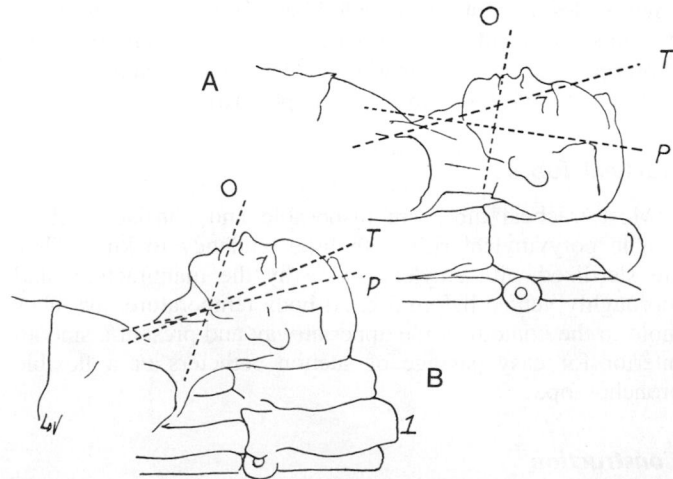

**FIGURE 24–17.** Position of the head for laryngoscopy and intubation of the trachea. *A,* Ordinary position. T, Axis of the trachea; P, axis of the pharynx; O, axis of the oral cavity. *B,* Modified position achieved with an extra headrest. Flexion of the cervical spine and extension at the atlantooccipital joint bring the three axes more nearly into line. (From Dripps RD, Eckenhoff JE, Vandam LD. *Introduction to Anesthesia: The Principles of Safe Practice.* 7th ed. Philadelphia, Pa: WB Saunders; 1988.)

### Straight-Blade Technique

Intubation with a straight blade (see Fig. 24–16) involves the same maneuvers but with one major difference. The blade is slipped beneath the epiglottis, and exposure of the larynx is accomplished by an upward and forward lift at a 45° angle. Again, leverage on the teeth must not be applied.

### Failure to Intubate

With either technique, the common causes of failure to intubate are as follows: inadequate position of the head; misplacement of the laryngoscope blade; inadequate muscle relaxation; insufficient depth of general anesthesia; allowing the tongue to obscure the glottis; and lack of familiarity with the anatomy, especially where there are pathologic changes. Inserting a laryngoscope blade too deeply results in lifting of the entire larynx and esophagus if the tip of the blade is not placed in the vallecula.

## Nasotracheal Intubation

Nasotracheal intubation is commonly used in oral and maxillofacial operations and in emergency situations outside the operating room. Although nasotracheal intubation is indicated in a patient with trismus or a fractured jaw, it is avoided in patients with a basilar skull fracture, a fractured nose, or nasal obstruction. It is also contraindicated in the presence of acute sinusitis or mastoiditis because the infection may spread to the rest of the airway. The technique may be applied either with a well-sedated, awake patient or after induction of general anesthesia and use of a neuromuscular blocker. Nasal intubation may be performed blindly or under direct vision using a laryngoscope or flexible fiberoptic bronchoscope.

### Blind Nasal Intubation

The procedure for blind nasal intubation is as follows:

- The patient's occiput rests on a firm pillow, somewhat higher than that used for oral intubation, with the chin further elevated. Prior topical application of 2- to 4-mL of lidocaine 4% with phenylephrine, 0.25% is used to shrink mucous membranes. Gentle exploration should be carried out with cotton swabs to detect nasal obstruction, particularly at the posterior choanae.
- A tube, smaller in diameter than required for oral intubation, should be soft and pliable to avoid injuring the nasal mucosa or turbinates but of a consistency to resist compression and to maintain a reasonable curvature. These conditions can be met by warming the plastic tube in hot water just before intubation.
- The well-lubricated tube is introduced with its concavity forward and bevel directed laterally; advancement is slow and gentle, with rotation when resistance is met. Tough maneuvers, large-bore rigid tubes, poor lubrication, and use of force against obstruction easily induce epistaxis. Guides to ultimate success during intubation include the following:
  Increase or decrease in breath sounds, heard by listening at the proximal end of the tube in spontaneously breathing patients
  Resistance to passage

Rotation of the tube and manual depression or elevation of

the larynx may be required. Voluntary hyperpnea helps if the patient is awake, as does hyperpnea produced by hypercapnia, because maximal abduction of the cords is present during inspiration. Entry into the trachea is signified by consistent breath sounds transmitted through the tube and inability to speak in the conscious patient as well as by lack of resistance, often accompanied by cough. One can then feel the inflation of the tracheal cuff below the larynx, followed by connecting the tube to the rebreathing system and expanding the lungs.

### Direct Vision

Nasotracheal intubation under direct vision is accomplished during laryngoscopy with or without the help of Magill forceps. The tube is inserted through one nostril into the oropharynx, with the bevel pointing laterally. The vocal cords are then exposed, and the tube is advanced under direct vision into the trachea. If it does not progress, Magill forceps are used to direct the tip toward the glottis, with an assistant then advancing the tube. Magill forceps may also be useful during conscious nasotracheal intubation under direct vision.

Advantages of nasotracheal over oral intubation are as follow:

- The tube is easily secured, with less tendency for accidental extubation.
- It is more comfortable in awake patients and eliminates the possibility of occlusion by biting on the tube.
- Oral feeding is possible during long-term nasotracheal intubation.

Disadvantages include the following:

- Damage to nasal tissues (epistaxis, dislodgment of adenoidal tissue) is possible.
- Infection can be transmitted from nose to trachea and lungs.
- The need for smaller tubes results in increased resistance to breathing.
- Secretions are not easily suctioned.

## When Is Tracheal Intubation Performed in the Conscious Patient?

An anesthesiologist should be able to intubate the trachea with a patient awake when induction of general anesthesia is considered unsafe, as in the absence of an assured airway. Indications for "awake" intubation are listed in Table 24–2. Preanesthetic preparation should include a detailed explana-

**TABLE 24–2.** Indications for Intubation in a Conscious Patient

Threat of aspiration of gastric contents during induction of general anesthesia
Ventilation after induction of anesthesia that is anticipated to be difficult or impossible because of pathologic changes in the pharynx, larynx, neck, or mediastinum
Inflammatory swelling encroaching on the mouth or pharynx
Malformation of the jaws
Scar tissue resulting from burns or operations around the head and neck
Congenital abnormalities of the upper airway
Morbid obesity

tion of the procedure to ensure maximal cooperation by patients.

## Requirements

### Sedation

Intubation of conscious patients can be performed either orally or nasally. Patients require sedation for relaxation and to minimize unpleasant recollections. Sedation is best achieved with incremental intravenous doses of sedatives or opioids, such as diazepam, midazolam, and fentanyl. Topical anesthesia of the airway is necessary.

### Topical Anesthesia

Topical anesthesia of the upper airway can be accomplished by means of a nebulizer, application of cotton swabs, superior laryngeal nerve block, transtracheal injection of local anesthetic through the cricothyroid membrane, or spraying with a topical anesthetic under direct laryngoscopic vision. The structures are anesthetized in the following order: oropharynx, base of tongue, epiglottis, pyriform fossae, vocal cords, and finally the larynx and upper trachea by instillation of 2 mL of local anesthetic through the glottis.

For nasotracheal intubation, the mucosa should also be thoroughly anesthetized. A minimal amount of anesthetic is used to prevent untoward reactions—not more than 4 mL of 4% lidocaine—using wrung-out swabs.

### Risk for Aspiration

The uses of topical anesthesia and heavy sedation for tracheal tube placement are controversial in patients with a full stomach. Sedation, opioids, and topical anesthesia may result in an incompetent larynx and thus risk for aspiration should regurgitation or vomiting occur. The Sellick maneuver[22] is usually employed. In the awake patient, tracheal intubation is generally less traumatic and more often successful if performed with a flexible fiberoptic bronchoscope.

### Care After Intubation

The first steps after intubation include the following:

- Cuff inflation using the minimal leak method to seal off the trachea and to avoid excessive cuff pressure
- Observation of chest movement as the lungs are inflated with $O_2$
- Observation of the repetitive presence of exhaled $CO_2$ and listening for breath sounds bilaterally high in the axillae and over the epigastrium to make certain that the trachea, and not the esophagus or a bronchus, has been entered

As noted, a tube enters the right mainstem bronchus more easily than the left because of their relative angles at the bifurcation. Failure of one side of the chest to move with ventilation and absence of breath sounds suggest bronchial intubation, in which case the tube should be withdrawn several centimeters beyond where breath sounds are bilaterally and equally audible.

## Tube Stabilization and Fixation

After orotracheal intubation, an oropharyngeal airway or soft bite block is placed between the teeth to prevent biting on the tube. The tube is secured with adhesive or umbilical tape tied around the patient's neck; suturing to the teeth or gums may be required during maxillofacial operations. In cases of excessive secretions, as in the face-down position, or when solutions used to prepare the operative field loosen the adhesive, preparation of the skin with tincture of benzoin before taping is useful. Nasotracheal tubes should also be fixed securely, with the connector at the level of the nares, so as not to deform the nasal cartilages.

## Why Does Coughing Occur, and How Is It Treated?

Coughing after intubation frequently occurs when topical anesthesia is inadequate, during light planes of general anesthesia, and when the tube touches the carina. If the coughing is mild, only transient hypertension and tachycardia result. In the more severe reaction, thoracic muscle spasm and bronchospasm may be difficult to overcome while ventilation is impaired, resulting in hypoxia. If the tube touches the carina, it should be withdrawn slightly. If coughing persists, intravenous injection of a small amount of lidocaine or neuromuscular blocker followed by controlled ventilation usually relieves chest wall spasm.

## What Factors Affect Tube Movement?

When a patient's position on the operating table is subsequently changed, the position of the tube must again be verified. Flexion of the head, shortening the distance from teeth to carina, and steep Trendelenburg position, which causes the abdominal contents to elevate the hila of the lungs and carina, may direct a tube into a mainstem bronchus.

## How Is Esophageal Intubation Detected?

### Clinical Signs

A tracheal tube inadvertently placed in the esophagus is suggested by absence of clear breath sounds and exhaled $CO_2$, progressive distention of the stomach with attempted ventilation, deterioration in $O_2$ saturation as seen on pulse oximetry, and development of cyanosis. While listening over the stomach with a stethoscope, the anesthetist may detect air entry as the reservoir bag is compressed. When in doubt, one should immediately remove the tracheal tube and ventilate the lungs with a face mask. After tracheal intubation has been successful, the stomach should be emptied of gas by orogastric or nasogastric suctioning.

Capnography is essential in detecting esophageal intubation; absence of $CO_2$ in exhaled air is diagnostic and minimizes the time for corrective action. Unrecognized esophageal intubation is one of the common causes of anoxia and death and not an infrequent factor in medicolegal action. When standard capnography is unavailable, portable devices may be used.[24]

## How Is Extubation Performed?

### Preparation

Before extubation, the oropharynx is suctioned, neuromuscular blockade is reversed, and the adequacy of spontaneous ventilation is ensured. Routine tracheal suctioning is unnecessary; however, when indicated, a sterile suction catheter should be used. Although it is essential to rid the trachea or pharynx of secretions before extubation, one should not persist if coughing is protracted and the $SpO_2$ drops.

### Oxygen Administration

Before and after tracheal suctioning, $O_2$ is administered. Tape or other fixation devices are removed, the cuff is deflated, and the tube is withdrawn as the lungs are inflated with $O_2$. A tube should not be removed with the aspirating catheter in place because this technique depletes the lungs of $O_2$; this maneuver is not effective in preventing aspiration. If the catheter brushes against the vocal cords, bleeding or laryngospasm may occur.

### Technique

After the tube is removed, the patient is given $O_2$ by mask; if necessary, the oropharynx is again suctioned. If laryngospasm develops, it is now less threatening because the lungs have been inflated with $O_2$ before extubation. To avoid laryngospasm, extubation can be carried out at a relatively deep plane of anesthesia during spontaneous ventilation or when a patient has reacted sufficiently to have regained airway control. Laryngospasm and cough may be minimized by injection of lidocaine, 50 to 100 mg intravenously, 1 or 2 minutes before extubation.

## Why Is Extubation Sometimes Difficult?

Removal of a tracheal tube is occasionally difficult or impossible. The common causes are failure to deflate the cuff or unintentional suturing of a nasotracheal tube to the tissues during maxillofacial surgery. Also, a patient may have bitten on the tube.

## What Precautions Are Necessary?

A tracheal tube should not be removed in the presence of $O_2$ desaturation and cyanosis, when respiratory exchange is inadequate or uncontrollable with mask and bag, or when the operation has compromised the airway. In patients with a full stomach, a tube is left in place until the patient is fully awake; extubation is then accomplished with the patient in the lateral decubitus position. When maxillofacial operations result in a compromised airway, elective tracheostomy may be necessary before extubation. If respiratory exchange is inadequate, the tube is left in place, the patient transported to the recovery room with assisted breathing, and ventilation continued mechanically until adequate.

**TABLE 24–3.** Untoward Sequelae of Tracheal Intubation

**Immediate**

Esophageal or bronchial intubation
Tube kinking, mucus plug
Occlusion by distended cuff
Bevel against tracheal wall
Sympathetic responses

**Delayed and Postextubation**

Overdistention of the cuff (nitrous oxide)
Secretions
Laryngospasm
Inadequate oxygenation
Full stomach
Postoperative compromised airway

**Trauma**

Dental damage
Lacerations, bleeding
Mediastinal emphysema
Aspiration of gastric contents
Vocal cord paralysis
Polyp formation
Laryngeal edema and tracheitis

## What Are the Complications of Tracheal Intubation?

Complications related to tracheal intubation are many and must be carefully weighed against the benefits (Table 24–3; Fig. 24–18).

### Immediate Sequelae

#### Trauma

Intubation may result in lacerated or bruised lips and tongue; chipped, loosened, or dislodged teeth; laceration of

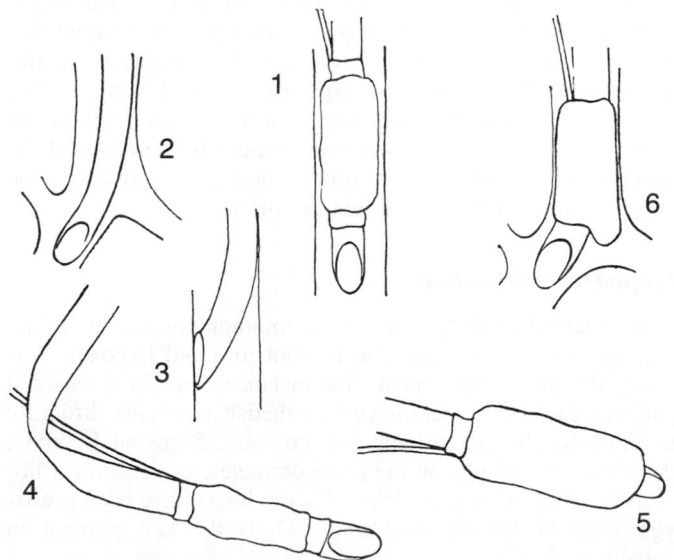

**FIGURE 24–18.** Accidents with tracheal intubation. 1, Normal position of the tube. 2, Intubation of the right main bronchus. 3, Tube opening against side of trachea, resulting in one-way valve effect. 4, Kinked tube. 5, Endotracheal cuff inflated with partial occlusion of opening. 6, Inflated cuff partially occluding left main bronchus. (From Dripps RD, Eckenhoff JE, Vandam LD. *Introduction to Anesthesia: The Principles of Safe Practice.* 1st ed. Philadelphia, Pa: WB Saunders; 1957.)

the pharyngeal wall; dislodged adenoidal tissue; or epistaxis. Rupture of the hypopharynx, esophagus, or trachea may result in mediastinal or subcutaneous emphysema and pneumothorax, perhaps more often encountered when a stylet has been used. Pneumothorax requires immediate diagnosis, insertion of chest drainage tubes, and reexpansion of the lungs.

### Cardiovascular Response

Hypertension and tachycardia almost always accompany laryngoscopy and tracheal intubation, the so-called stress response. Dysrhythmias may also be precipitated. Perhaps a shorter period during laryngoscopy may minimize the magnitude and duration of these changes. In patients with coronary artery disease, hypertension and tachycardia may cause myocardial ischemia and infarction. Dysrhythmias such as polymorphic ventricular tachycardia and premature ventricular contractions more often occur with agents (halothane) that sensitize the myocardium to the action of catecholamines. Deepening anesthesia and hyperventilation usually eliminate the dysrhythmias. Additional drug therapy may be necessary as follows:

**Lidocaine.** Laryngotracheal spray with 4% lidocaine immediately preceding placement of a tracheal tube often does not prevent the circulatory reaction. Lidocaine, 1 mg/kg, given intravenously 1 minute before laryngoscopy, may modify the response by depressing airway reflexes and by deepening the level of anesthesia, but a significant cardiovascular response may still occur.

**Opioids and β-Adrenergic Blockers.** Intravenous injection of one of the ultrapotent opioids or a short-acting β-adrenergic blocker may be the treatment of choice.

### Spinal Cord and Vertebral Column Injury

Patients with cervical spinal fractures and dislocations, osteoporosis, osteolytic lesions, and congenital malformations of the spine are susceptible to spinal cord and cervical vertebral injury during laryngoscopy and attempted tracheal intubation. Both flexion and hyperextension of the neck, as usually practiced during laryngoscopy with a rigid laryngoscope, should be avoided. Alternate techniques, such as fiberoptic or "blind" nasotracheal intubation, should be considered. In most of these patients, fiberoptic intubation can easily be accomplished without manipulating the neck.

### Esophageal Intubation

Esophageal intubation is a more common complication than realized; recognition must be prompt to avoid hypoxia. It is easily detected under most circumstances, but in occasional patients, even an experienced anesthetist may have difficulty in immediately recognizing the problem. Signs of hypoxia, desaturation readings on the pulse oximeter, and electrocardiographic changes may be delayed if the lungs have been preoxygenated. Monitoring end-tidal $CO_2$ is the key element in detection.

### Aspiration of Gastric Contents

Special precautions should be taken in patients at high risk for aspiration. Awake tracheal intubation or rapid-sequence induction and intubation with Sellick maneuver[22] are the two most commonly used techniques. Fiberoptic tracheal intubation may be of value in awake patients. Partial airway obstruction, distention of the stomach during mask anesthesia, and spontaneous breathing against an obstructed airway facilitate regurgitation and aspiration. Extubation before protective reflexes return increases the risk during emergence from anesthesia.

### Laryngospasm

Painful stimulation of the patient during anesthesia, attempts at tracheal intubation with inadequate anesthesia or without a neuromuscular blocker, and the presence of blood or secretions in the airway after extubation can result in laryngeal spasm.

### Bronchial Intubation

Bronchial intubation may take place during intubation or subsequent positioning when flexing the neck or when a steep Trendelenburg position is used.

## Delayed Sequelae

### Vocal Cord Paralysis

The mechanism of vocal cord paralysis following intubation is unknown.[25] Paralysis may be unilateral, presenting as hoarseness, or bilateral, causing inspiratory obstruction because the relaxed cords are drawn to the midline. Pressure exerted by an overinflated cuff on branches of the recurrent laryngeal nerve has been implicated as a cause, as have poorly aerated tubes after ethylene oxide sterilization. Most often, the occurrence is unexplained. The paralysis is usually transient.

### Laryngeal Edema, Tracheitis, and Infection

Subglottic edema, the gravest of the laryngeal edemas, occurs mostly in children younger than 3 years of age; onset is apparent within 1 to 2 hours after extubation. Treatment includes inhalation of humidified $O_2$. Dexamethasone is helpful, as is nebulized racemic epinephrine, to reduce vascular engorgement. Reintubation or tracheotomy may be necessary in refractory cases. Maxillary sinusitis and retropharyngeal abscess may follow nasotracheal intubation. Bacteremia has been shown to be more common after nasotracheal than after oral intubation.

### Sore Throat

Sore throat is the most common sequel of tracheal intubation. It is sometimes severe, and the incidence is high after head and neck operations. Laryngitis, as manifested by hoarseness and a sore throat, appears in a small percentage of patients but is transient. Recovery is usual, and special treatment is not needed.

### Failed Intubation

Inability to obtain a secure airway often results in disaster. To minimize the consequences, the emergency must be detected early and prearranged maneuvers immediately applied. For such emergencies outside the operating suite, an emergency supply cart stocked with necessary equipment and supplies should be available. An interesting technique that can be used in unanticipated difficult intubation involves placement of an LTA stylet (LTA 360 Kit, Abbott Laboratories, North Chicago, Ill) through the Murphy eye of the ETT, using it as a guide to tracheal placement.[26] The glass syringe barrel of the kit is removed and the lidocaine discarded. Next, the capnograph sampling tubing is attached to a three-way stopcock inserted into the hole in the blue rubber plunger. In this study, a $P_{CO_2}$ plateau of $>12$ mm Hg confirmed tracheal placement of the ETT with 90% accuracy.

## References

1. Caplan RA, Posner KL, Ward RJ, et al. Adverse respiratory events in anesthesia: a closed claims analysis. *Anesthesiology.* 1990;72:828.
2. Negus VE. *The Comparative Anatomy and Physiology of the Larynx.* New York, NY: Grune & Stratton; 1949.
3. Bramble DM, Carrier DM. Running and breathing in mammals. *Science.* 1983;219:25.
4. Lewin R. Four legs bad, two legs good. *Science.* 1987;235:969.
5. Kaban LB. Dental and oral problems. In: Vandam LD, ed. *To Make The Patient Ready for Anesthesia.* 2nd ed. Menlo Park, Calif: Addison-Wesley; 1984:208.
6. Proctor DF. Form and function of the upper airways and larynx. In: Macklem PT, Mead J, eds. *Handbook of Physiology.* Section 3. Bethesda, Md: American Physiological Society; 1982. *Mechanics of Breathing.* Part I. Vol 3.
7. Courtiss EH, Gorgon TJ, Courtiss GB. Nasal physiology. *Ann Plast Surg.* 1984;13:214.
8. Klein HC. Why can't physicians examine the larynx? *JAMA.* 1982;247:2111.
9. Mallampati SR, Gugino LD, Desai SP, et al. A clinical sign to predict difficult tracheal intubation: a prospective study. *Can Anaesth Soc J.* 1985;32:429.
10. Pollard R, Lobato EB. Endotracheal tube location verified reliably by cuff palpation. *Anesth Analg.* 1995;81:135.
11. Stirt JA. Endotracheal tube misplacement. *Anaesth Intensive Care.* 1982;10:274.
12. Sugiyama K, Yokoyama K, Satoh K-I, et al. Does the Murphy eye reduce the reliability of chest auscultation in detecting endobronchial intubation? *Anesth Analg.* 1999;88:1380.
13. Kubota Y, Magaribuchi T, Toyoda Y, et al. Selective bronchial suctioning in the adult using a curve-tipped catheter with a guide mark. *Crit Care Med.* 1982;10:767.
14. Eckenhoff JE. Some anatomic considerations of the infant larynx influencing endotracheal anesthesia. *Anesthesiology.* 1951;12:401.
15. Warner JA, Finlay WEI. Fulminating epiglottitis in adults: report of three cases and a review of the literature. *Anaesthesia.* 1985;40:348.
16. Fink BR. The etiology and treatment of laryngeal spasm. *Anesthesiology.* 1956;17:569.
17. Mushin WW. Bilateral vagus nerve block. *Proc R Soc Med.* 1944;38:308.
18. Labat G. *Regional Anesthesia: Its Technical and Clinical Application.* 2nd ed. Philadelphia, Pa: WB Saunders; 1928:143.
19. Bartlett D Jr. Respiratory functions of the larynx. *Physiol Rev.* 1989;69:33.
20. Dripps RD, Eckenhoff JE, Vandam LD. *Introduction to Anesthesia: The Principles of Safe Practice.* 7th ed. Philadelphia, Pa: WB Saunders; 1988.
21. Tu HN, Saidi N, Lieutaud T, et al. Nitrous oxide increases endotracheal cuff pressure and the incidence of tracheal lesions in anesthetized patients. *Anesth Analg.* 1999;89:187.
22. Sellick BA. Cricoid pressure to control regurgitation of stomach contents during induction of anaesthesia. *Lancet.* 1961;2:404.
23. Bannister FB, Macbeth RG. Direct laryngoscopy and tracheal intubation. *Lancet.* 1944;2:651.
24. Cardoso MMSC, Banner,MJ, Melker RJ, et al. Portable devices used to detect endotracheal intubation during emergency situations: a review. *Crit Care Med.* 1998;26:957.
25. Halley HS, Gildea JE. Vocal cord paralysis after tracheal intubation. *JAMA.* 1971;215:281.
26. Bourke DL, Biehl J. The laryngotracheal topical anesthesia kit with capnography for difficult intubation. *Anesth Analg.* 1999;88:943.

## General Reading

Benumof JL. Management of the difficult airway. *Anesthesiology.* 1991;75:1087.

Fink BR, Demaret RJ. *Laryngeal Biomechanics.* Cambridge, Mass: Harvard University Press; 1978.

Finucaine BT, Santura AH. *Principles of Airway Management.* Philadelphia, Pa: FA Davis; 1988.

Negus VE. *The Comparative Anatomy and Physiology of the Larynx.* New York, NY: Grune & Stratton; 1949.

Snell RS, Katz J. *Clinical Anatomy for Anesthesiologists.* Norwalk, Conn: Appleton & Lange; 1988.

Vandam LD. Functional anatomy of the larynx. *Wkly Anesth Update.* 1977;1:95.

CHAPTER

# 25

# The Spine

Edward T. Crosby

Anne C. P. Lui

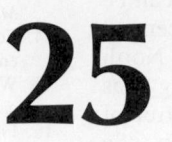

## EMBRYOLOGIC DEVELOPMENT

## VERTEBRAL ANATOMY

*What Are the Normal Characteristics?*

*What Are the Major Joints?*

*What Are the Important Ligamentous Structures?*

*How Is the Spine Linearly Oriented?*

*What Are the Subdivisions Within the Neural Canal?*

## THE CERVICAL SPINE

*What Are the Relevant Anatomic Features?*

*How Does Cervical Spinal Anatomy Differ in the Pediatric Age Group?*

*What Important Anatomic Changes Occur With Advancing Age?*

*What Are Common Congenital Anomalies of the Cervical Spine?*

*What Factors Control Cervical Spinal Movement?*

*How Is Cervical Spinal Movement Affected by Advancing Age?*

*How Do Inflammatory Arthropathies Alter Cervical Spine and Airway Anatomy?*

*What Anatomic Structures Determine Cervical Spine Stability?*

*How Is the Cervical Spine Rendered Unstable by Injury?*

*What Are the Characteristics of Pediatric Cervical Spine Injury?*

*What Are the Effects of Airway Maneuvers on the Injured Neck?*

*What Effect Does Previous Cervical Spine Surgery Have on the Airway?*

## THE THORACIC SPINE

*What Are the Relevant Anatomic Characteristics?*

*How Is Thoracic Epidural Catheter Placement Achieved?*

*How Are Abnormal Curvatures of the Thoracic Spine Described?*

*What Problems Are Associated With Scoliosis?*

*Does the Cause of Scoliosis Matter?*

*What Are the Mechanisms of Injury to the Thoracolumbar Spine?*

*When Is the Thoracic Spine Unstable?*

## THE LUMBAR SPINE

*What Are the Relevant Anatomic Characteristics?*

*What Are the Unique Characteristics of the Epidural Space in the Lumbar Spine?*

*Is It the Plicae Mediana Dorsalis, a Posterior Dural Fold, or a Posterior Epidural Fat Pad?*

*What Are the Common Congenital Anomalies of the Lumbar Spine?*

*What Age-Related Changes Occur in the Lumbar Spine That Affect Neuraxial Blockade?*

*How Deep Is the Lumbar Epidural Space?*

*What Are the Considerations for the Paramedian Approach in the Lumbar Spine?*

*What Changes in Lumbar Spine Anatomy and Function Occur With Pregnancy?*

*Why Does Low Back Pain Occur?*

*What Makes Back Pain Chronic?*

*What Are the Effects of Spinal Injury and Surgery on the Epidural Space?*

*Is Regional Anesthesia Feasible After Spinal Surgery?*

*What Are the Etiologic Factors Implicated in Postoperative or Postpartum Backache?*

## THE SACRAL SPINE

*What Are the Relevant Anatomic Considerations?*

*How Likely Is Dural Puncture During Caudal Anesthesia?*

*Where Do Misplaced Injections Go?*

*What Sacral Abnormalities Are Significant?*

The ability to assess spinal function and to appreciate the impact of altered anatomy and biomechanical function on anesthetic techniques should be part of every anesthesiologist's clinical repertoire. This review is intended to help the reader gain such an appreciation by highlighting important aspects of the anatomy and function of the spine and noting the implications of both congenital and acquired processes. For discussion purposes, the spine is divided into cervical, thoracic, lumbar, and caudal portions. The clinical focus of the discussion of the cervical spine is on tracheal intubation and airway maneuvers; that of the thoracic spine is on the effects of thoracic spinal deformity on anesthesia; and that of the lumbosacral spine is on regional anesthesia.

## EMBRYOLOGIC DEVELOPMENT

Beginning at about 3 weeks' gestational age, mesodermal somites begin to appear along each side of the neural groove. Each somite differentiates into a dorsolateral myotome (muscle plate) and a ventromedial sclerotome (vertebral plate). Growth of the sclerotomes occurs in 3 directions: medially to surround the notochord and establish the vertebral body, dorsally to enclose the neural tube and produce the vertebral arch and spinous process, and laterally to give rise to the transverse processes. Chondrification centers arise in the arch rudiments and in the primitive body. In the third month of gestation, ossification centers replace the chondrogenous centers.

At birth, each hemiarch and its corresponding body is separated by cartilaginous plates. Hemiarches unite dorsally during the first postnatal year, and the completed arches join the vertebral bodies during the third to sixth years of life. Absence of an ossification center in the vertebral body may result in formation of a hemivertebra. Failure of closure of the neural arch results in spina bifida. Finally, failure of the arch to fuse with the ossified vertebral body results in spondylolysis.

## VERTEBRAL ANATOMY

### What Are the Normal Characteristics?

The spine is composed of 33 vertebrae (7 cervical, 12 thoracic, 5 lumbar, 5 fused sacral, and 4 coccygeal) and describes 4 curves (Fig. 25–1). The cervical and lumbar curves are convex anteriorly (lordotic), and the thoracic and sacral curves are convex posteriorly (kyphotic).

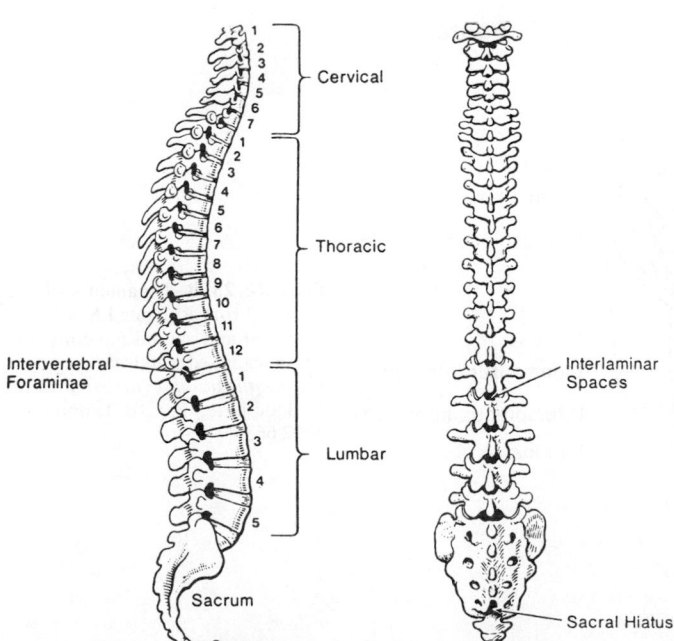

**FIGURE 25–1.** The vertebral column, lateral and posterior views.

A typical vertebra (C3-L5) consists of a body anteriorly and a neural arch posteriorly (Fig. 25–2).

### The Body

The heavy body resembles a short long bone, and its principal function is to support weight. The bodies of the vertebrae from C3 to L5 become progressively larger to bear incrementally greater weight.

### Neural Arch

The dorsal neural arch serves to shelter and protect the neural elements. It is formed by two pedicles rising from the vertebral body to constitute the side walls of the arch, which is closed superiorly by the laminae.

### Articular Processes

Four articular processes (two superior and two inferior), two laterally placed transverse processes, and a dorsal spinous process arise from the neural arch. The pedicles are notched both inferiorly and superiorly.

### What Are the Major Joints?

The vertebrae from C2 to S1 articulate with each other through three joints: one anterior nonsynovial joint; the intervertebral disk; and two posterior synovial joints, the facet joints.

### Intervertebral Disks

The intervertebral disks account for about 25% of total spinal length. They are composed of peripheral fibrous tissue and fibrocartilage arranged in concentric rings (the annulus fibrosus), surrounding a soft central core (the nucleus pulposus). They adhere above and below to hyaline cartilage, which covers the articular surfaces of the vertebral bodies.

### Facet Joints

The facet joints are true synovial joints. Their articular surfaces are covered with hyaline cartilage, and each joint is surrounded by an articular capsule. These capsules are longer and looser in the cervical region than in the subcervical spine, allowing for greater range of joint motion.

### What Are the Important Ligamentous Structures?

The spinal column is bound together, through its length, by several ligaments that give it stability and elasticity (Fig. 25–3).

### Supraspinous Ligament

The supraspinous ligament is a strong fibrous cord that connects the apices of the spinous processes from the sacrum to C7, above which it continues to the external occipital protuberance as the ligamentum nuchae.

## Posterior-superior view

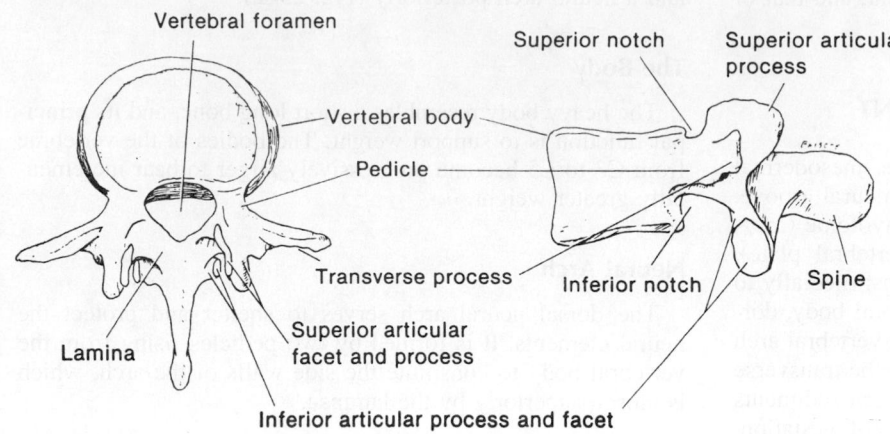

## Lateral view

**FIGURE 25–2.** Typical vertebral body. (From Levinson G. Spinal anesthesia. In: Benumof JL, ed. *Clinical Procedures in Anesthesia and Intensive Care*. Philadelphia, Pa: JB Lippincott; 1992:646.)

### Interspinous Ligament

The interspinous ligament is a thinner, more membranous structure that connects the spinous processes, blending ventrally with the ligamentum flavum and dorsally with the supraspinous ligament.

### Ligamentum Flavum

The ligamentum flavum lies deep to the interspinous ligament and connects the laminae of adjacent vertebrae. It covers the interlaminar space and forms the roof of the epidural space.

### Longitudinal Ligaments

The anterior and posterior longitudinal ligaments bind the vertebral bodies together. The anterior ligament inserts on the intervertebral disks and adjacent vertebrae and ascends along the anterior surface of the spine. The posterior longitudinal ligament courses upward along the dorsal surface of the vertebral bodies, forming the floor of the neural canal.

### How Is the Spine Linearly Oriented?

In the supine position, the median highest points of the lumbar spinal canal in men and women is located at L4.[1] The lowest point of the thoracic spinal canal is at T7 through T9 in both men and women. The highest point of the lumbar spinal canal changes with pregnancy to a lower lumbar region, L4 through L5.[2] The lowest point of the thoracic spinal canal is located at a higher thoracic region in pregnant patients (T6-T7). The apex of lumbar lordosis is more caudad, and thoracic kyphosis is reduced in the supine position in the later stages of pregnancy. These changes in the curvature of the spinal column may explain, in part, the enhanced cephalad spread of

## Anterior

## Posterior

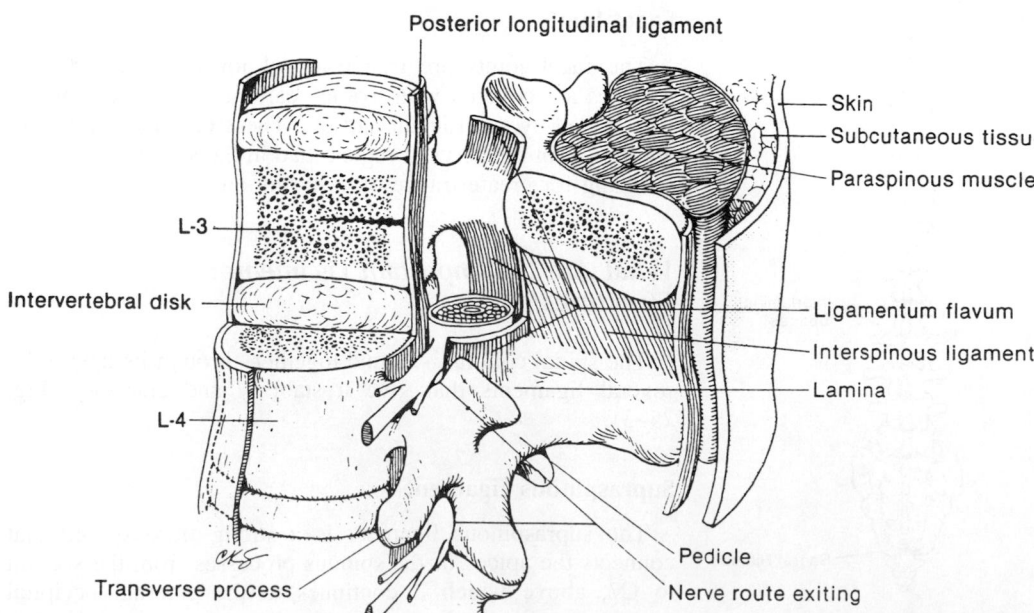

**FIGURE 25–3.** Ligaments of the spine. (From Reisner LS, Ellis J. Epidural and caudal puncture. In: Benumof JL, ed. *Clinical Procedures in Anesthesia and Intensive Care*. Philadelphia, Pa: JB Lippincott; 1992:663.)

subarachnoid hyperbaric anesthetic solutions in the later stages of pregnancy.[2]

## What Are the Subdivisions Within the Neural Canal?

### The Epidural Space

The epidural space is the outermost division of the neural canal. It extends from the foramen magnum, where the dura is fused to the base of the skull, to the sacral hiatus, where it is covered by the sacrococcygeal ligament. Its boundaries are the posterior longitudinal ligament anteriorly, the pedicles laterally, and the anterior surfaces of the lamina and the ligamentum flavum posteriorly.

The anterior epidural space is narrow because of the close proximity of the dura to the posterior longitudinal ligament. The epidural contents are found in circumferentially and metamerically segmented compartments, rather than in a uniform layer.[3] Trabeculations between the dura and the posterior ligament are common, rendering this space discontinuous across the midline. Large areas of the dura are directly in contact with the spinal canal wall. The steeply arched ligamenta flava are fused in the midline to a variable degree. The space anterior to the dura is filled with veins and is isolated from the rest of the epidural space by a membranous lateral extension of the posterior longitudinal ligament. This membrane and a midline posterior fat pedicle are the only observed potential barriers to the spread of epidural solutions.[3]

As compared with the lumbar level, there are diminished epidural contents at the thoracic and cervical levels, and the ligamentum flavum is more frequently discontinuous. Although the epidural contents are typically divided into compartments, there is incomplete segmentation of the posterior compartments during early childhood and often at thoracic levels in adults. Several changes occur with aging: at the thoracic and cervical levels, there are diminished epidural contents, and the ligamentum flavum is frequently discontinuous. In addition, degenerative disk and joint changes and distortion and compression of the epidural space are typical.[4]

The epidural space is widest in its sagittal plane posteriorly and varies with the vertebral level, ranging from 1 to 1.5 mm at C5; 2.5 to 3 mm at T6; and, at its widest point, 5 to 6 mm at L2. In addition to the nerve roots that cross it, the contents of the epidural space include fat, areolar tissue, lymphatics, arteries, and an extensive internal vertebral venous plexus.

### The Subdural Space

The subdural space is a potential space, bounded by the dura externally and the pia-arachnoid membranes internally, and containing a small amount of serous fluid.[5] It extends laterally over the nerve roots and ganglia and is greater in its posterior aspects. Both intentional and accidental subdural injections have been reported.[6–8] Injections into the subdural space tend to localize primarily in its posterior aspects; a predominantly sensory (dorsal root) blockade results.

### The Subarachnoid Space

The subarachnoid space is bound internally by the pia and externally by the arachnoid and is filled by the cerebrospinal fluid (CSF), brain, spinal cord, and nerve roots. It has three divisions: cranial, spinal, and nerve root, all of which are in free communication with one another. Little is known about CSF volume, including its variability among individuals, longitudinal distribution, or the influence of body habitus on volume. CSF volume was measured in volunteers by fast spin-echo sequence magnetic resonance imaging (MRI), which highlights CSF.[9] From the T11-12 disk to the sacral terminus of the dural sac, the mean volume for all subjects is 49.9 ± 12.1 mL (mean ± SD), with a considerable range of 28 to 81 mL. CSF volume was significantly less in relatively obese subjects (42.9 ± 9.5 mL) than in nonobese subjects (53.5 ± 12.9 mL). Abdominal compression decreased CSF and nerve root volume. The decreased CSF volume that results from increased abdominal pressure, such as with obesity or pregnancy, may produce more extensive neuraxial blockade through diminished dilution of local anesthetic. The mechanism by which increased abdominal pressure decreases CSF volume is not associated with venous distention as traditionally believed but is more likely due to the inward movement of soft tissue in the intervertebral foramen, which displaces CSF.[9]

CSF volume correlates with pinprick assessments of peak sensory block height and duration of surgical anesthesia (as assessed by the duration of tolerance to transcutaneous electrical stimulation at the ankle). Variability in lumbosacral CSF volume is the most important factor identified to date that contributes to the variability in the spread of spinal sensory anesthesia.[10] Neither weight gain during pregnancy (6-22 kg), height (152-185 cm), weight (56-98 kg) nor body mass index (BMI) (20.2-31.8 kg/m$^2$) correlates with the cephalad spread of sensory blockade.[11]

## THE CERVICAL SPINE

### What Are the Relevant Anatomic Features?

#### The Atlas

The first cervical vertebra, the atlas (C1), has thick anterior and posterior arches that blend laterally into large masses (Fig. 25–4). The occipital condyles of the skull articulate with large kidney-shaped depressions on the superior aspects of these lateral masses. The flatter inferior surfaces of the lateral masses transmit the weight of the skull onto the superior facet joints of the axis, the C2 vertebra (Fig. 25–5). On the inner aspects of the anterior arch of the atlas, arising bilaterally and projecting inward, two bony tubercles give rise to the transverse ligament.

#### The Axis

Laterally placed on the superior surface of the axis (C2) are circular facets that articulate with the lateral masses of the atlas (see Fig. 25–5). The body of the axis extends upward to form the odontoid process. The space between the posterior border of the anterior ring of the atlas and the anterior border of the odontoid process is the atlas-dens interval (ADI). In the adult, measured on a lateral radiograph, the ADI is <3 mm in both flexion and extension. The narrowed waist of the odontoid process is compressed by the transverse ligament of the atlas. Alar and apical ligaments fan upward from the odontoid process to insert on the anterior margins of the

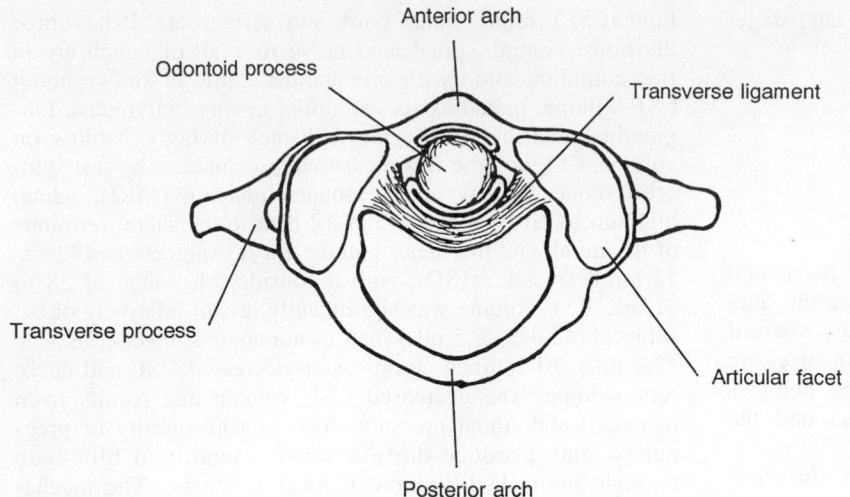

FIGURE 25–4. The atlas. Superior view of the atlantoaxial articulation (skull removed) detailing superior surface anatomy of the atlas. (From Crosby ET, Lui A. The adult cervical spine: implications for airway management. *Can J Anaesth*. 1990;37:77.)

foramen magnum (Fig. 25–6). The spinous process of the axis is large and heavy, allowing muscle and ligamentous insertion.

## The Lower Cervical Vertebrae

The lower five cervical vertebrae are anatomically more typical. The transverse processes are the unique features, with laterally projecting costal processes and the foramen transversarium, transmitting the vertebral artery through most of the cervical spine. The arches of the C2 through C7 vertebrae articulate by means of horizontally oriented facet joints. There is an intervertebral disk between C2 and C3 and each subjacent pair of vertebrae.

## The Longitudinal Ligaments

Anterior and posterior longitudinal ligaments extend the length of the cervical spine. The anterior ligament terminates over the anterior arch of the atlas, forming the anterior atlantooccipital ligament, which inserts on the base of the skull (see Fig. 25–6). The posterior ligament courses upward along the dorsal surface of the vertebral bodies, fans over the body of the axis and the odontoid process, and terminates as the tectorial membrane, which inserts into the basiocciput.

## How Does Cervical Spinal Anatomy Differ in the Pediatric Age Group?

Many of the anatomic differences in the pediatric cervical spine relative to that of an adult result from variances in the ossification centers, unfused synchondroses, and laxity of the ligamentous structures.[12] Anterior wedging of the incompletely ossified vertebral body in young children can produce the appearance of a compression fracture. Anterior pseudosubluxation, especially at or above C3, and an increase in the ADI are due to laxity of the spinal ligaments and are normal anatomic variants in young children. Secondary ossification centers appear during puberty at the superior and inferior borders of the vertebral bodies and may not close until into the third decade. These secondary centers may be confused with chip fractures of the vertebral body.

## What Important Anatomic Changes Occur With Advancing Age?

Degeneration of the cervical spinal joints and disk spaces is radiologically demonstrable in 80% to 90% of the popula-

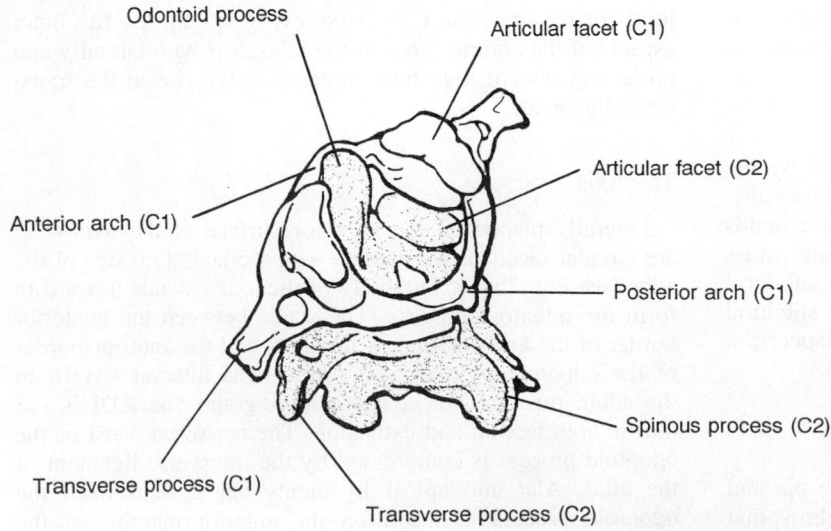

FIGURE 25–5. The atlantoaxial joint. Details of the articulating surfaces of the atlantoaxial joint.

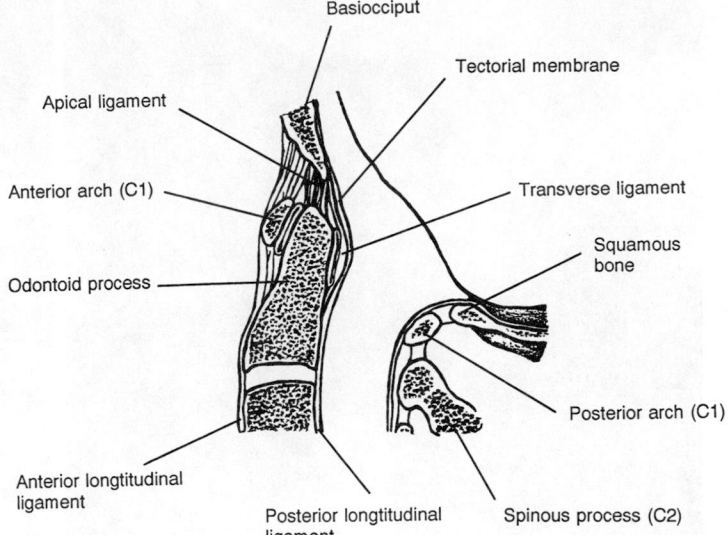

Basiocciput

Apical ligament

Tectorial membrane

Anterior arch (C1)

Transverse ligament

Odontoid process

Squamous bone

Posterior arch (C1)

Anterior longtitudinal ligament

Posterior longtitudinal ligament

Spinous process (C2)

**FIGURE 25–6.** The occipitoatlantoaxial articulation. Lateral view, sagittal section. (From Crosby ET, Lui ACP. The cervical spine: fundamental considerations. In: Lui ACP, Crosby ET, eds. *Anesthesia and Musculoskeletal Disorders. Problems in Anesthesia*. Philadelphia, Pa: JB Lippincott; 1991;5:1.)

tion by 40 years of age and is the result of normal aging. The radiologic changes of cervical spondylosis are listed in Table 25–1. These changes are thought to result from the accumulated effects of years of weight bearing on the joints and desiccation of the disk. An age-associated reduction in normal lordosis, loss of joint cartilage and intervertebral disk height, and increased new bone formation in the cervical spine occur. These changes are common throughout the aging population, although in some patients, they become apparent at an earlier age and follow a more rapidly progressive course.

Osteophyte formation is common, and new bone may encroach on the spinal foramina or the canal, giving rise to root or cord compression, respectively. These changes usually do not interfere with tracheal intubation, although difficulties related to hypertrophic bony changes on the anterior aspects of the cervical vertebral bodies are reported.[13,14] Rotation and displacement of the trachea and difficulty achieving intubation were noted.

## Ossification of the Posterior Longitudinal Ligament

*Ossification of the posterior longitudinal ligament* is a condition of unknown etiology, usually occurring in the midcervical spine. The ligament is evident on a lateral radiograph as an ossified plaque of variable thickness along the posterior margins of the vertebral bodies and disks. The ossified ligament may encroach on the spinal canal, producing cord or root lesions. Associated anterior osteophyte formation is common.

## Diffuse Idiopathic Skeletal Hyperostosis

*Diffuse idiopathic skeletal hyperostosis* (DISH; also called *ankylosing hyperostosis* or *Forestier disease*) is an ossifying diathesis in elderly patients that leads to spinal and extraspinal new bone formation as well as ligament calcification and ossification (Fig. 25–7). Prevalence, in adults older than 40 years of age, is estimated at 3.8% for men and 2.6% for women.[15] The prevalence increases in men older than 50 years of age to 25% and in women older than 50 years of age to 15%. It climbs to 28% in men over 80 years of age and to more than 35% in men older than 70 years of age. In women older than 80 years of age, the prevalence is 26%. DISH is less common in black, Native American, and Asian populations.[16] Signs and symptoms include stiffness and pain in the back, dysphagia due to direct esophageal compression and distortion, pain related to associated tendinitis, myelopathy related to cord compression (associated with ossification of the posterior longitudinal ligament), and pain related to vertebral complications, including fractures and subluxations.[17]

Isolated or predominant cervical spine involvement has been reported, but thoracic and lumbar segments are more typically involved. Abnormalities are more common in the lower cervical region and begin with cortical hyperostosis along the anterior surface of the vertebral body. Forestier described three stages in the evolution of the disease.[18] Initially, there is a laminated thickening across the intervertebral disk space anteriorly. The prevertebral thickening is accentuated and, eventually, there is fusion and ossification of the prediscal space and ossification of the anterior longitudinal ligament. The bony spread across the space is much greater than is typical in ankylosing spondylitis. In patients with severe and extensive disease (≥5 contiguous spaces involved), the spine may fracture as a long bone with relatively minor trauma in a fashion analogous to ankylosing spondylitis.

Anterior bone deposition in the cervical spine in patients with DISH has variable effects on the anatomy of the airway,

**TABLE 25–1.** Bony Anomalies Involving the Cervical Spine

**Cranio-occipital Anomalies**

Occipitalization of vertebrae
Occipital dysplasia
Condylar hypoplasia
Assimilation of the atlas
Arnold–Chiari malformation
Foramen magnum stenosis (achondroplasia)

**Anomalies of the Atlas and Axis**

Arch aplasias—atlas
Odontoid anomalies
  Aplasia
  Hypoplasia
  Os odontoideum
  Ossiculum terminale

**Anomalies Below C2**

Failure of segmentation (Klippel-Feil syndrome)
Failure of fusion (spina bifida, spondylolisthesis)
Cervical ribs

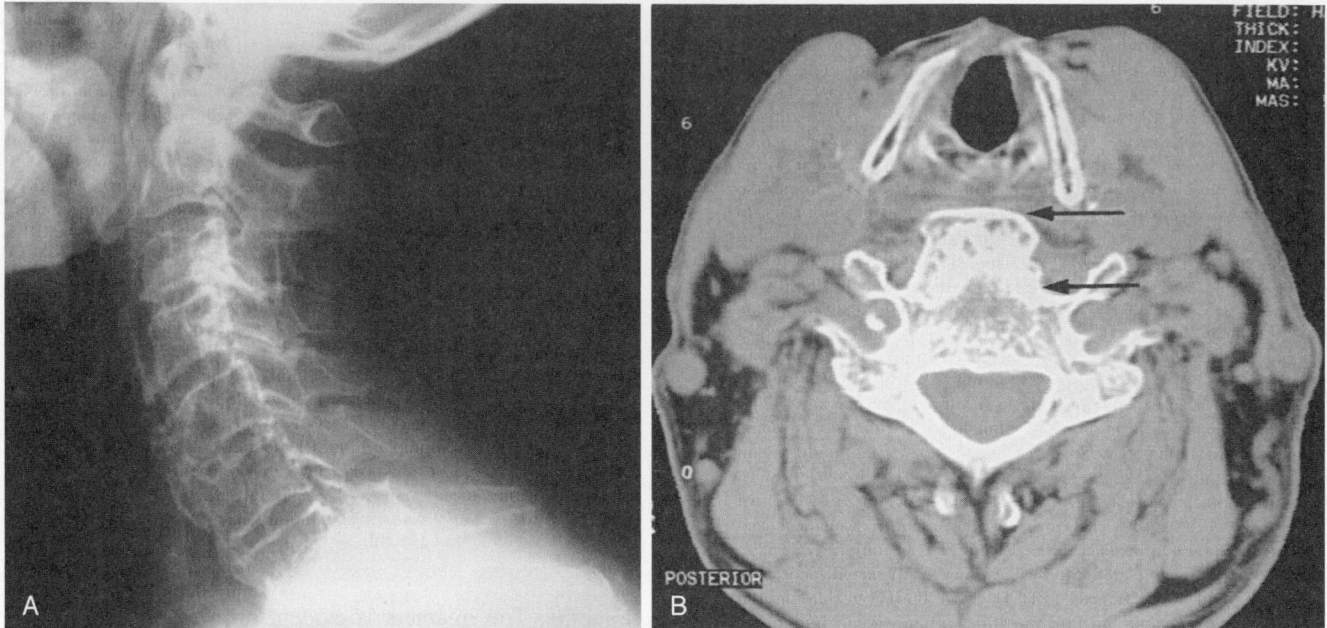

**FIGURE 25–7.** Diffuse idiopathic skeletal hyperostosis. *A,* Lateral view of the cervical spine. There is a large anterior osteophyte at C4 as well, bridging osteophytes at C5 through C6 and C6 through C7. There is anterior bowing of the trachea over the osteophytes at the C5 through C7 levels. *B,* Magnetic resonance image of the same patient demonstrating a large anterior osteophyte at C4 with resultant forward displacement of the trachea (*arrows*).

depending not only on the levels involved but also on the amount and orientation of the bone deposited. Bony outgrowths eventually extend across the anterior intervertebral disk. Apophyseal joint narrowing is common, as is ossification of the ligamentum nuchae. Skipped areas of involvement along the anterior spine are frequent; the posterior aspects of the vertebral bodies and the intervertebral disks are usually spared. In a controlled study, patients with DISH had greater reduction in neck rotation and thoracic movements than either patients with spondylosis or healthy controls and had a greater reduction in lumbar movement than healthy controls.[19]

The more limited bony bridging of DISH, coupled with the lack of involvement of the facet joints, typically causes loss of motion and allows greater spinal flexibility than does ankylosing spondylitis. Therefore, tracheal intubation is not usually more difficult in patients with DISH of the cervical spine. However, large anterior osteophytes may result in distortion of the airway and interfere with both upper airway function and intubation. Recurrent right-sided aspiration pneumonia was reported in an 80-year-old man with DISH involving the cervical spine, characterized by a giant cervical osteophyte.[20] A case of DISH was reported in which excessively enlarged cervical osteophytes led to edema of the laryngeal inlet and consequent severe dyspnea, necessitating emergency tracheotomy.[21] Another case was reported in which prominent osteophytes at the midcervical level, in combination with subglottic tracheal stenosis, resulted in unexpected difficulties during tracheal intubation.[14]

## What Are Common Congenital Anomalies of the Cervical Spine?

A large number of bony anomalies involve the cervical spine (Table 25–2).

## The Odontoid Process

The odontoid process of the axis is formed from paired centers that appear in the fifth gestational month. An additional center appears above the cleft tip of the odontoid. Between the third and sixth years of life, the separate components of the axis meet and fuse, and ossification is completed during puberty. Failure of the ossification centers in the odontoid process results in an aplastic or hypoplastic process (Fig. 25–8).

### Hypoplasia of the Odontoid Process

If the paired centers fail to fuse, a bifid odontoid process results. If these centers fail to fuse to the body of the axis, an os odontoideum develops. Hypoplasia of the odontoid process is encountered in a number of syndromes and may occur as an isolated anomaly (Table 25–3). Both odontoid hypoplasia and os odontoideum result in loss of the buttressing action of the dens during extension of the head and neck. The atlas subluxates anteriorly on the axis, reducing the space available for the spinal cord (SAC), and results in compression of the neural elements. Patients with both Morquio syndrome and disproportionate dwarfism are at risk for odontoid hypoplasia, with resultant atlantoaxial subluxation (AAS) and decreased joint stability; therefore, spinal cord injury may result after even minor trauma.[22,23]

**TABLE 25–2.** Radiologic Changes of Cervical Spondylosis

Narrowing of the disk space
Osteophyte formation at the anterior and posterior margins of the vertebral bodies
Vertebral endplate sclerosis
Osteoarthritic changes of the synovial joints
Ossification of the longitudinal ligaments
Narrowing of the sagittal diameter of the spinal canal

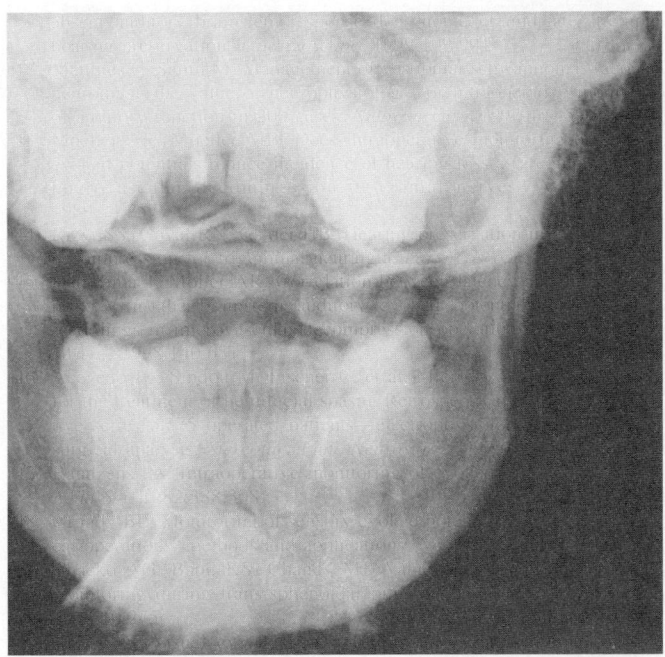

**FIGURE 25–8.** Aplasia of the odontoid process. Anteroposterior view of the atlantoaxial joint. The odontoid process is absent.

## Down Syndrome

Laxity of the transverse ligament and atlantoaxial instability are encountered in 14% to 22% of children with Down syndrome.[24–26] Extension of the head may subluxate the atlas anteriorly on the axis, with resultant compression of the cord by the odontoid process. Case reports in the anesthesiology literature have documented both rotatory subluxation of the atlantoaxial joint and posterior subluxation of the axis as new postoperative findings.[25,26]

Excessive laxity of other joints correlates well with the presence of AAS in Down syndrome. It is thought that such patients have an intrinsic defect of the collagen fibers that form their ligamentous structures. Other cervical spine abnormalities noted in Down syndrome include spina bifida of the atlas, vertebral occipitalization, os odontoideum, and Klippel-Feil syndrome.

## Klippel-Feil Syndrome

Klippel-Feil syndrome is characterized by ankylosis of the cervical spine and has also been noted in trisomy 18, Turner syndrome, and other less common syndromes, as well as being described as an isolated anomaly[27] (Fig. 25–9). Fusion of several cervical vertebrae into an osseous mass is encountered, as are other abnormalities of the cervical spine.[28] In severely affected individuals, a single slender block vertebra

**TABLE 25–3.** Syndromes Associated With Odontoid Hypoplasia

| | |
|---|---|
| Morquio's syndrome | Disproportionate dwarfism |
| Klippel-Feil syndrome | Congenital scoliosis |
| Down's syndrome | Osteogenesis imperfecta |
| Spondyloepiphyseal dysplasia | Neurofibromatosis |

From Crosby ET, Lui A. The adult cervical spine: implications for airway management. *Can J Anaesth.* 1990;37:77.

replaces the lower cervical spine. Neck movements are severely limited in all planes. Neurologic symptoms are variable and are predicted by associated anomalies rather than by the fusion itself.[27]

Tracheal intubation may be made variably more difficult, both by the reduction in neck movement and, also by the fact that the neck may be quite short (Fig. 25–10). The sniffing position, with alignment of the oral and pharyngeal axes, may be impossible to achieve yielding a persistently anterior trachea.

### Other Congenital Connective Tissue Disorders

In an unselected group of 104 consecutive patients with Marfan syndrome, the prevalence of focal kyphosis was 16%, and 54% had increased atlantoaxial translation.[29] The preadolescent Marfan population has a greater range of motion than either the adolescent or adult populations. There is also an increased radiographic prevalence of basilar impression (36%), and the odontoid height (3.69 ± 0.53 cm) was larger than reported norms (2.34 ± 0.22 cm). Cervical stenosis was rare, with 3% demonstrating stenosis at C3 and 2% at C6.

AAS is reported to be more common in patients with Ehlers-Danlos syndrome type IV than types I, II, or III.[30]

### Clinical Significance

The clinical significance of an anomaly in the cervical spine is related to its effect on movement and stability of the spine. Clinically important anomalies are usually a result of failed fusion, excess ossification, or ligamentous laxity. Many congenital abnormalities of the cervical spine result in an actual

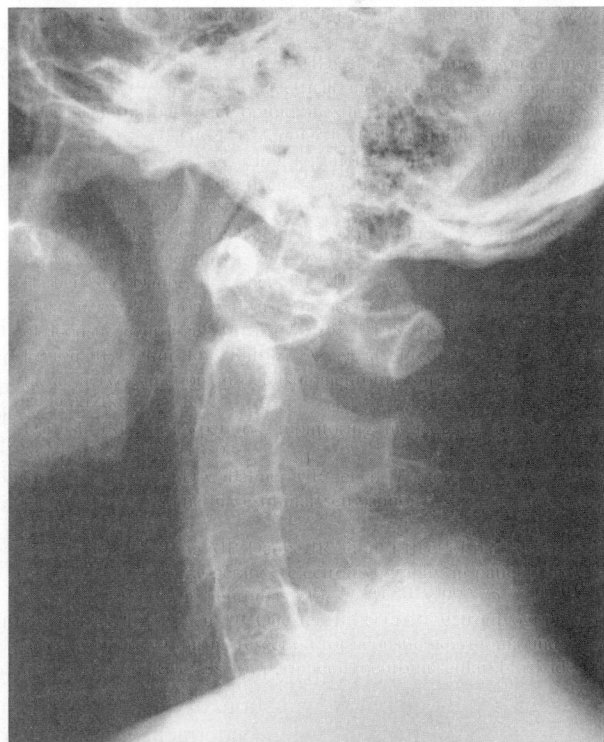

**FIGURE 25–9.** Klippel-Feil syndrome. Lateral view of the cervical spine. The cervical spine is fused into a single block of vertebrae, and the odontoid process is absent.

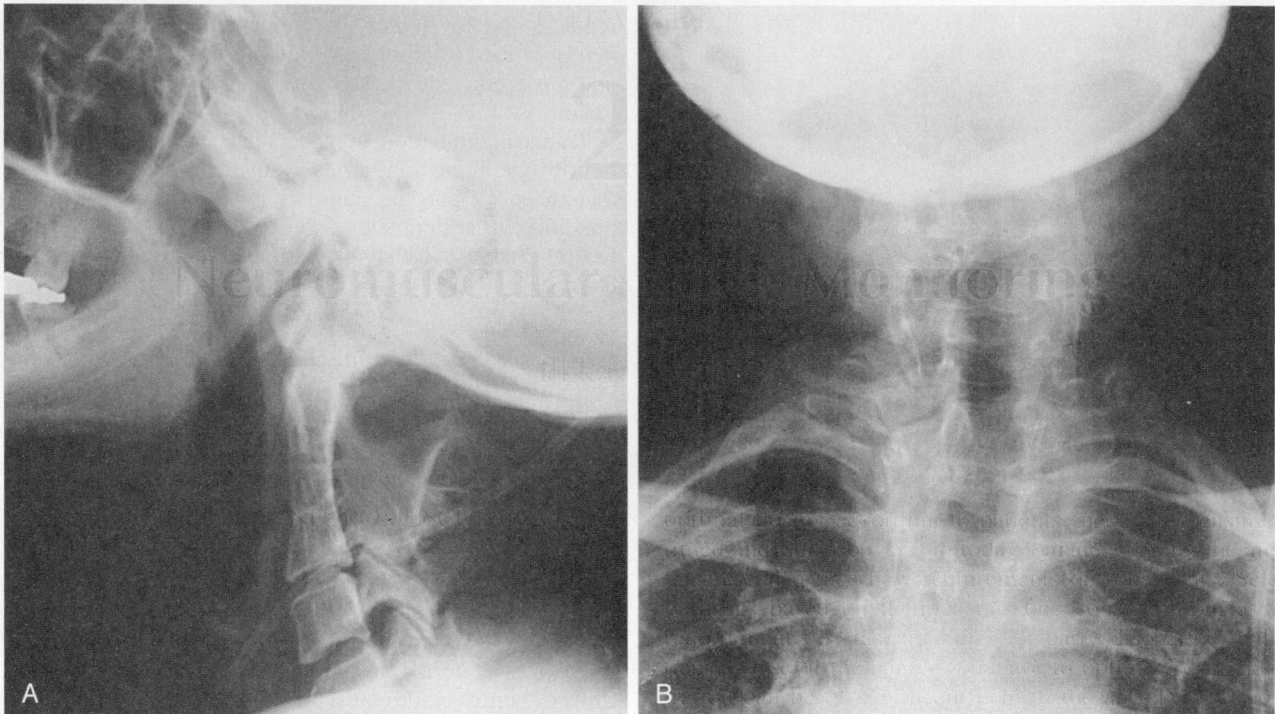

**FIGURES 25–10.** Klippel-Feil syndrome. *A,* Lateral view of the cervical spine demonstrating the absence of an ossified odontoid process and fusion of multiple vertebrae. The neck is shortened, the patient is obese, and the sniffing position is unattainable. Laryngoscopy would be predictably difficult and was reported to be grade IV. *B,* Anteroposterior view of the cervical spine demonstrating absence of neural arches throughout the midcervical spine (cervical spina bifida).

or potential reduction in the lumen of the spinal canal. Thus, the SAC is reduced, and the neural elements are at risk. A dynamic component to the luminal reduction may be present, as in AAS, with symptoms precipitated in some patients only by movement. Other congenital anomalies, such as odontoid hypoplasia, often reduce the threshold tolerance for traumatic injury and spinal instability; cord damage may result from seemingly trivial trauma. Conditions that result in decreased spinal movements typically result in a more anteriorly positioned larynx during laryngoscopy and thus may present difficulties in tracheal intubation if it is facilitated by direct laryngoscopy.

### Preanesthetic Evaluation

Patients with congenital syndromes associated with significant cervical spinal anomaly should have both clinical and radiographic evaluation before receiving an anesthetic. Adequate assessment includes a review of the lateral cervical spine radiographs in the neutral, flexed, and extended positions for evidence of AAS. Measurement of the SAC, rather than the ADI, may be of greater clinical relevance in an abnormal cervical spine. A difficult intubation should be anticipated in patients with ankylosis and decreased neck mobility. Postoperatively, neck symptoms or altered neurologic status should be assessed. If present, they should prompt an urgent clinical and radiographic evaluation.

Asymptomatic patients with Down syndrome do not routinely require radiographic evaluation of the cervical spine before anesthesia. However, when endotracheal intubation is expected to be difficult, preoperative radiographic assessment is recommended, possibly requiring neck positioning at the extremes of the ranges of motion, or when the surgical proce-

dure involves unusual head positioning or repeated manipulations of the head and neck. Gentle manipulations of the head and neck are necessary to minimize the risk for injury during anesthesia.

### What Factors Control Cervical Spinal Movement?

Flexion-extension occurs in the upper cervical spine at both the atlantooccipital and atlantoaxial articulations; a combined 35° of motion may be achieved.[31] Flexion is limited by contact between the odontoid process and the anterior border of the foramen magnum at the atlantooccipital articulation and by the tectorial membrane and posterior elements at the C1 to C2 level. Extension is limited by the contact of the posterior arch of the atlas with the occiput superiorly and with the arch of the axis inferiorly. A further 66° of flexion-extension may be achieved in the lower cervical spine, with the C5 through C7 segments contributing the largest component.[31]

### Implications for Tracheal Intubation

The distance from the posterior arch of the atlas to the occiput is termed the *atlantooccipital gap* (AOG); a narrow AOG has been cited as a common cause of difficult intubation.[32] With the head in the sniffing position, the lower cervical spine is relatively straight. Curvature increases from C4 to C2, and the atlantoaxial complex is at or near full extension. Attempts to extend the head farther in patients with a narrow AOG result in anterior bowing of the cervical spine, forward displacement of the larynx, and difficulty visualizing the larynx during laryngoscopy.[32] If difficulty in laryngeal visualization is encountered, additional neck flexion may facilitate intubation. A short interspace between the posterior arches of the atlas and the axis may result in the same phenomenon, although to a lesser degree.

Calder and colleagues[33] assessed 253 patients presenting for cervical spine surgery. The prevalence of difficulty during laryngoscopy (Cormack and Lehane grades 3-4) was 20%. Patients with disease that involves the occipitoatlantoaxial complex were more likely to have difficult laryngoscopy than those with disease below the axis vertebra. The best single predictor of difficulty was reduced separation of the posterior elements of the C1 and C2 vertebrae on lateral radiographs.

## Clinical Evaluation

Bedside evaluation of atlantooccipital extension may be performed by having the patient sit straight and face directly to the front, with the head held erect. In this position, the occlusal surface of the upper teeth is horizontal and parallel to the ground. The patient extends the atlantooccipital joint as much as possible, and the examiner estimates the angle traversed by the occlusal surface of the upper teeth. A reduction in extension can be expressed as a fraction of normal. This information may be used, in conjunction with other clinical information, to predict the probability of difficulty in both obtaining a line of vision during laryngoscopy and achieving endotracheal intubation.[34]

## *How Is Cervical Spinal Movement Affected by Advancing Age?*

As age increases, cervical mobility decreases. Hayashi compared three groups of healthy volunteers aged 20 to 40, 40 to 60, and 60 to 82 years.[35] A 25% reduction in maximum flexion-extension occurred in the 60- to 82-year-old group compared with the 20- to 40-year-old group. Much of the lost range of motion occurs in the lower cervical spine and is not likely to result in difficult intubation. However, calcification of the anterior longitudinal ligament resulting in limitation of spinal movement has been reported as a rare cause of difficult intubation in elderly patients.

## *How Do Inflammatory Arthropathies Alter Cervical Spine and Airway Anatomy?*

The cervical spine is commonly involved in both adult- and juvenile-onset rheumatoid arthritis, with 43% to 70% of patients having symptoms referable to the neck and 17% to 86% demonstrating radiologic evidence of neck involvement.[36,37]

## Rheumatoid Arthritis

### *Atlantoaxial Subluxation*

AAS is the most common radiographic finding in rheumatoid arthritis, occurring in 25% of patients. It results from attenuation or disruption of the transverse ligament, allowing for anterior movement of C1 on C2 during neck flexion. Radiographically, AAS is marked by an increase in the ADI. This change is best demonstrated on a lateral cervical spine radiograph with the neck flexed (Fig. 25–11).

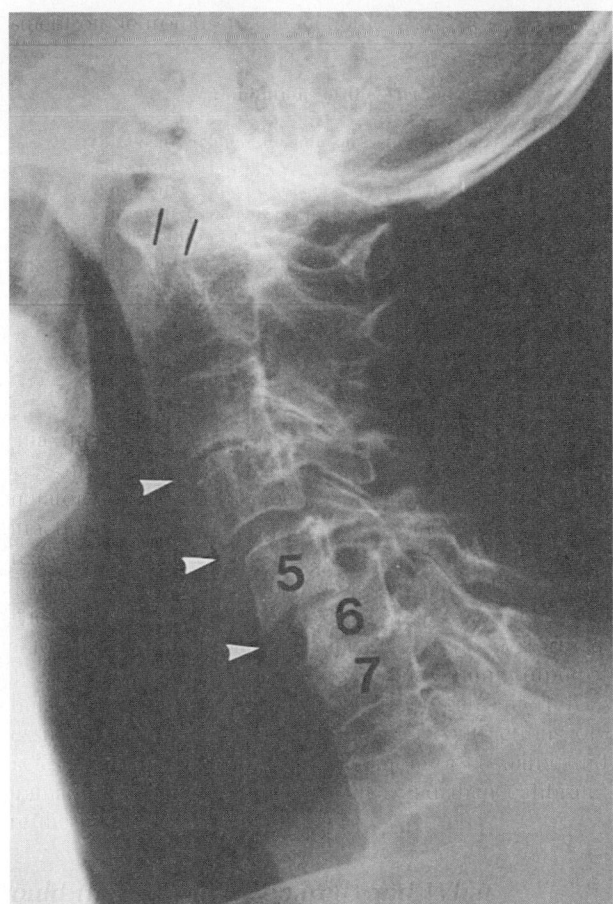

**FIGURE 25–11.** Rheumatoid arthritis. Lateral view of the cervical spine. There is generalized osteoporosis. Six millimeters of atlantoaxial subluxation is measured from the posterior aspects of the anterior arch of the atlas (at) and the anterior aspects of the odontoid process of the axis (ax). A subaxial subluxation is at C4 through C5, and vertebral endplate erosions are at C2 through C3 and C6 through C7.

### *Odontoid Subluxation*

Vertical subluxation of the odontoid process through the foramen magnum and into the posterior fossa may occur in 4% to 35% of patients with rheumatoid arthritis. This is far more common in elderly patients with severe and long-standing disease and usually occurs in conjunction with anterior AAS.[38] As the odontoid process migrates superiorly and posteriorly, a severe reduction in the lumen of the spinal canal results (Figs. 25–12 and 25–13). Consequently, 10% to 50% of patients with the combined subluxation develop cord compression.[38,39]

### Ankylosing Spondylitis

Ankylosing spondylitis is an inflammatory arthropathy marked by increasing calcification and ankylosis of the axial skeleton. Complete ankylosis of the cervical spine, characteristically in the flexed position, is the end result (Fig. 25–14).

### Clinical Implications

Many patients with inflammatory arthropathies manifest a decrease in the safe range of neck motion, and spinal cord compromise can result from inappropriate neck manipulation.

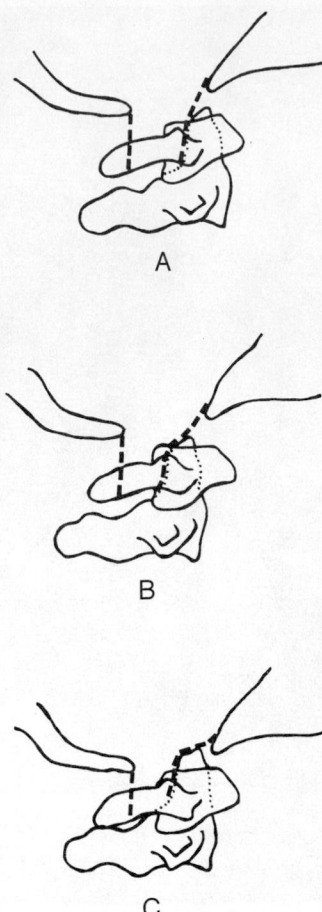

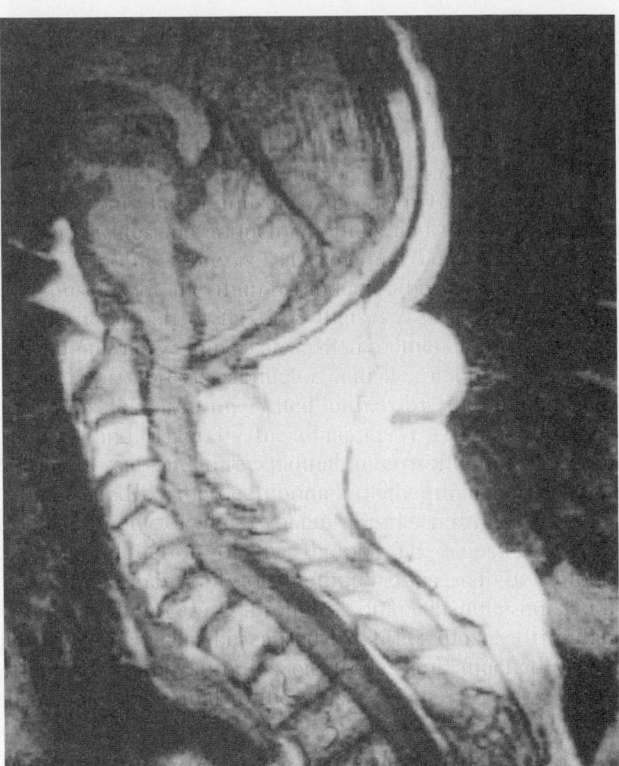

**FIGURE 25–13.** Vertical subluxation. Preoperative magnetic resonance image of the same patient as in Figure 25–18*C*, demonstrating vertical subluxation of the odontoid process through the foramen magnum with upward displacement of the brainstem.

**FIGURE 25–12.** Atlantoaxial subluxation. Lateral views, occipitoatlantoaxial complex. The space available for the cord (SAC) is outlined by the *bold, dashed line*. The odontoid process is outlined by the *smaller dashed line*. *A,* Normal complex. *B,* Anterior subluxation. The SAC is decreased in the anteroposterior plane. *C,* Combined anterior and vertical subluxation. The SAC is severely reduced, with the potential for brainstem compression by the odontoid process. (From Crosby ET, Lui A. The adult cervical spine: implications for airway management. *Can J Anaesth.* 1990;37:77.)

In addition, the mandibular space may be reduced by temporomandibular joint involvement, resulting in relative anterior positioning of the larynx and difficulty in obtaining a line of vision for intubation.

A scoliotic deformity of the trachea and larynx secondary to neck shortening from vertical subluxation has been reported in patients with long-standing rheumatoid arthritis.[40] Laryngeal deviation may result, and a rotational malalignment of the larynx relative to the sternal notch is noted, resulting in difficult intubation (Fig. 25–15).

Increasing difficulties are experienced during laryngoscopy with progression of ankylosis in ankylosing spondylitis. At the extreme, direct laryngoscopy is virtually impossible, and alternatives to direct laryngoscopy are required for tracheal intubation.

### What Anatomic Structures Determine Cervical Spine Stability?

Although the neck muscles exert some stabilizing forces, the high incidence of secondary neurologic injury in trauma

victims not initially recognized to be at risk for a spinal injury suggests that this muscle splint is insignificant. Conversely, the role of the ligamentous structures, intervertebral disks, and osseous articulations in determining stability has been

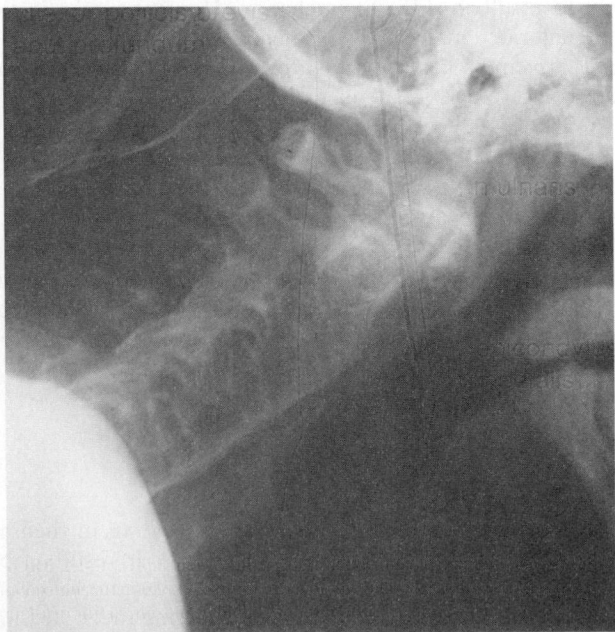

**FIGURE 25–14.** Ankylosing spondylitis. Lateral view of the cervical spine. There is fusion of the cervical spine as well as marked and generalized osteoporosis.

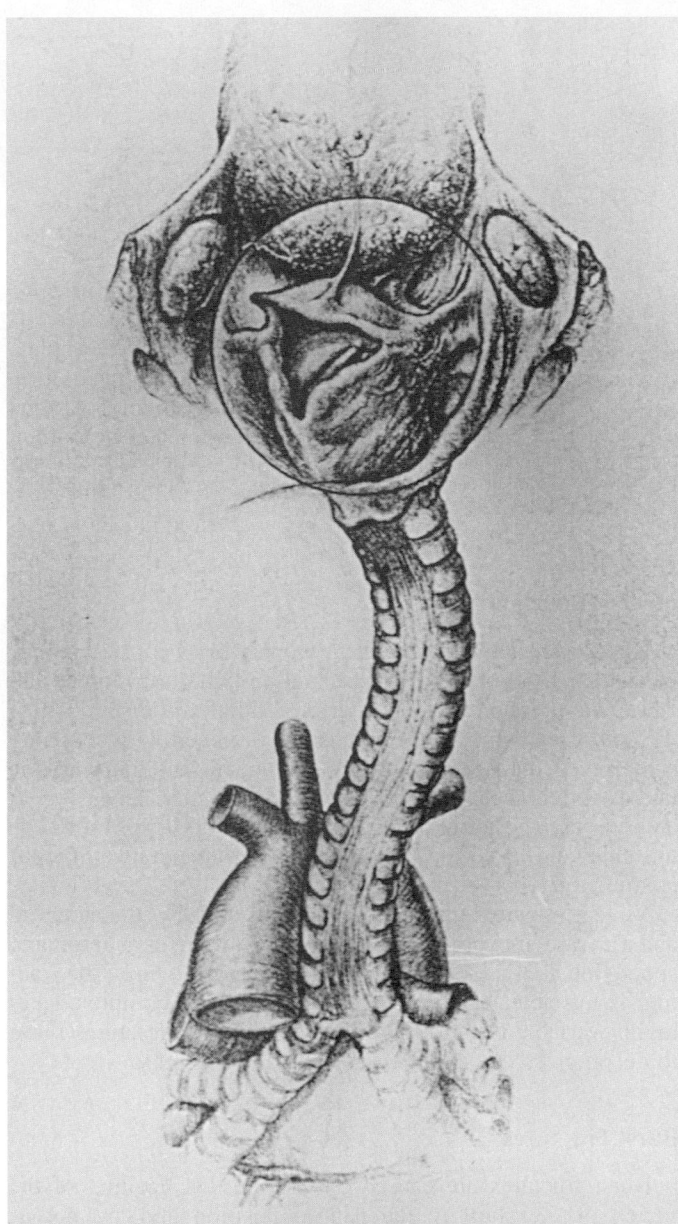

FIGURE 25–15. The airway in severe cervical spinal arthritis. The larynx is displaced anterolaterally, tilted forward, and rotated. (From Keenan MA, Stiles CM, Kaufman RL. Acquired laryngeal deviation associated with cervical spine disease in erosive polyarticular arthritis. *Anesthesiology.* 1983;58:441.)

demonstrated repeatedly. Conditions associated with instability of the cervical spine are listed in Table 25–4.

## Upper Cervical Spinal Stability

Contributing to the stability of the upper cervical spine complex are the transverse, apical, and alar ligaments and the superior terminations of the anterior and posterior longitudinal ligaments.[41] In adults, the transverse ligament normally allows no more than 3 mm of anteroposterior translation between the odontoid and the anterior ring of the atlas (the ADI). If the transverse ligament is disrupted but the alar and apical ligaments remain intact, as much as 5 mm of movement may be

seen on a lateral radiograph in flexion. If all the ligaments are disrupted, 10 mm or more of displacement may result.

Significant posterior displacement of the dens reduces the SAC in the vertebral column. In a normal spine, the SAC at C1 is about 20 mm. Cord compression does not occur when the SAC is >18 mm but may occur if it is <14 mm.[42] Steel defined a rule of thirds.[43] The area of the vertebral canal at C1 may be divided into one third odontoid, one third cord, and one third "space." The one third that is space allows some encroachment of the spinal lumen without cord compromise. However, once this margin of safety is compromised, compression of neural elements occurs.

## Lower Cervical Spinal Stability

In the lower cervical spine, structures contributing to stability, from anterior to posterior, include the anterior longitudinal ligament, the intervertebral disks, the posterior longitudinal ligament, the facet joints with their capsular ligaments, the interspinous ligament, and the supraspinous ligaments.[44]

The posterior longitudinal ligament and the structures anterior to it are grouped as the anterior elements or anterior column. The posterior elements or posterior column comprises those elements behind the posterior ligament. The anterior

**TABLE 25–4.** Conditions Associated With Cervical Spinal Instability

**Congenital**

Isolated bony malformations
Klippel-Feil syndrome
Chromosomal anomalies
Transverse ligament laxity

**Inflammatory**

Rheumatoid arthritis
Juvenile rheumatoid arthritis
Seronegative arthritides
Ankylosing spondylitis

**Infectious**

Tuberculosis
Osteomyelitis
Grisel's disease

**Neoplastic, Benign**

Bone cysts
Histiocytosis X
Osteoid osteoma
Osteoblastoma
Giant cell tumors

**Neoplastic, Malignant**

Multiple myeloma
Sarcomas
Chordomas

**Neoplastic, Metastatic**

Lung
Breast
Prostate
Kidney
Thyroid

**Degenerative Disorders**

Cervical spondylosis
Diffuse idiopathic skeletal hyperostosis
Ossification of the posterior longitudinal ligament

**Trauma**

column contributes more to the stability of the spine in extension, and the posterior column exerts its major forces in flexion.

One element in an injured column must be preserved to achieve spinal stability. If a single column is disrupted, a small amount of movement in the opposite column is permissible, but none in the disrupted column. If both columns are likely to have been disrupted, no movement is permissible.

## How Is the Cervical Spine Rendered Unstable by Injury?

Spinal injuries may be classified according to the mechanism of injury (Table 25–5; Fig. 25–16).

### Flexion

Flexion injuries usually result from blows to the back of the head or forceful decelerations; they cause compression of the anterior column and distraction of the posterior column. Pure flexion trauma may result in wedge fracture of the vertebral body without ligamentous injuries. These injuries are stable and are rarely associated with neurologic injuries. With more extreme trauma, elements of the posterior column are disrupted as well, and bilateral facet joint dislocation may result. These injuries are unstable and are associated with a high incidence of cord damage.

### Flexion-Rotation

Flexion-rotation injuries disrupt the posterior ligamentous complex and may produce unilateral facet joint dislocation. They tend to be stable and are not usually associated with spinal cord injury. However, cervical root injury is common.

**TABLE 25–5.** Classification of Spinal Injuries by Mechanism of Injury

**Hyperflexion**
Anterior subluxation
Bilateral interfacetal dislocation
Wedge compression fracture
Flexion teardrop fracture

**Hyperflexion and Rotation**
Unilateral interfacetal dislocation

**Hyperextension**
Hyperextension fracture-dislocation
Fracture of posterior arch of atlas
Traumatic spondylolisthesis (hangman's fracture)
Laminar fracture

**Vertical Compression**
Wedge compression fracture
Burst fracture
Jefferson's burst fracture (C1)

**Mixed Mechanism**
Atlantooccipital dislocation
Odontoid fractures
Total ligamentous disruption

From Crosby ET, Lui A. The adult cervical spine: implications for airway management. *Can J Anaesth.* 1990;37:77.

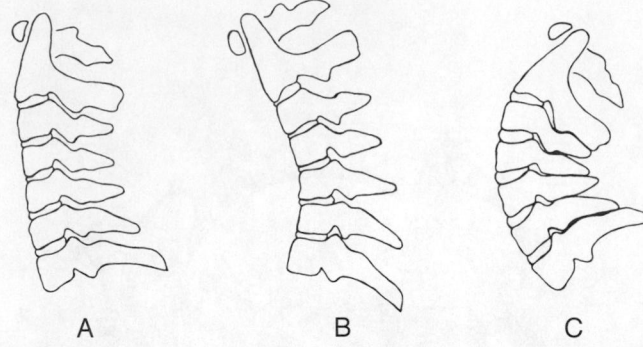

**FIGURE 25–16.** Mechanisms of injury. Lateral view, cervical spine. *A,* Normal. *B,* Hyperflexion with compression of the anterior elements and distraction in the posterior column. *C,* Hyperextension with compression of the posterior elements and distraction in the anterior column. (From Crosby ET, Lui A. The adult cervical spine: implications for airway management. *Can J Anaesth.* 1990;37:77.)

### Hyperextension

Hyperextension injuries result from a blow to the anterior part of the head or from an acceleration (whiplash) injury and cause compression of the posterior column and distraction of the anterior column. Hyperextension combined with compressive forces (eg, diving injury) may result in injury to the lateral vertebral masses, pedicles, and laminae. Because both anterior and posterior columns are disrupted, this injury is unstable and is associated with a high incidence of cord dysfunction.

Violent hyperextension, with fracture of the pedicles of C2 and forward movement of C2 on C3, produces a traumatic spondylolisthesis of the axis, or *hangman's fracture.* The fracture is unstable, but the degree of neurologic compromise is highly variable because the bilateral pedicular fractures serve to decompress the spinal cord at the site of injury.

### Burst Fractures

Burst fractures are caused by compressive loading of the vertex of the skull in the neutral position and are not as common as flexion-extension injuries. Compressive forces in the lower cervical spine result in the explosion of compressed disk material into the vertebral body. Depending on the magnitude of the compression loading and associated angulating forces, the resulting injury ranges from loss of vertebral body height with relatively intact margins to complete disruption of the vertebral body. Posterior displacement (retropulsion) of comminuted fragments may result, producing cord injury (Fig. 25–17). Despite cord injury, the spine is usually stable.

## What Are the Characteristics of Pediatric Cervical Spine Injury?

Cervical spine injury is a rare occurrence in children.[12] About 60% to 70% of pediatric spinal injuries occur in children older than 12 years of age, result largely from the same traumatic events that lead to adult injuries, and have a similar distribution. In children younger than 8 years of age, injuries are primarily restricted to the upper cervical spine. Children

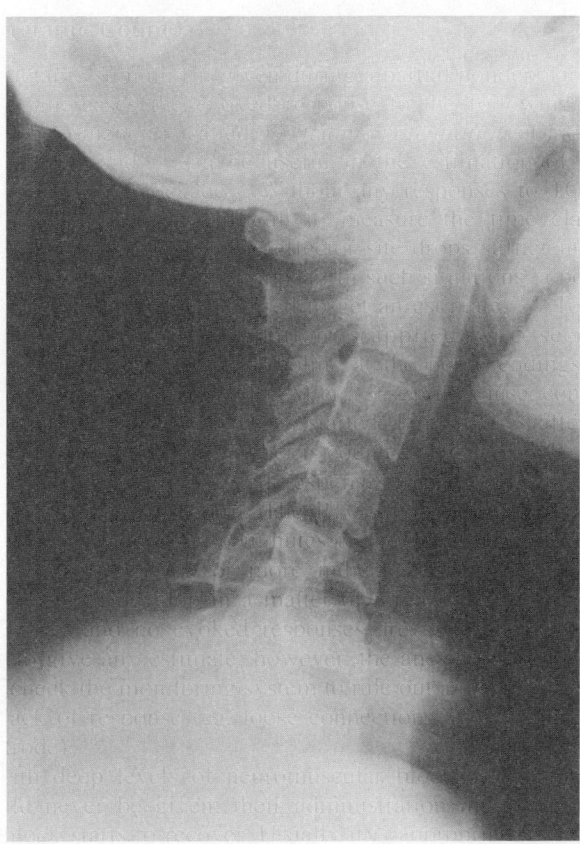

**FIGURE 25–17.** Burst fracture of C5. Lateral view of the cervical spine demonstrating burst fracture of C5 with disruption of the posterior spinal line and spinal canal compromise.

aged 8 to 12 years have a distribution of injuries ranging from that of young children to adults.

An unusual pattern of cord injury in children is that of spinal cord injury without radiographic abnormalities (SCIWORA).[12] It is most common in children younger than 8 years of age and is thought to result from mechanisms that lead to a disruption in the microvascular blood supply of the spinal cord. Ligamentous laxity in an immature cervical spine may allow longitudinal distraction and flexion-compression of the spinal cord and has been cited as a possible explanation for SCIWORA.

### Radiographic Assessment in Children

Interpretation of pediatric cervical spine radiographs may be perplexing. A number of normal variants that mimic spinal injury result from incomplete ossification and ligamentous laxity. Anterior wedging is sometimes seen in adjacent vertebrae in younger children and may represent incompletely ossified vertebrae. Pseudosubluxations are common in young children. An ADI of up to 5 mm may be seen in normal individuals, owing to normal laxity of the transverse ligament.[12] Finally, the indirect signs of injury, including loss of lordosis and increased retropharyngeal and retrotracheal soft tissue spaces, are even less specific in children than they are in adults.

## What Are the Effects of Airway Maneuvers on the Injured Neck?

After surgical disruption of the anterior and most of the posterior column in a human cadaver, the effects of airway maneuvers were studied with lateral cervical spine radiographs.[45] Basic maneuvers included chin lift, jaw thrust, head tilt, and placement of oral and esophageal airways. Advanced maneuvers included placement of an esophageal obturator airway, insertion of an orotracheal tube using both straight and curved laryngoscope blades, and blind placement of a nasotracheal tube.

Chin lift and jaw thrust resulted in expansion of the disk space >5 mm at the site of injury. When blind nasotracheal intubation was effected with anterior pressure to stabilize the airway, 5 mm of posterior subluxation occurred at the site of injury. The other advanced airway maneuvers produced 3 to 4 mm of disk space enlargement. Maneuvers were then repeated after the application of soft and semirigid cervical collars. Neither type of collar immobilized the neck effectively and consistently.

### Manual In-Line Stabilization During Airway Maneuvers

The application of manual in-line stabilization (MILS) during airway maneuvers in patients with, or at risk for, cervical spine trauma reduces the amount of neck movement resulting from airway care and is an accepted and expected intervention.[46] The optimal method for performing MILS has not been described, but published data provide some insight concerning techniques to avoid.

Bivins and colleagues studied the effects of in-line traction in deceased victims of blunt trauma.[47] Twenty-two kilograms of traction was applied across the neck using a head halter device. In cadavers without spinal column injury, in-line traction resulted in lengthening of the spinal column. When unstable spinal injuries were present, traction resulted in average distraction at the fracture site of 7.75 mm, with up to 4 mm of posterior subluxation. Although the amount of force exerted during this study was far in excess of what would normally be applied during conventional MILS during intubation, the use of traction forces during MILS is discouraged. Sufficient MILS forces should be exerted, in the appropriate directions, only to offset and minimize movement resulting from the physician performing airway interventions.

## What Effect Does Previous Cervical Spine Surgery Have on the Airway?

All fusion results in some loss of neck movement. However, considerable loss of spinal movement must result before it becomes a major factor in predicting difficult intubation.[34] For this reason, fusion involving 2 to 3 levels rarely leads to subsequent difficulties with direct laryngoscopy, whereas fusion involving multiple levels of the entire cervical spine predictably does so (Fig. 25–18). Anterior approach cervical spine procedures are associated with airway compromise requiring reintubation in as many as 2 of 125 cases within 24 hours of surgery. Airway abnormalities include pharyngeal edema and vocal cord paralysis. Severe pharyngeal lesion

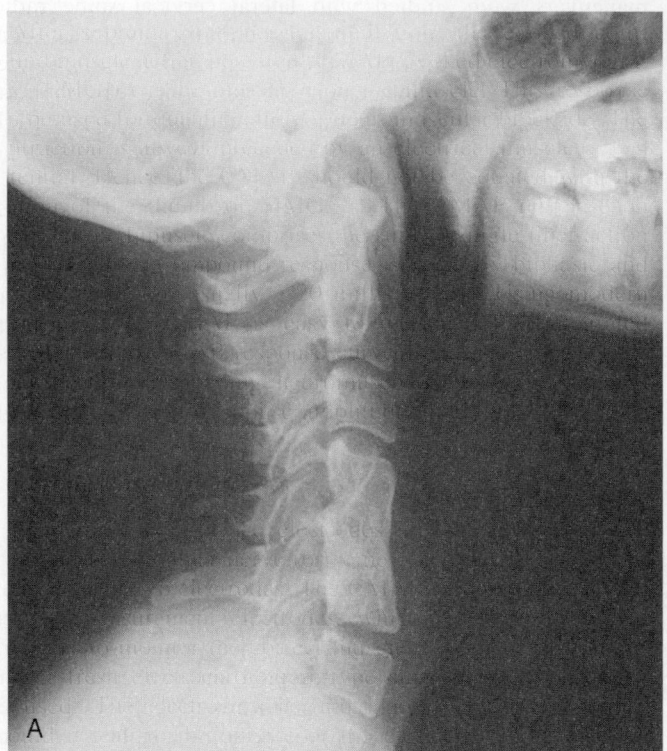

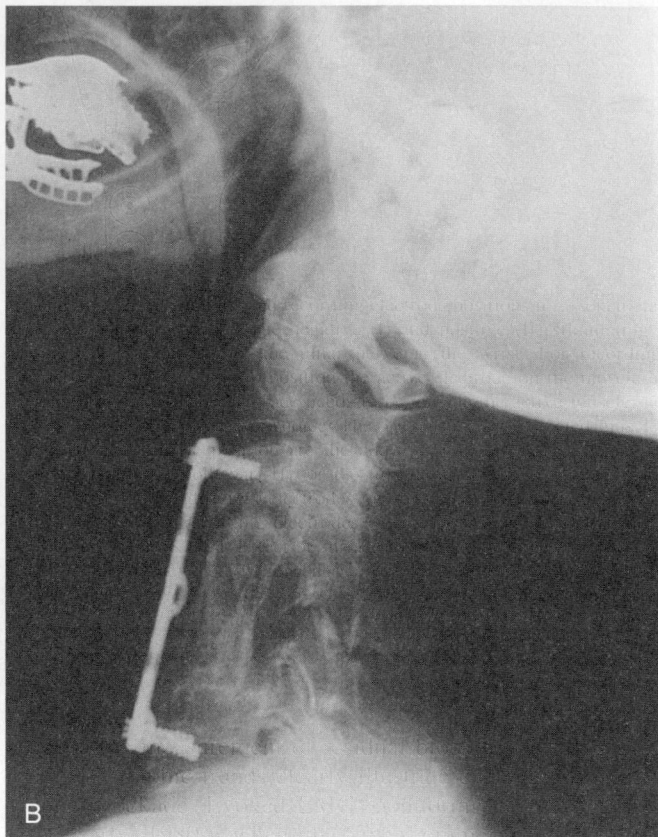

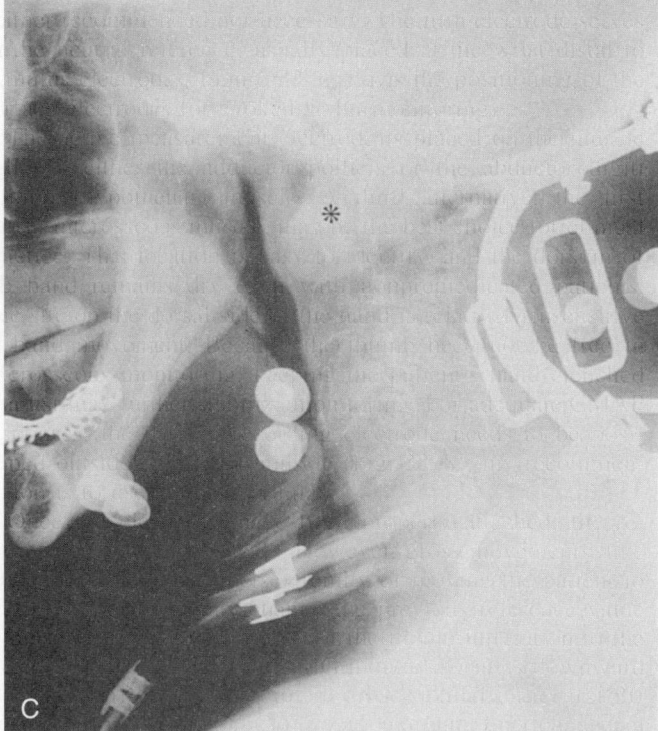

**FIGURE 25–18.** Movement in the cervical spine after surgery. *A,* Lateral view of the cervical spine demonstrating healed fusion involving the C4 through C6 elements. Spinal mobility is diminished only slightly, and laryngoscopy remains grade 1. *B,* Lateral view of the cervical spine demonstrating fusion with interbody graft involving the C3 through C7 elements. Although the mobility of the subaxial cervical spine is markedly diminished, occipitoatlantoaxial movement is preserved, the sniffing position can be achieved, and laryngoscopy has been consistently grade 1. *C,* Lateral view of the cervical spine demonstrating occipitocervical fusion performed to arrest vertical subluxation of the odontoid process through the foramen magnum (*asterisk*). The patient undergoes fusion in a neutral position and has no residual neck movement; laryngoscopy would be predictably difficult.

correlated with duration of surgery, the number of levels of fusion, and the age of the patient.[48]

## THE THORACIC SPINE

### *What Are the Relevant Anatomic Characteristics?*

#### Spinous Processes

The spinous processes of the 12 thoracic vertebrae are long and directed caudally. From T1 to T4, they are bladelike and project backward at an angle of about 40° from the perpendicular. The middle 4 spinous processes are longer and are directed at an angle of 60°, with the spines completely overlapping the subjacent vertebrae. The spines of the four most inferior thoracic vertebrae resemble the first four in direction and shape.

#### Flexion-Extension

Rib attachments to the upper segments of the thoracic spine limit flexion-extension of this area; these movements become freer in the lower thoracic segments. Flexion increases the interlaminar distance, allowing easier access to the intraspinal space. A slight cephalad displacement at the termination of the spinal cord occurs with flexion, allowing safe insertion of a spinal needle, even at the level of L2 to L3.

#### Spinal Cord

The spinal cord is enlarged in two regions of the thoracic spine. The cervical enlargement includes the C3 to T2 cord segments and is found at the corresponding vertebral levels. The lumbar enlargement is composed of the L1 to S3 cord segments and extends from the body of T11 to that of L1. The spinal cord is widest in the upper thorax (9 mm), narrows through the midthorax (6.5-8 mm), and is expanded again in the lower thorax (7-9 mm) before terminating in the conus medullaris in the upper lumbar spine.

#### Epidural Space

At the thoracic level, epidural contents are diminished, segmentation of the posterior compartment is incomplete, and patency of the epidural space at the thoracic level is increased.[4,49] This may account for the reduced resistance encountered during threading of the epidural catheter as compared with the lumbar level.

The dorsal epidural space is narrowest in its midsagittal dimension in the upper thorax (3-4 mm), increases through the midthorax (3-5 mm), and is largest at the thoracolumbar junction (4-6 mm). At the midthoracic spine, the narrowest portion of the spinal cord is associated with a relatively wide epidural space, allowing for safe administration of epidural anesthesia. However, this is the site of the most extreme angulation of the spinous processes, and the midline approach may be difficult. The arterial supply is more tenuous in the midthoracic region and is most sluggish at T4. If a compressive lesion such as an epidural hematoma develops, the risk for ischemia in this region increases.

### *How Is Thoracic Epidural Catheter Placement Achieved?*

#### Midline Approach

The advantage of the midline approach for an anesthesiologist experienced with lumbar epidural blocks is that it provides the security and "feel" associated with traversing the usual ligamentous structures. Because the ligamentum flavum may be discontinuous at the thoracic level, however, the epidural space may occasionally be entered without encountering the ligament.[4]

In the midthorax, between T4 and T8, the midline approach is feasible only with the needle directed at an angle of 60° or more from the perpendicular (Fig. 25–19). The needle may enter the epidural space at 7 cm or more from the skin. The midline approach becomes more straightforward below T8, where the spines are shorter and less acutely angulated, and the vertebral segment can be flexed to optimize access to the interlaminar space (see Fig. 25–19).

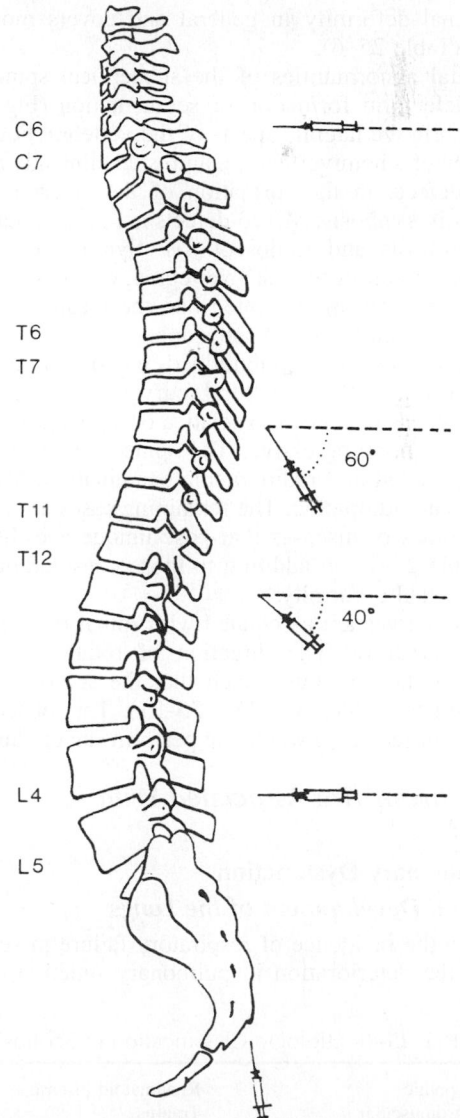

**FIGURE 25–19.** Lateral aspect of the vertebral column illustrating the angle of needle entry required with the midline approach to access the intraspinal space.

### Paramedian Approach

The paramedian approach avoids the extremely angled approach in the midthorax and the longer distance to the epidural space. This technique may provide the only access to the epidural space when the bony elements deter midline access. A key to success in using the paramedian approach is to enter immediately beside the spinous process. This method avoids being so far lateral that the needle never encounters the ligamentous structures and reduces the likelihood of entering the epidural space in its narrow lateral aspects.

## How Are Abnormal Curvatures of the Thoracic Spine Described?

The terms *scoliosis, kyphosis, lordosis,* and combinations of *kyphoscoliosis* or *lordoscoliosis* are often encountered. *Scoliosis* (derived from the Greek word *skoliosis,* meaning "crookedness") refers to a lateral curvature of the spine. *Kyphosis,* meaning "humpback," describes a backward convexity of the spine, and *lordosis* describes a forward convexity of the spine. For the purpose of this discussion, only the classification of scoliosis is presented because it is representative of spinal deformity in general and covers most of the etiologies (Table 25–6).

Congenital abnormalities of the subcervical spine are the result of defects in formation or segmentation (Fig. 25–20). Failure to form the lateral aspects of the vertebral body results in formation of a hemivertebra, manifested clinically as scoliosis. Pure defects in the formation of the anterior vertebral body result in kyphosis. Mixed defects are common and result in kyphoscoliosis and lordoscoliosis. Symmetric defects of segmentation result in "block" vertebrae, whereas asymmetric defects result in an unsegmented bar, the location and lesion determining the curvature of the spine.

Scoliotic curves can be subdivided into structural and non-structural variants. Nonstructural curves are those seen in postural scoliosis or related to sciatica or leg length discrepancies; they are nonprogressive. The spine appears completely normal on clinical and radiographic examination. Most structural curves are idiopathic. The remaining cases are associated with syndromes or diseases that pose unique anesthetic challenges (Table 25–7), in addition to those considerations relating to the spinal deformity.

Structural curves are associated with spinal rotation as well as lateral curvature. The direction of rotation is into the convexity of the curvature, such that the spinous processes point toward the concavity (Fig. 25–21). This observation is of obvious consequence when one performs an epidural block.

## What Problems Are Associated With Scoliosis?

### Cardiopulmonary Dysfunction

### Growth and Development of the Lungs

Although the incidence of respiratory failure in scoliosis is unknown, the deterioration in pulmonary function correlates

**TABLE 25–6.** Etiologic Classification of Scoliosis

| | |
|---|---|
| Idiopathic | Rheumatoid disease |
| Neuromuscular | Trauma |
| Congenital | Osteochondrodystrophies |
| Neurofibromatosis | Metabolic disorders |
| Mesenchymal disorders | Tumors |

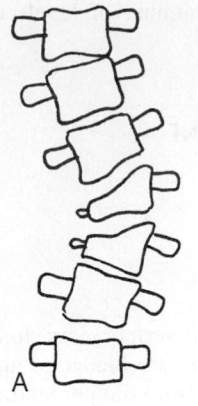
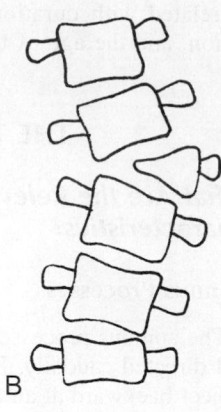

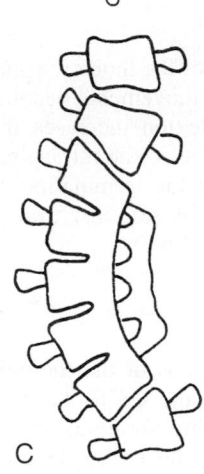
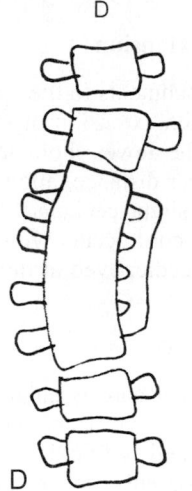

**FIGURE 25–20.** Congenital deformities of the spine, mechanisms for failed development. *A,* Partial unilateral failure of formation. *B,* Complete unilateral failure of formation. *C,* Unilateral failure of segmentation. *D,* Bilateral failure of segmentation.

with the severity of the curvature. Scoliosis interferes with the formation, growth, and development of the lungs. Because the number of alveoli increases by a factor of 10 between birth and 8 years of age, the occurrence of scoliosis before lung maturity may reduce the number of alveoli formed. The pulmonary vasculature forms in parallel with the alveoli and is likewise affected, resulting in increased pulmonary resistance and, in severe cases, right heart failure.

### Ventilation-Perfusion Abnormalities

The most common blood gas abnormality is an increased alveolar-to-arterial oxygen partial pressure gradient. The reduction in arterial oxygen content, coupled with normal levels of carbon dioxide, suggests ventilation-perfusion mismatch with venoarterial shunting and altered regional perfusion.

### Mechanical Function

The pulmonary pathophysiology of scoliosis also includes the effects of the vertebral and rib cage deformity on the

**TABLE 25–7.** Anesthetic Considerations in Patients With Scoliosis

| Syndrome | Anesthetic Considerations |
| --- | --- |
| Idiopathic scoliosis (>65°) | Mitral valve prolapse, pulmonary hypertension, right ventricular hypertrophy, restrictive respiratory defect |
| Neuropathic disorders (cerebral palsy) | Recurrent pneumonia, upper airway obstruction, malnutrition, difficult vascular access, positioning difficulties |
| Myopathic disorders (muscular dystrophy, myotonia, central core disease) | Cardiomyopathy, mitral valve prolapse, arrhythmias, respiratory failure, upper airway obstruction, altered responses to neuromuscular blockers, hyperkalemia with succinylcholine, malignant hyperthermia |
| Neurofibromatosis | Pulmonary valvular stenosis, fibrosing alveolitis, airway obstruction, pheochromocytoma |
| Mesenchymal disorders (Marfan syndrome) | Aortic: dissection and valve incompetence |
| Rheumatoid disease (rheumatoid arthritis) | Pericarditis, valvular involvement, pulmonary fibrosis, pleural effusions, atlantoaxial subluxation, Felty's syndrome, positioning difficulties |
| Osteochondrodystrophies (Morquio syndrome) | Aortic valvular incompetency, heart failure, atlantoaxial instability |
| Metabolic disorders (osteogenesis imperfecta) | Aortic valvular incompetence, abnormal platelets, positioning difficulties |

mechanical function of the lungs. The most common pulmonary function abnormality is a restrictive pattern with reduction in vital capacity, total lung capacity, and lung compliance. This pattern is encountered in virtually all patients with thoracic curves of >65°. The rotation of the spine and thoracic cage puts the lungs at a mechanical disadvantage, and the work of breathing may increase fivefold from normal.

Other factors that may impair lung function in patients with scoliosis include associated lordosis, poor muscle function, and reduced distensibility of the lungs.

### Associated Cardiac Abnormalities

In adolescent scoliosis, the incidence of mitral valve prolapse exceeds 25%.[50] Children with congenital heart disease have an increased incidence of scoliosis. A high incidence of right ventricular hypertrophy and hypertensive pulmonary vascular changes is found at autopsy in patients with thoracic scoliosis. A wide variety of disease processes, ranging from neuromuscular disorders to inborn errors of metabolism, are associated with scoliosis. With each disease or syndrome, associated cardiovascular abnormalities may also be present.[51]

### Does the Cause of Scoliosis Matter?

Typically, when scoliosis occurs as a result of a primary neurologic or myopathic disorder, the curve severity is greater than in idiopathic forms of the disease. Abnormal respiratory function is not only due to the skeletal deformity of scoliosis, it is also a result of abnormalities in both the central control of respiration and the supraspinal innervation muscles as well as the loss of muscle function due to lesions of the motor neurons and peripheral nerves or myopathy. Respiratory function may be further compromised by impairment of the de-

fense mechanisms of the airways caused by loss of control of the pharynx and the larynx, by ineffective cough mechanism, and by infrequent or reduced large breaths. Recurrent aspiration pneumonitis results from compromised airway protective reflexes. In general, the prognosis of scoliosis caused by neuromuscular disease is worse than that of idiopathic scoliosis; it is determined predominantly by progression of the primary disorder and results in irreversible respiratory failure at a younger age.

### What Are the Mechanisms of Injury to the Thoracolumbar Spine?

The basic mechanisms of injury to the thoracolumbar spine are flexion, extension, rotation, and shear. Flexion accounts for almost 85% of injuries. Because the natural curvature of the thoracic spine is predominantly one of flexion, a vertical force acting on the spine increases the flexion. The resultant injury is a wedge fracture of the vertebral body. As the vertical compressive force is increased, the likelihood of a comminution injury to the vertebral body is presented. Retropulsion of a comminuted fragment into the canal may result in cord injury.

### When Is the Thoracic Spine Unstable?

As with the cervical spine, stability of the thoracic column depends on the integrity of not only the skeletal components but also the ligaments, intervertebral disks, and facet joints. Thoracic instability is defined by Denis's three-column con-

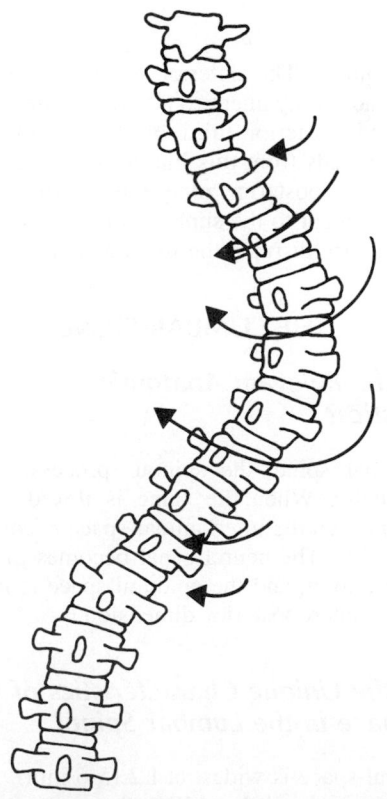

**FIGURE 25–21.** Idiopathic scoliosis. Both lateral curvature and rotation of the spine occur. The direction of the rotation is such that the spinous processes rotate into the concavity of the lateral curve.

EXTENSION

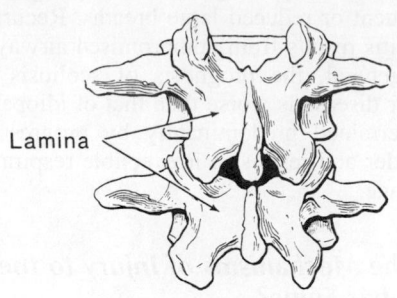

Lamina

FLEXION

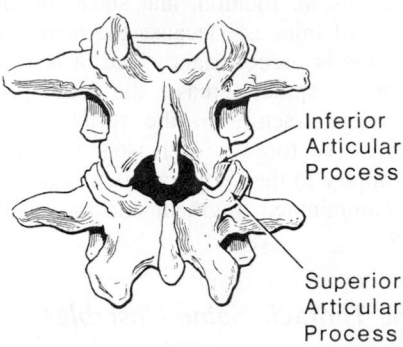

Inferior
Articular
Process

Superior
Articular
Process

**FIGURE 25–22.** Interlaminar space, lumbar region, in flexion and extension. In extension, the boundaries are the roots of spinous processes and the laminae. With flexion, the space is widened in both dimensions, and the new lateral boundaries are the articular processes. (From Cousins MJ. Epidural neural blockade. In: Cousins MJ, Bridenbaugh PO, eds. *Neural Blockade in Clinical Anesthesia and Management of Pain.* Philadelphia, Pa: JB Lippincott; 1980:192.)

cept of the spine.[52] The anterior column extends from the anterior longitudinal ligament to a vertical line drawn through the middle and posterior third of the vertebral body. The middle zone extends from this line to the posterior longitudinal ligament. The posterior zone extends from the posterior longitudinal ligament to the supraspinous ligament. Instability occurs when injury disrupts the middle zone.

## THE LUMBAR SPINE

### What Are the Relevant Anatomic Characteristics?

In the lumbar spine, the spinous processes are oriented more horizontally. When the spine is flexed, access to the spinal canal through the interlaminar space becomes relatively easy (Fig. 25–22). The neural canal becomes more triangular in the lumbar region, and the epidural space is increased to 5 to 6 mm in its anteroposterior dimension.

### What Are the Unique Characteristics of the Epidural Space in the Lumbar Spine?

The epidural space is widest at L2 (5-6 mm). As compared with the thoracic level by MRI, there are more epidural contents, and the ligamentum flavum is more frequently continuous.[4] Extraduroscopic examination confirms that the

amount of fatty and fibrous connective tissue is greater in the lumbar than in the thoracic spine.[49] The differences between the structure of these two vertebral regions may affect the spread of local anesthetics in the extradural space. Along with the amount of fatty tissue, a large amount of fibrous connective tissue in the lumbar epidural space may decrease the longitudinal spread of anesthetic solution.[49] At each segmental level, the extradural region narrows abruptly at its cranial end as the lamina becomes adjacent to the dura.[53] If the Tuohy needle enters the space in this superior part, attempts at introducing the catheter may meet with almost immediate obstruction as it strikes the inferior surface of the laminae.[53]

### Is It the Plicae Mediana Dorsalis, a Posterior Dural Fold, or a Posterior Epidural Fat Pad?

Dissection and injection studies have demonstrated a midline connective tissue membrane, the plicae mediana dorsalis, as well as a posterior dural fold in the lumbar epidural space.[52–54] Both the plicae and the median dural fold tend to be consistent through several successive lumbar vertebral levels and have the effect of dividing the posterior lumbar epidural space into two dorsolateral compartments. These structures have been cited as the etiologic factors responsible for unilateral epidural blockade[9,55,56] (Fig. 25–23).

Hogan, using cryomicrotome technology, was unable to demonstrate the posterior midline epidural septa but did describe the consistent presence of a posterior epidural fat pad

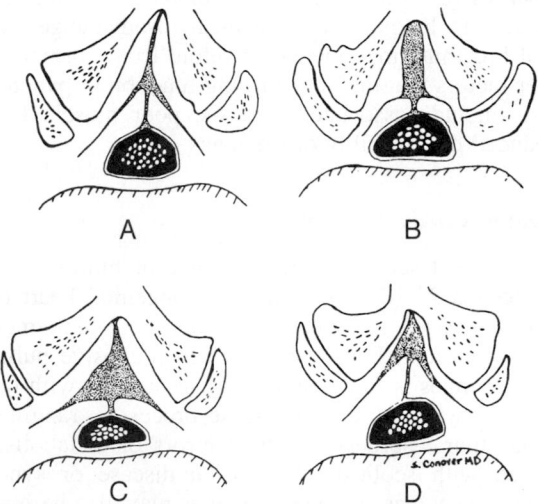

A

B

C

D

**FIGURE 25–23.** The plicae mediana dorsalis. The anatomic configuration of both the plicae and the posterior epidural space approximates one of the four general patterns determined by the amount and location of fatty material deposited between the membranes. *A,* Seven of 40 patients showed thin linear membranes with minimal fatty content. *B,* Two of 40 patients showed a somewhat thicker configuration of the plica but still retained a linear orientation. *C,* Eighteen of 40 patients showed a large triangular junction of membranes, with copious fat contributing to the extra bulk of the midline structure. Such a configuration might impede or deflect an epidural catheter or, perhaps, even receive injection of solutions within the midline structure itself. *D,* Thirteen of 40 patients demonstrated a smaller triangular membrane junction located posteriorly on the plica. The junction produced less bulk but, by virtue of its location, could possibly interfere with catheter introduction through a Tuohy needle. (From Savolaine ER, Pandya JB, Greenblatt SH, et al. Anatomy of the human lumbar epidural space: new insights using CT-epidurography. *Anesthesiology.* 1988;68:217.)

and a midline pedicle for the pad.[3] It is likely that these structures represent the same structure labeled the plicae mediana dorsalis. A recent study using computed tomography suggested that posterior midline structures play a minimal role in impeding the distribution of epidural injectate. Lateral catheter position is a more likely cause of unilateral blocks.[57]

### Anterior Epidural Space

A consistent feature that may be responsible for unilateral blockade is the small and discontinuous anterior epidural space. When the tip of the catheter is positioned in the anterolateral aspects of the epidural space, inadequate block may result as the injected local anesthetic solution spreads predominantly ipsilaterally[58] (Fig. 25–24). Bilateral blockade is dependent on retrograde flow around the dura in the posterior epidural space. Large volumes of local anesthetic solution that approach or exceed the recommended safe dose may be required for some patients.

## What Are the Common Congenital Anomalies of the Lumbar Spine?

### Spina Bifida

Spina bifida results from the failure of the bony vertebrae to enclose the neural elements in a bony canal completely. There is a wide spectrum with respect to the severity of the deformity and its implications. *Spina bifida occulta* is defined as failed fusion of the neural arch without herniation of meninges or neural elements. A defect limited to a single vertebra, usually L5 or S1, is so common (occurring in 5%-36% of the population) that it can be considered a normal variant.[59] Superficial signs of this lesion may include a tuft of hair, cutaneous angioma, lipoma, or a skin dimple, but such signs are not common in patients with isolated vertebral arch

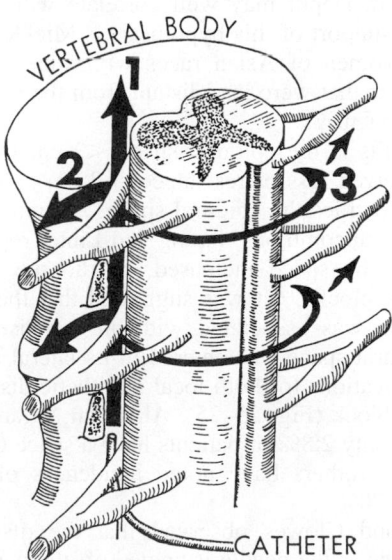

**FIGURE 25–24.** With the tip of the catheter in the anterior or anterolateral epidural space, longitudinal (1) and ipsilateral transverse (2) spread of the local anesthetic solution predominates. The magnitude of the circumferential spread around the dura (3) determines the quality of contralateral blockade. (From Usubiaga JE, Dos Reis A, Usubiaga LE. Epidural misplacement of catheters and mechanisms of unilateral blockade. *Anesthesiology.* 1970;32:158.)

anomalies and an underlying normal cord. Patients with spina bifida occulta rarely have symptoms related to this anomaly, although they may have a higher incidence of posterior disk herniation.[59]

*Spina bifida cystica* occurs when there is herniation of the meninges (ie, meningocele) or of both the meninges and neural elements (ie, myelomeningocele) through the vertebral defect. These conditions are relatively uncommon and occur with an incidence of 1 to 3 per 1000 births.[60–65] Neurologic deficits involving the lower extremities and sphincters occur in almost all patients and vary only in degree of severity. Hydrocephalus is present in most patients, and shunting of the ventricular system is often required. Early and aggressive surgical treatment of the lesion increased survival rates from 45% in the early 1970s to 70% to 90% by the mid-1980s.[63,64] Myelomeningocele is a progressive neurologic disease, eventually producing orthopedic, neurologic, and genitourinary complications. Kyphoscoliosis is common in patients with a thoracic lesion and occurs in 20% of patients with a lumbosacral defect.[65] Paralytic scoliosis is the most common type and results from an imbalance of paravertebral muscle tone; it also undergoes rapid progression with growth.

There is an intermediate group of conditions wherein the bony defect is associated with one or more anomalies of the spinal cord, including intraspinal lipomas, dermal sinus tracts, dermoid cysts, fibrous bands, and diastematomyelia (split cord). These are termed *occult spinal dysraphism* to differentiate them from the more benign occulta lesions described previously.[66] These patients may have no neurologic symptoms or may have minor motor and sensory deficits of the lower limbs, bowel, and bladder. Patients with cord abnormalities have cutaneous stigmata in 50% to 70% of cases. The association of cutaneous stigmata with underlying spina bifida increases the likelihood of a cord anomaly.

### Tethered Cord

The spinal cord may be attached to a congenitally abnormal structure in the lumbar spine, resulting in a tethered spinal cord.[66,67] This condition is marked by a low-lying (L2-L3) conus medullaris anchored by a thick filum terminale. MRI studies suggest that tethering is present in virtually all patients with spina bifida cystica and myelomeningocele.[67] Tethered cord is also common in patients with occult spinal dysraphism.[68] It is not clear what proportion of patients with spina bifida occulta have a tethered cord, but the incidence appears low. The presence of a low-lying tethered cord may be associated with a more caudal termination of the subarachnoid space.

### Regional Anesthesia and Spina Bifida

The epidural space may be incomplete or discontinuous across the level of occulta lesions because of the absent lamina and variable formation of the ligamentum flavum at this site. An attempt to identify the epidural space at the site of this lesion will likely result in unintentional dural puncture.[60] However, successful epidural analgesia has been reported with the catheter placed within the zone of the lesion.[61] Flow of local anesthetic solution through the lateral and anterolateral epidural space may be sufficient to extend a block beyond the level of the lesion.

Despite its common occurrence in the population and the

inevitability of dural puncture if epidural analgesia is attempted at affected spinal levels, spina bifida occulta rarely complicates the administration of regional anesthesia for two reasons. First, the lesion typically occurs at the L5 to S1 segments, below the level at which most epidural and spinal anesthetics are administered.[61] Second, the most common anomaly is a simple midline split in the lamina; this defect rarely interferes with either the performance or development of spinal or epidural anesthesia. More extensive lesions involving multiple vertebral segments are less common.

There are published reports of the use of epidural and spinal anesthesia in patients with spina bifida cystica.[61–64,69,70] Unfortunately, the experience is limited, and most published series of patients (usually parturients) with spina bifida cystica report neither the type of anesthesia provided nor the complications experienced. It seems appropriate to administer epidural or spinal anesthesia in patients with well-preserved neurologic function. The anesthesiologist should be aware that the terminal portion of the spinal cord lies at a vertebral level lower than normal. Therefore, subarachnoid injection should be performed in the lower lumbar spine or avoided in favor of epidural anesthesia. Inadequate epidural anesthesia is more likely because of the abnormal, discontinuous epidural space.

In most patients with negligible function of the extremities and sphincters, the presence of a low-lying tethered cord is clinically irrelevant, and it need not alter the level of subarachnoid injection. In these patients, spinal anesthesia may be easier technically, and it may provide anesthesia more reliably. A subarachnoid hematoma after spinal anesthesia in an elderly woman with occult spinal dysraphism and a tethered cord (L4) has been reported.[70] Dural puncture was made at the L3 to L4 level and was complicated initially by blood in the CSF, which cleared. At laminectomy, a bleeding vessel was identified on the surface of the cord.

### Scoliosis and Epidural Anesthesia

A rotatory component is associated with the scoliotic curve, as was noted earlier, and the axial rotation of the vertebral body is always into the convexity of the lateral curve, so that the spinous process rotates back into the concavity (see Fig. 25–21). Hence, the midline of the epidural space is deviated toward the convexity of the curve relative to the spinous process palpable at the skin level. The needle should enter the selected interspace and be directed toward the convexity of the curve. An experienced clinician can track the resistance and feel both the interspinous ligament and the ligamentum flavum to maintain a true course into the epidural space. Minor functional curves, such as those commonly seen in term pregnant women, rarely result in significant rotatory deviation of the vertebrae. Little, if any, accommodation in technique is required for successful needle or catheter placement. As the curves become more extreme, greater degrees of difficulty are experienced, and attempts should ideally be made in areas least affected by the curve, including the lumbosacral junction.

### What Age-Related Changes Occur in the Lumbar Spine That Affect Neuraxial Blockade?

With advancing age, desiccation of the intervertebral disks and loss of disk height occur. Osteoporosis, occurring especially in women, leads to compression fractures that are common to the weight-bearing vertebrae of the lumbar spine. Both processes tend to diminish separation of the posterior elements of the lumbar spine and result in smaller interlaminar spaces. In addition, osteophyte formation and ligamentous ossification lead to encroachment of foramina and interspaces and may, similarly, produce smaller interlaminar spaces. The net result is greater difficulty as attempts are made to pass a needle into either the epidural or subarachnoid spaces. Igarashi and associates, using a flexible extraduroscope, demonstrated that the extradural space becomes widely patent and the fatty tissue within diminishes with increasing age.[71] In patients of advanced age with degenerative disk and joint changes, distortion and compression of the epidural space are typical.[4]

More cephalad spread of local anesthetic injected into the epidural space has been documented in the elderly. It was hypothesized that this occurred, in part, because of decreased loss through the intervertebral foramina, compared with younger patients. However, Saitoh and colleagues, although confirming that a correlation exists between longitudinal spread of iohexol and age, noted no relation between leakage of iohexol through the intervertebral foramina and age.[72] Saitoh's data suggest that longitudinal extradural spread of local anesthetics in elderly patients may not be attributed to decreased leakage through the intervertebral foramina. The decrease in epidural content may account for the increased cephalad spread.

### How Deep Is the Lumbar Epidural Space?

In most adults, the epidural space lies 4 to 6 cm below the skin.[73–77] The depth increases from L2-3 to L4-5, but the difference is not great.[73–75] Increasing weight and BMI correlate with increasing depth, but maternal height reportedly does not.[73,74,78] This difference is likely an artifact of small study population size, with few patients at the extremes of height being assessed. Depth may well correlate with height at its extremes. In support of this hypothesis is Mieklejohn's observation that women of Asian races with smaller stature had epidural spaces that were less distant from the skin than taller European women.[77]

In few adults is the epidural space <3 cm from the skin. Thus, a perceived loss of resistance at 3 cm or less from the skin rarely identifies the epidural space. A depth of >7 cm is also relatively uncommon. Narang and Linter reported that as the depth of the space increased, so did the incidence of unsatisfactory blocks.[76] It was suggested that the greater distance traveled was associated with an increased likelihood that the epidural space was entered in its lateral aspects, with obvious implications for both local anesthetic distribution and the resultant block (Fig. 25–25). Although Narang and Linter reported that only 2.8% of patients have a space 6 cm or more from the skin, others have noted incidences of such depth from 13% to 20%.

Harrison and Clowes observed that the distance to the space increases as the needle is angled off the perpendicular.[75] However, the error introduced is relatively small and is likely to increase the depth of the space by only 2 to 3 mm. The distance from the skin to the epidural space was also greater in 2123 term parturients when epidural puncture was performed in the lateral position as compared with the sitting position.[78]

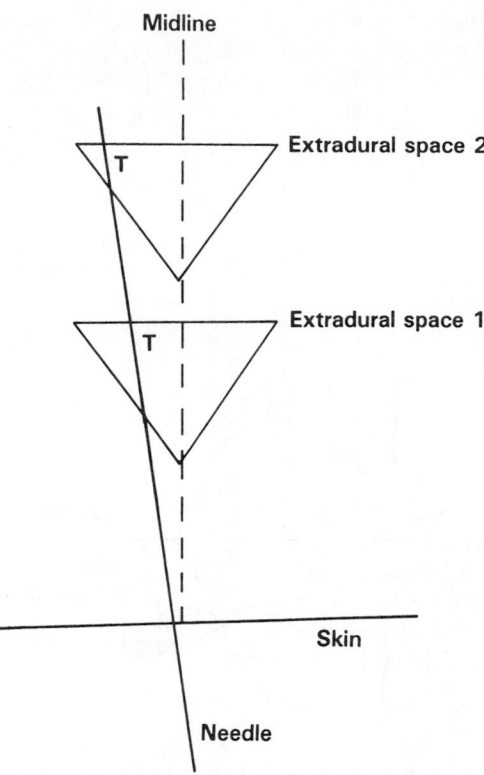

Midline

Extradural space 2

T

Extradural space 1

T

Skin

Needle

**FIGURE 25–25.** Diagram showing increasing lateral displacement of the tip of the needle (T) as the skin-to-extradural space distance increases from extradural space 1 to extradural space 2. (From Narang VPS, Linter SPK. Failure of extradural blockade in obstetrics. *Br J Anaesth.* 1988;60:402.)

The skin-epidural distance in children between 6 months and 10 years of age can be estimated at 1 mm per kg.[79] The mean depth to the epidural space in neonates is 1 cm (range, 0.4-1.5 cm), and the depth of epidural space in older infants and children correlates with age and weight.[80]

## What Are the Considerations for the Paramedian Approach in the Lumbar Spine?

Blomberg and colleagues compared the median and paramedian approaches to the epidural space using fiberoptic epiduroscopy[81] (Fig. 25–26). In the 14 subjects studied, the epidural space was an average 9.3 mm farther from the skin with the paramedian approach than with the midline approach. Once loss of resistance to air was recognized, the needle could travel another 3.9 mm until dural contact with the midline approach, compared with 7.6 mm with the paramedian approach. On this basis, accidental dural puncture was concluded to be more likely with the midline approach. With the midline technique, the catheters entered the space at right angles, causing dural tenting in all subjects. By comparison, with the paramedian approach, the catheter entered the space at 120° to 135° to the dura and did not cause dural tenting. It was concluded that the risk for dural puncture was greater with the midline technique. The catheter moved in a cephalad direction in all cases in the paramedian trial but in only 29% of the median attempts. It moved laterally in the epidural space in 64% of the midline insertions, theoretically increasing the risk for blood vessel trauma with this technique.

Although this study highlights the advantages cited for the paramedian approach—a lower incidence of accidental dural puncture, blood vessel cannulation, and paresthesia and a straighter, predictable course for the catheter in the epidural space—comparisons of the techniques do not demonstrate a consistent, clinically important advantage for the paramedian technique.[82,83] Blomberg and colleagues reported a higher incidence of difficult insertions and difficulty encountered in identifying the epidural space, as well as catheter-related problems with the midline approach.[81] However, his reported incidence of difficulties with the median approach is much higher than that reported by others, thus skewing their comparison. Jaucot, reporting more than 1000 epidural anesthetic procedures, described no important differences between midline and paramedian techniques.[83] A slightly increased incidence of paresthesias, blood vessel puncture, and inability to pass the catheters was recorded in the midline approach group, but the overall incidence of these events was small. The success rate on the first attempt was 94.5% with the midline approach and 98% with the paramedian approach, not a significant difference.

Griffin and Scott reported similar success with catheter placement, difficulty locating the space, analgesia on the first attempt, the incidence of passing the catheter, and blood vessel cannulation.[83] A higher incidence of pain was observed with the paramedian approach but was attributed to the small volumes of local anesthetic used to provide anesthesia.

Despite the touted advantages of the paramedian approach, only 2% of British anesthetists surveyed used the paramedian route, and 85% of anesthetists preferred the midline approach for routine use.[84]

## What Changes in Lumbar Spine Anatomy and Function Occur With Pregnancy?

An increase in the lumbar lordotic curve occurs during pregnancy as the pelvis rotates forward. This alteration exaggerates the normal loads borne by the posterior aspects of the intervertebral disks and the zygapophyseal joints. Back pain is common, occurring in about half of all parturients at some point during their pregnancy.[85] The pain is usually related to softening of the sacroiliac and pubic ligaments, with resultant mechanical instability in these joints. True pathology (ie, herniated disk) related to pregnancy is uncommon; it should be recognized and distinguished from the more benign forms of gestational back problems.

### Spinal Canal and Epidural Venous Plexus

As a result of caval obstruction caused by a gravid uterus, enhanced blood flow occurs through the vertebral venous plexus, with engorgement of the epidural venous plexus (Fig. 25–27). The result is a decrease of the CSF volume, smaller relative spinal canal volume, and lower volume requirements for local anesthetics during major regional blockade.[53] Additionally, an increased risk for epidural vascular trauma occurs in parturients, compared with nonpregnant patients. This risk may be reduced by using softer catheters and perhaps by injecting a volume of saline or local anesthetic through the epidural needle before attempting to pass the catheter.[86,87]

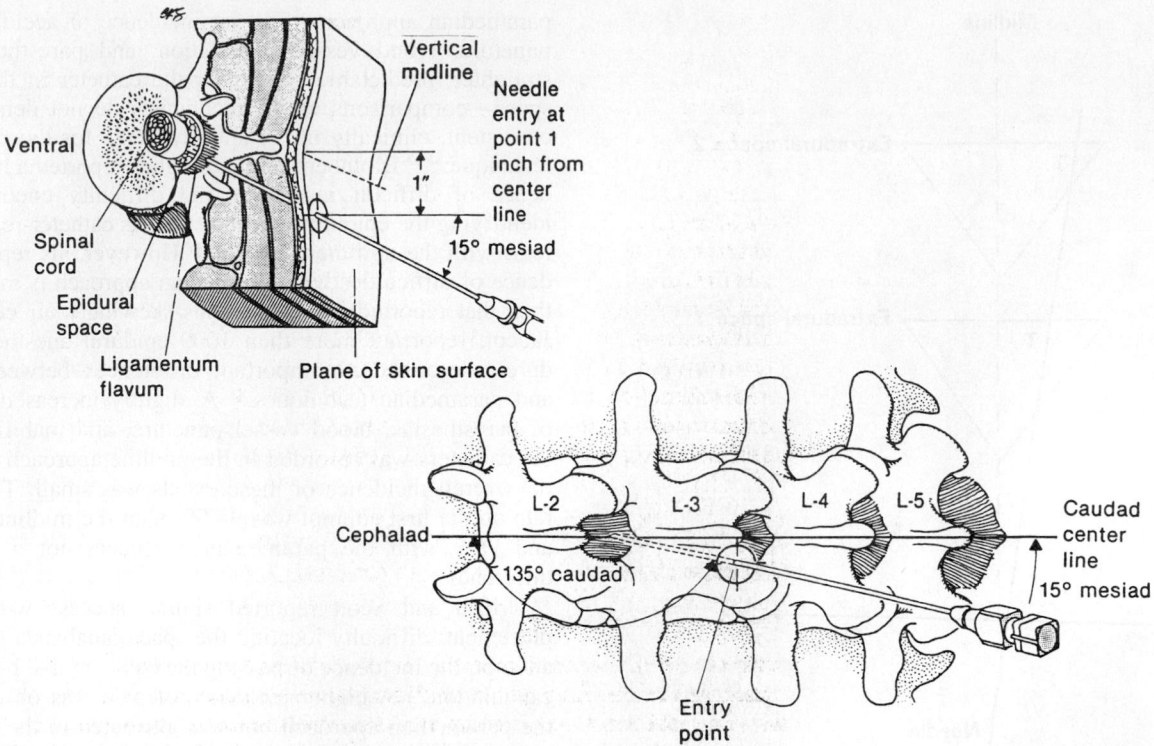

**FIGURE 25–26.** Epidural venous plexus. The large epidural venous plexus may become engorged with increased intraabdominal pressure and during pregnancy. (From Reisner LS, Ellis J. Epidural and caudal puncture. In: Benumof JL, ed. *Clinical Procedures in Anesthesia and Intensive Care*. Philadelphia, Pa: JB Lippincott; 1992:663.)

## Why Does Low Back Pain Occur?

Pain may arise from three distinct anatomic areas in the spinal column, each of which gives rise to a characteristic pain syndrome[88] (Fig. 25–28). Type A pain is most common and originates in the motion segments and associated ligamen-tous and muscular structures. It is a dull, deep, aching pain that is poorly localized and not associated with neurologic findings. Type B pain arises in the superficial structures of the vertebral column and is usually well localized to the area of injury. Type C pain is caused by involvement of nerve trunks associated with the vertebral column. It is a sharp radiating pain that is often referred and is associated with neurologic findings.

Spinal pain may originate from one anatomic structure, but injuries may not be limited to one source; various degrees of overlap of pain type do occur. Most instances of acute low back pain are types A and B or combinations thereof and

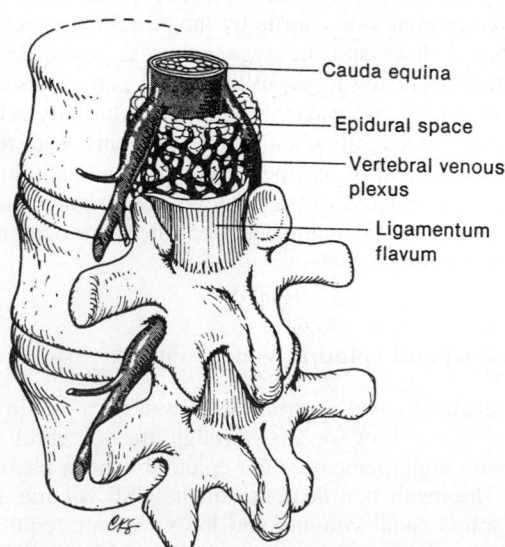

**FIGURE 25–27.** Epidural puncture, paramedian approach. The paramedian approach avoids the overlap of spinous processes but is not characterized by the same feel as the midline approach because the supraspinous and interspi-nous ligaments are avoided. (From Reisner LS, Ellis J. Epidural and caudal puncture. In: Benumof JL, ed. *Clinical Procedures in Anesthesia and Intensive Care*. Philadelphia, Pa: JB Lippincott; 1992:663.)

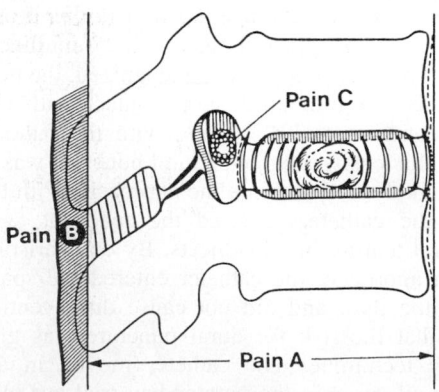

**FIGURE 25–28.** Low back pain. Back pain may arise from three distinct anatomic areas in the spinal column, each area giving rise to a characteristic pain syndrome (see text). (From O'Brien JP. Mechanisms of spinal pain. In: Wall PD, Melzack R, eds. *Textbook of Pain*. New York, NY: Churchill Livingstone; 1984:240.)

**TABLE 25–8.** Anatomic Irregularities Correlating With Chronic Low Back Pain

**Likely Causes**

Spondylolisthesis (moderate to severe)
Spinal stenosis
Multiple narrowed disk spaces
Diffuse idiopathic skeletal hyperostosis
Inflammatory spondyloarthropathies
Congenital kyphosis
Scoliosis (severe)

**Questionable Causes**

Spondylolisthesis (mild)
Scoliosis (mild to moderate)
Retrolisthesis of vertebral body
Lumbar scoliosis
Single-level disk space narrowing

represent minor self-limited injuries to the motion segments and adjacent structures. The pain of these acute injuries may be reproduced by injection of hypertonic saline into supraspinous, interspinous, and longitudinal ligaments; ligamenta flava; and the facet joint capsules.[89,90]

In about 1% of these cases, prolapse of the nucleus pulposus occurs with compression of neural elements, resulting in type C pain (sciatica). This injury most commonly occurs in the L4 to L5 or L5 to S1 motion segments in patients 20 to 50 years of age.[91]

## What Makes Back Pain Chronic?

Three months after an episode of acute low back pain, only about 5% of patients have persistent symptoms. A number of conditions are associated with chronic low back pain[91] (Table 25–8). Anatomic features common to many of these conditions are hypertrophic bony changes and disk degeneration. The bony changes may reduce the lumen of the spinal or nerve root canal and result in chronic compression of neural elements and pain.

When the disk degenerates, changes occur throughout the motion segment, any or all of which may result in pain. Load bearing of the facet joints is increased; distribution of stress concentration is altered in the endplates and in the subchondral bone of the vertebrae; and encroachment on the nerve root canal occurs. Finally, an increased demand is placed on intersegmental muscles and ligaments to stabilize the motion segments.[92]

The association between abnormal anatomy and pain is not entirely clear because these pathologic conditions, including disk degeneration and herniation, are found in many asymptomatic patients.[91] Ruiz and associates noted a higher incidence of the following findings in patients with mechanical lumbar pathology: degenerative facet joint disease with posterior capsule and lateral or capsular extension calcifications, lumbarized vertebra with lateral or capsular extension and upper attachment calcifications, and isthmic spondylolisthesis with lateral or capsular extension calcification.[93] In a significant proportion of patients with chronic low back pain, however, no anatomic pathology is demonstrable.

## What Are the Effects of Spinal Injury and Surgery on the Epidural Space?

The onset of epidural anesthesia is delayed in patients with back pain or sciatica, with the affected roots being blocked 10 to 70 minutes later than contralateral roots at the same level.[94] Central disk herniations also result in delayed onset of block distal to the level of the lesion. Delay in block onset likely results from the inability of local anesthetic to diffuse into the area of the injured root; contrast material placed during epidurograms fails to reach the nerve root in many patients with disk prolapse and does not move beyond the affected disk space in others.[55] The contrast material escapes the epidural space through the foramina below the affected level. Prolapse of the intervertebral disk thus may result in relative or total obstruction to local anesthetic flow within the epidural space. The unblocked area includes the affected segment but may also include all segments distal to the affected level in an ipsilateral or bilateral distribution. Either a double catheter technique or, more reliably, a subarachnoid injection of local anesthetic could be used to manage the unblocked segments.

## Is Regional Anesthesia Feasible After Spinal Surgery?

Some distinction should be made between the more limited decompressions (laminotomy, foraminotomy) and fusion undertaken in the lumbar area for disk disease and the more extensive fusion involving the thoracolumbar spine (Table 25–9). Not surprisingly, even with relatively minor surgery, the extent of the intervention correlates with the residual anatomic pathology. The development of degenerative spondylosis after successful operative decompression of the affected nerve root was prospectively evaluated in a comparative case series of 100 patients with a herniated lumbar nucleus pulposus.[95] At an average postoperative follow-up of 65 months, the incidence of a one-grade increase in degenerative spondylosis was 80% of the laminotomy and diskectomy patients as compared with 39% of the posterolateral diskectomy patients.

Patients with more limited spinal operations have been reported to have high rates (91.2%) of successful epidural anesthesia when the block was performed by experienced clinicians.[96] However, the success rate was lower than that experienced by the same clinicians in a population not previously subjected to back surgery (98.7%). The investigators attributed the increased rate of failures to the distortion of surface anatomy and the tethering of the dura to the ligamentum flavum by scar formation, rendering the epidural space discontinuous.

**TABLE 25–9.** Technical Considerations in Postsurgical Epidural Blocks

Reliable surface landmarks may be absent.
Epidural needle insertion may not be possible through the mass of osseous graft material.
False loss of resistance is common.
Degenerative changes occur in the spine below the lower level of the fusion at a greater rate in nonscoliotic patients. Both retrolisthesis and spondylolisthesis are increased.
The ligamentum flavum may be injured during surgery, resulting in adhesions in the epidural space and partial or total obliteration of the epidural space; this may interfere with local anesthetic spread.
Obliteration of the epidural space may make accidental dural puncture inevitable. It may not be possible to perform an epidural blood patch if postdural puncture headache results.

Support for this latter hypothesis of block failure was provided by LaRocca and Macnab's description of the laminectomy membrane.[97] After laminectomy, they noted the formation of an organized fibrous tissue surrounding the dura and, at times, binding the nerves to the posterior aspects of the disk and adjacent vertebral body. The fibrous response was proportional to the extent of the surgical trauma, being more marked with wider operative exposures. Peridural fibrosis extended beyond the laminectomy defect in the more extensive exposures, obliterating the epidural space at that level.

## Spinal Fusion

Lumbar epidural anesthesia has also been reported in patients who have undergone extensive spinal fusion for kyphoscoliosis or after traumatic spinal injury.[98–101] The major factor determining successful outcome appears to be the persistence of lumbar interspaces not involved in the fusion. When the fusion terminates in the upper lumbar spine, successful outcome is likely (Fig. 25–29). Some difficulties may be experienced, including multiple attempts before successful catheter placement, catheter-induced blood vessel trauma, difficulties defining the epidural space, and patchy or ineffective blocks.[98,100,101]

About 20% of fusion cases include L4 and below; in these patients, lower success rates are reported (Fig. 25–30). Hub-

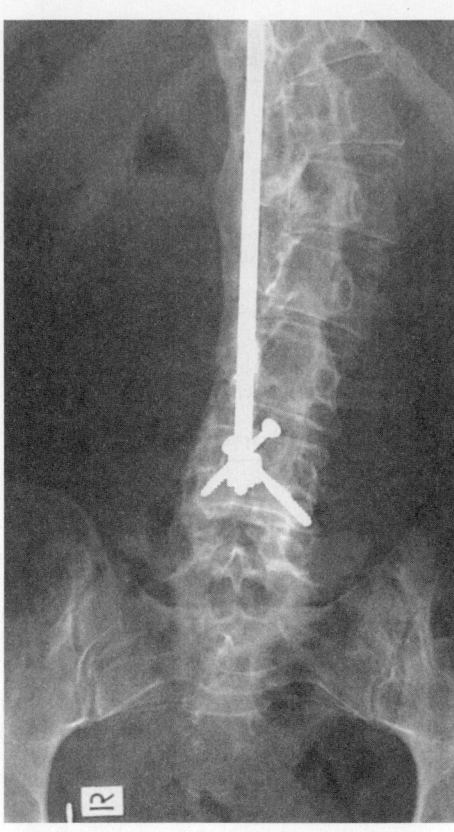

**FIGURE 25–30.** Spinal fusion for scoliosis. Anteroposterior view of the thoracolumbar junction and lumbar spine demonstrating fusion that involves the entire lumbar spine. There is rotation of the lumbar spinous processes into the concavity of the lateral curve, and the transverse processes are seen in the midline of the midlumbar vertebrae.

bert noted an 80% rate of successful epidural blockade in obstetric patients with fusion ending above L4 and sparing the lower lumbar interspaces but only a 41% success rate in patients with fusion involving the entire lumbar spine.[101]

## What Are the Etiologic Factors Implicated in Postoperative or Postpartum Backache?

### Postoperative Backache

Back pain after surgery had been reported to be unrelated to the type of anesthesia. Retrospective studies, however, have reported an increased incidence of postoperative backache in patients who received epidural or subarachnoid anesthesia compared with patients who had general anesthesia.[102,103] Hiller and colleagues randomly allocated 60 patients to receive spinal anesthesia with hyperbaric lidocaine or balanced general anesthesia with neuromuscular block.[104] Pain in the back, buttocks, or legs occurred more commonly in patients receiving spinal anesthesia (27%) compared with those provided general anesthesia (3%).

Transient postoperative backache occurred in 26% of patients receiving subarachnoid block (26-gauge needle) for knee arthroscopy but in only 4% of those who received general anesthesia.[102] The backaches were characterized as mild and lasted an average of 2 days. In 22% of patients, multiple attempts were required for dural puncture, a factor that may have had some influence on the incidence. Typically,

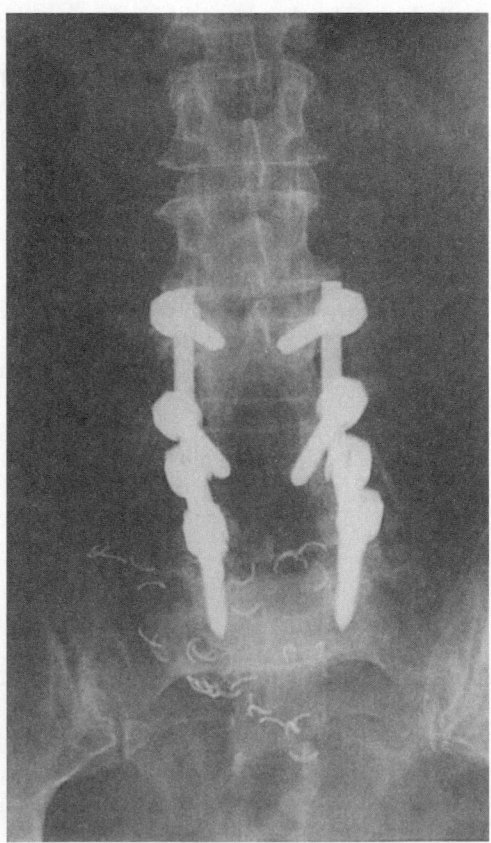

**FIGURE 25–29.** Decompression fusion of the lumbar spine. Anteroposterior view of the lumbar spine demonstrating decompression and fusion of the lumbar spine with bilateral rods held in place by screws placed in the vertebral bodies. The neural arch has been removed from the elements involved in the fusion. The patient has had successful subarachnoid anesthesia on two occasions, with the puncture being made in the space immediately above the fusion (L2-L3).

patients' satisfaction with the course of their anesthetics is not diminished by the occurrence of mild, transient backache.[102,103]

## Postpartum Backache

Postpartum backache (PPB) is a common complaint. MacArthur, citing data obtained from a postal survey of 11 701 women who had delivered 1 to 9 years previously, reported that PPB starting within 3 months of delivery and persisting for 6 weeks or longer occurred in 23% of women.[105,106] About 25% of these had experienced backache before delivery, but 14% reported new PPB. In many, the pain was persistent: 70% had had it for more than 2 years, and 65% had it at time of questioning 1 to 9 years later. Back pain was more common in women who delivered vaginally with labor epidural analgesia (18.9%) compared with those who did not have epidural analgesia (10.5%). Women who had epidural analgesia were also more likely to have had induced labor; abnormal presentations; multiple pregnancies; longer first stage; longer second stage; forceps deliveries; cesarean section; episiotomy; postpartum hemorrhage; and larger babies (height, weight, and head circumference). PPB, headache, neck ache, and tingling in the hands and fingers were commonly associated and considered to be an "epidural-associated symptom complex." MacLeod and colleagues also performed a postal survey of 2065 patients 1 year postpartum and found a 26.2% incidence of PPB in parturients who had epidural analgesia compared with 1.7% in those who did not.[107] The latter incidence of PPB is the lowest reported, by far, for any group of women in the first year postpartum.

A number of authors have carried out prospective evaluations to eliminate the potential for reporting bias confounding the retrospective surveys. Breen and associates carried out a 6-month prospective assessment of 1042 parturients.[108] Although 44% of women experienced PPB, there was no difference between those who had epidural anesthesia and those who did not. The most significant predictor of PPB was antenatal back pain. Weight gain was greater in patients with PPB and new-onset back pain. Groves and associates assessed the incidence of late (12-18 months) PPB in this same cohort of patients.[109] The incidence of late PPB was 49%, and there was no difference in the incidence in patients who had epidural analgesia (49%) and those who did not (50%). The incidence was greater in women who had reported early PPB (66%) than in those who did not (33%). The incidence of late-onset PPB, not present in the first 2 months postpartum, was 21%. Macarthur and colleagues also prospectively studied the association between epidural analgesia and early, new-onset PPB in 329 parturients.[110] In patients who labored without epidural analgesia, the incidence of PPB was 43% at 1 day, 23% at 7 days, and 7% at 6 weeks. The incidence of PPB in patients who had epidural analgesia was higher on the first postpartum day (53%), but this increase was not persistent. At 1 year postpartum, 12% had back pain—9.9% in the epidural analgesia group, and 13.8% in the nonepidural group. The numeric rating score for the intensity of back pain was the same in both groups.

Although both transient and more persistent PPBs are common, there is little evidence that they are related to the provision of epidural anesthesia for labor analgesia. Similarly, there is no evidence that denying a parturient epidural analgesia will result in a lower incidence of back troubles in the postpartum period. Factors that are associated with more persistent PPB include the presence of back pain before pregnancy, the presence of gestational backache, performance of physically heavy work, and multiparity.[111]

## Transient Radicular Irritation

Transient radicular irritation (TRI), also referred to as *transient neurologic symptoms,* is a relatively newly described symptom complex occurring most typically after subarachnoid anesthesia. It is defined as back pain, with radiation down one or both buttocks or legs occurring within 24 hours after surgery. It is most commonly seen after the use of hyperbaric lidocaine, with or without added epinephrine, and less commonly after bupivacaine, mepivacaine, and prilocaine.[112–115] The incidence of TRI is not affected by the concentration of hyperbaric lidocaine, being as common (16%) with the use of 2% solution as it is with the use of 5% solution.[112]

The duration of the symptom complex is short, with symptoms typically resolving over 24 to 48 hours. Thus, the timing of the follow-up may influence the incidence. A prospective, blinded, randomized study was conducted to compare the incidence of TRI after spinal anesthesia with that of hyperbaric lidocaine 5% or prilocaine 5% in 200 patients.[116] Three to 5 days after spinal anesthesia, all patients were interviewed by an anesthesiologist using a standardized symptom checklist. The incidence of TRI in both groups was low (4% in the lidocaine group and 1% in the prilocaine group), and differences were not found.

To evaluate the role of other factors such as the loss of strength of the supportive structures of the spine in the development of transient neurologic symptoms, Hiller and colleagues randomly allocated 60 patients to receive either spinal anesthesia with hyperbaric lidocaine or balanced general anesthesia with neuromuscular block.[104] Transient neurologic symptoms, consisting of pain in the buttocks or pain radiating symmetrically to the lower extremities, occurred more commonly in patients receiving spinal anesthesia (27%) than in those receiving general anesthesia (3%).[104]

Freedman and associates conducted a multicenter, prospective data collection to assess the role of multiple factors in TRI.[117] Patients given lidocaine were at higher risk for symptoms compared with those receiving bupivacaine (relative risk, 5.1; 95% CI, 2.5-10.2) or tetracaine (relative risk, 3.2; 95% CI, 1.04-9.84). For patients who received lidocaine, the relative risk for transient neurologic symptoms was 2.6 (95% CI, 1.5-4.5) with the lithotomy position compared with other positions; 3.6 (95% CI, 1.9-6.8) for outpatients compared with inpatients; and 1.6 (95% CI, 1-2.5) for obese (BMI >30) compared with nonobese patients.[117] Pollock and associates also reported that the incidence of TRI was greater in patients undergoing arthroscopy than in those undergoing hernia repair (13% versus 5%, respectively).[112]

These results indicate that transient neurologic symptoms commonly follow lidocaine spinal anesthesia but are relatively uncommon with bupivacaine or tetracaine. The data also identify the lithotomy position, arthroscopy, and outpatient status as important risk factors in patients who receive lidocaine. Both the lithotomy position and arthroscopy occur with the patient in a flexed-knee position, which appears to be a contributing factor. Among other factors postulated to increase risk, obesity had an effect of borderline statistical significance, whereas age, gender, history of back pain, needle type, and lidocaine dose and concentration have failed to affect risk.[117]

We inform patients regarding TRI when lidocaine is considered for subarachnoid anesthesia.

## THE SACRAL SPINE

### What Are the Relevant Anatomic Considerations?

The sacrum is a large triangular wedge-shaped bone, usually composed of five fused vertebrae. In some patients, the first sacral vertebra is not fused to the sacrum; this variant is termed *lumbarization. Sacralization* (fusion to the sacrum) of the fifth lumbar vertebra occurs in a similar proportion of the population. These conditions have been related to low back pain, although this association is disputed.[91] The spinous processes of the upper sacral vertebrae are fused to form the median sacral crest. This crest ends at the sacral hiatus as an upside down V and is covered by the thick, fibrous sacrococcygeal ligament. Using MRI, the sacrococcygeal membrane (SCM) could not be detected in 10.8% of patients.[118] The maximal depth (mean depth, 4.6 mm; range, 1-8 mm) of the caudal space adjacent to the SCM was beneath the upper third of the SCM in >90% of patients. The shortest linear distance from the dura to the upper limit of the SCM varied considerably (mean, 60.5 mm; range, 34-80 mm), as did the volume of the caudal space excluding the foramina and dural sac (mean, 14.4 mL; range, 9.5-26.6 mL).

### The Sacral Hiatus

The sacral cornua are found on either side of the hiatus and provide useful landmarks to identify it during the performance of a caudal block. The hiatus varies widely in size and shape, ranging from longitudinal to horizontal slits, and is absent in up to 7.7% of the population. The apex of the hiatus is usually below the lower third of S4 but can be higher; complete sacral spina bifida is found in about 1% of specimens.

The fused sacral transverse processes form the lateral sacral crest. They can form a sufficient bump to be confused with the sacral cornua, creating a "decoy" hiatus. Injection into a decoy hiatus covered by ligament is usually met with resistance.

### The Sacral Canal

The "dry" volume of the sacral canal is commonly quoted to be between 12 and 65 mL. Recent MRI studies of the canal filled with the dural sac and its contents (nerves, blood vessels, fat, and connective tissue) estimated the volume to be 9 to 27 mL in adult patients.[118] The variable volume of the sacral canal and the range in size and patency of the sacral foramina, which determine the amount of extravasation out of the sacral canal, make the volume of local anesthetic necessary for effective caudal analgesia unpredictable.

### How Likely Is Dural Puncture During Caudal Anesthesia?

The risk for dural puncture during a caudal block is very real because the distance between the bottom of the dural sac

and the top of the sacral hiatus can vary between 16 and 75 mm (average, 45 mm). In 5% of the population, the anteroposterior diameter of the sacral canal may be <2 mm, barely wide enough to admit a 21-gauge needle.

To increase the chances of performing a successful caudal block with minimal risk of dural puncture, the needle or cannula should enter the SCM in its upper third at 90°, followed by caudal depression through an angle of 55° to 60° and advancement along the canal no more than is necessary.[118] An absent hiatus and SCM should be considered if the block proves difficult or impossible to perform.

### Where Do Misplaced Injections Go?

The needle can be easily misplaced during attempts to perform caudal epidural block (Fig. 25–31). Lateral needle placement can result in injection into the S4 foramen. Subcutaneous injections occur, particularly in obese patients, in whom palpable landmarks may be difficult to appreciate. Injections into the presacral soft tissues are also possible, and injection into the fetal scalp has been reported during caudal blockade for labor analgesia.[119] Entry into the thin cortical

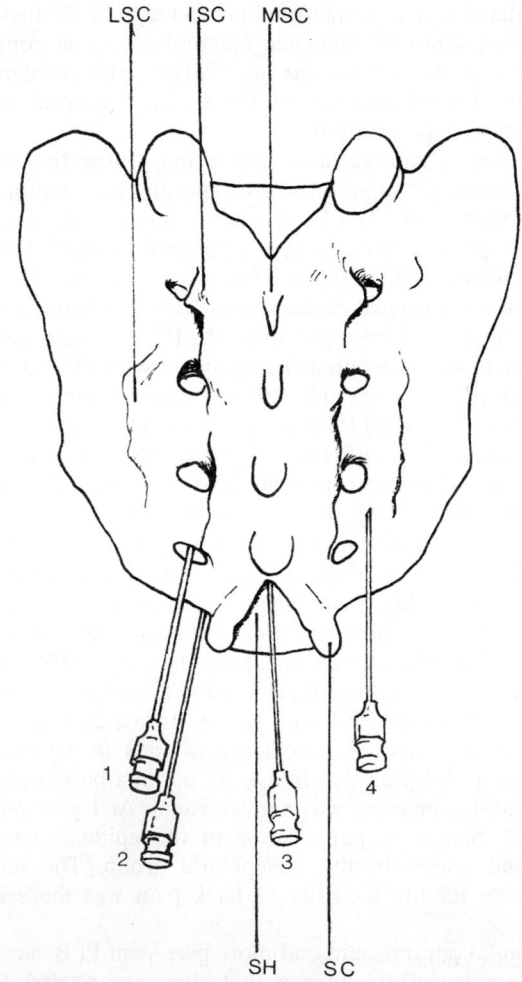

**FIGURE 25–31.** The sacrum and misplacements of attempted caudal blocks. 1, Entry into the S4 foramen. 2, Entry into the presacral area. 3, Correct needle placement for caudal block. 4, Entry into "decoy" hiatus. LSC, lateral sacral crest; ISC, intermediate sacral crest; MSC, median sacral crest; SH, sacral hiatus; SC, sacral cornua.

bone overlying the anterior wall of the sacral canal can have a similar feel to traversing the sacrococcygeal ligament but results in injection into the bone marrow.

## What Sacral Abnormalities Are Significant?

Sacral agenesis and congenital absence of the sacrum is rare and associated with maternal diabetes. Other anomalies in the remainder of the spine are often associated with the agenesis and include scoliosis, spina bifida, vertebral fusion, tethered cord, lipoma, dermoid cyst, and diastematomyelia. A low-lying tethered cord may be associated with a more caudal termination of the subarachnoid space. Sacral agenesis is also often associated with important anomalies of the digestive and genitourinary tracts as well as other musculoskeletal malformations.

Congenital lumbosacral spinal anomalies do not represent an absolute contraindication to epidural anesthesia. However, preoperative evaluation of the lumbosacral spine in order to delineate the anatomy and an awareness of the implications of these anomalies for major regional anesthesia are necessary to ensure safe performance.

## References

1. Hirabayashi Y, Shimizu R, Saitoh K, et al. Anatomical configuration of the spinal column in the supine position, I: a study using magnetic resonance imaging. *Br J Anaesth*. 1995;75:3.
2. Hirabayashi Y, Shimizu I, Fukuda H, et al. Anatomical configuration of the spinal column in the supine position, II: comparison of pregnant and non-pregnant women. *Br J Anaesth*. 1995;75:6.
3. Hogan QH. Lumbar epidural anatomy: a new look by cryomicrotome technology. *Anesthesiology*. 1991;75:767.
4. Hogan QH. Epidural anatomy examined by cryomicrotome section. Influence of age, vertebral level, and disease. *Reg Anesth*. 1996;21:395.
5. Blomberg RG. The lumbar subdural extraarachnoid space of humans: an anatomical study using spinaloscopy in autopsy cases. *Anesth Analg*. 1987;66:177.
6. Reynolds F, Speedy HM. The subdural space: the third place to go astray. *Anaesthesia*. 1990;45:120.
7. Lubenow T, Keh-Wong E, Kristof K, et al. Inadvertent subdural injection: a complication of an epidural block. *Anesth Analg*. 1988;67:175.
8. Morgan B. Unexpectedly extensive conduction blocks in obstetric epidural analgesia. *Anaesthesia*. 1990;45:148.
9. Hogan QH, Prost R, Kulier A, et al. Magnetic resonance imaging of fluid volume and the influence of body habitus and abdominal pressure. *Anesthesiology*. 1996;84:1341.
10. Carpenter RL, Hogan QH, Liu SS, et al. Lumbosacral cerebrospinal fluid volume is the primary determinant of sensory block extent and duration during spinal anesthesia. *Anesthesiology*. 1998;89:24.
11. Ekeløf NP, Jensen E, Poulsen J, et al. Weight gain during pregnancy does not influence the spread of spinal analgesia in the term parturient. *Acta Anaesth Scand*. 1997;41:884.
12. Fesmire FM, Luten RC. The pediatric cervical spine: developmental anatomy and clinical aspects. *J Emerg Med*. 1989;7:133.
13. Lee HC, Andree RA. Cervical spondylosis and difficult intubation. *Anesth Analg*. 1979;58:434.
14. Crosby ET, Grahovac S. Diffuse idiopathic skeletal hyperostosis: an unusual cause of difficult intubation. *Can J Anaesth*. 1993;40:54.
15. Mata S, Fortin PR, Fitzcharles MA, et al. A controlled study of diffuse idiopathic skeletal hyperostosis: clinical features and functional status. *Medicine (Baltimore)*. 1997;76:104.
16. Weinfeld RM, Olson PN, Maid DD, et al. The prevalence of diffuse idiopathic skeletal hyperostosis (DISH) in two large American Midwest metropolitan hospital populations. *Skeletal Radiol*. 1997;26:222.
17. Cammisa M, De Serio A, Guglielmi G. Diffuse idiopathic skeletal hyperostosis. *Eur J Radiol*. 1998;27(suppl 1):S7.
18. Forestier J, Lagier R. Ankylosing hyperostosis of the spine. *Clin Orthop*. 1971;74:65.
19. Mata S, Fortin PR, Fitzcharles MA, et al. A controlled study of diffuse

idiopathic skeletal hyperostosis: clinical features and functional status. *Medicine (Baltimore)*. 1997;76:104.
20. Babores M, Finnerty JP. Aspiration pneumonia secondary to giant cervical osteophyte formation (diffuse idiopathic skeletal hyperostosis or Forrestier's disease): a case report. *Chest*. 1998;14:1481.
21. Marks B, Schober E, Swoboda H. Diffuse idiopathic skeletal hyperostosis causing obstructing laryngeal edema. *Eur Arch Otorhinolaryngol*. 1998;25:256.
22. Lipson SJ. Dysplasia of the odontoid process in Morquio's syndrome causing quadriparesis. *J Bone Joint Surg Am*. 1977;59:340.
23. Herrick IA, Rhine EJ. The mucopolysaccharidoses and anaesthesia: a report of clinical experience. *Can J Anaesth*. 1988;35:67.
24. Pueschel SM, Scola FH. Atlantoaxial instability in individuals with Down's syndrome: epidemiologic, radiographic and clinical studies. *Pediatrics*. 1987;80:555.
25. Moore RA, McNicholas KW, Warran SP. Atlantoaxial subluxation with symptomatic spinal cord compression in a child with Down's syndrome. *Anesth Analg*. 1987;66:89.
26. Williams JP, Somerville GM, Miner ME, et al. Atlantoaxial subluxation and trisomy-21: another perioperative complication. *Anesthesiology*. 1987;67:253.
27. Pizzutillo PD. Klippel-Feil syndrome. In: Cervial Spine Research Society, Editorial Committee. *The Cervical Spine*. 2nd ed. Philadelphia, Pa: JB Lippincott; 1989:258.
28. Naguib M, Farag H, Ibrahim AEW. Anaesthetic considerations in Klippel-Feil syndrome. *Can Anaesth Soc J*. 1986;33:66.
29. Hobbs WR, Sponseller PD, Weiss Air, et al. The cervical spine in Marfan syndrome. *Spine*. 1997;22:983.
30. Halko GJ, Cobb R, Abeles M. Patients with type IV Ehlers-Danlos syndrome may be predisposed to atlantoaxial subluxation. *J Rheumatol*. 1995;22:152.
31. Jofe MH, White AA, Panjabi MM. Clinically relevant kinematics of the cervical spine. In: Cervical Spine Research Society, Editorial Committee. *The Cervical Spine*. 2nd ed. Philadelphia, Pa: JB Lippincott; 1989:57.
32. Nichol HC, Zuck D. Difficult laryngoscopy: the "anterior" larynx and the atlanto-occipital gap. *Br J Anaesth*. 1983;55:141.
33. Calder I, Calder J, Crockard HA. Difficult direct laryngoscopy in patients with cervical spine disease. *Anaesthesia*. 1995;50:756.
34. Bellhouse CP, Dore C. Criteria for estimating likelihood of difficulty of endotracheal intubation with the Macintosh laryngoscope. *Anaesth Intensive Care*. 1988;16:329.
35. Hayashi H, Okada K, Hamada M, et al. Etiologic factors of myelopathy: a radiographic evaluation of the aging changes in the cervical spine. *Clin Orthop*. 1987;214:200.
36. Komusi T, Munro T, Harth M. Radiologic review: the rheumatoid cervical spine. *Semin Arthritis Rheum*. 1985;14:187.
37. Grantham SA. Rheumatoid arthritis and other noninfectious inflammatory diseases: atlantoaxial instability. In: The Cervical Spine Research Society, Editorial Committee. *The Cervical Spine*. 2nd ed. Philadelphia, Pa: JB Lippincott; 1989:564.
38. Weissman BNW, Aliabadi P, Weinfeld MS, et al. Prognostic features of atlantoaxial subluxation in rheumatoid arthritis patients. *Radiology*. 1982;114:745.
39. Pellicci PM, Ranawat CS, Tsairis P, et al. A prospective study of the progression of rheumatoid arthritis of the cervical spine. *J Bone Joint Surg*. 1981;63A:342.
40. Keenan MA, Stiles CM, Kaufman RL. Acquired laryngeal deviation associated with cervical spine disease in erosive polyarticular arthritis. *Anesthesiology*. 1983;58:441.
41. Johnson RM, Wolf JW. Stability. In: Cervical Spine Research Society, Editorial Subcommittee. *The Cervical Spine*. 1st ed. Philadelphia, Pa: JB Lippincott; 1983:35.
42. Hensinger RN. Congenital anomalies of the atlantoaxial joint. In: Cervical Spine Research Society, Editorial Subcommittee. *The Cervical Spine*. 2nd ed. Philadelphia, Pa: JB Lippincott; 1989:236.
43. Steel HH. Anatomical and mechanical considerations of the atlantoaxial articulations. *J Bone Joint Surg*. 1968;50:14.
44. White AA, Southwick WO, Panjabi MM. Clinical instability in the lower cervical spine. *Spine*. 1976;1:15.
45. Aprahamian C, Thompson BM, Finger WA, et al. Experimental cervical spine injury model: examination of airway management and splinting techniques. *Ann Emerg Med*. 1984;13:584.
46. Majernick TG, Bieniek R, Houston JB, et al. Cervical spine movement during orotracheal intubation. *Ann Emerg Med*. 1986;15:417.
47. Bivins HG, Ford S, Bezmalinovic Z, et al. The effect of axial traction

during orotracheal intubation of the trauma victim with an unstable cervical spine. *Ann Emerg Med.* 1988;17:25.

48. Francois JM, Castagnera L, Carrat X, et al. Etude prospective des complications ORL de la chirurgie du rachis cervical par voie anterieure. *Rev Laryngol Otol Rhinol (Bord).* 1998;119:95.

49. Igarashi T, Hirabayashi Y, Shimizu K, et al. Thoracic and lumbar extradural structure examined by extraduroscope. *Br J Anaesth.* 1998;81:121.

50. Hirschfeld SS, Ruder C, Nasch CL, et al. The incidence of mitral valve prolapse in adolescent scoliosis and thoracic hypokyphosis. *Pediatrics.* 1982;40:451.

51. Sullivan PJ, Miller DR, Wynands JE. Cardiovascular manifestations of musculoskeletal diseases. In: Lui ACP, Crosby GT, eds. *Anesthesia and Musculoskeletal Disorders. Problems in Anesthesia.* Philadelphia, Pa: JB Lippincott; 1991;5:107.

52. Denis F. Spinal instability as defined by the three column spine concept in acute spinal trauma. *Clin Orthop.* 1984;189:65.

53. Westbrook JL, Renowden SA, Carrie LE. Study of the anatomy of the extradural region using magnetic resonance imaging. *Br J Anaesth.* 1993;71:495.

54. Husemeyer RP, White DC. Topography of the lumbar epidural space. *Anaesthesia.* 1980;35:7.

55. Luyendijk W, Van Voorthuisen AE. Contrast examination of the spinal epidural space. *Acta Radiol.* 1966;5:1051.

56. Savolaine ER, Pandya JB, Greenblatt SH, et al. Anatomy of the lumbar epidural space: new insights using CT-epidurography. *Anesthesiology.* 1988;68:217.

57. Boezaart AP. Computerized axial tomo-epidurographic and radiographic documentation of unilateral epidural analgesia. *Can J Anaesth.* 1989;36:697.

58. Hogan Q. Epidural catheter tip position and distribution of injectate evaluated by computed tomography. *Anesthesiology.* 1999;90:964.

59. Aavrahami E, Frishman E, Fridman Z, et al. Spina bifida occulta of S1 is not an innocent finding. *Spine.* 1994;19:12.

60. McGrady EM, Davis AG. Spina bifida occulta and epidural anaesthesia. *Anaesthesia.* 1988;43:867.

61. Cooper MG, Sethna NF. Epidural analgesia in patients with congenital lumbosacral spinal anomalies. *Anesthesiology.* 1991;75:370.

62. Vaagenes P, Fjaerestad I. Epidural block during labor in a patient with spina bifida cystica. *Anaesthesia.* 1981;36:299.

63. Evans RC, Tew B, Thomas MD, et al. Selective surgical management of neural tube malformations. *Arch Dis Child.* 1985;60:415.

64. Charney EB, Weller SC, Sutton LN, et al. Management of the newborn with myelomeningocele: time for the decision making process. *Pediatrics.* 1985;75:58.

65. Muller EB, Nordwall A. Prevalence of scoliosis in children with myelomeningocele. *Spine.* 1992;17:1097.

66. Page LK. Occult spinal dysraphism and related disorders. In: Wilkins RH. Rengachary SS, eds. *Neurosurgery.* New York, NY: McGraw-Hill; 1985:2053.

67. Rekate HL. Neurosurgical management of the child with spina bifida. In Rekate HL, ed. *Comprehensive Management of Spina Bifida.* Boca Raton, Fla: CRC Press; 1991:93.

68. James CCM, Lassman LP. Tight filum terminale and tethered cord syndromes. In: James CCM, Lassman LP, eds. *Spina Bifida Occulta.* London, United Kingdom: Academic Press; 1981:202.

69. Nuyten F, Gielen M. Spinal catheter anaesthesia in a patient with spina bifida. *Anaesthesia.* 1990;45:846.

70. Wood GG, Jacka MJ. Spinal hematoma following spinal anesthesia in a patient with spina bifida occulta. *Anesthesiology.* 1997;87:983.

71. Igarashi T, Hirabayashi Y, Shimizu R, et al. The lumbar extradural structure changes with increasing age. *Br J Anaesth.* 1997;78:149.

72. Saitoh K, Hirabayashi Y, Shimizu R, et al. Extensive extradural spread in the elderly may not relate to decreased leakage through intervertebral foramina. *Br J Anaesth.* 1995;75:688.

73. Crosby ET. Epidural catheter migration during labor: a hypothesis for inadequate analgesia. *Can J Anaesth.* 1990;37:789.

74. Palmer SK, Abram SE, Maitra AM, et al. Distance from the skin to the lumbar epidural space in an obstetric population. *Anesth Analg.* 1983;62:944.

75. Harrison GR, Clowes NWB. The depth of the lumbar space from the skin. *Anaesthesia.* 1985;40:685.

76. Narang VPS, Linter SPK. A failure of extradural blockade in obstetrics. *Br J Anaesth.* 1988;60:402.

77. Meiklejohn BH. Distance from skin to the epidural space in an obstetric population. *Reg Anesth.* 1990;15:134.

78. Hamza J, Smida M, Benhamou D, et al. Parturient's posture during epidural puncture affects the distance from skin to epidural space. *J Clin Anesth.* 1995;7:1.

79. Bosenberg AT, Gouws E. Skin-epidural distance in children. *Anaesthesia.* 1995;50:895.

80. Hasan MA, Howard RF, Lloyd-Thomas AR. Depth of epidural space in children. *Anesthesia.* 1994;49:1085.

81. Blomberg RG, Jaanivald A, Walther S. Advantages of the paramedian approach for lumbar epidural analgesia with catheter technique: a clinical comparison between midline and paramedian approaches. *Anaesthesia.* 1989;44:742.

82. Jaucot J. Paramedian approach of the peridural space in obstetrics. *Acta Anaesthesiol Belg.* 1986;37:187.

83. Griffin RM, Scott RPF. A comparison between the midline and paramedian approaches to the extradural space. *Anaesthesia.* 1984;39:584.

84. Davies MW, Ryan TDR. Current practice of epidural analgesia during normal labour: a survey of maternity units in the United Kingdom. *Anaesthesia.* 1993;48:63.

85. Ostgaard HC, Anderson GBJ, Karlsson K. Prevalence of back pain in pregnancy. *Spine.* 1991;16:549.

86. Rolbin SH, Hew E, Ogilvie G. A comparison of two types of epidural catheters. *Can J Anaesth.* 1987;34:459.

87. Verniquet AJW. Vessel puncture with epidural catheters. *Anaesthesia.* 1980;35:660.

88. O'Brien JP. Mechanisms of spinal pain. In: Wall PD, Melzack R, eds. *Textbook of Pain.* New York, NY: Churchill Livingstone; 1984:240.

89. McCall IW, Park WM, O'Brien JP. Induced pain referral from posterior lumbar elements in normal subjects. *Spine.* 1979;4:441.

90. Hirsch C, Ongelmark B-E, Miller M. The anatomical basis for low back pain: studies on the presence of sensory nerve endings in ligamentous, capsular and intervertebral disc structures in the human lumbar spine. *Acta Orthop Scand.* 1963;33:1.

91. Frymoyer JW. Back pain and sciatica. *N Engl J Med.* 1988;318:291.

92. White AA III, Panjabi MM. The clinical biomechanics of spine pain. In: White AA III, Panjabi MM, eds. *Clinical Biomechanics of the Spine.* 2nd ed. Philadelphia, Pa: JB Lippincott; 1990:379.

93. Ruiz SF, Alcazar RPP, Lopez ME, et al. Calcification of lumbar ligamentum flavum and facet joints capsule. *Spine.* 1997;22:1730.

94. Benzon HT, Braunschweig R, Molloy RE. Delayed onset of epidural anesthesia in patients with back pain. *Anesth Analg.* 1981;60:874.

95. Kambin P, Cohen LF, Brooks M, et al. Development of degenerative spondylosis of the lumbar spine after partial discectomy: comparison of laminotomy, discectomy, and posterolateral discectomy. *Spine.* 1995;20:599.

96. Sharrock ME, Urqhart B, Mineo R. Extradural anaesthesia in patients with previous lumbar spine surgery. *Br J Anaesth.* 1990;65:237.

97. LaRocca H, Macnab I. The laminectomy membrane: studies in its evolution, effects and prophylaxis in dogs. *J Bone Joint Surg.* 1974;56:545.

98. Crosby ET, Halpern SH. Obstetric epidural anaesthesia in patients with Harrington instrumentation. *Can J Anaesth.* 1989;36:693.

99. Feldstein G, Ramanathan S. Obstetrical lumbar epidural anesthesia in patients with previous posterior spinal fusion for kyphoscoliosis. *Anesth Analg.* 1985;64:83.

100. Daley MD, Morningstar BA, Rolbin SH, et al. Epidural anesthesia for obstetrics after spinal surgery. *Reg Anesth.* 1990;15:280.

101. Hubbert CH. Epidural anesthesia in patients with spinal fusion. *Anesth Analg.* 1985;64:843.

102. Dahl JB, Schultz P, Anker-Moller E, et al. Spinal anaesthesia in young patients using a 29-gauge needle: technical considerations and an evaluation of postoperative complaints compared with general anaesthesia. *Br J Anaesth.* 1990;64:178.

103. Sarma VJ, Lundstrom J. Epidural anaesthesia for day care surgery: a retrospective study. *Anaesthesia.* 1989;44:683.

104. Hiller A, Karjalainen K, Balk M, et al. Transient neurological symptoms after spinal anaesthesia with hyperbaric 5% lidocaine or general anaesthesia. *Br J Anaesth.* 1999;82:575.

105. MacArthur C, Lewis M, Crawford S. Epidural anaesthesia and longterm backache after childbirth. *BMJ.* 1990;301:9.

106. MacArthur C, Lewis M, Crawford S. Investigation of longterm problems after obstetric epidural anaesthesia. *BMJ.* 1992;304:1279.

107. MacLeod J, Macintyre C, McClure JH, et al. Backache and epidural analgesia: a retrospective survey of mothers 1 year after childbirth. *Int J Obstet Anesth.* 1995;4:21.

108. Breen TW, Ransil BJ, Groves PA, et al. Factors associated with back pain after childbirth. *Anesthesiology.* 1994;81:29.

109. Groves PA, Breen TW, Ransil BJ, et al. The natural history of postpar-

tum back pain and its relationship with epidural anesthesia. *Anesthesiology*. 1994;81:A1167.

110. Macarthur A, Macarthur C, Weeks S. Epidural anaesthesia and low back pain after delivery: a prospective cohort study. *BMJ*. 1995;311:1336.

111. Ostgaard HC, Andersson GBJ. Postpartum low-back pain. *Spine*. 1992;17:53.

112. Pollock JE, Neal JM, Stephenson CA, et al. Prospective study of the incidence of transient radicular irritation in patients undergoing spinal anesthesia. *Anesthesiology*. 1996;84:1361.

113. Hampl KF, Heinzmann-Wiedmer S, Luginbuehl I, et al. Transient neurologic symptoms after spinal anesthesia: a lower incidence with prilocaine and bupivacaine than with lidocaine. *Anesthesiology*. 1998;88.629.

114. Liguori GA, Zayas VM, Chisholm MF. Transient neurologic symptoms after spinal anesthesia with mepivacaine and lidocaine. *Anesthesiology*. 1998;88:619.

115. Salmela L, Aromaa U. Transient radicular irritation after spinal anesthesia induced with hyperbaric solutions of cerebrospinal fluid-diluted lidocaine 50 mg/ml or mepivacaine 40 mg/ml or bupivacaine 5 mg/ml. *Acta Anaesthesiol Scand*. 1998;42:765.

116. Martinez-Bourio R, Arzuaga M, Quintana JM, et al. Incidence of transient neurologic symptoms after hyperbaric subarachnoid anesthesia with 5% lidocaine and 5% prilocaine. *Anesthesiology*. 1998;88:624.

117. Freedman JM, Li D, Drasner K, et al. Transient neurologic symptoms after spinal anesthesia. An epidemiologic study of 1,863 patients. *Anesthesiology*. 1998;89:633.

118. Crighton IM, Barry BP, Hobbs GJ. A study of the anatomy of the caudal space using magnetic resonance imaging. *Br J Anaesth*. 1997;78:391.

119. Finster M, Poppers PJ, Sinclair JC, et al. Accidental intoxication of the fetus with local anesthetic drug during caudal anesthesia. *Am J Obstet Gynecol*. 1965;92:922.

CHAPTER

# 26

# Autonomic Nervous System and Sympathetic Blockade

Thomas J. Ebert

Robert E. Kettler

## ANATOMIC AND FUNCTIONAL CHARACTERISTICS

*What Factors Distinguish the Autonomic and Somatic Nervous Systems?*

*How Is Sympathetic Control Regulated?*

## SYMPATHETIC BLOCKADE

*What Are the Indications?*

*What Agents and Techniques Are Applicable?*

*What Preparation Is Needed?*

*How Is a Block Evaluated?*

*What Should You Know About Paravertebral Block?*

*What Should You Know About Ganglionic Block?*

*How Are Sympathetic Blocks Performed?*

*What Does Radiologic Assistance Contribute?*

*Can Peripheral Nerve or Neuraxial Block Techniques Be Used to Achieve Sympathetic Blockade?*

*What Are the Complications?*

*How Are These Complications Managed?*

## AUTONOMIC DYSFUNCTION: DYSREFLEXIA

*What Patients Are at Risk?*

*Why Does It Occur?*

*What Are the Stimuli, Signs, and Symptoms?*

*Who Needs Preventive Treatment?*

*What Therapeutic Modalities Are Useful?*

*What Special Considerations Apply to the Quadriplegic Parturient?*

The autonomic nervous system (ANS) consists of a network of neural connections that maintains body homeostasis by regulating tissue and organ function. Autonomic outflow arises in the medullary vasomotor centers and is modulated by ascending input from peripheral sensors and by descending signals from higher brain centers. The ANS is segmental and, to some degree, parallels the somatic distribution to skeletal muscle. Sympathetic control is from thoracolumbar segments,

and parasympathetic control is from the cranial and sacral segments (Fig. 26–1). The ANS is primarily an effector system that is tonically active and maintains visceral organs in a state of intermediate function. This activity permits central control and peripheral reflex mechanisms to augment or diminish autonomic outflow in order to adjust blood flow and visceral organ function in response to environmental changes.

## ANATOMIC AND FUNCTIONAL CHARACTERISTICS

### *What Factors Distinguish the Autonomic and Somatic Nervous Systems?*

#### Function and Organization

The ANS is sometimes referred to as the *visceral* motor system, in contrast to the *somatic* motor system. Two characteristics distinguish it from the somatic nervous system. First, the ANS essentially is under involuntary control. Second, the majority of somatic motor neurons are located within the central nervous system (CNS), and their efferent pathway to skeletal muscle is monosynaptic. In contrast, all autonomic motor neurons are peripherally located within ganglia that lie outside the CNS (*postganglionic neurons*). Preganglionic neurons that originate in the brainstem and the spinal cord synapse with these peripheral ganglia and activate postganglionic neural fibers. Thus, the ANS is a disynaptic system.

#### Nerves

The autonomic nerves are composed of small myelinated and unmyelinated fibers. Preganglionic B fibers are generally myelinated, have diameters of less than 3 μm, and conduct impulses at a speed of 2 to 14 m/s. Postganglionic C fibers are largely unmyelinated, have a diameter that ranges from 0.3 to 1.3 μm, and conduct impulses at less than 2 m/s.

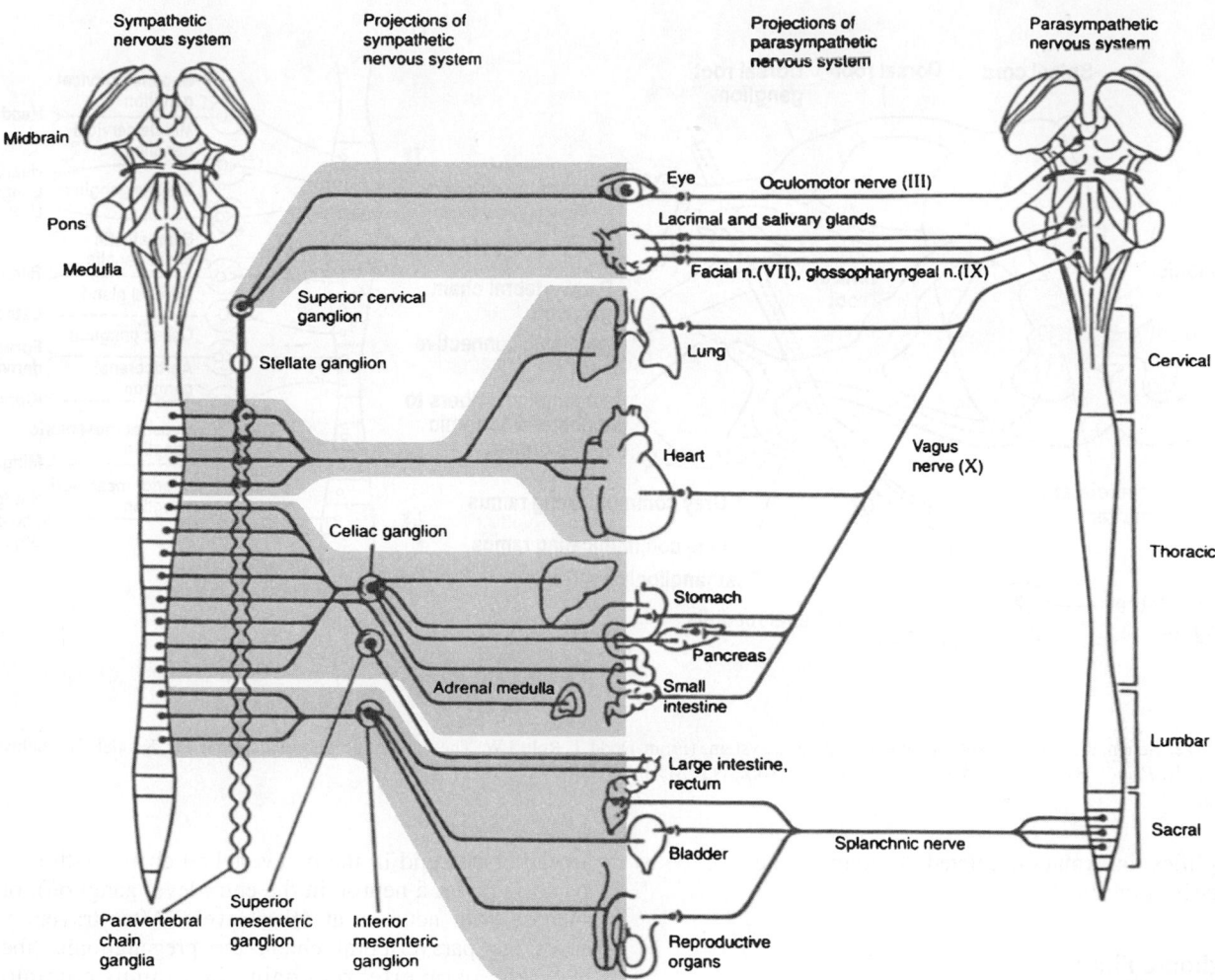

**FIGURE 26–1.** Sympathetic and parasympathetic divisions of the autonomic nervous system. Preganglionic neurons of the sympathetic division extend from the first thoracic spinal segment to lower lumbar segments. Parasympathetic ganglionic neurons are located within the brainstem and from segments S2 to S4 of the spinal cord. This figure also illustrates the coordinate innervation of a subset of targets by these two divisions of the autonomic nervous system. (From Dodd J, Role LW. The autonomic nervous system. In: Kandel ER, Schwartz JH, Jessell TM, eds. *Principles in Neural Science.* 3rd ed. New York, NY: McGraw-Hill; 1991:763.)

## Sympathetic

The sympathetic divisions of the ANS consist of preganglionic fibers that exit the spinal cord from the first thoracic to the third lumbar vertebral levels. Most of these fibers make synaptic connections in the lateral sympathetic chain, but some extend to peripheral ganglia before synapsing. In addition, preganglionic fibers make direct connections with the adrenal medulla (Figs. 26–1 and 26–2).

## Parasympathetic

In the parasympathetic system, preganglionic fibers terminate in ganglia close to or within specific organs. Short postganglionic fibers extend into the organ tissue. No interconnections are present between the cranial and sacral components. Furthermore, the parasympathetic system innervates only selected smooth muscle tissue, and visceral organs (see Fig. 26–1).

## Enteric

A third division is the enteric system, which is composed of local sensory neurons that respond to alterations in the tension and chemical environment of gut walls in order to regulate gastrointestinal, pancreatic, and gallbladder activity. The enteric system can function autonomously, although its activity normally is regulated by CNS reflexes.

## Activity

The sympathetic nervous system (SNS) is the "fight or flight" division, whereas the parasympathetic system functions to "rest and digest." Activation of the SNS under stress (eg, in the presence of blood loss, temperature change, or exercise) increases sympathetic neural activity to the heart and other viscera, peripheral vasculature, sweat glands, ocular muscles, and piloerector muscles. The results are increases in cardiac output, blood glucose, pupillary dilation, and body temperature. In contrast, activation of the parasympathetic system slows heart rate, respiration, and metabolism while increasing digestion and gastrointestinal motility.

## How Is Sympathetic Control Regulated?

A useful principle to facilitate an understanding of the pertinent neuroanatomy of the SNS is that it disseminates

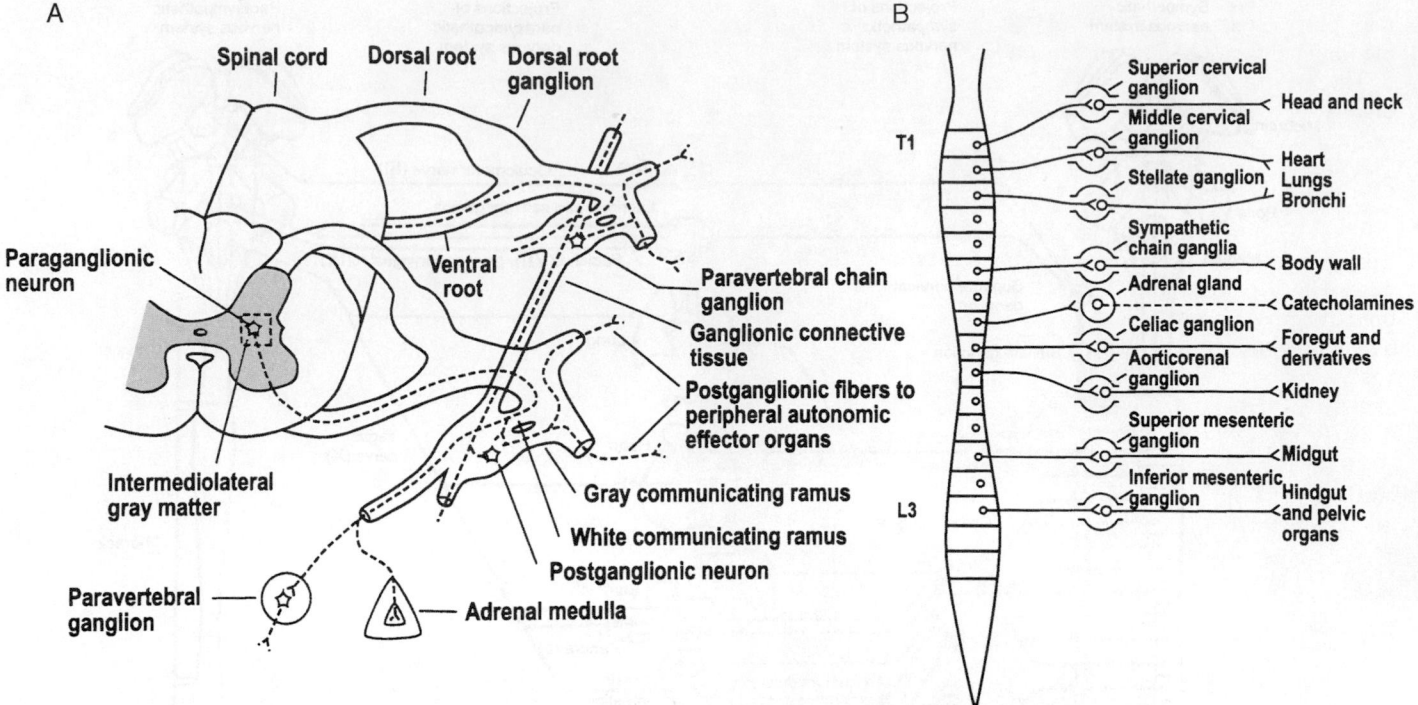

**FIGURE 26–2.** Schematic representation of the sympathetic system. (From Dodd J, Role LW. The autonomic nervous system. In: Kandel ER, Schwartz JH, Jessell TM, eds. *Principles in Neural Science*. 3rd ed. New York, NY: McGraw-Hill; 1991:764.)

and amplifies information related to maintenance of body homeostasis (Fig. 26–3).[1–3]

## Preganglionic Fibers

The preganglionic sympathetic neurons lie in the intermediolateral cell columns of the spinal cord gray matter, extending from T1 to L2. Axons of the sympathetic neurons are small and myelinated. They leave the spinal cord in the ventral spinal roots along with somatic alpha motor neurons and gamma motor neurons; they then branch off into the white (myelinated) rami communicantes and enter the paravertebral ganglia.

The preganglionic fiber can synapse with one or more sympathetic neurons in the ganglion that it has entered; it can

ascend or descend in the paravertebral chain (with or without synapsing with a neuron in the entry level ganglion); or it can synapse with neurons at other levels. After traveling up or down the paravertebral chain, the preganglionic fiber may leave the paravertebral chain via a ramus communicans griseus. It can then join a somatic nerve and travel to an effector site (eg, the blood vessels), synapse with an intermediate ganglion cell, or synapse with a prevertebral ganglion cell.

Although *preganglionic fibers* are present in the various sympathetic ganglia and, in fact, sometimes exit from them, they are so named because they have not yet synapsed with a ganglion cell. Likewise, *postganglionic fibers* are so named because they are the terminal fibers of a ganglion cell and synapse with the appropriate end organ.

### Sympathetic Ganglia

There are four types of sympathetic ganglia: paravertebral, prevertebral, intermediate, and terminal (see Fig. 26–2).

The paravertebral ganglia are arranged in a bilateral vertical chain running the length of the spinal column and located on the anterolateral aspect of the vertebral bodies. Some examples of paravertebral ganglia are the superior and middle cervical ganglia, the stellate ganglion (*cervicothoracic ganglion*), and the lumbar sympathetic chain (see Fig. 26–2B).

Prevertebral ganglia are composed of a network of preganglionic and postganglionic sympathetic fibers, parasympathetic fibers, and ganglion cell bodies. Those of most significance to an anesthesiologist performing nerve blocks are the celiac and superior hypogastric ganglia (see Fig. 26–2B).

The intermediate ganglia are small structures, occasionally microscopic, that are located near the paravertebral chain. Their significance for the anesthesiologist is unclear, but they

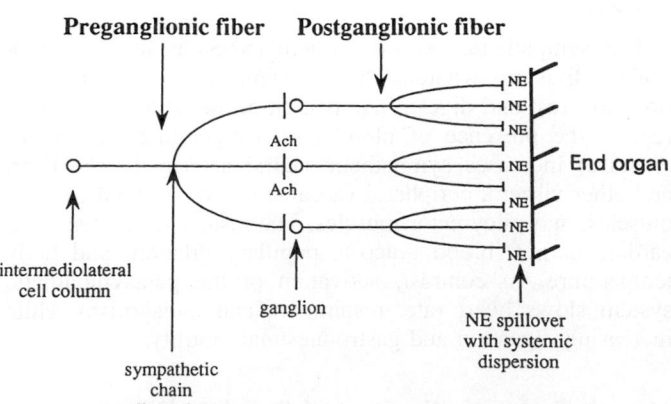

**FIGURE 26–3.** Schematic drawing of the organization of the sympathetic nervous system that results in dispersion and amplification of efferent signals. Ach, acetylcholine; NE, norepinephrine.

may play a role in surgical sympathectomies that result in an incomplete physiologic sympathectomy.

The terminal ganglia lie in close proximity to their end organs (eg, the urinary bladder and the rectum).

### Postganglionic Fibers

The postganglionic sympathetic fibers are not myelinated. Like preganglionic fibers, one postganglionic fiber can synapse with a number of effector cells; however, a postganglionic fiber synapses with only one type of end organ. For example, one postganglionic fiber might synapse with several vascular smooth muscle cells but would not simultaneously synapse with a sweat gland and a piloerector muscle. The important end organs include the eye, the secretory structures (including the sweat glands), the heart, the blood vessels, the adrenal medulla, the abdominal and pelvic viscera, and the piloerector muscles.

### Dispersion and Amplification With Regionalization

Historically, activation of the SNS has been considered a "mass reflex" or response. Current understanding is that there is selectivity of a sympathetic response, although the site of differentiation or regulation of the selectivity is not known.

One clear example of the selectivity of the SNS response can be observed in the neural activity recorded from the skin compared with the muscle sympathetic nerves in human beings. The efferent sympathetic nerves to blood vessels, sweat glands, and piloerector muscles in the skin are generally silent during quiet resting conditions and during blood pressure (BP) perturbations, but these nerves are activated when a sudden noise is imposed or an embarrassing question is asked. In contrast, the efferent sympathetic nerves that supply skeletal muscle blood vessels show significant tonic activity that is inversely modified by changes in BP via the baroreflex. This sympathetic activity is not altered by startle maneuvers.

Despite this regional selectivity, the SNS has evolved so that its efferent outflow is amplified by dispersion. This process is accomplished by preganglionic and postganglionic fibers that synapse with multiple effector cells. With a burst of sympathetic activity, the release of the postganglionic neurotransmitter norepinephrine may exceed the capacity of the local uptake system and enzymatic breakdown that terminates its action. This excess (or overflow) norepinephrine can be dispersed by the circulatory system and result in widespread effects (see Fig. 26–3).

## SYMPATHETIC BLOCKADE

### What Are the Indications?

Sympathetic blockade can benefit surgical anesthesia through its vasodilating effects or its ability to reduce postoperative sympathetically induced pain.[4–6] However, some practitioners believe that sympathetic blockade is not beneficial and suggest that anesthetic and surgical outcome may actually be worsened when it is used.[7,8] Their discussions usually focus on the beneficial or harmful effects of the resultant hypotension. However, hypotension from a sympathetic block can be significantly reduced with the use of selective techniques.

Sympathetic blockade also has been recommended for the treatment of sympathetically maintained pain,[9] acute herpes zoster (*shingles*),[10] vascular insufficiency,[11] neuropathic pain,[12] and a number of miscellaneous conditions.[13–17] Celiac plexus blockade has been used in the management of pain due to upper abdominal malignancy[18] and chronic pancreatitis.[19] Likewise, superior hypogastric plexus blockade has been suggested for pain from pelvic malignancy.[20]

Much of the rationale for sympathetic blockade has resulted from extrapolation of what is known of the neurophysiology of the SNS. However, many practitioners question the benefit of blocks carried out for traditional indications, partly because of a lack of randomized clinical trials establishing the efficacy and effectiveness of these techniques in pain management as well as in surgical anesthesia.[21–24] Despite the lack of convincing clinical studies, many of the blocks have become a traditional component of the solution for various pain management problems (Table 26–1).[21–24]

### What Agents and Techniques Are Applicable?

#### Parenteral Drugs

Blockade of the ANS can be performed with parenteral agents that block the parasympathetic muscarinic receptor (eg, atropine); that inhibit sympathetic outflow by central mechanisms (eg, clonidine); or that inhibit sympathetic end-organ responses (eg, α- and β-blockers). In addition, sympathetic ganglia can be blocked with intravenous agents such as hexamethonium.

#### Regional Block

Regional anesthetic techniques that use local anesthetics and neurolytic agents can also be employed. Central neuraxial anesthetic techniques, such as spinal or epidural anesthesia, provide sympathetic block of the preganglionic fibers; these techniques and their pertinent anatomy are discussed in Chapter 29. Note, however, that epidural anesthesia commonly results in incomplete block of the sympathetic nerves.

Selective regional sympathetic blockade can also be performed by injecting pharmacologic agents in proximity to the paravertebral and prevertebral ganglia. Such techniques provide a postganglionic block. Finally, intravenous regional

**TABLE 26–1.** Indications for Sympathetic Blocks

**Vasodilation**

Vascular surgery
Replantation surgery
Rest pain of lower extremities
Intra-arterial injection of caustic substances (eg, thiopental)

**Pain Management**

Sympathetically maintained pain
Shingles
Neuropathic pain
Intractable visceral pain

**Prognostic**

Before surgical sympathectomy

approaches have been used to perform sympathetic blocks at an end-organ level.

## Local Agents

Lidocaine (1%-2%), bupivacaine (0.25%-0.5%), and chloroprocaine (2%-3%) are frequently used. Bretylium, reserpine, and guanethidine have been used for intravenous regional anesthesia to interrupt synaptic nerve function. With many sympathetic blocks, the duration of local anesthetic action is not important; rather, the goal is to perform a series of blocks in an effort to achieve progressive improvement in pain through transient interruptions of SNS activity.

## Neurolytic Drugs

Various neurolytic agents have been used to provide long-lasting sympathetic block; the most common are ethanol and phenol. Both agents work by disruption of myelin and precipitation of protein elements. They do not always provide a permanent block because neural fibers can regenerate; however, if the neural cell bodies in the ganglion are destroyed, permanent loss of neural function can be achieved. In patients who are not expected to survive more than 6 to 12 months, these blocks may be effectively permanent because the patient will not survive long enough for neural regeneration to occur.

Controversy exists regarding the exact role of neurolytic agents in sympathetically mediated pain. However, a neurolytic celiac plexus block for treatment of pain secondary to upper abdominal malignancy is accepted therapy; the patient's life expectancy is often less than the time required for neural regrowth. The techniques of neurolytic blockade and the pharmacology of ethanol, phenol, and other neurolytic agents are covered in a number of pain management texts.[25-27]

## What Preparation Is Needed?

The practitioner must assess each situation in terms of the patient's general condition, the expected ease of intravenous catheter placement, and the likelihood of a complication. Preparation for a sympathetic block can be largely inferred from the information contained in the discussion of complications. The operating room table provides a useful surface for performing the block because it can be used to place the patient in the Trendelenburg position and provides a firm surface for cardiopulmonary resuscitation, if needed. Suction equipment to clear an obstructed airway, an apparatus to provide oxygen and positive-pressure ventilation, and an assortment of airway equipment (eg, laryngoscopes, endotracheal tubes, and pharyngeal airways) must be immediately available.

In addition to monitoring equipment for assessment of the block, an electrocardiograph and sphygmomanometer are commonly employed. Intravenous access should be available to administer anxiolytic agents and emergency drugs, even though specific recommendations to this effect are absent in the literature. Resuscitative drugs include thiopental sodium, benzodiazepines, succinylcholine, epinephrine, atropine, lidocaine, bretylium, and amiodarone.

## How Is a Block Evaluated?

The success of a block is assessed similarly in most procedures: symptoms are elicited, a physical examination is performed, and data from special studies are evaluated. For example, after stellate ganglion block, the patient can be queried about nasal congestion, a warm sensation in the extremity, or relief of pain. Signs of Horner syndrome or increased temperature of the extremity can be noted. Postblock change in the patient's pain is commonly evaluated with a visual analogue pain scale.[28] Pain relief alone is not an indicator of sympathetic blockade but is an important part of the assessment. A number of special studies can be performed.[29]

### Physical Characteristics

The obvious findings present on physical examination can be predicted based on one's knowledge of ANS anatomy. Several end organs have special significance.

#### Skin

A careful skin examination should reveal that the skin has become smooth and dry because of piloerector muscle and sweat gland inactivation.

#### Vascular Bed

Venous dilation may be obvious because of anesthetic denervation of the venular smooth muscle. This sign may be present even when the arteriolar system is too diseased to respond to sympathetic blockade (eg, in patients with peripheral vascular disease). When arteriolar dilation is present, the pressure at the arteriolar side of the capillary circulation is decreased; with simultaneous venous dilation and facilitated drainage, the pressure on the venous side is reduced. This combination results in increased blood flow to the capillary bed, which is apparent as a rapid filling (relative to baseline) time after blanching beneath a fingernail.

#### Horner Syndrome

Probably the most striking set of physical findings are those of Horner syndrome produced by a stellate ganglion block. The classic triad consists of ptosis, miosis, and anhidrosis. These are apparent on the side of the face ipsilateral to the block.

#### Temperature

Following a sympathetic block, the volume of blood in the capillaries increases, bringing skin surface temperature closer to core body temperature. This increase in temperature can be measured by placement of a temperature probe on the skin in the anatomic distribution of the block. Bilateral temperature probes can be used to compare the blocked and unblocked sides.

#### Plethysmographic Waveforms

The waveform obtained from a photoplethysmograph can also be used to evaluate a successful sympathetic block. In its simplest application, a pulse oximeter is placed on a digit of the extremity to be blocked. Because most pulse oximeters incorporate an automatic gain control to create a prominent waveform, unless the gain setting can be fixed, this approach can be misleading.[30] A control pulse tracing should be com-

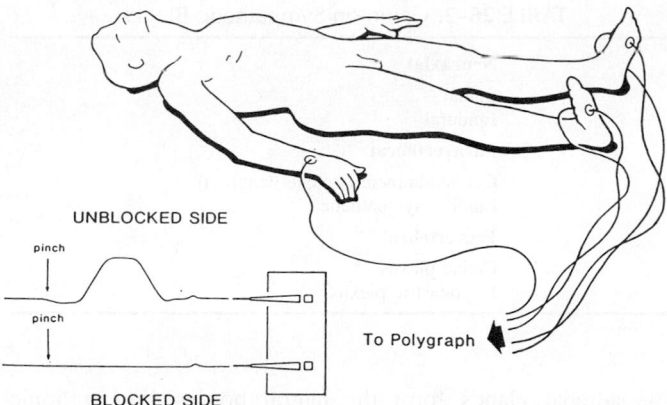

**FIGURE 26–4.** Sympathogalvanic response. Electrodes are placed on the front and back of hands or feet, and a ground electrode is placed elsewhere on the body. Changes in baseline level on an electrocardiographic recorder indicate changes in sweat gland activity. (From Lofstrom JB, Cousins MJ. Sympathetic neural blockade of upper and lower extremity. In: Cousins MJ, Bridenbaugh PO, eds. *Neural Blockade in Clinical Anesthesia and Management of Pain.* 2nd ed. Philadelphia, Pa: JB Lippincott; 1988:475.)

pared with the postblock tracing. A successful sympathetic block results in an increase of amplitude and area beneath the pulse waveform.

Successful blockade also can be evaluated by a cold pressor test (typically the immersion of an unblocked extremity in ice water for 60 seconds). This preblock maneuver causes a reduction in the pulse amplitude. When a sympathetic block has been successfully performed, the waveform, which has increased in size owing to the block, should not change during the cold stimulus.

### Sympathogalvanic Reflex

In patients with severe peripheral vascular disease, the aforementioned tests may not be positive despite the presence of successful blockade. In this situation, the sympathogalvanic reflex is useful. A 2-lead electrocardiographic monitoring system is employed. The positive and negative leads are placed on the patient's skin in the area to be blocked; a ground electrode is placed elsewhere. The waveform displayed is a representation of cutaneous electrical current.

When sympathetic activity to the skin increases (eg, in response to a noxious stimulus, such as loud noise, skin pinch, or startle response), a positive deflection of the waveform occurs in response to the increased sympathetic discharge. After a successful sympathetic block, the increase in cutaneous conductance during a noxious stimulus is absent, and the waveform deflection is not apparent (Fig. 26–4).

### Sweat Tests

Finally, tests of sweat gland function can assess sympathetic activity. In the triketohydrindene hydrate (Ninhydrin), cobalt blue, and starch iodide tests, color changes in specific dyes occur with increased skin surface moisture (sweat). A successful block eliminates sweating in the affected areas. These tests are used infrequently because they are less convenient and are messy compared with those previously mentioned.

### Critique

The utility of any of the tests mentioned, including the subjective sensation of pain relief, has proponents and critics.

Individual tests and combinations of tests have been used in numerous studies of sympathetic blockade.[17,31–34] However, none of the commonly used methods to evaluate end-organ function has been rigorously studied for utility (specificity and sensitivity). A thorough evaluation of these tests should include the variability inherent in each, the variability of results in normal subjects, the establishment of a gold standard with which the tests can be compared, and determination of each test's diagnostic discrimination.[35,36] Perhaps the best approach is to combine physical assessment, a practical test for the given clinical setting, and a therapeutic goal.[37]

## What Should You Know About Paravertebral Block?

### Anatomic Features

Stellate ganglion and lumbar sympathetic blocks are performed fairly frequently. The thoracic sympathetic chain is less commonly blocked. In the neck, the paravertebral ganglia lie against the vertebral transverse processes; they are more anterior in the thorax, lying in front of the heads of the rib insertions. The lumbar paravertebral chain lies along the anterolateral aspect of the lumbar vertebral bodies. In the pelvis, the sympathetic chains are anterior to the sacrum and terminate as a single ganglion located anterior to the coccyx (Fig. 26–5).

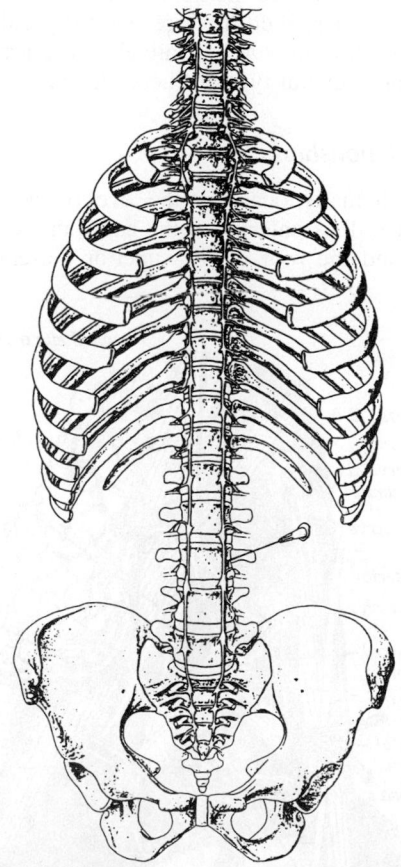

**FIGURE 26–5.** Anatomic location of the thoracic sympathetic ganglia increases the likelihood of a pneumothorax when a block in this region is attempted. The lumbar sympathetic chain is more easily accessed and with fewer complications. (From Scott DB. *Techniques of Regional Anaesthesia.* Norwalk, Conn: Appleton & Lange; 1989:205.)

## Potential Complications

The location of the thoracic sympathetic ganglia means that a pneumothorax is a potential complication of an attempt to block this portion of the paravertebral chain. A thoracic epidural or intercostal nerve block is an alternative, although each technique has potential complications as well.

The paravertebral chain in the neck also lies in close proximity to a number of structures that, when pierced, can give rise to complications. These include the dural sleeves that invest the cervical nerve roots, the vertebral artery, and the dome of the pleura. Other nearby structures are the phrenic and vagus nerves, carotid artery, jugular vein, esophagus, trachea, and cervical discs. Lumbar sympathetic chains are also close to structures of importance, including the kidneys, lumbar nerve roots and their dural sleeves, genitofemoral nerves, and major blood vessels (Figs. 26–6 and 26–7).

Despite the potential for complications owing to needle puncture or injection of local anesthetics into nearby structures along the paravertebral chain, the cervical and lumbar portions of the chain are more safely approached and thus more frequently blocked than are the thoracic elements (Table 26–2).

## What Should You Know About Ganglionic Block?

### Celiac Plexus

Celiac plexus blocks are the most common of the prevertebral blocks. These procedures are typically called *plexus blocks* because they involve a relatively large area that contains ganglia and several types of nerve fibers.

### Anatomic Relationships

The celiac plexus is located at the level of the T12 and L1 vertebral bodies. It is anterior to the aorta and surrounds the celiac artery and the root of the superior mesenteric artery.

**TABLE 26–2.** Common Sympathetic Blocks

| |
|---|
| **Neuraxial** |
| Spinal |
| Epidural |
| **Paravertebral** |
| Cervicothoracic (stellate ganglion) |
| Lumbar sympathetic |
| **Prevertebral** |
| Celiac plexus |
| Hypogastric plexus |

The adrenal glands form the lateral border. Preganglionic fibers penetrate the crura of the diaphragm and synapse in the plexus. The greater splanchnic nerve (T5-10), the lesser splanchnic nerve (T9-11), and the least splanchnic nerve (T12) are the preganglionic nerves that join with branches of the vagus and phrenic nerves and with postganglionic fibers to form the neural network of the plexus. Also contained in the plexus are the celiac ganglia and the aorticorenal ganglia.

Interestingly, the target of a local anesthetic or neurolytic block of the celiac plexus is the visceral afferent fibers, which carry nociceptive information from the abdominal viscera. These fibers do not synapse in the preaortic ganglia and, in fact, are not part of the SNS. They are like other primary nociceptive afferents in that their cell bodies are in the dorsal root ganglion, and they synapse in the dorsal horn of the spinal cord gray matter.

### Superior Hypogastric Plexus

The superior hypogastric plexus is located in a more caudal direction by several lumbar levels.[26] It is composed of branches of the aortic plexus, the third and fourth lumbar splanchnic nerves, and the superior hypogastric ganglia. The plexus is anterior to the aortic bifurcation, from the body of L5 to the sacral promontory, and between the iliac arteries. It

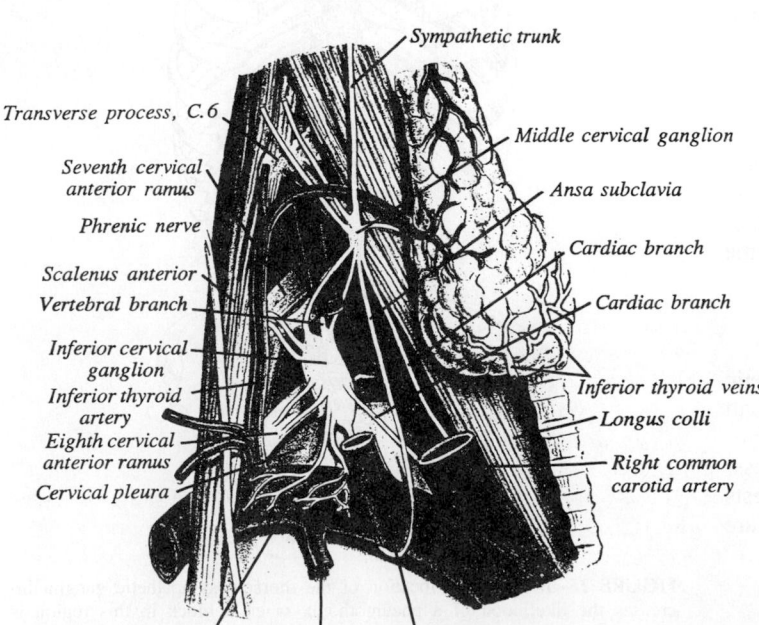

Sympathetic trunk

Transverse process, C.6

Seventh cervical anterior ramus

Phrenic nerve

Scalenus anterior

Vertebral branch

Inferior cervical ganglion

Inferior thyroid artery

Eighth cervical anterior ramus

Cervical pleura

Middle cervical ganglion

Ansa subclavia

Cardiac branch

Cardiac branch

Inferior thyroid veins

Longus colli

Right common carotid artery

Right subclavian artery  Internal thoracic artery  Vertebral artery, cut

**FIGURE 26–6.** Anterior view of the inferior cervical (or stellate) ganglion. Part of the vertebral artery has been excised to show the inferior cervical ganglion. Surrounding structures could be inadvertently penetrated during needle placement. (From Williams PL, Warwick R, Dyson M, et al, eds. *Gray's Anatomy.* 37th ed. New York, NY: Churchill Livingstone; 1989:1161.)

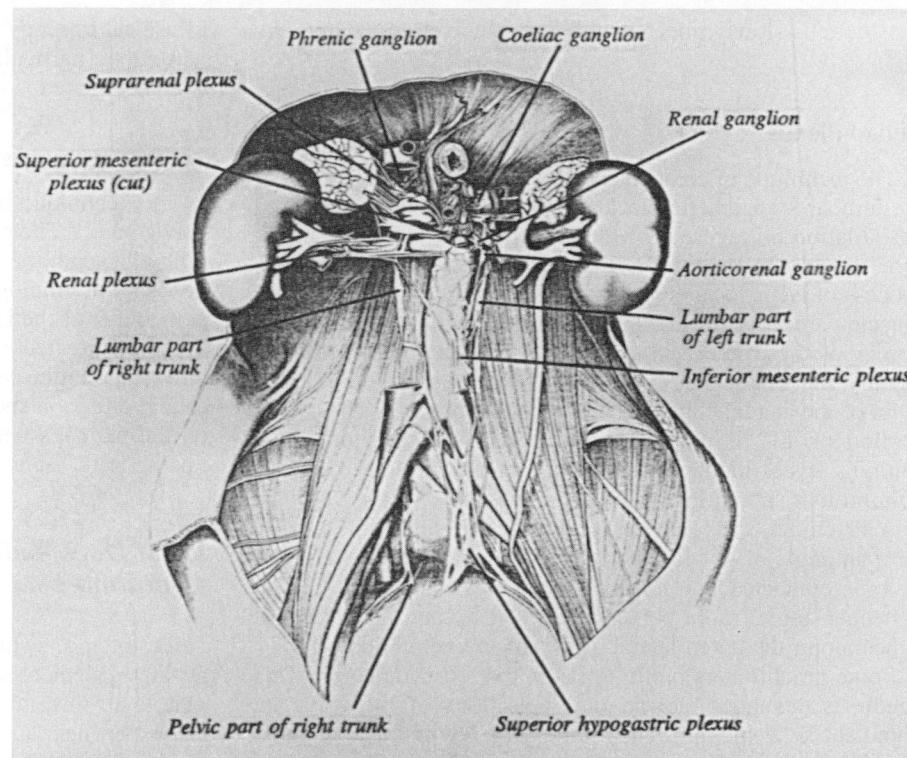

**FIGURE 26–7.** The abdominal part of the sympathetic system. Structures adjacent to the ganglia could be penetrated during needle placement. (From Williams PL, Warwick R, Dyson M, et al, eds. *Gray's Anatomy.* 37th ed. New York, NY: Churchill Livingstone; 1989:1163.)

is continuous with the inferior hypogastric plexus in a more caudal direction.

Because the pelvic viscera have a dual afferent innervation that consists of nociceptive fibers traveling with both the sympathetic fibers and the sacral parasympathetic fibers, a superior hypogastric plexus block may not provide complete pelvic analgesia.

## How Are Sympathetic Blocks Performed?

### Intravenous Regional

A capped intravenous catheter is placed in the distal portion of the extremity to be blocked with a tourniquet positioned on the proximal limb. The extremity is exsanguinated by elevation and an Esmarch bandage wrap, and the arterial inflow is occluded by inflation of the tourniquet above systolic pressure. A sympatholytic agent (eg, guanethidine, reserpine, or bretylium, usually with 0.5% lidocaine) is slowly injected through the intravenous catheter. After a minimum of 20 minutes, the tourniquet can be released in stepwise fashion.[31]

### Stellate Ganglion

The patient is placed in a supine position. The cricoid cartilage is identified by palpation. A 22-gauge, short-bevel needle is inserted just lateral to the cricoid cartilage in a slight medial direction but otherwise toward the surface on which the patient is lying. When the transverse process of C6 is contacted by the needle tip, the needle is withdrawn slightly. Aspiration to check for intravascular or subarachnoid placement is performed. If the aspiration is negative, 5 to 10 mL of local anesthetic is slowly injected with repeated attempts at aspiration after every few milliliters of injection.[29]

An alternative technique is to perform the block at the level of the C7 transverse process. The insertion site is located two fingerbreadths lateral and cephalic to the suprasternal notch. Again, the needle is inserted until the transverse process is contacted and is then withdrawn slightly.

The approach at C6 has several anatomic advantages[3]:

1. At the C6 level, the needle is more distant from the dome of the pleura, which lowers the risk of pneumothorax.
2. At the C6 level, the vertebral artery passes through the transverse process (in contrast to its superficial location at C7).
3. The bifid transverse process of C6 protects the roots of the brachial plexus, whereas the transverse process of C7 does not.

### Lumbar Sympathetic

The patient is placed with a pillow beneath the hips to flex the lumbar spine. The spinous process of L2 is identified by palpation, and a point 8 to 12 cm lateral to its cephalic position is marked. The variability in distance from the midline depends on the body habitus. In general, the insertion site is just lateral to the border of the paraspinous muscle.

A 12-cm, 20-gauge needle is inserted toward the vertebral body at a 45° angle to the horizontal plane of the patient's back (the cephalic tip of the spinous process usually corresponds to a midpoint level of the vertebral body). When the vertebral body is contacted, the needle is withdrawn, and its angle is increased to about 60° (from the horizontal toward the perpendicular); it is then advanced again. The tip of the needle should slide off the anterolateral portion of the vertebral body and lie in proximity to the lumbar sympathetic chain. After a negative aspiration, 10 to 20 mL of local anesthetic is slowly injected with frequent aspiration (Fig. 26–8).[38]

## Celiac Plexus

The technique of celiac plexus blockade is a modification of the lumbar sympathetic block technique.[39] Because of marked vasodilation, intravascular volume expansion is important before the block. A point 8 to 10 cm lateral to the spinous process of L1 is located on both flanks. Again, the paraspinous muscles are a useful landmark; the intersection of the lateral border of these muscles and the caudal edge of the 12th rib usually marks the insertion site. This site should lie at the level of the caudal edge of the L1 spinous process. The caudal portion of T12 is palpated and marked. Be sure to form a "mind's eye" picture of a point anterior to the vertebral column that should locate the celiac plexus.

A 12-cm, 20-gauge needle is advanced to this point, initially with an angle of 45° to a horizontal plane. Once the vertebral body is contacted, the needle is withdrawn and redirected to a steeper angle (more perpendicular); it is then inserted until it lies along the anterolateral aspect of the vertebral body.

Some practitioners prefer to insert the left needle first. This needle is advanced slowly until pulsations of the aorta are noted at the needle hub. The needle is then withdrawn slightly, and the right-sided needle placed in a similar direction and to a similar depth.

After aspiration and use of a test dose to check for intravascular and subarachnoid placement, 20 to 25 mL of local anesthetic or neurolytic agent is slowly injected through each needle. If only a single, left-sided needle is used, 40 to 50 mL of anesthetic are injected slowly. Most practitioners prefer to use fluoroscopy or computed tomography to guide needle placement, particularly when a neurolytic celiac plexus block is contemplated.

## Superior Hypogastric Plexus

This technique has been described for the management of pelvic pain.[20] The patient is placed in the prone position with a pillow beneath the hips. Like celiac plexus blockade, bilateral needles are employed. The needle insertion sites are located at the level of the L4-5 interspace, 5 to 7 cm from the midline. They are directed in a medial and caudal direction. The medial direction should be at a 45° angle to the sagittal plane. The caudal direction should be at a 30° angle to a horizontal plane on the patient's back. The needles are positioned so that the tips lie at the anterolateral aspect of the L5-S1 interspace.

## *What Does Radiologic Assistance Contribute?*

Radiologic techniques can be used to assist or confirm needle placement in any of the blocks just described. Various radiologic imaging procedures have added to our knowledge of the pertinent anatomy but have generated controversy about the proper needle placement. Considerable discussion has focused on whether radiologic techniques help to reduce complications.[40–50] For some of the procedures, there is no consensus as to the most useful radiologic technique.

Our opinion is that good outcome from these procedures is based on a combination of anatomic knowledge, experience, the use of test doses, and careful monitoring and follow-up of

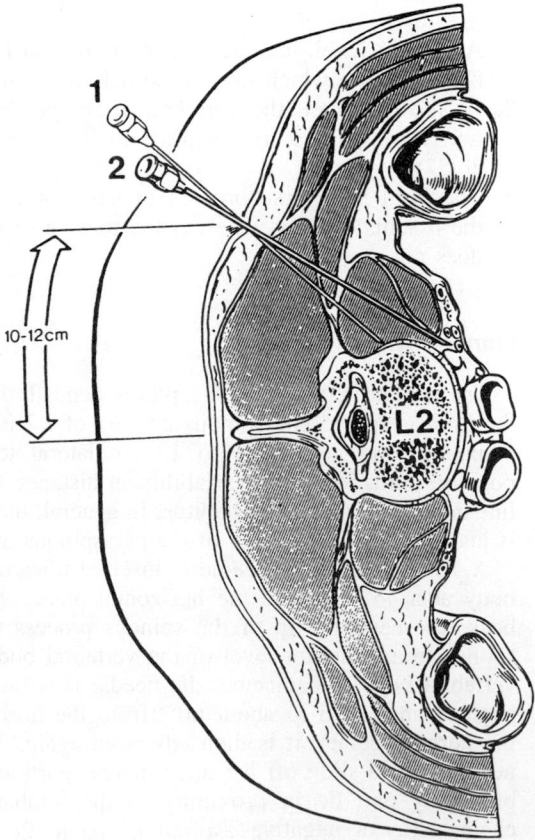

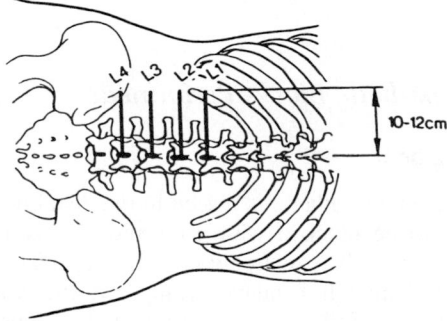

**FIGURE 26–8.** Technique of lumbar sympathetic block. Note location of skin marks for L1 and L5 spinous processes; these marks permit identification of L2 and L3. A line is drawn through the center of the spinous processes. Needle insertion is at the lateral margin of the erector spinae muscle (≈10-12 cm from midline). If the depth of the transverse process is to be checked, the needle must be angled cephalad. Otherwise, the needle is inserted at approximately 45° toward the vertebral body until this structure is located. The needle is then angled more steeply until it slips just past the vertebral body and through the psoas fascia (2). A single needle can be used instead of 2 or 3 needles; however, with a single needle, an increased volume must be injected. (From Lofstrom JB, Cousins MJ. Sympathetic neural blockade of upper and lower extremity. In: Cousins MJ, Bridenbaugh PO, eds. *Neural Blockade in Clinical Anesthesia and Management of Pain.* 2nd ed. Philadelphia, Pa: JB Lippincott; 1988:487.)

the patient's clinical course. If the patient's body habitus makes palpation of landmarks difficult, radiologic imaging can facilitate needle placement. When a neurolytic procedure is performed, radiographic visualization of needle placement may reduce the likelihood of serious neurologic complications. However, controlled studies that employ rigorous methodology and compare the success of blind techniques to those performed with imaging techniques have not been done.

## Can Peripheral Nerve or Neuraxial Block Techniques Be Used to Achieve Sympathetic Blockade?

Any block of a nerve containing sympathetic fibers can provide sympathetic blockade. There may be instances when a spinal anesthetic is more appropriate than a lumbar sympathetic block, or an axillary block is more appropriate than a stellate ganglion block. The practitioner must understand the goals of the block and what is most appropriate in the clinical situation.

Techniques that may be more specific for a sympathetic block, either because they are anatomically selective (eg, a stellate ganglion block instead of an axillary block) or pharmacologically selective (eg, 0.5% lidocaine instead of 2.0% lidocaine), may be more useful for prognostic or diagnostic blocks. However, the practitioner should realize that this is a controversial issue.[51]

## What Are the Complications?

The potential complications are of two general types: (1) complications related to needle trauma; and (2) those related to the substance injected. Trauma to neural structures is possible with any regional anesthetic technique. However, a review of the literature does not reveal the frequency with which this problem occurs in clinical practice. Trauma to proximate structures is also possible; most can be surmised from a review of the regional anatomy pertinent to each ganglion.

During a stellate ganglion block, the following structures are at risk of needle trauma: the vertebral artery, the cervical nerve roots (and the accompanying dural sleeve), the pleura, the trachea, and the esophagus. With celiac plexus and lumbar sympathetic blocks, nerve roots and dural sleeves, the major abdominal vessels, the kidneys, the bowel, and the pleura (celiac plexus block) are at risk (Table 26–3).

## How Are These Complications Managed?

### Puncture of Abdominal Viscera

Some of the potential complications are not of great clinical significance, and routine follow-up may be all that is necessary. If bowel perforation occurs with an anterior celiac plexus block using a 22-gauge or smaller needle, adverse outcome is rare.[52,53] The technique of lumbar sympathetic block has been modified to reduce the likelihood of renal puncture. Patients should be alerted to the possibility that hematuria may develop if it occurs. Hematuria is usually transient and of little clinical consequence. If the patient develops flank pain with a mass, persistent or heavy hematuria, or hypertension, urologic con-

**TABLE 26–3.** Complications of Sympathetic Blockade

**Needle Trauma**

Nerves and dura
Blood vessels
Viscera (kidney, bowel)
Pleura

**Effect of Injected Substance**

Local anesthetic toxicity
Extensive sympathetic blockade (hypotension)
Extensive spread of neurolytic solution, causing somatic nerve injury or bowel or bladder dysfunction

**Miscellaneous**

Infection (very rare)
Vasovagal response
Allergic reaction to contrast dye or local anesthetic

sultation should be ordered. Many of the complications are self-limited and do not require further anesthesia or surgical management.[54]

### Vascular Trauma and Bleeding

Serious needle-induced vascular trauma also seems to be a relatively rare event. In fact, the lumbar approach for aortography is similar to that used for lumbar sympathetic block and celiac plexus block. Serious hemorrhage is rare with both blocks if small-gauge needles are used and if the patient has a normal blood coagulation profile. The advisability of nerve block techniques in the presence of some degree of pathologic or therapeutic coagulation dysfunction has been a long-standing controversy. A recent monograph reviews this issue.[55] Probably the most prudent approach is to weigh the benefits to be gained from the block against the risk of hemorrhage (unquantified) and to observe the patient carefully for signs or symptoms of hematoma formation or other hemorrhage.

### Pneumothorax

Puncture of the pleura can result in a pneumothorax; this complication is associated with celiac plexus block or stellate ganglion block (especially if performed at C7). Chest pain, dyspnea, cyanosis, loss of fremitus over the chest wall, hyperresonance of the ipsilateral hemithorax, and loss of breath sounds are pertinent findings.[56] Inspiratory and expiratory chest radiographs facilitate the diagnosis. A thoracic surgery consult for chest tube placement should be considered if the pneumothorax is more than 20%. If a pneumothorax results in rapid deterioration, a large-bore intravenous catheter (14- to 16-gauge) can be inserted in the second intercostal space in the midclavicular line.

### Esophageal Perforation

Puncture of the esophagus with subsequent osteitis of the transverse process or mediastinitis is a potential, but apparently very rare, complication.[10]

### Neural Injury

The incidence of neural injury from needle trauma during sympathetic blockade has not been studied. Appropriate management should include careful documentation of symptoms and neurologic deficit (if present) and careful follow-up to ensure resolution of the problem. Most symptoms gradually diminish over several months. Neuropathic syndromes can be managed with nonsteroidal antiinflammatory drugs, antidepressants, anticonvulsants, injections of local anesthetics or steroids, and physical therapy.

## Intravascular Injection

Unrecognized injection of local anesthetics into a blood vessel can result in local anesthetic toxicity. The likelihood of a seizure depends on the quantity and rapidity of local anesthetic delivered to the brain. During an attempted lumbar sympathetic block, 20 mL of 0.5% lidocaine (100 mg) could be injected into the inferior vena cava with a relatively low risk of toxicity. However, during an attempted stellate ganglion block, less than 1 mL of local anesthetic injected into the vertebral artery likely will result in a seizure because of direct delivery to the brain.

Before injection, perform careful aspiration to identify intravascular positioning. All injections should be made in small (2- to 5-mL) increments. The patients must be observed for signs of local anesthetic toxicity (tinnitus, perioral numbness, blurred vision, slurred speech, seizure) during and after injection.

If a seizure occurs, a patent airway, adequate ventilation, and circulatory stability need to be maintained. Hyperventilation with 100% oxygen is always indicated. Administration of a benzodiazepine or other CNS depressant (eg, thiopental) to terminate the seizure and a muscle relaxant to facilitate airway management may be necessary. The decision to use these agents must be based on the practitioner's assessment of each situation.

## Subarachnoid Injection

The accidental injection of anesthetic solution into the subarachnoid space can result in extensive sympathetic blockade, respiratory arrest, and, if untreated, cardiovascular collapse. Profound hypotension secondary to arterial vasodilation, impaired venous return, and cardiac sympathectomy (T1-4) with reduced cardiac rate and contractile function often occur. Reduced venous return can also result from celiac plexus or lumbar sympathetic block owing to sequestration of venous blood in the viscera or lower extremities. Appropriate management of this problem is the immediate restoration of venous return by leg elevation, rapid infusion of intravenous fluids, and administration of temporizing drugs such as ephedrine, atropine, or phenylephrine.[57]

## Neurolytic Agent Spread

Unexpected extensive spread of neurolytic agents can lead to neurologic damage of a prolonged nature. The best management of this problem is prevention. In all cases, an analysis of risk versus benefit is in order. The procedures must be done with care; a test dose of local anesthetic and radiographic confirmation of needle placement are indicated.

## AUTONOMIC DYSFUNCTION: DYSREFLEXIA

Patients with spinal cord injury are frequently seen in the operating room for plastic reconstruction and for orthopedic, genitourinary, and neurologic surgery. For each patient, the degree of derangement of sympathetic control systems is a function of the level, completeness, and duration of the spinal cord injury.

Acute spinal cord trauma is a medical emergency. The major cause of morbidity and mortality is impaired respiratory function. Patients may be unable to protect their airway and clear bronchial secretions; therefore, prevention of aspiration of gastric contents is a recurring concern. Pulmonary edema and bronchopneumonia frequently occur.

In addition, these acute status patients are functionally hypovolemic and frequently require intravenous fluids and vasopressors to support BP. This relative hypovolemia stage is due to low systemic vascular resistance that is caused by disruption of sympathetic vasoconstrictor mechanisms. The vasodilated state of the acute spinal cord injury patient also leads to significant heat loss and a predisposition to hypothermia.

Autonomic dysreflexia (AD) is a hypertensive crisis that occurs in paraplegic and quadriplegic patients. It is due to massive sympathetic vasoconstriction that is initiated below the segmental level of the spinal cord lesion (Fig. 26–9).

## *What Patients Are at Risk?*

Two to 3 weeks following acute spinal cord trauma, sweating and the appearance of reflex flexor activity in the legs coincide with the return of autonomic responsiveness below the cord lesion. From this point forward, many spinal cord injured patients are at risk for AD. About 65% to 85% of spinal cord injury patients with lesions at or above the T7 level have hypertensive episodes in their daily activities.[58] Patients with lesions between T5 and T10 may have only mild elevations in BP during AD-triggering episodes. With cord lesions below T10, the occurrence rate is relatively low (<10%).[59] In patients with an infarcted spinal cord or a cord that has otherwise been damaged, a minimal risk of AD episodes is present because spinal reflexes are generally abolished.

## *Why Does It Occur?*

The gradation of hypertensive responses relative to the level of spinal cord lesion is due to neurophysiologic mechanisms. Most commonly, visceral stimuli (eg, bowel and bladder distention) and, less commonly, somatic and cutaneous stimuli can trigger AD (Fig. 26–10). C-fiber afferent nerves from bladder and bowel are involved with neurogenic hyperreflexive responses. Afferent signals are believed to travel to the spinal cord through sacral routes via the pudendal (somatic, S2-4), hypogastric (sympathetic, T9-L2), and pelvic (parasympathetic, S2-4) nerves. They proceed up the spinal cord via the spinothalamic tracts and dorsal columns.[59,60] These signals can trigger both ipsilateral and contralateral increases in sympathetic outflow at each spinal level below the cord lesion (see Fig. 26–10).[61]

In normal individuals, this outflow is inhibited by descending signals from higher CNS centers. This descending inhibition is interrupted in the spinal cord injury patient. If splanchnic sympathetic outflow is included in the sympathetic response (cord lesions at or above T7), the ensuing vasoconstriction can precipitate large increases in BP that cannot be

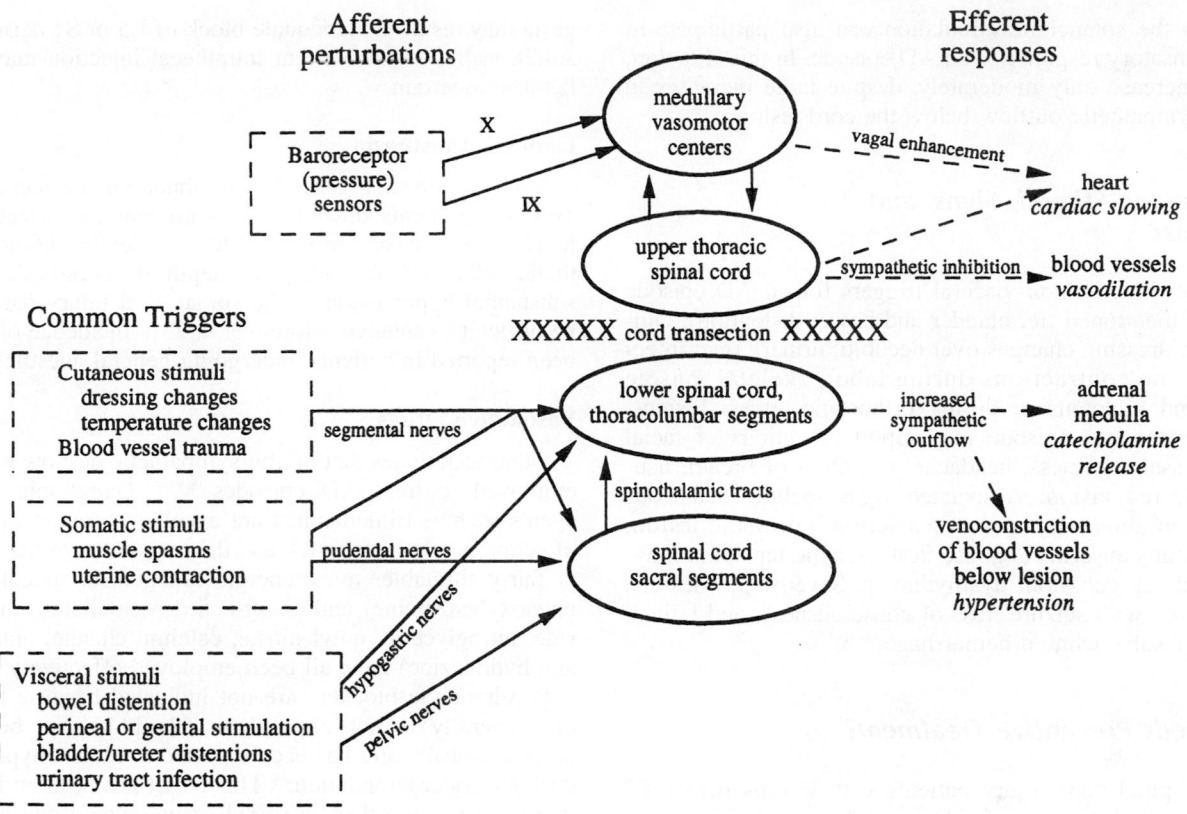

**FIGURE 26–9.** Autonomic dysreflexia. Neural pathways involved in autonomic dysreflexia. Triggering stimuli below the lesion lead to increased sympathetic outflow and hypertension. The baroreceptors sense the pressure elevation and elicit increases in vagal (parasympathetic) outflow and decreases in sympathetic outflow.

adequately compensated for by baroreflex-mediated cardiac slowing and sympathoinhibition to vascular sites above the lesion. The neurally intact adrenal medulla can also participate in the response. In addition, the denervated blood vessels of spinal cord injury patients appear to be hypersensitive to sympathetic stimulation and catecholamines.[60]

Spinal cord transection does not interfere with afferent neural connections from the carotid and aortic arch baroreceptors (cranial nerves IX and X) to the brainstem. These receptors are activated by systemic hypertension during an AD episode. They promote reflex slowing of the heart through an intact vagus and reduced sympathetic activity to the vasculature above the level of the cord lesion. In patients with low cord injuries (T10 or below), reflex inhibition of sympathetic

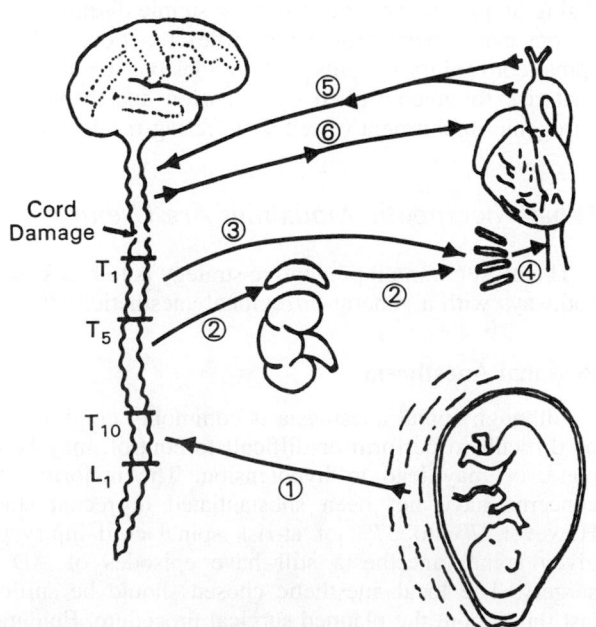

**FIGURE 26–10.** Mechanism of cardiovascular changes in autonomic hyperreflexia. *1,* Afferent impulses from contracting uterus to spinal cord segments T10 through L1. *2,* Efferent impulses from segments T5 to T9 to adrenal medulla causing discharge of catecholamines. *3,* Efferent impulses from sympathetic centers T1 through L1 directly to vascular bed causing vasoconstriction. *4,* Increase in arterial blood measure as a result of stimuli by 2 and 3. *5,* Afferent impulses from carotid sinus and aortic arch to cardiac centers in medulla oblongata. *6,* Efferent impulses through vagus nerves to heart causing bradycardia. (From Abouleish EI, Hanley ES, Palmer SM. Can epidural fentanyl control autonomic hyperreflexia in a quadriplegic parturient? *Anesth Analg.* 1989;68:523–526.)

outflow to the splanchnic circulation can also participate in the compensatory response to an AD episode. In this situation, BP may increase only moderately, despite large increases in regional sympathetic outflow below the cord lesion.

## What Are the Stimuli, Signs, and Symptoms?

Many of the common visceral triggers for an AD episode have been mentioned (ie, bladder and bowel distention). Others include dressing changes over decubiti, urinary tract infections, uterine contractions during labor, skeletal muscle spasms, and hypotension during orthostatic stress. Patients who experience an episode may report sensations of facial tingling, nasal stuffiness, headache, shortness of breath, nausea, or blurred vision. Associated signs include cutaneous vasodilation above and vasoconstriction below the lesion, sweating, cutis anserina ("goose flesh"), hypertension, bradycardia, and, on occasion, dysrhythmias. Severe episodes can be associated with seizure, loss of consciousness, and retinal, cerebral, or subarachnoid hemorrhage.[58-60]

## Who Needs Preventive Treatment?

Should spinal cord injury patients with lesions below T7 and no previous history of AD receive preventive therapy during surgical procedures below the lesions (where sensations are absent)? Because of the potential morbidity of an unablated episode, the answer probably is "Yes."

An important consideration is that autonomic responses are proportional to the strength of the stimulus. In daily activities, the strength and duration of potential triggering stimuli for AD may be much less than those of the stimuli that occur during surgical procedures. Thus, a patient with a low spinal cord transection and a negative history for AD might still have a major episode during a stimulating surgical procedure.

An additional consideration is that during an AD episode, reflex compensatory responses above the level of the cord lesion are dependent on intact baroreceptor mechanisms. Aging, hypertension, and various systemic diseases and medications can impair baroreceptor reflex function.[62] Thus, many spinal cord injury patients with low lesions are still at significant risk for uncontrolled hypertension due to pathologic or iatrogenic impairment of reflex buffering mechanisms.

## What Therapeutic Modalities Are Useful?

The most common preventive strategy is to block the neural pathways with a general or regional anesthetic.[62-66]

### Regional Anesthesia

Although spinal anesthesia is commonly employed, it may be difficult to perform or difficult to control, may be incomplete, or may lead to hypotension. The majority of these concerns have not been substantiated in recent studies.[4,66] However, 7% to 27% of at-risk spinal cord injury patients given spinal anesthesia still have episodes of AD during surgery. The local anesthetic chosen should be sufficient to last throughout the planned surgical procedure. Epidural anal-gesia may result in inadequate block of L5 or S1 dermatomes. Additionally, an inadvertent intrathecal injection may be difficult to ascertain.

### General Anesthesia

Many anesthesiologists choose inhalation anesthetics. However, these agents do not always prevent AD because deep levels of anesthesia are needed to sufficiently obtund sympathetic reflexes.[66] An adequate depth of anesthesia without substantial hypotension in the spinal cord injury patient may be difficult to achieve. Moreover, a 23% incidence of AD has been reported in patients undergoing general anesthesia.[66]

### Vasoactive Drugs

Other techniques that inhibit sympathetic outflow have been employed to treat AD episodes.[58,59,67] Ganglionic blocking agents such as trimethaphan are excellent because their onset of action is relatively quick and the magnitude of the response is fairly titratable. α-Adrenergic antagonists (phentolamine, phenoxybenzamine) and direct-acting vasodilators (nitroprusside, nitroglycerin, amyl nitrite, calcium channel antagonists, and hydralazine) have all been employed effectively.

β-Adrenergic blockers are not indicated because tachycardia generally is not a problem. Clonidine has been used prophylactically and has been reported to reduce hypertension during bladder stimulation.[68] This effect has been attributed to its ability to act either on spinal preganglionic neurons or on peripheral presynaptic $\alpha_2$-adrenoceptors. Clonidine may also reduce skeletal muscle spasms.[60]

## What Special Considerations Apply to the Quadriplegic Parturient?

The uterus has a capacity to contract normally during labor despite complete interruption of its efferent neural regulation.[69] When the spinal cord is completely severed, labor is painless but can be associated with AD. Recurring episodes of AD may, in fact, be the only indication of the onset of labor.[69-71] In this situation, the nociceptive stimulus originates from the contracting uterus.

Epidural opioids have been employed to attenuate AD activity owing to their ability to modulate nociceptive transmission at the posterior horn cells. Meperidine (100 mg) has also been reported to be successful in controlling AD in the quadriplegic parturient.[70] However, epidural fentanyl (75-μg bolus; 10-μg/h infusion) has failed in this application, perhaps owing to incomplete suppression of cord transmission of neural signals and to the use of such a low dose.[71] Meperidine may have been more effective because it has both opioid receptor and local anesthetic effects in human beings.

Higher doses of other opioids may also be effective; however, they carry the usual risk of opioid side effects, including nausea, vomiting, pruritus, urinary retention, sedation, and respiratory depression. The optimal choice of epidural anesthetic for the quadriplegic patient in labor may be a combination of a low dose (<0.125%) of bupivacaine and an opioid.

### References

1. Lykowitz RJ, Hoffman BB, Taylor P. Neurohumoral transmission: the autonomic and somatic motor nervous system. In: Gilman AG, Rall TW, Nies AS, et al, eds. *Goodman and Gilman's The Pharmacological Basis of Therapeutics.* 8th ed. New York, NY: Pergamon Press; 1990:84.

2. Livingston RB. Visceral control mechanisms. In: West JB, ed. *Best and Taylor's Physiological Basis of Medical Practice.* 12th ed. Baltimore, Md: Williams & Wilkins; 1991:1053.

3. Williams PL, Warwick R, Dyron M, et al, eds. *Gray's Anatomy.* 37th ed. New York, NY: Churchill Livingstone; 1989:1154.

4. Shanahan PT. Replantation of extremities. *Anesth Clin North Am.* 1989;7:675.

5. Hobelmann CF Jr, Delon AL. Use of prolonged sympathetic blockade as an adjunct to surgery in the patient with sympathetic-maintained pain. *Microsurgery.* 1989;10:151.

6. Ladd AL, DeHaven KE, Thanik J, et al. Reflex sympathetic imbalance: response to epidural blockade. *Am J Sports Med.* 1989;17:660.

7. Gamulin Z, Forster A, Simonet F, et al. Effects of renal sympathetic blockade on renal hemodynamics in patients undergoing major aortic abdominal surgery. *Anesthesiology.* 1986;65:688.

8. VanTwisk R, Gielen JM, Pavlov PW, et al. Is additional epidural sympathetic block in microvascular surgery contraindicated? A preliminary report. *Br J Plast Surg.* 1988;41:37.

9. Bonica JJ. Causalgia and other reflex sympathetic dystrophies. In: Bonica JJ, ed. *The Management of Pain.* 2nd ed. Philadelphia, Pa: Lea & Febiger; 1990:220.

10. Colding A. The effect of regional sympathetic blocks in the treatment of herpes zoster. *Acta Anaesthesiol Scand.* 1969;13:133.

11. Bonica JJ. Pain due to vascular disease. In: Bonica JJ, ed. *The Management of Pain.* 2nd ed. Philadelphia, Pa: Lea & Febiger; 1990:502.

12. Tasker RR, Dostrovsky JO. Deafferentation and central pain. In: Wall PD, Melzak R, eds. *Textbook of Pain.* Edinburgh, United Kingdom: Churchill Livingstone; 1989:154.

13. Bengsston A, Bengsston M. Regional sympathetic blockade in primary fibromyalgia. *Pain.* 1988;33:161.

14. DeWitt RFE, Remme JJ. A report on the efficacy of regional intravenous sympathetic blocks (RIS-blocks) with guanethidine (Ismelin) in long-standing and complicated leg ulcers. *Arch Dermatol Res.* 1989;281:206.

15. Dyson A, Henderson AM. Continuous axillary brachial plexus blockade following intra-arterial injection of nicotinic acid. *Anaesth Intensive Care.* 1987;15:462.

16. Floyd JB. Traumatic cerebral edema relieved by stellate ganglion anesthesia. *South Med J.* 1987;80:1328.

17. Sanchez V, Segedin ER, Moses M, et al. Role of lumbar sympathectomy in the pediatric intensive care unit. *Anesth Analg.* 1988;67:794.

18. Bonica JJ, Ventafridda V, Twyerors RG. Cancer pain. In: Bonica JJ, ed. *The Management of Pain.* 2nd ed. Philadelphia, Pa: Lea & Febiger; 1990:400.

19. Bell S, Cole R, Robert-Thompson IC. Coeliac plexus block for control of pain in chronic pancreatitis. *BMJ.* 1980;281:1604.

20. Plancarte R, Amescua C, Patt RB, et al. Superior hypogastric plexus block for pelvic cancer pain. *Anesthesiology.* 1990;73:236.

21. Leung JWC, Bowen-Wright M, Aveling W, et al. Coeliac plexus block for pain in pancreatic cancer and chronic pancreatitis. *Br J Surg.* 1983;70:730.

22. Nurmikko T, Wells C, Bowsher D. Pain and allodynia in postherpetic neuralgia: role of somatic and sympathetic nervous systems. *Acta Neurol Scand.* 1991;84:146.

23. Sharfman WH, Walsh TD. Has the analgesic efficacy of neurolytic celiac plexus block been demonstrated in pancreatic cancer pain? *Pain.* 1990;41:267.

24. Yanagida H, Suwa K, Corssen G. No prophylactic effect of early sympathetic blockade on postherpetic neuralgia. *Anesthesiology.* 1987;66:73.

25. Bonica JJ, Buckley FP, Moricca G, et al. Neurolytic blockade and hypophysectomy. In: Bonica JJ, ed. *The Management of Pain.* 2nd ed. Philadelphia, Pa: Lea & Febiger; 1990:1980.

26. Verrill P. Sympathetic ganglion lesions. In: Wall PD, Melzak R, eds. *Textbook of Pain.* 2nd ed. Edinburgh, United Kingdom: Churchill Livingstone; 1989:773.

27. Wood KM. Peripheral nerve and root chemical lesions. In: Wall PD, Melzak R, eds. *Textbook of Pain.* 2nd ed. Edinburgh, United Kingdom: Churchill Livingstone; 1989:768.

28. Reading AE. Testing pain mechanisms in persons in pain. In: Wall PD, Melzak R, eds. *Textbook of Pain.* 2nd ed. Edinburgh, United Kingdom: Churchill Livingstone; 1989:269.

29. Lofstrom JB, Cousins MJ. Sympathetic neural blockade of upper and lower extremity. In: Cousins MJ, Bridenbaugh PO, eds. *Neural Blockade in Clinical Anesthesia and Management of Pain.* 2nd ed. Philadelphia, Pa: JB Lippincott; 1988:461.

30. Wahr JA, Tremper KK. Pulse oximetry. In: Blitt CD, Hines RL, eds. *Monitoring in Anesthesia and Critical Care Medicine.* 3rd ed. New York, NY: Churchill Livingstone; 1995:392.

31. Rosenberg PR. Intravenous regional anesthesia. In: Brown DL, ed. *Regional Anesthesia and Analgesia.* Philadelphia, Pa: WB Saunders; 1996:385.

32. Diaz P. Use of liquid crystal thermography to evaluate sympathetic blocks. *Anaesthesia.* 1976;44:443.

33. Higa K, Dan K, Manabe H, et al. Factors influencing the duration of treatment of acute herpetic pain with sympathetic nerve block: importance of severity of herpes zoster assessed by the maximum antibody titers to varicella-zoster virus in otherwise healthy patients. *Pain.* 1988;32:147.

34. Malmquist L-A, Tryggvasm B, Bengtsson M. Sympathetic blockade during extradural analgesia with mepivacaine or bupivacaine. *Acta Anaesthesiol Scand.* 1989;33:444.

35. Riegelman RK, Hirsch RP. *Studying a Study and Testing a Test: How to Read the Medical Literature.* 2nd ed. Boston, Mass: Little, Brown & Co; 1989:127.

36. Haynes RB. How to read clinical journals, II: to learn about a diagnostic test. *Can Med Assoc J.* 1981;124:703.

37. Hannington-Keff JG. Pharmacological target blocks in painful dystrophic limbs. In: Wall PD, Melzak R, eds. *Textbook of Pain.* 2nd ed. Edinburgh, United Kingdom: Churchill Livingstone; 1989:754.

38. Brown DL. *Atlas of Regional Anesthesia.* 2nd ed. Philadelphia, Pa: WB Saunders; 1999:275.

39. Brown DL. *Atlas of Regional Anesthesia.* 2nd ed. Philadelphia, Pa: WB Saunders; 1999:282.

40. Brown DL, Bulley CK, Quiel EL. Neurolytic celiac plexus block for pancreatic cancer pain. *Anesth Analg.* 1987;66:869.

41. Brown EM, Kunjappen V. Single needle lateral approach for lumbar sympathetic block. *Anesth Analg.* 1975;54:725.

42. Fujita Y, Takaori M. Pleural effusion after CT-guided alcohol celiac plexus block. *Anesth Analg.* 1987;66:911.

43. Hardy PAJ, Wells JDC. Coeliac plexus block and cephalic spread of injectate. *Ann R Coll Surg Engl.* 1989;71:48.

44. Hogan QH, Erickson SJ, Haddox JD, et al. The spread of solutions during stellate ganglion block. *Reg Anaesth.* 1992;17:78.

45. Kirvela O, Svedstrom E, Lundblom N. Ultrasonic guidance of lumbar sympathetic and celiac plexus block: a new technique. *Reg Anaesth.* 1992;17:43.

46. Lieberman RP, Waldman SD. Celiac plexus neurolysis with the modified transaortic approach. *Radiology.* 1990;175:274.

47. Moore DC, Bush WH, Burnett LL. Celiac plexus block: a roentgenographic anatomic study of technique and spread of solution in patients and corpses. *Anesth Analg.* 1981;60:369.

48. Moore DC, Bush WH, Burnett LL. An improved technique for celiac plexus block may be more theoretical than real. *Anesthesiology.* 1982;57:347.

49. Singler RC. An improved technique for alcohol neurolysis of the celiac plexus. *Anesthesiology.* 1982;56:137.

50. Sprague RS, Ramamurthy S. Identification of the anterior psoas sheath as a landmark for lumbar sympathetic block. *Reg Anaesth.* 1990;15:253.

51. Hogan QH, Abram SE. Diagnostic and prognostic neural blockade. In: Cousins MJ, Bridenbaugh PO, eds. *Neural Blockade in Clinical Anesthesia and Management of Pain.* 3rd ed. Philadelphia, Pa: Lippincott-Raven; 1998:837.

52. Lieberman RP, Nance PN, Cuka DJ. Anterior approach to celiac plexus block during interventional biliary procedures. *Radiology.* 1988;167:562.

53. Matamala AM, Lopez FV, Sanchez JLA, et al. Percutaneous anterior approach to the coeliac plexus using ultrasound. *Br J Anaesth.* 1989;62:637.

54. Wheatly JK, Motamedi F, Hammonds WD. Page kidney resulting from massive subcapsular hematoma: complication of lumbar sympathetic nerve block. *Urology.* 1984;24:361.

55. Heit JA, Horlocker TT. Neuraxial anesthesia and anticoagulation. *Reg Anesth Pain Med.* 1998;23(suppl 2):129.

56. DeGowin RL. *DeGowin and DeGowin's Bedside Diagnostic Examination.* 5th ed. New York, NY: Macmillan Publishing; 1987:948.

57. Greene NM. *Physiology of Spinal Anesthesia.* 3rd ed. Baltimore, Md: Williams & Wilkins; 1981:63.

58. Schonwald G, Fish KJ, Perkash I. Cardiovascular complications during anesthesia in chronic spinal cord injured patients. *Anesthesiology.* 1981;55:550.

59. Johnson B, Thomason R, Pallares V, et al. Autonomic hyperreflexia: a review. *Mil Med.* 1975;140:345.

60. Mathias CJ, Frankel HL. Cardiovascular control in spinal man. *Ann Rev Physiol.* 1988;50:577.

61. Fagius J, Karhuvaara S. Sympathetic activity and blood pressure increases with bladder distension in humans. *Hypertension.* 1989;14:511.

62. Ebert TJ, Stowe DF. Peripheral circulation: recent insights into autonomic

nervous control and endothelial factors relevant to cardiovascular disease and anesthesia. *Curr Opin Anaesth.* 1991;3.

63. Lambert DH, Deane RS, Mazuzan JE. Anesthesia and the control of blood pressure in patients with spinal cord injury. *Anesth Analg.* 1982;61:344.

64. Broecker BH, Hranowski N, Hackler RH. Low spinal anesthesia for the prevention of autonomic dysreflexia in the spinal cord injury patient. *J Urol.* 1979;122:366.

65. Katz RL, Thorp JM, Cefalo RC. Epidural analgesia and autonomic hyperreflexia: a case report. *Am J Obstet Gynecol.* 1990;162:471.

66. Stowe DF, Bernstein JS, Madsen KE, et al. Autonomic hyperreflexia in spinal cord injured patients during extracorporeal shock wave lithotripsy. *Anesth Analg.* 1989;68:788.

67. Dykstra DD, Sidi AA, Anderson LC. The effect of nifedipine on cystoscopy-induced autonomic hyperreflexia in patients with high spinal cord injuries. *J Urol.* 1987;138:1155.

68. Mathias CJ, Frankel HL. Autonomic failure in tetraplegia. In: Banister R, ed. *Autonomic Failure.* 2nd ed. Oxford, United Kingdom: Oxford University Press; 1988:453.

69. Robertson DNS. Pregnancy and labor in the paraplegic. *Paraplegia.* 1972;10:209.

70. Baraka A. Epidural meperidine for control of autonomic hyperreflexia in a paraplegic parturient. *Anesthesiology.* 1985;62:688.

71. Abouleish EI, Hanley ES, Palmer SM. Can epidural fentanyl control autonomic hyperreflexia in a quadriplegic parturient? *Anesth Analg.* 1989;68:523.

# Vascular Access

Felipe Urdaneta
Emilio B. Lobato
Nikolaus Gravenstein

Vascular cannulation (peripheral or central) remains one of the most common procedures performed by anesthesiologists.

In the adult population (absent a mask induction), no other anesthetic procedure can be performed until intravenous access is established. Recent advances, especially in regard to the technique for central venous cannulation with the aid of ultrasound (US) guidance, have been made since the first edition of this book. Despite these advances, major problems can still occur when accessing the circulatory system, and controversies persist regarding vascular catheterization.

## EQUIPMENT

### What Is Necessary?

#### Peripheral Catheter

A peripheral vein is usually the first choice for intravenous infusion. In adults, catheterization of arm veins is safer than that of the head, neck, or lower extremity veins and, therefore, should be attempted first. A good place to look for veins is in the dorsum of the hand or on the forearm. If possible, the nondominant extremity is used. The veins of the antecubital fossa should ideally be reserved for venipuncture and percutaneously inserted central venous catheters (CVCs) and used for other intravenous access only in emergencies or when other sites cannot be identified or cannulated. If excessive hair is present over the insertion site, its removal should be considered.

In general, the smallest gauge catheter that is appropriate for the clinical situation should be used. Factors that guide catheter choice include the condition of available veins and skin sites and the types and duration of intravenous therapy. Alert patients can often recommend the best site based on their prior experience. The most commonly used method for venous distention is application of a tourniquet proximal to the intended cannulation site. Other useful distention methods include placing the limb in the dependent position, milking the vein from proximal to distal, and applying moist heat or a thin film of nitroglycerin ointment. Vigorous tapping over the vein is also helpful because it causes a temporary neura-

**TABLE 27–1.** Equipment for Peripheral Vascular Cannulation

Clean gloves
Antiseptic solution (chlorhexidine, povidone-iodine, or 70% isopropyl alcohol swabs)
Venous tourniquet
Intravenous cannulas
Tape of occlusive dressings
Flush syringe or intravenous tubing set
Syringe with 0.5–1 mL of 1% lidocaine without epinephrine with the smallest needle available for local infiltration
Sterile 2 × 2- or 4 × 4-cm gauze

praxia of the nervi vasorum, allowing venodilation. When distention by these methods is inadequate, a small-bore catheter may be placed and used to infuse fluid to effect venous distention so that a larger catheter may be inserted via a guidewire exchange technique.

A list of the equipment necessary for peripheral vascular catheterization is provided in Table 27–1. Wearing gloves is standard for all invasive procedures as part of the universal precautions. Chlorhexidine has become quite popular and is the most efficacious antiseptic solution for preparation of the vascular access site, both in peripheral and central cannulation as well for arterial catheterization.[1]

Of the different choices of needles and catheters available today, over-the-needle plastic catheters are used most commonly. They are typically 2 inches or less in length. The Centers for Disease Control and Prevention recommends that stainless steel cannulas be used for temporary peripheral access to reduce the incidence of phlebitis.[2] If plastic catheters are used for cannulation, replacement every 48 to 72 hours is recommended.[3] The National Intravenous Therapy Association recommends steel catheters for single or short-term use and plastic catheters for long-term access.[4] Stainless steel cannulas have the disadvantage of predisposing to venous perforation and extravasation and are not suitable for intraoperative application.

### Procedure

After the necessary equipment has been assembled and the limb is positioned, the intended vein is distended by one of the previously mentioned methods, and the site is cleansed. Local anesthetic is infiltrated, and the vein is stabilized by applying distal traction.

The needle is inserted at a 30° to 45° angle to the skin with the bevel up. Of note is that it is probably counterproductive to loosen the catheter from the needle stylet before venipuncture because the manufacturer goes to considerable effort to build a smooth transition between catheter and stylet. Loosening the catheter defeats this effort and makes threading more difficult. Entry may be from the side or directly over the vein. Once blood return is noted, the needle is advanced slightly such that the bevel is completely within the vessel. Thus, large-bore needles need to be advanced farther into the vein than smaller ones before advancing the catheter off the needle stylet. The needle is then brought down parallel to the skin, and the catheter is rotated and advanced (threaded) off the needle.

After satisfactory placement, the tourniquet (if used) is released and the stylet is withdrawn and disposed of. The catheter is flushed or an intravenous infusion tubing is attached, and the site is dressed in a way that allows periodic evaluation of the puncture site. If swelling occurs around the intravenous site, the catheter must be removed and a new site chosen. If it is not clear that the cannula is intravascular, an easy test to confirm proper placement is to observe the intravenous drip chamber with the roller clamp open and obstruct the venous circulation proximal to the intravenous cannulation site with digital pressure or a tourniquet. If the drip in the chamber slows down, then the catheter is intravascular; if it does not slow down, the location is extravascular. It is recommended that a loop of tubing be attached to the skin to minimize inadvertent extraction of the intravenous catheter and tubing or line if it gets caught on some object. The use of an armboard is recommended in cases in which the immobilization of a limb is necessary to prevent flexion and extension of the limb that causes movement of the catheter within the vein and increases the incidence of phlebitis, extravasation, and/or dislodgment of the catheter.

### Arterial Catheter

Direct monitoring of arterial pressure is often necessary in critically ill or hemodynamically unstable patients. Patients requiring frequent blood analysis benefit from an arterial catheter as well. Procedures under cardiopulmonary bypass require the placement of an arterial catheter because this is the only feasible way available to monitor blood pressure during bypass because automated noninvasive methods require pulsatile flow.

The insertion of an arterial catheter requires considerably more skill and patience than peripheral venous cannulation. All patients who have arterial catheters should be under close supervision because inadvertent disconnection of the system can have disastrous consequences.

In theory, any superficial artery can be chosen for cannulation; but, in practice, the radial artery is the one most commonly chosen, owing to ease of placement. Lower extremity, axillary, and brachial catheters should be reserved for cases in which the benefit of placement outweighs the risks, and catheterization should be performed by practitioners with experience in placing catheters in such locations. The advantages and disadvantages of common arterial cannulation sites are listed in Table 27–2.[5]

### Allen Test

The Allen test is used by many practitioners to assess collateral ulnar arterial flow. To perform the test, the practitioner compresses the radial and ulnar arteries as the patient opens and closes his or her hand. Once the hand is blanched, the ulnar artery is released and the time it takes for the blush to reappear is measured. Normally, the blush should reappear in <7 seconds. Seven to 15 seconds is considered borderline, and >15 seconds is considered to reflect an absence of adequate collateral flow through the ulnar artery.

The reliability of this test as a predictor of good collateral flow is questionable because neither the presence nor the absence of a normal Allen test response reliably predicts absence or occurrence, respectively, of thrombotic complications.[6]

### Equipment

Arterial catheterization can be performed with much of the same equipment used for peripheral venous access. This

**TABLE 27–2.** Peripheral Arterial Cannulation Sites: Advantages and Disadvantages

| Site | Advantages | Disadvantages |
|---|---|---|
| Radial | Highly accessible<br>Easily visible<br>No adjacent nerve | Relatively high complication rate<br>High degree of disability if complication occurs |
| Femoral | Relatively low complication rate<br>Longer catheter function<br>More accurate readings<br>High cannulation success rate | Decreased mobilization of patient<br>Possibly higher contamination rate<br>Occult bleeding |
| Axillary | Low complication rate<br>Longer catheter function<br>More accurate readings | Low accessibility and visibility<br>High degree of disability if complication occurs<br>Adjacent nerves<br>Occult bleeding |
| Dorsalis pedis | Easily visible<br>Highly accessible | Congenital absence in 12% of population<br>High rate of cannulation failure<br>Decreased mobilization of patient |
| Temporal | Low thrombotic complication rate<br>A preductal site | Difficult cannulation<br>Short catheter function<br>Significant risk of cerebral embolization |
| Brachial | Highly accessible | Inadequate collateral circulation<br>High degree of disability if complication occurs<br>Adjacent median nerve<br>Not recommended by most authors |

Modified from Venus B, Mallory DL. Vascular cannulation. In: Civetta JM, Taylor RW, Kirby RR, eds. *Critical Care.* Philadelphia, Pa: JB Lippincott; 1988:165.

equipment and additional items are listed in Table 27–3. For distal extremities, 1.25- to 1.5-inch 20-gauge Teflon catheters are usually used. Some are available with a built-in guidewire.

For femoral artery catheterization, a 0.35-mm guidewire fed through an 18-gauge cannulating needle may be used. The catheter should be 3.75 to 4.5 inches long, depending on the

**TABLE 27–3.** Arterial Catheterization Equipment

Antiseptic preparation solution: chlorhexidine, povidone-iodine, 70% isopropyl alcohol
Gloves
1% lidocaine (Xylocaine) without epinephrine or alternative for local anesthesia
20- or 22-gauge catheter or smaller (with or without guidewire) for peripheral artery
18-gauge thin-walled needle for femoral artery
3.125- or 4.75-inch 20-gauge catheter for femoral artery
0.021-mm guidewire
5-mL syringe
Heparin-flushed tubing, transducer, flushing system, and pressure monitor
2-0 or 3-0 silk suture on cutting needle if femoral artery is cannulated
Needle holder (sterile) if curved needle is used
Sterile dressing

*Recommended*

Sterile drapes and several 4 × 4 gauze pads
Armboard
Towel roll
Tape
15-cm flushed extension tubing with three-way stopcock and 10-mL syringe containing heparinized saline
Pencil probe Doppler monitor for dorsalis pedis artery in children

patient's body size. Larger cannulas are used for procedures such as cardiac catheterization but are not recommended for routine monitoring. In children, particularly in infants, the use of a Doppler pulse monitor on the dorsalis pedis artery may assist with artery localization and guide arterial compression for hemostasis.[7]

## ARTERIAL CATHETERIZATION TECHNIQUES

### How Is the Radial Artery Approached?

To cannulate the radial artery, the wrist is gently hyperextended 30° to 60° and the hand supinated. Rolled gauze or a washcloth can be placed beneath the wrist and the arm immobilized by taping the hand and forearm to an armboard. It is also helpful to tape along the thumb to provide additional skin immobilization during cannulation. After gloves have been placed, the radial area is cleansed and anesthetized using a small-gauge needle. Lidocaine serves two purposes: it decreases the patient's discomfort and reduces arterial vasospasm.[8] If the pulse is lost while the local anesthetic is injected, massaging the wheal should restore it. The catheter device may be flushed with heparinized saline before use to reduce clotting during placement.

It is helpful to palpate the artery with two fingers alongside, and not over, the pulse to fix it in place and to help the operator visualize the path of the vessel. The needle is introduced, bevel up, through the skin at a 15° to 30° angle and advanced toward the palpated pulse until blood return is noted. Once again, the needle is advanced sufficiently so that the entire bevel is within the vessel. If threading is unsuccessful, the technique may be changed to one of transfixation, in which the needle and catheter are passed through both walls of the artery, after which the needle is completely withdrawn. The catheter is then slowly withdrawn until pulsatile blood flow is observed, and the needle is gently reinserted three fourths of its length to act as a stylet. Usually the catheter can then be easily advanced with a rotating (spinning) motion as the needle is held still. Inconsistent blood return may be resolved by rotating the bevel of the needle 90° or more to exclude partial occlusion by an intimal flap.

### Liquid Stylet

Alternatively, the radial artery can be cannulated using a liquid stylet. The catheter over the needle is advanced through the far side of the artery. A syringe filled with heparinized saline is attached and the needle and catheter withdrawn until blood return is noted. The needle is removed, and the catheter is advanced while the heparinized saline solution is gently flushed.[9]

### Guidewire Technique

Some catheters have a guidewire that, after blood return is noted, is advanced through the needle into the artery, after which the catheter is threaded over it. This is an especially useful approach when other techniques have failed.

### Pressure Monitoring

Another technique for cannulating difficult radial arteries uses the pressure-monitoring system while the catheter is placed. The system is connected directly to the catheter-over-needle. As the needle enters the arterial lumen, an arterial pressure curve is displayed on the screen. The catheter is advanced while observing the screen. Once it is in place, the needle is removed, and the tubing to the monitor is re-connected to the catheter, which is then secured and the site dressed after removing the thumb tape and placing the wrist back in neutral position to avoid nerve injury.[10]

### How Is the Femoral Artery Approached?

To cannulate the femoral artery, the leg is extended and slightly abducted. Folded towels are placed under the ipsilateral hip of obese individuals to help elevate the inguinal area. Large abdominal folds may be taped out of the working field, or an assistant may hold them away from the inguinal area. Once the leg is positioned, the inguinal region is cleansed, preferably with a chlorhexidine-based solution. Clipping the hair is optional. Local anesthesia is infiltrated using a small-gauge needle.

The artery is palpated 0.3 to 1.5 cm below the inguinal fold, and the needle is advanced toward the pulse at a nearly perpendicular 75° angle. Once pulsatile flow is obtained, the needle and syringe are lowered against the skin while maintaining blood flow. The syringe is removed, and a flexible guidewire is inserted through the needle into the vessel. If difficulty advancing the wire is encountered, the needle may be advanced 1 mm or rotated to free the bevel if it is covered by an intimal flap. The needle is withdrawn, and, if necessary, the skin at the site of wire entry may be nicked to create a larger opening. A 5-cm or longer catheter is then advanced over the wire by rotating it in to its full length. The wire is removed, and the catheter is connected to the monitoring equipment. In distinction to other arterial catheter sites, the femoral catheter is sutured in place and the site cleansed and dressed.

### How Is the Axillary Artery Approached?

The left axillary artery is preferred over the right because the risk of inadvertent cerebral embolization is higher with right axillary artery catheterization. Any retrograde emboli that enter the adjacent central aortic circulation by way of the right axillary and subclavian artery traverse the aortic arch and the origins of the vertebral and carotid arteries, but any that enter through the left axillary and subclavian arteries do not.

The arm is extended and externally rotated. The elbow may be flexed, with its head resting in the patient's hand. The artery is located at its highest palpable point and entered at a 30° to 45° angle. Once adequate flow is confirmed, the catheter is connected to the monitoring system, secured, and dressed. Because it is difficult to immobilize this site, it is also advantageous to wire a longer (eg, 5-cm) catheter and suture it in place. Only small volumes of solution at slow flush rates should be used, thus lowering the risk of cerebral embolization.

### How Is the Brachial Artery Approached?

Brachial artery catheterization is generally avoided because of concern for inadequate collateral flow and an assumed

**TABLE 27–4.** Complications of Peripheral Arterial Cannulation

Local ischemia, inflammation, or infection
Arterial spasm
Hematoma formation and infection
Bleeding from cannula disconnection
Thrombosis
Proximal or distal embolization
Limb ischemia and necrosis
Sepsis
Pseudoaneurysm
Arteriovenous fistula
Peripheral neuropathy

Modified from Venus B, Mallory DL. Vascular cannulation. In: Civetta JM, Taylor RW, Kirby RR, eds. *Critical Care*. Philadelphia, Pa: JB Lippincott; 1988:167.

increased risk of complications. If one chooses to use the brachial artery, the arm is positioned fully extended. The artery is palpated above the antecubital fossa medial to the bicipital tendon. In an adult, a 2-inch 20-gauge catheter-over-needle is inserted using the same technique as for the radial artery; a modified Seldinger technique may also be used. Once the artery is cannulated, the arm must be splinted in the extended position.

After the artery has been cannulated and the catheter gently flushed, the system is then secured to the skin in a way that allows periodic monitoring of the site and prevents accidental disconnection and/or inadvertent loss of the line due to the tubing getting caught on any external obstacle.

### What Factors Predispose to Complications?

Complications of arterial cannulation are summarized in Table 27–4. Factors predisposing to complications are summarized in Table 27–5. This section addresses some of the more common or serious complications.

### Bleeding, Thrombosis, and Retrograde Cerebral Embolization

Risk of bleeding is increased in anticoagulated patients or after multiple puncture attempts. The risk of thrombosis is increased with large-gauge catheters and with a duration of

**TABLE 27–5.** Factors Increasing the Chance of Complications After Peripheral Arterial Cannulation

Low perfusion state
Use of vasopressors
Intrinsic vascular disease
Female gender
Cannula/vessel diameter ratio near unity
Tapered catheters
Catheter material (non-Teflon)
Long duration of cannulation
Repeated cannulation attempts
?Abnormal Allen test results
Insertion by cutdown
Presence of bacteremia
Bleeding diathesis or hypercoagulable states
Use of dextrose solutions for flush systems
Flush system close to insertion site

Modified from Venus B, Mallory DL. Vascular cannulation. In: Civetta JM, Taylor RW, Kirby RR, eds. *Critical Care*. Philadelphia, Pa: JB Lippincott; 1988:167.

catheterization of >48 hours.[11] Repeated catheterization attempts also increase the risk of thrombosis.[12]

Vessel size appears to directly correlate with the incidence of thrombosis. Because the femoral and axillary arteries have a larger radius, thrombosis is relatively rare.[10] Continuous heparin flush systems reduce the overall incidence of thrombosis, whereas intermittent flushing is ineffective.[12]

Factors that increase the risk of retrograde cerebral embolization include small stature; use of (in decreasing order) the temporal, right axillary, left axillary, right radial, or left radial site; and rapid flush rate or large flush volumes. The flush or irrigation flow rate should be kept at <1 mL/s, especially in infants or children or when a proximal site is cannulated.

### Infection and Sepsis

Arterial catheter infection occurs infrequently as a complication of catheterization if the site is used for <96 hours.[13] Guidewire exchange is a safe alternative if new sites are not available. Sepsis secondary to nosocomial bacteremia is an important but uncommon complication of arterial cannulation. It does not occur in the absence of catheter-related infection. Conversely, preexisting bacteremia may not resolve until a colonized arterial catheter is removed.[14] Local inflammation as a predictive sign of catheter infection is not consistent.[15-17] Local inflammation may be the result of irritation by the dressing, topical antibiotics, or reaction to the catheter.

Skin flora are usually the source of catheter-related infections, although contaminated infusate and monitoring equipment have also been implicated.[8] Organisms isolated from arterial catheter infections are usually gram negative and include *Pseudomonas*, *Serratia*, *Enterobacter*, and *Flavobacterium*. *Candida* is occasionally isolated. Catheter-related infection causing delayed radial artery rupture has also been described.[18] Such complications are infrequent but can lead to hemorrhage or pseudoaneurysm formation.[19]

## CENTRAL VENOUS CATHETERIZATION

The percutaneous insertion of a CVC was originally described over 40 years ago. Since this first description, the indications for and number of placements of CVCs have proliferated. Central venous cannulation is associated with a number of significant complications, some of them potentially fatal; therefore, it is not surprising that safer techniques are being developed to minimize the chances of adverse outcomes during placement of a CVC.

### What Techniques Are Used?

Currently, the most common technique is the modified Seldinger (over the guidewire) external anatomic landmark-guided approach. Some studies have actually shown that there may not be a direct correlation between landmarks and vessel location, and minor and major complications as well as a reported failure of cannulation in as many as 19% of patients have been described. During the 1980s, Doppler-assisted CVC placement was introduced. Subsequent improvements in technology and increasing availability have made two-dimensional US the preferred method for vessel location.

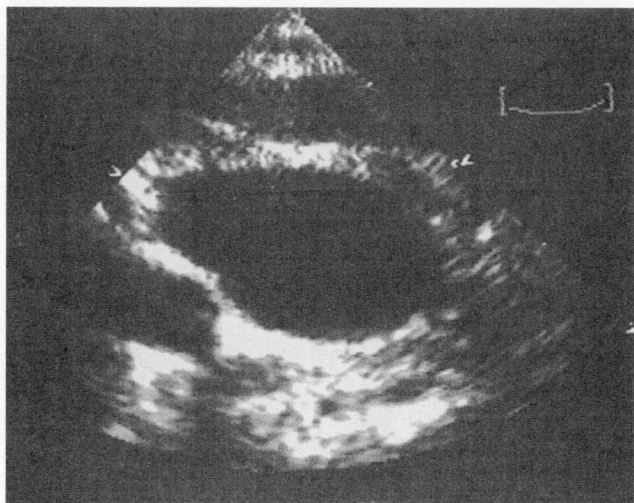

**FIGURE 27–1.** Note the relationship between the internal jugular vein on top and the carotid artery on the bottom left of the picture. Each dot on the sector scan represents 1 cm of distance or depth.

The advantages of US are noninvasive detection of the target vessel location, depth, and related structures and determination of vessel caliber and patency, both of which ultimately steer cannulation strategy (Figs. 27–1 to 27–3). US as an aid to CVC placement has been consistently found to decrease the following:

1. The failure and complication rate
2. The number of cannulation attempts required to access the desired vein
3. The time to cannulation
4. The incidence of accidental carotid puncture[20-22]

We believe that the single most important advance in the field of CVC placement has been the introduction of US for CVC placement and positioning, specifically when using the internal jugular vein (IJV) approach.

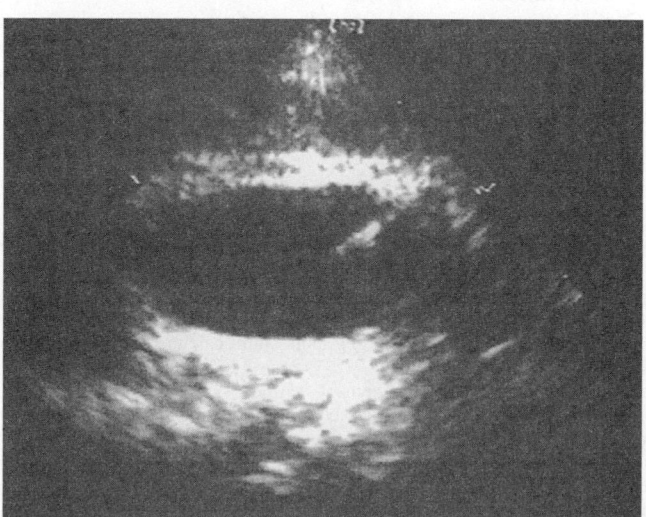

**FIGURE 27–2.** Position of the guidewire inside the internal jugular is confirmed by the presence of the echogenic shadow inside the vessel.

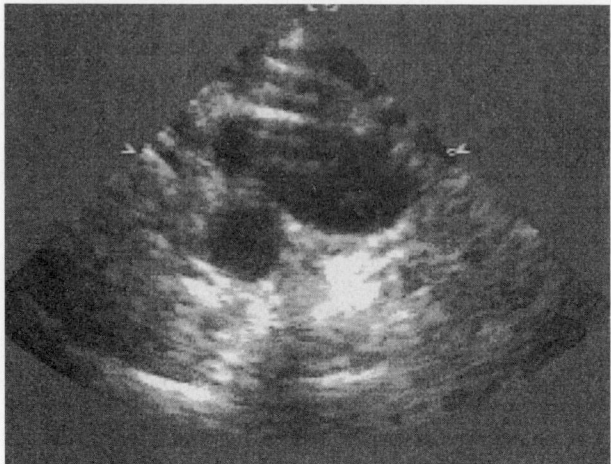

**FIGURE 27–3.** Note the relationship between the compressible internal jugular vein on top and the noncompressible pulsatile carotid artery on the bottom left of the picture. Each dot on the sector scan represents 1 cm of distance or depth.

## What Equipment Is Necessary?

Table 27–6 summarizes the indications for CVC placement.[23] Equipment for cannulation is available in sterile prepackaged kits. Most adult kits include an 18-gauge thin-walled needle or a 16-gauge catheter over a 20-gauge needle, a 0.89-mm (0.036-inch) diameter soft tipped J-wire, and a single-lumen or multilumen CVC. Table 27–7 lists the recommended equipment. Masks, caps, and sterile gloves and gowns should be used. The use of full-barrier precautions during CVC placement has been one of the key strategies in the prevention of intravascular-related infections.[24]

## How Is It Done?

The essential equipment is gathered before beginning the procedure to avoid delay. The patient is placed supine, and if the patient is nervous or uncomfortable, a sedative or narcotic may be administered.

Once a venous site is selected, positioning the patient is a key to success. For clavicular or jugular approaches, the Trendelenburg position (head down) is recommended unless contraindicated by elevated intracranial pressure or cardiores-

**TABLE 27–6.** Common Indications for Central Venous Cannulation

Hemodynamic evaluation and management (eg, central venous pressure or pulmonary artery pressure monitors)
The need for multiple concomitant intravenous catheters
Infusion of thrombogenic material (eg, potassium, calcium chloride, hyperalimentation solutions)
Inability to cannulate peripheral veins
Immediate or potential need for massive fluid resuscitation
Diagnostic techniques (eg, cardiac catheterization, endomyocardial biopsy)
Emergency transvenous pacing
Treatment of air embolism (eg, sitting craniotomy)
Temporary venous access (eg, hemodialysis, plasmapheresis)

From Novak RA, Venus B. Clavicular approaches for central vein cannulation. *Probl Crit Care.* 1988;2:248.

**TABLE 27–7.** Central Venous Catheterization Equipment

Central venous catheter
Chlorhexidine or povidone-iodine and applicator
Mask with sterile gown and gloves
Sterile drapes and several 4 × 4 gauze pads
5-mL syringe with 1.5-inch 21- or 23-gauge locator needle (for use with internal jugular vein cannulation)
Flexible tip guidewire 10 cm longer than the cannula to be inserted
Scalpel
Vessel dilator
Heparinized saline for catheter flush
2-0 or 3-0 silk suture on cutting needle
Needle holder (sterile) if curved needle is used
Sterile dressing

***Optional Equipment***

Sterile pencil probe Doppler and gel
Sterile tubing for manometry
Ultrasound equipment

piratory insufficiency. Ventilation and oxygenation must be monitored at all times during the procedure.

Historically, the patient's head has been turned to the contralateral side for the IJV approach, and for the subclavian vein (SCV) approach, the shoulders are retracted by placing a towel roll vertically between the scapulae. These recommendations should be reconsidered in view of data that show that head rotation moves the IJV over the carotid artery, predisposing it to incidental puncture if the vein is transfixed, as is usually the case during cannulation (Table 27–8).[25]

Our current recommendation is to leave the head in as neutral a position as possible.[25] This is also ideal for subclavian catheterization because in both instances, turning the head away from the side of catheterization reduces the acute angle between the IJV and SCV, thereby predisposing the guidewire and catheter going into the SCV from the IJV, and vice versa.[26] In point of fact, turning a patient's head toward the side of subclavian catheterization makes passage of the catheter into the neck least likely. Use of a shoulder roll is similarly counterproductive in that it actually decreases the dimension of the SCV by compressing it between the clavicle and the first rib.[26]

Operator preparation is also essential; adequate lighting should be available and all possible obstructions removed. For supraclavicular approaches, we suggest that the operator be positioned at the head of the bed on the side of the procedure. For infraclavicular approaches, the operator is ideally positioned lateral to the patient's shoulder on the side of the cannulation site. A qualified assistant with training and experience should be in attendance.

**TABLE 27–8.** Percentage Overlap of the Carotid Artery by the Internal Jugular Vein as Shown by Ultrasound With Different Degrees of Head Rotation

| Side of Neck | 0° | 40° | 80° |
|---|---|---|---|
| Right | 1.5 ± 0.8 | 6.5 ± 2.8 | 27.5 ± 7.4* |
|  | 0 to 17.4 | 0 to 48 | 0 to 100 |
| Left | 5.2 ± 2.9 | 11.5 ± 4.9 | 44.7 ± 7.2* |
|  | 0 to 54 | 0 to 76.5 | 0 to 100 |

*$P<.05$ compared with 0% and 40% on the same side of the neck.
Modified from Sulek CA, Weiss L, Gravenstein N, et al. Influence of head position on relationship between internal jugular vein and carotid artery. *Anesth Analg.* 1996;82:125.

The insertion site must be scrubbed with an appropriate antimicrobial solution. Choices include chlorhexidine, povidone-iodine in 70% isopropyl alcohol, 70% alcohol, and tincture of iodine. Chlorhexidine and 70% isopropyl alcohol are ideal alternatives for those patients allergic to iodine. Whichever solution is used, standard surgical protocol must be followed. Operators must wash their hands with an antimicrobial soap and wear sterile gloves before sterilizing the skin. From the intended site of insertion, scrubbing is done in a continuous, outward circular motion to cover a margin of approximately 5 cm peripheral to the area of fenestration in the drapes used. This approach allows coverage over the external jugular vein (EJV), IJV, and SCV sites. Final preparation may be completed at this time.

In the awake patient, infiltration of the skin and catheter path with a local anesthetic is advisable. Lidocaine 1% without epinephrine is most commonly used. With a 25-gauge needle, a 1-cm skin wheal is made at the site of insertion. A 1.5-inch 22-gauge needle is used for infraclavicular approaches, and subsequent 0.2-mL boluses are injected after advancing the needle in 2-mm increments. The syringe is aspirated before injection to exclude free-flowing blood, and injection is done slowly to minimize burning and pain from tissue distention in sensitive patients; between 2 and 4 mL is usually adequate for analgesia. If large volumes and deep infiltration are used for IJV cannulation, it is possible to anesthetize the ipsilateral phrenic nerve.

In general, if the procedure is supplemented with sedatives, it is preferable to use either benzodiazepines or narcotics because specific pharmacologic antagonists are available. Midazolam, a short-acting benzodiazepine, is favored for patients with substantial anxiety. Doses of 0.5 to 1 mg titrated intravenously over a 2-minute period are generally effective.

## What Placement Sites Are Used?

Table 27–9 summarizes the advantages and disadvantages of various central venous insertion sites.[23] Table 27–10 lists central venous insertion sites in a proposed order of preference for common clinical situations.[23]

Supraclavicular sites interfere less with cardiopulmonary

**TABLE 27–9.** Advantages and Disadvantages of Various Central Venous Approaches

| Approach | Advantages | Disadvantages |
|---|---|---|
| External jugular vein | Part of surface anatomy<br>Clotting abnormalities do not prohibit<br>Pneumothorax avoided<br>Head-of-table access<br>Often prominent in elderly | High failure rate<br>Not ideal for prolonged central venous access<br>Dressing and maintenance are difficult<br>Poor landmarks in obese patients<br>Unsuccessful in young patients<br>Difficult approach for threading central venous catheters |
| Internal jugular vein | Pneumothorax rate<br>High success rate<br>Head-of-table access (general anesthesia)<br>Control of bleeding is easier<br>Right internal jugular straight path to superior vena cava (easier to pass catheters, fewer malpositions) | Not ideal for prolonged central venous access (eg, total parenteral nutrition)<br>Uncomfortable<br>Dressing and catheter difficult to maintain<br>Left internal jugular approach increases risk of thoracic duct injury and central vein perforation<br>Poor landmarks in obese or edematous patients<br>Difficult access with tracheostomies<br>Contraindicated with intracranial hypertension<br>Vein more prone to collapse with volume depletion or shock<br>Not ideal for temporary hemodialysis<br>Difficult access during emergencies when airway control is being established<br>Carotid artery puncture incidence is relatively frequent (4%) |
| Supraclavicular | Low incidence of pneumothorax<br>High success rate<br>Easier to pass catheters<br>Head-of-table access<br>Good landmarks<br>No interference with CPR<br>Anatomic landmarks constant<br>Short path from skin to vein | Control of bleeding is difficult<br>Pneumothorax possible<br>Not ideal for prolonged venous access<br>More uncomfortable<br>Dressing and catheter maintenance difficult<br>Thoracic duct puncture possible on the left<br>Not ideal for temporary hemodialysis |
| Infraclavicular | Easier to maintain dressing and more comfortable for patients<br>Better landmarks in obesity<br>Large vein does not collapse during volume depletion or shock<br>Better access when airway control is being established simultaneously<br>Multiple catheter insertions easier when massive volume resuscitation needed | Higher risk of pneumothorax<br>Compression of bleeding site difficult<br>Decreased success rate with inexperience<br>Long distance from skin to vein<br>Catheter malposition common<br>Relatively inaccessible from head of table<br>Interference with chest compressions during CPR |
| Femoral | Fast, easy access; high success rate<br>Does not interfere with chest compressions<br>Does not interfere with airway management<br>No risk of pneumothorax<br>Supine or head-down position not necessary during insertion | Delayed circulation of drugs during CPR<br>Higher risk of complications in patients with abdominal pathology<br>Prevents patient mobilization<br>Arteriovenous fistula possible<br>Difficult to keep the site sterile<br>Greater difficulty with pulmonary artery catheter flotation |

CPR, cardiopulmonary resuscitation.
Modified from Novak RA, Venus B. Clavicular approaches for central vein cannulation. *Probl Crit Care*. 1988;2:249–250.

**TABLE 27–10.** Preferred Techniques for Specific Clinical Situations

| Clinical Situation | Choices (Order of Preference) | | | | |
| | 1st | 2nd | 3rd | 4th | 5th |
| --- | --- | --- | --- | --- | --- |
| Bleeding diathesis | EJ | Femoral* Peripheral large-vein cannulation | IJ† | High clavicular notch‡ | SC |
| Obesity or edema | SC | IC | IJ | Femoral | EJ |
| Decreased pulmonary reserve; hyperinflation or PEEP | EJ | IJ† | Femoral | SC | IC |
| TPN | IC | SC | IJ | EJ | Short term |
| Hypovolemia; shock | IC or SC | Femoral | IJ | Peripheral large-vein cannulation | EJ |
| Cardiopulmonary resuscitation | IJ | SC | EJ | IC | Femoral |
| Emergency airway management§ | Femoral | IC | SC | IJ | EJ |
| Temporary hemodialysis | IC | Femoral | IJ | SC | EJ |
| Multiple catheter insertion | IC | SC | IC or SC | IC or IJ | SC or IJ |
| Pulmonary artery catheter insertion | IC or RIJ | SC or IJ | IJ | EJ | Femoral |
| Temporary pacemaker‖ | RIJ | RSC | LIC | EJ | Femoral |
| Tracheotomy or sternal wounds | EJ | IJ | Femoral | SC | IC |
| Short diagnostic techniques | IJ/femoral | SC | IC | | |
| Inability to lower head | Femoral | EJ | SC | IC | |

*Femoral approach is most useful for emergency large-vein access for volume resuscitation and rarely used for hemodynamic monitoring or temporary pacing.

†Higher (ie, nearer the cricoid than the clavicle) IJ approaches recommended.

‡High clavicular notch refers to skin puncture 1-2 cm above clavicle, thereby allowing easier tamponade for arterial bleeding. The skin puncture site is close to that in the central IJ technique.

§Situations where airway is unstable and control is highest priority. Simultaneous large-vein access is next to highest priority; however, interference with airway control is contraindicated.

‖Order of vein preference would be the same as for pulmonary artery catheterization if balloon-tipped Swan or Paceport Swan is used. The semirigid pacing catheter using fluoroscopy increases the preferability of the femoral approach. If SC or IJ is used, the preferred site is the right side.

EJ, external jugular; IC, infraclavicular; IJ, internal jugular; L, left when one is preferred; PEEP, positive end-expiratory pressure; R, right; SC, supraclavicular; TPN, total parenteral nutrition.

Modified from Novak RA, Venus B. Clavicular approaches for central vein cannulation. *Probl Crit Care* 1988;2:249–250.

resuscitation than infraclavicular or jugular sites and therefore should be considered during resuscitation. A long (30-cm) femoral catheter inserted so that its tip lies above the diaphragm is an acceptable alternative.

Patients who have a chest tube in place and who need a CVC should have a site chosen on the same side as the chest tube, if possible, to reduce the risk of iatrogenic pneumothorax. Those with severe unilateral lung disease should be catheterized on the ipsilateral side. A pneumothorax on the nonaffected side severely compromises the already marginal pulmonary status.

Subclavian sites are best avoided in patients with chronic obstructive lung disease or in those receiving high-level positive end-expiratory pressure. These patients are at high risk for pneumothorax. An EJV, if prominent, would be the first choice in this group. It is also the first site choice in patients with a bleeding diathesis because the subclavian sites are avoided in this circumstance because compression is impossible if the subclavian artery is inadvertently punctured. The use of US systems to visualize target veins and aid CVC placement has proved of tremendous value in this field and has added a new dimension of safety.[20–22]

## TECHNIQUES OF CENTRAL VENOUS CATHETERIZATION

### What Considerations Are Generally Applicable?

Strict aseptic technique must be used. The site is prepared as previously described. If a finder needle is used, blood

return is confirmed with the finder needle, the angle and depth of the finder needle are carefully noted, and the needle is removed. A catheter-over-needle is then inserted using the same angle and depth at the exact site. Alternatively, the needle may be left in place with the syringe attached to prevent air embolism and the catheter-over-needle advanced directly behind it at the same angle to the same depth.

Once free-flowing venous blood is obtained, the catheter-over-needle is advanced 2 to 3 mm with the needle in a plane parallel to the vein. The catheter is advanced into the vein, the needle/syringe apparatus is removed, and blood return is confirmed. The hub of the catheter should be occluded at all times if the patient is breathing spontaneously to prevent air embolism.

A J-tipped guidewire is then advanced (with the J-tip leading) to a maximal distance of 20 cm (many CVC guidewires are 60 cm long). The short catheter is removed, and a small skin cut is made at the lateral side of the guidewire entry site. The dilator should then be passed smoothly through the skin and the subcutaneous tissues. It should not be advanced farther than necessary to dilate the path to the vessel itself (ie, 1-2 cm beyond the depth of the previous needle insertion). With skin traction held over the incision, the catheter is advanced over the guidewire, taking care not to allow the guidewire to migrate into the heart during this maneuver. The catheter is then advanced to the desired depth. After removal of the guidewire, blood return is confirmed from each port before flushing with heparinized saline. The ports should be flushed within 1 to 2 minutes of insertion to prevent catheter thrombosis. The catheter is held in place until it is securely sutured at a depth chosen to ensure superior vena cava and not intra-atrial placement, after which a dressing is applied. The catheter site is dressed according to protocol after suturing the catheter.

## How Is the External Jugular Vein Catheterized?

The patient's head is positioned facing 30° to 45° away from the EJV selected. The right EJV is generally preferred because of easier catheter passage. The vein may be better visualized if the patient performs the Valsalva maneuver or is placed in a Trendelenburg position. If the vein cannot be visualized or palpated, another site should be selected.

The large-bore needle or catheter-over-needle is inserted at a 15° to 20° angle above the skin along the vein course. Slight negative pressure is kept on the syringe while the vein is sought. As the vein is entered, blood return is noted. The needle is then advanced 1 to 2 mm. If a catheter-over-needle is used, the catheter is advanced into the vein. If a longer catheter is to be inserted, a guidewire is passed through the catheter or a large-bore needle is used. The guidewire is easiest to pass if the J-tip is advanced and the wire is rotated during passage to allow the J-tip to find its way. Several attempts may be necessary to advance the guidewire beyond the EJV-SCV junction.

## How Is the Internal Jugular Vein Catheterized?

The patient's head is positioned facing no more than 20° away from the selected site. The following landmarks are identified and palpated: the sternal notch, carotid artery, cricoid cartilage, and the two heads of the sternocleidomastoid (SCM) muscle.

The course of the IJV is from the apex of the triangle outlined by the clavicle inferiorly, the sternal head of the SCM medially, and the clavicular head of the SCM laterally through the middle or medial portion of this triangle just lateral to the carotid artery and 1 to 3 cm deep to the skin.

Three basic approaches—anterior, medial, and posterior—are used for IJV cannulation. A high or low site may be selected for each approach. Higher sites have a lower risk of pneumothorax or hemothorax but also have slightly lower success rates because the vein is smaller at the entry site.

### Anterior Approach

In an anterior approach, the finder needle (22-gauge 1.5-inch) is placed medial to the sternal head of the SCM between the apex of the triangle and the cricoid cartilage and lateral to the carotid artery. The needle is advanced at a 10° to 20° angle to the skin toward the ipsilateral shoulder. Negative pressure is applied to the syringe until blood return is noted. If the first pass is unsuccessful after insertion to 3 cm depth, the needle is slowly withdrawn while aspirating. If blood is still not encountered, it is redirected medially 10° to 15° and advanced again. The procedure is repeated until blood appears in the syringe. The needle path should not cross the sagittal plane nor enter the area where the carotid artery is palpated. The carotid should not be palpated during actual venipuncture because this action decreases the IJV diameter. If multiple

passes with the finder needle are unsuccessful, venipuncture with a larger needle should not be attempted. Instead, a new site approximately halfway down the SCM should be selected.

### Median Approach

For the median approach, the finder needle is placed at the apex of the triangle formed by the two bellies of the SCM. The apex is easiest to locate by palpation. The needle is advanced at a 30° angle to the skin toward the ipsilateral nipple. The vein is usually <2.5 cm deep, but the needle may occasionally have to be advanced up to 4 cm. If the first pass is unsuccessful after insertion to 3 cm, the needle is slowly withdrawn while continuing to aspirate with the syringe. If blood is not encountered, the needle is redirected 10° to 15° medially. This approach may be repeated up to five times before choosing a lower site. As with the anterior approach, to avoid complications the needle should not be directed across the sagittal plane to lessen the chance of carotid artery puncture.

### Posterior Approach

The posterior approach theoretically poses an increased risk of carotid artery, tracheal, and sympathetic chain puncture; however, these complications have not been reported frequently.[27] The finder needle is positioned 4 cm above the clavicle and lateral to the clavicular head of the SCM. The needle is advanced beneath the SCM toward the contralateral nipple. Venous return is usually noted before a maximum depth of 4 to 5 cm is reached. Deeper insertion angles may be necessary to pass the needle beneath the SCM. If unsuccessful, the process may be repeated at a point along the lateral border of the SCM closer to the clavicle.

### Carotid Artery Puncture

The incidence of unintentional carotid artery puncture is at least 4%, even in experienced hands. It is, therefore, important to verify that the vessel entered is not the artery. We have found that when using a pencil probe Doppler, the artery is reliably avoided. If a landmark and palpation technique is used, it is wise to attach a piece of intravenous tubing to the needle, aspirate blood into the tubing, elevate the tubing, remove the syringe, and verify that blood flows back into the vessel. We routinely perform this manometry because the absence of pulsatile blood does not preclude arterial puncture since the needle bevel may be against the artery wall, blood color is unreliable, and the consequences of dilation and catheterization of the carotid artery can be devastating.[28]

## How Is the Subclavian Vein Catheterized?

### Infraclavicular Approach

The SCV is usually approached by the infraclavicular approach; other approaches are described in the following paragraphs for the sake of completeness. The patient is positioned supine. A towel between the scapulae may actually decrease the size of the SCV by compressing it between the clavicle and first rib.[25] The head is left in a neutral position or turned toward the side being catheterized to decrease the angle be-

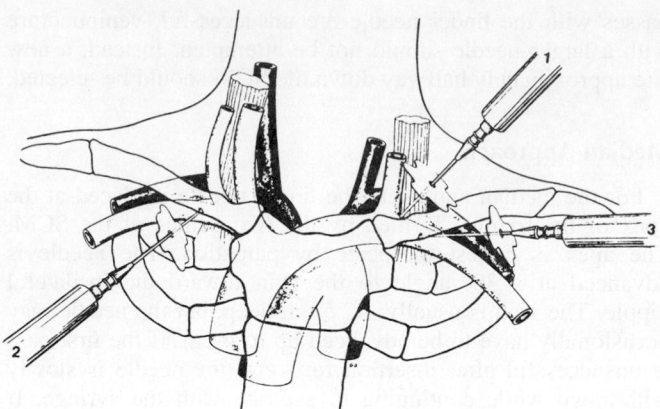

**FIGURE 27–4.** 1, Supraclavicular, modified junctional approach (Helm-kamp); 2, infraclavicular, midclavicular approach—scalene tubercle orientation; 3, infraclavicular, lateral approach. (From Novak RA, Venus B. Clavicular approaches for central vein cannulation. *Probl Crit Care.* 1988;2:256.)

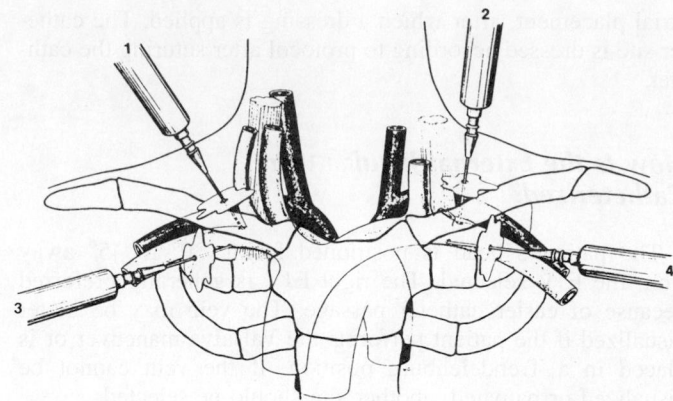

**FIGURE 27–5.** 1, Supraclavicular, junctional approach (Yoffa); 2, supraclavicular, anterior scalene-first rib approach; 3, midclavicular approach, sternal notch orientation; 4, infraclavicular, medial approach—sternal notch orientation. (From Novak RA, Venus B. Clavicular approaches for central vein cannulation. *Probl Crit Care.* 1988;2:254.)

tween the subclavian and ipsilateral jugular vein to make it more difficult for the guidewire to find its way into the IJV. The following landmarks are identified: the inferior border of the clavicle, the sternal notch, and the SCM-clavicular triangle. Infraclavicular approaches may be divided into three basic insertion points.

## Lateral Approach

The lateral insertion point is lateral to the midclavicular line at the junction of the lateral and middle thirds of the clavicle (Fig. 27–4). A large-bore needle is directed beneath the clavicle by "marching" it down the clavicle or by inserting it 1 to 2 cm inferior to the clavicle and slipping beneath it. The needle/syringe assembly is kept parallel to the skin surface as it is gently advanced toward the sternal notch. The index finger of the nondominant hand is kept on the sternal notch as a guide during venipuncture, and the thumb is held over the needle to help guide it under the clavicle. It is often helpful to bend (curve) the needle gently to facilitate passing it under the clavicle. Once venous return is noted, the bevel of the needle is oriented caudad to minimize guidewire malposition.

## Midclavicular and Medial Approach

The procedure is the same for the second subclavian insertion point (midclavicular) (Figs. 27–4 to 27–6) and for the third point (medial) (see Figs. 27–5 and 27–6), which is at the junction of the middle and medial thirds of the clavicle. If venipuncture is unsuccessful on the first pass at any point, the needle path may be redirected 5° to 10° above the sternal notch and advanced, keeping the needle/syringe assembly parallel to the skin surface. No more than five passes at each insertion point should be attempted.

After successful venipuncture, the basic procedure outlined earlier is used to insert the introducer and then the catheter.

## Supraclavicular Approach

Patients are positioned either with the head turned slightly to the contralateral side or neutral. The right side is preferred to avoid the thoracic duct and because catheter placement is

easier. Three supraclavicular approaches are determined by landmarks and skin puncture sites. The anatomic relationships and proper and improper needle insertions for supraclavicular and inferior clavicular approaches are shown in Figures 27–4 to 27–8.

## Junctional Approach

The finder needle is placed at a 45° angle between the lateral border of the clavicular head of the SCM and the clavicle and is advanced beneath the clavicle toward the sternal notch (see Figs. 27–4 to 27–6). The depth of puncture is usually between 0.5 and 5 cm. If the first pass is unsuccessful, the needle may be redirected in three ways: (1) 2 to 3 cm superior to the clavicle, close to the lateral border of the SCM; (2) 1 to 1.4 cm above the junction of the clavicle and the lateral border of the SCM; or (3) 1 cm above the clavicle and 1 cm lateral to the lateral border of the SCM.

In a variation of the technique, after venipuncture, the large-bore needle or catheter-over-needle and syringe are "swung" laterally 35° from the sagittal plane and depressed slightly before passage of the guidewire or cannula.[29]

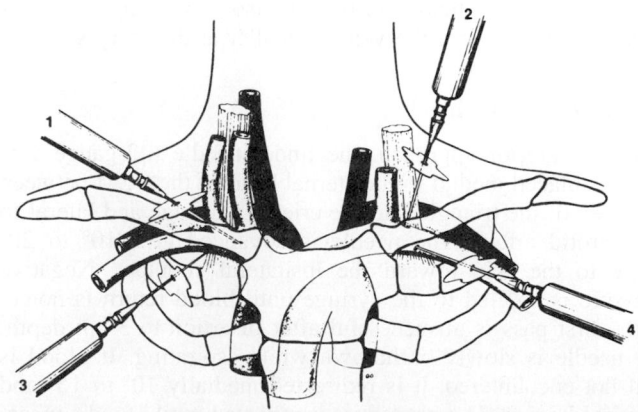

**FIGURE 27–6.** 1, Supraclavicular, modified junctional approach (Brahos); 2, supraclavicular, modified junctional approach (Haapaenimi and Slatis); 3, infraclavicular, midclavicular approach—clavicular sternocleidomastoid triangle orientation. (From Novak RA, Venus B. Clavicular approaches for central vein cannulation. *Probl Crit Care.* 1988;2:255.)

the course of the vein, and the catheter or guidewire is advanced into the vein.

A modification of this technique is described by Parsa and Tabora.[30] The needle is directed perpendicular to the scalene tubercle and advanced until venipuncture is achieved. The needle/syringe is aligned with the course of the vein before catheter or guidewire passage.

## Clavicular Notch Approach

For the clavicular notch approach, a patient is positioned with a towel roll placed under the shoulders to extend the neck slightly. The head is turned away from the site. The clavicular notch is located by palpating the sternal notch and sliding a finger along the anterior superior edge of the clavicle. It may also be palpated just lateral to the carotid artery along the anterosuperior edge of the clavicle.

The finder needle is advanced at a 30° to 45° angle to the skin parallel to the sagittal plane (see Fig. 27–8). The vein is usually located between 2 and 4 cm below the skin. Venipuncture is noted by a click and venous blood return. If the first attempt is unsuccessful, the needle is redirected and advanced in a slightly more lateral plane.

Alternatively, the insertion point may be extended 1 to 2 cm above the notch. With the same angle and direction of insertion, the needle is "marched" down the clavicle and advanced as it slips beneath the clavicle until blood return is noted.

## How Is the Femoral Vein Catheterized?

The patient is positioned supine, with slight external rotation of the leg. In an obese individual, an assistant may be needed to retract abdominal folds away from the inguinal field. Placing a folded towel under the hip may help elevate the inguinal field into better view.

The finder needle is positioned at a 45° angle above the skin medial to the femoral artery (Fig. 27–9). The skin site should be distal enough so that the tip of the needle does not traverse the inguinal ligament (ie, enter the abdominal cavity) as it is advanced cephalad. The needle may be directed slightly toward the palpable artery as it is advanced. Gentle negative

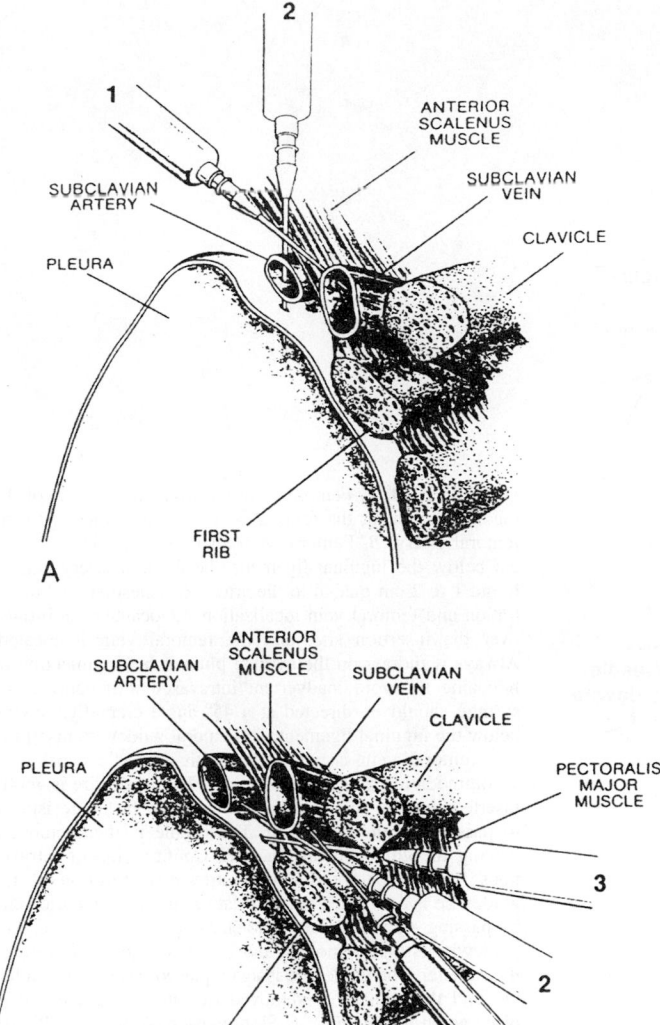

**FIGURE 27–7.** Sagittal view of subclavian vein and pertinent superficial and deep perivascular anatomy. Safe and unsafe insertions are demonstrated for supraclavicular and infraclavicular approaches. *A,* Supraclavicular approaches. 1, Safe angle and depth of insertion, anterior to the anterior scalenus muscle; 2, unsafe angle and depth of insertion prone to arterial and pleural puncture after traversing the anterior scalenus muscle. *B,* Infraclavicular approaches. 1, Safe angle and depth of insertion; 2, unsafe depth and angle predispose to arterial puncture; 3, insertion prone to pleural puncture. (From Novak RA, Venus B. Clavicular approaches for central vein cannulation. *Probl Crit Care.* 1988;2:245.)

## Anterior Scalene–First Rib Approach

For the anterior scalene–first rib approach, a patient's head is turned 45° to the opposite side and the neck flexed approximately 15° (see Fig. 27–5). The ipsilateral arm may be crossed over the abdomen. These maneuvers enlarge the costoclavicular space. The landmarks are identified by placing the nondominant index finger on the scalene tubercle located behind the insertion point of the clavicular head of the SCM.

The finder needle is inserted lateral to the scalene tubercle over the first rib and advanced until blood appears in the syringe. The process is repeated using the catheter-over-needle. When venipuncture is accomplished, the catheter-over-needle is lowered toward the shoulder to align the needle with

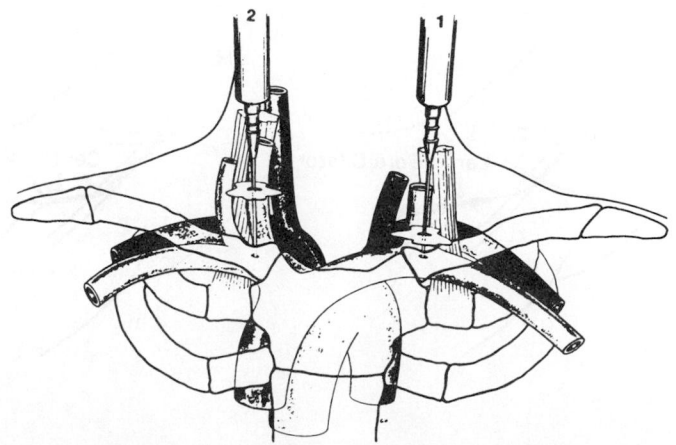

**FIGURE 27–8.** 1, Supraclavicular, clavicular notch approach; 2, supraclavicular, modified clavicular notch approach. (From Novak RA, Venus B. Clavicular approaches for central vein cannulation. *Probl Crit Care.* 1988;2:257.)

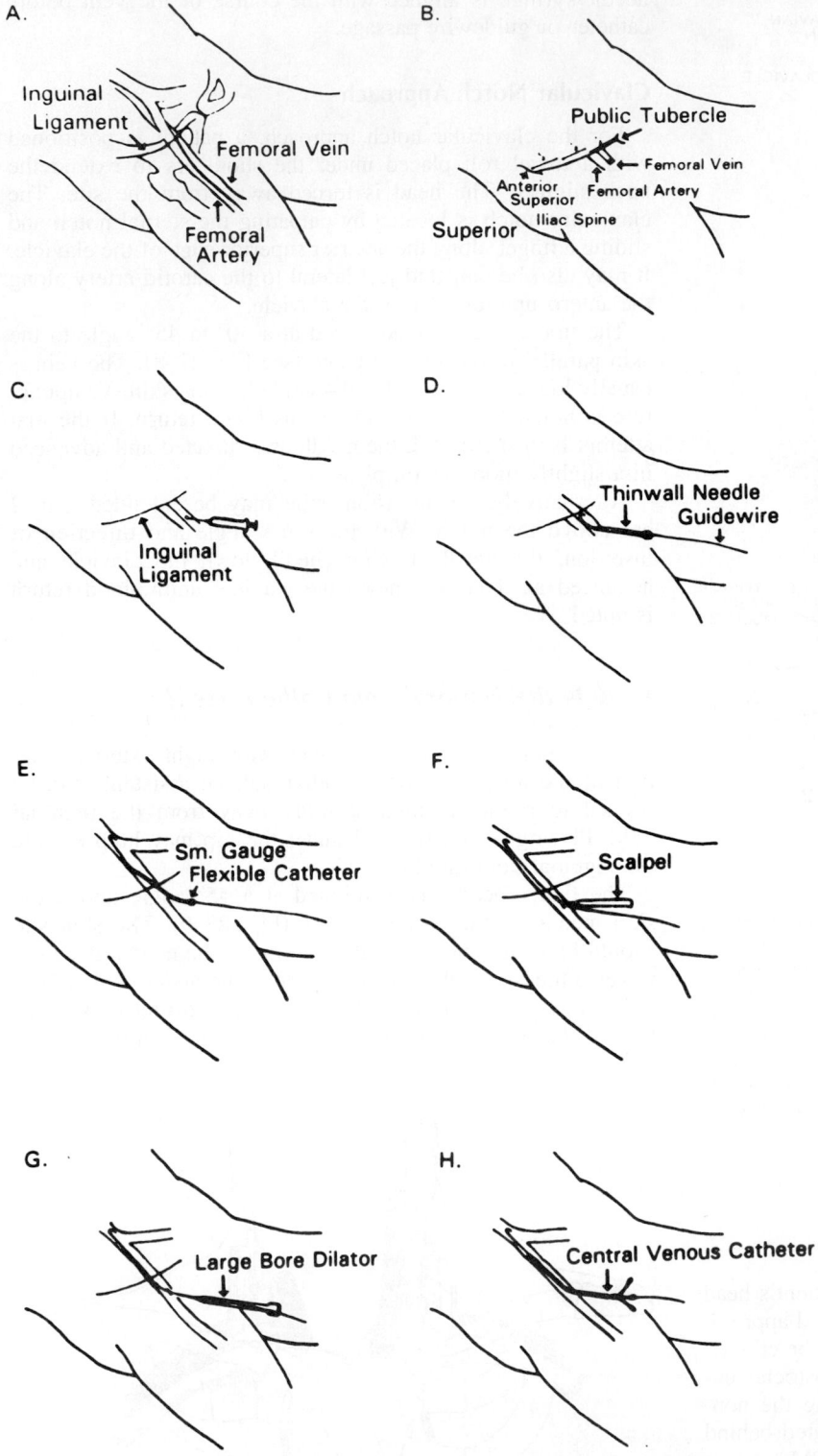

**FIGURE 27–9.** *A,* Femoral vein location. At the level of the inguinal ligament, the femoral vein is located medial to the femoral artery. *B,* Femoral vein anatomy. At a level 2 to 3 cm below the inguinal ligament, the femoral artery can be found 1 to 2 cm medial to the artery. *C,* Anesthetic administration and femoral vein localization. Lidocaine is infiltrated over the insertion site, and the femoral vein is located. Always withdraw on the syringe plunger before injection of lidocaine to avoid inadvertent intravascular injection. The syringe should be directed at a 45° angle cranially, staying below the inguinal ligament. *D,* Femoral guidewire insertion. The femoral vein is cannulated with a needle capable of accommodating a flexible guidewire. The guidewire is gently inserted through the needle. There should be no resistance to passage of the guidewire. The needle is then removed, leaving the guidewire in place. *E,* Confirmation of intravenous location before dilation. Intravenous location of the guidewire is confirmed before dilation of the cannulation site by passing a small flexible catheter over the guidewire. The guidewire is then removed, and blood is withdrawn through the catheter. The guidewire is again placed through the catheter, and the catheter is removed (leaving the guidewire in place again in the vein). *F,* Skin incision. A small (0.25-cm) skin incision is made adjacent to the site of entry of the guidewire. *G,* Insertion of venous dilator. A large-bore dilator is passed over the guidewire. The dilator is then removed, leaving the guidewire in place in the vein. *H,* Insertion of venous catheter. The central venous catheter is placed over the guidewire. The guidewire is removed, and the catheter is sutured securely in place. (From Tribett D, Brenner M. Peripheral and femoral vein cannulation. *Probl Crit Care.* 1988;2:279.)

pressure is applied on the syringe while advancing the needle. If venipuncture is unsuccessful on the first pass, the needle is redirected a few degrees closer to the femoral artery as it is advanced. As many as five passes may be necessary.

Once the vein is located, a large-bore needle is introduced at the same site and inserted to the same depth. After confirmation of adequate venous flow, a guidewire is introduced and the needle removed. The skin is nicked at the site of guidewire entry and the vein dilated. The catheter is inserted to its full length and secured.

## How Far Should a Central Venous Catheter Be Advanced?

Catheter tip position is of utmost importance after CVC placement. Cardiac tamponade and vessel perforation are well-known, potentially lethal complications of catheter tip malposition.[31,32] Both are preventable by ensuring proper positioning. Erosion and perforation occur either when the catheter tip is perpendicular to the vessel wall or when the tip enters the right atrium or ventricle.[27,32–34] This problem is particularly likely with left-sided approaches.[32] The critical angle of incidence between catheter tip and superior vena cava is probably 40°.

The catheter tip should lie within the superior vena cava but outside the right atrium. The distance between the puncture site and the superior vena cava-atrial junction can vary considerably, depending on the site selected and the patient's height and body habitus. CVCs should be inserted 13 to 16 cm for right SCV and jugular vein approaches and 15 to 20 cm for left-sided approaches. Thus, it makes little sense to use a 20-cm or longer catheter from the right side. One may approximate the insertion distance by placing the catheter over the chest, traveling over the envisioned path from the insertion site to a point 2 to 3 cm below the sternoclavicular joint. Several formulas based on a patient's height and the insertion site have been proposed to provide a potentially more accurate method for determining insertion distance. We have found that for right IJV placements, the catheter can be placed to a depth that is equal to the patient height in centimeters, divided by 10, minus 2. A chest film is necessary to reliably assess and predict catheter tip position and orientation.[35]

Right atrial electrocardiography is an alternative method to determine catheter position.[36,37] An exploring electrocardiographic electrode is placed on the end of a saline-filled catheter during insertion, and lead II is monitored. An increase in P wave size occurs as the catheter enters the right atrium. Withdrawing the catheter 1 cm beyond the point where the P wave size becomes normal ensures correct placement outside the heart, unless a patient's neck is subsequently flexed or the shoulder is adducted with jugular and subclavian catheters, respectively.

The risk of vessel perforation is minimized by positioning the catheter tip so that it lies parallel to the superior vena cava. This is most easily accomplished with right-sided placements. Left-sided catheterizations are more prone to result in acute impingement of the catheter tip against the vena cava (Fig. 27–10).[37] A review of reported cases and in vitro data suggests that any catheter tip that is at a >40° impingement angle to the superior vena cava should be repositioned.[38,39]

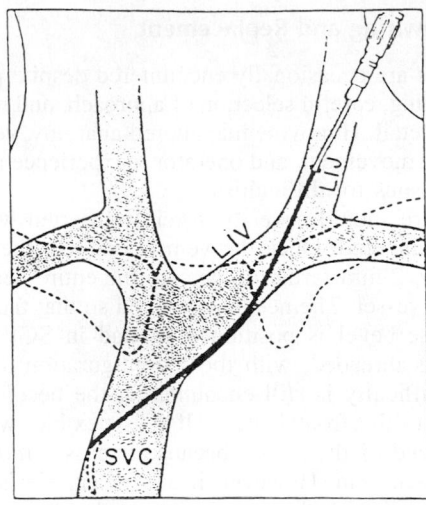

**FIGURE 27–10.** Schematic drawing of central venous catheter. Course is along the left internal jugular vein (LIJ), left innominate vein (LIV), and superior vena cava (SVC). The sharp angle of the catheter tip against the SVC may lead to perforation of the vessel. Dotted lines at bottom demonstrate proper position of catheter tip, which lies parallel to the vessel wall. (From Iberti TJ, Katz B, Reiner MA. Hydrothorax as a late complication of central venous indwelling catheters. *Surgery.* 1983;94:845.)

## Is a Chest Radiograph Necessary After Central Venous Catheter Placement?

Controversy surrounds the use of a chest radiograph because it exposes patients to radiation, is relatively expensive, and is potentially not cost effective, considering the low complication rate with jugular vein approaches. However, chest radiographs are used not only to rule out immediate complications such as pneumothorax but also to confirm that the catheter is not lying in the heart or at an unacceptable angle to the wall of the superior vena cava.[40] We recommend immediate chest radiography after subclavian catheterization out of concern for pneumothorax. Chest radiographs after uncomplicated IJV catheterization can be delayed until the end of the operative procedure because their primary utility is to allow catheter position to be assessed.

## If a Catheter Is Malpositioned, Can It Be Repositioned Without Contamination?

Malpositioning is a well-known complication of central venous catheterization. Catheters are malpositioned in the ipsilateral IJV or contralateral SCV 11% to 19% of the time.[40] Placement in the brachiocephalic, azygos, and pericardiophrenic veins, among others, has been reported. The only way to safely reposition a CVC without removal is if it can be done by partial withdrawal. Otherwise, it should be replaced unless extenuating circumstances such as hypovolemia, poor landmarks, and coagulopathy, as well as exposing patients to further risk, make such attempts less desirable. To reduce these risks during the initial attempt, electrocardiographic and US real-time guidance, fluoroscopic placement, and flow-directed techniques can be used.[41–43] However, additional equipment is required and may not be immediately available.

## Catheter Rewiring and Replacement

Difficulties are occasionally encountered despite proper patient positioning, careful selection of approach, and meticulous attention to detail. Hypovolemia, altered anatomy, vein thrombosis, patient movement, and operator inexperience are among the many reasons for difficulties.

A guidewire should never be forcibly inserted when resistance is encountered. Once the vein is entered, the needle is advanced 1 to 2 mm farther to be sure the entire needle bevel is within the vessel. The needle is rotated so that the proximal portion of the bevel is positioned caudad in SCV attempts. The J-wire is threaded, with the J configuration also facing caudad. If difficulty is still encountered, the needle is maintained close to the frontal plane. If it is flexible, we also try the straight end of the J-wire because it passes more readily through a small vein. However, if any resistance is met, this method is abandoned, the wire is removed, and the needle is repositioned. Several unsuccessful attempts suggest that the needle is in a small neck vein, and a new puncture is performed at an adjacent or different site. Guidewires are available separately and in various diameters. When possible, a smaller, flexible angiographic wire can also be used to advantage.

Subclavian guidewire placement from the EJV can also be difficult. Maneuvers such as medial and lateral flexion of the neck, abduction and adduction, plus external and internal rotation of the ipsilateral arm provide some help. Withdrawal of the J-wire approximately 1 cm followed by concomitant rotation of the wire medially by 90° during readvancement is occasionally useful. If resistance is met when the J-wire is retracted, be sure that the needle/cannulas and wire are removed simultaneously to prevent shearing the wire.

## Duration of Catheterization

Studies of when a catheter should be changed have been either inconclusive or conflicting. Maki and colleagues showed that the potential for infection increases after 72 hours with catheters not used for hyperalimentation in critically ill patients.[44] A study by Gil and associates revealed that colonization and bacteremia increase significantly after 6 days.[45] Others maintain a catheter to a later date or until a complication develops. Individuals and institutions should evaluate their patient populations, type and number of catheters placed, and incidence of infection to determine policies for replacement. The use of antibiotic-bonded catheters coupled with daily site care might allow extension of catheter use beyond our current standard, and a study is undergoing at our institution to determine the optimal duration of catheterization with these types of catheters. Based on our experience and that of others, we recommend the following protocol:

1. In critically ill patients with adequate access available, a catheter change using a different site after 72 hours appears reasonable for infection control unless an antibiotic or antiseptic catheter is used. Low infection rates using single-lumen or multilumen catheters have been reported with this approach.[18,46–49]
2. If access is limited (eg, obesity, extreme burns, scar tissue), an option is to leave the catheter for an extended period with close daily observation or to change the catheter after 72 hours over a J-wire and culture the tip. If the culture result is positive, a new site and catheter should be chosen. If the catheter is to be left in for an extended period, it should be replaced before signs of infection are evident. A maximum of 6 days is suggested unless otherwise indicated.
3. CVCs placed through the antecubital fossa should be removed after 72 hours. Studies report a higher frequency of complications (12.5%-23%) at this site.[49]
4. Both pulmonary artery catheters and their introducers should be replaced after 72 hours. The risk of infection is reported to increase for those catheters left for >3 days.[49,50]
5. CVCs are discontinued as soon as they are no longer required.

## Complications

Complications are many, varied, and potentially lethal. They, together with those associated with pulmonary artery catheterization, are listed in Table 27–11. Most can be avoided by meticulous attention to detail, careful preparation, and a sound knowledge of the involved anatomy. Table 27–11 lists early and late complications of central venous and pulmonary artery catheterization.[51–56] Sustained ventricular dysrhythmias with CVCs are usually due to catheter overinsertion and should be treated by withdrawing the catheter. The postplacement chest radiograph can be somewhat misleading in this regard because it is a portable film done with the patient supine and with the neck somewhat extended, thereby projecting the catheter to be more proximal in the SVC than when it is in a neutral position. A knotted catheter usually can be removed in a cardiac catheterization laboratory without much difficulty. The incidence of pulmonary artery rupture is low but has a high mortality. Rupture should be suspected whenever hemoptysis occurs, especially if it is temporally related to balloon inflation. Factors predisposing to pulmonary artery rupture are listed in Table 27–12. Mechanical damage to the

**TABLE 27–11.** Complications of Central Venous and Pulmonary Artery Catheterization

**Immediate**

Multiple puncture
Pneumo/hemo/hydro/chylothorax-mediastinum
Arterial puncture—hematoma or bleeding
Air embolism
Cardiac dysrhythmias
Catheter malposition
Catheter knotting
Subcutaneous and mediastinal emphysema
Tracheal puncture or laceration

**Late**

Pulmonary artery rupture
Pulmonary infarction
Catheter-related sepsis
Balloon rupture
Endocardial or valvular damage
Venous thrombosis
Infections (cellulitis, osteomyelitis, endocarditis, thrombophlebitis)
Nerve injury
Cerebrovascular compromise
Cardiac or vena cava perforation and pleural effusion or cardiac tamponade
Arteriovenous fistula
Thrombocytopenia

Modified from Venus B, Mallory DL. Vascular cannulation. In: Civetta JM, Taylor RW, Kirby RR, eds. *Critical Care.* Philadelphia, Pa: JB Lippincott; 1988:157.

**TABLE 27–12.** Factors Predisposing to Pulmonary
Artery Rupture

Age >60 y
Female gender
Cardiopulmonary bypass
Hypothermia
Anticoagulation
Pulmonary hypertension
Peripheral catheter tip location (ie, >5 cm lateral to mediastinum)
Multiple wedge pressure determinations
Atypical pulmonary artery pressure waveform (mitral valve disease)

From Gravenstein N, ed. *Manual of Complications During Anesthesia.* Philadelphia,
Pa: JB Lippincott; 1991:290.

cardiac valves and endocardium may occur as a result of prolonged catheterization. Valvular ruptures have been reported when the catheter is entrapped in the trabeculae. The balloon must always be deflated before withdrawing the catheter.

## PULMONARY ARTERY CATHETERIZATION

Since its introduction more than three decades ago, no other monitor has attracted more controversy than the pulmonary artery catheter. Indications for pulmonary artery cannulation are outlined in Table 27–13. The catheter is designed to provide information about pressures in the pulmonary circuit and assess cardiac function. In addition, some catheters allow continuous mixed venous oxygen saturation monitoring, atrial or ventricular pacing, calculation of right ventricular volumes and ejection fractions, and continuous cardiac output determination. Equipment for pulmonary artery catheterization is similar to that used for CVC placement, in addition to an introducer sheath and pulmonary artery catheter. Special introducers made from polyurethane or polyethylene have been developed for easier passage of the pulmonary artery catheter and are available with a side port that can be used as an additional infusion site. Pulmonary artery catheters are made from polyvinyl chloride with heparin bonding. The catheter softens somewhat at body temperature. They are

**TABLE 27–13.** Indications for Pulmonary Artery Cannulation

**Cardiovascular**

Complicated cardiac surgery
Dissecting abdominal aneurysm
Thoracic aorta aneurysmectomy
Emergency or extensive surgery
Cardiogenic shock

**Respiratory**

Pneumonectomy
Acute pulmonary edema
Acute lung injury
Complicated mechanical ventilation

**Miscellaneous**

Severe burns
Multiple trauma
Septic shock
Research
Preoperative optimization (eg, pheochromocytoma)

Modified from Venus B, Mallory DI. Vascular cannulation. In: Civetta JM, Taylor
RW, Kirby RR, eds. *Critical Care.* Philadelphia, Pa: JB Lippincott; 1988:164.

available in sizes ranging from 5 to 8 French and are approximately 110 cm long. A sterile plastic sleeve to protect the external portion of the catheter is available in the introducer kits. An additional pulmonary artery pressure transducer and monitoring system are also needed, as is a connection for the thermistor used for cardiac output determination.[57,58]

### What Technique Is Used?

The technique for accessing the central circulation is the same as described with placement of CVCs. Once the guidewire is introduced in the vein, the assembled dilator-sheath apparatus is advanced gently to avoid venous perforation. The dilator is not advanced below the collar bone; rather, the sheath is slid over it. The dilator is then removed, and the sheath is sutured to the skin.

The pulmonary artery catheter is then introduced through the sheath. Before insertion and after the catheter is introduced in the sterile sleeve, meticulous attention is placed to maintaining sterility throughout the catheter setup. The catheter is then flushed by a second person and calibrated and placed in a pressure transducer assembly. All lumina are flushed and filled with sterile heparinized saline solution, and the balloon is tested.

The balloon remains deflated until the catheter tip is beyond the end of the introducer. Once the tip is advanced to approximately 20 cm, the balloon is inflated with 1.5 mL of air or carbon dioxide. The catheter is then slowly advanced, with continuous observation of electrocardiographic and pressure waveform across the tricuspid valve and into the pulmonary artery through the right ventricle. The right ventricular tracing should appear about 45 to 55 cm from the antecubital fossa, 40 to 55 cm from the femoral vein, 35 to 40 cm from the IJV, and 30 to 40 cm from the SCV (lower numbers represent right-sided approaches). Characteristic pressure changes accompany passage from the right ventricle to the pulmonary artery and into the occlusion position. The occlusion position should be obtained when the balloon is inflated with 1.5 mL of air. If occlusion is obtained with <1 mL inflation, the catheter is too far in the pulmonary artery and needs to be retracted to a distance where 1.5 mL is required to wedge the tip. Once the catheter is in position, it is secured in place.

Placement may be difficult in the presence of right atrial or ventricular dilatation, low cardiac output, pulmonary hypertension, or tricuspid regurgitation. Passage during deep spontaneous inspiration in the sitting position may facilitate entrance to the right ventricle.[59] Catheter passage is also facilitated by placing the patient in a 5° head-up position with a right lateral tilt.[60] Transesophageal echocardiography offers another approach to help achieve pulmonary artery catheterization in difficult cases. Stiffening the catheter by irrigating in a cold solution before passage or use of a guidewire (length 120 cm, outer diameter 0.021 inches) under fluoroscopy can help as well. Distal migration of the catheter tip subsequent to initial placement must be anticipated as the catheter warms and softens. If it migrates to a wedge position, it should again be withdrawn. Because of the anticipated distal migration, it is critical to inflate the balloon gradually any time a wedge pressure determination is made during continuous pulmonary artery pressure waveform monitoring.

## What Are the Complications?

In addition to the complications associated with CVC placement, the pulmonary artery catheter is associated with some unique problems that can be potentially life threatening. Sustained ventricular dysrhythmias are usually due to catheter slack and should be treated by withdrawing the catheter to relieve any slack. Pulmonary artery rupture should be suspected whenever hemoptysis occurs, especially if it is temporally related to balloon inflation (see earlier). Factors predisposing to pulmonary artery rupture are listed in Table 27–12.

Pulmonary artery catheters also predispose to bacterial colonization and systemic infection. The degree of catheter manipulation and the length of time it is in place are important factors. In critically ill patients, entrapment of platelets by the catheter may also cause clinically significant thrombocytopenia, which responds to removal of the catheter.

## SUMMARY

Vascular access is a common feature of patient care. With proper care and consideration it can be done effectively, efficiently, and safely to improve patient care.

## References

1. Garland JS, Buck RK, Maloney P, et al. Comparison of 10% povidone-iodine and 0.5% chlorhexidine gluconate for the prevention of peripheral intravenous catheter colonization in neonates: a prospective study. *Pediatr Infect Dis J.* 1995;14:510.
2. Forber B. Infection control in intensive care. In: *Centers for Disease Control Guidelines for the Prevention of Intravascular Infections.* New York, NY: Churchill Livingstone; 1987:50.
3. US Department of Health and Human Services. Guidelines for prevention of intravascular device-related infections. *Am J Infect Control.* 1996;24:262.
4. National Intravenous Therapy Association. *Intravenous Nursing Standards of Practice.* Vol 4. Cambridge, Mass: National Intravenous Therapy Association; 1981:9.
5. Venus B, Mallory DL. Vascular cannulation. In: Civetta JM, Taylor RW, Kirby RR, eds. *Critical Care.* Philadelphia, Pa: JB Lippincott; 1992:149.
6. Slogoff A, Keats AS, Arlund BS. On the safety of radial artery cannulation. *Anesthesiology.* 1983;59:42.
7. Becher C, Toulin RB. Doppler flow monitoring of the dorsal artery of the foot facilitates puncture of the femoral artery in children. *AJR Am J Roentgenol.* 1990;155:131.
8. Seneff M. Arterial line placement and care. In: Rippe JM, Irwin RS, Alpert JS, et al, eds. *Intensive Care Medicine.* Boston, Little, Brown & Co; 1991:37.
9. Stirt JA. "Liquid stylet" for percutaneous radial artery cannulation. *Can Anaesth Soc J.* 1982;29:492.
10. Kondo K. Percutaneous radial artery cannulation using a pressure-curve-directed technique. *Anesthesiology.* 1984;61:639.
11. Mallory DL, Sapienza R, McGee WT, et al. "State-of-the-art" vascular cannulation in the ICU. *Res Medica.* 1988;4:5.
12. Sladen A. Complications of invasive hemodynamic monitoring in the intensive care unit. In: Ravitch MM, ed. *Current Problems in Surgery.* Chicago, Ill: Year Book Medical; 1988:69.
13. Norwood SH, Cormier B, McMahon NG, et al. Prospective study of catheter-related infection during prolonged arterial catheterization. *Crit Care Med.* 1988;16:836.
14. Clark CA, Harman EM. Hemodynamic monitoring: arterial catheters. In: Civetta JM, Taylor RW, Kirby RR, eds. *Critical Care.* Philadelphia, Pa: JB Lippincott; 1988:289.
15. Moyer MA, Edwards LD, Farley L. Comparative culture methods on 101 intravenous catheters. *Arch Intern Med.* 1983;143:66.
16. Thomas F, Burke JP, Parker J, et al. The risk of infection related to radial vs femoral sites for arterial catheterization. *Crit Care Med.* 1983;11:807.
17. Ducharme FM, Gauthier M, Lacroix J, et al. Incidence of infection related to arterial catheterization in children: a prospective study. *Crit Care Med.* 1988;16:272.
18. Arnow PM, Costas CO. Delayed rupture of the radial artery caused by catheter-related sepsis. *Rev Infect Dis.* 1988;10:1035.
19. Russell RC, Steichen JB, Sook EG. Radial artery pseudoaneurysms: their diagnosis, treatment and prevention. *Orthop Rev.* 1979;8:49.
20. Randolph AG, Cook DJ, Gonzalez CA, et al. Ultrasound guidance for placement of central venous catheters: a meta-analysis of the literature. *Crit Care Med.* 1996;24:2053.
21. Gordon AC, Saliken JC, Johns D, et al. US-guided puncture of the internal jugular vein: complications and anatomic considerations. *J Vasc Interv Radiol.* 1998;9:333.
22. Koski EM, Suhonen M, Mattila MA. Ultrasound facilitated central venous cannulation. *Crit Care Med.* 1992;20:424.
23. Novak RA, Venus B. Clavicular approaches for central vein cannulation. In: Venus B, Mallory DL, eds. *Problems in Critical Care.* Philadelphia, Pa: JB Lippincott; 1988:242.
24. Mermel LA. Prevention of intravascular catheter related infections. *Ann Intern Med* 2000;132:391.
25. Sulek CA, Gravenstein N, Blackshear RH, et al. Head rotation during internal jugular vein cannulation and the risk of carotid artery puncture. *Anesth Analg.* 1996;82:125.
26. Jesseph JM, Conces DJ, Agustyn GT. Patient positioning for subclavian vein catheterization. *Arch Surg.* 1987;122:1207.
27. McGee WT, Mallory DL. Cannulation of the internal and external jugular veins. In: Venus B, Mallory DL, eds. *Problems in Critical Care.* Philadelphia, Pa: JB Lippincott; 1988:217.
28. Schwartz AJ, Jobes DR, Greenhow DE, et al. Carotid artery puncture with internal jugular cannulation using the Seldinger technique: incidence, recognition, treatment, and prevention. *Anesthesiology.* 1979;51:S160.
29. Haapaniemi L, Slatis P. Supraclavicular catheterization of the superior vena cava. *Acta Anaesthesiol Scand.* 1974;18:12.
30. Parsa MH, Tabora F. Central venous access in critically ill patients in the emergency department. *Emerg Med Clin North Am.* 1986;4:709.
31. Ellis L, Vogel S, Copeland E. Central venous catheter vascular erosions: diagnosis and clinical course. *Ann Surg.* 1989;209:475.
32. Sheep R, Guiney W. Fatal cardiac tamponade: occurrence with other complications after left internal jugular vein catheterization. *JAMA.* 1982;248:1632.
33. Dane TE, Kreig EG. Fatal cardiac tamponade and other mechanical complications of central venous catheters. *Br J Surg.* 1975;62:6.
34. Purdue GF, Hunt JL. Placement and complications of monitoring catheters. *Surg Clin North Am.* 1991;71:4.
35. Peres PW. Positioning central venous catheters—a prospective survey. *Anaesth Intens Care.* 1990;18:4.
36. McGee WT, Mallory DL, Johans TG, et al. Safe placement of central venous catheters is facilitated using right atrial electrocardiography. *Crit Care Med.* 1988;16:4.
37. Iberti TJ, Katz B, Reiner MA. Hydrothorax as a late complication of central venous indwelling catheters. *Surgery.* 1983;94:842.
38. Blackshear RH, Gravenstein N. Critical angle of incidence for delayed vessel perforation by central venous catheter: a study of in vivo data [abstract]. *Ann Emerg Med.* 1992;21:659.
39. Gravenstein N, Blackshear RH. In vitro evaluation of relative perforating potential of central venous catheters: comparison of materials, selected models, number of lumens, and angle of incidence to simulated membrane. *J Clin Monit.* 1991;7:1.
40. Deital M, McIntyre J. Radiographic confirmation of site of central venous pressure catheters. *Can J Surg.* 1971;14:42.
41. Nolsoe C, Nielsen J, Korstrup S, et al. Ultrasonically guided subclavian vein catheterization. *Acta Radiol.* 1989;30:108.
42. Babikian G, Byron R, Hassett J Jr. Redirection of central venous catheters using a flow-directed technique. *Surg Gynecol Obstet.* 1986;163:482.
43. Tryba M, Kleine P, Zeng M. Sonographic studies for optimizing cannulation of the internal jugular vein. *Anaesthetist.* 1982;31:626.
44. Maki DG, Goldman DA, Rhome RS. Infection control in intravenous therapy. *Ann Intern Med.* 1973;79:867.
45. Gil RT, Krause JA, Thill-Baharozian MC, et al. Triple versus single lumen central venous catheters. *Arch Intern Med.* 1989;149:1139.
46. Kelly CS, Ligas JR, Smith CA, et al. Sepsis due to triple lumen central venous catheters. *Surg Gynecol Obstet.* 1986;14:163.
47. Hilton E, Haslett T, Borenstein M, et al. Central catheter infections: single versus triple lumen catheters. *Am J Med.* 1988;84:667.
48. Elliott TS. Intravascular-device infections. *J Med Microbiol.* 1988;27:161.

49. Myers M, Austin T, Sibbold W. Pulmonary artery catheter infections: a prospective study. *Ann Surg.* 1985;201:237.
50. Miller J, Venus B, Mathru M. Comparison of the sterility of long-term central venous catheterization using single lumen, triple lumen, and pulmonary artery catheters. *Crit Care Med.* 1984;12:634.
51. Childs D, Wilkes RG. Puncture of the ascending aorta: a complication of subclavian venous cannulation. *Anesthesia.* 1986;41:331.
52. Herbst CA. Indications, management, and complications of percutaneous subclavian catheters. *Arch Surg.* 1978;113:1421.
53. Brown CQ. Inadvertent prolonged cannulation of the carotid artery. *Anesth Analg.* 1982;61:150.
54. Bernard RW, Stahl WM. Subclavian vein catheterization: a prospective study, I: non-infectious complications. *Ann Surg.* 1971;173:184.
55. Jay AWL, Aldridge HE. Perforation of the heart or vena cava by central venous catheters inserted for monitoring or infusion therapy. *Can Med Assoc J.* 1986,135.1143.
56. Aldridge HE, Jay AWL. Central venous catheters and heart perforation. *Can Med Assoc J.* 1986;135:1143.
57. Chatterjie K, Swan J, Ganz W, et al. Use of a balloon-tipped flotation electrode catheter for cardiac monitoring. *Am J Cardiol.* 1975;36:56.
58. Baele P, McMechan J, Marsh H, et al. Continuous monitoring of mixed venous oxygen saturation in critically ill patients. *Anesth Analg.* 1982;61:513.
59. Venus B, Mathru M. A maneuver for bedside pulmonary artery catheterization in patients with right heart failure. *Chest.* 1982;82:803.
60. Keusch DJ, Winters S, Thys DM. The patient's position influences the incidence of dysrhythmias during pulmonary artery catheterization. *Anesthesiology.* 1989;70:582.

# Positioning the Surgical Patient

Robert C. Morell

Nikolaus Gravenstein

## GENERAL CONSIDERATIONS

*How Should the Patient Be Moved and Positioned?*

*What Are the Effects of Preexisting Medical Problems?*

*Why Does Postoperative Backache Occur?*

*Can Positioning Cause Cardiorespiratory Compromise?*

*When Is Neurovascular Compromise a Problem?*

*How Are Pressure Points Managed?*

*How Can Nerve Stretch Be Minimized?*

*What Documentation Is Important?*

*What Is the Incidence of Perioperative Nerve Injuries?*

*What Is the Double-Crush Syndrome?*

## SPECIFIC CONSIDERATIONS

*What Considerations Are Associated With the Supine Position?*

*How Should the Arms Be Positioned for the Supine Patient?*

*What Is the Beach Chair or Lawn Chair Position?*

*What Considerations Are Associated With the Prone Position?*

*What Is a Way to Move the Patient From Supine to Prone?*

*What Considerations Are Associated With the Lateral Decubitus Position?*

*What Is a Way to Move the Patient From Supine to the Lateral Decubitus Position?*

*What Considerations Are Associated With the Head-Up or Semisitting Position?*

*What Contributes to the Risk of Air Embolism?*

*What Considerations Are Associated With the Lithotomy Position?*

*How Can Compartment Syndrome Occur?*

*What Problems Are Associated With the Trendelenburg Position?*

## PERIPHERAL NERVE INJURIES

*How Is a Postoperative Peripheral Nerve Complaint Evaluated?*

*Why Is the Brachial Plexus Commonly Injured?*

*Why Is the Radial Nerve Vulnerable?*

*How Is the Median Nerve Traumatized?*

*How Does Ulnar Nerve Damage Occur?*

Positioning the patient for surgery is an important aspect of anesthetic care and patient safety. Several goals should be kept in mind. The patient's position should (1) facilitate the surgery and optimize access to the surgical anatomy; (2) minimize the potential for pressure, stretch, or friction-induced injuries; and (3) preserve the anesthesiologist's access to the patient's airway, monitoring devices, and intravascular catheters. The responsibility for proper positioning is shared by the anesthesiologist, surgeon, and operating room nurse.

Anesthesia usually renders the patient insensible to pain and pressure and unable to alter his or her position. Care should always be taken to position the patient in a fashion designed to minimize pressure, stretch, traction, and friction. The use of muscle relaxants can also enable an anesthetized patient to be placed in a position he or she would ordinarily not be able to assume. Long surgical procedures can be associated with a higher risk of positioning-related injury and may necessitate extra care and vigilance. The American Society of Anesthesiologists (ASA) Closed Claims database indicates that approximately 16% of closed malpractice claims related to anesthesia care involved peripheral nerve injuries.[1] Such perioperative nerve injuries are frequently attributed to the patients' positioning during operation. However, in many cases (≈66%), a mechanism of injury cannot be identified and positioning was deemed appropriate.[2] It is therefore difficult to make concrete and absolute recommendations for specific optimal positioning strategies, largely due to limited objective data.

## GENERAL CONSIDERATIONS

### How Should the Patient Be Moved and Positioned?

When practical, the patient should position himself or herself by moving to the operating table from the stretcher or wheelchair. The patient may then assume the position for the surgical procedure while still awake. Any aspects of the trial position that are uncomfortable can thus be corrected. If the required position is not assumed until *after* induction of anesthesia, the anesthesiologist should verify that the patient can assume the intended position. For example, if the arms are to be abducted, it is a good idea to determine if arm abduction can be accomplished without pain or discomfort. This can be accomplished by questioning or by having the patient assume the position during the preoperative evaluation or before the induction of general anesthesia. Documentation of awake positioning or tolerance of the expected intraoperative position in the medical record is important to record the care taken to minimize the chance of postoperative positioning-related injury.

### What Are the Effects of Preexisting Medical Problems?

Preexisting anatomic or medical conditions may influence surgical positioning. The ability to assume a given position may be compromised by skeletal deformities, excessive bulk, morbid obesity, cardiac disease, pulmonary disease, or rheumatoid arthritis. Conditions such as congestive heart failure (CHF), ascites, and morbid obesity may limit a patient's ability to lie flat and may necessitate elevating the head of the bed.

### Why Does Postoperative Backache Occur?

Postoperative backache is often attributed to positioning, but this problem is more likely a function of the duration of surgery; the use of muscle relaxants, which may contribute to the loss of normal lumbar lordosis; and the stretching of intervertebral ligaments.[3] The incidence of postoperative backache ranges from 12% to 37%.[3,4] Slightly flexing the hips and knees, placing a pillow under the knees, using a semireclining beach chair (modified Fowler) position, or inserting a small lumbar support may minimize backache. We know of no definitive preventive measures at this time.

### Can Positioning Cause Cardiorespiratory Compromise?

Potential compromise of cardiorespiratory function may result from specific positions. Positions that minimize respiratory compromise (eg, the head-elevated position) may aggravate circulatory insufficiency, and vice versa. Use of the kidney rest, prone positioning, lateral positioning with marked flexion, and exaggerated lithotomy positioning may interfere with venous return from the lower body. Pulmonary compliance and functional residual capacity may also be significantly decreased.

### When Is Neurovascular Compromise a Problem?

Neurovascular compromise can occur by compression or stretching of the intraneural vasa nervorum and can result in nerve ischemia.[5] This complication can occur when a nerve or neural plexus has a long and superficial course between two points of fixation (Fig. 28–1). Another mechanism can involve compression of a nerve between bony internal struc-

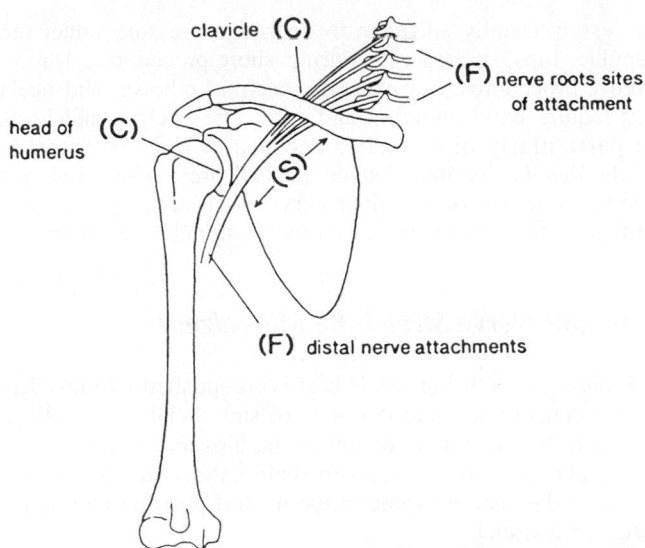

**FIGURE 28-1.** Schematic diagram of brachial plexus injury. Positioning may stretch (S) the plexus between points of fixation (F), increasing the likelihood of compression injury at several sites (C). (From Mahla ME. Nervous system. In: Gravenstein N, ed. *Manual of Complications During Anesthesia.* Philadelphia, Pa: JB Lippincott; 1991:384.)

tures and external rigid objects such as the operating table or stirrups. The most detrimental circumstances occur when stretching and compression are combined; a stretched nerve is exquisitely vulnerable to ischemic compression.[6] The administration of large amounts of fluid may cause tissue edema, which may contribute to neurovascular compression.

Compression of tissue may be more likely to produce injury when it occurs in a small area. The duration of such compression is also important.[6] As a general rule, at least 20 minutes of ischemic compression is required for a nerve injury to occur. For example, consider how long an arm or leg takes to become numb when the nerve supply to either is compressed. A stretch or crush injury, in contrast, can occur instantaneously (eg, brachial plexus avulsion). The etiology of perioperative nerve injuries is multifactorial. Contributing factors include compression, stretch, ischemia, patient insensibility, preexisting medical conditions, and exposure to certain medications. Perioperative nerve injuries may *not* always be preventable, and the mechanisms of such injuries often are not identifiable.[2]

### How Are Pressure Points Managed?

Careful padding of pressure points and attention to changes from the initial surgical position are important. Pressure points vary with patient position (Table 28–1). The operating table

**TABLE 28–1.** Pressure Points

| Supine | Prone | Decubitus |
|--------|-------|-----------|
| Occiput | Forehead | Ear |
| Scapula | Eyes | Axilla |
| Elbows | Chest | Hip |
| Hips | Elbows | Knee (peroneal nerve) |
| Sacrum | Iliac crests | Ankle |
| Heels | Knees | |

mattress is usually adequate to distribute pressure under the scapulae, hips, and sacrum during short procedures. During lengthy procedures, however, the occiput, elbows, and heels may require extra attention and care. The occiput and heels are particularly problematic because of the considerable weight that is distributed over a small area. The fixed, yet superficial course of the ulnar nerve at the ulnar groove can predispose the ulnar nerve to injury by stretch or pressure.

### How Can Nerve Stretch Be Minimized?

Avoiding stretch injuries is best accomplished by considering the course and fixation points of superficial nerves (Figs. 28–2 and 28–3). Gentle flexion of the hips and knees, limitation of abduction of the arms to <90° extension, and conformance of the cervical spine to the neutral position may minimize nerve stretch.

### What Documentation Is Important?

Patient positioning should be documented on the anesthesia record to indicate that care was used in determining and ensuring proper positioning. The patient's response to the position should be indicated on the chart if he or she was awake during positioning. A description of the padding should also be included. The use of a stick figure drawing of the position and associated padding is useful. Figure 28–4 is an example of such a drawing for a supine patient. Relative angles should be indicated. For example, note the identification of specific padding and arm abduction, which is clearly <90°. Such a figure is intended to be schematic and not

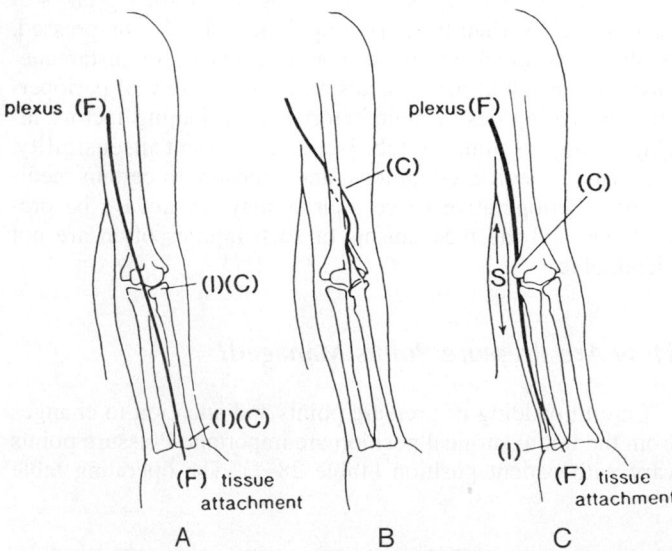

FIGURE 28–2. Schematic diagram of selected upper extremity nerve injuries. *A,* Median nerve. Injuries may occur by direct damage from intravenous catheter insertion (I) or intravenous infiltration with resultant compression (C). Stretching may occur between points of fixation (F) by dorsiflexion of the wrist. *B,* The radial nerve is susceptible to compression against the posterior surface of the humerus (C). *C,* The ulnar nerve is susceptible to stretching (S) between fixation points (F). In addition, it may be vulnerable to compression at the elbow (C). (From Mahla ME. Nervous system. In: Gravenstein N, ed. *Manual of Complications During Anesthesia.* Philadelphia, Pa: JB Lippincott; 1991:387.)

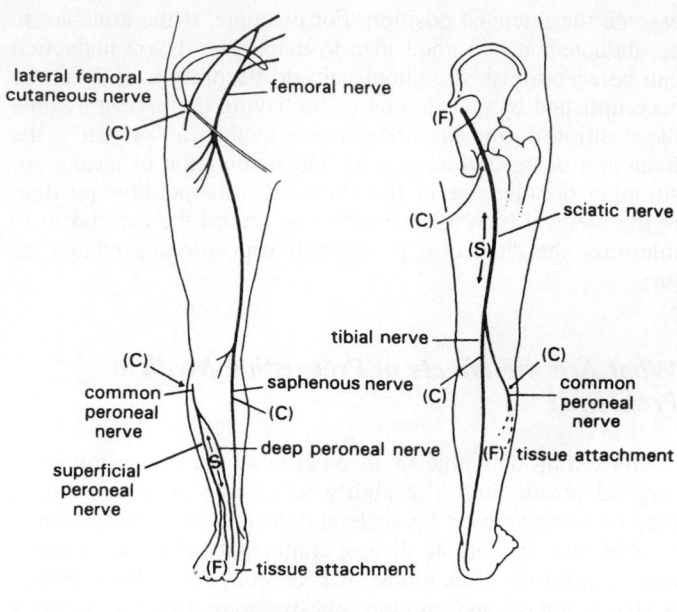

**ANTERIOR VIEW**     **POSTERIOR VIEW**

FIGURE 28–3. Schematic diagram of selected lower extremity nerve injuries. *A,* Anterior view. The lateral femoral cutaneous nerve may be compressed (C) between an external appliance and the iliac spine. The common peroneal nerve may be compressed (C) between the head of the fibula and an external appliance. Pressure against the medial aspect of the upper one third of the tibia may compress (C) the saphenous nerve. The superficial and deep peroneal nerves may be stretched (S) if the foot is plantar flexed. *B,* Posterior view. The sciatic nerve may be stretched (S) between its fixation points by flexion of the hip without flexion at the knee. It may also be compressed (C) at the ischial tuberosity. The tibial nerve is susceptible to compression (C) at the popliteal fossa. (From Mahla ME. Nervous system. In: Gravenstein N, ed. *Manual of Complications During Anesthesia.* Philadelphia, Pa: JB Lippincott; 1991:388.)

precise, that is, it is intended to show that the arms were abducted to <90° or tucked at the patient's side and not that they were abducted precisely the number of degrees determined by placing a protractor over the figure.

### What Is the Incidence of Perioperative Nerve Injuries?

According to Kroll and coworkers, of the 1541 claims reviewed up to 1990 and recorded in the ASA Closed Claims study database, 227 were for anesthesia-related nerve injury.[1] The most frequent claimed injury was ulnar neuropathy, which represented 34% of all nerve injuries. Less frequent were brachial plexus (23%) and lumbosacral (16%) injuries. More recently, Cheney and colleagues analyzed 4183 claims for anesthesia-related nerve injuries: 28% were ulnar nerve injur-

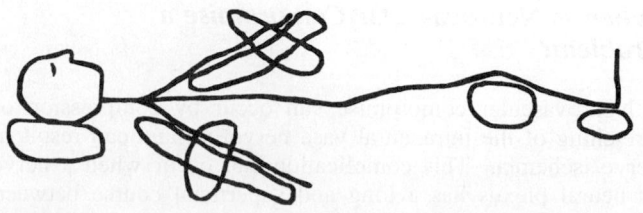

FIGURE 28–4. Schematic representation of position and pressure point documentation of a patient in the supine position.

ies, 20% involved the brachial plexus, 16% involved the lumbosacral roots, and 13% were spinal cord injuries.[2] Of interest were the authors' conclusions that although nerve damage is a significant source of anesthesia-related claims, most often it cannot be explained. In particular, ulnar nerve injuries seem to occur without any identifiable mechanism.[1,7] Gender and body habitus may also be important variables. For example, in the Closed Claims analysis, 75% of the ulnar nerve damage claims were made by men, even though the overall gender distribution of claims was equal.[1]

### What Is the Double-Crush Syndrome?

The double-crush syndrome is a type of nerve injury whereby a relatively mild injury to a nerve may potentiate the severity of a second injury. This may be due to a cumulative effect on axoplasmic flow. A clinical example is that of carpal tunnel syndrome occurring in patients with a cervical or brachial plexus lesion. Coexisting diseases may work in a similar fashion to potentiate nerve injuries.[8]

## SPECIFIC CONSIDERATIONS

### What Considerations Are Associated With the Supine Position?

#### Padding

When the patient is placed in a supine position, the weight is borne by the occiput, scapulae, elbows, sacrum, calves, and heels (see Table 28–1). Appropriate padding should be ensured to protect each pressure point to prevent pressure injuries, especially in older patients undergoing prolonged procedures. We advocate the use of soft foam or gel-filled padding. Consideration should be given to padding the sacrum in patients undergoing lengthy procedures, particularly if lower perfusion pressures are anticipated.

Another pressure point is the occiput; a number of cases describe pressure alopecia secondary to poor occipital circulation that causes an obliterative vasculitis when the occiput is allowed to rest on a hard surface.[4] Although the scalp is vascular, the occiput is still vulnerable because of the head's weight and the small area that is in contact with the bed or table. Padding serves not only to soften the contact point but also to allow the weight to be distributed over a greater area.

Additional means to optimize supine positioning include the placement of pillows under the knees to prevent hyperextension of the leg and the knee and resultant tibial and peroneal nerve stretch. Positioning of the safety belt above the knees and below the hips can also avoid compressing the peroneal and lateral femoral cutaneous nerves, respectively.

### How Should the Arms Be Positioned for the Supine Patient?

There is significant debate about the limits for safe positioning of the patient's arms. Surgical considerations frequently dictate if the arms must be tucked at the patient's side, extended on an arm board, or flexed and wedged. The literature is contradictory with respect to the incidence of brachial plexus injury and ulnar neuropathy when the arms are tucked, abducted to an angle of <90°, or flexed and supported over the head.[9,10] Similarly, the relative advantages of having the forearms supinated, prone, or in an in-between position are unclear. Prielipp and associates determined that pressure directly over the ulnar nerve is minimized in awake volunteers by having the arm placed in supination in all (30°, 60°, and 90°) degrees of abduction[11] (Fig. 28–5). These observations reflect only pressure and do not address the contribution of stretch.

If a patient's arms are positioned out and to the sides on arm boards, the practitioner must ensure that they are not abducted >90° relative to the plane of the body. Feeling the degree of tension placed on the pectoral muscle in the axilla can help to ensure that the brachial plexus is not being stretched. The height of the arm board padding should be matched to that of the mattress so that the humerus does not lie behind the plane of the body. Should this occur, the head of the humerus moves anteriorly and can result in pressure and stretch on the axillary portion of the brachial plexus. A rigid stepoff (or unusual height) from the operating table to the arm board can also place direct pressure on the radial nerve as it passes below the humerus (Fig. 28–6).

If the patient's arms are tucked at the side, they should be padded and secured. A shield or "toboggan" placed under the mattress prevents the arm from falling off the table and protects it from being leaned against by surgeons. If a shield is used, it, too, should be padded. An alternative approach is to secure the arms to the bed by encircling them with the draw sheet, which is then tucked underneath the patient.

Regardless of which position is selected, the ulnar nerve—or at least the ulnar groove—should be palpated to ensure that it is not being compressed. A final consideration is to verify that the patient's fingers are protected from hinges in the bed so that they are not injured if the foot/leg portion of the bed is raised or if the table is flexed.

### What Is the Beach Chair or Lawn Chair Position?

The contoured supine position is also called the *beach chair* or *lawn chair* position. The back of the bed is elevated 10° to 20°, and the table is contoured so that the hips and knees are slightly flexed. A conscious patient lying flat supine and motionless can usually maintain a normal distribution of tissue perfusion for approximately 1 hour before he or she notices increasing discomfort that necessitates moving. This "lying-at-attention" position, also known as the *rigid supine position*, results in significant discomfort to the patient who is awake while undergoing a protracted procedure.

In contrast, the lawn chair position adds to patient comfort by more uniformly distributing his or her weight and by providing support along the full length of the dorsal body surface. It also permits gentle flexion of the hips and knees, which helps to put these joints into more anatomically neutral positions (Fig. 28–7). Because the horizontal axis of the trunk is not changed, pulmonary blood volume is usually not redistributed; thus, venous congestion in the poorly ventilated pulmonary apices, as would typically occur in a patient in the Trendelenburg position, is avoided.

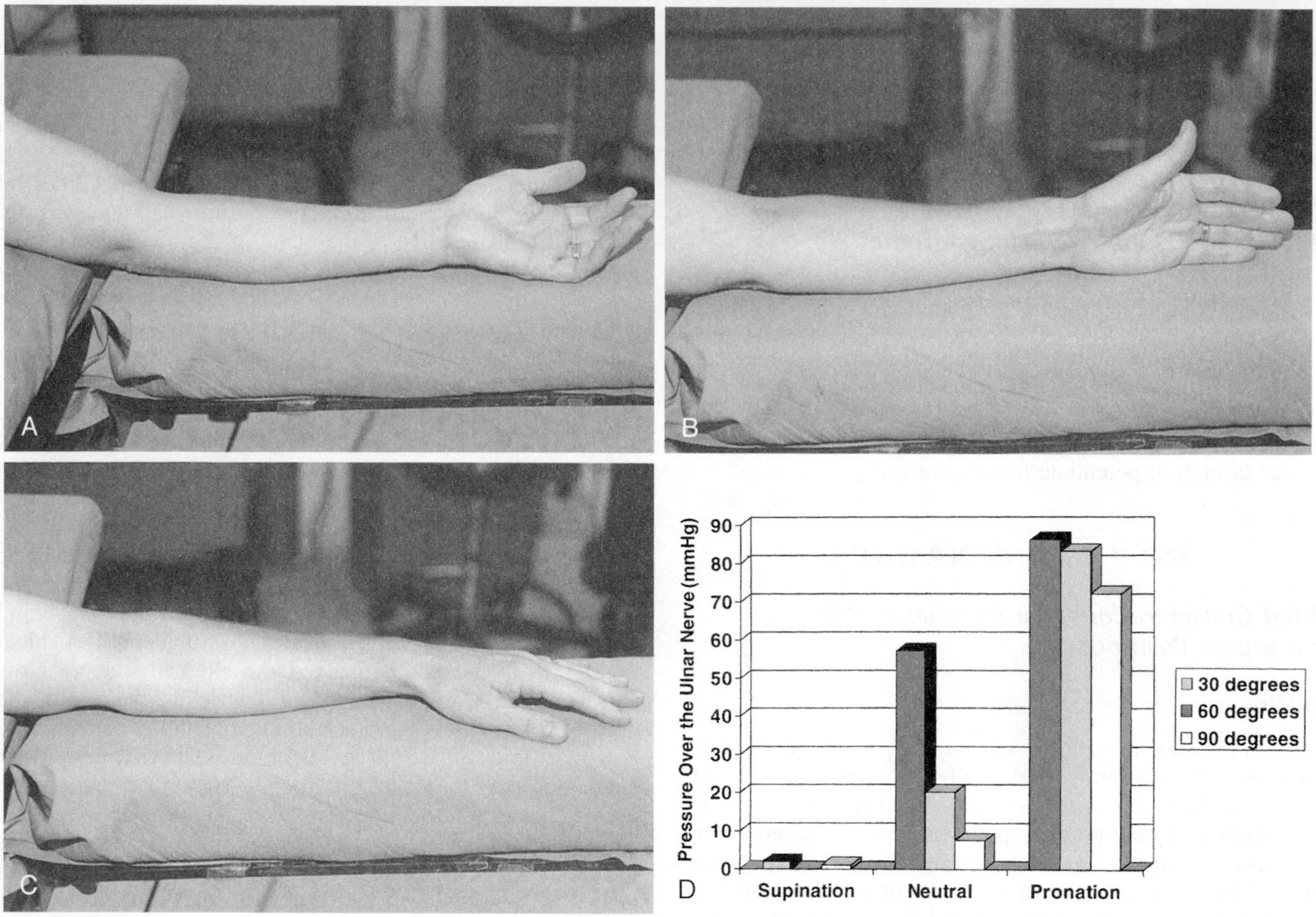

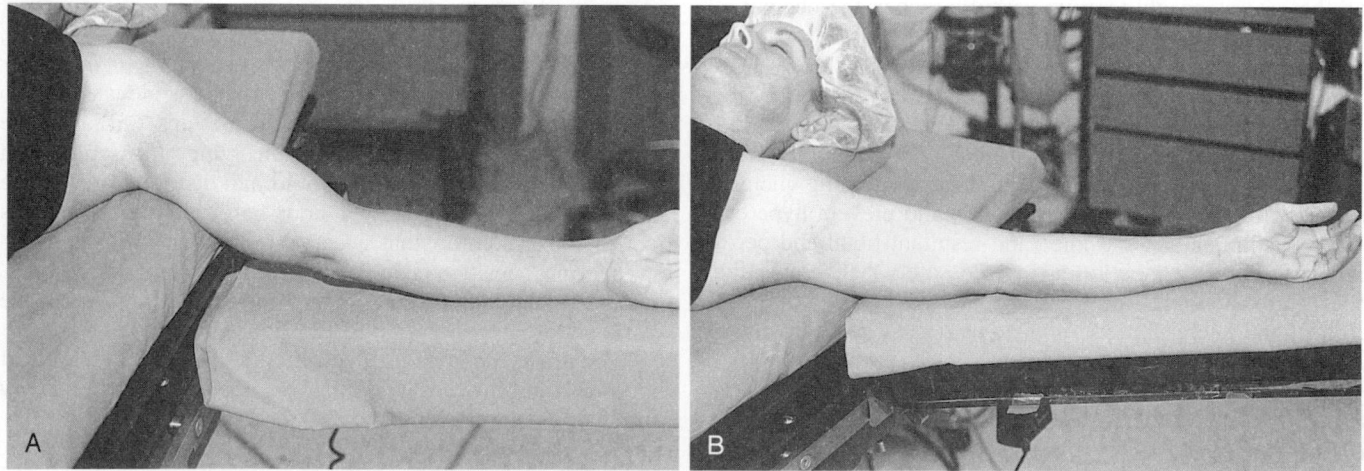

**FIGURE 28–5.** *A,* Arm in supination. *B,* Arm in neutral position. *C,* Arm in pronation. *D,* Pressure under ulnar nerve in each of these positions.

**FIGURE 28–6.** *A,* Mismatched arm board height with stepoff from operating table placing pressure on radial nerve. *B,* Excessive abduction of arm >90°.

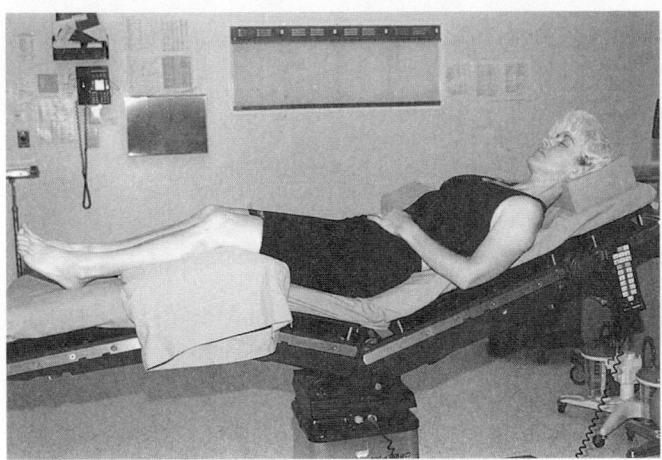

**FIGURE 28–7.** Lawn chair or modified Fowler position with gentle flexion of hips and knees.

## What Considerations Are Associated With the Prone Position?

The prone position is useful for operations involving the rectum, spine, or back. When this position is used, attention should be focused on several areas to protect them from direct pressure and resultant ischemia: the eyes, ears, and nose. Pressure on the eyes can result in retinal and optic nerve injury and permanent blindness. The patient's breasts or genitalia may also be at risk for compression against a hard surface or may become pinched by the mechanism of the operating table. Monitoring may be interfered with during the actual turn—from supine to prone position—and vigilance must remain high.

Respiratory problems result mainly from restriction of the diaphragm during inspiration by abdominal contents or by the weight of the patient against the thorax. Both can create a restrictive defect, compromise chest expansion, and increase the work of breathing in the spontaneously ventilating patient. Positive pressure ventilation may be effective in overcoming the decreased lung-thorax compliance. Increased peak inspiration pressure may occur particularly with improper positioning. High peak pressures can cause pulmonary barotrauma, which in turn can result in pneumothorax or mediastinal, subcutaneous, or interstitial emphysema.[12] The cardiovascular system may be affected by compression of the abdomen, which obstructs flow in the inferior vena cava and decreases preload to the right heart. Such compression may also increase perivertebral venous pressure and increase surgical bleeding, particularly during spinal surgery. Chest rolls and positioning frames (Relton-Hall, Andrews, and Wilson frames) can lessen this problem by minimizing abdominal or thoracic compression. The prone position may actually improve oxygenation and ventilation-perfusion ($\dot{V}/\dot{Q}$) matching when the abdomen is allowed to hang free.[12] When the abdomen is hanging free, epidural-perivertebral venous pressure is also lowest.

## What Is a Way to Move the Patient From Supine to Prone?

### Technique

An effective way to place the patient in the prone position after induction of anesthesia is to align the patient's torso (with the arms at the patient's sides) with the padding on the frame that is to be used. The anesthesiologist is responsible for the head and neck and a second person for the feet and legs. A third person rolls the patient into the arms of a fourth who is leaning across the padding or support frame. This "catcher" secures the patient's arms while the stretcher is moved out of the way. The patient's torso is centered over the frame, and the arms are positioned and padded, either at the sides or on arm boards. In the latter situation, the arms are abducted with the elbows flexed and padded so that the hands are near the head in front of the plane of the body. A sufficient number of people must be available if injury, not only to the patient but also to the personnel helping in the lifting process, is to be avoided. All accessories (eg, arm boards, pillows, support for the patient's head) should be prepositioned at their appropriate locations and conveniently available to ensure rapid, safe, and effective positioning.

### Head

The head may be kept neutral or rotated gently to the side if a patient is placed in the prone or three quarter prone position for neurosurgical procedures in which the head is to be supported by pins. The anesthesiologist should be directly involved and should verify that no undue flexion or extension of the neck occurs and that the endotracheal tube (ETT) is adequately secured once the new position is achieved. At least two fingerbreadths of space should be present between the chin and sternum to avoid excessive flexion and the potential for kinking or biting the ETT or obstructing the jugular veins.

In some cases, a horseshoe headrest may be used in the prone (or supine) position (Fig. 28–8). This headrest may be used with tongs and weights intended to provide cervical traction. Horseshoe headrests should be well padded, adjustable, and carefully fitted to the patient's face. The anesthesiologist should be aware that slippage and shifting of the face relative to the horseshoe can occur during surgery. This necessitates frequent checking and repositioning if necessary (with adequate warning to the surgeon if head or neck movement is anticipated). Pressure on the horseshoe should be distributed over the forehead and the malar regions. Care must be taken to ensure that no pressure is applied to the eyes or orbits. Three quarter–inch or 1-inch umbilical tape can be placed around the padding to compress it where the padding might

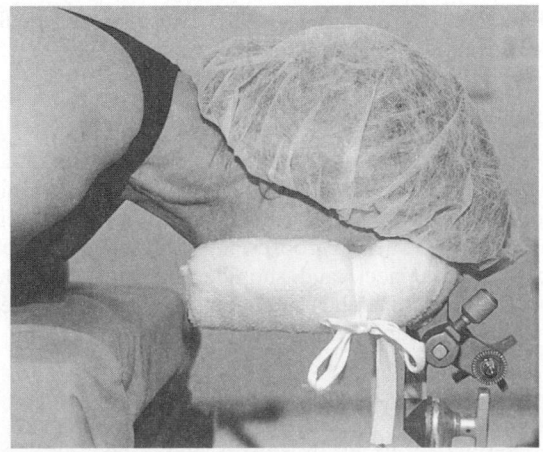

**FIGURE 28–8.** Horseshoe headrest in the prone position.

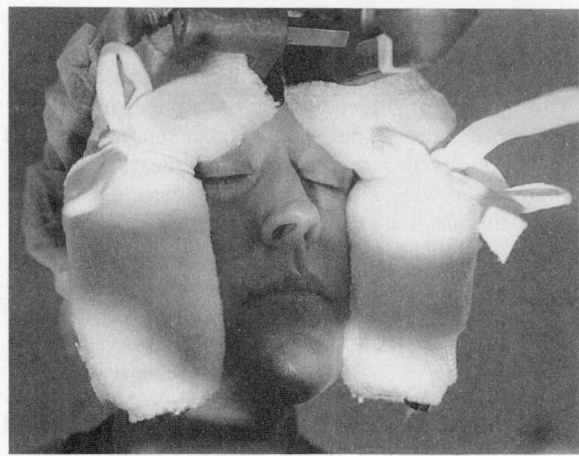

**FIGURE 28–9.** Umbilical tape compressing padding to prevent direct pressure on the eyes.

otherwise place pressure on the eyes (see Fig. 28–8; Fig. 28–9).

Positioning the head in the prone position is done with strict attention devoted to the eyes, orbits, cervical spine, ears, and the ETT. Pressure on the eyes can result in retinal artery thrombosis and postoperative blindness, and can be prevented by use of a soft foam headrest with a cutout for the face and ETT. As previously noted, care must be taken to prevent shifting of the face on the headrest. Use of supplemental rigid plastic eye goggles is discouraged because they have a rigid frame that may focus pressure on the face if they are not completely out of contact with the foam cushion. Pressure against a folded external ear when the head is turned to the side can cause cartilaginous damage.[4]

### Endotracheal Tube

ETT management in the prone patient can be problematic. It may be difficult to assess tube position and identify possible kinking. Secretions may also cause a loss of tape adherence. Administration of an antisialagogue can help to minimize secretions. A contoured foam head support with an opening for the ETT and cutouts for the eyes is both useful and effective. If the tube is secured with tape that encircles the neck, it should be loose enough to ensure that cerebral venous drainage is not obstructed. The eyes, ears, and nose should be individually inspected and verified to be free of any externally applied pressure from the padding. These areas should be rechecked at intervals throughout the case.

### Cervical Spine

The head may be turned to the side or kept neutral. The cervical spine is usually maintained in a neutral to slightly flexed position during the procedure. Neutrality of the cervical spine is easily verified by observing symmetry of the skin folds between the neck and shoulder on each side and by ensuring that several inches of space are present between the mandible and the suprasternal notch.

### Arms

Arm position in the prone patient should also be assessed. All efforts should be made to limit arm abduction to a 90°

angle to the sagittal plane of the body to minimize stretch of the brachial plexus. The presence of a skin crease visible over the posterior shoulder may indicate that the arm is in an overly abducted position. It is better to see both arms somewhat abducted slightly in front of the coronal plane of the body. This position is made possible by use of a chest support of sufficient height.

### Chest/Abdomen

Chest rolls, a Wilson-type laminectomy frame, or a Relton-Hall frame may be used to facilitate prone positioning. However, complications can result from the use of any frame. One known complication is the occurrence of pressure ulcers on that portion of the chest wall that is in contact with the chest roll or frame. This problem is related to the duration of surgery and may occur despite careful and diligent efforts. These skin injuries likely represent a combination of traction and pressure. Despite attempts to eliminate traction on the skin and to pad the weight-bearing areas (see Table 28–1), areas of pressure are still common, especially in procedures that last several hours.

The chest rolls or laminectomy frame should be placed so that the iliac crests and lateral hemithoraces bear the weight (Figs. 28–10 through 28–12). Support should not be borne by the clavicles; otherwise, the brachial plexus may become compressed between the clavicle and the underlying ribs. Either support system allows the abdomen to hang freely. Care should also be taken to verify that breast tissue and genitalia are not trapped; once the patient is draped, reassessment and repositioning are extremely difficult. Knee and chest positioning (Fig. 28–13) or positioning on the Andrews frame can result in decreased venous pressure at the surgical site because of abdominal venous pooling. The possibility of air entrainment or venous air embolism exists, particularly with spontaneous ventilation. Use of compression stockings, fluid loading, or positive pressure ventilation may decrease this risk.

### Bony Prominences

Sufficient padding of bony prominences should be considered, especially in the ulnar nerve region on the medial aspects

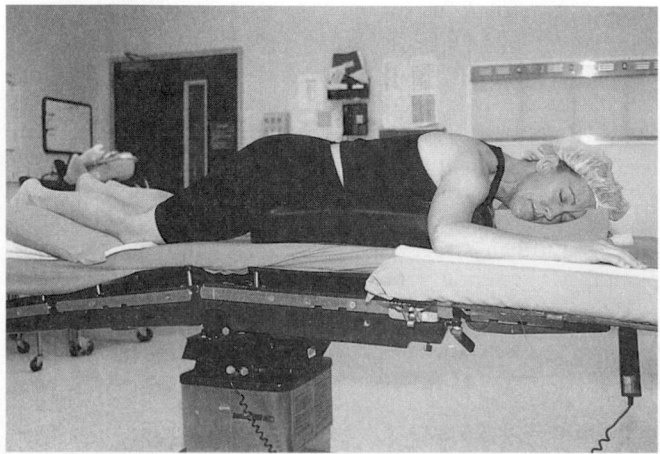

**FIGURE 28–10.** Prone position on gel-filled chest rolls. Note padding under arms and knees. Arm abduction is limited to 90°.

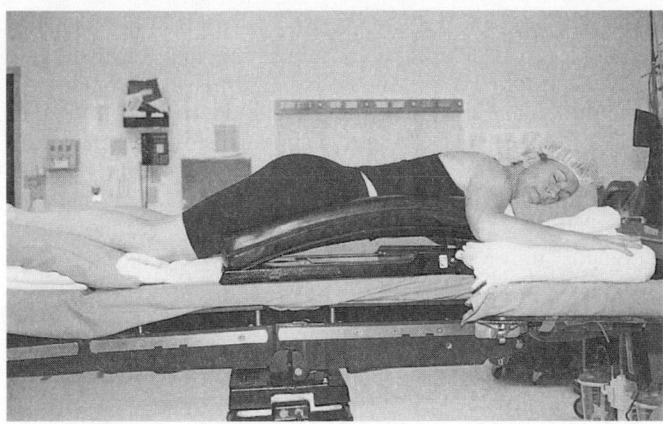

**FIGURE 28–11.** Prone position on Wilson frame with mild leg flexion and knee and arm padding.

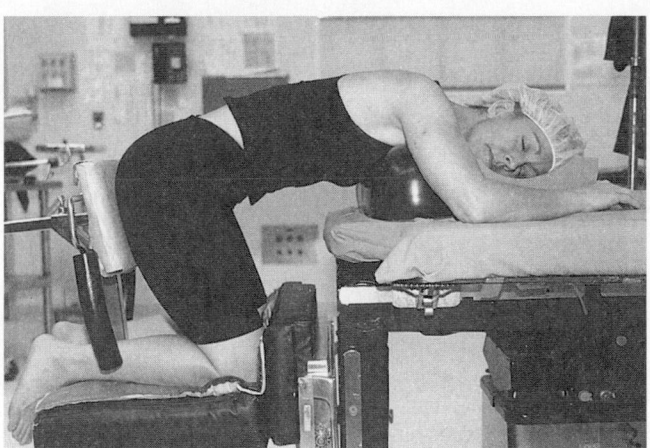

**FIGURE 28–13.** Andrews frame for laminectomy allowing abdomen to hang free. Note knee and chest gel-filled padding.

of the arms. The iliac crests, knees, ankles, and tibial portions of the lower legs should also be padded.

## Cervical Instability

Surgery may be performed on a patient with an unstable cervical spine or a severe myelopathy. In such a case, preoperative discussion with the surgeon is prudent. Several options exist:

1. Awake intubation, which can permit a neurologic examination after intubation or positioning
2. Asleep fiberoptic intubation
3. Conventional laryngoscopy with in-line cervical stabilization
4. Alternative techniques such as lightwand or intubating laryngeal mask airway

The specific technique depends on the clinical circumstances and the collaboration of the anesthesiologist and surgeon. Such techniques and precautions should be carefully documented on the record. This documentation can help to limit subsequent liability, should a neurologic complication occur.

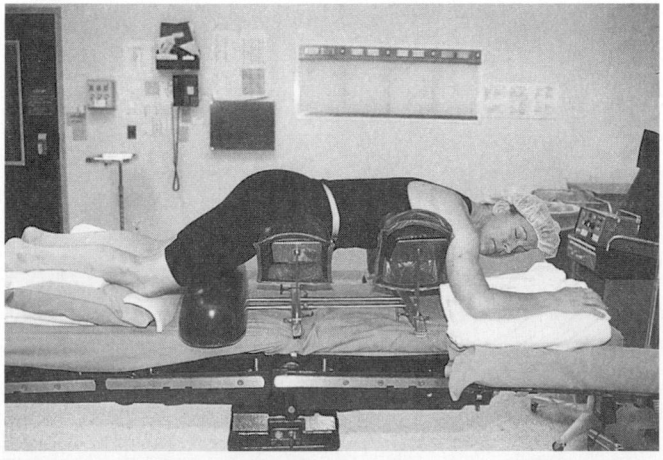

**FIGURE 28–12.** Prone position on Relton-Hall frame. Note iliac crest and thoracic support. Pillows and padding allow mild flexion and arm and leg support.

## What Considerations Are Associated With the Lateral Decubitus Position?

The lateral decubitus position is most often used for hip, chest, or renal procedures. It is designated as left or right to identify the side of the patient *in contact* with the operating table. $\dot{V}/\dot{Q}$ mismatches may be significant. The dependent lung receives most of the pulmonary blood flow and is compressed by mediastinal contents and a cephalad shift of the diaphragm. The nondependent lung receives most of the ventilation (during positive pressure ventilation). This $\dot{V}/\dot{Q}$ mismatch can lead to hypoxemia and a larger than usual arterial to end-tidal $CO_2$ gradient. During spontaneous ventilation, the cephalad displacement of the dependent diaphragm may result in a mechanical advantage. This can result in better ventilation of the dependent lung and an improved $\dot{V}/\dot{Q}$ match.

### Precautions

#### Dependent Arm and Axilla

The dependent arm should be well padded and a chest roll placed just *below* the axilla to support the upper part of the rib cage to ensure decompression of the axillary neurovascular bundle and remove pressure from the head of the humerus (Figs. 28–14 and 28–15). If the chest roll is placed too cephalad, brachial plexus compression can occur. If an open space is present between the axilla and the chest roll and if the pulse in that arm is palpable, the arm and axilla are likely in appropriate position. The usual considerations apply for protecting the ulnar nerve. The nondependent arm is positioned over the dependent one, and pillows, blankets, or an overhead arm board are placed between them.

#### Head and Neck

The patient's head should be kept in a neutral cervical spine position, and the ear must be checked to minimize folding and cartilaginous pressure. Our experience is that a pad thicker than might be expected is usually required to support the head in a normal position. Neutrality is easily checked by comparing the posterior neck skin creases for symmetry. The dependent eye should also be checked to ascertain that it is free from pressure. Use of an antisialogogue, as mentioned previously,

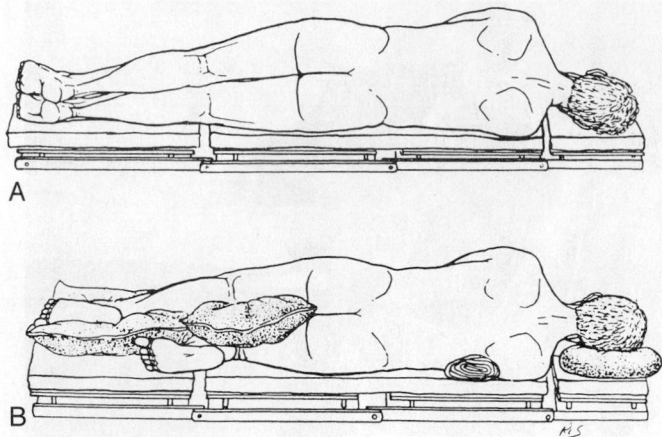

**FIGURE 28–14.** The standard right lateral decubitus position. *A,* Improper head position and inadequate padding. *B,* Proper padding is present over bone prominences, a chest roll is placed to protect the axilla, and the cervical spine is properly aligned. A flexed lower leg stabilizes the torso and relaxes the lower extremity. (From Lawson NW, Meyer JD. Lateral positions. In: Martin JT, Warner MA, eds. *Positioning in Anesthesia and Surgery.* 3rd ed. Philadelphia, Pa: WB Saunders; 1996:127.)

minimizes oral secretions that may otherwise cause loosening of the tape used to secure the ETT in this position.

### Hip and Leg

Considerable pressure is exerted on the dependent iliac crest, greater trochanter, and knee. A foam (eggcrate) pad or gel-filled pad can be placed between the mattress and the patient to protect these points. The dependent leg is also flexed, and the safety strap is placed so that it is across the waist or the thigh rather than the hip or knee. The peroneal nerve at the dependent knee is especially vulnerable; padding should be checked so that no pressure is exerted over the peroneal nerve as it courses around the head of the fibula.

### What Is a Way to Move the Patient From Supine to the Lateral Decubitus Position?

When the patient is placed in the lateral decubitus position, there must be an adequate number of people to assist in lifting. Each person is assigned a task. The patient is usually anesthetized on the operating table rather than on a gurney. The anesthesiologist continues to be responsible for control of the head and ETT. The head, shoulders, and body are turned as a unit under the anesthesiologist's direction, and the patient is, in effect, log-rolled into position. This maneuver requires at least three and preferably four people. If an ether screen is used, the patient's arms should not be allowed to rest against it.

After the chest roll is in place, an easy (although imperfect) test for vascular compromise to the dependent arm and hand is to place the pulse oximeter on one of the dependent fingers. Although a palpable pulse and normal oxygen saturation alone are not adequate to verify acceptable positioning, when used in conjunction with visual inspection and palpation of pressure points, they complete the assessment process.

### What Considerations Are Associated With the Head-Up or Semisitting Position?

The head-up position is used to facilitate exposure and enhance venous drainage for posterior fossa craniotomies and some operations on the cervical spine, face, neck, and shoulders. The position, however, may predispose the patient to venous air embolism. Initially, the patient is supine for anesthetic induction and then is moved into the lawn chair position. The neck is flexed, and the head may be placed in a three-point head holder by the neurosurgeon, with the anesthesiologist having control of the airway at all times. The back of the table is raised to create the sitting position while the table is tilted downward (Fig. 28–16).

Neck flexion is limited to allow at least two fingerbreadths between the sternum and the chin to prevent kinking or biting the ETT, jugular venous obstruction, and cervical spinal cord ischemia. This should also prevent stretch of the cervical musculature. Gluteal padding should be ensured with foam, and the knees should be flexed with the feet in the slightly dorsiflexed position. The patient's arms are either secured to padded arm boards at the sides, or they are placed across the chest. In both instances, the courses of the ulnar nerves should be inspected.

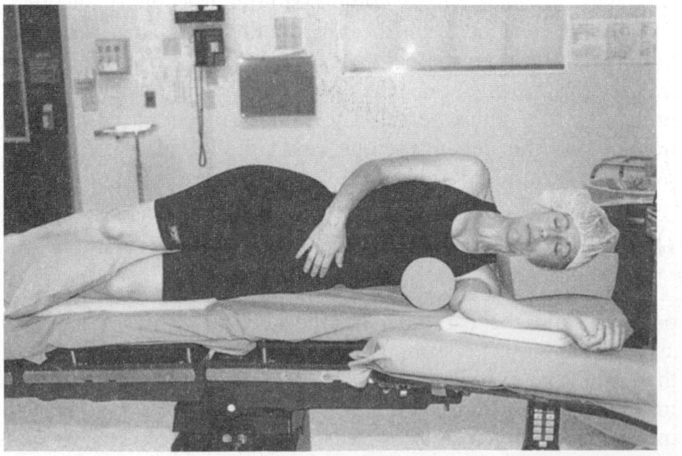

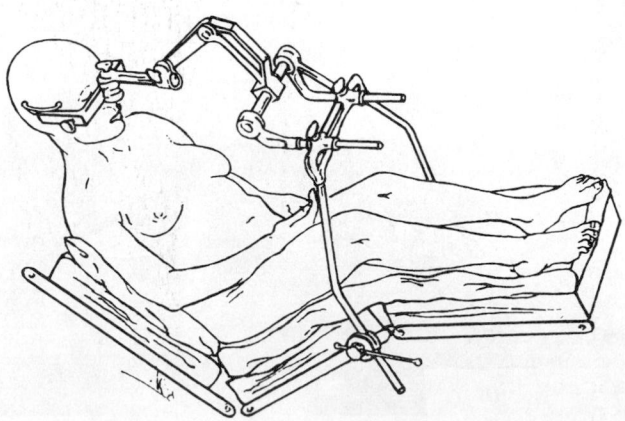

**FIGURE 28–15.** Lateral decubitus position showing axillary roll and padding of head, dependent arm, and dependent leg.

**FIGURE 28–16.** Patient in position using a 3-pin clamp. (Reproduced with permission from Anderton JM, Keen RI, Neave R. *Positioning the Surgical Patient.* London, United Kingdom: Butterworth-Heinemann; 1988:68.)

## What Contributes to the Risk of Air Embolism?

The risk of air embolism from the surgical field is always present when the surgical field is higher than the right atrium. Holes made in the skull with pin-type head holders that open venous sinuses or bony canals can allow air to be entrained into the vascular system, thus causing a venous air embolism. Patients in the sitting position should be routinely monitored for early detection of air embolism.

Continuous monitors include (1) a precordial Doppler ultrasound probe, which is secured over the heart in a position that is known to detect air; and (2) capnography, which identifies any sudden decrease in expired carbon dioxide. A central venous catheter located at the junction of the superior vena cava and right atrium can assist in confirming the diagnosis of venous air embolism and, if needed, in the removal of entrained air.

Clinical indicators of air embolism include dysrhythmias, hypotension, and the late, relatively uncommon, pathognomonic "mill-wheel" murmurs. If the patient has a patent foramen ovale, air embolism can be extremely hazardous. Air can pass from the right side of the heart to the left side (paradoxically) and enter the coronary or cerebral circulation, causing ischemia and permanent injury.

A patient with physical findings or history suggestive of an intracardiac defect or patent foramen ovale preferably should be operated in a non—head-elevated position (eg, in the prone or three quarter prone position) to minimize (but not eliminate) the likelihood of venous and paradoxical air embolism. If this approach is not feasible, a transesophageal echocardiography probe is the most sensitive indicator of venous air embolism and should be considered for use in conjunction with the other monitors.

An additional consideration in head-elevated cases is transducer positioning. Blood pressure (BP) transducers are referenced to the external auditory meatus and central venous pressure transducers to the heart. If BP is referenced to the heart, as it is in the supine position, the hydrostatic pressure difference between the heart and the brain may be such that the brain may be hypoperfused, even though cardiac perfusion is adequate.

## What Considerations Are Associated With the Lithotomy Position?

The lithotomy position is most commonly used for gynecologic and urologic surgery. The first consideration for lithotomy positioning is to make sure that the equipment fits the patient. A leg support system is preferable (Fig. 28–17). An ankle strap system can also be used. When using either system, attention should be given to the patient's height, age, and weight and to estimates of the knee-to-ankle and thigh lengths.

If the patient is properly positioned supine, the gluteal folds are at the hinge, or break, in the operating table before anesthesia is induced. This preparation avoids the need to move the patient toward the foot of the bed after induction of anesthesia, but it may require that the headpiece of the table be attached to the foot of the bed so that the patient's feet do not hang over the end. The patient's arms are then secured to the armrests in a comfortable position that allows surgical and equipment access. During laparoscopic procedures, an arm is

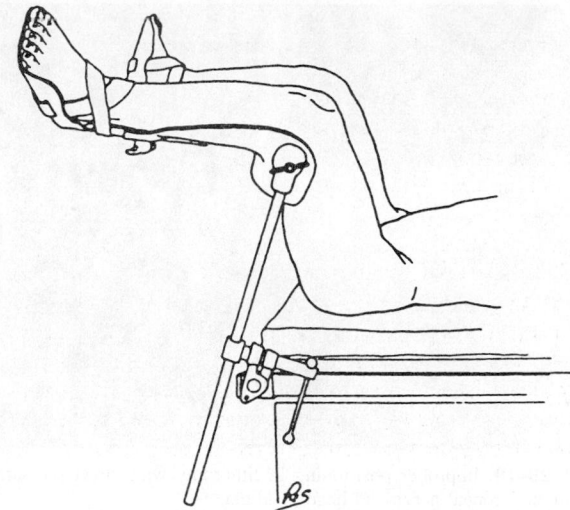

**FIGURE 28–17.** Proper lithotomy position. There is minimal external rotation of the legs, the thighs are minimally flexed toward the abdomen, and the legs symmetrically positioned. Protective padding is not shown. (From Martin JT, Lithotomy positions. In: Martin JT, Warner MA. *Positioning in Anesthesia and Surgery.* 3rd ed. Philadelphia, Pa: WB Saunders; 1996:47.)

often tucked and padded at the patient's side to allow equipment positioning while the other is abducted. Care must be taken to ensure that fingers do not become pinched where the table is hinged (Fig. 28–18).

Once anesthesia commences, the legs are simultaneously elevated, flexed at the hips and knees, and then positioned in either the stirrups or leg supports. Care should be taken to cushion both ankles and knees with soft foam padding or gel-filled foam padding to prevent pressure injury to the peroneal nerve where it crosses the head of the fibula (Fig. 28–19). The lithotomy position may be associated with positioning-related complications, including nerve injuries and compartment syndromes, in the lower extremities.[13]

### Specific Nerves

#### Obturator Nerves

Injury to the obturator nerve results in weakness or paralysis of the adductors of the thigh. Injury to the obturator nerve is

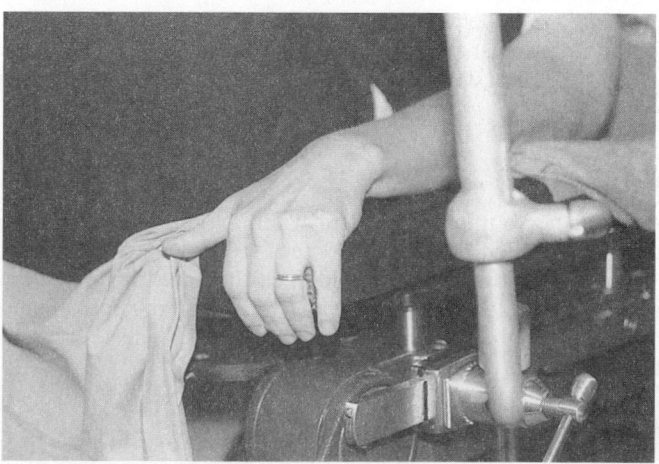

**FIGURE 28–18.** Fingers hanging in hinged area of operating table may become pinched when the foot of the bed is raised.

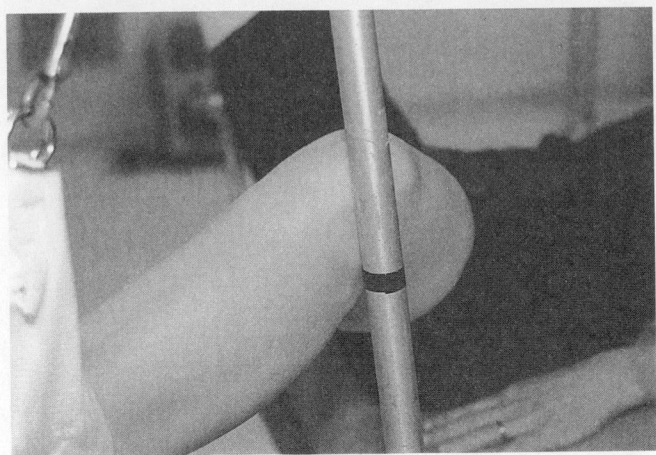

**FIGURE 28–19.** Improper positioning in lithotomy with direct pressure on the common peroneal nerve and head of fibula.

best prevented by avoiding acute flexion (>90°) of the thigh onto the groin, especially in obese patients; otherwise, this position risks stretching and compression of the obturator nerve at the inguinal ligament.

### Saphenous Nerves

The saphenous nerve is sensory to the medial portion of the leg, and its compression at the medial portion of the thigh can lead to loss of sensation along its distribution.

### Femoral Nerves

More common than obturator or saphenous nerve injury is trauma to the femoral nerve as it is trapped under the inguinal ligament after acute flexion and angulation of the thigh.[14] Injury to this nerve is manifested by abnormal gait, loss of quadriceps sensation, numbness, and hyperesthesia over the quadriceps. This complication can be lessened by avoiding excess abduction of the thigh and external rotation of the hip by lateral thigh supports.

### Lateral Femoral Cutaneous Nerve

Injury to the lateral femoral cutaneous nerve can cause a condition known as *meralgia paresthetica* that manifests as numbness or hyperesthesia of the anterior lateral thigh. This condition has been associated with wearing tight-fitting pants or belts and even with nerve compression from wallets or pagers.

### Sciatic Nerves

Sciatic nerve injury can occur when the thighs and legs are externally rotated or when the knees are extended. Clinically, all muscles below the knee, and even the hamstrings, may be paralyzed, and numbness of the lateral half of the calf and almost all of the foot occurs, except at the inner border of the arch.

### Common Peroneal Nerves

The most common injury to the lower extremity associated with the lithotomy position involves the superficial peroneal

nerve (see Figs. 28–3 and 28–19). It is vulnerable to compression along the lateral aspects of the knee by the leg support rods or by the supports themselves. Superficial peroneal nerve injury is manifested by weakness to the intrinsic muscles of the foot, sensory deficit to the sole of the foot, and footdrop.

### How Can Compartment Syndrome Occur?

Compartment syndrome of the lower extremity is a rare but serious complication that is caused by direct pressure on calf muscle tissue. Close attention to adequacy of padding and uniform weight distribution over weight-bearing areas may minimize the likelihood of compartment syndrome. Remember that the perfusion pressure in the legs, especially in the calves and feet, is reduced in proportion to the height to which they are elevated above the heart (0.7 mm Hg for every 1 cm of elevation).

### What Problems Are Associated With the Trendelenburg Position?

The Trendelenburg, or head-down, position, is commonly used to improve exposure of pelvic organs during gynecologic or urologic surgery. Historically, this position was characterized by a steep 30° to 40° tilt and necessitated shoulder braces to prevent the patient from sliding off the table. These braces were often implicated in brachial plexus injury.

In modern practice, the tilt is usually limited to 10° to 15°, and thus it does not require any additional patient restraints. With the Trendelenburg position, arterial pressure in the legs is decreased while relative engorgement occurs in the vessels of the mediastinum and head. Preload to the heart is increased. Intracranial pressure may increase because of the interference with cerebral venous drainage. This can result in decreased cerebral perfusion pressure and is particularly to be avoided in patients with increased intracranial pressure.

Use of the head-down position to treat hypotension and shock has not been shown to provide any consistent beneficial effect.[15,16] When hypovolemia is present, this position does not improve BP but may improve cardiac output slightly. Simple elevation of the patient's legs to increase preload is a more prudent measure. In addition to increasing intracranial pressure, placing a patient with CHF in the head-down position may also result in increased left ventricular end-diastolic pressure, which can exacerbate acute CHF, produce myocardial ischemia, or both.[17] The head-down position also decreases functional residual capacity, decreases pulmonary compliance, and increases the work of breathing. Atelectasis is aggravated, and hypoxemia may follow, especially when the patient is obese or elderly. Because of the cephalad shift of the mediastinum, ETT position should be reconfirmed when an intubated patient is placed in the head-down position. This shift can displace the lungs and the carina cephalad, causing the tip of the ETT to migrate distally into a mainstem bronchus.

## PERIPHERAL NERVE INJURIES

The principal cause of peripheral nerve injury in anesthetized patients is ischemia of the intraneural vasa nervorum.

This can result from nerve stretch, compression, or both. Stretching and compression is more likely to occur in anesthetized rather than awake patients because muscle tone is reduced, and the patients are unable to complain of pain or paresthesias.

In the conscious patient, abduction of the arm >90° may quickly become painful and intolerable. After a few minutes, the radial pulse disappears in 83% of volunteers.[18] However, cases of upper extremity nerve injury have occurred in awake patients having lower extremity surgery under monitored anesthesia care or regional anesthesia. This is contrary to the argument often put forth that "had the patient been awake, the injury would not have occurred." In addition, bilateral abnormalities in nerve conduction velocities were found in 12 of 14 patient presenting with postoperative unilateral ulnar nerve symptoms.[19] Factors that contribute to the likelihood of peripheral nerve injury include hypotension, diabetes mellitus, peripheral vascular disease, vasoconstriction, and smoking, among others (Table 28–2).

### How Is a Postoperative Peripheral Nerve Complaint Evaluated?

#### Assessment of Injury Mechanism

The differential diagnosis for a postoperative peripheral nerve injury should consider trauma sustained before surgery and anesthesia, compression by a hematoma from a preexisting disease, prior injection injury, preexisting medical conditions, drugs, and toxins, as well as intraoperative positioning or direct surgical trauma. For example, the femoral nerve is prone to damage by pressure, lateral deflection, and direct trauma during lower abdominal procedures that use self-retaining retractors. On examination, loss of hip flexion, knee extension, and musculus quadriceps femoris palsy are noteworthy. In the early 1900s, the incidence of postpartum femoral neuropathy was reported to be as high as 4.7%.[20] Although the condition is less common now, it still occurs as a result of prolonged lithotomy positioning and the exertion of undue pressure on the patient's legs by surgeons performing pelvic and perineal surgery.[20]

#### Neurologic Consultation

When a postoperative nerve injury is suspected, a neurologist should be consulted. Electrophysiologic testing can be performed to obtain information concerning the injury site and to give some indication of the duration of the injury (ie, whether it was present before the procedure). A patient's electromyogram does not become abnormal until at least 1 week after the injury.[7]

In many instances, nerve conduction studies allow the location of the nerve injury to be delineated. They may also give an indication of its severity (eg, conduction delay versus absence). Thus, a patient with a perioperative nerve injury would initially have normal electromyographic study results, but several weeks later would manifest abnormal electromyographic responses consisting of reduced amplitude of the evoked motor and sensory responses.

### Why Is the Brachial Plexus Commonly Injured?

The brachial plexus apparently is susceptible to perioperative injury for two reasons. First, the plexus has a relatively long and mobile superficial course in the axilla between two firm points of fixation: the vertebrae and prevertebral fascia above and the axillary fascia below. Second, the plexus lies in proximity to a number of freely movable bone structures (see Fig. 28–1).

#### Mechanism of Injury

The chief cause of injury is thought to be stretching from dorsal extension and lateral flexion of the humeral head. This problem can best be avoided by maintaining the arm on an arm board that is level with the plane of the body and by never abducting the arm to an angle >90° from the sagittal plane.

#### Clinical Presentation

Brachial plexus injury is characterized by shoulder pain and tenderness in the supraclavicular area from one to several days after surgery. If the entire plexus is involved, the arm hangs flaccidly, and the skin of the whole limb is numb. If only the upper roots (C5-C7) are injured, Erb's paralysis (internal rotation of the arm, extension of the forearm, and pronation of the hand) results. Rarely, the lower roots (C8 and T1) are affected, and a Klumpke paralysis (loss of finger flexion, paralysis of the hand muscles, and perhaps Horner syndrome) result.

### Why Is the Radial Nerve Vulnerable?

The radial nerve may be traumatized if it is compressed as it passes in the spiral groove around the lateral border of the middle of the humerus. Radial nerve palsy is characterized by wrist drop, inability to extend the metacarpal joints, and inability to abduct the thumb. Sensation may be lost over the lateral 3½ fingers and the hand. The superficial radial nerve is also vulnerable to injury during intravenous catheter insertion into the cephalic vein at the proximal wrist.

### How Is the Median Nerve Traumatized?

The median nerve, which lies adjacent to the medial cubital and basilic veins in the antecubital fossa, may be traumatized

**TABLE 28–2.** Factors Associated With Polyneuropathies

| Drugs | Toxins | Diseases |
|---|---|---|
| Cisplatin | Diphtheria | Diabetes |
| Hydralazine | Lead | Uremia |
| Metronidazole | Arsenic | Liver disease |
| Phenytoin | Organophosphates | Porphyria |
| Vincristine | Thallium | Vitamin deficiencies |
| Amiodarone | | Amyloidosis |
| Pyridoxine | | Obstructive lung disease |
| Isoniazid | | Polycythemia vera |
| | | Lymphoma |
| | | Acromegaly |
| | | Malabsorption states |
| | | Hypothyroidism |

by direct needle penetration or by drug extravasation. The median nerve may also become compressed as it passes within the carpal tunnel at the wrist. Edema from intravenous fluid administration may contribute to nerve compression within the carpal tunnel. The patient is unable to oppose the thumb and little finger, has decreased ability to abduct the thumb, and loses flexion of the distal phalanx of the second finger. Sensation and sweating are diminished over the palmar surface of the lateral 3½ digits and the adjacent palm.

## How Does Ulnar Nerve Damage Occur?

The ulnar nerve may be injured by compression, stretch, or a combination of the two. The relative contribution of each is unknown. However, cases of postoperative ulnar nerve palsy occur in which, based on all available information, appropriate padding and positioning were used.[1,2] Therefore, as previously noted, the specific etiology of most ulnar neuropathies is unknown.[10]

The result of ulnar nerve injury is the decreased ability to grip with the hand and inability to abduct or oppose the little finger to the thumb. Decreased sensation occurs over both surfaces of the medial 1½ fingers in the hand. In severe cases,

the intrinsic hand muscles atrophy and contractures develop, resulting in the characteristic "claw hand."

The ulnar nerve may also be injured at the wrist during ulnar artery puncture or catheterization. Unlike the radial nerve, which becomes separate from the radial artery proximal to the wrist, the ulnar artery and nerve lie in close proximity at this location. Distal placement and frequent cycling of a noninvasive BP cuff near the elbow has also been implicated in a case of ulnar nerve injury.[21]

In summary, careful and safe positioning requires knowledge of anatomy, physiology, and attention to detail. Despite the best and appropriate efforts of careful and competent anesthesiologists, position-related injuries may still occur. In an attempt to guide clinicians better and delineate our understanding of mechanisms and prevention of perioperative nerve injuries, the ASA, in April 2000, issued a practice advisory for the prevention of perioperative peripheral neuropathies.[22] The consultant survey of evidence linkage and positioning interventions thought to decrease peripheral neuropathy is given in Table 28–3. It is clear that, with the exception of protecting the fibular head from contact pressure, there is no unanimity of opinion. It is noteworthy to be reminded that practice advisories are intended to "assist in decision-making areas of patient care where scientific evidence is insuffi-

**TABLE 28–3.** Consultant Survey of Evidence Linkages

| Type of Neuropathy | Positioning Intervention to Decrease Risk of Peripheral Neuropathy (Does the Use of the Intervention Impact the Risk of Neuropathy?) | N | % Agreement | | |
| --- | --- | --- | --- | --- | --- |
| | | | Agree | Disagree | Don't Know |
| Any | A focused preoperative history | 84 | 93 | 6 | 1 |
| Any | A focused preoperative examination | 82 | 88 | 5 | 7 |
| Upper extremity | Periodic assessment of upper extremity position during procedures | 83 | 92 | 5 | 3 |
| Brachial plexus | Limiting abduction of the arm(s) in a supine patient | 82 | 92 | 1 | 7 |
| Brachial plexus | Limiting abduction of the arm(s) in a prone patient | 81 | 88 | 5 | 7 |
| Ulnar | Specific forearm position(s) in a supine patient with an arm(s) tucked at the side | 83 | 72 | 11 | 17 |
| Ulnar | Specific forearm position(s) in a supine patient who has an arm(s) abducted on an armboard | 83 | 74 | 16 | 10 |
| Ulnar | Flexion of the elbow | 81 | 52 | 20 | 28 |
| Radial | Pressure in the spiral groove of the humerus from prolonged contact with a hard surface | 82 | 89 | 2 | 9 |
| Median | Extension of the elbow in an anesthetized, supine patient beyond the normal range of extension that is comfortable during the preoperative exam | 82 | 59 | 7 | 34 |
| Sciatic | In a patient who is positioned in a lateral or lithotomy position, stretching of the hamstring muscle group beyond a range that is comfortable during a preoperative evaluation | 81 | 48 | 9 | 43 |
| Femoral | Extension of the hip in a supine patient beyond a range that is comfortable during a preoperative evaluation | 83 | 40 | 10 | 50 |
| Peroneal | Pressure near the fibular head from contact with a hard surface or a rigid support | 83 | 92 | 0 | 8 |
| Upper extremity | Padded armboards | 83 | 89 | 1 | 10 |
| Brachial plexus | A chest roll placed under the "downside" (dependent) lateral thorax in a patient who is positioned laterally | 83 | 78 | 7 | 15 |
| Ulnar | Specific padding (eg, foam or gel pads) at the elbow | 83 | 67 | 10 | 23 |
| Peroneal | Specific padding to prevent contact of the peroneal nerve (at the fibular head) with a hard surface | 81 | 9 | 1 | 5 |
| | Padding in some circumstances may increase peripheral neuropathy | 81 | 68 | 14 | 18 |
| Brachial plexus | Shoulder braces to prevent a patient from sliding cephalad when placed in a steep head-down position | 83 | 66 | 9 | 25 |
| Ulnar | Automated blood pressure cuff on the arm | 82 | 39 | 26 | 35 |
| Radial | Automated blood pressure cuff on the arm | 83 | 39 | 21 | 40 |
| Median | Automated blood pressure cuff on the arm | 82 | 29 | 29 | 42 |
| Any | Examining a patient in the postanesthesia care unit | 83 | 72 | 17 | 11 |
| Any | Documentation on an anesthetic record of specific positioning actions | 84 | 88 | 8 | 4 |

From American Society of Anesthesiologists. Practice advisory for the prevention of perioperative peripheral neuropathies: a report by the American Society of Anesthesiologists Task Force on Prevention of Perioperative Peripheral Neuropathies. *Anesthesiology.* 2000;92:1177.

cient."[23] It is obvious that further research regarding perioperative nerve injuries is needed.

## References

1. Kroll DA, Caplan RA, Posner K, et al. Nerve injury associated with anesthesia. *Anesthesiology.* 1990;73:202.
2. Cheney FW, Domino KB, Caplan RA, et al. Nerve injury associated with anesthesia: a closed claims analysis. *Anesthesiology.* 1999;90:1062.
3. Brown EM, Elman DS. Postoperative backache. *Anesth Analg.* 1961;40:683.
4. Courington FW, Little DM. The role of posture in anesthesia. *Clin Anesth.* 1968;3:24.
5. Denny-Brown D, Doherty MM. Effects of transient stretching of peripheral nerve. *Arch Neurol Psychiatr.* 1945;54:116.
6. Britt BA, Gordon RA. Peripheral nerve injuries associated with anaesthesia. *Can Anaesth Soc J.* 1964;11:514.
7. Dawson DM, Krarup C. Perioperative nerve lesions. *Arch Neurol.* 1989;46:1355.
8. Nakata DA, Stoelting RK. Positioning. In: Morell RC, Eichhorn JH, eds. *Patient Safety in Anesthetic Practice.* New York, NY: Churchill Livingstone; 1997:293.
9. Vander Salm TJ, Cereda J-M, Cutler BS. Brachial plexus injury following median sternotomy. *J Thorac Cardiovasc Surg.* 1980;80:447.
10. Stoelting RK. Postoperative ulnar nerve palsy: is it a preventable complication? *Anesth Analg.* 1993;76:7.
11. Prielipp RC, Morell RC, Walker FO, et al. Ulnar nerve pressure: influence of arm position and relationship to somatosensory evoked potentials. *Anesthesiology.* 1999;91:345.
12. Martin JT. The ventral decubitus (prone) positions. In: Martin JT, Warner MA, eds. *Positioning in Anesthesia and Surgery.* 3rd ed. Philadelphia, Pa: WB Saunders; 1996:155.
13. Martin JT. Compartment syndromes: concepts and perspectives of the anesthesiologist. *Anesth Analg.* 1992;75:275.
14. Tondare AS, Nadkarni AV, Sathe CH, et al. Femoral neuropathy: a complication of lithotomy position under spinal anaesthesia *Can Anaesth Soc J.* 1983;30:84.
15. Sibbald WJ, Patterson NAM, Holliday RL, et al. The Trendelenburg position: hemodynamic effects in hypotensive and normotensive patients. *Crit Care Med.* 1979;7:218.
16. Gentili DR, Benjamin E, Berger SR, et al. Cardiopulmonary effects of the head-down tilt position in elderly postoperative patients: a prospective study. *South Med J.* 1988;81:1258.
17. Kubal K, Komatsu T, Sonchala V, et al. Trendelenburg position used during venous cannulation increases myocardial oxygen demand [abstract]. *Anesth Analg.* 1984;63:239.
18. Wright S. The neurovascular syndrome produced by hypertension of the arms. *Am Heart J.* 1945;29:1.
19. Alvine FG, Schurrer ME. Postoperative ulnar-nerve palsy: are there predisposing factors? *J Bone Joint Surg Am.* 1987;69:255.
20. Vargo MM, Robinson LR, Nicholas JJ, et al. Postpartum femoral neuropathy: relic of an earlier era. *Arch Phys Med Rehabil.* 1990;71:591.
21. Sy W. Ulnar nerve palsy possibly related to use of automatically cycled blood pressure cuff. *Anesth Analg.* 1981;60:687.
22. American Society of Anesthesiologists. Practice advisory for the prevention of perioperative peripheral neuropathies: a report by the American Society of Anesthesiologists Task Force on Prevention of Perioperative Peripheral Neuropathies. *Anesthesiology.* 2000;92:1168
23. Caplan RA. Will we ever understand perioperative neuropathy? A fresh approach offers hope and insight. *Anesthesiology.* 1999;91:335.

Anesthetic prescription is often made with more thought toward institutional tradition than individualization of technique for a specific patient. General anesthetic proponents often suggest that in most patients, no measurable outcome differences can be demonstrated between general and regional anesthesia. If the focus of anesthetic prescription and clinical outcome simply includes the intraoperative period, likely they are correct.

Nevertheless, when anesthesiologists are questioned about their preference for anesthetic prescription, they overwhelmingly choose regional anesthesia for themselves.[1,2] Perhaps they recognize there is more to anesthetic prescription than just a consideration of the intraoperative period. Experimental and clinical evidence is increasingly accumulating that preventing painful intraoperative neural impulses from adversely affecting patients is a position that minimizes pain transmission in the immediate as well as distant postoperative period.[3-5]

## PHILOSOPHY OF REGIONAL ANESTHESIA

### When Is It Indicated?

If anesthetic prescriptions take into consideration the prevention of dorsal horn wind-up and central sensitization of pain pathways, almost every surgical patient is a candidate for some form of regional anesthesia. If an anesthetic is

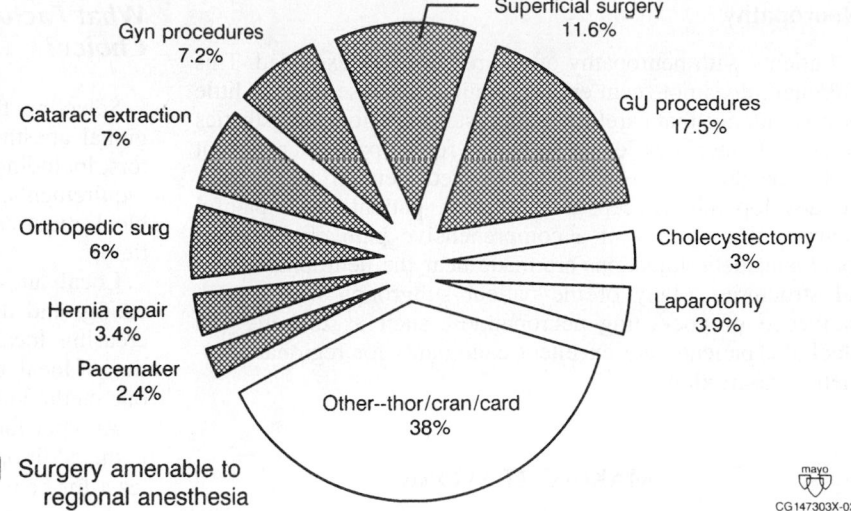

**FIGURE 29–1.** Proportion of surgical procedures performed in patients over age 65 years. card, cardiac; cran, cranial; Gyn, gynecologic; GU, genitourinary; thor, thoracic. (Modified from *Sourcebook of Aging.* Chicago, Ill: Marquis Academica Media; 1979:422.)

selected on the basis of other factors, such as the applicability of regional anesthesia to the surgical procedure in question, the group of patients may be slightly different.

Kopacz and Nickel suggested that almost 60% of patients older than 65 years of age are candidates for regional anesthesia.[6] They developed this estimate by calculating the number of Medicare patients undergoing specific operations in the United States (Fig. 29–1). Because those more than 65 years of age undergo most of the surgical procedures in many practices, the possibility for widespread use of regional anesthesia seems evident.

## When Is It Contraindicated?

### Patient Refusal or Inability to Cooperate

Are there situations in which regional anesthesia is contraindicated? One obvious and absolute contraindication to regional anesthesia is patient refusal. Often, however, such refusal results because the technique is presented to them in an unfavorable light by anesthesiologists uncomfortable with their own abilities.[7]

Many patients are concerned because they are led to believe they will be "awake" during the surgical procedure. In my experience, it is a rare adult who is unwilling to receive a regional block if it is presented as an option with confidence, if it is administered humanely and comprehensively, and if anxiolytics and opioids are titrated according to the patient, surgical procedure, and anesthetic technique chosen.

Another absolute contraindication to regional anesthesia is a patient's inability to cooperate. Risks are unnecessarily increased by attempting a regional block in a patient who is either unable or unwilling to hold still while the regional anesthetic is induced.

### Aortic Stenosis

Patients in whom regional anesthetics should be cautiously prescribed are those with significant aortic stenosis. This condition is not an absolute contraindication to a neuraxial block. However, the pathophysiologic process of aortic stenosis (thickened left ventricle requiring higher perfusion pressures)

needs to be seriously considered before a neuraxial block is considered.[8] There is evidence that use of spinal or epidural anesthesia in selected patients with aortic stenosis is acceptable.[9] This approach appears possible only if the cardiovascular physiologic changes accompanying aortic stenosis are taken into account in the treatment of cardiovascular perturbations after induction of the neuraxial anesthetic.

### Coagulopathy

Other patients who often are excluded from regional anesthetic prescription are those with any signs of coagulopathy. Automatic exclusion of anyone receiving drugs that may affect the coagulation system may be convenient; however, appropriate risk-benefit partitioning needs to be considered if regional anesthesia is to be appropriately prescribed. For example, most orthopedic surgical patients undergoing total joint replacement have received platelet-active drugs, and regional anesthetics are often safely used. Some patients receiving oral preoperative anticoagulants, such as warfarin, have prothrombin times not yet returned to a normal range. They still may be candidates for expertly performed regional anesthetics.

My preference is to consider small-gauge, midline, "single-shot" spinal anesthetics when prothrombin times are up to 1.5 times normal (approximately 16-17 seconds, international normalized ratio ≈1.4), and the anesthetic provides clear advantages. Such patients include people with significant reactive airway disease or those with a pertinent history of deep venous thrombosis after prior surgical procedures. Each anesthesiologist must develop a risk-benefit equation to suit his or her practice and patient subgroups.

### Sepsis

Patients who are considered septic are often excluded from consideration for spinal or epidural blocks because the needle may allow infected blood to enter either the epidural or subarachnoid space,[10] resulting in either epidural abscess or meningitis. If a patient has received antibiotic therapy and shows a positive response, and the risk-benefit calculation of spinal or epidural versus a general anesthetic favors a regional technique, it is acceptable.[11]

## Neuropathy

Patients with neuropathy often are similarly excluded. This judgment does not seem entirely logical because there is little or no evidence that carefully administered regional anesthetics carry a higher risk of neuropathy for a particular patient and procedure than well administered general anesthetics. To develop this concept even further, patients with painful neuropathies often visit a comprehensive pain clinic where local anesthetic injections are made near the neuropathic neural structures. Many of the patient subgroups with a high incidence of coexisting neuropathies, such as diabetic and alcoholic patients, are excellent candidates for regional anesthetic prescription.

## MAKING IT WORK

### Why Should an Induction Area Be Available?

Performance of regional anesthesia demands an integrated approach to its induction if the anesthesiologist is to successfully incorporate varied techniques into a daily practice. An essential component of comprehensive regional anesthesia is an area of the operating suite that can be used for induction. Many regional blocks can be administered while the operating room is still being readied.

If dedicated areas for regional anesthesia induction are not available in the operating suite, an area of the postanesthesia care unit or a partitioned area in the preoperative holding area can be used. Any area that is chosen must be equipped with the full array of resuscitative aids.

If one's practice involves teaching regional anesthesia, an induction area is even more essential than for a person in private practice. My clinical impression is that trainees are able to remember and incorporate more aspects of regional anesthesia in a nonstressful induction area than in a hectic operating theater with an audience of impatient surgeons in attendance.

### What Factors Govern Local Anesthetic Choice?

Selecting the appropriate local anesthetic for a given regional anesthetic requires consideration of a number of factors, including the duration of surgery, postoperative analgesia requirements, the operative site (including the degree of motor block required), and a patient's status (outpatient versus inpatient).

Local anesthetics range from short, to medium, to long acting, and the degree of motor blockade increases with increasing local anesthetic concentration. Thus, individualization of local anesthetic choice is possible. Figure 29–2 outlines one method of "walking across the local anesthetic time line."

Another factor that affects the duration of local anesthetics is the addition of vasoconstrictors or α-adrenergic agonists (at least for neuraxial blocks). Epinephrine or phenylephrine may prolong useful local anesthetic action by 30% to 50%.[12] A patient's weight, the volume of anesthetic needed to achieve the block, and avoidance of toxic doses are additional factors to consider (Table 29–1).

### What Constitutes a Successful Block?

Perhaps the most important concept in successful use of regional anesthesia is an understanding of what constitutes a successful block. For too many practitioners, a regional anesthetic is considered successful only if no additional sedative drugs are administered.[13] This concept needs rethinking. Supplementation of a regional anesthetic with intravenous or inhaled agents should not be considered a marker of a failed block but rather an appropriate use of balanced anesthesia. Anxiolysis is an extremely important part of any perioperative anesthetic experience, and patients undergoing regional anesthesia are no different from patients undergoing general anesthetic techniques.

The following analogy may help to focus this issue. An anesthesiologist would not be expected to select an arbitrary concentration of isoflurane before administering a general

## LOCAL ANESTHETIC TIME LINE (in minutes)

|  | Procaine | Chloroprocaine | Lidocaine | Mepivacaine | Tetracaine | Etidocaine | Bupivacaine |
|---|---|---|---|---|---|---|---|
| Infiltration | 45-60 |  | 75-90 |  |  |  | 180-360 |
| + epi | 60-90 |  | 90-180 |  |  |  | 200-400 |
| Peripheral |  |  | 90-120 | 100-150 |  |  | 480-780 |
| + epi |  |  | 120-180 | 120-220 |  |  | 600-900 |
| SAB* | 60-75 |  | 60 |  | 70-90 |  | 90-110 |
| + epi | 75-90 |  | 75-100 |  | 100-150 |  | 100-150 |
| phenylephrine† | 90-120 |  |  |  | 200-300 |  |  |
| Epidural |  | 45-60 | 80-120 | 90-140 |  | 120-200 | 165-225 |
| + epi |  | 60-90 | 120-180 | 140-200 |  | 150-225 | 180-240 |

*Subarachnoid block, † For lower extremity surgery

**FIGURE 29–2.** Local anesthetic timeline. Understanding the length of time that specific local anesthetics can be expected to provide surgical anesthesia can be extremely helpful in matching local anesthetic choice to patient, procedure, surgeon, and so on.

CG 147303B-01

**TABLE 29–1.** Comparative Pharmacology of Local Anesthetics

| Classification | Potency | Maximum Single Dose | | | Toxic Plasma Concentration (μg/mL) |
| | | *(mg)* | Plain *(mg/kg)* | With Epinephrine *(mg/kg)* | |
|---|---|---|---|---|---|
| *Esters* | | | | | |
| Procaine | 1 | 500 | 7–8 | 10–12 | |
| Chloroprocaine | 4 | 600 | 8–9 | 10–12 | |
| Tetracaine | 16 | 100 | | 2 | |
| *Amides* | | | | | |
| Lidocaine | 1 | 300 | 4–5 | 7–8 | >5 |
| Mepivacaine | 1 | 300 | 4–5 | 7–8 | >5 |
| Prilocaine | 1 | 400 | 5–6 | 8–9 | >5 |
| Bupivacaine | 4 | 175 | 2–3 | 3–4 | ~1.5 |
| Etidocaine | 4 | 300 | 4–5 | 5–6 | ~2 |

Data from Covino BG, Vassalo HL. *Local Anesthetics: Mechanisms of Action and Clinical Use.* New York, NY: Grune & Stratton: 1976:151.

anesthetic and, on discovering that the concentration needed to be altered during the anesthetic, consider the technique a failure. Regional anesthesia is no different; after its initial induction, supplementation should be administered to provide optimal operating conditions for the patient, surgeon, and anesthesiologist. The intravenous agents that are available for appropriate regional anesthesia sedation include benzodiazepines, opioids, propofol, and barbiturates.

## NEURAXIAL BLOCKS: SPINAL ANESTHESIA

### How Is a Spinal Anesthetic Performed?

Spinal anesthesia is unrivaled in the way a small amount of drug, almost devoid of systemic pharmacologic effect, produces profound, reproducible surgical anesthesia. Furthermore, by altering the drug choice, different levels of spinal anesthesia can be produced. Low spinal anesthesia, a block below T10, carries with it a different physiologic impact than does a block performed to produce higher spinal anesthesia (above T5).

The block is unsurpassed for lower abdominal or lower extremity surgical procedures. However, for operations in the middle to upper abdomen, "light" general anesthesia may be needed to supplement the spinal block. Stimulation of the diaphragm during upper abdominal procedures often causes patient discomfort. The area is difficult to block completely through high spinal anesthesia (to do so requires blockade of the phrenic nerve, not a desirable goal).

### Patient Selection

Patient selection for spinal anesthesia often places too much focus on a side effect—spinal headache—than on the applicability of the technique.[14] The incidence of spinal headache increases with decreasing age and female sex; however, with proper technique and needle selection, it should not preclude spinal anesthesia in young, healthy patients if the block has advantages over epidural anesthesia.[15] Almost any patient who is to have a lower extremity operation is a potential candidate for spinal anesthesia, as are most patients scheduled for lower abdominal surgery (gynecologic, urologic, and obstetric procedures and inguinal herniorrhaphy).

### Drug Choice

In North America, three local anesthetics are commonly used to produce spinal anesthesia: lidocaine, tetracaine, and bupivacaine. Lidocaine produces a short- to intermediate-acting spinal anesthetic; tetracaine and bupivacaine provide intermediate- to long-duration block.

### Lidocaine

Lidocaine, without epinephrine, is often chosen for procedures that can be completed in 1 hour or less. The mixture most commonly used is a 5% solution in 7.5% dextrose. When epinephrine (0.2 mg) is added, the useful length of clinical anesthesia in the lower abdomen and lower extremities is approximately 90 minutes.[10]

### Tetracaine

Tetracaine is packaged as both niphanoid crystals (20 mg) and as a 1% solution (2-mL ampule). When dextrose is added to make the solution hyperbaric, tetracaine usually produces effective clinical anesthesia for procedures lasting up to 1.5 to 2 hours in the plain form, for up to 2 to 3 hours when epinephrine (0.2 mg) is added, and up to 5 hours for lower extremity procedures when phenylephrine (5 mg) is added as a vasoconstrictor.[11]

### Bupivacaine

Bupivacaine spinal anesthesia is commonly carried out with 0.5% or 0.75% solution, either plain or in 8.25% dextrose. My impression is that the clinical difference between 0.5% tetracaine and 0.75% bupivacaine as hyperbaric solutions is minimal.[16] Bupivacaine is useful for procedures lasting from 2 to 2.5 hours.

### Hypobaric Techniques

Local anesthetics can be mixed to produce hypobaric spinal anesthesia. The most common method of formulating a hypobaric solution is to mix tetracaine in a 0.1% to 0.33% solution with sterile, preservative-free water. Lidocaine also can be mixed to provide useful hypobaric spinal anesthesia.[17] This drug is diluted from a 2% solution with sterile, preservative-free water to make a 0.5% solution, and a total of 30 to 40 mL is used.

## Anatomic Considerations

The spinous processes of the lumbar vertebrae have an almost perpendicular relationship to the long axis of their respective vertebral bodies. When a needle is inserted between lumbar vertebrae, it should be placed almost perpendicular to the long axis of the back. To facilitate spinal anesthesia, an anesthesiologist must constantly keep in mind the relationship of the midline of the patient (neuraxial) and the needle.[18] As illustrated in Figure 29–3, the needle must puncture skin, subcutaneous tissue, supraspinous ligament, interspinous ligament, ligamentum flavum, epidural space, and finally the dura and arachnoid mater to reach the cerebrospinal fluid (CSF).

## Positioning

Induction of spinal anesthesia is carried out in three positions: lateral decubitus, sitting, and the prone jackknife. In both the lateral decubitus and sitting positions, a well trained assistant is essential if the block is to be easily and safely administered in a time-efficient manner.

### Lateral Decubitus

The assistant should help the patient to assume the position with the legs flexed on the abdomen and chin flexed on the chest. This goal is most effectively accomplished by pulling the head toward the chest, placing an arm behind the patient's knees, and pushing the head and knees together. The position is facilitated by an appropriate amount of sedation that permits a patient to be relaxed yet cooperative.

### Sitting

The sitting position can make location of the midline easier in obese patients or those with scoliosis. The patient should assume a comfortable sitting position with legs placed over

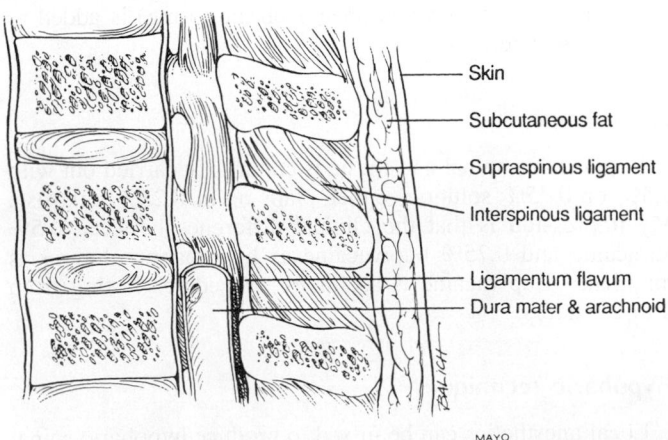

**FIGURE 29–3.** Spinal block; sagittal lumbar anatomy. From the surface inward, a spinal needle must puncture skin, subcutaneous fat, supraspinous ligament, interspinous ligament, ligamentum flavum, epidural space, dura mater, and arachnoid mater.

the edge of the operating table and feet supported by a stool. A pillow should be placed in the lap, and the arms should be allowed to drape over the pillow, resting on the flexed lower extremities. An assistant should be positioned immediately in front of the patient, supporting the shoulders and allowing the patient to minimize lumbar lordosis, while ensuring that the vertebral midline remains in a vertical position.

### Prone Jackknife

It is sometimes more time efficient to place a patient in a prone jackknife position before administering the spinal anesthetic. An assistant is not as essential for this technique as for the lateral decubitus and sitting positions. However, to improve efficiency, an assistant can position the patient while the anesthesiologist readies the equipment and drugs.

## What Factors Govern Needle Choice?

One of the first choices with spinal anesthesia is to decide what kind of needle to use. Although many eponyms are applied to spinal needles, they are divided into two main types: those that cut the dura and those that spread dural fibers. The former category includes the traditional, disposable, Quincke-Babcock needle; the latter category contains the Whitacre, Greene, and Sprotte needles (Fig. 29–4). If a continuous spinal technique is chosen, a Tuohy or other thin-walled needle facilitates passage of the catheter.

To make a logical choice of spinal needle, the anesthesiologist must understand the risks and benefits of each. Small needles reduce the incidence of postdural puncture headache. Larger needles improve the tactile sense of needle placement, thus increasing operator confidence. However, these risk-benefit ratios are relative. For example, a small, 26-gauge needle does not decrease headache incidence in younger patients if a number of passes through the dura are required until CSF flow is recognized. Likewise, a larger needle, such as a 22-gauge Whitacre, may result in a lower postdural puncture headache incidence if subarachnoid needle localization occurs on the first pass. Different needle tip designs likely are a factor in postdural puncture headache incidence, even when needle sizes are comparable. The most recent data suggest that the pencil-point, dural, fiber spreading-type needles are associated with the lowest incidence of postdural puncture headache.[15]

To avoid multiple passes through the dura with the smaller gauge needles, it is probably advantageous to perform the block with the patient sitting up to increase hydrostatic pressure and thereby assist CSF flow into the needle. If flow is not spontaneous, the needle should be intermittently aspirated with a small syringe to overcome surface tension and tissue plug effects that inhibit CSF flow.

## How Is the Needle Placed?

### Midline Approach

With a patient positioned properly, the palpating hand identifies the intervertebral space and midline. As illustrated in Figure 29–5, this important maneuver is carried out by moving the fingers in an alternating cephalocaudal direction, as well

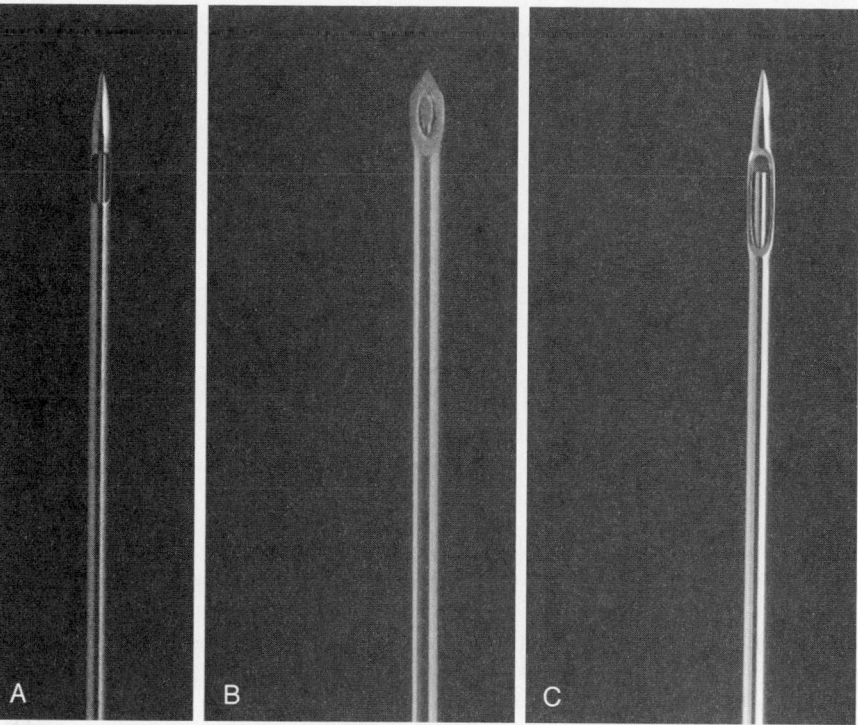

**FIGURE 29–4.** Collage of spinal needles in oblique and anteroposterior views. *A,* No. 25 Whitacre needle designed to spread dura fibers. *B,* No. 25 Quincke needle designed to cut dural fibers. *C,* No. 24 Sprotte needle designed to spread dural fibers.

as rolling them side to side. The latter maneuver confirms midline positioning. Once the appropriate intervertebral space has been clearly identified, a skin wheal is raised over it.

Next, an introducer needle is inserted into the substance of the interspinous ligament, taking care to seat it firmly in the midline. The introducer is grasped and steadied with the palpating fingers, while the other hand holds the spinal needle, somewhat like a dart (see Fig. 29–5). With the fifth finger of the needle hand used as a tripod against the patient's back, the needle, with the bevel (if present) parallel to the longitudinal dural fibers, is advanced slowly to heighten the sensation of tissue planes traversed, as well as to avoid skewering nerve roots. A characteristic change in resistance is noted as the needle passes through the ligamentum flavum and again as it passes through the dura.

The stylet is then removed, and CSF should appear at the needle hub. If it does not, the needle should be rotated in 90° increments until CSF appears. If CSF does not appear in any quadrant, the needle should be advanced a few millimeters and rechecked in all four quadrants. If CSF still has not appeared and the needle is at an apparently appropriate depth, it should be gently aspirated. If this maneuver is unsuccessful, the needle and introducer should be withdrawn and insertion steps repeated. The most common reason for lack of CSF return is needle insertion off the midline. Another common error is needle insertion at too great a cephalad angle.

Once CSF flows freely, the dorsum of the anesthesiologist's nondominant hand steadies the spinal needle against the patient's back while the syringe containing the therapeutic dose is attached. CSF is again freely aspirated into the syringe, and the dose injected.

## Paramedian Approach

The midline approach to subarachnoid block is the technique of first choice because it requires anatomic projection in only two planes and is relatively avascular. When difficulties with needle insertion are encountered, however, the paramedian route, which does not require the same level of patient cooperation or reversal of lumbar lordosis, may be used.

As illustrated in Figure 29–6, the paramedian approach exploits the larger subarachnoid target that exists if a needle is inserted slightly lateral to the midline. The palpating fingers should identify the caudal edge of the cephalad spinous process of the intervertebral space chosen; a skin wheal is raised 1 cm lateral and 1 cm caudad to this point. A 4-cm, 22-gauge short-beveled needle is then used to infiltrate deeper tissues in a cephalomedial plane. The spinal introducer and needle

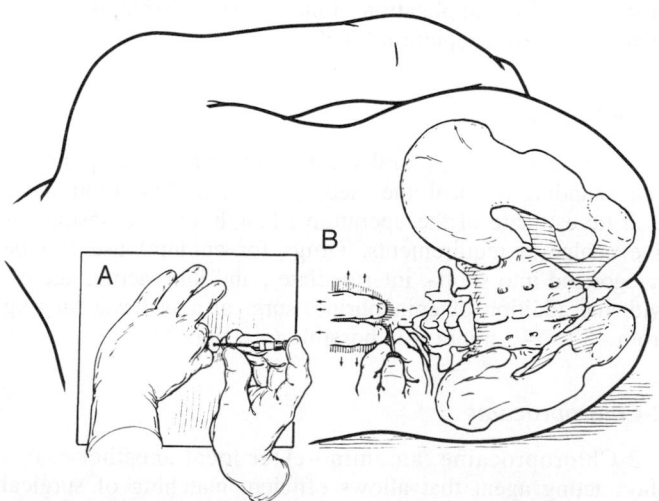

**FIGURE 29–5.** Spinal needle insertion. *A,* During needle insertion, the needle should be stabilized in a tripod fashion while held in the hand (as if it were a dart to be thrown). *B,* The palpating fingers are "rolled" in both a side-to-side and cephalic-to-caudal direction to identify interspinous space.

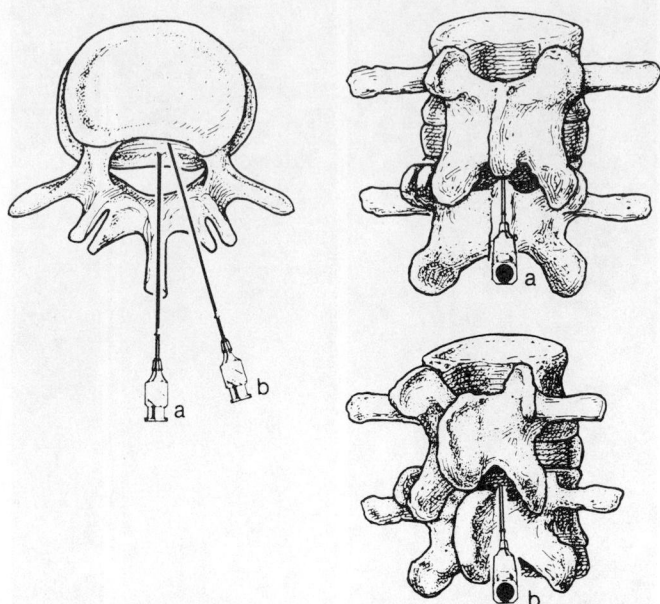

**FIGURE 29–6.** The advantage of a larger paramedian target (b) with the neuraxial technique compared with the midline approach (a).

are then inserted 10° to 15° off the sagittal plane in a cephalomedial plane. The most common error with this technique is also to angle the needle either too cephalad or too medial on the initial insertion. In the latter case, it encounters either the contralateral vertebral lamina or paraspinous muscles.

Once the needle contacts bone, it is redirected in a slightly cephalad or medial direction. If bone is again contacted but at a deeper level, incremental redirection is continued because it is likely that the needle is being walked up the lamina toward the intervertebral space. When CSF is obtained, the block is similar to that described for the midline approach.

## Lumbosacral Approach

A modification of the paramedian approach is the lumbosacral approach of Taylor.[19] The technique is carried out at the L5-S1 interspace, the largest interlaminal interspace of the vertebral column. As illustrated in Figure 29–7, the skin insertion site is 1 cm medial and 1 cm caudal to the ipsilateral posterior superior iliac spine. Through this point, a 12- to 15-

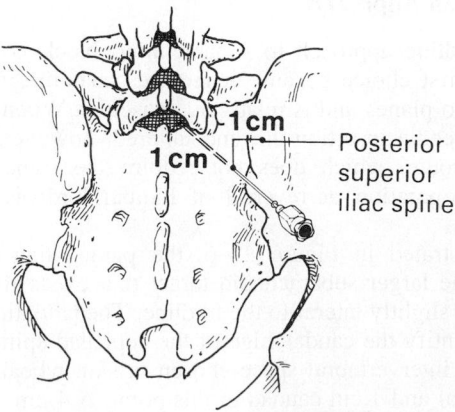

**FIGURE 29–7.** Anatomy of the Taylor approach, which is really a paramedian approach at the L5-S1 level.

cm spinal needle is inserted in a cephalomedial direction toward the midline. If bone is encountered on the first insertion, the needle is walked off the sacrum into the subarachnoid space, similar to the method for a lumbar paramedian approach.

## NEURAXIAL BLOCKS: EPIDURAL ANESTHESIA

### How Is an Epidural Anesthetic Performed?

Epidural anesthesia is the second major type of neuraxial block. In contrast to spinal anesthesia, epidural block requires pharmacologic doses of local anesthetics, making local anesthetic systemic toxicity a concern. In skilled hands, the incidence of postdural puncture headache should be lower with epidural anesthesia than with spinal anesthesia. Most commonly, spinal anesthesia is a single-shot technique, whereas frequent intermittent injection often is performed through an epidural catheter, allowing prolongation of the block. Another difference is that epidural block, unlike spinal block, permits segmental anesthesia. Thus, if a thoracic injection is made with an appropriate amount of local anesthetic, a band of anesthesia can be produced that does not block the lower extremities.

### Patient Selection

Epidural block is appropriate for virtually the same patients as is spinal anesthesia, with the exception that it can be used in the cervical and thoracic areas—levels at which spinal anesthesia is not often performed. As with spinal anesthesia, if epidural block is to be used for intraabdominal procedures involving the upper abdomen, it is advisable to combine the technique with a light general anesthetic; diaphragmatic irritation can make the patient, surgeon, and anesthesiologist uncomfortable.

Other patients for whom epidural anesthesia is useful are those receiving a continuous technique, which is maintained with local anesthetic or opioid analgesia after major surgical procedures. This application alone probably explains the increased interest in epidural block.[20]

### Drug Choice

Effective use of epidural local anesthesia also requires an understanding of local anesthetic potency and duration and a realistic estimate of the operation's length and the postoperative analgesia requirements. Drugs for epidural use can be categorized into short-, intermediate-, and long-acting agents; with the addition of epinephrine, surgical anesthesia ranging from 45 to 240 minutes is possible (see Fig. 29–2).

### 2-Chloroprocaine

2-Chloroprocaine, an amino-ester local anesthetic, is a short-acting agent that allows efficient matching of surgical procedure length and duration of epidural analgesia, even in outpatients. It is available in 2% and 3% concentrations, with the latter preferable for surgical anesthesia and the former for techniques not requiring muscle relaxation.

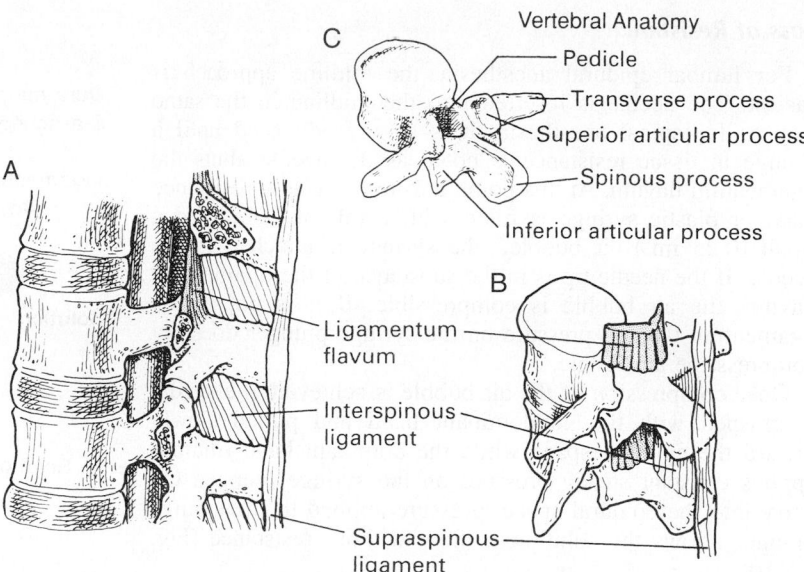

**FIGURE 29–8.** Vertebral anatomy. *A,* Sagittal view. *B,* Oblique view of lumbar vertebra showing ligamentum flavum thickening in the caudad extent of intervertebral space and in the midline. *C,* Oblique view of a single lumbar vertebra.

### Lidocaine and Mepivacaine

Lidocaine is the prototypical amide local anesthetic and is used in 1.5% and 2% concentrations. Mepivacaine concentrations are similar to lidocaine but last from 15 to 30 minutes longer at equivalent dosages. Epinephrine significantly prolongs the duration of surgical anesthesia with 2-chloroprocaine, lidocaine, and mepivacaine (ie, ≈50%).

### Bupivacaine

Bupivacaine, an amide provided in 0.5% and 0.75% concentrations, is the most widely used long-acting drug for epidural anesthesia. Analgesic techniques can be performed with concentrations from 0.125% to 0.25%. Its duration of action is not as consistently prolonged by the addition of epinephrine, although up to 240 minutes of surgical anesthesia can be obtained when epinephrine is added.

### Anatomic Considerations

The key to carrying out successful epidural anesthesia is an understanding of midline neuraxial anatomy. The anesthesiologist should create a cross-sectional image of the neuraxial midline structures underlying the palpating fingers (Fig. 29–8). When a lumbar approach is used, the depth from the skin to the ligamentum flavum commonly is 4 cm; 80% of patients have their epidural space cannulated between 3.5 and 6 cm from the skin. In the lumbar region, the ligamentum flavum is 5 to 6 mm thick in the midline; in the thoracic region, it is somewhat thinner, 3 to 5 mm thick. If needles are kept in the midline, the ligamentum flavum is perceived as thicker than if it is inserted off the midline.

### Positioning

Positioning for epidural anesthesia is similar to that for spinal anesthesia, with lateral decubitus, sitting, and prone jackknife approaches all applicable. The lateral decubitus position is applicable to both lumbar and thoracic techniques, whereas the sitting position allows lumbar and thoracic as well as cervical epidural anesthesia to be administered. The prone jackknife position permits access to the caudal epidural space.

### Needle Placement

A palpation technique similar to that used for spinal anesthesia should be used to identify midline structures. If a single-shot technique is chosen, a Crawford needle is appropriate; if a continuous catheter technique is indicated, a Tuohy or other needle with lateral face opening is appropriate (Fig. 29–9).

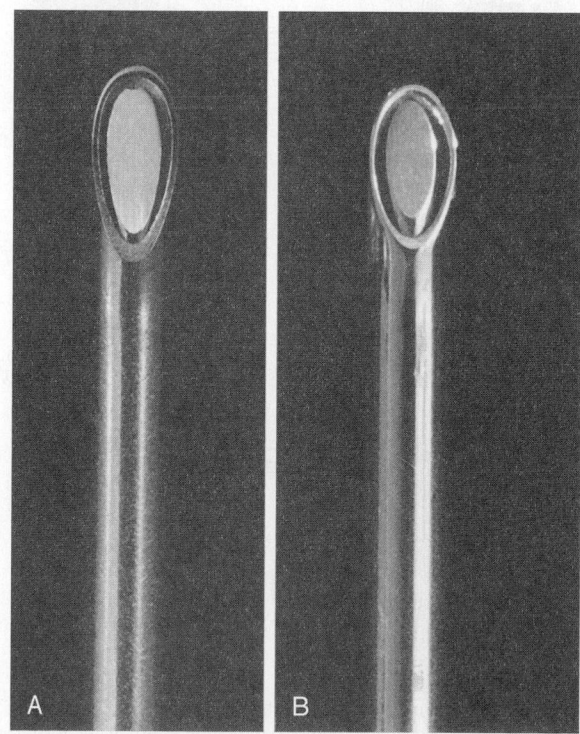

**FIGURE 29–9.** Collage of epidural needles in oblique and anteroposterior views. *A,* No. 17 Tuohy needle designed with a laterally facing opening. *B,* No. 18 Hustead needle designed with a laterally facing opening.

## Loss of Resistance

For lumbar epidural anesthesia, the midline approach is easiest. The needle is inserted into the midline in the same way as for spinal anesthesia. It is slowly advanced until a change in tissue resistance is noted as the needle abuts the ligamentum flavum. At this point, a 3- to 5-mL low-resistance glass or plastic syringe is filled with 2 mL of saline and a small (0.25 mL) air bubble. The syringe is attached to the needle. If the needle tip is in the substance of the ligamentum flavum, the air bubble is compressible. If it is not in the ligamentum flavum, pressure on the syringe plunger does not compress the air bubble.

Once compression of the air bubble is achieved, the needle is grasped with the nondominant hand and pulled slowly toward the epidural space while the dominant hand (thumb) applies constant steady pressure on the syringe plunger. On entry into the epidural space, pressure applied to the syringe plunger allows the solution to flow without resistance (Fig. 29–10).

## Hanging Drop

Another technique (although I believe with a less precise endpoint) is the hanging drop identification of entry into the epidural space. When the needle is inserted into the ligamentum flavum, a drop of solution is placed in the hub. As the needle is slowly advanced into the epidural space, the solution should be "sucked in" as the dura is tented away from the ligament, creating negative pressure in the epidural space (Fig. 29–11).

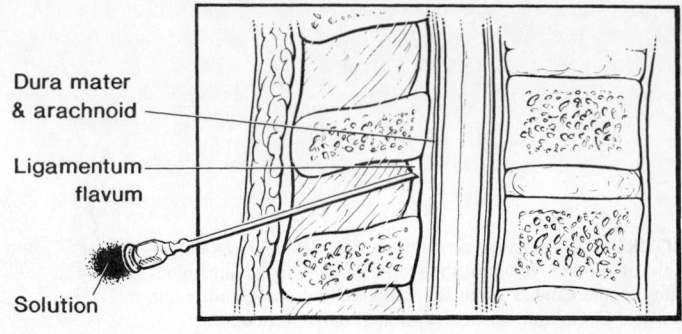

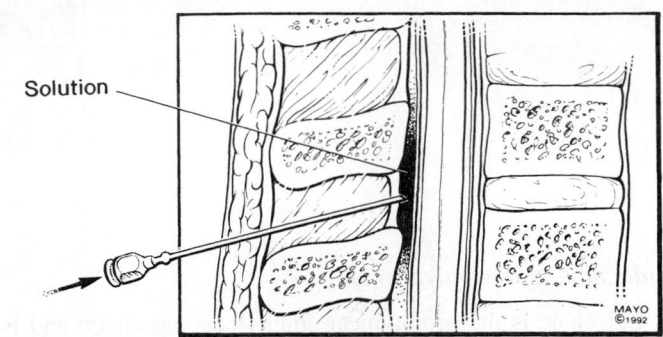

**FIGURE 29–11.** Hanging drop technique of epidural block needle insertion. Once the epidural needle tip enters the epidural space, the solution placed in the hub will be sucked into the needle.

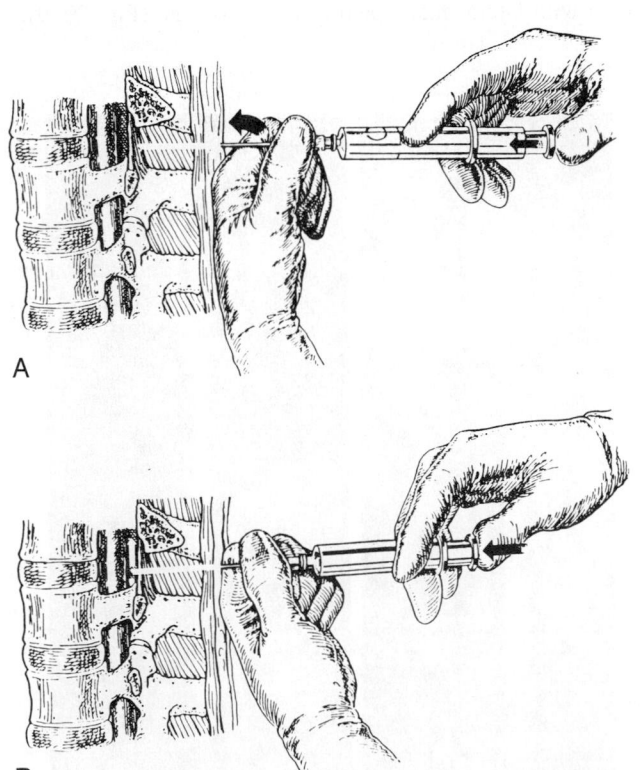

**FIGURE 29–10.** Loss of resistance technique. *A*, Needle is "seated" in interspinous ligament and ligamentum flavum while constant, steady pressure is applied to the syringe plunger. *B*, Entry of the needle into epidural space is confirmed by the loss resistance to syringe plunger pressure and by the easy entry of the solution into the space.

## Catheter Insertion

When the epidural space is cannulated, the frequency of successful catheter insertion may be increased by advancing the needle an additional 1 to 2 mm. In addition, the incidence of unintentional intravenous cannulation with an epidural catheter may be lessened by distending the epidural space by injecting 5 to 10 mL of solution before threading the catheter.[21–23]

The catheter should be inserted only 2 to 3 cm into the epidural space to decrease the likelihood of catheter malposition. If analgesia is the primary indication for an epidural catheter and the surgical procedure is primarily upper abdominal or thoracic, thoracic catheter placement may be necessary. If this is the case because of the longer, overlapping thoracic spinous processes, a paramedian approach at T6-7 often allows a more time-effective placement than a midline approach. My preference is to use a loss-of-resistance technique for thoracic catheter placements as well, although others recommend the hanging drop technique.

## What Are Potential Problems?

### Intravascular Injection

One of the most feared complications of epidural anesthesia is systemic toxicity resulting from intravenous injection of the intended epidural anesthetic dose. One way to identify intravenous injection is to administer a test dose of 3 mL of local anesthetic solution containing 1:200 000 epinephrine (ie, 15 μg of epinephrine). If a tachycardiac response occurs, either the needle or catheter tip should be considered to be in an epidural vein and repositioned. Subsequently, the anesthesiologist should inject incrementally, be vigilant for unintentional intravascular injection, and have all necessary equipment and drugs available to treat local anesthetic-induced systemic toxicity.

### Unintentional Spinal

Another problem is unintentional administration of an epidural dose into the CSF through either needle or catheter. Aspirating before injecting any anesthetic usually identifies CSF. As with any neuraxial block that reaches high sensory levels, blood pressure (BP) and heart rate should be supported pharmacologically and ventilation assisted as required. Atropine and ephedrine usually suffice or at least provide the time to administer more potent catecholamines. If the entire dose (20-25 mL) of local anesthetic is administered into the CSF, tracheal intubation and mechanical ventilation are indicated. Approximately 1 to 2 hours pass before a patient can consistently maintain adequate spontaneous ventilation after such an event.

When epidural anesthesia is performed and a higher-than-expected block develops only after a delay of 15 to 30 minutes, subdural placement of the local anesthetic must be considered. Treatment is symptomatic, and the most difficult aspect is recognizing that a subdural injection may have occurred.

## NEURAXIAL BLOCKS: CAUDAL ANESTHESIA

### *How Is a Caudal Anesthetic Performed?*

Caudal anesthesia can be effectively used for anorectal, perineal, and some lower extremity operations.

### Patient Selection

Patient selection should be determined by the anatomy of the sacral hiatus. In approximately 5% of patients, the sacral hiatus is nearly impossible to cannulate with a needle or catheter; thus, in 1 of 20 patients the technique is impractical.[24] In some patients, the tissue mass overlying the sacrum makes the technique difficult; if another technique is applicable, caudal block should be deferred. Probably more so than for any other block, experience and confidence with the technique are necessary to carry it out effectively.

### Drug Choice

When local anesthetics are prescribed for caudal anesthesia, the same considerations as those for epidural anesthesia apply. Volumes of local anesthetic of 25 to 35 mL are necessary to provide a sensory level of T12 to T10.

### Anatomic Considerations

The sacral hiatus can be localized by finding the posterior superior iliac spines bilaterally, drawing a line to join them, and then completing a caudally directed equilateral triangle, the tip of which overlies the hiatus (Fig. 29–12). Overlying the sacral hiatus is a fibrous elastic membrane, which is the functional equivalent of the ligamentum flavum.

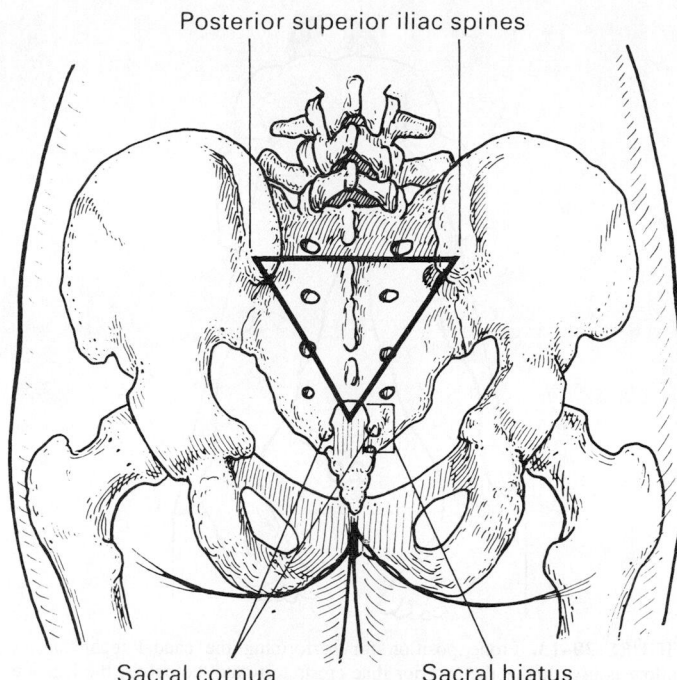

Posterior superior iliac spines

Sacral cornua          Sacral hiatus

**FIGURE 29–12.** Sacral surface anatomy. An equilateral triangle can be drawn to connect the posterior superior iliac spines and the sacral hiatus. This can be useful in confirming palpation of the sacral hiatus.

### Positioning

Caudal block is carried out in a lateral decubitus position or prone position. In adults, the prone position, with a pillow placed beneath the lower abdomen, seems most effective. Localization of the sacral hiatus in a prone patient is aided by having the legs abducted to a 20° angle and the toes rotated inward. This maneuver helps to relax the gluteal muscles and allows easier identification of the sacral hiatus (Fig. 29–13). Patients can be sufficiently sedated to make the block comfortable, and midline identification is easier than in the lateral position.

In contrast, pediatric caudal anesthesia is commonly carried out with a child in the lateral decubitus position. Because most pediatric caudal blocks are performed after induction with general anesthesia, the lateral position is almost mandatory. Identification of the midline and performance of the block are less complicated in pediatric patients.

### Needle Placement

If a single-shot caudal anesthetic is to be performed, almost any needle of sufficient length to reach the caudal canal is appropriate. In adults, a needle at least 22 gauge or larger is recommended because it is large enough to allow sufficiently rapid injection of solution to help detect a misplacement. If a through-the-needle catheter is to be used, a needle of sufficient size to allow catheter passage is required; otherwise, a 1.5-inch, 20-gauge intravenous catheter is adequate.

After the sacral hiatus is identified, the index and middle fingers of the palpating hand are placed on the sacral cornu, and the caudal needle is inserted at an angle of approximately 45° to the sacrum. While the needle is advanced, a decrease in resistance should be appreciated as it enters the caudal

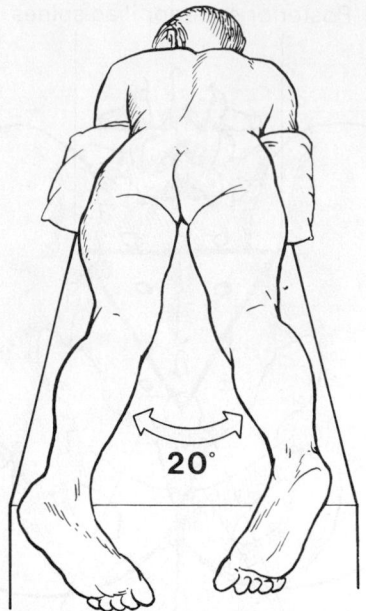

**FIGURE 29–13.** Prone position for performing the caudal technique. A pillow is used under the anterior iliac crests to rotate the pelvis, the legs are spread 20° to ease identification of the sacral hiatus, and the heels are rotated laterally to relax the gluteal musculature.

canal. It is then further advanced until the dorsal aspect of the ventral plate of the sacrum is contacted.

Next, the needle is withdrawn slightly and redirected so that the angle of insertion relative to the skin surface is decreased. In male patients, this angle ends up almost parallel to the skin; in female patients, a slightly steeper angle is necessary (Fig. 29–14). During redirection after loss of resistance, the needle should be advanced approximately 1 to 1.5 cm into the caudal canal. Further advancement is not suggested because dural puncture and unintentional intravascular cannulation become more likely.

### Testing Needle Location

Before administration of the therapeutic dose of local anesthetic, aspiration and a test dose injection should be performed. A helpful technique that confirms needle location during caudal anesthesia is a test injection of preservative-free saline. Once the needle has been placed into what is thought to be the caudal canal, the anesthesiologist applies a palpating hand across the dorsal sacral region and injects 5 mL of saline rapidly through the caudal needle. Subcutaneous needle positioning overlying the sacrum is immediately apparent because a bulge during injection develops over the midline during injection. If the needle is correctly positioned in the caudal canal, no midline bulge should be palpable.

In thin patients, accurate needle placement in the caudal canal followed by rapid injection of solution may cause small pressure waves more laterally overlying the sacral foramina. These smaller pressure waves should not be confused with those associated with a misplaced subcutaneous needle.

### What Are Potential Problems?

Caudal anesthesia embodies most of the same complications that can accompany lumbar epidural anesthesia. One distinct difference, however, is that the incidence of subarachnoid puncture is exceedingly low with caudal techniques. The dural sac ends at approximately the S2 level; thus, unless a needle is inserted deeply within the caudal canal, subarachnoid puncture is unlikely. In children, the dural sac extends more distally in the caudal canal; this fact should be considered when carrying out pediatric caudal anesthesia.

## UPPER EXTREMITY BLOCKS

### What Is the Relevant Anatomy?

The brachial plexus is formed by the ventral rami of the fifth to eighth cervical nerves and the greater part of the ramus of the first thoracic nerve (Fig. 29–15). Small contributions also may be made by the fourth cervical and the second thoracic nerves.

#### Trunks

After the cervical nerve roots pass the lateral margin of the scalene muscles, they reorganize into brachial plexus trunks: superior, middle, and inferior.

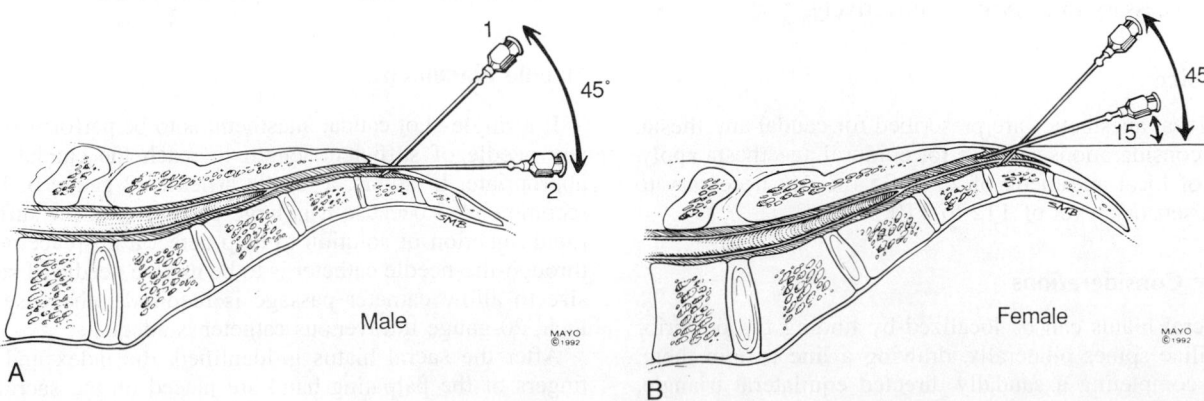

**FIGURE 29–14.** Caudal block anatomy and technique. The initial needle insertion angle for both male and female patients is 45° from the horizontal plane with the patients in a prone position. *A,* In males, the final needle position within the caudal canal will often end in the horizontal plane. *B,* In females, the final needle position within the caudal canal will often end approximately 15° off the horizontal plane.

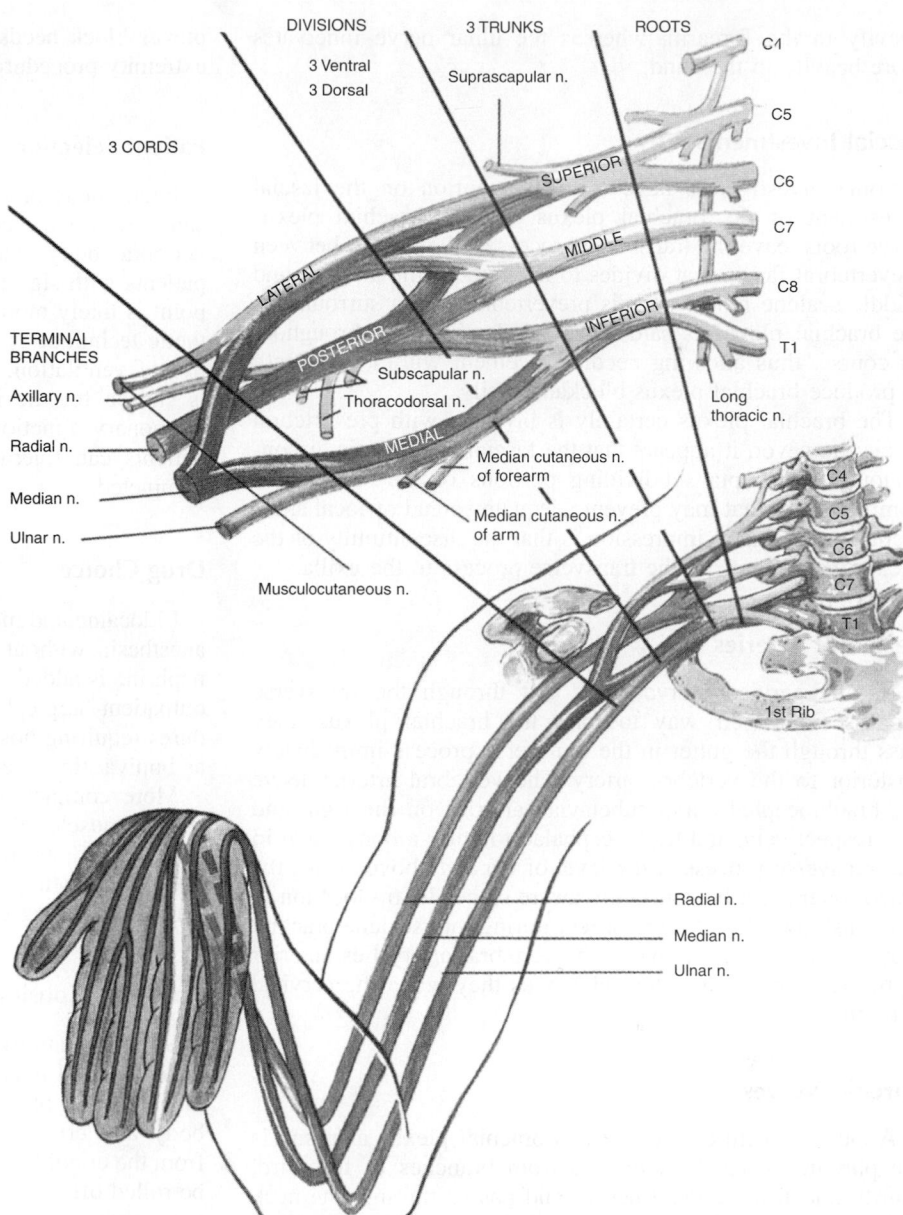

DIVISIONS   3 TRUNKS   ROOTS

3 Ventral
3 Dorsal

Suprascapular n.

C4
C5
C6
C7
C8
T1

SUPERIOR

MIDDLE

INFERIOR

3 CORDS

LATERAL

POSTERIOR

MEDIAL

TERMINAL
BRANCHES

Axillary n.

Radial n.

Median n.

Ulnar n.

Subscapular n.
Thoracodorsal n.

Median cutaneous n.
of forearm

Median cutaneous n.
of arm

Musculocutaneous n.

Long
thoracic n.

C4
C5
C6
C7
T1

1st Rib

Radial n.
Median n.
Ulnar n.

**FIGURE 29–15.** The brachial plexus anatomy. (From Brown DL. *Atlas of Regional Anesthesia.* 2nd ed. Philadelphia, Pa: WB Saunders; 1998:15.)

## Divisions

The trunks continue toward the first rib, at the lateral edge of which they undergo a primary separation into ventral and dorsal divisions. This is also the point at which an understanding of brachial plexus anatomy frequently gives way to frustration and unnecessary descriptive complexity. Nevertheless, this anatomic division is functionally significant because nerves destined to supply the originally ventral part of the upper extremity separate from those that supply the dorsal part.

## Cords

As these divisions enter the axilla, they give way to cords. The posterior divisions of all three trunks unite to form the posterior cord; the anterior divisions of the superior and middle trunks form the lateral cord; and the medial cord is the nonunited, anterior division of the inferior trunk. These cords

are named according to their relationship to the second part of the axillary artery.

## Peripheral Nerves

At the lateral border of the pectoralis minor muscle, the three cords reorganize to give rise to the peripheral nerves of the upper extremity. The branches of the lateral and medial cords are all ventral nerves to the upper extremity. The posterior cord, in contrast, provides all dorsal innervation to the upper extremity. Thus, the radial nerve supplies all the dorsal musculature in the upper extremity below the shoulder. The musculocutaneous nerve supplies muscular innervation in the arm and cutaneous innervation to the forearm.

In contrast, the median and ulnar nerves are nerves of passage in the arm, but in the forearm and hand they provide the ventral muscles with motor innervation. These nerves can be further categorized: the median nerve innervates more heavily in the forearm, whereas the ulnar nerve innervates more heavily in the hand.

## Fascial Investments

Some investigators have focused attention on the fascial investment of the brachial plexus. As the brachial plexus nerve roots leave the transverse processes, they do so between prevertebral fascia that divides to invest both the anterior and middle scalene muscles. This prevertebral fascia surrounding the brachial plexus is said to be tubular in form throughout its course, thus allowing needle placement within the sheath to produce brachial plexus blockade easily.

The brachial plexus certainly is invested with prevertebral fascia; however, it appears that the fascial covering is discontinuous, with septa subdividing portions of the sheath into compartments that may prevent adequate spread of local anesthetics. My clinical impression is that the discontinuity of the sheath increases from the transverse process to the axilla.

## Vertebral Arteries

As the cervical nerve roots exit through the transverse processes on their way to form the brachial plexus, they pass through the gutter in the transverse process immediately posterior to the vertebral artery. The vertebral arteries leave the brachiocephalic and subclavian arteries on the right and left, respectively, and travel cephalad to enter a bony canal in the transverse process at the level of C6 and above. Thus, the practitioner must be constantly aware of needle tip location in relationship to the vertebral artery during interscalene brachial plexus blocks. For emphasis, the vertebral artery lies anterior to the roots of the brachial plexus as they leave the cervical vertebrae.

## Phrenic Nerves

Another structure of interest to brachial plexus anatomy is the phrenic nerve. It is formed from branches of the third, fourth, and fifth cervical nerves and passes through the neck on its way to the thorax on the ventral surface of the anterior scalene muscle. It is almost always blocked during interscalene anesthesia and less frequently with supraclavicular techniques. Avoidance of phrenic blockade is important in only a small percentage of patients, although the phrenic nerve's functional location should be kept in mind for those with significantly decreased pulmonary function, that is, those whose day-to-day activities are limited by their pulmonary impairment.

## *How Is an Interscalene Block Performed?*

Interscalene block is indicated for surgery of the shoulder or upper arm because the upper roots of the brachial plexus are most easily blocked with this technique.[25,26] The ulnar nerve is often spared, unless a special effort is made to inject local anesthetic caudad to the site of the initial paresthesia.

The block is ideal for reduction of a dislocated shoulder and often can be achieved with as little as 10 to 15 mL of local anesthetic. It can also be performed with a patient's arm in almost any position and thus can be useful when brachial plexus block needs to be repeated during a prolonged upper extremity procedure.

## Patient Selection

Interscalene block is appropriate in almost all patients because even obese people usually have identifiable scalene and vertebral body anatomy. However, it should be avoided in patients with significantly impaired pulmonary function. This point is likely moot if a combined regional and general anesthetic technique is planned, which allows intraoperative control of ventilation. Even when a long-acting local anesthetic is chosen for the interscalene technique, phrenic nerve and pulmonary function usually have returned to a level that patients can tolerate by the time the surgical procedure is completed.

## Drug Choice

Lidocaine and mepivacaine produce 2 to 3 hours of surgical anesthesia without epinephrine and 3 to 5 hours when epinephrine is added. These drugs are useful for less involved or outpatient surgical procedures. For extensive surgical procedures requiring hospital admission, a longer acting agent such as bupivacaine is appropriate.

More complex surgical procedures on the shoulder often require muscle relaxation; thus, bupivacaine concentrations of at least 0.5% are needed. Plain bupivacaine produces surgical anesthesia lasting from 4 to 6 hours; the addition of epinephrine may prolong this to 8 to 12 hours.

## Anatomic Considerations

Surface anatomy of importance involves the larynx, sternocleidomastoid muscle, and external jugular vein. Interscalene block is most often performed at the level of the C6 vertebral body and cricoid cartilage.[26] By projecting a line laterally from the cricoid cartilage, the level at which the fingers should be rolled off the sternocleidomastoid muscle onto the belly of the anterior scalene and then into the interscalene groove can be identified. With firm pressure, it is possible to feel the transverse process of C6 in most people, and in some, it is possible to elicit a paresthesia by deep palpation. The external jugular vein often overlies the interscalene groove at the level of C6, although this relationship should not be relied on.

The anesthesiologist should always create a mental image of what lies under the palpating fingers. The key to success is identifying the interscalene groove. The closeness of the lateral border of the anterior scalene muscle and the posterior border of the sternocleidomastoid should be constantly kept in mind.

## Positioning

The patient lies supine, with the neck in the neutral position and the head turned slightly opposite the site to be blocked, and is asked to lift the head off the table. This movement tenses the sternocleidomastoid and allows identification of its lateral border. The fingers are rolled onto the belly of the anterior scalene and subsequently into the interscalene groove in the horizontal plane through the cricoid cartilage.

## Needle Placement

When the fingers are firmly pressing into the interscalene groove, the needle is inserted in a slightly caudad and posterior direction. If a paresthesia is not elicited on insertion, the needle is walked (maintaining the same angulation) in a plane joining the cricoid cartilage to the C6 transverse process. Because the brachial plexus is traversing the neck at virtually a right angle to this plane, a paresthesia is almost certain if small enough steps of needle reinsertion are carried out (Fig. 29–16).

In anesthetic procedures for shoulder surgery, this probably is the one brachial plexus block in which a large volume of local anesthetic, coupled with a single needle position, allows effective anesthesia. From 30 to 40 mL of lidocaine, mepivacaine, or bupivacaine can be used.

## Potential Problems

Problems that can arise from interscalene block are related to subarachnoid injection, epidural block, intravascular injection (especially in the vertebral artery), pneumothorax, and phrenic block.

If the operation requires ulnar nerve block, this is not my choice of brachial plexus block. The ulnar nerve is difficult to anesthetize with the interscalene approach because it is derived from the eighth cervical nerve, which is seldom blocked by injection at a more cephalad site. Also, caution is necessary in a patient with significant pulmonary impairment because phrenic blockade is almost guaranteed to occur. If an epidural block occurs, the anesthesiologist should consider that it is likely to result in a bilateral phrenic nerve block and be prepared to ventilate the patient.

## *How Is a Supraclavicular Block Performed?*

Supraclavicular block provides anesthesia of the entire upper extremity in the most consistent, time-efficient manner of any brachial plexus technique.[25] It is the most effective block for all portions of the upper extremity and is carried out at the division level of the brachial plexus, explaining why limited sparing of peripheral nerves may occur even if an acceptable paresthesia is obtained. If this block is to be used for shoulder surgery, it should be supplemented with a superficial cervical plexus technique to block the cutaneous innervation of the shoulder.[27]

## Patient Selection

Almost all patients are potential candidates for this block, with the exception of those who are uncooperative. In addition, in less experienced hands, it may be inappropriate for outpatients. Although pneumothorax is an infrequent complication, it often becomes apparent only after a delay of several hours, when an outpatient might already be at home.

## Drug Choice

As with other brachial plexus blocks, the prime consideration of drug selection should be the length of the procedure and the degree of motor blockade desired. Mepivacaine (1%-1.5%), lidocaine (1%-1.5%), and bupivacaine (0.5%) all are applicable. Lidocaine and mepivacaine produce from 2 to 3 hours of surgical anesthesia without epinephrine and 3 to 5 hours when epinephrine is added. These drugs can be useful for less involved or outpatient surgical procedures.

For more involved surgical procedures requiring hospital admission, a longer acting agent like bupivacaine can be chosen. Plain bupivacaine produces surgical anesthesia lasting from 4 to 6 hours, and adding epinephrine may prolong this period to 8 to 12 hours.

## Anatomic Considerations

The relevant anatomy involves the relationship between the brachial plexus and the first rib, subclavian artery, and cupula

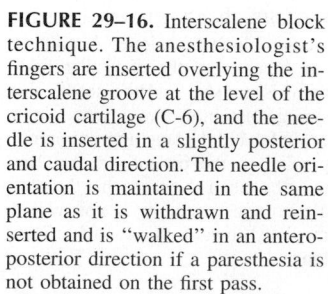

**FIGURE 29–16.** Interscalene block technique. The anesthesiologist's fingers are inserted overlying the interscalene groove at the level of the cricoid cartilage (C-6), and the needle is inserted in a slightly posterior and caudal direction. The needle orientation is maintained in the same plane as it is withdrawn and reinserted and is "walked" in an anteroposterior direction if a paresthesia is not obtained on the first pass.

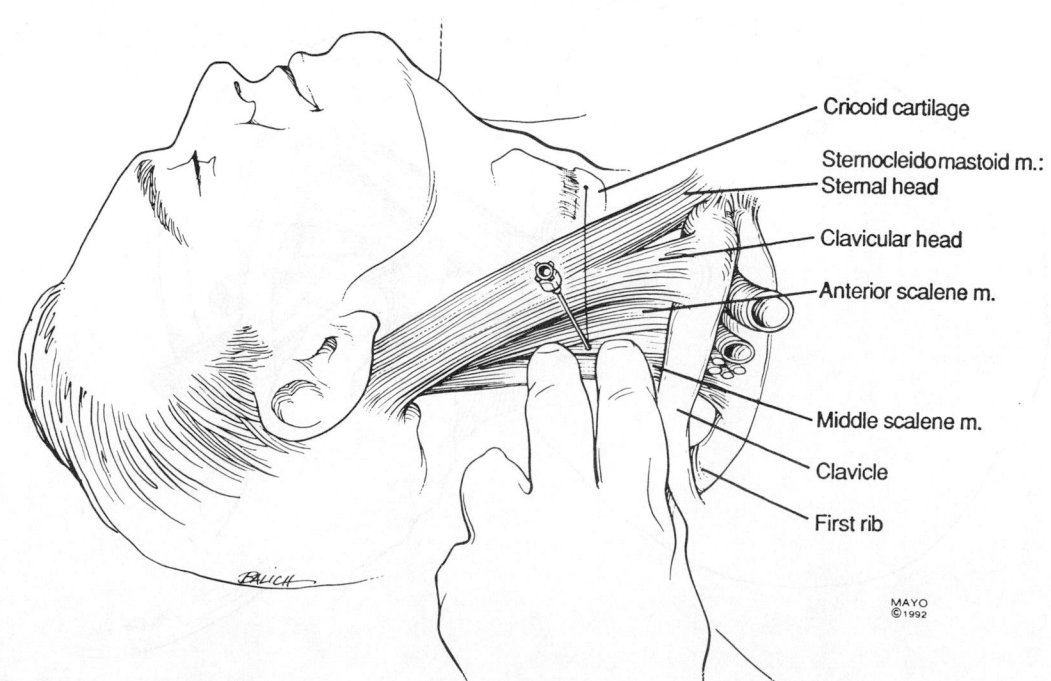

Cricoid cartilage

Sternocleidomastoid m.:
Sternal head
Clavicular head

Anterior scalene m.

Middle scalene m.

Clavicle

First rib

MAYO
©1992

of the lung. My experience suggests that this block is more difficult to teach than many of the other regional blocks, and for that reason, two approaches to the supraclavicular block are illustrated: the classic Kulenkampff approach and the plumb bob approach. The plumb bob approach has been developed in an attempt to overcome the difficulty and prolonged learning curve that seems attendant to the classic supraclavicular block approach. Despite that caution, either of the techniques is clinically useful, once mastered.

The subclavian artery and brachial plexus pass over the first rib between insertion of the anterior and middle scalene muscles onto the first rib. The nerves lie in a cephaloposterior relationship to the artery; thus, paresthesia may be elicited before the needle contacts the rib. At the point where the artery and plexus cross the first rib, it is broad and flat, sloping in a caudad direction as it moves from posterior to anterior. Although the rib is a curved structure, a needle can be walked in an anterior-posterior direction for a distance of 1 to 2 cm. Remember, immediately medial to this first rib is the cupula of the lung; when the needle is angled too medially, pneumothorax may result.

### Classic Approach

#### Positioning

The patient is supine without a pillow, with the head turned opposite to the side to be blocked. The arms are at the sides, and the anesthesiologist can stand either at the head of the table or at the patient's side near the arm to be blocked.

#### Needle Puncture

The needle insertion site is approximately 1 cm superior to the clavicle at the clavicular midpoint (Fig. 29–17). This entry site is closer to the middle of the clavicle than to the junction of the middle and medial third, as is often described. In addition, if the artery is palpable in the supraclavicular fossa, it can be used as a landmark.

The needle and syringe are inserted in a plane approximately parallel to the patient's neck and head, with care taken that the axis of syringe and needle does not aim medially toward the cupula of the lung.[25] The needle should be a 22-gauge, 5-cm length that typically contacts the rib at a depth of 3 to 4 cm, although it sometimes requires a depth of 6 cm in a large patient.

Initial needle insertion should not be carried out past 3 to 4 cm until a careful search in an anteroposterior plane does not identify the first rib. During insertion, the assembly should be controlled with the hand, as illustrated in Figure 29–17. The hand rests lightly against a patient's supraclavicular fossa to prevent unintentional deeper insertion because with elicitation of a paresthesia, patients often move their shoulder.

### Plumb Bob Supraclavicular Block

#### Positioning

The plumb bob approach resulted from efforts to simplify the anatomic projections necessary for the block.[28] A patient is positioned similarly to that for the classic approach, lying supine without a pillow, with the head turned slightly away from the side to be blocked. The anesthesiologist should stand lateral to the patient at the level of the upper arm. This block involves inserting the needle and syringe assembly at approximately a 90° angle to the classic approach.

#### Needle Puncture

Patients should raise their head slightly off the table so that the lateral border of the sternocleidomastoid muscle can be marked as it inserts onto the clavicle. From that point, a mental plane is imagined running parasagittally. Through a skin mark, the needle-syringe assembly is then inserted in the parasagittal plane at a 90° angle to the table top.

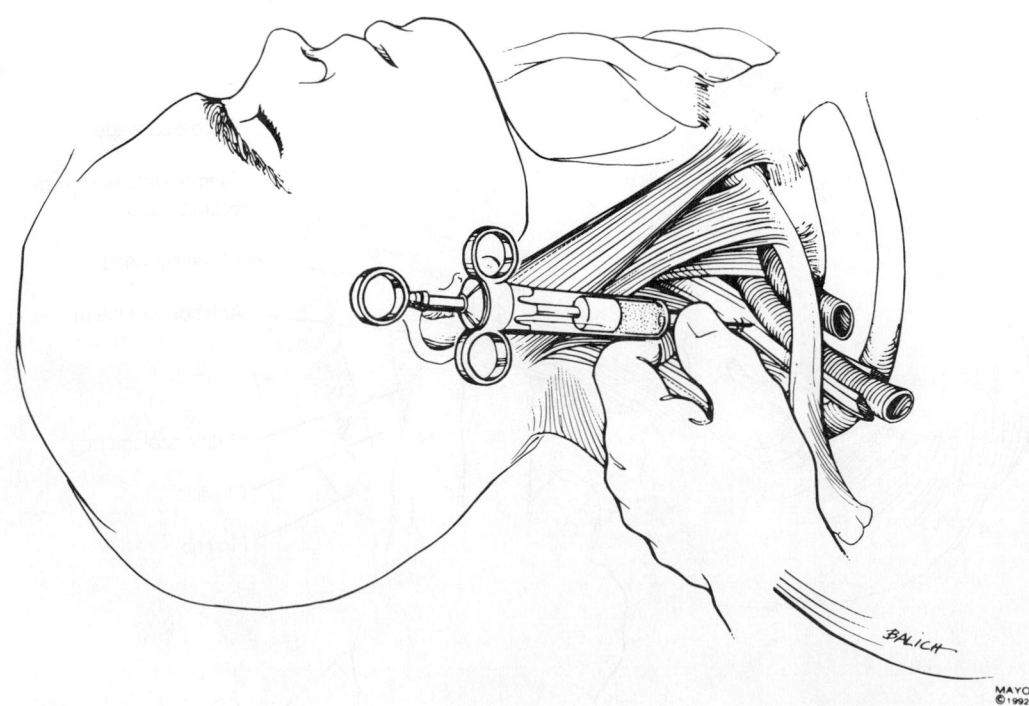

**FIGURE 29–17.** Classic supraclavicular block technique. A point 1 cm superior to the clavicular midpoint is marked, and the needle and syringe assembly are inserted in a cephalocaudal plane approximately parallel to the patient's neck. Care must be taken to ensure that the needle-syringe assembly is not angled medially toward the cupula of the lung.

**FIGURE 29–18.** Plumb bob (vertical) supraclavicular block technique. A point is marked at the junction of the lateral border of the sternocleidomastoid muscle as it attaches onto the clavicle. Patient should be instructed to turn his or her head slightly opposite of the side to be blocked. The needle-syringe assembly is then inserted in the parasagittal plane of the skin entry site and at 90° to the tabletop (position 1). If paresthesia is not obtained on the initial needle insertion, the needle-syringe assembly is withdrawn and reinserted in small steps through an arc of 30° cephalad (position 2). If a paresthesia is still not obtained, this process is repeated in a caudad direction through another 30° arc (position 3). Again, it is important to avoid angling the needle-syringe assembly medially toward the cupula of the lung.

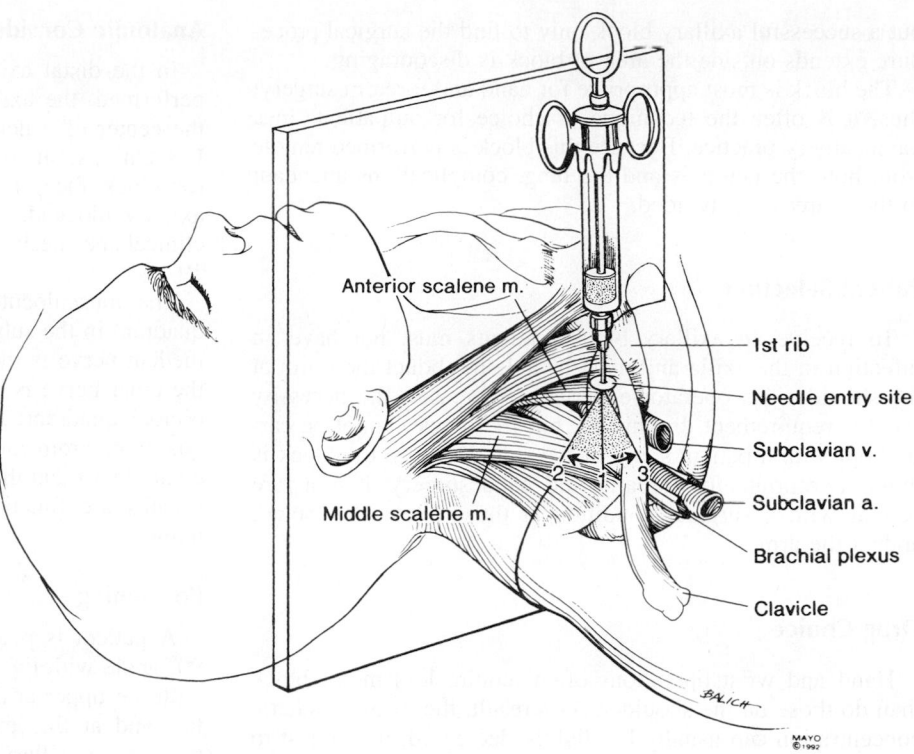

If paresthesia is not elicited on the first pass, the needle and syringe are redirected cephalad in small steps through an arc of approximately 30°. If a paresthesia still has not been obtained, they are reinserted at the starting position and then moved in small steps through an arc of approximately 30° in a caudal direction (Fig. 29–18).

Because the brachial plexus lies cephaloposterior to the artery as it crosses the first rib, a paresthesia often can be elicited before contacting either the artery or the first rib. If that occurs, approximately 30 mL of local anesthetic is inserted at this single site.

If a paresthesia is not elicited with the maneuvers described but the first rib is contacted, the block is carried out just like in the classic approach—walking along the first rib until paresthesia is elicited. As in the classic approach, care should be taken not to aim the syringe and needle assembly medially toward the cupula of the lung.

## Potential Problems

### Pneumothorax

The most feared complication of these blocks is pneumothorax. The principal cause of this problem is needle-syringe angles that drift medially toward the cupula of the lung. Special attention should be directed toward walking the needle in a strict anteroposterior direction. Pneumothorax often takes a number of hours to develop; thus, it is likely related to impingement of the needle on the lung rather than air entering the pleural space as the needle is inserted.

If a pneumothorax does occur after supraclavicular block, it can most often be observed while the patient is reassured. If the pneumothorax is large enough to cause dyspnea or discomfort, aspiration through a small-gauge catheter often is all the treatment that is necessary. The patient should be admitted for observation; however, it is the exceptional patient who needs tube thoracostomy for reexpansion of the lung.

### Phrenic Nerve Blockade

Phrenic nerve blockade does occur, probably in 30% to 50% of cases, and the block's use in patients with significantly impaired pulmonary function must be weighed individually.

### Subclavian Artery Puncture

The development of hematoma after supraclavicular block, as a result of puncture of the subclavian artery, usually requires only observation.

### Applicability

The predictability and rapid onset of this block allow its use even in a busy practice. As previously outlined, a longer learning curve is associated with it than with most other regional blocks. For that reason, anesthesiologists should develop a system for its use. Unfocused probing at the root of the neck is not the way to approach this block. The practitioner should choose either the classic or plumb bob approach early, and give each a fair trial before abandoning it.

## How Is an Axillary Block Performed?

Axillary brachial plexus block is most useful for surgical procedures distal to the elbow.[25] In selected patients, procedures on the elbow or distal humerus can be carried out with an axillary block, but strong consideration should be given to supraclavicular block for more proximal operations. To carry out a successful axillary block only to find the surgical procedure extends outside the area of block is discouraging.

The block is most appropriate for hand and forearm surgery; thus, it is often the technique of choice for outpatients in a hand surgery practice. Because this block is performed remote from both the neuraxis and the lung, complications attendant to those areas are avoided.

## Patient Selection

To receive an axillary block, patients must not have an infection in the axilla and must be able to abduct their arm at the shoulder. As operator experience increases, the necessity for this requirement diminishes, but the block cannot be carried out with a patient's arm at the side. Because the block is most appropriate for forearm and hand surgery, it is a rare patient with a surgical condition at those sites who cannot abduct the arm.

## Drug Choice

Hand and wrist operations often require less motor block than do those on the shoulder. As a result, the local anesthetic concentration can usually be slightly decreased, in contrast to supraclavicular or interscalene block. Appropriate drugs are lidocaine (1%-1.5%), mepivacaine (1%-1.5%), and bupivacaine (0.5%).

Lidocaine and mepivacaine produce from 2 to 3 hours of surgical anesthesia without epinephrine and 3 to 5 hours when epinephrine is added. These drugs are useful for less involved or outpatient surgical procedures. For more extensive procedures requiring hospital admission, a longer acting agent such as bupivacaine can be chosen. Plain bupivacaine produces surgical anesthesia lasting from 4 to 6 hours; the addition of epinephrine may prolong this to 8 to 12 hours.

## Anatomic Considerations

In the distal axilla or upper arm, where axillary block is performed, the axillary artery can be imagined as indicating the center of a neurovascular bundle divided into quadrants. It seems useful to conceptualize these nerves in a quadrant (or clock face) manner because multiple injections during axillary blockade may result in more predictable and rapid clinical anesthesia than does injection at a single site (Fig. 29–19).

The musculocutaneous nerve is in the 9- to 12-o'clock quadrant in the substance of the coracobrachialis muscle. The median nerve is most often in the 12- to 3-o'clock quadrant; the ulnar nerve is inferior to the median nerve in the 3- to 6-o'clock quadrant; and the radial nerve is in the 6- to 9-o'clock quadrant. From radiographic and anatomic study of the brachial plexus and the axilla, it is clear that separate and distinct sheaths are functionally associated with the plexus at this point.

## Positioning

A patient is placed supine with the upper arm forming a 90° angle with the trunk and the forearm forming a 90° angle with the upper arm. This position allows the anesthesiologist to stand at the level of the patient's upper arm and easily palpate the axillary artery or neurovascular cord. A line should be drawn tracing the course of the artery from the midaxilla to the lower axilla. The anesthesiologist's fingers overlying this line identify the artery and displace the subcutaneous tissue surrounding the neurovascular bundle. In this manner, a sense of the longitudinal course of the artery can be developed, which is essential for axillary block.

## Needle Puncture

Undue expenditure of time and patient discomfort should not occur during attempts to elicit a paresthesia. As illustrated

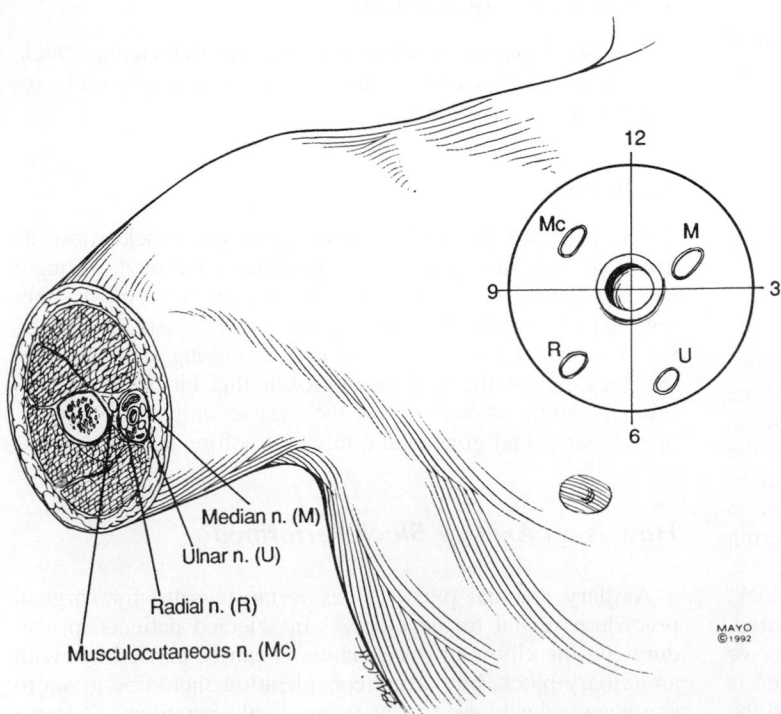

**FIGURE 29–19.** Axillary block anatomy; functional quadrant anatomy. It is useful to imagine the perivascular axillary anatomy in a cross-sectional plane of the upper arm as if it were the face of a clock. In a patient's right arm, the median, ulnar, radial, and musculocutaneous nerves are found approximately in the 12- to 3-o'clock, 3- to 6-o'clock, 6- to 9-o'clock, and 9- to 12-o'clock quadrants, respectively.

Median n. (M)

Ulnar n. (U)

Radial n. (R)

Musculocutaneous n. (Mc)

MAYO
©1992

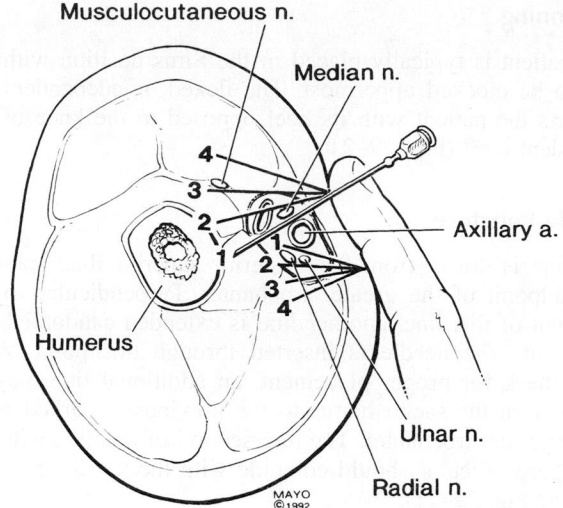

**FIGURE 29–20.** Needle placement for performance of axillary block. Numbers refer to the fanlike infiltration pattern to block the several nerves listed, using the axillary artery as the point of reference.

in Figure 29–20, this technique of axillary block is produced by using the axillary artery as an anatomic landmark and infiltrating in a fanlike manner around it. Anesthesia of the musculocutaneous nerve is best achieved by identifying the coracobrachialis muscle and injecting into its substance or by inserting a longer needle until it contacts the humerus and injecting in a fanlike manner.

For axillary block to be as effective as possible, an understanding of the organization of the peripheral nerves at the level of the lower axilla is necessary. The axillary sheath at this level is discontinuous. A single injection may produce useful surgical anesthesia; however, I believe the most consistently effective axillary block results from depositing smaller amounts of local anesthetic in multiple sites.

### How Is Intravenous Regional Anesthesia Performed?

Intravenous regional anesthesia, also called *Bier block,* can be used for various upper extremity operations, including both soft tissue and orthopedic procedures, primarily in the hand and forearm. It also has been used for foot procedures with a calf tourniquet.

### Patient Selection

Intravenous regional anesthesia is best suited for patients with no disruption in the involved upper extremity because the technique relies on an intact venous system. It can be used for distal orthopedic fractures and soft tissue operations. It may not be appropriate for patients in whom movement of the upper extremity causes significant pain because such movement is required to exsanguinate the venous system adequately.

### Drug Choice

The agent most commonly used for an upper extremity block is a dilute (0.5%) concentration of lidocaine, approxi-

mately 50 mL. Because of the risk of toxic reaction, bupivacaine is not an appropriate drug for this technique.

### Anatomic Considerations

The only requirement for intravenous regional anesthesia is access to a peripheral vein in the involved extremity.

### Positioning

A patient should be resting supine on the operating table with an intravenous infusion established in the nonoperative arm. The involved arm should be extended on an arm board.

### Needle Puncture, Exsanguination, and Tourniquet Inflation

A double or single tourniquet should be placed around the operative upper arm. An intravenous cannula is inserted in the operative extremity, as distally as possible. Two methods are acceptable for exsanguination of venous blood from the operative extremity: the traditional technique requires the wrapping of an Esmarch bandage from distal to proximal. When an Esmarch bandage is not available or a patient has too much pain to allow its placement, another method is to raise the arm for 3 to 4 minutes, allowing gravity to produce venous exsanguination.

After exsanguination, the tourniquet is inflated. If a single tourniquet is used, it is inflated. If a double tourniquet is used, the upper tourniquet is inflated at this point. Recommendations for tourniquet inflation vary and include 50 mm Hg above systolic BP with a wide cuff; a cuff pressure double the systolic BP; or 300 mm Hg pressure regardless of BP. A calibrated tourniquet manometer should be used, and regardless of technique, pressures >300 mm Hg should not be used.

If an Esmarch bandage has been wrapped and the tourniquet is inflated, the elastic bandage is then unwrapped, and 50 mL of 0.5% lidocaine without a vasoconstrictor is slowly injected in an average adult. Onset of the block is usually within 5 minutes. When a double tourniquet is used, the lower (distal) one is now inflated, after which the upper one is deflated. This usually affords an additional 20 minutes of relief before tourniquet pain again is an issue. It is my clinical impression that use of propofol to provide conscious sedation during intravenous regional anesthesia postpones the onset of tourniquet pain. The intravenous cannula is removed before preparation for operation. The block persists as long as the cuff is inflated and disappears shortly after deflation.

### Potential Problems

The major potential problem of intravenous regional anesthesia is that associated with premature accidental tourniquet release, causing local anesthetic-induced systemic toxicity. The tourniquet should not be deflated for at least 20 minutes after an anesthetic injection, even if the operation is completed before that; otherwise, the risk of toxicity is excessive. After that, the tourniquet can be cycled with several deflation-reinflation cycles to allow redistribution of the anesthetic. During upper extremity intravenous regional anesthesia, many patients complain about tourniquet pressure even when a double tourniquet is used; this often is the clinically limiting feature of this technique. Important for patients' acceptance is appropriate use of intravenous sedatives.

## LOWER EXTREMITY BLOCKS

### How Is a Sciatic Nerve Block Performed?

The sciatic nerve is one of the largest nerves in the body, yet few surgical procedures can be performed with sciatic block alone. It is most often combined with femoral, lateral femoral cutaneous, or obturator nerve blocks to produce analgesia or surgical anesthesia of the lower leg.

### Patient Selection

Sciatic nerve block may be indicated for patients requiring analgesia before transport for definitive repair of lower leg or ankle fractures. In selected patients, it may be desirable to avoid the sympathectomy accompanying spinal or epidural block. Sciatic block, combined with femoral nerve block, often allows ankle and foot procedures to be carried out. It is also useful in patients undergoing distal amputations of the lower extremity if their vascular compromise is based on diabetes or peripheral vascular disease.

### Drug Choice

Sciatic nerve block requires 20 to 25 mL of local anesthetic solution. When this volume is added to that required for other lower extremity peripheral nerve blocks, the total may reach the upper end of the acceptable local anesthetic dose range (see Table 29–1). If motor block is needed, either 1.5% mepivacaine or lidocaine is necessary; 0.5% bupivacaine also is effective.

### Anatomic Considerations

The sciatic nerve is derived from the L4 through S3 spinal nerve roots (sacral plexus) on the anterior surface of the lateral sacrum. The *medial sciatic nerve* functionally is the tibial nerve, which forms from the ventral branches of the anterior rami of L4 to L5 and S1 to S3. The posterior branches of the ventral rami of these same nerves form the *lateral sciatic nerve,* which functionally is the peroneal nerve.

As the sciatic nerve exits from the pelvis, it is anterior to the piriformis muscle and is joined by the posterior cutaneous nerve of the thigh. At the inferior border of the piriformis muscle, the nerve is approximately equidistant from the ischial tuberosity and the greater trochanter. It continues on a downward course through the thigh to lie along the posterior medial aspect of the femur.

At the cephalad portion of the popliteal fossa, it usually divides to form the tibial and common peroneal nerves. This division occasionally occurs much higher, and the tibial and peroneal nerves sometimes are separate through their entire course.

In the popliteal fossa, the tibial nerve continues its downward course into the lower leg, and the common peroneal nerve travels laterally along the medial aspect of the short head of the biceps femoris muscle.

### Positioning

A patient is typically placed in the Sims position with the side to be blocked uppermost. The flexed, nondependent leg supports the patient with its heel opposed to the knee of the dependent leg[29] (Fig. 29–21).

### Needle Puncture

A line is drawn from the posterior superior iliac spine to the midpoint of the greater trochanter. Perpendicular to the midpoint of this line, another line is extended caudomedially for 5 cm. The needle is inserted through this point. As a cross-check for proper placement, an additional line may be drawn from the sacral hiatus to the previously marked point on the greater trochanter. The intersection of this line with the 5-cm perpendicular should coincide with the needle insertion site (see Fig. 29–21).

A 22-gauge, 10- to 12-cm needle is inserted and directed toward an imaginary point where the femoral vessels cross the inguinal ligament. The needle is inserted until a paresthesia is elicited or bone is contacted. If bone is encountered before eliciting a paresthesia, the needle is redirected along the line joining the sacral hiatus and the greater trochanter until paresthesia is elicited or neurostimulation is produced.

During this needle redirection, the needle should not be inserted >2 cm past the depth at which bone was originally contacted, or it will be anterior to the sciatic nerve. Once a paresthesia to the lower leg is elicited, 20 to 25 mL of local anesthetic is injected.

### Potential Problems

When sciatic nerve block is used after injury to the lower extremity, the Sims position is sometimes difficult to achieve. This block can be long lived, and patients should be warned of this possibility before surgery to prevent undue concern after surgery about slow return of function.

### How Is a Femoral Block Performed?

Superficial and deep surgical procedures may be carried out on the anterior thigh with this block. It is most frequently combined with other lower extremity peripheral blocks to provide anesthesia for operations on the lower leg and foot. It is useful as an analgesic technique for femoral fractures.

### Patient Selection

Because a patient is in the supine position when femoral block is performed, virtually anyone undergoing a surgical procedure of the lower extremity is a candidate. Paresthesias are not necessary for this block; therefore, in selected circumstances even anesthetized patients are candidates.

### Drug Choice

As with all lower extremity blocks, a decision must be made about the desired extent of sensory and motor block. If motor blockade is essential, higher concentrations of local anesthetic are necessary. The requirement for motor block must be considered in light of the total volume of local

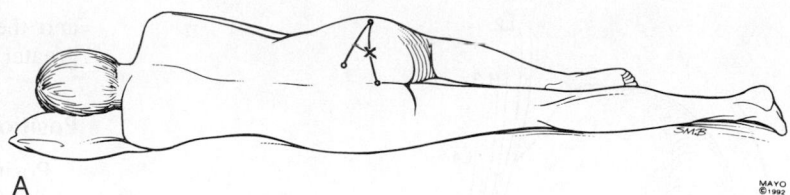

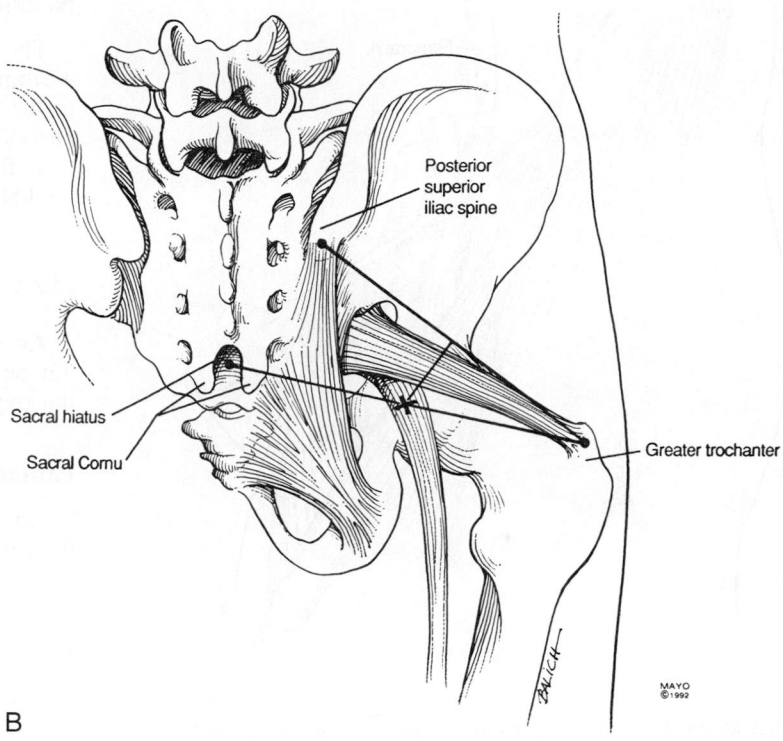

**FIGURE 29–21.** Sciatic nerve block technique. *A,* The patient is positioned in Sims position, rotated slightly away from the anesthesiologist and the side to be blocked. The patient's nondependent heel should oppose his or her dependent knee. *B,* Surface markings for sciatic block are made by joining the posterior-superior iliac spine and the greater trochanter with a line. At the midpoint of this line, a second line is drawn caudomedially, and a point 5 cm off the original line is marked. The needle is then inserted through this point toward an imaginary point where the femoral vessels cross under the inguinal ligament. As a cross-check for the needle insertion site, a line is drawn from the sacral hiatus to the greater trochanter. It should cross the caudomedially directed line at the previously marked needle site.

anesthetic necessary if femoral, sciatic, lateral femoral cutaneous, and obturator blocks are combined. Approximately 20 mL of local anesthetic should be adequate to produce femoral block.

### Anatomic Considerations

The femoral nerve traverses the pelvis in the groove between the psoas and iliac muscles. It becomes more superficial beneath the inguinal ligament, posterolateral to the femoral vessels. It frequently divides into its branches at or above the level of the inguinal ligament.

### Needle Puncture

The patient is in a supine position, and the anesthesiologist should stand at the side to palpate the femoral artery. A line is drawn connecting the anterosuperior iliac spine and the pubic tubercle. The femoral artery is palpated on this line, and a 22-gauge, 4-cm needle is inserted (Fig. 29–22). The initial insertion should abut the femoral artery in a perpendicular fashion and then produce a "wall" of local anesthetic in a fanlike manner, by redirecting the needle in progressive steps. Because the injection is made adjacent to two large vessels, the anesthesiologist must aspirate repeatedly to allow immediate identification of intravascular needle placement. Approximately 20 mL of local anesthetic is injected incrementally in

this fashion. The needle entry can also be directed laterally 1 cm and aimed immediately posterior to the femoral artery; an additional 2 to 5 mL of drug is then injected to block those nerve fibers that may be more posterior to the femoral artery.

### Potential Problems

Unilateral lower extremity blocks are often indicated for patients with peripheral vascular disease. If a patient has recently undergone placement of a prosthetic femoral artery graft, efforts should be made to avoid the prosthesis.

### *How Is a Lateral Femoral Cutaneous Block Performed?*

If a lateral femoral cutaneous block is used together with other lower extremity blocks, procedures can be carried out with fewer complaints of tourniquet pain. It also allows superficial procedures on the lateral thigh, including skin graft harvesting. The diagnosis of meralgia paresthetica, a neuralgia involving the lateral femoral cutaneous nerve, can be made if the pain resolves when the nerve is blocked.

### Patient Selection

The lateral femoral cutaneous block also is carried out with the patient in the supine position. Thus, almost all patients are candidates.

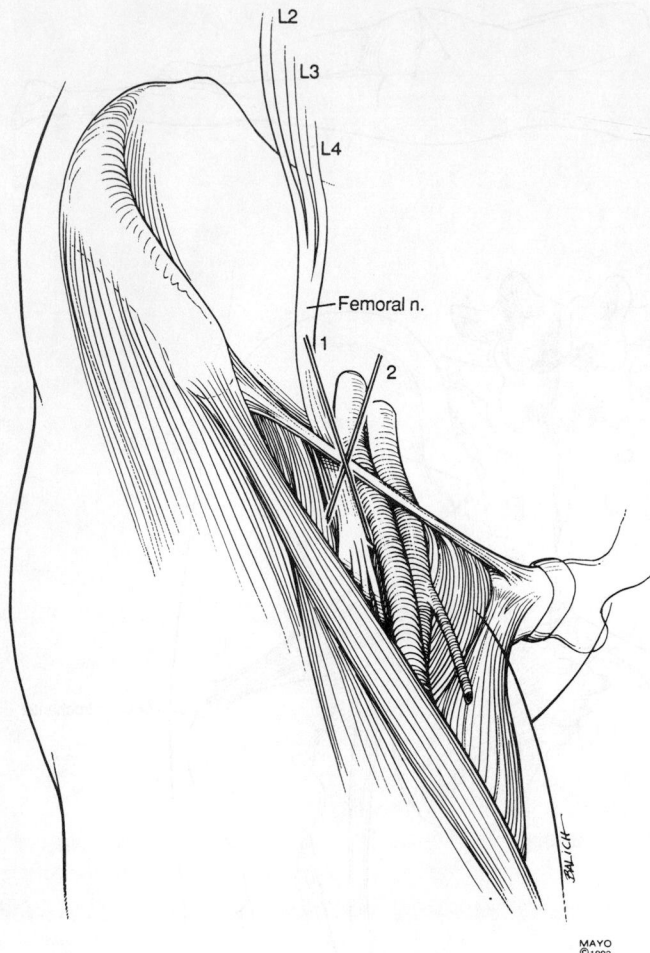

**FIGURE 29–22.** Femoral nerve block technique. The femoral artery should be located and the needle-syringe assembly inserted to abut the femoral artery in the sagittal plane (position 1). During local anesthetic injection, the needle is withdrawn and reinserted in small steps to build a "wall of anesthesia" through an arc ending at position 2.

## Drug Choice

The same concerns about total local anesthetic dose outlined in the sciatic and femoral sections apply to the lateral femoral cutaneous block. If multiple nerves to the lower extremity are to be anesthetized, the practitioner must be aware of the total mass of drug administered. Because this nerve does not have motor components, a lower concentration of 10 to 15 mL is effective.

## Anatomic Considerations

The lateral femoral cutaneous nerve emerges along the lateral border of the psoas muscle immediately caudad to the ilioinguinal nerve. It courses deep to the iliac fascia and anterior to the iliac muscle to emerge from the fascia immediately inferior and medial to the anterior superior iliac spine. After passing beneath the inguinal ligament, it crosses or passes through the origin of the sartorius muscle and travels beneath the fascia lata, dividing into anterior and posterior branches at variable distances below the inguinal ligament. The anterior branch supplies skin over the anterolateral thigh,

and the posterior branch supplies the skin laterally from the greater trochanter to midthigh.

## Positioning

Positioning is the same for lateral femoral cutaneous block as for femoral nerve block.

## Needle Puncture

The anterior superior iliac spine is marked, and a 22-gauge, 4-cm needle is inserted at a site 2 cm medial and 2 cm caudal to the mark. The needle is advanced until a pop is felt as it passes through the fascia lata. Local anesthetic is then injected in a fanlike manner above and below the fascia lata, from medial to lateral (Fig. 29–23).

## *How Is an Ankle Block Performed?*

An ankle block is useful for surgical procedures carried out on the foot, especially when high tourniquet pressure is not required.

## Patient Selection

An ankle block is principally an infiltration block, not demanding elicitation of paresthesia. A patient's cooperation is not mandatory for success.

## Drug Choice

Because motor block is not often needed for procedures carried out during ankle block, lower concentrations of local anesthetics may be used. Practical choices are 1% lidocaine, 1% mepivacaine, and 0.25% to 0.5% bupivacaine. Epinephrine should not be used, especially if injection is circumferential.

The peripheral nerves requiring block during ankle block all are derived from the sciatic nerve, except for the saphenous nerve (the only branch of the femoral nerve below the knee). It courses superficially anterior to the medial malleolus, providing cutaneous innervation to an area of the medial ankle and foot. The remaining nerves requiring block are the common peroneal and tibial. The tibial nerve divides into posterior tibial and sural nerves, and the common peroneal nerve divides into its terminal branches, the superficial and deep peroneal nerves, in the proximal portion of the lower leg.

## Needle Puncture

Ankle block can be performed with a patient in the supine position if the foot is placed on a padded support (Fig. 29–24).

### *Deep Peroneal, Superficial Peroneal, and Saphenous Nerves*

The anterior tibial artery pulsation is located at the superior level of the malleoli. A 22-gauge, 4-cm needle is advanced posteriorly and immediately lateral to this point. Alternatively, the needle is inserted between the tendons of the anterior tibial and extensor hallucis longus muscles. Approximately 3

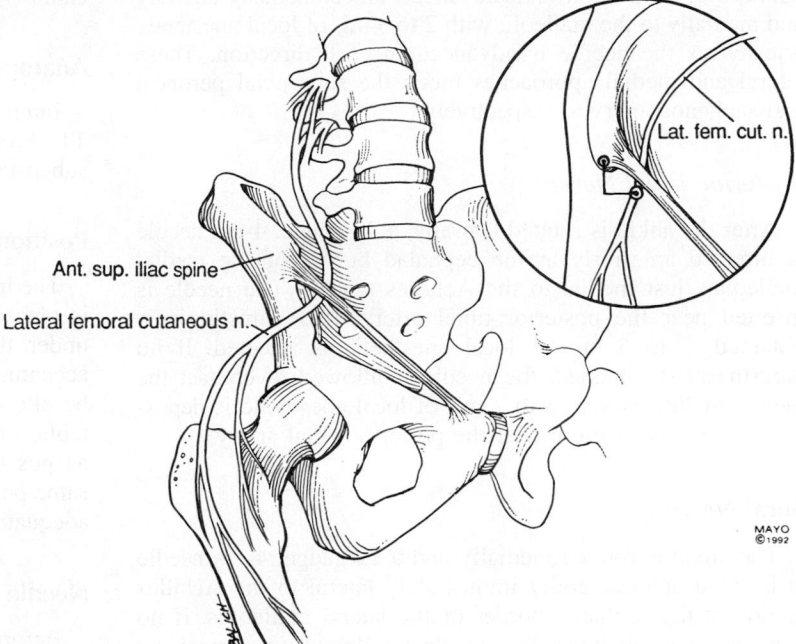

**FIGURE 29–23.** Lateral femoral cutaneous nerve block technique. The lateral femoral cutaneous nerve emerges from beneath the inguinal ligament immediately inferior and medial to the anterior superior iliac spine. A point is marked 2 cm inferior and 2 cm medial to the anterior superior iliac spine, and the needle is inserted through this site to develop a wall of anesthetic above and below the fascia lata.

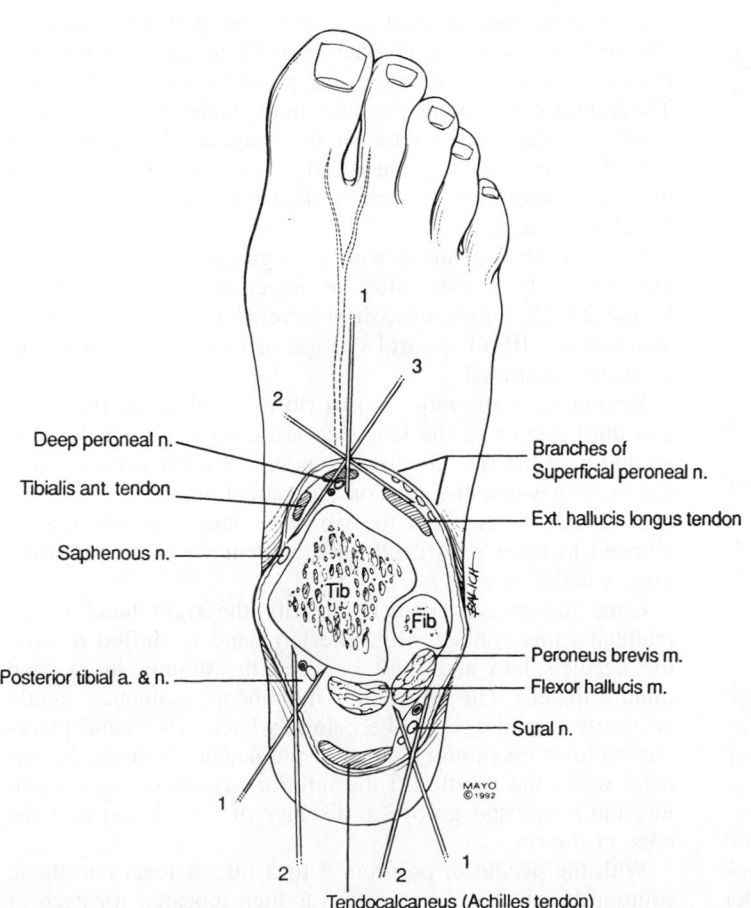

**FIGURE 29–24.** Ankle block technique. This block can be performed with the patient in the supine position if the ankle is supported, or it can be performed in 2 stages with the patient in both the supine and prone positions. In either case, 3 injections are made. First, the deep and superficial peroneal and saphenous nerves are blocked by inserting a needle between the anterior tibial and extensor hallucis longus tendons (position 2) and by developing a wall of local anesthetic from tibia to skin. The needle is then inserted subcutaneously both medial and lateral from the original skin insertion site to anesthetize the subcutaneous branches of superficial peroneal (position 2) and saphenous nerves (position 3). Second, the tibial nerve is anesthetized by inserting a needle immediately medial to the Achilles tendon (position 1) at the level of the medial malleolus and by developing a wall of anesthesia through an arc (position 2). Third, the sural nerve is anesthetized by inserting a needle immediately lateral to the Achilles tendon (position 1) at the level of the lateral malleolus and by developing a wall of anesthesia through an arc (position 2).

to 5 mL of local anesthetic is injected in this area. From this midline skin wheal, using the same or a longer 22-gauge, 8-cm needle, the infiltration is advanced subcutaneously laterally and medially to the malleoli, with 2 to 3 mL of local anesthetic injected as the needle is advanced in each direction. These lateral and medial approaches block the superficial peroneal and saphenous nerves, respectively.

### Posterior Tibial Nerve

After the ankle is rotated laterally, a 22-gauge, 4-cm needle is directed anteriorly at the cephalad border of the medial malleolus, just medial to the Achilles tendon. The needle is inserted near the posterior tibial artery; if a paresthesia is obtained, 3 to 5 mL of local anesthetic is injected. If no paresthesia is obtained, the needle is allowed to contact the medial malleolus, and 5 to 7 mL of local anesthetic is deposited in a fanlike pattern near the posterior tibial artery.

### Sural Nerve

The ankle is rotated medially and a 22-gauge, 4-cm needle is inserted anterolaterally immediately lateral to the Achilles tendon at the cephalad border of the lateral malleolus. If no paresthesia is obtained, the needle is allowed to contact the lateral malleolus, and 5 to 7 mL of local anesthetic is injected in a fanlike manner.

## Potential Problems

The ankle block can be painful if a patient is not adequately sedated. This problem should be infrequent because an alert patient is not essential for the block.

## TRUNCAL BLOCKS

## How Is an Intercostal Nerve Block Performed?

Intercostal nerve block provides excellent body wall analgesia. Thus, the technique is appropriate for relieving pain after unilateral upper abdominal and thoracic surgery or for rib fracture analgesia. Minor surgical procedures can be performed on the chest or abdominal wall using only intercostal blocks, but in general, some supplementation is most often appropriate. This block can also be used when chest tubes or feeding gastrostomy tubes are inserted.

## Patient Selection

All patients are candidates for intercostal nerve block, although it is more difficult in obese patients.

## Drug Choice

If intercostal nerve block is combined with light general anesthesia for intraabdominal surgery and the intercostal block is expected to provide abdominal muscle relaxation, a higher concentration of local anesthetic is needed. In this setting, 0.5% bupivacaine, 1.5% lidocaine, or 1.5% mepivacaine is an appropriate choice. Conversely, if only sensory analgesia is required, 0.25% bupivacaine, 1% lidocaine, or 1% mepivacaine is appropriate.

## Anatomic Considerations

Intercostal nerves are formed from the ventral rami of T1 through T11. The 12th thoracic nerve is technically a subcostal nerve.

## Positioning

The intercostal nerves are most easily blocked if the patient is placed in the prone position. A pillow should be inserted under the midabdomen to reduce the lumbar lordosis and accentuate the intercostal spaces posteriorly. The arms should be allowed to hang dependently from the edge of the block table (or gurney) to allow the scapula to rotate as far laterally as possible. If the block is for postoperative analgesia, the same positions used for performing a lumbar puncture provide adequate access.

## Needle Puncture

Before needle puncture, appropriate intravenous sedation should be administered to produce amnesia and analgesia during the multiple injections needed for the block. Barbiturates, benzodiazepines, ketamine, or short-acting opioids can be combined.

A marking pen is used to outline the pertinent anatomy. The midline should be marked from T1 to L5. Two paramedian lines should be drawn at the posterior angle of the ribs. These lines should angle medially in the upper thoracic region, paralleling the medial edge of the scapula. By successfully palpating and marking the inferior edge of each rib along these two paramedian lines, a diagram like that in Figure 29–25 is created.

Skin wheals are raised with a 30-gauge needle at each of the previously marked sites of injection. As illustrated in Figure 29–25, a 22-gauge, short-beveled 3- to 4-cm needle is attached to a 10-mL control syringe, using the hand and finger positions illustrated.

Beginning at the most caudal rib to be blocked, the index and third fingers of the left hand are used to retract the skin up and over the rib. The needle should be introduced through the skin between the tips of the retracting fingers and advanced until it contacts the rib. The needle should not be allowed to enter to a depth greater than what the palpating fingers define as rib.

Once the needle contacts the rib, the right hand firmly maintains this contact while the left hand is shifted to hold the needle's hub and shaft between the thumb, index, and middle fingers. The left hand's hypothenar eminence should be firmly placed against the patient's back. This hand placement allows maximum control of the needle depth as the left hand walks the needle off the inferior margin of the rib and into the intercostal groove, a distance of 2 to 3 mm past the edge of the rib.

With the needle in position, 3 to 5 mL of local anesthetic solution is injected. The process is then repeated for each of the nerves to be blocked. In certain patients with cachexia or severe barrel chest deformity, the intercostal injection can be

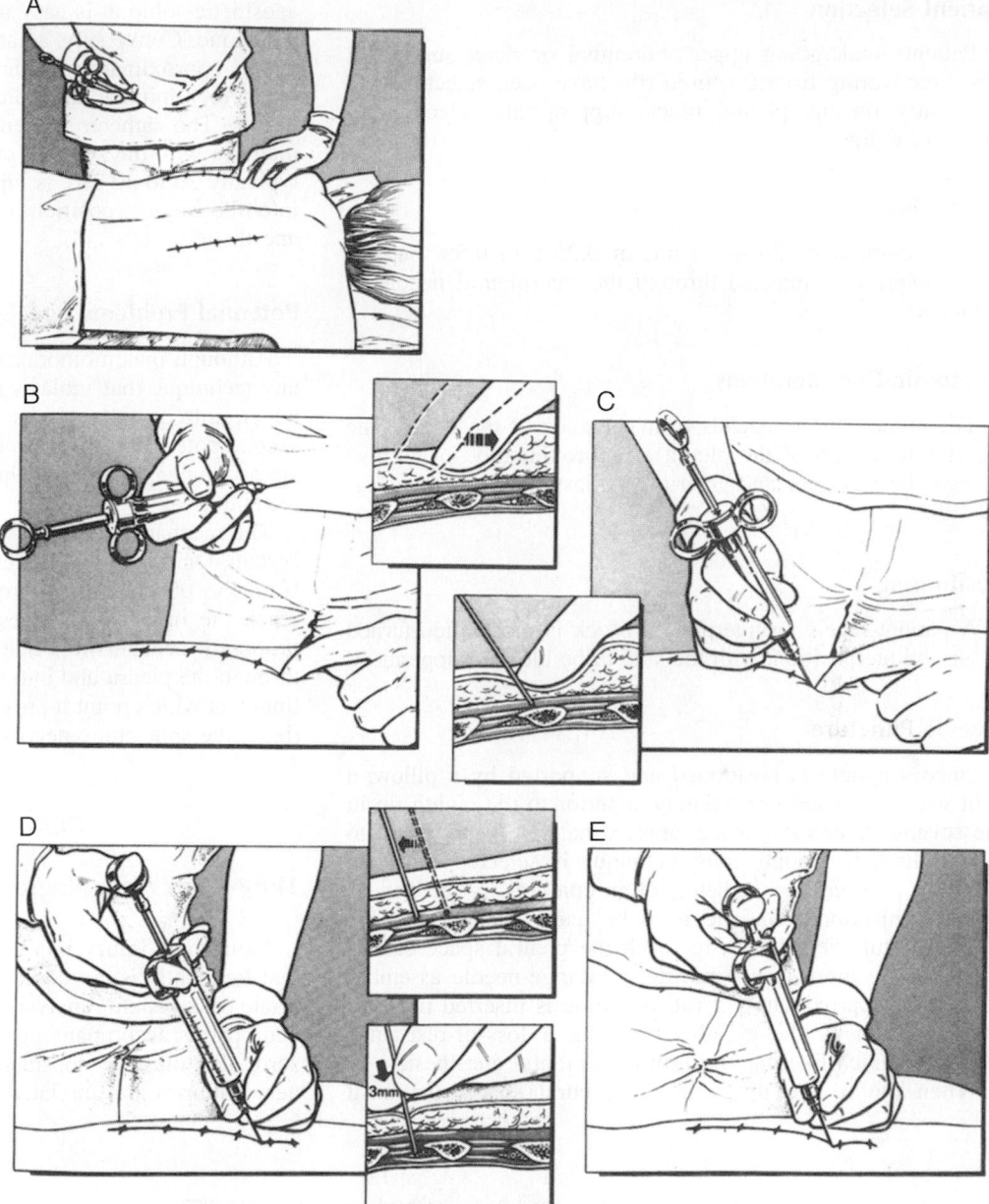

**FIGURE 29–25.** Technique for intercostal block and corresponding deep anatomy (see text). *A,* Skin markings at lateral edge of sacrospinalis muscle (6-8 cm from midline). Note the medial curve of the line superiorly to avoid the scapulae. Ribs and interspaces are palpated. The lowest (most inferior) intercostal nerve is blocked first because the lower ribs are easy to palpate. (Diagrams A-E show the second last intercostal nerves to be blocked in this patient.) *B,* Skin at the lower edge of the rib is retracted superiorly onto the rib. *C,* The needle is inserted onto rib (see also inset). Note that the finger palpating the rib is still in place and that the hand holding the syringe is firmly braced against the back. *D,* The position of the hands now changes. Note that the left hand now rests against the back and holds the needle as it is walked off the inferior edge of the rib and advanced 3 mm. The right hand is free to aspirate and inject. *E,* Injection is completed with the left hand still firmly braced against the patient's back while the needle is controlled.

most effectively carried out with an even shorter 23- or 25-gauge needle.

## Potential Problems

The principal concern with intercostal nerve block is pneumothorax. Many physicians avoid this block because of the imagined high frequency and seriousness of this complication. Data suggest that the incidence of pneumothorax is <0.5%, and even when it occurs, careful clinical observation is usually all that is necessary.[30]

The incidence of symptomatic pneumothorax after intercostal block is even lower, approximately 1:1000. If treatment is deemed necessary, needle aspiration can often be carried out with successful lung reexpansion. Chest tube drainage should be performed only after failure of lung reexpansion after observation or percutaneous aspiration.

As a result of the vascularity of the intercostal space, local anesthetic blood levels are higher for multiple-level intercostal block than for any other regional anesthetic technique. Because these peak blood levels may be delayed for 15 to 20 minutes, patients should be closely monitored after the completion of a block for at least that interval.

## *How Is an Interpleural Block Performed?*

Interpleural anesthesia is a technique to provide body wall and visceral analgesia after upper abdominal or thoracic surgery. Accurate stratification of the risks and benefits of interpleural anesthesia currently remains elusive, perhaps in large part because of the success and popularity of epidural opioid analgesia.

## Patient Selection

Patients undergoing upper abdominal or flank surgery or those recovering from fractured ribs have been selected most frequently for interpleural block. Appropriate selection remains ill defined.

## Drug Choice

Most commonly, 20 to 30 mL of 0.25% to 0.5% bupivacaine solution is injected through the interpleural needle or catheter.

## Anatomic Considerations

The pleural space extends from the apex of the lung to the inferior reflection of the pleura at approximately L1. It also invests the posterior and anterior mediastinal structures (Fig. 29–26).

## Positioning

A patient receiving interpleural block is most often turned to an oblique position, with the side to be blocked uppermost.

## Needle Puncture

Once a patient is positioned and supported by a pillow, a skin wheal is raised immediately superior to the eighth rib in the seventh intercostal space, approximately 10 cm lateral to the midline. If a continuous technique is selected, a needle allowing passage of a catheter (often epidural) is selected. If a single-injection technique is to be used, a short, beveled needle of sufficient length to reach the pleural space can be used. Before inserting the needle, a syringe-needle assembly containing approximately 2 mL of saline is inserted immediately superior to the eighth rib, using a loss-of-resistance technique much like that used during epidural anesthesia.

When the needle tip is in the pleural space, the local anesthetic solution is easy to inject, if it is to be a single-shot technique. Conversely, a catheter can be threaded through the needle approximately 10 cm into the pleural space, with care taken to minimize the volume of air entrained through the needle. The catheter is then taped in a position that does not interfere with the surgical procedure, and the local anesthetic, typically 20 to 30 mL, is injected. Finally, the patient is rolled into the supine position to allow distribution of the local anesthetic.

## Potential Problems

Although pneumothorax would seem to be associated with any technique that violates the pleural space, it is reported to be an infrequent problem with interpleural anesthesia.[30] A second potential problem is the unpredictable nature of analgesia accompanying what otherwise seems to be an acceptable technique.

The mechanism behind interpleural anesthesia remains uncertain. One theory proposes that the local anesthetic diffuses from the pleural space through the intercostal membrane to reach the intercostal nerves along the chest wall. A second proposed mechanism is that the local anesthetic is distributed through the pleura and into the region of the posterior mediastinum, at which point it provides visceral analgesia by anesthetizing the splanchnic nerves.

## COMPLICATIONS

### Why Does Neurologic Injury Occur?

Neurologic injury is a complication of regional anesthesia that frequently is not comprehensively evaluated. If an appropriate risk-benefit analysis is undertaken, the incidence of neuropathy accompanying general anesthesia, which is not zero, also must be considered. Similarly, many perioperative nerve injuries are unrelated to anesthetic care. Some of these

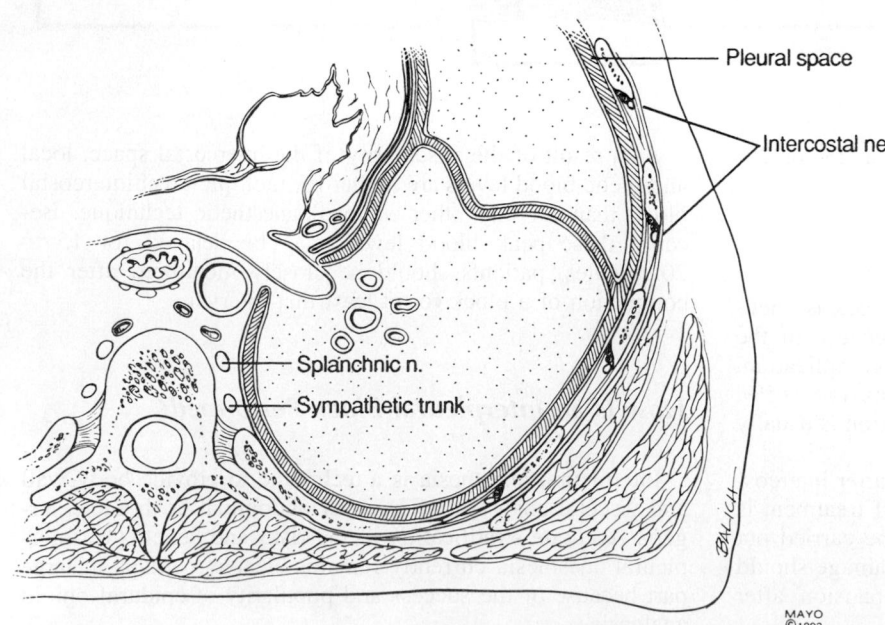

Pleural space

Intercostal nerves

Splanchnic n.

Sympathetic trunk

**FIGURE 29–26.** Interpleural block cross-sectional anatomy. The block likely results in both intercostal nerve block and block of deep splanchnic nerves.

include surgical positioning problems, surgical trauma, tourniquet sequelae, pressure from extremity casts, preexisting neurologic conditions, and postoperative nerve injury.[31,32]

## Do Paresthesias Have a Role?

Some have suggested that paresthesia-seeking techniques are more likely to cause nerve injury. This impression needs perspective. The original report by Selander and colleagues concluding that paresthesia should be avoided during regional block was a nonrandomized, unblinded study in which no statistical difference between paresthesia-seeking and nonparesthesia-seeking patient groups was found.[33]

It might be supposed that if regional anesthesia can be successfully conducted without elicitation of a paresthesia, the occasional needle-induced nerve injury can be avoided. Nevertheless, even in situations in which paresthesias were not being sought, a paresthesia was obtained unintentionally in almost half of the patients.[33] Persistent neuropathy after peripheral nerve block is usually temporary and resolves with time. A number of large series demonstrate the relative neurologic safety of these techniques.[34,35]

## Are Neuraxial Blocks Problematic?

Large series of neuraxial blocks also highlight the relative neurologic safety of these techniques.[36,37] Reports have focused attention on neurologic injury after continuous spinal anesthesia[38] and after low molecular weight heparin (LMWH).[39]

Neuraxial neurologic complications have a long and colorful history. Many Medicare-age patients remember the publicity in the lay press associated with the well publicized Wooley and Roe case in England in the late 1940s.[40] What most are unaware of is the report by Marinacci from Los Angeles shortly after that era in which 99% of the neurologic lesions believed due to postspinal anesthetic changes were found on neurologic and electromyographic (EMG) examination to be related to other factors.[41]

It is clear that a new risk has evolved with neuraxial anesthetic and analgesia techniques—it is the combination of LMWH with neuraxial techniques. As Horlocker and colleagues suggested, a cautious approach to this combination of LMWH prophylaxis and neuraxial techniques is required[39] (Table 29–2).

Neurologic injury can occur with neuraxial blocks, but a rational risk-benefit analysis requires that those neurologic injuries associated with general anesthesia be included in the equation.

## Continuous Spinal Catheters

Continuous spinal anesthesia with small-bore catheters resulted in a sufficient number of cases of cauda equina syndrome to prompt the US Food and Drug Administration (FDA) to issue a safety alert on May 29, 1992, "advising against the use of any small-bore catheter for continuous spinal administration of any local anesthetic agent."[42] The mechanism by which this problem occurs is uncertain but may relate to the slow rate at which drug is injected through

**TABLE 29–2.** Recommendations for Patients Receiving Low Molecular Weight Heparin and Neuraxial Anesthesia

1. Monitoring of anti-factor Xa level is not recommended. The anti-Xa level is not predictive of the risk of bleeding and is, therefore, not helpful in the management of patients undergoing neuraxial blocks.
2. Antiplatelet or oral anticoagulant medications administered in combination with LMWH may increase the risk of spinal hematoma. Concomitant administration of medications affecting hemostasis, such as antiplatelet drugs, standard heparin, or dextran, represents an additional risk of perioperative hemorrhagic complications, including spinal hematoma. Education of the entire patient care team is necessary to avoid potentiation of the anticoagulant effects.
3. Presence of blood during needle and catheter placement does not necessitate postponement of surgery. However, initiation of LMWH therapy in this setting should be delayed for 24 h after surgery. Traumatic needle or catheter placement may signify an increased risk of spinal hematoma, and it is recommended that this consideration be discussed with the surgeon.
4. Patients on preoperative LMWH can be assumed to have altered coagulation. A single-dose spinal anesthetic may be the safest neuraxial technique in patients receiving preoperative LMWH. In these patients, needle placement should occur at least 10 to 12 h after the LMWH dose, whereas patients receiving higher doses of LMWH (eg, enoxaparin 1 mg/kg twice daily) require longer delays (24 h). Neuraxial techniques should be avoided in patients administered a dose of LMWH 2 h before surgery (general surgery patients), because needle placement would occur during peak anticoagulant activity.
5. Patients with postoperative initiation of LMWH thromboprophylaxis may safely undergo single-dose and continuous catheter techniques. The first dose of LMWH should be administered no earlier than 24 h after surgery and only in the presence of adequate hemostasis. In addition, it is recommended that indwelling catheters be removed before initiation of LMWH thromboprophylaxis. If a continuous technique is selected, the epidural catheter may be left indwelling overnight and removed the following day, with the first dose of LMWH administered 2 h after catheter removal.
6. The decision to implement LMWH thromboprophylaxis in the presence of an indwelling catheter must be made with care. Extreme vigilance with regard to the patient's neurologic status is warranted. An opioid or dilute local anesthetic solution is recommended in these patients to allow frequent monitoring of neurologic function. If epidural analgesia is anticipated to continue for more than 24 h, LMWH administration may be delayed (in selected cases) or an alternate method of thromboprophylaxis may be selected (eg, external pneumatic compression) based on the risk profile for the individual patient. These decisions should be made before surgery to allow optimal management of both postoperative analgesia and thromboprophylaxis.
7. For any LMWH prophylaxis regimen, the timing of catheter removal is of paramount importance. Catheter removal should be delayed for at least 10 to 12 h after a dose of LMWH. A true normalization of the patient's coagulation status could be achieved if the evening dose of LMWH was not given and the catheter was removed the following morning (24 h after the last dose). Again, subsequent dosing should not occur for at least 2 h after catheter removal.

LMWH, low molecular weight heparin.

these catheters, resulting in poor mixing (dilution) of the anesthetic in the CSF and thereby creating pockets of toxic concentrations of local anesthetic.[43,44]

One additional concern I have about potential neuraxial nerve injury involves the use of continuous spinal catheters for postoperative analgesia. Many substances are used in the subarachnoid space to improve postoperative analgesia. Nevertheless, I believe this is a risk-filled endeavor.

We have found that if a continuous epidural catheter is in place out of the immediate operating theater, various unintentional drug injections occur.[45] The epidural space is likely more forgiving of misapplied drugs than is the subarachnoid space. For these reasons, anesthesiologists should be extremely cautious about continuing subarachnoid catheters in a setting where drug swaps and unintentional drug injection may be more likely to occur.

## When Should Neurologic Consultation Be Obtained?

If neurologic injury occurs after regional anesthesia, an important decision that needs to be made involves the request for a neurologic consultation. Anesthesiologists who use regional anesthesia should have a close working relationship with at least a few neurologists in their practice setting.

A frequent dilemma is caused by a neurologist who provides a well focused consultation but then suggests that an EMG would not be useful immediately after surgery because "all physicians know the neurologic changes may take from 14 to 21 days to develop after injury." That is exactly the point. As noted previously, Marinacci found that 99% of the neurologic lesions believed related to spinal anesthesia that were found (often with EMG help) actually represented preexisting neurologic deficits.[41]

If a neurologic deficit develops after operation, a baseline EMG may help to outline that neurologic abnormalities were present before operation, rather than being solely attributable to the anesthetic technique. Neurologic injury related to anesthesia has been well outlined in a report formatted from the American Society of Anesthesiologists Closed Claims database; the concluding statement in that report suggests that for most perioperative nerve injuries, the cause is not apparent.[31]

## What Are the Cardiovascular Effects of Regional Anesthesia?

The most frequent cause of cardiovascular side effects is autonomic blockade. Reduced BP and heart rate during central neuraxis blocks are primarily attributable to the vasodilation (especially venous) produced by sympathetic blockade. The second major mechanism for cardiovascular side effects is direct actions of the local anesthetic (or its additives) on the cardiovascular system.

One of the advantages of peripheral regional blocks is that they have minimal cardiovascular side effects because they are most often administered at sites remote from autonomic neural pathways. Therefore, the cardiovascular side effects attributed to peripheral blocks are almost exclusively a result of local anesthetic or vasoconstrictor side effects.

## Should Epinephrine Be Used?

In planning a peripheral block, a decision that needs to be made is whether to add epinephrine to the local anesthetic mixture. An epinephrine dilution of 1:200 000 (5 μg of epinephrine per milliliter of local anesthetic solution) provides adequate prolongation of the local anesthetic block without undue side effects.[46]

In situations when >45 mL of local anesthetic solution is administered during a peripheral regional block, the total dose of epinephrine should be limited to 0.25 mg (250 μg) to minimize epinephrine-related side effects.[27]

## How Is Hypotension Defined?

Although neuraxial blocks almost always routinely lower BP, what level of lowered BP should be defined as hypotension? Arterial BP decreases should approximate 15% of preblock levels, if euvolemia is maintained.[47]

Complicating clinical decisions about the augmentation of BP during neuraxial block is the recognition that for many of the patients we are most concerned about, those with ischemic heart disease, reduction of BP normally is a desirable long-term goal to minimize myocardial oxygen demands. In one sense, a neuraxial block is similar to β-adrenergic blockade; that is, BP is lowered, as is heart rate, albeit acutely.

Clinical judgment and tradition, as well as some experimental evidence, suggest that mean arterial BP should not be allowed to decline >30% after a neuraxial block. Most anesthesiologists aim to keep mean arterial BP at or above 65 mm Hg even in nonhypertensive patients. If patients have preexisting hypertension, this minimum level is necessarily shifted upward. A contrarian and clinically successful technique was carried out by Sharrock and Salvati, who combined a hypotensive epidural anesthetic with an epinephrine infusion for orthopedic patients.[48]

## What Is Profound Bradycardia?

Considerable attention has been focused on what has been described as an unrecognized entity: profound bradycardia after neuraxial blockade.[49] When viewed over time, this problem is neither new nor unrecognized by most anesthesiologists performing regional anesthesia.[36,50,51] Symptomatic bradycardia and even asystole are possible after autonomic interruption by neuraxial block.

Appropriate therapy usually includes an anticholinergic drug, such as atropine, and verification that the bradycardia is not secondary to hypoxemia. If atropine is not successful in raising the heart rate to an acceptable level, epinephrine, 25 to 100 μg, is indicated. If these treatment options, together with adequate volume replacement, are used, profound bradycardia is manageable.[52]

## What Is Local Anesthetic Toxicity?

Local anesthetic systemic toxicity usually results from unintentional intravascular injection or use of an excessive dose during regional block. Manifestations are primarily reflected in the central nervous system (CNS) and cardiovascular system. Approximately 4 to 7 times as much local anesthetic is required to produce cardiovascular collapse as to initiate convulsions[53] (Table 29–3). Systemic effects occur on a continuum (Fig. 29–27).

### Central Nervous System Effects

The CNS toxic effects of local anesthetic range from sedation to seizure. They are plasma concentration dependent. In general, the CNS toxic-to-therapeutic ratio of local anesthetics is quite similar after intravenous administration. Convulsions result from inhibitory fiber depression in the subcortical brain structures, probably the amygdala, with subsequent amplification to grand mal seizures.[54] Modification of CNS toxicity can

**TABLE 29–3.** Comparative Central Nervous System and Cardiovascular Toxicity of Local Anesthetics in Dogs

| Drug | Cumulative Convulsive Dose (mean ± SEM) | Cumulative Lethal Dose (mean ± SEM) | CV/CNS |
|------|------|------|------|
| Lidocaine | 22.0 ± 6.7 | 76.2 ± 15.1 | 3.5 |
| Etidocaine | 8.0 ± 2.2 | 40.4 ± 6.0 | 5.1 |
| Tetracaine | 4.0 ± 2.2 | 26.9 ± 4.6 | 6.7 |
| Bupivacaine | 5.0 ± 0 | 20.4 ± 2.4 | 4.1 |

CNS, central nervous system; CV, cardiovascular; SEM, standard error of the mean.

be achieved by the use of barbiturates, benzodiazepines, and even inhalational anesthetics.[55–59]

The decision to administer benzodiazepines prophylactically before regional block affects the risk-benefit relationship of systemic toxicity in two ways. CNS toxicity is less likely in a patient who has received benzodiazepines. Conversely, the early signs of CNS toxicity may be observed in a patient who has not been so "prophylaxed," allowing earlier intervention before the cardiovascular effects become apparent.

## Cardiotoxic Effects

The sodium-blocking action of local anesthetics produces dose-related decreases of myocardial contractility and cardiac conduction. At low concentrations, a small increase in mean arterial pressure often occurs, whereas at high concentrations, vasodilation or vasoconstriction can be noted.[60–64]

For many years, the potential for cardiac toxicity related to local anesthetics was believed to parallel their anesthetic potency.[65] It now has become apparent, however, that the long-acting local anesthetics, bupivacaine and etidocaine, are proportionally more cardiotoxic than their relative anesthetic potencies suggest.[66,67] This increase in cardiac toxicity appears to result from proportionally more and longer lasting sodium channel blockade.

Sodium channel block typically develops during systole and resolves during diastole. However, the long-acting agents such as bupivacaine do not leave the sodium channels as rapidly

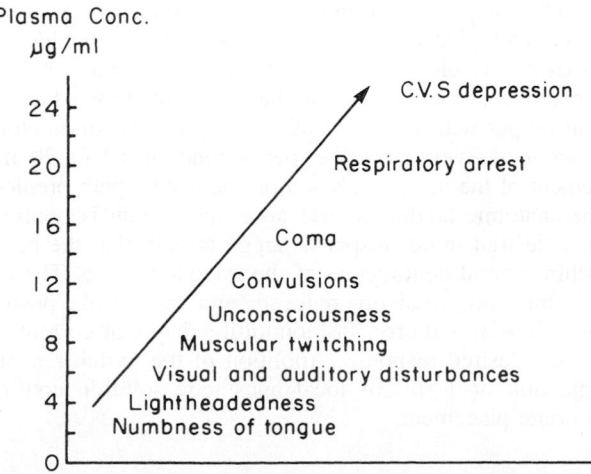

**FIGURE 29–27.** Local anesthetic systemic toxicity continuum. Symptoms begin with changes in sensorium and with perioral numbness. They progress along the continuum to seizures and eventually cardiovascular depression.

during diastole, and the sodium channel block accumulates.[68] CNS activity also may influence cardiac toxicity.[69,70]

## Treatment

Local anesthetic-induced systemic toxicity ranges from minor alterations in sensorium to significant tonic-clonic seizures that result in profound hypoxemia, hypercarbia, and acidosis. These metabolic and acid-base changes can develop quite rapidly (seconds to minutes) and can significantly increase toxicity.[71–73] If it is suspected that toxicity is developing, the first drug to administer is oxygen. Oxygen alone occasionally is sufficient treatment,[74] but positive-pressure breathing with a bag and mask may be necessary.

A CNS depressant (barbiturate or benzodiazepine) is usually all that is necessary to treat local anesthetic-induced seizures. If a CNS depressant and rapid-acting neuromuscular relaxant, such as succinylcholine, are deemed necessary, the latter should be administered first to prevent seizure-induced muscle activity and the accompanying acidosis. Furthermore, after administration of succinylcholine, the airway is more easily managed and oxygen more effectively delivered.

Most anesthesiologists encounter local anesthetic-induced toxicity rarely during their entire career. Hence, they should practice a local anesthetic-induced seizure management drill, much like the recommendations for failed intubation drills.

As outlined earlier, local anesthetic systemic toxicity progresses to cardiovascular toxicity. The ABCs of resuscitation should be followed in this setting, recognizing that larger than usual doses of epinephrine may be needed. Ventricular dysrhythmias (especially those related to the long-acting local anesthetics, bupivacaine and etidocaine) are likely more effectively treated with bretylium than lidocaine.[75–77]

A fundamental modification of local anesthetic use that may reduce the number of systemic toxic reactions is to use a test dose whenever possible or techniques to inject local anesthetics incrementally. If an intravascular injection occurs, only a small mass of drug is injected at any one time.

## Why Do Spinal Headaches Occur?

One of the principal reasons anesthesiologists recommend epidural over spinal anesthesia in patients for whom either technique is an option is concern that spinal anesthesia will lead to a significant incidence of position-related headaches. The loss of CSF through the dural puncture site is the principal cause of postdural puncture headache.[78] Why certain patient subgroups are more or less likely to have headaches after spinal anesthesia remains speculative. The factors listed in Table 29–4 seem to be associated with an increased incidence.

## Characteristics

The onset of headaches typically ranges from immediate to approximately 1 week after the spinal anesthetic. The peak incidence appears to be on postoperative day 2 or 3, often just when a surgeon would like to discharge an inpatient from the hospital.[79] Postdural puncture headaches developing more than 1 week after spinal anesthesia are unusual, and additional reasons for the headaches should be sought. The diagnosis is supported if the headache is most pronounced in an upright or sitting position; it should lessen or be significantly relieved

**TABLE 29–4.** Factors in Spinal Headaches

| Factors increasing incidence of headache | Age |
| --- | --- |
| | Gender (female) |
| | Needle size |
| | Needle bevel |
| | Younger > older |
| | Female > male |
| | Larger > smaller |
| | Cutting bevel > "spreading" bevel greater when dural |
| | Fibers cut transversely |
| | Pregnancy |
| | Number of dural passes |
| | Greater when pregnant |
| | Greater with multiple punctures |
| Factors unrelated to incidence of headache | Continuous epidural |
| | Timing of ambulation |

in the supine position. As with all medical conditions, spinal headache symptoms exist on a continuum that must be kept in mind when a diagnosis is made or ruled out.

Before the development of epidural blood patch therapy, typical headaches lasted from 2 to 3 days to approximately a week. On rare occasions, they persisted for weeks to months.[80–82]

### Prevention

The most important means to minimize the incidence of postdural puncture headache is appropriate matching of patients, equipment, and techniques. Postdural puncture headaches are more frequent in women (especially parturients) and are two times more common in women than men in the under 50 age group.[83] Younger patients have headaches more frequently than older patients.

A critical factor is an operator's skill. If the anesthesiologist is able to identify the subarachnoid space easily with one pass of the spinal needle, a lower headache incidence likely results than when a novice is unable to recognize subarachnoid placement and perforates the dura a number of times before achieving obvious subarachnoid placement.

One clinical dictum that seems unrelated to the incidence of postdural puncture headache is the prescription for bed rest after spinal anesthesia. This approach may delay the onset of the headache, but it does not appear to reduce the incidence.[80,84]

Increasing evidence suggests that splitting dural fibers by using pencil-point side-hole needles rather than cutting them with conventional needle points reduces the incidence. In addition, for similar-tipped needles, the incidence of headache decreases as needle size decreases.[85] It may also be decreased by using a paramedian rather than a midline approach.[86]

Incidence of postdural puncture headache after continuous spinal anesthesia may be lower than would be anticipated from the needle size used to perform the dural puncture.[87–89] For this reason, I am concerned about the push to develop increasingly smaller spinal catheters. Their appropriate use (and indications) need much further clarification as well as resolution of the issues leading to the FDA Safety Alert[42] before we introduce them widely into our practices, especially for postoperative analgesia.

### Treatment

Finally, if spinal anesthesia is to be used successfully and postdural puncture headaches are not allowed to limit our

choice, epidural blood patch therapy must be provided in a time-efficient manner. Although bed rest is often an appropriate short-term treatment, it should not be unnecessarily prolonged before undertaking an epidural blood patch.

The prescription for hydrating (possibly overhydrating) patients intravenously needs rethinking. Little evidence supports the concept that hydration actually treats postdural puncture headaches.

Caffeine (7 mg/kg) relieves some headaches but often needs to be repeated, and thus seems to be a temporizing treatment.[90] Any question about the efficacy of caffeine also should not delay definitive epidural blood patch therapy.

## Is There a Role for Nerve Stimulator-Assisted Regional Anesthesia?

Clearly, regional anesthesia is routinely and successfully implemented based on knowledge of the local anatomy and occasionally also elicitation of paresthesias. In some circumstances, however, a patient is unable to respond adequately to interrogation about either onset of block or occurrence of paresthesia. There are also patients whose anatomic landmarks are indistinct and occasions when the anesthesiologist is asked to place an infrequently performed block. In such instances, a nerve stimulator is quite helpful to verify that the tip of the block needle is located precisely adjacent to the desired nerve. This localization is manifested as an evoked motor response, that is, a twitch for a motor nerve or a burning sensation if it is a sensory nerve referable to the intended nerve. If the nerve is a mixed sensory and motor nerve, then the motor response predominates because large myelinated fibers (motor) are stimulated by lower currents than their smaller unmyelinated sensory nerve counterparts.

### Needle Placement

To obtain maximum use of nerve stimulator-assisted peripheral nerve identification, an insulated or shielded needle should be used first. The insulation serves to localize the densest current at the needle tip, compared with an insulated needle, which emits some current along its entire shaft. A conducting portion of this needle is then connected to the negative terminal of the nerve stimulator, usually by an alligator clamp. The positive terminal is connected to an electrocardiograph pad placed on the lateral ipsilateral shoulder for upper extremity block or buttock for lower extremity block.

The nerve stimulator should have a discretely adjustable current output with a display of the output. The stimulator is then set to deliver one pulse per second of 10 to 20 mA. Placement of the needle is based on the needle path predicted by the anatomic landmarks. Because this current is relatively large, a desired motor response suggests only that the needle is within several centimeters of the intended nerve. The current is then progressively reduced, and the needle position adjusted in trial-and-error fashion until <1 mA of current still elicits the desired response. Abolition of the twitch response on injection of 1 mL of local anesthetic solution confirms appropriate placement.

### References

1. Katz JA. A survey of anesthetic choice among anesthesiologists. *Anesth Analg.* 1973;52:373.

2. Broadman LM, Mesrobian R, Ruttimann U, et al. Do anesthesiologists prefer a regional or general anesthetic for themselves? *Reg Anesth.* 1986;11:A57.

3. Bach S, Noreng MF, Tjellden NU. Phantom limb pain in amputees during first 12 months following limb amputation, after preoperative lumbar epidural blockade. *Pain.* 1988;33:297.

4. Dickenson AH, Sullivan AF. Subcutaneous formalin-induced activity of dorsal horn neurones in the rat: differential response to an intrathecal opiate administered pre or post formalin. *Pain.* 1987;30:349.

5. Tverskoy M, Cozacov C, Ayache M, et al. Postoperative pain after inguinal herniorrhaphy with different types of anesthesia. *Anesth Analg.* 1990;70:29.

6. Kopacz DJ, Nickel P. Regional anesthesia in the elderly patient. *Probl Anesth.* 1989;3:602.

7. Bridenbaugh LD. Are anesthesia resident programs failing regional anesthesia? *Reg Anesth.* 1982;7:26.

8. O'Keefe JH, Shub C, Rettke SR. Risk of noncardiac surgical procedures in patients with aortic stenosis. *Mayo Clin Proc.* 1989;64:400.

9. Torsher LC, Shub C, Rettke SR, et al. Risk of patients with severe aortic stenosis undergoing noncardiac surgery. *Am J Cardiol.* 1998;81:448.

10. Moore DC, Chadwick HS, Ready LB. Epinephrine prolongs lidocaine spinal: pain in the operative site the most accurate method of determining local anesthetic duration. *Anesthesiology.* 1987;67:416.

11. Chestnut DH. Spinal anesthesia in the febrile patient. *Anesthesiology.* 1992;76:667.

12. Caldwell C, Nielsen C, Baltz T, et al. Comparison of high-dose epinephrine and phenylephrine in spinal anesthesia with tetracaine. *Anesthesiology.* 1985;62:804.

13. Palve H, Kirvela O, Olin H, et al. Maximum recommended doses of lignocaine are not toxic [see comments]. *Br J Anaesth.* 1995;74:704.

14. Gielen M. Post dural puncture headache (PDPH): a review. *Reg Anesth.* 1989;14:101.

15. Seeberger MD, Lang ML, Drewe J, et al. Comparison of spinal and epidural anesthesia for patients younger than 50 years of age. *Anesth Analg.* 1994;78:667.

16. Moore DC. Spinal anesthesia: bupivacaine compared with tetracaine. *Anesth Analg.* 1980;59:743.

17. Greene NM. Hypobaric, isobaric, and hyperbaric spinal anesthesia. *Curr Rev Clin Anesth.* 1985;5:99.

18. Brown DL. *Atlas of Regional Anesthesia.* 2nd ed. Philadelphia, Pa: WB Saunders; 1998.

19. Taylor JA. Lumbosacral subarachnoid tap. *J Urol.* 1940;43:561.

20. Brown DL, Carpenter RL. Perioperative analgesia: a review of risks and benefits. *J Cardiothorac Anesth.* 1990;4:368.

21. Philip BK. Effect of epidural air injection on catheter complications: experience in obstetric patients. *Reg Anesth.* 1985;10:21.

22. Verniquet AJW. Vessel puncture with epidural catheters. *Anaesthesia.* 1980;35:660.

23. Mannion D, Walker R, Clayton K. Extradural vein puncture—an avoidable complication. *Anaesthesia.* 1991;46:585.

24. Trotter M. Variations of the sacral canal: their significance in the administration of caudal anesthesia. *Anesth Analg.* 1947;26:192.

25. Lanz E, Theiss D, Jankovic D. The extent of blockade following various techniques of brachial plexus block. *Anesth Analg.* 1983;62:55.

26. Winnie AP. Interscalene brachial plexus block. *Anesth Analg.* 1970;49:455.

27. Moore DC. *Regional Block: A Handbook for Use in the Clinical Practice of Medicine and Surgery.* 4th ed. Springfield, Ill: Charles C Thomas; 1965.

28. Brown DL, Cahill DR, Bridenbaugh LD. Supraclavicular nerve block: anatomic analysis of a method to prevent pneumothorax. *Anesth Analg.* 1993;76:530.

29. Labat G. *Regional Anaesthesia: Its Technique and Clinical Application.* Philadelphia, Pa: WB Saunders; 1923.

30. Moore DC, Bridenbaugh LD. Pneumothorax: its incidence following intercostal nerve block. *JAMA.* 1960;174:842.

31. Kroll DA, Caplan RA, Posner K, et al. Nerve injury associated with anesthesia. *Anesthesiology.* 1990;73:202.

32. Warner MA, Warner DO, Matsumoto JY, et al. Ulnar neuropathy in surgical patients. *Anesthesiology.* 1999;90:54.

33. Selander D, Edshage S, Wolff T. Paresthesia or no paresthesia. *Acta Anaesthesiol Scand.* 1979;23:27.

34. Winchell SW, Wolfe R. The incidence of neuropathy following upper extremity nerve blocks. *Reg Anesth.* 1985;10:12.

35. Thompson AM, Newman RJ, Semple JC. Brachial plexus anaesthesia for upper limb surgery: a review of 8 years experience. *J Hand Surg [Br].* 1988;13:195.

36. Moore DC, Bridenbaugh LD. Spinal (subarachnoid) block: a review of 11,574 cases. *JAMA.* 1966;195:907.

37. Vandam LD, Dripps RD. Long-term follow-up of 10,098 spinal anesthetics: incidence and analysis of minor sensory neurological defects. *Surgery.* 1955;38:463.

38. Rigler M, Drasner K, Yelich S, et al. Cauda equina syndrome after continuous spinal anesthesia. *Anesth Analg.* 1991;72:275.

39. Horlocker TT, Wedel DJ. Neuraxial block and low-molecular-weight heparin: balancing perioperative analgesia and thromboprophylaxis. *Reg Anesth Pain Med.* 1998;23(suppl 2):164.

40. Cope RW. The Wooley and Roe case: Wooley and Roe versus the Ministry of Health and others. *Anesthesia.* 1954;9:247.

41. Marinacci AA. Neurologic aspects of complications of spinal anesthesia. *Los Angeles Neurol Soc Bull.* 1960;25:170.

42. US Food and Drug Administration. FDA safety alert: cauda equina syndrome associated with use of small-bore catheters in continuous spinal anesthesia. Rockville, Md: US Food and Drug Administration; 1992.

43. Ross BK, Coda B, Heath CH. Local anesthetic distribution in a spinal model: a possible mechanism of neurologic injury after continuous spinal anesthesia. *Reg Anesth.* 1992;17:69.

44. Rigler ML, Drasner K: Distribution of catheter-injected local anesthetic in a model of the subarachnoid space. *Anesthesiology.* 1991;75:684.

45. Bickler P, Spears R, McKay W. Intralipid solution mistakenly infused into epidural space [letter]. *Anesthesiology.* 1990;71:712.

46. Tucker GT, Moore DC, Bridenbaugh PO, et al. Systemic absorption of mepivacaine in commonly used regional block procedures. *Anesthesiology.* 1972;37:277.

47. Greene NM. *Physiology of Spinal Anesthesia.* 3rd ed. Baltimore, Md: Williams & Wilkins; 1981.

48. Sharrock NE, Salvati EA. Hypotensive epidural anesthesia for total hip arthroplasty: a review. *Acta Orthop Scand.* 1996;67:91.

49. Caplan RA, Ward RJ, Posner K, et al. Unexpected cardiac arrest during spinal anesthesia: a closed claims analysis of predisposing factors. *Anesthesiology.* 1988;68:5.

50. Wetstone DL, Wong KC. Sinus bradycardia and asystole during spinal anesthesia. *Anesthesiology.* 1974;41:87.

51. Thompson KW. Fatalities from spinal anesthesia. *Anesth Analg.* 1934;13:75.

52. Mackey DC, Carpenter RL, Thompson GE, et al. Bradycardia and asystole during spinal anesthesia: a report of three cases without morbidity. *Anesthesiology.* 1989;70:866.

53. Liu PL, Feldman HS, Giasi R, et al. Comparative CNS toxicity of lidocaine, etidocaine, bupivacaine, and tetracaine in awake dogs following rapid IV administration. *Anesth Analg.* 1983;62:375.

54. Wagman IH, de Jong RH, Prince DA. Effects of lidocaine on the central nervous system. *Anesthesiology.* 1967;28:155.

55. de Jong RH, Wagman IH, Prince DA. Effect of carbon dioxide on the cortical seizure threshold to lidocaine. *Exp Neurol.* 1967;17:221.

56. Ausinsch B, Malagodi MN, Munson ES. Diazepam in the prophylaxis of lignocaine seizures. *Br J Anaesth.* 1976;48:309.

57. de Jong RH, Heavner JE. Local anesthetic seizure prevention: diazepam vs. pentobarbital. *Anesthesiology.* 1972;36:449.

58. Feinstein MB, Lenard W, Mathias J. The antagonism of local anesthetic induced convulsions by the benzodiazepine derivative diazepam. *Arch Int Pharmacodyn Ther.* 1970;187:144.

59. de Jong RH, Heavner JE, de Oliveira LF. Effects of nitrous oxide on the lidocaine seizure threshold and diazepam protection. *Anesthesiology.* 1972;37:299.

60. Gibbs CP, Noel SC. Response of arterial segments from gravid human uterus to multiple concentrations of lignocaine. *Br J Anaesth.* 1977;49:409.

61. Johns RA, DiFazio CA, Longnecker DE. Lidocaine constricts or dilates rat arterioles in a dose-dependent manner. *Anesthesiology.* 1985;62:141.

62. Johns RA, Seyde WC, DiFazio CA, et al. Dose-dependent effects of bupivacaine on rat muscle arterioles. *Anesthesiology.* 1986;65:186.

63. Fleisch JH, Titus E. Effect of local anesthetics on pharmacologic receptor systems of smooth muscle. *J Pharmacol Exp Ther.* 1973;186:44.

64. Klein SW, Sutherland RI, Morch JE. Hemodynamic effects of intravenous lidocaine in man. *CMAJ.* 1968;99:472.

65. Block A, Covino B. Effect of local agents on cardiac conduction and contractility. *Reg Anesth.* 1981;6:55.

66. de Jong RH, Ronfeld RA, DeRosa R. Cardiovascular effects of convulsant and supraconvulsant doses of amide local anesthetics. *Anesth Analg.* 1982;61:3.

67. Kotelko DM, Shnider SM, Dailey PA, et al. Bupivacaine-induced cardiac arrhythmias in sheep. *Anesthesiology.* 1984;60:10.

68. Clarkson CW, Hondeghem LM. Mechanism for bupivacaine depression

of cardiac conduction: fast block of sodium channels during the action potential with slow recovery from block during diastole. *Anesthesiology.* 1985;62:396.

69. Thomas RD, Behbehani MM, Coyle DE, et al. Cardiovascular toxicity of local anesthetics: an alternative hypothesis. *Anesth Analg.* 1986;65:444.

70. Heavner JE. Cardiac dysrhythmias induced by infusion of local anesthetics into the lateral cerebral ventricle of cats. *Anesth Analg.* 1986;65:133.

71. Munson ES, Tucker WK, Ausinsch B, et al. Etidocaine, bupivacaine, and lidocaine seizure thresholds in monkeys. *Anesthesiology.* 1975;42:471.

72. Moore DC, Crawford RD, Scurlock JE. Severe hypoxia and acidosis following local anesthetic-induced convulsions. *Anesthesiology.* 1980;53:259.

73. Morishima HO, Covino BG. Toxicity and distribution of lidocaine in nonasphyxiated and asphyxiated baboon fetuses. *Anesthesiology.* 1981;54:182.

74. Moore DC, Bridenbaugh LD. Oxygen: the antidote for systemic toxic reactions from local anesthetic drugs. *JAMA.* 1960;174:842.

75. Kendig JJ. Clinical implications of the modulated receptor hypothesis: local anesthetics and the heart. *Anesthesiology.* 1985;62:382.

76. Kasten GW, Martin ST. Bupivacaine cardiovascular toxicity: comparison of treatment with bretylium and lidocaine. *Anesth Analg.* 1985;64:911.

77. Kasten GW, Martin ST. Comparison of resuscitation of sheep and dogs after bupivacaine-induced cardiovascular collapse. *Anesth Analg.* 1986;65:1029.

78. Kunkle EC, Ray BS, Wolf HG. Experimental studies on headaches: analysis of the headache associated with changes in intracranial pressure. *Neurol Psychiatr.* 1943;49:323.

79. Vandam LD, Dripps RD. A long-term follow-up of patients who received 10,098 spinal anesthetics, II: incidence and analyses of minor sensory neurologic defects. *Surgery.* 1955;38:463.

80. Jones RJ. The role of recumbency in the prevention and treatment of postspinal headache. *Anesth Analg.* 1974;53:788.

81. Driessen A, Mauer W, Fricke M, et al. Prospective studies of the postspinal headache. *Reg Anesth.* 1980;3:38.

82. Kortum K, Nolte H, Kenkmann HJ. Beschwerden nach Spinalanaesthesie. Sex difference related complication rates after spinal anesthesia. *Reg Anesth.* 1982;5:1.

83. Gielen M. Postdural puncture headaches: a review. *Reg Anesth.* 1989;14:101.

84. Thornberry EA, Thomas TA. Posture and post-spinal headache: a controlled trial in 80 obstetric patients. *Br J Anaesth.* 1988;60:195.

85. Mulroy MF. Spinal headaches: management and avoidance. *Probl Anesth.* 1987;1:602.

86. Ready LB, Culpin S, Haschke RH, et al. Spinal needle determinants of rate of transdural fluid leak. *Anesth Analg.* 1989;69:457.

87. Denny N, Masters R, Pearson D, et al. Postdural puncture headache after continuous spinal anesthesia. *Anesth Analg.* 1987;66:791.

88. Peterson DO, Borup JL, Chestnut JS. Continuous spinal anesthesia. Case review and discussion. *Reg Anesth.* 1983;8:109.

89. Kallos T, Smith TC. Continuous spinal anesthesia with hypobaric tetracaine for hip surgery in lateral decubitus. *Anesth Analg.* 1972;51:766.

90. Sechzer PH, Abel L. Post spinal anesthesia headache treated with caffeine. *Curr Ther Res.* 1978;24:307.

# Pharmacologic Considerations and Anesthetic Administration

CHAPTER

# 30

# Basic Pharmacologic Applications in Anesthesia

Lisette Volckmar

Roderic G. Eckenhoff

Pharmacology is a basic and clinical science that involves the study of the interactions between drugs and living systems. In this chapter, the terms *drug level* or *drug concentration* refer to a concentration of a medication in blood, serum, or plasma, and the assumption is made that this value is related to the physiologic or behavioral response. This chapter focuses on the following three major areas of pharmacology as they relate to the practice of anesthesia:

- *Pharmacokinetics* is a term derived from the Greek words for "drug" and "motion." It refers to the movement of drugs throughout the body and what the body does to the drug.
- *Pharmacodynamics* is a term derived from the Greek words for "drug" and "action" and refers to the effects of drugs on the body. These drug effects involve the relationship between drug concentration and pharmacologic responses. Pharmacodynamic effects are frequently mediated by the interaction between drugs and their receptors.
- *Pharmacogenetics* is the study of genetic factors that alter and affect drug disposition.

We do not intend this chapter to be a comprehensive resource document. Rather, it is written as a primer for the clinician wishing to refamiliarize himself or herself with basic pharmacologic concepts, and to prepare for more detailed reading.

## DRUG DISPOSITION: PHARMACOKINETICS

### What Happens After a Patient Receives a Medication?

Whether administered enterally or parenterally, medications are usually first absorbed or deposited into the systemic circulation. They are then distributed throughout the body, reach a site of action, and produce a response of some sort. Finally, they are cleared or removed from the body by biotransformation or elimination (Fig. 30–1).

Medications can also be administered in a more selective fashion to sites such as the epidural or subarachnoid (intrathecal) spaces, the pleural or peritoneal spaces, skin, muscle, peripheral nerves, and corneal or mucosal surfaces. Even infiltration of wounds with a local anesthetic can be useful in blocking nociception. Drugs can also be introduced intraarterially in a few select situations. For example, phentolamine mesylate or heparin can be selectively administered intraarterially to relieve arterial vasospasm or thrombosis, respectively.

Even though medications are frequently administered near their site of action, systemic absorption still occurs and may produce unwanted side effects. For example, eye drops containing phenylephrine or timolol may produce clinically significant hemodynamic effects.[1] Also, eye drops containing echothiophate result in the inhibition of pseudocholinesterase, which is responsible for the metabolism of ester local anesthetics and succinylcholine. Echothiophate eye drops, when systemically absorbed, may cause potentiation and prolongation of these drugs.

### How Does the Route of Administration Affect Drug Disposition?

The route of drug administration affects:

1. Amount of drug entering the systemic circulation
2. Time of onset and duration of drug effect
3. Peak drug concentration and consequently the intensity of the drug effect

For example, medications given subcutaneously (eg, insulin, terbutaline, or epinephrine) or intramuscularly (eg, ephedrine) provide a more sustained effect than does a single intravenous bolus, although more must be given. Topical drug administration, such as use of fentanyl, clonidine, or nitroglycerin patches, also results in sustained release of drug. Duration of effect can also be influenced by the drug itself or other drugs administered concomitantly. Vasoconstriction caused by the addition of epinephrine to local anesthetics reduces the absorption and prolongs the effects of these drugs.

Drugs administered by the pulmonary route, such as the volatile agents or bronchodilators, are quickly absorbed into the systemic circulation, avoiding the first-pass effect by the liver. The effect of the route of administration on drug concentration is demonstrated for local anesthetics in Figure 30–2.[2] As shown, tracheal administration of a drug can result in a high peak plasma concentration. Thus, the administration of certain resuscitative drugs (eg, epinephrine, atropine, or lidocaine) through an endotracheal tube during cardiopulmonary resuscitation can be a useful temporizing measure before venous access is established. However, this measure also provides undesirable topical anesthesia of the airway because of the rapid absorption of local anesthetics into the circulation, as previously mentioned. Cumulative doses of aerosolized and topical lidocaine should be kept within therapeutic, nontoxic levels and vigilance maintained for signs of local anesthetic toxicity. Many clinicians include a benzodiazepine for seda-

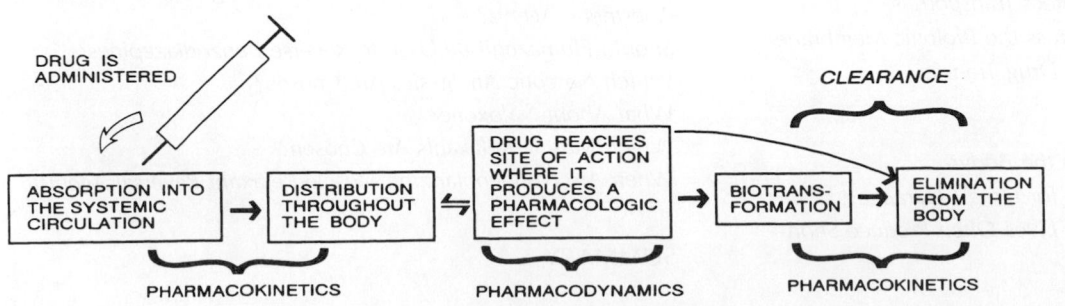

**FIGURE 30–1.** Pathway of drug distribution and elimination.

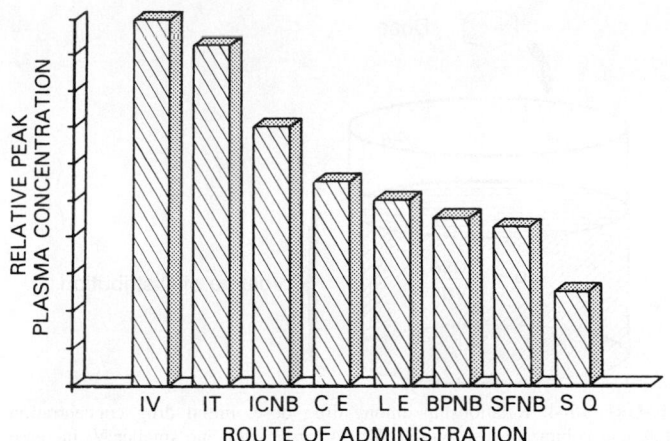

**FIGURE 30–2.** Effect of route of administration of local anesthetics on peak plasma concentration. BPNB, brachial plexus nerve block; CE, caudal epidural; ICNB, intercostal nerve block; IT, intratracheal; IV, intravenous; LE, lumbar epidural; SFNB, superficial nerve block; SQ, subcutaneous.

tion in procedures requiring extensive topical anesthesia in the hope of protecting against local anesthetic-induced seizures.

Drugs administered orally or topically may be incompletely absorbed or may be metabolized by the liver before reaching the systemic circulation. Consequently, only a fraction of a given dose of medication may reach the systemic circulation. To describe this, *bioavailability* (F) has been defined:

$$F = \frac{\text{Amount of Medication Reaching the Systemic Circulation}}{\text{Amount of Medication Administered}}$$

(Equation 1)

Thus, the bioavailability describes the extent to which a drug is available to reach its site of action.

The *extraction ratio* (ER) is the ratio of a dose that is cleared from the body before reaching the systemic circulation. This concept applies to drugs that are given enterally and exhibit a first-pass effect by the liver. Drugs given sublingually (eg, nitroglycerin or nifedipine) bypass the liver initially on absorption. Drugs given per rectum (eg, rectal acetaminophen [Tylenol] in pediatric patients) exhibit varying first-pass effects. The following equation illustrates the relationship between extraction ratio and bioavailability:

$$ER = 1 - F$$

(Equation 2)

### How Is Bioavailability Measured?

Measurements of bioavailability involve administering a medication on separate days by different routes (eg, orally and parenterally). Multiple drug levels are then measured and plotted against time after administration. The areas under the plasma concentration versus time curves (AUCs) are then determined and corrected for any differences in dose. Bioavailability is determined by comparing the ratio of these two areas (Fig. 30–3). For instance, if the AUC after oral administration is 25% of that after parenteral administration, the bioavailability is 25%. The bioavailability of parenterally administered drugs is typically considered to be 100%.

### Why Are Extraction Ratio and Bioavailability Clinically Important?

Consider the following hypothetical problem:

**Problem.** A patient taking the antihypertensive medication labetalol must fast for several days before and after surgery. During this period, you wish to maintain a parenteral dose of labetalol that is comparable with her usual oral dose of 300 mg/d. You refer to a pharmacology reference and note that the extraction ratio is 0.75 (ie, three fourths of a dose of orally administered labetalol is extracted by the liver before it reaches the systemic circulation because of a high first-pass effect by the liver). Therefore, if this patient responds like an average patient, of the 300 mg of labetalol administered orally, approximately 225 mg (75%) is cleared during the first pass through the liver, and 75 mg (25%) reaches the systemic circulation. A reasonable intravenous dose for this patient would, therefore, be 75 mg/d given in divided doses.

### What About Interindividual Variability?

Considerable interindividual variability is usually noted in pharmacokinetic parameters such as bioavailability. Bioavailability can be altered by factors that alter liver enzyme function or splanchnic blood flow. Interindividual pharmacokinetic differences are influenced by factors such as smoking, alcohol or drug intake, nutritional status, age, disease processes, race, or hormonal status. Surgery and anesthesia may also alter bioavailability. For example, abdominal surgery, the use of volatile agents, and hypotension all result in diminished blood flow to the liver and therefore increase the bioavailability of drugs that are highly extracted by the liver.

Bioavailability is also affected by factors that influence absorption from the intestine, such as local blood flow, gastric emptying time, pH conditions, and absorptive area. The appropriate drug dose may change over time for a given individual, depending on the influence of these other variables. Also, drug responses in typical surgical patients may be quite different from those seen in young, healthy, unanesthetized volunteers who are often the subjects of drug studies.

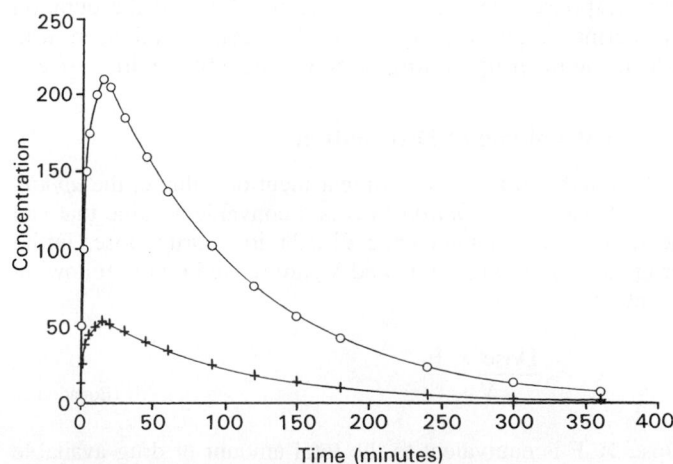

**FIGURE 30–3.** Plasma concentrations following parenteral (o) and oral (+) drug administration. Bioavailability is determined by the ratio of the areas under the curves.

## Intravenous Administration

Traditionally, multicompartment pharmacokinetic models have been used to study the distribution and elimination of intravenously administered anesthetic drugs. These models include the central or initial volume of distribution ($V_C$), in which the drug instantaneously appears after intravenous administration and before redistribution to other tissues. Intercompartmental clearance thus describes the distribution of drug to fast and slowly equilibrating volumes of distribution, which are determined by blood flow and transcapillary permeability. Elimination describes drug metabolism or removal from the body. These concepts are useful in understanding drug dosing in patients when a drug is given by continuous infusion or multiple doses.[3]

Multicompartment models do not readily explain individual variability in response to a single rapid intravenous dose such as occurs during induction. Front-end kinetics best describe the pharmacokinetics of early drug distribution when given by rapid intravenous administration. Studies reveal that cardiac output is a major determinant of how quickly and extensively a drug distributes to the brain. Low cardiac output results in higher peak concentrations of drug because of dilution of the initial bolus by blood. Further dilution occurs by peripheral distribution to active and other tissues.[3] Therefore, when determining an intravenous induction dose, consideration should be given to factors that alter cardiac output (eg, obesity, sympathomimetics, gender, age, and hypovolemia), as well as factors that affect subsequent peripheral distribution of the drug (eg, hemorrhagic shock or sepsis where blood flow to peripheral tissues is diminished).

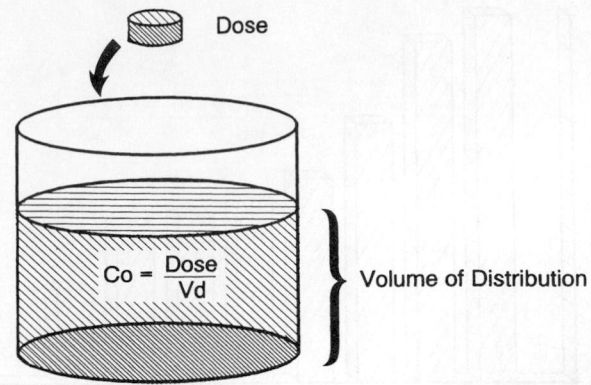

**FIGURE 30–4.** Relationship among drug dose, initial drug concentration ($C_0$), and volume of distribution ($V_d$). A larger dose and smaller $V_d$ increase the $C_0$.

Under steady-state conditions, $V_d$ is affected by both drug and patient characteristics. A large $V_d$ occurs under conditions that favor tissue uptake, resulting in a lower plasma concentration. Drug features that favor tissue uptake include low molecular weight and high lipid solubility; patient features are hypoalbuminemia and hypovolemia. The calculated $V_d$ may even exceed body volume because of the one-compartment assumption (plasma). A smaller $V_d$ occurs when drug or patient features favor retention of drug in the plasma; this includes drugs of high molecular weight, those that are highly water soluble, and drugs with avid plasma protein-binding capacity.

# DRUG DISTRIBUTION

## Why Should We Be Concerned About Drug Distribution?

Once in the systemic circulation, a medication distributes throughout the body. Drug distribution is affected by factors such as body composition, regional blood flow, protein binding, tissue diffusion, and the physicochemical characteristics of a drug. Clinicians are interested in the process of drug distribution because it influences two critical determinants of drug response: the peak drug concentration and the duration of pharmacologic response. Peak drug concentration, in turn, affects the intensity of drug response and adverse drug effects.

## Apparent Volume of Distribution

Although not an actual compartment or volume, the *apparent volume of distribution* ($V_d$) is a convenient value that can be used to understand drug distribution. Drug dose, initial drug concentration ($C_0$), F, and $V_d$ are related by the following equation:

$$C_0 = \frac{Dose \times F}{V_d}$$

(Equation 3)

Dose $\times$ F is equivalent to the total amount of drug available at its site of action. The implication of Equation 3 is that $C_0$ is increased when a larger dose is given, and the $V_d$ is decreased (Fig. 30–4).

## How Do Changes in Volume of Distribution Affect Water-Soluble Drugs?

When corrected for weight (ie, when expressed as volume per kilogram), the $V_d$ of water-soluble drugs is generally

- Larger in men than in women
- Larger in children than in adults
- Larger in younger than in older adults
- Larger in lean than in obese people

The differences relate to body composition. In particular, changes in the ratio of body fat to body water may change the $V_d$ of a hydrophilic medication. From the relationship illustrated in Equation 3, it is predicted that as $V_d$ increases, peak drug levels should decrease. The maximum intensity of pharmacologic response parallels changes in peak drug levels and, therefore, the maximum drug effect usually decreases as the $V_d$ increases. In addition, half-lives ($t_{1/2}$s) change with the $V_d$ (see the section, How Do Changes in Volume of Distribution Affect Fat-Soluble Drugs?).

For example, ethanol and succinylcholine are hydrophilic drugs that distribute primarily in body water. After a given dose of alcohol, blood levels usually are higher in older than in younger adults[4] (Fig. 30–5) and higher in women than in men. This fact explains why women or the elderly may appear to be more sensitive to alcohol than young adult men.

Similarly, in the case of succinylcholine, a given dose (in milligrams per kilogram) usually is associated with lower blood levels in young children than in adults.[5] Hence, the

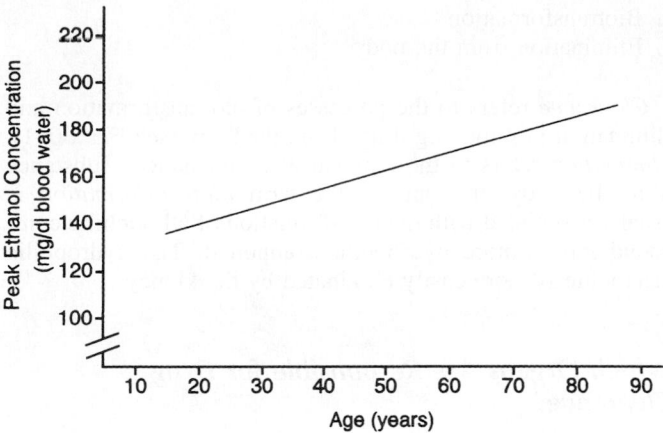

**FIGURE 30–5.** A given dose of a water-soluble drug such as ethanol produces a higher blood level in older adults because their ratio of body water to body fat is reduced. Thus, the volume of distribution for water-soluble drugs is reduced.

intubating dose of succinylcholine is higher in infants than in adults.

## How Do Changes in Volume of Distribution Affect Fat-Soluble Drugs?

In general, the $t_{1/2}$ of lipophilic medications increases as body fat composition increases (in part because of an increased $V_d$; see Equation 7). Peak drug levels, and hence the intensity of drug effect, decrease as body fat composition increases (see Equation 3).

> **Example.** The $t_{1/2}$ of the lipophilic benzodiazepine diazepam increases with age secondary to age-related changes in body fat composition[6] (Fig, 30–6). Similarly, the $t_{1/2}$ of midazolam has been found to be prolonged in obese patients.

## How Does Protein Binding Affect Volume of Distribution?

A drug in the bloodstream may be present as free, unbound drug in plasma taken up into red blood cells and other cellular

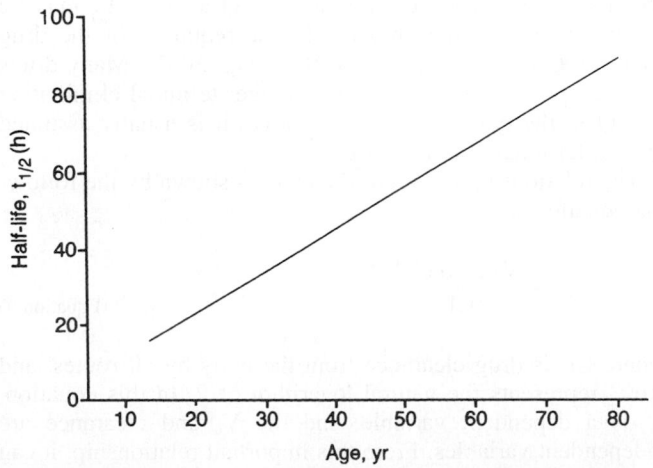

**FIGURE 30–6.** Increased half-life of diazepam (a lipophilic drug) because of increased fat stores associated with aging. Similar findings apply in obese patients.

blood elements or bound to plasma proteins, typically serum albumin or $\alpha_1$-acid glycoprotein. The latter is an acute-phase reactant protein that binds many *basic* drugs, such as propranolol and many of the local anesthetics. Its concentration may be increased after trauma, infection, myocardial infarction, or inflammation. Albumin, on the other hand, binds many *acidic* drugs such as benzodiazepines, warfarin, and thiopental. Albumin concentrations are lower in malnutrition, cirrhosis, and old age.

As the degree of binding to plasma proteins increases, more drug stays within the intravascular space, and therefore the $V_d$ decreases.[7] In addition, a smaller fraction of drug exists in plasma in the free, unbound form. It can be expected, therefore, that drug concentrations in other organs, such as the central nervous system (CNS), would be decreased as protein binding increases. The net effect of these changes is that the response to a medication decreases as the amount of protein binding increases. Conversely, as protein binding decreases, the $V_d$ increases and the free fraction increases.[8]

> **Example.** Thiopental is highly bound to albumin. If albumin levels are decreased, we can expect a large fraction of this drug to be in the free, unbound form in the circulation.[9] Thus, more thiopental is able to leave the circulation and enter the CNS. It can be predicted, therefore, that hypoalbuminemic patients will be extremely sensitive to the sedative-hypnotic effects of thiopental.

## DIFFUSION AND TRANSPORT OF DRUGS

### What Is Fick's Law of Diffusion?

This important law relates the rate of drug diffusion (D) to the temperature-dependent permeability coefficient (P), the area across which diffusion occurs (A), and the concentration gradient of unbound drug across the membrane ($\Delta C$):

$$D = P \times A \times \Delta C \qquad \text{(Equation 4)}$$

The permeability coefficient is inversely proportional to the thickness of the membrane and the size of the drug molecule and is directly proportional to the degree of lipophilicity of the drug.

The degree of protein binding also affects drug transport across a membrane. Because only the free or unbound form of a drug is available to cross a membrane, the rate of drug diffusion decreases as protein binding increases. For highly ionized or highly protein-bound drugs to cross a membrane, a large concentration gradient must exist.

### How Do Acid-Base Changes Affect Transport?

Most drugs enter cells by diffusion in the nonionized state through a lipid membrane. Because medications often are either weak acids or weak bases, the degree of ionization depends on the dissociation constant (pKa) of the medication and the pH of the medium. The *Henderson-Hasselbalch* equation demonstrates the relationship between pKa, pH, and the ratio of charged to uncharged forms of a molecule:

$$pKa = pH + \log [acid/base] \qquad \text{(Equation 5)}$$

## How Does Transport Occur Across the Biologic Membrane?

Drugs may penetrate cellular membranes by passive diffusion, facilitated diffusion, active transport, or endocytosis. Passive diffusion relies on a concentration gradient and permeability, and requires no additional energy. In both active transport and facilitated diffusion, drug transport is mediated by a macromolecule, so it is saturable and specific for certain molecules. In active transport, energy is required and is used to move drugs "uphill" against the drug's concentration gradient. Energy is not a requirement in facilitated diffusion, which does not move a drug against its concentration gradient. The source of energy for active drug transport is frequently a sodium-potassium adenosine triphosphatase enzyme.

*Endocytosis* refers to intracellular drug transportation by a vacuolar apparatus. An example of this relatively minor process of drug transport is the intracellular transport of insulin.

## What Factors Control Placental Drug Transfer?

The same principles can be applied to drug transport across the placenta. Many drugs cross the placenta by simple diffusion. Most analgesic and anesthetic drugs are lipid soluble and highly permeable and thus readily cross to the fetus following a concentration gradient from the maternal circulation.[10]

For example, during cesarean section, large amounts of thiopental (lipophilic), but not succinylcholine (hydrophilic), cross the placenta to the fetus.[11] Another example illustrates the importance of protein binding as a consideration when choosing a local anesthetic for use during epidural analgesia. Bupivacaine is acceptable for analgesia during labor because it is highly protein bound in the maternal circulation and thus less available as the free form for diffusion to the fetus.[12] Fetal acidosis increases the accumulation of some weak basic drugs (like local anesthetics) in the fetal compartment[10] because a larger proportion of molecules become charged at low pH and can no longer cross the placenta by simple diffusion.

### Fetal Protection

Several important mechanisms help to protect a fetus from drugs present in the maternal circulation. First, the human placenta contains enzymes that are involved in drug biotransformation. In addition, drugs that cross the placenta pass initially through the umbilical vein and fetal liver before entering the fetal circulation. As a result of these two mechanisms, many drugs present in the maternal circulation are transformed to less active forms before entering the fetal circulation.

## DRUG CLEARANCE

### How Are Drugs Removed From the Body?

Drug levels in blood or plasma decrease because of the following:

1. Distribution into other body compartments

2. Biotransformation
3. Elimination from the body

*Clearance* refers to the processes of biotransformation and elimination in removing drugs from the body (see Fig. 30–1). *Elimination* refers to the removal of an unchanged substance from the body. In contrast, the term *biotransformation* is usually associated with the transformation of a lipophilic compound into a more hydrophilic compound. The hydrophilic metabolite is more easily eliminated by the kidneys.

## Which Organs Are Responsible for Drug Clearance?

The major organs responsible for drug clearance are the liver, kidneys, and lungs. Nonetheless, other organs may have a role in clearing drugs from the body, including the gastrointestinal tract, sweat glands, and breasts (milk secretion). For drugs that are metabolized, the amount of drug that may be cleared from the blood by an organ is limited by the blood flow to the organ and the intrinsic capacity of the enzymes in the organ to biotransform that drug. By applying Fick's principle to drug clearance, the following can be said:

$$\text{Clearance} = \text{Blood Flow} \times \text{ER} \qquad \text{(Equation 6)}$$

where ER is the extraction ratio (see Equation 2). During surgery, drugs also may be removed from the body by nonphysiologic clearance mechanisms, such as blood loss, loss through washing in a Cell Saver, and absorption or adsorption to the cardiopulmonary bypass circuit.[13]

Clearance values are given in units of volume divided by time. Clearance signifies the volume of blood or plasma that is cleared of drug per unit time. The total body clearance is the sum of all the individual clearances. For example, if a drug is removed from the blood by the kidney and liver at rates of 100 mL/min and 500 mL/min, respectively, the total clearance is 600 mL/min.

### Half-Life

As indicated, drug distribution also affects the duration of pharmacologic response, often expressed as a $t_{1/2}$. $t_{1/2}$ may be defined simply as the amount of time required for the drug concentration to be reduced by 50% (Fig. 30–7). Many drugs have a rapid distribution $t_{1/2}$ and a longer terminal elimination $t_{1/2}$. When the type of $t_{1/2}$ is unspecified, it is usually assumed to be a terminal elimination $t_{1/2}$.

The relationship between $t_{1/2}$ and $V_d$ is shown by the following equation:

$$t_{1/2} = \frac{V_d \times 0.693}{\text{CL}} \qquad \text{(Equation 7)}$$

where CL is drug clearance from the body by all routes, and 0.693 represents the natural logarithm of 2. In this equation, $t_{1/2}$ is a dependent variable, and the $V_d$ and clearance are independent variables. From this important relationship, it can be inferred that the only ways to alter the $t_{1/2}$ of a medication are to change the $V_d$ or the clearance. The following examples illustrate the clinical importance of this relationship.

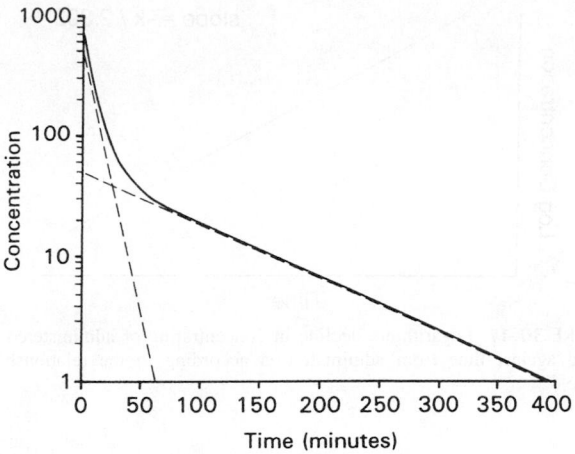

**FIGURE 30–7.** The half-life of a drug can be represented by a log plot of plasma concentration against time and is defined as the amount of time for the drug concentration to be reduced by 50%.

**Example 1.** Alfentanil and fentanyl are structurally similar narcotic analgesics that have markedly different pharmacokinetic profiles. Specifically, the $t_{1/2}$ values for alfentanil and fentanyl are approximately 90 and 220 minutes, respectively.[14,15] For $t_{1/2}$ to be smaller, clearance must be increased or $V_d$ decreased. In this case, the large difference in $t_{1/2}$ is due to alfentanil having a much smaller $V_d$.

**Example 2.** The $t_{1/2}$ of midazolam is prolonged in obese compared with nonobese patients. This increase in $t_{1/2}$ is due to an increased $V_d$[16] (Fig. 30–8). The $V_d$ is increased because midazolam is a lipophilic drug with a larger volume in which to distribute in obese patients.

**Example 3.** The $t_{1/2}$ of atropine is longer in infants and the elderly than in young adults[17] (Fig. 30–9) The increased $t_{1/2}$ of infants is due to a larger $V_d$ of this drug in these patients. In contrast, the $t_{1/2}$ is prolonged in the elderly because the clearance of atropine is also decreased.

## Why Do Drugs With Long Half-Lives Often Produce Short-Lived Biologic Effects?

The key to this question is distribution. After administration, drugs rapidly distribute to well-perfused organs such as

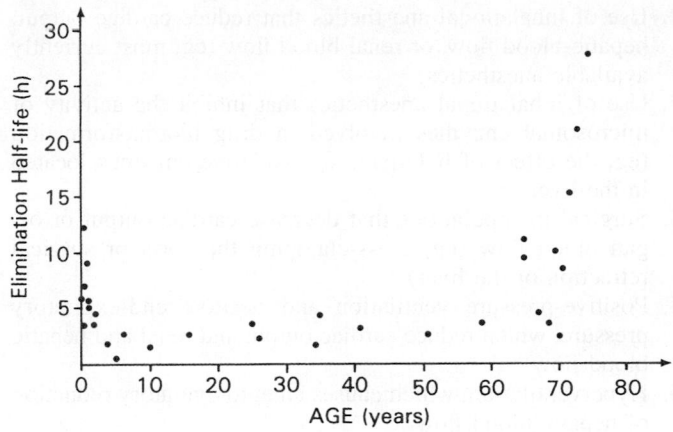

**FIGURE 30–9.** Increase in elimination half-life in infants (increased volume of distribution) and in the elderly (decreased clearance).

the brain, heart, lungs, kidneys, and liver. Redistribution then occurs. As a rule, lipophilic medications rapidly redistribute to adipose tissue. Adipose tissue constitutes a large storage volume for lipid-soluble drugs such as thiopental, midazolam, or fentanyl. Only a small portion of the dose remains as unbound (ie, active or free) drug in plasma. The effect of redistribution is most pronounced for the first dose of a medication and for relatively small doses in relation to the $V_d$.

**Example.** Thiopental is a lipophilic drug with an elimination $t_{1/2}$ of approximately 5 to 12 hours. The minimum blood concentration that produces a hypnotic effect is higher than the concentration reached after rapid redistribution for a small but not a large dose[18,19] (Fig. 30–10). Therefore, a small dose of thiopental produces a short-lived effect, whereas a large dose or repetitive small doses produce long-lasting effects.

## What Factors Decrease Clearance?

Clearance is decreased by reducing organ blood flow or inhibiting enzymes that are involved in drug biotransformation (see Equation 6). The following factors may reduce drug clearance in surgical patients:

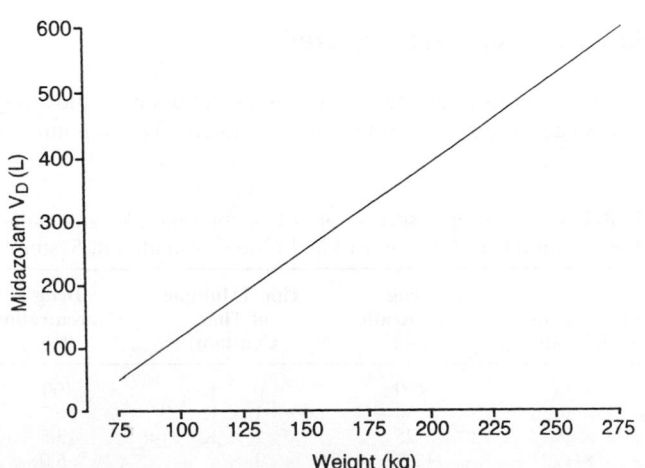

**FIGURE 30–8.** Prolonged half-life of midazolam with increasing weight owing to increased volume of distribution ($V_d$).

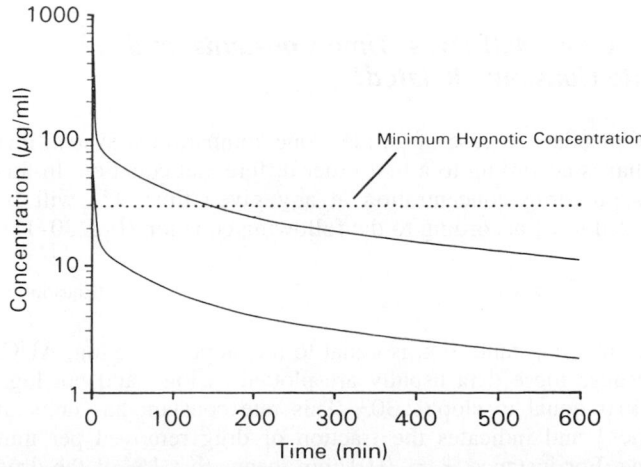

**FIGURE 30–10.** The effect of rapid redistribution of thiopental (a lipophilic drug) on small and large doses. A small dose quickly falls below the minimum hypnotic concentration, whereas a large dose maintains plasma levels above this concentration for a longer time.

1. Use of inhalational anesthetics that reduce cardiac output, hepatic blood flow, or renal blood flow (eg, most currently available anesthetics)[20]
2. Use of inhalational anesthetics that inhibit the activity of microsomal enzymes involved in drug biotransformation (eg, the effect of halothane on oxidative enzymes located in the liver)[21,22]
3. Surgical manipulations that decrease cardiac output or organ blood flow (eg, cross-clamping the aorta or surgical retraction of the liver)
4. Positive-pressure ventilation and positive end-expiratory pressure, which reduce cardiac output and renal and hepatic blood flow[23]
5. Hyperventilation, which causes an autoregulatory reduction of hepatic blood flow
6. Histamine receptor type 2 blockers reduce clearance by either reduction of hepatic blood flow (eg, cimetidine) or by competitive inhibition of certain enzymes. For example, cimetidine inhibits certain hepatic microsomal $P_{450}$ enzymes, and ranitidine inhibits the activity of the enzyme alcohol dehydrogenase.[24]
7. Congestive heart failure, which reduces hepatic blood flow
8. Advanced age, which causes alterations in hepatic and renal function
9. Malnutrition, which results in reduced levels of certain enzymes that are involved in drug biotransformation (eg, pseudocholinesterase)

## What Factors Increase Clearance?

Drug clearance occasionally may be increased when enzymes involved in biotransformation are induced. For example, theophylline clearance is increased by cigarette smoking[25,26]; thus, cigarette smokers require higher maintenance doses of theophylline compared with nonsmokers. Other examples include the increased biotransformation of enflurane in patients receiving isoniazid,[27] which may result in a potentially nephrotoxic concentration of free fluoride ion, and the enhanced biotransformation of certain muscle relaxants by phenytoin. Thus, larger maintenance doses of nondepolarizing relaxants may be required.

## How Are Half-Lives, Time Constants, and Rate Constants Related?

Consider the case of an ideal one-compartment system that behaves according to a first-order differential equation. In this system, drug concentration at any given time ($C_t$) will be related to $C_0$ according to the following equation (Fig. 30–11):

$$C_t = C_0 e^{-kt}$$ (Equation 8)

The rate constant, $-k$, is equal to the slope of the $\log_e$ AUC. Because these data usually are plotted as $\log_{10}$ and not $\log_e$, $-k$ is equal to slope/2.303. This rate constant has units of time$^{-1}$ and indicates the fraction of drug removed per unit time. For instance, $k = 0.01$/min means that 1% of the drug is removed from the body every minute. By definition, if $t = t_{1/2}$, then $C_t/C_0 = 0.5$. Therefore, $0.5 = e^{-kt_{1/2}}$, and $t_{1/2} = \ln 2/k$, or the following:

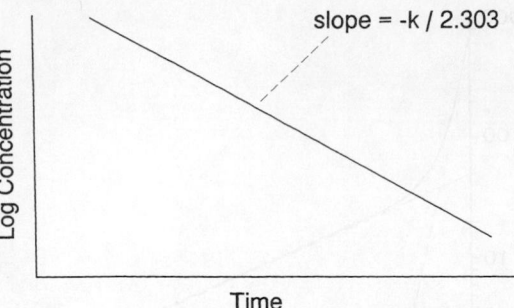

**FIGURE 30–11.** Logarithmic decline in concentration of administered drug plotted against time from administration according to the relationship $C_t = C_0 e^{-kt}$.

$$t_{1/2} = 0.693/k$$ (Equation 9)

Thus, $t_{1/2}$ is inversely related to the rate constant.

**Example.** If the elimination $t_{1/2}$ of thiopental is 12 hours, how much is removed from the body each hour? Solve this problem by substituting 12 hours for $t_{1/2}$ into Equation 9, and $k = 0.06$/h. Therefore, 6% of the amount of thiopental in the body is cleared each hour.

In this model, the time constant, K, is the amount of time equal to $1/k$. (Note the upper and lower cases: rate constant $= k$, time constant $= K$.) From Equation 8, at time $= K$, $C_K = C_0 e^{-1} = C_0 \times 0.37$. (Recall that e is a number roughly equal to 2.7.) From this relationship, it can be seen that approximately 63% of a drug is removed from this system after a period of time equal to one time constant. To summarize (Table 30–1) this information:

1. This one-compartment system may be used to model the pharmacokinetics of some but not all drugs.
2. The rate constant indicates the fraction of drug removed per unit time.
3. The rate constant is mathematically related to both $t_{1/2}$ and K.
4. After each $t_{1/2}$, drug concentration is reduced by 50%.
5. After each K, drug concentration is reduced by 63%.
6. The K for a given medication is always greater than the corresponding $t_{1/2}$.

## How Do Drugs Accumulate?

After repetitive dosing, all drugs accumulate in the body until steady-state conditions are obtained. The amount of

**TABLE 30–1.** Comparison of Drug Concentration Versus Half-Life or Time Constant for an Ideal One-Compartment System

| Time (Multiple of Half-Life) | Drug Concentration (%) | Time (Multiple of Time Constant) | Drug Concentration (%) |
|---|---|---|---|
| $0 \times t_{1/2}$ | 100 | $0 \times K$ | 100 |
| $1 \times t_{1/2}$ | 50 | $1 \times K$ | 36.7 |
| $2 \times t_{1/2}$ | 25 | $2 \times K$ | 13.5 |
| $3 \times t_{1/2}$ | 12.5 | $3 \times K$ | 5.0 |
| $4 \times t_{1/2}$ | 6.25 | $4 \times K$ | 1.8 |
| $5 \times t_{1/2}$ | 3.125 | $5 \times K$ | 0.7 |

**TABLE 30–2.** Degree of Accumulation After Multiple Dosing Based on the Ratio of the Dosing Interval to the Elimination Half-Life (DI/$t_{1/2}$)

| DI/$t_{1/2}$ | Degree of Accumulation |
|---|---|
| 0.5 | 3.41 |
| 1.0 | 2.00 |
| 2.0 | 1.33 |
| 5.0 | 1.03 |

From Thompson GA. Dosage regimen design: a pharmacokinetic approach. *J Clin Pharmacol.* 1992;32:210.

accumulation is determined principally by the dose, the *dosing interval* (DI), the apparent $V_d$, and clearance. Fortunately, if only the DI and elimination $t_{1/2}$ are combined, the degree of accumulation after multiple dosing can be predicted[28] (Table 30–2).

### What Are the Primary Determinants of Drug Accumulation?

The following generalizations are useful in understanding drug accumulation:

1. The time to reach steady state is independent of the DI and solely determined by the elimination $t_{1/2}$.[28]
2. For practical purposes, steady state is reached after a time equal to 3 to 5 elimination $t_{1/2}$s.
3. As the ratio of the DI to elimination $t_{1/2}$ increases, the degree of accumulation decreases (see Table 30–2).

   **Example.** Consider a patient who receives 10 mg of morphine intravenously every 3 hours. Assume that the $t_{1/2}$ of morphine is 3 hours. Three hours after the initial dose, 5 mg of morphine remains (half has been cleared from the body). Immediately after the second dose, 15 mg of morphine is present. Similarly, just before and after the third dose, 7.5 mg and 17.5 mg of morphine are present, respectively. After steady state has been achieved, 10 mg of morphine will be present before and 20 mg of morphine will be present after each dose is given.

Note that the degree of accumulation in this case is 2.0 (see Table 30–2). Accordingly, if a 10-mg dose is administered every 90 minutes (ie, DI/$t_{1/2}$ = 0.5), approximately 34 mg of morphine will accumulate when steady state has been achieved.

### How Are Appropriate Intravenous Regimens Devised?

Three steps are involved in developing a dosing regimen for an intravenously administered medication. Values of the three pharmacokinetic parameters required for this process (target concentration, clearance, and $V_d$) may be obtained from a pharmacology reference text or the package insert.

### Step 1. *Select a target drug concentration.*

The tacit assumption here is that beneficial and adverse drug effects are related to plasma drug concentrations. Therefore,

consider the minimum drug concentration that will produce a therapeutic response and the minimum concentration that will likely produce a unacceptable toxic response. This range of acceptable plasma drug concentrations defines a *therapeutic window* (Fig. 30–12) and presupposes a knowledge of the dose-response effects of a given drug. From the therapeutic window, we can determine the acceptable amount of fluctuations in plasma drug levels.

### Step 2. *Determine the loading dose.*

The loading dose may be calculated from Equation 3. For drugs administered intravenously, bioavailability is typically considered to be equal to 1. Therefore, loading dose equals target plasma concentration multiplied by the $V_d$. Never give this dose as a single bolus. It assumes that the processes of distribution and redistribution have already occurred.

### Step 3. *Calculate the maintenance dose.*

Under steady-state conditions, the amount of drug entering the body is equivalent to the amount being removed from the body and can be written as follows:

$$X_0 = CL \times C_{ss} \qquad \text{(Equation 10)}$$

where $X_0$ is the amount of drug given per unit time, and $C_{ss}$ is the mean steady-state drug concentration. Equation 10 is used to calculate the maintenance dose of a medication. Note that rearrangement of this equation gives the more familiar relationship:

$$C_{ss} = \frac{X_0}{CL} \qquad \text{(Equation 11)}$$

   **Example.** Consider the case of lidocaine. Values for therapeutic concentration (3 mg/L), clearance (0.95 L/min), and $V_d$ (90 L) determine the loading and the maintenance doses. Specifically, the loading dose is 3 mg/L times 90 L = 270 mg; the maintenance infusion rate is 3 mg/L times 0.95 L/min = 2.9 mg/min ($\approx$3 mg/min). This loading dose should be given over 15 to 30 minutes and then the infusion started when initiating therapy. While a patient is maintained with a constant infusion of lidocaine, the steady-state concentration may be measured after 3 to 5 $t_{1/2}$s (ie,

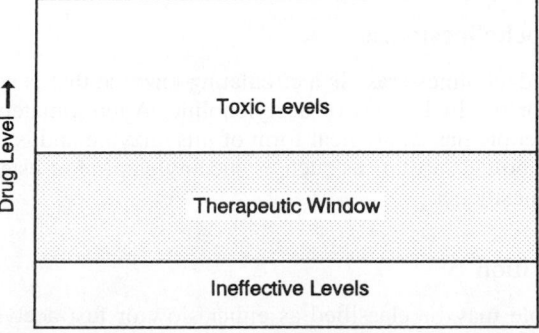

**Therapeutic Window**

Drug Level →

Toxic Levels

Therapeutic Window

Ineffective Levels

**FIGURE 30–12.** Schematic representation of the therapeutic window above which an unacceptable toxic response will occur and below which the drug will likely be ineffective.

after 4.5-7.5 h), and appropriate dosage adjustments may then be made.

Note that Equation 6 relates the determinants of clearance. Equations 10 and 11 illustrate the effect of clearance on the steady-state concentration of a substance.

### In What Other Area Are These Principles Used?

Other examples of these principles include the following:

1. Oxygen uptake (ie, CL) by the body is the familiar application of Equation 6 (ie, oxygen uptake is the product of cardiac output and oxygen extraction ratio).
2. The removal (ie, CL) of carbon dioxide ($CO_2$) by the lungs is analogous to Equation 11 (ie, the fraction of $CO_2$ in blood can be obtained by dividing $CO_2$ production by minute alveolar ventilation).
3. Glomerular filtration rate (GFR) can be determined from creatinine clearance by application of Equation 10. For example, if steady-state serum creatinine concentration is 1 mg/100 mL, and the amount of creatinine collected is 1 mg/min (or 1440 mg/d), then from Equation 10, the GFR must be 100 mL/min. However, if the GFR is then reduced by 50% but no change in creatinine production occurs, then the serum creatinine concentration must double after steady-state conditions are achieved.

### How Do Genetic Differences Affect Drug Regimens?

Drug response may be affected by age, smoking, disease processes, other medications, nutritional status, surgery, anesthesia, and even mechanical ventilation. Besides these factors, genetically determined differences in drug response also play an important role in affecting the manner in which a given individual responds to anesthesia. Most genetic differences affecting drug response can be accounted for by differences in certain enzymes or proteins. For example, 5% to 10% of all patients do not have the cytochrome $P_{450}$ microsomal enzyme that biotransforms codeine to its active metabolites. Consequently, approximately 1 of every 10 to 20 patients does not have a therapeutic response to this particular narcotic analgesic.[29] Other examples of pharmacogenetic conditions that may alter response to anesthesia follow.

### Pseudocholinesterase

Pseudocholinesterase is a circulating enzyme that is responsible for the hydrolysis of acetylcholine. Approximately 1 in 3000 people has an atypical form of this enzyme and is unable to metabolize substances such as succinylcholine or ester-type local anesthetics.

### Acetylation

People may be classified as either slow or fast acetylators. The manner in which a person acetylates certain compounds explains the relatively selective toxicity of medications such as procainamide, isoniazid, and hydralazine.[30]

### Cytochrome $P_{450}$ Enzymes

Cytochrome $P_{450}$ enzymes are a family of hepatic microsomal enzymes that are involved in specific oxidative reactions. These reactions normally transform lipophilic compounds into more hydrophilic substances that may be eliminated by the kidneys. As noted previously, the presence or absence of these enzymes may have an important role in controlling the way people metabolize medications. Besides codeine, other drugs that may be affected by genetically impaired cytochrome $P_{450}$ activity include dextromethorphan, caffeine, propranolol, debrisoquin, and mephenytoin.[31]

### Ethnic Differences

Many examples of altered drug response due to ethnic differences exist. For instance, Chinese people are known to have enhanced sensitivity to β-adrenergic agonists and antagonists.[32,33] Also, black men are more prone to have essential hypertension.[34,35] In addition, the low incidence of alcoholism among Japanese may be due in part to reduced activity of enzymes that are involved in alcohol metabolism.[36]

### Malignant Hyperthermia

See Chapter 48 for a complete discussion of malignant hyperthermia and its effects on response to anesthesia.

### Glucose-6-Phosphate Dehydrogenase Deficiency

This is one of the most common disorders in the world, with a prevalence of up to 10% among black men and people from the Mediterranean coast.[37] In patients with this disorder, red blood cells are susceptible to drug-induced hemolysis.

### Intermittent Porphyria

This condition is inherited in an autosomal dominant pattern and is associated with the absence of porphobilinogen deaminase. Barbiturates may trigger abdominal pain, polyneuropathies, and acute psychiatric disturbances.

## PHARMACODYNAMICS

Most drugs produce their pharmacologic effects by binding reversibly to saturable, stereospecific, membrane-bound receptors. However, for the much less potent inhaled anesthetics, the mode of action is less clear.

### What Is Affinity?

The degree to which a compound binds to a receptor at a specific concentration is roughly termed *affinity*. The importance of drug affinity may be demonstrated by the antihypertensive agent, labetalol.[38] Labetalol is a compound with two chiral centers. As a consequence, racemic labetalol consists of four stereoisomers. Two of these isomers are pharmacologically inactive. One stereoisomer has affinity for β-adrenergic receptors and the other for α-adrenergic receptors. The β-receptor effect dominates, however, because the β receptor binds its stereoisomer with greater affinity than the α receptor binds its stereoisomer.

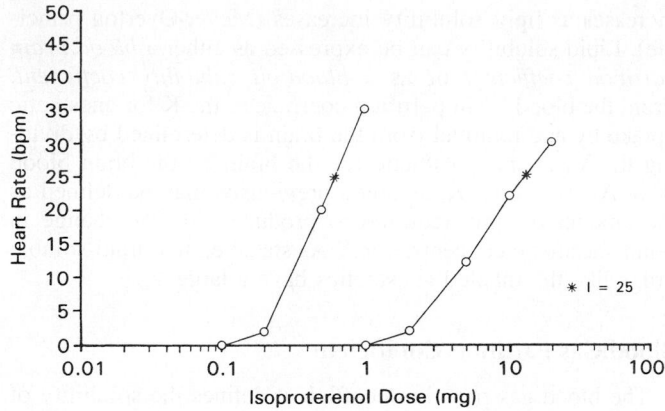

**FIGURE 30–13.** Efficacy of β-adrenergic blockade based on response to increasing doses of isoproterenol. *Left,* Responses before blockade. *Right,* Responses after blockade. In these examples, the dose to produce a 25-beat/min (bpm) increase in heart rate is the endpoint.

## What Is Efficacy?

Not all drugs that bind to a given receptor produce the same degree of response. Some drugs produce a maximum response and are said to have high *efficacy.* Other drugs produce only a partial response, and some drugs produce no response. Drugs are either agonists, partial agonists, or antagonists, depending on whether they produce a maximum, partial, or negligible response, respectively. The degree of response produced by various doses of medication can be depicted by dose-response curves, in which the intensity of drug effect is plotted against the logarithm of the dose (Fig. 30–13).

> **Example.** Suppose you wished to know whether a patient was adequately β blocked. You could administer progressively larger doses of isoproterenol and note the dose that produces a given increase in heart rate (such as the I-25, or a 25-beat-per-minute increase in heart rate).[39] Figure 30–14 compares log isoproterenol dose versus heart rate dose-response curves in a patient before and after β blocker administration. The degree of β blockade is related to how far the dose-response curve is shifted to the right. The antagonism of a pharmacologic effect by an antagonist or partial agonist is illustrated in Figure 30–14. Clinically, isoproterenol is rarely used to counteract β blockade.

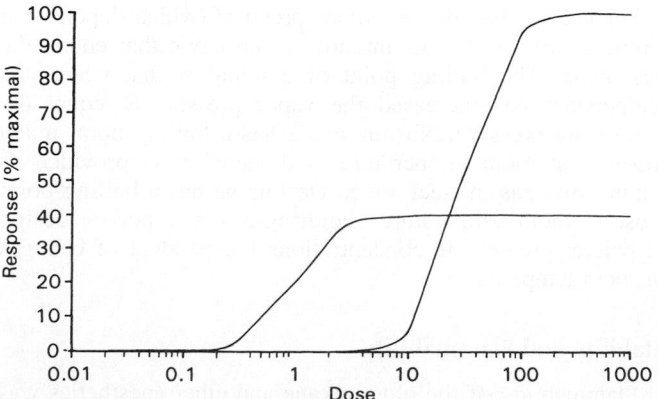

**FIGURE 30–14.** Antagonism of pharmacologic effect by an antagonist (*left*) or a partial agonist (*right*).

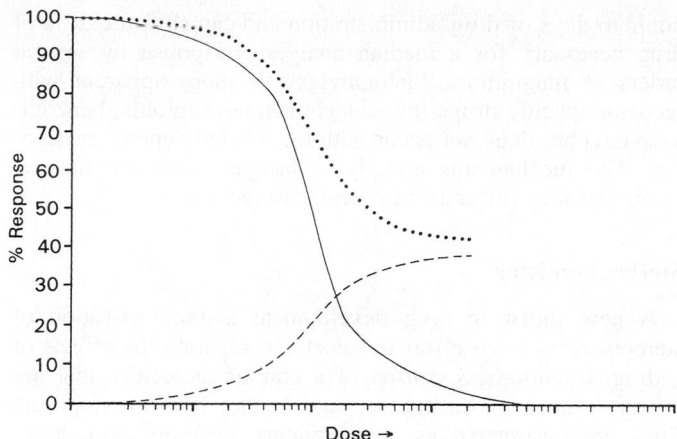

**FIGURE 30–15.** Pharmacologic responses to some drugs may vary greatly with logarithmic changes in dose.

## Pharmacologic Responses

For most drugs, the pharmacologic response is related to the logarithm of the dose or concentration (Fig. 30–15). Thus, clinically significant changes in drug response are often related to orders-of-magnitude change in dose. The typical receptor with a single binding site requires almost a 100-fold increase in drug concentration to go from no response to maximal response, and this is important to take into consideration when titrating intravenous drug to effect. However, the same is not true for many of the general anesthetics, where the concentration-effect curves are much steeper.

As noted, drug dosage should be titrated to response. For example, the response to a peripheral nerve stimulator may be used to guide the dosing of muscle relaxants. However, it is important that the response be a *direct* reflection of receptor occupancy by that drug, not an indirect downstream effect. Thus, blood pressure is a poor physiologic marker on which to base opioid dosing, whereas respiratory rate and depth is fairly reliable. In cases where physiologic responses are unreliable, an alternative may be to base dosing on measured drug levels, such as the measurement of end-tidal inhaled anesthetic concentrations.

> **Problem.** What doses of orally administered morphine might be comparable with an intravenously administered dose of 24 mg/d? From a pharmacology reference source, you find that the bioavailability of morphine varies between 10% and 40%.[40] Consequently, for 24 mg of a daily oral dose to reach the systemic circulation, an administered oral dose ranging between 60 and 240 mg/d could be required (ie, 24 mg divided by 0.40 or 0.10, respectively; refer to Equation 1).

## Tolerance and Tachyphylaxis

Living organisms have evolved the ability to adapt to their environment and reduce the effect of toxins and drugs. Thus, enzyme systems can be upregulated, enhancing the clearance of some compounds, and thereby the physiologic effect. The induction of alcohol dehydrogenase by chronic ethanol ingestion is one example. Alternatively, the pharmacodynamic response to a given concentration of drug can be modulated, such that a much smaller effect is noted without an increase in clearance, termed *tachyphylaxis.* Opioids constitute a classic example. Tachyphylaxis to the opioids develops within several hours to days of drug administration and can shift the dose of drug necessary for a median analgesic response by several orders of magnitude. Tachyphylaxis is more apparent with receptor-specific drugs (eg, catecholamines, opioids, benzodiazepines) but does not occur with the inhaled general anesthetics. The mechanisms underlying tachyphylaxis are not yet clear, and may differ from receptor to receptor.

## Stereochemistry

A new thrust in drug development is the separation of stereoisomers in an effort to select and separate the effects of a drug. Enantiomers consist of a pair of molecules that are mirror images of each other and cannot be superimposed. They are designated as dextrorotatory ($+$) or levorotatory ($-$), depending on how they rotate polarized light. Enantiomers demonstrate differences in absorption and distribution, metabolism and clearance, toxicity, and affinity for receptors. Racemic mixtures consist of two enantiomers present in equal proportion.[41] Pharmacologically, enantiomers may act like two different drugs.

For example, the *N*-methyl-D-aspartate (NMDA) receptor may be an important target for the anesthetic and analgesic action of ketamine. The S($+$) enantiomer is a more potent inhibitor of NMDA receptors than the S($-$) enantiomer and can be used in lesser doses. Thus, use of the S($+$) enantiomer allows for a more rapid emergence and fewer psychotomimetic emergence reactions than does the racemic mixture.[42] Cisatracurium is a stereoisomer of atracurium that has much lower potency for releasing histamine than its enantiomer. Ropivacaine is an isomer of bupivacaine that has reduced cardiotoxicity.[43]

## ANESTHETIC DRUG SELECTION

Choice of anesthetic drugs is highly subjective and is based as much on practitioner experience and philosophy as on pharmacologic principles. The clinical status of a patient, as well as concomitant medications, needs to be considered when tailoring an individual patient's anesthetic. It is essential to have an understanding of drug metabolism and elimination, as well as an understanding of how a patient's pathologic process may alter these processes. Cost and availability are also factors guiding choice. In this section, we primarily relate our discussion to the pharmacologic principles presented previously.

## What Factors Guide the Choice of Inhalational Anesthetics?

The choice of inhaled anesthetics frequently simplifies to that with which the anesthetist has the most experience. There are, however, a few pharmacokinetic and pharmacodynamic considerations that also may guide choice. Other factors, such as the spectrum of side effects, are covered in other chapters.

## Lipid Solubility

The potency of anesthetic agents is related to lipid solubility. For both inhalational and intravenous agents, the potency increases as lipid solubility increases (Meyer-Overton principle). Lipid solubility can be expressed as either a *blood:brain partition coefficient* or as a *blood:oil solubility coefficient*. From the blood:brain partition coefficient, the K for anesthetic uptake by and removal from the brain is determined by dividing the $V_d$ of the anesthetic for the brain by the brain blood flow. Alternatively, K, as noted previously, may be defined as the amount of time required to produce a 63.2% change in brain anesthetic concentration.[44] As stated earlier, lipid-soluble drugs like the inhaled anesthetics have a large $V_d$.

## Blood:Gas Partition Coefficient

The blood:gas partition coefficient defines the solubility of an anesthetic, that is, how much of an anesthetic gas will move into blood at equilibrium. It also has implications for the rate of equilibration. Thus, a low blood:gas partition coefficient (eg, nitrous oxide) indicates that little anesthetic has to move from the gas (alveoli) to the blood to achieve equilibrium, so equilibration is more rapid, and anesthesia can occur more rapidly. A compound with high blood:gas partitioning, such as diethyl ether, equilibrates more slowly because many molecules must transfer to blood to reach equilibration. A similar situation occurs on emergence; less soluble compounds are eliminated more rapidly, and emergence is rapid. This underlies the common use of nitrous oxide in the last hour of prolonged operations; a compound of lower solubility is substituted for a compound of greater solubility. It is also the basis for promoting desflurane and sevoflurane in ambulatory care settings; their low solubility in blood tends to produce faster induction and emergence and permits the rapid turnover desired in this setting. Elimination depends on more than blood:gas partitioning, however, as shown by the slower elimination of desflurane compared with nitrous oxide, despite the lower blood:gas partitioning. This is explained by the much higher tissue:blood partitioning of desflurane compared with nitrous oxide.

Solubility also has implications for closed gas spaces in the body such as the gut, middle ear, or a vascular embolus. Because nitrous oxide is 34 times more soluble in blood than nitrogen (presumably the dominant initial gas in these spaces), nitrous oxide can be delivered to the space faster than the nitrogen can leave, resulting in a transient expansion of the space.

## Vapor Pressure

For volatile liquids, the vapor pressure (which depends on temperature) affects the amount of anesthetic that enters the gas phase. The boiling point of a liquid is that where the temperature has increased the vapor pressure to equal the barometric pressure. Nitrous oxide has a boiling point much lower than room temperature, and therefore is provided as compressed gas in steel tanks. Desflurane has a boiling point close to room temperature, requiring a new vaporizer design to deliver predictable concentrations independent of changes in room temperature.

## Stability and Flammability

Flammability of the older alkane and ether anesthetics was eliminated by halogenation, which also increased their potency. The danger of flammable anesthetics and the expense of equipping surgical areas for their use have essentially eliminated them from practice. Halogenation with the light halogens (principally fluorine) has enhanced the stability of these compounds so that they react less with light, metal, and soda lime and are also less metabolized. Thus, isoflurane, an extensively fluorinated methyl ethyl ether with a single chlorine atom, is more stable and less metabolized than methoxyflurane, with fewer fluorines and two chlorine atoms. Desflurane is simply isoflurane with the chlorine atom replaced by a fluorine, again leading to an increase in stability and a decrease in metabolism.

## Minimum Alveolar Concentration

Minimum alveolar concentration (MAC) is a convenient unit for expressing the potency of anesthetic agents. Essentially, an $EC_{50}$ MAC is defined as the alveolar concentration of a volatile agent at one atmosphere that prevents movement in response to a painful stimulus in 50% of subjects. Although MAC is highly conserved in the overall population, it can be altered to a small degree by age[45,46] and other drugs, especially those having CNS effects.[47] MAC is an equilibrium, pharmacodynamic measure and, thus, is independent of features influencing kinetics, such as cardiac output or minute ventilation.

## How Is the Speed of Induction Changed When Using Inhalational Agents?

During the induction of anesthesia, the anesthetic partial pressure in the lungs exceeds that in the blood, which in turn exceeds that in the brain. Increasing the alveolar concentration of an anesthetic increases this gradient, and therefore increases the onset of action. This may be achieved by the following:

1. Increased minute ventilation[48]
2. Rapid uptake of nitrous oxide, producing a second gas or concentrating effect[49,50]
3. High inspired anesthetic concentration (ie, overpressure)
4. Decreased functional residual capacity (eg, infants, pregnant or obese patients)

Cardiac output also influences the speed of induction in much the same way as mentioned earlier for intravenously administered drugs. Low cardiac output enhances equilibration of blood with alveolar anesthetic, and therefore the rate of onset of anesthesia. The influence of anesthetic blood and lipid solubility on both pharmacodynamics (Meyer-Overton behavior) and pharmacokinetics has been addressed previously.

## What Factors Are Important When Choosing Intravenous Anesthetic Agents?

Intravenous drugs can be used for both the induction and maintenance of general anesthesia. In general, because of the broader spectrum of action and shorter, controllable elimination rates, the inhaled drugs seem to be preferred for the maintenance of general anesthesia and the intravenous drugs for induction.

## Induction Agents

The action of most intravenous induction agents is terminated not by elimination, but by redistribution to body compartments not contributing to the anesthetic response. Thiopental and propofol may act by potentiating inhibitory neurotransmission, whereas drugs such as ketamine may preferentially inhibit excitatory transmission. Among these drugs, propofol is popular for outpatient surgery, for surgical cases lasting <1 hour, or for intravenous infusion anesthesia because its unusually large $V_d$ promotes rapid and extensive redistribution, hastening emergence. Also, propofol has a slightly slower onset of action than thiopental, perhaps because it must first distribute out of the lipid emulsion vehicle in which it is injected. Most induction agents should be used in reduced doses in patients with low cardiac output and hypovolemia because peak concentrations are higher, as discussed, and many produce cardiovascular depression.

## Benzodiazepines

Benzodiazepines produce anxiolysis and sedation, probably by potentiating inhibitory neurotransmission. Commonly used as preoperative sedatives and as adjuncts for local or regional anesthesia, benzodiazepines have a better safety profile than do other CNS depressants, primarily because they are associated with less respiratory and cardiovascular depression. However, the respiratory depressant effects of opiates are dramatically potentiated by the addition of an otherwise trivial amount of benzodiazepine. Midazolam is one of the most frequently administered medications during anesthesia because it has a shorter duration of action than diazepam or lorazepam, is water soluble, and does not produce pain on injection like the previous diazepam formulations. Midazolam's short duration can be attributed to the small $V_d$ and relatively rapid terminal elimination $t_{1/2}$.

Lorazepam is an oral anxiolytic with a slow onset and a long duration of effect. Because lorazepam does not have active metabolites and undergoes glucuronidative (as opposed to oxidative) metabolism, its pharmacokinetic profile is preserved in elderly patients or patients with liver disease.[51] In addition, fewer drug-drug interactions occur with lorazepam than with most other benzodiazepines. The onset of action is much longer than that of many other benzodiazepines. Diazepam is less potent but longer acting than midazolam. Both lorazepam and diazepam are erratically absorbed after intramuscular injection, the oral or intravenous routes being preferred.

In addition to sedation and anxiolysis, benzodiazepines are used to prevent and treat seizure activity and delirium tremens. Dosage should be reduced in the elderly, again because of their smaller $V_d$, and therefore higher peak concentrations.

## Should Flumazenil Be Used to Reverse Benzodiazepines?

Flumazenil is a specific benzodiazepine receptor antagonist indicated for the reversal of benzodiazepine overdose. Benzodiazepines rarely require reversal, and such therapy is not benign. Acute withdrawal reactions and seizures may occur after flumazenil administration.[52] Furthermore, the risk of resedation after premature discharge from the recovery area is a potential problem.

Flumazenil is approved for reversal of the sedating but not the respiratory depressant effects of benzodiazepines. Physostigmine and aminophylline have also been used to reverse the effects of benzodiazepines with varying degrees of success.[53]

## Which Narcotic Analgesics Are Chosen?

### Fentanyl

Fentanyl, a preferential μ receptor agonist, is the most commonly used opiate in anesthetic practice. Opioids stabilize hemodynamics during maintenance and provide for less pain, coughing, and delirium during emergence. Fentanyl is frequently used in conjunction with midazolam for intravenous sedation. Its $V_d$ is relatively large (4 L/kg), translating to a brief duration of effect through redistribution despite a fairly long $t_{1/2}$ of approximately 4 hours. It is of intermediate potency and approximately 85% protein bound.

### Morphine

Morphine is more water soluble (and therefore has a lower $V_d$) and less potent than fentanyl. More rapidly cleared and eliminated, the overall pharmacokinetics of morphine are changed less by obesity, liver disease, and aging than with the other opioids. For these reasons and because of low cost, morphine is also the agent of choice for patient-controlled intravenous analgesia.

### Alfentanil

Alfentanil, a fentanyl derivative, is the least potent, with the smallest $V_d$ of the currently used opioids. For these reasons, bolus doses have a rapid onset of effect. However, despite the small $V_d$ and slow clearance (relative to fentanyl), termination of action is relatively quick, primarily because of redistribution.

### Remifentanil

Remifentanil, a newer fentanyl derivative, incorporates an ester structure so it can be rapidly metabolized by blood and tissue nonspecific esterases.[54] Because of this additional, widespread metabolic clearance pathway, it can be administered in large doses to achieve a rapid onset, yet still demonstrate rapid recovery. These qualities make it well suited for the outpatient setting and for total intravenous anesthesia techniques. However, in procedures where emergence and persistent pain are anticipated, the use of this drug implies that a longer-acting opioid will be necessary at the end to provide postoperative analgesia.[55]

## What About Naloxone?

Naloxone is a μ receptor antagonist; thus, it can antagonize the analgesic and respiratory effects of opioids. It has proven extremely effective for perioperative narcotic overdose, but its pharmacokinetics must be kept in mind. It has a shorter $t_{1/2}$ than most of the currently used opioids, owing to a high clearance rate and an intermediate $V_d$. Thus, close monitoring

for renarcotization is essential after bolus administration of naloxone, or the drug should be given by continuous infusion.

## Which Muscle Relaxants Are Chosen?

Muscle relaxants are commonly used as adjuncts for tracheal intubation and to facilitate abdominal and thoracic surgery. A variety of drugs are now available with different rates of onset and offset; choice is often made by virtue of the spectrum of side effects. These drugs are often divided into depolarizing and nondepolarizing agents. The former bind and depolarize nicotinic acetylcholine receptors but dissociate more slowly than acetylcholine, producing an inactive, desensitized state. Nondepolarizers also bind the same receptor and prevent normal agonist binding, but do so without causing depolarization. The latter drugs tend to act much longer than depolarizing drugs.

### Succinylcholine

Succinylcholine is a depolarizing relaxant, used primarily for its rapid onset and $t_{1/2}$ of only a few minutes. It is used mostly to facilitate tracheal intubation but has application wherever brief and complete relaxation is required. Because of the generalized depolarization and release of cellular potassium, succinylcholine is typically avoided in patients with elevated potassium or any disorder likely to exaggerate the release or cause greater sensitivity to it. The generalized but discoordinated muscle contraction may transiently elevate pressure in the eye, head, or abdomen and may be responsible for the myalgias commonly experienced after its use, particularly in younger patients.

### Pancuronium

Pancuronium bromide is an aminosteroid, nondepolarizing muscle relaxant with a $t_{1/2}$ of >2 hours. Having a small $V_d$, it is mostly excreted through the kidney. The antimuscarinic effects of pancuronium are manifest by an increased heart rate, but it does not result in release of histamine.

### Atracurium

For shorter procedures or for patients with renal insufficiency, atracurium is chosen because of its predictable pharmacokinetic profile. Atracurium is metabolized by Hoffman degradation and nonspecific ester hydrolysis, and thus has a $t_{1/2}$ of approximately 20 minutes. Large boluses of atracurium are associated with histamine release, but cisatracurium, an isomer of atracurium, has a much lower potency for this side effect.

### Rocuronium

Rocuronium is another aminosteroid with an intermediate duration of action, but with a more rapid onset of action than pancuronium. It is an appropriate choice in patients requiring a rapid-sequence induction in whom succinylcholine (see earlier) is contraindicated. It is non-histamine releasing and has minimal cardiovascular effects.

## Vecuronium

Vecuronium is a drug of intermediate duration with a $t_{1/2}$ of approximately 1.5 hours. Eliminated mostly through the liver, its duration is extended in those with liver disease or reduced hepatic blood flow (eg, during upper abdominal surgical procedures).[56] Its use is associated with few hemodynamic side effects.

## *When Are Nondepolarizing Muscle Relaxant Reversal Agents Used?*

Because of the extreme vulnerability of paralyzed patients, reversal of neuromuscular blockade is routinely considered and commonly used. Because the relaxants themselves are considered competitive antagonists of the nicotinic acetylcholine receptors, the reversal strategy is to increase the neuromuscular junction concentration of the natural agonist, acetylcholine, through the use of acetylcholinesterase antagonists. Thus, drugs such as neostigmine or edrophonium are typically given, but only when clear evidence of recovery from the relaxant is apparent. This strategy prevents reparalysis after the shorter $t_{1/2}$ anticholinesterase wears off. Anticholinergics are given in combination with the anticholinesterase to block unwanted muscarinic effects (bradycardia, salivation).

## SUMMARY

Anesthesiology is one of the few medical disciplines capable of directly discerning the pharmacokinetics and pharmacodynamics of the drugs used. Indeed, the immediate feedback from therapy is one of the major features attracting physicians to the field. Some straightforward but fundamental principles govern the behavior of drugs in people, and this chapter has made an attempt to summarize them in a readable fashion. Knowing some key parameters, such as the mechanism of action, $V_d$, potency, and elimination rate, allows reasonable formulation of a plan for administration of a new drug or a drug with which the practitioner is unfamiliar. A crucial aspect of drug delivery in a perioperative setting is the application of feedback into modification of therapy. Vigilance and titration are the hallmarks of a successful anesthetic.

## *References*

1. Mishra P, Calvey TN, Williams NE, et al. Intraoperative bradycardia and hypotension associated with timolol and pilocarpine eye drops. *Br J Anaesth.* 1983;55:897.
2. Covino BG, Vasallo HL. *Local Anesthetics: Mechanisms of Action and Clinical Use.* New York, NY: Grune & Stratton; 1976.
3. Krejcie TC, Avram MJ. What determines anesthetic induction dose? It's the front end kinetics, doctor! *Anesth Analg.* 1999;89:541.
4. Vestal RE, McGuire EA, Tobin JD, et al. Aging and ethanol metabolism. *Clin Pharmacol Ther.* 1977;21:343.
5. Cook DR, Fischer CG. Neuromuscular blocking effects of succinylcholine in infants and children. *Anesthesiology.* 1975;42:662.
6. Greenblatt DJ, Abernethy DR, Locniskar A, et al. Effect of age, gender, and obesity on midazolam kinetics. *Anesthesiology.* 1984;61:27.
7. Wood M. Plasma binding and limitation of drug access to site of action. *Anesthesiology.* 1991;75:721.
8. Marathe PH, Shen DD, Artru AA, et al. Effect of serum protein binding on the entry of lidocaine into brain and cerebrospinal fluid in dogs. *Anesthesiology.* 1991;75:804.
9. Burch PG, Stanski DR. The role of metabolism and protein binding in thiopental anesthesia. *Anesthesiology.* 1983;58:146.
10. Carson R. The administration of analgesics [review]. *Mod Midwife.* 1996;6:12.
11. Kosaka Y, Takahashi T, Mark LC. Intravenous thiobarbiturate anesthesia for caesarean section. *Anesthesiology.* 1969;31:489.
12. Thomas J, Long G, Moore G, et al. Plasma protein binding and placental transfer of bupivacaine. *Clin Pharmacol Ther.* 1976;19:426.
13. Holley FO, Ponganis KV, Stanski DR. Effects of cardiac surgery with cardiopulmonary bypass on lidocaine disposition. *Clin Pharmacol Ther.* 1984;35:617.
14. Alfenta [package insert]. Piscataway, NJ: Janssen Pharmaceuticals; 1987.
15. Shafer SL, Varvel JR. Pharmacokinetics, pharmacodynamics, and rational opioid selection. *Anesthesiology.* 1991;74:53.
16. Greenblatt DJ, Allen MD, Harmatz JS, et al. Diazepam disposition determinants. *Clin Pharmacol Ther.* 1980;27:301.
17. Virtanen R, Kanto J, Usalo E, et al. Pharmacokinetic studies on atropine with special reference to age. *Acta Anaesthesiol Scand.* 1982;26:297.
18. Becker KE Jr. Plasma levels of thiopental necessary for anesthesia. *Anesthesiology.* 1978;49:192.
19. Christensen JH, Andersen F, Jansen JA. Pharmacokinetics and pharmacodynamics of thiopentone: a comparison between young and elderly patients. *Anaesthesia.* 1982;37:398.
20. Reilly CS, Merrell J, Wood AJJ, et al. Comparison of the effects of isoflurane or fentanyl-nitrous oxide anaesthesia on propranolol disposition in dogs. *Br J Anaesth.* 1988;60:791.
21. Pessayre D, Allemand H, Benoist C, et al. Effect of surgery under general anaesthesia on antipyrine clearance. *Br J Clin Pharmacol.* 1978;6:505.
22. Reilly CS, Wood AJJ, Koshakji RP, et al. The effect of halothane on drug disposition: contribution of changes in intrinsic drug metabolizing capacity and hepatic blood flow. *Anesthesiology.* 1985;63:70.
23. Perkins MW, Dasta JF, DeHaven B, et al. A model to decrease hepatic blood flow and cardiac output with pressure breathing. *Clin Pharmacol Ther.* 1989;45:548.
24. DePadova C, Roine R, Frezza M, et al. Effects of ranitidine on blood alcohol levels after ethanol ingestion. *JAMA.* 1992;267:83.
25. Vestal RE, Wood AHH. Influence of age and smoking on drug kinetics in man. *Clin Pharmacokinet.* 1980;5:309.
26. Bukowskyj M, Nakatsu K, Munt PW. Theophylline reassessed. *Ann Intern Med.* 1984;101:63.
27. Mazze RI, Woodruff RE, Heerdt ME. Isoniazid-induced enflurane defluorination in humans. *Anesthesiology.* 1982;57:5.
28. Thompson GA. Dosage regimen design: a pharmacokinetic approach. *J Clin Pharmacol.* 1992;32:210.
29. Chen ZR, Somogyi AA, Reynolds G, et al. Disposition and metabolism of codeine after single and chronic doses in one poor and seven extensive metabolisers. *Br J Clin Pharmacol.* 1991;31:381.
30. Uetrecht JD, Woosley RL. Acetylator phenotyped and lupus erythematosus. *Clin Pharmacokinet.* 1981;6:118.
31. Gonzalez FJ, Meyer UA. Molecular genetics of the debrisoquin-sparteine polymorphism. *Clin Pharmacol.* 1991;50:233.
32. Zhou HH, Koshakji RP, Silberstein DJ, et al. Racial differences in drug response: altered sensitivity to and clearance of propranolol in men of Chinese descent as compared with American whites. *N Engl J Med.* 1989;320:565.
33. Wood AJJ, Zhou HH. Ethnic differences in drug disposition and responsiveness. *Clin Pharmacokinet.* 1991;20:350.
34. Talmers FN, Cushman WC, Schnaper H, et al. Comparison of propranolol and hydrochlorothiazide for the initial treatment of hypertension. *JAMA.* 1982;248:1996.
35. Falkner B. Differences in blacks and whites with essential hypertension: biochemistry and endocrine. *Hypertension.* 1990;15:681.
36. Guttendorf RJ, Wedlund PJ. Genetic aspects of drug disposition and therapeutics. *J Clin Pharmacol.* 1992;32:107.
37. Schrier SL. Anemia: hemolysis. In: Rubenstein E, Federman DD, eds. *Scientific American Medicine.* New York, NY: Scientific American; 1988:5:10.
38. Louis WJ, McNeil JJ, Drummer OH. Pharmacology of combined alpha-beta-blockade. *Drugs.* 1984;28S:16.
39. Coltart DJ, Shand DG. Plasma propranolol levels in the quantitative assessment of beta-adrenergic blockade in man. *BMJ.* 1970;26:731.
40. Gilman AG, Rall TW, Nies AS, et al, eds. *Goodman and Gilman's The Pharmacological Basis of Therapeutics.* 8th ed. New York, NY: Pergamon Press; 1991.

41. Stoelting RK. *Pharmacology and Physiology in Anesthetic Practice.* 3rd ed. Philadelphia, Pa: Lippincott Williams & Wilkins, 1999.

42. Kohrs R, Durieux ME. Ketamine: teaching an old drug new tricks. *Anesth Analg.* 1998;87:1186.

43. Markham A, Faulds D. Ropivacaine: a review of its pharmacology and therapeutics in regional anesthesia. *Drugs.* 1996;52:429.

44. Lowe HJ, Ernst EA. *The Quantitative Practice of Anesthesia.* Baltimore, Md: Williams & Wilkins; 1981.

45. Gregory GA, Eger EI II, Munson ES. The relationship between agent and halothane requirement in man. *Anesthesiology.* 1969;30:488.

46. Stevens WC, Dolan WM, Gibbons RT, et al. Minimum alveolar concentrations (MAC) of isoflurane with and without nitrous oxide in patients of various ages. *Anesthesiology.* 1975;42:197.

47. Orkin LR, Chen CH. Addiction, alcoholism, and anesthesia. *South Med J.* 1977;70:1172.

48. Stoelting RK, Eger EI II. The effects of ventilation and anesthetic solubility on recovery from anesthesia: an in vivo and analog analysis before and after equilibrium. *Anesthesiology.* 1969;30:290.

49. Eger EI II. Effect of inspired anesthetic concentration on the rate of rise of alveolar concentrations. *Anesthesiology.* 1963;24:153.

50. Epstein RM, Rackow H, Salanitre E. Influence of the concentration effect on the uptake of anesthetic mixtures: the second gas effect. *Anesthesiology.* 1964;25:364.

51. Kraus JW, Desmond PV, Marshall JP, et al. Effects of aging and liver disease on disposition of lorazepam. *Clin Pharmacol Ther.* 1978;24:411.

52. Klotz U, Kanto J. Pharmacokinetics and clinical use of flumazenil (Ro 15-1788). *Clin Pharmacokinet.* 1988;14:1.

53. Gallen JS. Aminophylline reversal of midazolam sedation [letter]. *Anesth Analg.* 1989;69:268.

54. Lemmens HJ. Pharmacokinetic-pharmacodynamic relationships for opioids in balanced anaesthesia [review]. *Clin Pharmacokinet.* 1995;29:231.

55. Burkle H, Dunbar S, Van Aken H. Remifentanil: a novel, short-acting, mu-opioid [review]. *Anesth Analg.* 1996;83:646.

56. Lebrault C, Berger JL, D'Hollander AA, et al. Pharmacokinetics and pharmacodynamics of vecuronium (ORG NC 45) in patients with cirrhosis. *Anesthesiology.* 1985;62:601.

# 31

# The Preoperative Visit and Premedication

## Sno E. White

## PSYCHOLOGIC PREPARATION

The preoperative visit allows anesthesia personnel to prepare patients for surgery mentally as well as physically. Numerous studies suggest that patients benefit from a preoperative interview.[1-3] Personal interviews, even when conducted by nonanesthetists, are more effective than printed instructional booklets.[2] Does this mean the human factor is important? Or is the significant factor the individualization of comments and the response to specific questions?

### What Do Patients Fear?

Most patients face surgery with some trepidation. Certain procedures are particularly anxiety-provoking. In one group of 218 patients, 86% of those undergoing cancer operations and 79% of those anticipating major genitourologic surgery were anxious as compared with 57% of patients having other types of procedures.[1] In another study of 260 patients who ranked their concerns, the number one fear was loss of sight. Diagnosis of cancer and loss of an organ ranked second and third. The absence of a diagnosis and anxiety about pain followed close behind.[4]

Klafta and Roizen summarized studies of patient concerns specifically related to anesthesia.[5] In the four largest series,[6-9] fear of "not waking up" (death) was acknowledged by 25% to 45% of patients and 20% to 50% worried about "waking up during surgery." Postoperative pain was feared by 35%, nausea and vomiting by 20%.[7]

### How Much Do Patients Really Want to Know?

This question was addressed by Roizen and colleagues in an editorial and subsequent review article.[5,10] Studies have shown wide variations in patient preferences. Ninety-two percent of Australian patients,[11] as compared with 43% of Scottish patients,[12] wanted to be informed of all possible complications, including life-threatening risks. Litman and associates polled parents following ambulatory surgery on their healthy children.[13] Eighty-eight percent of these parents whose preanesthetic counseling included death as a risk stated they wanted this information. However, 38% of parents whose preanesthetic counseling *did not* mention death as a risk said they did not want to hear about it. Perhaps more importantly, 47% to whom death was not mentioned wished they had been told.

**TABLE 31–1.** Association of Different Levels of Preoperative Fear With Different Coping Mechanisms*

| | Level of Preoperative Fear | | |
| Coping Mechanism | Low (N = 15) | Moderate (N = 21) | High (N = 27) |
| --- | --- | --- | --- |
| 1. Adopted a joking or facetious attitude | 40% | 10% | 0% |
| 2. Thought that operation would be of a very minor or trivial nature | 27% | 10% | 15% |
| 3. Felt confident in surgeon or gained reassurance from talking with him or her | 27% | 48% | 26% |
| 4. Made effort to learn about the operative procedure or its effects | 13% | 29% | 11% |
| 5. Thought that pains and discomforts would be of short duration or that he or she would be free from medical complications | 7% | 19% | 4% |
| 6. Concentrated on anticipated gains from the operation | 7% | 19% | 4% |
| 7. Plunged into distracting games or fantasies | 7% | 5% | 22% |
| 8. Adopted an attitude of resignation, fatalism, or trust in God | 0% | 5% | 15% |
| 9. Miscellaneous contents | 7% | 10% | 7% |

*The data are based on a content analysis of written answers obtained in a questionnaire survey of 63 major surgery cases.

Note: The percentages add up to more than 100% because some subjects mentioned more than one type of anesthesia.

From Janis IL. *Psychological Stress: Psychoanalytic and Behavioral Studies of Surgical Patients.* New York, NY: John Wiley & Sons; 1958.

Many years ago, Janis did extensive psychologic evaluation and follow-up of patients undergoing elective surgery.[14] The points he made are worth remembering (summarized in Table 31–1 and Fig. 31–1). His patients in the "low fear" group, characterized by their joking or facetious attitude and their trivialization of the surgery and its effects, had a significantly higher incidence of dissatisfaction. These patients may have had unrealistic expectations. Preoperative counseling should include not only presentation of major risks but also reasonable expectations.

A more recent study showed an inverse relationship between patient anxiety and the degree to which patients were satisfied with the amount of information they had received.[15] Conversely, there was no relationship between the actual amount of information provided and subsequent patient anxiety. It seems most efficient, once the basics have been covered, to simply ask patients if they have any further questions.

### Should Pain Be Discussed Preoperatively?

Egbert and coworkers achieved a significant reduction in postoperative narcotic requirement with a combination of preoperative counseling concerning postoperative pain and its management with postoperative follow-up and encouragement.[16] At least one third of patients are already concerned about pain.[7] Patients who do not seem concerned about pain should at least be made aware of its possibility. As long as pain continues to be a part of normal recovery, it is important to inform patients in order to avoid an unnecessary fear that pain means a complication has occurred (Fig. 31–2). Further, it is reassuring for patients when anesthesia personnel express

their dedication to pain control. The preoperative interview allows the practitioner to determine which methods of pain management will be most appropriate: continuous epidural infusion with patient-controlled bolus, single-shot regional anesthetic, patient-controlled intravenous analgesia, or oral medication. Contraindications to regional anesthesia must be discovered and a plan made and discussed with the patient (see Chapters 13 and 14).

### What Coping Mechanisms Are Useful?

Langer and associates presented patients with simple cognitive coping techniques in addition to information during preoperative interviews.[17] This combination improved postoperative coping. In this study, patients were told that although most people are somewhat anxious before an operation, they can learn to control their thoughts by focusing their attention on subjects that evoke pleasant thoughts or feelings. Other benefits were suggested, such as "the rare opportunity to relax, and to have a vacation from outside pressures." Not only was postoperative anxiety diminished but also sedative and analgesia requirements were reduced as well.

### Active Participation and Control

Patients function better if they consider themselves active participants in their health care team rather than helpless victims of their condition or disease. Exercise of control is an effective tool in stress tolerance. Perceived control over the

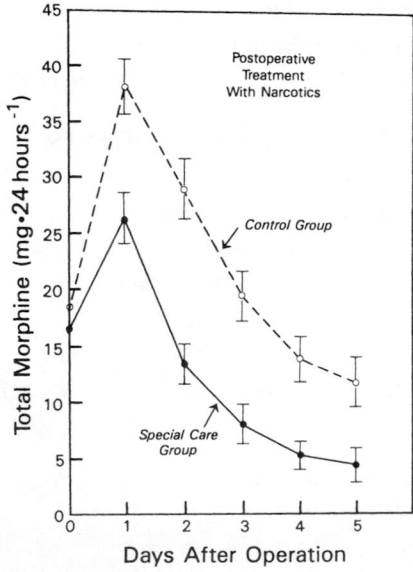

**FIGURE 31–1.** Ninety-seven patients who were to undergo abdominal surgery were divided into two groups. Each patient in the control group had a preoperative visit during which the anesthesiologist discussed his or her medical condition but did not explain postoperative events. Patients in the special care group were given a careful preoperative explanation about postoperative pain that addressed its character, intensity, and management; it was also stressed that pain was a normal occurrence. The special care group required significantly less morphine for pain relief than did the control group. This finding emphasizes the importance of the preoperative visit in postoperative care. (Reprinted from Egbert LD, Battit GE, Welch CE, et al. Reduction of postoperative pain by encouragement and instruction of patients: a study of doctor-patient rapport. *N Engl J Med.* 1964;270:825, by permission of the *New England Journal of Medicine.*)

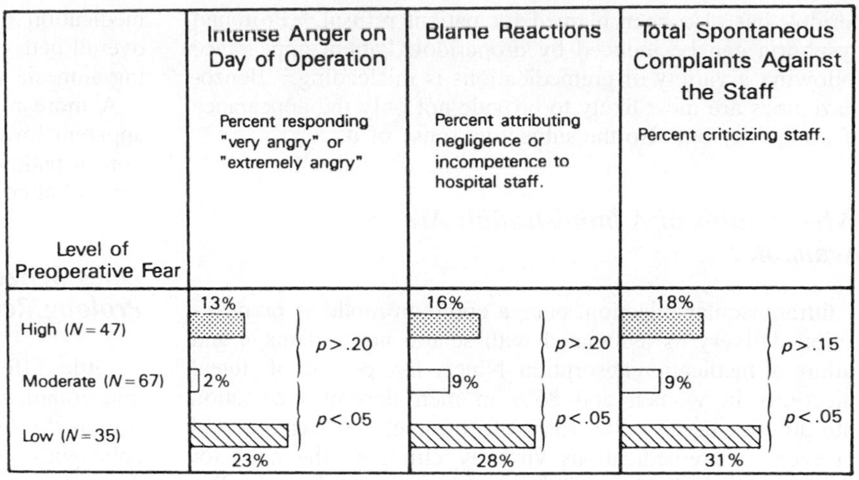

**FIGURE 31–2.** Relationship between the level of preoperative fear and subsequent aggressive reactions. (From Janis IL. *Psychological Stress: Psychoanalytic and Behavioral Studies of Surgical Patients.* New York, NY: John Wiley & Sons; 1958.)

delivery of aversive stimuli renders stimuli more tolerable.[18,19] Control over details can be important to patients, especially because many aspects of their disease or dysfunction are out of their hands. The functions that patients *can* control should be emphasized. No matter what the circumstances, patients have the ability to choose what to think about and how they view events that occur.

Patients can control the rate and depth of their breathing (much of the time). Panting (*rapid ventilation*) is commonly used to lessen labor pains. Control of breathing supports the implications that other physiologic processes can be controlled as well. Psychologists recommend encouragement such as, "You are in control. Take a deep breath. You can relax now."[20] The deep breath that the patient takes reinforces the credibility of the suggestion that the patient is in control and can relax. This sequence of sentences is superior to the simple command "Relax," which may cause the patient to think, "I can't relax." Anesthetizing personnel are generally highly attuned to the consequences of specific word choice, as exemplified by their avoidance of the phrase "put to sleep" (which evokes euthanasia).

Control, in addition to immediacy, is probably a key factor in the success of patient-controlled analgesia infusion devices. Control is essential for children and even more crucial for adolescents. Whenever possible, children should be given choices such as which finger to monitor with the pulse oximeter. Challenges such as "How high can you make those green (end-tidal carbon dioxide) mountains?" and "How big can you blow up the balloon?" are usually well received, as is encouragement such as "I'll help by adding some extra air."

A word of warning, however, is in order. In some areas, giving control to the child can increase his or her distress. For example, the sentence, "Tell me when you are ready" has been associated with increased child distress.[21] The child may never *feel* ready. Further, he or she may not know what to do in order to become ready. Other adult behaviors associated with increased child distress include apologizing, reassuring, and being overly sympathetic.[21,22] Adult behaviors associated with decreased child distress were distraction and coaching (eg, deep breathing).[22]

## Mental Distraction

Subjects given a means of mental distraction have a higher level of tolerance for adverse conditions.[23] Distraction can take the form of selective attention, guided imagery, music, or progressive relaxation. A stress management adage states, "Don't think about fear, just think about what you have to do."[20] It may be helpful to review with a patient just what he or she does have to do. For example, on emergence, a patient needs to wake up, breathe deeply, and communicate his or her needs.

Guided imagery can be facilitated by helping patients mentally envision a scene in which they can best relax. Patients may want to bring a tape of some favorite music or programmed relaxation (Table 31–2).

## When Are Pharmacologic Anxiolytics Indicated?

Patients with extremely high levels of anxiety may benefit greatly from anxiolytics. Small children given benzodiazepines are more likely to find a face mask acceptable. Anxiolytics can ease invasive catheter placement before induction and prevent anxiety-induced myocardial ischemia. Sedative premedication is generally not used, or used only cautiously, in patients younger than 1 and older than 80 years of age. Similarly, extra caution is indicated when it is given to patients who are hypoxic or have carbon dioxide retention because they are particularly vulnerable and sensitive to the associated acute respiratory depressant effects of sedatives. Pharmacologic depression of mental status is disadvantageous for the patient undergoing carotid endarterectomy or intracranial surgery, after which immediate postoperative neurologic status influences further management.

Lack of premedication may contribute to last-minute refusal of surgery. Conversely, premedication, particularly with dro-

**TABLE 31–2.** Psychologic Approach

1. Determine expectations
2. Assess anxiety, its level, and its cause
3. Correct information deficits
4. Describe pain relief modalities
5. Solicit active participation
   Induction: Select "escape," music
   Emergence: Spirometry, ambulation
6. Demonstrate areas of control (breathing, thoughts, muscle tension)

peridol, has also been blamed for patient refusal.[24] Profound dysphoria can be induced by droperidol. Patient appearance following a variety of premedications is misleading.[25] Benzodiazepines are most likely to provide not only the appearance of tranquility but also the subjective sense of it.

## What Routes of Administration Are Available?

Intramuscular injection, once a common mode of premedication delivery, is associated with sciatic nerve damage and failure of medication absorption. Ninety-five percent of gluteal injections in women and 85% in men deposit medication into adipose tissue rather than into muscle.[26] Newer oral and intravenous premedications virtually eliminate the need for intramuscular injections. Children in particular hate needles of any kind, usually citing them as the most distressing aspect of hospitalization.

In the days when children were accustomed to having their temperature measured rectally, rectal administration seemed rational. Today, many children have their temperature measured with infrared devices. These children may find rectal administration disturbing.

The intranasal approach in children is effective, does not require complete patient cooperation, and has a much more rapid onset than does oral administration of drugs such as midazolam. Nasal application of midazolam is too noxious for routine use but may be greatly appreciated when the oral route fails and sedation is still desired. Sublingual administration of midazolam allows lower dosing because the drug is directly absorbed into the bloodstream and does not undergo first-pass elimination.[27]

## When Are Benzodiazepines Useful?

The main adverse effects of benzodiazepines are depression of ventilation and interference with normal cognitive and fine motor functions. For inpatients whose neurologic function is not required to return immediately to normal at the end of the surgical procedure and whose memory of the postoperative period can be ablated, oral lorazepam can be given the morning of surgery in addition to or instead of its dosing the night before. For outpatients, oral diazepam or intravenous midazolam are more appropriate.

Kain and associates found that midazolam premedication was more effective than parental presence in reducing child and parental anxiety during induction of anesthesia.[28] They also found that premedication with midazolam was associated with less negative behavioral changes in the first week postoperatively.

Anxiolytics can ease catheter placement in adults before induction. In a double-blind study of 200 adult outpatients, 5 mg of oral diazepam 30 minutes before intravenous catheter placement was associated with improved vein quality as well as placement of larger gauge catheters.[29] The subjects who received diazepam also had a significant reduction in their anxiety scores.

Benzodiazepines improve patient satisfaction with needle localization and breast biopsy.[30] Midazolam, in a dose as low as 3.75 mg orally, has been documented to significantly lower the endocrine response to stress.[31] Sublingual lorazepam pre-

medication (1 mg) before peribulbar anesthesia enjoys an overall better patient response than placebo, mostly by inducing amnesia without unnecessary sedation.[32]

A more recent observation that bears consideration is the apparent lower incidence of postoperative cognitive dysfunction in patients who receive benzodiazepines. This finding is somewhat counterintuitive and merits further study.[33]

## Does Benzodiazepine Premedication Prolong Recovery?

Little difference in recovery times has been found between midazolam and placebo premedication of children in many studies.[34–36] Other investigators have reported delays. Cray and colleagues showed a 30-minute delay in discharge from the day surgery unit following an oral midazolam dose of 0.75 mg/kg (as opposed to 0.5 mg/kg in other studies).[37] Bevan and coworkers also demonstrated a delay in recovery with oral midazolam premedication (0.5 mg/kg) followed by propofol.[38] Here, the increased sedation was attributed to synergistic γ-aminobutyric acid receptor interactions between propofol and midazolam.[39,40] Viitanen and associates found that midazolam, 0.5 mg/kg, delayed recovery when given before sevoflurane anesthesia.[41] Spontaneous eye opening occurred in 15 minutes in the midazolam group and 11 minutes in the placebo group. Full recovery took 9 minutes longer in the midazolam group. Interestingly, 30% of the placebo group had sleep disturbance at home, as compared with only 4% of those who received midazolam.[41] Nine minutes of prolonged recovery time is a relatively small price to pay for easier parental separation, better mask acceptance, and less postoperative sleep disturbance.

In adult patients undergoing laparoscopic tubal ligation, midazolam increased postoperative sedation but did not delay recovery or time-to-discharge readiness.[42] Anesthesia for these patients, although induced with propofol, was maintained with isoflurane and nitrous oxide. Elwood and colleagues also found no delay in discharge related to midazolam use during brief propofol anesthesia.[43]

## How Do Midazolam and Diazepam Differ?

The elimination half-life of midazolam is short (1-4 hours) compared with that of diazepam (20-100 hours). Although aging can increase the half-life of midazolam by as much as 8 hours, advanced age can prolong the half-life of diazepam by several days. Midazolam, like diazepam, is almost completely metabolized by microsomal oxidative enzymes in the liver.

Midazolam and diazepam both have active byproducts, but those of midazolam are relatively weak. Both metabolites of diazepam—oxazepam and desmethyldiazepam—clinically prolong sedation. Desmethyldiazepam is only slightly less potent than its parent compound and accounts for the exacerbation of drowsiness that occurs 6 to 8 hours after diazepam administration.

Such facts suggest that midazolam may be the better benzodiazepine for the outpatient who not only needs a sedative but also needs to be free of residual sedation as soon as possible. In one study, 50 patients undergoing at least two outpatient dental procedures served as their own controls, receiving

**TABLE 31–3.** Dosing and Characteristics of Midazolam,*
Diazepam, and Lorazepam

|  | Midazolam | Diazepam | Lorazepam |
|---|---|---|---|
| Peroral dose | 0.3–0.75 mg/kg | 0.15–0.2 mg/kg | 0.03–0.05 mg/kg |
| Peak effect | 0.5–1 h | 1–1.5 h | 2–4 h |
| Duration | 1–2 h | 2–2.5 h | 4–6 h |
| Elimination half-life | 1–4 h | 20–100 h | 8–24 h |
| Apparent volume of distribution | 1.1–1.7 L/kg | 0.7–1.7 L/kg | 0.8–1.3 L/kg |
| Protein binding | 94%–97% | 97%–99% | — |
| Active metabolites | Weak | Strong | None |
| Metabolism | Hydroxylation Conjugation | Methylation Conjugation | Conjugation Less effect (age/ hepatic) |
| Clearance | 6–11 mL/kg/ min (50% of hepatic blood flow) | 0.2–0.5 mL/kg/ min | 0.7–1.0 mL/kg/ min |
| Lipid solubility | High | High | Moderate |
| Elderly | ↓ dose 15% per decade | Hours half-life = years of age | Little change |

*Intravenous midazolam latency is 2 to 3 minutes; frequency of amnesia is 70% to 80%, with duration of 20 to 30 minutes.

intravenous midazolam sedation for one procedure and intravenous diazepam for the other. Significantly greater amnesia and quicker recovery were associated with midazolam use (Table 31–3, Figs. 31–3 and 31–4).[44]

## Why Have So Many Deaths Been Associated With Midazolam?

Inattention to ventilation and oxygenation has been cited since 83 of 86 deaths reported to the US Department of Health and Human Services occurred outside of the operating room. In 38% of the patients who died, opioids had been given in

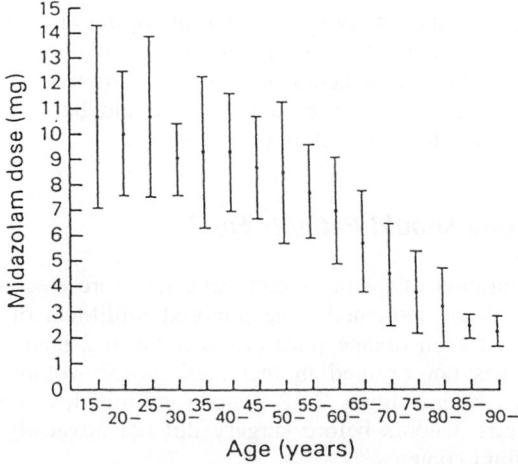

**FIGURE 31–3.** Relationship between age of patient and the mean dose (± 1 SD) of intravenous midazolam required to produce adequate sedation before upper gastrointestinal endoscopy. (From Bell GD, Spickett GP, Reeve PA, et al. Intravenous midazolam for upper gastrointestinal endoscopy: a study of 800 consecutive cases relating dose to age and sex of patient. *Br J Clin Pharmacol.* 1987;23:242.)

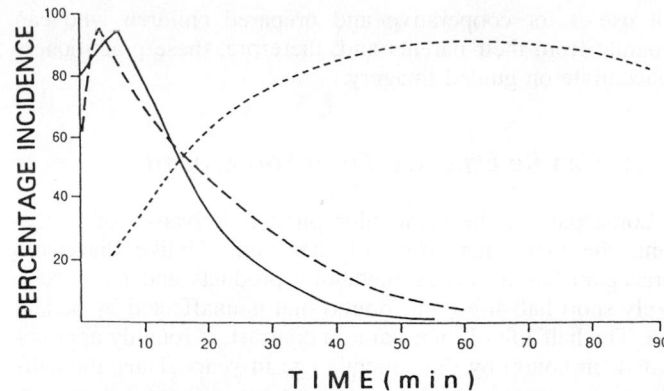

**FIGURE 31–4.** The extent and duration of amnesia following equipotent intravenous doses of 5 mg of midazolam *(solid line)*, 10 mg of diazepam *(large dashed line)*, and 4 mg of lorazepam *(small dashed line)*. (From Dundee JW, Halliday NJ, Harper KW, et al. Midazolam: a review of its pharmacological properties and therapeutic use. *Drugs.* 1984;28:520.)

addition to midazolam.[45] These observations emphasize the importance of monitoring oxygenation and ventilation after the parenteral administration of midazolam[45] and suggest that special caution be exercised when opioids are used concurrently with midazolam.

## How Is Midazolam Used in Children?

### Oral

Midazolam has revolutionized pediatric induction. No longer present is the worry that the cheerful cooperative child seen preoperatively will develop acute face mask phobia. In the past, intramuscular ketamine offered an alternative solution; now, oral midazolam, 0.5 mg/kg, usually prevents the problem. In 80% of cases, 30 minutes after the oral administration of midazolam (0.5 mg/kg), the pediatric patient easily separates from the parents and accepts monitor placement and face mask. When the dose of oral midazolam is increased to 0.75 mg/kg, 91% of patients undergo induction without crying or combativeness. The effects of oral midazolam start to dissipate in an hour.[46]

Oral midazolam is quite useful in situations in which crying and stress may worsen the underlying condition, such as congenital heart disease associated with "tet spells." Many children with congenital heart disease show improvement in oxyhemoglobin saturation following midazolam use. Some, however, may undergo oxyhemoglobin desaturation (3 of 17 children with cyanotic heart disease had a decrease of >10% in saturation)[47]; thus, pulse oximetry monitoring is critical if midazolam use is contemplated in these children.

### Nasal

Intranasal midazolam, 0.3 mg/kg, requires less patient cooperation and has a quicker onset than does oral midazolam. In one study, only 3% of children younger than 5 years of age were crying or combative during induction of anesthesia 15 minutes after intranasal instillation of midazolam.[48] Intranasal administration may be helpful after an oral dose fails.

Rarely, midazolam can cause a hyperexcitability reaction. However, because of this possibility, some practitioners do not use it for cooperative and prepared children who can separate from their parents and, therefore, these practitioners concentrate on guided imagery.

### What Can Be Expected From Lorazepam?

Lorazepam is the orthochlorophenyl derivative of oxazepam, the main metabolite of diazepam. Unlike diazepam, lorazepam has no active metabolic products and has a relatively short half-life ($\approx$12 hours) that is unaffected by patient age. The half-life of diazepam, in contrast, is roughly approximated (in hours) by the patient's age in years. Thus, the half-life of diazepam in a 72-year-old patient is about 3 days.

### Why Is Lorazepam Longer Lasting Than Diazepam?

Lorazepam is less lipophilic than is diazepam; thus, it traverses the blood-brain barrier more slowly. However, with oral administration, the onset of action of both diazepam and lorazepam is between 30 and 60 minutes.[49] Lorazepam has less tissue affinity than does diazepam; thus, its effects are not dissipated as rapidly by tissue redistribution as are the effects of diazepam. Psychomotor impairment persists 12 hours after a single dose of lorazepam.[50] Lorazepam undergoes glucuronidation and is then renally excreted. Glucuronide conjugation is faster than oxidation (the elimination pathway of diazepam) and is more resistant to the effects of both aging and hepatocellular disease.

Lorazepam, 2 mg orally (about equal in potency to 10 mg diazepam), produces sedation that lasts 4 to 6 hours. Increasing the dose to 5 mg reliably adds antegrade amnesia that lasts up to 8 hours.[51] Most references suggest limiting the dose to 4 mg because 40% of patients who received 5 mg were disoriented for as long as 17 hours.[50]

Lorazepam is superior to diazepam in preventing recall. Ten milligrams of oral diazepam provides almost no amnesia. Twenty milligrams of diazepam prevents recall in 30% of patients, whereas 4 mg of oral lorazepam prevents recall in 72%.[51] With intravenous administration, 3 mg of lorazepam impairs recall significantly, whereas 10 mg of intravenous diazepam does not.[50]

Lorazepam use may not be advisable for outpatients, but it can be quite beneficial for patients undergoing major procedures followed by intensive care unit monitoring. An advantage for the critically ill patient is that lorazepam causes no myocardial depression or relaxation of vascular smooth muscle, even at dosages as high as 9 mg.[51] When a traditional premedication for adult patients with heart disease—intramuscular morphine (0.1 mg/kg) and scopolamine—was compared with lorazepam, 0.06 mg/kg, given orally 90 minutes before surgery, no difference in the levels of anxiolysis and sedation was detected.[52]

### MODIFICATION OF GASTRIC CONTENTS

Physiologic preparation for surgery includes pharmacologic emptying and modification of gastric contents. The association of aspiration of gastric contents with maternal mortality represented an anesthetic breakthrough. Intubation of the trachea to protect the lungs from gastric acid has improved the outcome of obstetric anesthesia.

### What Drugs Are Useful?

Animal experiments have shown that both large volume and low pH of gastric secretions exacerbate the pneumonitis caused by aspiration. Hence, the goals of reducing gastric volume below 0.3 mL/kg and elevating gastric pH above 2.5 have been proposed.[53]

Particulate antacids have detrimental pulmonary effects. Nonparticulate antacids such as sodium citrate are recommended. Histamine receptor blockade decreases gastric acidity without increasing volume.

### Who Is at Greatest Risk of Aspiration?

To answer this question, gastric pH and volume were measured in many groups of patients. Alarming results were reported. Gastric volumes >0.4 mL/kg with pH <2.5 were identified in 75% of pediatric patients[54] and in 50% of adult outpatients.[55,56] Various regimens were investigated, as was the recommendation that all outpatients receive some pharmacologic prophylaxis. However, despite the magnitude of the at-risk population, numerous practitioners noted that the actual incidence of aspiration was low. One review of 40 240 anesthetic procedures in children revealed only four episodes of aspiration, two of which occurred intraoperatively and two postoperatively.[57]

In a review of 185 358 anesthetic procedures, only 83 cases of aspiration were noted, an incidence of 1 per 2000 cases. Furthermore, in 68 of these 83 cases, conditions associated with delayed gastric emptying (increased intracranial pressure, obesity, history of gastritis or ulcer, pregnancy, extreme pain or stress, emergency surgery, or upper abdominal surgery) were present.[58] Of the 15 cases in which no risk factors existed, 10 involved difficulties with the airway. Timing of surgery was important as well. Operations performed at night carried six times the risk of those performed during daylight hours (Fig. 31–5).

Because of the relatively low risk of aspiration in healthy patients without risk factors who are undergoing elective procedures, routine pharmacologic aspiration prophylaxis is not recommended. However, each patient should be scrutinized preoperatively for risk factors (Table 31–4).

### How Long Should Patients Fast?

The duration of fasting recommended before elective surgery has been shortened. One hundred milliliters of water, coffee, and even orange juice (without pulp) 2 hours before surgery has not resulted in increased gastric volumes.[59] In pediatric patients (ages 2-12 years), unlimited volumes of clear fluids 3 hours before surgery did not adversely affect gastric fluid contents.[60]

Note that although the stomach can be expected to empty itself of clear fluids within 2 hours of ingestion, gastric function is arrested by trauma. Hence, if a patient sustains an injury 1 hour after dinner, there is no known period of time after which one can be sure that the stomach will be empty.

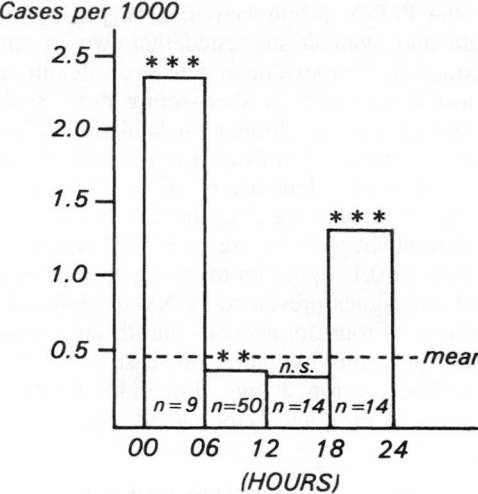

**FIGURE 31–5.** Incidence of aspiration during anesthesia according to the hour of day. n.s., Difference between this group and the other groups not significant; *, $P < .05$; **, $P < .01$; ***, $P < .001$. (From Olsson GL, Hallen B, Hambraeus-Jonzon K. Aspiration during anaesthesia: a computer-aided study of 185,358 anaesthetics. *Acta Anaesthesiol Scand.* 1986;30:86. © 1986 Munksgaard International Publishers Ltd, Copenhagen, Denmark.)

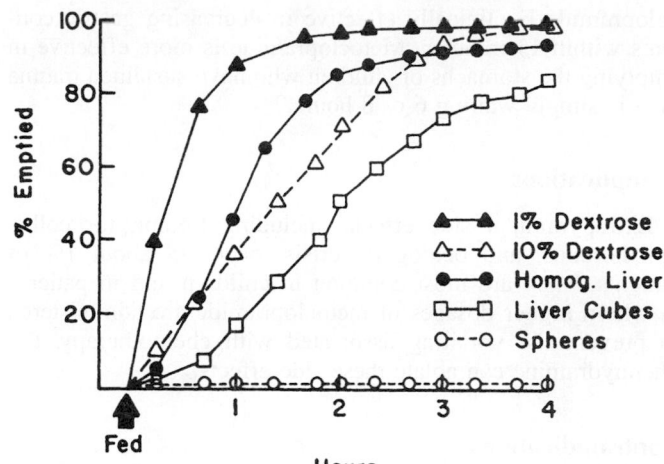

**FIGURE 31–6.** The rate of gastric emptying is influenced considerably by the makeup of any given meal. Note the large difference in emptying times between 1% dextrose and cubes of liver. Solid plastic spheres pass very slowly if at all. Experiments performed in dogs. (From Hinder RA, Kelly KA. Canine gastric emptying of solids and liquids. *Am J Physiol.* 1977;233:335.)

Because gastric function ceases at the time of injury, solids can remain in the stomach for prolonged periods of time, even more than 24 hours (Fig. 31–6).

Sodium citrate, a nonparticulate antacid, works immediately upon ingestion by alkalinizing the contents of the stomach. It is probably useful for any patient whose stomach may not be empty. However, if there is a large volume of fluid in the stomach, a small amount of antacid (30 mL) will be ineffective.

### What Are the Current Nil Per Os Guidelines?

The current nil per os guidelines are listed in Table 31–5.[61]

### What Is the Role of Metoclopramide?

Gastroparesis is common in patients with diabetes, chronic renal failure, and a variety of other conditions. Metoclopram-

ide, a dopamine antagonist, stimulates gastrointestinal motility in an organized fashion. It lowers the pressure threshold required for initiation of the peristaltic reflex, relaxes the pyloric sphincter as it increases antral contractions, and enhances duodenal and jejunal peristalsis. Metoclopramide does not increase gastric secretions.

In addition to emptying the stomach, metoclopramide increases lower esophageal sphincter tone and decreases reflux into the hypopharynx. All its actions decrease the risk of aspiration. Many commonly used anesthetic drugs decrease esophageal sphincter tone, as do the antiemetics: droperidol and prochlorperazine maleate (Compazine).

Oral metoclopramide should be given 90 to 120 minutes preoperatively in a dose of 0.3 mg/kg. Intravenous delivery decreases the onset of action to 3 minutes. Even without intravenous access, the onset of action occurs within 20 minutes of oral administration. In emergency situations, oral met-

**TABLE 31–4.** Which Patients Need Aspiration Prophylaxis?

Anticipated difficult airway
Emergency surgery
Trauma
Depressed level of consciousness (eg, drug ingestion, head trauma)
Intestinal obstruction
Increased intracranial pressure (edema or mass lesion)
Impaired laryngeal reflexes (bulbar palsy, cerebrovascular accident, multiple sclerosis, Shy-Drager syndrome, amyotrophic lateral sclerosis, vocal cord paralysis)
Obesity (or history of gastric stapling)
History of ulcer disease, partial gastrectomy, or vagotomy (gastric paresis)
Gastroesophageal reflux
Pregnancy
Upper abdominal surgery
Abdominal tumor or ascites
Other causes of gastric paresis (diabetes, chronic renal failure)

**TABLE 31–5.** Summary of Fasting Recommendations to Reduce the Risk of Pulmonary Aspiration*

| Ingested Material | Minimum Fasting Period† (h) |
|---|---|
| Clear liquids‡ | 2 |
| Breast milk | 4 |
| Infant formula | 6 |
| Nonhuman milk§ | 6 |
| Light meal‖ | 6 |

*These recommendations apply to healthy patients who are undergoing elective procedures. They are not intended for women in labor. Following the guidelines does not guarantee complete gastric emptying.

†The fasting periods noted above apply to all ages.

‡Examples of clear liquids include water, fruit juices without pulp, carbonated beverages, clear tea, and black coffee.

§Because nonhuman milk is similar to solids in gastric emptying time, the amount ingested must be considered when determining an appropriate fasting period.

‖A light meal typically consists of toast and clear liquids. Meals that include fried or fatty foods or meat may prolong gastric emptying time. Both the amount and type of foods ingested must be considered when determining an appropriate fasting period.

From American Society of Anesthesiologists Task Force. Practice guidelines for preoperative fasting and the use of pharmacologic agents to reduce the risk of pulmonary aspiration: application to healthy patients undergoing elective procedures. *Anesthesiology.* 1999;90:896.

oclopramide is clinically effective in decreasing gastric contents within 15 minutes. Metoclopramide is more effective in emptying the stomachs of children who have sustained trauma than is simply waiting 6 or 8 hours.[58]

### Complications

Extrapyramidal side effects, including tremor, torticollis, opisthotonos, and oculogyric crisis, occur in about 1% of patients. They are most common in children and in patients in whom higher dosages of metoclopramide are administered to prevent the vomiting associated with chemotherapy. Diphenhydramine can ablate these side effects.

### Contraindications

Patients taking other dopamine antagonists, monoamine oxidase inhibitors, tricyclic antidepressants, or sympathomimetics should not receive metoclopramide. Metoclopramide has caused hypertensive crises in patients with undiagnosed pheochromocytomas.

### *How Are Histamine-2 Receptor Blockers Useful?*

Histamine-2 receptor blockers like cimetidine and ranitidine work by decreasing gastric acid secretion. Hence, they do not improve pH immediately and do not chemically empty the stomach. Ranitidine may be preferred over cimetidine due to its longer duration of action (8 hours) and its lower incidence of side effects and drug interactions.[62] Ranitidine given at least an hour before surgery will raise pH over 2.5 in 88% of patients undergoing elective surgery when an intravenous dose of 50 mg is used. Doubling the dose to 100 mg raises pH over 2.5 in 93% of patients.[63]

If one drug is good, are three better? Maltby and coworkers answered this question, showing no advantage of double or triple prophylaxis (citrate, metoclopramide, and ranitidine) over ranitidine alone.[64]

### *What Can Be Done to Prevent Postoperative Nausea and Vomiting?*

Postoperative nausea and vomiting (PONV) are particularly detrimental to patient satisfaction. Certain procedures, anesthetic agents, and patient conditions are associated with a higher incidence of PONV. Investigators have developed risk scores for predicting PONV.[65,66] Procedures associated with increased PONV include breast surgery (both mastectomy and breast augmentation); laparoscopy; shoulder surgery; ear, nose, and throat operations (especially middle ear surgery and tonsillectomy); strabismus correction; and orchiopexy.[67,68] A prospective evaluation of almost 18 000 outpatients showed that a 30-minute increase in duration of anesthesia increased the likelihood of PONV by 60%.[68] In this study, women developed PONV twice as often as men. Every decade increase in age decreased the risk of PONV by 13%.

Other studies have emphasized that a history of PONV or motion sickness is a strong predictor of PONV.[65] Patients at high risk need to be identified preoperatively so that their anesthetic and PONV prophylaxis can be planned appropriately. White and Watcha suggested that two or three drug combinations (eg, droperidol-ondansetron-dexamethasone) may be most beneficial.[68] A short-acting drug, such as ondansetron (which has an elimination half-life of 3 hours) is most efficacious when administered at the end of surgery.[69,70] Dexamethasone, with a half-life of 36 to 72 hours, has suppressed delayed emesis (ie, beyond 24 hours) in patients receiving chemotherapy.[71] Its use in PONV was reviewed in 2000.[72] A dose of 0.1 mg/kg up to 10 mg appears efficacious. Scuderi and colleagues prevented PONV in high-risk patients with a regimen of total intravenous anesthesia (propofol and remifentanil), generous hydration (at least 25 mL/kg), triple antiemetics (ondansetron 1 mg, droperidol 0.625 mg, and dexamethasone 10 mg), and ketorolac 30 mg.[73]

## MISCELLANEOUS DRUGS

### *What Are the Indications?*

#### Anticholinergics

Anticholinergics are useful for drying secretions in preparation for awake intubation, procedures for which the upper airway must be topically anesthetized, and bronchoscopies. It also prevents the bradycardia that results from laryngeal stimulation in infants.[74]

Critically ill adult patients, such as those with dead bowel or ruptured aortic aneurysm who cannot tolerate an anesthetic of any sort, may benefit from intravenous scopolamine, 0.4 mg. A patient who is already maximally catecholamine-stimulated and tachycardic usually tolerates scopolamine without further clinically significant increments in heart rate. If anticholinergic administration (atropine or scopolamine) results in postoperative delirium (because, unlike glycopyrrolate, both compounds cross the blood brain barrier), it may be treated with physostigmine (Antilirium) titrated in 0.5-mg increments.

#### Narcotics

Narcotics are necessary for patients who are in pain. The rapidity of action of intravenous narcotics is useful in patients for whom the move from stretcher to operating room table will likely be painful (patients with burns, fractures, and ischemic bowels or extremities). Alternatively, anesthesia can be induced while the patient is still on the stretcher.

#### Clonidine

The centrally acting α-agonist clonidine has been promoted as a premedication for hypertensive patients. Clonidine effectively reduces sympathetic nervous system activity and diminishes cardiovascular responses to intubation and other noxious stimuli.[75,76] Clonidine may be useful for the patient with uncontrolled hypertension who requires urgent surgery. However, irreversibly impaired sympathetic responses can interfere both with the identification of hidden volume loss and its compensation.

## SUMMARY

Historically, a premedication was an intramuscular injection of narcotic and sedative administered to facilitate induction.

With less noxious modern anesthetics, other goals and approaches have emerged. Optimization of the psychologic and physiologic states of the patient requires careful assessment, active patient participation, pain management planning, and selective medication use.

## References

1. Egbert LD, Battit GE, Turndorf H, et al. The value of the preoperative visit by an anesthetist. *JAMA.* 1963;185:553
2. Leigh JM, Walker J, Janaganathan P. Effect of preoperative anaesthetic visit on anxiety. *BMJ.* 1977;2:987
3. Arellano R, Cruise C, Chung F. Timing of the anesthetist's preoperative outpatient interview. *Anesth Analg.* 1989;68:645
4. Volicer BJ, Bohannon MW. A hospital stress rating scale. *Nurs Res.* 1975;24:352
5. Klafta JM, Roizen MF. Current understanding of patients' attitudes toward and preparation for anesthesia: a review. *Anesth Analg.* 1996;83:1314.
6. Hume MA, Kennedy B, Asbury AJ. Patient knowledge of anesthesia and perioperative care. *Anaesthesia.* 1994;49:715.
7. Shevde K, Panagopoulos G. A survey of 800 patients' knowledge, attitudes, and concerns regarding anesthesia. *Anesth Analg.* 1991;73:190.
8. Ramsay MA. A survey of preoperative fear. *Anaesthesia.* 1972;27:396.
9. McCleane GJ, Cooper R. The nature of pre-operative anxiety. *Anaesthesia.* 1990;45:153.
10. Roizen MF, Klock A, Klafta J. How much do they really want to know? Preoperative patient interviews and the anesthesiologist. *Anesth Analg.* 1996;82:443.
11. Farnill D. Patients' desire for information about anaesthesia: Australian attitudes. *Anaesthesia.* 1993;48:162.
12. Lonsdale M, Hutchison GL. Patients' desire for information about anaesthesia: Scottish and Canadian attitudes. *Anaesthesia.* 1991;46:410.
13. Litman RS, Perkins FM, Dawson SC. Parental knowledge and attitudes toward discussing the risk of death from anesthesia. *Anesth Analg.* 1993;77:256.
14. Janis IL. *Psychological Stress. Psychoanalytic and Behavioral Studies of Surgical Patients.* New York, NY: John Wiley & Sons; 1958.
15. Williams OA. Patient knowledge of operative care. *J R Soc Med.* 1993;86:328.
16. Egbert LD, Battit GE, Welch CE, et al. Reduction of postoperative pain by encouragement and instruction of patients. *N Engl J Med.* 1964;270:825.
17. Langer EJ, Janis IL, Wolfer JA. Reduction of psychological stress in surgical patients. *J Exp Soc Psychol.* 1975;11:155.
18. Corah NL, Boffa J. Perceived control, self-observation and response to aversive behavior. *J Pers Soc Psychol.* 1970;16:1.
19. Kanfer FH, Seidner ML. Self-control: factors enhancing tolerance of noxious stimulation. *J Pers Soc Psychol.* 1973;25:381.
20. Meichenbaum D, Cameron R. Stress inoculation training. In: Meichenbaum D, Jaremko ME, eds. *Stress Reduction and Prevention.* New York, NY: Plenum Press; 1983;115.
21. Dahlquist LM, Power TG, Carlson L. Physician and parent behavior during invasive pediatric cancer procedures: relationships to child behavioral distress. *J Pediatr Psych.* 1995;20:477.
22. Blount RL. The relationship between adults' behavior and child coping and distress during BMA/LP procedures: a sequential analysis. *Behavior Therapy.* 1989;20:585.
23. Kanfer FH, Goldfoot DA. Self-control and tolerance of noxious stimulation. *Psychol Rep.* 1966;18:79.
24. Lee CM, Yeakel AE. Patient refusal of surgery following Innovar premedication. *Anesth Analg.* 1975;54:224.
25. Forrest WH, Brown CR, Brown BW. Subjective responses to six common preoperative medications. *Anesthesiology.* 1977;47:241.
26. Cockshott WP, Thompson GT, Howlett LJ. Intramuscular or intralipomatous injection? *N Engl J Med.* 1982;307:356.
27. Lim TW, Thomas E, Choo SM. Premedication with midazolam is more effective by the sublingual than oral route. *Can J Anaesth.* 1997;44:723.
28. Kain ZN, Mayes LC, Caramico LA. Parental presence during induction of anesthesia: a randomized controlled trial. *Anesthesiology.* 1996;84:1060.
29. Wittenberg MI, Lark TL, Butler CL, et al. Effects of oral diazepam on intravenous access in same-day surgery patients. *J Clin Anesth.* 1998;10:13.
30. van Vlyman JM, Sa Rego MM, White PF. Benzodiazepine premedication:

31. Kiefer RT, Weindler J, Ruprecht KW. The endocrine stress response after oral premedication with low-dose midazolam for intraocular surgery in retrobulbar anaesthesia. *Eur J Ophthalmol.* 1998;8:239.
32. Ghanchi FD, Khan MY. Sublingual lorazepam as a premedication in peribulbar anesthesia. *J Cataract Refract Surg.* 1997;23:1581.
33. Moller JT, Cluitmans P, Rasmussen LS, et al, for the ISPOCD Investigators. Long-term postoperative cognitive dysfunction in the elderly: ISPOCDI study. *Lancet.* 1998;351:857.
34. Weldon BC, Watcha MF, White P. Oral midazolam in children: effect of time and adjunctive therapy. *Anesth Analg.* 1992;75:51.
35. Vetter TR. A comparison of midazolam, diazepam, and placebo as oral anesthetic premedicants in younger children. *J Clin Anesth.* 1993;5:58.
36. McMillan CO, Spahr-Schopfer IA, Sikich N, et al. Premedication of children with oral midazolam. *Can J Anaesth.* 1992;39:545.
37. Cray SH, Dixon JL, Heard CMB, et al. Oral premedication for paediatric day case patients. *Paediatr Anaesth.* 1996;6:265.
38. Bevan JC, Veall GR, Mcnab AJ, et al. Midazolam premedication delays recovery after propofol without modifying involuntary movements. *Anesth Analg.* 1997;85:50.
39. McClune S, McKay AC, Wright PM, et al. Synergistic interaction between midazolam and propofol. *Br J Anaesth.* 1992;69:240.
40. McAdam LC, MacDonald JF, Orser BA. Midazolam increases the affinity of the GABA A receptor for propofol. *Can J Anaesth.* 1996;43(suppl):A49.
41. Viitanen H, Annila P, Viitanen M, et al. Premedication with midazolam delays recovery after ambulatory sevoflurane anesthesia in children. *Anesth Analg.* 1999;89:75.
42. Richardson M, Wu C, Hussain A. Midazolam premedication increases sedation but does not prolong discharge times after brief outpatient general anesthesia for laparoscopic tubal sterilization. *Anesth Analg.* 1997;85:301.
43. Elwood T, Hutchcroft S, MacAdams C. Midazolam conduction does not delay discharge after very brief propofol anaesthesia. *Can J Anaesth.* 1995;42:114.
44. Barker I, Butchart DGM, Gibson J, et al. IV sedation for conservative dentistry: a comparison of midazolam and diazepam. *Br J Anaesth.* 1986;58:371.
45. Bailey PL, Pace NL, Ashburn MA, et al. Frequent hypoxemia and apnea after sedation with midazolam and fentanyl. *Anesthesiology.* 1990;73:826.
46. Feld LH, Negus JB, White PF. Oral midazolam preanesthetic medication in pediatric outpatients. *Anesthesiology.* 1990;73:831.
47. DeBock TL, Davis PJ, Tome J, et al. Effect of premedication on arterial oxygen saturation in children with congenital heart disease. *J Cardiothorac Anesth.* 1990;4:425.
48. Wilton NCT, Leigh J, Rosen DR, et al. Preanesthetic sedation of preschool children using intranasal midazolam. *Anesthesiology.* 1988;69:972.
49. Kothary SP, Brown ACD, Pandit UA, et al. Time course of antirecall effect of diazepam and lorazepam following oral administration. *Anesthesiology.* 1981;55:641.
50. Heisterkamp DV, Cohen PJ. The effect of intravenous premedication with lorazepam (Ativan), pentobarbitone or diazepam on recall. *Br J Anaesth.* 1975;47:79.
51. Ameer B, Greenblatt DJ. Lorazepam: a review of its clinical pharmacological properties and therapeutic uses. *Drugs.* 1981;21:161.
52. Thomson IR, Bergstrom RG, Rosenbloom M, et al. Premedication and high-dose fentanyl anesthesia for myocardial revascularization: a comparison of lorazepam versus morphine-scopolamine. *Anesthesiology.* 1988;68:194.
53. Olsson GL, Hallen B, Hambraeus-Jonzon K. Aspiration during anaesthesia: a computer-aided study of 185,358 anaesthetics. *Acta Anaesthesiol Scand.* 1986;30:84.
54. Coté CJ, Gouldsouzian NG, Liu LMP, et al. Assessment of risk factors related to the acid aspiration syndrome in pediatric patients: gastric pH and residual volume. *Anesthesiology.* 1982;56:70.
55. Manchikanti L, Colliver JA, Marrero TC, et al. Ranitidine and metoclopramide for prophylaxis of aspiration pneumonitis in elective surgery. *Anesth Analg.* 1984;63:903.
56. Ong BY, Palahniuk RJ, Cumming M. Gastric volume and pH in outpatients. *Can Anaesth Soc J.* 1978;25:36.
57. Tiret L, Nivoche Y, Hatton F, et al. Complications related to anaesthesia in infants and children: a prospective survey of 40,240 anaesthetics. *Br J Anaesth.* 1988;61:263.
58. Olsson GL, Hallén B. Pharmacological evacuation of the stomach with metoclopramide. *Acta Anesth Scand.* 1982;26:417.
59. Hutchinson A, Maltby JR, Reid CRG. Gastric fluid volume pH in elective

inpatients, I: coffee or orange juice versus overnight fast. *Can J Anaesth.* 1988;35:12.

60. Splinter WM, Schaefer JD, Zunder IH. Clear fluids three hours before surgery do not affect the gastric fluid contents of children. *Can J Anaesth.* 1990;37:498.

61. American Society of Anesthesiologists Task Force. Practice guidelines for preoperative fasting and the use of pharmacologic agents to reduce the risk of pulmonary aspiration: application to healthy patients undergoing elective procedures. *Anesthesiology.* 1999;90:896.

62. Smith SR, Kendall MJ. Ranitidine versus cimetidine a comparison of their potential to cause clinically important drug interactions. *Clin Pharmacol.* 1988;15:44.

63. Maile CJD, Francis RN. Pre-operative ranitidine: effect of a single intravenous dose on pH and volume of gastric aspirate. *Anaesthesia.* 1983;38:324.

64. Maltby JR, Elliott RH, Warnell I, et al. Gastric fluid volume and pH in elective surgical patients: triple prophylaxis is not superior to ranitidine alone. *Can J Anaesth.* 1990;37:650.

65. Apfel CC, Greim CA, Haubitz I, et al. The discriminating power of a risk score for postoperative vomiting in adults undergoing various types of surgery. *Acta Anaesthesiol Scand.* 1998;42:5028.

66. Sinclair DR, Chung F, Mezei G. Can postoperative nausea and vomiting be predicted? *Anesthesiology.* 1999;91:109.

67. Watcha MF, White PF. Postoperative nausea and vomiting [review article]. *Anesthesiology.* 1992;77:162.

68. White PF, Watcha MF. Postoperative nausea and vomiting: prophylaxis versus treatment. *Anesth Analg.* 1999;89:1337.

69. Sun R, Klein KW, White PF. The effect of timing of ondansetron administration in outpatients undergoing otolaryngologic surgery. *Anesth Analg.* 1997;84:331.

70. Tang J, Wang B, White PF, et al. The effect of timing of ondansetron administration on its efficacy, cost-effectiveness, and cost-benefit as a prophylactic antiemetic in the ambulatory setting. *Anesth Analg.* 1998;86:274.

71. Tavorath R, Hesketh PJ. Drug treatment of chemotherapy-induced delayed emesis. *Drugs.* 1996;52:639.

72. Henzi I, Walder B, Tramer MR. Dexamethasone for the prevention of postoperative nausea and vomiting: a quantitative systematic review. *Anesth Analg.* 2000;90:186.

73. Scuderi PE, James RL, Hams L, et al. Multimodal management eliminates postoperative nausea and vomiting (PONV) following outpatient laparoscopy. *Anesthesiology.* 1999;91:A6.

74. Miller BR, Friesen RH. Oral atropine premedication in infants attenuates cardiovascular depression during halothane anesthesia. *Anesth Analg.* 1988;67:180.

75. Ghignone M, Calvillo O, Quintin L. Anesthesia and hypertension: the effect of clonidine on perioperative hemodynamics and isoflurane requirements. *Anesthesiology.* 1987;67:3.

76. Pouttu J, Scheinin B, Rosenberg PH, et al. Oral premedication with clonidine: effects on stress responses during general anaesthesia. *Acta Anaesthesiol Scand.* 1987;31:730.

# General Anesthesia: Induction, Maintenance, and Emergence

Joachim S. Gravenstein

Robert R. Kirby

## ANESTHETIC CHOICE

### How Is the Anesthetic Chosen?

Ideally, the choice of anesthetic management should be based on controlled studies that identify the anesthetic procedure and agent that provide the best outcome for the patient. The fact that many different agents and procedures are in common use for similar patients and operative procedure demonstrates that we lack data that would firmly guide us in selecting one or the other anesthetic approach. Consequently, we must rely on what our common sense suggests and, importantly, on techniques and drugs with which we are most familiar.

Common sense is not easily defined. Common sense dictates not to use high spinal anesthesia in a patient in hemorrhagic shock. That type of common sense is not based on controlled studies in human beings but on an understanding of the consequences of sympathetic blockade in a patient relying on high sympathetic tone to maintain circulation. However, if we were to list all anesthesia practices based on common sense, we would soon discover that the foundation covers a wide spectrum of common sense, from well established to rather tenuous.

In a study conducted in 1992, 27% of 2800 patients showed features that common sense suggested to be important for the anesthetist to know about before he or she started a routine general anesthetic.[1] The proposed anesthetic included sodium thiopental and succinylcholine for induction; tracheal intuba-

**TABLE 32–1.** Common Findings During Preanesthetic Evaluation That Can Affect Anesthetic Technique

| Findings | Precautions to Be Taken |
|---|---|
| Hiatal hernia | Use rapid-sequence induction to prevent aspiration. |
| Asthma | Intubate under deep anesthesia to prevent bronchospasm. |
| Difficult airway | Prepare for alternative to routine orotracheal intubation under direct visualization. |
| Rheumatoid arthritis | Rule out ligamentous instability at C1-2 with flexion-extension radiograph of cervical spine before submitting patient to routine orotracheal intubation. |
| | Anticipate in 26% of patients the possibility of involvement of the cricoarytenoid joint,[2] which may hinder intubation.[3] |
| Stroke | Prevent changes in cerebral perfusion and intracranial pressure. |

tion; and nitrous oxide ($N_2O$), oxygen ($O_2$), and isoflurane for maintenance. The most common relevant historical findings are listed in Table 32–1.[2,3] Other, rarer findings that can influence the choice of technique and drugs include conditions such as allergies, diabetes, and hypertension, all of which may require special consideration in the anesthetic management. A review of the data contained in the preoperative evaluation also includes an assessment of the drugs a patient has been given or should have received before he or she is to be anesthetized (see Chapter 1).

## PRELIMINARY CONCERNS

### What Is Needed Before Inducing General Anesthesia?

#### A Few Preliminaries

A patient should be asked how long he or she has been fasting (but a patient should not be asked, "When did you have your last meal?"). Examine his or her face and check to see whether intubation is likely to present difficulties. Many patients are now seen preoperatively by someone who likely will not be providing the anesthetic. During the preanesthetic examination, a patient may have been sitting and facing the examiner; in the operating room, he or she is lying down, and such positioning may alter the appearance of the airway and the estimation of how easy or difficult intubation will be. In children and mentally retarded patients, make sure that nothing is in the mouth before inducing anesthesia. Chewing gum or the rubber cap from the plunger of a plastic syringe has been found at the last-minute check.

#### Dentures

Many patients come to the operating room holding a blanket in front of their mouths because they are embarrassed to be seen without their dental prostheses. In modern anesthesia, it is rather unlikely that the patient will swallow or aspirate a prosthesis. Often, we find it acceptable to leave the false teeth in place (to the considerable comfort of the patient) if we believe that keeping the teeth in place will not hinder anesthetic management. During intubation, dental prostheses often become dislodged and must be taken out, an acceptable procedure at this point because the patient is asleep. However, special precautions must be taken to ensure that the false teeth are not lost and that they are safely stored after surgery. Admittedly, it is more convenient for the clinical team if the patient comes without removable teeth. However, before the removal of false teeth becomes a routine preanesthetic requirement, thought should be given to a patient's comfort and dignity.

### Personal Interaction

Always address a patient by his or her name. If a patient prefers, and relatively few adults object, you can use the first name. Whether you are a man or a woman, do not call a female patient "honey" or other similar casual informality. Remember, patients are likely to be afraid; anything you can do to make them feel that they are in competent, professional hands helps to allay their fears.

Just before induction is not the time to present a patient with options. Patients expect you to have a firm plan. Explain to him or her what you will do; do not ask for his or her opinion (even if the patient is a professor of anesthesiology). Anesthesia, even though you administer it daily, is something special for the individual patient. Options should have been discussed during the preoperative visit, not before the induction of anesthesia.

Tell patients that you will obtain blood pressure (BP) and heart rate measurements and other information before you collect it. Comment that the BP is fine (if it is) or that the $O_2$ saturation is excellent (assuming that it is). Talk with patients so that they do not feel as if they are lying in a factory awaiting their turn in some impersonal and awful process. When you are about to apply the mask or inject the first drug, do not ask the patient if he or she is ready. This is a well-meaning phrase on your part, but it leaves some individuals with the unsettling feeling that you expect an intellectual contribution to an undertaking that should be entirely in your expert hands.

Requesting a patient to swallow everything in his or her mouth before starting anesthesia should be omitted if the patient has come dry-mouthed to the operating room. Let those patients with a productive cough clear their throats to remove phlegm poised to drop into the glottis and trigger laryngospasm on induction of anesthesia. Let them clear their throats to spit out what is lodged in the pharynx while they are sitting up, or at least let them turn a little to the side; expectoration is difficult for one who is lying in the supine position.

### Equipment Check

Although this subject is discussed elsewhere in this book, it cannot be overly stressed that a last look at the anesthesia equipment is essential before it is used. Think about every step you are about to take and about the equipment you will use, from drug injection to intubation; from BP recording to reversal of muscle relaxant; and from tongue blade insertion to emergency drug use. Check the light on the laryngoscope and the cuff on the endotracheal tube (ETT). You should have a flashlight ready should the main *and* emergency power fail (this problem can and does happen occasionally). Also, you should have emergency equipment handy to insufflate $O_2$ into the trachea, should this be necessary. If you do not have such equipment ready but find you need it, you will not have time to send someone to get it; it must be within easy reach at all times.

### Monitoring Before Induction

The anesthesiologist requires baseline data before beginning induction (and the Joint Commission on Accreditation of Health Care Organizations mandates documentation on the anesthetic record that the patient's overall condition has not changed from the baseline preanesthetic assessment). The patient may have a pulse oximeter-monitored $O_2$ saturation ($SpO_2$) of only 90%, electrocardiographic evidence of a silent myocardial infarction, or some other unexpected problem that has not yet been detected. The anesthesiologist also needs reference data for comparison should something go wrong during anesthesia and again for comparison when the patient is discharged from the postanesthesia care unit.

## PREOXYGENATION

### Why Preoxygenate?

The rationale for preoxygenation or denitrogenation is simple: filling the lungs with $O_2$ gains time should a patient's airway become obstructed during induction of anesthesia.[4] A simple calculation shows that a functional residual capacity of 2500 mL filled with air contains roughly 250 mL of water vapor and carbon dioxide ($CO_2$); 2250 mL of air contains approximately 470 mL of $O_2$. Assuming that adult patients at complete rest consume 300 mL of $O_2$ per minute (and much more, should they struggle), it is not long before they become quite hypoxemic and stop breathing. Eliminating the nitrogen increases the reservoir of $O_2$ five-fold and thus generates a grace period of several minutes before a patient becomes hypoxic.

This grace period may be short. In the presence of a completely obstructed airway, the $O_2$ saturation may drop below 85% in a child or an obese patient within 3 minutes, as was shown by Benumof and colleagues.[4] Because of their relatively low alveolar volume (compared with weight), desaturation occurs more quickly the smaller the child and the more obese the adult. Shunts, increased $O_2$ consumption, and decreased $O_2$ carrying capacity are other factors that influence the duration of the grace period, that is, the time until the $SpO_2$ drops after preoxygenation.

Finally, the anesthesiologist may not assume that breathing $O_2$ for 2 or 3 minutes will accomplish denitrogenation of the lungs in all patients. A leak around the mask, a fresh gas flow too low to prevent rebreathing of exhaled nitrogen, and slow washout of nitrogen from poorly ventilated areas of lungs may all conspire to prevent adequate denitrogenation.

Preoxygenation may have a drawback. Breathing high concentrations of $O_2$ by some patients may contribute to the development of atelectasis, particularly if the functional volume is restricted, as is likely to occur in upper abdominal and thoracic procedures.[5] However, the brief period involved is unlikely to produce long-lasting deleterious effects. Only in an occasional patient should circumstances dictate avoidance of extensive denitrogenation. Clinical experience suggests that preoxygenation is well tolerated and that the benefits outweigh the disadvantages.

### Techniques

Do not start preoxygenation until you are ready to devote your full attention to the task. Some anesthesiologists like to strap the mask to a patient's face and then complete other chores, leaving the patient on his or her own during the preoxygenation. If the mask fits tightly and comfortably, this approach may be acceptable. However, it is even better if you can talk during the preoxygenation period, holding the mask yourself rather than strapping it on the patient. Patients welcome the human contact during this time of high anxiety. More likely than not, a mask held in a hand cradling the patient's face is more comfortable than one secured with the help of a head strap. Finally, when you hold the mask properly, your fourth finger supports the mandible, and the fifth finger rests gently to detect motion of the floor of the mouth should the patient talk, swallow, or retch (Fig. 32–1).

### Fresh Gas Flows

Preoxygenation proceeds most quickly if you can provide the $O_2$ without having the patient rebreathe any expired gas. This approach necessitates a high flow rate of $O_2$. Figure 32–2 shows computer-generated depictions of body compartments. Observe how long it takes to wash out the alveolar nitrogen to <10% of its original value if a fresh gas flow of 6 L/min is administered with a semiclosed system and if the patient is breathing normally. Compare this value with that obtained with an open system (no rebreathing at all) and with hyperventilation. (Figure 32–2 assumes an average adult without lung disease.)

Make sure there is no leak around the mask. If the breathing bag does not fill completely with every exhalation, a leak is present around the mask until proven otherwise (of course, you had prechecked the breathing circuit and the mask and you know that they were tight). When a leak is present, the

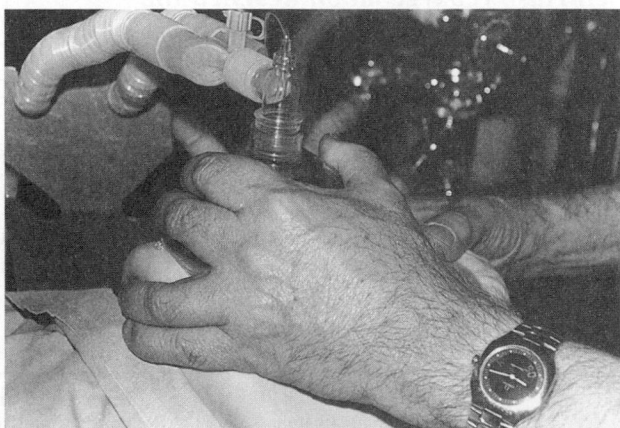

**FIGURE 32–1.** Photograph showing the position of the hand of the anesthesiologist as it holds a face mask. Observe that the fourth finger supports the chin, whereas the fifth rests gently to feel motion of the floor of the mouth; thus, the fifth finger can detect swallowing, which is often the forerunner to retching and vomiting. Thumb, index, and middle fingers adjust pressure to provide a comfortable but tight fit of the mask to the patient's face.

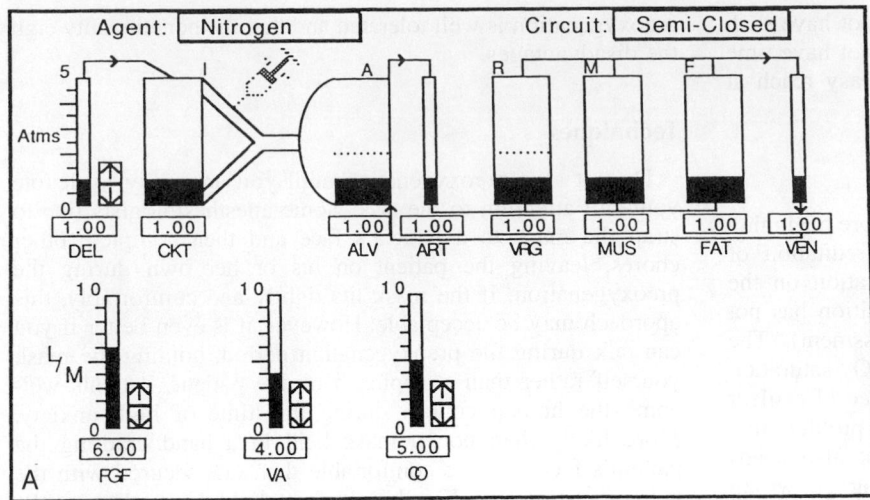

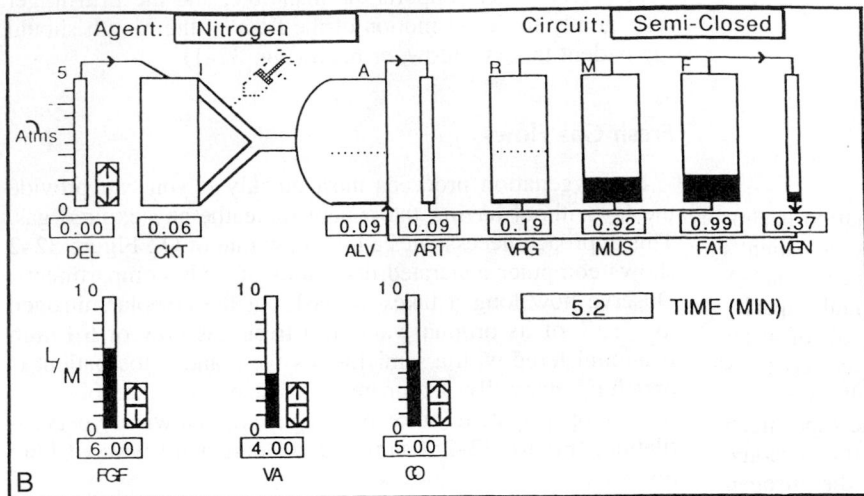

**FIGURE 32–2.** *A and B,* All panels are based on GasMan, a computer simulation of the uptake and distribution of gases in an average adult. The interconnected boxes at the *top* represent different compartments of the anesthesia machine and body; the numbers under the boxes represent the concentrations of the gases in the compartments. Boxes are blackened according to the concentration of gas in each. From *left to right:* DEL, the concentration of gases delivered into the anesthesia machine; CKT, the breathing circuit, the volume of which is assumed to be approximately 7 L; ALV, the functional residual capacity (FRC), 2.5 L, showing the alveolar concentration of the gas; ART, the arterial concentration of the gas; VRG, the concentration of the gas in the vessel-rich group (≈6 L), which receives 76% of the cardiac output; MUS, the concentration of gas in the muscle group (≈33 L), which receives only 18% of the cardiac output; FAT, a fat compartment (14.5 L), which receives only approximately 0.06% of the cardiac output. The *lower row* of icons: FGF, fresh gas flow chosen by the anesthesiologist; VA, the effective alveolar ventilation; CO, the cardiac output. The box on the *right* shows the time from the start of the simulation.

*A,* Before the simulation is started, nitrogen is in equilibrium in all compartments in the body.

*B,* The FGF is 6 L/min. The patient is assumed to breathe normally with an effective VA of approximately 4 L/min.

After 5.2 minutes, preoxygenation is stopped because the concentration of nitrogen in the ALV is <10% of the starting value. Observe that muscle and fat, in particular, still show significant partial pressures of nitrogen.

In a system in which the patient would not rebreathe at all and at the same time would hyperventilate, the washout of nitrogen from the lungs would be even faster than shown for *B.*

patient inhales some air (with a large amount of nitrogen) in addition to the O₂ from the breathing circuit.

### When Has Preoxygenation Reached the Desired Goal?

Do not be satisfied if the pulse oximeter shows 100% O₂ saturation. Check the *exhaled* O₂ concentration. Once it is >90%, you know this indicates that most of the nitrogen has been washed out from the lungs. If you cannot monitor exhaled O₂, have patients take at least three vital capacity breaths (if their lungs are healthy), or allow at least 3 minutes for patients with obstructive lung disease.[6,7] More recent work

suggests that eight deep breaths within 60 seconds achieves the same PaO₂ as does 3 minutes of oxygen breathing, but is associated with a decreased rate of oxyhemoglobin desaturation.[8] The reason for this finding is unclear, but it may involve enhanced denitrogenation in patients who breathe deeply during the preoxygenation period as opposed to normal tidal volume breathing with the more traditional 3-minute period.

### INDUCTION OF ANESTHESIA

Table 32–2 gives a general overview of different patterns of inducing general anesthesia. All of these patterns may be

**TABLE 32–2.** Common Patterns of Inducing General Anesthesia

| Mask | Intravenous and Endotracheal Inhalation | Intravenous and Relaxant: Endotracheal Inhalation | Narcotic/Relaxant | Rapid-Sequence Induction |
|---|---|---|---|---|
| Start inhalation anesthetic | Small dose of thiopental, methohexital, or propofol Start inhalation anesthetic Intubation under deep anesthesia | Large dose of thiopental, methohexital, or propofol Inflate lungs Relaxant Intubation | Large dose of narcotic/tranquilizer Inflate lungs Relaxant Intubation | After thorough preoxygenation, large dose of thiopental, methohexital, or propofol Relaxant Intubation |

modified by borrowing from one another or by substituting other drugs.

## When Is Mask Anesthesia Acceptable?

Mask anesthesia is a rational option for relatively brief anesthesia if it is administered to a patient with a freely patent airway, who is breathing spontaneously, who is not at risk of aspirating stomach content, and who is positioned so that tracheal intubation can be accomplished with the slightest provocation. In other words, never rely on mask anesthesia when a muscle relaxant (even in a dose that enables the patient to breathe spontaneously) has been given; when the patient has respiratory insufficiency and requires assisted ventilation; when the upper airway is obstructed; or when the patient is in a position other than flat on his or her back with the face in easy reach of the anesthesiologist.

Long anesthetic procedures can be conducted using mask anesthesia, but maintenance of the airway becomes a chore. With fatigue, the clinician may slacken his or her support of the airway, and optimal ventilation is thus jeopardized.

## When Is the Laryngeal Mask Airway Acceptable?

The laryngeal mask airway (LMA) has secured a place for itself in anesthetic practice. It can take the place of the face mask once the patient is sufficiently anesthetized to accept manipulation of the upper airway and insertion of a foreign body into the hypopharynx. The LMA should not be used in the patient at risk of vomiting because it does not protect against aspiration; nor should it be used in the paralyzed patient in need of mechanical ventilation. Although it is true that a well-seated LMA may enable positive pressure ventilation with peak airway pressures up to 20 cm $H_2O$, safety during mechanical ventilation rests with the properly placed ETT. The LMA does not prevent insufflation of the esophagus and stomach, in addition to or instead of the trachea. This is particularly true in patients with poor pulmonary compliance. The LMA technique also demands an open glottis and thus levels of anesthesia deep enough to prevent laryngospasm.

Despite these limitations, the LMA has become the friend of the anesthesiologist because its placement does not require a laryngoscope and it does not cause a sore throat. Up to 50% of patients, however, do complain of pharyngeal discomfort on the day of surgery, complaints that disappear over 1 to 2 days. Some report that the incidence of discomfort can be decreased by inserting the LMA with the cuff inflated, an insertion technique apparently as easy (or difficult) as the traditional technique with the cuff collapsed.[9]

## Are Inhalation Induction Techniques Still Useful?

Induction of anesthesia by inhalation through a face mask is the oldest technique and is still used often in children, who abhor needle sticks. This method is discussed in greater detail in Chapter 57. Here is a tip concerning inhalation induction in adults, which is occasionally necessary if the patient has no accessible veins, and if a surgical cut-down seems the greater of two evils: *If you induce by mask and inhalation, do not ask the patient to hyperventilate during preoxygenation; subsequent minute ventilation will be reduced, and uptake of the inhalation anesthetic will be delayed.*

### Slow Inhalation Induction

After completing preoxygenation (but before removing the mask), select a high flow of $N_2O$ and $O_2$ (eg, 6 L/min of $N_2O$ and 2 L/min of $O_2$). Do not administer the $N_2O$ for too long because the patient might become excited. After just a few breaths, begin to add a halogenated inhalation agent. Halothane and sevoflurane are the least irritating of these agents, but induction can be accomplished with any agent. Starting $N_2O$ and the halogenated agent together exploits the second gas effect (see Chapter 34). Warn the patient that the gas will smell a little strong. Talk, but do not ask questions; it is not easy for the patient to answer with a mask over his or her face.

### Three-Breath Rule

With every third breath, increase the concentration of the inhalation anesthetic by approximately 0.125%. The *three-breath rule* can help: the first breath gives the gas a chance to reach the patient; the second gives him or her an opportunity to react to it; and the third shows you whether he or she will breath-hold, cough, or retch in response to the irritating vapor. If the patient does tolerate the concentration, increase it. If the patient breath-holds, do not take the mask off; instead, wait until he or she once again is breathing normally, and then increase the concentration.

Do not encourage the taking of deep breaths. The patient is able to do so while he or she is responsive (ie, when the concentration of the anesthetic is still low). However, by the time the anesthetic concentration is sufficiently increased, the patient will have hyperventilation-induced shallow breathing that slows gas uptake.

### Manual Ventilation

Do not push on the breathing bag during the induction. You are likely to trigger a cough or laryngospasm. Once you think the patient is anesthetized (ie, he or she has regular and perhaps depressed ventilation, no eye movement, and pupils that are moderately dilated [unless you have given a narcotic] and unresponsive to light), manually inflate the lungs with gas containing the high anesthetic concentration. If the patient tolerates this process without breath-holding, he or she is likely to be ready for the placement of an LMA or even intubation and certainly for the insertion of an intravenous catheter.

### Tracheal Intubation

If you now intubate, remember that the patient is early in the process of distributing the anesthetic into the different body compartments. Depth of anesthesia therefore rapidly decreases as the anesthetic in the vessel-rich group is redistributed to the other compartments that have not yet reached high anesthetic partial pressures. When you remove the mask (remember to turn off the gas delivery so as not to fill the operating room), the depth of anesthesia quickly decreases.

Be swift with intubation. As a rule, if you cannot intubate after one quick exposure of the larynx, do not persist in your attempts; otherwise, the patient may develop laryngospasm. Take the laryngoscope out while the patient is still breathing spontaneously, reapply the mask, and reinstitute the delivery of high gas concentrations, once again deepening anesthesia. Then repeat laryngoscopy and intubation.

## Rapid Induction

Alternatively, you can induce inhalation anesthesia directly with a high concentration of a vapor, such as 5% isoflurane in $O_2$. For this technique, you need two systems, one for preoxygenation (eg, a Mapleson D system with a high flow of $O_2$) and the other to provide anesthesia (ie, the anesthesia machine, which stands ready with its system already filled with the desired high concentration of the anesthetic in $O_2$).

After preoxygenation, ask the patient to take a single vital capacity breath and blow it out down to the residual volume. At this point, switch systems so that the next vital capacity breath that the patient takes fills his or her lungs with the high concentration of the anesthetic. To lessen the likelihood of coughing, it may be useful (but not essential) to premedicate the patient with a narcotic.[10]

## *What Are the Characteristics of Intravenous Induction?*

All other induction techniques use intravenous agents. Intravenous agents have three advantages:

1. The patient is spared the discomfort of having to breathe a smelly vapor.
2. General anesthesia can be applied—alone or in conjunction with other drugs.
3. The patient is rendered quickly ready for tracheal intubation.

They have two disadvantages:

1. Venous access is required, although this route is usually available.
2. They are not as readily controlled as inhalation agents, which can be accurately measured in inhaled and exhaled gas and, if necessary, can be removed actively by the lungs.

## *When Is a Combination Intravenous and Mask Induction Useful?*

This technique slightly modifies slow mask induction. Patients with significant reactive airway disease benefit if intubation is delayed until the bronchial smooth muscles are relaxed and bronchoconstrictive airway reflexes are obtunded. However, the use of an intravenous agent to ease the transition from the inhalation of $O_2$ to that of halogenated anesthetic is acceptable.

You need give only small amounts of sodium thiopental or other short-acting intravenous agent, such as propofol. A large, intubating dose of the agent (or narcotics) depresses ventilation and slows the inhalation induction. A typical dose

for the average patient might be thiopental, 1 to 2 mg/kg, or propofol, 200 to 400 μg/kg. These doses can be repeated and must be adjusted to each patient's tolerance.

Once a patient is in the surgical stage of anesthesia and still breathing spontaneously, you can intubate. If necessary, you can now use muscle paralysis to facilitate intubation; however, instead of giving a usual intubating dose, such as 1 mg/kg succinylcholine, you now need only one half to one third of this dose. Remember that halogenated inhalation anesthetics reduce the need for large doses of relaxants.

## *What Is a Standard Intravenous Induction?*

This is by far the most common technique in use. A relatively (ie, adjusted for the patient's physical condition) large dose of thiopental, 4 to 5 mg/kg, propofol, 2 mg/kg, or methohexital, 2 mg/kg, is injected rapidly. Within one circulation period ($\approx$20 seconds), the patient feels the drug's effect and perhaps yawns. Approximately 1 minute after injection, the lid reflex (gently touch the eyelashes to check it) is absent, ventilation is depressed, and arterial BP is reduced. At this time, test the patency of the airway by inflating the patient's lungs with a few deep breaths (either of $O_2$ or of $O_2$ and a potent inhalation agent).

Alternatively, propofol (either 20- to 30-mg boluses until the lid reflex disappears, or an infusion with 50 to 100 μg/kg/min or more as needed, is acceptable) can be used to ease the patient to sleep before starting an inhalation agent.

## Airway Obstruction

Management of airway obstruction depends on whether the obstruction is due to laryngospasm or to soft tissue obstruction. The two cannot always be easily distinguished. Laryngospasm often comes on suddenly, secondary to irritation of the vocal cords. When the patient can get a little air through the vocal cords, a typical stridorous noise often occurs. High airway pressures often lead to inflation of the stomach. Soft tissue obstruction of the hypopharynx, if complete, prevents gas entry into the lungs or the stomach. Obstruction of the larynx or trachea due to tumor, trauma, a foreign body, or swelling may be impossible to distinguish from laryngospasm. Either form of airway obstruction can be associated with postobstructive (negative-pressure) pulmonary edema in spontaneously breathing patients.[11]

## *Soft Tissue*

If the airway obstruction is caused by soft tissue, try simple maneuvers first. Sometimes, insertion of an oral airway is all that is required. However, caution should be exercised: if you insert the airway before adequate anesthesia is established, you may trigger a laryngospasm. A nasal airway may serve equally well, but do not force the nasal tube into the nose; to do so may cause troublesome bleeding, particularly in patients at increased risk of nasal bleeding.

If neither of these benign attempts helps, and if you cannot visualize the larynx and you cannot intubate, stop all efforts and let the patient awaken from the single dose of the induction agent. Provided you have not had a heavy hand in selecting your dosages, the patient is likely to recover muscle tone and, at about the same time, spontaneous ventilation before sustaining harm. Remember that the grace period is short in the obese, the child, and in sick patients. A well-conducted preoxygenation demonstrates its benefit by delaying hypoxemia. You will appreciate having used the lowest effective dose of succinylcholine ($\leq$1 mg/kg), the effect of which dissipates quickly (provided the patient's cholinesterases are functioning properly). And you will appreciate not having complicated the picture and prolonged the paralysis by pretreating, unnecessarily, with a depolarizing agent (see Should a Defasciculating Drug Be Given Before Succinylcholine Is Injected?, later).

### Laryngospasm

If the obstruction is due to laryngospasm, administer succinylcholine to relax the striated muscle of the mouth and pharynx to enable tracheal intubation. Do not expect a relaxant to reestablish the ease of manual ventilation if any of the following is true:

1. Bronchospasm exists. Neuromuscular blocking drugs do not relax the airway smooth muscle or any other smooth muscle. Indeed, some relaxants may contribute to bronchospasm by releasing histamine. Start treating the bronchospasm. If it is so severe that you need high airway pressures to deliver gas into the patient's lungs, let him or her wake up. Then optimize therapy for bronchospasm, and start again when better conditions are present.
2. The obstruction is attributed to anatomic abnormalities or to edema or a tumor that blocks the upper airway. The prudent decision is to let the patient wake up and then to reassess the anesthetic approach. Ordinarily, such problems are discovered during a careful preanesthetic evaluation, and an awake intubation is chosen.

### How Is Anesthesia Induced Without a Halogenated Inhalation Drug?

A technique that is gaining favor relies on $O_2$ and intravenous drugs, including muscle relaxants, and avoids inhalation agents altogether or uses them only as adjuvants. It calls for titration of the intravenous drug until the patient becomes sleepy, usually with concomitant depression of ventilation. The patient may still respond to commands to take deep breaths.

Doses of one of the major tranquilizers (eg, midazolam) are used in preparation and are followed by sufentanil, 1 $\mu$g/kg; fentanyl, 10 $\mu$g/kg; or alfentanil, 100 $\mu$g/kg. In some patients, muscle rigidity develops after the administration of narcotics. Neuromuscular blocking drugs (eg, succinylcholine) can be given to overcome this "tight chest" syndrome. Although small doses suffice to relax the rigid chest, this usually is the time to intubate.

Administration of a small dose of thiopental, 2 mg/kg, or an alternative intravenous induction agent to ensure amnesia, may be necessary for intubation.

Instead of induction with narcotics, propofol can be used alone with $O_2$ or can be supported by narcotics and muscle relaxants as needed. Alternatively, propofol can be given with $N_2O$, other inhalation agents, and muscle relaxants as required. A typical amount for induction is approximately 2 to 2.5 mg/

**TABLE 32–3.** Risk Factors for Pulmonary Aspiration of Gastric Contents

| Perioperative | Laryngeal Incompetence |
|---|---|
| Pregnancy | Bulbar dysfunction |
| Obesity | Multiple sclerosis |
| Gastrointestinal dysfunction | Stroke |
| Intestinal obstruction | Muscular dystrophy |
| Emergency surgery | Myasthenia gravis |
| **Depressed Level of Consciousness** | Amyotrophic lateral sclerosis |
| | Vocal cord trauma |
| Head injury | |
| Drug overdose | |
| Coma | |
| Central nervous system infections | |
| Seizures | |

kg, given in divided doses. In elderly or debilitated patients, lower doses are used.

### When Is a Rapid-Sequence Induction Indicated?

A rapid-sequence induction (sometimes inelegantly called a *crash induction*) is indicated in certain situations (Table 32–3).

### Patients at Risk of Aspiration

### Patients With Full Stomach

The patient who aspirates stomach contents may suffocate on the spot, or a piece of food may occlude a bronchus, with the likelihood of causing first atelectasis and later an abscess. Signs and symptoms are listed in Table 32–4. All patients who, because of an emergency, have not fasted and all women in labor must be suspected of having a full stomach.

Typically, we ask the adult patient not to take anything by mouth after midnight, if the operation is scheduled for the early morning. In children, we are prepared to accept a shorter fast. A survey published in 1996 shows that a more tolerant approach is widely adopted.[12] A reasonable compromise for the adult patient is to continue with the prescription of no solid food for 6 hours before the anesthetic but to permit clear liquids (water or apple juice) up to 4 hours before the anesthetics. In children, these times are shortened, allowing

**TABLE 32–4.** Characteristics of Various Types of Aspiration

| Particulate Obstruction | Acidic (Liquid pH <2.5) |
|---|---|
| *Total ("café coronary")* | Tachypnea |
| Inability to speak or breathe | Dyspnea |
| Cyanosis | Wheezing |
| Rapidly fatal | Hypotension, often profound |
| *Partial* | Pulmonary edema |
| Stridor | |
| Tachypnea | |
| Wheezing | |
| **Particulate Nonobstructive** | |
| Tachypnea | |
| Wheezing | |
| Cyanosis | |
| Cough | |
| Cardiovascular collapse | |

solids (including milk) for up to 3 hours before the anesthetic and clear liquids up to 2 hours (and infants even 1 hour) before the anesthetic.

### Patients With Gastric Juice of Low pH

Patients who give a history of regurgitation, heartburn, or hiatal hernia fall into this category. All have an incompetent gastroesophageal sphincter and are at risk of bringing the gastric juice (often silently, ie, without retching or vomiting) into the hypopharynx, from where it can trickle into the larynx or can be aspirated. If enough material reaches the lungs and if it is sufficiently acidic (pH <2.5), lung tissue will sustain a chemical burn, and the so-called Mendelson syndrome develops[13] (see Table 32–4).

### Technique

For a rapid-sequence induction, the Sellick maneuver is used. We do not give a defasciculating dose of a nondepolarizing neuromuscular blocking drug. Such a dose might reduce the patient's ability to deal with reflux while still awake and delays the onset of the effect of succinylcholine. To counteract that possibility and the antagonistic effects of succinylcholine and the nondepolarizing agent, one would have to give a large dose of succinylcholine, thereby increasing the duration of relaxation.

After preoxygenation, inject an intubating dose (adjusted to the patient's status but given here for a healthy and vigorous adult) of thiopental, 5 mg/kg, or ketamine, 1.5 mg/kg, or propofol 2.5 mg/kg, or etomidate 0.4 mg/kg, or methohexital 1.5 mg/kg and immediately follow it with an intubating dose of succinylcholine, 1 mg/kg (other relaxant drugs can be used, but none works as fast as succinylcholine).

As soon as the drugs are injected and before the patient loses consciousness, pressure is applied over the cricoid cartilage (the patient should be warned) and maintained until the cuff of the ETT is inflated and the correct position of the tube is confirmed by capnography (preferably) or by auscultation and other, less reliable methods.

### The Sellick Maneuver

The method of pressing on the cricoid cartilage to obstruct (not really occlude) the esophagus is not new.[14] It was originally used to prevent the inflation of the stomach with air during mechanical ventilation of the lungs by mask. It is therefore acceptable to ventilate the lungs during the seconds of apnea and before intubation. There is some worry that the putative benefits of cricoid pressure are bought at a price that may at times be too high.[15] On the one hand, the maneuver may not prevent gastric insufflation or regurgitation; on the other hand, it makes laryngoscopy and intubation more difficult. Esophageal rupture during vomiting or damage to the spinal cord in patients with neck fractures are rare and devastating complications of the Sellick maneuver.

Many anesthesiologists do not ventilate during the period of apnea with a rapid-sequence induction because of their fear of pushing gas into the stomach. We believe that gentle manual ventilation is not only acceptable but preferable, as long as unusual pressures (eg, >20 mm Hg) are not required to inflate the lungs and thus potentially the stomach.

### Patients Who Are Easy to Intubate

The technique of injecting the intubating doses of thiopental and succinylcholine in rapid succession can be used in most routine anesthetic procedures. Indeed, an argument can be advanced in favor of the rapid sequence (with or without the Sellick maneuver): if thiopental and succinylcholine are injected together (do not mix them in the same syringe—the thiopental will precipitate), their duration of action is likely to be approximately as long as the duration of either one given alone, provided that the patient has normal pseudocholinesterase activity. Hemodynamically, patients seem to fare best if the intubation is accomplished while the peak effects of thiopental and succinylcholine coincide.

### Should a Defasciculating Drug Be Given Before Succinylcholine Is Injected?

No. Yet we are aware that many anesthesiologists are strong advocates of giving the average adult 3 mg of *d*-tubocurarine or an equivalent dose of another nondepolarizing agent approximately 3 minutes before injecting the intubating dose of succinylcholine. They point to studies showing that patients have less muscle pain if a defasciculating dose is used. However, almost as many studies report that pretreatment with a defasciculating dose failed to prevent so-called succinylcholine myalgia. Indeed, even the association between fasciculation and postoperative myalgia is in question.[16] Other reasons why we do not favor pretreatment with a nondepolarizing agent are summarized in Table 32–5.[17]

### What Should Be Done When the Patient Cannot Be Intubated and Ventilated?

If you have tried all the "tricks of the trade" (see Chapter 53) and absolutely cannot intubate the trachea orally, nasally, blindly, or fiberoptically and cannot ventilate the lungs, even with an oral or nasal airway in place, then:

1. Ask for help. Two people may be required to ventilate using bag and mask: one to hold the mask with two hands while lifting the patient's chin, and the other to squeeze the bag. Positioning of the jaw is important. Sometimes it helps to lift and push the mandible forcefully forward, thus allowing the lower incisor teeth to be anterior to the upper incisors.

**TABLE 32–5.** Defasciculating Pretreatment

| Pro | Cons |
|---|---|
| In many patients, it reduces postsuccinylcholine myalgia | In many patients, it fails to reduce postsuccinylcholine myalgia<br>Nondepolarizing relaxants are antagonistic to depolarizing agents; therefore, succinylcholine dose has to be increased<br>Onset of succinylcholine action is slowed<br>Duration of succinylcholine is prolonged<br>Unpleasant effects of defasciculating dose include diplopia, inability to swallow, and sometimes dyspnea |

2. If the $O_2$ saturation begins to drift downward into unacceptable ranges <80%, depending on the patient's physical condition, take steps at once to insufflate $O_2$ percutaneously into the trachea. The necessary techniques are described in detail in Chapter 53.

## MAINTENANCE OF ANESTHESIA

A wise Creator has surrounded our vital organs with sensitive coverings. Thus, cutting through skin, dura, and peritoneum or scraping periosteum hurts more than does surgery on muscle, brain, gut, or bone. Consequently, a patient requires more analgesia (anesthesia) during incision and closure than he or she does during the middle of a procedure.

### How Should Agents Be Administered?

Because we never fully equilibrate the anesthetic agents across all body compartments, anesthesia should be maintained as lightly as possible during the phases in which only moderate analgesic requirements must be met. The less time the patient spends in deep anesthesia (with high blood levels of anesthetic agents), the faster he or she recovers from the drugs, be they inhalation or intravenous agents.

Figure 32–3 presents a comparison of two computer-simulated anesthetic procedures with isoflurane lasting 2 hours. All variables (fresh gas flow, ventilation, cardiac output, and induction concentrations) were kept the same for both cases, but in one case, isoflurane concentration was decreased to 1.5% during the maintenance phase. In the other case, it was kept at 2%.

For the painful closure, anesthesia was deepened: in the first case to 4% for 5 minutes, and in the second case only to 3% (because the patient was already more deeply anesthetized). Once the isoflurane administration was discontinued and the "patients" had breathed room air for 5 minutes, the one who had been under light anesthesia during the maintenance phase had approximately one-fifth less anesthetic (1.4 L versus 1.7 L of isoflurane vapor dissolved in the tissues) than did the other who had been kept in a deeper stage during the maintenance phase.

For intraabdominal procedures, the requirement for muscle relaxation is also greatest during exposure and closure. Again, recovery from relaxation is faster the less drug given.

### How Are Fluids Regulated?

Although drug requirements may be fairly small during the maintenance phase of anesthesia, fluid requirements are likely to be greatest at this time. While the wound is open to room air (fluid loss by evaporation); while the surgeon works on the tissue, which causes edema to form and fluids to be sequestered in traumatized tissue (third space losses); and while outright bleeding occurs, losses must be replaced (see Chapters 38 and 40).

### When and Why Should Patients Be Allowed to Breathe Spontaneously?

Allowing spontaneous ventilation once was common during the maintenance phase of anesthesia, even for thoracic and upper abdominal operative procedures. With the introduction of the LMA, spontaneous ventilation during the maintenance phase of anesthesia is making a comeback, if not for thoracic and upper abdominal procedures. As soon as muscle relaxants are used or whenever the airway must be protected from potential aspiration, an ETT is needed and mechanical ventilation becomes necessary.

### Monitoring of Anesthetic Depth

Many operative procedures do not require relaxants before incision of the fascia and after its closure. Many more require no relaxants whatsoever when an LMA is used and even after tracheal intubation. Spontaneous ventilation provides an elegant means to assess the clinical depth of anesthesia; in many ways, the rate and volume of the patient's tidal ventilation are superior to conventional measurements of pulse and BP. If a paralyzed patient is tachycardic during an isoflurane anesthetic procedure, is it because the anesthesia is too light or because this is simply a normal, autonomic response to the agent? However, if the spontaneously breathing patient doubles the respiratory rate and the tidal volume increases by 50% after incision (or if the patient moves), valuable information has been obtained.

The introduction of the bispectral index monitor has made available an objective assessment of depth of anesthesia.[18] It may not enable the clinician to pinpoint the actual depth of anesthesia, but it has proven helpful in monitoring changes of anesthetic level in individual patients.[19]

### Maintenance of Arterial Carbon Dioxide Partial Pressure and pH

If large doses of narcotics are administered, spontaneous ventilation will be inadequate to maintain acceptable $Pa_{CO_2}$ levels. An ETT reduces physiologic dead space by 50% or more. Thus, what would be marginal or unsatisfactory ventilation during mask anesthesia may be adequate in the intubated patient. Because it is impossible to predict what is adequate, we recommend continuous monitoring of exhaled gases and pulse oximetry to maintain acceptable blood gas and pH values.

### Ventilation-Perfusion Relationships

Spontaneous breathing during general anesthesia is advantageous in maintaining more normal ventilation-perfusion relationships.[20] In contrast, manual or mechanical ventilation increases dead space in nondependent lung areas and increases shunting in dependent ones. If you do not agree with this statement, ask yourself how many patients have a normal, predicted $Pa_{O_2}$ for any given inspired $O_2$ concentration? Then, consider why tidal volumes of 10 to 15 mL/kg are necessary to maintain normal $Pa_{CO_2}$ and pH during mechanical ventilation when volumes of 6 to 8 mL/kg suffice in awake, spontaneously breathing people.

Finally, consider that positive pressure manual or mechanical ventilation decreases venous return and cardiac output and thus exacerbates the myocardial depressant effects of many anesthetics. Spontaneous breathing, however, enhances venous return and thus helps cardiovascular function.

Spontaneous breathing has much to offer in terms of maintaining cardiopulmonary integrity. It also provides satisfaction

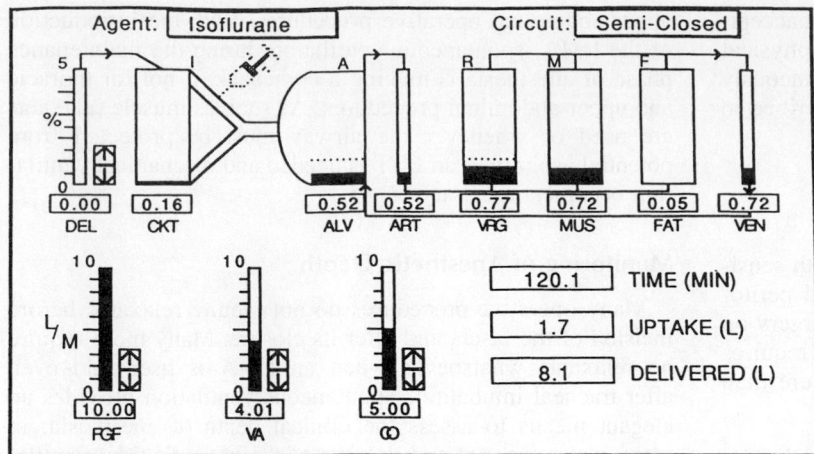

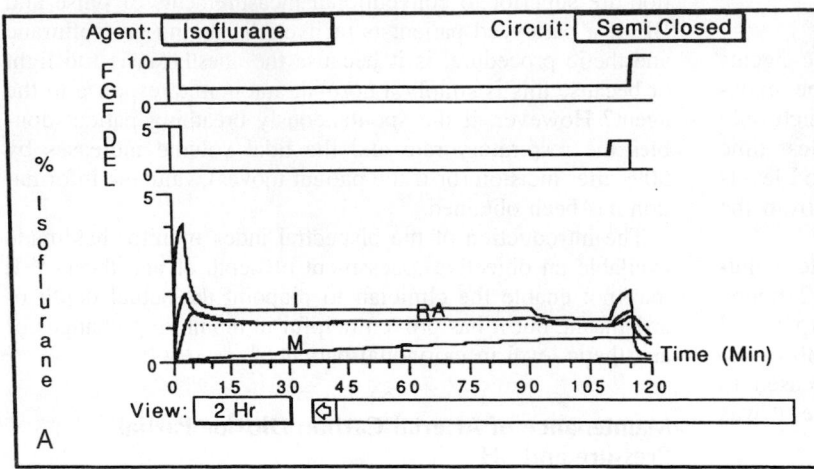

**FIGURE 32–3.** All panels are based on GasMan, a computer simulation of the uptake and distribution of gases in an average adult. *A and B, upper frames,* The boxes on the *lower right* show the elapsed time since the start of the simulation, the total volume of isoflurane vapor dissolved in the body (UPTAKE), and the volume of isoflurane (in liters) delivered since the beginning of the simulation. *A and B, lower frames,* Graphic representations of the course of anesthesia with fresh gas flow (FGF) on *top* (10 L/min for induction and emergence, 3 L/min for maintenance) and the setting of the vaporizer. The effective alveolar ventilation (VA) and cardiac output (CO) are constant. The curves show the concentration of isoflurane (in volume %) in the different compartments. A and R, artery- and vessel-rich group; F, fat group; I, inspired; M, muscle group. Two anesthetic procedures are simulated: *A,* Keeping the patient fairly deeply anesthetized.

to the anesthesiologist who titrates anesthetic depth based on a patient's needs rather than using a "cookbook" approach or by reading the exhaled anesthetic concentration on a gas analyzer. When the operative procedure allows, spontaneous breathing should be attempted.

## EMERGENCE AND EXTUBATION

### *When Should Analgesics Be Administered?*

Should you administer an analgesic before the end of the operation to cover the early postoperative period? The answer to this question depends largely on the operation and on what type of anesthesia the patient had received. If the primary anesthetic was an inhalation agent of low solubility or propofol with $N_2O$, you may want to give an intramuscular analgesic approximately 45 minutes before admission to the recovery room. Medication that has a longer plasma concentration plateau than that obtainable with a single intravenous dose is preferable. For the average adult, 10 mg morphine or 60 mg ketorolac is a reasonable choice. If the anesthesia included large intermittent doses or a continuous infusion of narcotics, do not administer more at the end of the case. Even the so-called short-acting narcotics have long elimination times.

In contrast, remifentanil, with its short half-life of <10 minutes, presents the opposite problem. A patient given remi-

fentanil as the main analgesic during the operation may be in severe pain soon after the operation because the drug so quickly vanishes secondary to its hydrolysis in plasma. In that case, it is useful to give a prophylactic dose of a longer-lasting narcotic, such as morphine, 10 mg intramuscularly, to the average adult before the patient leaves the operating room. An alternate is to continue an infusion of remifentanil between 0.05 and 0.23 µg/kg/min into the early postoperative period.[21,22]

### *When Should the Patient Be Extubated?*

In the days when diethyl ether was the primary agent, all patients were slow to awaken. Extubation of patients still in surgical levels of anesthesia was common. This is no longer necessary because we now use inhalation and intravenous agents that are more rapidly eliminated. In general, the trachea can be extubated if the patient is capable of protecting the airway and maintaining adequate ventilation. The latter can be tested by asking him or her to take a deep breath ($\approx$15 mL/kg). Muscle power needs to be checked by verifying that the patient can raise his or her head off the pillow for 5 seconds.

A patient who can execute these tasks can be safely extubated. However, a patient who received large doses of narcotics and relaxants may be able to lift his or her head, take a

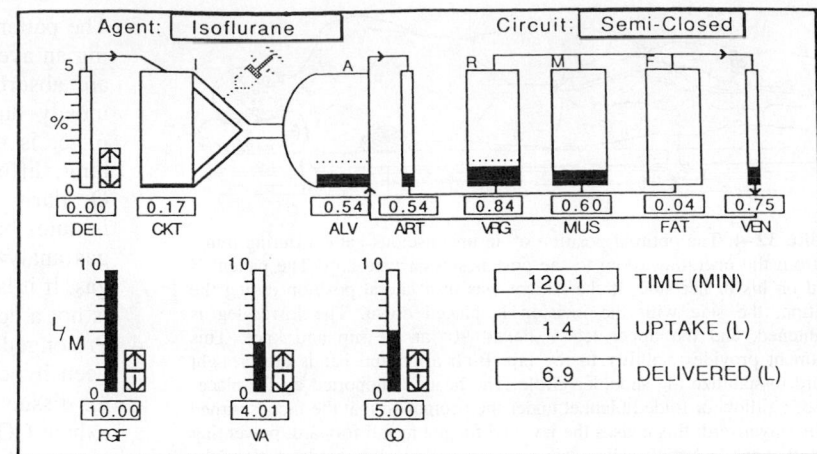

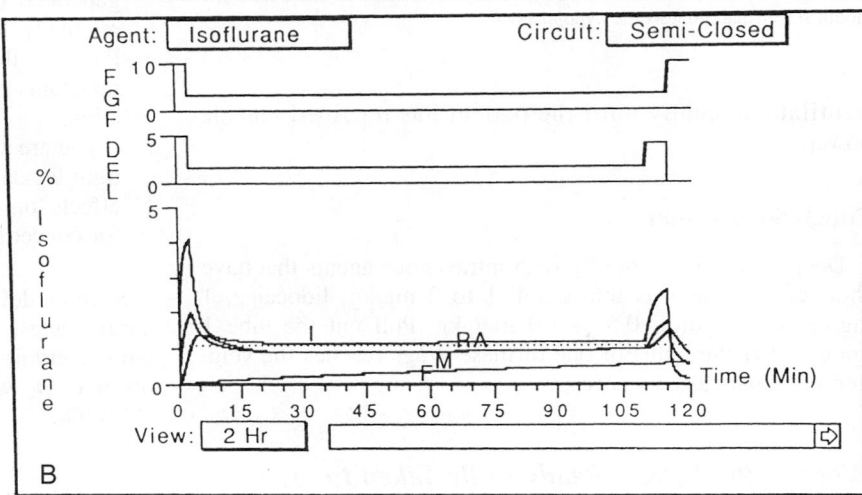

**FIGURE 32–3** *Continued. B,* Keeping the patient fairly lightly anesthetized. Observe that at the end of operation, there is *(A)* 1.7 L of dissolved isoflurane vapor in the tissues and *(B)* 1.4 L of dissolved isoflurane vapor in the tissues (approximately one-fifth less). For a rapid recovery, it is worth adjusting the anesthetic administration to the minimal patient requirements.

deep breath on command, and even answer questions after extubation, but 10 to 30 minutes later the same person may sustain respiratory arrest in the postanesthesia care unit (PACU). We assume that this sequence results when the respiratory depressant effect of the narcotic lingers while the respiratory stimulating effects of pain begin to subside in the PACU. Beware of the insidious "tail" effect of some intravenous anesthetics.

Be careful not to remove the bite block or oral airway before extubation. Once the patient begins to respond, he or she may bite down on the ETT and occlude the airway. If the bite block or oral airway has fallen out, and if the patient bites on the tube, try to pry the teeth apart using tongue blades. Insert one followed by another between the teeth. Even in patients with clenched teeth, this maneuver is usually possible. Then, wedge additional tongue blades between the first two, and in this way separate the incisors far enough that the ETT is protected.

Alternatively, you may slide the gloved index fingers of each hand posteriorly, *very carefully,* lateral to the premolar and molar teeth, hooking them between the upper and lower gums *behind* the last molars. This maneuver is extremely painful (try it on yourself, then attempt to bite down), and even a semiconscious, uncooperative patient seldom fails to open his or her mouth wide enough to permit the anesthesiologist to relieve the obstructed tube, or to extract it, and remove or insert a bite block or other device.

### How Is Extubation Done If the Patient Should Not Cough or Struggle?

After regaining their reflexes, many patients strain and cough during extubation. This activity is occasionally undesirable, such as in a patient with an eye injury (straining → increased venous pressure → increased intraocular pressure → loss of vitreous). Three techniques can be used to abolish straining during extubation. All require preoxygenation (because once again the patient's airway may be jeopardized right after the tube is removed) and preparation for reintubation (should the patient lose his or her airway).

#### Deep Anesthesia

Keep the patient well anesthetized, and extubate under deep anesthesia. Then, put the patient on his or her side (Fig. 32–4) so that the tongue falls forward, preventing obstruction. Should the patient regurgitate or vomit, the gastric material will follow gravity and drain from the mouth instead of pooling in the hypopharynx.

#### Extubation-Like Intubation

Repeat the induction sequence and extubate after the patient has been paralyzed with a small dose of succinylcholine.

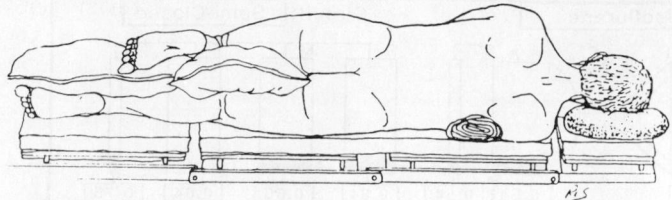

**FIGURE 32–4.** The optimal position of an unconscious patient during transport from the operating room to the postanesthesia care unit. The patient is placed on his or her side. If the patient was in a lateral position during the operation, the side with the incision is placed down. The lower leg is straightened, and the upper leg is flexed 90° at the hip and knee. This adjustment provides stability to the hip. Both arms and hands are brought forward to stabilize the shoulder girdle. The head is supported by the placement of a pillow or folded blanket under the occiput so that the face is turned slightly downward; this causes the jaw and tongue to fall forward, preventing obstruction while letting saliva, gastric juice, or vomitus to drain from the mouth rather than pool in the hypopharynx.

Ventilate manually until the patient has regained muscle power.

### Cough Suppression

Deepen anesthesia briefly with intravenous agents that have short effects, such as thiopental, 1 to 2 mg/kg; lidocaine, 1 mg/kg; or propofol, 0.5 to 1.0 mg/ kg. Pull out the tube 1 minute after the bolus of one of these drugs reaches the vein. Ventilate manually as necessary.

### *When Is the Patient Ready to Be Taken to the Postanesthesia Care Unit?*

We are sometimes too casual when taking a patient to the PACU. During general anesthesia, the patient breathed a gas mixture enriched with $O_2$. Now the patient is breathing room air, and he or she may be exhaling $N_2O$ by the liter, presenting the real risk of diffusion hypoxia. During surgery, the patient stayed in one position; now, he or she is being moved and turned. Compensatory vascular reflexes may still be depressed by anesthetic after-effects; with sudden turning, the patient may become hypotensive. Make sure that ventilation and circulation are adequate before leaving the operating room. If necessary, encourage deep breaths during transport and give $O_2$.

### *When Should Oxygen Be Given During Transport?*

Oxygen should be given if any of the following circumstances are applicable:

1. The patient's trachea is still intubated. This should be the case if muscle relaxants and lingering anesthetic or narcotic effects depress ventilation.
2. The patient is extubated, awake, and breathing normally, but the pulse oximeter shows values that are reduced by about 3% (more or less, depending on the patient's condition and control values) below the preanesthetic values. Lung dysfunction (shunting) should be expected.

3. The patient continues to exhale $N_2O$. Remember that during an average case of $N_2O$ anesthesia, many liters of $N_2O$ are absorbed. When large volumes of $N_2O$ are exhaled, mostly during the first few minutes after the $N_2O$ flow meter is turned off, they replace $O_2$ and nitrogen in the lung; diffusion hypoxia is the consequence. Therefore, give $O_2$ during transport if $N_2O$ was given up until a few minutes before transport to the postanesthesia care unit. A gas analyzer shows how much $N_2O$ is left in the expired gas. If it is less than approximately 10%, diffusion hypoxia is not a concern.
4. Prolonged hyperventilation was used. A patient who had been hyperventilated for several hours will have depleted his tissue stores of dissolved $CO_2$. Instead of having to exhale $CO_2$ to maintain normal $PaCO_2$ values, much of the generated $CO_2$ is absorbed by the tissue.[23] Consequently, relatively low minute ventilation suffices to maintain the $PaCO_2$ within a normal range. Although this adjustment maintains normal $PaCO_2$, it may lead to inadequate oxygenation.
5. If you are aware of lung disease, surgery (eg, thoracotomy), tight bandages, or splinting secondary to pain and of their effects on ventilation. Give $O_2$ if you have any reason for concern.

Several devices are available. Most commonly used are nasal prongs, $O_2$ masks (not assuming a tight fit), and masks with reservoir bags. Table 32–6 shows approximate values of inspired $O_2$ with these devices for different flow rates of 100% $O_2$.

### *How Should Ventilation Be Supported?*

A patient who is apneic or hypoventilating should not simply be supplied with $O_2$ but should have ventilation actively controlled or assisted. For this purpose, several devices are available. Commonly used is the Mapleson D system, which requires a source of compressed $O_2$ (Fig. 32–5). Gas flow rates should be twice the patient's normal minute ventilation. In adults, this value is often not obtained: the patient's

**TABLE 32–6.** Approximate Values of Inspired Oxygen for Different Devices

| | 100% Oxygen (L/min) | Oxygen in Inspired Gas (%) |
|---|---|---|
| Nasal cannula or catheter | 1 | 24 |
| | 2 | 28 |
| | 3 | 32 |
| | 4 | 36 |
| | 5 | 40 |
| | 6 | 44 |
| Oxygen mask | 5-6 | 40 |
| | 6-7 | 50 |
| | 7-8 | 60 |
| Mask with reservoir | 6 | 60 |
| | 7 | 70 |
| | 8 | 80 |
| | 9 | 90 |
| | 10 | 99 |

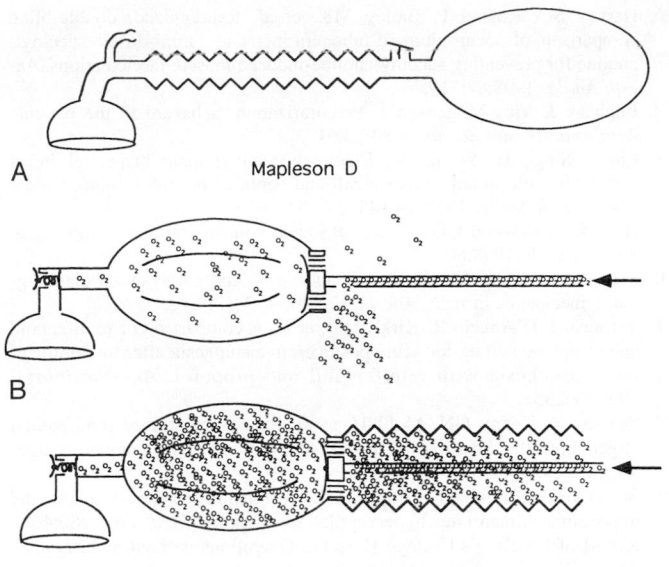

A    Mapleson D

B

C    Self-inflating  Resuscitation  Bag

**FIGURE 32–5.** Bags and mask used for manual ventilation during transport, shown at end of exhalation. *A,* The Mapleson D system requires relatively high flow rates of oxygen to prevent rebreathing. Without a source of compressed gas, this system cannot be used. *B and C,* The self-inflating devices can be used to ventilate a patient's lungs with ambient air. If the patient's inspired gas is to be enriched with oxygen, it is necessary to have the extension bellows (*C*) attached because the oxygen delivered by the oxygen tube does not blow directly into the bag; instead, it deposits in front of the intake valve, where it accumulates during expiration. Without the extension bellows, little extra oxygen is made available to the patient (*B*).

alveoli contain enough $O_2$, but some rebreathing of expired gas occurs, and the $Paco_2$ rises.

Alternatively, you can use a self-inflating resuscitation bag. This bag can be used without $O_2$ because it fills itself with air. However, patients with pulmonary disease may require an $O_2$-enriched atmosphere. To obtain significant concentrations of $O_2$ with such devices, the self-inflating bag must have a reservoir in which $O_2$ accumulates. Figure 32–5 shows this principle.

## AWARENESS DURING GENERAL ANESTHESIA

Many problems and some complications are associated with the administration of general anesthetics. One in particular, however, has been of particular interest almost since the first demonstration of the anesthetized state: awareness of intraoperative events by patients who supposedly were anesthetized.[24] The problem is not only medical, but medicolegal and has been the subject of ongoing study in the American Society of Anesthesiologists Closed Claims Project.[25] Two percent (69) of the first 3533 analyzed claims were related to patient recall of events (54 claims) and inadvertent paralysis of awake patients (15 claims). This incidence was similar to the rate of claims for myocardial infarction, aspiration pneumonia, back pain, and hepatic dysfunction after anesthesia.

### Why Does Awareness Occur?

Factors include failure to turn on the halogenated agent vaporizer, vaporizer malfunction, and failure to administer appropriate amounts of induction agents, all of which were thought to represent substandard care. However, cases of awareness also occurred in which the standard of care appeared to have been met. Risk factors in cases that resulted in malpractice claims included female sex, gynecologic/obstetric procedures, the intraoperative use of muscle relaxants and opioids, and the lack of a volatile anesthetic agent.[26] Hypertension and tachycardia, conditions that might be assumed to indicate the possibility of recall, although occasionally present, were absent in most cases.

### Can Recall Be Mistaken?

The aforementioned risk factors of female sex and gynecologic or obstetric procedures have been noted for more than 150 years and were described in an early anesthesiology textbook.[27] Apparently, medicolegal and criminal prosecution of anesthesia providers occurred not infrequently as a result of many perceived improprieties on their female patients. The following description of such a case appears to be typical of those that were reported[2]:

*The Boston Med. And Surg J, p. 287, November, 1858 gives an account of a case in Montreal, in which a dentist was tried for an alleged attempt to commit rape upon one of his patients to whom he had given chloroform. One of the witnesses for the defense testified that his own wife was fully impressed with the belief that she had been violated by the prisoner under the influence of chloroform, and she persisted in this delusion notwithstanding the fact that her husband was present during the whole period of anaesthesia. In spite of this and other testimony, the jury brought in a verdict of guilty of an attempt to commit rape, though they had the grace to join with it a recommendation to mercy.[27]*

In another case the following description appeared:

*A young woman had chloroform anesthesia administered to her by a doctor in the presence of a dentist and of the young lady's mother and father. After a tooth had been extracted, and the patient had become conscious, she steadfastly affirmed that she had been criminally assaulted by the dentist, and to this statement she adhered, although the 4 persons present in the room strove to disabuse her mind.[28]*

Cases such as this might be considered to be of historical interest only, if it were not for the fact that they still occur. One of us (RRK) served as an expert witness for the defense in an Air Force court martial of a male nurse anesthetist who was accused of almost identical criminal acts on female patients recovering from the effects of general anesthesia in the PACU. The defendant was found not guilty, but his career effectively was ruined.

Although it is clear that assault and rape of female patients by anesthesia personnel and other caregivers has occurred, it is disturbing to find that altered perception or dreaming in a "semianesthetized" state can result in accusations of malpractice and criminal activity that have no basis in fact. Although this problem has been addressed in numerous publications in the past,[27–29] it appears to have received less attention in recent years.[30]

## References

1. Gibby GL, Gravenstein JS, Layon AJ, et al. How often does the preoperative interview change anesthetic management? [abstract]. *Anesthesiology.* 1992;77:1174.
2. Lofgren RH, Montgomery WW. Incidence of laryngeal involvement in rheumatoid arthritics. *N Engl J Med.* 1962;267:193.
3. Gardner DL, Homes F. Anaesthetic and postoperative hazards in rheumatoid arthritis. *Br J Anaesth.* 1961;33:259.
4. Benumof JL, Benumof R. Critical hemoglobin desaturation will occur before return to an unparalyzed state following 1 mg/kg intravenous succinylcholine. *Anesthesiology.* 1997;87:979.
5. Baker AB, McGinn A, Joyce CJ. Effect on lung volumes of oxygen concentration when breathing is restricted. *Br J Anaesth.* 1993;70:259.
6. Preoxygenation: physiology and practice [editorial]. *Lancet.* 1992;339:31.
7. Valentine SJ, Marjot R, Monk CR. Preoxygenation in the elderly: a comparison of the four-maximal breath and three minute techniques. *Anesth Analg.* 1990;71:516.
8. Baraka A, Taha SK, Aouad M, et al. Preoxygenation: comparison of maximal breathing and tidal volume breathing techniques. *Anesthesiology.* 1999;91:612.
9. Wakeling HG, Butler PJ, Baxter PJC. The laryngeal mask airway: a comparison between two insertion techniques. *Anesth Analg.* 1997; 85:687.
10. Loper K, Reitan J, Bennet H, et al. Comparison of halothane and isoflurane for rapid anesthetic induction. *Anesth Analg.* 1987;66:766.
11. Sulek CA. Negative-pressure pulmonary edema. In: Gravenstein N, Kirby RR, eds. *Complications in Anesthesiology.* 2nd ed. Philadelphia, Pa: Lippincott-Raven; 1996:191.
12. Green CR, Pandit SK, Schork MA. Preoperative fasting time: is the traditional policy changing? Results of a national survey. *Anesth Analg.* 1996;83:123.
13. Mendelson CL. The aspiration of stomach contents into the lungs during obstetric anesthesia. *Am J Gynecol.* 1946;52:191.
14. Sellick BA. Cricoid pressure to control regurgitation of stomach contents during induction of anaesthesia. *Lancet.* 1961;2:404.
15. Brimacombe JR, Berry AM. Cricoid pressure: review article. *Can J Anaesth.* 1997;44:414.
16. Harvey SC, Roland P, Bailey MK, et al. Randomized, double-blind comparison of rocuronium, d-tubocurarine, and "mini-dose" succinylcholine for preventing succinylcholine-induced muscle fasciculations. *Anesth Analg.* 1998;87:719.
17. Engbeak J, Viby-Mogensen J. Precurarization: a hazard to the patient? *Acta Anaesthesiol Scand.* 1984;28:61.
18. Liu J, Singh H, White PF. Electroencephalographic bispectral index correlates with intraoperative recall and depth of propofol-induced sedation. *Anesth Analg.* 1997;84:185.
19. Hall JD, Lockwood GG. Bispectral index: comparison of two montages. *Br J Anaesth.* 1998;80:342.
20. Froese AB, Bryan AC. Effects of anesthesia and paralysis on diaphragmatic mechanics in man. *Anesthesiology.* 1974;41:242.
21. Yarmush J, D'Angelo R, Kirkhart B, et al. A comparison of remifentanil and morphine sulfate for acute postoperative analgesia after total intravenous anesthesia with remifentanil and propofol. *Anesthesiology.* 1997;87:235.
22. Schraag S, Kenny GN, Mohl U, et al. Patient-maintained remifentanil target-controlled infusion for the transition to early postoperative analgesia. *Br J Anaesth.* 1998;81:365.
23. Salvatore AJ, Sullivan SF, Papper EM. Postoperative hypoventilation and hypoxemia in man after hyperventilation. *N Engl J Med.* 1968;280:467.
24. Report of the King's College Hospital. Operations without pain. *Lancet.* 1847;1:77.
25. Domino KB, Posner KL, Caplan RA, et al. Awareness during general anesthesia: a closed claims analysis [abstract]. *Anesthesiology.* 1999;90:1053.
26. Domino KB. Closed malpractice claims for awareness during anesthesia. *ASA Newsletter.* 1996;60:14.
27. Lyman HM. *Artificial Anaesthesia and Anaesthetics.* New York, NY: William Wood & Co; 1881:93.
28. Gwathmey JT. *Anesthesia.* New York, NY: Macmillan; 1925:675.
29. Buxton DW. The medico-legal status of the anesthetist. In: Lewis HK, ed. *Anaesthetics: Their Use and Administration.* Philadelphia, Pa: P. Blakiston's Son & Co; 1920:636.
30. Jastak JT, Malamed SF. Nitrous oxide sedation and sexual phenomena. *J Am Dent Assoc.* 1980;101:38.

CHAPTER

# 33

# Intravenous Anesthetic Agents

Richard J. Rogers

Intravenous anesthetic agents are used in practically every anesthetic delivered by physicians, nurses, and physician-assistants in the United States—almost 27 million times per year. Therefore, knowledge of the special properties and indications of these agents is mandatory.

## PHARMACOKINETIC PROPERTIES OF INTRAVENOUS AGENTS

### What Pharmacokinetic Factors Affect Dosing of Intravenous Anesthetic Agents?

#### Volume of Distribution

By the nature of administration, intravenous anesthetic agents represent the simplest pharmacokinetic drug form because no absorption phase occurs, only distribution and elimination. The volume of distribution ($V_d$) of a drug is a hypothetical, apparent volume obtained in the following fashion. If a known amount of drug is injected into a patient, a sampling of the blood, after sufficient time for distribution, would produce a specific drug concentration by assay. Dividing the original drug dose by the measured drug concentration yields the $V_d$. Note that this calculation is predicated on the assumption that the drug distributes equally to all parts of the body.

The actual distribution of the administered drug within the body depends on other chemical and biologic features. Some of the salient features are inherent to the drug itself, whereas others are characteristics of the patient. Perhaps the most important factor determining distribution is the lipid solubility of the drug. Highly lipid-soluble drugs distribute more widely to lipid membranes and fatty tissues. At equilibrium, the concentration of a highly lipid-soluble drug (eg, fentanyl) in the blood is much lower than would be expected if its distribution were limited to the blood volume alone, as would be the case for a much more water-soluble drug (eg, atracurium). Thus, the apparent $V_d$ is many times larger than the predicted blood volume.

#### Protein Binding

The distribution of intravenous agents is a dynamic process dependent on the degree of protein binding. Recall that within the circulation, the principal proteins that bind drugs are albumin and $\alpha_1$-acid glycoprotein. High degrees of protein binding of a drug can outweigh fat solubility for lipid-soluble drugs, causing the $V_d$ to decrease because the drug does not easily leave the circulation.

## Redistribution and Equilibrium

Redistribution is the movement of drug from bound sites to unbound sites. This is usually considered to be a dynamic process in which drug moves away from sites of action (receptors) into the extracellular space and other tissues, usually through the blood. An equilibrium is eventually reached between bound and unbound drug (in both the tissues and blood). Movement from blood to tissues takes time, during which, if blood samples are analyzed, a higher concentration of the drug is found than would be predicted based simply on its $V_d$ and the dose administered. This movement is referred to as the *distribution phase* ($\alpha$-phase).

Figure 33–1 depicts two drugs given intravenously. Drug A is highly distributed, as evidenced by the long, sloping, initial part of the curve. Because we measure drug concentration in the blood compartment, we would expect that as the drug moves from the blood into other tissues, its concentration in the blood would decrease rapidly at first and then more slowly as tissue equilibrium is approached.

## Elimination: Clearance and Half-Life

Once blood and tissue equilibrium occurs, drug elimination by either metabolism or excretion accounts for the remainder of the curve. The elimination phase is the linear part of the log concentration versus time curve in Figure 33–1. The common log or natural log value is usually plotted against time. Because the decay is rapid, the decrease in concentration is an exponential function given by the following equation:

$$C_t = C_0 e^{-kt}$$

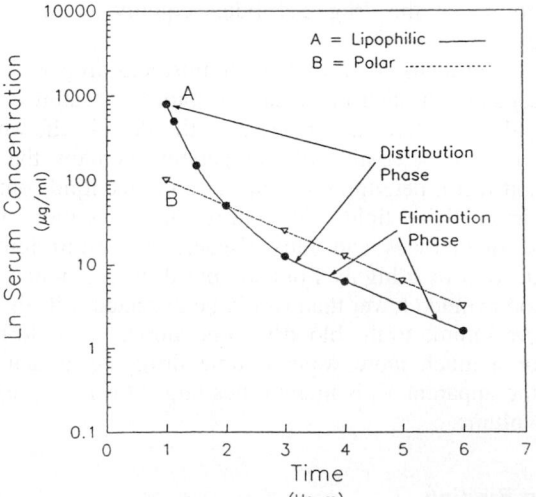

**FIGURE 33–1.** Lipophilic versus polar drug level profiles. *A*, Hypothetical lipophilic drug profile, with distribution phase and elimination phase. *B*, Polar drug profile with only elimination phase.

**TABLE 33–1.** Dose Range, Lipid Solubility, and Half-Life of Several Intravenous Anesthetic Agents

| Agent | Dose Range (mg/kg) | Lipid Solubility | Half-Life (h) |
|---|---|---|---|
| Thiopental | 3–5 | High | 6.4–7.6 |
| Methohexital | 1–1.5 | High | 1.8–6 |
| Propofol | 1–2 | High | 1.1–6.6 |
| Etomidate | 0.3–0.5 | High | 1.8–4 |
| Ketamine | 0.5–1.5 | High | 2–3 |
| Midazolam | 0.1–0.4 | Medium | 1.9–3.5 |
| Diazepam | 0.3–0.6 | Medium | 32.4–60.8 |
| Lorazepam | 0.5–1 | Medium | 11–22 |
| Morphine | 0.1–0.5 | Low | 1–2.2 |
| Meperidine | 1–5 | High | 3.2–4.4 |
| Fentanyl | 0.001–0.075 | High | 3.1–4.4 |
| Sufentanil | 0.0001–0.005 | High | 2.7 |
| Alfentanil | 0.0005–0.1 | Low | 0.5–1 |
| Remifentanil | 0.0005–0.001 | High | 0.2–0.8 |

where $C_t$ represents the concentration of a drug at a given time, $C_0$ is the initial concentration, $-k$ is a rate constant, and $t$ is the half-life. By plotting the common log or natural log values of these concentrations, we convert a curve to nearly a straight line. The slope of the latter part of this line then represents the elimination constant for the drug, which is inversely proportional to the half-life.

Drug B has little or no distribution (see Fig. 33–1), as might occur with a water-soluble agent. Table 33–1 lists several commonly used intravenous anesthetic agents, their usual dose ranges for single-bolus administration, their relative lipid solubility, and the half-life of their terminal elimination phase ($\beta$ – phase).

## *What Factors Alter Clearance?*

### Ionization

Clearance is dependent on the $V_d$ elimination constant. As mentioned earlier, the $V_d$ of a drug is dependent on its relative lipid solubility, the degree of protein binding, and its ionization. Ionization has an important role. Drugs are generally more soluble in the ionized state; however, they are usually not cleared from the body as well because they have difficulty crossing cell membranes. They also tend to be more protein bound and are thus less available to their target tissues.

Weak acids, such as sodium thiopental, are more ionized and more protein bound in a basic medium. Because a smaller amount of the drug is able to cross cell membranes, the drug effect is diminished. For example, patients maintained in an alkalotic state during hyperventilation therapy for closed head injury have less effect from similar levels of sodium thiopental than do nonalkalotic subjects. Increased ionization results in less drug available to cross into the brain. Conversely, on termination of hyperventilation therapy, as the blood becomes less alkalotic, more drug is available for both therapeutic effect and clearance. Table 33–2 gives the measure of acid strength ($pK_a$), protein binding, and acid-base characteristics of several commonly used intravenous agents.

**TABLE 33–2.** Chemical Properties of Several Intravenous Anesthetic Agents

| Agent | pKa | Type | Protein Bound (%) |
|---|---|---|---|
| Thiopental | 7.6 | Acid | 85 |
| Methohexital | 7.9 | Acid | 73 |
| Propofol | 11.0 | Acid | 98 |
| Etomidate | 4.2 | Base | 75 |
| Ketamine | 7.5 | Base | 12 |
| Midazolam | 6.2 | Base | 96 |
| Diazepam | 3.5 | Base | 98 |
| Lorazepam | 11.5 | Base | 97 |
| Morphine | 7.9 | Base | 36 |
| Meperidine | 7.9 | Base | 82 |
| Fentanyl | 8.4 | Base | 87 |
| Sufentanil | 8.0 | Base | 93 |
| Alfentanil | 6.5 | Base | 92 |
| Remifentanil | 7.07 | Base | Not available |

## Drug Interactions

Several other factors should be considered when assessing or predicting drug clearance. Considerable potential exists for drug interactions during the administration of anesthesia. First, patients often have concomitant medical conditions requiring medications. The conduct of anesthesia is by its nature polypharmacy. Finally, by acutely depressing central nervous system (CNS) responses, anesthetics may inhibit protective reflexes.

Drug interactions come in many forms. Adverse interactions may result from physicochemical incompatibilities between drugs or intravenous fluids. Acidic drugs (eg, barbiturates) dissolved in a basic solution may precipitate as the free acid if mixed with a drug in a basic medium (ie, nondepolarizing muscle relaxants).

Anesthetic agents may affect the elimination of other drugs by altering the delivery of drug to the liver (ie, hepatic blood flow) or hepatic enzymes (ie, enzymatic induction or inhibition). For example, potent inhalational anesthetics are known to reduce liver blood flow and to prolong the clearance of drugs such as lidocaine, which is metabolized primarily by the liver and may have a prolonged duration of action in hepatic failure.

Drug interactions may affect pharmacodynamics when one drug increases (or decreases) the reactivity to another, owing to actions on similar membrane receptors or organ systems. Interactions involving CNS depressant drugs, such as intravenous anesthetic agents (eg, narcotics and benzodiazepines), are among the most commonly seen by the anesthesiologist.

## Metabolism

Drug metabolism may be increased by enzyme induction. Certain enzymes are modulated and can increase their function, thus increasing clearance of some agents. An example of this type is the accelerated clearance of muscle relaxants when a patient takes anticonvulsants such as phenobarbital or phenytoin. These agents increase the metabolic rate of the cytochrome $P_{450}$ enzymes in the liver, which is responsible for metabolizing vecuronium and thus shortening its duration of action for any given dose. Enzyme induction generally takes days to weeks to occur; hence, it is not usually a concern after the acute administration of barbiturates.

## INTRAVENOUS ANESTHETIC AGENTS

### What Are the Properties of an "Ideal" Intravenous Anesthetic?

If the ideal intravenous anesthetic agent were to exist, it would likely have the following properties. It would be stable in aqueous solution with an unlimited shelf-life. Parenteral injection would cause no tissue or organ injury owing to its solubility in the innocuous vehicle, water. It would also be nonallergenic. After intravenous injection, the ideal anesthetic agent would provide rapid, smooth onset of hypnosis, amnesia, and analgesia, all reversible with a specific antagonist. Metabolism to inactive products would be rapid and complete. Adverse effects, such as cardiopulmonary depression and postoperative side effects (nausea and vomiting), would be negligible. In addition, the drug itself would offer cerebral protection by decreasing cerebral metabolic rate of oxygen consumption ($CMRo_2$), cerebral blood volume, and intracranial pressure (ICP).

None of the intravenous anesthetic drugs described in this chapter qualify as an ideal agent. All have qualities, however, which can be used to achieve the desired anesthetic results, when chosen properly.

### What Are the Different Classes of Available Intravenous Anesthetics?

The available intravenous anesthetics can be divided as follows: barbiturates, benzodiazepines, ketamine, etomidate, propofol, and narcotics. None of the available intravenous anesthetic agents provides the five characteristics of a complete anesthetic: hypnosis, amnesia, analgesia, muscle relaxation, and modulation of autonomic hemodynamic and endocrine responses. Many of these agents, however, have characteristics that are optimum in certain patients under certain situations. The real challenge is to match the patient with the correct dose of the best anesthetic agent.

### How Does One Choose Among All the Different Agents?

For most healthy patients, any of the available intravenous agents could be used for the induction of anesthesia. For many patients with coexisting disease states, however, it may be crucial to choose the correct drug. Typically, diseases of the cardiac or pulmonary system influence the choice of anesthetic. Other conditions, such as an intracranial mass with increased ICP or a surgical procedure particularly prone to cause postoperative nausea and vomiting, may make the anesthesiologist avoid or favor an individual intravenous agent. A thorough knowledge of the available pharmacologic agents is the basis for sorting out the answer to this question.[1]

## Why Have Barbiturates Been Used in Clinical Practice So Long?

Despite being used in clinical practice since the 1950s, barbiturates are still considered by many to be the gold standard against which all new agents are compared. The combination of their desirable anesthetic effects and safety record make it unlikely that barbiturates will be completely replaced in the anesthesiologist's drug cart anytime soon.

## Mechanism of Action

It appears there are multiple sites and more than one mechanism of action. The actions of barbiturates can be summarized as two general types of effects at specific synapses: (1) facilitation of enhancement of the synaptic actions of inhibitory neurotransmitters (eg, γ-aminobutyric acid [GABA]); and (2) blockade of the synaptic actions of excitatory neurotransmitters (eg, acetylcholine and L-glutamate). The end result of these effects is the depression of the reticular activating system and, thus, hypnosis and amnesia.

## Physicochemical Properties and Pharmacokinetics

Barbiturates in clinical practice can be subdivided into two major groups: the oxybarbiturates and the thiobarbiturates, based on the substitution of the oxygen at the C2 position with a sulfur. The substitution with a sulfur atom confers higher lipid solubility and a more rapidly acting drug (eg, thiopental). Addition of a methyl group in the C3 position of methohexital creates a fairly rapidly acting drug with fairly rapid recovery but with a high incidence of excitatory phenomenon.

Barbiturates are weak acids (thiopental $pK_a$, 7.6; methohexital, $pK_a$, 7.9) that are also highly protein bound (70%-80%). They are both lipid soluble with a short distribution (α-phase) half-life (thiopental, 8 minutes; methohexital, 5 minutes) but with different elimination (β-phase, hepatic metabolism) half-lives (thiopental, 11 hours; methohexital, 4 hours). Drug redistribution is the basis for the short duration of effect and is most responsible for the clinical utility of barbiturates.[2]

## Pharmacodynamics

In sufficient doses, barbiturates produce CNS depression that is termed *general anesthesia* and is attended by loss of consciousness (hypnosis) and amnesia. Although the response to pain and other noxious stimulation during general anesthesia appears to be obtunded, results of pain studies (tibial pressure in human beings) reveal that barbiturates may actually decrease the pain threshold.[3] This antianalgesic effect occurs only at low blood levels of barbiturates, such as with small induction doses of thiopental or after emergence from thiopental when the blood levels are low.

When given as a bolus, barbiturates decrease the mean arterial pressure (MAP) and cardiac output, primarily owing to depression of the medullary vasomotor center with a reflex increase in heart rate, but also increase the systemic vascular resistance (SVR). The effect on central venous pressure is variable, but most agree that peripheral venous dilation causes venous pooling and a reduction in venous return, which in turn reduces cardiac output and MAP.

Barbiturates depress the medullary ventilatory center, resulting in a reduction of tidal volume and apnea. The depth of narcosis at which apnea occurs depends not only on the dose of barbiturate but also, to a great extent, on any premedication used and any painful stimulus at the time.

Induction doses of thiopental may suppress the adrenal cortex and decrease plasma cortisol levels. Unlike etomidate, however, the adrenal suppression is rapidly reversible and responds to adrenocorticotropic hormone stimulation.

### Methohexital Sodium (Brevital)

Methohexital is supplied as a freeze-dried, sterile, nonpyrogenic mixture of methohexital sodium with 6% anhydrous sodium carbonate added as a buffer in vials of 500 mg, which can be reconstituted in 50 mL of sterile water, 5% dextrose in water ($D_5W$), or normal saline for a concentration of 10 mg/mL. It is recommended that reconstituted vials not be used after 24 hours.

Methohexital is used as an induction agent, for supplementation of regional anesthesia, and as the sole anesthetic for minimally painful procedures (eg, cardioversion).

**Suggested Dosing**
- Sedation
  IV, 0.25 to 1 mg/kg
- Induction
  IV, 1.5 to 2.5 mg/kg
  IM, 7 to 10 mg/kg
  Rectal, 20 to 30 mg/kg; 5% aqueous solution for children (500 mg injectate powder in 10 mL sterile water given through a well-lubricated catheter)
- Infusion
  50 to 150 μg/kg/min (0.2% solution; 500 mg in 250 mL of $D_5W$ or NS for a concentration of 2 mg/mL). Do not administer intravenously in a concentration >1% (10 mg/mL).

### Thiopental Sodium (Pentothal)

Thiopental is supplied as a mixture of sterilized, yellow-white, hygroscopic powder of thiopental sodium (91.7%) with anhydrous sodium carbonate as a buffer. When reconstituted in sterile water as a 2.5% weight per volume (w/v) solution, it is strongly alkaline (pH 10.5) and stable at room temperature for 24 hours. Thiopental should not be used intravenously in concentrations exceeding 25 mg/mL.

Thiopental is used as an induction agent, for supplementation of regional anesthesia, as an anticonvulsant, for reduction of elevated ICP, and for cerebral protection (barbiturate narcosis).

**Suggested Dosing**
- Induction
  IV, 3 to 5 mg/kg (children, 5-6 mg/kg; infants, 7-8 mg/kg)
- Anesthesia supplementation
  IV, 0.5 to 1 mg/kg
- Anticonvulsant
  IV, 0.5 to 2 mg/kg, repeat as necessary
- Reduction in ICP
  IV, 1 to 4 mg/kg
- Barbiturate narcosis
  IV bolus, 8 mg/kg as needed to maintain electroencepha-

logram (EEG) burst suppression (mean total dose, 40 mg/kg)

Infusion, 0.05 to 0.35 mg/kg/min; inotropic support required at high doses

### Adverse Effects and Precautions

Premedication with opioids decreases the incidence of excitatory phenomena associated with induction doses of barbiturates, particularly with methohexital.[4] It is recommended that the dosage be reduced in elderly, hypovolemic, hypertensive, uremic, septicemic, and high-risk surgical patients, especially when used concomitantly with narcotics or other sedative hypnotics.

Extravascular injection of barbiturates may cause necrosis, and intraarterial injection may cause gangrene. It is advised to treat inadvertent intraarterial injection by injecting the artery with 10 mL of 1% procaine, 40 to 80 mg of dilute solution of papaverine, or local infiltration of phentolamine (2.5-5 mg in 10 mL) to produce vasodilation. Sympathectomy may be necessary and can be achieved by stellate ganglion block or brachial plexus block.

Barbiturates are contraindicated in patients with latent or manifest porphyria (acute intermittent porphyria, variegate porphyria, and hereditary coproporphyria).

## How Can Benzodiazepines Be Used for Induction of Anesthesia?

Unlike barbiturates, which are used principally to cause hypnosis, benzodiazepines are used in clinical practice for their anxiolytic and amnestic properties. Alone, benzodiazepines would need to be used in large doses to obtain the level of anesthesia similar to an equipotent dose of sodium thiopental. Benzodiazepines are usually used as a premedicant to take advantage of the powerful amnesia and anxiolysis obtained with even small doses. When combined with narcotics, benzodiazepines can be part of a complete anesthetic, causing hypnosis, amnesia, and analgesia as a consequence of their synergism.

### Mechanism of Action

Benzodiazepines act on specific receptor sites throughout the brain and spinal cord. Radioisotope-binding studies have shown these to be most dense in the cerebral cortex, the hippocampus, and the cerebellum. Their effect is produced by the potentiation of certain inhibitory interneurons, which use the neurotransmitter GABA. On release of GABA in the synapse, an increase in the flow of $Cl^-$ ions into the target neuron occurs, resulting in hyperpolarization. The nerve cell is thus made more refractory to any excitatory impulse. In the spinal cord, benzodiazepines cause increased availability of glycine, which acts as an inhibitory neurotransmitter. Benzodiazepines cause dose-related cerebral depression with increasing doses. All of these drugs can cause mild sedation, drowsiness, and even hypnosis. Certain pharmacokinetic differences determine the time of onset of intravenous benzodiazepines, but in anesthetic practice, these are less important than their metabolism, particularly their breakdown to active metabolites and the duration of action of both the parent compound and the metabolite.

### Physicochemical Properties and Pharmacokinetics

Benzodiazepines are all weak bases (diazepam $pK_a$ 3.5; lorazepam $pK_a$, 11.5; diazolam $pK_a$, 6.2) with high degrees of protein binding (diazepam, 98.7%; lorazepam, 97%; midazolam, 96%). The distribution ($\alpha$-phase) half-lives (diazepam, 30-60 minutes; lorazepam, 15-20 minutes; midazolam, 3-5 minutes) and the elimination ($\beta$-phase) half-lives of benzodiazepines in clinical practice vary considerably (diazepam, 20-50 hours [3 active metabolites]; lorazepam, 11-22 hours [no active metabolites]; midazolam, 1.7-2.6 hours [4 inactive metabolites] all metabolized in the liver with renal excretion).

Because the metabolism of lorazepam is not entirely dependent on the hepatic microsomal enzymes, its elimination is less likely (compared with diazepam) to be prolonged by alterations in hepatic function, age, or drugs such as cimetidine.

### Pharmacodynamics

All benzodiazepines produce in dose-related fashion anxiolytic, sedative, hypnotic, amnesic, muscle relaxant, and anticonvulsant effects, presumably by facilitation of the inhibitory action of GABA or glycine on neuronal transmission. All also decrease the $CMRO_2$, cerebral blood flow (CBF), and ICP.

Benzodiazepines decrease MAP slightly as a result of a decrease in SVR with a modest increase in heart rate. More dramatic changes are seen with midazolam, possibly because of its high potency and rapid onset. It is recommended to reduce doses in elderly, hypovolemic, high-risk patients and in those with concomitant use of other sedatives or narcotics. Unexpected hypotension and respiratory depression may occur when given with opioids, particularly in the elderly or patients with other medical conditions; hence, smaller doses should be considered.

Modest respiratory depression occurs with all of the benzodiazepines; patients with chronic obstructive pulmonary disease are unusually sensitive to the respiratory depressant effects.

### Diazepam (Valium)

Diazepam is a colorless, crystalline base that is insoluble in water. The formulation available for intravenous injection (Valium) contains 5 mg/mL in an aqueous vehicle composed of organic solvents consisting mainly of propylene glycol, ethyl alcohol, and sodium benzoate. Inject slowly through large veins to reduce the incidence of thrombophlebitis. Do not mix or dilute with other solutions or drugs.

Diazepam is used for premedication and amnesia, as a sedative-hypnotic, as an induction agent, for skeletal muscle relaxation, as an anticonvulsant, and for treatment of acute alcohol withdrawal.

#### Suggested Dosing
- Premedication and sedation
    IV, IM, PO, and rectal, 2 to 10 mg (0.1-0.2 mg/kg)
- Induction
    IV, 0.3 to 0.5 mg/kg
- Anticonvulsant
    IV, 0.05 to 0.2 mg/kg every 10 to 15 minutes; maximal dose, 30 mg
    PO and rectal, 2 to 10 mg 2 to 4 times daily

- Withdrawal
    IV, 5 to 10 mg (0.15-0.2 mg/kg) every 3 to 4 hours
    PO, 5 to 10 mg 3 or 4 times daily

### Lorazepam (Ativan)

Lorazepam is a nearly white powder almost insoluble in water. Each milliliter of injection contains either 2 or 4 mg of lorazepam and 0.18 mL polyethylene glycol in propylene glycol with 2.0% benzyl alcohol as a preservative. Refrigerate the injection at 2° to 8°C and protect from light and freezing.

Lorazepam is used for premedication and amnesia, as an induction agent, as an anticonvulsant, for treatment of acute alcohol withdrawal, and for chemotherapy-induced or postoperative nausea and vomiting.

#### Suggested Dosing
- Sedation
    IV and IM, 1 to 4 mg (0.002-0.08 mg/kg); it is recommended to dilute before IV administration with equal volume of $D_5W$ or NS. For IM injection, use undiluted solution.
    PO, 2 to 3 mg 2 or 3 times a day (elderly patients, 1-2 mg in divided doses)
- Induction
    IV, 0.5 to 1 mg/kg
- Antiemetic
    IV, 0.5 to 0.1 mg (0.01-0.02 mg/kg)
    PO, 1 to 2 mg 2 or 3 times a day

### Midazolam HCl (Versed)

Midazolam is unique among the benzodiazepines in that it possesses the chemical property of a pH-dependent solubility. At a pH of <4.0, midazolam exists in an open-ring, water-soluble configuration. At pH values above 4.0, however, the ring closes, and the drug becomes highly lipid soluble. The drug is formulated in aqueous solution buffered to a pH of about 3.5 (may burn when injected in a small-caliber intravenous catheter). Because its $pK_a$ is 6.0, at the physiologic pH of 7.4, midazolam is largely un-ionized, as well as highly lipid soluble, and thus rapidly crosses the blood-brain barrier and other blood-tissue barriers.

Midazolam is used for premedication and amnesia, for conscious sedation, as an induction agent, and for supplementation of anesthesia.[5]

#### Suggested Dosing
- Premedication
    IM, 2.5 to 10 mg (0.05-0.2 mg/kg)
    PO, 0.5 mg/kg (maximum, 10 mg). Use high-potency injectate solution (5 mg/mL). Dilute in 3 to 5 mL of clear juice (may need extra sugar; solution is bitter) or 5 mL of ibuprofen (Pediaprofen) for postoperative analgesia. Some may add atropine, 0.03 mg/kg PO, to reduce secretions.
    Intranasal, 0.2 to 0.3 mg/kg. Use high-potency injectate solution (5 mg/mL).
    Rectal, 0.3 to 0.35 mg/kg. Dilute in 5 mL of NS.
- Conscious sedation
    IV, 0.5 to 5 mg (0.025-1.0 mg/kg). Titrate slowly to the desired effect (eg, slurred speech), monitoring cardiac and respiratory function continuously. Infusion, 1 to

15 mg/h (20-300 µg/kg/h) with same monitoring; respiratory support may be required.
- Induction
    IV, 50 to 350 µg/kg
    Infusion, 0.25 to 5 µg/kg/min
- Anticonvulsant
    IV/IM, 2 to 5 mg (0.025-0.1 mg/kg) every 10 to 15 minutes as needed

#### Adverse Effects and Precautions

Benzodiazepines are contraindicated in patients with acute narrow-angle or open-angle glaucoma unless they are receiving the appropriate therapy.

Respiratory depression and arrest may occur when used for conscious sedation, especially when combined with other agents (opioids, propofol), particularly in elderly, hypovolemic, high-risk surgical patients and in patients with chronic obstructive pulmonary disease.

### Flumazenil (Romazicon)

Flumazenil is a benzodiazepine receptor antagonist with little or no agonist activity. It competitively inhibits the binding of benzodiazepines at the benzodiazepine recognition site on the GABA-benzodiazepine receptor complex and reverses sedation, respiratory depression, amnesia, and psychomotor effects of benzodiazepines. The administration of flumazenil to patients given agonists is remarkably free of cardiovascular effects, unlike opioid reversal with naloxone. Resedation may occur and is more common with larger doses of benzodiazepines and long procedures. Flumazenil produces withdrawal symptoms (seizures, emergent confusion, and agitation) in the presence of physical dependence.

#### Suggested Dosing
- IV bolus, 0.2 to 1 mg (4-20 µg/kg) at a rate of 0.2 mg/min. Titrate to patient response. May repeat at 20-minute intervals. Maximal single dose, 1 mg. Maximal total dose, 3 mg in any one hour. Lack of patient response at 5 minutes after cumulative dose above 5 mg implies that the major cause of sedation is unlikely to be benzodiazepines.

## Why Has Propofol Become So Popular in Ambulatory Anesthesia?

Ambulatory surgery and anesthesia continue to account for an increasing amount of the cases performed in the United States. With the need to have patients ready to leave the hospital or surgical center within hours of surgery, newer anesthetic agents were necessary to meet this need. Propofol combines the right mix of anesthetic characteristics to fulfill many of these needs.

Propofol is a hindered phenol, which is chemically dissimilar to any other compounds used in anesthesia. It is insoluble in water and is currently available as a 1% w/v aqueous emulsion containing 10% w/v soy bean oil, 1.2% w/v egg phosphatide (lecithin), and 2.25% w/v glycerol with a pH of 6 to 8.5. It should be stored at 4° to 22°C. Refrigeration is not recommended. Shake well before use. The soybean-fat emulsion vehicle of propofol supports rapid growth of bacteria, and thus strict aseptic technique must be maintained during handling. The ampule should be discarded after a single use and the drug administered within 6 hours after the ampule has been opened. There is no preservative.

Propofol may be used for conscious sedation, as an induction agent, and for maintenance of anesthesia.[6,7]

## Mechanism of Action

Several studies have demonstrated that propofol enhances synaptic inhibition mediated by $GABA_A$, much like barbiturates and benzodiazepines. However, each individual anesthetic agent causes qualitatively different patterns of $GABA_A$-mediated synaptic inhibition and consequently on the firing pattern of neurons. Although the $GABA_A$ receptor-ion channel complex is involved in the anesthetic state, no uniform action of anesthetics at the molecular level can explain the anesthetic action. Thus, it would appear that the actions of general anesthetics are amazingly complex.

## Physicochemical Properties and Pharmacokinetics

Propofol is a weak acid ($pK_a$, 11) with a significant amount of protein binding (98%). The distribution ($\alpha$-phase) half-life is 2 to 8 minutes, and the elimination ($\beta$-phase) half-life is 4 to 7 hours, with propofol undergoing hepatic and extrahepatic (pulmonary) metabolism. In extremely hypoalbuminemic patients, propofol (much like any drug with a high degree of protein binding) has an enhanced effect. The key pharmacokinetic parameter responsible for the rapid offset of the action of propofol, compared with sodium thiopental or methohexital, is its faster clearance,[8] demonstrated in Figure 33–2.

### Suggested Dosing
- Sedation
  IV bolus, 25 to 50 mg (0.5-1 mg/kg); titrate slowly to the desired effect (eg, onset of slurred speech).

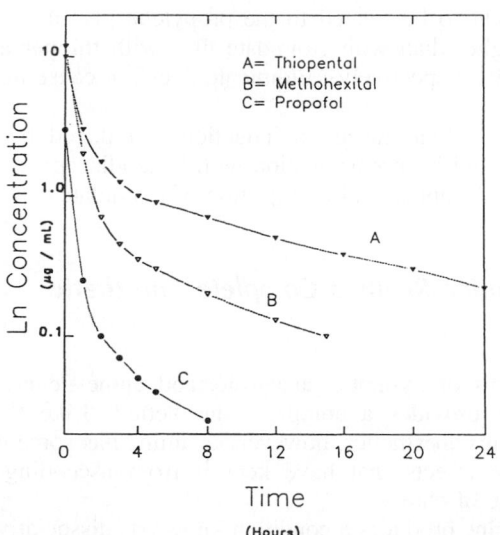

**FIGURE 33–2.** Thiopental, methohexital, and propofol level profiles. *A*, Thiopental level profile for a single dose, 6.1 mg/kg, intravenous (IV). *B*, Methohexital level profile for a single dose, 2.9 mg/kg, IV. *C*, Propofol level profile for a single dose, 2.5 mg/kg, IV. (Adapted from Cockshott ID. Propofol pharmacokinetics and metabolism: an overview. *Postgrad Med J*. 1985;61:45–50 and Hudson RJ, Stanski DR, Burch PG. Pharmacokinetics of methohexital and thiopental in surgical patients. *Anesthesiology*. 1981;59:215–219.)

Infusion, 20 to 75 $\mu$g/kg/min, monitoring respiratory and cardiac function continuously
- Anesthetic induction
  IV, 2 to 2.5 mg/kg (give slowly over 30 seconds in 2-3 divided doses)
- Anesthetic maintenance
  IV bolus, 25 to 50 mg
  Infusion, 100 to 200 $\mu$g/kg/min
- Antiemetic
  IV, 10 mg

## Pharmacodynamics

Propofol decreases the $CMR_{O_2}$, CBF, and ICP but may significantly decrease cerebral perfusion pressure owing to its effect on MAP. It causes minimal excitatory activity (myoclonus) compared with etomidate. The proconvulsant effects of propofol may represent activation of epileptogenic foci, whereas the anticonvulsant effects are most likely due to nonspecific cortical depression, rather than elevation of seizure threshold.

Propofol directly depresses myocardial contractility and decreases SVR, resulting in hypotension (decreased MAP 15%-31%, even in patients without cardiovascular disease) as a result of the decreased cardiac output and decreased SVR.[9]

Single induction doses of propofol (2 mg/kg) cause a profound reduction of tidal volume with a period of apnea varying from 30 to 60 seconds. The incidence of apnea approaches 100% when administered with premedication (narcotics or benzodiazepines). Propofol has no effect on resting bronchomotor tone but does significantly depress laryngeal reflexes much more than barbiturates or etomidate.

Propofol does not cause significant hepatic enzyme derangements and, compared with other agents (particularly etomidate), causes less nausea and vomiting. In fact, propofol probably has intrinsic antiemetic effects. Similar to thiopental, propofol has no significant effect on adrenocortical function.

### Adverse Effects and Precautions
As with other intravenous agents, it is recommended that the doses be reduced in elderly, hypovolemic, and high-risk surgical patients with concomitant use of narcotics and sedative hypnotics.

Pain frequently occurs on injection into small veins (especially on the dorsum of the hand). Methods to minimize the pain include injecting into a large vein, mixing intravenous lidocaine (0.1 mg/kg) with the dose of propofol, or both. Other premedicants, such as small doses of fentanyl (50-100 $\mu$g) or ketamine (50 $\mu$g), can lessen the pain on injection. The incidence of venous thrombophlebitis is much less common with the current formulation (previous Cremophor preparation was much more irritating).

Histamine release may occur with rapid injection, and allergic reactions may likely manifest as anaphylaxis. The use of propofol is contraindicated in patients allergic to eggs or soybeans.

Compared with thiopental, induction doses of propofol may be associated with high umbilical vein concentrations, muscular hypotonia, and lower neonatal Apgar scores at 1 and 5 minutes. Therefore, it should be used with caution during cesarean section.

## Why Has Etomidate Not Become the Intravenous Agent of Choice?

When etomidate was initially released, many thought that it would become the anesthetic induction agent of choice principally because of its lack of cardiovascular or pulmonary adverse effects[10]; however, the drug has enough negative adverse effects to have kept it from dislodging sodium thiopental from the premier spot.

Etomidate, chemically unrelated to any other induction agent used in anesthesia, is a pure hypnotic with no analgesic properties. It is supplied as a white crystalline salt powder, which is soluble in water but unstable in aqueous solution. Only the dextro (+) isomer is pharmacologically active as a hypnotic. The only formulation currently available in the United States is a 2 mg/mL solution in a 35% propylene glycol vehicle. This formulation has a pH of 6.9. Etomidate appears to be compatible in intravenous solution with all medications commonly used during induction, except for vecuronium.

### Mechanism of Action

Etomidate emulates the CNS inhibitory neurotransmitter, GABA, and depresses the reticular activating system. It has disinhibitory effects on parts of the CNS that control extrapyramidal motor activity.

Etomidate can be used for induction and supplementation of anesthesia.

### Physicochemical Properties and Pharmacokinetics

Etomidate is a weak base ($pK_a$, 4.2) with a moderate degree of protein binding (75%). The distribution ($\alpha$-phase) half-life is 3 minutes, and the elimination ($\beta$-phase) half-life is 3 to 5 hours.

#### Suggested Dosing

- IV induction, 0.1 to 0.4 mg/kg
- Infusion, 0.25 to 1 mg/min (5-20 $\mu$g/kg/min)
- Rectal, in children 6 months to 6 years old, 6.5 mg/kg produces reliable hypnosis in 4 minutes but maintains a rapid recovery without any untoward effects. The manufacturer's package insert does not recommend use in children younger than 10 years old because of the lack of adequate data for dosage recommendations.

### Pharmacodynamics

Etomidate decreases the $CMR_{O_2}$, CBF, and ICP. Because of its minimal effect on systemic blood pressure, it is more successful than thiopental or propofol in maintaining cerebral perfusion pressure. Etomidate appears to lower the seizure threshold in individuals with focal seizure disorders, but acts similar to thiopental as a protectant against generalized seizure activity. Myoclonic movements occur in about one third of patients during induction and are due to disinhibition of subcortical suppression of extrapyramidal activity. A potentially significant disadvantage of etomidate is its lack of analgesic efficacy; thus, it does not blunt any transient sympathetic response to endotracheal intubation.

Etomidate causes the least hemodynamic changes of any induction agent, with minimal decreases in heart rate, MAP, and SVR.

Induction doses of etomidate usually do not result in apnea unless other drugs (narcotics or sedatives) are administered, even in poor-risk patients with cardiac and pulmonary disease.[11] The mean duration of apnea after an induction dose of 0.3 mg/kg is 20 seconds. Excitatory effects of coughing, vocalization, and hiccoughing are seen in about 10% of patients given etomidate.

Postoperative nausea and vomiting can occur in up to 30% to 40% of patients. This incidence compares with an incidence of 10% to 20% with methohexital and thiopental and even less with propofol. The diffusible fraction of etomidate increases in hepatic and renal disease; thus, the induction dose may need to be decreased.

Adrenocortical suppression of both cortisol and aldosterone production, which may occur after a single induction dose, is predominantly due to etomidate-induced inhibition of the enzyme, 11-$\beta$ — hydroxylase.[12] The relative reduction of cortisol and aldosterone levels starts about 30 minutes after a single induction dose and lasts 5 to 15 hours. However, a single dose use of etomidate has not been shown to have adverse clinical effects as a result of its transient inhibition of corticosteroid synthesis. The only reports of clinically important consequences of etomidate on corticosteroid production have been when used by continuous infusion for days or weeks in the intensive care unit setting.[13] If concern exists regarding adrenal suppression by etomidate, cortisone can be administered to protect against ongoing stress.

#### Adverse Effects and Precautions

It is recommended to use large veins for injection of etomidate because pain frequently occurs (up to 62% of patients) and is more likely if etomidate is injected rapidly into small veins. Comparative studies have demonstrated that propofol and methohexital have a similar or slightly lower incidence of pain on injection, whereas pain with thiopental injection is much less common. The incidence of venous thrombophlebitis, thought to be related to the propylene glycol vehicle, is much higher than with etomidate than with thiopental (24% versus 4%, respectively). Etomidate does not cause histamine release.

The myoclonus seen on induction is reduced by slower injection and by premedication with benzodiazepines or opioids 1 to 2 minutes before injection of etomidate.

## Is Ketamine Really a Complete Anesthetic Agent?

In terms of hypnotic, analgesic, and amnestic properties, ketamine provides a complete anesthetic.[14] Like the other intravenous anesthetics, however, ketamine has some undesirable side effects that have kept it from ascending to the anesthetic of choice.

Ketamine produces a condition known as dissociative anesthesia, which is quite different from conventional anesthesia. It is characterized by catalepsy, light sedation, amnesia, and marked analgesia. This state has been described as "a dissociation of the limbic from the thalamoneocortical systems."[15]

Ketalar is supplied as a solution for injection in concentrations of 10 mg/mL, 50 mg/mL, and 100 mg/mL. It should be stored at room temperature (15°-30°C) and protected from light and heat. Avoid mixing with barbiturates in same syringe because precipitates may form.

Ketamine is used for induction and maintenance of anesthesia, especially in the hypovolemic or high-risk patient, as well as the sole anesthetic for short surgical procedures.[16]

## Mechanism of Action

Ketamine likely interacts with more than one type of pharmacologic receptor to produce its effects. The analgesia appears to be at least partially mediated by opioid receptors at the brain, spinal cord, and peripheral sites. Ketamine binds preferentially to the μ, rather than the δ, opioid receptor. Ketamine has been shown to interact with σ, which may mediate the dysphoria that can be induced by ketamine. Ketamine has been shown to be a potent, noncompetitive, N-methyl-D-aspartate (NMDA) receptor antagonist. NMDA inhibition produces catalepsy, consistent with the effect of ketamine administration. It is suggested that this may be the mechanism for its anesthetic and behavioral effects.

## Physicochemical Properties and Pharmacokinetics

Ketamine is a weak base ($pK_a$, 7.5) with minimal protein binding (12%). It is, however, highly lipid soluble (5-10 times more than thiopental). The distribution ($\alpha$ − phase) half-life is 15 minutes, and the elimination ($\beta$ − phase) half-life is 2 to 3 hours.

### Suggested Dosing

- Sedation and analgesia
  IV, 0.5 to 1 mg/kg
  IM and rectal, 2.5 to 5 mg/kg
  PO, 5 to 6 mg/kg. Dilute injectate solution in 5 to 10 mL (0.2 mL/kg) of flavored drink.
- Induction
  IV, 1 to 2.5 mg/kg
  IM and rectal, 5 to 10 mg/kg
- Infusion
  15 to 80 μg/kg/min (augment with 2-5 mg IV diazepam or 1-2 mg IV midazolam as needed). Dilution for infusion, 250 mg ketamine in 250 mL $D_5W$ or NS (1 mg/mL)[17]
- Epidural and caudal, 0.5 mg/kg; dilute (preservative-free) NS or local anesthetic (1 mL/kg)

## Pharmacodynamics

The major effects of ketamine administration involve the CNS. The term *dissociative state* refers to a functional and electrophysiologic separation of the thalamoneocortical and limbic systems. In this state, it is believed that the brain fails to transduce afferent impulses correctly because of disruption in normal communication between the sensory cortex and the association areas. The result resembles catalepsy, in which the eyes may remain open with slow nystagmus and intact corneal reflexes. Patients are generally noncommunicative, although they may appear to be awake.

Ketamine poses a unique problem when assessing the level of sedation or anesthesia because it is often difficult to assess a clear endpoint when ketamine is administered. Although ketamine can activate epileptiform foci in patients with known seizure disorders, it paradoxically appears to possess anticonvulsant properties. Ketamine potently vasodilates cerebral blood vessels, increasing CBF by 62% to 80%, and thus increases ICP. In addition, ketamine causes an increase in $CMRO_2$. This effect is reduced if diazepam, midazolam, or thiopental is administered before the ketamine. Nevertheless, increased cerebrospinal fluid pressure contraindicates the use of ketamine.

Ketamine also differs from most anesthetic agents in that it appears to stimulate the cardiovascular system, producing increases in MAP, pulmonary artery pressure, central venous pressure, heart rate, and CO. The central sympathetic stimulation, neuronal release of catecholamines, and inhibition of neuronal uptake of catecholamines usually override the direct myocardial depressant effects of ketamine. Hemodynamic effects (which depend on intact sympathetic responses) include increases in systemic and pulmonary arterial pressure, heart rate, and CO. The sympathomimetic effects of ketamine administration tend to increase myocardial oxygen demand, and thus are contraindicated in patients with significant ischemic heart disease. α-Blockers, β-blockers, and calcium-channel blockers may unmask the direct myocardial depressant effect of ketamine.

Ketamine appears to be unique in its ability to maintain functional residual capacity on induction of anesthesia. In spontaneously breathing patients, the minute ventilation may be maintained at the same level as in the awake state. Because skeletal muscular tone is maintained during ketamine anesthesia, atelectasis and changes in ventilation-perfusion and functional residual capacity do not occur. Ketamine has other beneficial effects on the respiratory apparatus, including increased lung compliance and decreased airway resistance. Bronchodilation induced by ketamine is not affected by histamine, acetylcholine, potassium chloride, propranolol, or indomethacin.

Although ketamine is reported to maintain laryngeal tone and reflexes with lower doses, there are reported cases of pulmonary aspiration. Ketamine is a potent stimulator of salivary and tracheobronchial secretions, and diligent suction of the oral cavity is required in the nonintubated patient to decrease the possibility of coughing and aspiration and to prevent laryngospasm, especially in children. The antisialagogue effects of glycopyrrolate and atropine are effective in reducing these secretions.

### Adverse Effects and Precautions

Emergence reactions are more common in adults (15-65 years of age) who have received rapid administration of high doses of ketamine. The incidence of these reactions can be reduced by premedication with benzodiazepines and droperidol.

As mentioned previously, critically ill patients with catecholamine depletion may respond to ketamine with unexpected reductions in blood pressure and CO. Ketamine should be used with caution in patients with severe hypertension, ischemic heart disease, or aneurysms.

It is also advised that one avoid the use of ketamine after topical nasal cocaine, in acute cocaine intoxicated, chronic alcoholic, and acutely alcohol-intoxicated patients or with concomitant administration of sympathomimetics. Hypertension, dysrhythmias, and myocardial ischemia may occur.

Ketamine-induced increases in ICP may be attenuated by hyperventilation and benzodiazepine pretreatment.

## *How Can the Analgesic Effects of Narcotics Be Used for Intravenous Anesthesia?*

The term *narcotic* (derived from the Greek word ναρκω? for "stupor") is interchangeably used with the word *opioid* (referring to drugs, which were originally derived from opium, but now also includes synthetic drugs). Opium is composed of more than 20 alkaloids, one of which, morphine, has been used for its analgesic effects for more than a century. The properties that make narcotics part of the vast majority of delivered anesthetics include the tremendous analgesia (particularly with the newer synthetic drugs), preservation of blood flow autoregulation (CNS, heart, kidneys), minimal cardiac depression with maintenance of hemodynamics, and blunting of autonomic responses to airway manipulation or surgical stress.[18] The variety of agents available allows the anesthesiologist to match the surgical and postoperative pain requirements with the pharmacokinetic and pharmacodynamic characteristics of the drug in a highly efficacious manner.[19]

### Receptor Activation and Mechanism of Action

All narcotic analgesics activate specific cell surface opioid receptors in both the central and peripheral nervous systems. It is this receptor activation that is responsible for both the desirable and the undesirable pharmacologic effects. Five receptor classes (μ, δ, κ, σ, and ε) have been identified on the basis of pharmacologic studies. Subtypes of the μ, δ, and κ receptors have not only been characterized pharmacologically but also successfully cloned in the laboratory. A newer nomenclature classifies the opioid receptors as OP1 (δ), OP2 (κ), and OP3 (μ).

The different receptors activated by the opioid agents account for the spectrum of responses that are seen clinically. μ-Receptor activation by opioids within the brain is responsible not only for the analgesia but also for the ventilatory depression, euphoria, and physical dependence. κ-Receptor occupation in the spinal cord results in analgesia as well as depression of ventilation, sedation, and miosis when supraspinal κ-receptors are activated. σ-Receptor activation results in dysphoria, hallucinations, and vasomotor and ventilatory stimulation. The δ-receptor modulates the effect on the μ-receptor, which may account for some of the tolerance seen when narcotics are administered over a prolonged period.

Although knowledge of the different receptors may not seem to have direct clinical application, it may help to understand how the various agents might interact. For example, if epidural morphine is administered to obtain analgesia by activating κ-receptors in the spinal cord, nalbuphine can be administered intravenously to attenuate the undesirable side effects of pruritus or nausea. The side effects are activated by peripheral receptors, which can be blocked, whereas the centrally mediated analgesia is unimpaired.

### Physicochemical Properties and Pharmacokinetics

For highly lipid-soluble drugs (eg, fentanyl), the onset of action reflects their circulation time to the CNS because they can rapidly penetrate all biologic membranes. Much less lipid-soluble drugs (eg, morphine) have a slower onset due to the relatively slow penetration of the blood-brain barrier.

Opioids in blood are bound to proteins, such as albumin and $\alpha_1$-acid glycoprotein. Chronic changes in plasma proteins, such as those seen in debilitated, malnourished patients or those with congestive heart failure (CHF), can result in higher concentrations of free opioid for a given dose, and the dose required for a given intensity of effect will be less. Protein binding varies considerably between the different narcotic agents. Morphine is 36% protein bound, whereas sufentanil is 92% protein bound.

At lower doses, redistribution plays a significant role in the short duration of effect for several opioids. As higher doses are given, particularly for longer periods of time, the peripheral tissues accumulate the opioid, with a lower concentration gradient between blood and the peripheral tissues. Hence, less drug moves into the tissues, and the decline in plasma (blood) concentrations due to redistribution is of progressively less importance. At that point, most of the decline depends on the elimination processes: metabolism and excretion. After a 4-hour infusion, the time required for a 50% reduction in concentration is markedly prolonged for fentanyl but only moderately prolonged for sufentanil and alfentanil, while it remains short for remifentanil.[20] For long cases with continuous infusions, this difference may be significant.

Most opioids are metabolized in the liver. Morphine is conjugated with glucuronic acid, resulting in active (morphine-6-glucuronide) and relatively inactive (morphine-3-glucuronide) metabolites. Meperidine is *N*-demethylated to normeperidine, which is also hydrolyzed to meperidinic acid. Normeperidine has an elimination half-life that is 5 to 6 times that of meperidine, and it can accumulate, producing CNS excitation manifested as tremors, muscular twitching, and seizures. Fentanyl, sufentanil, and alfentanil are also metabolized in the liver (*N*-dealkylation, hydroxylation, and conjugation), and their pharmacokinetics are altered by changes in liver blood flow. Their metabolites are excreted by the kidneys, but because they are pharmacologically inactive, changes in renal function do not prolong the duration of action of these three opioids. Remifentanil is unique in its metabolism, which is mainly produced by ester-hydrolysis catalyzed by nonspecific esterases present in the blood and other tissues. Because remifentanil is metabolized in multiple tissues, its elimination is essentially independent of hepatic or renal function. The metabolite produced by the hydrolysis of remifentanil is pharmacologically active, but its potency is extremely low and does not affect the duration of action of the parent drug. A small portion of remifentanil is also metabolized by *N*-dealkylation.

### Pharmacodynamics

Activation of μ-type opioid receptors in the brain and spinal cord produces analgesia, sleep, suppression of cough (antitussive), and obtundation of somatic autonomic and endocrine responses to noxious stimulation. Actions on μ-type opioid receptors in other parts of the CNS lead to ventilatory depression to the point of apnea; nausea at small doses, owing to stimulation of the chemoreceptor trigger zone (large doses depress the vomiting center); bradycardia (mediated by the vagal nerves); and hypotension (probably related to inhibition of certain reflexes modulating sympathetic nervous system activity, thereby reducing sympathetic outflow to vascular smooth muscle in veins and arterioles). Outside the CNS, μ-type opioid receptors mediate the constriction of smooth muscle (eg, sphincter of Oddi [biliary colic], gastrointestinal tract [constipation], and ureter [renal colic]).

Morphine and some of its derivatives, as well as meperidine, enter mast cells and displace histamine, which can produce hypotension, cutaneous erythema, and pruritus. The latter can also result from effects on the CNS by an unknown mechanism involving sympathetic nerves.

Another CNS action that is incompletely understood is the increase in skeletal muscle activity that is most prominent with relatively large doses of μ-receptor agonists. It has a variety of manifestations, including glottic closure, truncal rigidity, flexion, and occasionally flapping of the extremities (seizure-like movement with no EEG manifestations of seizures). This so-called rigidity typically occurs at doses that induce apnea and may interfere with positive pressure ventilation (eg, glottic closure, decreased thoracic compliance, or both).

## Induction of Anesthesia

Narcotics have been used for induction of anesthesia, but this typically requires extremely high doses of narcotics: 25 to 100 μg/kg of fentanyl, 10 to 20 μg/kg of sufentanil, or 50 to 250 μg/kg or alfentanil. With such large doses, hormonal (cortisol or epinephrine release) and hemodynamic responses to surgical stimulation are blunted or prevented.[21,22]

Although analgesia with such doses is excellent, high-dose narcotic techniques have associated problems. Muscle rigidity, particularly of the thoracic cage, is common, with the incidence of occurrence directly related to the potency of the narcotic used (sufentanil > alfentanil > fentanyl > morphine). Neuromuscular blocking agents are often necessary to inhibit this effect and allow ventilation.

Another substantial problem with high-dose narcotic techniques is recall. Addition of small doses of benzodiazepines or inhalational agents virtually eliminates this problem.

## Agonists

Although activation of a specific opioid receptor produces a specific effect, all available narcotic agents can variably activate all receptors. Some opioids, like fentanyl, are more pure receptor agonists; that is, they activate primarily one receptor and produce a positive response without activating multiple receptors or blocking other drug effects.

### Morphine Sulfate

The oldest opioid available for clinical use, morphine is an alkaloid extract of opium, which exerts its primary effects on the CNS and organs containing smooth muscle. Morphine produces analgesia, drowsiness, euphoria, dose-related respiratory depression, blockade of adrenocortical response to stress at high doses,[21] and reduction in peripheral resistance due to arteriolar and venous dilation.

Morphine can be used for premedication as a potent analgesic, during induction of anesthesia and for treatment of myocardial ischemic pain and dyspnea associated with CHF.

#### Suggested Dosing
- Analgesia
    IV, 2.5 to 15 mg (children 0.05-0.2 mg/kg, maximum 15 mg)

Epidural, 2 to 5 mg (40-100 μg/kg) diluted in 10 mL preservative-free saline or local anesthetic can be given as a bolus with 0.1 to 1 mg/h (2-20 μg/kg/h) infusion. Spinal, 0.1 to 1 mg (4-20 μg/kg) in preservative-free solution

#### Adverse Effects and Precautions
Epidural or intrathecal morphine may cause delayed respiratory depression (up to 24 hours after a single dose).

Morphine, as well as other opioids, may cause spasm at the sphincter of Oddi in the biliary tract (highest with fentanyl). This opioid-induced biliary tract spasm may be reversed with naloxone (intravenously or intramuscularly, 0.2-0.4 mg) or glucagon (intravenously or intramuscularly, 0.25-2 mg).

Depression of the cough and gag reflex is a direct effect on the cough center in the medulla. It may also produce vomiting by activating the chemoreceptor trigger zone.

Morphine induces the release of histamine and can cause erythema and pruritus along the vein draining from the site of injection. This should not be confused with an allergic reaction. Direct binding of morphine (and other opioids) to opiate receptors in the medulla oblongata alter sensory modulation and may be the mechanism for pruritus after epidural or intrathecal administration. Antihistamines (eg, diphenhydramine, 12.5-25 mg intravenously or intramuscularly every 6 hours as needed) are usually effective to alleviate symptoms.

As with all narcotic agents, it is recommended that doses be reduced in elderly, hypovolemic, and high-risk surgical patients as well as when used concomitantly with sedatives or other narcotics.

All narcotics tend to cross the placental barrier. The use of these agents during labor and delivery may produce respiratory depression and hypotonia in the neonate. Naloxone may be necessary, and resuscitation may be required.

Urinary retention that does not respond to naloxone may require bladder catheterization.

### Meperidine HCl (Demerol)

Meperidine is a synthetic opioid agonist and is about one tenth as potent as morphine but with a slightly more rapid onset and shorter duration of action. It can be used as a premedication, as an analgesic, and for treatment of postoperative shivering.

#### Suggested Dosing
- Analgesia
    IV, 25 to 100 mg (0.5-2 mg/kg)
- Treatment for shivering, 25 to 75 mg (0.5-2 mg/kg)

#### Adverse Effects and Precautions
Because of the direct myocardial depressant effect at high doses, meperidine is not recommended for high narcotic technique anesthesia.

The other undesirable effects of narcotics (respiratory depression, pruritus, nausea and vomiting, biliary spasm, urinary retention) may occur with meperidine as well.

### Fentanyl (Sublimaze)

Fentanyl is a synthetic phenylpiperidine derivative, which is a potent opioid agonist with analgesic properties about 100 times more potent than morphine.[23] The greater lipid solubility of fentanyl is responsible for its rapid onset and shorter duration of action.

### Suggested Dosing
- Analgesia

  IV, 25 to 100 µg (0.7-2 µg/kg) as a single bolus
- Supplemental anesthesia, 0.5 to 20 µg/kg as a bolus or 0.25 to 10 µg/kg/h as an infusion
- Induction of anesthesia, 5 to 40 µg/kg as a bolus (to avoid chest wall rigidity, a muscle relaxant should be administered simultaneously with induction dose).
- Epidural, bolus 50 to 100 µg (1-2 µg/kg) in 10 mL of preservative-free saline or local anesthetic or an infusion of 0.5 to 0.7 µg/kg/h
- Spinal, 5 to 20 µg (0.1-0.4 µg/kg) as a bolus

### Adverse Effects and Precautions
Cardiovascular stability is maintained when used as the sole anesthetic; however, doses may need to be reduced in elderly, hypovolemic, and high-risk surgical patients as well as when used concomitantly with sedatives or other narcotics.

## Sufentanil Citrate (Sufenta)

Sufentanil, also a synthetic opioid, is a thiamyl analogue of fentanyl with 5 to 10 times the analgesic potency. Sufentanil may be used for the very same indications as fentanyl.

### Suggested Dosing
- Analgesia, IV 10 to 30 µg (0.2-0.6 µg/kg) as a single bolus
- Supplemental anesthesia, 0.6 to 4 µg/kg as a bolus or 0.02 to 3 µg/kg/h as an infusion
- Induction of anesthesia, 2 to 10 µg/kg as a bolus (to avoid chest wall rigidity, a muscle relaxant should be administered simultaneously with induction dose).
- Epidural, bolus 5 to 30 µg (0.2-0.7 µg/kg) in 10 mL of preservative-free saline or local anesthetic or in an infusion of 0.1 to 0.6 µg/kg/h
- Spinal, 1 to 10 µg (0.02-0.08 µg/kg) as a bolus

### Adverse Effects and Precautions
The cardiovascular effects of sufentanil are similar to fentanyl, but sufentanil may produce a dose-dependent bradycardia (possibly due to stimulation of the vagus nucleus in the medulla), especially when combined with nonvagolytic muscle relaxants (eg, vecuronium).

## Alfentanil HCl (Alfenta)

Alfentanil is a synthetic opioid with characteristics of rapid onset and short duration but is about 50 times less potent than fentanyl.[24]

### Suggested Dosing
- Analgesia, IV 250 to 500 µg (5-10 µg/kg) as a single bolus
- Supplemental anesthesia, 10 to 100 µg/kg as a bolus or 3-75 µg/kg/h as an infusion
- Induction of anesthesia, 50 to 300 µg/kg as a bolus (to avoid chest wall rigidity, a muscle relaxant should be administered simultaneously with induction dose).
- Epidural, bolus 500 to 1000 µg (10-20 µg/kg) in 10 mL of preservative-free saline or local anesthetic or an infusion of 2 to 5 µg/kg/h

### Adverse Effects and Precautions
The analgesia of alfentanil is enhanced and prolonged by $\alpha_2$-agonists (eg, clonidine). The serum levels of alfentanil are increased with the concomitant administration of propofol, and the clearance is reduced in patients taking erythromycin.

As with all narcotics, doses should be reduced in elderly, hypovolemic, high-risk surgical patients or when used with sedatives or other narcotics.

## Remifentanil (Ultiva)

Remifentanil is the first agent in a new class of short-acting, synthetic, 4-anilidopiperidine derivatives with potent and selective µ-opioid receptor agonist activity.[25] Remifentanil contains an ester linkage, which makes it susceptible to rapid metabolism by esterase hydrolysis in the blood and other tissues. It appears to have similar pharmacodynamic properties to other potent µ-agonists.

Initial studies in human volunteers revealed that remifentanil had a rapid onset, a small volume of distribution, rapid redistribution, and clearance with an elimination half-life of 8.8 minutes, whereas alfentanil is 61 minutes.[20] Regardless of the duration of infusion, the time for the plasma concentration of remifentanil to decrease by 80% is 15 minutes. In addition, a single bolus dose of remifentanil is 20 to 30 times as potent as a similar dose of alfentanil.

Remifentanil is a titratable opioid that is useful for brief or prolonged painful procedures that require potent analgesia but rapid recovery. It is not as useful for postoperative analgesia because it is so rapidly metabolized.

### Suggested Dosing
- IV induction of anesthesia, 0.5 to 1 µg/kg as a bolus over >30 seconds followed by an infusion at 1.5 to 120 µg/kg/h when used with 66% $N_2O$, up to 1.5 minimum alveolar concentration (MAC) isoflurane, or 100 to 200 µg/kg/min with propofol. Supplemental doses of remifentanil (1 µg/kg) may be administered for transient episodes of intense surgical stress.

### Adverse Effects and Precautions
The most common adverse events associated with remifentanil are characteristic of µ-opioid receptor agonists and include bradycardia, hypotension, skeletal muscle rigidity, respiratory depression, shivering, and nausea and vomiting. However, because of the pharmacokinetic characteristics of this drug, these adverse reactions resolve within minutes of discontinuing or decreasing the rate of administration.

## Agonist-Antagonists

The agonist-antagonist drug group is a heterogeneous group of partially or totally synthetic opioids that are moderate to strong analgesics. They were introduced primarily because of the need for increased safety when administering opioids for the treatment of pain. This group of drugs differs from pure opioid agonists principally by the way in which they act as opioid receptors. A pure opioid agonist has both affinity and efficacy at the receptor; whereas, a partial agonist has affinity but reduced intrinsic activity. Therefore, the dose-response curve is relatively flat and does not provide the same maximal effect. The major clinical advantage of this group of drugs is to limit respiratory depression. The respiratory depressant effects also tend to parallel analgesic efficacy, thus limiting the clinical advantages.

## Pentazocine (Talwin)

Pentazocine produces its analgesic effects primarily by agonistic activity at κ-receptors. It is only one fourth as potent as morphine and exhibits a ceiling to both its respiratory depressant and analgesic effects. Pentazocine is of little utility to the anesthesiologist because of its limited analgesia and its dysphoric and cardiac effects (increased systemic and pulmonary artery pressures). In addition, sufficient doses of pentazocine can precipitate withdrawal symptoms in narcotic-dependent patients.

### Butorphanol Tartrate (Stadol)

Butorphanol is a moderately potent analgesic (about 5 times more potent than morphine) with weak antagonistic effects at $\mu$-receptors. Use of butorphanol with morphine-like drugs does not alter their analgesic properties. The potential cardiovascular and dysphoric side effects of butorphanol are similar to those of pentazocine.

### Nalbuphine HCl (Nubain)

Nalbuphine, structurally related to $\mu$-oxymorphone (agonist) and naloxone (antagonist), produces analgesic effects at $\kappa$-receptors and moderately potent antagonist effects at $\mu$-receptors. It is about equipotent to morphine for analgesic doses. Like other agonist-antagonists, nalbuphine demonstrates a ceiling effect for analgesia and ventilatory depression. Unlike pentazocine or butorphanol, nalbuphine produces neither deleterious hemodynamic effects in patients with cardiac disease nor psychic side effects.

### Buprenorphine (Buprenex)

Buprenorphine is a partial $\mu$-agonist that is highly lipophilic. It is 25 to 50 times more potent than morphine and produces analgesia and other CNS effects comparable to morphine. Although hemodynamic effects are mild, significant ventilatory depression has been reported. The incidence of psychomimetic effects is low.

### Dezocine (Dalgan)

Dezocine is slightly more potent than morphine, with a more rapid onset and shorter duration of action. Side effects are similar to morphine, although dezocine does not appear to release histamine. Dezocine appears to be considerably more effective than other agonist-antagonists as an anesthetic supplement.

### Antagonists

The pure antagonists are oxymorphone derivatives that are competitive antagonists at $\mu$-, $\delta$-, $\kappa$-, and $\sigma$-opioid receptors. Even at moderately high doses, antagonists have no discernible intrinsic activity except when administered with opioid agonists, which stimulate opioid receptors.

### Naloxone HCl (Narcan)

Naloxone is administered intravenously to reverse opioid agonist side effects, specifically, ventilatory depression, sedation, and pruritus. Unfortunately, all opioid effects are reversed in parallel, including analgesia. If large doses of naloxone (0.1-0.4 mg) are used, the unmasked pain may result in significant sympathetic and cardiovascular stimulation, leading to hypertension, atrial and ventricular dysrhythmias, pulmonary edema, and cardiac arrest. Naloxone should be titrated intravenously in small incremental doses (20-40 $\mu$g) to achieve the desired effect without sudden onset of pain. In addition, the half-life of naloxone (45-60 minutes) is shorter than the half-lives of many of the available opioids. Therefore, renarcotization may occur when naloxone is used to reverse longer-acting opioids. Prolonged reversal of opioid agonist activity may be achieved by administering an intramuscular dose of naloxone after titrating to effect intravenously. A more efficient method involves the use of a naloxone infusion (5-15 $\mu$g/kg/h) after a loading dose (1-4 $\mu$g/kg), with infusion rates being adjusted according to patient response.

### Naltrexone (Revia)

Naltrexone is a longer-acting antagonist (half-life of 10 hours) available for oral administration ($\geq$100 mg) that can be used to counteract the side effects of spinal opioids used for chronic pain.

## What Are the Alternatives to Narcotic Analgesics?

### Nonsteroidal Antiinflammatory Drugs

Nonsteroidal antiinflammatory drugs (NSAIDs) act by inhibiting the enzyme cyclooxygenase, which is crucial for prostaglandin synthesis. This inhibition is responsible for decreasing the swelling and pain associated with prostaglandin production. Best results are obtained when these agents are administered before the surgical insult. The most frequently used intravenous NSAID is ketorolac.[26]

NSAIDs are not narcotics and as such possess no respiratory depressant activity. However, they do inhibit prostaglandin-mediated renal blood flow, particularly in patients with intrinsic renal disease or CHF and thus must be used with caution. They also inhibit prostaglandin-mediated platelet aggregation, but, unlike aspirin, the effect is reversible when the drug concentration diminishes.

### Ketorolac (Toradol)

Ketorolac is an NSAID with analgesic, antiinflammatory, and antipyretic activity. The analgesic potency of 30 mg of ketorolac is equivalent to 9 mg of morphine with less drowsiness, less nausea and vomiting, and no significant respiratory depression.

#### Suggested Dosing
- IV/IM
  Loading, 30 to 60 mg. IV doses should be infused slowly (>15 seconds) to reduce the risk for phlebitis.
  Maintenance, 15 to 30 mg every 6 hours as needed

## What Are the Advantages of a Continuous Intravenous Anesthetic Infusion?

Intravenously administered anesthetic agents require frequent dosing to maintain the minimal drug effect and concentration at the site of action because they undergo redistribution

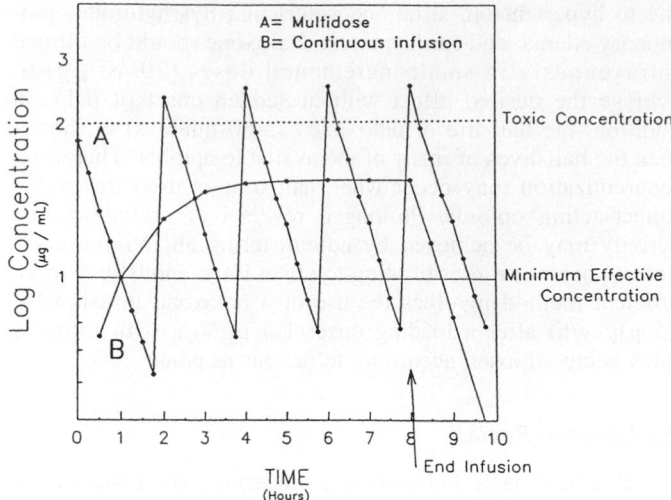

**FIGURE 33–3.** Multidose versus continuous infusions. *A*, Drug levels from multiple doses of a hypothetical drug. *B*, Continuous infusions of same hypothetical drug. Note repetitive decay below minimum effective concentration with intermittent dosing.

and elimination according to the physicochemical properties of the drug. To eliminate the peak and valley effect of frequent intermittent administration, a continuous infusion technique is preferable.[27] Figure 33–3 shows the relationship of multiple injections versus a continuous infusion of a drug with rapid clearance. It should be noted how continuous infusion dampens the oscillations in serum drug levels that may cause toxicity at the peak or inadequate effect at the trough (valley).

## When Should a Continuous Drug Infusion Be Used?

The decision about whether an intermittent bolus or continuous infusion technique is appropriate should be based on several key elements.

### Therapeutic Index

The therapeutic index is the ratio of the lethal dose to the effective dose of a drug. Agents with a high therapeutic index can be safely administered in large intermittent doses because concern about overshooting the target concentration is less significant. If, however, the therapeutic index of an agent is small, continuous infusions minimize the overshoot that occurs with periodic boluses (see Fig. 33–3).

### Saturable Effects

If the desired effect sought with a particular drug is saturable (maximal) with a single dose, no advantage will be obtained with continuous infusion. An example of this behavior would be histamine-2 blockers (eg, cimetidine, ranitidine). At the maximal effective drug concentration, no further blockade of acid production occurs, regardless of additional drug administration. However, if the process is not saturable (as is the case for most of the intravenous anesthetic agents), providing the minimal effective concentration with a continuous infusion will maintain the desired pharmacologic effect.

## Offset of Action

With the emergence of more intravenous agents with short half-lives, the concept of offset of action—the time for resolution of pharmacologic effect once drug administration is discontinued—becomes more important. If the drug concentration is maintained just above the minimal effective concentration, discontinuing the infusion quickly allows the concentration to fall below the minimal effective concentration. If an intermittent bolus technique is used, prolonged distribution and elimination would be required for a recently administered bolus dose.

Administration of propofol or remifentanil are good examples of this approach. Maintenance of the drug level just high enough to provide anesthesia allows rapid emergence once the infusion is discontinued. However, much more delayed arousal would follow administration of a large bolus (see Fig. 33–3).

## Half-Life of Drug

As previously mentioned, continuous infusions are best suited to drugs with short half-lives and rapid clearance.[28] Because these drugs are eliminated from the blood rapidly, they would require numerous intermittent boluses. Clearly, remifentanil, with a half-life of 5 to 12 minutes, is much better administered by continuous infusion than by intermittent boluses. Alternatively, morphine, with a half-life of 1.7 to 2.2 hours, can be delivered by intermittent bolus effectively.

Continuous infusions are also more cost-effective. Because only enough drug is delivered to maintain the desired effect, less total drug is administered, resulting in savings for the patient. The decrease in costs can be substantial in the case of the newer, more expensive drugs.

Finally, continuous infusions of drugs can be less labor intensive because once the infusion is started, less effort is required to maintain the pharmacologic effects.

## How Is the Correct Infusion Rate Determined?

Maintenance of a particular steady-state drug level is required to sustain the desired pharmacologic effect.[27] To achieve this, the amount of drug entering the body must equal the amount of drug being removed (cleared) from the body. We know that the concentration at steady state ($C_{ss}$) is determined by the following relationship:

$$C_{ss} = X_o/CL$$

where $X_o$ is the amount of drug given per unit time and *CL* is the volume of blood cleared of the drug per unit time. Thus, for example, fentanyl (clearance of 12.7 mL/kg/min), administered by continuous infusion at a rate of 2 µg/kg/h or 0.033 µg/kg/min, yields a steady-state concentration of 0.0026 µg/mL (2.6 ng/mL). This value is within the minimal effective concentration range (1 to 5 ng/mL for analgesia and minimal respiratory depression). Knowledge of the clearance of a drug and the approximate minimal effective concentration in the blood allows prediction of the infusion rate necessary to achieve a particular level (Table 33–3).

A steady-state drug concentration can be achieved with a

**TABLE 33–3.** Pharmacokinetic and Pharmacodynamic Parameters of Several Intravenous Anesthetic Agents

| Agent | Clearance Rate (mL/kg/min) | Volume of Distribution (L/kg) | Minimal Effective Concentration (µg/mL) |
|---|---|---|---|
| Thiopental | 3–3.8 | 1.92–5 | 12.9–25.5 |
| Methohexital | 7–13 | 3.68 | 10 |
| Propofol | 33.8–36.6 | 1.8–3.04 | 0.96–1.14 |
| Etomidate | 12.3–24.5 | 2–6.72 | 0.231–0.383 |
| Ketamine | 16.6–21.6 | 4.4–5.8 | 0.43–0.85 |
| Midazolam | 5.1–9.9 | 1.29–1.91 | 0.78–0.236 |
| Diazepam | 0.4 | 1.53 | N/A |
| Morphine | 15–23 | 3.2–3.4 | 0.02–0.2 |
| Fentanyl | 11–21 | 3.2–5.9 | 0.001–0.005 |
| Alfentanil | 5–7.9 | 0.5–1 | 0.05–1.5 |
| Sufentanil | 9–14 | 2.86 | 0.0005–0.001 |
| Meperidine | 8–18 | 2.8–4.2 | 0.1–0.5 |
| Remifentanil | 50–60 | 6.3–0.5 | N/A |

constant infusion, but this is a slow process (see curve B in Figure 33–3). This can be overcome by administering a loading dose (LD) as bolus or as a rapidly priming infusion. The loading dose (LD) equals the target plasma concentration (Cp) multiplied by the $V_d$:

$$LD = Cp \times V_d$$

Thus, from the previous example, the loading dose of fentanyl (in a 70-kg patient using a $V_d$ of 3.2 L/kg) would be as follows:

$$LD = (0.0026\ \mu g/mL) \times (70\ kg) \times (3.2\ L/kg) \times (1000\ mL/L) = 582\ \mu g$$

## What Other Factors Affect the Amount of Drug Needed?

The minimal serum level of an intravenous agent for a particular procedure varies with the type and degree of surgical stimulus. Titration of the agent according to vital sign changes after surgical stimulus is necessary to fine-tune the requisite dose. This adjustment of the dose to the desired effect provides the best method of reaching steady-state levels that are appropriate for the stimuli provided. Pharmacokinetic parameters alone may lead to insufficient levels but do serve as a starting point from which one can increase the dose to provide the desired effect.

## What Is Total Intravenous Anesthesia?

Before the development of shorter-acting intravenous drugs, it was difficult to provide a complete anesthetic with an onset and recovery comparable to the inhalational anesthetics. The advantages of the newer intravenous agents (better pharmacokinetic and pharmacodynamic properties) allow their use not only during induction but also during maintenance of anesthesia, particularly with continuous intravenous infusion.[29–31] The release of propofol made the practice of total intravenous anesthesia a much more viable alternative to inhalational anesthesia.[32]

Although progress in the development of better intravenous agents has been significant, the impact would be limited were it not for the simultaneous development of better delivery systems. The advances in pharmacokinetic model-driven drug-delivery systems or computer-assisted continuous infusion devices allow intravenous agents to be administered with an ease similar to inhalational agents.[33]

Now that better intravenous agents and infusion systems exist, all that remains for the establishment of automated closed-loop drug delivery is the development of reliable monitors of depth and adequacy of anesthesia. Although monitoring the effects of drugs that affect arterial blood pressure or muscle relaxation is fairly standard, monitoring the effects of other intravenous drugs, such as anesthetics, is difficult. Presently, various derivatives of processed EEGs may be used to provide a relatively consistent measure of anesthetic depth,[34] especially with hypnotics. However, there are no methods available to monitor anesthetic drug levels noninvasively, which would allow correlation with EEG measurements. Further studies need to be done to determine whether there is a linear relationship between anesthetic depth and median EEG frequency; if there is consistency among patients and across drugs; and finally, if the delivery method is equally effective for drug combinations.

## References

1. Heath PJ, Kennedy DJ, Ogg TW, et al. Which intravenous induction agent for surgery? A comparison of propofol, thiopentone, methohexitone and etomidate. *Anaesthesia*. 1988;43:365.
2. Seltzer JL, Gerson JI, Allen FB. Comparison of the cardiovascular effects of bolus vs incremental administration of thiopentone. *Br J Anaesth*. 1980;52:527.
3. Briggs LP, Dundee JW, Bahar M, et al. Comparison of the effect of diisopropyl phenol (ICI 35,868) and thiopentone on response to somatic pain. *Br J Anaesth*. 1982;54:307.
4. Barron DW. Effect of rate of injection on incidence of side effects with thiopental and methohexital. *Anesth Analg*. 1968;47:171.
5. Reves JG, Fragen RJ, Vinik HR, et al. Midazolam: pharmacology and uses. *Anesthesiology*. 1985;62:310.
6. Bryson HM, Fulton BR, Faulds D. Propofol. An update of its use in anaesthesia and conscious sedation. *Drugs*. 1995;50:513.
7. Sebel PS, Lowdon JD. Propofol: a new intravenous anesthetic. *Anesthesiology*. 1989;71:260.
8. Shafer A, Doze VA, Shafer, SL, et al. Pharmacokinetics and pharmacodynamics of propofol infusions during general anesthesia. *Anesthesiology*. 1988;69:348.
9. Hug CC, McLeskey CH, Nahrwald ML, et al. Hemodynamic effects of propofol: data from over 25,000 patients. *Anesth Analg*. 1993;77(suppl):521.
10. Gooding JM, Corssen G. Effect of etomidate on the cardiovascular system. *Anesth Analg*. 1977;56:717.
11. Bergen JM, Smith DC. A review of etomidate for rapid sequence intubation in the emergency department. *J Emerg Med*. 1997;15:221.
12. Wagner RL, White PF. Etomidate inhibits adrenocortical function in surgical patients. *Anesthesiology*. 1984;61:647.
13. Fellows IW, Bastow MD, Byrne AJ, et al. Adrenocortical suppression in multiply injured patients: a complication of etomidate treatment. *BMJ*. 1983;287:1835.
14. White PF, Way WL, Trevor AJ. Ketamine: its pharmacology and therapeutic uses. *Anesthesiology*. 1982;56:119.
15. Corssen G, Domino EF. Dissociative anesthesia: further pharmacologic studies and first clinical experience with the phencyclidine derivative CI-581. *Anesth Analg*. 1966;45:29.
16. Haas DA, Harper DG. Ketamine: a review of its pharmacologic properties and use in ambulatory anesthesia. *Anesth Prog*. 1992;39:61.
17. Idvall J, Ahlgren I, Aronsen KF, et al. Ketamine infusions: pharmacokinetics and clinical effects. *Br J Anaesth*. 1979;51:1167.
18. Moldenhauer CC, Hug CC. Use of narcotic analgesics as anesthetics. *Clin Anesthesiol*. 1984;2:107.

19. Shafer SL, Varvel JR. Pharmacokinetics, pharmacodynamics, and rational opioid selection. *Anesthesiology.* 1991;74:53.

20. Westmoreland CL, Hoke JF, Sebel PS, et al. Pharmacokinetics of remifentanil (GI87084B) and its major metabolite (GI90291) in patients undergoing elective inpatient surgery. *Anesthesiology.* 1993;79:893.

21. George JM. Morphine anesthesia blocks cortisol and growth hormone response to surgical stress in humans. *J Clin Endocrinol Metab.* 1974;38:736.

22. Philbin DM, Coggins CH. Plasma antidiuretic hormone level in cardiac surgical patients during morphine and halothane anesthesia. *Anesthesiology.* 1987;49:95.

23. Stanley TH, Philbin DM, Coggins CH. Fentanyl-oxygen anesthesia for coronary artery surgery: cardiovascular and antidiuretic hormone responses. *Can Anaesth Soc J.* 1979;26:168.

24. White PF, Coe V, Shafer A, et al. Comparison of alfentanil with fentanyl for outpatient anesthesia. *Anesthesiology.* 1986;64:99.

25. Burkle H, Dunbar S, Van Aken H. Remifentanil: a novel, short-acting, μ-opioid. *Anesth Analg.* 1996;83:646.

26. Buckley MM, Brogen RN. Ketorolac: a review of its pharmacodynamic and pharmacokinetic properties, and therapeutic potential. *Drugs.* 1990;30:86.

27. White PF. Clinical uses of intravenous anesthetic and analgesic infusions. *Anesth Analg.* 1989;68:161.

28. Raftery S, Sherry E. Total intravenous anaesthesia with propofol and alfentanil protects against postoperative nausea and vomiting. *Can J Anaesth.* 1992;39:37.

29. Wessen A, Persson PM, Nilsson A, et al. Concentration-effect relationships of propofol after total intravenous anesthesia. *Anesth Analg.* 1993;77:1000.

30. Dahaba AA, von Klobucar F, Rehak PH, et al. Total intravenous anesthesia with remifentanil, propofol and cisatracurium in end-stage renal failure. *Can J Anaesth.* 1999;46:696.

31. Gray C, Swinhoe CF, Myint Y, et al. Target controlled infusion of ketamine as analgesia for TIVA with propofol. *Can J Anesth.* 1999;46:957.

32. Glass PSA. Prevention of awareness during total intravenous anesthesia. *Anesthesiology.* 1993;78:399.

33. Cook RI, Woods DD. Implications of automation surprises in aviation for the future of total intravenous anesthesia (TIVA). *J Clin Anesth.* 1996;8:29S.

34. Stanski DR. Monitoring depth of anesthesia. In: RD Miller, ed. *Anesthesia.* 4th ed. New York, NY: Churchill Livingstone; 1994:1127.

CHAPTER

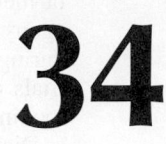

# Inhalation Agents

Michael Seropian
Wendell C. Stevens

*Is the Use of Nitrous Oxide Appropriate?*
*When is Recall a Problem?*

## PROLONGED ANESTHESIA

*Will Recovery Be Prolonged if an Inhaled Agent is Used?*

## PREGNANCY AND THE PUERPERIUM

*Should Inhalation Agents Be Used for Cervical Cerclage?*
*What Are the Fetal Effects of Inhalation Agents?*
*Is Any Potent Agent Preferable for Operative Deliveries?*

## AMBULATORY SURGERY

*What Role Do New Agents Play in Ambulatory Surgery and at What Cost?*

*How Long Do Changes in Mental Function Persist After Anesthesia?*

*Are Inhaled Agents Associated With Postoperative Nausea and Vomiting?*

Inhalation agents were the foundation of general anesthesia and were used without adjuvants for many decades. This practice changed in the 1920s, when Lundy[1] introduced the concept of *balanced anesthesia*, an approach to anesthesia care that involves the use of several techniques or agents simultaneously. Since that time, and increasingly since about 1970, general anesthesia has been performed with combined inhalation, intravenous, and regional anesthetics.

Inhalation agents have become one alternative among many to provide analgesia and amnesia, to control reflex responses to noxious stimuli, and to induce muscle relaxation. Inhalation agents provide parts of these components of anesthesia but ordinarily not all of them. The context of this chapter assumes that one wants to provide as much of the anesthetic state as possible with inhalation agents, while recognizing that this may not be the way in which most anesthetics are given. Data are not available to demonstrate superior outcomes for a pure inhalation approach in comparison with the various balanced techniques, or vice versa. Clearly, general anesthesia can be provided safely with any one of several techniques.[2]

Nevertheless, roles for pure inhalation techniques do exist. One is to allow gradual, breath-by-breath change in anesthetic level as the anesthesiologist assesses airway adequacy and circulatory changes that accompany anesthetic induction. Another is to improve the simplicity of anesthesia management, to allow one to ascribe more clearly a cause-and-effect relationship to intraanesthetic events than might occur if multiple drugs were used. The use of inhalation agents provides a logical way to learn and to maintain airway management skills. These skills are the hallmark of capable anesthesiologists who must maintain a high level of proficiency if they are to manage the patient's airway successfully. Finally, if venous access cannot be obtained, the patient can usually be anesthetized with inhalation agents.

## HISTORY OF INHALED ANESTHETICS

### Why Were They Developed and Introduced?

Early experiments with drugs that became anesthetics were directed more toward scholarly explication of their chemical or physical properties, their application as medical therapies, or their use for pleasurable purposes than toward relief of the agony of surgery.[3] Sedation, sleep, and analgesia that occurred during medicinal or exhilarating uses of the drugs triggered trials of their use as anesthetics by physicians who had been looking for some ways to make surgery pain-free.[4]

Diethyl ether, nitrous oxide ($N_2O$), and chloroform—drugs introduced into clinical practice almost simultaneously in the 1840s—were the only anesthetics used regularly for nearly half a century. Around 1930, efforts were directed toward *biochemomorphology*,[5] which is the design of drugs based on structure-activity relationships. The first widely used anesthetic developed by this process was divinyl ether (Vinethene). Analysis of structure-activity relationships guided the explorations of fluorinated hydrocarbons by Robbins,[6] Van Poznak and Artusio,[7] and Krantz,[8] and the analysis of hundreds of fluorinated ethylmethyl ethers by Terrell and coworkers.[9] Table 34–1 lists 20 inhalation anesthetics that have been given to human beings. Some are of only historical interest, and some are in the developmental process.

### Why Does the Search for New Agents Continue?

Although there have been vast improvements in inhaled anesthetic agents since the mid-20th century, there currently is no ideal agent. Such an agent should be rapidly titratable and predictable, should be easy to administer, and should include pharmacologic properties that make it attractive for use in patient care. It should produce amnesia and analgesia, control reflex responses to noxious stimuli, and induce muscle relaxation and immobility. Even the most current inhaled agents (such as desflurane) do not provide all of these charac-

**TABLE 34–1.** Chronology of Use of Inhaled Anesthetics

| Drug | Date Use Reported in Human Beings | Status or Reason If Not Current |
|---|---|---|
| Diethyl ether | 1842 | Current (developing countries) |
| Nitrous oxide | 1844 | Current |
| Chloroform | 1847 | Hepatotoxicity |
| Ethyl chloride | 1894 | Flammability; cardiac dysrhythmias |
| Ethylene | 1923 | Flammability |
| Divinyl ether (Vinethene) | 1923 | Flammability |
| Cyclopropane | 1933 | Flammability |
| Trichloroethylene (Trilene) | 1935 | Reacts with soda lime |
| Metopryl | 1946 | Flammability |
| Ethyl vinyl ether (Vinamar) | 1947 | Flammability |
| Trifluoroethyl vinyl ether (Fluroxene) | 1953 | Flammability; toxic metabolites |
| Halothane | 1956 | Current |
| Methoxyflurane (Penthrane) | 1960 | Nephrotoxicity; high tissue solubility |
| Teflurane | 1961 | Cardiac arrhythmias |
| Halopropane | 1962 | Cardiac arrhythmias |
| Enflurane (Ethrane) | 1966 | Current, but disappearing; seizures |
| Isoflurane (Forane) | 1971 | Current |
| Aliflurane | 1979 | In development |
| Sevoflurane (Ultane) | 1981 | Current |
| Desflurane (Suprane) | 1990 | Current |

teristics without associated adverse effects. Improvements in efficacy and safety are paramount considerations in the ongoing search for new drugs and account for loss of interest in older ones. It is therefore imperative that research continue to refine the current inhaled anesthetic solutions. Testing must be exhaustive and is, therefore, expensive because government approval of a drug must be obtained before widespread clinical use is permitted. Commercial goals definitely have a role in the search for new anesthetics.

## PHARMACOKINETICS AND PHARMACODYNAMICS: CLINICAL IMPLICATIONS

### Why Are Inhalational Agents Useful?

A significant feature of inhalation agents is the ease and predictability with which changes in anesthetic depth can be achieved with their use. Because these anesthetics are entirely administered and chiefly eliminated through the lungs, the alveolar concentration of these drugs governs concentrations in all tissues. Anesthesiologists can increase or decrease the alveolar concentration by changing the inspired concentration and ensuring adequate alveolar ventilation in an otherwise healthy individual.

Furthermore, inhalational agents produce predictable changes in respiratory and cardiovascular function that allow for a safe and effective anesthetic. Anesthetic effects can be rapidly reversed or produced through titration of these agents. Few intravenous agents possess this unique property.

### What Factors Determine the Delivery of Inhaled Agent to the Brain?

A key factor determining the depth of anesthesia is the tissue anesthetic concentrations. Once the agent is delivered to the alveoli, it must dissolve into the blood and then be delivered to, and dissolve into, the brain tissue. It is useful to consider this concept in multiple parts. The determinants of delivery to the lung include alveolar ventilation and the inspired partial pressure. The inspired partial pressure is determined primarily by the vaporizer concentration setting, total gas flow, and volume of the anesthetic circuit. The anesthetic agent must then be taken up into the blood and delivered to the brain tissue.

Uptake of the inspired agent into the blood is determined by (1) the blood solubility of the gas (the blood and gas partition coefficient), (2) cardiac output, and (3) the alveolar and blood partial pressure difference of the gas. Once uptake at the lungs has occurred, the agent is delivered to brain tissue, where the tissue solubility (blood and brain partition coefficient) determines the rate of uptake by the brain. As long as the mixed venous anesthetic is lower than the alveolar concentration, uptake and deepening of anesthesia occurs. The uptake is rapid for tissues whose blood flow is high (eg, brain) in relation to their capacity for the anesthetic. For these tissues, the equilibrium of concentrations occurs rapidly, and the alveolar concentration accurately reflects tissue concentration after only a few minutes have passed. For example, the anesthetic concentration in the brain is about 95% of the alveolar concentration within about 5 minutes, presuming that

stable alveolar concentration, normal cardiac output, and distribution of output exist.

### Is the Rapidity of Equilibration Always an Advantage?

It is usually desirable to be able to adjust the anesthetic dose rapidly and see a fast response. However, substantial risk of rapid overdose occurs if techniques such as *overpressurization* are used in combination with either insoluble or soluble agents. The use of overpressurization for induction with sevoflurane has gained considerable acceptance. Data from recent studies suggest that induction with high-dose sevoflurane may in fact be preferable to incremental dose inductions. These studies showed fewer side effects and induction times of less than 1 minute.[10]

The clinician must remain alert to the potential for rapid establishment of supranormal anesthetic levels when using controlled ventilation. The combination of hyperventilation and high inspired anesthetic concentration of all inhalation agents results in rapidly increasing alveolar anesthetic concentrations. A positive feedback occurs as cardiac output and anesthetic uptake decrease, further accelerating the rate of rise of alveolar concentration as agent continues to be delivered to the lung[11] (Fig. 34–1). At times of rapid increase in delivered anesthetic concentration, one probably should preserve spontaneous breathing or avoid a high-inspired anesthetic concentration and make an effort not to hyperventilate the patient.

### What Is Overpressurization?

*Overpressurization* is the use of supranormal anesthetic concentrations (above those required for anesthetic mainte-

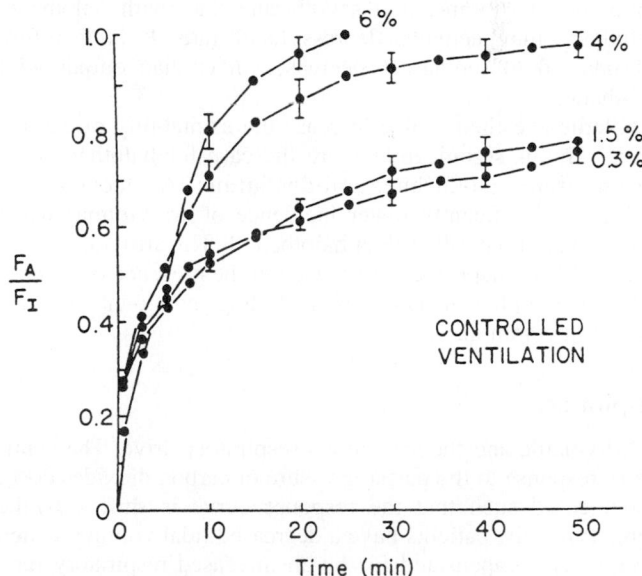

**FIGURE 34–1.** The rates of rise of $F_A/F_I$ (ratio of alveolar fraction of halothane to inspired fraction of halothane) over time at various inspired halothane concentrations. After the first 5 minutes, the rates were more rapid at the higher inspired halothane concentrations in dogs receiving constant controlled ventilation. This is due to depression of cardiac output and decreased anesthetic uptake. (From Gibbons RT, Steffey EP, Eger EI II. The effect of spontaneous versus controlled ventilation on the rate of rise of alveolar halothane concentrations in dogs. *Anesth Analg.* 1977;56:32–34. © International Anesthesia Research Society.)

nance) to achieve desired anesthetic concentrations rapidly. Overpressurization increases the alveolar and venous partial pressure difference and therefore increases the uptake of agent into the blood. It is used to increase the rapidity of induction; however, it also introduces the dangers of overdosage. If the inspired concentration is not reduced appropriately over time, the patient will be at increased risk for adverse effects related to high anesthetic concentrations. As noted previously, this possibility is especially likely in mechanically ventilated patients.

## Do Inhalation Agents Have Significant Side Effects?

All of the potent inhaled anesthetic agents can produce the desired effects for surgical anesthesia (analgesia, amnesia, immobility or muscle relaxation, and decreased autonomic response to noxious stimuli). However, each has a side effect profile that must be understood to use these agents effectively and safely. The main side effects relate to the cardiovascular and respiratory systems.

### Cardiovascular

Cardiac output depends on stroke volume and heart rate. Stroke volume depends mainly on preload, cardiac contractility, and afterload. All volatile anesthetic agents decrease cardiac contractility to some degree (halothane > enflurane > isoflurane ≈ sevoflurane ≈ desflurane). Systemic vascular resistance (SVR) affects afterload. Volatile anesthetics cause vasodilation and a decreased SVR with a resulting redistribution of blood flow. Under normal physiologic conditions, a decrease in SVR is compensated by an increase in heart rate. This physiologic response appears better maintained with isoflurane, desflurane, and sevoflurane than with halothane. Halothane may actually depress heart rate. It is therefore not unusual to see larger decreases in cardiac output with halothane.

Volatile anesthetics also increase the excitability of cardiac tissue. This is significantly more the case for halothane than for enflurane, isoflurane, and desflurane. A recent study showed a significantly lower incidence of arrhythmias when using sevoflurane rather than halothane.[12] The arrhythmogenic potential of epinephrine is increased in the presence of volatile anesthetics. Other arrhythmias, including junctional rhythms, are not uncommon.

### Respiratory

All volatile anesthetics depress respiratory drive. The ventilatory response to the partial pressure of carbon dioxide ($PCO_2$) is decreased such that the response curve is shifted to the right. Typically, patients have a decreased tidal volume, which is partially compensated for by an increased respiratory rate. However, total minute ventilation is decreased. This effect increases with increased anesthetic concentrations. Hypoxic ventilatory drive is depressed or ablated by inhaled anesthetic agents. This depression may occur even at subanesthetic doses, underscoring the importance of postoperative monitoring in patients who have been exposed to inhaled agents; their hypoxic ventilatory drive may remain depressed for some time after the anesthetic is concluded.

## Which Inhaled Agents Interact With Soda Lime?

Several anesthetic agents have been implicated in the production of byproducts when exposed to soda lime and barium hydroxide lime (Baralyme). Carbon monoxide has been isolated in several studies and case reports[13,14] using desflurane, enflurane, and isoflurane. Halothane and sevoflurane showed minimal or no degradation to carbon monoxide. The clinical implication of this is not known; however, factors such as temperature, absorbent material dryness, absorbent type, flow rates, anesthetic choice, and anesthetic concentration may play a role in the carbon monoxide concentration.

Sevoflurane has also been implicated in the production of degradation products. In a recent study, methanol, compound A, formaldehyde, and fluoride were all detected when sevoflurane was exposed to dry soda lime.[15,16] Only compound A and fluoride were detected with the use of sevoflurane and fresh soda lime. Halothane showed only small amounts of degradation to fluoride. The clinical implications of these byproducts are also uncertain, but they present a source of potentially toxic inhaled substances. The use of "wet" soda lime appears to decrease the concentration of these byproducts.

## Is Anesthetic Elimination as Controllable as Uptake?

Anesthetic gases are almost entirely eliminated through the lungs. The concepts introduced for uptake and delivery to the brain apply for elimination except that the partial pressure gradients are reversed. Elimination depends on agent solubility, cardiac output, ventilation, and tissue and alveolar partial pressure differences. The tissue partial pressure represents the driving pressure for agent into the blood to be delivered to the lungs. Alveolar partial pressure approaches zero over time as agent is eliminated with ventilation and replaced with fresh gas. Overpressurization is an excellent example of the use of alveolar and venous partial pressure difference to allow inductions to occur rapidly and in a controllable manner. No similar assist can occur during emergence because the inspired anesthetic concentration cannot be less than zero.

Cardiac output and its distribution are not easily controlled by the anesthesiologist. As with uptake, elimination also depends on cardiac output. When the cardiac output is low during emergence, smaller than usual amounts of anesthetic are delivered to the lungs. The rate at which tissue anesthetic concentration decreases is slowed. Although continued ventilation rapidly lowers the alveolar anesthetic concentrations, the tissue-to-alveolar partial pressure gradients may still be large. The low alveolar concentration may lead one to think arousal should occur quickly. However, the patient may still be anesthetized because of high tissue concentration of anesthetic.

Persistent tissue anesthetic levels may result in the continuation of drug-induced respiratory depression at a time when spontaneous ventilation is desired. The apneic threshold for carbon dioxide may be high despite low alveolar anesthetic concentrations, so that the patient fails to breathe as expected. This situation leads to a dilemma in the management of emergence: hypoventilation required to increase the arterial $CO_2$ partial pressure ($PaCO_2$) delays the removal of anesthetic from blood and tissues. A way to avoid this problem is to maintain end-tidal carbon dioxide ($CO_2$) at or only slightly below the $CO_2$ apneic threshold throughout the anesthetic procedure.

## How Much Anesthetic Is Required for Surgery?

### Assessment of Depth

Anesthetic depth can be considered in terms of the body's response to various alveolar or tissue levels of anesthetic drugs. The Guedel stages and planes of anesthesia and the correlation of electroencephalogram (EEG) patterns with blood anesthetic levels are examples of this approach. Another approach is analysis of the anesthetic concentration required to block responses to stimuli.[17] The stimuli can be non-noxious, such as verbal commands, or noxious, such as skin incision or traction on abdominal viscera. The anesthetic doses required to block responses to various stimuli have been quantified[18-21] (Table 34–2). The data provide guidelines by which the anesthesiologist predicts the amount of anesthetic to administer or when awakening is to be expected. It is important to keep in mind that as the delivered concentration of inhaled agents is increased to ensure appropriate depth of anesthesia, the likelihood of complications and side effects also increases.

### External Determinants of Depth

Provision of an anesthetic is a dynamic process. The amount of anesthetic drug required varies with the type of stimulus encountered. A dynamic relationship is present among the stimuli, the anesthetic, and the patient. Patient factors, such as age, ongoing drug regimens, and body temperature, alter anesthetic requirement. Large differences in anesthetic requirement probably occur during different stages of the operation and for operations in different sites. This phenomenon has been shown clearly with intravenous agents,[22] but data are not as well developed for inhaled agents.

### Inadequate or Excessive Anesthetic Depth

Achieving the appropriate depth of anesthesia in the face of so many variables can indeed be challenging. Inadequate levels of anesthesia can lead to preventable complications in a patient. Of particular importance are the autonomic responses to noxious stimuli. Inadequate levels of anesthesia

**TABLE 34–2.** Alveolar Halothane Concentrations (F$_A$) Required to Prevent Responses to Various Stimuli in 50% of Subjects

| Stimulus | Response | F$_A$ (%) |
|---|---|---|
| Verbal | Open eyes | 0.41[12] |
| Skin incision | Gross muscle response | 0.77[13] |
| Laryngoscopy | Extremity movement; relaxation of vocal cords | 1.12[14] |
| Endotracheal intubation | Coughing | 1.46[14] |
| Skin incision | Norepinephrine level | 1.12[15]* |

*Plus 60% nitrous oxide.

may fail to blunt exaggerated responses to stimuli. For example, an inadequate level of anesthesia may allow undesirable increases in blood pressure (BP) or heart rate to pose significant threats to the patient with underlying cardiac pathology. High concentrations of inhaled agents may be required to blunt autonomic responses. Clinicians often use narcotics in combination with inhaled agents to decrease the inhaled anesthetic requirement. Narcotics may, in fact, be more effective in blocking cardiovascular responses than potent inhaled agents.

Movement may at times be particularly hazardous with procedures such as open eye surgery. The degree of muscle relaxation and immobility required during some surgical procedures may require high delivered anesthetic concentrations. It is common practice to use intravenous muscle relaxants in these cases to ensure immobility, thus avoiding high inhaled concentrations and associated side effects.

Careful attention must also be given to ensuring adequate anesthesia to prevent recall during an anesthetic (see Chapter 32). This consideration is especially relevant when muscle relaxants are used and when patients are immobilized, irrespective of their level of awareness. Explicit recall in most cases is entirely preventable and may be avoided by the appropriate use of adequate concentrations of inhaled agents or other potent amnestics such as midazolam. Studies have shown that recall may or may not be painful or disturbing to the patient.[23,24] Devices using bispectral analysis are being assessed for their role in preventing surgical awareness. Their relationship to various phenomena such as movement and autonomic response have yet to be clarified.

Excessive anesthesia can cause severe cardiac and respiratory depression and collapse.[25] Such outcomes reflect our inability to determine with certainty the appropriate depth of anesthesia for all patients at all times. Often, attention is focused on the maintenance of circulatory variables within chosen ranges because a better approach is lacking. Assuming the establishment of adequate oxygenation and ventilation, it is generally accepted that tissue perfusion should be maintained above all else. Satisfactory management involves constant review of clinical signs and monitored data.

## CENTRAL NERVOUS SYSTEM CONSIDERATIONS

The effects of inhalation anesthetics on the central nervous system (CNS) include alteration of the cerebral metabolic rate for oxygen ($CMR_{O_2}$), direct effects on blood vessels, vascular effects by interaction with $CO_2$, effects on cerebrospinal fluid (CSF) dynamics, and alteration of neuronal function and electrical activity.

## Does the Alteration of CMR$_{O_2}$ Have Clinical Significance?

All potent inhaled agents decrease $CMR_{O_2}$[26] primarily by decreasing brain functional activity as reflected by EEG changes.[27] The effect of $N_2O$ on $CMR_{O_2}$ is not predictable and probably depends on the level of CNS depression produced by diseases or other drugs.[28] Decrease in electrical activity, characterized as burst suppression, occurs with all potent inhaled anesthetics. Of special significance is the finding that isoflurane and desflurane begin to produce burst suppression

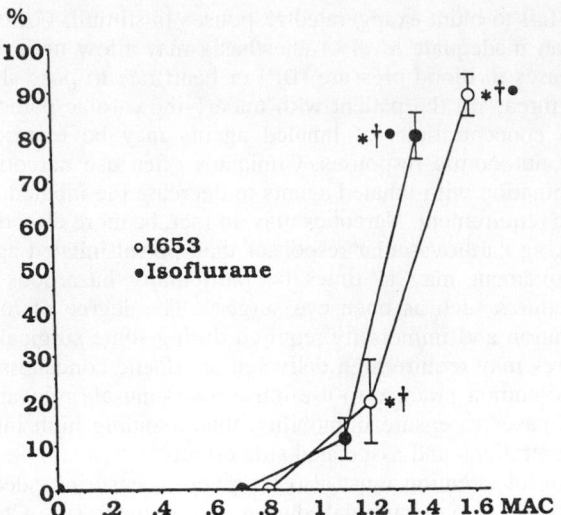

**FIGURE 34–2.** Burst suppression ratios for I653 (desflurane) and isoflurane at various multiples of minimal alveolar concentration (MAC). Burst suppression ratio is the percentage of time in 4-second epochs during which the electroencephalogram voltage did not exceed 5 μV. (From Rampil IJ, Weiskopf RB, Brown JG, et al. I653 and isoflurane produce similar dose-related changes in the electroencephalogram of pigs. *Anesthesiology.* 1988;69:298.)

at moderate levels of anesthesia, between 0.5 and 1.0 times the minimal alveolar concentration (MAC) (Fig. 34–2). When doses of these agents equivalent to 1.5 MAC are given, the EEG demonstrates burst suppression over 90% of the time.[29]

The electrical suppression produced by isoflurane is probably of clinical significance. Greater decreases in cerebral blood flow (CBF) are tolerated with isoflurane before cerebral ischemia occurs than with halothane or enflurane. This observation may reflect the electrical effects of isoflurane (Fig. 34–3). The relationship between blood flow and EEG changes defines the critical regional CBF at which cerebral ischemia is detected.[30,31]

Although reliance on cerebral protection from inhaled agents is not warranted,[27] isoflurane, and perhaps desflurane, offer the advantage of maximal depression of $CMRo_2$ at moderate commonly used levels of anesthesia. Other evidence

of the favorable effect of isoflurane is better preservation of cerebral welfare during deliberate hypotension compared with halothane.[32]

## How Are Cerebral Blood Volume and Intracranial Pressure Affected?

### Anesthetic-Induced Cerebrovasodilation

The potent agents produce cerebrovasodilation (halothane > enflurane > isoflurane = desflurane).[33,34] The smaller effect of isoflurane may be due to its prominent effect of decreasing $CMRo_2$.[35] $N_2O$ produces vasodilation to a degree similar to that with an equivalent MAC multiple of potent agent.[36] Cerebrovasodilation increases CBF and therefore increases intracranial pressure (ICP). The benefits of the use of inhaled agents must be weighed against the risks in patients with raised ICP. The newer agents, desflurane and sevoflurane, both appear to leave $CMRo_2$ and CBF coupling intact.[37,38]

### Hypocapnia-Induced Cerebrovasoconstriction

Cerebrovasodilation is modified by changes in $Paco_2$. This physiologic mechanism remains intact with all inhaled anesthetics. Cerebrovascular resistance increases as $Paco_2$ decreases to hypocapnic levels, resulting in decreased CBF. Control of ICP by this mechanism is better with isoflurane than with halothane[39] or desflurane.[40] Hyperventilation must precede halothane administration if increases in ICP are to be attenuated in patients with intracranial tumors.[39] Hypocapnia effectively decreases CBF and ICP over a broad range of anesthetic depths.[41] Decreases in CBF from hypocapnia may decrease ICP less than expected because the anesthetics may cause cerebrovenodilation that is not responsive to change in $Paco_2$.

### Cerebrospinal Fluid Production and Reabsorption

The finding of increased ICP despite adequate depth of anesthesia and hypocapnia led to consideration of CSF dy-

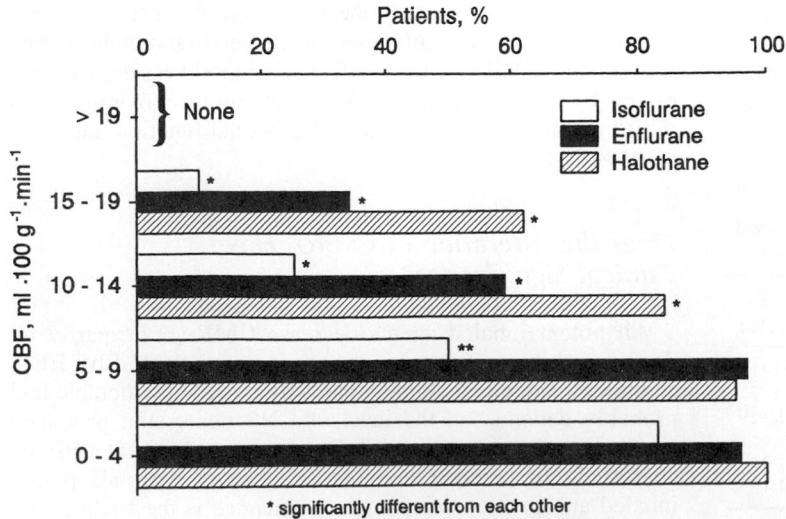

**FIGURE 34–3.** Percentage of patients who manifested electroencephalographic evidence of cerebral ischemia after carotid occlusion during carotid endarterectomy. Cerebral blood flow (CBF) was measured by xenon washout. (From Michenfelder JD, Sundt TM, Fode N, et al. Isoflurane when compared to enflurane and halothane decreases the frequency of cerebral ischemia during carotid endarterectomy. *Anesthesiology.* 1987;67:336.)

**TABLE 34–3.** Effect of Inhaled Anesthetics on Cerebrospinal Fluid Dynamics

| Drug | Cerebrospinal Fluid Production | Resistance to Resorption |
|---|---|---|
| Enflurane[34] | Increased | Increased |
| Halothane[35, 36] | Decreased | Increased |
| Isoflurane[37] | Unchanged | Unchanged |

namics as a factor governing ICP. The potent agents affect CSF production, reabsorption, or both[42–45] (Table 34–3). Enflurane is unfavorable in both respects.

### Do the Inhaled Agents Have Predictable Electroencephalographic Effects?

EEG patterns have long been recognized as an indicator of anesthetic depth.[46] A pattern of progressive cortical depression occurs as depth increases; that is, wave frequency decreases while amplitude increases.[47] The amount of time that the EEG is electrically silent progressively increases with the anesthetic dose.[48] Despite the predictability of these changes, the EEG is not yet used routinely to monitor depth of anesthesia, perhaps because burst suppression is a nonstationary event. New adaptations of this technology (eg, bispectral analysis) may become beneficial in the future to predict depth of anesthesia. EEG suppression may be highly variable[48] at any given time because it is determined not only by anesthetic concentration but also by other factors such as stimulation.

Many agents cause EEG epileptiform activity.[49] At higher concentrations and with hypocapnia, enflurane causes EEG and muscular epileptiform activity.[49,50] However, enflurane is not contraindicated in patients who exhibit seizure foci preoperatively.[51]

### Can Inhaled Agents Be Used With Evoked Potential Monitoring?

Inhalation anesthetics have a greater effect on cortical responses than on subcortical recordings.[52] They cause dose-related decreases in amplitude and increases in latency of cortical somatosensory-evoked potentials.[53] The decreasing order of depression is enflurane to isoflurane to halothane. Of paramount importance is maintenance of stable alveolar concentration of all anesthetics throughout the period of recording, so that changes are less likely to be due to anesthetic agents.

### Is Complete Central Nervous System Recovery to Be Expected After Elimination of the Agent?

Cerebral elimination of inhaled agents resembles the pattern of their elimination from alveoli. As predicted from blood and tissue solubility, the decreasing order of elimination rates is desflurane to sevoflurane to isoflurane to halothane.[54] This ranking parallels the ranking of speed of recovery of animals from anesthesia.[55] Although CNS recovery is complete after

elimination of inhaled anesthetics, several days may be required for all behavioral or mental effects to disappear. Neurologic signs, including transient hyperreflexia or Babinski reflex, commonly exist in the first several minutes of recovery.[56] Their presence early in recovery is not necessarily or even usually a sign of CNS damage.

## MANAGEMENT OF BREATHING

Inhalation agents affect breathing in multiple ways[57] (Table 34–4). In some instances, variables are changed toward more satisfactory gas exchange. Decreased $CO_2$ production and total body $O_2$ demand[58] reduce the ventilatory requirement. Another favorable effect is decreased bronchomotor tone, which reduces airway resistance.[59] Airway maintenance is a problem, however, because inhaled anesthetics relax upper airway muscles and disrupt reflexes intended to maintain patency.[60] Functional residual capacity nearly always decreases with induction of anesthesia; increased intrapulmonary shunting of blood and increased airway resistance may result.[61] Intrapulmonary shunting may also increase if the anesthetic agent attenuates hypoxic pulmonary vasoconstriction[62] or if lowered pulmonary artery pressure favors distribution of blood to less well-ventilated parts of the lung.

### How Do These Factors Influence the Management of Ventilation?

One may need to preserve the patient's respiratory efforts when dealing with upper airway obstruction from supraglottitis and tumors or with more distal obstruction from cervical or mediastinal masses. A number of problems are likely to occur during inhalation induction in such instances. Anesthetics probably abolish reflexly maintained phasic pharyngeal muscle activity, which preserves upper airway patency in the awake state.[63] Loss of airway patency may require manipulation of head position, use of increased airway pressure, and insertion of an oropharyngeal or nasopharyngeal airway to overcome upper airway obstruction. If inhalation induction is chosen, isoflurane and desflurane induce more airway reflex responses than does halothane.[64] Sevoflurane has now gained favor as an inhalational induction agent partially because of its non-noxious characteristics.[10]

Inhalation inductions with spontaneous breathing may provide more satisfactory gas exchange than controlled breathing in patients with obstruction of the intrathoracic trachea; transpulmonary pressure and nonturbulent gas flow are probably better maintained with this approach.[65] Children may also benefit from inhalation inductions. Intravenous placement is often difficult and frightening to children. Sevoflurane and

**TABLE 34–4.** Influence of Inhalation Anesthetics on Respiration

Decrease whole body or individual organ metabolism
Obtund upper airway reflexes affecting airway patency
Depress peripheral chemoreceptors
Depress the central respiratory control center
Alter mechanical properties of the chest wall and diaphragm
Decrease bronchomotor tone
Alter volume and distribution of pulmonary blood flow

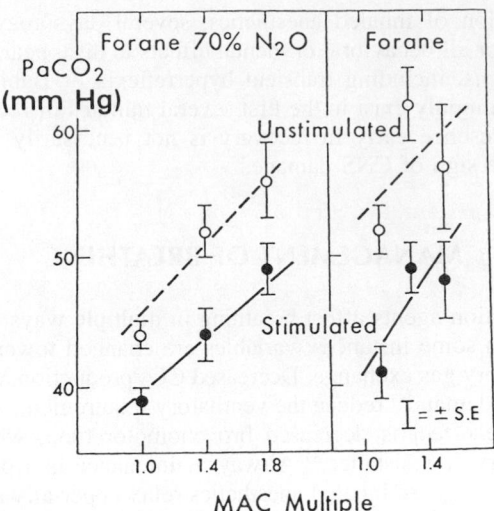

**FIGURE 34–4.** $Pa_{CO_2}$ before and during operations (unstimulated and stimulated, respectively). Results are shown for several minimal alveolar concentration (MAC) multiples of nitrous oxide with isoflurane (Forane) and isoflurane alone. (From Eger EI II, Dolan WM, Stevens WC, et al. Surgical stimulation antagonizes the respiratory depression produced by Forane. *Anesthesiology.* 1972;36:544.)

halothane provide less noxious characteristics for an inhalation induction than do desflurane and isoflurane. Sevoflurane may have several advantages over halothane as an induction agent. It does not appear to be more noxious at higher concentrations than at lower ones.[10] In addition, the cardiovascular side effects characteristic of high concentration halothane are considerably decreased or absent with sevoflurane. However, with careful avoidance of supranormal concentrations of halothane, both agents have been shown to produce similar cardiovascular effects on induction.[66] One would expect induction with sevoflurane to be much more rapid than with halothane based on solubility differences. The literature to date does not clearly show this.[66]

## Is Spontaneous Breathing Useful During Maintenance?

Anesthetic dose-dependent depression of the ventilatory $CO_2$ response and increase in the apneic threshold are common to the potent agents.[67,68] Consequently, $Pa_{CO_2}$ is elevated during spontaneous breathing. Substitution of some of the potent agent with $N_2O$ lessens the respiratory depression and leads to a lower $Pa_{CO_2}$.[69] The depression is antagonized by surgical stimulation such that $Pa_{CO_2}$ returns toward (but ordinarily not to) normal levels when surgery begins[70] (Fig. 34–4).

Changes in ventilatory variables provide reliable guides to anesthetic depth.[71] Tidal volume decreases and frequency of breathing commonly increases as alveolar anesthetic concentration increases.[67] When the patient and anesthesiologist must be separated by some distance, monitors of breathing provide a useful indicator of anesthetic depth. Also, if a mechanical problem such as an airway disconnection occurs, the patient continues to breathe. A commonly used technique includes mechanical ventilation to just below the patient's apneic threshold. If a decrease in ventilation should occur (as in disconnection), the patient begins to breathe shortly thereafter as the $Pa_{CO_2}$ reaches the apneic threshold.

The functional residual capacity decreases with onset of general anesthesia regardless of the anesthetic drugs selected or the mode of ventilation used.[61,72] A major cause of the decrease is thought to be compression atelectasis. Similar amounts of atelectasis occur with spontaneous or controlled breathing.[72] Studies suggest that occasional inflation of the lung up to 40 cm $H_2O$ for 7 to 8 seconds may reexpand atelectasis and improve oxygenation.[73]

## Will Increased Airway Resistance Affect Spontaneous Ventilation?

Anesthetics depress the normal immediate response to imposed resistance that is characterized by prolonged inspiration and maintained tidal volume and respiratory frequency.[74] During halothane anesthesia, less inspiratory compensation occurs than during anesthesia with other agents, and that which develops is delayed until the central hypercapnic drive is augmented. The anesthetized patient compensates poorly for weight placed on the chest.[75]

An inverse relationship exists between preoperative forced expiratory volume in 1 second ($FEV_1$) and intraoperative $Pa_{CO_2}$. Although few data document this effect, those that do exist are convincing.[76,77] Whether this effect is due only to impairment of mechanics of breathing or results in part from altered chemical control of respiration is unknown. In any event, allowing spontaneous ventilation in patients with chronic obstructive pulmonary disease and low $FEV_1$ almost certainly results in elevated $Pa_{CO_2}$, sometimes to inordinate levels (Fig. 34–5).

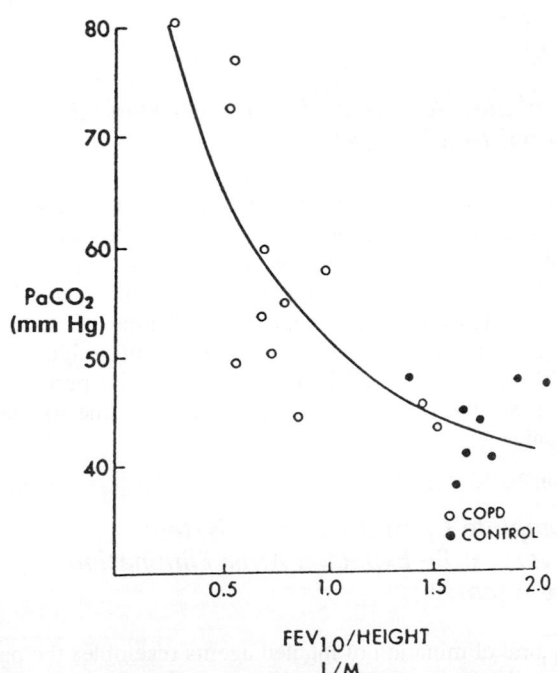

**FIGURE 34–5.** Relationship between $Pa_{CO_2}$ levels during anesthesia with spontaneous ventilation and preoperative $FEV_1$ expressed in terms of body height. (From Pietak S, Weenig CS, Hickey RF, et al. Anesthetic effects on ventilation in patients with chronic obstructive pulmonary disease. *Anesthesiology.* 1975;42:160.)

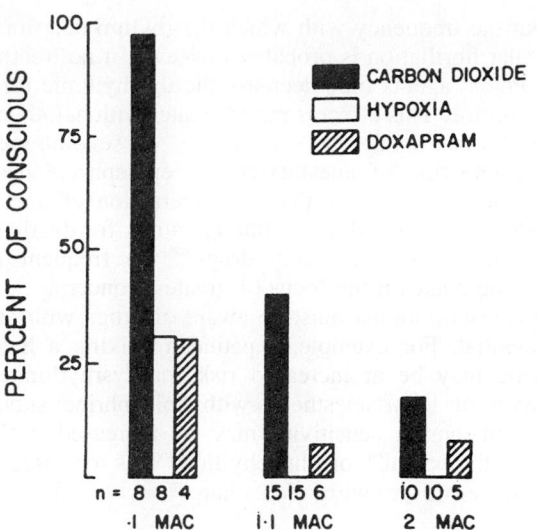

**FIGURE 34–6.** Relative activity of respiratory chemoreflexes in human beings during various levels of halothane anesthesia. Responses are shown as a percentage of the ventilatory responses that occurred in subjects during the control state. n, number of patients. (From Knill RL, Gelb AW. Ventilatory responses to hypoxia and hypercapnia during halothane sedation and anesthesia in man. *Anesthesiology.* 1978;49:244.)

### Is Halothane the Preferred Agent in Reactive Airway Disease?

The answer to this question is predicated on the accepted concept that tracheal intubation should not be attempted until deep anesthesia has been obtained.[78] Inhalation induction appears to be most easily accomplished with halothane or sevoflurane. Once induction is completed, however, halothane, enflurane, and isoflurane are equally effective in preventing or reversing bronchoconstriction.[79,80]

### Should Inhalation Agents Be Avoided During One-Lung Ventilation?

The potent inhalation agents depress hypoxic pulmonary vasoconstriction and increase the alveolar-to-arterial oxygen partial pressure difference.[62,72] In the clinical setting, when relatively low doses of inhaled agents are used, intrapulmonary shunting is not increased by these drugs over the amount that occurs during primarily intravenous anesthesia.[81]

### Do Inhalation Agents Suppress Ventilatory Hypoxic Drive?

The ventilatory hypoxic drive mediated through peripheral chemoreceptors is attenuated at subanesthetic doses of potent agents and obliterated when the drugs are given at anesthetizing concentrations[82] (Fig. 34–6). The clinical significance of this effect is that a small increase or no increase in breathing might occur if hypoxia develops during anesthesia and recovery.

## MANAGEMENT OF THE CIRCULATION

It is rare in clinical practice for an inhaled agent to be used as the sole anesthetic, especially in adults. Consequently, the impact of inhaled agents on the circulation is modified by interaction with other drugs. In some circumstances, inhaled agents may be a favorable choice. The effects of inhaled agents alone on circulatory variables are listed in Table 34–5. Note that arterial pressure decreases with all agents except $N_2O$.

These effects can be expected to occur when inhaled agents are given concomitantly with other drugs. The specific properties of the agents can be used to advantage if an inhalation anesthetic is a component of a multidrug-balanced technique. For example, isoflurane decreases SVR when added to a narcotic-based regimen.[83] If myocardial depression is desired, halothane reliably produces it and maintains heart rate at near control levels.[84] The careful titration of inhaled agents provides the practitioner with a valuable tool to control hemodynamics while providing a margin of safety through predictability.

### Why Has the Use of Inhaled Agents as Sole Anesthetic Drugs Decreased?

The dose of anesthetic required to attenuate circulatory responses to stimulation from surgery or anesthetic procedures may be large, leading to undesirable effects on multiple systems, such as apnea or inordinate cardiovascular depression. For example, the dose of halothane required to prevent movement during tracheal intubation is 1.33 MAC,[85] and the dose required to block the adrenergic response to skin incision is 1.45 MAC.[22] On average, these doses lead to at least a 25% to 30% decrease in arterial pressure, even in healthy patients,[86] and probably to greater decreases in patients with vascular or cardiac diseases. The adrenergic or laryngeal responses can be blocked in part by narcotics[87] or local anesthetics.[88] Use of adjuvants to allow lower doses of the inhaled agents during these procedures is preferred by many anesthesiologists.

### Are Inhaled Agents Useful in Patients With Coronary Artery Disease?

Although agreement is not universal, the anesthetic drug by itself is probably of minor importance as a determinant of

**TABLE 34–5.** Changes From Awake Values of Circulatory Variables Produced by Inhalation Anesthetics*

| Value | Desflurane[93, 94] | Enflurane[95] | Halothane[77] | Isoflurane[96] | Nitrous Oxide[85] | Sevoflurane[93] |
|---|---|---|---|---|---|---|
| Arterial pressure | Decreased | Decreased | Decreased | Decreased | Unchanged or increased | Decreased |
| Cardiac output | Decreased | Decreased | Decreased | Unchanged | Unchanged or increased | Unchanged |
| Heart rate | Increased | Increased | Unchanged | Decreased | Unchanged or increased | Decreased |
| Systemic vascular resistance | Decreased | Decreased | Unchanged | Decreased | Unchanged or increased | Decreased |
| Central venous pressure | Increased | Increased | Increased | Unchanged or increased | ? | ? |

*The effects of nitrous oxide are those occurring when it is added to anesthesia with a volatile agent.

outcome from surgery and anesthesia in patients with coronary artery disease.[89-91] Research has increased the knowledge about coronary and myocardial physiology and the effects of anesthetic drugs on the heart. Much more is now known about the relative importance of factors affecting cardiac $O_2$ supply-and-demand relationships. The importance of inhaled agents in the setting of coronary artery disease lies in the thorough and careful understanding of the inhaled agent's effects on the cardiovascular system. The manipulation and alteration from baseline may adversely effect a patient with coronary artery disease. A classic example is a patient with coronary artery disease and severe or critical aortic stenosis. In this patient, the introduction of excessive systemic vasodilation increases the likelihood of ischemia to the myocardium secondary to decreased perfusion pressure.

Despite concern that anesthesia-induced coronary vasodilation (the *steal phenomenon*) from isoflurane may lead to myocardial ischemia, this problem simply has not been clinically significant. Anesthesia-induced negative inotropism actually may prevent the steal phenomenon.[92]

### Are Inhaled Anesthetics Appropriate in Patients With Valvular Disease?

The use of potent agents in the setting of valvular disease presupposes two things: first, that the practitioner understands fully the altered physiology of the patient with valvular disease; and second, that similar to the patient with coronary artery disease, the practitioner must understand the pharmacologic effects of the agents being used. For mitral regurgitation, the relatively rapid heart rate and decrease in SVR seen with isoflurane correspond well to the requirements for maintained myocardial performance. These same factors make isoflurane, desflurane, and to some extent, enflurane weak choices for management of patients with aortic stenosis or idiopathic hypertrophic subaortic stenosis. Such statements apply fully only if anesthesia is managed with inhalation agents alone. In practice, balanced anesthesia is commonly used. The inhalation agents provide an attractive component when myocardial depression (halothane) or vasodilation (isoflurane, enflurane) is needed in addition to somewhat deeper anesthesia.

#### Nitrous Oxide

The appropriate role for $N_2O$ in patients with coronary artery or valvular disease is uncertain. The inspired $O_2$ concentration must necessarily be decreased when $N_2O$ is used. Infants with high pulmonary vascular resistance may have further increases caused by $N_2O$.[93] Its direct myocardial effects are negligible, but SVR may increase.[94] The major advantage of $N_2O$ is the prompt onset and emergence from anesthesia that it provides. $N_2O$ may also be useful by blunting the cardiovascular effects that would occur if potent agents were used alone.

### Can Volatile Agents Be Used Safely During Catecholamine Administration?

All potent agents may induce arrhythmias, including junctional rhythms or premature ventricular contractions. Arrhythmias associated with catecholamine administration are not

rare, but the frequency with which the rhythm deteriorates to ventricular fibrillation is probably low, even if no treatment is given. Potent agents may decrease the dysrhythmic threshold of epinephrine. This effect is much greater with halothane than with enflurane, isoflurane, desflurane, or sevoflurane.[12,95-97]

The interaction of anesthetics and epinephrine has been studied more extensively than the interaction of anesthetics with other vasoactive drugs. Although a risk for dysrhythmias exists with the use of many drugs,[98] the frequent use of epinephrine makes it the focus of greatest concern.

The anesthesiologist must be aware of drugs with arrhythmic potential. For example, a patient receiving a halothane anesthetic may be at increased risk for dysrhythmias after infiltration of local anesthetic with epinephrine subcutaneously. Epinephrine sensitivity may be increased with such drugs as thiopental[99] or theophylline,[100] as opposed to no change in sensitivity with midazolam.[101]

## NEUROHUMORAL RESPONSE TO SURGERY

### Do Inhaled Agents Alone Effectively Attenuate the Stress Response?

Anesthesia alone results in significant increases in plasma cortisol, growth hormone, and norepinephrine levels.[102] Sufficient levels of inhaled agents block the adrenergic response to surgical incision. The results of a study by Roizen and coworkers[21] suggest that a reliable relationship exists between anesthetic dose and blockade of the response. However, other work with halothane[103] and isoflurane[104] indicates that the hormonal responses to 0.5 to 1.2 MAC, as well as to doses approximately twice as large, were similar. Thus, inhaled anesthetics can decrease the hormonal response to surgery,[105] but the dose required to do so reliably may be large.

In current practice, adjuvants, including adrenergic antagonists and narcotics, are often used to decrease the sympathetic nervous system response to surgery.[101] Although the response can be prevented by the use of inhaled agents alone, much experience supports the current practice of using combinations of drugs.[106] Lower doses of inhaled agents can then be used, and the suppression of stress response may extend into the postoperative period.[107]

## RENAL FUNCTION

### Are Enflurane and Sevoflurane Contraindicated in Renal Disease?

This question arises because increases of inorganic fluoride to nephrotoxic levels can occur with the use of both of these drugs as a consequence of their metabolism.[108,109] With both agents, the duration of the peak levels appears to be so brief that kidney injury does not occur. Studies suggest that intrarenal metabolism of anesthetics may contribute to nephrotoxicity and that intrarenal fluoride levels may be more important that plasma fluoride concentrations.[110] Prudence suggests their use should be, at least, questioned in patients with renal disease because alternatives to their use are available.[111]

## Renal Perfusion

Disturbance of renal function in the perioperative period is related far less to toxicity of anesthetic metabolites than to changes in renal perfusion. The direct effects of anesthetic drugs on the kidney are small compared with the indirect effects of combined anesthesia and surgery acting through the renin-angiotensin system.[112,113] In dog studies, when halothane was delivered at concentrations of 1% to 1.5%[114] and enflurane at doses as high as 1.75 MAC,[115] renal blood flow was preserved by autoregulation. If the anesthetic dose is high enough, however, decreases in cardiac output may exceed the ability of the kidney to compensate, and renal blood flow decreases.

Anesthetics may attenuate the response to activation of the renin-angiotensin system caused by surgery or tracheal intubation, but they do not obliterate it. This response leads to intraoperative oliguria,[112] may be an appropriate response to anesthesia and surgery, and does not necessarily mean kidney injury is present.[116,117] On the other hand, anuria that is not due to a simple problem, such as an occluded urinary catheter, is an ominous sign.

## LIVER AND INHALED AGENTS

### What Is the Role of Hepatic Perfusion and Metabolism?

Hepatic effects are related more to impairment of hepatic perfusion than to a cellular toxic effect of the anesthetics. Cellular toxicity is believed to be connected to anesthetic metabolism.[118,119] The fraction of an administered dose that is metabolized is in the decreasing order of halothane to enflurane to isoflurane to desflurane. Sevoflurane is metabolized, but the implication of this process in hepatic damage is unknown.

The oxidative pathway of halothane metabolism can yield products that bind to proteins and lipids, leading to cellular damage.[118] The anesthetic metabolite-protein complex stimulates antibody formation, so that future contact with halothane may produce hepatic injury. Christ and colleagues[120] recently showed that enflurane and possibly isoflurane metabolism can produce covalently bound adducts that are recognized by antibodies from patients who had halothane hepatitis. This mechanism of toxicity has provoked great interest in desflurane, which is minimally metabolized, is largely insoluble in body tissues, and is rapidly removed from the body. Whether this agent is truly less hepatotoxic than the more widely used anesthetics is unknown at this time.

### Why Do Alterations in Hepatic Function Occur?

As with renal function, alterations in hepatic function occur after most anesthetic procedures and appear to be related to the effects of anesthesia and surgery, and not to those of anesthesia alone. This general statement, however, obscures the differences among agents.[121–124] For example, hepatic artery flow is preserved during isoflurane but not halothane anesthesia.[125,126] Hepatic artery perfusion in the presence of hemorrhage is better preserved during isoflurane than during halothane anesthesia.[127] The decrease in perfusion pressure

caused by inhaled agents may have negative effects on hepatic function, especially in the diseased liver.

If the surgical procedure also interferes with hepatic blood flow, liver function may be further decreased. Thus, alterations in liver function are greatest with upper abdominal operations.

### Should Halothane Be Used in Adults or Patients With Hepatic Insufficiency?

Although rare, severe hepatic injury can result from halothane use (halothane hepatitis).[128] As described earlier, the process is thought to be autoimmune in nature. This phenomenon is mainly found in the adult population. Because alternatives are available, halothane use ordinarily is avoided in adult patients, especially those with damaged livers. Data on this subject are not uniform and may in part result from the low incidence of halothane hepatitis.

Halothane may have a negative perfusion profile as compared with other agents such as isoflurane. The use of halothane in patients with underlying hepatic disease should be carefully weighed against the benefits of its use. For example, one may use halothane as an induction agent but then change to isoflurane for maintenance. Data, however, are not uniform, as demonstrated by Zinn and associates,[129] who did not detect a difference in hepatic effects of several anesthetic regimens in patients with alcoholic hepatitis. A study by Tiainen and Rosenberg also found no significant difference between halothane and isoflurane hepatic effects.[122]

## ENDOCRINE EFFECTS

### Will Inhalation Anesthetics Affect Diabetes?

Blood sugar increases during anesthesia, from both decreased insulin secretion and decreased tissue response to insulin.[130–132] There is no evidence, however, that any one inhaled agent controls the diabetic state best. Few experimental data explore the impact of diabetes on anesthesia, a surprising fact in view of the frequency with which diabetic patients are anesthetized. One of the few research reports addressing this topic showed that diabetic patients with autonomic neuropathy have significantly wider swings in circulatory variable measurements than do diabetic patients without neuropathy.[133] The patients did not receive purely inhalation agents, however. The response is similar regardless of the inhalation agent used and only underscores the effect of all inhaled agents on the abnormal autonomic nervous system.

Diabetic patients pose a unique problem of considerable end-organ dysfunction that may have significant implications when inhaled agents are used. All major systems, including cardiovascular, respiratory, renal, hepatic, and gastrointestinal, may be affected and must be considered.

### Are Other Endocrine Effects Significant?

Increase of adrenal cortical secretion during anesthesia was alluded to earlier.[102] Antidiuretic hormone output does not change significantly in response to the use of inhalation anesthetics alone, but these drugs may modify the output of antidiuretic hormone in response to surgery.[134] The direct effect of inhaled anesthetics on thyroid function is small or insignificant.[135]

## OBESITY

### Should Inhaled Agents Be Used in Obese Patients?

#### Potential Disadvantages

Evidence is lacking to show advantage of one technique over another in obese patients. Any anesthetic drug with significant lipid solubility, whether intravenous or inhaled, accumulates in body fat. Adipose tissue is a reservoir for many anesthetic drugs and empties slowly when anesthesia is terminated. This effect does not significantly delay awakening, but it does impede total removal of anesthetic from the body. As a result, subclinical concentrations in the blood persist for long periods and lead to continued metabolism of the anesthetic. There is evidence that morbidly obese patients receiving desflurane recover more quickly than with isoflurane.[136]

Levels of metabolites are higher for longer periods of time in obese patients.[137,138] This fact may explain in part the greater incidence of hepatic injury from halothane in obese patients. Obese patients may also be more liable to hypoxic episodes, which lead to the combined effects of larger amounts of reductive metabolites in obese than in nonobese patients.

#### Potential Advantages

No evidence demonstrates that pure inhalational anesthesia offers any advantage over other techniques. However, advantages can be proposed for the use of inhaled agents over fixed anesthetics. First, smaller amounts of muscle relaxants should be required because the inhaled agents potentiate the effects of neuromuscular blocking drugs.[139] Return of full skeletal muscle function should be more easily accomplished. Second, removal of anesthetic can be accomplished actively by ventilating the patient, perhaps simplifying the assessment of respiratory and mental function.

## MUSCLE RELAXATION

### Are Inhalation Agents Contraindicated in Patients With Neuromuscular Disease?

Selection of an inhalation agent is logical in the management of patients with neurodegenerative disease because the anesthetic dose can be increased or decreased at will (providing relaxation as needed) and reversed simply by ventilating the drug away. In patients with muscle weakness, the additional relaxation needed for surgery may be small and provided easily by the use of inhalation agents. In contrast to intravenous anesthetics, inhaled drugs depress skeletal muscle function.[140,141] Greater relaxation is produced by isoflurane, enflurane, and desflurane than by halothane, and the effect is related to the anesthetic dose.[142]

Certain myopathies, however, have possible associations with malignant hyperthermia (eg, Duchenne-type muscular dystrophy). In these cases, potent inhalational agents should not be used because they may act as triggers for malignant hyperthermia. Other myopathies also may have weak associations with malignant hyperthermia.

### Can Volatile Anesthetics Potentiate Muscle Relaxation?

Volatile agent–induced muscle relaxation can be used to advantage when profound relaxation is needed. Volatile drugs potentiate the effects of depolarizing and nondepolarizing neuromuscular blocking drugs. As a result, smaller doses of blocking drugs are needed to provide equivalent conditions during anesthesia with inhalation agents than with intravenous anesthetics[143] (Fig. 34–7). There may be a difference in relaxation potentiation among inhaled agents.[144–146] Similarities have been found between sevoflurane and isoflurane and desflurane and isoflurane. Halothane may prolong recovery when compared with sevoflurane.

The implications of this potentiation are twofold: (1) addition or removal of the inhaled anesthetic supplements or reverses the neuromuscular blockade in part; and (2) less anticholinesterase reversal should be required to reverse the relaxant effect, thus decreasing side effects such as nausea and vomiting. Work by Wright and associates convincingly showed that inhalation agents can be used to titrate the degree of muscle relaxation in the setting of a constant level of neuromuscular blocking agent.[147]

## BONE MARROW TRANSPLANTATION

### Are Effects on Hematopoiesis of Concern?

Concern exists for $N_2O$ use because detectable decreases in liver methionine synthetase level occur when this drug is

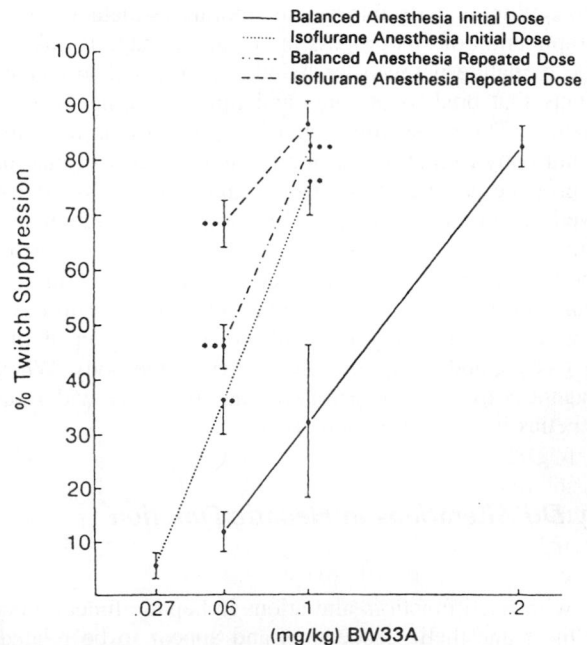

**FIGURE 34–7.** Twitch depression as a function of dose of atracurium (BW33A) during balanced and isoflurane anesthesia. Repeated doses were given after twitch tension had returned to 95% of the control level. Significantly greater blockade occurred with isoflurane than with balanced anesthesia (*) and repeated doses of atracurium (**). (From Sokoll MO, Gergis SD, Mehta M, et al. Safety and efficacy of atracurium (BW33A) in surgical patients receiving balanced or isoflurane anesthesia. *Anesthesiology.* 1983;58:450.)

administered to human beings in a concentration of 60% for 1.2 hours.[148] However, $N_2O$ has not been shown to be detrimental to marrow survival. If $N_2O$ at a concentration of 40% or greater is inspired for 3 to 5 days, predictable leukopenia occurs.[149] This event precludes the use of $N_2O$ for prolonged anesthesia or analgesia in the intensive care setting. Despite these findings, no evidence shows that inhaled agents affect the survival or function of transplanted bone marrow.

## TRAUMA

### How Do Inhaled Agents Affect the Circulation?

The incidence of hypovolemia and other major cardiovascular pathology is high in trauma. The use of inhaled anesthetics may be precluded by the patient's cardiovascular status. If inhaled anesthetics are to be used, careful consideration must be given to the effect of interaction of anesthesia and hypovolemia on the cardiovascular and respiratory systems.

The use of inhaled anesthetics in the presence of hypovolemia may accentuate or unmask cardiovascular instability. The inhaled agents are vasodilators and therefore may inhibit some of the physiologic responses necessary to maintain adequate BP in the setting of hypovolemia. Circulatory baroreflex responses are also blunted by volatile agents; thus, heart rate may not increase with hypovolemia.[150] Small amounts of blood loss can be tolerated during halothane, isoflurane, or enflurane anesthesia, with an insignificant effect on systemic arterial pressure.[151] In animal studies, after blood loss exceeded 10% of estimated blood volume, BP decreased in relation to the amount of blood lost.[151] With each of the anesthetics, loss of blood short of exsanguination in animals was tolerated well for short periods of time without development of metabolic acidosis. The use of inhaled agents in the setting of hypovolemia must be considered carefully and titrated to effect. Other drugs with fewer cardiovascular effects may be appropriate as adjuncts or as sole agents. Other injuries associated with trauma, such as myocardial and lung contusions, may also predispose the patient to exaggerated negative hemodynamic effects when potent agents are used.

### Is the Use of Nitrous Oxide Appropriate?

$N_2O$ should be avoided in patients with pneumothorax or pneumocranium for fear of tension pneumothorax and tension pneumocranium. $N_2O$ is more soluble in blood than nitrogen. Therefore, when exposed to a closed space containing air (eg, pneumothorax) $N_2O$ diffuses into the closed space faster than the nitrogen dissolves into the blood. This results in an increase in volume of gas in the closed space. The increase in volume occurs quickly in spaces surrounded by highly perfused tissues, such as lung or brain tissue.[152] In like fashion, the volume of an air embolus also increases in the presence of high concentrations of $N_2O$.[153]

### When Is Recall a Problem?

The incidence of awareness is high in trauma patients. The anesthesiologist is placed in a precarious situation of balanc-

ing the need for anesthetic agents against their negative effects on the cardiovascular system. At times, anesthesia may be withheld from the patient with inadequate circulation until function is restored. The incidence of explicit recall, which included awareness of pain, was 43% in one group of patients who had 20-minute or longer periods of no anesthetic delivery.[23]

In patients whose hemodynamic status may be tenuous, even small doses of inhaled anesthetics may produce severe hypotension and may be deleterious to the overall condition of the patient. The use of other agents, such as scopolamine or midazolam (to avoid recall), may be better choices to avoid recall. They, too, have their side effects, so that treatment must be individualized to each patient. The reader should note, however, that recall is not always a painful experience (especially in the presence of narcotics), but one does need to discuss it openly with patients after surgery to avoid ongoing anxiety and possible medicolegal issues.[154] All personnel in the operating theater should use gentle and encouraging language, especially in the setting just described.

## PROLONGED ANESTHESIA

The requirements for procedures necessitating prolonged anesthesia, such as extremity reimplantation, include maintenance of arterial pressure at near-awake values, preservation of body temperature, and immobility of the operative site. Among the possible regimens to accomplish these goals is the use of inhalation agents with or without adjuvants.

### Will Recovery Be Prolonged If an Inhaled Agent Is Used?

The major determinants are the solubility of the anesthetic and the depth and duration of anesthesia. The greater the total dose of anesthetic, that is, the concentration delivered multiplied by the duration of delivery, and the greater the blood solubility of the drug, the longer the recovery time.[155]

If anesthesia is to be provided by the inhalation route alone, the alveolar anesthetic concentration must be about 1.25 times the MAC or greater to ensure nonmovement. Prolonged anesthesia at this level requires at least 30 to 40 minutes for awakening if halothane is used, and 15 to 20 minutes if isoflurane is used. With newer agents such as desflurane and sevoflurane, whose solubilities are similar to the solubility of $N_2O$, duration of anesthesia has little effect on recovery time.[55,156] Recovery time is nearly the same for both brief and prolonged anesthesia with desflurane and sevoflurane.

## PREGNANCY AND THE PUERPERIUM

Inevitably, inhalation agents are given to some patients during pregnancy or the puerperium despite the popularity of regional anesthesia for obstetric care. Choosing the best parameters for anesthesia care of the mother may be at odds with optimal care of the fetus. The potent inhalation agents have at least one advantage over other general anesthetic agents in this setting: they provide unconsciousness and uterine relaxation simultaneously. Hence, they offer a method to relax the uterus reversibly when manipulations such as cervical cerclage, delivery of an after-coming head, and manual removal of the placenta are required. The use of inhalation agent above 1.0 MAC may also pose dangers in that uterine contraction may be inhibited at a time when it is needed (eg, immediately postpartum) and lead to significant blood loss. Similarly, hypotension accompanying inhalation anesthesia may decrease blood flow to the uterus and thus to the fetus.

### Should Inhalation Agents Be Used for Cervical Cerclage?

Although concern about teratogenicity or fetal loss may be a reason to avoid these agents during the earliest stages of pregnancy,[157,158] this concern no longer exists by the time cerclage is ordinarily performed. Uterine relaxation provided by inhalation agents may be an advantage. A quiet, comfortable, nonstraining patient is probably more important than the technique used to provide these conditions.

### What Are the Fetal Effects of Inhalation Agents?

Transfer of agent to the fetus is rapid.[159,160] The umbilical vein–to–maternal artery anesthetic concentration ratio increases throughout the anesthetic procedure. When the anesthetic procedure is completed, the anesthetic drugs are removed quickly as well. Laboratory studies show that $N_2O$ is fetotoxic to rats and may lead to increased reproductive loss when given at a specific time in the gestation.[161] The potent agents have not shown the same effects.[157]

In another study, the presence of $N_2O$ did not affect in vitro fertilization success rates.[162] It does not appear that inhalation anesthetic drugs by themselves influence fetal welfare when surgery must be done during pregnancy.[163] Once the gestation has progressed sufficiently for the mother to be certain that she is pregnant, probably only intervening complications such as hypotension and hypoxia have a detrimental effect on the fetus, uterus, or placenta.[164]

### Is Any Potent Agent Preferable for Operative Deliveries?

The agents are so similar in their ability to relax the uterus that no agent is preferable to the others.[165] In doses equivalent to 1.0 MAC, all of the agents significantly relax the uterus. When doses of 0.5 MAC or less were compared with respect to their effects on blood loss at cesarean section, no differences were found.[165,166] In most studies, no greater loss occurred with inhalation agents compared with regional techniques.[167]

The maximal discrepancy in anesthetic goals for the mother and fetus exists during emergency cesarean section, when fetal welfare may already be compromised and anesthesia still must be provided. One study demonstrated that the stressed fetus may have an exacerbation of metabolic and respiratory acidosis when exposed to anesthetizing concentrations of isoflurane.[168] Anesthetizing the mother with an inhalation agent may be necessary, but the cost may include worsening the condition of the already depressed baby.

## AMBULATORY SURGERY

As the indications for operations in the ambulatory setting are extended, rapid recovery of cognitive and psychomotor skills is increasingly relevant.[169] All inhalational agents can be used in this setting. However, some of the newer agents may deserve a special role in ambulatory anesthesia given their low blood solubility. The ability to titrate quickly the effect of these newer agents makes them ideal for this setting. There remains some controversy, however, regarding the clinical significance of these relatively insoluble potent agents. For anesthetics of short duration given at low doses, anesthetic solubility may not be of great significance in determining speed of recovery.[55]

### What Role Do New Agents Play in Ambulatory Surgery and at What Cost?

Desflurane is truly the only new agent introduced in the 1990s. Sevoflurane was actually developed in the early 1980s and has been gaining wider acceptance since the 1990s. Both agents possess characteristics that make them well suited for ambulatory surgery (low blood solubility [desflurane < sevoflurane]) leading to rapid onset and offset as compared with isoflurane.[170] Considering only the pharmacokinetic properties of the inhaled agents, the rate of elimination of desflurane and sevoflurane is similar to that of $N_2O$ (desflurane more so than sevoflurane) and is more rapid than enflurane, isoflurane, or halothane.[156,171] Hence, return of consciousness after anesthesia with desflurane and sevoflurane should be more rapid than with the more soluble drugs.

Data suggest that patients receiving desflurane may actually have more rapid emergence than patients receiving sevoflurane.[172] Although initial awakening may be more rapid with desflurane and other drugs of low solubility, discharge from the postanesthesia care unit and hospital may be influenced more by administration of analgesics or sedatives or administrative activities than by recovery from the inhaled agents.[173]

Low-flow anesthesia is rapidly gaining acceptance in the setting of ambulatory surgery. Traditionally, rapid changes in anesthetic concentration have been achieved in part by increasing total gas flow as well as the inspired concentration of the potent agent. The low blood solubility of desflurane permits somewhat more rapid changes in anesthetic concentration at low flows. Economic and environmental benefits accrue from this characteristic. Desflurane, however, does act as an airway irritant and may possess sympathomimetic effects at higher concentrations. Thus, it has not gained wide acceptance for inhalation inductions secondary to its airway-irritant characteristics.

Desflurane and sevoflurane are considerably more expensive per unit than older, traditional agents, such as isoflurane. Direct and indirect costs and savings, such as decreased time to discharge or decreased side effects, must be evaluated to assess the economic soundness of using these newer agents. Patient satisfaction must also weigh heavily in the decision process. A recent study showed significant differences in patient satisfaction measures when comparing sevoflurane with propofol.[174] A greater proportion of patients reported dissatisfaction with sevoflurane as compared with propofol.

## How Long Do Changes in Mental Function Persist After Anesthesia?

The greatest fractional recovery occurs in the first few minutes after anesthesia. Recovery is slower after prolonged anesthesia than after brief exposures.[156,169] N[2]O is not likely to have an important influence on psychomotor skills 1 hour after anesthesia. Recommended time periods that patients do not drive after anesthesia have varied from 24 to 48 hours.[169] Sedatives, hypnotics, and analgesic drugs given concomitantly with inhaled agents delay full recovery of cognitive and psychomotor skills.[169,175]

## Are Inhaled Agents Associated With Postoperative Nausea and Vomiting?

Persistence of emetic symptoms prolongs hospitalization and prevents resumption of activity. Premedicant, intraoperative, or postoperative administration of narcotics increases the incidence of nausea.[176,177] Of all the currently used inhaled agents, N[2]O has been singled out as a cause of postoperative nausea. However, any enhancement caused by N[2]O must be small, if it exists at all.[169,178,179]

## References

1. Lundy JS. Balanced anesthesia. *Minn Med.* 1926;9:399.
2. Forrest JB, Cahalan MK, Rehder K, et al. Multicenter study of general anesthesia, II: results. *Anesthesiology.* 1990;72:262.
3. Keys TE. The early pneumatic chemists and physicians: their influence on the development of surgical anesthesia. *Anesthesiology.* 1969;30:447.
4. Keys TE. The development of anesthesia. *Anesthesiology.* 1941;2:552.
5. Leake CD. The role of pharmacology in the development of ideal anesthesia. *JAMA.* 1934;102:1.
6. Robbins BH. Preliminary study of the anesthetic activity of fluorinated hydrocarbons. *J Pharmacol Exp Ther.* 1946;86:197.
7. Van Poznak A, Artusio JF Jr. Anesthetic properties of a series of fluorinated compounds, I: fluorinated hydrocarbons. *Toxicol Appl Pharmacol.* 1960;2:363.
8. Krantz JC Jr. The rationale of the use of fluorinated hydrocarbons and ethers as volatile anesthetic agents. *Anesth Analg.* 1965;44:260.
9. Terrell RC, Speers L, Szur AJ, et al. General anesthetics, 1: halogenated methylethyl ethers as anesthetic agents. *J Med Chem.* 1971;14:517.
10. Epstein RH, Stein AL, Marr AT, et al. High concentrations versus incremental induction of anesthesia with sevoflurane in children: a comparison of induction times, vital signs and complications. *J Clin Anesth.* 1998;10:41.
11. Gibbons RT, Steffey EP, Eger EI II. The effect of spontaneous versus controlled ventilation on the rate of rise of alveolar halothane concentration in dogs. *Anesth Analg.* 1977;56:32.
12. Paris ST, Cafferkey M, Tarling M, et al. Comparison of sevoflurane and halothane for outpatient dental anaesthesia in children. *Br J Anaesth.* 1997;79:280.
13. Berry PD, Sessler DI, Larson MD. Severe carbon monoxide poisoning during desflurane anesthesia. *Anesthesiology.* 1999;90:613.
14. Fang ZX, Eger EI, Laster MJ, et al. Carbon monoxide production from degradation of desflurane, enflurane, isoflurane, halothane, and sevoflurane by soda lime and Baralyme. *Anesth Analg.* 1995;80:1187.
15. Funk W, Gruber M, Wild K, et al. Dry soda lime markedly degrades sevoflurane during simulated inhalation induction. *Br J Anaesth.* 1999;82:193.
16. Bito H, Ikeda K. Effect of total flow rate on the concentration of degradation products generated by reaction between sevoflurane and soda lime. *Br J Anaesth.* 1995;74:667.
17. Prys-Roberts C. Anaesthesia: a practical or impractical construct? *Br J Anaesth.* 1987;59:1341.
18. Stoelting RK, Longnecker DE, Eger EI II. Minimum alveolar concentration in man on awakening from methoxyflurane, halothane, ether and fluroxene anesthesia: MAC awake. *Anesthesiology.* 1970;33:5.
19. Saidman LJ, Eger EI II, Munson ES, et al. Minimum alveolar concentrations of methoxyflurane, halothane, ether and cyclopropane in man: correlation with theories of anesthesia. *Anesthesiology.* 1967;28:994.
20. Yakaitis RW, Blitt CD, Angiulo JP. End-tidal halothane concentration for endotracheal intubation. *Anesthesiology.* 1977;47:386.
21. Roizen MF, Horrigan RW, Frazer BM. Anesthetic doses blocking adrenergic (stress) and cardiovascular responses to incision-MAC BAR. *Anesthesiology.* 1981;54:390.
22. Ausems ME, Hug CC Jr, Stanski DR, et al. Plasma concentrations of alfentanil required to supplement nitrous oxide anesthesia for general surgery. *Anesthesiology.* 1986;65:362.
23. Bogetz MS, Katz JA. Recall of surgery for major trauma. *Anesthesiology.* 1984;61:6.
24. Breckenridge JL, Aitkenhead AR. Awareness during anaesthesia: a review. *Ann R Coll Surg Engl.* 1983;65:93.
25. Keenan RL, Boyan CP. Cardiac arrests due to anesthesia: a study of incidence and causes. *JAMA.* 1985;253:2372.
26. Stullken EH Jr, Milde JH, Michenfelder JD, et al. The non-linear responses of cerebral metabolism to low concentrations of halothane, enflurane, isoflurane, and thiopental. *Anesthesiology.* 1977;46:28.
27. Warner DS. Volatile anesthetics and the ischemic brain. *J Neurosurg Anesth.* 1989;1:290.
28. Warner DS, Zhou J, Ramani R, et al. Nitrous oxide does not alter infarct volume in rats undergoing reversible middle cerebral artery occlusion. *Anesthesiology.* 1990;73:686.
29. Rampil IJ, Weiskopf RB, Brown IG, et al. I653 and isoflurane produce similar dose-related changes in the electroencephalogram of pigs. *Anesthesiology.* 1988;69:298.
30. Michenfelder JD, Sundt TM, Fode N, et al. Isoflurane when compared to enflurane and halothane decreases the frequency of cerebral ischemia during carotid endarterectomy. *Anesthesiology.* 1987;67:336.
31. Messick JM, Casement B, Sharbrough FW, et al. Correlation of regional cerebral blood flow (CBF) with EEG changes during isoflurane anesthesia for carotid endarterectomy. *Anesthesiology.* 1987;66:344.
32. Newberg LA, Milde JH, Michenfelder JD. Systemic and cerebral effects of isoflurane-induced hypotension in dogs. *Anesthesiology.* 1984;60:541.
33. Smith AL, Wollman H. Cerebral blood flow and metabolism: effects of anesthetic drugs and techniques. *Anesthesiology.* 1972;36:378.
34. Lutz LJ, Milde JH, Milde LN. The cerebral functional, metabolic, and hemodynamic effects of desflurane in dogs. *Anesthesiology.* 1990;73:125.
35. Drummond JC, Todd MM, Scheller MS, et al. A comparison of the direct cerebral vasodilating potencies of halothane and isoflurane in the New Zealand white rabbit. *Anesthesiology.* 1986;65:462.
36. Hansen TD, Warner DS, Todd MM, et al. Effects of nitrous oxide and volatile anaesthetics on cerebral blood flow. *Br J Anaesth.* 1989;63:290.
37. Mielck F, Stephan H, Weyland A, et al. Effects of one minimum alveolar anesthetic concentration sevoflurane on cerebral metabolism, blood flow and CO[2] reactivity in cardiac patients. *Anesth Analg.* 1999;89:364.
38. Mielck F, Stephan H, Buhre W, et al. Effects of 1 MAC desflurane on cerebral metabolism, blood flow and carbon dioxide reactivity in humans. *Br J Anaesth.* 1998;81:155.
39. Adams RW, Gronert GA, Sundt TM, et al. Halothane, hypocapnia, and cerebrospinal fluid pressure in neurosurgery. *Anesthesiology.* 1972;37:510.
40. Muzzi DA, Losasso TJ, Dietz NM, et al. The effect of desflurane and isoflurane on cerebrospinal fluid pressure in humans with supratentorial mass lesions. *Anesthesiology.* 1992;76:720.
41. McPherson RW, Brian JE Jr, Traystman RJ. Cerebrovascular responsiveness to carbon dioxide in dogs with 1.4% and 2.8% isoflurane. *Anesthesiology.* 1989;70:843.
42. Artru AA, Nugent M, Michenfelder JD. Enflurane causes a prolonged and reversible increase in the rate of CSF production in the dog. *Anesthesiology.* 1982;57:255.
43. Artru AA. Effect of halothane and fentanyl on the rate of CSF production in dogs. *Anesth Analg.* 1983;62:581.
44. Maktabi MA, Elboki FF, Faraci FM, et al. Halothane decreases the rate of production of cerebrospinal fluid: possible role of vasopressin V[1] receptors. *Anesthesiology.* 1993;78:72.
45. Artru AA. Isoflurane does not increase the rate of CSF production in the dog. *Anesthesiology.* 1984;60:194.
46. Courtin EF, Bickford RG, Faulconer A Jr. The classification and significance of electroencephalographic patterns produced by nitrous oxide-ether anesthesia during surgical operation. *Proc Staff Meet Mayo Clin.* 1950;25:197.

47. Eger EI II, Stevens WC, Cromwell TH. The electroencephalogram of man anesthetized with Forane. *Anesthesiology.* 1981;35:504.

48. Rampil IJ, Lockart SH, Eger EI II, et al. The electroencephalographic effects of desflurane in humans. *Anesthesiology.* 1991;74:434.

49. Joas TA, Stevens WC, Eger EI II. Electroencephalographic seizure activity in dogs during anesthesia. *Br J Anaesth.* 1973;43:739.

50. Neigh JL, Garman JK, Harp JR. The electroencephalographic pattern during anesthesia with Ethrane: effects of depth of anesthesia, PaCO$_2$ and nitrous oxide. *Anesthesiology.* 1971;35:482.

51. Opitz A, Brechts B, Stenzel E. Enflurane anesthesia for epileptic patients. *Anaesthetist.* 1977;26:329.

52. Peterson DO, Drummond JC, Todd MM. Effects of halothane, enflurane, isoflurane and nitrous oxide on somatosensory evoked potentials in humans. *Anesthesiology.* 1986;65:35.

53. Grundy BL. Intraoperative monitoring of sensory evoked potentials. *Anesthesiology.* 1983;58:72.

54. Lockhart SH, Cohen Y, Yasuda N, et al. Cerebral uptake and elimination of desflurane, isoflurane and halothane from rabbit brain: an in vivo NMR study. *Anesthesiology.* 1991;74:575.

55. Eger EI II, Johnson BH. Rates of awakening from anesthesia with I-653, halothane, isoflurane and sevoflurane: a test of effect of anesthetic concentration and duration in rats. *Anesth Analg.* 1987;66:977.

56. Rosenberg H, Clofine R, Bialik O. Neurologic changes during awakening from anesthesia. *Anesthesiology.* 1981;54:125.

57. Keats AS. The effect of drugs on respiration in man. *Annu Rev Pharmacol Toxicol.* 1985;25:41.

58. Theye RA, Tuohy GF. Oxygen uptake during light halothane anesthesia in man. *Anesthesiology.* 1964;25:627.

59. Heneghan CPH, Bergman NA, Jordan C, et al. Effect of isoflurane on bronchomotor tone in man. *Br J Anaesth.* 1986;58:24.

60. Jones JG. Mechanisms of some pulmonary effects of general anaesthesia. *Br J Hosp Med.* 1987;38:472.

61. Bergman NA. Distribution of inspired gas during anesthesia and artificial ventilation. *J Appl Physiol.* 1963;18:1085.

62. Domino KB, Borowec L, Alexander CM, et al. Influence of isoflurane on hypoxic pulmonary vasoconstriction in dogs. *Anesthesiology.* 1986;64:423.

63. Rodenstein DO, Stanescu DC. The soft palate and breathing. *Am Rev Respir Dis.* 1986;134:311.

64. Taylor RH, Lerman J. Induction, maintenance and recovery characteristics of desflurane in infants and children. *Can J Anaesth.* 1992;39:6.

65. Sibert KS, Biondi JW, Hirsch NP. Spontaneous respiration during thoracotomy in a patient with mediastinal mass. *Anesth Analg.* 1987;66:904.

66. Black A, Sury MRJ, Hemington L, et al. A comparison of the induction characteristics of sevoflurane and halothane in children. *Anesthesia.* 1996;51:539.

67. Fourcade HE, Stevens WC, Larson CP Jr, et al. The ventilatory effects of Forane, a new inhaled anesthetic. *Anesthesiology.* 1971;35:26.

68. Hickey RF, Fourcade HE, Eger EI II, et al. The effects of ether, halothane and Forane on apneic thresholds in man. *Anesthesiology.* 1971;35:32.

69. Wahba WM. Analysis of ventilatory depression by enflurane during clinical anesthesia. *Anesth Analg.* 1980;59:103.

70. Eger EI II, Dolan WM, Stevens WC, et al. Surgical stimulation antagonizes the respiratory depression produced by Forane. *Anesthesiology.* 1972;36:544.

71. Cullen DJ, Eger EI II, Stevens WC, et al. Clinical signs of anesthesia. *Anesthesiology.* 1972;36:21.

72. Hedenstierna G. Causes of gas exchange impairment during general anaesthesia. *Eur J Anaesthesiol.* 1988;5:221.

73. Rothen HU, Neumann P, Berglund JE, et al. Dynamics of re-expansion of atelectasis during general anesthesia. *Br J Anaesth.* 1999;82:551.

74. Lindahl SGE, Charlton AJ, Hatch DJ, et al. Ventilatory responses to inspiratory mechanical loads in spontaneously breathing children during halothane anaesthesia. *Acta Anaesthesiol Scand.* 1986;30:122.

75. Nunn JF, Ezi-Ashi TI. The respiratory effects of resistance to breathing in anesthetized man. *Anesthesiology.* 1961;22:174.

76. Pietak S, Weenig CS, Hickey RF, et al. Anesthetic effects of ventilation in patients with chronic obstructive pulmonary disease. *Anesthesiology.* 1975;42:160.

77. Wahba WM. Influence of airway resistance and ventilatory pattern in PaCO$_2$ during enflurane anaesthesia. *Br J Anaesth.* 1979;51:123.

78. Kingston HGG, Hirshman CA. Perioperative management of the patient with asthma. *Anesth Analg.* 1984;63:844.

79. Hirshman CA, Bergman NA. Halothane and enflurane protect against bronchospasm in an asthma dog model. *Anesth Analg.* 1978;57:629.

80. Hirshman CA, Edelstein G, Peetz S, et al. Mechanism of action of inhalational anesthesia on airways. *Anesthesiology.* 1982;56:107.

81. Benumof JL. One-lung ventilation and hypoxic pulmonary vasoconstriction: implications for anesthetic management. *Anesth Analg.* 1985;64:821.

82. Knill RL, Kieraszewicz HT, Dodgson BG, et al. Chemical regulation of ventilation during isoflurane sedation and anaesthesia in humans. *Can J Anaesth.* 1983;30:607.

83. Hess W, Arnold B, Schulte-Sasse U, et al. Comparison of isoflurane and halothane when used to control intraoperative hypertension in patients undergoing coronary artery bypass surgery. *Anesth Analg.* 1983;62:15.

84. Hamilton WK. Do let the blood pressure drop and do use myocardial depressants! *Anesthesiology.* 1976;45:273.

85. Yakaitis RW, Blitt CD, Angiulo JP. End-tidal halothane concentration for endotracheal intubation. *Anesthesiology.* 1977;47:386.

86. Eger EI II, Smith NT, Stoelting R, et al. Cardiovascular effects of halothane in man. *Anesthesiology.* 1970;32:396.

87. Crawford DC, Fell D, Achola KJ, et al. Effects of alfentanil on the pressor and catecholamine responses to tracheal intubation. *Br J Anaesth.* 1987;59:707.

88. Henderson PS, Cohen JI, Jarnberg PO, et al. A canine model for studying laryngospasm and its prevention. *Laryngoscope.* 1992;102:1237.

89. Tuman KJ, McCarthy RJ, Spiess BD, et al. Does choice of anesthetic agent significantly affect outcome after coronary artery surgery. *Anesthesiology.* 1989;70:189.

90. Slogoff S, Keats AS. Randomized trial of primary agents on outcome of coronary artery bypass operations. *Anesthesiology.* 1989;70:179.

91. Thomson IR, Bowering JB, Hudson RJ, et al. A comparison of desflurane and isoflurane in patients undergoing coronary artery surgery. *Anesthesiology.* 1991;75:776.

92. Lillehaug SL, Tinker JH. Why do "pure" vasodilators cause coronary steal when anesthetics don't (or seldom do)? *Anesth Analg.* 1991;73:681.

93. Hickey PR, Hansen DD, Strafford M, et al. Pulmonary and systemic hemodynamic effects of nitrous oxide in infants with normal and elevated pulmonary vascular resistance. *Anesthesiology.* 1986;65:374.

94. Eger EI II. Cardiovascular effects of nitrous oxide. In: Eger EI II, ed. *Nitrous Oxide.* New York, NY: Elsevier; 1985:125.

95. Johnston R, Eger EI II, Wilson C. A comparative interaction of epinephrine with enflurane, isoflurane, and halothane in man. *Anesth Analg.* 1976;55:709.

96. Weiskopf RB, Eger EI II, Holmes MA, et al. Epinephrine-induced premature ventricular contractions and changes in arterial blood pressure and heart rate during I-653, isoflurane, and halothane anesthesia in swine. *Anesthesiology.* 1989;70:293.

97. Imamura S, Ikeda K. Comparison of the epinephrine-induced arrhythmogenic effect of sevoflurane with isoflurane and halothane. *J Anesth.* 1987;1:62.

98. Tucker W, Rackstein A, Munson E. Comparison of arrhythmic doses of adrenaline, metaraminol, ephedrine and phenylephrine during isoflurane and halothane anesthesia in dogs. *Br J Anaesth.* 1974;46:392.

99. Atlee JL, Malkinson CE. Potentiation by thiopental of halothane-epinephrine-induced arrhythmias in dogs. *Anesthesiology.* 1982;57:285.

100. Roizen MF, Stevens WC. Multiform ventricular tachycardia due to interaction of aminophylline and halothane. *Anesth Analg.* 1978;57:738.

101. Court MH, Dodman NH, Greenblatt DJ, et al. Effect of midazolam infusion and flumazenil administration on epinephrine arrhythmogenicity in dogs anesthetized with halothane. *Anesthesiology.* 1993;78:155.

102. Werder KV, Stevens WC, Cromwell TH, et al. Adrenal function during long-term anesthesia in man. *Proc Soc Exp Biol Med.* 1970;135:854.

103. Lacoumenta S, Paterson J, Burrin J, et al. Effects of two different halothane concentrations on the metabolic and endocrine responses to surgery. *Br J Anaesth.* 1986;58:844.

104. Gelman S, Rivas J, Erdemir H, et al. Hormonal and haemodynamic responses to upper abdominal surgery during isoflurane and balanced anaesthesia. *Can J Anaesth.* 1984;31:509.

105. Hamberger B, Jarnberg PO. Plasma catecholamines during surgical stress: difference between neurolept and enflurane anaesthesia. *Acta Anaesthesiol Scand.* 1983;27:307.

106. Bovill JG, Sebel PS, Stanley TH. Opioid analgesics in anesthesia: with special reference to their use in cardiovascular anesthesia. *Anesthesiology.* 1984;61:731.

107. Campbell B, Parikh R, Naismith A. Comparison of fentanyl and halothane supplementation to general anesthesia on the stress response to upper abdominal surgery. *Br J Anaesth.* 1984;56:257.

108. Frink EJ Jr, Ghantous H, Malan TP, et al. Plasma inorganic fluoride with sevoflurane anesthesia: correlation with indices of hepatic and renal function. *Anesth Analg.* 1992;74:231.

109. Mazze RI, Woodruff RE, Heerdt ME. Isoniazid-induced enflurane defluorination in humans. *Anesthesiology.* 1982;57:5.

110. Kharasch ED, Hankins DC, Thummel KE. Human kidney methoxyflurane and sevoflurane metabolism: intrarenal fluoride production as a possible mechanism of methoxyflurane nephrotoxicity. *Anesthesiology.* 1995;82:689.

111. Mazze RI. Fluorinated anaesthetic nephrotoxicity: an update. *Can J Anaesth.* 1984;31:S16.

112. Mirenda JV, Grissom TE. Anesthetic implications of the renin angiotensin system and angiotensin-converting enzyme inhibitors. *Anesth Analg.* 1991;72:667.

113. Miller ED Jr, Longnecker DE, Peach MJ. The regulatory function of the renin-angiotensin system during general anesthesia. *Anesthesiology.* 1978;48:399.

114. Priano LL. Effect of halothane on renal hemodynamics during normovolemia and acute hemorrhagic hypovolemia. *Anesthesiology.* 1985;63:357.

115. Bernard JM, Doursout MF, Wouters P, et al. Effect of enflurane and isoflurane on hepatic and renal circulations in chronically instrumented dogs. *Anesthesiology.* 1991;74:298.

116. Priano LL, Smith JD, Cohen JI, et al. IV fluid administration and urine output during radical neck surgery. *Head Neck.* 1993;15:208.

117. Sweny P. Is postoperative oliguria avoidable? *Br J Anaesth.* 1991;67:137.

118. Brown BR. Hepatotoxicity and inhalation anesthetics: views in the era of isoflurane. *J Clin Anesth.* 1989;1:368.

119. Koblin DD. Characteristics and implications of desflurane metabolism and toxicity. *Anesth Analg.* 1992;75:S10.

120. Christ DD, Kenna JG, Kammerer W, et al. Enflurane metabolism produces covalently bound liver adducts recognized by antibodies from patients with halothane hepatitis. *Anesthesiology.* 1988;69:833.

121. Eger EI II, Johnson BH, Strum DP, et al. Studies of the toxicity of I-653, halothane, and isoflurane in enzyme-induced, hypoxic rats. *Anesth Analg.* 1987;66:1227.

122. Tiainen P, Rosenberg PH. Hepatocellular integrity during and after isoflurane and halothane anaesthesia in surgical patients. *Br J Anaesth.* 1996;77:744.

123. O'Riordan J, O'Beirne HA, Young Y, et al. Effects of desflurane and isoflurane on splanchnic microcirculation during major surgery. *Br J Anaesth.* 1997;78:95.

124. Nishiyama T, Yokoyama T, Hanaoka K. Liver function after sevoflurane or isoflurane anaesthesia in neurosurgical patients. *Can J Anaesth.* 1998;4:753.

125. Gelman S, Dillard E, Bradley E. Hepatic circulation during surgical stress and anesthesia with halothane, isoflurane and fentanyl. *Anesth Analg.* 1987;66:936.

126. Gelman S, Fowler KC, Smith LR. Liver circulation and function during isoflurane and halothane anesthesia. *Anesthesiology.* 1984;61:726.

127. Seyde WC, Longnecker DE. Anesthetic influences on regional hemodynamics in normal and hemorrhaged rats. *Anesthesiology.* 1984;61:686.

128. Subcommittee on the National Halothane Study. Summary of the National Halothane Study. *JAMA.* 1966;197:775.

129. Zinn SE, Fairley HB, Glenn JD. Liver function in patients with mild alcoholic hepatitis, after enflurane, nitrous oxide-narcotic, and spinal anesthesia. *Anesth Analg.* 1985;64:487.

130. Hirsch I, McGill J, Cryer P, et al. Perioperative management of surgical patients with diabetes mellitus. *Anesthesiology.* 1991;74:346.

131. Desborough JP, Knowles MG, Hall GM. Effects of isoflurane-nitrous oxide anaesthesia in insulin secretion in female patients. *Br J Anaesth.* 1998;80:250.

132. Iwasaka H, Itoh K, Miyakawa H, et al. Glucose intolerance during prolonged sevoflurane anaesthesia. *Can J Anaesth.* 1996;43:1059.

133. Burgos LG, Ebert TJ, Asiddao C, et al. Increased intraoperative cardiovascular morbidity in diabetics with autonomic neuropathy. *Anesthesiology.* 1989;70:591.

134. Philbin D, Coggins C. Plasma antidiuretic hormone levels in cardiac surgical patients during morphine and halothane anesthesia. *Anesthesiology.* 1978;49:95.

135. Oyama T, Matsuki A, Kudo T. Effect of halothane, methoxyflurane anaesthesia and surgery on plasma thyroid-stimulating hormone (TSH) levels in man. *Anaesthesia.* 1972;27:2.

136. Vadam C, Juvin PH, Malek L, et al. Recovery from desflurane, isoflurane or propofol anesthesia in morbidly obese patients. *Anesthesiology.* 1999;91(suppl):A378.

137. Young SR, Stoelting RK, Peterson C, et al. Anesthetic biotransformation and renal function in obese patients during and after methoxyflurane or halothane anesthesia. *Anesthesiology.* 1975;42:451.

138. Bentley JB, Vaughan RW, Gandolfi AJ, et al. Halothane biotransformation in obese and non-obese patients. *Anesthesiology.* 1982;57:94.

139. Miller RD, Eger EI II, Way W, et al. Comparative neuromuscular effects of Forane and halothane alone and in combination with d-tubocurarine in man. *Anesthesiology.* 1971;35:38.

140. Ali HA, Savarese JJ. Monitoring of neuromuscular function. *Anesthesiology.* 1976;45:216.

141. Waud BE, Waud DR. Effects of volatile anesthetics on directly and indirectly stimulated skeletal muscle. *Anesthesiology.* 1979;50:103.

142. Caldwell JE, Laster MJ, Magorian T, et al. The neuromuscular effects of desflurane, alone and combined with pancuronium or succinylcholine in humans. *Anesthesiology.* 1991;74:414.

143. Sokoll MD, Gergis SD, Mehta M, et al. Safety and efficacy of atracurium (BW33A) in surgical patients receiving balanced or isoflurane anesthesia. *Anesthesiology.* 1983;58:450.

144. Morita T, Kurosaki D, Tsukagoshi H, et al. Sevoflurane and isoflurane impair edrophonium reversal of vecuronium-induced neuromuscular block. *Can J Anaesth.* 1996;43:799.

145. Kaplan RF, Garcia M, Hannallah RS. Mivacurium-induced neuromuscular blockade during sevoflurane and halothane anaesthesia in children. *Can J Anaesth.* 1995;42:16.

146. Kumar N, Mirakhur RK, Symington MJ, et al. A comparison of the effects of isoflurane and desflurane on neuromuscular effects of mivacurium. *Anaesthesia* 1996;51:547.

147. Wright PM, Hart P, Lau M, et al. The magnitude and time course of vecuronium potentiation by desflurane versus isoflurane. *Anesthesiology.* 1995;82:404.

148. Koblin DD, Waskell L, Watson JE, et al. Nitrous oxide inactivates methionine synthetase in human liver. *Anesth Analg.* 1982;61:75.

149. Lassen HCA, Henriksen E, Neukirch F, et al. Treatment of tetanus: severe bone-marrow depression after prolonged nitrous-oxide anaesthesia. *Lancet.* 1956;i:527.

150. Kotrly K, Ebert T, Vucins E, et al. Baroreceptor reflex control of heart rate during isoflurane anesthesia in humans. *Anesthesiology.* 1984;60:173.

151. Weiskopf RB, Townsley MI, Riordan KK, et al. Comparison of cardiopulmonary responses to graded hemorrhage during enflurane, halothane, isoflurane and ketamine anesthesia. *Anesth Analg.* 1981;60:481.

152. Eger EI II, Saidman LJ. Hazards of nitrous oxide anesthesia in bowel obstruction and pneumothorax. *Anesthesiology.* 1965;26:61.

153. Munson ES, Merrick HC. Effect of nitrous oxide on venous air embolism. *Anesthesiology.* 1966;27:783.

154. Blacher RS. Awareness during surgery [editorial]. *Anesthesiology.* 1984;61:1.

155. Eger EI II. Recovery from anesthesia. In: Egar EI II, ed. *Anesthetic Uptake and Action.* Baltimore, Md: Williams & Wilkins; 1974:228.

156. Smiley RM, Ornstein E, Matteo RS, et al. Desflurane and isoflurane in surgical patients: comparison of emergence time. *Anesthesiology.* 1991;74:425.

157. Lane GA, Nahrwold M, Tait A, et al. Anesthetics as teratogens: nitrous oxide is fetotoxic, xenon is not. *Science.* 1980;210:899.

158. Mazze RI, Fujinaga M, Rice SA, et al. Reproductive and teratogenic effects of nitrous oxide, halothane, isoflurane and enflurane in Sprague-Dawley rats. *Anesthesiology.* 1986;64:339.

159. Marx GF, Joshi CW, Orkin LR. Placental transmission of nitrous oxide. *Anesthesiology.* 1970;32:429.

160. Gregory GA, Wade JG, Beihl DR, et al. Fetal anesthetic requirement (MAC) for halothane. *Anesth Analg.* 1983;62:9.

161. Fink BR, Shepherd TH, Blandau RJ. Teratogenic activity of nitrous oxide. *Nature.* 1967;214:146.

162. Rosen MA, Roizen MF, Eger EI II, et al. The effect of nitrous oxide on in-vitro fertilization success rates. *Anesthesiology.* 1987;67:42.

163. Aldridge LM, Tunstall ME. Nitrous oxide and the fetus. *Br J Anaesth.* 1986;58:1348.

164. Duncan PE, Pope WDB, Cohen MM, et al. Fetal risk of anesthesia and surgery during pregnancy. *Anesthesiology.* 1986;64:790.

165. Warren TM, Datta S, Ostheimer GW, et al. Comparison of the maternal and neonatal effects of halothane, enflurane, and isoflurane for cesarean delivery. *Anesth Analg.* 1983;62:516.

166. Moir DD. Anaesthesia for cesarean section. *Br J Anaesth.* 1970;42:136.

167. Gilstrap LC III, Hauth JC, Hawkins GDV, et al. Effect of type of anesthesia on blood loss at cesarean section. *Obstet Gynecol.* 1987;69:328.

168. Baker BW, Hughes SC, Shnider SM, et al. Maternal anesthesia and the

stressed fetus: effects of isoflurane on the asphyxiated fetal lamb. *Anesthesiology.* 1990;72:65.

169. Korttila K. Postanesthetic cognitive and psychomotor impairment. *Int Anesth Clin.* 1986;24:59.

170. Beaussier M, Hugues D, Abdelahim Z, et al. Comparative effects of desflurane and isoflurane on recovery after long lasting anaesthesia. *Can J Anaesth.* 1998;45:429.

171. Van Hemelrijck J, Smith I, White PF. Use of desflurane for outpatient anesthesia. *Anesthesiology.* 1991;75:197.

172. Eger EI, Gong D, Koblin DD, et al. The effect of anesthetic duration on kinetic and recovery characteristics of desflurane versus sevoflurane, and on the kinetic characteristics of compound A, in volunteers. *Anesth Analg.* 1998;86:414.

173. Ghouri AF, Bodner M, White PF. Recovery profile after desflurane-nitrous oxide in outpatients. *Anesthesiology.* 1991;74:419.

174. Thwaites A, Edmends S, Smith I. Inhalation induction with sevoflur-ane: a double blind comparison with propofol. *Br J Anaesth.* 1997;78:356.

175. Fletcher JE, Sebel PS, Murphy MR, et al. Psychomotor performance after desflurane anesthesia: a comparison with isoflurane. *Anesth Analg.* 1991;73:260.

176. Rising S, Dogson MS, Steen PA. Isoflurane versus fentanyl for outpatient laparoscopy. *Acta Anaesthesiol Scand.* 1985;29:251.

177. Hackett GH, Harris MNE, Plantevin OM, et al. Anaesthesia for outpatient termination of pregnancy: a comparison of two anaesthetic techniques. *Br J Anaesth.* 1982;54:865.

178. Wrigley SR, Fairfield JE, Jones RM, et al. Induction and recovery characteristics of desflurane in day case patients: a comparison with propofol. *Anaesthesia.* 1991;46:615.

179. Hovorka J, Korttila K, Erkola O. Nitrous oxide does not increase nausea and vomiting following gynaecological laparoscopy. *Can J Anaesth.* 1989;36:145.

CHAPTER

# 35

# Local Anesthetics

## Jay S. Ellis

MECHANISMS OF ACTION

*How Do Local Anesthetics Work?*

*Are All Nerves Equally Susceptible to Local Anesthetics?*

*What Are the Important Chemical Properties of Local Anesthetics?*

*How Are Local Anesthetics Metabolized?*

CLINICAL APPLICATIONS

*How Should a Local Anesthetic Be Chosen?*

*How Can Local Anesthetics Be Made to Work Better?*

*Can Local Anesthetic Solutions Be Modified to Improve Performance?*

*What Are the Differences Between Agents?*

TOXICITY

*What Are the Central Nervous System Effects of Local Anesthetic Overdose?*

*How Is Cardiovascular Toxicity Manifested?*

*How Is Local Anesthetic Toxicity Avoided?*

*How Can Inadvertent Intravenous Injection Be Avoided?*

*What Is the Treatment?*

*Do Local Anesthetics Cause Allergic Reactions?*

*Do Local Anesthetics Cause Tissue Toxicity?*

Local anesthetics provide anesthetists with the ability to render patients insensible to pain without having to render them unconscious. This characteristic permits many procedures to be performed with minimal physiologic challenge. Such drugs significantly expand the number of anesthetic choices and contribute a great deal to the art of our specialty. Like all therapeutic agents, local anesthetics have their risks. This chapter discusses the rational use of these drugs, with particular attention paid to their anesthetic properties, toxicity, and therapeutic uses.

The chemical structure of clinically useful local anesthetics consists of three parts: an aromatic group, an intermediate chain, and an amine group (Fig. 35–1). Local anesthetics are classified into major groups depending on the presence of the amide or ester linkage of the intermediate chain. The amide local anesthetics include lidocaine, mepivacaine, prilocaine,

bupivacaine, and etidocaine (remember the amide local anesthetics as those drugs having an "i" in the drug name before the *caine*). The ester local anesthetics are cocaine, procaine, chloroprocaine, and tetracaine.

## MECHANISMS OF ACTION

### *How Do Local Anesthetics Work?*

**Physiology of Nerve Conduction**

A review of the physiology of nerve conduction is necessary before discussing the mechanism of action of local anesthetics. The resting nerve fiber maintains a transmembrane potential between $-70$ and $-80$ mV. This transmembrane potential results from the high concentration of potassium ions

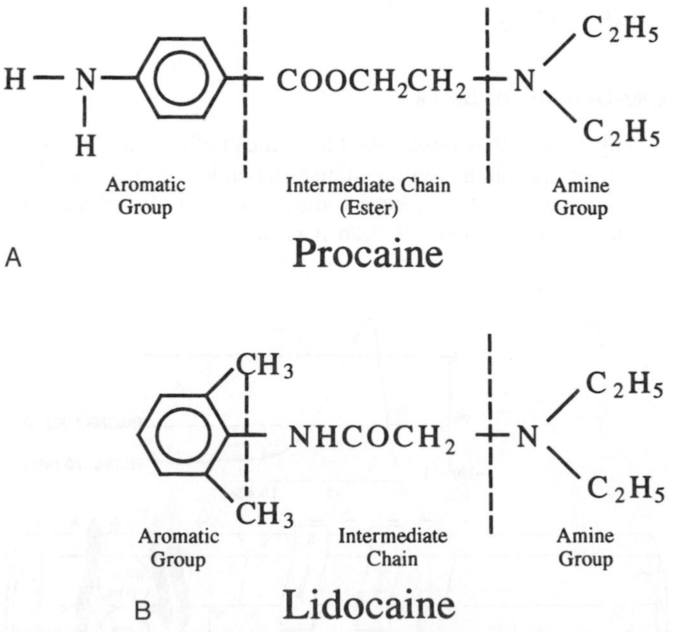

**FIGURE 35–1.** Chemical structure of (*A*) ester local anesthetic procaine and (*B*) amide local anesthetic lidocaine. Local anesthetics in clinical use all consist of an aromatic element, an intermediate element, and an amine element. Modification of the chemical structure of the three parts affects the clinical properties of the local anesthetic agent.

---

All material in this chapter is in the public domain, with the exception of any borrowed figures or tables.

inside the nerve relative to the surrounding extracellular fluid. A concentration gradient also exists for sodium ions, the extracellular concentration of which is much higher than the intracellular concentration.

When a nerve is stimulated, sodium ion channels in the nerve cell membrane undergo a voltage-dependent conformational change that opens the channel, allowing rapid influx of sodium ions into the cell. This movement changes the transmembrane potential. When a certain level (the threshold potential) is exceeded, an action potential is generated and an impulse is conducted down the fiber. The change in potential opens adjacent sodium channels, allowing propagation of the action potential and generation of the impulse.

The nerve reacquires its resting membrane potential through the efflux of potassium ions. The relative concentrations of sodium and potassium ions are then restored by the energy-dependent sodium-potassium adenosine triphosphatase pump.[1] Figure 35–2 summarizes these events.

### Effect on the Action Potential

Local anesthetics bind to the sodium channels in the nerve cell membranes and inhibit the influx of sodium ions.[2] The limited influx of ions reduces the rate of rise of the action potential. If enough sodium channels are blocked, the action potential fails to reach the threshold level and no impulses are conducted. As a result, local anesthetics do not affect the resting membrane potential, but they do affect the rate of rise and the maximum level of the action potential.

The exact mechanism by which local anesthetics affect the sodium channels remains to be determined. Several theories have been proposed,[3] the most popular of which suggests that local anesthetics bind to the protein subunits of the sodium channel and inhibit the previously mentioned voltage-dependent conformational changes that allow sodium influx into the cell (Fig. 35–3).

### Use-Dependent Block

Any theory that describes local anesthetic action must account for the phenomenon of use-dependent block, in which the local anesthetic effect is much more pronounced after repeated action potentials than it is in resting nerves.

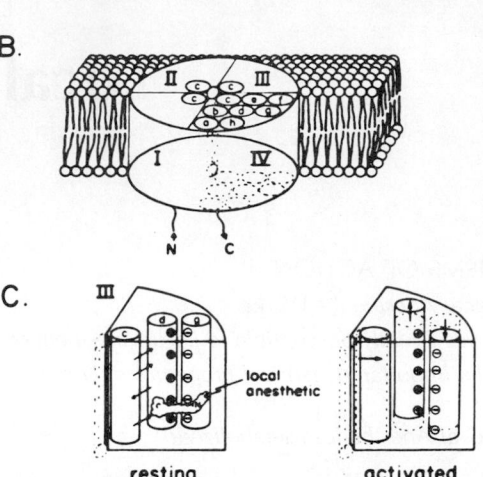

**FIGURE 35–3.** Speculative model for the molecular mechanism of local anesthetic action. *A,* The large protein subunit of the Na⁺ channel has four regions of six to eight repeating amino acids. *B,* The four regions align themselves with the polar edges, forming the lining of the ion pod. *C,* The amino acids form a strip of positive or negative charge owing to their arrangement in α-helical structures. When the membrane depolarizes, it causes movement in one helix that then causes movements in adjoining helices, resulting in the opening of the ion channel. Butterworth and Strichartz speculate that the local anesthetic molecule prevents the movement of these helices, impeding Na⁺ channel opening. (*A,* from Butterworth JF IV, Strichartz GR. Molecular mechanisms of local anesthesia: a review. *Anesthesiology.* 1990;72:729. *B,* adapted, reprinted from *FEBS Letters*, Volume 193, Greenblatt RE, Blatt Y, Montal M. The structure of the voltage sensitive sodium channel: inferences derived from computer aided analysis of the *electrophorus electricus* channel primary structure, page 125, Copyright 1985, with permission of Elsevier Science.)

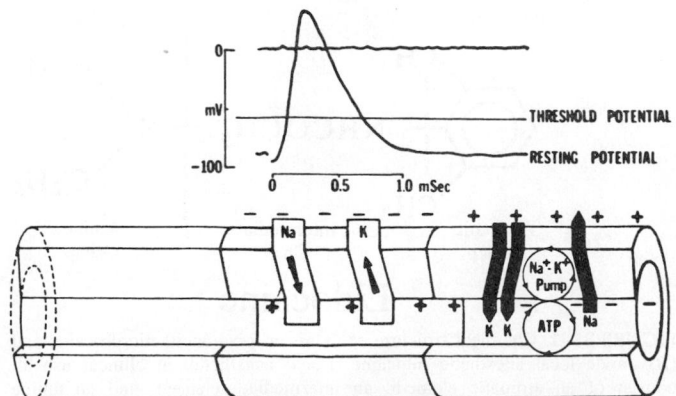

**FIGURE 35–2.** Summary of the ion and membrane potential changes during nerve conduction. (From Covino BG, Vassallo HG. *Local Anesthetics: Mechanisms of Action and Clinical Use.* New York, NY: Grune & Stratton; 1976:20.)

One explanation for this phenomenon is the modulated receptor hypothesis, which states that local anesthetics bind more tightly to the sodium channel during the open or inactive states than they do during resting states. An alternative proposal is the guarded receptor hypothesis. According to this hypothesis, the affinity of the local anesthetic for the sodium channel does not change. However, the channel itself limits the access of local anesthetic to its binding site during the resting state and allows more access to the binding site after an action potential (Fig. 35–4).

The differences between these theories are small. Both theories indicate that the interaction between the drug and the sodium channel is a dynamic one in which local anesthetic molecules are moving in and out of the sodium channels, rather than acting as a simple plug that physically obstructs the sodium ion as it enters.

### *Are All Nerves Equally Susceptible to Local Anesthetics?*

For many years, the conventional teaching was that large, myelinated nerves such as the A alpha and A beta fibers required greater amounts of local anesthetic to effect a block

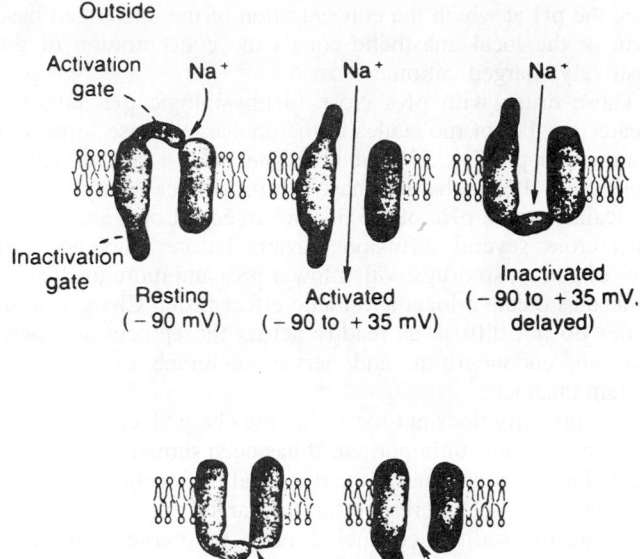

Outside

Activation
gate    Na⁺          Na⁺          Na⁺

Inactivation
gate

Resting        Activated        Inactivated
(−90 mV)      (−90 to +35 mV)   (−90 to +35 mV,
                                  delayed)

K⁺            K⁺

Resting        Slow activation
(−90 mV)      (−90 to +35 mV)
Inside

**FIGURE 35–4.** Representation of the voltage-dependent conformational changes of Na⁺ and K⁺ channel protein subunits. Note that during the resting phase, access of molecules to the interior of the Na⁺ channel is limited by the activation gate. This is not true during the activated and inactivated states. This is one theoretic explanation for use-dependent block, with which local anesthetics are more effective after repeated stimulations of the nerve. Repeated stimulation leaves fewer Na⁺ channels in the resting state. (From Guyton AC. *Human Physiology and Mechanisms of Disease.* 8th ed. Philadelphia, Pa: WB Saunders; 1991:56.)

than did the smaller A, B, or C fibers. This differential sensitivity to local anesthetic agents was thought to be due to the greater diameter of the large fibers. Gissen and colleagues[4–6] demonstrated that the margin of safety for nerve transmission in vitro was greater for small fibers, such as the pain-carrying A delta and C fibers, but that the larger fibers had more barriers to diffusion than did the smaller fibers. These barriers account for the clinical finding that small fibers are blocked more readily than large fibers. Fiber diameter is not a factor.

## Differential Blockade

Although this information refuted conventional wisdom, it did not explain the phenomenon of differential block encountered with epidural and spinal anesthesia. With spinal anesthesia, the loss of temperature discrimination extends approxi-

mately two dermatomes higher than the loss of sharp-dull sensation, which is in turn approximately two dermatomes higher than the loss of sensation to light touch. With epidural anesthesia, similar effects are noted during the initial phases of the block, and dilute solutions of local anesthetic can block pain while preserving motor and some sensory function.

### Nodes of Ranvier

Fink attributes differential block to differences in the number of nodes of Ranvier bathed by the local anesthetic solution.[7] If a 2-mm segment of nerve is bathed by local anesthetic, the small nerve fibers, which have more nodes of Ranvier per millimeter, have more nodes bathed than do larger nerve fibers. Conducted impulses can skip two blocked nodes of Ranvier but not three. Therefore, the large nerves have fewer nodes exposed to the local anesthetic and are better able to conduct impulses than are the small fibers. Characteristics of nerve fibers are shown in Table 35–1.

### Partial Blockade of Multiple Nodes

This explanation works well for epidural anesthesia, when a nerve segment of a few millimeters is bathed by local anesthetic, but not for spinal anesthesia, when larger segments are involved. Fink explained differential block for spinal anesthesia with the theory that multiple partially blocked nodes decrementally reduce conduction sufficiently so that the impulse ultimately fails to conduct.[7] The number of nodes to be blocked varies inversely with the concentration of the local anesthetic solution. High-concentration solutions need to bathe fewer nodes to block conduction.

At the extremes of local anesthetic diffusion in spinal anesthesia, large nerve fiber nodes would be blocked to the same degree as small fiber nodes. Because small nerve fibers have more nodes per millimeter, the small fibers are more likely to reach the critical combination of number of nodes blocked plus intensity of block to effect decremental conduction.[8]

## What Are the Important Chemical Properties of Local Anesthetics?

The four key chemical properties of local anesthetics are lipid solubility, protein binding, capacity to produce vasodilation, and degree of ionization (Table 35–2).

### Lipid Solubility

Local anesthetics that are more lipophilic than hydrophilic tend to be more potent. For example, tetracaine and bupiva-

**TABLE 35–1.** Physical Characteristics of Nerve Fibers

| Fiber | Diameter (µm) | Conduction Velocity (m/s) | Internodal Distance (mm) | Function |
|---|---|---|---|---|
| C | 0.5-1.3 | 0.5-2.0 | Unmyelinated | Pain, temperature |
| B | 1-3 | 3-14 | 0.1 | Preganglionic, sympathetic |
| A delta | 2-5 | 12-30 | 0.2 | Pain, touch, temperature |
| A gamma | 3-6 | 30-70 | 0.5 | Motor to muscle spindle |
| A beta | 5-12 | 30-70 | 0.8 | Touch, pressure |
| A alpha | 12-20 | 70-120 | 1.2 | Proprioception, somatic motor |

**TABLE 35–2.** Physical Properties of Local Anesthetics and Their Local Effects

| Physical Property | Clinical Effect |
| --- | --- |
| Lipid solubility | Potency |
| Protein binding | Duration of action |
| Vasodilator activity | Duration of action |
| pKa | Onset time |

caine differ from their congeners, procaine and mepivacaine, by having an additional butyl group on the molecule. This extra butyl group increases the lipid solubility of tetracaine 80-fold and the lipid solubility of bupivacaine 28-fold over the less potent drugs procaine and mepivacaine, respectively. Tetracaine is roughly 8 times more potent than procaine, and bupivacaine is 4 times more potent than mepivacaine.

## Protein Binding

Drugs that are highly protein bound have a longer duration of action than do drugs of low protein binding. The shortest acting local anesthetic, procaine, is only 6% bound by plasma protein. The long-acting local anesthetics, tetracaine, bupivacaine, and etidocaine, have protein binding levels of 76%, 96%, and 94%, respectively. Although high levels of plasma protein binding mean that less drug is available to diffuse across nerve membranes, the highly protein-bound drugs appear to bind to cell membrane proteins with much higher affinity once they reach the binding sites and therefore produce a much longer duration of block.

Changes in protein binding due to the presence of other drugs or in hypoproteinemic states may substantially affect the amount of free drug available to exert its effect. Such alterations not only change the potency of the drug and its local anesthetic effect but also may result in toxic reactions at lower than expected doses.[9,10]

Finally, protein binding may have some relation to toxicity. The three drugs that are most highly protein bound are bupivacaine, ropivacaine, and etidocaine. These drugs are associated with higher degrees of cardiovascular toxicity than the agents with lower levels of protein binding.[11] Whether this difference is related to the drug's high degree of protein binding or some other chemical characteristic is unclear.

## Vasodilation

Vasodilation is another factor that affects duration of action. All local anesthetics except cocaine are vasodilators, but the relative ability to produce vasodilation differs among specific agents. For example, lidocaine shows protein-binding properties similar to those of mepivacaine and prilocaine. In isolated nerve preparations, these three drugs have a similar duration of action. In vivo, lidocaine has a shorter duration of action than prilocaine or mepivacaine because of the greater vasodilation produced by lidocaine. When a vasoconstrictor such as epinephrine is added, the duration of action of the three drugs is the same.[12]

## Ionization

The degree of ionization determines the time to onset of action for a local anesthetic. It is determined by the drug's pKa, the pH at which the concentration of the uncharged base form of the local anesthetic equals the concentration of the positively charged cationic form.

Those drugs with pKa close to physiologic pH have the greater number of molecules in the uncharged, base form. For example, at pH 7.4, 35% of lidocaine, with a pKa of 7.9, is present in the uncharged base form, whereas only 5% of tetracaine, with a pKa of 8.5, is uncharged.[12] Local anesthetics must cross several diffusion barriers before reaching their sites of action, so drugs with a lower pKa and more uncharged molecules create a local anesthetic effect faster. Charged molecules do not diffuse as readily across the epineurium, perineurium, endoneurium, and nerve membrane to reach the sodium channels.

This property does not mean that the charged, cationic form of the molecule is unimportant. It has been shown to bind with the sodium channel and to exert a local anesthetic effect.[13] A binding site also is present for uncharged molecules. They penetrate the sodium channel through the nerve membrane, not the cytoplasm, making both forms important for successful channel blockade.[13] Uncharged ions cross the numerous barriers to diffusion to reach the cytoplasm. Once they are in the cytoplasm, the intracellular pH establishes a new equilibrium of ionized and nonionized molecules. The ionized molecules then move into the sodium channel to prevent channel opening.

### Acidic Environments

The phenomenon of ionization due to pKa also explains why local anesthetics work poorly in acidic environments such as those associated with abscesses or cellulitis. Because the local tissue pH surrounding an abscess is <7.4, more drug exists in the cationic form. Fewer local anesthetic molecules are available for diffusion across the nerve structures, resulting in a block that is slow to set up and of less intensity than would otherwise be expected.

## How Are Local Anesthetics Metabolized?

### Esters

Ester local anesthetics undergo ester hydrolysis in the plasma, red blood cells, and liver. The products of hydrolysis do not exert any significant pharmacologic effect, with the exception of *para*-aminobenzoic acid, which may be a source of allergic reactions associated with ester local anesthetic use.[14]

Procaine, chloroprocaine, and tetracaine undergo rapid hydrolysis in blood; the half-lives of chloroprocaine and procaine in plasma are <1 minute.[15] Chloroprocaine in particular appears to be a safe drug. Case reports of massive overdoses of chloroprocaine failed to show any serious effect despite high serum levels detected 10 minutes after injection.[16]

### Atypical Cholinesterase

Some patients possess an atypical cholinesterase enzyme that is less efficient in drug hydrolysis. In theory, delayed metabolism of ester local anesthetics should result, depending on the severity of the atypical cholinesterase disorder. However, red blood cell esterases and liver metabolism may compensate for atypical cholinesterase deficiencies, and thus even patients with an atypical cholinesterase may not manifest a prolonged effect.

### Liver Disease

Liver disease may also affect the metabolism of ester local anesthetics because the plasma cholinesterase enzyme is produced in the liver. However, red blood cell esterase activity remains normal, and overall plasma hydrolysis is probably affected only at the extremes of liver disease, making ester-type local anesthetics possibly even safer than the amide drugs for these patients.

### Neostigmine, Echothiophate, and Acetazolamide

Drugs that inhibit plasma pseudocholinesterase, such as neostigmine and echothiophate, a drug used in treatment of glaucoma, can decrease the clearance of the ester local anesthetics. Acetazolamide can also decrease ester local anesthetic clearance because of inhibition of hydrolysis by red blood cell esterase enzymes[17] (Table 35–3). A prudent anesthetist exercises caution in using ester local anesthetics in these patients.

### Amides

The amide local anesthetics undergo biotransformation in the liver by aromatic hydroxylation, N-dealkylation, and amide hydrolysis. The importance of each route of transformation varies greatly among the different drugs.

### Lidocaine

Lidocaine primarily undergoes N-dealkylation to monoethylglycinexylidide (MEGX). MEGX is important because it has local anesthetic effects comparable with those of lidocaine.[18] In long-term infusions of lidocaine, MEGX may add to the potential toxicity of the parent drug.

### Prilocaine

Prilocaine is metabolized to o-toluidine. If the total dose of prilocaine exceeds 600 mg in adults, methemoglobinemia can develop. In normal adults with normal oxygen-carrying capacity, prilocaine in doses <600 mg may be the safest amide local anesthetic because of its rapid hydrolysis and low level of central nervous system (CNS) toxicity[12]; these unique properties also may make it the ideal drug for intravenous regional anesthesia. Other amide local anesthetics have metabolic products with some of the pharmacologic activity of the parent drug.[14]

**TABLE 35–3.** Drugs Reducing Local Anesthetic Clearance

| Drug | Local Anesthetic |
| --- | --- |
| Anticholinesterase agents | Ester agents |
| Echothiophate | Ester agents |
| Acetazolamide | Ester agents |
| Propranolol | Lidocaine* |
| Cimetidine | Lidocaine* |

*Other amides may also be affected.

### Liver and Renal Disease

Because of the dependence of amide local anesthetics on metabolism in the liver, any process that affects liver function or liver blood flow can dramatically alter their metabolism. Disease states that are known to result in increased drug levels include congestive heart failure, severe hepatic cirrhosis, and the acute phase of viral hepatitis.

Renal disease does not appear to affect metabolism.[19] However, metabolites of local anesthetics that depend on renal excretion, such as glycinexylidide, another metabolite of lidocaine, may accumulate in the blood. Evidence that such accumulation contributes significantly to drug toxicity is lacking.[20]

### Drug Interactions

Like all therapeutic agents, local anesthetics are subject to interaction with other drugs. β-Adrenergic blockers, propranolol in particular, decrease the clearance of lidocaine by inhibiting the mixed-function oxidase enzymes and decreasing liver blood flow.[21] β-Blockers with intrinsic sympathomimetic activity (pindolol) and low lipid solubility (atenolol) tend to affect lidocaine metabolism less than propranolol.[22]

Cimetidine can reduce the clearance of lidocaine by 30%.[23,24] This effect also appears to be due primarily to inhibition of the mixed-function oxidase enzyme system of the liver, although some reports suggest that cimetidine also reduces hepatic blood flow. Ranitidine, another $H_2$ antagonist, does not affect lidocaine clearance.[25]

Because lidocaine is predominantly metabolized by the cytochrome $P_{450}$ 3A4 enzyme, any drug that is similarly metabolized may affect lidocaine elimination.[26] Such drugs include erythromycin, ketoconazole, and selective serotonin reuptake inhibitor antidepressants.

## CLINICAL APPLICATIONS

### How Should a Local Anesthetic Be Chosen?

#### Type of Block

The choice of a local anesthetic agent depends on several factors. First is the type of block to be performed. Some agents, such as bupivacaine, are used in almost all local anesthetic procedures, including peripheral, spinal, and epidural anesthesia. Others, because of their slow onset of action and limited potential to diffuse across anatomic barriers surrounding peripheral nerves, are used only for spinal anesthesia. Tetracaine and dibucaine have limited usefulness in peripheral nerve blocks but are excellent spinal anesthetic agents.

#### Duration of Procedure

The second important factor is the duration of the procedure, which needs to be well matched to the duration of action of the local anesthetic. Local anesthetics can be categorized into three broad classes based on duration of action (Table 35–4). The duration of action of the drug varies with the technique and use of adjunctive agents (discussed later).

A good rule of thumb is to choose an agent with a duration of action at least 50% greater than the expected duration of the procedure. If the expected duration of the procedure is

**TABLE 35–4.** Local Anesthetics Classified by Duration of Action

| Short-Acting Agents | Long-Acting, High-Potency Agents |
|---|---|
| Procaine | Tetracaine |
| Chloroprocaine | Bupivacaine (levobupivacaine) |
| **Intermediate-Acting Agents** | Etidocaine |
| Lidocaine | Ropivacaine |
| Mepivacaine | |
| Prilocaine | |

unknown or unpredictable, two choices are available. The first is use of the longest-acting agents, such as bupivacaine or etidocaine. A bupivacaine brachial plexus block can last 12 hours or more. However, to keep a patient anesthetized for many hours after the completion of a procedure may be undesirable. The second choice is to use a catheter technique that allows either continuous infusion or repetitive dosing of local anesthetics.

### Motor Blockade

The third factor to be considered is the need for motor block. For some procedures (orthopedic joint surgery, intraabdominal surgery, gynecologic surgery), motor blockade is desirable or necessary. In other situations, such as epidural analgesia for vaginal delivery, motor blockade is undesirable.

Of the long-acting local anesthetics, bupivacaine and ropivacaine appear to have less propensity for motor blockade than etidocaine.[12] Why these agents permit selective sensory nerve block with less motor block is unclear, but it may be related to a unique relationship between their pKa and lipid solubility.[6] Etidocaine, on the other hand, causes dense motor blockade. As a result, it is much better suited for intraabdominal and orthopedic procedures, whereas bupivacaine and ropivacaine are more useful to provide analgesia without interrupting motor function.

### Toxicity

The last factor to consider is the potential for toxicity with a particular technique. Local anesthetic toxicity is discussed in detail later in the chapter, but a few words about toxicity and anesthetic selection are appropriate.

For special techniques such as intravenous regional anesthesia, certain drugs have specific advantages. Prilocaine has a low potential for toxicity, and the amount of prilocaine needed for intravenous regional anesthesia is usually 200 to 400 mg, well below the 600 mg usually associated with methemoglobinemia.

Chloroprocaine, which is probably the safest of the ester local anesthetics, might seem to be another ideal choice for intravenous regional anesthesia based on its extremely short serum half-life. However, chloroprocaine can cause phlebitis on intravenous injection.[27]

Bupivacaine, which has a potential for serious cardiovascular toxicity, is not approved for intravenous regional anesthesia. The 0.75% concentration is not approved for obstetric anesthesia because of potentially severe cardiovascular toxicity that resulted in several maternal deaths.[12]

## How Can Local Anesthetics Be Made to Work Better?

The ideal local anesthetic would have a rapid onset of action, predictable duration of action, reliable depth of anesthesia, and low toxicity. As with all things in life, the ideal seldom exists, and local anesthesia is no exception. Fortunately, a wide selection of local anesthetics can be tailored to meet virtually all requirements for anesthesia and analgesia. To make the best use of these agents, the important principles that determine time of onset, quality of anesthesia, duration of action, and toxicity must be considered (Table 35–5).

### Dosage

The single most important factor in determining time of onset, duration of action, and intensity of nerve blockade is the total dose of local anesthetic used. A study comparing the anesthetic effects of epidural prilocaine randomized patients to receive either 30 mL of a 2% solution or 20 mL of a 3% solution for a total dose of 600 mg with both techniques.[28] Time of onset, duration of anesthesia, and intensity of motor blockade were the same with both solutions.

The extent of anesthesia varies with increasing volumes; 30 mL of local anesthetic solution provides anesthesia over a greater area than does 20 mL of solution.[29] This characteristic can be used to advantage to provide intense anesthesia over a limited number of dermatomes. For example, a highly concentrated solution in low volumes is useful in thoracic epidural techniques. Intense anesthesia is needed over the thoracic dermatomes with concomitant sparing of motor function in the lower extremities.

Other work with epidural bupivacaine showed that increasing the dose of local anesthetic produced more rapid onset of anesthesia, increased motor blockade, and lengthened duration of action.[30] Clearly, increasing the mass (milligrams) of drug used magnifies the overall anesthetic effects.

### Vasoconstrictors

Vasoconstrictors, epinephrine in particular, are added to local anesthetic solutions to increase the duration of action, serve as markers for intravascular injection, and reduce peak serum levels. The optimal dose of epinephrine appears to be a 1:200 000 solution or 5 µg/mL.[31] Vasoconstrictors are thought to produce local vasoconstriction and reduce the vascular uptake of anesthetic solution.[12] This action leaves more local anesthetic molecules available to exert their effect locally and reduces the peak plasma levels (potential toxicity). In the spinal canal, epinephrine also may have actions of its own, directly modulating pain transmission in the spinal cord.[32]

Other vasoconstrictor drugs such as norepinephrine and phenylephrine are also used, but they are not more effective than epinephrine when used in equivalent doses.[33] Phenylephrine may produce less tachycardia than epinephrine, and some practitioners use phenylephrine in patients thought to be especially sensitive to the β-adrenergic effects of epinephrine.

### Epidural and Peripheral Blocks

Vasoconstrictors do not work for all local anesthetics in all situations (Table 35–6). Epinephrine prolongs the duration of

**TABLE 35–5.** Clinical Properties of Local Anesthetics

| Agent | Concentration (%) | Clinical Use | Onset | Usual Duration | Recommended Maximum Single Dose (mg) | Comments | pH of Plain Solutions* |
|---|---|---|---|---|---|---|---|
| *Amides* | | | | | | | |
| Lidocaine | 0.5-1.0 | Infiltration | Fast | 1.0-2.0 h | 300 | Most versatile agent | 6.5 |
| | 0.25-0.5 | IV regional | | | 500 + epinephrine | | |
| | 1.0-1.5 | Peripheral nerve block | Fast | 1.0-3.0 h | 500 + epinephrine | | |
| | 1.5-2.0 | Epidural | Fast | 1.0-2.0 h | 500 + epinephrine | | |
| | 4 | Topical | Moderate | 0.5-1.0 h | 500 + epinephrine | | |
| | 5 | Spinal | Fast | 0.5-1.5 h | 100 | | |
| Prilocaine | 0.5-1.0 | Infiltration | Fast | 1.0-2.0 h | 600 | Least toxic amide agent | 4.5 |
| | 0.25-0.5 | IV regional | | | 600 | Methemoglobinemia usually occurs | |
| | 1.5-2.0 | Peripheral nerve block | Fast | 1.5-3.0 h | 600 | | |
| Mepivacaine | 2.0-3.0 | Epidural | Fast | 1.0-3.0 h | 400 | Duration of plain solutions longer than lidocaine without epinephrine | 4.5 |
| | 0.5-1.0 | Infiltration | Fast | 1.5-3.0 h | | Useful when epinephrine is contraindicated | |
| Bupivacaine (levobupivacaine same as bupivacaine, except with less potential for cardiac toxicity) | 1.0-1.5 | Peripheral nerve block | Fast | 2-3 h | 500 + epinephrine | Lower concentrations provide differential sensory/motor block | 4.5-6 |
| | 1.5-2.0 | Epidural | Fast | 1.5-3 h | 100 | Ventricular arrhythmias and sudden cardiovascular collapse reported after rapid IV injection | |
| | 4.0 | Spinal | Fast | 1.5 | 175 | | |
| | 0.25 | Infiltration | | 2-4 h | | | |
| | 0.25-0.5 | Peripheral nerve block | Slow | 4-12 h | 225 + epinephrine | | |
| | 0.25-0.5 | Obstetric epidural | Moderate | 2-4 h | 225 + epinephrine | | |
| | 0.5-0.75 | Surgical epidural | Moderate | 2-5 h | 225 + epinephrine | | |
| | 0.5-0.75 | Spinal | Fast | 2-4 h | 20 | | |
| | 0.5 | Infiltration | Fast | 2-4 h | 300 | | |
| Etidocaine | 0.5-1.0 | Peripheral | Fast | 3-12 h | 400 + epinephrine | Profound motor block useful for surgical anesthesia but not for obstetric analgesia | 4.5 |
| | 1.0-1.5 | Surgical epidural | Fast | 2-4 h | 400 + epinephrine | | |

*Table continued on following page*

**TABLE 35–5.** Clinical Properties of Local Anesthetics *Continued*

| Agent | Concentration (%) | Clinical Use | Onset | Usual Duration | Recommended Maximum Single Dose (mg) | Comments | pH of Plain Solutions |
|---|---|---|---|---|---|---|---|
| Ropivacaine | 0.5-1.0 | Brachial plexus block | Slow | 9-11 h | No recommended* maximum dose | Less cardiovascular toxicity and less motor block than bupivacaine | |
| Dibucaine | 0.25-0.5 hyperbaric | Spinal | Fast | 2-4 h | 10 | Recommended only for spinal and topical use | |
| | 0.00067 hyperbaric | Spinal | Fast | 2-4 h | 10 | | |
| | | Topical | Slow | 0.5-1.0 h | 50 | | |
| *Esters* Procaine | 1.0 | Infiltration | Fast | 0.5-1.0 h | 1000 | Used mainly for infiltration and differential spinal blocks; allergic potential after repeated use | 5-6.5 |
| | 1.0-2.0 | Peripheral nerve block | Slow | 0.5-1.0 h | 1000 | | |
| | 2.0 | Epidural | Slow | 0.5-1.0 h | 1000 | | |
| | 10.0 | Spinal | Moderate | 0.5-1.0 h | 200 | | |
| | 1.0 | Infiltration | Fast | 0.5-1.0 h | 800 | Lowest systemic toxicity of all local anesthetics | 2.7-4 |
| Chloroprocaine | 2.0 | Peripheral nerve block | Fast | 0.5-1.0 h | 1000 + epinephrine | Intrathecal injection may be associated with sensory/motor deficits. Occasional back pain with epidural use | 2.7-4 |
| Tetracaine | 2.0-3.0 | Epidural | Fast | 0.5-1.0 h | 1000 + epinephrine | Use is primarily limited to spinal and topical anesthesia | 4.5-6.5 |
| | 0.5 | Spinal | Fast | 2-4 h | 20 | | |
| | 2.0 | Topical | Slow | 0.5-1.0 h | 20 | Use is primarily limited to spinal and topical anesthesia | 4.5-6.5 |
| Cocaine | 4.0-10.0 | Topical | Slow | 0.5-1.0 h | 150 | Topical use only, addictive, causes vasoconstriction, CNS toxicity, initially features marked excitation ("fight or flight") response. May cause cardiac arrhythmias | |
| Benzocaine | Up to 200 | Topical | Slow | 0.5-1.0 h | 200 | Useful only for topical anesthesia | |

*No maximum recommended dose is currently available. Doses of 3.1 mg/kg for brachial plexus block and 200 mg for epidural use are reported without any signs of toxicity.

CNS, central nervous system; IV, intravenous.

TABLE 35–6. Effects of Epinephrine on Duration of Action of Different Local Anesthetics

| Local Anesthetic | Spinal | Epidural | Peripheral Nerve Block |
|---|---|---|---|
| Tetracaine | + | 0 | + |
| Chloroprocaine | 0 | + | + |
| Lidocaine | − (dose <0.6 mg) | + | + |
| Mepivacaine | 0 | + | + |
| Prilocaine | 0 | − | + |
| Bupivacaine | − | − | + |
| Etidocaine | 0 | − | + |
| Ropivacaine | 0 | 0 | − |

+, prolongation; −, no effect; 0, not used.

action of all agents used for peripheral nerve blocks except ropivacaine.[34] Ropivacaine has weak intrinsic vasoconstrictor activity. Epinephrine also prolongs the duration of action of chloroprocaine, lidocaine, and mepivacaine in epidural blockade, but not prilocaine, etidocaine, or bupivacaine.[35,36]

The reasons for these differences are unclear, but there are plausible explanations. The uptake of prilocaine, which is a less potent vasodilator than lidocaine, is not significantly prolonged by epinephrine. Etidocaine and bupivacaine, which are highly lipid soluble, are thought to be taken up by epidural fat, which then acts as a depot for prolonged slow release of these local anesthetics. Because they are quickly absorbed into the local tissues and then slowly released, their duration of action may be so long that it is not extended by a vasoconstrictor.

Adding epinephrine does not significantly alter blood levels of epidural etidocaine and bupivacaine. Nor does epinephrine affect the blood levels of ropivacaine when it is used in brachial plexus block.[37] Epinephrine appears to improve the incidence of satisfactory analgesia with low concentrations of epidural bupivacaine (0.125% and 0.25%) in labor analgesia, but it does not alter the effect of solutions of higher concentration.[38] It also enhances etidocaine and bupivacaine motor blockade in epidural anesthesia.[39]

### Subarachnoid Block

The effect of epinephrine when used as an adjunct for subarachnoid anesthesia is somewhat confusing. If the duration of anesthesia is defined as the time for the sensory level to regress by two dermatomes from its maximum level of anesthesia, epinephrine does not prolong the effects of subarachnoid lidocaine or bupivacaine. However, it significantly extends the duration of action of tetracaine.[40–42] The effect on lidocaine spinal anesthesia may be dose dependent. A study comparing the effects of 0.6 mg of epinephrine added to hyperbaric lidocaine found that this larger dose prolonged the time to regression of the block by two dermatomes in the thoracic region compared with the plain solution; lower doses did not delay regression. All epinephrine solutions delayed full recovery from lidocaine spinal anesthesia.[43]

This observation is of most importance when spinal anesthesia is used for prolonged intraabdominal procedures. The regression of the level of anesthesia could cause a patient to become uncomfortable. However, anesthesia at the site of injection, specifically in the sacral areas and lower lumbar segments, is prolonged for all three local anesthetic agents. The explanation for this phenomenon may be a difference

between the three agents and their effects on spinal cord blood flow. Subarachnoid tetracaine increases spinal cord blood flow in dogs.[44] Hence, a vasoconstrictor such as epinephrine may block the increase in blood flow, reduce tetracaine uptake, and increase the duration of anesthesia.

The key point of this discussion is that epinephrine prolongs a tetracaine spinal anesthetic used for an intraabdominal procedure but does not affect lidocaine or bupivacaine used in the same fashion, unless it is used in a dose of at least 0.6 mg. However, epinephrine prolongs the effects of all three agents when they are administered in the subarachnoid space for procedures on the lower extremities.

### Physiologic Consequences

Addition of a vasoconstrictor not only changes the quality of nerve block but also may alter its physiologic effects. Epinephrine affects the hemodynamic characteristics of a nerve block compared with the same block performed without epinephrine. Epidural anesthesia performed with epinephrine-containing solutions results in greater decreases in mean arterial pressure than do plain solutions.[45] This response is due to the predominantly β-adrenergic effects of epinephrine in the low doses (1:200 000) used with epidural solutions. When used in local anesthetic solutions for brachial plexus block, epinephrine also causes dose-related changes in pulse and mean arterial pressure, whereas brachial plexus block without vasoconstrictors produces no significant change.[31]

### Precautions

When using epinephrine, many find it desirable to add it to the solution just before use. Commercial preparations of local anesthetics contain antioxidants that reduce the solution pH. This change results in a solution with slower time to onset. Epinephrine added just before use does not significantly change pH, but it does create the potential for a drug dosage error.

## Can Local Anesthetic Solutions Be Modified to Improve Performance?

The answer is "Yes." Another method to improve local anesthetic performance is to modify the standard preparations with selected additives. Commercial preparations of local anesthetics are prepared as hydrochloride salts with pH values from 3.6 to 5.6. This pH range increases the charged, cationic molecular form.

### Alkalization

Sodium bicarbonate ($NaHCO_3$) added immediately before injection of the local anesthetic increases the solution pH and the percentage of local anesthetic molecules in the uncharged base form. This approach should improve the onset of action and possibly the quality of anesthesia, and clinical evidence supports this practice in many, but not all, situations.

### Bupivacaine

Alkalization of bupivacaine for epidural analgesia during labor appears to reduce the onset time of sensory anesthesia and the duration of nerve block as well.[46] However, other studies of alkalized bupivacaine failed to demonstrate any benefit over the plain solution.[47,48]

The addition of $NaHCO_3$ to solutions of bupivacaine for brachial plexus block improved onset time in one study[49] but not in another.[50] The study showing no improvement used 0.1 mL of 8.4% $NaHCO_3$ solution per 20 mL of local anesthetic; the other study used 0.1 mL per 10 mL of solution. However, the final pH in both was at least 6.4 to 7.15.

### Lidocaine and Mepivacaine

Alkalized lidocaine and mepivacaine for epidural anesthesia showed improved onset time and improved the quality of anesthesia.[51–54] The dose of $NaHCO_3$ was 1.0 mL of an 8.4% solution per 10 mL of anesthetic solution. A prospective study evaluating the effect of alkalization of lidocaine used for brachial plexus block failed to show significant improvement in the time to onset or the quality of sensory or motor blockade.[55]

In summary, alkalization of local anesthetics decreases the onset time and improves the quality of lidocaine and mepivacaine epidural anesthesia. Evidence supporting the value of $NaHCO_3$ for lidocaine peripheral nerve blocks is equivocal. Available information suggests that alkalization of bupivacaine is of little value for epidural anesthesia.

## Effects of Carbonation

When carbonated local anesthetics are injected near a nerve, carbon dioxide is believed to diffuse rapidly out of the solution, through the nerve and into the cytoplasm, to lower the intracellular pH and raise the pH of the local anesthetic solution. When local anesthetic molecules subsequently diffuse into the cytoplasm, the lowered intracellular pH results in a higher proportion of ionized molecules. Because they diffuse poorly across the nerve membrane, these molecules are trapped inside the cell, providing a larger number to bind to their sites of action in the sodium channels.

### Lidocaine

Lidocaine carbonate appears to have a more rapid onset when used for brachial plexus anesthesia.[56] Studies comparing the onset of carbonated lidocaine anesthesia in epidural blockade yield conflicting data.[57,58] A randomized, double-blind comparison of carbonated lidocaine to plain lidocaine and lidocaine with sodium bicarbonate found no difference between the plain solution and the carbonated lidocaine with regard to time of onset, spread, or intensity of epidural block.[54]

### Bupivacaine

Carbonated bupivacaine appears to improve the depth of sensory and motor blockade during epidural anesthesia and may improve quality and spread of anesthesia in brachial plexus block.[59,60]

## Dextran

In a randomized study of intercostal nerve blockade, the mean duration of the intercostal nerve block was not significantly altered by the use of dextran.[61] Conflicting data on dextran result from the fact that it may alter the local anesthetic pH. One study compared bupivacaine and dextran at pH 8.0 with bupivacaine and dextran at a pH of 4.5 to 5.5 during coccygeal nerve block in rats.[62] The pH 8.0 solution significantly prolonged the duration of nerve block, but the more acidic solution did not, suggesting that the change of pH, not the dextran molecule, imparts the therapeutic benefit.

### Hyaluronidase

Hyaluronidase breaks down extracellular hyaluronic acid, a component of connective tissue, to improve the diffusion of local anesthetic between tissue planes. It is commonly used for retrobulbar block[63] but also has been described for leg and upper extremity nerve blocks and epidural blockade. Hyaluronidase does not improve epidural anesthesia, and its advantages in peripheral nerve block are questionable.[64]

### Clonidine

A review of clonidine use concluded "clonidine added to local anesthetics for epidural, spinal, or peripheral block prolongs and intensifies anesthesia for surgery."[65] Clonidine is an $\alpha_2$-adrenergic agonist and it has effects in both the CNS and peripheral nerves. It has intrinsic analgesic effects when used alone and an additive effect when used in combination with a local anesthetic. When added to an epidural local anesthetic in a dose of 150 µg or more, the analgesia time is doubled. Clonidine does cause sedation in a dose-related manner and a slight reduction in blood pressure when used as an epidural analgesic.

Clonidine prolongs the analgesia from peripheral nerve block by 50% to 100% when used in a dose of 1 µg/kg. Clonidine also provides postprocedure analgesia and reduces tourniquet pain when added to an intravenous regional block in a dose of 150 µg.[66] The biggest disadvantage of clonidine is its expense. The current injectable preparation contains 0.1 mg/mL of clonidine. Unless this preparation is fractionated for use in multiple patients, the cost per treatment is prohibitive.

### Local Anesthetic Mixtures

Some investigators combine two local anesthetics in an attempt to develop a solution with the rapid onset characteristic of the short-acting component drug and the long duration characteristic of the more potent but slower onset component drug.

#### Chloroprocaine and Bupivacaine

One study combined 10 mL of 3% chloroprocaine with 20 mL of 0.5% bupivacaine for brachial plexus block. This mixture had quicker time to complete anesthesia, a similar duration of action, and a more intense block than 30 mL of 0.5% bupivacaine.[67] Other studies using mixtures of chloroprocaine and bupivacaine for epidural anesthesia reported no advantage of the mixture over either drug alone, and further found that chloroprocaine may reduce the effectiveness of bupivacaine during labor.[68,69]

Two studies suggest why chloroprocaine may inhibit the effectiveness of bupivacaine. In one study, a mixture of the drugs was applied to isolated nerves and the pH varied.[70] At a pH of 3.6, the block had the characteristics of chloroprocaine alone, whereas at a pH of 5.5, the block resembled bupivacaine alone. In another study of isolated nerves, a metabolite of chloroprocaine, 4-amino-2-chlorobenzoic acid, completely blocked the effects of bupivacaine.[71] In general, a mixture of chloroprocaine and bupivacaine has no advantage over either solution alone.

### Lidocaine and Bupivacaine

In a randomized study of lidocaine and bupivacaine in various proportions for epidural anesthesia, no significant difference between bupivacaine alone and any of the other solutions of bupivacaine and lidocaine was observed.[72]

To summarize, no benefit accrues to mixtures of local anesthetics for epidural anesthesia. In brachial plexus block, a slight advantage in terms of time of onset may result from a mixture of chloroprocaine and bupivacaine compared with bupivacaine alone. However, large studies in support of this conclusion are lacking. The toxicity of local anesthetics is additive, and mixing of agents does not allow an increase in the total dose.

## What Are the Differences Between Agents?

The most useful clinical division of local anesthetic agents is by duration of action and ability to produce a dense anesthetic block with adequate muscle relaxation. They can be divided into three categories: short-acting agents of low potency; agents with intermediate duration and potency; and agents with long duration and high potency (see Table 35–4).

### Short-Acting Agents

#### Procaine

Before the discovery of lidocaine, procaine was the most commonly used local anesthetic; it now has limited clinical use. Procaine is available as a 1% or 2% solution for skin infiltration and peripheral nerve block. Blocks have a relatively slow onset and short duration of 30 to 60 minutes. Procaine is also available in a 10% solution for spinal anesthesia. It is still occasionally used as a spinal anesthetic for the diagnosis of chronic pain disorders and occasionally for vaginal delivery.

#### Chloroprocaine

Chloroprocaine is the least toxic local anesthetic agent.[12] It is used in concentrated solutions ranging from 1% to 3%, has a fast onset of action, and a duration of 30 to 60 minutes. It is used extensively in cesarean section; its low toxicity, rapid onset, and short duration make it ideal for epidural anesthesia.

**Neurotoxicity.** Prolonged and sometimes permanent neurologic deficits have been reported after inadvertent massive subarachnoid injections during attempted epidural anesthesia.[73,74] These deficits were thought to result from the combination of low pH and the preservative sodium bisulfite.[75] The chloroprocaine molecule is not neurotoxic in clinically used solutions.

**Back Pain.** Current solutions of chloroprocaine avoid the combination of sodium bisulfite and low pH. However, the new solutions have been associated with severe back pain after epidural anesthesia.[76–78] This pain is described as a dull, deep lumbar ache, occasionally associated with spasm of the erector spinae muscles. The hypothesized cause of low backache is the new preservative agent, ethylenediaminetetraacetic acid (EDTA).

EDTA is a chelator of calcium and may affect localized skeletal muscle calcium activity. One patient received calcium chloride in graduated doses to a total of 300 mg to relieve what was thought to be chloroprocaine-induced back pain after an epidural anesthetic.[79] In another report, 10 volunteers who received epidural chloroprocaine as part of a clinical investigation had back pain as the anesthetic resolved. Epidural fentanyl, 100 to 200 μg, effectively treated the back pain.[78]

Factors thought to contribute to chloroprocaine-induced back pain are the large volumes of chloroprocaine and its use to infiltrate the intraspinous ligaments before insertion of the epidural needle.

### Cocaine

Cocaine, which was the first clinically used local anesthetic, is now used almost exclusively for mucous membrane topical anesthesia. Unlike the other local anesthetics, cocaine blocks norepinephrine reuptake and has significant vasoconstrictor properties. The 4% solution is used as a topical anesthetic and vasoconstrictor for ear, nose, and throat surgery. However, the potential for abuse and serious toxic reactions, including hypertension and cardiac arrhythmias, limits its clinical usefulness.

### Intermediate-Acting Agents

#### Lidocaine

Lidocaine is the most versatile and widely used of all local anesthetics. Solutions of 0.5% are useful for skin infiltration, with a rapid onset and a duration of 1 to 2 hours. In 1% to 2% solutions, it provides excellent anesthesia for peripheral nerve blocks. The duration of action is 1 to 1.5 hours for plain solutions and 2 to 2.5 hours for solutions with epinephrine. Lidocaine is also used for epidural anesthesia (2% solution), as a topical anesthetic (4% solution), and for spinal anesthesia (5% solution).

#### Prilocaine

Prilocaine can be used for any technique. It may be advantageous for intravenous regional anesthesia because of its lower systemic toxicity. Prilocaine without epinephrine also has a longer duration of action than lidocaine without epinephrine, making it a useful agent when epinephrine is contraindicated. Because prilocaine in doses of 600 mg can cause methemoglobinemia, its use has been discouraged in obstetric anesthesia. Otherwise, its spectrum of activity is equivalent to that of lidocaine.

#### Mepivacaine

Mepivacaine also has the same spectrum of action as lidocaine, although it is not effective as a topical anesthetic. Like prilocaine, solutions without a vasoconstrictor have a longer duration of action than solutions of lidocaine without a vasoconstrictor. Thus it is useful when epinephrine is contraindicated, as in patients with unstable angina or other cardiac conditions. Mepivacaine with epinephrine has the same duration of action as lidocaine with epinephrine. It is not used for obstetric anesthesia because the fetus cannot metabolize it as well as the other local anesthetics.[12]

## Long-Acting, High-Potency Anesthetics

### Tetracaine

Tetracaine is the most potent ester local anesthetic. Because of its slow onset of action, its use is virtually confined to spinal anesthesia as a 1% solution or as lyophilized crystals. The crystals allow tetracaine to be made into hypobaric, isobaric, or hyperbaric solutions, making it a versatile agent. A 2% solution is an effective topical anesthetic agent. However, because of its high potency, the maximum recommended single dose is 20 mg. Case reports of deaths associated with tetracaine used as a topical anesthetic agent have been published. Thus, careful attention to dose and symptoms of toxicity is essential.[12]

### Bupivacaine

Bupivacaine is a useful and versatile local anesthetic. It is available in 0.25%, 0.5%, and 0.75% solutions. The solutions of low concentration can be used to provide a differential block for analgesia during labor. Solutions of 0.125% combined with narcotic provide satisfactory labor analgesia with almost no motor block.[80] High concentrations of bupivacaine for peripheral nerve blocks provide anesthesia lasting 12 to 24 hours when used with a vasoconstrictor.

A 0.75% solution of epidural bupivacaine provides rapid onset of surgical anesthesia, and a commercially available hyperbaric spinal solution of 0.75% bupivacaine is an extremely effective anesthetic, with a duration of action of 2 to 4 hours.

Bupivacaine's only drawback is its tendency to cause severe cardiovascular toxicity when administered inadvertently as a large intravenous dose (see section on Toxicity, later). Because of the risk of cardiovascular toxicity, bupivacaine is not recommended for intravenous regional anesthesia in any concentration, and the 0.75% solution is not recommended for use in obstetrics.

### Etidocaine

Etidocaine is a long-acting local anesthetic characterized by profound motor block. This feature makes the agent extremely useful for surgical anesthesia but much less so as an analgesic in obstetrics. It is approximately half as potent as bupivacaine. Surgical anesthesia is achieved with a 1.5% solution. Etidocaine's duration of action is similar to that of bupivacaine. Cases of profound motor block without sensory anesthesia have been reported, a fact that has dampened the enthusiasm for this otherwise useful agent.

### Ropivacaine

Ropivacaine has a chemical structure similar to that of bupivacaine and mepivacaine. It appears to be just slightly less potent than bupivacaine for sensory block but provides less motor block. It is prepared as the pure $S-(-)$ isomer, which enhances the clinical properties of the drug compared with the racemic mixture.[81]

**Cardiovascular Toxicity.** Ropivacaine appears to have less cardiovascular toxicity than bupivacaine, but more toxicity than lidocaine.[80] The dose producing CNS toxicity is the same for ropivacaine and bupivacaine, but ropivacaine causes fewer arrhythmias and less myocardial depression.[82–85]

**Clinical Properties.** The drugs have nearly equivalent potency and time to onset.[86] Compared with bupivacaine, ropivacaine has a slightly shorter duration of action (333 versus 394 minutes) and less motor block when used as an epidural anesthetic.[87,88] Ropivacaine does not appear to have increased toxicity in pregnant animal models, another advantage over bupivacaine.[89]

**Comparative Features.** Ropivacaine appears to be an equally effective yet less toxic drug than bupivacaine. However, cardiovascular toxicity from bupivacaine is still a rare event that usually occurs only when a large amount of bupivacaine is injected intravenously.

Bupivacaine has been used widely for many years. Many anesthetists are reluctant to trade a tried-and-true drug for a relative newcomer, although the near-equipotent dose of ropivacaine makes transition from bupivacaine that much easier. The determining factor regarding use may be the cost of ropivacaine relative to bupivacaine and the type of procedure performed. When small amounts of local anesthetic are used in continuous epidural infusion, the risk of systemic toxicity is low and the advantage of ropivacaine lies in its tendency to provide less motor block. When large amounts of drug are used, as in brachial plexus block, ropivacaine has a clear advantage because it has less risk of serious toxicity, and its anesthetic effect is clinically indistinguishable from bupivacaine's when using the 0.5% concentration.

### Levobupivacaine

Levobupivacaine is the $S-(-)$ enantiomer of bupivacaine. The advantage of levobupivacaine over the racemic mixture of bupivacaine is a reduced risk of both cardiac and CNS toxicity. Levobupivacaine may have less affinity for certain myocardial ion receptor subunits, which would explain its lower risk of myocardial toxicity. Otherwise, it is clinically indistinguishable from the racemic mixture of bupivacaine containing both the $R-(+)$ and the $S-(-)$ enantiomers. This drug provides all of the advantages of traditional bupivacaine with a dramatically reduced risk of toxicity.[90]

## TOXICITY

Toxicity due to local anesthetics is rare but can be life threatening. It may take the form of systemic and local reactions. Systemic toxicity results from allergic reactions, drug overdose, and drug metabolites (eg, prilocaine-induced methemoglobinemia). Tissue toxicity occurs at the site of injection because of drug irritation.

### What Are the Central Nervous System Effects of Local Anesthetic Overdose?

Signs and symptoms of CNS toxicity appear before those of cardiovascular toxicity[91] (Fig. 35–5). The ability of any

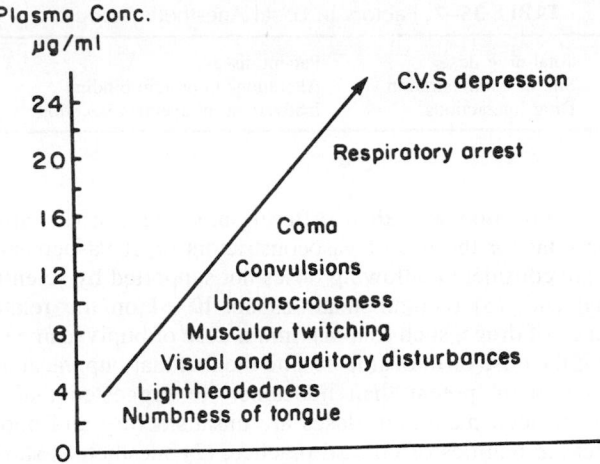

**FIGURE 35–5.** Relationship of signs and symptoms of local anesthetic toxicity to plasma concentrations of lidocaine. C.V.S., cardiovascular system. (From Covino BG. Clinical pharmacology of local anesthetic agents. In: Cousins MG, Bridenbaugh PO, eds. *Neural Blockade in Clinical Anesthesia and Management of Pain.* 2nd ed. Philadelphia, Pa: JB Lippincott; 1988:122.)

local anesthetic to produce CNS toxicity is related directly to the potency of the drug. For example, tetracaine, which is 8 times more potent than procaine, requires only one eighth the amount of drug to produce an equivalent amount of CNS toxicity. This relationship is not always true for cardiovascular toxicity.

CNS toxicity is remarkably similar for all drugs. Test subjects who received intravenous infusions of local anesthetics reported initial circumoral numbness, numbness of the extremities and trunk, a lightheaded sensation, and tinnitus.[15,91] Other visual and auditory disturbances were also reported. As the dose of infused local anesthetic becomes larger, more pronounced effects result. They include muscle twitching and, if doses are high enough, unconsciousness, seizures, coma, and respiratory arrest.[91]

## How Is Cardiovascular Toxicity Manifested?

The cardiovascular toxicity of local anesthetics manifests in three possible ways: direct action on cardiac muscle, affecting myocardial contractility; disturbance of the conduction system of the heart; and direct effects on peripheral vascular smooth muscle.[92]

### Contractility

Local anesthetics exert a negative inotropic effect on cardiac muscle that is dose and potency related.[93] As with CNS toxicity, the negative inotropic effect of tetracaine is approximately 8 times that of procaine, reflecting the relative potency of the two drugs. Drug levels associated with the usual clinical doses of local anesthetics do not significantly affect myocardial contractility. However, the blood levels achieved with a rapid intravenous injection or from an absolute overdose of local anesthetics can result in decreased cardiac output.

### Conductivity

The myocardial conduction system also has ion channels that are susceptible to the effects of local anesthetics. Antiar-

rhythmic effects of lidocaine are well known. Lidocaine decreases the action potential duration and, to a lesser degree, the effective refractory period. It increases the ratio of effective refractory period to action potential duration in ventricular muscle Purkinje fibers.[94]

Not all local anesthetics are equal in their effects on the cardiac conduction system. In animal studies of massive intravenous overdoses of lidocaine, the sequence of events is a prolongation of conduction time in the heart followed by a decrease in spontaneous pacemaker activity, profound bradycardia, and eventual cardiac standstill.[95]

Case reports of cardiac arrest after inadvertent intravenous administration of bupivacaine during epidural anesthesia led to a number of studies investigating its potential cardiac toxicity.[91,92,94] Bupivacaine and, to a lesser degree, etidocaine and ropivacaine produce cardiovascular effects that are quantitatively and qualitatively different from those of the local anesthetics of low and intermediate potency. Bupivacaine at toxic doses results in ventricular tachycardia and fibrillation in a significant percentage of animals.[96,97] Similar effects occur to a lesser extent with etidocaine and ropivacaine, but not with intermediate-potency local anesthetics such as lidocaine[85,98] (Fig. 35–6). Resuscitation of animals with ventricular arrhythmias is difficult, as it is in humans who receive inadvertent overdoses of bupivacaine.[11,99]

### Mechanisms

The reason why bupivacaine is more prone to cause ventricular arrhythmias is unclear. Protein binding alone is not a factor because etidocaine, which is more protein bound than bupivacaine, has a lower incidence of ventricular arrhythmias. The piperidine ring is not responsible because mepivacaine and ropivacaine also possess one. Mepivacaine does not cause ventricular arrhythmias in animal models.[98] The incidence of ventricular arrhythmias with ropivacaine is much less than with bupivacaine, despite the fact that the drugs are almost equipotent.[85]

**Electrophysiologic Changes.** Electrophysiologic studies in cardiac muscle show that bupivacaine binds to ion channels for much longer periods than do other local anesthetics.[100]

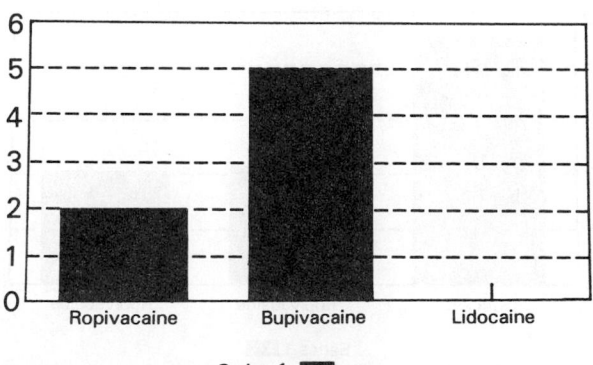

**FIGURE 35–6.** Six sheep in each of these groups received toxic doses of three different local anesthetic agents (ropivacaine, bupivacaine, or lidocaine). Almost all of the sheep in the bupivacaine-treated group had ventricular arrhythmias, whereas none of the lidocaine-treated sheep did. (From Nancarrow C, Rutten AJ, Runciman WB, et al. Myocardial and cerebral drug concentrations and the mechanisms of death after fatal intravenous doses of lidocaine, bupivacaine, and ropivacaine in the sheep. *Anesth Analg.* 1989; 69:276.)

Even at relatively slow heart rates, ion channels may not fully recover from bupivacaine-induced blockade, resulting in conditions that favor reentrant-type cardiac arrhythmias.

**Serum Levels.** An important feature of bupivacaine myocardial toxicity is the relatively low serum levels necessary. Morishima and colleagues[101,102] studied the infusion rates of lidocaine, bupivacaine, and etidocaine needed to cause cardiovascular collapse (CC) and convulsions (CNS) in sheep. For lidocaine, the CC/CNS ratio was 7.1:1 (ie, 7 times more lidocaine was required to cause cardiovascular collapse than convulsions). Ratios for bupivacaine and etidocaine were 3.7:1 and 4.4:1, respectively. The CC/CNS ratio of blood levels of bupivacaine and etidocaine was also half that of lidocaine.

In a separate study evaluating the ratio of fatal doses to convulsive doses for the three drugs,[86] the values were lidocaine 4.5:1, bupivacaine 2.2:1, and ropivacaine 2.1:1 (Fig. 35–7). These studies demonstrate that the margin for error is less with the potent, long-acting agents than with the agents of intermediate potency. Inadvertent intravenous injections of the long-acting potent agents can result in rapid progression from CNS toxicity to cardiovascular collapse. If a patient is sedated or the dose injected is relatively large, no premonitory CNS symptoms may be noted before cardiac arrest occurs.

Although bupivacaine toxicity is a real and potentially dangerous problem, the drug remains one of the most widely used local anesthetics. If steps are taken to avoid inadvertent large intravenous doses, the chances of serious toxicity remain extremely small.

## How Is Local Anesthetic Toxicity Avoided?

The key to avoiding local anesthetic toxicity is to identify those factors that contribute to high levels in the blood (Table 35–7) and then to take steps to minimize them (Table 35–8).

### Total Dose

Scott pointed out many of the problems associated with currently accepted maximum recommended doses of local anesthetics.[103] They include (1) failure to account for different

**TABLE 35–7.** Factors in Local Anesthetic Toxicity

| | |
|---|---|
| Total drug dose | Patient disease |
| Site of administration | Alterations in protein binding |
| Drug interactions | Inadvertent intravenous injection |

sites of injection with their differing blood levels; (2) failure to account for the use of vasoconstrictors or, if vasoconstrictors are considered, allowing doses not supported by scientific study; and, (3) recommendations not based on the relative potency of drugs, such as a maximum dose of bupivacaine that is half the dose of lidocaine despite the fact that bupivacaine is 4 times more potent than lidocaine. He suggested that (1) recommended maximum doses are unsatisfactory and poorly reflect the realities of clinical practice; (2) anesthetists should use recommended doses only as broad guidelines in the total perspective of patient health and anesthetic technique; and (3) the greatest threat to patients is a rapid, direct intravenous injection of local anesthetics, which can cause serious reactions even at recommended "safe" doses.

### Site of Administration

Blood levels of local anesthetics vary greatly with site of administration.[104] Intercostal nerve blocks are associated with the highest levels of local anesthetic, followed by caudal, epidural, brachial plexus, and sciatic-femoral nerve blocks (Fig. 35–8). Spinal anesthesia produces low levels in the blood. Anesthetic techniques with the highest blood levels usually require the highest drug doses to achieve effective anesthesia and are associated with high vascularity at the site of injection. An acceptable dose of local anesthetic for brachial plexus anesthesia could prove toxic if administered for intercostal nerve blocks. When feasible, lower concentrations of local anesthetics with vasoconstrictors should be used in highly vascular areas.

One striking example of the large variation in recommended doses of local anesthetic is the use of lidocaine for tumescent liposuction. Some studies support lidocaine doses of 55 mg/kg.[105] Tumescent liposuction uses large volumes of a dilute solution injected over an extended period into the subcutaneous tissue. Then, some of that tissue is suctioned out of the body, most likely taking a significant amount of the local anesthetic with it. Despite the widespread safety of this technique, there are reports of bad outcomes that may involve local anesthetic toxicity.[106] A case report of lidocaine toxicity associated with tumescent liposuction and concurrent use of serotonin reuptake inhibitors poses the possibility that patients

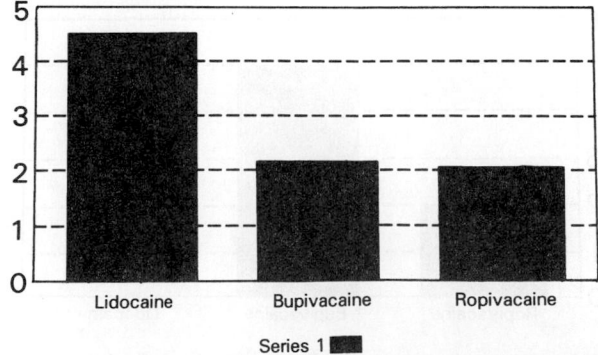

**FIGURE 35–7.** Bupivacaine and ropivacaine both demonstrate a lower ratio of fatal to convulsive doses of local anesthetics compared with lower potency agents such as lidocaine. This indicates a lower margin of safety for toxic reactions from the onset of central nervous system symptoms to development of serious cardiovascular toxicity. (Extrapolated from Nancarrow C, Rutten AJ, Runciman WB, et al. Myocardial and cerebral drug concentrations and the mechanisms of death after fatal intravenous doses of lidocaine, bupivacaine, and ropivacaine in the sheep. *Anesth Analg.* 1989;69:276. © International Anesthesia Research Society.)

**TABLE 35–8.** Prevention of Local Anesthetic Toxicity

Prepare emergency equipment
    Airway equipment
    Intravenous line
    Resuscitative drugs
Adjust drug dose for patient's disease
Monitor pulse, blood pressure, and oxygenation
Aspirate needle before injecting
Consider using a vasoconstrictor
    Reduces blood levels
    Marker for intravenous injection
Fractionate dose

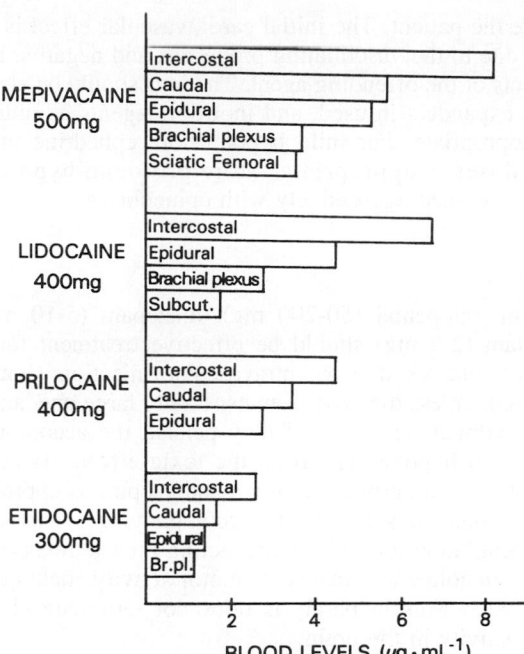

**FIGURE 35–8.** Comparative peak levels of various local anesthetic agents after administration for different local anesthetic techniques. Br. pl., brachial plexus; Subcut., subcutaneous. (From Covino BG, Vassallo HG. General pharmacological and toxicological aspects of local anesthetic agents. In: *Local Anesthetics: Mechanisms of Action and Clinical Use.* New York, NY: Grune & Stratton; 1976:97.)

receiving such large doses of local anesthetics may be at much greater risk for toxicity due to drug interactions.[26] The authors of this case report recommend great caution when using doses >35 mg/kg because of the significant interindividual variations in lidocaine metabolism due to age, gender, body habitus, and concurrent medication use.

## Drug Interactions

Interactions with other medications a patient may be using can be important. Propranolol and cimetidine decrease local anesthetic metabolism; both drugs increase blood levels of lidocaine. Patients with severe liver disease and congestive heart failure are also more prone to development of amide local anesthetic toxicity because of impaired metabolism. Patients with atypical plasma cholinesterase enzymes may have some impairment of ester local anesthetic metabolism.

## Pregnancy

Pregnancy affects the body's susceptibility to local anesthetic toxicity. Pregnant patients require a lower dose of local anesthetics for effective nerve blocks and reduced doses of local anesthetics for epidural and spinal anesthesia.[107,108] The recommended dose of local anesthetics for spinal and epidural anesthesia during pregnancy is approximately 25% to 30% lower than in nonpregnant patients.[109] The altered response to local anesthetics in pregnancy may be related to increased levels of progesterone.[110]

Pregnant animals also are more susceptible to cardiovascular toxicity with bupivacaine but not lidocaine and ropivacaine.[89,111] This susceptibility does not appear to be related to increased myocardial uptake of bupivacaine. It may result

from the increase in circulating progesterone levels. Progesterone-treated animals show more depression of the maximum rate of Purkinje fiber depolarization than do nontreated animals.[112] Progesterone has no effect on the electrophysiologic changes occurring with lidocaine.

## Protein Binding

Protein binding of local anesthetics can affect the blood levels required to produce toxicity. The free local anesthetic drug, not the protein-bound form, crosses the blood-brain barrier to cause CNS toxicity.[113] Therefore, anything that alters protein binding also alters the amount of free drug.

## $\alpha_1$-Acid Glycoprotein

Unfortunately, predicting which patients will have alterations in protein binding is not simple. The primary binding protein for local anesthetics is $\alpha_1$-acid glycoprotein.[113] This substance is an acute-phase reactant that is increased during sepsis, other acute illnesses, and cancer. Because $\alpha_1$-acid glycoprotein is an acute-phase reactant, it is elevated in almost all clinical situations in which local anesthetics are used, including surgery, trauma, and chronic pain states. This rise is theorized to protect patients from local anesthetic toxicity, especially during local anesthetic infusions.

Support for this theory was provided by patients who received long-term infusions of epidural local anesthetics for postoperative pain relief.[114–116] In one group of 9 patients, 4 had bupivacaine levels exceeding 4.0 μg/mL. Despite these high serum levels, no patient experienced symptoms of toxicity. Given the slow rate of rise of the drug levels, increased protein binding conceivably kept free drug levels low, despite the relatively high total values. Because the free drug is responsible for toxic symptoms, postsurgical patients may have some degree of CNS protection from toxicity due to the increased levels of $\alpha_1$-acid glycoprotein.

## Vasoconstrictors

Vasoconstrictor agents are useful in preventing local anesthetic toxicity. They reduce the peak blood levels of local anesthetics by causing local vasoconstriction at the injection site and reducing vascular uptake of the drug. An additional benefit is their role as a marker for intravascular injection. A 3-mL solution of local anesthetics with 1:200 000 epinephrine contains 15 μg of epinephrine. This solution, when administered intravenously, augments the pulse by 20 to 30 beats per minute within 20 seconds of administration,[117] can be reliably detected, and should prevent the subsequent administration of larger amounts of local anesthetic intravenously. Other β-agonist drugs, such as isoproterenol and ephedrine, have also been used as markers for intravascular injection, although none is convincingly superior to epinephrine.[118]

### Pros and Cons of Vasoconstrictor Use

Certain patients do not respond reliably to standard test doses of epinephrine, including those taking β-adrenergic antagonist agents,[119] children under halothane general anesthesia,[120] and pregnant patients in labor. In the latter group, Leighton and colleagues could not reliably identify heart rate changes in women given 15 μg of epinephrine intravenously.[121] The wide changes in pulse and blood pressure associated with labor make detection of transient changes in heart rate difficult.

Some practitioners believe that epinephrine test doses may cause dangerous reductions in uterine blood flow in all pregnant patients and severe hypertension in preeclamptic patients. Because a test dose is unreliable, they conclude it is dangerous and is of little use.[118]

The alternative opinion is that 15 μg of intravenous epinephrine has never been shown to cause adverse human fetal or maternal outcomes despite animal studies showing reductions in uterine blood flow. Even if epinephrine does not detect all intravenous injections, it detects some of them and does prevent more serious problems associated with subsequent inadvertent intravenous injections of local anesthetics.

## How Can Inadvertent Intravenous Injection Be Avoided?

To avoid intravenous injection, the anesthetist should (1) aspirate before injecting to ensure there is no blood return, and (2) give the local anesthetic in fractional incremental doses over time. Negative results on aspiration tests do not ensure the prevention of intravenous injections. Therefore, fractionation of the dose is important, usually in 3- to 5-mL increments every 30 seconds or more. This procedure allows detection of the early symptoms of toxicity before they progress to seizures and cardiovascular collapse.

## What Is the Treatment?

The key to treatment of local anesthetic toxicity is early recognition. Any alteration in a patient's mental status should be viewed as local anesthetic toxicity until proved otherwise. The classic symptoms such as a metallic or strange taste, circumoral numbness, tinnitus, and numbness of the trunk or extremities are almost diagnostic. Treatment follows that of virtually all anesthetic emergencies: (1) maintain a patent airway, (2) ventilate the patient, and (3) support the circulation (Table 35–9).

## Hypoxia and Acidosis

Hypoxia and acidosis aggravate toxicity.[122] If breathing ceases, the anesthetist must administer 100% oxygen and

**TABLE 35–9.** Treatment of Local Anesthetic Toxicity

| |
|---|
| Establish an airway |
| Ventilate with 100% oxygen |
| Support circulation |
|   Elevate legs |
|   Administer volume expanders |
|   Ephedrine, 5-25 mg |
| Treat seizures |
|   Diazepam, 5-10 mg |
|   Midazolam, 2-5 mg |
|   Thiopental, 50-200 mg |
| Treat cardiovascular collapse |
|   Epinephrine |
|   Atropine |
|   Bretylium for ventricular arrhythmias* |

*As of this writing, bretylium is unavailable (2000).

ventilate the patient. The initial cardiovascular effect is hypotension due to the vasodilating properties and negative inotropic effects of the offending agent. The legs should be elevated, volume expanders infused, and inotropic agents administered when appropriate. For mild hypotension, ephedrine in 5- to 25-mg doses is appropriate. More profound hypotension should be treated aggressively with epinephrine.

### Seizures

Sodium thiopental (50-200 mg), diazepam (5-10 mg), or midazolam (2-5 mg) should be effective treatment for most seizures. Seizures due to intravascular injection should be short lived, unless the dose is an especially large one, and may subside without treatment. If they persist, the accompanying acidosis and hypoxia aggravate the toxic effects. Hence, administration of a barbiturate or benzodiazepine is appropriate.

Tonic-clonic muscle activity accompanying seizures often makes ventilation difficult. A fast-acting muscle relaxant such as succinylcholine terminates the motor activity, making ventilation easier. Muscle paralysis does not terminate electrical seizure activity in the brain.

### Cardiovascular Collapse

Profound cardiovascular collapse requires aggressive treatment with epinephrine and atropine. If malignant ventricular arrhythmias result, immediate defibrillation is essential. Bupivacaine-induced ventricular arrhythmias are especially difficult to convert. Animal models suggest that large doses of epinephrine, atropine, and bretylium increase the chance of successful resuscitation.[123] Lidocaine should not be administered as an antiarrhythmic for ventricular arrhythmias associated with local anesthetic toxicity. Bupivacaine-induced cardiovascular collapse may require prolonged resuscitation for several hours. In some instances, heroic steps such as the use of cardiopulmonary bypass to maintain circulation may be considered.

## Do Local Anesthetics Cause Allergic Reactions?

Local anesthetics can cause allergic reactions, but such reactions are rare. Allergic reactions are more common with the ester class of drugs.

### Incidence

Esters are derivatives of *para*-aminobenzoic acid, a substance to which a percentage of the population has demonstrated allergic reactions. The number of patients who relate a history of local anesthetic allergy and actually demonstrate allergic phenomena during skin testing or subcutaneous challenge is extremely low. deShazo and Nelson reviewed their experience with 90 patients reported to be allergic to local anesthetics.[124] Of these 90 patients, only 14 had histories consistent with immediate hypersensitivity reactions, and 12 of these 14 patients had negative skin test responses and negative subcutaneous challenge to lidocaine. The investigators concluded that "the vast majority of patients labeled allergic to local anesthetics are, in fact, not."[124] Gall evaluated 177 patients with a history of local anesthetic hypersensitivity.[125] The evaluation included prick, intracutaneous tests, provocative challenges and immunoglobulin E (IgE) radioimmunoassay. Two patients had immediate-type reactions to articaine and lidocaine, but no IgE was detected. A literature review also concluded that hypersensitivity reactions to local anesthetics is extremely rare.[126]

## Evaluation

In evaluating patients with an alleged allergy to "cain" drugs, taking a history is the first step in determining the presence of true immediate hypersensitivity reactions (Table 35–10). Symptoms consistent with this diagnosis are wheezing, hives, angioedema, rhinorrhea, shock, and tachycardia.[127] Manifestations of vasoconstrictor effect may also be misinterpreted as allergy. Most commonly, these are described as palpitations and a sense of nervousness or anxiety. Bradycardia usually is not a symptom of anaphylaxis and can aid in differentiating immediate hypersensitivity from other toxic reactions such as intravenous injections of local anesthetics and local anesthetic overdose. Patient-generated symptoms such as vasovagal reactions and anxiety-hyperventilation syndrome can also masquerade as allergic reactions.

If the history is suggestive of allergy to local anesthetics, two approaches are open (Fig. 35–9). First, if the local anesthetic causing the reaction is known, an agent from the other class can be used. If the agent is unknown or if it is not possible to use an agent from the other class, skin testing should be performed, followed by subcutaneous challenge with the agent to be used.[124,127,128] Skin testing should be carried out by a consultant knowledgeable about local anesthetic allergy. False-negative skin test results are rare, but false-positive rates may be as high as 10%.[128]

Patients must be challenged with the local anesthetic solution proposed for use in the procedure. If the solution contains preservatives such as parabens and bisulfites, challenge with the drug including preservatives should be performed because preservatives are also responsible for allergic reactions.

If the skin test results are negative and graded subcutaneous challenges, including 1 mL of undiluted drug, produce no response, the risk of allergic reaction to that drug is no greater than the risk in the general population.[124] With this approach, a safe local anesthetic agent can be identified for every patient.[124,126,127]

## Do Local Anesthetics Cause Tissue Toxicity?

Standard solutions of local anesthetics rarely cause permanent nerve injury. Prolonged neurologic deficits after local

**TABLE 35–10.** Differential Diagnosis of Local Anesthetic Reactions

| Diagnosis | Signs and Symptoms |
| --- | --- |
| *Local Anesthetic Toxicity* | Central nervous system toxicity, |
| Intravenous injection | convulsions, bradycardia or tachycardia, |
| Drug overdose | rapid onset |
| *Vasoconstrictor Reaction* | Tachycardia, hypertension, palpitations, |
| | nervousness |
| *Patient Disease* | Bradycardia |
| Vasovagal | Chest pain |
| Myocardial infarction | |
| Bronchospasm | |
| *Allergic Reactions* | Tachycardia, urticaria, bronchospasm |

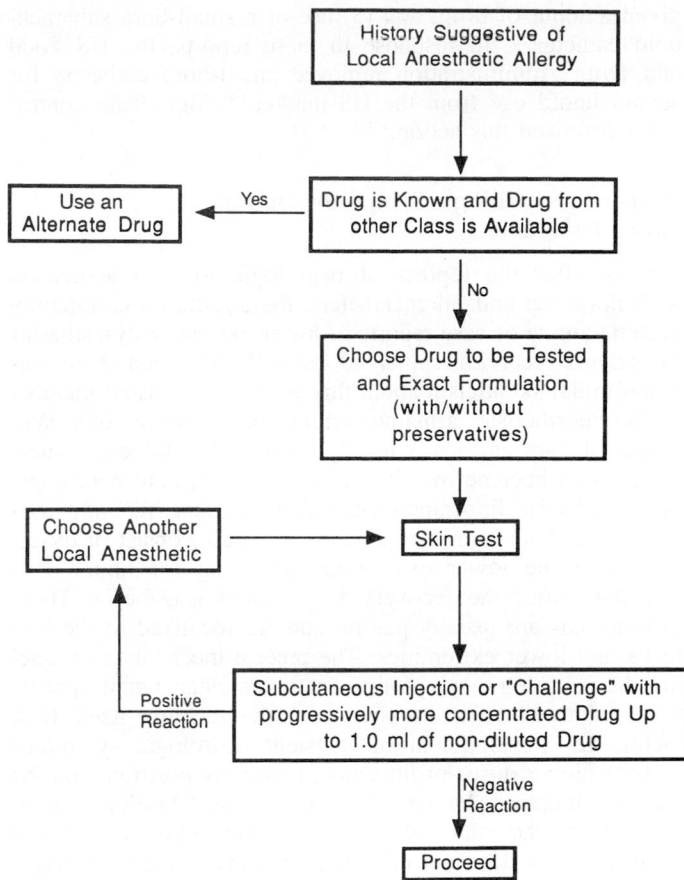

**FIGURE 35–9.** Algorithm for management of the patient with a history suggestive of local anesthetic allergy. If the patient has a history of reaction to a specific drug, then a drug from the other class (ester or amide) can be used safely. If the drug is unknown or if there is no acceptable alternative, then skin testing followed by subcutaneous injection of progressively more concentrated solutions of drug can help identify a local anesthetic for safe use. Skin tests are best done by a consultant experienced in allergy testing.

anesthetic techniques are much more likely to be due to direct trauma to the nerves as a result of the anesthetic infiltration or the accompanying surgery.

## Chloroprocaine Neurotoxicity

As was mentioned previously, chloroprocaine solutions were associated with permanent neurologic deficits after inadvertent administration of large amounts of drug into the subarachnoid space during attempted epidural anesthesia. The manufacturer subsequently altered the solution to avoid the combination of the low pH and bisulfite solution that was the etiologic factor in chloroprocaine toxicity.

## Spinal Microcatheters and High-Concentration Lidocaine Neurotoxicity

Another reported cause of prolonged neurologic deficits involves the use of microcatheters and large doses of 5% lidocaine in 7.5% dextrose for continuous spinal anesthesia. Several reports of cauda equina syndrome revealed the following elements common to these cases: (1) 5% lidocaine in 7.5% dextrose, with initial or total doses exceeding 100 mg; (2) unusually low or inadequate levels of anesthesia for a given amount of drug; and (3) use of a small-bore subarachnoid catheter.[129] In response to these reports, the US Food and Drug Administration removed small-bore catheters for subarachnoid use from the US market.[130] Significant controversy followed this action.[131]

## Transient Neurologic Symptoms Due to Spinal Lidocaine

Soon after the reports of neurologic toxicity associated with lidocaine and microcatheters, the anesthesia community became aware of case reports of lower extremity dysesthesias in patients receiving spinal lidocaine.[132] Although there was much initial skepticism about this attack on a trusted member of the anesthetists' armamentarium, the evidence for a syndrome of transient neurologic symptoms after lidocaine anesthesia soon became overwhelming.[133,134] Transient neurologic symptoms after lidocaine (also called *transient radicular irritation*), as this syndrome came to be called, consist of dysesthesias in the lower extremities persisting for hours or a few days after the recovery from spinal anesthesia. These dysesthesias are usually painful and are localized to the buttocks and lower extremities. The precise mechanism producing the neurologic symptoms remains unclear, but it appears to be due to a localized toxicity from the lidocaine itself. Risk factors for development of transient neurologic symptoms include higher doses of lidocaine, lithotomy position, and the use of epinephrine in the lidocaine solution. Dilution of lidocaine from the standard 5% hyperbaric solution to lower concentrations does not eliminate the development of dysesthesias.[135,136] Removal of glucose from the lidocaine solution does not appear to affect its toxicity.[135] Transient neurologic symptoms occur less frequently with prilocaine and bupivacaine.[137,138]

Transient neurologic symptoms are self-limiting and usually subside within a few days. Patients receiving spinal lidocaine must be counseled as to the risk for development of some aches and pains for a few days after the spinal anesthetic. Prilocaine, bupivacaine, and procaine remain alternatives to spinal lidocaine, but they have their own drawbacks. Procaine has a slow onset, bupivacaine has a long duration of action, and prilocaine is not commercially available worldwide in a solution approved for intrathecal use.

## Skeletal Muscle Damage

Local anesthetics may cause damage to skeletal muscle. With bupivacaine in particular, intramuscular injections cause local skeletal muscle fiber reaction.[12] This damage is almost never associated with clinical symptoms, and muscle regeneration is complete within several weeks after the injection.

## References

1. Wildsmith JAW. Peripheral nerve and local anaesthetic drugs. *Br J Anaesth.* 1986;58:692.
2. Taylor RE. Effect of procaine on electrical properties of squid axon membrane. *Am J Physiol.* 1959;196:1071.
3. Butterworth JF IV, Strichartz GR. Molecular mechanisms of local anesthesia: a review. *Anesthesiology.* 1990;72:711.
4. Gissen AJ, Covino BG, Gregus J. Differential sensitivity of fast and slow fibers in mammalian nerve fibers to local anesthetic drugs. *Anesthesiology.* 1980;53:467.
5. Gissen AJ, Covino BG, Gregus J. Differential sensitivity of fast and slow fibers in mammalian nerve, II. *Anesth Analg.* 1982;61:561.
6. Gissen AJ, Covino BG, Gregus J. Differential sensitivity of fast and slow fibers in mammalian nerve, III: effects of etidocaine and bupivacaine on fast and slow fibers. *Anesth Analg.* 1982;61:570.
7. Fink BR. Mechanisms of differential axial blockade in epidural and subarachnoid anesthesia. *Anesthesiology.* 1989;70:851.
8. Raymond SA, Steffenson SC, Gugino LD, et al. The role of length of nerve exposed to local anesthetics in impulse blocking action. *Anesth Analg.* 1989;68:563.
9. Marathe PH, Shen DD, Artru AA, et al. Effect of serum protein binding on the entry of lidocaine into brain and cerebrospinal fluid in dogs. *Anesthesiology.* 1991;75:804.
10. Tucker GT. Pharmacokinetics of local anesthetics. *Br J Anaesth.* 1986;58:717.
11. Albright GA. Cardiac arrest following regional anesthesia with etidocaine and bupivacaine. *Anesthesiology.* 1979;51:285.
12. Covino BG. Clinical pharmacology of local anesthetic agents. In: Cousins MG, Bridenbaugh PO, eds. *Neural Blockade in Clinical Anesthesia and Management of Pain.* 2nd ed. Philadelphia, Pa: JB Lippincott; 1988:111.
13. Courtney KR. Local anesthetics. *Int Anesthesiol Clin.* 1988;26:239.
14. Tucker GT, Mather LE. Properties, absorption, and disposition of local anesthetics. In: Cousins MG, Bridenbaugh PO, eds. *Neural Blockade in Clinical Anesthesia and Management of Pain.* 2nd ed. Philadelphia, Pa: JB Lippincott; 1988:47.
15. Foldes FF, Davidson GN, Duncalf D, et al. The intravenous toxicity of local anesthetic agents in man. *Clin Pharmacol Ther.* 1965;6:328.
16. Gross TL, Kuhnert PM, Kuhnert BR. Plasma levels of 2-chloroprocaine and lack of sequelae following an apparent intravenous injection. *Anesthesiology.* 1981;54:173.
17. Calvo R, Carlos R, Erill S. Effects of disease and acetazolamide on procaine hydrolysis by red cell enzymes. *Clin Pharmacol Ther.* 1980;27:175.
18. Blumer J, Strong JM, Atkinson AJ. The convulsant potency of lidocaine and its N-dealkylated metabolites. *J Pharmacol Exp Ther.* 1973;186:31.
19. Thompson P, Melmon KL, Richardson JA, et al. Lidocaine pharmacokinetics in advanced heart failure, liver disease, and renal failure in humans. *Ann Intern Med.* 1973;78:499.
20. Collinsworth KA, Strong JM, Atkinson AJ, et al. Pharmacokinetics and metabolism of lidocaine in patients with renal failure. *Clin Pharmacol Ther.* 1975;18:59.
21. Bax NDS, Tucker GT, Lennard MS, et al. The impairment of lignocaine clearance by propranolol—major contribution from enzyme inhibition. *Br J Clin Pharmacol.* 1985;19:597.
22. Tucker GT, Bax NDS, Lennard MS, et al. Effects of beta-adrenoreceptor antagonists on the pharmacokinetics of lignocaine. *Br J Clin Pharmacol.* 1984;17:21S.
23. Feely J, Wilkinson GR, McCallister CB, et al. Increased toxicity and reduced clearance of lidocaine by cimetidine. *Ann Intern Med.* 1982;96:592.
24. Webb TD, Ward DS. Elimination of lidocaine following regional block is inhibited by cimetidine. *Anesthesiology.* 1983;59:A213.
25. Feely J, Guy E. Lack of effect of ranitidine on the disposition of lignocaine. *Br J Clin Pharmacol.* 1983;15:378.
26. Klein JA, Kassarjdian N. Lidocaine toxicity with tumescent liposuction. *Dermatol Surg.* 1997;23:1169.
27. Harris WH. Choice of anesthetic agents for intravenous regional anesthesia. *Acta Anaesthesiol Scand Suppl.* 1969;36:47.
28. Crawford OB. Comparative evaluation in peridural anesthesia of lidocaine, mepivacaine and L-67, a new local anesthetic agent. *Anesthesiology.* 1964;25:321.
29. Erdemir HA, Soper LE, Sweet RB. Studies of factors affecting peridural anesthesia. *Anesth Analg.* 1965;44:400.
30. Scott DB, McClure JH, Giasi RM, et al. Effects of concentration of local anesthetic drugs in extradural block. *Br J Anaesth.* 1980;52:1033.
31. Kennedy WF Jr, Bonica JJ, Ward RJ, et al. Cardiorespiratory effects of epinephrine when used in regional anesthesia. *Acta Anaesthesiol Scand Suppl.* 1966;23:320.
32. Yaksh TL. Pharmacology of spinal adrenergic systems which modulate spinal nociceptive processing. *Pharmacol Biochem Behav.* 1985;22:845.
33. Concepcion M, Maddi R, Francis D, et al. Vasoconstrictors in spinal anesthesia with tetracaine: a comparison of epinephrine and phenylephrine. *Anesth Analg.* 1984;63:134.
34. Hickey R, Candido KD, Ramamurthy S, et al. Brachial plexus block with a new local anaesthetic: 0.5 percent ropivacaine. *Can J Anaesth.* 1990;37:732.
35. Buckley FP, Littlewood DG, Covino BG, et al. Effects of adrenaline

and the concentration of solution on extradural block with etidocaine. *Br J Anaesth.* 1978;50:171.

36. Kier L. Continuous epidural analgesia in prostatectomy: comparison of bupivacaine with and without adrenaline. *Acta Anaesthesiol Scand.* 1974;18:1.

37. Hickey R, Blanchard J, Hoffman J, et al. Plasma concentrations of ropivacaine given with or without epinephrine for brachial plexus block. *Can J Anaesth.* 1990;37:878.

38. Littlewood DG, Buckley P, Covino BG, et al. Comparative study of various local anesthetic solutions in extradural block in labor. *Br J Anaesth.* 1979;51:47.

39. Sinclair CJ, Scott DB. Comparison of bupivacaine and etidocaine in extradural blockade. *Br J Anaesth.* 1984;56:147.

40. Chambers WA, Littlewood DG, Scott DB. Spinal anesthesia with hyperbaric bupivacaine: effect of added vasoconstrictors. *Anesth Analg.* 1982;61:49.

41. Chambers WA, Littlewood DG, Logan MR, et al. Effect of added epinephrine on spinal anesthesia with lidocaine. *Anesth Analg.* 1981;60:417.

42. Concepcion M, Maddi R, Francis D, et al. Vasoconstrictors in spinal anesthesia with tetracaine: a comparison of epinephrine and phenylephrine. *Anesth Analg.* 1984;63:134.

43. Kito K, Kato H, Shibata M, et al. The effect of varied doses of epinephrine on the duration of lidocaine spinal anesthesia in the thoracic and lumbosacral dermatomes. *Anesth Analg.* 1998;86:1018.

44. Kozody R, Palahniuk RJ, Cumming MO. Spinal cord blood flow following subarachnoid tetracaine. *Can Anaesth Soc J.* 1985;32:23.

45. Cousins MJ, Bromage PR. Epidural neural blockade. In: Cousins MG, Bridenbaugh PO, eds. *Neural Blockade in Clinical Anesthesia and Management of Pain.* 2nd ed. Philadelphia, Pa: JB Lippincott; 1988:253.

46. McMorland GH, Douglas MJ, Jeffery WK, et al. Effect of pH adjustment of bupivacaine on onset and duration of epidural analgesia in parturients. *Can Anaesth Soc J.* 1986;33:537.

47. Benhamou D, Labaille T, Bonhomme L, et al. Alkalinization of epidural 0.5% bupivacaine for cesarean section. *Reg Anesth.* 1989;14:240.

48. Stevens RA, Chester WL, Gruetter JA, et al. The effect of pH adjustment of 0.5% bupivacaine on the latency of epidural anesthesia. *Reg Anesth.* 1989;14:236.

49. Hilgier M. Alkalinization of bupivacaine for brachial plexus block. *Reg Anesth.* 1985;10:59.

50. Bedder MD, Kozody R, Craig DB. Comparison of bupivacaine and alkalinized bupivacaine in brachial plexus anesthesia. *Anesth Analg.* 1988;67:48.

51. Sweeney N, Denson D, Juneja MM, et al. The effect of pH on the onset and duration of epidural lidocaine in the parturient. *Reg Anesth.* 1989;14:21.

52. Difazio CA, Carron H, Grosslight KR, et al. Comparison of pH adjusted lidocaine solutions for epidural anesthesia. *Anesth Analg.* 1986;65:760.

53. Galindo A. pH adjusted local anesthetics: clinical experience. *Reg Anesth.* 1983;8:35.

54. Curatolo M, Petersen-Felix S, Arendt-Nielsen L, et al. Adding sodium bicarbonate to lidocaine enhances the depth of epidural blockade. *Anesth Analg.* 1998;86:341.

55. Chow MY, Sia AT, Koay CK, et al. Alkalinization of lidocaine does not hasten the onset of axillary brachial plexus block. *Anesth Analg.* 1998;86:566.

56. Bromage PR. An evaluation of two new local anesthetics for major conduction blockade. *Can Anaesth Soc J.* 1970;17:557.

57. Bromage PR. A comparison of the hydrochloride and carbon dioxide salts of lidocaine and prilocaine in epidural analgesia. *Acta Anaesthesiol Scand Suppl.* 1965;16:55.

58. Morrison DH. A double blind comparison of carbonated lidocaine and lidocaine hydrochloride in epidural anaesthesia. *Can Anaesth Soc J.* 1981;28:387.

59. Brown DT, Morrison DH, Covino BG, et al. Comparison of carbonated bupivacaine and bupivacaine hydrochloride for extradural anaesthesia. *Br J Anaesth.* 1980;52:419.

60. McClure JH, Scott DB. Comparison of bupivacaine hydrochloride and carbonated bupivacaine in brachial plexus block by the interscalene technique. *Br J Anaesth.* 1981;53:523.

61. Bridenbaugh LD. Does the addition of low molecular weight dextran prolong the duration of action of bupivacaine? *Reg Anesth.* 1978;3:6.

62. Rosenblatt RM, Fung DL. Mechanism of action of dextran prolonging regional anaesthesia. *Reg Anesth.* 1980;5:3.

63. Feitl ME, Krupin T. Neural blockade for ophthalmologic surgery. In: Cousins MG, Bridenbaugh PO, eds. *Neural Blockade in Clinical Anes-*

*thesia and Management of Pain.* 2nd ed. Philadelphia, Pa: JB Lippincott; 1988:577.

64. Bromage PR, Burfoot MF. Quality of epidural blockade, II: influence of physio-chemical factors. Hyaluronidase and potassium. *Br J Anaesth.* 1966;38:857.

65. Eisenach JC, De Klock M, Klimsch W. Alpha-2-adrenergic agonists for regional anesthesia. *Anesthesiology.* 1996;85:655.

66. Gentili M, Bernard JM, Bonnet F, et al. Adding clonidine to lidocaine for intravenous regional anesthesia prevents tourniquet pain. *Anesth Analg.* 1999;88:1327.

67. Cunningham NL, Kaplan JA. A rapid onset, long-acting regional anesthetic technique. *Anesthesiology.* 1974;41:509.

68. Cohen SE, Thurlow A. Comparison of a chloroprocaine-bupivacaine mixture with chloroprocaine and bupivacaine used individually for obstetric epidural analgesia. *Anesthesiology.* 1979;51:288.

69. Hodgkinson R, Husain FJ, Bluhm C. Reduced effectiveness of bupivacaine 0.5% to relieve labor pain after prior injection of chloroprocaine 2%. *Anesthesiology.* 1982;57:3A201.

70. Galindo A, Wichter T. Mixtures of local anesthetics bupivacaine-chloroprocaine. *Anesth Analg.* 1980;59:683.

71. Corke BC, Carlson LG, Dettbarn WD. The influence of 2-chloroprocaine on the subsequent analgesic potency of bupivacaine. *Anesthesiology.* 1984;60:25.

72. Seow LT, Lipps FJ, Cousins MJ, et al. Lidocaine and bupivacaine mixtures for epidural blockade. *Anesthesiology.* 1982;56:177.

73. Ravindran RS, Bond VK, Tasch MD, et al. Prolonged neural blockade following regional anesthesia with 2-chloroprocaine. *Anesth Analg.* 1980;58:447.

74. Moore DC, Spierdijk J, VanKleef JD, et al. Chloroprocaine neurotoxicity: four additional cases. *Anesth Analg.* 1982;61:155.

75. Gissen AJ, Datta S, Lambert D. The chloroprocaine controversy, II: is chloroprocaine neurotoxic? *Reg Anesth.* 1984;9:135.

76. Fibuch EF, Opper SE. Back pain following epidurally administered Nesacaine-MPF. *Anesth Analg.* 1989;69:113.

77. Levy L, Randall GI, Pandit SK. Does chloroprocaine (Nesacaine MPF) for epidural anesthesia increase the incidence of backache? *Anesthesiology.* 1989;71:476.

78. Stevens RA, Chester WL, Artuso JD, et al. Back pain after epidural anesthesia with chloroprocaine in volunteers: preliminary report. *Reg Anesth.* 1991;16:199.

79. Dikes WE. Treatment of Nesacaine-MPF induced back pain with calcium chloride. *Anesth Analg.* 1990;70:461.

80. van Steenberge A, DeBroux HC, Noorduin H. Extradural bupivacaine with sufentanil for vaginal delivery: a double blind trial. *Br J Anaesth.* 1987;59:1518.

81. Brown DL, Carpenter RL, Thompson GE. Comparison of 0.5% ropivacaine and 0.5% bupivacaine for epidural anesthesia in patients undergoing lower extremity surgery. *Anesthesiology.* 1990;72:633.

82. Hickey R, Hoffman J, Ramamurthy S. Comparison of ropivacaine 0.5% and bupivacaine 0.5% for brachial plexus block. *Anesthesiology.* 1991;74:639.

83. Ackerman B, Hellberg IB, Trassvik C. Primary evaluation of the local anesthetic properties of the amino amide agent ropivacaine (LEA 103). *Acta Anaesthesiol Scand.* 1988;32:571.

84. Moller R, Covino BG. Cardiac electro-physiologic properties of bupivacaine and lidocaine compared with those of ropivacaine, a new amide local anesthetic. *Anesthesiology.* 1990;72:322.

85. Feldman HS, Arthur GR, Covino BG. Comparative systemic toxicity of convulsant and supraconvulsant doses of intravenous ropivacaine, bupivacaine, and lidocaine in the conscious dog. *Anesth Analg.* 1989;69:794.

86. Nancarrow C, Rutten AJ, Runciman WB, et al. Myocardial and cerebral drug concentrations and the mechanisms of death after fatal intravenous doses of lidocaine, bupivacaine, and ropivacaine in the sheep. *Anesth Analg.* 1989;69:276.

87. Scott DB, Lee A, Fagan D, et al. Acute toxicity of ropivacaine compared with that of bupivacaine. *Anesth Analg.* 1989;69:563.

88. Concepcion M, Arthur GR, Steele SM, et al. A new local anesthetic, ropivacaine: its epidural effects in humans. *Anesth Analg.* 1990;70:80.

89. Pederson H, Santos A, Morishima HA. Systemic toxicity of ropivacaine in pregnant and non-pregnant ewes. *Anesthesiology.* 1988;69:A344.

90. McClellan KJ, Spencer CM. Levobupivacaine. *Drugs.* 1998;56:355.

91. Covino BG, Vassallo HG. *Local Anesthetics: Mechanisms of Action and Clinical Use.* New York, NY: Grune & Stratton; 1976:123.

92. Covino BG. Toxicity of local anesthetic agents. *Acta Anaesthesiol Belg.* 1988;39:159.

93. Courtney KR. Potentially toxic actions of local anesthetics in cardiac

tissue. In: Roth SH, Miller KW, eds. *Molecular and Cellular Mechanisms of Anesthetics.* New York, NY: Plenum Medical Books; 1986:377.

94. Reiz S, Nath S. Cardiotoxicity of local anesthetic agents. *Br J Anaesth.* 1986;58:736.

95. Feldman HS, Arthur RG, Covino BG. Toxicity of intravenously administered local anesthetic agents in the dog: cardiovascular and central nervous system effects. In: Roth SH, Miller KW, eds. *Molecular and Cellular Mechanisms of Anesthetics.* New York, NY: Plenum Medical Books; 1986:395.

96. Kotelko DM, Shnider SM, Daily PA, et al. Bupivacaine induced cardiac arrhythmias in sheep. *Anesthesiology.* 1984;60:10.

97. Sage D, Feldman H, Arthur GR, et al. Cardiovascular effects of lidocaine and bupivacaine in the awake dog. *Anesthesiology.* 1983;59:A210.

98. Feldman HS, Arthur GR, Norway SB, et al. Cardiovascular effects of mepivacaine and etidocaine in the awake dog. *Anesthesiology.* 1984;61:A229.

99. Thigpen JW, Kotelko DM, Shnider SM, et al. Bupivacaine cardiotoxicity in hypoxic-acidotic sheep. *Anesthesiology.* 1983;59:A204.

100. Hondeghem LM, Clarkson CW. Modulated receptor theory and cardiac toxicity of local anesthetics. In: Roth SH, Miller SW, eds. *Molecular and Cellular Mechanisms of Anesthetics.* New York, NY: Plenum Medical Books; 1986:385.

101. Morishima HO, Pederson H, Finster M, et al. Is bupivacaine more cardiotoxic than lidocaine? *Anesthesiology.* 1983;59:A409.

102. Morishima HO, Pederson H, Finster M, et al. Etidocaine toxicity in the adult, newborn and fetal sheep. *Anesthesiology.* 1983;58:342.

103. Scott DB. "Maximum recommended doses" of local anaesthetic drugs. *Br J Anaesth.* 1989;63:373.

104. Tucker GT, Moore DC, Bridenbaugh LD, et al. Systemic absorption of mepivacaine in commonly used regional block procedures. *Anesthesiology.* 1972;37:277.

105. Ostad A, Kageyama N, Moy RL. Tumescent anesthesia with a lidocaine dose of 55 mg/kg is safe for liposuction. *Dermatol Surg.* 1997;22:921.

106. Rao RB, Ely SF, Hoffman RS. Deaths related to liposuction. *N Engl J Med.* 1999;340:1471.

107. Datta S, Lambert DH, Gregus J, et al. Differential sensitivities of mammalian nerve fibers during pregnancy. *Anesth Analg.* 1983;62:1070.

108. Flanagan HL, Datta S, Lambert DH, et al. Effects of pregnancy on bupivacaine-induced conduction blockade in the isolated rabbit vagus nerve. *Anesth Analg.* 1987;66:123.

109. Shnider SM, Levinson G. Anesthesia for cesarean section. In: Shnider SM, Levinson G, eds. *Anesthesia for Obstetrics.* 2nd ed. Baltimore, Md: Williams & Wilkins; 1987:159.

110. Flanagan HL, Datta S, Moller RA, et al. Effect of exogenously administered progesterone on susceptibility of rabbit vagus nerves to bupivacaine. *Anesthesiology.* 1988;69:A676.

111. Morishima HO, Pederson H, Finster M, et al. Bupivacaine toxicity in pregnant and nonpregnant ewes. *Anesthesiology.* 1985;63:134.

112. Moller RA, Datta S, Fox J, et al. Effects of progesterone on the cardiac electrophysiologic action of bupivacaine and lidocaine. *Anesthesiology.* 1992;76:604.

113. Marathe PH, Shen DD, Artru AA, et al. Effect of serum protein binding on the entry of lidocaine into brain and cerebrospinal fluid in dogs. *Anesthesiology.* 1991;75:804.

114. Ross RA, Clarke JE, Armitage EN. Postoperative pain prevention by continuous epidural infusion. *Anaesthesia.* 1980;35:663.

115. Richter O, Glein K, Abel J, et al. The kinetics of bupivacaine Carboste-sin) plasma concentrations during epidural anesthesia following intraoperative bolus injection and subsequent infusion. *Int J Clin Pharmacol Ther Toxicol.* 1984;22:611.

116. Thomas JM, Schug SA. Recent advances in the pharmacokinetics of local anaesthetics. *Clin Pharmacokinet.* 1999;36:67.

117. Moore DC, Batra M. The components of an effective test dose prior to epidural block. *Anesthesiology.* 1981;55:693.

118. Mulroy MF. Epidural test doses. *Anesthesiol Clin North Am.* 1992;10:45.

119. Guinard JP, Mulroy MF, Carpenter RL, et al. Optimal epinephrine content with and without acute beta-adrenergic blockade. *Anesthesiology.* 1990;73:386.

120. Desparmet J, Mateo J, Ecoffey C, et al. Efficacy of an epidural test dose in children anesthetized with halothane. *Anesthesiology.* 1988;69:A774.

121. Leighton BL, Norris MC, Sosis M, et al. Limitations of epinephrine as a marker of intravascular injection in laboring women. *Anesthesiology.* 1987;66:688.

122. Thigpen JW, Kotelko DM, Shnider MS, et al. Bupivacaine cardiotoxicity in hypoxic-acidotic sheep. *Anesthesiology.* 1983;59:A204.

123. Kasten GW, Martin ST. Successful resuscitation after massive intravenous bupivacaine overdose in the hypoxic dog. *Anesthesiology.* 1984;61:A206.

124. deShazo RD, Nelson HS. An approach to the patient with a history of local anesthetic hypersensitivity: experience with 90 patients. *J Allergy Clin Immunol.* 1979;63;387.

125. Gall H, Kaufmann R, Kalveram CM. Adverse reaction to local anesthetics: analysis of 197 cases. *J Allergy Clin Immunol.* 1996;97:933.

126. Eggleston ST, Lush LW. Understanding allergic reactions to local anesthetics. *Ann Pharmacother.* 1996;30:851.

127. Glinert RJ, Zachary ZB. Local anesthetic allergy: its recognition and avoidance. *J Dermatol Surg Oncol.* 1991;17:491.

128. Schatz M. Drug allergy. In: Patterson R, ed. *Allergic Diseases Diagnosis and Management.* 3rd ed. Philadelphia, Pa: JB Lippincott; 1985:622.

129. Hurley RJ, Lambert D. Cauda equina syndrome after continuous spinal anesthesia. *Anesth Analg.* 1991;72:817.

130. Benson JS. *FDA safety alert: cauda equina syndrome associated with the use of small bore catheters in continuous spinal anesthesia.* Rockville, Md: US Food and Drug Administration; 1992.

131. Special Edition. FDA safety alert. *ASRA News.* 1992;July:1.

132. Schneider M, Ettlin T, Kaufmann M. Transient neurological toxicity after hyperbaric subarachnoid anesthesia with 5% lidocaine. *Anesth Analg.* 1993;76:1154.

133. Snyder R, Flugstad P, Hui G, et al. More cases of possible neurologic toxicity associated with single subarachnoid injections of 5% hyperbaric lidocaine [letter]. *Anesth Analg.* 1994;78:411.

134. Hampl KF, Schneider MC, Ummenhofer W, et al. Transient neurologic symptoms after spinal anesthesia. *Anesth Analg.* 1995;81:1148.

135. Hampl KF, Schneider MC, Pargger H, et al. A similar incidence of transient neurologic symptoms after spinal anesthesia with 2% and 5% lidocaine. *Anesth Analg.* 1996;83:1051.

136. Morisaki H, Masuda J, Kaneko S, et al. Transient neurologic syndrome in one thousand forty one patients after 3% lidocaine spinal anesthesia. *Anesth Analg.* 1998;86:1023.

137. Hampl KF, Wiedmer S, Harms C, et al. Incidence of transient neurologic symptoms after spinal anesthesia with prilocaine, lidocaine and bupivacaine [abstract]. *Anesthesiology.* 1997;87:A778.

138. Sakura A, Chan VW, Ciriales R, et al. The addition of 7.5% glucose does not alter the neurotoxicity of 5% lidocaine administered intrathecally in the rat. *Anesthesiology.* 1995;82:236.

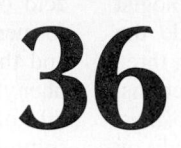

# 36

# Drug Interactions

Mark Veerman

Salvatore R. Goodwin

## DRUG COMPATIBILITY

*What Types of Incompatibilities Occur?*

*What Is the Major Cause of Physical Incompatibilities?*

*How Is the Anesthesiologist Alerted to Incompatibilities?*

*How Can Incompatible Drugs Be Administered Concurrently?*

*Can Intravenous Drug Incompatibilities Cause Harm to the Patient?*

## PHARMACOKINETIC DRUG INTERACTIONS

*How Is Absorption Altered by Other Drugs?*

*What Factors Alter Drug Distribution?*

*Can Other Medications Affect the Elimination of Anesthetic Agents?*

*What Are the Effects of Drug Metabolism?*

*How Are Drugs Eliminated?*

## PHARMACODYNAMIC INTERACTIONS

*How Are Inhalation Anesthetics Involved?*

*How Do Adrenergic Agents Interact With Volatile Anesthetics?*

*What Are the Effects of Antipsychotic Medications?*

*What Problems May Be Associated With Antidepressants?*

*Should Antidepressant Administration Be Discontinued Before Anesthesia?*

*Does Lithium Administration Alter Neuromuscular Blockade?*

*Should Monoamine Oxidase Inhibitors Be Discontinued Before Surgery?*

*Should Antihypertensive Agents Be Discontinued Before Surgery?*

*Do Centrally Acting Antihypertensive Agents Decrease Minimum Alveolar Concentration?*

*Is Clonidine Useful for Spinal Anesthesia and Nerve Blocks?*

*Do Special Considerations Apply to Patients Taking β-Blockers?*

*Do Calcium Channel Blockers Affect Cardiovascular Function During Anesthesia?*

*Do Other Antihypertensive Agents Have Potential Interactions?*

*Are There Any Effects in Patients Administered Transdermal Nitroglycerin and Anesthetic Agents?*

*What Medications Interact With Neuromuscular Blocking Agents?*

*Can Different Neuromuscular Blockers Be Used Sequentially to Take Advantage of the Kinetics of Each Drug?*

*Have Drug Interactions Occurred With Propofol?*

*What Are Significant Benzodiazepine Interactions?*

*What Is the Role of Flumazenil?*

## SUMMARY

In 1984, Levy[1] published a multicenter study on isoflurane that listed preoperative medications and included the smoking history of patients. Figure 36–1 shows the percentage of these patients receiving any of five classes of medications, the percentage of smokers, and the percentage of those who did not smoke or take any medications. Significantly, 45% of the patients were either smokers or were taking the listed medications, as well as other unlisted medications, before surgery. Considering that five or more drugs are commonly used during a typical anesthetic procedure, the potential for possible drug interactions, both desired and undesired, is significant.

Drug interactions can be beneficial or harmful. Although

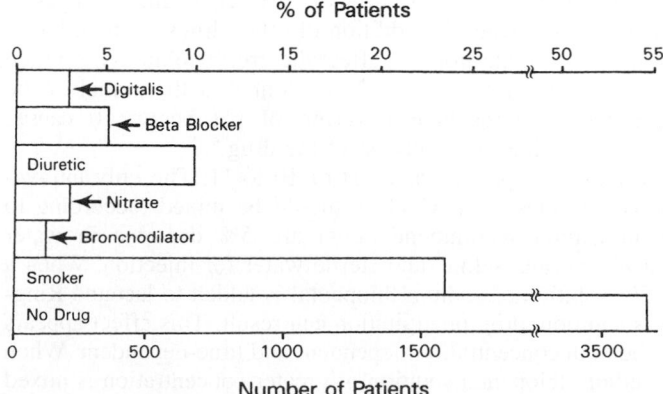

**FIGURE 36–1.** The incidence of preoperative medication with any of five classes of drugs, the percentage of smokers, and the percentage of those who did not smoke or take any medication. Almost half of the patients in this study were either smokers or took at least one of the listed medications. (From Levy WJ. Clinical anesthesia with isoflurane. *Br J Anaesth.* 1984;56:101s.)

not all interactions must be avoided, the possible effects of combining drugs should be known by the anesthesiologist before surgery. This chapter asks questions that guide the reader into discussions of important drug interactions in three categories: drug compatibility, pharmacokinetic interactions, and pharmacodynamic interactions. The terms *pharmacokinetics* and *pharmacodynamics* refer to the effects of the body on drugs and the effects of drugs on the body. Questions apply to drug interactions during not only anesthesia but also the perioperative period. Included in this chapter are expanded tables that list many of the potential drug interactions important to anesthesiologists.

## DRUG COMPATIBILITY

The physical compatibility or, conversely, incompatibility of drugs often is not considered a drug interaction; in fact, incompatibility is significant and can lead to a diminished response or an increase in adverse effects. Drug interactions of this type primarily involve the physical properties of injectable medications.

### What Types of Incompatibilities Occur?

Drug incompatibilities are of two types. *Physical incompatibilities* result when a drug is no longer soluble. Visible examples include precipitation, haze, color change, and evolution of a gas from a drug. However, microcrystalline formation, which cannot be seen, can also occur; thus, the interaction is not observable. *Chemical inactivation* is the second form of incompatibility. This process results in chemical degradation of the active drug, prevents any pharmacologic response, and cannot be detected visually.[2–4] An example is physicochemical inactivation of gentamicin by complex formation with ticarcillin or carbenicillin.[5]

### What Is the Major Cause of Physical Incompatibilities?

The solubility of many drugs is pH-dependent. Changes in pH that result from the addition of other drugs or the dilution of the drug in question can affect the drug's solubility.[3,4] When injectable phenytoin (pH 12) is diluted with normal saline (pH 5-6), the resultant lowering of pH below 10 causes microcrystalline precipitation of the drug.[6]

Sodium thiopental has a pH of 10 to 11. The only intravenous solutions with which it should be mixed (according to manufacturer recommendations) are 5% dextrose in water ($D_5W$), normal saline, and sterile water for injection. When a 2.5% solution of sodium thiopental is added to lactated Ringer's solution, drug precipitation can result. This effect appears to be both concentration-dependent and time-dependent. When a sodium thiopental solution of greater concentration is mixed with lactated Ringer's solution, the rate of precipitation increases. The longer the sodium thiopental–lactated Ringer's solution is allowed to stand before use, the greater the probability that precipitation will occur.[7] Sodium thiopental also is incompatible with other medications, including morphine sulfate, fentanyl citrate, succinylcholine, atracurium, vecuronium, and especially rocuronium.

Most drugs are the salts either of a weak base and a strong acid or of a weak acid and a strong base. Examples of the former are morphine sulfate and midazolam hydrochloride, and those of the latter are sodium phenobarbital and sodium phenytoin. Midazolam hydrochloride has a solubility >22 mg/mL of water at a pH of 2.8, whereas at a pH of 6.2, its solubility decreases to 0.24 mg/mL. Thus, in a high pH intravenous solution such as lactated Ringer's solution, it is both chemically and physically stable for only 4 hours at a concentration of 0.5 mg/mL.[4,8]

In contrast, injectable diazepam is even less soluble than midazolam because diazepam is only available as a weak base rather than as a salt. Diazepam is soluble in propylene glycol but is only sparingly soluble in aqueous solutions. Thus, midazolam hydrochloride is the better of the two benzodiazepines to mix with intravenous solutions because it is less likely to precipitate.

### How Is the Anesthesiologist Alerted to Incompatibilities?

The package insert supplied by the manufacturer of a drug often contains information pertaining to intravenous solution compatibility. Most hospital pharmacies have several reference books that list drug compatibility information. We recommend the *Handbook of Injectable Drugs* by Lawrence Trissel[9] and *Guide to Parenteral Admixtures* by James C. King[10] as useful references for compatibility information. Most of the information in these sources pertains to physical compatibility, not to chemical stability. The concentrations of drugs described in these references also may be different from those that are being used. Therefore, if one fails to observe the expected response, compatibility and stability problems are potential explanations.

When no compatibility information is available, comparing the salt types of the drugs to be combined may give some information on the compatibility. Drugs of the same salt type, such as morphine sulfate and midazolam hydrochloride (both of which are weak base and strong acid salts), are more likely to be compatible than are drugs of different salt types, such as morphine sulfate and sodium phenobarbital (which are strong base and weak acid salts, respectively). Infusion of drugs via the same catheter lumen or in solutions that may be incompatible should be avoided whenever possible. Figure 36–2 lists compatibility information for common medications used in the operating room, postanesthesia care unit, and intensive care unit.

### How Can Incompatible Drugs Be Administered Concurrently?

Incompatible drugs can be given in the same intravenous infusion if, after the first drug is administered, the tubing is flushed with a compatible solution having a volume equal to twice the volume from the site of drug administration to the infusion site in the patient. Gauger and coworkers[11] determined that if a flush volume less than twice the tubing volume is used, residual amounts of the drug will remain in the tubing. Typical normal bore intravenous tubing extension sets with stopcocks have 3.5- to 4-mL volumes and thus ideally require at least an 8-mL flush volume between incompatible drugs.

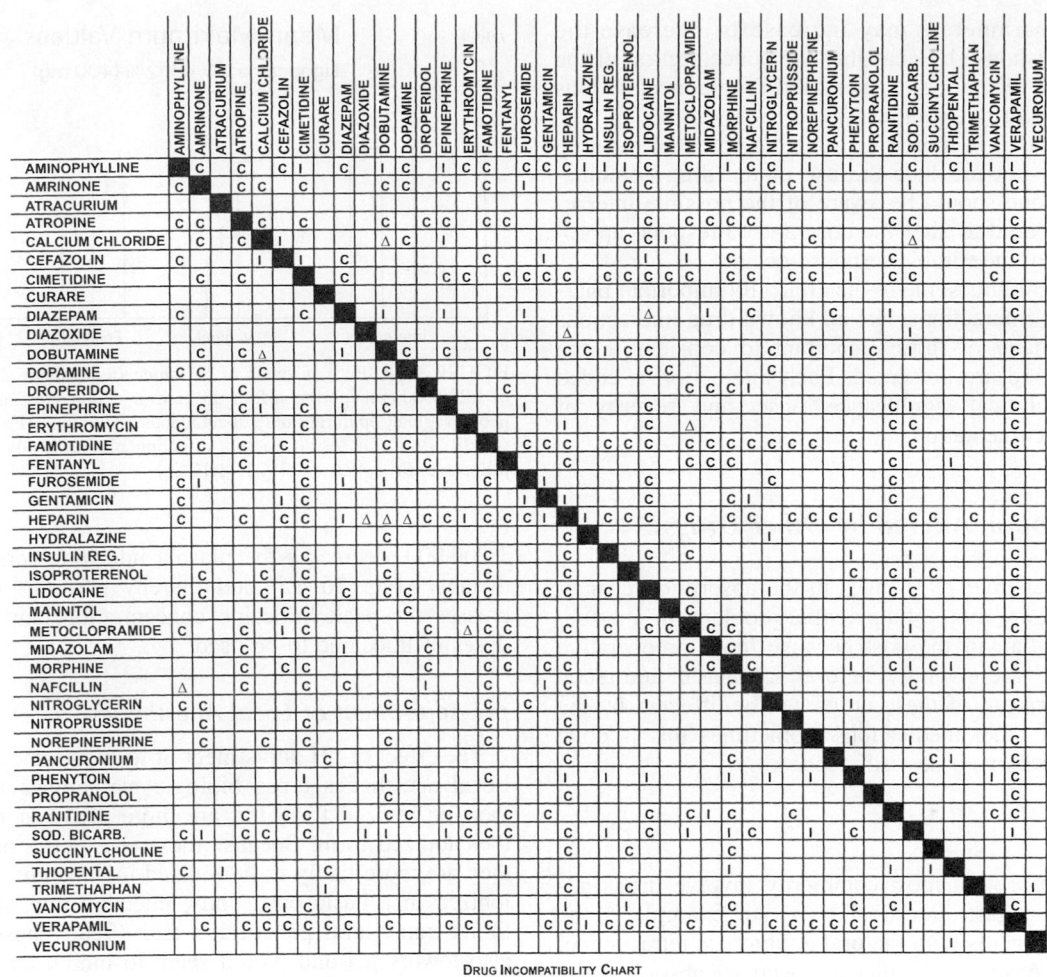

DRUG INCOMPATIBILITY CHART
I = INCOMPATIBILITY
C = COMPATIBLE
Δ = CONCENTRATION DEPENDENT

**FIGURE 36–2.** Drug compatibility chart.

## Can Intravenous Drug Incompatibilities Cause Harm to the Patient?

Intravenous mixtures that form a precipitate can cause venous irritation, embolism, and granuloma formation.[3] Notably, precipitation can also cause occlusion of the catheter or the infusion tubing, or both. This is especially likely with small-gauge catheters. Also, drugs that are chemically inactivated likely will not yield the desired pharmacologic response.[12] Thus, care should be taken not to infuse the precipitate into the patient. All anesthesiologists have observed the precipitate that forms when even a small amount of sodium thiopental comes into contact with succinylcholine, atracurium, or rocuronium. No observable untoward reactions have been reported as a consequence of these precipitates; however, it has been shown that thiopental-atracurium precipitates are prone to cause histamine release and may lead to serious systemic reactions as a result of aggregate anaphylaxis.[4] The precipitate that forms with pentothal and rocuronium is particularly solid and often results in immediate occlusion of the intravenous catheter at a crucial time during the induction sequence. Thus, it is important to flush the stopcock and tubing between administration of these two drugs.

## PHARMACOKINETIC DRUG INTERACTIONS

Pharmacokinetic interactions are the effects of coadministered drugs on absorption, distribution, metabolism, and elimination. Figure 36–3 illustrates these interrelationships. Varia-

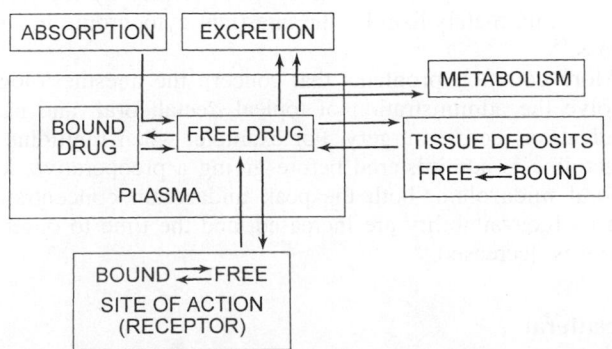

**FIGURE 36–3.** Schematic representation of drug disposition. (From Goodwin SR. Drugs and drug reactions. In: Gravenstein N, ed. *Manual of Complications During Anesthesia.* 1st ed. Philadelphia, Pa: JB Lippincott; 1991:479–508.)

tions in these parameters may increase or decrease the pharmacologic response by changing the concentration of the active drug at the receptor site. Increased drug concentrations may also increase drug toxicities.[4,13]

We emphasize that in most situations the potential for drug interactions does not preclude the use of the drug combinations. However, one should be aware of the possible interactions and be prepared to alter the dose and to respond appropriately should an undesirable response occur.

Table 36–1 highlights some of the clinically important pharmacokinetic drug interactions. Not all known drug interactions are listed, but many of those important to consider in the perioperative period are presented. Each interaction is coded to indicate its clinical significance, onset and severity of response, and documentation.

## How Is Absorption Altered by Other Drugs?

Interactions that involve changes in the absorption characteristics of a drug are more of a potential problem for anesthesiologists today than in the past because more preoperative medications today are given by the oral, intranasal, and rectal routes. The absorption of these drugs can be affected by the administration of other medications (sometimes this is done intentionally to achieve a desired response).

### Enteral

Changes in absorption most commonly involve drugs administered via the gastrointestinal tract. An example is the combination of antacids with the oral antibiotics, tetracycline, or ciprofloxacin. Antacids significantly decrease absorption by forming complexes with these antibiotics.[13–15] Histamine$_2$ (H$_2$) blockers also may be more poorly absorbed when they are administered with antacids. However, their effectiveness does not appear to be affected significantly.

The absorption of orally administered cyclosporin can also be altered by several medications. Erythromycin increases the rate and extent of cyclosporin absorption in two ways: (1) it inhibits the cytochrome P$_{450}$-dependent metabolism of cyclosporin within the gastrointestinal mucosa, and (2) it decreases cyclosporin metabolism by the liver.[16]

Metoclopramide also can increase the rate of cyclosporin absorption in the small bowel, probably by accelerating the gastric emptying rate.[17] Conversely, phenytoin significantly reduces the absorption of cyclosporin, possibly by increasing presystemic metabolism by the intestinal cytochrome P$_{450}$ enzymes.[18]

More common problems that concern the anesthesiologist involve the administration of topical, rectal, oral, and nasal medications before surgery. For example, when ranitidine or cimetidine is administered before giving a preoperative dose of oral midazolam, both the peak midazolam concentration and its bioavailability are increased, and the time to onset of action is decreased.[19]

### Parenteral

#### Epinephrine

The addition of epinephrine to local anesthetics results in vasoconstriction, which delays drug absorption. Epinephrine,

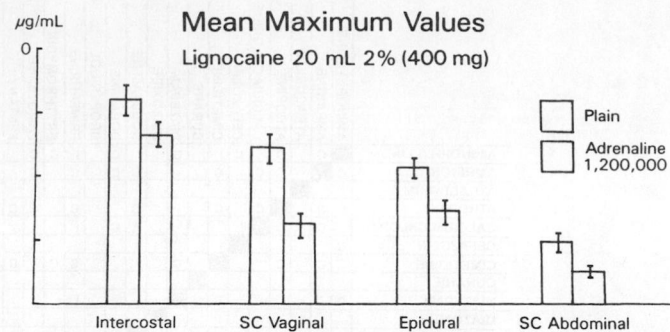

**FIGURE 36–4.** Plasma levels of lidocaine (lignocaine) showing the effects of 1:200 000 epinephrine at four different injection sites: intercostal, subcutaneous vaginal, epidural, and subcutaneous abdominal. (From Scott DB, Jebson JR, Braid DP, et al. Factors affecting plasma levels of lignocaine and prilocaine. *Br J Anaesth.* 1972;44:1043.)

1:200 000, decreases the plasma lidocaine concentration predictably (Fig. 36–4)[20] and thereby prolongs the block, decreases the peak lidocaine concentration, and allows higher doses of lidocaine to be used.

### pH Adjustment of Local Anesthetics

The effect of pH adjustment of local anesthetics is complex. Local anesthetics cross biologic membranes more easily in their un-ionized form but are more active at the receptor in their ionized form. Because these anesthetics are weak bases, they are more likely to be ionized in an acidic milieu and un-ionized in a basic one. Thus, injection into an acid abscess limits transneural penetration and effectiveness. Carbonation also lowers pH and would seem to inhibit absorption. However, efficacy may be enhanced by other mechanisms. Carbon dioxide may have local anesthetic properties; its diffusion may reduce intracellular pH and thereby decrease pH and cause ion trapping intracellularly. Alkalinization of local anesthetics has also been shown to speed onset of action, although opinions regarding this practice and its efficacy have been mixed.

## What Factors Alter Drug Distribution?

*Distribution* is a pharmacokinetic term that describes the process of drug movement from plasma to tissue spaces or binding sites. The distribution process is quantified by the volume of distribution (Vd) in liters per kilogram as expressed by the following formula:

$$Cp = Dose/Vd$$

where Cp is the plasma concentration of the drug and dose is the number of milligrams administered per kilogram. The greater the Vd, the lower the serum concentration for a given dose of a drug. The Vd may be greater or smaller than either the total body or plasma volume, depending on the drug's solubility and partition coefficient. Consider that sodium thiopental has a Vd of approximately 2.3 L/kg.

### Lipid and Water Solubility

Lipid-soluble drugs usually have a greater Vd than do water-soluble drugs. They also distribute more readily across

*Text continued on page 691*

**TABLE 36–1.** Pharmacokinetic Drug Interactions

### Inhaled Anesthetics

**Halothane**

| | Barbiturates | Rifampin / Isoniazid (INH) |
|---|---|---|
| Significance: | Anticipate | Avoid |
| Onset: | >24 h | <24 h |
| Effect: | Increased metabolism to hepatotoxic metabolites in presence of hypoxia | Rifampin plus isoniazid with halothane anesthesia may lead to hepatotoxicity |
| Severity: | Major | Major |
| Documentation: | Possible | Possible |

**Isoflurane**

| | |
|---|---|
| Significance: | Be aware of |
| Onset: | <24 h |
| Effect: | Reported to increase fluoride concentration, but no adverse effects noted |
| Documentation: | Suspected |

### Benzodiazepines (BZDs)

| | Cimetidine | Theophylline | Oral Contraceptives | Ethanol | Omeprazole | Erythromycin |
|---|---|---|---|---|---|---|
| Significance: | Be aware of | Be aware of | Be aware of | Anticipate | Be aware of | Be aware of |
| Onset: | <24 h | <24 h | >24 h | <24 h | >24 h | <24 h (rapid) |
| Effect: | Inhibition of metabolism by cimetidine may increase BZD concentration, prolonging effect | Sedative effect may be antagonized by theophylline, possibly through binding to intracerebral receptors | Inhibition of BZD metabolism may prolong effect | Increased central nervous system effects from acute to chronic alcohol ingestion and decreased elimination secondary to impaired liver function | Decreased hepatic metabolism of BZD increases serum concentrations, prolonging effect | Decreased metabolism of BZD, increasing BZD effects and prolonging sedation |
| Severity: | Minor | Minor | Minor | Minor | Minor | Moderate |
| Documentation: | Probable | Suspected | Suspected | Established | Suspected | Suspected |

### Anticonvulsants

**Phenytoin**

| | Theophylline | Anticoagulants (Warfarin, Dicumarol) | Barbiturates | Benzodiazepines (BZDs) | Carbamazepine (CBZ) | Cimetidine | Disulfiram | Fluconazole |
|---|---|---|---|---|---|---|---|---|
| Significance: | Be aware of | Anticipate | Clinical changes unlikely | Clinical changes unlikely | Be aware of phenytoin effect on CBZ; clinical changes unlikely for CBZ effect on phenytoin | Anticipate | Anticipate | Be aware of |
| Onset: | >24 h | >24 h | >24 h | >24 h | >24 h | >24 h | <24 h | >24 h |
| Effect: | Increased metabolism of phenytoin by theophylline and vice versa, decreasing serum concentrations of both | Increased phenytoin concentration and increased prothrombin times, with increased bleeding | Addition of barbiturates results in unpredictable phenytoin changes; seldom requiring changes, but phenytoin may increase phenobarbital concentration | Increase in phenytoin concentrations due to decreased metabolism | Decreased CBZ concentration from increased metabolism; variable changes of phenytoin concentration | Inhibits phenytoin metabolism, increasing phenytoin concentration | Inhibits phenytoin metabolism, increasing phenytoin concentration | May inhibit phenytoin metabolism, increasing phenytoin concentration |
| Severity: | Moderate | Moderate | Minor | Minor | Moderate | Moderate | Moderate | Moderate |
| Documentation: | Probable | Suspected | Possible | Possible | Suspected | Established | Established | Suspected |

**Phenytoin**

| | Isoniazid (INH) | Omeprazole | Rifampin | Nondepolarizing Muscle Relaxants (NDMRs) |
|---|---|---|---|---|
| Significance: | Anticipate | Clinical changes unlikely | Anticipate | Anticipate |
| Onset: | >24 h | >24 h | >24 h | <24 h |
| Effect: | Inhibits hepatic metabolism of phenytoin; increases phenytoin concentrations | May inhibit phenytoin metabolism | Increases metabolism of phenytoin | Patients taking phenytoin increase NDMR metabolism, decreasing duration of muscle relaxant effects |
| Severity: | Moderate | Moderate | Moderate | Moderate |
| Documentation: | Established | Possible | Suspected | Suspected |

*Table continued on following page*

**TABLE 36–1.** Pharmacokinetic Drug Interactions *Continued*

**Barbiturates (Pentobarbital, Phenobarbital)**

| | Theophylline | β-Blockers (Propanol, Metoprolol only) | Valproic Acid | Cimetidine |
|---|---|---|---|---|
| Significance: | Be aware of | Anticipate | Anticipate | Clinical changes unlikely |
| Onset: | >24 h | <24 h | >24 h | >24 h |
| Effect: | Barbiturates may increase theophylline metabolism, decreasing theophylline concentration | Barbiturates increase metabolism, possibly decreasing duration and effect | Inhibits barbiturate metabolism, increasing concentration | May inhibit metabolism of thiopental and phenobarbital, increasing serum concentrations of both |
| Severity: | Moderate | Minor | Moderate | Minor |
| Documentation: | Suspected | Probable | Established | Unlikely |

**Carbamazepine**

| | Cimetidine | Erythromycin | Barbiturates | Calcium Channel Blockers (Verapamil, Diltiazem) | Valproic Acid | Nondepolarizing Neuromuscular Blocking Agents (NMDRs) |
|---|---|---|---|---|---|---|
| Significance: | Anticipate | Anticipate | Be aware of | Anticipate | Anticipate | Anticipate |
| Onset: | >24 h | <24 h | >24 h | >24 h | >24 h | <24 h |
| Effect: | Inhibits CBZ metabolism, increasing CBZ concentration | Inhibits CBZ metabolism, increasing CBZ concentration | May increase clearance of CBZ, decreasing CBZ concentration | May inhibit CBZ metabolism, increasing CBZ concentration | Both drugs may enhance metabolism of each other, decreasing serum concentrations of both | NMDRS may have shorter than expected duration in patients receiving CBZ |
| Severity: | Moderate | Moderate | Minor | Moderate | Moderate | Moderate |
| Documentation: | Suspected | Established | Suspected | Suspected for verapamil; less likely for diltiazem | Suspected | Probable |

**Anticoagulants / Warfarin**

| | Amiodarone | Barbiturates | β-Blockers | Cephalosporins (Cefoperazone, Cephamandole, Cefotetan, Moxalactam) | Cephalosporin (Cefazolin, Cefoxitin, Ceftriaxone) | Corticosteroids | Erythromycin | Cimetidine |
|---|---|---|---|---|---|---|---|---|
| Significance: | Avoid | Avoid | Clinical changes unlikely | Avoid | Be aware of | Clinical changes unlikely | Anticipate | Avoid |
| Onset: | >24 h | >24 h | >24 h | >24 h | >24 h | >24 h | >24 h | >24 h |
| Effect: | Inhibits metabolism, increasing anticoagulant effect | Increases the metabolism by induction, decreasing anticoagulant effect | Increases the anticoagulant effect | Anticoagulant effects may increase due to warfarin-like activity of these cephalosporins | Increased anticoagulant effect by an unknown mechanism | Increase and decrease in coagulability have been reported | Increase anticoagulant effect of warfarin probably due to decreased warfarin metabolism | Increased anticoagulant effect due to inhibition of warfarin metabolism |
| Severity: | Major | Major | Moderate | Major | Moderate | Minor | Major | Major |
| Documentation: | Established | Established | Possible | Suspected | Possible | Possible | Established | Established |

**Warfarin**

| | Furosemide | Metronidazole | Rifampin | Salicylates | Trimethoprim and Sulfamethoxazole (Bactrim, Septra) |
|---|---|---|---|---|---|
| Significance: | Clinical changes unlikely | Avoid | Anticipate | Avoid | Anticipate |
| Onset: | >24 h | >24 h | >24 h | >24 h | >24 h |
| Effect: | Possible displacement of protein-bound warfarin may occur | Increased anticoagulant effect due to decreased warfarin metabolism | Increases the metabolism of warfarin, decreasing its anticoagulant effect | Increases the anticoagulant effect of warfarin | Increased anticoagulant effect of warfarin due to decreased warfarin metabolism |
| Severity: | Moderate | Major | Moderate | Major | Major |
| Documentation: | Possible | Established | Established | Established | Established |

## Heparin

**Cephalosporins (Parenteral)**
- Significance:
- Onset: Clinical changes unlikely; >24 h
- Effect: Increased bleeding tendencies have been reported
- Severity: Moderate
- Documentation: Possible

**Nitroglycerin (IV)**
- Significance:
- Onset: Clinical changes unlikely; <24 h
- Effect: Decreased anticoagulation effects may occur
- Severity: Moderate
- Documentation: Possible

**Carbamazepine**
- (see under carbamazepine)

## Anti-Infective Agents
### Erythromycin

**Theophylline**
- Significance: Anticipate
- Onset: <24 h
- Effect: Decreases metabolism by inhibiting cytochrome $P_{450}$ system
- Severity: Major
- Documentation: Established

**Warfarin**
- (see under warfarin)

## Ciprofloxacin

**Theophylline**
- Significance: Anticipate
- Onset: >24 h
- Effect: Inhibits the liver metabolism of theophylline by inhibition of cytochrome $P_{450}$ system
- Severity: Moderate
- Documentation: Probable

**Cyclosporin**
- Be aware of
- >24 h
- May inhibit the metabolism of cyclosporin
- Moderate
- Possible

## β-Blockers

**Theophylline**
- Significance: Anticipate
- Onset: <24 h
- Effect: Propranolol may inhibit metabolism, increasing concentrations of theophylline
- Severity: Moderate
- Documentation: Probable

**Cimetidine**
- Anticipate
- <24 h
- Decreases first pass elimination of oral propranolol, increasing propranolol effects
- Moderate
- Probable

**Ranitidine**
- No interaction
- >24 h
- May increase β-blocker effects
- Minor
- Unlikely

## β-Blockers

**Hydralazine**
- Significance: Anticipate
- Onset: >24 h
- Effect: Serum concentration of propranolol is increased by decreasing first pass effect of orally administered propranolol
- Severity: Moderate
- Documentation: Probable

## Digoxin

**Acetylcholine Esterase Inhibitors (Captopril, Enalapril, Lisinopril)**
- Significance:
- Onset: Clinical changes unlikely; >24 h
- Effect: Plasma concentrations of digoxin may be increased or decreased
- Severity: Minor
- Documentation: Possible

**Anticholinergics**
- Clinical changes unlikely
- >24 h
- Digoxin concentrations may increase owing to increased absorption of tablets
- Moderate
- Possible

**Esmolol**
- Clinical changes unlikely
- <24 h
- Serum digoxin concentration may increase for unknown reasons
- Moderate
- Possible

**Quinidine**
- Avoid
- >24 h
- Quinidine decreases both the volume of distribution and elimination, increasing digoxin concentrations
- Major
- Established

**Verapamil**
- Avoid
- <24 h
- Decreases digoxin elimination, increasing concentrations
- Major
- Established

*Table continued on following page*

**TABLE 36–1.** Pharmacokinetic Drug Interactions *Continued*

### Digoxin

| Interacting Drug | Significance | Onset | Effect | Severity | Documentation |
|---|---|---|---|---|---|
| Loop Diuretics (Furosemide, Bumetanide, Ethacrynic Acid) | | Anticipate >24 h | Increased potassium loss, potentially increasing the risk of digoxin toxicity | Moderate | Established |
| Thiazide and Other Miscellaneous Diuretics (Chlorothiazide, Hydrochlorothiazide, Chlorothalidone, Metolazone, Acetazolamide) | | Anticipate >24 h | Increased potassium loss, potentially increasing the risk of digoxin toxicity | Moderate | Established |

### Cyclosporine (CSA)

| Interacting Drug | Significance | Onset | Effect | Severity | Documentation |
|---|---|---|---|---|---|
| Barbiturates | Clinical changes unlikely | >24 h | Induce hepatic enzymes, increasing clearance of CSA, decreasing CSA concentrations | Moderate | Possible |
| Carbamazepine (CBZ) | Clinical changes unlikely | >24 h | Induces metabolism, decreasing CSA concentration | Moderate | Possible |
| Diltiazem | | Anticipate >24 h | Inhibits metabolism, increasing CSA concentrations | Moderate | Established |
| Erythromycin | | Anticipate >24 h | Inhibits metabolism, increasing CSA concentration; erythromycin may also increase oral absorption of CSA | Moderate | Established |
| Phenytoin | | Anticipate >24 h | Decrease in CSA concentrations by either decreased elimination or metabolism, or both | Major | Probable |
| Ketoconazole | | Anticipate >24 h | Probably inhibits metabolism, increasing the CSA concentration | Moderate | Probable |
| Ciprofloxacin (Quinolones) | Clinical changes unlikely | >24 h | Some reports of increased concentrations caused by inhibiton of cytochrome $P_{450}$ system | Minor | Possible |
| Nondepolarizing Neuromuscular Blocking Agents (NMDRs) | Clinical changes possible | <24 h | Prolonged neuromuscular blockade | Moderate | Possible |

### Succinylcholine

| Interacting Drug | Significance | Onset | Effect | Severity | Documentation |
|---|---|---|---|---|---|
| Echothiophate | | Anticipate <24 h | Systemic absorption of echothiophate inhibits pseudocholinesterase, the enzyme responsible for metabolizing succinylcholine | Moderate | Established |
| Cyclophosphamide | | Anticipate <24 h | Inhibits plasma pseudocholinesterase, the enzyme responsible for metabolizing succinylcholine | Moderate | Probable |
| Anticholinesterases (eg, Edrophonium, Neostigmine) | | Anticipate <24 h | Inhibits pseudocholinesterase, increasing the duration of neuromuscular blockade | Moderate | Probable |

### Succinylcholine

| Interacting Drug | Significance | Onset | Effect | Severity | Documentation |
|---|---|---|---|---|---|
| Metoclopramide | | Anticipate <24 h | Metoclopramide may inhibit plasma cholinesterase, prolonging neuromuscular blockade | Anticipate | Suspected |
| Quinidine, Quinine | | Anticipate <24 h | Neuromuscular blockade may be prolonged secondary to decreases in plasma cholinesterase activity | Avoid | Suspected |

### Propofol

| Interacting Drug | Significance | Onset | Effect | Severity | Documentation |
|---|---|---|---|---|---|
| Alfentanil/Sufentanil | | Beware of <24 h | Propofol may affect alfentanil/sufantanil concentration by inhibiting their metabolism | Moderate | Probable |

the blood-brain barrier than do water-soluble drugs. Diazepam passes readily into the central nervous system (CNS), and this is followed by its rapid distribution out of the CNS into lipid tissues; it has an unbound Vd of about 1.33 L/kg. This property leads to a rapid onset of action but also to a decreased duration of effect. The large Vd for diazepam compared with that of lorazepam is a result of its almost fourfold greater degree of lipophilicity.[20-25] Lorazepam, a more water-soluble benzodiazepine with an unbound Vd of only 12 L/kg, penetrates less readily into the CNS but has a longer duration of effect.

Homer and Stanski[26] found that thiopental rapidly affects electroencephalographic recordings and has a mean pharmacodynamic half-life effect of 1.2 minutes. This observation indicates an almost immediate distribution of thiopental to brain tissue by rapid perfusion and partitioning from the blood. In fact, the distribution of thiopental to brain tissue is so rapid that it cannot be effectively measured pharmacokinetically; therefore, it can be considered to be instantaneous following administration. The redistribution of thiopental from brain tissue to muscle and fat is also rapid and is nearly complete after about 10 minutes.

## Protein Binding

Plasma protein binding also represents a site of drug distribution. Changes in plasma protein binding can increase or decrease the unbound portion of the drug. The unbound or "free" drug is the active portion that is capable of diffusing across membranes and interacting with receptor sites.[3,27,28] Table 36–2 lists factors that influence drug plasma and tissue distribution.

Certain characteristics are necessary for an interaction to be of practical importance. The drug should be highly protein bound (>85%), have a narrow therapeutic range, and have a small Vd.[28] A good example is phenytoin, which is 90% bound to albumin, has a narrow therapeutic range (10-20 µg/L), and has a Vd of 0.7 L/kg.[29]

### Albumin

Albumin constitutes 60% of the plasma proteins and is capable of binding drugs of different charges. Hypoalbuminemia is associated with burns, cancer, inflammatory diseases, liver disease, malnutrition, nephrotic syndrome, renal disease, premature and term infant birth, and extensive intraabdominal surgery.[30]

Thiopental and phenytoin are usually at least 90% albumin-bound. The percentage of unbound or free phenytoin is higher than normal in patients with renal failure and hypoalbuminemia and in patients receiving drugs such as valproic acid, which displaces phenytoin from albumin. If the phenytoin concentration (unbound and protein-bound) remains constant,

**TABLE 36–2.** Physiologic Determinants of Drug Partition or Distribution Ratios Between Plasma and Tissue

| | |
|---|---|
| Active transport | Plasma protein binding |
| Donnon ion effect | Tissue binding |
| pH difference | Lipid partitioning |

Reprinted by permission from *Applied Pharmacokinetics: Principles of Therapeutic Drug Monitoring.* 3rd ed. edited by William E. Evans, Jerome J. Schentag, and William J. Jusko, published by Applied Therapeutics, Inc, Vancouver, Washington; © 1992.

a higher unbound percentage results in an increase in effects just as if the total serum phenytoin concentration were elevated in a patient with normal protein binding or albumin stores.

Patients suspected of having a higher percentage of unbound phenytoin should have their serum unbound phenytoin levels monitored to determine whether they are in the therapeutic range of 1 to 2 µg/mL.[29] In the analogous case of thiopental administration, it is wise to start with a reduced dose.

### α₁-Acid Glycoprotein

The $\alpha_1$-acid glycoprotein is an acute phase reactant that increases in concentration in response to stresses such as trauma, inflammation, and acute myocardial infarction.[28,30] Drugs that may have a decreased effect in response to an increase in $\alpha_1$-acid glycoprotein include bupivacaine, lidocaine, meperidine, methadone, and propranolol. Phenytoin, quinidine, and meperidine displace bupivacaine in vitro; this increases its unbound fraction three- to fivefold. This effect may increase the toxicity of systemically absorbed bupivacaine from epidural administration, and possibly that of other local anesthetics, if the same interaction occurs in vivo.[31,32]

## Can Other Medications Affect the Elimination of Anesthetic Agents?

Narcotic agents depress alveolar ventilation; this leads to delayed excretion of inhaled anesthetics and prolongs their effects in spontaneously breathing patients.[27] Probenecid can increase the duration of thiopental-induced anesthesia. Kaukinen and colleagues examined the effects of pretreatment with 0.5 to 1 g of probenecid on thiopental-induced anesthesia (4-7 mg/kg).[33] The mean duration of anesthesia was prolonged by 109%.

The mechanism by which probenecid prolongs thiopental anesthesia may be related to increased penetration to the sites of action in the brain or to displacement of thiopental from plasma proteins. Thus, reduced doses of thiopental may be indicated for patients receiving probenecid.[33,34]

## What Are the Effects of Drug Metabolism?

Metabolism is primarily a function of the liver, which biotransforms drugs to more readily excretable metabolites through a series of chemical reactions. Phase I reactions involve oxidation, reduction, or hydrolysis to a more polar compound. Further metabolism by conjugation, a phase II reaction, results in a more highly polar metabolite that can be excreted by the kidneys.

Metabolites generally have decreased or absent pharmacologic activity. However, some drugs, such as chloral hydrate, are transformed to an active metabolite. Also, although metabolized drug forms are generally less toxic than unmetabolized forms, in certain circumstances, some drugs become more toxic, such as acetaminophen taken in overdose.[35]

Drug metabolism occurs within the hepatocyte. Cytochrome $P_{450}$ and NADPH (nicotinamide-adenine dinucleotide phosphate) cytochrome $P_{450}$ reductase are the responsible enzyme systems. Their induction or inhibition is affected by genetic factors, age, hormones, disease, nutrition, stress, and exogenous chemicals. Drugs initially metabolized by the body are more variably eliminated than are those excreted unchanged in the urine. Therefore, the effect of hepatic enzyme induction or inhibition on drug interactions varies considerably.[27,35,36] Table 36–1 lists drug interactions that result from changes in metabolism.

## Volatile Anesthetics and Enzyme Induction

### Halothane Hepatitis

Enzyme induction may play a role in halothane-induced hepatitis. Models in which animals were given hypoxic gas mixtures with halothane after phenobarbital pretreatment have caused liver injury. The proposed mechanism is a change from the normal oxidative pathway to a reductive pathway for halothane metabolism.[27,37,38] Although the exact mechanism is still a subject of controversy and may also be immune-mediated, the following factors seem to be required: drug-related enzyme induction; poor nutritional status; halothane anesthesia; reduced hepatic oxygenation associated with an anesthetic-related decrease in splanchnic blood flow; and a reduced concentration of oxygen during abdominal surgery.[27,39]

### Methoxyflurane Nephrotoxicity

Methoxyflurane metabolism yields a free fluoride ion that is nephrotoxic when present in sufficient concentrations. Patients taking phenobarbital may have enhanced metabolism of methoxyflurane, which increases the formation of fluoride ions to potentially toxic concentrations.[27,40] Enflurane metabolism also releases fluoride ions but probably only results in increased nephrotoxicity after prolonged exposure in obese patients or in patients taking isoniazid who also acetylate rapidly. Enflurane metabolism and free fluoride ion release is not enhanced by other enzyme-inducing drugs such as phenobarbital.[41]

## Drug Class Similarities and Differences

Often, the members of a given drug class alter metabolism similarly, but notable exceptions do occur.[42] The $H_2$ blockers—cimetidine, famotidine, and ranitidine—are available in the United States. Cimetidine is a consistent inhibitor of the cytochrome $P_{450}$ system and can lead to increased concentrations of other drugs that are dependent on this system for metabolism.[43] These drugs include theophylline, cyclosporin, phenytoin, carbamazepine, and warfarin.

In a study comparing the inhibition of theophylline elimination, Powell and colleagues found that cimetidine, but not ranitidine, statistically decreased mean theophylline clearance.[43] Ranitidine inhibited theophylline metabolism in some subjects, but the magnitude of this effect was not as great as with cimetidine. Famotidine, the newest of the $H_2$ blockers, appears to be relatively free of effects on the cytochrome $P_{450}$ system.[44] Because efficacy among the $H_2$ blockers is thought to be equivalent, famotidine may have some advantages in patients who are taking other medications subject to inhibition.[45,46]

## Time to Onset of Induction or Inhibition

The metabolic induction of drugs is most likely due to increased synthesis of cytochrome $P_{450}$ system enzymes.[43,47,48]

Studies of warfarin have demonstrated that phenobarbital and rifampin induction can be detected within 6 to 7 days and within 2 days, respectively. The maximum effect is seen at 14 to 21 days with phenobarbital and at 4 days with rifampin. Upon discontinuation of the inducing drug, the same time course is followed to the return of normal status.[49,50]

## Competitive and Noncompetitive Inhibition

Drug inhibition can be competitive or noncompetitive. In competitive inhibition, the inhibitor is an alternate substrate for the metabolizing enzyme, whereas in noncompetitive inhibition, the drug inactivates the enzyme. Most drugs that inhibit drug metabolism do so by inhibiting the cytochrome $P_{450}$ system. Drug inhibitors that act directly on enzyme synthesis generally have a rapid onset of inhibition. Cimetidine reversibly binds to cytochrome $P_{450}$ enzymes in a competitive or noncompetitive manner. It inhibits drug metabolism within 24 hours after administration of a single dose. As a general rule, inhibitory drugs exert their effect within a short period of time compared with those drugs that induce liver microsomal enzymes.[35]

## Practical Considerations

An anesthesiologist must know when a drug treatment was begun (or discontinued) to determine whether it will affect his or her ministrations. If a drug capable of changing liver metabolism is administered for several weeks before anesthesia, its effect can be seen during anesthesia. Dosage requirements of those drugs metabolized by the liver may change, depending on whether an inhibitor or inducer is used. Erythromycin inhibits cytochrome $P_{450}$ microsomal enzymes and augments the action of drugs that undergo similar metabolism. Prolonged respiratory depression has been demonstrated with alfentanil in patients who have received erythromycin.[51]

Drug inducers given simultaneously with anesthetics, such as sodium thiopental, have no lasting effects unless they are continued for extended periods of time. In contrast, if cimetidine is given preoperatively, it can decrease the metabolism of drugs that were given several hours later, resulting in an exaggerated or prolonged response.

Echothiophate (Phospholine Iodide) is an organophosphate anticholinesterase that is used for the treatment of glaucoma. It is capable of depleting plasma pseudocholinesterase. Despite extraocular administration, sufficient amounts of echothiophate may be absorbed systemically, preventing succinylcholine metabolism by pseudocholinesterase. Glaucoma patients are thus at risk for prolonged neuromuscular blockade from succinylcholine. Discontinuation of echothiophate several weeks before surgery would be necessary to allow pseudocholinesterase activity to return to normal.[52,53]

## How Are Drugs Eliminated?

Drug elimination is primarily by renal excretion, but it can also proceed through the biliary and respiratory systems. Remarkably, few drugs interact to alter the elimination of other drugs. Diuretic administration can not only enhance the elimination of other renally excreted medications but also can impede elimination. Drugs that bind bile salts (cholestyramine) can enhance the elimination of those agents that undergo reabsorption via the enterohepatic circulation. Examples of such drugs include digoxin, thyroid compounds, and propranolol.

## Diuretics and Lithium Excretion

Lithium elimination by renal excretion is decreased by diuretic therapy. The result is increased serum lithium concentrations. This interaction can occur perioperatively and requires careful monitoring of serum lithium concentrations.[54,55]

## PHARMACODYNAMIC INTERACTIONS

The changes in the effect of a drug brought about by the concurrent use of another drug or drugs represents a pharmacodynamic interaction. Changes in drug responsiveness or an adverse effect may result. Pharmacodynamic interactions may be additive, synergistic, potentiating, or antagonistic. A purist might argue justifiably that additive drug interactions are not interactions; however, they are included for completeness (Table 36–3).

Pharmacodynamic drug interactions often prove important during anesthesia. Because many anesthetics have narrow therapeutic ranges, combining drugs produces an additive or synergistic response. With this approach, the same desired pharmacologic effect can result but with lesser risk to the patient. This goal is accomplished by decreasing the individual side effects of each agent. Obviously, certain combinations of agents can result in an increase in adverse effects.

Pharmacodynamic interactions can be grouped into drug categories or classes. Table 36–4 lists many of the classes that are important in the operating room and intensive care environments. The remainder of this chapter addresses some of the important aspects of these drug interactions.

## How Are Inhalation Anesthetics Involved?

The combination of inhaled anesthetic agents with other medications is frequently used in balanced anesthesia techniques. Pharmacodynamic interactions between inhaled anesthetic agents and other CNS depressants usually decrease the minimal alveolar concentration (MAC) of the inhaled agents. Sometimes, however, they lead to antagonism of the inhaled anesthetic.[38]

## How Do Adrenergic Agents Interact With Volatile Anesthetics?

### Epinephrine

The volatile anesthetics sensitize the myocardium to the arrhythmogenic effects of endogenous or exogenous cate-

**TABLE 36–3.** Mathematic Examples of Additive, Synergistic, Potentiating, and Antagonistic Interactions

| | |
|---|---|
| Additive | $2 + 2 = 4$ |
| Synergistic | $2 + 2 > 4$ |
| Potentiation | $0 + 2 > 2$ |
| Antagonism | $2 + 2 < 4$ |

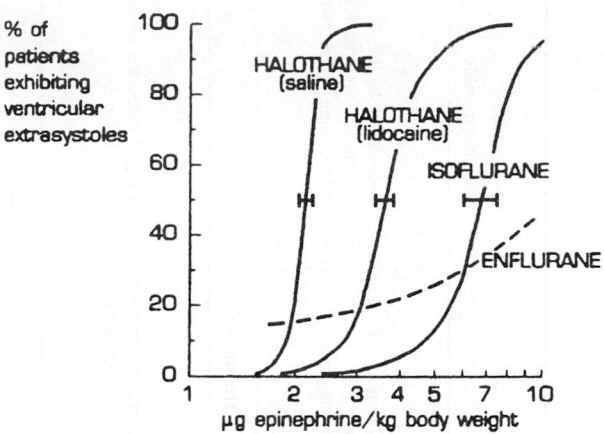

**FIGURE 36–5.** Results of a statistical analysis of the dose response curve for epinephrine-induced cardiac arrhythmias during anesthesia. The ED50 is significantly lower during halothane than during isoflurane anesthesia ($P <$ 0.01). The bars indicate the standard deviation from the ED50. (From Johnston RR, Eger EI II, Wilson CA. A comparative interaction of epinephrine with enflurane, isoflurane, and halothane in man. *Anesth Analg.* 1976;55:709–712.)

cholamines.[56] Coadministration of lidocaine attenuates this effect while coadministration of thiopental potentiates this effect. As can be seen in Figure 36–5, halothane is the most sensitizing, with 50% of patients experiencing ventricular extrasystoles at doses of approximately 2 μg/kg body weight. When lidocaine is added, this increases to about 3 μg/kg. Isoflurane is less sensitizing, with 50% of patients experiencing arrhythmias at 6 μg/kg. Sevoflurane is similar to isoflurane in arrhythmogenic potential.[57] In one study, premature ventricular contractions were absent when epinephrine doses of less than 5 μg/kg were used and were present in 4 of 12 patients when doses of 5 μg/kg or higher were used.

### Cocaine

With nearly 4 million Americans admitting to the regular use of cocaine, this agent has become one of the most widely abused drugs. Cocaine inhibits the uptake of norepinephrine both centrally and peripherally. It may stimulate presynaptic release of catecholamines and blocks serotonin reuptake. The catecholamine reuptake blockade results in postsynaptic stimulation. However, it also leads to metabolism and eventual depletion of catecholamines and serotonin. Thus, one may see varying responses with drug interactions, depending on acute versus chronic use. To complicate the issue even further, most cocaine abusers also abuse other drugs. The intravenous use of cocaine and heroin, so-called speedballing, is associated with an estimated 12% to 15% of toxic cocaine episodes in the emergency department. The combination of ethanol and cocaine increases the risk of sudden death from cocaine 21.5 times compared to cocaine alone.[58]

The lists of cardiovascular, respiratory, neurologic, and other complications associated with cocaine use are legion. The anesthesiologist is faced with a patient who is likely to respond unpredictably to anesthetic agents as well as all other autonomic nervous system medications. Hypertension, hypotension, dysrhythmias, and changes in heart rate have all been reported with acute and chronic use. Patients may have an exaggerated response to vasopressors. In animals, acute cocaine ingestion increases the MAC of halothane and decreases

*Text continued on page 698*

**TABLE 36–4.** Pharmacodynamic Interactions

### Barbiturate Anesthetics (Thiopental, Methohexital, Thiamylal)

| | Benzodiazepines | Narcotic Analgesics (eg, Alfentanil, Fentanyl, Morphine, Pentazocine) | Phenothiazines (eg, Chlorpromazine, Promethazine) | Metoclopramide |
|---|---|---|---|---|
| Significance: | Anticipate | Anticipate | Be aware of | Anticipate |
| Onset: | <24 h | <24 h | <24 h | <24 h |
| Effect: | Synergistic central nervous system effects | Narcotic analgesics reduce the anesthetic dose of thiopental | Phenothiazines may increase frequency of neuromuscular excitation and hypotension with barbiturate analgesia | Metoclopramide decreases the thiopental hypnotic requirement probably by blocking $D_2$ receptors |
| Severity: | Moderate | Moderate | Minor | Moderate |
| Documentation: | Established | Suspected | Suspected | Probable |

### Ketamine

| | Theophylline | Halothane |
|---|---|---|
| Significance: | Be aware of | Anticipate |
| Onset: | <24 h | <24 h |
| Effect: | Increased extensor-type seizures have occurred when patients taking theophylline received ketamine | Hypotension and decreased cardiac output can occur when ketamine and halothane are given together. Also reduces minimum alveolar concentration (MAC) of halothane. |
| Severity: | Moderate | Moderate |
| Documentation: | Possible | Established |

### Nondepolarizing Muscle Relaxants (NDMRs)

| | Trimethaphan | Verapamil | Lithium |
|---|---|---|---|
| Significance: | Anticipate | Anticipate | Clinical changes unlikely |
| Onset: | <24 h | <24 h | <24 h |
| Effect: | Trimethaphan can prolong the neuromuscular blockade of NDMRs | Verapamil may prolong the neuromuscular blockade of NDMRs | Patients taking lithium may have prolonged effect from NDMRs |
| Severity: | Moderate | Moderate | Moderate |
| Documentation: | Suspected | Suspected | Possible |

### Nondepolarizing Muscle Relaxants (NDMRs)

| | Aminoglycosides | Benzodiazepines (BZDs) | β-Blockers | Carbamazepine (CBZ) | Clindamycin |
|---|---|---|---|---|---|
| Significance: | Anticipate | Clinical changes unlikely | Clinical changes possible | Anticipate | Be aware of |
| Onset: | <24 h | <24 h | <24 h | <24 h | <24 h |
| Effect: | Have synergistic effects on neuromuscular blockade | May have a variable effect on neuromuscular blockade | May potentiate, counteract, or have no effect on the action of NDMRs | May cause shorter duration of action of neuromuscular blockade by nondepolarizing muscle relaxants | Potentiates neuromuscular blockade of NDMRs probably by inhibiting acetylcholine release |
| Severity: | Major | Moderate | Moderate | Moderate | Moderate |
| Documentation: | Established | Possible | Established | Suspected | Suspected |

### Nondepolarizing Muscle Relaxants (NDMRs)

| | Inhalation Anesthetics | Ketamine | Magnesium Sulfate (Parenteral) | Phenytoin | Polypeptide Antibiotics (Bacitracin, Polymyxin B, Vancomycin) |
|---|---|---|---|---|---|
| Significance: | Anticipate | Anticipate | Anticipate | Be aware of | Anticipate |
| Onset: | <24 h | <24 h | <24 h | <24 h | <24 h |
| Effect: | Potentiate the neuromuscular blockade of NDMRs | Potentiates the neuromuscular blockade | Can potentiate the neuromuscular blockade | Neuromuscular blockade may be shortened in patients receiving phenytoin | Enhance neuromuscular blockade by affecting presynaptic and postsynaptic blockade |
| Severity: | Major | Moderate | Moderate | Moderate | Moderate |
| Documentation: | Established | Probable | Suspected | Suspected | Probable |

**Nondepolarizing Muscle Relaxants (NDMRs)**

| | Quinidine, Quinine | Theophylline | Azathioprine | MAOI (Phenelzine) | Phenytoin | Metoclopramide | Propofol |
|---|---|---|---|---|---|---|---|
| Significance: | Anticipate | Be aware of | Be aware of | Be aware of | Anticipate | Anticipate | Be aware of |
| Onset: | <24 h | <24 h | <24 h | <24 h | <24 h | <24 h | <24 h |
| Effect: | May enhance neuromuscular blockade of NDMRs | May antagonize the neuromuscular blockade | May inhibit phosphodiesterase at the nerve terminal and, increase cAMP, thereby antagonizing the neuromuscular blockade | Phenelzine may decrease plasma pseudocholinesterase to subnormal range, leading to enhanced effects of succinylcholine | May prolong succinylcholine block | Metoclopramide may inhibit plasma cholinesterase interfering with inactivation of succinylcholine | Severe bradycardia has occurred with co-administration of both agents |
| Severity: | Moderate | Moderate | Moderate | Moderate | Moderate | Moderate | Moderate |
| Documentation: | Suspected | Suspected | Suspected | Possible (note: effects could persist 2 wks after discontinuation of phenelzine) | Established | Suspected | Possible |

**Succinylcholine**

| | Aminoglycosides | Cimetidine | Lithium | Ketamine | Lidocaine |
|---|---|---|---|---|---|
| Significance: | Anticipate | Clinical changes unlikely | Clinical changes unlikely | Be aware of | Anticipate |
| Onset: | <24 h | <24 h | <24 h | <24 h | <24 h |
| Effect: | Can be additive or synergistic neuromuscular block with succinylcholine | May potentiate the neuromuscular blocking effects of succinylcholine by inhibiting metabolism of succinylcholine | May potentiate neuromuscular blocking effects of succinylcholine | May prolong the neuromuscular block of succinylcholine | May prolong the neuromuscular block |
| Severity: | Moderate | Moderate | Moderate | Moderate | Moderate |
| Documentation: | Probable | Possible | Possible | Possible | Suspected |

**Succinylcholine**

| | Trimethophan | Azathioprine | Phenytoin | Metoclopramide |
|---|---|---|---|---|
| Significance: | Anticipate | Anticipate | Anticipate | Anticipate |
| Onset: | <24 h | <24 h | <24 h | <24 h |
| Effect: | Inhibits pseudocholinesterase by decreasing succinylcholine metabolism | May potentiate neuromuscular block of succinylcholine, probably by inhibiting phosphodiesterase | May prolong the neuromuscular block of succinylcholine | May prolong the neuromuscular block |
| Severity: | Major | Major | Major | Moderate |
| Documentation: | Probable | Suspected | Suspected | Suspected |

**Benzodiazepines (BZDs)**

| | Narcotics (eg, Morphine, Fentanyl) | Barbiturates | Halothane |
|---|---|---|---|
| Significance: | Anticipate | Anticipate | Anticipate |
| Onset: | <24 h | <24 h | <24 h |
| Effect: | May cause hemodynamic depression; synergistic enhancement of BZD effect | Synergistic central nervous system effects occur when used concurrently | Decreases the MAC of halothane |
| Severity: | Moderate | Moderate | Moderate |
| Documentation: | Established | Established | Suspected |

**Propofol**

| | Benzodiazepines | Theophylline | Alfentanil/Fentanyl | ACE Inhibitors |
|---|---|---|---|---|
| Significance: | Clinical changes unlikely (synergistic) | Clinical changes unlikely | Be aware of | Be aware of |
| Onset: | <24 h | <24 h | <24 h | <24 h |
| Effect: | Increase effects of propofol (synergistic) | May antagonize effects of propofol | Alfentanil/fentanyl may reduce the propofol requirement, but may not have a corresponding stable induction of anesthesia | Severe hypotension may occur when used together |
| Severity: | Moderate | Minor | Moderate | Moderate |
| Documentation: | Established | Possible | Possible | Possible |

*Table continued on following page*

**TABLE 36–4.** Pharmacodynamic Interactions *Continued*

| Drug | Interacting agent | Significance | Onset | Effect | Severity | Documentation |
|---|---|---|---|---|---|---|
| Halothane | Labetalol | Anticipate | <24 h | Synergistic cardiodepressant effects, which also occur with enflurane and isoflurane | Moderate | Probable |
| Halothane | Theophylline | Anticipate | >24 h | Catecholamine-induced arrhythmias in patients taking theophylline | Major | Probable |
| Desflurane | Labetalol | | >24 h | Clinical changes unlikely | | |
| Desflurane | Tetracyclines | | | ? | | Possible |
| Desflurane | Aminoglycosides | | | Nephrotoxicity of aminoglycosides may be increased | Moderate | |
| Isoflurane, Sevoflurane | Tetracyclines | Avoid | <24 h | Synergistic renal toxicity from both agents may occur | Major | Possible |
| Isoflurane, Sevoflurane | Aminoglycosides | Avoid | <24 h | May have synergistic nephrotoxicity when both agents are given together | Major | Possible |
| Narcotic Analgesics (Morphine, Fentanyl, Sufentanil, Meperidine, Alfentanil, Remifentanil) | Benzodiazepines (BZDs) | Anticipate | <24 h | Decreased mean arterial pressure and systemic vascular resistance synergistic of BZD effects | Moderate | Established |
| Narcotic Analgesics | Nitrous Oxide | Anticipate | <24 h | Decreased cardiac output | Moderate | Probable |
| Narcotic Analgesics | Inhalation Anesthetics | Anticipate | >24 h | Decreases the MAC requirement for anesthesia | Moderate | Established |
| Narcotic Analgesics | Naloxone | Anticipate | <24 h | Reverse respiratory depression, analgesia, and other narcotic effects | Moderate | Established |
| β-Blockers | Epinephrine | Avoid | <24 h | Restrict epinephrine's effect to α-receptor stimulation | Major | Established |
| β-Blockers | Ketamine | Avoid | <24 h | Hypotension may occur secondary to the heart's inability to respond to sympathetic stimulation | Major | Probable |
| β-Blockers | Halothane (also Desflurane, Sevoflurane) | Be aware of | <24 h (rapid) | Hypotension can occur secondary to cardiac depression | Moderate | Probable |
| Digoxin | Loop Diuretics | Anticipate | >24 h | May induce electrode losses of $K^+$ and $Mg^{2+}$, which predispose to digoxin-related arrhythmias | Moderate | Established |
| Digoxin | Succinylcholine | Be aware of | <24 h | Increased potential for cardiac arrhythmias when succinylcholine is given to digitalized patients | Moderate | Possible |

| Drug | Interacting Agent | Significance | Onset | Effect | Severity | Documentation |
|---|---|---|---|---|---|---|
| Methyldopa | β-Blockers | Be aware of | <24 h | Clinical changes unlikely. Severe hypertension may occur due to unopposed vasoconstriction from α-methylnorepinephrine owing to β-blockade | Major | Possible |
| Methyldopa | Sympathomimetics | Anticipate | <24 h | Methyldopa may potentiate the pressor response of sympathomimetics | Major | Possible |
| Methyldopa | Inhaled Anesthetics | Be aware of | <24 h | MAC reduced | Moderate | Established |
| Reserpine | Sympathomimetics | Anticipate | <24 h | Reserpine may potentiate the vasopressor response of direct-acting sympathomimetics | Moderate | Suspected |
| Reserpine | Inhaled Anesthetics | Be aware of | <24 h | A decrease in MAC may occur in reserpine-treated patients | Moderate | Established |
| Clonidine | β-Blockers | Avoid | >24 h | Blockade of β-receptor-mediated vasodilation may result in unopposed vasoconstriction | Major | Suspected |
| Clonidine | Inhaled Anesthetics | Anticipate | <24 h | Decreases the MAC requirement for inhaled anesthetics | Moderate | Established |
| Clonidine | Narcotics | Be aware of | <24 h | Clonidine may potentiate the effects of narcotics | Moderate | Suspected |
| Prazosin | β-Blockers | Anticipate | <24 h | May have increased postural hypotension | Moderate | Probable |
| Prazosin | Verapamil | Be aware of | <24 h | May have increased postural hypotension | Moderate | Suspected |
| Angiotensin-Converting Enzyme Inhibitors (Captopril, Enalapril, Lisinopril) | Propofol | Be aware of | <24 h | Prolonged hypotension has occurred with these agents | Minor | Possible |
| Monoamine Oxidase Inhibitors (Phenelzine, Nialamide, Isocarboxazid, Pargyline, Tranylcypromine) | Meperidine | Avoid | <24 h | Seizures, agitation, fever, coma, apnea, and death have occurred for unknown reasons | Major | Established |
| Monoamine Oxidase Inhibitors (Phenelzine, Nialamide, Isocarboxazid, Pargyline, Tranylcypromine) | Sympathomimetics (Epinephrine, Dopamine, Ephedrine, Pseudoephedrine, Metaraminol) | Avoid | <24 h | Inhibition of the enzyme monoamine oxidase decreases the breakdown of biogenic amines, increasing their activity | Major | Established |

the sedative effect of benzodiazepines. Chronic use of cocaine also resulted in an increase of the MAC of isoflurane.[59]

Although a drug history is important for all patients, anesthesiologists may need to specifically ask about cocaine use especially in the trauma patient.

## Nitrous Oxide

The combination of nitrous oxide ($N_2O$) and a potent volatile agent results in an additive drug interaction. If $N_2O$ is delivered at 50% MAC, a 50% reduction in the MAC of the inhalation agent is to be expected. Furthermore, because the initial uptake of $N_2O$ is extremely rapid, the alveolar concentration of a coadministered volatile anesthetic is increased by the loss of alveolar gas volume. This phenomenon is known as the *second gas effect*[60,61] and results in increased speed of induction. Discontinuation of $N_2O$ and its rapid elimination reverses this process, increasing minute ventilation and thereby also elimination of the inhaled volatile agent.

The addition of $N_2O$ decreases respiratory depression to a lesser degree than would be expected from higher concentrations of the volatile anesthetic alone. It also decreases cardiovascular depression. Bahlman studied the effects of 1.2 and 2.4 MAC equivalents of halothane-oxygen compared with those of halothane-$N_2O$.[62] Depression of cardiac output, mean arterial pressure, and ventricular work was greater with halothane alone than with halothane combined with $N_2O$. The lesser degree of cardiovascular depression at the same MAC level when $N_2O$ is added makes this an appealing drug combination.

The effects of $N_2O$ combined with chloral hydrate was studied by Litman and associates.[63] Chloral hydrate at a dose of 70 mg/kg was studied alone and with the addition of 30% and 50% $N_2O$ in 32 children undergoing a pediatric dentistry procedure. In patients receiving chloral hydrate alone, 25% were not sedated, 31% were consciously sedated, and 44% were deeply sedated. That compares with the 30% $N_2O$ group in which 6% were not sedated, 0% consciously sedated, and 94% deeply sedated; and with the 50% $N_2O$ group in which 3% were not sedated, 0% consciously sedated, 94% deeply sedated, and 3% were anesthetized.

The authors concluded the addition of $N_2O$ frequently causes deep sedation, and not conscious sedation, in children. In this study, the end-tidal carbon dioxide measurements for chloral hydrate alone, with 30% $N_2O$ and 50% $N_2O$ were 48.8 ± 5.2, 52.4 ± 4.8, and 52.1 ± 5.1, respectively.

## What Are the Effects of Antipsychotic Medications?

Antipsychotic medications include phenothiazines, thioxanthenes, and butyrophenones. They are used for the treatment of a variety of problems, including schizophrenia and psychoses associated with organic brain syndromes. The antipsychotic mechanism of action of these drugs includes blocking of dopaminergic receptors within the CNS and other effects, some of which may be adverse. Table 36–5 lists the relative differences in sedative, cardiovascular, and extrapyramidal side effects of the various agents. Patients taking antipsychotics at the time of surgery may have exaggerated respiratory depression, sedation, and analgesia.[62,64]

$\alpha$-Adrenergic blockade caused by many antipsychotic

**TABLE 36–5.** Pharmacologic Profile of the Adverse Effects of Antipsychotic Agents

| Class | Sedative | Cardiovascular* | Extrapyramidal† |
|---|---|---|---|
| *Phenothiazine* | | | |
| Aliphatic | 3‡ | 3 | 2 |
| Piperidine | 2 | 2 | 1 |
| Piperazine | 1 | 1 | 3 |
| *Butyrophenone* | 1 | 1 | 3 |
| *Thioxanthene* | | | |
| Aliphatic | 3 | 3 | 2 |
| Piperazine | 1 | 1 | 3 |
| *Dihydroindolone* | 1 | 1 | 3 |
| *Dibenzoxazepine* | 2 | 2 | 3 |

*Orthostatic hypotension (2° to $\alpha$-blockade) and electrocardiogram changes.
†Refers to dystonia, akathisia, and pseudoparkinsonism, but not to tardive dyskinesia.
‡Greatest relative incidence = 3.
From Perry PJ, Alexander B, Liskow BI. *Psychotropic Drug Handbook.* Cincinnati, Ohio: Harvey Whitney Books; 1988:17.

agents is commonly associated with orthostatic hypotension.[65] This action theoretically can attenuate the pressor effects of norepinephrine and epinephrine or even lead to unopposed $\beta$-effects with subsequent hypotension, as demonstrated in dogs receiving epinephrine (0.005 mg/kg) and chlorpromazine.[66] Additionally, dopaminergic blockade by phenothiazine and butyrophenones may decrease the vasopressor effect of dopamine infusions.[67]

Enflurane and isoflurane administration with chlorpromazine has resulted in hypotension that is disproportionate to that which might have been expected from the administration of each drug separately.[68] Should hypotension occur with any of the halogenated anesthetic and antipsychotic agents, treatment with sympathetic amines that possess $\alpha$-adrenergic activity (norepinephrine, phenylephrine) or fluids is recommended.[4]

## What Problems May Be Associated With Antidepressants?

### Tricyclic Agents

The tricyclic antidepressants are thought to work by increasing CNS concentrations of serotonin or norepinephrine, or both, through blockade of their reuptake in presynaptic nerve terminals.[69] Chronic use (ie, >10-20 days) leads to significant receptor changes. Downregulation of presynaptic $\alpha_2$-adrenergic receptors occurs; this increases the release of norepinephrine from storage vesicles. Increased neuronal responsiveness of postsynaptic $\alpha_1$-adrenergic receptors also occurs, as does increased sensitivity of the postsynaptic receptors to serotonin. The number of $\beta$-adrenergic binding sites and CNS responsiveness to $\beta$-adrenergic agonists are either reduced or downregulated.[64] The overall result is that the $\beta$-receptors have increased sensitivity to drugs that stimulate postsynaptic $\alpha_1$-receptors (eg, ephedrine, epinephrine, and norepinephrine).

Tricyclic antidepressants also possess anticholinergic activity, which, along with the increase in adrenergic tone that they produce, can cause problems during anesthesia. Patients who are taking tricyclic antidepressants may be at greater risk for developing cardiac dysrhythmias. Edwards and associates found that dogs that received chronic imipramine therapy manifested a higher frequency of cardiac dysrhythmias during halothane anesthesia after they had received pancuronium.[70] They recommended the avoidance of pancuronium in patients who are treated with chronic tricyclic antidepressants and are anesthetized with halothane. Enflurane did not provoke cardiac dysrhythmias under the same conditions in this animal study.

Sympathomimetics, especially indirect-acting agents (eg, ephedrine) may result, at worst, in an exaggerated or, at best, unpredictable response from increased norepinephrine at the receptor site.[71,72] Other potential problems in patients receiving tricyclic antidepressants include potentiation of opioid analgesics, decreased seizure threshold, and increased barbiturate sedative and depressant effects.[66,73]

## Other Antidepressants

In addition to the tricyclic antidepressants, other antidepressants are amoxapine, maprotiline, trazodone, and the specific serotonin reuptake inhibitor (SSRI) family of antidepressants including fluoxetine, fluoxamine, paroxetine, and sertraline. The mechanisms of action of amoxapine and maprotiline are similar to those of the tricyclic antidepressants, with the exception that maprotiline does not block reuptake of serotonin.[7] Because of similar actions of amoxapine and maprotiline, anesthetic concerns for patients taking these drugs are the same as those for patients taking tricyclic agents. To date, however, no interactions have been reported. Amoxapine does not have as many cardiovascular side effects as does maprotiline. Maprotiline has significant adverse side effects in overdose situations. Maprotiline can also lower seizure threshold, which is a consideration in patients receiving enflurane or ketamine anesthetics.

Trazodone does not affect the reuptake of norepinephrine or dopamine and is thought to have a more benign effect than do the tricyclics.[74] No interactions with anesthetic agents have been reported. Fluoxetine and other SSRIs primarily inhibit the reuptake of serotonin in the CNS and have little effect on other neurotransmitters. The SSRIs do not have significant cardiotoxicity. The only major drug interaction that may affect the anesthetized patient is inhibition of diazepam metabolism; this possibility necessitates a reduction in diazepam dosage.[7]

## Should Antidepressant Administration Be Discontinued Before Anesthesia?

No answer to this question is universally accepted. We feel that antidepressant use should be discontinued 72 hours before elective surgeries in nonsuicidal patients. In emergency situations or in suicidal patients, the anesthesiologist should be aware of the potential interactions and treat the patient accordingly (ie, avoid halothane and pancuronium and, if a vasopressor is required, use titrated phenylephrine rather than ephedrine).

## Does Lithium Administration Alter Neuromuscular Blockade?

Several case reports published in the 1970s suggested prolonged neuromuscular blockade followed the use of pancuronium and succinylcholine in lithium-treated patients.[75,76] A follow-up study conducted in lithium-treated dogs showed prolonged neuromuscular blockade with succinylcholine, decamethonium, and pancuronium but not with gallamine or d-tubocurarine. Therapeutic lithium concentrations in the guinea pig model showed no significant effect of pancuronium.[77] In a retrospective review of 17 lithium-treated patients who had received succinylcholine before electroconvulsive therapy, prolonged recovery from succinylcholine did not occur.[78]

Although the information is conflicting, therapeutic concentrations of lithium do not appear to prolong neuromuscular blockade significantly.

## Should Monoamine Oxidase Inhibitors Be Discontinued Before Surgery?

Six monoamine oxidase inhibitors (MAOIs) are available for use, two of which are not available in the United States. They are used either as antidepressants (isocarboxazid, phenelzine, tranylcypromine, moclobemide), antiparkinsonism agents (selegiline), or antihypertensive agents (pargyline). There are three types of MAOIs: selective inhibitors of either MAO-A or MAO-B and nonselective inhibitors, which inhibit both MAO-A and MAO-B enzymes (Table 36-6).[79] These groups of medications inhibit oxidative deamination of the naturally occurring monoamines: serotonin, dopamine, tyramine, norepinephrine, and epinephrine. The resultant catecholamine accumulation at the receptor site produces increased sympathetic stimulation.[3,27] Sympathomimetics administered to patients taking MAOIs may cause the release and persistence of excessive amounts of neurotransmitters, resulting in cardiovascular instability, tachycardia, hypertensive crisis, severe headache, and hyperpyrexia.[80]

Meperidine is uniquely contraindicated in patients receiving MAOIs. The interaction resulting from administration of meperidine to a patient taking an MAOI has two distinct forms. Type I (*excitatory*) reactions can be severe, and include agitation, hypertension or hypotension, seizures, hyperthermia, coma, and even death. Type II (*depressive*) are characterized by hypotension, respiratory depression, and coma.[79] Other drugs that should be avoided in MAOI-treated patients include phenothiazines, other antidepressants, and tyramine-containing food and cheese products.[27,66]

The nonselective MAOIs fall into either the hydrazine or nonhydrazine class (see Table 36-6). This is of consequence because the nonhydrazine compounds are considered to be reversible blockers devoid of pharmacologic effect 24 hours after discontinuation. The hydrazine compounds, however, bind to the enzyme irreversibly; thus, the recommendation is to discontinue therapy at least 2 weeks before elective surgery.[81] If this is not possible or if hemodynamic instability

**TABLE 36-6.** Monoamine Oxidase Inhibitors

| Generic Name | Brand Name | Type | Selectivity |
|---|---|---|---|
| Isocarboxazid* | Marplan | Hydrazine | Nonselective |
| Pargyline | Eutonyl | Nonhydrazine | Nonselective |
| Phenelzine | Nardil | Hydrazine | Nonselective |
| Tranylcypromine | Parnate | Nonhydrazine | Nonselective |
| Moclobemide* | Manerex | Nonhydrazine | MAO-A Selective |
| Selegiline | Eldepryl | Nonhydrazine | MAO-B Selective |

*Not available in the United States.

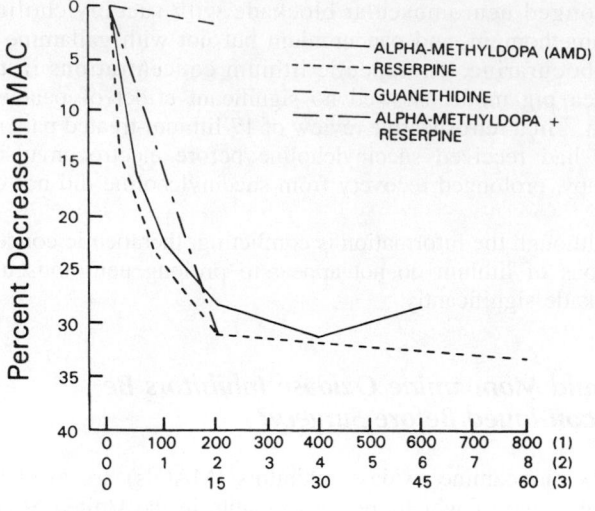

**FIGURE 36–6.** Percentage decreases in halothane minimal alveolar concentration associated with prior administration of α-methyldopa, reserpine, guanethidine, and α-methyldopa in combination with reserpine. (From Miller RD, Way WL, Eger EI. The effects of α-methyldopa, reserpine, guanethidine, and iproniazid on minimum alveolar anesthetic [MAC] requirement. *Anesthesiology.* 1968;29:1156.)

occurs despite drug discontinuation according to the recommended protocol, labetalol or sodium nitroprusside are recommended for hypertension, and fluid or titrated quantities of a direct-acting vasopressor (phenylephrine) or both, are suggested for treatment of hypotension. Moclobemide, a selective and reversible inhibitor of MAO-A, has a short half-life (4 hours). Case reports by Martyr and Orlikowski[82] and McFarlane[79] suggest the MAOI effect disappears after 24 hours and may allow discontinuation 24 hours before surgery.

## Should Antihypertensive Agents Be Discontinued Before Surgery?

The extensive number of antihypertensives on the market today present the anesthesiologist with many potential drug interactions. Understanding the interactions of these agents can affect the choice of anesthetic drugs.

Discontinuation of antihypertensive agents may lead to rebound hypertension from withdrawal. Unless specific circumstances dictate otherwise, antihypertensive therapy should not be discontinued before surgery.[76,77]

## Do Centrally Acting Antihypertensive Agents Decrease Minimum Alveolar Concentration?

Methyldopa, clonidine, and reserpine act centrally to treat hypertension. Abrupt discontinuation of methyldopa or clonidine use also can lead to rebound hypertension. Methyldopa and reserpine deplete central catecholamine stores, whereas clonidine is a central α-adrenergic agonist. Because of their central effects, each is capable of decreasing the MAC of anesthetic agents.[83,84] A decrease in the MAC of halothane in dogs has been noted for both methyldopa and reserpine (Fig. 36–6).[85] The authors hypothesized that CNS norepinephrine depletion was responsible for the MAC decrease.

Clonidine decreases the MAC of inhalation agents and has been administered preoperatively to reduce the requirements for these agents and for narcotics.[86–88] Table 36–7 compares the different requirements for isoflurane and fentanyl in patients not receiving clonidine (group 1) and in patients who received a 5 μg/kg dose preoperatively (group 2). The requirements for both isoflurane and fentanyl were markedly reduced in the clonidine-treated patients.[87]

In a randomized, double-blind, controlled trial, intravenous clonidine was compared with placebo to determine the thiopental dosage requirements used for anesthesia.[89] Intravenous doses of 2.5 μg/kg and 5 μg/kg clonidine were administered 15 minutes before beginning thiopental. Clonidine reduced the thiopental dosage by 25% and 36%, respectively, for the two clonidine groups compared to the placebo group ($P < 0.05$). Further investigation may allow determination of the useful effects of clonidine in general anesthesia.

Clonidine given preoperatively to children, at an oral dose of 4 μg/kg, decreased the MAC for tracheal intubation of sevoflurane from 3.2% to 2.4%. When $N_2O$ was added to preoperatively administered clonidine, the reduction of the MAC of sevoflurane was found to be larger than if either drug is given alone.[90] Clonidine, 0.6 mg, given preoperatively also reduces the dosage requirements of propofol during surgery.[91]

Discontinuation of antihypertensive agents may lead to rebound hypertension from withdrawal. Clonidine is an excellent example of this. The α-agonist stimulation results in decreased sympathetic outflow from the CNS. Abrupt with-

**TABLE 36–7.** Drug Requirements*

| | Intraoperative | | | | Postanesthesia Recovery Room (Morphine [mg]) |
| | *Isoflurane (End-Expiratory %)* | *Fentanyl (μg)* | *Thiopental (mg)* | *Nitrous Oxide (%)* | |
|---|---|---|---|---|---|
| Group 1† | 1.03 ± 16 | 250 ± 345 | 353 ± 93 | 51 ± 3.5 | 7.0 ± 7.7 |
| Group 2‡ | 0.62 ± .2 | 61 ± 99 | 302 ± 112 | 49 ± 5 | 9 ± 5 |
| *P* | $P < 0.01$ | $P < 0.005$ | Not significant | Not significant | Not significant |

*Mean ± SD.
†No clonidine.
‡Received clonidine (5 μg/kg preoperatively).
From Ghignone M, Calvillo O, Quintin C. Anesthesia and hypertension: the effect of clonidine on perioperative hemodynamics and isoflurane requirements. *Anesthesiology.* 1987;67:7.

drawal is often associated with profound rebound hypertension. Patients who must be in the nil per os status should have an alternate antihypertensive regimen instituted and their blood pressure (BP) monitored frequently. Clonidine patches can be used under these circumstances, but their effects must be monitored closely. Transition from oral to patch delivery of clonidine must be titrated to effect as it is not completely predictable.

## Is Clonidine Useful for Spinal Anesthesia and Nerve Blocks?

Tschernko and colleagues[92] compared three groups: (1) 2 mg/kg of 0.5% bupivacaine as intercostal nerve blockade (ICB) mixed with a 2 μg/kg dose of clonidine (block group); (2) ICB bupivacaine and an intramuscular dose of clonidine (intramuscular group); or (3) ICB bupivacaine and no clonidine (control group). The block group had significantly higher $PaO_2$ for the first 4 hours after surgery than both the control and the intramuscular group. This would suggest that clonidine mixed with bupivacaine improves pain control and alveolar ventilation and oxygenation.

In a study by Goyagi and associates,[93] the response to bolus injections of 0.2 mg/kg of ephedrine, as manifested by BP and heart rate changes, were compared in patients randomized to receive clonidine or placebo. Oral clonidine at a dose of 5 μg/kg was administered 90 minutes before spinal anesthesia with tetracaine, compared with spinal anesthesia with tetracaine alone. In this randomized controlled trial, patients receiving clonidine before spinal anesthesia had greater increases in BP response to ephedrine than patients not receiving clonidine. The authors concluded 0.2 mg/kg of ephedrine effectively counteracted hypotension from spinal anesthesia even when patients were pretreated with clonidine. Also, the pressor effect of patients treated with ephedrine was augmented with clonidine. A similar increase in arterial BP was found with clonidine premedication in response to phenylephrine and increased heart rate from isoproterenol in 60 patients undergoing general anesthesia.[94]

## Do Special Considerations Apply to Patients Taking β-Blockers?

Currently, 15 β-adrenergic blockers are available in the United States as intravenous, oral, and ophthalmic preparations. These drugs have different indications, selectivity, pharmacokinetics, and other receptor site actions. Pharmacodynamic interactions of β-blockers with anesthetics result in changes in cardiac output and BP.

β-Blockers limit the heart's ability to respond to endogenous or exogenous catecholamines. If epinephrine is used in patients with β-blockade, unopposed alpha constriction can result and potentially lead to hypertension and myocardial ischemia. Agents with β-agonist activity—such as dobutamine and isoproterenol or calcium, glucagon, and digoxin—can be used to counteract the effects of β-blockade.[4,95,96]

Some inhalation anesthetics can produce myocardial depression that may be intensified by β-blockers.[97–100] Animal studies have shown that methoxyflurane, cyclopropane, ether, and trichloroethylene produce significant myocardial depression when combined with β-blockers, a fact that obviously is of historical interest only. Enflurane in high concentrations also produces increased circulatory depression in dogs administered β-blockers.[98] Although halothane and isoflurane are better tolerated in this situation, additive myocardial depression is still seen in patients receiving β-blockers. Use of these drugs should be continued up to the time of surgery, but the anesthesiologist should be prepared to adjust the dosage of volatile anesthetics to account for the aforementioned effects and to treat them if they occur.

Esmolol, when added to the analgesic, alfentanil, further reduced the MAC of isoflurane. Johansen[101] showed that the MAC for isoflurane decreased in patients receiving alfentanil as a computer-controlled infusion to a target concentration of 50 ng/mL and esmolol as a bolus dose of 1 mg/kg followed by a constant infusion of 250 μg/kg/min. The mechanism of action is unclear, but the combination may be useful from a hemodynamic standpoint in some patients.

## Do Calcium Channel Blockers Affect Cardiovascular Function During Anesthesia?

Calcium channel blockers are useful in the treatment of hypertension, angina, dysrhythmias, and migraine headaches. They have significant interactions with a number of drugs used in general medical practice, and thus knowledge of their potential interactions with other drugs is important. Hypotension, bradycardia, negative inotropic activity, and peripheral vasodilation may occur as a result of their use.

Inhalation and narcotic anesthetics can have additive adverse effects.[102,103] In animal studies, verapamil, nifedipine, or diltiazem produces marked ventricular depression when given with isoflurane or halothane. More importantly, those animal studies that were conducted with open chest instrumentation showed left ventricular depression that was greater than that which occurred in other acutely anesthetized animals.[104–107] Patients with good ventricular function who are taking calcium channel blocking agents should be able to tolerate anesthetic agents well. However, those requiring open chest surgery could have a pronounced decrease in ventricular function with inhalation anesthetics.[108]

Calcium channel blocking agents can also affect neuromuscular blockade. Verapamil potentiates depolarizing and nondepolarizing blocking drugs. It may also inhibit the antagonism of neuromuscular blockade with neostigmine.[109,110]

## Do Other Antihypertensive Agents Have Potential Interactions?

Only one interaction of angiotensin-converting enzyme inhibitors, such as captopril or enalapril, has been reported (a case of prolonged hypotension with propofol,[111] which was thought to be due to decreased preload and systemic vascular resistance). Peripheral vasodilators, such as hydralazine or minoxidil, have no known interactions with anesthetic agents. Prazosin, an α-adrenergic blocker, may offer some protection against dysrhythmias produced as a result of halothane-epinephrine interaction. When prazosin is used for the first time, a low dose must be administered to minimize the first dose phenomenon that often results in exaggerated hypotension.[4]

**TABLE 36–8.** Interaction of Antibiotics, Muscle Relaxants, Neostigmine, and Calcium

| | Neuromuscular Block From Antibiotic Alone, Antagonized by | | Increase in Neuromuscular Block of | | Neuromuscular Block From Antibiotic and d-Tubocurarine, Antagonized by | |
|---|---|---|---|---|---|---|
| | *Neostigmine* | *Calcium* | *d-Tubocurarine* | *Succinylcholine* | *Neostigmine* | *Calcium* |
| Neomycin | Sometimes | Sometimes | Yes | Yes | Usually | Usually |
| Streptomycin | Sometimes | Sometimes | Yes | Yes | Usually | Usually |
| Gentamicin | Sometimes | Yes* | Yes | † | Sometimes | Yes* |
| Kanamycin | Sometimes | Sometimes | Yes | Yes | Sometimes | Sometimes |
| Paromomycin | Yes* | Yes* | Yes | † | Yes* | Yes* |
| Viomycin | Yes* | Yes* | Yes | † | Yes* | Yes* |
| Polymyxin A | No | No | Yes | † | No | No |
| Polymyxin B | No‡ | No | Yes | Yes | No‡ | No |
| Colistin | No | Sometimes | Yes | Yes | No | Sometimes |
| Tetracycline | No | † | Yes | No | Partially | Partially |
| Lincomycin | Partially | Partially | Yes | † | Partially | Partially |
| Clindamycin | Partially | Partially | Yes | † | Partially | Partially |

*Despite this, difficulty with antagonizing the block from these antibiotics is still likely to occur.
†Not studied.
‡Block augmented by neostigmine.
From Miller RD, Smith NT. Neuromuscular blocking agents. In: *Drug Interactions in Anesthesia.* 2nd ed. Philadelphia, Pa: Lea & Febiger; 1986:366.

## Are There Any Effects in Patients Administered Transdermal Nitroglycerin and Anesthetic Agents?

Transdermal nitroglycerin, when placed 20 to 30 minutes after spinal injection of sufentanil, was able to enhance the spinal effects of sufentanil. Fifty-six patients following orthopedic surgery were randomized to receive one of four different regimens, including transdermal nitroglycerin and spinal sufentanil. This combination resulted in 13 hours of postoperative analgesia.[112]

## What Medications Interact With Neuromuscular Blocking Agents?

### Antidysrhythmic Agents

Many of the antidysrhythmic medications can potentiate neuromuscular blockade because they act at the prejunctional membrane.[113–115] This effect has occurred with quinidine in both nondepolarizing and depolarizing blockade, and with lidocaine and procainamide during nondepolarizing blockade.

Quinidine has significant anticholinergic and α-adrenergic blockade activity, and, thus, can potentially produce additive responses when combined with other similarly acting agents. Other concerns regarding the use of quinidine and procainamide are the ability to enhance conduction through the A-V node, which can potentially lead to ventricular tachycardia. If these agents are to be used to treat or suppress supraventricular tachydysrhythmias, pretreatment with digoxin should prevent ventricular tachycardia.[116]

### Antibiotics

Aminoglycoside antibiotics (amikacin, gentamicin, tobramycin, neomycin, streptomycin, kanamycin) can produce synergistic neuromuscular blockade when used with nondepolarizing agents.[117,118] This effect can occur if the aminoglycoside is given intraoperatively or preoperatively.[4,118]

Other antibiotics (clindamycin, tetracycline, polymyxin B, vancomycin) may produce additive effects or potentiation of neuromuscular blockade. This enhanced blockade may not be antagonized by neostigmine and calcium. Table 36–8 lists the effects that neostigmine or calcium may have when used to antagonize the neuromuscular blockade caused by various anti-infective agents.[4,119,120]

## Can Different Neuromuscular Blockers Be Used Sequentially to Take Advantage of the Kinetics of Each Drug?

There are many circumstances where the ideal neuromuscular blocking agent is one which has rapid onset, rapid metabolism, no side effects and is inexpensive. When such a drug is not available, clinicians often combine drugs to maximize the desired effects and minimize the undesired ones. Drugs acting on similar receptors, such as the neuromuscular endplate, can have additive, synergistic, or antagonistic effects. When steroidal neuromuscular blockers (pancuronium, rocuronium, vecuronium, rapacuronium, pipecuronium) are combined with benzylisoquinoline (mivacurium, d-tubocurarine, metocurine, atracurium, doxacurium, cisatracurium), synergism occurs. Thus, combining rocuronium with mivacurium yields the advantage of rapid onset and cardiovascular stability of the rocuronium with the shorter acting and less costly mivacurium (less rocuronium needed per dose). This potentiation is more pronounced in the elderly, followed by young adults, adolescents, and children, in whom it is the least pronounced.[121] It is tempting to use this property by using rocuronium for intubation and mivacurium for subsequent dosing to permit rapid return of neuromuscular function. However, data suggests the duration of action of the neuromuscular block depends more on the kinetics of the initial drug than the subsequent agent. Thus, there does not seem to be an advantage of using mivacurium for subsequent dosing after either rocuronium or vecuronium have been administered.[122]

## Have Drug Interactions Occurred With Propofol?

Propofol is a short-acting anesthetic agent with an effective half-life of a few minutes. Only a few possible drug interactions have been reported. Hendley[123] noted convulsions following the use of topical cocaine and propofol but stated that it was unclear whether the convulsions were caused by propofol alone. Halothane may prolong the elimination of propofol by decreasing hepatic blood flow, thereby decreasing the rate of metabolism of propofol.[124,125] Fentanyl, 1.5 $\mu$g/kg, combined with propofol did *not* affect anesthetic duration, eye opening time, or the time to repeat the correct birth date. It also did not affect propofol elimination.[126] In a subsequent study, propofol reduced the intraoperative analgesic requirements of fentanyl. The study by Kazama and colleagues[127] suggested a synergistic interaction of propofol and fentanyl between the somatic and hemodynamic responses after surgical stimulation. Propofol can inhibit the metabolism of alfentanil and sufentanil. Pharmacodynamically, propofol and opioids have a synergistic interaction that is greatest with remifentanil.[128] The combination of propofol and benzodiazepines is synergistic (the combination of the two drugs has 1.44 times the potency of the use of the agents in isolation).[129] This observation can be used to advantage, that is, the propofol dose can be decreased during either conscious sedation or general anesthesia applications when fentanyl is also used.

## What Are Significant Benzodiazepine Interactions?

Benzodiazepines have been found to interact synergistically with barbiturates, narcotics, and propofol.[126,130,131] Table 36–9 illustrates the dramatic effect of the coadministration of midazolam and alfentanil. Analogous effects occur with any—and probably all—narcotic, benzodiazepine, propofol, and barbiturate combinations and should be considered, especially during concomitant administration in the induction of conscious sedation. A case report of 8-year-old child who lost consciousness after being premedicated with midazolam, followed shortly thereafter with an intravenous erythromycin dose, illustrates another potential interaction.[132] This carries implications for patients given midazolam either for conscious sedation or as part of general anesthesia, who are currently receiving or will receive erythromycin shortly after the midazolam is administered. The result may be an increased effect from midazolam

or increased duration of action. Patients receiving cimetidine would also have the potential for this interaction.[132]

## What Is the Role of Flumazenil?

Flumazenil was approved for use in 1991 by the US Food and Drug Administration for the complete or partial reversal of benzodiazepine sedation. This drug acts by competitively binding to the benzodiazepine receptor.[130,131] Flumazenil rapidly reverses sedation and antagonizes the effect of midazolam on tidal volume but does not correct the depressant effect of midazolam on the slope of the carbon dioxide response curve.[131]

In a manner similar to narcotic reversal with naloxone, the antagonistic effects of flumazenil may dissipate before the effects of the benzodiazepine are reversed, particularly when high doses of benzodiazepines have been given. Flumazenil should also be used with caution in patients with a long-term history of benzodiazepine therapy or with a seizure disorder treated with a benzodiazepine, as they are more likely to develop withdrawal symptoms and seizure activity if given flumazenil.[133]

Flumazenil also has been shown to be an effective antidote in benzodiazepine poisoning or mixed drug overdosage. It may prevent other, more invasive interventions.[130] Flumazenil is effective in reversing sedation and some aspects of respiratory depression during or following conscious sedation, general anesthesia, and benzodiazepine poisoning. It does not have proven pharmacodynamic antagonistic properties for other medications.

## SUMMARY

The drug interactions that the anesthesiologist can expect in clinical practice include not only the frequently considered pharmacokinetic and pharmacodynamic drug interactions but also physical incompatibilities. Tables 36–1 and 36–4 list many of the selected drug interactions of interest to anesthesiologists.

Whenever the administration of two or more drugs results in an unexpected effect, the anesthesiologist should consider a drug interaction as a potential explanation. Because of the myriad drug combinations that can occur during the perioperative period, all possible interactions cannot be known or predicted. Knowledge of drug classes, mechanisms of action,

**TABLE 36–9.** Equieffective Doses (ED$_{50}$)

| Groups | Alfentanil Component | | Midazolam Component | | Sum of Fractional Doses | Ratio* |
|---|---|---|---|---|---|---|
| | Fraction of ED$_{50}$ | Dose (mg/kg) | Fraction of ED$_{50}$ | Dose (mg/kg) | | |
| Alfentanil | 1.00 | 0.13 (0.11, 0.19) | 0.00 | 0.00 | 1.00 | — |
| Midazolam | 0.00 | 0.00 | 1.00 | 0.22 (0.15, 0.50) | 1.00 | — |
| Alfentanil and midazolam | 0.21 | 0.028 (0.018, 0.036) | 0.33 | 0.07† | 0.54 ($P < 0.0001$)‡ | 1.85 |

*Ratio of single drug fractional dose to combined fractional dose.
†Dose was kept constant.
‡$P$ = Significance of deviation from additivity.
From Vinik HR, Bradley EL Jr, Kissin I. Midazolam-alfentanil synergism for anesthetic induction in patients. *Anesth Analg.* 1989;69:216. © International Anesthesia Research Society.

and potential adverse effects is helpful to predict possible drug interactions.

## References

1. Levy WJ. Clinical anaesthesia with isoflurane. *Br J Anaesth.* 1984;56(suppl):101.
2. Zeller FP, Anders RJ. Compatibility of intravenous drugs in a coronary intensive care unit. *Drug Intell Clin Pharm.* 1986;20:349.
3. Davie IT. Specific drug interactions in anaesthesia. *Anaesthesia.* 1977;32:1000.
4. Goodwin SR. Drugs and drug reactions. In: Gravenstein N, ed. *Manual of Complications During Anesthesia.* 1st ed. Philadelphia, Pa: JB Lippincott; 1991:479.
5. Schentag JJ, Simons GW, Schultz RW, et al. Complexation versus hemodialysis to reduce elevated aminoglycoside serum concentrations. *Pharmacotherapy.* 1984;4:374.
6. Bauman JL, Sieplen JK, Fitzloff J. Phenytoin crystallization in intravenous fluids. *Drug Intell Clin Pharm.* 1977;11:646.
7. Finch ME. Sodium thiopental in 5% dextrose in lactated Ringer's precipitate. *Hosp Pharm.* 1979;14:559.
8. McEvoy GK, ed. *American Hospital Formulary Service Drug Information.* 9th ed. Bethesda, Md: American Society of Hospital Pharmacists; 1992:1345.
9. Trissel LA. *Handbook of Injectable Drugs.* 10th ed. Bethesda, Md: American Society of Health System Pharmacists; 1998.
10. King JC. *Guide to Parenteral Admixtures.* Napa, California: Kings Guide Publications; 2000.
11. Gauger LJ, Gibboney ER, Nordin BJ. Flow dynamics of a retrograde IV drug infusion system. *Am J Hosp Pharm.* 1984;41:492.
12. Horrow JC, Digregorio GJ, Barbieri EJ, et al. Intravenous infusions of nitroprusside, dobutamine, and nitroglycerin are compatible. *Crit Care Med.* 1990;18:858.
13. Evans WE. General principles of applied pharmacokinetics. In: Evans WE, Schentag JJ, Jasko WJ, eds. *Applied Pharmacokinetics.* 2nd ed. Spokane, Wash: Applied Therapeutics; 1986:1.
14. Höffken G, Borner K, Glatzel PD. Reduced enteral absorption of ciprofloxacin in presence of antacids. *Eur J Clin Microbiol.* 1985;4:345.
15. Garty M, Hurwitz A. Effect of cimetidine and antacids on gastrointestinal absorption of tetracycline. *Clin Pharmacol Ther.* 1980;28:203.
16. Yee GC, McGuire TR. Pharmacokinetic drug interactions with cyclosporin (part 1). *Clin Pharmacokinet.* 1990;19:319.
17. Wadhwa NK, Schroeder TJ, O'Flaherty E, et al. The effect of oral metoclopramide on the absorption of cyclosporine. *Transplant Proc.* 1987;19:1730.
18. Freeman DJ, Laupacis A, Keown PA, et al. Evaluation of cyclosporin-phenytoin interaction with observations on cyclosporin metabolites. *Br J Clin Pharmacol.* 1984;18:887.
19. Fee JPH, Collier PS, Howard PJ, et al. Cimetidine and ranitidine increase midazolam bioavailability. *Clin Pharmacol Ther.* 1987;41:80.
20. Scott DB, Jebson PJR, Braid DO, et al. Factors affecting plasma levels of lignocaine and prilocaine. *Br J Anaesth.* 1972;44:1040.
21. DiFazio CH, Carron H, Grosslight KR. Comparison of pH-adjusted solutions for epidural anesthesia. *Anesth Analg.* 1986;65:760.
22. Greenblatt DJ, Allen MD, Harmatz JS, et al. Diazepam disposition determinants. *Clin Pharmacol Ther.* 1980;27:301.
23. Greenblatt DJ, Divoll M. Diazepam versus lorazepam: relationship of drug distribution to duration of clinical action. *Adv Neurol.* 1983;34:487.
24. Ameer B, Greenblatt DJ. Lorazepam: a review of its clinical pharmacological properties and therapeutic uses. *Drugs.* 1981;21:161.
25. Lacey DJ, Singer WD, Horwitz J, et al. Lorazepam therapy of status epilepticus in children and adolescents. *J Pediatr.* 1986;108:771.
26. Homer TD, Stanski DR. The effect of increasing age on thiopental disposition and anesthetic requirement. *Anesthesiology.* 1985;62:714.
27. Cullen BF, Miller MG. Drug interactions and anesthesia: a review. *Anesth Analg.* 1979;58:413.
28. Wood M. Plasma drug binding: implications for anesthesiologists. *Anesth Analg.* 1986;65:786.
29. Winter ME, Tozen TN. Phenytoin. In: Evans WE, Schentag JJ, Jusko WJ, eds. *Applied Pharmacokinetics.* 2nd ed. Spokane, Wash: Applied Therapeutics; 1986:493.
30. Svensson CK, Woodruff MN, Lalka D. Influence of protein binding and use of unbound drug concentrations. In: Evans WE, Schentag JJ, Jusko WJ, eds. *Applied Pharmacokinetics.* 2nd ed. Spokane, Wash: Applied Therapeutics; 1986:187.
31. Munson ES. Local anesthetics. In: Smith NJ, Corbascio AN, eds. *Drug Interactions in Anesthesia.* 2nd ed. Philadelphia, Pa: Lea & Febiger; 1986:391.
32. Ghoeneim MM, Pandya H. Plasma protein binding of bupivacaine and its interaction with other drugs in man. *Br J Anaesth.* 1974;46:435.
33. Kaukinen S, Eerola M, Ylitalo P. Prolongation of thiopentone anaesthesia by probenecid. *Br J Anaesth.* 1980;52:603.
34. McMurray JJ, Dundee JW, Henshaw JS. The influence of probenecid on the induction dose of thiopentone. *Br J Clin Pharmacol.* 1984;17:224.
35. Powell JR, Cate EW. Induction and inhibition of drug metabolism. In: Evans WE, Schentag JJ, Jusko WJ, eds. *Applied Pharmacokinetics.* 2nd ed. Spokane, Wash: Applied Therapeutics; 1986:139.
36. Rawling MD. General mechanisms of drug interactions. In: Grahame-Smith DG, ed. *Drug Interactions.* Baltimore, Md: University Park Press; 1977:35.
37. Brown BR, Sipes JC. Biotransformation and hepatotoxicity of halothane. *Biochem Pharmacol.* 1977;26:2091.
38. Halsey MJ. Drug interactions in anaesthesia. *Br J Anaesth.* 1987;59:112.
39. Neigh JL. Inhalation anesthetic agents. In: Smith NT, Corbascio AN, eds. *Drug Interactions in Anesthesia.* 2nd ed. Philadelphia, Pa: Lea & Febiger; 1986:340.
40. Mazze RI, Trudell JR, Cousins MJ. Methoxyflurane metabolism and renal dysfunction: clinical correlation in man. *Anesthesiology.* 1971;35:247.
41. Dooley JR, Mazze RI, Rice SA, et al. Is enflurane defluorination inducible in man? *Anesthesiology.* 1979;50:213.
42. Powell JR, Donn KH. Histamine H$_2$-antagonist drug interactions in perspective: mechanistic concepts and clinical implications. *Am J Med.* 1984;77(suppl SB):57.
43. Powell JR, Rogers JF, Wargin WA, et al. Inhibition of theophylline clearance by cimetidine but not ranitidine. *Arch Intern Med.* 1984;144:484.
44. Feldman M, Barton ME. Histamine$_2$-receptor antagonists: standard therapy for acid-peptic diseases. *N Engl J Med.* 1990;323:1672.
45. Teem WR, Davis PM, Hyams JS. Suppression of gastric acid secretion by intravenous administration of famotidine in children. *J Pediatr.* 1991;118:812.
46. Feldman M, Barton ME. Histamine$_2$-receptor antagonists: standard therapy for acid-peptic diseases. *N Engl J Med.* 1990;323:1749.
47. Conney AH. Pharmacological implications of microsomal enzyme induction. *Pharmacol Rev.* 1967;19:317.
48. Gelehrter TD. Enzyme induction. *N Engl J Med.* 1976;294:522.
49. Breckenridge AM, Orme MLE. Clinical implications of enzyme induction. *Ann N Y Acad Sci.* 1971;179:421.
50. Dossing M, Pilsgaard H, Rasmassen B, et al. Time course of phenobarbital and cimetidine mediated changes in hepatic drug metabolism. *Eur J Clin Pharmacol.* 1983;25:215.
51. Bartkowski RR, McDonnell TE. Prolonged alfentanil effect following erythromycin administration. *Anesthesiology.* 1990;73:566.
52. Pantuck EJ. Ecothiophate iodide eye drops and prolonged response to suxamethonium. *Br J Anaesth.* 1966;38:406.
53. Eildenton TE, Farmati O, Zsigmond EK. Reduction in plasma cholinesterase levels after prolonged administration of echothiophate iodide eyedrops. *Can Anaesth Soc J.* 1968;15:291.
54. Himmelhoch JM, Poust RI, Mallinger AG, et al. Adjustment of lithium dose during lithium-chlorothiazide therapy. *Clin Pharmacol Ther.* 1977;22:225.
55. Hartig HI, Dyson WL. Lithium toxicity enhanced by diuresis [letter]. *N Engl J Med.* 1974;290:748.
56. Johnston RR, Eger EI II, Wilson C. A comparative interaction of epinephrine with enflurane, isoflurane and halothane in man. *Anesth Analg.* 1976;55:709.
57. Navaro R, Weiskop RB, Moore MA. Humans anesthetized with sevoflurane or isoflurane have similar arrhythmic response to epinephrine. *Anesthesiology.* 1994;80:545.
58. Albertson TE, Marelich GP, Tharratt RS. Cocaine. In: Haddad LM, Shannon MW, Winchester JF, eds. *Clinical Management of Poisoning and Drug Overdose.* Philadelphia, Pa: WB Saunders; 1998:542.
59. Bernards CM, Kern C, Cullen BF. Chronic cocaine administration reversibly increases isoflurane minimal alveolar concentration in sheep. *Anesthesiology.* 1996;85:91.
60. Stoelting RK, Eger EI. An additional explanation for the second gas effect. *Anesthesiology.* 1969;30:273.
61. Eyer EI. Surgical stimulation antagonizes the respiratory depression produced by Forane. *Anesthesiology.* 1972;36:544.
62. Bahlman SH. The cardiovascular effects of nitrous oxide: halothane anesthesia in man. *Anesthesiology.* 1974;35:274.
63. Litman RS, Kottra JA, Verga KA, et al. Chloral hydrate sedation: the

additive sedative and respiratory depressant effects of nitrous oxide. *Anesth Analg.* 1998;86:724.

64. Perry PJ, Alexander B, Liskow BI. *Psychotropic Drug Handbook.* Cincinnati, Ohio: Harvey Whitney Books; 1988.

65. Lambertsen CJ, Wendel H, Longenhagen JB. The separate and combined respiratory effects of chlorpromazine and meperidine in normal men controlled at 46 mm Hg alveolar Pco$_2$. *J Pharmacol Exp Ther.* 1961;131:381.

66. Eggers GWN, Corssen G, Allen CR. Comparison of vasopressor responses in the presence of phenothiazine derivatives. *Anesthesiology.* 1959;20:261.

67. Stoelting RK. Drugs used in treatment of psychiatric disease. *Pharmacology and Physiology in Anesthetic Practice.* Philadelphia, Pa: JB Lippincott; 1991:365.

68. Gold MI. Profound hypotension associated with preoperative use of phenothiazines. *Anesth Analg.* 1974;53:844.

69. Baldessarin RJ. Drugs and the treatment of psychiatric disorders. In: Gilman AG, Rall TW, Nies AS, et al, eds. *Goodman and Gilman's the Pharmacological Basis of Therapeutics.* 8th ed. New York, NY: Pergammon Press; 1990:383.

70. Edwards RP, Miller RD, Roizen MF, et al. Cardiac responses to impromine and pancuronium during anesthesia with halothane or enflurane. *Anesthesiology.* 1979;50:421.

71. Boakes AJ, Laurene DR, Teoh DC, et al. Interactions between sympathomimetic amines and antidepressant agents in man. *BMJ.* 1973;1:311.

72. Wong KC, Puerto AX, Puerto BA, et al. Influence of imipramine and pargyline on the arrythmogenicity of epinephrine during halothane, enflurane, or methoxyflurane anesthesia in dogs. *Anesthesiology.* 1980;53(suppl):25.

73. Dobkin AB. Potentiation of thiopental anaesthesia with tigan, panectyl, benadryl, gravol, marzine, histadyl, librium, and haloperidol. *Can Anaesth Soc J.* 1961;8:265.

74. Janowsky EC, Risch SC, Janowsky DS. Psychotropic agents. In: Smith NT, Corbascio AN, eds. *Drug Interactions in Anesthesia.* 2nd ed. Philadelphia, Pa: Lea & Febiger; 1986:261.

75. Borden H, Clarke M, Katz H. The use of pancuronium bromide in patients receiving lithium carbonate. *Can Anaesth Soc J.* 1974;21:79.

76. Hill GE, Wong KL, Hodges MR. Potentiation of succinylcholine neuromuscular blockade by lithium carbonate. *Anesthesiology.* 1976;44:439.

77. Waud BE, Farrell C, Waud DR. Lithium and neuromuscular transmission. *Anesth Analg.* 1982;61:399.

78. Martin BA, Kramer PM. Clinical significance of the interaction between lithium and neuromuscular blocker. *Am J Psychiatry.* 1982;139:1326.

79. McFarlane HJ. Anaesthesia and the new generation monoamine oxidase inhibitors. *Anaesthesia.* 1994;49:597.

80. Prys-Roberts C. Hypertension and anesthesia: fifty years on. *Anesthesiology.* 1979;50:281.

81. Hurt GR, Anderson RJ. Withdrawal syndromes and the cessation of antihypertensive therapy. *Arch Intern Med.* 1981;141:1125.

82. Martyr JW, Orlikowski CE. Epidural anaesthesia, ephedrine and phenylephrine in a patient taking moclobemide, a new monoamine oxidase inhibitor. *Anaesthesia.* 1996;51:1150.

83. Stoelting RK. Antihypertensive drugs. *Pharmacology and Physiology in Anesthetic Practice.* 2nd ed. Philadelphia, Pa: JB Lippincott; 1991:311.

84. Stoelting RK. Antihypertensives and alpha-blockers. In: Smith NT, Corbascio AN, eds. *Drug Interactions in Anesthesia.* 2nd ed. Philadelphia, Pa: Lea & Febiger; 1986:147.

85. Miller RD, Woy WL, Eger EI. The effects of alpha-methyldopa, reserpine, guanethidine, and iproniazid on minimum alveolar anesthetic requirement (MAC). *Anesthesiology.* 1968;29:1153.

86. Engelman E, Lipszyc M, Gilbert ES, et al. Effects of clonidine on anesthetic drug requirements and hemodynamic response during aortic surgery. *Anesthesiology.* 1989;71:178.

87. Ghignone M, Calvillo O, Quintin L. Anesthesia and hypertension: the effect of clonidine on perioperative hemodynamics and isoflurane requirements. *Anesthesiology.* 1987;67:3.

88. Flacke JW, Bloor BL, Flacke WE, et al. Reduced narcotic requirements by clonidine with improved hemodynamic and adrenergic stability in patients undergoing coronary bypass surgery. *Anesthesiology.* 1987;67:11.

89. Leslie K, Mooney PH, Sibert BS. Effect of intravenous clonidine on the dose of thiopental required to induce anesthesia. *Anesth Analg.* 1992;75:530.

90. Nihina K, Mikawa K, Shiga M, et al. Oral clonidine premedication reduces minimum alveolar concentration of sevoflurane for tracheal intubation in children. *Anesthesiology.* 1997;87:1324.

91. Richards MJ, Skaes MA, Jarcuis AP, et al. Total IV anaesthesia with

propofol and alfentanil: dose requirements for propofol and the effect of premedication of clonidine. *Br J Anaesth.* 1990;65:157.

92. Tschernko EM, Klepetko H, Gruber E, et al. Clonidine added to the anesthetic solution enhances analgesia and improves oxygenation after intercostal nerve block for thoracotomy. *Anesth Analg.* 1998;87:107.

93. Goyagi T, Tanaka M, Nishikawa T. Oral clonidine premedication enhances the pressor response to ephedrine during anesthesia. *Anesth Analg.* 1998;87:1336.

94. Watanabe Y, Iida H, Tanabe K, et al. Clonidine premedication modifies responses to adrenoceptor agonists. *Can J Anaesth.* 1998;45:1084.

95. Stoelting RK. Alpha- and beta-adrenergic receptor antagonists. *Pharmacology and Physiology in Anesthetic Practice.* 2nd ed. Philadelphia, Pa: JB Lippincott; 1991:295.

96. Lowenstein E, Foey P. Beta-adrenergic blockers. In: Smith NT, Corbascio AN, eds. *Drug Interactions in Anesthesia.* 2nd ed. Philadelphia, Pa: Lea & Febiger; 1986:119.

97. Foey PL. Alpha- and beta-adrenoreceptor antagonists. *Br J Anaesth.* 1984;56:751.

98. Horan BJ, Prys-Roberts C, Hamilton WK, et al. Haemodynamic responses to enflurane anaesthesia and hypovolemia in the dog and their modification by propranolol. *Br J Anaesth.* 1977;49:1184.

99. Roberts JG, Foey P, Clarke TNS, et al. Haemodynamic interactions of high-dose propranolol pre-treatment and anaesthesia in the dog, III: the effects of haemorrhage during halothane and trichloroethylene anaesthesia. *Br J Anaesth.* 1976;48:411.

100. Saner CA, Foey P, Roberts JG, et al. Methoxyflurane and practolol: a dangerous combination. *Br J Anaesth.* 1975;47:1025.

101. Johansen JW, Schneider G, Windson AM, et al. Esmolol potentiates reduction of minimum alveolar isoflurane concentration by alfentanil. *Anesth Analg.* 1998;87:671.

102. Bosnjak ZJ, Kampine JP. Effects of halothane, enflurane, and isoflurane on the SA node. *Anesthesiology.* 1983;58:314.

103. Nussmeier NA, Curling PE, Murphy DA, et al. Nifedipine: cardiovascular effects after sublingual administration during fentanyl-pancuronium anesthesia in man. *Anesthesiology.* 1983;59:A34.

104. Tosone SR, Reves JG, Kissin I, et al. Hemodynamic response to nifedipine in dogs anesthetized with halothane. *Anesth Analg.* 1983;62:903.

105. Ramsay JG, Cutfield GR, Francis CM, et al. Halothane-verapamil causes regional myocardial dysfunction in the dog. *Br J Anaesth.* 1986;58:321.

106. Kapur PA, Bloor BC, Flacke WE, et al. Comparison of cardiovascular responses to verapamil during enflurane, isoflurane, or halothane anesthesia in the dog. *Anesthesiology.* 1984;61:156.

107. Priebe HJ, Skarvan K. Cardiovascular and electrophysiologic interactions between diltiazem and isoflurane in the dog. *Anesthesiology.* 1987;66:114.

108. Merin RG. Calcium channel blocking drugs and anesthetics: is the drug interaction beneficial or detrimental [editorial]. *Anesthesiology.* 1987;66:111.

109. Jones RM, Cashman JN, Casson WR, et al. Verapamil potentiation of neuromuscular blockade: failure of reversal with neostigmine, but prompt reversal with edrophonium. *Anesth Analg.* 1985;64:1021.

110. Lawson NW, Kraynack BJ, Gintantas J. Neuromuscular and electrocardiographic responses to verapamil in dogs. *Anesth Analg.* 1983;62:50.

111. Littler C, McConachie I, Healy JEJ. Interaction between enalapril and propofol [letter]. *Anaesth Intens Care.* 1989;17:514.

112. Lauretti GR, de Oliveira R, Reis MP, et al. Transdermal nitroglycerine enhances spinal sufentanil postoperative analgesia following orthopedic surgery. *Anesthesiology.* 1999;90:734.

113. Harrah MD, Way WL, Katzung BG. The interaction of d-tubocurarine with antiarrhythmic drugs. *Anesthesiology.* 1970;33:406.

114. Miller RD, Way WL, Katzung BG. The potentiation of neuromuscular blocking agents by quinidine. *Anesthesiology.* 1967;28:1036.

115. Miller RD, Way WL, Katzung BG. The neuromuscular effects of quinidine. *Proc Soc Exp Biol Med.* 1968;129:215.

116. Atlee JL III. Antidysrhythmic agents. In: Smith NT, Corbascio AN, eds. *Drug Interactions in Anesthesia.* 2nd ed. Philadelphia, Pa: Lea & Febiger; 1986:225.

117. Waterman PM, Smith RB. Tobramycin-curare interaction. *Anesth Analg.* 1988;56:587.

118. Pittinger C, Adamson R. Antibiotic blockade of neuromuscular function. *Ann Rev Pharmacol.* 1972;12:169.

119. Burkett L, Bikhazi GB, Thomas KC, et al. Mutual potentiation of the neuromuscular effects of antibiotics and relaxants. *Anesth Analg.* 1979;58:107.

120. Fogdall RP, Miller RD. Prolongation of a pancuronium-induced neuromuscular blockade by clindamycin. *Anesthesiology.* 1974;41:407.

121. Goudsouzian N, Martyn JA. Potentiation of mivacurium by rocuronium

is age and time-dependent: a study in children, adolescents, and young and elderly adults. *J Clin Pharmacol.* 1997;37:649.

122. Kim DW, Joshi GP, White PF, et al. Interactions between mivacurium, rocuronium, and vecuronium during general anesthesia. *Anesth Analg.* 1996;83:818.

123. Hendley BJ. Convulsions after cocaine and propofol [letter]. *Anaesthesia.* 1990;45:788.

124. Nies AS, Shand DG, Wilkinson GR. Altered hepatic blood flow and drug disposition. *Clin Pharmacokinet.* 1976;1:135.

125. Cockshott ID, Douglas EJ, Prys-Roberts C, et al. Pharmacokinetics of propofol during and after IV infusion in man. *Br J Anaesth.* 1987;59:941P.

126. Gill SS, Wright EM, Reilly CS. Pharmacokinetic interaction of propofol and fentanyl: single bolus injection study. *Br J Anaesth.* 1990;65:760.

127. Kazama T, Ikeda K, Morita K. The pharmacodynamic interaction between propofol and fentanyl with respect to the suppression of somatic or hemodynamic responses to skin incision, peritoneum incision, and abdominal wall retraction. *Anesthesiology.* 1998;89:894.

128. Vuyk J. Pharmacokinetic and pharmacodynamic interactions between opioids and propofol. *J Clin Anesthesia.* 1997;9:23S.

129. Short TG, Chui PT. Propofol and midazolam act synergistically in combination. *Br J Anaesth.* 1991;67:539.

130. Brogden RN, Goa KL. Flumazenil: a reappraisal of its pharmacological properties and therapeutic efficacy as a benzodiazepine antagonist. *Drugs.* 1991;42:1061.

131. Amnein R, Leishman B, Bentzingen C, et al. Flumazenil in benzodiazepine antagonism, actions and clinical use in interactions and anesthesiology. *Med Toxicol.* 1987;2:411.

132. Christensen LQ, Bonde J, Kampmann JP. Drug interactions with intravenous and local anaesthetics. *Acta Anaesthesiol Scand.* 1994;38:15.

133. Gross JB, Weller RS, Conard P. Flumazenil reversal of midazolam. *Anesthesiology.* 1991;75:179.

# 37

# Muscle Relaxants

## Antoni M. Nejman

Neuromuscular blocking agents (NMBAs) interrupt the transmission of impulses from the motor nerve to the muscle fiber, thus achieving a decrease in muscle activity. Lessening muscular activity enables the surgeon to operate in a quiet field, providing good surgical exposure and doing so without the need for deep anesthesia that might compromise the cardiovascular stability of the patient. It is crucial to remember that NMBAs have no anxiolytic, amnestic, sedative, or analgesic properties.

## PHARMACODYNAMICS

### How Do Neuromuscular Blocking Drugs Work?

Acetylcholine (ACh) is synthesized in the nerve and stored in the endings of the motor nerve. ACh is released by the arrival of a nerve impulse, diffuses across the neuromuscular junctional cleft, and binds to the nicotinic ACh receptors on the postsynaptic membrane (motor endplate). This receptor binding causes a momentary change in the membrane's permeability to sodium ions, which in turn causes a decline in the resting membrane potential from $-90$ to $-45$ mV. Once this threshold potential is reached, the propagated action potential spreads over the surface of the muscle fiber, causing contraction.

Two types of postjunctional nicotinic ACh receptors respond to NMBAs: those found on the postjunctional membrane and those found extrajunctionally. The extrajunctional receptors proliferate and appear throughout skeletal muscle after denervation or muscle trauma.[1] These receptors are responsible for many of the complications seen when succinylcholine is given to patients with denervated muscles.

Prejunctional nicotinic receptors found on motor nerves influence the release of neurotransmitters and may facilitate mobilization of ACh from the site of synthesis to the site of release. NMBAs may interfere with ACh function both presynaptically and postsynaptically.

The postsynaptic ACh receptor comprises five glycoprotein subunits, forming a channel for ion passage. These subunits are designated $\alpha$, $\beta$, $\gamma$, and $\delta$ (there are two $\alpha$ subunits). This complex extends through the skeletal muscle cell membrane into the cytoplasm.

### What Is a Depolarizing Blockade?

Succinylcholine (diacetylcholine) is the primary depolarizing NMBA in use today. It attaches itself to the postjunctional nicotinic receptor at the $\alpha$ subunits and mimics the action of ACh, thus depolarizing the membrane, which can then no longer respond to the release of endogenous ACh. When both $\alpha$ subunits are occupied, the receptor ion channel remains open, causing muscle depolarization and fasciculations. A sustained configurational change in the receptor allows the leakage of potassium ion from the muscle cell, causing an increase in serum $K^+$ of approximately 0.5 mEq/L.

In patients with an increased number of extrajunctional receptors (after denervation, prolonged immobilization, burns, sepsis), this $K^+$ increase can be pronounced, reaching serum levels up to 8 to 10 mEq/L, which may cause life-threatening cardiac dysrhythmias.[2] Second and third doses of succinylcholine given within minutes of a previous dose are frequently associated with sinus bradycardia, junctional rhythms, and

**TABLE 37–1.** Side Effects Produced by Succinylcholine

| Side Effect | Probable Cause |
|---|---|
| Hyperkalemia | Normally, serum $K^+$ increased by up to 0.5 mEq/L secondary to potassium leaking from the depolarized muscle. In patients after crush injuries, burns, denervating injuries, or malignant hyperthermia, $K^+$ levels may rise much higher. |
| Dysrhythmias | Secondary to hyperkalemia or ganglionic effects of succinylcholine. Wide electrocardiographic complexes leading to cardiac arrest have been seen in children with dystrophin-deficient muscular dystrophies, Duchenne muscular dystrophy, and Becker muscular dystrophy.[*] |
| Myalgia | Secondary to fasciculation, even though some patients complain of muscle pain without having shown evidence of fasciculation. |
| Myoglobinemia | A rare complication after extensive fasciculation or in malignant hyperthermia. |
| Elevated intragastric pressure | Secondary to contraction of abdominal muscles during fasciculation.[†] However, the elevations of intragastric pressure seen after succinylcholine are less significant than occur with $CO_2$ insufflation during laparoscopic procedures. |
| Elevated intracranial pressure | This is postulated to be secondary to fasciculation and increased central venous pressure. There is doubt that succinylcholine has much of an effect.[‡] A traumatic intubation by itself may cause increased intracranial pressure. |
| Elevated intraocular pressure | The mechanism is not known. It appears not to be related to the contraction of ocular muscles during succinylcholine-induced fasciculation.[§] |
| Malignant hyperthermia | A genetic predisposition. The mechanism by which succinylcholine triggers the syndrome is not understood. |
| Masseter spasm | Seen more often in children than in adults, perhaps more so when succinylcholine is used with halothane than with thiopental[‖]; sometimes followed by malignant hyperthermia. |

[*]Sullivan M, Thompson WK, Hill GD. Succinylcholine-induced cardiac arrest in children with undiagnosed myopathy. *Can J Anaesth.* 1994;41:497.

[†]Smith G, Dalling R, Williams TIR. Gastroesophageal pressure gradient changes produced by induction of anaesthesia and suxamethonium. *Br J Anaesth.* 1978;50:1137.

[‡]Kovarik WD, Mayberg TS, Lam AM, et al. Succinylcholine does not change intracranial pressure, cerebral blood flow velocity, or the electroencephalogram in patients with neurologic injury. *Anesth Analg.* 1994;78:469.

[§]Kelly RE, Dinner M, Turner LS, et al. Succinylcholine increases intraocular pressure in the human eye with the extraocular muscles detached. *Anesthesiology.* 1993;79:948.

[‖]Lazzell VA, Carr AS, Lerman J, et al. The incidence of masseter muscle rigidity after succinylcholine in infants and children. *Can J Anaesth.* 1994;41:475.

even sinus arrest. Therefore, the patient should be pretreated with atropine or glycopyrrolate before repeating the dose of succinylcholine, such as during a difficult intubation.

One other characteristic of a succinylcholine-induced blockade is the intense nerve-muscle activity—often visible as fasciculations—heralding the onset of blockade. Muscle pain after succinylcholine administration may be related to these fasciculations. The fasciculations are probably mediated by the prejunctional ACh receptors and are blocked by small doses of nondepolarizing muscle relaxants. See Table 37–1 for a summary of potential side effects produced by succinylcholine.

## How Is the Action of Succinylcholine Terminated?

Plasma cholinesterase (also called *pseudocholinesterase*) rapidly terminates the effect of succinylcholine. Indeed, most (up to 90%) of an intravenously injected dose of succinylcholine undergoes hydrolysis, and only a small percentage actually reaches the effector site. Therefore, in patients with cholinesterase abnormalities, succinylcholine has a prolonged effect. Atypical cholinesterases are found in approximately 1:2000.

Several genetic variations of the plasma cholinesterases have been described, and the gene loci have been identified. Most patients are homozygous for plasma cholinesterase. After an intubating dose of approximately 1 mg/kg body weight, muscle paralysis lasts approximately 3 minutes. In patients heterozygous for plasma cholinesterase, the paralysis may last two or three times as long. In patients homozygous for atypical cholinesterase, the paralysis can last 5 or more hours after an intubating dose of 1 mg/kg. The treatment of a patient with a prolonged paralysis after succinylcholine is focused on symptoms. The patient may be awake but paralyzed and should, therefore, be mechanically ventilated until muscle power has returned. To a conscious patient, the pro-

longed paralysis is most alarming, and the patient should be sedated as long as ventilation must be supported.

## How Is Atypical Cholinesterase Detected?

The quality of the plasma cholinesterase activity can be assessed with the help of the dibucaine number. Dibucaine, a local anesthetic, strongly inhibits normal plasma cholinesterase.[3] The percentage of cholinesterase inhibition measured in vitro is expressed as the dibucaine number. A dibucaine number of approximately 80 confirms the patient's blood as being homozygous for normal plasma cholinesterase. In a patient homozygous for atypical cholinesterase, the dibucaine number may be 20 or 30; for the heterozygous patient, it is in the midrange between these extreme values. The dibucaine number does not measure the quantity of pseudocholinesterase, which may be decreased in patients with liver disease or who are taking anticholinesterase drugs, such as those treated for myasthenia gravis (long-acting cholinesterase inhibitors) or glaucoma (echothiophate), or in patients poisoned from exposure to insecticides.

The normal $ED_{90}$ (the dose causing 90% blockade) for succinylcholine is approximately 0.27 mg/kg.[4] The dosing of succinylcholine at 1.0 mg/kg (1.5 to 2.0 mg/kg in patients pretreated with a nondepolarizing drug) is common, and onset times of 30 to 60 seconds and peak effect in 60 to 90 seconds are the norm, with a duration of action in the 3- to 5-minute range. Dosing of succinylcholine as an infusion or as multiple-bolus doses often results in a prolonged blockade that resembles that seen with a nondepolarizing drug. Similar to a nondepolarizing block, this type II blockade can be reversed by acetylcholinesterase inhibitors; however, most clinicians prefer to treat the prolonged paralysis with mechanical ventilation without recourse to cholinesterase inhibitors because their effect may be unpredictable in patients with atypical cholinesterases.

## Why Use Succinylcholine?

At my center, we usually pick succinylcholine as our agent of choice for tracheal intubation in situations requiring rapid onset of action *and* rapid return of muscle function. These circumstances include any rapid-sequence intubations (eg, trauma, full stomach, pregnancy, diabetes, bowel obstruction). The short duration of blockade has been promoted as a reason to use succinylcholine in patients in whom establishing an airway may be problematic. A rapid return of consciousness and muscle power can be life-saving in the dreaded situation of "can't ventilate, can't intubate." Any paralysis in the face of a difficult airway should be considered a major risk. With the advent of new, short-acting nondepolarizers, we now have choices for rapid-onset paralysis other than succinylcholine. The risks and benefits of succinylcholine need to be weighed, and it should be given only with a rational indication, as is true for all medications.

## Can Succinylcholine Be Given for Short-Lasting Relaxation After the Administration of a Cholinesterase Inhibitor?

This question arises not infrequently when the surgeon needs "just a little more relaxation" during closure of an abdomen and when the anesthesiologist has already given a cholinesterase inhibitor to reverse the effect of a nondepolarizing NMBA. At that point, can the anesthesiologist give succinylcholine, which might be ideal because of its rapid onset of relaxation and short duration of action? Or would the pharmacologic features of the different drugs interact and produce undesirable consequences?

The question was tested in an interesting study by Fleming and colleagues, who found that 15 minutes after neostigmine, 0.05 mg/kg, or pyridostigmine, 0.24 mg/kg, had been given, the duration of action of a bolus (1 mg/kg) of succinylcholine was doubled, lasting approximately 20 minutes.[5] Such a drug interaction was not observed after edrophonium, 0.75 mg/kg. This drug interaction could not be explained solely by changes in the observed plasma cholinesterase levels brought about by the cholinesterase inhibitors. The clinical lesson: once a cholinesterase inhibitor has been given and relaxation of short duration is desired, succinylcholine may be used, but only very little, perhaps 20% of an intubating dose. When such a possibility can be anticipated, edrophonium may be the drug of choice for reversal of a nondepolarizing block.

## What Is Nondepolarizing Neuromuscular Blockade?

Nondepolarizing reversible blockade takes place when an NMBA without agonist activity binds reversibly to the postsynaptic nicotinic receptor. These drugs compete for the binding sites with endogenous ACh. At high doses, the drug molecules may actually block the receptor channels, as opposed to just binding to the receptor. Up to 75% of the receptors may be blocked without producing neuromuscular blockade, as evidenced by monitoring with a nerve stimulator (twitch monitor).[6] The degree of blockade also varies depending on the muscle group, with the diaphragm being one

of the most resistant (Table 37–2). Because they act competitively at the neuromuscular receptor, increasing levels of ACh antagonize the nondepolarizing agents. This is accomplished by the administration of acetylcholinesterase inhibitors, primarily edrophonium and neostigmine.

The nondepolarizing NMBAs are subdivided into two main groups: the benzylisoquinolinium and the steroid nucleus groups. These groups are then further subdivided into short-, intermediate-, and long-acting drugs. The duration of action given in the Table 37–3 refers to averages observed when a single ED$_{95}$ of the drug is administered. When larger doses are given, as is typically the case, for instance to accelerate the onset of relaxation in preparation for tracheal intubation, the duration of action is proportionally prolonged. Table 37–3 (classification and duration of action), Table 37–4 (clinical pharmacology), and Table 37–5 (cost) present summaries of currently used NMBAs.

## What Are the Benzylisoquoliniums?

### Mivacurium

Mivacurium is a short- to intermediate-acting NMBA with an ED$_{95}$ of 0.08 mg/kg. It is metabolized by plasma cholinesterase. Administration of three times the ED$_{95}$ over 10 to 15 seconds for rapid relaxation for intubation causes enough histamine release to lower blood pressure transiently. The duration of effect is 12 to 18 minutes.

**TABLE 37–2.** Reduction in Train-of-Four Response With Two Different Doses of Vecuronium

| Muscle | 0.04 mg/kg | 0.07 mg/kg |
|---|---|---|
| Adductor pollicis | 84% | 95% |
| Diaphragm | 78% | 95% |
| Orbicularis oculi | 62% | 82% |

**TABLE 37–3.** Classification and Duration of Action of Neuromuscular Blocking Agents

| Classification | | |
|---|---|---|
| **Benzylisoquinolines** | **Steroid Nucleus** | |
| Atracurium | Rapacuronium | |
| Cisatracurium | Rocuronium | |
| Doxacurium | Pancuronium | |
| *d*-Tubocurarine | Pipecuronium | |
| Metocurine | Vecuronium | |
| Mivacurium | | |
| **Duration of Action** | | |
| *<0.5 h* | *Intermediate* | *>1 h* |
| Rapacuronium | Atracurium | Doxacurium |
| Mivacurium | Cisatracurium | Pancuronium |
| | Rocuronium | Pipecuronium |
| | Vecuronium | |

The table can assist in selecting a suitable drug for a short or long operation. The magnitude of a single dose and, even more so, the effect of cumulative doses markedly influence the duration of action. The duration also varies depending on how the endpoint of action is defined. Do not rely on the listed duration of action, but treat the patient guided by an assessment of the patient's neuromuscular integrity.

**TABLE 37–4.** Summary of Neuromuscular Blocking Agents

| Drug | Intubating Dose (mg/kg) | Minutes to Peak Effect | Infusion ($\mu$g/kg/h) | Metabolism | Percentage Unchanged in Urine | Remarks |
|---|---|---|---|---|---|---|
| Succinylcholine | 1 | 1-1.5 | 1-200 | Plasma cholinesterase | | Phase II block with infusion |
| *Benzylisoquinolines* | | | | | | |
| Mivacurium | 0.2-0.3 | 2 | 1-15 | Plasma cholinesterase | <10 | Histamine release |
| Atracurium | 0.3-0.5 | 3 | 2-15 | Hoffman elimination and plasma cholinesterase | 10 | Histamine release; laudanosine metabolite |
| Cisatracurium | 0.2-0.3 | 3-4 | 1-8 | Mostly Hoffman elimination | Little | Laudanosine metabolite |
| *d*-Tubocurarine | 0.3-0.6 | 3-5 | | Hepatic | 45 | Histamine release |
| Doxacurium | 0.05-0.08 | 4-5 | | Mostly renal | 70 | |
| *Steroid Nucleus* | | | | | | |
| Rapacuronium | 1.5 | 1-2 | 40-60 | | | Mild hypotension/ tachycardia |
| Rocuronium | 0.6-1.2 | 1-3 | 5-15 | Hepatic | 30 | |
| Vecuronium | 0.2-0.3 | 3-4 | 1-2 | Mostly renal | 20 | |
| Pancuronium | 0.04-0.1 | 3-5 | | Mostly renal | 80 | Tachycardia |
| Pipecuronium | 0.07-0.85 | 3-5 | | Mostly renal | 70 | |

No infusion rates are given for the long-acting drugs.

## Atracurium

Atracurium is an intermediate-acting NMBA, with an $ED_{95}$ of 0.2 mg/kg. It undergoes ester hydrolysis and spontaneous degradation (Hoffman elimination) in vivo to laudanosine and electrophilic acrylates. This degradation depends on pH and temperature, being slowed by acidosis and cold, whereas the opposite is true of alkalosis and increased temperature. Ester hydrolysis contributes to a lesser degree to the production of laudanosine. At 10 $\mu$g/kg plasma concentration, laudanosine can cause epileptic spikes on the EEG; at 17 $\mu$g/kg, it can trigger seizures.[7] These concentrations are not reached clinically; the laudanosine level seen with a paralyzing dose of atracurium approaches approximately 0.3 $\mu$g/kg, which is 30 times lower than the plasma concentration causing epileptiform activity. Atracurium releases histamine when injected rapidly. The drug does not depend on renal elimination, an advantage in patients in renal failure.

## Cisatracurium

Cisatracurium resembles atracurium in duration of action but has an $ED_{95}$ of 0.05 mg/kg. It also undergoes degradation by the Hoffman pathway but differs in that it undergoes little nonspecific esterase hydrolysis. Cisatracurium does not cause histamine release, which makes it an attractive alternative to its sibling, atracurium. The drug has become popular in the critical care community because it does not accumulate to a significant degree. Metabolites include laudanosine and a monoquaternary acrylate.

## *d*-Tubocurarine

*d*-Tubocurarine is the prototype nondepolarizing NMBA. It is no longer used because of its marked propensity to release histamine on rapid injection of a bolus.[8] It is predominantly excreted by the kidneys, with a minor biliary component to elimination. The $ED_{95}$ is 0.51 mg/kg.

## Metocurine

Metocurine is a trimethylated derivative of *d*-tubocurarine. Although it is twice as potent ($ED_{95}$ = 0.28 mg/kg), it releases far less histamine. It is renally excreted with no hepatic

**TABLE 37–5.** Relative Costs* of Paralyzing Medications

| Neuromuscular Blocking Agent | Bottle | Amount in Bottle (mg) | Cost ($/mg) | Average Dose (mg/h) | 24-h Infusion Cost |
|---|---|---|---|---|---|
| Atracurium | $28.12 | 100 | $0.28 | 40 | $269.95 |
| Cisatracurium | $14.36 | 20 | $0.72 | 8.5 | $146.47 |
| Doxacurium | $14.82 | 5 | $2.96 | 1 | $ 71.13 |
| Pancuronium | $ 1.17 | 10 | $0.12 | 2 | $ 5.61 |
| Pipecuronium | $10.60 | 10 | $1.06 | 2 | $ 50.88 |
| Rapacuronium† | $11.08 | 100 | $0.11 | — | — |
| Rocuronium | $27.09 | 100 | $0.27 | 50 | $325.08 |
| Succinylcholine | $ 0.31 | 100 | $0.0031 | — | — |
| Vecuronium | $12.74 | 10 | $1.27 | 4 | $122.30 |

*Prices as of 1999.
†Not yet approved for infusion.

metabolism. It, too, has been replaced by newer agents of intermediate duration of action.

### Doxacurium

Doxacurium is a long-acting, potent NMBA without histamine-releasing properties. It has an $ED_{95}$ of 25 to 30 µg/kg, and its metabolism is dependent on renal clearance. It has a slow onset time and a duration of action similar to pancuronium.

## What Are the Steroid Nucleus Neuromuscular Blocking Agents?

### Rocuronium

Rocuronium, a recent addition to this family of drugs, has an $ED_{95}$ of 0.25 to 0.3 mg/kg. It has an onset of action that almost rivals that of succinylcholine when given in doses four to five times the $ED_{95}$. It is becoming a popular choice for rapid-sequence intubations when succinylcholine is contraindicated. Its duration of action is comparable with that of vecuronium. Because its metabolism is primarily hepatic, it is not affected by renal failure. It does not cause an increase in serum histamine levels.[9] It readily precipitates when exposed to thiopental and can then obstruct small-bore intravenous catheters.

### Vecuronium

Vecuronium, an aminosteroid NMBA with little cardiovascular effect, has been one of the most popular agents for paralysis. It has an $ED_{95}$ of 50 µg/kg and can be used either intermittently or by infusion. It is metabolized by the liver to 3-desacetyl, 17-desacetyl, and 3,17-desacetyl vecuronium, with the 3-desacetyl form being 50% as active as the original compound. The metabolites are renally excreted and, as such, tend to accumulate in patients with renal failure.

### Pancuronium

Pancuronium, the oldest member of the aminosteroid nucleus group, is a long-acting NMBA. Its $ED_{95}$ is 70 µg/kg. It is associated with tachycardia and increases in blood pressure. Pancuronium has a metabolite, 3-OH-pancuronium, which is 50% as active as the parent drug. Both the original and the metabolic byproduct are primarily excreted by the kidney and also tend to accumulate when the kidneys fails.

### Pipecuronium

Pipecuronium, an aminosteroid NMBA with a duration of action somewhat longer than that of pancuronium, has an $ED_{95}$ of 50 µg/kg. It is not associated with cardiovascular side effects or histamine release. Pipecuronium and its metabolites are renally excreted.

### Rapacuronium

Rapacuronium is the newest aminosteroid relaxant. It has a low potency ($ED_{95}$ = 1 mg/kg), a rapid onset, and a short duration of action. Tracheal intubating conditions are good to excellent 60 seconds after 1.5 mg/kg is given, followed by relaxation lasting approximately 10 to 15 minutes. With large or repeated doses, the recovery index gradually increases, probably as a result of accumulation of the 3-OH metabolite, which is cleared more slowly than the parent compound.

Schiere and colleagues compared equipotent doses of vecuronium and rapacuronium and showed, as expected, that rapacuronium has a more rapid onset and shorter duration than vecuronium. Also, the duration of maintenance doses of rapacuronium is shorter than those of vecuronium, whether preceded by rapacuronium or by vecuronium. The onset time is only slightly shorter than that of rocuronium.[10,11] With its rapid onset and short duration, it can replace succinylcholine for tracheal intubation in short operative procedures requiring neuromuscular relaxation. It can be pharmacologically reversed minutes after an intubating dose.[12]

Unfortunately, the status of rapacuronium is unclear. On March 27, 2001, the manufacturer (Organon, Inc., West Orange, NJ) sent a letter to the FDA and to all anesthesiologists, hospital pharmacists, and other drug consignees, announcing the voluntary market withdrawal of the drug. Organon had received reports of mild to severe cases of bronchospasm, including five deaths, during or following the administration of rapacuronium.[13]

A summary of NMBAs can be found in Table 37–3.

## PARALYSIS

Reports of prolonged paralysis with NMBAs have become more frequent in the literature.[14,15] It is thus necessary to understand some of the causes of NMBA potentiation. The problem is of less concern in the operating room and a greater worry in the intensive care unit (ICU).

## How Much Paralysis Is Enough?

Just as in the operating room, the degree of muscle relaxation used in the ICU should be tailored to the indication. Complete obliteration of ventilatory response is usually unnecessary. If $O_2$ consumption must be minimized, it may be necessary to aim for more than merely the control of a patient's dangerous and uncontrolled thrashing.

In the ICU, we usually titrate the infusion of a muscle relaxant so as to maintain a 1- to 2-twitch response of the adductor pollicis. If a greater degree of neuromuscular blockade is needed, the posttetanic count can guide the clinician. To ensure the maintenance of normal neuromuscular function, at least twice a day the patient should recover to between 1 and 2 twitches without tetanic potentiation.

## What Are the Common Causes of Prolonged Paralysis in the Intensive Care Unit?

Some causes of prolonged paralysis are listed in Table 37–6, whereas Table 37–7 shows the much shorter list of factors that enhance the effect of NMBAs. Overdose of NMBAs explains most cases of prolonged paralysis. The excessive administration of NMBAs and accumulation of their active metabolites is best avoided with the continuous infusion of the chosen agent in concert with neuromuscular blockade monitoring.

Segredo and coworkers described a group of 7 of 16 ICU patients with prolonged paralysis after the discontinuation of vecuronium infusions.[15] These patients all had extensive renal failure and metabolic acidosis, with the probable accumulation of the active metabolite of vecuronium (3-desacetyl vecuronium).

**TABLE 37–6.** Factors That Prolong Paralysis

| Pathophysiologic Causes | Pharmacologic Causes |
|---|---|
| Acid maltase deficiency | Aminoglycoside toxicity |
| Adrenocortical dysfunction | Penicillin toxicity |
| Acute intermittent porphyria | Steroid myopathy |
| Amyotrophic lateral sclerosis | ***Antihypertensives*** |
| Anoxia/ischemia | |
| Carcinomatous polyneuropathy | Ganglionic blockers |
| Compressive neuropathy | Calcium channel blockers |
| Critical illness polyneuropathy | β-Blockers |
| Diphtheria | Furosemide |
| Eaton-Lambert syndrome | ***Antidysrhythmics*** |
| Guillain-Barré syndrome | Quinidine |
| Hypokalemia and hypocalcemia | Bretylium |
| Hypomagnesemia | Procainamide |
| Hypophosphatemia | Local anesthetics in large doses |
| Hypothermia | |
| Motor neuron disease | ***Antibiotics*** |
| Multiple sclerosis | Aminoglycoside antibiotics |
| Muscular dystrophy | Polymyxin B |
| Myasthenia gravis | Clindamycin |
| Myotonic syndromes | Tetracycline |
| Neurofibromatosis | ***Miscellaneous Drugs*** |
| Nonspecific nutritional deficiency | |
| Poliomyelitis | Cyclosporine |
| Porphyria | Steroids |
| Pyridoxine abuse | Volatile anesthetics |
| Polymyositis | Dantrolene |
| Renal failure (variable | Magnesium |
| prolongation) | Lithium |
| Respiratory acidosis | Azathioprine |
| Sepsis | Organophosphate poisoning |
| Thiamine deficiency | |
| Tick bite paralysis | |
| Trauma | |
| Vitamin E deficiency | |
| Wound botulism | |

Prolonged paralysis has been reported in asthmatic patients treated with both steroids and muscle relaxants. The interaction of muscle relaxants and the acute myopathy observed after high doses of corticosteroids may explain this adverse effect.[16–18] There are fewer reports of prolonged paralysis when atracurium or cisatracurium was administered in the ICU to patients who were also given steroids. The atracurium quaternary ammonium molecule differs structurally from the vecuronium/pancuronium aminosteroid nucleus. The structural similarity of vecuronium-like drugs to the steroids may play a role in the myopathy seen with vecuronium and pancuronium.

In summary, the ICU patients we choose to paralyze, for whatever reason, are at risk for prolonged neuromuscular malfunction. At particularly high risk are the following types of patients:

**TABLE 37–7.** Factors That Enhance the Effect of Neuromuscular Blocking Agents

| Pathophysiologic Factors | Pharmacologic Factors |
|---|---|
| Alkalosis | Phenytoin |
| Extensive burns | Carbamazepine |
| Diabetes | Sympathomimetics |
| Hepatic failure with ascites | Chronic exposure to neuromuscular |
| Hemiplegia | blocking agents |
| Denervation syndromes | |
| Hyperkalemia | |
| Hypercalcemia | |

1. Those with sepsis and multiorgan system dysfunction (critical illness polyneuropathy)
2. Those with renal failure (accumulation of renally excreted active metabolites)
3. Those with hepatic failure (for hepatically metabolized agents)
4. Those concomitantly receiving corticosteroids

The evaluation of these patients with prolonged blockade should include, along with a review of their history, an assessment of their neuromuscular function with physical examination, nerve stimulators, and electromyography. Occasionally, a muscle or nerve biopsy may be indicated if a dysregulation of the ACh receptor secondary to excessive exposure to NMBAs is suspected.[19] There is no specific treatment for the condition. In mild cases, the paralysis usually clears in a matter of weeks; the more severe cases may take months. Occasionally, the patient may be left with a permanent disability and must receive both physical and mental support throughout this difficult period. These potentially serious complications compel us to monitor the level of neuromuscular integrity whenever a blocking agent is used in the critical care population.

## Antagonism of Residual Blockade

Pharmacologic antagonism of neuromuscular blockade must take into account the duration of action of the NMBA and interindividual variations. Long-acting drugs are less completely antagonized than intermediate-acting NMBAs, given the same starting level of blockade (ie, train-of-four ratio) and using equivalent doses of neostigmine. Bartkowski showed that anticholinesterases do not have an unlimited capacity to antagonize curare-like drugs.[20] It has also been demonstrated that some NMBAs are better antagonized by specific anticholinesterases, with atracurium and mivacurium better antagonized by edrophonium.[21,22]

The anticholinesterase agents act by decreasing acetylcholinesterase activity, which results in an increase in the available ACh for competitive postjunctional receptor stimulation. Ideally, the anticholinesterase should have a longer duration of action than the NMBA that is being reversed, lest there be a return of paralysis. The anticholinesterase also promotes increased ACh activity at the muscarinic receptors of the body and thus unwanted side effects (ie, increased secretions, bronchoconstriction, miosis, increased tone in the gastrointestinal and urinary tracts, and, in particular, bradycardia). This is avoided by administering a muscarinic blocking agent along with the reversal agent. I prefer to use atropine with edrophonium, and glycopyrrolate with neostigmine and pyridostigmine. Common clinical doses are shown in Table 37–8. I like to match neostigmine, 0.05 mg/kg, or edrophonium, 0.5 mg/kg, with atropine, 0.02 mg/kg, or glycopyrrolate, 0.01 mg/kg. The peak effect of neostigmine and pyridostigmine is not reached for up to 10 minutes, whereas the peak effect of atropine and glycopyrrolate occurs in less than half that time. With short-acting nondepolarizing NMBAs, a significant delay of activity can be expected while the cholinesterase inhibitors develop their full effect. Table 37–8 summarizes the dosages and duration of action of drugs used in the reversal of a clinical neuromuscular block.

Clinical judgment must dictate whether to give a full reversal dose, a reduced dose, or no reversal at all. After the use

**TABLE 37–8.** Dosing of Neuromuscular Blockade Reversing Agents

| Drug | IV Dose | Time to Peak | Duration |
|---|---|---|---|
| Edrophonium | 0.5-1 mg/kg | 1 min | 45 min |
| Neostigmine | 0.05 mg/kg to ≤5 mg total | 10 min | 60 min |
| Pyridostigmine | 0.25 mg/kg | 12 min | 100 min |
| Atropine | 15 μg/kg | 70 s | 1-2 h |
| Glycopyrrolate | 10-20 μg/kg | 2 min | 2-4 h |

IV, intravenous.

of short-acting NMBAs and if long intervals have passed after the last dose with no evidence of muscle weakness by nerve stimulation and clinical signs, reversal agents need not be given. A reversal dose should be given if there is any evidence of paralysis. Some clinicians always give a full reversal dose as long as there is any evidence of muscle paralysis, however minor. Others administer less than a full reversal dose in the face of waning paralysis. When in doubt, the clinician should err on the side of full reversal because the complications of inadequate spontaneous ventilation are more dangerous than the side effects of the reversal regimen.

## THE ANTICHOLINESTERASES

### What Is the Toxicity of the Anticholinesterases?

#### Carbamates

Neostigmine, edrophonium, physostigmine, ambenonium, and demecarium are all classified as reversible anticholinesterase agents of the carbamate variety. The last three drugs find use in the treatment of myasthenia gravis. These five drugs differ in their potency and duration of action and in how well they are absorbed from the gastrointestinal tract. They all delay or block the hydrolysis of ACh, which can explain many of their side effects and toxicity.

However, they exhibit effects that are not simply related to increased ACh activity. Instead, these drugs may exert direct agonistic or antagonistic effects on ganglia and the muscles themselves. For example, neostigmine has effects on the spinal cord and the neuromuscular junction brought about by direct cholinergic stimulation. Large doses of neostigmine or edrophonium can weaken muscles through such direct effects, complications not likely to arise with the dosages used in routine clinical practice. Relatively high doses or inadequate concomitant cholinergic blockade are more likely to result in side effects of bradycardia, salivation, intestinal cramps, and, particularly in asthmatic patients, bronchoconstriction.

#### Organophosphorus Agents

Other cholinesterases are characterized by their organophosphorus structure. In this group, we find one drug of great clinical use, namely echothiophate, which is used in the treatment of glaucoma. Miosis (but usually still responding to light) and reduced intraocular pressure indicate effective drug levels in the eye. When this is observed, the possibility of systemic cholinesterase inhibition should be considered. The toxic potential of the organophosphorus compounds is exploited by a group of insecticides, including parathion and malathion. Up to 80% of pesticide-related hospital admissions may be attributed to organophosphorus insecticides.

Far grimmer are the homicidal agents commonly referred to as *nerve gases*. These include Tabun and Sarin, both of which have made headlines in recent years. These extremely potent poisons can be absorbed through the skin. Cholinesterase inhibition and direct effects through nicotinic and muscarinic stimulation account for the symptoms. Their high lipid solubility gives them access to the central nervous system. Symptoms of toxicity can appear within minutes of exposure or can develop over hours with continuous slow absorption from the skin. Miosis, ciliary spasm, rhinorrhea, sweating, bronchospasm, bradycardia, and intestinal cramps suggest organophosphorus poisoning. In severe cases, these signs and symptoms are accompanied by hypotension, vomiting, diarrhea, muscle fasciculation, weakness, confusion, slurred speech, convulsions, and coma.

The treatment is directed against the overactivity of ACh. Atropine is the drug of choice, not only because it inhibits the muscarinic effect in the periphery but also because it penetrates into the central nervous system. Atropine has to be injected in large intravenous doses, titrated to effect. However, atropine does not antagonize peripheral neuromuscular effects and paralysis. To combat the direct and indirect effects of the poisons, a cholinesterase reactivator is used. Pralidoxime (1-2 g intravenously injected no more rapidly than 500 mg/min) or obidoxime must be given as early after exposure as possible.

## References

1. Pumplin DW, Fambrough DM. Turnover of acetylcholine receptors in skeletal muscle. *Annu Rev Physiol.* 1982;44:319.
2. Cooperman LH, Strobel GE Jr, Kennell EM. Massive hyperkalemia after administration of succinylcholine. *Anesthesiology.* 1970;32:161.
3. Kalow W, Genest K. A method for the detection of atypical forms of the human serum cholinesterase: determination of dibucaine numbers. *Can J Biochem.* 1957;35:339.
4. Smith CE, Donati F, Bevan DR. Dose response curves for succinylcholine: single versus cumulative techniques. *Anesthesiology.* 1988;69:338.
5. Fleming NW, Macres S, Antognini JF, et al. Neuromuscular blocking action of suxamethonium after antagonism of vecuronium by edrophonium, pyridostigmine or neostigmine. *Br J Anaesth.* 1996;77:492.
6. Paton WDM, Waud DR. The margin of safety of neuromuscular transmission. *J Physiol (Lond).* 1967;191:59.
7. Chapple DJ, Miller AA, Ward JB, et al. Cardiovascular and neurological effects of laudanosine: studies in mice and rats, and in conscious and anaesthetized dogs. *Br J Anaesth.* 1987;59:218.
8. Basta SJ, Savarese JJ, Ali HH. Histamine-releasing potencies of atracurium and dimethyl-tubocurarine. *Br J Anaesth.* 1983;55:105S.
9. Levy JH, Davis GK, Duggan J, et al. Determination of the hemodynamics and histamine release of rocuronium (Org9426) when administered in increasing doses under N₂O/O₂-sufentanil anesthesia. *Anesth Analg.* 1994;78:318.
10. Bevan DR. Neuromuscular relaxants—1997. *Can J Anaesth.* 1997;44:1135.
11. Schiere S, van den Broek L, Proost JH, et al. Comparison of vecuronium with ORG 9487 and their interaction. *Can J Anaesth.* 1997;44:1138.
12. Purdy R, Bevan DR, Donati F, et al. Early reversal of rapacuronium with neostigmine. *Anesthesiology.* 1999;91:51.
13. United States Food and Drug Administration (FDA). Talk paper: injectable anesthesia drug being withdrawn from market. Available at: http://www.fda. gov/bbs/topics/ANSWERS/2001/AN501072.html Accessed March 29, 2001.
14. Kupfer Y, Namba T, Kaldawi E, et al. Prolonged paralysis after long term infusion of vecuronium. *Ann Intern Med.* 1992;117:484.

15. Segredo V, Caldwell JE, Miller R. Persistent paralysis in critically ill patients after long term administration of vecuronium. *N Engl J Med.* 1992;327:524.

16. Hanson-Flaschen J, Cowen J, Raps EC. Neuromuscular blockade in the intensive care unit. *Am Rev Respir Dis.* 1993;147:234.

17. Hirano M, Ott B, Raps E, et al. Acute quadriplegic myopathy: a complication of treatment with steroids, nondepolarizing blocking agents, or both. *Neurology.* 1992;42:2082.

18. Williams TJ, O'Hehir RE, Czarny D, et al. Acute myopathy in severe acute asthma treated with intravenously administered corticosteroids. *Am Rev Respir Dis.* 1988;137:460.

19. Lee C. Intensive care unit neuromuscular syndrome? [editorial]. *Anesthesiology.* 1995;83:237.

20. Bartkowski RR. Incomplete reversal of pancuronium neuromuscular blockade by neostigmine, pyridostigmine, and edrophonium. *Anesth Analg.* 1987;66:594.

21. Cook DR, Chakravorti S, Brandom BW, et al. Effects of neostigmine, edrophonium, and succinylcholine on the in vitro metabolism of mivacurium: clinical correlates. *Anesthesiology.* 1992;77:A948.

22. Kopman AF. Tactile evaluation of train-of-four count as an indicator of reliability of antagonism from vecuronium or atracurium-induced neuromuscular blockade. *Anesthesiology.* 1991;75:588.

# Physiologic Aberrations and Their Control

CHAPTER

# 38

# Trauma and Shock

Scott H. Norwood

Van L. Vallina

Injury is the leading cause of death and functional limitation in individuals younger than 45 years of age.[1] The most common cause of death from injury in 1995 was motor vehicle crashes, causing 16.2 deaths/100 000 population. Deaths from firearms ranked second at 13.7/100 000 population.[2] Injury treatment and prevention presents complex medical and economic problems at the community, state, and national levels in both developed and undeveloped countries. Injuries were responsible for 5.1 million deaths worldwide in 1990, accounting for >10% of all deaths worldwide.[3] Motor vehicle crashes, falls, war injuries, self-inflicted injuries, and violence account for a significant number of global disability-adjusted life years, which takes into consideration not only years lost to death but also years lost from disability.[3] By the year 2020, a significant increase in the total number of global deaths from motor vehicle crashes, violence, and wars is anticipated.[3]

It has been estimated that the cost to society of each injury-related death in the United States is $335 000.[4] This cost is over 2.5 times higher than the combined costs to society of deaths from cancer and cardiovascular disease. These data emphasize the considerable economic benefit of developing prevention strategies for injury-related deaths and disability.

Improvements in emergency medical services in the United States have been instrumental in reducing immediate mortality from injury. Injured patients who previously died at the scene of injury are now being rapidly transported to trauma centers for definitive care. Advancements during warfare have contributed to major improvements in prehospital care and emergency resuscitation. Despite these advances, however, trauma continues to take an appalling toll in terms of morbidity and mortality globally. Successful management of severely injured patients is dependent on rapid transport, early definitive resuscitation, operative intervention, comprehensive critical care, and early, comprehensive rehabilitation.

# EPIDEMIOLOGY

## How Is Trauma Categorized?

Mechanism of injury categorization is familiar to most physicians. The conventional categories are *blunt* (motor vehicle crashes, falls) and *penetrating* (gunshot wounds, stab wounds). Another method focuses on the motive responsible for the injury, that is, *intentional* (deliberate) versus *unintentional* (accidental). This latter classification is often used by legal, statistical, and insurance systems. A third, geographic method (*urban* versus *rural*) is useful in planning trauma care systems.

## How Significant Is Trauma?

The overall age-adjusted injury death rate in the United States was 51.5 deaths/100 000 population in 1995.[2] The death rate from motor vehicle crashes was 16.2/100 000, followed by deaths from firearms at 13.7/100 000.[2] Fatal injuries involving motor vehicles (including motorcycles, bicycles, and vehicle-pedestrian mechanisms) are highest in the 15- to 24-year age group (29.5/100 000). The second highest incidence, emphasizing the increasing death rate from trauma in the elderly, is in the 65 and older group (22.6/100 000).[2] Firearm deaths were highest in the 15- to 24-year age group at 27.2/

100 000.[2] Falls are the most common mechanism of injury leading to death in patients over 65 years old, accounting for 23.5/100 000 population.[2] Mortality from injury increases dramatically with age and, despite the traditional correlation with youth, trauma in the elderly is increasing.[5]

### What Injury Patterns Occur in the Urban Setting?

Urban trauma is characterized by intentional, penetrating, and vehicle-pedestrian injuries. Penetrating trauma outnumbers blunt trauma by 2:1.[6] Homicides, assaults, burns, and pedestrian fatalities are highest among the poor,[7,8] and socioeconomic differences among urban populations increase the risk of intentional injury. In 1991, 38 317 people were killed from firearm injuries,[9] and from 1988 to 1991 the firearms death rate for teenagers age 15 to 19 years increased by 77%.[10] Urban trauma centers treat more patients than rural centers because of the large population base and tertiary care referral.

### How Does Rural Trauma Care Differ?

Rural trauma is predominantly nonpenetrating. Blunt trauma outnumbers penetrating by 9:1. Although only 25% of motor vehicle crashes occur in rural areas, they account for two thirds of all traffic deaths.[11,12] The five states with the highest death rates per 100 000 population from trauma in 1992 were Alaska, Mississippi, New Mexico, Wyoming, and Alabama.[13] Rural trauma presents unique obstacles to care, including long transport distances, varied terrain, a smaller population base, predominance of basic and intermediate level prehospital personnel, and limited access to professional and institutional resources. All of these factors tend to isolate the injured patient in an environment where access to definitive care is limited.

### What Is a Trauma System?

A network of professionals working cooperatively to achieve optimal care for injured patients defines a trauma system. Trauma system goals are to reduce mortality and morbidity by recognizing significant injury and integrating both prehospital emergency medical services and hospital resources to rapidly reverse the effects of injury. Up to 40% of trauma deaths occur within hours after injury,[6,14] and 70% of deaths at Level I centers occur within the first 24 hours of admission.[15] Prevention, early identification, and treatment of potentially lethal injuries are the focus of trauma system personnel.

The concept of an inclusive trauma system was first developed in the early 1990s and implemented under the auspices of the Health Resources Services Administration in 1992.[16] This written plan clearly outlines the basic system components and is used throughout the United States for trauma system implementation.

## ASSESSMENT OF INJURY SEVERITY

Accurately identifying severe injury is essential for appropriate utilization of trauma system resources. Equally im-

**TABLE 38–1.** The Revised Trauma Score

| | Value | Score | |
|---|---|---|---|
| Systolic blood pressure (mm Hg) | >89 | 4 | Points |
| | 76–89 | 3 | |
| | 50–75 | 2 | |
| | 1–49 | 1 | |
| | 0 | 0 | |
| Respiratory rate (breaths per minute) | 10–29 | 4 | Points |
| | >29 | 3 | |
| | 6–9 | 2 | |
| | 1–5 | 1 | |
| | 0 | 0 | |
| **Glasgow Coma Scale (GCS)*** | | | |
| *Eye Opening* | | | |
| Spontaneous | | 4 | Points |
| To voice | | 3 | |
| To pain | | 2 | |
| None | | 1 | |
| *Verbal Response* | | | |
| Oriented | | 5 | Points |
| Confused | | 4 | |
| Inappropriate words | | 3 | |
| Incomprehensible words | | 2 | |
| None | | 1 | |
| *Motor Response* | | | |
| Obeys commands | | 6 | Points |
| Localizes to pain | | 5 | |
| Withdraw (pain) | | 4 | |
| Flexion (pain) | | 3 | |
| Extension (pain) | | 2 | |
| None | | 1 | |

*Total GCS points = Trauma Points:

$$13 - 15 = 4$$
$$9 - 12 = 3$$
$$6 - 8 = 2$$
$$4 - 5 = 1$$
$$3 = 0$$

A coded value <4 in any area should suggest transport to a trauma center.
From Boyd CR, Tolson MA, Copes WS. Evaluating trauma care: the TRISS method. *J Trauma.* 1987;27:370.

portant is a standardized method for evaluating injury severity so that individual system performance may be compared with other systems and standard models of care.

### What Defines a Severely Injured Trauma Victim?

A number of scoring systems that assign numeric values to physiologic and anatomic indicators of injury are useful for identifying severe injury. The Revised Trauma Score (RTS) is commonly used by prehospital and emergency department (ED) personnel (Table 38–1).[17] This score uses systolic blood pressure (BP), respiratory rate, and neurologic function (with the Glasgow Coma Scale [GCS]) to determine injury severity. A Pediatric Trauma Score has also been developed and tested by Tepas and colleagues.[18]

Scoring systems allow standardized injury severity classifications by both prehospital and trauma care providers. A threshold score can be determined to identify those patients who require full trauma team evaluation.

### How Are Injuries and Outcomes Compared?

Certain scoring systems allow for comparison among different patient groups, institutions, and trauma systems.[9-22] The

Injury Severity Score (ISS) numerically describes the overall severity of anatomic injury and may be applied to victims with multiple or isolated injuries.[20] Several limitations of the ISS are well recognized. Because the ISS gives equal weight to each body region, multiple injuries to the chest or abdomen may result in underscoring of these anatomic regions.[23] Short-term mortality risk may therefore be underestimated by ISS.[24]

The TRISS (Trauma Injury Severity Score) score uses the ISS, age, RTS, and mechanism of injury (blunt or penetrating) to quantify probability of survival.[21] This methodology, and the more recent ASCOT (A Severity Characterization of Trauma) score[25] were developed to reduce the limitations of the ISS. The TRISS method, although limited when used for penetrating trauma,[26] is the mainstay of retrospective probability of survival analyses. TRISS is the most common method for determining probability of survival in most trauma registry data systems. Other proposed methods include an artificial intelligence technique developed by McGonigal and colleagues[27] and a system based on the *International Classification of Diseases, Ninth Revision (ICD-9)* by Rutledge.[28]

Regardless of the method used, one should examine the deaths that occur in patients with predicted survival of >50% through a continuous quality improvement process to identify problems with patient care delivery.

## Which Patients Activate the System and Who Goes to a Trauma Center?

Criteria for each trauma system may vary depending on unique characteristics and resources. The major criteria include mechanism of injury and physiologic, anatomic, and comorbid factors such as respiratory or cardiac disease, age, transport distances, and prehospital personnel expertise. The American College of Surgeons Committee on Trauma has developed and endorsed a general field triage plan to determine which patients should be transported to a trauma center (Table 38–2).[29] These criteria should be used in the beginning stages of trauma system development and modified as the system matures and trauma patient data and outcomes are analyzed.[30–33]

## EMERGENCY DEPARTMENT LOGISTICS AND OPERATING ROOM PREPARATION

Optimal trauma care requires a team effort and rapid team response to the resuscitation area when necessary. System criteria that direct patients to a trauma center are usually similar to the trauma team activation criteria.

## How Is the Trauma Team Activated?

An activation system for trauma team members must be reliable and periodically tested (usually every 8–12 hours). Key areas (operating room [OR], blood bank, radiology, and laboratory services) are also notified. All team members have a predetermined time frame for arrival, generally 5 to 10 minutes based on institutional size and inhospital personnel requirements. Any effective system is carefully monitored and tested frequently. Continuous quality improvement monitoring

**TABLE 38–2.** Field Triage Decision Scheme

| | Measure vital signs and level of consciousness. | |
|---|---|---|
| **Step 1** | Glasgow Coma Scale | <14 *or* |
| | Systolic blood pressure (mm Hg) | <90 *or* |
| | Respiratory rate (breaths per minute) | <10 *or* >29 *or* |
| | Revised trauma score | <11 *or* |
| | Pediatric trauma score | <9 |
| | YES | NO |
| | Take to trauma center. | Assess anatomy of injury. |
| **Step 2** | All penetrating injuries to head, neck, torso, and extremities proximal to elbow and knee | |
| | Flail chest | |
| | Combination trauma with burns | |
| | 2 or more proximal long bone fractures | |
| | Pelvic fractures | |
| | Open and depressed skull fractures | |
| | Paralysis | |
| | Amputation proximal to wrist and ankle | |
| | Major burns | |
| | YES | NO |
| | Take to trauma center. | Evaluate for evidence of mechanism of injury and high-energy impact. |
| **Step 3** | Ejection from automobile | |
| | Death in same passenger compartment | |
| | Extrication time >20 min | |
| | Falls >20 ft | |
| | Rollover | |
| | High-speed auto crash | |
| |   Initial speed >40 mph | |
| |   Major auto deformity >20 in. | |
| |   Intrusion into passenger compartment >12 in. | |
| | Auto-pedestrian/auto-bicycle injury with significant (>5 mph) impact | |
| | Pedestrian thrown or run over | |
| | Motorcycle crash >20 mph or with separation of rider from bike | |
| | YES | NO |
| | Contact medical director and consider transport to a trauma center. | |
| **Step 4** | Age <5 or >55 y | |
| | Cardiac disease; respiratory disease | |
| | Insulin-dependent diabetes; cirrhosis; obesity or coagulopathy | |
| | YES | NO |
| | Contact medical director and consider transport to trauma center. | Reevaluate with medical control. |

**WHEN IN DOUBT TAKE TO A TRAUMA CENTER**

From The Committee on Trauma, American College of Surgeons. *Resources for Optimal Care of the Injured Patient, 1999.* Chicago, Ill: American College of Surgeons; 1999:14.

and action on variances are important in preventing delays in care.

## What Is the Trauma Team?

The composition and key roles of the trauma team are listed in Table 38–3. Resuscitation protocols are developed for major trauma victims, including delineation of specific team member's roles.

### The Anesthesiologist's Role

The anesthesiologist or certified registered nurse anesthetist is responsible for maintaining the patient's airway during a

**TABLE 38–3.** Trauma Team Members and Their Roles

| Personnel | Key Role |
| --- | --- |
| Trauma surgeon | Team leader; performs primary and secondary surveys and necessary procedures; directs resuscitation efforts and follow-through care |
| Emergency physician | Fulfills role of team leader if trauma surgeon not present; assists with procedures |
| Anesthesiologist/anesthetist | Assesses, establishes, and/or assists in maintaining airway while maintaining cervical spine integrity; assists with line access and hemodynamic monitoring, if necessary |
| Private nurse | Performs primary and secondary survey along with team leader; establishes intravenous access on left; assists team leader with procedures; maintains patient contact |
| Secondary nurse | Establishes intravenous access on right; monitors vital signs and cardiac monitoring; places nasogastric tube/Foley catheter; provides wound care; splints; acts as family liaison |
| Respiratory care technician | Assists with airway management; performs arterial blood gas analysis; sets up ventilator; assists during transport |
| Laboratory technician | Procures, labels, and transports blood specimens |
| Radiography/computed tomography technician | Procures radiographic studies; evacuates and prepares computed tomography scanner |
| Nursing supervisor | Documents all activities and interventions; initiates bed assignment |
| Operating room backup/operating room team | Ensures preparation for potential surgery |
| Chaplain | Notifies and provides support for family and significant others |
| Security officer | Secures valuables; maintains crowd control |
| Trauma coordinator | Provides supervision/supportive assistance; assists with direct care when necessary |

major resuscitation. Circumstances, preexisting protocols, and experience of other team members determine what techniques are used and who performs endotracheal intubation.

The anesthesiologist's critical care background provides a solid base for decision making within the trauma resuscitation framework. Positioned at the head of the patient, anesthesia personnel have the best view of the progress in patient resuscitation and assist with patient monitoring. This role may continue during diagnostic testing (angiography, computed tomography [CT]) and, of course, into the OR.

Many anesthesiologists contribute significantly to the critical care aspects of trauma patient care, and a basic knowledge of the initial resuscitation, as presented in the Advanced Trauma Life Support (ATLS) Course, is strongly recommended.[34–36]

## Must the Entire Team Always Respond?

Many trauma centers conserve resources by activating the entire team only when life-threatening injury is probable. Fewer resources are needed to manage patients with lesser injuries. Gomez and colleagues, using a two-tiered system, demonstrated an equally safe level of care, a 70% reduction

in patient resuscitation charges, and incalculable savings in manpower.[37] Tiered response systems must be continually monitored to ensure that appropriate resources are always available when needed.

## What Should the Operating Room Personnel Do to Prepare During Trauma Team Activation?

Advanced notice of a patient's arrival is accomplished in most systems by including the OR in the trauma paging system. Depending on the trauma case mix, the OR response may have two tiers. Initial preparation includes ensuring that there is an available OR and that staff are preparing for the patient's arrival. In many systems, a second call is made to the OR confirming the need for surgery. With the second call the OR personnel rapidly open the room. In centers treating primarily blunt trauma victims, a two-tiered system is effective and economical. A dedicated OR for trauma patients and in-house OR personnel are essential criteria for Level I and Level II trauma centers.[38] The necessity of this requirement has been questioned for Level II trauma centers[39] and for Level I trauma centers where victims of blunt trauma are primarily treated.[40] A dedicated OR may not be economically feasible or medically necessary in certain situations,[39,40] but alternative methods for providing immediate OR access must be available and continually monitored.

Some investigators support direct transport to the OR for resuscitation of severely injured patients.[41] In centers treating predominantly penetrating trauma or when specific criteria are met (Table 38–4), all preparations commence with the prehospital call. The ED is bypassed, and the patient is transported directly to the OR for evaluation and resuscitation. This approach may require dispatching an ED nurse to the OR or additional training of the OR staff because they now assume responsibilities for diagnosis and initial stabilization in addition to definitive surgery.

## What Factors Modify the Ideal Situation?

There are many variances from ideal situations, and the following suggestions may help resolve some problems.

### Patient Volume

A small trauma patient volume does not have to equate with inadequate preparation. Commitment and a constant state of awareness are keys to avoiding problems. The trauma staff is accountable for checking the availability and working order

**TABLE 38–4.** Criteria for Direct Admission to Operating Room

Penetrating trauma with cardiac arrest
Witnessed cardiac arrest
Hypovolemic shock unresponsive to fluid resuscitation
Penetrating trauma to the torso
Major nonguillotine amputation or degloving injury
Evisceration of abdominal contents
Severe maxillofacial injuries
Interhospital transfer with known need for immediate surgery

of trauma room equipment and supplies at the beginning of each work shift. The degree of personal accountability correlates directly with the amount of essential supplies available during an emergency resuscitation or operation.

### Supervisory Personnel

Injured patients frequently arrive during the off hours when the on-call crew lacks full supervisory and support personnel. Continuous training and education are essential to maintain familiarity with patient preparation and essential policies such as emergency blood procurement. Continuous training and reassessment of the system by individual practitioners are essential in maintaining readiness.

## What Can Be Done to Speed Up the System?

A working knowledge of system resources and a little creativity can produce a more efficient system. The trauma team activation system described earlier saves considerable time in notifying appropriate personnel.

### Patient Identification

A reliable patient identification system is crucial because multiple patients often arrive unidentified. Our system uses prearranged aliases and computer-generated medical record numbers. When proper identification is obtained, the correct name is applied along with the alias to the medical record number. The patient is thus identified with the same medical record number throughout hospitalization regardless of the name change.

### Enhanced Communication

Communication is improved with fax machines between the laboratory, radiology department, ED, and OR. Fax machines are also useful in rural systems with prolonged interhospital transport times. Our system supports immediate patient transfer once the necessity is determined. Awaiting laboratory results and radiographic interpretations should not delay transfer. Patients who may need blood transfusions are sent with uncrossmatched O-negative blood. Laboratory data and radiographic interpretations are faxed to the trauma center when available.

### Documentation

Information control and documentation are essential. Resuscitation procedures are concurrently recorded to document and assist with each phase of care. The recorder is preferably a nurse or paramedic. Most important is that the person selected for recording be a trained observer familiar with the terminology, personnel, and procedures involved in trauma resuscitation.

A trauma resuscitation flow sheet reduces the amount of narrative documentation and is useful to the recorder, primary nurse, and quality improvement auditor. All data including the flow sheet, laboratory results, radiographs, and any other pertinent information remains with the patient throughout re-

**TABLE 38–5.** Blunt Trauma Series of Radiographs*

| | |
|---|---|
| Lateral cervical spine | AP pelvis |
| Supine AP chest† | AP cervical spine |
| Lateral thoracic spine | Swimmer's view lower cervical spine |
| Lateral lumbar spine | |

*Any study may be deleted by the team leader based on a patient's presentation and stability.
†May be delayed until after spinal films are obtained if the patient is stable and an upright film is desired.
AP, anteroposterior.

suscitation. This eliminates errors of mistaken identity and provides readily available data to consulting physicians.

### Radiology

The radiology department has a crucial role, particularly following blunt trauma. Placing cassettes for chest and pelvic radiographs on the stretcher before patient arrival is a simple maneuver to save time. Developing a predetermined series and order for obtaining radiographs minimizes diagnostic time.

Radiology technicians are trained to anticipate the common machine settings necessary (settings by weight are posted in the trauma room and on the portable radiograph machine for easy reference). A blunt trauma series is ordered for over 90% of the severely injured patients in our facility (Table 38–5). Adding extremity films or deleting unnecessary films from the blunt trauma series is a simple process.

### Computed Tomography

CT has become a standard of care for trauma victims. Maximum benefit is achieved if the scanner is rapid, readily available, and in close proximity to the resuscitation area. If the CT suite is occupied, evacuation occurs as soon as possible after trauma team activation. CT is reserved until trauma patient evaluation is complete or the scanner is released by the attending trauma surgeon.

### Subspecialist Response

Subspecialty surgeon response should not be a source of delay. A formal call list of subspecialty surgeons needed for trauma care must be accurate and readily available.

### Environment and Leadership

The final components to expedite care are complementary: environment and leadership. The environment in the resuscitation room must be calm and controlled, allowing clear communication and coordination of team efforts.

The trauma surgeon is usually responsible for providing direction and maintaining control. Philosophic arguments are unacceptable, create inefficiency, and detract from the resuscitation. The individual with the most experience in treating critically injured trauma patients—surgeon, anesthesiologist, emergency physician, or other—should assume a leadership role.

# INITIAL PATIENT ASSESSMENT AND RESUSCITATION STRATEGY

## What Is Advanced Trauma Life Support?

The Committee on Trauma of the American College of Surgeons through the ATLS Course has developed guidelines for the initial assessment and resuscitation of critically injured patients.[42] Many of the recommendations and guidelines for therapy outlined in this chapter are derived from our experience using the techniques and recommendations so described.

## Why Is Initial Assessment Critical?

Most injured patients are not life threatened. The difficulty is in differentiating those 10% to 15% of critically injured patients who can rapidly deteriorate and die without proper care. Initial physiologic parameters may be misleading, and the mechanism of injury must be considered during triage and evaluation.

Assessment and resuscitation occurs simultaneously in unstable patients. Effective management requires knowledge of cardiopulmonary physiology, injury kinematics, and performance of certain manual tasks. Understanding how to deal with patients and families during stressful situations is helpful.

### Diagnostic and Therapeutic Priorities

Definitive diagnosis is low priority during initial resuscitation and may delay lifesaving resuscitative measures. For example, it is important to determine quickly the presence of hemoperitoneum but not the actual source of bleeding, and recognizing that ventilation or oxygenation is inadequate is the only prerequisite for starting appropriate therapy. A systematic approach provides the best results because rapid assessment and resuscitation are crucial for survival.

### Primary Survey

The primary survey is a process for evaluating the ABCs of life support:

**A.** Airway assessment (with cervical spine immobilization)
**B.** Breathing assessment
**C.** Establishment of circulation and control of major hemorrhage
**D.** Disability assessment, with a brief neurologic examination
**E.** Environmental control and exposure of the patient by removing all clothing for complete evaluation[42]

Correction of physiologic abnormalities related to the ABCs occurs as they are identified.

### Secondary Survey

The secondary survey is a complete head-to-toe examination with further neurologic assessment once stabilization is achieved. Diagnostic studies such as cervical spine radiographs, CT scans, abdominal ultrasonography (US), and angiography are performed at this time.

**TABLE 38–6.** AMPLE History

| | |
|---|---|
| A | Allergies |
| M | Medications (current) |
| P | Past medical and surgical history, pregnancy |
| L | Last meal, last tetanus booster, last menses |
| E | Events and environment related to the injury |

Modified from The Committee on Trauma, American College of Surgeons. *Advanced Trauma Life Support for Doctors.* Chicago, Ill: American College of Surgeons; 1997:35.

### Definitive Care

The definitive care phase usually occurs in the OR or the intensive care unit (ICU). Continuous reassessment during the first 24 hours of hospitalization is crucial. Reevaluation often identifies other less serious injuries that were not initially apparent.

## What Historical Information Is Important?

A patient's history is obtained from any available source. Prehospital personnel are helpful with mechanism of injury and describing important prognostic parameters such as initial neurologic status and vital signs. Witnesses to the accident or other injured patients may be helpful. Family members are often needed to provide the patient's medical history. A rapid AMPLE history is all that is required (Table 38–6). These data may be obtained by any member of the trauma team during the initial resuscitation (eg, a social worker or chaplain) while the physicians and nursing staff are treating the patient.

## What If the Patient Is Combative or Uncooperative?

The approach to evaluating an awake, alert, cooperative patient is less complicated than the global evaluation needed for patients with multiple injuries arriving comatose, combative, or uncooperative. If a patient can answer appropriately, proper questioning can direct the examination to identify potentially serious injuries.

Initial questions are directed toward identifying life-threatening or debilitating injuries. Alcohol- or drug-intoxicated patients give unreliable responses and evaluation must be guided by other factors. Combative, uncooperative behavior should not be considered secondary to alcohol or drug intoxication if the mechanism of injury supports a reasonable probability of head injury. Although drugs or alcohol may cause such behavior, closed head injury and hypoxemia may also be contributing factors. Rapid control of these patients with sedation, paralysis, and orotracheal intubation can expedite the evaluation process. The incidence of significant intracranial pathology in our combative patient population is 42%.[43]

## What Are the Components of the Primary Survey?

Injured patients are assessed and treatment priorities are established based on physiologic parameters. Vital signs (pulse, respiratory rate, oxygen saturation, and BP) are quickly assessed, and treatment is initiated with the goals of improving physiologic parameters, alleviating hypoxia, and eliminating hypercarbia.

## Airway and Cervical Spine Protection

Prehospital endotracheal intubation improves survival in patients with severe head injury.[44] Establishing a patent airway is the first priority of resuscitation. Failure to respond appropriately to verbal questioning may indicate an airway problem or brain injury. Hypoxia may cause severe agitation, and hypercarbia can cause extreme obtundation.

Unconscious and obtunded patients are intubated to protect the airway, deliver supplemental oxygen, and support ventilation. Proper oxygenation and adequate ventilation reduce the risk of secondary brain injury. Indeed, in the prehospital setting the only skill that consistently improves outcome in trauma patients is the ability to provide an airway.[45]

### Clinical Signs of Airway Obstruction

Various noninvasive forms of airway control are helpful, including chin lift, jaw thrust, and oropharyngeal or nasopharyngeal airways. A "tonsil" suction tip should be available to clear the upper airway of secretions and foreign bodies. Stridor, gurgling, or sonorous respirations indicate airway obstruction. Hoarseness or inability to speak clearly suggests a laryngeal fracture. Immediate airway control is obtained if these findings are present or if the patient is extremely anxious or combative.

Fiberoptic-guided placement of an orotracheal tube is preferred for patients with laryngeal fractures if the equipment and expertise are available. This technique guards against false passage of the tube or aggravation of the injury. Tracheostomy is the only alternative if orotracheal intubation fails, because cricothyroidotomy is contraindicated for laryngeal fracture. Victims of falls, motor vehicle crashes, and isolated head injuries are at high risk for associated cervical spine injury, and the cervical spine must be protected during maneuvers used for airway control. Techniques to protect the cervical spine while obtaining airway control must be mastered by personnel involved in the care of trauma patients. Delaying intubation while the cervical spine is cleared with roentgenograms is not acceptable.

### Techniques of Intubation

**Orotracheal.** A growing body of knowledge supports planned neuromuscular blockade in the emergency setting for orotracheal intubation. This technique is now the preferred method of airway control in most trauma patients.[42] In emergency situations, cervical spine evaluation and nasogastric tube insertion should not be done before orotracheal intubation. Stimulating the oropharynx during passage of a nasogastric tube may induce vomiting and cause aspiration of gastric contents.[46]

**Nasotracheal.** Nasotracheal intubation is avoided in patients with suspected maxillofacial injuries. Any patient with suspected head injury may have an anterior fossa basilar skull fracture. Potential complications of nasotracheal intubation include inadvertent placement of the tube through the cribriform plate into the brain.[47] Other potential problems include bacteremia from nasal bacteria and mucosal abrasion[48] and later complications of maxillary sinusitis[49] and otitis media.[50]

Nasotracheal intubation is more difficult to perform in intoxicated or combative patients. A smaller endotracheal tube (ETT) is usually required, causing increased work of breathing during spontaneous ventilation. ETT insertion may also increase intracranial pressure (ICP) if a patient is not adequately sedated. In combative trauma victims, adequate sedation is often not achieved without dangerously high doses of sedatives, which can severely depress spontaneous ventilation, a requirement for successful nasotracheal intubation. This method of intubation is more difficult to master unless frequently performed.

### Emergency Cricothyroidotomy

Emergency cricothyroidotomy is reserved for patients with severe facial injuries or upper airway obstruction in which orotracheal intubation is prohibitive. It is performed by making either a vertical or horizontal skin incision over the area of the cricothyroid membrane. A scalpel blade (No. 11 or 15) is used to incise directly through the cricothyroid membrane, and either a curved hemostat or Trousseau's tracheal dilator is inserted to open the cricothyroid membrane for passage of a 7- to 8-mm endotracheal or tracheostomy tube.

The neck is kept in neutral position during this procedure. Cricothyroidotomy is not recommended in children younger than 12 years of age because of potential damage to the cricoid cartilage, the only totally circumferential support for the upper trachea in children.

Cricothyroidotomy is recommended over tracheotomy because the technique is relatively simple, easy to learn by individuals with a nonsurgical background, and, theoretically, is performed in a bloodless plane. Under emergency conditions, however, it is frequently a bloody procedure. Little and colleagues[51] studied the region anterior to the cricothyroid membrane in 34 adult cadavers; 79% of the cadavers had vascular structures within the area of cricothyroidotomy. Other potential complications of cricothyroidotomy include permanent voice change, bleeding at the surgical site, wound infection, and the most serious complication, subglottic stenosis.

### Emergency Tracheotomy

Tracheotomy has no place in the emergency setting for airway control except in patients with an obstructing laryngeal fracture in whom fiberoptic-guided orotracheal intubation is unsuccessful. Cricothyroidotomy is not recommended in cases of laryngeal fracture.

### Other Methods of Emergency Airway Control

Difficulty with endotracheal intubation in the prehospital setting led to the development and promotion of a number of different methods for airway control. These include the esophageal obturator airway (EOA), the esophageal gastric tube airway (EGTA), and the pharyngotracheal lumen airway (PTLA). Another addition to this armamentarium is the esophageal tracheal Combitube (ETC) (Combitube, Sheridan Catheter Corp, Argyle, NY). Physicians and personnel involved in the management of trauma patients should be familiar with these tubes because of their use in the prehospital setting. These tubes should be exchanged for an orotracheal tube on arrival in the ED. One study suggested that the ETC may be useful in the ED for trauma patients who fail rapid sequence intubation.[52]

## Breathing-Ventilation Assessment

Tension pneumothorax, flail chest, open pneumothorax, and massive hemothorax are conditions that interfere with ventilation and cardiac preload. These conditions must be rapidly diagnosed and treated during the primary survey.

### Tension Pneumothorax

Tension pneumothorax is often a clinical rather than a radiologic diagnosis if a patient presents with severe respiratory distress and hypotension.

**Pathophysiology.** This abnormality occurs when a bronchial injury or a parenchymal lung injury allows air movement into the pleural space. As the amount of air in the pleural space increases, the lung collapses, causing inadequate ventilation. Increasing pressure on mediastinal structures causes decreased blood return to the heart and diminished cardiac output.

**Diagnosis.** The noisy ED environment makes chest examination difficult. The reported signs of tracheal deviation to the unaffected hemithorax, distended neck veins, unilateral absent breath sounds, and cyanosis are not always present, especially in hypovolemic patients. More commonly, patients present with grunting respirations, respiratory distress, a decrease in pulse pressure, and extreme agitation.

**Treatment.** Tension pneumothorax requires immediate treatment. Documentation of the abnormality with a chest radiograph is unnecessary and potentially dangerous in unstable patients. Rapid insertion of a 14- or 16-gauge intravenous catheter into the second intercostal space at the midclavicular line of the affected hemithorax is the initial emergency treatment. A sudden rush of air from the chest cavity confirms the clinical diagnosis. A large-bore chest tube (36-40 French) is inserted through the fifth intercostal space in the midaxillary line and directed posteriorly and superiorly after initial decompression. This tube position adequately removes both air and blood. Small-bore tubes frequently become obstructed with blood clots and are not recommended in adults.

### Open Pneumothorax

Large chest wall defects associated with pulmonary parenchymal injuries can create an open pneumothorax (*sucking chest wound*).

**Pathophysiology.** Chest wounds that are at least two thirds the diameter of the trachea create preferential air movement through the chest wall with each respiratory effort. This abnormal equilibration between intrathoracic and atmospheric pressure causes poor ventilation and hypoxia.

**Treatment.** The defect is covered with air- and water-resistant bandages (such as petroleum jelly gauze) and tube thoracostomy is performed to prevent tension pneumothorax.

### Flail Chest

**Pathophysiology.** Flail chest occurs when a segment of the chest wall becomes completely disconnected from the remainder of the bony thorax. This problem occurs when two or more ribs are fractured in at least two places. The chest wall segment moves paradoxically in the opposite direction of the thorax during spontaneous breathing.

**Management.** Hypoxemia and hypercapnia can occur with flail chest. Immediate tracheal intubation and mechanical ventilation are usually necessary. Ventilatory dysfunction is caused by decreased vital capacity, functional residual capacity, and total lung volume. The degree of underlying pulmonary contusion determines the severity of ventilation-perfusion mismatch and anatomic shunting.

Therapy consists of prolonged mechanical ventilation with continuous positive airway pressure until the underlying pulmonary abnormality resolves. Splinting, traction, or operative stabilization of the chest wall is usually unnecessary.

### Massive Hemothorax

**Pathophysiology.** Massive hemothorax, defined as >1500 mL of blood in the chest cavity, presents as signs and symptoms similar to tension pneumothorax, although distended neck veins are not present. Massive hemothorax is usually caused by penetrating chest trauma, but it may also be due to blunt force injury.

**Management.** One or more large-bore (36-40 French) chest tubes are inserted posteriorly through the fifth intercostal space along with rapid volume resuscitation.

Thoracic exploration is determined by the rate of continued blood loss rather than the initial volume removed. A persistent blood loss rate of 200 mL/h usually requires operative intervention because the bleeding is frequently from a lacerated intercostal or internal mammary artery, a branch of the pulmonary vein, or the aorta.[42] Parenchymal lung bleeding usually subsides with lung reexpansion because the pulmonary vasculature is a relatively low pressure system.

## Circulation Assessment

Level of consciousness, rate and quality of peripheral pulses, and identification of bleeding sources are important assessment features. A quick assessment of BP, pulse, mental status, respiratory rate, and urine output allows classification of the level of circulatory dysfunction (Table 38–7). In young adults and children, mental status and BP may remain nearly normal until massive blood loss occurs. Children and young adults have tremendous hemodynamic reserve and a capacity for prolonged vasoconstriction. Hypotension may not develop until 30% to 40% of blood volume is lost.

### Immediate Care Priorities

Immediate control of any external bleeding with direct pressure is initiated. Vascular clamps are not used on open wounds because inadvertent nerve injury may occur. Bleeding from most wounds is adequately controlled with sterile compressive dressings secured by either an air splint or elastic wrap until further definitive management is possible. Exceptions are major scalp and facial lacerations, which are difficult to control with direct pressure. These are better managed with either temporary large mattress sutures or disposable Raney clips. Cosmetic closure is accomplished after life-threatening problems are resolved.

**Restoration of Perfusion.** The initial goal is to restore tissue perfusion to vital organs. Sophisticated monitoring in the ED is usually unavailable and unnecessary. Persistent

**TABLE 38–7.** Classes of Hypovolemic Shock With Estimated Fluid and Blood Requirements (70-kg Man)

|  | Class I | Class II | Class III | Class IV |
|---|---|---|---|---|
| Blood loss (mL) | Up to 750 | 750-1500 | 1500-2000 | 2000 or more |
| Blood loss (% blood volume) | Up to 15% | 15-30% | 30-40% | 40% or more |
| Pulse rate | <100 | >100 | >120 | 140 or higher |
| Blood pressure | Normal | Normal | Decreased | Decreased |
| Pulse pressure (mm Hg) | Normal or increased | Decreased | Decreased | Decreased |
| Respiratory rate | 14-20 | 20-30 | 30-40 | >35 |
| Urine output (mL/h) | 30 or more | 20-30 | 5-15 | Negligible |
| CNS—mental status | Slightly anxious | Mildly anxious | Anxious and confused | Confused, lethargic |
| Fluid replacement (3:1 rule) | Crystalloid | Crystalloid | Crystalloid + blood | Crystalloid + blood |

Modified from The Committee on Trauma, American College of Surgeons. *Advanced Trauma Life Support for Doctors.* Chicago, Ill: American College of Surgeons; 1997:98.

tachycardia (>120 beats per minute [BPM]) after infusion of 2 L crystalloid suggests continued bleeding. Tachycardia may be blunted in patients who are prescribed β-blockers or digitalis and in patients with cervical spinal cord injuries.

Diminished pulse pressure is a frequent early sign of significant blood loss or pericardial tamponade. Muffled heart sounds, jugular venous distention, hypotension, and pulsus paradoxus are pathognomonic of pericardial tamponade, but the signs are frequently absent in hypovolemic patients. US is the most rapid noninvasive method for confirming the diagnosis.[53]

**Intravenous Catheter Sites.** Two large-bore (12-16 gauge) peripheral intravenous catheters are inserted immediately on arrival in the ED. The antecubital fossa is a reliable site for rapid venous access. Central venous catheters are usually avoided during the initial resuscitation because of potential complications.

The femoral veins are useful and usually accessible if burns or injury prohibits upper extremity access. An 8.5 or 9.0 French pulmonary artery (PA) catheter introducer is useful for femoral access if rapid volume resuscitation is needed. A flow rate of 1 L/min is possible if a pressure infusion device is used. Successful resuscitation through the femoral vein can be done even if intraabdominal injuries are present.

The subclavian or internal jugular routes are cannulated if necessary. In hypovolemic patients the subclavian vein may be easier to cannulate because of its fascial attachments, but iatrogenic pneumothorax can significantly complicate resuscitation efforts.

**Blood Pressure.** Systolic BP can be estimated by palpating pulses at various levels. A palpable radial pulse usually indicates a systolic BP of at least 80 mm Hg; a femoral pulse, 70 mm Hg; and a carotid pulse, 60 mm Hg. Compensatory mechanisms maintain cerebral blood flow until systolic pressure falls to <60 mm Hg.

**Fluid-Transfusion Therapy.** Initial fluid resuscitation is both therapeutic and prognostic. Two liters of Ringer's injection, lactated, or normal saline is infused over 5 to 10 minutes (thus the need for large-bore catheters). If BP and heart rate improve, hypovolemia is the probable cause of shock.

A blood sample is obtained during intravenous catheter insertion for type and screen or crossmatch, serum electrolytes, and a complete blood cell count. If appropriate, a blood alcohol level and urine toxicology screen are also obtained. Type-specific blood is usually available within 15 to 30 minutes. Fully crossmatched blood requires up to 1 hour to prepare for infusion.

Patients who are severely hypovolemic and unresponsive to initial crystalloid resuscitation may need uncrossmatched O-negative blood. Emergency thoracotomy or exploratory laparotomy may be necessary if the patient fails to respond. Appropriate red blood cell–saving devices can aid in the recovery of ongoing blood loss.

There is clinical evidence to support delayed fluid and blood resuscitation in patients with penetrating trauma where prehospital transport times are short (<10 minutes) and immediate access to the OR is available.[54,55] Volume resuscitation is mandatory, however, when prehospital times are >10 minutes, OR availability is not immediate, and blunt force is the mechanism of injury.

**Pneumatic Antishock Garment.** Prospective randomized studies have shown that a pneumatic antishock garment (PASG) is not indicated when prehospital transport times are short.[56] Currently the only strong indication for using a PASG is for splinting extremity and pelvic fractures to control bleeding. The PASG inflated to high pressures increases systemic vascular resistance, elevates systolic BP, and may reduce cardiac output by increasing afterload and stimulating bleeding at levels above the PASG application. Inflating the abdominal compartment may impair venous return by compressing the inferior vena cava.[56]

The PASG has been associated with compartment syndrome and limb loss in patients with either multiple injuries or isolated extremity injuries.[57] Despite these potential problems, the PASG is still useful in situations in which prehospital transport times may be prolonged (>20 minutes).

**Emergency Department Thoracotomy.** Primary therapy may include ED thoracotomy under certain clinical conditions. This procedure is performed only by physicians experienced in the technique and only when access to an OR is immediately available.

A study by Branney and associates[58] showed that ED thoracotomy was both efficacious and cost-effective in select patient populations. The patients most likely to benefit from ED thoracotomy are those with stab wounds to the chest and abdominal gunshot wounds.[58] Overall survival after ED thoracotomy in 868 patients over a 23-year period was 4.4%, with 3.9% surviving functionally intact.[58] ED thoracotomy after blunt trauma is generally not indicated. However, these investigators showed that the functional survival after ED thoracotomy was 2.5% in blunt trauma patients with either a palpable pulse or a recorded BP in the field.

Other investigators[30,59] recommended that strict prehospital criteria be met before submitting a pulseless patient with penetrating trauma to an ED thoracotomy. Battistella and coworkers reviewed 604 victims of prehospital traumatic cardiopulmonary arrest. There were no survivors in the 212 patients who had either asystole or agonal electrical cardiac activity (heart rate <40 BPM) despite aggressive resuscitation efforts. They recommended that these patients should be pronounced dead at the scene of injury.[30] Local hospital resources, the overall incidence of penetrating trauma, and individual surgical expertise with ED thoracotomy dictates whether this procedure becomes a part of the primary resuscitation.

## Disability-Neurologic Assessment

Neurologic assessment is limited to level of consciousness, pupillary reflexes, and extremity motor response. This assessment should take no more than 1 minute. The AVPU method[42] is a simple technique to describe level of consciousness (Table 38–8). Pupillary size and reaction are also recorded.

The GCS is used during the primary assessment or later during the secondary survey (see Table 38–1). If a patient requires neuromuscular blockade and tracheal intubation, a rapid neurologic assessment including extremity motor strength and GCS is performed. Extremity movement is documented before giving paralytic agents. Sluggish or absent movement of one or both lower extremities in response to painful stimulation may be a sign of spinal cord injury. Remember, however, that local spinal reflexes may be present with complete spinal cord injuries.

Therapeutic neurosurgical interventions are frequently performed based on an accurate GCS.[60] Uniform and accurate scoring is essential before treatment algorithms, trauma scoring, therapeutic interventions, and outcome prediction are based on GCS.[61] Other studies suggest that the GCS, particularly the motor component, may be the best field predictor of the need for trauma center care and trauma team activation.[62,63]

## Exposure and Environmental Control

The patient is completely undressed and carefully logrolled to examine the posterior torso. Complete exposure is essential to assess for other injuries during the secondary survey.

It is important to keep the patient warm by increasing room temperature and using warm blankets or other external warming devices to prevent hypothermia. Warm intravenous fluids are given to maintain normal core body temperature.

Normothermia reduces the risks of coagulopathy and wound infection.[64]

## *What Is Done During the Secondary Survey?*

The secondary survey is a complete but rapid head-to-toe physical assessment to identify other nonimmediate but potentially life- or limb-threatening injuries. The secondary survey is performed after resuscitation efforts have been initiated, the primary survey has been completed, and the patient's condition has stabilized.[42]

## Radiologic Studies

Further radiologic evaluation is performed during the secondary survey. In those patients with high-velocity blunt force mechanisms, a blunt trauma series of radiographs is helpful to screen for major chest, pelvic, and spinal injuries (see Table 38–5). Certain films in the series may not be needed in awake patients who can give a reliable history and physical examination. Radiographs in cooperative patients can be directed to symptomatic areas identified on physical examination. Further extremity evaluation may identify other injuries that require radiographic confirmation.

## Focused Assessment for the Sonographic Examination of the Trauma

Focused assessment for the sonographic examination of the trauma patient (FAST) is a reliable screening test for diagnosing blunt intraabdominal and intrathoracic trauma.[65,66] The inaccuracy of physical examination alone for blunt abdominal trauma has encouraged trauma physicians to use abdominal US, which can be performed simultaneously with ongoing resuscitation measures in the ED. This modality is safe, noninvasive, and inexpensive and may be repeated frequently.[66] A FAST examination is performed primarily to identify free fluid (blood or enteric fluid) within the abdominal and thoracic cavities and to diagnose pericardial tamponade. A specific sequence for the examination has been described previously.[65,66] FAST is performed either during the initial resuscitation phase immediately after the primary survey or later during the secondary survey. Immediate identification of a large hemoperitoneum may eliminate the need for further investigation until definitive operation is performed.

## Cervical Spine

Patients with severe maxillofacial or head trauma and all combative, uncooperative, or unconscious patients must be evaluated for cervical spine injuries. Initial assessment consists of anteroposterior, lateral, and odontoid cervical spine radiographs. If any question of cervical spine injury remains after these studies are completed, immobilization must be maintained.

The absence of neck symptoms does not completely eliminate the possibility of cervical spine injury. Obtunded or comatose patients are maintained in proper cervical immobilization until further definitive studies are performed regardless of whether plain radiographs are normal. Definitive evaluation consists of either a reliable clinical examination when the patient is awake and alert,[67] flexion-extension radiographs, preferably under fluoroscopy to rule out instability,[68] cervical CT with sagittal reconstruction imaging, or magnetic resonance imaging.

Immobilization is maintained in patients wearing a sports or motorcycle helmet while the helmet is removed.[42]

## Blunt Carotid and Vertebral Artery Injuries

Patients presenting with hemiparesis or hemiplegia may have blunt carotid or vertebral artery injuries. Early recogni-

---

**TABLE 38–8.** Brief Neurologic Assessment During the Primary Survey: AVPU

| | |
|---|---|
| A | Alert |
| V | Responsive to vocal stimuli |
| P | Responsive to painful stimuli |
| U | Unresponsive to all stimuli |

Modified from The Committee on Trauma, American College of Surgeons. *Advanced Trauma Life Support for Doctors.* Chicago, Ill: American College of Surgeons; 1997:30.

tion and diagnosis of this devastating injury are crucial for meaningful recovery. Treatment may be operative or nonoperative with anticoagulation depending on angiographic or magnetic resonance angiography findings and on associated injuries. Once believed to be rare, recent evidence suggests that these devastating injuries are increasing in incidence.[69] Brain CT is of limited value immediately after the injury, and only a heightened suspicion of this potentially life-threatening injury followed by emergency angiography (or magnetic resonance angriography) and rapid treatment will improve outcome and survival.

## Pericardial Tamponade and Tension Pneumothorax

Closer examination of the chest may reveal subtle changes that were not initially apparent during the primary survey. Distant heart sounds and distended neck veins signify possible pericardial tamponade or tension pneumothorax. Pericardiocentesis or needle decompression of the chest may be needed if the clinical condition deteriorates. These procedures may have already been performed during the primary survey if the patient arrived in a severely compromised state. Subxiphoid sagittal views of the heart, performed during the FAST examination, are helpful in diagnosing acute pericardial tamponade.[53]

## Pulmonary Contusion

Pulmonary contusions may cause severe hypoxia and are usually associated with chest wall trauma. Arterial blood gas analysis is obtained if multiple rib fractures or chest wall contusions are identified. Patients may be tachypneic if hypoxemia is significant. Early management is supportive with tracheal intubation and mechanical ventilation. Treatment with positive end-expiratory pressure is beneficial in reducing the physiologic shunt fraction and work of breathing.

## Blunt Cardiac Injury

Blunt cardiac injury (BCI) is often difficult to diagnose because most patients present with multiple injuries. BCI may be overlooked except in the severe cases in which victims present with multiple arrhythmias or cardiogenic shock. The clinical manifestations are variable and dependent on the magnitude of myocardial muscle injury. One should suspect BCI with any high-energy blow to the chest. Sternal fracture should increase the suspicion. The most common mechanism of injury is a direct blow when the anterior chest wall strikes a steering wheel.

Diagnosing BCI after blunt thoracic trauma is controversial and occasionally difficult.[70]

### Physical Findings

Conscious patients may develop angina with severe injuries. The clinical spectrum of symptoms found with myocardial infarction (MI) and occasionally cardiogenic shock may be present.[71,72] Cardiogenic shock after isolated BCI is rare and usually indicates ventricular septal or valve injury. In addition to myocardial contusion, other BCIs include myocardial rupture, septal perforation, coronary artery dissection, pericardial rupture (with potential for cardiac herniation), ruptured valve cusps, and papillary muscle or chordae tendineae rupture.[70]

Biffl and associates, using multivariate analysis of risk factors for BCI, found that an abnormal electrocardiogram was the most significant independent predictor of complications after BCI.[71] Two-dimensional echocardiography should be performed as soon as possible when significant dysrhythmias or other electrocardiographic abnormalities are present. Abnormal segmental heart wall motion, cardiac wall thinning, myocardial hematomas, chamber dilation, intracavitary filling defects (from hematomas), valvular dysfunction, and increased pericardial fluid are some of the findings considered diagnostic for BCI.[70–72]

### Laboratory Testing

Creatine kinase (CK)-MB is the most commonly used laboratory test for diagnosing BCI, but small amounts of the CK-MB isoenzyme are found in skeletal muscle and other body tissues, making the test nonspecific. More recently, a new enzyme assay, cardiac troponin I, has been recommended as more specific for cardiac injury. We have found this enzyme to be as nonspecific as CK-MB in diagnosing myocardial injury.

No single laboratory test absolutely confirms the diagnosis, and CK-MB elevation alone is not a reliable predictor of complications after BCI.[71] Biffl and coworkers have recommended that cardiac enzyme determinations be eliminated in the evaluation of patients for BCI.[71] The prognosis for most patients with BCI is excellent. Superficial or limited full-thickness contusions usually heal without permanent disability.

## Thoracic Aortic Disruption

Patients injured from severe deceleration mechanisms (falls, motor vehicle crashes, vehicle-pedestrian accidents) are at increased risk for thoracic aortic injury. A portable supine anteroposterior 36-inch chest radiograph is obtained in any patient with chest trauma. Stable patients who can tolerate the sitting position receive a 72-inch erect anteroposterior chest radiograph for better evaluation of the mediastinum.

### Physical Findings

Some patients with thoracic aortic disruption may have minimal or no physical findings. Major chest wall contusions and sternal fractures are all indications for further evaluation. Diminished breath sounds in the left side of the chest due to massive hemothorax may indicate aortic injury or other great vessel injury. Upper extremity hypertension compared with the lower extremities is an unusual but diagnostic sign. Awake patients may complain of severe chest and back pain or dyspnea.

### Radiographic Findings

The chest radiograph may be normal. Loss of aortic knob contour on an anteroposterior supine or upright chest radiograph indicates possible mediastinal hematoma. A widened superior mediastinum >8 cm at the aortic isthmus, depression of the left main stem bronchus of >140°, a left apical hematoma (apical cap), and massive left hemothorax all suggest aortic injury.

Recent clinical studies support the use of contrast medium–enhanced spiral CT to diagnose thoracic aortic injury.[73,74] Demetriades and associates[75] recommend that all trauma patients with high-risk deceleration injuries undergo chest CT because 44% of patients with aortic rupture in their study had a normal chest radiograph. If the enhanced spiral CT is negative for mediastinal hemorrhage or aortic abnormality, then no further work-up is necessary. However, aortography is required if CT is positive for aortic injury or if mediastinal blood is present.

### Important Prognostic Factors

Thoracic aortic injuries are associated with a high prehospital mortality rate. Survival in patients who reach the hospital alive is <50%.[76] Most patients who survive to the ED have a tear in the descending aorta just distal to the left subclavian artery. Patients who are unstable at the scene or during the first 4 hours of hospitalization have a mortality rate >90%.[76] Stable patients who are treated nonoperatively with afterload reducing agents and β-blockers (assuming other injuries are survivable) have a >90% survival rate.[76] Evidence suggests that delaying operative repair of descending aortic injuries in stable patients may improve outcome with less risk of paraplegia from spinal cord ischemia.[73]

### Preoperative Treatment

Initial medical management of aortic injury may include the use of both α- and β-blockers to lower systolic BP and reduce afterload. Such drugs are contraindicated if the patient is hypovolemic from other injuries. Management is challenging and difficult, because many of these patients present with multiple injuries.

### Diaphragmatic Injuries

Diaphragmatic injuries are usually the result of blunt torso trauma or penetrating stab wounds. These injuries occur in 1% to 5% of hospitalized patients after motor vehicle crashes and in 10% to 15% of patients with penetrating trauma to the lower chest.[77] Rapid deceleration against a malpositioned lap belt restraint is a common cause. Crush injuries and falls are also common mechanisms. Eighty-five percent of injuries affect the left hemidiaphragm because the right hemidiaphragm is somewhat protected by the liver, which often absorbs the force generated by compression of the right upper abdomen.

### Physical Findings

Patients may present with severe tachypnea, hypoxemia, and hypercarbia. Diminished breath sounds may be present on the affected side, simulating a pneumothorax. The diagnosis is usually made by chest radiography or CT. Findings on physical examination are rarely pathognomonic because many of these patients have multiple injuries.

### Radiographic Findings

A torn left hemidiaphragm can be diagnosed with a chest radiograph if the stomach, bowel, or other abdominal organ is seen within the left chest. Injury to the right hemidiaphragm is less obvious, appearing as an elevated hemidiaphragm be-cause of herniation of the liver. In this situation, the diagnosis may be confirmed by either fluoroscopy or CT.

### Treatment

Diaphragm injuries require immediate surgery. Initial management includes gastric tube decompression and endotracheal intubation for treatment of respiratory compromise. There are cases of delayed diagnosis. In one study, researchers reported 10 patients with posttraumatic diaphragmatic hernia diagnosed 20 days to 28 years after the initial injury.[77] These patients should undergo urgent diaphragmatic hernia repair as soon as the diagnosis is made. The operative approach for a missed diaphragmatic hernia may be through either the chest or the abdomen.

## Tracheobronchial Injuries

Direct trauma to the trachea may cause life-threatening upper airway obstruction. Stridorous respirations indicate partial airway obstruction. Establishing a patent airway is crucial. Injury to the left or right mainstem bronchus or one of the major bronchioles is an unusual but frequently fatal injury.

These injuries are caused by blunt chest trauma, with the most life-threatening injuries occurring within 1 inch of the carina. Patients present with severe respiratory failure, subcutaneous emphysema, tension pneumothorax, hypotension, and mediastinal shift. Tube thoracostomy is usually diagnostic because a massive air leak is identified after placement. Immediate surgery to repair the defect is required.

## Esophageal Injuries

Most injuries to the esophagus result from penetrating trauma and are usually diagnosed during thoracic exploration for other injuries. Blunt esophageal trauma is rare but frequently lethal if not rapidly diagnosed. The mechanism of injury from blunt trauma to the upper abdomen is a forceful ejection of gastric contents that cause a linear tear in the lower esophagus. Mediastinal air or a left pneumothorax without pulmonary injury or rib fracture suggests this injury. Diagnosis is confirmed by an esophageal contrast study or esophagoscopy.

## Abdominal Injuries

Abdominal trauma ranks third behind head and chest injuries as the most common cause of death from injury. Abdominal stab wounds in stable patients can be treated by local wound exploration to diagnose peritoneal penetration before subjecting the patient to celiotomy. Many abdominal stab wounds do not cause major intraabdominal injury, and nonoperative observation has gained wide acceptance in the absence of hypotension or obvious peritoneal signs on physical examination. A nonoperative approach has also gained some acceptance for management of abdominal gunshot wounds in major trauma centers treating large numbers of penetrating trauma victims. Initial evaluation with abdominal CT followed by selective nonoperative management and careful clinical follow-up has become accepted practice for some injuries.[78–80]

Penetrating chest injuries below the nipple line may cause intraabdominal injury. Diaphragmatic injuries are especially difficult to diagnose. CT may be helpful, although false-negative rates of 40% for small penetrating injuries have been reported.[81] Diagnostic peritoneal lavage (DPL) may be helpful, but this procedure also has reported false-negative rates of 12% to 40%.[81] Diagnostic laparoscopy and thoracoscopy are useful under certain conditions.

## Diagnosis

**Ultrasonography.** Abdominal US evaluation is considered effective in screening for blunt abdominal trauma in adults and pediatric patients.[65,66,82–86] A negative FAST mandates further evaluation either with DPL or abdominal CT if no other explanation for hemodynamic instability is determined.

**Diagnostic Peritoneal Lavage.** DPL is sensitive for detecting intraabdominal blood. Unfortunately, a positive DPL may identify self-limited, solid parenchymal injuries that can often be treated nonoperatively. Henneman and colleagues,[87] in a retrospective review of 994 patients with blunt and penetrating trauma, reported an overall DPL accuracy of 93%, with a positive predictive value of 80% and a negative predictive value of 98% for intraabdominal injury requiring surgical repair.

Any of the following criteria are considered positive after blunt injury: aspiration of >10 mL of gross blood, red blood cell (RBC) count >100 000/mm³, white blood cell (WBC) count >500/mm³, amylase >200 U/L, or bacteria present on microscopic examination of the lavage fluid.

DPL has been recommended for penetrating flank wounds and for through and through gunshot wounds, which may be tangential to the peritoneal cavity.[88] For stab wounds to the lower chest and abdomen, and tangential abdominal gunshot wounds, the following values are considered positive: aspiration of >1 mL of gross blood, RBC count >5000/mm³, WBC >500/mm³, amylase >200 U/L, or the presence of bacteria in the lavage fluid.

**Abdominal Computed Tomography.** Contrast medium–enhanced abdominal CT provides the most comprehensive information in the stable patient. The lower chest is also well visualized, providing diagnostic information for occult pneumothoraces, hemothoraces, and pulmonary contusions. The retroperitoneum, pelvic organs, and skeletal structures are readily visualized. Abdominal CT is considered the gold standard by which other diagnostic modalities (eg, abdominal US) are compared.

A recent study of 2299 patients at four Level I trauma centers presenting with suspected abdominal injury found a 22% incidence of positive findings on abdominal CT in those patients with abdominal tenderness or bruising (a total of 1380 patients). Nineteen percent of patients with positive CT scans had no abdominal tenderness. Free intraperitoneal fluid without solid visceral injury was present in 90 patients, but only 7 patients had intestinal injuries. In this series, CT detected 22 of the 25 blunt intestinal injuries. These data indicate the unreliability of abdominal tenderness for predicting abdominal injury, and in patients with normal abdominal CT scans, hospital admission and observation in the absence of other extraabdominal injuries may not be necessary.[89]

## Intestinal Injuries

Intestinal injuries are difficult to diagnose after blunt abdominal trauma. Inappropriately applied seat belts are associated with intestinal injuries and fractures of the thoracolumbar spine (Chance fractures)[90–92] after high-speed motor vehicle crashes. Rapid deceleration during high-speed crashes can cause sudden flexion around a fixed lap belt with severe compression of abdominal viscera. Children restrained in rear seats with adult lap belts are at high risk for such injuries.[92]

Abdominal US, abdominal CT, and DPL may all give false-negative results. Patients treated nonoperatively for solid organ injuries may have intestinal injuries that are difficult to detect because of the presence of intraabdominal blood. Although oral contrast solution with CT has been recommended in the past, a recent randomized study found oral contrast unhelpful in diagnosing bowel injury.[93] Intraabdominal fluid collections without solid organ injury on abdominal CT are also nondiagnostic. Controversy exists concerning whether these patients should undergo exploratory celiotomy.[94–96] CT findings associated with bowel injury include free fluid, a thickened bowel wall, and extraluminal air.[97] Because of the difficulty in diagnosing bowel injury, and because of the variety of acceptable diagnostic tests, a variety of algorithms to identify bowel injury may be used. Ultimately, repeated clinical evaluation and the patient's overall clinical status will direct care.

## Orthopedic Injuries

Orthopedic injuries are occasionally overlooked in patients with multiple injuries. Fractures may be missed even after a well-performed secondary survey. Identifying open fractures is a crucial first step in management because these require more immediate attention.[98]

Fracture stabilization contributes significantly to the overall recovery of injured patients. Early mobilization and rehabilitation not only reduces orthopedic morbidity but also reduces the risk of pneumonia and deep venous thrombosis.

All fractures are temporarily splinted after the initial resuscitation phase until orthopedic consultation can be arranged. All open fractures require immediate orthopedic consultation. Attention to tetanus prophylaxis and antibiotic therapy is crucial. Patients with open fractures are given a first-generation cephalosporin preoperatively. ED management consists of cleaning the wound with an antiseptic solution and placement of a dry sterile gauze dressing and a light pressure bandage.

### Physical Findings

The secondary survey includes examination of the extremities, spine, and pelvis. Inspection and palpation of the thoracolumbar and cervical spine can identify areas of deformity and tenderness. Inspection and palpation of the extremities may identify areas of edema, deformity, or crepitance, indicating a possible fracture or joint dislocation. Simultaneous neurovascular evaluation distal to the fracture is also performed. Any areas in question undergo radiographic evaluation when the patient is stabilized.

### Radiographic Findings

Patients with potentially unstable cervical spine injuries require immobilization with a rigid cervical collar until further definitive evaluation with a full cervical spine series (including flexion and extension views) can be obtained. Cervical spine CT may be needed to rule out cervical fracture. Unconscious or intoxicated patients are left in the cervical collar until a reliable examination can be performed. Normal antero-posterior, lateral, and odontoid radiographs do not completely rule out cervical spine injury unless accompanied by a normal physical examination.

Patients who are unable to provide adequate histories or respond appropriately to physical examination should have at a minimum screening lateral thoracic and lumbar spine radiographs to identify any major fractures. Any evidence of thoracic or lumbar spine fracture requires orthopedic or neurosurgical evaluation. The upper thoracic spine is especially difficult to evaluate with plain radiographs. This area frequently harbors unstable fractures, and careful evaluation of the thoracic spine both clinically and by the anteroposterior chest and lateral thoracic spine radiograph, along with a swimmer's view of the cervical and upper thoracic spine, may be helpful.

Neurosurgical consultation is obtained immediately after hemodynamic stabilization if signs of spinal cord injury are present.

### Critical Fracture Complications

Fractures and dislocations of the hip or knee, displaced fractures of the tibia and fibula, and fractures or dislocations of the ankle can cause acute compartment syndrome. Permanent neurovascular injuries or skin sloughing may result. Delays beyond 24 hours in reducing a dislocated hip are associated with a nearly 100% risk of aseptic femoral head necrosis.

Upper extremity fractures and dislocations, particularly at the elbow, can be devastating. Diagnosing and correcting or preventing vascular and neurologic injury from extremity fractures and dislocations are crucial. Open fractures are emergencies requiring surgical treatment within 8 hours of injury to minimize infection risks.

**Acute Compartment Syndrome.** Extremity edema and blood loss from closed fractures below the knee or elbow can cause acute compartment syndrome. Severe extremity pain distal to the fracture (eg, in the foot or hand), often described as burning or deep throbbing unrelenting pressure, is the first sign of compartment syndrome. The pain is often disproportional to the clinical findings and is unrelieved by rest or immobilization. Sensory and motor changes are late clinical findings.

Extremity compartment pressure is measured by various methods. A pressure transducer attached to fluid-filled extension tubing and a needle is one technique. Commercially available portable compartmental pressure gauges are more convenient.

Patients with compartmental pressures >30 mm Hg are decompressed surgically unless conservative measures such as elevation and ice packs reduce the swelling within 1 to 2 hours.[99] Surgical decompression is performed immediately if the initial compartment pressure is >40 mm Hg or the pressure exceeds 30 mm Hg for more than 1 hour.[99]

### Burns

Burn patients are treated early and aggressively using the principles of ATLS.[29] Principles outlined in the primary survey are followed with a high index of suspicion for smoke inhalation and upper airway compromise from edema.

Patients with facial burns are at particularly high risk for upper airway edema even if the initial assessment is unremarkable. These patients are best treated with early intubation, particularly if prolonged transport to a burn center is anticipated. There are a number of methods to determine the percentage of body surface area burn.

Anatomic burn charts indicating the body surface area for both adults and children are available in most EDs. If burn charts are not available, the *rule of nines* is a handy technique for determining the percent of body surface area involved. In adults, the anterior lower extremity surface represents 9%, the posterior lower extremity surface 9%, the anterior torso 18%, the posterior torso (including the buttocks) 18%, the entire surface of each upper extremity 9%, the head and face 9%, and the genitalia 1%.[29] These percentages change in children, with the head comprising 18% of the body surface area and each lower extremity only 14%.

Another method is to use the patient's palm size (not including the fingers), which correlates to 1% of the body surface area. High-voltage electrical injuries and victims of lightning strike are at particular risk for cardiac dysrhythmia and injury.[100,101] The extent of burn tissue in patients with electrical injury may not be apparent on initial examination. Entrance and exit wounds indicate the path of electrical current and may be the only finding on physical examination. Underlying tissue damage may be extensive, and these patients are best treated at a burn center.

The guiding principles for burn care include early airway control, aggressive volume resuscitation to maintain urine output at approximately 1 mL/kg/h, and early transfer to a burn center for patients with 15% or greater total body surface second- or third-degree burns. If there is any question concerning whether a patient should be transferred, early consultation with a burn center surgeon is obtained.

### What Is a Tertiary Trauma Survey?

The concept of a tertiary trauma survey (standardized repeat clinical assessment) within 24 hours of admission has been proposed by some trauma surgeons.[102,103]

Missed injuries are inevitable in the blunt force trauma victim. The most important aspect of the primary and secondary survey is to rapidly identify life-threatening and potentially disabling injuries. Other injuries can become evident at any stage of the management process. At some point within the first 24 to 48 hours of admission, mandatory review of all radiographic reports and films, along with a repeat physical examination, will often identify injuries that were not initially apparent.

We find it helpful to record all diagnoses and procedures on a Diagnostic and Procedural Summary Sheet placed in the front of the chart. Active medical problems and ongoing injuries causing disability are recorded daily in the critical care progress note. This prompts team members to ensure that appropriate therapy for each diagnosis is being rendered daily. Alert trauma patients may often have severe distracting injuries that can minimize symptoms from other minor injuries. For example, it is not unusual for patients with femur fractures to overlook the pain associated with an isolated metacarpal fracture until pain relief from the femur fracture defers attention to the other minimal injury.

Patients and families are informed early in the care process that missed injuries are frequent and expected. This simple

**TABLE 38–9.** Diagnostic Features of Commonly Abused Drugs

| Drugs | Pupils | Respiratory | Central Nervous System | Seizures | Initial Evaluation | Withdrawal |
|---|---|---|---|---|---|---|
| Opioids | Pinpoint | Depressed | Lethargy, coma | + | Respiratory depression; drug-altered LOC | Withdrawal |
| Barbiturates | Small, reactive (not pinpoint) | Depressed | Lethargy, coma | + | Respiratory depression; hypotension; drug-altered LOC | Withdrawal (severe) |
| Anxiolytics | Normal, reactive | May be depressed | Lethargy, coma | − | Drug-altered LOC; respiratory depression (in elderly and when combined with ETOH) | Withdrawal |
| Amphetamines and cocaine | Dilated, reactive | Stimulated | Confusion, delusions, disorientation, paranoia | + | Seizures; ventricular arrhythmias; lack of cooperation | Withdrawal (mild); rhabdomyolysis (cocaine) |
| Marijuana | Dilated, reactive | No consistent changes | Euphoria, drowsiness, decreased attention span, paranoia | − | Dilated pupils; lack of cooperation | — |
| LSD | Dilated, reactive | No consistent changes | Euphoria, hallucinations, drowsiness | + | Lack of cooperation; altered mental status; combativeness | — |
| PCP | Dilated, reactive | No consistent changes | Aggressive, violent behavior | + | Lack of cooperation; altered mental status; combativeness | Rhabdomyolysis |
| ETOH | Dilated, reactive | Depressed with high levels | Variable (initial aggressiveness, then somnolence) | − | Lack of cooperation, aggressiveness, or somnolence/lethargy | Withdrawal (mild to severe); seizures |

ETOH, ethanol; LOC, level of consciousness; LSD, lysergic acid diethylamide; PCP, phencyclidine HCl.
From Norwood SH, Dellinger RP. Managing substance abuse in the trauma patient. *Probl Crit Care.* 1987;1:117.

acknowledgment often reduces anxiety and loss of confidence in the trauma team when an injury is later identified. Nurses and physical therapists are also helpful in identifying injuries after the initial phase of treatment, especially in comatose patients.

## ALCOHOL AND DRUG INTOXICATION

Patients intoxicated with alcohol or drugs may present with a broad range of mental status changes ranging from violent behavior to depression and coma.[104]

Although cautious observation may be safe in nontrauma patients, this approach can lead to disastrous consequences in patients with major injuries. Alcohol and drugs are powerful respiratory depressants that can exacerbate hypoxemia and respiratory acidosis. Alcohol and barbiturates are cardiac depressants at higher doses, further enhancing the hemodynamic instability of hypovolemic shock.

### What Are Findings on Physical Examination?

Needle tracks, subcutaneous abscesses, skin ulcerations, or draining sinuses from deeper subcutaneous tissues may be found. These signs signify chronic, heavy drug abuse. Recent needle tracks suggest narcotic or cocaine abuse, although amphetamines and occasionally barbiturates are abused intravenously.[104]

Neurologic assessment is difficult and unreliable in these patients, but it may help to determine the type of drug used. Clinical signs associated with the more frequently abused

drugs are outlined in Table 38–9. These clinical findings may not be helpful in patients with head injury. Despite a positive drug or alcohol history, intracranial injury must always be considered before implicating substance abuse as the sole reason for a patient's altered mental status.

Head CT is obtained after stabilization. In a series of 229 patients who underwent emergency tracheal intubation, 76 were paralyzed and intubated because of combative or uncooperative behavior. In this group, 42% had significant intracranial injury detected by CT and 22% had other life-threatening injuries requiring expedient therapy.[43]

### What Are the Effects of Alcohol?

Animal studies of alcohol intoxication during hypovolemic shock show a significant increase in mortality compared with shock without alcohol intoxication.[105] Depression of the respiratory response to shock and a reduction in the quantity of blood loss needed to cause severe hypovolemic shock also have been demonstrated.[106] This lack of normal physiologic response is associated with a higher mortality rate. Presumably, these same abnormalities occur in intoxicated patients after traumatic shock.

### Cardiovascular

Peripheral vasodilation combined with diuresis from diminished antidiuretic hormone can cause significant hypovolemia with minimal blood loss. High serum alcohol levels exert negative inotropic effects, reducing mean arterial BP out of proportion to the actual volume of blood lost.[107]

Peripheral vasodilation also contributes to hypothermia. Patients may present with decreased pain perception, making physical examination unreliable. Cirrhotic patients often have a relatively low systolic BP (90-110 mm Hg), a high cardiac output, and a low systemic vascular resistance. These physiologic changes must be considered when evaluating injured cirrhotic patients.

### Coagulation

Coagulation disorders may complicate the management of alcoholic patients. Coagulopathy is a common problem in cirrhotic patients. Acute alcohol intoxication can also cause significant platelet abnormalities.[108]

### Alcohol Withdrawal Syndrome

Prompt recognition and management of alcohol withdrawal in trauma patients are crucial. The syndrome usually begins after 12 to 36 hours of abstinence. Prophylactic benzodiazepines are recommended to prevent alcohol withdrawal in its most severe form, delirium tremens.

## THE FULL STOMACH

### How Can Aspiration Be Avoided?

Trauma victims often arrive with an unsavory concoction of undigested food, alcohol, and blood distending their stomachs. Anxiety, pain, and the metabolic response to injury can delay or completely arrest gastric emptying.[109] Head-injured patients are also prone to vomiting.

The most dangerous immediate complication of aspiration is obstruction of the upper airway by large food particles. Although various suggestions about management of a full stomach have been proposed, the most reliable method in obtunded trauma victims is to apply cricoid pressure followed by rapid paralysis and airway intubation. The estimated risk of aspiration in patients with full stomachs during intubation for emergency surgery is approximately 5%.[109,110]

### Are Prophylactic Measures Helpful?

Administering agents such as metaclopromide and histamine receptor type II ($H_2$) blockers to decrease the risk of aspiration is usually not possible, owing to the need for urgent intubation. Nasogastric tube insertion may induce retching and is generally ineffective in preventing vomiting. Such maneuvers increase ICP and must be avoided in head-injured patients.

## CERVICAL SPINE INJURY

Approximately one third of patients with cervical spine injuries will present with moderate to severe brain injuries.[110] The potential for serious iatrogenic injury is high with manipulation of an unstable cervical spine during the acute management and evaluation phase. Aggressive cervical manipulation can convert an unstable fracture with no neurologic injury into quadriplegia. Thus, every precaution is taken to immobilize the cervical spine until injury is ruled out.

### How Should the Trachea Be Intubated?

Patients can be safely intubated orotracheally with in-line cervical traction.[43,109,111] Concern for a cervical spine injury must not, under any circumstances, delay airway control, but proper precautions must be followed. Cervical flexion and extension are avoided during intubation.

### Is Methylprednisolone of Value?

High-dose methylprednisolone is administered for 24 hours after spinal cord injury with motor deficits (30 mg/kg in the first hour, followed by 5.4 mg/kg/h for 23 hours). A 24-hour infusion is recommended for patients whose therapy begins within 3 hours after injury. The infusion is extended to 48 hours for patients whose treatment begins within 3 to 8 hours after the injury.[112,113] Although improvement in neurologic outcome with methylprednisolone has been reported,[112,113] these studies have been criticized.[114] Treatment with high-dose corticosteroids is not without risk. A higher incidence of sepsis and pneumonia is reported with extended use of methylprednisolone.[113] Despite these risks, and because of the devastating nature of spinal cord injury, any slight improvement in function is considered worth the added risk of infection during the acute recovery period.

### How Is the Diagnosis of Blunt Cervical Arterial Injury Made?

The incidence (or identification) of blunt cervical vessel injuries has increased over the past decade. Studies document an incidence of 0.1% to 0.86%.[69,115–119] The mortality rate is high in these patients because of the difficulty with early diagnosis. Mortality ranges from 15% to 31% in most recent studies.[69,115,116]

Delayed recognition of blunt carotid and vertebral artery injury is common. Many patients present with multisystem trauma and head injury that precludes accurate neurologic examination. Head CT is often normal after this injury, and early clinical signs of cerebral ischemia may be subtle. Further diagnostic studies are indicated for patients with cervical bruits, signs or history of external cervical trauma with altered mental status, and lateralizing neurologic deficits including hemiparesis, transient ischemic attacks, amaurosis fugax, or Horner syndrome.[69] Neurologic deficits that do not correlate with CT findings, or evidence of cerebral infarction on CT, indicate possible carotid or vertebral artery injury. Patients with suspected cervical arterial injuries require immediate angiography to establish the diagnosis. Other potential diagnostic modalities include magnetic resonance angiography[117] and CT angiography.[119]

### What Is the Treatment?

Lesions accessible to surgical repair are best treated operatively. Many injuries occur at the skull base or more distally and are not amenable to operative repair. Full anticoagulation with heparin is the treatment of choice for surgically inaccessible injuries.[69,116] The complication rate from anticoagulation is significant and may be as high as 54%.[69] Whether heparinization is necessary in all cases has been questioned.[118] For surgically inaccessible lesions providers must weigh the risks of heparinization versus the risk of no therapy, which often leads to a devastating neurologic outcome or death.

## RETROPERITONEAL INJURIES

The retroperitoneal space can sequester several liters of blood and fluid without causing symptoms. Massive retroperitoneal hemorrhage leads to irreversible shock in <1% of blunt trauma patients.

### What Are the Presenting Signs and Symptoms?

The most serious bleeding is associated with sacral and pelvic fractures causing venous plexus injuries. This area is obscured from examination by the abdomen ventrally and musculoskeletal structures dorsally.

Conscious patients may complain of abdominal, back, or perineal pain, but specific symptoms are frequently absent. Flank ecchymosis (Grey Turner sign) and periumbilical ecchymosis (Cullen sign) are absent initially and may not appear until 48 hours after injury. Pelvic instability on physical examination is frequently the first clue that significant retroperitoneal hemorrhage exists. Hematuria from associated genitourinary injuries may also be an early sign.

### Is Computed Tomography Helpful?

Retroperitoneal hemorrhage is confirmed either at laparotomy or by abdominal and pelvic CT. CT is helpful in determining the nature of the retroperitoneal injury. Abdominal-pelvic CT with intravenous contrast is more sensitive for detecting retroperitoneal injuries and genitourinary injuries than intravenous pyelogram.

### How Urgent Is Surgical Intervention?

The urgency of intervention depends primarily on the retroperitoneum's tamponading effect in limiting blood loss. Large retroperitoneal hematomas can displace intraperitoneal organs ventrally, causing vascular compromise of the bowel. The need for operative intervention depends on the retroperitoneal organ injured, the extent of bleeding, and hemodynamic instability. Most renal injuries are managed nonoperatively unless urinary extravasation is identified. Angiographic embolization of retroperitoneal arterial bleeding is frequently beneficial.

## HEAD INJURIES

Brain injury is the major cause of disability, death, and economic loss to society after trauma. As the understanding of the pathophysiology of head injury has improved, clinicians have become more aware that not all neurologic damage occurs at the moment of impact but evolves over the ensuing hours and days.[120] Developing guidelines for head injury was intensified when a study by Ghajar and associates[121] documented considerable variability in brain injury management throughout the United States. This study showed that only 28% of trauma centers routinely used ICP monitoring.[121] Routine hyperventilation and osmotic diuretics were used in 83% of trauma centers, with 64% reporting corticosteroid use for closed head injury. Hyperventilation was empirically and aggressively used with a target $PaCO_2$ <25 mm Hg at 29% of trauma centers. A similar study in the United Kingdom documented a lack of ICP monitoring and routine use of hyperventilation.[122]

Recommendations for treatment based on an extensive review of the existing literature were published as *Practice Guidelines* by the American Association of Neurological Surgeons Joint Section on Neurotrauma and Critical Care and by the Brain Trauma Foundation.[120] These guidelines assessed the degree of certainty associated with a particular form of therapy for head injury using a system that has been widely accepted for practice guideline development in other medical disciplines. The following discussion and recommendations are based in part on these practice guidelines.

### What Are the Treatment Priorities?

Treatment begins at the accident scene. Airway control and hypotension are important in preventing secondary brain injury. Hypotension, anemia, and hypercarbia significantly increase mortality and morbidity after head injury. Over 25% of patients with severe head injury are exposed to secondary insults from hypotension and hypoxia from the time of injury until resuscitation.[123] Hypotension occurred in 34.6% of patients in one study and was associated with a 150% increase in mortality.[124]

Patients with severe head injury are immediately intubated using techniques that avoid increasing ICP. Most patients with clinical signs of head injury will have positive findings on CT; 15% of patients with abnormal head CT scans require emergent neurosurgical intervention.[125]

### Is Hyperventilation Beneficial?

Routine hyperventilation of head-injured patients is no longer recommended.[120] Muizelaar and associates[126] showed that hyperventilation is deleterious in patients with Glasgow Motor Scale scores of 4 to 5. The theoretic advantages of hyperventilation are cerebral vasoconstriction to reduce ICP and reversal of brain and cerebrospinal fluid acidosis. The concern, however, is that cerebral vasoconstriction may cause cerebral ischemia of both injured and noninjured areas of the brain. In addition, the cerebrospinal fluid effects of hyperventilation in reducing acidosis are short lived.[126] Hyperventilation to a $PaCO_2$ <30 mm Hg is recommended only if other forms of ICP control fail.[120]

### Are Diuretics Helpful?

Intravenous bolus doses of 0.25 to 1.0 g/kg of mannitol intravenously are frequently used to reduce ICP. Mannitol exerts beneficial effects by 2 mechanisms: (1) immediate reduction of hematocrit and blood viscosity, effects that increase cerebral blood flow and improve cerebral oxygen delivery,[120] and (2) delay of the osmotic diuretic effect for 15 to 30 minutes until gradients are established between plasma and brain cells. This delayed osmotic diuresis prolongs the reduction in ICP.[120] A recent study suggested that isolated severe traumatic brain injury may cause hypotension.[127] The overuse of diuretics, however, may have been a contributing factor. The temptation to treat head-injured patients with around-the-clock diuretics to "keep them dry" is unfounded and contraindicated. Mannitol is used only when ICP exceeds 20 to 25 mm Hg and other forms of therapy are unsuccessful.[120]

### What Is Recommended Current Therapy?

Intravascular volume expansion combined with inotropic support to improve mean arterial pressure and maintain cerebral perfusion pressure (CPP) >70 mm Hg may improve outcome.[128] It is our practice to routinely use ICP monitoring by ventriculostomy for patients with a GCS lower than 9. Ventriculostomy is not only diagnostic for intracranial hypertension but also may be therapeutic because cerebrospinal fluid drainage reduces ICP possibility.

Other benefits of ICP monitoring include (1) earlier detection of intracranial mass lesions, (2) avoidance of indiscriminate potentially harmful therapies, (3) possibly helping determine prognosis, and (4) possibly improving outcome.[120] ICP monitoring is helpful in patients with multiple injuries, especially those patients with acute lung injury in whom increased positive airway pressure is needed. ICP monitoring in these critically injured patients will ensure early recognition of adverse effects of mechanical ventilation. Persistent elevation of ICP mandates a repeat head CT to identify mass lesions. If no mass lesion is present, then various second-tier therapies may be considered, including standard hyperventilation to a $Paco_2$ of 25 to 30 mm Hg, hypothermia, barbiturate therapy, decompressive craniectomy, and hypertensive therapy.[120] Early enteral nutritional support is also recommended.

### Are Penetrating Head Wounds Treated Differently?

Gunshot wounds to the head (GSWH) are the most lethal of all major head injuries, with overall mortality rates >90%. Most patients do not survive long enough for neurosurgical evaluation. Those who reach the ED have a mortality rate of 75% to 80%. Because the majority of patients with GSWH do not survive, it is important to develop strategies to determine which patients warrant aggressive medical and surgical intervention.

There is little enthusiasm for operating on patients with GCS scores of 3 to 5.[129] Variables that correlate with poor outcome include suicide attempts, posterior fossa wounds, through-and-through wounds, increased ICP, and hypotension.[130] CT findings associated with high mortality include bihemispheric injury, transventricular injury, subarachnoid and intraventricular hemorrhage, midline shift, compression of mesencephalic cisterns, and intracerebral hematoma.[131]

Grahm and colleagues[132] prospectively evaluated 100 consecutive patients with GSWH who arrived in the ED with at least two neurologic signs of life after initial resuscitation (eg, brainstem reflexes and positive response to pain). All patients received head CT scans followed by surgical débridement if they survived initial evaluation. Aggressive postoperative care was provided to all patients. In this series no patient with a postresuscitation GCS score lower than 6 had a satisfactory outcome (defined as disabled but independent or better). There were also no satisfactory outcomes in patients with GCS scores of 6 to 8 with bihemispheric or multilobar dominant hemispheric injuries. Based on these results the authors recommended no aggressive surgical intervention for patients with a GCS score lower than 6 after resuscitation unless a significant mass lesion was present. The authors also questioned the role of aggressive therapy in many GSWH patients with GCS scores of 6 to 8.[132]

### What Should Be Done If Only a Loss of Consciousness Is Reported?

Many patients present with a history of questionable or brief loss of consciousness. Findings on neurologic examination and the GCS score are frequently normal. A study of 1170 patients with a history of loss of consciousness or amnesia for the traumatic event found that 3.3% had abnormalities detected by head CT.[133] A total of 1.8% had therapeutic changes resulting from CT findings, including four operative procedures. No patient with a negative head CT scan deteriorated during observation. The authors concluded that CT is indicated in patients with a history of loss of consciousness or amnesia for the event because the results may lead to therapeutic changes in a small but significant group of patients. Hospitalization for patients with a normal head CT scan is not necessary based on this study.[133]

## TRAUMA AND PREGNANCY

Injury occurs to about 7% of pregnant women, with hospitalization required in 0.4%. Trauma is the leading cause of nonobstetric deaths in women aged 14 to 44 years.[134] Motor vehicle crashes, followed by violent assault, are the most common mechanisms of injury.

### What Physiologic Changes Complicate Diagnosis and Resuscitation?

Pregnancy alters physiologic parameters and imposes demands on the mother that confuse and complicate evaluation, resuscitation, and definitive management after injury.[134] Alterations in hemodynamic function and blood volume occur. These changes can obscure injuries to both mother and fetus. Physiologic changes in other organ systems are listed in Table 38–10.

Pregnancy does not increase mortality in women after injury. However, its rare prevalence as an associated condition, trauma team members' unfamiliarity with the physiologic changes, and the emotional overtones of the situation may lead to serious delays in diagnosis and treatment.[135] Pregnancy alters the pattern of injury; severe abdominal trauma is more common than severe head injury when compared with nonpregnant female patients.[134]

**TABLE 38–10.** Physiologic Changes Associated With Pregnancy

| **Hemodynamic** | |
| --- | --- |
| Cardiac output | ↑ 1.0-1.5 L/min |
| Heart rate | ↑ 15-20 beats per minute |
| Systolic/diastolic pressure* | ↑ 5-15 mm Hg |
| **Blood** | |
| Blood volume (34 weeks' gestation) | ↑ 40-50% |
| Hematocrit | ↓ to 30-35% |
| Leukocyte count | ↑ to 20 000/mL |
| Serum fibrinogen | ↑ |
| Clotting factors | ↑ |
| Serum albumin | ↓ to 2.2-2.8 g/dL |
| **Respiratory** | |
| Tidal volume | ↑ 40% |
| $Paco_2$ | ↓ to 30 mm Hg |
| **Gastrointestinal** | |
| Delayed gastric emptying | |
| Intestines displaced cephalad | |

*Vena cava compression by the uterus when patient is in the supine position may cause severe hypotension and decreased cardiac output.

Modified from The Committee on Trauma, American College of Surgeons. *Advanced Trauma Life Support for Doctors.* Chicago: American College of Surgeons, 1997:315–323.

## What Are the Causes of Fetal Death After Trauma?

Risk factors for fetal death include maternal death, a high injury severity score, abdominal injury, hemorrhagic shock, and vaginal bleeding.[136] Direct uteroplacental injury, direct fetal trauma, and the indirect effects of maternal trauma, including hypoxia and hypovolemia, are potential causes of fetal death. Sympathetic nervous system stimulation and increased maternal serum norepinephrine and epinephrine levels cause decreased uterine blood flow in hypovolemic and normovolemic mothers. Isolated maternal head injury may also lead indirectly to fetal injury by increasing levels of thromboxane $A_2$ and prostaglandins. These powerful vasoconstrictors can decrease uterine blood flow.[137]

Placental abruption presents as vaginal bleeding, abdominal pain, uterine irritability, shock, and fetal distress.[138] The incidence of placental abruption is 1% to 5% after minor trauma and up to 50% after major trauma. Most abruptions occur within the first 6 hours after injury.[138]

Trauma affects the fetus primarily in the short term. If there is no placental abruption, premature rupture of uterine membranes, or urgent delivery, then no difference occurs in pregnancy outcome when factors such as birth weight, Apgar scores, premature delivery, and the need for cesarean section are compared with those of pregnant nontrauma patients.[134]

## How Does Management Differ?

The initial evaluation and treatment of pregnant trauma victims are identical to those of nonpregnant patients. Because of the increased blood volume, a normal BP and pulse may be present even with severe blood loss. Pregnant patients whose history suggests severe injuries should be aggressively evaluated and resuscitated.

### Supine Hypotension

The supine position reduces venous return and aortic outflow because of uterine vascular compression. Unless a spinal injury is suspected, transportation and evaluation should occur with the patient positioned on her left side. If she must remain supine, the right hip is elevated (unless injured) and the uterus manually displaced to the left to relieve pressure on the inferior vena cava.[42]

### Fetal Monitoring

There are no well-developed guidelines or recommendations for fetal monitoring after trauma. Tocography is not routinely employed if the gestational age of the fetus is <26 weeks.[134] Firm conclusions on the usefulness of prolonged fetal monitoring after trauma have not been determined.

In our institution, fetal US is performed as soon as possible to evaluate fetal viability and to determine gestational age. Obstetric consultation is obtained to guide decisions concerning fetal monitoring and the need for observation or hospitalization in those situations where the mother has only minimal injuries.

### Fetal Risks From Diagnostic Studies

Teratogenic risks to the fetus from radiation exposure during diagnostic testing can be an emotionally charged and irrational subject. Appropriate diagnostic and therapeutic procedures must not be withheld from the mother, regardless of pregnancy status. Abdominal US and DPL using a supraumbilical approach are both safe procedures.[135] Correction of hypovolemia and hypoxemia along with aggressive management of maternal injuries provide the best chance for fetal survival.[134,135]

## PEDIATRIC TRAUMA VICTIMS

Nothing is more emotionally distressing to medical personnel than treating a severely injured child. Although pediatric trauma centers have significantly improved the care of critically injured children in urban areas, the majority of injured children are still initially managed in local hospital EDs. Children, like adults, are approached in a systematic fashion so that proper and timely assessment and resuscitation occur.

## How Are Children Different?

Head injuries are common after blunt trauma. Because a child's head is large relative to the trunk, it is often the leading contact point in falls and high-speed motor vehicle crashes.[139] Children also develop hypothermia much earlier because of their larger body surface area in relation to body mass.

### Airway Considerations

The glottis lies in a more anterosuperior position in the pharynx, favoring orotracheal over nasotracheal intubation. Infants are obligate nasal breathers. Nasal fractures, soft tissue injuries, and blood can occlude the upper airway. Oral insertion of gastric tubes and ETTs are preferred over the nasal route in infants and younger children.

ETT size is gauged by the approximate diameter of the child's external nares or the diameter of the small finger. The following formula is also useful:

$$\text{Internal Diameter (mm) of Tube} = \frac{[16 + \text{Age (Years)}]}{4}$$

The airway is narrowest at the cricoid level in children. Therefore, uncuffed ETTs are used until the child is approximately 8 years of age.[139]

### Normative Data

Because of age-related differences in size and physiologic parameters, published normal ranges for pulse, BP, and respiratory rate should be available in the ED for each age group. The Broselow system is frequently used to estimate a child's weight and drug dosages based on height.[140]

The following relationships are useful in establishing dosage ranges and resuscitation measures. A child's weight in kilograms is approximately the age in years plus 8.[139] Blood volume is approximately 80 mL/kg. Systolic BP is estimated at approximately 70 mm Hg plus twice the age in years.[139]

## What Factors Suggest Severe Injury?

Children with Pediatric Trauma Scores <8,[18] or with an RTS <11, are extensively evaluated for serious injury or transferred to a facility capable of performing an evaluation.[139] Any child whose mechanism of injury involves high blunt force, such as a fall from a height >10 feet and pedestrian or motor vehicle accidents, must be carefully assessed for possible life-threatening injuries. Young adults and children have tremendous hemodynamic reserve, and normal vital signs do not eliminate the possibility of severe injury. Liberal use of CT and other diagnostic modalities is imperative. A wait and see approach is unacceptable.

## How Is Venous Access Achieved?

Two percutaneous intravenous catheters are placed in the upper extremities if possible. If this approach is unsuccessful, lower extremity intravenous catheters are used. If cutdowns are necessary, the venous anatomy that the operating physician is most familiar with is used. Subclavian central venous catheters can be used but are often difficult to place under emergency situations and are generally reserved for children older than 2 years.[141]

## When Is Intraosseous Infusion Useful?

Cannulation of a long bone medullary cavity in an uninjured extremity is safe and effective for emergency vascular access.[142] The intraosseous route should be considered early when a child is not in extremis. It is considered after two unsuccessful attempts at peripheral venous cannulation.[142]

### Technique

Intraosseous infusion is achieved by placing a rigid needle (preferably a 16-gauge disposal bone marrow aspiration needle) through the bony cortex into the medullary cavity of spongy bone. The proximal tibia and distal femur are the two

**TABLE 38-11.** Fluids and Medications Given by Intraosseous Infusion

| Fluids | Medications |
|---|---|
| 5-10% dextrose | Antibiotics |
| Packed red blood cells | Anticonvulsants |
| Plasma | Atropine |
| Ringer's injection, lactated | Catecholamines |
| Saline solution | Dextrose |
| Whole blood | Mannitol |
| | Sodium bicarbonate |

most commonly used sites.[142] Fluid instilled into the marrow cavity is rapidly dispersed through the extensive network of venous sinusoids into the systemic circulation. Various fluids, blood products, and medications can be given successfully by this route (Table 38-11).

### Contraindications

The only contraindications to intraosseous infusion are bone disorders, such as osteogenesis imperfecta and osteopetrosis, and the presence of infected burns, cellulitis, or recent fractures in the area of catheter insertion.[142]

## APPROACH TO VICTIMS OF MULTIPLE TRAUMA

Isolated injuries are uncommon after high blunt force mechanisms of injury. Information must be assimilated shortly after arrival in the ED. The trauma team leader assigns priorities to life-threatening injuries and addresses each one definitively. Patients undergo a rapid primary survey with resuscitation as previously described in this chapter. Only those patients who become hemodynamically stable progress to the secondary survey, which focuses on a complete physical examination and further diagnostic studies.

Unstable patients may require emergency surgery. The minimal diagnostic studies performed in unstable patients are chest, lateral cervical spine, and anteroposterior pelvic radiographs.[143] A FAST examination is useful for determining hemoperitoneum.

## What Are the Immediate Priorities?

Our approach is to obtain immediate airway control using neuromuscular blockade and orotracheal intubation. Two large-bore peripheral intravenous catheters are immediately placed by nursing personnel while the primary survey is being performed by the trauma surgeon. Combative and uncooperative patients are controlled with neuromuscular blockade because a high percentage of these patients have severe injuries.[43] If the patient's condition stabilizes, progression to the secondary survey along with a blunt trauma series of radiographs are performed. A FAST examination is performed during this time if it was not performed earlier.

## When a Patient's Condition Does Not Stabilize, What Follows?

If the patient does not respond to volume resuscitation with stabilization of vital signs, then recognition of hemoperitoneum by FAST examination mandates exploratory laparotomy. If the FAST is nondiagnostic, DPL may also be performed. We prefer using the quicker percutaneous technique for DPL because the complication rate is similar to the open technique.

If the patient's condition stabilizes despite findings of hemoperitoneum by FAST or DPL, then abdominal CT is performed to further delineate the nature of the intraabdominal injuries. The majority of these patients will also need a head CT.

## When Is Aortography or Chest Computed Tomography Appropriate?

If the initial chest radiograph shows a widened mediastinum or a large hemothorax, a decision to proceed with immediate aortography versus chest CT must be made. Unless aortic injury is obvious, chest CT with intravenous contrast medium enhancement is first performed. If aortic injury is obvious by chest radiograph, or if the CT does not definitely rule out aortic injury, then aortography is the next step.

## What Surgical Intervention Is Required?

### Subdural and Epidural Hematomas

Large subdural and epidural hematomas require immediate treatment in most cases. If severe shock from intraabdominal injury is also present, then exploratory laparotomy and craniotomy may be done simultaneously. Patients with nonsurgical intracranial injuries are best monitored with a ventriculostomy placed before or during other operative procedures.

### Combined Abdominal and Thoracic Injuries

Patients with abdominal and thoracic injuries, particularly those with thoracic aortic rupture, require a well-coordinated resuscitative effort. The ABCs of resuscitation are more complicated because of the risk of aortic rupture during routine resuscitative maneuvers.

Unstable patients with intraabdominal bleeding and thoracic aortic injury should undergo immediate exploratory laparotomy. Townsend and colleagues[144] advocate a quick laparotomy using simple maneuvers to control major bleeding and gross contamination. A temporary towel clip abdominal closure is performed. The aortic injury is then addressed with angiography followed by aortic repair. The laparotomy incision is reopened and definitive repair of all abdominal injuries is completed after thoracotomy.[144]

### Other Procedures

Peripheral vascular injuries are assigned the next priority for surgery after head and torso injuries. Orthopedic injuries are the fourth priority. Early fixation of most orthopedic injuries (within the first 24 hours) is recommended because of the benefits of early mobilization.[143] Maxillofacial injuries generally constitute the fifth priority of care.[144]

## POSTOPERATIVE COMPLICATIONS

## What Are the Goals of Management?

The fundamental goal of critical care in the postoperative or postresuscitative period is to maintain adequate oxygen delivery to vital tissues. The secondary survey may be delayed until arrival in the ICU if emergency surgery was needed for resuscitation. A tertiary survey is also performed within the next 24 hours.

A good knowledge of potential complications of surgically repaired injuries is important. Understanding the adverse effects of trauma on organ physiology is also important. Sepsis and multiple organ failure (MOF) are the leading causes of death in the postoperative period. A logical approach for evaluating sepsis must be developed.

## What Are the Causes of Sudden Unexplained Hypotension?

Common causes are listed in Table 38–12. Immediate resuscitative efforts, rapid evaluation to rule out mechanical causes, and immediate notification of the surgical team are crucial for patients who develop sudden unexplained postoperative hypotension. Hypotension associated with bradycardia indicates severe hypoxemia unless cervical spine injury is present. Loss of airway, tension pneumothorax, or cardiac tamponade must be quickly ruled out if hypotension and bradycardia occur as an acute event.

### Tension Pneumothorax

Decreased breath sounds, tracheal deviation, and a sharp rise in peak inspiratory pressure during mechanical ventilation are signs of tension pneumothorax. A chest radiograph is obtained if time permits. However, if systolic pressure falls below 70 mm Hg or severe bradycardia develops, aspiration of the chest with a 14- or 16-gauge catheter is performed. Surgical decompression is performed immediately with a tube thoracostomy if air is withdrawn. A previously placed chest tube does not eliminate the possibility of ipsilateral tension pneumothorax. The old tube may be occluded with blood, or the lung may become adherent to the tube openings. The diagnosis of pneumothorax is often difficult in the ICU setting.

### Hemothorax

Hemothorax can develop after the initial evaluation and resuscitation. This problem may be diagnosed and treated in a manner similar to that for pneumothorax. Persistent bleeding may require further surgery.

### Cardiac Tamponade

Muffled heart sounds, jugular venous distention, hypotension, increased systolic pressure variation with mechanical ventilation, and equalization of left and right atrial chamber pressures indicate cardiac tamponade. These signs can also occur with tension pneumothorax. If bilateral chest decom-

**TABLE 38–12.** Common Causes of Sudden Hypotension in Critically Ill Patients

| | |
|---|---|
| Loss of airway | Intraabdominal hemorrhage |
| Tension pneumothorax | Acute myocardial infarction |
| Pericardial tamponade | Bacteremia and sepsis |
| Hemothorax (massive) | Reaction to medication |

pression does not improve clinical status, pericardiocentesis or pericardiotomy may be necessary. A subxiphoid US view of the pericardium may be diagnostic. US is also helpful during placement of a pericardial catheter.

## Intraabdominal Bleeding

Intraabdominal or retroperitoneal bleeding should be strongly considered in patients with blunt trauma or previous abdominal exploration if all extraabdominal sources have been eliminated. This is especially pertinent with the trend toward increased nonoperative management of many solid organ injuries. The abdomen is rapidly assessed for any obvious signs of distention or bloody drainage through the incision or from abdominal drains.

Other catastrophic abdominal problems include ischemic bowel from embolization or volvulus, missed or subsequent perforation of the alimentary tract, pancreatitis, and streptococcal or clostridial wound infections. These complications require immediate surgical intervention. Intravascular volume resuscitation is the most important therapy while preparing for abdominal reexploration.

## What Is Abdominal Compartment Syndrome?

The term *abdominal compartment syndrome* (ACS) was first used by Kron to describe the pathophysiology from elevated intraabdominal pressure (intraabdominal hypertension) after abdominal aortic aneurysm surgery.[145] ACS now refers to the cardiovascular, pulmonary, renal, splanchnic, abdominal wall (and wound), and intracranial disturbances resulting from elevated intraabdominal pressure, regardless of the cause.[146] Increasing evidence also supports extending the syndrome to include isolated impairment of gut perfusion, because this abnormality has adverse effects on outcome even in the absence of other organ system abnormalities.[146,147]

ACS can develop after isolated abdominal trauma and major burns and from massive volume/blood resuscitation in the absence of abdominal trauma. Urinary bladder pressure measurement is the most common method of confirming the diagnosis,[145–147] although neurogenic bladder and intraperitoneal adhesions may cause unreliable measurements.[146] Chronic increases in intraabdominal pressure from obesity, pregnancy, or ascites must also be considered when making the diagnosis of ACS.

ACS is suspected if a patient's clinical condition deteriorates in the presence of a distended tense abdomen. A low urine output, increased peak airway pressures, diminished gas exchange, and a low pHi combined with intraabdominal pressures >25 mm Hg confirms the diagnosis. These abnormalities with an associated intraabdominal pressure >35 mm Hg mandate reexploration or decompressive celiotomy, which improves outcome when ACS develops.[145–147]

## What Is Iatrogenic Posttraumatic Hypothermia?

Hypothermia frequently complicates massive volume resuscitation in trauma patients. Anatomic and metabolic abnormalities inhibit temperature homeostasis. This disrupts the skin/

**TABLE 38–13.** Organ System Dysfunction Associated With Hypothermia

| | |
|---|---|
| Skin | Vasoconstriction (>32.2°C), vasodilation (≤32.3°C) |
| Kidneys | ↓ Reabsorption Na⁺ and H₂O (cold diuresis) |
| Mental status | Confusion, ↓ reflexes (<31.7°C), coma (<26.7°C) |
| Respiration | Progressive depression of respiratory center |
| Gastrointestinal | ↓ Gastrointestinal motility; stress ulcers, pancreatitis (<26.7°C) |
| Lungs | Pulmonary edema (<26.7°C) |
| Cardiac | Progressive bradycardia |
| O₂ consumption | Progressive decrease (4%/0.5°C) |
| Blood pressure | ↑ Initially, then progressively ↓ |
| Cardiac output | ↑ Initially, then progressively ↓ |
| Serum electrolytes | Hyponatremia, hyperkalemia, hyperglycemia |
| Acid-base status | Progressive metabolic acidosis |
| Coagulation | Impaired coagulation; occasional disseminated intravascular coagulation |

Modified from Fisher RP, Souba WP, Ford EG. Temperature-associated injuries and syndromes. In: Feliciano DV, Moore EE, Mattox KL, eds. Trauma. 3rd ed. Stamford, Conn: Appleton & Lange, 1996:951–958.

central nervous system/core negative feedback mechanisms for temperature control. Patients become passive responders to ambient temperature and the physics of heat loss.[148] Children and patients with head or spinal cord injury are particularly susceptible to hypothermia with or without associated hypovolemia and massive fluid resuscitation.

Cellular enzymatic systems fail as core temperature falls. Recent evidence in adult trauma patients suggests that hypothermia independent of hemorrhage causes coagulopathy in patients with core temperatures <34°C.[149] This coagulopathy occurs as a result of enzymatic activity slowing and decreased platelet function.[149]

Mild hypothermia increases the incidence of wound infections in patients after elective colorectal surgery.[64]

Iatrogenic posttraumatic hypothermia is categorized into three groups: mild (35°-32.3°C [95°-90°F]), moderate (32.2°-26.7°C [90°-80°F]), and severe (<25.7° [<80°F]). A summary of organ system dysfunction associated with hypothermia is presented in Table 38–13.

## Treatment

### Standard Measures

The best treatment is prevention. For mildly hypothermic patients, passive rewarming can be accomplished with warming blankets. Aluminum space blankets trap and reflect body heat to the patient. Resuscitation areas in the ED and OR should be kept warm. Patients should receive warm fluid and blood during resuscitation, intraoperatively and postoperatively.

Crystalloids and blood are warmed to 37.7° to 40°C (100°-104°F) with fluid-warming and blood-warming devices. Each liter of room temperature fluid (70°C) decreases body temperature by approximately 0.2°C in a 70-kg individual. In the OR, a heating blanket under the patient is helpful and a heated humidifier circuit for the ventilator should be used.

### Core Warming

If moderate to severe hypothermia develops despite these preventive measures, active core warming is performed. Warm lavage of the thoracic and peritoneal cavities is effective but gives slow results. Extracorporeal bypass is occasionally needed for severe hypothermia. The most effective, easily managed, and readily available technique of active core warming is by inhalation. Intubation and ventilation with warmed humidified oxygen effectively and rapidly warm the heart and brain. The maximal inspired temperature should be 43.3° to 50°C (110°-122°F) to prevent thermal injury to the respiratory system. In an awake patient, the inspiratory temperature must be reduced to approximately 40°C (104°F).

## What Are the Homeostatic Responses to Injury?

Severe injury causes complex homeostatic responses secondary to acute volume loss and inadequate hemoperfusion.

### Hormonal Interplay

Acute volume reduction stimulates pressor receptors in the carotid artery and the aortic arch as well as volume (stretch) receptors in the left atrium. Increased aldosterone secretion from the zona glomerulosa of the adrenal gland and antidiuretic hormone (ADH) from the posterior pituitary gland occurs in response to afferent input from these receptors.[150]

Painful stimuli from injured areas also stimulate ADH secretion. Aldosterone and ADH, respectively, stimulate reabsorption of sodium and water by the kidneys. Afferent nerve stimulation causes increased levels of adrenocorticotropic hormone, which increases aldosterone release.[150]

### Continued Hypoperfusion

Decreased hemoperfusion results in elevated lactic acid production, which stimulates hyperventilation. Severe cellular damage and membrane dysfunction ensues if inadequate hemoperfusion persists. Membrane permeability defects are manifested by increased requirements for larger volumes of fluid to achieve adequate resuscitation. Reperfusion is associated with the generation of oxygen free radicals, further tissue injury, and cellular disruption.[150]

## Why Are Metabolic Demands Increased?

Severely injured patients have increased metabolic demands because of elevated levels of catabolic hormones and catecholamines (epinephrine and norepinephrine) that initially stimulate catabolism and accelerate loss of body fat and protein.

### Protein and Fat Metabolism

The hypermetabolic response is characterized by increased lipolysis, fat oxidation, and proteolysis. Dramatic loss of body cell mass from fat stores, skeletal muscle protein, and acute phase reactant proteins occurs if the metabolic response to injury persists. Activated polymorphonuclear leukocytes and macrophages release various mediator substances, including cytokines such as tumor necrosis factor (TNF) and the interleukins. Further activation of the cyclo-oxygenase pathway produces various prostaglandins that may cause adverse systemic effects.[150]

### Thermoregulation

Hypothalamic alterations cause changes in thermoregulation. At any ambient temperature, core and skin temperatures of injured or septic patients are greater than those in normal individuals.[150] Pharmacologic agents that affect the temperature set point generally are not effective in reducing the hypermetabolism and hyperpyrexia that occur after injury.

### Stress Hormones

A marked rise in glucagon, cortisol, growth hormone, adrenocorticotropic hormone, and the catecholamines occurs with injury. In contrast, plasma levels of insulin are initially low but return to normal or become elevated after patient stabilization. Insulin is inhibited, even with hyperglycemia, by α-adrenergic stimulation.[150] Insulin inhibition accounts in part for the posttraumatic hyperglycemia that is commonly observed.

## SHOCK

Understanding the various causes and pathophysiology of shock and the current modes of treatment is necessary for anesthesiologists who are frequently involved in the management of critically injured patients.

## What Is Shock?

The answer to this question is analogous to asking the Inuit of the Arctic Circle, "What is ice?" For the layman, ice is frozen water, but to the Inuit whose lives depend on an accurate description of their environment, there are 20 different words that the layman would translate to "ice." The term *shock* also has numerous definitions. The traditional classification of shock into various categories may aid in its understanding. The best definition of shock is "a profound and widespread reduction in the effective delivery of oxygen and other nutrients that first results in reversible and then, if prolonged, to irreversible cellular injury."[151]

The concept of shock and its causes has evolved over the past century with an increased understanding of the molecular cascades and their effects. The first medical use of the term *shock* appeared in the translation of LeDran's work into English in 1743. Describing his extensive experience with gunshot wounds, he observed that blood vessels became constricted during shock as if they were surrounded with a ligature causing "the stream of animal spirits to become intercepted or entirely suspended—with a universal coldness due to interception of the fluids."[152] James Latta, in 1795, used the term *shock* to describe an epileptic patient treated with electricity by Benjamin Franklin.[153]

In 1831, Thomas Latta was the first to use intravenous saline to treat shock secondary to cholera. Writing in the *Lancet,* he stated, "Having no precedent to direct me, I decided to throw the fluid (saline) directly into the circulation."[154] The use of blood transfusions in the treatment of shock, banned in 1678 by a special edict of the pope, was resurrected by Hunter in 1776. The scientific basis for the success of these treatments for shock was not elucidated until the end of the 19th century, when George Crile established reproducible experimental models of hemorrhagic shock, documenting that the central venous pressure dropped after hemorrhage and that survival increased with saline infusions.[155]

Utilizing their observations of patients injured during World War I, Cannon and Bayliss were able to document various biochemical and physiologic changes occurring in shock. Cannon stated in 1923 in regard to the use of sodium bicarbonate, "The important matter is not to increase the sodium bicarbonate of the blood in the late stages of shock, but to restore early the essential lack—the needed oxygen—by a better blood supply."[156] By examining traumatic extremity injuries in an animal model, Cannon hypothesized that traumatic shock was mediated by a toxin produced at the time of injury.[157] This hypothesis was challenged by Alfred Blalock in 1930 when he demonstrated that hypovolemia was the primary mechanism in the pathophysiology of shock.[158] Blalock's observations became the cornerstones for further study and treatment of shock. Interestingly, it is only in the latter part of this century that many of the previously discounted hypotheses have been partially or completely validated and a general theorem of shock has emerged.

## What Are the Traditional Categories of Shock?

Shock is divided, based on etiology, into four categories: hypovolemic, cardiogenic, neurogenic, and vasogenic (or distributive). Vasogenic shock includes the subgroups septic, traumatic, and anaphylactic. Although generally accepted, this classification is misleading in its simplicity. Frequently, a combination of causes may cause shock in a single patient. One increasingly common example is the elderly patient involved in a motor vehicle crash, with hypovolemia from multiple injuries causing blood loss that precipitates an acute MI, causing cardiogenic shock. Despite the limitations of such a classification system, a basic description of the various causes is needed to better understand the complicated pathophysiology of shock.

### Hypovolemic Shock

Hypovolemic shock occurs when intravascular fluid losses from either hemorrhage (trauma) or plasma volume losses (burns) result in significant tissue hypoperfusion.

### Neurogenic Shock

Neurogenic shock occurs after spinal cord injury and is the result of the loss of sympathetic input to maintain normal vascular tone.

### Cardiogenic Shock

Cardiogenic shock results when the heart is unable to provide an adequate cardiac output to maintain tissue perfusion. This may be the result of primary pump failure that can occur with MIs or congestive heart failure or of secondary mechanisms such as pericardial tamponade (cardiac compressive shock).

### Vasogenic (Distributive) Shock

Vasogenic shock incorporates a variety of causes in which numerous vasoactive mediators cause tissue hypoperfusion and/or hypoxia. Septic, traumatic, and anaphylactic shock are classified under this category.

## What Are the Common Pathophysiologic Features?

All four types of shock share the common feature of inadequate cellular oxygenation for existing metabolic demands. Whether it is the result of limited tissue perfusion or increased metabolic demands, the imbalance causes tissue hypoxia, organ dysfunction, organ failure, and death. Cellular hypoxia alone does not cause immediate cell death. Hypoxia alters cellular metabolism by utilizing anaerobic pathways that initiate various metabolic cascades. These changes alter the intracellular milieu and eventually cause changes in the microcirculation and macrocirculation.

## How Do Aerobic and Anaerobic Metabolism Differ?

Mammals normally utilize aerobic metabolism for energy, and it is the circulatory redistribution, with preferential flow to the heart and brain, that initially provides a survival advantage for the organism. Under usual aerobic conditions, pyruvate, the metabolite of glycolysis, enters the mitochondria via the Krebs cycle, producing 38 molecules of adenosine triphosphate (ATP)/glucose molecule. Anaerobic metabolism, which precedes circulatory redistribution, results in the production of lactate, yielding only two molecules of ATP/glucose molecule (Fig. 38–1). Lactate production increases as hypoxia worsens.

## Are Serum Lactate Levels Beneficial?

Numerous studies document using lactate levels to detect both the presence and the severity of shock.[159–162] Siegel and

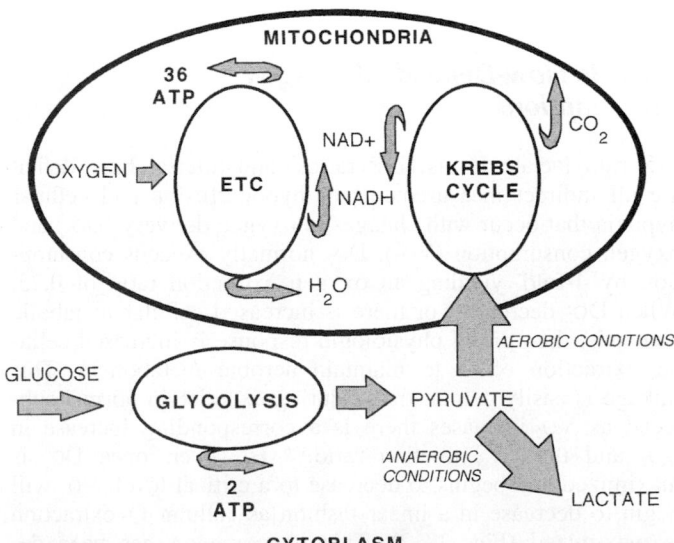

**FIGURE 38–1.** Cellular metabolism comparing aerobic and anaerobic processes.

associates examined multiple variables that might differentiate survivors from nonsurvivors of blunt trauma. Lactate levels on admission and at 48 hours after admission were predictive for discriminating survivors from nonsurvivors.[163] Another prospective study in trauma patients documented a 100% survival rate if excess serum lactate cleared within 24 hours. Survival was only 14% if lactate clearance was not achieved by 48 hours.[164]

A randomized prospective study of surgical patients by Boyd and associates[165] examined mortality rates after deliberate attempts to increase oxygen delivery and demonstrated that clearance of lactate was a reasonable goal of resuscitation.

It is important to consider lactate production as well as lactate clearance. Cohen and Woods divided lactic acidosis into two categories: type A, secondary to hypoperfusion, and type B, lactic acidosis in the absence of hypoperfusion that occurs with hepatic failure and decreased clearance.[166] Other causes of type B lactic acidosis are diabetes, methanol, ethanol, and inherent errors of metabolism such as glucose-6-phosphatase deficiency.

## What Is the Lactate/Pyruvate Ratio?

The lactate/pyruvate (L/P) ratio and base deficit are considered more specific for monitoring cellular hypoxia and recovery from shock than serum lactate levels alone. Huckabee postulated that serum L/P ratios >10:1 were indicative of an anaerobic state.[167] Others have documented that the L/P ratio, when normal, despite elevated lactate levels, indicates adequate oxygenation.[168–170] Because lactate levels and L/P ratios take time to procure, the arterial-based deficit is advocated as a more readily available alternative. The arterial base deficit is rapidly calculated from easily measured values of arterial pH and $Paco_2$. Davis demonstrated a strong correlation between arterial base deficit and serum lactate levels in an animal model[171] and showed that the base deficit predicted survival in injured patients.[172–174] Siegel and associates demonstrated that blunt trauma patients with an initial base deficit of 0 mmol/L had an 8% mortality rate and that 95% of those patients with a base deficit >26 mmol/L died. The $LD_{50}$ occurred with a base deficit of 11.8 mmol/L.[175]

## What Is Flow-Dependent Oxygen Consumption?

Serum lactate levels, L/P ratios, and arterial base deficit are all indirect measurements of hypoperfusion and cellular hypoxia that occur with changes in oxygen delivery ($Do_2$) and oxygen consumption ($Vo_2$). $Do_2$ normally exceeds consumption by 4-fold, yielding an oxygen extraction ratio of 0.25. When $Do_2$ decreases, or there is increased cellular metabolic demands, the normal physiologic response is increased cellular extraction of $O_2$ to maintain aerobic metabolism. This linkage is easily demonstrated during exercise in normal subjects; as $Vo_2$ increases there is a corresponding increase in $Do_2$ and the $O_2$ extraction ratio.[176] However, once $Do_2$ is maximized and begins to decrease to a critical level, $Vo_2$ will begin to decrease in a linear fashion as cellular $O_2$ extraction is maximized (Fig. 38–2). This phenomenon has been described as flow-dependent oxygen consumption. With the development of modern PA catheters with oximetry capabilities,

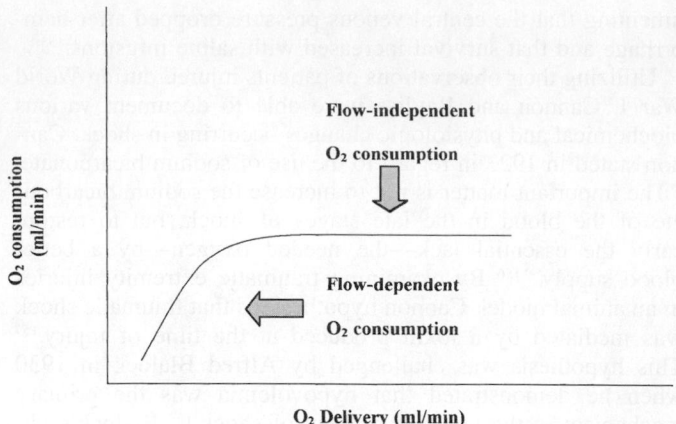

**FIGURE 38–2.** Relationship between oxygen consumption and oxygen delivery.

$Do_2$ and $Vo_2$ can be measured and differences between survivors and nonsurvivors of shock can be determined. Shoemaker demonstrated in 1993 that whereas nonsurvivors maintained normal values for cardiac index, $Do_2$, and $Vo_2$, these values were significantly lower than those of survivors.[177] This led to the concept of achieving supranormal values for these physiologic measurements and encouraged many investigators to conduct studies with the hypothesis that attaining these supranormal values would increase survival.

Investigators have confirmed increased survival rates in a mixed population of ICU patients requiring PA catheters,[178] high-risk surgery patients,[165,179] peripheral vascular patients,[180] elderly blunt trauma patients,[181] and severely injured trauma patients.[182,183] Bishop and associates[184] prospectively randomized trauma patients to receive therapy with the goal of achieving either supranormal or normal $Do_2$ and $Vo_2$ values within 24 hours after admission. The objective was also to maintain these values for a total of 48 hours. Survival in the supranormal group was 76% versus 56% in the normal group. Other authors have been unable to demonstrate any survival benefit in prospective randomized trials.[185,186] In 1996 Heyland and coworkers[187] attempted a meta-analysis of randomized clinical trials concerned with interventions to achieve supranormal values for $Do_2$ and $Vo_2$ and concluded that while this hypothesis could not undergo meta-analysis due to study variability, current evidence did not support attempts at achieving supranormal oxygenation values in all critically ill patients. There may be subgroups, specifically surgical and trauma patients, that may benefit.

## What Is Circulatory Redistribution?

Hypoperfusion and cellular hypoxia result initially in macrocirculatory changes at the organ level to maximize perfusion to the heart and brain. This is done by sacrificing blood flow to skin, muscle, and gut as a result of the effects of a circulating milieu of hormones, catecholamines, and metabolites, whose net effects are vasoconstriction. The unique microcirculatory arrangement of the intestine, with its countercurrent blood flow exchange system and high concentration of vasoconstrictor receptors, makes the intestinal mucosa extremely disposed to hypoperfusion. The predominant intestinal vasoconstrictors contributing to splanchnic hypoperfusion are angiotensin II and vasopressin. To a lesser extent thromboxane A$_2$, the catecholamines, and thyrotropin-releasing hormone are involved. This complex response of the intestinal microvasculature consists of vasoconstriction of larger arterioles and vasodilation of smaller arterioles, resulting in preservation of mucosal blood flow and decreased perfusion of the muscularis propria. Prolonged ischemia causes increased mucosal permeability to macromolecules within 1 hour and obvious morphologic injury to the small intestinal villi at 2 hours.[188] Although this response initially protects vital organs (brain, heart), prolonged hypoperfusion will produce significant, potentially irreversible changes in the affected organ. The pathogenesis of gut dysfunction results from both the initial hypoxia as well as reperfusion injury if hypoxia is prolonged.

Carrico and colleagues described the gut as the motor of irreversible shock.[189] Reperfusion injury aggravates the increased mucosal permeability that occurred during ischemia. Reperfusion injury is believed to be secondary to generation of free oxygen radicals and other metabolic products. Under normal conditions of perfusion and oxygenation, xanthine dehydrogenase catalyzes the formation of ATP via oxidative phosphorylation. Under anaerobic conditions, both xanthine dehydrogenase and the degradation products of ATP accumulate. Xanthine dehydrogenase is converted to xanthine oxidase, which converts the final degradation product of ATP, hypoxanthine, to xanthine. During the irreversible conversion to uric acid, various oxygen and hydroxyl radicals are formed. The irreversible nature of these reactions depletes the cell of substrate for later ATP regeneration. These radicals cause lipid peroxidation with cell membrane disruption, nucleic acid degeneration, and the attraction and activation of polymorphonuclear leukocytes that release proteases.[190–193] Reperfusion allows for these reactive substances to be washed out, resulting in further mucosal injury. Subsequently, bacterial or endotoxin translocation may initiate the systemic inflammatory response syndrome (SIRS) and contribute to the beginning of multiple organ dysfunction syndrome (MODS). Bacterial translocation as a cause for SIRS, however, is controversial.[194–196]

### What Are the Neuroendocrine Responses to Shock?

After injury the body initiates several processes to maintain homeostasis, to prevent further injury, and to begin healing. Many of the initial clinical signs of shock are caused by these neuroendocrine responses. The overall effects achieve two goals: maintaining perfusion to vital organs (heart and brain) and decreasing perfusion to those areas most commonly injured (skin, muscle, extremities, and splanchnic bed). A second effect of this neuroendocrine response is to mobilize energy stores so that increased glucose is available for metabolism. Hypovolemia causes decreased venous return to the heart, diminished cardiac output, and a drop in BP. This decrease in BP initiates responses at the baroreceptors of the aortic arch and the carotid sinus, as well as stretch receptors in the atria. The resultant diminished afferent stimulation of the vasomotor center of the medulla causes a reflex increase in sympathetic activity, increased arterial and venous constriction, increased systemic vascular resistance, increased venous blood return to the heart, and finally increased cardiac output and BP. Sympathetic stimulation also causes increased secretion of epinephrine and norepinephrine from the adrenal medulla,[150] which increases heart rate, myocardial contractility, and vascular constriction.

The response of the posterior pituitary gland to hypotension is the release of antidiuretic hormone (ADH), which produces vasoconstriction, particularly in the splanchnic circulation, and increased water reabsorption in the distal renal tubules. Hypoperfusion of the kidneys' juxtaglomerular apparatus initiates the renin-angiotensin-aldosterone pathway, releasing angiotensin II, the most potent endogenous vasoconstrictor, and aldosterone, which promotes sodium reabsorption in the renal tubule to increase circulatory volume. Renal microcirculatory regulation consists of postglomerular vasoconstriction with increased reabsorption of both water and sodium in the proximal renal tubule.[197]

The second arm of the neuroendocrine response to hypovolemia increases glucose production for metabolism. The anterior pituitary gland secretes adrenocorticotropic hormone, which increases cortisol production by the adrenal medulla. The overall effect is one of catabolism with cortisol initiating proteolysis, lipolysis, and gluconeogenesis.[150] Increased epinephrine levels stimulate glucagon secretion by the pancreas and inhibit insulin secretion. The hyperglycemia that develops not only provides glucose substrate for fuel but also increases serum osmolality, which enhances reabsorption of fluid from the interstitial space into the vascular space. This homeostatic response to hypovolemia will ultimately fail with continued blood loss, and inadequate perfusion to vital organs causing cellular hypoxia will begin. Failure of this response to hypovolemia develops in patients with normal cardiac status at a loss of 25% to 30% of blood volume (class III shock; see Table 38–7).

### What Are the Cellular Responses to Hypovolemia?

Several common pathways can be defined even though the cellular response to hypoperfusion differs among cell types and by duration and degree of hypoperfusion. Connett used the term *dysoxia* in describing the alterations of cell function from hypoxia.[198] The dysoxic cell has oxygen-limited mitochondrial cytochrome turnover. As ATP is depleted, the sodium-potassium ATPase pump is unable to maintain normal electrolyte and water balance. Cellular edema develops from increased cellular sodium concentrations. Mitochondria become edematous if the cellular ion changes are not corrected by volume resuscitation. With mitochondrial failure, calcium influx begins and irreversible cellular changes are initiated.

Some investigators have used calcium antagonists to improve cellular and organ function. Increased calcium levels activate phospholipases, endonucleases, and proteinases.[199] Lysozymes degenerate, and with the release of degradative enzymes intracellular digestion further damages the cell. The cells are now primed to cause a reperfusion injury. As described previously, a variety of metabolic byproducts may now be distributed throughout the body as circulation is restored, initiating a systemic inflammatory response and organ dysfunction. Hypoxia also has cellular effects at the gene level. Hypoxia alone increases interleukin 8 (IL-8) gene expression in human cells.[200] Hypoxia stimulates the production of nuclear factors that control the inducible expression of a variety of genes in cytokine production, acute phase protein production, and cytokine receptors.[201]

## What Are the Organ Responses to Hypovolemia?

Organ response to hypovolemia also varies depending on the organ type, duration, and degree of shock. The role of the gut has been previously discussed.

### The Lungs

The decrease in oxygen delivery to the carotid bodies results in early stimulation of the respiratory drive causing respiratory alkalosis. Lung parenchymal fluid increases secondary to the previously described mechanisms, but oxygen diffusion is only affected minimally. If the shock state persists, release of a variety of proinflammatory mediators from circulating polymorphonuclear leukocytes, macrophages, alveolar cells, and the vascular endothelium can lead to alveolar flooding and progress to the acute respiratory distress syndrome.

### The Heart

The heart is one of the critical organs affected by the homeostatic responses to hypotension. Coronary blood flow is not diminished initially because of autoregulation. As the duration and degree of shock increase, myocardial oxygen requirements also increase. It is not completely understood if increased oxygen extraction can compensate for this increased demand.[202,203] Shock also produces a myocardial depressant factor that was initially described in 1966.[204] Recent evidence implicates TNF-$\alpha$ and IL-1 as the mediators that initiate myocardial depression. These mediators act both alone and synergistically to diminish myocardial contractility.[205] Their synergism increases the availability of nitric oxide, which decreases the availability of calcium to the myocardium.[206–208] As shock progresses, the heart becomes recalcitrant to the effects of volume loading and inotropic support.

### The Kidneys

The kidneys, like the heart and brain, are directly involved in the neuroendocrine response to hypoperfusion. Persistent shock results in intrarenal shunting of blood from the renal cortex to the renal medulla. If nephron ischemia occurs, cellular changes as previously described occur and cellular sloughing, known as acute tubular necrosis, begins. Tubular obstruction secondary to hyaline casts results in further injury. Although irreversible renal failure secondary to isolated hypovolemic shock is now uncommon, dialysis may be temporarily required for support.

### The Brain

The brain also benefits from an autoregulatory mechanism to maintain blood flow during hypovolemia. As mean arterial BP drops below 50 mm Hg, these autoregulatory mechanisms become overwhelmed. This becomes a significant problem when head injury coexists with other injuries that cause hypotension. Several studies support using hypertonic saline for resuscitation in patients with head injuries.[209–213]

### The Liver

The liver, similar to the gut, suffers from decreased blood flow during shock to support flow to vital organs. With persistent shock, the hepatocyte, like the enterocyte, is a major contributor to the proinflammatory cascade. The reticuloendothelial system is the major source of TNF-$\alpha$ in humans. Unfortunately, unlike the kidneys, heart, and lungs, the ability to support hepatic function through a period of failure and recovery is not often successful. "Shock liver," however, is rare after hypovolemic shock, and massive hepatic necrosis is unusual in patients with previously normal liver function.

The previously described cellular and organ changes initiate various shifts in body fluid compartments. The degree of initial extracellular fluid compartment contraction is directly related to the degree of blood loss. If appropriately resuscitated, this fluid contraction persists for about 24 hours. After the fluid sequestration phase, intracellular fluid is mobilized and diuresed as body fluid compartments are restored to normal.

## What Are the Traditional and Limited Fluids Approaches to Hypovolemic Shock?

The traditional approach to resuscitating a trauma patient is volume loading with crystalloids to achieve and maintain a near-normal BP and heart rate. Restoring intravascular volume is achieved with fluid boluses (10 mL/kg of crystalloid), observing the response, and repeating the bolus as needed, while attempts are made to diagnose and correct the cause of shock. Blood products may be needed if the patient's vital signs do not stabilize. Fluid resuscitation continues until the source of hypotension is identified and corrected.

In the past decade, clinical and laboratory evidence has led to questions concerning the logic of this traditional approach to fluid resuscitation in some hypovolemic patients. The concept of limited fluid resuscitation is based on the hypothesis that before control of the bleeding site, aggressive resuscitation causes hemodilution, increased BP, and increased blood loss through the injury site.

In an animal model, controlled hypotension to a mean arterial pressure of 40 mm Hg lessened acidemia and improved survival compared with resuscitation to a mean arterial pressure of 80 mm Hg.[214] Other animal studies have shown similar results,[215–218] with one suggesting that traditional fluid resuscitation after head injury with hemorrhagic shock worsened cerebral hemodynamics.[219] Based on these data and an animal model of ruptured abdominal aortic aneurysm,[220] several clinical trials have been conducted. Bickell and co-workers[54] prospectively examined nearly 600 patients with penetrating trauma to the torso who presented with systolic BPs $\leq$90 mm Hg to determine whether delaying fluid resuscitation until surgery changed outcome. Survival (70% versus 62%) and length of hospital stay (11 versus 14 days) were improved in the delayed resuscitation group. In 1997, Sampalis and associates[221] performed an observational study in two matched groups comparing initiation of intravenous fluids at the accident scene with no intravenous placement. This study showed that for patients with prehospital times of 30 minutes or less, providing on-site intravenous fluids was nonbeneficial. For those patients with prehospital times of 30 minutes or more, prehospital intravenous fluid administration was actually associated with an increase in mortality rate. Critics of both studies believe that design flaws hinder their conclusions and that further randomized control trials will be required to appropriately address these issues. A logical analysis of these studies and an understanding of the pathophysiology of hypovolemia lend some credence to limited fluid resuscitation before operative control of bleeding. Which groups of patients will benefit remains to be elucidated.

## What Type of Fluid Is Best for Resuscitation?

The controversy of crystalloids versus colloids has persisted for decades. Recently, the issue of hypertonic crystalloid solutions for resuscitation has further complicated matters. A review analyzed 37 prospective randomized controlled trials examining crystalloid versus colloid resuscitation in critically ill patients and found a 4% increased mortality rate associated with colloid resuscitation.[222]

The effectiveness of hypertonic saline for resuscitation depends on the type of trauma patient. While several studies have demonstrated the advantages of hypertonic saline in the resuscitation of head-injured patients,[209,210,212] its use in burn patients is associated with higher renal failure and mortality rates.[223]

## What Is Neurogenic Shock?

Neurogenic shock develops whenever spinal cord injury, severe head trauma, or sympathetic blockade (high spinal anesthesia) produces a loss of sympathetic stimulation and vasomotor tone. The decrease in systemic vascular resistance significantly increases venous capacitance, which decreases venous return, reducing cardiac output. Clinically, the patient is hypotensive, but unlike hypovolemic patients, the skin is warm and dry. As with hypovolemic shock, initial therapy is volume resuscitation. It is imperative in the trauma patient that other sources of hypotension are ruled out. α-Adrenergic agonists such as phenylephrine administered at 0.1 to 3.0 μg/kg/min may be useful if fluid resuscitation alone does not correct hypotension. If pathologic vasodilation persists, norepinephrine may be needed beginning at 0.01 μg/kg/min and titrated as needed. Patients with high spinal cord lesions are also usually bradycardic, and small doses of atropine may be needed for heart rates of ≦50 BPM if BP is rate dependent.

## What Is Traumatic Shock?

Traumatic shock is a subtype within the traditional category of vasogenic (or distributive) shock. The injuries associated with traumatic shock also frequently cause simple hypovolemic shock, but the amount of volume needed for resuscitation is significantly magnified. Patients with burns, substantial soft tissue trauma, major fractures with vascular compromise, or crush injuries develop severe local cellular damage significant enough to initiate inflammatory mediator cascades, leading to severe systemic inflammation and organ failure. Microvascular permeability is increased, leading to massive fluid requirements that are much greater than expected if estimated based solely on blood loss. Rhabdomyolysis from skeletal muscle trauma releases cellular contents into the plasma, particularly myoglobin, which can cause renal failure. Treatment includes adequate, often massive, fluid resuscitation, alkalinization of the urine, mannitol, and/or loop diuretics. The risk of developing organ failure is greater with traumatic shock when compared with simple hypovolemic shock. PA catheters, mechanical ventilation, dialysis, and inotropic support may be required.

## What Is Septic Shock?

Septic shock is a subtype of vasogenic (or distributive) shock. This form of shock occurs when an infection initiates the inflammatory mediator cascades that cause a systemic response that includes fever, hypotension, hypoperfusion, and cellular hypoxia. In 1992, the American College of Chest Physicians/Society of Critical Care Medicine Consensus Conference Committee attempted to standardize the various terms associated with septic shock.[224]

### Systemic Inflammatory Response Syndrome

*SIRS* is defined as the systemic inflammatory response to a variety of severe clinical insults. SIRS is characterized by two or more of the following:

1. Temperature ≥38°C (100.4°F) or ≦36°C (96.8°F)
2. Heart rate ≥90 BPM
3. Respiratory rate ≥20 breaths per minute or $Paco_2$ <32 mm Hg
4. WBC count >12 000/mm³, <4000 mm³, or >10% band forms.

### Sepsis

Sepsis is defined as the presence of SIRS in association with culture-proven infection.

### Septic Shock

Septic shock is defined as sepsis with hypotension despite adequate fluid resuscitation, along with manifestations of hypoperfusion, including, but not limited to, lactic acidosis, oliguria, or an acute alteration in mental status.

### Multiple Organ Dysfunction Syndrome

*MODS* is defined as the presence of altered organ function in an acutely ill patient such that homeostasis cannot be maintained without intervention.

A significant number of patients, particularly trauma patients, develop SIRS without infection. The shared systemic manifestations of fever, leukocytosis, hypermetabolism, and a hyperdynamic circulatory state are commonly seen in septic patients but are also common with other forms of vasogenic shock as well as prolonged hypovolemic shock followed by resuscitation. Goris and colleagues[225] demonstrated that only one third of trauma patients who died of MOF had an untreated focus of infection. A continuum exists when injury and/or infection combined with hypoperfusion and ischemia, followed by reperfusion injury with resuscitation, initiates one or more inflammatory mediator cascades that result in the clinical signs of SIRS. The duration and severity of SIRS will determine whether the patient progresses to MODS and MOF. The epidemiology for the development of SIRS has been studied in a prospective trial, which also demonstrated that the criteria for SIRS are not specific enough to predict which

**TABLE 38–14.** Multiple Organ Dysfunction Score

| | Score | | | | |
| Organ System | 0 | 1 | 2 | 3 | 4 |
|---|---|---|---|---|---|
| Respiratory* (PaO₂/FIO₂ ratio) | >300 | 226-300 | 151-225 | 76-150 | ≤75 |
| Renal† (serum creatinine) | ≤100 | 101-200 | 201-350 | 351-500 | >500 |
| Hepatic‡ (serum bilirubin) | ≤20 | 21-60 | 61-120 | 121-240 | >240 |
| Cardiovascular§ (PAR) | ≤10.0 | 10.1-15.0 | 15.1-20.0 | 20.1-30.0 | >30.0 |
| Hematologic‖ (platelet count) | >120 | 81-120 | 51-80 | 21-50 | ≤20 |
| Neurologic¶ (Glasgow Coma Scale score) | 15 | 13-14 | 10-12 | 7-9 | ≤6 |

*The PaO₂/FIO₂ ratio is calculated without reference to the use or mode of mechanical ventilation and without reference to use of the level of positive end-expiratory pressure.

†The serum creatinine concentration is measured in micromoles per liter without reference to the use of dialysis.

‡The serum bilirubin concentration is measured in micromoles per liter.

§The pressure-adjusted heart rate (PAR) is calculated as the product of the heart rate (HR) multiplied by the ratio of the right atrial (central venous) pressure (RAP) to the mean arterial pressure (MAP): PAR = HR × RAP/mean blood pressure.

‖The platelet count is measured in platelets per cubic milliliter.

¶The Glasgow Coma Scale score is preferably calculated by the patient's nurse and is scored conservatively (for patients receiving sedation or muscle relaxants, normal function is assumed unless there is evidence of intrinsically altered mentation).

From Marshall JC, Cook DJ, Christou NV, et al. Multiple organ dysfunction score: a reliable descriptor of a complex clinical outcome. *Crit Care Med.* 1995;23:1638-1652.

patients will progress further to MODS.[226] Using the Consensus definitions, mortality rates for patients with two, three, and four SIRS criteria were 6%, 9%, and 18%, respectively.[227] The same study showed that severe SIRS with positive cultures (indicating infection) had a mortality rate of 20% when there were no clinical signs of shock and 46% when shock was present.

MOF is a systemic disorder involving the disruption of the normal complex immunologic, inflammatory, endothelial, and metabolic programming that is supposed to result in the reinstatement of normal physiology. First described in 1973 by Tilney and coworkers,[228] MOF may be primary or secondary.[224] Primary MOF is the direct result of the initiating event (ie, renal failure from rhabdomyolysis). The organ dysfunction resulting from the initial hypotension, ischemia, and reperfusion also constitute primary MOF. Secondary MOF results from a persistent hyperinflammatory state (ie, SIRS) that involves organ dysfunction remote from the initial injury.

Marshall and associates[229] developed a MODS score that predicts ICU mortality (Table 38–14). As an outcome measure, the ICU mortality rate was about 25% at 9 to 12 points, 50% at 13 to 16 points, 75% at 17 to 20 points, and 100% with >20 points. The common pathway leading to SIRS, septic shock, MODS, and MOF is comprised of the various mediators that function as immunologic and inflammatory messengers.

## What Are the Important Mediators of Shock, Systemic Inflammatory Response Syndrome, and Multiple Organ Dysfunction Syndrome?

### Endotoxin

In septic shock, the initiating factor is the stimulation of macrophages by bacterial endotoxin to begin the inflammatory pathway, initially with TNF-α. Endotoxin, or lipopolysaccharide, is a complex molecule located in the walls of gram-negative bacteria that consists of three distinct areas: the lipid A moiety, a core polysaccharide (R core antigen), and the oligosaccharide (O)-specific side chains. The lipid A area initiates the production of TNF-α by binding to the CD-14 receptor on monocytes and macrophages. Treatment with antiendotoxin antibodies has produced indeterminate results in two large clinical trials.[230,231] Certain patient populations may benefit, but further studies are needed.

### Cytokines

This large diverse group of soluble proteins is produced by a variety of cell lines in response to injury, infection, tumor, inflammation, and hypoperfusion. TNF-α, IL-1, and IL-6 are the most active cytokines mediating the hyperinflammatory response in sepsis and injury (Fig. 38–3). TNF-α is secreted primarily by monocytes and macrophages but also to a lesser degree by lymphocytes, Kupffer cells, and other cell types.[205] The initial cytokine detected in the serum, TNF-α induces further cytokine cascade formations, hypotension, fever, disseminated intravascular coagulopathy, and increased systemic vascular permeability. These effects are initiated at the tissue level through oxidant release, nitric oxide, and eicosanoid production. Macrophages, monocytes, and the endothelium all produce IL-1.[205] Secreted in response to both TNF-α and endotoxin, IL-1 produces fever, skeletal muscle proteolysis, other cytokine release, endothelial cell procoagulant release, and T and B lymphocyte stimulation. IL-6 is also elaborated by similar inflammatory cell types and is a major stimulant for hepatic production of acute phase proteins.[205]

### Complement Fragments

Complement activation occurs via the alternative pathway when initiated by endotoxin or antigenic protein aggregates.

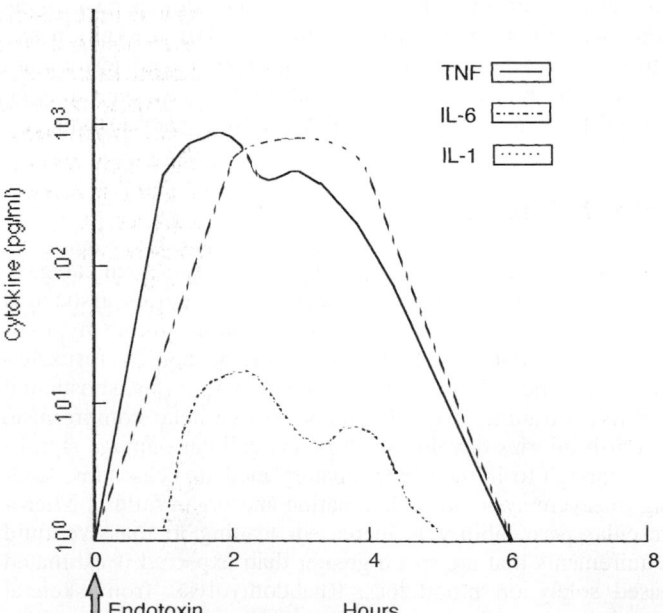

**FIGURE 38–3.** A single intravenous bolus of *Escherichia coli* endotoxin was administered to human volunteers; shown here are the changes in plasma tumor necrosis factor (TNF), interleukin 1 (IL-1), and IL-6 concentrations that ensued. Peak TNF levels occurred first during endotoxemia, followed by rises in IL-1 and IL-6.

With sequential proteolysis of complement substrate, various complement fragments occur. C3 and C5a exert the greatest physiologic effects, being potent *chemoattractants* for neutrophils and macrophages, as well as causing histamine release from basophils and mast cells. Histamine's effects include vasodilation and increased vascular permeability. Increased concentrations of activated complement are associated with higher mortality in septic patients.[232]

### Eicosanoids

Eicosanoids are a large group of compounds that have arachidonic acid as the primary precursor. They include the leukotrienes, prostaglandins, and thromboxanes.[233] The prostaglandins, which are produced via the cyclo-oxygenase pathway, are potent vasodilators and bronchodilators produced locally by vascular endothelium. They also inhibit platelet aggregation. Thromboxane $A_2$, produced by a similar pathway in platelets, has the opposite effect, causing vasoconstriction and platelet aggregation.[233]

The leukotrienes are produced via the lipoxygenase pathway by a variety of inflammatory cells and vascular endothelium. These are potent chemoattractants, vasoconstrictors, and mediators of increased vascular permeability. They may play a major role in the development of acute respiratory distress syndrome.[233]

### Platelet-Activating Factor

Platelet-activating factor (PAF) is a lipid compound first described by Benveniste and associates[234] and is the most potent lipid mediator identified thus far. It is released by a variety of cell types, including mast cells, macrophages, neutrophils, and basophils. PAF's in vivo function was believed to be mediation of platelet aggregation. It is now known that when exposed to endotoxin, PAF activates phagocytes, promotes increased vascular permeability, and stimulates oxygen free radical production.

### Kinins

Bradykinin is a major product of the plasma contact activation system and mediates vasodilation locally while activating coagulation, the complement cascade, and fibrinolysis. Bradykinin can also activate phospholipase, which increases eicosanoid formation.[205]

### Nitric Oxide

Also known as endothelial-derived relaxing factor, NO is the most potent vasodilator produced in vivo. Endotoxin and TNF-α induce the enzyme NO synthase, which is produced by vascular endothelial cells, neutrophils, and Kupffer's cells.[235] Limited production of NO may produce local vasodilation, as in the lungs, but pathologic production leads to severe vasodilation and hypotension. Groeneveld and coworkers[236] demonstrated a significant correlation between MODS scores and serum nitrate levels, a marker for NO production.

### Endogenous Opioids

Injury and infection stimulate the production of endorphins, which are vasodilators.[237] Various studies have tried to determine whether endorphin antagonists could ameliorate the hypotension of shock.[238] Many of the previously discussed mediators have been targeted with antagonists in clinical trials. Various anti–TNF-α regimens,[239–245] anti–IL-1,[246] bradykinin antagonist,[247] PAF antagonist,[248,249] and the eicosanoid antagonist ibuprofen[250] have failed to improve survival.

## Why Has Inflammatory Mediator Modulation Been Unsuccessful?

The explanation for failure of proinflammatory mediator modulation is unclear. Many of the same therapies have been successful in animal models. Failures in human trials are related to studying inappropriate patient populations, inappropriate initiation and duration of therapy, and dose-related issues. Two new theories have been proposed to explain SIRS and its continuum to MODS and MOF. Both hypotheses use the term *chaos* in their explanations of the events leading to SIRS and MODS. Bone[251] hypothesized that the reason these new therapies for sepsis have failed was because of discounting the natural balance between inflammatory and antiinflammatory mediators. He introduced the mnemonic CHAOS, in which the "C" stands for cardiovascular compromise, the "H" for homeostasis, the "A" for apoptosis, the "O" for organ dysfunction, and the "S" for suppression of the immune system. Godin and Buchman[252] in a more complex hypothesis used the concept of chaos to explain MODS as an uncoupling of biologic oscillators.

Dynamics is the study of change in a system over time. A dynamic system is deterministic if each future state of the system can be determined from a single prior state. A system is linear if the change is linearly proportional to the system variables. A nonlinear system is one whose behavior is not a simple sum or multiple of the initial prior state. Deterministic, nonlinear systems are present throughout nature.

Chaos is defined as the irregular behavior of some deterministic nonlinear systems, but this behavior is dependent on the initial conditions. The initial conditions, which may be altered by a small simple change in rules, can, over time, result in a progressive divergence in the system. Thus, chaos is not a random series of events but actually implies underlying structure and determinism. The advantage that chaos confers on a biologic system is the ability for chaotic systems to associate with one another and therefore create spontaneous order that can adapt more readily to external influences. "The stability of the system depends on the number, bias, and type of the interconnections among the systems' constituents."[252] The authors hypothesize that while the changes in coupling (interactions) are a consequence of SIRS they are a cause of MODS. They cite three articles that examine the chaos of the heart. Normally, the heart has chaotic electrical signaling, which leads to subtle but measurable variability in the RR interval. Increases in morbidity and mortality were associated with loss of variability of the RR interval.[253–255] Although these studies described the loss of variability as a consequence of the disease process, the increased regularity of the heart rate may be a result of uncoupling of the heart from other organ systems.

Winchell and Hoyt examined heart rate variability in a large series of patients in ICUs and found that a low variability in heart rate, in noncardiac patients, had a 13-fold increased risk of death.[256] The prolonged recovery from MODS is attributed to the body's search to establish the appropriate organ interconnections.

In a follow-up article, Godin and associates[257] examined in a prospective, randomized, blinded study infusion of endotoxin into human volunteers. A significant reduction in heart rate variability occurred in those subjects receiving endotoxin. The chaos theory is attractive in its ability to explain the dichotomy between animal and human antiinflammatory mediator studies, as well as why some of the human studies may show significance in small subsets of studies.

In animal studies, the initiating factors are identical in genetically identical animals and the sensitivity of chaotic systems to initiating events allows for reproducible outcomes. In human shock studies, both the initial events as well as individual human variability allow for vastly different scenarios. Unfortunately, to date, the chaos theory offers few suggestions regarding the treatment of shock. However, this theory may in the future allow for better detection of the early shock state.

## How Is Sepsis From Infection Differentiated From Systemic Inflammatory Response Syndrome?

In trauma patients, the diagnosis of sepsis versus SIRS can be difficult. In the presence of a hyperdynamic cardiac state with other signs of infection, such as leukocytosis and fever, a diligent search for an infectious source must be undertaken. Death after trauma 1 to 2 weeks after injury is usually due to sepsis and MODS.[258,259]

### The Lungs

Pneumonia remains the most common infectious complication following injury, often secondary to aspiration at the time of injury. Pneumonia within the first week is often from community-acquired organisms, whereas late pneumonia is usually secondary to gram-negative organisms indigenous to the ICU. Making the diagnosis may be simple, as in an isolated closed head injury patient with a new infiltrate on a chest radiograph, to complex, as in a trauma patient with multiple injuries and acute respiratory distress syndrome.

### Device-Related Sources

Other sources for sepsis include the urinary tract, central nervous system, and intravascular access. Each of these is usually related to invasive indwelling devices, closed drainage systems for the urinary bladder, ventriculostomy for ICP monitoring, and vascular catheters for venous access and hemodynamic monitoring. Eighty percent of patients requiring urinary catheters for >10 days have bacterial colonization. Central venous catheters were previously associated with about 32 infections per 1000 catheter-days, but the introduction of antiseptic- and antibiotic-impregnated catheters has decreased this to less than 2 infections per 1000 catheter-days.[260,261]

### Other Sources

Paranasal sinuses, soft tissue injuries, surgical wounds, and intraabdominal sources of sepsis are often difficult to diagnose. CT is the preferred test for diagnosing sinusitis and intraabdominal infections. When the diagnosis of an abdominal source can be established with CT, treatment ranges from percutaneous drainage of abscesses to laparotomy. The problem arises when abdominal CT fails to identify a source in a patient with impending MODS. Norwood and Civetta reported, in 1985, that abdominal CT was only helpful in 24% of their surgical ICU patients.[262] The decision to perform a nondirected laparotomy, however, must be based on the chance of finding a missed injury, a history of previous laparotomy, and the temporal relationship of MODS onset to previous laparotomy.

MODS occurring earlier than 2 weeks after laparotomy is more likely to be from an abdominal source. Similarly, intraabdominal sources of sepsis are more likely when clinical sepsis precedes the onset of pulmonary failure.[263] Even for patients with MODS there is clinical evidence that a negative laparotomy does not change survival.

To date, there has been no magic bullet that can prevent the sequelae of severe shock, SIRS, and MODS.[264] The treatment remains early recognition of shock, aggressive resuscitative efforts, removal and treatment of septic sources, and support of failing organ systems.

Scalea and colleagues[181] found that when hemodynamic monitoring with PA catheters was initiated within 2 hours of hospital admission in geriatric blunt trauma patients, the mortality rate was reduced to 47% compared with 93% when monitoring did not begin until at least 6 hours after hospital admission. The initial presence or achievement of normal clinical vital signs should not be accepted as the only endpoints in determining the adequacy of resuscitation. Shoemaker and coworkers[177] found no difference in the postoperative BP and heart rate of high-risk surgical patients who survived versus nonsurvivors. Although optimizing $\dot{V}o_2$ and $\dot{D}o_2$ as described by Bishop and coworkers[182] remains controversial for improving survival, improving these variables quickly seems prudent to optimize perfusion of both vital and "nonvital" organs.

Volume loading with blood components and crystalloid to achieve a normal intravascular volume, stable hemoglobin, and normal coagulation parameters with observed improvements in lactate clearance, base deficit, and organ perfusion parameters remain the standard of care for resuscitation. Inotropic agents may be necessary as volume status is normalized to enhance $\dot{D}o_2$ if preselected goals are not met.

The continued poor outcomes observed in patients who initially survive the shock state have led to questions concerning the survival benefits of the body's response to shock. Two recent studies examined the genetics involved in the expression of TNF-α and IL-1.[265,266]

The Pulitzer Prize–winning author Edward O. Wilson has observed that evolutionary pressures work toward species survival, occasionally at the expense of the individual. Perhaps, thousands of years ago, SIRS and MODS endowed a survival benefit to the group by ensuring that severely injured individuals die quickly so that species energy and resources are not wasted to keep a severely injured individual alive. Thousands of years later, in the ICU setting, we are struggling against these complex systems that conferred species survival long ago.

### References

1. Holbrook TL, Anderson JP, Sieber WJ, et al. Outcome after major trauma: discharge and 6-month follow-up results from the trauma recovery project. *J Trauma*. 1998;45:315.

2. McLoughlin E, McGuire A. Injury prevention. In: Trunkey DD, Lewis FR, eds. *Current Therapy of Trauma.* 4th ed. St Louis, Mo: CV Mosby; 1999:3.

3. Meyer AA. Death and disability from injury: a global challenge. *J Trauma.* 1998;44:1.

4. Murray C, Lopez A. Alternative projections of mortality and disability by cause 1990-2020: global burden of disease study. *Lancet.* 1997;349:1498.

5. Tornetta P, Mostafavi H, Riina J, et al. Morbidity and mortality in elderly trauma patients. *J Trauma.* 1999;46:702.

6. Baker CC. Epidemiology of trauma: the civilian perspective. *Ann Emerg Med.* 1986;15:1389.

7. National Research Council and Institute of Medicine. *Injury in America.* Washington, DC: National Academy Press; 1985.

8. Centers for Disease Control. Leads from the MMWR: differences in death rates due to injury among blacks and whites, 1984. *JAMA.* 1989;261:214.

9. Webster DW. The unconvincing case for school-based conflict resolution programs for adolescents. *Health Affairs.* 1993;12:226.

10. Hammond WR, Yung BR. Preventing violence in at risk African-American youth. *J Health Care Poor Underserved.* 1991;2:359.

11. Committee on Trauma, American College of Surgeons. *Resources for Optimal Care of the Injured Patient: 1999.* Chicago, Ill: American College of Surgeons; 1998:49.

12. Baker SP, Whitfield RA, O'Neill B. Geographic variations in mortality from motor vehicle crashes. *N Engl J Med.* 1987;316:1384.

13. Bennett-Jacobs B, Jacobs LM. Epidemiology of trauma. In: Feliciano DV, Moore EE, Mattox KL, eds. *Trauma.* 3rd ed. Stamford, Conn: Appleton & Lange; 1996:15.

14. Uzych L. Trauma care systems. *Am J Emerg Med.* 1990;8:71.

15. Acosta JA, Yang JC, Winchell RJ, et al. Lethal injuries and time to death in a Level I trauma center. *J Am Coll Surg.* 1998;186:528.

16. Committee on Trauma, American College of Surgeons. *Resources for Optimal Care of the Injured Patient: 1999.* Chicago, Ill: American College of Surgeons; 1998:5.

17. Champion HR, Sacco WJ, Copes WS, et al. A revision of the Trauma Score. *J Trauma.* 1989;29:623.

18. Tepas JJ, Mollitt DL, Talbert JL. The pediatric trauma score as a predictor of injury severity in the injured child. *J Pediatr Surg.* 1987;22:14.

19. Champion HR, Copes WS, Sacco WJ, et al. The major trauma outcome study: establishing national norms for trauma care. *J Trauma.* 1990;30:1356.

20. Baker SP, O'Neill B, Haddow W, et al. The injury severity score: a method for describing patients with multiple injuries and evaluating emergency care. *J Trauma.* 1974;14:187.

21. Boyd CR, Tolson MW, Copes WS. Evaluating trauma care: the TRISS method. *J Trauma.* 1987;27:370.

22. Copes WS, Champion HR, Sacco WJ, et al. Progress in characterizing anatomic injury. *J Trauma.* 1990;30:1200.

23. Brenneman FD, Boulanger BR, McLellan BA, et al. Measuring injury severity: time for a change? *J Trauma.* 1998;44:580.

24. Copes WS, Champion HR, Sacco WJ, et al. The Injury Severity Score revisited. *J Trauma.* 1988;28:69.

25. Champion HR, Copes WS, Sacco WJ, et al. A new characterization of injury severity. *J Trauma.* 1990;30:539.

26. Cornwell EE, Velmahos GC, Berne TV, et al. Lethal abdominal gunshot wounds at a Level I trauma center: analysis of TRISS fallouts. *J Am Coll Surg.* 1998;187:123.

27. McGonigal MD, Cole J, Schwab W, et al. A new approach to probability of survival scoring for trauma quality assurance. *J Trauma.* 1993;34:863.

28. Rutledge R. Injury severity and probability of survival assessment in trauma patients using a predictive hierarchical network model derived from ICD-9 codes. *J Trauma.* 1995;38:590.

29. Committee on Trauma, American College of Surgeons. *Resources for Optimal Care of the Injured Patient: 1999.* Chicago, Ill: American College of Surgeons; 1998:13.

30. Battistella FD, Nugent W, Owings JT, et al. Field triage of the pulseless trauma patient. *Arch Surg.* 1999;134:742.

31. Huei-Ming M, MacKenzie EJ, Alcorta R, et al. Compliance with prehospital triage protocols for major trauma patients. *J Trauma.* 1999;46:168.

32. Helling TS, Watkins M, Evans LL, et al. Low falls: an underappreciated mechanism of injury. *J Trauma.* 1999;46:453.

33. Goodacre S, Than M, Goyder EC, et al. Can the distance fallen predict serious injury after a fall from a height? *J Trauma.* 1999;46:1055.

34. Grande CM, Stene JK, Bernhard WN, et al. Trauma anesthesia and critical care: the concept and rationale for a new subspecialty. *Crit Care Clin.* 1990;6:1.

35. de Mello W, Griffiths C. Anesthetists and trauma. *Anesthesia.* 1991;46:151.

36. Emergency Nurses Association. *Trauma Nursing Core Course Provider Manual.* Park Ridge, Ill: Emergency Nurses Association; 1995.

37. Gomez MJ, Ferraro CA, Charlson DA, et al. The cost effectiveness of a two-tier trauma response [abstract]. *J Trauma.* 1991;31:1716.

38. Committee on Trauma, American College of Surgeons. *Resources for Optimal Care of the Injured Patient: 1999.* Chicago, Ill: American College of Surgeons; 1998:100.

39. Barone JE, Ryan MC, Cayten CG, et al. Is 24-hour operating room staff absolutely necessary for Level II trauma center designation? *J Trauma.* 1993;34:878.

40. Brasel KJ, Akason J, Weigelt JA. Dedicated operating room for trauma: a costly recommendation. *J Trauma.* 1998;44:832.

41. Hoyt DB, Shackford SR, McGill T, et al. The impact of in-house surgeons and operating room resuscitation on outcome of traumatic injuries. *Arch Surg.* 1989;124:906.

42. Committee on Trauma, American College of Surgeons. *Advanced Trauma Life Support for Doctors: Student Course Manual.* Chicago, Ill: American College of Surgeons; 1997.

43. Norwood SH, Myers MB, Butler J. The safety of emergency neuromuscular blockade and orotracheal intubation in the acutely injured patient. *J Am Coll Surg.* 1994;179:646.

44. Winchell RJ, Hoyt DB. Endotracheal intubation in the field improves survival in patients with severe head injury. *Arch Surg.* 1997;132:592.

45. Rhodes M, Brader AH. Organization of a trauma resuscitation system. In: Maul KI, Cleveland HC, Strauch GO, et al, eds. *Advances in Trauma.* Vol 4. Chicago, Ill: Year Book Medical; 1989:19.

46. Ligier B, Buchman TG, Breslow MJ, et al. The role of anesthetic induction agents and neuromuscular blockade in the endotracheal intubation of trauma victims. *Surg Gynecol Obstet.* 1991;173:477.

47. Seebacher J, Nozik D, Mathieu A. Inadvertent intracranial introduction of a nasogastric tube, a complication of severe maxillofacial trauma. *Anesthesiology.* 1975;42:100.

48. Dinner M, Tjeuw M, Artusio JF. Bacteremia as a complication of nasotracheal intubation. *Anesth Analg.* 1987;66:460.

49. Bos AP, Tibboel D, Hazebroek FWJ, et al. Sinusitis: hidden source of sepsis in postoperative pediatric intensive care patients. *Crit Care Med.* 1989;17:886.

50. Dauphinee K. Nasotracheal intubation. *Emerg Med Clin North Am.* 1988;6:715.

51. Little CM, Parker MG, Tarnopolsky R. The incidence of vasculature at risk during cricothyroidostomy. *Ann Emerg Med.* 1986;15:805.

52. Blostein PA, Koestner AJ, Hoak S. Failed rapid sequence intubation in trauma patients: esophageal tracheal Combitube is a useful adjunct. *J Trauma.* 1998;44:534.

53. Rozycki GS, Feliciano DV, Ochsner MG, et al. The role of ultrasound in patients with possible penetrating cardiac wounds: a prospective multicenter study. *J Trauma.* 1999;46:543.

54. Bickell WH, Wall MJ, Pepe PE, et al. Immediate versus delayed fluid resuscitation for hypotensive patients with penetrating torso injuries. *N Engl J Med.* 1994;331:1105.

55. Demetriades D, Chan L, Cornwell E, et al. Paramedic vs private transportation of trauma patients. *Arch Surg.* 1996;131:133.

56. Mattox KL, Bickell W, Pepe PE, et al. Prospective MAST study in 911 patients. *J Trauma.* 1989;29:1104.

57. Aprahamian C, Gessert G, Bandy KD, et al. MAST-associated compartment syndrome (MACS): a review. *J Trauma.* 1989;29:549.

58. Branney SW, Moore EE, Feldhaus KM, et al. Critical analysis of two decades of experience with post injury emergency department thoracotomy in a regional trauma center. *J Trauma.* 1998;45:87.

59. Stratton SJ, Brickett K, Crammer T. Prehospital pulseless, unconscious penetrating trauma victims: field assessments associated with survival. *J Trauma.* 1998;45:96.

60. Servadei F, Nasi MT, Cremonini AM, et al. Importance of a reliable admission Glasgow Coma Scale Score for determining the need for evacuation of post traumatic subdural hematomas: a prospective study of 65 patients. *J Trauma.* 1998;44:868.

61. Buechler CM, Blostein PA, Koestner A, et al. Variation among trauma centers' calculation of Glasgow Coma Scale Score: results of a national survey. *J Trauma.* 1998;45:429.

62. Meredith W, Rutledge R, Hansen AR, et al. Field triage of trauma patients based upon the ability to follow commands: a study in 29,573 injured patients. *J Trauma.* 1995;38:129.

63. Ross SE, Leipold C, Terregino C, et al. Efficacy of the motor component of the Glasgow Coma Scale in trauma triage. *J Trauma.* 1998;45:42.

64. Kurz A, Sessler DI, Lenhardt R, et al. Perioperative normothermia to reduce the incidence of surgical-wound infection and shorten hospitalization. *N Engl J Med.* 1996;334:1209.

65. Ballard RB, Rozycki GS, Newman PG, et al. An algorithm to reduce the incidence of false-negative FAST examinations in patients at high risk for occult injury. *J Am Coll Surg.* 1999;189:145.

66. Fernandez L, McKenney MG, McKenney KL, et al. Ultrasound in blunt abdominal trauma. *J Trauma.* 1998;45:841.

67. Gonzalez RP, Fried PO, Holevar MR, et al. Role of clinical examination in screening for blunt cervical spine injury. *J Am Coll Surg.* 1999;189:152.

68. Sees DW, Rodriguez LR, Flaherty SF, et al. The use of bedside fluoroscopy to evaluate the cervical spine in obtunded trauma patients. *J Trauma.* 1998;45:768.

69. Biffl WL, Moore EE, Ryu RK, et al. The unrecognized epidemic of blunt carotid arterial injuries. *Ann Surg.* 1998;228:462.

70. Feliciano DV, Mattox KL, Trunkey DD. Heart injury. In: Trunkey DD, Lewis FR, eds. *Current Therapy of Trauma.* 4th ed. St Louis, Mo: CV Mosby; 1999:205.

71. Biffl WL, Moore FA, Moore EE, et al. Cardiac enzymes are irrelevant in the patient with suspected myocardial contusion. *Am J Surg.* 1994;169:523.

72. Maenza RL, Seaberg D, D'Amico F. A meta-analysis of blunt cardiac trauma: ending myocardial confusion. *Am J Emerg Med.* 1996;14:237.

73. Fabian TC, Davis KA, Gavant ML, et al. Prospective study of blunt aortic injury. *Ann Surg.* 1998;227:666.

74. Mirvis SE, Shanmuganathan K, Buell J, et al. Use of spiral computed tomography for the assessment of blunt trauma patients with potential aortic injury. *J Trauma.* 1998;45:922.

75. Demetriades D, Gomez H, Velmahos G, et al. Routine helical computed tomographic evaluation of the mediastinum in high-risk blunt trauma patients. *Arch Surg.* 1998;133:1084.

76. Mattox KL, Wall MJ, LeMaire SA. Thoracic great vessel injury. In: Trunkey DD, Lewis FR, eds. *Current Therapy of Trauma.* 4th ed. St Louis, Mo: CV Mosby; 1999:216.

77. Reber PU, Seiler CA, Baer HU, et al. Missed diaphragmatic injuries and their long-term sequelae. *J Trauma.* 1998;44:183.

78. Demetriades D, Velmahos G, Cornwell E, et al. Selective nonoperative management of gunshot wounds of the anterior abdomen. *Arch Surg.* 1997;132:178.

79. Grossman MD, May AK, Schwab CW, et al. Determining anatomic injury with computed tomography in selected torso gunshot wounds. *J Trauma.* 1998;45:446.

80. Demetriades D, Gomez H, Chahwan S, et al. Gunshot injuries to the liver: the role of selective nonoperative management. *J Am Coll Surg.* 1999;188:343.

81. Karmy-Jones R, Wagner JW, Lewis JW. Diaphragmatic injury. In: Trunkey DD, Lewis FR, eds. *Current Therapy of Trauma.* 4th ed. St Louis, Mo: CV Mosby; 1999:224.

82. Partrick DA, Bensard DD, Moore EE, et al. Ultrasound is an effective triage tool to evaluate blunt abdominal trauma in the pediatric population. *J Trauma.* 1998;45:57.

83. Yoshii H, Sato M, Yamamoto S, et al. Usefulness and limitations of ultrasonography in the initial evaluation of blunt abdominal trauma. *J Trauma.* 1998;45:45.

84. Scalea TM, Rodriguez A, Chiu WC, et al. Focused assessment with sonography for trauma (FAST): results from an International Consensus Conference. *J Trauma.* 1999;45:466.

85. Rozycki GS, Oshsner MG, Schmidt JA, et al. A prospective study of surgeon-performed ultrasound as the primary adjuvant modality for injured patient assessment. *J Trauma.* 1995;39:492.

86. Han DC, Rozycki GS, Schmidt JA, Feliciano DV. Ultrasound training during ATLS: an early start for surgical interns. *J Trauma.* 1996;41:208.

87. Henneman PL, Marx JA, Moore EE, et al. Diagnostic peritoneal lavage: accuracy in predicting necessary laparotomy following blunt and penetrating trauma. *J Trauma.* 1990;30:1345.

88. Keleman JJ, Martin RR, Obney JA, et al. Evaluation of diagnostic peritoneal lavage in stable patients with gunshot wounds to the abdomen. *Arch Surg.* 1997;132:909.

89. Livingston DH, Lavery RF, Passannante MR, et al. Admission or observation is not necessary after a negative abdominal computed tomographic scan in patients with suspected blunt abdominal trauma: results of a prospective, multi-institutional trial. *J Trauma.* 1998;44:273.

90. Asbun HJ, Irani H, Roe EJ, et al. Intra-abdominal seat belt injury. *J Trauma.* 1990;30:189.

91. Anderson PA, Rivara FP, Maier RV, et al. The epidemiology of seat belt-associated injuries. *J Trauma.* 1991;31:60.

92. Newman KD, Bowman LM, Eichelberger MR, et al. The lap belt complex: intestinal and lumbar spine injuries in children. *J Trauma.* 1990;30:1133.

93. Stafford RE, McGonigal MD, Weigelt JA, et al. Oral contrast solution and computed tomography for blunt abdominal trauma. *Arch Surg.* 1999;134:622.

94. Brasel KJ, Olson CJ, Stafford RE, et al. Incidence and significance of free fluid on abdominal computed tomographic scan in blunt trauma. *J Trauma.* 1998;44:889.

95. Cunningham MA, Tyroch AH, Kaups KL, et al. Does free fluid on abdominal computed tomographic scan after blunt trauma require laparotomy? *J Trauma.* 1998;44:599.

96. Hulka F, Mullins RJ, Leonardo V, et al. Significance of peritoneal fluid as an isolated finding on abdominal computed tomographic scans in pediatric trauma patients. *J Trauma.* 1998;44:1069.

97. Frick EJ, Pasquale MD, Cipolle MD. Small bowel and mesentery injuries in blunt trauma. *J Trauma.* 1999;46:920.

98. Trafton PG. Fractures. In: Trunkey DD, Lewis FR, eds. *Current Therapy of Trauma.* 4th ed. St Louis, Mo: CV Mosby; 1999:282.

99. Houin HP. Lower extremity and degloving injuries. In: Trunkey DD, Lewis FR, eds. *Current Therapy of Trauma.* 4th ed. St Louis, Mo: CV Mosby; 1999:279.

100. Rai J, Jeschke MG, Barrow RE, et al. Electrical injuries: a 30-year review. *J Trauma.* 1999;46:933.

101. Fahmy FS, Brinsden MD, Smith J, et al. Lightning: the multisystem group injuries. *J Trauma.* 1999;46:937.

102. Enderson BL, Reath DB, Meadors J, et al. The Tertiary Trauma Survey: a prospective study of missed injury. *J Trauma.* 1990;30:666.

103. Jahangir KJ, Sugrue M, Deane SA. Prospective evaluation of early missed injuries and the role of tertiary trauma survey. *J Trauma.* 1998;44:1000.

104. Norwood SH, Dellinger RP. Managing substance abuse in the trauma patient. *Prob Crit Care.* 1987;1:115.

105. Gettler DT, Allbritten FF. Effect of alcohol intoxication on the respiratory exchange and mortality rate associated with acute hemorrhage in anesthetized dogs. *Ann Surg.* 1963;158:151.

106. Malt SH, Bawe AE. The effects of ethanol as related to trauma in the awake dog. *J Trauma.* 1971;11:76.

107. Swan KG, Vidaver RM, Lavigne JE, et al. Acute alcoholism, minor trauma, and "shock." *J Trauma.* 1977;17:215.

108. Straus DJ. Hematologic aspects of alcoholism. *Semin Hematol.* 1973;10:183.

109. Stene JK, Grande CM, Barton CR. Airway management for the trauma patient. In: Steve JK, Grande CM, eds. *Trauma Anesthesia.* Baltimore, Md: Williams & Wilkins; 1991:64.

110. Iida H, Tachibana S, Kitahara T, et al. Association of head trauma with cervical spine injury, spinal cord injury, or both. *J Trauma.* 1999;46:450.

111. Majernick TG, Bieniek R, Houston JB, et al. Cervical spine movement during orotracheal intubation. *Ann Emerg Med.* 1986;15:417.

112. Bracken MB, Shepard MJ, Collins WF, et al. A randomized, controlled trial of methylprednisolone or naloxone in the treatment of acute spinal cord injury. *N Engl J Med.* 1990;322:1405.

113. Bracken MR, Shepard MJ, Holford TR, et al. Administration of methylprednisolone for 24 or 48 hours or tirilazad mesylate for 48 hours in the treatment of acute spinal cord injury. *JAMA.* 1997;277:1597.

114. Nesathurai S. Steroids and spinal cord injury: revisiting the NASCIS2 and NASCIS3 trials. *J Trauma.* 1998;45:1088.

115. Carrillo EH, Osborne DL, Spain DA, et al. Blunt carotid artery injuries: difficulties with the diagnosis prior to neurological event. *J Trauma.* 1999;46:1120.

116. Fabian TC, Patton JH Jr, Croce MA, et al. Blunt carotid injury: importance of early diagnosis and anticoagulant therapy. *Ann Surg.* 1996;2223:513.

117. Weller SJ, Rossitch E, Malek AM. Detection of vertebral artery injury after cervical spine trauma using magnetic resonance angiography. *J Trauma.* 1999;46:660.

118. Eachempati SR, Vaslef SN, Sebastian MW, et al. Blunt vascular injuries of the head and neck: is heparinization necessary? *J Trauma.* 1998;45:997.

119. Rogers FB, Baker EF, Osler TM, et al. Computed tomographic angiography as a screening modality for blunt cervical arterial injuries: preliminary results. *J Trauma.* 1999;46:380.

120. Bullock R, Chesnut RM, Clifton G, et al. *Guidelines for the Management of Severe Head Injury 1995.* Park Ridge, Ill: Brain Trauma Foundation and the American Association of Neurological Surgeons; 1995.

121. Ghajar J, Hariri RJ, Narayan RK, et al. Survey of critical care management of comatose, head-injured patients in the United States. *Crit Care Med.* 1995;23:560.

122. Matta B, Menon D. Severe head injury in the United Kingdom and Ireland: a survey of practice and implications for management. *Crit Care Med.* 1996;24:1743.

123. Chesnut RM. Secondary brain insults after head injury: clinical perspectives. *New Horizons.* 1995;3:366.

124. Chesnut RM, Marshall LF, Klauber MR, et al. The role of secondary brain injury in determining outcome from severe head injury. *J Trauma.* 1993;34:216.

125. Redan JA, Livingston DH, Tortella BJ, et al. The value of intubating and paralyzing patients with suspected head injury in the emergency department. *J Trauma.* 1991;31:371.

126. Muizelaar JP, Marmarou A, Ward JD, et al. Adverse effects of prolonged hyperventilation in patients with severe head injury: a randomized clinical trial. *J Neurosurg.* 1991;75:731.

127. Chesnut RM, Gautille T, Blunt BA, et al. Neurogenic hypotension in patients with severe head injuries. *J Trauma.* 1998;44:958.

128. Rosner MJ, Rosner SD, Johnson AH. Cerebral perfusion pressure: management protocol and clinical results. *J Neurosurg.* 1995;83:949.

129. Kaufman HH, Schwab K, Salazar AM. A national survey of neurosurgical care for penetrating head injury. *Surg Neurol.* 1991;36:370.

130. Polin RS, Shaffrey ME, Phillips CP, et al. Multivariate analysis and prediction of outcome following penetrating head injury. *Neurosurg Clin North Am.* 1995;6:689.

131. Trask T, Narayan RK. Head and brain. In: Ivatury RR, Cayten CG, eds. *Textbook of Penetrating Trauma.* Baltimore, Md: Williams & Wilkins; 1996;241.

132. Grahm TW, Williams FC Jr, Harrington T, et al. Civilian gunshot wounds to the head: a prospective study. *Neurosurgery.* 1990;27:696.

133. Nagy KK, Joseph KT, Krosner SM, et al. The utility of head computed tomography after minimal head injury. *J Trauma.* 1999;46:268.

134. Shah KH, Simons RK, Holbrook T, et al. Trauma in pregnancy: maternal and fetal outcomes. *J Trauma.* 1998;45:83.

135. Esposito TJ, Gens DR, Smith LG, et al. Trauma during pregnancy: a review of 79 cases. *Arch Surg.* 1991;126:1073.

136. Morris JA, Rosenbower TJ, Jurkovich GJ, et al. Infant survival after cesarean section for trauma. *Ann Surg.* 1996;223:481.

137. Kissinger DP, Rozycki GS, Morris JA, et al. Trauma in pregnancy: predicting pregnancy outcome. *Arch Surg.* 1991;126:1079.

138. Dahmus MA, Sibai BM. Blunt abdominal trauma: are there any predictive factors for abruptio placentae or maternal-fetal distress? *Am J Obstet Gynecol.* 1993;169:1054.

139. Jaffe D, Wesson D. Emergency management of blunt trauma in children. *N Engl J Med.* 1991;324:1477.

140. Lubitz DS, Seidel JS, Chameides L, et al. A rapid method for estimating weight and resuscitation drug dosages from length in the pediatric age group. *Ann Emerg Med.* 1998;17:576.

141. Tepas JJ. Pediatric trauma. In: Feliciano DV, Moore EE, Mattox KL, eds. *Trauma.* 3rd ed. Stamford, Conn: Appleton & Lange; 1996:879.

142. Spivey WH. Intraosseous infusion. *J Pediatr.* 1987;111:639.

143. Trunkey D. Initial treatment of patients with extensive trauma. *N Engl J Med.* 1991;324:1259.

144. Townsend RN, Colella JJ, Diamond DL: Traumatic rupture of the aorta: critical decisions for trauma surgeons. *J Trauma.* 1990;30:1169.

145. Kron IL, Harmon PK, Nolan SP. The measurement of intra-abdominal pressure as a criteria for abdominal re-exploration. *Ann Surg.* 1984;199:28.

146. Saggi BH, Sugerman HJ, Ivatury RR, et al. Abdominal compartment syndrome. *J Trauma.* 1998;45:597.

147. Ivatury RR, Porter JM, Simon RJ, et al. Intra-abdominal hypertension after life-threatening penetrating abdominal trauma: prophylaxis, incidence, and clinical relevance to gastric mucosal pH and abdominal compartment syndrome. *J Trauma.* 1998;44:1016.

148. Reuler JB. Hypothermia: pathophysiology, clinical settings, and management. *Ann Intern Med.* 1978;89:519.

149. Daywatts D, Trask A, Soeken K, et al. Hypothermic coagulopathy in trauma: effect of varying levels of hypothermia on enzyme speed, platelet function, and fibrinolytic activity. *J Trauma.* 1998;44:846.

150. Wilmore DW. Homeostasis: bodily changes in trauma and surgery. In: Sabiston DC, Lyerly HK, eds. *Textbook of Surgery.* 15th ed. Philadelphia, Pa: WB Saunders; 1997:55.

151. Parillo JE. Shock: new concepts. Paper presented at: 65th Clinical Congress on Diseases of the Chest; November 1999; Chicago, Ill.

152. LeDran HF. *A Treatise or Reflections, Drawn From Practice on Gunshot Wounds.* Translated from the French. London, United Kingdom: 1743.

153. Latta J. *A Practical System of Surgery.* London, United Kingdom: 1795.

154. Latta T. Malignant cholera: documents communicated by the Central Board of Health, London, relative to the treatment of cholera by the copious injection of aqueous and saline fluids into the veins. *Lancet.* 1831–1832;2:274.

155. Crile GW. *Hemorrhage and Transfusion: Experimental and Clinical Research.* New York, NY: D Appleton; 1909.

156. Cannon WB. *Traumatic Shock.* New York, NY: D Appleton; 1923.

157. Cannon WB. Some characteristics of shock induced by tissue injury. *Great Br Med Res Committee.* 1919;26:27.

158. Blalock A. Trauma to the intestines: the importance of the local loss of fluid in the production of low blood pressure. *Arch Surg.* 1931;22:214.

159. Broder G, Weil MH. Excess lactate—an index of reversibility of shock in human patients. *Science.* 1964;143;145.

160. Weil MH, Afifi AA. Experimental and clinical studies on lactate and pyruvate as indicators of the severity of acute circulatory failure. *Circulation.* 1970;41:989.

161. Scalea TJ, Holman M, Fuortes M, et al. Central venous blood oxygen saturation: an early, accurate measurement of volume during hemorrhage. *J Trauma.* 1988;28:725.

162. Siegel JH, Fabian M, Smith JA, et al. Use of recombinant hemoglobin solution in reversing lethal hemorrhagic hypovolemic oxygen debt shock. *J Trauma.* 1997;42:199.

163. Siegel JH, Rivkind A, Dale S, et al. Early physiologic predictors of injury severity and death in blunt multiple trauma. *Arch Surg.* 1990;125:498.

164. Abramson D, Scalea TM, Hitchcock R, et al. Lactate clearance and survival following injury. *J Trauma.* 1993;35:584.

165. Boyd O, Grounds M, Bennett D, et al. Preoperative increase of oxygen delivery reduces mortality in high risk surgical patients. *JAMA.* 1993;270:2699.

166. Cohen RD, Woods HF. *Clinical and Biochemical Aspects of Lactic Acidosis.* Boston, Mass: Blackwell Scientific; 1976.

167. Huckabee WE. Relationships of pyruvate and lactate during anaerobic metabolism. *J Clin Invest.* 1985;37:244.

168. Relman AS. Lactic acidosis. In: Brenner BM, Stein JH, eds. *Acid-Base and Potassium Homeostasis.* New York, NY: Churchill Livingstone; 1978:65.

169. Park R, Arieff AI. Lactic acidosis. *Adv Intern Med.* 1980;25:33.

170. Kreisberg RA. Lactate homeostasis and lactate acidosis. *Ann Intern Med.* 1980;92:227.

171. Davis J. The relationship of base deficit to lactate in porcine hemorrhagic shock and resuscitation. *J Trauma.* 1994;36:168.

172. Davis JW, Shackford SR, Holbrook TL. Base deficit as a sensitive indicator of compensated shock and tissue oxygen utilization. *Surg Gynecol Obstet.* 1991;173:473.

173. Davis JW, Parks SN, Kaups KL, et al. Admission base deficit predicts transfusion requirements and risk of complications. *J Trauma.* 1996;41:769.

174. Davis JW, Kaups KL. Base deficit in the elderly: a marker of severe injury and death. *J Trauma.* 1998;45:873.

175. Siegel JH, Rivkind A, Dalal S, et al. Early physiologic predictors of injury severity and death in blunt multiple trauma. *Arch Surg.* 1990;125:498.

176. Astrand P, Cuddy TE, Saltin B, et al. Cardiac output during submaximal and maximal work. *J Appl Physiol.* 1964;19:268.

177. Shoemaker WC, Appel PL, Kram HB. Hemodynamic and oxygen transport responses in survivors and nonsurvivors of high risk surgery. *Crit Care Med.* 1993;21:977.

178. Yu M, Takanishi D, Myers SA, et al. Frequency of mortality and myocardial infarction during maximizing oxygen delivery: a prospective, randomized trial. *Crit Care Med.* 1995;23:1025.

179. Shoemaker WC, Appel PL, Kram HB, et al. Prospective trial of supranormal values of survivors as therapeutic goals in high-risk surgical patients. *Chest.* 1988;94:1176.

180. Berlauk JF, Abrams JH, Gilmour IJ, et al. Preoperative optimization of cardiovascular hemodynamics improves outcome in peripheral vascular surgery. *Ann Surg.* 1991;214:289.

181. Scalea TM, Simon HM, Duncan AO, et al. Geriatric blunt multiple trauma: improved survival with early invasive monitoring. *J Trauma.* 1990;30:129.

182. Bishop MH, Shoemaker WC, Kram HB, et al. Prospective randomized trial of survivor values of cardiac index, oxygen delivery, and oxygen consumption as resuscitation endpoints in severe trauma. *J Trauma.* 1995;38:780.

183. Bishop MW, Shoemaker WC, Appel PI, et al. Relationship between

supranormal values, time delays and outcome in severely traumatized patients. *Crit Care Med.* 1993;21:56.

184. Bishop MH, Shoemaker WC, Kram HB, et al. Prospective randomized trial of survivors values of cardiac index, oxygen delivery, and oxygen consumption as resuscitation endpoints in severe trauma. *J Trauma.* 1996;38:780.

185. Barone J. Maximization of oxygen delivery: a plea for moderation, part II. *J Trauma.* 1994;37:337.

186. Gattinoni L, Brazzi L, Pelosi P, et al. A trial of goal oriented hemodynamic therapy in critically ill patients. *N Engl J Med.* 1995;333:1025.

187. Heyland DK, Cook DJ, King D, et al. Maximizing oxygen delivery in critically ill patients: a methodological appraisal of the evidence. *Crit Care Med.* 1996;24:517.

188. Haglund U. Systemic mediators released from the gut in critical illness. *Crit Care Med.* 1993;21:S15.

189. Carrico CJ, Meakins JL, Marshall JC, et al. Multiple organ failure syndrome. *Arch Surg.* 1986;121:196.

190. Rice-Evans C, Diplock AT. Current status of antioxidant therapy. *Free Radic Biol Med.* 1993;15:77.

191. Machlin LJ, Bendich A. Free radical tissue damage: protective role of antioxidant nutrients. *FASEB J.* 1987;1:441.

192. Yagihashi A, Tsuruma T, Tarumi K, et al. Prevention of small intestinal ischemia-reperfusion injury in rats by anticytokine-induced neutrophil chemoattractant monoclonal antibody. *J Surg Res.* 1998;78:92.

193. Rossman JE, Caty MG, Zheng S, et al. Mucosal protection from intestinal ischemia-reperfusion reduces oxidant injury to the lung. *J Surg Res.* 1997;73:41.

194. Rush BF Jr, Sori AJ, Murphy TF, et al. Endotoxemia and bacteremia during hemorrhagic shock: the link between trauma and sepsis. *Ann Surg.* 1988;297:549.

195. Peitzman AB, Edekwu AO, Ochoa J, et al. Bacteria translocation in trauma patients. *J Trauma.* 1991;31:1083.

196. Moore FA, Moore EE, Poggetti R, et al. Gut bacterial translocation via the portal vein: a clinical perspective with major torso trauma. *J Trauma.* 1991;31:629.

197. Gann DS, Wright HK. Effects of trauma on sodium metabolism and urinary concentrating ability. *J Surg Res.* 1966;6:93.

198. Connett R, Honig C, Gayeski T, et al. Defining hypoxia: a systems view of $Vo_2$, glycolysis, energetics, and intracellular $Po_2$. *J Appl Physiol.* 1990;68:833.

199. Wang P, Ba ZF, Meldrum DR, et al. Diltiazem restores cardiac output and improves renal function after hemorrhagic shock and crystalloid resuscitation. *Am J Physiol.* 1992;262:H1435.

200. Karukurum M, Shreeniwas R, Chen J, et al. Hypoxic induction of interleukin-8 gene expression in human endothelial cells. *J Clin Invest.* 1994;93:1564.

201. Schulze-Osthoff K, Beyeart R, Vandevoorde V, et al. Depletion of the mitochondrial electron transport abrogates the cytotoxic and gene-inductive effects of TNF. *EMBO J.* 1993;12:3095.

202. Davis JW, Shackford SR, Mackersie RC, et al. Base deficit as a guide to volume resuscitation. *J Trauma.* 1988;28:1464.

203. Llundsgaard-Hansen P. Oxygen supply and anaerobic metabolism of the heart in experimental shock models. *Ann Surg.* 1966;163:10.

204. Baxter CR, Cook WA, Shires GT. Serum myocardial depressant factor in burn shock. *Surg Forum.* 1966;17:1.

205. Vedder NB, Harlan JM. Neutrophil-endothelial cell interactions. In: Grenvik A, Ayres SM, Holbrook PR, et al, eds. *Textbook of Critical Care.* 4th ed. Philadelphia, Pa: WB Saunders; 2000:570.

206. Kumar A, Kosuri R, Thota V, et al. Nitric oxide and cyclic GMP generation mediates human septic serum-induced in-vitro cardiomyocyte depression [abstract]. *Chest.* 1993;104:12S.

207. Kumar A, Kosuri R, Kandula R, et al. Tumor necrosis factor-induced myocardial cell depression in-vitro is mediated by nitric oxide generation [abstract]. *Crit Care Med.* 1993;21:S278.

208. Gulick T, Chung MK, Pieper SJ, et al. Interleukin-1 and tumor necrosis factor inhibit cardiac myocyte adrenergic responsiveness. *Proc Natl Acad Sci U S A.* 1989;86:6753.

209. Anderson JT, Wisner DH, Sullivan PE, et al. Initial small-volume hypertonic resuscitation of shock and brain injury: short- and long-term effects. *J Trauma.* 1997;43:592.

210. Battistella FD, Wisner DH. Combined hemorrhagic shock and head injury: effects of hypertonic saline (7.5%) resuscitation. *J Trauma.* 1991;31:182.

211. Krausz MM. Controversies in shock research: hypertonic resuscitation—pros and cons. *Shock.* 1995;3:69.

212. Prough DS, Johnson JC, Poole GVJ, et al. Effects on intracranial

213. Schmoker JD, Zhuang J, Shackford SR. Hypertonic fluid resuscitation improves cerebral oxygen delivery and reduces intracranial pressure after hemorrhagic shock. *J Trauma.* 1991;31:1607.

214. Capone AC, Safar P, Stezoski W, et al. Improved outcome with fluid restriction in treatment of uncontrolled hemorrhagic shock. *J Am Coll Surg.* 1995;180:49.

215. Kowalenko T, Stern S, Dronen S, et al. Improved outcome with hypotensive resuscitation of uncontrolled hemorrhagic shock in a swine model. *J Trauma.* 1992;33:349.

216. Bickell WH, Bruttig SP, Wade CE, et al. The detrimental effects of IV crystalloid after aortotomy in the swine [abstract]. *Ann Emerg Med.* 1989;18:476.

217. Gross D, Landau EH, Assalia A, et al. Is hypertonic saline resuscitation safe in "uncontrolled" hemorrhagic shock? *J Trauma.* 1989;29:79.

218. Gross D, Landau EH, Klin B, et al. Quantitative measurement of bleeding following hypertonic saline therapy in "uncontrolled" hemorrhagic shock. *J Trauma.* 1989;29:79.

219. Bourguignon PR, Shackford SR, Shiffer C, et al. Delayed fluid resuscitation of head injury and uncontrolled hemorrhagic shock. *Arch Surg.* 1998;133:390.

220. Crawford ES. Ruptured abdominal aortic aneurysm. *J Vasc Surg.* 1991;13:348.

221. Sampalis JS, Tamim H, Denis R, et al. Ineffectiveness of on-site intravenous lines: is prehospital time the culprit? *J Trauma.* 1997;43:608.

222. Schierhout GRI. Fluid resuscitation with colloid or crystalloid solutions in critically ill patients: a systematic review of randomized trials. *BMJ.* 1998;316:961.

223. Huang PP, Stucky FS, Dimick AR, et al. Hypertonic sodium resuscitation is associated with renal failure and death. *Ann Surg.* 1995;221:543.

224. ACCP/SCCM. American College of Chest Physicians/Society of Critical Care Medicine Consensus Conference. Definitions for sepsis and organ failure and guidelines for the use of innovative therapies in sepsis. *Crit Care Med.* 1992;20:864.

225. Goris RJA, te Boekhorst TP, Nuytinck JK, et al. Multiple organ failure. Generalized autodestructive inflammation? *Arch Surg.* 1985;120:1109.

226. Pittet D, Rangel-Frausto S, Li N, et al. Systemic inflammatory response syndrome, sepsis, severe sepsis and septic shock: incidence, morbidity and outcomes in surgical ICU patients. *Intensive Care Med.* 1995;21:302.

227. Rangel-Fransto M, et al. The natural history of the systemic inflammatory response syndrome (SIRS): a prospective study. *JAMA.* 1995;273:117.

228. Tilney NL, Bailey GL, Morgan AP. Sequential system failure after rupture of abdominal aortic aneurysms: an unsolved problem in postoperative care. *Ann Surg.* 1973;178:117.

229. Marshall JC, Cook DJ, Christou NV, et al. Multiple organ dysfunction score: a reliable descriptor of a complex clinical outcome. *Crit Care Med.* 1995;23:1638.

230. Zeigler EJ, Fisher CJ, Sprung CL, et al. Treatment of gram negative bacteremia and septic shock with HA-1A human monoclonal antibody against endotoxin. *N Engl J Med.* 1991;324:429.

231. Greenman RL, Schein RM, Martin MA, et al. A controlled clinical trial of E5 murine monoclonal IgM antibody to endotoxin in the treatment of gram-negative sepsis. *JAMA.* 1991;266:1097.

232. Hack CE, Nuijens JH, Felt-Bersma RJ, et al. Elevated plasma levels of the anaphylatoxins C3a and C4a are associated with fatal outcome in sepsis. *Am J Med.* 1989;86:20.

233. Cook JA, Halushka PV. Prostaglandins, thromboxanes, leukotrienes, and other products of arachidonic acid. In: Grenvik A, Ayres SM, Holbrook PR, et al, eds. *Textbook of Critical Care.* 4th ed. Philadelphia, Pa: WB Saunders; 2000:596.

234. Benveniste J, Henson PM, Cochrane CG. Leukocyte-dependent histamine release from rabbit platelets, I: the role of IgE, basophils and a platelet activating factor. *J Exp Med.* 1972;136:1356.

235. Moncada S, Palmer RMJ, Higgs EA. Nitric oxide: physiology, pathophysiology, and pharmacology. *Pharmacol Rev.* 1991;43:109.

236. Groeneveld PHP, Kwappenberg KMC, Langermans JAM, et al. Nitric oxide (NO) production correlates with renal insufficiency and multiple organ dysfunction syndrome in severe sepsis. *Intensive Care Med.* 1996;22:1197.

237. Gurll NG, Vargish T, Reynolds DG, et al. Opiate receptors and endorphins in the pathophysiology of hemorrhagic shock. *Surgery.* 1981;80:364.

238. Hinshaw LB, Archer LT, Beller BK, et al. Evaluation of naloxone

therapy for *Escherichia coli* sepsis in the baboon. *Arch Surg.* 1988;123:700.

239. Abraham E, Wunderink R, Silverman H, et al. Efficacy and safety of monoclonal antibody to human tumor necrosis factor alpha in patients with sepsis syndrome: a randomized, controlled, double-blind, multicenter clinical trial. *JAMA.* 1995;273:934.

240. Dhainaut JF, Vincent JL, Richard C, et al. CDP571, a humanized antibody to human tumor necrosis factor-α: safety, pharmacokinetics, immune response, and influence of the antibody on cytokine concentrations in patients with septic shock. *Crit Care Med.* 1995;23:1461.

241. Fischer CJ, Opal SM, Dhainaut J, et al. Influence on an anti-tumor necrosis factor monoclonal antibody on cytokine levels of patients with sepsis. *Crit Care Med.* 1993;21:318.

242. Agosti JM, Fisher CJ, Opal SM, et al, and sTNFR Sepsis Study Group. Treatment of patients with sepsis syndrome with soluble receptor (sTNFR). In: *Proceedings of the 34th Interscience Conference on Antimicrobial Agents and Chemotherapy, October 4–7, 1994.* p 65.

243. Reinhart K, Wiegand-Lohnert C, Grimminger F, et al. Assessment of the safety and efficacy of the monoclonal anti-tumor necrosis factor antibody-fragment, MAK 195F, in patients with sepsis and septic shock: a multicenter, randomized, placebo-controlled, dose-ranging study. *Crit Care Med.* 1996;24:733.

244. Fisher CJ Jr. Treatment of septic shock with the tumor necrosis factor receptor: Fc fusion protein. *N Engl J Med.* 1996;334:1697.

245. Abraham E. p55 tumor necrosis factor receptor fusion protein in the treatment of patients with severe sepsis and septic shock: a randomized controlled multicenter trial. *JAMA.* 1997;277:1531.

246. Fisher CJ, Dhainaut JF, Opal SM, et al. Recombinant human interleukin-1 receptor antagonist in the treatment of patients with sepsis syndrome: results from a randomized, double-blind, placebo controlled trial. *JAMA.* 1994;271:1836.

247. Fein AM. Treatment of severe systemic inflammatory response syndrome and sepsis with a novel bradykinin antagonist, deltibant (CP-0127): results of a randomized, double-blind, placebo-controlled trial. *JAMA.* 1997;277:482.

248. Dhainaut JF, Tenaillon A, Hemmer M, et al. Confirming phase III clinical trial to study the efficacy of a PAF antagonist, BN 52021, in reducing mortality of patients with severe Gram-negative sepsis [abstract]. *Am J Respir Crit Care Med.* 1995;151:A447.

249. Dhainaut JFA, Tenaillon A, Le Tulzo Y, et al. Platelet-activating factor receptor antagonist BN 52021 in the treatment of severe sepsis: a randomized, double-blind, placebo-controlled, multicenter clinical trial. *Crit Care Med.* 1994;22:1720.

250. Bernard GR. The effects of ibuprofen on the physiology and survival of patients with sepsis. *N Engl J Med.* 1997;336:912.

251. Bone RC. Sir Isaac Newton, sepsis, SIRS and CARS. *Crit Care Med.* 1996;24:1125.

252. Godin PJ, Buchman TG. Uncoupling of biological oscillators: a complementary hypothesis concerning the pathogenesis of multiple organ dysfunction syndrome. *Crit Care Med.* 1996;24:1107.

253. Woo M, Stevenson W, Moser D, et al. Patterns of beat-to-beat heart rate variability in advanced heart failure. *Am Heart J.* 1992;123:704.

254. Fleisher L, Pincus S, Rosenbaum S. Approximate entropy of heart rate as a correlate of postoperative ventricular dysfunction. *Anesthesiology.* 1993;78:683.

255. Singer D, Martin G, Magid N, et al. Low heart rate variability and sudden cardiac death. *J Electrocardiol.* 1998;21:S46.

256. Winchell RJ, Hoyt DB. Spectral analysis of heart rate variability in the ICU. *J Surg Res.* 1996;63:11.

257. Godin PJ, Fleisher LA, Eidsath A, et al. Experimental human endotoxemia increases cardiac regularity: results from a prospective, randomized, crossover trial. *Crit Care Med.* 1996;24:1117.

258. Villard J, Slutsky AS, Hew E, et al. Oxygen transport and oxygen consumption in critically ill patients. *Chest.* 1990;98:687.

259. McGuire GP, Pearl RG. Sepsis and the trauma patient. *Crit Care Clin.* 1990;6:121.

260. Norwood S. Catheter colonization and catheter-related bacteremia. In: Grenvik A, Ayres SM, Holbrook PR, Shoemaker WC, eds. *Textbook of Critical Care.* 4th ed. Philadelphia, Pa: WB Saunders; 2000:674.

261. Richet H, Hubert B, Nitemberg G, et al. Prospective multicenter study of vascular-catheter-related complications and risk factors for positive central-catheter cultures in intensive care unit patients. *J Clin Microbiol.* 1990;28:2520.

262. Norwood SH, Civetta JM. Abdominal CT scanning in critically ill surgical patients. *Ann Surg.* 1985;202:166.

263. Fry DE, Pearlstein L, Fulton RL, et al. Multiple system organ failure: the role of uncontrolled infection. *Arch Surg.* 1980;115:136.

264. Deitch EA. Animal models of sepsis and shock: a review and lessons learned. *Shock.* 1998;9:1.

265. Fang XM, Schroder S, Hoeft A, et al. Comparison of two polymorphisms of the interleukin-1 gene family: interleukin-1 receptor antagonist polymorphism contributes to susceptibility to severe sepsis. *Crit Care Med.* 1999;27:1330.

266. Majetschak M, Flohe S, Obertacke U, et al. Relation of a TNF gene polymorphism to severe sepsis in trauma patients. *Ann Surg.* 1999;230:207.

# Thermal Injuries: Pathophysiology and Anesthetic Considerations

Maximilian W. B. Hartmannsgruber

David W. Mozingo

A. Joseph Layon

Major burns pose a challenge both to patients and members of the burn team. Anesthesiologists are involved throughout the resuscitation and recovery phases of the burn in the emergency department, burn intensive care unit (ICU), and operating room. Increasingly, we are asked to provide consultations for pain control as well.

Since the early 1990s, there has been a 50% decline in deaths attributed to fire and burns, as well as acute hospitalization for burn injury,[1] thought to result from research advances and prevention.[2] Many centers now report survival after burns involving as much as 70% to 80% total body surface area (TBSA).[3,4] In 1991, the number of deaths in the United States from fire and burns totaled 5500; about 51 000 burn patients were acutely admitted to hospitals, and 1.25 million total burn injuries were treated.[1,5] Children younger than 5 years of age and adults older than 65 years of age have the highest fire and burn death rates; about three fourths of fire deaths occur in the home.[1,6]

The single biggest advance in burn care has been the ability to débride and graft the burn wound promptly before it becomes infected. Infected wounds cannot be grafted and can lead to sepsis. Extensive perioperative monitoring, provision of adequate nutrition, pain control, meticulous wound care techniques, and a safe blood supply, all provided by the burn team led by an experienced surgeon, not only allow the successful treatment of extensive burns but also make it possible to judge results by function rather than by survival alone.[7]

## PATHOLOGY

### What Is a Burn?

The most significant factor that determines the prognosis of an area of burned skin is the depth of skin destruction at the time of injury. Excessive thermal exposure causes characteristic changes in the damaged tissues.[8] Three distinct zones of tissue injury have been described[9]:

1. The *zone of coagulation* is the area closest to the site of heat. Blood flow has ceased, vessels are thrombosed, and the tissue is nonviable.
2. The *zone of stasis* includes tissue that is seriously damaged but, at least initially, is still viable and represents an area that shows signs of increasing vascular occlusion. This zone is of concern because of the possibility of intervening therapeutically, thereby preventing cell death.[10] This injury zone is thought to be capable of recovery for up to 48 hours after a burn. Topical or systemic administration of local anesthetics may prevent progressive dermal ischemia after injury through inhibition of burn-induced plasma albumin extravasation by direct action on vascular permeability and inhibition of the pathophysiologic response after burn injury.[11,12] The zone of stasis can be further subdivided into two subzones.
   a. A *zone of early stasis* (the upper one third of the zone of stasis) results from formation of early edema within the first 4 hours.
   b. A *zone of delayed stasis* (the deeper two thirds of the zone of stasis) results from delayed edema formation. It develops 4 to 24 hours after a burn as a result of vascular occlusion. The zone of hyperemia is reactive, responding to damage in the first 2 zones; thus, it is not directly injured. Only in relatively small burns is the zone of hyperemia restricted to the immediate site of injury. Burn injuries of >20% TBSA are more appropriately viewed as a whole-body inflammatory response to injury.[13] Even in the noninjured skin sites, tissue fluid translocation increases significantly up to 6 days after the burn. Acute therapy of large burns is initially concerned with resuscitation from hypovolemic shock and treatment of concurrent injuries. Subsequently, treatment of the integumentary defects, multiple-system organ dysfunction, and psychiatric needs must be addressed. Many of these problems are potentially lethal and are discussed in detail later.

### What Are the Effects of Electrical Injury?

Although electrical burns constitute only about 5% of admissions to burn centers in the United States, they can be more devastating injuries than one might initially suspect. For current to flow, a closed pathway (circuit) and a difference in potential (voltage) must exist between two points. Bone and skin offer relatively high resistance to current flow, but skin resistance can be decreased by moisture. Blood, muscle, and nerve, on the other hand, are good conductors.

### Cardiovascular

The pathway of current through the body is unpredictable. If the heart is involved, dysrhythmias are possible. Low-voltage death may result from relatively small amounts of current that produce ventricular fibrillation. High-intensity current can result in cardiac asystole and respiratory arrest, probably due to injury of medullary centers in the brain. Echocardiographic study of survivors of electrical injury has demonstrated wall motion abnormalities.[14] In patients with a history of electrical injuries who present with electrocardiographic (ECG) abnormalities, echocardiographic determination of cardiac function may be indicated before elective operative procedures are planned.

### Soft Tissue

Extensive carbonification of the skin and underlying tissues may obscure damage to striated muscle and blood vessels. The current may also travel through blood vessels and muscles. Thus, thromboses may result at sites distant from the body surface. *In general, one should always be suspicious that the injury from an electrical burn is more extensive than appreciated on first inspection.*

### Neuromuscular

Fractures of bone may result from convulsive muscle contractions or falls after an electric shock. Nervous system injuries are frequent and include partial or complete transection of the spinal cord due to vertebral fractures. The latter injuries may result from tetanic muscular contractions produced by alternating current or are sustained in falls (eg, from utility poles, transmitter towers, and so forth). A careful neurologic evaluation must be performed before manipulation or tracheal intubation of these patients. If this is not possible, as in comatose patients, patients should be treated as though a spinal column or cord injury is present.

### Renal

Renal tubular damage from myoglobin liberated during massive muscle necrosis and hemolysis may lead to acute renal failure. Although the mechanism by which myoglobinuria causes renal damage is not entirely clear, it likely involves more than mechanical obstruction of the tubules by precipitated myoglobin.[15] Intravenous administration of sodium bicarbonate (eg, 100 mEq in a liter of $D_5W$ run at maintenance rate) to alkalinize the urine protects the kidneys by preventing myoglobin precipitation. A urine pH of between 7.0 and 8.0 produces a myoglobin solubility of about 80% and is a reasonable goal.

If myoglobinuria is present, hydration and the use of mannitol, initially 25 g intravenously or about 0.5 g/kg, followed by 12.5 g/h (about 0.25 g/kg/h) are indicated. A urine output of 50 to 100 mL/h ($\geq$1.5 mL/kg/h) should be maintained.[16–18]

If mannitol alone is insufficient to establish diuresis, furosemide is added. Hammond and Ward reported an 8% incidence of renal complications even when this aggressive therapy was used in patients who suffered high-voltage electrical injury.[18]

## What Are the Effects of Chemical Injury?

Chemical burns pose additional problems to those previously mentioned because of the possibility of systemic absorption of the caustic agent through the injured skin. For example, an alkali injury may continue until all the agent is combined with tissue. Phosphorus burns require immediate débridement and washing under regional or general anesthesia to avoid further particle spread. Serum calcium and phosphorus levels may be seriously deranged after a phosphorus burn because the increased phosphate level induces a decrease in serum calcium.[19]

## CLASSIFICATION

### What Is the Depth of Injury?

#### First-Degree Burns

First-degree burns are superficial injuries involving the outer epidermis. The significant pain, evident after such injuries, is thought to be caused by local prostaglandin production. Healing usually occurs within 5 to 10 days.

#### Second-Degree Burns

Second-degree burns involve the epidermis and variable portions of the dermis. Superficial second-degree burns are also known as *superficial partial-thickness* burns. These burns include the epidermal and upper one third of the dermal layers of the skin, usually healing in 7 to 10 days with minimal to no scarring. Deep second-degree burns are also referred to as *deep partial-thickness* burns and extend further into the dermis. Keratinocytes from epidermal remnants in hair follicles and sweat and sebaceous glands are spared. They are an important source from which skin regenerates over 3 to 5 weeks, albeit with significant scarring.[20] Grafting is performed both to speed recovery and to minimize scarring.

#### Third-Degree Burns

In third-degree, or *full-thickness*, burns, skin is destroyed down to the subcutaneous tissue. Reepithelialization does not occur, and grafting must be done to cover the defect.[21] With full-thickness burns, destruction of the nerve endings usually results in the absence of pain. An exception is the severe pain of a chemical burn in which the burning process continues for minutes to hours.

Increasing evidence suggests that early excision and coverage of full-thickness burns with autograft skin are desirable. The estimation of burn wound depth is difficult and is often possible only in retrospect. Burn wound depth has been determined by histologic examination of biopsy specimens. This examination is most accurate by 3 days after a burn. Admission laser Doppler flowmetry, which noninvasively measures the rate and volume of blood cells moving through tissues,

**TABLE 39–1.** Calculation of Percentage of Body Surface Area Burned

| Patient | Area Burned | Percentage Burned |
|---|---|---|
| Adult burn patient: body surface area (rule of nines) | Head and neck | 9 |
| | Left arm | 9 |
| | Right arm | 9 |
| | Anterior chest | 9 |
| | Posterior chest | 9 |
| | Anterior abdomen | 9 |
| | Posterior lower back | 9 |
| | Anterior left leg | 9 |
| | Posterior left leg | 9 |
| | Anterior right leg | 9 |
| | Posterior right leg | 9 |
| | Perineum | 1 |
| Infant burn patient: body surface area (rule of elevens) | Anterior head and neck | 11 |
| | Posterior head and neck | 11 |
| | Left arm | 11 |
| | Right arm | 11 |
| | Anterior torso | 11 |
| | Posterior torso | 11 |
| | Left leg | 11 |
| | Right leg | 11 |
| | Buttocks | 11 |
| | Perineum | 1 |

has also been used.[22] The assessment is, however, usually a clinical one.

## What Is the Body Surface Area Involved?

The *rule of nines* approximates the size of burn wounds in adults. The relative percentages of the TBSA differ between adults and infants (Table 39–1). In infants, the *rule of elevens* is a better approximation. The surface of a patient's hand approximates 1% of the patient's TBSA. The TBSA burn is the arithmetic sum of the burned areas. It is convenient to use a diagram to depict the involved area and make the calculation (Fig. 39–1).

## How Is Severity Assessed?

Major burns are categorized as in Table 39–2. Prediction of burn mortality is closely approximated by the abbreviated burn severity index developed by Tobiasen and colleagues[23] (Table 39–3). Gender, age, inhalation injury, depth of burn, and TBSA are correlated with survival.

**TABLE 39–2.** Categorization of Major Burns

| | |
|---|---|
| Total body surface area | Adults: ≥25% |
| | Children: ≥20% |
| | Children <2 y: ≥10% |
| Full thickness | Adults: ≥15% |
| | Children 2-15 y: >10% |
| | Children <2 y: >2% |
| Miscellaneous | Burns on the face, hands, feet, perineum |
| | Electrical burns |
| | Burns with inhalation injuries |
| | Burns with associated injuries |
| | Burns of patients with major chronic illnesses |

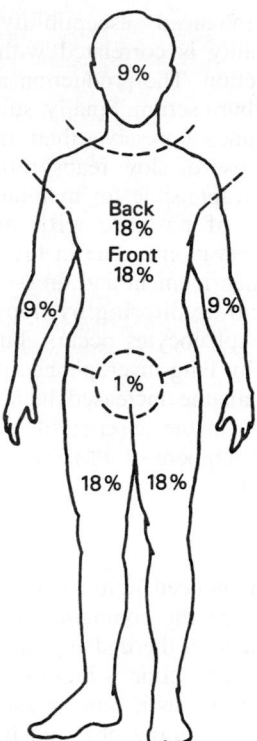

**FIGURE 39–1.** Burn total body surface area picture from burn unit. (From Demling RH. Fluid resuscitation. In: Boswick JA Jr, ed. *The Art and Science of Burn Care.* Rockville, Md: Aspen; 1987.)

**TABLE 39–3.** Burn Severity Index and Calculated Threat to Life

| Measure | Score |
|---|---|
| **Gender** | |
| Female | 1 |
| Male | 0 |
| Age | |
| <20 y | 1 |
| 21–40 y | 2 |
| 41–60 y | 3 |
| 61–80 y | 4 |
| >80 y | 5 |
| **Inhalation Injury** | 1 |
| **Full-Thickness Burn** | 1 |
| **Total Body Surface Area Involved (%)** | |
| ≤10 | 1 |
| 11–20 | 2 |
| 21–30 | 3 |
| 31–40 | 4 |
| 41–50 | 5 |
| 51–60 | 6 |
| 61–70 | 7 |
| 71–80 | 8 |
| 81–90 | 9 |
| >90 | 10 |

| Total Burn Score | Threat to Life | Probability of Survival (%) |
|---|---|---|
| 2–3 | Very low | 99 |
| 4–5 | Moderate | 98 |
| 6–7 | Moderate to severe | 80–90 |
| 8–9 | Serious | 50–70 |
| 10–11 | Severe | 20–40 |
| 12–13 | Maximal | <10 |

Modified from Tobiasen J, Hiebert JH, Edlich RF. Prediction of burn mortality. *Surg Gynecol Obstet.* 1982;154:711. By permission of *Surgery, Gynecology, & Obstetrics.*

# PATHOPHYSIOLOGY

## How Are Hypermetabolic States Manifested?

### Endocrine Response

Immediately after a burn, cellular nutrient and oxygen ($O_2$) deliveries to the injured area are decreased. The adrenal medulla and the autonomic nervous system release large amounts of catecholamines, leading to increased systemic vascular resistance. Glucagon and corticosteroid release, coupled with decreased responsiveness of peripheral tissues to insulin, lead to hyperglycemia.[24] Renin and aldosterone production are increased due to burn-induced hypovolemia, leading to decreased free water clearance and increased urine concentration. Hypothermia due to heat loss through the injured skin, as well as pain and anxiety, potentiates the stress response.

### Metabolic Rate

The metabolic rate, which initially decreases, begins to increase after resuscitation and usually peaks between days 7 and 12 after injury. It increases linearly in patients with thermal injuries of <40% TBSA. For those with injuries of >40% TBSA, basal metabolic rate and $O_2$ consumption may reach values twice normal.[25]

### Nutritional Changes

The hypermetabolic state results in catabolic protein loss, impaired immune function, and delayed wound healing. To offset this metabolic demand, wound closure (débridement and grafting) and enteral feeding are crucial. Although we prefer to feed using a duodenojejunal feeding tube, nonbolus enteral feeding through a nasogastric tube is safe and may be instituted rapidly after injury.[26] This approach not only provides nutrients but also may help to maintain intestinal barrier function, thus preventing bacterial and fungal translocation. Early feeding of a burned patient may enhance the patient's ability to control a septic insult.[27] Wound healing may be further improved if the morbid catabolic response following thermal injury is modified with human growth hormone or the testosterone analogue oxandrolone. When administered 7 to 10 days after the burn, both significantly decrease weight loss while improving wound healing. Oxandrolone was noted to achieve this without side effects, whereas human growth hormone may cause hyperglycemia.[28]

Enteral diets that include fatty acids of the ω-3 series, nucleotides, and arginine, may be beneficial.[28–31] These are thought to improve immunologic function and, thus, may decrease infectious complications.[32–35] Although it is not always clear whether cellular immune function changes alter, or even affect, outcome, the data of Herndon and colleagues suggest that enterally fed burned patients have a survival rate about twice that of patients supplemented with parenteral nutrition.[36] This may be due to an increase in secretory immunoglobulin production, with a resultant decrease in bacterial translocation across the gut wall. Decisions for early feeding must be weighed against the increased risk for aspiration in case of emergent intubation or surgery. Tube feedings may be initiated within the first 12 hours after burn injury.[37] In the future, we will likely see thermally injured patients coming to the operating room with continuous small bowel feeds infusing.

## What Are the Systemic Effects of Thermal Injury?

### Immune Function

Once dermal integrity is compromised, the body may become substrate to many infectious agents. In most patients with burns of >40% TBSA, virtually all specific (cell-mediated and humoral) and nonspecific (polymorphonuclear leukocyte [PMNL], macrophage) immune functions are deranged. These patients should be treated as immunocompromised.

### Histamine Release and Complement Activation

At the local site of thermal injury, histamine release and complement activation lead to increased vascular permeability. Interaction of histamine with xanthine oxidase leads to formation of toxic OH⁻ radicals and hydrogen peroxide.[38] It has been speculated that increased vascular permeability may be attenuated by xanthine oxidase inhibitors (allopurinol) or cromolyn sodium, an inhibitor of histamine release.

The complement cascade and xanthine oxidase cause activation of PMNLs, mast cells, and endothelial cells, further increasing histamine and xanthine oxidase activity. Release of cytokines, such as tumor necrosis factor (TNF) and interleukin 1 (IL-1), also occurs.[39] TNF is implicated in the hyperdynamic hypermetabolic state after burns,[39] whereas IL-1 acts as a primary mediator of the acute phase organ response to infection and injury.[39]

### Sepsis and Multiple-System Organ Failure

The effects of IL-1 and TNF are additive. These cytokines have properties that mimic the clinical presentation of sepsis and multiple-system organ failure (MSOF). Sepsis and MSOF have many characteristics in common with thermal injuries; indeed, sepsis, MSOF, and the adult respiratory distress syndrome (ARDS) remain major causes of death after burn injury.[40] Secretion of these cytokines results in responses that are detailed in Table 39–4.[41–43]

### Later Changes

Continuing through the second to fourth postburn weeks, the activation, proliferation, and differentiation processes of B lymphocytes are impaired in severely injured patients. This

**TABLE 39–4.** Effects of Release of Interleukin 1 (IL-1) and Tumor Necrosis Factor

Fever
Production of hepatic acute-phase reactants
T- and B-lymphocyte activation
Fibroblast proliferation
Cyclo-oxygenase gene expression
Shock
Induction of IL-6 and IL-8
Complement system activation
Coagulation and fibrinolytic activation
Further release of IL-1 and tumor necrosis factor

may contribute to enhanced susceptibility to infection and sepsis.[44] Burn mortality is correlated with failure of T-cell function and IL-2 action. The production and action of IL-2 are inhibited by postburn serum. Finally, subeschar tissue fluid is even more immunosuppressive than is the serum of a burned patient. Because of slow reabsorption, this fluid may be at least partially responsible for maintaining the immunocompromised state of patients with nondébrided burn wounds.[45] These observations argue in favor of early, aggressive, and repetitive débridement and dressing changes.

Decreased particulate filtering by hepatic macrophages (Kupffer cells) and splenocytes occurs, but accumulation of particulate material by lung macrophages is increased.[46] This alteration may explain the increased incidence of ARDS in burned patients, even in the absence of an inhalation injury. Although increased numbers of PMNLs are noted, they are functionally impaired.[47]

### Blood Transfusion

Blood transfusion–induced immunosuppression appears to be an additional nonspecific component of the immune dysfunction encountered with thermal injuries.[48,49] The observed impairment of immune function is indomethacin sensitive and is possibly induced by series E prostaglandins. Increased risk may result when large volumes of donor blood are used over a short period of time.[50] However, successful coverage of the integumentary defect may require the use of blood and blood products. Careful attention to hemostasis, as well as tourniquet use whenever possible during débridement and grafting, will help decrease the patient's exposure to donor blood products. Finally, there is no single "transfusion trigger." The "lowest acceptable" hemoglobin depends on age and underlying pathophysiology.

### Neurologic and Immunologic Coupling

Increasing evidence suggests a coupling of neurologic and immunologic functions. Endogenous opioids play a role in the altered immune response after injury, and morphine sulfate has been linked to altered cell-mediated immune response. In vitro morphine sulfate–induced impairment of lymphocyte function, as measured by delayed-type hypersensitivity assay, was prevented by concurrent treatment with the opioid antagonist naloxone.[51] The relevance of this in vitro study to the clinical setting in the burn ICU is unclear, but clearly merits further study.

### Conclusions

Given the immunocompromised state of burned patients, it is no surprise that sepsis remains a major cause of death despite significant improvements in burn survival rates and antibiotic therapy. Of those who die after a burn, infection is the cause of death in most children and adults.[52] In addition to focused, specific intravenous and topical antibiotic coverage and aseptic technique, immune function may be improved by early enteral nutrition and early excision of burn wounds.[53,54]

## CARDIOVASCULAR INJURY

### How Is Cardiovascular Function Affected?

Immediately after a significant burn, cardiac output falls to about 50% to 60% of the normal resting value. This decrease is likely due to a combination of reduced preload, impaired contractility, and increased arterial resistance.[55] Although some controversy exists, impaired contractility has been attributed to a low-molecular-weight myocardial depressant factor.[56] Increased arterial resistance is due to increased plasma catecholamines.

In the untreated thermally injured animal, cardiac output falls to about 20% of normal resting values. This observation underscores the need for aggressive fluid resuscitation, despite which cardiac output still remains below normal until the beginning of the hyperdynamic phase, which peaks between days 7 and 12 after injury. It may then climb to values as high as 200% of normal.

## Why Do Fluid Shifts Occur?

The marked tissue swelling observed in the burned area is due to leaky capillaries and should be essentially complete within 12 hours of resuscitation. Diffuse edema (anasarca) is also frequently encountered after fluid resuscitation of patients with >30% TBSA burns. The processes that lead to edema formation are not entirely understood and cannot be blamed entirely on fluid resuscitation, which is necessary to restore intravascular volume. The prudent practice is to err on the side of too much rather than too little fluid because of the more serious sequelae of inadequate fluid resuscitation.

### Microvascular Injury

Edema occurring within the first few minutes of a thermal injury is thought to be secondary to direct injury of the microvasculature. Endothelial gaps form and lead to transvascular loss of fluid, electrolytes, and proteins; this fluid shift results in increased volume of both the interstitial and intracellular compartments at the expense of the intravascular compartment.

### Cell Membrane Dysfunction

Vasoactive agents, such as prostaglandins, leukotrienes, histamine, and kinins, promote continued fluid loss from the intravascular to the interstitial and intracellular compartments. Cellular swelling most likely results from a generalized impairment in cell membrane function with subsequent sodium and water movement into the cells. This initial defect is reversed within about 12 hours of the thermal injury. Further fluid shifts and edema are a result of burn- and resuscitation-induced hypoproteinemia.[57] After the initial 12-hour period has elapsed, the use of a colloid-containing fluid may be considered.

## What Are the Effects of Fluid Translocation?

Extracellular fluid shifts from the circulating plasma volume result in decreased venous return and preload. If the resulting hypovolemia and hypotension are not reversed, conversion of a viable, but ischemic (zone of stasis), deep partial-thickness burn to one that is full thickness and nonviable may occur. Unfortunately, even carefully managed fluid resuscitation may be followed by massive edema formation, resulting in increased tissue pressure and a decreased tissue partial pressure

of oxygen. Increased work of breathing may also occur from edema of the thorax imposing a *restrictive* load, whereas upper respiratory tract edema imposes a *resistive* load. The latter may be quite serious. Edema formation at sites other than those that were burned may be due to overhydration, decreased oncotic pressure, or a vascular leak linked to circulating vasoactive mediators, adherence of leukocytes to vascular endothelium, and activation of the alternate complement pathway.[58]

## Can Edema Formation Be Controlled?

Cyclo-oxygenase inhibitors, such as 5% ibuprofen or 5% flurbiprofen creams, applied topically, have been shown to reduce local lymph flow about 3.5-fold in a sheep model of treated scald burns.[59] Flurbiprofen, a much longer acting agent than ibuprofen, additionally inhibits leukocyte migration. Interestingly, although topical flurbiprofen decreases burn hypermetabolism, much like early excision and closure of burn wounds, it does not attenuate local burn wound vascular permeability.[60] Burn-induced thromboxane release enhances permeability edema and can be decreased, at least in an experimental model, by thromboxane synthetase inhibition.[61]

Despite these data, pharmacologic manipulation of the previously mentioned vasoactive mediators has not resulted in reproducible modification of edema.[62] As with much of life, this process is likely more complicated than we presently understand.

## PULMONARY INJURY

Inhalation injury is a significant contributor to mortality.[63] Airway mucosal sloughing and pulmonary edema, with atelectasis caused by increased microvascular permeability, result in progressive pulmonary deterioration.[64] The extent of direct injury due to smoke inhalation is less than that due to steam. Smoke is usually only hot enough to injure just the larynx and upper trachea. Steam, on the other hand, has a heat content that is sufficiently high to injure the alveoli directly.

Nonsteam smoke injury in small airways is usually due to chemical irritation or toxic inhalation. Early decreased $Pao_2$ results from direct injury of the alveoli by the products of combustion. The chemical components of smoke may lead to airway irritation and severe bronchospasm. This problem may be treated by albuterol or other bronchodilator by nebulizer or metered dose inhaler. Prophylactic steroids in inhalational injury are controversial and in general have not proved beneficial.[65]

Early increases in extravascular lung water occur only with severe inhalation injury or as a result of toxic inhaled gases. Major increases in extravascular lung water are more frequently noted 4 to 24 days after injury and are usually due to wound or pulmonary sepsis.[66] The impact of smoke inhalation on later complications may be significant. Wroblewski and Bower found that 85% of patients with facial burns developed pneumonia, compared with only 12% of patients with burns without facial injury.[67] Patients with thermal injury and concomitant inhalation injury require fluid volumes in the early resuscitation phase in excess of those required in noninhalation injury cases.[68,69] Intrabronchial treatment with bovine surfactant of severely burned patients with inhalational injury

**TABLE 39–5.** Comparison of Ventilatory Parameters: Conventional Ventilation With High-Frequency Percussive Ventilation*

| Measure | CV | HFPV | P |
|---|---|---|---|
| Mean PIP | $50.1 \pm 6.8$ | $30.6 \pm 5.2$ cm $H_2O$ | <.001 |
| PEEP | $10.5 \pm 1.2$ | $10.5 \pm 2.1$ cm $H_2O$ | NS |
| $Pao_2/Fio_2$ | $85.7 \pm 21.6$ | $303.4 \pm 55.3$ | <.001 |
| $Paco_2$ | $53.4 \pm 6.2$ | $34.3 \pm 4.6$ mm Hg | <.001 |

*10 hours treatment, $N = 11$ patients.

CV, conventional ventilation; HFPV, high-frequency percussive ventilation; PEEP, positive end-expiratory pressure; PIP, peak inspiratory pressure.

and ARDS shows promise as an approach to improving survival.[70] High-frequency percussive ventilation, delivered by a pulse generator to the severely inhalation-injured burn patient, represents an interesting and useful alternative to conventional ventilation. It likely induces a more efficient gas distribution, with lower peak airway and transpulmonary pressures and less circulatory compromise, and allows ventilation at a lower inspired oxygen concentration[71] (Table 39–5). Cioffi and colleagues presented data suggesting that complications were decreased when high-frequency percussive ventilation was used to ventilate patients with inhalational injury.[72]

### What Are the Effects of Smoke Inhalation?

Most deaths (80%) resulting from smoke inhalation are due to asphyxia or carbon monoxide intoxication.[73] Cellular respiration may be impaired by carbon monoxide or cyanide intoxication associated with smoke inhalation. Carbon monoxide, with 200 times greater affinity for hemoglobin than $O_2$, displaces the latter and produces a leftward shift in the oxyhemoglobin ($HbO_2$) dissociation curve. Further, it likely causes direct cellular damage by interference with the cytochrome oxidase system.

### Treatment

#### Carbon Monoxide Intoxication

The half-life of carbon monoxide during room air breathing is about 250 minutes; this time can be shortened to 40 to 60 minutes by breathing 100% $O_2$, and to 20 minutes in a hyperbaric chamber. Carbon monoxide poisoning should always be suspected in thermal injury, especially if a patient demonstrates even subtle neurologic changes. A blood sample subjected to co-oximeter analysis for carboxyhemoglobin is diagnostic if the level is $\geq 10\%$ and should be part of the routine laboratory screen for any smoke-associated burn injury.

In suspected intoxication, 100% $O_2$ (or treatment in a hyperbaric chamber if availability and patient stability allow) should be used until the carboxyhemoglobin level is less than about 3%. It is our preference to treat all stable carbon monoxide (CO) intoxication victims in the hyperbaric chamber until symptoms have resolved, the arterial CO level is in the normal range, and neuropsychologic testing variables have returned to normal values.[74]

#### Cyanide Intoxication

After other differential diagnostic possibilities are excluded, unless prolonged exposure to carbon monoxide has occurred, cyanide intoxication should be suspected when a patient remains comatose with carboxyhemoglobin levels of <30% to 40%. Empiric therapy should begin with inhalation from amyl nitrite ampules held under the patient's nose and mouth for 15 to 30 seconds every 1 to 3 minutes until sodium nitrite and sodium thiosulfate are available. Ten milliliters of 3% sodium nitrite and 50 mL of 25% sodium thiosulfate should then be infused slowly. If symptoms persist, one half of the original dose may be repeated 30 minutes later. Pediatric doses are 3% sodium nitrite, 6 to 8 mL/m² or 0.2 mL/kg; and 25% sodium thiosulfate, 7 g/m² to a dose of no more than 12.5 g.

The presence of combined CO and cyanide intoxication is seriously problematic. Because the treatment of cyanide intoxication results in the formation of methemoglobin, which is also incapable of carrying oxygen, these patients are treated in the hyperbaric chamber.[75]

## INITIAL THERAPY

### When Is Hospitalization Required?

Not all burned patients require hospitalization. Minor non-electrical burns, defined as a partial-thickness (<15% TBSA) or full-thickness (<2% TBSA) burn, unless the face, genitalia, hands, or feet are involved, may be treated in an outpatient facility. In small children, a short period of observation may be appropriate even in cases of minor injury.

Moderate burns, defined as partial-thickness injury of 15% to 25% TBSA or full-thickness injury between 2% and 10% TBSA, require hospitalization. A community hospital is adequate for the care of these injuries as long as experienced and interested nursing and medical personnel are available.

A major burn is one with a burn severity index (BSI) of >8. BSI is related to the patient's age, gender, presence of absence of inhalational injury, TBSA involved, and the proportion that is full thickness (see Table 39–3). A BSI of >6 requires care in a designated burn unit as soon as possible.

Patients with a thermal injury classified as minor to moderate but with serious underlying medical problems such as diabetes mellitus, ischemic heart disease, and obstructive or restrictive lung disease should be treated as if they had more severe burns. These individuals do not easily withstand the stresses imposed by thermal injury.

### What Should Be Done in the Emergency Department?

#### History and Physical Examination

For a severely burned patient, as for any acute trauma victim, the initial care provided involves special attention to the airway to ensure that it is patent and that oxygenation, ventilation, and circulation are not compromised. The cervical spine must be considered at risk until proved otherwise, especially if a fall or trauma was involved.

As soon as a patient is moved into the emergency department treatment room, while the initial evaluation is ongoing, a focused history must be obtained. Necessary information includes details of the burn (where it occurred, how it started, whether the area was open or closed, what the patient did to extinguish the fire), underlying medical problems, allergies, and medicinal or recreational drug use. If the patient is unable to provide the necessary information, one of the health team member must obtain the history from a family member, the police, firefighters, or a paramedic or emergency medical technician.

A history of fire in a closed space has important implications when considering the possibility of major airway or inhalation injury. Symptoms and signs include burnt facial hair or eyebrows, face and neck burns, hoarseness, stridor, wheezing, bronchorrhea, carbonaceous sputum, and mental changes. Dyspnea and cyanosis are late findings.

### Fiberoptic Bronchoscopy and Direct Laryngoscopy

If a patient is not in respiratory distress upon admission, yet has one or more of the previously mentioned findings suggestive of an airway or inhalation injury, we consider fiberoptic bronchoscopy. Positive findings include erythema and edema in superficial burns; blister formation, hemorrhage, and ischemia in partial-thickness injury; and ulceration and necrosis of the mucous membrane in full-thickness burns.[76-78] Although these findings do not correlate with later mortality, severity of respiratory failure, or subsequent requirement for mechanical ventilatory support, they allow identification of patients who may have significant upper airway injury and require intubation out of concern for edema.[79]

Fluid resuscitation of patients with large burns may result in such tracheal edema as to jeopardize intubation. Thus, even when we determine that fiberoptic bronchoscopy is not required, direct laryngoscopy is performed to evaluate for erythema and edema; only rarely is this procedure contraindicated.

#### Protecting the Airway

The decision about whether to intubate a thermally injured patient on arrival in the emergency department or simply to observe may be difficult. We have often been impressed with the extent of airway changes within 24 hours of admission. When in doubt, our policy is to opt for intubation. We do not hesitate to intubate a patient prophylactically for 2 to 4 days if upper airway erythema or edema is evident. In any patient with upper airway erythema or blisters, *not* intubating imposes substantial risk because upper airway injury may not become apparent until almost complete occlusion takes place.

The use of muscle relaxants to facilitate intubation of a patient with upper airway edema is fraught with risks and may be fatal because bag-mask ventilation and intubation may be extremely difficult after neuromuscular paralysis. Awake intubation or intubation over a bronchoscope is the safest approach if there is any question about the ease of airway exposure. An emergent cricothyrotomy is only rarely required. After intubation, we document the endotracheal tube cuff volume necessary to just occlude the endotracheal tube cuff. This value or volume serves as an indicator of progressive or residual airway edema. A cricothyrotomy, using, for example, the Melker cricothyrotomy kit (Cook Catheter Co, Bloomington, Ind), or an emergent bedside tracheotomy may be performed if needed. The former, rather than the latter, procedure may be more helpful if the airway is lost acutely. Even in the hands of an experienced surgeon, an emergent tracheotomy in an edematous burned patient may require 15 minutes because of the distorted anatomy.

### Fluid Resuscitation

As soon as the airway has been secured, with ventilation endpoints usually being a $Paco_2$ of 38 to 45 mm Hg, and an oxygen saturation as measured by pulse oximetry ($SpO_2$) of >93%, attention is turned to the circulation. Several large-bore peripheral intravenous catheters should be placed and infusions of warmed lactated Ringer's solution, or other solutions begun. Appropriate fluid resuscitation must be ensured. An indwelling urethral catheter should be placed as well. Resuscitation is adequate, all other things being equal, when urine output approximates 0.5 mL/kg/h and the patient is oriented and lucid. Invasive monitoring may be required if cardiopulmonary disease is present. The placement of an arterial and central venous catheter is often helpful in patients with moderate to severe burns to guide the fluid and hemodynamic resuscitation.

### Miscellaneous Considerations

With the airway secured and volume infusion begun, attention may be turned to a more detailed physical examination, tetanus prophylaxis, sedation and analgesia, and cleansing of the burn wound. A nasogastric tube should be placed to decrease gastric volume and in anticipation of the ileus that commonly accompanies significant burns. Preliminary baseline laboratory studies should be ordered (hematocrit, electrolytes, blood urea nitrogen, creatinine, arterial blood analysis, co-oximetry to determine the carboxyhemoglobin level, and a chest radiograph).

## DEFINITIVE THERAPY

### How Should Resuscitation Be Managed?

Prevention of hypovolemic shock and renal failure pose a major challenge in the first 24 hours after a burn is sustained. Fluid requirements tend to decrease after this time. Early work by Kilgore and colleagues suggested that the origin of edema fluid in thermal injuries <24 hours old was the extracellular rather than the intracellular compartment.[80] This determination was made using $^{51}Cr$-labeled red blood cells (RBCs), $^{131}I$-labeled serum, $^{35}S$-labeled sodium sulfate ($Na_2SO_4$), and the $Na^+$-to-$K^+$ ratio in rhesus monkeys with 35% to 40% TBSA burns caused by flame (kerosene gauze for 25 seconds) or scald (70°C for 15 seconds). These investigators found decreases in the RBC mass (10.5%), plasma volume (25%), and functional extracellular volume (44%) 18 hours after injury. Loss of RBC mass is likely due to lysis. Electrolytic concentration of the edema fluid suggested that its origin was from the extracellular fluid compartment.

### Replacement Formulas

Numerous fluid formula recommendations have been suggested for initial replacement guidance; these are shown, primarily for historic interest, in Table 39–6. The crucial issue with each of these formulations is that they are approximations. The actual volume administered may be increased or

**TABLE 39–6.** Resuscitation Formulas*

| Fluid Type | Evans Formula | Brooke Formula | Parkland Formula |
|---|---|---|---|
| **First 24 h** | | | |
| Colloid | 1 mL/kg/% TBSA (2800) | 0.5 mL/kg/% TBSA (1400) | None |
| Electrolyte solution (lactated Ringer's or normal saline) | 1 mL/kg/% TBSA | 1.5 mL/kg/% TBSA (4200) | 4 mL/kg/% TBSA (11 200) |
| Glucose ($H_2O$) ($D_5W$) | (2000) | (2000) | None |
| **Second 24 h** | | | |
| Colloid | 0.5 mL/kg/% TBSA (1400) | 0.25 mL/kg/% TBSA (700) | As needed for urine output (70-100 mL/h) |
| Electrolyte solution | 0.5 mL/kg/% TBSA (1400) | 0.75 mL/kg/% TBSA (2100) | None |
| Glucose ($H_2O$) | (2000) | (2000) | Urine output tested as needed |

*Assumes a 70-kg male with a 40% TBSA thermal injury. Number in *parentheses* is volume (mL) for that particular fluid; total volume for each 24-h period may be calculated by summation of numbers in parentheses in each column.

TBSA, total body surface area.

decreased depending on a patient's mental status and urine output.

The Evans and Brooke formulas call for increasing fluid as needed to keep the urinary output between 30 and 50 mL/h. The Parkland formula requires administration of fluid to keep a urine output of 50 to 100 mL/h. Each of these regimens assumes that urine output is a reliable indicator of volume status. Although this maxim generally holds true, in some clinical situations (eg, patients with uncontrolled blood sugar and a resultant diuresis, or after mannitol therapy), it does not. In these circumstances or when urine output is inadequate despite apparently adequate fluid administration, invasive monitoring may be used to monitor and guide fluid resuscitation.

## Why Are Hypertonic Solutions Inappropriate?

In the past, several investigators demonstrated a significant reduction in fluid requirement and maintenance of adequate urine output after the administration of concentrated sodium solutions.[81,82] Although about the same amount of sodium was administered (0.5-0.6 mEq/kg per TBSA percentage), the decreased water load was thought to decrease edema. This was believed to be a significant advantage because excessive edema, as noted previously, has been implicated in increasing burn depth. Evidence suggests that hypertonic sodium resuscitation is associated with renal failure[83] and that hypernatremia worsens burn depth progression.[84,85]

Under hypernatremic conditions, the leukocytic chemotactic function is depressed, and leukocyte mobility is inhibited at the limiting sodium concentration. Leukocytes cease to migrate when the limiting point in the osmotic gradient of the dermis is reached. The highest point of this gradient occurs at the surface of the burn wound; the lowest point, similar to the serum sodium concentration, occurs at the deep zone of the dermis where an almost normal blood circulation is maintained. In burns treated with hypertonic saline, leukocytes reaching the point at which migration is inhibited begin to damage the surrounding tissue and increase burn depth. Burn wounds facilitate free water loss more easily than sodium loss because of the increasing evaporative water loss from the burn wound surface. Serum hypernatremia accelerates the hypernatremic tendency near the wound surface. The use of

hypertonic solutions in burn resuscitation can, therefore, no longer be endorsed.

## When Is Pulmonary Artery Catheterization Helpful?

Data suggest that urine output and vital sign changes may be inadequate for optimal resuscitation. Dries and Waxman studied 14 patients with burns averaging 61% TBSA.[86] Flow-directed balloon-tipped pulmonary artery (PA) catheters were placed in all patients. Measured wedge pressure, cardiac output, and calculated systemic vascular resistance, $O_2$ delivery ($Do_2$), and $O_2$ consumption ($\dot{V}o_2$) parameters were obtained during resuscitation. They found that within the first 48 hours, urine output and vital signs, as assessed by heart rate and mean arterial pressure, did not correlate with the invasively determined physiologic parameters. In some patients, fluid boluses increased $\dot{V}o_2$, further suggesting that despite other clinical parameters being normal, $O_2$ delivery was not optimized. These individuals could not be predicted based on clinical criteria. The investigators suggested that PA catheters may be helpful in the resuscitation of patients with $\geq$28% TBSA burns.

A shortcoming of this study was that no control group was reported, so that readers could not determine whether the discrepancy in vital signs and urine output, and therefore fluid management, affects outcome. We do not, as a matter of course, place PA catheters in our thermally injured patients, but rather have a low threshold when there are any questions regarding the fluid status of a patient or in patients with other significant medical problems. Esophageal Doppler ultrasonography and partial $CO_2$ rebreathing techniques (NICO system, Novametrix Medical Systems Inc, Wallingford, Conn) for cardiac output determination are newer and less invasive than either the PA catheter or transesophageal echocardiography for facilitating fluid resuscitation.[87,88]

## How Are Compartment Syndromes Assessed?

Full-thickness injury is associated with almost complete loss of skin elasticity, leading to encasement of tissue compartments. This change can impede venous outflow, arterial inflow, or both. Physical assessment of peripheral pulses and skin temperature is unreliable in severely vasoconstricted patients with edema due to burn wounds and resuscitation fluids; hence, distal extremity blood flow, arterial and venous, should be assessed hourly with an ultrasonic Doppler probe. A pressure transducer connected to an appropriately placed needle or catheter may also be used to evaluate tissue pressures, as elucidated next.

### Indications for Decompression

Even if distal Doppler pulses are present, nutrient flow into the muscle compartments may be inadequate. Indications for surgical decompression, aside from the loss of distal pulses, include delayed capillary refilling; paresthesias or motor weakness; cyanosis of distal, uninjured skin; and tense edema with rigid muscle compartments.[89] Intracompartmental pressure is easily measured by sterile placement of a fluid-filled hollow needle attached to a pressure transducer zeroed to the middle of the compartment. Interstitial pressure—that is, subescharotic or compartmental pressure—consistently >25 mm Hg warrants escharotomy; pressures >40 mm Hg require immediate decompression by escharotomy or fasciotomy. One option is to reassess compartment pressure after escharotomy. If it is <25 mm Hg, escharotomy was therapeutic; if it remains >25 mm Hg, consider proceeding to fasciotomy.[90] Elevation of the extremities may reduce edema formation, but an escharotomy is indicated when vascular impairment is apparent.

### Escharotomy

An escharotomy is an incision through the full depth of the burn eschar. These incisions are usually performed on the lateral and medial aspects of the extremity and should be continued across the joints. Once performed, return of peripheral perfusion is to be expected. Continued absence of peripheral blood flow requires reassessment of intravascular fluid status and the extent and depth of the escharotomies. Rarely, fasciotomy is necessary after swelling in the muscle compartment. Electrical burns may be more prone to compartment edema, requiring fasciotomy, than thermal injuries.

## What Is the Burn Wound Sepsis?

Surface microflora of the skin changes after burn injury, with eventual predominance of more pathogenic organisms. Immediately after thermal injury, the burn wound may be sterile, but within 48 hours, it becomes colonized. Subsequent growth into the burn wound (supraeschar, intrafollicular, and intraeschar colonization) may lead to invasion of viable nonburned tissue, termed *burn wound sepsis*.[91] This condition is diagnosed pathologically from biopsy samples of skin (including eschar and subcutaneous fat). Microscopic invasion into viable tissue is seen, and culture of the specimen demonstrates $\geq 10^5$ bacterial colonies per gram of tissue.

### Offending Organisms

Many organisms cause burn wound colonization and infection, including *Pseudomonas* species, β-hemolytic *Streptococcus* species, *Staphylococcus aureus*, *Enterobacter cloacae*, and *Klebsiella*, *Proteus*, *Escherichia*, and *Providencia* species. Yeast, fungal, and viral pathogens may also be present. Topical antimicrobial therapy is an important component of wound care before and after débridement of nonviable tissue.

### Therapeutic Agents

#### Silver Sulfadiazine

Silver sulfadiazine is a bacteriostatic material synthesized from silver nitrate and sodium sulfadiazine. It is available as a 1% cream and has a broad antimicrobial spectrum of activity. Treatment failures occur, especially in burns of >50% TBSA. Eschar penetration is intermediate between the relatively poor penetration of silver nitrate and the deep penetration of mafenide. This agent is painless on application and is generally used in the initial hours after injury. When treatment failure occurs, another agent, such as mafenide, is used.

Transient leukopenia 2 to 3 days after initiation of therapy is often noted. This change, however, may well be an intrinsic response to the burn injury itself rather than an untoward effect of drug therapy. A maculopapular rash may also be seen. It usually does not require cessation of the agent.

#### Mafenide

Mafenide is a broad-spectrum bacteriostatic topical agent with superior eschar-penetrating properties. It is helpful for early treatment of a burn wound; a significant drawback is the pain it causes on application. Mafenide is available as an 11% cream in a water-soluble base. Side effects include inhibition of carbonic anhydrase, which may result in hyperchloremic metabolic acidosis.

The drug is highly absorbed within about 3 hours of application. Metabolism of the parent drug results in the presentation of a large osmotic load to the kidneys, with resultant osmotic diuresis. The diuresis is enhanced by the drug's carbonic anhydrase effect. The metabolic acidosis and diuretic effects generally become clinically important in thermal injuries of ≥40% TBSA and serve to confound fluid management further.

#### Cerium Nitrate–Silver Sulfadiazine

Cerium nitrate–silver sulfadiazine primarily enhances control of enteric flora in a burn wound. It apparently is not as useful in control of staphylococci. In addition to superior control of enteric bacteria compared with silver sulfadiazine, it may enhance cell-mediated immunity. The untoward effects occurring with silver sulfadiazine may be complicated further by methemoglobinemia. It should be suspected if the skin or blood appears cyanotic or gray and the pulse oximeter identifies a desaturation in the presence of a normal $Pao_2$.

#### Honey

We have no experience with using honey to treat burns. Nevertheless, when honey was compared with silver sulfadiazine in patients with 21% to 40% TBSA burns, 91% of wounds were rendered sterile within 7 days when treated with honey, whereas only 7% showed control of infection within 7 days when treated with silver sulfadiazine. Healthy granulation tissue in the honey-treated group was observed in 7.4

days, versus 13.4 days in the silver sulfadiazine–treated patients. Finally, 87% of the honey-treated group healed within 15 days, compared with only 10% in the group treated with silver sulfadiazine. Relief of pain and a lower incidence of hypertrophic scar and postburn contracture were observed with honey.[92] A histologic study revealed that in honey-dressed wounds, early subsidence of acute inflammatory changes, better control of infection, and quicker wound healing were observed, whereas in the silver sulfadiazine–treated wounds, a sustained inflammatory reaction was noted even on epithelialization of raw areas.[93]

### Silver Nitrate

Although effective against most strains of *S. aureus, Staphylococcus epidermidis*, and *Pseudomonas aeruginosa*, silver nitrate is infrequently used today because of poor eschar penetration and the association of electrolyte disturbances secondary to its hypotonicity. Rarely, methemoglobinemia occurs through bacterial reduction of nitrate to nitrite, which is subsequently absorbed.[94]

### Biologic Dressings and Skin Substitutes

In severely burned patients, the disparity between donor site area and burn wound area may require the use of temporary skin substitutes or biologic dressings to close the wound temporarily while awaiting donor site availability.[95] Biologic dressings and skin substitutes prevent desiccation of the wound bed, decrease protein and fluid losses, promote angiogenesis of granulation tissue, and reduce pain. The most commonly used temporary skin substitute is in the form of cadaver allograft. Allograft becomes vascularized from the underlying wound bed and remains adherent until surgically excised or immunologically rejected by the patient. As a result of the immunosuppression imparted by thermal injury, the allograft may remain intact and viable for several weeks after application. The same risks for disease transmission associated with solid organ donation, such as hepatitis, HIV infection, and so forth, apply to the use of cadaveric allografts and require the same detailed tissue-banking procedures, such as donor screening and tissue tracking.

Several synthetic skin substitutes have been developed in an attempt to avoid the problems of disease transmission and storage requirements common to biologic dressings.[96] The most successful materials have been composed of a bilaminate structure with an outer layer mimicking the epidermis and an inner dermal layer designed to promote adherence and fibrovascular ingrowth from the wound bed.

At present, Biobrane (Dow Hickam Pharmaceuticals, Inc, Sugar Land, Tex) is the most commonly used synthetic skin substitute. The epidermal layer is composed of pliable Silastic, and the dermal component is derived from porcine collagen on a nylon scaphoid. The elastic nature allows freedom of motion and is well adapted to body contours. Application of this material promotes healing of second-degree burns and may provide adequate short-term coverage for excised wounds, although submembrane infection, fluid accumulation, and lack of adherence remain problems.

TransCyte (Smith & Nephew, Inc, Largo, Fla) is a composite skin substitute composed of Biobrane and cultured neonatal fibroblasts.[97] In culture, the fibroblasts proliferate on the dermal surface of the Biobrane and secrete matrix components, such as collagen and glycosaminoglycans. Many growth factors have also been identified within the dermal component. This skin substitute may have the advantage of better wound adherence owing to the presence of the allogeneic matrix proteins. TransCyte may provide a suitable replacement for cadaver allografts, thus eliminating the current donor screening requirements and problems with allograft availability and quality. Also, it may allow more superior healing of intermediate-depth partial-thickness wounds.

### Dermal Replacements

Several products are available that may be used to augment the dermal thickness lost in deep partial-thickness or full-thickness burns. Split-thickness skin grafting transfers only a thin layer of dermis to the recipient bed, which, in part, accounts for the decreased pliability of grafted burns.

Integra (Integra Life Sciences Corporation, Plainsboro, NJ; Johnson & Johnson Medical, Arlington, Tex) is a synthetic dermal substitute that is unique in that a neodermis is formed by fibrovascular ingrowth of the wound bed into a 2-mm thick glycosaminoglycan matrix dermal analogue.[98] The epidermal component is a Silastic sheet and may be removed after the dermal analogue is vascularized in about 3 weeks. Ultrathin split-thickness autografts are then placed on the neodermis. This permits more rapid healing of donor sites, where repeated autograft harvesting is required. The dermal replacement provides a more elastic and functional skin cover after complete healing and wound maturation occurs.

## What Are the Effects of Burn Débridement and Skin Grafting?

Open burn wounds initiate and perpetuate tissue oxidant changes and hypermetabolism. Early removal and closure of a wound minimize these effects. Early excision and grafting of burn wounds, rather than allowing separation over 2 to 6 weeks, was popularized in the early 1970s and was shown to decrease the duration of hospitalization, pain, and the need for future reconstructive procedures.[99] Extensive wound excision in the acute shock stage (24 $\pm$ 14 hours postburn), rather than 4 to 5 days postburn, has also proved beneficial in reducing blood loss as well as shortening wound healing time by 7 days.[100]

## How Is Operative Blood Loss Managed?

Major burn débridement may be a bloody procedure, even requiring replacement of an entire blood volume in the first 30 minutes after incision. Loss of between 200 and 600 mL ($\approx$5%-10% of blood volume) of blood for every 1% of the TBSA excised by tangential excision technique has been estimated.[101,102] Adequate amounts of crossmatched blood must be in the operating room before incision.

Blood and blood products, in addition to being immunosuppressive, carry a 1 in 300 000 to 1 000 000 risk for hepatitis C or HIV transmission. They should be used judiciously. Careful attention to hemostasis and the use of tourniquets whenever possible should be the rule. Hypertension should be meticulously avoided during débridement, as well as postoperatively, in order to decrease oozing. In those patients with significant blood loss, intraoperative monitoring of coagulation status (ie, prothrombin time, partial thromboplastin time, platelets, fibrin degradation products, fibrinogen, and even thromboelastography) and appropriate replacement therapy help to decrease blood product requirements. Burn patients appear to recover to preoperative levels of fibrinogen, platelets, and Factors V, VIII, and IX within 48 hours after surgery, suggesting that they may safely undergo reoperation at 48-hour intervals for successive débridement if clinically indicated.[103]

## Topical Vasoconstrictors and Reduction of Blood Loss

Immediately after débridement, significant reduction in blood loss is obtained by application of topical vasoconstrictors. Epinephrine-soaked towels or sponges, 1:200 000 concentration, are superior to thrombin when applied to the donor site.[104] Although rarely a problem, if ventricular dysrhythmogenicity becomes an issue, epinephrine may be replaced by phenylephrine solution (1 mL of 1% phenylephrine in 1000 mL normal saline). Sponges or towels soaked with vasoconstrictive agents are placed on the bleeding wound site after excision. Blood volume loss may be estimated (Table 39–7).

The delay of some seconds before the vasoconstrictive agent has its effect on the cut and bleeding vessel within the wound surface has been criticized as leading to inferior control of blood loss, when compared with a method whereby the skin is wetted with epinephrine from a hand pump spray bottle before harvesting skin grafts. The donor site is prepared by removing any traces of the disinfectant agent. Application of 1:100 000 epinephrine-to-saline solution by spraying the skin and dermatome blade with solution from the bottle can provide a smooth gliding surface for the dermatome. During the process of harvesting the graft, the assistant continues to spray along the cutting head and immediately behind the path of the dermatome. With this technique for obtaining thin or medium split-thickness grafts, hemostasis is reported to be achieved within 10 minutes of harvesting the skin, with no additional need for cauterization of the vessels.[105] For the débridement of burned tissue, the use of blood products can be reduced more than 50% by subcutaneous injections of saline-epinephrine (0.5 mg in 1000 mL) or saline-phenylephrine (50 mg in 1000 mL) before tangential excision, and avoidance of vasodilating anesthetics or medications.[106] No adverse graft results have been described with this technique.[107] The median (range) of blood loss when this type of subeschar infiltration technique is used is 0.9% (0.3%-4%) of the blood volume for each percentage of the body surface excised and grafted (blood loss from donor sites included).[108] Even with extensive wound débridement, neither concentrated topical epinephrine (1 mg/10 mL) nor subcutaneous injected

dilute epinephrine (0.5 mg/1000 mL lactated Ringer's injection) lead to detectable increases in plasma levels of epinephrine or norepinephrine.[109,110] Both techniques are considered safe under general anesthesia.

## Miscellaneous Regimens

Major burns have been successfully managed without blood or blood products using a high-calorie, high-protein diet, iron supplementation, and pediatric blood sampling techniques and allowing spontaneous eschar separation rather than performing early débridement.[111] We have used this approach successfully, together with the administration of recombinant erythropoietin, when treating Jehovah's Witnesses.

# ANESTHETIC MANAGEMENT

## *What Are the Vascular Access Requirements?*

We do not anesthetize patients for wound débridement without adequate vascular access. Because temperature regulation is often problematic after significant thermal injuries, we prefer to have all catheters placed at the bedside, before moving a patient to the operating room.

The decision about what constitutes adequate venous access is subjective. In our experience, whenever a patient with a major thermal injury ($\geq$20%-25%) is taken to the operating room for anything more than the final touch-up work (ie, débridement and grafting of small areas of eschar after all of the major débridement has been performed), significant blood loss is possible. We use, at a minimum, two large-bore (16- to 14-gauge) catheters. A 9 French catheter placed in a central vein and an arterial catheter may be necessary for critically ill thermally injured patents.

In critically ill patients, a central venous catheter is useful for several reasons. Vasoactive drugs may be needed, and these are preferably infused into the central circulation. Calcium chloride may be required to counteract myocardial depression attendant to rapid transfusion of citrate-containing blood[112] and may cause serious soft tissue damage if it extravasates when administered peripherally. Because catheter sepsis is a problem in these patients, we fully gown, glove, mask, and drape when placing central catheters and remove the catheter as soon as it is no longer considered necessary. We use antibiotic-coated catheters and replace them every 12 days.[113]

## *What Should Be Monitored During Anesthesia?*

Monitoring of patients about to undergo débridement and split-thickness skin grafting requires consideration of several factors.

## Electrocardiography

Monitoring for rhythm and ischemia is made difficult in severely burned patients because unburned skin may be unavailable for placement of ECG electrode pads. Commercially

---

**TABLE 39–7.** Estimation of Blood Volume Lost Onto Various Absorbent Materials*

| Material | Dry | Epinephrine-Wetted |
|---|---|---|
| 4 × 4 pad | 20 mL | 10 mL |
| Laparotomy pad | 200 mL | 100 mL |
| Bath towel | 500 mL | 250 mL |

*Assumes absorbent material is soaked with blood.

available needle or back pad electrodes may be used. Serious dysrhythmias are fortunately less frequent now, most likely because of the use of rapid infusion and warming devices for the administration of blood products and fluids.

Continuous ECG recording allows rapid diagnosis of hypocalcemia, which causes prolongation of the QT interval. Myocardial depression due to rapid transfusion of citrate-containing blood can be rapidly corrected by intravenous administration of calcium chloride. Our practice is to administer as an intravenous bolus 500 mg to 1 g of calcium chloride when blood products are administered at a rate of $\geq 1$ unit every 5 minutes.

## Pulse Oximetry

Pulse oximetry is essential; the probe may be applied to fingers, toes, ears, the nose, or even the cheek or tongue when suitable extremity sites are unavailable.

## Temperature

Temperature monitoring is also essential. Because patients with significant thermal injuries have difficulty with temperature regulation and because hypothermia can cause severe dysrhythmias, we monitor temperature in all patients. We stop the operative procedure if a patient's core temperature decreases to <35°C or falls by >2°C below baseline. The operating room temperature is monitored as well and usually is kept >29°C.

## Exhaled Gases

Monitoring of the inhaled and exhaled gases is vital. In our burn unit operating room, we have identified low cardiac output syndromes, partial endotracheal tube obstruction, and inadequate minute ventilation by virtue of continuous gas analysis.

## Urine Output

Output from an indwelling catheter provides an indication of renal perfusion. Provided the urine output is >0.5 mL/kg/h and an osmotic diuresis does not contribute to urine flow, this is usually an indication of adequate intravascular volume status. An indwelling urethral catheter is most frequently placed in patients with thermal injuries of more than about 25% TBSA.

## Neuromuscular Blockade

Monitoring of neuromuscular blockade provides useful information. The ulnar nerve may be used for this purpose. However, if both wrists are burned, we use the facial or posterior tibial nerves. After induction and intubation, we do not strive for complete neuromuscular blockade because it is usually unnecessary for débridement and split-thickness skin grafting, but more importantly because deep anesthesia may be unsafe secondary to the tenuous hemodynamic status of these patients. The usual signs of light anesthesia—tachycardia, hypertension, and diaphoresis—are common and therefore nondiagnostic in these patients. Thus, a patient's movement or attempted movement is an excellent monitor of

**TABLE 39–8.** Resuscitation Drug Use During Débridement and Skin Grafting

| Drug | Concentration | Volume |
|---|---|---|
| Atropine | 0.4 mg/mL | 30 mL |
| Ephedrine | 5 mg/mL | 10 mL |
| Epinephrine | 10 µg/mL | 10 mL |
| | 100 µg/mL | 10 mL |
| Calcium chloride | 100 mg/mL | 10 mL |
| Phenylephrine | 40 µg/mL | 1-mL ampule of 10% concentration taped to 250-mL bag of lactated Ringer's |

inadequate anesthesia and can almost always safely be followed up by deepening the anesthetic.

## Which Resuscitation Drugs Are Essential?

A thermally injured patient undergoing débridement must be considered hemodynamically unstable. Accordingly, we have available for use the drugs listed in Table 39–8.

## When Is Air Embolization Problematic?

Rapid-infusion warming devices help maintain hemodynamic and temperature stability when large amounts of warmed blood, blood products, and fluids are needed. Despite the obvious usefulness of these devices, our experience is that the air eliminator may be overwhelmed by residual air in fluid bags or by entrained air during fluid bag exchange.[114] Crystalloid bags contain about 60 mL of air when you take them out of their wrapper. If no effort has been made to vent this air during spiking, and the fluid infusion rate is augmented by pressurization of the fluid bag, air emboli readily occur despite these air filters. One must, therefore, remove air from bags during the spiking maneuver and maintain vigilance so that air is not infused intravenously.

## How Is Body Temperature Maintained Intraoperatively?

Because maintenance of body temperature is a problem in thermally injured patients and because there is the potential for multiple problems in hypothermic patients (ie, ineffective coagulation, dysrhythmias, increased myocardial $O_2$ consumption secondary to postoperative shivering), the operating room should be kept warm (29°C) during débridement. Although the efficacy of an actively warmed airway humidifier has been questioned,[115] its use should be considered along with use of a low fresh gas flow rate, covering all body parts not involved in the surgical procedure, and warming all fluids going into the patient. Overhead warming lights and a warming blanket are useful during operative procedures in thermally injured children.

## How Is Ventilation Supported?

Edema of the chest and abdominal walls and ARDS may result in a noncompliant lung-thorax unit, requiring high inspiratory pressures to maintain adequate gas exchange. Preoperative evaluation of mechanically ventilated burned patients must include a measurement of the peak inspiratory pressures and minute ventilation. Many operating room ventilators cannot predictably generate peak pressures of >50 cm $H_2O$ or minute ventilations of >15 L/min.[116] If the patient requires higher pressure or minute ventilation, the ICU ventilator should be brought to the operating room.

## What Factors Govern the Choice of Anesthetic?

When anesthetic agents have to be administered within the first 24 postburn hours, circulatory instability should be anticipated owing to the previously described marked vasoconstriction and depressed cardiac output. Acute fluid resuscitation should be continued in the operating room in addition to the appropriate replacement of intraoperative fluid and blood losses. Establishment of large-bore intravenous catheters, especially in children or obese patients, may be difficult. Intravenous access without penetrating burn eschar is optimal but cannot always be avoided.

### General Considerations

Intravenous drug and inhaled anesthetic agent administration need careful titration. An increase in the anesthetic dose requirement is common once the acute stage of a thermal injury is survived. Sodium thiopental, narcotic, and ketamine requirements may be increased for months after burn injury.[117,118] Ketamine, at a dose of 0.25 to 1 mg/kg intravenously, is frequently used for bedside dressing changes. We often coadminister an anticholinergic drug (glycopyrrolate, 0.2-0.4 mg intravenously) to minimize salivation and midazolam or lorazepam to minimize the potential for emergence hallucinations. We avoid the use of nitrous oxide because of its potentially adverse effect on hematopoiesis and wound healing by inhibition of methionine synthase activity in patients who undergo multiple procedures.[119]

## Why Do We Prefer Intravenous Techniques?

Inhaled volatile anesthetic agents allow rapid adjustments in the depth of anesthesia and have been used successfully and safely in many burned patients. However, for débridement of burns of 20% TBSA or more, we feel hemodynamic stability is better maintained with intravenous anesthetic techniques. Although controversial, there are data suggesting immunosuppressive effects of the inhaled agents,[120] but it is unclear whether these in vitro studies have any significant in vivo implications. One of two major intravenous techniques is used (Table 39–9). We have found hemodynamic function with these techniques to be stable, provided blood loss is adequately corrected. An additional advantage is that continued sedation or analgesia in the postoperative period is provided by either technique by simply titrating the infusion rate downward.

### Avoidance of General Anesthesia in High-Risk Thermally Injured Patients

Patients with significant coexisting medical problems requiring skin grafting of small-size full-thickness burns (<10% TBSA) may benefit from local anesthesia application of EMLA cream about 2 hours before the procedure on the donor site and 1 hour before surgery on the burn wound. In one study, even though up to 145 g of EMLA cream was applied topically, which is the equivalent of 3625 mg lidocaine and 3625 mg prilocaine, no central nervous system side effects were observed.[121] Dose limits for topical application of local anesthetic agents to burn wounds have not been established, but there is evidence that surprisingly little systemic absorption occurs.[122]

**TABLE 39–9.** Intravenous Anesthetic Regimens Used at the University of Florida, Shands Hospital Burn Operating Room

| Period | Ketamine-Based Regimen | Narcotic-Based Regimen |
|---|---|---|
| *Preoperative Medication* (8 AM case) | Lorazepam, 1-3 mg (7 AM)<br>Famotidine,* 20 mg (6 AM) | Lorazepam, 1-3 mg (7 AM)<br>Famotidine,* 20 mg (6 AM) |
| *Induction* | Lorazepam, 0.05-0.1 mg/kg<br>Ketamine, 1-2 mg/kg<br>Vecuronium, 0.2 mg/kg; *or* atracurium, 1 mg/kg; or mivacurium, 0.3 mg/kg | Lorazepam, 0.05-0.1 mg/kg<br>Fentanyl, 5-10 μg/kg<br>Vecuronium, 0.2 mg/kg; *or* atracurium, 1 mg/kg; *or* mivacurium, 0.3 mg/kg |
| *Maintenance*<br>Ketamine infusion<br>    1000 mg in 100 mL 0.9% saline = 10 mg/mL<br>Fentanyl infusion<br>    2500 μg in 250 mL 0.9% saline = 10 μg/mL<br><br>Mixture of a remifentanyl infusion usually involves diluting a 1-, 2-, or 5-mg vial with 20 mL diluent, giving a concentration of, respectively, 50, 100, or 250 μg/mL | Ketamine 1-4 mg/kg/h infusion | Fentanyl, 1-5 μg/kg/h infusion<br><br>Sufentanil (may be used in place of fentanyl, if desired), 0.5-1 μg/kg load, followed by 0.1-0.5 μg/kg/h<br>Remifentanyl may be used in those relatively minor burn débridements in which rapid onset and offset are desired.<br>Loading dose (0.5-5 μg/kg) is given after a small dose (2-3 mg/kg) of thiopental; thereafter, an infusion of between 1 and 5 μg/kg/min is used with $N_2O$. |

*Ranitidine and cimetidine are equally effective; famotidine is less expensive in our institution.
OCOR, on-call to the operating room.

## When Is Continuation of Anesthesia and Surgery Contraindicated?

Of crucial importance in providing anesthesia for burn débridement is good rapport with the surgical team. The team needs to be informed when blood loss due to débridement is approaching or exceeding either replacement availability or capability. Interruption of further débridement to focus attention on control of bleeding for a few minutes is often all that is required to catch up with blood and fluid replacement.

Surgical duration probably has a significant impact on outcome in large burns. Thus, we usually limit our surgical colleagues to about 2 hours of operative time. We recommend discontinuation of surgery even before this time period has expired if more than two blood volumes have been lost or, as noted previously, the body temperature falls to 35°C or by >2°C from baseline. Even with adherence to these limits, massive postoperative resuscitation and correction of continued bleeding problems may require the continued involvement of the anesthesiologist long after the patient has left the operating room.

## Which Neuromuscular Blockers Are Used?

### Succinylcholine

Succinylcholine in burned patients can cause massive potassium efflux from the muscle cells and result in lethal acute hyperkalemia. The mechanism of the hyperkalemia is thought to be due to a denervation phenomenon, with proliferation of acetylcholine receptors throughout the muscle membranes. This hyperkalemic response is related to the dose of succinylcholine, time elapsed since injury, and severity of the burn injury.[123] The hyperkalemia and subsequent cardiac arrest usually occur within minutes of the administration of a paralyzing dose of succinylcholine.[124] Although the hyperkalemic response is usually seen between 20 and 60 days after the burn injury, we simply do not use this agent, *ever*, in thermally injured patients. In fact, succinylcholine is not allowed in the burn operating room.

### Nondepolarizing Agents

In thermal injury, resistance to nondepolarizing neuromuscular blockers, proportional to the TBSA involved (from 25% TBSA upward) has been demonstrated. Resistance is not observed in the first postburn week; maximum resistance occurs between 15 and 40 days after the initial thermal injury.[125] To achieve a given level of paralysis, a longer onset time is required; both the dose administered and serum concentrations required are increased twofold to threefold.

Early *local* resistance to atracurium in muscles under thermally injured skin in rats (2% TBSA burn) was shown by Pavlin and colleagues.[126] Ligand binding with bungarotoxin showed that at 2 weeks, acetylcholine receptors in the gastrocnemius muscle under the burned skin were 4 times denser than in the gastrocnemius in the contralateral uninjured leg. This group suggested that facial burns might be associated with unexpected resistance to nondepolarizing neuromuscular blockers due to the nature of the muscles in the area. Using facial nerve rather than ulnar nerve stimulation to assess adequacy of relaxation for intubation may be of value in the setting of a facial burn.

### Tracheal Intubation

For intubation, we commonly use vecuronium, 0.3 mg/kg; pancuronium, 0.3 mg/kg; or atracurium, 1 mg/kg. With any of these dose regimens, relaxation sufficient for intubation is achieved within about 60 seconds.

Although hypotension is a concern with an atracurium dose of >0.5 mg/kg, it was not noted when 0.8 mg/kg was used in burned patients.[127] We have also used mivacurium, 0.3 mg/kg, to facilitate rapid airway control.[128] Hemodynamic stability is preserved, and the drug onset is rapid. Frequent monitoring with a nerve stimulator is necessary if continued muscle relaxation is desired. Débridement and grafting, however, usually do not require profound muscle relaxation.

## THE CHRONIC PHASE OF BURNS

### How Are Repetitive Anesthetics Managed?

#### Pain Control

Pain control is of critical importance during the acute and chronic phases of burn injury. Enlisting the help of a pain management service to assist members of the burn care team must be considered. As mentioned earlier, use of ketamine during dressing changes and whirlpool procedures is critical. Drug options for control of pain are detailed in Table 39–10. Psychologic support during the period of acute, chronic, and rehabilitative care must be considered as important as volume resuscitation and débridement.

A critical stage in the treatment of patients with burns is control of the hypertrophic scarring that is responsible for deformities and contractures. With burns that involve the face, hypertrophic scarring can be disfiguring and painful. This problem can be ameliorated by the use of a contoured pressure mask. Fabrication of this mask in children often requires sedation or general anesthesia.

Intravenous anesthesia with ketamine, in which tracheal intubation is not performed, has been used frequently. However, apnea may occasionally occur, engendering significant risk if the alginate mold material completely covers the face.[129] Because rapid-sequence induction with succinylcholine is contraindicated in these patients secondary to potential problems with hyperkalemia, we recommend inhalation anesthesia and nasotracheal intubation, with or without nondepolarizing muscle relaxants.[130]

**TABLE 39–10.** Intravenous Pain Control Regimens Used at the University of Florida, Shands Hospital Burn Center

| Regimen | Dose |
|---|---|
| *Amnesia* | |
| Lorazepam | 0.01-0.03 mg/kg/h |
| Midazolam | 0.05-0.1 mg/kg/h |
| *Analgesia* | |
| Morphine sulfate | 0.1-2 mg/kg/h |
| Fentanyl | 0.5-10 μg/kg/h |
| Ketamine | 0.5–3 mg/kg/h |

# References

1. National Safety Council. *Accident Facts*. Chicago, Ill: National Safety Council; 1990.
2. Demling R. Burns. *N Engl J Med*. 1985;313:1389.
3. Burke JF. From desperation to skin regeneration: progress in burn treatment. *J Trauma*. 1990;30:S36.
4. Zhou YP, Zhou ZH, Zhou WM, et al. Successful recovery of 14 patients afflicted with full-thickness burns for more than 70 per cent body surface area. *Burns*. 1998;24:162.
5. Brigham PA, McLoughlin E. Burn incidence and medical care use in the United States: estimates, trends, and data sources. *J Burn Care Rehabil*. 1996;17:95.
6. Barillo DJ, Goode R. Fire fatality study: demographics of fire victims. *Burns*. 1996;22:85.
7. Heimbach D. Burn patients, then and now. *Burns*. 1999;25:1.
8. Zimmermann TJ, Krizek TJ. Thermally induced dermal injury: a review of pathophysiologic events and therapeutic intervention. *J Burn Care Rehabil*. 1984;5:193.
9. Jackson DM. The diagnosis of depth of burning. *Br J Surg*. 1953;40:588.
10. Zawacki BE. Reversal of capillary stasis and prevention of necrosis in burns. *Ann Surg*. 1974;180:98.
11. Jönsson A, Brofeldt BT, Nellgard P, et al. Local anesthetics improve dermal perfusion after burn injury. *J Burn Care Rehabil*. 1998;19:50.
12. Jönsson A, Mattson U, Tarnow P, et al. Topical local anesthetics (EMLA) inhibit burn-induced plasma extravasation as measured by digital image colour analysis. *Burns*. 1998;24:313.
13. Lindahl OA, Zdolsek J, Sjöberg F, et al. Human postburn oedema measured with the impression method. *Burns*. 1993;19:479.
14. Homma S, Gillam L, Weyman A. Echocardiographic observations in survivors of acute electrical injury. *Chest*. 1990;97:103.
15. Gabrielli A, Caruso L, Weiner ID, et al. Postoperative acute renal failure secondary to rhabdomyolysis from exaggerated lithotomy position (Case Conferences of the University of Florida). *J Clin Anesth*. 1999;11:257.
16. Dixon GF. The evaluation and management of electrical injuries. *Crit Care Med*. 1983;11:384.
17. Bingham H. Electrical burns. *Clin Plast Surg*. 1986;13:75.
18. Hammond JS, Ward CG. High-voltage electrical injuries—management and outcome of 60 cases. *South Med J*. 1988;81:1351.
19. Kaufman T, Yehuda U, Yaron H-S. Phosphorus burns: a practical approach to local treatment. *J Burn Care Rehabil*. 1988;9:474.
20. Dziewulski P. Burn wound healing (James Ellsworth Laing Memorial Essay for 1991). *Burns*. 1992;18:466.
21. Demling RH, Lalonde C. *Burn Trauma*. New York, NY: Thieme Medical Publishers; 1989:43.
22. O'Reilly TJ, Spence RJ, Taylor RM, et al. Laser Doppler flowmetry evaluation of burn wound depth. *J Burn Care Rehabil*. 1989;10:1.
23. Tobiasen J, Hiebert JH, Edlich RF. Prediction of burn mortality. *Surg Gynecol Obstet*. 1982;154:711.
24. Parker CR Jr, Baxter CR. Divergence in adrenal secretory pattern after thermal injury in adult patients. *J Trauma*. 1985;25:508.
25. Wilmore DW. Metabolic changes after thermal injury. In: Boswick JA Jr, ed. *The Art and Science of Burn Care*. Rockville, Md: Aspen; 1987:137–144.
26. McDonald WS, Sharp CW, Deitch EA. Immediate enteral feeding in burn patients is safe and effective. *Ann Surg*. 1991;213:177.
27. Saito H, Trocki O, Alexander JW. The effect of route of nutrient administration on the nutritional state, catabolic hormone secretion, and gut mucosal integrity after burn injury. *J Paren Enter Nutr*. 1986;11:1.
28. Demling R. Comparison of the anabolic effects and complications of human growth hormone and the testosterone analog, oxandrolone, after severe burn injury. *Burns*. 1999;25:215.
29. Alexander JW, MacMillan BG, Stinnett JD, et al. Beneficial effects of aggressive protein feeding in severely burned children. *Ann Surg*. 1980;192:505.
30. Alexander JW, Peck MD. Future prospects for adjunctive therapy—pharmacological and nutritional approaches to immune system modulations. *Crit Care Med*. 1990;18:S159.
31. Madden HP, Breslin RJ, Wasserkrug HL, et al. Stimulation of T-cell immunity by arginine enhances survival in peritonitis. *J Surg Res*. 1988;44:658.
32. Daly JM, Weintraub FN, Shou J, et al. Enteral nutrition during multimodality therapy in upper gastrointestinal cancer patients. *Ann Surg*. 1995;221:327.
33. Furukawa K, Tashiro T, Yamamari H, et al. Effects of soybean oil emulsion and eicosapentaenoic acid on stress response and immune function after a severely stressful operation. *Ann Surg*. 1999;229:255.
34. Moore FA, Moore EE, Kudsk KA, et al. Clinical benefits of an immune-enhancing diet for early postinjury enteral feeding. *J Trauma*. 1994;37:607.
35. Atkinson S, Sieffert E, Bihari D, et al. A prospective, randomized, double-blind, controlled clinical trial of enteral immunonutrition in the critically ill. *Crit Care Med*. 1998;26:1164.
36. Herndon DN, Barrow RE, Stein M, et al. Increasing mortality with intravenous supplemental feeding in severely burned patients. *J Burn Care Rehabil*. 1989;10:309.
37. Raff T, Hartmann B, Germann G. Early intragastric feeding of seriously burned and long-term ventilated patients: a review of 55 patients. *Burns*. 1997;23:19.
38. Ward PA, Till GO. Pathophysiologic events related to thermal injury of skin. *J Trauma*. 1990;30:S75.
39. DeCamp MM, Demling RH. Posttraumatic multisystem organ failure. *JAMA*. 1988;260:530.
40. Pitman JM III, Thurman GW, Anderson BO, et al. WEB2170, a specific platelet-activating factor antagonist, attenuates neutrophil priming by human serum after clinical burn injury. *J Burn Care Rehabil*. 1991;12:411.
41. Dinarello CA. The proinflammatory cytokines interleukin-1 and tumor necrosis factor and treatment of the septic shock syndrome. *J Infect Dis*. 1991;163:1177.
42. Barton R, Cerra FB. The hypermetabolism multiple organ failure syndrome. *Chest*. 1989;96:1153.
43. Cerra FB. The systemic septic response: concepts of pathogenesis. *J Trauma*. 1990;30:S169.
44. Schlüter B, König W, Köller M, et al. Studies on B-lymphocyte dysfunctions in severely burned patients. *Trauma*. 1990;30:1380.
45. Ferrara JJ, Dyess DL, Luterman A, et al. The suppressive effect of subeschar tissue fluid upon *in vitro* cell-mediated immunologic function. *J Burn Care Rehabil*. 1988;9:584.
46. Trop M, Schiffrin EJ, Jung WK, et al. Effect of acute burn trauma on phagocytic activity of the reticuloendothelial system in rats. *J Burn Care Rehabil*. 1989;10:388.
47. Gruber DF, D'Alesandro MM. Alteration of rat polymorphonuclear leukocyte function after thermal injury. *J Burn Care Rehabil*. 1989;10:394.
48. Schriemer PA, Longnecker DE, Mintz PD. The possible immunosuppressive effects of perioperative blood transfusion in cancer patients. *Anesthesiology*. 1988;68:422.
49. Waymack JP, Miskell P, Gonce S. Alterations in host defense associated with inhalation anesthesia and blood transfusion. *Anesth Analg*. 1989;69:163.
50. Shelby J. Transfusion-induced immunosuppression. *J Burn Care Rehabil*. 1987;8:546.
51. Hendrickson M, Shelby J, Sullivan JJ, et al. Naloxone inhibits the *in vivo* immunosuppressive effects of morphine and thermal injury in mice. *J Burn Care Rehabil*. 1989;10:494.
52. Alexander JW: The body's response to infection. In: Artz CP, Moncrief JA, Pruitt BA Jr, eds. *Burns: A Team Approach*. Philadelphia, Pa: WB Saunders; 1979:107–119.
53. Deitch EA, Berg R. Bacterial translocation from the gut: a mechanism of infection. *J Burn Care Rehabil*. 1987;8:475.
54. Dobke MK, Simoni J, Ninnemann JL, et al. Endotoxemia after burn injury: effect of early excision on circulating endotoxin levels. *J Burn Care Rehabil*. 1989;10:107.
55. Suzuki K, Nishina M, Ogino R, et al. Left ventricular contractility and diastolic properties in anesthetized dogs after severe burns. *Am J Physiol*. 1991;260:H1433.
56. Moncrief JA. Burns. *N Engl J Med*. 1973;288:444.
57. Demling RH, Kramer GC, Gunther R, et al. Effect of non-protein colloid on post-burn edema formation in soft tissues and lung. *Surgery*. 1984;95:593.
58. Zimmerman TJ, Krizek TJ. Thermally induced dermal injury: a review of pathophysiologic events and therapeutic intervention. *J Burn Care Rehabil*. 1984;5:193.
59. Demling RH, Lalonde C. Topical ibuprofen decreases early postburn edema. *Surgery*. 1987;102:857.
60. Lalonde C, Knox J, Daryani R, et al. Topical flurbiprofen decreases burn wound–induced hypermetabolism and systemic lipid peroxidation. *Surgery*. 1991;109:645.
61. Alexander F, Mathieson M, Teoh KHT, et al. Arachidonic acid metabolites mediate early burn edema. *J Trauma*. 1984;24:709.
62. Deitch EA. The management of burns. *N Engl J Med*. 1990;323:1249.
63. Haponik EF, Crapo RO, Herndon DN, et al. Smoke inhalation. *Am Rev Respir Dis*. 1988;138:1060.

64. Herndon DN, Traber DL, Linares H, et al. Etiology of the pulmonary pathophysiology associated with inhalation injury. *Resuscitation.* 1986;14:43.

65. Moylan JA, Chan CK. Inhalation injury: an increasing problem. *Ann Surg.* 1978;188:34.

66. Tranbaugh RF, Elings VB, Christensens JM, et al. Effect of inhalation injury on lung water accumulation. *J Trauma.* 1983;23:597.

67. Wroblewski DA, Bower GC. The significance of facial burns in acute smoke inhalation. *Crit Care Med.* 1979;7:335.

68. Navar PD, Jeffrey RS, Glenn DW. Effect of inhalation injury on fluid resuscitation requirements after thermal injury. *Am J Surg.* 1985;150:716.

69. Dai NT, Chen TM, Cheng TY, et al. The comparison of early fluid therapy in extensive flame burns between inhalation and noninhalation injuries. *Burns.* 1998;24:671.

70. Pallua N, Warbanow K, Noah EM, et al. Intrabronchial surfactant application in cases of inhalation injury: first results from patients with severe burns and ARDS. *Burns.* 1998;24:197.

71. Reper P, Dankaert R, Van Hille F, et al. The usefulness of combined high-frequency percussive ventilation during acute respiratory failure after smoke inhalation. *Burns.* 1998;24:34.

72. Cioffi WG Jr, Rue LW III, Graves TA, et al. Prophylactic use of high-frequency percussive ventilation in patients with inhalational injury. *Ann Surg.* 1991;213:575.

73. Zikria BA, Budd DC, Floch F, et al. What is clinical smoke poisoning? *Ann Surg.* 1975;181:151.

74. Gabrielli A, Gallagher TJ, Caruso L, et al. Psychometric tests (PSYTs) are a sensitive marker of persistent carbon monoxide poisoning after hyperbaric oxygen (HBO) treatment [abstract]. *Crit Care Med.* 1999;27:A118.

75. Kern K, Langevin PB, Dunn BM. Methemoglobinemia after topical anesthesia with lidocaine and benzocaine for a difficult intubation. *J Clin Anesth.* 2000;12:167.

76. Moylan JA. Diagnostic techniques and steroids. *J Trauma.* 1979;19:11S.

77. Vossmann H. Das Inhalationstrauma beim Brandverletzten Handchirurgie, Mikrochirurgie. *Plast Chir.* 1988;20:229.

78. Zellner PR. The 1990 Everett Idris Evans Memorial Lecture: the inhalation injury. *J Burn Care Rehabil.* 1990;11:487.

79. Bingham HG, Gallagher TJ, Powell MD. Early bronchoscopy as a predictor of ventilatory support for burned patients. *J Trauma.* 1987;27:1286.

80. Kilgore E, Baxter CR, Shires GT. Changes in body fluid compartments in full thickness burns. *Surg Forum.* 1965;16:29.

81. Monafo WW, Halverson JD, Schechtman K. The role of concentrated solutions in the resuscitation of patients with severe burns. *Surgery.* 1984;95:129.

82. Moylan JA, Reckler JM, Mason AD. Resuscitation with hypertonic lactate saline in thermal injury. *Am J Surg.* 1973;125:580.

83. Caldwell FT, Bowser BH. Critical evaluation of hypertonic and hypotonic solutions to resuscitate severely burned children—a prospective study. *Ann Surg.* 1979;189:546.

84. Huang PP, Stucky FS, Dimick AR, et al. Hypertonic sodium resuscitation is associated with renal failure and death. *Ann Surg.* 1995;221:543.

85. Kuroda T, Harada T, Tsutsumi H, et al. Hypernatremia deepens the demarcating borderline of leukocytic infiltration in the burn wound. *Burns.* 1997;23:432.

86. Dries DJ, Waxman K. Adequate resuscitation of burn patients may not be measured by urine output and vital signs. *Crit Care Med.* 1991;19:327.

87. Sinclair S, James S, Singer M. Intraoperative intravascular volume optimization and length of hospital stay after repair of proximal femoral fracture: randomised controlled trial. *BMJ.* 1997;315:909.

88. Jaffe MB. Partial $CO_2$ rebreathing cardiac output: operating principles of the NICO system. *J Clin Monit.* 1999;15:387.

89. DiVincenti FC, Moncrief JA, Pruitt BA. Electrical injuries: a review of 65 cases. *J Trauma.* 1969;9:497.

90. Monafo WW, Freedman BM. Electrical and lightning injury. In: Boswick JA, ed. *The Art and Science of Burn Care.* Rockville, Md: Aspen; 1987:247.

91. Teplitz C. The pathology of burns and the fundamentals of burn wound sepsis. In: Artz CP, Moncrief JA, Pruitt BA Jr, eds. *Burns: A Team Approach.* Philadelphia, Pa: WB Saunders; 1979:45.

92. Subrahmanyam M. Topical application of honey in treatment of burns. *Br J Surg.* 1991;78:497.

93. Subrahmanyam M. A prospective randomised clinical and histological study of superficial burn wound healing with honey and silver sulfadiazine. *Burns.* 1998;24:157.

94. Monafo WW, West MA. Current treatment recommendations for topical burn therapy. *Drugs.* 1990;40:364.

95. Hansbrough JF. Current status of skin replacement for coverage of extensive burn wounds. *J Trauma.* 1990;30(suppl 12):S155.

96. Pruitt BA Jr. The evolutionary development of biologic dressing and skin substitutes. *J Burn Care Rehabil.* 1997;18:S2.

97. Hansbrough JF, Mozingo DW, Kealey GP, et al. Clinical trials of a biosynthetic temporary skin replacement, Dermagraft: transitional covering compared with cryopreserved human cadaver skin for temporary coverage of excised burn wounds. *J Burn Care Rehabil.* 1997;18:43.

98. Heimbach D, Luterman A, Burke J, et al. Artificial dermis for major burns: a multicenter, randomized clinical trial. *Ann Surg.* 1988;208:313.

99. Schiozer WA, Hartinger A, von Donnersmarck GH, et al. Composite grafts of autogenic cultured epidermis and glycerol-preserved allogeneic dermis for definitive coverage of full thickness burn wounds: case reports. *Burns.* 1994;20:503.

100. Janzekovic Z. A new concept in the early excision and immediate grafting of burns. *J Trauma.* 1970;10:1103.

101. Guo ZR, Sheng CY, Diao L, et al. Extensive wound excision in the acute shock stage in patients with major burns. *Burns.* 1995;21:139.

102. Moran KT, O'Reilly TJ, Furman W, et al. A new algorithm for calculation of blood loss in excisional burn surgery. *Am Surg.* 1988;54:207.

103. Goodwin CW, Maguire MS, McManus WF, et al. Prospective study of burn wound excision of the hands. *J Trauma.* 1983;23:510.

104. Chang P, Murray DJ, Olson JD, et al. Analysis of changes in coagulation factors after postoperative blood loss in burn and non-burn patients. *Burns.* 1995;21:432.

105. Brezel BS, McGeever KE, Stein JM. Epinephrine vs thrombin for split-thickness donor site hemostasis. *J Burn Care Rehabil.* 1987;8:132.

106. Smoot EC, Kucan JO. Epinephrine spray-bottle technique for harvesting skin grafts. *J Burn Care Rehabil.* 1992;13:221.

107. Kahalley L, Dimick AR, Gillespie RW. Methods to diminish intraoperative blood loss. *J Burn Care Rehabil.* 1991;12:160.

108. Hughes WB, DeClement FA, Hensell DO. Intradermal injection of epinephrine to decrease blood loss during split-thickness skin grafting. *J Burn Care Rehabil.* 1996;17:243.

109. Janezic T, Prezelj B, Brcic A, et al. Intraoperative blood loss after tangential excision of burn wounds treated by subeschar infiltration of epinephrine. *Scand J Plast Reconstr Hand Surg.* 1997;31:245.

110. Missavage AE, Bush RL, Kien ND, et al. The effect of clysed and topical epinephrine on intraoperative catecholamine levels. *J Trauma.* 1998;45:1074.

111. Schlagintweit S, Snelling CFT, Germann E, et al. Major burns managed without blood or blood products. *J Burn Care Rehabil.* 1990;11:214.

112. Coté CJ, Drop LJ, Hoaglin DC, et al. Ionized hypocalcemia after fresh frozen plasma administration to thermally injured children: effects of infusion rate, duration, and treatment with calcium chloride. *Anesth Analg.* 1988;67:152.

113. Raad I, Darouiche R, Dupuis J, et al. Central venous catheters coated with minocycline and rifampin for the prevention of catheter-related colonization and bloodstream infections. *Ann Intern Med.* 1997;127:267.

114. Hartmannsgruber MW, Gravenstein N. Very limited air elimination capability of the Level 1 A fluid warmer. *J Clin Anesth.* 1997;9:233.

115. Hynson JM, Sessler DI. Intraoperative warming therapies: a comparison of three devices. *J Clin Anesth.* 1992;4:194.

116. Marks JA, Schapera A, Kraemer RW, et al. Pressure and flow limitations of anesthesia ventilators. *Anesthesiology.* 1989;71:403.

117. Coté CJ, Petkau AJ. Thiopental requirements may be increased in children reanesthetized at less than one year after recovery from extensive thermal injury. *Anesth Analg.* 1985;64:1156.

118. Martyn J. Clinical pharmacology and drug therapy in the burned patient. *Anesthesiology.* 1986;65:67.

119. Royston BD, Nunn JF, Weinbren HK, et al. Rate of inactivation of human and rodent hepatic methionine synthase by nitrous oxide. *Anesthesiology.* 1988;68:213.

120. Layon AJ, Peck AB. Anesthetic effects on immune function: where do we stand? In: Stoelting RK, Barash PG, Gallagher TJ, eds. *Advances in Anesthesia.* St Louis, Mo: Mosby-Year Book; 1993;10:69.

121. Janezic TF. Skin grafting of full thickness burns under local anaesthesia with EMLA cream. *Burns.* 1998;24:259.

122. Alvi R, Jones S, Burrows D, et al. The safety of topical anaesthetic and analgesic agents in a gel when used to provide pain relief at split skin donor sites. *Burns.* 1998;24:54.

123. Schaner PJ, Brown RL, Kirksey TD, et al. Succinylcholine hyperkalemia in burned patients. *Anesth Analg.* 1969;48:764.

124. Tolmie JD. Succinylcholine danger in the burned patient. *Anesthesiology.* 1967;28:467.

125. Dwersteg JF, Pavlin EG, Heimbach DM. Patients with burns are resistant to atracurium. *Anesthesiology.* 1986;65:516.

126. Pavlin EG, Haschke RH, Marathe P, et al. Resistance to atracurium in thermally injured rats: the role of time, activity, and pharmacodynamics. *Anesthesiology.* 1988;69:696.

127. Marathe PH, Dwersteg JF, Pavlin EG, et al. Effect of thermal injury on the pharmacokinetics and pharmacodynamics of atracurium in humans. *Anesthesiology.* 1989;70:752.

128. Layon AJ, Pratt B II, Mizutani T, et al. Mivacurium: comparison of three doses and comparison with vecuronium in burned patients [abstract]. *Anesthesiology.* 1995;83:A895.

129. White PF, Way WL, Trevor AJ. Ketamine: its pharmacology and therapeutic uses. *Anesthesiology.* 1982;56:119.

130. Layon AJ, Vetter TR, Hanna PG, et al. An anesthetic technique to fabricate a pressure mask for controlling scar formation from facial burns. *J Burn Care Rehabil.* 1991;12:349.

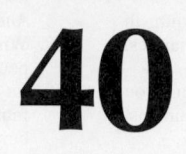
# Fluids, Electrolytes, Blood, and Blood Substitutes

Lawrence J. Caruso

Robert R. Kirby

NEUROSURGERY

*Is Glucose Contraindicated?*

*How Should Cerebral Edema Be Minimized?*

*How Is Diabetes Insipidus Controlled?*

PEDIATRIC PATIENTS

BURN PATIENTS

Abnormalities of fluid and electrolyte balance are extremely common in surgical patients. These disorders are significant contributors to inpatient hospital morbidity and mortality, whether they occur as a result of a disease process or as a consequence of medical interventions. Understanding the principles that govern fluid balance and the distribution of solutes among the various body compartments is of paramount importance to maintaining or restoring homeostasis. This chapter describes the homeostatic mechanisms that keep the balance of body water and electrolytes constant, despite internal and external influences; alterations in the various pathophysiologic states leading to electrolyte imbalance; differential diagnosis; and therapy. Aspects of fluid and colloid therapy are also discussed, as is the administration of hypertonic solutions.

The human body is 60% to 70% water. In obese patients, the percentage of water decreases, whereas in thin patients, it increases. The body's percentage of water is also affected greatly by disease states such as renal failure, hepatic failure, congestive heart failure (CHF), and sepsis as well as by age. Body water is divided into various compartments (Fig. 40–1). A means to remember this division is the "rule of thirds." Two thirds of total body weight (in a lean patient) is water; of this quantity, two thirds is intracellular, and one third is extracellular. Of the extracellular water, two thirds to three fourths is extravascular (*interstitial*), and the remaining one third to one fourth is intravascular. Although this rule is only an approximation, it presents an easy way to remember body water composition.

## FLUID COMPARTMENTS

The intracellular and extracellular compartments are separated by cell membranes. These membranes are permeable

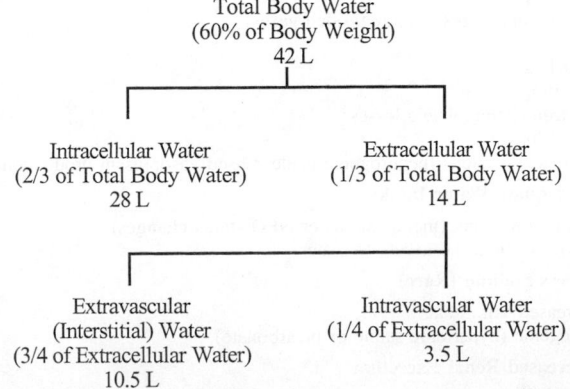

**FIGURE 40–1.** Distribution of body water in an "ideal" 70-kg man.

**TABLE 40–1.** Approximate Electrolyte Concentrations

| Electrolyte | Extracellular Fluid* (mEq/L) | Intracellular Fluid (mEq/L) |
|---|---|---|
| Sodium | 140 | 10 |
| Potassium | 4.5 | 150 |
| Calcium | 5 | 1 |
| Magnesium | 2 | 40 |

*Plasma and interstitial.

to water but are relatively impermeable to ionized particles (electrolytes). Therefore, water crosses membranes freely. The equilibrium between the intracellular and extracellular body compartments is determined by osmotic gradients. These osmotic differences determine the size of each compartment. Intravascular and extravascular spaces are separated by capillary endothelium that is freely permeable not only to water but also to electrolytes and other small molecules. However, it is normally less permeable to large molecules such as albumin. Permeability to ions and proteins varies from organ to organ, being least in the brain (blood-brain barrier) and highest in the liver.

## How Do the Fluid Compartments Differ?

Each of the fluid compartments has a different composition (Table 40–1). The intravascular compartment contains water and electrolytes, a high concentration of proteins, and the formed blood elements (red blood cells [RBCs], white blood cells, and platelets). This fluid space is accessible to the anesthesiologist for drug administration and for the measurement of various body components, and it is essential for oxygen transport. The principal difference between the intravascular and interstitial fluid compartments is the absence of much of the protein and most of the formed blood elements in the latter.

Because fluids and electrolytes pass freely between these compartments, the electrolyte composition is about the same. However, because of the previously described, relatively impermeable cellular membranes and the membrane-bound sodium-potassium pump, the concentration of electrolytes in the intracellular compartment is different from that in the extracellular compartment (see Table 40–1). The importance of some of these differences is discussed in the section on electrolyte disturbances.

### Regulation of Body Fluid Composition

Normally, the body's fluid composition is carefully regulated. Figure 40–2 represents the major factors of importance. Water balance is intimately associated with solute balance. The human kidneys can produce urine with a solute concentration of between 50 and 1400 mOsm/L.[1] These changes in concentration are caused by changes in the level of antidiuretic hormone (ADH; also known as *arginine-vasopressin*).

The production of ADH is controlled by extracellular fluid volume, osmoreceptors, and perfusion to various organ systems, including the central nervous system and the kidneys. In awake patients, thirst and drinking control the intake of both solutes and water. However, during anesthesia, thirst is eliminated. Furthermore, during major operative procedures,

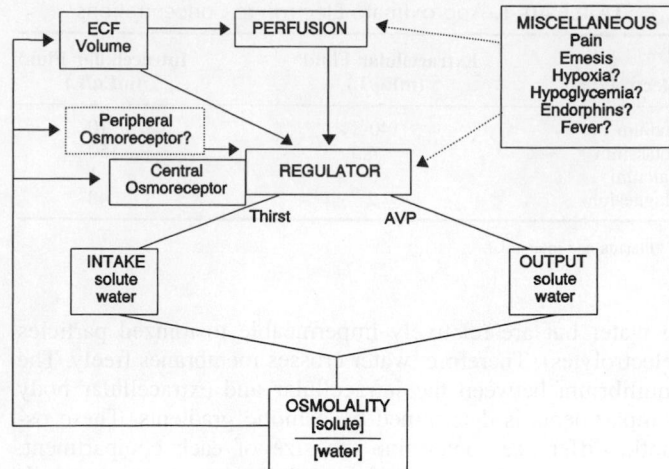

**FIGURE 40–2.** Factors affecting water balance. *Question marks* and *dashed lines* indicate factors that are not clearly understood. AVP, arginine-vasopressin; ECF, extracellular fluid. (From Tonneson AS. Water balance and control of osmolality. In: Askanazi J, Starker PM, Weissman C, eds. *Fluid and Electrolyte Management in Critical Care*. Boston, Mass: Butterworth; 1986:99.)

the fluid shifts and blood loss that occur are often much greater than could be corrected by the usual drinking response and oral intake.

The observation of urine output provides a rough but often imprecise indication of fluid balance; this topic is discussed later in this chapter in the section on monitoring of adequacy of replacement. For a more complete description of the regulation of body water, the reader is referred to other sources.[2]

## PERIOPERATIVE ELECTROLYTE AND GLUCOSE MANAGEMENT

### *What Are Common Sodium Disorders?*

Sodium is the predominant extracellular cation (see Table 40–1). Total body sodium content is about 5000 mEq. The average daily requirement for sodium is 1 to 2 mEq/kg. However, the kidneys can compensate for a wide range of intake, from about 0.25 mEq/kg/d to >6 mEq/kg/d. Sodium is also one the major cations involved in intravascular volume regulation. Disorders in sodium concentration often reflect disorders of intravascular volume status more than actual changes in total body sodium. Normally, the intake of sodium by the diet is adequate to meet the body's needs. Therefore, the kidneys regulate sodium concentration in relation to water balance.

Sodium and its accompanying cations account for about 93% of serum osmolality, which may be approximated by the following formula:

$$\text{Osmolality (mOsm/kg } H_2O) = 2 \times [Na^+] + [\text{Glucose}]/18 + [\text{BUN}]/28$$

where BUN is serum urea nitrogen.

### Hypernatremia

Patients with hypernatremia present a wide range of signs and symptoms, including mental status changes, increased thirst, peripheral edema, myoclonus, and possibly cardiovascular decompensation. Most commonly, hypernatremia is caused by excess renal excretion of free water or extrarenal free water losses such as sweating, diarrhea, fever, and increased respiratory evaporation (Table 40–2).

### *Treatment*

In the patient with hypernatremia, hypotonic fluids (eg, 0.45%-0.20% saline), administered at a rate sufficient to reduce serum $Na^+$ concentration by about 2 mEq/h, restores volume and electrolyte status to normal. The total free water deficit can be calculated as follows:

$$\text{Free Water Deficit (mL)} = 0.6 \times \text{Weight (kg)} \times (\text{Plasma } Na^+/140 - 1)$$

In case of excess total body sodium, as might be seen after the administration of large amounts of sodium bicarbonate or hypertonic saline solutions, administration of a loop diuretic, such as furosemide, and fluid replacement with hypotonic solutions restores equilibrium.

### Hyponatremia

Hyponatremia is more often caused by a water excess than a sodium deficit. Common causes include renal failure, CHF, and replacement of fluid losses (vomiting or diarrhea) with sodium-deficient solutions (Table 40–3). Patients with the syndrome of inappropriate antidiuretic hormone have inappropriate water retention, a decrease in serum osmolality, and an increase in urine osmolality.

When evaluating patients with hyponatremia, one must be certain to exclude possible laboratory error. Laboratories calculate the sodium concentration based on the total volume of plasma rather than on the volume of water in the plasma. In patients with extreme hyperlipidemia or hyperproteinemia, a significant portion of the plasma is occupied by these interfering substances so that the *measured* sodium concentration is much lower than the *effective* sodium concentration,[3] a condition known as *pseudohyponatremia*. In addition, hyperosmolarity (hyperglycemia or mannitol intoxication) causes an osmotic shift of water into the intravascular compartment,

**TABLE 40–2.** Causes of Hypernatremia

**Excess-Free Water Loss**

Sweating
Respiratory losses (nonhumidified gases)
Fever
Diarrhea
Vomiting
Gastrointestinal fistula losses
Renal losses
Diabetes insipidus (nephrogenic or decreased vasopressin production)

**Inadequate Water Intake**

Inability to drink (mental status or NPO status changes)
Environmental (no access to water)

**Excess Sodium (Rare)**

Increased salt intake
Iatrogenic (hypertonic saline or bicarbonate)

**Decreased Renal Excretion**

Renal failure

**TABLE 40–3.** Causes of Hyponatremia

**Free Water Excess**

Congestive heart failure
Hepatic failure
Renal failure
Excessive antidiuretic hormone (vasopressin)
Pain, blood loss, dehydration, hypotension
Syndrome of inappropriate antidiuretic hormone (SIADH)
Replacement of fluid losses (eg, sweating, vomiting, diarrhea) with
   hypotonic fluid (eg, beer, soda, tea, plain water)
Inappropriate intravenous fluids
Psychogenic water drinkers
Syndrome of transurethral resection of the prostate (TURP syndrome)

**Sodium Deficit**

Renal losses (eg, with use of diuretics)
Excessive losses (eg, sweating, vomiting, diarrhea)
Inadequate intake
Inappropriate intravenous fluids

creating hyponatremia with normal or elevated serum osmolality.

### Treatment

In patients with mild hyponatremia (an absolute serum sodium level greater than about 125 mEq/L, and normal mental status), treatment is usually conservative. Evaluation of the patient's volume status and restriction of fluid intake suffice. If patients are significantly hypervolemic, diuretic use may be indicated. Sodium intake can be increased by administering isotonic or slightly hypertonic fluids. The management of severe, *acute,* symptomatic hyponatremia is much different. Absolute sodium values of <110 to 120 mEq/L may represent a true medical emergency. All but the most urgent surgical procedures should be canceled, the patient should be admitted to the intensive care unit, and the hyponatremia should be corrected in a careful and controlled manner.

Debate regarding the speed of correction is widespread.[4–9] An increase in sodium level to 120 to 125 mEq/L can proceed relatively rapidly (1-2 mEq/L/h) in cases of acute, symptomatic hyponatremia, followed by a slower increase into the low-normal range. Normal or hypertonic saline is used while intravascular volume status is carefully monitored. Diuretics are useful to increase the excretion of free water.

Rapid correction of severe hyponatremia is believed by some to predispose the patient to central pontine myelinolysis, a myelin degenerative disease that is associated with paraparesis or quadriparesis. A cause and effect relationship, however, is not well established. Nevertheless, a 1992 paper by Sterns[10] suggested that rapid correction of even severe *chronic* hyponatremia (serum sodium as low as 98 mEq/L) is seldom, if ever, indicated and may lead to an osmotic demyelination syndrome. In such cases, Sterns recommended correction by no more than 0.5 mEq/L/h.

## What Are Common Potassium Disorders?

Total body potassium averages 3500 mEq, most of which is intracellular (see Table 40–1). Therefore, measurements of serum potassium concentration represent a small fraction of total body potassium. However, potassium equilibrium is im-

portant in the maintenance of cell membrane potentials, particularly in excitable cells, such as those of the myocardium.

Normal regulation of potassium concentration occurs in the kidneys, which can alter urinary potassium from <5 to >100 mEq/L under the influence of aldosterone. As is to be expected, most abnormalities of potassium concentration occur when the kidneys' ability to regulate potassium is compromised by renal failure or by the administration of diuretics. Other nonrenal losses include excessive sweating and diarrhea.

### Hyperkalemia

Hyperkalemia can be life-threatening. Common causes are listed in Table 40–4. Hemolysis of RBCs in a laboratory specimen may cause an artifactually high reported serum potassium concentration. Thus, a patient's clinical status must be correlated with the laboratory value. In patients with chronic renal failure, a potassium concentration of 5 to 6 mEq/L may have few physiologic effects. The same level of potassium in patients who are not chronically exposed to such high levels may cause arrhythmias. The most sensitive indicator of hyperkalemia is the electrocardiogram (ECG). Peaked T waves are often followed by a prolonged PR interval and absent P waves. In severe hyperkalemia, a widened QRS complex precedes a sine wave pattern, ventricular tachycardia, and ventricular fibrillation.

### Treatment

Initial treatment includes intravenous glucose (25 g) and regular insulin (10 U), which induce a rapid extracellular-to-intracellular potassium shift. Alkalization with sodium bicarbonate has a slower onset but may be synergistic with insulin and glucose. Hyperventilation also is effective. Inhaled albuterol (20 µg) also has been shown to shift potassium intracellularly.[11] Finally, calcium chloride should be administered with ECG monitoring to counteract the cellular membrane effects of hyperkalemia. which induces an extracellular-to-intracellular potassium shift.

None of these measures decreases total body potassium content. A potassium-binding resin, diuretics, or dialysis must be used for this purpose. However, these approaches are much slower than the acute interventions that are necessary in an

**TABLE 40–4.** Common Causes of Hyperkalemia

**"False" Cases**

Hemolysis of blood sample

**Inadequate Excretion**

Renal failure
Potassium-sparing diuretics
Angiotensin-converting enzyme inhibitors

**Excessive Intake**

Salt substitutes
Intravenous administration
Rapid, massive blood transfusion

**Extracellular Redistribution**

Acidosis
Hemolysis
Cellular destruction (electrical burns, rhabdomyolysis)
Succinylcholine
β-Blockers   •

**TABLE 40–5.** Common Causes of Hypokalemia

**Increased Losses**
Diuretics
Vomiting
Sweating
Diarrhea, bowel preparation, enemas
Magnesium deficiency
Alcoholism
Amphotericin B therapy

**Redistribution**
Alkalosis (metabolic or hyperventilation)
Insulin activity
Glycogen

**Inadequate Intake**
Iatrogenic (chronic intravenous fluids with no K$^+$)
Inadequate postoperative intake (rare)

emergent situation. Succinylcholine should be avoided in patients with preexisting, significant hyperkalemia (>5.5 mEq/L).

## Hypokalemia

Hypokalemia is frequently an iatrogenic problem (Table 40–5) most commonly caused by the chronic use of diuretics with inadequate potassium replacement. Patients with chronic hypokalemia often have significant total body potassium depletion. The initial volume of distribution of intravenously administered potassium, however, is the extracellular volume. Therefore, correction of large potassium deficits must take place over several days to avoid acute hyperkalemia.

### Delay of Elective Surgery

A few years ago, patients with potassium levels of 3 to 3.5 mEq/L would have their operations canceled and their potassium levels corrected to the normal range because of the perceived risk for increased intraoperative arrhythmias. However, studies from the middle and late 1980s[12,13] indicate that chronic hypokalemia as low as 2.5 to 3 mEq/L, if without side effects, is not associated with increased risk. Current recommendations suggest that patients receiving diuretic therapy have their potassium levels checked on the day before surgery.

Intraoperatively, hypokalemia may be exacerbated by hyperventilation-induced respiratory alkalosis. This situation represents an intracellular shift of potassium and should not be corrected with potassium administration. Instead, ventilation should be adjusted to a normal value, using arterial pH as the primary guideline.

### Treatment

In patients with severe hypokalemia, an associated magnesium deficiency can be inferred. These patients may receive large amounts of supplemental potassium with limited increase in the serum level. Administration of supplemental magnesium sulfate usually corrects the deficit. The link between potassium and magnesium movements is unclear, but cellular levels tend to rise and fall together during periods of a deficiency in either. It may be that magnesium deficiency prevents cells from establishing a normal transcellular gradient for potassium. Magnesium deficiency perhaps selectively affects membrane-bound magnesium, which, in turn, regulates permeability to potassium. In hypokalemia, replacement of magnesium, even in the absence of potassium replacement, often corrects the deficiency.

Because potassium is irritating to peripheral vessels, it normally should be administered through a central vein unless it is diluted. In adults, up to 40 mEq of potassium chloride diluted in a volume of 100 mL or greater is given over about 1 hour when rapid correction is deemed necessary. A dilute solution (eg, 40 mEq/L) can be administered peripherally. The rate of potassium administration to children should not exceed 0.5 mEq/kg/h and should be followed by continuous ECG monitoring.

## What Are Common Chloride Disorders?

Chloride is the major extracellular anion. Its chief importance is in acid-base regulation. Primary disorders of chloride without associated acid-base disorders are unusual. Hyperchloremia is commonly associated with metabolic (nonrespiratory) acidosis, and hypochloremia is associated with metabolic alkalosis.

### Hyperchloremia

Hyperchloremic metabolic acidosis is often seen in conjunction with renal tubular acidosis or as a result of the administration of excessive amounts of chloride. Therapy for renal tubular acidosis consists of evaluation of the underlying acid-base disorder and of the avoidance of solutions containing excessive chloride.

### Treatment

Substitution of phosphate, bicarbonate, or acetate for chloride as the major anions usually should be made in hyperalimentation fluids or other chronically administered solutions. In the operating room, the major concern is the potential hyperchloremic acidosis and whether it should be corrected with sodium bicarbonate.

### Hypochloremia

Hypochloremia and its associated alkalosis result from excessive loss of chloride after diuretic administration and nasogastric suction. It is seen frequently in patients with pyloric stenosis and small bowel or gastric outlet obstruction. It may also follow the administration of large-volume blood transfusions. The associated metabolic alkalosis can present significant problems when one attempts to wean patients from mechanical ventilation. Such individuals may hypoventilate as a compensatory response to the metabolic alkalosis.

### Treatment

Administration of an appropriate volume of saline and potassium or ammonium chloride usually corrects hypochloremia. At one time, dilute hydrochloric acid (0.1 N) was infused slowly through a central vein but is seldom used now. Acetazolamide (Diamox), a carbonic anhydrase inhibitor, can be given in a dose of 250 to 500 mg that is repeated once or twice at 4-hour intervals. This treatment corrects the alkalosis but not the hypochloremia. As long as the patient's acid-base status is acceptable, surgery need not be postponed because of moderate degrees of hyperchloremia or hypochloremia. However, a work-up for the basis of the disorder should be undertaken.

## What Are Common Calcium Disorders?

Ninety-nine percent of the body's calcium is contained in bone and is not immediately available to the circulation. Calcium's major function is the maintenance of cell membrane integrity, membrane excitability, and excitation-contraction coupling. It is also involved in the coagulation cascade. Calcium is highly protein bound; therefore, ionized calcium, which can be measured with ion-specific electrodes, is a more reliable indicator of activity than is the total serum calcium level.

Calcium binding is decreased by acidosis and increased by alkalosis. Normal calcium metabolism is under the control of parathyroid hormone and vitamin D. Fluid resuscitation in patients in shock tends to lower total and ionized calcium concentrations. Infused albumin, with its calcium-binding sites, and transfusion of large amounts of citrate-containing banked blood also decrease the level of ionized calcium.

### Hypercalcemia

Hypercalcemia is associated with a variety of conditions (Table 40–6). The primary signs are mental status changes, weakness, and renal failure.

### Treatment

Treatment must be directed at the underlying condition; otherwise, it is relatively ineffective. Diuresis and administration of large volumes of normal saline are the mainstays of supportive therapy. Patients with symptomatic hypercalcemia should have elective surgery postponed until the underlying condition can be evaluated and treated. Those with mild hypercalcemia and no symptoms may undergo surgical procedures, but the ionized calcium level should be sequentially determined.

**TABLE 40–6.** Causes of Hypercalcemia

**Redistribution**

Osteolysis
Malignancy
Sarcoidosis
Tuberculosis
Vitamin D excess
Parathyroid hormone excess (often seen with renal failure)
Immobilization
Adrenal insufficiency
Hypophosphatemia

**Excess Intake**

Vitamin D intoxication
Milk-alkali syndrome
Iatrogenic

**Decreased Excretion**

Parathyroid hormone excess
Renal failure

**TABLE 40–7.** Common Causes of Hypocalcemia

**Redistribution**

Alkalosis
Citrate (banked blood) infusion
Rapid albumin infusion
Phosphate infusion
Sepsis
Hemodialysis
Pancreatitis
Hypomagnesemia

**Inadequate Intake or Inability to Mobilize From Bone**

Vitamin D deficiency
Parathyroid hormone deficiency
Inadequate diet (rare)

### Hypocalcemia

Hypocalcemia (Table 40–7) is much more common in the operating room than is hypercalcemia. The major signs and symptoms relate to the irritability of electrically active cells and include mental status changes, tetany, Chvostek's and Trousseau's signs, and dysrhythmias. Abnormal excitation-contraction coupling, manifested by a prolonged QT interval on the ECG, depressed myocardial contractility, and associated hypotension may result. In the operating room, rapid infusion of citrated blood (usually in excess of 1.5 mL/kg/min) or albumin, coupled with acute hyperventilation, is the most common acute cause of symptomatic hypocalcemia.

### Treatment

Treatment with intravenous calcium chloride (15 mg/kg), through a central venous catheter, or with calcium gluconate (45 mg/kg), through a peripheral or central venous catheter, should be accompanied by careful and continuous ECG monitoring. Note that except in cases of documented hypocalcemia, recommendations for calcium salts during resuscitation from cardiac arrest have been virtually eliminated.[14]

## What Are Magnesium Disorders?

Magnesium is a predominantly intracellular cation that is involved in membrane excitability as well as in the regulation of potassium concentration. Patients receiving chronic diuretic therapy are sometimes severely magnesium depleted. Magnesium supplementation in the acute setting is indicated for arrhythmias associated with hypomagnesemia or hypokalemia, with uncorrectable hypokalemia or with preeclampsia or eclampsia.

Rapid administration of magnesium may cause symptomatic hypotension. High magnesium levels are associated with muscle weakness and potentiate neuromuscular blocking agents. Hypermagnesemia is usually iatrogenically induced and is associated with the treatment of preeclampsia or eclampsia. Intravenous calcium antagonizes the toxic effects of hypermagnesemia.

## What Are Phosphate Disorders?

Eighty-five percent of the body's phosphate is contained in bone. The remaining 15% is involved in energy flux (adenosine triphosphate) and in the production of nucleic acids and proteins. Hyperphosphatemia may induce hypocalcemia through calcium binding. Significant phosphate abnormalities are uncommon in the operating room. When seen, they are usually associated with chronic malnutrition or iatrogenic complications of hyperalimentation. Intravenous phosphate is infused slowly to avoid vascular tissue calcification or acute hypocalcemia.

## What Are Common Glucose Disorders?

Although glucose is not an electrolyte, disorders of glucose concentration can severely affect the perioperative fluid status. The most common cause of alterations in glucose status is diabetes mellitus. However, acute alterations in serum glucose level can result from fluid and electrolyte therapy as well.

### Hyperglycemia

Hyperglycemia is more common in the operating room than is hypoglycemia and usually follows the administration of large amounts of glucose in intravenous fluids. The stress response to surgery also increases serum glucose concentration. Transient, moderate hyperglycemia is less dangerous than hypoglycemia. However, glucose in excess of about 300 mg/dL places patients at increased risk for osmotic diuresis and for a worsened neurologic outcome after an anoxic or ischemic event.

#### Treatment

Because of unpredictable skin perfusion, the administration of subcutaneous insulin to control hyperglycemia is not recommended in the operating room. Small intermittent doses of intravenous regular insulin or a continuous insulin infusion should be used instead.

### Hypoglycemia

Hypoglycemia in normal adults, even after prolonged periods with no oral glucose intake, is uncommon. Exceptions include patients with severe liver disease, those undergoing major hepatic resections, and neonates, all of whom frequently are depleted of glycogen stores and therefore prone to hypoglycemia. Diabetic patients who have received long-acting (neutral protamine Hagedorn) insulin or oral antihyperglycemic agents are also at risk for significant intraoperative hypoglycemia. General anesthesia masks the usual clinical signs and symptoms of hypoglycemia but does not protect the central nervous system and other organ systems from its effects. Patients at increased risk for hypoglycemia should have frequent monitoring of their blood glucose levels.

## ORIGINS OF THERAPEUTIC MISCONCEPTIONS

### Does "Salt Intolerance" Exist?

Throughout the 1940s and 1950s, patients in the immediate postoperative period received salt-free solutions such as 5% dextrose in water ($D_5W$). This practice was derived from the hypothesis that these patients were salt intolerant, that is, that they were unable to excrete an administered sodium load. Most of these assumptions were based on small numbers of case reports in which patients were thought to have received sufficient amounts of intravenous saline but had major complications, including abdominal distention, somnolence, lethargy, coma, shock, and sometimes, death.[15] Salt intolerance was blamed. However, on later review, it was realized that the complications reported were those of hyponatremia and hyposmolarity associated with the administration of excess $D_5W$. Nevertheless, for years thereafter, surgical patients underwent forced sodium restriction in the immediate postoperative period, and as a result, severe hyponatremia and water intoxication continued to occur.

### Hormonal Fluxes

The identification and characterization of ADH, the 17-OH corticosteroids, and aldosterone, as well as more precise delineation of intraoperative fluid shifts and renal function, resulted in significant changes in the concepts underlying fluid and electrolyte therapy. Nonstressed patients can form as much as 10 mL of urine for each milliosmole of solute excreted by the kidneys. However, stressed surgical patients can only excrete 1.2 to 1.6 mL/mOsm of solute,[16] due, at least in part, to increased levels of aldosterone and ADH. Thus, when such patients are given a fluid such as $D_5W$ with minimal solute, they are unable to excrete a large water load and retain large amounts of free water; consequently, they develop a dilutional hyponatremia, hyposmolarity, and water intoxication.

Additionally, in the operative and postoperative periods, significant fluid losses occur. These include continued bleeding and so-called third space losses. The latter represents the loss of isotonic fluid, that is, fluid with the same electrolyte composition as that in plasma. Current recommendations are to replace these losses with fluid of a composition that is similar to that of the fluid being lost (ie, balanced electrolyte solutions, colloid solutions, or both).

Our better understanding of the hormonal control of fluid balance, improved invasive and noninvasive monitoring, and rapid measurements of serum and urine electrolytes and hematocrit allow more precise titration of fluid therapy than was ever possible when urine output was the primary determinant of fluid status and renal function.[17]

## FLUID BALANCE DURING SURGERY

### What Changes Occur With Regional Anesthesia?

If patients had no physiologic changes during anesthesia and surgery, there would be little need for fluid therapy other than to replace blood loss. However, physiologic alterations do occur. When spinal, epidural, or caudal anesthesia is induced, a variable degree of sympathetic blockade results. Peripheral vasodilation results in venous pooling and effectively removes circulating blood from the central intravascular compartment. Sufficient fluid must be administered to maintain venous return, blood pressure (BP), and cardiac output.

Most young patients tolerate this sympathectomy well if

they have been sufficiently hydrated before the induction of anesthesia. However, elderly patients with underlying heart disease or patients taking diuretics or antihypertensive drugs may not be able to mount the responses necessary to overcome the sympatholytic effects of regional anesthesia. Careful fluid administration and judicious use of anticholinergic drugs (atropine, glycopyrrolate) or vasopressors (dopamine, phenylephrine hydrochloride, ephedrine, epinephrine) are sometimes essential to the successful use of such techniques.

Regional anesthesia involving small areas of the body, such as brachial plexus blocks, requires much less fluid replacement. When spinal anesthesia is chosen, up to 1 L of fluid is usually administered before the start of the anesthesia because the onset of sympathetic blockade is rapid. With epidural techniques, especially when a catheter and incremental doses are used, the fluid administration can occur concomitantly with the slower onset of anesthesia.

## What Changes Occur With General Anesthesia?

General anesthesia has two components of importance to fluid management. First are the anesthetic effects, and second are the effects of positive pressure ventilation.

### Anesthetic Effects

No commonly used anesthetics cause increased fluid losses. Nevertheless, all anesthetics may blunt the normal response to absolute or relative hypovolemia, especially during induction. A moderately hypovolemic patient with a normal BP may suddenly become hypotensive after anesthesia has been induced. These effects are exaggerated when myocardial depressants, such as barbiturates or propofol, or agents with potent vasodilatory properties, such as isoflurane, are used. However, even a usually sympathomimetic agent such as ketamine can produce similar effects if the sympathetic response before induction is already maximum, thereby uncovering its myocardial depressant effect.

### Mechanical Ventilation

Mechanical ventilation also affects fluid balance by decreasing the release of atrial natriuretic hormone and, particularly when administered with positive end-expiratory pressure, by increasing the release of ADH. Thus, patients retain slightly more sodium and fluid. Of more importance are the reduction of venous return and BP, which, when added to the anesthetic-induced decreases, may be profound. In general, these changes are rapidly reversed upon discontinuation of the anesthetic and resumption of spontaneous breathing. They rarely lead to prolonged postoperative fluid shifts and decrease in urine output.

## What Surgical Factors Are Important?

The major fluid and electrolyte shifts result from the trauma of surgery. In addition to blood replacement, third space losses (edema, intracellular translocation, ascites, and so forth) must be replenished. Such losses are not easily quantified and do not exist in nor move to specific anatomic areas. The involved fluid, although still physically present in the body, is no longer functional in terms of its contribution to intravascular volume, oxygen and nutrient delivery, and waste removal.

### Trauma-Induced Fluid Loss

A convenient way to think about this problem is to consider the fluid that is lost from the area of surgical trauma. An increase of capillary permeability and localized swelling (edema) occurs much the same as is seen when one's thumb is struck with a hammer. The leaked fluid is still present but is in a new location and is obviously no longer functional in fluid homeostasis. If the area of involvement is sufficiently large, as it is with bowel resection, retroperitoneal exploration, radical prostatectomy or hysterectomy, or major trauma, several liters of fluid are lost and must be replaced so that functional activity is maintained. Successful management results in an obligatory increase in total body water in order to restore the functional component to normal.

### Bleeding and Third Space Fluid Loss

Third space fluid loss also occurs with major bleeding. In a classic resuscitation experiment, Shires and coworkers[18] showed that replacement of all lost blood in a dog model of hemorrhagic shock produced only 30% survival. When a quantity of lactated Ringer's solution equal to 5% of the body weight was given with the shed blood, survival increased to 70% (Fig. 40–3). Simple restoration of shed blood volume alone is insufficient to restore function and ensure survival when major blood loss and large fluid shifts have occurred.

Patients undergoing major surgery, therefore, need fluid replacement in addition to that required for the lost blood. This additional fluid must eventually be excreted, usually between the second and the fifth postoperative days in uncomplicated cases. The third space losses are mobilized at this time into the intravascular compartment, and a brisk spontane-

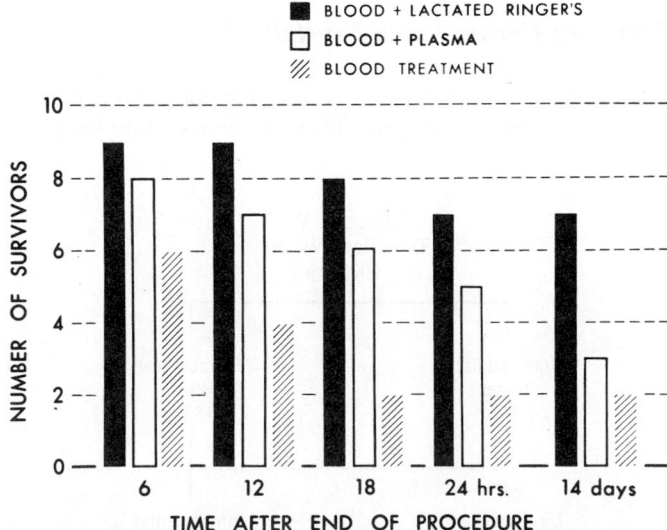

**FIGURE 40–3.** Survival from hemorrhagic shock following resuscitation with blood alone; with blood and plasma; and with blood and Ringer's injection, lactated. (Redrawn from Shires T, Cohn D, Carrico J, et al. Fluid therapy in hemorrhagic shock. *Arch Surg.* 1964;88:688. Copyright 1964, American Medical Association.)

**TABLE 40–8.** Composition of Selected Intravenous Fluids

| | Na⁺ (mEq/L) | Cl⁻ (mEq/L) | K⁺ (mEq/L) | Mg²⁺ (mEq/L) | Ca²⁺ (mEq/L) | Lactate (mEq/L) | Other | Approximate pH | Calculated mOsm/L |
|---|---|---|---|---|---|---|---|---|---|
| D₅W | | | | | | | Dextrose (5 g/L) | 5.0 | 253 |
| 0.9% Sodium chloride | 154 | 154 | | | | | | 4.2 | 308 |
| Lactated Ringer's solution | 130 | 109 | 4.0 | | 3.0 | 28 | | 6.5 | 273 |
| PlasmaLyte | 140 | 98 | 5.0 | 3.0 | | | Acetate, 27 mEq/L; gluconate, 23 mEq/L | 7.4 | 294 |
| Hespan | 154 | 154 | | | | | Hydroxyethyl starch, 6 g/dL | 5.5 | 310 |
| Dextran 70 | 154 | 154 | | | | | | 5.5 | 308 |
| 5% Albumin | 145 | 145 | | | | | Albumin, 5 g/dL | | 308 |
| 3% NaCl | 513 | 513 | | | | | | 5.0 | 1027 |
| 5% NaCl | 855 | 855 | | | | | | 5.6 | 1710 |

ous diuresis ensues. Patients with tenuous cardiac or renal function may not tolerate this mobilization, and CHF sometimes results. Such a complication, although undesirable, is often a necessary consequence of appropriate fluid administration in the operative and immediate postoperative periods. Careful fluid restriction and diuretic use in this phase is indicated in such cases.

## FLUID THERAPY

In addition to blood, commonly used fluids for intraoperative use are divided into three categories:

1. Conventional crystalloids
2. Colloids
3. Hypertonic solutions

Some less commonly used fluids include blood substitutes. In this section, the choice of initial fluids and the question of glucose use are addressed.

### What Are Conventional Crystalloids?

Conventional crystalloids are fluids that contain a combination of water and electrolytes. They are divided into balanced salt solutions and hypotonic salt solutions. Balanced salt solutions include Ringer's injection, lactated; Plasma-Lyte; and Normosol (Table 40–8). Either their electrolyte composition approximates that of plasma, or they have a total calculated osmolality that is similar to that of plasma.

Normal saline (0.9%) is frequently considered to be balanced but is actually hypertonic with respect to sodium and especially to chloride, if the osmolality is calculated. However, when normal saline is subjected to a freezing point depression test in an osmometer, its osmolality is about 285 mOsm/L. The *calculated* value is derived by simple addition of its ionic constituents, whereas the *measured* value is affected by ionic association and dissociation. Thus, sodium chloride has a relative osmolality of 1 compared with that of Na⁺ and Cl⁻, the value of which is 2. Other balanced electrolyte solutions are slightly hypotonic in vitro (~265 mOsm/L) in comparison with their calculated values and normal plasma. Solutions that contain less than the concentration of electrolytes found in lactated Ringer's solution are not used as often intraoperatively.

### How Are Crystalloids Distributed?

The distribution of water after the administration of D₅W, lactated Ringer's solution, hypertonic saline, and albumin is shown in Figures 40–4 to 40–7. Note that when an electrolyte-free solution such as D₅W is administered, <10% stays

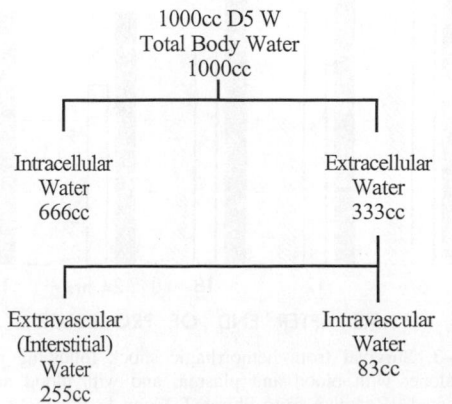

**FIGURE 40–4.** Distribution of 1 L of an administered solution of D₅W in an "ideal" 70-kg man (in cubic centimeters).

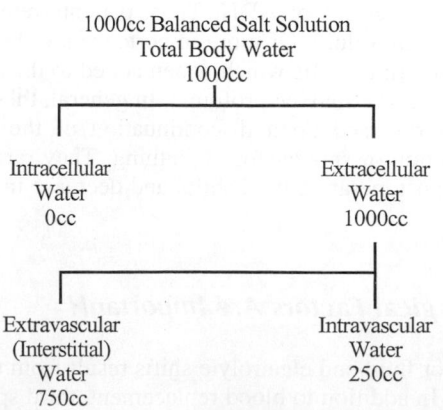

**FIGURE 40–5.** Distribution of 1 L of an administered balanced salt solution, such as lactated Ringer's solution or normal saline.

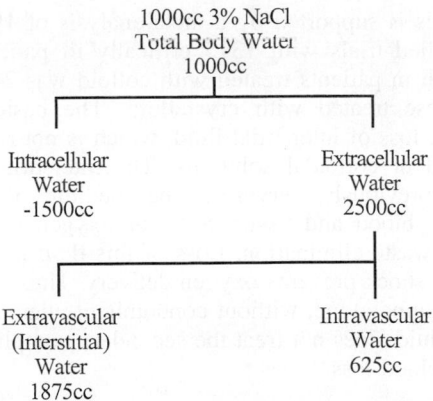

**FIGURE 40–6.** Distribution of 1 L of an administered solution of hypertonic saline (3% sodium chloride) in an "ideal" 70-kg man.

intravascular. A large amount of fluid, about two thirds, is distributed to the intracellular space. Thus, intravascular resuscitation is minimal, and cellular swelling occurs. The administered free water causes a decrease in the serum and interstitial electrolyte concentrations (dilutional effect) and may lead to symptomatic hyponatremia.

When solutions such as 0.2% or 0.45% saline are administered, similar although slightly less pronounced redistribution occurs. Therefore, a balanced salt solution with a sodium concentration of 130 mEq/L is normally chosen when major operative procedures are performed and when excessive blood loss is anticipated. Hypotonic solutions and $D_5W$ should be restricted to minor procedures and pediatric surgery (see Chapters 56 and 57).

## What Are Colloids?

Colloids commonly used in the United States include albumin, hydroxyethyl starch (HES; also known as Hetastarch) and dextran. In Europe, gelatin derivatives are available as well. Colloid molecules are sufficiently large that they normally do not cross capillary membranes in significant numbers. Therefore, under normal conditions, most of an administered colloid remains intravascular (see Fig. 40–4). Distribution of fluid throughout the body is dependent on the forces represented in the Starling equation:

$$JV = K(P_{MV} - P_T) - \sigma(COP_{MV} - COP_T)$$

where JV represents the rate of filtration of fluid across the capillaries; K is the ultrafiltration coefficient (a measure of permeability); $P_{MV}$ is the hydrostatic pressure within the microvasculature (ie, the capillaries); $P_T$ is the hydrostatic pressure in the interstitial space (the tissues); $\sigma$ is the reflection coefficient, which is a relative value expressing the ability of the semipermeable membrane to prevent movement of a given solute (in this case, the colloids of interest); $COP_{MV}$ is the colloid oncotic pressure in the microvasculature; and $COP_T$ is the colloid oncotic pressure in the tissue.

## How Are Colloids Distributed?

For colloids to work, $\sigma$ must be large (approaching 1), that is, the colloids must not cross the capillary membranes into

the extravascular space. The value of $\sigma$ varies greatly among tissues; for example, the lungs are moderately permeable ($\sigma = 0.6$); muscle is moderately impermeable ($\sigma = 0.9$); and the brain and glomeruli are essentially impermeable to protein entry ($\sigma = 0.99$ and 1, respectively). The $\sigma$ value for other tissues, such as liver, is low ($\sigma = 0$).[19]

### Changes in Capillary Permeability

During trauma or sepsis, these $\sigma$ values may change significantly. A classic example is the increase in capillary permeability to albumin in the lungs during the adult respiratory distress syndrome. In such a case, administered colloid may freely move across what ordinarily would be moderately permeable membranes in much the same fashion as does a balanced electrolyte solution. Increased capillary permeability (a *capillary leak*) also occurs at the site of surgical trauma, and administered colloid moves out of the capillaries into the involved interstitium. In this setting, colloids are less effective than would otherwise be expected for intravascular expansion and may actually increase interstitial edema.

### Oncotic Pressure Gradients

Once colloid molecules have leaked into the interstitial space, they must be removed or they will exert a reverse oncotic pressure gradient, resulting in further swelling of the involved tissue. Rarely, if ever, does a concentration gradient exist for colloid movement from the interstitial space back into the capillaries. Instead, it must be removed by the lymphatic system. Although many tissues, especially lung tissue, have a large capacity for lymphatic drainage, others, including skeletal muscle tissues, do not. Removal of colloid is much slower than that of crystalloids, and persistent edema, even to the point of blood flow interruption, sometimes results. This situation is particularly problematic in major trauma and burns.

## Are Colloids or Crystalloids Preferable?

Few topics in anesthesia and surgery have generated as much controversy as the relative merits of colloids and crystalloids for intraoperative fluid replacement and resuscitation. Numerous animal and human studies have been undertaken to

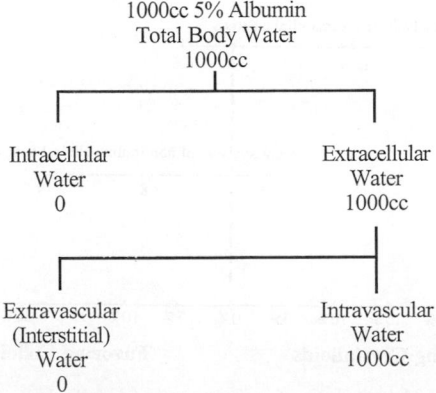

**FIGURE 40–7.** Distribution of 1 L of an administered 5% albumin solution in an "ideal" 70-kg man.

attempt to prove that one or the other is superior.[20–25] In many cases, the choice is based more on personal opinion and dogma rather than on scientific merit. The most comprehensive evaluation of colloid therapy was presented in a recent workshop on the assessment of plasma volume expanders.[26] All of the pertinent clinical trials involving albumin, dextran, and HES were carefully evaluated in terms of efficacy, cost, indications for use, and complications. Little evidence was found for either a short-term or long-term benefit from the use of supplemental colloidal agents in the clinical situations listed (blood loss, burns, cardiopulmonary bypass, pulmonary edema, trauma, and nutrition). No evidence suggested that serum albumin levels as low as 3 g/dL were deleterious, and even values as low as 2 g/dL have not been clearly shown to be problematic.

One noteworthy attempt to sort out this controversy was undertaken by Valanovich.[20] He performed a meta-analysis of mortality for eight previously published human trials in patients receiving either crystalloid or colloid for resuscitation. These pooled data showed an overall 5.7% decrease in the mortality rate in patients who were resuscitated with crystalloid rather than colloid solutions. When the data were divided into subgroups of trauma/sepsis and elective surgery, a 12.3% decrease in mortality rate in the former group was demonstrated. Conversely, a 7.8% increase in mortality rate was found in the crystalloid group undergoing elective surgical procedures (Fig. 40–8).

Valanovich believed that patients with trauma and sepsis have an increase in capillary permeability that allows the administered colloid to leak out of the vasculature, to be less effective as an intravascular volume expander, and to slow resolution of edema from the affected tissues (mentioned earlier). In patients undergoing elective procedures, the amount of capillary leak, in contradistinction to that in major trauma, is more discretely limited to the surgical site; thus, the use of colloids may be more efficacious in increasing intravascular volume, but this advantage has not been translated into improvement in outcome.

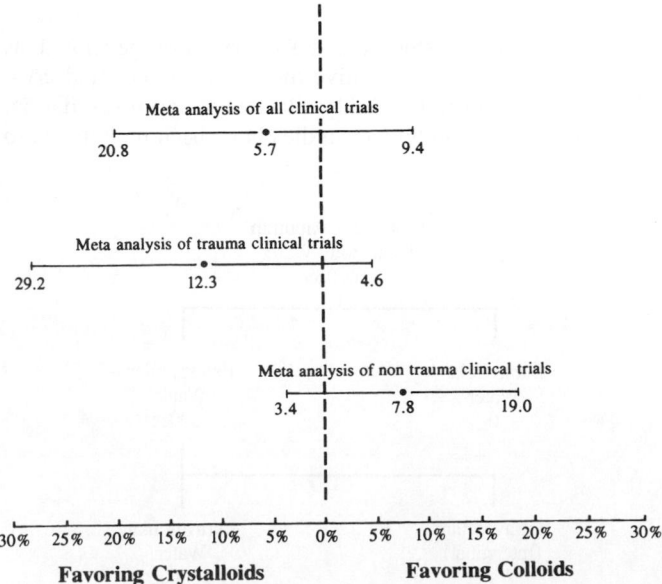

**FIGURE 40–8.** Meta-analysis of mortality rates for colloid versus crystalloid fluid resuscitation. (From Valanovich V. Crystalloid vs. colloid fluid resuscitation: a meta-analysis of mortality. *Surgery.* 1989;105:70.)

This thesis is supported by a meta-analysis of 19 randomized controlled trials with 1315 critically ill patients.[27] The risk of death in patients treated with colloid was 24% versus 20% in those treated with crystalloid. The basic problem involves the loss of interstitial fluid, which is not replaced by either blood or colloidal solutions. The interstitial fluid, as mentioned previously, serves as the medium of exchange between the blood and tissue cells for oxygen and nutrient supply and waste elimination. Loss of this fluid in prolonged or profound shock prevents oxygen delivery. Thus, restoration of blood volume alone, without concomitant augmentation of interstitial fluid, does not treat the secondary complications of significant blood loss.

## How Are Comparisons Made?

Most advocates of colloid use do not recommend colloid substances as the sole resuscitative fluid. The usual protocol involves the initial administration of crystalloids, followed by the administration of colloid solutions when large volumes are necessary to reduce the amount of crystalloid. In general, crystalloid needs to be administered in volumes that are about 2 to 3 times that of colloid to obtain the same hemodynamic effect when iso-oncotic colloid solutions such as 5% albumin or HES are used. When more concentrated colloid solutions, such as 25% albumin, are used, this ratio is no longer valid.

This fact is often not taken into account during comparison studies. For example, investigators analyzed the effects of colloid and crystalloid administration on gastric intramucosal pH (pHi) to patients undergoing open heart surgical procedures.[28] The control and protocol study patients received crystalloid and colloid according to the usual practice of the anesthesiologists involved. In addition, the protocol study patients were given 200-mL boluses of 6% HES every 15 minutes throughout surgery, except while they were on cardiopulmonary bypass. Prebypass colloid administration averaged 250 mL and 900 mL of colloid in the control and protocol groups, respectively. Total colloid administration equaled about 750 mL in the control group and 1350 mL in the protocol group. Total crystalloid equaled about 1100 mL in the control group and 850 mL in the protocol group. The pHi, as might be expected, was significantly better in the protocol group. However, the equivalency of fluid administration between the two groups is clearly suspect, and the alleged superiority of colloid solutions in maintaining pHi is not established by this study.

### Pulmonary Edema

Administration of albumin in hypoalbuminemic patients, by abruptly increasing pulmonary artery perfusion pressure, may produce the very complication it is designed to prevent—interstitial and alveolar flooding.[29]

### Renal Function

Raising the colloid oncotic pressure a remarkably small amount above normal significantly impairs renal salt and water excretion. No congenital hyperalbuminemic states are known, and the body reacts to transient elevations of albumin by immediately stopping production and accelerating catabolism. The adverse renal effects may be associated with the absence of naturally occurring states of excess albumin, whereas those in which albumin level is low are common. However, toxic effects of albumin therapy have not been demonstrated. The effects of colloidal products on bleeding and clotting are discussed in detail later.

## HYPERTONIC SOLUTIONS

### What Are Hypertonic Saline Solutions?

Hypertonic saline solutions (sodium concentration greater than that found in normal saline) include 1.8%, 3%, 5%, 7.5%, and 10% sodium chloride solutions. Other anions such as lactate and acetate may be incorporated. They are sometimes mixed with colloids such as dextran.

### How Are These Fluids Distributed?

Figure 40–6 shows what happens when 1 L of 3% sodium chloride solution is administered to a normal 70-kg adult. Because the osmolality of the administered solution exceeds that of intracellular water and because sodium and chloride ions cannot freely cross cell membranes, the extracellular fluid becomes slightly hyperosmolar. A gradient for water to pass from the cells into the extravascular compartment is established, and the extracellular volume is expanded by about 2.5 L.

Because electrolytes freely cross capillary membranes, the fluid is divided between the intravascular and extravascular compartments according to their relative volumes. Although hypertonic saline solutions increase the intravascular volume more than would the same volume of a balanced salt solution, they do so at the expense of a decreased intracellular volume. If large volumes of previously administered balanced electrolyte solutions have already increased intracellular volume (remember that most are, in effect, slightly hypotonic), hypertonic saline is therapeutic. If not, cellular dehydration can result.

### What Are Potential Complications?

Hypertonic saline solution use is not widespread. However, there has been a resurgence of interest in these solutions for both intraoperative administration and trauma resuscitation.[30–34] A major concern is the potential development of hypernatremia. However, complications associated with hypernatremia have not been reported in the clinical trials. Hypernatremia, when it occurs, is usually transient, especially when these solutions are used with balanced electrolyte or colloid solutions.[30]

### What Other Hypertonic Solutions Are Useful?

Hyperosmotic solutions, such as 20% mannitol or urea, are used as osmotic diuretics and to reduce cerebral edema, most commonly during neurosurgical procedures. In the latter case, an osmotic gradient must be established between the intravas-cular and extravascular compartments. This goal is easily accomplished in the brain, where the normally functioning blood-brain barrier with its tight intercellular junctions excludes passive ion transport. However, in tissues such as muscle and lung that are more permeable, an effective gradient cannot be established or is only transient, and little or no edema fluid is removed.

## BLOOD SUBSTITUTES

Discovery of the human immunodeficiency virus and recognition of transfusion complications have prompted the search for alternatives to blood administration. Oxygen-carrying solutions that can be stored without refrigeration for long periods of time and stocked in large amounts have been investigated. Such substances could be carried in ambulances and used for mass trauma resuscitation in times of war or civil disasters.

### What Types Are Available?

#### Perfluorochemical Emulsions

Perfluorochemical emulsions have a linear oxygen-carrying capability as opposed to the sigmoid affinity of naturally occurring RBCs.[35] The oxygen-carrying capacity of the first-generation compounds was insufficient to support cellular respiration at concentrations that can be tolerated in human beings.[35–38] Second-generation compounds can be infused at higher concentrations, allowing much greater oxygen-carrying capacity. However, high inspired oxygen concentrations are required.[37]

#### Stroma-Free Hemoglobin

The second class of RBC substitutes includes stroma-free hemoglobin solutions that are produced by processing human or animal RBCs.[39–42] After polymerization of the hemoglobin molecules and addition of pyridoxal phosphate, a solution with a reasonable colloid oncotic pressure and an oxygen-carrying capacity that approximates that of normal hemoglobin is obtained. Initial clinical studies of stroma-free hemoglobin substances suggested a detrimental effect on renal function after their administration.[39,40] However, development of polymerized hemoglobin appears to have solved this problem. In a recent study in traumatized patients, polymerized hemoglobin reduced the amount of allogenic blood required over the 3 days following traumatic injury, with no significant toxicity.[42]

#### Synthetic Hemoglobin

Synthetic hemoglobin, manufactured using recombinant DNA technology, is still undergoing clinical trials.

## BLOOD

### When Is Blood Indicated?

Historically, a hemoglobin level of 10 g/dL was considered necessary for patients in the perioperative period. Recently, however, consensus panels have recommended allowing the hemoglobin to decrease to 6 or 7 g/dL before transfusing RBCs. Indeed, many patients tolerate these low levels without adverse effects. However, some patients require much higher levels.

## Why Is Anemia a Problem?

The major risk for anemia is an imbalance between myocardial supply and demand, which leads to myocardial ischemia and, if prolonged, infarction. The myocardium normally extracts about 70% of the oxygen delivered by each hemoglobin molecule, leaving little reserve for further extraction in the face of inadequate supply. Therefore, in the presence of anemia, the only means of increasing oxygen transport into the myocardial cells is by increasing coronary blood flow, coronary vasodilation, and increased cardiac output. Because increasing cardiac output increases myocardial work and hence oxygen demand, coronary vasodilation remains the most efficient way to restore the balance between myocardial oxygen supply and demand.

Patients with normal coronary arteries have significant coronary vascular reserve; that is, they can significantly increase myocardial blood flow through vasodilation. However, patients with significant coronary artery disease (CAD) have fixed stenosis of their coronaries and little coronary vascular reserve. These are the patients most at risk from anemia.

## What Clinical Data Are Available?

The available data, while limited, support the view that comorbid disease, particularly CAD and left ventricular dysfunction, determine the extent to which anemia is tolerated. In a study by Nelson and colleagues,[43] patients undergoing vascular surgery (a group known to be at high risk for CAD), had a higher incidence of morbid cardiac events if the hematocrit was <28%. In another study of patients at risk for CAD, Christopherson and associates showed an association between postoperative cardiac ischemia and hematocrit lower than 29%.[44]

On the other hand, several studies have shown that intraoperative hemodilution to a hematocrit of 20% to 26% is well tolerated in otherwise healthy patients, including elderly patients.[45–47] However, many of these patients were given back their own blood at the end of surgery, making their postoperative hematocrit higher. Because oxygen consumption is generally lower intraoperatively, anemia during this period may be better tolerated than when the patient is awake and oxygen demand increases.

## INDICATIONS FOR GLUCOSE IN WATER

Routine fluid administration in the operating room frequently includes $D_5W$ combined with a balanced electrolyte solution. The logic behind this approach is that patients usually are in nil per os (NPO) status for variable lengths of time before arrival in the operating room and are thus prone to intraoperative hypoglycemia. However, many nondiabetic patients on entry to the operating room are actually hyperglycemic.[48] Addition of glucose to the intravenous infusions results in further hyperglycemia that may exceed the kidney's ability to reabsorb glucose, leading to a forced osmotic diuresis. Routine use of dextrose in intravenous solutions for nondiabetic adults is, therefore, discouraged.

## How Should Diabetic Adults Be Managed?

Diabetic adults present special problems. The continuation of oral antihyperglycemic agents or insulin may cause significant hypoglycemia if glucose is not administered. Several approaches are commonly used in caring for these patients.

### Non–Insulin-Dependent Diabetic Adults

Oral hypoglycemic agents are discontinued at midnight the night before surgery. A nonglucose intravenous infusion is started, and blood sugar measurements are obtained on arrival to the hospital for outpatients or in the operating room for inpatients. Insulin (glucose >300 mg/dL), intravenous glucose (glucose <100 mg/dL), or both are added based on the patient's serum glucose concentration.

For most patients maintained on an oral antihyperglycemic agent, this approach is simple and safe. However, some of the oral hyperglycemic agents have long half-lives; therefore, patients who are scheduled for surgery late in the afternoon require periodic glucose monitoring throughout the day and need to be cautioned about the possibility of hypoglycemia.

### Insulin-Dependent Diabetic Adults

Management of insulin-dependent diabetic patients is more complicated. One standardized approach is to administer half of the usual morning dose of regular insulin and to start an intravenous infusion of a glucose solution at either midnight the night before surgery or early in the day upon arrival in the hospital. Sequential monitoring of serum glucose follows, and the appropriate quantity of dextrose or insulin is added as needed. The limits of serum glucose fluctuation are broad; most recommendations suggest no treatment for serum glucose levels of <200 to 300 mg/dL.

Although this approach is simple, it does not provide tight glucose control. Outpatients scheduled for surgery late in the day may remain on NPO status for a prolonged period of time after taking insulin in the morning. This situation is especially problematic for particularly diabetic patients. Scheduling surgery early in the day for such patients is prudent.

Another approach is more complicated but provides for tighter blood glucose control. Patients are maintained on NPO status from midnight and do not take insulin in the morning. Two infusions, one containing dextrose and one containing insulin, are started, and frequent serum glucose determinations are made. The insulin infusion is adjusted to maintain euglycemia. This approach is preferred by some clinicians because of its ability to maintain tight glucose control. However, because of the difficulty and labor intensiveness of the continuous glucose and insulin infusions, this technique is not popular. Furthermore, tight glucose control has not been shown to be of benefit in the short-term operative management of most diabetic adults.[49]

## Should Glucose Solutions Be Used in Children?

The management of glucose infusions in children differs from that in adults in several ways. Young children have limited glycogen stores and do not tolerate long periods with no oral intake. In these situations, the use of intravenous glucose, combined with a balanced salt solution, may be indicated.

$D_5W$ often induces hyperglycemia.[48] Therefore, formula can be given by mouth until midnight, and clear glucose-containing solutions can be given orally until about 3 to 6 hours before surgery. In young patients, a 2.5% glucose *maintenance* infusion should be provided. Glucose should *not* be included in the *replacement* balanced electrolyte solution because large glucose loads may result from glucose-containing fluid boluses.

## ESTIMATION OF FLUID REQUIREMENTS

When considering patients undergoing surgery, it is helpful to divide fluid needs into several categories and, at least in theory, to deal with each category separately. Four areas of major concern are as follows:

1. Preoperative fluid deficit
2. Intraoperative blood loss
3. Third space needs
4. Other (unusual) needs

In practice, a unified approach is necessary despite the need for individual considerations.

### What Is the Preoperative Fluid Deficit?

Most patients scheduled for elective surgical procedures have a simple preoperative fluid deficit equal to the amount of fluid that would have been required during the NPO period. In children who weigh 20 kg or less, the hourly fluid requirement is calculated by taking the first 10 kg of the patient's weight and multiplying it by 4 mL/h and then by the number of hours; the second 10 kg of the patient's weight is multiplied by 2 mL/h, multiplied by the number of hours. Thus, a 17-kg child on NPO status for 6 hours would have a preoperative fluid deficit of 10 kg × 2 mL/h × 6 hours, or 324 mL.

For patients who weigh >20 kg, the hourly requirement in milliliters is equal to the weight in kilograms plus 40. A 60-kg adult on NPO status for 8 hours would have a fluid requirement of 60 plus 40, or 100 mL × 8 hours, or 800 mL. Normally, half of this preoperative fluid deficit is replaced during the first hour of surgery and the remainder over the next 2 hours.

Other preoperative deficits may result from chronic diuretic use, nasogastric suction, vomiting, diarrhea, bleeding, a bowel preparation, intravenous contrast agents, fever, or losses from gastrointestinal fistulas.

### Clinical Evaluation

Because the deficit in each of these situations is different, no prediction can quantify it precisely.

### Urine Output

A workable estimate may be made using urine output as a guide. A urine volume of <0.5 mL/kg/h suggests a significant deficit. An adult who has not voided in the preceding 6 to 8 hours often has a 1- to 3-L overall deficit. A urine specific gravity of <1.020 indicates a normally hydrated patient, whereas specific gravity of >1.030 to 1.040 suggests a 1- to 3-L deficit. Urine-specific gravity of >1.040 indicates a severe dehydration fluid deficit in excess of 3 L.

### Vital Signs

Pulse and BP measurements with the patient lying supine provide useful information. If a >20% change in either parameter occurs when the patient stands, significant dehydration is indicated. However, the reliability of orthostatic changes is interfered with by many commonly used antihypertensive drugs (β-blockers or direct-acting vasodilators).

One useful piece of information obtained from continuous, direct BP monitoring is the amount of change in the patient's BP during the respiratory cycle. This phenomenon is often referred to as *cycling* or *systolic pressure variation*[50,51] (Fig. 40–9). In patients who are hypovolemic, the decrease in venous return may be significant. A >10-mm Hg reduction in systolic pressure associated with each mechanical breath is presumptive but indirect evidence of relative hypovolemia.

### Physical Assessment

Other signs and symptoms are helpful. Dry mucous membranes and significant thirst indicate dehydration and may still be helpful in patients whose urine output or orthostatic changes are questionable. Patients with jugular venous distention probably are not significantly dehydrated, whereas those with flat jugular veins, especially when they are supine or in a slightly head-down tilt, may be.

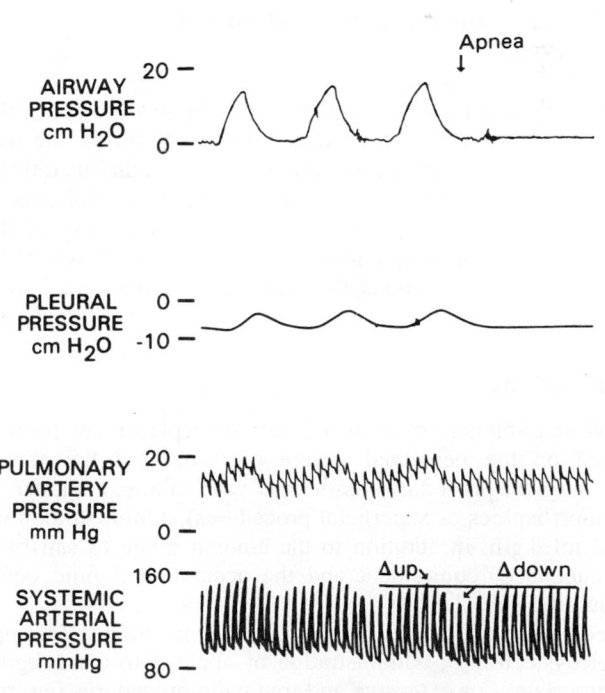

**FIGURE 40–9.** Variations in airway, pleural, pulmonary artery, and systemic pressures with positive pressure ventilation after a 10% hemorrhage. (Reproduced with permission from Perel A, Pizov R, Cotev S. Systolic blood pressure variation is a sensitive indicator of hypovolemia in ventilated dogs subjected to graded hemorrhage. *Anesthesiology.* 1987;67:498.)

### Invasive Monitoring

When all else fails, placement of a central venous or pulmonary artery catheter may be indicated to assess fluid status perioperatively. However, significantly fewer of such invasive devices should be used than are in reality, at least for this purpose.

### Anesthetic Effects

Marked dehydration is associated with hypotension and hemodynamic instability. Young, healthy patients often compensate for hypovolemia while they are awake. However, most induction agents blunt these compensatory reflexes, predisposing patients to significant hypotension. The administration of 1 to 2 L of a balanced electrolyte solution often alleviates this problem.

### How Should Intraoperative Blood Loss Be Replaced?

If significant amounts of blood are lost, the anesthesiologist has two choices. The first is to administer fresh or stored autologous or homologous blood in the form of reconstituted packed RBCs. The second is to eschew the use of blood and to give instead crystalloid solutions, colloid solutions, or both. With colloid solutions, an equal volume of an iso-oncotic solution, such as 5% albumin or HES, is indicated. If a balanced electrolyte solution is used, a volume at least equal to 3 times that of the lost blood is necessary to maintain a euvolemic state. In general, blood loss should be replaced by such solutions as it occurs.

### When Are Third Space Fluid Losses Replaced?

During major surgical procedures, a large third space fluid loss occurs that, as was noted, is not anatomic in the usual sense. Replacement of this loss necessitates administration of a fluid with an electrolyte profile similar to that of plasma and interstitial fluid. The protein concentration in third space fluid is variable and usually unknown but is probably less than that of plasma. The volume of fluid required to replace such losses varies considerably.[52]

#### Calculations

Most clinicians recommend various replacement formulas based on the perceived degree of trauma of the surgery. For surgical procedures associated with minimal trauma (eg, herniorrhaphies or superficial procedures), administration of 1 to 3 mL/kg/h, in addition to the amount given to satisfy the maintenance requirement and the accumulated fluid deficit, should be sufficient.

For those operations involving moderate trauma (eg, open cholecystectomy), administration of about 4 to 6 mL/kg/h is appropriate. For extensive and traumatic procedures (eg, radical intraperitoneal resections, or in the presence of severe peritonitis), infusion rates of 7 to 9 mL/kg/h or greater are necessary.

These recommendations represent an initial estimate of third space losses. Patients must be carefully monitored, and the rate of replacement must be adjusted up or down based on their clinical response.

### What Other Fluid Losses Occur?

During surgery, exposure of peritoneal or pleural surfaces to the operating room environment predisposes the patient to major evaporative loss. Anesthetic gases are anhydrous, and respiratory water loss occurs unless adequate humidification is provided. Patients treated with diuretics, acutely or chronically, may have continued urinary losses that must be replaced with appropriate fluids. Intravenous contrast agents, mannitol, and large glucose loads often induce an osmotic diuresis, even in the presence of relative hypovolemia, thus further increasing the fluid requirements.

## FLUID THERAPY AND COAGULATION

### How Do Colloids Affect Hemostasis?

Patients who undergo surgery with significant blood loss often have problems with coagulation. However, not all coagulation deficits seen in surgical patients can be related to the use of blood. Colloid solutions have been reported to be responsible in many settings. These deficits are in addition to those expected purely from the dilution associated with large-volume resuscitation.

#### Albumin

Johnson and coworkers[53] treated severely injured patients with a standardized resuscitation protocol. About half of the patients received 150 g/d of additional albumin for 3 to 5 days. The patients given supplemental albumin required greater volumes of whole blood and fresh frozen plasma to obtain normal clotting studies than did those who were resuscitated with crystalloid solutions. Albumin-treated patients had a significant decrease in fibrinogen concentration and prolongation of the prothrombin time that could not be explained by dilution. In contrast, the prolonged thromboplastin time and decreased platelet counts that also occurred in the albumin-treated group were ascribed to dilution.

The amount of albumin administered in this study was much greater than that usually given in clinical settings. Other investigators, using smaller doses of albumin, reported clotting abnormalities that could be explained solely on the basis of dilution.[54] In addition, in vitro studies found that albumin did not adversely influence clotting, nor did it affect the structure of fibrin clots.[55] Overall, albumin may exert some mild effects on hemostasis; however, these effects seem to be primarily dilutional as a result of volume expansion. When large amounts of albumin are infused, the degree of volume expansion exceeds that obtained with a comparable amount of crystalloid solutions. Therefore, a more pronounced coagulation defect is likely.

#### Dextran

Dextran is used not only for volume expansion but also as a form of antiaggregant in patients undergoing vascular and microvascular surgical procedures. Clotting deficits associated with dextran are probably related to defects in platelet interaction and to an antithrombotic effect. The platelet-vascular interaction is believed to be primarily associated with an effect on factor VIII.[56–58] Dextran also appears to be incorporated into the polymerizing fibrin clot so that it alters clot structure and enhances fibrinogenolysis.[59–62]

### Types

Dextran is commonly supplied in two forms: dextran 70 and dextran 40. The numbers 70 and 40 refer to the average molecular weights (70 000 and 40 000, respectively) of the molecules in solution. Dextran 40 appears to have greater inhibitory effects on coagulation than does dextran 70. It is used in vascular surgery to prevent thrombosis but is rarely employed as a primary volume expander. Dextran 70, on the other hand, is used as a primary volume expander, alone or in combination with hypertonic saline.

### Hydroxyethyl Starch

HES is derived from carbohydrate (usually corn). It is available in the United States as a 6% solution in 0.9% sodium chloride (Hespan).

### Clotting Factors

The effects of HES have been studied in two major groups of patients. The first group consists of healthy patients undergoing leukapheresis for donation of white blood cells. These patients usually receive small amounts (about 500 mL) of HES. In one study, 10 donors who received HES during leukapheresis had slight but significant prolongation of their prothrombin time and prolonged thromboplastin time (mean increases of 0.6 and 2.5 seconds, respectively).[63] Levels of fibrinogen, factor VIIIc, and factor V were similarly reduced but remained within the normal range. In another report, no defects in platelet function were noted.[64] The second group of patients includes those who receive larger doses of HES for trauma and surgery. In these patients, a prolonged partial thromboplastin time and up to a 50% decrease in factor VIIIc occurs with an infusion of 1 L HES.

### Clot Formation

In addition to its effect on levels of factor VIII, HES appears to cause changes in fibrin clot formation and fibrinogenolysis. This characteristic may be related to incorporation of the HES molecules into the clot, with subsequent prevention of solid clot formation.

### Pentastarch

Pentastarch is a lower-molecular-weight version of HES that has fewer hydroxyethyl groups per molecule. The anticoagulant effects of pentastarch are under investigation.

### Summary

All of the synthetic colloids have some adverse effects on clotting, especially when administered in large quantities. Albumin appears to have a purely dilutional effect that is less than that of any of the synthetic agents. If the latter are to be used for volume expansion, HES is recommended in a maximal volume between 1 and 1.5 L. If additional colloid is desired, a switch to albumin is probably indicated.

The synthetic colloids are relatively contraindicated in patients in whom small amounts of bleeding would be potentially devastating (eg, neurosurgical patients). Dextran 40 is not commonly used for volume expansion but may be used for its anticoagulant effects in vascular surgery patients and other patients prone to thrombosis.

## COMPLICATIONS OF FLUID THERAPY

### Why Do Electrolyte Changes Occur?

When balanced electrolyte solutions are administered, minimal electrolyte changes should occur because the composition of the fluids approximates that of normal plasma (see Tables 40–1 and 40–2). However, when solutions that contain nonbalanced electrolytes are used (0.25%, 0.5%, or 0.9% saline, hypertonic saline, or colloid), significant changes can occur. All products that are suspended in 0.9% saline (albumin and synthetic colloids) have a chloride composition higher than that of normal plasma (see Table 40–8). Patients who are given large volumes of these solutions often develop a transient hyperchloremic acidosis that, although usually mild, may worsen other acidotic conditions (see Chapter 41).

### Should Hypotonic Solutions Be Used?

If hypotonic solutions, such as 0.45% or 0.2% saline or $D_5W$ are used, patients can develop significant hyponatremia and hyposmolar states. Although isosmotic when administered, $D_5W$ provides a large free water excess as the glucose is metabolized. These complications are much more common and severe than is the transient hyperchloremia associated with normal saline. As noted previously, hypotonic solutions are not recommended for major surgical procedures. They are acceptable for minor surgery with minimal fluid shifts.

### Should Glucose Solutions Be Used?

Glucose-containing solutions can produce hyperglycemia with resultant electrolyte abnormalities. Hyperglycemia, if untreated, may lead to a hyperosmolar state in susceptible patients. In addition, it promotes an osmotic diuresis. Because of these problems, routine use of glucose-containing solutions during major surgery in adults, as has been noted repeatedly throughout this chapter, is not recommended.

### Why Does Renal Failure Occur?

Physiologic responses attempt to correct hypovolemia. The kidney is one of the major organs that is affected. If patients are inadequately volume resuscitated in the operating room, urine output will fall. Significant hypotension for as little as 10 minutes has resulted in acute renal failure.[65] Mortality associated with acute postoperative renal failure, even with dialysis, is high. The cornerstone of prevention is to provide adequate fluid replacement in patients undergoing surgical procedures. There are many therapeutic interventions for fluid overload and CHF but relatively few for renal insufficiency. When in doubt, one should err on the side of too much fluid rather than too little. Both the type and volume of fluid are important. As long as patients produce at least 0.5 to 1 mL/kg/h of urine, renal function generally is preserved.

### When Is Congestive Heart Failure Likely?

Healthy patients can usually receive large volumes of fluid with no change in cardiac function. However, postoperative pulmonary edema as the presenting finding leading to death has been described in patients receiving >67 mL/kg/d within the first 36 hours.[66] Whether this finding represents only fluid overload, without comorbid factors has been questioned.[67] Nevertheless, the problem, whatever its cause, is potentially a serious one that appears to be overlooked in many instances. In contrast, elderly patients and patients with underlying cardiac disease may suffer significant cardiac complications from even moderate amounts of fluid. Because these patients have limited cardiac reserve, increasing their intravascular volume may overdistend the heart, or the heart may not be able to compensate for the increased volume, leading to CHF. In addition, these patients have difficulty in the postoperative mobilization phase of edema and other third space fluids.

Advocates of colloid therapy suggest that because the total volume of fluid administered is lower than that with crystalloid resuscitation, less stress is placed on a compromised heart. However, no good experimental studies back up this claim, and the problems encountered with such therapy have been discussed.

### Which Factors Lead to Pulmonary Dysfunction?

Pulmonary dysfunction after large volume resuscitation is multifactorial. Fluid overload and an increase in pulmonary capillary permeability (sepsis, anaphylaxis, or other inflammatory reactions) place patients at much greater risk for this phenomenon. Those with limited myocardial reserve or impaired renal function are also at increased risk.[15,16]

### Is Peripheral Edema a Problem?

Massive peripheral edema sometimes accompanies large-volume fluid resuscitation, particularly after trauma and burns. It represents a classic example of third space loss. A frequently posed question is whether this edema is detrimental. It is certainly cosmetically unappealing, but the medical implications are unclear. A major consideration involves wound healing and burn conversion. If edema is significant, the distance between capillaries and cells increases, and cellular hypoxia is a distinct possibility.

Another potential but fortunately uncommon complication is the development of a compartment syndrome. When edema in a closed space such as an extremity increases sufficiently, interstitial pressure rises; this pressure eventually exceeds the venous pressure, at which time ischemia follows. This problem occurs in circumferential burns and extremity trauma.

### How Is Hypothermia Produced?

Fluids stored at room temperature are actually cool compared with body temperature. One liter of room-temperature

fluid decreases a 70-kg patient's body temperature by about 0.2%. Even if warmed before infusion, these fluids may undergo significant cooling while passing through the intravenous tubing. Cold fluids such as stored blood can induce hypothermia when infused rapidly. Therefore, large volume infusions should be passed through fluid warming devices. However, although important, warming of fluids is a relatively inefficient means to prevent, and especially to treat, hypothermia (see Chapter 48).

## TRANSURETHRAL RESECTION OF THE PROSTATE

### What Problems Arise?

Transurethral resection of the prostate (TURP) entails the infusion of large volumes of electrolyte-free irrigation fluid through the surgical resectoscope to provide a clear field of view for the surgeon. Multiple prostatic sinuses are opened, and significant volumes of this irrigation fluid, up to 20 to 30 mL/min, are absorbed into the circulation. Patients can develop severe hyponatremia, hypotonicity, and hypervolemia.[68] In addition, if glycine is used in the irrigating solution, glycine intoxication, which presents as transient blindness, may result (see Chapter 66).

### Presentation

Major aberrations in the TURP syndrome involve mental status changes, which result from hyponatremia, and CHF, which results from fluid overload. This syndrome usually occurs only after large or prolonged (>30-45 minutes) prostatic resections. Spinal anesthetics for TURP are recommended, in part so that mental status can be assessed. Sequential measurement of serum sodium is indicated in longer procedures.

## SEPSIS

### How Is Fluid Therapy Altered?

Patients with sepsis develop widespread increases in capillary permeability. They often translocate so much fluid into the third space that they are severely hypovolemic, even when their total body water is increased. Fluid therapy is a challenge, particularly when urgent or emergent surgery is performed to drain abscesses or look for a source of infection. This, in combination with the myocardial depressant factors that are present, underscores the complexity of the situation.[69] These problems are mentioned again to emphasize their importance and ubiquity. As was stated previously, colloids offer no definitive advantage over crystalloids and may even worsen outcome in this setting.

## LIVER FAILURE

### What Are the Effects on Fluid Requirements?

Complications of end-stage liver disease include ascites, severe hypoproteinemia, and the hepatorenal syndrome. When patients with massive ascites undergo intraabdominal surgery, several liters of protein-rich fluid are drained. During surgery, ascitic fluid continues to form and is lost. This combination of events means higher fluid requirements than in a patient with no liver disease undergoing the same type of surgical procedure. Because of the severe associated hypoproteinemia, these patients are prone to a hypo-oncotic state and, therefore, are subject to increased peripheral edema. However, as was discussed previously, colloid administration does not appear to ameliorate this situation.

### When Is Hypervolemia a Problem?

Some patients with uncontrollable ascites may undergo insertion of a peritoneovenous shunt, allowing fluid to be siphoned from the abdomen and returned to the vasculature. Initially, this procedure results in a hypervolemic state. After a period of several days to weeks, the kidneys will excrete the additional fluid load, and a new equilibrium will be established. Intraoperatively and perioperatively, therefore, these patients should receive minimal amounts of fluid and may be candidates for the use of diuretics in the immediate postoperative period.

## NEUROSURGERY

### Is Glucose Contraindicated?

Human and animal studies suggest that recovery from a central nervous system ischemic event is worse when hyperglycemia is present before the development of the ischemia.[70] Because of the possibility of localized (and occasionally generalized) ischemia related to surgical retraction and the operative procedure, glucose solutions are believed by many to be contraindicated in neurosurgical patients. Glucose monitoring and aggressive control of stress-induced hyperglycemia are indicated in these patients. This approach is different from that used two to three decades ago, when electrolyte solutions were believed to be contraindicated in such cases and when $D_5W$ or $D_{10}W$ was advocated as the fluid of choice.

### How Should Cerebral Edema Be Minimized?

Normally, the blood-brain barrier excludes translocation of fluid and prevents the formation of cerebral edema. However, during neurosurgical procedures or in the presence of trauma and tumors, this barrier function is often abnormal. Mannitol or another osmotic agent is often administered in an attempt to induce some degree of cerebral dehydration and to prevent edema formation. Intraoperative fluid management should be tailored to produce mild hypovolemia to minimize additional cerebral swelling. Because of the osmotic diuretics, urine output may not be an accurate indicator of overall fluid status.

In a human study of potentially great significance, Suarez and associates[71] were able to lower intracranial pressure (ICP) significantly after the administration of 30 mL of 23.4% saline (8008 mOsm/L) over a 15- to 20-minute period. Eight patients with a variety of lesions (subarachnoid hemorrhages, head trauma, tumor) had a median ICP of 41.5 mm Hg. One hour, 2 hours, and 3 hours following the bolus dose (240 mmol of saline), ICP decreased to 17, 16, and 14 mm Hg, respectively. In 80% of cases, the ICP was reduced by >50% of the pretreatment value within 21 ± 10.3 minutes. It fell below 20 mm Hg in 65% of the patients, and the mean time before it rose above 20 mm Hg was 6.3 ± 4.9 hours. Associated with the decrease in ICP was a significant increase in cerebral perfusion pressure, which increased from a 66 mm Hg baseline value to 87 mm Hg at 1 hour. No complications of therapy were noted, and serum $Na^+$ was unchanged. An accompanying editorial[72] suggested that mannitol, long a standby for osmotherapy of increased ICP, eventually may be relegated to the category of historical interest with respect to this particular application.

### How Is Diabetes Insipidus Controlled?

Patients undergoing pituitary surgery often develop diabetes insipidus because of a lack of ADH. Large volumes of dilute urine may result in a postoperative hyperosmolar state. Measurement of serum sodium and urine and serum osmolality is indicated. The administration of adequate volumes of 0.25% saline or, when possible, allowing the patient to drink large volumes of liquids, maintains a euvolemic state and electrolyte balance. In severe cases, aqueous vasopressin, 5 to 10 U given subcutaneously or intramuscularly, or DDAVP, 2 to 4 μg given subcutaneously or intravenously, may be indicated.

## PEDIATRIC PATIENTS

Chapters 56 and 57 deal with neonatal and pediatric surgical patients. The newborn's kidneys have limited capability for concentrating or diluting urine; as a result, electrolyte balance may be more difficult to achieve during and after surgery. Invasive monitoring in these patients is often more problematic than in adults. Clinical examination is essential to determine the adequacy of perioperative hydration, but orthostatic changes in vital signs are unreliable, and an age-related baseline tachycardia is present. Changes in moisture of the mucous membranes and skin turgor are important signs.

## BURN PATIENTS

Patients who sustain thermal or electrical burns present special problems with respect to fluid therapy; these are discussed in Chapter 39. Few situations present greater problems in management than burns, including their potential for producing severe and often life-threatening complications.[73]

### References

1. Pitts RF. *Physiology of the Kidney and Body Fluids.* 3rd ed. Chicago, Ill: Year Book Medical; 1974.
2. Askanazi J, Starker PM, Weissman C. *Fluid and Electrolyte Management in Critical Care.* Boston, Mass: Butterworth; 1986.
3. Alpern RJ, Saxton CR, Seldin DW. Clinical interpretation of laboratory values. In: Kokko JP, Tannen RL, eds. *Fluids and Electrolytes.* 2nd ed. Philadelphia, Pa: WB Saunders; 1990:3.
4. Arieff AI. Hyponatremia, convulsions, respiratory arrest, and permanent

brain damage after elective surgery in healthy women. *N Engl J Med.* 1986;314:1529.

5. Sterns RH, Riggs JE, Schochet SS. Osmotic demyelination syndrome following correction of hyponatremia. *N Engl J Med.* 1986;314:1535.

6. Narins RG. Therapy of hyponatremia: does haste make waste? [editorial]. *N Engl J Med.* 1986;314:1573.

7. Ayus JC, Krothapalli RK, Arieff AI. Treatment of symptomatic hyponatremia and its relation to brain damage. *N Engl J Med.* 1987;317:1190.

8. Chung HM, Kluge R, Schrier RW, et al. Postoperative hyponatremia: a prospective study. *Arch Intern Med.* 1986;146:333.

9. Sterns RH. Severe symptomatic hyponatremia: treatment and outcome. A study of 64 cases. *Ann Intern Med.* 1987;107:656.

10. Sterns RH. Severe hyponatremia: the case for conservative management. *Crit Care Med.* 1992;20:534.

11. Tannen RL. Potassium disorders. In: Kokko JP, Tannen RL, eds. *Fluids and Electrolytes.* 3rd ed. Philadelphia, Pa: WB Saunders; 1996:111.

12. Vitez TS, Soper LE, Wong KC, et al. Chronic hypokalemia and intraoperative dysrhythmias. *Anesthesiology.* 1985;63:130.

13. Hirsch IA, Tomlinson DL, Slogoff S, et al. The overstated risk of preoperative hypokalemia. *Anesth Analg.* 1988;67:131.

14. American Heart Association. Guidelines for cardiopulmonary resuscitation and emergency cardiac care. *JAMA.* 1992;268:2209.

15. Coller FA, Campbell KN, Vaughan HH, et al. Postoperative salt intolerance. *Ann Surg.* 1944;119:533.

16. Hayes MA, Goldenberg IS. Renal effects of anesthesia and operation mediated by endocrines. *Anesthesiology.* 1963;24:487.

17. Bernards WC, Kirby RR. A brief history of fluid and electrolyte therapy in the surgical patient. *Prob Crit Care.* 1991;5:331.

18. Shires T, Cohn D, Carrico J, et al. Fluid therapy in hemorrhagic shock. *Arch Surg.* 1964;88:688.

19. Gabel JC, Drake RE. Plasma proteins and protein osmotic pressure. In: Staub NC, Taylor AE, eds. *Edema.* New York, NY: Raven Press; 1984:371.

20. Valanovich V. Crystalloid versus colloid fluid resuscitation: a meta-analysis of mortality. *Surgery.* 1989;105:65.

21. Gammage GW. Crystalloid versus colloid: is colloid worth the cost? *Int Anesthesiol Clin.* 1987;25:32.

22. Vincent JL. Fluids for resuscitation. *Br J Anaesth.* 1991;67:185.

23. Nearman HS, Herman ML. Toxic effects of colloids in the intensive care unit. *Crit Care Clin.* 1991;7:713.

24. Falk JL, Rackow EC, Astiz M, et al. Fluid resuscitation in shock. *J Cardiothorac Anesth.* 1988;2(suppl):33.

25. London MJ. Plasma volume expansion in cardiovascular surgery: practical realities, theoretical concerns. *J Cardiothorac Anesth.* 1988;2(suppl):39.

26. Center for Biologics, Food and Drug Administration and National Heart, Lung, Blood Institute, Division of Blood Diseases and Resources. Workshop on Assessment of Plasma Volume Expanders; March 25-26, 1991; Bethesda, Md.

27. Schierhout G, Roberts I. Fluid resuscitation with colloid or crystalloid solutions in critically ill patients: a systematic review of randomized trials. *BMJ.* 1998;316:961.

28. Mythen MG, Webb AR. Perioperative plasma volume expansion reduces the incidence of gut mucosal hypoperfusion during cardiac surgery. *Arch Surg.* 1995;130:423.

29. Lucas CE, Ledgerwood AM, Higgins RF. Impaired pulmonary function after albumin resuscitation from shock. *J Trauma.* 1980;20:446.

30. Holcroft JW, Vassar MJ, Turner JE, et al. 3% NaCl and 7.5% NaCl/dextran 70 in the resuscitation of severely injured patients. *Ann Surg.* 1987;206:279.

31. Maningas PA, Mattox KL, Pepe PE, et al. Hypertonic saline-Dextran solutions for the prehospital management of traumatic hypotension. *Am J Surg.* 1989;157:528.

32. Jelenko C, Williams JB, Wheeler ML, et al. Studies in shock and resuscitation, I: use of a hypertonic, albumin-containing, fluid demand regimen (HALFD) in resuscitation. *Crit Care Med.* 1979;7:157.

33. Cross JS, Gruber DP, Gann DS, et al. Hypertonic saline attenuates the hormonal response to injury. *Ann Surg.* 1989;209:684.

34. Committee on Fluid Resuscitation for Combat Casualties Division of Health Sciences Policy. Protocols of Care at the Site of Injury. In: Pope A, French G, Longnecker DE, eds. *Fluid Resuscitation: State of the Science for Treating Combat Casualties and Civilian Injuries.* Washington, DC: National Academy Press, 1999:103.

35. Gould SA, Rosen AL, Sehgal LR, et al. Red cell substitutes: hemoglobin solution or fluorocarbon? *J Trauma.* 1982;22:736.

36. Spence RK, McCoy S, Costabile J, et al. Fluosol DA-20 in the treatment of severe anemia: randomized, controlled study of 46 patients. *Crit Care Med.* 1990;18:1227.

37. Goodnough LT, Scott MG, Monk TG. Oxygen carriers as blood substitutes: past, present, and future. *Clin Orthop Relat Res.* 1998;357:89.

38. Gould SA, Rosen AL, Sehgal LR, et al. Fluosol-DA as a red-cell substitute in acute anemia. *N Engl J Med.* 1986;314:1653.

39. Savitsky JP, Doczi J, Black J, et al. A clinical safety trial of stroma-free hemoglobin. *Clin Pharmacol Ther.* 1978;23:73.

40. Moss GS, Gould SA, Sehgal LR. Hemoglobin solution-from tetramer to polymer. *Surgery.* 1984;95:249.

41. Gould SA, Moss GS, Rosen AL, et al. Red cell substitutes. In: Civetta JM, Taylor RW, Kirby RR, eds. *Critical Care.* Philadelphia, Pa: JB Lippincott; 1992:1719.

42. Gould SA, Moore EE, Hoyt DB, et al. The first randomized trial of human polymerized hemoglobin as a blood substitute in acute trauma and emergent surgery. *J Am Coll Surg.* 1998;187:113.

43. Nelson AH, Fleisher LA, Rosenbaum SH. Relationship between postoperative anemia and cardiac morbidity in high-risk vascular patients in the intensive care unit. *Crit Care Med.* 1993;21:860.

44. Christopherson R, Frank S, Norris E, et al. Low postoperative hematocrit is associated with cardiac ischemia in high-risk patients. *Anesthesiology.* 1981;75:A39.

45. Rose D, Forest R, Coutsoftiedes T. Acute normovolemic hemodilution. *Anesthesiology.* 1979;51:S91.

46. Fahmy NR, Chandler HP, Patel DG, et al. Hemodynamics and oxygen availability during acute hemodilution in conscious man. *Anesthesiology.* 1980;53:S84.

47. Spahn DR, Zollinger A, Schlump RB, et al. Hemodilution tolerance in elderly patients without known cardiac disease. *Anesth Analg.* 1996;82:681.

48. Welborn LG, McGill WA, Hannallah RS, et al. Perioperative blood glucose concentrations in pediatric outpatients. *Anesthesiology.* 1986;54:543.

49. Roizen MF. Anesthetic implications of concurrent disease. In: Miller RD, ed. *Anesthesia.* 4th ed. New York, NY: Churchill Livingstone, 1994:903.

50. Perel A, Pizov R, Cotev S. Systolic blood pressure variation is a sensitive indicator of hypovolemia in ventilated dogs subjected to graded hemorrhage. *Anesthesiology.* 1987;67:498.

51. Perel A, Segal E, Pizov R. Assessment of cardiovascular function by pressure waveform analysis. In: Vincent JL, ed. *Update in Intensive Care and Emergency Medicine.* Berlin, Germany: Springer-Verlag; 1989:541.

52. Shires T, Williams J, Brown F. Acute change in extracellular fluids associated with major surgical procedures. *Ann Surg.* 1961;154:803.

53. Johnson SD, Lucas CE, Gerrick SJ, et al. Altered coagulation after albumin supplements for treatment of oligemic shock. *Arch Surg.* 1979;114:279.

54. Strauss RG. Volume replacement and coagulation: a comparative review. *J Cardiothorac Anesth.* 1988;2(suppl 1):24.

55. Carr ME. Turbidimetric evaluation of the impact of albumin on the structure of thrombin-mediated fibrin gelation. *Haemostasis.* 1987;17:189.

56. Aberg M, Hedner U, Bergentz S. Effects of dextran on factor VIII (antihemophilic factor) and platelet function. *Ann Surg.* 1979;189:243.

57. Aberg M, Hedner U, Bergentz S. The antithrombotic effect of dextran. *Scand J Haematol.* 1979;34:61.

58. Battle J, del Rio F, Lopez-Fernandez F, et al. Effect of dextran on factor VIII/von Willebrand factor structure and function. *Thromb Haemost.* 1985;54:697.

59. Carr ME, Gabriel DA. The effect of dextran 70 on the structure of plasma derived fibrin gels. *J Lab Clin Med.* 1980;96:985.

60. Katsuda K, Maeno H. Mechanism for the inhibitory effect of dextran on $\alpha_2$ plasmin inhibitor activity. *Thromb Res.* 1980;19:655.

61. Carlin G, Saldeen T. On the interaction between dextran and the primary fibrinolysis inhibitor $\alpha$-antiplasmin. *Thromb Res.* 1980;19:103.

62. Carlin G, Bang NU. Enhancement of plasminogen activation and hydrolysis of purified fibrinogen and fibrin by dextran 70. *Thromb Res.* 1980;19:535.

63. Kisker CT, Strauss RG, Kaepke JA, et al. The effects of combined platelet and leukopheresis on the blood coagulation system. *Transfusion.* 1978;19:173.

64. Maguire LC, Henriksen RA, Strauss RG, et al. Platelet function in donors undergoing intermittent-flow centrifugation plateletpheresis or leukapheresis. *Transfusion.* 1980;20:549.

65. Beck C. Disordered renal function. In: Civetta JM, Taylor RW, Kirby RR, eds. *Critical Care.* Philadelphia, Pa: JB Lippincott; 1988:1315.

66. Arieff AI. Fatal postoperative pulmonary edema: pathogenesis and literature review. *Chest.* 1999;115:1371.

67. Kirby RR. Perioperative fluid therapy and postoperative pulmonary edema: cause-effect relationship? *Chest.* 1999;115:1224.
68. Berger JJ. Transurethral resection of the prostate. *Probl Crit Care.* 1991;5:376.
69. Schuster DP, Lefrak SS. Shock. In: Civetta JM, Taylor RW, Kirby RR, eds. *Critical Care.* Philadelphia, Pa: JB Lippincott; 1992:407.
70. Sieber FE, Traystman RJ. Special issues: glucose and the brain. *Crit Care Med.* 1992;20:104.
71. Suarez JI, Qureshi AI, Bhardwaj A, et al. Treatment of refractory intracranial hypertension with 23.4% saline. *Crit Care Med.* 1998;26:1118.
72. Prough DS, Zornow MH. Mannitol: an old friend on the skids? *Crit Care Med.* 1998;26:997.
73. Hartmannsgruber M, Angel JJ. Burn therapy. In: Kirby RR, ed. *Critical Care.* Philadelphia, Pa: Current Medicine; 1997:11.1. Miller RR, series ed. *Atlas of Anesthesia;* vol 1.

### Additional Reading

Zaloga GP, Kirby RR, Bernards W, et al. Fluids and electrolytes. In: Civetta JM, Taylor RW, Kirby RR, eds. *Critical Care.* 3rd ed. Philadelphia, Pa: Lippincott-Raven; 1997:413.

# Clinical Applications of Acid-Base Chemistry and Physiology

David R. Bevan

Interpretation of laboratory acid-base values is difficult, largely because of the confusing nomenclature that developed from the difficulty of measurement. It is not possible to measure hydrogen ion concentration ($[H^+]$) or its activity in biologic systems directly. Instead, measurements are made of the differences in electrical potential generated between unknown and standard buffered solutions to which pH numbers have been assigned at fixed temperatures.[1] These numbers are considered to be equivalent to assessments of $H^+$ activity and concentration.

The relationship between $[H^+]$ and the partial pressure of carbon dioxide ($P_{CO_2}$) has been expressed with a multiplicity of simplified diagrams and equations in an attempt to make interpretation easy. The diagrams gave rise to an associated jargon (buffer base, base excess, base deficit, standard bicarbonate, and so forth) with the intention of simplifying therapeutic actions.

Unfortunately, some of these diagrams were based on erroneous interpretation of the complicated physicochemical concepts underlying acid-base data. For example, it was believed that the relationship between $[H^+]$ and $P_{CO_2}$ was similar in blood (in vitro) to that in the whole body (in vivo). In fact, the values differ considerably in a number of clinical settings. The roles of the kidneys and the liver in the maintenance of acid-base homeostasis in health and disease have undergone considerable re-evaluation since the 1980s. Also, interpretation of acid-base variables has shifted from a graphic to a mathematical format, giving a false appearance of accuracy to the evaluation. Opinions differ about the optimal sampling site for acid-base evaluation (venous, central venous, arterial) in certain conditions and whether the values should be "corrected" according to a patient's temperature.

The purpose of this chapter is to provide a current review of the pathophysiology of acid-base balance, to explain current nomenclature, to produce a framework for the recognition of acid-base disorders, and to suggest a rational approach to their management.

## PHYSIOLOGY

### What Is an Acid?

An acid ionizes in solution to produce $H^+$ and anions ($A^-$). The more $H^+$ produced, the stronger the acid. Acids are proton donors, and bases are proton acceptors. Each day, the body produces 50 to 100 mmol (50 000 000–100 000 000 nmol) $H^+$, whereas the amount of free $H^+$ at any one time is limited to 4000 nmol because of the action of buffers.

## What Are Buffers?

When acids or bases are added to solutions, they tend to cause a change in $H^+$ of the solution. Buffers are substances that limit the change in $H^+$. When an acid is presented to the body, the change in $H^+$ is titrated by intracellular (proteins and polypeptides) and extracellular (hemoglobin, plasma proteins, and bicarbonate [$HCO_3^-$]) buffers. The arterial blood pH (pHa) is normally maintained within fairly close limits: 7.35 to 7.45. For venous blood, the range is 7.32 to 7.42. When the pHa is <7.35, *acidemia* is present; when it is >7.45, *alkalemia* is present.

### The Henderson-Hasselbalch Equation

The key to the understanding of acid-base terminology lies in the relationship among changes in $H^+$, $Pco_2$, and $HCO_3^-$ as expressed in the Henderson-Hasselbalch equation[2,3]:

$$pH = pK + \log [HCO_3^-]/H_2CO_3$$

$H_2CO_3$ is carbonic acid and pK equals the pH (6.1) at which the $HCO_3^-$ and $H_2CO_3$ are present in equal amounts.

## How Does Buffering Occur?

Buffering of $H^+$ in the extracellular fluid is achieved by $HCO_3^-$, which is also responsible for 50% of the buffering in the blood; hemoglobin (35%), plasma protein (6%), and phosphates are also important. The activity of a buffer is greatest when the pH is at the pK of the particular system, which for $HCO_3^-/H_2CO_3$, as noted previously, is 6.1. The buffer reaction follows:

$$H^+ + HCO_3 \rightleftarrows H_2CO_3 \rightleftarrows H_2O + CO_2$$

At physiologic pH (7.4), this system is relatively weak. Its importance lies in the ability of the lungs to excrete $CO_2$ so that the addition of $H^+$ or elimination of $CO_2$ drives the equation to the right. $H_2CO_3$ can be formed by the addition or failure of elimination of either $CO_2$ (respiratory load) or nonvolatile acids (nonrespiratory, metabolic load).

## What Are Metabolic and Respiratory Compensation?

In situations in which the tendency to develop acidemia by either a respiratory or metabolic component is matched, at least in part, by metabolic or respiratory compensation, the disorders are known, respectively, as *respiratory acidosis with metabolic compensation* or *metabolic acidosis with respiratory compensation*. Such compensations make acidemia and alkalemia uncommon.

The Henderson-Hasselbalch equation may be rearranged to relate the $H^+$ (but not pH) to $Pco_2$ and $HCO_3^-$[4]:

**TABLE 41–1.** Conversion of Hydrogen Ion Concentration ($H^+$) to pH Units

| [H+] nmol/L | [H+] mol/L | pH |
|---|---|---|
| 1 000 000 | 001 = $10^{-3}$ | 3 |
| 10 000 | 0.000 01 = $10^{-5}$ | 5 |
| 100 | 0.000 000 1 = $10^{-7}$ | 7 |
| 10 | 0.000 000 0001 = $10^{-9}$ | 9 |

$$H^+ \text{ (nmol/L)} = 24 \times Pco_2/HCO_3^-$$

This rearrangement facilitates mathematic manipulation of acid-base data and demonstrates that changes in $H^+$ are determined by the ratio of $Pco_2$ to $HCO_3^-$, not by either alone.

## How Is Acidity Measured?

$[H^+]$ in body fluids ranges from $10^{-1}$ to $10^{-15}$ mol/L. For convenience, these values are expressed by exponential arithmetic so that pH is the negative logarithm of the $[H^+]$ (Table 41–1).

### The Relationship Between pH and [H+]

Within the pH range of 7.10 to 7.50, an almost linear relationship exists between pH and $[H^+]$.

#### Mathematical Point 1
*For each 0.01 unit change in pH from 7.4, the $[H^+]$ changes by 1 nmol/L.*

For example, a decrease in pH from 7.4 to 7.2 increases by 20 nmol/L. A more precise estimate is obtained by multiplying the $[H^+]$ at a pH of 7.4 (40 nmol/L) by 1.25 for each 0.1 decrease in pH. Thus, the $[H^+]$ at pH 7.2 is $40 \times 1.25 \times 1.25 = 63$ nmol/L. For each 0.1 increase in pH, the $[H^+]$ is multiplied by 0.8 so that at pH 7.6, the $[H^+]$ is $40 \times 0.8 \times 0.8 = 26$ nmol/L.

### Temperature Correction

The $Pco_2$ and pH of a blood sample are temperature dependent. As the sample is warmed, the pH decreases and the $Pco_2$ increases as it comes out of solution, but the total $CO_2$ content of the sample does not change. Most laboratories maintain the measurement electrodes at 37°C; they may correct the values according to a patient's temperature in certain situations such as hypothermic cardiopulmonary bypass.

It has been suggested that the uncorrected values should be used in the ventilatory management of hypothermic patients.[5] This practice, alpha-stat ($\alpha$-stat) management, has some physiologic merit because in nonhomeothermic animals, the pHa varies inversely with temperature.[6]

### Cerebral Perfusion and Cerebral Metabolic Rate of Oxygen With Temperature Correction

In practice, it is difficult to demonstrate much advantage with respect to cerebral or myocardial function with either approach. However, during hypothermic cardiopulmonary bypass, if the values are corrected for temperature (pH stat management), then administering $CO_2$ induces hypercapnia and produces cerebral vasodilation despite a decrease in cerebral metabolic rate of oxygen uptake ($CMRO_2$). In contrast, the decrease in $CMRO_2$ is matched by a decrease in cerebral perfusion so that coupling of blood flow and metabolism is preserved when the values are not corrected (α-stat). Neurological outcome, in infants undergoing deep hypothermic (26°C) circulatory arrest, is improved by pH-stat acid-base management probably because of more rapid brain cooling and greater reduction in cerebral oxygen ($O_2$) consumption.[7] However, in adults undergoing cardiopulmonary bypass at moderate hypothermia (32°C), α-stat management improves outcome probably because it reduces cerebral embolization.[8]

### Should Arterial or Venous Sample Be Used?

Usually, arterial blood is sampled for acid-base analysis, in part because this practice enables the simultaneous measurement of partial pressure of arterial oxygen ($PaO_2$). However, arterial blood may also be viewed as easily obtained "arterialized" mixed venous blood. Blood from warm, vasodilated peripheral veins (arterialized capillary blood) has been used as a close estimate of arterial blood, at least for the measurement of pH and $PCO_2$ during inhalation anesthetics (Table 41–2).

### Advantages to Using Venous Blood

The acid-base status of most body tissue is best reflected in the blood draining that tissue. (The brain is an exception because lactate, from anaerobic metabolism, is confined to the brain cells and cerebrospinal fluid by the blood-brain barrier.) Arterial and mixed venous acid-base variables may differ considerably in states of impaired tissue perfusion or cardiac arrest.[9,10] In this situation, mixed venous (pulmonary artery) or central venous sampling may be more representative than arterial for acid-base evaluation.

### What Is the Intracellular pH?

The measurement of intracellular pH (pHi), although desirable, is not possible in clinical practice. The methods available (insertion of microelectrodes, calculations from the distribution of weak acids, examination of pH-dependent reactions) are neither robust nor repeatable. Normally, pHi is less than

**TABLE 41–2.** Differences in Arteriovenous Values During Anesthesia With Three Inhalation Anesthetics*

| | Isoflurane (N = 15) | Enflurane (N = 16) | Halothane (N = 17) |
|---|---|---|---|
| $PCO_2$ | −1.2 ± 1.6 | −1.5 ± 2.1 | −1.6 ± 1.6 |
| pH | 0.01 ± 0.01 | 0.01 ± 0.01 | 0.02 ± 0.02 |
| BE (mEq/L) | 0.09 ± 0.56† | 0.03 ± 0.75† | 0.20 ± 0.33 |
| $PO_2$ | 49.5 ± 36.9 | 39.4 ± 29.1 | 56.9 ± 52.1 |
| $O_2$ (mL/dL) | 0.65 ± 0.98 | 0.57 ± 0.44 | 0.69 ± 0.45 |

*Values are mean ± SD.
†With these exceptions, all arteriovenous values were significantly different at the 0.05 level.
BE, base excess.
From Williamson DG, Munson ES. Correlation of peripheral venous and arterial blood gas values during general anesthesia. *Anesth Analg.* 1982;61:951.

extracellular pH, but the magnitude of the difference may change considerably in acid-base disorders. $CO_2$ but not highly ionized acids or alkalis is permeable across cell membranes.

Indirect estimates of intramucosal pH have been made by measuring gastric lumen $PCO_2$ by tonometry, $[HCO_3^-]$ in blood, and calculating pH from the Henderson-Hasselbalch equation in an attempt to detect gastric, small and large intestinal ischemia in ICU patients,[11] but there is considerable debate about their clinical utility.

### What Is the Anion Gap?

**Mathematical Point 2**
*The anion gap (AG) is estimated as the difference between serum sodium and the sum of chloride and $HCO_3^-$ concentrations[12]:*

$$AG = Na^+ - (Cl^- + HCO_3^-)$$

The normal range is 12 ± 2 mmol/L and is a reflection of anions other than chloride that balance the positive charge of sodium. $HCO_3^-$ may be replaced with endogenous (lactate, keto acids) or exogenous (salicylate, paraldehyde, formate, glycolate) organic and inorganic acids and toxins. An AG that is >30 mmol/L is usually indicative of significant organic acid acidosis.

Stewart defined a similar *strong ion difference* (SID) as the difference between the concentrations of the cations sodium and potassium and the anions chloride and lactate.[13] A positive SID is indicative of acidosis and an increase in $H^+$. Infusion of large amounts of 0.9% saline causes a hyperchloremic metabolic acidosis and a concomitant reduction in the SID.[14] The resulting decrease in pH does not appear to be clinically significant. However, this form of acidosis must be differentiated from other types such as lactic acidosis or diabetic ketoacidosis in order to judge whether corrective therapy is necessary and in what amount.[15]

### What Is Lactic Acidosis?

Lactic acidosis is defined as the combination of pH <7.25 and blood lactate concentration >5 mmol/L and may result from either increased production or decreased metabolism of lactic acid. High levels of lactic acid (>9 mmol/L) are associated with a high mortality rate. Lactic acidosis is discussed later.

## VENTILATION AND ACID-BASE STATUS

### What Happens When the Body Carbon Dioxide Changes?

The Henderson-Hasselbalch equation enables the change in pH following an acute alteration in $PCO_2$ to be predicted. An in vivo $CO_2$ titration curve can be constructed when a steady state has been reached after a step increase or decrease in $PCO_2$ (Fig. 41–1).

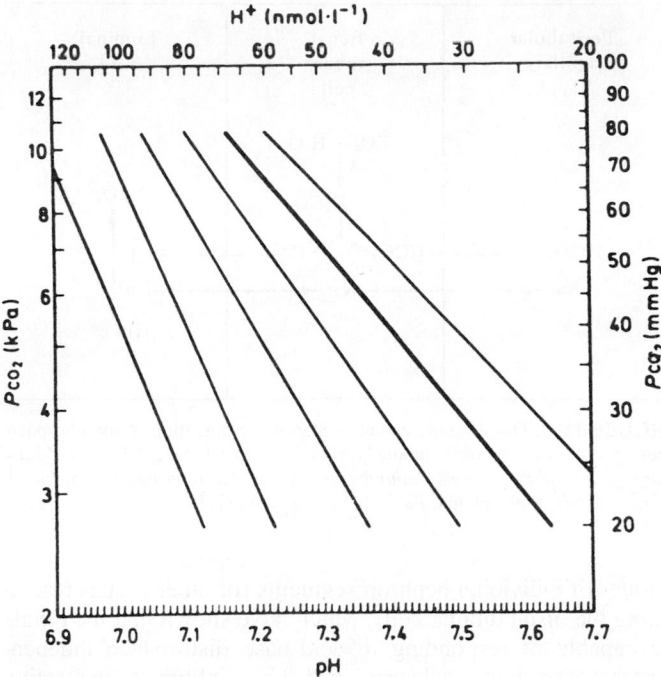

**FIGURE 41–1.** Family of in vivo $CO_2$ titration curves after addition of acid or alkali.

## Mathematical Point 3

$\Delta[H^+](nmol/L)$ is approximately $0.8 \times \Delta P_{CO_2}$ (mm Hg).

In addition, $\Delta[HCO_3^-]$ can be predicted: the $[HCO_3^-]$ increases by 1 mmol/L for every 10 mm Hg increase in $P_{CO_2}$ above 40 mm Hg and decreases by 2 mmol/L for each 10 mm Hg decrease in $P_{CO_2}$ below 40 mm Hg.

When the change in $[H^+]$ or $[HCO_3^-]$ differs from that predicted, an additional metabolic (nonrespiratory) disorder is implied.

## How Can These Changes Be Displayed?

When such $P_{CO_2}$ titrations are performed in acidotic subjects or in animals made acid by the infusion of increasing amounts of hydrochloric acid (HCl), a family of in vivo $CO_2$ titration curves is produced parallel and to the left of the normal curve. Similarly, in alkalotic situations, the curves are shifted to the right. The more acid or alkaline the subject, the more the lines are shifted from normal (see Fig. 41–1).[16]

## What Happens When the Blood $P_{CO_2}$ Changes?

A similar $CO_2$ titration may be performed by changing the $P_{CO_2}$ of a blood sample rather than $P_{CO_2}$ of the whole body. Such an in vitro $CO_2$ titration curve formed the basis of the early assessment of acid-base status using a pH electrode before the availability of the $CO_2$ electrode.

The $CO_2$ titration lines lie to the left of the normal in acidotic and to the right of the normal in alkalotic conditions. Also, the slope of the line is modified by a change in hemoglobin concentration. A number of indices were introduced to account for these variations in an attempt to produce a numeric indication of the metabolic disturbance.

## Base Excess

The most common of these indices, which is still in use, is the *base excess*.[17] This is easily calculated from a nomogram (Fig. 41–2) after measuring pH and $P_{CO_2}$ or $HCO_3^-$.

## Buffer Base and Standard Bicarbonate

Earlier indices of acid-base status included the calculation of the sum of all the buffer anions ($HCO_3^-$, plasma proteins, and hemoglobin), the *buffer base*.[18] The influence of hemoglobin was also estimated by *standard bicarbonate*, which was the $[HCO_3^-]$ in plasma equilibrated to a $P_{CO_2}$ of 40 mm Hg.[19]

## *How Should Acid-Base Changes Be Assessed?*

Base excess, standard bicarbonate, and buffer base are outdated and should no longer be used. The terminology is confusing and seldom understood. More important, the indices are based on the in vitro titration of blood and do not reflect the changes in pH that might be expected when the whole body $P_{CO_2}$ is changed: in vitro $CO_2$ titration curves have a steeper slope than in vivo curves and, thus, may introduce errors into the assessment. It is recommended that acid-base assessment be based on predictions from the Henderson-

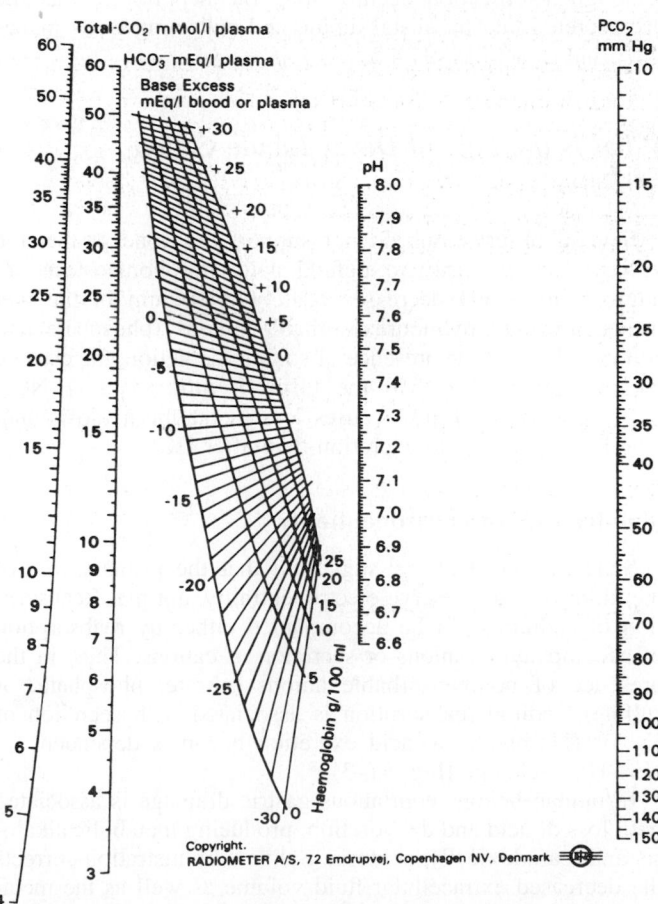

**FIGURE 41–2.** Base excess curve. (From Astrup P, Jorgensen K, Siggaard-Andersen O, et al. The acid-base metabolism: a new approach. *Lancet.* 1960;1:1035. Copyright RADIOMETER A/S, Emdrupvej, Copenhagen NV, Denmark.)

Hasselbalch equation using either a graphic (see Fig. 41–2) or mathematical representation for the calculation of actual bicarbonate.

## RENAL RESPONSES TO ACID-BASE DISTURBANCE

Classically, renal control of acid-base homeostasis has been explained in terms of reabsorption of bicarbonate (5000 mmol/d), which reduces systemic acidity and the excretion of nonvolatile acid (50-100 mmol/d) by trapping $H^+$ with phosphate buffers and ammonium salts. However, there are several confusing observations that do not fit with these simple explanations.

### What Is Bicarbonate Reabsorption?

$H^+$ is produced in the renal tubular cells in the presence of carbonic anhydrase (CA):

$$CO_2 + H_2O \rightleftarrows H_2CO_3 \rightleftarrows H^+ + HCO_3^-$$

The $H^+$ neutralizes the filtered $HCO_3^-$, and the $CO_2$ diffuses back into the tubular cell to recapture the $HCO_3^-$. $HCO_3^-$ reabsorption takes place primarily in the proximal tubule, although acidification occurs along the nephron so that the $H^+$ secreted into the distal tubule and collecting ducts makes the urine as acid as pH 4.5.

### What Is the Role of Distal Tubule Cation Exchange?

Several observations do not support the concept that the kidneys act primarily to defend acid-base homeostasis. In animals, urine pH decreases acutely if sodium in the diet is accompanied by nonreabsorbable anions (phosphate and sulfate). Also, in the presence of sodium depletion, the chronic administration of $H^+$ in the form of nitric acid ($H_2NO_3$) or sulfuric acid ($H_2SO_4$) causes less metabolic acidosis and, therefore, greater acid excretion than after HCl.

#### Maintenance of Electroneutrality

Schwartz and Cohen[20] suggested that the primary role of the kidneys is to preserve electroneutrality, not pH. Reabsorption of sodium must be accompanied either by reabsorption of accompanying anions or secretion of cations. Thus, in the presence of nonreabsorbable anions (nitrate, phosphate, or sulfate), sodium reabsorption is associated with secretion of $H^+$ or $K^+$, and renal acid excretion becomes dependent on $Na^+$-$H^+$ exchange (Fig. 41–3).[18]

In human beings, continuous gastric drainage is associated with loss of acid and dehydration, producing metabolic alkalosis and, paradoxically, aciduria. Saline administration corrects the decreased extracellular fluid volume as well as the metabolic acidosis by decreasing urine acid excretion. Again, $Na^+$-$H^+$ exchange is invoked as the cause of the aciduria and its correction with volume replacement.

This hypothesis is not supported by micropuncture tech-

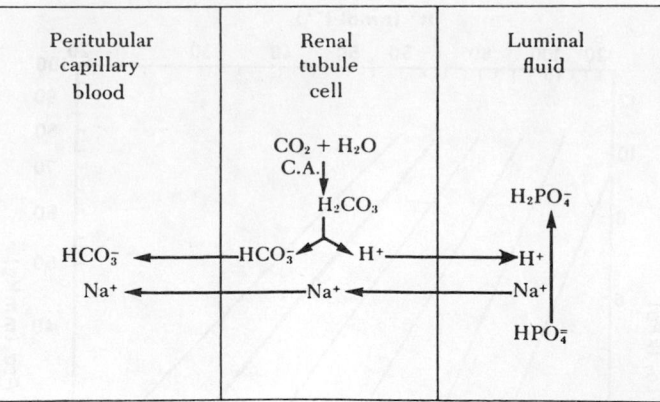

**FIGURE 41–3.** Distal tubule cation exchange; acidification of the phosphate buffer system in the renal tubule. (From Masoro EJ, Seigel PD. *Acid-Base Regulation: Its Physiology, Pathophysiology, and the Interpretation of Blood-Gas Analysis.* Philadelphia, Pa: WB Saunders; 1977:75.)

niques of individual nephron segments (or other tissues resembling the distal tubular cell), which have shown that the tubule is capable of responding to acid-base disturbance independently of sodium reabsorption.[19] Thus, although the cation exchange mechanism may account for some chronic acid-base disturbances, renal acid excretion is not solely a byproduct of electrolyte homeostasis.

### Are Phosphate Buffers Important?

Approximately 30 to 40 mmol/d of $H^+$ is excreted as *titratable acid* bound to monohydrogen phosphate (see Fig. 41–3):

$$HPO_4^{-2} + H^+ \rightleftarrows H_2PO_4^-$$

At pH 6.8, the phosphate buffer is only 50% titrated, but it is nearly fully titrated at pH 5.

### How Are Ammonium Salts Used?

Similarly, $H^+$ is buffered by ammonia ($NH_3$) (Fig. 41–4):

$$NH_3 + H^+ \rightleftarrows NH_4^+$$

The rate of excretion of ammonium ($NH_4^+$) may be increased 5 to 10 times in diabetic ketoacidosis.[21] It has been suggested that this equation represents a fundamental error. Urinary $NH_4^+$ is formed from glutamine, but at the pH in the tubule, glutamine already is ionized to $NH_4^+$ and cannot further buffer $H^+$.[22] Thus, the increased excretion of $NH_4^+$ in acidosis should not be regarded as a means to excrete additional $H^+$ but rather as a means of depriving the liver of a source of $NH_3$ for urea synthesis and the consequent increase in $H^+$ production.[23] The importance of this observation requires further evaluation.

## THE LIVER AND ACID-BASE REGULATION

Each day, approximately 20 mmol/kg of lactate and its accompanying cation are produced. The $H^+$ is titrated with

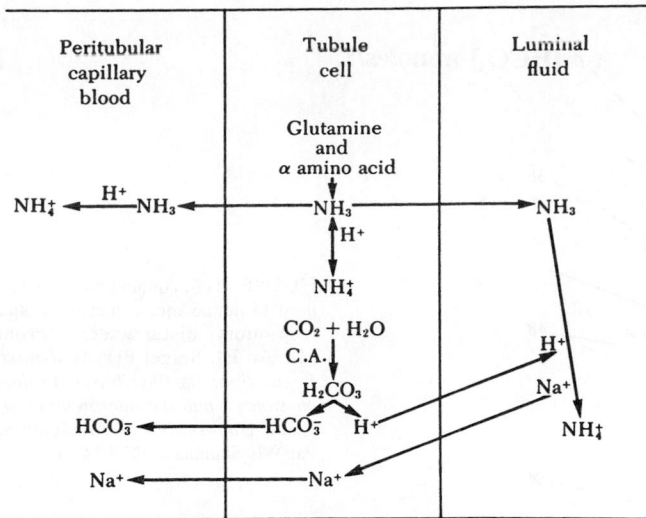

**FIGURE 41–4.** Suggested mechanism for the secretion of $NH_3$ by tubular cells and the excretion of $NH_4^+$ in urine. (From Masoro EJ, Seigel PD. *Acid-Base Regulation: Its Physiology, Pathophysiology, and the Interpretation of Blood-Gas Analysis.* Philadelphia, Pa: WB Saunders; 1977:76.)

$HCO_3^-$, as described earlier, and the lactate is metabolized mainly in the liver (70%) but also in the kidneys by gluconeogenesis or oxidation. Either pathway consumes 1 mol $H^+$ for each mole of lactate that is metabolized. In effect, this process leads to the generation of 1 mol $HCO_3^-$.

## Why Is Urea Synthesis Important?

Urea is synthesized in the liver:

$$CO_2 + 2NH_4^+ \rightleftarrows CO(NH_2)_2 + H_2O + H^+ \text{ (urea)}$$

Each mole of urea produces 2 mol of $H^+$, which are used to neutralize $HCO_3^-$ generated from the metabolism of amino acids. A decrease in the availability of $NH_4^+$ resulting from the increased renal $NH_4^+$ excretion associated with diabetic ketoacidosis reduces $H^+$.[24] In addition, acidosis decreases urea synthesis directly.

### Alterations in Liver Disease

Liver disease is often associated with decreased urea synthesis and metabolic alkalosis. The acidosis of uremia is a consequence not only of decreased $NH_4^+$ excretion but also of increased urea synthesis. Compensation for acute respiratory acidosis may result from depression of urea synthesis and a failure to titrate the $HCO_3^-$ from amino acid metabolism.[25] The disposal of lactate is impaired by acidosis, high lactate concentrations (>3-5 mmol/L), and decreased hepatic perfusion.[26] However, metabolism is increased through stimulation of gluconeogenesis by the stress hormones (catecholamines, angiotensin, vasopressin, glucagon).[27]

## ACID-BASE DISTURBANCES

## If Ventilation Changes, What Happens?

### Respiratory Acidosis

When the elimination of $CO_2$ is less than its production, the $P_{CO_2}$ increases.

### Mathematical Point 4

*Apnea results in an increase of $P_{CO_2}$ of 3 mm Hg/min at normal metabolic rate.*

In surgical patients, the most common causes are respiratory center depression by anesthetic agents or narcotics, as well as persistent neuromuscular blockade; these changes may be augmented by pulmonary disease or instability of the rib cage.

### Compensation

The change in pH in response to an increase in $P_{CO_2}$ can be predicted according to the in vivo $CO_2$ titration curve (see Fig. 41–1). Renal and hepatic compensation is slow and is not complete for 48 hours. In chronic respiratory acidosis, the increase in $H^+$ averages only 0.3 times the increase in $P_{CO_2}$, compared with 0.8 times the increase in $P_{CO_2}$ during acute disturbances (Fig. 41–5). An increase in extracellular $H^+$ is associated with $H^+$-$K^+$ exchange across the cell membrane so that hypercapnia is commonly associated with hyperkalemia.

### Appropriate Treatment

Correction of respiratory acidosis, as for all acid-base disturbances, should be achieved slowly and, primarily, by correcting the underlying cause, particularly when the persistent effects of respiratory depressant or neuromuscular blocking drugs are responsible.

Chronic $CO_2$ retention is associated with decreased central drive to ventilation, which then becomes dependent on peripheral chemoreceptors. If the $P_{CO_2}$ is reduced rapidly in these patients, the sudden increase in cerebrospinal fluid pH may produce convulsions and unconsciousness.[28] Thus, $P_{CO_2}$ should be reduced slowly (eg, over 48 hours).

### Respiratory Alkalosis

Hypocapnia occurs when the effective pulmonary ventilation is increased. The most common cause seen by anesthesiologists is mechanical hyperventilation. However, the condition occurs frequently when the respiratory center is stimulated by pain, anxiety, fear, pregnancy, salicylate intoxication, and numerous other entities (Table 41–3). Peripheral hypoxic chemoreceptor stimulation occurs at high altitude and probably also accounts for the hypocapnia of sepsis, anemia, and heart failure. Although $CO_2$ depletion is common in hepatic failure, decreased lactate and urea metabolism causes more important metabolic than respiratory disturbances of acid-base status, as noted previously.

### Compensation

The initial change in $H^+$ and $HCO_3^-$ can be predicted from the in vivo $CO_2$ titration curves (see Fig. 41–1).

### Mathematical Point 5

*In acute respiratory disturbances, each 1 mm Hg decrease in $P_{CO_2}$ decreases $[H^+]$ by 0.8 nmol/L and decreases $HCO_3^-$ by 0.2 mmol/L.*

### Mathematical Point 6

*In chronic respiratory disturbances, $H^+$ decreases by 0.4 nmol/L and $HCO_3^-$ by 0.4 mmol/L for each 1 mm Hg decrease in $P_{CO_2}$.*[29]

Within hours, renal and hepatic mechanisms counteract the

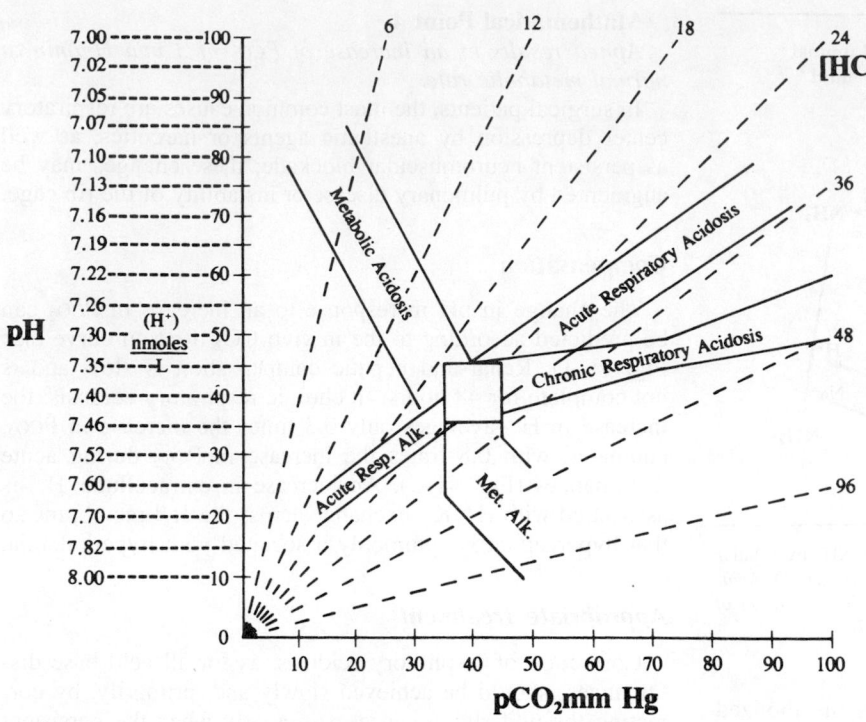

**FIGURE 41–5.** An acid-base "map" used to define mixed metabolic and respiratory disturbances. (From Masoro EJ, Seigel PD. *Acid-Base Regulation: Its Physiology, Pathophysiology, and the Interpretation of Blood-Gas Analysis.* Philadelphia, Pa: WB Saunders; 1977:142.)

change in pH so completely that the hypocapnia of altitude is accompanied by a normal or nearly normal pH. Respiratory alkalosis appears to be the only acid-base disturbance in which compensation restores pH to normal.[12]

### Appropriate Treatment

Respiratory alkalosis is better prevented than treated by avoiding increased central or peripheral ventilatory drive. In

**TABLE 41–3.** Causes of Respiratory Alkalosis

**Drugs**

Salicylates
Analeptics
Doxapram

**Hormones**

Progesterone
Epinephrine

**Hypermetabolic State**

Fever
Exercise
Thyrotoxicosis

**Hypoxia/Anoxia**

Hypovolemia
Hypoxemia
Decreased tissue perfusion

**Central Nervous System Lesions**

Meningitis
Encephalitis
Hemorrhage
Trauma

**Hepatic Failure, Shock, Gram-Negative Bacteremia (without fever or shock), Systemic Inflammatory Response Syndrome**

**Interstitial Pulmonary Disease**

**Iatrogenic Hyperventilation**

particular, mechanical ventilation should be guided by end-tidal or arterial $P_{CO_2}$ monitoring.

It may be difficult to maintain $Pa_{O_2}$ when ventilation is reduced to correct profound hypocapnia, because the depletion in $CO_2$ stores causes an apparent reduction in the respiratory quotient (R). Consequently, as predicted from the alveolar air equation,

$$PA_{O_2} = FI_{O_2} (PB = PH_{2O}) - PaCO_2 [FI_{O_2} + (1 - FI_{O_2})/R]$$

$PA_{O_2}$ and hence $Pa_{O_2}$ decrease, providing further justification for additional $O_2$ when patients are weaned from mechanical ventilation.[30] ($FI_{O_2}$ is fraction of inspired $O_2$ and PB is barometric pressure.)

Respiratory alkalosis results in hypokalemia from both $H^+$-$K^+$ exchange across the cell membrane and an increase in renal potassium excretion.

### If Metabolic Changes Occur, What Happens?

#### Metabolic Acidosis

Metabolic acidosis is commonly classified according to the AG (Table 41–4). Those conditions associated with an increased AG may be further divided, depending on the presence or absence of hypoxia, and this subdivision may have important therapeutic implications. The toxic causes listed are the result of the addition of organic acids or substances that produce acid by their metabolism (paraldehyde, ethylene glycol, methanol).

Alternatively, some conditions may result from an increased loss of base (diarrhea, biliary/pancreatic fistulas). Creation of an ileal bladder results in chloride reabsorption and $HCO_3^-$ secretion.[31] Administration of large volumes of stored blood,

**TABLE 41–4.** Causes of Metabolic Acidosis

| Increased Anion Gap | Normal Anion Gap |
| --- | --- |
| Lactic acidosis* | Renal tubular acidosis |
| Circulatory arrest* | Diarrhea |
| Pulmonary edema* | Biliary/pancreatic fistulas |
| Gram-negative sepsis* | Ileal bladder |
| Ketoacidosis | Saline excess |
| Toxins | |
| Nitroprusside | |
| Fructose | |
| Acid-citrate-dextrose blood | |

*Associated with hypoxia.

particularly when acid-citrate-dextrose was used as an anticoagulant, produced an acute metabolic acidosis that was converted into a metabolic alkalosis during the next 2 to 3 days as the citrate was metabolized to $HCO_3^-$. Infusion of several liters of saline during resuscitation may result in a mild metabolic acidosis from dilution of extracellular $HCO_3^-$ and an increase in the SID.[32] Although the pH of saline is decreased compared with the normal blood value, the titratable acidity (actual acid load) is small. The pH is low because there are no buffers in saline; thus a small amount of acid causes a significant reduction of pH.

### Lactic Acidosis

Type A lactic acidosis is the result of tissue hypoxia and anaerobic metabolism and is more common than type B, which results from other causes[33] (Table 41–5). In shock, if the blood lactate concentration is >5 mmol/L , the mortality is >75%; mortality is reduced to 18% at a concentration of 1.3 to 4.4 mmol/L.[34]

**Type A Lactic Acidosis.** Lactic acidosis is commonly associated with hypoxia because the available $O_2$ is inadequate for a patient's needs. In shock, hypovolemia, and sepsis, overall $O_2$ consumption may not be altered because the decrease in cardiac output is offset by an increase of $O_2$ extraction. However, the distribution of $O_2$ uptake is modified: extraction by the liver, muscle, kidneys, and gut decreases while that of the heart and brain increases. Decreased $O_2$ availability in the affected tissues leads to anaerobic glycolysis and the accumulation of lactate. In addition, as previously noted, decreased lactate uptake by the liver leads to decreased clearance.

After cardiac arrest, the increase in myocardial $H^+$ is the result of $CO_2$ accumulation and failure of sufficient adenosine triphosphate generation to drive the $Na^+$-$H^+$ exchange.[35,36] If sodium bicarbonate ($NaHCO_3$) is given to correct the acidosis, the result is liberation of $CO_2$, which causes further increase in intracellular $H^+$ and acidosis.[37] In this regard, Forsythe and Schmidt[38] concluded,

**TABLE 41–5.** Causes of Type B Lactic Acidosis

| Systemic Disease B1 | Drugs and Toxins B2 | Inherited B3 |
| --- | --- | --- |
| Diabetes mellitus | Biguanides | Glycogen storage |
| Renal failure | Salicylates | Fructose-1, 6-diphosphate deficiency |
| Hepatic failure | Parenteral nutrition | Methylmalonic acidemia |
| Leukemia | | Pyruvate dehydrogenase deficiency |

*The oft-cited rationale for bicarbonate use, that it might ameliorate the hemodynamic depression of metabolic acidemia, has been disproved convincingly. . . . Given the current lack of evidence supporting its use, we cannot condone bicarbonate administration for patients with lactic acidosis. We extend this to those with pH < 7.2 on vasoactive drugs, inasmuch as bicarbonate has no measurable beneficial effects even in these sickest patients. Indeed, we do not give or advise bicarbonate infusion regardless of the pH.*

**Type B Lactic Acidosis.** The lactic acid in type B lactic acidosis originates from metabolic causes and is not associated with hypoxia (see Table 41–4). Severe renal and hepatic disease is associated with lactate accumulation. Acidosis may cause rapid lactic acidosis in uremia; hepatic gluconeogenesis is decreased, but renal gluconeogenesis, which increases lactic acid production, is increased.

Biguanides (oral hypoglycemic agents) act by reducing alimentary absorption of glucose and amino acids; they increase glycolysis and decrease hepatic gluconeogenesis. Normally, lactate concentrations are <2 mmol/L, but they may increase considerably in the presence of renal or hepatic disease.

Fructose, sorbitol, and xylitol all have been used in parenteral nutrition as a source of carbohydrate because they are metabolized in the absence of insulin and produce less venous irritation. However, all lead to an increase in lactate production; consider that 30% to 40% of a fructose load is converted to lactate.

Finally, several congenital diseases of the liver, such as pyruvate dehydrogenase deficiency, are associated with impaired hepatic lactate metabolism.

### Compensation

Metabolic acidosis stimulates ventilation, producing hypocapnia, which limits the decrease in pH. The $P_{CO_2}$ decreases slowly to reach its nadir at 12 to 24 hours. Although the change in $P_{CO_2}$ is variable, it is related to the $\Delta HCO_3^-$ and to the pH.

**Mathematical Point 7**
*Anticipated $P_{CO_2}$ (mm Hg) = 1.5 ($\Delta HCO_3$ mmol/L) + 8.*

**Mathematical Point 8**
*Anticipated $P_{CO_2}$ is approximately equal to the last two numbers of the pH (eg, at pH 7.20, the anticipated $P_{CO_2}$ is 20 mm Hg).*

### Appropriate Treatment

**Sodium Bicarbonate.** Traditionally, metabolic acidosis has been treated by $NaHCO_3$ titration. The quantity required can be estimated from the numeric expression of the Henderson-Hasselbalch equation, assuming that the $HCO_3^-$ is distributed through the extracellular fluid volume (20% body weight). Half the estimated deficit was given slowly over 10 minutes, and subsequent therapy was dictated by frequent acid-base assessment.

For example, a 70-kg patient has a 14-kg extracellular fluid volume. If normal $HCO_3^-$ is 24 mmol/L and the patient's $HCO_3^-$ is 14 mEq/L, each kilogram (liter) of extracellular fluid has a deficit of 10 mmol/L, or a total deficit of 140 mmol. One half of this value (70 mmol) would be infused slowly over 10 minutes, followed by assessment.

Although such therapy may be appropriate for some causes of metabolic acidosis (uremia, diarrhea and fistulas, renal tubular acidosis), administration of $NaHCO_3$ in the presence of hypoxia neither corrects the acidosis nor improves the cardiovascular status. In experimental metabolic acidosis, $NaHCO_3$ leads to an *increase* in intracellular $H^+$ in the heart, liver, muscle, and red blood cells.[11] In addition, $NaHCO_3$ promotes cerebrospinal fluid acidosis, hypoxia, circulatory depression, hyperosmolality, and hypernatremia.

$NaHCO_3$ has no place in the treatment of diabetic ketoacidosis. It does not decrease ketone body concentration, increase pH or improve patients' survival. Management is with fluid and insulin to restore glucose metabolism, which has the additional advantage of improving hepatic metabolism of accumulated lactate, itself a store of $HCO_3^-$.

Several promising alternatives to $NaHCO_3$ have been tried experimentally.

**Sodium Dichloroacetate.** Sodium dichloroacetate (DCA) has been shown to decrease lactate concentration and to improve cardiovascular function in several hypoxic states without an increase in $PCO_2$ and thus, presumably, without an increase in intracellular $H^+$. It acts by stimulating pyruvate dehydrogenase, which encourages the conversion of lactate to pyruvate for eventual removal via the Krebs cycle in the liver. DCA has also been used prophylactically, 40 mg/kg infused over 1 hour, to reduce lactate acidosis during the anhepatic phase of liver transplantation.[39]

**Carbicarb.** An equimolar mixture of $NaHCO_3$ and sodium carbonate, this substance buffers acid in a similar manner to $NaHCO_3$ but without an increase in $PCO_2$. It produces little hemodynamic effect but improves acid-base status and decreases intracellular $H^+$ and lactate production.

**THAM.** This substance (tromethamine) is unusual in that it crosses cell membranes and buffers, intracellular as well as extracellular $H^+$, again without an increase in $PCO_2$.

**Tribonat.** A mixture of tromethamine, sodium bicarbonate, acetate, and phosphate, Tribonat also is alleged to overcome many of the perceived problems of bicarbonate administration.[40,41] However, almost no evidence of efficacy is published. Large-scale, prospective studies are necessary to establish its utility.

Sodium DCA, Carbicarb, THAM, and Tribonat do not possess the problems associated with $NaHCO_3$, particularly with regard to intracellular $H^+$ increase, and are currently undergoing clinical evaluation. However, they also have not been shown to improve outcome from conditions associated with prolonged hypoxia and acidosis (ie, cardiac arrest). At present, it appears that the safest treatment of hypoxia-induced metabolic acidosis in hypoxia is removal of the cause and aggressive cardiorespiratory support. Survival depends on the ability of the individual to increase cardiac output and $O_2$ delivery in the presence of tissue hypoxia and anaerobic metabolism.

## Metabolic Alkalosis

Severe metabolic alkalosis has a mortality as high as 65% when the pH is >7.65.[42] The causes of metabolic alkalosis include loss of gastrointestinal fluid, adrenal hyperplasia, and administration of loop diuretics, cortisone, or alkali (Table 41–6).

**TABLE 41–6.** Causes of Metabolic Alkalosis

| Saline Responsive | Saline Unresponsive |
| --- | --- |
| Gastrointestinal losses | Aldosterone |
| Diuretics | Cortisone |
| | Alkali |

### Compensation

The in vivo $CO_2$ titration curve (see Fig. 41–1) is shifted to the right in metabolic alkalosis. Respiratory compensation does occur but often is variable. The resulting $PCO_2$ is seldom >50 mm Hg but can be predicted.

**Mathematical Point 9**
*In metabolic alkalosis, $PCO_2$ (mm Hg) = 0.9 × $HCO_3^-$ + 9 mmol/L.*

### Appropriate Treatment

The management of metabolic alkalosis is removal of the cause. Many patients respond to rehydration with saline, suggesting that the principal abnormality was related to loss of $Cl^-$ and not $H^+$. Ammonium chloride, one-sixth molar, may act as a source of acid by the production of urea and $H^+$, but normal hepatic function is required. Ammonium chloride should be avoided in hypokalemic patients because further potassium loss may be induced. Infusion of HCl has been attempted, but it is not part of conventional therapy.

### Mixed Disturbances

The acid-base disturbances previously discussed placed considerable emphasis on the ability to predict the compensatory changes that are induced by a primary alteration in $PCO_2$, $H^+$, or $HCO_3^-$. Such predictions may be made using mathematic or graphic representations of the in vivo $CO_2$ titration curves. An acid-base map plots the 95% confidence limits of the relationship between pH and $PCO_2$ in various acute and chronic respiratory and metabolic disorders (see Fig. 41–5).[43] In some situations, this approach may make it easier to determine the cause of the disturbance.

For example, using such a map, the finding of a pH of 7.25 and a $PCO_2$ of 25 mm Hg suggests metabolic acidosis. However, a pH of 7.25 and $PCO_2$ of 80 mm Hg could represent either acute *respiratory acidosis* and slight *metabolic alkalosis* or chronic *respiratory acidosis* and slight *metabolic acidosis*. Clearly, a clinical history is essential in making a correct diagnosis; acid-base values cannot be evaluated in isolation.

### Metabolic and Respiratory Acidosis

The most common disturbance is metabolic and respiratory acidosis. It is frequently encountered when the presence of chronic lung disease prevents the appropriate ventilatory compensation for a metabolic acidosis (eg, cardiac arrest, pulmonary edema, chronic lung disease with hypoxia). Some substances (sodium nitroprusside, carbon monoxide, ethylene glycol) depress ventilation and induce metabolic acidosis. The importance of the combination is that administration of $NaHCO_3$ leads to further increase in $PCO_2$, which cannot be removed because of impaired ventilation. Such patients require mechanical ventilatory support.

### Metabolic Alkalosis and Respiratory Acidosis

Administration of diuretics to patients with chronic lung disease induces potassium loss and metabolic alkalosis that results in a compensatory respiratory acidosis. Treatment with ammonium chloride corrects the alkalosis and reduces $P_{CO_2}$.

### Respiratory Alkalosis and Metabolic Acidosis

The combination of respiratory alkalosis and metabolic acidosis may be induced by salicylate poisoning. It also occurs in critically ill patients when the ventilatory response to lactic acidosis is excessive. This condition is difficult to recognize, although a normal pH with an increased AG may be suggestive. Again, the clinical history is important in making the diagnosis.

## EFFECTS OF ACID-BASE DISTURBANCES

### Is the Circulation Impaired?

The effects of acid-base disturbance on the circulation depend on the origin. For respiratory disturbances, the direct depressant actions of $P_{CO_2}$ may be offset by the associated sympathetic stimulation. $CO_2$ acts as a peripheral vasodilator and a pulmonary vasoconstrictor. However, in the presence of an intact autonomic system, its secondary sympathetic stimulation leads to vasoconstriction of those organs such as the kidneys with a rich sympathetic innervation. Thus, hypoventilation induces renal vasoconstriction and cerebral vasodilation. Also, sympathetic activation leads to increases in stroke volume, heart rate, and cardiac output.

When the $P_{CO_2}$ is maintained constant, the cardiovascular effect of pH depends on the source and distribution of $H^+$. In general, a decrease in pH leads to myocardial depression with decreased stroke volume and cardiac output. However, in the presence of myocardial ischemia, intracellular $H^+$ decreases from hydrolysis of adenosine triphosphate and the local production of $CO_2$. In this situation, the heart is particularly vulnerable to attempts at correcting the acidosis with $NaHCO_3$. The resulting increase in $P_{CO_2}$ leads to further increase in intracellular $H^+$, myocardial depression, and impaired tissue oxygenation.

### How Is Ventilation Affected?

Hypercapnia stimulates central and peripheral chemoreceptors maximally at a $P_{CO_2}$ of about 80 mm Hg. Above that level, ventilation is depressed. Elevated $P_{CO_2}$ induces a rapid increase in ventilation from stimulation of the aortic and carotid bodies. The accompanying decrease in pH produces a slower but additional central stimulus to ventilation. $CO_2$ and $H^+$ produce separate and additive rightward shifts of the oxyhemoglobin dissociation curve. The $P_{50}$ (normal 26 mm Hg) is increased by about 2 mm Hg per 0.1 pH unit reduction.

Tissue $O_2$ delivery is the product of cardiac output and arterial $O_2$ content. To some extent, the shift in the $O_2$ dissociation curve induced by hypercapnia and acidosis compensates for the hemodynamic depression. Consequently, it is preferable, in the correction of metabolic acidosis, to produce a slight under-correction rather than over-correction because metabolic alkalosis has a detrimental effect on both cardiac output and the $O_2$ dissociation curve.

### What Neurologic Changes Occur?

$CO_2$ and $H^+$ have no direct effect on cerebral metabolism except as a consequence of altered cerebral perfusion. Hypocapnia has been shown to have some effect on increasing pain threshold. Tetany, in alkalotic states, is secondary to a decrease in the ionized calcium concentration.

### Are Pharmacologic Actions Altered Significantly?

Drug activity is modified by pH as a result of the degree of ionization. This has some therapeutic application: absorption of drugs is increased in the un-ionized state. At the pH of the stomach, salicylates (weak acids) are mainly un-ionized and, consequently, well absorbed. Conversely, absorption of quinidine (weak base) is enhanced by alkalization of the gastric pH. Similarly, alkalization of the urine increases the ionization of weak acids (salicylates, phenobarbitone), decreases their tubular reabsorption, and increases renal excretion.

The extent of ionization also modifies protein binding and the amount of active free drug. The duration of action of $d$-tubocurarine, but not other neuromuscular blocking drugs, is prolonged by acidosis. Curare normally has a single quaternary $NH^+_4$ grouping, but in acidotic situations it becomes a bis-quaternary compound, which increases its potency.[44]

Although metabolism of atracurium by Hoffman elimination is pH dependent, hypercapnia induces only a small increase in its duration of action, and recovery is only marginally more rapid in alkalotic conditions.[45] Thus, the effect of acid-base disturbances on pharmacologic activity is multifactorial and difficult to predict.

## CONCLUSION

Acid-base disturbances are common in clinical practice. Interpretation of laboratory values may be difficult. However, when the compensatory responses to primary disturbances can be predicted, either graphically or mathematically, it is usually possible to determine the initiating mechanisms.

The effects of the disturbances are wide-ranging and include major organ dysfunction and abnormal responses to several drugs. Correction should be directed primarily at reversing the underlying defect. Respiratory disturbances are usually managed by appropriate mechanical ventilation. Metabolic disturbances are more difficult. Although $NaHCO_3$ has been used for more than 50 years to correct metabolic acidosis, it appears that its use has been excessive. In particular, it is ineffective in hypoxia-induced acidosis and may actually worsen the disturbance. The most important goal of therapy is to improve tissue $O_2$ delivery.

### References

1. Bates RG. Determination of pH. *Theory and Practice*. New York, NY: John Wiley & Sons; 1964.

2. Henderson LJ. The theory of neutrality regulation in the animal organism. *Am J Physiol.* 1908;21:427.

3. Hasselbalch KA. Die Berechnung der Wasserstoffzahl des Blutes aus der freien und gebundenen Kohlensäure desselben und die Sauerstoffbindung des Blutes als Funktion der Wasserstoffzahl. *Biochemie.* 1917;78:112.

4. Kassirer JP, Bleich HL. Rapid estimation of plasma carbon dioxide tension from pH and total carbon dioxide content. *N Engl J Med.* 1965;272:1067.

5. Ream AK, Reitz BA, Silverberg G. Temperature correction of $P_{CO_2}$ and pH in estimating acid-base status. *Anesthesiology.* 1982;56:41.

6. Rahn H, Reeves RB, Howell BJ. Hydrogen ion regulation, temperature, and evolution. *Am Rev Respir Dis.* 1975;112:165.

7. du Plessis AJ, Jonas RA, Wypij D, et al. Perioperative effects of alpha-stat versus pH-stat strategies for deep hypothermic cardiopulmonary bypass in infants. *J Thorac Cardiovasc Surg.* 1997;114:991.

8. Murkin JM, Martzke JS, Buchan AM, et al. A randomized study of the influence of perfusion technique and pH management strategy in 316 patients undergoing coronary artery bypass surgery, II: neurologic and cognitive outcomes. *J Thorac Cardiovasc Surg.* 1995;110:349.

9. Androgue HJ, Rashad MN, Gorin AB, et al. Assessing acid-base status in circulatory failure. *N Engl J Med.* 1989;320:1312.

10. Weil MH, Rackow EC, Trevino R, et al. Difference in acid-base state between venous and arterial blood during cardiopulmonary resuscitation. *N Engl J Med.* 1986;315:153.

11. Fiddian-Green RG. Gastric intramucosal pH, tissue oxygenation and acid-base balance. *Br J Anaesth.* 1995;74:591

12. Narins RG, Emmett M. Simple and mixed acid-base disorders: a practical approach. *Medicine.* 1987;56:161.

13. Stewart PA. *How to Understand Acid-Base: A Quantitative Acid-Base Primer for Biology and Medicine.* New York, NY: Elsevier; 1981.

14. Scheingraber S, Rehm M, Schmisch C, et al. Rapid saline infusion produces hyperchloremic metabolic acidosis in patients undergoing gynecologic surgery. *Anesthesiology.* 1999;90:1265.

15. Prough D. Hyperchloremic metabolic acidosis is a predictable consequence of intraoperative infusion of 0.9% saline [editorial]. *Anesthesiology.* 1999;90:1247.

16. Kappagoda CT, Linden RJ, Snow HM. An approach to the problems of acid-base balance. *Clin Sci.* 1970;39:169.

17. Astrup P, Jorgensen K, Siggaard-Andersen O, et al. The acid-base metabolism. A new approach. *Lancet.* 1960;1:1035.

18. Singer RB, Hastings AB. An improved method for the estimation of disturbances of the acid-base balance of human blood. *Medicine.* 1948;27:223.

19. Jorgensen K, Astrup P. Standard bicarbonate: its clinical significance, and a new method for its determination. *Scand J Clin Lab Invest.* 1957;9:122.

20. Schwartz WB, Cohen JJ. The nature of the renal response to chronic disorders of acid-base equilibrium. *Am J Med.* 1978;64:417.

21. Levine DZ, Jacobson HR. The regulation of renal acid secretion: new observations from studies of distal nephron segments. *Kidney Int.* 1986;29:1099.

22. Pitts RF. *Physiology of the Kidney and Body Fluids.* 3rd ed. Boston, Mass: Year Book Medical Publishers; 1974.

23. Oliver J, Bourke E. Adaptations in urea and ammonium excretion in metabolic acidosis in the rat. *Clin Sci Mol Med.* 1975;48:515.

24. Atkinson DE, Bourke E. Metabolic aspects of the regulation of systemic pH. *Am J Physiol.* 1987;252:F947.

25. Cohen RD. Roles of the liver and kidney in acid-base regulation and its disorders. *Br J Anaesth.* 1991;67:154.

26. Oliver J, Koelz AM, Costello J, et al. Acid-base alterations in glutamine metabolism and ureagenesis in perfused muscle and liver of the rat. *Eur J Clin Invest.* 1977;7:445.

27. Pilkis SJ, El-Maghrabi MR, Claus TH. Fructose-2, 6-diphosphate in control of hepatic gluconeogenesis. *Diabetes Care.* 1990;13:582.

28. Cotev S, Severinghaus JW. Role of cerebrospinal fluid pH in management of respiratory problems. *Anesth Analg.* 1969;48:42.

29. Krapf R, Beeler I, Hertner D, et al. Chronic respiratory alkalosis: the effect of sustained hyperventilation on renal regulation of acid-base equilibrium. *N Engl J Med.* 1991;324:1394.

30. Sykes MK, McNicol MW, Campbell EJM. *Respiratory Failure.* 2nd ed. Oxford, United Kingdom: Blackwell Scientific; 1976.

31. Azzam FJ, Steinhardt GF, Tracey TF, et al. Transient preoperative metabolic acidosis in a patient with ileal bladder augmentation. *Anesthesiology.* 1995;83:198.

32. Mathes DD, Maxwell RC, Rohr MS. Dilutional acidosis: is it a real clinical entity? *Anesthesiology.* 1997;86:501.

33. Cohen RD, Woods HF. *Clinical and Biochemical Aspects of Lactic Acidosis.* Oxford, United Kingdom: Blackwell Scientific; 1976.

34. Peretz DL, Scott HM, Duff J. The significance of lactic acidemia in the shock syndrome. *Ann N Y Acad Sci.* 1965;119:1133.

35. Johnson DG, Alberti KGMM. Acid-base balance in metabolic acidosis. *Clin Endocrinol Metabol.* 1983;12:267.

36. Zilva JF. The origin of acidosis in hyperlactaemia. *Ann Clin Biochem.* 1978;15:40.

37. Graf H, Leach W, Arieff AI. Evidence for detrimental effect of bicarbonate therapy in hypoxic lactic acidosis. *Science.* 1985;227:754.

38. Forsythe SM, Schmidt GA. Sodium bicarbonate for the treatment of lactic acidosis. *Chest.* 2000;117:260.

39. Shangraw RE, Winter R, Hromco J, et al. Amelioration of lactic acidosis with dichloroacetate during liver transplantation in humans. *Anesthesiology.* 1994;81:1127.

40. Bjerneroth G. Tribonat—a comprehensive summary of its properties. *Crit Care Med.* 1999;27:1009.

41. Gazumi RJ. Buffer treatment for cardiac resuscitation: putting the cart before the horse. *Crit Care Med.* 1999;27:875.

42. Wilson RF, Gibson D, Percinel AK, et al. Severe alkalosis in critically ill surgical patients. *Arch Surg.* 1972;105:197.

43. Goldberg M, Green SB, Moss ML, et al. Computer-based instruction and diagnosis of acid-base disorders. *JAMA.* 1973;223:269.

44. Hughes R. The influence of changes in acid-base balance on neuromuscular blockade in cats. Br J Anaesth. 1970;42:658.

45. Hughes R, Chapple DJ. The pharmacology of atracurium: a competing neuromuscular blocking agent. *Br J Anaesth.* 1981;53:31.

## General Reading

Masoro EJ, Seigel PD. *Acid-Base Regulation: Its Physiology, Pathophysiology, and the Interpretation of Blood-Gas Analysis.* Philadelphia, Pa: WB Saunders; 1977.

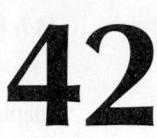

# Allergy and Immunology

## Jerrold H. Levy

An allergic reaction is one form of an adverse drug reaction that can occur in human beings. Often, however, patients complain of being "allergic" to a drug when what they actually have experienced is a form of predictable adverse drug reaction.[1] For example, patients often state they are allergic to an opioid because it causes nausea. Opioids, however, are known to produce nausea as one of their side effects by stimulating receptors in the chemotrigger zones. True allergy to a drug is an untoward response that is mediated by an immune mechanism (Table 42–1).[1]

An immune reaction involves activation of either cellular or humoral processes that can interact with many different types of foreign molecular structures called *antigens* to provide host defense. Immunologic mechanisms involve interaction of antigens with either antibodies or specific effector cells, or both. If a patient has antibodies against a specific drug or protein, exposure to that agent activates the patient's immune system.[1]

The immune system normally functions to protect the body against external microorganisms and toxins and internal threats from neoplastic cells.[2] However, the immune system can also respond inappropriately and cause allergic reactions. Clinically observed life-threatening allergic reactions to drugs and other foreign substances may represent different types of immune responses.[1,3] This chapter reviews the life-threatening allergic reactions an anesthesiologist may encounter.

## ANTIGENS AND ANTIBODIES

### What Are Antigens?

Molecules capable of stimulating an immune response when injected are called *antigens*. Only a few drugs administered by anesthesiologists, such as large polypeptides (chymopapain, latex) and other large macromolecules (dextrans), are complete antigens (Table 42–2).

Neuromuscular blocking agents are one of the few small molecular weight compounds or drugs that are complete antigens. The presence of biquarternary ammonium structures allows for bridging of two immunoglobulin E (IgE) antibodies to trigger mast cell activation.[1]

### Haptens

Most commonly used drugs are simple organic compounds of low molecular weight, usually <1000. For such a small molecule to become a complete antigen capable of sensitizing a patient, it must bind to circulating host proteins such as albumin or cellular membranes. Such anesthetic drugs or drug metabolites are called *haptens* and, by themselves, are not antigenic.[4] Some reactive drug metabolites (eg, the penicilloyl derivative of penicillin) are thought to bind with macromole-

**TABLE 42–1.** Characteristics of an Allergic Reaction

| |
|---|
| Adverse response of host |
| Produced after injection of a foreign drug/blood product |
| Mediated by antibodies or sensitized cells |
| Can be reproduced if foreign substance reinjected |

**TABLE 42–2.** Drugs and Macromolecules That Can Be Foreign Antigens

| | |
|---|---|
| Chymopapain | Protamine |
| Latex | Dextrans |
| Muscle relaxants | |

cules to become antigens, but for most drugs this relationship has not been proved.

## What Are Antibodies?

Antibodies are proteins with a molecular weight of approximately 150 000. They are also called *immunoglobulins* and can recognize and bind with specific antigens.[1] The basic structure of the antibody molecule is illustrated in Figure 42–1. Each antibody has at least two heavy chains and two light chains that are bound together by disulfide bonds. The Fab fragment has the ability to bind antigen. The Fc fragment is responsible for the unique biologic properties of the different classes of immunoglobulins (cell binding and activation of the complement system).[5,6] Once antibodies bind with antigens, they undergo conformational changes to activate either mast cells or the complement cascade.

Antibodies have been developed in the laboratory and used clinically to treat nonimmunologic disorders. Monoclonal antibodies with binding sites directed against endotoxin are clinically available for use in combating septic shock. Fab antibody fragments are also clinically available for treating digoxin overdose. Because digoxin cannot be dialyzed, the only current therapy in overdoses is to administer Fab fragments that selectively bind to digoxin to inactivate its biologic activity.

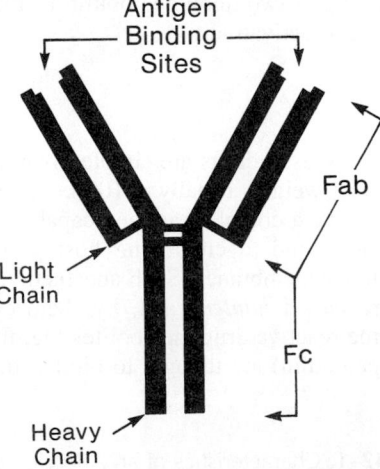

Antigen
Binding
Sites

Fab

Light
Chain

Fc

Heavy
Chain

**FIGURE 42–1.** Simplified basic structural configuration of an antibody molecule representing human immunoglobulin G. Immunoglobulins are composed of 2 heavy chains and 2 light chains bound by disulfide linkages (represented by *cross bars*). Papain cleaves the molecule into 2 Fab fragments and 1 Fc fragment. Antigen binding occurs on the Fab segments; the Fc segment is responsible for membrane or complement activation. (From Levy JH. *Anaphylactic Reactions in Anesthesia and Intensive Care.* 2nd ed. Boston, Mass: Butterworth-Heinemann; 1992, with permission.)

## ANAPHYLAXIS

### What Is the Pathophysiology?

Acute cardiovascular and pulmonary collapse occurs in anaphylaxis, the most severe form of allergic reaction.[1] Studies suggest approximately 1 in every 2700 hospitalized patients experiences drug-induced anaphylaxis.[7] In 1902, Portier and Richet first used the word *anaphylaxis* (*ana*, "against," and *prophylaxis*, "protection") to describe the profound shock and subsequent death that sometimes occurred in dogs immediately after a second parenteral challenge with a foreign antigen.[8]

Life-threatening allergic reactions mediated by antibodies are described as anaphylactic. When antibodies are not responsible for the reaction, when other antibody-independent mechanisms of mast cell or complement activation occur, or when we are unable to prove antibody involvement, the reaction is called *anaphylactoid*.[1] One cannot distinguish between anaphylactic and anaphylactoid reactions on the basis of clinical observation.

### Immunoglobulin-Mediated Reactions

Antigen binding with IgE antibodies initiates anaphylaxis (Fig. 42–2).[6,9,10] Prior exposure to the antigen or to a substance of similar structure is required to produce sensitization, although an allergic history may be unknown to the patient. When the foreign substance is reintroduced in the patient, the antigen binds with and bridges two IgE antibodies located on the surfaces of mast cells and basophils. Antigen-antibody binding on these cell surfaces releases stored mediators.[1,5,10]

Other chemical mediators, including the lipid-derived compounds, arachidonic acid metabolites (leukotrienes and prostaglandins), platelet activating factors, peptide-derived mediators, and kinins, subsequently are synthesized and released in response to cellular activation.[11–18] The liberated mediators produce a unique symptom complex of bronchospasm and upper airway edema in the respiratory system; vasodilation and increased capillary permeability in the cardiovascular system; and urticaria in the cutaneous system. Various mediators are released from mast cells and basophils after activation.

### What Are the Cardiopulmonary Effects of the Chemical Mediators?

#### Histamine

Histamine is the most commonly studied mediator of anaphylaxis (Fig. 42–3). Stored in mast cell granules before release, it stimulates histamine$_1$ (H$_1$) and histamine$_2$ (H$_2$) receptors. H$_1$ receptor binding activates the vascular endothelium to release endothelium-derived relaxing factor and prostacyclin, potent short-acting mediators that produce vasodilation.[1] H$_1$ receptor stimulation also causes increased capillary permeability, bronchoconstriction, and smooth muscle contraction.[11,12]

H$_2$ receptor activation causes gastric secretion and inhibits mast cell activation.[19] Vasodilation results from the interaction of both H$_1$ and H$_2$ receptors. When injected into skin, histamine produces the classic wheal (increased capillary permeability producing tissue edema) and flare (cutaneous vasodilation) response in human beings.[20]

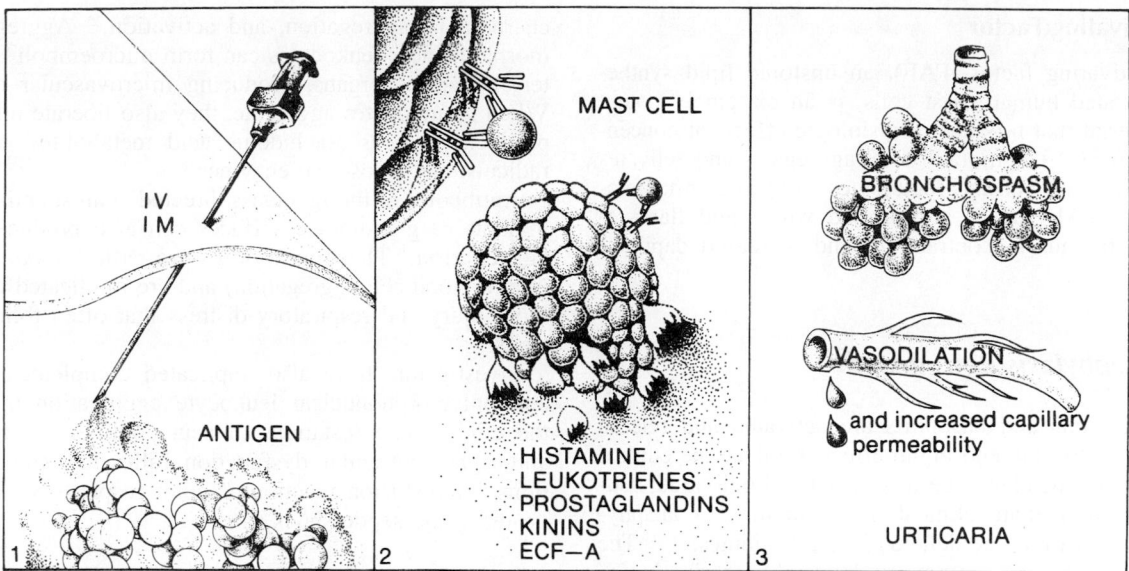

**FIGURE 42–2.** Immunoglobulin E (IgE) anaphylaxis (type I immediate hypersensitivity reaction). When an antigen enters a patient parenterally—either intravenously or intramuscularly—it bridges 2 IgE antibodies on the surface of the mast cells and basophils. In a calcium- and energy-dependent process, cells release various substances (histamine, eosinophilic and other chemotactic factors, lipid mediators [including prostaglandins and leukotrienes], and bradykinin), producing the characteristic pulmonary, cardiovascular, and cutaneous effects. The most severe and life-threatening effects of these vasoactive mediators occur in the respiratory and cardiovascular systems. (Reprinted from Levy JH. Identification and treatment of anaphylaxis. In: *Chemonucleolysis Anaphylaxis: Mechanisms of Action and Strategies for Treatment Under General Anesthesia.* Chicago, Ill: Smith Laboratories; 1982, with permission.)

Histamine has a very short half-life and undergoes rapid metabolism in human beings, catalyzed by the enzymes histamine *N*-methyltransferase and diamine oxidase located in endothelial cells.[1]

## Chemotactic Factors of Anaphylaxis

Peptide and lipid products are released from mast cells and basophils, causing granulocyte migration (chemotaxis) and collection at the site of the inflammatory stimulus. Eosinophilic and neutrophilic chemotactic factors of anaphylaxis are small molecular weight peptides that produce chemotaxis and activation of polymorphonuclear leukocytes. Eosinophils release enzymes that can inactivate histamine. Granulocyte activation may be responsible for recurrent manifestations of anaphylaxis. Other lipid mediators, including leukotrienes and prostaglandins, may cause activation and directed migration of polymorphonuclear leukocytes.[15,21]

## Leukotrienes

Various leukotrienes are synthesized from arachidonic acid metabolism of phospholipid cell membranes via the lipoxygenase pathway following mast cell activation.[1] The slow-reacting substance of anaphylaxis is a combination of leukotrienes $C_4$, $D_4$, and $E_4$.[13] Leukotrienes produce bronchoconstriction, increased capillary permeability, vasodilation, coronary vasoconstriction, and myocardial depression.[21]

## Prostaglandins

Prostaglandins are the products of arachidonic acid metabolism synthesized by the cyclooxygenase pathway.[22] They are potent mast cell mediators that produce vasodilation, bronchospasm, pulmonary hypertension, and increased capillary permeability.[15,21] Prostaglandin $D_2$, the major metabolite of mast cells, produces bronchospasm and vasodilation.[21] Elevated plasma levels of thromboxane $B_2$ (the metabolite of thromboxane $A_2$), also a prostaglandin synthesized by mast cells as well as polymorphonuclear leukocytes, have been demonstrated after protamine reactions associated with pulmonary hypertension.[1,16]

## Kinins

Small peptides called *kinins* are synthesized in mast cells to produce vasodilation, increased capillary permeability, and bronchoconstriction. The exact part that kinins play in anaphylaxis is not well understood. Bradykinin, a potent activator of vascular endothelium, stimulates the release of endothelium-derived relaxing factor and prostacyclin in a manner analogous to $H_1$ receptor stimulation.[1]

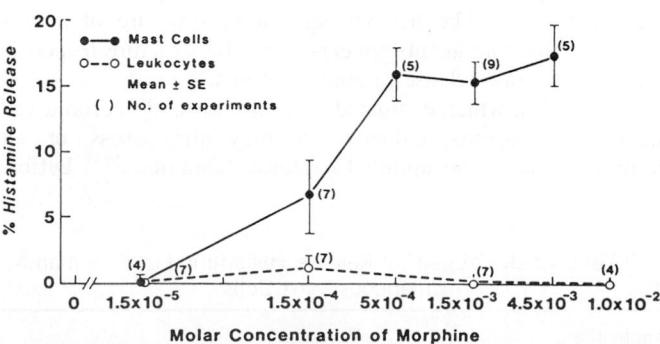

**FIGURE 42–3.** Percentage of histamine release from plasma leukocytes and human skin at increasing concentrations of morphine sulfate. Morphine sulfate induces dose-related histamine release from skin mast cell preparations but not from leukocyte preparations. (From Hermens JM, Eberty JM, Hanifan JM, et al. Comparison of histamine release in human skin mast cells by morphine, fentanyl, and oxymorphone. *Anesthesiology.* 1985;62:124.)

## Platelet-Activating Factor

Platelet-activating factor (PAF), an unstored lipid synthesized in activated human mast cells, is an extremely potent biologic material that produces physiologic effects at concentrations as low as $10^{-10}$ molar.[15] PAF aggregates and activates human platelets and perhaps leukocytes to release inflammatory products. PAF causes a profound wheal and flare response, smooth muscle contraction, and increased capillary permeability.[21]

## *How Is Anaphylaxis Recognized?*

When mast cells and basophils are activated and release mediators, their specific end-organ effects produce the clinical syndrome. Antigenic challenge in a sensitized individual usually produces immediate clinical manifestations of anaphylaxis, but the onset may be delayed 2 to 20 minutes.[1,22,23] The reaction may include symptoms and signs primarily in the cardiovascular and pulmonary systems.

The manifestations and course of anaphylaxis vary greatly from one affected individual to another.[1] A spectrum of reactions exists, ranging from minor clinical changes through acute cardiovascular or pulmonary dysfunction to cardiopulmonary arrest and death.[1] The problems clinicians face when anaphylactic reactions develop in the perioperative period are (1) the unpredictability of an attack, (2) the severity of the attack, and (3) the improbability that the patient will be aware of a prior allergy to an implicated drug.

## *What Are Non–IgE-Mediated Reactions?*

Other immunologic and nonimmunologic mechanisms liberate many of the mediators previously discussed, independent of IgE, creating a clinical syndrome identical to anaphylaxis. Specific pathways important in producing the same spectrum of clinical manifestations are considered later.

## *What Is Complement Activation?*

### Triggering Mechanisms

Complement activation can be triggered by either immunologic (antibody-mediated, ie, classic pathway) or nonimmunologic (alternative) pathways. The complement system is a series of multimolecular, self-assembling proteins that resemble the coagulation cascade. Activation of either pathway can liberate biologically active complement fragments of C3 and C5.[24]

### Effects

C3a and C5a are called *anaphylatoxins* because they release histamine from mast cells and basophils, contract smooth muscle, and increase capillary permeability.

### *Granulocytes*

In addition, C5a interacts with specific receptors on polymorphonuclear leukocytes and platelets, initiating granulocyte chemotaxis, aggregation, and activation.[25] Aggregated polymorphonuclear leukocytes can form microemboli that sequester in various organs, producing microvascular obstruction. When granulocytes aggregate, they also liberate inflammatory products such as arachidonic acid metabolites, oxygen-free radicals, and lysosomal enzymes.

Antibodies of the IgG class directed against antigenic determinants or granulocyte surfaces can also produce leukocyte aggregation.[1] These antibodies are called *leukoagglutinins* (white blood cell aggregation) and are implicated in the acute lung injury and respiratory distress that often follow transfusions.[1]

Investigators have also implicated complement activation and polymorphonuclear leukocyte aggregation in producing the clinical manifestations of acute pulmonary hypertension and right ventricular dysfunction following protamine reactions,[16] transfusion reactions,[26] adult respiratory distress syndrome,[27] and septic shock.[27]

## NONIMMUNOLOGIC RELEASE OF HISTAMINE

Various drugs administered during the perioperative period release histamine in a dose-dependent, nonimmunologic fashion (Table 42–3).[28-33] Intravenous administration of morphine, thiopental, atracurium, or vancomycin can release histamine, producing vasodilation, systemic hypotension, and urticaria along the vein of administration.[28,30,33]

## *What Are the Mechanisms?*

The mechanisms involved in nonimmunologic histamine release are not well understood but appear to represent noncytotoxic degranulation of mast cells (but not basophils).

### Opioids and Neuromuscular Blocking Agents

The opioids, morphine, meperidine, and codeine release histamine in human skin equipotently.[20,32] However, sufentanil, fentanyl, and alfentanil, all μ-receptor agonists, do not appear to release histamine when administered intravenously.[20]

Different molecular structures release histamine in human beings, suggesting that both opioid and nonopioid receptors are involved.[20,33] The benzylisoquinoline structure of neuromuscular blocking agents appears to be the structure responsible for histamine release in human beings.[33]

Our studies, which evaluated both opioids and neuromuscular blocking agents, indicate that they all possess, on an equimolar basis, the ability to release histamine.[20,33] Differ-

**TABLE 42–3.** Drugs That Release Histamine From Human Cutaneous Mast Cells

| | |
|---|---|
| Antibiotics | Vancomycin |
| Hyperosmotic agents | Mannitol, ionic radiocontrast media |
| Induction agents | Sodium thiopental, thiamylal |
| Muscle relaxants | Atracurium, *d*-tubocurarine, mivacurium, doxacurium |
| Opioids | Morphine, meperidine, codeine |
| Polybasic compounds | Protamine |

**TABLE 42–4.** Initial Therapy for Anaphylactic or Anaphylactoid Reactions

Stop administration of antigen if known or suspected
    Blood products
    Muscle relaxants
    Narcotics
    Antibiotics
Secure airway; administer 100% oxygen
Discontinue *all* anesthetic drugs
Infuse volume rapidly
Administer epinephrine

ences in histamine release reported represent different doses administered and not different abilities to release histamine (see Fig. 42–3).

## Precautions During Administration

Because mast cells reside in the perivascular spaces of the skin and other tissues, any drug known to release histamine should be given slowly and in a diluted solution (eg, vancomycin). Prior administration of antihistamines before injecting drugs that are known to release histamine in human beings does not directly inhibit histamine release but rather competes with histamine at the receptor and may attenuate decreases in systemic vascular resistance.[34] However, the effect of any drug on systemic vascular resistance may be dependent on other factors in addition to histamine release.[35,36]

## What Is the Appropriate Treatment for Anaphylaxis?

A plan for the treatment of anaphylactic or anaphylactoid reactions is outlined in Table 42–4. These life-saving interventions are essential to treat the hypotension and hypoxia that result from vasodilation, increased capillary permeability, and bronchospasm.[1] The treatment plan is the same for life-threatening anaphylactic or anaphylactoid reactions.

Drugs must be titrated with careful monitoring. Severe reactions require aggressive therapy and may be associated with refractory shock, pulmonary vasoconstriction and right heart failure, lower respiratory obstruction, or laryngeal obstruction that persists 5 to 32 hours despite appropriate and aggressive therapy.[37] All patients who have had an anaphylactic reaction should be admitted to a postanesthesia care unit (PACU) or intensive care unit for 24 hours of monitoring because they can develop a recurrence of manifestations after successful treatment.[1,37]

## Initial Therapy

### Stop Antigens

Blood products, antibiotics, protamine, or any other infusion should be stopped immediately at the first sign of anaphylactic reaction. Limiting antigen administration may prevent further recruitment of activated mast cells and basophils.

### Oxygenation, Ventilation

Profound hypoxemia, airway obstruction, and air trapping can occur during anaphylaxis, as well as ventilation-perfusion abnormalities producing hypoxemia.[1,38] Always administer 100% oxygen along with airway and ventilatory support as needed. Pulse oximetry, end-tidal carbon dioxide, and arterial blood gases should be monitored during the reaction resuscitation and into the intensive care unit or PACU.[1]

### Discontinue All Anesthetic Drugs

Inhalation anesthetic drugs are not the drugs of choice in treating allergy-mediated bronchospasm following anaphylaxis, especially when hypotension is present. These drugs interfere with the body's compensatory response to cardiovascular collapse. Furthermore, halothane sensitizes the myocardium to catecholamines, which must be administered in severe reactions.

### Volume Expansion

Hypovolemia rapidly ensues during anaphylactic shock. Fisher reported a loss of up to 40% of intravascular fluid into the interstitial space during reactions, as demonstrated by hemoconcentration.[39] Therefore, volume expansion is extremely important, in conjunction with epinephrine, in correcting the acute hypotension.

**Hypotension.** Initially, 2 to 4 L of lactated Ringer's solution, normal saline, or colloid solutions should be administered, keeping in mind that an additional 25 to 50 mL/kg may be necessary with persistent hypotension. Refractory hypotension following volume and epinephrine administration requires additional hemodynamic monitoring, including pulmonary and radial arterial catheterization for accurate assessment of intravascular volume and to guide rational therapeutic interventions.

**Pulmonary Edema.** Fulminant noncardiogenic pulmonary edema due to acute increases in pulmonary capillary permeability volume can occur after anaphylaxis.[1,38] This condition is due to loss of intravascular volume into pulmonary interstitial spaces in tissue and requires peak end-expiratory pressure (PEEP) or continuous positive airway pressure (CPAP), as well as intravascular volume repletion with careful hemodynamic monitoring until the capillary defect improves.

### Epinephrine

Epinephrine is the drug of choice in the initial resuscitation of patients during anaphylactic shock. Epinephrine stimulates $\alpha$-, $\beta_1$-, and $\beta_2$-adrenergic receptors. $\alpha$-Adrenergic effects constrict both venous capacitance and arterial resistance vessels to reverse hypotension; $\beta_2$-receptor stimulation bronchodilates and inhibits mediator release by increasing cyclic adenosine monophosphate (cAMP) in mast cells and basophils; and $\beta_1$-receptor stimulation increases myocardial contractility.

Epinephrine dosage and method of administration depend on the patient's condition. Rapid and timely intervention using common sense is crucial when treating anaphylaxis. During regional or general anesthesia, patients may have altered sympathoadrenergic responses to acute anaphylactic shock. Spinal or epidural anesthesia may partially sympathectomize patients, necessitating earlier intervention with larger doses of catecholamines.[40]

**Dosage.** In hypotensive patients, 5- to 10-$\mu$g intravenous boluses of epinephrine should be titrated to restore blood pressure. Additional volume and incrementally increased

**TABLE 42–5.** Secondary Therapy for Anaphylactic or Anaphylactoid Reactions

| | |
|---|---|
| Antihistamines | Corticosteroids |
| Catecholamine infusions | Sodium bicarbonate |
| Phosphodiesterase inhibitors | Airway evaluation |

doses of epinephrine should be administered until hypotension is corrected.[1] Although an infusion is the ideal method to administer epinephrine, it is usually impossible to infuse the drug through peripheral intravenous routes during acute volume resuscitation.

With cardiovascular collapse, full intravenous cardiopulmonary resuscitative doses of epinephrine, 0.5 to 1.0 mg, should be administered and repeated until hemodynamic stability occurs. In patients without intravenous access, epinephrine can be administered into the endotracheal tube. Epinephrine should not be administered intravenously to patients with normal blood pressure.[1,41]

## Secondary Treatment

After initial treatment, additional therapy may be useful (Table 42–5).

### Antihistamines

Because $H_1$ receptors mediate many of the adverse effects of histamine, intravenous administration of 0.5 to 1 mg/kg of an $H_1$ antagonist, such as diphenhydramine, may be useful in treating acute anaphylaxis. The $H_1$ antagonists currently available for parenteral administration may have antidopaminergic effects and should be given slowly to prevent precipitous hypotension in potentially hypovolemic patients.[1] The indication for administering an $H_2$ antagonist once anaphylaxis has occurred remains unclear.

### Catecholamine Infusions

Catecholamines are important first- and second-line therapeutic agents in the treatment of anaphylaxis. Specific direct-acting catecholamines—epinephrine, norepinephrine, and isoproterenol—should be administered as needed for their $\alpha$-, $\beta_1$-, and $\beta_2$-adrenergic effects. Indirect acting catecholamines, such as dopamine, should not be first-line therapeutic agents.

**Epinephrine.** Epinephrine infusions may be useful in patients with persistent hypotension or bronchospasm after initial resuscitation.[1] Epinephrine infusions should be started at 4 to 8 $\mu$g/min and titrated to correct hypotension.

**Norepinephrine.** Norepinephrine infusions of 4 to 8 $\mu$g/min may be required in patients with refractory hypotension due to decreased systemic vascular resistance. They should be adjusted to correct hypotension.[1]

**Isoproterenol.** Isoproterenol infusions can be used in patients with refractory bronchospasm, pulmonary hypertension, or right ventricular dysfunction. The usual starting dose is 0.5 to 1 $\mu$g/min. Isoproterenol has profound $\beta_2$-adrenergic effects that can produce systemic vasodilation; therefore, it must be used cautiously in hypotensive or hypovolemic patients.[1]

### Phosphodiesterase Inhibitors

Phosphodiesterase inhibitors prevent the catabolism of cyclic nucleotides in cells. The net effect is to increase intracellular levels of cAMP and cyclic guanosine monophosphate.[42] These drugs also act additively with catecholamines to augment the production of intracellular nucleotides.

**Aminophylline.** Aminophylline is the most commonly used phosphodiesterase inhibitor. Its therapeutic effectiveness in patients with asthma and chronic obstructive pulmonary disease may be due to improvements in diaphragmatic contractility, augmentation of right and left ventricular ejection fraction, and reduction in pulmonary vascular resistance.

**Amrinone, Milrinone, Enoximone.** The newer cAMP-specific phosphodiesterase inhibitors—drugs such as amrinone, milrinone, and enoximone—also increase biventricular contractility and decrease pulmonary and systemic vascular resistance.

In patients with persistent pulmonary hypertension and right ventricular dysfunction following anaphylactic reactions, these drugs are important therapeutic considerations and should be administered in addition to the catecholamines.

### Corticosteroids

**Mechanisms of Action.** Although corticosteroids are not first-line therapeutic agents, they help to correct anaphylaxis by mechanisms that include decreasing arachidonic acid metabolites, inhibiting phospholipid membrane breakdown, and preventing or attenuating the activation and migration of polymorphonuclear leukocytes.[43,44]

Corticosteroids may require from 12 to 24 hours to work and, despite their unproven usefulness in treating acute reactions, they often are administered as adjuncts to therapy when refractory bronchospasm or shock occurs after anaphylaxis.

**Dosage.** The appropriate corticosteroid dose and preparation are not established to treat anaphylaxis; however, 0.25 to 1 g of hydrocortisone appears to be an appropriate dose for IgE-mediated reactions. Alternatively, 1 to 2 g of methylprednisolone (30-35 mg/kg) may be useful in treating reactions that are thought to be complement mediated, such as acute pulmonary hypertension following protamine administration or transfusion reactions.[44] Administering corticosteroids after an anaphylactic reaction may also be important in attenuating the late-phase reactions reported to occur 12 to 24 hours after anaphylaxis.[37]

### Sodium Bicarbonate

During anaphylactic shock, acidosis develops rapidly, diminishing the beneficial effects of epinephrine on the heart and systemic vasculature. With refractory hypotension or acidemia, sodium bicarbonate, 0.5 to 1 mEq/kg, should be given and repeated every 5 minutes or as indicated by arterial blood gas and pH analysis. (For a detailed analysis of new guidelines for bicarbonate therapy, see Chapter 47.)

### Airway Evaluation

Laryngeal edema and airway obstruction can occur after anaphylactoid reactions; therefore, the airway should be evaluated before extubation of the trachea.[1,37] In patients with persistent facial edema, underlying airway edema can also occur; they should remain intubated until the edema subsides. The development of a significant air leak after endotracheal tube cuff deflation is useful in assessing airway patency before extubation of the trachea. If there is any question of airway

**TABLE 42–6.** Agents Most Often Implicated in
Perioperative Anaphylaxis

| | |
|---|---|
| Antibiotics | Latex |
| Blood products | Neuromuscular blocking agents |
| Chymopapain | Protamine |
| Induction agents | |

edema, direct laryngoscopy should be performed before extubation.

## PERIOPERATIVE ANAPHYLAXIS

### What Drugs Are Implicated?

Many of the potentially offending agents have already been discussed. Almost every drug, at some time, has been implicated in producing an anaphylactic reaction.[1,45–61] The incidence of perioperative anaphylaxis varies, depending on the country reporting, but appears to be approximately 1 in 5000 to 25 000 anesthetized patients.

Agents most often implicated are listed in Table 42–6. Latex (rubber) is an environmental antigen that is ubiquitous in anesthetic, intravenous, and operative equipment. Patients who have spina bifida and who have undergone multiple surgical procedures, as well as health workers, are potentially at increased risk for anaphylaxis to latex. These individuals appear to be sensitized from repeated exposure to this large foreign plant antigen.

Drugs that are nonimmunologic histamine releasers may cause a higher incidence of adverse drug reactions and produce acute cardiovascular dysfunction with rapid intravenous administration. Vancomycin, which produces its adverse effects by histamine release, is a noteworthy example. Slow administration of a diluted solution is important to prevent severe reactions.

### How Is an Allergic Reaction Recognized?

Only a small percentage of adverse drug reactions are allergic in nature (Table 42–7).

#### Signs and Symptoms

Observed clinical signs and symptoms of the allergic reaction do not resemble known pharmacologic actions of the drug. The temporal relationship between exposure to the drug and clinical manifestations of the adverse drug reaction is the most important information to determine which administered drugs were the cause of a suspected allergic reaction.[62]

Although the reaction may produce a life-threatening response in the cardiopulmonary system (anaphylaxis), other clinical presentations of drug allergy include cutaneous eruptions, fever, and pulmonary reactions.[62] The reaction can usually be reproduced by giving very small doses of the suspected drug or other agents possessing similar or cross-reacting chemical structures.

On occasion, drug-specific antibodies or lymphocytes that react with the suspected drug have been identified, although this test is seldom diagnostically useful in practice. As with adverse drug reactions in general, the reaction usually subsides within several days after discontinuation of the drug.[62]

#### Historical Factors

Life-threatening allergic reactions are more likely to occur in patients with a history of allergy, atopy, or asthma.[46] Nevertheless, because the incidence is low, the presence of such a history is not a reliable predictor that an allergic reaction will occur and does not mandate that these patients should be investigated or pretreated or that specific drugs be selected or avoided. Drugs and foreign substances implicated in producing adverse drug reactions may have both immunologic and nonimmunologic mechanisms.

### How Should Patients Be Evaluated?

Identification of the drug responsible for a suspected allergic reaction still depends on a high degree of clinical suspicion implicating the temporal sequence of drug administration. Conventional in vivo and in vitro methods to diagnose allergic reactions to most anesthetic drugs are either unavailable or not applicable to supporting the diagnosis of an allergic reaction.

The most important factor in diagnosis is a physician's awareness that an untoward event may be related to a drug that a patient received.[1,62] Always be aware that any drug may produce a life-threatening anaphylactic reaction.

A clinical history is extremely important when evaluating whether an adverse drug reaction is allergic and whether the drug can be readministered. Although a prior allergic reaction to the drug in question is important, it is rarely ascertained. Although an anesthesiologist commonly administers small test doses of anesthetic drugs, these doses represent large numbers of molecules and have nothing to do with immunologic doses.[1]

#### Specific Tests

The demonstration of drug-specific IgE antibodies is generally accepted as evidence that a patient may be at risk for anaphylaxis if the drug is administered.[62] Different clinically available tests to confirm or diagnose drug allergy have been reported and are individually considered in Table 42–8.

For a patient who has had a suspected anaphylactic reaction, the causative agent should be identified to prevent readministration. When one particular drug has been administered and a clear correlation between time of administration and occurrence of reaction can be demonstrated, then testing may be

**TABLE 42–7.** Characteristics of an Allergic Reaction

Occur in a small percentage of patients
Unrelated to known pharmacologic drug actions
Temporally related to the suspected drug administration
Produced by the presence of an immunospecific antibody

**TABLE 42–8.** Tests Used to Evaluate Patients After Anaphylaxis

Radioallergosorbent testing
Enzyme-linked immunosorbent assay testing
Intradermal testing (skin testing)

unnecessary and the drug should not be readministered. However, when patients simultaneously receive multiple drugs (eg, induction agent, opioid, muscle relaxant, and antibiotic), determining which particular drug caused the reaction is more difficult.

When patients want to know which drug was the culprit or when patients are scheduled for several other procedures, some degree of allergy evaluation should be undertaken to determine the implicated drug. Unfortunately, few in vitro tests exist for anesthetic drugs. Currently available allergy tests are discussed.

### Radioallergosorbent Test

The radioallergosorbent test detects specific IgE antibodies directed toward particular antigens.[63] In this test, antigens are linked to an insoluble matrix such as sepharose, cellulose, or paper to make an immunoabsorbent and are then incubated with the serum from the patient to be evaluated so that immunospecific antibodies directed toward the antigen can bind. After washing, the antigen-antibody complex on the immunoabsorbent is incubated with radioactive iodine-labeled antibodies directed against human IgE, and the complex is counted in a scintillation counter to evaluate the concentration of specific IgE.

The radioallergosorbent test is more quantitative than skin tests and avoids the risk of re-exposure of an antigen to a patient who had a life-threatening anaphylactic reaction. However, it is more expensive, and the antigens available for anesthetic drug testing are limited. Radioallergosorbent testing has been used to detect the presence of IgE antibodies to meperidine, protamine, muscle relaxants, propofol, and thiopental.[1,64,65] Two major limitations of this test are the commercial unavailability of a drug prepared as an antigen and potential false-positive test results.

### Enzyme-Linked Immunosorbent Assay

The enzyme-linked immunosorbent assay also measures antigen-specific antibodies. The basis of this test is similar to the radioallergosorbent test. IgE antibodies directed against the antigen in question are determined by the addition of an anti-IgE coupled to peroxidase, an enzyme that acts as a chromogen. A colorless substrate is converted by peroxidase to produce a colored byproduct.

The enzyme-linked immunosorbent assay has been used to demonstrate IgE antibodies to chymopapain and protamine and has been developed to screen patients for other antibodies to infectious agents such as HIV, but no tests for anesthetic drugs are clinically available.[1]

### Intradermal Testing (Skin Testing)

Skin testing is the method most widely used to confirm specific sensitivity in patients who have had anaphylactic reactions to anesthetic drugs.[66–69] After intradermal antigen injection, histamine released from cutaneous mast cells causes flare and wheal.

Fisher has used this technique extensively, and multiple reports from his group and others suggest that it is a safe and useful method for establishing a diagnosis in most cases of suspected anaphylactic reactions.[66,67] Intradermal testing can determine cross-sensitivity among drugs of similar structures,

an especially important factor when evaluating patients after reactions to the neuromuscular blocking agents.

Skin testing for local anesthetics is considered a direct challenge or provocative dose testing.[69] Local anesthetic drugs are injected in increasing quantities under controlled circumstances. This test determines if an individual can safely receive amide derivatives (eg, lidocaine), and it can also be used to determine sensitivity to the *para*-aminobenzoic ester agents (eg, tetracaine or procaine).

## SUMMARY

Allergic reactions are adverse drug reactions that are produced by pathologic activation of the immune system. The most life-threatening form of allergic reaction is anaphylaxis, which can manifest as acute cardiovascular and pulmonary dysfunction produced by physiologic responses to the mediators released from mast cells and basophils. Other immune and nonimmune pathways may also be activated to produce a similar clinical syndrome of cardiopulmonary dysfunction.

Recognition and appropriate therapy are important clinical considerations. Because any drug can potentially produce anaphylaxis, anticipation that a drug may be implicated in perioperative cardiovascular collapse is important. Certain drugs and environmental antigens are more likely to be implicated.

Although different tests have been studied to evaluate patients after anaphylaxis, skin testing is the most often reported and readily available method.

### References

1. Levy JH. *Anaphylactic Reactions in Anesthesia and Intensive Care.* 2nd ed. Boston, Mass: Butterworth-Heinemann; 1992.
2. Stevenson GW, Hall SC, Rudnick S, et al. The effect of anesthetic agents on the human immune response. *Anesthesiology.* 1990;72:542.
3. Walton B. Anaesthesia, surgery, and immunology. *Anaesthesia.* 1978;33:322.
4. Roitt I, Brostoff J, Male D, eds. *Immunology.* St Louis, Mo: CV Mosby; 1989.
5. Metcalf DD. Effector cell heterogeneity in immediate hypersensitivity reactions. *Clin Rev Allergy.* 1982;1:311.
6. Ishizaka T. Analysis of triggering events in mast cells for immunoglobulin E-mediated histamine release. *J Allergy Clin Immunol.* 1981;67:90.
7. Porter J, Jick H. Drug-induced anaphylaxis, convulsions, deafness, and extrapyramidal symptoms. *Lancet.* 1977;1:587.
8. Portier MM, Richet C. De l'action anaphylactique de certains venins. *CR Soc Biol.* 1902;54:170.
9. Gomez E, Corrado OJ, Baldwin DL, et al. Direct in vivo evidence for mast cell degranulation during allergen-induced reactions in man. *J Allergy Clin Immunol.* 1986;78:637.
10. Kazimierczak W, Diamant B. Mechanisms of histamine release in anaphylactic and anaphylactoid reactions. *Prog Allergy.* 1978;4:295.
11. Ginsburg R, Bristow MR, Stinson EB, et al. Histamine receptors in the human heart. *Life Sci.* 1980;26:2245.
12. Majno G, Palade GE. Studies on inflammation, I: the effect of histamine and serotonin on vascular permeability: an electron microscopic study. *J Biosphys Biochem Cytol.* 1961;11:571.
13. Parker CW. Leukotrienes: their metabolism, structure, and role in allergic responses. In: Samuelsson B, Paoletti R, eds. *Leukotrienes and Other Lipoxygenase Products.* New York, NY: Raven Press; 1982:115–126.
14. Oflaherty JT, Wylde RL: Mediators of anaphylaxis. *Clin Lab Med.* 1983;3:619.
15. Schulman ES, Newball HH, Demers LM, et al. Anaphylactic release of thromboxane A$_2$, prostaglandin D$_2$, and prostacyclin from human lung parenchyma. *Am Rev Respir Dis.* 1981;124:402.
16. Morel DR, Zapol WM, Thomas SJ, et al. C5a and thromboxane generation associated with pulmonary vaso- and bronchoconstriction during protamine reversal of heparin. *Anesthesiology.* 1987;66:597.

17. Meier HL, Kaplan AP, Lichtenstein LM, et al. Anaphylactic release of a prekallikrein activator from human lung in vitro. *Clin Invest.* 1983;72:574.

18. Weiss ME, Adkinson NF, McFadden R Jr, et al. Airway constriction in normal humans produced by inhalation of leukotriene D. *JAMA.* 1983;249:2814.

19. Reinhardt D, Borchard V. H$_1$ receptor antagonists: comparative pharmacology and clinical use. *Klin Wochenschr.* 1982;60:983.

20. Levy JH, Brister NW, Shearin WA, et al. Wheal and flare responses to opioids in humans. *Anesthesiology.* 1989;70:756.

21. Pavek K, Wegmann A, Nordström L, et al. Cardiovascular and respiratory mechanisms in anaphylactic and anaphylactoid shock reactions. *Klin Wochenschr.* 1982;60:941.

22. Goldberg M. The allergic response and its treatment. *Curr Rev Clin Anesth.* 1985;5:153.

23. Delage C, Irey NS. Anaphylactic deaths: a clinicopathologic study of 43 cases. *J Forensic Sci.* 1972;17:525.

24. Frank MM. Complement: a brief review. *J Allergy Clin Immunol.* 1988;84:411.

25. Dubois M, Lotze MT, Diamond WI, et al. Pulmonary shunting during leukoagglutinin-induced noncardiogenic pulmonary edema. *JAMA.* 1989;244:2186.

26. Teissner B, Brandslund I, Grunnet N, et al. Acute complement activation during an anaphylactoid reaction to blood transfusion and the disappearance rate of C3c and C3d from the circulation. *J Clin Lab Immunol.* 1983;12:63.

27. Hammerschmidt DE, Weaver LJ, Hudson LD, et al. Association of complement activation and elevated plasma-C5a with adult respiratory distress syndrome. *Lancet.* 1980;1:947.

28. Rosow CE, Moss J, Philbin DM, et al. Histamine release during morphine and fentanyl anesthesia. *Anesthesiology.* 1982;56:93.

29. Hirshman CA, Edelstein RA, Eastman CL. Histamine release by barbiturates in human mast cells. *Anesthesiology.* 1985;63:353.

30. Levy JH, Kettlekamp N, Goertz P, et al. Histamine release by vancomycin: a mechanism for hypotension in man. *Anesthesiology.* 1987;67:122.

31. Hermens JM, Ebertz JM, Hanifin JM, et al. Comparison of histamine release in human skin mast cells by morphine, fentanyl, and oxymorphone. *Anesthesiology.* 1983;62:124.

32. Casale TB, Bowman S, Kaliner M. Induction of human cutaneous mast cell degranulation by opiates and endogenous opioid peptides: evidence for opiate and nonopiate receptor participation. *J Allergy Clin Immunol.* 1984;73:775.

33. Levy JH, Adelson DM, Walker BF. Wheal and flare responses to muscle relaxants in humans. *Agents Actions.* 1991;34:302.

34. Philbin DM, Moss J, Akins CW, et al. The use of H$_1$ and H$_2$ histamine antagonists with morphine anesthesia: a double-blind study. *Anesthesiology.* 1981;55:292.

35. Hirshman CA, Downes H, Butler J. Relevance of plasma histamine levels to hypotension. *Anesthesiology.* 1982;57:424.

36. Levy JH, Hug CC. Cardiopulmonary bypass as a model to study the effects of drugs on myocardial function. *Br J Anaesth.* 1988;60:35S.

37. Stark BJ, Sullivan TJ. Biphasic and protracted anaphylaxis. *J Allergy Clin Immunol.* 1986;78:76.

38. Levy JH, Rockoff MR. Anaphylaxis to meperidine. *Anesth Analg.* 1982;61:301.

39. Fisher MM. Blood volume replacement in acute anaphylactic cardiovascular collapse related to anaesthesia. *Br J Anaesth.* 1977;49:1023.

40. Barnett A, Hirshman CA. Anaphylactic reaction to cephapirin during spinal anesthesia. *Anesth Analg.* 1979;58:337.

41. Levy JH. Cardiovascular changes during anaphylactic/anaphylactoid reactions in man. *J Clin Anesth.* 1989;1:426.

42. Levy JH, Ramsay JM, Bailey JM. Pharmacokinetics and pharmacodynamics of phosphodiesterase III inhibitors. *J Cardiothorac Anesth.* 1990;4(S):7.

43. Hammerschmidt DE, White JG, Craddock PR, et al. Corticosteroids inhibit complement-induced granulocyte aggregation. A possible mechanism for their efficacy in shock states. *J Clin Invest.* 1979;63:798.

44. Sheagren JN. Septic shock and corticosteroids [editorial]. *N Engl J Med.* 1981;305:456.

45. Laxenaire MC, Moneret-Vautrin DA, Vervloet D, et al. Accidents anaphylactoides graves peranesthétiques. *Ann Fr Anesth Reanim.* 1985;4:30.

46. Fisher MM, Outhred A, Bowey CJ. Can clinical anaphylaxis to anaesthetic drugs be predicted from allergic history? *Br J Anaesth.* 1987;59:690.

47. Fisher MM, Munro I. Life-threatening anaphylactoid reactions to muscle relaxants. *Anesth Analg.* 1983;62:559.

48. Laxenaire MC, Moneret-Vautrin DA, Watkins J. Diagnosis of the causes of anaphylactoid anaesthetic reactions. *Anaesthesia.* 1983;38:147.

49. Vervloet D, Nizankowska E, Arnaud A, et al. Adverse reactions to suxamethonium and other muscle relaxants under general anesthesia. *J Allergy Clin Immunol.* 1983;71:552.

50. Assem ESK, Frost PG, Levis RD. Anaphylactoid-like reaction to suxamethonium. *Anaesthesia.* 1981;36:405.

51. Bennet MJ, Anderson LK, McMillan JC, et al. Anaphylactic reaction during anesthesia associated with positive intradermal skin test to fentanyl. *Can Anaesth Soc J.* 1986;33:75.

52. Hilgard P. Immunological reactions to blood and blood products. *Br J Anesth.* 1979;51:45.

53. Sheffer AL, Pennoyer DS. Management of adverse drug reactions. *J Allergy Clin Immunol.* 1984;74:580.

54. Levy JH, Zaidan JR, Faraj B. Prospective evaluation of risk of protamine reactions in NPH insulin-dependent diabetics. *Anesth Analg.* 1986;65:739.

55. Doolan L, McKenzie I, Krafchek J, et al. Protamine sulphate hypersensitivity. *Anesth Intensive Care.* 1981;9:147.

56. Goldberg M. Systemic reactions to intravascular contrast media. A guide for the anesthesiologist. *Anesthesiology.* 1984;60:46.

57. Isbister JP, Fisher MM. Adverse effects of plasma volume expanders. *Anesth Intensive Care.* 1980;8:145.

58. Colman WR. Paradoxical hypotension after volume expansion with plasma protein fraction. *N Engl J Med.* 1978;299:97.

59. Ring K, Messmer K. Incidence and severity of anaphylactoid to colloid volume substitutes. *Lancet.* 1977;1:466.

60. Gold M, Swartz JS, Braude BM, et al. Intraoperative anaphylaxis: an association with latex sensitivity. *J Allergy Clin Immunol.* 1991;87:662.

61. Nguyen DH, Burns MW, Shapiro GG, et al. Intraoperative cardiovascular collapse secondary to latex allergy. *J Urol.* 1991;146:571.

62. De Swarte RD. Drug allergy-problems and strategies. *J Allergy Clin Immunol.* 1984;74:209.

63. Johansson SGO. In vitro diagnosis of reagin-mediated allergic diseases. *Allergy.* 1978;33:292.

64. Baldo BA, Fisher MM. Detection of serum IgE antibodies that react with alcuronium and tubocurarine after life-threatening reactions to muscle relaxants. *Anaesth Intensive Care.* 1983;11:194.

65. Harle DG, Baldo BA, Smal MA, et al. Detection of thiopentone-reactive IgE antibodies following anaphylactoid reactions during anesthesia. *Clin Allergy.* 1986;16:493.

66. Fisher MM. Intradermal testing after anaphylactoid reaction to anaesthetic drugs: practical aspects of performance and interpretation. *Anaesth Intensive Care.* 1984;12:115.

67. Fisher MM, Munro I. Life threatening, anaphylactoid reactions to muscle relaxants. *Anesth Analg.* 1983;62:559.

68. Sage D. Intradermal drug testing following anaphylactoid reactions during anesthesia. *Anaesth Intensive Care.* 1981;9:381.

69. Shatz M. Skin testing and incremental challenge in the evaluation of adverse reactions to local anesthetics. *J Allergy Clin Immunol.* 1984;74:606.

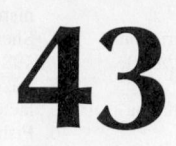

# Myocardial Ischemia and Dysfunction

Martin J. London

Kathryn Rouine-Rapp

## PERIOPERATIVE MYOCARDIAL ISCHEMIA

*What Is It and What Are Its Hemodynamic Causes?*

*What Is the Ischemic Cascade?*

*What Is the Most Useful Clinical Tool to Detect Ischemia?*

*How Is Transesophageal Echocardiography Used to Detect Ischemia?*

*What Are the Major Types of Ischemia and Their Effects on Ventricular Function?*

*What Characteristics of Ischemia Are Unique to Patients With Coronary Artery Disease?*

*Does Treatment of Perioperative ST Segment Changes Alter Outcome?*

*When Is a Patient With Coronary Artery Disease Ready for Surgery?*

## ANESTHESIA AND INTRAOPERATIVE ISCHEMIA

*Is There a Best Technique?*

## MYOCARDIAL DYSFUNCTION

*What Are the Determinants of Stroke Volume?*

*How Is Myocardial Dysfunction Assessed?*

*What Are the Effects of Inhalational Anesthetics?*

*What Are the Effects of Narcotics?*

*Is Regional Anesthesia Safer Than General Anesthesia for At-Risk Patients?*

## INTRAOPERATIVE ISCHEMIA

*How Should It Be Treated?*

*How Is Cardiogenic Shock Managed?*

## POSTOPERATIVE MYOCARDIAL INFARCTION

*What Is the Clinical Presentation and Timing?*

*What Is the Incidence?*

*What Are the Suspected Perioperative Etiologic Factors?*

*When and How Should a Patient Be Ruled Out for Myocardial Infarction?*

*How Is Myocardial Dysfunction Assessed and Quantitated?*

*Which Patients Are at Greatest Risk?*

## TREATMENT OF PERIOPERATIVE MYOCARDIAL DYSFUNCTION

*What Are the Pharmacologic Options?*

*How Should Actual or Potential Perioperative Dysfunction Be Monitored?*

## PREOPERATIVE OPTIMIZATION OF PATIENTS WITH MYOCARDIAL DYSFUNCTION

*How Should It Be Done?*

Perioperative myocardial ischemia presents a complex and often frustrating series of diagnostic and therapeutic problems for an anesthesia practitioner. An increasing number of clinical studies suggest that vigorous detection and therapy of perioperative ischemia significantly improve patients' outcome. Although patients with manifest or occult coronary artery disease (CAD) are the largest group at risk for development of ischemia and postoperative infarction, clinical situations also occur in which ischemia may develop *in the absence* of CAD. ST segment changes consistent with ischemia are common in patients with aortic stenosis (ie, subendocardial ischemia), in otherwise healthy women undergoing cesarean section, and even in neonates undergoing cardiac surgery for congenital lesions (eg, arterial switch operation). However, the implications of ischemia in patients with CAD are emphasized and discussed in detail in this chapter.

## PERIOPERATIVE MYOCARDIAL ISCHEMIA

### What Is It and What Are Its Hemodynamic Causes?

In the simplest pathophysiologic terms (ie, assuming normal coronary arteries and myocardium), ischemia results from a significant imbalance of myocardial oxygen ($O_2$) supply and demand (Fig. 43–1). The key determinants of myocardial $O_2$ consumption are depicted in Figure 43–2. Although the basic determinants appear to be straightforward, the relations between them are not. Recall that they are components of a complex homeostatic system; they exert either negative or

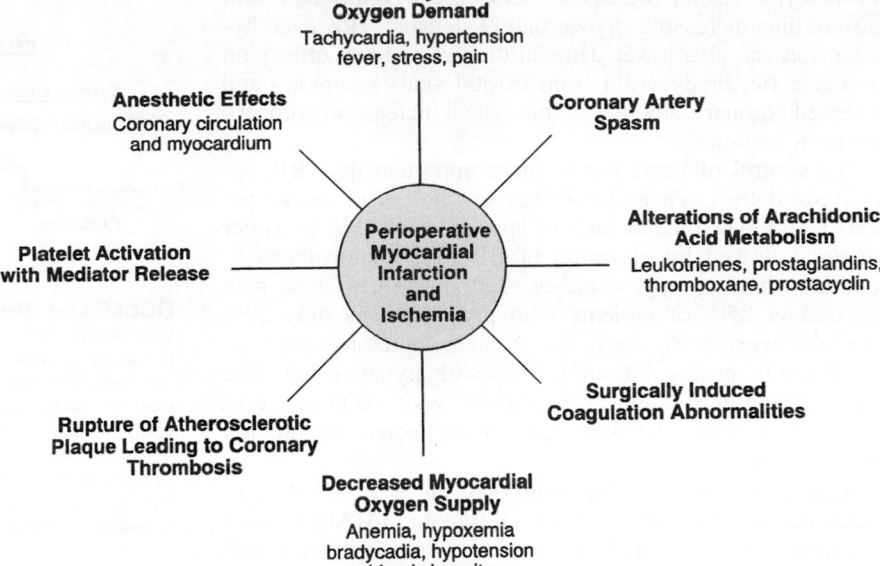

FIGURE 43–1. Many factors, both morphologic and physiologic, influence myocardial oxygen balance. The anesthesiologist can effectively manipulate most of the physiologic and hemodynamic factors. However, our ability to influence the many factors involved in the pathogenesis of ischemia directly related to coronary artery disease is very limited. (From London MJ. Silent ischemia and postoperative infarction. *J Cardiothorac Vasc Anesth*. 1990;4[suppl 1]:60.)

positive gains within the system; and they act in varying combinations. Thus, a clinician must strive to dissect the system to its simplest level first. This process may be straightforward, although in sicker patients, complex interactions are more likely to occur.

## Heart Rate

Although indices derived from various parameters—either noninvasive (eg, rate pressure product, the product of heart rate and systolic blood pressure [BP]) or invasive (eg, tension-time index, the product of mean systolic pressure and systolic duration)—have been used to estimate myocardial $O_2$ consumption ($M\dot{V}O_2$), the bulk of evidence suggests that tachycardia is the most important clinical variable.[1]

There is a distinct trend in clinical practice emphasizing the control of heart rate as a major goal of perioperative hemodynamic management with increasing evidence in the literature suggesting an etiologic role for tachycardia in perioperative non–Q-wave infarction. Heart rate is a key determinant not only of myocardial $O_2$ demand but also of myocardial $O_2$ supply, moderating the time during which coronary blood flow occurs (diastolic perfusion time). In the left ventricle (LV), blood flow is restricted almost exclusively to diastole because systolic compression of intramural coronary arteries "throttles" forward blood flow. The relationship between heart rate and diastolic time is nonlinear, with small changes in rate producing large increases in diastolic time, especially at lower heart rates[2] (Fig. 43–3).

## Blood Pressure

Alteration in systemic BP alters the myocardial supply-demand equation in a more complex manner than heart rate.

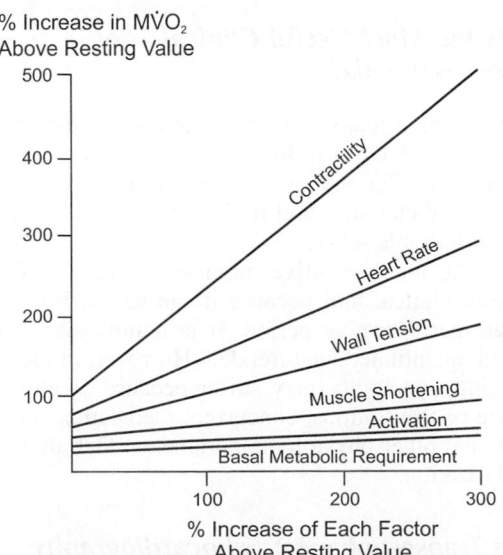

FIGURE 43–2. A stylized depiction of the relative importance of various physiologic parameters and myocardial oxygen consumption. (From Marcus ML. *The Coronary Circulation in Health and Disease*. New York, NY: McGraw-Hill; 1983:70.)

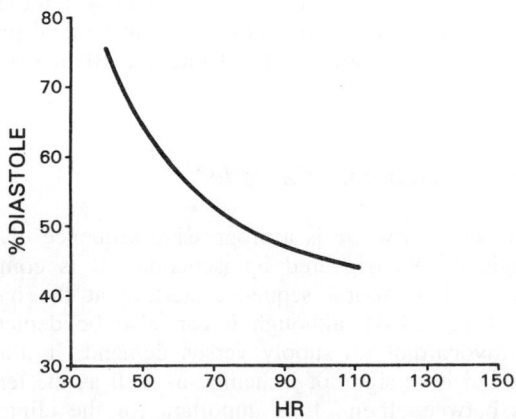

FIGURE 43–3. The relation between heart rate and percentage of the cardiac cycle spent in diastole is shown. Note the nonlinear relationship, in which small changes in heart rate produce large increases in diastolic time, especially at low heart rates (eg, 15% increase from 70 to 50 bpm). HR, heart rate in beats per minute. (From Boudoulas H, Rittgers SE, Lewis RP, et al. Changes in diastolic time with various pharmacologic agents. *Circulation*. 1979;60:165.)

Severe hypertension increases afterload and ventricular wall tension, thus increasing myocardial $O_2$ demand. However, hypertension can also lower demand through indirect effects on heart rate (ie, bradycardia from carotid sinus receptors) and increased coronary blood flow through an increase in coronary perfusion pressure.

That control of heart rate is more important than BP was emphasized by Loeb and colleagues, who paced awake patients with CAD to heart rates of approximately 140 beats per minute, followed by elevation of BP with methoxamine to systolic values of approximately 200 mm Hg.[3] Chest pain occurred in 85% of patients with pacing versus only 30% with hypertension. Similarly, ST segment depression occurred in 70% with pacing but only 15% with hypertension. The critical lesson here is that hypertension (with maintenance of a normal preload) increases rather than decreases coronary perfusion pressure.

Buffington, using a highly controlled canine model, demonstrated that the ratio of mean arterial pressure (MAP) to heart rate, rather than their product, is more closely correlated with regional ischemia.[4] Between MAPs of 60 and 120 mm Hg, ischemia occurred only when heart rate exceeded the MAP (MAP/heart rate ratio <1.0). This observation is a useful rule of thumb to consider when treating ischemia believed to be related to hemodynamic insufficiency, rather than that mediated by local factors, vasomotor tone, or vascular factors (eg, thrombus). Despite these laboratory findings, clinical studies have been conflicting and this index has not seen widespread clinical acceptance.

### Contractility, Wall Tension, and Other Factors

As noted in Figure 43–2, contractility is a primary determinant of myocardial $O_2$ demand. Practitioners are well aware that sudden catecholamine surges due to light anesthesia or unexpected surgical stimulation can cause myocardial ischemia. This is usually accompanied by simultaneous elevation of BP, heart rate, and contractility. In this situation, volatile anesthetics, with their dose-related depressant effects on contractility, may exert a beneficial effect. However, the sympathetic-stimulating properties of desflurane (noted primarily with a rapid increase in end-tidal concentration) may exacerbate the situation. Measurement of contractility, wall tension, and other minor determinants is difficult in clinical practice, hence the greater reliance on heart rate and BP management in routine practice.

### *What Is the Ischemic Cascade?*

The *ischemic cascade* is a progressive sequence of pathophysiologic events triggered by ischemia.[5] It is commonly displayed as a temporal sequence starting at the onset of ischemia (Fig. 43–4), although it can also be depicted by plotting myocardial $O_2$ supply versus demand. It illustrates the most sensitive signs of ischemia, as well as the temporal relations between them. It is important for the clinician to appreciate the steps of the cascade because they constitute the functional clinical outcomes of ischemia that may eventually lead to myocardial infarction (MI). The clinician may (or may not) be able to intervene at various stages of the cascade, depending on the ultimate cause (ie, morphologic versus functional physiologic).

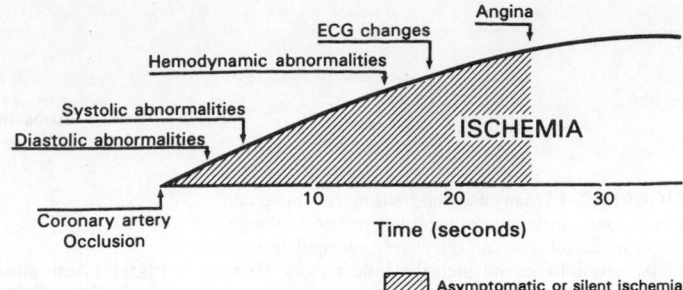

**FIGURE 43–4.** The ischemic cascade depicted as the approximate temporal sequence of physiologic abnormalities after onset of ischemia. Note that the exact sequence is variable, particularly with regard to the onset of electrocardiographic (ECG) changes, hemodynamic changes, and angina. In most instances, ECG changes occur earlier than depicted here. Hemodynamic changes (eg, decreased cardiac output) occur only after compensatory mechanisms (eg, hyperkinesis of adjacent nonischemic myocardium) fail. In many patients, angina does not occur (silent myocardial ischemia). (From Kennedy HL, Wiens RD. Ambulatory [Holter] electrocardiography and myocardial ischemia. *Am Heart J.* 1989;117:165.)

The earliest steps of the cascade include alterations of diastolic compliance with an increase in LV end-diastolic pressure (LVEDP). As ischemia worsens, systolic function is altered, and regional wall motion abnormalities (WMAs) occur. The latter may be observed with echocardiography. Subsequently, surface electrocardiographic (ECG) changes occur and later still, anginal chest pain in awake patients. A global reduction in ventricular function occurs only if the compensatory response of adjacent nonischemic myocardium is inadequate or if the ischemia is global (ie, subendocardial ischemia due to severe hypotension, reducing coronary blood flow in all perfusion territories).

Although the cascade is best considered a continuum, in certain instances, various signs may not occur (eg, no angina with silent myocardial ischemia [SMI]). Also, the signs of ischemia may not reverse in the same temporal order in which they occurred (eg, the persistence of WMAs despite resolution of ECG changes with stunned myocardium).

### *What Is the Most Useful Clinical Tool to Detect Ischemia?*

There are three major clinical tools used to detect myocardial ischemia: ECG, two-dimensional transesophageal echocardiography (TEE), and pulmonary artery (PA) catheterization.[6] The characteristics and limitations of these monitors are considered in Table 43–1.

TEE is the most sensitive monitor. However, ECG is the most useful clinical tool because it can be used continuously during the perioperative period. It is noninvasive and easily automated, quantitated, and trended. However, in the perioperative setting, specificity may suffer because of alterations of electrolyte concentrations, concurrent medication (particularly digoxin), and other physiologic parameters that alter ventricular repolarization.[7]

### *How Is Transesophageal Echocardiography Used to Detect Ischemia?*

Given the rapid growth in the use of intraoperative TEE along with development of practice guidelines and a formal

**TABLE 43–1.** Clinical Assessment of Perioperative Myocardial Ischemia

|  | ECG | TEE | PAOP |
|---|---|---|---|
| Ischemia detection | Electrical: QRST abnormalities | Wall motion, compliance changes (Doppler) | Compliance changes |
| Other uses | Rhythm, conduction | Assessment of cavitary volume, contractility, CO, valve function | CO, pressures, resistances, mixed venous oxygen saturation |
| Invasiveness | Low | Medium | High |
| Limitations | Bundle branch and other conduction blocks, Q wave leads, open chest | Esophageal disease, technical factors (spatial relations of heart to esophagus) | Valvular pathology, severe pulmonary hypertension |
| Sensitivity for ischemia | Medium | High | Low |
| Specificity for ischemia | High | Medium | Low |
| Analysis | Easy, automated | Difficult, not automated | Medium |
| Expense | $5000–$10 000/unit | $100 000–$200 000/unit | $50–$250/catheter |
| Utility | Perioperative | Intraoperative | Perioperative |

CO, cardiac output; ECG, electrocardiography; PAOP, pulmonary artery occlusion pressure; TEE, transesophageal echocardiography.

certification mechanism, anesthesiologists must be familiar with the basics of echocardiographic detection of ischemia.[8] Although more complex than recognition of common ECG changes, recognition of basic WMAs is rapidly learned by anesthesia practitioners.

Rapid depression of regional contractile function is associated with reduction in regional coronary blood flow. Reduction in the normal degree of thickening that occurs across the ventricular wall during systole (systolic wall thickening) is the most sensitive marker of ischemia. The most recognizable sign is a reduction in movement of the ventricular wall toward the center of the ventricle. This is easily assessed by movement of the endocardial border (endocardial excursion). Although segment shortening may decline with as little as a 10% to 20% reduction in coronary blood flow, akinesis is usually present only when flow decreases by >90% and dyskinesis at a >95% reduction.

A semiquantitative scoring system is most commonly used to evaluate WMAs using visual analysis of endocardial excursion and wall thickening (Table 43–2). Both variables are used despite experimental findings that wall thickening declines earlier and more closely defines the actual boundaries of an ischemic area[9] (Fig. 43–5). *Tethering* of the ischemic myocardium or differences in *tissue stress* may account for this discrepancy. However, this scoring system correlates well with perfusion measured by thallium scintigraphy. Variation in wall motion in normal population samples, ventricular hypertrophy, or other abnormalities (ie, myocardial infiltrative disorders) must be considered when diagnosing WMAs.

The American Society of Echocardiography recommends classification of the LV into 16 segments for scoring WMAs

(Fig. 43–6). The LV is subdivided into basal, middle, and apical segments in each of the major anatomic surfaces (anterior, inferior, lateral, and posterior). The most common view for intraoperative monitoring is the short-axis view at the level of the papillary muscles.[10] In this view, a limited portion of the perfusion zones of all of the three major coronary arteries can be assessed (Fig. 43–7). This view is easy to maintain and also provides information on loading conditions (ie, volume).

The type of TEE probe (monoplane, biplane, or omniplane) is important. Several studies document the increment in sensitivity afforded by the biplane or omniplane probe. Rouine-Rapp and colleagues evaluated 12 ventricular segments in nine different imaging planes and found that only 17% were present in the midpapillary short-axis view.[11] Using multiple planes, this was increased to 65%.

The observation that WMAs are not always specific for acute ischemia may result from reading of wall motion during either hypovolemic or hypervolemic states. This is clearly an

**TABLE 43–2.** Clinical Scoring of Wall Motion Abnormalities Based on Visual Observation of Endocardial Excursion and Systolic Wall Thickening

| Grade | Endocardial Excursion | Wall Thickening |
|---|---|---|
| Normal | >30% | 30%–50% |
| Hypokinesis |  |  |
|   Mild | 10%–30% | 30%–50% |
|   Severe | <10% | <30% |
| Akinesis | Absent | Absent |
| Dyskinesis | Outward bulging | Absent, systolic thinning |
| Hyperkinesis | >Normal | >Normal |

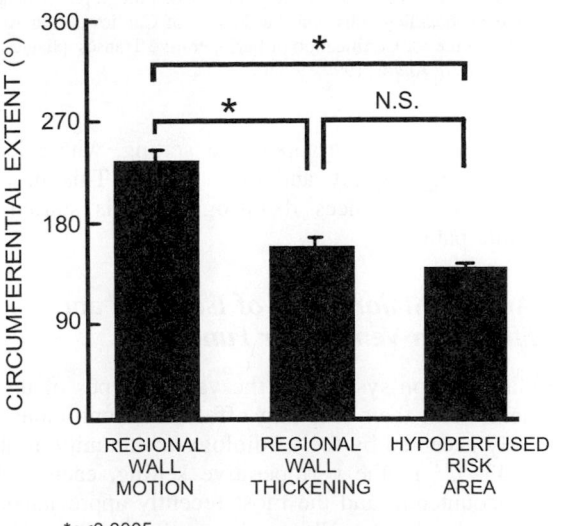

*p<0.0005

**FIGURE 43–5.** Correlation of endocardial excursion with systolic wall thickening with area at risk as measured by radioactive microspheres in a canine model of regional ischemia. Endocardial excursion significantly overestimates the actual degree of ischemia. (From Buda AJ, Zotz RJ, Pace DP, et al. Comparison of two-dimensional echocardiographic wall motion and wall thickening abnormalities in relation to the myocardium at risk. *Am Heart J.* 1986;111:587.)

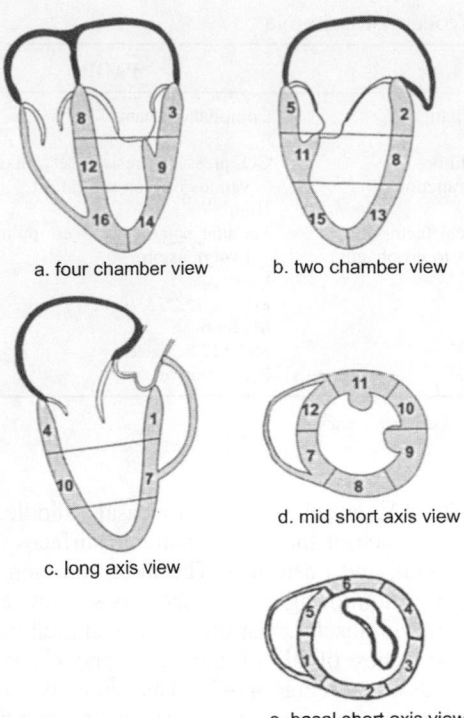

a. four chamber view     b. two chamber view

c. long axis view

d. mid short axis view

e. basal short axis view

| Basal Segments | Mid Segments | Apical Segments |
| --- | --- | --- |
| 1 = Basal Anteroseptal | 7 = Mid Anteroseptal | 13 = Apical Anterior |
| 2 = Basal Anterior | 8 = Mid Anterior | 14 = Apical Lateral |
| 3 = Basal Lateral | 9 = Mid Lateral | 15 = Apical Inferior |
| 4 = Basal Posterior | 10 = Mid Posterior | 16 = Apical Septal |
| 5 = Basal Inferior | 11 = Mid Inferior | |
| 6 = Basal Septal | 12 = Mid Septal | |

**FIGURE 43–6.** Sixteen-segment model of the left ventricle adopted by the American Society of Echocardiography for localizing abnormalities of wall motion with transesophageal echocardiography. (From Shanewise JS, Cheung AT, Aronson S, et al. ASE/SCA guidelines for performing a comprehensive intraoperative multiplane transesophageal echocardiography examination: recommendations of the American Society of Echocardiography Council for Intraoperative Echocardiography and the Society of Cardiovascular Anesthesiologists Task Force for Certification in Perioperative Transesophageal Echocardiography. *Anesth Analg.* 1999;89:870.)

important issue in the intraoperative setting, where loading conditions change rapidly and dramatically. This may also have serious consequences if nitroglycerin is started in a hypovolemic patient!

## What Are the Major Types of Ischemia and Their Effects on Ventricular Function?

The classification system for the various types of myocardial ischemia and their resulting effects on ventricular function, widely accepted by the cardiology community, is shown in Table 43–3.[12] In the perioperative setting, each of these may be encountered, and the most recently appreciated, preconditioning, is now actually used as a therapeutic maneuver in patients undergoing "off-pump" coronary artery bypass graft (CABG) surgery.

### Conventional Ischemia

This group, the oldest clinical class, is the simplest to understand given its basic construct linking coronary blood

flow to ischemia in a monotonic (although not necessarily linear) fashion. It may be completely reversible, assuming prompt restoration of coronary blood flow by hemodynamic (eg, treatment of tachycardia) or anatomic-morphologic interventions (eg, rapid thrombolysis in the setting of acute coronary thrombosis). It is subdivided into subendocardial or transmural ischemia based on the degree of alteration of flow across the myocardial wall. The subendocardium, having a higher $O_2$ demand than the outer epicardial layers of the heart, is usually the first area to manifest ischemia with graded reduction of coronary blood flow.

Given that many MIs are caused by thrombosis of one of the larger epicardial or subepicardial vessels, the first manifestation may be transmural ischemia. However, accumulating literature evidence suggests that subendocardial (non-Q wave) infarction is the now the most common perioperative manifestation of infarction and may be linked to a sustained increase in $O_2$ demand due to sustained postoperative tachycardia.[13,14]

### Subendocardial Ischemia

Subendocardial ischemia, manifested as ST segment depression (horizontal or downsloping of >1 mm at 60-80 msec after the J point, or slowly upsloping depression of >1.5-2.0 mm), is the most common type of perioperative ischemia.[7]

### Transmural Ischemia

With more profound imbalance of the supply-demand ratio, transmural ischemia may occur, manifested as an ST segment elevation of similar magnitude to one another (in leads without a preexisting Q wave). In patients undergoing cardiac surgery,

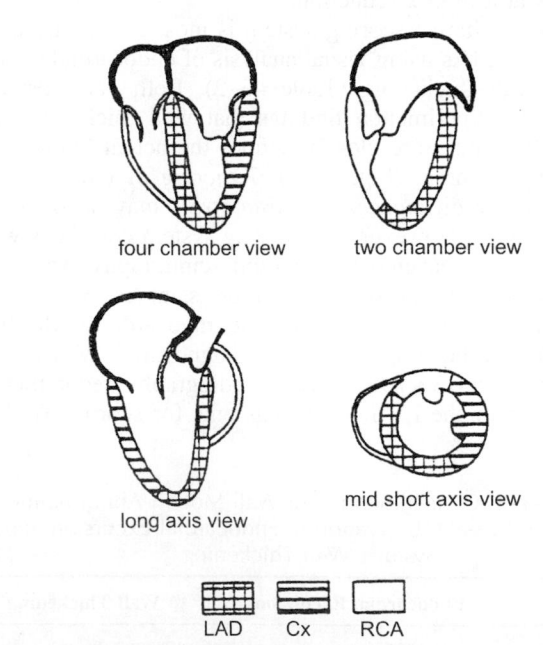

four chamber view     two chamber view

long axis view     mid short axis view

LAD     Cx     RCA

**FIGURE 43–7.** Predominant patterns of coronary perfusion by each of the major coronary arteries. Different patterns may be observed with variants and with collateral circulation. (From Shanewise JS, Cheung AT, Aronson S, et al. ASE/SCA guidelines for performing a comprehensive intraoperative multiplane transesophageal echocardiography examination: recommendations of the American Society of Echocardiography Council for Intraoperative Echocardiography and the Society of Cardiovascular Anesthesiologists Task Force for Certification in Perioperative Transesophageal Echocardiography. *Anesth Analg.* 1999;89:870.)

**TABLE 43–3.** Opie Types of Myocardial Ischemia

| Parameter | Conventional Ischemia | Acute Stunning | Chronic Stunning | Hibernation | Preconditioning |
|---|---|---|---|---|---|
| Myocardial function | Reduced | Reduced | Reduced | Reduced | Protected during repeat ischemia by prior ischemia |
| Coronary blood flow | Severely reduced | Postischemic; fully restored | Partially restored | Modestly reduced or possibly normal at rest and repetitively reduced during exercise | Brief ischemia |
| Myocardial energy metabolism | Reduced; increasingly severe as ischemia proceeds | Normal or excessive | Unknown, possibly depressed | Reduced in relation to contractile decrease | Reduced ATP demand in test ischemic period |
| Duration | Minutes to hours | Hours to days | Days to weeks | Days to months | Protection may last for hours; may return with "second window" |
| Outcome | Infarction if severe ischemia persists | Full recovery | Incomplete recovery | Recovery with revascularization | Decreased postischemic infarct size; decreased surrogate damage |
| Proposed changes in regulation of calcium | Insufficient glycolytic ATP to control cell calcium and prevent irreversibility | Cytosolic overload and excess oscillations of calcium ions in early reperfusion | Prolonged calcium overload may have led to partial necrosis | Just enough glycolytic ATP to prevent contracture; chronic downregulation of ATP demand | Role of calcium not elucidated |

ATP, adenosine triphosphate.

particularly CABG, transmural ischemia is common and may result from various processes, including coronary vasospasm and coronary embolism (air or particulate debris) (Fig. 43–8).

## Stunned Myocardium

In certain patients, after return of normal coronary blood flow to a previously ischemic region, ST segment changes, regional WMAs, or impaired ventricular function may persist for up to several days (Fig. 43–9). This interesting phenomenon is termed *stunned myocardium* and is most common after brief, repetitive episodes of ischemia.[15] It may occur during a stormy surgical procedure, such as thoracic aortic aneurysm repair or repetitive high aortic cross-clamping. The latter procedure markedly increases afterload and wall stress, decreases

coronary perfusion pressure, and increases myocardial $O_2$ demand. Hypovolemia due to hemorrhage or vasodilation distal to the clamp decreases preload, markedly reducing cardiac output and systemic pressure and further compromising coronary perfusion.

That myocardial stunning occurs clinically is suggested by an early clinical study using continuous TEE wall motion monitoring in which we observed that most patients who had new akinetic segments persisting at the conclusion of surgery did not sustain infarction.[16] However, such a process is not likely entirely benign, either, because it may result in significant postoperative ventricular dysfunction. Studies in patients undergoing CABG surgery suggest that TEE evaluation of myocardial perfusion (perfusion contrast echocardiography)

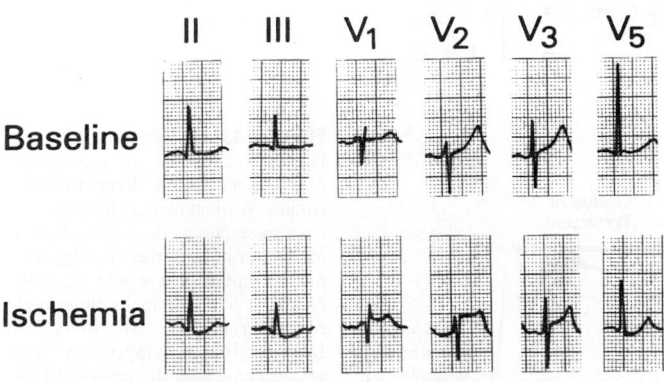

**FIGURE 43–8.** Ischemic episode diagnostic of transmural ischemia in the distribution of the left anterior descending artery with ST segment elevation in $V_1$ to $V_3$ (verified by anterior wall akinesis on transesophageal echocardiography). Changes in the routine monitoring leads (II and $V_5$) are reciprocal and of much lower magnitude, and do not engender the same degree of clinical concern. (From London MJ, Hollenberg M, Wong MG, et al. Intraoperative myocardial ischemia: localization by continuous 12 lead electrocardiography. *Anesthesiology.* 1988;69:233.)

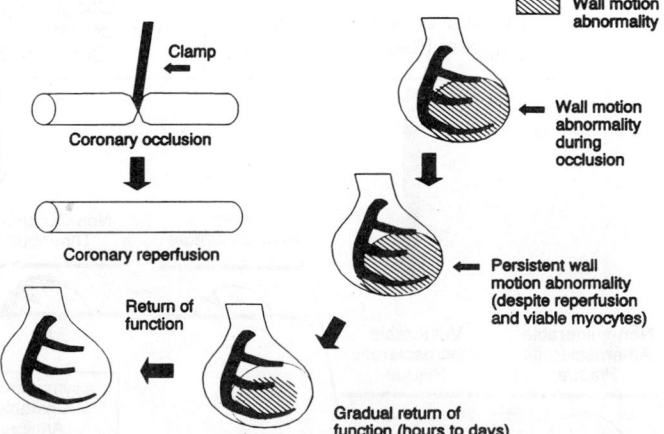

**FIGURE 43–9.** Schematic representation of stunned myocardium after coronary reperfusion. This syndrome is now well recognized as a common clinical event. It may have significant prognostic implications for postoperative myocardial dysfunction. (From Kloner RA, Przyklenk K, Patel B. Altered myocardial states: the stunned and hibernating myocardium. *Am J Med.* 1989;86[suppl 1A]:15.)

holds promise in distinguishing between stunning and infarction. However, current methods of administration are limited to the invasive aortic root injection. Active work on contrast agents capable of myocardial imaging through venous injection is ongoing.

More recently, stunning has been categorized as either acute or chronic, based on the temporal recovery profile (see Table 43–3). Given the prolonged, incomplete recovery defining chronic stunning, it has been euphemistically termed *maimed myocardium*. It is likely that both types can occur perioperatively.

## Hibernating Myocardium

Hibernating myocardium is chronic regional dysfunction (ie, severe hypokinesis or akinesis) distal to a significant coronary stenosis.[15] This process, occurring in the absence of infarction, is considered an adaptive response to chronic ischemia. Wall motion frequently normalizes after myocardial revascularization or with reduction in myocardial $O_2$ demand during anesthesia. Thus, wall motion assessed by intraoperative TEE may appear substantially better than that observed by preoperative precordial echocardiography, multigated angiography, or contrast ventriculography. Preoperative dobutamine stress echocardiography is often used to verify whether the myocardium is hibernating. An increase in regional function with dobutamine correlates well with recovery after CABG surgery.

## Preconditioning

Preconditioning is the most recently appreciated and probably the most complex ischemic phenomenon. In contrast to stunning, in which repetitive episodes of ischemia cause cumulative damage, preconditioning involves short episodes of severe ischemia before a prolonged insult that actually protect the myocardium against postischemic dysfunction or may greatly limit the size of an MI (in the case of a prolonged occlusion).[15] This phenomenon is thought to be mediated by tissue release of adenosine, which activates guanine regulatory proteins (G proteins), or by stimulation of protein kinase C. Both of these pathways appear to involve the stimulation of adenosine triphosphate-regulated potassium ($K_{ATP}$) channels as the end-mediator.

This has sparked a resurgence of interest in volatile anesthesia, given evidence that all volatile anesthetics exert preconditioning properties not only in the myocardium, but in other vascular endothelium. Preconditioning with volatile agents involves an *acute memory phase* because the protection remains active for several hours after the initial stimulus.[17]

Given the recent appreciation of the laboratory mechanisms of preconditioning, clinical applications are still limited. Preconditioning is commonly used in patients undergoing off-pump CABG where a 2- to 3-minute occlusion is performed before the prolonged occlusion (15-20 minutes) required for anastomosis of the diseased vessel. A few studies suggest it is also effective before global ischemic arrest with conventional cardiopulmonary bypass. However, it does not appear to be widely applied. Once a reliable pharmacologic mediator is available to mimic the occlusive stimulus, it most likely will lead to more common use.

## What Characteristics of Ischemia Are Unique to Patients With Coronary Artery Disease?

In patients with CAD, a unique set of factors may complicate the straightforward $O_2$ supply-demand schema. CAD is a complex morphologic process; thus, an understanding of how its pathophysiologic process can result in various clinical presentations (ie, chest pain, unstable angina, subendocardial or transmural infarction) is essential[18] (Fig. 43–10).

### Silent Myocardial Ischemia

SMI is relatively common in patients with CAD ($\approx40\%$) and is manifested by ST segment depression on prolonged

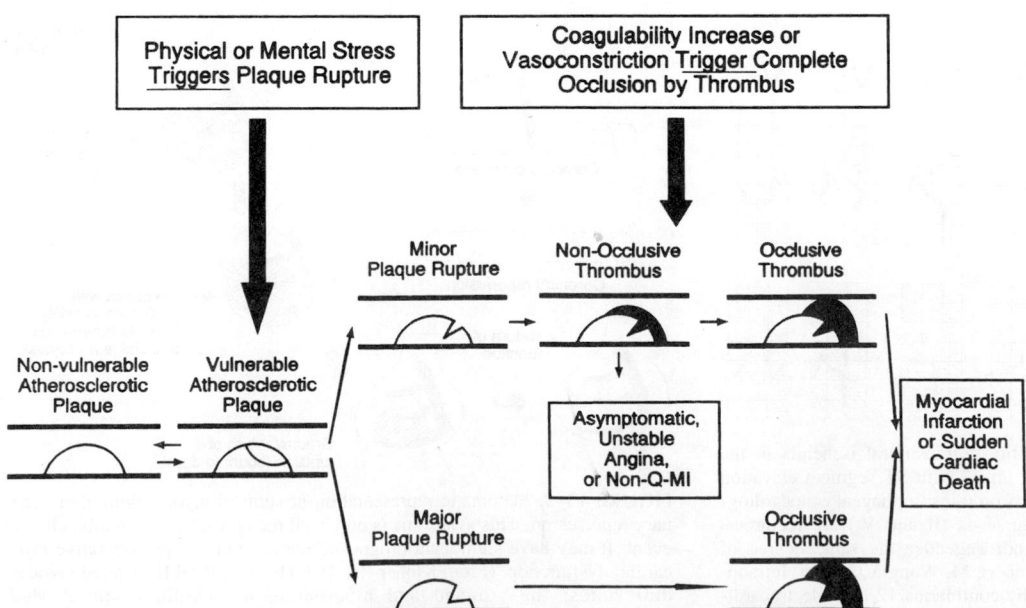

**FIGURE 43–10.** Sequence of events leading to clinical syndromes of coronary artery disease. Recent clinical studies on silent myocardial ischemia have more clearly delineated the major role of mental stress in triggering plaque rupture that would place the patient at risk for a major thrombotic event. (From Muller JE, Tofler GH. Introduction: a symposium: triggering and circadian variation of onset of acute cardiovascular disease. *Am J Cardiol.* 1990;66[suppl]:4G.)

**TABLE 43–4.** Cardiac Morbidity and Mortality in Patients With Silent Myocardial Ischemia

| Study | N | Monitor Leads/ Duration | Ischemia (% Patients) | Events—Ischemic Group | Events—Nonischemic Group | Predictors of Outcome |
|---|---|---|---|---|---|---|
| Pasternack et al[21] | 200 Vasc | Q-Med 1 lead/18 h pre, 37 h intra/ post | 64%, >post | 10/127 (8%) | None | Preoperative ischemia, rest angina |
| Raby et al[22] | 176 Vasc | Holter 2 leads/pre only | 18%, pre only | 12/32 (38%) | 1/144 (<1%) | Preoperative ischemia: RR 24.4 |
| Mangano et al[23] | 172 Vasc | Holter 2 leads/48 h pre, 48 h intra/ post | 20% pre, 25% intra, 41% post | Post: 12/167 (7%) | 0–2 (<1%) | Postoperative ischemia: RR 9.2 |
| | 474 Total | | | | | |

Holter, standard analog recorder; Q-Med, real-time digital Holter monitor; RR, relative risk; Vasc, vascular surgery.

ambulatory monitoring, in the absence of chest pain, with only minor or no alterations in heart rate and BP.[19] The underlying mechanism of SMI is a transient reduction in regional coronary artery blood flow due to increased vasomotor tone at the site of an already significant coronary lesion (ie, >70% reduction in cross-sectional area). Increased α-adrenergic tone is probably responsible, although other hormonal mediators may be important. In the past, SMI was believed to be unique to diabetic patients, in whom painless infarction was well recognized. However, it is now a well-accepted clinical phenomenon in patients with stable or unstable anginal syndromes.

### Stable and Unstable Angina

A number of clinical studies using different diagnostic modalities, including exercise treadmill testing, ambulatory ST segment monitoring, invasive catheterization (ie, coronary sinus sampling), and radionuclear perfusion scanning, have conclusively proved the existence of SMI in patients with CAD.[7] It is prognostic of adverse outcomes in certain subgroups of patients with CAD, particularly those with unstable angina and in those recovering from a recent MI.

However, its significance in patients with stable angina pectoris, the extent to which various cardiac medications are effective in suppressing it, and how aggressively it should be treated remain controversial. In this regard, the largest study available is the Asymptomatic Cardiac Ischemia Pilot (ACIP) Study in which 558 patients with SMI during treadmill testing and ambulatory Holter monitoring (with coronary anatomy amenable to bypass on previous catheterization) were randomized to one of three treatment strategies: medical therapy titrating to either anginal symptoms or SMI, or interventional therapy with revascularization (either percutaneous transluminal coronary angioplasty or CABG).[20] Medical therapy was continued for 1 year. After 2 years of follow-up, the frequency of death or MI was 4.7% with revascularization, 8.8% for ischemia-guided therapy, and 12.1% for anginal therapy. Although the findings of this study are striking, it was designed only as a pilot trial, and thus the investigators urge caution in its generalization. However, the impressive results suggest that short of revascularization, aggressive medical therapy of SMI may be indicated.

### Silent Perioperative Myocardial Ischemia

Recent perioperative studies using various ECG techniques for perioperative monitoring (eg, ambulatory ST segment

monitors, routine operating room ECG monitors, computerized 12-lead monitors) have confirmed the presence of SMI in the surgical population, documenting that it is at least as common as hemodynamically mediated ischemia. In this setting, SMI may not be entirely benign, and patients who have it are at significantly increased risk for postoperative cardiac morbidity or mortality (Table 43–4). Its role as an independent risk factor is underscored by its similar frequency in patients with and without preoperative clinical markers of CAD.

### Does Treatment of Perioperative ST Segment Changes Alter Outcome?

Despite the finding that patients with ischemia are at a statistically increased risk for morbidity (high sensitivity), the percentage of those who actually sustain an infarct is small. This observation poses significant logistical problems for clinical management because aggressive intraoperative and early postoperative monitoring of large numbers of patients would be necessary to detect a single patient who will have an infarct (low positive predictive value).

Probably the most important information from these studies is that patients without perioperative ischemia are at exceedingly low (or no) risk for morbidity (very high negative predictive value). This finding has particular significance in guiding the length of intensive care unit (ICU) stay necessary for postoperative cardiac monitoring of high-risk patients. It should be remembered, however, that these studies have not yet answered the most important question: Does treatment of perioperative ST segment changes alter adverse outcome, or is it simply a marker of a pathophysiologic process over which we may have little control? Although several groups have reported abstract data on immediate therapy of silent perioperative ischemia using continuous-telemetry ST segment monitoring, as of yet there are no peer-reviewed publications on this important topic. It is likely that there are patients in whom treatment is important and others in whom it is of little consequence.

### When Is a Patient With Coronary Artery Disease Ready for Surgery?

Deciding whether a patient with CAD is ready for surgery is a continually evolving science. In many practice settings, it is left up to an internist or cardiologist to clear a patient for surgery. Before the late 1970s, there were several cardinal principles: first, no patient should undergo elective surgery within 6 months of an MI; second, no patient should go to the operating room with any degree of heart failure; and third, no patient should go to the operating room while taking β-adrenergic blockers because of their myocardial depressant effects.

However, starting with the landmark work of Goldman and colleagues, the first to develop a widely used scoring system, these rules have been substantially modified.[24] Patients now commonly undergo elective surgical procedures within 6 months of an MI; patients with heart failure undergo surgery after they are optimized with afterload reduction, diuresis, and the like; and withdrawal of β-blockade before surgery is well recognized as contraindicated. In fact, it is now recommended that perioperative β-blockers be administered to patients at risk for perioperative MI.[25,26]

The American Heart Association and the American College of Cardiology have jointly published guidelines for perioperative cardiovascular evaluation of patients undergoing noncardiac surgery that contain detailed decision algorithms outlining what diagnostic tests are needed for various subgroups of patients with or at risk for ischemic heart disease.[27] Although there are a wide variety of risk stratification schemes and diagnostic modalities available, the presence of easily inducible myocardial ischemia on provocative testing or poor functional capacity indicative of poor cardiac function are the two most important predictors of perioperative cardiac morbidity and mortality.

### Ischemic Burden

A newly evolving issue that relates closely to the third question mentioned earlier deals with a patient's *ischemic burden,* that is, how much and how easily a patient experiences reversible ischemia, either as angina pectoris or as SMI. It is being closely examined as a risk factor.

### ß-Blockers

Clinical evidence suggests that patients who are β-blocked before surgery have less ischemia than those who are not or who are receiving calcium channel blockers only. This difference appears to be related to lower heart rates or, more precisely, less tachycardia in β-blocked patients, a supposition that is supported by the results of several major studies of postinfarction β-blockade in medical patients.

One long-term, randomized, placebo-controlled study of 200 men undergoing noncardiac surgery suggests that perioperative administration of atenolol (intravenous preinduction and immediately after surgery, and orally or intravenously for the first 7 days after surgery) was associated with a significant reduction in the 2-year mortality rate, primarily because of a reduction in cardiac-related deaths during the first 6 to 8 months after surgery.[25,28] Although these findings have been incorporated into the practice guidelines for perioperative management of the American College of Physicians, the findings of this study remain controversial because of safety concerns in the larger population of patients outside of this study, as well as logistical considerations.

More recently, Poldermans and associates have reported striking randomized, multicenter data on perioperative β-blockade in 112 patients undergoing vascular surgery identi-

fied to be at high risk based on positive results on preoperative dobutamine stress echocardiographic testing.[26] In contrast to Mangano and coworkers, they noted a striking reduction (91%) in cardiac death and complications *within 30 days after surgery* (3.4% versus 34%). This study (performed in Europe) will raise additional controversy because of several flaws, the most notable of which was nonblinded treatment. The strikingly high rate of complications in the placebo group is not consistent with most US centers, even in high-risk patients. However, a randomized (but nonblinded) study of β-blockade in elderly patients (>65 years of age) undergoing primarily intraabdominal surgery demonstrated better hemodynamic control, decreased analgesic requirements, and faster recovery with perioperative β-blockade.[29] Therapy was well tolerated with no adverse events. Curiously, levels of hormonal markers of stress were no different between patients receiving β-blockers and those who did not. Although this study was too small (63 patients total) to detect differences in outcomes, intraoperative ischemia was not detected in any patient, although subclinical release of troponin-I was present in 20% to 45% of patients, with the greatest release in those not receiving β-blockers.

### Calcium Channel Antagonists

In similar epidemiologic studies, short-acting preparations of calcium channel antagonists have resulted in worse outcome, perhaps related to their negative inotropic effects. Newer, nondepressant and sustained-release agents may yield better results. However, calcium channel antagonists may have beneficial effects by preventing stunned myocardium.

### Nitrates

Curiously, no firm data on the value of preoperative nitrate therapy are available, and results of studies of its prophylactic (intravenous) intraoperative use are conflicting.[30–32] As a result, both anesthesiologists and consulting cardiologists seem rarely to recommend or use it except in the highest-risk patients (ie, patients with acute unstable angina requiring emergency noncardiac surgery). The value of prophylactic nitrates in medical patients with known CAD but no angina (ie, remote MI or SMI only) remains controversial (see discussion of ACIP Study, earlier).

## ANESTHESIA AND INTRAOPERATIVE ISCHEMIA

### Is There a Best Technique?

In few areas of anesthesiology does clinical art diverge so far from academic science as in that concerning the relationship between anesthesia and intraoperative ischemia. The literature is replete with carefully controlled, invasive animal studies and clinical trials rigorously evaluating the effects of different anesthetic agents on hemodynamic function and signs of ischemia. In these highly controlled studies, a significant number of agents have been shown to precipitate ischemia, either through direct myocardial effects (coronary steal with isoflurane) or peripheral effects (vagolytic effects of pancuronium causing tachycardia).

Despite these studies, there is little conclusive evidence that any anesthetic agent is more likely to precipitate ischemia than any other when it is used by experienced clinicians. More important, no evidence shows that one technique is associated with better outcome. The basic adage, "It's not what you use, but how you use it," remains the most important rule for anesthetic management. This generalization does not imply that any agent can be used with impunity; rather, it suggests that a clinician must properly dose agents to achieve the desired physiologic endpoints despite varying effects on the myocardium and autonomic nervous system.

## Control of Heart Rate

Despite the multiplicity of factors involved in the development of ischemia, particularly in patients with CAD, the heart rate should be maintained at the lowest level consistent with adequate cardiac output to meet peripheral and myocardial $O_2$ demands. This is most often a heart rate of <70 beats per minute.

## Control of Blood Pressure

Recommendations for maintenance of BP are more controversial, including which pressure is most important: systolic, diastolic, or mean. Some authorities vigorously recommend maintaining BPs within 20% of the preoperative mean.

This approach suffers from several problems. The first is a lack of validation of what constitutes a representative mean value for hospitalized patients. Second, during a well-conducted anesthetic, $O_2$ demands of all organs are significantly reduced. Thus, autoregulatory responses should allow adequate perfusion at a lower pressure.

Although autoregulatory responses distal to a significant coronary lesion may be markedly impaired or even abolished because maximal vasodilation is already present, other moderating factors influence ischemia.[33] Obviously, elevated heart rate at a low pressure places a patient at greater risk than lower heart rate at an equivalent pressure. Also, the effects of BP on afterload and wall stress (direct relation) must be considered. A factor of particular importance in today's clinical milieu, with the ever-present risk of transfusion-associated infections, is that higher BPs result in greater blood loss, increasing the probability of transfusion.

### Magnitude and Duration of Hypotension

Although Goldman and colleagues suggested that profound hypotension (>50% decrease below control) was a major risk factor, the duration also was shown to be important. Reductions of pressure >33% for periods >10 minutes were statistically related to adverse postoperative cardiac outcome.[24] However, in healthy patients, even cardiac arrest on induction, if treated promptly, is rarely associated with adverse sequelae.

## MYOCARDIAL DYSFUNCTION

Myocardial dysfunction is commonly equated with an abnormally low cardiac output, resulting in impaired systemic $O_2$ delivery. However, cardiac output is modulated by both myocardial and peripheral vascular factors. To diagnose and treat low cardiac output, clinicians must have a firm grasp of normal cardiac physiology.[34] The temporal relation between

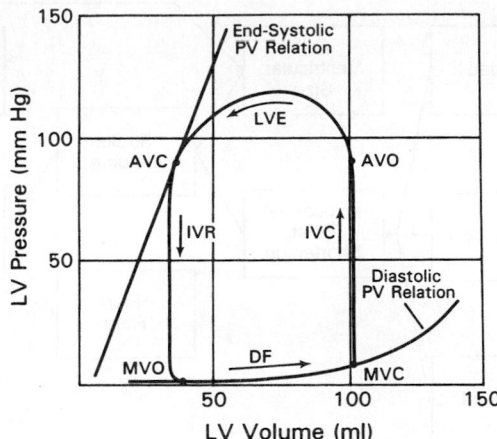

**FIGURE 43–11.** Pressure-volume loop illustrating the change in left ventricular pressure and volume during a single cardiac cycle in a normal ventricle. A point of significant importance in assessing myocardial contractility is the pressure-volume relation at end-systole. AVC, aortic valve closure; AVO, aortic valve opening; DF, diastolic filling; IVC, isovolumic contraction; IVR, isovolumic relaxation; LV, left ventricular; LVE, left ventricular ejection; MVC, mitral valve closure; MVO, mitral valve opening; PV, pressure-volume. (From Hutter AM. Congestive heart failure. In: Rubenstein E, ed. *Scientific American Medicine.* New York, NY: Scientific American; 1988:4. Scientific American Medicine, Section I, Subsection II. © 1988 Scientific American, Inc. All rights reserved.)

ventricular pressure and volume throughout the cardiac cycle can be effectively displayed as a pressure-volume loop (Fig. 43–11). From this plot, both stroke volume (the volume ejected during systole) and stroke work (the energy expended to eject it) can be visualized by examining the difference between the end-systolic and end-diastolic volumes (for stroke volume) and the area enclosed by the loop (for stroke work).

## What Are the Determinants of Stroke Volume?

The major determinants of stroke volume are preload, afterload, and contractility.[1] Alterations of one or more of these factors alter cardiac output (Fig. 43–12). Under most clinical conditions, *preload*, the stretch on the myofibrils at end-diastole, and *afterload*, the force resisting systolic shortening of the myofibrils, are modulated primarily by the peripheral vasculature: venous return and aortic impedance, respectively. *Contractility* (inotropy), the intrinsic property of the cardiac muscle cells to generate force, is modulated by hormonal catecholamine and drug (eg, digoxin) effects. Heart rate (*chronotropy*) is also modulated by hormonal and chemical effects, as well as direct and indirect autonomic innervation (ie, sinoatrial node automaticity and peripheral baroreceptors).

Stroke volume and preload are directly related. The Frank-Starling relation (or ventricular function curve) illustrates this point. In humans, throughout a physiologic range of pressures, little evidence of a distinct plateau portion of the curve is seen. The relationship between stroke volume and afterload is inverse. A ventricle with significant depression of contractile function may generate normal cardiac output if preload is optimized and afterload reduced (Fig. 43–13).

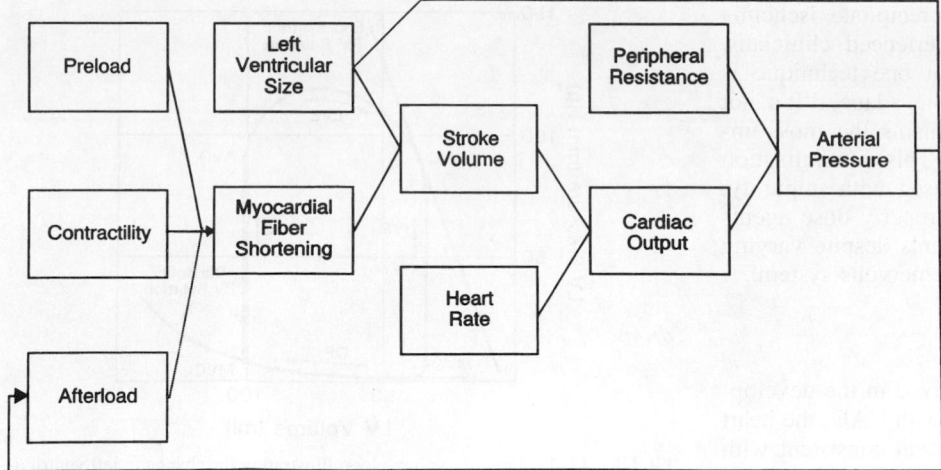

**FIGURE 43–12.** Relation between major factors modulating cardiac function. The *solid line* indicates positive effect, and the *dashed line* indicates negative effect. Left ventricular size influences both stroke volume and preload. (From Braunwald E. Regulation of the circulation. *N Engl J Med.* 1974;290:1129, reprinted by permission of the *New England Journal of Medicine.*)

## How Is Myocardial Dysfunction Assessed?

When approaching a patient with abnormal hemodynamics, a clinician must first attempt to localize the problem to the appropriate component of the cardiovascular system (ie, the peripheral vasculature or the cardiac pump). If the cardiac pump appears to be primarily affected (the focus of this discussion), the abnormality should be characterized as either systolic or diastolic. Systolic dysfunction is by far the more common clinical problem and is characterized by abnormalities of one or more of the determinants of stroke volume.

### Diastolic Dysfunction

Recognition of diastolic dysfunction as a clinical entity has increased in recent years, especially with the use of calcium

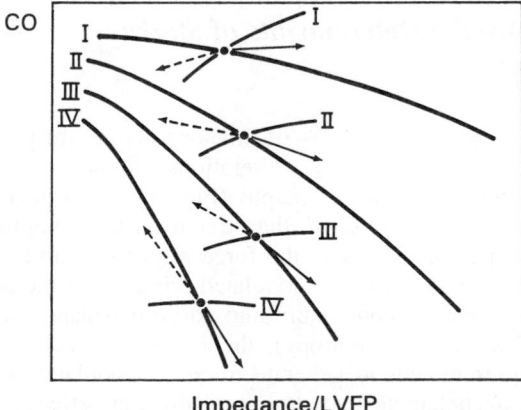

**FIGURE 43–13.** Relation between preload (*short segments*) and afterload effects (*longer segments*) on ventricular function. The classic Frank-Starling curve for either parameter is the relation of the parameter (either left ventricular filling pressure/volume for preload or outflow resistance/impedance for afterload) to a measure of ventricular output (eg, cardiac output, stroke volume, or stroke work). A balanced arteriolar and venous vasodilator such as nitroprusside reduces both preload and afterload. In patients with normal ventricular function (*curves I and II*), the effects of preload reduction predominate over those of afterload reduction, and cardiac output may fall (*hatched arrows*). With impaired function (*curves III and IV*), afterload reduction predominates and cardiac output increases. CO, cardiac output; LVFP, left ventricular filling pressure. (From Cohn JN, Franciosa JA. Vasodilator therapy of cardiac failure [part II]. *N Engl J Med.* 1977;297:28, reprinted by permission of the *New England Journal of Medicine.*)

entry blockers. Pulmonary edema or congestion develops in certain patients despite normal systolic function. In these patients, abnormalities of ventricular relaxation (lusitropy) or filling are present. A number of diseases have been associated with diastolic dysfunction (Table 43–5). The pathophysiologic hallmark of this disorder—impaired ventricular filling—is significantly worsened by tachycardia because it dramatically decreases diastolic filling time[35] (see Fig. 43–3).

As complex forms of cardiovascular monitoring such as PA catheterization (invasive) and TEE (noninvasive) become almost routine in clinical practice, the emphasis on the interrelations between hemodynamic variables has increased. End-diastolic wall stress (EDWS), an estimate of the force stretching the myocardial fibers at end-diastole, can be assessed. It is derived from wall thickness (h), ventricular radius (R), and end-diastolic pressure or preload (P):

$$EDWS = PR/2h \qquad \text{(Equation 1)}$$

The EDWS is a critical variable modulating systolic ejection; end-systolic wall stress is a critical determinant of afterload effects.

## What Are the Effects of Inhalational Anesthetics?

The older volatile agents—isoflurane, halothane, and enflurane—differ in their circulatory and myocardial effects, with halothane and isoflurane representing the two ends of the spectrum of effects on contractility. The circulatory and myocardial effects of the newer volatile agents—desflurane and sevoflurane—have in general been compared with those of isoflurane. Enflurane is intermediate between isoflurane and

**TABLE 43–5.** Diseases Associated With Diastolic Dysfunction

Myocardial ischemia
Hypertrophic cardiomyopathies
Systemic hypertension with left ventricular hypertrophy
Infiltrative systemic disorders
Diabetes mellitus
Hypothyroidism

halothane in many of its effects and is not considered further because of its infrequent use in the United States.

## Halothane

Halothane has significant negative inotropic effects that are either desirable or dangerous, depending on a clinician's perspective. These effects reduce myocardial and peripheral $O_2$ demand, decreasing the risk of ischemia unless the decrement in cardiac output is severe. If end-diastolic volume and pressure increase, however, an increase in wall tension and $O_2$ demand may result, together with decreased coronary perfusion pressure.

The heart rate is usually unchanged or may decline. However, a greater potential for atrioventricular dissociation and junctional rhythm exists, owing to slowing throughout the conduction system. Cardiac output is decreased from the negative inotropic and chronotropic effects, as well as from loss of the atrial kick if a nodal rhythm ensues. The coronary vasculature is unaffected, although coronary blood flow falls in proportion to the lower myocardial $O_2$ demand.

## Isoflurane

The negative inotropic effects of isoflurane are much less than those of halothane, although in the elderly the differences are not as marked (ie, both exert significant effects). It is a potent peripheral and coronary vasodilator.[36–39] The heart rate is unchanged or may increase and, in rare instances, frank tachycardia may occur. Because isoflurane has no effect on the cardiac conduction system, sinus rhythm is usually maintained.

## Desflurane

A rapid increase in inhaled concentration of either isoflurane or desflurane can cause sympathetic nervous system stimulation with resultant hypertension and tachycardia.[40] However, this effect is greatest with desflurane. During induction, administration of 1.0 to 1.5 minimum alveolar concentration (MAC; corresponding to an end-tidal concentration or value of 7.5%-10.9%) may cause sympathetic hyperactivity that can lead to myocardial ischemia in patients with CAD. However, at lower anesthetic concentrations in the range of 0.55 to 0.83 MAC (end-tidal of 4%-6%), this effect usually is not clinically significant.

Although sympathetic stimulation can precipitate myocardial ischemia in at-risk patients, this is rarely a significant problem when other anesthetic agents (eg, opioids, propofol) or adrenergic blocking agents (eg, esmolol, clonidine) are given to blunt sympathetic response to increased catecholamines. This agent is clearly a valuable one for either short or lengthy cases because of its rapid washout.

## Sevoflurane

In contrast to desflurane, sevoflurane does not appear to increase heart rate, arterial BP, or plasma norepinephrine concentrations at anesthetic concentrations in the range of 1.5 to 2.7 MAC. In fact, at 1.5 MAC, it significantly lowers the heart rate. Its effect on cardiac contractility appears comparable with the effects of isoflurane and desflurane. The incidence of myocardial ischemia in patients with or at high risk for

CAD undergoing noncardiac surgery does not appear to be different from that with isoflurane.[41] The authors prefer this agent over desflurane in patients with hypertension and normal ventricular function because of its lack of sympathetic stimulation.

## Coronary Steal

The clinical significance of isoflurane's coronary vasodilating properties has been hotly debated. A few well-publicized clinical and animal studies suggested a *coronary steal syndrome*[36,37]; other studies have not.[38,39] More important, epidemiologic studies and widespread clinical use have confirmed its safety. These properties should be considered more properly *luxury perfusion* because in most instances, global $M\dot{V}O_2$ is significantly reduced. Desflurane and sevoflurane do not appear to cause clinically significant maldistribution of coronary blood flow.[42]

## Myocardial Depression

The lesser myocardial depressant properties of isoflurane compared with halothane are occasionally a liability. Control of hemodynamic function is often difficult during acute hyperadrenergic states. Thus, myocardial ischemia may occur as a result of elevated demand. In this situation, concurrent administration of a β-blocker and an opioid may be indicated. The myocardial depressant properties of desflurane and sevoflurane appear comparable with those of isoflurane.

## *What Are the Effects of Narcotics?*

The narcotics are commonly cited as the best agents for at-risk patients because of their lack of intrinsic myocardial depression. Their vagotonic effects cause bradycardia, improving diastolic perfusion time. The decrease in BP is minor, consistent with a reduction in sympathetic tone.

## Recall and Amnesia

As sole anesthetic agents, narcotics must be administered in high doses to ensure unconsciousness. However, even at these doses, recall can occur. Administration of other agents to ensure amnesia, most commonly benzodiazepines, can cause significant hypotension owing to peripheral vasodilation. In the authors' experience, a low-dose propofol infusion (25 μg/kg/min), especially with low end-tidal concentrations of a volatile agent, is a good alternative to the use of benzodiazepines, especially for fast-tracking of CABG patients.

## Adrenergic Responses

The dose-response relationship between plasma levels of opioid and suppression of adrenergic responses is extremely variable. Thus, breakthrough hypertension and tachycardia can occur, placing patients at risk for myocardial dysfunction and ischemia. This effect is less likely with the more potent agent, sufentanil.

Use of narcotics in a balanced technique with a benzodiazepine (particularly midazolam) or a low-dose potent inhaled anesthetic, a nondepolarizing muscle relaxant (particularly those lacking vagolytic effects), and nitrous oxide is appealing because a low $O_2$ demand state can be achieved. This technique is also associated with improved early postoperative analgesia.

## Is Regional Anesthesia Safer Than General Anesthesia for At-Risk Patients?

The merits of spinal or epidural anesthesia compared with general anesthesia have been debated vigorously in the specialty for many years. An early study suggesting dramatic improvement in cardiac outcome with lumbar epidural anesthesia and detailed analyses of the protective effect of postoperative epidural analgesia on the stress response have fueled the controversy.[43,44]

More recently, the use of thoracic epidural anesthesia, long popular outside of the United States, has become increasingly popular for a variety of abdominal, thoracic, and even cardiac procedures. Proponents of this technique claim better control of the stress response and even improvements in coronary blood flow autoregulation.[45] In the noncardiac surgical setting, most studies to date have not resolved the controversy; therefore, it is not known if intraoperative epidural anesthesia, postoperative epidural analgesia, or both significantly reduce perioperative morbidity and mortality rates in patients undergoing high-risk surgical procedures.[46,47]

### Advantages

The potential advantages of regional anesthesia alone in the case of amenable peripheral surgery, or in combination with general anesthesia for major intraabdominal or thoracic surgery, are many. Relatively small doses of drug, particularly with spinal anesthesia, provide predictable and long-lasting surgical anesthesia and muscle relaxation.

The stress response during a well-performed regional anesthetic is reliably attenuated or completely blocked. Vasodilation during vascular surgery with lumbar epidural anesthesia can facilitate surgical anastomoses and graft perfusion. The propensity for deep venous thrombosis is attenuated, although few surgeons rely on this approach. In patients with compromised cardiac function, thoracic epidural anesthesia may suppress the stress response to surgery and reduce the myocardial $O_2$ demand better than lumbar epidural anesthesia.[45] Evidence for enhanced patient outcome (ie, decreased incidence of MI, stroke, death) has been advanced but remains controversial.

### Disadvantages

As was noted, a poorly performed regional (or local) anesthetic in which placement of the block causes considerable discomfort, as well as one in which spontaneous ventilation is allowed during lengthy surgery in a compromised patient, can induce much greater stress than a well-performed general anesthetic and increase cardiac morbidity. Hypotension and bradycardia from a high sympathectomy may be a significant hazard if excessive doses of intrathecal or epidural anesthetic are used or if appropriate supportive therapy is not rapidly provided. The clinician must consider the small but present risk of epidural hematoma in both the vascular and cardiac settings. Preoperative and intraoperative administration of a variety of anticoagulants (ie, aspirin, nonsteroidal antiinflammatory drugs, long-acting and short-acting heparin preparations, warfarin, platelet inhibitors) pose logistical problems that must be carefully considered.

The evidence for improved outcome and patient comfort with postoperative epidural analgesia (narcotic or narcotic-local anesthetic combinations) is rapidly accumulating. In the authors' opinion, this fact provides ample reason for preoperative placement of epidural catheters for major surgery whenever feasible. The use of intraoperative epidural anesthesia, in combination with a light general anesthetic, may maximize the benefits of both techniques.

## INTRAOPERATIVE ISCHEMIA

### How Should It Be Treated?

#### ß-Blockers

Effective treatment of intraoperative ischemia entails a rapid assessment of the clinical situation and a decision about which determinants of myocardial $O_2$ balance have been compromised. In most instances, tachycardia, elicited through excessive adrenergic activity from a host of factors (eg, light anesthesia, hypercarbia, hypovolemia, or acute anemia), is the offending factor.

Although treatment is most effective when directed at the underlying cause, management of tachycardia can be enhanced by the judicious use of β-blockers (Table 43–6), initially with the ultrashort-acting agent esmolol. Inappropriate use of β-blockers can be disastrous, especially in the setting of unrecognized hypovolemia (thus the rationale for starting with esmolol). However, they are invaluable when myocardial $O_2$ demand and adrenergic tone are clearly increased.

Although additional anesthesia or analgesia is indicated in many instances, most commonly with opioids, poor correlation of plasma opioid levels with adrenergic suppression demonstrated by Philbin and colleagues supports the use of both analgesia and β-blockade.[48]

**TABLE 43–6.** Cardiovascular Effects of Nitrates, β-Blockers, and Calcium Entry Blockers

| Agent | Coronary Vasodilation | Peripheral Vasodilation | Myocardial Contractility | Heart Rate | Atrioventricular Conduction |
|---|---|---|---|---|---|
| Nitrates | ↑ | ↑ | 0/↑ | 0/↑ | 0 |
| β-Blockers | 0 | ↓ | ↓↓ | ↓↓ | ↓ |
| Calcium entry blockers | | | | | |
|   Verapamil | ↑ | ↑ | 0/↓ | 0/↓ | ↓ |
|   Diltiazem | ↑ | ↑ | ↓ | 0/↓ | 0/↓ |
|   Nifedipine | ↑ | ↑↑ | ↓ | ↑ | 0 |
|   Nicardipine | ↑↑ | ↑↑ | 0 | ↑ | 0 |

## Nitroglycerin

Assessment of preload is also crucial. Coronary perfusion pressure decreases with increased preload, especially if severe ischemia impairs global ventricular function, cardiac output, and MAP, a major variable influencing coronary perfusion pressure. The adverse effects of ischemia on diastolic function include decreased ventricular compliance due to impaired relaxation, and thus increased LVEDP. β-Blockers also can decrease contractility enough to increase LVEDP, especially if the dose is excessive (ie, bradycardia and hypotension occur).

The most effective agent to lower preload is nitroglycerin. Its potent venodilating effects lower end-diastolic volume and pressure. If a PA catheter is in place, the PA occlusion pressure (PAOP) should be reduced to a level just adequate to maintain cardiac output. Reduction below this level predisposes to a significant increase in heart rate in a normal ventricle. Hypotension results from an excessive dose in a normal ventricle or at low doses in an impaired one.

Because hypovolemia, relative or absolute, is common in the perioperative period, cautious intravascular volume expansion is almost always indicated during nitroglycerin administration. When ischemia has resulted in significant impairment of ventricular function, with acute ventricular dilation causing altered geometry of the mitral valve apparatus and a significant reduction in atrial compliance, acute mitral regurgitation is common (Fig. 43–14). Nitroglycerin, through its salutary effect on end-diastolic volume, is effective in reducing the degree of regurgitation. In this situation, intravascular volume expansion may be contraindicated.

Although technically complex, TEE can provide similar information. Assessment of ventricular cross-sectional area is achieved with short-axis views of the LV, and mitral function is analyzed with color flow Doppler imaging and spectral Doppler tracings of diastolic inflow velocities (E/A ratio).

## Sodium Nitroprusside

A primary reduction in afterload may also be indicated, especially during severe uncontrolled hypertension. Several arteriolar vasodilators are available. Sodium nitroprusside (SNP) is most commonly used but has a relatively low therapeutic index, especially at high doses (ie, cyanide toxicity or cardiovascular collapse). An uncommon effect of SNP is acute coronary steal, either between two coronary perfusion zones or from the subendocardium to the epicardium.

## Calcium Channel Antagonists

The so-called second-generation dihydropyridine calcium channel antagonists include amlodipine, felodipine, isradipine, nicardipine, and nisoldipine. Whereas the prototype of the dihydropyridines, nifedipine, has little direct myocardial action, newer dihydropyridines have almost none. The newer agents are potent systemic and coronary vasodilators that lack negative inotropic effects. Their principal clinical effect is to reduce arterial BP with minimal changes in heart rate or cardiac output. The sustained-release formulations reduce arterial BP gradually, thereby eliminating a trigger of the sinoaortic baroreflex and subsequent reflex tachycardia.[49] However, their onset of action and half-lives are much longer than those of SNP, and thus they are more difficult to titrate clinically.

NTG Effects on Abnormal PCWP "V" Waves

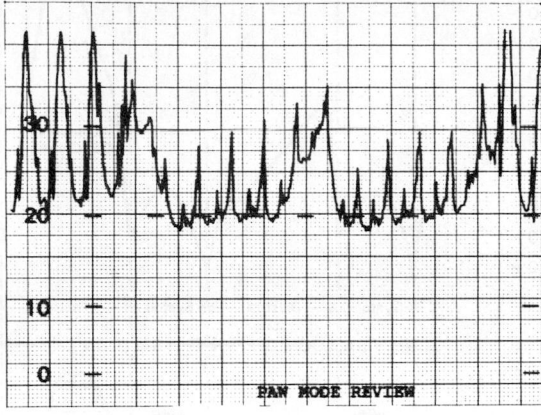

Pre-NTG

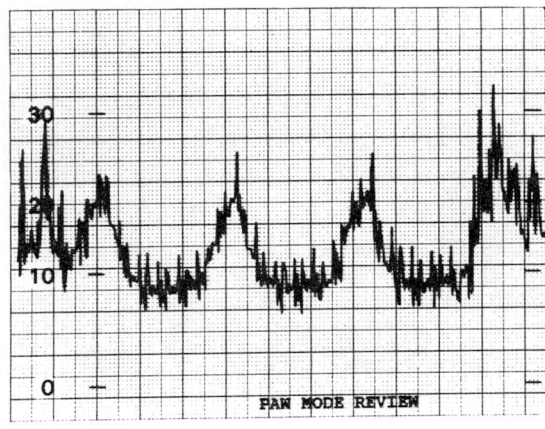

Post-NTG

**FIGURE 43–14.** Compressed pulmonary capillary wedge pressure (PCWP) tracings from a patient with severe, inoperable coronary artery disease undergoing aortofemoral bypass grafting. Elevated PCWP with 10-mm Hg V waves is indicative of impaired ventricular function, most likely resulting from chronic ischemia, mitral regurgitation, and decreased left atrial compliance. After intravenous institution of low-dose nitroglycerin (NTG), PCWP fell dramatically, V waves resolved, and cardiac output increased. (From London MJ. Monitoring for myocardial ischemia. In: Kaplan JA, ed. *Vascular Anesthesia.* New York, NY: Churchill Livingstone; 1991:281.)

## *How Is Cardiogenic Shock Managed?*

An uncommon situation, but one in which failure to act appropriately and aggressively may be disastrous, occurs when ischemia depresses global ventricular function and cardiac output to such a degree that severe hypotension results from cardiogenic shock. Nitroglycerin is still helpful, although it may be contraindicated with severe hypotension.

### Inotropic Support

In this case, there is no consensus about the best inotropic agent, and inotropic support with epinephrine, dopamine, dobutamine, amrinone, or milrinone is indicated. The dose should be carefully titrated to a point where BP and cardiac output are sufficiently elevated that nitroglycerin can be started. The dose of the selected inotrope should be continuously monitored to avoid arrhythmias or worsening the ubiquitous tachycardia that accompanies low cardiac output states.

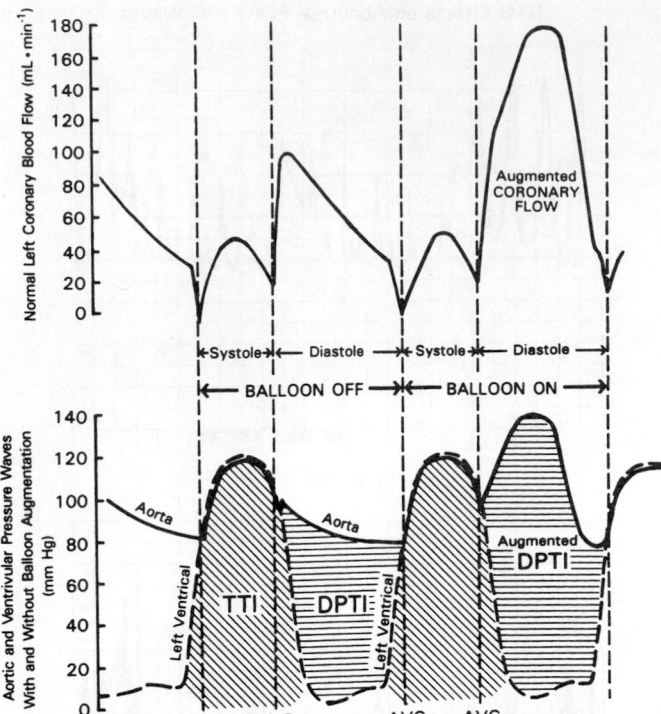

**FIGURE 43–15.** Effects of intraaortic balloon counterpulsation on coronary blood flow and intracardiac pressures. *Top panel*, Coronary flow tracings during diastolic augmentation. *Bottom panel*, Augmentation of diastolic pressure time index (DPTI; a measure of myocardial oxygen supply) versus systolic tension-time index (TTI; a measure of myocardial oxygen demand). (From Maccioli GA, Lucas WJ, Norfleet EA. The intraaortic balloon pump: a review. *J Cardiothorac Vasc Anesth.* 1988;2:369.)

## Intraaortic Balloon Counterpulsation

If inotropic therapy alone fails to increase cardiac output, or if the doses used produce adverse effects, such as oliguria or severe tachycardia, intraaortic balloon counterpulsation therapy should be instituted.

Balloon counterpulsation acts in several different, mutually beneficial ways to improve coronary perfusion and decrease myocardial O₂ demand.[50] Its most important function is to augment diastolic coronary perfusion. This goal is accomplished by inflating the balloon in the thoracic aorta during diastole and pushing blood in the aortic root from the preceding systolic ejection into the coronary vessels.

With rapid deflation of the balloon during early systole (isovolumic contraction), afterload is significantly reduced, allowing more efficient systolic ejection (ie, end-systolic volume is diminished; Fig. 43–15). This effect, in turn, reduces end-diastolic volume (ie, preload). Despite these beneficial effects, the use of this device must be tempered by its high cost and its propensity for major vascular complications.

## POSTOPERATIVE MYOCARDIAL INFARCTION

### What Is the Clinical Presentation and Timing?

As noted previously, ischemic syndromes span a wide physiologic spectrum. Early epidemiologic studies identified a peak incidence of perioperative infarction on or by the third postoperative day. Intraoperative infarction is reported much less commonly than early postoperative infarction, emphasizing the significant degree of stress that patients undergo after surgery compared with the well-controlled and relatively stress-free intraoperative period. The incidence of Q-wave and non–Q-wave infarction is similar in earlier studies, as was the associated mortality rate of roughly 50%. Chest pain is relatively uncommon, occurring in <50% of patients. Most patients, however, manifest a significant change in their clinical picture—particularly new or worsened heart failure, hypotension, or significant ventricular dysrhythmias.

A more recent screening of 323 patients with known ischemic heart disease (12-lead ECGs, creatine kinase (CK), CK isoenzymes, and troponin-T assays for the first 7 days after surgery) undergoing noncardiac surgery suggests a changing presentation relative to older studies.[14] In the 5.6% of patients meeting criteria for perioperative MI, 44% occurred on the first postoperative night. Non–Q-wave MI (56%) was more common than Q-wave MI (33%, with the remainder indeterminate). Chest pain was distinctly unusual (17%), although 56% of patients had a change in clinical status. In contrast to older studies, the acute mortality rate was only 17%. It is likely that the progressive sophistication of cardiovascular care, from preoperative management and therapy of ischemic heart disease to intraoperative monitoring and more aggressive use of pain management modalities to postoperative ICU monitoring, is responsible for improving statistics. However, the greater likelihood that surgical therapy will be used on sicker and older patients acts as a constant counterbalance.

### What Is the Incidence?

Infarction after noncardiac surgery in the general surgical population is a rare event, with an incidence of 0% to 0.7%. In patients with documented CAD or those with risk factors, the incidence is markedly higher and most closely related to the type of surgery. Patients undergoing major vascular surgery are at greatest risk. Statistics vary substantially depending on the type and size of the study; however, general estimates of between 4% and 6% for nonvascular surgery and 6% and 12% for vascular surgery (again depending on the type, with aortic vascular and peripheral limb revascularization the highest) appear to reflect the latest studies.[51]

### What Are the Suspected Perioperative Etiologic Factors?

A variety of etiologic factors have been proposed. A prolonged hyperadrenergic state induced by surgical stress and postoperative pain, associated with sustained sinus tachycardia with increased myocardial O₂ demand, has been described.[13] A prothrombotic state, precipitated by the stress response and direct activation of the coagulation system by surgical trauma, may precipitate intracoronary thrombosis.[52] Mild degrees of early postoperative hypothermia (<35.4°C) are associated with a doubling of cardiac morbidity rates relative to normothermic patients.[53] A postoperative hematocrit <28% has been identified as a threshold below which cardiac morbidity is significantly increased.[54]

**TABLE 43–7.** Reinfarction After Anesthesia in Patients With Myocardial Infarction

| Interval Between Infarction and Anesthesia (mo) | Patients With Postoperative Reinfarction (%) | |
| --- | --- | --- |
| | Group I* | Group II* |
| 0 - 3 | 36 | 5.8† |
| 4 - 6 | 26 | 2.3† |
| 7 - 12 | 5 | 1 |
| 13 - 24 | 5 | 1.6 |
| 25 | 5 | 1.7 |
| Total | 7.7 | 1.9‡ |

*Group I, historical control group (1973-1976); group II, prospective study group (1977–1982).
†$P < .05$.
‡$P < .005$.
From Rao T, Jacobs K, El-Etr A. Reinfarction following anesthesia in patients with myocardial infarction. *Anesthesiology.* 1983;59:499.

## Prior Myocardial Infarction

Patients with prior MI are at significantly increased risk over those with stable angina alone. The time interval between the initial (or latest) infarction and the surgical procedure was previously considered to be a major prognostic factor. Patients undergoing surgery within 6 months of infarction were thought to be at markedly elevated risk.

However, several studies, starting with that by Rao and coworkers, have documented significant reduction in reinfarction and mortality rates in these patients[55] (Table 43–7). These early investigators suggested that aggressive intraoperative and early postoperative invasive pressure monitoring and therapy with β-blockers and nitrates were critical. This study was performed before the advent of TEE and did not consider ST segment monitoring.

Because most clinicians are able to accomplish this goal without as aggressive a routine as Rao's group proposed, better preoperative management, as well as lighter, less depressant anesthetic regimens, may be more important. Significant improvement in postoperative pain management, especially routine patient-controlled analgesia or epidural opioids, is also likely to be of significance based on measured reductions in postoperative hormonal stress responses.

## When and How Should a Patient Be Ruled Out for Myocardial Infarction?

Ruling out an MI because of intraoperative findings suggestive of ischemia or infarction is a common clinical exercise, especially in the geriatric surgical population. In many in-

stances, the anesthesiologist triggers an algorithm based on suspect intraoperative ECG findings or abnormal hemodynamics (eg, unexplained hypotension with elevated PAOP). This observation leads to the patient being admitted directly to an ICU for monitoring of vital signs and cardiac rhythm, performance of serial 12-lead ECGs, and obtaining blood for assay of biochemical markers of injury or infarction (Table 43–8).

Until recently, CK-MB was the most commonly used assay. Although sensitive for myocardial injury, it suffers from relatively low specificity in the perioperative period because of increased MB production after surgical skeletal muscle injury (so-called return to ontogeny phenomenon due to fetal gene expression).[56] With the widespread introduction of troponin assays and striated regulatory muscle proteins that modulate muscle contraction, clinicians now have available a marker (troponin-I) that is 100% sensitive and specific for cardiac muscle. Troponin-T may be slightly less specific than troponin-I. The time course of elevation of the troponins and CK-MB is similar, although the duration of elevation of the troponins is significantly longer. Though rare, this may make it impossible to distinguish between unrecognized preoperative and postoperative MI. Other markers listed in Table 43–8 have a much quicker onset, although they suffer from substantially lower specificity.

### Indications

Most of these decisions are based on a clinician's bias and experience. Different clinicians may have various levels of concern about the intraoperative findings, how long they were present, and to what magnitude. The most common indications for ruling out MI are intraoperative ECG changes, particularly ST segment depression, T-wave inversions, and frequent premature ventricular contractions. ST segment elevation is rarely encountered in patients undergoing noncardiac surgery. It should be considered diagnostic of infarction until proven otherwise.[7]

### Diagnostic Measures

For accurate diagnosis, the change should be observed in the diagnostic mode (0.05-Hz low-frequency response) rather than the monitoring mode (0.5-Hz response) of the ECG monitor.[57] The monitoring mode exaggerates ST segment responses (Fig. 43–16). If the particular monitor does not have a diagnostic mode, a common deficiency of small 3-lead monitors used in older operating rooms, the change must be carefully compared with a 12-lead ECG done in the immediate postoperative period.

**TABLE 43–8.** Biochemical Markers of Myocardial Infarction and Injury

| Marker | Molecular Weight (daltons) | First Elevation (h) | Peak Elevation (h) | Duration (d) |
| --- | --- | --- | --- | --- |
| Myoglobin | 17 800 | 1 - 4 | 6 - 7 | 1 |
| Myosin light chain | 19 - 27 000 | 6 - 12 | 24 - 48 | 6 - 12 |
| CK-MB | 86 000 | 3 - 12 | 24 | 2 - 3 |
| CTn-I | 23 500 | 3 - 12 | 24 | 5 - 10 |
| CTn-T | 33 000 | 3 - 12 | 12 - 48 | 5 - 14 |
| LDH | 135 000 | 10 | 24 - 48 | 10 - 14 |

CK-MB, MB isoenzyme of creatine kinase; CTn-I, cardiac troponin-I; CTn-T, cardiac troponin-T; LDH, lactate dehydrogenase.

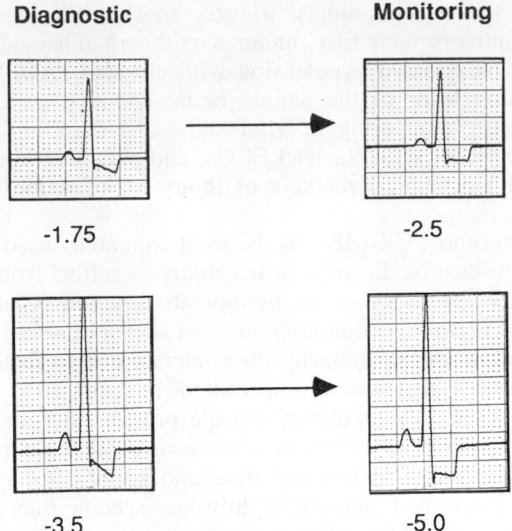

**Diagnostic**                    **Monitoring**

−1.75                             −2.5

−3.5                              −5.0

**FIGURE 43–16.** Effects of monitoring versus diagnostic mode on ST segment morphology (PC2 monitor; SpaceLabs, Inc, Redmond, Wash). Note change in slope and augmentation of ST segment depression. This occurs with any monitor when the low-frequency response is altered. Fortunately, all segment-trending devices default to the diagnostic mode during analysis. (From London MJ. Ischemia monitoring: ST segment analysis versus TEE. In: Kaplan JA, ed. *Cardiothoracic and Vascular Anesthesia Update.* Vol 3. Philadelphia, Pa: WB Saunders; 1993:5.)

Careful consideration of lead placement is essential. Although standard torso mounting of the limb leads provides a lead II similar to the 12-lead ECG, many clinicians fail to take the time to locate the precordial leads properly, particularly $V_5$.[58] Placement of the precordial $V_5$ is often several interspaces above or below and far to the right or left of the true position. Correct placement is the fifth intercostal space in the anterior axillary line. The sensitivity and specificity of a response in an aberrantly placed precordial lead, particularly in cases involving changes in the axis of the heart (ie, thoracotomy or upper abdominal surgery), are dubious.

### Sensitivity and Specificity of Electrocardiographic Changes

In many instances, transient intraoperative ECG changes, particularly minor ST depression, are likely to be false-positive responses or transient episodes of subendocardial ischemia and need not be ruled out. T-wave changes are less specific for ischemia, given their marked sensitivity to various autonomic stimuli. However, when symmetrically inverted, particularly in the anterior precordial leads, they are likely to represent ischemia.

Frequent ventricular ectopy that accompanies ECG changes is particularly worrisome and probably represents ischemia. Significant intraoperative ischemia is likely to manifest on the postoperative 12-lead ECG, although intraoperative therapy may have attenuated or aborted it. Thus, at times, a clinician may have to recommend a rule-out protocol despite a normal postoperative 12-lead ECG.

### *How Is Myocardial Dysfunction Assessed and Quantitated?*

### Preload

Precise quantitation of the determinants of stroke volume is difficult, and clinical estimations are, to various degrees, imprecise. Preload is the easiest to estimate using central venous pressure or PAOP measurements. However, these pressures provide only indirect assessment of left or right ventricular end-diastolic volume, the relation being defined by ventricular compliance (dV/dP). Although this approximation is useful in most instances, marked abnormalities of compliance commonly occur (eg, LV hypertrophy, after cardiopulmonary bypass). In these instances, compliance is usually reduced. Thus, to obtain a similar ventricular volume, a significantly higher intraventricular pressure is necessary and may reduce coronary perfusion pressure and lead to subendocardial ischemia.

### Afterload

Afterload is often equated with systemic vascular resistance. This approximation is a gross oversimplification of a complex phenomenon. In fact, a precise definition of afterload has yet to be universally accepted by physiologists. Some equate afterload with end-systolic wall stress, whereas others relate it to instantaneous aortic impedance during ventricular ejection. A more recent approach involves estimating arterial elastance, defined as end-systolic pressure divided by stroke volume.

### Contractility

Contractility, the variable of most interest to clinicians, is also the most difficult to quantitate. It must be assessed at known loading conditions (ie, constant preload and afterload). A number of indices unique to each phase of systole (isovolumetric contraction and systolic ejection) have been proposed to quantitate contractility.

### dP/dt

The maximum rate of rise of systolic pressure during isovolumic contraction (dP/dt) has been widely used by cardiologists because it can be easily measured during cardiac catheterization. However, its use is limited by its dependence on preload (increasing by 5%-10% with an acute increase in preload). The rate of rise of systolic wall stress is more robust because it takes into account LV geometry and mass, factors that vary greatly between individuals.

### Ejection Fraction

The most commonly used ejection phase index is the ejection fraction, the percentage of change in ventricular volume from end-diastole to end-systole. This noninvasive measurement is easily made using radionuclide or echocardiographic techniques and is widely used clinically.[34] It also depends on loading conditions and may remain normal despite deteriorating contractility, especially if preload is augmented or afterload is reduced. Conversely, preload may be low, despite normal contractile function, with increased afterload (so-called afterload mismatch).[59] However, in an intact organism, preload and afterload do not vary independently. An increase in preload simultaneously increases afterload, counterbalancing the theoretic increase in ejection fraction.

### End-Systolic Pressure-Volume Relation

During the 1990s, the end-systolic pressure-volume relation, a series of pressure-volume measurements at end-systole

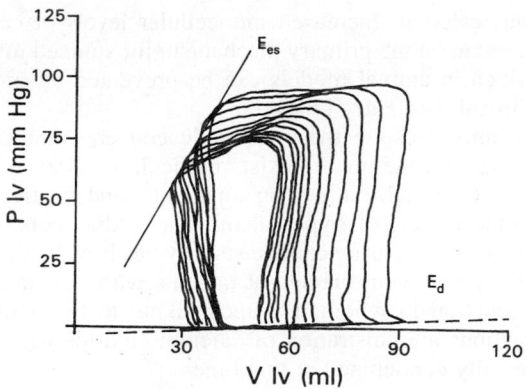

**FIGURE 43–17.** Pressure-volume loops from a patient undergoing cardiac surgery as measured by an intraventricular catheter capable of determining pressure (micromanometer tip) and volume (electrical impedance). The slope of the line joining a series of end-systolic pressure-volume points (obtained by a rapid decrease in preload during inferior vena cava occlusion), termed *end-systolic elastance* (Ees), is a measure of contractility unaffected by alteration in loading conditions. End-diastolic elastance (Ed) is determined from the same series of points at end-diastole and changes with alterations of ventricular stiffness. P lv, left ventricular pressure; V lv, left ventricular volume. (From Schreuder JJ, Biervliet JD, van der Velde ET, et al. Systolic and diastolic pressure-volume relationships during cardiac surgery. *J Cardiothorac Vasc Anesth.* 1991;5:543.)

from a series of cardiac cycles obtained by rapidly reducing preload, became widely accepted as a useful model to characterize contractility independent of loading conditions (Fig. 43–17). These points lie on a straight line, the slope of which is end-systolic elastance (Ees). Ees is the reciprocal of compliance and is proportional to contractility. It is unaffected by changes in preload or afterload. In a similar fashion, end-diastolic elastance (Ed) is determined from the same series of points at end-diastole and changes with alterations of ventricular stiffness. Although complex and invasive, this assessment has been used during cardiac surgery through a specialized ventricular catheter capable of measuring both pressure (micromanometer tip) and volume (electric conductance).[60]

## Which Patients Are at Greatest Risk?

Clinical signs of congestive heart failure (CHF), or a significant reduction in ejection fraction after acute MI, are important predictors of short- and long-term survival. In patients with heart failure secondary to nonischemic causes such as hypertension and infiltrative diseases, the degree of functional impairment assessed by the New York Heart Association (NYHA) classification is also predictive.

### Outcome Analysis

Goldman and colleagues prospectively evaluated patient outcomes after noncardiac surgery, finding preoperative $S_3$ gallop and jugular venous distention to be the most important multivariate predictors.[24,61] Not unexpectedly, the preoperative NYHA classification was also predictive. Patients with significant valvular disease were at increased risk as well.

Preoperative cardiomegaly in the absence of clinical signs, however, was not significant. More than half of the patients with postoperative pulmonary edema had no preoperative signs of failure, although almost all were >60 years of age,

underwent either major vascular or abdominal surgery, and had abnormal ECGs. These patients fared poorly, with 40% dying of cardiac causes. In contrast, no cardiac deaths occurred in patients with new postoperative heart failure but no pulmonary edema.

Other clinical studies using various techniques to quantitate ventricular function have confirmed many of these findings. However, with the trend in anesthesiology toward less depressant anesthetic techniques, frequent intraoperative monitoring of PA pressures or ventricular function (using TEE), and more effective postoperative pain management, these patients can be anesthetized with low morbidity and mortality rates. At the time of Goldman and colleagues' 1975 study, halothane was the primary anesthetic agent for most cases, PA catheterization with thermodilution cardiac output measurements was a specialized procedure, TEE did not exist, intravenous nitroglycerin was not widely available, and epidural narcotics were not used. Clearly, these advances have had a substantial impact on patient safety and outcome.

## TREATMENT OF PERIOPERATIVE MYOCARDIAL DYSFUNCTION

### What Are the Pharmacologic Options?

The treatment of intraoperative myocardial dysfunction involves proper diagnosis of the underlying problem and correction of reversible etiologic or exacerbating physiologic abnormalities (ie, acid-base disorders, particularly acidosis, impaired oxygenation or ventilation, severe anemia, sepsis, acute dysrhythmias). If these interventions are insufficient, pharmacologic or mechanical support of the circulation is indicated.

Therapy is tailored to a patient's pathophysiologic state. In most clinical situations encountered perioperatively, it requires augmentation of contractility; reduction of preload to decrease ventricular dimensions, wall stress, and myocardial $O_2$ demand; and optimization of diastolic filling, primarily by maintaining or establishing sinus rhythm and controlling heart rate. In certain instances, afterload reduction is indicated (eg, regurgitant valves and severe cardiomyopathy), whereas in others (eg, aortic stenosis), it is hazardous.

### Inotropes

Inotropic agents include the catecholamines, either endogenous (epinephrine, norepinephrine, and dopamine) or synthetic (isoproterenol, dobutamine), that act on adrenergic receptors. A noncatecholamine inotrope such as ephedrine acts on adrenergic receptors as well but lacks the catecholamine structure (catechol nucleus and amine side chain) or works through nonadrenergic mechanisms (ie, amrinone or milrinone by phosphodiesterase inhibition; digoxin by inhibition of sodium-calcium countertransport; or calcium chloride by direct augmentation of excitation-contraction coupling).

### Mechanisms of Action

Catecholamines and other adrenergic agonists act to stimulate the enzyme, adenyl cyclase adenosine triphosphate, which converts to cyclic adenosine monophosphate (cAMP), thereby increasing intracellular calcium concentration. Phosphodiesterase inhibitors achieve a similar effect through a different mechanism, inhibiting phosphodiesterase, the enzyme responsible for inactivation of cAMP.

### Adrenergic Receptors

Three major classes of adrenergic receptors, α, β, and dopaminergic (Table 43–9), modulate the diverse physiologic functions of the autonomic nervous system.[62] Receptor concentration is dynamic in number and responds to various physiologic factors, particularly plasma catecholamine concentrations and neural innervation of an organ. This upregulation or downregulation markedly affects the response of a particular organ to exogenous catecholamines. Almost all of the catecholamines—endogenous or synthetic—activate both α and β receptors, although affinity varies with the particular agent and its concentration. Phenylephrine and isoproterenol are notable exceptions with exclusive α and β affinity, respectively.

### Calcium Chloride

Calcium chloride has long been used for acute management of myocardial dysfunction in the operating room, particularly during cardiac surgery and cardiopulmonary resuscitation. Severe depression of extracellular *ionized* calcium levels causes myocardial depression and peripheral vasodilation.

Ionized calcium may be reduced after massive transfusion with citrated blood products. It is also reduced during cardiopulmonary bypass because of hemodilution from the pump prime and calcium binding by citrate, albumin, and heparin. However, considerable controversy exists over the level at which hemodynamic effects occur and, curiously, what hemodynamic effects are associated with its acute administration.

Studies performed after cardiopulmonary bypass have shown that small doses (5 mg/kg) increase MAP but not cardiac output.[63] Also, administration before β-adrenergic inotropes (particularly epinephrine) significantly attenuates their hemodynamic effects.[64] Calcium chloride also has been implicated in the development of acute coronary spasm.

**Advanced Cardiac Life Support.** Routine administration of calcium chloride has been eliminated from the advanced cardiac life support protocols of the American Heart Association. As the cellular role of calcium has become more clearly defined during the past decade, theoretic arguments against its use have been advanced. A major consideration is the adverse role of increased intracellular calcium levels during ischemic reperfusion on subsequent cellular viability and function. Diastolic relaxation, an energy-requiring process involving transport of calcium out of the cell, may be adversely affected by exogenous calcium. Increased intracellular levels of calcium are believed to be the primary mechanism for stunned myocardium, which in animal models can be prevented by pretreatment with calcium entry blockers.

**Indications.** Despite these theoretic concerns, indications for the use of calcium do exist, particularly after massive transfusion (especially in pediatric patients) and for treatment of the acute effects of hyperkalemia on cardiac conduction. Although its value during cardiac surgery has been challenged, studies have not been directed at patients with impaired ventricular function in whom it is most likely to be of benefit. Thus, cautious administration of calcium chloride should not be universally condemned at this time.

### Choice of Agent

When choosing an inotrope, the clinician must consider the net effect of a particular agent with regard to its direct inotropic actions and its effects on arteriolar and venous resistance, heart rate (chronotropy) and conduction velocity (dromotropy), lusitropy (ventricular relaxation), and renal dopaminergic receptors (Table 43–10). The actual high and low dose ranges in Table 43–10 are arbitrary owing to relatively wide variability between patients.

Note that potent physiologic modifiers of expected responses exist based on receptor affinity alone. In anesthetized patients, baroreceptor-mediated vagal bradycardia due to marked increase in MAP ($\alpha_1$ stimulation) may not occur, although it often does, particularly during narcotic or isoflurane anesthesia.

**Dopaminergic Effects.** Dopaminergic stimulation, in the absence of strong α stimulation, causes increased renal blood flow (usually preserving urine output). At high doses or with other α-adrenergic agents, effects on renal blood flow are controversial. At least one animal study suggests that when administered concomitantly with norepinephrine, dopamine maintains renal blood flow (ie, prevents norepinephrine-mediated vasoconstriction). However, in clinical use, few data support these findings, and oliguria is common during high-dose α-adrenergic therapy, even when used together with low-dose dopamine.

**α-Receptor Stimulation.** An additional factor to be considered is the difference between arterial and venous α-receptor activation. Venoconstriction has direct effects on preload (increasing it), whereas arteriolar constriction has effects on afterload. In general, most α-adrenergic agents cause venoconstriction at lower doses than are necessary for arteriolar effects.

**Clinical Application.** Since the early 1980s, there has been a shift away from rigorous maintenance of a normal MAP, as

**TABLE 43–9.** Adrenergic Receptors

| Receptor Type | Location | Actions |
|---|---|---|
| $\alpha_1$ | Postsynaptic—vascular smooth muscle | Vasoconstriction |
| $\alpha_2$ | Presynaptic | Inhibition of norepinephrine release, decreased central sympathetic outflow |
| $\beta_1$ | Postsynaptic—myocardium | Increased inotropy, chronotropy, dromotropy |
| $\beta_2$ | Postsynaptic—vascular bronchial, uterine smooth muscle | Vasodilation, bronchodilation, uterine relaxation |
| $D_1$ | Postsynaptic—renal mesenteric smooth muscle | Renal, mesenteric vasodilation |
| $D_2$ | Presynaptic | Inhibition of norepinephrine release |

D, dopamine.

**TABLE 43–10.** Inotropes

| Inotrope | Dose Range | Receptor | | | | Dose (Titrate to Effect) | Clinical Effects |
|---|---|---|---|---|---|---|---|
| | | $\alpha_1$ | $\beta_1$ | $\beta_2$ | *Dopaminergic* | | |
| *Catecholamines* | | | | | | | |
| Epinephrine | Low | 0/+ | + + + | + + | 0 | 0.025-0.15 μg/kg/min | Natural hormone; increased CO, SVR, HR; may increase PVR (rare) |
| | High | + + + + | + + + + | + + + | 0 | | |
| Norepinephrine | Low | + + + + | + | 0 | 0 | 0.025-0.15 μg/kg/min | Natural neurotransmitter; preserves cerebral and coronary flow; may be effective in combination with "inodilators" |
| | High | + + + + | + + | 0 | 0 | | |
| Dopamine | Low | 0/+ | + | + | + + + + | 1-3 μg/kg/min | Enhanced renal flow |
| | High | + + + | + + + + | + + | + + + + | 4-20 μg/kg/min | Effects of DA stimulation unclear at high doses |
| Isoproterenol | Low | 0 | + + + + | + + + + | 0 | 0.025-0.05 μg/kg/min | Use restricted to refractory bradydysrhythmias and elevated PVR; expect ventricular dysrhythmias |
| | High | 0 | + + + + | + + + + | 0 | | |
| Dobutamine | Low | 0 | + + | + | 0 | 1-10 μg/kg/min | So-called inodilator may be helpful in right and left ventricular failure due to afterload reduction |
| | High | + | + + + + | + + + | 0 | 10-20 μg/kg/min | |
| *Noncatecholamines* | | | | | | | |
| Ephedrine | | + + + | + + | + | 0 | 5-10 mg bolus | Mixed α and β agonist; bronchodilator, preserves uterine blood flow |
| Phenylephrine | | + + + + | 0 | 0 | 0 | 50-100 μg bolus or as infusion | Pure α agonist, potent baroreceptor effects on heart rate |
| Amrinone | 0 | 0 | 0 | 0 | | 0.75-1.5 mg/kg bolus load; 2–20 μg/kg/min infusion | Inodilator; phosphodiesterase inhibitor; peripheral vasodilation more potent than inotropic action |

CO, cardiac output; DA, dopaminergic; HR, heart rate; PVR, pulmonary vascular resistance; SVR, systemic vascular resistance.

was done previously with primary vasoconstrictors such as norepinephrine, and toward optimization of cardiac output. MAP is then titrated to the minimum level consistent with major organ perfusion. Dopamine and dobutamine are the most widely used agents, although the mechanism of increase in cardiac output by dobutamine, a dose-dependent increase in heart rate, can limit its use in patients who undergo coronary revascularization.[65] Many clinicians rely on epinephrine because it is the natural agent; however, this property is also a limitation because of its other noncardiac physiologic effects (hyperglycemia, hypokalemia, and type B lactic acidosis).

The phosphodiesterase inhibitor, amrinone, has received substantial attention and promotion. Its inotropic actions result from an increase in the concentration of intracellular cAMP and are comparable to those of dobutamine in patients with a low cardiac output state after coronary artery revascularization, whereas its peripheral vasodilating effects are greater.[66] A newer analogue of amrinone, milrinone, has similar inotropic effects but is less likely to cause thrombocytopenia with chronic administration.[67] In addition, milrinone can decrease pulmonary capillary wedge pressure and increase cardiac index significantly in patients with acute or decompensated heart failure.[68] Because the vasodilating effects of amrinone and milrinone can reduce MAP substantially, some clinicians believe that concurrent administration of primary vasoconstrictors such as phenylephrine or even norepinephrine, with its own potent inotropic effects, provides an optimal combination.

## How Should Actual or Potential Perioperative Dysfunction Be Monitored?

An intraarterial catheter should be placed in patients with myocardial dysfunction for beat-to-beat monitoring of arterial pressure. Indirect assessment of contractility is also possible by observation of the systolic upstroke and pulsus alternans, when it occurs.

### Pulmonary Artery Catheterization

In patients who have marginally impaired function and are undergoing minor surgery, a central venous catheter is usually adequate, especially if the dysfunction is predominantly right-sided (ie, cor pulmonale). However, in patients with significant LV dysfunction and in any at-risk patient undergoing major surgery involving significant blood loss or high aortic cross-clamping, a PA catheter is mandatory. Such monitoring also allows measurement of cardiac output by thermodilution.

Although the clinical signs of low cardiac output may be obvious in awake patients, they are difficult to assess during anesthesia. For example, anesthetic-induced alterations of renal autoregulation may reduce urine output unrelated to cardiac output. Further, the increased work of breathing associated with increased pulmonary extravascular fluid is not obvious during controlled ventilation. Thus, direct measurement of cardiac output and calculation of cardiac index for diagnosis and precise titration of therapeutic agents are essential. Noninvasive technologies for measuring cardiac output are available (ie, esophageal or tracheal Doppler probes, bioelectric impedance), although none is as reliable as thermodilution measurement.

Continuous mixed venous $O_2$ saturation measurement provides additional assessment of cardiovascular function (ie, $O_2$-carrying capacity and consumption) but is primarily used as a continuous warning system for changes in cardiac output, hematocrit, or $O_2$ consumption.

### Transesophageal Echocardiography

TEE can be used to evaluate systolic and diastolic ventricular function in the perioperative period. The transgastric short-axis cross-sectional view at the level of the midpapillary muscles can be used to evaluate changes in intracavitary size and shape, providing a real-time qualitative evaluation of systolic function. New technology allows continuous tracking of the LV endocardial borders with automated estimation of LV end-diastolic area and end-systolic area (automated boundary detection) and calculation of fractional area of change (FAC), which correlates well with radionuclide-determined ejection fraction.[69] The fractional area of change is calculated by the following formula:

$$FAC = (EDA - ESA)/EDA \times 100\% \qquad \text{(Equation 2)}$$

where EDA is LV end-diastolic area and ESA is LV end-systolic area. However, technical factors (ie, poor endocardial resolution) may limit accuracy underestimating LV ejection fraction. When compared with pressure-dimension indices used to measure LV contractility, automated boundary detection is not as sensitive.[70]

TEE can be used to measure cardiac output using pulsed-wave spectral Doppler, which quantitates blood flow velocity through a specific area of the heart. The blood flow velocity curve is integrated (velocity time integral [VTI]), which represents the distance traveled by red blood cells with each heartbeat and multiplied by the cross-sectional area (CSA) to estimate stroke volume. Stroke volume is then multiplied by heart rate (HR) to estimate cardiac output (CO), represented by the following formula:

$$\text{Doppler CO} = VTI \times CSA \times HR \qquad \text{(Equation 3)}$$

Doppler cardiac output can be measured at the mitral valve, aortic valve, and PA-right ventricular outflow tract, each with varying accuracy relative to thermodilution cardiac output measurements.[71] The best correlations have been obtained using the deep transgastric view which, when obtainable (in the authors' experience, >80% of the time), allows nearly parallel interrogation of the LV outflow tract and aortic root.[72] The opening of the aortic valve in the basal aortic root view is traced and used in the VTI equation.

TEE can also be used to assess diastolic ventricular function, providing important clinical information for patients with heart disease. In patients with CHF, diastolic dysfunction can occur with normal systolic function. Diseases associated with diastolic ventricular dysfunction are listed in Table 43–2.

Doppler measurements of transmitral and pulmonary venous blood inflow direction and velocity are associated with abnormalities in LV relaxation and compliance.[35,73] At the onset of diastole, the LV relaxes without change in LV volume

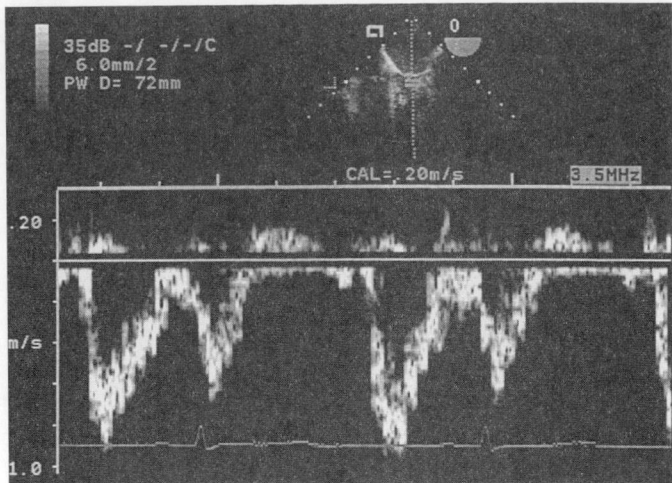

**FIGURE 43–18.** Normal transmitral inflow velocity profile with normal E/A ratio obtained by pulsed-wave Doppler at the level of the mitral valve leaflets.

and the isovolumetric relaxation time occurs. The initial transmitral blood inflow velocity accelerates to a rapid early-filling velocity, represented by the E wave. Velocity then decelerates at a measured rate known as the *deceleration time,* considered an important measure of LV stiffness or decreased compliance. Next, atrial contraction occurs and causes the late-filling A wave of the mitral inflow velocity pattern. The normal pattern has a broad and predominant E wave (Fig. 43–18). The isovolumetric relaxation time, E/A ratio, and deceleration time are used together to evaluate diastolic function. Pulmonary venous inflow occurs during ventricular systole and diastole, and the inflow velocity pattern is also used to evaluate diastolic function. A typical pulmonary venous inflow velocity pattern includes a systolic (S) and diastolic (D) peak velocity wave and sometimes a flow reversal wave as the left atrium fills or atrial contraction occurs (Fig. 43–19). Thorough TEE evaluation of diastolic ventricular function is possible but time consuming and limited by technical factors, alteration in loading conditions, and other physiologic factors (eg, age, arrhythmias, respiratory factors). Changes in the pattern of mitral inflow, such as a reversal of the E/A ratio, may be used to detect short-term changes in ventricular compliance (Fig. 43–20).

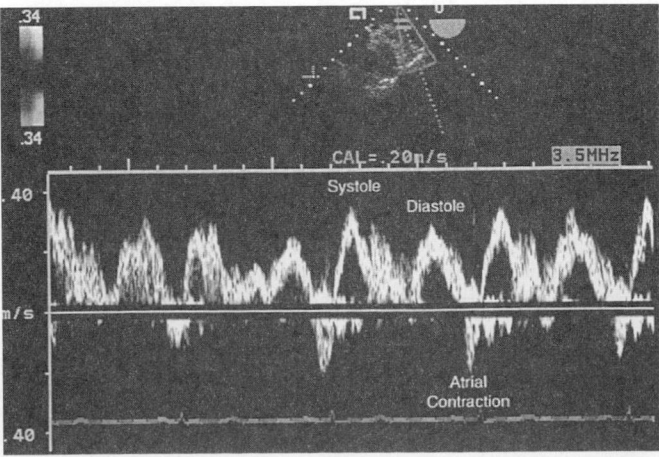

**FIGURE 43–19.** Normal inflow velocity profile from the left upper pulmonary vein obtained by pulsed wave Doppler.

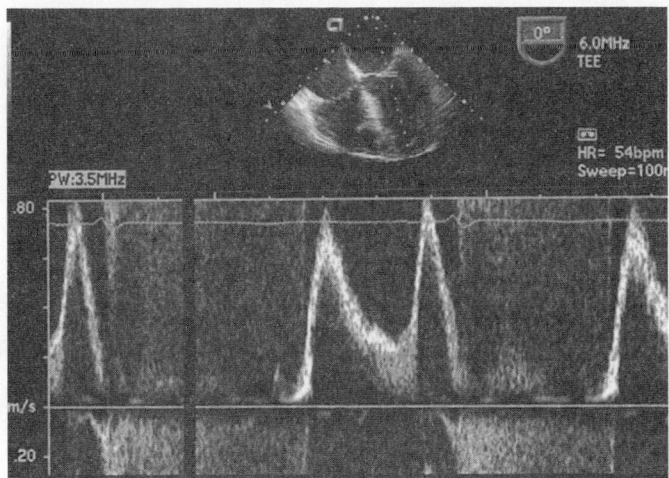

**FIGURE 43–20.** Abnormal transmitral inflow velocity profile with accentuation of A wave consistent with previously documented diastolic dysfunction and abnormal ventricular compliance.

Transmitral and pulmonary venous blood inflow patterns also can be used to estimate PAOP. In patients with decreased LV systolic function (ejection fraction <35%), PAOP correlates well with the deceleration time of the E wave ($r^2$ = 0.899).[74] In addition, a pulmonary venous blood inflow pattern with predominance of the peak diastolic velocity (S/D ratio <1) indicates a PAOP of >15 mm Hg.[75] An experienced anesthesiologist may use TEE to estimate PAOP instead of placing a PA catheter, but this practice is controversial because of unexpected technical limitations and physiologic variations.

## PREOPERATIVE OPTIMIZATION OF PATIENTS WITH MYOCARDIAL DYSFUNCTION

### How Should It Be Done?

Because of the significant risk of postoperative infarction in patients with preoperative dysfunction, optimization of ventricular function before surgery is crucial. In recent years, medical management of chronic CHF has focused on pharmacologic afterload reduction rather than digoxin and diuretics alone. More efficacious oral inotropic agents, such as the phosphodiesterase inhibitors, amrinone and milrinone, will eventually replace digoxin, which has a comparatively low therapeutic index.

Hydralazine has been used with good results. However, angiotensin-converting enzyme (ACE) inhibitors are now used almost exclusively. Although it is believed that all preoperative surgical candidates with CHF should be treated with ACE inhibitors, prospective study of the issue is clearly indicated. To what degree ACE inhibitors impair compensatory vasoconstrictive reflexes, particularly during weaning from cardiopulmonary bypass, with its attendant vasodilation during rewarming, is unclear.

### Preoperative Admission to the Intensive Care Unit

For elective surgical patients with CHF, outpatient evaluation with serial ejection fractions (precordial echocardiogra-phy or multigated angiography) and medical management with ACE inhibitors for a period of weeks are all that is usually required to optimize a patient's condition before surgery. In urgent or emergent cases or in patients with significant decompensation due to intercurrent surgical illness, admission to an ICU for PA catheterization is frequently recommended to assess filling pressures, cardiac output, and the response to a fluid challenge.

### Therapeutic Interventions

If the PAOP is elevated, nitroglycerin should be used to lower it while the corresponding cardiac index is assessed. In general, PAOP should be maintained in the range of 10 to 15 mm Hg. Lower pressures may result in a precipitous decline in cardiac index if intravascular volume falls during surgery. Higher pressures are likely to result in a significant decline in coronary perfusion pressure and pulmonary vascular congestion. However, selected patients may tolerate lower or higher wedge pressures based on their particular pathophysiologic process.

In patients with profound degrees of dysfunction, inotropic augmentation, diuretics, and afterload reduction should be used to increase cardiac index above the range of 2.0 to 2.2 L/m². A common approach is to use low-dose dopamine (3 µg/kg/min) to improve renal perfusion and facilitate diuresis. An inotropic agent with predominant β effects and a low dose of an arteriolar vasodilator such as SNP are frequently added. Increased emphasis also has been placed on inodilator agents such as milrinone and amrinone. However, their superiority over a primary inotrope such as epinephrine or dopamine, plus a primary vasodilator such as nitroglycerin or SNP, has not been demonstrated conclusively.

### Hazards

A word of caution about preoperative placement of catheters and optimization of hemodynamics is necessary. These techniques and assessments are often performed by surgeons or cardiologists. Many permutations of this approach are recognized, ranging from helpful to nearly destructive. Patients frequently are stressed and are given little if any sedation or analgesia during invasive catheterization. Curiously, little attention is paid to the hemodynamic changes or significant tachycardia that may be induced by this stress.

Surgeons usually prefer the subclavian approach to PA catheterization, with its attendant hazards. Many cardiologists prefer femoral cannulation, which is not accessible to the anesthesiologist during surgery, thereby placing the patient at risk of PA perforation if the catheter cannot be manipulated during hypovolemic states or cardiopulmonary bypass. In some instances, adapters, tubing, fittings, and the like differ from those used in the operating room, presenting additional problems to the anesthesiologist, who must then make on-the-spot adjustments or changes.

### References

1. Buckberg GD, Robertson JM, McConnell DH, et al. Determinants of myocardial performance and the adequacy of subendocardial blood flow. In: Utley JR, ed. *Perioperative Cardiac Dysfunction.* Baltimore, Md: Williams & Wilkins; 1985:139.
2. Boudoulas H, Rittgers SE, Lewis RP, et al. Changes in diastolic time with various pharmacologic agents. *Circulation.* 1979;60:164.

3. Loeb HS, Saudye A, Croke RP, et al. Effects of pharmacologically induced hypertension on myocardial ischemia and coronary hemodynamics in patients with fixed coronary obstruction. *Circulation.* 1978;57:41.

4. Buffington CW. Hemodynamic determinants of ischemic myocardial dysfunction in the presence of coronary stenosis in dogs. *Anesthesiology.* 1985;63:651.

5. London MJ. Monitoring for myocardial ischemia. In: Kaplan JA, ed. *Vascular Anesthesia.* New York, NY: Churchill Livingstone; 1991:249.

6. London MJ. Ischemia monitoring: ST segment analysis versus TEE. In: Kaplan JA, ed. *Cardiothoracic and Vascular Anesthesia Update.* Philadelphia, Pa: WB Saunders; 1993:1.

7. London MJ, Kaplan JA. Advances in electrocardiographic monitoring. In Kaplan JA, ed. *Cardiac Anesthesia.* 4th ed. Philadelphia, Pa: WB Saunders; 1998:413.

8. American Society of Anesthesiologists and the Society of Cardiovascular Anesthesiologists Task Force on Transesophageal Echocardiography. Practice guidelines for perioperative transesophageal echocardiography: a report by the American Society of Anesthesiologists and the Society of Cardiovascular Anesthesiologists Task Force on Transesophageal Echocardiography. *Anesthesiology.* 1996;84:986.

9. Buda AJ, Zotz RJ, Pace DP, et al. Comparison of two-dimensional echocardiographic wall motion and wall thickening abnormalities in relation to the myocardium at risk. *Am Heart J.* 1986;111:587.

10. Shanewise JS, Cheung AT, Aronson S, et al. ASE/SCA guidelines for performing a comprehensive intraoperative multiplane transesophageal echocardiography examination: recommendations of the American Society of Echocardiography Council for Intraoperative Echocardiography and the Society of Cardiovascular Anesthesiologists Task Force for Certification in Perioperative Transesophageal Echocardiography. *Anesth Analg.* 1999;89:870.

11. Rouine-Rapp K, Ionescu P, Balea M, et al. Detection of intraoperative segmental wall-motion abnormalities by transesophageal echocardiography: the incremental value of additional cross sections in the transverse and longitudinal planes. *Anesth Analg.* 1996;83:1141.

12. Opie LH. The multifarious spectrum of ischemic left ventricular dysfunction: relevance of new ischemic syndromes. *J Mol Cell Cardiol.* 1996;28:2403.

13. Landesberg G, Luria MH, Cotev S, et al. Importance of long-duration postoperative ST-segment depression in cardiac morbidity after vascular surgery. *Lancet.* 1993;341:715.

14. Badner NH, Knill RL, Brown JE, et al. Myocardial infarction after noncardiac surgery. *Anesthesiology.* 1998;88:572.

15. Kloner RA, Bolli R, Marban E, et al. Medical and cellular implications of stunning, hibernation, and preconditioning: an NHLBI workshop. *Circulation.* 1998;97:1848.

16. London MJ, Tubau JF, Wong MG, et al. The "natural history" of segmental wall motion abnormalities in patients undergoing noncardiac surgery. *Anesthesiology.* 1990;73:644.

17. Kersten JR, Schmeling TJ, Pagel PS, et al. Isoflurane mimics ischemic preconditioning via activation of K(ATP) channels: reduction of myocardial infarct size with an acute memory phase. *Anesthesiology.* 1997;87:361.

18. Théroux P, Fuster V. Acute coronary syndromes: unstable angina and non-Q-wave myocardial infarction. *Circulation.* 1998;97:1195.

19. Mulcahy D, Husain S, Zalos G, et al. Ischemia during ambulatory monitoring as a prognostic indicator in patients with stable coronary artery disease. *JAMA.* 1997;277:318.

20. Davies RF, Goldberg AD, Forman S, et al. Asymptomatic Cardiac Ischemia Pilot (ACIP) study two-year follow-up: outcomes of patients randomized to initial strategies of medical therapy versus revascularization. *Circulation.* 1997;95:2037.

21. Pasternack PF, Grossi EA, Baumann FG, et al. The value of silent ischemia monitoring in the prediction of perioperative myocardial infarction in patients undergoing peripheral vascular surgery. *J Vasc Surg.* 1989;10:617.

22. Raby KE, Goldman L, Creager MA, et al. Correlation between preoperative ischemia and major cardiac events after peripheral vascular surgery. *N Engl J Med.* 1989;321:1296.

23. Mangano DT, Browner WS, Hollenberg M, et al. Association of perioperative myocardial ischemia with cardiac morbidity and mortality in men undergoing noncardiac surgery. *N Engl J Med.* 1990;323:1781.

24. Goldman L, Caldera D, Nussbaum S, et al. Multifactorial index of cardiac risk in noncardiac surgical procedures. *N Engl J Med.* 1977;297:845.

25. Mangano DT, Layug EL, Wallace A, et al. Effect of atenolol on mortality and cardiovascular morbidity after noncardiac surgery: multicenter study of Perioperative Ischemia Research Group. *N Engl J Med.* 1996;335:1713.

26. Poldermans D, Boersma E, Bax JJ, et al. The effect of bisoprolol on perioperative mortality and myocardial infarction in high-risk patients undergoing vascular surgery. *N Engl J Med.* 1999;341:1789.

27. Eagle KA, Brundage BH, Chaitman BR, et al. Guidelines for perioperative cardiovascular evaluation for noncardiac surgery: report of the American College of Cardiology/American Heart Association Task Force on Practice Guidelines (Committee on Perioperative Cardiovascular Evaluation for Noncardiac Surgery). *J Am Coll Cardiol.* 1996;27:910.

28. Wallace A, Layug B, Tateo I, et al. Prophylactic atenolol reduces postoperative myocardial ischemia: McSPI Research Group. *Anesthesiology.* 1998;88:7.

29. Zaugg M, Tagliente T, Lucchinetti E, et al. Beneficial effects from beta-adrenergic blockade in elderly patients undergoing noncardiac surgery. *Anesthesiology.* 1999;91:1674.

30. Coriat P, Daloz M, Bousseau D, et al. Prevention of intraoperative myocardial ischemia during noncardiac surgery with intravenous nitroglycerin. *Anesthesiology.* 1984;61:193.

31. Thomson IR, Mutch WA, Culligan JD. Failure of intravenous nitroglycerin to prevent intraoperative myocardial ischemia during fentanyl-pancuronium anesthesia. *Anesthesiology.* 1984;61:385.

32. Dodds TM, Stone JG, Coromilas J, et al. Prophylactic nitroglycerin infusion during noncardiac surgery does not reduce perioperative ischemia. *Anesth Analg.* 1993;76:705.

33. Bradley JA, Alpert JS. Coronary flow reserve. *Am Heart J.* 1991;122:1116.

34. Grossman W. Evaluation of systolic and diastolic function of the myocardium. In: Grossman W, ed. *Cardiac Catheterization and Angiography.* Philadelphia, Pa: Lea & Febiger; 1986:301.

35. Cohen GI, Pietrolungo JF, Thomas JD, et al. A practical guide to assessment of ventricular diastolic function using Doppler echocardiography. *J Am Coll Cardiol.* 1996;27:1753.

36. Reiz S, Balfors E, Sorenson MB, et al. Isoflurane: a powerful coronary vasodilator in patients with coronary artery disease. *Anesthesiology.* 1983;59:91.

37. Buffington CW, Romson JL, Levine A, et al. Isoflurane induces coronary steal in a canine model of chronic coronary occlusion. *Anesthesiology.* 1987;66:280.

38. Cason BA, Verrier ED, London MJ, et al. Effects of isoflurane and halothane on coronary vascular resistance and collateral myocardial blood flow: their capacity to induce coronary steal. *Anesthesiology.* 1987;67:665.

39. Priebe HJ. Isoflurane and coronary hemodynamics. *Anesthesiology.* 1989;71:960.

40. Weiskopf RB, Moore MA, Eger EIN, et al. Rapid increase in desflurane concentration is associated with greater transient cardiovascular stimulation than with rapid increase in isoflurane concentration in humans. *Anesthesiology.* 1994;80:1035.

41. Ebert TJ, Kharasch ED, Rooke GA, et al. Myocardial ischemia and adverse cardiac outcomes in cardiac patients undergoing noncardiac surgery with sevoflurane and isoflurane: Sevoflurane Ischemia Study Group. *Anesth Analg.* 1997;85:993.

42. Kitahata H, Kawahito S, Nozaki J, et al. Effects of sevoflurane on regional myocardial blood flow distribution: quantification with myocardial contrast echocardiography. *Anesthesiology.* 1999;90:1436.

43. Yeager MP, Glass DD, Neff RK, et al. Epidural anesthesia and analgesia in high-risk surgical patients. *Anesthesiology.* 1987;66:729.

44. Breslow MJ, Jordan DA, Christopherson R, et al. Epidural morphine decreases postoperative hypertension by attenuating sympathetic nervous system hyperactivity. *JAMA.* 1989;261:3577.

45. Meissner A, Rolf N, Van Aken H. Thoracic epidural anesthesia and the patient with heart disease: benefits, risks, and controversies. *Anesth Analg.* 1997;85:517.

46. Baron JF, Bertrand M, Barré E, et al. Combined epidural and general anesthesia versus general anesthesia for abdominal aortic surgery. *Anesthesiology.* 1991;75:611.

47. Dodds TM, Burns AK, DeRoo DB, et al. Effects of anesthetic technique on myocardial wall motion abnormalities during abdominal aortic surgery. *J Cardiothorac Vasc Anesth.* 1997;11:129.

48. Philbin DM, Rosow CE, Schneider RC, et al. Fentanyl and sufentanil anesthesia revisited: how much is enough? *Anesthesiology.* 1990;73:5.

49. Silvestry FE, St John Sutton MG. Sustained-release calcium channel antagonists in cardiovascular disease: pharmacology and current therapeutic use. *Eur Heart J.* 1998;19(suppl I):I8.

50. Maccioli GA, Lucas WJ, Norfleet EA. The intra-aortic balloon pump: a review. *J Cardiothorac Vasc Anesth.* 1988;2:365.

51. Oliver MF, Goldman L, Julian DG, et al. Effect of mivazerol on perioperative cardiac complications during non-cardiac surgery in patients with

coronary heart disease: the European Mivazerol Trial (EMIT). *Anesthesiology*. 1999;91:951.

52. Rosenfeld BA, Beattie C, Christopherson R, et al. The effects of different anesthetic regimens on fibrinolysis and the development of postoperative arterial thrombosis: Perioperative Ischemia Randomized Anesthesia Trial Study Group. *Anesthesiology*. 1993;79:435.

53. Frank SM, Fleisher LA, Breslow MJ, et al. Perioperative maintenance of normothermia reduces the incidence of morbid cardiac events: a randomized clinical trial. *JAMA*. 1997;277:1127.

54. Nelson AH, Fleisher LA, Rosenbaum SH. Relationship between postoperative anemia and cardiac morbidity in high- risk vascular patients in the intensive care unit. *Crit Care Med*. 1993;21:860.

55. Rao T, Jacobs K, El-Etr A. Reinfarction following anesthesia in patients with myocardial infarction. *Anesthesiology*. 1983;59:499.

56. Adams JE, Sicard GA, Allen BT, et al. Diagnosis of perioperative myocardial infarction with measurement of cardiac troponin I. *N Engl J Med*. 1994;330:670.

57. London MJ, Ahlstrom LD. Validation testing of the SpaceLabs PC2 ST-segment analyzer. *J Cardiothorac Vasc Anesth*. 1995;9:684.

58. London MJ, Hollenberg M, Wong MG, et al. SPI Research Group: intraoperative myocardial ischemia: localization by continuous 12 lead electrocardiography. *Anesthesiology*. 1988;69:232.

59. Ross JJ. Afterload mismatch in the perioperative period. In: Utley JR, ed. *Perioperative Cardiac Dysfunction*. Baltimore, Md: Williams & Wilkins; 1985:139.

60. Schreuder JJ, Biervliet JD, van der Velde ET, et al. Systolic and diastolic pressure-volume relationships during cardiac surgery. *J Cardiothorac Vasc Anesth*. 1991;5:539.

61. Goldman L. Multifactorial index of cardiac risk in noncardiac surgery: ten year status report. *J Cardiothorac Vasc Anesth*. 1987;1:237.

62. Breslow MJ, Ligier B. Hyperadrenergic states. *Crit Care Med*. 1991;19:1566.

63. Royster RL, Butterworth J, Prielipp RC, et al. A randomized, blinded, placebo-controlled evaluation of calcium chloride and epinephrine for inotropic support after emergence from cardiopulmonary bypass. *Anesth Analg*. 1992;74:3.

64. Zaloga GP, Strickland RA, Butterworth J, et al. Calcium attenuates epinephrine's beta-adrenergic effects in postoperative heart surgery patients. *Circulation*. 1990,81.196.

65. Romson JL, Leung JM, Bellows WH, et al. Effects of dobutamine on hemodynamics and left ventricular performance after cardiopulmonary bypass in cardiac surgical patients. *Anesthesiology*. 1999;91:1318.

66. Dupuis JY, Bondy R, Cattran C, et al. Amrinone and dobutamine as primary treatment of low cardiac output syndrome following coronary artery surgery: a comparison of their effects on hemodynamics and outcome. *J Cardiothorac Vasc Anesth*. 1992;6:542.

67. Rathmell JP, Prielipp RC, Butterworth JF, et al. A multicenter, randomized, blind comparison of amrinone with milrinone after elective cardiac surgery. *Anesth Analg*. 1998;86:683.

68. Seino Y, Momomura S, Takano T, et al. Multicenter, double-blind study of intravenous milrinone for patients with acute heart failure in Japan: Japan Intravenous Milrinone Investigators. *Crit Care Med*. 1996;24:1490.

69. Liu N, Darmon PL, Saada M, et al. Comparison between radionuclide ejection fraction and fractional area changes derived from transesophageal echocardiography using automated border detection. *Anesthesiology*. 1996;85:468.

70. Declerck C, Hillel Z, Shih H, et al. A comparison of left ventricular performance indices measured by transesophageal echocardiography with automated border detection. *Anesthesiology*. 1998;89:341.

71. Maslow A, Comunale ME, Haering JM, et al. Pulsed wave Doppler measurement of cardiac output from the right ventricular outflow tract. *Anesth Analg*. 1996;83:466.

72. Darmon PL, Hillel Z, Mogtader A, et al. Cardiac output by transesophageal echocardiography using continuous-wave Doppler across the aortic valve. *Anesthesiology*. 1994;80:796.

73. Rakowski H, Appleton C, Chan KL, et al. Canadian consensus recommendations for the measurement and reporting of diastolic dysfunction by echocardiography: from the Investigators of Consensus on Diastolic Dysfunction by Echocardiography. *J Am Soc Echocardiogr*. 1996;9:736.

74. Nomura M, Hillel Z, Shih H, et al. The association between Doppler transmitral flow variables measured by transesophageal echocardiography and pulmonary capillary wedge pressure. *Anesth Analg*. 1997;84:491.

75. Kuecherer HF, Kusumoto F, Muhiudeen IA, et al. Pulmonary venous flow patterns by transesophageal pulsed Doppler echocardiography: relation to parameters of left ventricular systolic and diastolic function. *Am Heart J*. 1991;122:1683.

CHAPTER

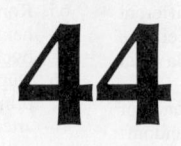

# Intracranial Pressure

## Cheri A. Sulek

Intracranial pressure (ICP) is determined by the volumes of blood, cerebrospinal fluid (CSF), and brain tissue contained within the calvarium. The regulation of the intracranial contents and pressure becomes compromised when pathology is introduced. Structural components of the intracranial compartment that limit expansion are well defined. However, the concept of abnormal ICP and management goals continue to evolve as we gain a better understanding of the primary and secondary pathophysiologic processes involved in producing brain injury. It is now well recognized that ICP is not always uniform within the intracranial compartment. For instance, local differences in ICP and cerebral blood flow (CBF) may exist after head injury or in the region surrounding a brain tumor.[1-3] Although the management goals may differ between local and global alterations in ICP or blood flow, there exists the potential for ischemic insult that may affect ultimate neurologic outcome.

Secondary neuronal injury after a traumatic or ischemic insult ultimately may be more important in determining neurologic outcome than the primary pathology after head injury. For this reason, the use of monitors to measure cerebral hemodynamics and oxygenation is more commonplace in the perioperative management of head-injured patients with increased ICP. In the near future, treatment of head-injured patients with abnormal elastance may be directed not only toward the primary event but also toward initiation of therapy that may attenuate or prevent secondary neuronal injury.[4]

Additionally, the introduction of new anesthetic agents in clinical practice prompts the anesthesiologist to recognize the impact of these agents on ICP to provide a safe intraoperative course and optimal operating conditions. This pharmacologic knowledge is also important to apply to those patients with suspected or documented intracranial hypertension undergoing nonneurosurgical procedures.

The goals of this chapter are to provide the following:

1. A basic understanding of ICP
2. The regulation of ICP and impact on cerebral perfusion
3. The impact of anesthetic agents on ICP
4. The perioperative management of patients with intracranial hypertension secondary to acute or chronic pathologic processes.

## DETERMINANTS AND REGULATION OF INTRACRANIAL PRESSURE

### What Are the Intracranial Contents That Determine Intracranial Pressure?

Brain tissue, CSF, blood, and meninges comprise the intracranial contents and are responsible for ICP and its regulation. The calvarium is a nondistensible, semiclosed container that strictly limits intracranial volume and the expansion of any acute or chronic process. It is no longer considered closed in the presence of a fracture, during a craniotomy after bone flap removal, or in infancy before suture and fontanelle closure. Internally, the superior and inferior intracranial compartments are separated by the tentorium and communicate through the tentorial incisura. The cranial and spinal contents also remain in continuity through the foramen magnum.

Brain tissue alone accounts for 88% of the total intracranial volume. The meninges and other structures supporting the brain contribute minimally and have limited distensibility. Eighty percent of brain volume is water, 20% of which is sequestered in the extracellular space.[5] Expansion of brain volume is either secondary to an increase in water content, as occurs with disruption of the blood-brain barrier, or caused by growth of the solid substance itself (ie, brain tumor). CSF constitutes 9% of the total intracranial volume. Although the intracranial blood volume contributes only 2% to 3% of total volume, it is an important determinant of ICP and is the parameter most commonly manipulated by an anesthesiologist.

The intracranial volume remains constant until the addition of a new volume (eg, hematoma) or expansion of an existing volume (eg, tumor) occurs. The maintenance of a normal ICP requires a mandatory, reciprocal reduction in volume of one of the intracranial components to offset the effects of the new volume added. These concepts embody the basic principles of the Monro-Kellie doctrine and its modifications.[6–8]

### What Are Normal and Abnormal Values for Intracranial Pressure?

In adults, normal ICP measured in the horizontal position is 5 to 15 mm Hg. Values recorded in infants and young children are lower. In the horizontal position, the lumbar subarachnoid pressures should reflect the ICP as long as the two compartments freely communicate. Lumbar pressure can be misleading when local ICP elevation (eg, peritumor edema) exists because the "global" ICP is often recorded in the normal range.

Intracranial pressure is considered abnormal and classified as intracranial hypertension when values exceed 15 to 20 mm Hg. Neurologic outcome in head-injured patients appears to correlate well with the degree and duration of intracranial hypertension, making it prudent to treat ICP elevations aggressively.[9,10] Recent data support maintenance of ICP <20 mm Hg and a cerebral perfusion pressure (CPP) >70 mm Hg.[10,11] Sustained ICP elevations exceeding 25 to 30 mm Hg that are refractory to treatment are often fatal. The detrimental effects of intracranial hypertension result from cerebral ischemia and direct compressive effects on vital brain structures.

### How Is Normal Intracranial Pressure Maintained in Pathologic States?

ICP is closely regulated, even in the presence of a space-occupying lesion, as long as compensatory mechanisms are functional and the pathologic process evolves slowly. If rapid volume expansion occurs, as with an epidural hematoma, ICP rises abruptly because compensatory mechanisms are limited in the acute situation. Conversely, a chronic pathologic process ultimately increases brain volume, but the chronicity of the disease allows reductions in cerebral blood volume (CBV) and CSF to maintain normal intracranial dynamics, often for many years.

The reduction of CBV, particularly from the low-pressure venous side, can be easily manipulated and reduced to provide additional space for an expanding lesion. In the situation of acute volume expansion, the only operative compensatory mechanism is displacement of intracranial blood; unfortunately, reserve is limited, and spatial exhaustion occurs early. The greatest buffering capacity is afforded by the CSF system and is most effective in a chronic situation. The rate of CSF absorption increases in the presence of a space-occupying lesion; the rate of CSF production is minimally affected. When maximal CSF reabsorption capacity is reached, spatial exhaustion occurs, and ICP rises acutely. Brain atrophy may also occur from chronic water and electrolyte loss.

#### Intracranial Pressure-Volume Curve

The pressure-volume curve depicts the ideal relationship between ICP and volume with chronic volume expansion. (Fig. 44–1). During the period of spatial compensation, ICP increases minimally, even with relatively large changes in intracranial volume. When the buffering capacity of the intracranial space is exhausted, small increases in volume (dV) are followed by abrupt rises in ICP (dP). The dP/dV of the pressure-volume curve defines the elastance of the system and reflects its stiffness or resistance to deformation exerted by the intracranial contents with the addition of volume.[12] Along the horizontal portion of the curve, the elastance of the intracranial compartment is low, whereas the opposite relationship exists for the vertical portion of the curve.

## CEREBRAL PHYSIOLOGY

### How Does Intracranial Pressure Affect Cerebral Perfusion Pressure?

Elevated ICP alters the perfusion of cortical and subcortical structures. CPP is the pressure gradient that drives CBF and

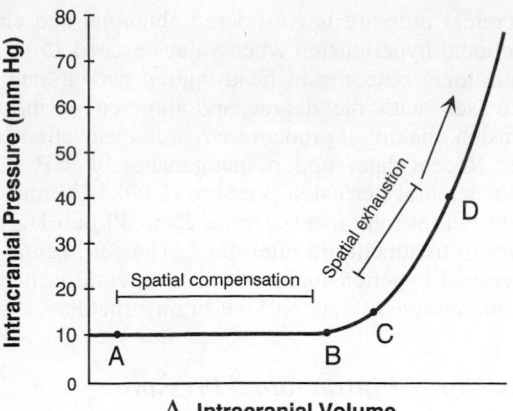

**FIGURE 44–1.** Intracranial pressure (ICP)-volume curve. Spatial compensation with increasing intracranial volume occurs between points A to B. The elastance of the system is low and ICP normal. At point C, compensatory mechanisms fail, spatial exhaustion occurs, and ICP rises. Between points C and D, small changes in intracranial volume result in large changes in ICP. (From Sulek CA. Intracranial pressure. In: Cucchiara RF, Black S, Michenfelder JD, eds. *Clinical Neuroanesthesia.* 2nd ed. New York, NY: Churchill Livingstone; 1998:76.)

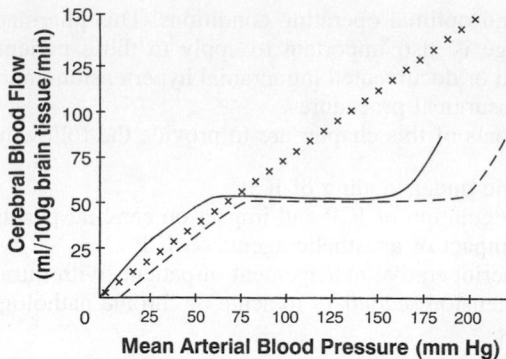

**FIGURE 44–2.** Cerebral autoregulation curves in normotensive and chronic hypertensive states and with loss of autoregulation. Cerebral blood flow (CBF) remains constant in normotensive individuals when mean arterial pressure (MAP) ranges from 60 to 160 mm Hg. The upper and lower limits of autoregulation shift to higher values when the MAP is chronically elevated. With loss of autoregulation, CBF passively follows changes in MAP. Cerebral autoregulation in normotensive individual = (——); cerebral autoregulation in a chronically hypertensive individual = (-----); loss of autoregulation = (xxx). (From Sulek CA. Intracranial pressure. In: Cucchiara RF, Black S, Michenfelder JD, eds. *Clinical Neuroanesthesia.* 2nd ed. New York, NY: Churchill Livingstone; 1998:77.)

metabolite delivery. The relationship between ICP and CPP is defined: CPP = MAP − ICP or CVP (central venous pressure) when ICP is not available (MAP, mean arterial pressure). The lower limit of CPP acceptable in adults without intracranial pathology is 50 mm Hg; it is much lower in infants. In the presence of intracranial pathology, effective perfusion pressure declines as ICP rises. Previously, maintenance of CPP >50 mm Hg was considered acceptable in head-injured patients. However, at least 30% of patients with severe head injury have regional or global cerebral ischemia (CBF <18 mL/100 g/min).[1] Of those patients who die of traumatic brain injury, a significant percentage have histologic evidence of ischemic injury.[13] In accordance with new guidelines for severely head-injured patients, CPP should be maintained >70 mm Hg to minimize the risk for cerebral ischemia.[11,14,15] A decrease in MAP or an elevation in ICP deleteriously alters the effective perfusion pressure.

## How Is Cerebral Blood Flow Regulated?

Cerebral autoregulation involves the maintenance of a constant CBF when the MAP is between 60 and 160 mm Hg (CPP, 50-150 mm Hg under normal conditions) and is accomplished by the adjustment of cerebrovascular resistance (CVR) (Fig. 44–2). Cerebral autoregulation protects the brain from abrupt changes in arterial blood pressure (BP). As MAP decreases, the cerebral resistance vessels (arterioles) dilate to increase CBV and to maintain constant CBF. In contrast, CVR increases with acute elevations in MAP to prevent abrupt rises in CBF. CBF passively follows MAP when the limits of autoregulation are exceeded or impaired.

Autoregulation frequently is impaired globally or focally after acute stroke; subarachnoid hemorrhage (SAH) or head injury; in association with arteriovenous malformation (AVM), tumors, hypoxia ($PaO_2$ <50 mm Hg), extreme hypercarbia, or acidosis; and iatrogenically with high doses of potent inhalational anesthetic agents. The exact mechanism of autoregulation is unknown but likely reflects the response of resistance

vessels to the local metabolic environment or to changes in transmural pressure.

## What Disease Processes Can Be Associated With Elevated Intracranial Pressure?

A multitude of disease processes have the potential to increase intracranial elastance (Table 44–1). The pathophysiology involved affects the acuity or chronicity of symptom development, treatment options, and prognosis. Pathophysiologic processes that can lead to an increase in ICP, alone or in combination, include growth of the solid substance of the brain, formation of cerebral edema with disruption of the blood-brain barrier, hemorrhage, axonal disruption, and disruption of CSF regulatory pathways. The diagnosis of intracranial hypertension is determined clinically. When intracranial hypertension develops, regardless of etiology, there is the threat of cerebral ischemia, direct or indirect distortion of brain tissue, initiation of secondary cellular injury and neuronal loss, and herniation of brain tissue.

## Why Is Intracranial Hypertension Dangerous?

### Ischemia of Cortical or Subcortical Structures

As ICP rises and compensatory mechanisms become exhausted, the risk for brain tissue ischemia increases signifi-

**TABLE 44–1.** Disease Processes Associated With Intracranial Hypertension

| | |
|---|---|
| Brain tumors | Venous sinus thrombosis |
| Head injury | Eclampsia |
| Subdural or epidural hematoma | Pseudotumor cerebri |
| Subarachnoid hemorrhage | Hepatic encephalopathy |
| Arteriovenous malformation | Inflammatory processes |
| Hydrocephalus | Hypoxic injury |
| Stroke | Reye syndrome |

From Sulek CA. Intracranial pressure. In: Cucchiara RF, Black S, Michenfelder JD, eds. *Clinical Neuroanesthesia.* 2nd ed. New York, NY: Churchill Livingstone; 1998:79.

cantly. Ischemia may occur regionally or globally depending on the etiology of the intracranial hypertension. Peritumor edema, for example, may cause localized ICP elevation and a regional decrease in blood flow near the tumor bed, whereas traumatic brain injury is frequently associated with sustained global or transient diffuse ischemia.[1,2,4] If ICP continues to rise and is not successfully treated, the low-resistance venous system collapses and prevents vascular outflow. When ICP approaches diastolic arterial pressure levels, the brain is only perfused during systole. If this problem is not corrected, cerebral circulatory arrest may be imminent. As ICP reaches systolic arterial pressure levels, cerebral circulatory arrest develops and is usually fatal unless ICP is rapidly reduced.

### Secondary Neuronal Injury

Cerebral ischemia occurs commonly after severe head injury and has even been documented after mild to moderate head injury, particularly when associated with systemic injuries.[1,4] Secondary ischemic insults contribute significantly to poor neurologic outcome in those patients with moderate to severe head injury. Elevated ICP, systemic hypotension, and hypoxia contribute to cerebral ischemia in the traumatically injured brain. Even the mildly injured brain appears more susceptible to small insults than the uninjured brain. Regardless of the inciting event (traumatic or ischemic), secondary neuronal injury reflects a common final pathway of insult at a cellular and biochemical level. The primary cascade of events leading to either acute or delayed programmed cell death include energy failure, ionic fluxes, neurotransmitter release (glutamate), and calcium influx.

### Herniation of Brain Tissue

Herniation of brain tissue represents maximal spatial exhaustion, is associated with marked intracranial hypertension until decompensation occurs, and usually denotes a poor prognosis unless corrected with aggressive ICP-reducing maneuvers. Herniation of brain tissue can occur upward or downward depending on the site of the lesion; it can even be transcalvarial if a bony defect exists (eg, postoperative craniectomy, skull fracture, during craniotomy) (Fig. 44–3). Neurologic deterioration from supratentorial lesions progresses in a rostral-to-caudal direction and, if left untreated, results in central, uncal, or tonsillar herniation. Expansion of an infratentorial mass lesion causes tonsillar or upward cerebellar herniation. Subfalcine or cingulate herniation is associated with supratentorial lesions and often remains asymptomatic unless the anterior cerebral artery is compromised.

## How Is Intracranial Hypertension Diagnosed Clinically?

The symptoms and signs of elevated ICP are relatively nonspecific and depend on the location and chronicity of the underlying pathologic process. Clinical presentation of a slow-growing brain tumor is markedly different from an acute, rapidly expanding epidural hematoma with impending herniation. Symptoms reflect the direct distortion or ischemia of brain tissue secondary to increased ICP.

The classic clinical manifestations of intracranial hypertension are headache, nausea, vomiting, visual disturbances, and

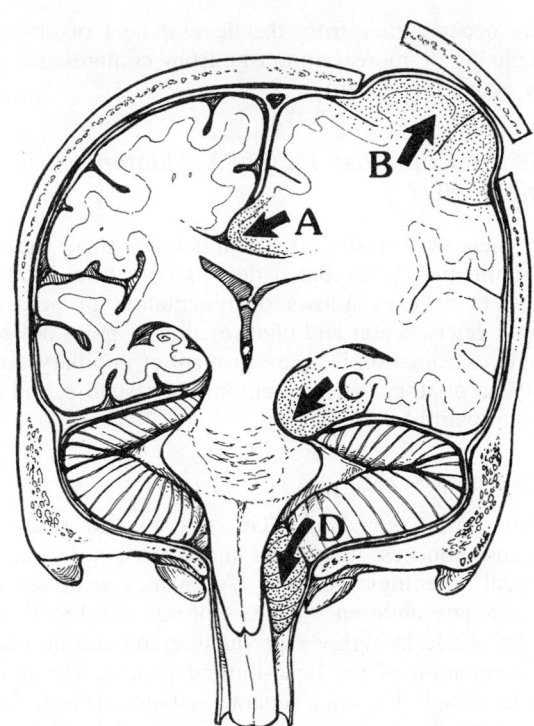

**FIGURE 44–3.** Sites of herniation: A, subfalcine; B, transcalvarial; C, uncal; D, Tonsillar. (From Sulek CA. Intracranial pressure. In: Cucchiara RF, Black S, Michenfelder JD, eds. *Clinical Neuroanesthesia.* 2nd ed. New York, NY: Churchill Livingstone; 1998:81.)

altered mentation.[16–18] Although headache is suggestive of elevated ICP, it is not diagnostic. Headache, nausea, and vomiting typically occur in the morning, and headache is relieved with emesis. Dural stretching or traction on vessels at the base of the brain caused by the mass lesion contribute to the headache. Intracranial hypertension is more difficult to assess in infants and children but most often manifests as irritability, somnolence, poor oral intake, nausea, and vomiting. Papilledema, ocular palsies, or focal neurologic deficits may be detected on neurologic examination.

## How Do Supratentorial and Infratentorial Lesions Differ?

### Supratentorial Pathology

The initial clinical presentation and progression of neurologic deterioration depends on the location of the mass lesion. Neurologic deterioration progresses in a rostral-to-caudal direction in the presence of a supratentorial lesion. Brainstem dysfunction is typically a late finding, except with acute pathology. Loss of consciousness with a supratentorial mass is ominous in the absence of a metabolic disturbance and suggests bilateral cerebral hemispheric or diencephalic dysfunction. With severe head injury, loss of consciousness occurs abruptly as a result of axonal disruption.

### Infratentorial Pathology

Brainstem dysfunction is frequently an early manifestation of an infratentorial mass lesion owing to the proximity of the pathologic process to the brainstem. Depressed mental status may also occur earlier from the development of obstructive hydrocephalus or more ominously from compression of the reticular activating system.

## How Is the Comatose Patient Evaluated Neurologically?

Assessment of brainstem function is the basis of the neurologic examination when the patient is comatose. Evaluation of brainstem reflexes allows documentation of progressive neurologic deterioration and confirmation of brain death. The neurologic examination is an assessment of pupillary size and reactivity, respiratory pattern, oculomotor response, and motor response to painful stimuli.

### Glasgow Coma Scale

The Glasgow Coma Scale (GCS) is used to evaluate the level of consciousness after head injury but is not designed to assess focal neurologic deficits.[19] A separate scale should be used to evaluate children <4 years of age (Children's Coma Scale). The scale is highly reproducible and can be used for serial examination of the head-injured patient. The maximal obtainable score is 15, and a separate notation (t) is designated for intubated patients. Severe head injury is defined as a GCS <8. The initial GCS is used to determine the need for ICP monitoring and provides prognostic information for the head-injured patient.

### Evaluation of Brainstem Function

#### Midbrain

Neurologic findings differ depending on the site of herniation (central versus uncal); nevertheless, prognosis is grim in the late stages of midbrain involvement. Central herniation differs initially from uncal herniation because (1) it usually results from chronic pathology, and (2) it initially manifests as diencephalic dysfunction before midbrain involvement.

In central herniation, the pupils become fixed and dilated in midposition; pupil changes are unilateral in early uncal herniation. As progressive third cranial nerve compromise occurs, complete oculomotor palsy develops. Oculovestibular and oculocephalic reflexes are preserved in early midbrain compression but impaired or absent as herniation progresses. Hyperventilation replaces a normal or Cheyne-Stokes respiratory pattern (diencephalic involvement). Central neurogenic hyperventilation is exceedingly rare, but when it occurs, it results from the loss of descending inhibitory control of ventilation by the cerebral cortex.[20] Decorticate posturing is rare in uncal herniation; ultimately, decerebrate rigidity characterizes both central and uncal herniation.

#### Pons

Central and uncal herniation are indistinguishable when deterioration to the pontine level occurs. Distortion of the pons is characterized by the following:

1. Dilated and fixed pupils in the midposition
2. Absence of the oculovestibular and oculocephalic reflexes
3. Flaccid motor response

Prognosis at this stage is grave, and reversibility depends on the primary pathologic process and efficacy of aggressive medical treatment, surgical intervention, or both. For example, a rapidly expanding epidural hematoma may result in life-threatening herniation that can be reversed by emergent surgical decompression.

#### Medulla

Herniation to the medullary stage is a terminal event in which the following occur:

1. Pupils fully dilate
2. Respiratory pattern is irregular with sighs, gasps, and ultimately apnea
3. Hemodynamic function is unstable

The Cushing triad (hypertension, bradycardia, and respiratory irregularity) is rarely observed and has been most commonly reported with infratentorial mass lesions.[21]

Tonsillar herniation from supratentorial or infratentorial pathology is a rapid, often fatal event if not promptly recognized and treated. The cerebellar tonsils descend through the foramen magnum, compressing the lower brainstem; this results in fatal respiratory arrest. Tonsillar herniation is differentiated from central or uncal herniation by the rapidity of events and narrow window for intervention to prevent death.

## Is Neuroradiologic Testing Helpful in Diagnosing Intracranial Hypertension?

Computed tomography (CT) or magnetic resonance imaging (MRI) studies of the brain are performed routinely in patients with suspected intracranial pathology and increased ICP. CT remains the radiographic study of choice for the detection of acute intracranial pathology. It is a highly sensitive imaging modality for the diagnosis of acute hemorrhage, mass lesions, and osseous injury (skull fracture); it is ideal for hemodynamically unstable patients who benefit from a rapid imaging time. Routine CT scanning remains controversial in patients with minor head injury. In a recent study of 520 patients with minor head injury but normal admission GCS, and neurologic examination, 6.9% had evidence of intracranial pathology by CT scan.[22] Of the patients with an abnormal scan, all could be predicted (100% sensitivity) if the patient had one or more of the following clinical findings: short-term memory deficit, drug or alcohol intoxication, evidence of trauma above the clavicles, age >60 years, seizure, headache, and vomiting. CT imaging is still recommended for head-injured patients with GCS <15.

MRI is used to detect subacute collections of blood, to evaluate chronic intracranial pathology, and to detect subtle pathology after head injury. It is more sensitive than CT imaging for diagnosing milder forms of diffuse axonal injury (punctate areas of edema) after head trauma.

Peritumor edema, diffuse cerebral edema, subarachnoid blood, hydrocephalus, compressed ambient cisterns, midline shift, and the presence of a mass lesion suggest elevated ICP but do not provide quantitative information (Fig. 44–4). In severely head-injured patients, the presence of midline shift and compressed ambient cisterns is highly predictive of intracranial hypertension.[23] When diagnosing herniation or degree of ICP elevation, CT or MRI findings must be correlated with the neurologic examination. A radiographic study may suggest

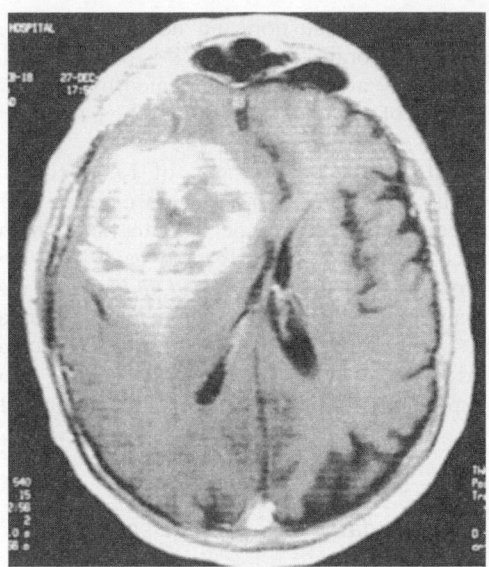

**FIGURE 44–4.** T1-weighted magnetic resonance imaging study of a glioblastoma multiforme of the right frontal lobe with associated mass effect and subfalcine herniation, suggesting elevated intracranial pressure. (From Sulek CA. Intracranial pressure. In: Cucchiara RF, Black S, Michenfelder JD, eds. *Clinical Neuroanesthesia*. 2nd ed. New York, NY: Churchill Livingstone; 1998:83.)

elevated ICP, but because of the chronicity of the disease process, the patient may not have symptoms.

## *How Is Intracranial Pressure Measured?*

### Indications for Monitoring

An ICP monitor does not replace the neurologic examination in a comatose patient but can be used to measure ICP quantitatively and to guide treatment when intracranial hypertension is present. In patients with severe head injury (GCS, 3-8) and an abnormal CT scan, ICP monitoring is warranted.[11] The need for monitoring is not only dictated by severity of head injury and CT scan findings but also determined by the patient age, neurologic examination, and presence of hypotension. Monitoring should be initiated in severely head-injured patients with a normal CT scan if two of the following conditions are met at the time of admission: age >40 years, unilateral or bilateral motor posturing, and systolic BP <90 mm Hg. A significant percentage of patients with severe head injury and a normal admission CT scan develop intracranial hypertension at some time during their hospitalization.[23,24]

One caveat is that ICP monitoring may be misleading in patients with head injury and focal lesions. In a recent study of 50 head-injured patients with bilateral frontal intraparenchymal ICP monitoring, a supratentorial interhemispheric ICP gradient existed in 50% of patients with a focal lesion, and a significant percentage of patients required adjustment in therapy based on ICP values recorded.[3] Recorded ICP was higher in the hemisphere with greatest volume. Considering the results of this study and others, the underlying pathology may dictate the more appropriate location for placement of the ICP monitor to optimize treatment strategies.

Therapy that may alter ICP (ie, mechanical ventilation and positive end-expiratory pressure [PEEP]) in a patient with abnormal intracranial elastance may warrant ICP monitoring.

Intraventricular catheters (ventriculostomy) are commonly placed in patients with hydrocephalus associated with brain tumors and in patients after aneurysmal SAH with hydrocephalus or Hunt-Hess grade of 3 or greater (suspected ICP elevation). The decision to place an ICP monitoring device perioperatively is generally at the discretion of the neurosurgeon and may be influenced by institutional protocols.

### Intracranial Pressure Monitoring Sites and Complications

Intracranial pressure can be recorded from epidural, subdural, subarachnoid, ventricular, or intraparenchymal sites, and several different monitoring devices are commercially available (catheters, bolts, screws, fiberoptic cables, microchip pressure transducers). A supratentorial location is the most common and safest site for ICP recording; monitoring from the posterior fossa is feasible but poses the additional risk for cranial nerve or brainstem injury.

The incidence of complications associated with ICP monitors is reported at 1% to 7.7%.[25] The most frequently encountered complications include infection, hemorrhage, brain injury, seizures, CSF leaks, brainstem or cranial nerve injury, and technical problems.

### Intracranial Pressure Monitoring Devices

The intraventricular catheter (or ventriculostomy) remains the gold standard in monitoring devices and is the only one that can be used both diagnostically and therapeutically for the treatment of intracranial hypertension. The ability to drain CSF has become an integral part of the treatment strategy for head-injured patients with intracranial hypertension. Relative to other monitoring devices, its placement requires considerably more skill and is associated with a higher incidence of infection and a greater risk for brain injury during insertion.

The subarachnoid bolt or screw is associated with a lower incidence of infection and brain injury but does not provide the therapeutic benefit of CSF drainage. It requires less skill to place but is less accurate than the subarachnoid or intraventricular catheter for ICP monitoring.[26] Subarachnoid bolts have the added disadvantage of producing falsely low readings when ICP is high, owing to obstruction of the lumen of the bolt by brain tissue.

Fiberoptic ICP monitoring devices are popular and have accuracies comparable to the intraventricular catheter. Recordings can be made from an intraparenchymal, subdural, or intraventricular site. Technical problems associated with this type of monitor include significant drift, inability to recalibrate in vivo, and fragility of the fiberoptic cable. A cumulative drift of ± 6 mm Hg has been observed over a 5-day period.[27] They require replacement every 5 days to minimize false readings and to reduce the risk for infection.

A newer ICP monitoring device uses a microchip pressure transducer in place of a fiberoptic cable. Laboratory data from animals have demonstrated improved durability over the fiberoptic system with similar accuracy and drift, but clinical experience and validation studies in humans remain limited.[28]

### Intracranial Pressure Waveforms

The physiologic ICP waveform is made up of small pulsations that correlate with the systolic arterial pressure wave

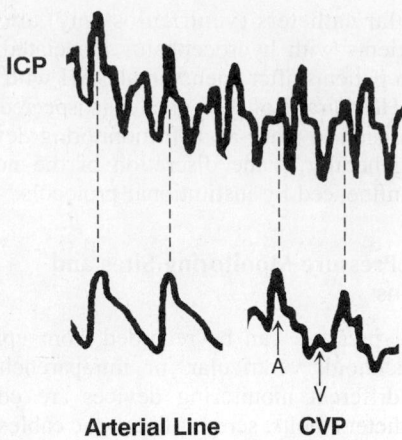

## Normal Elastance

**FIGURE 44–5.** Correlation of pulsations of the ICP waveform with components of the arterial and CVP tracings. The initial peak of the ICP waveform corresponds to the systolic component of the systemic arterial waveform. The second peak corresponds to the central venous A wave from the right atrium. CVP, central venous pressure; ICP, intracranial pressure. (From Sulek CA. Intracranial pressure. In: Cucchiara RF, Black S, Michenfelder JD, eds. *Clinical Neuroanesthesia.* 2nd ed. New York, NY: Churchill Livingstone; 1998:87.)

and the central venous A wave and is influenced by the normal respiratory pattern[29] (Fig. 44–5). Pulsations of the ICP waveform reflect transmission of the systemic BP to the intracranial compartment. The initial, larger peak is 1 to 2 mm Hg in amplitude with a dicrotic notch, correlates with the systolic arterial pressure wave, and increases in amplitude when systemic arterial pressure is elevated.[30] A smaller distinct peak follows the initial peak and corresponds to the central venous A wave from the right atrium. When cannon A waves are detected on the CVP tracing, the ICP waveform becomes more venous appearing. As ICP increases to 20 to 30 mm Hg, the ICP waveform becomes "arterialized" in shape as the pulsations of venous origin disappear.

Lundberg was the first to describe pathologic pressure waves in patients with brain tumors and intracranial hypertension.[31] These waves have been named *Lundberg A* (plateau), *B*, and *C waves*. *Plateau waves* are abrupt in onset and defined by an amplitude increase of 50 to 100 mm Hg above baseline with a duration of 5 to 20 minutes or longer[31] (Fig. 44–6).

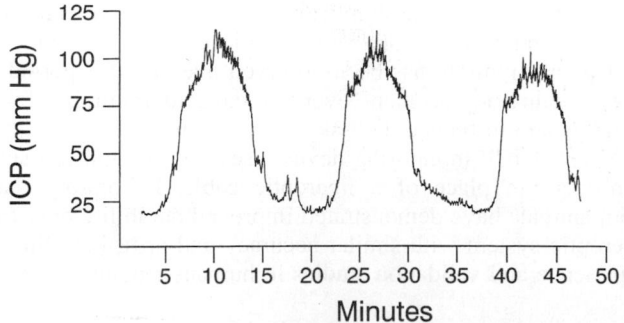

**FIGURE 44–6.** Plateau waves in a patient with head injury and intracranial hypertension. ICP, intracranial abressure. (From Sulek CA. Intracranial pressure. In: Cucchiara RF, Black S, Michenfelder JD, eds. *Clinical Neuroanesthesia.* 2nd ed. New York, NY: Churchill Livingstone; 1998:87.)

They signal spatial exhaustion and herald a life-threatening event (herniation of brain tissue) if ICP is not acutely lowered. When present, they are often accompanied by headache, nausea, altered level of consciousness, hyperpnea, and decerebrate rigidity.[30,32]

The clinical significance, if any, of Lundberg B and C waves remains unclear. Lundberg B, or *1-per-minute waves*, occur at a frequency of 0.5 to 2 per minute, range in amplitude from imperceptible to 50 mm Hg, and have been associated with abnormal respiratory patterns. *Lundberg C waves* are smaller in amplitude (usually <30 mm Hg), occur at a frequency of 4 to 8 per minute, and may be associated with Traube-Hering-Mayer variations of systemic BP.[33] Lundberg C waves superimposed on the plateau wave signal a terminal event.

## *What Other Modalities Can Be Used?*

### Transcranial Doppler Ultrasonography

Transcranial Doppler ultrasonography (US) can be used as an adjunct for diagnosing intracranial hypertension and brain death; however, the findings must be correlated with the clinical examination and other information available. It is an inexpensive, noninvasive US technique that determines blood flow velocity and direction through major cerebral arteries and provides indirect measurement of vascular resistance or tone of the vessel insonated.

As ICP increases and approaches diastolic arterial pressure, diastolic flow velocity decreases, approaches zero, and then reverses flow[34] (Fig. 44–7). Until cerebral circulatory arrest occurs, there is still forward flow during systole. According to recently published international guidelines, brain death can be confirmed by transcranial Doppler if two separate examinations document the presence of oscillating flow (forward and reverse components must be equal or symmetric) or systolic spikes in both intracranial and extracranial vessels.[35] When these criteria are applied, the diagnosis of cerebral circulatory

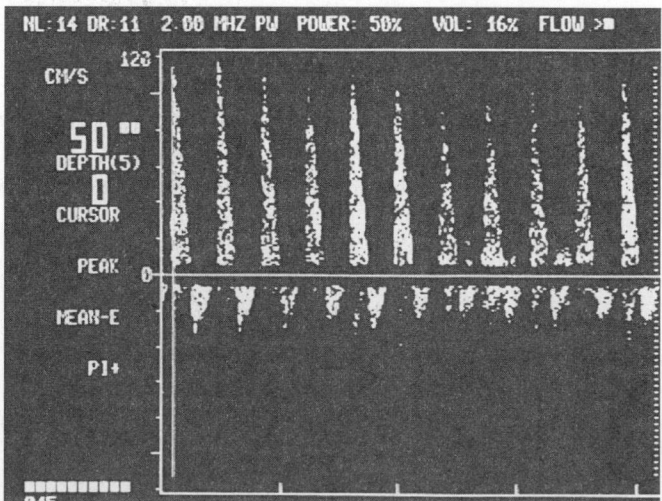

**FIGURE 44–7.** Transcranial Doppler ultrasonography image of diastolic flow reversal in a patient with intracranial hypertension and ultimate brain death. (From Sulek CA. Intracranial pressure. In: Cucchiara RF, Black S, Michenfelder JD, eds. *Clinical Neuroanesthesia.* 2nd ed. New York, NY: Churchill Livingstone; 1998:89.)

arrest can only be made in conjunction with the neurologic examination. An absent signal should always be interpreted cautiously and verified in other vessels, as signals can be difficult to detect in older women and when the temporal bone is ossified.

## ANESTHETIC AND SUPPLEMENTAL AGENTS

The selection of an anesthetic technique and supplemental drugs for a patient with intracranial hypertension should be tailored as follows:

1. To maintain adequate CBF
2. To minimize ICP elevation
3. To provide cerebral protective measures if necessary
4. To actively reduce ICP

The anesthesiologist must recognize the impact that anesthetic agents or pharmacologic interventions have on CBF, CBV, and ICP.

### What Are Their Effects on Intracranial Pressure?

#### Potent Inhalational Agents

#### Halothane

In animals and humans, halothane is a potent cerebral vasodilator that increases CBF by reducing CVR and has a deleterious effect on ICP, especially in the presence of an intracranial mass.[36–38] Halothane increases CBF in a dose-related fashion, and it increases the ratio of CBF to cerebral metabolic rate for oxygen ($CMRO_2$) to a greater extent than other volatile agents.[39] Halothane decreases $CMRO_2$, yet it has powerful vasodilating properties that predominate except at low agent concentrations. The initiation of hyperventilation ($PaCO_2$ <30 mm Hg) before the institution of halothane has been shown to attenuate or prevent elevations in CSF pressure (CSFP) in patients with intracranial pathology.[36] When hyperventilation and halothane are instituted simultaneously, rises in CSF pressure are not consistently prevented, and elevations are clinically significant.

The effects of halothane on ICP result from increased CBV, alterations in CSF dynamics, or both. The mechanism of cerebral vasodilation is not well understood, but it is not dependent on membrane-bound receptors or presence of endothelium. Direct smooth muscle relaxation or response of the vasculature to a second messenger have been proposed as mechanisms. Alteration of the normal CSF pathway (resistance to reabsorption) probably contributes to the late sustained increase in CSFP recorded with prolonged halothane exposure.

The reactivity of the cerebral circulation to $CO_2$ is preserved with 1.0 minimal alveolar concentration (MAC) of halothane. Cerebral autoregulation is impaired to a greater extent with halothane than with isoflurane or enflurane.[38–40] Autoregulation may be impaired but not abolished with halothane concentrations as low as 0.5%.[41]

In neuroanesthesia practice, halothane should be used cau-

tiously, if at all, in patients with suspected or documented intracranial hypertension, particularly with the availability of safer alternative inhalational agents (isoflurane and sevoflurane). If used, halothane should be administered in low concentrations with hyperventilation established before its use.

#### Isoflurane

Isoflurane has profound, nonlinear, dose-related cerebral metabolic depressant properties (at <1.0 MAC anesthesia) compared with equipotent doses of halothane or enflurane. With 2.0 MAC isoflurane in dogs, an isoelectric electroencephalogram (EEG) is produced, and $CMRO_2$ reduction is maximum.[42,43]

In humans, minimal changes in CBF occur with isoflurane concentrations of 1% to 2%.[44–46] A reduction in CVR accounts for the change in CBF and CBV. Profound changes in CBF have been observed when nitrous oxide is substituted for an equipotent concentration of isoflurane, validating concerns that nitrous oxide is a potent cerebral vasodilator.[44,47,48] Nitrous oxide is often used clinically to reduce the concentration of isoflurane; however, its substitution for an equipotent dose of volatile agent is contraindicated in patients with intracranial hypertension.

Isoflurane possesses cerebral vasodilating properties and, as such, may elevate ICP in patients with increased intracranial elastance. Establishing hyperventilation ($PaCO_2$, 25-30 mm Hg) simultaneously with the initiation of isoflurane prevents elevation of CSFP in patients with intracranial pathology.[49] Unlike the case with halothane, hyperventilation is unnecessary before isoflurane administration. When isoflurane and nitrous oxide are used together, hyperventilation does not consistently prevent increases in CBF.[47] The effect of isoflurane on ICP is small and results from cerebral vasodilation alone. Resistance to CSF reabsorption is lowered and rate of CSF production is unaffected by isoflurane.[50,51] Cerebrovascular reactivity to $CO_2$ is well preserved with isoflurane anesthesia in humans. Cerebral autoregulation remains intact at 1.0 MAC of isoflurane but is significantly attenuated or abolished at 2.0 MAC of isoflurane.[52,53] Isoflurane remains a safe potent inhalational agent for patients with intracranial pathology and has a long proven safety record in neuroanesthesia.

#### Sevoflurane

Sevoflurane is a relatively new fluorinated ether anesthetic that possesses a low blood gas partition coefficient that facilitates rapid induction and emergence. In animal and human studies, sevoflurane has cerebrovascular and metabolic properties similar to isoflurane. Recent data, however, suggest that sevoflurane may be a weaker cerebral vasodilator than other volatile agents in clinical practice.[54]

Sevoflurane has comparable effects on CBF and ICP as isoflurane.[55–57] In a study of patients undergoing spine surgery, the effects of 0.5 and 1.5 MAC isoflurane or sevoflurane on middle cerebral artery blood flow velocity (Vmca) were evaluated after an isoelectric EEG was produced with propofol.[54] Under stable hemodynamic conditions, Vmca was increased to a much greater degree with isoflurane than sevoflurane at equipotent concentrations.

Reduction in $CMRO_2$ appears dose related and declines by 50% at 1.0 MAC of sevoflurane.[55] Burst suppression of the EEG is observed at 2.15 MAC sevoflurane in animals.[56] Of concern are reports of seizure activity associated with sevoflurane anesthesia in animals and children.[58-60] Although limited data exist, sevoflurane obviously is a less than ideal agent for neurosurgical patients if it possesses epileptogenic properties. Cerebrovascular reactivity to alterations in $Paco_2$ and autoregulation is similar to that observed for isoflurane.

Sevoflurane closely resembles the cerebral hemodynamic profile of isoflurane; although, a few differences may exist. Sevoflurane may be an acceptable alternative to isoflurane in patients with intracranial pathology, but more data are needed to assess the risk for seizures with its use. ICP elevations probably can be prevented with simultaneous hyperventilation. In long-duration cases, emergence is similar to that with isoflurane, making it a more suitable agent for shorter cases. Because of its advantageous effects on CBF, sevoflurane is preferable to halothane for inhalational induction.

### Desflurane

Desflurane is another relatively new volatile anesthetic with a blood gas partition coefficient similar to that of nitrous oxide. It is a potent cerebral vasodilator and has the potential to produce adverse effects on CBF and CBV, particularly when intracranial elastance is increased.[61-64] Reductions in $CMRo_2$ are similar to those with isoflurane. Response of the cerebral vasculature to $CO_2$ remains intact in animals and humans at clinically relevant concentrations.[63,65]

The effect of desflurane on ICP is controversial. In a study of hyperventilated patients with supratentorial lesions and associated mass effect, CSFP progressively increased with desflurane compared with isoflurane.[61] ICP elevations also have been documented in animals. Limited human data contradict this finding; therefore, desflurane should be used cautiously in patients with abnormal intracranial elastance.

### Nitrous Oxide

For decades, nitrous oxide has been used as a supplemental anesthetic during neurosurgical procedures, but its safety in this setting is now challenged. CBF studies have often been difficult to interpret owing to species differences, CBF techniques, or the use of supplemental anesthetics that confound the effects of nitrous oxide on the cerebral vasculature. However, considerable evidence suggests that nitrous oxide is a powerful cerebral vasodilator.

CBF increases with nitrous oxide alone or in combination with volatile anesthetics in animals and humans.[66-69] Nitrous oxide alone can substantially elevate CBF; however, it has been speculated that such increases reflect light planes of anesthesia rather than direct cerebral vasodilation.[66,69] In humans, nitrous oxide increases blood flow in all brain regions except the cerebellum and pons.[69] A combination of nitrous oxide and isoflurane produces a greater elevation in CBF than equipotent concentrations of the volatile agent alone.[44,47,48] Combinations of nitrous oxide and halothane result in CBF levels that are similar to equipotent concentrations of halothane alone.[48] The effects on CBF result from direct vasodilatory actions or indirectly by changes in $CMRo_2$. The vasodilatory effect predominates at increased depths of anesthesia when $CMRo_2$ is maximally suppressed by the volatile agent in use.

ICP elevations have been reported in patients with abnormal elastance.[70,71] For many years, it was generally agreed that nitrous oxide–induced ICP increases could be prevented or abolished by the administration of concurrent drugs (ie, sodium thiopental) and hyperventilation. Recent studies demonstrate that hyperventilation does not consistently prevent increases in CBF, even if established before nitrous oxide administration.[47,68,69]

Nitrous oxide is acceptable for neurosurgical procedures as long as intracranial elastance is normal. It probably should be avoided in patients with increased intracranial elastance because alternative anesthetic agents are available that allow prompt emergence.

## Intravenous Anesthetics

### Barbiturates

Barbiturates have powerful effects on the cerebral vasculature and metabolism that, unlike potent inhalational agents, are coupled. Sodium thiopental is the most widely used barbiturate in neuroanesthesia. It is consistently shown to lower CBF, $CMRo_2$, and spinal cord blood flow in a dose-dependent fashion.[72-74] Methohexital in small doses possesses epileptogenic properties that can increase CBF and $CMRo_2$. Cerebral oxygen consumption is reduced by 55% when the EEG becomes isoelectric after thiopental administration.[73] Similar dose-dependent $CMRo_2$ reductions have been reported with phenobarbital and pentobarbital.[75,76] Thiopental suppresses neuronal synaptic transmission but preserves metabolic function necessary for the maintenance of cellular integrity and homeostasis.

ICP is consistently and effectively lowered with thiopental in patients with intracranial hypertension.[77] Barbiturates have minimal effect on ICP in individuals with normal elastance. They remain an important part of the anesthetic induction technique for patients with increased ICP, are useful in the treatment of intractable intracranial hypertension, and can be used as cerebral protectant agents.

### Etomidate

Etomidate lowers $CMRo_2$ and CBF, but in contrast to barbiturates, blood flow changes are independent of changes in metabolism.[78-80] Etomidate effectively lowers ICP, reflecting its powerful vasoconstrictor effects.[81] Because CBF changes occur more rapidly than reductions in $CMRo_2$, ischemia can occur. The cerebrovascular response to $CO_2$ remains intact.[79,80]

Etomidate is not commonly used in neuroanesthesia practice in patients with abnormal elastance because barbiturates effectively control ICP. It is used preferentially for patients with hemodynamic instability or myocardial dysfunction. Although etomidate is associated with greater hemodynamic stability, it has several undesirable side effects, including myoclonic activity with induction and prolonged use, adrenocortical suppression, and epileptogenic properties.

### Propofol

Propofol decreases CBF and $CMRo_2$; its ability to reduce CBF has been attributed to parallel changes in metabolism.[82,83] It can suppress neuronal function to produce an isoelectric EEG much like barbiturates, etomidate, and potent inhalational agents.

Propofol reduces or has minimal effects on ICP. The largest

reductions have been observed in patients with intracranial hypertension.[82,84] Significant reductions in MAP, even in young healthy patients, are observed with anesthetic doses of propofol. They should be aggressively treated to prevent deleterious reductions in CPP.

This agent is used in neuroanesthesia primarily for conscious sedation in the operating room and intensive care unit and for cases of short duration. Patients receiving propofol have a clearer sensorium and better cognitive function postoperatively than those receiving traditional inhalational anesthetic techniques. Alternatively, propofol can be used as an anesthetic induction agent in patients with intracranial hypertension.

### Lidocaine

Lidocaine has been used in neuroanesthesia during induction, before placement of the pinion system, for extubation, and for endotracheal tube suctioning. It has a biphasic effect on CBF and $CMRo_2$. At low doses sufficient to produce sedation and general anesthesia, $CMRo_2$ and CBF are reduced. At higher doses, seizures are precipitated, causing increases in $CMRo_2$ and CBF.

Lidocaine has been reported to either decrease or have no effect on ICP.[85,86] In some studies, it was shown to prevent elevations in ICP if used before pinion placement, intubation, or endotracheal suctioning. Intratracheal lidocaine may be more effective than intravenous lidocaine in similar doses during tracheal suctioning.[86]

### Ketamine

Ketamine is a phencyclidine derivative with N-methyl-D-aspartate antagonist properties that are responsible for its production of hallucinations and seizure activity.[87-89] It causes marked increases in both CBF and $CMRo_2$. The CBF changes result from direct vasodilation, reduction of CVR, and perhaps accompanying metabolic alterations. In humans, ketamine selectively increases CBF in the frontotemporal and parieto-occipital regions of the brain.[90]

Ketamine consistently and substantially elevates ICP and CSFP when it is used as the primary anesthetic agent in patients with normal and abnormal elastance.[91,92] Ketamine-induced ICP elevations can be attenuated or prevented by thiopental administration and hyperventilation.[87,91] However, ketamine use should be restricted in patients with documented or suspected intracranial hypertension. If hemodynamic instability is present, etomidate is a reasonable alternative for the induction of anesthesia.

### Benzodiazepines

The cerebral effects of benzodiazepines are variable depending on the animal model, background anesthetic, and neurologic status. In general, benzodiazepines can be regarded as metabolic depressants that possess vasoconstrictive properties but are less potent than barbiturates. In animals, diazepam lowers CBF; $CMRo_2$ is either reduced or unchanged.[93-96] In diazepam-treated neurosurgical patients, no significant changes in ICP were observed.[97] Reactivity of the cerebral vasculature to $CO_2$ is preserved with diazepam.

Midazolam decreases $CMRo_2$ and CBF in humans and animals.[95,98,99] A ceiling effect on CBF and $CMRo_2$ changes may reflect maximal occupancy of benzodiazepine receptors. The effect of midazolam on ICP is variable and depends on the neurologic status of the patient and whether the drug is administered as a large bolus or infusion. In severely head-injured patients sedated with midazolam, a significant number of patients with intracranial hypertension had increases in ICP after drug administration, and most were attributed to reductions in MAP.[100]

Benzodiazepines are safe when administered to ventilated neurosurgical patients as long as the BP is supported. They should be used cautiously in unintubated patients with intracranial hypertension because oversedation may lead to respiratory depression and hypercarbia.

## Narcotics

### Synthetic Opioids

Fentanyl, sufentanil, and alfentanil have either no effect or increase ICP in humans.[101-107] When observed, ICP elevations are often small and transient and are associated with large bolus doses and reductions in MAP. Remifentanil has minimal effect on ICP in patients with space-occupying lesions but is associated with greater reductions in MAP than the other synthetic opioids.[107-109]

Synthetic opioids have a long-standing history of safety in neurosurgical patients; however, some studies contend that fentanyl, sufentanil, and alfentanil may cause ICP elevations. This increase likely is attributable to the use of large bolus doses, influence of the background anesthetic, opioid-induced chest wall rigidity, hypotension that reduces CPP, and respiratory depression with hypercapnia, hypoxia, or both. When increases in ICP occur, they are transient and not associated with adverse outcome. Synthetic opioids remain an integral part of anesthetic induction and maintenance to provide hemodynamic stability and smooth emergence.

## Neuromuscular Blockers

### Succinylcholine

Succinylcholine consistently produces dramatic elevations in CBF and ICP in humans and animals, even in the absence of fasciculations.[110-113] These increases in CBF and ICP are thought to reflect (1) afferent muscle spindle activation with stimulation of portions of the motor and somatosensory cortex and (2) secondary increases in $Paco_2$ from enhanced muscle oxygen consumption.[110,111] Pretreatment with a defasciculating dose of nondepolarizing muscle relaxant may prevent fasciculations but does not prevent CBF elevations unless intubating doses of nondepolarizing agents are used as pretreatment.[112] Succinylcholine causes significant ICP elevations in patients with both normal and abnormal intracranial elastance.

### Nondepolarizing Muscle Relaxants

Current nondepolarizing muscle relaxants have no effect on ICP and are safe in neuroanesthesia practice. Although atracurium and mivacurium have been associated with histamine release, no significant change in ICP occurs when they are used in usual clinical doses.[114-116] If histamine release occurs, any associated declines in MAP should be treated.

## VASOACTIVE AGENTS

### What Are Their Effects on Intracranial Pressure?

The cerebral vasculature is innervated by $\alpha$- and $\beta$-receptors, but their role in the brain is unclear. No significant changes in CBF, $CMR_{O_2}$, or CVR occur with phenylephrine, epinephrine, dopamine, or norepinephrine.[117,118] The cerebral vasculature is also unaffected by $\alpha$- or $\beta$-blockade; reactivity to $CO_2$ and autoregulation remain intact despite blockade.[119-121] It is predominantly affected by local metabolic and transmural pressure changes.

### Nitroglycerin

Nitroglycerin is an antihypertensive, antianginal agent that is contraindicated for use in neurosurgical patients with abnormal elastance because of its potent venodilating effects. Nitroglycerin produces deleterious increases in ICP within seconds of administration to humans and animals in the absence or presence of space-occupying lesions.[122-124] It appears to have greater effects on ICP than does sodium nitroprusside. ICP elevations result from dilation of venous capacitance vessels, causing increases in CBV. Barbiturates do not attenuate nitroglycerin-induced ICP changes.[123] Unlike sodium nitroprusside, CBF is not preserved when CPP reaches 50 mm Hg.

### Sodium Nitroprusside

Sodium nitroprusside is an antihypertensive agent commonly used in neuroanesthesia that causes significant ICP elevations, similar to but less profound than nitroglycerin. It has rapid onset and offset and the ability to control the BP "tightly." It consistently increases ICP in humans and animals by dilating capacitance, not resistance, vessels.[125,126] Even with significant levels of hypotension, CBF is preserved.[127,128] Sodium nitroprusside does not mask the hemodynamic signs of intracranial hypertension. Tachyphylaxis to the drug is often seen when ICP increases.

Nitroglycerin and sodium nitroprusside are potent dilators of capacitance vessels and are unsafe in patients with abnormal elastance. The dramatic rise in CBV with either agent can result in spatial exhaustion and intracranial hypertension. Trimethaphan, phentolamine, and $\beta$-blockade agents are acceptable alternative antihypertensives that have minimal effects on the cerebral vasculature.

## SURGICAL MANAGEMENT

### When Is Surgical Intervention Warranted?

#### Intracranial Bleeding

The need for surgical intervention after an intracranial hemorrhage is dictated by the etiology of the bleeding and the patient's neurologic status. Surgical intervention may be warranted for an epidural hematoma, acute or chronic subdural hematoma, intracerebral hemorrhage, life-threatening hematoma associated with an AVM or aneurysm, bleeding into a tumor bed, or postoperative hemorrhage after carotid endarterectomy or AVM resection. Emergent surgical decompression is required when there is a rapid deterioration in neurologic status, increase in ICP, or signs of impending herniation. Prompt ICP-reducing maneuvers (ie, mannitol) and surgical intervention must be instituted immediately to decrease neurologic morbidity and improve outcome. Postoperatively, ICP monitoring may be necessary owing to underlying brain injury from the primary insult (ie, subdural hematoma) or risk for reaccumulation of blood.

### Head Injury

Early surgical intervention to evacuate mass lesions may be mandatory to lower ICP, increase CPP, and improve neurologic outcome. Unfortunately, many patients with closed head injury and intracranial hypertension do not have operable lesions and require medical therapy in the intensive care unit to control ICP. If ICP is uncontrollable with maximal medical therapy, removal of a portion of the calvaria or temporal or frontal lobectomy may be considered.[129] The surgical removal of brain tissue is only considered an option for ICP reduction when all other measures have failed.

### Brain Tumors

Surgical removal is often the treatment of choice for supratentorial and infratentorial brain tumors, but adjunctive treatment may be required, such as radiation therapy, embolization, or chemotherapy. Supratentorial and infratentorial tumors often differ in their initial clinical presentation as well as their time course for development of intracranial hypertension. Clinical manifestations also depend on the type of tumor: malignant, benign, infiltrative, localized, primary, metastatic, aggressive, or slow growing. For instance, a patient with a slow-growing meningioma may remain symptom-free for years until spatial exhaustion occurs, whereas a patient with an aggressive glioblastoma multiforme may develop neurologic deficits and symptoms of intracranial hypertension early in the course of the disease.

The initial presentation of a patient with an infratentorial mass may be related to symptoms of elevated ICP due to hydrocephalus or neurologic deficits secondary to brainstem compression or infiltration (ie, cranial nerve or cerebellar findings). In contrast to supratentorial lesions, hydrocephalus is more frequently an early finding owing to obstruction of the cerebral aqueduct, fourth ventricle, or foramina of Magendie or Luschka. A colloid cyst (supratentorially located) is an exception because its most common presentation is acute hydrocephalus (occasionally leading to sudden death) from obstruction of the foramen of Monro. When acute obstructive hydrocephalus develops from supratentorial or infratentorial pathology, initial treatment may be directed toward decreasing ICP through placement of a ventriculostomy followed by tumor resection. Long-term management may require insertion of a ventriculoperitoneal shunt for chronic hydrocephalus.

### Hydrocephalus

Hydrocephalus usually causes a gradual rise in ICP but may occasionally cause symptoms acutely, as observed in patients with a colloid cyst or in patients with chronic hydrocephalus following multiple shunt insertions (small scarred ventricles with reduced compliance). A multitude of etiologies are responsible for the development of hydrocephalus, including congenital, postinfectious, posthemorrhagic, brain tumors, and others. Hydrocephalus may develop from obstruction at any point along the CSF pathway and may be communicating or noncommunicating. A brain tumor, for instance, may obstruct the CSF pathway, and hydrocephalus development is referred to as noncommunicating or obstructive. In contrast, a patient sustaining an aneurysmal SAH may develop acute hydrocephalus from obstruction of the arachnoid granulations by blood, thereby reducing CSF reabsorption (communicating hydrocephalus).

Treatment of hydrocephalus and the location of placement of a ventriculostomy or ventriculoperitoneal or ventriculoatrial shunt depend on the underlying etiology. CSF drainage may be needed for a limited period of time or for a lifetime.

### Aneurysmal Subarachnoid Hemorrhage

Subarachnoid hemorrhage from a ruptured intracranial aneurysm may lead to elevated ICP if acute hydrocephalus develops or a life-threatening hematoma is present. Acute ICP elevation occurs in all patients at the time of the hemorrhage but decreases rapidly unless the conditions mentioned previously are present. Acute lowering of the ICP should proceed cautiously because the transmural pressure (MAP − ICP) across the aneurysm sac is increased when MAP is increased or ICP reduced. An increase in transmural pressure may result in aneurysmal rebleed, associated with a high morbidity and mortality.

Emergent surgery may be warranted if a life-threatening hematoma exists to evacuate the clot, reduce ICP, and surgically clip the aneurysm if feasible. If a hematoma is not present, surgical clipping or endovascular embolization is usually performed on an urgent basis within 72 hours of the hemorrhage. The trend in the United States is early surgical or neuroradiologic intervention to eliminate the risk for rebleeding and to allow the safe and aggressive treatment of cerebral vasospasm.[130] Emergent ventriculostomy placement is also warranted to lower ICP when acute hydrocephalus develops. When CSF drainage is employed, it must be done cautiously to avoid dramatic reductions in ICP leading to increases in transmural pressure. For this reason, during patient transport to the operating room or radiology suite, a ventriculostomy catheter should always be closed to avoid inadvertent CSF drainage.

## ANESTHETIC MANAGEMENT

To safely anesthetize a patient with suspected or documented intracranial hypertension requires an understanding of the primary pathologic process involved, an estimate of intracranial reserve, and knowledge of the impact of anesthetic agents, mechanical ventilation, and hemodynamic manipulations on ICP. Patients with intracranial pathology and elevated ICP may present directly for neurosurgical intervention or for nonneurosurgical procedures, as frequently occurs with head-injured patients with multiple systemic injuries (ie, abdominal or orthopedic). Regardless of the planned procedure, the anesthetic management goals are the same: (1) to maintain an effective CPP and oxygenation, and (2) to minimize alterations in ICP. In head-injured patients, it is particularly important to avoid ischemic insults that may lead to potentiation of secondary neuronal injury.

## What Information Is Important?

### Preoperative Evaluation

A detailed history of the current intracranial disease process, symptoms suggestive of elevated ICP, and the baseline neurologic examination are essential for planning the intraoperative management. Documentation of the neurologic examination also allows the detection of new deficits on emergence from anesthesia. Additionally, determination of coexisting medical illnesses, concurrent injuries, or both is important for optimizing the perioperative care of the patient with elevated ICP. Given the importance of maintaining an adequate CPP, it is imperative to document the range of baseline BP values for a patient. This information is of particular importance for the hypertensive patient in whom cerebral autoregulation may be shifted to higher MAP, and it becomes mandatory to maintain higher BPs intraoperatively to avoid ischemic insults. In many instances, the patient's actual ICP is not known preoperatively, making it important to maintain arterial BP in the normal range for that patient.

Patients with a space-occupying lesion often manifest overt symptoms of increased ICP only when compensatory mechanisms are near exhaustion or are exhausted. The ICP may be known if a monitoring device is in place preoperatively. If ICP values are available, documentation of the range of ICP, CPP, and successful therapeutic interventions is important for continuity of care intraoperatively. However, more frequently than not, only a *probable* ICP can be ascertained from patient symptoms or radiographic data. Often, the neurosurgeon providing care for the patient can provide valuable information regarding probable ICP. Although it is not performed routinely, a patient with limited intracranial reserve will probably not tolerate the Trendelenburg position.

A CT or MRI study of the brain not only localizes the intracranial pathology but also may provide evidence suggestive of increased ICP. Midline shift and obliteration of the ambient cisterns strongly suggests the presence of intracranial hypertension.[23] Diffuse cerebral edema, hydrocephalus, subarachnoid blood, peritumor edema, and presence of a space-occupying lesion also suggest abnormal intracranial elastance.

### Intraoperative Monitoring

The need for ICP monitoring, CSF drainage, or both should be established by the neurosurgeon and anesthesiologist. Input from the anesthesiologist is important, particularly during a nonneurosurgical procedure in a patient with elevated ICP, when the brain cannot be observed for tenseness or bulging and the neurologic examination will be lost after induction of general anesthesia. During a nonneurosurgical procedure, placement of an ICP monitoring device is prudent for effective management of patients with head injury and a GCS score <8. An intraventricular catheter may be selected in some cases, not only to assess the impact of anesthetic and hemodynamic interventions on ICP but also to provide a therapeutic measure to actively lower ICP. Additionally, as the number of liver transplant recipients with encephalopathy and coagulopathy increases, the decision to place an ICP monitor must be balanced against the risk for intracranial hemorrhage.

CSF drainage should only be performed at the request of the neurosurgeon or with his or her guidance because deleterious effects can occur depending on the ICP-producing pathology (ie, aneurysmal SAH). In institutions routinely providing care to head-injured patients, monitoring of jugular venous oxygen saturation and arterial-jugular venous difference for oxygen (Ca − vo$_2$) may be commonplace preoperatively and extended into the perioperative period.

Invasive intraoperative monitoring should, at a minimum, include arterial cannulation either before induction or as soon after as is feasible. Arterial cannulation allows constant BP monitoring to maintain an effective CPP and frequent arterial blood gas and pH measurement to optimize Paco$_2$. Additional hemodynamic monitoring, such as central venous or pulmonary arterial cannulation, is dictated by the underlying intracranial pathology, planned surgical procedure, anticipated blood loss, position during surgery (ie, sitting), concurrent systemic injuries, or coexisting medical illnesses.

## General Versus Regional Anesthesia

The anesthetic technique usually is most dictated by the planned surgical procedure, and less frequently by any coexisting illnesses or systemic injuries. Most intracranial procedures, except for ICP monitoring device placement, require a general anesthetic. ICP monitor placement can often be performed at the bedside in the intensive care unit using local anesthesia and judicious intravenous sedation. In selected nonneurosurgical procedures (ie, orthopedics), regional anesthesia is ideal to allow frequent assessment of the neurologic examination. Unfortunately, regional anesthesia is often not a feasible alternative to general anesthesia for the following reasons:

1. Uncooperative patient
2. Presence of an intracranial mass precluding spinal anesthesia
3. Presence of hemodynamic or pulmonary instability due to concomitant injuries
4. Coagulopathy
5. Unprotected airway if neurologic deterioration occurs
6. Less precise control over ventilation

## How Is the Patient With Elevated Intracranial Pressure Managed Intraoperatively?

### Preoperative Medications and Sedation

Maintenance of anticonvulsants, steroids, calcium-channel blockade agents, and osmotic diuretics is mandatory in the perioperative period, and those administered depend on the underlying pathologic process. Other preoperative medications, such as antihypertensive and cardiac agents, should be continued as for any other patient undergoing anesthesia.

Premedication with anxiolytics or narcotics should either be avoided or titrated carefully by the anesthesiologist when the patient is in the operating room with hemodynamic and pulse oximetry monitoring established. Premedication is frequently avoided to prevent oversedation and decreased level of consciousness, resulting in hypoventilation, hypercarbia, and deleterious rises in CBF and ICP. As ICP rises, consciousness deteriorates further. Preoperative sedation should be individualized, and, if employed, the dosages should be small, narcotics should be preferentially avoided, and drug effects should be noted before further administration. When the

planned procedure is of short duration, preoperative benzodiazepine administration may delay emergence or alter mental status postoperatively. Reversal of benzodiazepines may not be safe in some patients because flumazenil has been associated with development of seizures in high-risk populations.[131-133]

### Special Considerations for the Patient With Acute Pathology

ICP-reducing measures are frequently instituted in the field or emergency room in patients with an acute pathologic process and associated intracranial hypertension. If the patient was intubated preoperatively, sedatives, narcotics, and neuromuscular blockade agents may have been given to treat agitation, pain, or struggling against the endotracheal tube and positive pressure ventilation. Although sedation, pain control, and neuromuscular blocking agents are accepted as part of the global treatment of elevated ICP, the neurologic examination, except for pupillary findings, is lost, particularly after the administration of muscle relaxants. If muscle relaxants have been used preoperatively, they should be accompanied by sedatives, narcotics, or both, and the degree of relaxation should be closely monitored to ensure reversibility at the end of the surgical procedure.

Steroid therapy is not part of the treatment strategy for head-injured patients. However, for patients with concomitant spinal cord injury, high-dose methylprednisolone is a standard of care of treatment within 8 hours of injury. Steroids do not improve outcome or lower ICP in head-injured patients. In two independent studies, dexamethasone failed to alter neurologic outcome in head-injured patients.[134,135] When high-dose methylprednisolone was administered to severely head-injured patients, there were no significant reductions in ICP.[136] Steroids are associated with significant complications, including hyperglycemia, infections, and gastrointestinal bleeding. They have no role in the treatment of head-injured patients and should be reserved for the management of edema formation associated with an intracranial tumor.

Initial clinical trials using calcium channel antagonists have not yielded promising results and currently are not part of the treatment strategy for head-injured patients. Calcium channel antagonists, particularly the dihydropyridine derivatives, are hypothesized to improve outcome and decrease infarct volume by improving blood flow and preventing calcium influx. A randomized, placebo-controlled trial of nimodipine initiated within 12 hours of injury in 852 patients with severe head injury did not demonstrate improved outcome in treated patients.[137] Nimodipine-treated patients with traumatic SAH had a better outcome than placebo-treated patients, but results did not reach statistical significance. Until further data become available, calcium channel antagonists do not appear beneficial for head-injured patients unless they can be shown to provide benefit to a specific group of patients. In contrast, nimodipine remains a mainstay of prophylactic treatment for cerebral vasospasm in patients with aneurysmal SAH.

### Special Considerations for the Patient With Chronic Pathology

Steroids have a beneficial role in reducing peritumor edema and midline shift, improving intracranial elastance, and are considered a cornerstone of treatment.[138-140] The effect is not immediate; hence, steroid therapy is often initiated days or weeks before surgery. Although the patient may or may not have symptoms after the initiation of steroids, intracranial elastance likely is still abnormal.

### The Infant or Child With Elevated Intracranial Pressure

Anesthetizing an infant or child with intracranial pathology and elevated ICP is challenging but warrants the same considerations as anesthetizing an adult patient. The development of intracranial hypertension is possible even in infants with open fontanelles and sutures and should be suspected when the fontanelles are bulging or tense. Valuable information may be gained from the neurosurgeon regarding intracranial reserve that may guide the perioperative management of the infant or child.

The same considerations for preoperative sedation of adults are operative for the infant and child. Benzodiazepines and narcotics are often avoided, but each case should be individualized and at the discretion of the anesthesiologist. The anesthesiologist must also decide whether to proceed with intravenous or mask induction. Intravenous catheter insertion, even after local anesthetic cream application, often results in crying and transient ICP elevation, which can be further exacerbated by difficult intravenous placement. However, infants and children with intracranial pathology and elevated ICP often cry or become agitated at home but do not have herniation of brain tissue. If mask induction is chosen, sevoflurane is the potent inhalational agent of choice but poses additional risk for laryngospasm (less than with halothane) or loss of the airway before placement of the intravenous catheter. Many neuroanesthesiologists prefer to place an intravenous catheter in infants or children with intracranial hypertension. If a mask induction technique is chosen, rapid intravenous placement after induction, administration of thiopental and neuromuscular blockade agent, and control of the airway with hyperventilation are recommended.

## How Is Intracranial Pressure Managed During the Induction of Anesthesia?

### Considerations Before Anesthetic Induction

The patient should be positioned with the head neutral and elevated 30° to improve cerebral venous drainage; this 30° head elevation has been shown to lower ICP without compromising CPP.[141] The safety of head elevation, however, has been challenged by some investigators. In limited studies, 0° head position has been found to improve CPP through the maintenance of MAP without a significant increase in ICP.[142] Nevertheless, until more data exist, current recommendations are to maintain head elevation perioperatively for those patients with abnormal intracranial elastance.

The arterial catheter and ICP monitor, if available, should be zeroed to the level of the external auditory canal to reflect accurately ICP and CPP. Voluntary hyperventilation is initiated before the induction of anesthesia in cooperative children and adults. If voluntary hyperventilation is not possible, ICP will be rapidly reduced if sodium thiopental is used as an anesthetic induction agent. Adequate preoxygenation is important because hypoxia will lead to increases in CBF and ICP. CBF decreases to a small degree with $Pao_2$ >300 mm Hg.

### Selection of Induction Agents and Intubation

Selection of the anesthetic induction technique should be made with the following goals in mind:

1. Maintenance of hemodynamic stability to preserve CPP and minimize ICP elevations
2. Rapid airway control and initiation of mild hyperventilation (if indicated)
3. Laryngoscopy time <15 seconds to decrease the hemodynamic response to tracheal intubation

Barbiturates remain the induction agents of choice when the patient is hemodynamically stable and cardiac status permits. Etomidate is preferable to ketamine when the patient is hemodynamically unstable, hypovolemic, or has significant myocardial dysfunction. Ketamine should be avoided in patients with elevated ICP.

Despite reports of ICP elevation with synthetic opioids, they remain an important adjunct for the induction and maintenance of anesthesia and have a long history of proven safety in neuroanesthesia. Although any narcotic can be used, sufentanil and fentanyl are frequently preferred for procedures of long duration, owing to ease of titration, stable hemodynamic profile, and rapid emergence when titrated properly. Narcotics are safe for use in patients with increased ICP as long as the following considerations are kept in mind:

1. Avoidance of large bolus doses
2. Attenuation of chest wall rigidity by pretreatment with a small priming dose of neuromuscular blockade agent
3. Aggressive treatment of narcotic-induced hypotension
4. Use of barbiturates during induction
5. Institution of mild hyperventilation

The hemodynamic response to tracheal intubation can be attenuated with the use of intravenous lidocaine or short-acting β-blockade agents, such as esmolol.

### Tracheal Intubation

The choice of neuromuscular blockade agent depends on the urgency of the procedure, nil per os (NPO) status, airway examination, and presence of concomitant facial or cervical injuries. Nondepolarizing muscle relaxants are preferable because those used in current clinical practice have no effect on ICP. When using a nondepolarizing agent, be sure to document loss of the train-of-four response to avoid precipitous rises in BP and ICP associated with coughing or bucking against the endotracheal tube.

Succinylcholine can be used if a difficult airway is anticipated or a rapid sequence induction is needed. Although some nondepolarizing muscle relaxants can be used when rapid intubating conditions are required (ie, rocuronium, mivacurium, rapacuronium), none replaces the rapid onset and offset of succinylcholine. If succinylcholine is chosen, pretreatment with a defasciculating dose of a nondepolarizing muscle relaxant is recommended in conjunction with barbiturates and initiation of hyperventilation after the airway is secured. Intravenous lidocaine may also be used to attenuate ICP elevations associated with the administration of succinylcholine. Although succinylcholine administration transiently elevates ICP, it is safer and less detrimental than loss of an airway or aspiration of gastric contents with resultant hypercarbia and hypoxemia.

If cervical spine injuries are suspected or documented, neutral head position with inline stabilization (no traction) should be maintained by the neurosurgeon during tracheal intubation. If the patient is awake and cooperative, an awake intubation technique may be desirable in this scenario for documentation of the neurologic examination after final positioning. When a difficult airway is anticipated or facial injuries preclude intubation under general anesthesia, awake intubation or creation of a surgical airway is acceptable as long as the airway is well topicalized with local anesthesia, and sedation is administered judiciously. Awake tracheal intubation may also be required for adult patients with brain tumors undergoing stereotactic craniotomy, unless the base ring with a removable mouthpiece is available or frameless stereotaxy is used. For children requiring stereotactic intracranial procedures, general anesthesia and tracheal intubation are performed before placement of the base ring.

## What Are the Goals for Anesthetic Maintenance?

Maintenance of anesthesia in patients with abnormal intracranial elastance should be performed with the same goals as for induction. Halothane should be used cautiously in patients with intracranial hypertension, and hyperventilation should be established before its administration. Low concentrations of isoflurane or sevoflurane have minimal effects on CBF and ICP and are safe in conjunction with concomitant hyperventilation. When intracranial hypertension is suspected preoperatively, nitrous oxide should not be used because other, safer anesthetic agents exist. A continuous infusion of narcotic is preferable to promote hemodynamic stability, ensure steady-state plasma levels, and provide for a smooth emergence at the conclusion of surgery. Neuromuscular blockade is maintained, unless cranial nerve monitoring is employed, to prevent movement in the pinion system that can result in scalp lacerations or cervical spine injuries. Maintenance of neuromuscular blockade during light planes of anesthesia prevents an increase in cerebral venous pressure associated with increased abdominal and thoracic tone.

## How Should Ventilation Be Controlled?

The cerebral resistance vessels, predominantly the end-arterioles, are exquisitely sensitive to alterations in $PaCO_2$. Hypocapnia is characterized by vasoconstriction of arterioles that results in decreased CBV, CBF, and ICP; hypercapnia influences the vascular tone in the opposite manner. CBF is increased by approximately 2 mL/100 g/min, or a 4% change for each 1 mm Hg increase in $PaCO_2$.[143,144]

Ventilation is controlled in all patients with intracranial hypertension, and the decision to lower $PaCO_2$ or to maintain normocarbia during the procedure is dependent on the intracranial pathology and quality of the operating conditions. For those patients with a chronic pathologic process, mild hypocarbia ($PaCO_2$ in low 30s) is frequently maintained until the time of dural closure to improve surgical exposure and to decrease the amount of brain retraction. For those patients with aneurysmal SAH, any acute ICP-reducing maneuvers are avoided until the dura is open and ICP is zero. Once the dura is opened, hyperventilation may be initiated, if needed, to optimize operating conditions. Regardless of the pathology, when hyperventilation is induced, $PaCO_2$ should be maintained ≥25 mm Hg to avoid cerebral ischemia.

Historically, hyperventilation was the mainstay of treatment for lowering ICP in head-injured patients. Published guidelines for the management of head injury advocate maintenance of normocarbia ($PaCO_2$ >35 mm Hg).[11] Global or regional cerebral ischemia (CBF <18 mL/100 g/min) has been documented in at least 30% of head-injured patients within 4 to 6 hours of injury.[1,2] Hyperventilation can reduce CBF even further when cerebral ischemia is present. If ICP elevations persist despite general maneuvers (ie, head elevation), ventricular drainage, and mannitol, ventilation should be increased to achieve $PaCO_2$ levels of 30 to 35 mm Hg. Jugular venous oxygen saturation and CBF monitoring are recommended by some if hyperventilation to a $PaCO_2$ of less than 30 mm Hg is required to lower ICP.[11]

Concomitant pulmonary injuries often accompany head injury and result in hypoxemia that warrants the use of PEEP. When PEEP of 10 cm $H_2O$ or less is used and accompanied by frequent determinations of $PaCO_2$, no significant elevations in ICP occur.[145] With increasing PEEP, dead space ventilation rises and causes an increase in $PaCO_2$ and ICP. When a PEEP value of more than 10 cm $H_2O$ is used, ICP elevations result not only from increased dead space ventilation but also from obstruction of cerebral venous return as CVP increases. Low PEEP values can be used safely as long as arterial blood gas determinations are made. If oxygenation worsens, increase PEEP or use pressure-control ventilation. Hypoxemia before initial resuscitation and during the hospitalization adversely affects neurologic outcome in head-injured patients.[146]

## How Should Blood Pressure Be Managed?

When ICP monitoring is not used, MAP should be maintained in the range of preoperative values for that patient to avoid cerebral ischemia. Hypotension should always be aggressively treated to maintain CPP. If cerebral autoregulation is intact, hypotension lowers CPP, causing cerebral vasodilation and exacerbation of intracranial hypertension, which in turn decreases CPP and initiates a vicious cycle. In the absence of cerebral autoregulation, CBF decreases dramatically with systemic hypotension. In head-injured patients, CPP should be maintained >70 mm Hg with volume expansion or vasopressors.[11] This goal may be difficult to achieve in head-injured patients with severe systemic injuries and significant blood loss. The number of hypotensive episodes (defined as systolic BP <90 mm Hg) worsens neurologic outcome in head-injured patients.[4]

Marked hypertension is treated, unless it is suspected that elevations are a protective measure to preserve CPP in the presence of severe intracranial hypertension. In this scenario, the bleeding risk is increased, but the BP should not be decreased until decompression occurs. In many instances, decompression will lead to profound hypotension as a result of rapid reduction in ICP and loss of the driving force maintaining the BP. Systemic hypertension is not always related to intracranial hypertension and is often the result of light anesthesia, surgical stimulation, or preexisting hypertension. Hypertension is frequently associated with placement of the pinion system and with incision until the dura is opened. Under these circumstances, hypertension may lead to increases in ICP and should be treated. The expected increases in BP can be attenuated or prevented by the administration of supplemental narcotics, barbiturates, inhalational agent, or β-blockade agents. If not effective, phentolamine or trimethaphan can be used, often combined with β-blockade to prevent reflex tachycardia. Trimethaphan, however, exerts its effects through ganglionic blockade and produces mydriasis that interferes with the neurologic examination postoperatively.

## How Should Intravenous Fluids Be Managed Intraoperatively?

Intraoperative fluid management is directed toward maintenance of euvolemia. Aggressive resuscitation with crystalloids, hypertonic saline, colloids, and blood products is often needed for the head-injured patient in hemorrhagic shock. Historically, volume restriction was employed to reduce brain water but often resulted in hypotension. Hypovolemia is no longer recommended because of the danger of associated hypotension.

In the intact brain, movement of fluid across the brain is dictated by the plasma osmolality, not plasma oncotic pressure as was previously thought.[147] Isotonic fluids (ie, normal saline) are the mainstay of fluid replacement intraoperatively. Considerable data support their safety in patients with intracranial pathology. Normal saline use did not promote increases in brain water in rats with cryogenic lesions, even though plasma oncotic pressure was significantly reduced.[148] Although colloids increase plasma oncotic pressure, no difference in brain water content is seen in animals with cryogenic injury treated with lactated Ringer's injection or 6% dextran 70.[149] Hypotonic fluids, including lactated Ringer's, can exacerbate cerebral edema by lowering plasma osmolality and should not be used in patients with intracranial pathology.

Glucose-containing solutions are avoided, particularly when the risk for cerebral ischemia exists. The exception may be in infants at risk for hypoglycemia. If the decision is made to use a non–dextrose-containing fluid in infants, serum glucose is monitored closely during the intraoperative period. Elevated plasma glucose levels provide substrate for anaerobic metabolism during periods of ischemia. Increased lactate and intracellular acidosis result, both of which adversely affect neurologic outcome. In a recent study of 267 head-injured patients (GCS, 3-12), higher admission glucose levels were found in patients with severe head injury compared with those with moderate injury.[150] Glucose levels >200 mg/dL in severely head-injured patients were associated with worse neurologic outcome and could be correlated with abnormal pupillary reaction and intracranial hypertension. From the data available, serum glucose should be maintained at 200 mg/dL or less; more aggressive control can result in hypoglycemia that also has detrimental effects on the brain.

Hypertonic saline reduces ICP consistently similar to mannitol, improves regional CBF, and improves hemodynamic status during early resuscitation without the use of large volumes of conventional crystalloids.[151–155] Ideally, hypertonic saline can be used in head-injured patients with hemorrhage to reduce ICP and stabilize hemodynamics. Adverse effects from hypertonic saline include the development of hypernatremia and hyperchloremic metabolic acidosis. Serum sodium

levels can be safely increased to 155 mEq/L or to a calculated plasma osmolality <320 mOsm/kg. The rapid elevation of serum sodium from previously normal levels has not been associated with pontine myelinolysis.

## How Should Temperature Be Managed?

The use of mild hypothermia to lower ICP, reduce secondary neuronal injury, and improve neurologic outcome in head-injured patients appeared efficacious in phase II trials; however, many phase III trials have yielded disappointing results.[156] Hypothermia decreases $CMRo_2$ and CBF, inhibits excitatory amino acid release, and stabilizes cell membranes. It has been shown to reduce infarct volume and to improve outcome in animal models of focal cerebral ischemia.[157,158] Even moderate to mild degrees are protective in animal models.[157]

Hypothermia has been used in human clinical trials to lower ICP and improve neurologic outcome, although results have been variable. Mild to moderate hypothermia (33°-35°C) effectively lowers ICP in patients with severe ischemic stroke and with severe head injury.[159,160] Whether this effect translates into improved clinical outcome remains unclear and demands further investigation and redesigning of neuroprotective trials.[156,159,161]

Although limited human data support hypothermia, most neuroanesthesiologists employ it to some degree intraoperatively as a cerebral protective measure, particularly when the risk for cerebral ischemia is high (ie, intracranial aneurysm surgery). Considering the complications and lack of proven benefit in humans, only mild degrees of hypothermia (ie, no lower than 34°C) should be used intraoperatively to minimize systemic complications. The theoretical benefits should be weighed against the risks. Mild hypothermia may act as a cerebral protectant in humans, but large clinical trials are warranted to study its efficacy in ICP reduction and improvement in outcome.

## How Are Intracranial Pressure Elevations Managed Intraoperatively?

A plan should be formulated preoperatively to address ICP elevations that occur intraoperatively. Systemic hypertension and bradycardia may signal an increase in ICP. When acute ICP elevations or hemodynamic changes occur, an acute intracranial process, such as bleeding, must be suspected and surgical opening expedited. If an ICP monitor is not in place, the dura and brain can be inspected for tenseness when the bone flap is removed. Although the ICP is zero after the dura is open, the brain can still protrude through the craniotomy site, resulting in ischemia or edema with difficult closure.

### Mannitol

Mannitol 20% (0.5-1.0 g/kg) is routinely administered before removal of the bone flap during neurosurgical procedures and is an important treatment modality for head-injured patients with intracranial hypertension. It is a hypertonic, hyperosmotic agent that reduces brain water by establishing an osmotic gradient, favoring movement of water from the brain interstitium into the vasculature. Mannitol is only effective in areas of intact blood-brain barrier. Onset of action occurs within 10 to 20 minutes of administration. Initially, ICP increases in response to direct vasodilation, followed by a decrease in ICP and increase in CPP that often lasts for 90 minutes.[162] Mannitol use is limited by the plasma osmolality, which should be maintained at <320 mOsm/kg. It has the added benefit of free radical scavenging ability.

If the diuretic response to mannitol is not adequate and ICP elevations persist, a loop diuretic, such as furosemide, can be used as long as the patient is euvolemic. The combination of mannitol and furosemide has an additive effect on ICP reduction and duration of diuresis.[163] However, a danger of profound hypovolemia is present when the drugs are administered in combination.

## Hyperventilation

In patients with chronic pathology, additional hyperventilation may be instituted to improve operating conditions and lower ICP. In severely head-injured patients at high risk for cerebral ischemia, hyperventilation can be initiated to lower ICP acutely but should only be considered when all other measures are ineffective. The long-term impact of even short periods of hyperventilation in severely head-injured patients remains unknown.

## Head Position

Maintenance of head elevation should be verified and increased further to improve cerebral venous drainage as long as MAP is not significantly reduced. In most neurosurgical cases, the head cannot be stabilized in a neutral position because of operating requirements. Occasionally, positioning the head and neck in extreme flexion or lateral rotation compromises cerebral venous return, requiring intraoperative repositioning. Cerebral venous return can also be impaired with neck compression that results from an electrocardiographic lead crossing the neck tightly or with circumferential taping of the endotracheal tube.

## Treatment of Hypotension or Hypertension

As was discussed previously, hypotension should always be aggressively treated to maintain an effective perfusion pressure. When systemic hypertension is significant enough to increase ICP and is not considered a protective measure, therapy should also be directed at its etiology. If the anesthetic depth is considered adequate, BP should be lowered with an antihypertensive with neutral effects on ICP.

## Cerebrospinal Fluid Drainage

Drainage of CSF can improve spatial compensation and is a rapid and effective measure to reduce ICP. CSF drainage can be accomplished through an intraventricular catheter, lumbar drain, or at the time the sylvian fissure is split. In the presence of a space-occupying lesion, lumbar CSF drainage is contraindicated. A lumbar drain may be placed before surgical incision in patients with posterior circulation aneurysms (ie, basilar tip) to drain CSF and improve exposure of the aneurysm. When a significant amount of CSF is drained, a large pneumocephalus may develop and interfere with patient emergence.

## Hypertonic Saline

Hypertonic saline reduces ICP to a similar degree as mannitol and should be considered when intracranial hypertension develops intraoperatively. If the brain appears tight, hypertonic saline may be selected over crystalloids as long as serum sodium and acid-base status permit.

## Anesthetic Agents

Although volatile agents in low concentrations have minimal effects on ICP, they may need to be discontinued if intracranial hypertension persists or brain conditions are not improved with other maneuvers. Nitrous oxide should be discontinued if in use. The degree of muscle relaxation should be verified and a train-of-four response of one or less confirmed.

## Barbiturates

Barbiturates are highly effective in reducing ICP by lowering $CMRO_2$ and CBF and should be administered if intracranial hypertension persists despite ventricular drainage (if available), mannitol, general maneuvers, or hyperventilation ($PaCO_2$, 30-35 mm Hg). Barbiturates also appear to possess cerebral protective properties mediated through $CMRO_2$ reduction, alteration of vascular tone, and inhibition of free radical–mediated lipid peroxidation. High-dose barbiturates are effective in reducing ICP and may decrease mortality in patients with intracranial hypertension that is uncontrollable by medical and surgical interventions.[11,164–166] The impact of barbiturates on quality of survival in severely head-injured patients requires further investigation.

Sodium pentothal is the barbiturate most frequently used intraoperatively to lower ICP. Pentobarbital remains the barbiturate of choice when long-term use is anticipated. If EEG monitoring is available, barbiturates are titrated to >90% suppression of total EEG activity and not to isoelectricity, in order to control the amount of drug administered. $CMRO_2$ reduction from 90% EEG suppression to isoelectricity is insignificant. Vasopressors are usually needed to maintain an adequate CPP. Once barbiturates are administered, postoperative neurologic assessment may be impossible, depending on the amount required to lower ICP or improve operating conditions.

## How Is Intracranial Pressure Controlled During Emergence?

Prior to closure at surgery, if ICP is normal, the $PaCO_2$ should be normalized to minimize the degree of pneumocephalus. Pneumocephalus can be large after CSF drainage or posterior fossa procedures. Nitrous oxide should never be instituted after dural closure in order to prevent enlargement of a pneumocephalus. In patients with subdural hematoma, normalization of $PaCO_2$ after evacuation of the clot is necessary to prevent reaccumulation of blood. If ICP elevations are expected to persist or develop postoperatively, the patient should remain intubated postoperatively, and some degree of hyperventilation may be required.

Extubation is planned at the conclusion of surgery unless hyperventilation may be needed to lower ICP, mental status was impaired preoperatively, cranial nerve injury (eg, cranial nerves IX and X) is suspected, or large doses of barbiturates have been administered during the case. Even if extubation is not planned, emergence should be directed to permit an early neurologic examination, when possible. During emergence, antihypertensive agents are often needed to control blood pressure. A significant number of patients develop hypertension during emergence from a neurosurgical procedure and should be aggressively treated if ICP elevations are still of concern and to decrease the risk for postoperative bleeding. Nitroglycerin and sodium nitroprusside are not recommended for emergence unless a large mass lesion has been removed and there is no danger of increased ICP. The anesthesiologist should tailor the anesthetic to provide for a rapid, smooth emergence without coughing against the endotracheal tube. Postoperatively, frequent neurologic assessments are mandatory to detect any changes in the examination that may signal elevated ICP, increased cerebral edema, or bleeding.

## OUTCOME

### What Factors Are Important?

#### Pathologic Considerations

The outcome of patients with intracranial hypertension largely depends on the underlying pathologic process. For a patient with an epidural hematoma, prognosis may be favorable if evacuation of the clot is performed expeditiously and there is minimal or no underlying brain injury. The prognosis of patients with brain tumors depends on the histopathology of the mass lesion. Only 30% of patients with aneurysmal SAH have a good functional outcome. The outcome of head-injured patients is predicted by the following[2,9,167–169]:

1. Age of the patient
2. Degree and type of intracranial pathology
3. Initial GCS
4. Number of episodes of hypoxemia and hypotension
5. Degree and duration of ICP elevation
6. $CMRo_2$
7. Presence of cerebral ischemia

#### Physiologic Changes

The frequency of hypoxemia and hypotension, especially during resuscitation, worsens neurologic outcome after head injury and may lead to diffuse cerebral swelling that independently alters prognosis.[146] Children with diffuse swelling have a higher mortality rate than adults.[146] Mortality increases with CT evidence of midline shift more than 3 mm, compressed ambient cisterns, masses with volumes >15 mL, and the presence of an extracerebral mass.[23] The presence of cerebral ischemia at any time during the hospital course or the persistence of a low-flow state is associated with increased morbidity and mortality in head-injured patients.[2,170] Secondary neuronal injury significantly influences not only the extent of injury but also the overall outcome.

Patients with head injury continue to improve after discharge; functional status 6 months after injury correlates well with final neurologic outcome.[171] The most common neurobehavioral finding at 1 year after injury is impairment of memory and information processing.[172]

## CONCLUSION

The fundamental processes controlling normal intracranial dynamics and pressure have not changed over time. However, our understanding of the impact of pathologic processes on global or regional CBF, cerebral autoregulation, and potentiation of secondary injury has evolved at a rapid pace. In patients with brain tumors, advancements in stereotaxis have revolutionized the diagnosis, surgical treatment, and radiation therapy in these patients. For some patients with intracranial aneurysms, endovascular embolization is a viable option and associated with considerably less surgical stress and fluid shifts than a craniotomy for surgical clipping.

In head-injured patients, improvements in ICP and cerebral hemodynamic monitoring have led to more accurate medical and surgical interventions to reduce ICP, improve CPP, and ultimately positively affect neurologic outcome. To prevent further neurologic injury, the anesthesiologist must understand not only the underlying pathologic process but also the impact that anesthetic agents, pharmacologic interventions, and hemodynamic manipulations have on ICP and promotion of secondary injury. In the future, improved monitoring techniques that can accurately and continuously assess CBF, brain oxygenation, and biochemical markers of ischemia are likely to become available. For head-injured patients, medical therapy is likely to be directed not only toward the primary brain injury but also toward active prevention of secondary injury.

## References

1. Bouma GJ, Muizelaar JP, Stringer WA, et al. Ultra-early evaluation of regional cerebral blood flow in severely head-injured patients using xenon-enhanced computerized tomography. *J Neurosurg.* 1992;77:360.
2. Bouma GJ, Muizelaar P, Choi SC, et al. Cerebral circulation and metabolism after severe traumatic brain injury: the elusive role of ischemia. *J Neurosurg.* 1991;75:685.
3. Sahuquillo J, Poca M-A, Arribas M, et al. Interhemispheric supratentorial intracranial pressure gradients in head-injured patients: are they clinically important? *J Neurosurg.* 1999;90:16.
4. Teasdale GM, Graham DI. Craniocerebral trauma: protection and retrieval of the neuronal population after injury. *Neurosurgery.* 1998;43:723.
5. Rowland LP, Fink ME, Rubin L. Cerebrospinal fluid: blood-brain barrier, brain edema, and hydrocephalus. In: Kandel ER, Schwartz JH, Jessell TM, eds. *Principles of Neural Science.* 3rd ed. New York, NY: Elsevier;1991:1050.
6. Wilkinson HA. Intracranial pressure. In: Youmans JR, ed. *Neurological Surgery.* 3rd ed. Vol 2. Philadelphia, Pa: WB Saunders; 1990:662.
7. Marmarou A, Shulman K, LaMorgese J. Compartmental analysis of compliance and outflow resistance of the cerebrospinal fluid system. *J Neurosurg.* 1975;43:523.
8. Kuncz A, Dóczi T, Bodosi M. The effect of skull and dura on brain volume regulation after hypo- and hyperosmolar fluid treatment. *Neurosurgery.* 1990;27:509.
9. Jaggi JL, Obrist WD, Gennarelli TA, et al. Relationship of early cerebral blood flow and metabolism to outcome in acute head injury. *J Neurosurg.* 1990;72:176.
10. Juul N, Morris GF, Marshall SB, et al, and the Executive Committee of the International Selfotel Trial. Intracranial hypertension and cerebral perfusion pressure: influence on neurological deterioration and outcome in severe head injury. *J Neurosurg.* 2000;92:1.
11. Bullock R, Chesnut RM, Clifton G, et al. Guidelines for the management of severe head injury. *J Neurotrauma.* 1996;13:638.
12. Löfgren J, von Essen C, Zwetnow NN. The pressure-volume curve of the cerebrospinal fluid space in dogs. *Acta Neurol Scand.* 1973;49:557.
13. Graham DI, Ford I, Adams JH, et al. Ischaemic brain damage is still common in fatal non-missile head injury. *J Neurol Neurosurg Psychiatry.* 1989;52:346.
14. Rosner MJ, Daughton S. Cerebral perfusion pressure management in head injury. *J Trauma.* 1990;30:933.

15. Muizelaar JP, Schröder MI. Overview of monitoring of cerebral blood flow and metabolism after severe head injury. *Can J Neurol Sci.* 1994;21:S6.

16. Shapiro HM. Intracranial hypertension: therapeutic and anesthetic considerations. *Anesthesiology.* 1975;43:445.

17. Langfitt TW, Weinstein JD, Kassell NF. Cerebral vasomotor paralysis produced by intracranial hypertension. *Neurology.* 1965;15:622.

18. Brain WR. A clinical study of increased intracranial pressure in sixty cases of cerebral tumour. *Brain.* 1925;48:105.

19. Jennett B, Teasdale G. Aspects of coma after severe head injury. *Lancet* 1977;1:878.

20. Hodge CJ, Primrose D. Physiological considerations. In: Apuzzo MLJ, ed. *Brain Surgery: Complication Avoidance and Management.* New York, NY: Churchill Livingstone; 1993:1574.

21. Cushing H. Concerning a definite regulatory mechanism of the vasomotor centre which controls blood pressure during cerebral compression. *Bull Johns Hopkins Hosp.* 1901;12:290.

22. Haydel MJ, Preston CA, Mills TJ, et al. Indications for computed tomography in patients with minor head injury. *N Engl J Med.* 2000;343:100.

23. Eisenberg HM, Gary HE, Aldrich EF, et al. Initial CT findings in 753 patients with severe head injury. *J Neurosurg.* 1990;73:688.

24. O'Sullivan MG, Statham PF, Jones PA, et al. Role of intracranial pressure monitoring in severely head-injured patients without signs of intracranial hypertension on initial computerized tomography. *J Neurosurg.* 1994;80:46.

25. Rosenwasser RH, Kleiner LI, Krzeminski JP, et al. Intracranial pressure monitoring in the posterior fosse: a preliminary report. *J Neurosurg.* 1989;71:503.

26. Mollman HD, Rockswold GL, Ford SE. A clinical comparison of subarachnoid catheters to ventriculostomy and subarachnoid bolts: a prospective study. *J Neurosurg.* 1988;68:737.

27. Crutchfield JS, Narayan RK, Robertson CS, et al. Evaluation of fiberoptic intracranial pressure monitor. *J Neurosurg.* 1990;72:482.

28. Fernandes HM, Bingham K, Chambers IR, et al. Clinical evaluation of the Codman microsensor intracranial pressure monitoring system. *Acta Neurochir Suppl (Wien).* 1998;71:44.

29. Hamer J, Alberti E, Hoyer S, et al. Influence of systemic and cerebral vascular factors on the cerebrospinal fluid pulse waves. *J Neurosurg.* 1977;46:36.

30. Kjallquist A, Lundberg N, Pontén U. Respiratory and cardiovascular changes during rapid spontaneous variations of ventricular fluid pressure in patients with intracranial hypertension. *Acta Neurol Scand.* 1964;40:291.

31. Lundberg N. Continuous recording and control of ventricular fluid pressure in neurosurgical practice. *Acta Psychiatr Neurol Scand (Suppl).* 1960;149:1.

32. Czosnyka M, Smielewski P, Piechnik S, et al. Hemodynamic characterization of intracranial pressure plateau waves in head-injured patients. *J Neurosurg.* 1999;91:11.

33. Lundberg N, Troupp N, Lorin H. Continuous recording of the ventricular-fluid pressure in patients with severe acute traumatic brain injury. *J Neurosurg.* 1965;22:581.

34. Feri M, Ralli L, Felici M, et al. Transcranial Doppler and brain death diagnosis. *Crit Care Med.* 1994;22:1120.

35. Ducrocq X, Hassler W, Moritake K, et al. Consensus opinion on diagnosis of cerebral circulatory arrest using Doppler-sonography. Task Force Group on cerebral death of the Neurosonology Research Group of the World Federation of Neurology. *J Neurol Sci.* 1998;159:145.

36. Adams RW, Gronert GA, Sundt TM, et al. Halothane, hypocapnia, and cerebrospinal fluid pressure in neurosurgery. *Anesthesiology.* 1972;37:510.

37. Albrecht RF, Miletich DJ, Rosenberg R, et al. Cerebral blood flow and metabolic changes from induction to onset of anesthesia with halothane or pentobarbital. *Anesthesiology.* 1977;47:252.

38. Albrecht RF, Miletich DJ, Madala LR. Normalization of cerebral blood flow during prolonged halothane anesthesia. *Anesthesiology.* 1983, 58:26.

39. Drummond JC, Todd MM, Toutant SM, et al. Brain surface protrusion during enflurane, halothane, and isoflurane anesthesia in cats. *Anesthesiology.* 1983;59:288.

40. Brussel T, Fitch W, Brodner G, et al. Effects of halothane in low concentrations on cerebral blood flow, cerebral metabolism, and cerebrovascular autoregulation in the baboon. *Anesth Analg.* 1991;73:758.

41. Lee JG, Hudetz AG, Smith JJ, et al. The effects of halothane and isoflurane on cerebrocortical microcirculation and autoregulation as assessed by laser-Doppler flowmetry. *Anesth Analg.* 1994;79:58.

42. Cucchiara RF, Theye RA, Michenfelder JD. The effects of isoflurane on canine cerebral metabolism and blood flow. *Anesthesiologyy.* 1974;40:571.

43. Newberg LA, Milde JH, Michenfelder JD. The cerebral metabolic effects of isoflurane at and above concentrations that suppress cortical electrical activity. *Anesthesiology.* 1983;59:23.

44. Lam AM, Mayberg TS, Eng CC, et al. Nitrous oxide-isoflurane anesthesia causes more cerebral vasodilation than an equipotent dose of isoflurane in humans. *Anesth Analg.* 1994;78:462.

45. Bisonnette B, Leon JE. Cerebrovascular stability during isoflurane anaesthesia in children. *Can J Anaesth.* 1992;39:128.

46. Algotsson L, Messeter K, Nördstrom CH, et al. Cerebral blood flow and oxygen consumption during isoflurane and halothane anesthesia in man. *Acta Anaesthesiol Scand.* 1988;32:15.

47. Algotsson L, Messeter K, Rosen I, et al. Effects of nitrous oxide on cerebral haemodynamics and metabolism during isoflurane anaesthesia in man. *Acta Anaesthesiol Scand.* 1992;36:46.

48. Hansen TD, Warner DS, Todd MM, et al. Effects of nitrous oxide and volatile anaesthetics on cerebral blood flow. *Br J Anaesth.* 1989;63:290.

49. Adams RW, Cucchiara RF, Gronert GA, et al. Isoflurane and cerebrospinal fluid pressure in neurosurgical patients. *Anesthesiology.* 1981;54:97.

50. Artru AA. Effects of enflurane and isoflurane on resistance to reabsorption of cerebrospinal fluid in dogs. *Anesthesiology.* 1984;61:529.

51. Artru AA. Isoflurane does not increase the rate of CSF production in the dog. *Anesthesiology.* 1984;60:193.

52. Hoffman WE, Edelman G, Kochs E, et al. Cerebral autoregulation in awake versus isoflurane-anesthetized rats. *Anesth Analg.* 1991;73:753.

53. McPherson RW, Brain JE, Traystman RJ. Cerebrovascular responsiveness to carbon dioxide in dogs with 1.4% and 2.8% isoflurane. *Anesthesiolgy.* 1989;70:843.

54. Matta B, Heath K, Tipping K, et al. Direct cerebral vasodilator effects of sevoflurane and isoflurane. *Anesthesiology.* 1999;91:677.

55. Scheller MS, Tateishi A, Drummond JC, et al. The effects of sevoflurane on cerebral blood flow, cerebral metabolic rate for oxygen, intracranial pressure, and the electroencephalogram are similar to those of isoflurane in the rabbit. *Anesthesiology.* 1988;68:548.

56. Scheller MS, Nakakimura K, Fleischer JE, et al. Cerebral effects of sevoflurane in the dog: comparison with isoflurane and enflurane. *Br J Anaesth.* 1990;65:388.

57. Artru AA, Lam AM, Johnson JO, et al. Intracranial pressure, middle cerebral artery flow velocity, and plasma inorganic fluoride concentrations in neurosurgical patients receiving sevoflurane or isoflurane. *Anesth Analg.* 1997;85:587.

58. Osawa M, Shingu K, Murakawa M, et al. Effects of sevoflurane on central nervous system electrical activity in cats. *Anesth Analg.* 1994;79:52.

59. Komatsu H, Taie S, Endo S, et al. Electrical seizures during sevoflurane anesthesia in two pediatric patients with epilepsy. *Anesthesiology.* 1994;81:1535.

60. Woodforth IJ, Hicks RG, Crawford MR, et al. Electroencephalographic evidence of seizure activity under deep sevoflurane anesthesia in a nonepileptic patient. *Anesthesiology.* 1997;87:1579.

61. Muzzi DA, Losasso TJ, Dietz NM, et al. The effect of desflurane and isoflurane on cerebrospinal fuid pressure in humans with supratentorial mass lesions. *Anesthesiology.* 1992;76:720.

62. Lutz LJ, Milde JH, Milde LN. The cerebral functional, metabolic, and hemodynamic effects of desflurane in dogs. *Anesthesiology.* 1990;73:125.

63. Lutz LJ, Milde JH, Milde LN. The response of the canine cerebral circulation to hyperventilation during anesthesia with desflurane. *Anesthesiology.* 1991;74:504.

64. Young WL. Effects of desflurane on the central nervous system. *Anesth Analg.* 1992;75:S32.

65. Ornstein E, Young WL, Fleischer LH, et al. Desflurane and isoflurane have similar effects on cerebral blood flow in patients with intracranial mass lesions. *Anesthesiology.* 1993;79:498.

66. Baughman VL, Hoffman WE, Miletich DJ, et al. Cerebrovascular and cerebral metabolic effects of $N_2O$ in unrestrained rats. *Anesthesiology.* 1990;73:269.

67. Drummond JC, Scheller MS, Todd MM. The effect of nitrous oxide on cortical cerebral blood flow during anesthesia with halothane and isoflurane, with and without morphine, in the rabbit. *Anesth Analg.* 1987;66:1083.

68. Kaieda R, Todd MM, Warner DS. The effects of anesthetics and $Paco_2$ on the cerebrovascular, metabolic, and electroencephalographic responses to nitrous oxide in the rabbit. *Anesth Analg.* 1989;68:135.

69. Reinstrup P, Ryding E, Algotsson L, et al. Effects of nitrous oxide on

human regional cerebral blood flow and isolated pial arteries. *Anesthesiology*. 1994;81:396.

70. Phirman JR, Shapiro HM. Modification of nitrous oxide-induced intracranial hypertension by prior induction of anesthesia. *Anesthesiology*. 1977;46:150.

71. Henriksen HT, Jörgensen PB. The effect of nitrous oxide on intracranial pressure in patients with intracranial disorders. *Br J Anaesth*. 1973;45:486.

72. Stullken EH, Milde JH, Michenfelder JD, et al. The nonlinear responses of cerebral metabolism to low concentrations of halothane, enflurane, isoflurane, and thiopental. *Anesthesiology*. 1977;46:28.

73. Michenfelder JD. The interdependency of cerebral functional and metabolic effects following massive doses of thiopental in the dog. *Anesthesiology*. 1974;41:231.

74. Pierce EC, Lambertsen CJ, Deutsch S, et al. Cerebral circulation and metabolism during thiopental anesthesia and hyperventilation in man. *J Clin Invest*. 1962;41:1664.

75. Hodes JE, Soncrant TT, Larson DM, et al. Selective changes in local cerebral glucose utilization induced by phenobarbital in the rat. *Anesthesiology*. 1985;63:633.

76. Nilsson L, Siesjo BK. The effect of phenobarbitone anaesthesia on blood flow and oxygen consumption in the rat brain. *Acta Anaesth Scand (Suppl)*. 1975;57:18.

77. Shapiro HM, Galindo A, Wyte SR, et al. Rapid intraoperative reduction of intracranial pressure with thiopentone. *Br J Anaesth*. 1973;45:1057.

78. Milde LN, Milde JH, Michenfelder JD. Cerebral functional, metabolic, and hemodynamic effects of etomidate in dogs. *Anesthesiology*. 1985;63:371.

79. Renou AM, Vernhiet J, Macrez P, et al. Cerebral blood flow and metabolism during etomidate anaesthesia in man. *Br J Anaesth*. 1978;50:1047.

80. Cold GE, Eskesen V, Eriksen H, et al. CBF and $CMRO_2$ during continuous etomidate infusion supplemented with $N_2O$ and fentanyl in patients with supratentorial cerebral tumour: dose-response study. *Acta Anesthesiol Scand*. 1985;29:490.

81. Prior JGL, Hinds CJ, Williams J, et al. The use of etomidate in the management of severe head injury. *Intensive Care Med*. 1983;9:313.

82. Pinaud M, Lelausque JN, Chetanneau A, et al. Effects of propofol on cerebral hemodynamics and metabolism in patients with brain trauma. *Anesthesiology*. 1990;73:404.

83. Vandesteene A, Trempont V, Engelman E, et al. Effect of propofol on cerebral blood flow and metabolism in man. *Anaesthesia Suppl*. 1988;43:42.

84. Ravussin P, Thorin D, Guinard JP, et al. Effect of propofol on cerebrospinal fluid pressure in patients with and without intracranial hypertension. *Anesthesiology*. 1989;71:A120.

85. Bedford RF, Persing JA, Pobereskin L, et al. Lidocaine or thiopental for rapid control of intracranial hypertension? *Anesth Analg*. 1980;59:435.

86. Yano M, Nishiyama H, Yokota H, et al. Effect of lidocaine on ICP response to endotracheal suctioning. *Anesthesiology*. 1986;64:651.

87. Dawson B, Michenfelder JD, Theye RA. Effects of ketamine on canine cerebral blood flow and metabolism: modification by prior administration of thiopental. *Anesth Analg*. 1971;50:443.

88. Kayama Y, Iwama K. The EEG, evoked potentials, and single-unit activity during ketamine anesthesia in cats. *Anesthesiology*. 1972;36:316.

89. Ferrer-Allado T, Brechner VL, Dymond A, et al. Ketamine-induced electroconvulsive phenomena in the human limbic and thalamic regions. *Anesthesiology*. 1973;38:333.

90. Hougaard K, Hansen A, Brodersen P. The effect of ketamine on regional cerebral blood flow in man. *Anesthesiology*. 1974;41:562.

91. Sari A, Okuda Y, Takeshita H. The effect of ketamine on cerebrospinal fluid pressure. *Anesth Analg*. 1972;51:560.

92. Gibbs JM. The effect of intravenous ketamine on cerebrospinal fluid pressure. *Br J Anaesth*. 1972;44:1298.

93. Carlsson C, Hagerdal M, Kaasik AE, et al. The effects of diazepam on cerebral blood flow and oxygen consumption in rats and its synergistic interaction with nitrous oxide. *Anesthesiology*. 1976;45:319.

94. Maekawa T, Sakabe T, Takeshita H. Diazepam blocks cerebral metabolic and circulatory responses to local anesthetic-induced seizures. *Anesthesiology*. 1974;41:389.

95. Nugent M, Artru AA, Michenfelder JD. Cerebral metabolic, vascular, and protective effects of midazolam maleate. *Anesthesiology*. 1982;56:172.

96. Roald OK, Steen PA, Milde JH, et al. Reversal of the cerebral effects of diazepam in the dog by the benzodiazepine antagonist Ro15-1788. *Acta Anesthesiol Scand*. 1986;30:341.

97. Tateishi A, Maekawa T, Takeshita H, et al. Diazepam and intracranial pressure. *Anesthesiology*. 1981;54:335.

98. Forster A, Juge O, Morel D. Effects of midazolam on cerebral blood flow in human volunteers. *Anesthesiology*. 1982;56:453.

99. Hoffman WE, Miletich DJ, Albrecht RF. The effects of midazolam on cerebral blood flow and oxygen consumption and its interaction with nitrous oxide. *Anesth Analg*. 1986;65:729.

100. Papazian L, Albanese J, Thirion X, et al. Effect of bolus doses of midazolam on intracranial pressure and cerebral perfusion pressure in patients with severe head injury. *Br J Anaesth*. 1993;71:267.

101. Tobias JD. Increased intracranial pressure after fentanyl administration in a child with closed head trauma. *Pediatr Emerg Care*. 1994;10:89.

102. Sperry RJ, Bailey PL, Reichman MV, et al. Fentanyl and sufentanil increase intracranial pressure in head trauma patients. *Anesthesiology*. 1992;77:416.

103. Jung R, Shah N, Reinsel R, et al. Cerebrospinal fluid pressure in patients with brain tumors: impact of fentanyl versus alfentanil during nitrous oxide-oxygen anesthesia. *Anesth Analg*. 1990;71:419.

104. Marx W, Shah N, Long C, et al. Sufentanil, alfentanil, and fentanyl: impact on cerebrospinal fluid pressure in patients with brain tumors. *J Neurosurg Anesth*. 1989;1:3.

105. Herrick IA, Gelb AW, Manninen PH, et al. Effects of fentanyl, sufentanil, and alfentanil on brain retractor pressure. *Anesth Analg*. 1991;72:359.

106. From RP, Warner DS, Todd MM, et al. Anesthesia for craniotomy: a double-blind comparison of alfentanil, fentanyl, and sufentanil. *Anesthesiology*. 1990;73:896.

107. Guy J, Hindman BJ, Baker KZ. Comparison of remifentanil and fentanyl in patients undergoing craniotomy for supratentorial space-occupying lesions. *Anesthesiology*. 1997;86:514.

108. Warner DS. Experience with remifentanil in neurosurgical patients. *Anesth Analg*. 1999;89:S33.

109. Ostapkovich ND, Baker KZ, Fogarty-Mack P, et al. Cerebral blood flow and $CO_2$ reactivity is similar during remifentanil/$N_2O$ and fentanyl/$N_2O$ anesthesia. *Anesthesiology*. 1998;89:358.

110. Lanier WL, Iaizzo PA, Milde JH. Cerebral function and muscle afferent activity following intravenous succinylcholine in dogs anesthetized with halothane: the effects of pretreatment with a defasciculating dose of pancuronium. *Anesthesiology*. 1989;71:87.

111. Lanier WL, Milde JH, Michenfelder JD. Cerebral stimulation following succinylcholine in dogs. *Anesthesiology*. 1986;64:551.

112. Minton MD, Grosslight K, Stirt JA, et al. Increases in intracranial pressure from succinylcholine: prevention by prior nondepolarizing blockade. *Anesthesiology*. 1986;65:165.

113. Cottrell JE, Hartung J, Giffin JP, et al. Intracranial and hemodynamic changes after succinylcholine administration in cats. *Anesth Analg*. 1983;62:1006.

114. Rosa G, Orfei P, Sanfilippo M, et al. The effects of atracurium bresylate (Tracrium) on intracranial pressure and cerebral perfusion pressure. *Anesth Analg*. 1986;65:381.

115. Minton MD, Stirt JA, Bedford RF, et al. Intracranial pressure after atracurium in neurosurgical patients. *Anesth. Analg*. 1985;64:1113.

116. Cafiero T, Razzino S, Mastronardi P, et al. Mivacurium in patients with intracranial pathology. *Minerva Anestesiol*. 1999;65:81.

117. Strebel SP, Kindler C, Bissonnette B, et al. The impact of systemic vasoconstrictors on the cerebral circulation of anesthetized patients. *Anesthesiology*. 1998;89:67.

118. Myburgh JA, Upton RN, Grant C, et al. A comparison of the effects of norepinephrine, epinephrine, and dopamine on cerebral blood flow and oxygen utilization. *Acta Neurochir Suppl (Wien)*. 1998;71:19.

119. Hoff JT, Sengupta D, Harper M, et al. Effect of alpha-adrenergic blockade on response of cerebral circulation to hypocapnia in the baboon. *Lancet*. 1972;2:1337.

120. Waltz AG, Yamaguchi T, Regli F. Regulatory responses of cerebral vasculature after sympathetic denervation. *Am J Physiol*. 1971;221:298.

121. Van Aken H, Puchstein C, Schweppe ML, et al. Effect of labetalol on intracranial pressure in dogs with and without intracranial hypertension. *Acta Anesthesiol Scand*. 1982;26:615.

122. Cottrell JE, Gupta B, Rappaport H, et al. Intracranial pressure during nitroglycerin-induced hypotension. *J Neurosurg*. 1980;53:309.

123. Dohi S, Matsumoto M, Takahashi T. The effects of nitroglycerin on cerebrospinal fluid pressure in awake and anesthetized humans. *Anesthesiology*. 1981;54:511.

124. Rogers MC, Hamburger C, Owen K, et al. Intracranial pressure in the cat during nitroglycerin-induced hypotension. *Anesthesiology*. 1979;51:227.

125. Marsh ML, Shapiro HM, Smith RW, et al. Changes in neurologic

status and intracranial pressure associated with sodium nitroprusside administration. *Anesthesiology.* 1979;51:336.

126. Cottrell JE, Patel K, Turndorf H, et al. Intracranial pressure changes induced by sodium nitroprusside in patients with intracranial mass lesions. *J. Neurosurg.* 1978; 48:329.

127. Michenfelder JD, Milde JH. The interaction of sodium nitroprusside, hypotension, and isoflurane in determining cerebral vasculature effects. *Anesthesiology.* 1988; 69:870.

128. Candia GJ, Heros RC, Lavyne MH, et al. Effect of intravenous sodium nitroprusside on cerebral blood flow and intracranial pressure. *Neurosurgery.* 1978;3:50.

129. Guerra WK-W, Gaab MR, Dietz H, et al. Surgical decompression for traumatic brain swelling: indications and results. *J Neurosurg.* 1999;90:187.

130. Haley EC Jr, Kassell NF, Torner JC, et al. The International Cooperative Study on the Timing of Aneurysm Surgery: the North American experience. *Stroke.* 1992; 23:205.

131. Spivey WH. Flumazenil and seizures: analysis of 43 cases. *Clin Ther.* 1992;14:292.

132. Davis CO, Wax PM. Flumazenil associated seizure in an 11-month-old child. *J Emerg Med.* 1996;14:331.

133. Schulze-Bonhage A, Elger CE. Induction of partial epileptic seizures by flumazenil. *Epilepsia.* 2000;41:186.

134. Dearden NM, Gibson JS, McDowall DG, et al. Effect of high-dose dexamethasone on outcome from severe head injury. *J Neurosurg.* 1986;64:81.

135. Cooper PR, Moody S, Clark WK, et al. Dexamethasone and severe head injury: a prospective double-blind study. *J Neurosurg.* 1979;51:307.

136. Gudeman SK, Miller JD, Becker DP. Failure of high-dose steroid therapy to influence intracranial pressure in patients with severe head injury. *J Neurosurg.* 1979;51:301.

137. The European Study Group on Nimodipine in Severe Head Injury. A multicenter trial of the efficacy of nimodipine on outcome after severe head injury. *J Neurosurg.* 1994;80:797.

138. Andersen C, Astrup J, Gyldensted C. Quantitative MR analysis of glucocorticoid effects on peritumoral edema associated with intracranial meningiomas and metastases. *J Comput Assist Tomogr.* 1994;18:509.

139. Ito U, Reulen HJ, Tomita H, et al. A computed tomography study on formation, propagation, and resolution of edema fluid in metastatic brain tumors. *Adv Neurol.* 1990;52:459.

140. Rommel T, Bodsch W. Glucocorticosteroid treatment of vasogenic oedema. *Acta Neurochir Suppl (Wien).* 1988;43:145.

141. Feldman Z, Kanter MJ, Robertson CS, et al. Effect of head elevation on intracranial pressure, cerebral perfusion pressure, and cerebral blood flow in head-injured patients. *J Neurosurg.* 1992;76:207.

142. Rosner MJ, Coley IB. Cerebral perfusion pressure, intracranial pressure and head elevation. *J Neurosurg.* 1986;65:636.

143. Lassen NA, Christensen MS. Physiology of cerebral blood flow. *Br J Anaesth.* 1976;48:719.

144. Grubb RL, Raichle ME, Eichling JO, et al. The effects of changes in $Pa_{CO_2}$ on cerebral blood volume, blood flow, and vascular mean transit time. *Stroke.* 1974;5:630.

145. Cooper KR, Boswell PA, Choi SC. Safe use of PEEP in patients with severe head injury. *J Neurosurg.* 1985;63 552.

146. Aldrich EF, Eisenberg HM, Saydjari C, et al. Diffuse brain swelling in severely head-injured children: a report from the NIH Traumatic Coma Data Bank. *J Neurosurg.* 1992;76:450.

147. Zornow MH, Prough DS. Fluid management in patients with traumatic brain injury. *New Horizons.* 1995;3:488.

148. Zornow MH, Scheller MS, Todd MM, et al. Acute cerebral effects of isotonic crystalloid and colloid solutions following cryogenic brain injury in the rabbit. *Anesthesiology.* 1988;69:180.

149. Zhuang J, Shackford SR, Schmoker JD, et al. Colloid infusion after brain injury: effect on intracranial pressure, cerebral blood flow, and oxygen delivery. *Crit Care Med.* 1995;23:140

150. Rovlias A, Kotsou S. The influence of hyperglycemia on neurological outcome in patients with severe head injury. *Neurosurgery.* 2000;46:335.

151. Battistella FD, Wisner DH. Combined hemorrhagic shock and head injury: effects of hypertonic saline (7.5%) resuscitation. *J Trauma.* 1991;31:182.

152. Prough DS, Whitley JM, Taylor CL, et al. Regional cerebral blood flow following resuscitation from hemorrhagic shock with hypertonic saline. *Anesthesiology.* 1991;75:319.

153. Schmoker JD, Zhuang J, Shackford SR. Hypertonic fluid resuscitation improves cerebral oxygen delivery and reduces intracranial pressure after hemorrhagic shock. *J Trauma.* 1991;31:1607.

154. Freshman SP, Battistella FD, Matteucci M, et al. Hypertonic saline (7.5%) versus mannitol: a comparison for treatment of acute head injuries. *J Trauma.* 1993;35:344.

155. Gemma M, Cozzi S, Tommasino C, et al. 7.5% Hypertonic saline versus 20% mannitol during elective neurosurgical supratentorial procedures. *J Neurosurg Anesthesiol.* 1997;9:329.

156. Bullock MR, Lyeth BG, Muizelaar JP. Current status of neuroprotection trials for traumatic brain injury: lessons from animal models and clinical studies. *Neurosurgery.* 1999;45:207.

157. Karibe H, Chen J, Zarow GJ, et al. Delayed induction of mild hypothermia to reduce infarct volume after temporary middle cerebral artery occlusion in rats. *J Neurosurg.* 1994;80:112.

158. Karibe H, Zarow GJ, Weinstein PR. Use of mild intraischemic hypothermia versus mannitol to reduce infarct size after temporary middle cerebral artery occlusion in rats. *J Neurosurg.* 1995; 83:93–98.

159. Schwab S, Schwarz S, Spranger M, et al. Moderate hypothermia in the treatment of patients with severe middle cerebral artery infarction. *Stroke.* 1998;29:2461.

160. Tateishi A, Soejima Y, Taira Y, et al. Feasibility of the titration method of mild hypothermia in severely head-injured patients with intracranial hypertension. *Neurosurgery.* 1998;42:1065.

161. Marion DW, Penrod LE, Kelsey SF, et al. Treatment of traumatic brain injury with moderate hypothermia. *N Engl J Med.* 1997;336:540.

162. Donato T, Shapira Y, Artru A, et al. Effect of mannitol on cerebrospinal fluid dynamics and brain tissue edema. *Anesth Analg.* 1994;78:58.

163. Pollay M, Fullenwider C, Roberts PA, et al. Effect of mannitol and furosemide on blood-brain osmotic gradient and intracranial pressure. *J Neurosurg.* 1983;59:945.

164. Lobato RD, Sarabia, Cordobes C, et al. Post traumatic cerebral hemispheric swelling: analysis of 55 cases studied with computerized tomography. *J Neurosurg.* 1988;68:417.

165. Nordstrom CH, Messeter K, Sundbarg G, et al. Cerebral blood flow, vasoreactivity, and oxygen consumption during barbiturate therapy in severe traumatic brain lesions. *J Neurosurg.* 1988;68:424.

166. Marshall LF, Smith RW, Shapiro HM. The outcome with aggressive treatment in severe head injuries. *J Neurosurg.* 1979;50:260.

167. Hamm RJ, Jenkins LW, Lyeth BG, et al. The effect of age on outcome following traumatic brain injury in rats. *J Neurosurg.* 1991;75:914.

168. Cruz J. On-line monitoring of global cerebral hypoxia in acute brain injury. *J Neurosurg.* 1993;79:228.

169. Sheinberg M, Kantner MJ, Robertson CS, et al. Continuous monitoring of jugular venous oxygen saturation in head-injured patients. *J Neurosurg.* 1992;76:212.

170. Sioutos PJ, Orozco JA, Carter LP, et al. Continuous regional cerebral cortical blood flow monitoring in head-injured patients. *Neurosurgery.* 1995;36:943.

171. Choi SC, Barnes TY, Bullock R, et al. Temporal profile of outcomes in severe head injury. *J Neurosurg.* 1994;81:169.

172. Levin HS, Gary HE, Eisenberg HM, et al. Neurobehavioral outcome 1 year after severe head injury: experience of the Traumatic Coma Data Bank. *J Neurosurg.* 1990;73:699.

# Hypoxemia

Roy D. Cane
Scott Bullard

*Hypoxemia* is defined as a relative deficiency of oxygen ($O_2$) in the arterial blood. In clinical practice, arterial $O_2$ is quantified by measurement of the partial pressure exerted by the $O_2$ dissolved in plasma ($PaO_2$) or by the relative $O_2$ saturation of hemoglobin present in the blood as measured by pulse oximetry ($SpO_2$). In terms of these measurements, the classic definition of hypoxemia is a $PaO_2$ of <80 mm Hg or an $SpO_2$ of <95% when a patient breathes room air. Because the content of $O_2$ is minimally changed by increases in oxyhemoglobin ($HbO_2$) saturation above 90%, many clinicians consider hypoxemia as a $PaO_2$ of <60 mm Hg or an $SpO_2$ of <90%.

## HYPOXEMIA, ARTERIAL OXYHEMOGLOBIN SATURATION, AND OXYGEN CONTENT

Most blood $O_2$ is in combination with hemoglobin. The affinity of hemoglobin for $O_2$ varies with the degree of oxygenation of the hemoglobin molecule. Thus, the relationship between the partial pressure of $O_2$ ($PO_2$) and $HbO_2$ saturation ($SaO_2$) is not linear. Figure 45–1 illustrates the relationship between $PO_2$ and $SaO_2$.

### What Factors Control the Affinity of Oxygen for Hemoglobin?

The affinity of hemoglobin for $O_2$ is increased (leftward shift of the $HbO_2$ dissociation curve) by reductions in temperature, partial pressure of carbon dioxide ($PCO_2$, hydrogen ion concentration (alkalemia), and red blood cell concentration of 2,3-diphosphoglycerate (2,3-DPG); increases in these factors decrease the $HbO_2$ affinity (rightward shift of the $HbO_2$ dissoci-

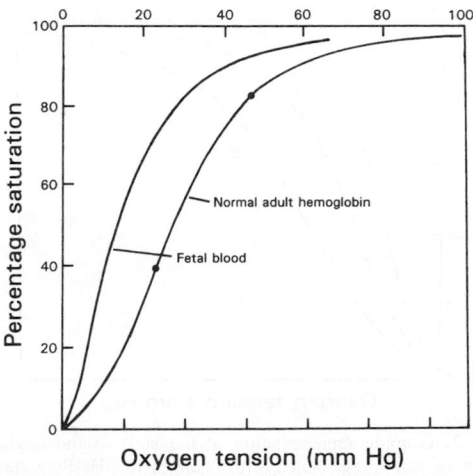

**FIGURE 45–1.** Graphic depiction of the relationship between $PaO_2$ and oxyhemoglobin saturation for adult and fetal hemoglobin.

ation curve) (Fig. 45–2). These alterations in hemoglobin-$O_2$ affinity have the potential to impair tissue $O_2$ availability significantly under conditions of acute severe acidemia or hypercarbia.

## How Do $PaO_2$ and $SpO_2$ Correlate?

Pulse oximetry measures the $SpO_2$ in vivo and is an indirect reflection of the $PaO_2$. Note that the magnitude of change in $SpO_2$ secondary to changes in $PaO_2$ is greater at $PaO_2$ levels of <60 mm Hg ($SpO_2$ <90%) and decreases with increasing $PaO_2$ levels >60 mm Hg. Thus, pulse oximetry is a sensitive monitor of arterial oxygenation in critical $PaO_2$ levels of <60 mm Hg but is a relatively insensitive monitor at higher and supranormal $PaO_2$ levels.

## How Do $PaO_2$ and Arterial Blood Oxygen Content Correlate?

The actual volume content of $O_2$ in the arterial blood ($CaO_2$) is the sum of the amount of $O_2$ in combination with hemoglobin and the amount dissolved in the plasma. The $O_2$ content of an arterial blood sample (mL/dL) can be calculated as follows:

$$CaO_2 = Hb \times 1.34 \times SaO_2 + PaO_2 \times 0.003$$

(Equation 1)

Assuming a $PaO_2$ of 100 mm Hg and a hemoglobin concentration of 15 g/100 mL, the $CaO_2$ is about 20.3 mL/dL, 20 mL of which is in combination with hemoglobin and 0.3 mL of which is in solution in the plasma. Because of the nonlinear relationship between $PaO_2$ and $SaO_2$, increasing $PaO_2$ >60 mm Hg ($SpO_2$ >90%) results in small increases in $CaO_2$. Figure 45–3 shows the relative amounts of dissolved $O_2$ and $HbO_2$ relative to $PaO_2$ and $SaO_2$.

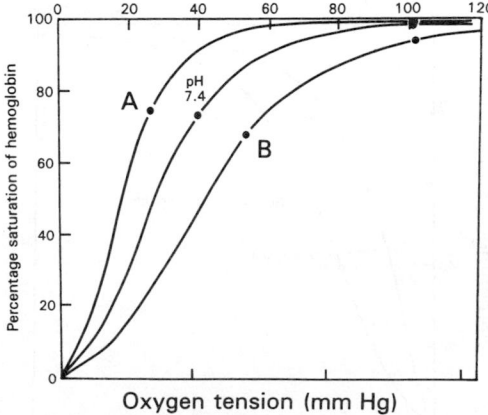

**FIGURE 45–2.** Graphic representation of the shift in the oxyhemoglobin ($HbO_2$) saturation curve associated with changes in pH, $PCO_2$, temperature, and 2,3-diphosphoglycerate (2,3-DPG). The *center curve* is the normal curve under standard conditions; the other two curves show the leftward displacement (*curve A*) caused by a decrease and the rightward shift (*curve B*) caused by an increase in hydrogen ion concentration, temperature, $PCO_2$, and 2,3-DPG concentration.

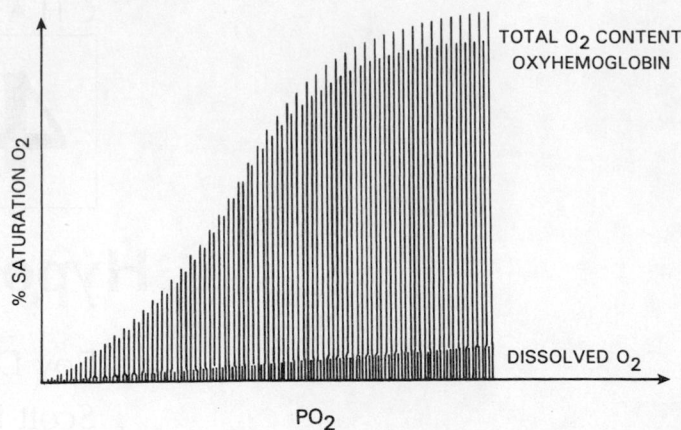

**FIGURE 45–3.** Graphic depiction of the contributions of the dissolved oxygen ($O_2$) and the oxyhemoglobin content to the total $O_2$ content of blood at different oxyhemoglobin saturations and $PO_2$. (From Shapiro BA, Harrison RA, Cane RD, et al. Arterial oxygenation. In: *Clinical Application of Blood Gases.* 4th ed. Chicago, Ill: Year Book Medical; 1989:66.)

## Dyshemoglobinemias

Pathologic forms of hemoglobin (eg, carboxyhemoglobin, methemoglobin) that are unable to combine reversibly with $O_2$ reduce the $CaO_2$ even when the $PaO_2$ is normal. Calculation of $CaO_2$ should be based on direct measurement of the $SaO_2$ by co-oximetry rather than obtained from values derived from nomograms if any form of abnormal hemoglobin is suspected.

## What Are the Causes of Hypoxemia?

Six factors have been identified: low fraction of inspired oxygen ($FIO_2$); hypoventilation; decreased barometric pressure (high altitude); ventilation-perfusion ($\dot{V}/\dot{Q}$) mismatch (worsened by decreased mixed venous oxygen saturation [$SO_2$], which is affected by anemia, decreased cardiac output, and increased oxygen consumption); left-to-right shunt; and diffusion defect.

$O_2$ moves from the alveolar gas to the plasma by diffusion down a partial pressure gradient. When $O_2$ dissolves in the plasma, it is almost immediately taken up by combination with hemoglobin. $O_2$ continues to move from alveolar gas to pulmonary capillary blood until the partial pressure gradient no longer exists. At this equilibrium point, the hemoglobin is maximally saturated for that $PO_2$.

Development of adequate $PO_2$ in the pulmonary capillary blood is dependent on maintenance of an adequate alveolar $O_2$ partial pressure ($PAO_2$); given that the $PO_2$ at the end of a pulmonary capillary should be equal to the $PAO_2$, inadequate oxygenation of the pulmonary capillary blood occurs if the $PAO_2$ is <80 mm Hg.

Appropriate matching of alveolar ventilation ($\dot{V}A$) and perfusion ($\dot{Q}$) is also essential for adequate gas exchange. Hypoxemia commonly develops because of pulmonary abnormalities that impair $\dot{V}A$ or $\dot{Q}$.

### Pulmonary Mechanisms

Alveolar gas is a mixture of $O_2$, nitrogen ($N_2$), water vapor, carbon dioxide ($CO_2$), and various trace inert gases. The partial pressure of the individual gases in a mixture of gases contained in a closed space is equal to the total pressure within that space. The total pressure of gas in an alveolus is equal to barometric pressure (PB).

## Ventilation

The $PaO_2$ is determined by $\dot{V}A$, the $FIO_2$, and alveolar $O_2$ uptake. Ideal alveolar gas cannot be sampled; however, the ideal $PaO_2$ may be calculated as follows:

$$PaO_2 = PB \times (FIO_2 - [O_2 \text{ Uptake}/\dot{V}A]) \qquad \text{(Equation 2)}$$

The alveolar $CO_2$ partial pressure ($PaCO_2$) is determined by the level of $\dot{V}A$ (see Chapter 46). Assuming that the $PaCO_2$ is equal to the $PaCO_2$ and that the $O_2$ in the inspired gas is exchanged for the $CO_2$ in exhaled gas, the $PaO_2$ can be approximated by the following equation:

$$PaO_2 = \text{Inspired } PO_2 - PaCO_2 \qquad \text{(Equation 3)}$$

Application of correction factors to compensate for the fact that $CO_2$ production is less than $O_2$ consumption (reflected by the respiratory quotient [RQ]) produces the following clinically practical relationship:

$$PaO_2 = \text{Inspired } PO_2 - (PaCO_2/RQ) \qquad \text{(Equation 4)}$$

Note that although equation 4 does not account for the difference between inspired and expired gas volumes, it allows bedside calculations of the ideal $PaO_2$. The inspired $PO_2$ is equal to the PB minus the partial pressure of $N_2$ and water vapor (47 mm Hg); that is, $PIO_2 = (PB - PH_2O) \times FIO_2$. A clinically useful form of the equation follows:

$$PaO_2 = [(PB - 47) \times FIO_2] - [PaCO_2/0.8] \qquad \text{(Equation 5)}$$

Thus, lower PB (high altitude) or $FIO_2$, and higher $PaCO_2$ (hypoventilation) result in reduced $PaO_2$. Figure 45–4 graphically represents the relationship between $PaO_2$, $FIO_2$, and $\dot{V}A$. What is the acute physiologic response to altitude-associated hypoxemia, and how does it enhance $PaO_2$? Hyperventilation decreases $PaCO_2$ (and $PaCO_2$), which increases the fraction of oxygen within the alveolus.

> **Example:** At the top of Pike's Peak at an altitude of roughly 14 000 feet, PB = 450 mm Hg, and $PaO_2 = (450 - 47) \times 0.21 - (40/0.8) = 37$ mm Hg, without hyperventilation. Increasing ventilation and reducing $PaCO_2$ by half would result in a $PaO_2$ of 60 mm Hg.

## Ventilation-Perfusion Mismatching

For any given level of $\dot{V}A$, the distribution of ventilation relative to the distribution of pulmonary perfusion determines the effective gas exchange, which thus has a role in determining the $PaO_2$.

A normal pulmonary gas exchange unit consists of an alveolus and an associated pulmonary capillary. Normal gas exchange between blood and alveolar gas depends on matching of relatively equal $\dot{V}A$ and $\dot{Q}$ (ie, a $\dot{V}A/\dot{Q}$ ratio of $\approx$1). Figure 45–5 depicts the spectrum of alveolar ventilation and pulmonary perfusion relationships.

**Dead Space Ventilation.** Ventilation in excess of $\dot{Q}$ results

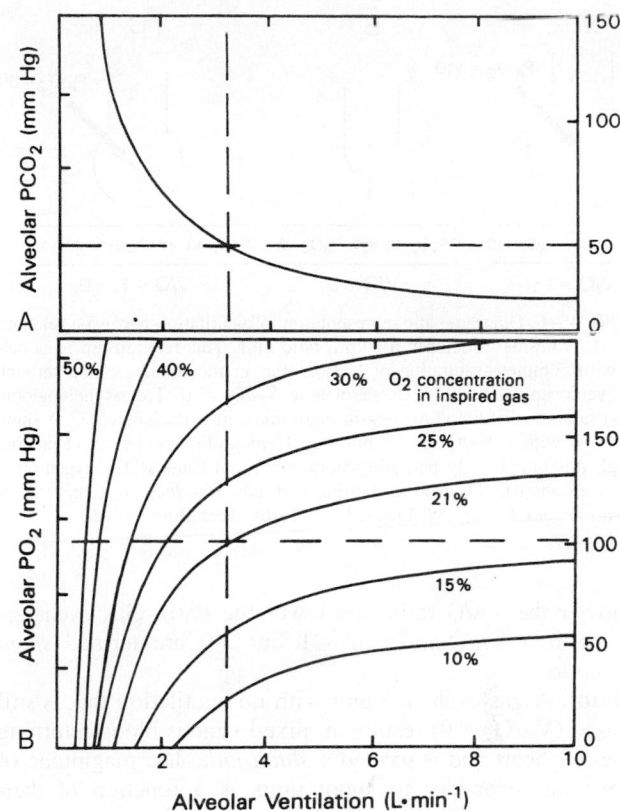

**FIGURE 45–4.** Alveolar gas tensions produced by different levels of alveolar ventilation. *A,* The hyperbolic relationship between alveolar $PaCO_2$ and $\dot{V}A$. *B,* The relationship between the partial pressure of oxygen in the alveoli ($PaO_2$) and $\dot{V}A$ for different levels of oxygen concentration in the inspired gas. The *broken vertical line* indicates a $\dot{V}A$ of 3.2 L/min. Dry barometric pressure = 713 mm Hg; $CO_2$ output = 180 mL/min (BTPS); oxygen uptake = 225 mL/min (BTPS). No allowance has been made for the difference between inspired and expired minute volumes. BTPS, body temperature and ambient pressure saturated with water vapor; $\dot{V}A$, alveolar ventilation. (From Nunn JF. Pulmonary ventilation. In: Nunn JF, ed. *Applied Respiratory Physiology.* 3rd ed. London, United Kingdom: Butterworth-Heinemann; 1987:111.)

in increased dead space ventilation ($\dot{V}DS$) and primarily impairs $CO_2$ excretion (see Chapter 46).

**Shunt Effect.** Diminished $\dot{V}A$ relative to $\dot{Q}$ results in a reduced $PaO_2$ and, hence, a reduced $PO_2$ in the pulmonary capillaries. Figure 45–6 demonstrates the incomplete oxygenation of pulmonary capillary blood in regions of lung with $\dot{V}A/\dot{Q}$ of <1 but >0, and zero.

When the partial pressure of pulmonary capillary blood $O_2$ ($Pc'O_2$) is reduced, a lower $O_2$ content ($Cc'O_2$) results. This change, in turn, reduces the $CaO_2$ in left heart blood and results in hypoxemia. The magnitude of hypoxemia is a function of the amount and degree of lung with reduced $\dot{V}A/\dot{Q}$ matching;

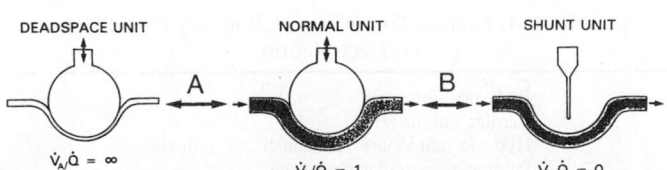

**FIGURE 45–5.** Ventilation-perfusion relationships. *A,* The spectrum of ventilation in excess of perfusion. *B,* The spectrum of perfusion in excess of ventilation. The true dead space unit is represented by $\dot{V}A/\dot{Q} = \alpha$; the normal unit is represented by $\dot{V}A/\dot{Q} = 1$; the shunt unit is represented by $\dot{V}A/\dot{Q} = 0$.

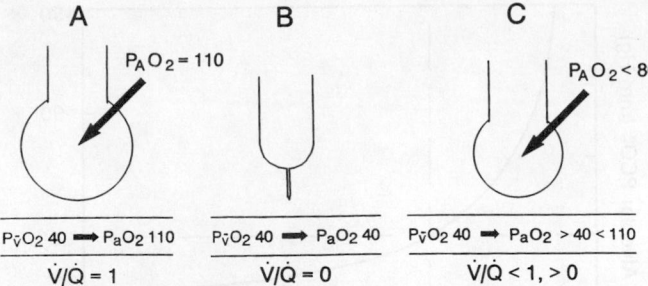

**FIGURE 45–6.** Diagrammatic representation of ventilation-perfusion relationships. *A*, A normal relationship with a ratio of 1. This relationship is associated with complete saturation of hemoglobin in the blood passing through this alveolocapillary unit. *B*, A shunt unit, $\dot{V}_A/\dot{Q} = 0$. The oxyhemoglobin ($HbO_2$) saturation of blood passing through this unit is unchanged. *C*, A shunt effect unit with a $\dot{V}_A/\dot{Q}$ of <1 but >0. Hemoglobin in the blood passing through this unit is only partially saturated. (From Cane RD. Oxygen challenge. In: Cane RD, Davison R, Albrink MH, eds. *Handbook of Critical Care Procedures and Therapy.* St Louis, Mo: Mosby–Year Book; 1992.)

the lower the $\dot{V}_A/\dot{Q}$ ratio, the lower the $P_{AO_2}$. Gas exchange units with a $\dot{V}_A/\dot{Q}$ ratio of <1 but >0 are termed *shunt effect units.*

**Shunt.** A gas exchange unit with no ventilation that is still perfused ($\dot{V}_A/\dot{Q} = 0$) results in mixed venous blood returning to the left heart and is termed a *shunt unit.* The magnitude of hypoxemia secondary to shunt units is a function of their number and the $O_2$ content of the shunted mixed venous blood.

### Cardiopulmonary Pathology

Cardiopulmonary pathology results in various degrees of $\dot{V}_A/\dot{Q}$ mismatching. The magnitude of hypoxemia depends on the relative ratio of shunt to shunt effect units and the amount of lung tissue with abnormal $\dot{V}_A/\dot{Q}$ relationships. Factors that affect the distribution of pulmonary blood flow and ventilation are summarized in Table 45–1. Maldistribution of ventilation secondary to regional differences in airway resistance and lung compliance associated with pulmonary disease is the most common cause of mismatch.

### Diffusion Block

Oxygen moves from alveolar gas to capillary blood by a process of diffusion. The rate of diffusion is determined by the factors listed in Table 45–2. Whether a diffusion block is a cause of hypoxemia is controversial. However, a $\dot{V}_A/\dot{Q}$ mismatch can result in reduction of $P_{AO_2}$ and in the surface area across which gas diffusion occurs. Thus, impairment of

**TABLE 45–1.** Factors That Affect Pulmonary Blood Flow and Ventilation

> Body position
> Cardiac output
> Hypoxic pulmonary vasoconstrictor reflexes
> Pulmonary vascular resistance
> Alveolar ventilation
> Regional variations in airway resistance
> Regional variations in lung compliance
> Inspired oxygen concentrations

**TABLE 45–2.** Factors That Determine the Rate of Oxygen Diffusion

> The tension gradient between alveolar gas and pulmonary capillary plasma ($P_{AO_2} - Pc'_{O_2}$)
> The surface area across which gas exchange occurs
> The length of the diffusion pathway (ie, thickness of the alveolar-capillary membrane)
> The solubility of oxygen in the plasma
> The rate at which hemoglobin takes up oxygen from the plasma
> The transit time of blood in the capillary bed

diffusion may be a factor in the hypoxemia associated with $\dot{V}_A/\dot{Q}$ mismatching.

Electron microscopic studies of the alveolar-capillary membrane in pulmonary edema and fibrosis have not revealed appreciable thickening of the area of membrane across which gas exchange occurs, suggesting that lengthening of the diffusion pathway is not a clinical reality.

**Mean Transit Time.** The mean transit time of blood in the pulmonary capillary is about 0.8 seconds, although the range around the mean is great. An average transit time of 0.3 seconds is thought to be necessary to develop a maximum $Pc'_{O_2}$. Blood from capillaries with short transit times (<0.2 second) will be desaturated and may contribute to hypoxemia. Capillary transit times vary throughout the lungs, and a wide spread of transit times increases the gradient between the $P_{AO_2}$ and $Pa_{O_2}$.[1,2]

**Hemoglobin-Oxygen Uptake.** The rate at which hemoglobin takes up $O_2$ from the pulmonary capillary plasma is sufficiently slow so that at normal pulmonary capillary transit times, $HbO_2$ uptake is the rate-limiting factor for diffusion of $O_2$.

### Nonpulmonary Mechanisms

#### Changes in Cardiac Output and Oxygen Consumption

The relationship between cardiac output, $O_2$ consumption ($\dot{V}_{O_2}$), and the $O_2$ content difference between arterial and mixed venous blood, $C(a - \bar{v})_{O_2}$ may be represented by Fick's equation:

$$\text{Cardiac Output} = \dot{V}_{O_2}/C(a - \bar{v})_{O_2} \qquad \text{(Equation 6)}$$

If cardiac output remains unchanged and $\dot{V}_{O_2}$ increases or $\dot{V}_{O_2}$ remains constant but cardiac output decreases, the amount of $O_2$ extracted from the arterial blood increases. A decrease in the $C\bar{v}_{O_2}$ and an increase in $C(a - \bar{v})_{O_2}$ result. Table 45–3 shows the relationship of cardiac output to $O_2$ extraction.

Intrapulmonary shunting of mixed venous blood results in hypoxemia, the magnitude of which varies directly with the amount of shunt and inversely with the $C\bar{v}_{O_2}$. For any given intrapulmonary shunt ($\dot{Q}sp/\dot{Q}t$), a lower $C\bar{v}_{O_2}$ increases the degree of hypoxemia.

Cardiac output normally is adjusted to meet the tissue $O_2$ demand. However, in patients with limited myocardial function, this physiologic mechanism fails, and hypoxemia results in response to an increase in tissue $O_2$ demand. Primary myocardial failure (cardiogenic shock) causes hypoxemia because of the low $C\bar{v}_{O_2}$. Table 45–4 shows the relationship between cardiac output and $Pa_{O_2}$.

**TABLE 45–3.** Relationship of Cardiac Output to Oxygen Extraction

|  | Oxygen Consumption (mL/min) | Cardiac Output (L/min) | Oxygen Extraction C (a − v̄) o₂ (mL/dL) |
|---|---|---|---|
| Normal cardiac output | 250 | 5 | 5 (50) |
| Increased cardiac output | 250 | 10 | 2.5 (25) |
| Decreased cardiac output | 250 | 2.5 | 10 (100) |

### Anemia

Anemia reduces $CaO_2$. Tissue $O_2$ delivery is the product of cardiac output and $CaO_2$. Normally, a decrease in $CaO_2$ is compensated for by an increase in cardiac output, thus maintaining delivery. If cardiac output cannot be increased and $\dot{V}O_2$ remains constant, the net result is a reduction in $C\bar{v}O_2$ with the potential for hypoxemia described earlier.

Anemia is likely to be a factor in hypoxemia if limited myocardial function or an increase in $\dot{V}O_2$ exceeds a patient's ability to increase cardiac output. In patients with good myocardial function, hemoglobin concentrations as low as 7 g/100 mL are well tolerated. When myocardial failure is present, consideration should be given to maintaining $\dot{D}O_2$ by increasing the $O_2$-carrying capacity and $CaO_2$; hemoglobin concentrations of 10 to 11 g/100 mL may be necessary.

### Right-to-Left Intracardiac Shunting

Right-to-left intracardiac shunts result in mixed venous blood entering the left heart and a reduction in the $CaO_2$. The magnitude of hypoxemia that results depends on the size of the shunt and the $C\bar{v}O_2$.

## ASSESSMENT OF HYPOXEMIA

### What Are Conventional Blood Gas Measurements?

Modern blood gas analyzers incorporate electrodes that measure pH, $PCO_2$, and $PO_2$.[3] Bicarbonate concentration and base deficit are derived from nomograms based on the Henderson-Hasselbalch equation.

### pH

If two solutions of different pH are separated from each other by a pH-sensitive glass membrane, a potential difference develops across the glass membrane and can be measured as a voltage. If the pH of one solution is known, that of the second solution can be determined from the measured potential difference.

### $PCO_2$

When a $CO_2$-containing solution is separated from an aqueous bicarbonate solution by a semipermeable membrane, $CO_2$ diffuses across the membrane and undergoes the following chemical reaction:

$$CO_2 + H_2O \rightleftarrows H_2CO_3 \rightleftarrows H^+ + HCO_3^- \quad \text{(Equation 7)}$$

The hydrogen ion concentration ($H^+$) developed is proportional to the $PCO_2$ of the $CO_2$-containing solution. This principle is applied in the Severinghaus electrode.

### $PO_2$

The polarographic $PO_2$ electrode (Clark's electrode) consists of a silver anode and a platinum cathode in a potassium chloride solution. Oxidation of the anode to form silver chloride results in a flow of electrons and a measurable current.

At the cathode, $O_2$ is reduced to hydroxyl ions, a reaction that consumes electrons and, in turn, accelerates the oxidation reaction at the anode. The electrode is separated from the blood sample by a polypropylene membrane that allows slow diffusion of $O_2$ into the electrode.

The change in the current flow from cathode to anode is related to the number of electrons consumed at the cathode, which in turn is proportional to the amount of $O_2$ reduced. Thus, the $PO_2$ in the blood is proportional to the change in current measured at the anode.

## What Are the Alternatives to Conventional Analysis?

Conventional blood gas analysis has the disadvantage of being an interval monitor that requires collection of an arterial blood sample for analysis at a remote site with a significant time delay. Newer developments in blood gas monitoring allow continuous online monitoring at the patient's bedside.

### Optical Fluorescent Techniques

Pulse oximetry and transcutaneous blood gas measurements are well defined and characterized. Optical fluorescence techniques enable bedside blood gas analyzers to perform intermittent, on-demand, ex vivo arterial blood gas (ABG) measurement with response times of <2 minutes. Continuous

**TABLE 45–4.** Comparison Effect of Cardiac Output on Arterial Oxygen Partial Pressure

| $\dot{Q}sp/\dot{Q}t$ (%) | $\dot{V}O_2$ (mL/min) | $\dot{Q}$ (L/min) | C(a − v̄) o₂ (mL/dL) | Pao₂ (mm Hg) |
|---|---|---|---|---|
| 25 | 250 | 10 | 2.5 | 127 |
| 25 | 250 | 5 | 5.0 | 84 |
| 25 | 250 | 2.5 | 10.0 | 55 |
| $PAO_2$ = 335 mm Hg | $FIO_2$ = .50 | Hemoglobin = 15 g/100 mL | $Cc'O_2$ = 2.17 mL/dL | |

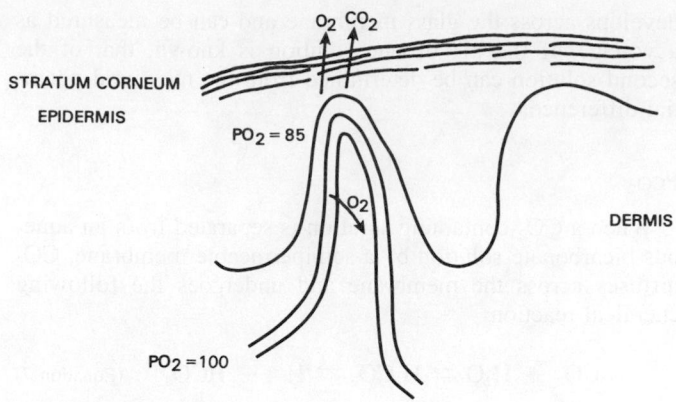

**FIGURE 45–7.** Diagrammatic representation of the countercurrent flow of $O_2$ in a capillary of a dermal papilla. The $P_{O_2}$ at the base of the capillary loop is about 100 mm Hg; as blood ascends in the capillary loop, $O_2$ diffuses across to the descending limb of the capillary loop, resulting in a $P_{O_2}$ at the tip of the loop of only about 85 mm Hg.

intraarterial monitors are technically feasible.[4] These optical fluorescence-based techniques have just become available for routine clinical application.

## Transcutaneous Gas Measurement

Transcutaneous $P_{O_2}$ ($P_{tcO_2}$) electrodes (modified Clark's electrodes) measure the flux of $O_2$ across the skin.[5] Perfusion of the dermis involves capillary loops that extend up into the epidermal papillae.

### Arterial Venous Mixing

As well-oxygenated arterial blood flows up the loop, $O_2$ diffuses out of the ascending limb of the capillary into the less well-oxygenated blood in the descending limb of the loop. Thus, the blood at the skin surface has a $P_{O_2}$ that is about 15% less than the $Pa_{O_2}$. Figure 45–7 illustrates this principle.

### Skin Perfusion

The $P_{tcO_2}$ is also dependent on skin perfusion and is a reliable reflector of $Pa_{O_2}$ only when the cardiac index is $>2$ L/min/m². Available transcutaneous monitors all use heated electrodes that raise the skin temperature to 40°C to 44°C. Blood flow rate and transcutaneous flow of $O_2$ are thereby enhanced.

Although transcutaneous monitoring of $P_{O_2}$ provides reliable trend information in patients with adequate cardiovascular function, pulse oximetry is the more widely used technique for continuous monitoring of the arterial oxygenation status.

## Oximetry

Oximetry describes various spectrophotometric techniques that determine the $HbO_2$ saturation. If blood is exposed to light of a particular wavelength and intensity, measurement of the light absorbed by the $HbO_2$ moiety is proportional to the relative amount of $HbO_2$ present. This relationship can be expressed mathematically as follows:

$$A = alc \qquad \text{(Equation 8)}$$

where A is the amount of light absorbed, a is the absorption of $HbO_2$ at a given wavelength, l is the length of the light path, and c is the concentration of $HbO_2$. Rearranging this equation gives the following mathematical relationship for absorption:

$$a = A/lc \qquad \text{(Equation 9)}$$

A calibration constant can be derived by comparison of absorption between two substances with identical absorption at a given wavelength:

$$A/lc \text{ (Standard [st])} = A/lc \text{ (Unknown[u])} \qquad \text{(Equation 10)}$$

If the light path length is held constant, the concentration of the unknown substance is determined by the following relationship:

$$C_u = A_u \times C_{st}/A_{st} \qquad \text{(Equation 11)}$$

Application of these principles to patient monitoring assumes that the measured change in absorption is a function of the different forms of hemoglobin present in the blood only. The presence of other substances with spectral activity in the light wavelengths used results in erroneous measurements. Two applications of these principles are routinely used in the clinical management of anesthetized and critically ill patients: pulse oximetry and mixed venous oximetry.

### Pulse Oximetry

**Principles of Operation.** Pulse oximeters are dual-wavelength spectrophotometers that use light-emitting diodes as a light source and photodiodes for light detection. When the light source and detector are separated by a pulsating arterial vascular bed, the degree of change in the transmitted light (light emitted minus light absorbed) is proportional to the size of the arterial pulse, the wavelengths of light, and the $HbO_2$ concentration. If the pulse is considered to be entirely due to the passage of arterial blood and the appropriate light wavelengths (660 and 940 nm) are used, the $Sp_{O_2}$ can be continuously measured.

**Accuracy.** The clinical accuracy of pulse oximeters compared with laboratory co-oximeters is excellent for $HbO_2$ saturations of $>80\%$.[6-14] At saturations of $<80\%$, agreement between the pulse oximeter and co-oximeter is diminished; however, the pulse oximeter still reliably trends the changes in $HbO_2$ saturation.

Table 45–5 shows the range of bias and precision of four different commercially available pulse oximeters. Note that the precision is best at $HbO_2$ saturations of $>95\%$ and deteriorates at lower levels.

**Applicability.** The noninvasive nature, almost universal applicability, and real time measurements of pulse oximetry, coupled with the lack of any calibration routine and sensor site preparation, have resulted in widespread use of this monitor for continuous assessment of patients' arterial oxygenation status in the operating room and intensive care unit.

**Reliability.** Pulse oximetry may be unreliable under the following circumstances.

*Spectrophotometric Limitations.* Substances other than reduced hemoglobin and $HbO_2$ with spectral activity in the light wavelengths used for pulse oximetry give spurious results.

**TABLE 45–5.** Ranges of Bias and Precision of $SpO_2$ Measured With Four Different Pulse Oximeters

| Range of $SaO_2$ | <85% | 85%–89% | 90%–95% | >95% |
|---|---|---|---|---|
| Bias | 0.02–2.41 | ±0.12–1.12 | 0.35–1.45 | −0.16–1.09 |
| Precision | ±2.7–±4.5 | ±1.97–±3.68 | ±1.55–±2.1 | ±0.98–±1.95 |

Unpublished data courtesy of David Thrush.

Methylene blue, indocyanine green, and indigo carmine have been reported to interfere.[15] Intralipid has spectral activity in the wavelengths used for co-oximetry and may interfere with pulse oximetry.[16]

Significant amounts of other hemoglobin moieties (carboxyl-hemoglobin; methemoglobin) may impair pulse oximetry. The algorithm used in most pulse oximeters contains a correction factor that compensates for fetal hemoglobin; thus, pulse oximetry can be reliably used to monitor neonates and infants.

*Severe anemia* (hemoglobin <5 g/100 mL) results in unreliable pulse oximeter readings. High levels of ambient infrared light from heating lamps used in pediatric care can interfere with pulse oximetry if the sensor is not properly shielded.[17]

***Absence of Pulsatile Flow.*** Absence of arterial pulsation, as may occur with cardiopulmonary arrest, severe hypotension, cardiopulmonary bypass, and significant hypothermia, renders pulse oximetry unreliable.[18,19] Similarly, significant venous pulsations can impair the validity of pulse oximetry readings. Clinical circumstances in which this aberration may occur include severe right ventricular failure, obstruction to venous drainage, tricuspid incompetence, markedly increased intrathoracic pressures, and placement of a pulse oximetry probe on a dependent limb.[19]

**Interference Artifact.** Motion of the digit to which the sensor is applied may be interpreted as pulsatile motion and lead to spurious readings. Electrocautery can interfere with the instrument, a problem readily overcome by having the electrocautery device on a separate alternating current circuit or running the pulse oximeter from an internal battery.[18]

## Mixed Venous Oximetry

Incorporating fiberoptic techniques in flow-directed pulmonary artery catheters enables continuous measurement of the $HbO_2$ concentration of mixed venous blood in the pulmonary artery. Mixed venous oximetry is an application of reflectance spectrophotometry, in which light of appropriate wavelengths is flashed down a fiberoptic path; the resultant reflected light from the hemoglobin passes back up the fiberoptic path. The ratio of reflected light between the different wavelengths is proportional to the mixed venous $HbO_2$ saturation ($S\bar{v}O_2$).[20]

**Calibration.** The catheter must be calibrated. Stability of the calibration is unaffected by temperature variations and by hemoglobin concentration, provided the hematocrit is >40%.[21] Calibration curves are shifted by 1% for every 0.1 change in pH.[21] Thus, calibration, either against a standard sample of known $HbO_2$ saturation before insertion[22] or against a measured $S\bar{v}O_2$ obtained from a blood sample taken after catheter placement,[20] is feasible and reliable. Technical limitations of mixed venous oximetry are listed in Table 45–6.[20,23]

Mixed venous fiberoptic oximetry correlates well with co-oximetric measurement of $S\bar{v}O_2$.[23,24] Clinically acceptable accuracy is unaffected by body temperature, hemoglobin concentration, cardiac index, and method of calibration.

**Clinical Significance.** The $S\bar{v}O_2$ is proportional to the $C\bar{v}O_2$ and thus reflects the balance between tissue oxygen delivery and $\dot{V}O_2$. Because tissue oxygenation depends on cardiac output, $CaO_2$, tissue perfusion, and tissue $\dot{V}O_2$, any change in these factors may alter the $S\bar{v}O_2$.

**Changes in Cardiac Output.** Significant decreases in $CaO_2$ secondary to reductions in $PaO_2$ or hemoglobin concentration usually result in an increase in cardiac output and no change in $S\bar{v}O_2$. If a patient's cardiovascular function is limited, a reduction in $PaO_2$ or hemoglobin concentration may result in a fall in $S\bar{v}O_2$. If hemoglobin concentration and pulmonary gas exchange remain constant, changes in $S\bar{v}O_2$ readings reflect changes in cardiac output, $\dot{V}O_2$, or both.

Table 45–7 lists average values for measurements of the oxygenation of mixed venous blood under different conditions

**TABLE 45–6.** Limitations of Mixed Venous Oximetry

Catheter breakage.
Vessel wall interference secondary to the catheter's tip lying against the vessel wall.[23] Repositioning of the catheter usually corrects this problem.
Thrombus formation over the catheter tip; appropriate continuous flushing of the catheter minimizes this problem.
Presence of other substances with spectrophotometric activity in the light wavelengths used. In vivo calibration of the catheter against a co-oximeter–measured $S\bar{v}O_2$ corrects this problem, provided the concentrations of carboxyhemoglobin and methemoglobin remain relatively constant.[20]
Hemodilution. Hematocrits between 40% and 30% result in $S\bar{v}O_2$ readings that vary by about 3%.

**TABLE 45–7.** Reference Values Relating to Pulmonary Artery Oxygenation in the Critically Ill

| Cardiovascular Status | $P\bar{v}O_2$ (mm Hg) | $S\bar{v}O_2$ (%) | $C(a - \bar{v})O_2$ (mL/dL) |
|---|---|---|---|
| Healthy resting human volunteer | 40 (37–43) | 75 (70–76) | 5.0 (4.5–6.0) |
| Critically ill, adequate cardiovascular status | 37 (35–40) | 70 (68–75) | 3.5 (2.5–4.5) |
| Critically ill, borderline cardiovascular status | 32 (30–35) | 60 (56–68) | 5.0 (4.5–6.0) |
| Critically ill, inadequate cardiovascular status | <30 | <56 | >6.0 |

**TABLE 45–8.** Relationship Between Ranges of $S\bar{v}O_2$ and Reserve of Oxygen Available to the Tissues

| $S\bar{v}O_2$ (%) | Oxygen Reserve |
| --- | --- |
| >65 | Adequate |
| 51-65 | Limited |
| 35–50 | Inadequate |
| <35 | Tissue hypoxia |

of cardiovascular function. These guidelines are rendered unreliable by anemia, hypoperfusion, acidemia, and sepsis.

**Adequacy of Tissue Perfusion.** Any change in $S\bar{v}O_2$ requires complete evaluation of the patient's cardiopulmonary function.[25] However, the ranges of $S\bar{v}O_2$ reflecting the adequacy of $O_2$ reserves if the $\dot{V}O_2$ demand increases are reliable (Table 45–8).

## When Is Physiologic Shunt Calculation of Value?

The foregoing discussion has demonstrated the interrelated aspects of cardiopulmonary function and the multiple factors that affect $PaO_2$. Evaluation of the relative contribution of cardiac and pulmonary dysfunction to hypoxemia is frequently useful in guiding management of disorders of tissue oxygenation in critically ill patients. Assessment of how well the lungs are functioning as an oxygenator is best accomplished by calculation of the $\dot{Q}sp/\dot{Q}t$.

The concept behind this calculation is best stated as a question: How much of the cardiac output would have to pass directly from the right heart to the left heart to produce this degree of hypoxemia?

## Methodology

Calculation of the $\dot{Q}sp/\dot{Q}t$ requires simultaneous arterial and mixed venous blood gas measurements. The formula for the calculation is as follows:

$$\dot{Q}sp/\dot{Q}t = Cc'O_2 - CaO_2/Cc'O_2 - C\bar{v}O_2 \quad \text{(Equation 12)}$$

The $Cc'O_2$ is calculated assuming that $Pc'O_2$ equals $PAO_2$ and the $O_2$ saturation of pulmonary capillary blood equals 100% (generally true if the $PAO_2$ is at least 150 mm Hg). If the $PAO_2$ is <150 mm Hg, correction factors can be applied to enable calculation of $Cc'O_2$.[26] Figure 45–8 illustrates the $O_2$ content relationships expressed in the $\dot{Q}sp/\dot{Q}t$ calculation.

The $\dot{Q}sp/\dot{Q}t$ incorporates both the true shunt ($\dot{V}A/\dot{Q} = 0$) and the shunt effect ($\dot{V}A/\dot{Q} >0$ but <1) contributions to hypoxemia.

## Limitations

The $\dot{Q}sp/\dot{Q}t$ originally was calculated from blood gas measurements made with a patient breathing 100% $O_2$ in an attempt to separate the relative contribution of true shunt and shunt effect. Unfortunately, breathing of $O_2$ in concentrations of >50% is associated with iatrogenic increases in shunt[27,28] (Fig. 45–9).

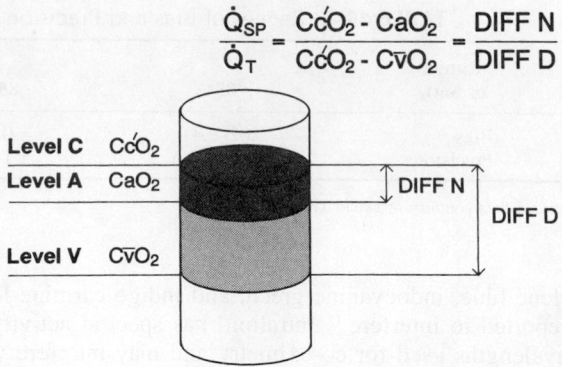

$$\frac{\dot{Q}_{SP}}{\dot{Q}_T} = \frac{Cc'O_2 - CaO_2}{Cc'O_2 - C\bar{v}O_2} = \frac{\text{DIFF N}}{\text{DIFF D}}$$

**FIGURE 45–8.** Diagrammatic representation of the oxygen content levels of end-pulmonary capillary ($Cc'O_2$), arterial ($CaO_2$), and mixed venous ($C\bar{v}O_2$) blood. The relationship of these contents to each other as expressed by the equation for calculation of the intrapulmonary shunt, $\dot{Q}sp/\dot{Q}t$, is shown. D, denominator; N, numerator. (From Shapiro BA, Harrison RA, Cane RD, et al. Applying the physiologic shunt. In: *Clinical Application of Blood Gases*. 4th ed. Chicago, Ill: Year Book Medical; 1989:152.)

## Practical Considerations

Calculation of $\dot{Q}sp/\dot{Q}t$ with a patient breathing a maintenance $FIO_2$ (other than 1.0) provides a reliable means of assessing the degree of lung dysfunction and of tracking progression of the disease and the effect of therapy. Intrapulmonary shunt fractions of <0.1 (10%) are normal; shunts of >0.19 (19%) are associated with significant pulmonary dysfunction. Shunts of >0.30 (30%) are potentially life-threatening and usually require aggressive cardiopulmonary supportive care.

## Effect of the $FIO_2$

Calculation of the $\dot{Q}sp/\dot{Q}t$ theoretically considers the $FIO_2$ and cardiac output. However, the $\dot{Q}sp/\dot{Q}t$ does vary with the $FIO_2$. Figure 45–9 reveals that increasing $FIO_2$ up to 0.4 to 0.5 corrects for the component due to shunt effect by increasing $PAO_2$ and thereby reduces the calculated total. At an $FIO_2$ of >0.5, this value increases, probably because of loss of hypoxic pulmonary vasoconstriction (HPV) or denitrogenation atelectasis.

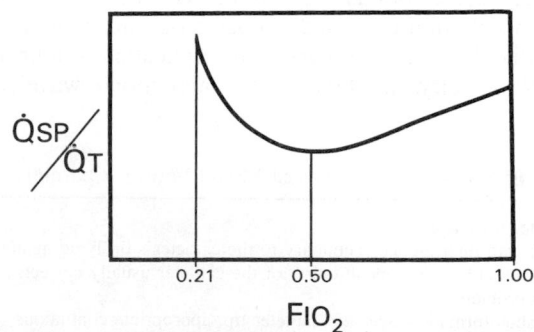

**FIGURE 45–9.** Graphic depiction of the relationship between $\dot{Q}sp/\dot{Q}t$ and the fraction of inspired oxygen ($FIO_2$). As the $FIO_2$ is increased from 0.21 (room air) toward 0.50, $\dot{Q}sp/\dot{Q}t$ decreases because the hypoxemic effect of shunt effect units ($\dot{V}A/\dot{Q}$ <1 but >0) decreases as the partial pressure of oxygen in the alveoli ($PaO_2$) increases. As the $FIO_2$ is increased from 0.50 toward 1.0, the shunt fraction increases. (From Shapiro BA, Harrison RA, Cane RD, et al. Hypoxemia and oxygen therapy. In: *Clinical Application of Blood Gases*. 4th ed. Chicago, Ill: Year Book Medical; 1989:120.)

The HPV reflexes reduce blood flow to those areas of the lungs with decreased or absent ventilation. These reflexes are initiated by a low $P_{AO_2}$ (areas of lung with low but finite $\dot{V}_A/\dot{Q}$) and low $P\bar{v}_{O_2}$ (areas of lung with $\dot{V}_A/\dot{Q} = 0$).

### Cardiovascular Changes

Intrapulmonary shunting tends to change directly with cardiac output. It usually increases with the administration of vasoactive drugs (eg, sodium nitroprusside, dopamine, dobutamine).

## What Are Oxygen Partial Pressure–Based Indices?

The major drawback to $\dot{Q}_{sp}/\dot{Q}_t$ calculation is the need to obtain a mixed venous blood sample. Several alternative means of assessing the degree of lung dysfunction based on $P_{AO_2}$ have been described.

### Estimated Shunt

The shunt equation can be mathematically manipulated to enable substitution of an assumed value for $C(a - \bar{v})_{O_2}$ as follows:

$$\dot{Q}_{sp}/\dot{Q}_t = (Cc'_{O_2} - Ca_{O_2})/$$
$$[(Cc'_{O_2} - Ca_{O_2}) + C(a - \bar{v})_{O_2}] \quad \text{(Equation 13)}$$

Most critically ill patients with good cardiovascular function have a $C(a - \bar{v})_{O_2}$ of 3.5 mL/dL.[29] Thus, the estimated shunt is calculated as follows:

$$\dot{Q}_{sp}/\dot{Q}_t \text{ (Est)} = (Cc'_{O_2} - Ca_{O_2})/$$
$$[(Cc'_{O_2} - Ca_{O_2}) + 3.5] \quad \text{(Equation 14)}$$

### Alveolar-to-Arterial Oxygen Partial Pressure Gradient

When the $Pa_{O_2}$ is $>150$ mm Hg, the $Pc_{O_2}$ must also be $>150$ mm Hg, and the arterial and pulmonary capillary $HbO_2$ is fully saturated with $O_2$. Under these circumstances, the difference between $Cc'_{O_2}$ and $Ca_{O_2}$ reflects the amounts of dissolved $O_2$. Because the $Pc_{O_2}$ is assumed to be equal to the $P_{AO_2}$, to the extent that the $Pa_{O_2}$ is less, disruption of pulmonary $O_2$ transfer is indicated.[30]

The alveolar to arterial $O_2$ partial pressure gradient, $P(A - a)_{O_2}$, is a useful index in patients who have stable cardiac function and are breathing room air. However, because this value varies directly with changes in the $F_{IO_2}$, $Sa_{O_2}$, and $S\bar{v}_{O_2}$, and because many critically ill patients have a $Pa_{O_2}$ of $<100$ mm Hg, it is frequently unreliable.[31,32]

### Arterial-to-Alveolar Oxygen Partial Pressure Ratio

The arterial to alveolar $O_2$ partial pressure ratio ($Pa_{O_2}/P_{AO_2}$) is less affected by $F_{IO_2}$ changes than is the $P(A - a)_{O_2}$[33] and is more reliable at an $F_{IO_2}$ of $<0.55$.[34] Oxygen transfer

**TABLE 45–9.** Comparison of Gas Exchange Indices

| Parameter | (Mean ± SD) | Range (Min–Max) | $r^2$ Value |
|---|---|---|---|
| $\dot{Q}_{sp}/\dot{Q}_t$ | 22.3 (11.2) | 3.0–5 | 3.0 |
| Estimated shunt | 27.6 (11.3) | 2.7–62.3 | +0.88 |
| Respiratory index | 3.1 (2.6) | 0.3–14.0 | +0.55 |
| $Pa_{O_2}/P_{AO_2}$ | 0.3 (0.2) | 0.06–0.77 | −0.52 |
| $Pa_{O_2}/F_{IO_2}$ | 1.8 (0.9) | 0.1–4.3 | −0.50 |
| $P(A - a)_{O_2}$ | 222.8 (141.7) | 32–611 | +0.38 |

abnormalities secondary to true shunts are better reflected by the $Pa_{O_2}/P_{AO_2}$ than are those secondary to shunt effect.[35]

### Arterial Oxygen Partial Pressure–to–$F_{IO_2}$ Ratio

The $Pa_{O_2}$-to–inspired $F_{IO_2}$ ratio ($Pa_{O_2}/F_{IO_2}$) varies with changes in $Pa_{CO_2}$.[36] It correlates poorly within patients with burns and respiratory tract disease and in critically ill children.[37–39]

### Respiratory Index

The respiratory index is a modification of the $P(A - a)_{O_2}$ gradient. It is intended to improve accuracy in the presence of $F_{IO_2}$ changes and is calculated by dividing the $P(A-a)_{O_2}$ by the $Pa_{O_2}$.[40]

Table 45–9 shows the correlations between $\dot{Q}_{sp}/\dot{Q}_t$ and the previously described $P_{O_2}$-based indices in a large heterogeneous group of critically ill patients.[41] Only the estimated shunt correlates acceptably with $\dot{Q}_{sp}/\dot{Q}_t$.

## What Is Dual Oximetry?

Simultaneous pulse and mixed venous oximetric monitoring (dual oximetry) includes changes in $Pa_{O_2}$ as measured by pulse oximetry, thus allowing greater discrimination of the underlying reason for changes in $S\bar{v}_{O_2}$. Furthermore, dual oximetry enables continuous real-time measurements of $O_2$ extraction and a $\dot{V}/\dot{Q}$ index.

### Oxygen Extraction Index

Oxygen extraction from arterial blood is reflected by the $C(a - \bar{v})_{O_2}$. If the small amount of $O_2$ dissolved in the plasma ($P_{O_2} \times 0.003$) is ignored, the $C(a - \bar{v})_{O_2}$ can be expressed as $Sa_{O_2}$ minus $S\bar{v}_{O_2}$ or by substituting $Sp_{O_2}$ for $Sa_{O_2}$: $Sp_{O_2}$ minus $S\bar{v}_{O_2}$. Dividing this value by the $Sp_{O_2}$ gives the $O_2$ extraction index ($O_2EI$):

$$O_2EI = (Sp_{O_2} - S\bar{v}_{O_2})/Sp_{O_2} \quad \text{(Equation 15)}$$

Because the $Sp_{O_2}$ is a reliable reflection of $Sa_{O_2}$ at values of $>90\%$, it is not surprising that the $O_2EI$ correlates well with total body $O_2$ use.[42]

What value of the $O_2EI$ is normal? What is worrisome? Normal oxygen extraction generates values of 0.25 to 0.3. At values of 0.5 to 0.6, maximum extraction for the average human being is occurring. Beyond this level, oxygen supply does not meet demand, and anaerobic metabolism with resultant lactic acidosis ensues. Consequently, maneuvers designed to increase the $S\bar{v}_{O_2}$ are typically undertaken, such as the enhancement of arterial saturation, transfusion, or augmentation of cardiac output, resulting in increased oxygen delivery.

### Ventilation-Perfusion Index

If the dissolved $O_2$ in the plasma is ignored and the hemoglobin concentration, common to all parts of the equation, is deleted, the calculation of $\dot{Q}sp/\dot{Q}t$ can be rendered in terms of $Sao_2$ and $S\bar{v}o_2$:

$$\dot{Q}sp/\dot{Q}t = (Sc'o_2 - Sao_2)/(Sc'o_2 - S\bar{v}o_2) \quad \text{(Equation 16)}$$

Assuming complete saturation of pulmonary capillary blood (reasonable assumption at $Fio_2$ of 0.3 or greater) and substituting $Spo_2$ for $Sao_2$, the equation becomes the following:

$$\dot{Q}sp/\dot{Q}t = (1 - Spo_2)/(1 - S\bar{v}o_2) \quad \text{(Equation 17)}$$

This form of the equation has been termed the shunt index (VQI).[43]

Close correlations between $\dot{Q}sp/\dot{Q}t$ and VQI have been reported in a large heterogeneous group of critically ill patients.[43,44] The continuous real-time nature of the VQI enables more rapid, cost-effective titration of positive end-expiratory pressure (PEEP) therapy than does serial calculation of $\dot{Q}sp/\dot{Q}t$.[45]

## Why Is Hypoxemia a Problem?

Hypoxemia potentially affects normal physiologic processes by increasing cardiopulmonary work and impairing the maintenance of tissue oxygenation. Hypoxemia stimulates the peripheral chemoreceptors of the carotid bodies, resulting in increased ventilation. An increase in ventilation may increase the $Pao_2$, thereby correcting or improving the $Pao_2$. This compensatory mechanism is inefficient, however, because it only improves hypoxemia that is secondary to a reduced $Pao_2$ ($\dot{V}a/\dot{Q} <1, >0$). Furthermore, the increase in $\dot{V}o_2$ by the increased ventilatory muscle work may exceed the additional $O_2$ uptake by the arterial blood. The cardiac response to hypoxemia and reduced $Cao_2$ is an increase in temperature.

### Tissue Oxygenation

Tissue oxygenation depends on the delivery of an amount of $O_2$ sufficient to meet the tissue $O_2$ demands. Hypoxemia results in a reduced $Cao_2$, which can lead to reduced tissue oxygenation. The usual physiologic response to a reduced $Cao_2$ is an increase in cardiac output and maintenance of oxygenation. If the patient is unable to increase cardiac output sufficiently to compensate for the reduced $Cao_2$, inadequate $O_2$ delivery leads to tissue hypoxia.

Figure 45–10 illustrates the changes in $O_2$ content of pulmonary capillary, arterial, and mixed venous blood consequent to changes of cardiac output and $Fio_2$.

## How Is Hypoxemia Corrected?

### Increasing the $Fio_2$

Breathing of gas mixtures with an increased $Fio_2$ may correct hypoxemia and reduce the work of breathing required to maintain a given $Pao_2$. The myocardial work necessary to maintain a given $Pao_2$ may also be decreased.

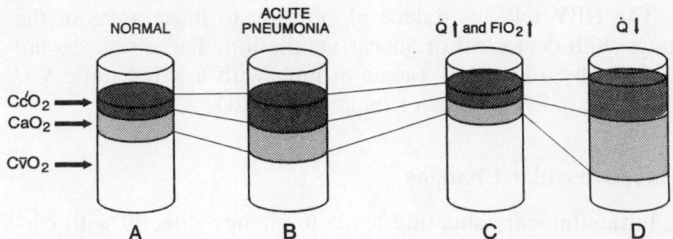

**FIGURE 45–10.** *A and B,* Diagrammatic representation of the relative changes in $O_2$ contents from normal (*A*) with the development of pneumonia (*B*). *C,* The changes in $O_2$ content secondary to the physiologic response of an increase in CO and provision of $O_2$ therapy. *D,* What would happen if the CO were to fall. Note that although the $Cc'o_2$ in *D* remains unchanged because of the $O_2$ therapy, the $Cao_2$ falls as the CO declines. (From Shapiro BA, Harrison RA, Cane RD, et al. Applying the physiologic shunt. In: *Clinical Application of Blood Gases.* 4th ed. Chicago, Ill: Year Book Medical; 1989:154.)

### Change in the Shunt Effect

Figure 45–11 illustrates the effect of breathing 100% $O_2$ on the hypoxemia associated with shunt effect. Alveolus A represents a shunt effect unit ($\dot{V}a/\dot{Q} <1$ but $>0$), whereas alveolus B is normal ($\dot{V}a/\dot{Q} = 1$). Denitrogenation associated with breathing 100% $O_2$ increases $Pao_2$ in the underventilated alveolus to a level sufficient to ensure complete $HbO_2$ saturation; thus, hypoxemia is corrected.

The $Fio_2$ needed to elevate $Pao_2$ enough to saturate the hemoglobin to $>80$ mm Hg depends on the magnitude of $\dot{V}a/\dot{Q}$ discrepancy; the lower the $\dot{V}a/\dot{Q}$, the higher the required $Fio_2$. For practical purposes, hypoxemia secondary to shunt effect is responsive to $O_2$ therapy and is usually corrected with an $Fio_2$ up to 0.5.

### Effect on True Shunt

Hypoxemia caused by true shunt ($\dot{V}a/\dot{Q} = 0$) is barely responsive to an increased $Fio_2$. Blood passing through shunt units is *not* exposed to alveolar gas; therefore, it is unaffected by an increase in $Fio_2$. The $Pao_2$ in undiseased lung areas usually is $>80$ mm Hg, even with breathing room air; therefore, little additional $O_2$ can be added to the exposed blood by an increase in $Pao_2$. Overall, then, shunt-induced hypoxemia is refractory to $O_2$ therapy. The possibility that a refractory hypoxemia is present should be considered when the $Pao_2$ is $<55$ mm Hg and the $Fio_2$ is $>0.35$.

### Oxygen Challenge

Most hypoxemia results from combinations of shunt and shunt effect mechanisms. Because an $Fio_2$ of $>0.5$ is potentially harmful, identification of hypoxemic states that are relatively refractory to $O_2$ therapy is important. The $O_2$ challenge is a useful clinical technique that helps to differentiate between those patients with refractory hypoxemia (predominantly caused by shunt) and those with hypoxemia that is responsive to $O_2$ therapy (predominantly caused by shunt effect).

To perform an $O_2$ challenge, obtain baseline ABG values, then increase the $Fio_2$ by 0.2; repeat the ABG measurements after about 30 minutes. If the $Pao_2$ has increased by $>10$ mm Hg from baseline, the patient has responsive hypoxemia; if the change in $Pao_2$ is $<10$ mm Hg, the hypoxemia is refractory.

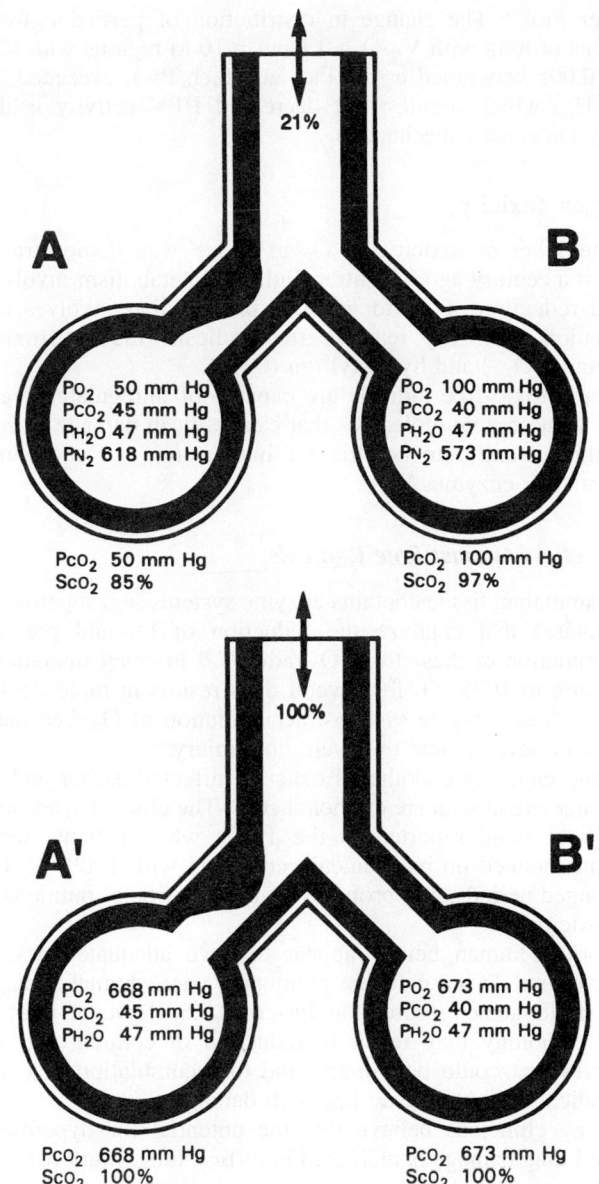

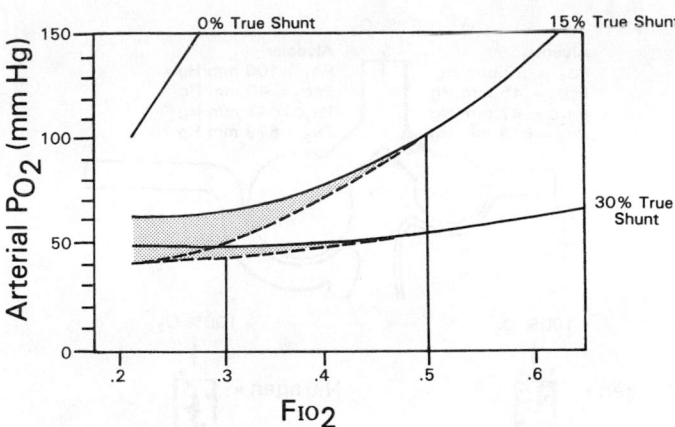

**FIGURE 45–12.** Representation of two patients with a PaO$_2$ of 40 mm Hg while breathing room air. Patient A's hypoxemia is due to a 0.30 shunt with a small additional component of shunt effect. Patient B's hypoxemia is due to a shunt of 0.15 with a large additional component of shunt effect. The *broken lines* represent the PaO$_2$ and fraction of inspired oxygen (FIO$_2$) relationships from both the shunt and shunt effect, whereas the *solid lines* represent the PaO$_2$ and FIO$_2$ relationships from the shunt alone. The O$_2$ challenge (increasing FIO$_2$ from 0.3-0.5) results in an increase in PaO$_2$ of <10 mm Hg for patient A (refractory hypoxemia) and of >10 mm Hg for patient B (responsive hypoxemia).

**FIGURE 45–11.** Alveoli A and A′ represent diminished ventilation with normal perfusion; alveoli B and B′ represent normal ventilation and perfusion. After 15 minutes of breathing 100% O$_2$, the lung is denitrogenated (A′ and B′). Note that any meaningful PaO$_2$ difference is ablated after denitrogenation. (From Shapiro BA, Harrison RA, Cane RD, et al. Hypoxemia and oxygen therapy. In: *Clinical Application of Blood Gases*. 4th ed. Chicago, Ill: Year Book Medical; 1989:113.)

Figure 45–12 illustrates the O$_2$ challenge. Patients with responsive hypoxemia can usually be managed with increases in FIO$_2$ up to 0.5, with or without low levels of positive airway pressure (+5 to +10 cm H$_2$O). Table 45–10 lists the common pathologic entities that are associated with refractory hypoxemia.

## What Are the Adverse Effects of Oxygen Therapy?

### Denitrogenation Atelectasis

Increases in PaO$_2$ secondary to increased FIO$_2$ result in a reduction of the alveolar N$_2$ partial pressure. In alveoli with reduced ventilation but good perfusion, the volume of O$_2$ removed by the blood may be greater than the volume of gas that enters with each tidal ventilation. In this circumstance, reduction of N$_2$ may allow the alveolar volume to decrease below a critical value, resulting in collapse.

Figure 45–13 illustrates the development of denitrogenation atelectasis. Patients with low but finite (V̇A/Q̇) ratios who breathe a high FIO$_2$ (>0.5) can develop this problem in as little as 15 to 30 minutes.[46,47] The higher the FIO$_2$, the greater is the degree of denitrogenation and the more likely is the development of denitrogenation atelectasis.

### Effect of Low V̇A/Q̇ Ratio

The lower the ratio, the lower the alveolar volume following significant denitrogenation and the more likely is the collapse of that alveolus. Thus, an additional factor contributing to denitrogenation atelectasis is a high FIO$_2$ that reduces HPV reflex activity. In turn, blood flow to underventilated or nonventilated regions is increased.

Recent studies have confirmed the role of inspired oxygen concentration in reducing lung volume and increasing intrapulmonary shunting. Baker and colleagues demonstrated a persistent reduction in functional residual capacity (FRC) and residual volume associated with breathing of >25% oxygen in normal volunteers with and without restriction of lung.[48] In a canine model, Cane and associates showed that breathing

**TABLE 45–10.** Common Pathologies Producing Refractory Hypoxemia

| | |
|---|---|
| Cardiovascular | Right-to-left intracardiac shunt |
| | Pulmonary arteriovenous fistula |
| Pulmonary | Consolidated pneumonitis |
| | Lobar atelectasis |
| | Large neoplasm |
| | Adult respiratory distress syndrome |

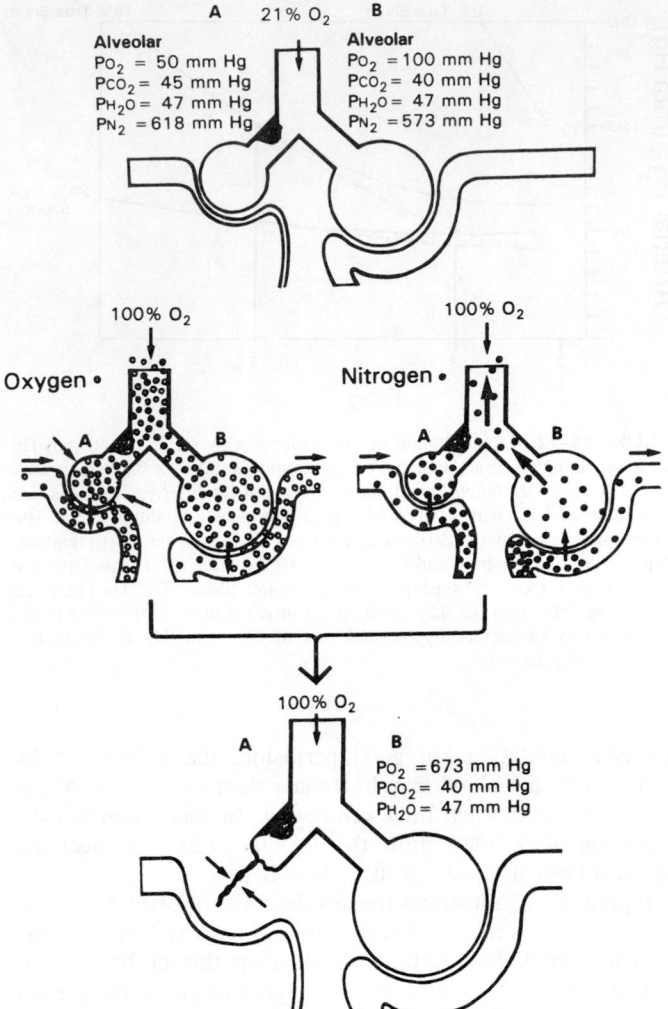

**FIGURE 45–13.** Diagrammatic representation of the mechanism of denitrogenation absorption atelectasis. Alveolus A has low relationships (minimal ventilation); alveolus B has normal relationships. The *top panel* shows the alveolar partial pressures on breathing room air. The *center panel* shows the effect of breathing 100% oxygen. The high fraction of inspired oxygen ($F_{IO_2}$) results in a loss of hypoxic pulmonary vasoconstriction (HPV), and blood flow to alveolus A increases. The increased blood flow to this poorly ventilated alveolus results in significantly increased $O_2$ extraction, which in turn results in a diminished gas volume in alveolus A. *Black circles* represent nitrogen, which is rapidly depleted from all units because the inspired nitrogen concentration is now zero. Initially, more nitrogen leaves the blood and the body through unit B because it is better ventilated. As the blood $PN_2$ level progressively decreases, however, nitrogen starts to leave alveolus A through the blood. This process results in further loss of gas volume from alveolus A because it remains poorly ventilated but well perfused. Thus, nitrogen is depleted from all units within 5 to 15 minutes. The *bottom panel* represents the final steady state in which increased $O_2$ and nitrogen extraction has caused alveolus A to collapse. Thus, a poorly ventilated, poorly perfused unit, A, becomes a nonventilated, poorly perfused unit after administration of 100% inspired oxygen. (From Shapiro BA, Harrison RA, Cane RD, et al. Hypoxemia and oxygen therapy. In: *Clinical Application of Blood Gases.* 4th ed. Chicago, Ill: Year Book Medical; 1989:121.)

35% and 50% oxygen resulted in an increase in perfusion to regions of lung with low $\dot{V}A/\dot{Q}$ (<0.1) mainly due to increased perfusion of lung with $\dot{V}A/\dot{Q}$ of <0.005.[49] This effect was greater with 50% than with 35% oxygen and was magnified by external restriction of lung to a compliance of half of baseline value. After cardiopulmonary bypass, increased perfusion to regions of lung with low $\dot{V}A/\dot{Q}$ was associated with

higher $F_{IO_2}$.[50] The change in distribution of perfusion from regions of lung with $\dot{V}A/\dot{Q}$ >0.1 but <10 to regions with $\dot{V}A/\dot{Q}$ <0.005 was noted at the $F_{IO_2}$ at which $P\bar{v}O_2$ exceeded 36 mm Hg, which implies that decreased HPV activity is the likely underlying mechanism.

## Oxygen Toxicity

The inherent toxicity of $O_2$ to tissue was demonstrated almost a century ago.[51,52] Intracellular $O_2$ metabolism involves serial reduction of $O_2$ to water, a process that involves the formation of highly reactive free radicals, the superoxide molecule ($O_2^-$) and hydroxyl ion ($OH^-$).

These toxic free radicals are capable of unregulated reactions with organic molecules that can result in damage to cell membranes and mitochondria and inactivation of cytoplasmic and nuclear enzymes.[53]

### Protection Against Free Radicals

Mammalian tissue contains enzyme systems (eg, superoxide dismutase) that catalyze the reduction of $O_2$ and prevent accumulation of these toxic $O_2$ radicals.[54] In small mammals, exposure to 100% $O_2$ for several days results in rapid depletion of these enzyme systems, accumulation of $O_2$–free radicals, and development of severe lung injury.[55]

Lung capillary endothelial cells are affected earlier and to a greater extent than are epithelial cells. The clinical syndrome ventilator lung, reported in the 1950s when patients were first maintained on mechanical ventilation with 100% $O_2$ for prolonged periods, was probably a manifestation of pulmonary $O_2$ toxicity.[56]

Normal human beings appear to have adequate enzyme reserves and do not manifest pulmonary parenchymal damage after prolonged exposure to an $F_{IO_2}$ of <0.6. However, pulmonary pathology may result in reduction of cellular enzyme reserves that could potentially lead to accumulation of toxic $O_2$ radicals and hyperoxic lung cell damage.

Many clinicians believe that the potential for hyperoxia-related lung damage is increased in diffuse lung injury (eg, the adult respiratory distress syndrome) and attempt to maintain a patient's arterial oxygenation with an $F_{IO_2}$ of <0.5. Given that responsive hypoxemia, associated with shunt effect, is usually fully corrected by increases in $F_{IO_2}$ to 0.4 to 0.5, this approach seems prudent.

### Retinopathy of Prematurity

A special case of $O_2$ toxicity is the retinopathy that develops in premature neonates when the $PaO_2$ is >100 mm Hg. $O_2$ therapy must be carefully titrated to prevent this disastrous consequence of hyperoxia.

### What $F_{IO_2}$ Should Be Used?

In emergent situations (during cardiopulmonary resuscitation), when a patient manifests acutely unstable cardiopulmonary function, or while transporting patients, administration of 100% $O_2$ is advisable. Remember that $O_2$ toxicity develops only after significant periods of exposure to a high $F_{IO_2}$ (>72-96 h).

In all other circumstances, the therapeutic efficacy of $O_2$

generally is limited to $FIO_2$ from 0.21 to 0.5 for the following reasons:

1. $O_2$-responsive hypoxemia secondary to shunt effect is usually reversed with an $FIO_2$ of 0.5 or less.
2. Denitrogenation atelectasis developing at an $FIO_2$ of $>0.5$ increases true $\dot{Q}sp/\dot{Q}t$ and results in worsening hypoxemia that is refractory to $O_2$ therapy.

Hypoxemia due to true shunting ($\dot{V}A/\dot{Q} = 0$) requires therapy to improve $\dot{V}A/\dot{Q}$ matching. Hypoxemia due to nonpulmonary causes (low cardiac output, with or without high $\dot{V}O_2$ or severe anemia) is improved by correction of the underlying pathology in conjunction with an $FIO_2$ of $<50\%$.

## How Should Oxygen Be Administered?

$O_2$ may be delivered by rebreathing or nonrebreathing systems. Modern anesthesia machines commonly use a rebreathing circle circuit in which exhaled $CO_2$ is scrubbed by soda lime. For discussion of the gas delivery circuits, see Chapter 15.

### The Postanesthesia Care Unit

$O_2$ for critically ill patients or patients in a postanesthesia care unit (PACU) is properly administered by nonrebreathing systems.

### High-Flow Systems

High-flow $O_2$ systems supply the total inspired gas (patients breathe only gas supplied by the apparatus). They provide a warmed and humidified consistent $FIO_2$, irrespective of a patient's ventilatory pattern. Adequate flows are achieved by inclusion of some form of inspiratory reservoir that supplies additional amounts of gas during the transient times when a patient's inspiratory flow demand exceeds the uniform flow delivered by the apparatus. Alternatively, an extremely high flow of gas may be provided, but this approach is wasteful

**TABLE 45–11.** Approximate Air Entrainment Ratios for Different Oxygen Concentrations

| Oxygen Concentration (%) | Air/Oxygen (L/min) |
| --- | --- |
| 24 | 25/1 |
| 28 | 10/1 |
| 34 | 5/1 |
| 40 | 3/1 |
| 60 | 1/1 |
| 70 | 0.6/1 |

and expensive. A total gas flow at least three times a patient's measured minute volume usually ensures that the peak inspiratory flow demand is met.

Many systems use air entrainment to provide a specific $FIO_2$ and gas flow. Air entrainment is achieved by constant pressure jet mixing, in which a rapid velocity of gas passing through a restricted orifice creates viscous shearing forces that entrain air into the main gas stream. The air entrainment ratio (and hence $FIO_2$) depends on orifice and entrainment port sizes. Variation in the $O_2$ flow rate through the orifice determines the total gas flow delivered by the device.

Table 45–11 lists approximate air entrainment ratios for different $O_2$ concentrations. An $FIO_2$ from 0.24 to 0.35 is most frequently provided by air entrainment devices. Higher values are best provided by systems that deliver adequately high flows of gas at known $FIO_2$ values.

Commonly used high-flow $O_2$ delivery systems include T-piece circuits, face masks with wide-bore gas delivery circuits, and air entrainment masks (often referred to as *Venturi masks*) (Fig. 45–14).

### Low-Flow Systems

Low-flow $O_2$ systems do not provide sufficient gas flow to supply the entire inspired atmosphere; thus, part of each breath is received from the room air. $FIO_2$ values from 0.21 to 0.8 can be provided by a low-flow system. The $FIO_2$ is determined by the size of the available $O_2$ reservoir (usually the nose,

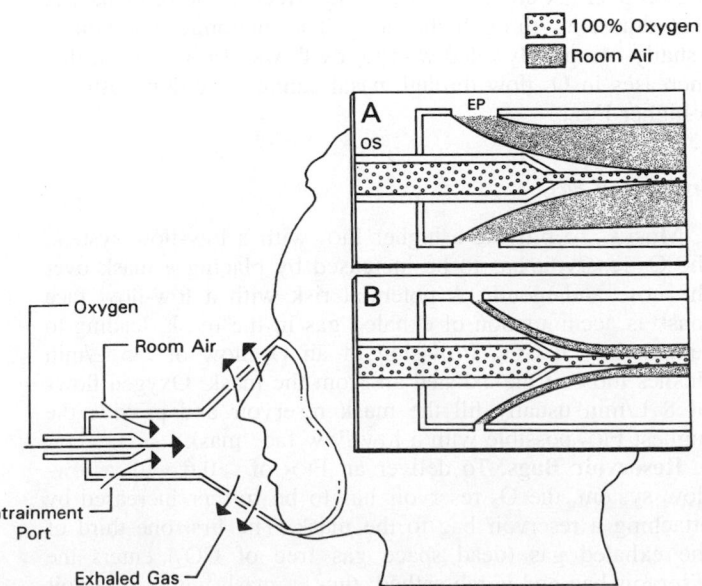

**FIGURE 45–14.** Operational principle of a Venturi mask. A high-pressure jet of $O_2$ is directed down the center of the mask. Entrained air is drawn into the mixing tube by viscous interaction with the jet flow. The percentage of $O_2$ is determined by the size of the entrainment ports controlling the flow of ambient air. In some masks, these are fixed; in others, they are variable.

**TABLE 45–12.** Approximate $F_{IO_2}$ Delivered by Different Low-Flow Oxygen Delivery Systems*

| Nasal Cannula | | Oxygen Mask | | Mask With Reservoir Bag | |
|---|---|---|---|---|---|
| $O_2$ Flow (L/min) | $F_{IO_2}$ | $O_2$ Flow (L/min) | $F_{IO_2}$ | $O_2$ Flow (L/min) | $F_{IO_2}$ |
| 1 | 0.24 | 5–6 | 0.4 | 6 | 0.6 |
| 2 | 0.28 | 6–7 | 0.5 | 7 | 0.7 |
| 3 | 0.32 | 7–8 | 0.6 | 8 | 0.8 |
| 4 | 0.36 | | | | |
| 5 | 0.4 | | | | |
| 6 | 0.44 | | | | |

*Assumes a normal ventilatory pattern.

nasopharynx, and oropharynx), the $O_2$ flow (L/min), and ventilatory pattern.

## Practical Applications

With a preset $O_2$ flow, the $F_{IO_2}$ varies inversely with minute ventilation. Larger tidal volume (VT) or faster respiratory rate decreases the $F_{IO_2}$; the smaller the VT or the slower the respiratory rate, the higher the $F_{IO_2}$. Critically ill patients frequently manifest an unstable ventilatory pattern. If delivery of a consistent $F_{IO_2}$ is deemed important, a high-flow system should be used.

## Equipment

Commonly used systems for low-flow $O_2$ delivery include nasal cannulas, simple $O_2$ masks, and $O_2$ masks with a reservoir bag. Table 45–12 shows the approximate $F_{IO_2}$ that will be achieved with commonly used low-flow $O_2$ delivery systems (provided a patient has a relatively normal ventilatory pattern).

### Anatomic Reservoir

Mouth breathing does not affect the $F_{IO_2}$ delivered by nasal cannulas, provided the nasal passages are patent. Airflow in the oropharynx creates a jet mixing effect in the nasopharynx that draws air through the nose. The anatomic reservoir is usually completely filled with $O_2$ by flows of 6 L/min; further increases in $O_2$ flow through nasal cannulas seldom result in a higher $F_{IO_2}$.

### Increased $F_{IO_2}$

**Masks.** To provide a higher $F_{IO_2}$ with a low-flow system, the $O_2$ reservoir has to be increased by placing a mask over the nose and mouth. A potential risk with a low-flow face mask is accumulation of exhaled gas in the mask, leading to rebreathing of $CO_2$. Provision of an $O_2$ flow of >5 L/min flushes most of the exhaled air from the mask. Oxygen flows of 8 L/min usually fill the mask reservoir and provide the highest $F_{IO_2}$ possible with a low-flow face mask.

**Reservoir Bags.** To deliver an $F_{IO_2}$ of >0.6 with a low-flow system, the $O_2$ reservoir has to be further increased by attaching a reservoir bag to the mask. The first one third of the exhaled gas (dead space gas free of $CO_2$) enters the reservoir bag and is rebreathed; thus, a mask with a reservoir

bag is a partial rebreathing system. For proper function, the mask should be close fitting and the flow of $O_2$ sufficient to prevent the reservoir bag from totally emptying during inspiration (>6 L/min).

## What Are the Clinical Guidelines for Oxygen Therapy?

### Patients Without Chronic Lung Disease and Hypoventilation

Provision of an $F_{IO_2}$ of 0.4 through a high-flow delivery system is a reliable starting point. The adequacy of therapy must be evaluated by patient assessment *and* measurement of arterial oxygenation status. The $F_{IO_2}$ should be adjusted to maintain a $PaO_2$ of 60 to 80 mm Hg or an $SpO_2$ of 90% to 94%. When a patient's arterial oxygenation and cardiopulmonary function have stabilized and an appropriate pattern of breathing with an $F_{IO_2}$ of <0.4 is achieved, switch to a low-flow $O_2$ delivery system can be considered. Performance of an $O_2$ challenge before initiation of therapy is strongly recommended to identify patients with predominant shunt and refractory hypoxemia.

### Patients With Chronic Lung Disease and Chronic Elevation of $PaCO_2$

Patients with chronic $CO_2$ retention represent a particular challenge with respect to $O_2$ therapy. First, they may hypoventilate in response to arterial hyperoxia. The mechanism of hyperoxia-induced hypoventilation is not understood.

Second, worsening hypoxemia is difficult to assess because these patients often have a markedly reduced $PaO_2$ (usually <60 mm Hg) when they are "well." Suspect acute hypoxemia if examination reveals acute respiratory distress in the early phase of an acute cardiopulmonary problem. ABG analysis often shows acute alveolar hyperventilation superimposed on chronic alveolar hypoventilation ($PaCO_2$ elevated, with pH > 7.40). Careful monitoring of respiratory rate, heart rate, and a patient's subjective feelings of ease or difficulty in breathing provides the best indicators of oxygenation.

Third, because the hypoxemia usually is due to shunt effect and is responsive to increases in the $F_{IO_2}$, do not perform an $O_2$ challenge. Finally, recall that the $F_{IO_2}$ of a low-flow system varies inversely with minute ventilation. Hence, transient and inadvertent hyperoxia resulting in hypoventilation leads to an increase in $F_{IO_2}$ that potentially results in further hypoventilation.

Because these patients seldom require a high $F_{IO_2}$ or high minute ventilation, air entrainment masks are reliable. Start with an $F_{IO_2}$ of 0.24 and evaluate the patient's response. Titrate the $F_{IO_2}$ in increments of 0.04 to 0.05. The desirable end point is best determined by normalization of the respiratory rate, heart rate, and pHa.

Patients usually state that their breathing feels easier when appropriate arterial oxygenation is restored. The actual value of $PaO_2$ or $SpO_2$ depends on the degree of underlying lung disease and, invariably, is <60 mm Hg or 90%, respectively. Prior knowledge of a patient's usual ABG values is of considerable benefit.

### When Is Mechanical Ventilation Indicated?

Airway pressure therapy includes the application of positive pressure to the airway during the inspiratory phase only (mechanical ventilation) or during the entire ventilatory cycle (ie, continuous positive airway pressure). Hypoxemia that is secondary to hypoventilation and acute ventilatory failure is readily corrected by mechanical ventilatory support. If the $O_2$ cost of breathing is extremely high, ventilatory support may also be beneficial. However, increased work of breathing is associated with various causes, and alternative therapeutic options can be used.[57]

### When Is Continuous Positive Airway Pressure Indicated?

Hypoxemia in anesthetized and critically ill surgical patients is most frequently associated with an acute process. Restriction of lung function and volume, particularly the FRC, results. Maintenance of airway pressure above ambient pressure increases FRC. If a patient can maintain adequate spontaneous breathing, hypoxemia secondary to $\dot{V}A/\dot{Q}$ mismatching is best treated with increase of the $FIO_2$ and continuous positive airway pressure (CPAP), not with mechanical ventilation.

### Mechanism of Action

CPAP increases the FRC by expansion of patent alveoli or reexpansion of collapsed alveoli, a process termed *alveolar recruitment*. Lower levels of CPAP ($+5$ to $+15$ cm $H_2O$) improve shunt effect. Higher levels ($>15$ cm $H_2O$) are required to recruit collapsed alveoli. Reexpansion of collapsed alveoli converts true shunt into shunt effect units, thereby changing hypoxemia from refractory to responsive.

### Benefits

Judicious use of CPAP, when it is indicated, invariably enables reduction of the $FIO_2$, minimizing the risks associated with high $FIO_2$. It provides the additional benefit of improved lung compliance that was reduced by a loss of intrathoracic gas volume. Improvement of compliance reduces the inspiratory work of breathing.

### Techniques of Administration

CPAP can be provided by face mask, nasal prongs, nasal mask, or endotracheal tube. In patients with particularly severe restrictive lung pathology (eg, adult respiratory distress syndrome), augmentation of ventilation may be required despite improved lung function secondary to CPAP therapy. Improvement in the FRC with intermittent positive pressure ventilation (IPPV) is achieved by the addition of PEEP.

### How Is Hypoxemia Prevented During Apnea?

In anesthetic practice, patients are frequently rendered apneic by the administration of neuromuscular blocking agents to facilitate tracheal intubation and surgery. Gas exchange across the alveolocapillary membrane continues, resulting in a rise in $PACO_2$ and a fall in the $PAO_2$. If the pulmonary $O_2$ reserve is augmented by increasing the $PAO_2$, arterial oxygenation can be maintained; hypercarbia and acidosis then become the limiting factors. An apneic patient with a patent airway connected to a high-flow 100% $O_2$ delivery circuit can maintain arterial oxygenation for at least 20 minutes.[58]

### Preoxygenation

Preoxygenation increases the $PAO_2$ and minimizes apnea-induced hypoxemia. Complete denitrogenation of the lungs requires breathing of 100% $O_2$ for at least 15 minutes. However, to protect against hypoxemia during intubation, 3 to 5 minutes of $O_2$ breathing is usually sufficient. Alternatively, having a patient take four maximum breaths of pure $O_2$ provides similar protection to 3 minutes of preoxygenation with normal ventilation.[59]

### Rate of Rise of Carbon Dioxide

Table 45–13 shows the approximate rate of rise of $PaCO_2$ with apnea.[60] These data suggest that up to 5 minutes of apnea can occur before acidosis becomes significant.

### Why Does Hypoxemia Occur During Anesthesia?

Several factors may contribute to the development of hypoxemia during anesthesia.

### Reduction of the Functional Residual Capacity

#### Supine Positioning

Induction of anesthesia in supine patients is associated with a reduction of about 15% to 20% in the FRC.[61] This reduction occurs within minutes of induction, irrespective of the anesthetic agents used, is not progressive, and appears to be unaffected by neuromuscular blocking drugs and a high $FIO_2$.

The supine position clearly is a factor because the FRC is unchanged by anesthesia administration to patients in the sitting position. Active expiration secondary to increased expiratory muscle tone in anesthetized patients may contribute in nonparalyzed patients. The reduction in FRC persists into the first 4 to 6 hours after emergence.

#### Diaphragmatic Tone

Loss of end-expiratory diaphragmatic tone during anesthesia results in a cephalad diaphragmatic shift.[62] The reduction

**TABLE 45–13.** Predicted $PaCO_2$–pH Relationships With Apnea

| Apnea Time (min) | $PaCO_2$ (mm Hg) | pH (Units) |
|---|---|---|
| 0 | 40 | 7.400 |
| 1 | 52 | 7.340 |
| 2 | 55.5 | 7.323 |
| 3 | 59 | 7.305 |
| 4 | 62.6 | 7.288 |
| 5 | 66 | 7.260 |
| 10 | 83.5 | 7.183 |
| 15 | 101 | 7.095 |

in FRC correlates with the observed increase in the $P(A-a)O_2$ gradient and as such probably has a role in the development of hypoxemia under anesthesia.

### Shunt Increases

A reduction in FRC may reduce the end-expiratory lung volume below the closing capacity, particularly in older patients. Premature airway closure, absorptive collapse, and shunting can result. The closing capacity equals the FRC in the supine position on average in individuals in their mid-40s; whereas, in the sitting position, this occurs at a later age, usually in the mid-60s.

Whether significant increase of $\dot{Q}sp/\dot{Q}t$ occurs under anesthesia is controversial. Atelectasis in dependent lung, associated with up to 17% shunt after only 15 minutes of halothane anesthesia, has been documented using multiple inert gas elimination technique and computed tomography scanning.[63] Patients undergoing lower abdominal surgery, remote from the diaphragm, with an inhalational agent plus muscle relaxant anesthetic, manifested a one-third reduction in FVC and a one-fifth reduction in $PaO_2$, corresponding to a mean atelectatic area of 2%. Not surprisingly, this degree of atelectasis was not readily apparent on standard chest radiograph.[64] Anesthesia-associated shunting is probably related to changes in HPV and not simply to changes in the FRC–closing capacity relationships. Unlike $\dot{V}A/\dot{Q}$ mismatch, the degree of shunt and atelectasis are considered to be age independent.[65]

### Tube Malpositioning

Esophageal and bronchial intubation lead to profound hypoxemia and a potentially lethal outcome if not detected early and corrected immediately.

### Ablation of Hypoxic Pulmonary Vasoconstriction

Inhalation but not intravenous anesthetics[66,67] depresses HPV in an isolated lung and may contribute to increased $\dot{V}/\dot{Q}$ mismatching and hypoxemia. Because HPV is modulated by the partial pressure of $O_2$ in mixed venous blood ($P\bar{v}O_2$) as well as $PaO_2$, concomitant decrements in cardiac output with reduction in $P\bar{v}O_2$ may override the effect of inhalation agents on HPV in intact animals and human beings.[68]

### Intermittent Positive Pressure Ventilation

IPPV is a common adjunct to anesthesia delivery. It is associated with increased volume of gas distribution to nondependent lung areas. Reduced dependent lung ventilation increases the number of lung regions with low $\dot{V}A/\dot{Q}$ relationships. A high $FIO_2$ may exaggerate this effect by inhibiting HPV. Preexisting $\dot{V}A/\dot{Q}$ relationships are important; lower values before administration of a high $FIO_2$ make the development of increased shunting secondary to denitrogenation more likely.

### Equipment Malfunction

Disconnection of a patient from the anesthesia circuit and $O_2$ supply probably is the most common technical mishap that results in hypoxemia. A wide variety of errors related to anesthesia machine, gas supply, and machine-patient interface have been described.[69,70]

### Oxygen Administration

For patients without preexisting cardiopulmonary disease, an $FIO_2$ between 0.25 and 0.3 is usually sufficient. A higher $FIO_2$ is required for patients with preexisting cardiopulmonary disease or for specific surgical procedures that impair ventilation (eg, airway endoscopy or one-lung anesthesia). Patients maintained with CPAP or IPPV plus PEEP preoperatively should receive similar support intraoperatively and postoperatively.

How much PEEP should be used has been a topic of controversy since the 1970s. In the 1970s, recommendations were made for levels of 18 mm Hg or higher ($\geq 25$ cm $H_2O$) in refractory adult respiratory distress syndrome.[71] By the 1980s and into the 1990s, considerably lower PEEP and peak inspiratory pressure (PIP) were advocated to avoid barotrauma,[72,73] although this concept was not substantiated in later prospective and randomized work.[74] Recent work also suggests that failure to maintain the lungs inflated with sufficient PEEP is injurious because of cyclical alveolar collapse and reexpansion with each PIP.[75–77] The open lung concept currently in vogue suggests that higher PIP and PEEP are acceptable therapeutic modes but that tidal volume should be reduced to prevent volutrauma.[78–81] The important point for anesthesiologists to keep in mind is that patients who are treated with high PIP, PEEP, or both in the intensive care unit should have the same levels maintained in the operating room if they require surgery. Unfortunately, operating room ventilators are not always up to this task.

### Why Does Hypoxemia Occur Postoperatively?

In the immediate postanesthetic period, patients may develop hypoxemia. The previously discussed mechanisms productive of intraoperative hypoxemia often persist into the postanesthetic period. Additional factors that have a role include residual anesthesia, neuromuscular blockade, induced hypoventilation, and increased $\dot{V}O_2$ secondary to shivering.

### Diffusion Hypoxia

When nitrous oxide is discontinued, large amounts enter the alveoli and dilute the alveolar $O_2$ concentration. This so-called diffusion hypoxia is short-lived and easily corrected by maintaining an $FIO_2$ of 0.5 to 1.0 for 3 to 5 minutes. However, if this period of high $O_2$ delivery is prolonged (>15 minutes), lung denitrogenation may predispose to atelectasis. This problem is of particular significance if a patient hypoventilates. The risk is reduced by washing out the nitrous oxide with an $FIO_2$ of about 0.5 in nitrogen (ie, 4 L $O_2$ in 6 L air).

### What Is the Value of Pulse Oximetry in the Postanesthesia Care Unit?

Monitoring a patient's oxygenation status with pulse oximetry is a standard practice in modern anesthesia. The ease of application and the low cost, coupled with the continuous real-time nature of $SpO_2$ monitoring, make it an ideal monitor for the PACU.

As discussed previously, the sensitivity of pulse oximetry is greatest when the $SaO_2$ is 95% or less. Thus, the almost routine practice of administering 30% to 40% $O_2$ to all postoperative patients in the PACU reduces the sensitivity by increasing the $Pao_2$ to >100 mm Hg. Pulse oximetry removes the need for routine $O_2$ therapy in the PACU.

We recommend that routine $O_2$ therapy not be used in the PACU, that all patients be monitored with pulse oximetry, and that significant hypoxemia (persistent $SpO_2$ <90%) be appropriately investigated. The indicated therapy must be based on the underlying cause.

## References

1. Piiper J. Variations of ventilation and diffusing capacity to perfusion determining the alveolar-arterial $O_2$ difference: theory. *J Appl Physiol.* 1961;16:507.
2. Piiper J, Haab P, Rahn H. Unequal distribution of pulmonary diffusing capacity in the anesthetized dog. *J Appl Physiol.* 1961;16:499.
3. Shapiro BA, Harrison RA, Cane RD, et al, eds. Blood gas analyzers. In: *Clinical Application of Blood Gases.* 4th ed. Chicago, Ill: Year Book Medical; 1989:265.
4. Shapiro BA, Cane RD, Chomka CM, et al. Preliminary evaluation of an intra-arterial blood gas system in dogs and humans. *Crit Care Med.* 1989;17:455.
5. Tremper KK, Waxman KS, Bowman R. Continuous transcutaneous oxygen monitoring during respiratory failure, cardiac decompensation, cardiac arrest and CPR. *Crit Care Med.* 1980;8:377.
6. Hess D, Kochansky M, Hassett L, et al. An evaluation of the Nellcor N-10 portable pulse oximeter. *Respir Care.* 1986;31:796.
7. Yelderman M, New W. Evaluation of pulse oximetry. *Anesthesiology.* 1983;59:349.
8. Mihm FG, Halperin BD. Non-invasive detection of profound arterial desaturations using a pulse oximetry device. *Anesthesiology.* 1985;62:85.
9. Fait CD, Wetzel RC, Dean JM, et al. Pulse oximetry in critically ill children. *J Clin Monit.* 1985;1:232.
10. Taylor MB, Whitham JG. The current status of pulse oximetry. *Anesthesiology.* 1986;41:943.
11. Fanconi S, Doherty P, Edmonds JF, et al. Pulse oximetry in pediatric intensive care: comparison with measured saturations and transcutaneous oxygen tension. *J Pediatr.* 1985;107:362.
12. Ramanthan R, Durand M, Larrazabal C. Pulse oximetry in very low birth weight infants with acute and chronic lung disease. *Pediatrics.* 1987;79:612.
13. Jenni MS, Peabody JL. Pulse oximetry: an alternative method for the assessment of oxygenation in newborn infants. *Pediatrics.* 1987;79:524.
14. Durand M, Ramanathan R. Pulse oximetry for continuous oxygen monitoring in sick newborn infants. *J Pediatr.* 1986;109:1052.
15. Scheller MS, Unger RJ, Kelner MJ. Effects of intravenously administered dyes on pulse oximetry readings. *Anesthesiology.* 1986;65:550.
16. Cane RD, Harrison RA, Shapiro BA, et al. The spectrophotometric absorbance of Intralipid. *Anesthesiology.* 1980;53:53.
17. Brooks TD, Paulus DA, Winkle WE. Infrared heat lamps interfere with pulse oximeters. *Anesthesiology.* 1984;61:630.
18. New W. Pulse oximetry. *J Clin Monit.* 1985;1:126.
19. Kim J-M, Arakawa, K, Benson KT, et al. Pulse oximetry and circulatory kinetics associated with pulse volume amplitude measured by photoelectric plethysmography. *Anesth Analg.* 1986;65:1333.
20. Martin WE, Cheung PW, Johnson CC, et al. Continuous monitoring of mixed venous oxygen saturation in man. *Anesth Analg.* 1973;52:784.
21. Johnson CC, Palm D, Stewart DC, et al. A solid state fiberoptics oximeter. *J Assoc Adv Med Instrument.* 1971;5:77.
22. Taylor JB, Lown B, Polanyi M. In-vivo monitoring with a fiber optic catheter. *JAMA.* 1972;221:667.
23. Divertie MB, McMichan JC. Continuous monitoring of mixed venous oxygen saturation. *Chest.* 1984;85:423.
24. Baele PL, McMichan JC, Marsh HM, et al. Continuous monitoring of mixed venous oxygen saturation in critically ill patients. *Anesth Analg.* 1982;61:513.
25. Shapiro BA, Harrison RA, Cane RD, et al. Oximetric measurement. In: *Clinical Applications of Blood Gases.* 4th ed. Chicago, Ill: Year Book Medical; 1989:283.
26. Shapiro BA, Harrison RA, Cane RD, et al. Applying the physiologic shunt. In: *Clinical Application of Blood Gases.* 4th ed. Chicago, Ill: Year Book Medical; 1989:157.
27. Douglas ME, Downs JB, Dannemiller FJ, et al. Changes in pulmonary venous admixture with varying inspired oxygen. *Anesth Analg.* 1976;55:688.
28. Shapiro BA, Cane RD, Harrison RA, et al. Changes in intrapulmonary shunting with the administration of 100% oxygen. *Chest.* 1980;77:138.
29. Harrison RA, Davison R, Shapiro BA, et al. Reassessment of the assumed A-V oxygen content difference in the shunt calculation. *Anesth Analg.* 1975;54:198.
30. Liliental JL, Riley RL, Proemmel DD, et al. An experimental analysis in man of the oxygen pressure gradient from alveolar air to arterial blood. *Am J Physiol.* 1946;147:199.
31. Peris LV, Boix JH, Salom JV, et al. Clinical use of the arterial/alveolar oxygen tension ratio. *Crit Care Med.* 1983;11:888.
32. Kanber GJ, King FW, Eshchar YR, et al. The alveolar-arterial oxygen gradient in young and elderly men during air and oxygen breathing. *Am Rev Respir Dis.* 1968;97:376.
33. Hess D, Maxwell C. Which is the best index for oxygenation: $P(A-a)O_2$, $PaO_2/PAO_2$ or $PaO_2/FIO_2$? *Respir Care.* 1985;30:961.
34. Gilbert R, Keighley JF. The arterial/alveolar oxygen tension ratio: an index of gas exchange applicable to varying inspired oxygen concentrations. *Am Rev Respir Dis.* 1974;109:142.
35. Gilbert R, Auchincloss JH, Juppinger M, et al. Stability of the arterial/alveolar oxygen partial pressure ratio: effects of low ventilation/perfusion regions. *Crit Care Med.* 1979;7:267.
36. Lawrence M. Abbreviating the alveolar gas equation: an argument for simplicity. *Respir Care.* 1985;30:964.
37. Cohen A, Taeusch HW Jr, Stanton C. Usefulness of the arterial/alveolar oxygen tension ratio in the care of infants with respiratory distress syndrome. *Respir Care.* 1983;28:169.
38. Martyn JAJ, Aikawa N, Wilson RS, et al. Extrapulmonary factors influencing the ratio of arterial oxygen tension to inspired oxygen concentration in burn patients. *Crit Care Med.* 1979;7:492.
39. Wallfisch HK, Tonnesen AS, Huber P. Respiratory indices compared to venous admixture. *Crit Care Med.* 1981;9:147.
40. Sjanga G, Seigal JH, Coleman W, et al. Physiologic meaning of the respiratory index in various types of critical illness. *Circ Shock.* 1985;17:179.
41. Cane RD, Shapiro BA, Templin R, et al. The unreliability of oxygen tension based indices in reflecting intrapulmonary shunting in the critically ill. *Crit Care Med.* 1988;16:1243.
42. Räsänen J, Downs JB, Seidman P, et al. Estimation of oxygen utilization by dual oximetry. *Crit Care Med.* 1987;15:404.
43. Räsänen J, Downs JB, Malec DJ, et al. Oxygen tensions and oxyhemoglobin saturations in the assessment of pulmonary gas exchange. *Crit Care Med.* 1987;15:1058.
44. Bandala LC, Cane RD, Shapiro BA. Validation of the VQI in critically ill patients. *Crit Care Med.* 1989;17:S21.
45. Räsänen J, Downs JB, Dehaven B. Titration of continuous positive airway pressure by real time dual oximetry. *Crit Care Med.* 1987;15:395.
46. Suter PM, Fairley HB, Schlobohm RM. Shunt, lung volume and perfusion during short periods of ventilation with oxygen. *Anesthesiology.* 1975;43:617.
47. Markello P, Winter P, Olszowka A. Assessment of ventilation-perfusion inequalities by arterial-venous nitrogen differences in intensive care patients. *Anesthesiology.* 1972;37:4.
48. Baker AB, McGinn A, Joyce C. Effect on lung volumes of oxygen concentration when breathing is restricted. *Br J Anaesth.* 1993;70:259.
49. Cane RD, O'Lenic T, Downs JB. Ventilation:perfusion relationships are adversely affected by breathing oxygen concentrations below 50%. *Anesthesiology.* 1994;81:A273.
50. Murdoch CG, Gill P, Cane RD, et al. Changes in perfusion, not ventilation mediate $\dot{V}A/\dot{Q}$ responses to augmented $FIO_2$. *Crit Care Med.* 1996;24:A28.
51. Smith JL. The influence of pathological conditions on active absorption of oxygen by the lungs. *J Physiol.* 1897;22:307.
52. Smith JL. The pathological effects due to increase of oxygen tension in the air breathed. *J Physiol.* 1899;24:19.
53. Crapo J, Tierney D. Superoxide dismutase and pulmonary oxygen toxicity. *Am J Physiol.* 1974;226:1401.
54. Stevens JB, Autor AP. Oxygen induced synthesis of ethylene oxide. *Anesthesiology.* 1969;30:349.
55. Kistler GS, Caldwell PRB, Weibel ER. Development of fine structural damage to alveolar and capillary lining cells in oxygen-poisoned rat lungs. *J Cell Biol.* 1967;32:605.
56. Winter P. The toxicity of oxygen. *Anesthesiology.* 1972;37:210.
57. Cane RD. Detrimental work of breathing. In: Cane RD, Shapiro BA, Davison R, eds. *Case Studies in Critical Care Medicine.* 2nd ed. Chicago, Ill: Year Book Medical; 1990:30.

58. Frumin MJ, Epstein RM, Cohen G. Apneic oxygenation in man. *Anesthesiology.* 1959;20:789.

59. Gambee, AM, Hertzka RE, Fisher DM. Preoxygenation techniques: comparison of three minutes and four breaths. *Anesth Analg.* 1987;66:468.

60. Stock MC, Schisler JQ, McSweeney TD. The $Pa_{CO_2}$ rate of rise in anesthetized patients with airway obstruction. *J Clin Anesth.* 1989;1:328.

61. Don H. The mechanical properties of the respiratory system during anesthesia. *Int Anesth Clin.* 1977;15:113.

62. Muller N, Volgyesi G, Becker L, et al. Diaphragmatic muscle tone. *J Appl Physiol.* 1979;47:279.

63. Hedenstierna G, Tokics L, Strandberg A, et al. Correlation of gas exchange impairment to development of atelectasis during anesthesia and muscle paralysis. *Acta Anaesthesiol Scand.* 1986;30:183.

64. Lindberg P, Gunnarson L, Tocis L, et al. Atelectasis and lung function in the postoperative period. *Acta Anaesthesiol Scand.* 1992;36:546.

65. Hedenstierna G. Atelectasis formation and gas exchange impairment during anaesthesia. *Monaldi Arch Chest Dis.* 1994;49:315.

66. Sykes MK, Loh L, Seed RF, et al. The effect of inhalational anesthetics on hypoxic pulmonary vasoconstriction and pulmonary vascular resistance in the perfused lungs of the dog and cat. *Br J Anesth.* 1972;44:776.

67. Bjertnaes LJ. Hypoxia-induced vasoconstriction in isolated lungs exposed to injectable or inhalation anesthetics. *Acta Anaesthesiol Scand.* 1977;21:133.

68. Marshall BE, Marshall C. Anesthesia and pulmonary circulation. In: Covino BG, Fozzard HA, Rehder K, et al, eds. *Effects of Anesthesia.* Bethesda, Md: American Physiological Society; 1985.

69. Eger EI, Epstein RM. Hazards of anesthetic equipment. *Anesthesiology.* 1964;25:490.

70. Ward CS. The prevention of accidents associated with anesthetic apparatus. *Br J Anaesth.* 1968;40:692.

71. Kirby RR, Downs JB, Civetta JM, et al. High level positive end-expiratory pressure (PEEP) in acute respiratory insufficiency. *Chest.* 1975;67:156.

72. Albert RK. Least PEEP: *primum non nocere. Chest.* 1985;87:2.

73. Hickling KG, Henderson SJ, Jackson R. Low mortality associated with low volume pressure limited ventilation with permissive hypercapnia in severe adult respiratory distress syndrome. *Intensive Care Med.* 1990;16:372.

74. Brower RG, Shanholtz CB, Fessler HE, et al. Prospective, randomized, controlled clinical trial comparing traditional versus reduced tidal volume ventilation in acute respiratory distress syndrome patients. *Crit Care Med.* 1999;27:1492.

75. Amato MBP, Barbas CSV, Medeiros DM, et al. Effect of a protective ventilation strategy on mortality in the acute respiratory distress syndrome. *N Engl J Med.* 1998;338:347.

76. Weg JG, Anzueto A, Balk R, et al. The relation of pneumothorax and other air leaks to mortality in the acute respiratory distress syndrome. *N Engl J Med.* 1998;338:341.

77. Stewart TE, Meade MO, Cook DJ, et al. Evaluation of a ventilation strategy to prevent barotrauma in patients at high risk for acute respiratory distress syndrome. *N Engl J Med.* 1998;338:355.

78. Lachmann B. Open up the lung and keep the lung open. *Intensive Care Med.* 1992;18:319.

79. Hudson LD. Protective ventilation for patients with acute respiratory distress syndrome [editorial]. *N Engl J Med.* 1998;338:385.

80. Hoyt JW. The shifting sands of mechanical ventilation [editorial]. *Crit Care Med.* 1998;26:1162.

81. The Acute Respiratory Distress Syndrome Network. Ventilation with lower tidal volumes as compared with traditional tidal volumes for acute lung injury and the acute respiratory distress syndrome. *N Engl J Med.* 2000;342:1301.

CHAPTER

# 46

# Abnormal Ventilation

Roy D. Cane
Scott Bullard

## CHARACTERISTICS OF VENTILATORY WORK
*What Is It?*

## ALVEOLAR HYPOVENTILATION
*What Are the Consequences?*
*What Are the Central Nervous System Effects?*
*What Are the Effects on Cardiac Rhythm?*
*What Electrolyte Changes Occur?*
*What Is the Effect on Oxyhemoglobin Affinity?*
*How Are Pulmonary Vascular Resistance and Bronchomotor Tone Affected?*
*Why Does Hypoventilation Occur?*
*What Is the Effect of Failed Carbon Dioxide Transport?*
*What Are the Causes of Respiratory Center Depression?*
*What Role Do Abnormalities of Impulse Conduction Play?*
*When Is Ventilatory Muscle Dysfunction Problematic?*
*What Are the Effects of Structural Derangement?*
*How Should Hypoventilation Be Corrected?*

## ALVEOLAR HYPERVENTILATION
*What Are the Consequences?*
*What Are the Central Nervous System Effects?*
*How Is Cardiovascular Activity Affected?*
*What Is the Effect on Oxyhemoglobin Affinity?*
*How Are Pulmonary Vascular Resistance and Bronchomotor Tone Affected?*
*Why Does Alveolar Hyperventilation Occur?*
*How Is Hyperventilation Corrected?*

## VENTILATORY WORK
*What Are the Consequences?*
*Why Does Ventilatory Work Occur?*
*What Are the Effects of Airway Obstruction?*
*What Are the Effects of Decreased Respiratory System Compliance?*
*What Are the Effects of Increased Dead Space?*
*What Factors Increase Carbon Dioxide Production?*

## "ABNORMAL" VENTILATORY THERAPY
*When Is It Indicated?*

Hypoventilation is present when a patient's alveolar ventilation ($\dot{V}A$) is insufficient to maintain $Paco_2$ at or below the upper limit of the normal range (45 mm Hg). Hyperventilation is defined as excessive $\dot{V}A$ that lowers the $Paco_2$ below the lower limit of the normal range (35 mm Hg). By definition, hypoventilation is associated with hypercapnia and respiratory acidosis, and hyperventilation is linked to hypocapnia and respiratory alkalosis.

The terms *hypoventilation* and *hyperventilation* are sometimes used incorrectly to denote low minute ventilation and high minute ventilation, respectively. However, a patient with a slow ventilatory rate (bradypnea) or low tidal volume (hypopnea) does not necessarily have hypoventilation; similarly, hyperventilation may not be present even if a patient's ventilatory rate is fast (tachypnea) or tidal volume ($V_T$) is high (hyperpnea). An unusually high or low minute ventilation may be appropriate for maintaining carbon dioxide ($CO_2$) homeostasis when the $CO_2$ output or the ratio of dead space to tidal volume ($V_{DS}/V_T$) is altered.

## CHARACTERISTICS OF VENTILATORY WORK

### What Is It?

Ventilatory work is required to maintain minute ventilation. The physical definition of work as the product of force and distance or pressure and volume is only applicable to situations in which a change in distance or volume occurs. Therefore, an isovolemic change in intrathoracic pressure during inspiration against a closed airway or respiratory circuit does not constitute work in the physical sense, even though it may be associated with forceful muscle contraction and considerable energy expenditure.

### Respiratory Effort

To account for isovolemic work, the total muscle activity of breathing is sometimes referred to as *respiratory effort*.

Inspiratory work is stored as potential energy in the respiratory system, to be expended during the following exhalation, or is used to overcome resistive forces during lung inflation.

Exhalation usually occurs passively using the energy stored in inspiratory deformation of the lungs and the chest wall. However, when increased resistance to exhalation or increased expiratory flow requirement calls for additional energy expenditure, the expiratory muscles are recruited and contribute to the respiratory work.

## Assessment

If changes in lung volume and the pressure differential distending the lungs or the lung-thorax combination can be measured, ventilatory work can be calculated. During spontaneous breathing or full mechanical ventilatory support, work to inflate the lungs can be separated from work to displace the chest wall and the diaphragm.[1]

During partial ventilatory support, when the ventilatory muscles and the mechanical ventilator are simultaneously active, total ventilatory work can be calculated, but ventilator work and spontaneous work of breathing have been difficult to separate accurately. Various techniques, such as calculation of time-tension relationships of airway and transdiaphragmatic pressure and measurement of total body oxygen ($O_2$) consumption ($\dot{V}_{O_2}$), have been used. The utility of these estimates is questionable at best.

A portable monitor that measures airway and esophageal pressures, gas flow, and $V_T$ and that provides automated pressure-volume loops has been introduced. Published work indicates that patient and ventilator work differentiation is easily determined with this device under most clinical circumstances.[2] At least some work of breathing is expended whenever spontaneous breathing is present, even with mechanical ventilatory support.[2] Whether the patient should be subjected to this work must be evaluated clinically.

## Clinical Correlates

The presence or absence of ventilation is determined clinically by listening to breath sounds, observing chest wall movement, and feeling gas movement at the airway. When the patient is intubated and connected to an anesthesia circuit, observation of inspiratory deflation of the reservoir bag and expiratory fogging of the transparent tracheal tube wall provides additional proof of ventilation.

Alveolar hypoventilation and hyperventilation are assessed with arterial blood gas analysis. Their presence may be inferred from capnography data, but because of the virtually inevitable arterial versus end-tidal $CO_2$ differences that occur with this method, blood gas analysis remains the gold standard.

### Signs and Symptoms

Clinical signs and symptoms of these conditions vary widely, depending on their etiology and modifying factors. However, tachycardia, hypertension, wide pulse pressure, and arrhythmias during acute hypercapnia, as well as tachycardia, hypotension, carpopedal spasms, chest discomfort, and paresthesias in acute hypocapnia, are seen with some consistency.

An acute increase in the patient's $Pa_{CO_2}$ by >10 mm Hg from baseline that is accompanied by a fall in arterial blood

pH by at least 0.1 unit below normal represents acute ventilatory failure. These values should lead to consideration of pharmacologic intervention (eg, muscle relaxant antagonism) or of mechanical ventilatory support.

### Capnography and Pulse Oximetry

Under most circumstances, the $Pa_{CO_2}$ can be estimated from a capnogram or from the output of a transcutaneous $CO_2$ monitor, taking into account the limitations of these devices (see Chapter 20). Monitoring of oxygenation with a pulse oximeter can be used to indicate ventilatory adequacy only when the patient is breathing room air. An oxyhemoglobin ($Hb_{O_2}$) saturation of 90% suggests hypoventilation and a $Pa_{CO_2}$ and $Pa_{O_2}$ of about 60 mm Hg each (in the absence of other factors that produce hypoxemia).[3]

This approximation arises out of the prediction made by the alveolar gas equation and assumes a physiologic degree of shunting. The simplified form of this equation states the following:

$$Pa_{O_2} = P_{I_{O_2}} - Pa_{CO_2}/R \qquad \text{(Equation 1)}$$

where $P_{I_{O_2}}$ is inspired $O_2$ partial pressure; $Pa_{CO_2}$ is alveolar $CO_2$ partial pressure; and R is the respiratory exchange ratio (normally, 0.8).

If the $Pa_{O_2}$ is 85 mm Hg, a 20-mm Hg increase in $Pa_{CO_2}$ decreases the $Pa_{O_2}$ by 20/0.8, or about 25 mm Hg. However, even minimal $O_2$ supplementation compensates for such hypoventilation-induced hypoxemia and invalidates the pulse oximeter as a monitor of ventilation (Fig. 46–1).

### Respiratory Mechanics

Ventilatory work is evaluated by studying the patient's respiratory mechanics (chest wall expansion, use of accessory ventilatory muscles, intercostal and suprasternal retractions, ventilatory rate, and the ratio of inspiratory time to expiratory

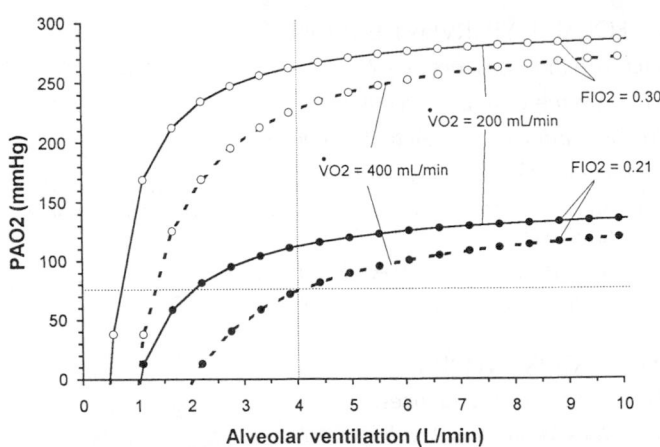

**FIGURE 46–1.** The effect of fraction of inspired oxygen ($FI_{O_2}$) and $O_2$ consumption per unit time ($\dot{V}_{O_2}$) on the relationship between alveolar ventilation and partial pressure of $O_2$ in the alveoli ($PA_{O_2}$). The *dotted vertical line* represents normal alveolar ventilation (4 L/min) and a $PA_{O_2}$ that produced an arterial blood oxyhemoglobin saturation of 90% in the absence of pulmonary pathology. $O_2$ supplementation (*open circles*) corrects hypoventilation-induced hypoxemia unless ventilation is reduced to a low level. Increased $O_2$ consumption may cause hypoxemia during room-air breathing even when alveolar ventilation is only slightly depressed.

**TABLE 46–1.** Clinical Signs of Increased Ventilatory Work

Tachypnea
Anxiety
Tachycardia
Hypertension
Sitting, forward-leaning position
Intercostal and suprasternal retractions during inspiration
Use of accessory respiratory muscles
Refusal of oxygen mask
Erratically variable $V_T$

time). Additional clues to increased ventilatory work are tachycardia, hypertension, anxiety, and the patient's refusal of an $O_2$ mask, which he or she feels is an added resistance to breathing (Table 46–1).

Patients often attempt to assume a sitting, forward-leaning position with the arms supported to minimize inspiratory effort. When increased ventilatory work is secondary to increased airway flow resistance, the ventilatory rate is decreased and the $V_T$ increased to minimize turbulent airflow. In contrast, a reduction in respiratory system compliance usually leads to rapid, shallow breathing.[4]

Impending ventilatory failure from excessive work is characterized by an erratically variable rate and depth of breathing that rapidly progress to bradypnea and apnea if mechanical ventilatory support is not instituted.

## ALVEOLAR HYPOVENTILATION

### What Are the Consequences?

Hypoxemia develops during hypoventilation when $O_2$ transfer into the alveoli is insufficient to maintain the alveolar $O_2$ partial pressure ($P_{AO_2}$) for a given $O_2$ uptake. The interdependence of $P_{AO_2}$ and $P_{ACO_2}$ is expressed in the alveolar air equation, the long version of which is as follows:

$$P_{AO_2} = (PB - PH_2O) \times F_{IO_2} - P_{ACO_2}\left[F_{IO_2} + \frac{1 - F_{IO_2}}{R}\right]$$

(Equation 2)

where PB is barometric pressure; $PH_2O$ is water vapor pressure; and $F_{IO_2}$ is the fraction of inspired $O_2$. Given a stable metabolic rate and unchanged composition of inspired gas, the inverse and linear relationship between $P_{AO_2}$ and $P_{ACO_2}$ is evident. The $P_{ACO_2}$ is dependent on $CO_2$ production ($\dot{V}_{CO_2}$) and on alveolar ventilation ($\dot{V}_A$)

$$P_{ACO_2} = (PB - PH_2O) \times \dot{V}_{CO_2}/\dot{V}_A \qquad \text{(Equation 3)}$$

$\dot{V}_{CO_2}$ can be derived from $O_2$ consumption ($\dot{V}_{O_2}$) and R, as follows:

$$\dot{V}_{CO_2} = \dot{V}_{O_2} \times R \qquad \text{(Equation 4)}$$

Thus, $P_{AO_2}$ can be expressed as a function of $\dot{V}_A$ and $\dot{V}_{O_2}$, as follows:

$$P_{AO_2} = (PB - PH_2O) \times [F_{IO_2} - \dot{V}_{O_2}/\dot{V}_A] \times \left[F_{IO_2} + \frac{1 - F_{IO_2}}{R}\right]$$

(Equation 5)

which defines a hyperbolic relationship between $P_{AO_2}$ and $\dot{V}_A$ (see Fig. 46–1). This relationship is shifted by changes in the $F_{IO_2}$ and $\dot{V}_{O_2}$. Consequently, hypoventilation-induced hypoxemia is easily masked by $O_2$ supplementation, and dangerous hypoxemia may be precipitated in a hypercapnic patient if the inspired $O_2$ concentration is suddenly lowered.

Alveolar hypoventilation leads inevitably to respiratory acidemia. However, the consequences of hypercapnia and acidosis vary, depending on the effects of compensatory mechanisms on intracellular and extracellular pH and on factors that modify the normal response of the various organ systems.

### What Are the Central Nervous System Effects?

Hypercapnia has profound direct and indirect effects on the central nervous system (CNS).[5] In experimental animals, the anesthetic effect of $CO_2$ becomes apparent when the $P_{aCO_2}$ reaches 90 to 100 mm Hg. With increasing hypercapnia, the minimum anesthetic concentration of inhalation anesthetics is reduced, and the ventilatory stimulant effect of $CO_2$ decreases.

$CO_2$ narcosis likely is a consequence of intraneuronal acidosis, which interferes with normal cellular processes. Alone, 30% $CO_2$ alone produces general anesthesia with an isoelectric electroencephalogram. However, the use of $CO_2$ as an anesthetic in human beings has been abandoned because it frequently produces seizures at anesthetic concentrations.

### Cerebral Blood Flow

Increasing the $P_{aCO_2}$ from its normal range up to 100 mm Hg is associated with a nearly linear increase in cerebral blood flow secondary to cerebral arteriolar vasodilation. This effect is accentuated by inhalation anesthetics that have a cerebral vasodilating effect of their own. Hypercapnia-induced augmentation of cerebral blood flow and volume cause an immediate rise in intracranial pressure, which may be detrimental to patients with space occupying intracranial lesions or generalized cerebral edema.

### Sympathetic Nervous System

The sympathetic nervous system is stimulated by hypercapnia both directly and by way of increased release of epinephrine and norepinephrine from the adrenal medulla. This sympathomimetic response almost completely reverses the direct effects of hypercapnia on circulatory function. Although $CO_2$ has negative myocardial inotropic and chronotropic effects, the net effect of moderate hypercapnia in humans with a functioning autonomic nervous system is an increase in heart rate, blood pressure, pulse pressure, and cardiac output as well as a slight decrease in systemic vascular resistance.

In the elderly, in patients with cardiovascular disease, and in individuals receiving β-adrenergic antagonists, respiratory acidosis may impair circulatory function both directly and by attenuating the circulatory response to circulating catecholamines.

### What Are the Effects on Cardiac Rhythm?

Arrhythmias, most commonly ventricular premature contractions, may occur in hypercapnic patients as a result of a direct effect of $CO_2$ and low pH on the heart, elevated catecholamine levels, or electrolyte abnormalities, particularly hyperkalemia. The likelihood of hypercapnia-induced dysrhythmias increases during halothane anesthesia.[6]

## What Electrolyte Changes Occur?

Acute respiratory acidemia is accompanied by an increase in serum potassium concentration by an average of 0.1 mEq/L for every 0.1-unit decrease in pH.[7] This change is variable but generally smaller than that seen in metabolic acidosis of similar magnitude. In chronic ventilatory failure, the serum potassium level is normal or slightly decreased.

## What Is the Effect on Oxyhemoglobin Affinity?

The decrease in blood pH during alveolar hypoventilation decreases $HbO_2$ affinity. Therefore, unloading of $O_2$ into the peripheral tissues is facilitated because a lower $HbO_2$ saturation can be reached at tissue $O_2$ partial pressures. However, simultaneous impairment of $O_2$ loading in the lungs may decrease the $O_2$ content of arterial blood, resulting in a net reduction in tissue $O_2$ delivery. Compromise in tissue $O_2$ delivery is accentuated if hypoventilation leads to a concurrent decrease in $Pa_{O_2}$ (see Fig. 46–1 and Equation 2).

## How Are Pulmonary Vascular Resistance and Bronchomotor Tone Affected?

In the lungs, respiratory acidemia effects an increase in the tone of both the pulmonary vasculature and small airways. After cardiopulmonary bypass, the increase in pulmonary vascular resistance with rising $Pa_{CO_2}$ is markedly accentuated and can be demonstrated even within the range of normal ventilation.[8] A combination of hypercapnia and hypoxemia may elevate pulmonary vascular resistance sufficiently to cause right ventricular failure in a compromised patient. A coexisting reduction in airway caliber further aggravates respiratory failure by increasing ventilatory work and ventilation-perfusion ($\dot{V}A/\dot{Q}$) mismatching.

## Why Does Hypoventilation Occur?

The causes of hypoventilation may lie at one level or at more than one level in the chain of events that maintain and control spontaneous breathing (Table 46–2). In a patient rendered apneic during anesthesia, a host of potential iatrogenic causes of hypoventilation require attention.

When ventilatory problems are suspected in an intubated patient, a useful differential diagnostic procedure entails manual ventilation of the lungs with an $FI_{O_2}$ equivalent to or higher than that previously used. If the patient is receiving positive end-expiratory pressure (PEEP), it too should be continued.

### Equipment Malfunction or Misuse

Manual ventilation with simultaneous auscultation of breath sounds and observation of chest wall motion and the response

**TABLE 46–2.** Factors Contributing to Respiratory Acidosis

Equipment malfunction and misuse
Impaired transport of carbon dioxide to the alveoli
   Hypoperfusion of ventilated lung
   Right-to-left shunting of blood
   Diffusion block
Inadequate respiratory drive
   Metabolic alkalosis
   Respiratory depressant drugs
   Injury to the respiratory center
   Altered responsiveness of the respiratory center
Failure of neuromuscular transmission
   Injury to the neural pathway
   Disease of the neuromuscular junction
   Neuromuscular blockade
Respiratory muscle dysfunction
   Muscular dystrophy
   Poor muscle strength and fatigue
   Excessive ventilatory load
Structural abnormality of the respiratory system
   Inability to generate negative intrathoracic pressure
   Restriction of lung or chest wall expansion

of the pulse oximeter and capnograph usually allow one to distinguish between ventilatory problems associated with the ventilator and those caused by the artificial airway or a change in the patient's clinical condition. "Feeling" the mechanics of manual ventilation usually directs attention appropriately to tracheal tube misplacement, airway obstruction, or reduction in respiratory system compliance.

### Tracheal Tube Malpositioning

Misplacement of the tracheal tube should always be suspected as a cause of a ventilatory problem until correct placement is confirmed.

**Physical Findings.** Manual ventilation and auscultation of breath sounds bilaterally below the clavicles frequently detect esophageal intubation. However, ventilation of the stomach may feel and sound deceptively similar to ventilation of the lungs. Therefore, confirmation of tracheal intubation should be sought whenever possible with capnography, by direct visualization of the larynx and of the tracheal tube passing between the vocal cords, or using fiberoptic bronchoscopy.

**Capnography.** A stable, normal capnogram during positive pressure ventilation indicates that the tip of the tracheal tube is in the trachea or a bronchus. $CO_2$ may be present in the stomach as a result of earlier mask ventilation or ingestion of $CO_2$-releasing material. However, the end-tidal concentration of $CO_2$ is low and decreases rapidly during continued ventilation of the stomach.[9,10]

During spontaneous ventilation, exhaled $CO_2$ can be detected at the tracheal tube even when the tube is not in the trachea as long as its tip is at or above the laryngeal opening. In this situation, exhalation around the tracheal tube, low insertion depth of the tube, and unsuccessful manual ventilation usually indicate tube misplacement.

Bronchial intubation may not produce alveolar hypoventilation if the ventilated lung is normal, but it can do so in patients with pulmonary disease. Signs alerting to bronchial intubation include an increase in peak airway pressure and asymmetric motion of the chest during inspiration. Inadvertent advancement of the tracheal tube below the carina can usually be detected by bilateral auscultation of the lungs. However, in pediatric and obese patients, auscultation is often unreliable.

**TABLE 46–3.** Causes of Equipment-Related Hypoventilation

Misplaced artificial airway
Power or gas supply failure
Inadequate ventilator settings
   Ventilator turned off
   Failure to adjust to changes in pulmonary mechanics
Failure to adjust to changes in metabolic rate
Circuit leak
Rebreathing of exhaled gas
   Inadequate fresh gas flow in a rebreathing circuit
   Carbon dioxide absorber off or not functioning
   Circuit valve dysfunction
Misinterpretation or calibration of the capnogram

### Circuit Problems

If manual ventilation is possible without difficulty, the cause of ventilatory problems should be sought in the breathing circuit or in the ventilator (Table 46–3). Anesthesiologists should be thoroughly familiar with how to troubleshoot the equipment they use and should know how to obtain technical assistance or acquire replacement parts so that a problem can be quickly located and corrected.

**Leaks and Disconnections.** The multiple connections between the different parts of an anesthesia machine allow leaks and disconnections to develop easily in the breathing circuit (see Chapter 16). Equipment-related mishaps tend to occur during times of cardiopulmonary instability, when the activity level is high and multiple tasks require simultaneous attention from the anesthesiologist. During these periods, it is particularly important to maintain vigilance and to ensure that a combination of alarm systems can signal failure of adequate ventilation, whatever its cause may be. A backup plan that allows continuation of anesthesia and cardiopulmonary support, regardless of failure of electrical or pneumatic equipment, should always be formulated before inducing anesthesia.

**Mechanical Ventilation.** The operating principle of the mechanical ventilator may contribute to the development of alveolar hypoventilation during changing clinical circumstances. The $V_T$ delivered by a pressure-cycled ventilator at a given peak airway pressure decreases if lung compliance is reduced or if airway resistance is increased.

The $V_T$ delivered by time-cycled and volume-cycled ventilators is also affected by changes in lung compliance and airway resistance but only to the extent that the increased peak airway pressure results in inspiratory circuit distention and gas compression within the breathing circuit.

**Metabolic and Mechanical Interactions.** Factors that produce an increase in $CO_2$ output may cause alveolar hypoventilation during anesthesia. Decreasing the depth of anesthesia or level of neuromuscular blockade and the development of hypermetabolic states such as septicemia and malignant hyperthermia cause profound respiratory acidosis unless the increased $CO_2$ output is promptly compensated for with an adjustment in minute ventilation.

**Standard Circle Systems.** Equipment-related causes of alveolar hypoventilation during anesthesia vary between different types of breathing circuits. A standard circle system that incorporates a functioning in-line $CO_2$ absorber prevents rebreathing of $CO_2$ as long as minute ventilation and gas volume in the circuit are adequate. However, incompetence of the one-way valves that are intended to ensure unidirectional flow of exhaled gas through the absorber quickly leads to hypercapnia secondary to rebreathing.

If the inspiratory unidirectional valve seats permanently in the closed position, ventilation is impossible, and the canister pressure rises while pressure in the patient's airway remains low. An obstructed expiratory valve or closed overflow (pop-off) valve increases pressure in the breathing circuit and in the patient's airway.

**Partial Rebreathing Circuits.** In circuits that allow rebreathing of exhaled gas, the fresh gas flow rate relative to the patient's $CO_2$ output is an essential factor in determining $CO_2$ removal. Insufficient fresh gas flow in these circuits results in increased $PaCO_2$ owing to rebreathing. As with the circle system, a combination of hypercapnia and dangerous hyperinflation occurs if the fresh gas flow is allowed to accumulate in the system owing to excessive closure of the pop-off valve.

**Interpretive Errors.** An equipment-related cause of pseudoalveolar hypoventilation is related to misinterpretation of the capnogram. Although abnormally high exhaled $CO_2$ concentrations virtually always indicate alveolar hypoventilation, the end-tidal $CO_2$ partial pressure ($P_{ETCO_2}$) may be low for several reasons, including low blood flow to the lungs, increased dead space ventilation, inadequate expiratory time, or sensor calibration and function. These conditions result in a change in the difference between end-tidal and arterial $CO_2$ concentrations. Responding to low $P_{ETCO_2}$ by reducing minute ventilation without appropriate differential diagnostic attention may subject the patient to serious underventilation and respiratory acidemia.

## What Is the Effect of Failed Carbon Dioxide Transport?

Excretion of $CO_2$ is possible only if sufficient blood flow can be maintained through the ventilated lungs. The efficiency of $CO_2$ transport and considerable ventilatory reserve suggest that only extreme impairment of pulmonary blood flow will result in increased $PaCO_2$ if ventilation is not depressed.

### Causes

#### Reduced Pulmonary Blood Flow

Severe reduction in pulmonary blood flow may result from right or left ventricular failure, blood volume loss, obstructed venous return, or pulmonary artery obstruction. Hypoperfused but ventilated alveoli (zone I units) constitute alveolar dead space and require a compensatory increase in minute ventilation.

Zone I lung units can also be created from the alveolar side by excessive lung inflation (ventilation with high tidal volume, inappropriately high PEEP, or a rapid ventilatory rate that does not allow complete emptying of the alveoli during exhalation). Increased expiratory flow resistance from bronchoconstriction or technical problems that cause increased flow resistance in the expiratory limb of the breathing circuit may lead to dynamic hyperinflation of the lungs, even with a normal ventilatory rate.

#### Increased Shunting

Right-to-left shunting of blood constitutes another potential mechanism for failure of $CO_2$ to reach the alveoli. Shunting may occur through nonventilated lung units in patients with pulmonary disease, or it may be extrapulmonary, making part of the cardiac output bypass the lungs completely.

The effect of shunting must be compensated for by functioning lung units to maintain normoventilation. Because $CO_2$ diffuses rapidly through the alveolocapillary membranes, areas of low but finite $\dot{V}A/\dot{Q}$ ratio have less effect on $CO_2$ excretion than they do on oxygenation.

## What Are the Causes of Respiratory Center Depression?

Several acute and chronic disease processes result in ventilatory failure, particularly in patients receiving anesthetics or analgesics.

### Chronic Lung Disease

Chronic ventilatory failure associated with many types of pulmonary disease causes respiratory depression by poorly understood mechanisms that resemble depression of the respiratory center. Hypoxemia, not hypercarbia, becomes the major driving force of ventilation. Correction of chronic hypoxemia with $O_2$ therapy in such patients may lead to severe acute hypoventilation and respiratory acidemia.

### Morbid Obesity

Patients with morbid obesity or chronic upper airway obstruction also frequently have abnormalities of ventilatory drive and may be particularly prone to developing alveolar hypoventilation during recovery from anesthesia or on receiving narcotic analgesics.

### Respiratory Center Impairment

Any acute condition that results in the compression of the respiratory center or impairs its blood supply (eg, hypotension) may lead to ventilatory failure of central origin. Although impairment of ventilatory control by neoplasms, vascular disease, or CNS trauma frequently is known when a patient presents for surgery, the possibility of CNS catastrophe developing during anesthesia must be considered in the differential diagnosis of postanesthetic ventilatory failure.

### Metabolic Alkalosis

Metabolic alkalosis produces alveolar hypoventilation as a compensatory change to attenuate the increase in blood pH. The response is variable, ranging between a 0.4- and 0.9-mm Hg increase in $Paco_2$ for each 1 mEq/L increase in plasma bicarbonate concentration. Respiratory compensation for metabolic alkalosis occurs slowly, reaching its maximum in 12 to 24 hours. Alveolar hypoventilation to a $Paco_2$ of >50 mm Hg occurs rarely in conscious and alert patients but may be encountered in patients with depressed consciousness.

### Drug Effects

Respiratory depression is one of the most common and serious side effects of drugs used by anesthesiologists. There-

fore, the severity and expected duration of the respiratory effects of each drug that one uses in practice must be known, and modifying factors in individual patients must be taken into account. Monitoring of ventilatory function after anesthesia and during the administration of postoperative pain medication must be arranged to cover the period of respiratory depression with a sufficient margin of safety.

## What Role Do Abnormalities of Impulse Conduction Play?

Conduction of the electrical impulse from the respiratory center to the ventilatory muscles can be interrupted by several conditions.

### Spinal Cord Trauma

Spinal cord trauma below the C5 level spares the phrenic nerves but results in a degree of paralysis of the intercostal muscles, which depends on the extent, type, and level of injury. Transection of the spinal cord above the C3 level results in the permanent inability of a patient to maintain spontaneous ventilation.

### Nontraumatic Problems

Several nontraumatic conditions, including infections, demyelinating CNS diseases, poliomyelitis, and Guillain-Barré syndrome, may lead to ventilatory failure secondary to impaired neural impulse conduction at different levels of the efferent neural pathway.

### Phrenic Nerve Damage

The phrenic nerves are subject to damage from neoplastic disease, regional anesthesia (interscalene block in particular), and surgery that involves the neck and thorax. Topical cooling and distention of mediastinal structures during cardiac surgery may render one or both phrenic nerves nonfunctional for several months and may result in the need for prolonged postoperative ventilatory support.[11]

### Intercostal Muscle Function

Regional anesthesia extending to the thoracic nerve roots may compromise intercostal muscle function sufficiently to reduce ventilatory reserve and contribute to ventilatory failure when other abnormalities such as airway obstruction or parenchymal lung injury are present.

### Neuromuscular Coupling

The neuromuscular junction is a common target of anesthetic management and, therefore, a frequent site of derangements that lead to ventilatory failure. Incomplete reversal of neuromuscular blockade is a common problem in the postanesthesia recovery period, especially in patients with preexisting disorders of neuromuscular function such as myasthenia gravis, the Eaton-Lambert syndrome, and muscular dystrophies.

## Uncommon Problems

Rare, acute disorders that disable the neuromuscular junction include botulism, organophosphate insecticide poisoning, and exposure to some nerve gases. Infection with *Clostridium tetani* may cause ventilatory failure by inducing spasm of ventilatory and laryngeal muscles.

**Inability to Reverse Relaxants.** Reversal of nondepolarizing neuromuscular blockade may be difficult in patients who are receiving large doses of some antibiotics (particularly the aminoglycosides) and in those with electrolyte and acid-base abnormalities (hypokalemia, hypocalcemia, hypermagnesemia, and acidosis).[12]

**Inadequate or Atypical Pseudocholinesterase.** Succinylcholine and mivacurium may effect prolonged muscle relaxation in patients with inadequate levels of pseudocholinesterase or a hereditary condition that results in production of an atypical form of this enzyme. A partially paralyzed patient exhibits a characteristic discoordinated breathing pattern in which diaphragmatic contraction pushes the flaccid abdominal muscles outward while the anterior chest wall moves paradoxically inward.

## Tests of Neuromuscular Function

Several tests of neuromuscular function have been proposed to predict when a patient will be able to maintain spontaneous ventilation. A forced vital capacity of 15 mL/kg, a negative inspiratory pressure of <25 cm $H_2O$, and the patient's ability to keep the head elevated for 5 seconds while he or she is lying supine are commonly considered indications of the presence of adequate muscle strength for spontaneous breathing. However, these tests do not ensure normal muscle strength. Endurance and ventilatory muscle failure may still ensue if the work of breathing is increased.

## When Is Ventilatory Muscle Dysfunction Problematic?

Ventilatory muscle weakness may be a primary cause of hypoventilation in patients with muscular dystrophies or hypothyroidism. More commonly, ventilatory muscle weakness contributes to the development of alveolar hypoventilation. Strength can be compromised by disuse atrophy after long periods of mechanical ventilation, by malnutrition, or by imbalances in nutritional homeostasis, particularly hypokalemia and hypophosphatemia.[13,14]

## Fatigue

Ventilatory muscle fatigue is defined as loss of ventilatory muscle contractile force during exercise. Because a VT of 500 mL in a normal individual only requires a 4- to 6-cm $H_2O$ decrease of intrathoracic pressure, fatigue is usually caused by abnormal muscle loading, deranged lung or chest wall mechanics, or high ventilatory demand.

Exposure to conditions requiring prolonged development of 40% or more of maximum transdiaphragmatic pressure from a normal functional residual capacity (FRC) eventually leads to fatigue and ventilatory failure.[15] If muscle contraction is started from a volume higher than the normal FRC, as may be the case in patients with chronic obstructive lung disease,

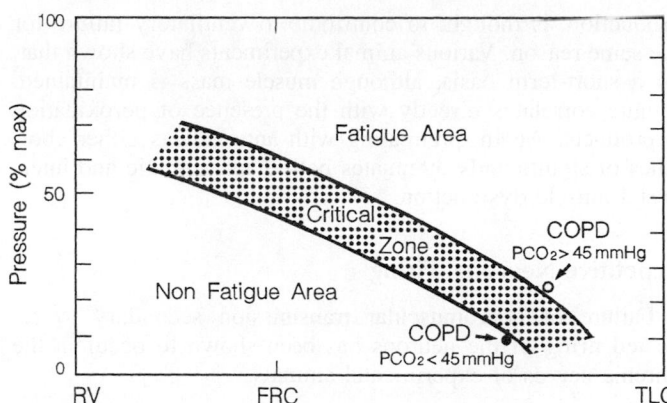

**FIGURE 46–2.** A schematic diagram of respiratory system pressure and volume demonstrating the dependence of critical intrathoracic or transdiaphragmatic pressure at which respiratory muscle fatigue occurs on expiratory lung volume. At normal functional residual capacity, the critical zone is 40% to 60% of maximum load. If the inspiratory phase is started at higher lung volume, fatigue occurs at much smaller load. Patients with chronic obstructive lung disease (COLD) and chronic alveolar hypoventilation are placed in the fatigue area. COPD, chronic obstructive pulmonary disease; FRC, functional residual capacity; RV, residual volume; TLC, total lung capacity. (Redrawn from Roussos C. Respiratory muscle fatigue and ventilatory failure. *Chest.* 1990;97:89S, with permission.)

the initial overstretching of the ventilatory muscles at the start of the contraction puts them at a disadvantage for pressure development (Fig. 46–2). Fatigue in such patients develops at lower workloads than it does in patients with normal resting lung volume. Patients with conditions that impair neuromuscular function may not tolerate any increase in ventilatory load.

Controversy exists regarding the extent of diaphragmatic impairment after upper abdominal surgery, with some authorities concluding that impaired ventilation occurs from abnormal abdominal wall movement,[16] changes in phrenic nerve output,[17] or diaphragm dysfunction and decreased muscle strength. It would appear, however, that diaphragmatic dysfunction is associated with a >50% reduction in maximum transdiaphragmatic pressure, with effects lingering for about one week.[18–21]

## Energy Supply and Demand Imbalance

Muscles may fail to contract because of an imbalance between energy supply and demand. Fatigue occurs more readily when patients with diminished systemic blood flow or blood $O_2$ content are subjected to an increased respiratory workload. In fact, ventilatory muscle fatigue and ventilatory failure can be induced in experimental animals by reducing $O_2$ even when lung mechanics are normal.[22] When muscle cells revert to anaerobic metabolism, the accumulation of lactic acid further impairs contractile function and accelerates the development of fatigue.

Much attention has focused recently on elucidating the biochemical basis for muscle fatigue. Ischemia and reperfusion of diaphragmatic muscle has implicated $O_2$-derived free radicals as causative agents because pretreatment with antioxidants attenuates the muscle fatiguability.[23] Fatigue may represent direct muscle damage (membrane or contractile protein), activation of proteolysis, or endothelial damage that alters blood and nutrient supply.

Similarly, sepsis, with its associated increased free radical production, is thought to contribute to ventilatory failure for the same reason. Various animal experiments have shown that, on a short-term basis, although muscle mass is maintained, fatigue correlates directly with the presence of peroxidation byproducts. Again, pretreating with antioxidants either abolishes or significantly attenuates both diaphragmatic and intercostal muscle dysfunction.[24–27]

## Repetitive Neuronal Firing

Failure of neuromuscular transmission secondary to repeated firing of the neurons has been shown to occur in the phrenic nerves of experimental animals.[15,28]

## Inhibition of Muscle Stimulation

Evidence suggests that afferent impulses from the ventilatory muscles, when transmitted to the respiratory center, inhibit the electrical stimulation of the muscles before actual muscle contractile failure sets in.[29] This CNS "fatigue" may be a mechanism by which the ventilatory muscles are protected from exhaustion. The exact role of transmission fatigue and respiratory center failure in human beings is not known.

## What Are the Effects of Structural Derangement?

Adequate ventilation requires that contraction of ventilatory muscles results in lung inflation. If intrathoracic pressure fails to decrease during spontaneous inspiration, movement of gas into the lungs will not occur despite adequate respiratory drive, neural and neuromuscular impulse transmission, and muscle strength.

## Pneumothorax

Equilibration of intrathoracic and ambient pressure after an open pneumothorax and the loss of chest wall rigidity after multiple rib fractures may disrupt the structural integrity of the respiratory system sufficiently to impair spontaneous ventilation. Conditions such as pneumothorax or hemothorax restrict inspiratory lung expansion, making breathing difficult or impossible until the air or fluid is evacuated from the pleural space.

## Pulmonary Contusion

A crushing injury to the chest wall that produces these conditions usually also decreases the distensibility of the lung parenchyma (pulmonary contusion), requiring large increases in transpulmonary pressure to provide a normal $V_T$.

## Pendelluft

Unilateral disruption of chest wall integrity may lead to a *pendelluft* phenomenon in which the functioning lung receives a large part of its $V_T$ by deflating the contralateral lung. During exhalation, gas returns into the traumatized lung from which it is rebreathed during the next inspiration. Rebreathing of exhaled gas results in inefficient removal of $CO_2$ and in respiratory acidemia.

## Congenital Deformities and Abdominal Distention

Restriction of lung expansion leads to chronic alveolar hypoventilation in patients with congenital or acquired chest wall or thoracic spine deformities. In pulmonary interstitial fibrosis, minimal lung expansion is accomplished despite increased effort. Distention of the abdominal cavity during laparoscopy or in patients with large amounts of ascites may restrict diaphragmatic movement sufficiently to cause ventilatory failure.

## Diffusion Block

Reduction in the gas-exchanging area of the lung eventually leads to impaired excretion of $CO_2$. Because $CO_2$ moves through the alveolocapillary membrane much more readily than does $O_2$, conditions that affect transfer of $CO_2$ from capillary blood to alveolar gas usually present first with hypoxemia (see Chapter 45).

Because of the rapid diffusion of $CO_2$, intrapulmonary shunting of blood and an increase in dead space volume, rather than diffusion block, are the predominant mechanisms impairing removal of $CO_2$ during acute lung injury.

## How Should Hypoventilation Be Corrected?

When acute ventilatory failure with respiratory acidemia is evident, mechanical ventilatory assistance should be instituted without further delay. In less severe cases, correction with measures directed at the cause of hypoventilation and without mechanical ventilatory support often suffice.

## Postanesthetic Depression

Mild postanesthetic respiratory depression can frequently be corrected by verbal and tactile stimulation. Ventilation may be improved by having the patient assume a semisitting position that allows the diaphragm to move with less impedance from the abdominal organs. However, patients who have been extubated after deep inhalation anesthesia should be placed in a lateral recumbent position to maintain patency of the upper airway and to allow drainage of the pharynx should regurgitation of gastric contents occur.

Opiate-induced respiratory depression can be reversed with opiate antagonists or with doxapram. Neuromuscular blockade should be evaluated in any patient with alveolar hypoventilation during recovery from anesthesia involving muscle relaxants. In patients with chronic lung disease, $O_2$ therapy must be planned and conducted carefully to avoid loss of the hypoxic drive to breathe.

## Pneumothorax and Hydrothorax

A pneumothorax or hydrothorax may require immediate needle or chest tube drainage before positive pressure ventilation is instituted. Tracheal intubation and mechanical ventilation delay definitive treatment and, in the case of a pneumothorax, may result in further cardiopulmonary compromise.

## Airway Management

Several measures can be taken to reduce increased work before mechanical ventilatory support is initiated if ventilatory fatigue is not imminent. Components of the circuit should be checked and changed to minimize equipment-related dead space and resistance. Airway obstruction to the midtrachea can frequently be alleviated with an artificial airway without mechanical ventilation.

### Continuous Positive Airway Pressure

**Decreased Compliance.** When increased ventilatory work is caused by decreased lung compliance, an increase in end-expiratory lung volume by continuous positive airway pressure (CPAP) often improves lung mechanics and decreases the work of breathing sufficiently to obviate mechanical ventilatory support (Fig. 46–3). CPAP can be applied with a face mask, even for prolonged periods of time.[30,31] The beneficial effects probably result from recruitment of previously collapsed alveoli, increase in the distensibility of patent lung units, increase in the caliber of conducting airways, reduced intrapulmonary shunting of blood, and correction of hypoxemia.[32,33]

The improvement in lung mechanics is instantaneous and can easily be recognized in the responding patient by a reduction in respiratory rate, less inspiratory intercostal retraction, absence of accessory ventilatory muscle contraction, and subjective relief of breathing effort (Fig. 46–4). Simplicity of the equipment and the rapid onset of a favorable effect make a trial of CPAP therapy applicable, even in patients with overt ventilatory failure, unless respiratory exhaustion is imminent.[34,35]

Mask CPAP should not be used in patients with obtunded protective laryngeal reflexes because of the possibility of

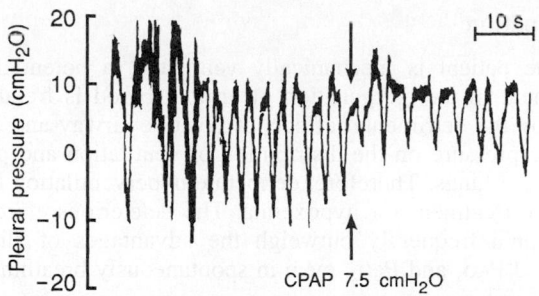

**FIGURE 46–4.** A tracing of directly measured intrathoracic pressure in a patient with cardiogenic pulmonary edema before and after application of 7.5 cm $H_2O$ continuous positive airway pressure (CPAP). Within one respiratory cycle from the institution of CPAP therapy, the ventilatory rate and the inspiratory fall in intrathoracic pressure decrease dramatically.

regurgitation and aspiration of gastric contents. In hypovolemic patients, CPAP may decrease stroke volume and require restoration of venous return with fluid therapy.

**Cardiogenic Ventilatory Failure.** In patients with cardiogenic ventilatory failure, decreased muscle work, alleviation of hypertension and tachycardia, and augmentation of left ventricular function secondary to decreased afterload are also important advantages of CPAP.[36,37]

**Relief of Airway Obstruction.** Airway obstruction due to accumulation of secretions can be alleviated by thorough bronchial suctioning using a tracheal tube with a catheter or a flexible bronchoscope. Obstructive pulmonary disease may require the use of topical or systemic bronchodilators.

When bronchoconstriction occurs during anesthesia, the bronchodilating effects of inhalation anesthetics and ketamine may be useful. In fact, inadequate anesthesia is a frequent cause of operative bronchoconstriction and wheezing, particularly in children.

### Mechanical Ventilation

Mechanical ventilation must be instituted if ventilatory failure is caused by a factor for which another immediate remedy is not available. It is also indicated if increased ventilatory work is likely to lead to ventilatory failure before its cause can be removed. Several techniques are available to provide total or partial ventilatory support. The reader is referred to specific texts for detailed description of their application.[38]

### Extracorporeal Carbon Dioxide Removal

Severe reduction in the gas-exchange area after acute lung injury may not allow matching of $\dot{V}A$ and $\dot{V}CO_2$. Extracorporeal removal of $CO_2$, with or without simultaneous extracorporeal oxygenation, has been used in children and adults in this rare and extreme case.[39,40]

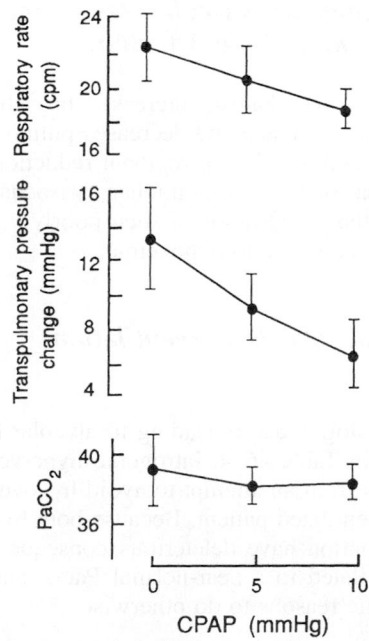

**FIGURE 46–3.** Changes in ventilatory rate, inspiratory fall in transpulmonary pressure, and $PaCO_2$ on application of up to 10 mm Hg continuous positive airway pressure (CPAP) in 14 patients with respiratory failure secondary to acute myocardial infarction. Improvement in pulmonary mechanics results in an almost linear decrease in ventilatory rate and transpulmonary pressure change and normalization of $PaCO_2$. cpm, counts per minute. (Redrawn from Rägänen J, Väisänen I, Heikkila J, et al. Acute myocardial infarction complicated by left ventricular dysfunction and respiratory failure: the effects of continuous positive airway pressure. *Chest*. 1985;87:158, with permission.)

## ALVEOLAR HYPERVENTILATION

### What Are the Consequences?

The sequelae of alveolar hyperventilation depend on whether the patient is hyperventilating spontaneously or is mechanically hyperventilated. In all patients, a reduction in $PaCO_2$ will increase $PaO_2$ (see Equation 2).

## Oxygenation

If the patient is mechanically ventilated, a potential improvement in the oxygenation of arterial blood is frequently offset by the detrimental effects of positive airway and intrathoracic pressure on the distribution of ventilation and perfusion in the lungs. Therefore, deliberate hyperventilation is not effective treatment for hypoxemia. The deleterious effects of hypocapnia frequently outweigh the advantages of slightly increased $PAO_2$ and $PaO_2$, even in spontaneously breathing patients.

## Carbon Dioxide

An increase in alveolar ventilation beyond the needs of $CO_2$ production produces hypocapnia and respiratory alkalosis. When induced with artificial ventilation, hypocapnia usually results in apnea when the $PaCO_2$ decreases below 32 mm Hg.

## What Are the Central Nervous System Effects?

Respiratory alkalemia generally increases CNS excitability and lowers the threshold for seizures.

### Tetany

Tetany in patients with severe respiratory alkalemia has been attributed to decreased ionized calcium ion ($Ca^{2+}$) concentrations in the plasma. However, tetany is seen at higher $Ca^{2+}$ concentrations in patients with respiratory alkalemia than in those in other hypocalcemic states, suggesting that the $Ca^{2+}$ level alone is not responsible for this problem.[41]

### Cerebral Vasoconstriction

A decrease in $PaCO_2$ produces cerebral vasoconstriction, reduces the cerebral blood flow and volume, and lowers intracranial pressure (ICP). The decrease in cerebral blood flow is nearly linear down to a $PaCO_2$ of 20 mm Hg. Below this level, further vasoconstriction probably is limited by concurrent hypoxia effected by reduced $O_2$ delivery.

Induction of cerebral vasoconstriction with hypocapnia can be used to reduce ICP when it is elevated by intracranial disease and to counteract the vasodilatory properties of inhalation anesthetics in patients who cannot tolerate a perioperative rise in ICP.

## How Is Cardiovascular Activity Affected?

### Myocardial Function

Although mild hyperventilation has little effect on cardiovascular function, moderate to severe respiratory alkalemia may indirectly depress myocardial contractility by reducing the $Ca^{2+}$ concentration in the blood and by causing coronary artery vasoconstriction.[42,43]

### Systemic Vascular Resistance

The systemic vascular resistance is increased by the peripheral effects and lowered by the central effects of hypocapnia.

If hyperventilation is accomplished with positive pressure ventilation, the increased intrathoracic pressure decreases right and left ventricular filling and causes a reduction in cardiac output. This effect is magnified by hypovolemia. On the other hand, in cardiac failure, positive pressure ventilation can actually unload the left ventricle.

### Arrhythmias

Respiratory alkalemia is associated with electrical irritability of the myocardium and with an increased incidence of cardiac dysrhythmias. The arrhythmogenicity of increased blood pH is further accentuated by a fall in serum potassium concentration that is effected by intracellular translocation in exchange for hydrogen ions. The likelihood of serious hypokalemia-induced dysrhythmias is of particular concern in patients who receive digitalis glycosides.[22]

## What Is the Effect on Oxyhemoglobin Affinity?

An increase in blood pH during alveolar hyperventilation increases the $HbO_2$ affinity. Consequently, $O_2$ uptake by hemoglobin in the lungs is facilitated, whereas unloading of $O_2$ from blood to tissues is impeded. Concurrently, alkalosis increases $\dot{V}O_2$ by uncoupling oxidative phosphorylation. Diminished systemic blood flow, shifting of the $HbO_2$ dissociation curve to the left, and increased $\dot{V}O_2$ produces a potentially deleterious impairment in the matching of $O_2$ supply ($\dot{D}O_2$) and demand.

## How Are Pulmonary Vascular Resistance and Bronchomotor Tone Affected?

Acute respiratory alkalosis increases bronchomotor tone and airway flow resistance and decreases pulmonary vascular resistance. The combination of regional reductions in ventilation and reversal of hypoxic pulmonary vasoconstriction further decreases the $\dot{V}A/\dot{Q}$ ratios of such poorly ventilated lung units and may contribute to hypoxemia.

## Why Does Alveolar Hyperventilation Occur?

Common etiologic factors leading to alveolar hyperventilation are listed in Table 46–4. Iatrogenic hyperventilation frequently follows from an attempt to avoid hypoventilation in a mechanically ventilated patient. Because both hypoventilation and hyperventilation have deleterious consequences, patients should be ventilated to a near-normal $PaCO_2$ and pH, unless there are specific reasons to do otherwise.

### Equipment Malfunction or Misuse

#### Mechanical Ventilation

Modern mechanical ventilators rarely deliver excess minute ventilation when properly used. However, in anesthesia breathing circuits, an increase in fresh gas flow during mechanical ventilation may lower the $PaCO_2$ to a hypocapnic

**TABLE 46–4.** Factors Contributing to Alveolar Hyperventilation

Equipment malfunction and misuse
   Mechanical overventilation
   Excessive fresh gas flow
Increased central stimulation of the respiratory center
   Anxiety
   Injury to the respiratory center
   Pain
   Fever
   Liver failure
   Pharmacologic agents
   Gram-negative septicemia
   Hormonally mediated (catechols, thyroxine)
   Pregnancy (hyperprogesteronemia)
Hypoxia
Hypotension
Metabolic acidosis

level because the fresh gas flow augments the ventilator-delivered $V_T$. This is most commonly an issue immediately after induction and before emergence, when the highest fresh gas flows are used.

**Volume-Cycled and Time-Cycled Ventilators.** Conventional volume-cycled or time-cycled, patient-triggered mechanical ventilatory support may produce hypocapnia and respiratory alkalemia as a side effect because the $V_T$ is controlled by the ventilator and not by the patient.[44] The ventilator delivers the set $V_T$ and eventually lowers the $CO_2$ partial pressure below the apneic threshold. When, after a period of apnea, the patient again triggers the ventilator, the fixed $V_T$ again lowers the $Pa_{CO_2}$. Thus, the $Pa_{CO_2}$ ultimately fluctuates slightly above and below the apneic threshold, and hypocapnia is predictable.

**Pressure-Cycled Ventilators.** Failure to adjust the settings of a pressure-cycled ventilator may also lead to inadvertent hyperventilation if the patient's respiratory system compliance increases or if airway resistance decreases during recovery.

**Changes in Dead Space and Carbon Dioxide Production.** Decrease in respiratory $V_{DS}$ or $CO_2$ production during mechanical ventilation leads to alveolar hyperventilation if ventilator settings are maintained unchanged. $CO_2$ production may decrease significantly with increasing depth of anesthesia, neuromuscular blockade, or decreasing body temperature.

## Respiratory Center Stimulation

Respiratory center stimulation may be induced by higher-level centers (ie, cerebral cortex), by neural feedback mechanisms that affect it directly, or by blood-borne chemical or pharmacologic effectors. Many factors act simultaneously in some clinical situations; others are counteracted by respiratory center depressants. Therefore, the ventilatory status in a given clinical setting may vary.

## Anxiety

Anxiety-related primary hyperventilation syndrome is a common cause of emergency room admission. Although this condition is usually characterized by the absence of signs of illness other than those related to the anxiety and alveolar hyperventilation, the associated chest discomfort, dyspnea, and ST-segment changes in the electrocardiogram sometimes produce differential diagnostic problems. Alveolar hyperventi-

lation is also a common response to stimuli that cause physical pain and discomfort.

## Central Nervous System Factors

CNS lesions such as tumors, infections, hemorrhage, or loss of blood supply in the brainstem region may produce alveolar hyperventilation by direct mechanical or chemical stimulation.

### Central Hyperventilation

Central hyperventilation may take the form of a stable increase in ventilatory rate and $V_T$, or it may present as a periodic fluctuation in the rate and depth of ventilation (Cheyne-Stokes respiration). The former is more likely to result from localized disease, whereas the latter is usually caused by diffuse CNS lesions. Periodic hyperventilation may also accompany conditions in which the circulation time is prolonged sufficiently to prevent efficient control of blood $CO_2$ tension.[45]

### Hypoxemia

The most important respiratory center chemical stimulants are hypoxemia and acidosis. When the $Pa_{O_2}$ falls below 55 to 60 mm Hg for any reason, minute ventilation begins to increase until a maximum stimulating effect is reached at a $Pa_{O_2}$ of about 40 mm Hg.[46] The stimulating effect of hypoxemia overrides the normal controlling effects of pH and $Pa_{CO_2}$ and results in respiratory alkalosis.

### Plasma Bicarbonate

A 1-mEq/L fall in plasma bicarbonate concentration, that is, a metabolic acidosis, produces a compensatory 1- to 1.4-mm Hg decrease in $Pa_{CO_2}$. The last two digits of blood pH provide a rough estimate of the expected $Pa_{CO_2}$.[47] Ventilatory changes in response to acidosis occur relatively slowly (over 12–24 hours). The reversal of this compensation occurs equally slowly, which explains the respiratory alkalosis seen after rapid correction of metabolic acidosis.

### Fever

Fever produces alveolar hyperventilation by directly stimulating the respiratory center neurons through neural connections from the hypothalamus or by causing the release of neurotransmitters. Fever-induced hyperventilation may lead to chronic respiratory alkalosis if the fever persists for a long period of time.

### Mechanoreceptors

Feedback from pulmonary mechanoreceptors frequently causes alveolar hyperventilation in the early stages of acute pulmonary diseases such as asthma, acute lung injury, pulmonary embolus, pulmonary edema, and pneumonia. Anxiety, hypoxemia, acidosis, pain, and fever provide further stimuli for such patients. As pulmonary gas exchange deteriorates and ventilatory work increases, the initial alveolar hyperventilation is replaced by ventilatory failure and respiratory acidemia.

Stimulation of baroreceptors by hypotension and circulating

mediators, the nature of which is poorly defined, has been implicated in alveolar hyperventilation by critically ill patients with systemic infections.

### Drugs

Alveolar hyperventilation can be induced pharmacologically by doxapram hydrochloride through peripheral chemoreceptor stimulation. The increase in minute ventilation results mainly from an augmentation of $V_T$, although an increase in ventilatory rate is also seen.

Epinephrine, norepinephrine, and theophylline cause alveolar hyperventilation but only when they are used in very large doses. Administration of >12 g of salicylate within a 24-hour period produces respiratory alkalemia in the average adult.[48] The mechanism is unclear but probably is related, at least in part, to the anion gap acidosis that results from salicylate intoxication.

## How Is Hyperventilation Corrected?

Mechanical overventilation is corrected by decreasing ventilator rate, $V_T$, or both. Spontaneous hyperventilation usually resolves when the underlying cause of the abnormality is corrected. If respiratory alkalemia is detrimental to a critically ill patient with spontaneous hyperventilation, correction can be accomplished by inducing deep sedation or neuromuscular blockade in conjunction with a gradual return to normal ventilation with mechanical ventilatory support.

The time-honored treatment of psychogenic hyperventilation is rebreathing of exhaled gas to increase the $Pa_{CO_2}$. This treatment is effective and safe in patients with true anxiety-related hyperventilation, but it is not effective and may be hazardous in patients who hyperventilate in response to other stimuli, such as hypoxemia.

## VENTILATORY WORK

### What Are the Consequences?

Increased ventilatory work may lead to ventilatory failure and respiratory acidemia when the ventilatory muscles are no longer able to maintain adequate $\dot{V}_A$. However, even in the absence of overt failure, increased ventilatory work has considerable deleterious effects, particularly on cardiovascular function[49] (Table 46–5).

**TABLE 46–5.** Factors Contributing to Development of Left Ventricular Dysfunction During Increased Ventilatory Work

| | |
|---|---|
| Anxiety | Respiratory muscle fatigue |
|   Hypertension |   Lactic acidosis |
|   Tachycardia |   Hyperkalemia |
|   Myocardial ischemia |   Arrhythmias |
| Negative intrathoracic pressure |   Myocardial ischemia |
|   Increased muscle work | Ventilatory fatigue |
|   Increased cardiac output requirement |   Respiratory acidosis |
|   Redistribution of blood flow |   Hypoxemia |
|   Left ventricular distention |   Hyperkalemia |
|   Increased left ventricular afterload |   Arrhythmias |
|   Myocardial ischemia |   Myocardial ischemia |

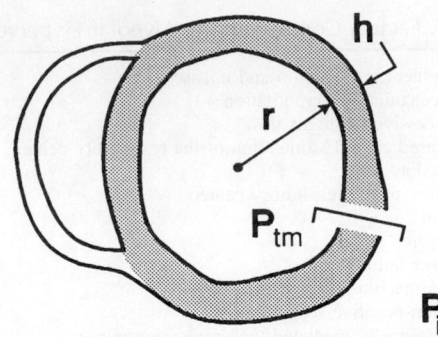

**FIGURE 46–5.** A schematic cross-section of the left ventricle (*shaded*). A decrease in intrathoracic pressure (Pit) increases the transmural chamber pressure (Ptm) and the chamber radius and decreases wall thickness (h). These three factors change in a direction that will increase wall stress (W) according to Laplace's law: W = Ptm × r/2h. An elevation in wall stress (afterload) will increase myocardial oxygen consumption and may produce ischemia and wall motion abnormalities in a susceptible patient.

### Increased Ventilatory Muscle Work

The increased muscle effort during respiratory distress not only requires an increase in cardiac output (CO) but also diverts blood flow to the ventilatory muscles at the expense of other organ tissues, including the myocardium.[38] Consequently, myocardial $O_2$ demand is increased in the face of reduced supply. The tachycardia and hypertension associated with the anxiety of suffocation and acidosis secondary to anaerobic muscle metabolism further load the circulation.[50,51]

### Pleural Pressure Fluctuations

Increased respiratory effort is always associated with "negative" (subambient) fluctuations of intrathoracic pressure that have additional direct effects on cardiac function.[52] The negative pressure surrounding the left ventricle raises transmyocardial pressure, increases the ventricle's size, and effects a reduction in wall thickness (Fig. 46–5). These changes are related according to the law of Laplace:

$$Ptm = 2h\,W/r \qquad \text{(Equation 6)}$$

where Ptm is transmural chamber pressure, W is wall stress, r is chamber radius, and h is wall thickness. Rearrangement of these terms results in the following expression:

$$W = Ptm \times r/2h \qquad \text{(Equation 7)}$$

A patient with normal left ventricular function can tolerate the increase in afterload because the function of a normal heart is primarily dependent on preload. However, myocardial ischemia, left ventricular failure, and cardiogenic pulmonary edema may be induced by negative intrathoracic pressure secondary to increased ventilatory work in patients with preexisting left ventricular dysfunction.[53,54] Further impairment in lung mechanics and gas exchange from pulmonary vascular congestion may trigger a vicious cycle of cardiopulmonary failure and quickly lead to the patient's demise unless ventilatory work is reduced effectively and promptly.

### Why Does Ventilatory Work Occur?

Common causes of increased ventilatory work are listed in Table 46–6. Work imposed by the breathing circuit is in

**TABLE 46–6.** Sources of Increased Ventilatory Work

Breathing circuit-related work
    Demand valve resistance
    Circuit resistance
    Tracheal tube size and length
    Resistance of the exhalation valve and
        positive end-expiratory pressure valve
    Type of positive airway pressure therapy
    Maximum inspiratory flow
Airway obstruction
Lung compliance
Chest wall compliance
Volume of functional dead space
Carbon dioxide production

addition to that required to effect pulmonary ventilation in the absence of the circuit. The most important characteristics in terms of added work of breathing are the mechanisms by which inspiratory gas flow is made available; the flow resistance of the circuit; the tracheal tube; and the exhalation valve. When PEEP is used during spontaneous breathing, two additional factors must be taken into account: the flow resistance of the PEEP valve and the stability of airway pressure during the respiratory cycle (Fig. 46–6).

## Generation of Inspiratory Flow

Inspiratory flow and volume can be made available from a continuous, free flow of gas or by the patient's triggering of the opening of a demand valve in the inspiratory limb.

### Continuous Gas Flow

Continuous flow circuits usually incorporate a reservoir to collect gas during exhalation for the subsequent inspiratory phase. This arrangement allows the fresh gas flow to be reduced considerably and to be immediately available at all times.

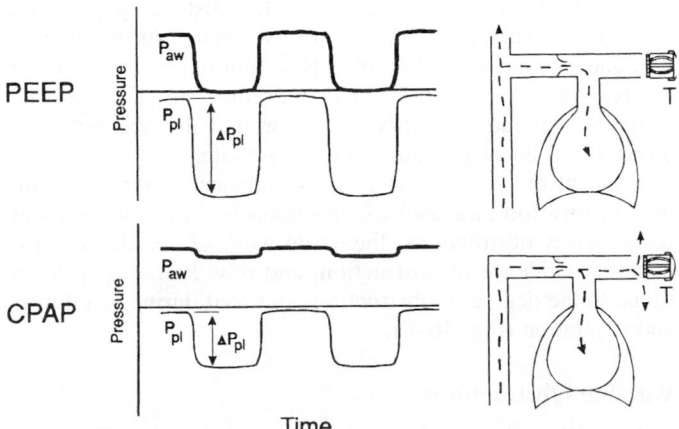

**FIGURE 46–6.** Changes in airway (Paw) and pleural (Ppl) pressure during spontaneous breathing with positive end-expiratory pressure (PEEP) and continuous positive airway pressure (CPAP) circuits. Positive circuit pressure is created by the threshold resistor valve (T) only when gas flows through it. The necessity of bringing airway pressure to ambient status before start of lung inflation during breathing with PEEP as compared with CPAP increases the required change in intrathoracic pressure and ventilatory work.

### Demand Valves

In a demand valve circuit, no gas is available to the patient unless inspiratory effort activates the flow. The signal to open the demand valve is usually the initial fall in airway pressure at the beginning of inspiration. These circuits supply gas with minimal inspiratory effort as long as the fresh gas flow and the reservoir volume are sufficient to meet the patient's demand. However, if the VT and inspiratory flow rate exceed the capacity of the breathing circuit, gas flow stops. The patient continues the inspiratory effort against what amounts to a closed airway.

Breathing with a demand valve circuit requires additional effort, the magnitude of which depends on the time required to initiate flow from the ventilator, the trigger sensitivity, and the valve design. The maximum inspiratory flow and volume available after the valve opens are also important determinants of inspiratory work. Considerable differences reflect the functional characteristics of commercially available circuits.[55] Some have been shown to impose a significantly larger inspiratory load on the spontaneously breathing patient than do continuous-flow circuits.[56,57]

### Circuit Flow Resistance

Components of the anesthesia circuit, tubing, elbow connectors, valves, and humidifiers may offer significant flow resistance. Such resistance must be overcome by the patient during spontaneous breathing and by the ventilator during mechanical ventilation.

When turbulent gas flow occurs, flow resistance is directly proportional to the flow rate. Therefore, a rapid ventilatory frequency and high flow rate increase the resistive effect of a given circuit configuration. Although the resistance of a single component may not appear significant, the additive effect of the different components arranged in series may contribute to ventilatory fatigue and failure.

### The Tracheal Tube

The size and length of the tracheal tube have a significant effect on the resistance of the breathing circuit. Depending on gas flow, each 1-mm decrease in an adult-size tracheal tube diameter increases ventilatory work by 34% to 154%, depending on the ventilatory flow rate.[58]

Fiastro and coworkers[59] reported that the mechanically generated inspiratory pressure required to overcome resistance from the ventilator circuit and tracheal tube was 6 cm $H_2O$ for a 9-mm diameter tube and 15 cm $H_2O$ for a 7-mm diameter tube at a gas flow rate of 40 L/min. Tube resistance also increases with length, which is usually alterable and therefore should be minimized.

Christie and Leon[60] reported that spontaneous breathing through an endotracheal tube and standard circle system without positive airway pressure during inhalational anesthesia was associated with a twofold increase in the work of breathing. A demand-flow circuit was associated with a work of 690 mJ/L, which decreased to 170 mJ/L after the application of 5 cm $H_2O$ inspiratory pressure support.

This amount of work represents only 0.5% to 1% of the resting total body energy expenditure; therefore, the changes are not significant for a healthy person. However, minimizing the extrinsic, equipment-related work may be of considerable importance in patients with pulmonary insufficiency, for whom intrinsic ventilatory work already represents significant energy expenditure.

## The Exhalation Valve

The flow resistance of the exhalation valve can increase inspiratory and expiratory ventilatory work.[61,62] Resistance to exhalation is overcome first by increasing $V_T$ so that more elastic energy is available for subsequent exhalation. As the load increases further, expiratory muscles are recruited to contract actively during exhalation.[63]

### Spontaneous Breathing With Positive Pressure

When positive airway pressure is applied with a continuous flow system, the pressure and flow characteristics of the valve that generates the positive circuit pressure become important (see Fig. 46–6).[64] During exhalation, the valve must accommodate a patient's expiratory flow and the continuous flow; an increase in pressure above the baseline occurs when a flow-resistor valve is used.

If the valve has significant flow resistance, a reduction in flow through the valve as it is diverted into the patient's lungs leads to a fall in circuit pressure (Fig. 46–7). This drop in pressure must be generated by the patient and, therefore, requires increased respiratory effort.[65]

Conversely, a threshold resistor valve does not depend on flow to generate pressure. Therefore, airway pressure does not fluctuate significantly during the respiratory cycle, and the valve-induced work of breathing is reduced.

**Positive End-Expiratory Pressure.** The technique used to apply PEEP also has implications for ventilatory work during spontaneous breathing.[66] PEEP can be applied to a spontaneously breathing patient by attaching a PEEP valve to the expiratory limb of a nonrebreathing circuit (ie, a resuscitator bag equipped with a nonrebreathing valve). This valve pressurizes the airway and the expiratory limb as long as expiratory flow is present.

At the beginning of the next inspiration, the airway pressure must fall by an amount equivalent to the applied PEEP before

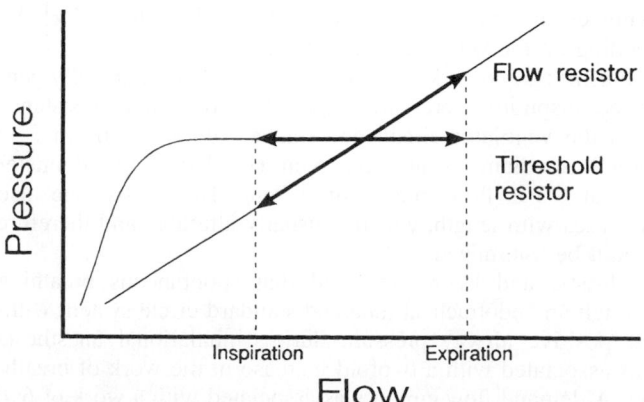

**FIGURE 46–7.** The mechanism by which inspiratory work is increased by the resistance of the positive-pressure valve during continuous-flow continuous positive airway pressure therapy. Fluctuation in flow through a flow resistor positive end-expiratory pressure (PEEP) valve causes fluctuations in airway pressure that increase ventilatory effort. A threshold resistor PEEP valve does not increase effort because it can accommodate variation in flow without a change in circuit pressure.

gas flows into the lungs. A tidal breath requires an even greater reduction of intrathoracic pressure, the amount of which is dependent on the $V_T$, respiratory system compliance, and airway resistance.

The fall in intrathoracic pressure necessary to bring the airway pressure down from the PEEP level to ambient represents additional energy expenditure and increases the magnitude of negative intrathoracic pressure fluctuations (see Fig. 46–6). Both of these effects are detrimental, particularly to patients with compromised left ventricular function.

**Continuous Positive Airway Pressure.** If the entire circuit is pressurized to the prescribed level throughout the respiratory cycle, CPAP results. The early inspiratory drop in airway and intrathoracic pressure is avoided, and ventilatory work decreases (see Fig. 46–6). Therefore, when positive airway pressure is indicated for a spontaneously breathing patient and work of breathing is a concern, CPAP should be used. If only a PEEP circuit is available as, for example, during transport of a patient supported with a PEEP-equipped resuscitator bag, controlled ventilation should be applied or the PEEP valve removed, whichever is less detrimental to the patient's overall cardiopulmonary function.

## What Are the Effects of Airway Obstruction?

Airway obstruction increases ventilatory work in a variety of conditions characterized by pathologic airway reactivity, altered structure of the air passages, or reduced lung volume. Localized airway obstruction may occur at any level secondary to external compression by tumors and hematomas or to intraluminal narrowing from scarring, edema, secretions, and foreign bodies. Reduction in airway caliber imposes an abnormal load to ventilation during inspiration, expiration, or throughout the entire respiratory cycle, depending on the degree, localization, and dynamic characteristics of the obstruction.

### Fixed Obstructions

A fixed resistance in the airway does not change in diameter or length regardless of changes in the distending pressure. Therefore, a similar resistance to flow occurs during inspiration and expiration, and its effects do not depend on whether the resistance is intrathoracic or extrathoracic. The pressure differential required to drive flow through the obstruction is directly and linearly related to the flow rate.

Tracheal or bronchial stenosis secondary to fibrosis or tumor infiltration and mediastinal masses represents typical fixed airway obstructions. Increased work of ventilation, auscultatory evidence of obstruction, and flow limitation proportional to the degree of obstruction are noted during inspiration and expiration (Fig. 46–8).

### Variable Obstructions

A variable airway obstruction allows the distending pressure of the airway to modify flow resistance.

#### Intrathoracic

Intrathoracic variable airway obstruction, which is seen for example in a patient with bronchial asthma or bronchomalacia,

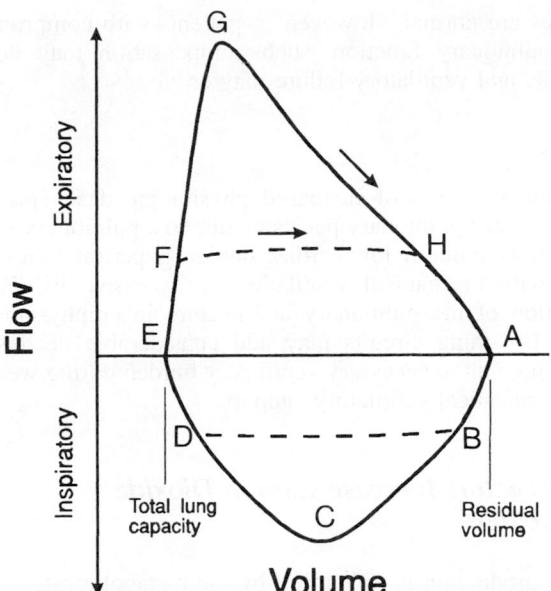

**FIGURE 46–8.** Maximum flow-volume curve under normal conditions (*continuous line*, ACEGA) and during fixed airway obstruction (*broken line*, ABDEFHA). With variable intrathoracic airway obstruction, the curve follows the *broken line* during expiration, whereas inspiratory flow-volume characteristics may be nearly normal (ACEFHA). During variable extrathoracic airway obstruction, inspiratory flow is limited, whereas expiratory flow may be unobstructed (ABDEGA).

is alleviated during inspiration; the negative intrathoracic pressure increases the distending pressure and the diameter of the obstructed segment. This effect opposes the decrease in intraluminal pressure effected by gas flow through the narrow airway segment, which promotes airway collapse (the Bernoulli effect).

During exhalation, the flow-related decrease in intraluminal pressure is not opposed by intrathoracic pressure, and the obstruction worsens. In fact, forced positive intrathoracic pressure may contribute to increased obstruction, even though the intraluminal pressure distal (upstream) to the obstruction may be positive.

### Extrathoracic

Extrathoracic variable airway obstruction, which is seen, for example, with laryngomalacia, is not affected by changes of intrathoracic pressure. Therefore, the inspiratory fall in intraluminal pressure worsens the obstruction. During expiration, positive intraluminal pressure distal (upstream) to the obstruction promotes gas flow, making expiration less obstructed than inspiration.

The differences in gas flow limitation between respiratory phases, depending on the location of the obstruction, are evident in flow-volume loop studies (see Fig. 46–8) and during clinical examination. Regardless of the type of airway obstruction, a functioning respiratory center "attempts" to make an adjustment toward a slow ventilatory rate with an increase in $V_T$ to minimize the work of breathing. Because low flow allows gas to pass through the obstruction with a smaller pressure differential (less turbulence), the phase in which the obstruction is worse is prolonged.

## What Are the Effects of Decreased Respiratory System Compliance?

The remarkably small effort required for normal breathing is largely a result of the high distensibility of the lung-thorax combination.

In a normal, upright adult, lung compliance ($C_L$) is 200 mL/cm $H_2O$, and chest wall compliance ($C_{CW}$) is 200 mL/cm $H_2O$. Total respiratory system compliance ($C_{RS}$) is determined according to the following equation:

$$1/C_{RS} = 1/C_L + 1/C_{CW} \qquad \text{(Equation 8)}$$

Solving for $C_{RS}$, $1/C_{RS} = 1/200 + 1/200 = 1/100$; $C_{RS} = 100$ mL/cm $H_2O$.

However, in a normal supine anesthetized adult, the $C_L$ is reduced to about 150 mL/cm $H_2O$ because of pressure from the abdominal viscera and cephalad displacement of the diaphragm. Chest wall compliance is unchanged. The result is a reduction of $C_{RS}$ to 85 mL/cm $H_2O$. A $V_T$ of 500 mL can be achieved by applying 8 cm $H_2O$ positive pressure to the airway or by decreasing intrathoracic pressure by an additional 6 cm $H_2O$ beyond the −2 cm $H_2O$ baseline level[67] (Fig. 46–9).

Any process that reduces lung compliance necessitates a larger change in intrathoracic pressure during spontaneous breathing or a higher positive airway pressure during mechanical ventilation. Increased ventilatory work results. If chest wall compliance is reduced, the transpulmonary pressure change during tidal breathing is not increased, but more muscle work is required to generate a given change in intrathoracic pressure.

### Causes of Reduced Lung Compliance

Lung compliance is reduced by factors that effect a decrease in the volume or distensibility of inflated lung tissue, or both. Most acute parenchymal lung diseases are associated with decreased lung compliance and increased ventilatory work.

Regardless of whether the acute lung injury is caused by infection, by damage to the alveolocapillary membranes, or by hydrostatic vascular congestion and edema, a mixture of inflated, recruitable, and nonrecruitable lung parenchyma is present. The distensibility of the lungs and the impact of the injury on ventilatory work at different lung volumes depend on the relative magnitude of these components and on the mechanical characteristics of gas-containing areas of the lung.[68,69]

### Causes of Reduced Chest Wall Compliance

Chest wall compliance is reduced by the prone position, obesity, abdominal distention, chest deformities, and chronic disease states that alter the structure and configuration of the thoracic cage.

### Morbid Obesity

Ventilatory function in morbidly obese patients is often markedly sensitive to position. Such patients may only be able to breathe spontaneously in the upright or semisitting position because abdominal pressure in the supine position limits diaphragmatic descent.

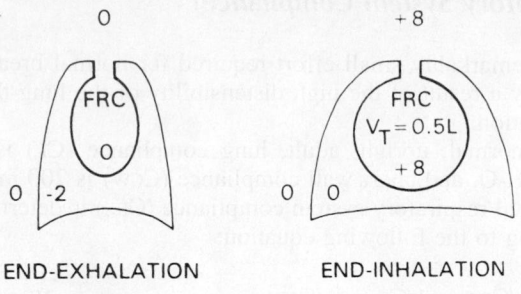

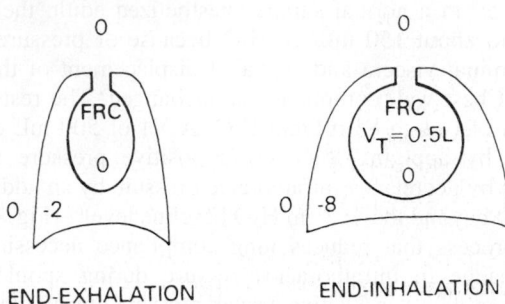

**FIGURE 46–9.** Changes in airway and intrathoracic pressure in a supine, anesthetized adult whose respiratory system compliance (CRS) is 85 mL/cm H₂O. The initial end-exhalation transpulmonary pressure (airway pressure minus intrathoracic pressure) is $0 - (-2 \text{ cm H}_2\text{O}) = 2 \text{ cm H}_2\text{O}$. With positive-pressure inflation, airway pressure increases to 8 cm H₂O, and intrathoracic pressure increases to 0. The transthoracic pressure is now $8 \text{ cm H}_2\text{O} - 0 = 8 \text{ cm H}_2\text{O}$ at end inhalation. The *change* in transpulmonary pressure (end inhalation minus end exhalation) is $8 \text{ cm H}_2\text{O} - 2 \text{ cm H}_2\text{O} = 6 \text{ cm H}_2\text{O}$. Tidal volume (VT) is calculated as follows:

$$V_T = \text{transpulmonary pressure} \times C_{RS}$$

$$= 6 \text{ cm H}_2\text{O} \times 85 \text{ mL/cm H}_2\text{O}$$

$$= 510 \text{ mL}$$

$$= 0.5 \text{ L}$$

With a spontaneous breath, the change in transpulmonary pressure is also 6 cm H₂O, the same value as that achieved with intermittent positive-pressure ventilation (IPPV). An identical VT of about 0.5 L results. FRC, functional residual capacity.

### Hyperinflation

Hyperinflation of the lungs leads to reduced respiratory system compliance when the lung-thorax combination approaches the limits of its expansion. This factor is significant in patients with chronic lung disease and asthma.

## What Are the Effects of Increased Dead Space?

Increase in physiologic dead space (ie, the ventilated but not perfused parts of the respiratory system) requires augmentation of minute ventilation and increased ventilatory work for effective V̇A. An increase in minute ventilation to compensate for moderate increases in dead space can easily be accomplished if the respiratory mechanics and ventilatory muscle reserves are normal. However, in patients with compromised cardiopulmonary function, such compensation may not be possible, and ventilatory failure may ensue.

### Causes

Common causes of increased physiologic dead space include reduced pulmonary perfusion due to a pulmonary embolus, hypovolemia or low cardiac output, hyperinflation of the lungs with mechanical ventilation or excessive PEEP, and disruption of the pulmonary architecture in emphysematous lungs. Breathing circuits may add considerable dead space and impose an unnecessary ventilatory burden during weaning from mechanical ventilatory support.

## What Factors Increase Carbon Dioxide Production?

CO₂ production is influenced by the metabolic rate and by the nature of metabolic processes that determine CO₂ production (V̇CO₂) and V̇O₂. Maintenance of CO₂ and pH homeostasis requires matching changes in V̇A with V̇CO₂. Factors associated with increased V̇CO₂ include fever, decreasing depth of anesthesia, rapid administration of bicarbonate-containing solutions, and overfeeding.

Because ventilation normally requires little work, fluctuations in metabolic rate are generally well tolerated. However, in patients with borderline ventilatory function, a nutrition-related increase in V̇CO₂ and rapid correction of metabolic acidosis with sodium bicarbonate may lead to acute ventilatory failure.

## "ABNORMAL" VENTILATORY THERAPY

### When Is It Indicated?

#### Control of Intracranial Pressure

The physiologic effects of alveolar hyperventilation can be used for therapeutic purposes in specific clinical circumstances. The most common example is to control ICP. Because hyperventilation is the most rapid method available to reduce ICP consistently, it can be used as first-line therapy without monitoring when life-threatening intracranial hypertension is suspected. However, such monitoring should be instituted as soon as possible to allow accurate titration of this and other forms of therapy.

### Acceptable Limits

When continued control of ICP is attempted, the minimum level of hyperventilation that produces the desired effect should be used. This strategy allows further lowering of PaCO₂ to counteract tachyphylaxis and to control sudden further elevations in ICP with minimum side effects.

The effect of respiratory alkalosis on ICP is probably mediated both by changes in pH and by a direct effect of hypocapnia. The primary mechanism is cerebral arterial vasoconstriction, which decreases cerebral blood flow. Such therapy may prevent herniation and other pressure-related detrimental sequelae inside the cranium, but it does not necessarily improve brain tissue oxygenation, even when it results in an increase in the calculated cerebral perfusion pressure.

To prevent cerebral ischemia, the $Paco_2$ should not be reduced below 20 mm Hg. If ICP monitoring is not available, the $Paco_2$ should be maintained between 25 and 30 mm Hg and verified by arterial blood gas analysis. Equilibration of pH between blood and cerebrospinal fluid causes an attenuation of hypocapnic cerebral vasoconstriction within 24 to 72 hours. Subsequent return to normal ventilation then has a vasodilating effect. Therefore, hyperventilation should be discontinued gradually to avoid a sudden rise in ICP.

## Reduction of Pulmonary Vascular Resistance

The pulmonary vasculature is also sensitive to changes in blood pH and $Paco_2$. Increases of blood pH up to 7.50 are frequently helpful in infants with pulmonary hypertension; resistance to pulmonary blood flow is decreased without systemic hypotension.[70]

Considerable sensitivity to alveolar hypoventilation has been demonstrated in the adult pulmonary circulation after open heart operations requiring cardiopulmonary bypass.[8] Even though these data suggest the importance of avoiding hypoventilation in such patients, deliberate hyperventilation with respiratory alkalemia has not been consistently successful in reducing the pulmonary vascular resistance.

## Hyperventilatory Compensation for Metabolic Acidosis

The hazards of treating metabolic acidosis with sodium bicarbonate emphasize the importance of maintaining adequate oxygenation and slight to moderate hyperventilation.[71] $CO_2$ diffuses readily in and out of cells; thus, changes in $Paco_2$ rapidly translate into similar directional changes in intracellular $CO_2$ tension and pH. The hyperventilatory response to metabolic acidosis is, therefore, a key element in compensating for metabolic acidosis inside the cell.

### Sodium Bicarbonate

If blood pH is corrected rapidly with sodium bicarbonate administration and if compensatory hyperventilation decreases simultaneously, the resultant increase of intracellular $Pco_2$ may lower intracellular pH significantly. Worsening intracellular acidosis has detrimental effects, particularly in the CNS and the myocardium. These considerations favor slow correction of metabolic acidosis, preferably by eliminating its cause; partial compensation for acidosis with hyperventilation; and avoidance of aggressive sodium bicarbonate therapy unless the acidosis is severe (pH $<$ 7.10) or other reasons (eg, hyperkalemia) require rapid correction.

## References

1. Annat G, Viale JP. Measuring the breathing workload in mechanically ventilated patients. *Intensive Care Med.* 1990;16:418.
2. Banner MJ, Kirby RR, Blanch PB, et al. Decreasing imposed work of the breathing apparatus to zero using pressure support ventilation. *Crit Care Med.* 1993;21:1333.
3. Räsänen J, Cane RD. Continuous oximetry: is it beneficial? [commentary]. *Perspect Crit Care.* 1991;4:133.
4. McIlroy MB, Eldridge FL, Thomas JP, et al. The effect of added elastic and non-elastic resistances on the pattern of breathing in normal subjects. *Clin Sci.* 1956;15:337.
5. Nunn JF. The effects of changes in the carbon dioxide tension. In: Nunn JF, ed. *Applied Respiratory Physiology.* 3rd ed. London, United Kingdom: Butterworths; 1987:460.
6. Black GW, Linde HW, Dripps RD, et al. Circulatory changes accompanying respiratory acidosis during halothane anesthesia in man. *Br J Anaesth.* 1959;31:238.
7. Molony DA, Jacobson HR. Respiratory acid-base disorders. In: Kokko JP, Tannen RL, eds. *Fluids and Electrolytes.* Philadelphia, Pa: WB Saunders; 1986:305.
8. Salmenperä M, Heinonen J. Pulmonary vascular responses to moderate changes in $Paco_2$ after cardiopulmonary bypass. *Anesthesiology.* 1986;64:311.
9. Linko K, Paloheimo M, Tammisto T. Capnography for detection of accidental oesophageal intubation. *Acta Anesthesiol Scand.* 1983;69:199.
10. Sum-Ping ST, Mehta MP, Anderton JM. A comparative study of methods of detection of esophageal intubation. *Anesth Analg.* 1989;27:627.
11. Curtis JJ, Nawarawong W, Walls JT, et al. Elevated hemidiaphragm after cardiac operations: incidence, prognosis, and relationship to the use of topical ice slush. *Ann Thorac Surg.* 1989;48:764.
12. Cronnelly R. Muscle relaxant antagonists. In: Katz RL, ed. *Muscle Relaxants: Basic and Clinical Aspects.* Orlando, Fla: Grune & Stratton; 1985:197.
13. Roussos C, Macklem PT. The respiratory muscles. *N Engl J Med.* 1982;307:786.
14. Aubier M, Murciano D, Lecocguic Y, et al. Effect of hypophosphatemia on diaphragmatic contractility in patients with acute respiratory failure. *N Engl J Med.* 1985;313:420.
15. Roussos C. Respiratory muscle fatigue and ventilatory failure. *Chest.* 1990;97:89S.
16. Nimmo A, Drummond G. Respiratory mechanics after abdominal surgery measured with continuous analysis of pressure, flow and volume signals. *Br J Anaesth.* 1996;77:317.
17. Dureuil B, Viires N, Cantineau J, et al. Diaphragmatic contractility after upper abdominal surgery. *J Appl Physiol.* 1986;61(5):1775.
18. Erice F, Fox G, Salib Y, et al. Diaphragmatic function before and after laparoscopic cholecystectomy. *Anesthesiology.* 1993;79:966.
19. Simmoneau G, Vivien A, Sartene R, et al. Diaphragm dysfunction induced by upper abdominal surgery: role of postoperative pain. *Am Rev Respir Dis.* 1983;128:899.
20. Dureuil B, Cantineau J, Desmonts J. Effects of upper or lower abdominal surgery on diaphragmatic function. *Br J Anaesth.* 1987;59:1230.
21. Ford G, Whitelaw W, Rosenal T, et al. Diaphragm function after upper abdominal surgery in humans. *Am Rev Respir Dis.* 1983;127:431.
22. Aubier M, Trippenbach T, Roussos C. Respiratory muscle fatigue during cardiogenic shock. *J Appl Physiol; Respir Environ Exerc Physiol.* 1981;51:499.
23. Supinski G, Renston J, DiMarco A. Free radical mediated diaphragmatic injury following ischemia/reperfusion [abstract]. *Am Rev Respir Dis.* 1992;145:A672.
24. Supinski G, Nethery D, DiMarco A. Effect of free radical scavengers on endotoxin-induced respiratory muscle dysfunction. *Am Rev Respir Dis.* 1993;148:1318.
25. Van Surell C, Boczkowski J, Pasquier C, et al. Effects of N-acetylcysteine on diaphragmatic function and malondialdehyde content in *Escherichia coli* endotoxemic rats. *Am Rev Respir Dis.* 1992;146:730.
26. Boczkowski J, Dureuil B, Branger C, et al. Effects of sepsis on diaphragmatic function in rats. *Am Rev Respir Dis.* 1988;138:260.
27. Anzueto A, Supinski GS, Levine SM, et al. Mechanisms of disease: are oxygen-derived free radicals involved in diaphragmatic dysfunction? *Am J Respir Crit Care Med.* 1994;149:1048.
28. Aubier M, Farkas G, De Troyer A, et al. Detection of diaphragmatic fatigue in man by phrenic nerve stimulation. *J Appl Physiol.* 1981;50:538.
29. Bellemare F, Bigland-Ritchie B. Central components of diaphragmatic fatigue assessed from bilateral phrenic nerve stimulation. *J Appl Physiol.* 1987;62:1307.
30. Räsänen J, Heikkilä J, Downs JB, et al. Continuous positive airway pressure by face mask in the treatment of cardiogenic pulmonary edema. *Am J Cardiol.* 1985;55:296.
31. Branson RD, Hurst JM, DeHaven CB. Mask-CPAP: state of the art. *Respir Care.* 1985;30:846.
32. Kirby RR, Downs JB, Civetta JM, et al. High level positive end-expiratory pressure (PEEP) in acute respiratory insufficiency. *Chest.* 1975;67:156.
33. Katz JA, Marks JD. Inspiratory work with and without continuous positive airway pressure in patients with acute respiratory failure. *Anesthesiology.* 1985;63:598.
34. Perel A, Williamson DC, Modell JH. Effectiveness of CPAP by mask

for pulmonary edema associated with hypercarbia. *Intensive Care Med.* 1983;9:17.

35. Bersten AD, Holt AW, Vedig AE, et al. Treatment of severe pulmonary edema with continuous positive airway pressure delivered by face mask. *N Engl J Med.* 1991;325:1825.

36. Räsänen J, Väisänen I, Heikkilä J, et al. Acute myocardial infarction complicated by left ventricular dysfunction and respiratory failure: the effects of continuous positive airway pressure. *Chest.* 1985;87:158.

37. Väisänen I, Räsänen J. The cardiopulmonary effects of continuous positive airway pressure and supplemental oxygen in patients with acute cardiogenic pulmonary edema. *Chest.* 1987;92:481.

38. Kirby RR, Banner MJ, Downs JB, eds. *Clinical Applications of Ventilatory Support.* New York, NY: Churchill Livingstone; 1990.

39. Gattinoni L, Pesenti A, Bombino M, et al. Extracorporeal carbon dioxide removal. In Grenvik A, Downs JB, Räsänen J, et al, eds. *Mechanical Ventilation and Assisted Respiration: Contemporary Management in Critical Care.* New York, NY: Churchill Livingstone; 1990:591.

40. Dalton HJ, Thompson AE. Extracorporeal membrane oxygenation. In: Grenvik A, Downs JB, Räsänen J, et al, eds. *Mechanical Ventilation and Assisted Respiration: Contemporary Management in Critical Care.* New York, NY: Churchill Livingstone; 1990:5.

41. Edmondson JW, Brashear RE, Li TK. Tetany: quantitative interrelationships between calcium and alkalosis. *Am J Physiol.* 1975;228:1082.

42. Coetzee A, Holland D, Foëx P, et al. The effect of hypocapnia on coronary blood flow and myocardial function in the dog. *Anesth Analg.* 1984;63:991.

43. Rasmussen K, Bagger JP, Bottzauw J, et al. Prevalence of vasospastic ischaemia induced by the cold pressor test or hyperventilation in patients with severe angina. *Eur Heart J.* 1984;5:354.

44. Downs JB, Douglas ME, Ruiz BC, et al. Comparison of assisted and controlled mechanical ventilation in anesthetized swine. *Crit Care Med.* 1979;7:5.

45. Brown HW, Plum F. The neurologic basis of Cheyne-Stokes respiration. *Am J Med.* 1961;30:849.

46. Hey EN, Loyd BB, Cunningham DJC, et al. Effects of various respiratory stimuli on the depth and frequency of breathing in man. *Respir Physiol.* 1966;1:193.

47. Narins RG, Emmett M. Simple and mixed acid-base disorders: a practical approach. *Medicine.* 1980;59:161.

48. Farber HR, Yiengst MJ, Shock NW. The effect of therapeutic doses of aspirin on the acid-base balance of the blood in normal adults. *Am J Med Sci.* 1949;217:256.

49. Lemaire F, Teboul JL, Cinotti L, et al. Acute left ventricular dysfunction during unsuccessful weaning from mechanical ventilation. *Anesthesiology.* 1988;69:171.

50. Viires N, Sillye G, Rassidakis A, et al. Effect of mechanical ventilation on respiratory muscle blood flow during shock. *Physiologist.* 1980;23:1.

51. Mason DT, Spann JF Jr, Zelis R, et al. Alterations of hemodynamics and myocardial mechanics in patients with congestive heart failure: pathophysiologic mechanism and assessment of cardiac function and ventricular contractility. *Prog Cardiovasc Dis.* 1970;12:507.

52. Pinsky MR, Matuschak GM, Klain M. Determinants of cardiac augmentation by elevations in intrathoracic pressure. *J Appl Physiol.* 1985;58:1189.

53. Scharf SM, Bianco JA, Tow DE, Brown R. The effects of large negative intrathoracic pressure on left ventricular function in patients with coronary artery disease. *Circulation.* 1981;63:871.

54. Weber KT, Janicki JS, Hunter WC, et al. The contractile behavior of the heart and its functional coupling to the circulation. *Prog Cardiovasc Dis.* 1982;24:375.

55. Katz JA, Marks JD. Inspiratory work with and without continuous positive airway pressure in patients with acute respiratory failure. *Anesthesiology.* 1985;63:598.

56. Beydon L, Chasse M, Harf A, et al. Inspiratory work of breathing during spontaneous ventilation using demand valves and continuous flow systems. *Am Rev Respir Dis.* 1988;138:300.

57. Christopher KL, Neff TA, Bowman JL, et al. Demand and continuous flow intermittent mandatory ventilation systems. *Chest.* 1985;87:625.

58. Bolder PM, Hedy TEJ, Bolder AR, et al. The extra work of breathing through adult endotracheal tubes. *Anesth Analg.* 1986;65:853.

59. Fiastro JF, Habib MP, Quan SF. Pressure support compensation for inspiratory work due to endotracheal tubes and demand continuous positive airway pressure. *Chest.* 1988;93:499.

60. Christie JM, Smith RA. Pressure support ventilation decreases inspiratory work of breathing during general anesthesia and spontaneous ventilation. *Anesth Analg.* 1992;75:167.

61. Banner MJ, Downs JB, Kirby RR, et al. Effects of expiratory flow resistance on inspiratory work of breathing. *Chest.* 1988;93:795.

62. Marini JJ, Culver BH, Kirk W. Flow resistance of exhalation valves and positive end-expiratory pressure devices used in mechanical ventilation. *Am Rev Respir Dis.* 1985;131:850.

63. Abbrecht PH, Rajagopal KR, Kyle RR. Expiratory muscle recruitment during inspiratory flow-resistive loading and exercise. *Am Rev Respir Dis.* 1991;144:113.

64. Pinsky MR, Hrehocik D, Culpepper JA, et al. Flow resistance of expiratory positive-pressure systems. *Chest.* 1988;94:788.

65. Mecklenburgh JS, Latto IP, Al-Obaidi TAA, et al. Excessive work of breathing during intermittent mandatory ventilation. *Br J Anaesth.* 1986;58:1048.

66. Downs JB, Mitchell LA. Pulmonary effects of ventilatory pattern following cardiopulmonary bypass. *Crit Care Med.* 1976;4:295.

67. Nunn JF. Elastic forces and lung volumes. In: Nunn JF, ed. *Applied Respiratory Physiology.* 3rd ed. London, United Kingdom: Butterworths; 1987:23.

68. Gattinoni L, Pesenti A, Torresin A, et al. Adult respiratory distress syndrome profiles by computed tomography. *J Thorac Imaging.* 1986;1:25.

69. Gattinoni L, Pesenti A, Bombino M, et al. Relationships between lung computed tomographic density, gas exchange, and PEEP in acute respiratory failure. *Anesthesiology.* 1988;69:824.

70. Drummond WH, Gregory GA, Heymann MA, et al. The independent effects of hyperventilation, tolazoline and dopamine on infants with persistent pulmonary hypertension. *J Pediatr.* 1981;93:603.

71. Grekin RJ. Ketoacidosis, hyperosmolar states and lactic acidosis. In: Kokko JP, Tannen RL, eds. *Fluids and Electrolytes.* Philadelphia, Pa: WB Saunders; 1986:688.

# 47

# Cardiopulmonary Resuscitation

Richard J. Melker
Robert R. Kirby

Desperate measures long have been used to try to restore life to the dead and dying.[1] Early techniques included placing burning materials on the chest and abdomen to restore warmth to a cold body and flagellating with whips or stinging nettles to revive the victim. Carrying the person on the back of a trotting horse or rolling him or her over a barrel was thought to mimic a normal respiratory pattern. Not until the 19th century were true anatomic and physiologic principles incorporated into resuscitative techniques.

Cardiopulmonary resuscitation (CPR) has been widely accepted since its introduction in 1961. Initially, enthusiasm was high for this new technique, which combined artificial ventilation with closed chest cardiac compression.[2] It was predicted that this technique would replace open chest cardiac massage and improve survival rates dramatically. Predictions suggested that 70% of out-of-hospital victims of witnessed ventricular fibrillation (VF) or tachycardia would be saved with effective bystander CPR and paramedic response time of less than 4 minutes.[3] Further, 80% of cardiac arrest patients admitted to a coronary care unit (CCU) were estimated to survive with the immediate availability of a defibrillator and adequately trained personnel.

In fact, survival rates for both the prehospital[4] and in-hospital settings have been dramatically lower.[5,6] Prehospital

**TABLE 47–1.** Patient and Cardiopulmonary Resuscitation (CPR) Variables Related to Outcome

| Variable | Poor Outcome | Favorable Outcome |
|---|---|---|
| Prearrest | Malignancy, sepsis; end-stage renal, neurologic, respiratory disease | Absence of these variables |
| Intraarrest | Prolonged CPR (>30 min); initial asystole or pulseless electrical activity; unwitnessed arrest | Short duration (<15 min); initial ventricular fibrillation and ventricular tachycardia; witnessed arrest |
| Postarrest | Coma >48 h; Glasgow Coma Score (GCS) ≤4 at 24 h; absent brainstem reflexes | Absence of coma; GCS ≥10 at 24 h; return of pupillary, light, corneal reflexes |

and in-hospital resuscitation frequently is performed on victims with comorbid noncardiac conditions and noncardiac origins of arrest. Prehospital survival is determined primarily by the etiology of arrest. For primary cardiac arrest resulting in VF or ventricular tachycardia (VT), critical determinants of success include whether the arrest is witnessed and how much time elapses from arrest to arrival of a defibrillator.[3]

Survival rates for cardiac arrest secondary to other etiologies (eg, drowning, drug overdose, trauma) remain low and have not changed significantly in the almost three decades since the introduction of emergency medical systems. Likewise, survival rates for both noncritically ill (floor)[5,6] and critically ill (intensive care)[7] hospitalized patients have never met early expectations and have not improved significantly since the introduction of CPR. Several factors affect in-hospital survival rates[5] (Table 47–1).

Survival in children has not been demonstrated to be higher than in adults. Early studies suggested that children in intensive care units were more likely to respond (with meaningful survival) to high-dose epinephrine than adults.[8,9] However, research does not confirm that routine use of initial and repeated or escalating doses of epinephrine can improve survival in cardiac arrest (class indeterminate) and does not improve neurologic outcomes. Cardiac arrest survivors who receive high-dose epinephrine may have more postresuscitation complications than survivors who received the standard dose. Because of the potential for harm, high-dose epinephrine (0.1 mg/kg) is not recommended (class indeterminate).[10]

Patients with multiple organ failure or critical illness unrelated to heart disease have a poor prognosis. The question is how to distinguish patients who have a good prognosis for meaningful survival and might benefit from CPR from the considerable number with poor expected outcome in whom CPR can be confidently withheld. Early involvement of the patient's family and, when possible, the patient, in decision-making precludes unnecessary resuscitative attempts. This problem is particularly acute in the operating room (OR) for patients who require surgery but who have do-not-resuscitate orders in effect. When and how to handle this particular situation is receiving increased attention in anesthesiology.[11]

## GOALS

CPR is intended to support or restore respiration and, in cardiac arrest, to provide some perfusion of the brain and heart. It consists of basic, intermediate, and advanced life support techniques.

### What Is Basic Life Support?

Basic life support (BLS) includes creating a patent airway, using mouth-to-mouth ventilation, and, in the setting of cardiac arrest, performing closed chest cardiac massage. These techniques were introduced in the early 1960s. The ABC steps of CPR

**A,** Airway
**B,** Breathing
**C,** Circulation

constitute the initial management of unconscious patients. Proper execution of these skills in the prescribed sequence is essential.

### What Is Intermediate Life Support?

Intermediate life support constitutes a situation in which some adjuncts of advanced life support (ALS) are available but not others. This scenario is frequently the case in prehospital care, when emergency medical service personnel may be trained to ventilate with a bag-valve-mask but not to perform tracheal intubation, or they may be trained to use an automatic external defibrillator but not to start intravenous infusions or give drugs.

### What Is Advanced Life Support?

ALS, the techniques of which are in a state of constant revision, comprises additional methods of airway management plus the prompt diagnosis and, when appropriate, treatment of life-threatening arrhythmias. Definitive management of these arrhythmias may require defibrillation, cardioversion, pacemaker insertion, and pharmacologic therapy. Interim recommendations (advisory statements) have been published by the International Liaison Committee on Resuscitation (ILCOR) and are available at the American Heart Association (AHA) website: http://www.americanheart.org/scientific/statements/index.html. In 2000, new AHA guidelines for CPR and emergency cardiac care were published.[10]

## AIRWAY

### How Should Support Be Provided?

#### Patency

After establishing that a patient is unconscious, the rescuer must evaluate airway patency. If possible, the patient should be placed in the supine position, preferably on a firm surface, with the neck slightly flexed at the shoulders and extended at the atlantoaxial joint in the so-called sniffing position (Fig. 47–1). This position can be maintained by placing a towel or roll under the victim's occiput.

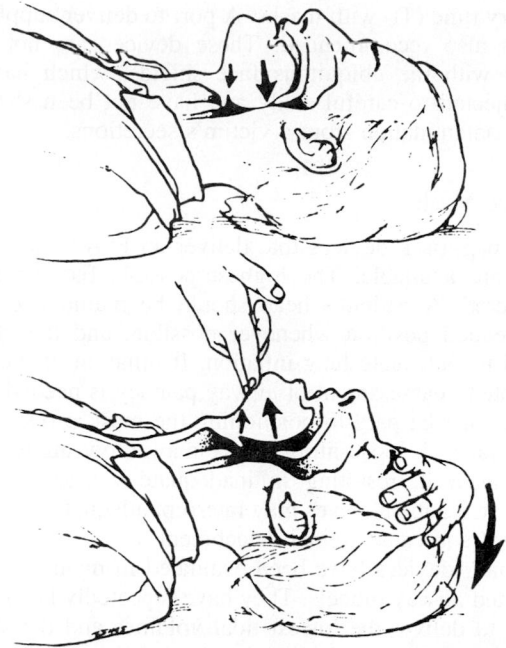

**FIGURE 47–1.** A patent airway is best created by extending the head and lifting the mandible anteriorly. (Reproduced with permission from Adjuncts for airway control, ventilation, and supplemental oxygen. In: *Textbook of Advanced Cardiac Life Support.* 2nd ed. Dallas, Tex: American Heart Association; 1987:27.)

Observe the chest and abdomen for signs of spontaneous respiration or evidence of airway obstruction, such as paradoxical movement of the chest and abdomen, intercostal retraction, and absent or noisy upper airway respiratory sounds. The tongue, epiglottis, and soft tissues of the posterior pharynx may completely obstruct the upper airway of an unconscious patient unless the head is maintained in the sniffing position. This simple maneuver, which often is all that is necessary to establish a patent airway, must be executed carefully so that the cervical vertebrae, spinal cord, and nerves are not injured. When unconscious patients are spontaneously breathing, rolling them on their side into the recovery position is now recommended to decrease the likelihood of obstruction and aspiration.

### Cervical Fractures

If cervical fractures are suspected (eg, in a trauma victim), the head should not be hyperextended because of an even greater chance of damaging the spinal cord. Lifting or thrusting the jaw forward may move the tongue anteriorly and create a patent airway without hyperextension of the head (Fig. 47–2). When the patient's condition allows both maneuvers to be used, however, the combination of jaw lift and hyperextension usually is more successful.

### Infants

The upper airway is most patent in infants when the head is maintained in the sniffing position. Hyperextension may collapse the soft trachea, which does not have well-formed rigid cartilaginous rings. Spontaneously breathing unconscious infants and children can also be placed in the recovery position.

## What Is the Role for Nasal and Oropharyngeal Airways?

When airway adjuncts are available, additional procedures may be performed if the patient shows signs of airway obstruction despite proper positioning of the head or lifting the jaw. Any obvious foreign materials that obstruct the airway, such as food, vomitus, or a loose dental prosthesis, should be removed. A nasal or oropharyngeal airway may relieve the obstruction caused by soft tissue. Insertion of a nasal airway, however, may traumatize the nasal mucosa and cause bleeding, which exacerbates the existing obstruction.

Semiconscious patients may tolerate a nasal airway better than an oral airway, which predisposes to gagging and vomiting. On the other hand, an oral airway is probably more effective in unconscious patients. When improperly inserted, however, it can push the tongue back into the pharynx and worsen, the airway obstruction.

## How Is a Foreign Body Removed?

Since 1976, subdiaphragmatic abdominal thrusts (the Heimlich maneuver) have been recommended to dislodge and expel a foreign body that is not readily visible. Slapping blows with the open palm on the midposterior thorax, which may increase airway pressure enough to dislodge the object, are recommended only in infants. Midsternal chest thrusts, in erect or supine patients, may generate enough expulsive air movement from the chest to expel the foreign body and can be used in pregnant or obese people or in children. Abdominal thrusts should not be used in these patients because they increase the risk for injury to the fetus or the abdominal organs.

After these maneuvers are completed, the mouth should be gently probed for any dislodged materials. A child's mouth should not be probed for foreign objects because they can easily be forced more deeply into the airway. Instead, the pharynx can be examined if the rescuer places his or her

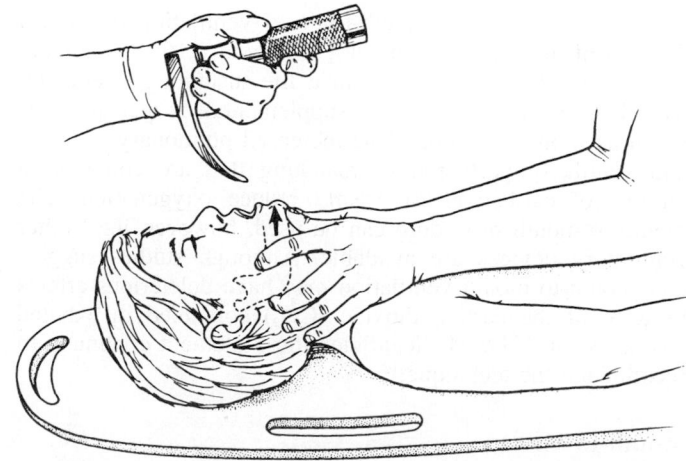

**FIGURE 47–2.** Cervical spine stabilization and intubation. One person holds the head and neck with both hands, lifting the jaw and immobilizing the neck. The other performs the intubation. (From Emergency Cardiac Care Committee and Subcommittee, American Heart Association. Guidelines for cardiopulmonary resuscitation and emergency cardiac care, VII: neonatal resuscitation. *JAMA.* 1992;268:2271. Copyright 1992, American Medical Association.)

thumb over the child's tongue and lifts the jaw forward. The foreign body, once visualized, should be removed.

## BREATHING

In some situations, a patient's life may be saved by simply creating a patent airway. In many cases, however, it is necessary to assist or to control a patient's ventilation. This is the second step in the resuscitation plan.

### Is the Victim Apneic?

If a victim is not breathing, give two slow lung inflations (ie, the inflation takes at least 2 seconds) of about 800 mL with sufficient time for exhalation between breaths. Positive airway pressure increases the chance of gastric inflation in patients with an unprotected airway and greatly increases the incidence of regurgitation and aspiration. One should strive, therefore, to keep it as low as possible by using long inspiratory times. Gastric inflation may also cause restriction of diaphragmatic excursion, and thus ventilation, particularly in infants. Ventilation should then continue with inflation of the lungs about every 5 to 6 seconds (10-12 per minute) in adults and every 3 seconds (20 per minute) in infants.

The 2000 ventilation guidelines recommended a reduction in the ventilation tidal volume to about one half of that recommended previously for patients not in cardiovascular collapse.[10] Volume should approximate 6 to 7 mL/kg over 1.5 to 2 seconds in adults (class IIa) and 1 second in children. The "chest rise" sign can be used as a rough indication of ventilation tidal volumes that are in the range of 6 to 7 mL/kg. Smaller tidal volumes increase the risk for inducing hypoxia and hypercarbia. Therefore, supplemental oxygen ($O_2$) should be provided whenever possible.

### What Methods Are Available?

#### Mouth-to-Mouth

Mouth-to-mouth (or mouth-to-nose) ventilation delivers a fraction of inspired oxygen ($FIO_2$) of about 0.16; this amount is usually sufficient to maintain a life-sustaining arterial $O_2$ partial pressure. Nevertheless, supplemental oxygen must be given as soon as possible. The increased pulmonary shunting and ventilation-perfusion mismatching that are common in victims of cardiac arrest greatly reduce oxygenation. The mouth-to-mouth procedure can be used, however, until other ventilatory devices are available. Although studies suggest that mouth-to-mouth ventilation may have deleterious effects because of the carbon dioxide ($CO_2$) contained in exhaled gas, a recent AHA Medical/Scientific Statement continued to recommend the technique.[12]

#### Mouth-to-Mask

Studies have demonstrated the superiority of mouth-to-mask ventilation over bag-valve-mask ventilation. Most masks are fitted with one-way valves to prevent rebreathing of exhaled gas by the rescuer. Mannequin studies show that all groups of rescuers (emergency medical technicians, paramedics, physicians) deliver higher tidal volume ($VT$) with longer

inspiratory time ($TI$) with masks. A port to deliver supplemental $O_2$ is also recommended. These devices are not to be confused with the ubiquitous face shields, which have not been subjected to careful study and have not been shown to prevent contamination from a victim's secretions.

### Bag-Valve-Mask

Many bag-mask devices that deliver an $FIO_2$ between 0.21 and 1.0 are available. The highest possible $FIO_2$ should be administered. A patient's head should be maintained in the hyperextended position whenever possible, and the chest is observed for adequate lung inflation. If inflation of the stomach is noted, reassessment of airway patency is needed. Close attention must be paid to positioning the mask properly on a patient's face. A loose-fitting mask may allow air to escape from beneath it, resulting in inadequate ventilation. Mask pressure on a patient's eyes may interrupt adequate blood flow to the eyes and cause retinal detachment.

Bag-mask devices have been evaluated in mannequins and unprotected airway models. They have repeatedly been shown not only to deliver the lowest tidal volumes and the shortest $TI$ of all devices but also to result in the greatest magnitude of gastric insufflation. Whenever possible, they should be used by two rescuers to ensure adequate mask seal, and two hands should squeeze the bag.[13] Additionally, cricoid pressure should be used during ventilation of unintubated patients to reduce the risk for gastric insufflation, regurgitation, and pulmonary aspiration.

### Tracheal Intubation

Tracheal intubation is indicated for patients with an otherwise difficult to manage airway and for patients who remain unconscious. The new guidelines suggest that only ACLS providers with 6–12 intubations per year should attempt intubation.[13]

A critically important recommendation is contained in the 2000 guidelines: *tracheal tube position must be confirmed by using nonphysical examination techniques.*[10] Included in this category are esophageal detector devices and qualitative or quantitative end-tidal $CO_2$ devices. In patients not in full cardiac arrest, these devices are class IIa. In patients in cardiac arrest and with conditions of low pulmonary flow, the class is lowered to IIb because the devices may falsely indicate esophageal placement, leading to unnecessary removal of a properly placed tube.

### Airway Adjuncts

Recommended devices for emergency use include the esophageal-tracheal double-lumen Combitube (Kendall-Sheridan Catheter Corp, Argyle, NY) (Fig. 47–3). This device has been classified as IIb by National Institutes of Health (NIH) criteria and is, therefore, considered to be acceptable and possibly helpful; however, the full extent of complications is not yet known, nor have they been well studied.

A recent report showed that the hemodynamic stress response (increased plasma epinephrine and norepinephrine levels) after insertion of this device was significantly greater than that associated with tracheal intubation or insertion of a laryngeal mask airway.[14] What the implication of these findings might be to a patient in cardiac arrest is unclear. However,

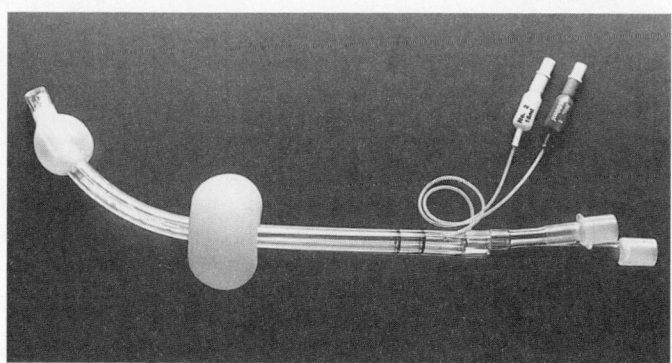

**FIGURE 47–3.** The Combitube (esophageal-tracheal double-lumen airway) can be used as an esophageal blocker or an endotracheal tube. It is particularly useful as a bridge to a definitive airway in patients with congenital or acquired facial and cervical spine abnormalities in whom conventional tracheal intubation is difficult or impossible.

such a response in an already stressed patient, who has not yet arrested, might be deleterious. Endotrol endotracheal tubes (ETTs) (Mallinckrodt Medical-Anesthesia Division, St Louis, Mo), a prepackaged cricothyrotomy set such as the Melker percutaneous dilational cricothyrotomy set (Amplatz extra stiff wire guide, Cook Critical Care, Bloomington, Ind) (Fig. 47–4), equipment for transtracheal jet ventilation, ETT changers, and laryngeal mask airways should be available in an emergency airway cart.

## When Are Emergency Percutaneous or Surgical Techniques Indicated?

Cricothyroidotomy[15] and transtracheal catheter ventilation[16] may be required in patients who cannot be ventilated with a mask or cannot be intubated, as may occur after face and neck trauma.

## Cricothyroidotomy

Cricothyroidotomy is performed by puncturing the cricothyroid membrane with either a cricothyroidotomy blade and tube or a knife blade. Percutaneous cricothyroidotomy sets for the placement of tubes by the Seldinger technique are available[15] (see Fig. 47–4). Once a tube has been placed through the cricothyroidotomy, a patient should be able to breathe spontaneously or with controlled ventilation through this opening.

## Transtracheal Catheter Ventilation

For transtracheal catheter ventilation, a 14-gauge catheter-over-needle is inserted in a caudal direction through the cricothyroid membrane into the larynx.[17,18] A high-pressure jet of $O_2$ (at least 20 pounds per square inch gauge) introduced through this catheter into the trachea inflates the lungs. The pressure generated in the airway with this technique is dissipated (ie, exhaled) through the glottis and mouth. If upper airway obstruction occludes this escape route, extremely high intrapulmonary pressures with resulting barotrauma can occur.

These procedures can be life saving, but they are not without hazards. They should be used only when other, less traumatic methods are not feasible and should be performed only by trained individuals. Potential complications include hemorrhage, creation of a false passage, subcutaneous or mediastinal emphysema, perforation of the esophagus, infection, pneumothorax, and subsequent tracheal stenosis.

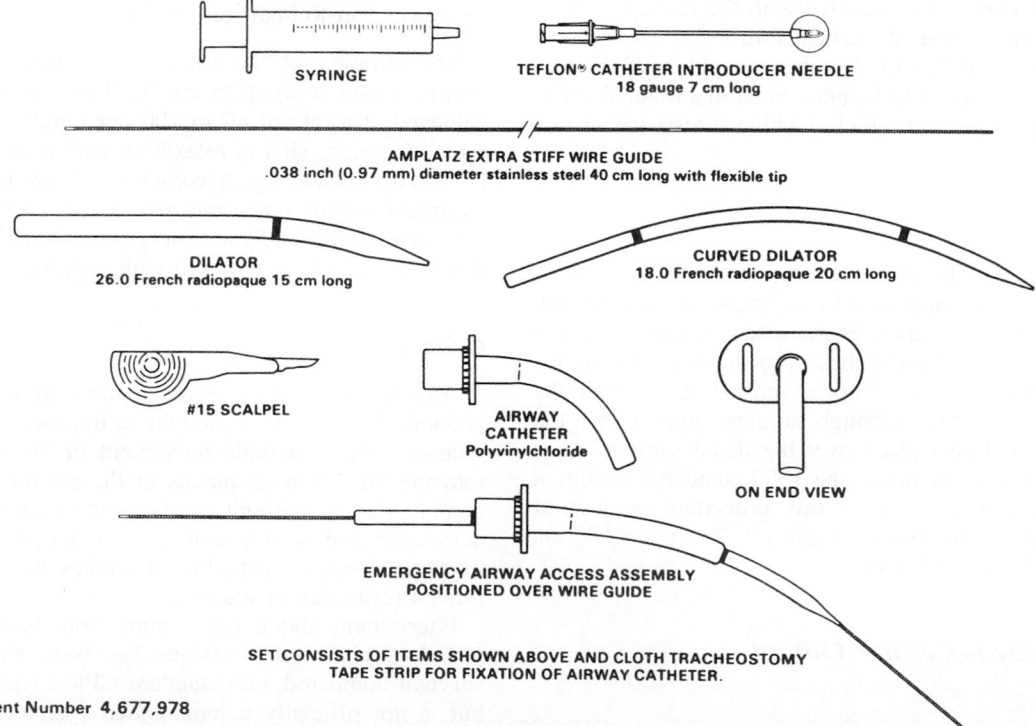

**FIGURE 47–4.** Melker emergency cricothyrotomy catheter set. Airway access is gained by percutaneous entry through the cricothyroid membrane. Subsequently, dilation of the trachea and tracheal entrance site permits insertion of 6-mm internal diameter airway. Positive pressure ventilation and spontaneous breathing are permitted. (Courtesy of Cook Critical Care, Bloomington, Ind.)

## CIRCULATION

If a patient has respiratory arrest only, creating a patent airway for life support or providing adequate ventilation may be all that is necessary. In many situations, however, respiratory arrest occurs in conjunction with cardiac arrest or life-threatening arrhythmia. After establishing a patent airway and giving an apneic patient the initial lung inflations, the rescuer should evaluate cardiac function by feeling for a carotid pulse. The carotid pulse can easily be palpated just lateral to the thyroid cartilage. Because of peripheral vasoconstriction associated with a shock state, the radial pulse may be difficult to palpate. The femoral pulse may also be difficult to locate in some patients because of body habitus.

In children, the precordial impulse or the brachial or temporal artery pulse may be more easily monitored. If the pulse is absent and the patient is unconscious, external cardiac compression should be initiated. In cases with significant hypovolemia (hemorrhagic shock), no benefit accrues to the Trendelenburg (head-down) position. Instead, the legs should be elevated to enhance venous return.

### *How Is Closed Chest Cardiac Massage Performed?*

#### Adults

External cardiac compression is a relatively simple technique that can be performed after appropriate training. However, it may be totally ineffective or even hazardous if performed improperly. After positioning at the side of the patient, the rescuer should place the heel of one hand over the lower half of the sternum about 1 to 1.5 inches above the tip of the xiphoid. The heel of the second hand is then placed on top of the first. The arms must be extended with the rescuer's finger tips off the patient's chest. A vertical thrust that displaces an adult's sternum about 1.5 to 2 inches should be delivered. Closed cardiac massage must be performed in a regular, deliberate, uninterrupted manner; quick, jabbing thrusts are far less effective.[19]

#### Infants

In infants, the middle and index finger tips of one hand traditionally were recommended to compress the midsternum a distance of 0.5 to 0.75 inch. Some rescuers prefer to place their hands around an infant's chest, positioning both thumbs on the midsternum and exerting a vertical thrust with the thumb tips (Fig. 47–5). Although studies suggest that the compression should take place over the distal sternum, as is the case in adult resuscitation,[20] the 1992 standards for infant resuscitation do not recommend this procedure because of potential damage to abdominal organs.[21] In small children, only the heel of one hand is used.

### *How Effectively Is Cardiac Output Maintained?*

Under ideal circumstances of CPR and drug therapy, a cardiac output of about 30% of pre-arrest blood flow can be maintained with effective external compression; therefore,

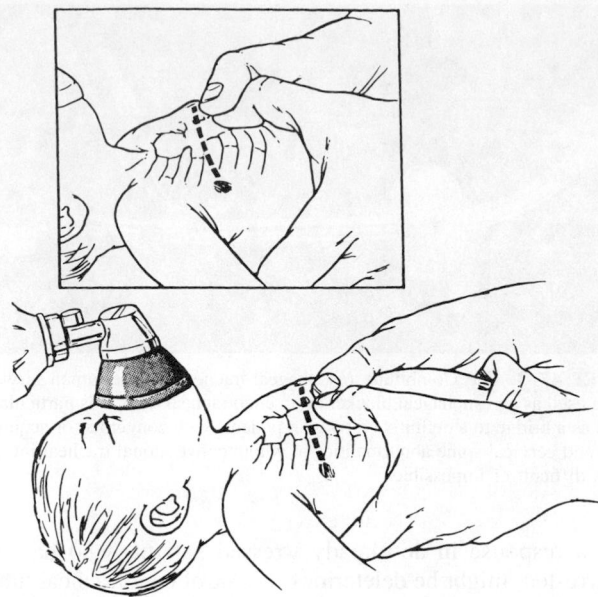

**FIGURE 47–5.** Method of external cardiac compression in neonates and small infants. (From Emergency Cardiac Care Committee and Subcommittee, American Heart Association. Guidelines for cardiopulmonary resuscitation and emergency cardiac care, VII: neonatal resuscitation. *JAMA.* 1992;268:2279. Copyright 1992, American Medical Association.)

only minimal interruptions are tolerated. Both the compression of the heart between the sternum and vertebral column (chest pump model) and the increase in intrathoracic pressure during compression (thoracic pump model) may cause the forward flow of blood from the chest in some instances; in others, one mechanism or the other predominates.

### Compression-Relaxation Cycle

The duration of the compression should be 50% of the compression-relaxation cycle. This ratio is most easily achieved at a rate of 80 to 100 per minute. Maintaining this ratio of compression to relaxation with a manual technique is physically exhausting. A commercially available $O_2$-powered automatic compression unit may be more effective and is not subject to human fatigue. These portable units provide effective compressions interposed with appropriate ventilation.[22]

### G-Suits

An additional adjunct is the application of a G-suit over the abdominal cavity. It is thought to improve cardiac output by retarding the retrograde movement of blood from the heart into the large venous plexus in the peritoneal cavity during compression.[23] This suit can be used in combination with the automatic compression unit for an even greater improvement in cardiac output, but clinical studies have not shown improved resuscitation success.

Intermittent abdominal compression during the relaxation phase of chest compressions has been shown to improve survival compared with standard CPR on in-hospital patients but is not officially recommended.[24] A recent animal study suggested that aortic occlusion in conjunction with epinephrine improves myocardial and coronary blood flow and can lead to spontaneous restoration of circulation.[25] Although this technique will not have broad application, it might be considered in the OR setting if aortic occlusion is possible.

## Compression Rate

### Two Rescuers

If two rescuers are present, one can perform cardiac compressions while the second ventilates the patient. The rate of cardiac compression in this case is 80 to 100 per minute for adults, with a compression-to-ventilation ratio of 15 compressions for every two breaths no matter how many rescuers are on hand.[10] Exhalation occurs during chest compression.

Simultaneous compression and ventilation previously was evaluated as a means of further increasing cardiac output; it did not improve survival[26] and is not currently recommended. However, application of continuous positive airway pressure (CPAP) without mechanical ventilation has been shown in animals to reduce $PaCO_2$, increase $SaO_2$, and increase arteriovenous $O_2$ content difference during chest compressions without positive pressure ventilation.[27] The investigators hypothesized that this approach might be useful to reduce the risk for gastric insufflation and presumably the potential for aspiration of gastric contents in unintubated patients undergoing CPR. Furthermore, use of CPAP, as opposed to manual or mechanical positive pressure ventilation, might eliminate the need for a second rescuer.

Although close attention must be paid to both the rate of compression and the ratio of compression to relaxation, the latter probably has a greater influence on cardiac output. The second rescuer must periodically check the carotid pulse to evaluate the effectiveness of the cardiac compressions and to note the return of spontaneous cardiac activity. Bear in mind, however, that a palpable carotid pulse may reflect only external, not internal, carotid artery flow; thus, it does not guarantee effective cerebral circulation.

### One Rescuer

Fifteen chest compressions are performed at a rate of 80 to 100 per minute, followed by two breaths of 1.5 to 2 seconds each. This cycle is repeated four times, followed by reassess-

**TABLE 47–2.** Complications Associated With Closed Chest Compression

| |
|---|
| Fracture of the xiphoid and sternum |
| Costochondral separation |
| Pneumothorax |
| Hemothorax |
| Lung contusion |
| Laceration of the liver, stomach, heart, and lungs |
| Fat embolization |
| Cardiac contusion |

ment. If CPR is continued, the rescuer should reassess for pulse and spontaneous breathing every few minutes. In infants, compressions are performed at about 100 to 120 per minute, with one breath interposed after every fifth compression. BLS should be continued until the patient has recovered, the rescuers are exhausted, relief rescuers have arrived, or a medical decision to discontinue resuscitative efforts has been made.

## Complications

Complications related to closed chest compression are listed in Table 47–2.

## How Is the Efficacy of Cardiopulmonary Resuscitation Monitored?

No reliable prognostic indicator exists for the efficacy of ongoing CPR efforts. Experimental studies suggest that aortic diastolic and coronary perfusion pressures correlate with successful resuscitation.[28] These findings have been corroborated in a small number of human beings. When arterial catheters are present, the diastolic pressure should be optimized, and in instances in which a pulmonary artery catheter is available, arterial minus right atrial diastolic pressure may be an indicator of CPR efficacy and survival.

Capnography is promising to evaluate blood flow during CPR[29,30] and for confirming ETT placement (Fig. 47–6). Un-

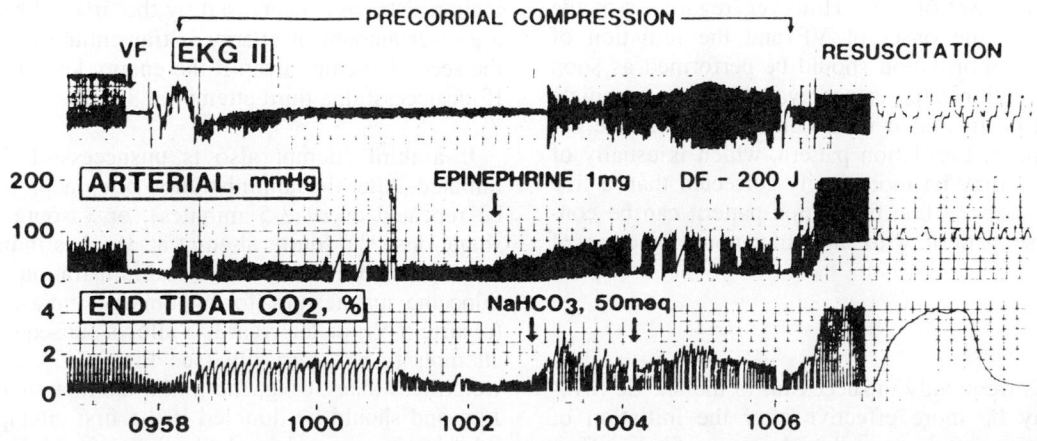

**FIGURE 47–6.** Serial changes in the end-tidal carbon dioxide concentration ($ETCO_2$), arterial blood pressure, and electrocardiograph in a patient before and immediately after a cardiac arrest, during precordial compression, and after defibrillation (DF) and resuscitation. The transient increase in the $ETCO_2$ after the administration of sodium bicarbonate ($NaHCO_3$) is also demonstrated. The original tracing has been modified because of space limitations. (Modified from Falk JL, Rackow EC, Weil MH. End-tidal carbon dioxide concentration during cardiopulmonary resuscitation. *N Engl J Med.* 1988;318:607–611, with permission from *The New England Journal of Medicine.*)

fortunately, many drugs given during resuscitation, and a variable minute ventilation, unless a patient is mechanically ventilated, interfere with the interpretation of end-tidal $CO_2$ measurements during CPR. Despite these caveats, a sudden increase in end-tidal $CO_2$ is generally the earliest sign of return of spontaneous ventilation, unless sodium bicarbonate ($NaHCO_3$) has just been given[31] (see Fig. 47–6). Recent studies support this limited value of capnography during CPR and suggest that patients with higher end-tidal $CO_2$ during CPR are more likely to be resuscitated successfully.[32]

## What Is the Role of the Precordial Thump?

### Indications

A precordial thump is most effective when it is performed as soon as possible after the onset of VT or fibrillation and when the arrhythmia is not secondary to hypoxia.[33] This technique is used only when the rescuer observes the onset of the arrhythmia and a defibrillator is not immediately available, as may occur in monitored patients in the OR, postanesthesia care unit, or intensive care unit or in unmonitored patients who suffer an arrest in the presence of someone who can initiate therapy immediately.

### Technique

A precordial thump is performed by delivering a single blow to the midsternum with the fleshy portion of the clenched fist from a distance of 8 to 12 inches. Repeated precordial thumps are not indicated. An effective precordial thump interrupts VT and VF by causing ventricular depolarization. The cardiac activity may then return with a coordinated contraction, frequently of supraventricular origin. Performing the thump in a patient with VT can, unfortunately, also cause conversion to VF, asystole, or pulseless electrical activity.

## How Is Ventricular Defibrillation Performed?

Defibrillation is most successful when it is performed immediately after the onset of VF.[34] However, regardless of the time lapse between the onset of VF and the initiation of therapy, electrical defibrillation should be performed as soon as possible. If a defibrillator is not available for immediate use, BLS should be instituted until defibrillation can be accomplished. A coarse fibrillation pattern, which is usually of more recent onset, may be more easily corrected than a fine pattern. In many cases, a fine fibrillation pattern can be converted to a coarse pattern with an intravenous injection of epinephrine.

### Precautions

Defibrillation is frequently unsuccessful in the anoxic myocardium and may be more effective after the initiation of CPR. This situation often prevails when a patient suffers cardiac arrest outside the hospital or when it is secondary to hypoxia, as may occur in drug overdose, asphyxiation, or near-drowning. Defibrillation is also less successful when it is performed in a patient who is acidotic. However, immediate defibrillation should be attempted in all situations if feasible, even before initiating BLS or administering drugs.[34] Electrical defibrillation is not indicated in the treatment of asystole unless there is uncertainty about whether the rhythm is fine VF or asystole.[35] More than one electrocardiogram (ECG) lead tracing should be viewed to make this determination.

### Technique

Before the paddles are placed on a patient's chest, conductive electrode paste or saline sponges should be applied. Skin impedance is thereby decreased, and the efficiency of current passage through the thorax is increased. The risk for skin burns is also reduced. The electrode paste or saline of one paddle must not come into contact with the conductive material of the other paddle. Otherwise, the amount of current delivered through the myocardium will be reduced and the effectiveness of the defibrillation minimized. The risk for skin burns will also be increased. Alcohol-soaked sponges should never be used as conductive material because the current may cause them to burst into flames.

### Paddle Placement

Two 8- to 12-cm diameter paddles should be placed on the patient's chest, with one paddle to the right of the upper sternum just below the clavicle and the other to the left of the left nipple in the midaxillary line.[36] If the design permits, one paddle may be placed anteriorly over the heart and the other posteriorly.[36,37] This positioning is preferred by some rescuers, but it is not practical in most emergencies. The paddles should be firmly placed against the patient's skin, using an estimated 20 to 25 lb of pressure on each. Smaller paddles should be used in children: 4.5 cm diameter for infants and 8.0 cm for older children.

### Energy Level

The initial defibrillation should be attempted with 200 J of delivered energy.[38] If unsuccessful, a second shock at 200 to 300 J should be attempted immediately. Because the transthoracic resistance is decreased by the first defibrillation attempt, a greater amount of energy is transmitted to the heart during the second attempt, even if the energy level is not increased.[39] If unsuccessful, a third attempt at 360 J is performed (Fig. 47–7).

If a third attempt also is unsuccessful, BLS should be initiated. After the administration of epinephrine, 1.0 mg (may be repeated every 3-5 minutes), or vasopressin, 40 U as a single dose,[10] a fourth attempt at 360 J is indicated. If it, too, is unsuccessful, intravenous administration of amiodarone, lidocaine, magnesium (for hypomagnesemia), or procainamide (recurrent VF or tachycardia) allows subsequent defibrillation attempts to be successful (see Fig. 47–7). For patients who weigh less than 50 kg, the initial attempt should be with two J/kg and should be doubled if the first attempt is unsuccessful.[40] During open chest defibrillation in adults (such as during cardiac surgery), defibrillation should be attempted with 10 J of delivered energy through paddles specifically designed for internal use.[41] The energy may be increased stepwise, if necessary.

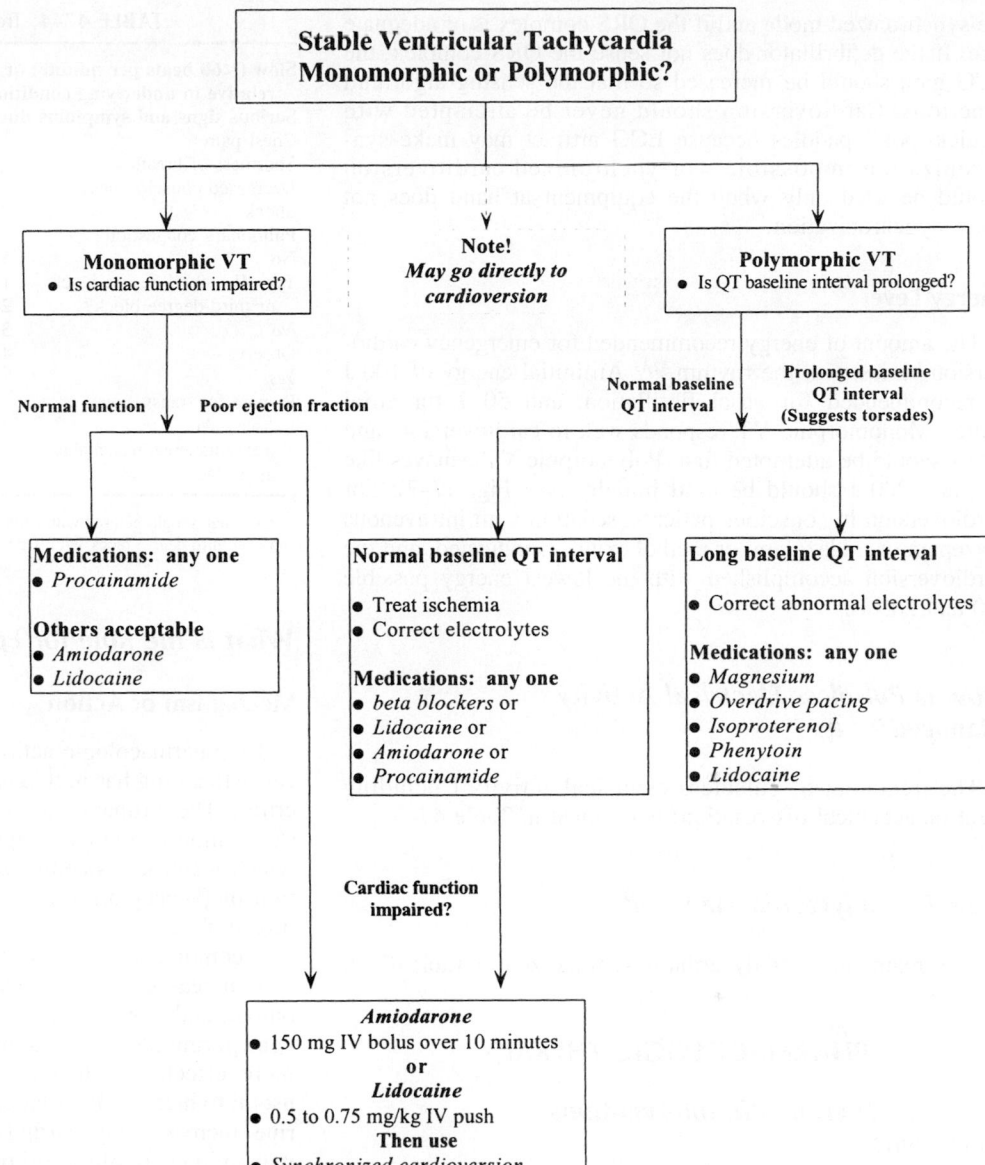

**FIGURE 47–7.** Algorithm for treatment of stable ventricular tachycardia. (Modified from American Heart Association. International Guidelines 2000 for CPR and ECC. *Circulation.* 2000;102[suppl I]:I-1–I-370.)

## Complications

Damage to the myocardium is related to the following factors:

**Energy Level.** The higher the energy level, the greater the potential for myocardial damage. Delivered energy may not be the same as the energy level selected on the defibrillator dials, however. Because internal energy loss may occur in the machine, all defibrillators must be tested periodically for the amount of energy actually delivered through a 50-Ω resistance (the approximate resistance of the body).

**Frequency of Shocks.** Multiple defibrillation attempts in quick succession may be associated with a higher incidence of myocardial damage.

**Electrode Paddle Size.** Large paddles are associated with less myocardial and skin damage than small paddles. Internal paddles, which have a small surface area, should never be used for external defibrillation.

## When Is Electrical Cardioversion Performed?

### Indications

Electrical cardioversion, rather than pharmacologic therapy, may be the treatment of choice for life-threatening arrhythmias causing rapid cardiovascular deterioration. These include VT (see Fig. 47–7) and supraventricular tachycardias (ie, paroxysmal atrial tachycardia, atrial flutter, or atrial fibrillation with a rapid ventricular response).

### Technique

Unlike defibrillation, cardioversion must be synchronized with the patient's ECG. The ideal discharge point is during the upstroke of the R wave of the QRS. Delivery of the energy during the T wave of the QRS may result in VF. Most commercially available defibrillators automatically coordinate the discharge to the patient's ECG if the machine is placed in the synchronized mode and if the QRS complex is of adequate size. If the defibrillator does not sense the QRS complex, the ECG gain should be increased so that the sensing algorithm functions. Cardioversion should never be attempted with "quick-look" paddles because ECG artifact may make synchronization impossible. Unsynchronized cardioversion should be used only when the equipment at hand does not allow synchronization.

### Energy Level

The amount of energy recommended for emergency cardioversion varies with the rhythm.[42,43] An initial energy of 100 J is recommended for atrial fibrillation, and 50 J for atrial flutter. Monomorphic VT responds well to cardioversion, and 100 J should be attempted first. Polymorphic VT behaves like VF, and 200 J should be used initially (see Fig. 47–7). For cardioversion in conscious patients, sedation with intravenous diazepam or midazolam, or methohexital, is indicated, and the cardioversion accomplished with the lowest energy possible (50 and 200 J).

### *How Is Pulseless Electrical Activity Managed?*

The treatment of pulseless electrical activity (including electromechanical dissociation) is outlined in Table 47–3.

### *How Is Bradycardia Managed?*

The treatment of bradycardia is summarized in Table 47–4.

## PHARMACOLOGIC THERAPY

### *How Are Therapeutic Interventions Classified?*

The 1992 National Conference on Cardiopulmonary Resuscitation and Emergency Cardiac Care classified therapeutic interventions according to the scheme in Table 47–5. The AHA adopted the NIH classification system and adapted it for drugs and other interventions.

**TABLE 47–3.** Treatment of Pulseless Electrical Activity*

Check responsiveness, call for defibrillator.
Initiate CPR: intubate, deliver 100% oxygen, start IV, epinephrine 1 mg IV or 2.5 mg via endotracheal tube. (Consider bicarbonate and calcium chloride, but not through endotracheal tube.)
Continue CPR (consider volume infusion).
Consider cause secondary to hypovolemia, cardiac tamponade, acute coronary syndrome, tension pneumothorax, cardiac rupture, pulmonary embolism, hypoxemia, or acidosis.
Repeat epinephrine, 1 mg every 3–5 min.*
Atropine, 1 mg IV, if PEA is slow; repeat every 3–5 min as needed to a total dose of 0.04 mg/kg.

*If this approach fails, epinephrine in escalating doses (1-3-5 mg IV, 3 min apart); intermediate doses (2–5 mg IV every 3–5 min); or high doses (0.1 mg/kg IV every 3–5 min) may be used.
CPR, cardiopulmonary resuscitation; IV, intravenously; PEA, pulseless electrical activity.

**TABLE 47–4.** Treatment of Bradycardia

**Slow (<60 beats per minute) or Relatively Slow (rate less than expected relative to underlying condition or cause)**
**Serious signs and symptoms due to the bradycardia?**

| | |
|---|---|
| Chest pain | |
| Shortness of breath | |
| Decreased consciousness | |
| Shock | |
| Pulmonary congestion | |
| **No** | **Yes** |
| Type II second-degree block or third-degree block? | 1. Atropine, 0.5–1.0 mg* |
| *No* | 2. Transcutaneous pacemaker if available |
| Observe | 3. Dopamine, 5–20 μg/kg/min |
| *Yes* | 4. Epinephrine, 2–10 μg/min |
| Prepare for transvenous pacemaker; use transcutaneous pacemaker as bridge | |

*Atropine should be used with caution in type II second-degree atrioventricular block and new third-degree block with wide QRS complexes.

### *What Is the Role for Epinephrine?*

#### Mechanism of Action

The pharmacologic actions of epinephrine are complex because this drug has both α-stimulating and β-stimulating properties. The primary cardiovascular effect mediated through stimulation of the $\alpha_1$-receptors is peripheral vasoconstriction, which increases systemic vascular resistance (SVR). Stimulation of β-receptors increases heart rate and myocardial contractile force.

A combination of increased contractile force, increased rate, and increased SVR increases blood pressure (BP), cardiac output, and work of the heart. Most important, large doses of epinephrine have been thought to promote cerebral perfusion more effectively than any other drug and are particularly useful to increase internal carotid artery blood flow.[44] Epinephrine increases myocardial irritability and automaticity and may initiate rhythms originating from various ectopic foci, especially the ventricles.

#### Indications

#### *Pulseless Electrical Activity*

Epinephrine effectively improves cardiac output in a failing myocardium. Such is the case in patients with pulseless electrical activity due to poor cardiac output (see Table 47–3). In these patients, even though the ECG may appear normal, ventricular contractility is so impaired that an effective pulse or BP is lacking.

**TABLE 47–5.** Classification of Therapeutic Interventions in Cardiopulmonary Resuscitation and Emergency Cardiac Care

| Class | Therapeutic Intervention |
|---|---|
| I | Indicated, always acceptable; considered useful and effective |
| II | Acceptable, of uncertain efficacy; may be controversial |
| IIa | Weight of evidence is in favor of usefulness and efficacy |
| IIb | Not well established, but may be helpful; probably not harmful |
| III | Inappropriate and without scientific support; may be harmful |

**TABLE 47–6.** Treatment of Cardiac Standstill

Check unresponsiveness, call for defibrillator, initiate CPR.
Continue CPR, intubate, deliver 100% oxygen; start IV, epinephrine, 1 mg
  IV or 2.5 mg by endotracheal tube.
Transcutaneous pacing (if considered, perform immediately).
Epinephrine, 1.0 mg IV push; repeat every 3–5 min.
Atropine, 1.0 mg IV; repeat every 3–5 min as necessary to total dose of
  0.04 mg/kg.

CPR, cardiopulmonary resuscitation; IV, intravenously.

## Cardiac Standstill

Epinephrine's ability to increase automaticity is useful when one attempts to convert cardiac standstill to spontaneous contractions (Table 47–6). Even though the rhythm it produces may be another life-threatening arrhythmia (which can be treated appropriately), the alternative (a dead heart) is less acceptable.

## Fine Ventricular Fibrillation

Epinephrine, as noted previously, may also be useful in converting a fine VF pattern to a coarse pattern, which is more responsive to electrical defibrillation. This effect may be less significant than originally thought. The exact mechanism of this change in rhythm is not known.

## Symptomatic Bradycardia

In symptomatic bradycardia, epinephrine at a constant infusion of 2 to 10 μg/min is considered class IIb (atropine, class I and IIa, is preferred for initial treatment).

## Recommended Dosage

Current guidelines recommend an epinephrine dose of 1.0 mg (10 mL of a 1:10 000 solution) every 3 to 5 minutes.[10,45–47] Each peripheral injection should be followed by a 20-mL flush of intravenous fluid to ensure that it is delivered to the central circulation. Studies suggest that an even higher dose of epinephrine is needed for tracheal administration. Although the optimal dose is unknown, it is at least 2.5 times greater than the intravenous dose. The dose should be drawn up from a 1:1000 solution, diluted to 10 mL with sterile water, and administered by a catheter to the tip of the ETT.

Results of several large multicenter trials on more than 5000 combined patients in cardiac arrest clearly have demonstrated the futility of using high-dose epinephrine (0.07-0.2 mg/kg). They show no statistically significant difference in survival compared with patients treated with standard doses of epinephrine.[45–48] Thus, higher doses of epinephrine are no longer recommended.[10] One should keep in mind the fact that most patients studied represented victims of "out-of-hospital" cardiac arrest. Whether the data are directly applicable to in-hospital arrest patients is unclear. However, an additional study failed to demonstrate a survival value of epinephrine, in either normal or high doses, when compared with placebo after in-hospital resuscitation of 194 patients with in-hospital and out-of-hospital cardiac arrest.[49] Equally sobering is a recent report on in-hospital cardiac arrest that found no association between advanced cardiac life support (ACLS) drug protocols and survival.[50] However, this study specifically ex-

cluded patients whose cardiac arrest occurred in the OR, labor and delivery, or postanesthesia care unit. Thus, its relevance to anesthesiologists is questionable.

## Route of Administration

Epinephrine is best administered through a central venous catheter. It may be given into the tracheobronchial tree through an ETT if an intravenous route is not available, but this technique is not nearly as efficient and requires 2.5 to 10 times the intravenous dose.[45] If the tracheal route is used, peripheral bronchial administration through a catheter is much more efficient than endotracheal administration.[51] An intracardiac injection of epinephrine may be indicated in a patient in asystole who is unresponsive to intravenous or endotracheal administration. However, the needle piercing the myocardium may be more of a cardiac stimulant than the epinephrine itself. Possible hazards of this route of administration are listed in Table 47–7.

## Are Alternative Drug Interventions Applicable?

Vasopressin (arginine vasopressin) may be a more effective pressor agent than epinephrine in cardiac arrest. The evidence from prospective clinical trials in human beings is limited but consistently positive (class IIb).[52–58] Vasopressin (40 U intravenously, not repeated) may be substituted for epinephrine.

## Mechanism of Action

Catecholamines, corticotropin, cortisol, renin, and vasopressin are released during cardiac arrest. One study demonstrated a direct correlation between vasopressin levels and the potential for return of spontaneous circulation.[57] This observation is the converse of what was found for endogenous catecholamines. Although the mechanism of action during cardiac arrest is poorly understood, vasopressin causes profound shunting of blood to the heart and brain. The effect may be mediated by nitric oxide. In the brain, vasopressin administration provides significantly more perfusion during CPR than epinephrine and continues to cause intense vasoconstriction of greater duration even in the presence of profound acidosis.

## Indications

Vasopressin use must be considered to be experimental at this time, but a preliminary out-of-hospital study randomized to vasopressin or epinephrine for VF showed that a significantly greater proportion of patients treated with vasopressin were resuscitated initially and survived for 24 hours.[51]

**TABLE 47–7.** Hazards of Intracardiac Epinephrine Injection

Interruption of cardiac compression and ventilation
Pneumothorax
Coronary artery laceration
Cardiac tamponade
Intramyocardial injection and intractable ventricular fibrillation

**TABLE 47–8.** Indications for Sodium Bicarbonate During Cardiopulmonary Resuscitation

| Class | Indications for Sodium Bicarbonate |
|---|---|
| Class I | In known preexisting hyperkalemia |
| Class IIa | In known preexisting bicarbonate-responsive acidosis (eg, diabetic ketoacidosis); tricyclic antidepressant overdose; to alkalinize urine in aspirin overdose |
| Class IIb | In prolonged resuscitation with effective ventilation upon return of spontaneous circulation after long arrest interval |
| Class III | In hypoxic lactic acidosis (eg, cardiac arrest and CPR with inadequate ventilation)* |

*Adequate ventilation and CPR, not NaHCO₃, are the major "buffers" in cardiac arrest. Sodium bicarbonate is not recommended for routine use in cardiac arrest.
CPR, cardiopulmonary resuscitation.

## Recommended Dose and Route of Administration

Human studies to date compared 1.0 mg of epinephrine intravenously to 40 U of vasopressin intravenously. No other routes have been studied.

## Should Sodium Bicarbonate Be Used?

Sodium bicarbonate is a controversial drug in CPR. In other clinical settings, it may have efficacy. Indications and contraindications are summarized in Table 47–8. Both respiratory and metabolic acidosis usually develop during cardiac arrest. All patients maintained with external cardiac compression have decreased tissue perfusion and tissue hypoxia. Lactic acid is generated through anaerobic metabolism, producing metabolic acidosis. At the same time, inadequate ventilation, as well as the administration of NaHCO₃, which causes the release of >1 L of $CO_2$ per 50 mEq NaHCO₃, leads to hypercarbia and respiratory acidosis. Respiratory acidosis is best treated through improved ventilation by reducing $CO_2$; metabolic acidosis is best managed by a combination of bicarbonate administration, if the arterial pH is <7.10, and hyperventilation.

An elevated $CO_2$ is probably more detrimental to myocardial performance than is metabolic acidosis. Because $CO_2$ diffuses readily, it enters the myocardial cells rapidly; intracellular acidosis quickly develops, causing life-threatening derangements of myocardial function. Likewise, cerebrospinal fluid acidosis may occur secondary to the diffusion of $CO_2$ across the blood-brain barrier, producing postarrest cerebral acidosis. Therefore, administration of NaHCO₃ without sufficient ventilation and circulation to remove the $CO_2$ that it produces is more detrimental than helpful.[59]

## Mechanism of Action

Administration of NaHCO₃ results in a simple acid-base reaction, as follows:

$$H^+ + HCO_3^- \rightleftharpoons H_2CO_3 \rightleftharpoons H_2O + CO_2$$

The carbonic acid dissociates into water and $CO_2$, which is eliminated through the lungs, thereby elevating the pH of the blood and surrounding tissues. However, if ventilation is marginal and widespread abnormalities are present, as is usu-

ally the case during resuscitation efforts, the $CO_2$ cannot be eliminated and increases to as much as 300 to 400 mm Hg in the mixed venous blood and the myocardial cells. Profound intramyocardial acidosis then develops.

## Indications

Untreated acidosis causes the suppression of spontaneous cardiac activity. It decreases the electrical threshold required for the onset of VF, decreases ventricular contractile force, and may decrease cardiac responsiveness to catecholamines, such as epinephrine. Under these circumstances, bicarbonate therapy may be useful but should only be used after confirmed interventions, such as defibrillation, cardiac compression, intubation, ventilation, and more than one trial of epinephrine, have been used.[60,61] Evidence suggests that whatever effectiveness bicarbonate therapy may have is related to augmentation of intravascular volume (it is hypertonic, and draws fluid into the intravascular space from the interstitial space), rather than to any beneficial role in correcting acid-base disturbances.[62] A comprehensive review of the detrimental effects of bicarbonate therapy is highly recommended to those interested in the subject.[63]

## Recommended Dose

If arterial blood gas measurements are not available, the recommended initial dose of NaHCO₃ is 1 mEq/kg intravenously; half this dose may be repeated at 10-minute intervals. For children, this 1 mEq/kg dose should be diluted 1:1 with sterile water to reduce the osmolality. During the initial stage of patient management, when NaHCO₃ is given empirically, the rescuer must be careful to avoid an excessive dose. As soon as possible, arterial blood gas measurements should be obtained as a guide to further therapy.

## Route of Administration

Sodium bicarbonate should be given as incremental bolus injections rather than as a continuous infusion. This method allows better minute-to-minute control of the quantity administered. It also reduces the possibility of inactivating other drugs, such as calcium chloride and the catecholamines, that cannot be mixed directly with bicarbonate.

## Complications

Administration of excessive amounts of NaHCO₃ results in the problems listed in Table 47–9. These problems to a large extent can be offset by the use of agents such as Tribonat,[7,64] a mixture of THAM, NaHCO₃, and phosphate as an alkalinizing agent. However, proof of its efficacy in cardiac arrest awaits further study.

**TABLE 47–9.** Effects of Excess Sodium Bicarbonate

Metabolic alkalosis; leftward shift of oxyhemoglobin dissociation curve; interference with tissue oxygenation
Hypernatremia, hyperosmolality
Hypokalemia
Worsening of respiratory, myocardial acidosis if adequate ventilation cannot be maintained
Intracranial hemorrhage in neonates

### When Is Atropine Useful?

#### Mechanism of Action

Atropine is a drug that long has been used for its vagolytic actions. A reduced vagal influence on the heart improves both the rate of firing of the sinoatrial node and impulse conduction through the atrioventricular (AV) conduction system, with a resulting increase in heart rate.

#### Indications

With absolute (<60 beats per minute [bpm]) or relative symptomatic bradycardia, atropine is considered class I and IIa. Atropine is most useful in treating sinus bradycardia when it occurs with hypotension or frequent premature ventricular contractions (PVCs) secondary to unsuppressed ectopic electrical activity arising in the area of injured tissue during the prolonged period after repolarization (see Table 47–3). Sinus bradycardia after a myocardial infarction (MI) may predispose the heart to the onset of VF.[65] When profound bradycardia is present, acceleration of the heart rate >60 bpm may improve cardiac output and reduce the incidence of VF. Atropine may also be useful for treating a high-degree AV block with a slow ventricular rate. However, in type II AV block and third-degree block with new wide-QRS complexes, atropine is considered class III (possibly harmful) by some investigators.

Asystole subsequent to increased parasympathetic tone that results in suppression of the electrical activity to the heart also frequently responds to atropine. Because heart rate is a major determinant of myocardial $O_2$ consumption, however, any excessive increase in heart rate in an ischemic myocardium may result in frank infarction. Therefore, care should be taken in selecting the proper dose.

#### Recommended Dosage

The recommended dose for bradycardia is 0.5 to 1.0 mg intravenously repeated every 5 minutes until the desired pulse rate is obtained or a maximum of 0.04 mg/kg has been given.[66,67] A larger dose has little therapeutic value, and a smaller dose may actually slow the heart rate. Atropine may also be given intratracheally, in which case the dose is 2 to 2.5 mg. In the treatment of asystole, incremental doses of 1 mg are preferred.

#### Complications

VT and VF after intravenous administration have been reported. In second-degree type II heart block, a paradoxical decrease in ventricular response may result.[65]

### When Should Lidocaine Be Given?

#### Mechanism of Action

By raising the electrical stimulation threshold of the ventricle during diastole, lidocaine renders the myocardial tissue less prone to ectopic electrical activity. In ischemic myocardial tissue after infarction, it may also suppress reentrant arrhythmias such as VT or VF. This effect occurs by an induced delay of conduction through damaged myocardial tissue in the ischemic areas until the surrounding normal tissue is depolarized and refractory to the propagation of an abnormal impulse.

#### Indications

Lidocaine, an amide local anesthetic, is the drug of choice for the treatment and prevention of arrhythmias of ventricular origin. Because of its reliability, relatively low incidence of side effects, and ease of administration, lidocaine appears in the algorithm for stable monomorphic or polymorphic VT. It is acceptable for all four possible VT scenarios:

1. Stable, monomorphic VT with normal cardiac function
2. Stable, monomorphic VT with impaired cardiac function
3. Polymorphic VT with normal baseline QT interval
4. Polymorphic VT with prolonged QT interval

However, in all of these indications, other drugs such as amiodarone have replaced it as the drug of choice[10] (Fig. 47–8).

#### Recommended Dosage

The recommended loading dose is 1 to 1.5 mg/kg given as an intravenous bolus. To control the arrhythmia and to prevent its recurrence, the bolus dose may have to be repeated, up to a total of 3 mg/kg, followed by a continuous infusion of 20 to 40 μg/kg/min (2-4 mg/min in a 70-kg patient). Only bolus therapy should be used during cardiac arrest.

#### Complications

Used in the recommended doses, lidocaine has no significant effect on myocardial contractility, arterial BP, or AV and intraventricular conduction. On the other hand, excessive doses may induce heart block or depression of sinus node discharge, especially in patients with preexisting conduction disturbances.

#### Overdose

An overdose can occur either from administration of too large a dose or from high plasma levels because of reduced redistribution, metabolism, or excretion of the drug. A decreased lidocaine dose may be indicated in patients with hepatic dysfunction, such as occurs with cirrhosis, or in patients with compromised hepatic blood flow secondary to reduced cardiac output or congestive heart failure. These conditions result in decreased metabolism of lidocaine by the liver, producing a gradual accumulation of the circulating drug, if an infusion is instituted.

#### Toxicity

Likewise, toxicity may occur more easily in oliguric or anuric patients because the degradation products of lidocaine, which also have pharmacologic effects and toxic potential, cannot be adequately eliminated from the plasma. Early clinical signs of lidocaine toxicity are related to the drug's central nervous system (CNS) effects (Table 47–10). They may be followed by collapse of the cardiovascular system. If CNS irritability occurs, lidocaine therapy should be withdrawn. A barbiturate or a benzodiazepine may be administered if

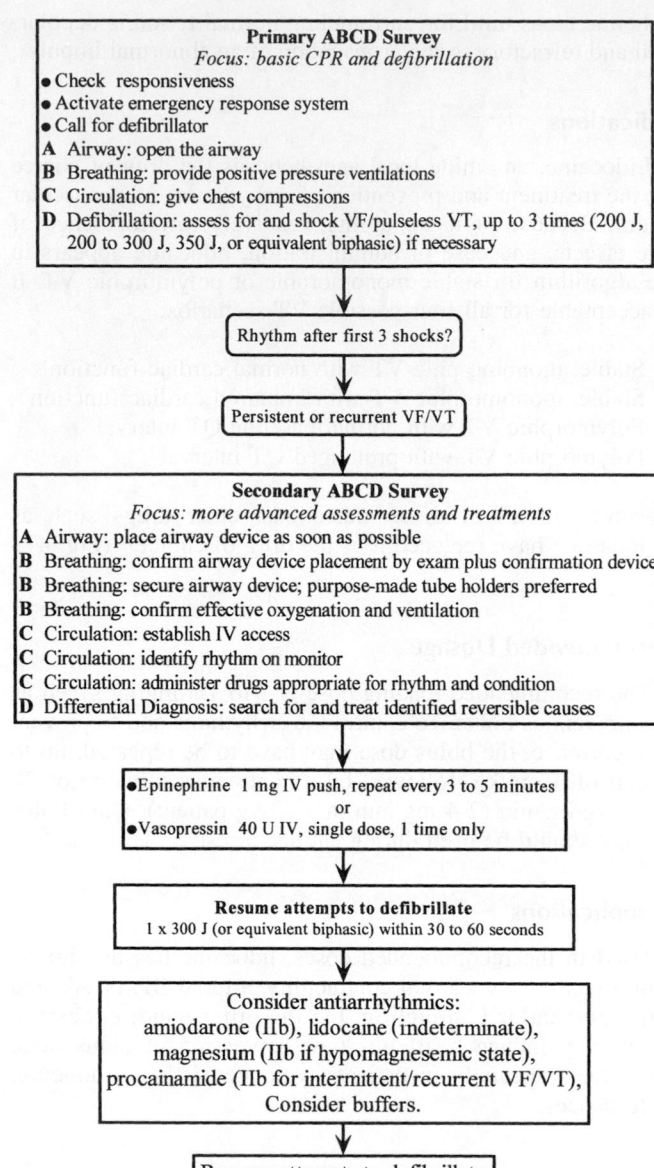

**FIGURE 47–8.** Algorithm for treatment of ventricular fibrillation or pulseless ventricular tachycardia. (Modified from American Heart Association. International Guidelines 2000 for CPR and ECC. *Circulation.* 2000;102[suppl I]:I-1–I-370.)

deemed necessary and if a patient's circulatory status is sufficiently stabilized.

## When Is Procainamide Useful?

### Mechanism of Action

The mechanism of action of procainamide is similar to that of lidocaine. It may decrease the rate of discharge of an

**TABLE 47–10.** Lidocaine Toxicity

| | |
|---|---|
| Drowsiness | Paresthesias |
| Slurred speech | Muscle twitching |
| Disorientation | Focal or grand mal seizures |

ectopic irritable focus. It also blocks reentrant arrhythmias by slowing electrical conduction in the damaged myocardial tissue and by creating a bidirectional block.

### Indications

A second-line agent, procainamide is used in the management of PVCs, VT, and persistent VF (class IIa) unresponsive to lidocaine or when lidocaine is contraindicated.

### Recommended Dosage

Incremental bolus injections are slowly infused at 20 mg/min until one of the following occurs:

1. The arrhythmia is controlled.
2. Hypotension occurs.
3. The QRS complex is widened 50%.
4. A total dose of 17 mg/kg has been given.

After initial control of the arrhythmia with the bolus injection, a continuous infusion of 1 to 4 mg/min may be required to prevent recurrent arrhythmias. Other effective administration schedules have been tested and approved, but all are designed to maintain a therapeutic plasma level of 4 to 8 µg/mL.

### Complications

Because of the profound myocardial depressant effects that may occur during administration of procainamide, continuous ECG and arterial BP monitoring are mandatory. Patients may be especially prone to these side effects after an MI, and their treatment requires extreme caution. End points of therapy include hypotension and >50% widening of the QRS complex.

## When Should Bretylium Tosylate Be Used?

### Mechanism of Action

The pharmacologic effects of bretylium tosylate, a quaternary ammonium compound, are complex. It has both postganglionic adrenergic-blocking properties and a positive inotropic action. After the administration of an initial dose, catecholamine release may increase peripheral resistance and central inotropy. This response is followed by adrenergic blockade and a decrease in peripheral resistance, which frequently produces postural hypotension when the drug is administered to a conscious patient.

A large body of data documents the antifibrillatory effect of bretylium in animals, but this concept has been challenged. Clinically, bretylium has been found to be useful in the treatment of both VT and VF. In direct comparisons, it has been found to be no better than lidocaine; thus, it is considered to be a second-line drug.[68] Moreover, bretylium is now essentially eliminated as a consideration for therapy, and references to bretylium have been dropped from the VF/pulseless VT algorithm. In 1998 through 2000, severe problems with obtaining the raw materials to produce bretylium stopped the supply for a number of months, and it appears that the world's natural sources of bretylium are nearly exhausted. The drug remains acceptable to use, but it is no longer recommended.

## Indications

Bretylium is recommended (class IIa) if (1) lidocaine and defibrillation fail to convert VF, (2) VF recurs despite lidocaine therapy, or (3) lidocaine and procainamide fail to control VT associated with a pulse.

## Recommended Dosage

In refractory VF, 5 mg/kg is given intravenously as a bolus, followed by attempts at electrical defibrillation. If VF persists, the dose may be increased to 10 mg/kg and repeated every 5 minutes up to a maximum dose of 35 mg/kg. In persistently recurring VT, 5 to 10 mg/kg can be diluted to 50 mL with 5% dextrose in water and given intravenously over 8 to 10 minutes. After the loading dose, bretylium can be administered as a continuous infusion at a rate of 1 to 2 mg/min.[67]

## *Is Calcium Chloride Useful?*

### Mechanism of Action

Calcium chloride has long been used for improving myocardial contractility, but the mechanisms of its effects on the myocardium are still poorly understood. Research into the part that calcium plays in malignant hyperthermia has shown that calcium ions enter the sarcoplasm of muscle from the extracellular space through an intracellular tubular network called the *sarcoplasmic reticulum.*

On spread of the excitation impulse in cardiac muscle, the calcium ions travel from the sarcoplasmic reticulum to the points of interaction between the actin and myosin filaments of the sarcomere. Calcium interacts there with troponin, a regulatory protein that inhibits the formation of cross-bridges between actin and myosin. When this inhibition is terminated by the action of calcium on troponin, cross-bridges form between the contractile elements of the muscle, and contraction ensues. It is probably through this mechanism that calcium has its positive inotropic effect.

### Indications

Calcium chloride is most beneficial in reversing the cardiac effects of hyperkalemia, hypocalcemia, and toxicity due to the administration of calcium channel blockers. It is considered class IIa in these situations. In all others, it is considered class III (harmful).

### Recommended Dosage

The use of calcium chloride is controversial because of the fear that it may produce a tetanic contraction of an irritable myocardium or depression of the sinus node, resulting in asystole. It has been hypothesized that the drug may pass through the cell membranes of cells with marginal viability, denaturing intracellular proteins and hastening cell death. This effect is particularly worrisome because the brain is so sensitive to hypoxia.

If it is to be used, the recommended dose is 2 mL of a 10% solution of calcium chloride (2-4 mg/kg). A bolus may be repeated at 10-minute intervals, if necessary. Calcium salts cannot be mixed directly with bicarbonate solution because they precipitate as calcium carbonate. Several calcium preparations are available for intravenous use; calcium chloride, calcium gluceptate, and calcium gluconate are the most popular. Calcium gluceptate can be given in a dose of 5 to 7 mL, and calcium gluconate in a dose of 6 to 8 mL.

### Complications

Rapid administration of a large bolus of calcium chloride, especially through a central venous catheter, may produce severe sinus bradycardia or sinus arrest. Undiluted calcium chloride given through a peripheral vein causes sclerosis and tissue injury; therefore, if a central site is not available, it should either be markedly diluted or be given in a less irritating form (eg, calcium gluconate). Calcium must also be used cautiously in digitalized patients because it can produce or accentuate digitalis toxicity. Much controversy surrounds the issue of whether calcium is indicated at all in the management of cardiac arrest, unless documented hypocalcemia is present or a calcium channel blocking drug is known to have been taken. Otherwise, it should not be used.[69,70]

## *When Should β-Adrenergic Blockers Be Used?*

### Mechanism of Action

Three β-blockers (atenolol, metoprolol, and propranolol) have been shown to reduce significantly the incidence of VF in post-MI patients who did not receive thrombolytic agents. Studies suggest a potential benefit in patients receiving thrombolytics as well. β-Blockers act to control rate and to limit infarct size. They also have a role in chronic therapy after MI to reduce mortality rates.

### Indications

β-Blockers are used in paroxysmal supraventricular tachycardia (PSVT) after the rate is initially controlled, as well as in uncomplicated MI.

### Recommended Dosage

In patients who have had an MI and are not receiving thrombolytic agents, the recommended dose of atenolol is 5 to 10 mg intravenously over 5 minutes. Alternatively, metoprolol can be used. Doses of 5 to 10 mg are given as slow intravenous boluses at 5-minute intervals to a total of 15 mg; an oral regimen can then be initiated. Propranolol, in a dose of 0.1 mg/kg, divided into three equal, slowly administered doses, can also be used, as can esmolol in a dose of 1 to 2 mg/kg, followed by an infusion titrated to maintain the heart rate at the desired level. Oral therapy can then be initiated.

### Complications

Side effects that should be monitored include bradycardia, AV conduction delays, and hypotension. Cardiovascular decompensation to cardiogenic shock is rarely observed. Contraindications include bradyarrhythmias, greater than first-degree heart block, conduction delays, hypotension, overt congestive heart failure, and lung disease caused by bronchospasm.

## What Is the Role of Calcium Channel Blocking Agents?

### Mechanism of Action

Verapamil and diltiazem are the calcium channel blocking agents of choice in emergency cardiac care. Both agents slow conduction and increase refractoriness in the AV node. These actions may terminate reentrant arrhythmias requiring the AV node for their continuation. Verapamil and diltiazem may also be used to control ventricular response rate in atrial fibrillation and flutter. Because these agents decrease myocardial contractility, they may exacerbate congestive heart failure in patients with severe left ventricular dysfunction, despite their vasodilatory effects.

### Indications

Intravenous verapamil is effective in terminating narrow-complex PSVT and can be used to control the ventricular rate in atrial fibrillation. It may not be as effective in controlling atrial flutter. In wide-complex tachycardia of uncertain type, verapamil is class III. Diltiazem appears to be equally efficacious and may produce less myocardial depression than verapamil.

### Recommended Dosage

The initial dose of verapamil is 2.5 to 5 mg given intravenously over 2 minutes. In the absence of a response or a drug-induced adverse event, repeated doses of 5 to 10 mg may be administered every 15 to 30 minutes to a maximum of 20 mg. Diltiazem is given at a dose of 0.25 mg/kg, followed by a second dose of 0.35 mg/kg.

### Complications

Verapamil may produce significant hypotension, which can be reversed with calcium chloride, 0.5 to 1 g, given slowly through a central catheter, or 1.5 to 3 g calcium gluconate, given slowly via a peripheral vein.[71]

## When Is Adenosine Indicated?

### Mechanism of Action

Adenosine, available in the United States only since 1990, is an endogenous purine nucleoside that depresses AV node and sinus node activity. It is effective in terminating common forms of PSVT because they involve a reentry pathway including the AV node. It does not terminate arrhythmias that are not due to reentry involving the AV node (eg, atrial flutter, atrial fibrillation, atrial or ventricular tachycardia) but may produce transient AV or ventriculoatrial block that clarifies the diagnosis.

### Indications

Adenosine is indicated in PSVT and may also be used to differentiate PSVT from other tachyarrhythmias, including VT. Adenosine is class I in PSVT. In wide-complex tachycardia of uncertain type, it is class IIa.

### Recommended Dosage

The recommended initial dose is 6 mg given as a bolus over 3 to 5 seconds, followed by a 20-mL saline flush. If no response is observed in 1 to 2 minutes, a 12-mg dose should be given. Larger doses have not been well studied.

### Complications

Side effects are common but transient. Flushing, dyspnea, and chest pain are frequently encountered. These side effects rarely last more than 1 to 2 minutes. Sinus bradycardia and ventricular ectopy are common transiently after termination of PSVT. Because the half-life of adenosine is less than 5 seconds, PSVT may recur and require additional adenosine or calcium channel blocker. Adenosine produces few hemodynamic effects because of its short duration of action. However, its use should be reserved for situations in which suppression of AV nodal activity will be of therapeutic or diagnostic value. Adenosine interacts with methylxanthines, which block the receptor responsible for adenosine's effects. Dipyridamole blocks adenosine uptake and potentiates its effects. Alternative therapy is warranted for patients receiving these drugs.

## When Should Nitroglycerin Be Used?

### Mechanism of Action

Nitroglycerin relaxes vascular smooth muscle. It is the nitrate of choice for acute angina pectoris. In patients with congestive heart failure, intravenous nitroglycerin produces hemodynamic effects similar to those of sodium nitroprusside. Low doses (30-40 μg/min) produce predominantly venodilation; high doses (150-500 μg/min) lead to arteriolar dilation as well.

### Indications

Indications for the use of nitroglycerin in emergency cardiac care include congestive heart failure and unstable angina associated with MI.

### Recommended Dosage

For suspected angina pectoris, one nitroglycerin tablet is administered sublingually. It may be repeated at 3- to 5-minute intervals if discomfort is unrelieved. Safe administration of intravenous nitroglycerin usually requires hemodynamic monitoring. The initial intravenous dosage is 10 to 20 μg/min, and the dosage may be increased by 10 μg/min until the desired response occurs.

### Complications

The principal toxic side effect of nitroglycerin is hypotension, which may exacerbate myocardial ischemia. Other potential complications include tachycardia, paradoxical bradycardia, hypoxemia due to increased ventilation-perfusion mismatch, increased intracranial pressure, and headache.

## When Should Magnesium Sulfate Be Used?

Magnesium deficiency is associated with cardiac arrhythmias, cardiovascular insufficiency, and sudden cardiac death.

**TABLE 47–11.** Indications for Magnesium Sulfate in Cardiac Arrest

Arrest associated with torsades de pointes (class IIa)
Suspected hypomagnesemia
Refractory ventricular fibrillation (after lidocaine and bretylium) (class IIa)
Torsades de pointes with a pulse (class IIa)
Life-threatening ventricular arrhythmias associated with digitalis toxicity or tricyclic antidepressant overdose
Prophylactic administration in hospitalized patients with acute myocardial infarction (class IIa)

It can lead to refractory VF and hinder the replacement of intracellular potassium. Hence, hypomagnesemia should be corrected. Indications for magnesium therapy are summarized in Table 47–11.

### Recommended Dosage

For acute administration during VT, 1 or 2 g of magnesium sulfate (2-4 mL of a 50% solution) is diluted in 10 mL of $D_5W$ and administered intravenously over 1 to 2 minutes. If VF is present, the drug should be given as an intravenous bolus. For torsades de pointes, doses up to 5 to 10 g can be used.

### Complications

Toxicity is rare. Side effects include flushing, diaphoresis, bradycardia, and hypotension. Hypermagnesemia can result in depressed reflexes, flaccid paralysis, and cardiorespiratory collapse.

## What Are the Roles of Vasoconstrictor Drugs?

Norepinephrine is one of a number of α-stimulators that produce vasoconstriction by acting directly on peripheral vessels. (Isoproterenol, in contrast, is a purely α-stimulating drug that causes peripheral vasodilation and increased heart rate, electrical conduction, and contractility.)

Drugs such as ephedrine have both a direct α-stimulating effect and an indirect effect through the release of catecholamines, which in turn stimulate the α- and β-receptors. Dopamine, a precursor of norepinephrine, has direct α effects. It also stimulates dopamine receptors in low dosages (3-5 µg/kg/min) and improves renal blood flow.

### Indications

Much debate centers on the indications for the use of vasoconstrictors in patients in shock, particularly those with coronary artery disease. Potent vasoconstrictors predispose to ischemic damage of vital organs. Although an elevation in systemic BP may improve cerebral, coronary, and renal perfusion, this beneficial effect is frequently accompanied by increased cardiac work and $O_2$ consumption. These opposing effects must be considered in any decision to use vasoconstrictor therapy. It is probably better to have a low cardiac output with centralization from α-stimulation-induced peripheral vasoconstriction than a low cardiac output without preferable

shunting of flow to the brain and heart. α-Stimulation is generally reserved until after an inotrope has been tried.

## LIFE-THREATENING ARRHYTHMIAS

## How Are Atrial Fibrillation and Paroxysmal Supraventricular Tachycardia Managed?

Atrial fibrillation or PSVT with a rapid ventricular response may be associated with such a fast ventricular rate that diastolic filling time is shortened and ventricular volume is markedly reduced. The result is decreased cardiac output and decreased coronary artery perfusion. If the patient does not develop life-threatening cardiovascular decompensation, pharmacologic therapy is recommended.

### Calcium Channel Blockers and Digitalis

A calcium channel blocker (verapamil or diltiazem) or digitalis is usually the first therapeutic intervention for atrial fibrillation or atrial flutter. Sufficient drug is given so that an AV block is created, thereby reducing the ventricular response to atrial stimulation. These drugs do not convert the arrhythmia. Verapamil and diltiazem may decrease myocardial contractility and precipitate congestive heart failure. Diltiazem is less of a myocardial depressant than is verapamil.

### β-Blockers and Adenosine

β-Blockers can be used to slow the ventricular rate if calcium channel blockers or digitalis is not effective. They also slow the atrial rate in PSVT. However, adenosine is the choice for narrow complex PSVT.

### Cardioversion

Patients who are refractory to pharmacologic therapy or who have symptoms may require elective cardioversion. In compromised patients with hypotension or pulmonary edema, sinus rhythm must be restored rapidly. In this situation, cardioversion is the indicated initial therapy.

## How Are Ventricular Arrhythmias Controlled?

### Premature Ventricular Contractions

PVCs can be monomorphic and polymorphic, and they can occur in salvos. The proximity of a PVC to the preceding T wave is critical; if it falls on the T wave, it can initiate VT or VF. When PVCs in a patient with suspected MI are frequent, occur in salvos, or are closely coupled to a previous T wave, intravenous lidocaine, 1 to 1.5 mg/kg, is the recommended initial therapy. Procainamide, propranolol, or quinidine can also be used. If bradycardia is present, the heart rate should be maintained above 60 bpm with intravenous atropine in 0.5-mg increments.

### Ventricular Tachycardia

VT is defined as three or more consecutive beats of ventricular origin at a rate usually exceeding 100 bpm. Management is outlined in Figure 47–8. Drug therapy includes intravenous lidocaine, procainamide, and bretylium, in order of priority. If no response occurs or if a patient's condition is critical, cardioversion or insertion of a transvenous pacemaker and overdrive pacing may be beneficial.

Although lidocaine remains acceptable as an antiarrhythmic to use for the treatment of shock-refractory VF and pulseless VT, the evidence supporting its efficacy is poor. Many investigators feel that amiodarone should be used before lidocaine. Lidocaine can be used for VF/VT and merits only an indeterminate class of recommendation (class indeterminate). Lidocaine has not been recommended for routine prophylaxis of ventricular arrhythmias in the setting of acute MI for many years. However, available data do not justify changing the classification of lidocaine to a class III (evidence-of-harm) agent.

The 2000 AHA guidelines now recommend amiodarone (class IIb) and procainamide (class IIb) ahead of lidocaine and adenosine for the initial treatment of hemodynamically stable wide-complex tachycardia, especially in patients with compromised cardiac function. Amiodarone is recommended as a class IIa drug for the treatment of stable monomorphic and polymorphic VT.

PSVT with aberrant conduction is often difficult to differentiate from VT. Guidelines for differentiating these arrhythmias are useless in acutely ill patients and divert attention from appropriate care. Critical points to remember include the following:

1. *Do not* administer verapamil because it can accelerate heart rate and lower BP, especially in Wolff-Parkinson-White syndrome.
2. *Do not* rely on clinical criteria to distinguish PSVT from VT. Many patients with VT may appear stable.
3. Treat hemodynamically significant, wide-complex tachycardias as VT.
4. Adenosine may have a role in distinguishing PSVT from VT in hemodynamically stable patients, but further study is necessary.

### Ventricular Fibrillation

VF is the most common cause of cardiac arrest. It is classified as *coarse* or *fine,* terms that describe the amplitude and the frequency of the ECG waveform. Coarse fibrillation (high-amplitude, slow-frequency waveforms) is usually of recent onset and frequently is more responsive to therapy. Fine fibrillation (low amplitude, fast frequency) may be refractory to defibrillation. Epinephrine administration sometimes converts the fine pattern to coarse VF, which is more responsive to defibrillation.

If the onset is observed, a defibrillator is not available, and hypoxia is not the precipitating event, a precordial thump may be effective. If not, defibrillation should be performed as quickly as possible. BLS must be administered until defibrillation can be accomplished or until an effective rhythm supervenes (see Fig. 47–7).

### Ventricular Asystole

Ventricular asystole, or cardiac standstill, is a total absence of ventricular electrical or mechanical activity and usually results from extensive myocardial ischemia, hypoxia, hyperka-lemia, severe acidosis, extreme parasympathetic activity (eg, drug overdose), or hypothermia. CPR must be initiated immediately. Pharmacologic measures that should be considered include intravenous administration of epinephrine, $NaHCO_3$ when the arterial pH is <7.10, and atropine. If response to these modalities does not occur, a transvenous or transcutaneous pacemaker is necessary. Because fine VF may appear as asystole, an attempt at electrical defibrillation should be considered (see Table 47–5).

### How Is Sinus Bradycardia Managed?

Sinus bradycardia is characterized by a heart rate below 60 bpm. Unless hypotension or ventricular ectopic beats are present, therapy is unnecessary. However, intravenous atropine in 0.5-mg increments is used when patients develop symptoms or if ectopy appears. A dopamine infusion or a transvenous or transcutaneous pacemaker may be needed in the absence of a response to atropine (see Table 47–3).

### How Is Second-Degree Atrioventricular Block Managed?

Mobitz type II second-degree AV block usually occurs in the conductive pathway below the AV node. Because it is frequently associated with myocardial damage rather than increased vagal tone, the prognosis is usually poor. Temporary pacer placement followed by a permanent pacemaker is often required for a patient with this form of second-degree AV block because a complete heart block commonly ensues (see Table 47–4).

### How Is Third-Degree Atrioventricular Block Managed?

Third-degree AV block is characterized by complete cessation of electrical conduction between the atria and ventricles. The conduction block may occur at or below the AV node. A block at the node is frequently associated with acute inferior MI, increased vagal tone, or toxic drug effect. In this instance, the prognosis is usually favorable, and the block may be corrected with intravenous atropine. If no response is seen, a temporary pacer is used. When the block occurs below the AV node, it is often secondary to an extensive anterior MI. A pacemaker or intravenous atropine or epinephrine may be used (see Table 47–4).

### How Is Pulseless Electrical Activity Managed?

Pulseless electrical activity is characterized by ineffective ejection of blood even though myocardial electrical activity is normal. The result is a pulseless patient with a normal ECG pattern. The prognosis for these patients is poor. If the etiology is myocardial failure, the patient may respond to CPR and the intravenous administration of epinephrine or to dobutamine infusion. In the absence of a response, hypovolemia should be considered and a fluid bolus given. Other causes include tension pneumothorax, cardiac tamponade, cardiac rupture, pulmonary embolism, hypoxemia, acidosis, massive MI, drug overdose, and hypothermia.

## References

1. Mörch ET. Mechanical ventilation. In: Kirby RR, Banner MJ, Downs JB, eds. *Clinical Applications of Ventilatory Support.* 2nd ed. New York, NY: Churchill Livingstone; 1990:1.

2. Kouvenhoven WB, Jude JR, Knickerbocker GG. Closed-chest cardiac massage. *JAMA.* 1960;173:1064.

3. Eisenberg M, Hollstrom A, Bergner L. The ACLS score: predicting survival from out-of-hospital cardiac arrest. *JAMA.* 1981;246:50.

4. Becker LB, Ostrander MP, Barrett J, et al. Survival from cardiopulmonary resuscitation in a large metropolitan area: where are the survivors? *Ann Emerg Med.* 1991;20:355.

5. Erb D, Nowak RM. Resuscitation in the in-hospital setting: special considerations. In: Paradis NA, Halperin HR, Nowak RM, eds. *Cardiac Arrest: The Science and Practice of Resuscitation Medicine.* Baltimore, Md: Williams & Wilkins; 1996:597.

6. Berger R, Kelley M. Survival after in-hospital cardiopulmonary arrest of non critically ill patients: a prospective study. *Chest.* 1994;106:872.

7. Landry FJ, Parker JM, Phillips YY. Outcome of cardiopulmonary resuscitation in the intensive care setting. *Arch Intern Med.* 1992;152:2305.

8. Goetting MG, Paradis NA. High-dose epinephrine improves outcome from pediatric cardiac arrest. *Ann Emerg Med.* 1991;20:22.

9. Nadkarni V, Hazinski MF, Zideman D, et al. An Advisory Statement from the Pediatric Working Group of the International Liaison Committee on Resuscitation, 1997.

10. American Heart Association. International Guidelines 2000 for CPR and ECC. *Circulation.* 2000;102(suppl I):I-1.

11. Trough RD, Waisel DB, Burns JP. DNR in the OR: a goal-directed approach. *Anesthesiology.* 1999;90:289.

12. Becker LB, Berg RA, Pepe PE, et al. A reappraisal of mouth-to-mouth ventilation during bystander-initiated cardiopulmonary resuscitation. A Statement for Healthcare Professionals From the Ventilation Working Group of the Basic Life Support and Pediatric Support Subcommittees, American Heart Association. Dallas, Tex: American Heart Association; 1997.

13. Kern KB, Halperin HR, Field J. New guidelines for cardiopulmonary resuscitation and emergency cardiac care. *JAMA.* 2001;285:1267.

14. Oczenski W, Krenn H, Dahaba AA, et al. Hemodynamic and catecholamine stress responses to insertion of the Combitube, laryngeal mask airway or tracheal intubation. *Anesth Analg.* 1999;88:1389.

15. Walls RM. Cricothyroidotomy. *Emerg Clin North Am.* 1986;6:725.

16. Melker RJ, Banner MJ. Work imposed by breathing through cricothyrotomy tube. Paper presented at: Sixth World Congress on Emergency and Disaster Medicine; September 1989; Hong Kong.

17. Scuderi PE, McLeskey CH, Comer PB. Emergency percutaneous transtracheal ventilation during anesthesia using readily available equipment. *Anesth Analg.* 1982;61:867.

18. Gammage G. Airway management. In: Civetta JM, Taylor RW, Kirby RR, eds. *Critical Care.* Philadelphia, Pa: JB Lippincott; 1988:197.

19. Babbs CF, Voorhees WD, Fitzgerald KR, et al. Relationship of blood pressure and flow during CPR to chest compression amplitude: evidence for an effective compression threshold. *Ann Emerg Med.* 1983;12:527.

20. Orlowski JP. Optimum position for external cardiac compression in infants and young children. *Ann Emerg Med.* 1986;15:667.

21. Emergency Cardiac Care Committee and Subcommittee, American Heart Association. Guidelines for cardiopulmonary resuscitation and emergency cardiac care, VII: neonatal resuscitation. *JAMA.* 1992;268:2276.

22. McDonald JL. Systolic and mean arterial pressures during manual and mechanical CPR in humans. *Ann Emerg Med.* 1982;11:292.

23. Halperin HR, Tsitlik JE, Guerci AD, et al. Determinants of blood flow to vital organs during cardiopulmonary resuscitation in dogs. *Circulation.* 1986;73:539.

24. Sack JB, Kesselbrenner MB, Bregman D. Survival from in-hospital cardiac arrest with interposed abdominal counterpulsation during cardiopulmonary resuscitation. *JAMA.* 1992;266:379.

25. Gedeborg R, Rubertsson S, Wiklund L. Improved haemodynamics and restoration of spontaneous circulation with constant aortic occlusion during experimental cardiopulmonary resuscitation. *Resuscitation.* 1999;40:171.

26. Krischer JP, Fine EG, Weisfeldt ML, et al. Comparison of prehospital conventional and simultaneous compression-ventilation cardiopulmonary resuscitation. *Crit Care Med.* 1989;17:1263.

27. Hevesi ZG, Thrush DN, Downs JB, et al. Cardiopulmonary resuscitation: effect of CPAP on gas exchange during chest compressions. *Anesthesiology.* 1999;90:1078.

28. Paradis NA, Martin GB, Rivers EP, et al. Coronary perfusion pressure and the return of spontaneous ventilation in human cardiopulmonary resuscitation. *JAMA.* 1990;263:1106.

29. Falk JL, Rackow EC, Weil MH. End-tidal carbon dioxide concentration during cardiopulmonary resuscitation. *N Engl J Med.* 1988;318:607.

30. Callaham M, Barton C. Prediction of outcome of cardiopulmonary resuscitation from end-tidal carbon dioxide concentration. *Crit Care Med.* 1990;18:358.

31. Nakatani K, Yukioka H, Fujimori M, et al. Utility of colorimetric end-tidal carbon dioxide detector for monitoring during prehospital cardiopulmonary resuscitation. *Am J Emerg Med.* 1999;17:203.

32. Martin GB, Gentile NT, Paradis NA, et al. Effect of epinephrine on end-tidal carbon dioxide monitoring during CPR. *Ann Emerg Med.* 1990;19:396.

33. Befeler B. Mechanical stimulation of the heart: its therapeutic value in tachyarrhythmias. *Chest.* 1978;73:832.

34. Kerber RE. Statement on early defibrillation. American Heart Association: Medical Scientific Statement from the Emergency Cardiac Care Committee. *Circulation.* 1991;83:2233.

35. Ewy GA, Dahl CF, Zimmerman M, et al. Ventricular fibrillation masquerading as ventricular standstill. *Crit Care Med.* 1981;9:841.

36. American Heart Association standards and guidelines for cardiopulmonary resuscitation (CPR) and emergency cardiac care (ECC). *JAMA.* 1992;268:2212.

37. Kerber KE, Grayzel J, Kennedy J, et al. Elective cardioversion: influence of paddle-electrode location and size on success rates and energy requirements. *N Engl J Med.* 1981;305:658.

38. Weaver WD, Cobb LA, Copass MK, et al. Ventricular defibrillation: a comparative trial using 176-J and 320-J shocks. *N Engl J Med.* 1982;307:1101.

39. Sirna SJ, Ferguson DW, Charbonnier F, et al. Electrical cardioversion in humans: factors affecting transthoracic impedance. *Am J Cardiol.* 1988;62:1048.

40. Gutgesall LHP, Zacker WP, Geddes LA, et al. Energy dose for ventricular defibrillation of children. *Pediatrics.* 1976;58:898.

41. Kerber RE, Carter J, Klein S, et al. Open-chest defibrillation during cardiac surgery: energy and current requirements. *Am J Cardiol.* 1980;46:393.

42. Kerber RE, Martins JB, Kienzle MG, et al. Energy, current, and success in defibrillation and cardioversion: clinical studies using an automated impedance-based energy adjustment method. *Circulation.* 1988;77:1038.

43. Kerber RE, Kienzle MG, Olshansky B, et al. Ventricular tachycardia rate and morphology determine energy and current requirements for transthoracic cardioversion. *Circulation.* 1992;85:158.

44. Brown CG, Werman HA, Davis EA, et al. Comparative effects of graded doses of epinephrine or regional brain blood flow during CPR in a swine model. *Ann Emerg Med.* 1986;15:1138.

45. Emergency Cardiac Care Committee and Subcommittee, American Heart Association. Guidelines for cardiopulmonary resuscitation and emergency cardiac care, III: adult advanced cardiac life support. *JAMA.* 1992;268:2208.

46. Cummins RO, ed. Cardiovascular pharmacology I (epinephrine). In: American Heart Association. *Advanced Cardiac Life Support.* Dallas, Tex: American Heart Association; 1997:7-2.

47. Kloeck W, Cummins RO, Chamberlain D, et al. The universal advanced cardiac life support algorithm. An Advisory Statement from the Advanced Life Support Working Group of the International Liaison Committee on Resuscitation. International Liaison Committee on Resuscitation; 1997.

48. Gueugniaud PY, Mols P, Goldstein P, et al. A comparison of repeated high doses and repeated standard doses of epinephrine for cardiac arrest outside the hospital. European Epinephrine Study Group. *N Engl J Med.* 1998;339:1595.

49. Woodhouse SP, Cox S, Boyd P, et al. High dose and standard dose adrenaline do not alter survival, compared with placebo, in cardiac arrest. *Resuscitation.* 1995;30:243.

50. Van Walraven C, Stiell IG, Wells GA, et al. Do advanced cardiac life support drugs increase resuscitation rates from in-hospital cardiac arrest? The OTAC Study Group. *Ann Emerg Med.* 1998;32:544.

51. Mazkereth R, Paret G, Ezra D, et al. Epinephrine blood concentrations after peripheral bronchial versus endotracheal administration of epinephrine in dogs. *Crit Care Med.* 1992;20:1582.

52. Lindner KH, Dirks B, Strohmenger HU, et al. Randomised comparison

of epinephrine and vasopressin in patients with out-of-hospital ventricular fibrillation. *Lancet.* 1997;349:535.

53. Chugh SS, Lurie KG, Lindner KH. Pressor with promise: using vasopressin in cardiopulmonary arrest. *Circulation.* 1997;96:2453.

54. Wenzel V, Lindner KH, Prengel AS, et al. Vasopressin combined with epinephrine decreases cerebral perfusion compared with vasopressin alone during cardiopulmonary resuscitation in pigs. *Stroke.* 1998;29:1462.

55. Wenzel V, Lindner KH, Mayer H, et al. Vasopressin combined with nitroglycerin increases endocardial perfusion during cardiopulmonary resuscitation in pigs. *Resuscitation.* 1998;38:13.

56. Wenzel V, Lindner KH, Krismer AC, et al. Repeated administration of vasopressin but not epinephrine maintains coronary perfusion pressure after early and late administration during prolonged cardiopulmonary resuscitation in pigs. *Circulation.* 1999;99:1379.

57. Lindner KH, Strohmenger HU, Ensinger H, et al. Stress hormone response after cardiopulmonary resuscitation. *Anesthesiology.* 1992;77:662.

58. Eichinger MR, Walker BR. Enhanced pulmonary arterial dilation to arginine vasopressin in chronically hypoxic rats. *Am J Physiol.* 1994;267:H2413.

59. Kette F, Weil M, Gazmuri R, et al. Buffer solutions may compromise cardiac resuscitation by reducing coronary perfusion pressure. *JAMA.* 1991;266:2121.

60. Emergency Cardiac Care Committee and Subcommittee, American Heart Association. Guidelines for cardiopulmonary resuscitation and emergency cardiac care, III: adult advanced cardiac life support. *JAMA.* 1992;268:2210.

61. Cummins RO, ed. Cardiovascular pharmacology I (sodium bicarbonate). In: American Heart Association. *Advanced Cardiac Life Support.* Dallas, Tex: American Heart Association; 1997:7-14.

62. Benjamin E, Oropello JM, Abalos AM, et al. Effects of acid-base correction on hemodynamics, oxygen dynamics, and resuscitability in severe canine hemorrhagic shock. *Crit Care Med.* 1994;22:1616.

63. Forsythe SM, Schmidt GA. Sodium bicarbonate for the treatment of lactic acidosis. *Chest.* 2000;117:260.

64. Bjerneroth G. Tribonat—a comprehensive summary of its properties. *Crit Care Med.* 1999;27:1009.

65. Gunnar RM, Passamani ER, Bourdillon PD, et al. American College of Cardiology/American Heart Association Guidelines for the early management of patients with acute myocardial infarction. Report of the ACC/AHA Task Force on Assessment of Diagnostic and Therapeutic Cardiovascular Procedures. *Circulation.* 1990;82:664.

66. Emergency Cardiac Care Committee and Subcommittee, American Heart Association. Guidelines for cardiopulmonary resuscitation and emergency cardiac care, III: adult advanced cardiac life support. *JAMA.* 1992;268:2206.

67. Cummins RO, ed. Cardiovascular pharmacology I (atropine). In: American Heart Association. *Advanced Cardiac Life Support.* Dallas, Tex: American Heart Association; 1997:7-4.

68. Haynes RE, Chinn TL, Copass MK, et al. Comparison of bretylium tosylate and lidocaine in management of out of hospital ventricular fibrillation: a randomized clinical trial. *Am J Cardiol.* 1981;48:353.

69. Emergency Cardiac Care Committee and Subcommittee, American Heart Association. Guidelines for cardiopulmonary resuscitation and emergency cardiac care, III: adult advanced cardiac life support. *JAMA.* 1992;268:2209.

70. Cummins RO, ed. Cardiovascular pharmacology I (calcium chloride). In: American Heart Association. *Advanced Cardiac Life Support.* Dallas, Tex: American Heart Association; 1997:7-16.

71. Weiss AT, Lewis BS, Halon DA, et al. The use of calcium with verapamil in the management of supraventricular tachyarrhythmias. *Int J Cardiol.* 1983;4:275.

# C H A P T E R

# 48

# Temperature Management and Aberrations

Richard Lilly, Jr
Thomas C. Mort

Assuming the care of both healthy and critically ill patients requires a basic knowledge and understanding of human physiology. As such, routine temperature monitoring to detect hypothermia and hyperthermia during anesthesia administration can assist in formulating a more streamlined differential diagnosis of problems that may arise.

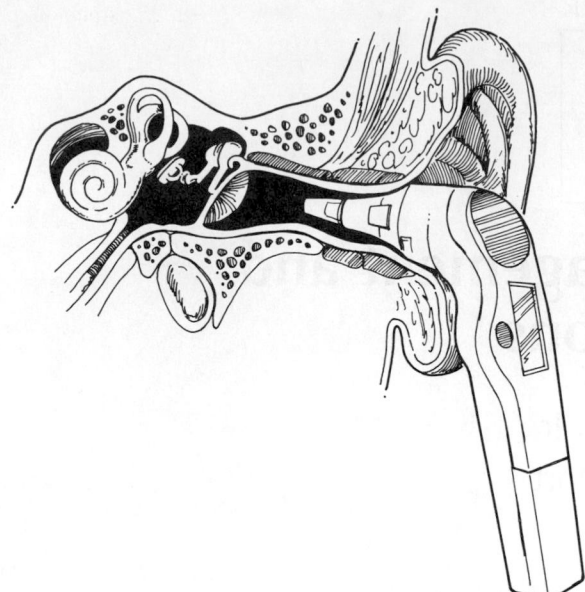

FIGURE 48–1. An infrared detector of tympanic membrane temperature. It is excellent for making single determinations, especially during recovery, but not for use as a continuous monitor. The detector must be acurately aimed at the tympanic membrane rather than at the wall of the ear canal.

## MEASURING TEMPERATURE

### What Is Normal Temperature Gradient?

There is always a temperature gradient from the core of the body to the peripheral tissues to the skin. Typically, in awake human beings, core temperature is 37°C, peripheral tissue is 31° to 35°C, and skin is 28° to 32°C. One usually wants to measure core temperature.

### What Type of Measuring Devices Are Available?

#### Thermistors and Thermocouples

Thermistors measure temperature change by changing electrical resistance. In a thermocouple, two dissimilar metals in proximity produce electric current, which varies with temperature. Thermocouples can be made cheaply and may be disposable. This is the technology behind most axillary, esophageal, and tympanic membrane probes that we use today.

#### Liquid Crystal Probes

Liquid crystal probes change color as a function of temperature. As such, they are measuring only skin temperature. Some manufacturers make a scale adjustment so that the temperature indicated is "corrected" to reflect core temperature. However, as discussed in this chapter, there are wide-ranging differences in skin and core temperatures that may vary throughout the course of anesthetic administration. Skin temperature has been shown to be an unreliable predictor of malignant hyperthermia in swine.[1] Therefore, liquid crystal probes applied to the skin are not an ideal temperature monitor for anesthesia.

#### Tympanic Membrane Probes

Infrared temperature probes detect electromagnetic heat radiation from the body. The typical probe looks like an otoscope and takes instant ear temperatures (Fig. 48–1). However,

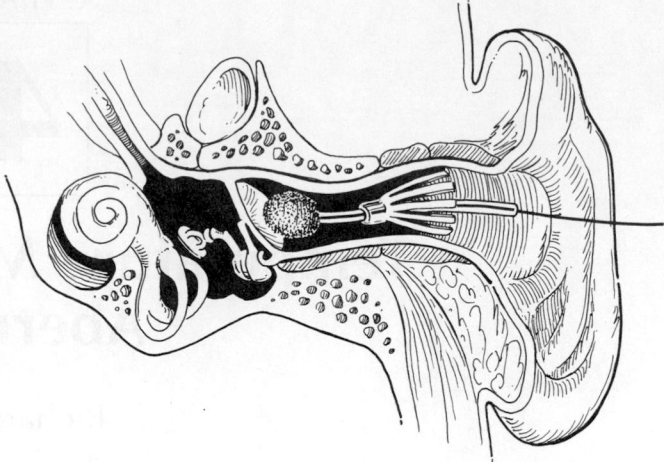

FIGURE 48–2. Probe designed for monitoring of tympanic membrane temperature. It should only be placed in the awake patient before anesthesia to minimize risk for tympanic membrane injury.

they are accurate only if carefully aimed directly at the tympanic membrane, which is often not done. A true tympanic probe (Fig. 48–2) is a thermistor or thermocouple placed carefully in the external auditory canal so that it is gently in contact with the tympanic membrane—this is the gold standard of temperature monitoring.

### What Sites Are Appropriate for Temperature Monitoring?

Core temperature is the temperature of the brain and highly perfused organs. That is the temperature one wants to measure because perturbations of temperature have the most effect on these vital organs. In general, temperature monitoring sites in close proximity to the brain, heart, or high arterial blood flow are most reliable.

According to Sessler, the four most reliable sites are tympanic membrane, nasopharynx (Fig. 48–3), distal esophagus (Fig. 48–4), and pulmonary artery.[2] All of these sites reflect brain temperature accurately. An open chest during cardiac

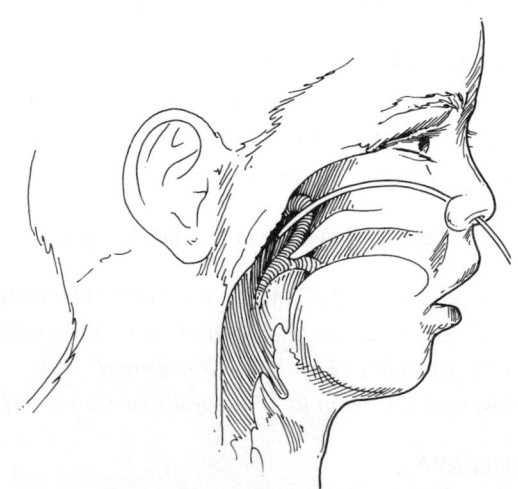

FIGURE 48–3. The nasopharyngeal probe should be inserted only as far as the posterior nasopharynx. This is about the same distance as from the tragus of the ear to the ala nasi.

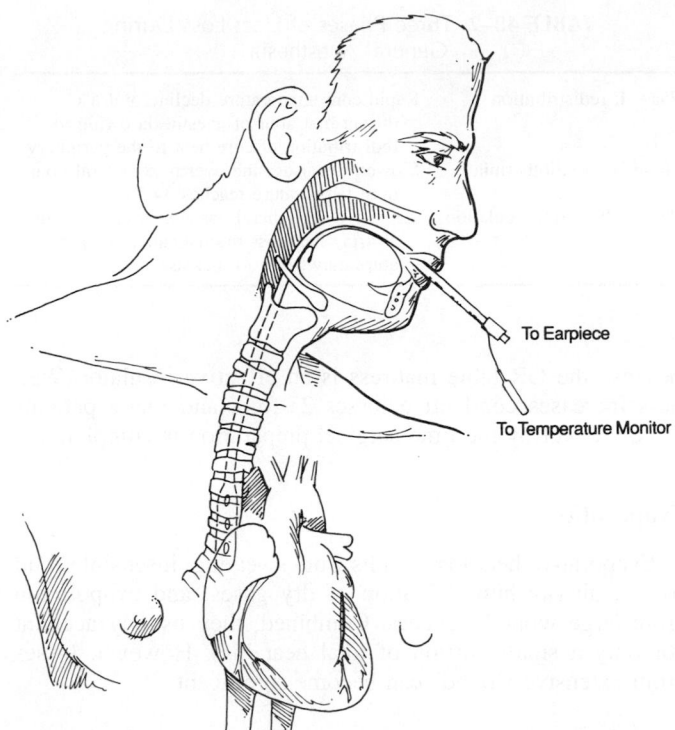

To Earpiece

To Temperature Monitor

**FIGURE 48–4.** The esophageal temperature probe can be combined with the esophageal stethoscope. It is best placed where the heart sounds are loudest or just beyond that.

surgery may make pulmonary artery temperature read low because of cool ambient temperature. In the esophagus, the proximal two thirds are considerably affected by airway temperature, but the distal one third reflects core temperature because of its proximity to the heart and great vessels. The most accurate temperature usually correlates with where the loudest heart tones are heard or with the esophageal probe inserted just deep to that. It is instructive to do the experiment: Place the probe where best airway sounds are heard. Record the temperature and then compare with the temperature obtained with the probe sited at or beyond the loudest heart sounds. Usually, the difference is >0.5°C. A nasopharyngeal probe should be inserted to a depth equal to the distance from the nostril to the ear to measure brain temperature. Other depths may be influenced by ambient or airway temperature.

Bladder temperature accurately reflects core temperature; some Foley catheters include a thermistor probe. Rectal temperature is unreliable and has slow response time because feces act as an insulator. Rectal temperature, like skin temperature, has been shown to be an unreliable predictor of malignant hyperthermia (MH) in swine.[1]

Oral and axillary temperatures are less reflective of core temperature than are temperatures of other areas discussed. Great toe temperature is a poor reflection of core temperature but a good gauge of sympathetic tone in that leg. Toe temperature has been suggested to correlate with cardiac output.[3] The higher the cardiac output, the better the peripheral perfusion, and thus the higher the toe temperature.

## American Society of Anesthesiologists Temperature Monitoring Guidelines

Present guidelines require that the ability to monitor temperature be available at all anesthetizing locations. At the

1999 meeting of the American Society of Anesthesiologists (ASA) House of Delegates, a proposal was debated that would have required temperature monitoring in all cases over 1 hour long. However, that proposal was not approved. The thinking behind the proposal stresses that hypothermia is a common problem that deserves routine monitoring to identify, prevent, and treat optimally. Malignant hyperthermia is expected to be diagnosed by other means before the temperature begins to go up. Thus, new temperature monitoring guidelines, when they are adopted, will be aimed at preventing hypothermia and not at diagnosing malignant hyperthermia.

## THERMOREGULATORY RESPONSES IN ANESTHETIZED PATIENTS

Classic teaching suggests that anesthetized patients become poikilothermic, that is, their body temperature passively approaches ambient temperature. Thus, in a cool operating room (OR) environment, hypothermia is to be expected. In the past few years, Sessler and associates published a series of reports[4-11] that greatly improve our understanding of thermoregulation during anesthesia.

In awake human beings, body temperature is maintained within a narrow range of 37°C ± 0.4°C. When temperature rises above that range, the body responds by vasodilation and sweating and with behavioral changes such as removing a sweater. When temperature falls, the normal response is behavioral changes, vasoconstriction, shivering, and, in babies, nonshivering thermogenesis.

During anesthesia, initial cooling is not accompanied by a thermoregulatory response (Fig. 48–5). However, once the temperature reaches 34.5°C, significant peripheral vasoconstriction occurs, and the rate of temperature decline decreases. This observation led to the description of an expanded interthreshold range under anesthesia. The normally tight 36.6° to 37.4°C range in awake human beings expands more than fivefold from 34.5° to 39°C (see Fig. 48–5). Within that range, an anesthetized patient is, indeed, poikilothermic. Once the range is exceeded, thermoregulatory responses *do* occur in anesthetized patients.

In fully anesthetized adults, shivering is unlikely, especially when muscle relaxants are used; nonshivering thermogenesis is confined to neonates; and behavorial changes are impossible. Therefore, vasoconstriction is the only response to hypothermia. Once temperature falls below 34.5°C, vasoconstriction decreases cutaneous heat loss by 25%.[9] Sweating and vasodilation manifest in response to hyperthermia just as in awake patients, but they are not apparent until hypothalamic temperature approaches 39°C.[10]

## HEAT LOSS

### What Are the Mechanisms?

Four mechanisms of heat loss occur in anesthetized patients (Table 48–1).

### Radiation

Radiation is loss of heat in the form of electromagnetic radiation to cooler objects in the room. It is responsible for

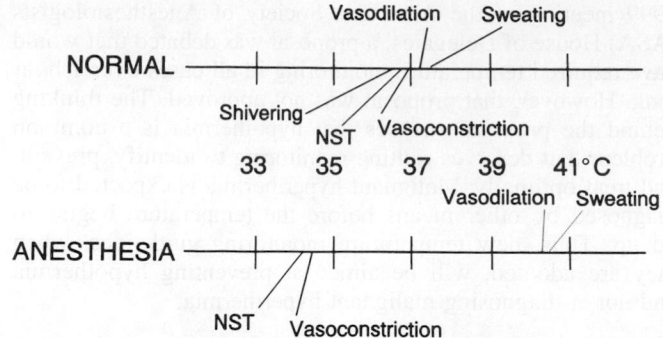

**FIGURE 48–5.** A schematic drawing illustrating thresholds and gains for common thermoregulatory responses in awake and anesthetized human beings. The *angled lines* represent different effector responses, and the *thick horizontal lines* show mean body temperature. The intersection of each line with the temperature scale is the threshold, and the slope indicates the gain of that response. Thermoregulatory sensitivity is shown as the distance between the first cold response (vasoconstriction) and the first warm response (active vasodilation); temperatures within this range do not elicit thermoregulatory compensation. Actual thresholds in unanesthetized individuals are closer than illustrated (ie, about 0.4°C), and the gains are higher. The slope of the line that represents shivering is relatively small because there is a broad range of shivering intensity and because intensity increases in proportion to hypothermia. Nonshivering thermogenesis (NST) is not triggered until vasoconstriction is nearly complete. The slope of the line that represents vasoconstriction is large because the response is an "all-or-nothing" phenomenon. Because each thermoregulatory effector has its own threshold and gain, there is an orderly progression of responses, with response intensities in proportion to need. During general anesthesia *(bottom part of figure)*, shivering is not shown because it is inhibited by muscle relaxants and local effects of inhaled anesthetics. The thresholds for vasoconstriction and nonshivering thermogenesis are shifted down to about 34.5°C (depending on anesthetic type and dose). The effects of anesthetics on active vasodilation and sweating are unknown, but the thresholds are probably several degrees above normal. (From Sessler DI. Temperature monitoring. In: Miller RD, ed. *Anesthesia.* 3rd ed. New York, NY: Churchill Livingstone; 1990:1227–1242.)

70% of the body's heat loss but can be greatly reduced by any simple covering.

## Convection

Convection is the loss of heat to air currents flowing over the body—the *wind-chill effect.* In an OR with high air turnover rates and poorly designed air vents, a significant breeze may blow over a patient. Again, simply covering patients dramatically reduces convective losses.

## Conduction

Conduction represents loss of heat to cooler objects that the body is touching. This source of loss is usually much less

**TABLE 48–1.** Mechanism of Heat Loss in Order of Importance

| Radiation | 70% of heat loss | Prevented by simple covering |
|---|---|---|
| Convection | Wind chill effect of cool, drafty operating room | Prevented by simple covering |
| Conduction | Small losses unless patient is wet. Wetness increases conduction loss 25-fold. | Keep patient dry. |
| Evaporation | Sweating, insensible loss, humidification of gases; normally a small factor | Use heat and moisture exchanger or humidifier. |

**TABLE 48–2.** Three Phases of Heat Loss During General Anesthesia

| Phase I: redistribution | Rapid core temperature decline of 1.5°C during first hour of anesthesia owing to redistribution of core heat to the periphery |
|---|---|
| Phase II: poikilothermia | Slower, linear decline over next several hours until temperature reaches 34.5°C |
| Phase III: thermoregulation | At 34.5°C, peripheral vasoconstriction occurs, slowing heat loss dramatically. Temperature may begin to increase. |

because the OR table mattress is an effective insulator. Wetness increases conductive losses 25-fold, and many patients are quite wet by the time surgical preparation is completed.

## Evaporation

Evaporative heat loss results from sweating, insensible fluid losses, airway humidification of dry gases, and evaporation from large wound surfaces. Combined, they usually account for only a small portion of total heat loss. However, losses from extensive wounds can become significant.

## *How Does Hypothermia Develop Under Anesthesia?*

Three predictable phases occur in the development of hypothermia under anesthesia[9] (Table 48–2).

## Phase I: Redistribution

Phase I is a rapid linear temperature decrease of 1.5°C during the first hour of anesthesia. The greatest heat loss occurs during this period. Heat production decreases because of decreased muscle tone and metabolism. Heat loss increases because of anesthesia-induced vasodilation at a time when most of a patient's clothing is removed in a cold, drafty room, and wet preparation solution is poured over the body surface. It is no wonder patients get cold.

Interestingly, measurements of heat loss during the first hour show that heat loss alone is not enough to explain the decrease of core temperature. In fact, much of this temperature decline is caused by redistribution of core heat to the periphery.[11] Phase I temperature decline is hard to prevent because of this redistribution phenomenon. The best way to control temperature loss is to warm the periphery actively, thereby decreasing the core to the periphery temperature gradient. To accomplish this requires about 30 minutes of convective blanket heating to bring the peripheral temperature to 38°C before anesthesia induction. This is generally not practical but is a consideration for sickle cell patients in whom prevention of hypothermia is important.

## Phase II: Poikilothermia

Phase II is a steady decline of 0.5°C per hour for 3 to 4 hours until the temperature approaches 34.5°C. This is the period of poikilothermia, in which body temperature passively drifts toward ambient temperature.

## Phase III: Return of Thermoregulation

Phase III occurs when the lower limit of the interthreshold range (ie, 34.5°C) is reached, and active *thermoregulation* (vasoconstriction) resumes. At this point, temperature decline diminishes, and temperature may even begin to increase.

### How Is Temperature Regulated During Spinal or Epidural Anesthesia?

The thermoregulatory set-point is located in the hypothalamus, but about 20% of thermal sensory input comes from skin sensors. Spinal or epidural anesthesia can have several effects on thermoregulation. Vasodilation below the level of the block causes heat redistribution and loss; motor block reduces the muscle mass available for heat production; and sensory block of thermal afferents occurs as well. Thus, patients who receive spinal or epidural anesthetics, not surprisingly, are also at risk for developing hypothermia.

Spinal or epidural vasodilation increases cutaneous heat loss about 16%, but shivering generates more than enough heat to offset this loss.[12] Nevertheless, central hypothermia develops because of redistribution of core heat to the cooler periphery, analogous to phase I during general anesthesia.

Tremor occurring during epidural anesthesia meets all of the criteria for thermoregulatory shivering. No other tremor patterns or etiologies have been identified. Shivering during epidural anesthesia is less vigorous than after general anesthesia and, therefore, has fewer hemodynamic and metabolic consequences.

Patients' perception of cold does not correlate with central hypothermia. Hynson and colleagues' volunteers perceived a feeling of warmth despite maximal central hypothermia and shivering.[12] They speculated that the conflicting signals of central hypothermia and subjective peripheral warmth may delay the onset of thermoregulatory shivering.

### Does the Temperature of the Epidural Drug Cause Shivering?

No clear answer can be given to this question. In Hynson's nonpregnant volunteers, injectate temperature had no influence on the incidence of shivering.[12] However, others studying parturients have suggested that cool epidural injectate was more likely to cause shivering than drug injected at body temperature.[13,14]

Epidural narcotics may reduce the shivering associated with epidural anesthesia. Epidural sufentanil in large doses of up to 100 μg is so effective in blocking shivering that it may cause patients to develop significant hypothermia.[15] As discussed later, intravenous meperidine, 12.5 to 25 mg, may be effective in controlling shivering during spinal or epidural anesthesia. Cutaneous heating with radiant heat lamps or a convective blanket may also help.

### What Is the Clinical Significance of This Information?

Hypothermia and shivering are as much of a problem during spinal and epidural anesthesia as they are during general anesthesia. Patients having similar procedures under general or regional anesthesia arrive in the postanesthesia care unit (PACU) at the same temperature, but those who received regional anesthesia take twice as long to rewarm. Obviously, the mechanisms of heat loss persist in the regional anesthesia group until the block wears off, whereas the general anesthesia group begins to rewarm immediately on emergence. The skin should be kept warm in patients having regional anesthesia until the block wears off.

### Which Patients Are at Particular Risk for Hypothermia?

From 60% to 80% of all patients arriving in the PACU are hypothermic. Because the greatest core heat loss (redistribution) is during the first hour of surgery, as previously mentioned, virtually all patients are at risk. Conahan and colleagues studied a group of patients undergoing laparoscopy in an ambulatory surgery setting.[16] They showed that heated humidification during the procedure allowed them to bring patients to the recovery room 0.5°C warmer and, more important, to discharge them 1 hour sooner. In a busy facility, this practice can have significant economic benefit. Ikeda showed more core-to-peripheral heat redistribution with propofol induction than with sevoflurane induction.[17] Therefore, even patients having short ambulatory procedures can benefit from heat conservation measures. We have reduced shivering in our ambulatory surgery PACU by using convective heating blankets on all major knee and shoulder ambulatory cases.

### Infants

Infants are clearly at high risk for developing hypothermia because of the large surface area (for heat loss) relative to their small body mass. Because nonshivering thermogenesis is a real factor in infants, it can cause significant increases in oxygen ($O_2$) consumption in hypothermic infants even when muscle relaxants prevent shivering.

### Elderly Patients

Elderly or debilitated patients are also at increased risk because they have less insulating subcutaneous tissue and less muscle mass available for heat generation. On the other hand, they shiver less vigorously than younger patients and, therefore, may suffer fewer hypothermia-induced metabolic consequences.

### Burn Victims

Burn victims lack insulating subcutaneous tissue in areas of full-thickness wounds; tremendous evaporative heat loss often results.

### Trauma Victims

Trauma victims often become hypothermic in the field before they are rescued. Large-volume room temperature fluid resuscitation further contributes to heat loss unless fluids are warmed. These patients present some of the most severe cases of hypothermia. Patients subjected to large volumes of room-

**TABLE 48–3.** Influence of the Response to Hypothermia on Oxygen Consumption

| | |
|---|---|
| Temperature decrease of 0.3°C | Increases O₂ consumption 7% |
| Temperature decrease of 0.3°–1.2°C | Increases O₂ consumption 92% |
| Violent shivering | Increases O₂ consumption 200%–500% |

temperature irrigating solution and those with large abdominal wounds also lose heat rapidly.

## PATHOPHYSIOLOGY OF HYPOTHERMIA

### Are There Any Benefits of Hypothermia?

In the physiologic temperature range, each 1°C decrease in temperature reduces metabolism and oxygen consumption by about 7%. Thus, dropping a patient's temperature from 37° to 30°C, as is often done in cardiac surgery, reduces O₂ consumption by 50% and helps protect organs during times of lower perfusion. Minimal reductions in temperature of 1° to 3°C to provide organ protection from ischemia in animal models[18] (Table 48–3). Marion and colleagues showed that maintaining a core temperature of 32°C improved outcome in moderately severe (Glasgow Coma Scale, 5–7) head injuries.[19] Villar and Slutsky similarly showed reduced mortality from septic adult respiratory distress syndrome in patients who were cooled to 34°C.[20] It seems logical to let a patient's temperature drift down 2° to 3°C whenever there is a risk for organ ischemia, for example, in intracranial or carotid artery surgery. In doing so, one must, however, be prepared to deal with the adverse consequences of hypothermia discussed in this chapter.

### What Are the Adverse Effects of Hypothermia?

#### Increased Oxygen Consumption During Rewarming

The beneficial effects of hypothermia noted previously presuppose that the patient is anesthetized and not shivering. In awake hypothermic patients, even small degrees of hypothermia can significantly increase O₂ consumption (see Table 48–3). The most serious consequences of perioperative hypothermia are attributed to this increased O₂ consumption, which occurs on awakening. Other physiologic consequences are discussed later and outlined in Table 48–4.

#### The Cardiovascular System

In the awake patient, hypothermia causes vasoconstriction and perhaps hypertension. Increased cardiac output is needed because of the increased metabolic demand caused by shivering. In anesthetized patients, as discussed previously, vasoconstriction does not occur until core temperature is about 34.5°C. As a patient's temperature declines below 34°C, bradycardia and myocardial depression occur, leading to hypotension. Fluid also shifts out of the vascular space; with severe hypothermia (25°C), the hematocrit may increase 150%. The ensuing increase in blood viscosity and reduction in blood volume further contribute to decreased cardiac output.

**TABLE 48–4.** Pathophysiology of Hypothermia

| Organ or System | Major Effects |
|---|---|
| Heart | Bradycardia, myocardial depression, ventricular irritability lead to fibrillation at 28°C. |
| Vascular system | Initial vasoconstriction and hypertension, hemoconcentration, late hypotension |
| Coagulation | Decreased activity of humoral clotting factors, but more important, reversible sequestration of platelets and decreased platelet function |
| Kidney | Vasoconstriction may lead to antidiuretic hormone suppression and diuresis. Depressed tubular reabsorptive function with normal glomerular filtration rate also promotes diuresis of dilute urine. |
| Metabolism | Decreases 7% per 1°C if not shivering |
| Minute alveolar concentration | Decreases 7% per 1°C if not shivering |
| Neurologic system | Short-term memory decline at 35°C; semiconsciousness at 33°C. Shivering stops at 33°C; coma at 30°C. |

The initial electrocardiogram (ECG) changes are sinus bradycardia with prolonged PR, QRS, and QT intervals. As body temperature approaches 30°C, about 30% of patients develop a J wave after the QRS (Fig. 48–6). This event is a precursor to ventricular fibrillation, which occurs between 28°C and 25°C. At temperatures <30°C, mechanical stimulation of the heart may also provoke ventricular fibrillation.

#### Coagulation and Surgical Blood Loss

Hypothermia may cause coagulopathy. Decreasing temperature reduces the activity of humoral clotting factors. More important as temperature falls, the liver sequesters platelets, causing relative thrombocytopenia.[21] As a patient rewarms, these platelets are released back into the circulation and function normally within an hour. Valeri and colleagues showed that wound cooling depresses platelet function and that wound rewarming restores platelet functions to normal.[22] These findings support warming the OR and directing a radiant heat source at large operative wounds.

#### Immune System

Mild perioperative hypothermia (2°C) can directly impair white blood cell immune functions such as chemotaxis, phagocytosis, motility, and antibody production.[23,24] Hypothermia causes vasoconstriction, which, in turn, may reduce tissue partial presence of O₂, especially in peripheral skin and subcutaneous areas where surgical wounds may start. This hypothermia-induced vasoconstriction and reduced tissue oxygenation

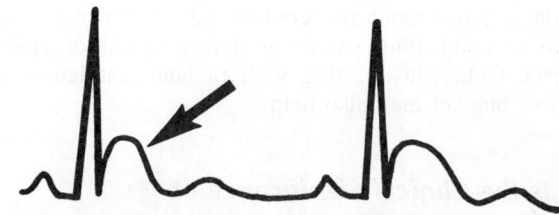

**FIGURE 48–6.** Osborne J wave *(arrow)* after the QRS complex (pathognomonic for hypothermia). (From Farmer JC. Temperature-related injuries. In: Civetta JM, Taylor RW, Kirby RR, eds. *Critical Care.* 2nd ed. Philadelphia, Pa: JB Lippincott; 1988:695.)

occur in 78% of hypothermic patients but in only 22% of normothermia controls. Mild tissue hypoxia impairs function of white blood cells. Decreased tissue oxygenation may also slow wound healing and actually delay time until a wound is clinically ready for suture removal.

### The Kidneys

Cold-induced vasoconstriction can mimic volume overload, leading to antidiuretic hormone (ADH) suppression and diuresis. Hypothermia also depresses tubular reabsorptive functions but not glomerular filtration, factors that also cause diuresis.

### Metabolic Functions

All metabolic processes slow by about 7% per 1°C fall in temperature, and liver blood flow decreases. Therefore, all drugs dependent on the liver for metabolism have prolonged effects during hypothermia. Nondepolarizing muscle relaxant clearance is prolonged by hypothermia. The minimum alveolar concentration of inhalation anesthetic agents also decreases 7% per 1°C; thus, anesthetic concentration must be decreased as a patient cools.

### Neurologic Function

Short-term memory declines at 35°C and is decreased 70% by 34°C. At 33°C, shivering ceases, and patients can no longer actively warm themselves. Reduction in consciousness begins at 33°C, and coma develops by 30°C. As a result, postoperative hypothermia causes delayed emergence from anesthesia that becomes clinically significant when the temperature is <34°C. A temperature decrease of 2° to 3°C increases the latency of somatosensory evoked potentials and complicates their interpretation.

### The Oxygen Dissociation Curve

Cold shifts the $O_2$ dissociation curve to the left, meaning that $O_2$ binds more tightly to hemoglobin and is not released as readily to tissues. The affinity of hemoglobin for $O_2$ increases 6% per every 1°C decrease. Cold-induced, peripheral vasoconstriction makes pulse oximeter readings difficult to obtain. If this phenomenon is suspected, and there is no contraindication, digital nerve block with 1% plain lidocaine frequently restores the signal within 10 minutes.

## SPECIAL POSTOPERATIVE PROBLEMS

The most serious consequences of intraoperative hypothermia occur not in the OR but in the PACU or intensive care unit (ICU) during rewarming (Table 48–5). The metabolic and cardiovascular changes caused by the body's response to hypothermia, shivering, and rewarming are potentially detrimental to patients with limited cardiorespiratory reserve.

### *Is Postanesthesia Shivering Always Caused by Hypothermia?*

The short answer is "no."[25] There are many examples of severe postanesthesia shivering (PAS) in normothermic pa-

**TABLE 48–5.** Problems Caused by Hypothermia in the Postanesthesia Care Unit

| | |
|---|---|
| Severe shivering | May cause venous and arterial hypoxemia and acidosis |
| Peripheral vasoconstriction | Can cause hypertension |
| Rewarming vasodilation | Can cause relative hypovolemia and hypotension |
| Ventilator adjustments | Shivering may interfere with ventilation. As rewarming occurs and metabolism increases, minute ventilation needs to increase as well. |

tients. Despite numerous studies, the etiology of normothermic PAS is unclear. Interestingly, in normal volunteers who have had anesthesia but no surgery, PAS occurs only when hypothermic. However, normothermic postsurgical patients shiver. Therefore, surgical stress or pain or the hormonal response to surgery must play a role in PAS.[26,27] PAS in normothermic patients is more common in those experiencing a great deal of postoperative pain.[27] Nevertheless, much of PAS is hypothermia related and can be prevented by appropriate intraoperative care to maintain normal temperature during and after surgery.

### *What Are the Consequences of Postanesthesia Shivering?*

Whatever the cause of PAS, the metabolic and cardiorespiratory consequences and treatment are the same (Table 48–6).[28] Shivering increases the metabolic $O_2$ requirement by up to 500%, in turn increasing the demand for cardiac output and ventilation to provide increased $O_2$ to the shivering muscles. If a patient is unable to increase ventilation because of disease or residual anesthesia, respiratory acidemia supervenes. Likewise, failure to increase cardiac output appropriately predisposes to venous desaturation and metabolic acidosis. Venous desaturation, when combined with ventilatory depression, ultimately leads to arterial hypoxemia. Furthermore, the demand for increased cardiac output in a patient with minimal myocardial reserve can precipitate congestive heart failure or myocardial ischemia.[29,30] In short, PAS can cause hypoxia and cardiac ischemia or congestive heart failure and must be treated aggressively.

### *What Problems Occur With Rewarming in the Postanesthesia Care Unit?*

Severely hypothermic patients have peripheral vasoconstriction and frequent postoperative hypertension. Fluid shifts,

**TABLE 48–6.** Practical Clinical Implications of Hypothermia

| Beneficial | Detrimental |
|---|---|
| Organ protection from ischemia | Preop and postop patient comfort |
| | Postanesthesia shivering (PAS) |
| | Hemodynamic consequences of PAS |
| | Increased cardiac morbidity |
| | Increased blood loss |
| | Increased wound infection |
| | Delayed discharge in both ambulatory and major cases |

combined with vasoconstriction, reduce intravascular volume. As a patient rewarms and vasodilation occurs, relative hypovolemia and hypotension may necessitate aggressive fluid therapy to prevent hypotension.

## Cardiac Surgery

After hypothermic cardiopulmonary bypass (CPB), patients tend to remain hypothermic. Their core temperature is often not fully restored even though the blood temperature may be 37°C when they are first weaned from bypass. When body temperature diminishes during wound closure and the early recovery period, several issues arise. If such patients are not fully paralyzed, they often shiver early in the postoperative period. Sladen and colleagues reported two ventilatory problems.[31,32] With shivering, mechanical ventilator function was compromised, and patients tended to be underventilated. Conversely, paralyzed hypothermic patients tended to be hyperventilated while cold and subsequently hypoventilated as they rewarmed, unless careful adjustment of the ventilator accompanied rewarming. The rewarming period for patients recovering after open heart surgery was 12 hours, with an overshoot to above normal temperatures at the end of the period.

Increased $O_2$ consumption, energy expenditure, carbon dioxide ($CO_2$) production, and venous desaturation have been reported during postoperative rewarming of patients after cardiac surgery.[33,34] Holtzclaw and Green noticed that masseter muscle fasciculations precede and are predictive of these deleterious respiratory and metabolic phenomena.[35] Patients undergoing cardiac surgery clearly are at increased risk for postoperative hypothermia and its attendant cardiorespiratory consequences. Prudence seems to dictate either warming these patients to a higher core (ie, bladder or rectal) temperature before separation from CPB (to prevent the delayed aftercooling) or keeping them paralyzed until they are fully warm.

Forced hot-air warmers, radiant heat sources, intravenous meperidine, and prolonging bypass to allow full core rewarming are effective measures to decrease postoperative increases in energy expenditure due to physiologic rewarming responses. These same principles also apply to any other cold, sick, intubated, mechanically ventilated postoperative patients.

## What Are the Effects of Shivering in Febrile Patients?

Fever represents a resetting of the body thermostat to a new, higher level. Shivering maintains temperature at that higher level. Violent fever-induced shivering has the same negative metabolic and cardiorespiratory consequences previously described. Active cooling of a febrile patient makes no sense if doing so serves only to increase shivering. Rather, one should administer antipyretics to restore the thermostat to normal before active cooling. Active cooling may be needed if the temperature reaches dangerous levels. However, its use should be monitored with an eye to the negative consequences of shivering.

## Other Practical Clinical Consequences of Hypothermia

Some of the most serious consequences of perioperative hypothermia occur in the PACU and have been discussed previously. Other major areas of practical clinical concern include preoperative patient comfort, perioperative cardiac morbidity, infection and wound healing, and surgical blood loss (see Table 48–6).

### Preoperative Patient Comfort

A nervous patient brought to a cold, drafty OR and uncovered for catheter and monitor placement may shiver violently from a combination of anxiety and feeling cold. At best, this sequence is acutely uncomfortable for patients and may make peripheral venous access more difficult. At worst, the hemodynamic and metabolic consequences of shivering can precipitate myocardial ischemia in a patient with minimum coronary reserve. Covering patients with a warmed blanket to keep the skin warm before induction helps prevent this scenario. Warming the OR until the patient is asleep is even better.

### Perioperative Cardiac Morbidity

There are now several studies that show increased postoperative cardiac morbidity in hypothermic patients. Steven and colleagues studied 300 patients with significant cardiac risk factors having major surgery.[29] They compared an aggressively warmed group to a control (hypothermic) group. The hypothermic group's average temperature at end of surgery was 35.4°C, compared with 36.7°C for the warmed group. Perioperative cardiac morbidity was 6.3% in the hypothermic group, compared with only 1.4% in the normothermic group. Cardiac morbidity was defined as myocardial ischemia, ventricular tachycardia, unstable angina, myocardial infarction, or cardiac arrest.

In another study of patients undergoing peripheral vascular surgery, 36% of the hypothermic group (temperature <35°C) developed myocardial ischemia, compared with only 13% of a normothermic group.[30]

### Blood Loss

Mechanisms of decreased coagulation attributable to hypothermia were discussed previously. There is now clinical evidence that even 1°C of hypothermia can significantly increase surgical blood loss. Schneid and associates estimated that mild hypothermia (35°C) would increase blood loss in patients undergoing total hip arthroplasty by an average of 500 mL.[36] Greher and colleagues, also working with total hip arthroplasty cases, showed that as little as 1°C of hypothermia increased blood loss by 400 mL.[37]

### Wound Infection and Healing

The theoretical considerations in wound healing and infection have been shown to have practical clinical implications. Two hundred patients having colectomies were studied. Patients with mild hypothermia (34.7°C) had 3-fold increase (6%–19%) in surgical wound infection compared with normothermic patients. Sutures were removed 1 day later in the hypothermic group. Discharge of the hypothermic group was prolonged by 2.6 days (20%).[38]

## PREVENTION AND TREATMENT OF HYPOTHERMIA

Minimizing heat loss should be a priority of the entire OR staff (Table 48–7). Nurses should learn that patients' skin

**TABLE 48–7.** Modalities to Prevent Heat Loss

| | |
|---|---|
| Warm the operating room until patients are draped. | A temperature of 25°C is ideal; even 21°C is better than the typical, which is 19°C. |
| Keep patients covered. | *Any* covering material reduces heat loss 30%. |
| Use radiant heat lamps. | Use during preparation and catheter placement when patients cannot be covered. |
| Apply forced hot air heating blankets. | Limited by need for surgical exposure; an upper body is available for use during abdominal surgery. |
| Use heat and moisture exchangers or heated humidifiers. | The former slows heat loss; the latter were effective in some studies in rewarming cold patients. |
| Use fluid warmers. | 1 L of 0.4°C blood product over 15 min decreases body temperature 0.5°C. |
| Apply water-circulating warming blankets. | These are of little or *no* value when placed under adults, but may be of value placed on top of patients and are worthwhile in infants. |

must never be unnecessarily exposed. They must consider getting the patient a warm blanket a higher priority than tying the surgeon's gown. Surgeons must learn to tolerate the temporary discomfort of a warm OR to avoid the unfavorable consequences of postoperative hypothermia.

Remember that the initial temperature decrease does not reflect heat loss to the environment but rather redistribution from a warm body core to a cooler periphery. This translocation is difficult to prevent. However, active peripheral warming helps to minimize the initial reduction in temperature. Most heat loss involves radiation from uncovered parts of the body. Keeping patients covered, including the head and shoulders, is an important factor in avoiding hypothermia.

### How Do I Get the Surgeons Interested in Heat Conservation?

Surgeons may be unenthusiastic about some heat conservation measures—especially warming the operating room. The whole OR team needs to be aware of the negative consequences of even mild hypothermia.[29,30] Everyone involved needs to make heat conservation a high priority. Although the surgeons may not care much about shivering in the PACU, risk factors such as perioperative cardiac morbidity, intraoperative bleeding, and wound infection may get their attention. The anesthesiologist has a responsibility as a perioperative physician to make the consequence of hypothermia well known to the entire surgical team.

### What Specific Modalities Should Be Considered?

#### Warm the Operating Room

Most OR temperatures are about 19°C. At least 21°C and preferably 25°C is needed to prevent heat loss. If surgeons cannot tolerate the warm room, it may be cooled again once a patient is draped.

#### Keep Patients Covered

Various covering materials, including simple cotton blankets, plastic wrap, aluminum foil, space blankets of aluminum and Mylar, and special reflective OR garments are available. Each reduces heat loss by about 30%, with no great difference in efficacy. The cheapest and most convenient is probably the best.[39]

#### Forced Hot Air Heating Systems

A plastic and paper disposable blanket with multiple openings placed on the patient allows warm air (up to 43°C) to be blown through the blanket and over the patient. This system is ideally suited to the PACU. An OR version covers the head, shoulders, chest, and outstretched arms of patients positioned for abdominal or lower extremity surgery. When the head and torso can be covered, the device is particularly useful, but special care must be paid to sealing the eyelids to prevent corneal drying.

Forced hot-air systems eliminate radiation and convection heat loss by surrounding a patient with a warmed microclimate. They provide a cutaneous heat source that is more effective than radiant heat lamps, reduce shivering, and enable earlier PACU discharge.[40] Prophylactic use after cardiac surgery also decreases shivering episodes. Sessler compared a forced hot air system (the Bair Hugger) with radiant heat sources and with a water-circulating blanket placed *over* a patient. The forced hot air system was most effective in warming. On the *high* setting, it raised body temperature 1.5°C per hour.[41] This has become the gold standard in both preventing and treating hypothermia.

#### Fluid Warmers

Administration of 1 L of room temperature fluid requires the patient to expend 15 kcal to warm the fluid to 37°C. This expenditure is 20% of a patient's hourly caloric production. Because the anesthetized patient cannot increase caloric production, body temperature falls approximately 0.2°C. One liter of blood at 4°C administered over 15 minutes reduces body temperature 0.5°C. Thus, fluid warmers are commonly used for blood administration and desirable for large fluid infusions if hypothermia is to be avoided. Use of a blood warmer should continue in the PACU if further transfusions are needed. The ideal fluid warmer must be easy to set up and to transport to the PACU. It should warm large volumes without reducing flow rate.

#### Heated Humidifiers or Heat and Moisture Exchangers

Only 10% of a patient's heat loss is through airway evaporation. A passive heat and moisture exchanger (HME) or active heated humidifier can prevent this loss. Increased humidity also maintains ciliary activity. Numerous studies show the dramatic effects of heated humidification in preventing heat loss and rewarming cold patients.[16,42,43] HMEs probably are as effective in preventing heat loss but do not actively transfer heat to patients to rewarm them. Sessler doubts the efficacy of heated humidification.[43]

#### Radiant Heat Lamps

Radiant heat lamps have long been popular in pediatric ICUs and ORs to help keep neonates warm. If several are used, they may be helpful for adults as well. They serve as a useful adjunct to warming the OR during extensive preparation and draping periods or while invasive catheters are placed.

The disadvantage of infrared heat lamps is that surgical draping usually prevents enough skin surface exposure to the heat source. Furthermore, convection and conduction losses persist in cold, drafty ORs. Radiant heat lamps are not as effective as forced hot air systems.[41] However, a radiant heat source on the skin can instantly stop PAS even without raising core temperature.[44,45]

### Water-Circulating Warming Blankets

Water-circulating warming blankets are of no value when placed under adults on the OR table. Reasons include limited contact of the body with the blanket, limited circulation through areas in contact with the body, and limited total circulation of water through the blanket (12-15 gallons per hour). However, they are effective when placed on top of a patient in the PACU. In this application, they are more effective than radiant heat lamps but less effective than forced hot air warmers.

### New Technologies

There are two new extracorporeal heat exchange devices available to rewarm severely hypothermic patients. Both depend on arteriovenous flow of blood by means of heparin-bonded tubing through an efficient heat exchanger. One depends on the patient's own circulation to drive the flow; the other uses a centrifugal pump. Because they use heparin-bonded tubing, systemic anticoagulation is not required.

Another new device places an extremity in a clear plastic "boot" with a vacuum applied to create vasodilation mechanically. The boot is heated, which in turn heats the blood flowing through the extremity; the manufacturer claims it may raise body temperature as much as 1°C every 10 minutes. Controlled studies on the use of either of these devices were not available at the time of this publication.

### How Is Shivering Treated in the Postanesthesia Care Unit?

Several measures can be used to minimize hypothermia and shivering (Table 48–8). The PACU should be comfortably warm, and patients should be kept covered. Supplemental O₂ must be provided to all hypothermic patients. Cutaneous warming stops shivering.[46,47] Rapid increase of cutaneous temperature, especially in the blush area of the face and chest, is most effective. Thermal comfort correlates with peripheral

**TABLE 48–8.** Treating Hypothermia and Shivering in the Postanesthesia Care Unit

---

Supplemental oxygen until patients are fully warm
Stop shivering
  Intravenous meperidine (12.5–25 mg)
  Intravenous clonidine (0.15 mg)
  Cutaneous heat source: forced hot air system warming blanket over the patient, radiant heat lamps
  Paralysis and mechanical ventilation in severely hypothermic, sick patients

---

rather than central temperatures. Cutaneous warming stops shivering before it raises core temperature. If the cutaneous heat source is removed, the patient shivers again.

### Meperidine and Clonidine

Intravenous meperidine, 12.5 to 25 mg, is effective in rapidly terminating or decreasing the severity of shivering after general anesthesia.[48] No other narcotic has this effect. The mechanism of action is unknown. This approach is the quickest, most efficacious, least costly, and most benign treatment for ordinary PAS. The efficacy of intravenous meperidine for shivering associated with epidural anesthesia is unclear. Clonidine, 0.15 mg intravenously, is as effective as meperidine.

### Intubation and Passive Warming

Finally, sick patients may not tolerate the hemodynamic consequences of shivering. Consideration should be given to keeping sick patients intubated, paralyzed, and on controlled ventilation while they are warmed with convective blankets to prevent the hemodynamic sequelae of vigorous shivering.

## HYPERTHERMIA

In ancient Greece, fever was viewed as a beneficial sign during infection, partly because of the humoral theory of disease. It was believed to promote purification and elimination of the evil body humors. In fact, considerable data support the hypothesis that temperature elevation can be beneficial in enhancing a host's defense mechanisms by promoting the mobility of leukocytes and their bactericidal and chemotactic properties and by enhancing lymphocyte transformation and interferon activity.[49,50] Fever may represent the body's response to viral, bacterial, or fungal infection; malignancy; drug toxicity; dehydration; connective tissue disease; hypersensitivity to foreign protein; endocrinopathy; and medication or substance withdrawal. However, regardless of its origin, fever is a costly metabolic process.

### What Is Hyperthermia?

*Hyperthermia* can be defined as a regulated elevation of central body temperature from a baseline temperature. In formulating this definition, consideration must be given to circadian rhythms, exercise, menstruation, and environment. Although not constant, an oral temperature of 37°C (98.6°F) can be considered normal under most circumstances. An evening increase to 38°C may be perfectly normal if multiple readings are scrutinized for a circadian trend.

The importance of temperature recording in anesthesia practice is to determine a baseline value and to investigate any acute trend that may develop (keeping in mind that body temperature typically decreases on commencement of anesthesia). The magnitude and rate of temperature elevation can lend helpful assistance in determining its source. For clarification, any acute rise of 2°C per hour merits rapid evaluation.

Extreme pyrexia with temperatures in excess of 41°C (106°F) is rare from an infection. Meningitis, pneumonia, AIDS, or bacteremia may be the culprit. High temperature is often caused by dysfunctional thermoregulation, represented by increased heat production (thyrotoxicosis, pheochromocytoma, exercise, neuroleptic malignant syndrome, and malignant hyperthermia); decreased heat dissipation (dehydration, heatstroke, autonomic dysfunction, excessive occlusive coverings, atropine); and hypothalamic influences (stroke, tumor, trauma, infection, and antipsychotic medications).[50]

## What Are the Physiologic Alterations Induced by Increased Temperature?

### Metabolic

A 1°C elevation of body temperature raises the basal metabolic rate by 10% to 12%, with a parallel increase in $O_2$ consumption, $CO_2$ production, and fluid and nutritional requirements. An alkalotic state due to respiratory compensation may be superseded by a cellular source of acid byproducts, leading to metabolic acidosis. This increased systemic demand can impose a great burden on a marginal cardiovascular system.

### Cardiovascular

Direct cardiovascular effects of extreme pyrexia include myocardial hemorrhages, myofibril degeneration, and occasional necrosis, especially in the left ventricular myocardium. Temperature-induced increases of catecholamine are primarily responsible for tachycardia, dysrhythmias, conduction changes, and demand-induced myocardial ischemia.

### Endocrine

The endocrine system may respond by increasing the release of ADH, aldosterone, growth hormone, corticosteroids, and thyroid hormone. Thus, further alterations in water and electrolyte balance, glucose, lipid and carbohydrate production and metabolism, and the body's overall metabolic rate can be directly or indirectly influenced by fever.

### Central Nervous System

Central nervous system (CNS) deterioration may be evidenced by alterations in sensorium and cognitive skills and by seizure activity. Microscopically, neuronal degeneration, cellular edema, and parenchymal hemorrhages have been noted at necropsy after hyperpyrexia.

### Hematologic

Hematologic changes may include decreases in platelets, prothrombin, fibrinogen, and coagulation factors (V, VI, VIII) as well as spontaneous fibrinolysis and a consumptive coagulopathy.

## What Is the Differential Diagnosis of Hyperthermia?

The vast array of causes can be narrowed to a manageable few by a quick review of a patient's medical history, medications and allergies, personal and family anesthetic history, current illness necessitating surgical intervention, and the anesthetic care rendered (Table 48–9). Although MH could be categorized under drug reactions, its importance in anesthetic practice is indisputable. The differential diagnosis of hypermetabolic states is summarized in Tables 48–9 and 48–10.

## What Metabolic Aberrations Lead to Hyperthermia?

### Acute Thyroid Crisis (Thyroid Storm)

Thyroid storm is a life-threatening state of decompensated thyrotoxicosis that can appear abruptly on induction of anesthesia, during the course of surgery, or postoperatively[51] (see Table 48–10). The usual manifestations of hyperthyroidism

**TABLE 48–9.** Differential Diagnosis of Hyperthermia

Metabolic imbalance
Excessive ambient, occlusive coverings
Drug reaction
Instrument malfunction or misuse
Central nervous system aberration
Malignant hyperthermia

**TABLE 48–10.** Hypermetabolic Syndromes—Differential Clinical Signs

| Clinical Sign | Malignant Hyperthermia | Neuroleptic Malignant Syndrome | Pheochromocytoma | Thyroid Crisis |
|---|---|---|---|---|
| Onset | Rapid, slow | Hours to days | Rapid | Rapid |
| Triggers | Succinylcholine, potent inhalation agents | Butyrophenones | Surgical stress | Surgical stress |
| Fever | Rapid, extreme | Slow, mild, moderate | Mild, moderate | Mild, moderate |
| Rigidity | 75%, rapid | Yes, slow | Rare or none | Rare or none |
| Tachycardia | Yes | Yes | Yes | Yes |
| Arrhythmias | Yes | Yes | Yes | Yes |
| Labile blood pressure | Yes | Yes | Yes | Yes |
| Hypermetabolic | Extreme | Yes | Yes, moderate | Yes, moderate |
| Rhabdomyolysis | Yes | Often | Rare | Rare |
| Diaphoresis | Yes | Yes | Yes | Yes |
| Creatine kinase elevation | Yes, extreme | Often | Unlikely | Unlikely |
| Familial or genetic | Yes | Doubtful | Often | Possible |
| Altered central nervous system | Yes | Yes | Possible | Often |
| Therapy (plus supportive treatment) | Dantrolene | Dantrolene or bromocriptine | α-, β-Blockers; surgical excision | β-Blockers, iodide, propylthiouracil |

are coupled with an extreme hypermetabolic and adrenergic-like state, leading to marked increases in cardiac output, $O_2$ consumption, and $CO_2$ production. Thyroxine, in animal models, increases sodium-potassium-adenosine triphosphatase activity, enhances adenosine triphosphate–supported calcium transport, and maximizes calcium storage capacity in the sarcoplasmic reticulum.

Tachycardia, dysrhythmias, tachypnea, extreme pyrexia, diaphoresis, and mental status changes are hallmarks of this acute response to excess thyroid hormones. Fortunately, this presentation is rare as a consequence of adequate preoperative preparation. Acute thyroid crisis can promote muscle rigidity in its extreme form and mimic MH.[52] Dantrolene has been used successfully as an antipyretic to relieve rigidity and decrease the hypermetabolic state when acute thyroid crisis could not be clinically differentiated from MH.

## Pheochromocytoma

Pheochromocytoma and its extraadrenal variants, similar to thyroid storm, stimulate an increase in metabolism with acute onset of diaphoresis, extreme tachycardia and hypertension, dysrhythmias, and pyrexia. Paroxysmal signs and symptoms due to episodic release of catecholamines can be precipitated by anesthesia, surgery, physical activity, and labor. The elevated temperature may originate from the body's increased metabolic rate and the catecholamine-induced peripheral vasoconstriction that diminishes cutaneous heat loss, subsequently elevating the core temperature. As with thyroid storm, the constellation of clinical changes associated with these two metabolic derangements can masquerade as MH[53] (see Table 48–10).

## Preexisting Infection

Whether it is community acquired or nosocomial in origin, preexisting infection is a common denominator in many patients who present for anesthetic care. Superficial skin infections requiring débridement, intrathoracic or intraabdominal infectious processes, urinary tract contamination, pulmonary emboli and infection, pericarditis and infective endocarditis, and perforated viscus and biliary tract involvement are but a few of the many conditions that may necessitate surgical care or be present as a result of coexisting disease. Postoperative fever in a patient with active, known infection or an infection that is yet undisclosed may confuse the differential diagnosis of fever.

## Recipients of Blood or Blood Components

Recipients of blood or blood components can experience a wide array of transfusion-related reactions leading to temperature elevation. Allergic reactions based on leukocyte-antibody interaction (donor versus recipient) and febrile reactions, most likely due to recipient antibodies and surface antigens of the donor platelet and leukocyte populations, occur in up to 3% of transfusions. Incompatible blood may lead to a hemolytic reaction, resulting in a low- to moderate-grade fever, among other characteristic morbidities. Bacterial contamination of the blood product (even autologously donated blood), which can lead to sepsis, although quite uncommon, is another possibility to be keep in mind.[54]

## Bacterial Transfer

Bacteria infused from outdated or "set-up-in-advance" intravenous fluid may be a source, as is contaminated intravenous fluid (by a needle, dirty administration set, uncapped and contaminated stopcock sites, and ports). Cross-contamination between patients can result from the illegal and ill-advised practice of reusing single-use vials and infusion sets (continuous infusion propofol, short-acting opioids, and muscle relaxants) for multiple patients. Outdated medications and unused, yet clean, syringes saved from a previous case also increase the possibility of introducing contaminated material and causing an acute febrile episode. Propofol and its carrier medium have been noted to promote the growth of microorganisms and should be disposed of within a reasonable time after opening the vial (within 6 hours). Thus, when drawing up propofol, the syringe should have the time filled written on it.

## Osteogenesis Imperfecta

Several publications mention the observation that the pyrexia associated with osteogenesis imperfecta may be related to an inherent hypermetabolic state leading to increased heart rate, respiratory rate, temperature, and metabolic rate. These changes perhaps are coincidental, but the suggestion that osteogenesis imperfecta is related to MH should be recognized and appreciated.[55]

## What Drug Reactions Should Be Considered?

### Neuroleptic Malignant Syndrome

Neuroleptic malignant syndrome (NMS) is caused by a neuroleptic-induced alteration of dopamine action in the basal ganglia and hypothalamus. It occurs in up to 1.5% of patients who are treated chronically with psychotropic drugs such as phenothiazines, butyrophenones, and monoamine oxidase inhibitors (MAOIs). It has a less abrupt onset (days to weeks) and a longer duration (1-2 weeks) than MH. The problem is characterized by a slow onset of akinesia, muscle rigidity, hyperpyrexia, and mental status fluctuations that may last 5 to 10 days. Autonomic dysfunction leads to diaphoresis, labile hemodynamics, and tachycardia. The mortality of such an event (15%) may be precipitated by dysrhythmia, respiratory failure, myocardial ischemia or infarction, pulmonary embolism, rhabdomyolysis-induced renal failure, or a combination of these events (see Table 48–10). Despite a typical leukocytosis, elevated liver enzymes, and increased creatine kinase (CK) levels, no diagnostic tests exist.

Therapy includes discontinuation of neuroleptics and initiation of supportive measures to control temperature, acid-base imbalance, muscle tone, and fluid requirements. No consensus has been reached about specific therapy, yet combination therapy with centrally acting bromocriptine and peripherally acting dantrolene may have clinical usefulness. Despite similarities between MH and NMS, the relatively small clinical sample of patients tested has failed to demonstrate a clear relationship through muscle contracture evaluation.[56,57]

### Central Anticholinergic Syndrome

Central anticholinergic syndrome is an extreme complication of routine doses of anticholinergics. Presenting signs range from excitatory or agitated behavior to respiratory depression and coma. Mild pyrexia may exist in 25% of episodes, although temperature elevation to 41.3°C associated with scopolamine administration has been reported.[58] After routine administration of atropine, one must recognize the common response of temperature elevation because of diminished sweating and tachycardia, both of which should also raise suspicion of MH.

### Monoamine Oxidase Inhibitors

MAOIs used in the therapy of various psychotic-depressive disorders are a potential source of serious drug interactions when patients receiving them are anesthetized. Blockade of the MAO enzyme complex promotes the accumulation of catecholamines (norepinephrine, epinephrine, dopamine, 5-hydroxytryptamine). Excessive doses of MAOIs can induce hyperpyrexia by two possible pathways: (1) excessive sympathetic α-stimulation with peripheral vasoconstriction, leading to limited cutaneous heat transfer; and (2) central effects with altered hypothalamic influence. Meperidine in particular and morphine, which cause catecholamine and histamine release, respectively, can induce a hypertensive, hyperpyrexic, rigid state with marked CNS aberration. Meperidine is to be absolutely avoided and morphine avoided or severely restricted in patients receiving MAOI medications.

### Tricyclic Antidepressants

Tricyclic antidepressants block neuronal norepinephrine uptake both centrally and peripherally and promote anticholinergic activity. The potential to foster dysrhythmias, tachycardia, cardiac decompensation, and hyperpyrexia is evident.

### Cocaine and Amphetamines

Cocaine and amphetamines alter the presynaptic reuptake of neurotransmitters, leading to a myriad of cardiovascular and CNS effects. Acute toxicity may present as agitation, paranoia, hallucinations, or combative behavior. These are frequently coupled with severe hypertension, dysrhythmias, stroke, and myocardial ischemia, even in patients with no history of previous cardiovascular disease. Hyperthermia can occur in response to increased basal metabolic rate and decreased peripheral heat loss due to cutaneous vasoconstriction. Further, cocaine can initiate the central anticholinergic syndrome and its effect on thermoregulation.

### Drug Withdrawal

Withdrawal from drugs, prescribed or illicit, can elevate core temperature. Ethanol and opioid abstinence during the perioperative period can elicit tachycardia, hypertension, and hyperpyrexia. Clonidine withdrawal, theoretically, can lead to catecholamine-induced temperature changes. Abrupt discontinuation of levodopa in the parkinsonian population can lead to either an elevation in temperature alone or, more seriously, NMS.

### When Are Mechanical Factors a Problem?

Conductive and convective heat gain through radiant warmers, warm air convection systems, or a warmed mattress, when in excess of the actual heat loss, promotes heat gain and temperature elevation. Overindulgence of techniques that minimize heat loss, coupled with losses that are smaller than anticipated, can induce further elevations in body temperature.

Warming blankets or heated humidifying systems with an excessively high set-point may contribute to elevated temperatures. More important, the danger of cutaneous thermal burns at skin contact points and tracheal and bronchial mucosal drying may lead to damage, with subsequent edema, inflammation, and hemorrhage.

Automated rapid-infusion (warm fluid) devices are a useful adjunct to resuscitation and, although temperature maintenance is the goal, occasional temperature overshoot may take place. A more than 1°C central temperature elevation may rarely occur after significant fluid replacement incorporating a rapid-infusion device, for example, during a radical prostatectomy.

### When Is the Central Nervous System a Source of Fever?

The anterior hypothalamus contains the body's thermoregulatory center, which receives input from cutaneous skin receptors, the spinal cord, and the sympathetic nervous system. Each may contribute to alterations in central temperature. Various clinical conditions in neurosurgical patients exemplify central influence on body temperature. Any disruption of the blood-brain barrier that allows blood and cerebrospinal fluid to contact each other can initiate a febrile reaction, such as following a cerebral vascular accident, an intracerebral hemorrhage, or surgical and traumatic manipulation of the brain. Also, direct trauma to the hypothalamus or surrounding tissue, edema, or vascular compromise can initiate "brain storming," with profound elevations in body temperature.

## MALIGNANT HYPERTHERMIA

Ombrédanne noted the relationship of anesthesia and hyperthermia in 1929 (Ombrédanne's syndrome), yet it was not until 1960 that Denborough and Lovell published their classic description of a familial trend in anesthetic-induced death.[59] In 1966, Wilson coined the term *malignant hyperpyrexia*. The term *malignant* was appropriate at the time, owing to an incomplete understanding of the disease, the lack of a specific antidote, and the high mortality rate. Characteristic findings are listed in Table 48–10. Extensive research, data collection and analysis, and an ongoing educational effort has propelled MH to its current position of importance with the anesthesia care provider.

### What Is the Incidence?

The estimated incidence of fulminant MH is 1 in 250 000 anesthetics[60] (Table 48–11). A combination of succinylcholine (SCH) and potent inhaled anesthetics may increase the incidence to 1 in 60 000 exposures. A 15-fold increase (1 in 4200) is noted in cases of suspected MH with this combination (see Table 48–10). The presenting signs and symptoms can be so variable, singly or in combination, that the suspicion of MH differs among individual patients according to the

**TABLE 48–11.** Incidence of Different Forms of Malignant Hyperthermia (MH) in Relation to Type of Anesthesia

| Type of Anesthesia | Fulminant MH | Abortive MH (All Subgroups Included) | Overall Incidence of Suspected Malignant Hypothermia |
|---|---|---|---|
| Total number of anesthetics | 1:251 063 | 1:17 435 | 1:16 303 |
| General anesthesia | 1:221 811 | 1:15 404 | 1:14 403 |
| Anesthesia with administration of succinylcholine | 1:140 006 | 1:8819 | 1:8297 |
| Anesthesia with potent inhalation agent | 1:84 488 | 1:6653 | 1:6167 |
| With succinylcholine | 1:61 961 | 1:4506 | 1:4201 |
| Without succinylcholine | 1:174 597 | 1:20 541 | 1:18 379 |

From Ording H. Incidence of malignant hyperthermia in Denmark. *Anesth Analg.* 1985;64:704. © International Anesthesia Research Society.

practitioner's interpretation. Although all age groups can experience MH, the incidence appears higher in children aged 3 to 12 years. However, a case of severe muscle rigidity has been described in a premature infant born by cesarean section after a triggering general anesthetic.[61]

## How Is the Diagnosis Made?

### Clinical Assessment

One word is the key to diagnosis: *suspicion*. Survival from an MH episode requires early treatment. The crucial element in early treatment is heightened awareness of the possibility of MH and a keen suspicion based on clinical signs while other potential causes are excluded. The onset may occur immediately after induction with potent inhalation agents, SCH, or both, or it may be delayed by the use of nondepolarizing relaxants and barbiturates until later in the case or even for as long as 18 to 24 hours postoperatively. The appearance of tachycardia, tachypnea (increased metabolism of onboard relaxants), muscle rigidity, rising partial pressure of end-tidal $CO_2$ ($ETCO_2$) in the presence of constant ventilation, and fever (frequently with a delayed onset) should stimulate the evaluation of arterial and venous blood samples for respiratory or metabolic acidosis (Table 48–12).

Capnography is a sensitive indicator of an evolving hypermetabolic state, but other causes should be excluded. A single clinical sign does not usually implicate MH susceptibility (MHS) correctly, although generalized rigidity alone may be the only single sign that suggests susceptibility.[62,63] The maximum temperature attained during a MH episode has a direct correlation to the mortality rate (Table 48–13). Remember, however, that rapid temperature elevation may be delayed in onset and should not be the sole criterion to suggest or confirm a diagnosis of MH.

The North American MH Registry is currently attempting to clarify diagnostic criteria (clinical signs) and to formulate a grading system that assesses both the likelihood of a clinical case representing true MH and a patient's chances of being MH susceptible through contracture testing. The MH clinical grading system will use clinical information exclusively, without reference to the results of the MH muscle biopsy. This approach will allow researchers to compare patients continent-wide and to consolidate investigative efforts. It is suggested that any practitioner who is confronted with a clear-cut case of MH or any case with questionable clinical signs and symptoms contact the Malignant Hyperthermia Association of the United States (MHAUS) to receive an adverse metabolic reaction to anesthesia questionnaire. This can be completed and forwarded to MHAUS for inclusion in the database (see telephone number, website, and email address at the end of the chapter).

## What Anesthetic Agents Are Triggers?

Triggers are any of the inhalational volatile agents, in addition to SCH. MHS in swine can be triggered by nonanesthetic factors (eg, stress, exercise, fright). Evidence is accumulating that families with MHS may have a higher incidence of sudden death and a predisposition to a nonspecific cardiomyopathy. Additionally, although MH is rare in conscious human beings, associations linking MH to heatstroke, unusual stress states, and myalgias are surfacing.[64]

The list of potential triggering agents has been modified with continued clinical testing and experience. Because amide local anesthetics can raise intracellular calcium levels, they were once considered unsafe. Presently, after extensive testing

**TABLE 48–12.** Frequency of Early Clinical Signs

| Clinical Sign | Number of Patients | Percentage of Patients With Sign |
|---|---|---|
| Tachycardia | 409 | 91 |
| Hyperventilation | 209 | 83 |
| Muscle rigidity | 448 | 79 |
| Altered blood pressure | 254 | 78 |
| Fever | 201 | 72 |
| Cyanosis | 273 | 69 |

Data from Britt BA, Lwong FHF, Endrenyi L. The clinical and laboratory features of malignant hyperthermia management: a review. In: Henschel EO, ed. *Malignant Hyperthermia Syndrome.* New York, NY: Appleton-Century-Crofts; 1977:9–45.

**TABLE 48–13.** Maximum Temperature Attained and Mortality Rates

| Maximum Temperature | | Number of Patients | Mortality (%) |
|---|---|---|---|
| (°F) | (°C) | | |
| 99–100.9 | 37.2–38.2 | 57 | 3.5 |
| 101–102.9 | 38.3–39.3 | 79 | 8.9 |
| 103–104.9 | 39.4–40.5 | 103 | 16.5 |
| 105–106.9 | 40.6–41.6 | 99 | 38.4 |
| 107–108.9 | 41.7–42.7 | 159 | 66.7 |
| 109–110.9 | 42.8–43.8 | 57 | 86.0 |
| >110.9 | >43.8 | 19 | 94.7 |

Data from Britt BA, Lwong FHF, Endrenyi L. The clinical and laboratory features of malignant hyperthermia management: a review. In: Henschel EO, ed. *Malignant Hyperthermia Syndrome.* New York, NY: Appleton-Century-Crofts; 1977:9–45.

of swine with MHS and the common use of amide local anesthetic techniques in patients with MHS during biopsies for MH, they have been reclassified to the "safe" group (Table 48–14). However, it has been suggested that they be avoided during an acute episode, if possible, because of their induction of calcium shifts.

## How Is an Acute Episode of Malignant Hyperthermia Treated?

Alterations in the sarcoplasmic calcium flux induced by triggering agents can lead to increases in metabolism, heat production, and acidic waste generation. If exposure to the triggers persists, the regulation of energy production and enzymatic control is lost. Cellular demand for $O_2$ and energy substrates outstrips supply, culminating in acidosis, cellular and interstitial edema, loss of perfusion, and further membranous breakdown. Fulminant MH requires urgent therapy to ensure survival. The clinical signs can be noted within minutes and, despite appropriate and timely treatment, deterioration can be so rapid that death ensues. Conversely, the course may be less rapid, allowing resuscitative measures and dantrolene to prove their worth. A suggested clinical plan for therapy of an acute MH episode is presented in Table 48–15.

## What Are the Serious Late Complications?

Rhabdomyolysis, with its associated muscle breakdown and pigment-induced acute tubular necrosis, is preventable or can at least be limited with adequate and timely dantrolene therapy and supportive measures to ensure adequate urine output (fluid, diuretics, mannitol, alkalization). A consumptive coagulopathy can be induced by the release of mediators, endothelial thromboplastins, hemolysis, inadequate capillary blood flow, and tissue destruction.

Appropriate therapy includes supportive and therapeutic care during the MH episode, which may control or eliminate

**TABLE 48–14.** Safe Anesthetic Agents in Patients With Malignant Hyperthermia and Malignant Hyperthermia Susceptibility

| | |
|---|---|
| Barbiturates and intravenous anesthetics | Thiopental (Pentothal) |
| | Methohexital (Brevital) |
| | Thiamylal (Surital) |
| | Propofol (Diprivan) |
| | Etomidate (Amidate) |
| Narcotics (opioids) | Morphine |
| | Meperidine (Demerol) |
| | Hydromorphone (Dilaudid) |
| | Fentanyl (Sublimaze) |
| | Sufentanil (Sufenta) |
| | Alfentanil (Alfenta) |
| Tranquilizers | Diazepam (Valium) |
| | Midazolam (Versed) |
| Amides | Lidocaine (Xylocaine) |
| | Mepivacaine (Carbocaine) |
| | Bupivacaine (Marcaine) |
| | Etidocaine (Duranest) |
| | Prilocaine (Citanest) |
| Esters | Procaine (Novocain) |
| | Chloroprocaine (Nesacaine) |
| | Tetracaine (Pontocaine) |

**TABLE 48–15.** Emergency Therapy for Malignant Hyperthermia (Revised 1993)

1. Immediately discontinue all volatile inhalation anesthetics and succinylcholine. Hyperventilate with 100% oxygen at high gas flows; at least 10 L/min. The circle system and $CO_2$ absorbent need not be changed.
2. Administer dantrolene sodium, 2–3 mg/kg initial bolus rapidly with increments up to 10 mg/kg total. Continue to administer dantrolene until signs of MH (eg, tachycardia, rigidity, increased end-tidal $CO_2$, and temperature elevation) are controlled. Occasionally, a total dose greater than 10 mg/kg may be needed. Each vial of dantrolene contains 20 mg of dantrolene and 3 g mannitol. Each vital should be mixed with 60 mL of sterile water for injection USP without a bacteriostatic agent.
3. Administer bicarbonate to correct metabolic acidosis as guided by blood gas analysis. In the absence of blood gas analysis, 1–2 mEq/kg should be administered.
4. Simultaneous with the above, actively cool the hyperthermic patient. Use IV iced saline (not lactated Ringer's solution), 15 mL/kg q 15 min × 3.
   a. Lavage stomach, bladder, rectum, and open cavities with iced saline as appropriate.
   b. Surface cool with ice and hypothermia blanket.
   c. Monitor closely because overvigorous treatment may lead to hypothermia.
5. Dysrhythmias will usually respond to treatment of acidosis and hyperkalemia. If they persist or are life-threatening, standard antiarrhythmic agents may be used, with the exception of calcium channel blockers (which may cause hyperkalemia and cardiovascular collapse).
6. Determine and monitor end-tidal $CO_2$; arterial, central, or femoral venous blood gases; serum potassium; calcium; clotting studies; and urine output.
7. Hyperkalemia is common and should be treated with hyperventilation, bicarbonate, intravenous glucose and insulin (10 units regular insulin in 50 mL 50% glucose titrated to potassium level). Life-threatening hyperkalemia may also be treated with calcium administration (eg, 2–5 mg/kg of $CaCl_2$).
8. Ensure urine output of greater than 2 mL/kg/h. Consider central venous or pulmonary artery monitoring because of fluid shifts and hemodynamic instability that may occur.
9. Boys younger than 9 years of age who experience sudden cardiac arrest after succinylcholine administration in the absence of hypoxemia should be treated for acute hyperkalemia first. In this situation, calcium chloride should be administered along with other means to reduce serum potassium. They should be presumed to have subclinical muscular dystrophy.

**Postacute Phase**

1. Observe the patient in an intensive care unit setting for at least 24 h because recrudescence of MH may occur, particularly after a fulminant case resistant to treatment.
2. Administer dantrolene, 1 mg/kg IV q 6 h for 24–48 h postepisode. After that, oral dantrolene, 1 mg/kg q 6 h, may be used for 24 h as necessary.
3. Follow arterial blood gases, creatine kinase, potassium, calcium, urine and serum myoglobin, clotting studies, and core body temperature until such time as they return to normal values (eg, q 6 h). Central temperature (eg, rectal, esophageal) should be continuously monitored until stable.
4. Counsel the patient and family regarding MH and further precautions. Refer the patient to Malignant Hyperthermia Association of the United States. Fill out an Adverse Metabolic Reaction to Anesthesia (AMRA) report available through the North American Malignant Hyperthermia Registry (717) 531-6936. **CAUTION:** This protocol may not apply to every patient and must of necessity be altered according to specific patient needs.

Used with permission from Malignant Hyperthermia Association of the United States.

the instigating mediator. Treatment with intravenous heparin, blood components, and ∈-aminocaproic acid should be reserved for difficult cases unresponsive to standard MH resuscitative measures. Insufficient oxygenation and perfusion (hypermetabolic state) and loss of cell membrane integrity may lead to cerebral edema, cellular ischemia and destruction, increased intracranial pressure, coma, paralysis, and other serious neurologic sequelae.

### How Does Dantrolene Work?

Dantrolene inhibits calcium release from the sarcoplasmic reticulum without altering the reuptake mechanism. Hence, it can foster a reversal of the calcium accumulation that occurs in the skeletal muscle sarcoplasm during a triggered MH episode. Originally investigated as an antibiotic, dantrolene found use in spastic muscle disorders by virtue of its muscle relaxation properties. It is also a very effective antipyretic.

Various hypercatabolic disorders presenting with clinical signs similar to MH can be treated with dantrolene with marked improvement. Its use in NMS, heatstroke, and MAOI overdose for reversal of the hyperpyrexia and hypermetabolic signs suggests a potentially wider array of clinical applications.[65–67] Likewise, clinical signs that are suggestive of MH and that appear during anesthetic administration and are treated successfully with dantrolene have proved, on occasion, not to represent MH but rather cases of acute thyroid crisis and pheochromocytoma.[62,63]

### Prophylactic Use in Patients With Malignant Hyperthermia

MHAUS suggests that prophylactic dantrolene administration should be considered on an individual basis. Questions to be addressed when making this decision should include the following:

1. Is the surgery emergent, and will the added stress involved initiate an MH episode?
2. What coexisting disease is present, and how well will the patient tolerate a potential multifocal increase in $O_2$ consumption, lactate production, tachycardia, fever, and hypercatabolic problems?
3. Does the patient have a preexisting muscular disorder in which muscle weakness could be exacerbated by dantrolene administration (eg, muscular dystrophy or myasthenia gravis)?

Susceptible parturients should receive dantrolene, if indicated, preferably after cord clamping to minimize fetal and newborn exposure. A well-informed patient and individual practitioners may be reluctant to leave the patient unprotected, feeling more comfortable with pretreatment. However, no case of severe or fatal MH has been reported when the anesthesia team was informed of the patient's risk and a nontriggering technique was used either with or without dantrolene prophylaxis.[68]

If prophylactic therapy is instituted, 2.5 mg/kg should be given intravenously 30 minutes before induction of anesthesia.[69,70] This recommendation is based on the data collected from a multicenter study in which a mean dose of 2.5 mg/kg was shown to be sufficient to reverse MH reactions.[69] The current trend is away from dantrolene prophylaxis (except in the previously mentioned circumstances), depending instead on monitoring temperature, $ETCO_2$, blood gas analysis, and muscle tone.[71] Additionally, standard recommendations for intraoperative care should be followed (Table 48–16).

**TABLE 48–16.** Treatment of Malignant Hyperthermia (MH)-Susceptible Patients (Known or Suspected)

Anesthesia machine: Remove or drain/disconnect vaporizers. High-flow $O_2$ (10 L/min) for 20 min through circuit, 10 min if fresh gas line is replaced. Use a new or disposable breathing circuit.

Preoperative creatine kinase determination and complete blood count

Cooling blanket on operating room table, nearly iced fluids, a posted MH plan in a conspicuous site, and an MH cart or kit with necessary medications (ie, dantrolene, at least 36 vials)

Dantrolene prophylaxis (controversial) should be considered on an individual basis.

Technique of choice: regional or local: Avoid triggering agents. Monitor routine American Society of Anesthesiologists guidelines, capnography, temperature. Invasive monitoring as appropriate for surgery.

Uneventful anesthetic course: postoperative minimum 4 h electrocardiography, temperature monitoring. No further dantrolene is necessary.

MH episode postoperative: titrate dantrolene to normalize clinical signs continue for 36 h after stabilization (suggested dose of 1 mg/kg q 6 h). Monitor vitals, capnography, core temperature; check venous and arterial blood gases, baseline creatine kinase, electrolytes, calcium, lactate, blood urea nitrogen, creatinine, coagulation profile, platelets, urine for color, myoglobin.

Modified from Malignant Hyperthermia Association of the United States (MHAUS). Darien, Conn: MHAUS; 1991.

### Oral Dantrolene

Prophylactic coverage with dantrolene by the oral route is believed by some to be inadequate for patients with MHS. This opinion appears to be founded on case reports in which breakthrough MH episodes surfaced despite preoperative oral dose coverage. However, the dose given may have been inadequate, considering total dose and the time sequence of administration.[68] Based on studies of swine with MHS, Flewellen and colleagues suggested that a dose of dantrolene that produces at least 95% of the maximum muscle twitch depression (serum level, 2.8 µg/mL) provides protection against MH.[69]

Attainment of an adequate serum level with oral dantrolene may require the US Food and Drug Administration's recommended 5 mg/kg/d, with proper timing of the last preinduction dose. Allen and colleagues incorporated this amount in four divided doses, with the last given 4 hours preinduction.[70] Appropriate plasma levels were reached at induction and maintained for 6 to 18 hours thereafter.

Despite this study and the fact that oral dantrolene is less costly, requires no reconstitution, and avoids the large dose of mannitol required to make intravenous dantrolene solution isotonic, intravenous preparation prevents any uncertainty about adequacy of serum levels. It may also decrease the incidence of preoperative muscle weakness, lethargy, and gastrointestinal distress and negate lengthy preoperative hospitalization. Although no anesthetic regimen can guarantee immunity to MH, provision of adequate preoperative sedation and preparation with oral or intravenous dantrolene may allow the use of a nontriggering anesthetic.

### Dosing Recommendations

The initial dose of intravenous dantrolene, as discussed, is 2.5 mg/kg.[71] Subsequent dosing is based on clinical signs. After the initial dose, if objective clinical evidence does not support improvement (resolved dysrhythmias and hemodynamic stability, less rigidity, decreased $ETCO_2$, lower temperature), repeating the dose up to 20 mg/kg is recommended. Although most cases respond to 4 mg/kg or less, an occasional patient requires higher doses for control. Also, recrudescence is possible within a few hours to days after the episode. After reversal and stabilization, continued administration of intravenous dantrolene (1 mg/kg every 4-6 hours) is warranted for at least 24 and possibly 48 hours. Oral dosing may be used after successful treatment.

### Side Effects

The potential side effects or adverse reactions include lethargy, altered sensorium, and muscle weakness. Gastrointestinal distress with nausea and vomiting, skin rash, and phlebitis are other concerns. Concurrent dantrolene administration may potentiate the action of neuromuscular blocking agents. Likewise, significant hyperkalemia and cardiac depression can occur with concurrent calcium channel blocker therapy. Placental transfer with subsequent fetal and neonatal lethargy and weakness, and the association of dantrolene and uterine atony leading to postpartum hemorrhage, are concerns in obstetric cases.[65]

## What Preoperative Conditions Suggest Risk?

### General Considerations

Factors that suggest MH risk include a personal or family history of anesthetic problems (high fever, dark urine, or rigidity), unexplained anesthetic deaths, and masseter muscle spasm. Screening CK values are elevated in 70% of affected people but have proved less useful in predicting MHS than was previously thought. If a resting serum CK level is elevated in a close relative of a patient with MHS, that relative could be considered susceptible without a documenting contracture test. However, a normal CK level has less predictive value; therefore, a biopsy specimen should be secured for testing.

### Associated Characteristics

Other characteristics noted to occur with higher frequency in individuals with MHS include squinting, backache, muscle weakness and cramps, ptosis, strabismus, kyphoscoliosis, inguinal hernia, pectus abnormalities, and others. Smith suggested that a combination of 20 such variables was capable of predicting MHS with 61.5% reliability compared with muscle biopsy results (considered 95% reliable in estimating susceptibility).[72] Closer scrutiny of these characteristics on a single basis, not as a group, does not reliably reflect a significant difference between patients with MHS and control groups.[73]

### Related Disease Conditions

Many conditions and clinical signs have been suggested to have a higher incidence in patients with MHS. Central core disease and King-Denborough syndrome are related to MH, and patients with Duchenne's muscular dystrophy and other myopathies may develop any or all of the signs across the MH spectrum (Table 48–17).[74]

Fewer causal or coincidental relationships exist with osteogenesis imperfecta, NMS, glycogen storage diseases, lymphoma, and sudden infant death syndrome. Myotonic conditions that respond to SCH with rigidity and contracture can be confused with MH. However, they cause rigidity in the absence of serious metabolic derangements. Myotonic states may have positive results after MH contracture testing, further adding to the confusion and controversy.

**TABLE 48–17.** Disorders Associated With Malignant Hyperthermia

| | |
|---|---|
| Duchenne dystrophy | King-Denborough syndrome |
| Central core disease | Schwartz-Jampel syndrome |
| Neuroleptic malignant syndrome | Osteogenesis imperfecta |
| Myotonia congenita | |

### Duchenne-Type Muscular Dystrophy

Patients with Duchenne-type muscular dystrophy (MD) may respond to potent inhalation agents, with or without SCH, with sudden cardiac arrest or rhabdomyolysis. Although the incidence of MH in such patients is not confirmed, Sethna and Rockoff reported that 6 patients receiving a "safe" technique had no complications, whereas 5 of 19 patients who received volatile agents had problems (2 cardiac arrests, 3 unexplained fever or tachycardia responsive to withdrawal of the volatile agents).[74]

The Newington, Connecticut Children's Hospital, in a 10-year retrospective review of 84 anesthetics administered to 36 biopsy-diagnosed cases of Duchenne-type MD, reported that only 2 patients had premature ventricular contractions: 1 patient had a potassium level of 2.9 mEq/L; 1 had hyperthermia (skin temperature 102°F, responsive to discontinuation of a warming blanket and surface cooling measures). The remainder of the procedure was uneventful, and the patient's temperature in the PACU was 98°F. Of the 84 anesthetics, 83 were considered triggering (potent inhalation agents: 62% halothane, 26% isoflurane, 11% enflurane); SCH was used once without sequelae (A. Peluso and A. Bianchini, oral communication, 1992). Nonetheless, cautious handling of these cases is warranted.

## How Should Patients With Malignant Hyperthermia Be Anesthetized?

The key to success in anesthetizing a patient with MHS is preoperative preparation and perioperative heightened awareness for clinical clues suggestive of an MH episode in its early stages. To provide reassurance, one should discuss the perioperative management plan with the patient and family while emphasizing the anesthesia team's knowledge of MH recognition and its therapy.

### Techniques

The anesthetic technique is chosen on the basis of the surgical site and the patient's condition, understanding that local and regional methods are safe and recommended. Berkowitz and Rosenberg reported their success with femoral nerve block for muscle biopsy in patients with MH, eliminating the need for dantrolene pretreatment, even in high-risk patients.[75]

General anesthesia must consist of nontriggering agents. It

is no longer necessary to use a new or uncontaminated anesthetic machine (flushing high-flow $O_2$ for an extended period). Removing the vaporizers (or draining and disconnecting them), replacing the fresh gas hose, and using a new disposable circuit make the machine safe to use after 5 to 20 minutes of high-flow $O_2$.[76–78] Dantrolene prophylaxis is considered on an individual basis. Central temperature and ETCO$_2$ monitoring are essential, if applicable to the surgical case.

A written treatment plan, as suggested by the MHAUS, can conserve time and can be life-saving. During surgery, any unexpected tachycardia, tachypnea, dysrhythmia, muscle rigidity, or ETCO$_2$ elevation requires urgent evaluation. Postoperative care for an uneventful anesthetic course should consist of at least 4 hours of observation in the PACU, with continuous temperature and ECG monitoring.

## What Is the Relevance of Masseter Muscle Rigidity?

Although the appropriate management and the clinical significance of masseter muscle rigidity (MMR) are controversial, further confusion has surfaced because of differing definitions of what masseter muscle stiffness truly represents. To determine the incidence, one must first adequately define the meaning of the term *MMR*. The degree of masseter stiffness can vary among individual patients under various clinical conditions, as can the practitioner's assessment of the rigidity.

### Characteristic Responses

Kaplan elegantly categorized the spectrum of masseter stiffness into three areas[63] (Fig. 48–7). This relationship is pertinent to our clinical practice of anesthesia because MMR has been associated with MH and may herald its onset. The first category is characterized by a degree of masseter muscle stiffness that can be physically overcome (with some difficulty). With a special mastication traction device, Van Der Spek and colleagues determined that SCH, when combined with halothane, consistently reduces mouth opening and increases masseter muscle tone, most often to a subclinical degree.[79] This response may be regarded as a normal phenomenon in children given both halothane and SCH and apparently does not portend a marked increase in risk for MH.

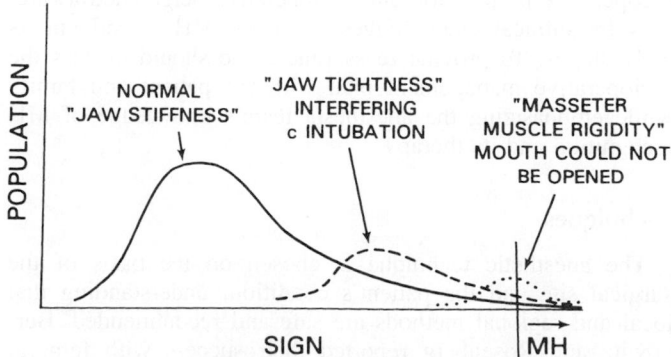

**FIGURE 48–7.** The spectrum of masseter muscle response to succinylcholine and the relationship to malignant hyperthermia. (From Kaplan RF. Hypothermia/hyperthermia. In: Gravenstein N, ed. *Manual of Complications During Anesthesia.* Philadelphia, Pa: JB Lippincott; 1991:138.)

**TABLE 48–18.** Suggested Therapy for Masseter Muscle Rigidity

1. Stop triggering agents.
2. Abort the procedure if elective (most conservative approach).
3. Ventilate with high-flow 100% oxygen; switch to a clean machine or Mapleson system.
    *Emergency case:* Hyperventilate, use a clean machine, alert for assistance.
4. Monitor vital signs, capnography, core temperature; check venous and arterial blood gases, baseline creatine kinase, electrolytes, calcium, lactate, blood urea nitrogen, creatinine, and urine for myoglobin, color.
5. If stable, hold dantrolene and observe in controlled setting (postanesthesia care unit, minimum of 4 h).
    *Emergency case:* Consider dantrolene to control a potential malignant hyperthermia crisis triggered by the emergency situation.
6. Give liberal fluids to force diuresis; creatine kinase determinations at 6, 12, 24 h. Additional laboratory studies as indicated.
7. Advise family counseling (noncontroversial), muscle biopsy (controversial).

The second category is a response to SCH in which jaw tightness interferes with the intubation process. Retrospective review suggests that the incidence is as high as 1% among children receiving both SCH and halothane. The precise risk for MH in patients who manifest this response is undetermined, yet it is considered to be small.

The third response can be described as "the mouth cannot be opened." This reaction to SCH most likely represents true MMR and may correspond to a high risk (~50%) for MHS, based on halothane contracture testing.[80,81] Other causes of limited jaw mobility should be excluded. Nevertheless, with any degree of perceived MMR, MH could follow immediately or after a delay of 20 minutes or more. Any patient experiencing MMR should be observed in the PACU for at least 4 hours, with attention paid to temperature, muscle tone, and hemodynamic alterations. After PACU discharge, periodic serum CK determinations (every 6–8 hours for 24 hours) and the urine should be checked for color and the presence of myoglobin.

### Cancellation of Operation

Three schools of thought have been published concerning this controversy. The most conservative approach suggests stopping the anesthetic and aborting the surgery if it is an elective procedure. If surgery must continue, switch to nontriggering agents with precautionary measures and monitoring for MH (Table 48–18). The second, less conservative plan is to switch to nontriggering agents (elective procedure) and continue with MH precautions and monitoring. The third approach is to continue the triggering agents while instituting appropriate MH monitoring.[82,83]

In the absence of another myopathy, all patients who were not receiving dantrolene for MMR and who had CK levels >20 000 IU/L after SCH use were MH positive by muscle biopsy.[80] In one review, all patients with MMR who had anesthesia halted after induction fared well whether or not they received dantrolene.[63]

Until these arguments are better supported with adequate data and contracture testing, prudence suggests handling this enigma in the most conservative manner, with follow-up serum CK determinations and urine evaluations. Providing patients with reassurance and education is essential.

## Anesthetic Management

Ideally, such patients will have undergone muscle contracture testing to determine their risk for MH; most, however, will likely not have had this procedure performed. Thus, SCH should definitely be omitted from the anesthetic plan. Until proved otherwise, all patients who experience MMR and their close relatives should be treated as MHS patients. Intraoperative $ETCO_2$ and temperature monitoring, muscle tone evaluation, close clinical scrutiny, heightened MH awareness, and a nontriggering anesthetic should suffice. Controversy exists about whether muscle biopsy testing for MH should be performed on all those experiencing MMR and their families and whether intravenous dantrolene should be administered after the occurrence of MMR in the absence of other signs of MH.

## What Should Be Known About the Biochemistry of Malignant Hyperthermia?

MH is a disease affecting seemingly all skeletal muscle membranes once a triggering agent initiates the calcium ($Ca^{2+}$)-related cascade. Excessive $Ca^{2+}$ in the myoplasm may result when the overly sensitive sarcoplasmic reticulum is exposed to halothane. Potentiation of $Ca^{2+}$ released by increased phospholipase $A_2$ activity and its effect on free unsaturated fatty acids from mitochondria have been linked with halothane exposure, leading to a further elevation of myoplasmic $Ca^{2+}$.

An abnormal $Ca^{2+}$-release channel protein in the sarcoplasmic reticulum, known as the *ryanodine receptor protein*, bridges the transverse tubules and the SR terminal cisternae membranes and may play a role in excitation-contraction coupling by promoting $Ca^{2+}$ release. Nelson suggested that human MHS muscle may have a defect in the ryanodine-sensitive $Ca^{2+}$ release channel.[84] Halothane causes inactive $Ca^{2+}$ channels to open, leads to an increase in channel conductance, and effects the activation and inactivation process of the $Ca^{2+}$ release from MHS muscle. Further investigations are evaluating the ryanodine receptor (through antibody-specific proteins) and its relationship to $Ca^{2+}$ release in MHS muscle. If this work bears fruit, a serum test for MHS may be possible.

## What Genetic Factors Influence the Occurrence of Malignant Hyperthermia?

Initial genetic testing in swine with MHS showed an autosomal dominant pattern of inheritance. Subsequent studies have suggested other patterns as well. McPherson and Taylor believed that an autosomal dominant pattern was the most typical pattern present in 93 families with MH.[85] An example of an MH-susceptible family tree is presented in Figure 48–8. It seems appropriate to assume that 50% of offspring of an individual with MHS are at risk. Relatives of individuals with MHS and elevated serum CK levels have a >70% chance of being at risk.[85] Remember that baseline CK levels may be of no predictive value, and likewise, offspring with normal levels may still be at risk for MH.

Ongoing research efforts are concentrating on the possibility that MH is caused by different genes in different families. Two possible gene candidates are the ryanodine receptor and the hormone-sensitive lipase. Determination of the genetic

**An MH susceptible family tree might look something like this:**

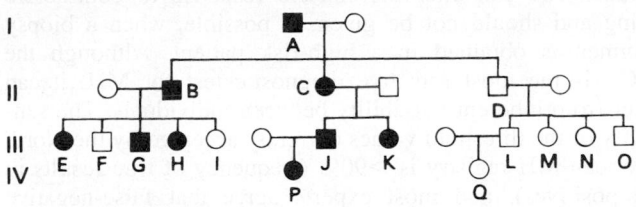

- ■ affected male
- ● affected female
- □ unaffected male
- ○ unaffected female

**FIGURE 48–8.** The father (A) in generation I is malignant hyperthermia (MH) susceptible. He passes the MH gene to his oldest son (B), who then transmits MH to three of his five children (E, G, and H). The father (A) also transmitted the MH gene to his daughter (C), who bore two children (J and K), both of whom were MH susceptible. The younger son (D) did not inherit the MH gene, so his children (L, M, N, and O) are unaffected, as is his granddaughter (Q).

mechanisms of regulation may provide further knowledge about MH and its link to familial transmission and muscle development.

## What Guidance and Counseling Are Available?

MHAUS and its counterpart in Canada are dedicated to the control of MH through several services available to families and physician caregivers. Ongoing education for physicians and patients and their families is a prime objective, as are encouragement of MH research and emotional support and guidance for affected families. A hotline is available to physicians who desire expert advice concerning their urgent MH needs. Telephone numbers, website, and email address are noted at the conclusion of the chapter.

## What Is the Basis of Contracture Testing?

The currently accepted standard for muscle contracture testing was suggested by Kalow and colleagues in 1970, when they noted that muscle from MHS patients exposed to caffeine responded abnormally.[86] Soon thereafter, other groups demonstrated similar striated muscle response abnormalities upon exposure to halothane.

### Methodology

One group of 4 to 8 strips of muscle with intact fascicles of appropriate length and weight, according to protocol typically from the vastus lateralis (thigh) group, is exposed to 3% halothane, and a second group is exposed to incremental caffeine concentration (hence the term *caffeine halothane contracture test* [CHCT]. A positive test for MHS occurs when at least one of the muscle strips undergoes contracture, thus generating a force greater than or equal to set protocol values (ie, halothane, 0.7 g within a 5-min exposure).[87,88]

## Sensitivity and Specificity

Dantrolene can alter the muscle response to contracture testing and should not be given, if possible, when a biopsy specimen is obtained in a high-risk patient. Although the CHCT is the most sensitive diagnostic test for MH, it can suffer from inherent variability between individuals. The sensitivity of the threshold values currently accepted by the North American MH registry is >90% (frequency of true results in true positives), and most experts agree that false-negative results are rare or absent when the standardized North American protocol has been followed.

Some myopathies express positive contracture test results with no direct relationship to MH.[88] A patient's true susceptibility is difficult to ascertain in such cases. To date, no patients with false-negative results have been reported to have experienced MH. Continued data collection may uncover a group of patients with false-negative results, possibly leading to an improved specificity rating of the CHCT for these patients if they undergo exposure to triggering agents.[87]

## Are Other Tests Useful in Predicting Malignant Hyperthermia Susceptibility?

Many tests have been suggested, tried, and ultimately discredited for human use. They include phosphorylase ratio, platelet adenosine triphosphate depletion, thin-strip muscle $Ca^{2+}$ uptake, assay of glutathione peroxidase, hypotonic red blood cell lysis, and abnormal protein in MH muscle.[89] More recent testing protocols for MH include a monocyte-$Ca^{2+}$ release test, intracellular inorganic phosphate-to-phosphocreatine ratio measured by magnetic resonance imaging, and measured intracellular $Ca^{2+}$ concentrations.[90] These tests require further evaluation to confirm or disclaim their applicability. The ideal test should be easily reproducible, inexpensive, noninvasive, highly reliable, and available at most large hospitals. Because MH is an inherited disorder, it was hoped that gene identification may prove useful, but to date, this has been unsuccessful.[90]

## When Should Muscle Biopsy Be Recommended?

Ideally, all patients who have had MH or an MH-like experience, those with an episode of MMR, and those siblings and offspring of MH-positive patients or patients with MMR should be tested. Considering that only 12 centers are accredited in the United States and Canada, where the logistics and expenses involved in travel and medical care are extreme, many patients will not undergo testing. Physicians should be cognizant and compassionate toward those many patients and their families who have emotional and financial difficulties when a family member is labeled MH positive.

The least that should be offered to patients and their families is referral to MHAUS for educational purposes. Relatives must be informed of the implications and risks as well. They then should communicate this potential risk with a medical bracelet, a physician's letter carried on their person, or an explanatory notation in their medical record. Testing should be performed on any person who will be reassured by it, as well as on anyone who is denied insurance, employment, or

other benefits on the basis of suspected but not biopsy-proven MH. If surgery is contemplated before proper testing can be completed, the patient and family members should be afforded a nontriggering anesthetic with the suggested perioperative monitoring as outlined.

For more information on MH, contact MHAUS at 800-986-4287, visit the website for additional information at *www.mhaus.org*, or send email to mhaus@norwich.net.

## References

1. Iazzo PA, Kehler CH, Zink RS, et al. Thermal response in acute porcine malignant hyperthermia. *Anesth Analg.* 1996;82:803–809.
2. Sessler DI. Temperature monitoring and management during neuraxial anesthesia. *Anesth Analg.* 1999;88:243–245.
3. Joly HR, Weil MH. Temperature of the great toe as an indicator of the severity of shock. *Circulation.* 1969;39:131.
4. Sessler DI, Moayeri A. Skin-surface warming: heat flux and central temperature. *Anesthesiology.* 1990;73:218.
5. Sessler DI, Olofsson CI, Rubinstein EH, et al. The thermoregulatory threshold in humans during halothane anesthesia. *Anesthesiology.* 1988;68:836.
6. Sessler DI, Olofsson CI, Rubinstein EH. Active thermoregulation during isoflurane anesthesia [abstract]. *Anesthesiology.* 1987;67:A405.
7. Sessler DI, Olofsson CI, Rubinstein EH. The thermoregulatory threshold in humans during nitrous oxide-fentanyl anesthesia. *Anesthesiology.* 1988;69:357.
8. Sessler DI, Ponte J. Disparity between thermal comfort and physiological thermoregulatory responses during epidural anesthesia [abstract]. *Anesthesiology.* 1989;71:A682.
9. Sessler DI, Rubinstein EH, Eger EI II. Core temperature changes during $N_2O$ fentanyl and halothane/$O_2$ anesthesia. *Anesthesiology.* 1987;67:137.
10. Sessler DI, Stoen R, Glosten B. Thermoregulatory vasoconstriction significantly decreases heat loss to the environment [abstract]. *Anesth Analg.* 1990;70:S362.
11. Sessler DI. Temperature monitoring. In: Miller RD, ed. *Anesthesia.* 3rd ed. New York, NY: Churchill Livingstone; 1990:1228.
12. Hynson JM, Sessler DI, Glosten BI, et al. Thermal balance and tremor patterns during epidural anesthesia. *Anesthesiology.* 1991;74:680.
13. Ponte J, Sessler DI. Extradurals and shivering. *Br J Anaesth.* 1990;64:731.
14. Walmsley AJ, Giesecke AH, Lipton JM: Contribution of extradural temperature to shivering during extradural anaesthesia. *Br J Anaesth.* 1986;58:1130.
15. Sevarine F, Johnson M, Lima M, et al. Effect of epidural sufentanyl on shivering and body temperature in the parturient. *Anesth Analg.* 1989;68:530.
16. Conahan TJ, Williams CD, Apfelbaum JL. Airway heating reduces recovery room time (cost) in outpatients. *Anesthesiology.* 1987;67:128.
17. Ikeda T, Sessler DI, Kikura M, et al. Less core hypothermia when anesthesia is induced with inhaled sevoflurane than with intravenous propofol. *Anesth Analg.* 1999;88:921.
18. Wass CT, Lanier WL, Hofer RE, Scheithauer BW, Andrews AG. Temperature changes of ≥1°C alter functional neurologic outcome and histopathology in a canine model of complete cerebral ischemia. *Anesthesiology.* 1995;83:325035.
19. Marion DW, Penrod LE, Kelsey SF, et al. Treatment of traumatic brain injury with moderate hypothermia. *N Engl J Med.* 1997;336:540.
20. Villar J, Slutsky AS. Effects of induced hypothermia in patients with septic adult respiratory distress syndrome. *Resuscitation.* 1993;26:183.
21. Thames J. Platelet function during and after deep surface hypothermia. *J Surg Res.* 1981;31:314.
22. Valeri R, Casidy G, Shabri K, et al. Hypothermia-induced platelet dysfunction. *Ann Surg.* 1987;205:175.
23. Sheffield CW, Sessler DI, Hunt TK. Mild hypothermia during isoflurane anesthesia decreases resistance to *E. coli* dermal infection in guinea pigs. *Acta Anaesthesiol Scand.* 1994;38:201–205.
24. Kurtz A, et al. Perioperative normothermia to reduce the incidence of surgical wound infection and shorten hospitalization. *N Engl J Med.* 1999;334:1209.
25. Sessler DI, Israel D, Pozoo RS. Spontaneous post anesthesia tremor does not resemble thermoregulatory shivering. *Anesthesiology.* 1988;68:843.
26. Horn E, Sessler D, Standle T, et al. Nonthermoregulatory shivering in patients recovering from isoflurane or desflurane anesthesia. *Anesthesiology.* 1998;89:878.

27. Horn E, Sessler D, Schroeder F, et al. Pain facilitates non-thermoregulatory shivering-like tremor. *Anesthesiology.* 1998:89:3AS.
28. Sessler DI, Rubenstein EH, Moayeri AM. Physiologic response to mild perianesthetic hypothermia in humans. *Anesthesiology.* 1991;75:594.
29. Steven M, Frank A, Fleisher L. Perioperative maintenance of normothermia reduces the incidence of morbid cardiac events. *JAMA.* 1997; 277:1127.
30. Frank SM, Beather C, Christopher R, et al. Unintentional hypothermia is associated with postoperative myocardial ischemia. The Perioperative Ischemia Randomized Trial study group. *Anesthesiology.* 1993;78:468.
31. Sladen R. Temperature changes and ventilation after hypothermic cardiopulmonary bypass. *Anesth Analg.* 1983;62:283.
32. Sladen R, Renaghan RRT, Ashton JP, et al. Effect of shivering on mechanical ventilation. *Anesthesiology.* 1985;63:A140.
33. Guffin A, Girad D, Kaplan J. Shivering following cardiac surgery: hemodynamic changes and reversal. *J Cardiothorac Anesth.* 1987;1:24.
34. Jachinsson PO, Nystrom SO, Tyden H. Extended rewarming during cardiopulmonary bypass. *Acta Anaesthesiol Scand.* 1987;31:543.
35. Holtzclaw BJ, Green RT. Shivering after heart surgery: assessment of metabolic effects. *Anesthesiology.* 1986;65:A18.
36. Schneid H, Kury A, Sessler D. Mild hypothermia increases blood loss and transfusion requirements during total hip arthroplasty. *Lancet.* 1996;347:289.
37. Greher M, Gold V, Harthanan T. Very mild hypothermia increases blood loss during hip arthroplasty. *Anesthesiology.* 1997;87(3S):55A.
38. Kury A, Sessler D, Lenhardt R. Perioperative normothermia to reduce the incidence of surgical wound infection and shorten hospitalization. *N Engl J Med.* 1996;334:1209.
39. Sessler DI, McGuire J, Sessler AM. Perioperative thermal insulation. *Anesthesiology.* 1991;74:875.
40. Lennon RL, Hosking MP, Conover MA, et al. Evaluation of forced hot air systems for rewarming hypothermic postoperative patients. *Anesth Analg.* 1990;70:424.
41. Sessler DI, Moayeri A. Skin surface warming, heat flux, and control of temperature. *Anesthesiology.* 1990;73:218.
42. Stone DR, Downs JB, Paul WL, et al. Adult body temperature and heated humidification. *Anesth Analg.* 1981;60:736.
43. Sessler DI. *Temperature Regulation and Anesthesia.* ASA 1991 Annual Refresher Course Lecture Series. Park Ridge, Ill: ASA; 1991.
44. Murphy MT, Lipton JM, Longhron MB, et al. Post anesthesia shivering in primates: inhibition by peripheral heating. *Anesthesiology.* 1985;63:161.
45. Sharkey A, Lipton JM, Murphy MT. Inhibition of post anesthetic shivering with radiant heat. *Anesthesiology.* 1987;66:249.
46. Lennon RL, Hosking MP, Conover MA, et al. Evaluation of forced hot air systems for rewarming hypothermic post operative patients. *Anesth Analg.* 1990;70:424.
47. Lilly RB. Significance and recovery room management of post anesthesia hypothermia and shivering. *Anesthesiol Clin North Am.* 1990;18:373.
48. Pauca AL, Savage RT, Simpson S, et al. Effect of pethedine, morphine and fentanyl on postoperative shivering in man. *Acta Anaesthesiol Scand.* 1984;28:138.
49. Kluger MJ, Kauffman CA. Biologic mechanisms of fever. In: Murray H, ed. *FUO, Fever of Undetermined Origin.* Mt Kisco, NY: Futura Publishing; 1983:1.
50. Isaac B, Kernbaum S, Burke M. *Unexplained Fever: A Guide to the Diagnosis and Management of Febrile States in Medicine, Surgery, Pediatrics, and Subspecialties.* Boca Raton, Fla, CRC Press; 1991.
51. Bennett MH, Wainwright AP. Acute thyroid crisis on induction of anaesthesia. *Anaesthesia.* 1989;44:28.
52. Stevens JJ. A case of thyrotoxic crisis that mimicked malignant hyperthermia. *Anesthesiology.* 1983;59:263.
53. Allen GC, Rosenberg H. Pheochromocytoma presenting as acute malignant hyperthermia: a diagnostic challenge. *Can J Anaesth.* 1990;37:593.
54. Stoelting R, Dierdorf S, McCammon R. Transfusion therapy. In: Stoelting RK, Dierdorf SF, McCammon RL, eds. *Anesthesia and Coexisting Disease.* 2nd ed. New York, NY: Churchill Livingstone; 1988:602.
55. Brownell AKW. Malignant hyperthermia: relationship to other diseases. *Br J Anaesth.* 1988;60:303.
56. Hermesh H, Aizenberg D, Lapidor M. The relationship between malignant hyperthermia and neuroleptic malignant syndrome. *Anesthesiology.* 1989;70:171.
57. Geiduschek J, Cohen S, Kahn A, et al. Repeat anesthesia for a patient with neuroleptic malignant syndrome. *Anesthesiology.* 1988;68:134.
58. Torline R. Extreme hyperpyrexia associate with central anticholinergic syndrome. *Anesthesiology.* 1992;76:470.
59. Denborough MA, Lovell RRH. Anesthetic deaths in a family. *Lancet.* 1960;2:45.
60. Ording H. Incidence of malignant hyperthermia in Denmark. *Anesth Analg.* 1985;64:700.
61. Sewall K, Flowerew R, Bromberger P. Severe muscular rigidity at birth: malignant hyperthermia syndrome? *Can J Anaesth Soc.* 1980;27:279.
62. Larach MG, Rosenberg H, Larach DR, et al. Prediction of malignant hyperthermia susceptibility by clinical signs. *Anesthesiology.* 1987; 66:547.
63. Kaplan RF. Hypothermia/hyperthermia. In: Gravenstein N, ed. *Manual of Complication During Anesthesia.* Philadelphia, Pa: JB Lippincott; 1991:121.
64. Brownell AKW. Malignant hyperthermia: relationship to other diseases. *Br J Anaesth.* 1988;60:303.
65. Ward A, Chaffman MO, Sorkin EM. Dantrolene. *Drugs.* 1986;32:130.
66. Malignant Hyperthermia Association of the United States. *Preventing Malignant Hyperthermia.* Darien, Conn: MHAUS; 1991.
67. Kolb ME, Horne ML, Martz R. Dantrolene in human malignant hyperthermia. *Anesthesiology.* 1982;56:254.
68. Wingard DW. Controversies regarding the prophylactic use of dantrolene for malignant hyperthermia. *Anesthesiology.* 1983;58:489.
69. Flewellen EH, Nelson TE, Jones WP, et al. Dantrolene dose response in awake man: implications for management of malignant hyperthermia. *Anesthesiology.* 1983;59:275.
70. Allen GC, Cattran CB, Peterson RG. Plasma levels of dantrolene following oral administration in malignant hyperthermia-susceptible patients. *Anesthesiology.* 1988;69:900.
71. Malignant Hyperthermia Association of the United States. *The Specific Treatment for Malignant Hyperthermia.* Darien, Conn: MHAUS; 1991.
72. Smith RJ. Preoperative assessment of risk factors. *Br J Anaesth.* 1988; 60:317.
73. Ording H. Diagnosis of susceptibility to malignant hyperthermia in man. *Br J Anaesth.* 1988;60:287.
74. Sethna NF, Rockoff MA. Cardiac arrest following inhalation induction of anesthesia in a child with Duchenne's muscular dystrophy. *Can Anaesth Soc J.* 1986;33:799.
75. Berkowitz A, Rosenberg H. Femoral block with mepivacaine for muscle biopsy in malignant hyperthermia patients. *Anesthesiology.* 1985;62:651.
76. Beebe JJ, Sessler DI. Preparation of anesthesia machines for patients susceptible to malignant hyperthermia. *Anesthesiology.* 1988;69:395.
77. Ritchie PA, Cheshire MA, Pearch NH. Decontamination of halothane from anaesthetic machines achieved by continuous flushing with oxygen. *Br J Anaesth.* 1988;60:859.
78. McGraw TT, Keon TP. Malignant hyperthermia and the clean machine. *Can J Anaesth.* 1988;36:530.
79. Van Der Spek AFL, Fang WB, Ashton-Miller JA, et al. The effects of succinylcholine on mouth opening. *Anesthesiology.* 1987;67:459.
80. Rosenberg H, Fletcher JE. Masseter muscle rigidity and malignant hyperthermia susceptibility. *Anesth Analg.* 1986;65:161.
81. Flewellen EH, Nelson TE. Masseter spasm induced by succinylcholine in children: contracture testing for malignant hyperthermia. Report of six cases. *Can J Anaesth.* 1982;29:42.
82. Gronert GA. Management of patients in whom trismus occurs following succinylcholine (with reply by Rosenberg H). *Anesthesiology.* 1988; 68:653.
83. Littleford JA, Patel LR, Bose D, et al. Masseter muscle spasm in children: implications of continuing the triggering anesthetic. *Anesth Analg.* 1991;72:151.
84. Nelson TE. Halothane effects on human malignant hyperthermia skeletal muscle single calcium-release channels in planar lipid bilayers. *Anesthesiology.* 1992;76:588.
85. McPherson EW, Taylor CA. The genetics of malignant hyperthermia: evidence for heterogenicity. *Am J Med Genet.* 1982;11:273.
86. Kalow W, Britt BA, Terreau ME, et al. Metabolic error of muscle metabolism after recovery from malignant hyperthermia. *Lancet.* 1970;2:895.
87. Malignant Hyperthermia Association of the United States. *The Communicator.* 1992;10(2).
88. Heiman-Patterson TD, Rosenberg H, Fletcher JE, et al. Halothane-caffeine contracture testing in neuromuscular diseases. *Muscle Nerve.* 1988;1:453.
89. Ording H. Diagnosis of susceptibility to malignant hyperthermia. *Br J Anaesth.* 1988;60:287.
90. Rosenberg H, Seitman D. Pharmacogenetics. In: Barash PG, Cullen BF, Stoelting RK, eds. *Clinical Anesthesia.* Philadelphia, Pa: JB Lippincott; 1989:459.

CHAPTER

# 49

# Occupational Hazards in the Operating Room

Paul Langevin

Salvatore LoPalo

A. Joseph Layon

*What Is the Narcotic Withdrawal Syndrome?*
*What Measures Are Useful for Prevention?*

TRACE GAS EXPOSURE
*What Are the Suspected Deleterious Effects?*
*What Are the Sources of Trace Gases?*
*How Are Anesthetic Agents Scavenged?*

The operating room (OR) environment is both the health provider's familiar workplace and an area replete with infectious, chemical, and psychologic threats. This chapter reviews what we consider the most significant of these threats and identifies methods to minimize risk while providing optimal patient care. Although we have no interest in hyperbole or portraying our work environment as more hostile than it actually is, our measured opinion is that the physicians and nurses who work in the OR may do so more safely if the hazards are known, understood, and, hence, avoided.

## HEPATITIS

### What Is the Relevant Epidemiology?

Concern about the possibility of HIV infection in the health care setting is appropriate, but we must be even more vigilant with regard to the hepatitides. HIV infects only with great difficulty apart from exchange of body fluids or blood-borne transmission. Hepatitis B virus (HBV), on the other hand, is approximately 100 times more infectious than HIV when blood-borne and is 10 times more prevalent among health care workers (HCWs) than HIV.[1] The Centers for Disease Control and Prevention (CDC*) reported 35 519 cases of hepatitis for 1998[2] with the following breakdown: 22 028 hepatitis A, 8651 hepatitis B, and 4840 hepatitis C/non-A, non-B hepatitis.[2] For comparison with the previous decade, in 1988 there were 56 800 cases of hepatitis reported, the break-

*The Centers for Disease Control and Prevention were formerly named the Centers for Disease Control. For consistency, we use the current title throughout this chapter, even though some references are from the period when the former title was used.

down of which was 28 500 hepatitis A, 23 200 hepatitis B, 2600 non-A, non-B hepatitis (including hepatitis C), and 2500 unspecified, a category that has now disappeared.[3]

Despite population growth in the 1990s, the incidence of hepatitis has decreased by 37.5%. This is likely a result of prevention through behavioral changes, vaccination, and blood donor policy. By the 35th week of 1999, 10 030 cases of hepatitis A, 4280 cases of hepatitis B, and 2259 cases of hepatitis C/non-A, non-B hepatitis were reported.[4,5] Summary statistics on hepatitides A, B, C/non-A, non-B are shown in Figures 49–1 and 49–2.

The hepatitides encountered in clinical practice may be divided into two main groups: primary and secondary. The *primary hepatitides* account for approximately 95% of cases of hepatitis; as the name suggests, these organisms have little effect other than on the liver. The *secondary hepatitides* account for only approximately 5% of cases of hepatitis and have clinical effects that are distant from the liver.

### What Are the Primary Hepatitides?

#### Hepatitis A

Hepatitis A virus (HAV) is an RNA virus found in the stool of acutely infected people.[6,7] In the United States, the seroprevalence increases with age so that by age 50 years, approximately 50% of people are seropositive. Acute hepatitis A may be diagnosed in the presence of HAV immunoglobulin (Ig) M antibody in conjunction with the appropriate clinical symptoms. Specific IgG is found in the plasma of previously infected people.

#### Clinical and Serologic Features

Symptoms of infection caused by HAV are seen 2 to 6 weeks after inoculation; for this reason, it has been termed *short-incubation hepatitis.* During this symptomatic period, elevated serum levels of aminotransferases are noted. Jaundice may follow several days after the initiation of symptoms, but anicteric disease is common. Just before the onset of symptoms, viral particles are noted in the stool and serum. This shedding of the virion, as well as infectiousness, stops with

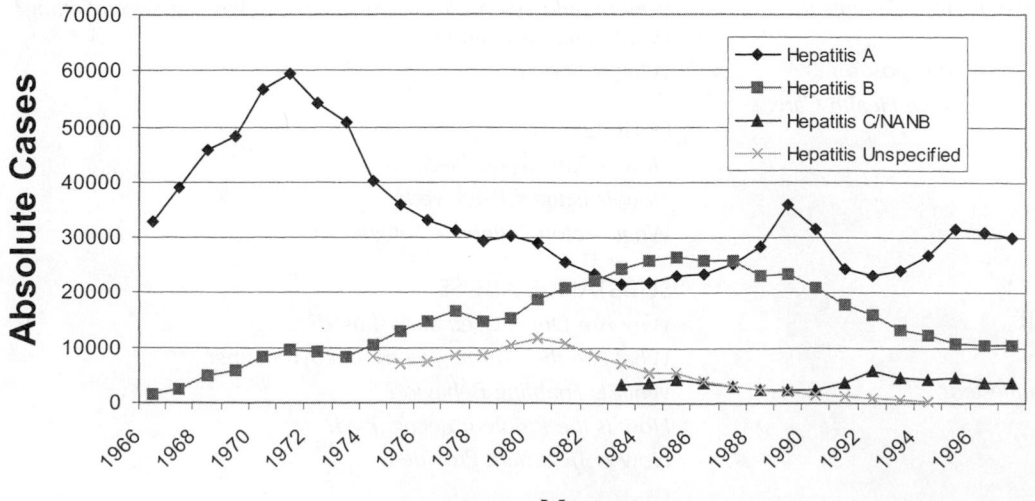

**FIGURE 49–1.** Summary of hepatitis A, B, and C/non-A, non-B cases from 1966 to 1997. Until 1973, hepatitis A was reported as *infectious hepatitis,* and hepatitis B was reported as *serum hepatitis.* Only beginning in 1974 was hepatitis non-A, non-B reported as *hepatitis, unspecified.* Beginning in 1982, hepatitis C/non-A, non-B was and hepatitis unspecified were reported. The anti-hepatitis C virus antibody test was available as of May 1990. Hepatitis unspecified was no longer nationally reportable as of 1995. (From Centers for Disease Control and Prevention. Summary of notifiable diseases, United States, 1997. *MMWR Morb Mortal Wkly Rep.* 1997;46:76.)

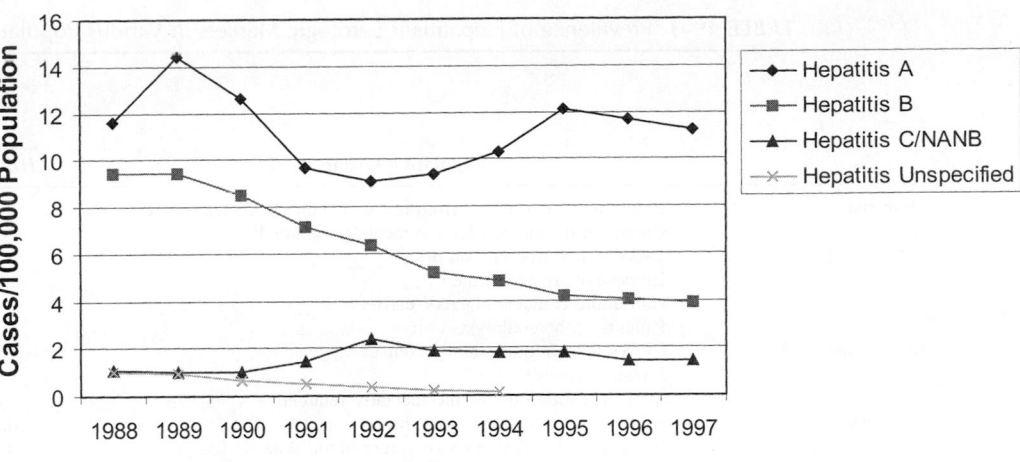

**FIGURE 49–2.** Cases of hepatitis per 100 000 population, 1988-1997. (From Centers for Disease Control and Prevention. Summary of notifiable diseases, United States, 1997. *MMWR Morb Mortal Wkly Rep.* 1997;46:73.)

the onset of jaundice. The clinical and serologic features of HAV infection are summarized in Figure 49–3.

### Transmission

HAV is transmitted by the fecal-oral route and parenterally, although the latter is uncommon. This agent is not considered of any significance in posttransfusion hepatitis. Although HAV only rarely causes fulminant hepatitis, one report noted that patients over 40 years of age were at risk for greater complications and, perhaps, death.[8] Complications in this series included acalculous cholecystitis, hemolysis, acute renal failure, reactive arthritis, new-onset diabetes mellitus, preterm labor, and pericardial and pleural effusions.

Chronic carrier states and chronic hepatitis are not thought to occur with HAV. The reservoir for this infectious process is believed to consist of the large number of clinically inapparent cases from which the organism is transmitted to uninfected people. Risk factors for HAV transmission may not be identified in 40% to 79% of cases.[8]

An increase in hepatitis A among homosexual men has been noted.[7] Passive or active immunization (vaccines as of 1997 were HAVRIX from SmithKline Beecham and VAQTA

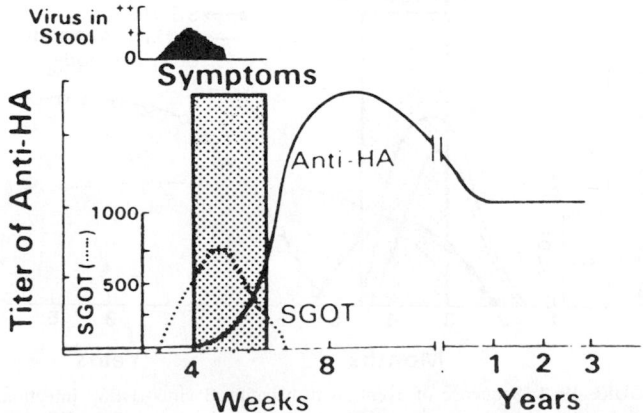

**FIGURE 49–3.** Sequence of events with hepatitis A virus (HAV) infection. Note that virus excretion in stool predates any symptom. The SGOT (aspartate transaminase) level is elevated before and anti-HAV is elevated after onset of symptomatology. (From LaMont JT. Viral hepatitis. In: Stein JH, ed. *Internal Medicine.* Boston, Mass: Little, Brown & Co; 1983.)

from Merck and Company) is now recommended for communities with high rates and periodic outbreaks of HAV infection.[9]

### Hepatitis B

HBV, discovered in 1966, infects more than 350 million people throughout the world. HBV infection is a major cause of acute and chronic hepatitis, cirrhosis, and primary hepatocellular carcinoma, causing approximately 1 million deaths per year. In the United States, Western Europe, and Australia, areas of low endemicity, the disease is spread horizontally by sexual activity, intravenous drug use, or occupational exposure. Less frequent causes of infection include household contact, hemodialysis, physician transmission, and organ/blood-mediated transmission; in 20% to 30% of cases, no clear risk factors are found. In areas of the world in which HBV infections are commonly seen—Southeastern Asia, China, and Africa—>50% of the population is infected at some time in their life, with approximately 8% of those infected becoming chronic carriers.[10]

Because an intact immune system is required both for hepatocellular injury and clearance of the virus, asymptomatic chronic carriage occurs in (1) 95% of neonatal infections with an immature immune system, (2) 30% of children infected after the neonatal period but before the age of 6 years, and (3) 3% to 5% of immunocompetent adults. This generally low incidence of viral carriage in immunocompetent people contrasts with the 10% incidence of people in the same populations who are positive for hepatitis B surface antibody (HBsAb). The implication is that most HBV infections are self-limited and followed by immunity; only occasionally does the chronic carrier state result. However, these chronic carriers appear to be the reservoir that perpetuates the virus.

### Viral Composition

HBV is a DNA virus of the family Hepadnavirus. The HBV genome is partially double-stranded DNA encoding four major genes: the S (envelope, surface) gene, the C (core) gene, the X (viral promoter and, questionably, hepatocellular carcinoma-promoting) gene, and the P (polymerase) gene.[10] The complete and infectious virus is a 42-nm sphere termed the *Dane particle.* An antigen, termed *e* (HBeAg), is most

**TABLE 49–1.** Prevalence of Hepatitis B Serologic Markers in Various Population Groups

| | Population Group | Prevalence of Serologic Markers of HBV Infection (%) | |
| --- | --- | --- | --- |
| | | *HBsAg* | *All Markers* |
| High risk | Immigrants or refugees from areas of high HBV endemicity | 13 | 70-85 |
| | Clients in institutions for the mentally retarded | 10-20 | 35-80 |
| | Users of illicit parenteral drugs | 7 | 60-80 |
| | Homosexually active men | 6 | 35-80 |
| | Household contacts of HBV carriers | 3-6 | 30-60 |
| | Patients on hemodialysis units | 3-10 | 20-80 |
| Intermediate risk | HCWs with frequent blood contact | 1-2 | 15-30 |
| | Prisoners (male) | 1-8 | 10-80 |
| | Staff of institutions for the mentally retarded | 1 | 10-25 |
| Low risk | HCWs with infrequent or no blood contact | 0.3 | 3-10 |
| | Healthy adults (first-time volunteer blood donors) | 0.3 | 3-5 |

For more information, see http://www.cdc.gov/nip/publications/pink/hepb.pdf.
HBsAg, hepatitis B surface antigen; HBV, hepatitis B virus; HCW, health care worker.
From Centers for Disease Control. Recommendations for protection against viral hepatitis. *Ann Intern Med.* 1985;103:395.

often present only in serum that contains circulating HBV DNA. HBeAg, perhaps because it resembles HBcAg—the nucleocapsid that encloses the viral DNA—is thought to act in a manner that promotes immunologic tolerance to the infection. Thus, it correlates well with infectivity. Antibody (HBsAb) to the proteins coded by the S gene (HBsAg) results in protective immunity. Indeed, it is recombinant HBsAg that provides the basis for the HBV vaccine.

### Risk of Infection

The risk of infection with HBV depends on individual activities (Table 49–1). Anesthesiologists, who as a group have frequent blood contact, are considered to be at intermediate risk for HBV, with 1% to 2% of that population being positive for HBsAg and approximately 10 times that many in the same population positive for any serologic marker of HBV infection. Data suggest that people with multiple sexual partners increase their risk of HBV infection.[11,12]

### Clinical and Serologic Features

The incubation period of HBV is variable, ranging between 6 and 24 weeks. The reason for this variable period of incubation relates to both the size of the inoculum and its portal of entry. For example, an infusion of 50 mL of infected blood may result in a patient becoming HBsAg-positive in a few weeks; a 50-μL inoculation most frequently results in surface antigenemia only after 3 to 4 months.

Serologic features are important in the diagnosis of this viral infection.[10,13] The first marker noted is HBsAg (Fig. 49–4), before any other clinical or laboratory findings are observable. The Dane particle markers, HBeAg, HBV DNA, and DNA polymerase, parallel the rise of HBsAg. Approximately 2 to 4 weeks after the appearance of these markers, aspartate and alanine aminotransferase levels begin to rise in the serum, peaking and then decreasing back to normal at 5 to 8 weeks. Six weeks after the onset of antigenemia, clinical symptoms may be noted.

### Antibody Formation

As HBV-associated DNA-polymerase becomes detectable, HBsAg levels peak. The first antibody against HBV, noted

within 2 to 4 weeks after initiation of antigenemia, is an IgM core antibody (HBcAb). The IgG isotype of HBcAb may persist for months to years after the antigenemia has cleared. Except in those patients in whom chronic viral disease eventually develops, HBsAb is noted several weeks after clearing of viral antigen. The presence of HBsAg indicates unequivocally either acute or chronic HBV infection. On the other hand, the presence of HBsAb generally implies a successful response to HBV and confers lifelong protection against further infection.

A small group of people with HBV infection are negative for both surface antigen and antibody but positive for HBcAb. These people are capable of transmitting HBV until HBsAb is produced. Most infected people, however, clear the viral antigen, which usually implies an eventual complete recovery.

### Chronic Carriers

Unfortunately, a small percentage of HBV-infected patients become chronic carriers. Carriers are, most frequently, patients who have a mild, anicteric acute hepatitis followed by gradual

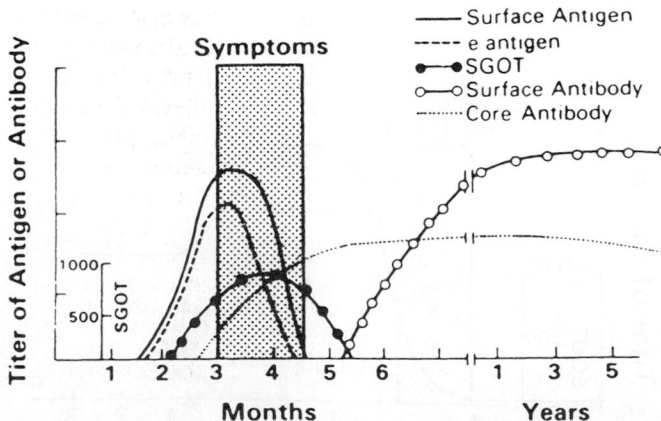

**FIGURE 49–4.** Sequence of events with hepatitis B virus (HBV) infection. Both hepatitis B surface antigen (HBsAg) and hepatitis B e antigen (HBeAg), which correlate with infectivity, are in relatively high concentrations before onset of symptoms. Note the late appearance of hepatitis B surface antibody (HBsAb), which usually implies a successful host response to HBV. (From LaMont JT. Viral hepatitis. In: Stein JH, ed. *Internal Medicine.* Boston, Mass: Little, Brown & Co; 1983.)

return to normal of liver function study results. Despite these normalizing biochemical parameters, patients are unable to clear the antigen and no HBsAb is detected. Of significance here is that chronic carriers are most frequently asymptomatic and are thus likely to infect others. Approximately 10% of HBV-infected patients have clinical manifestations for longer than 6 months and are classified as having chronic hepatitis. Treatment of chronic HBV infection with interferon alfa—5 to 10 million U/d, 3 times a week for 4 to 6 months—has been shown to induce long-term remission in 25% to 40% of these patients.[14] It also has been shown that use of the nucleoside analogue, lamivudine, in noncirrhotic patients with chronic HBV results in significant and sustained improvement in histologic and virologic parameters.[15]

### Epidemiology

The fecal-oral or urine-oral route of HBV transmission is thought unlikely because HBV particles are found least frequently in stool and urine. However, viral particles have been found in saliva, semen, vaginal secretions, tears, and breast milk. Thus, the major routes of transmission are thought to be parenteral and mucosal (including sexual transmission).

The parenteral route is most frequently identified in cases that are acquired in the hospital or in intravenous drug abusers. Only 10% of posttransfusion hepatitis cases are caused by HBV. In these cases, the viral antigen is present in such low titer that either the immunoassay used to screen blood cannot detect it, or the blood donor is a member of that small group with undetectable HBsAg and HBsAb but a positive titer for HBcAb.

HCWs are put at risk for HBV infection through accidental needle sticks. That the infection rate is only 10% seems to be due to the small amount of inoculated blood present on these sharp objects. Transmission may occur when inapparent cuts or abrasions are inoculated with infectious material; conjunctival contamination followed by infection may also occur.

When HCWs are compared with the general population, the serologic evidence of previous infection with HBV ranges from 15% to 30% for the former group, compared with only 3% to 5% in the latter.[6,16] Thus, distinctly unlike HIV infection, an excess prevalence of HBV infection occurs in HCWs. One study, in which sera of patients presenting to an inner-city emergency department were tested for HBV, HCV, and HIV, showed that the seroprevalence of HBsAg was 5%.[17] This incidence is more than 10 times the figure quoted for healthy adult, first-time blood donors[6] (see Table 49–1). One report noted the transmission of HBV to four patients from four infected surgeons, each of whom was negative for HBeAg,[18] usually thought to be associated with higher levels of circulating virus and, thus, infectivity.

### Hepatitis C/Non-A, Non-B Hepatitis

Although non-A, non-B hepatitis was thought to be due to more than one viral agent, it is caused primarily by a virus of the Flaviviridae family termed *hepatitis C virus* (HCV).[19–22] HCV has been the major cause of posttransfusion hepatitis, occurring at a rate of approximately 5 to 10 cases per 1000 transfusions.[23,24] However, since 1994, the rates of transfusion-transmitted HCV have decreased so much that the CDC's sentinel counties viral hepatitis surveillance system has been unable to detect any cases of transfusion-related HCV.[20] Con-

versely, intravenous drug abuse accounts for approximately 60% of HCV transmission.

The decreasing incidence of transfusion-associated HCV is likely due to our ability to test for anti-HCV. Before the advent of specific testing for HCV, there were data suggesting that HBcAb, and perhaps serum alanine aminotransferase, could serve as surrogate markers for hepatitis C to screen blood.[23–25] When these markers were used for equal numbers of units transfused, recipients of HBcAb-positive blood had an approximately twofold higher incidence of posttransfusion hepatitis. Specifically, the incidence was from 4% to 6% in HBcAb-negative blood and 8% to 14% in blood that was positive. Elimination of blood positive for HBcAb from the donor pool removed approximately 5% of the donated units and resulted in a decrement of approximately 20% of cases of non-A, non-B hepatitis. One study noted that the prevalence of anti-HCV was 18% in an inner-city population.[17]

The US Food and Drug Administration (FDA) has approved only serologic assays that measure anti-HCV. In a high-risk patient, the recommended testing sequence is the enzyme immunoassay (EIA); if positive, it is followed by the recombinant immunoblot assay (RIBA) for confirmation.[20] These tests have a sensitivity of ≥97% but do not differentiate among acute, chronic, and resolved infection. Assays using nucleic acid detection are available and in clinical use but are not FDA approved.[20]

### Clinical and Serologic Features

Although the viral agent may rarely be transmitted by the oral-fecal route, its epidemiologic pattern more commonly resembles that of HBV than HAV. Specifically, HCV is most commonly transmitted through needle sticks and transfusions. Symptoms range from mild to fulminant; non-A, non-B hepatitis is typically milder than HBV during the acute stage. Up to 70% of cases have no discernible symptoms; 20% to 30% may be jaundiced; and 10% to 20% have nonspecific symptoms such as anorexia, malaise, and abdominal pain. The average time from exposure to onset of symptoms is 6 to 7 weeks. The average time from exposure to anti-HCV seroconversion ranges from 8 to 9 weeks.[20] Spontaneous resolution occurs, but in a variable percentage of cases, ranging from 20% to 70%, biochemical and pathologic abnormalities are found suggestive of chronic disease; fulminant hepatic failure is rare. Within 30 years of acquiring HCV, hepatocellular carcinoma develops in 20% to 25% of patients.[26,27] HCWs do not appear to be at increased risk for HCV infection.[28]

Vertical transmission from mother to infant appears to occur with a frequency of 18% to 23%.[29] The highest risk mothers appear to be those who are either nonintravenous drug abusers with HCV RNA titers of >5 million copies/mL, or HIV-negative intravenous drug abusers. The highest transmission rate seems to occur in mothers who are both HIV and HCV positive. Although HCV RNA may be detected in breast milk, there are no data suggesting HCV transmission in this manner.[29]

Interferon-alfa, 2 to 3 × 10[6] units 3 times weekly for 12 months, has been shown to be effective in normalizing results of liver function and histologic studies in patients with HCV infection.[20,30] Using this regimen, approximately 50% of patients have normalization of biochemical abnormalities, and 33% have loss of HCV RNA from serum. Unfortunately, only 15% to 25% have a prolonged response (≥1 year) after the drug regimen is stopped.[20] Patients who do not respond after 12 months of therapy rarely respond to retreatment using standard interferon dosing. Use of interferon with the guanosine analogue ribaviron is reported to result in sustained response rates of 40% to 50%, compared with the 15% to 25% noted previously.[20,31,32]

## Hepatitis D

Delta hepatitis is an infection that occurs of necessity with HBV infection.[10,33] The agent, hepatitis D virus (HDV), is an incomplete/defective RNA virus requiring HBV assistance with both nucleocapsid assembly and envelope generation. HDV infection occurs most commonly in association with HBV or as a superinfection in an HBV carrier, most frequently encountered in intravenous drug abusers. A chronic carrier state and chronic hepatitis are known to occur, as does massive hepatic necrosis. Anti-HDV antibody is similar to HBcAb in that it signifies that infection has occurred but is not protective. Prevention is most important with regard to HDV disease. Without HBV, HDV does not occur.

## *What Protective and Therapeutic Measures Should Be Undertaken?*

Anesthesiologists are at intermediate risk for hepatitis infection as classified by the CDC[6] (see Table 49–1). A prevalence of approximately 1% to 2% of HBsAg is noted in anesthesiologists and other HCWs, with a 15% to 30% prevalence of all markers, such as HBsAb. Once again, the risk of patient-to-HCW transmission of HIV is much lower than that of HBV.

### Immunization

Based on the foregoing data, anesthesiologists (and, in our opinion, all HCWs) should be immunized with hepatitis B vaccine. In the United States, the vaccine is usually a recombinant product containing purified nonglycosylated HBsAg particles that are stabilized in aluminum hydroxide and preserved in thimerosal.[34] The vaccine is given as a 10- to 20-μg intramuscular injection, repeated 3 times, with the second and third doses 1 and 6 months after the first. Protective titers of anti-HBsAb (>10 mIU/mL) develop in 95% to 99% of healthy people who receive all 3 of the intramuscular injections.[34]

If blood exposure has occurred, the algorithm that should be followed depends on both the source of the exposure and the immunization status of the exposed HCW.

### Unknown Source

If the source of the needle stick is unknown, treatment of an exposed, nonimmunized HCW is initiation of the hepatitis B vaccine series immediately. If the worker already has been vaccinated against hepatitis B, no specific treatment is required.

### Known, Low-Risk Source

If the exposure is from a person at low risk of being HBsAg positive, an unvaccinated HCW should have the vaccine series initiated, and a vaccinated person, once again, requires no treatment.

### Known, High-Risk Source

If the exposure source is a person at high risk of being HBsAg positive, several things are done. In an unvaccinated person, the hepatitis B vaccine series is initiated. Further, the source of the exposure is tested for HBsAg status. If the source proves to be positive, a dose of hepatitis B immune globulin (HBIG) is immediately given to the exposed person. The dose for HBIG is 0.06 mL/kg, given intramuscularly.

If the exposed person has already been vaccinated and is a vaccine nonresponder, the source is tested for HBsAg status. If the source is indeed HBsAg positive, a dose of HBIG is given immediately, as well as a booster dose of hepatitis B vaccine.

### Known Serologic Positive Source

If the source is known to be HBsAg positive (as opposed simply to being high risk), the unvaccinated person is given a dose of HBIG immediately and the series of HBV vaccine immunizations begun. If the exposed person had been vaccinated, he or she is tested for anti-HBV antibody. An inadequate antibody level (<10 mIU/mL) necessitates a dose of HBIG immediately, plus a hepatitis B vaccine booster dose.

The risk of hepatitis B vaccine to the recipient is minimal. The doses for perinatal, sexual, percutaneous, and dialysis exposures and exposure of immunocompromised patients are listed in Table 49–2.

## *What Are the Secondary Hepatitides?*

In the differential diagnosis of viral hepatitis, the possibility of an agent that affects the liver secondarily rather than primarily must be considered. Such agents include cytomegalovirus (CMV), disseminated herpes simplex virus (HSV), coxsackieviruses A and B, Epstein-Barr virus, and yellow fever virus. These infectious agents account for approximately 5% of cases of clinical hepatitis and are termed *secondary hepatitides* because they only secondarily affect the liver. They are not discussed further.

## HIV INFECTION

Is disease caused by HIV an issue of concern for the anesthesiologist? If so, is it because we are at some greater risk than our colleagues or the general population for seroconversion? Although we have, in the past, taken the public position that HCWs might well be at increased risk,[35] our concerns have not, to date, been proven justified. Thus, our continued discussion of HIV disease (HIVD)/AIDS revolves around three specific points: (1) Where do we stand with this disease? (2) Should a different anesthetic technique be used for patients who are HIV infected? and (3) What are the risks of HIV transmission from patient to physician or from physician to patient?

## *What Is the Relevant Epidemiology?*

In 1998, there were 48 269 cases of AIDS reported in the United States, compared with 55 074 in 1997[36] (Fig. 49–5).

**TABLE 49–2.** Hepatitis B Virus Postexposure Recommendation

| | Hepatitis B Immunoglobulin | | Vaccine Dose | |
|---|---|---|---|---|
| Exposure | Dose | Recommended Timing | Recombivax HB | Engerix-B |
| Perinatal | 0.5 mL IM | Within 12 h | 5 μg | 10 μg |
| Sexual | 0.06/mL/kg IM | Single dose within 14 d of contact | 10 μg IM* | 20 μg IM* |
| Percutaneous | N/A | N/A | 10 μg IM† | 20 μg IM† |
| Dialysis and immunocompromised patients | N/A | N/A | 40 μg IM† | 40 μg IM |

*The first dose can be given at the same time as the dose of hepatitis B immune globulin but at a different site.

†Vaccine is recommended for homosexual men and for regular sexual contacts of hepatitis B virus carriers and is optional in initial treatment of heterosexual contacts of people with acute hepatitis B.

IM, intramuscular; N/A, not applicable.

Data from Centers for Disease Control and Prevention. Recommendations for protection against viral hepatitis. *Ann Intern Med.* 1985;103:399; *Facts and Comparisons.* Philadelphia, Pa: JB Lippincott; 1990;467; and Lemon SM, Thomas DL. Vaccines to prevent viral hepatitis. *N Engl J Med.* 1997;336:196.

Cases of HIV infection, as opposed to the end-stage of HIVD—AIDS—have not shown this same trend. These data are collected only from states with confidential HIV infection reporting and are admittedly incomplete because all states do not require this. The number of HIV infections increased from 12 438 to 19 393 cases from 1996 to 1998.[37,38] As of September 4, 1999, 30 285 cases of AIDS were reported in the United States, a decrease of 3.4% from the same time in 1998.[39] Worldwide, there are approximately 1 100 000 children infected with HIV, and something on the order of 1600 are infected each day; most of these new infections are in "developing" countries, and 90% are in sub-Saharan Africa.[40] Cases are seen predominantly in the following groups: (1) homosexual/bisexual men, about 35%; (2) intravenous drug abusers (heterosexual), 23%; and (3) heterosexuals, 14%.[36] The remaining 28% of cases occur in children, are transfusion related, or are of indeterminate cause.

### Pediatric AIDS

Cases of *pediatric AIDS* (defined as AIDS in children <13 years) have been of concern and, until recently, on the rise. In 1988, 574 cases were reported in the United States; this number was 648 (+13%), 788 (+22%), and 683 cases (−13%) in 1989, 1990, and 1991, respectively; by 1998 the number had decreased to 382 cases (−41%).[36,41] Overwhelmingly (89%), pediatric AIDS results from transmission from a mother who is HIV positive.[36] Most perinatal HIV transmission/AIDS transmission is thought to occur from mother to child by transplacental infection,[42] and thus prevention and prophylactic therapy for the pregnant woman are of great significance. Use of zidovudine during pregnancy decreases the infection rate by 70% to 80%.[43] A meta-analysis of 15 prospective, cohort studies found that cesarean section decreased the risk of vertical HIV transmission by approximately another 50%.[44]

### What Treatment Is Available?

Extensive work has resulted in the elucidation of the causative agent of AIDS. HIV is recognized as the etiologic agent for the immunocompromised state that results in the spectrum of complications we term *AIDS*,[45–47] although some controversy has existed on this point.[48] The molecular biology of this agent has been extensively detailed, including the steps by which the viral particle binds to and is incorporated into the CD4+ ("helper") lymphocyte.[49–57] More recent work on treatment of HIVD strongly suggests that highly active antiretroviral therapy using a combination of antiretroviral agents decreases morbidity and mortality rates in patients with HIV

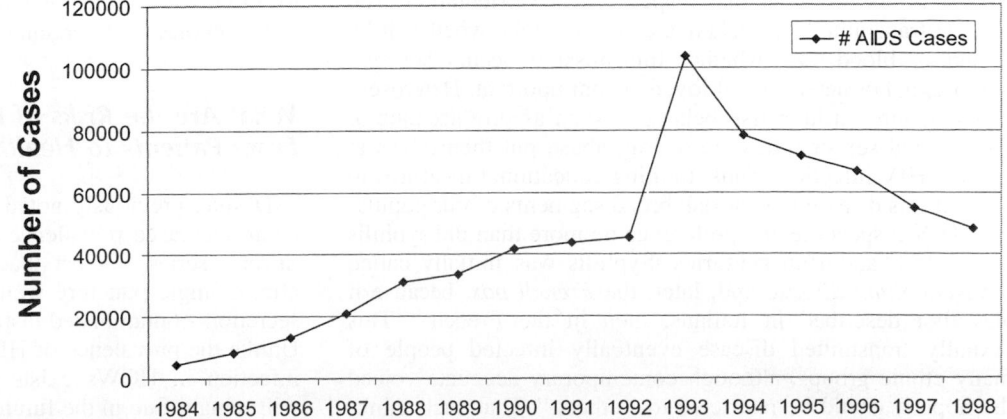

**FIGURE 49–5.** AIDS in the United States, 1984-1998. (From Centers for Disease Control and Prevention. Summary of notifiable diseases, United States, 1997. *MMWR Morb Mortal Wkly Rep.* 1997;46:74, 76; and Centers for Disease Control and Prevention. Provisional cases of selected notifiable diseases—United States weeks ending January 2, 1999 and December 27, 1997 [52nd week]. *MMWR Morb Mortal Wkly Rep.* 1999;47:1126, 1128.)

infection.[58–60] The drug combination most often consists of a protease inhibitor (eg, indinavir) and two nucleoside analogue reverse transcriptase inhibitors (eg, zidovudine and lamivudine). Unfortunately, up to 50% of treated patients do not have a sustained antiviral response and durable clinical benefit.[58–60] For this reason, clinical development of antiretroviral drugs continues. At least 23 new agents are in clinical development and could be available by 2003.

### Vaccine Development

Work continues in an effort to evaluate the feasibility of a vaccine against this viral agent.[61–64] Recombinant gp160 (a major envelope gene product) has been shown to induce antibody formation in both healthy and asymptomatic HIV-infected subjects; whether this effect is protective is unclear.[63,64] Although we continue to be cautiously optimistic, the availability of a vaccine—even one with only 40% to 50% efficacy—is still several years away.[61]

## *What Is the Role of Prevention?*

The advances alluded to previously have resulted in a significant decrease in the mortality rate from HIVD. Although HIV infection continues to take a significant toll, both worldwide and in the United States, HIV infection has now decreased from the 8th to the 14th leading cause of death among all age groups,[65,66] decreased from the 6th to the 7th leading cause of death in young adults 15 to 24 years of age,[67–69] and decreased from the leading cause to the 5th leading cause of death in 25- to 44-year-olds.[65,66]

### Education

Until recently, attempts to deal with HIV disease have placed significant emphasis on treatment. Prevention, specifically with regard to education and discussion of sexual behaviors, "safe sex," and needle exchange programs, received inadequate attention. This problem, recognized as a political rather than a medical one, is due to shortsighted leadership. Indeed, Donald P. Francis, who retired from the CDC's AIDS Division of the National Center for Prevention Services, stated emphatically in a 1992 article that the CDC was forced "to follow political dogma rather than sound public health principles."[70]

HIV is not an agent that respects sexual orientation. The virus is transmitted by exchange of body fluids; whether it be semen or blood, and whether transmission occurs between homosexual or heterosexual lovers, is unimportant. Heterosexuals engaging in high-risk behaviors such as promiscuous or unprotected sex or intravenous drug abuse put themselves at risk for HIV infection. Thus, limiting educational measures to prevent this disease puts at risk broad segments of our population. HIV respects sexual preference no more than did syphilis in the 15th and 16th centuries. Syphilis was initially called the *Neapolitan disease* and, later, the *French pox,* because it was first described in Italians, then in the French.[71] This sexually transmitted disease eventually infected people of many ethnic groups, although contemporary accounts voiced the hope it would be restricted to "others." That such thinking, now about HIV, still exists at the dawn of the 21st century is remarkable, sobering, and somewhat frightening.

## *How Is the Diagnosis Made?*

This is not the place to discuss, in significant detail, the techniques used for the diagnosis of HIVD. Notwithstanding this, however, the predictive value of any of the following studies is greater when coupled with a carefully taken history. Thus, when a test for HIV is to be performed, patients must be gently and nonjudgmentally queried about whether they engage in any high-risk behaviors such as intravenous drug use, sexual contact with an intravenous drug user, prostitution, or nonmonogamous homosexual or heterosexual contacts. Heterosexual promiscuity should be considered high-risk behavior.

Usually, tests using measurement of anti-HIV antibody are used for the initial and confirmatory studies for HIV. In adults, adolescents, and children ≥18 months of age, a reportable HIV case is diagnosed with EIA as the screening study and either Western blot or immunofluorescent antibody assays for confirmation. For people who engage in high-risk behavior, a strongly reactive enzyme-linked immunosorbent assay (ELISA) has a positive predictive value of 93%.[72] However, for people who do not practice high-risk behavior and thus have a relatively low disease prevalence, the positive predictive value for a strongly reactive specimen may be only 67%.[73] The importance of a confirmatory study is thus obvious.

Although the EIA tests for antibody to one of several viral antigens, the confirmatory test most commonly used is the Western blot. In this assay, viral antigen is electrophoretically dispersed, and a patient's serum specimen is then evaluated to determine if antibodies to the specific viral particles are present. To have a positive result, bands must be positive for any two of the following: p24 (core antigen), gp41 (envelope antigen), or gp120/gp160 (envelope antigen).[74] A negative result is the absence of all bands, and one that is indeterminate signifies the presence of bands on the Western blot that fail to meet the specific criteria for positivity.

A patient with an indeterminate test result for at least 6 months may, in the absence of any known risk factors or clinical symptoms, be considered negative for HIV. Such a person is almost certainly not infected with HIV, although no large-scale studies have confirmed this view.[72] Polymerase chain reaction, HIV p24 antigen, or HIV isolation are also used to make the diagnosis of HIV infection. The FDA approved a rapid HIV test that uses serum or plasma, has sensitivity similar to that of EIA, and produces results in 15 to 30 minutes.[75] This technique will likely become the initial test of choice in emergency departments and clinics.

## *What Are the Risks of HIV Transmission From Patients to Health Care Workers?*

Despite previously noted concern, there does not appear to be an increased prevalence of HIV infection among HCWs.[35] Several series suggest that the risk of HIV seroconversion after a single puncture wound with an HIV-positive blood or secretion–contaminated instrument is on the order of 0.5%.[76–79] Unlike the prevalence of HBV,[16] no excess prevalence of HIV infection in HCWs exists. Again, whether this observation will remain true in the future is unclear. At present, the HCWs with the highest number of HIV infections are nurses and laboratory technicians (Table 49–3).

**TABLE 49–3.** Health Care Workers With Documented and Possible Occupationally Acquired HIV Infection, Through 1998, United States

| Occupation | Transmission | Possible Occupational Transmission |
|---|---|---|
| Dental worker/dentist | 0 | 6 |
| Embalmer/morgue technician | 1 | 2 |
| Emergency medical technician/paramedic | 0 | 12 |
| Health aid/attendant | 1 | 14 |
| Housekeeper/maintenance | 1 | 12 |
| Clinical laboratory technician | 16 | 16 |
| Nonclinical laboratory technician | 3 | 0 |
| Nurse | 22 | 33 |
| Nonsurgical physician | 6 | 12 |
| Surgical physician | 0 | 6 |
| Respiratory therapist | 1 | 2 |
| Dialysis technician | 1 | 3 |
| Surgical technician | 2 | 2 |
| Other technician/therapist | 0 | 10 |
| Other health care workers | 0 | 4 |
| **Total** | **54** | **134** |

From Centers for Disease Control and Prevention. *HIV/AIDS Surveillance Report.* 1998;10(2):26.

## Prevention

Many, although not all, exposures to HIV infection are preventable if reasonable precautions are taken. We are cognizant that no matter how careful one is, the nature of surgical procedures is such that accidental punctures caused by bone fragments, scalpel blades, or unseen needles will occur. The best we can do is strive to minimize these incidents.

This approach becomes critically important because of an apparently asymptomatic pool of HIV-positive people who, depending on geography and age, comprise from 16% to 18% of the population studied.[80–83] Such information should make us ever more compulsive in preventing inadvertent inoculation with HIV-positive material, especially in the emergency department and OR. Thus, HCWs are at highest risk of inoculation with HIV-positive material, not from a patient who is known to have AIDS, but perhaps from a young, asymptomatic trauma victim or routine elective surgical patient for whom we are caring.

## Precautions

All patients and all blood and body fluid specimens *must be considered to be infectious at all times.* The CDC has promulgated precautions that we should strive to follow while caring for all patients:

1. Universal precautions (Table 49–4): those taken with all patients because HIV-infected people cannot reliably be identified by history and physical examination. Of particular significance are cases in emergency care settings, such as trauma resuscitation, when exposure to blood or body fluids is likely and the patient's infectious status is unknown.
2. Invasive precautions (Table 49–5): those taken in addition to the universal precautions when such a procedure is to be performed. An invasive procedure is defined by the CDC as any surgical entry into tissues, cavities, or an organ or repair of any traumatically induced lesions. These include but are not limited to lumbar puncture, traumatic

**TABLE 49–4.** Universal Precautions

| | |
|---|---|
| Barriers | Gloves, masks, eyewear as appropriate. |
| Needles | Do not resheathe, bend, or break. Dispose of in a puncture-proof container. |
| Dermatologic conditions | Weeping or exudative lesions as well as cuts and abrasions imply a breach in the integumentary barrier. This may increase risk if the area involved is not protected with a barrier. |
| Decontamination | Wash hands. |
| Pregnant health care workers | Be especially careful because intrauterine transmission occurs. |

lesions, cardiac catheterization and other angiographic procedures, vaginal or cesarean delivery, intravenous catheter placement, and dental surgical procedures. We also consider nasogastric and airway intubation to be invasive because of the possibility of blood contamination.[84]
3. Laboratory precautions (Table 49–6): those recommended for HCWs involved in clinical laboratories. Blood and body fluids from all patients, regardless of known HIV status, must be considered infectious until proven otherwise. The precautions noted supplement universal precautions.

If easy answers were available to the question of whether we are put at risk for HIV infection by our patients and at what degree, a separate section of this chapter would not be needed. Although only limited data exist, some of the following material represents nothing more than obvious good sense; the rest is our educated opinion.

Any integumentary contamination with a patient's blood must be washed with germicidal soap as soon as practical and safe. Gloves must be worn whenever patients are administered care. This practice, in our view, does not include the initial portion of the patient encounter, in which the anesthesiologist greets and shakes the patient's hand in the preoperative area, or when further contact is made in the OR before anesthetic induction. In addition to gloves, plastic eyewear or prescription glasses (preferably with side shields) are certainly appropriate in the prevention of mucous membrane contamination.

## Types of Injuries

Different types of exposures may carry different risks. Although cutaneous contaminations, barring breaks in the skin, are usually without great risk, they are nonetheless handled as noted previously.

### Needle Punctures

Exposure through hollow-tipped needles, such as those used to start intravenous infusions, is recognized to be responsible for approximately 61% of contamination events occurring in OR personnel; most of these occur in anesthesiologists.[85]

**TABLE 49–5.** Invasive Precautions

| | |
|---|---|
| Universal precautions plus additional barriers | Liquid-repellant gown over a repellant apron, repellant leggings and shoe covers. Consider double gloving. Watch for glove tears. |

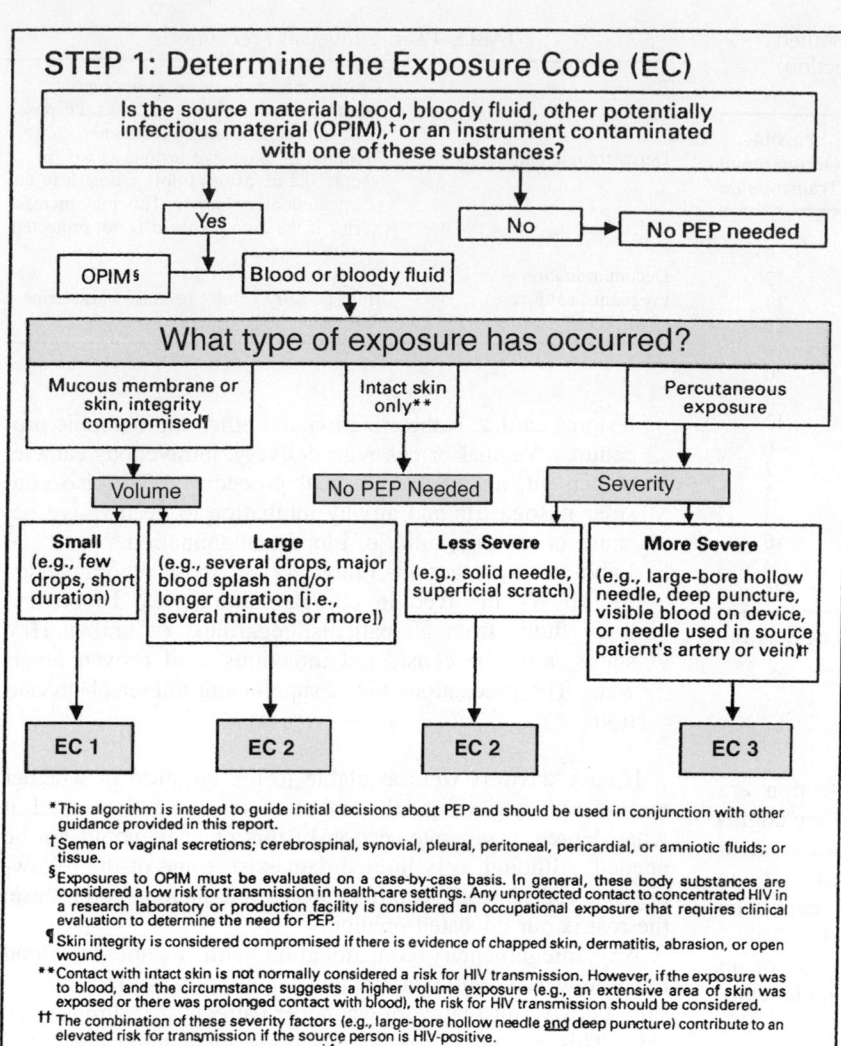

## STEP 1: Determine the Exposure Code (EC)

Is the source material blood, bloody fluid, other potentially infectious material (OPIM),† or an instrument contaminated with one of these substances?

Yes → No → No PEP needed

OPIM§ ← Blood or bloody fluid

### What type of exposure has occurred?

Mucous membrane or skin, integrity compromised¶ | Intact skin only** | Percutaneous exposure

Volume | No PEP Needed | Severity

**Small** (e.g., few drops, short duration) | **Large** (e.g., several drops, major blood splash and/or longer duration [i.e., several minutes or more]) | **Less Severe** (e.g., solid needle, superficial scratch) | **More Severe** (e.g., large-bore hollow needle, deep puncture, visible blood on device, or needle used in source patient's artery or vein)††

EC 1 | EC 2 | EC 2 | EC 3

\* This algorithm is inteded to guide initial decisions about PEP and should be used in conjunction with other guidance provided in this report.

† Semen or vaginal secretions; cerebrospinal, synovial, pleural, peritoneal, pericardial, or amniotic fluids; or tissue.

§ Exposures to OPIM must be evaluated on a case-by-case basis. In general, these body substances are considered a low risk for transmission in health-care settings. Any unprotected contact to concentrated HIV in a research laboratory or production facility is considered an occupational exposure that requires clinical evaluation to determine the need for PEP.

¶ Skin integrity is considered compromised if there is evidence of chapped skin, dermatitis, abrasion, or open wound.

\*\* Contact with intact skin is not normally considered a risk for HIV transmission. However, if the exposure was to blood, and the circumstance suggests a higher volume exposure (e.g., an extensive area of skin was exposed or there was prolonged contact with blood), the risk for HIV transmission should be considered.

†† The combination of these severity factors (e.g., large-bore hollow needle and deep puncture) contribute to an elevated risk for transmission if the source person is HIV-positive.

**FIGURE 49–6.** The Public Health Service's recommendations for postexposure prophylaxis. (From Centers for Disease Control and Prevention. Public Health Service guidelines for the management of health-care worker exposures to HIV and recommendations for postexposure prophylaxis. *MMWR Morb Mortal Wkly Rep.* 1998;47[RR-7]:1.)

## Sharp Injuries

Among surgical personnel, sharp injuries are more often inflicted by a solid instrument such as a scalpel or a sharp clamp. Wright and colleagues noted that three mechanisms accounted for almost 60% of sharp injuries: (1) those caused by instruments left on the surgical field but not in use (24%); (2) those caused to hands used in directly retracting tissue (17%); and (3) those of a stationary hand holding an instrument that was injured by a second instrument (16%).[86] Only 6% of sharp injuries occurred during passage of instruments between the scrub nurse and surgeon.

We cannot overemphasize that needles should never be resheathed, because this practice may lead to puncture wounds. All sharp objects should be discarded in a puncture-proof container immediately after use. This puncture-proof container should be placed as close to the procedure site as possible. Instruments not in use must be removed from the surgical field. The use of hands as retractors must be minimized, and double-gloving should be the norm.[87] Although we appreciate intellectually that these precautions should be followed, data suggest that these preventive measures are too frequently ignored by HCWs during patient care.[88,89] Of even more significance, up to 84% of blood contacts are preventable by barriers such as face masks or shields and fluid-resistant gowns and gloves.[90]

## Should Testing Be Performed After Possible Exposure?

The issue of testing after possible exposure to a person with HIV infection has been an even more difficult problem than prevention. Previously, we argued for a very careful

---

**TABLE 49–6.** Laboratory Precautions in Addition to Universal Precautions

**Material Handling**

Use a biologic safety hood.
Use only mechanical pipettes.
Use needle/syringes only if there is no alternative.
Use well-constructed containers with well-fitting lids.

**Cleanup**

Decontaminate work space after spills; household bleach works well.
Decontaminate/clean equipment before transport/repair.
Discarded liquids/solids should be appropriately neutralized (ie, by autoclave).

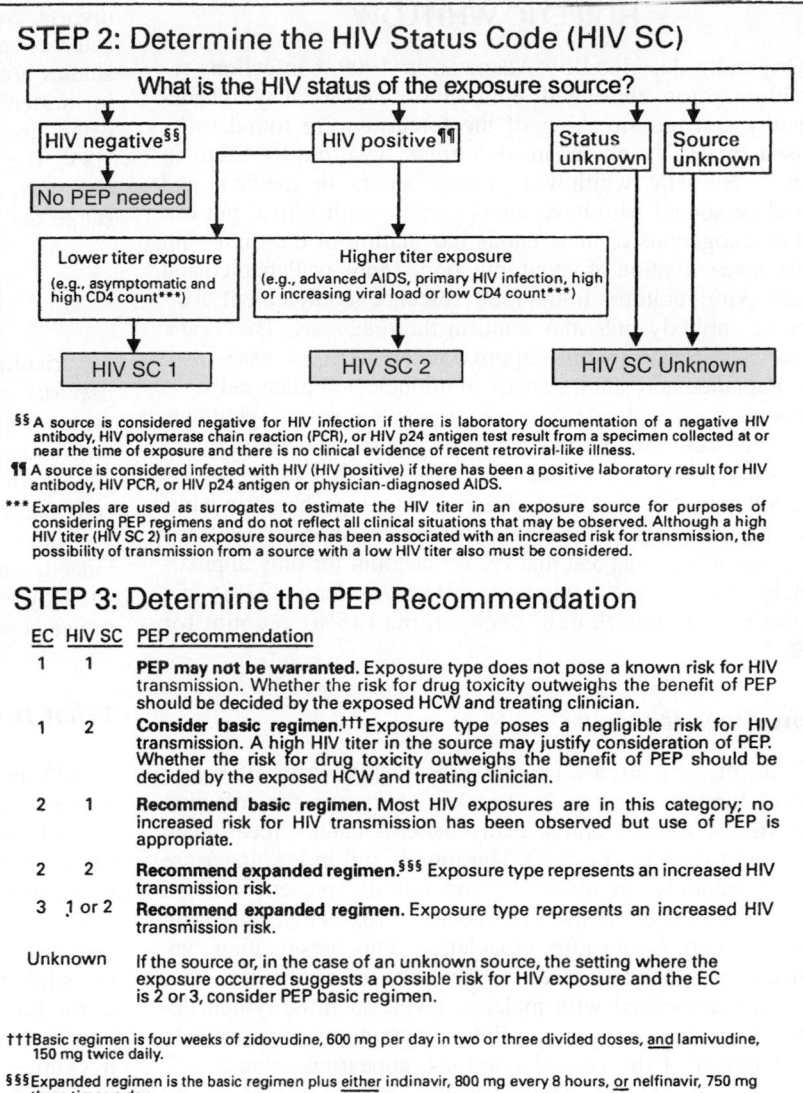

**FIGURE 49–6** *Continued.*

policy of testing, if for no other reason than because there were minimal data suggesting risk to patients from an HIV-positive HCW, and there was no effective therapy. The issue of prophylaxis and therapy has changed greatly since the first edition of this textbook. We suggest that after a percutaneous or mucous membrane exposure, the HCW be tested along with the patient, when possible. If the exposure fulfills the criteria for "high risk" then, despite the 14 or so instances in which zidovudine has failed to prevent HIV seroconversion,[91,92] we recommend following the Public Health Service's suggestions regarding postexposure prophylaxis.[92] This entails 4 weeks of either two nucleoside analogue reverse transcriptase inhibitors, or a protease inhibitor plus the two nucleoside analogues (Fig. 49–6). An incident report should be filed with the proper hospital or clinic personnel.

### Patient Testing

Patients should also be studied serologically. In Florida, this is done in one of two ways: (1) informed consent is given, the test result entered in the patient's chart, and the patient given pretest and posttest counseling; or (2) when

consent is not possible, as in the case of a comatose patient without family, the serologic study may be performed on a "leftover" blood specimen originally obtained for another reason. In this case, the result is not entered in the patient's chart. Clearly, the first of the two options is preferred.

### What Is the Risk to Patients From HIV-Positive Health Care Workers?

Cases studied by the CDC have suggested HIV transmission to patients from their dentist.[93,94] Precisely how infection occurred remains unknown. The dentist's office records are unclear about the precise technique used for instrument sterilization. Inadequate cleaning of instruments may have resulted in the transmission of the viral agent. The result of this case, however, was a very emotional and powerful call that all HCWs be serologically tested for HIV and that patients be informed about the worker's HIV status.[95] This approach has found little support from those of us providing health services.

## HERPETIC WHITLOW

Originally described by Adamson in 1909,[96] infections resembling paronychiae with epitrochlear and axial lymphadenopathy and red streaking of the forearm were found to be caused by HSV and renamed *herpetic whitlow* by Stern in 1959.[97] Herpetic whitlow typically occurs in medical and dental personnel who have direct contact with saliva, but can follow exogenous or autogenous inoculation of the digit with virus or reactivation of latent infection. Tzank or Papanicolaou smear, viral culture, immunofluorescence complement fixation, or antibody titer may confirm the diagnosis. The Tzank smear is accurate in only approximately 60% of cases and, like Papanicolaou stain, reveals multinucleated giant cells.

People positive for HSV antibody may not report symptoms during an acute infection. In fact, asymptomatic salivary excretion of HSV type 1 (HSV-1) is encountered in 2% to 9% of adults and 5% to 8% of children. Although herpetic whitlow has been reported as being more common in HCWs,[98] more recent data suggest that HCWs account for only approximately 8% of cases, whereas children/students (31%) and adults in non–health care occupations (45%) account for 76%.[99]

### How Does It Occur?

Typically, the disease begins with inoculation of HSV-1 or HSV-2 through a break in the skin. Although the infection may follow minor trauma, many patients cannot recall even the most trivial injuries.[97,100] The thumb and index finger are most commonly involved[101,102] and initially present with an area of painful erythema that radiates proximally, appearing approximately 4 days after inoculation. This presentation may indicate the secondary infection; primary infections, however, are often associated with malaise, fever, adenitis, lymphadenopathy, and other general flulike symptoms that precede development of the vesicular lesions, appearing some 5 to 7 days after inoculation. These vesicles usually appear around the nail bed and coalesce, but they may extend under the nail or more proximally up the digit. These vesicles initially contain clear serous fluid that may become thick, turbid, and yellow as the vesicles fill with debris from the destruction of soft tissue. This fluid may become frankly purulent if bacteria colonize the wound secondarily. The palmar surface of the distal phalanx is most often involved.

The vesicles may persist for more than 14 days, but usually are closed in approximately 2 weeks, at which point the dermis begins to peel and viral shedding ceases. Scarring and numbness may persist and hypersensitivity of the infected region may make work impossible. Twenty percent to 50% of the infections recur, even after several years.[103–105] Hypersensitivity and pain may continue unabated between episodes. HSV-1 and HSV-2 may be transmitted during examination of the oropharynx, genitalia, eyes, or skin around a tracheostomy site. Although the disease has a predilection for the chronically ill and immunologically challenged,[106] healthy people do contract this disease and should take appropriate precautions (wear gloves) to protect themselves.

### How Is It Treated?

Herpetic whitlow must be differentiated from paronychia because an attempted surgical drainage might systematize the disease. Surgical removal of the nail may, however, be indicated to relieve the pain of this viral process.[107] Although studies are few, oral acyclovir has been shown to be effective in shortening the duration of symptoms both in immunocompetent and immunocompromised patients with mucocutaneous HSV. The possibility of immunization is under investigation. For now, the most rational preventive measures are those suggested by universal precautions.[108]

## CHICKENPOX/HERPES ZOSTER

Varicella-zoster virus (VZV), sometimes referred to as *herpesvirus type III,* is a member of the herpesvirus family. The primary clinical form of VZV is chickenpox, and the reactive form is seen as herpes zoster, or shingles. The virion contains a core of double-stranded DNA. Once within the human cell, the virus induces specific enzymes collectively termed *thymidine kinase.* These act to phosphorylate nucleosides and, indeed, nucleoside analogues are preferentially phosphorylated by these enzymes. From this activity stems our ability to use acyclovir and ganciclovir against this agent.

### What Is the Relevant Epidemiology?

VZV is highly communicable. It is epidemic in large urban centers and, interestingly, in temperate climates. Humans are the only known species naturally infected; all races and both sexes are equally affected, although the attack rate for children is the highest of any population group.

The viral agent is spread by close contact with an infected person in the early stages of disease. Attack rates in susceptible siblings at home range from 70% to 87% and are lower in the school environment. VZV does not survive in scabs or crusts; thus, once the vesicles are crusted over, usually 5 to 7 days after their appearance in normal children, transmission is unlikely. Aerosol spread is documented, particularly in the hospital environment, because the virus is shed in respiratory secretions.

### Incidence

In the United States, approximately 3 million cases of this infection occur yearly, with the highest incidence of infection noted in children 5 to 9 years of age. Most people show evidence of infection by adulthood, and very sensitive antibody assays have shown that the seroprevalence of antibody to VZV ranges from 95% to 100%. Clinical varicella infection has been demonstrated by increases in antibody titer after exposure to VZV. Indeed, even though the subclinical attack rate is thought to be <5%, many who have protective titers of antibody have no history of clinical disease.[109]

For unclear reasons, in tropical regions, varicella has been noted to have higher morbidity and mortality rates, perhaps because childhood infection is less frequent. Infection thus occurs in an older population than is noted in temperate climates. Pregnant women from nontemperate regions may not be immune to VZV; they have a higher risk of bearing children with congenital varicella.[110]

Patients who have recurrent VZV in the form of herpes zoster may transmit the viral agent to previously uninfected people, thus resulting in primary varicella. Previously unexposed adults who have a negative varicella titer and are exposed to either a child with chickenpox or an adult with herpes zoster may acquire VZV infection. Therefore, recognition of the signs and symptoms of this infection is important.[111]

## How Is Varicella (Chickenpox) Manifested?

As noted previously, a history of exposure is common either in school or in the family. In a normal child, varicella is a relatively benign process. The incubation period ranges from 10 to 21 days, averaging 15 days. The prodromal stage, consisting of fever and malaise, is noted approximately 24 hours before the onset of rash. This stage is often more severe in adolescents and adults. The fever is usually ≤39°C, and affected children do not appear acutely ill; pruritus is common.

### Skin Lesions

Initially, the lesions may be seen on the scalp, mucous membranes, face, and neck. They often are most numerous on the trunk. The classic lesion of chickenpox is a superficial vesicle surrounded by a halo of erythema. The lesions may change very rapidly, within hours, from maculopapules to vesicles. With this change, the pruritus becomes intense. In an immunologically normal child, new lesions continue to form for approximately 5 days after the initial eruption, with the lower extremities often the last to be involved. Gradual healing of lesions occurs over a period of 3 weeks. Disfigurement is very uncommon with this process.

As a result of underreporting, the number of children hospitalized for varicella infection is unclear. Probably 2000 to 5000 hospitalizations occur annually. Approximately 10% of the children hospitalized for this process die, primarily from secondary bacterial infections or VZV CNS involvement.[108-110]

## How Is Infection Diagnosed?

Although the diagnosis of VZV infection is most frequently based on the history and clinical findings, isolation of the viral agent is definitive. Cells are obtained from vesicular lesions or from biopsy samples; the latter should be examined microscopically. The presence of multinucleated giant cells with eosinophilic intranuclear inclusions is suggestive of either HSV or VZV infection; studies with monoclonal antibody differentiate the two.

Measurement of specific antibody against VZV may be used to determine the susceptibility to infection. The most sensitive methods are either ELISA or indirect immunofluorescence against membrane antigen (IFAMA).[110]

## What Is the Prognosis?

In most immunologically normal children, varicella resolves without sequelae in 5 to 10 days. The complication rate in this group of patients is approximately 5%, with CNS involvement being the major cause of morbidity and mortality. Severity of infection and complications increase with age, including visceral dissemination of the virus resulting in,

among other things, respiratory failure. This progression is fairly common in either older adults or pregnant women.

Adults have a more serious complication rate with this infection, including visceral dissemination in otherwise healthy individuals. Thus, treatment with acyclovir may be instituted when the diagnosis of VZV is considered. Because varicella during pregnancy carries with it significant risk of maternal morbidity and mortality, treatment with acyclovir may also be necessary in this situation. Although this agent is not teratogenic in animal models, its use to decrease the risk of congenital varicella may be neither safe nor effective in humans[109]; nonetheless, its use should be considered. Antiviral therapy is likely to be necessary in immunocompromised individuals. Further, if a patient given steroids or other immunomodulating agents develops VZV, the dose should be decreased or, if possible, the agent discontinued.

## How Is It Prevented?

An attenuated varicella vaccine is under evaluation and may be available in the near future. Until then, VZV immune globulin may be used in high-risk patients. Although it has a failure rate of nearly 20%, it does appear to modify the ensuing infection. In addition, VZV immune globulin may prolong the incubation period for as long as 42 days after exposure to the virus.

### Immunization

Individuals at high risk should receive VZV immune globulin within 96 hours of exposure, at a dose of 125 units per 10 kg of body weight (minimum dose 125 units, maximum dose 625 units) via intramuscular injection. This agent is distributed by the Red Cross blood service. Before receiving VZV immune globulin, adults should be evaluated on an individual basis. This evaluation should take into consideration the possibility of exposure, the geographic background, the health status, and the likelihood of previous infection. HCWs with a negative history of VZV infection and significant exposure to children may benefit from laboratory testing to determine whether or not they have an antibody to VZV. Seronegative HCWs should not care for patients with varicella or herpes zoster.

### Isolation

Hospitalized patients with VZV infection should be isolated until their lesions have crusted. If possible, this isolation should be in a negative-pressure room to decrease or prevent the possibility of dissemination of viral particles to other patients.

## If I Have a Negative Varicella Titer and Am Exposed to Chickenpox, What Should I Do?

Seropositivity to VZV is extremely common in the United States. It is likely, even in an adult who has no recollection of symptoms, that exposure has occurred. However, for those who are unsure, testing for the antibody via either ELISA or IFAMA may be used to determine antibody titer. In a high-risk individual who has no titer, VZV immune globulin may be used to modify the attack rate and severity of symptoms. If visceral dissemination of this virus occurs, such as varicella pneumonia, acyclovir should be initiated. Until an adequate vaccine is available, an individual with a negative titer should not care for an infectious patient.

## CYTOMEGALOVIRUS INFECTION

### What Is the Relevant Epidemiology?

CMV is also a member of the herpesvirus group. In an intact person, CMV growth occurs in epithelial or endothelial cells and in macrophages. Because a very high titer of virus is produced in the salivary glands and kidneys, protracted CMV shedding is noted in oral secretions and urine; the viral agent can, however, be found in essentially all organs and body fluids.[112] CMV infection occurs commonly throughout the world; most patients are without symptoms. The incidence of infection in children ranges from 15% in Seattle to 99% in Tanzania.[113] The exact means of transmission has not been completely elucidated.

Young children asymptomatically shed the virus in urine and saliva. In daycare centers, for example, up to 69% of children may be so affected. Daycare workers and nurses caring for hospitalized children who shed CMV are infected at a rate that is similar to that of the general population. However, parents of children who are in daycare centers and are shedding acquire the infection at a very high rate. This observation may have implications for mothers of childbearing age, because serious congenital infection may occur in children born to infected mothers. Pregnant women infected with CMV transmit the virus to their children approximately 50% of the time.[114]

### Blood Transfusion

Transmission of the viral agent via blood transfusion occurs on occasion. The risk of infection from a single unit of blood may range from 3% to 6%. Although most of these infections are subclinical, in immune-suppressed patients or transplant recipients, infection with CMV may have catastrophic consequences. This can be avoided by using CMV-seronegative blood. Use of high-titer anti-CMV gamma globulin decreases the severity of an infection, although not the infection itself. The use of ganciclovir to treat infection or CMV vaccine to prevent it may be appropriate in the future.

### How Is Cytomegalovirus Infection Diagnosed?

The presence of circulating antibodies to CMV suggests prior infection, whereas seroconversion indicates more recent acquisition of the viral agent. Testing in this manner may be helpful in counseling pregnant women (eg, HCWs) who may have been exposed to CMV. This form of testing may not be helpful, however, to make the diagnosis in patients who are immunosuppressed. Detection of CMV IgM antibody is possible in up to 70% of infants who are infected with the agent in utero.

### What Is the Prognosis?

The prognosis for congenital CMV inclusion disease is relatively poor, because death or permanent institutionalization is frequently the result. Therapy for active infection is unsatisfactory, because CMV is resistant to agents such as vidarabine and acyclovir; ganciclovir is useful in some cases. Relapses are common, however, and multiple courses of therapy or prolonged maintenance therapy must be considered.

### Are Preventive Measures Effective?

Although prevention of the primary viral infection in seronegative women of childbearing age would be important to decrease morbidity and mortality, such measures are generally limited. From the epidemiologic data at hand, it appears that pregnant mothers are at greatest risk from their daycare-attending children, compared with the risk from infected HCWs. Nonetheless, although again the data are unclear, seronegative pregnant women should use extreme caution in caring for patients infected with CMV. Because one does not always know who is infected with CMV, universal precautions are appropriate. As always, transfusion should be minimized in all patients, but in those who are seronegative, only CMV-negative blood should be used.[115]

## TUBERCULOSIS

Since 1990, nosocomial (Florida and New York) and correctional system transmission of multidrug-resistant tuberculosis (MDR-TB) has been reported to the CDC.[116] All 8 of the correctional facility patients identified in a retrospective epidemiologic study died; 7 were HIV positive, and 1 was a state correctional facility employee who had recently been treated for cancer with radiation. All of these individuals had profoundly subnormal CD4+ (helper) lymphocyte counts, and all died before (mean, 25 days; range, 3-42 days) the hospital was notified that their isolates were positive for MDR-TB (mean time from collection of sputum to notification of the referring hospital, 18 weeks; range, 13-23 weeks). MDR-TB is reported to be resistant to isoniazid, rifampin, pyrazinamide, ethambutol, streptomycin, kanamycin, and ethionamide. The CDC identified no effective drug regimen to treat patients in this outbreak.

As a result of this outbreak, HCWs need to be aware of their tuberculin status. Annual tuberculin skin tests should be carried out on all staff who previously tested negative or do not know their tuberculin status. The HIV status of all patients with tuberculosis should be evaluated, because immunocompromised individuals with MDR-TB may die very rapidly. The role of anesthesia equipment in transmitting tuberculosis is unclear and deserves to be studied. Work we have recently published demonstrates that *Mycobacterium tuberculosis* is not killed in the carbon dioxide absorber and may be transmissible.[117] In addition, anesthesia technical support personnel responsible for changing the soda lime canisters in the machines may be at risk and should wear masks when doing so.

## STRESS

### Why Should We Address Stress in the Operating Room Setting? What Makes It Unique?

We all deal with stress in almost every aspect of life. There are some aspects of stress that distract us from the necessary vigilance required to conduct a safe anesthetic procedure. Stress can lead to fatigue, anxiety, depression, withdrawal, physical ailments, chemical dependency and, if not dealt with properly, it can confound and consume us.[118-120]

### What Is Stress?

It can be defined as a sense of pressure, strain, urgency or tension on one's physical or emotional well-being. If handled well, stress can be a mechanism for growth. We all are subject to physical, mental, and emotional stress daily. For the most part, there is no problem.

Stress comes from four basic origins:

1. Environmental factors: weather, noise, traffic, pollution must be endured. These factors deluge us and challenge our ability to adjust.
2. Social stressors: we are bombarded with conflicting demands on our time and attention, disagreements, financial problems, and arguments.
3. Physiologic changes: illness, aging, accidents, lack of exercise, pregnancy, menopause, poor nutrition, and disturbance of sleep patterns all strain the body. Our physiologic responses to environmental and social threats can result in such manifestations of stress as muscle tension, headaches, upset stomach, vomiting, diarrhea, and anxiety.
4. Thought processes: thoughts produce stress through interpretation and translation of changes in the environment and body and determine when to turn on the emergency (fight or flight) response.[121]

#### Stress Exposure and Response

Stress should be looked upon as two entities: stress exposure and stress response. Stress exposure is a very powerful stimulus for growth. People grow the most in areas in which they have been pushed to the limit. Stress exposure expands one's capacity to deal with stress. The *impact* of stress in life is determined not by the *exposure* to stress, but by the *response* to that exposure. The patient who is not completely evaluated, the emergent case that awaits as soon as this patient clears the recovery room, the evil-tempered surgeon with whom you are working today, the unprepared resident, the shortage of personnel, the colleague who called in sick leaving a room uncovered, among other events, are not what gets under our skin. Rather, it is our emotional response to these events that may devastate our whole being.[122-124]

There are two opposite extremes of the stress response[122]: karoshi and liming.

*Karoshi* is a Japanese word meaning "death from overwork." The Japanese Ministry of Health has identified five factors leading to the fatal *karoshi* syndrome:

1. Extremely long hours that interfere with normal recovery and rest patterns
2. Night work that interferes with normal recovery and sleep patterns
3. Working without holidays or breaks
4. High-pressure work, with no respite
5. Extremely demanding physical labor and continuously stressful work with no relief

The sequelae of such sustained patterns of stress appear as hypertension, stroke, myocardial infarction, carcinoma, suicide, and many stress-related degenerative and autoimmune diseases.[120] There is no question that these factors, and their deleterious results, are not unique to Japan. We see the same thing in our work environment.

The exact opposite of *karoshi* is the Caribbean practice of *liming*.[122] This is the art of doing absolutely nothing, remaining totally devoid of guilt. It is the culturally approved way of periodically breaking away from the stresses that consume us. Liming can take the form of any healthy pleasure that provides mental relief from the relentless stresses of everyday life.

There are many mechanisms for dealing with stress that are positive and strengthening. There are also many that may not be as good as might be desired. There are the standard ones: a double martini ("make that a triple, it's been a real bad day, I've been working like an animal"), a cigar or cigarette, double meat and cheese pizza, kicking the wall or the car, smoking a joint, doing a line of coke. Some are clearly worse from a social standpoint, such as smoking a joint, doing a line of coke, taking a cc of fentanyl, or abusing—either mentally or physically—one's spouse or children. Each of these may make us feel less stressed but all are deleterious in the long run. A person must endeavor to find a positive stress reducer[125] that fits into his or her lifestyle and do what works to reduce the negative effects of stress: swimming; running; gardening; bicycling; or playing the viola, violin, or piano.

## FATIGUE

### How Is Fatigue Defined?

In a dictionary, *fatigue* may be characterized as weariness and physical or mental exhaustion or as the cause of weariness, such as labor or toil. To fatigue is to tire out; to become weary with labor or any bodily or mental exertion; to harass with toil; to exhaust the strength and, finally, to weaken by continued use. Many factors add to fatigue, such as stress, both internal and external, and the ambiance within which a person functions.[126-130]

### How Is Fatigue Perceived?

Perceptions of fatigue in anesthesiology lie on a continuum that to some extent depends on professional status. Is the individual an actively practicing resident or a person close to retirement? In a residency setting, it is instructive to listen to the perceptions and attitudes about fatigue:

"They're not making residents like they used to."
"These kids have no stamina."
"They're coddled and are given every break in the world."
"When I was a resident (and dinosaurs walked the earth),

things were different. We were cut from a different cloth. We walked to and from the hospital in the snow (uphill both ways). We were on call 24 hours and then worked a full shift before going home for a few hours and came back to repeat the cycle. We never complained. We never fatigued."

The perception of one's own indefatigability is somewhat colored by the number of years that have passed since serving as a house officer.

## What Factors Influence Fatigue?

A number of factors influence fatigue in an anesthesia care provider.[127] First is individual variance. Some people simply tire more rapidly than others, and signs of fatigue are manifested in a shorter time. Factors such as physical and emotional well-being also enter into the picture. A common cold or influenza virus can sharply reduce effectiveness. Transient, slight depression often leads to disproportionate fatigue. Dealing with the day-to-day stresses of patient care responsibility also has an impact. Concerns about one's physical state, multisystem problems, psychologic well-being, family matters, and morbidity and mortality wear heavily on the psyche.

The surgical suite is an environment in which external stimuli such as daylight or darkness are not apparent. No windows allow confirmation of circadian rhythm. Trace gases may be in the inspired air.[128-130] Sleeplessness and long working hours are major factors that influence fatigue. Fatigue in the anesthesia provider can lead to abuse of alcohol and other substances.[131] The suicide rate among physicians is two to three times higher than among the general population.[132] Suicide is the most serious response to stress and fatigue.

### Workable Schedules

Collective bargaining units have negotiated workable schedules for house officers. What is fair, equitable, and safe has not been defined exactly, but a 12-hour workday with call every third night appears not to have any deleterious results that are measurable by current technology. Obviously, the central concern is patient safety. Because 95% of the reported problems in anesthesiology are related to human error, vigilance should be as nearly optimal as possible.[133] Fatigue factors can predispose to therapeutic misadventures with potentially disastrous results.

Parker[126] made the following suggestions to attenuate fatigue factors:

1. Any anesthesiologist involved in a procedure lasting >3 hours should be relieved every 2 hours for short periods.
2. No anesthesiologist should work longer than 17 hours without a full 12-hour recovery period.
3. No anesthesiologist should be on call more often than, on average, every third night.
4. One must not hesitate to say "no" to unreasonable workloads.

## SUBSTANCE ABUSE

No occupational hazard in the practice of anesthesiology has more devastating consequences than the abuse of

**TABLE 49–7.** Common Terms Defining Drug and Substance Use

| Term | Definition |
|------|-----------|
| Appropriate | Medication taken as prescribed by physician or manufacturer for specific indication |
| Misuse | Unintended or inappropriate drug use |
| Habituation | Continued taking of a drug after the initial reason for taking it has resolved. Intervals between taking drugs are sufficiently long to prevent dependence, but discontinuance of the drug causes anxiety. |
| Abuse | Intentional use of a psychoactive chemical to the extent that it interferes with a person's health or economic or social function |
| Dependence | An altered physiologic state produced by repeated exposure to a drug requiring continued administration to prevent the occurrence of withdrawal or abstinence syndrome characteristic of the particular drug |
| Addiction | Abuse characterized by compulsion, loss of control, and continued use despite adverse consequences. An overwhelming preoccupation with its use and securing its supply denotes increased tolerance and withdrawal reactions on cessation of drug intake. |
| Tolerance | Progressively larger doses of a drug are required to produce the same effect. |

drugs[131,134-151] (Table 49–7). Those who have been involved in anesthesiology for a few years can, almost without exception, relate at least one tragedy due to drug abuse. Abuse of chemical substances, both licit and illicit, can lead to addiction. Although addiction is considered to be a disease process in enlightened circles, sanctions—including criminal justice processes—potentially await abusers or addicts.[134] Loss of medical licensure and incarceration in state or federal penal institutions loom as possible legal measures levied by government bodies.

## Why Are Drugs Used and Abused?

The question must be asked, "Why would anyone use or abuse drugs?" Historical reasons are summarized in Table 49–8.[135]

### Occupational Factors

Many times, more than one reason lies behind the use or abuse of drugs by an anesthesia practitioner. Some common factors are cited by practitioners who abuse drugs.[131,134] First, drugs are easily available. Narcotics, a primary component in the armamentarium of most anesthesia practitioners, are easily available to the potential abuser. Second, many stresses are

**TABLE 49–8.** Reasons for Substance Use (and Abuse)

To stimulate artistic creativity and performance
To treat disease
To aid in religious practices
To explore the self
To alter moods
To promote and enhance social interactions
To stimulate artistic creativity and performance
To improve physical performance
To rebel
To go along with peer pressure
To establish an identity

involved in providing anesthesia care. Anesthesiology is one of the few specialties of medicine or nursing in which an act of omission or commission can lead to immediate catastrophe. The need to act quickly in many situations only increases the level of stress. Third, a common feeling among some anesthesia practitioners is that they are not held in the same esteem as other specialists.[131] This outlook has been called the *Rodney Dangerfield syndrome* because of this entertainer's famous saying, "I get no respect."

## What Are the Warning Signs and Symptoms?

A number of clues may give rise to suspicion that a practitioner is abusing chemical substances. The disease process has a predictable course, with progressive manifestations in certain settings.[131] Problems often arise first at home. Harmonious relations are replaced by those characterized by strife and a concomitant increase in fights and spousal or child abuse.

Behavior often becomes inappropriate and embarrassing. Vehicular accidents occur, as do arrests for driving while intoxicated. Withdrawal from friends, family, and social gatherings is common. Previously gregarious people isolate themselves from the closest of friends. A person's physical status changes. Numerous health complaints arise, and medical attention is sought more frequently. Prescription drug use increases dramatically. Emotional control becomes extremely difficult.

Finally, signs and symptoms become evident in the professional setting. When such changes are noted in the workplace, the disease process is in a very advanced stage. Evidence of addictive behavior and drug abuse is summarized in Tables 49–9 and 49–10.

## What Is Enabling Behavior?

A pattern that occurs at any or all levels in this progressive process has been termed *enabling behavior*.[131] Whether practiced by members of the family, friends, or professional colleagues, denial and rationalization of behavior enable an im-

**TABLE 49–9.** Signs of Addiction

**Social**

Withdrawal from leisure activities, friends, family; uncharacteristic or inappropriate behavior in social gatherings
Impulsive behavior (overspending, gambling)
Domestic turmoil (separation, spousal or child abuse, sexual dysfunction)
Change in behavior of spouse or children
Legal problems (arrests for driving while intoxicated)

**Health**

Deterioration of personal hygiene
Accidents
Numerous health complaints, frequent need for medical attention for unrelated conditions

**Professional**

Unreliability
Complaints by patients or staff; subject of hospital gossip
Unstable work history (frequent relocations)
Working at less than par performance

**TABLE 49–10.** Signs of Substance Abuse by Anesthesia Providers

Unusually heavy narcotic technique
Frequent breakage of ampules
Frequent illness and absence from work
Sloppy, illegible anesthesia records
Inappropriate temperature sensitivity
Need for a bathroom break (every 2 h); desire and request to work alone
Refusal of lunch breaks
Heavy use of adjunctive drugs
Hostility
Anesthetic mishaps (harm to patient at end stage of the disease)

paired professional to become more embroiled in a potentially fatal process. Having been involved personally with this process on a number of occasions, we trace it as follows.

Behavior that is out of the ordinary in a colleague with whom one has worked and socialized for several years is often justified as "just a bad day." As this behavior continues, it becomes clear that a problem exists, but it is often excused as the result of probable marital discord. As other symptoms surface, the rationale becomes, "Maybe he or she is drinking a bit too much." Not until one is slapped in the face with irrefutable proof, such as walking into a room and seeing the person with a needle in a vein, does everything coalesce.

The feelings that surface are devastating. Self-recrimination occurs as the observer asks, "Why did I not recognize it before?" The individual is frankly amazed that all of the signs, which should have been obvious much earlier, were recognized only when denial was no longer an option for dealing with the problem.[130,140]

## How Is the Problem Recognized?

For this problem to be recognized, the potential for its occurrence must be appreciated; signs and symptoms must be noted when they occur. Recognition is possible through education of hospital personnel, who need to be familiar with the nature of addictive disease and the appropriate responses to impaired colleagues. They also need to be aware that resources are available for prevention, treatment, and rehabilitation.

Drugs are rarely abused as single entities.[131,138,141] The drug that is the most commonly abused is alcohol. Fentanyl is also widely used, and its oral ingestion has been reported.[141] Even propofol, a noncontrolled substance, has been reported to cause chemical dependency.[142] Combinations of alcohol with other substances are extremely common. When an impaired colleague is confronted, he or she responds with denial, usually accompanied by belligerence and hostility. One person alone should not stage such a confrontation. The "platoon" technique, in which a number of people elicit an admission of use or abuse, may be necessary.[134]

## How Is Treatment Provided?

### Identification

Successful treatment depends on early recognition and identification of the impaired person. According to the disease model of chemical dependency, there is no cure for addiction.

However, successful treatment can lead to recovery, followed by social and occupational rehabilitation and an eventual return to a useful and productive career. Identification of addicted physicians is very important because they rarely seek help on their own. Denial is a key behavioral factor in addiction. Moreover, peers are reluctant to confront suspected abusers because they do not want to be responsible for the abuser's loss of license or job. Early intervention, however, may prevent serious or irreversible consequences for an addicted person.

## Intervention

Drug dependence and alcoholism are treatable, if not curable. First, the person must acknowledge his or her dependency and the need for treatment. A confrontational approach involving multidisciplinary chemical dependency specialists, psychiatrists, psychologists, and other health professionals is usually required to make impaired physicians realize the extent of their illness.[139] This intervention should be conducted in a caring, factual, nonjudgmental manner. Such confrontation is a very successful method for enrolling addicted physicians into recognized treatment programs.

## Referral

All states now have impaired physicians' assistance committees. The Medical Association of Georgia's Disabled Doctor Program[131,144] and the California Diversion Program[145] are examples of state medical society programs that have demonstrated great success in returning impaired physicians to productive careers. Recovery rates range from 60% to 80% in these types of programs. Recovery is a lifelong process, however, and relapses are common. Data from several programs demonstrate a relapse rate of approximately 40%; however, relapses do not necessarily predict a negative treatment outcome.

Methods of achieving long-term recovery are many and are shown in Table 49–11.

## Pharmacologic Measures

Pharmacologic manipulation of behavior is useful but must be undertaken only in the context of a multidisciplinary approach to the problem of substance abuse. Outside of this context, it is no panacea.

### Disulfiram

Disulfiram blocks the metabolism of ethanol, resulting in formation of the intermediate metabolite, acetaldehyde. It is relatively nontoxic when administered alone. However, when

**TABLE 49–11.** Achievement of Long-Term Recovery

Group psychotherapy sessions with other chemically dependent people
Individual and family therapy with a psychiatrist or psychologist
Participation in Alcoholics Anonymous (AA) or Narcotics Anonymous (NA)
Routine urine screening for alcohol and other drugs. Screening should be performed randomly and at least weekly for the first 6 mo, with a gradual reduction in frequency as therapy progresses
Use of specific blocking agents to prevent abuse

**TABLE 49–12.** Signs and Symptoms of Narcotic Withdrawal

**Early (first 10 h)**
Anxiety
Sweating
Tachypnea
Rhinorrhea
Dilated, reactive pupils

**Late (>10 h)***
Excessive lacrimation and rhinorrhea
Tachycardia
Hypertension
Tremor
Abdominal pain
Nausea, vomiting, diarrhea
Piloerection
Muscle spasms
Fever

*Symptoms can last 5 mo.
Adapted from Stimmel B. *Pain, Analgesia, and Addiction: The Pharmacological Treatment of Pain.* New York, NY: Raven Press; 1983; 120.

ethanol is ingested, the blood acetaldehyde concentration rises 5 to 10 times higher than normal, resulting in the acetaldehyde syndrome. This reaction is very unpleasant, producing intense vasodilation, headache, respiratory distress, sweating, blurred vision, nausea, copious vomiting, hypotension, vertigo, and confusion. A person treated with disulfiram usually does not ingest alcohol again after experiencing these adverse reactions.

### Naltrexone

This oral opiate antagonist with no agonist properties can block the effects of narcotics for 48 to 72 hours. If a narcotic is self-administered during this period, no unpleasant side effects occur, but the desired effect from the narcotic is not obtained either. Therefore, this agent may be a valuable adjunct in deterring physicians prone to the compulsive use of narcotics. Anesthesiologists in particular may benefit from such therapy, because they can continue to prescribe and administer narcotics to patients without the temptation to self-administer.

## What Is the Narcotic Withdrawal Syndrome?

Acute narcotic withdrawal can produce various signs and symptoms, some of which are very intense (Table 49–12). Addicts often resort to extreme measures to avoid this withdrawal syndrome. Treatment of acute withdrawal reactions relies substantially on the use of pharmacologic therapies. Once again, however, the use of drugs to "withdraw" a drug abuser is acceptable only in the context of a multidisciplinary approach to the treatment of the problem.

### Clonidine

An $\alpha_2$-adrenergic agonist, clonidine is an effective agent in controlling the excessive sympathetic response associated with acute opiate withdrawal. A total of 0.4 to 1.2 mg is given orally in divided doses on day 1, followed by the application of 2 Catapres-TTS-2 patches. The release of clonidine from the patches is constant and is equivalent to 0.4 mg/d orally for 7 days. The patches should be replaced once, for a total of 14 days of therapy.

## Methadone

Methadone is another effective drug used for detoxification and maintenance. In essence, it replaces the narcotic and thereby prevents the abstinence syndrome. A daily dose of 20 mg may be sufficient in alleviating symptoms to facilitate long-term rehabilitation. Most patients can be withdrawn completely from opioids in <10 days.

## *What Measures Are Useful for Prevention?*

Addiction and substance abuse have so many serious consequences that prevention is of prime importance. Several steps can be taken to help reduce the growing numbers of chemically dependent anesthesiologists and nurse anesthetists.

## Increased Control and Accountability of Narcotics

Many large hospitals have established OR satellite pharmacies. One of the many important functions provided by these pharmacies is greatly increased control of narcotics. Dispensing narcotics on a per case basis and issuing individual anesthesia drug boxes to each anesthesiologist are examples of greater narcotic control.[147] Documentation of administered doses is recorded, and unused drugs in syringes are returned to the satellite pharmacy rather than "wasted." Routine use of a refractometer or random assays on syringe contents can readily detect abusers.[148] Audit of individual practices can identify other prescribing patterns. Unfortunately, as has been well documented, control and accountability are anything but precise, uniform, and effective.[151,152]

## Reentry Into the Workplace

Reentry into the practice of anesthesia after a prolonged absence, for any reason, is stressful.[153] The return to a work environment after having been in a therapeutic milieu for an addictive disease, with the fears inherent in such a process, compounds the anxiety of readjustment. There is the real fear of rejection by one's colleagues.[118] After an appropriate therapeutic intervention, the recovering anesthesia practitioner is ready and willing to try to regain the trust and respect of his or her coworkers. The other members of the group must lend a sympathetic ear and a helping hand. The recovering person cannot rush into a full schedule, but must be allowed the time to develop a different lifestyle and new coping mechanisms. They have learned to deal with a heightened awareness of themselves, their feelings, and their weaknesses, and are better able to seek support from their peers. They have also set personal goals. The recovering addict also knows that chemical dependency is a disease process that remains throughout life and requires their conscious effort to prevent a relapse.

The other side of the coin is fear on the part of the other members of the group that there will be recidivism that will severely affect the corporate image. That fear is not without merit because studies show that recidivism rate in the first 2 years is 14% to 19%.[119,153]

The employing group or institution has a legal obligation to the public. Historically, groups have been very reticent to have a recovering practitioner return to their practice. With peer assistance programs, aftercare contracts, newer laboratory screening studies, and medications, these groups can protect themselves and the public.[118,154]

## *Issues*

A number of considerations must be addressed before reentry into a clinical practice can occur.[118,154] They include but are not limited to the following:

- Clinical competence
- Adequacy of the therapeutic intervention
- Legal constraints
- Pending medicolegal action
- Length of recovery/sobriety
- Job availability
- Documentation of drug screening, attendance at the required meetings, and aftercare[155]

Obstacles to reentry into practice include but are not limited to the following:

- A lack of a precedence in the group or institution
- No policy
- Resistant coworkers
- Institutional administrative obstruction
- Lack of structure in the group
- Loss of self-confidence
- Feared loss of competence
- Regulatory or legal constraints
- Probationary condition of license
- Other disciplinary measures
- Conviction for felonious theft or diversion of a controlled substance[120,154–156]

## Innovative Option

A research project is underway using the anesthesia patient simulator to assess the recovering anesthesia care provider's readiness to return to clinical practice. It is used to update skills with increasingly complex clinical scenarios that include the measured addition of role players and distracters to add realism to the setting. The purpose is to look for triggering mechanisms that elicit an anxiety response in the recovering provider. The challenges include preoperative setup, selection of anesthetic technique, anesthetic agents, and adjuncts, induction, intubation, monitoring, physiologic assessment, management of the anesthetic, documentation, and interpersonal interactions. The recovering practitioner is specifically observed for anxiety in his or her interface with the chosen drugs of abuse and the paraphernalia inherent in the illicit use of those drugs. Preliminarily, this process appears to play a positive role in placing the practitioner once again into the clinical milieu.[154]

## Summary

Early identification of substance abusers is critical. All anesthesia practitioners must look for warning signs and behavioral changes in coworkers. Not every resident who is a sloppy dresser or every partner who is short-tempered is an addict, but dismissing warning signs among peers can lead to disability or even death of an addicted person. Alerting the department chairperson or chief of staff about a potentially impaired colleague is the first step in intervention. Enrollment in a state-sponsored program for impaired physicians is a nonpunitive therapeutic alternative for ultimate rehabilitation without loss of license and career.[135,136]

## TRACE GAS EXPOSURE

Chronic low-level exposure to anesthetic agents has been a long-standing concern among anesthesia care providers.[128–130,147–170] Studies have suggested that carcinogenic and teratogenic hazards, spontaneous abortions, neurologic symptoms, miscarriages, hepatitis, renal disease, and decreased mental performance can result from chronic exposure to the potent inhaled anesthetic agents.[157–164] Because of these findings, the National Institute of Occupational Safety and Health (NIOSH) has recommended standards for occupational exposure to trace anesthetic gas contamination in the OR.[163]

Studies describing the hazards of chronic exposure to inhalation agents have often conflicted with one another. Many of the studies were epidemiologic surveys or animal series using extremely high concentrations of the potent inhaled anesthetic agents. Human studies have used health surveys of practicing anesthesiologists, nurse anesthetists, dentists, and OR nurses.[158,160–162]

### *What Are the Suspected Deleterious Effects?*

Dose-related bone marrow depression developing from chronic exposure to nitrous oxide was described by Eastwood and colleagues in 1963.[164] Increased mortality rates among anesthesiologists due to malignancies of the lymphoid and reticuloendothelial systems have been reported.[136] Knill-Jones and associates reported an 18.2% frequency of spontaneous abortions in married female nurse anesthetists versus a 13.7% rate in married female physician control subjects unexposed to anesthetic agents.[165] A survey of anesthesiologists and OR nurses, using similar control groups, revealed an abortion rate of 38% for anesthesiologists, 30% for OR nurses, and 10% for the control subjects.[166] It also revealed an increased incidence of congenital malformations in the live births of anesthesiologists working (6.5%) versus those not working (2.5%) during pregnancy.

A survey jointly conducted by the American Society of Anesthesiologists and NIOSH revealed a statistically greater incidence of spontaneous abortions, congenital anomalies, cancer, and hepatic disease among anesthesia practitioners than among control subjects.[167] The survey showed a 1.3- to 2-fold greater risk of spontaneous abortion in women exposed to the OR environment during the first trimester of pregnancy. An increase of 60% to 100% in the reported incidence of congenital anomalies in the offspring of exposed female anesthetists, as well as a 25% greater incidence of anomalies in the offspring of the wives of exposed male anesthetists, was noted.

The incidence of cancer was 1.3 to 2 times greater in exposed female respondents. The incidence of hepatic disease was also 1.3 to 2 times greater in exposed than in nonexposed women. A 1.2- to 1.4-fold increase in renal disease was noted among nurse anesthetists. These findings, although impressive, must be interpreted cautiously because of the voluntary and noncontrolled nature of the survey.[167] None has been verified by prospective, controlled, randomized studies.

### Performance Studies

Performance studies in human volunteers after exposure to nitrous oxide were conducted by Bruce and Bach.[129] Nitrous oxide alone at 500 ppm and at 500 ppm plus halothane or enflurane, 15 ppm, were studied. Also studied were patients exposed to nitrous oxide at 50 ppm plus halothane, 1 ppm, and 25 ppm of nitrous oxide plus 0.5 ppm of halothane. Significant deterioration of memory, recognition, decision-making ability, and action were demonstrated for concentrations as low as 50 ppm of nitrous oxide and 1 ppm of halothane.

These data were challenged by Smith and Shirley, who were unable to reproduce the reported findings.[130] A study of ambient concentrations of anesthetic gases in the ORs of 20 hospitals revealed nitrous oxide levels ranging from <10 to 3000 ppm.[168] The mean was 388.5 ppm, and halothane concentrations were <0.1 to 60 ppm, with a mean value of 2.8 ppm. As a result of this study, NIOSH recommended that levels be maintained at <25 ppm for nitrous oxide and <0.5 ppm for halothane.[163]

### *What Are the Sources of Trace Gases?*

The sources of trace gas exposure are well described. Leakage from high-pressure nitrous oxide tanks to the flowmeters on anesthesia machines can produce substantial ambient contamination. The most common leakage sites are the quick connect couplings on the central inflow lines, faulty threads and seals, or crimped joints. Leaks from the low-pressure side of the system, beginning with the flowmeters, can be so great that an otherwise effective control system is negated (Table 49–13). Even if no gas leaks result from mechanical malfunction, significant anesthetic agent pollution of the OR environment can still occur as a result of improper technique by the anesthesiologist or nurse anesthetist. Suggested measures that can avoid or significantly reduce gas contamination are noted in Table 49–14.

### *How Are Anesthetic Agents Scavenged?*

Control measures designed to capture gas overflow are incorporated in every modern anesthesia machine.[171–174] The central mechanism is the scavenging system. The system

**TABLE 49–13.** Common Low-Pressure Leak Sites

Improperly connected or leaking tubing
Improperly sealed valve domes
Deformed gas delivery lines or machine connection joints
Leaking delivery lines
Leaking Y-connector joints
Sidestream gas analyzer sampling volume vented into room

**TABLE 49–14.** Measures to Minimize Operating Room Pollution
With Anesthetic Agents

Ensure proper mask fit to patient.
Avoid turning on the nitrous oxide or the vaporizer until a tight mask seal
  is obtained or the patient is intubated and connected to the circuit.
Discontinue gas flows (while continuing oxygen) and empty the reservoir
  bag through the pop-off valve (not by emptying it into the room) before
  suctioning or intubation.
Administer oxygen as long as possible before extubation or removal of the
  mask.
Avoid spillage of volatile agents during vaporizer filling by using a
  vaporizer-specific filling device.
Do not disconnect and empty the reservoir bag into the room during
  emergence.
Return the sidestream gas analyzer's exhaust flow to the circuit or
  scavenger system.
Scavenge the oxygenator exhaust port from the cardiopulmonary bypass
  circuit if a vaporizer is in use.

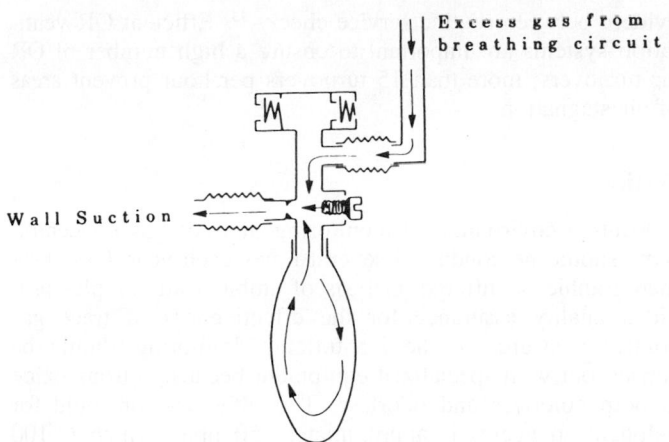

**FIGURE 49–8.** Anesthesia scavenger system. Note the incorporation of a
positive-pressure (overpressure) governor (*right*) and a negative-pressure
valve (*left*) to prevent the transmission of either positive or negative pressure
from the scavenger system to the ventilator or breathing circuit. (From
Gravenstein N, Lampotang S. Ventilation during anesthesia. In: Kirby RR,
Banner MJ, Downs JB, eds. *Clinical Applications of Ventilatory Support.*
New York, NY: Churchill Livingstone; 1990:282.)

connects to the expiratory limb of the breathing circuit and
consists of a gas-capturing assembly, an interface, and a disposal route[175] (Figs. 49–7 and 49–8). Excess gas from the
breathing circuit, ventilator, sidestream gas analyzer, or extracorporeal oxygenator is collected by the gas-capturing assembly and conducted to the disposal system.

Variation in anesthetic gas flow and effluent volumes requires that the scavenging system and the anesthesia circuit
be appropriately matched in terms of capacity and flow. The
interface is a pressure-regulating device designed to prevent
significant positive or negative pressures in the circuit (see
Fig. 49–8). It has two components: a reservoir to collect
transient overflow of gas that occurs when the outflow exceeds
the disposal rate, and a one-way valve designed to prevent
the suction of gas from the breathing circuit.

## Disposal

In ORs with a nonrecirculating ventilation system, disposal
is uncomplicated because waste gas can simply be directed to

the exhaust grill for elimination to the outside. ORs with
a recirculating ventilation system, however, should have an
alternate disposal route, such as an independent vacuum line
vented outside the hospital. Central vacuum lines are not used
because of fire code regulations. Charcoal absorbers are of
limited usefulness because they are expensive, have a short
life span, and do not remove nitrous oxide.

## Maintenance

Maintenance of anesthesia machines should be performed
by a factory-trained technician every 4 to 6 months. Nevertheless, anesthesia personnel should be vigilant for faulty connections, torn gaskets, and other potential flaws that can become

**FIGURE 49–7.** Schematic drawing
of gas supply and anesthesia machine
with a circle system. Anes-
thesia machine (1-13), breathing circuit (14-20),
scavenging system (21-24), anesthesia ventilator
(25-27), and patient interface (28-30). (From Gravenstein N, Lampotang S. Ventilation during anesthesia. In: Kirby RR, Banner MJ, Downs JB, eds.
*Clinical Applications of Ventilatory Support.* New
York, NY: Churchill Livingstone; 1990:282.)

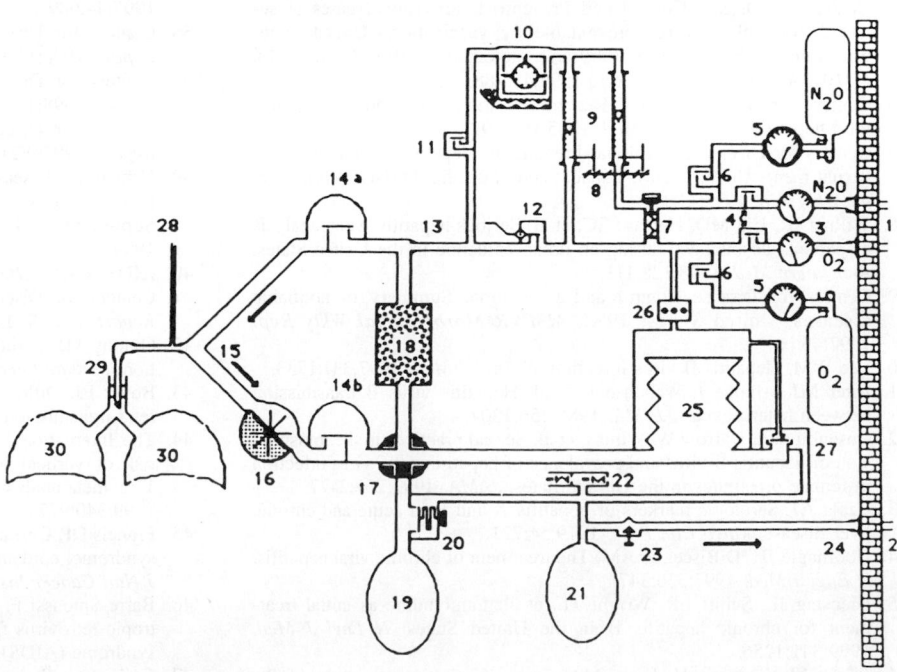

evident between routine service checks.[133] Efficient OR ventilation systems are important to ensure a high number of OR air turnovers; more than 15 turnovers per hour prevent areas of air stagnation.

## Testing

Routine environmental monitoring of trace gas concentrations should be conducted several times each year. Gas chromatographic or infrared analysis of ambient air samples provides quality assurance for the effectiveness of trace gas control measures in the institution. Monitoring should be carried out with specialized equipment because nitrous oxide is both colorless and odorless. The olfactory threshold for halogenated agents is approximately 50 ppm, which is 100 times greater than the NIOSH standard dictates.

In our institution, the clinical engineering department performs quarterly sampling of nitrous oxide concentrations using a time-weighted average method. Levels higher than 25 ppm are considered unacceptable by both our and NIOSH standards. All OR personnel should be educated about the potential hazards of trace anesthetic gases. Results of periodic monitoring under NIOSH conditions should be made available to all involved. Institutional guidelines for scavenging should be strictly followed by all personnel to minimize exposure.

## *References*

1. Centers for Disease Control. Summary of notifiable diseases—United States 1988. *MMWR Morb Mortal Wkly Rep.* 1988;37:3.
2. Centers for Disease Control and Prevention. Provisional cases of selected notifiable diseases—United States weeks ending January 2, 1999 and December 27, 1997 (52nd week). *MMWR Morb Mortal Wkly Rep.* 1999;47:1126, 1128.
3. Centers for Disease Control and Prevention. Summary of selected notifiable diseases—United States weeks ending June 27, 1992 (26th week). *MMWR Morb Mortal Wkly Rep.* 1992;41:471.
4. Centers for Disease Control and Prevention. Summary of selected notifiable diseases—United States weeks ending September 4, 1999 and September 5, 1998 (35th week). *MMWR Morb Mortal Wkly Rep.* 1999;48:785.
5. Centers for Disease Control and Prevention. Provisional cases of selected notifiable diseases preventable by vaccination—United States weeks ending September 4, 1999 and September 5, 1998 (35th week). *MMWR Morb Mortal Wkly Rep.* 1999;48:788.
6. Centers for Disease Control. Recommendations for protection against viral hepatitis. *Ann Intern Med.* 1985;103:391.
7. Centers for Disease Control and Prevention. Hepatitis A among homosexual men—United States, Canada, and Australia. *MMWR Morb Mortal Wkly Rep.* 1992;41:15.
8. Willner IR, Uhl MD, Howard SC, et al. Serious hepatitis A: an analysis of patients hospitalized during an urban epidemic in the United States. *Ann Intern Med.* 1998;128:111.
9. Centers for Disease Control and Prevention. Summary of notifiable diseases, United States, 1997. *MMWR Morb Mortal Wkly Rep.* 1997;46:ix.
10. Lee WM. Hepatitis B virus infection. *N Engl J Med.* 1997;337:1733.
11. Alter MJ, Ahtone J, Weisfuse I, et al. Hepatitis virus B transmission between heterosexuals. *JAMA.* 1986;256:1307.
12. Rosenblum L, Darrow W, Witte J, et al. Sexual practices in the transmission of hepatitis B virus and prevalence of hepatitis delta virus infection in female prostitutes in the United States. *JAMA.* 1992;267:2477.
13. Czaja AJ. Serologic markers of hepatitis A and B in acute and chronic liver disease. *Mayo Clin Proc.* 1979;54:721.
14. Hoofnagle JH, DiBisceglie AM. The treatment of chronic viral hepatitis. *N Engl J Med.* 1997;336:347.
15. Dienstag JL, Schiff ER, Wright TL, et al. Lamivudine as initial treatment for chronic hepatitis B in the United States. *N Engl J Med.* 1999;341:1256.
16. Berry AJ, Isaacson IJ, Kane MA, et al. A multicenter study of the prevalence of hepatitis B viral serologic markers in anesthesia personnel. *Anesth Analg.* 1984;63:738.
17. Kelen GD, Green GB, Purcell RH, et al. Hepatitis B and hepatitis C in emergency department patients. *N Engl J Med.* 1992;326:1399.
18. The Incident Investigation Teams and Others. Transmission of hepatitis B to patients from four infected surgeons without hepatitis B e antigen. *N Engl J Med.* 1997;336:178.
19. Aach RD, Stevens CE, Hollinger FB, et al. Hepatitis C virus infection in post-transfusion hepatitis: an analysis with first- and second-generation assays. *N Engl J Med.* 1991;325:1325.
20. Centers for Disease Control and Prevention. Recommendations for prevention and control of hepatitis C virus (HCV) infection and HCV-related chronic disease. *MMWR Morb Mortal Wkly Rep.* 1998;47:1.
21. Clarke B. Molecular virology of hepatitis C virus. *J Gen Virol.* 1997;78:2397.
22. Choo QL, Kuo G, Weiner AJ, et al. Isolation of a cDNA clone derived from a blood-borne non-A, non-B viral hepatitis genome. *Science.* 1989;244:359.
23. Stevens CE, Aach RD, Hollinger FB, et al. Hepatitis B virus antibody in blood donors and the occurrence of non-A non-B hepatitis in transfusion recipients. *Ann Intern Med.* 1984;101:733.
24. Czaja AJ, Davis GL. Hepatitis non-A non-B. *Mayo Clin Proc.* 1982;57:639.
25. Koziol DE, Holland PV, Alling DW, et al. Antibody to hepatitis B core antigen as a paradoxical marker for non-A non-B hepatitis agent in donated blood. *Ann Intern Med.* 1986;104:488.
26. Tillman HL, Manns MP. Hepatitis C virus infection—Diagnosis, natural course and therapy. *Kidney Blood Press Res.* 1996;19:215.
27. DiBisceglie AM. Hepatitis C. *Lancet.* 1998;351:351.
28. Howard RJ, Fry DE, Davis JM, et al. hepatitis C virus infection in healthcare workers. *J Am Coll Surg.* 1997;184:540.
29. Hunt CM, Carson KL, Sharara AI. Hepatitis C in pregnancy. *Obstet Gynecol.* 1997;89:883.
30. Baron S, Tyring SK, Fleischmann WR Jr, et al. The interferons: mechanisms of action and clinical applications. *JAMA.* 1991;266:1375.
31. Davis GL, Esteban-Mur R, Rustgi V, et al. Interferon alpha-2b alone or in combination with ribavirin for the treatment of relapse of chronic hepatitis C. *N Engl J Med.* 1998;339:1493.
32. McHutchinson JG, Gordon SC, Schiff EG, et al. Interferon alpha-2b alone or in combination with ribavirin as initial treatment for chronic hepatitis C. *N Engl J Med.* 1998;339:1485.
33. Lettau LA, McCarthy JG, Smith MH, et al. Outbreak of severe hepatitis due to delta and hepatitis B viruses in parenteral drug abusers and their contacts. *N Engl J Med.* 1987;317:1256.
34. Lemon SM, Thomas DL. Vaccines to prevent viral hepatitis. *N Engl J Med.* 1997;336:196.
35. Layon AJ, Rosenbaum SH, Dirk L. Human immunodeficiency virus and health care workers: risking livelihood as well as life. *Can J Anaesth.* 1997;44:689.
36. Centers for Disease Control and Prevention. *HIV/AIDS Surveillance Report.* 1998;10:14.
37. Centers for Disease Control and Prevention. *HIV/AIDS Surveillance Report.* 1998;10(2):9.
38. Centers for Disease Control and Prevention. *HIV/AIDS Surveillance Report.* 1997;9(2):32.
39. Centers for Disease Control and Prevention. Summary of selected notifiable diseases—United States weeks ending September 4, 1999 and September 5, 1998 (35th week). *MMWR Morb Mortal Wkly Rep.* 1999;48:784.
40. AIDS watch. *AIDS Clin Care.* 1999;11:63.
41. Centers for Disease Control and Prevention. *HIV/AIDS Surveillance Report.* 1992;9, 17.
42. Oxtoby MJ. Perinatally acquired human immunodeficiency virus infection. *Pediatr Infect Dis J.* 1990;9:609.
43. Boyer PJ, Dillon M, Navaie M, et al. Factors predictive of maternal-fetal transmission of HIV-1. *JAMA.* 1994;271:1925.
44. The International Perinatal HIV Group. The mode of delivery and the risk of vertical transmission of human immunodeficiency virus type 1: a meta-analysis of 15 prospective cohort studies. *N Engl J Med.* 1999;340:977.
45. Francis DP, Curran JW, Essex M. Epidemic acquired immune deficiency syndrome: epidemiologic evidence for a transmissible agent [editorial]. *J Natl Cancer Inst.* 1983;71:1.
46. Barre-Sinoussi F, Chermann JC, Rey F, et al. Isolation of a T-lymphotropic retrovirus from a patient at risk for acquired immune deficiency syndrome (AIDS). *Science.* 1983;220:868.
47. Gallo RC, Sarin PS, Gelmann EP, et al. Isolation of human T-cell

leukemia virus in acquired immune deficiency syndrome (AIDS). *Science.* 1983;220:865.

48. Duesberg PH. Human immunodeficiency virus and acquired immunodeficiency syndrome: correlation but not causation. *Proc Natl Acad Sci U S A.* 1989;86:755.

49. Klatzmann D, Champagne E, Chamaret S, et al. T-lymphocyte T4 molecule behaves as the receptor for human retrovirus LAV. *Nature.* 1984;312:767.

50. Dalgleish AG, Beverly PCL, Clapham PR, et al. The CD4 (T4) antigen is an essential component of the receptor for the AIDS retrovirus. *Nature.* 1984;312:763.

51. McDougal JS, Kennedy MS, Sligh JM, et al. Binding of HTLV-III/LAV to T4$^+$ T cells by a complex of the 110K viral protein and the T4 molecule. *Science.* 1986;231:382.

52. Ho DD, Pomerantz RJ, Kaplan JC. Pathogenesis of infection with human immunodeficiency virus. *N Engl J Med.* 1987;317:278.

53. Fauci AS. The human immunodeficiency virus: infectivity and mechanisms of pathogenesis. *Science.* 1988;239:617.

54. Levy JA. Human immunodeficiency viruses and the pathogenesis of AIDS. *JAMA.* 1989;261:2997.

55. El-Farrash MA, Masuda T, Harada S. Synergistic infectivity of highly and minimally infectious clones of human immunodeficiency virus in vitro. *J Infect Dis.* 1990;161:1010.

56. Greene WC. The molecular biology of human immunodeficiency virus type I infection. *N Engl J Med.* 1991;324:308.

57. Fauci AS, Schnittman SM, Poli G, et al. Immunopathogenic mechanisms in human immunodeficiency virus (HIV) infection. *Ann Intern Med.* 1991;114:678.

58. Murphy RL. New antiretroviral drugs, part I: PIs. *AIDS Clin Care.* 1999;11:35.

59. Carpenter C, Members of the NIH Panel to Define Principles of Therapy of HIV Infection. Report of the NIH Panel to Define Principles of Therapy of HIV Infection. *Ann Intern Med.* 1998;128:1057.

60. Fauci AS, Bartlett JG, the Panel on Clinical Practices for the Treatment of HIV Infection. Guidelines for the use of antiretroviral agents in HIV-infected adults and adolescents. *Ann Intern Med.* 1998;128:1079.

61. Berkeley S. An AIDS vaccine for all the world. *AIDS Clin Care.* 1999;11:55.

62. Javaherian K, Langlois AJ, LaRosa GJ, et al. Broadly neutralizing antibodies elicited by the hypervariable neutralizing determinant of HIV-1. *Science.* 1990;250:1590.

63. Dolin R, Graham BS, Greenberg SB, et al. The safety and immunogenicity of a human immunodeficiency virus type 1 (HIV-1) recombinant gp160 candidate vaccine in humans. *Ann Intern Med.* 1991;114:119.

64. Redfield RR, Birx DL, Ketter N, et al. A phase I evaluation of the safety and immunogenicity of vaccination with recombinant gp160 in patients with early human immunodeficiency virus infection. *N Engl J Med.* 1991;324:1677.

65. HHS News. AIDS falls from top ten causes of death; teen births, infant mortality, homicide all decline. Available at: http://www.cdc.gov/nchs/releases/98news/aidsmort.htm. Accessed April 12, 2001.

66. National Center for Health Statistics. *Natl Vital Stat Rep.* 1998;47:32.

67. Centers for Disease Control. The HIV/AIDS epidemic: the first 10 years. *MMWR Morb Mortal Wkly Rep.* 1991;40:357.

68. Chu SY, Buehler JW, Berkelman RL. Impact of the human immunodeficiency virus epidemic on mortality in women of reproductive age, United States. *JAMA.* 1990;264:225.

69. Centers for Disease Control and Prevention. Selected behaviors that increase risk for HIV infection among high school students—United States, 1990. *MMWR Morb Mortal Wkly Rep.* 1992;41:231.

70. Francis DP. Toward a comprehensive HIV prevention program for the CDCP and the nation. *JAMA.* 1992;268:1444.

71. Osler W, McCrae T. *The Principles and Practice of Medicine.* New York, NY: Appleton; 1920:269.

72. Weiss R, Their SO. HIV testing is the answer: what's the question? [editorial]. *N Engl J Med.* 1988;319:1010.

73. Meyer KB, Pauker SG. Screening for HIV: can we afford the false positive rate? *N Engl J Med.* 1987;317:238.

74. Centers for Disease Control. Interpretation and use of Western blot assay for serodiagnosis of human immunodeficiency virus type 1 infection. *MMWR Morb Mortal Wkly Rep.* 1989;38:1.

75. Rapid HIV tests: issues for laboratorians. *CDC Issues.* March 1998.

76. Lifson AR, Castro KG, McCray E. National surveillance of AIDS in health care workers. *JAMA.* 1986;256:3231.

77. McCray E. Occupational risk of the acquired immunodeficiency syndrome among health workers. *N Engl J Med.* 1986;314:1127.

78. Centers for Disease Control. Update: acquired immunodeficiency syndrome and human immunodeficiency virus infection among health care workers. *MMWR Morb Mortal Wkly Rep.* 1988;37:229.

79. Henderson DK, Fahey BJ, Willy M, et al. Risk for occupational transmission of human immunodeficiency virus type 1 (HIV-1) associated with clinical exposures: a prospective evaluation. *Ann Intern Med.* 1990;113:740.

80. Merigan TC, Skowron G, Bozzette SA, et al. Circulating p24 antigen levels and responses to dideoxycytidine in human immunodeficiency virus (HIV) infections: a phase I and II study. *Ann Intern Med.* 1989;110:189.

81. Wolinsky SM, Rinaldo CR, Kwok S, et al. Human immunodeficiency virus type 1 (HIV-1) infection median of 18 months before a diagnostic Western blot. *Ann Intern Med.* 1989;111:961.

82. Imagawa DT, Lee MH, Wolinsky SM, et al. Human immunodeficiency virus type 1 infection in homosexual men who remain seronegative for prolonged periods. *N Engl J Med.* 1989;320:1458.

83. Baker JL, Kelen GD, Silvertson KT: Unsuspected human immunodeficiency virus in critically ill emergency patients. *JAMA.* 1987;257:2609.

84. Kristensen MS, Sloth E, Jensen TK. Relationship between anesthetic procedure and contact of anesthesia personnel with patient body fluids. *Anesthesiology.* 1990;73:619.

85. Harrison CA, Rogers DW, Rosen M. Blood contamination of anesthetic and related staff. *Anaesthesia.* 1990;45:831.

86. Wright JG, McGeer AJ, Chyatte D, et al. Mechanisms of glove tears and sharp injuries among surgical personnel. *JAMA.* 1991;266:1668.

87. Matta H, Thompson AM, Rainey JB. Does wearing two pairs of gloves protect operating theatre staff from skin contamination? *BMJ.* 1988;297:597.

88. Hammond JS, Eckes JM, Gomez GA, et al. HIV, trauma, and infection control: universal precautions are universally ignored. *J Trauma.* 1990;30:555.

89. Gerberding JL, Schecter WP: Surgery and AIDS: reducing the risk [editorial]. *JAMA.* 1991;265:1572.

90. Panlilio AL, Foy DR, Edwards JR, et al. Blood contacts during surgical procedures. *JAMA.* 1991;265:1533.

91. Lange JMA, Boucher CAB, Hollak CEM, et al. Failure of zidovudine prophylaxis after accidental exposure to HIV-1. *N Engl J Med.* 1990;322:1375.

92. Centers for Disease Control and Prevention. Public Health Service guidelines for the management of health-care worker exposures to HIV and recommendations for postexposure prophylaxis. *MMWR Morb Mortal Wkly Rep.* 1998;47:1.

93. Centers for Disease Control. Update: transmission of HIV infection during an invasive dental procedure—Florida. *MMWR Morb Mortal Wkly Rep.* 1991;40:21.

94. Centers for Disease Control. Update: transmission of HIV infection during invasive dental procedures—Florida. *MMWR Morb Mortal Wkly Rep.* 1991;40:377.

95. Lo B, Steinbrook R. Health care workers infected with the human immunodeficiency virus: the next steps. *JAMA.* 1992;267:1100.

96. Haedicke, GJ, Grossman JAI, Fisher AE. Herpetic whitlow of the digits. *J Hand Surg [Br].* 1989;14:443.

97. Stern H, Elek SD, Millar DM, et al. Herpetic whitlow: a form of cross infection in hospitals. *Lancet.* 1959;2:871.

98. Goldberg ME, Brajer J, Seltzer JL. Herpetic whitlow: hazard for the anesthesiologist and an unusual complication. *Anesthesiol Rev.* 1985;12:26.

99. Gill MJ, Arlette J, Buchan K. Herpes simplex virus infection of the hand: a profile of 79 cases. *Am J Med.* 1988;84:89.

100. LaRossa D, Hamilton R. Herpes simplex infections of the digits. *Arch Surg.* 1971;102:600.

101. Knyvett AF. Herpetic whitlow. *Med J Aust.* 1966;13:601.

102. Kanaar P. Primary herpes simplex infection of fingers in nurses. *Dermatologica.* 1957;134:256.

103. Jarris RF, Kirkwood CR. Herpetic whitlow in family practice. *J Fam Pract.* 1984;19:797.

104. Eiferman RA, Adams G, Stover B, et al. Herpetic whitlow and keratitis. *Arch Ophthalmol.* 1979;97:1079.

105. Sehayik RI, Bassett FH. Herpes simplex infection involving the hand. *Clin Orthop.* 1982;166:138.

106. Logan WS, Tindall JP, Elson ML. Chronic cutaneous herpes simplex. *Arch Dermatol.* 1971;103:606.

107. Polayes IM, Arons MS. The treatment of herpetic whitlow: a new surgical concept. *Plast Reconstr Surg.* 1980;65:811.

108. Corey L, Spear PG. Infections with herpes simplex viruses. *N Engl J Med.* 1986;314:686.

109. England JA, Balfour HH Jr. Varicella and herpes zoster. In: Hoeprich

PD, Jordan MC, eds. *Infectious Diseases: A Modern Treatment of Infectious Processes.* 4th ed. Philadelphia, Pa: JB Lippincott; 1989:942.

110. Brunell PA. Varicella. In: Wyngaarden JB, Smith LH, eds. *Cecil Textbook of Medicine.* 18th ed. Philadelphia, Pa: WB Saunders; 1988:1788.

111. Weller TH. Varicella and herpes zoster. *N Engl J Med.* 1983;309:1362.

112. Lang DJ. Cytomegalovirus infection. In: Wyngaarden JB, Smith LH, eds. *Cecil Textbook of Medicine.* 18th ed. Philadelphia, Pa: WB Saunders; 1988:1784.

113. Weller TH. The cytomegaloviruses: ubiquitous agents with protean clinical manifestations. *N Engl J Med.* 1971;285:267.

114. Jordan MC. Cytomegalovirus infections. In: Hoeprich PD, Jordan MC, eds. *Infectious Diseases: A Modern Treatise of Infectious Processes.* 4th ed. Philadelphia, Pa: JB Lippincott; 1989:805.

115. Tegtmeier GE. Transfusion transmitted cytomegalovirus infections: significance and control. *Vox Sang.* 1986;51(suppl):22.

116. Centers for Disease Control and Prevention. Transmission of multidrug-resistant tuberculosis among immunocompromised persons in a correctional system—New York, 1991. *MMWR Morb Mortal Wkly Rep.* 1992;41:507.

117. Langevin PB, Rand KH, Layon AJ. The potential for dissemination of *Mycobacterium tuberculosis* through the anesthesia breathing circuit. *Chest.* 1999;115:1107.

118. Zacney JP, Galinkin JL. Psychotropic drugs used in anesthesia practice: abuse liability and epidemiology of abuse. *Anesthesiology.* 1999;90:269.

119. Seeley HF. The practice of anaesthesia: a stressor for the middle-aged? *Anaesthesia.* 1996;51:571.

120. Nauth-Misir RC. Anesthetists taking drugs: is overwork the cause? *CMAJ.* 1995;153:449.

121. Kam PC. Occupational stress in anesthesia. *Anaesth Intensive Care.* 1997;25:686.

122. Loehr JR. *Stress for Success.* New York, NY: Random House; 1997.

123. Selye H. *The Stress of Life.* New York, NY: McGraw-Hill; 1976.

124. Davis M, Robbins EE, McKay M. *The Relaxation and Stress Reduction Workbook.* New York, NY: MJF Books; 1995.

125. Bodger C. *Smart Guide to Relieving Stress.* New York, NY: John Wiley & Sons; 1999.

126. Parker JBR. The effects of fatigue on physician performance: an underestimated cause of physician impairment and patient risk. *Can J Anaesth.* 1987;34:489.

127. Hawkins MR, Vichick DA, Silsby HD, et al. Sleep and nutritional deprivation and performance of house officers. *J Med Educ.* 1985;60:530.

128. Bruce DL, Bach MJ, Arbit J. Trace anaesthetic gases on perceptual, cognitive, and motor skills. *Anesthesiology.* 1974;40:453.

129. Bruce DL, Bach MJ. Effects of trace anaesthetic gases on behavioral performance of volunteers. *Br J Anaesth.* 1976;48:871.

130. Smith G, Shirley AW. Failure to demonstrate effects of low concentrations of nitrous oxide and halothane on psychomotor performance [abstract]. *Br J Anaesth.* 1976;48:271.

131. Talbott GD, Benson EB. The impaired physician. *Postgrad Med.* 1980;68:56.

132. Blachly PH, Osterud HT, Josslin R. Suicide in professional groups. *N Engl J Med.* 1963;268:1278.

133. Cooper JB, Newbower RS, Kitz RJ. An analysis of major errors and equipment failures in anesthesia management: considerations for prevention and detection. *Anesthesiology.* 1984;60:34.

134. Spiegelman WG, Saunders L, Mazze RJ. Addiction and anesthesiology. *Anesthesiology.* 1984;60:335.

135. Weil A, Rosen W. *Chocolate to Morphine: Understanding Mind-Active Drugs.* Boston, Mass: Houghton Mifflin; 1976.

136. Bruce DL, Eide KA, Linde HW, et al. Causes of death among anesthesiologists: a 20 year survey. *Anesthesiology.* 1968;29:565.

137. Ward CF, Ward GC, Saidman LJ. Drug abuse in anesthesia training programs—a survey: 1970 through 1980. *JAMA.* 1983;250:922.

138. Herrington RE. The impaired physician: recognition, diagnosis and treatment. *Wisc Med J.* 1979;78:21.

139. Lew EA. Mortality experience among anesthesiologists, 1954–1976. *Anesthesiology.* 1979;51:195.

140. Gravenstein JS, Kory WP, Marks RG. Drug abuse by anesthesia personnel. *Anesth Analg.* 1983;62:467.

141. Hays LR, Stillner V, Littrell R. Fentanyl dependence associated with oral ingestion. *Anesthesiology.* 1992;77:819.

142. Follette JW, Farley WJ. Anesthesiologists addicted to propofol. *Anesthesiology.* 1992;77:817.

143. Herrington RE, Benzer DG, Jacobson GR, et al. Treating substance: use disorders among physicians. *JAMA.* 1982;247:2253.

144. Gualtieri AC, Dosentino JP, Becker JS. The California experience with a diversion program for impaired physicians. *JAMA.* 1983;269:226.

145. Talbott GD, Richardson AC, Mashburn JS, et al. The medical association of Georgia's disabled doctor program: a 5 year review. *J Med Assoc Ga.* 1981;70:545.

146. Adler GA, Potts FE, Kirby RR, et al. Narcotics control in anesthesia training. *JAMA.* 1985;253:3133.

147. Moleski RJ, Easley S, Barash PG, et al. Control and accountability of controlled substance administration in the operating room. *Anesth Analg.* 1985;64:989.

148. *Goodman and Gilman's the Pharmacologic Basis of Therapeutics.* 7th ed. New York, NY: Macmillan; 1985.

149. Johnson VE. *The Dynamics of Intervention: I'll Quit Tomorrow.* New York, NY: Harper & Row; 1980:43.

150. Garb S. Drug addiction in physicians. *Anesth Analg.* 1969;48:129.

151. Klein RL, Stevens WC, Kingston HGG. Controlled substance dispensing and accountability in United States anesthesiology residency programs. *Anesthesiology.* 1992;77:806.

152. Ward CF. Substance abuse: now and for some time to come [editorial]. *Anesthesiology.* 1992;77:619.

153. Paris R, Canavan D. Physician substance abuse impairment: anesthesiologists vs. other specialties. *J Addict Dis.* 1999;18:1.

154. Quinlan D. Innovative approaches to re-entry. *FANA Winter Syllabus.* January 1999.

155. Trimpey J. *The Rational Recovery.* New York, NY: Simon & Schuster; 1996.

156. Menk EJ, Baumgarten RK, Kingsley CP. Success of reentry into anesthesiology training programs by residents with a history of substance abuse. *JAMA.* 1990;264:2741

157. Lecky JH. Problems of trace anesthetic levels. In: Orkin FK, Cooperman LH, eds. *Complications in Anesthesia.* Philadelphia, Pa: JB Lippincott; 1980:715.

158. Axelsson G, Rylander R. Exposure to anesthetic gases and spontaneous abortion: response bias in a postal questionnaire study. *Int J Epidemiol.* 1982;11:250.

159. Lane GA, Nahrwold ML, Tait AR, et al. Nitrous oxide is teratogenic—xenon is not! *Anesthesiology.* 1979;51:S260.

160. Cohen EN, Brown BW, Wu ML, et al. Occupational disease in dentistry and chronic exposure to trace anesthetic gases. *J Am Dent Assoc.* 1980;101:21.

161. Vessey MP, Nunn JF. Occupational hazards of anesthesia. *BMJ.* 1980;281:696.

162. Ferstandig LL. Trace concentrations of anesthetic gases: a critical review of their disease potential. *Anesth Analg.* 1978;57:328.

163. National Institute for Occupational Safety and Health, DHEWC (NIOSH). *Criteria for a Recommended Standard: Occupational Exposure to Waste Anesthetic Gases and Vapors.* Publication 77-140. Washington, DC: 1977.

164. Eastwood DW, Green CD, Lamblin MA, et al. Effect of nitrous oxide on the white cell count in leukemia. *N Engl J Med.* 1963;268:297.

165. Knill-Jones RP, Moir DB, Rodrigues LV, et al. Anaesthetic practice and pregnancy: a controlled survey of women anaesthetists in the United Kingdom. *Lancet.* 1972;2:1326.

166. Cohen EN, Belville JW, Brown BW. Anesthesia, pregnancy, and miscarriage: a study of operating room nurses and anesthetists. *Anesthesiology.* 1971;35:343.

167. American Society of Anesthesiologists. Report of an ad hoc committee on the effect of trace anesthetics on the health of operating room personnel: occupational disease among operating room personnel—a national study. *Anesthesiology.* 1974;41:321.

168. Davenport HT, Halsey MJ, Wardley-Smith B, et al. Occupational exposure to anaesthetics in 20 hospitals. *Anaesthesia.* 1980;35:354.

169. Linde HW, Bruce DL. Occupational exposure of anesthetists to halothane, nitrous oxide, and radiation. *Anesthesiology.* 1969;30:363.

170. Corbett TH. Retention of anesthetic agents following occupational exposure. *Anesth Analg.* 1973;52:614.

171. Gravenstein JS, Paulus DA. *Monitoring Practice in Anesthesia.* Philadelphia, Pa: JB Lippincott; 1982:336.

172. Petty C. *The Anesthesia Machine.* New York, NY: Churchill Livingstone: 1987:108.

173. Dorsch JA, Dorsch SE. *Understanding Anesthesia Equipment.* 2nd ed. Baltimore, Md: Williams & Wilkins; 1984:254.

174. Bowie E, Huffman LM. *The Anesthesia Machine: Essentials for Understanding.* Madison, Wis: Ohmeda Corp; 1985:137.

175. Gravenstein N, Lampotang S. Ventilation during anesthesia. In: Kirby RR, Banner MJ, Downs JB, eds. *Clinical Applications of Ventilatory Support.* New York, NY: Churchill Livingstone; 1990:277.

# 50

# Anesthesia for Mass Casualty and Disaster Situations

John Casto

E. Stuart Cornett

Christopher M. Grande

## INTRODUCTION TO MASS CASUALTY AND DISASTER SITUATIONS

Most anesthesiologists are not accustomed to dealing with trauma patients in mass casualty and disaster situations. Indeed, it is usually experiences accumulated outside the practice of anesthesiology and subsequently brought to the profession that allow an anesthesiologist to function effectively when a mass casualty or disaster occurs. Although the conventional anesthesiologist will face this type of situation only occasionally, in an area where mass casualties have become more common, the anesthesiologist's skills will be demanded on a more routine basis.[1,2]

### How Are Mass Casualty and Disaster Situations Categorized?

Anesthesiologists encounter mass casualty and disaster situations typically in one of the following three categories:

1. Cataclysmic events: can be natural (eg, earthquake, tsunami, tornado) and man-made (eg, nuclear reactor meltdown, chemical spill)
2. War: is either full-scale or the more insidious type frequently found in a civil dispute within a nation (guerrilla warfare or low-intensity conflicts)
3. Terrorist actions: often lead to the development of either a cataclysmic event or war (eg, releasing a chemical or bacteriologic toxin, causing a cataclysmic event, or bombing an airliner, causing a man-made disaster)

The common thread running through the three categories is the fact that they are *predictably unpredictable*. Although there are similarities among these situations, there are also significant differences.

## Cataclysmic Events

During the past 20 years, disasters were the cause of more than 3 million deaths worldwide. Since 1900, more than 800 million people have been adversely affected by disasters.[3,4] Although there is no consensus definition, *disasters* are generally considered to be events that occur when destructive effects overwhelm the ability of a given community, state, or even country to meet the medical needs of its victims.

This inability to meet medical needs is particularly true in cases of cataclysmic events. Such events occur as complete surprises to those involved. However, they can be reasonably predicted and planned for by carefully evaluating the surrounding environment and performing a risk assessment or threat analysis. For example, being located in the vicinity of an earthquake fault portends the possibility of a disaster event occurring, which will not only result in a mass casualty situation but also severely compromise the ability of the local emergency medical services (EMS) system to respond and function as it would under normal conditions. In essence, any EMS response will be largely dependent on assistance from outside the general area, assuming that there is no persistent threat that prohibits outside assistance from accessing the disaster locale.

Certain types of cataclysmic events can be anticipated and prepared for in advance, and a direct relationship can be drawn between the existing risk and the disaster situation that can potentially result. The following are some examples:

- Airport → air crash → mass casualties, with many survivors suffering brain injury, smoke inhalation, and conventional trauma
- Chemical weapons development in laboratory → accidental release of agents → mass casualties, with victims ultimately suffering compromise of airway patency or respiratory, circulatory, and neurologic system failure
- Sports stadium → bleacher collapse → mass casualties, with victims experiencing multiple fractures, head and spine injuries, as well as crush syndromes

Although all of these situations are horrific, they can be anticipated with an accurate and complete appreciation of the risks, followed by realistic planning of both the local (immediate) and external (delayed) assistance available. Disaster planning, as well as simulations and drills, are covered more completely in the section, What Is the Prehospital Planning and Response?

## War

Caring for battlefield casualties during wartime differs from any other form of medicine. Overwhelming numbers of victims with casualties may present continuously over days or weeks. The health care infrastructure may be severely damaged or destroyed, and the health care providers may themselves be in danger or under direct attack. Treatment of casualties may have to be delayed or patients relocated in response to tactical situations. A provider may be called away from patient care in order to assist in the defense of the facility or unit. Tactical commanders have top priority in supply, communications, and manpower, at times resulting in severe shortages in all three areas.

Information can be scarce, and much of that information may be misinformation, in a phenomenon known as the *fog of war*.[5] Physicians may be expected to treat enemy soldiers. This presents the problem of preventing attacks from within and ensuring that injured enemy soldiers are disarmed of grenades, small arms, and other weapons that could injure or kill care providers. Fear, fatigue, and confusion among care providers create additional levels of stress. Practicing medicine on the battlefield requires more adaptability to changing conditions than in any other setting. Clinical examination skills learned in medical school, but often underused, become increasingly important under these conditions.

Military health care facilities and equipment designed for use in *forward locations* (close to combat) are generally simple, easy to maintain, mobile, lightweight, and able to function independent of local infrastructure. An anesthesiologist working under these conditions must be familiar with the equipment and be able to deliver a safe anesthetic with less technologic sophistication than in a typical peacetime operating room.[6] A modern anesthesia machine provides a wealth of information but is not realistically portable. Its sensitive electronics may not survive battlefield conditions nearly as well as a bag-valve-mask and an intravenous pump.

## Terrorism

In today's political climate, a terrorist attack can occur anytime and anywhere. Terrorist attacks can range from the conventional, such as small arms and bombs of varying strength and sophistication, to the unconventional, such as biologic, chemical, and even nuclear attacks. Conventional attacks can cause hundreds of casualties, and unconventional attacks may produce many thousands of casualties.

Because there is generally little advance warning of a terrorist attack, facilities, systems, and providers caring for the victims, to some extent, will be unprepared. If the number of victims is minimal, they can often be treated without invoking a contingency plan. However, when the number of casualties overwhelms the capabilities of the available treatment capacity, a *mass casualty* situation exists. Under mass casualty conditions, adequate contingency plans considered well in advance are essential to minimize loss of life and limb. These plans must adhere to the wartime mass casualty principles that will be discussed later in this chapter. Additionally, in the event of an unconventional attack, a system must be in place to prevent the health care providers themselves from becoming casualties.

Community disaster plans can work in a terrorist attack, provided they are well designed and practiced. However, other considerations are present during a terrorist attack that are not relevant during a natural disaster, including the potential for further attacks or acts of sabotage. Military assistance can be invaluable with respect to expertise regarding rescue, security, personal protective gear, decontamination, materiel, additional manpower, and organization of available resources. Contingency plans for a terrorist attack must include methods of activating and coordinating these resources.

*Terrorism* in its most fundamental form involves coercion through atrocity. Therefore, the maximal psychologic impact of a terrorist attack occurs when it is able to attract media coverage that reaches a large population. This makes terrorist actions much more likely during an event that has extensive media coverage, such as a visit from a dignitary, a sporting event, or any large gathering of people. Such situations require much more precise planning and training for a more specific threat. In these instances, it is advisable to obtain expert advice and professional help to minimize the inherent increased risks.

Anesthesia providers may be called on in the event of a terrorist attack.[7,8] Treating terrorist victims is not unlike treating war victims, although usually on a smaller and less extended scale. Often, there are more casualties than providers, mandating efficiency of triage. Because of the mechanisms of wounding, the injuries will be similar in nature and severity. It is not uncommon for anesthesiologists to be forced to work with equipment and monitoring not considered up to current standards and, indeed, to provide simultaneous care for more than one patient. To minimize the morbidity and mortality of patients with casualties, the anesthesiologist (and all other physicians) must be adaptable to changing conditions and able to improvise when necessary.

### What Is the Function of the Tactical Emergency Medical Services?

A more recent development in the arena of disaster management, and perhaps a blend of the response to war and terrorist actions, is the specialty of tactical emergency medical services (TEMS). Developed mainly to deal with high-risk warrant service, raids, and other dangerous law enforcement activities, TEMS has its origins in military counter-terrorist units and their activities. A complete discussion of the history and present applications of TEMS is provided elsewhere.[9] Only a few salient features are covered here.

TEMS's mission and environment involve high-powered firearms, explosives and other pyrotechnic devices, and chemical agents and contaminants. These weapons present the possibility of serious individual injuries and mass casualties. Immediate on-site stabilization is often important because evacuation could be protracted, depending on the tactical environment.

Components of TEMS that potentially involve anesthesiologists concern personnel issues, that is, the selection, training, and deployment of medical specialists. In the United States, the majority of these functions will be undertaken by nonphysician extenders; in Europe; the opposite situation exists:

- TACMED (tactical/medical): Tactical law enforcement and military personnel receive supplemental medical training to enable them to provide emergency care to the wounded.
- MEDTAC (medical/tactical): People with primarily medical backgrounds receive supplemental training in the tactical components of these activities. (Irrespective of which approach is adopted [TACMED or MEDTAC], it is essential that medical and tactical personnel have the opportunity for extensive training and drills together, are familiar with each other's role and equipment, and have integrated the hospital component of the TEMS system into the comprehensive response.[10])
- VIP/Executive Protection: This aspect involves the medical component of dignitary protection efforts, best typified by

the efforts of the US Secret Service to protect the President of the United States. A complex system has evolved over the years, primarily to prevent bodily harm to the protected individual but secondarily to deal with injuries if they occur. The same considerations apply in the selection and training of personnel in regard to MEDTAC skills, as well as working with the prehospital or EMS system and designated hospitals, which must be addressed in advance.[7-11]

## PRACTICAL ASPECTS OF MANAGING PREHOSPITAL MEDICAL CARE

In the United States, it is rare for physicians (including emergency medicine physicians) to practice actively in the field. Conversely, in Europe, anesthesiologists commonly serve in the field, on EMS helicopters, and on land ambulances, including mobile intensive care units (ICUs).[8] In true mass casualty and disaster situations and in situations requiring prolonged extrication of patients, many trauma centers use the concept of the "Go Team" to formulate operative teams to travel out of the hospital to the scene, sometimes performing emergency surgery and anesthesia procedures.

### How Is the Emergency Medical Services System Activated?

The first person on the scene quickly activates the EMS system, calling for help or assigning someone else to that task. It is important to avoid becoming committed to patient care until help is en route and the scene has been surveyed to make sure it is safe.[12]

In prehospital medicine, the first rule of thumb is *scene safety first*. Before the patient is approached, the rescuer should assess hazards such as collapsed electrical wires, broken glass, jagged metal, and unstable objects (such as a vehicle or something the vehicle struck); and ascertain imminent danger of fire, presence of toxic substances, existence of traffic hazards, and status of environmental conditions. If a hazardous situation exists, the area should not be entered until the hazards are secured and the scene is safe (Table 50–1).

### What Is the Prehospital Planning and Response?

Past experience has shown that the best way to manage a disaster is to be prepared.[3] Disaster simulations and drills

**TABLE 50–1.** Elements of a Proper Response to a Hazardous Materials Incident

Respond from uphill, upwind, or upstream
Use binoculars to observe for HAZMAT presence
Stop a safe distance away
Establish or report to the incident command post
Do not attempt rescue until the chemical is identified and responders have personal protective equipment
Isolate and secure the area from unauthorized entry
Establish a cold zone
Avoid low-lying areas
Remember that bystanders who stopped to assist may be contaminated

HAZMAT, hazardous materials

should be mandatory for all EMS providers. The Joint Commission on Accreditation of Healthcare Organizations (JCAHO) requires all hospitals to have a disaster plan and to test this plan twice a year. In fact, planning can be the most laborious part of disaster management.[13]

To a large degree, disaster planning involves incorporating a variety of simulations and drills.[1,14,15] Simulations can be staged at a variety of levels and with varying degrees of complexity and associated costs. Perhaps most simple and easy to execute are computer-based models that may employ a local area network to link participants.

One level up from using software developed for disaster modeling are *table-top* or *sand-table systems*. In these systems, miniaturized scale models of an area (often using materials from model railroad sets) are set up to demonstrate a threat and facilitate an interactive format. In this simulation, participants are able to view the situation in three dimensions, interactive discussion is possible, and a variety of scenarios can be played out.

The next level employs *full-scale* or *real-life* systems that involve life-size modeling, including moulage (or model) victims, actual response, and transport units such as ambulances, fire trucks, and helicopters. This simulation is expensive to conduct, requires a great deal of coordination in advance in order to maximize its value, and it is logistically intense. It may involve both prehospital and in-hospital components, as both must function for a disaster response to be effective.

*Drills* are mock alarms designed to test the readiness of a system, usually without advance warning. Drills may include various elements of the simulations described earlier.

Each year, the International Trauma Anesthesia and Critical Care Society (ITACCS) stages its International Chief Emergency Physician Training Course on Command Incident Management and Mass Casualty Disasters. This 3-day course employs all of the previously discussed simulations and culminates with a full-scale simulation on the last day. Candidates are typically senior physician members of trauma or EMS systems, including many anesthesiologists. It is assumed that they are already proficient in trauma patient management. The purpose of the course is to emphasize leadership and management skills on a broader scale.[16]

## What Are the Three Phases to Any Disaster Response?

Any disaster response has three phases: activation, implementation, and recovery.

### Activation

*Activation* is the initial response, followed by notification and the establishment of an incident command post. The first responder on the scene reports the nature of the incident; the number and types of injuries; the potential hazards for victims as well as rescuers; the extent of damage to the area; and possible access routes to and away from the scene. This relay of information is paramount and should be done before rendering any direct medical assistance.

Following the initial notification, the incident command post is established uphill and upwind in the event of a liquid or airborne hazard and as close to the scene as safety allows. The incident commander has overall authority on the scene

and, depending on the community, will be the fire chief or chief of police.

An inner hazard perimeter (*hot zone*) is established, and only fire and rescue personnel are permitted to enter it. Victims are brought from the inner perimeter to the decontamination area (*warm zone*), where the decontamination process ensues. Following their decontamination, victims are taken to the casualty collection point (CCP) for triage and stabilization. A staging area on the outer perimeter is designated in which transport crews, ambulances, and resources are readily available as needed to avoid congestion at the scene. Finally, a helicopter-landing zone is identified in the event air transport is needed (Fig. 50–1).

Scene safety is the primary concern and must be maintained by fire and police officials. Protection of the responders is the utmost priority. Rescues from contaminated areas are not attempted until the chemical is identified and proper personal protective equipment (PPE) and trained personnel are available. Another priority is crowd control. Police keep bystanders a safe distance from the scene to decrease their chance of becoming victims.

### Implementation

*Implementation* involves search and rescue (SAR), followed by triage and initial stabilization. SAR is carried out by specially trained, hazardous situation personnel. Medical personnel not trained in SAR should wait at the CCP to avoid becoming victims themselves. SAR is a variable procedure, depending on geographic location. Urban areas with large structures are very different from suburban areas. The rescue of victims trapped in thousands of tons of steel and concrete requires heavy equipment and skilled rescuers knowledgeable in large-scale extrication. Suburban and wilderness SAR is an entirely different entity. Knowledge of rope and vertical rescue is needed for mountainous terrain. Rescuers must be adept at conducting large-scale searches over vast areas in short amounts of time. Generally, SAR personnel are trained in the type of rescue they will most likely be performing in their particular community.

### Triage

Triage (from the French verb *trier,* meaning "to sort") is a crucial part of the implementation phase and deserves further elaboration. The process was originally developed by the military as a method of sorting large numbers of patients according to the priority with which they should be treated and transported. The goal of triage is to accomplish the greatest good for the greatest number of casualty victims.

During a time of mass casualties, conventional standards of care do not apply in all situations. Some seriously wounded people may not receive the same standard of care afforded a single admission. The concept of *reverse triage* is the exclusion of the patients with lethal injuries, thereby focusing available resource allocation on those with the greatest chance of survival. For example, a single, severely injured patient requiring 12 hours of surgery with a small chance of survival may inappropriately consume resources, resulting in the death of many patients with lesser injuries. Triage applies to both treatment and transport of patients to a higher echelon of care. Within the basic guidelines of these principles, triage must be adapted to the specific situation.[17] Logical categories to which

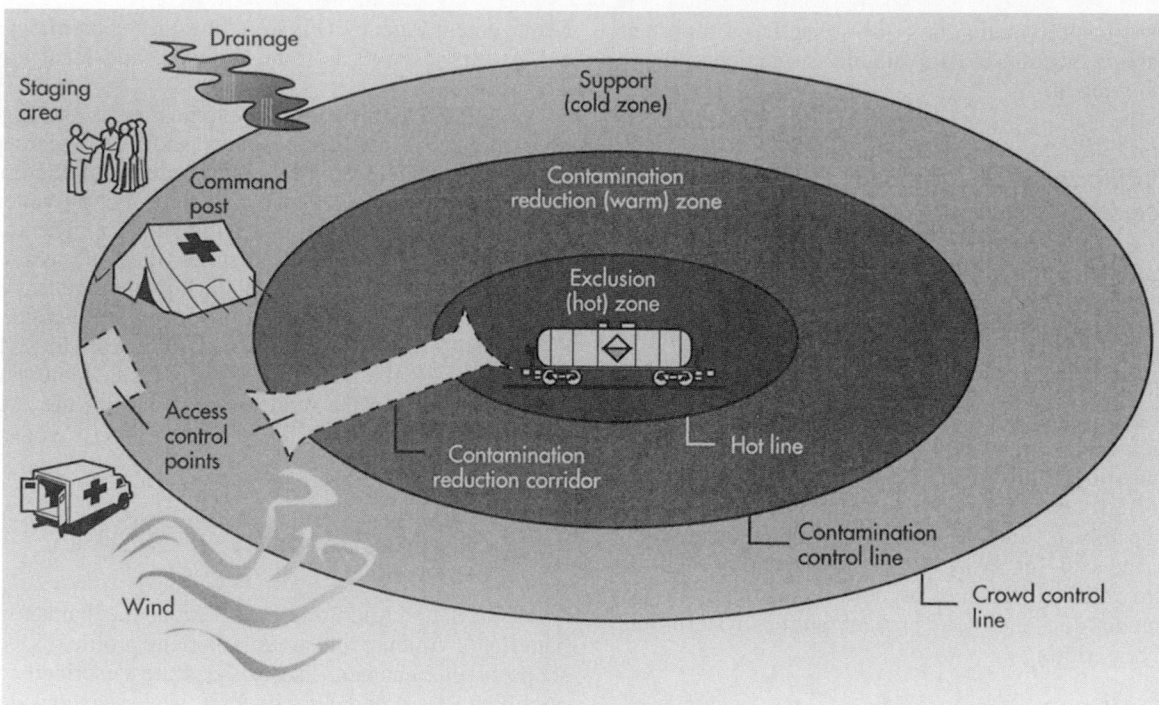

**FIGURE 50–1.** Basic layout of a chemically contaminated disaster area. Note special designated areas: hot, warm, and cold zones; casualty collection point; and incident command point. (From Currance PL, Bronstein A, eds. *Hazardous Materials for EMS: Practices and Procedures.* St Louis, Mo: Mosby; 1999:97.)

all casualties can be classified are referred to in the military as *minimal, delayed, immediate,* and *expectant* (Table 50–2). Anesthesia providers and other medical personnel may be called on to assist in the triage process. In military situations, anesthesiologists often assume the role of triage officers because they are often in the best position to make decisions regarding allocation of critical resources.[2,6]

An additional aspect of triage involves the immediate performance of any life-saving treatment that can be performed quickly (eg, application of a tourniquet, decompression of a tension pneumothorax) during the process of triage itself. This step may result in quick reclassification of an "immediate" patient to "delayed" status, thus conserving resources for other casualties. Triage is a process that needs to be ongoing and repeated according to the changing conditions and needs of the victims and to the treatment capability available.

### Priority of Care

Victims are first triaged by rescuers at the scene, followed by EMS personnel at the CCP, then by EMS personnel during

**TABLE 50–2.** Military Classifications of Casualties

| Classification | Injury Description | Action Taken |
|---|---|---|
| Minimal | Minor injuries not requiring prompt medical attention | Treated and transported after immediate and delayed patients |
| Delayed | Serious injuries requiring treatment but not immediately life-threatening | Treated and transported after immediate patients |
| Immediate | Injuries requiring immediate treatment to save life or limb | Treated and transported first |
| Expectant | Injuries sufficiently severe that survival under the current situation is unlikely | Comfort measures only |

transport, and finally by medical staff at the hospital, where definitive care is given.[18] Triage priority is as follows:

1. The highest priority is given to victims with severe injuries who will most likely survive if given initial stabilization and early transport but will probably die if not.
2. The next highest priority is given to victims with moderate injuries who would not likely die if treatment is withheld but who will eventually need definitive care.
3. The third highest priority is given to patients with minor injuries, the so-called walking wounded. These victims must wait at the scene until higher priority victims are transported.
4. The lowest priority is given to those who are hopelessly wounded or in cardiac arrest at the time of initial evaluation. This is difficult to accept for most medical personnel, but the goal of triage should always be remembered.

Once victims are brought to EMS personnel, triage is continued and initial stabilization is given. Medical care is limited to airway management, hemorrhage control, oxygen administration, and victim immobilization on backboards, as necessary. Victims are then transported to facilities that can provide definitive medical care.

### Recovery

*Recovery* is a three-step process. First is the systematic withdrawal of all personnel and equipment from the scene. Second is the return of all parties to normal operations. Third, *debriefing* occurs, which is the analysis of the event in an attempt to improve future responses as well as an opportunity for rescue personnel to discuss emotional difficulty concerning the disaster. The psychologic impact of disasters on rescue and medical personnel can be devastating, ranging from mild disturbances to posttraumatic stress disorder. It is important to have therapists or counselors available to members of the rescue team if needed.

## How Do Public Relations Affect the Disaster Scene?

Representatives of the media are present at all disasters. Their access to the scene must be limited, not only to protect the privacy of the victims but also to minimize the risk of reporters becoming victims themselves. A public relations officer should be appointed to give regular briefings about the event. A similar officer should be appointed at the receiving hospitals. Such designations will improve the flow of information from those in charge of the response and thus decrease the amount of erroneous information given to the public.

The media can be a valuable resource for announcing possible hazards, the call for evacuation, and even the need for additional fire, medical, rescue, or police personnel. Proper use of the media can also help prevent public hysteria and reactions such as rioting.

## What Is the Appropriate Hospital Disaster Response?

To conduct a JCAHO-mandated drill of a hospital disaster plan, a scenario is given to the hospital, and the hospital disaster response is initiated. Extra personnel are summoned, equipment and supplies are made available, and volunteer victims are brought to the emergency department. Moulage is used to make the drills appear as real as possible. To minimize waste of hospital supplies, either the supplies are not opened or out-of-date materials are used.

Most communities hold these disaster drills for EMS, fire, and police personnel. The drills are either planned or conducted at random. Planned drills are more beneficial in terms of training. The plan should involve every department and hospital employee.

In a true disaster situation, the decision to implement the hospital disaster response should not be delayed. In a brief period, the hospital could receive large numbers of victims, possibly critically injured. The emergency department should be cleared rapidly, and extra oxygen and crystalloid need to be readily available. Operating room personnel, including anesthesiologists, trauma surgeons, and support staff, must be prepared for emergent operations. Extra security will be needed to control family members and the media. A medical triage officer in the emergency department will be needed to prioritize care.

## What Is the Function of the National Disaster Medical System?

The National Disaster Medical System (NDMS) was created in 1984 to establish a way to care for large numbers of casualties from military as well as civilian disasters. This was a cooperative effort among the civilian hospital sector of the United States and the Department of Health and Human Services, the Department of Defense, the Federal Emergency Management Agency (FEMA), and the Department of Veterans Affairs, as well as state, regional, and local government agencies.

The NDMS is a two-part system. First is the organization of participating civilian hospitals and health care providers in 74 metropolitan areas. Large numbers of victims can be transported to any of these areas for definitive care. It is equivalent to mutual aid on a national scale. The second part of the NDMS consists of disaster medical assist teams—volunteer health care providers who, on request, will bring their own manpower and equipment to the disaster scene to assist local efforts. During civilian disasters, the NDMS can be employed if the governor of the affected state asks FEMA for assistance, and the request is granted by the President of the United States.

# MECHANISMS OF TRAUMA

A complete discussion of the various mechanisms of injury, patterns of trauma, and trauma patient profiles is beyond the scope of this chapter. These issues are described more thoroughly by Parr and Grande.[19] However, a consideration of several specific types of injury likely to be present in mass casualty and disaster situations is warranted.

## What Are the Major Categories?

### Blast Injuries

Because of the high likelihood of the use of explosive devices in many terrorist actions resulting in mass casualty or disaster situations, as well as the fact that pressure waves are a factor in many types of man-made and natural disasters, familiarity with the implications of a blast injury are important for the anesthesiologist.

Blast injuries result from explosions at atmospheric pressure in air, above atmospheric pressure under water, and below atmospheric pressure in space. Injuries result from a sudden release of energy that produces a localized increase in pressure and temperature. In addition, mechanical, electrical, or chemical injuries may comprise other trauma components (eg, an explosive device with shrapnel or a explosive device mixed with an injurious chemical).

When explosions occur in air, transformation of substances into gases takes place, resulting in a rapidly expanding sphere of high pressure, high temperature, and positive-pressure blast waves (*over-pressure* waves). Blast waves radiate from the source at approximately the speed of sound and are transmitted through the ground as a shock wave (Fig. 50–2). The duration of over-pressure can range from milliseconds to about 1 second. The longer the over-pressure, the longer the duration of exposure of bodies in its path, and the greater potential for injury (Table 50–3). However, at high pressures, duration becomes less critical.

Positive pressure is followed by a negative-pressure component (*under-pressure*). Resulting pressure changes cause mass movements of air that can create high-velocity blasts when directed toward or away from the source in an alternating fashion and may be as damaging as the initial over-pressure.

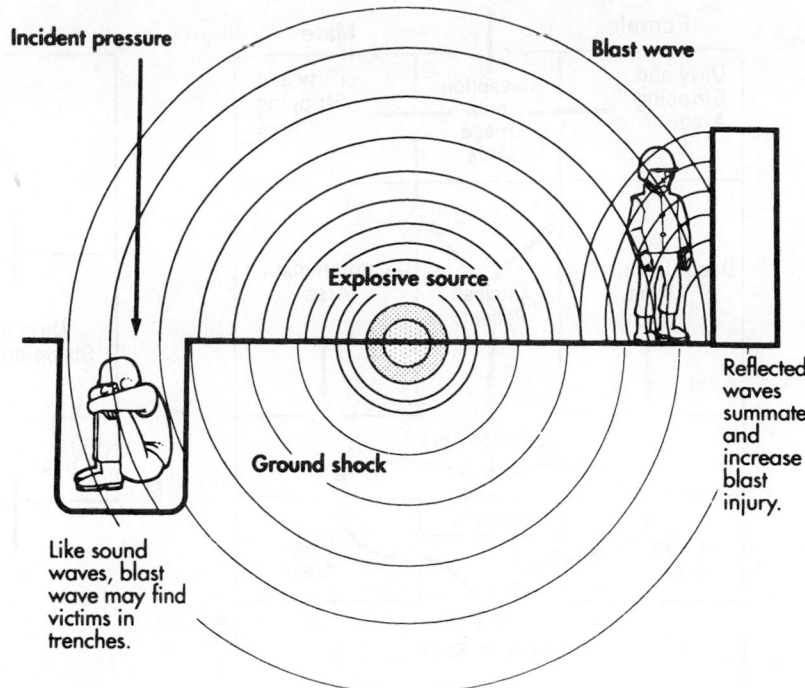

**FIGURE 50–2.** Diagram of explosion in air. Note direction of propagation of blast wave. As with sound waves, victims of blast waves may be found in holes. Pressure wave may also be reflected by walls and other obstacles, and the resulting summation of over-pressure may greatly increase wounding potential. (From Parr MJA, Grande CM. Mechanisms of trauma. In: Grande CM, ed. *Textbook of Trauma Anesthesia and Critical Care.* St Louis, Mo: Mosby–Year Book; 1993:337.)

## Classification

Blast injuries from explosions in air produce patterns of injury referred to as *primary, secondary, tertiary,* or *miscellaneous,* all of which may be encountered in the same patient.

Primary blast injury arises from direct exposure to the blast over-pressure. Secondary blast injury results from blunt, penetrating, or impalement from materials energized by the blast, arising either from the explosive device itself or from victims thrown a distance from the device. Tertiary blast injuries result from blast-induced whole or partial body displacement caused by the blast winds. Miscellaneous injuries include burns and inhalation injury from hot gases, dust, or other debris. Respiratory tract burns are uncommon, and inhalation of noxious fumes in these situations does not appear to be a problem in terms of inducing inhalation injury. Rather, secondary fires resulting from the explosions are more likely to be the cause of serious burns and inhalation injury.

### Toxic Trauma: Chemical or Biological Weapons

In the event of a nuclear, biological, or chemical attack, the prevention of additional casualties—particularly of health care providers—is of paramount importance. Of these three types of unconventional attack, we will focus on the issue of chemical agents because this has been a common theme in recent terrorist attacks perpetrated on civilian populations (eg, Sarin in the Tokyo subway incident).

Specialty equipment not normally required may be needed in certain disaster environments. Personal protective gear, such as the US military's Mission-Oriented Protective Posture, consists of a battle dress overgarment, gas mask, hood, overboots, and gloves. This equipment, although invaluable for personal protection outdoors, is cumbersome in a patient care facility. Care providers must practice with and adapt to performing in protective gear. In a hospital willing to accept victims of a chemical agent attack, provisions for decontamination of patients as well as a filtration system to provide decontaminated air to the interior of the sealed facility must be present (Figs. 50–3 and 50–4). The military maintains chemical protected vehicles for transport of casualties.

Most casualties of chemical agent incidents require supportive care only. Presently, there is no specific treatment for a specific agent,[20,21] with two notable exceptions: nerve agent and cyanide agent attack. Nerve agent prophylaxis and treatment kits are provided by the military. Nerve agents function by inhibiting cholinesterase, resulting in increased acetylcholine stimulation, (a familiar mechanism of action to anesthesiologists). Atropine (to block muscarinic cholinergic receptors) and pralidoxime chloride (2PAM) (to reactivate cholinesterase) are used to treat the effects of nerve agents. These drugs are prepackaged in autoinjectors in the military MARK I kit. Pyridostigmine has been used during research for prophylaxis against nerve agent exposure and is available in the military issued Nerve Agent Pyridostigmine Pretreatment kit. As the name implies, this kit is useful only before the nerve agent attack. Convulsive Antidote for Nerve Agent is a diazepam autoinjector used in the treatment of seizures that can result from nerve agent exposure (Fig. 50–5).

Exposure to a cyanide agent poisons cytochrome a3 in

**TABLE 50–3.** Relative Effects of Various Over-Pressures Lasting Four Milliseconds

| Over-Pressure (psi) | Effect |
|---|---|
| 1 | Damage to ordinary structures—flying glass and debris |
| 2 | Slight chance of perforation of tympanic membrane |
| 15 | 50% chance of perforation of tympanic membrane |
| 40 | Serious damage to reinforced concrete structures |
| 70 | 50% chance of severe pulmonary damage |
| 130 | 50% mortality |

From Mellor SG. The pathogenesis of blast injury and its management. *Br J Hosp Med.* 1988;39:536–539.

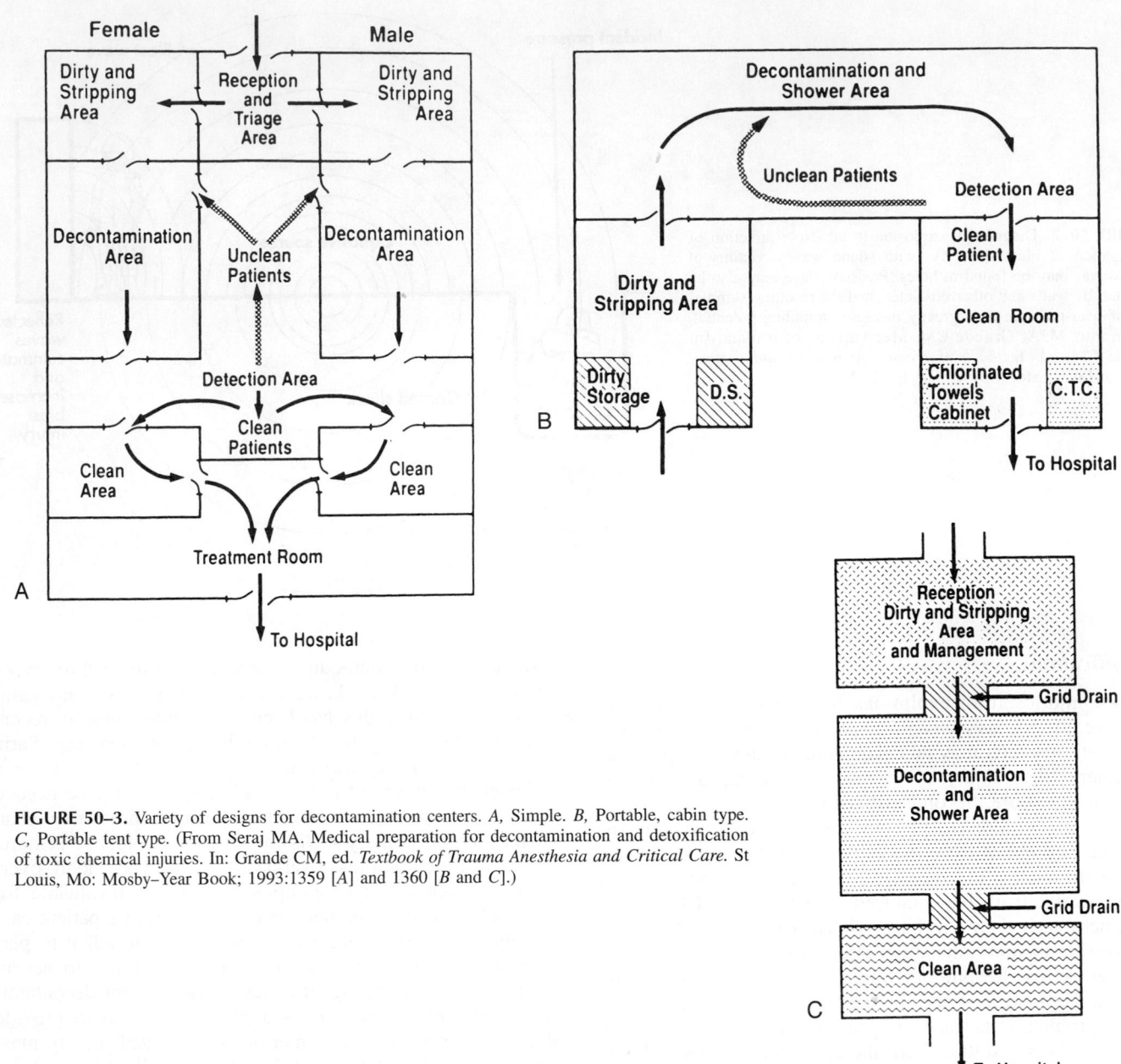

**FIGURE 50–3.** Variety of designs for decontamination centers. *A,* Simple. *B,* Portable, cabin type. *C,* Portable tent type. (From Seraj MA. Medical preparation for decontamination and detoxification of toxic chemical injuries. In: Grande CM, ed. *Textbook of Trauma Anesthesia and Critical Care.* St Louis, Mo: Mosby–Year Book; 1993:1359 [*A*] and 1360 [*B* and *C*].)

mitochondria, inhibiting cellular respiration. CNS cells are particularly susceptible. Methemoglobin converts cyanides into an inert compound. Thus, drugs that cause methemoglobinemia, such as amyl nitrite, 4-dimethylaminophenol hydrochloride, or *p*-aminopropiophenone, can be used as treatment. Cobalt edetate is a chelating agent for cyanide but should not be used if the patient has survived for longer than 5 minutes due to its extreme hepatotoxicity and nephrotoxicity.

It is impractical for civilian hospitals to maintain military combat hospital readiness for a nerve-biological-chemical attack. It is important, however, for hospitals to include the possibility of these types of attack in their contingency plans and to determine where to obtain specialty equipment in case the need arises (Table 50–4).

### Burns and Inhalation Injuries

Chemical and thermal burns are common types of injuries in mass casualty and disaster situations. Field care providers

must be able to quickly assess the extent and severity of burns, largely for the purpose of initial triage. The anesthetic and perioperative management of burned patients is discussed elsewhere,[22] but a general application of the heavy logistic demand created by their care is considered here.

Burn patients require heavy use of critical care resources such as intravenous fluids, airway management devices, and mechanical ventilation. Indeed, in austere situations and in nonmetropolitan areas that may be at some distance from tertiary referral centers, the issue of the number of available intensive care burn beds is a critical determinant that must be factored into the triaging process. That is to say, even many large cities only have a limited number of specifically designated burn beds. Secondary critical care transport will be required for possibly extended distances via sophisticated fixed-wing transport in order to successfully move large numbers of burn patients out of any given geographic area. In the personal experience of one of the authors (CMG), triage

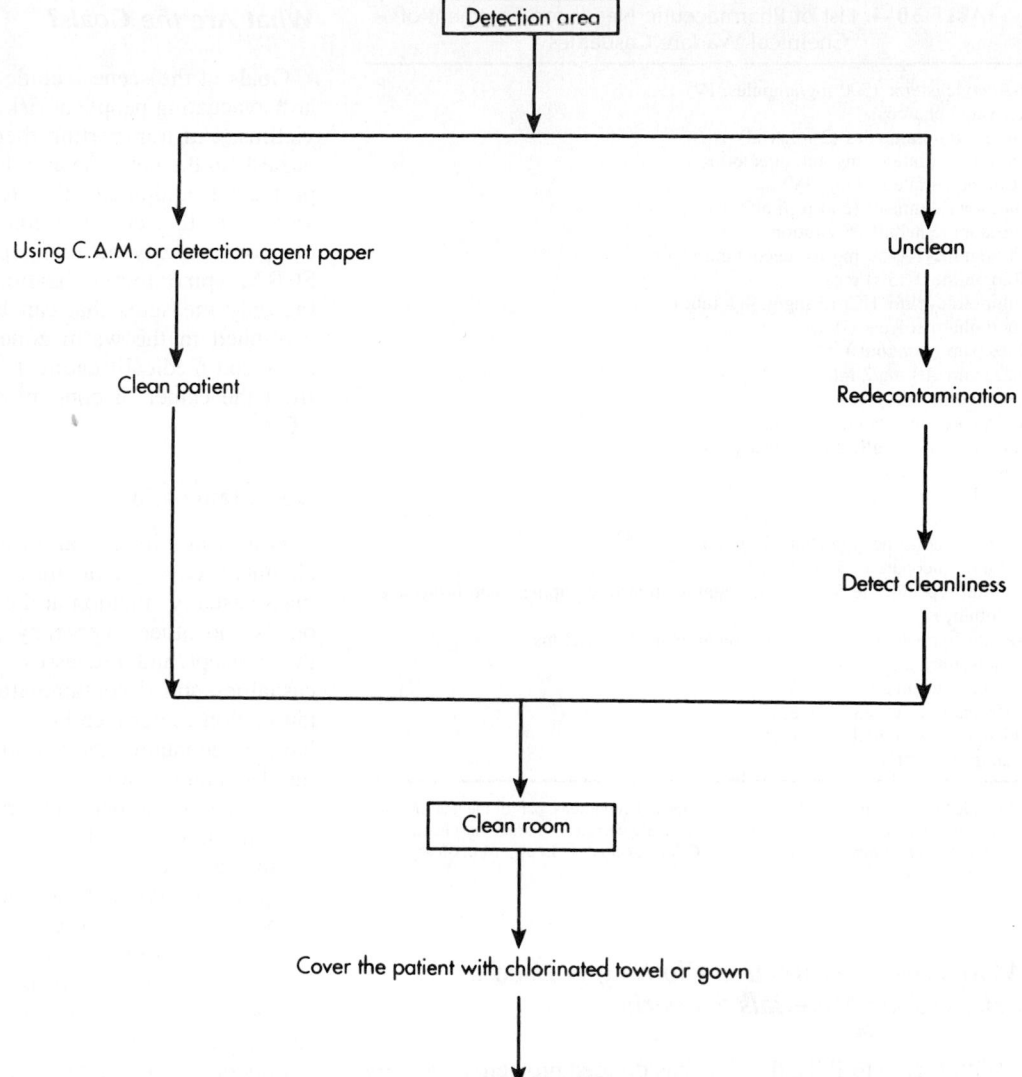

**FIGURE 50–4.** Procedure for allowing patients to proceed from detection area to clear room. CAM, chemical agents monitor. (From Seraj MA. Medical preparation for decontamination and detoxification of toxic chemical injuries. In: Grande CM, ed. *Textbook of Trauma Anesthesia and Critical Care.* St Louis, Mo: Mosby–Year Book; 1993:1362.)

considerations for burn patients in remote locations have required the use of extended critical care transport services (eg, from southeast Asia to locations as far away as Japan, Australia, and even the continental United States).

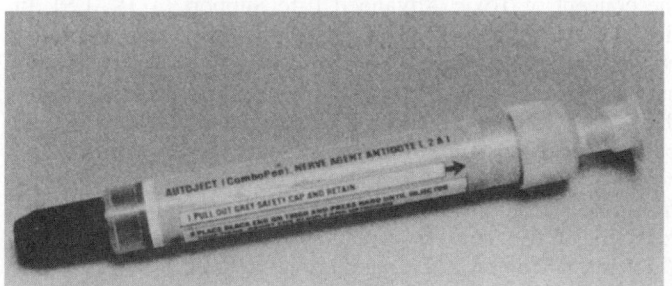

**FIGURE 50–5.** Autoinjector for immediate nerve agent treatment device delivers 2 mg of atropine, 500 mg of P2S (an oxime), and 10 mg of diazepam intramuscularly. (Courtesy of Combopen, Duphar, United Kingdom.) (From Baker DJ. Chemical and biologic warfare. In: Grande CM, ed. *Textbook of Trauma Anesthesia and Critical Care.* St Louis, Mo: Mosby–Year Book; 1993:1344.)

## MEDICAL PREPARATION FOR TOXIC CHEMICAL INJURIES

Hazardous materials (HAZMAT) pose one of the greatest threats for causing disasters. The rupture of a tanker carrying dangerous materials or a fire in a laboratory or industrial plant can cause large numbers of casualties. Thousands of deadly chemicals are transported through or manufactured near virtually every town in the United States. Because of this extreme potential risk, the US government passed the Superfund Amendments and Reauthorization Act of 1986, as well as regulations of the Environmental Protection Agency (EPA) and the Occupational Safety and Health Administration (OSHA). These regulations mandate that all personnel responding to hazardous materials incidents have the appropriate training and equipment necessary to manage a HAZMAT scene. Four levels of increasingly sophisticated training are available, and EMS providers must complete at least the first two. Scene safety is mandatory. Proper response actions for HAZMAT scenes include those listed in Table 50–1.

**TABLE 50–4.** List of Pharmaceutic Needs for Treatment of Chemical Warfare Casualties

*N*-Acetylcysteine (300 mg/ampules, IV)
Activated charcoal
Amyl nitrate ampules (2 mL/vial)
Atropine sulfate (2 mg autoinjectors)
Atropine sulfate (50 mg, IV)
Budesonide inhaler (200 μg/puff)
Budesonide nebulizer solution
Chloramine-T (250 mg for decontamination)
Chloramine-T (500 mg)
Chlortetracycline HCl (5 mg/g, 4 g tube)
Contrathion solvent (IV)
Diazepam (5 mg/mL)
Diazepam, 10 mg/2 mL
Hexamidine spray 0.2%
Hydrocortisone sodium succinate (IV)
Levocarnitine (2 g/L intragluteally, IV)
Magnesium sulfate
Potassium chloride
Pralidoxime
Silver sulfadiazine (Flamazine) cream
Sodium gluconate (2.5 g/10 mL)
Sodium hypochlorite 5% (for decontamination of equipment and protective clothing)
Sodium hypochlorite 5% (for decontamination of victims)
Sodium nitrate 3% (IV)
Sodium thiosulfate 10% (10 mL, IV)
Sulfacetamide 15% (4 g tube)
Thienamycins ampules (2 g, IV)
Vitamin C, 500 mg

Modified from Seraj MA. Extreme environmental conditions, part 3: medical preparation for decontamination and detoxification of toxic chemical injuries. In: Grande CM, ed. *Textbook of Trauma Anesthesia and Critical Care.* St Louis, Mo: Mosby–Year Book; 1993:1358.

## What Type of Protective Clothing Is Used in a Hazardous Materials Scenario?

With regard to PPE, the EPA has divided protective clothing and respiratory protection into four categories according to degree of protection afforded.

Level A offers the most protection and consists of self-containing breathing apparatus (SCBA), a fully encapsulating, vapor-tight, chemical-resistant suit; a hard hat; a cooling vest; and two-way radio communications. This level of protection should be worn when the highest level of respiratory, skin, eye, and mucous membrane protection is needed.

Level B should be worn when the highest level of respiratory protection is needed with less eye, skin, and mucous membrane protection. Level B has the same equipment as Level A, except the protective suit is not vapor-tight.

Level C equipment is the same as Level B, except for respiratory equipment. At this level, air-purifying respirators are used in place of SCBAs. Air-purifying respirators are air filters that can be used when atmospheric oxygen is >19.5%, the chemical substance and concentration is known and can be filtered, and no fire-fighting activities are underway.

Level D equipment is simply a work uniform with no special protective properties.

Possible HAZMAT scenes are surveyed initially with at least Level B PPE. They are then upgraded or downgraded as further information concerning the scene becomes available. Because of the tremendous cost of training and equipment, more sophisticated HAZMAT response teams are available on a regional basis and will assist local teams as needed.

## What Are the Goals?

Goals at the scene include isolating and confining the hazard, evacuating people at risk, decontaminating and stabilizing victims, and transporting them to definitive care. Because of hazards in the hot zone and the limitations of rescuers wearing protective equipment, the treatment that can be provided to victims in that area is limited. Airway control and isolation of spontaneously breathing patients with an escape mask or SCBA, spine immobilization, and hemorrhage control are the only measures that can be used. These interventions are continued in the warm zone during decontamination. More advanced medical treatment is started in the *cold zone* (away from the center of contamination) by EMS personnel at the CCP.

### Decontamination

Following the initial disaster situation resulting from a chemical-related toxic mass casualty incident is the second mass casualty situation at the definitive care site. Anesthesiologists and other emergency personnel must be familiar with the concept and processes of decontamination of chemical casualties and decontamination through a designated decontamination center (see Figs. 50–3 and 50–4). Hospitals should have a decontamination room as well as personnel trained in the decontamination process.[20,21]

In general, the decontamination process consists of removing all clothing and thoroughly washing the victims with warm water. Care is taken to avoid hypothermia. Signs and symptoms of hypothermia can resemble certain toxic exposure syndromes. Specific information about the chemicals in question can be obtained from the vehicle, Department of Transportation placard, material safety data sheet, the regional poison center, or by Chemtrec (800-424-9300). Certain chemicals require different decontamination protocols; therefore, it is imperative to ascertain the specific chemicals involved.

## What Is Toxic Advanced Life Support?

Conventional approaches to the management of contaminated patients consumes a substantial portion of the initial golden hour before basic and advanced life support maneuvers can be initiated.[23,24] With the advent of newer technologies in PPE and medical devices designed for use in contaminated environments (Figs. 50–6 and 50–7), ITACCS has developed the concept of Toxic Advanced Life Support (TOXALS). In the TOXALS paradigm, field care providers, using specially configured protective suits that allow interpersonal communications and the manual dexterity to perform life-saving procedures, can intervene earlier by assessing basic physiologic parameters (eg, respirations, pulse rate). Thus, patients in the hot and warm zones do not need to wait until being removed from the decontamination area before being intubated and receiving pharmacologic agents and fluid resuscitation.

Performance of tracheal intubation in chemical warfare gear has been evaluated, with substantial increase in the required time for successful completion of the procedure. Tube fixation after intubation was thought to be the most problematic component of the process.[25] These issues give rise to consideration of other alternatives for securing the airway, such as the laryngeal mask airway or Combitube (Kendall Healthcare

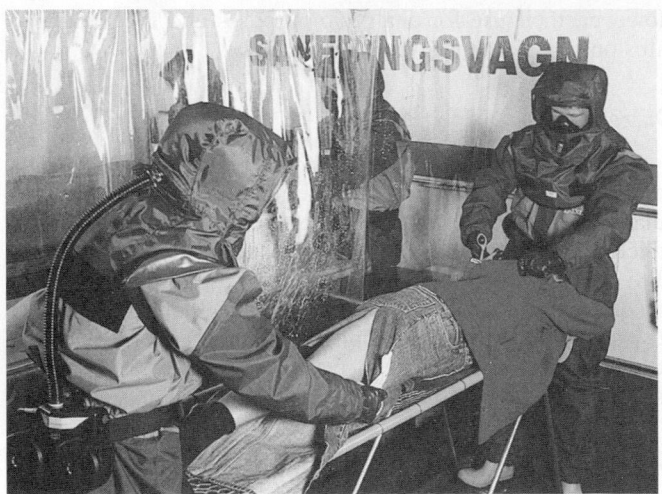

**FIGURE 50–6.** Personal protection equipment. (Courtesy of Swedish Emergency and Disaster Equipment [SWEDE], Stockholm, Sweden.)

Products, Mansfield, NH), which may require less dexterity and save time.

Ultimately, all toxic agents cause failure in the fundamental ABCs because massive secretions obstruct the airway; respiratory failure occurs as a result of direct lung pathology or neuromuscular weakness; or circulatory failure ensues. TOX-ALS allows the field provider to treat the root causes of death and thus enables more patients to survive until decontamination can be accomplished. Subsequently, more extensive definitive procedures can be undertaken.

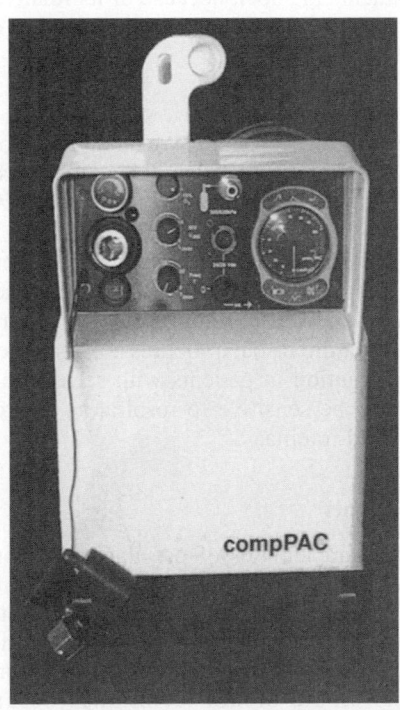

**FIGURE 50–7.** CompPAC portable ventilation system designed for use in chemically contaminated environments in which oxygen is in short supply or not available. The unit can be operated with a battery, fixed power, or compressed gas. Its capabilities include atmosphere filtering and variable frequency rate and minute volume. (Courtesy of SIMS PneuPAC Limited, London, United Kingdom.)

## PREHOSPITAL AND RESCUE EQUIPMENT

### What Is Available?

A wide range of specialized equipment for rescue and extrication exists, which is carried by most large-scale, well-supported EMS systems.[12] Sometimes this equipment is brought to the scene after the initial site survey. These include Jaws of Life (used to pry apart portions of automobiles) and lift bags (filled with air and used to elevate heavy objects).

Although a full discussion of the types and applications of this equipment is beyond the scope of this chapter,[12] it is useful for anesthesiologists who will interact with prehospital care providers and who may be activated in mass casualty and disaster situations to have some familiarity with the terminology and the types of equipment and their use. Equipment that has direct application to the medical component of prehospital emergency services will be discussed to some extent.

### Basic Life Support

Emergency equipment needed during disaster conditions varies in both type and quantity according to the specific situation. Basic equipment (**a, b, c**) that should always be available in the field includes the following:

**a**irway equipment (oral and nasal airways, masks, endotracheal tubes, laryngoscopes, and blades)
**b**reathing equipment (bag-valve masks, oxygen tanks, tubing, and regulators)
Equipment for maintenance of **c**irculation (intravenous fluids, blood, tubing, catheters, tape, drugs)

More sophisticated equipment may be required, depending on the level of care to be offered at a given location.[26]

### Anesthesia, Resuscitation, and Advanced Life Support

If anesthesia is to be administered on site, specialized equipment for that purpose is required.[27–29] Ideally, a state-of-the-art facility is available and fully functioning. However, the most basic equipment must include apparatus for delivering inhalational, intravenous, and regional anesthetics, as well as providing oxygenation and ventilatory support. This equipment can be simple and portable or sophisticated and stationary, depending on conditions.

#### Total Intravenous Anesthesia

Total intravenous anesthesia (TIVA) can be administered with an intravenous pump, airway or breathing equipment, and monitoring equipment. The equipment is extremely portable, and this technique can be used successfully in a variety of operative procedures. However, the patient must be monitored closely by trained personnel.

#### Regional Anesthesia

Regional anesthesia is another option for field anesthesia.[30,31] In a disaster situation, the ability to converse with a conscious patient can replace the need for extensive monitoring equipment. The equipment and materials needed for performing blocks is portable, simple, and reliable, and most blocks can be placed relatively quickly by trained personnel. Subarachnoid and epidural anesthesia, major nerve blocks (eg, femoral, axillary), and intravenous anesthesia (Bier block) used in appropriate circumstances offer the advantage of requiring minimal one-on-one monitoring after the initial placement and establishment of the block. A regional anesthetic that is functioning well can allow the anesthesiologist to monitor conscious patients with lesser trained personnel, freeing the anesthesiologist to tend to other patients in the immediate area.

## ANESTHETIC MANAGEMENT OF MASS CASUALTY AND DISASTER VICTIMS

### What Is the Anesthesiologist's Role?

Although the actual and specific perioperative and critical care management of trauma patients is covered elsewhere,[32] the anesthesiologist must be aware that the care of many patients can only be as good as the care provided for the single patient. Therefore, it follows that the anesthesiologist who might be involved in the response to a mass casualty incident caring for victims of injury must be familiar, hopefully on a routine basis, with the care of severely traumatized patients.

Important areas that the anesthesiologist must be aware of include a heightened awareness of the behavior of the hypovolemic patient; specific techniques and strategies for dealing with airway challenges common to the trauma patient (eg, the full stomach); cervical spine precautions; head injury and cerebral hemodynamics; the prevalence of hypothermia and its implications in trauma; and the impact of pneumothorax, its relationship to hemodynamics, and the implications of positive-pressure ventilation and nitrous oxide.

If one had to choose a single monitor to take to a disaster site, the pulse oximeter probably would be the device of choice. With its small size and low cost, it can supply the most physiologic data. With a decrease in perfusion pressure, disappearance of the pulse oximeter tracing signals an important clue. The Israeli Defense Force uses the pulse oximeter as the sole monitoring device for critically wounded patients during air evacuation.[2]

The capnograph also may be used to provide extended information other than the level of end tidal $CO_2$ and respiratory rate. Changes in the characteristics of the wave form and expired carbon dioxide level reflect issues of pulmonary dynamics and cardiac output.

### How Is Anesthesia and Analgesia Managed in Field Conditions?

Various agents and techniques are available and are examined in greater detail elsewhere.[33,34]

**Intravenous Agents**

#### Barbiturates

Barbiturates are popular as a low-cost induction agent, with particularly favorable effects on intracranial pressure.

However, their use for analgesic purposes and for prolonged infusion is not useful in austere conditions.

#### Diazepam

Diazepam has been described for use in a variety of field conditions and is given via both the intravenous and intramuscular route. One advantage is its longer elimination half-life, which allows it to be administered less frequently; this feature may be especially beneficial in mass casualty and disaster situations in which frequent re-dosing of patients is usually not feasible. Conversely, respiratory depression in moderate doses can be avoided and, in fact, is reversible if desired by using the specific benzodiazepine antagonist, flumazenil.

#### Midazolam

Midazolam is a water-soluble benzodiazepine with good cardiovascular stability that demonstrates variations in dose requirements. Concerns about humanitarian and medico-legal issues as related to perioperative awareness have increased the use of this agent in view of its promotion of hemodynamic stability in trauma patients. Its shorter acting profile, however, may be a relative disadvantage in the high-volume trauma scenarios encountered in mass casualty and disaster situations because more frequent dosing may be required. Like diazepam, it is also reversible with flumazenil.

#### Etomidate

Etomidate is an imidazole induction agent not recommended for prolonged infusion because of its adverse affects on steroid synthesis. It is frequently preferred for anesthetic induction in patients in shock because of its relative cardiostability.

#### Propofol

Propofol was introduced in the United Kingdom in 1986 and in the United States in 1988–1989. Suitable as a continuous infusion for sedation or as part of a TIVA regimen, propofol has a short redistribution half-life. Its volume of distribution is similar to that of thiopental and etomidate, but propofol has the highest clearance rate of all the induction agents. In hypovolemic patients, as with other induction agents, relative cardiovascular depression can be observed, thus warranting caution in patients with serious injury and in patients who may be sensitive to respiratory depression such as those with head trauma.

**Inhalational Agents**

The general characteristics of popular inhalation agents in use today, as well as their specific use in trauma, are described by Stene and Grande.[32] In patients with traumatic injuries, inhalants would be used largely for anesthetic maintenance. Because of full stomach considerations, inhalation induction (even with the single-breath techniques described with sevoflurane) would largely be avoided, unless other means are unavailable. Because of its tendency to induce airway irritability, desflurane is probably best avoided in trauma patients, leaving isoflurane and sevoflurane as the agents of choice.

## Analgesic Agents

A wide variety of new, nonsteroidal antiinflammatory agents and nonnarcotic synthetic agents are now available. Their mechanisms of actions vary widely. The drugs can be either additive or synergistic when used in combination with other agents. One of the primary benefits of these analgesics is the avoidance of central respiratory depression. This characteristic diminishes the requirements for close observation and monitoring and the need for respiratory support and mechanical ventilation, which are always at a premium in a mass casualty and disaster situation. Parenteral forms are preferred, particularly intravenous, although an intravenous-intramuscular combination regimen can be used as well, yielding immediate onset effects with a prolonged duration of action.

## Mixed Opioid Agonists and Antagonists

Buprenorphine, butorphanol, and nalbuphine are attractive for their ceiling effect on respiratory depression and relative cardiovascular and hemodynamic stability. The same benefits that apply to nonsteroidal agents (vis-à-vis avoiding the need for close monitoring and respiratory support) are attractive in the mass casualty and disaster setting. For these reasons, many military medical services have substituted mixed opioid agonist-antagonist agents for naturally occurring opium derivatives such as morphine for field use by medics.

## Opioids

Fentanyl is popular among anesthesiologists. Its onset of action and half-life are also attractive in comparison with the shorter acting agents, alfentanil and remifentanil, which would not be appropriate in mass casualty or disaster situations. The profound respiratory depression and chest wall rigidity experienced with sufentanil do not warrant its use in these scenarios. European anesthesiologists have made greater use of oxymorphone, propoxyphene, and other synthetic and semisynthetic opioid analgesics, which could have applications in these cases.

## Non-Opioid General Analgesics

### Ketamine

Ketamine, a phencyclidine derivative, functions as an intravenous anesthetic with analgesic activity. A controversial agent and variably popular in various trauma-related settings, ketamine is often thought to be the agent of choice in austere conditions because of its relative portability, extended shelf-life, high relative potency versus dose given, the ability to (relatively) preserve respiratory drive, and thus the avoidance of the need for close monitoring and respiratory support.[34-38]

Thought by some to represent the "ideal sole agent" for unfavorable situations, ketamine can be used in both anesthetic and subanesthetic doses and may be given intravenously, intramuscularly, or subcutaneously. Various regimens have also been described using it as part of a TIVA technique or as an intramuscular regimen with benzodiazepine in a large group of casualties.[35]

Conversely, others believe ketamine to be particularly unfavorable in situations such as military or mass casualty and disaster field situations because of its side effects such as involuntary muscle movements, vivid hallucinations, and hy-pertension. Moreover, its use in patients with head injuries is disputed because of concerns of increasing intracranial pressure.

### Nitrous Oxide

The inhalation analgesic, nitrous oxide, is generally avoided for in-hospital management of trauma patients. However, when administered as an analgesic by means of a portable apparatus such as the Entonox device (Air Liquid Gas AB, Edmonton, Alberta) (which provides a uniform 50:50 oxygen-nitrogen mixture), the agent has found some use as an analgesic for prehospital and emergency department use.[39] Nevertheless, the effects of expanding air-filled spaces, as commonly found in trauma patients (such as a pneumothorax or pneumocephalus), must be considered before use.

## Patient-Controlled Analgesia

Infusion pumps for use of patient-controlled analgesia will be at a premium and of limited availability in a mass casualty and disaster situation. However, various regimens, when used in a patient-controlled system, can alleviate the need for high nurse to patient ratios and thus help to make queuing for optimal services more tolerable.

# ANESTHESIA EQUIPMENT FOR AUSTERE CONDITIONS

## What Are the Requirements?

Anesthesia and critical care for trauma victims in out-of-hospital situations can be provided with the same level of sophistication as that found in hospital operating rooms and ICUs.[27-29] As a result of miniaturization of medical devices, extended battery life, increased durability, and multitasking of equipment, a wide range of capabilities can be found condensed within the same package (Fig. 50–8).

Equipment for providing anesthesia and critical care in austere conditions can be divided into those that *provide* a function and those that monitor or measure a function. In the first category are total anesthesia machines, ventilators, and infusion pumps. In the second category are electrocardiograph equipment and devices for noninvasive blood pressure measurement; arterial blood gas analysis; and blood analysis for electrolyte, hemoglobin, coagulation, and hemoglobin-hematocrit. Desirable characteristics of anesthesia equipment for use under austere conditions include portability, durability, serviceability, ease of operation and repair, and low cost. Electrical requirements should be minimal (or even optional), and, if possible, fresh gas requirements should also be minimized.

## Anesthesia Delivery Systems

Anesthesia delivery systems can be divided into three broad categories (which are covered elsewhere in this text): (1) demand flow equipment, (2) plenum or flow equipment, and (3) draw-over equipment. Standard operating room anesthesia machines use the first type.

*Closed circuit techniques* use standard plenum equipment

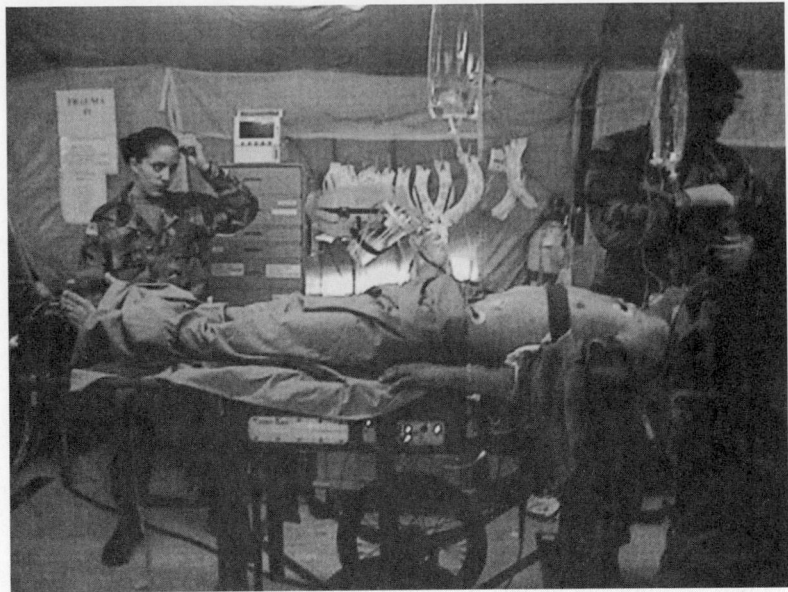

**FIGURE 50–8.** LSTAT: Life Support for Trauma and Transport. An individualized portable intensive care system and surgical platform provide resuscitation and stabilization capability. Features ventilation, suction, oxygen, infusion pump, physiologic monitor, clinical blood analyzer, and defibrillation, complemented by a fully network-capable on-board computer monitoring system and independent power system, packaged on a NATO litter form factor. (Courtesy of Integrated Medical Systems, Inc, Signal Hill, Calif.)

and a circle system, which conserves oxygen supplies and anesthetic agents but requires significant amounts of carbon dioxide absorbent. In addition, they require training and experience.

*Draw-over anesthetic systems* allow the administration of a known anesthetic concentration from a calibrated vaporizer using ambient air as the carrier gas. Supplemental oxygen can be added when available, but it is not essential for the operation of the system. A variety of draw-over systems and modifications exist today, primarily used by the United Kingdom commonwealth members (Britain, Australia, Canada)[40,41] (Fig. 50–9). Included in this range of devices is the basic draw-over anesthesia system, as in the Tri-Service Anesthesia apparatus (Penlon Ltd, Abingdon, England), as well as the Portable Anesthesia Complete unit (Ohmeda BOC, Madison, Wisc) (Fig. 50–10).

The Tri-Service Anesthesia and Portable Anesthesia Complete systems in their standard design do not incorporate any visual sign of the volume of spontaneous respiration. This can be provided by fitting an open-ended reservoir bag to the expiratory port of the one-way valve. Similarly, a scavenging hose for exhaled gases can be fitted to the expiratory port of this valve.

A more conventional, but still highly portable (86-lb), anesthetic delivery system is the Model 885-A Military Field Anesthesia Machine (Ohmeda BOC, Madison, Wisc) (Fig. 50–11) used by US forces (Tables 50–5 and 50–6). Although

it does not meet current American Society of Testing and Materials (ASTM) standards, thousands of anesthetics have been administered safely using this apparatus, which is a continuous flow, semiclosed circle system similar to the machines in common use in operating rooms throughout the world. Suction, a defibrillator, and monitoring equipment must also be available (Table 50–7) (Figs. 50–12 and 50–13).

## Monitoring Equipment

Monitoring equipment should always include pulse oximetry, if possible, as this is portable and provides a great deal of information (pulse, oxygenation status, sufficient arterial blood pressure for the machine to detect, and perfusion of extremities). Additional desirable monitoring equipment includes blood pressure monitor (automatic, manual, or invasive) and temperature monitors, capnography, gas analysis, electrocardiography, blood gas analysis, and basic laboratory tests. These monitors can vary significantly in sophistication and portability, and they may not all be available or required in every circumstance. The successful anesthesiologist in a disaster situation should be able to innovate with available equipment, improvise for what is not available, and provide a safe anesthetic.

## Oxygen Supply

Oxygen is perhaps the most essential "drug" administered to a trauma patient. Typically, in a conventional setting, it is

**TABLE 50–5.** Lower Section of the Model 885-A Military Anesthesia Medicine

| | |
|---|---|
| Caster | Cylinder holder |
| Cylinder adapters | Level |
| Masks and elbow | Absorber gasket replacement |
| Y connector | Flow calculator |
| Replacement parts | Scavenging tubes |
| Wrenches | Oxygen analyzer |
| Instrument tray | |

From Kingsley CP, Petty C, Olson K. Anesthesia equipment for austere conditions. In: Grande CM, ed. *Textbook of Trauma Anesthesia and Critical Care*. St Louis, Mo: Mosby–Year Book; 1993:1174.

**TABLE 50–6.** Upper Section of the Model 885-A Military Anesthesia Machine

| | |
|---|---|
| Cylinder regulator assemblies | Reservoir bags |
| Gas supply hoses | Head strap |
| Breathing tubes | Clipboard |
| Pediatric breathing system | Protective closure devices |

From Kingsley CP, Petty C, Olson K. Anesthesia equipment for austere conditions. In: Grande CM, ed. *Textbook of Trauma Anesthesia and Critical Care*. St Louis, Mo: Mosby–Year Book; 1993:1174.

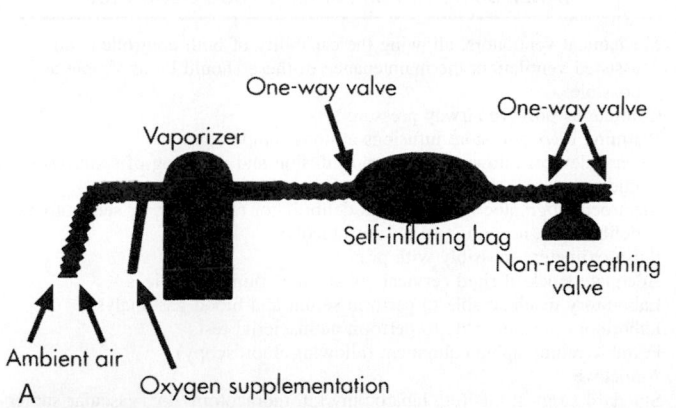

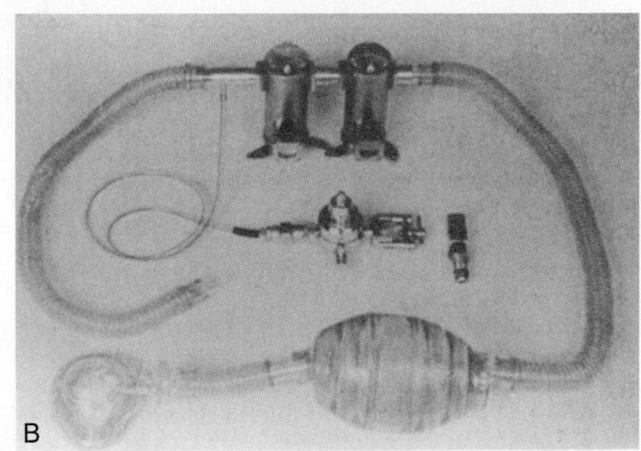

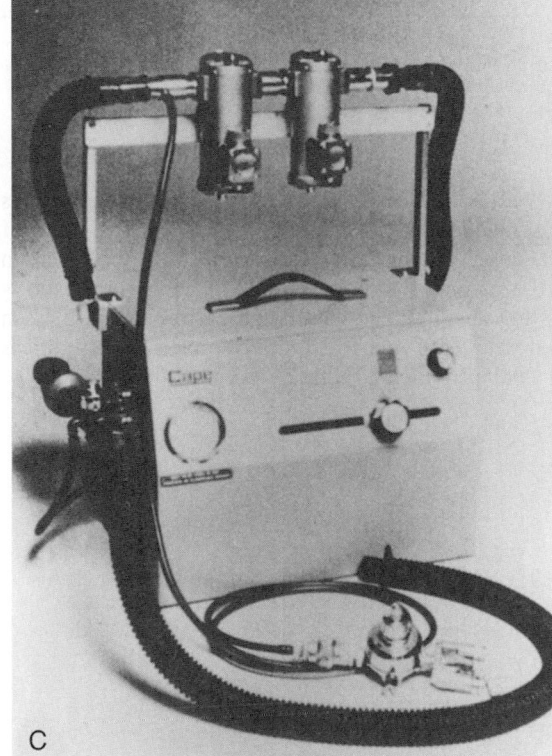

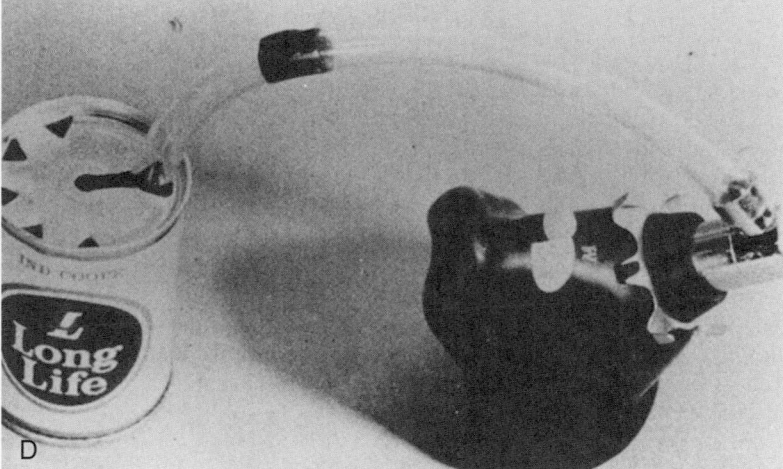

**FIGURE 50–9.** *A,* Components of draw-over anesthesia systems. *B,* Tri-Service anesthesia apparatus with Oxford Miniature vaporizer unit. *C,* Mounted on Cape TC50 ventilator. *D,* Field expedient system. (From Kingsley CP, Petty C, Olson K. Anesthesia equipment for austere conditions. In: Grande CM, ed. *Textbook of Trauma Anesthesia and Critical Care.* St Louis, Mo: Mosby–Year Book; 1993:1167 [*A* and *D*], 1314 [*B* and *C*]. *D,* Courtesy of Rob Calverly, MD.)

supplied by a direct pipe to operating rooms. In out-of-hospital situations, oxygen can be carried in a variety of tank sizes that are heavy and potentially dangerous to transport, particularly in the unstable situations frequently found in mass casualty and disaster scenarios.

Liquid oxygen is available in containers that weigh approximately 125 lb (56 kg) and will hold approximately 25 000 L. Using flows of 2 L/min, such containers will last for as long as 8 hours. However, liquid oxygen cannot drive a pneumatic ventilator because its operating pressure is too low. Instead, it is useful as a source of oxygen enrichment.

Alternatively, a variety of "oxygen concentrators" have been developed and miniaturized. These devices are usually more attractive for the mass casualty and disaster setting.

### Blood Transfusion

Trauma resuscitation often involves the need for transfusion or re-infusion of blood. Gaining increasing popularity are a variety of autotransfusion techniques. Many of these are fairly low tech and inexpensive. As long as sterility is maintained, they can be used in the prehospital setting, as well as inside the hospital operating room or ICU. Homologous blood transfusion, including screening and testing of donors for a variety of diseases, is frequently essential. In some locations, the physician must set a limit to the number of units of transfused blood. Commonly, in austere situations, the severity of injury and the requirement for blood equate determine survival.

## PSYCHOLOGIC IMPACT OF TRAUMA: ANESTHETIC IMPLICATIONS

The psychologic and emotional implications of injury on victims of trauma are often considered part of the holistic care plan; however, the psychologic impact that trauma may have on care providers is often neglected.[42] The anesthesiologist dealing with trauma patients, whether on an individual

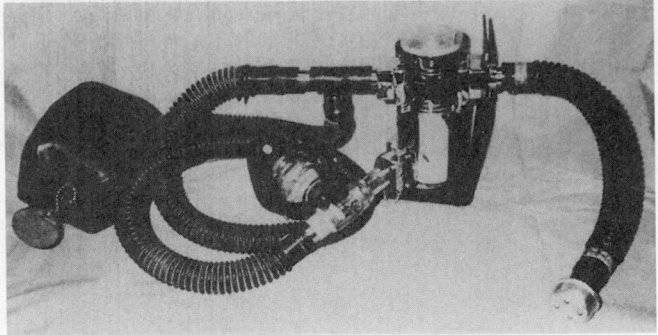

FIGURE 50–10. Portable anesthesia complete unit vaporizer system. (From Kingsley CP, Petty C, Olson K. Anesthesia equipment for austere conditions. In: Grande CM, ed. *Textbook of Trauma Anesthesia and Critical Care.* St Louis, Mo: Mosby–Year Book; 1993:1169.)

**TABLE 50–7.** Equipment for a 100-Person Crew

Mechanical ventilators, allowing the capability of both controlled and assisted ventilation; the maintenance of these should be as simple as possible

Continuous positive airway pressure sets

Warming device to store infusions at body temperature

Several devices allowing both rapid infusion and warming of solutions to be injected

Electrocardiographic machine with defibrillator (automatic or semiautomatic defibrillator, according to local protocols)

Pulse oximeters (possibly with printer)

Adequate stock of rigid cervical collars and splinting devices

Laboratory machine able to perform serum and blood gas analyses

Laboratory machine able to perform antibacterial tests

Portable radiographic equipment (allowing fluoroscopy)

Autoclave

Standard surgical kits (eg, laparotomy kit, thoracotomy kit, vascular surgery kit)

From Badiali S. Extreme environmental conditions, part 4: polar conditions. In: Grande CM, ed. *Textbook of Trauma Anesthesia and Critical Care.* St Louis, Mo: Mosby–Year Book; 1993:1368.

basis or in a mass casualty and disaster setting, needs to be aware of the psychologic and emotional impact of trauma both on the patient, on the themselves, and on colleagues (Table 50–8).

Steps must be taken to provide supportive care not only to the patient but also to relatives and others involved. Indeed, one focus unique to the anesthesiologist is perioperative awareness, which must be considered and, if possible, prevented by strategies such as early administration of benzodiazepines. However, benzodiazepines, per se, have not been proven to diminish the incidence or severity of perioperative awareness. A reliable dose-response curve that can be used as a guide is not available.[43]

Life-threatening traumatic stress can be a major event in the life of the care provider, potentially giving rise to posttraumatic stress disorder. A variety of strategies have been developed to deal with and to minimize posttraumatic stress disorder in care providers. Perhaps the most popular is the

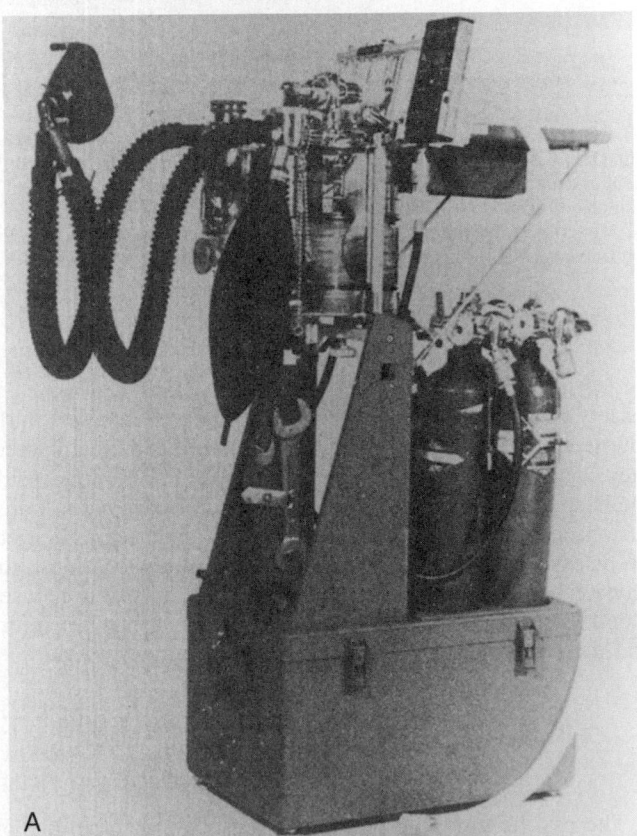

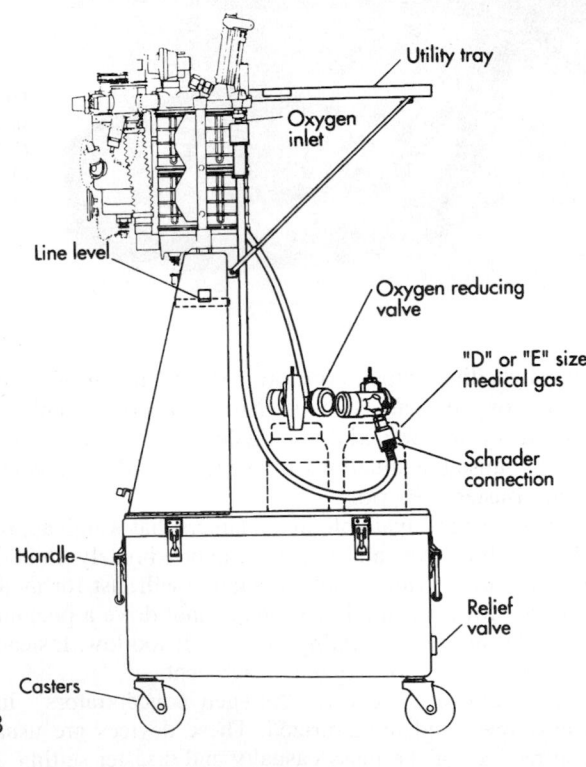

FIGURE 50–11. *A,* Model 885-A military field anesthesia machine (Ohmeda BOC). *B,* Side view: lower case casters provide mobility. Line level on side of support arm. Connection of size E gas cylinder to control head oxygen inlet. (From Kingsley CP, Petty C, Olson K. Anesthesia equipment for austere conditions. In: Grande CM, ed. *Textbook of Trauma Anesthesia and Critical Care.* St Louis, Mo: Mosby–Year Book; 1993:1174.)

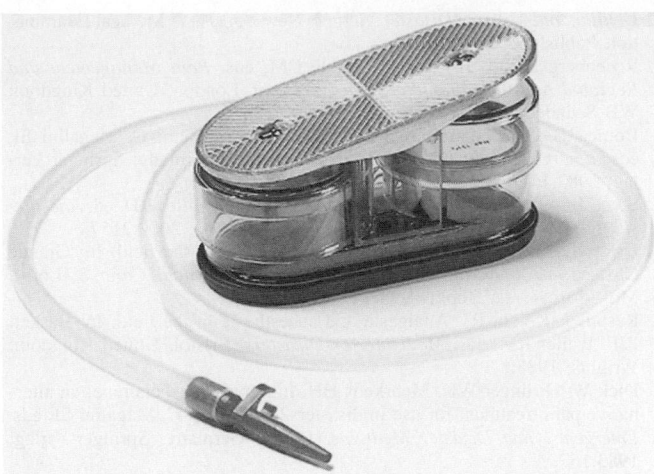

**FIGURE 50–12.** Ambu TwinPump. Manual emergency suction pump, for use in adverse weather conditions, can quickly and effectively aspirate 250 mL of thick fluid in 8 seconds. (Courtesy of Ambu International A/S, Brondby, Denmark.)

critical incident stress debriefing system, based on group discussions and talking out emotionally charged issues.

## SUMMARY

In this chapter, the background and overall management of mass casualty and disaster situations have been discussed. It is important for the anesthesiologist to have a basic appreciation for these instances because, frequently, the surgical man-

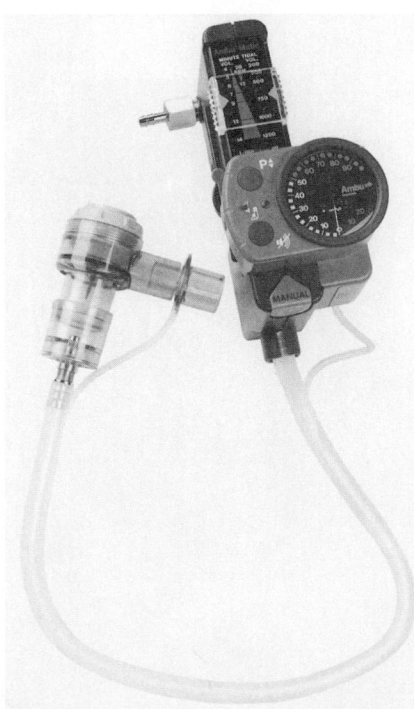

**FIGURE 50–13.** Ambu Matic with ventilation monitor. A compact and lightweight, pneumatically powered ventilator for emergency and transport situations. Ventilation monitor with mechanical and electronic pressure gauge indicating airway pressure (eg, disconnect, obstruction, leak). (Courtesy of Ambu International A/S, Brondby, Denmark.)

**TABLE 50–8.** Sequence of Panic Development

| Stage | Description |
|---|---|
| Preparation | Panic strikes dense concentrations of overwrought people, including many fragile individuals, without any organization or discipline |
| Emotional shock | The triggering event, which may be of modest proportion, causes an emotional block |
| Reaction | People become agitated and tension explodes in an uncontrolled behavior, the so-called true panic |
| Resolution | This stage may be spontaneous or may depend on an energetic outside intervention; resolution gives way to a state of profound prostration |

From Seidel MR. Psychologic impact of trauma: implications for the anesthesiologist. In: Grande CM, ed. *Textbook of Trauma Anesthesia and Critical Care.* St Louis, Mo: Mosby–Year Book; 1993:1292.

agement of trauma is a byproduct of the circumstances. As opposed to providing excellent care for a single victim of injury, in mass casualty and disaster situations, the anesthesiologist must now become adept at multitasking. Not only will simultaneous care of several patients be required, but it will be done under adverse and austere conditions. Nevertheless, with advance planning and training, as well as selection of program equipment and drugs, the same quality of care as is available in a conventional hospital setting can be achieved.

## References

1. Grande CM, Baskett PJF, Donchin Y, et al. Trauma anesthesia for disasters: anything, anytime, anywhere. *Crit Care Clin.* 1991;7:339.
2. Donchin Y, Wiener M, Grande CM, et al. Military medicine: trauma anesthesia and critical care on the battlefield. *Crit Care Clin.* 1990;6:185.
3. National Research Council. *Confronting Natural Disasters: An International Decade for Natural Disaster Reduction.* Washington, DC: Academy Press; 1987.
4. Office of US Foreign Disaster Assistance. *Disaster History: Significant Data on Major Disasters Worldwide, 1900–Present.* Washington, DC: Agency for International Development; 1994.
5. Von Clauswitz K, Howard M, Paret P. *On War.* New York, NY: Knopf; 1993. Everyman's Library Series.
6. Zajtchuk R, Grande CM, eds. *Textbook of Military Medicine: Part IV, Anesthesia and Perioperative Care of the Combat Casualty.* Falls Church, Va: Office of the Surgeon General of the Army; 1994.
7. LaCombe D, Grande CM. EMS support of executive protection and counter-terrorism operations. In: de Boer J, Dubolouz M, eds. *Handbook of Disaster Medicine.* Zeist, The Netherlands: VSP International Science Publishers; 2000:359.
8. Carmona R, Grande CM, Gonzales D. Trauma care support for mass events, counter-terrorism and VIP protection. In: Soreide E, Grande CM, eds. *Prehospital Trauma Care.* New York, NY: Marcel Dekker; In press.
9. Butler FK Jr, Hagmann JH, eds. Tactical management of urban warfare casualties in special operations. *Mil Med.* 2000;165(suppl):1.
10. Lavery RF, Addis MD, Doran JV, et al. Taking care of the "good guys": a trauma center-based model of medical support for tactical law enforcement. *J Trauma.* 2000;48:125.
11. Carrison D, Grande CM, eds. In sickness and in health. *Secur Manage.* 2000;44:65.
12. Olds M, Stocks G, Dauphinee K. Practical aspects of the prehospital medical care environment. In: Grande CM, ed. *Textbook of Trauma Anesthesia and Critical Care.* St Louis, Mo: Mosby–Year Book; 1993:309.
13. Orr SM, Robinson WA. The Hyatt Regency skywalk collapse: an EMS-based disaster response. *Ann Emerg Med.* 1982;12:601.
14. Auf der Heide E. The "paper" plan syndrome. In: Auf der Heide E, ed. *Disaster Response: Principles of Preparation and Coordination.* St Louis, Mo: CV Mosby; 1989:33.
15. Smith CE, Sinz E, Grande CM. New teaching and training methods in trauma care: present and future role of simulator technology. *Am J Anesthesiol.* 2000;27:186.
16. International Trauma Anesthesia and Critical Care Society. *International*

*Chief Emergency Physician Training Course in Command Incident Management in Disaster and Mass Casualty Incidents. Course Curriculum and Manual.* Baltimore, Md: ITACCS; 2000.

17. Bowen TE, Bellamy RF, eds. *Emergency War Surgery.* Washington DC: United States Government Printing Office; 1988.

18. Vayer JS, Ten Eyck RP, Cowan ML. New concepts in triage. *Ann Emerg Med.* 1986;15:927.

19. Parr JA, Grande CM. Mechanisms of trauma. In: Grande CM, ed. *Textbook of Trauma Anesthesia and Critical Care.* St Louis, Mo: Mosby–Year Book; 1993:335.

20. Baker DJ. Extreme environmental conditions, part 2: chemical and biologic warfare. In: Grande CM, ed. *Textbook of Trauma Anesthesia and Critical Care.* St Louis, Mo: Mosby–Year Book; 1993:1330.

21. Seraj MA. Extreme environmental conditions, part 3: medical preparation for decontamination and detoxification of toxic chemical injuries. In: Grande CM, ed. *Textbook of Trauma Anesthesia and Critical Care.* St Louis, Mo: Mosby–Year Book; 1993:1354.

22. Abdi S, Stiff J, Martyn JAJ. Emergency anesthesia and severe burns. In: Adams AP, Hewitt P, Grande CM, eds. *Emergency Anaesthesia.* 2nd ed. London, United Kingdom: Arnold; 1998:245.

23. Baker D, Grande CM. Current nerve agent policy could be poison for public. *Natl Defense.* 1997;81:38.

24. Baker DJ. The immediate care of casualties following the release of toxic chemicals. *Resuscitation.* 1999;42:101.

25. Hendler I, Nahtomi O, Segal E, et al. The effect of full protective gear on intubation performance by hospital medical personnel. *Mil Med.* 2000;165:272.

26. Badiali S. Extreme environmental conditions, part 4: polar conditions. In: Grande CM, ed. *Textbook of Trauma Anesthesia and Critical Care.* St Louis, Mo: Mosby–Year Book; 1993:1366.

27. Kingsley CP, Petty C, Olson K. Anesthesia equipment for austere conditions. In: Grande CM, ed. *Textbook of Trauma Anesthesia and Critical Care.* St Louis, Mo: Mosby–Year Book; 1993:1166.

28. Sanders CD. Anaesthetic equipment in disasters. *Br J Clin Equip.* 1977;2:5.

29. Mecca RS. Anesthesia in field situations. In: Burkle FM, ed. *Disaster Medicine; Application for the Immediate Management and Triage of Civilian and Military Disaster Victims.* New York, NY: Medical Examination Publishing; 1984:315.

30. Rosenberg AR, Bernstein R, Grande CM, eds. *Pain Management and Regional Anesthesia for the Trauma Patient.* London, United Kingdom: WB Saunders; 2001:1.

31. Bonica JJ. Pain control in mass casualties. In: Manni C, Magalini SI, eds. *Emergency and Disaster Medicine.* Berlin, Germany: Springer-Verlag; 1983:151.

32. Stene JK, Grande CM. Anesthesia for trauma. In: Miller RD, ed. *Anesthesia.* 5th ed. Philadelphia, Pa: Churchill Livingstone; 2000:2157.

33. Dow A, Baskett PJF. Anesthesia and analgesia in the field. In: Grande CM, ed. *Textbook of Trauma Anesthesia and Critical Care.* St Louis, Mo: Mosby–Year Book; 1993:297.

34. Restall J, Knight RJ. Analgesia and anaesthesia in the field. In: Baskett PJF, Weller RM, eds. *Medicine for Disasters.* Bristol, United Kingdom: Wrights; 1988:87.

35. Dick W, Hirlinger WK, Mehrkens HH. Intramuscular ketamine: an alternative pain treatment for use in disasters? In: Manni C, Magalini SI, eds. *Emergency and Disaster Medicine.* Berlin, Germany: Springer-Verlag; 1983:167.

36. Restall J, Tully AM, Ward PJ, et al. Total intravenous anaesthesia for military surgery: a technique using ketamine, midazolam and vecuronium. *Anaesthesia.* 1988;43:46.

37. Carson IW, Moore J, Balmer JP, et al. Laryngeal competence with ketamine and other drugs. *Anesthesiology.* 1973;38:128.

38. Grant IS, Nimmo WS, Clements JA. Lack of effect of ketamine analgesia on gastric emptying in man. *Br J Anaesth.* 1981;53:1321.

39. Baskett PJF, Withnell A. The use of Entonox in the ambulance service. *BMJ.* 1970;2:41.

40. Knight RJ, Houghton IT. Field experience with the Tri-Service Anaesthetic Apparatus in Oman and Northern Ireland. *Anaesthesia.* 1981;36:1122.

41. Houghton IT. The Tri-Service Anaesthetic Apparatus. *Anaesthesia.* 1981;36:1904.

42. Seidel MR. Psychologic impact of trauma: implications for the anesthesiologist. In: Grande CM, ed. *Textbook of Trauma Anesthesia and Critical Care.* St Louis, Mo: Mosby–Year Book; 1993:1290.

43. Lubke GH, Sebel PS. Awareness and different forms of memory in trauma anesthesia. *Curr Opin Anaesthesiol.* 2000;13:161.

CHAPTER

# Electrical Safety

Jan C. Horrow

## HISTORICAL CONSIDERATIONS

An explosion or fire requires the presence of three components: a fuel, an oxidizing substance, and an ignition spark. Several decades ago, anesthetic gases were explosive. Ether, cyclopropane, or one of the other flammable anesthetics constituted the fuel. They were almost always combined with oxygen or nitrous oxide, both oxidizing substances. Because this mixture leaked into the operating room atmosphere, prevention of sparks assumed great importance. Static electricity was the enemy.[1]

Hydraulics powered the anesthesia machine. Monitoring rarely used more than a manually operated blood pressure cuff, chest stethoscope, and finger on the pulse. Electrosurgery had not achieved universal use. Thus, operating rooms did not need extensive electric power. The few electric outlets permitted in operating rooms were placed 5 feet above floor level to limit their exposure to dense explosive gases. These special electric outlets ensured contact within an explosion-proof encasement. Personnel wore conductive shoes to dissipate any static charges through a conductive floor and tore adhesive tape above their heads in case that act generated static charge. A special power supply, isolated from ground, prevented sparks from line-powered devices.

Today, the environment of flammable anesthetics no longer exists. Static electric discharge carries no explosion risk, and conductive shoes are antiques. Nonflammable anesthetics permit free use of electrically powered devices, which have proliferated. What protective devices provide a safer electric environment? This chapter discusses electrical safety and the basis for protective devices.

## ELECTROCUTION

Forget about the operating room for the moment, and consider electrical safety in your own home or office. To understand what makes an environment electrically safe, let us first consider what makes the home environment hazardous. This understanding follows from a relatively painless review of physics.

## What Are the Laws of Current Flow?

An understanding of electrical safety does not require an in-depth review of the physical laws and equations governing electric energy. Only four principles pertain to this topic.

### Energy

First, electricity is energy, and energy performs work. Misapplied, this energy can be destructive. Uncontrolled electric energy harms property by starting fires. People may sustain burns or electrocution. The latter occurs when electric energy confounds the biopotentials that permit proper cardiovascular function.

### Circuit Components

Second, electric charges can flow only in an unbroken electric circuit. This circuit usually contains physically connected elements, such as wires, lamps, or speakers. Electrical hazards relate to unintentional flow of electric charge. The magnitude of this flow, measured in amperes, depends on the driving force for the electric charges (their voltage) and the resistance in their path, measured in ohms. Ohm's law defines this relationship:

$$\text{Potential Difference (V)} = \text{Current (I)} \times \text{Resistance (R)}$$

This equation is familiar to us in its cardiovascular analogy: pressure difference (mean arterial pressure minus central venous pressure) equals the product of cardiac output and systemic vascular resistance (Fig. 51–1). Note that just as the vascular bed with a smaller resistance receives greater blood flow, so does the limb of a circuit with less electric resistance receive greater current flow.

### Capacitance

The third physical principle needed to appreciate electrical safety is the operation of a capacitor. Conductive surfaces in close physical proximity separated by an insulator form a capacitor. Capacitance depends on the ability of the insulator between the conductive surfaces to block the flow of charge from one surface to the other despite a potential difference. Thus, the capacitor must tolerate a certain amount of electrical "stress."

### Direct Current

What happens when a constant voltage (as from a battery) is applied across a capacitor? Positive charges leave one conductive surface and travel toward the negative pole of the battery, and negative charges leave the opposite surface, being attracted by the positive pole of the battery. This nearly instantaneous flow occurs such that the potential difference

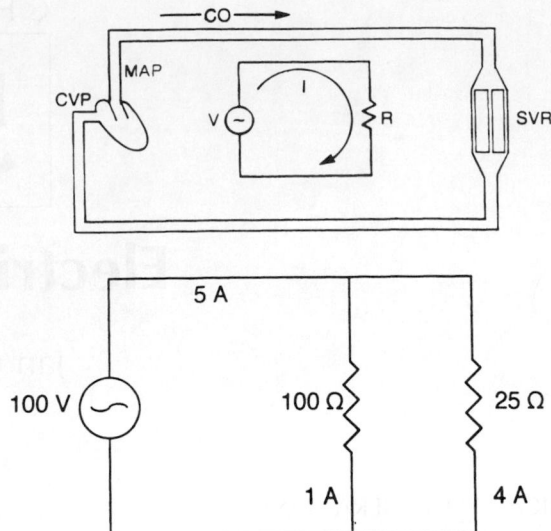

**FIGURE 51–1.** The *upper panel* displays the cardiovascular analogy of Ohm's law. The force driving blood through the systemic vasculature is the mean arterial pressure (MAP) less the central venous pressure (CVP). It is analogous to the potential difference (V) at the voltage source in the *lower panel*. The systemic vascular resistance (SVR) corresponds to the device resistive load (measured in ohms). Flow in the cardiovascular circuit (measured in liters per minute of cardiac output) corresponds to the flow of charge (I) in the electrical circuit (measured in amperes). The *lower panel* demonstrates Ohm's law. The 100-V potential difference produces a current of 1 A through the 100-Ω resistance, and 4 A through the 25-Ω resistance. Note that because a total of 5 A of current flows in the circuit, the equivalent resistance of the two parallel resistors is 20 Ω. (From Horrow JC, Seitman DT. Electrical safety and device calibration. *Anesthesiol Clin North Am.* 1988;6:699.)

appearing across the capacitor's surfaces equals that applied by the battery (Fig. 51–2). This equal and opposite potential difference creates a net driving force of zero voltage in the circuit, so that no current flows. Application of an unvarying voltage source such as a battery reveals that capacitors block direct current, just as if the circuit were open.

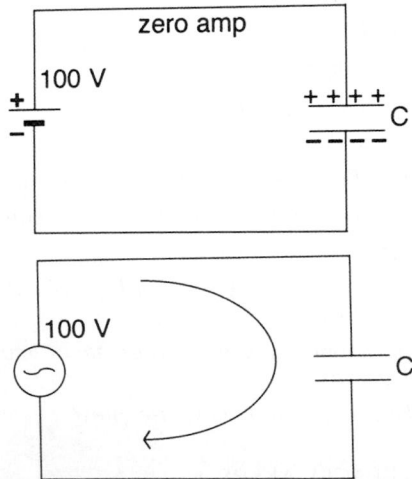

**FIGURE 51–2.** In the *upper panel*, a fixed voltage applied across the capacitor (C) yields zero current flow after a near-instantaneous equilibration. Charges move to the capacitor's plates to exactly oppose the applied voltage. However, a finite current flows with an alternating voltage source (depicted in the *lower panel*). The impedance to flow in this circuit (X) depends on the frequency of the applied voltage (f) and the capacitor's capacitance (C): $X = 1/(2\pi fC)$.

### Alternating Current

The behavior of alternating current differs. When the voltage applied across the capacitor varies with time, charges are continuously flowing between the capacitor's conductive surface and the voltage source. The voltage across the capacitor moves to oppose that of the changing voltage source. Although no current flows across the capacitor (between its conductive surfaces), current flows around it in the circuit. In fact, the more quickly the voltage source changes (ie, the higher its frequency), the more easily current flows. Should the circuit also contain resistive elements (which consume electric energy), this current produces work. Application of a varying voltage source reveals that capacitors permit the flow of alternating current.

## Capacitive Coupling

The fourth electrical concept is that of capacitive coupling. Because any two conductors in proximity form a capacitor, the wires carrying electricity from a power outlet form a weak capacitor. It is weak because they are separated by a poor conductor—in fact, an insulator. Air is also an effective insulator.

Such unintentional elements are termed *stray capacitors,* and the paths inadvertently formed are considered to be *capacitively coupled.* The extremely low capacitance and high resistance in these circuits determine extraordinarily small "leakage" currents. These leakage currents assume greater importance, however, when they pass through myocardium (discussed later).

## What Is a Grounded Electrical System?

Generating stations distribute electric power as alternating current at high voltage. This method minimizes the amount lost as heat during transmission. Power is the product of current and voltage (P = IV), but heat loss varies with the square of the current. Thus, optimal power transmission uses low current and high voltage. At a nearby utility pole or ground enclosure, a transformer decreases this 2400- to 8000-V supply to 110 V.[2] At the entrance of electrical service to a building, one (not both) of the two wires carrying this 110-V supply is permanently connected to a conductor that unmistakably contacts the earth[3] (ie, ground) (Fig. 51–3).

## Why Is a Ground Necessary?

The connection to ground prevents unwanted high voltages from residing in the end-user system. High voltages relative to ground are dangerous because they can overcome the insulating properties of air. The resulting spark may ignite a fire. High voltage in one conductor might occur from lightning or from insulation failure in the high-voltage transformer. Without this ground connection, high voltage, relative to ground, would usually occur in each of the two conductors. Even though the voltage between them remains 110 V, their source at the transformer is several thousand volts. Any conductive object connected to the earth in proximity to one of the conductors might then receive a voltage arc. The grounded system keeps these sources of high voltage away from the household conductors.

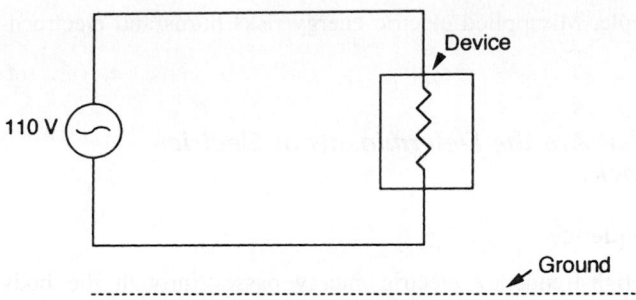

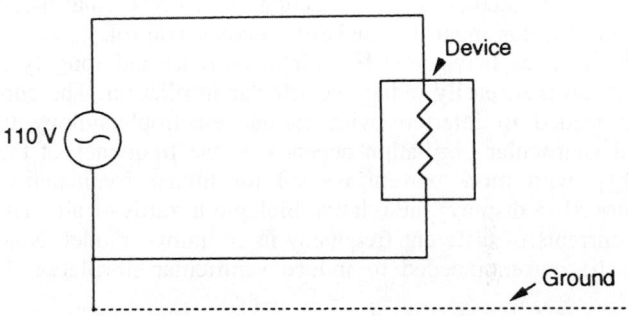

**FIGURE 51–3.** Ungrounded and grounded electrical systems. The *upper panel* depicts a typical electrical circuit in an ungrounded system. The *lower panel* shows the grounded system universally present in North America in which one of the power lines is connected to the ground. The ungrounded line is called *hot,* and the grounded line is described as *neutral* or *grounded.*

The grounded system also provides a low-resistance circuit when a live wire mistakenly contacts any conductor at ground potential, such as a water pipe (which is connected to ground) or the housing of any properly grounded device (Fig. 51–4). This low-resistance circuit is desirable because the resulting high current then triggers a fuse or circuit breaker, opening the circuit to protect the system from damage. Thus, the grounded system of electrical supply protects equipment and property, or in the case of the operating room, it protects

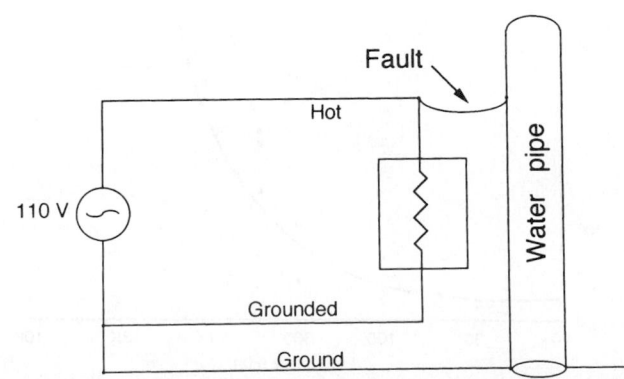

**FIGURE 51–4.** A fault situation in which the hot power line is connected to the ground by a conductor such as a metal water pipe. Current may flow uninterrupted from the voltage source through the connection between the ground and the other (grounded) power line. A large current will flow, causing a fuse to blow or a circuit breaker to trip, interrupting power to all devices grouped on that line.

people. Misapplied electric energy risks burns and electrocution.

## What Are the Determinants of Electric Shock?

### Frequency

High-frequency electric energy passes through the body harmlessly. Rapidly changing signals (>3 kHz) vary too quickly to confound the endogenous biopotentials that govern the orderly depolarization and repolarization of critical tissues (heart and nervous system). In contrast, direct current applied as a pulse to the chest wall can defibrillate the heart. In this situation, simultaneous depolarization of all myocardial tissue permits the dominant pacemaker to recover control.

Frequencies between 0 Hz (direct current) and roughly 1 kHz, however, easily induce ventricular fibrillation. The current needed to interfere with cardiac electrophysiology to yield ventricular fibrillation depends on the frequency of the energy, with more current needed for higher frequencies.[4] Figure 51–5 displays the relative biologic hazards of alternating currents of different frequency in an animal model. Note that the current needed to induce ventricular fibrillation is least when the frequency of the electric energy coincides with that of commercially supplied electric power (60 Hz), an unfortunate coincidence.

### Macroshock and Microshock

The current that induces fibrillation also depends on the point of entry. It is current density (flow per unit cross-sectional area) and not current itself that causes harm. Thus, 100 to 2500 mA applied across the trunk when the skin is wet induces fibrillation, but only 100 μA suffices when conducted by a saline-filled catheter in contact with the myocardium.[5] The latter current enters through a much smaller area and has no opportunity to disperse across additional tissue before reaching the organ at jeopardy. *Macroshock* describes the former situation, in which larger currents travel across the body, and *microshock* applies to minute currents entering myocardium directly.

Recent work[6] shed doubt on the national standard of 50 μA for maximal leakage current through intravascular catheters (microshock).[7] An alternating current of 32 μA at 60 Hz applied through a right ventricular pacing catheter causes a continuous capture (mean rate 213/min), appearing as ventricular tachycardia without pulsatile blood pressure. Currents as low as 20 μA cause intermittent capture.[6]

## What Are the Circuit Requirements for Electric Shock?

Figure 51–6 displays several possibilities. In the first, the victim interposes his body between the "hot" and "neutral" conductors. Should the natural barrier of intact skin be defeated by wet hands, its resistance falls to approximately 1 kΩ, yielding a current of 110 mA on application of 110 V.

The second case displays a more subtle opportunity for electrocution. Here, direct physical contact with only the "hot" conductor occurs. The connection to the neutral side arises from contact with ground because the neutral conductor is connected to ground at the entrance of power to the building. For this reason, shoes, which are electrical insulators, provide protection from electric shock. Likewise, the rubber tires of a car isolate the vehicle from ground, decreasing the likelihood that lightning will seek a path through the vehicle.

In the third case, an overt fault in the electrical system has not occurred. Rather, the device contains a capacitive coupling that enables flow of sufficient current to cause microshock. Pacemaker wires provide direct access to the myocardium for capacitively coupled currents.[8] Use of electrosurgery creates microshock-level currents in these wires or in the sensing wires of some pulmonary artery catheters.[9]

### Safety Measures

Can safety be provided for these three situations? Yes, in some cases. Unfortunately, no system currently provides the ability to differentiate between an electrical appliance and the human body when the latter is interposed between the two current-carrying conductors. Fortunately, few people create this situation.

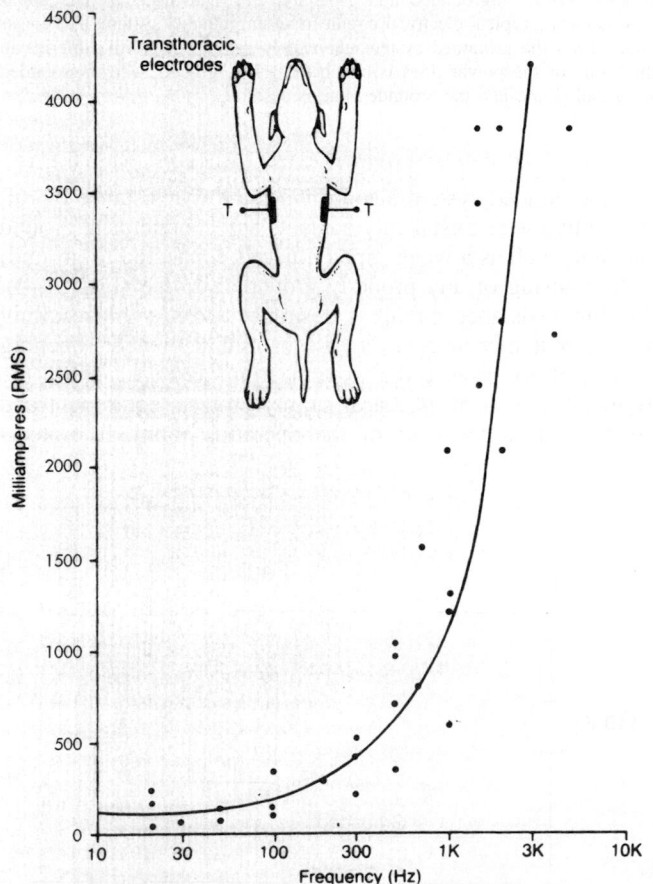

**FIGURE 51–5.** The hazard of alternating current applied across the thorax of a dog depends on the current's frequency, with lower-frequency signals requiring smaller currents to induce ventricular fibrillation. (From Geddes LA, Baker LE. Response to passage of electric current through the body. *J Assoc Adv Med Instrum.* 1971;5:13.)

In contrast, modern electrical wiring can avert electrocution in the second situation —that of line-to-ground contact. In the third case, complete safety does not accrue even with radical alteration of electric energy supply.

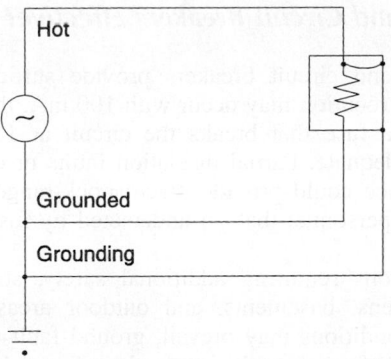

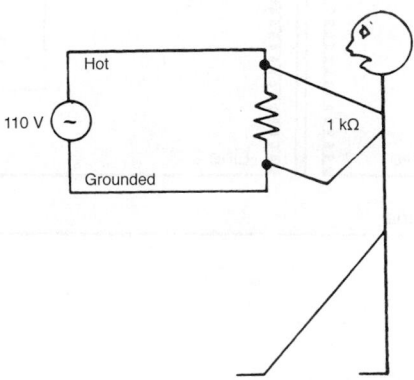

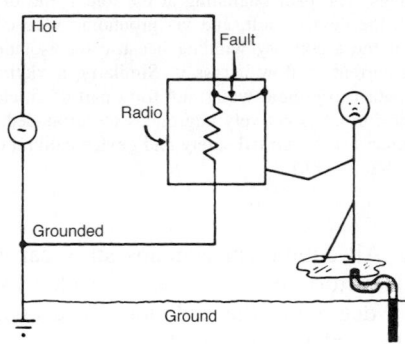

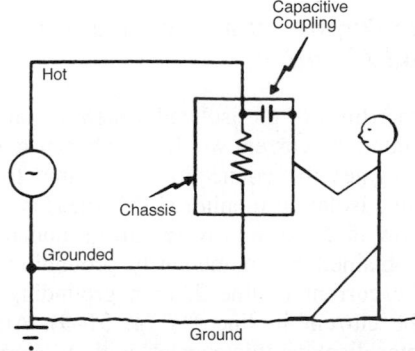

FIGURE 51–6. Three ways that electrocution can occur. In the *upper panel*, an ignorant victim simultaneously contacts both conductors, placing his or her body in parallel with the device supplied by the power cord. Regardless of the device's resistance, a current of 110 V ÷ 1 kΩ = 110 mA will flow across the trunk if the victim's hands are wet. The *middle panel* demonstrates how shock occurs in a grounded system when the victim contacts only one conductor. The insulation of the hot conductor of this radio has worn away so that the conductor contacts the radio's enclosure (*chassis*). Should the victim touch the chassis and be in electrical contact with ground, as easily happens in wet environments, he or she creates a parallel current path through his or her body to ground and back to the voltage source via the connection of the second power conductor to ground. The *lower panel* depicts a similar current path. In this case, the hot conductor insulation is intact. However, capacitive coupling permits a small current to flow through the device enclosure and through the victim as in the *middle panel*. The small current is of no consequence unless a direct path to the myocardium exists. (From Horrow JC, Seitman DT. Electrical safety and device calibration. *Anesthesiol Clin North Am.* 1988;6:699.)

## How Are Grounding and Grounded Systems Used?

Grounding provides protection from shock. It results from the practice of providing a third wire, usually green, in the power cord of an appliance. This wire, connected to ground at the service entrance of a building in a fashion similar to that of the neutral conductor, attaches to those parts of each appliance that should not be part of a current path, such as the covering (*chassis*).

Should defective insulation in the hot conductor cause contact of that wire with the chassis, current completes a circuit from the power source through the hot wire to the chassis and then through the grounding wire back to the power source (Fig. 51–7). As a result, a circuit breaker or fuse then breaks the circuit.

This design supplies safety by breaking the circuit before a person can touch the chassis, inadvertently providing a path through his or her body via ground. Without the grounding wire, the device chassis sits at hot wire potential, awaiting the victim.

## Why Are All Power Cords Not Three-Pronged?

A reader may note with some bewilderment that not all marketed appliances carry a three-prong grounding power cord. Some devices constructed with plastic or insulating materials obviate a grounding wire; they may or may not feature a polarized plug, which ensures that the neutral, grounded side of the circuit never becomes the hot side by inverting the plug.

If a device carries a three-prong grounding plug, interposed "cheater plugs," which interrupt contact with the grounding receptacle (the rounded hole), pose a risk of electrocution should a fault occur from the hot wire within the device. Such interruptions degrade safety.

## Are Fuses and Circuit Breakers Effective?

Do fuses and circuit breakers provide sufficient safety? Because electrocution may occur with 100 mA, the protection afforded by a fuse that breaks the circuit at 15 A appears woefully inadequate. Partial insulation faults or current leaks within a device could provide macroshock-range currents in contact with personnel that go undetected by fuses or circuit breakers.

For situations requiring additional safety, such as bathrooms, kitchens, basements, and outdoor areas, all places where wet conditions may prevail, ground fault circuit interrupters (GFCI) furnish further protection. These devices monitor the currents flowing in the hot and grounded wires. Faulty equipment draws extra current, returning it by the grounding wire instead of the grounded wire. When the currents in the hot (*supply*) and grounded (*return*) wires differ by at least 6 mA for at least 25 ms, the GFCI breaks the circuit.[3] The isolated power supply, originally used to prevent sparks, furnishes a solution superior to that of a GFCI.

## THE OPERATING ROOM

### What Is an Isolated System?

This approach to preventing electric shock by ground pathway nullifies the grounded electrical systems—that is, provides an isolated system. Transformers isolate electric circuits easily by converting electric energy to magnetic energy. If the number of windings on each limb of a transformer is equal, the output and input voltages will be equal. Energy transfer through the transformer occurs in the absence of a contiguous path for current flow.

Figure 51–8 demonstrates the placement of an isolation transformer to isolate a power supply from ground. Current flows separately in each part of the transformer (left and right), but not between them.[6] Energy, but not current, is transferred. Notice the lack of an unbroken path from the voltage source, via ground, back to the voltage source, despite the short circuit in a device, because current does not flow from the primary to the secondary limb of the transformer.

Why not, instead, simply omit the connection between the neutral power line and ground at the service entrance? This approach would risk supplying conductors with potentially high voltage with respect to ground. The step-down utility pole transformer secondary limb would then "float" at an average potential of 2400 to 8000 V relative to ground.[2] The isolation transformer primary and secondary limbs, however, contain 120 V relative to ground because they originate from a grounded system. The secondary limb conductors are termed *line 1* and *line 2*.

Isolation of the grounded system brings both the good and the bad. True, a solitary short circuit from hot to ground becomes harmless. The defect does not cause electrocution, nor is power interrupted, a valuable feature during critical operating room procedures. Unfortunately, the fault also remains undetected because a complete circuit via ground no longer exists. Thus, faulty equipment remains in service until a fault occurs from the other conductor to ground. In this case, electrocution becomes possible, and the fuse or circuit breaker interrupts service.

Another drawback of the isolated system arises from capaci-

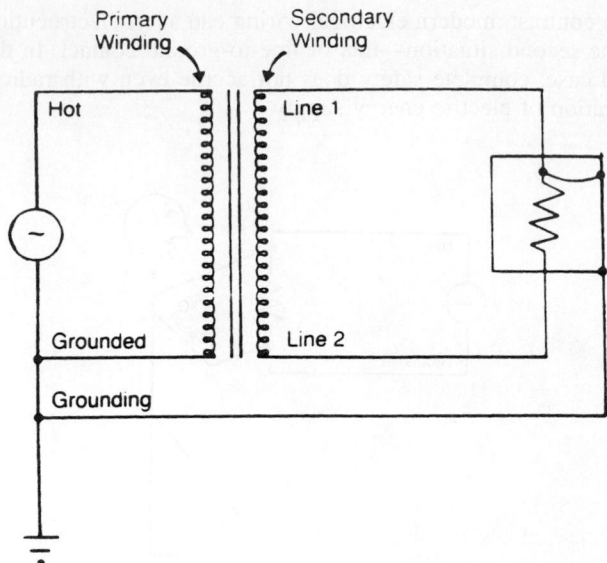

**FIGURE 51–8.** The isolated power supply. The isolation transformer permits electrical energy, but not electric current, to transfer from the primary to the secondary windings. The path beginning at the line 1 end of the secondary winding, through the device fault, and via grounding wire cannot return to the line 2 end of the secondary winding because the isolation transformer does not permit current to flow across it. Similarly, a victim touching the chassis and in contact to ground would not form part of an electrical circuit. The isolation transformer effectively ungrounds the grounded system. (From Horrow JC, Seitman DT. Electrical safety and device calibration. *Anesthesiol Clin North Am.* 1988;6:699.)

tive coupling. All equipment contains stray capacitances between the conductors and surfaces connected by grounding wires, thereby degrading the isolation. To account for these deficiencies, the isolated system also contains a special monitor that detects when a fault to ground occurs.

### What Is the Purpose of a Line Isolation Monitor and Alarm?

Should either limb of the isolated system contain a fault or leakage to ground, no current would flow because the isolation transformer negates the connection of ground to the power supply. The line isolation monitor (LIM) measures the current that would flow if the system were still grounded. This measurement is obtained by momentarily grounding line 1 and measuring the current in line 2, then grounding line 2 and measuring the current in line 1 (Fig. 51–9). An analog or digital ammeter displays this current, with an alarm sounding when it exceeds 2 mA.

To avoid nuisance alarms resulting from an accumulation of small leakage currents from the many electrically powered devices in the operating room, the National Fire Protection Association (NFPA) code increased the threshold from 2 to 5 mA in 1981. The most recent edition of the code also specifies that the monitor should not alarm for a fault current <3.7 mA, a condition not satisfied by systems with 2-mA thresholds.[7] Few clinicians, however, agree that the 2-mA level constitutes a nuisance. Thus, an LIM alarm may indicate that the last device plugged in has a serious electrical fault, or it may merely reflect "the straw that broke the camel's back"—namely, simultaneous use of many devices, each with a reasonable leakage current.

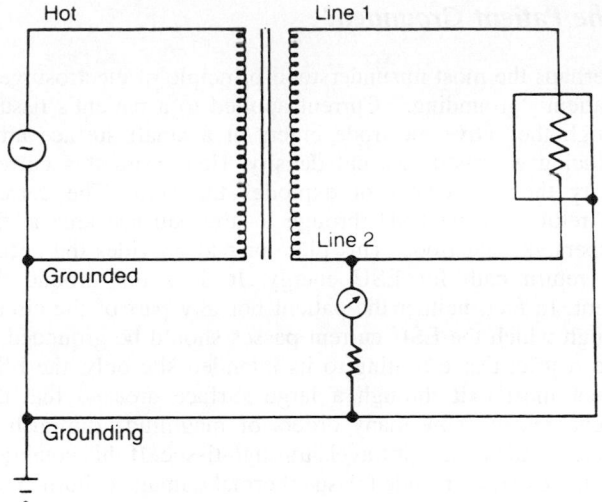

**FIGURE 51–9.** An isolated power system in which a line isolation monitor tests the current that would flow to ground from line 1 should line 2 be grounded. The ammeter displays the current that would flow back to the line 2 side of the secondary winding from the grounding conductor, whereas the series resistor limits the actual current flow. The line isolation monitor alternately tests each line by connecting its partner to ground through the ammeter, and displays the average leakage current. The current displayed does not actually flow but would flow had the isolation transformer not ungrounded the system. (From Horrow JC, Seitman DT. Electrical safety and device calibration. *Anesthesiol Clin North Am.* 1988;6:699.)

## What Are the Disadvantages and Limitations of Isolated Systems?

The isolation transformer allows a single fault to ground to occur without interrupting power or creating the potential for shock. The LIM warns of a situation that could cause electrocution or power interruption in a grounded system.

Does this isolated system with its monitor always provide protection? No system can protect from two-conductor contact (gripping line 1 in one hand and line 2 in the other). Furthermore, although the 2-mA threshold protects from macroshock (it is significantly below the 100 mA that induces ventricular fibrillation when applied across the trunk), but it is several orders of magnitude too large to protect from microshock ($\approx$100 $\mu$A).

### Thwarted Line-to-Ground Fault Detection

Some device circuit designs thwart line-to-ground fault detection. For example, if a device itself contains a transformer, it breaks the path of a complete circuit via grounding wire when a short occurs from the power line to ground. The LIM cannot detect the fault under those conditions. Devices with two-prong plugs (no grounding wires) provide no return path for stray currents to be measured by the LIM. The NFPA code (American National Standards Institutes/NFPA 99) forbids the use of two-prong devices in all patient care areas.[7]

### Expense

Expense constitutes another limitation of the isolated power supply. This factor, coupled with doubts about the need for an additional layer of electrical safety for patients and personnel, resulted in removal of the requirement for isolated power in

the NFPA guidelines. Facilities constructed after 1984 may omit isolated power in all patient care areas, including operating rooms and intensive care units. Immediate access to circuit breakers becomes imperative in the absence of an isolated system because power interruption may occur without warning in the course of critical procedures. Anesthesiologists need to know the kind of power supplied to their patient care area.

## Why Does the Isolated Power Debate Continue?

Because a grounded system cannot tolerate a single fault to ground, immediate access to replacement equipment becomes imperative. An isolated system clearly provides extra protection and should be preferred despite increasing the total cost of an operating room by approximately 1%.

Even when flammable agents became obsolete and special measures protecting from static electricity hazards such as conductive shoes and flooring disappeared, the isolated power system remained. Its final deletion from the NFPA code in 1984 occurred with great debate. The latest edition of the code requires labeling of receptacles as *grounded* or *isolated* in facilities having receptacles on isolated and grounded power.[7]

Some experts advocate continued use of isolated systems despite the NFPA code change.[10] In fact, current code requires use of GFCIs in hospitals only in established wet locations, which often do not include operating rooms or obstetric delivery areas. As a result, electric shock can (and does[11]) occur in these areas. This author implores hospitals and surgicenters to designate operating and delivery rooms as wet locations so that patients and health care workers can enjoy at least the same level of protection from electric shock afforded in their own kitchens.

Can a GFCI substitute for the isolated power supply? Although superior to the grounded system, the GFCI furnishes less protection than the isolated system: it breaks the circuit only after the hazardous current has flowed for 25 ms and then interrupts power. In contrast, the isolated system prevents that current from flowing, warns that it could flow, and maintains power all the while. For these reasons, a GFCI scheme ranks inferior to an isolated one in terms of safety.

## ELECTROSURGERY

### How Does It Work?

The industrial revolution of the late 19th century provided a substrate for many applications of alternating current that came of age in the early 20th century, including the transatlantic telegraph, transcontinental telephone service, and electrosurgery.

Initial successes in controlling surgical hemorrhage in Europe were rediscovered by the Philadelphia surgeon William L. Clark and published in 1910.[12] Independent of these events, Harvey Cushing, Surgeon-in-Chief at the Peter Bent Brigham Hospital in Boston, collaborated with the Harvard biologist and physicist William T. Bovie in an effort to control bleeding during neurosurgery. After their first operative success in 1905, the electrosurgical instrument took many years to gain

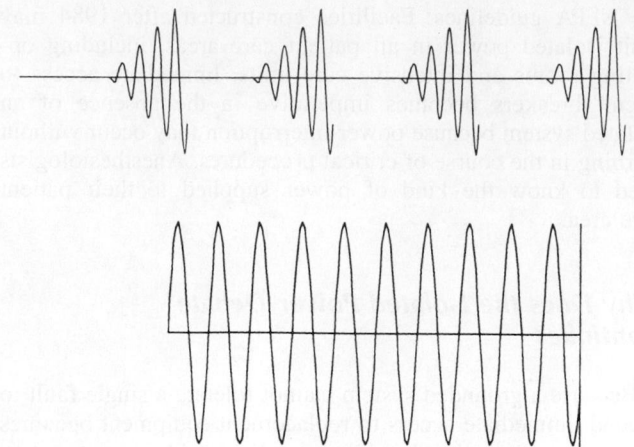

**FIGURE 51–10.** The current flowing from the electrosurgical unit during the cutting mode (*upper panel*) and during the coagulation mode (*lower panel*). The figure does not accurately reflect the actual time (<5% of a duty cycle) during which power output occurs in the coagulation mode because of artistic limitations.

popularity.[13] Electrosurgery now enjoys nearly universal application and the device has become known as the *Bovie.*

## What Is an Electrosurgical Unit?

Electrosurgery differs from electrocautery in that the latter uses electricity to heat a wire. Touching the hot wire to tissue transfers heat to the tissue. No current flows through the patient. With electrosurgery, however, the patient forms part of a circuit through which alternating current passes.

An electrosurgical unit (ESU) can cut or coagulate tissue. When tissue cutting is desired, voltage sufficiently high to generate a spark between electrode and tissue arcs into the cells. The high voltage instantly turns intracellular water to steam, exploding the cell and leaving a gap in the cellular matrix. The electrode travels on a blanket of steam, destroying cells as it moves. A continuous sinusoidal wave of constant amplitude provides the high power needed to vaporize intracellular water.[14]

## How Do Cutting and Coagulation Modes Differ?

In contrast, the coagulation mode provides electric output consisting of bursts of dampened sine waves (Fig. 51–10). These pulses are at a higher voltage, although the total power is less than that of the cutting current, because the pulsed nature of the output provides zero voltage more than 95% of the time.

Pulses of current desiccate the cells rather than exploding them. The resultant cellular debris clogs the vessels, providing hemostasis. Because desiccated cells provide higher resistance, the coagulation signal's peak voltage must be nearly twice as high as that of the continuous voltage supplied in the cutting signal.

Modern electrosurgery devices permit "blends" of cutting and coagulation waveforms, with both zero-power time and voltage increasing as the blend changes from pure cutting to pure coagulation.

## Is the Patient Grounded?

Perhaps the most misunderstood principle of electrosurgery is patient "grounding." Current applied to a patient's tissues through the active electrode enters at a small surface area, producing enormous current density. Heat from this current density then desiccates or explodes the cells. The current then returns to the ESU through a large surface area at the "dispersive" electrode. This plate or pad provides the necessary return path for ESU energy. It does not ground the patient. In fact, neither the patient nor any part of the circuit through which the ESU current passes should be grounded.

To restrict tissue heating to its intended site only, the ESU current must exit through a large surface area so that the current density, now many orders of magnitude diminished, produces little heat as it travels through tissue. If this condition does not exist, unintended tissue thermal damage ("burn") occurs.

As long as the current density remains low, high-frequency currents pass through the body without harm. In fact, D'Arsonval demonstrated nearly 100 years ago that radiofrequency current at 500 kHz can enter through one hand and power an electric light bulb held in the other.[12] These rapidly changing signals that do not confound endogenous biopotentials do not cause electrocution.

## Why Not Ground Both the Electrosurgical Unit and the Patient?

Under these circumstances, the ESU current can find many opportunities to return from the patient to the ESU: connections from patient to equipment and furniture and from equipment to ground are ubiquitous. Even though the current may be split into many paths, should a contact supply a small surface area, such as would occur with the head of the fibula touching a leg stirrup, or the back of the scalp on a conductive mattress, the resultant current density achieves sufficient intensity to burn the skin.

High-frequency signals easily form circuits by capacitive coupling; only moderate impedance exists at high frequency despite low capacitance (Fig. 51–11). High-frequency signals

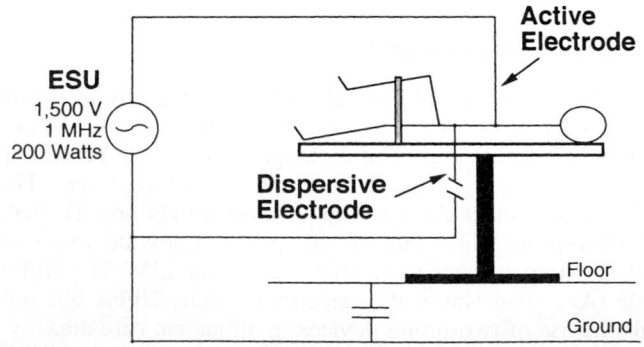

**FIGURE 51–11.** A patient undergoing surgery with the leg contacting a stirrup that is connected to ground by capacitive coupling to steel-reinforced concrete in the operating room floor. Should the dispersive electrode not supply a low-resistance path for current to return to the electrosurgery unit (ESU), current may flow from the active electrode into the patient, then out of the patient at the head of the fibula, through the stirrup, table, and floor to ground, back to the ESU. A skin burn at the contact point of the fibula results. For this reason, ESU devices with ungrounded circuits are safer.

can reach ground by traveling from the operating room table to the steel rods of the reinforced concrete of the operating room floor. Rather than grounding the patient and device, prevention of contact between patients and equipment and establishment of a reliable, dispersive electrode of large surface area maximize the current returning to the ESU through the desired dispersive electrode pathway.

### How Is Proper Dispersive Electrode Placement Verified?

Most dispersive electrodes contain not one but two wires that are connected at the pad applied to the patient. The device sends a small "interrogation" current out one wire and expects it to return on the other. If not, the wire is broken or the electrode is not plugged into the device. For this reason, the practitioner always plugs the electrode into the ESU *after* applying it to the patient. Otherwise, the device would sense electrode integrity, even though the pad may be nowhere near the patient.

A refinement of this scheme uses two separate surfaces in the dispersive electrode. The device sends a small high-frequency current into one and expects it to return from the other, traversing the patient in between. A pad connected to the device but not to the patient does not return the signal.

In yet a third attempt to prevent inadvertent tissue injury, one device compares the currents leaving and returning to the patient. If they are sufficiently different, the device shuts off current. Note that this feature mimics the operation of a GFCI. Devices provide the greatest safety by isolating the high-frequency ESU signal from ground.

### What Is a Bipolar Electrosurgical Unit?

If both active and return electrodes are placed in close proximity, the applicator is termed a *bipolar electrode*. Here, current enters through one electrode and returns to the ESU through the other, heating the tissue held between. This arrangement does not obviate a dispersive electrode, however. The tissue quickly desiccates, thus increasing the resistance of the current path enormously.

The low-resistance return path provided by a dispersive electrode prevents current from taking some unsuspected alternate pathway. Furthermore, a surgeon may not always touch both prongs of the bipolar electrode to tissue before activating the device. Finally, a bipolar electrode's return wire may have an undetected fault.

Fires,[15] shocks, and burns[16,17] ensuing from the proliferation of endoscopic surgery with monopolar electrosurgery have emphasized the safety of bipolar electrodes or use of active electrode monitoring.[18] (This same proliferation of endoscopic electrosurgery has also generated concerns regarding toxic effects of the smoke generated from electrosurgery in closed environments.[19])

### Why Are Electrosurgical Unit–Electrocardiographic Monitor Interactions Problematic?

In the past, an electrocardiographic (ECG) monitor served as a common partner with an ESU in causing unintended

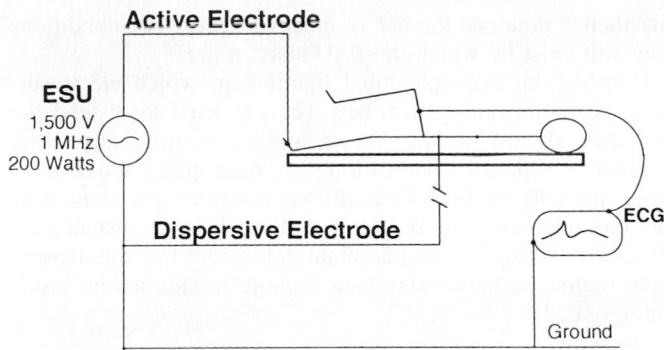

**FIGURE 51–12.** In this case, the right leg electrocardiogram (ECG) electrode provides a path to ground for electrosurgery unit (ESU) current that cannot return to the device because of a defective dispersive path. A skin burn at the electrode site results. The high-frequency ESU currents cannot be prevented by most ECG "isolated" circuits.

burns. Connection of the right leg lead of the ECG to ground explains this association: current entering a patient from the active electrode of the ESU could exit through the small surface area of the ECG electrode and return to the ESU through ground (Fig. 51–12). Early ECG designs featured circuitry to protect the ECG machine from large voltages such as defibrillating shocks. Unfortunately, these designs also provided a path for high-frequency signals through the ECG to ground.

### Do Electrocardiographic Devices With Isolated Circuits Prevent Electrosurgical Unit Burns?

Unfortunately, they do not. These isolated circuits filter out 60-Hz signals, not the radiofrequencies used in electrosurgery. When the ESU is activated, the ECG signal disappears from the monitor. It is possible to obtain ECG equipment with radiofrequency-squelching circuitry. In this way, ECG monitoring continues despite ESU use.

Even battery operation of a device does not obliterate the possibility of ESU current traveling through a device to ground. Any conductive material leading from a patient may capacitively couple to ground through mounting brackets or proximity to power cords. The most notable offenders in this category are temperature probes.[20-22]

To prevent unintended burns, the dispersive electrode should be placed over well-perfused, nonbony tissue, preferably a muscle mass. Electrodes contain a conductive gel that facilitates current flow and improves physical contact with skin. Dispersive electrodes with dried-out gel should be discarded. Never substitute ultrasound gel, which is not conductive, for the original gel.

ECG leads also require conductive gel. The same rules apply to placement of ECG electrodes as apply to placement of the ESU dispersive electrode. Failure of the latter may result in ESU current returning through the ECG electrodes. Isolated circuit ECG machines do not render safe the practice of placing ECG electrodes over bony prominences.

### How Can an Electrosurgical Unit Cause Fires?

By providing a spark, an ESU contributes one of the three requirements for a fire or explosion. Of course, flammable anesthetics preclude the use of electrosurgery. Yet, conditions may still exist by which the ESU starts a fire.[17]

Consider laparoscopic tubal ligation, in which electrosurgery closes the fallopian tubes. The gas used to distend the abdomen should not be nitrous oxide, as originally used, because it supports combustion.[23] A misapplied active electrode that cuts the bowel can release intestinal gas containing the fuel methane. Spark, fuel, and oxidizing substance all coexist, resulting in an abdominal explosion. For this reason, laparoscopic surgery today uses carbon dioxide as the insufflating gas.

## LIVING WITH PACEMAKERS

### *How Do They Work?*

Pacemakers are battery-powered devices that supply depolarizing pulses directly to the myocardium to correct or treat cardiac dysrhythmias. An external pacemaker resides outside the body, with only the wire electrodes entering the heart, usually through the vasculature. Internal pacemakers are implanted under the skin: both the device and the electrodes are physically inaccessible except when specifically approached during surgery.

Superlative engineering design has yielded reliable performance in even the most unfriendly electric environments. Sophisticated digital circuitry provides not only rhythm sensing, interpretation, and therapeutic responses but noise detection and elimination, as well as strategic responses to overwhelming interference and to battery depletion. Table 51–1 displays the code by which pacemakers are described and the common types likely to be encountered.

### Power Transmission

Battery power to permanent pacers derives from lithium cells, which last approximately 5 years. Plutonium-powered devices, popular many years ago, are now rarely used. Nuclear-powered devices undergo stringent regulatory control, and appropriately so. For example, what happens to the plutonium if the patient is cremated on death?

The wires attached to the control unit are used both to sense the endogenous rhythm (ie, provide incoming signal to the pacemaker) and pace the heart (ie, transmit the electric pulses output from the unit). Unipolar pacemakers, now uncommon, feature a single electrode to the target chamber (atrium or ventricle), using body tissues for return of current to the control unit.

With bipolar leads, two conductors terminate a few millimeters apart in the target chamber.[24] The latter arrangement eliminates much interference because the proximity of the two electrodes minimizes any potential difference between them.

### Sources of Interference

Oversensing and crosstalk are the major sources of interference in unipolar systems. Oversensing occurs when other signals such as pectoral muscle potentials (whether physiologic or succinylcholine induced) or myocardial repolarization (ECG T wave) become interpreted as the ECG R wave.

With crosstalk, an atrial stimulus sent out through an atrial electrode is sensed by the ventricular unipolar lead as an R

**TABLE 51–1.** Pacemaker Nomenclature*

| Position | Indicator | Choices |
|---|---|---|
| 1st | Chamber paced | O = none; A = atrium; V = ventricle; D = dual (A and V) |
| 2nd | Chamber sensed | O = none; A = atrium; V = ventricle; D = dual (A and V) |
| 3rd | Response to sensing | O = none; T = triggered; I = inhibited; D = dual (T and I) |
| 4th | Programmability | O = none; P = simple programmable†; M = multiprogrammable; C = communicating‡; R = rate modulation |
| 5th | Antitachydysrhythmia functions | O = none; P = pacing; S = shock; D = dual (P and S) |

*Examples*

*VOO*

Fixed-rate pacer. Used occasionally for temporary pacing.

*VVI*

Demand pacer. Stimulates ventricle when ventricular spike is not detected within set interval.

*VAT*

Atrial tracking pacer. Senses the atrium and stimulates the ventricle, thus supporting sinus rhythm with atrioventricular conduction block.

*DOO*

Fixed-rate atrioventricular sequential pacing. Often used after cardiopulmonary bypass in the absence of any intrinsic rhythm.

*DDD*

"Universal pacer." Can be set to perform most pacemaker functions, including atrial tracking.

*DDDR*

Rate-responsive pacemaker, in which the rate varies with some other input sensor, such as respiration rate, temperature, or movement. Useful to mimic the physiologic response to exercise.

*DDDMS*

An automatic implantable cardioverter/defibrillator (AICD).

*North American Society of Pacing Electrophysiology/British Pacing and Electrophysiology Group.
†Can reprogram parameters such as pulse width or atrioventricular interval.
‡Can be interrogated for summary historical rhythm and pacing data.

wave, thus inappropriately inhibiting the ventricular stimulus. Intelligent programming of the control unit easily overcomes each of these confounding influences.

### Circuit Protection

Modern pacemaker control units protect their integrated circuits from electrical harm, such as occurs when a patient receives countershock. Patients with pacemakers preferably receive countershock with the paddles applied in an anteroposterior direction rather than across the chest, so that the applied electricity is perpendicular to the plane of the electrodes.

These units effectively handle the electromagnetic interference from high-intensity electric fields such as power lines and from airport security magnetometers, microwave ovens, and automobile ignition systems. Only the ESU, with its intense radiofrequency output, can confound these clever devices. How and why this occurs is discussed after introducing the concept of the magnet.

### What Does a Magnet Do?

Historically, pacemakers began as fixed-output devices that sent pulses out at regular intervals, regardless of the underlying rhythm. Once component miniaturization permitted, the control units inhibited an output pulse when an endogenous depolarization (R wave) occurred. This process conserved battery power and obviated fibrillation from the R-on-T phenomenon.[25]

External interference that stimulated cardiac depolarization, however, would fool the control unit into inappropriately inhibiting output, resulting in cardiac asystole. The control unit design thus incorporated a safety feature: placing a magnet on the skin overlying the control unit caused the unit to revert to a fixed (VOO) mode (see Table 51–1), ensuring ventricular stimulation. (However, see later regarding magnet effects on modern pacemakers.)

For implantable defibrillators and pacemakers with this capability, a magnet disables the ability to sense lethal tachydysrhythmias. In the operating room, the feature proves both useful and hazardous.

### What Is the Impact of Electrosurgical Unit Interference?

When a patient with an implanted pacemaker becomes part of the high-voltage, high-frequency current electrosurgical circuit, the pacemaker senses enormous interference.[26] Is it imperative to use a magnet in this circumstance to prevent asystole? No, for several reasons that follow.

#### Pacing During Anesthesia

Few patients with implanted pacemakers actually depend on them during anesthesia and surgery. It is the exception rather than the rule for the pacemaker, in fact, to be pacing the patient. First, the patient is monitored to determine the underlying rhythm. A pulse oximeter or intra-arterial catheter (our modern equivalents of the traditional "finger on the pulse") is invaluable to determine the persistence of effective cardiac contraction when the ESU wipes out the monitored ECG waveform. Only asystole requires intervention.

#### Modern Pacemaker Design

Modern pacemaker design far surpasses that of older versions. Once they detect significant continuous electromagnetic interference, they automatically revert to either a fixed mode (VOO) or another specific preprogrammed mode, after pausing for several seconds in hopes that the interference will abate. Implantable defibrillators are an exception. Because they sense an ESU as a ventricular dysrhythmia, these devices *should* be disabled by programming before using an ESU. Although this approach prevents inappropriate defibrillator discharge during ESU use, it also incurs the additional hazard of disabling lethal dysrhythmia detection.

**TABLE 51–2.** How to Minimize Electrosurgical Unit–Induced Pacemaker Malfunction

Use a bipolar pacemaker.
Use a bipolar ESU.
Maintain the lowest ESU power output needed.
Keep the active electrode as remote from the pacer electrodes as possible.
Place the ESU dispersive electrode between the ESU active electrode and the pacemaker electrodes.
Limit the ESU duty cycle to bursts of several seconds of operation alternating with equal periods of inactivity.
If the ESU causes asystole, place a magnet over the control unit.
Arrange for someone to confirm intact programming following ESU exposure.

ESU, electrosurgical unit.

### Pacemaker Reprogramming

Some older pacemakers use a magnet to reprogram the unit.[27,28] Placing a magnet over the pacemaker not only induces fixed-mode VOO pacing but may direct the control unit to receive a manufacturer's password. The intense, erratic ESU radiofrequency environment could reprogram the pacemaker. Reprogramming of modern pacemakers requires information sufficiently complex to render this accidental reprogramming scenario absurdly unlikely. Nevertheless, many cardiologists recommend that patients with pacemakers undergo pacemaker evaluation after operative procedures to confirm that pacemaker programming is intact.

These considerations do not argue against preparing for the unexpected by having a magnet available, but its use usually should be avoided despite its presence.[29] ESU-pacemaker interaction can be minimized by the precautions listed in Table 51–2.

## HOW TO THINK ELECTRICALLY

### The Line Isolation Monitor Sounds— Now What?

Remember that the isolation transformer provides an added level of protection from electrical hazards. Although only one fault to ground can disable the grounded electrical system, two faults to ground are required in the isolated system. At worst, an LIM alarm indicates that the level of safety has reverted to that normally present with the grounded system.

#### What Not to Do

Most important is an understanding of what *not* to do.[30] Do not evacuate the operating room or discontinue the administration of any anesthetic gases. Indeed, surgery should not pause. Do not, under any circumstance, ground the patient, the surgeon, the anesthetist, or any other person, because that increases the risk of electrocution under any condition. Instead, think of the possible causes of the alarm.

#### What to Do

The most likely reason for an LIM alarm is recent connection to the power supply of a device with significant leakage current to ground. To verify the cause, simply unplug the last device plugged in while watching the LIM ammeter. If it drops substantially, the device is defective and should be sent for repair at the next convenient opportunity. If the device is absolutely indispensable at the moment, as would be true for a cardiopulmonary bypass machine, it should be removed for service only when doing so does not place the patient at risk. Remember, the isolated power supply protects the electric environment from this fault to ground.

A true fault to ground may not occur specifically within a device. In one case, intravenous fluid slowly leaking onto the face of a multiple-outlet extension cord triggered the LIM by shorting the power supply. Treatment involved drying the outlet and moving it away from the hazardous wet environment.

The second most likely reason for the LIM alarm is that a multitude of electrically powered devices have been plugged into a common receptacle. Although each of the devices carries an acceptable amount of leakage current, when combined they exceed the LIM threshold. In this case, the load should be redistributed among several outlets.

## How Can You Survive When the Lights Go Out?

Sudden interruption of the power supply to the operating room can be a frightening experience for all personnel. Remember, however, that almost no anesthesia machine in current use depends on electric power for delivery of a gas mixture or for hydraulic operation of the mechanical ventilator (although the ventilator timing circuits may require battery backup).

A battery backup may permit at least partial operation of monitors such as inspired oxygen concentration and ventilatory parameters. Battery backup commonly exists for independent pulse oximeters but not for integrated operating room monitors. Thus, despite loss of electric power, patient safety can be maintained. Even the anesthesia record can be continued: keep a flashlight in the drawer of the anesthesia machine.

The current NFPA code requires at least one battery-powered emergency lighting unit in every anesthetizing location.[7] Thus, total darkness will not hinder the anesthesiologist's efforts to maintain patient safety during this crisis. Are all anesthetizing locations at your facility so equipped?

## Why Does Sudden Power Loss Occur?

What causes sudden loss of power? Emergency power generators should enable recovery from global outages or an institution-wide loss of power. Because restoration of power occurs within a few minutes, drastic measures such as immediate closure of a surgical wound or postponement of surgery soon after induction of anesthesia should be avoided.

Locally, a short between conductors in a device activates the circuit breaker for that outlet, resulting in discrete power loss to a group of devices. (The isolated system prevents power interruption from a single fault to ground but not from contact of both conductors. Review Figure 51–8 to understand why.) In this case, the errant device is removed and the tripped circuit breaker reset to restore power.

## What Should Be Done When a Device Stops Working?

Even in the absence of a global or regional power failure, a device occasionally fails to work. Immediate replacement of the presumed defective device usually constitutes the first response. Unfortunately, this extreme reaction is often unnecessary. Minimal probing of the device commonly yields information that leads to prompt repair.

First, verify that failure has in fact occurred. Has the brightness to the output screen merely been adjusted too low, or has a secondary enabling switch been overlooked?

Second, turn the device off, wait a few seconds, and then turn it on again. Complex microprocessor-controlled instruments may "crash" from software malfunction. Resetting internal indicators by reapplication of power usually restores function, although at the risk of losing previously acquired data.

Finally, check the fuse. Many devices have a fuse that limits power consumption. Mechanical trespass (in whose operating room does this not occur?) can sever the delicate wire in the fuse, interrupting power to the device. Simply replacing the fuse restores function.

## SUMMARY

The household electric environment protects equipment but not people from live to ground faults. The operating room isolation transformer and LIM increase patient and personnel safety by warning of a potential fault to ground without interrupting power. The ESU cuts or coagulates tissue by purposefully making the patient part of a high-voltage, high-frequency electric circuit. Pacemakers enjoy sophisticated programming to filter out electric interference that confounds their ability to sense dysrhythmia and to restore effective cardiac function.

Knowledge of how these devices function enhances an anesthesiologist's ability to react and to direct the operating room team appropriately in an unexpected circumstance. Many readers benefit from presentation of the concepts of electrical safety and electrosurgery from multiple points of view. The author recommends that readers study specific additional materials.[30,31]

## References

1. Dripps RD, Eckenhoff JE, Vandam LD. *Introduction to Anesthesia: The Principles of Safe Practice.* 3rd ed. Philadelphia, Pa: WB Saunders; 1967:406.
2. Bruner JMR, Leonard PF. *Electricity, Safety, and the Patient.* Chicago, Ill: Year Book Medical Publishers; 1989:19.
3. Richter HP, Schwan WC. *Wiring Simplified.* 35th ed. St Paul, Minn: Park Publishing; 1986:47.
4. Geddes LA, Baker LE. Response to passage of electric current through the body. *J Assoc Adv Med Instrum.* 1971;5:13.
5. Bruner JMR. Hazards of electrical apparatus. *Anesthesiology.* 1967;28:396.
6. Swerdlow CD, Olson WH, O'Connor ME, et al. Cardiovascular collapse caused by electrocardiographically silent 60-Hz intracardiac leakage current. *Circulation.* 1999;99:2559.
7. National Fire Protection Association. *NFPA 99: Health Care Facilities.* Quincy, Mass: National Fire Protection Association; 1999:99-23.
8. Aggarwal A, Farber NE, Kotter GS, et al. Electrosurgery-induced ventricular fibrillation during pacemaker replacement: a unique mechanism. *J Clin Monit.* 1996;12:339.

9. McNulty SE, Cooper M, Staudt S. Transmitted radiofrequency current through a flow directed pulmonary artery catheter. *Anesth Analg.* 1994;78:587.

10. Bruner JMR, Leonard PF. *Electricity, Safety, and the Patient.* Chicago, Ill: Year Book Medical Publishers; 1989:310.

11. Day FJ. Electrical safety revisited: a new wrinkle. *Anesthesiology.* 1994;80:220.

12. Geddes LA. The beginnings of electromedicine. *IEEE Eng Med Biol Magazine.* 1984;3:8.

13. Cushing H. Electrosurgery as an aid to the removal of intracranial tumors: with a preliminary note on a new surgical current generator by W.T. Bovie. *Surg Gynecol Obstet.* 1928;47:751.

14. Bruner JMR, Leonard PF. *Electricity, Safety, and the Patient.* Chicago, Ill: Year Book Medical Publishers; 1989:229.

15. Lucarelli MJ, Lemke BN. Monopolar electrosurgical flash fire. *Ophthalmic Surg Lasers.* 1998;29:249.

16. Tucker RD. Laparoscopic electrosurgical injuries: survey results and their implications. *Surg Laparosc Endosc.* 1995;5:311.

17. Grosskinsky CM, Hulka JF. Unipolar electrosurgery in operative laparoscopy: capacitance as a potential source of injury. *J Reprod Med.* 1995;40:549.

18. Vancaillie TG. Active electrode monitoring: how to prevent unintentional thermal injury associated with monopolar electrosurgery at laparoscopy. *Surg Endosc.* 1998;12:1009.

19. Hensman C, Baty D, Willis RG, et al. Chemical composition of smoke produced by high-frequency electrosurgery in a closed gaseous environment: an in vitro study. *Surg Endosc.* 1998;12:1017.

20. Brock-Utne JG, Downing JW. Rectal burn after the use of an anal stainless steel electrode/transducer system for monitoring myoneural junction [letter]. *Anesth Analg.* 1984;63:1141.

21. Schneider AJL, Apple HP, Braun RT. Electrosurgical burns at skin temperature probes. *Anesthesiology.* 1977;47:72.

22. Wald AS, Mazzia VDB, Spencer FC. Accidental burns associated with electrocautery. *JAMA.* 1971;217:916.

23. Neufeld GR. Principles and hazards of electrosurgery including laparoscopy. *Surg Gynecol Obstet.* 1978;147:705.

24. Atlee JL. Cardiac pacing and electroversion. In: Kaplan JA, Reich DDL, Konstadt SN, eds. *Cardiac Anesthesia.* 4th ed. Philadelphia, Pa: WB Saunders; 1999:959.

25. Engle TR, Meister SG, Frankl WS. The "R-on-T" phenomenon: an update and critical review. *Ann Intern Med.* 1978;88:221.

26. Levine PA, Balady GJ, Lazard HL, et al. Electrocautery and pacemakers: management of the paced patient subject to electrocautery. *Ann Thorac Surg.* 1986;41:313.

27. Domino KB, Smith TC. Electrocautery-induced reprogramming of a pacemaker using a precordial magnet. *Anesth Analg.* 1983;62:609.

28. Goldberg ME, McSherry RT, O'Connor ME. Electrocautery and pacemaker reprogramming [letter]. *Anesth Analg.* 1984;63:541.

29. Shapiro WA, Roizen MF, Singleton MA, et al. Intraoperative pacemaker complications. *Anesthesiology.* 1985;63:319.

30. Horrow JC, Seitman DT. Electrical safety and device calibration. *Anesthesiol Clin North Am.* 1988;6:699.

31. Helfman SM, Berry AJ. Review of electrical safety and electrosurgery in the operating room. *Am J Anesthesiol.* 1999;26:313.

# 52

# Radiologic Procedures, Computed Tomography Scans, Magnetic Resonance Imaging, and Radiation Therapy

## Gordon L. Gibby

OPERATIONAL ISSUES

*What Are the American Society of Anesthesiologists' Guidelines for Procedures Performed in Nonoperating Room Locations?*

*What Issues Are Involved in the Preanesthetic Evaluation?*

*What Type of Team Effort Is Involved in Performing Radiologic Procedures?*

RISKS RELATED TO CONTRAST AGENTS

*How Are Contrast Agents Chosen?*

*What Effects Can Result From Injection of Iodinated Contrast Agents?*

*What Are the Mechanisms or Factors That Cause Adverse Reactions to Iodinated Contrast Agents?*

*What Can Be Done to Reduce the Risk of Untoward Reactions?*

RENAL IMPACT OF IODINATED CONTRAST AGENTS

*How Does Renal Damage Occur From Iodinated Contrast Agents?*

*What Alternative Radiographic Contrast Media Can Be Used for High-Risk Patients?*

RADIOLOGY-SPECIFIC PROCEDURES

*What Factors or Patient Conditions Require Customized Procedures?*

*What Are the Anesthesia Requirements?*

*What Is a "TIPS" Procedure?*

MAGNETIC RESONANCE IMAGING

*What Are the Magnetic Risks?*

Radiology is a dynamic and growing field of medicine. At the turn of the millennium, Margulis and Sunshine noted that in the 1995 Medicare data, 34% of radiologic imaging procedures and 73% of relative value units in radiology were in fields that were either new or only began a generation earlier.[1] These included computed tomography (CT), magnetic resonance imaging (MRI), ultrasonography, interventional radiology, and nuclear medicine. Innovations in radiology have been so tied to new computer technology that they cite Moore's Law about the continuous increase in the availability of computational hardware as pertinent to the growth of radiology.[1] Because many of these technologies require an absolutely motionless patient for either diagnosis or safe intervention, they often involve anesthesiologists as well. The key patient groups who require anesthesia for these procedures include pediatric patients, trauma or intubated intensive care unit patients, and those with claustrophobia.

When radiology and anesthesia are mixed, new issues involve the operational handling of the patient flow, impact of contrast agents, new procedures (eg, neuro-interventional, transjugular intrahepatic portosystemic stent-shunt procedures, and radiation therapy procedures), and unusual hazards from high magnetic or ionizing fields.

## OPERATIONAL ISSUES

The radiology staff, accustomed to a steady flow of conscious patients able to care for themselves without constant vigilance, may be confronted with new challenges when anesthetized patients, along with anesthesiologists, anesthesia equipment, evaluations, and consents, become part of their schedule. Anesthesiologists, likewise accustomed to the orderly flow of patient after patient through a single operating room, may find a collection of radiology cases to be a mixed blessing. The setting of the proposed procedure itself can be daunting. There may be tight quarters with radiology personnel who are not used to dealing with specialists other than radiologists and the anesthetized, and hence defenseless, patient (Fig. 52–1).

In addition, care may have to be delivered at a distance from the operating room, in areas that are not brightly lit,

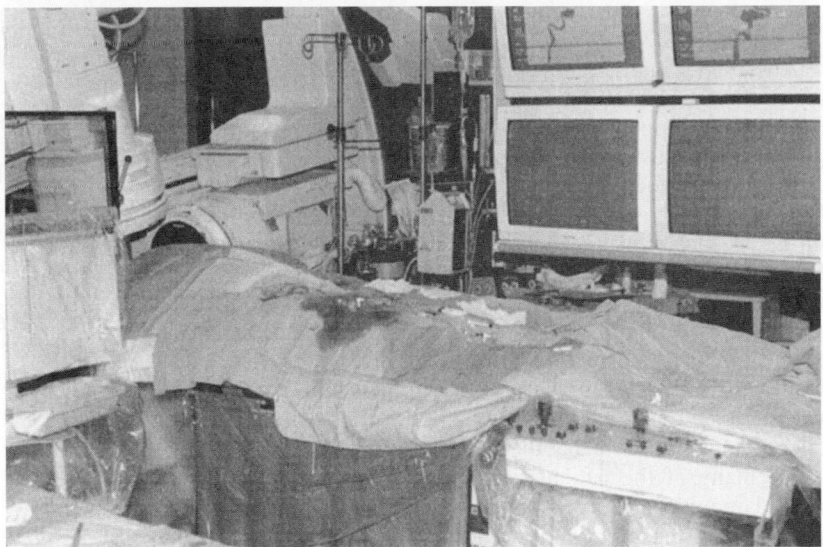

**FIGURE 52–1.** Radiology suites are often tight quarters for anesthesia equipment and personnel and may provide restricted access to the patient. In this photograph, the anesthesiologist is stationed behind the cathode ray tubes, and the patient's head is between two axis fluoroscopy cameras, an awkward reach for the anesthesiologist.

reducing the normal cues that guide anesthesiologists as to the progress of cases and instances of significant risks. Worse, the progress may only be visible on a dim monitor, understandable only by a trained radiologist and turned away from the anesthesiologist. There may be difficulty moving patients in and out of the room due to the mass and volume of the radiology equipment itself, and subsequent cases may be in different rooms, requiring movement and careful reconnection of heavy anesthesia equipment as well. Unusual patient positions, including the prone position, may be required. Furthermore, the ability to move the patient may be limited, the bed's abilities may be reduced, and few helpers may be available. Emergency access to the patient or the ability to bring in a bed and rotate a prone patient to supine may be limited.

### What Are the American Society of Anesthesiologists' Guidelines for Procedures Performed in Nonoperating Room Locations?

The American Society of Anesthesiologists (ASA) has issued guidelines that apply to nonoperating room locations. These guidelines include requirements for oxygen supplies, suction, waste anesthetic gas scavenging, self-inflating resuscitation equipment, required anesthetics and supplies, monitoring equipment to comply with the ASA Standards for Basic Anesthetic Monitoring,[2] an anesthesia machine (if inhalational anesthetics are used), sufficient electrical outlets, illumination, an immediately available defibrillator, 2-way communication, and compliance with all building and safety codes.[3]

### What Issues Are Involved in the Preanesthetic Evaluation?

The broader issues of the perioperative procedures that have contributed much to reduce risk in anesthesia are yet another problem. A comprehensive preanesthetic evaluation should be done, and informed consent for anesthesia obtained.[4] This may add an additional clinic visit to the outpatient's schedule or may be accomplished in the radiology holding area by a

mobile anesthesiologist, providing the hospital has sufficient coordination to provide all required past records to the holding area. The anesthesia consent is pivotal because for some procedures (such as MRI), there is virtually no risk other than anesthesia, nor benefit from the anesthetic alone without the radiologic imaging. Thus, to be properly informed, patients must be apprised of the benefits of imaging from their radiologists (or other physician ordering the study) and the risks of the anesthetic from an anesthesiologist.

### What Type of Team Effort Is Involved in Performing Radiologic Procedures?

To develop a successful, efficient system for providing anesthesia in the difficult environment of radiology suites requires an extraordinary commitment to quality on the part of the anesthesia department. Objective measurement of performance, including delay times, turnover times, and incidence of complications is extremely difficult to implement on an ongoing basis but is bedrock for process control (ie, the action taken to minimize variation in a process). To drive the objective measurements toward improvement will take cooperation among anesthesiologists, radiologists, and nurses. An oversight group dedicated to the improvement of anesthetic care within the radiology suites may wish to frame the quality improvement efforts in terms of the International Organization for Standardization (ISO) 9000 Quality Management System, which is used worldwide in many businesses and service systems since 1986.[5]

### Patient Education

Patient education, as required by the Joint Commission of Accreditation for Healthcare Organizations, is crucial to achieve quality and efficiency. There may already be a perioperative checklist in place documenting perioperative care including preoperative patient teaching as in the regular operating room suites. Such a system would optimally be adopted and fully used in the radiology area as well. The importance of patient preparation and insight into methods to best accomplish this goal have received considerable attention in the nursing literature.[6]

## Anesthetic Induction

Anesthetic induction may be an issue because the time required for induction reduces the throughput of expensive radiology equipment such as MRI or CT scanners. Although productivity must be considered, safety must be the primary concern. If induction occurs at a distance from the scanner for economic reasons, this will dictate the need for a transport monitor capable of meeting ASA Guidelines for Nonoperating Room Anesthetizing Locations (including capnography),[3] as well as the availability of required medications and equipment and possibly a complete second anesthesia machine and monitor setup in the destination radiology suite. Induction would ideally occur in a separate area equipped with piped gases, with privacy and full nursing support for the patient and telecommunications capability for emergency notification. Because many of the patients will be children, nursing support should include a plan for both conducting the parents to a pleasant waiting room and providing them with updates if the procedure is prolonged.

## Equipment

Each radiology suite and each major procedure type may require a different equipment setup or patient transport and monitoring plan. Written instructions and even floor markings are of great benefit.[7] Such basic issues as intravenous poles and infusion pumps may need to be addressed because anesthesia patients may have continuously running intravenous infusions far more frequently than conscious radiology patients. This becomes important for pediatric patients in whom smaller intravenous catheters are used with propofol to maintain total intravenous anesthesia; a cessation of "carrier" intravenous fluid flow could allow a patient to awaken.

## Staffing

Radiology suite staffing requires examination if quality is to be maintained. The perioperative nursing care required for an anesthetized patient is much greater than that normally required for ambulatory and conscious radiology patients. The hospital or radiology department may need to adjust their staffing to compensate. Issues such as the need for extra hands or communications in the event of an emergency during induction, maintenance, or emergence should be addressed. A chaperone, in the event that the genders of patient and anesthesiologist differ, may be required to prevent the possibility of allegations or events of abuse. Movement and positioning of anesthetized patients are familiar issues to the operating room suite but new and thus potentially challenging for the radiology area. To avoid lumbar spine injuries to professional providers, assistance in lifting patients will need to be provided. The "standard operating procedures" of the quality management expert are "clinical pathways" in nursing terminology and will greatly assist in the efficient movement of patients through the system. Effective communication with nursing resources to define the desired outcome, develop pathways, track variances, and repair problems will be of great value.[8]

## RISKS RELATED TO CONTRAST AGENTS

Just as the anesthesiologist must anticipate and treat the physiologic effects of conventional surgery, he or she must also anticipate the possible effects of one of the radiologist's most common interventions—the administration of contrast. Iodinated contrast agents (ICAs) are almost always involved if the patient is having a fluoroscopically guided intervention procedure or a CT scan, as well as some diagnostic radiographs. These agents principally affect the patient through cardiovascular effects or reactions, nephrotoxicity, or impact on coronary vasculature or coagulation.

## *How Are Contrast Agents Chosen?*

Contrast agents are chosen to have a high x-ray absorption relative to bone or soft tissue. Although gases may be used as negative contrast agents (exhibiting lower absorption), more commonly, dense substances are chosen that are relatively radiopaque compared with bone or tissue. Contrast effectiveness increases with the fourth power of the atomic number. Hence iodine, a halogen with a high atomic number (53), has traditionally been a component of radiographic contrast media because of its atomic weight and its relatively low toxicity and ease of chemical combination with organic molecules that can be excreted by the kidney. To further increase radiologic contrast while maintaining an acceptable osmolarity, multiple iodine atoms (3 atoms, for the cases of diatrizoic acid, iothalamic acid, and ipodate sodium) are covalently bound to a benzene ring as part of a complex benzoic acid or pyridone derivative. In the traditional ionic contrast, this forms the anion of a salt, with the cation potentially being sodium, calcium, magnesium, or a more complex organic molecule (eg, methylglucamine). The cation is normally unimportant in terms of physiologic impact or allergic potential, except in certain situations such as coronary angiography, where the choice of cation is made carefully to avoid arrhythmias. Only traces of iodine or iodide ion are found in solution. More than 99% of the iodine remains covalently bound to the ring, and excretion is primarily renal.[9]

## *What Effects Can Result From Injection of Iodinated Contrast Agents?*

### Cardiovascular

There are multiple cardiovascular responses resulting from the injection of ICAs. These may become severe and be considered reactions. ICAs are typically hypertonic, some exceeding 1000 mOsm/L. Rapid injection of hypertonic solutions are known to cause a brief hypertensive effect, followed by mild hypotension, with a decrease in systemic vascular resistance. Extracellular fluid will be drawn intravascularly by the increase in blood osmolarity—as much as 10%—leading to decreases in hematocrit of as much as 15%. Sickling is a risk in susceptible individuals who should be well hydrated before the administration of contrast media. Patients with multiple myeloma are at significant risk for renal damage related to proteinuria and potential dehydration. The resulting diuresis brought about after the glomerular filtration of the agent can also subsequently cause significant hypovolemia.[10]

Contrast agents compete for protein binding sites and may increase the effect of protein-bound drugs, thereby potentiating thiobarbiturates, warfarin, or isoniazid.[9]

Intravenous ionic contrast agents induce seizures in approximately 0.01% of the general population. In patients with a metastatic brain tumor, 15% may seize, and in those with a glioma, 16%. Five milligrams of intravenous diazepam, administered (over ~1 minute) immediately before the contrast agent has been found to greatly reduce, but not eliminate, the risk of contrast medium–induced seizures in both of these patient groups.[11]

## What Are the Mechanisms or Factors That Cause Adverse Reactions to Iodinated Contrast Agents?

There is a wide range of mechanisms responsible for adverse drug reactions to ICAs, including histamine release, complement activation, antibody-based true allergic response, increased sympathetic or parasympathetic tone, and anxiety. Many patients experience chills, fever, facial flushing, and slight mental status change described as a "peculiar feeling." Histamine levels may rise in 40% of patients, yet not all may consciously experience a reaction. Histamine-induced reactions may result in urticaria from disruption of normal capillary permeability. Anaphylactoid shock may begin as oral, lingual, and pharyngeal edema, followed by upper airway obstruction and bronchospasm with extremely difficult ventilation; death may result. Complement activation may occur in 63% of patients. This can result in degranulation of mast cells and basophils, releasing histamine and resulting in increased vascular permeability and its sequelae. Anaphylotoxin and chemotactic activators may be released, cell membranes disrupted, and thrombin activated; these effects may progress to anaphylactoid shock.[9]

### Allergic Reactions

Because of their small molecular weight, contrast media can only cause true antibody-mediated allergic reactions when they function as haptens. Both immunoglobulin G (IgG) and IgE antibodies have been produced in experimental animals using carrier proteins and ICAs. Patients may have been exposed to previous complex organic molecules that have similarities to the hapten protein, resulting from injection of contrast agents, and manifest an allergic response on their first usage. It has been difficult to correlate reactions with antibody-mediated allergic responses, both in the laboratory and in clinical practice. Further, patients sometimes fail to re-express the reaction on repeated treatments even without immunosuppressive pretreatment.[9]

### Central Nervous System

It is believed that many reactions are based on central nervous system toxicity because iodinated agents can cross the blood-brain barrier. Their intercisternal lethality is approximately 1000 times greater than intravenous, causing pulmonary edema and cardiac arrest. Sodium diatrizoate injected into the cerebrospinal fluid is well known for causing seizures in low doses. ICAs within the hypothalamus may cause fever or chills. Direct stimulation of the chemoreceptor trigger zone may explain the nausea and vomiting. Vagal stimulation through the hypothalamus, capable of causing bronchospasm and bradycardia, has been implicated in some reactions.[9]

### Patient History

The incidence of systemic reactions when ICAs are used is approximately 5% to 8%; most are mild. Intravenous cholangiography has twice the rate of reaction as excretory urography, which has twice the rate of intravenous angiography. Slower infusions lead to reduced incidences of reactions. A history of an allergy or atopic disease raises the risk severalfold. A 15% incidence of reaction was found in patients with a history of allergy to seafood or shellfish; asthmatics have an 11% incidence of reaction. Patients with a previous reaction may have a repeat risk from 17% to 35%, although some have no reaction. Patients with cardiac disease have both a more severe reaction and a 4 to 5 times higher incidence of reactions. Using <20 g of iodine results in a lower risk of reaction.[9]

## What Can Be Done to Reduce the Risk of Untoward Reactions?

### Testing

Patients with a known history of reaction or at high risk (based on allergic, atopic, or cardiac history) may be pretreated to reduce, but not eliminate, the risk. Skin and intradermal testing to determine if pretreatment is advised are considered useless. Intravenous testing may be more reliable but has significant risk.

There is benefit to simply pretreating patients who are at high risk. Prednisone, 150 mg, in divided doses was used in one study from 18 hours before to 12 hours after the study. Diphenhydramine alone may actually increase the incidence of minor reactions and is best combined with steroids.[9]

Once a reaction has occurred, the treatment is graded based on severity. The most common reactions—flushing, nausea, urticaria—are handled easily with reassurance by the radiologist or anesthesiologist if the patient is conscious. In darkened rooms with anesthetized patients, these cues will commonly be missed. The more severe reactions of bronchospasm and anaphylactoid shock require skillful treatment. Adrenergic agonists such as epinephrine (bolus or infusion), methylxanthines (eg, a loading dose of aminophylline) to treat bronchospasm, anticholinergics (atropine), antihistamines, steroids, and fluids will normally be considered and should be immediately available.[9] A sample protocol is given in Table 52–1.

## RENAL IMPACT OF IODINATED CONTRAST AGENTS

### How Does Renal Damage Occur From Iodinated Contrast Agents?

#### Renal Insufficiency and Failure

One of the well-known risks of ICAs is new onset or worsening of renal insufficiency or failure. ICAs are a leading cause of hospital-acquired acute renal failure.[12] Because we have so few easily obtainable measures of the complex function of kidneys, there is disagreement as to what constitutes failure or insufficiency, making it difficult to define the exact risk to a patient undergoing an ICA study. Isolated measurements of serum creatinine may vary substantially. The serum

**TABLE 52–1.** Treatment of Contrast Agent Reaction in Adults*

**Urticaria**

1. No treatment is required in most cases.
2. For $H_1$ receptor blockade, administer diphenhydramine PO/IM 50 mg of hydroxyzine PO/IM 25-50 mg; may add $H_2$ receptor blockade (eg, ranitidine).
3. If severe or widely disseminated, administer epinephrine SC (1:1000) 0.1-0.3 mL, if no cardiac contraindication.

**Facial/Laryngeal Edema**

1. Administer epinephrine SC (1:1000) 0.1-0.3 mL or, if SC route fails or if peripheral vascular collapse, then slowly IV (1:10 000) 1.0-3.0 mL.
2. Supply oxygen.
3. If patient has significant difficulty breathing, call for code assistance.

**Bronchospasm**

1. Supply oxygen; monitor pulse oximeter, BP, and ECG.
2. Administer epinephrine SC (1:1000) 0.1-0.3 mL or β-agonist inhalers (eg, albuterol). If SC route fails or if peripheral vascular collapse, then epinephrine slowly IV (1:10 000) 1.0-3.0 mL.
   Consider additional therapy: aminophylline 6 mg/kg IV over 10-20 min (loading dose) then 0.4-1.0 mg/kg/h prn; or terbutaline 0.25-0.5 mg IM/SC. If severe bronchospasm, call for code assistance.

**Hypotension With Tachycardia**

1. Put patient in Trendelenberg position. Monitor ECG, pulse oximeter, BP.
2. Supply oxygen.
3. Rapidly administer large volumes of isotonic lactated Ringer's solution (or similar).
4. If patient is poorly responsive, add IV therapy with epinephrine.

**Hypotension With Bradycardia (Vagal Reaction)**

1. Put patient in Trendelenberg position.
2. Supply oxygen; protect or secure airway.
3. Secure IV access, atropine 0.6-1.0 mg IV (if IV access is delayed, administer IM).
4. Monitor vital signs, repeat atropine up to 2.0 mg total dose.
5. Rapidly administer large volumes of isotonic lactated Ringer's solution (or similar).

**Seizure**

1. Supply oxygen.
2. Protect or secure airway.
3. Consider diazepam 5.0 mg or midazolam 2.5 mg IV.
4. If longer effect is needed, consider phenytoin 15-18 mg/kg administerd at 50 mg/min maximum.
5. Carefully monitor vital signs.

*Dosage adjustments will be required in children or small adults.
BP, blood pressure; ECG, electrocardiogram; $H_1$, histamine$_1$; $H_2$, histamine$_2$; IM, intramuscular; IV, intravenous; PO, by mouth; prn, as required; SC, subcutaneous.

creatinine is inversely related to the glomerular filtration rate so that small changes in creatinine may actually result from large decreases in filtration if the baseline creatinine was numerically small. Depending on the definition used, the frequency of renal damage caused by ICAs may reach 41% for patients with preexisting renal insufficiency.

There is no clear explanation of how this damage occurs. After the administration of ICA, there is an initial short-term rise in renal blood flow, followed by a much longer lasting decrease that slowly returns to baseline. Histologically, vacuolization in the glomerular tubules may be observed. Proteinuria may also occur. Medullary ischemia appears to result from decreased renal blood flow due to an alteration in the balance of vasodilating and vasoconstricting factors. In an animal model, histamine release is triggered by ionic contrast agents and appears to be the cause of a portion of renal segmental arterial vasoconstriction. A portion of the vasoconstriction can be blocked by diphenhydramine.[12] There may be multiple causes and risk factors. Even release of cholesterol

microemboli has been implicated.[13] The administration of theophylline may reduce the nephropathy associated with both iodinated and non-iodinated agents.[14] Atrial natriuretic peptide has not been found helpful in reducing renal injury when administered to patients with preexisting renal insufficiency.[15]

## Higher and Lower Osmolarity Agents

Older ICAs are extremely highly osmolar substances. Examples include diatrizoate meglumine 60% = 1400 mOsm/kg and diatrizoate meglumine 76% = 2016 mOsm/kg (Hypaque 60% and Hypaque 76%, respectively). In an attempt to reduce nephrotoxicity, manufacturers have pursued 2 fronts of new ICAs: lower osmolarity (LO) ionic agents and lower osmolarity non-ionic (LONI) agents. The ionic agents came first; osmolarity was reduced by enlarging the organic anion to include an additional ring capable of holding more iodine atoms. Although initially much more expensive, these newer, LO agents were tolerated by awake patients much better, with noticeably reduced pain on injection.[16] Histamine release is implicated in renal artery vasoconstriction, which is worse with ionic contrasts and less with the non-ionic agents.[12]

In two basic studies, LO agents exhibited lower amounts of renal artery constriction than older, higher osmolarity (HO) agents (Table 52–2). Phosphodiesterase inhibitors reduce renal artery constriction, which is generally worse with ionic contrast agents as compared with non-ionic agents. Inhibition of subtypes II and IV is most effective.[17]

The reduced pain on injection also raised hopes of reduced nephrotoxicity. Older HO agents were compared with the newer ionic, LO agents. Lautin and colleagues analyzed the renal function outcomes of patients undergoing femoral angiography.[18] For patients with normal baseline creatinine, the LO agents were statistically superior, resulting in a lower risk of renal damage, using 1 of the 6 renal deterioration criteria; however, trends were shown in 2 others. They concluded that it was not clear that the increased expense of LO agents was justified in patients with initially normal renal function. In all diabetic patients (both with and without preexisting renal insufficiency), LO agents had a lower incidence of renal damage than HO agents by all criteria, but there was no statistical significance. Diabetics with an elevated baseline creatinine showed a significantly increased risk for HO agent contrast-induced nephropathy for 5 of 6 criteria. For patients with a preexisting renal insufficiency denoted by an elevated initial creatinine, a statistically significant increased risk was shown for 3 of 6 criteria. Thus, although LO agents did not eliminate the risk of radiocontrast-induced renal damage, they

**TABLE 52–2.** Examples of Iodinated Contrast Agents

| Agent | Osmolarity (mOsm/kg) |
|---|---|
| *Traditional Agent* | |
| Diatrizoate meglumine 60% (Hypaque Meglomine 60%) | 1400 |
| *Ionic Lower Osmolarity Agents* | |
| Ioxaglate meglumine 320 (Hexabrix) | 600 |
| *Non-Ionic Lower Osmolarity Agents* | |
| Iohexol 300 (Omnipaque) | 672 |
| Iodixanol (Vispaque) | Iso-osmolar |

are indicated in patients with increasing degrees of renal insufficiency.[18]

Newer, non-ionic agents, also with lower osmolarity than the traditional agents, have been developed, although with even greater initial costs than the LO ionic agents. With these LONI agents, as well as with the LO ionic agents, pain and discomfort were reduced using the same amount of iodine (same radiopacity for studies). Both ionic and non-ionic agents are dialyzable, but the latter agents may be removed more quickly.[19] Animal[20] and in vitro[21] studies have suggested that renal damage is minimized by the use of non-ionic contrast agents. Both LO ionic and non-ionic agents demonstrated a reduction in incidence and severity of renal vasoconstriction and proteinuria, hemodynamic alteration, myocardial depression, and neurotoxicity in the case of an altered blood-brain barrier.[22, 23] They are certainly better than older HO ionic agents.[24] Iso-osmolar non-ionic agents in laboratory research have lower damage potential than LO agents.[25] Non-ionic agents effect less damage than those of approximately the same osmolarity, although there may be little clinical difference.[25, 26] Differences may be kept to a minimum with adequate hydration.[27] Reductions in costs for non-ionic agents have led to widespread use.

## Hydration

Hydration is probably the most important factor in reducing the risk of renal damage as a result of ICAs under the control of the anesthesiologist. It may be of approximately the same benefit as the switch from an HO agent to a LO agent. Solomon and associates showed that in patients with preexisting renal insufficiency (defined as serum creatinine exceeding 1.6 mg/dL or a creatinine clearance below 60 mL/min), the addition of half-normal saline infusions at 1 mL/kg of body weight per hour beginning 12 hours before scheduled angiography (using either HO or LO agents) and for 12 hours after had a lower rate of worsened *renal performance* (defined as an increase in serum creatinine concentration of at least 0.5 mg/dL within 48 hours of radiocontrast) than identically hydrated patients who additionally received either furosemide or mannitol as well.[28] The group with hydration alone had an 11% incidence of worsened renal damage compared to Lautin's observed 14% risk of a 0.3 mg/dL rise on day 1 or 2 for patients with preexisting renal damage, with LO agents, and the roughly 40% risk for patients receiving HO agents.[18]

The study by Solomon and coworkers has been criticized in that the patient receiving furosemide or mannitol may have been unexpectedly intravascularly depleted (due to the fixed hydration protocol).[28] Stevens and colleagues reported the results of the Prevention of Radiocontrast Induced Nephropathy Clinical Evaluation (PRINCE) study in which an attempt was made to maintain intravascular volume in patients with a baseline creatinine >1.8 mg/dL.[29] Half-normal saline was administered at 150 mL/h on arrival at the catheterization laboratory and continued throughout the procedure for 6 hours, followed by hourly adjustments to match the prior hours of urine output until 24 hours after the procedure. Patients were given furosemide as a single dose, 1 mg/kg (maximum 100 mg), and intravenous dopamine, 3 μg/kg/min. There was no statistical difference in the creatinine of patients treated with or without the medications. However, the degree of induced diuresis was predictive of the rise in serum creatinine; patients with urine flow rates >150 mL/h in the postprocedure period had a 21.6% rate of renal injury versus 45.9% ($P = .03$) in those with <150 mL/h.[29]

## Anticoagulation and Coronary Vasculature

Although primarily of concern during interventional cardiovascular procedures, the coagulation and coronary vasodilation-vasoconstriction effects of contrast media are important factors to anesthesiologists. The traditional HO ICAs are known to have significant anticoagulant properties. Non-ionic, LO contrast agents are weaker anticoagulants than LO ionic contrast agents; however, they do not increase the risk of thrombotic complications. Non-ionic iso-osmolar agents reduce the risk of reactions in patients undergoing coronary interventions compared to LO ionic agents.[30–32] In 1999, one non-ionic ICA, iopipiderol, was reported to have considerable anticoagulant impact. In vivo rat tests showed a prolongation of the activated partial thromboplastin time (aPTT) and thrombin time, with the aPTT prolonged significantly greater than for ioxaglate, an ionic contrast agent. There was no impact on the prothrombin time (PT). Platelet aggregation was also inhibited at clinically relevant concentrations. These effects would be beneficial during angioplasty, coronary angiography, and potentially interventional neuroradiology and appear to be local rather than systemic.[33] The systemic antiplatelet effects of aspirin far outweigh the impact of either the ionic agent, meglumine metrizoate, or the non-ionic agent, iohexol, in cerebral angiography.[34]

Although an older, high osmolarity ionic ICA would be expected to cause vasodilation when used for coronary angiography, a newer LO ionic agent (ioxaglate meglumine [Hexabrix] 320 mg/mL) was found not to change coronary dimensions. A non-ionic dimer iodixanol and iopromide exert vasodilation on normal coronary arteries with slight vasoconstriction on segments near coronary artery disease. The vasodilation of the non-ionic agents is blocked by cyclooxygenase inhibition by indomethacin (suggesting it may be mediated by prostacyclin) but not by an inhibitor of nitric oxide (indicating it is not mediated by nitric oxide). Because both a normal osmolar, non-ionic agent and a 770 mOsm/kg non-ionic agent had the same impact, it appears to be the chemical structure rather than the osmolarity that is causing these findings.

## *What Alternative Radiographic Contrast Media Can Be Used for High-Risk Patients?*

### Gadopentetate Dimeglumine

There are at least two alternatives to ICAs for patients with peripheral angiography and renal insufficiency. Kaufman and colleagues noted that gadopentetate dimeglumine (Magnevist) 0.5 mmol/mL, a gadolinium-based contrast agent developed for MRI, had no adverse impact on renal function in patients with renal insufficiency.[35] Although it is far less radiopaque than ICAs, with the added sensitivity of digital subtraction angiography (70 kilovolt [peak] [kVp], 6 mA) and with multiple injections of 10 mL of a 50:50 mixture of gadopentetate dimeglumine (undiluted osmolarity 1960 mOsm/kg) with normal saline, it has been used successfully. A total dose of 80 mL was used (~0.25 mm/kg). The cost of gadopentetate dimeglumine is approximately 4 times that of low osmolar contrast material which, in itself, is much more expensive than high contrast material.

## Carbon Dioxide

Carbon dioxide ($CO_2$), a negative contrast agent, is another appealing alternative for studies in patients at high risk for nephrotoxicity. In 1982, Back and colleagues described the use of intra-arterial $CO_2$ gas for peripheral angiography.[36] The mechanism is the forced replacement of blood by $CO_2$ gas, which has low viscosity and is compressible and able to fill most vessels. The method became successful with the availability of digital subtraction angiography and digital enhancement, which allowed the negative contrast effect to adequately delineate vessels. It actually has an advantage for displaying small distal vessels that the vascular surgeon may wish to use for runoff. A special syringe and care must be used to avoid the accidental insufflation of air; syringes of $CO_2$ left uncapped will relatively rapidly become filled with air. A bag-valve system has been developed that makes it much more difficult to accidentally insufflate air. Because $CO_2$ is extremely soluble in blood, and bubbles disappear quickly, there is a low risk of "vapor lock" in the right heart. However, it is not advised for studies above the diaphragm. With proper usage, there is no renal toxicity, and it is inexpensive,[36] although there can be some patient discomfort.[37] A small amount of iodinated contrast material or gadodiamide may, in some cases, be used to supplement the $CO_2$.[38]

## RADIOLOGY-SPECIFIC PROCEDURES

### What Factors or Patient Conditions Require Customized Procedures?

#### Intracranial Aneurysms

Intracranial aneurysms occur in as much as 2% of the population; the incidence of subarachnoid hemorrhage is 1 per 10 000 annually. Mortality is roughly 50%, due either to hemorrhage or vasospasm, occurring in 20% to 50% of cases. The rebleeding rate of a ruptured aneurysm, if left untreated, is approximately 4% in the first 24 hours and 19% in the first 2 weeks.

#### Treatment

The ideal treatment is to remove the aneurysm from the blood circulation as soon as possible; this avoids rebleeding and allows aggressive management of vasospasm with techniques that raise the blood pressure (BP) and cardiac output. Although surgical clipping of the aneurysm has been the treatment of choice, since the early 1980s, endovascular techniques have been gaining favor, beginning with patients whose aneurysms were less favorable for surgical treatment. Endovascular techniques were approved for use in surgically difficult aneurysms in September 1996.[39] Detachable balloons were the first of these and were used first to occlude the parent vessel and later to pack the aneurysm itself, resulting in aneurysm thrombosis. Subsequent recanalization of the lumen was a problem.

#### Guglielmi Detachable Coil

The development of the electrically detachable platinum coil (Guglielmi detachable coil [GDC]) has revolutionized endovascular treatment. The platinum GDC is soldered to a stainless steel delivery wire. Electrolysis induced by a small electrical current of only a milliampere or two, for a period of several minutes, is used to detach the platinum coil from the delivery wire at a relatively thin, exposed point. The coil itself is made of fine wire (typically 0.05 mm platinum) wound into a primary coil of approximately 0.375 mm diameter and a length of several centimeters. This coil is then re-coiled, with a diameter from 2 to 20 mm and a length of several millimeters to a few centimeters. When retracted into a delivery catheter, the tertiary structure straightens but remembers its circular memory and, when slid back out, resumes its tertiary structure, allowing it to remain packed in a ball once placed into the aneurysm sac (Fig. 52–2). Patients are usually heparinized for the duration of the procedure and given aspirin daily afterwards to avoid unwanted clotting elsewhere. Spasm of an intracranial vessel during or following deployment of a coil may be treated with papaverine (typically 60 mg) and possibly recombinant thromboplastin activator (eg, 15 mg). Usually, a large initial coil is placed so that several loops span the aneurysm neck, and then additional coils are placed within this basket. Neck size of the aneurysm is important in predicting the results. Wide necks predispose to recanalization after coil compaction over time inside the aneurysmal sac. Poor outcomes potentially include (1) underpacking of the aneurysm; (2) recanalization of lysed clot within the sac, allowing changes in architecture of the coils; and (3) reversion of the coils from the basket, allowing movement and potentially a portion of a coil to project from the aneurysm into the parent vessel or down the parent vessel.

### Complications

Complications include rupture of the aneurysm, in which case heparinization of the patient is reversed and clotting will (hopefully) occur rapidly. Conversely, microthrombi may result in some patients from the use of the guiding catheter

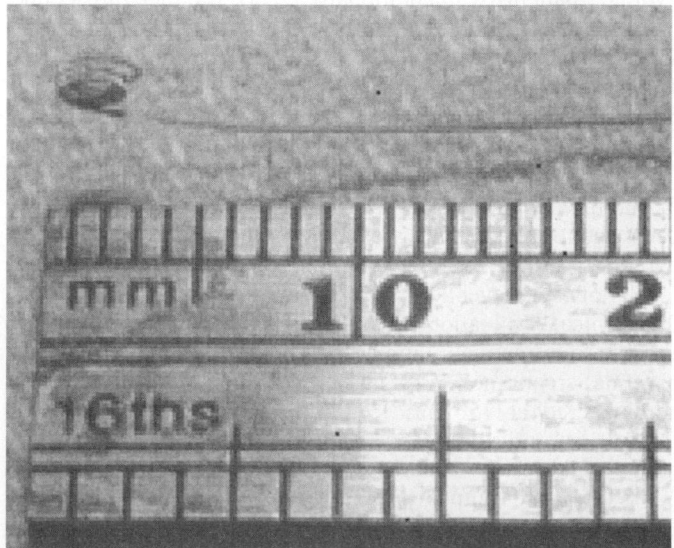

**FIGURE 52–2.** Close-up view of 3 mm Guglielmi detachable coil beside millimeter ruler. When extended from the sheath, the coil assumes its tertiary shape, as shown. The detachment site is not clearly visible but is just proximal to the coil. More than a dozen of these coils may be placed within one aneurysm.

and lead to neurologic outcomes such as a hemianopsia and hemiparesis. Post-procedure migration of a coil strand is considered most likely with middle cerebral artery (MCA) aneurysm where vessels arise at the base of the aneurysm. In one case,[40] right hemiparesis and dysphasia resulted 15 minutes after normal awakening from anesthesia, with a later extensive MCA territory infarct caused by migration of one of the coils into the MCA and anterior cerebral artery (ACA) with severe blood flow compromise. The mortality rate of the procedure in the first 200 cases was 1.5% but has decreased as the pool of patients has expanded to include those with initially more favorable neurologic status.[39, 40]

The success of the GDC endovascular system for treatment of intracranial aneurysms has begun to raise the issue of whether it is the treatment of choice for incidentally discovered aneurysms that have not yet ruptured. Endovascular treatment has low morbidity and mortality rates, which appear to be independent of location. It requires light general anesthesia or sedation and temporary heparinization. Hospital stays are approximately 3 days.

By contrast, the natural outcome of untreated aneurysms is poor, and worsens with larger aneurysms. Surgical treatment incurs a high risk and longer duration of stay, particularly with larger aneurysms. Patients with posterior circulation aneurysms may be particularly poor surgical candidates, with many "eloquent" perforating arteries and a requirement to manipulate cranial nerves to reach posterior fossa aneurysms. Advanced age and poor medical condition also may increase the risk of operative morbidity. In a series of 115 patients with 120 incidentally found aneurysms, complete or near complete occlusion by GDC endovascular treatment was achieved in 91% and was unsuccessful in only 5% of these patients; 94.8% remained neurologically intact or unchanged, and only 4.3% deteriorated. There were no deaths due to treatment, although one patient in severe symptomatic vasospasm developed a postangioplasty intraparenchymal hemorrhage and died. These results are comparable to the best expectations of surgical treatment.[41]

## Sedation and General Anesthesia

Sedation or general anesthesia may be required. Patients may become uncomfortable when placed for a long period of time on hard radiology tables which may not be as padded as operating room tables. Radiologists depend on near-motionless positioning of the head; if sedation is used, consider using tape to stabilize the forehead position. Perform a careful neurologic assessment before treatment of the patient and monitor oxygenation, ventilation, electrocardiograph, noninvasive BP (and possibly invasive BP), heart rate, and temperature. At times, the neuroradiologist may want higher BP due to concern about risk to parent vessel flow. This can be accomplished with a phenylephrine infusion (10 mg/250 mL saline titrated to effect). It is probably wise to avoid nitrous oxide to minimize the impact of any inadvertent introduction of air into the cerebral arterial circulation. If sedation is chosen, vigilance is required to detect the rare neurologic catastrophe with an abrupt change in mental status and the possibility of a respiratory or cardiac arrest. If a general anesthetic is used, be certain to assess mentation, strength, gag protection of the airway, and the possibility of ischemic stroke before extubation. In positioning the patient, check that the arm holders and other accessory equipment are adequately strong. Avoid being positioned too far from the patient.

If the femoral cannula is to be removed, keep the patient still for some time to allow clot to form. This may be done with the patient still anesthetized. If the cannula is to remain in place, the patient may be transported to the ICU.

## Intracranial Arteriovenous Fistulas

Arteriovenous fistulas (AVFs) of cranial vessels are rare. Causes include congenital and traumatic factors. Dural fistulas may be formed by phlebothrombosis. The size of the shunt determines whether they are high or low flow. If the flow is large, they may result in an arterial steal phenomenon with cerebral hypoperfusion. Increased flow in the cerebral veins results in increased intracranial pressure, headaches, bruit, tinnitus, or vertigo. If the cavernous sinus is the outflow tract, proptosis and chemosis are possible. Surgical clipping is being replaced by endovascular treatment. Detachable balloons, via the transarterial route, have been the usual treatment for traumatic carotid-cavernous fistula and vertebral AVF. When the orifice of the fistula or the venous compartment is small, it may be difficult to guide a balloon into such a position that the fistula can be occluded with preservation of the feeding artery. Moreover, the arterial route risks occlusion of the arterial anastomosis to the brain.

Often, there are multiple curved feeding arteries to the fistula, also making access difficult. Venous access is therefore safer. As a result, the transvenous approach with microcoil obstruction of dural fistulas is now the standard. Electrolytically detachable GDC coils can be used to occlude the fistula, with one study reporting 79% complete occlusions. The advantage of the GDC technique is that the coil can be placed multiple times until an ideal placement has been achieved before release. Coils are, however, less space-filling than balloons, and can result in incomplete occlusion if dense packing is not possible. They are also expensive; hence in some cases, the expensive detachable coils are used to build a "basket," which is then filled with less expensive microcoils.

Incomplete occlusion occurs in some cases. If the arterial wall is severely lacerated from trauma, it may be impossible to place any embolic material (either balloon or coil) in the cavernous sinus and preserve the internal carotid artery; this may require sacrifice of the internal carotid artery. Surgery may still be required in some cases in which the access is too tortuous or the vessels too small.[42]

## Arteriovenous Malformations

Endovascular treatment has become one of the recommended presurgical steps in the treatment of intracranial arteriovenous malformations (AVMs). When left untreated, the risk of hemorrhage is significant, perhaps 3% to 4% per year, with a mortality of 67%. Surgery also has considerable risk; one report demonstrated an overall mortality of 11%, rising to perhaps 25% in patients with large or deeply placed AVMs.

The alternative of radiosurgery is considered relatively safe but has a significant risk of radiation necrosis and a risk of bleeding until the nidus is obliterated.[43] Endovascular treatment may allow reduction of flow in the AVM before either surgery or radiosurgery by instillation of polyvinyl alcohol, silk, cyanoacrylate glues, or other agents. Cyanoacrylates have the longest lasting reduction of flow.[44]

Schumacher and Horton treated 35 patients with polyvinyl alcohol and, in some patients, also used silk, coils, Gelfoam, or detachable balloons.[45] In over half the patients, one third or more of the AVM can be obliterated. Two of 35 patients had subarachnoid and parenchymal bleeding; although the source could not be determined, it is assumed to be caused by vessel perforation after guidewire manipulation. Eight of 35 patients developed a mild to moderate neurologic deficit, with persistence in 3 of 35 (8.6%).

The development of neurologic deficits cannot be predicted based on the size or location of the tumor; they appear to be more related to the technique itself.[47] Given the high incidence of deficits, anesthesiologists should either secure the airway or be prepared to do so quickly, and the patient evaluated for neurologic status before extubation. If cyanoacrylates are used, the radiologist may need to rapidly remove the delivery catheter to prevent it becoming glued into the patient; this is usually a dramatic moment. In such patients, motion must be absolutely prevented, and relaxation is a wise choice.

## Intracranial Tumors

Hypervascular skull base tumors, including juvenile nasopharyngeal angiofibromas, glomus tumors, and hemangiopericytomas may be treated by direct tumor puncture and injection of glue (Histoacryl; Braun, Melsungen, Germany). However, there is a significant risk of glue extruding into undesired vessels. Casasco, in 1999, reported 2 cases out of 65 lesions where severe complications occurred; in one, a small portion entered the right internal carotid artery and polymerized in the right MCA, resulting in acute stroke and subsequent death. In the other, reflux into a collateral vessel reached the ophthalmic artery, resulting in acute loss of vision in one eye.[46] Anesthesiologists should be alert for sudden changes in consciousness in such cases. Guglielmi developed a crescent form of the GDC suitable for placement into the cavernous and petrous branches of the internal carotid artery that feed skull-based tumors, typically impossible to catheterize for placement of any other type of embolic agent because of their small size.[47] One or more of the crescent-shaped detachable coils can be inserted to embolize the tumor. This type of coil avoids the risk of reflux of embolic agents into the mainstream of the internal carotid artery.[47]

## Endovascular Treatment of Vasospasm

Endovascular techniques have some promise in the treatment of vasospasm, the dreaded complication of subarachnoid hemorrhage. Anesthesiologists may be called to assist because of complicated monitoring of hyperdynamic circulatory therapy used in such patients or due to a degraded mental status, which necessitated intubation. Angioplasty has been effective in treating vasospasm in large proximal cerebral vessels but is unable to reach smaller vessels, such as those distal to the MCA bifurcation, or sharply angled vessels, such as the ACA. It is more often used for the supraclinoid internal carotid artery and for the first segment of the MCA.[48]

Mathis and colleagues reported the intraarterial injection of papaverine in 36 patients in 48 vascular territories.[49] Papaverine, 300 mg, was diluted in 100 mL normal saline and administered via microcatheter over 20 to 30 minutes. The treatment was repeated if multiple areas required treatment. Six patients had transient neurologic events, including pupillary dilation

in 4, transient hemiparesis in 1, and respiratory arrest in 1. Pupillary dilation is related to flow into the ophthalmic artery and resolves after discontinuation of the papaverine infusion. Infusions into the posterior circulation have caused respiratory arrest and may cause cardiac dysfunction. The anesthesiologist should be prepared to provide resuscitation in such events. Even in the case of an unsecured ruptured aneurysm, a microcatheter can often be manipulated, with minimal risk, beyond the lesion to allow treatment of vasospasm without infusing the area of the aneurysm.[49] Schuknecht and associates, in 1999, reported the use of a combined approach of angioplasty and papaverine, which resulted in sustained clinical improvement in 73% of patients.[48] One patient had a transient hemiparesis following papaverine infusion into the MCA. Recurrent spasm is most common following treatment with papaverine alone, perhaps because of the short half-life of the drug. Retreatment was not required in any vessel treated by angioplasty alone or with a combination of angioplasty and papaverine; however, it was required due to spasm in some vessels treated with papaverine alone, with an incidence ranging from 12.5% (for ICA) to 21% (for a segment of the ACA).[48]

## Cerebral Angiography

Anesthesiologists will occasionally be called on to assist patients undergoing simple cerebral angiography. Although the newer non-ionic agents exhibit lower incidence of pain on injection, even in the external carotid artery circulation, there is significant risk. Transient neurologic impairment was seen in 1.7% (43 of 2509) of patients undergoing cerebral angiography, with insignificant differences between those in whom an ionic contrast agent was used and those given a non-ionic agent. Permanent neurologic sequelae were seen in 4 out of 2509 patients, one of whom sustained a minor scotoma and one who died after a brief radiologic examination.[34] Adequate monitoring and availability of resuscitative measures is mandatory for this procedure.

## Radiation Therapy

Radiation therapy can consist of either *radiosurgery* (delivery of a single large dose to small targets which may be close to sensitive structures) or *radiotherapy* (multiple smaller doses). A typical target for radiosurgery may be 24 mm in diameter. Precise positioning for either is important but more so for radiosurgery. The Kjellberg curve demonstrates that as the volume of brain exposed to radiation increases, the dose resulting in a 1% probability of radiation necrosis is dramatically reduced. This result indicates that maintaining accurate delivery of radiation, thus reducing the splatter volume, will greatly reduce unintended radiation necrosis. Two types of radiation generation system are in use: the Leksel Gamma Knife (Elekta Instruments, Inc, Atlanta, Ga), which uses multiple cobalt 60 beams focused on a point of interest, and the linear accelerator. Both the Gamma Knife and linear accelerators are used to produce gamma rays, which are high energy photons, more energetic than the photons produced by a radiograph machine.[50]

Precise positioning of the patient can be obtained by docking the patient into an isocentric subsystem, a rigid mechanical system allowing precision movements by vernier controls that can be physically attached to a target positioner, which in turn can be physically attached to a stereotactic ring rigidly fixed to the patient's skull with pointed pins driven into the skull under local or general anesthesia. Alternatively, patients may be held in a couch mount, employing three wall-mounted laser beams to align the patient.

Although the gantry rotation isocenter can maintain a precision of <0.5 mm, the couch system is prone to larger errors due to both rotation and translation of the couch while under patient load. At the University of Florida, an optical positioning system has been developed based on the use of a custom dental mold with rigidly attached infrared light-emitting diodes (LEDs). The dental mold provides a semi-rigid connection to an unchangeable feature of the patient's anatomy (the teeth), and using a commercially available Optotrak 3020 optical position sensor (Northern Digital, Inc, Ontario, Canada), the position of 6 infrared LEDs attached to the dental mold can be accurately (0.2-mm typical accuracy) determined. This allows precision positioning of the patient, even with roll rotation of the patient on the couch system, a situation in which the couch is particularly inaccurate.

The intracranial lesions that can be treated by fractionated stereotactic radiotherapy include many benign tumors (meningiomas, low-grade astrocytomas, craniopharyngiomas, pituitary adenomas, schwannomas, pineocytomas, chemodectomas, low-grade papillary neoplasms) and aggressive tumors (germinomas, primitive neuroectodermal tumors, chordomas, intermediate-grade pineal tumors, immature teratomas, undifferentiated sarcomas, anaplastic oligoastrocytomas, and metastatic tumors). Typically, tumors are <5 cm in the largest dimension. Reasons for preferring fractionated radiotherapy over one-time radiosurgery usually include proximity to the optic nerve or chiasm and lesion size. The daily dose received by the optic nerve is <1.9 Gy, whereas the benign tumor receives a daily fraction of 1.7 to 1.8 Gy and a total dose of 45 to 55 Gy. Benign tumors may be given an estimated 2 to 5 mm margin, smaller than the typical radiotherapy margins of systems without this exact positioning. Malignant tumors with poor prognosis may receive higher total doses (perhaps 60 Gy), with an addition of radiosurgery, perhaps 10 to 20 Gy. Radiation to approximately 5 mm is used in an attempt to cover all margins of aggressive tumors.[51]

Sequelae of this treatment may include edema, with an increase in lesion size, and neurologic compromise. Treatment with steroids will usually provide resolution of significant edema and neurologic symptoms. Progressive intracranial edema, signs of radiation necrosis, and neurologic deterioration are possible but have been limited. Mild fatigue and nausea and vomiting may also occur.[51]

## What Are the Anesthesia Requirements?

The physical setup for anesthetic monitoring may require special equipment. Because of the high radiation used for these treatments, treatment rooms are heavily lead-lined and have protective doors and corridors designed to avoid accidental exposure. The anesthesiologist should exit with the staff before each burst of radiation. This necessitates slaved monitors a short distance outside the treatment room. A television camera giving real time view of the patient is recommended. The ASA standards for intraoperative monitoring, as amended October 21, 1998, require capnography as part of ventilation monitoring for patients who are intubated or have a laryngeal mask airway (LMA). However, this requirement is one that can be waived in extenuating circumstances. The radiation therapy room is not a difficult environment in which to assemble anesthesia equipment, and hence capnography monitoring should be used.[52]

Anesthetic choices are based on the fact that repetitive radiotherapy sessions are brief, usually requiring only 5 minutes to position the patient and 5 minutes for therapy, and yet require guaranteed motionlessness because the physician may be out of the room. Older children may be able to remain sufficiently motionless with the assistance of modest restraints to allow therapy without anesthesia; typically children 3 years of age and younger will require an anesthetic. The anesthetic should provide rapid onset, brief duration, and quick recovery. Ketamine has been a long-standing favorite but sevoflurane and propofol are now replacing it. Because intracranial edema is one possible side effect of treatment, propofol may be preferable. Induction with intravenous agents is easier than in the past years where intravenous access was not so common. Many children receive indwelling catheters for chemotherapy—or, increasingly, for anesthesia when radiation therapy treatments of long duration are given. Particularly with repetitive handling of central catheters and the use of propofol, it is important to maintain asepsis to avoid infection. Fortney and coworkers noted an incidence of 15% of sepsis associated with the central venous catheter.[53]

Because the therapy sessions are typically short, the need for endotracheal intubation may be lessened. The natural airway or, in some cases, the LMA may be used. Nasal cannula, with one port used for continuous capnography, may suffice in thin children. Native- or steroid-induced obesity, or tumor involving the airway or respiratory control centers, may necessitate additional airway support. If the University of Florida upper dental mold is used, it may restrict ventilation through the mouth, but the LMA (for brief procedures) or endotracheal tube still functions beneath an upper mold. In most cases, different angles of incident radiation will be used, so the airway must be preserved through several cycles of staff and anesthesiologist re-entering the room to prepare for the next burst and then exiting again. The anesthesiologist should be alert for all actions of the staff as they reposition the equipment or patient for each new burst.

A simulation session may be required to allow planning of the radiation therapy or to create specific pillows, positioning devices, or mouthpieces. These sessions typically are considerably longer (hours) than the normal daily session (minutes), and it is common to use endotracheal intubation for these procedures. To allow calibration of the dental mold, one simulation session is required with the patient in a halo stereotactic positioning frame. The patient is anesthetized, an oral right angle endotracheal tube is used (because of the relative inconvenience of the LMA for longer sessions and possible multiple placement of the dental mold) and moved first to the CT scanner and then to the radiation therapy room. For safety purposes, there is an available frame with a removable front piece, which would allow emergent reintubation if required.

The nutritional needs of children must be considered. Many children will receive twice-daily radiation therapy, necessitating two anesthetics in one day. If excessively long nil per os (NPO) periods are deemed necessary, the child may be unable to eat both breakfast and lunch, allowing only the evening for nutritional requirements. 1999 guidelines from the ASA suggest a 6-hour NPO fast after light food (toast and clear liquid, or non-human milk), 4 hours after breast milk, and only 2 hours required after clear liquids.[54] These guidelines allow children to take in calories and liquid by way of clear liquids in between their anesthetics. However, these guidelines were intended only for healthy patients, and hence should be applied judiciously if signs of neurologic impairment are noted.

## What Is a "TIPS" Procedure?

The TIPS (transjugular intrahepatic portosystemic stent-shunt) procedure was developed as a minimally invasive method to lower the portal pressure in patients with end-stage liver disease and resulting portal hypertension. Initial experimental efforts to simply balloon-dilate tissue between the portal and hepatic veins were not successful because the tissue collapsed. The introduction of expandable stents to keep the shunt patent made the system successful.

From an entry point at the internal jugular, a catheter and needle are advanced through the vena cava into the right hepatic vein. Potentially, with ultrasound guidance, an intrahepatic branch of the portal vein is punctured; it is important for possible later liver transplant that this puncture and the stent path are entirely intrahepatic. If an extrahepatic puncture is made, the transplant surgeon may have difficulty finding a way to anastomose the remaining portal vein, and incurs the risk of laceration from the sharp wires of the expandable mesh of the stent. Measurement of the portal pressure can then be accomplished and compared with the right atrial pressure.

A significantly elevated baseline central venous pressure (perhaps >10 mm Hg) is a relative contraindication to the TIPS procedure because the right atrial pressure will become even more elevated. A tubular wire mesh mounted on a balloon catheter is then passed and dilated to bridge the tissue tract between the vessels. Typically, the stent is dilated to a diameter of 8 to 12 mm, which results in a shunt blood flow of approximately 2000 mL/min and reduces the portal pressure gradient above central venous pressure to approximately 10 mm Hg, effectively reducing variceal blood flow.

Successful placement of the shunt, in one study, was achieved in 93% of patients.[55] In that study, sedation was the only anesthesia used, and the procedure lasted an average of 1.2 ± 0.3 hours. Approximately 90% of patients with ascites will have improvement, with most not requiring diuretic agents. Shunt stenosis or occlusion (approximately 20% and 10%, respectively) are major problems. Complications that may occur include dislocation of the shunt, in which case it may be placed into a peripheral hepatic vein or the iliac vein. Catheters may become trapped in the shunt mesh and break. Clinical complications were encountered in 15% of patients including intraperitoneal hemorrhage, biliary hemorrhage, hematoma of the liver capsule, and migration of a stent into the pulmonary artery. If intraoperative hemodynamic instability occurs, these causes should be considered in the differential diagnosis.

Of those patients successfully stented, the overall 1-year survival rate was 87%—worse in the patients with Child-Pugh class C and better in healthier patients. Encephalopathy may develop because the shunt is designed to reduce portal pressure and therefore reduces flow through the cirrhotic liver. Bilirubin may rise in some patients; in one study, the rate of hepatic encephalopathy increased from 10% before treatment to 25% after treatment, predominately appearing in older patients. These results in encephalopathy are similar to those expected from surgery, with a reduction in morbidity and mortality. Sclerotherapy is associated with a relatively high rate of rebleeding and a 1-year survival rate comparable to that of the TIPS procedure.[55]

In addition to the treatment of patients with variceal bleeding, the TIPS procedure is effective in treating patients with bleeding from ruptured gastric varices, which can be difficult to treat with sclerotherapy. In such patients, the TIPS procedure can allow the establishment of hemostasis as well as prevent rebleeding. The complications are similar to those experienced in variceal bleeds.[56]

TIPS procedures for patients with ascites generally improve renal function after an early decrement in function related to contrast media (which may be so severe that they require hemodialysis temporarily). Urinary sodium excretion improved significantly in the first week after shunt in one study, and serum creatinine concentration and creatinine clearance improved significantly at 6 months. Patients with organic renal disease do not show improvements. It is not a cure for hepatorenal syndrome, thought to result from disturbances in the delicate balance between vasodilating and vasoconstricting substances in the renal cortex as a result of liver failure.[57] Vascular filling, as indicated by a rise in the central venous pressure, increases with a decrease in hyperaldosteronism. There may be improved absorption of nutrients and shunt induced hyperinsulinism—patients tend to gain weight after a successful shunt.[58]

Cardiac arrhythmias are a particular risk during the TIPS procedure, perhaps because the catheter traverses the right atrium. In institutions in which the procedure is done under local anesthesia with conscious sedation, there may be a risk of stress induced arrhythmias. One study of 12 patients undergoing the TIPS procedure under local anesthesia showed that 75% of patients had frequent episodes of unsustained ventricular tachycardias, as well as many unsustained supraventricular tachycardias; 1 of 12 had sustained supraventricular tachycardia.[59] Some patients undergoing liver transplantation will experience liver failure and return for a TIPS procedure, potentially as a bridge to retransplantation.[60] In one small study of such patients, ascites, hydrothorax, and variceal bleeding were controlled in all patients.

$CO_2$ angiography has been shown in an animal model to result in less damage to the liver than iodinated contrast studies.[61] $CO_2$ angiography, although reducing the risk to the patient from contrast agents, carries a special risk of accidental air embolus if air, rather than $CO_2$, is in the injector syringe. In such cases, 100% oxygen and resuscitative measures must be quickly instituted.

## MAGNETIC RESONANCE IMAGING

MRI is a noninvasive imaging method without ionizing radiation. Unfortunately, acquisition of images still takes considerable time, requiring the patient to remain motionless for 15 to 45 minutes, often inside a confined tubular structure. Anesthesiologists are increasingly involved to provide sedation or general anesthesia for children, adults with claustrophobia, or patients with pain or mental status changes who are unable to maintain the required degree of motionlessness.

### Anatomy of a Magnetic Resonance Imaging Scan

The MRI scanner consists of a strong magnet (typically 0.5-1.5 Tesla) that produces a combination of a static and dynamic magnetic field, as well as a relatively powerful variable frequency transmitter (in the tens of megahertz range) and a sensitive receiver. The dynamic magnetic field results in a noisy environment, essentially making the entire system a buzzing loudspeaker.

MRI is based on exploitation of the ability to magnetize the nucleus of some atoms. When an electric charge moves in a closed path (eg, a circle), it constitutes an electromagnet. Individual protons and neutrons within a nucleus contain electric charges, albeit small amounts. Because the protons and neutrons spin on their own axes, they constitute a tiny electromagnet. In atoms in which the spinning particles are paired, they normally cancel each other's effects; however, atoms with an odd number of either protons or neutrons (eg, hydrogen 1, carbon 13, fluorine 19, sodium 23) are unable to have complete cancellation, and hence display a net magnetic effect on an individual atom basis. Random orientation of these nuclei, however, results in no gross magnetization. When biologic tissues are exposed to an external magnetic field, their nuclear magnetic effects tend to line up either parallel or opposite to the field (with slightly more parallel), not unlike, but much weaker than what happens to iron atoms or even iron filings in a magnetic field. The energy state of nuclei anti-parallel is slightly higher than those parallel. By using a pulse of radiofrequency energy chosen to have photons of the correct energy equal to the difference between the parallel and anti-parallel energy states, the nuclei may be flipped. When the pulse ends, the nuclei will release the absorbed energy as a photon of radiated radiofrequency energy, the frequency determined by the applied magnetic field, and the type of nuclei. This resulting weak signal can be detected by a sensitive receiver and is the principle of nuclear magnetic resonance. The strength of the weak signal declines (within a few hundred milliseconds) as the matter returns to its previous state. The rate of decline is dependent on the speed at which energy can be transferred within the tissues. There are two possible methods:

1. The first method is characterized by T1, the spin-lattice relaxational or longitudinal relaxation time, and is based on transfer of energy between atoms and molecules via magnetic interactions. T1 is a constant describing the exponential decay of energy via this method.
2. A second method is described by T2, the spin-spin relaxation time, which is based on the fact that the nuclei, while lining up, do so with a wobble or precession, and spin coupling interactions cause the nuclei to dephase their precession.

T2 is always less than T1, and both can be measured. By using a gradient in the magnetic field and variations in the frequency of the applied radiofrequency pulses, the required geometric computations of the exact location of the bit of tissue emanating a particular received signal can be accomplished, thus allowing imaging. The mathematic computations are similar to those used by a CT scanner.

## What Are the Magnetic Risks?

Patients with embedded ferromagnetic particles or prostheses must not be allowed into the scanner area. The magnetic field may violently move the ferrous material, with any number of resulting injuries, including blindness or death. Check for history of metal splinters in the eye, ferrous intracranial clips, pacemakers, and shrapnel injury.

Ferrous anesthesia equipment may also be violently moved by the field, creating crushing or shrapnel injuries. Gas tanks, anesthesia machines, patient gurneys, and batteries must be non-ferrous. Typical laryngoscope batteries are not allowed. (Extension cord arrangements to power the non-ferrous laryngoscope may be used.)

Anesthesia monitors that include cathode-ray tube displays (CRT) will not function near the magnet because the electron beam of the CRT will be wildly deflected. Liquid crystal or LED displays will function properly. Even with the proper equipment, leads, and connections, electrocardiographic monitoring is likely to be useful only for gross measurements of QRS complex. ST-T wave changes and P wave changes have

---

**TABLE 52-3.** Standard Monitoring and Anesthesia Care

1. Train anesthesia personnel in risk management, and they should coordinate patient care with the technicians operating the MRI equipment, who should also be alert for possible risks.
2. Make sure patients undergoing anesthesia for MRI receive the same level of monitoring and care that is expected in the operating room; maintain careful compliance with the ASA Standards for Basic Intraoperative Monitoring. The design and construction of the MRI suite and the selection of monitoring equipment should be thoughtful.
3. Use an anesthesia machine that is constructed of nonferrous materials and, if necessary, physically stabilize it in the MRI suite.
4. If a table or tray is used that is not MRI-compatible, carefully mark it so that it is not brought within the magnetic field.
5. Use anesthesia electronic monitors (capnography, noninvasive blood pressure, inspired oxygen) that are MRI-compatible and that have low EMI emissions.
6. Maintain ECG leads that are high-resistance carbon fiber close to low-resistance patient connections in a small connection area. Use an MRI-certified ECG. The low patient footprint and closeness of the leads will reduce their enclosed area, reducing the resulting induced voltage. By using high-resistance leads, most of the voltage induced will be dropped along the leads themselves, not at the lower resistance of the patient's body or connections, hence, little heating power will be delivered to the patient.
7. Avoid coils in any conducting substance, including IV solutions.
8. Test or certify pumps, ventilators, and other devices that are electrically powered before use within the magnetic field. Additional lengths of IV tubing may be added to keep the pump well away from the field. Also, use fluidic ventilators.
9. Measure invasive pressures by extending the tubing as needed to bring transducers outside the magnetic field. Passageways may be brought out through radio frequency traps made of lengths of copper tubing through the wall.* There may be some degradation of the accuracy of systolic and diastolic blood pressures as a result of the length of tubing required.
10. Make temperature measurement readily available and, within the MRI suite, consider using liquid crystal skin measurement.
11. Remember that hypothermia is a considerable risk in smaller patients in the cool environment of the superconducting magnet.
12. Remember that unusual direct-current fluorescent lighting may make the recognition of hypoxia difficult and may be slow to turn back on if ever extinguished. Consider having additional incandescent lighting available.
13. Carefully plan the airway security because the patient may need to move to image certain areas.
14. Think through an emergency management plan for lost airway within the coil. This may involve a specially designed laryngoscope with an extension cord to a power source because typical laryngoscope batteries are ferromagnetic.

---

*Taber KH, Thompson J, Coveler LA, et al. Invasive pressure monitoring of patients during magnetic resonance imaging. *Can J Anaesth.* 1993;40:1092.

ASA, American Society of Anesthesiologists; ECG, electrocardiograph; EMI, electromagnetic interference; IV, intravenous; MRI, magnetic resonance imaging.

been observed. This may be due to the induction of electrical currents within the heart and (conductive) blood by the combination of motion of the heart and magnetic field or due to the motion of the blood itself within the magnetic field.[62]

Anesthesia connections to the patient that include conductive substances (saline solutions, wires) will develop unexpected currents due to the influence of the changing magnetic field on the conductive loops formed by these conductive substances (the functional equivalent of an electricity generator). Serious burns have been reported.[63]

Anesthesia monitors that emit radiofrequency energy may be detected by the sensitive receivers of the MRI scanner, with resulting degradation of the image.

Suggestions to accomplish standard monitoring and safe anesthesia care are listed in Table 52–3. At some centers, surgery is now being performed in "open coil" MRI suites. These typically involve a 0.5 Tesla superconductivity magnet with two coils separated by approximately 59 cm, allowing a region for the patient's body to be operated on. Surgically useful images can be obtained as fast as 14 seconds, allowing improvements in endoscopic sinus surgery, head and neck needle biopsies, as well as potential cryotherapy ablation of head and neck and abdominal and thoracic tumors. Caution should be exercised in making certain that the surgeon's tools are all MRI-compatible.[64, 65]

## References

1. Margulis AR, Sunshine JH. Radiology at the turn of the millennium. *Radiology.* 2000;214:15.
2. American Society of Anesthesiologists, House of Delegates. Standards for basic anesthetic monitoring, October 21, 1986, amended October 21, 1998. Available at: http://www.asahq.org/Standards/02.html#2. Accessed: March 22, 2001.
3. American Society of Anesthesiologists, House of Delegates. Guidelines for nonoperating room anesthesthetizing locations, October 19, 1994. Available at: http://www.asahq.org/Standards/14.html. Accessed: March 22, 2001.
4. American Society of Anesthesiologists, House of Delegates. Basic standards for preanesthesia care, October 14, 1987. Available at: http://www.asahq.org/Standards/02.html#1. Accessed: March 22, 2001.
5. Nevalainen DE. The quality systems approach. *Arch Pathol Lab Med.* 1999;123:566.
6. Posel N. Preoperative teaching in the preadmission clinic. *J Nurs Staff Dev.* 1998;14(1):52.
7. Hanson M. The "P's and Q's" of quality systems. *Arch Pathol Lab Med.* 1999;123:576.
8. Ibarra VL, Mueller T, Rossi N, et al. Interdisciplinary quality improvement from the perspective of a clinical pathway team. *J Nurs Care Qual.* 1998;12(3):19.
9. Goldberg M. Systemic reactions to intravascular contrast media. *Anesthesiology.* 1984;60:46.
10. Schwab SJ, Hlatky MA, Pieper KS, et al. Contrast nephrotoxicity: a randomized controlled trial of a nonionic and an ionic radiographic contrast agent. *N Engl J Med.* 1989;320:149.
11. Pagani JJ, Hayman LA, Bigelow RH, et al. Prophylactic diazepam in prevention of contrast media-associated seizures in glioma patients undergoing cerebral computed tomography. *Cancer.* 1984;54:2200.
12. Drescher P, Knes JM, Madsen PO. Histamine release and contrast media-induced renal vasoconstriction. *Acad Radiol.* 1998;5:785.
13. Cronin RE. Renal failure following radiologic procedures. *Am J Med Sci.* 1989;298:342.
14. Katholi RE, Taylor GJ, McCann WP, et al. Nephrotoxicity from contrast media: attenuation with theophylline. *Radiology.* 1995;195:17.
15. Kurnik BR, Allgren RL, Genter FC, et al. Prospective study of atrial natriuretic peptide for the prevention of radiocontrast-induced nephropathy. *Am J Kidney Dis.* 1998;31:674.
16. Smith DC, Yahiku PY, Maloney MD, et al. Three new low-osmolality contrast agents: a comparative study of patient discomfort. *AJNR Am J Neuroradiol.* 1988;9:137.
17. Drescher P, Knes JM, Madsen PO. Prevention of contrast medium-induced renal vasospasm by phosphodiesterase inhibition. *Invest Radiol.* 1998;33:858.
18. Lautin EM, Freeman NJ, Shoenfeld AH. Radiocontrast-associated renal dysfunction: a comparison of lower-osmolality and conventional high-osmolality contrast media. *AJR Am J Roentgenol.* 1991;157:59.
19. Furukawa T, Ueda J, Takahashi S, et al. Elimination of low-osmolality contrast media by hemodialysis. *Acta Radiol.* 1996;37:966.
20. Thomsen HS, Dorph S, Larsen S, et al. Urine profiles and kidney histology after ionic and nonionic radiologic and magnetic resonance contrast media in rats with cisplatin nephropathy. *Acad Radiol.* 1995;2:675.
21. Dascalu A, Peer A. Effects of radiologic contrast media on human endothelial and kidney cell lines: intracellular pH and cytotoxicity. *Acad Radiol.* 1994;1:145.
22. Swanson DP, Thrall JH, Shetty PC. Evaluation of intravascular low-osmolality contrast agents. *Clin Pharm.* 1986;5:877.
23. Heyman SN, Clark BA, Cantley L, et al. Effects of ioversol versus iothalamate on endothelin release and radiocontrast nephropathy. *Invest Radiol.* 1993;28:313.
24. Rudnick MR, Goldfarb S, Wexler L, et al. Nephrotoxicity of ionic and nonionic contrast media in 1196 patients: a randomized trial. The Iohexol Cooperative Study. *Kidney Int.* 1995;47:254.
25. Andersen KJ, Vik H, Eikesdal HP, Christensen EI. Effects of contrast media on renal epithelial cells in culture. *Acta Radiol Suppl.* 1995;399:213.
26. Harris KG, Smith TP, Cragg AH, et al. Nephrotoxicity from contrast material in renal insufficiency: ionic versus nonionic agents. *Radiology.* 1991;179:849.
27. Jakobsen JA, Berg KJ, Kjaersgaard P, et al. Angiography with nonionic x-ray contrast media in severe chronic renal failure: renal function and contrast retention. *Nephron.* 1996;73:549.
28. Solomon R, Werner C, Mann D, et al. Effects of saline, mannitol, and furosemide on acute decreases in renal function induced by radiocontrast agents. *N Engl J Med.* 1994;331:1416.
29. Stevens MA, McCullough PA, Tobin KJ, et al. A prospective randomised trial of prevention measures in patients at high risk for contrast nephropathy. Results of the PRINCE Study. *J Am Coll Cardiol.* 1999;33:403.
30. Bertrand ME, Esplugas E, Piessens J, et al. Influence of a nonionic, iso-osmolar contrast medium (iodixanol) versus an ionic, low-osmolar contrast medium (ioxaglate) on major adverse cardiac events in patients undergoing percutaneous transluminal coronary angioplasty: a multicenter, randomized, double-blind study. Visipaque in Percutaneous Transluminal Coronary Angioplasty VIP. *Circulation.* 2000;101:131.
31. Schrader R, Esch I, Ensslen R, et al. A randomized trial comparing the impact of a nonionic (Iomeprol) versus an ionic (Ioxaglate) low osmolar contrast medium on abrupt vessel closure and ischemic complications after coronary angioplasty. *J Am Coll Cardiol.* 1999;33:395.
32. Limburno U, Petronio AS, Amoroso G, et al. The impact of coronary artery disease on the coronary vasomotor response to nonionic contrast media. *Circulation.* 2000;101:491.
33. Valenti R, Motta A, Merlini S, et al. Iopiperidol: nonionic iodinated contrast medium with promising anticoagulant and antiplatelet properties. *Acad Radiol.* 1999;6:426.
34. Skalpe IO. Complications in cerebral angiography with iohexol (Omnipaque) and meglumine metrizoate (Isopaque cerebral). *Neuroradiology.* 1988;30:69.
35. Kaufman JA, Hu S, Geller SC, et al. Selective angiography of the common carotid artery with gadopentate dimeglumine in a patient with renal insufficiency. *AJR Am J Roentgenol.* 1999;172:1613.
36. Back MR, Caridi JG, Hawkins IF Jr, et al. Angiography with carbon dioxide ($CO_2$). *Surg Clin North Am.* 1998;78:575.
37. Culp W, Cowan TC, Hummel MM. Patient intolerance of $CO_2$ angiography. *AJR Am J Roentgenol.* 1999;173:240.
38. Spinosa DJ, Angle JF, Hagspiel KD, et al. Lower extremity arteriography with use of iodinated contrast material or gadodiamide to supplement $CO_2$ angiography in patients with renal insufficiency. *J Vasc Interv Radiol.* 2000;11:35.
39. Pruvo JP, Leclerc X, Ares GS, et al. Endovascular treatment of ruptured intracranial aneurysms. *J Neurol.* 1999;246:244.
40. Phatouros CC, McConachie NS, Jaspan T. Post-procedure migration of Guglielmi detachable coils and mechanical detachable spirals. *Neuroradiology.* 1999;41:324.
41. Murayama Y, Vinuela F, Duckwiler GR, et al. Embolization of incidental cerebral aneurysms by using the Guglielmi detachable coil system. *J Neurosurg.* 1999;90:207.
42. Jansen O, Dorfler A, Forsting M, et al. Endovascular therapy of arteriove-

nous fistulae with electrolytically detachable coils. *Neuroradiology.* 1999;41:951.

43. Chang HS, Nihei H. Theoretical comparison of surgery and radiosurgery in cerebral arteriovenous malformations. *J Neurosurg.* 1999;90:709.

44. Schweitzer JS, Chang BS, Madsen P, et al. The pathology of arteriovenous malformations of the brain treated by embolotherapy, II: results of embolization with multiple agents. *Neuroradiology.* 1993;35:468.

45. Schumacher M, Horton JA. Treatment of cerebral arteriovenous malformations with PVA. Results and analysis of complications. *Neuroradiology.* 1991;33:101.

46. Casasco A, Houdart E, Biondi A, et al. Major complications of percutaneous embolization of skull-base tumors. *AJNR Am J Neuroradiol.* 1999;20:179.

47. Guglielmi G. Use of the GDC crescent for emoblization of tumors fed by cavernous and petrous branches of the internal carotid artery. *J Neurosurg.* 1998;89:857.

48. Schuknecht B, Fandino J, Yuksel C, et al. Endovascular treatment of cerebral vasospasm: assessment of treatment effect by cerebral angiography and transcranial colour Doppler sonography. *Neuroradiology.* 1999;41:453.

49. Mathis JM, Jensen ME, Dion JE. Technical considerations on intra-arterial papaverine hydrochloride for cerebral vasospasm. *Neuroradiology.* 1997;39:90.

50. Meeks SL, Bova FJ, Friedman WA, et al. IRLED-based patient localization for LINAC radiosurgery. *Int J Radiat Oncol Biol Phys.* 1998;41:433.

51. Buatti JM, Bova FJ, Friedman WA, et al. Preliminary experience with frameless steriotactic radiotherapy. *Int J Radiat Oncol Biol Phys.* 1998;42:591.

52. American Society of Anesthesiologists, by House of Delegates. Standards for basic anesthetic monitoring. Approved on October 21, 1986 and last amended on October 21, 1998. Available at: http://www.asahq.org/Standards/02.htm. Accessed: March 22, 2001.

53. Fortney JT, Halperin EC, Hertz CM, et al. Anesthesia for pediatric external beam radiation therapy. *Int J Radiat Oncol Biol Phys.* 1999;44:587.

54. American Society of Anesthesiologists Task Force on Preoperative Fasting. Practice guidelines for preoperative fasting and the use of pharmacologic agents to reduce the risk of pulmonary aspiration: application to healthy patients undergoing elective procedures. *Anesthesiology.* 1999;90:896.

55. Rossle M, Haag K, Ochs A, et al. Transjugular intrahepatic protosystemic stent-shunt procedure for variceal bleeding. *N Engl J Med.* 1994;330:165.

56. Barange K, Peron JM, Imani K, et al. Transjugular intrahepatic portosystemic shunt in the treatment of refractory bleeding from ruptured gastric varices. *Hepatology.* 1999;30:1139.

57. Gentilini P, La Villa G, Casini-Raggi V, et al. Hepatorenal syndrome and its treatment today. *Eur J Gastroenterol Hepatol.* 1999;11:1061.

58. Ochs A, Rossle M, Haag K, et al. The transjugular intrahepatic portosystemic stent-shunt procedure for refractory ascites. *N Engl J Med.* 1995;332:1192.

59. Pidlich J, Peck-Radosavljevic M, Kranz A, et al. Transjugular intrahepatic portosystemic shunt and cardiac arrhythmias. *J Clin Gastroenterol.* 1998;26:39.

60. Lerut JP, Goffette P, Molle G, et al. Transjugular intrahepatic portosystemic shunt after adult liver transplantation: experience in eight patients. *Transplantation.* 1999;68:379.

61. Culp WC, Mladinich CR, Hawkins IF Jr. Comparison of hepatic damage from direct injections of iodinated contrast agents and carbon dioxide. *J Vasc Interv Radiol.* 1999;10:1265.

62. Jorgensen NH, Messick JM Jr, Gray J, et al. ASA monitoring standards and magnetic resonance imaging. *Anesth Analg.* 1994;79:1141.

63. Brown TR, Goldstein B, Little J. Severe burns resulting from magnetic resonance imaging with cardiopulmonary monitoring. Risks and relevant safety precautions. *Am J Phys Med Rehabil.* 1993;72:166.

64. Fried MP, Topulos G, Hsu L, et al. Endoscopic sinus surgery with magnetic resonance imaging guidance: initial patient experience. *Otolaryngol Head Neck Surg.* 1998;119:374.

65. Davis SP, Anand VK, Dhillon G. Magnetic resonance navigation for head and neck lesions. *Laryngoscope.* 1999;109:862.

CHAPTER

# 53

# Management of the Difficult Airway

Andrea Gabrielli

A. Joseph Layon

## TRAINING ISSUES IN MANAGING DIFFICULT AIRWAYS

*What Is the Best Way to Acquire Skill in Managing Difficult Airways?*

A systematic approach to difficult airway management has been shown to reduce the likelihood of an adverse outcome.[1-4] This chapter discusses guidelines for care of the difficult airway and offers practical suggestions to facilitate its management. Various stages of airway management are considered separately.

## INTRODUCTION

### What Are the Consequences of Hypoxia and Hypercapnia?

Oxygen delivery ($\dot{D}o_2$) in milliliters per minute represents the bulk movement of oxygen in the blood and is proportional to cardiac output and arterial oxygen content. It is described by the following equation:

$$\dot{D}o_2 = (\text{Cardiac Output} \times Cao_2) + 0.003\,(Pao_2)$$

The partial pressure of arterial oxygen ($Pao_2$) is an essential, but minor, component of $\dot{D}o_2$.

### Hypoxia

Bulk oxygen delivered to the tissue does not guarantee tissue oxygenation because passive movement of oxygen down the concentration gradient across tissue barriers to the mitochondria is ultimately responsible for cellular $\dot{D}o_2$. Nevertheless, when ventilation fails, both the $Pao_2$ and the level of systemic oxygenation rapidly fall; this decrement results in *hypoxemia* and *hypoxia*. As a consequence, progressive global hypoxia rapidly follows.

The tolerance of various tissues to hypoxia differs (Table 53–1).[5] In particular, when $Pao_2$ falls below about 30 mm Hg, hypoxia in most tissues follows in less than 3 minutes.[5] Although there is often a brief period of hypertension and tachycardia, because of sympathetic nervous system output, all cases of severe, uncorrected hypoxia trigger cardiac arrhythmias, culminating in severe bradycardia, peripheral vasodilation, systemic hypotension, severe metabolic acidosis, and death.

### Hypercapnia

Adequate ventilation is necessary to remove carbon dioxide ($CO_2$) from the tissues. The immediate consequence of hypoventilation is acute respiratory acidosis secondary to hypercapnia with acidemia (pH <7.35). In apneic patients and in patients who have not received intravenous administration of bicarbonate, the increase in partial pressure of $CO_2$ ($Paco_2$) is predictable with time, at about 3 mm Hg/min.

Respiratory acidosis in the absence of hypoxia may provoke sympathetic nervous system activity with consequent hypertension and tachycardia. When hypercapnia becomes severe (>80–100 mmHg), it may cause narcosis, severe acidemia, and cardiac arrest. In the presence of combined hypoventilation and hypoxia, the hemodynamic consequences of hypoxia prevail, and severe bradycardia rapidly develops.

## DEFINITION OF THE DIFFICULT AIRWAY

Both the American and the Canadian Societies of Anesthesiologists (ASA and CSA) have published recent guidelines regarding the difficult airway.[2,3] A *difficult airway* is defined as the following:

*the clinical situation in which a conventionally trained anesthesiologist experiences difficulties with mask ventilation, difficulty with tracheal intubation, or both.*[2, 3]

*Difficult mask ventilation* is defined as the following:

*a situation where it is not possible for the unassisted anesthesiologist to maintain an $Spo_2$ of >90% using 100% oxygen and positive pressure mask ventilation in a patient whose $Spo_2$ was more than 90% before instigating intervention; and/or it is not possible for the unassisted anesthetist/anesthesiologist to prevent or reverse signs of inadequate ventilation during positive pressure mask ventilation.*[2]

*Difficult laryngoscopy* is defined as the following:

(a situation in which) *it is not possible to visualize any portion of the vocal cords with conventional laryngoscopy.*

The task forces differ in defining difficult tracheal intubation. For the ASA, a *difficult endotracheal intubation* is defined as the following:

*proper insertion of the endotracheal tube with conventional laryngoscopy requiring more than three attempts or more than 10 minutes.*[3]

The CSA Task Force definition of difficult endotracheal intubation is more detailed:

*as when an experienced laryngoscopist, using direct laryngoscopy, requires*

- *More than one attempt with the same blade*
- *A change in the blade or adjunct to direct laryngoscopy*
- *Use of alternative devices or techniques when intubation has failed*[2]

The lack of consensus between the definitions presented by the ASA and CSA Task Forces may affect the epidemiologic data presented on difficult airway by the two societies. We agree with Benumof[6] that the Canadian definition of a difficult

**TABLE 53–1.** Tolerance to Hypoxia of Various Tissues

| Tissue | Survival Time |
|---|---|
| Brain | <3 min |
| Kidney and liver | 15-20 min |
| Skeletal muscle | 60-90 min |
| Vascular smooth muscle | 24-72 h |
| Hair and nails | Several days |

From Leach RM, Treacher DS. ABC of oxygen: oxygen transport, 2: tissue hypoxia. *BMJ*. 1998;317:1370.

**TABLE 53–2.** Preoperative Airway Examinations, Acceptable Endpoints, and Significance of Endpoints

| Preoperative Examination | Acceptable Endpoints | Significance of Endpoints |
| --- | --- | --- |
| **Dental** | | |
| Length of upper incisors with mouth fully open | Qualitative/short incisors | Long incisors; blade enters mouth in cephalad direction |
| Involuntary; maxillary teeth anterior to mandibular teeth (buck teeth) | No overriding of maxillary teeth anterior to the mandibular teeth | Overriding maxillary teeth; blade enters mouth in a more cephalad direction |
| Voluntary; protrusion of mandibular teeth anterior to the maxillary teeth | Anterior protrusion of the mandibular teeth relative to the maxillary teeth | Test of TMJ function; means good mouth opening and jaw, will displace anteriorly with laryngoscopy |
| Interincisor distance | >3 cm | 2-cm phalange on blade can be easily inserted between teeth |
| **Pharynx** | | |
| Oropharyngeal class Samsoon and Young | Class II | Tongue is small in relation to size of oropharyngeal cavity |
| Narrowness of palate | Should not appear very narrow or highly arched | A narrow palate decreases the oropharyngeal volume and room for both blade and ETT |
| MS length (thyromental distance) | 5 cm or 3 ordinary-sized fingerbreadths | Larynx is relatively posterior to other upper airway structures |
| MS compliance | Qualitative palpation of normal resistance/softness | Laryngoscopy retracts tongue into the MS; compliance of the MS determines if tongue fits into MS |
| **Neck** | | |
| Length of neck | Qualitative; a quantitative index is not yet available | A short neck decreases the ability to align the upper airway axes |
| Thickness of neck | Qualitative; a quantitative index is not yet available | A thick neck decreases the ability to align the upper airway axes |
| Range of motion of head and neck | Neck flexed and chest 35° + head extended on neck 80° = sniff position | The sniff position aligns the oral, pharyngeal, and laryngeal axes to create a favorable line of sight |

ETT, endotracheal tube; MS, mandibular space; TMJ, temporomandibular joint.
Modified from Benumof JL. The ASA difficult airway algorithm: new thoughts/considerations. *American Society of Anesthesiologists Refresher Course: 1998–1999;* October 1999. Lecture 134.

endotracheal intubation represents a closer picture of clinical reality inasmuch as it is independent of a preset number of attempts.

## How Is a Difficult Airway Predicted?

Systematic examination of the airway is the key to recognizing anatomy that may predispose to a difficult airway and planning for its safe management (Table 53–2).[7] A comprehensive noninvasive systematic review of the upper airway anatomy has been described.[8] Such a systematic approach resulted in a difficult intubation risk index, wherein the most important risk factors—weight, head and neck movement, jaw movement, receding mandible, and tooth angulation—were each scored from 0 to 2.[7] When this index was tested prospectively, a score of 1 was associated with a true positive difficult intubation of 92%; a score of 2, 72%; and a score of 3, 50%.[8]

## The Mallampati Classification

Anatomic observation of the upper airway should be integrated with knowledge of other possible airway-compromising, congenital, or acquired clinical conditions (Table 53–3). Mallampati and colleagues[9] described a clinical correlation between the anatomy of the oropharyngeal structures and the degree of difficulty of laryngeal exposure (Fig. 53–1). The basis of the Mallampati airway classification is the relative size of the tongue to the size of the oropharyngeal opening.

A subsequent modification of the Mallampati specification described by Samsoon and Young[10] is now in widespread use as the "modified Mallampati classification" (Fig. 53–2). This modification of the Mallampati classification represents a subdivision of the Mallampati class III airway into classes III and IV; class IV describes a condition in which the oropharynx is almost completely obscured by the tongue when the mouth is wide open.

**FIGURE 53–1.** Mallampati airway classification. Relative size of the tongue to the oropharyngeal opening. *A,* Class I. *B,* Class II. *C,* Class III. (From Mallampati SR, Gatt SP, Gugino LG, et al. A clinical sign to predict difficult tracheal intubation: a prospective study. *Can Anaesth Soc J.* 1985;32:429.)

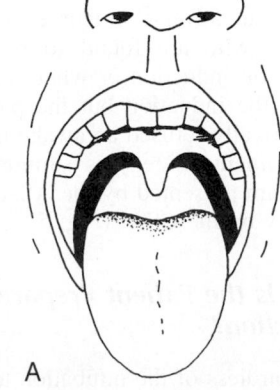

A

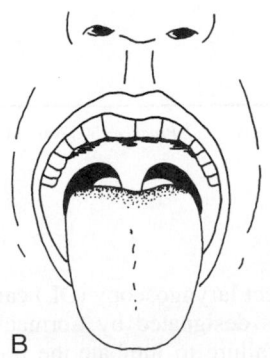

B

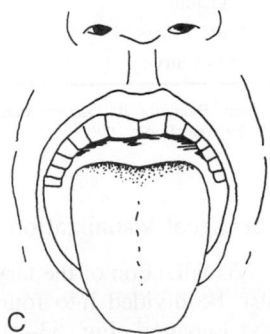

C

**TABLE 53–3.** Airway-Compromising Conditions

| Pathologic Condition | Principal Pathologic and Clinical Features |
|---|---|
| **A.  Supralaryngeal** | |
| 1.  Pierre Robin syndrome | Micrognathia, macroglossia, cleft soft palate |
| 2.  Treacher Collins syndrome | Auricular and ocular defects; malar and mandibular hypoplasia |
| 3.  Goldenhar's syndrome | Auricular and ocular defects; malar and mandibular hypoplasia; occipitalization of atlas |
| 4.  Down syndrome | Poorly developed or absent bridge of the nose; macroglossia |
| 5.  Klippel-Feil syndrome | Congenital fusion of a variable number of cervical vertebrae; restriction of neck movement |
| **B.  Sublaryngeal** | |
| 1.  Goiter | Compression of trachea, deviation of larynx-trachea |
| **C.  Infections** | |
| 1.  Supraglottis | Laryngeal edema |
| 2.  Croup | Laryngeal edema |
| 3.  Abscess (intraoral, retropharyngeal) | Distortion of the airway and trismus |
| 4.  Ludwig's angina | Distortion of the airway and trismus |
| **D.  Arthritis** | |
| 1.  Rheumatoid arthritis | Temporomandibular joint ankylosis, cricoarytenoid arthritis, deviation of larynx, restricted mobility of cervical spine |
| 2.  Ankylosing spondylitis | Ankylosis of cervical spine; less commonly, ankylosis of temporomandibular joints; lack of mobility of cervical spine |
| **E.  Benign tumors** | |
| 1.  Example: cystic hygroma, lipoma, adenoma, goiter | Stenosis or distortion of the airway |
| **F.  Malignant tumors** | |
| 1.  Example: carcinoma of tongue, larynx, or thyroid | Stenosis or distortion of the airway; fixation of larynx or adjacent tissues secondary to infiltration or fibrosis from irradiation |
| **G.  Trauma** | |
| 1.  Example: facial injury, cervical spine injury and laryngeal-tracheal trauma | Edema of the airway, hematoma, ongoing nose/sinus/laryngeal bleeding, unstable fracture(s) of the maxillae, mandible, and cervical vertebrae |
| **H.  Obesity** | |
| Short, thick neck; redundant tissue in the oropharynx; sleep apnea | |
| **I.  Acromegaly** | |
| Macroglossia; prognathism | |
| **J.  Acute Burns** | |
| Edema of airway | |

From Benumof JL. *Airway Management: Principles and Practice.* St Louis, Mo: Mosby–Year Book; 1996.

## Laryngeal Visualization

Visualization of the larynx by direct laryngoscopy (DL) can also be divided into four classes as designated by Cormack and Lehane[11] (Fig. 53–3). Overall failure to intubate the trachea after DL is observed in 1 to 3 cases per 1000 attempts,

and failure to bag-valve-mask (BVM) ventilate can be seen in 1 to 3 cases per 10 000 attempts.[2]

A clear clinical correlation exists between the Mallampati classification and the difficulty of DL in both prospective and retrospective studies.[9] However, if the patient has a known anatomic abnormality associated with difficult airway, serious consideration should be given to an awake intubation, regardless of the Mallampati classification. Similarly, we recommend considering an awake intubation in any patient with Mallampati class III or Samsoon and Young class 3 or 4 airway, as well as immediate access to a well-stocked difficult airway cart (discussed later).

### What Is the Risk of Aspiration?

Tracheobronchial aspiration of saliva or gastric contents has been described in 16% to 27% of all anesthetized patients.[12] Usually, the aspirated material is saliva or blood and has no clinical consequences. Aspiration of gastric contents may be seen secondary to regurgitation or vomiting in the patient with incompetent laryngeal reflexes or on induction of general anesthesia with or without muscle relaxation. The incidence of pulmonary aspiration of gastric contents ranged from 1.1% in a series of 10 000 elective anesthetics of ASA Physical Status Class I to 29% per 10 000 ASA Physical Status Classes IV and V emergency anesthetics.[13,14] Interestingly, one third of the aspirative events were observed during laryngoscopy and one third occurred at extubation. The final third were not witnessed.

Hypoxemia from severe ventilation-perfusion ($\dot{V}/\dot{Q}$) mismatch is the most severe consequence of pulmonary aspiration of gastric contents. As a consequence of the aspiration-induced alveolar capillary membrane damage, capillary leak occurs, with loss of circulating fluid volume into the lungs, increased extravascular lung water, resultant systemic hemoconcentration, hypotension, and tachycardia. Hypovolemic shock thus may aggravate hypoxemia. Pulmonary hypertension secondary to bronchospasm, loss of functioning alveoli, and left ventricular dysfunction may occur.[15]

## MANAGEMENT STRATEGIES

### Is a Management Strategy Necessary in Managing the Difficult Airway?

Absolutely yes. A management strategy organized in algorithm form facilitates a systematic approach to the difficult airway, decreases reaction time, and potentially decreases the risk of an adverse outcome. This approach is essential for patients who are found to have an unrecognized difficult airway on induction or when a difficult airway is recognized before the induction but the patient is uncooperative or has categorically refused an awake intubation. A good example of management strategy is summarized in the difficult airway algorithm presented by the ASA in 1993 (Fig. 53–4)[3] or more recently by the CSA[2] (Fig. 53–5).

### How Is the Patient Prepared Before Induction?

Regardless of the intubation technique planned, any patient undergoing an elective intubation should be fully preoxygen-

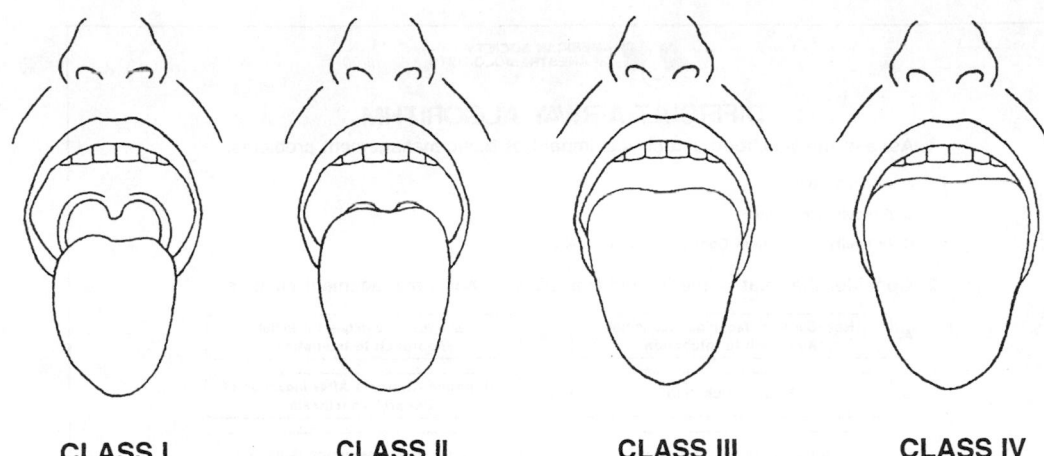

**FIGURE 53–2.** Samsoon and Young airway classification. (From Samsoon GLT, Young JRB. Difficult tracheal intubation: a retrospective study. *Anaesthesia.* 1987;42:487. Published by Blackwell Science Ltd.)

**CLASS I**          **CLASS II**          **CLASS III**          **CLASS IV**

ated because the apnea time necessary to reach critical $SpO_2$ (<90%) cannot always be mathematically predicted.[16] A fraction of inspired oxygen ($FIO_2$) of 1.0 is necessary for rapid and full tissue denitrogenation, and this may require several minutes to achieve. An $FIO_2$ of 1.0 is possible only with a tight mask fit, perhaps using a rubber mask-strap. Because the average time to critical desaturation (<90%) is usually shorter than the mean recovery time from an induction dose of succinylcholine (1 mg/kg)[16] (Fig. 53–6), the few extra minutes spent to explain both the discomforts and benefits of this technique are worthwhile even in the most uncooperative patient. This consideration is of particular importance in the categories of patients at risk for rapid desaturation after apnea, such as patients who are children, or those who are obese, have underlying chronic lung disease, and are critically ill.

## Preexisting Disease

Obese patients and those with underlying pulmonary disease have a decreased functional residual capacity (FRC)

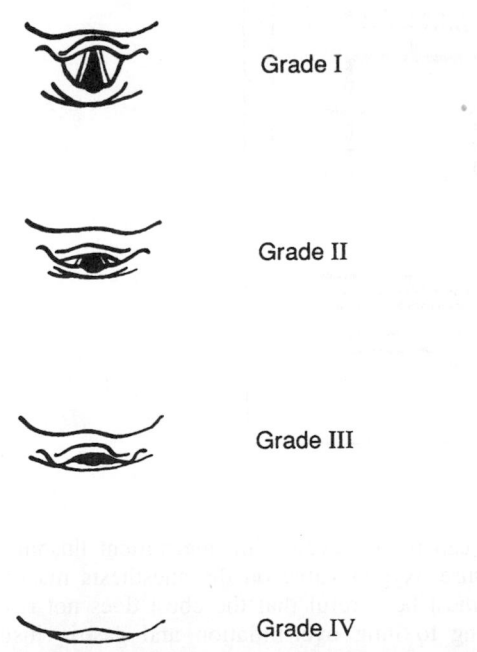

Grade I

Grade II

Grade III

Grade IV

**FIGURE 53–3.** Cormack and Lehane direct laryngoscopy classification. (From Cormack RS, Lehane J. Difficult tracheal intubation in obstetrics. *Anaesthesia.* 1984;39:1105. Published by Blackwell Science Ltd.)

and $\dot{V}/\dot{Q}$ mismatch. These changes are aggravated by supine positioning and paralysis. Metabolic rate and oxygen consumption are higher in the pediatric population. Critically ill patients combine increased oxygen consumption with $\dot{V}/\dot{Q}$ mismatch and decreased $\dot{D}O_2$. Again, the optimal duration of preoxygenation is unknown for an individual patient. We recommend a tight-fitting mask with 100% oxygen for several minutes or until (if gas analysis is available) $FIO_2$ equals fraction of expired oxygen ($FEO_2$).

## Aspiration Prophylaxis

Aspiration prophylaxis should be considered in all patients, not just those with predictable difficult airway or with a known history of or predisposition to gastroesophageal (GE) reflux (eg, obese or pregnant patients). Neutralization of gastric secretions can be achieved with sodium citrate (15-30 mL by mouth) shortly before induction of the anesthesia; oral ranitidine the evening before and 1 hour prior to surgery decreases acid production. Intravenous ranitidine can substitute for the oral preparation if the patient is on strict nil per os status. Metoclopramide, 10 mg intravenously, is added for all the patients at high risk of GE reflux unless a mechanical ileus is suspected.

## *What Is the Best Technique to Achieve Effective Mask Ventilation?*

Ventilation by face mask is a fundamental step in managing the airway after induction of general anesthesia. A high-flow, fresh gas source must be available to provide sufficient gas to compensate for face mask leaks and allow sufficient positive pressure to overcome respiratory system resistance. Jaw thrust and neck extension often are necessary to provide a patent airway. Proper seal of the adult face mask should be obtained by adjusting the cushion tension. With many masks, the cushion inflation volume can be adjusted by adding or removing air with a syringe via a valve in the mask.

The mask should be sized to cover the nose at the level of the nose bridge and the mouth just above the chin. In the edentulous patient, lateral seal may be a problem. Packing the inside of the cheeks with 4 × 4 gauze pads may help to compensate for the problem of a recessed chin or lack of teeth. Circumferential mask-straps may hold slack facial tissue against the mask cushion.

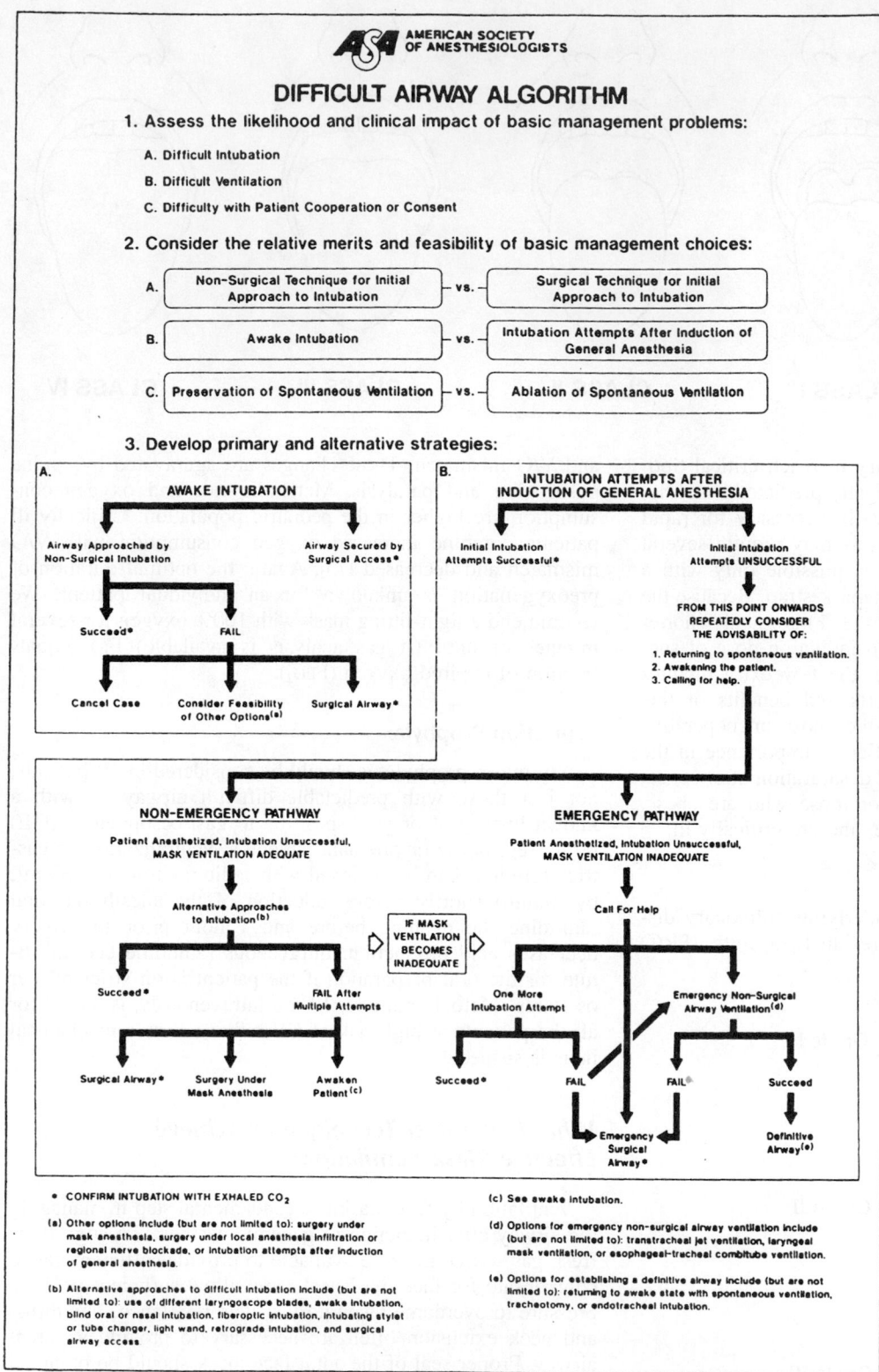

**FIGURE 53–4.** The Difficult Airway Algorithm presented by the American Society of Anesthesiology in 1993. The algorithm includes awake intubation. (From American Society of Anesthesiologists Task Force on Management of the Difficult Airway. Practice guidelines for management of the difficult airway. *Anesthesiology.* 1993;78:597.)

A number of alternative methods can be used to overcome lack of seal secondary to facial hair. Applying gauze soaked in petroleum jelly can help to fill facial contours under the mask cushion. Other homemade devices such as plastic film over the facial hair or even a defibrillator contact pad with a small hole cut in the middle at the level of the mouth opening may be helpful.[17] If the leak is massive, increased oxygen gas flow can be achieved with intermittent flushing of the high-pressure oxygen valve on the anesthesia machine. However, one must be careful that the chest does not rise excessively, leading to lung over-inflation and gastric insufflation. The incidence of gastric insufflation may also be minimized by ensuring airway pressure $<20$ cm $H_2O$ (often difficult to impossible) and an inspiratory time of 1.5 seconds.

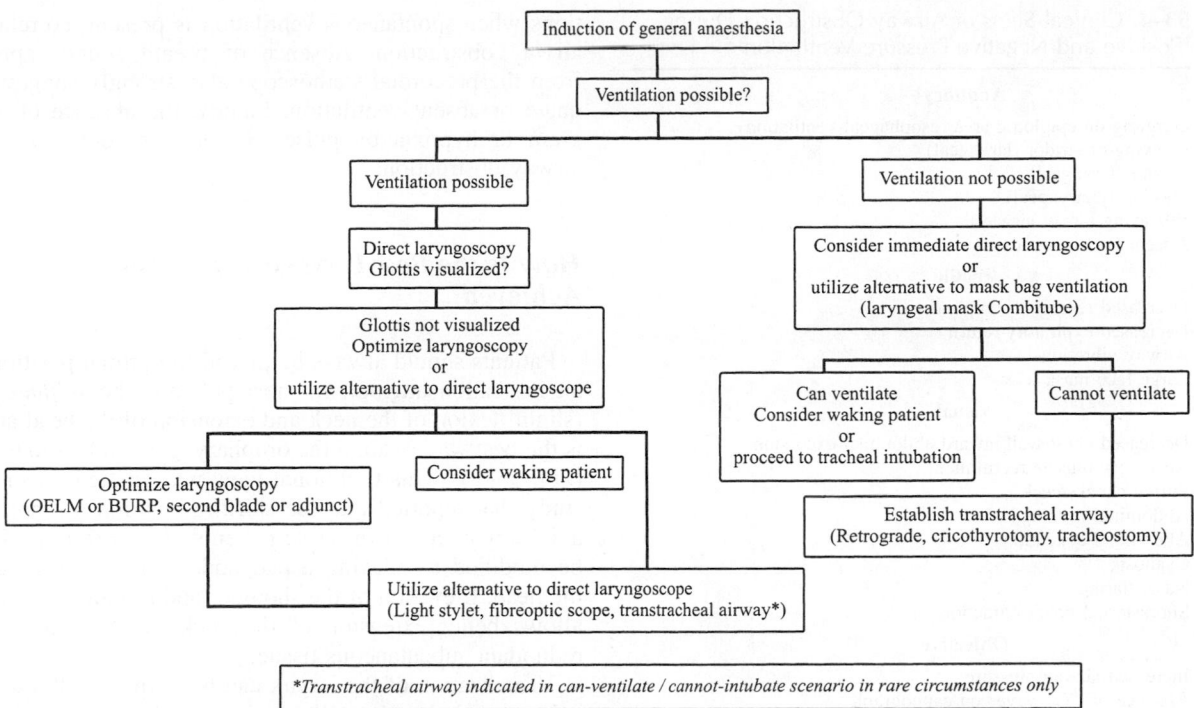

**FIGURE 53–5.** The Difficult Airway Algorithm presented by the Canadian Society of Anesthesiology in 1999, postinduction of general anesthesia. BURP, backward, upward, rightward laryngeal displacement; OELM, optimal external laryngeal manipulation. (From Crosby ET, Cooper RM, Douglas MJ, et al. The unanticipated difficult airway with recommendations for management. *Can J Anaesth.* 1998;45:757.)

## How Is Airway Obstruction Due to Soft Tissue Collapse Overcome?

The upper airway of an obese patient or of a patient with a history of sleep apnea or airway surgery may become totally obstructed after induction of the anesthesia. In obese patients, the combination of redundant oropharyngeal soft tissue, a bulky tongue, and a thick chin and neck pad may interfere with the ability to ventilate. Several methods may be used to overcome this obstruction. Lifting the chin pad while applying a jaw thrust can straighten the soft tissues of the anterior wall in the hypopharynx and facilitate ventilation. Inserting a plastic oral airway early or tilting the head laterally while ventilating may reduce the risk of the tongue falling backward against the soft palate of the posterior pharynx.

Before abandoning ventilation in any patient with a difficult airway, a two-person mask ventilation should be attempted. Two versions are displayed in Figure 53–7. The second version (see Fig. 53–7*B*) can be applied when the assistant has no expertise in airway management. A modification of this technique uses a pressure control anesthesia ventilator when a second assistant is not available. A pressure limit of 20 cm $H_2O$ is set to minimize risk of gastric insufflation. Tidal volume is adjusted to 1- to 2-cm chest rise at a rate between 15 to 20 breaths/minute.

**TIME TO HEMOGLOBIN DESATURATION WITH INITIAL $F_AO_2$ = 0.87**

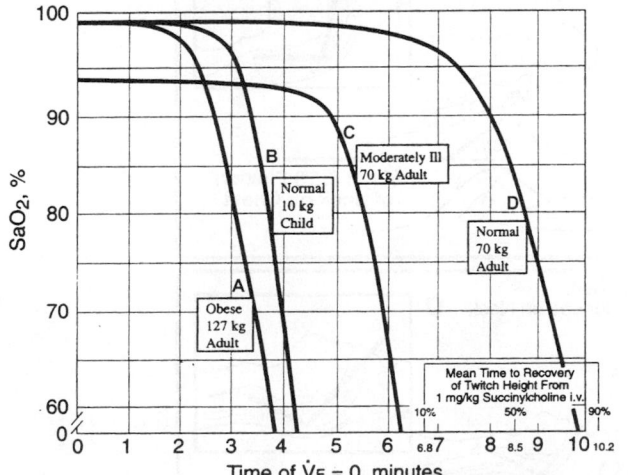

**FIGURE 53–6.** Mathematical extrapolations of arterial oxygen saturation post induction and paralysis with succinylcholine in (A) obese, (B) pediatric, (C) moderately critically ill, and (D) normal patients without ventilation. Critical desaturation precedes full recovery from succinylcholine in all the patients. (From Benumof JL, Dagg R, Benumof R. Critical hemoglobin desaturation will occur before return to an unparalyzed state following 1 mg/kg intravenous succinylcholine. *Anesthesiology.* 1997;87:979.)

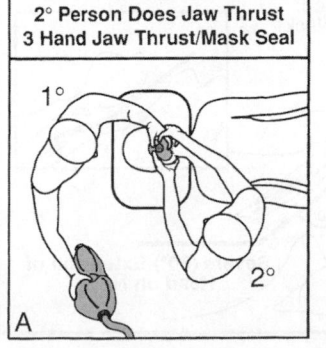

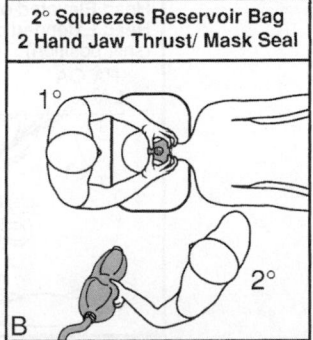

**FIGURE 53–7.** *A and B,* Two-person mask ventilation.

**TABLE 53–4.** Clinical Signs of Airway Obstruction During Positive and Negative Pressure Ventilation

**Auditory**

Gurgling on epiglottic area (esophageal ventilation)
Crowing or stridor (laryngeal)
Stridor (laryngeal)
Snoring (pharyngeal)
Wheezing (small airway)
Absent breath sounds

**Tactile**

Decreased reservoir compliance
Decreased expiratory return
Airway vibration
Large face mask leak

**Visual**

Decreased chest wall/inward abdominal excursion
Accessory muscle recruitment
Puffed cheeks/neck
Abdominal rocking
Abdominal distention
Cyanosis
Nasal flaring
Suprasternal notch retraction

**Objective**

Increased airway pressure
Absence of $CO_2$ waves on capnograph
Low measured expired volume
Hypoxemia (pulse oximeter)

### How Is an Obstructed Airway Recognized?

Various clinical signs may be noted during airway obstruction (Table 53–4). Gas passing through an obstructed airway may generate a characteristic bubbling noise. A rocking motion of the chest wall and abdomen, along with neck retrac-tions when spontaneous ventilation is present, correlates with airway obstruction. Absence of breath sounds appreciated from the precordial stethoscope also strongly suggests inade-quate or absent ventilation. Finally, the absence of a capno-gram or hypoxia by pulse oximeter are objective signs of airway obstruction.

### How Is the Best Laryngoscopic View Achieved?

Patients should always be placed in optimal position before an intubation attempt. In most patients, the *sniffing position* (slight flexion of the neck and extension of the head and neck) is the best way to align the oropharyngeal and laryngeal axes[18] (Fig. 53–8). (This traditional view was challenged in a recent study that reported that the sniffing position did not produce axial alignment.[19]) In obese patients, the sniffing position can be modified by placing a pad under both the shoulders and the head. Elevation of the shoulder and scapulae, in particular, allows better extension of the neck in obese patients with redundant subcutaneous tissue.

Visualization of the larynx can be optimized through exter-nal manipulations, usually applied by the right hand or by an assistant. The optimal external laryngeal manipulation (OELM)[19] and the backward, upward, rightward laryngeal displacement (BURP)[20] describe, respectively, the American and Canadian approaches to external manipulation of the larynx in order to improve vocal cord visualization during laryngoscopy.

OELM is described as posterior and cephalad pressure over the thyroid or cricoid cartilage. In the majority of cases, the best view is obtained simply by pressing the thyroid cartilage posteriorly. The BURP maneuver generates manual displace-

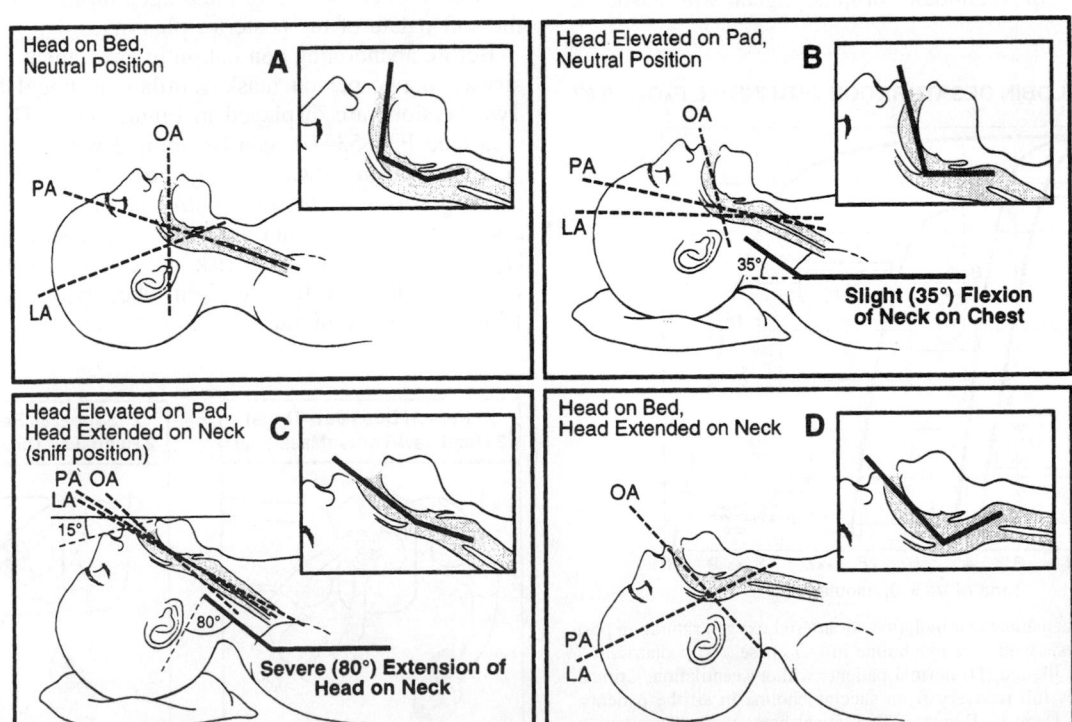

**FIGURE 53–8.** *A–D*, Head and neck position and the axes of the head, neck, and upper airway.

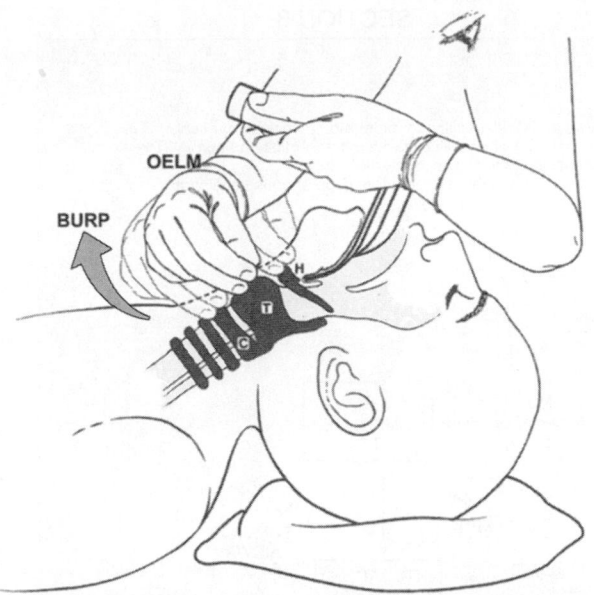

**FIGURE 53–9.** External manipulation to visualize the larynx during direct laryngoscopy optimal external laryngeal manipulation (OELM). Backward, upward, rightward external displacement of the larynx (BURP) (modified).

ment of the larynx posteriorly against the cervical vertebrae, then superiorly and as far as possible to the right. Both maneuvers are indicated in laryngoscopy grades 2 through 4, usually improving the view by at least one grade (Fig. 53–9).

### How Many Times Should Laryngoscopy Be Attempted Before Choosing an Alternative Approach?

Numerous attempts at DL may degrade the quality of the airway due to laryngeal edema and bleeding. Such conditions may render mask ventilation progressively more difficult or impossible. A degraded airway after numerous attempts at DL is the most common reason for the "cannot ventilate" scenario and adverse respiratory events in anesthesia.[1] Three to four attempts at DL usually are the maximum number before switching to an alternative plan or resuming mask ventilation.

To limit the possibility of adverse respiratory events, we recommend that inexperienced laryngoscopists not be allowed to perform laryngoscopy in patients with grade 3-4 laryngoscopic view until they have a track record of successfully intubating less challenging airways. During any manipulation of the airway, an expert laryngoscopist should always be present.

### What Laryngoscope Blade Should Be Used?

MacIntosh blades are recommended when a relatively small mouth opening, large tongue, or redundant subcutaneous tissue is present. A MacIntosh No. 4 is our blade of choice. On the other hand, the Miller blade may be optimal for visualization of the vocal cords in patients with a small mandibular space, large incisors, or a large, floppy epiglottis. The Miller blade remains the blade of choice for the pediatric population, owing to the relatively larger size of their epiglottis.

A commonly used adjunct device for DL in the unpredictable airway is the gum elastic stylet.[21] Under DL, the tip of the flexible stylet is blindly passed under the epiglottis into the trachea. The endotracheal tube (ETT) is then passed over the stylet, thereby allowing tracheal intubation. During insertion of the ETT, counter-clockwise rotation of the ETT by 90° to 180° is recommended to avoid impingement of the tip of the ETT on the right vocal cord.

A number of laryngoscopic blades have been introduced to improve access to the vocal cords when the larynx is anterior, all anecdotally advantageous in cases of difficult airway or limited mouth opening. A detailed review is available.[22]

## NAVIGATING THE DIFFICULT AIRWAY ALGORITHM

### How Can It Be Used Effectively?

The algorithm for difficult airway can be organized into three parts:

**Part One.** Predictable difficult intubation due to recognized difficult airway

**Part Two.** Unpredictable difficult airway with ability to ventilate by mask

**Part Three.** Unpredictable difficult airway, with inability to ventilate or oxygenate the patient, immediately after induction of anesthesia or after a short period of successful ventilation (Fig. 53–10)

### Part One: Fiberoptic Intubation for Recognized Difficult Airway

Perhaps the most optimal use of the fiberoptic bronchoscope (FOB) is in the awake patient with an established difficult airway. Because most of these patients are at high risk for aspiration, we administer histamine$_2$ (H$_2$) blocker the night before the scheduled operation and again early on the morning of surgery. One half-hour before surgery, we orally administer 15 to 30 mL of sodium citrate. Glycopyrrolate, 0.2 to 0.4 mg, is given intravenously 30 minutes, or intramuscularly 1 hour, before the surgery begins. The antisialagogue action of this agent minimizes secretions, improving visualization. Additionally, the tip of the instrument is wetted with an antifogging agent, and the ETT is preheated in warm saline for 5 to 10 minutes before the procedure to maximize visualization.

Our topical anesthetic of choice is 4% lidocaine (4-6 mL) nebulized into an aerosolized face mask 10 minutes before beginning the procedure. Bilateral superior laryngeal nerve and glossopharyngeal nerve blocks, using 2 to 3 mL of 1% lidocaine, are performed when feasible. Transtracheal block is not usually necessary if lidocaine nebulization by mask has been successful. The total amount of local anesthetic should not exceed the calculated toxic dose on a per kilogram basis. Local anesthesia may also be provided on a "spray as you go" basis, using aerosolized 2% lidocaine through the operative channel while advancing the FOB.

Gentle jaw thrust or pressure on the larynx with neck extension may facilitate the exposure of the vocal cords. Specialized airways such as the Berman, Ovassapian, and Williams can facilitate placement of the ETT in front of the vocal cords, deep into the hypopharynx. Concomitant con-

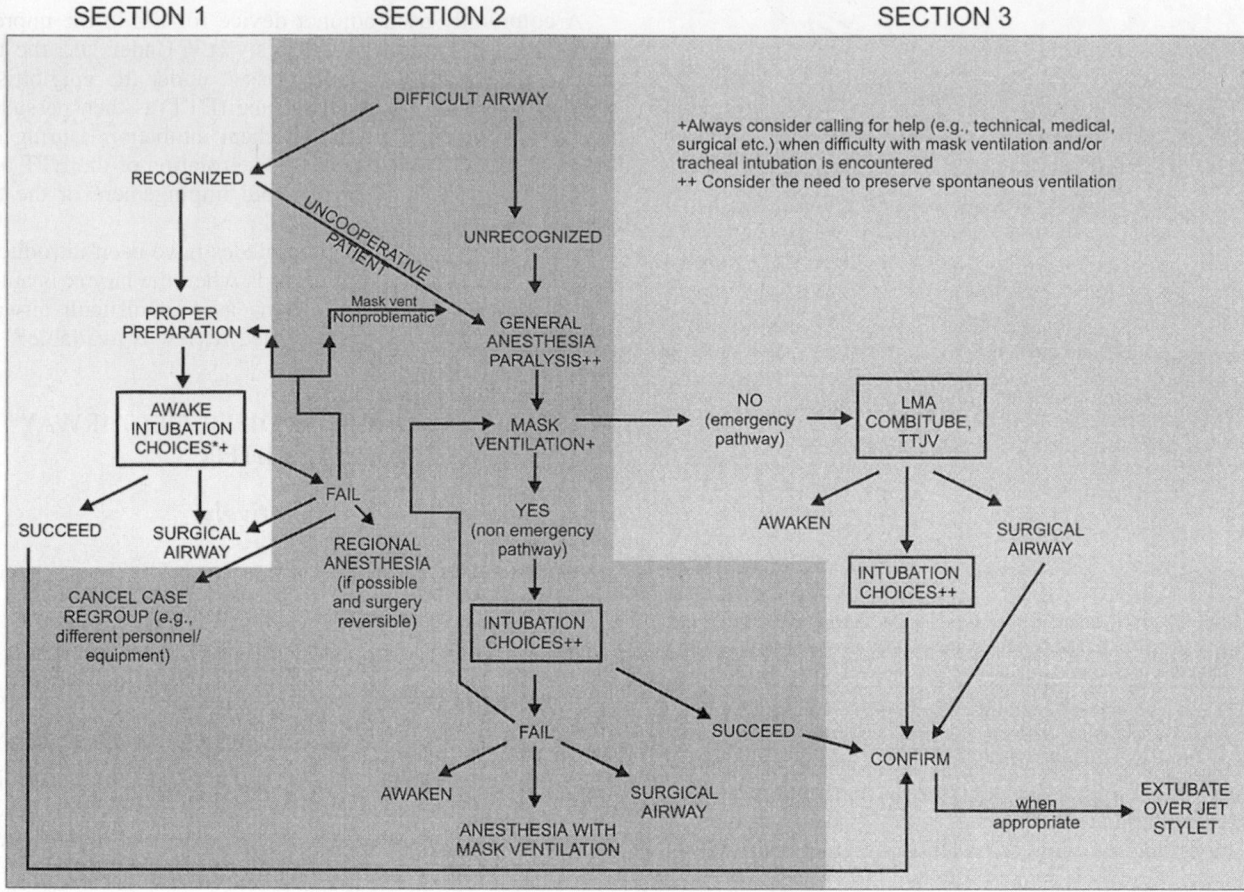

**FIGURE 53–10.** Navigating the Difficult Airway Algorithm. *Section 1,* The predictable difficult intubation approached awake. *Section 2,* The unpredictable difficult intubation with ability to ventilate by mask. *Section 3,* The unpredictable difficult intubation with inability to ventilate by mask. LMA, laryngeal mask airway; TTJV, transtracheal jet ventilation.

scious sedation may be provided to improve patient comfort. Although there is no cookbook drug regimen for this procedure, our preference is to use small doses of a short-acting benzodiazepine (midazolam) as an anxiolytic; low-dose propofol may also be used. Opiates are not required unless an independent source of pain is present because adequate topical anesthesia will provide airway analgesia.

Nasotracheal intubation is an alternative to the oral route for patients with a large tongue or edema of the oropharynx. We pretreat the mucosa of both nostrils with a solution of 0.1% phenylephrine, followed by progressive dilation using nasal trumpets lubricated with 2% lidocaine jelly. Four percent cocaine pledgets may be used as an alternative to phenylephrine HCl (Neo-Synephrine) in young individuals. Four percent cocaine is an excellent vasoconstrictor and topical analgesic for the nasopharynx, providing not only topical analgesia but also sphenopalatinum ganglion block. When using cocaine, one must keep in mind the potentiating effect of this drug on indirect sympathomimetic agents. Electrocardiographic monitoring should be used when administering cocaine anesthesia.

Fiberoptic intubation may be attempted orally after induction of anesthesia, if the patient can be ventilated by BVM, using the Patil-Syracuse mask (Fig. 53–11) or connecting a regular mask with a bronchoscope swivel adapter. However, the use of a flexible FOB after the patient has been rendered unconscious may be difficult owing to a collapse of the pharyngeal soft tissues. Fiberoptic intubation when the patient

is anesthetized should be performed by two experienced operators.

## Part Two: Strategy for the "Cannot Intubate" Patient When Bag-Valve-Mask Ventilation Is Still Possible

If laryngoscopy does not result in visualization of the glottis after multiple attempts, despite use of OELM or BURP, the safest alternative is to simply awaken the patient for fiberoptic intubation. Because prolonged manipulation of the airway may result in damage or edema to this normally soft tissue, surgery may need to be canceled. Nebulized racemic epinephrine and systemic steroids (dexamethasone, 5–20 mg/d) are indicated when edema of the hypopharynx results from laryngoscopic manipulation. If, instead of canceling the procedure, the decision to proceed with surgery is made, several alternatives to DL are available.

### Fiberoptic Intubation

FOB intubation, either as described previously or after laryngeal mask airway (LMA) placement, can be accomplished while the patient is anesthetized and breathing spontaneously. Ventilation may be provided during the procedure through a Portex right-angle adapter (Fig. 53–12).[14] To minimize air trapping and barotrauma, ventilation should be pro-

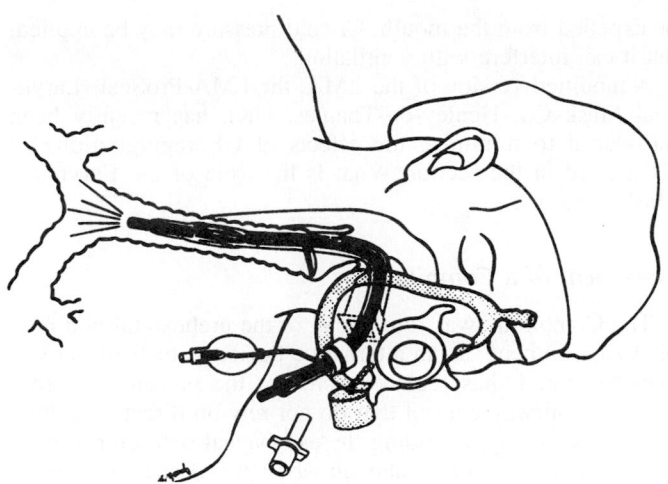

**FIGURE 53–11.** The intubating Patil-Syracuse mask.

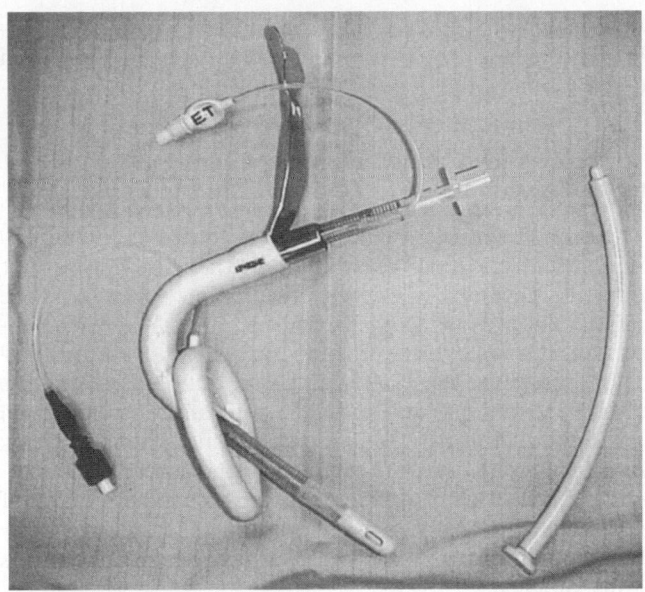

**FIGURE 53–13.** Fastrach intubating laryngeal mask airway (LMA). A silicone wire-reinforced cuffed endotracheal tube is placed in the LMA with the help of a silicone extension.

vided manually by an assistant using a self-inflating bag rather than a mechanical ventilator.

### Laryngeal Mask Airway-Fastrach

The LMA-Fastrach can facilitate placement of the ETT (Fig. 53–13). A straight, silicone wire–reinforced cuffed ETT up to 8 mm in internal diameter is available for placement through the Fastrach. The LMA-Fastrach is available in sizes 3, 4, and 5, for small, normal, and large adults, respectively. Wire-reinforced ETT is available in sizes 7 through 8 mm. The particular advantage of the LMA-Fastrach is that it permits single-handed insertion from any position without moving the head and neck from a neutral position and without placing fingers in the mouth (Fig. 53–14). The device is latex-free and reusable up to 40 times.

### Fiberoptic Bronchoscope Through Endoscopy Mask

The trachea can be intubated with an FOB using an endoscopy mask or connecting a regular mask to a bronchoscopy

swivel adapter (see Fig. 53–10). This technique requires an assistant to hold the mask and assist the patient with BVM ventilation. Inhalation anesthesia can be provided during the procedure. Fiberoptic intubation can be carried out while maintaining good airway seal because the port of entry for the FOB has a rubber or silicone diaphragm that minimizes leaks.

The main advantage of these techniques is that positive pressure ventilation, oxygen, and inhalation anesthetics can be provided continuously during the insertion of the ETT. As an alternative, an LMA or a mask can be used to provide an inhalation agent during a brief case using general anesthesia without attempting insertion of the ETT at all. However, this is a valid alternative only in patients with a low risk of pulmonary aspiration of gastric contents.

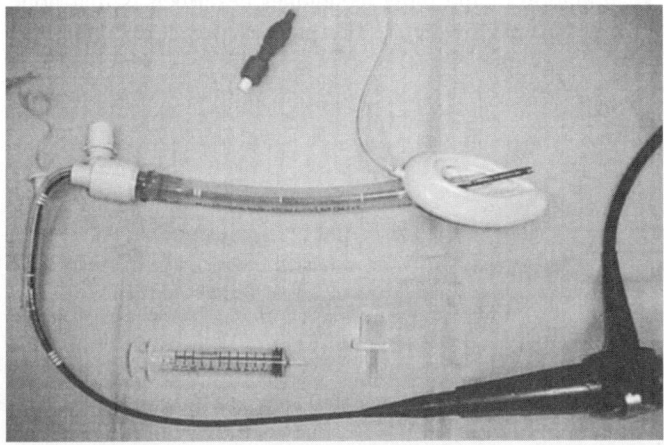

**FIGURE 53–12.** Fiberoptic intubation of a laryngeal mask airway with a Rae endotracheal tube. The swivel adapter in place allows ventilation during the procedure. (From Benumof JL. Laryngeal mask airway and the ASA difficult airway algorithm. *Anesthesiology.* 1996;84:686.)

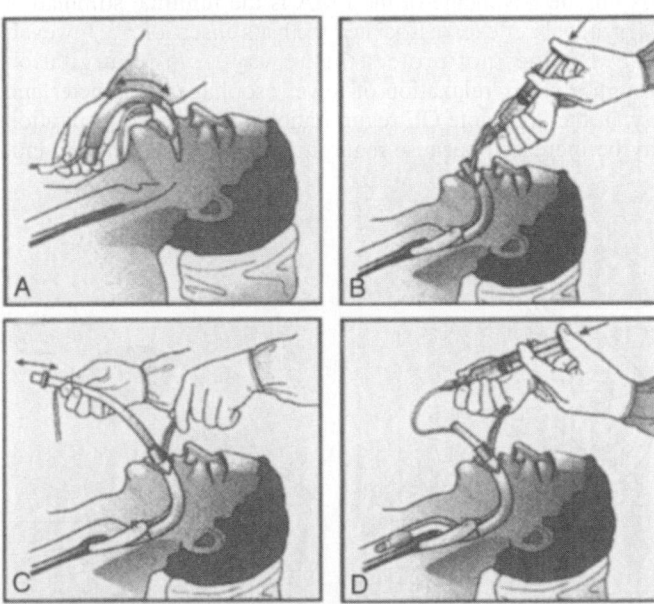

**FIGURE 53–14.** *A–D,* Placement of an endotracheal tube with the intubating laryngeal mask airway.

Other alternatives, discussed later in this chapter, are available. However, they do not allow simultaneous ventilation and intubation.

## Part Three: The "Cannot Ventilate, Cannot Intubate" Scenario

The cannot ventilate, cannot intubate scenario is an anesthesiologist's or certified registered nurse anesthetist's worst nightmare. The rate of oxygen desaturation depends on the length of the preoxygenation time, the patient's oxygen consumption, intrapulmonary shunting, and FRC. As noted previously, pediatric, obese, pregnant, and critically ill patients are particularly prone to early and significant desaturation. In this situation, the first step is to request more help. In many cases, this help may be life-saving. Two-person mask ventilation should be attempted before moving to another portion of the algorithm. Other personnel may be delegated to apply cricoid pressure, obtain supplies, or control hemodynamics pharmacologically.

The presence of severe pathology above the vocal cords (eg, tumor masses or facial trauma) may preclude the successful use of alternative airway techniques. This problem is reviewed in the paragraphs dedicated to the transtracheal approach to the airway.

In general, the cannot ventilate, cannot intubate scenario can be resolved only with placement of an LMA, a Combitube, or a cuffed oropharyngeal airway (COPA).

### Placement of a Laryngeal Mask Airway

Placing an LMA should be attempted first. In fact, the track record of the successful positioning of an LMA is excellent, even in nonexpert hands.[23] Paramedical personnel and students attempting to access known difficult airways were successful 94% of the time on first attempt with an LMA; none had prior experience.[24] The LMA has proved to be relatively easy to use in the case of difficult intubation, including class III and IV airways and laryngoscopy grade 3 or 4.[25]

A unique advantage of the LMA is the minimal stimulation of laryngeal reflexes associated with its insertion.[26] However, the LMA does not protect the airway from regurgitation through a reflex relaxation of lower esophageal sphincter and may, in fact, promote GE regurgitation.[27] The risk of aspiration may be increased because regurgitated gastric contents cannot

be expelled from the mouth. Cricoid pressure may be applied, but it can interfere with ventilation.[28]

A modified version of the LMA, the LMA-ProSeal (Laryngeal Mask Co, Henley-on-Thames, UK), has recently been introduced to minimize the effects of GE regurgitation.[29–32] (Discussed in the section What Is the Role of the Laryngeal Mask Airway?)

### Placement of a Combitube

The Combitube was introduced in the prehospital and hospital environments as an alternative device in difficult airway management. It has replaced some of the nonsurgical techniques for airway control that do not rely on direct visualization of the airway, including the esophageal obturator airway, the esophageal gastric tube airway,[33,34] and the pharyngeal lumen airway.[35]

The Combitube is a double-lumen tube with distal and proximal cuffs, presently available in sizes 37 French (women and young adults) and 41 French (men) (Fig. 53–15). Despite its bulky appearance, the Combitube has a good safety record with only rare case reports of esophageal rupture.[36,37] The device was initially introduced as a nonsurgical technique for airway control during cardiac and respiratory arrest.[38] It has been successfully used in hospitalized patients with sustained, nontraumatic cardiopulmonary arrest[39] and in patients undergoing elective surgery under general anesthesia.[40] Other indications for the Combitube are facial burn[41] and oropharyngeal hematoma.[42] The Combitube is a useful adjunct to facilitate airway control in trauma patients with possible cervical spine injury.[43–45]

### Placement of a Cuffed Pharyngeal Airway

Although limited information has been published about this device, the use of the COPA is intuitively easy (Fig. 53–16).[46–49] One of the main advantages with this device, once in place, is that the presence of a cuff in the pharyngeal space does not interfere with the advancement of the FOB. The cuff can lift the tongue, creating a space for a better bronchoscopy view. Unlike the LMA, the COPA does not limit the size of the ETT because the tube is passed not through it but laterally to it.

A limitation of the three techniques described is that none of them is effective when the difficult airway is secondary to

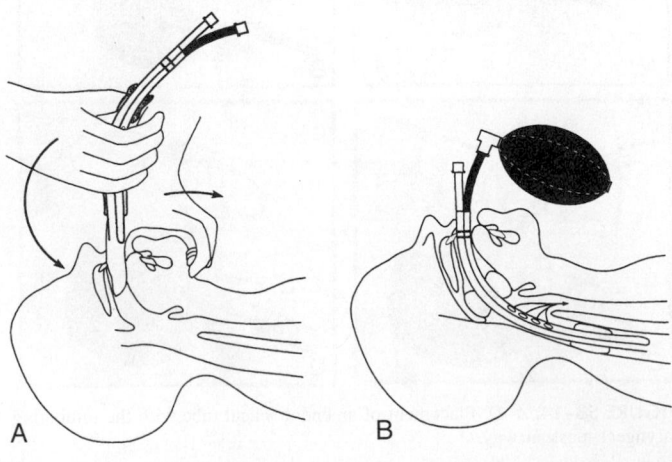

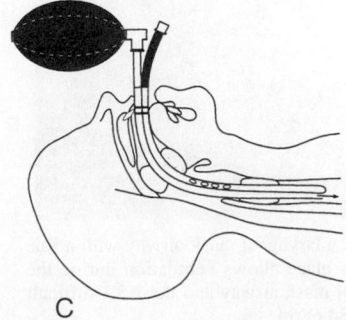

**FIGURE 53–15.** Placement of a Combitube. *A,* Minimal mouth opening required. *B,* Combitube in the esophagus, ventilation through the pharyngeal openings. *C,* Combitube in the trachea, ventilation through the distal opening.

A                    B                    C

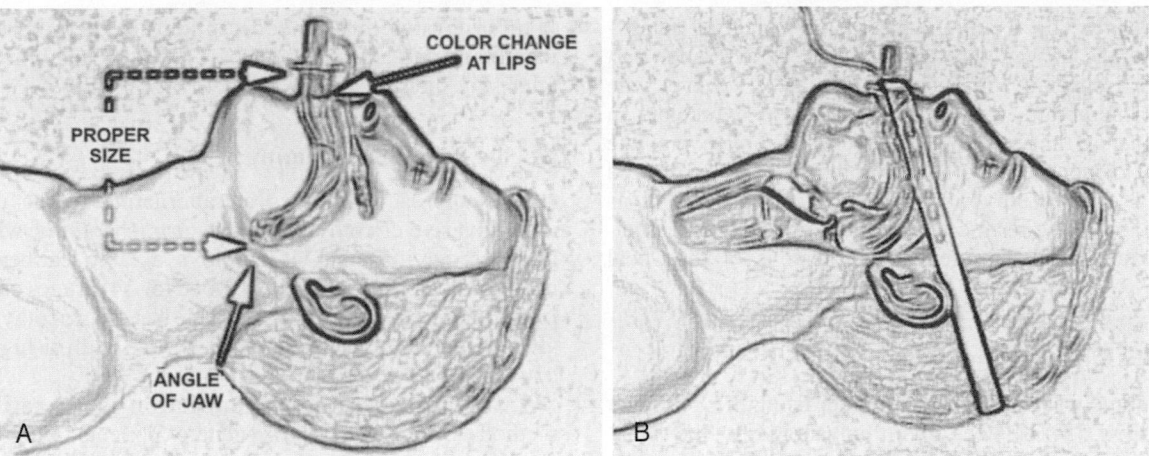

**FIGURE 53–16.** The cuffed oropharyngeal airway (COPA). *A,* In place. *B,* Cuff inflated to facilitate ventilation.

pathology above the vocal cords (eg, hematoma, pharyngeal abscess, neoplasia, airway edema, or massive facial trauma). In these cases, only two approaches are successful: transtracheal catheter placement and a surgical airway. Both are reviewed later.

## What Are the Alternatives for Supraglottic Pathology?

When the airway is compromised by trauma or when massive oropharyngeal or hypopharyngeal pathology is present, emergency access to the airway may be obtained through an emergency surgical airway (tracheotomy or cricothyroidotomy) or a percutaneous cricothyroidotomy.

### Tracheotomy

Emergency tracheotomy is usually performed using a vertical incision from the cricoid cartilage down, for approximately 1 cm, in the direction of the sternal notch. A No. 11 surgical blade, preferably, is used. A skilled, surgically trained operator can rapidly approach the trachea through this route. However, serious bleeding may occur via laceration of the anterior jugular and superior thyroid veins, the cricothyroid artery, and other vessels of the thyroid isthmus. If the procedure is successful and tracheal intubation is confirmed, as soon as the patient is stabilized, the next step is to immediately surgically revise the tracheotomy.

### Surgical Cricothyrotomy

Emergency cricothyrotomy is a valid alternative to the emergency tracheotomy for a physician not skilled or trained in the surgical approach to the airway (eg, emergency department physician, anesthesiologist, pulmonologist, or intensivist). This technique requires identification of the cricothyroid membrane, which is directly under the skin in the anterior neck between the thyroid cartilage superiorly and the cricoid cartilage inferiorly.[50] It covers the cricothyroid space, which averages 9 mm in height and 3 cm in width and consists of a central triangular portion (*conus elasticus*) and two lateral portions. It is often crossed horizontally in its upper third by the superior cricothyroid arteries.

Because the vocal cords are usually located a centimeter or more above the cricothyroid space, they are usually not injured, even during emergency cricothyrotomy. The anterior jugular veins run vertically in the lateral aspect of the neck and also are usually spared injury during the procedure. However, considerable variation is present in both the arterial and venous vessel patterns. Although the arteries are always located deep to the pretracheal fascia and are easily avoided during a skin incision, veins may be found in both the pretracheal fascia and between the pretracheal and superficial cervical fascias. To minimize the possibility of bleeding, the cricothyroid membrane should be incised at its inferior third.

To locate the cricothyroid membrane, external visible and palpable anatomic landmarks are used. The laryngeal prominence and the hyoid bone above it are readily palpable. The cricothyroid membrane usually lies 1 to 1½ fingerbreadths below the laryngeal prominence (Fig. 53–17). The cricoid cartilage is also easily felt caudal to the cricothyroid membrane. Usually, only a few seconds are required to identify these landmarks, but their importance must be emphasized. Conscious effort to identify these landmarks reduces the possibility of mistakenly placing the cricothyroid tube into the superiorly located thyroid space.

The incision is placed vertically, preferably with a No. 11 surgical blade, over the cricothyroid membrane. A small ETT, preferably armored, is placed through the membrane and

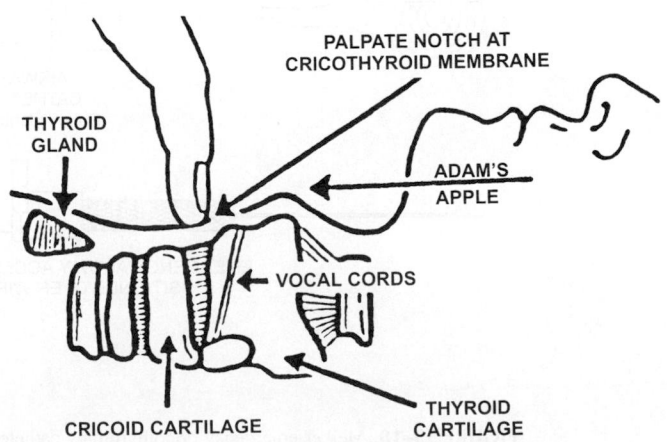

**FIGURE 53–17.** Anatomy of the cricothyroid membrane.

aimed downward. This technique has the advantage of achieving access to the airway through a relatively avascular part of the neck, especially in lean individuals. However, the cricothyroid membrane is not always easy to appreciate in obese patients or those with short necks. In any event, the successful placement of cricothyroidotomy should be followed by an elective tracheotomy or fiberoptic intubation as soon as possible, because long-term cricothyroidotomy may be associated with cricoid malacia, stenosis, or lesions of the vocal cords.

## Percutaneous Cricothyroidotomy

This technique was described by Melker using the Seldinger technique (Fig. 53–18). The main advantage is the blunt dissection of the subcutaneous tissues all the way to the cricothyroid membrane.[46] An airway catheter is then introduced over a dilator threaded over the guidewire. This technique allows the ultimate insertion of an airway considerably larger than the initial needle or catheter and often of sufficient internal diameter to allow ventilation with conventional ventilation devices, suctioning, and spontaneous ventilation (Fig. 53–19).

Although this technique is relatively atraumatic, it does require some knowledge of the anatomy of the neck and previously established proficiency in using the kit. It should not be used by physicians unfamiliar with this device. When established successfully, the airway placed is an uncuffed tracheotomy tube. To date, the manufacturers of cuffed tubes have been reticent to provide one for this kit.

A variation of this technique is the Patil cricothyroidotomy.

It incorporates direct needle puncture of the cricothyroid membrane and advancement of a dilator loaded on the needle after skin incision with a scalpel (Fig. 53–20).

## Needle Cricothyroidotomy

This approach provides an alternative to the use of the more invasive cricothyroidotomy or tracheotomy, whether surgical or percutaneous. It employs a large caliber over-the-needle catheter, usually No. 12 or No. 14 gauge, or a specialized armored version (Fig. 53–21). Needle cricothyroidotomy always requires the use of a jet device with a high-pressure oxygen source to provide ventilation.

Transtracheal catheter ventilation is a relatively easy method to *temporarily* oxygenate patients who cannot be mask-ventilated or intubated. We consider it to be a bridge technique that buys time until the patient is awakened or a definitive airway can be secured. The cricothyroid membrane is punctured percutaneously with a needle or, preferably, an over-the-needle catheter. In the latter case, the needle is removed and the catheter is attached to a high-frequency jet ventilator.

Although oxygenation may be adequate with transtracheal catheter ventilation, passive exhalation often is insufficient to sustain ventilation; hypercarbia and significant air trapping may result. Other complications include needle displacement into the subcutaneous tissue with massive subcutaneous emphysema, barotrauma with pneumothorax or tension pneumothorax; air trapping with severe hemodynamic instability due to impeded venous return to the right atrium; and right-to-left ventricular septal shift. The needle or catheter may break or

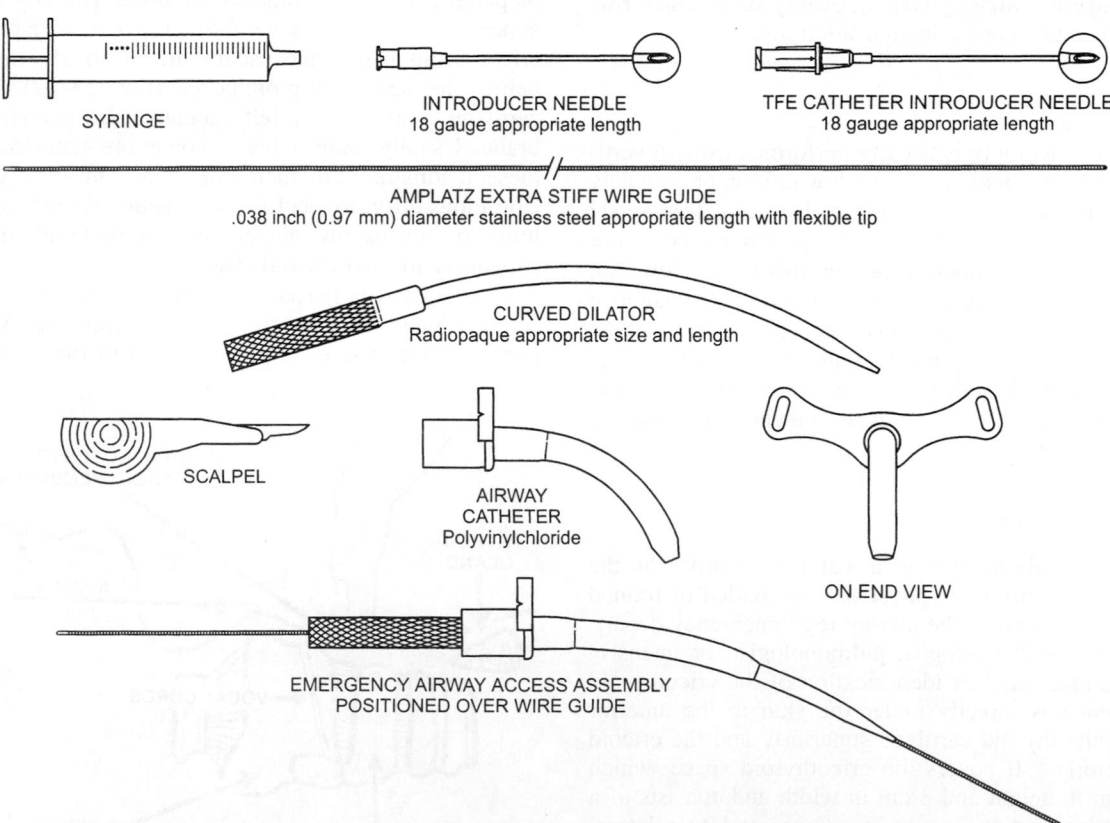

SYRINGE

INTRODUCER NEEDLE
18 gauge appropriate length

TFE CATHETER INTRODUCER NEEDLE
18 gauge appropriate length

AMPLATZ EXTRA STIFF WIRE GUIDE
.038 inch (0.97 mm) diameter stainless steel appropriate length with flexible tip

CURVED DILATOR
Radiopaque appropriate size and length

SCALPEL

AIRWAY
CATHETER
Polyvinylchloride

ON END VIEW

EMERGENCY AIRWAY ACCESS ASSEMBLY
POSITIONED OVER WIRE GUIDE

**FIGURE 53–18.** Melker emergency cricothyrotomy catheter kit. (Courtesy of Cook Critical Care, Inc, Bloomington, Ind.)

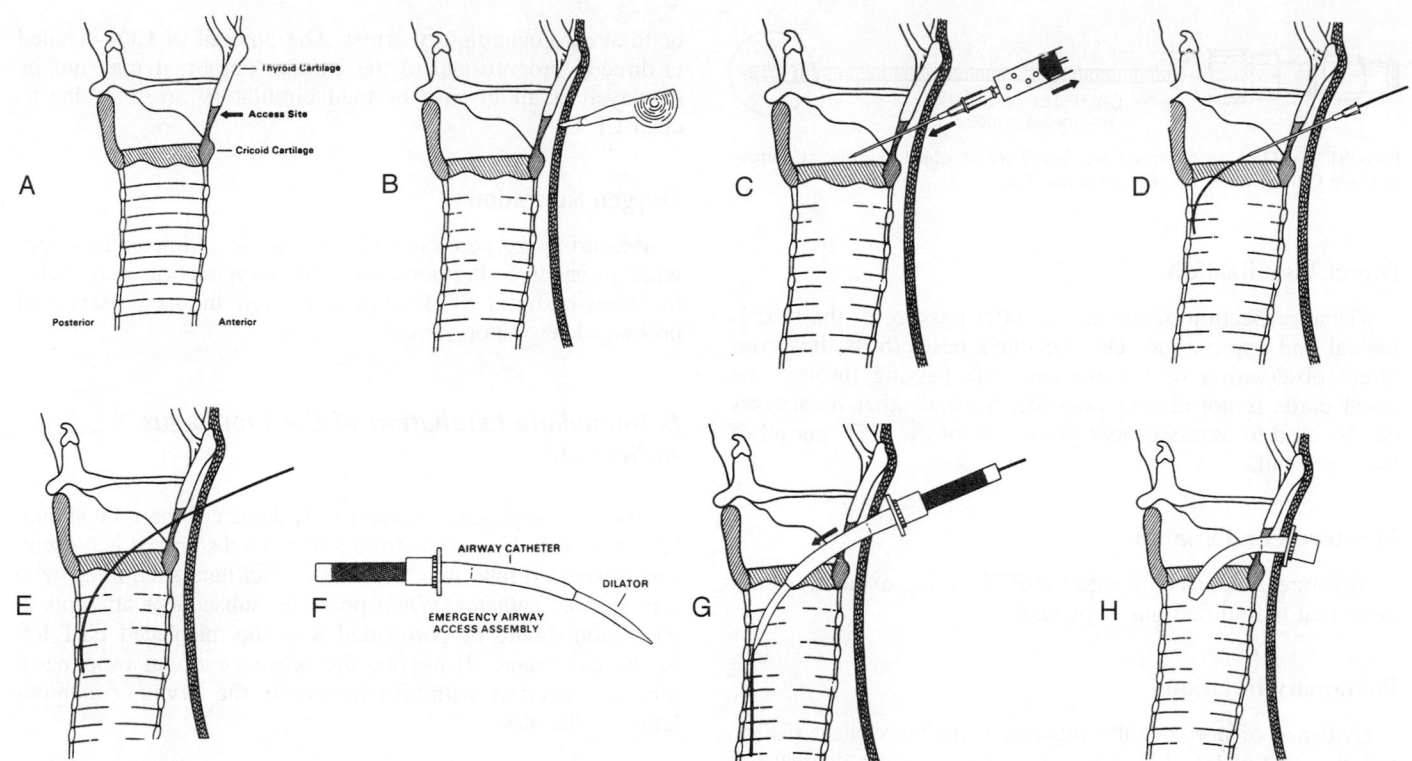

**FIGURE 53–19.** *A–H,* Percutaneous approach to the cricothyroid membrane with the Melker cricothyrotomy kit. (Courtesy of Cook Critical Care, Inc, Bloomington, Ind.)

bend if the patient coughs or moves, resulting in respiratory obstruction.

Of these complications, subcutaneous air injection—sometimes massive—with loss of anatomic landmarks and pneumothorax and catheter kinking appear to be the most serious and widely encountered. Use of this technique for more than short intervals is inappropriate with a needle or standard intravenous catheter because each is extremely difficult to secure and maintain in the proper position. In order to

minimize barotrauma, airway patency should be maintained with head extension, jaw thrust, and chin lift by an assistant.

## CONFIRMATION OF TRACHEAL INTUBATION

### How Is It Done?

Several methods to confirm tracheal intubation have been recommended.

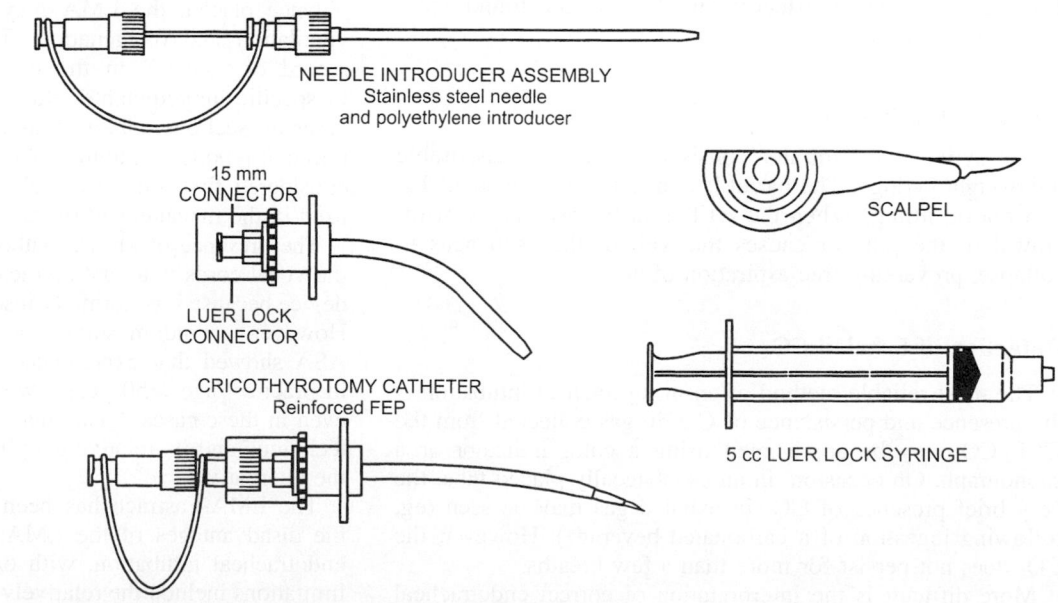

**FIGURE 53–20.** Patil cricothyrotomy kit. FEP, fluorinated ethylene-propylene. (Courtesy of Cook Critical Care, Inc, Bloomington, Ind.)

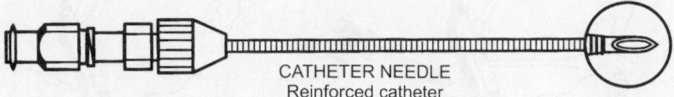

CATHETER NEEDLE
Reinforced catheter

**FIGURE 53–21.** Size 6 French reinforced transtracheal catheter. (Courtesy of Cook Critical Care, Inc, Bloomington, Ind.)

### Direct Visualization

Visual inspection of the airway after passage of the tube is logical and appropriate. Despite one's best efforts, however, direct observation of the tip and cuff passing through the vocal cords is not always possible. Several other maneuvers can be used to assess proper placement of the ETT, but all of them can fail.

### Moisture Condensation

Moisture condensation into the ETT during exhalation suggests that humidified gas is present.

### Pulmonary Inflation

Evidence of correct tube placement includes chest rise on inflation and bilateral breath sounds with a slight decrease in perceived compliance toward the end of expansion. These clues may be unreliable in obese patients or those with a rigid chest wall.

### Suction Bulb

A 75-mL self-inflating suction bulb connected with a plastic 15-mm plastic adapter to the proximal end of the ETT has been used to confirm tracheal intubation during cardiopulmonary resuscitation (CPR). Compression and release of the bulb, if the ETT is properly placed, results in the bulb filling with air. If the ETT is in the esophagus, the negative bulb pressure on release collapses the esophagus, and the bulb will not inflate. The device is disposable, small, and lightweight. The method, although effective in CPR, has not found widespread application.[51,52]

### Syringe Air Aspiration

The syringe air aspirator consists of a 60-mL disposable lightweight syringe. The barrel is connected to a standard 15-mm plastic fitting. When the ETT is in the esophagus, withdrawal of the plunger causes the wall of the esophagus to collapse, preventing free aspiration of air.[53]

### Detection of Exhaled CO$_2$

The most reliable method of ensuring tracheal intubation is the presence and persistence of CO$_2$ in gas collected from the ETT. CO$_2$ may be appreciated using a color indicator or a capnograph. On occasion, in an esophageally placed tube, the very brief presence of CO$_2$ in exhaled gas may be seen (eg, following ingestion of a carbonated beverage). However, the CO$_2$ does not persist for more than a few breaths.

More difficult is the interpretation of correct endotracheal intubation in patients with severe reduction of cardiac output

or total cardiocirculatory arrest. The amount of CO$_2$ exhaled is directly proportional to the cardiac output; it may not be displayed at all in case of total circulatory arrest or inefficient CPR.

### Oxygen Saturation

Measuring oxygen saturation by pulse oximeter is somewhat insensitive. Previous effective oxygenation may delay the time of onset of desaturation, even in the presence of prolonged respiratory arrest.

### *Is Immediate Extubation of the Esophagus Indicated?*

Once an esophageal intubation is detected, the tube should be left in place if vomitus from a distended stomach is present. The misplaced tube may be used to facilitate suctioning with a large bore catheter. When possible, subsequent attempts at intubation should be performed with the misplaced ETT left in the esophagus. However, the presence of an esophageal tube may interfere with visualization of the larynx or manipulation of the airway.

## ALTERNATIVES TO BAG-MASK VENTILATION AND DIRECT LARYNGOSCOPY

### *What Is the Role of the Laryngeal Mask Airway?*

The LMA now has a primary role in achieving airway control, oxygenation, and ventilation in an unpredictable difficult airway when general anesthesia, with or without paralysis, is induced. Several indications have been described. The LMA can be considered a temporary airway to facilitate the introduction of an ETT with the aid of FOB.[14]

Once placed, the LMA may be left in place to provide ventilation and oxygenation. The LMA has a solid track record of "saves" in the established difficult airway and in specific unpredictable situations, such as with emergency cesarean sections, airway trauma, and newborn infants, with minimal reports of failure.[54] At this time, the LMA should be considered first among the alternative airway devices to be used in the management of the difficult airway.

The presence of known pathology at the level of or above the vocal cords is a contraindication to the use of this airway device because it is normally inserted blindly into the pharynx. However, a random survey of 1000 active members of the ASA showed that experienced anesthesiologists (>10 years in practice, age >50 years) would consider use of the LMA even in these cases.[55] This may be due to familiarity with the technique and its relative simplicity to master compared with the alternatives.

The LMA-Fastrach has been developed to solve some of the disadvantages of the LMA when it is used to facilitate endotracheal intubation, with or without an FOB.[56–59] These limitations include the relatively small caliber of ETT allowed through the LMA (6-mm diameter), the difficulty of passing the ETT cuff through the grill of the LMA, and the possible laryngeal injury caused by an ETT inserted blindly through an off-centered LMA.[60]

The LMA-ProSeal has been designed to limit regurgitation and pulmonary aspiration of gastric contents while an LMA is being used. Furthermore, it is the first device of this type that specifically allows positive pressure ventilation in patients without spontaneous minute ventilation.[29,30] The LMA-ProSeal differs from previous versions of the LMA as follows: a rear cuff that improves the hypopharyngeal seal and a drainage tube that provides a conduit through the upper esophageal sphincter (Figs. 53–22 and 53–23). When the LMA-ProSeal is properly placed, the orifice of the drainage port is aligned with the upper esophageal sphincter; thus, a standard gastric tube can be inserted blindly into the esophagus to decompress the stomach and allow suctioning of liquid gastric contents.

The anti-esophageal reflex potential of the LMA-ProSeal has been studied in cadavers. When 40 mL of air was used to inflate the cuff, the LMA-ProSeal proved to be superior to the LMA in providing protection from esophageal regurgitation, although the LMA-ProSeal was also somewhat more difficult to insert.[31,32] Protection from esophageal reflux was even more striking when the gastric tube was correctly inserted into the LMA-ProSeal drainage port, advanced distally into the esophagus, and placed on continuous suction.

The increased protection from esophageal-gastric reflux is not due to higher sealing pressure but rather to the innovative design of the new airway (eg, a larger and different cuff). In

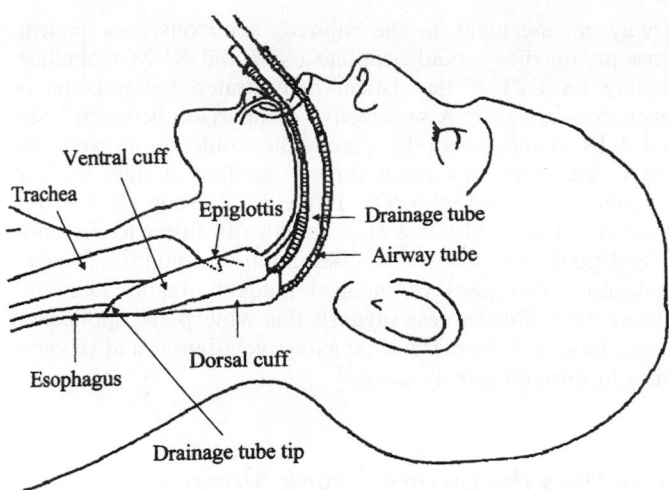

**FIGURE 53–23.** Schematic profile of the LMA-ProSeal laryngeal mask airway when correctly placed.

fact, when the pharyngeal pressure from an LMA-ProSeal was compared with that of the classic LMA, no significant changes could be demonstrated.[30]

Although the LMA-ProSeal may be inserted manually, a removable introducer is provided with this device to facilitate its insertion without the need for the operator to put fingers into the patient's mouth. The presence of a wire reinforced airway device and a built-in bite block minimizes the chance of tube occlusion or kinking. At the time of this writing, only sizes No. 5 (men), 4 (women), and 3 (young adults) are available.

## What Are the Main Contraindications to Use of the Laryngeal Mask Airway?

The LMA offers little or no protection against pulmonary aspiration of gastric contents. However, this complication has rarely been reported even in patients considered at risk.[23]

The incidence of regurgitation during insertion of the LMA is controversial. The LMA is associated with relaxation of the lower esophageal sphincter through distention of the hypopharyngeal muscles and prevention of the ejection of regurgitated food.[27] In other conditions, such as glottic edema, it is possible that the laryngeal mask's low-pressure cuff will seal around the laryngeal inlet, "adapting" to the edema. Experienced practitioners consider the LMA in selected difficult airway conditions only when no laryngeal obstruction, tumor, tonsil bleeding, epiglottitis abscess, or laryngeal abscess is present. In such situations, FOB should be used, if time allows. Nonetheless, we wish to emphasize that *there are no absolute contraindications to the LMA if the alternative is loss of the airway with its associated complications.*

## What Is the Role of the Laryngeal Mask Airway in Prehospital Difficult Airway Management?

In the United States, specially trained flight crews or paramedics perform airway management in the field. Although there is controversy as to what constitutes appropriate field

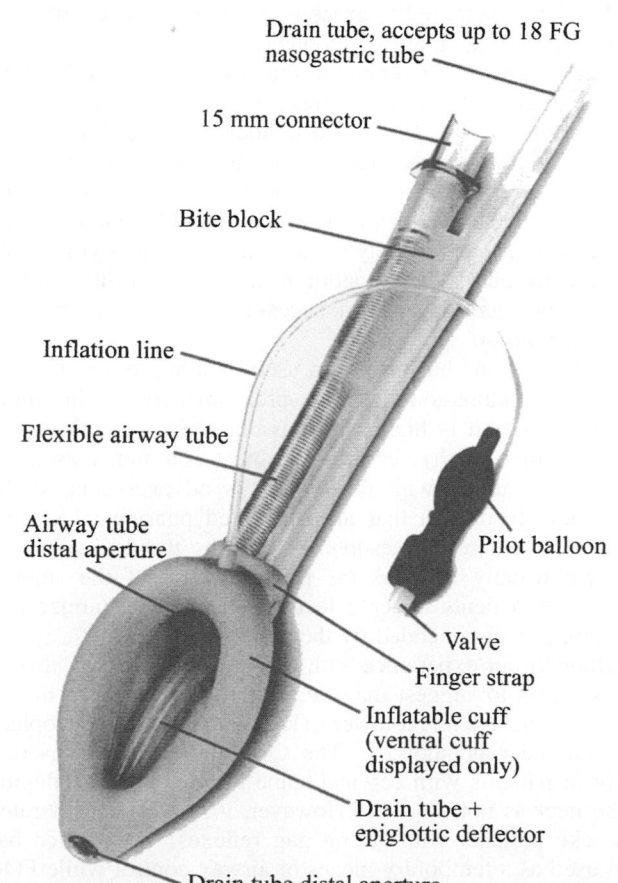

Drain tube, accepts up to 18 FG nasogastric tube

15 mm connector

Bite block

Inflation line

Flexible airway tube

Airway tube distal aperture

Pilot balloon

Valve

Finger strap

Inflatable cuff (ventral cuff displayed only)

Drain tube + epiglottic deflector

Drain tube distal aperture

**FIGURE 53–22.** Laryngeal mask airway ProSeal seen from the front.

airway management in the injured, semiconscious patient, most paramedics would ventilate using the BVM technique, placing an ETT if the patient deteriorated (deep coma or respiratory arrest).[61] A prospective comparison between LMA and ETT management by paramedic students showed that LMA placement was successful on the first attempt 94% of the time, compared with 69% in the ETT group ($P < 0.01$). Insertion of the LMA was also statistically faster to detection of end-tidal $CO_2$. The same observation was confirmed when respiratory therapists or medical students manipulated the airway.[24,62,63] This success suggests that widespread application in the field will increase satisfactory ventilation and oxygenation in difficult airway cases.[64]

## How Does the Laryngeal Mask Airway Facilitate Tracheal Intubation?

When clinically indicated, an emergently placed LMA may be used as a route for general anesthesia administration. However, the usual LMA pressure limitation is at about 15 to 20 cm $H_2O$. In a paralyzed patient who is mechanically ventilated with an LMA in place, incremental peak pressure increases of 15 to 30 cm $H_2O$ caused a progressive decrease in tidal volume of 13% to 27% and an increase in gastric esophageal inflation from 2% to 35%.[65]

In the majority of cases, the LMA should be replaced with an ETT. The blind passage of an ETT through the LMA has been associated with a low rate of success because the LMA can fail to negotiate the hypopharynx up to 65% of the time.[58] Therefore, the ETT usually is placed through the LMA using FOB. The rate of success in placement with this technique is close to 100%.[57]

Two limitations have been described: (1) cricoid pressure cannot be applied because it may further displace the LMA,[66,67] and (2) the size of the ETT that can be used is limited (3.5 mm for LMA size 1; 4.5 mm for LMA size 2; 5.0 mm for LMA size 2.5; 6 mm cuffed for LMA size 3 and 4; and 7.0 mm cuffed for LMA size 5). In adults, we recommend using a Rae tube because it is approximately 3 to 5 cm longer than the standard ETT and is thus easier to pass. We use a bronchoscopy elbow adapter on the ETT to allow ventilation and oxygenation during placement of the ETT using the fiberoptic technique (see Fig. 53–12). Several modifications of this technique have been described, each using the removal of the LMA after insertion of a gum elastic bougie, a tube exchanger, or a guidewire. This modification is less reliable than the technique described earlier.

The previously discussed LMA-Fastrach is a curved, short stainless steel tube with an LMA and guiding handle (see Fig. 53–13).[54-56] In a study of 31 modified Mallampati class III or IV patients, the success rate with blind intubation was 97%.[56] In some patients, the LMA-Fastrach can be placed with local anesthesia in the awake state.[68] The LMA-Fastrach is available in sizes 3, 4, and 5, corresponding respectively to the small, average, and large adult. The largest ETT that can be placed through the LMA-Fastrach is 8.0 mm; it can be placed both blindly or with an FOB. For safety, we recommend the use of the FOB, if the instrument is available, when an ETT is placed through the LMA-Fastrach in the hospital. The LMA-Fastrach is available with a cuffed silicone tracheal tube; the advantage of this is that it does not retain any significant curvature after

passing through the LMA. This design limits the possibility that the tip of the ETT will deviate from the vocal cords.

## What Is the Role of the Esophageal Tracheal Combitube?

The esophageal tracheal Combitube, an evolutionary step in the design of the esophageal obturator airway,[69] provides complete seal of the upper airway. Therefore, it can be used in patients at high risk of regurgitation and aspiration of gastric contents. The main indication for using the Combitube has been to rapidly establish an airway during CPR.[70,71]

The Combitube is essentially a double-lumen tube that is inserted blindly through the mouth into either the esophagus or the trachea; most of the time, blind insertion will result in esophageal intubation. Both lumens are color coded: blue for esophagus, clear for trachea. A proximal latex esophageal balloon (inflated first after placement) is filled with 100 cc of air and a distal plastic cuff is filled with 10 to 15 cc of air. These cuffs allow good seal of the hypopharynx and stability in the trachea or esophagus. The esophageal lumen is closed distally and perforated at the hypopharyngeal level with several small openings. The trachea lumen is open distally (see Fig. 53–15).

The Combitube has the same limitations as the LMA and thus may not be insertable in patients with hypopharyngeal pathology. In addition, although its safety record has been good, it can potentially exacerbate preexisting esophageal pathology such as tumor or esophageal varices.[37]

Until recently, the Combitube found its widest use in treatment of prehospital cardiac arrest.[70,71] In a prospective, randomized study, US Navy Seals, after brief training, were asked to intubate a mannequin with an ETT, a Combitube, and an LMA. Mean time to intubation with the Combitube compared with the ETT was similar.[72] The Combitube, however, can be inserted blindly without the use of a laryngoscope in poorly lit areas. These conditions may exist during military training and combat. DL is unnecessary and there is minimal risk of aspiration.

The Combitube has also been used with success in managing difficult intubations in obese pregnant patients, in whom risk of aspiration is high.[73] It is available in a standard size and SA (small adult) version. The most common reason for failure to ventilate with this device is advancement of the device too deeply, so that the perforated pharyngeal section has entirely entered the esophagus. Pulling the device back 3 to 4 cm usually resolves the problem. Use of the smaller version for patients under 5 feet in height, to minimize this problem, is recommended by the manufacturer.

Although our experience with this device is limited, that of others seems to suggest that the smaller version has a higher chance of success and a lower risk of damaging the hypopharynx and the esophagus.[74,75] The Combitube can be inserted safely in patients with cervical spine injuries because flexion of the neck is not required. However, it is not well tolerated in awake patients with strong gag reflexes. The device has been used as a temporary means of airway control while FOB placement of an ETT through the nose is carried out and for airway maintenance during percutaneous dilation tracheotomy.[76,77]

## How Is Ventilation Provided After Placement of a Transtracheal Airway?

Transtracheal ventilation can be a quick and inexpensive way to solve the problem of a cannot ventilate, cannot intubate difficult airway, but it contains many hidden dangers. The oxygen pressure from the wall is normally 50 psi. A direct connection from the wall to the transtracheal catheter is not acceptable because it may be associated with a large tidal volume breath and barotrauma. Additionally, whipping or displacement of the catheter in subcutaneous tissue may occur, with consequent massive subcutaneous emphysema. Several commercially available pressure down-regulators are available to titrate oxygen flow through a transtracheal airway[78] (Fig. 53–24).

Three alternative sources of high-pressure oxygen have been used: (1) fresh gas outlet on the anesthesia machine, with an average output of 20 L/min; (2) oxygen tank with a dual-stage regulator (low-flow regulators usually necessitate a longer inspiratory to inspiratory ratio); and (3) wall flow meter turned up to 15 to 20 L/min ("flush"). Although this procedure may be temporarily life-saving, we recommend moving to the operating room for a surgical airway as soon as possible after placement of the catheter.

If possible, two people should always perform transtracheal jet ventilation (TTJV): one holds the catheter in place, the other titrates the oxygen flow. The driving pressure of the regulator should be titrated slowly up from 5 psi to maintain a steady chest rise (1-2 cm) at each inhalation. Ventilation should be provided starting with an approximate inspiratory time of 0.5 sec, maintaining an inspiratory-expiratory (I:E) ratio of at least 1:1.[79] After this procedure has been initiated, a third person may be needed simply to try to maintain patency of the upper airway with energetic jaw thrust and chin lift. The result of transtracheal ventilation without a patent upper airway is progressive air trapping and barotrauma.[80–82]

We cannot overemphasize that in TTJV, the catheter must be kept steady and aimed slightly downward to avoid kinking at the posterior wall of the trachea. Accidental dislodgment of the catheter into the subcutaneous space or perforation of the posterior wall of the trachea results in several liters of oxygen being injected into the subcutaneous tissue and mediastinum in a fraction of a second.

Aspiration during TTJV is not well studied and is somewhat controversial. In dogs, no aspiration was noted if the respiratory frequency was maintained at more than 60 breaths/min. It has been speculated that a mechanism for preventing pulmonary aspiration could be the forceful continuous gas outflow through the larynx.[83,84] Although we have used TTJV, our preference, in an airway disaster in which an LMA or Combitube is not appropriate, is the immediate use of a percutaneous or surgical cricothyroidotomy, followed by insertion of a No. 5 or 6 ETT through the cricothyroid membrane. Despite the posterior tracheal wall perforations that have been described,[85] cricothyroidotomy has a long track record of success both in trauma victims and in house emergency use.[86–90]

## What Are the Roles of the Rigid Fiberoptic Laryngoscope, Lighted Stylet, and Retrograde Intubation?

Each of these three devices may be used in a "can ventilate, can't intubate" situation.

### Rigid Fiberoptic Laryngoscopes

The Bullard laryngoscope (Fig. 53–25), the UpsherScope, and the Wu scope are used to gain access to the trachea in the patient with limited mouth opening, morbid obesity, or a hypopharyngeal mass. The use and application of these devices in the difficult airway algorithm are still controversial,[91] and specific training similar to fiberoptic endoscopy is needed to acquire proficiency.[92]

The Bullard laryngoscope is more commonly used than the other rigid fiberoptic laryngoscopes and is available in three sizes: pediatric (newborn–2 years), pediatric long (up to 10 years), and adult.

### Illuminating Stylet

The illuminating stylet (*lightwand*) uses the principle of transillumination of the trachea and soft tissue to blindly guide the stylet beyond the vocal cords (Fig. 53–26).[93,94] This technique differs from the use of a gum elastic bougie because the blind intubation can be achieved with minimal mouth opening, relying on the transillumination of soft tissue. Indications for the device are a hypoplastic mandible, prominent upper incisors, restricted cervical spine movement or spinal immobilizations, glossomegaly, and restricted access to the airway (eg, presence of a halo frame). This technique is contraindicated for any condition in which pathology of the upper airway is known or suspected.

Common problems encountered while inserting the lighted stylet include the following:

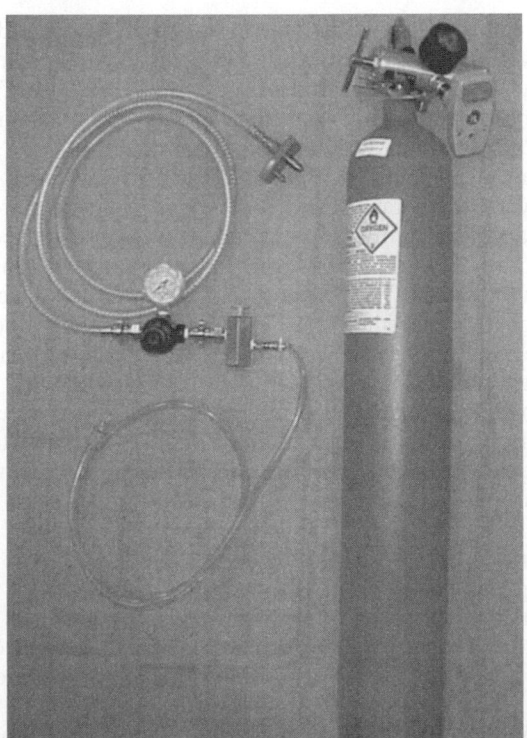

**FIGURE 53–24.** Manual jet ventilator with pressure regulator, which is to be connected to a wall oxygen source or to an oxygen tank regulator.

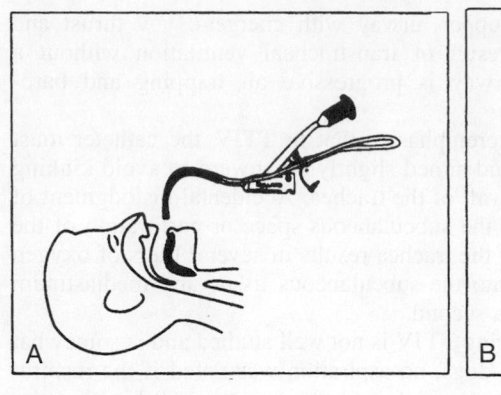
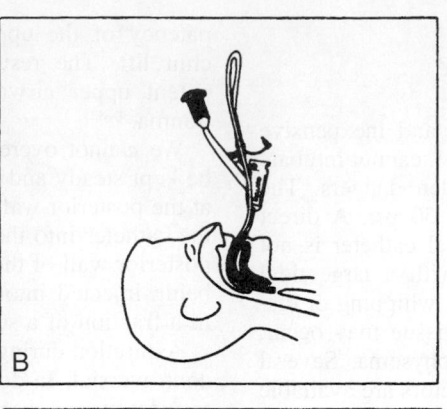
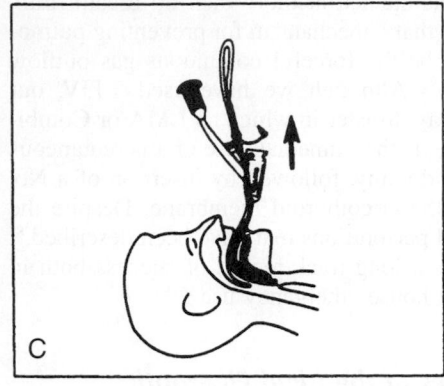
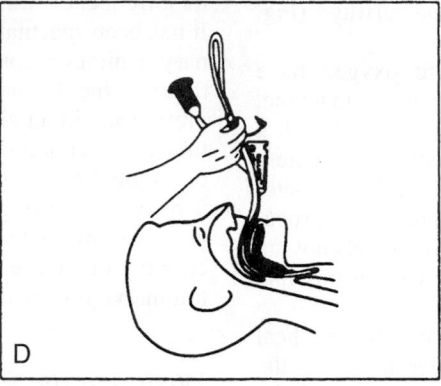

**FIGURE 53–25.** The Bullard rigid fiberoptic laryngoscope intubating sequence. *A and B,* Minimal airway opening required, no neck extension. *C,* Upward and anterior displacement of the tongue. *D,* Placement of the endotracheal tube under direct vision of the larynx.

- Failure to engage the tip in the hypopharynx. This can be obviated with gentle use of DL to displace the tongue, without attempting to achieve intubation conditions.
- Failure to advance the stylet once it is in the hypopharynx. This is usually due to entrapment of the tip in the pyriform sinuses. Gentle pressure on the pyriform sinuses from an assistant will reduce the risk that the lightwand will become lodged within these structures.
- Failure to transilluminate. This is usually due to the presence of neck edema or thick soft tissues (eg, in morbid obesity). In this situation, the procedure should be abandoned and an alternative substituted.
- Inability to advance the ETT beyond the lightwand, which is beyond the vocal cords. The most likely explanation for this problem is impingement of the ETT on the right vocal cord while it is advancing through the stylet. Gentle rotation

of the stylet 90° to 180° counterclockwise, along with anterior displacement of the tongue with tongue depressor or MacIntosh blade, and mild extension of neck, usually will resolve the obstruction.

## Retrograde Intubation

This can be achieved with the use of a long, J-tip guidewire (usually 100–120 cm in length), a flexible epidural catheter or a kit such as the Retrograde Guidewire Kit (Cook Critical Care, Inc, Bloomington, Ind) (Fig. 53–27). Known pathology above or below the vocal cords is a contraindication.[95] In the retrograde technique, the guidewire is inserted through the cricothyroid membrane similarly to cricothyroid puncture during dilational cricothyroidotomy. However, the needle is aimed upward at an angle of approximately 45° once inserted through the cricothyroid membrane. The wire is passed cephalad through the needle. Once secured through the mouth, it may be used directly to guide the ETT or indirectly through use of an intubating stylet.

A possible problem on insertion is failure to proceed beyond the vocal cords because the tube may impinge on the right vocal cord. Maneuvers recommended to overcome this problem follow:

- Twist the ETT 90° to 180° counterclockwise.
- Use gentle DL to displace the tongue anteriorly.
- When a simple guidewire or an epidural catheter is used, thread the guidewire through the Murphy eye end of the ETT instead of the distal opening to allow an additional 1 cm of the ETT to pass beyond the vocal cords and facilitate the passage of the tip of the ETT in the trachea (Fig. 53–28).

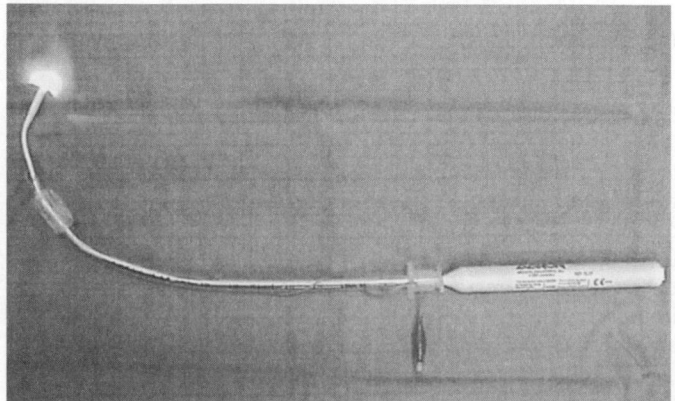

**FIGURE 53–26.** An endotracheal tube mounted on an illuminating stylet.

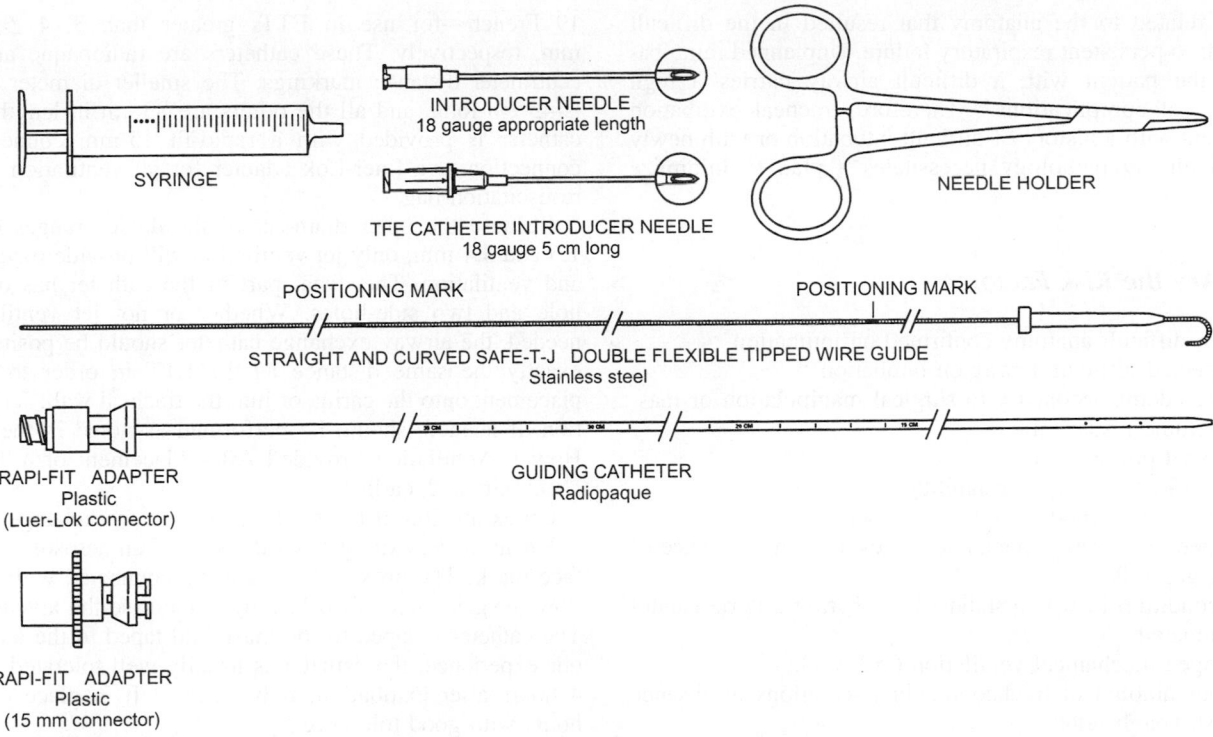

**FIGURE 53–27.** The cricothyroid membrane puncture retrograde guidewire kit. (Courtesy of Cook Critical Care, Inc, Bloomington, Ind.)

A modification of this technique passes the J-wire, once retrieved from the oropharynx, into the suction port of an FOB, then advancing the ETT through the FOB under direct vision. Use of the Patil-Syracuse mask allows ventilation to be continued during the procedure.

## EXTUBATION OF THE DIFFICULT AIRWAY

### *How Should Extubation Be Planned?*

The percentage of patients requiring reintubation following tracheal decannulation is unknown. The need to reintubate

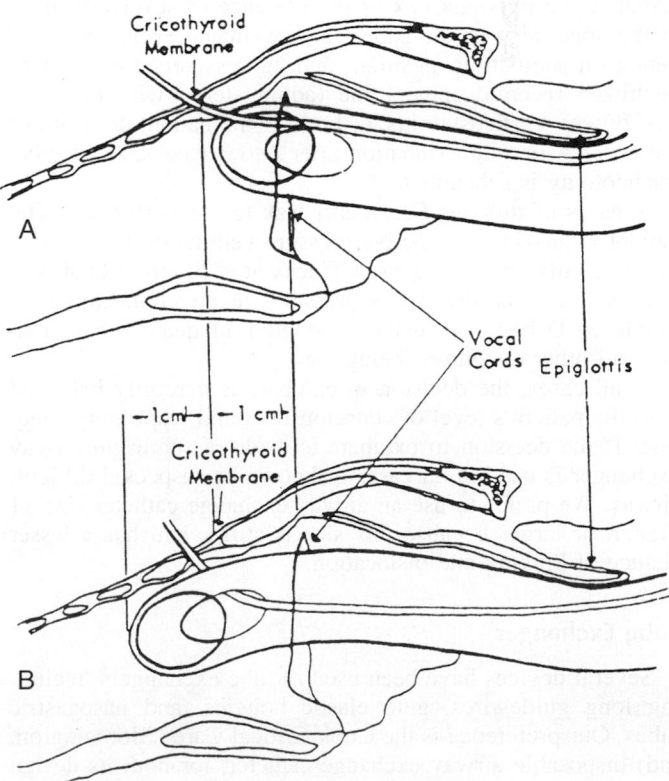

**FIGURE 53–28.** Retrograde guidewire passed through (*A*) the tip of the endotracheal tube and (*B*) the Murphy eye. *B*, Passage through the Murphy eye facilitates passage of the tip of the endotracheal tube beyond the vocal cords.

may be related to the anatomy that resulted in the difficult airway or to persistent respiratory failure. Unplanned reintubation in the patient with a difficult airway carries a high frequency of complications.[96] Therefore, tracheal extubation in a patient with a history of difficult intubation or with newly acquired airway pathology necessitates a plan to minimize this risk.

## What Are the Risk Factors?

- Known difficult anatomy confirmed on intubation
- Unexpected difficult airway on intubation
- Airway edema secondary to surgical manipulation or massive volume resuscitation
- Prolonged prone position
- Cervical immobility or instability
- Morbid obesity (body mass index >40)
- Postoperative altered mental status, even in the presence of strong gag reflex
- Any condition in which standard extubation criteria cannot be evaluated
- Prolonged mechanical ventilation (>2 weeks)
- Copious amount of tracheobronchial secretions in absence of brisk cough reflex
- Residual analgesia or anesthesia postsurgical procedure
- Residual neuromuscular paralysis and respiratory weakness

Overall, adverse outcomes from extubation have been reported in 7% of respiratory-related claims in the ASA Closed Claims study.[1,97] About 4% of these patients were in the intensive care unit.[1,97] DL precedes most of our difficult extubations, when the patient otherwise fits the criteria for extubation by respiratory strength and endurance parameters.

If the DL is judged inadequate due to the inability to visualize the hypopharynx or the presence of severe swelling of the upper airway, the patient is reevaluated every 48 hours, kept in a semisitting position, and aggressively treated with nebulized racemic epinephrine (administered with the ETT cuff down), corticosteroids, or both. If the patient does not fit the criteria for safe extubation after 2 to 3 weeks, an elective tracheotomy is scheduled.

In cases of dubious DL, a cuff leak test is performed. The patient is provided a positive pressure ventilation breath with the ETT cuff down. A good cuff leak at <20 cm $H_2O$ airway pressure, as recorded by a pressure gauge connected to a Mapleson-D bag, is usually considered adequate for extubation, all other conditions being met.

In all cases, the decision to extubate is carefully balanced with the patient's level of consciousness and respiratory function. If the decision to extubate is made, a semirigid airway exchanger is used in all cases of known or suspected difficult airway. We prefer to use an airway exchange catheter size 11 French or larger because this size is stiffer and has a lesser chance of kinking and dislocation.

### Tube Exchanger

Several devices have been used as tube exchangers, including long guidewires, gum elastic bougies, and nasogastric tubes. Our preference is the Cook Critical Care (Bloomington, Ind) disposable airway exchange catheter, for both its design and its material. Four sizes are manufactured—8, 11, 14, and 19 French—for use in ETTs greater than 3, 4, 5, and 7 mm, respectively. These catheters are radiopaque and have centimeter distance markings. The smaller diameter catheter is 45 cm long, and all the others are 83 cm in length. Every catheter is provided with a rapid-fit 15-mm connector for connection to a Luer-Lok adapter for jet ventilation or for a resuscitation bag.

Because the inner diameter of the device ranges between 1.6 and 3.4 mm, only jet ventilation will provide oxygenation and ventilation. The distal part of the catheter has one end-hole and two side-holes. Whether or not jet ventilation is needed, the airway exchange catheter should be positioned to exactly the same distance as the ETT in order to prevent placement onto the carina or into the tracheal wall. Jet ventilation, if needed, should be performed as noted in the section How Is Ventilation Provided After Placement of a Transtracheal Airway?, earlier.

On extubation of the trachea, the airway exchange catheter is left in place, exiting from the side of an aerosol or Venturi face mask. The proximal site can be connected with an low-flow oxygen source (4-6 L/min) to increase the alveolar $F_{IO_2}$. The catheter is taped to the mask and taped to the temple. In our experience, the catheter is usually well tolerated for 2 to 4 hours after extubation. It has been left in place up to 52 hours with good tolerance.[98]

If necessary, the one-time use of aerosolized 4% lidocaine (3-4 mL) may increase tolerance to the airway exchange catheter without compromising airway reflexes or increasing the risk of pulmonary aspiration. If reintubation is necessary, the use of a laryngoscope to displace the tongue and soft tissues forward and facilitate the passage of the tube into the hypopharynx may be needed.

Difficulty replacing the ETT may be due to impingement of the tube on the right vocal cord. This problem usually can be resolved with a gentle counterclockwise rotation of the ETT between 90° and 180°, better lubrication of the ETT, or gentle anterior displacement of the tongue with a laryngoscope. Before removal of the airway exchange catheter, successful tracheal intubation is confirmed with end-tidal $CO_2$.

### Exchange of Endotracheal Tubes

As a general rule, ETTs should be exchanged only when *strictly* necessary. Ineffective pulmonary toilet due to small ETT size or inability to perform positive pressure ventilation due to ETT balloon rupture are the most common indications. Increased imposed work of breathing due to small ETT size may be compensated through the appropriate use of pressure support ventilation.[99] An alternative to blind airway-catheter ETT exchange is to place a second ETT using FOB. With this procedure, the balloon of the in-place but defective ETT is deflated and an ETT-loaded pediatric FOB is advanced into the trachea parallel to and at the level of the ETT. The defective ETT is removed and a third ETT is placed using a tube changer as previously described. In case of accidental displacement of the tube changer, the second ETT-loaded FOB in place can be used for intubation of the trachea.

Exchange of an ETT or extubating a difficult airway can be dangerous, even in expert hands. The rate of complications is potentially high,[100,101] and specialized personnel (critical care nurse, intensivist, and surgeon familiar with cricothyroidotomy) should be readily available.

## THE DIFFICULT AIRWAY CART

### *What Should a Difficult Airway Cart Contain?*

Just as different physicians bring different preferences and skills to managing difficult airways, there is no standard difficult airway cart. However, because a difficult airway cart will be used in emergency conditions by personnel of differing skill levels, including those not involved with the preparation of the cart, some standard equipment should be stocked (Table 53–5).[102]

## THE PEDIATRIC DIFFICULT AIRWAY

### *What Are the Differences?*

The airway anatomy of a child progressively approaches that of the adult over the first several years of life. A newborn's airway anatomy, however, substantially differs from the adult. Common findings include a large tongue and epiglottis, large tonsils and adenoids, and a relatively anterior position of the larynx. The newborn's and child's airway anatomy, when associated with congenital abnormalities or other pathology involving the airways, represent formidable challenges to the physician attempting to obtain access. Other clinical concerns are a small FRC and high oxygen consumption leading to a faster rate of desaturation and an immature autonomic nervous system exquisitely sensitive to hypoxemia and airway manipulation, which may lead to acute bradycardia.

Adequate topical anesthesia of the airway for fiberoptic intubation of the trachea may be impractical or impossible in children, and inhalation anesthesia with spontaneous ventilation is often the only choice to control the airway. Nevertheless, a difficult airway cart should always be available and pediatric airway manipulation should be managed by personnel with appropriate *pediatric* airway skills.

The devices we think should be immediately available when dealing with pediatric difficult intubation follow:

- Flexible pediatric FOB
- Small size LMAs (1, 2, 3)[103]
- Pediatric lighted stylet (available as small as 2.5 mm outer diameter)[104]
- Pediatric Bullard laryngoscope[105]
- Pediatric retrograde endotracheal intubation kit (22-gauge catheter that will accommodate .018-inch guidewire)[106]

## DOCUMENTATION OF A DIFFICULT AIRWAY EXPERIENCE

### *What Are the Essential Elements?*

Access to the clinical information of patients with a difficult airway is strongly recommended in the published "Practice Guidelines for Management of the Difficult Airway."[3] A nonprofit organization, the Medic Alert Foundation was endorsed in 1979 by the ASA House of Delegates to build a national registry of patients with difficult airways and devise a visible

**TABLE 53–5.** Suggested Contents of the Difficult Airway Cart

**Adult**

*Nasal*

Nasopharyngeal airways: sizes 6, 7, 8
Nasal ETTs: sizes 6.0, 7.0, 8.0

*Oral*

Oropharyngeal airways: sizes 8, 9, 10, 11
Stylets and intubating guides
  ETT stylet
  Gum elastic bougies: sizes 10 French, 15 French
  Illuminating stylet
ETTs: cuffed sizes 5.0, 5.5, 6.0, 6.5, 7.0, 7.5, 8.0
Laryngoscope blades
  Curved: MacIntosh 3, 4
  Straight: Miller 3, 4
Laryngoscope handles: regular length, short length
Laryngeal masks: sizes 3, 4, 5
  Fastrach intubating laryngeal masks: sizes 3, 4
ETTs for laryngeal masks: sizes 6.0, 6.5, 7.0 cuffed
Combitubes: adult, small adult
Lung isolation
  Bronchial blockers: Fogarty occlusion catheter, sizes 8-14 French
  Double-lumen ETTs: sizes 35, 37, 39, 41 French

*Cricothyroid Membrane*

Transcricothyroid membrane jet ventilation
  IV catheters: 14, 12 gauge (length: 2 inches)
  Jet ventilation hose with controller handle pressure regulator and Luer-Lok connector
Retrograde transcricothyroid membrane kit
Melker percutaneous dilational cricothyroidotomy set: sizes 3, 4, 6
Patil cricothyroidotomy catheter
Surgical cricothyroidotomy
  3 scalpel handles, 11 blades, trachea retraction hook
  Size 6.0 ETT
  Shiley cuffed tracheostomy tubes: sizes 4, 6, 8

*Accessory Equipment*

Confirming position of ETT: ET$CO_2$ detector
Esophageal detector, self-inflating bulb
ETT exchange catheters: with jet ventilation capability
Patil-Syracuse mask
Bronchoscopy swivel adapter
Oxygen delivery
  Ambu manual resuscitation bag with masks
  Mapleson D with pressure gauge
  Oxygen tubing with nipple for connecting to oxygen wall outlet or tank
  Stethoscope
Suction
  Endotracheal suction catheters: sizes 10, 12, 14
  Yankauer oral suction tubing
Other
  Spare batteries and bulbs for laryngoscope
  Bite blocks
  Magill forceps
Local anesthetic and nasal vasoconstrictor
  Atomizer for spraying lidocaine 4% solution
  Benzocaine spray 20% solution
  1% Neo-Synephrine spray
Fiberoptic bronchoscope with intubating airway and defogger
Adult rigid fiberoptic laryngoscope of operator's choice

**Pediatric**

Laryngoscope Miller operator's 1 and 2
Esophageal airway 4, 5, 6, 7
Masks: neonatal, infant, toddler, child
Flexible pediatric FOB
Small size LMA: 1 and 2
Pediatric lighted stylet
Pediatric Bullard laryngoscope
Pediatric retrograde intubation kit

---

ETT, endotracheal tube; FOB, fiberoptic bronchoscope; IV, intravenous; LMA, laryngeal mask airway.
Modified from McGuire GP, Wong DT. Airway management: contents of a difficult intubation cart. *Can J Anaesth.* 1999;46:190.

alert emblem to be worn by the patient. At a nominal annual enrollment fee of US$15, the organization keeps information on individual patients, which may be accessed by telephone (209-634-4917 or 800-625-3480) 24 hours per day. General information on the organization is also available by telephone (800-432-5378). The physician who experiences difficulties in dealing with a patient's airway may provide the information by email or fax to the registry.

## TRAINING ISSUES IN MANAGING DIFFICULT AIRWAYS

### What Is the Best Way to Acquire Skill in Managing Difficult Airways?

The inability to successfully intubate the trachea is a leading cause of morbidity and mortality. Up to 30% of all deaths attributed to anesthesia are related to management of a difficult airway.[1] Therefore, each anesthesia trainee should be exposed, under supervision, to as many cases and techniques as possible involving patients with difficult airways. Supervision should always be provided in order to avoid unnecessary risk.[107,108] Training with mannequins and simulated drills of difficult airways in human cadavers are also recommended in order to improve skill level.[109–111] A retrospective study of 18 500 patients showed that 16% with grade 3-4 laryngoscopy experienced more than three laryngoscopy attempts before tracheal intubation was achieved, despite the ASA guidelines.[112] Continued use of DL in a difficult airway to achieve tracheal intubation clearly highlights the need for better training in difficult airway management. Nevertheless, a survey performed in 1995 showed that only 27% of anesthesiology residency programs require residents to participate in difficult airway rotation, and this exposure usually lasted less than a month.[113]

## References

1. Caplan RA, Posner KL, Ward RJ, et al. Adverse respiratory events in anesthesia: a closed claims analysis. *Anesthesiology.* 1990;72:828.
2. Crosby ET, Cooper RM, Douglas MJ, et al. The unanticipated difficult airway with recommendations for management. *Can J Anaesth.* 1998;45:757.
3. American Society of Anesthesiologists Task Force on Management of the Difficult Airway. Practice guidelines for management of the difficult airway. *Anesthesiology.* 1993;78:597.
4. Benumof JL. Management of the difficult adult airway: with special emphasis on awake tracheal intubation. *Anesthesiology.* 1991;75:1087.
5. Leach RM, Treacher DS. ABC of oxygen: oxygen transport: 2, tissue hypoxia. *BMJ.* 1998;317:1370.
6. Benumof JL. The unanticipated difficult airway [correspondence]. *Can J Anaesth.* 1999;46:510.
7. Benumof JL. The ASA difficult airway algorithm: new thoughts/considerations. *American Society of Anesthesiologists Refresher Course: 1998–1999.* October 1999 Lecture 134.
8. Wilson ME, Spiegelhalter D, Robertson JA, et al. Predicting difficult intubation. *Br J Anaesth.* 1988;61:211.
9. Mallampati SR, Gatt SP, Gugino LG, et al. A clinical sign to predict difficult tracheal intubation: a prospective study. *Can Anaesth Soc J.* 1985;32:429.
10. Samsoon GLT, Young JRB. Difficult tracheal intubation: a retrospective study. *Anaesthesia.* 1987;42:487.
11. Cormack RS, Lehane J. Difficult tracheal intubation in obstetrics. *Anaesthesia.* 1984;39:1105.
12. LoCicero J. Bronchopulmonary aspiration. *Surg Clin North Am.* 1989;69:71.
13. Warner MA, Warner ME, Weber JG. Clinical significance of pulmonary aspiration during the perioperative period. *Anesthesiology.* 1993;78:56.
14. Benumof JL. Laryngeal mask airway and the ASA difficult airway algorithm. *Anesthesiology.* 1996;84:686.
15. Kinni ME, Stout MM. Aspiration pneumonitis: predisposing conditions and prevention. *J Oral Maxillofac Surg.* 1986;44:378.
16. Benumof JL, Dagg R, Benumof R. Critical hemoglobin desaturation will occur before return to an unparalyzed state following 1 mg/kg intravenous succinylcholine. *Anesthesiology.* 1997;87:979.
17. Thomas DI. Overcoming the beard [letter]. *Anaesthesia.* 1999;54:100.
18. Benumof JL, Cooper SD. Quantitative improvement in laryngoscopic view by optimal external laryngeal manipulation. *J Clin Anesth.* 1996;8:136.
19. Adnet F, Borron S, Luc Dumas J, et al. Study of the "sniffing position" by magnetic resonance imaging. *Anesthesiology.* 2001;94:83.
20. Takahata O, Kubota M, Mamiya K, et al. The efficacy of the "BURP" maneuver during a difficult laryngoscopy. *Anesth Analg.* 1997;84:419.
21. Dogra S, Falconer R, Latto IP. Successful difficult intubation: tracheal tube placement over a gum-elastic bougie. *Anaesthesia.* 1990;45:774.
22. Cooper SD. The evolution of upper airway retraction: new and old laryngoscopy blades. In: Benumof JL, ed. *Airway Management.* St Louis, Mo: Mosby–Year Book; 1996:374.
23. Verghese C, Brimacombe JR. Survey of laryngeal mask airway usage in 11,910 patients: safety and efficacy for conventional and non-conventional usage. *Anesth Analg.* 1996;82:129.
24. Pennant JH, Walker MB. Comparison of the endotracheal tube and the laryngeal mask in airway management by paramedical personnel. *Anesth Analg.* 1992;74:531.
25. Mahiou P, Narchi P, Beyrac P, et al. Is laryngeal mask easy to use in case of difficult intubation? [poster]. *Anesthesiology.* 1992;77:a1228.
26. Akbar AN, Muzi M, Lopatka CW, et al. Neurocirculatory responses to intubation with either an endotracheal tube or a laryngeal mask airway in humans. *J Clin Anesth.* 1996;8:194.
27. Rabey PG, Murphy PJ, Langton JA, et al. Effect of laryngeal mask airway on lower oesophageal sphincter pressure in patients during general anaesthesia. *Br J Anaesth.* 1992;69:346.
28. Brimacombe JR, Berry AM. Cricoid pressure. *Can J Anaesth.* 1997;44:414.
29. Brain AIJ, Verghese C, Strube PJ. The LMA "ProSeal"—a laryngeal mask with an esophageal vent. *Br J Anaesth.* 2000;84:650.
30. Keller C, Brimacombe J. Mucosal pressure and oropharyngeal leak pressure with the ProSeal versus laryngeal mask airway in anaesthetized paralyzed patients. *Br J Anaesth.* 2000;85:262.
31. Brimacombe J, Keller C. The ProSeal laryngeal mask airway. A randomized, crossover study with the standard laryngeal mask airway in paralyzed, anesthetized patients. *Anesthesiology.* 2000;93:104.
32. Keller C, Brimacombe J, Kleinsasser A, Loeckinger A. Does the ProSeal laryngeal mask airway prevent aspiration of regurgitated fluid? *Anesth Analg.* 2000:91:1017.
33. Michael TAD. The esophageal obturator airway: a critique. *JAMA.* 1981;246:1098.
34. Hammargren Y, Clinton JE, Ruiz E. A standard comparison of esophageal obturator airway and endotracheal tube ventilation in cardiac arrest. *Ann Em Med.* 1985;14:953.
35. Bartlett RL, Martin SD, McMahon JM, et al. A field comparison of the pharyngeotracheal lumen airway and the endotracheal tube. *J Trauma.* 1992;32:280.
36. Klein H, Williamson M, Sue-Ling HM, et al. Esophageal rupture associated with the Combitube. *Anesth Analg.* 1997;85:937.
37. Vézina D, Lessard MR, Bussières J, et al. Complications associated with the use of the esophageal-tracheal Combitube. *Can J Anaesth.* 1998;45:76.
38. Atherton GL, Johnson JC. Ability of paramedics to use the Combitube in prehospital cardiac arrest. *Ann Emerg Med.* 1993;22:1263.
39. Frass M, Frenzer R, Zdrahal F, et al. The esophageal tracheal Combitube: preliminary results with a new airway for CPR. *Ann Emerg Med.* 1987;16:768.
40. Staudinger T, Brugger S, Watschinger B, et al. Emergency intubation with the Combitube: comparison with the endotracheal airway. *Ann Emerg Med.* 1993;22:1573.
41. Wagner A, Roeggla M, Roeggla G, et al. Emergency intubation with the Combitube in a case of severe facial burn [correspondence]. *Am J Emerg Med.* 1995;13:681.
42. Klauser R, Roeggla G, Pidlich J, et al. Massive upper airway bleeding after thrombolytic therapy: successful airway management with the Combitube. *Ann Emerg Med.* 1992;21:431.
43. Blostein PA, Koestner AJ, Hoak S. Failed rapid sequence intubation in

trauma patients: esophageal tracheal Combitube is a useful adjunct. *J Trauma*. 1998;44:534.

44. Mercer MH, Gabbott DA. Insertion of the Combitube airway with the cervical spine immobilised in a rigid cervical collar. *Anaesthesia*. 1998;53:971.

45. Mercer MH, Gabbott DA. The influence of neck position on ventilation using the Combitube airway. *Anaesthesia*. 1998;53:146.

46. Rogers SN, Benumof JL. New and easy techniques for fiberoptic endoscopy-aided tracheal intubation. *Anesthesiology*. 1983;59:569.

47. Hawkins M, O'Sullivan E, Charters P. Fiberoptic intubation using the cuffed oropharyngeal airway and Aintree intubation catheter. *Anaesthesia*. 1998;53:891.

48. Uezono S, Goto T, Nakata Y, et al. The cuffed oropharyngeal airway, a novel adjunct to the management of difficult airways. *Anesthesiology*. 1998;88:1677.

49. Charters P, O'Sullivan E. The "dedicated airway": a review of the concept and an update of current practice. *Anaesthesia*. 1999;54:778.

50. Caparosa RJ, Zavatsky AR. Practical aspects of the cricothyroid space. *Laryngoscope*. 1957;67:577.

51. Zaleski L, Abello D, Gould MI. The esophageal detector device: does it work? *Anesthesiology*. 1993;79:244.

52. Kasper CL, Deem S. The self-inflating bulb to detect esophageal intubation during emergency airway management. *Anesthesiology*. 1998;88:898.

53. Cardoso MMSC, Banner MJ, Melker RJ, et al. Portable devices used to detect endotracheal intubation during emergency situations: a review. *Crit Care Med*. 1998;26:957.

54. Brimacombe JR. Difficult airway management with the intubating laryngeal mask. *Anesth Analg*. 1997;85:1173.

55. Rosenblatt WH, Wagner PJ, Ovassapian A, et al. Practice patterns in managing the difficult airway by anesthesiologists in the United States. *Anesth Analg*. 1998;87:153.

56. Brain AIJ, Verghese C, Addy EV, et al. The Intubating laryngeal mask, I: development of a new device for intubation of the trachea. *Br J Anaesth*. 1997;79:699.

57. Joo H, Rose K. Fast-Trach—a new intubating laryngeal mask airway: successful use in patients with difficult airways. *Can J Anaesth*. 1998;45:253.

58. Brain AIJ, Verghese C, Addy EV, et al. The intubating laryngeal mask, II: a preliminary clinical report of a new means of intubating the trachea. *Br J Anaesth*. 1997;79:704.

59. Fukutome T, Amaha K, Nakazawa K, et al. Tracheal intubation through the intubating laryngeal mask airway (LMA) in patients with difficult airways. *Anesth Intensive Care*. 1998;26:387.

60. Lim SL, Tay DHB, Thomas E. A comparison of three types of tracheal tube for use in laryngeal mask assisted blind orotracheal intubation. *Anaesthesia*. 1994;49:255.

61. Rhee KJ, O'Malley RJ, Turner JE, et al. Field airway management of the trauma patient: the efficacy of bag mask ventilation. *Am J Emerg Med*. 1988;6:333.

62. Reinhart DJ, Simmons G. Comparison of placement of the laryngeal mask airway with endotracheal tube by paramedics and respiratory therapists. *Ann Emerg Med*. 1994;24:260.

63. Davies PRF, Tighe SQM, Greenslade GL, et al. Laryngeal mask airway and tracheal tube insertion by unskilled personnel. *Lancet*. 1990;336:977.

64. Baskett PJF, Parr MJA, Nolan JP. The intubating laryngeal mask: results of a multicentre trial with experience of 500 cases. *Anaesthesia*. 1998;53:1174.

65. Devitt JH, Wenstone R, Noel AG, et al. The laryngeal mask airway and positive-pressure ventilation. *Anesthesiology*. 1994;80:550.

66. Brimacombe J, White A, Berry A. Effect of cricoid pressure on ease of insertion of the laryngeal mask airway. *Br J Anaesth*. 1993;71:800.

67. Brimacombe J, Berry A. Cricoid pressure and the LMA: efficacy and interpretation [letter]. *Br J Anaesth*. 1994;73:862.

68. Shung J, Avidan MS, Ing DC, et al. Awake intubation of the difficult airway with the intubating laryngeal mask airway. *Anaesthesia*. 1998;53:645.

69. Schofferman J, Oill P, Lewis AJ. The esophageal obturator airway: a clinical evaluation. *Chest*. 1976;69:67.

70. Shea SR, MacDonald JR, Gruzinski G. Prehospital endotracheal tube airway or esophageal gastric tube airway: a critical comparison. *Ann Emerg Med*. 1985;14:102.

71. Rumball CJ, McDonald D. The PTL, Combitube, laryngeal mask and oral airway: a randomized prehospital comparative study of ventilatory device effectiveness and cost-effectiveness in 470 cases of cardiorespiratory arrest. *Prehosp Emerg Care*. 1997;1:1.

72. Calkins MD, Robinson TD. Combat trauma airway management: endo tracheal intubation versus a laryngeal mask airway versus Combitube. Use by Navy SEAL and reconnaissance combat corpsmen. *J Trauma*. 1999;46:927.

73. Wissler RN. The esophageal-tracheal Combitube. *Anesth Rev*. 1993;20:147.

74. Walz R, Davis S, Panning B. Is the Combitube a useful emergency airway device for anesthesiologists? [letter]. *Anesth Analg*. 1999;88:233.

75. Green KS, Beger TH. Proper use of the Combitube [letter]. *Anesthesiology*. 1994;81:513.

76. Gaitini LA, Vajda SJ, Fradis M, et al. Replacing the Combitube by an endotracheal tube using a fibre-optic bronchoscope during spontaneous ventilation. *J Laryngol Otol*. 1998;112:786.

77. Mallick A, Quinn AC, Bodenham AR, et al. The use of the Combitube for airway maintenance during percutaneous dilatational tracheostomy. *Anesthesiology*. 1998;53:249.

78. Benumof JL, Scheller MS. The importance of transtracheal jet ventilation in the management of the difficult airway. *Anesthesiology*. 1989;71:769.

79. Gaughan SD, Ozaki GT, Benumof JL. Comparison in a lung model of low- and high-flow regulators for transtracheal jet ventilation. *Anesthesiology*. 1992;77:189.

80. Benumof JL, Gaughan SD. Concerns regarding barotrauma during jet ventilation [letter]. *Anesthesiology*. 1992;76:1072.

81. Nicklaus TJ. Airway complications of jet ventilation in neonates. *Ann Otol Rhinol Laryngol*. 1995;104:24.

82. Peak DA, Roy S. Needle cricothyroidotomy revisited. *J Pediatr Emerg Care*. 1999;15:224.

83. Jawan B, Lee JA. Aspiration in transtracheal jet ventilation. *Acta Anesth Scand*. 1996;40:684.

84. Gaughan SD, Benumof JL, Ozaki GT. Quantification of the jet function of a jet stylet. *Anesth Analg*. 1992;74:580.

85. Trottier SJ, Hazard PB, Sakabu SA, et al. Posterior tracheal wall perforation during percutaneous dilational tracheostomy: an investigation into its mechanism and prevention. *Chest*. 1999;115:1383.

86. Salvino CK, Dries D, Gamelli R, et al. Emergency cricothyroidotomy in trauma victims. *J Trauma*. 1993;34:503.

87. Leibovici D, Fredman B, Gofrit ON, et al. Prehospital cricothyroidotomy by physicians. *Am J Em Med*. 1997;15:91.

88. Jacobson LE, Gomez GA, Sobieray RJ, et al. Surgical cricothyroidotomy in trauma patients: analysis of its use by paramedics in the field. *J Trauma*. 1996;41:15.

89. Isaacs JH Jr, Pederson AD. Emergency cricothyroidotomy. *Am Surg*. 1997;63:346.

90. Barrachina F, Guardiola JJ, Añó T, et al. Percutaneous dilatational cricothyroidotomy: outcome with 44 consecutive patients. *Intensive Care Med*. 1996;22:937.

91. Fridrich P, Frass M, Krenn CG, et al. The UpsherScope in routine and difficult airway management: a randomized, controlled clinical trial. *Anesth Analg*. 1997;85:1377.

92. MacQuarrie K, Hung OR, Law JA. Tracheal intubation using a Bullard laryngoscope for patients with a simulated difficult airway. *Can J Anaesth*. 1999;46:760.

93. Hung OR, Stewart RD. Lightwand intubation, I: a new lightwand device. *Can J Anaesth*. 1995;42:820.

94. Hung OR, Pytka S, Morris I, et al. Lightwand intubation, II: clinical trial of a new lightwand for tracheal intubation in patients with difficult airways. *Can J Anaesth*. 1995;42:826.

95. Sanchez TF. Retrograde intubation. *Anesth Clin North Am*. 1995;13:439.

96. Lee PJ, O'Reilly M, Tremper K, et al. An analysis of reintubations from a quality assurance database of 47,000 cases [abstract]. *Anesth Analg*. 1996;82:S270.

97. Miller KA, Harkin CP, Bailey PL. Postoperative tracheal extubation. *Anesth Analg*. 1995;80:149.

98. Hartmannsgruber MWB, Loudermilk EP, Stoltzfus DP. Prolonged use of a Cook airway exchange catheter obviated the need for postoperative tracheostomy in an adult patient. *J Clin Anesth*. 1997;9:496.

99. Banner MJ, Kirby RR, Blanch PB, et al. Decreasing imposed work of the breathing apparatus to zero using pressure-support ventilation. *Crit Care Med*. 1993;21:1333.

100. Dworkin R, Benumof JL, Benumof R, et al. The effective tracheal diameter that causes air trapping during jet ventilation. *J Cardiothorac Anesth*. 1990;4:731.

101. Benumof JL. Airway exchange catheters: simple concept, potentially great danger [editorial]. *Anesthesiology*. 1999;91:342.

102. McGuire GP, Wong DT. Airway management: contents of a difficult intubation cart. *Can J Anaesth*. 1999;46:190.

103. Nath G, Major V. The laryngeal mask in the management of a paediatric difficult airway. *Anaesth Intens Care.* 1992;20:518.

104. Holzman RS, Nargozian CD, Florence SB. Lightwand intubation in children with abnormal upper airways. *Anesthesiology.* 1988;69:784.

105. Borland LM, Casselbrant M. The Bullard laryngoscope: a new indirect oral laryngoscope (pediatric version). *Anesth Analg.* 1990;70:105.

106. Audenaert SM, Montgomery CL, Stone B, et al. Retrograde-assisted fiberoptic tracheal intubation in children with difficult airways. *Anesth Analg.* 1991;73:660.

107. Goldberg JS, Bernard AC, Marks RJ, et al. Simulation technique for difficult intubation: teaching tool or new hazard? *J Clin Anesth.* 1990;2:21.

108. Mason RA. Learning fiberoptic intubation: fundamental problems [editorial]. *Anaesthesia.* 1992;47:729.

109. From RP, Pearson KS, Albanese MA, et al. Assessment of an interactive learning system with "sensorized" manikin head for airway management instruction. *Anesth Analg.* 1994;79:136.

110. Orlowski JP, Kanoti, GA, Mehlman MJ. The ethics of using newly dead patients for teaching and practicing intubation techniques [editorial]. *N Engl J Med.* 1988;319:439.

111. Cooper SD, Benumof JL. Teaching the management of the difficult airway: the USCD airway rotation [abstract]. *Anesthesiology.* 1994;81:A1241.

112. Rose DK, Cohen MM. The airway: problems and predictions in 18,500 patients. *Can J Anaesth.* 1994;41:372.

113. Koppel JN, Reed AP. Formal instructions in difficult airway management: a survey of anesthesiology residency programs. *Anesthesiology.* 1995;83:1343.

## Acknowledgment

Special thanks to Ms. Poppy Smith for her determination, patience, and unflagging good humor.

# Anesthesia for Patients With Bronchial Asthma and Chronic Obstructive Lung Disease

Sreenivasa S. Moorthy

## PATHOPHYSIOLOGY

### What Is Bronchial Asthma?

*Bronchial asthma* is a chronic lung disease with episodic manifestations of signs and symptoms of airway obstruction.

Between the episodes, the patient is generally free of symptoms. The incidence of bronchial asthma ranges from 4% to 5% and is increasing still. Fifty percent of the patients develop their disease during childhood, and 75% of patients are <40 years of age.[1,2] Although the mortality is low (0.3 deaths in 10 000 patients), evidence suggests an increase.[3] Bronchial asthma does not produce progressive deterioration of pulmonary functions.

## What Is Chronic Obstructive Lung Disease?

Chronic obstructive lung disease (COLD) includes chronic bronchitis, emphysema, asthmatic bronchitis, and bronchiolitis.[3,4] In addition to airway obstruction, each disease has other distinguishing features (Table 54–1).[1] *Chronic bronchitis* is associated with cough, excessive mucus expectoration, and varying patterns of obstruction to airflow. *Emphysema* produces chronic enlargement of air spaces distal to terminal bronchioles, loss of lung elastic recoil, airflow obstruction, hyperinflation, and gas trapping. *Asthmatic bronchitis* is chronic persistent asthma with no symptom-free interval, airway inflammation, and hypertrophic, desquamative eosinophilic changes in bronchi. *Bronchiolitis* is usually a childhood viral disease characterized by small airway narrowing secondary to inflammation. Respiratory syncytial virus, influenza, rhinovirus, and mumps can produce bronchiolitis. COLD is more common in men than women (100:1) because of their genetic predisposition, exposure to causative factors, and cigarette smoking. Inhaling passive smoke and smoking marijuana or opium can also lead to emphysema. Air pollution, chronic lower respiratory infections, climatic factors, and heredity are associated with COLD. Also, people with blood types A and O are at increased risk. A deficiency of $\alpha_1$-antitrypsin produces a specific type of emphysema: *centrilobular emphysema*. It has an incidence of 1:2000 to 1:4000 in homozygous individuals, and 1:100 to 4:100 in heterozygous individuals.

## How Does the Pathophysiology of Bronchial Asthma Manifest?

The characteristic features of bronchial asthma include the following:

1. Reversible or partially reversible airway obstruction
2. Airway inflammation
3. Hyperreactivity of airways to a variety of stimuli

After repeated exposure to inciting stimuli, the bronchial tree becomes responsive to even nonspecific stimuli such as cold anesthetic gases, tracheal tubes, or tracheobronchial tree suctioning.

## What Factors Cause Airway Hyperreactivity?

The mechanisms by which the airways become sensitized and hyperreactive are not well known. However, once present, hyperreactivity persists. Airway reactivity varies markedly during the day. Bronchospasm or overt asthmatic attacks usually occur at night and in the early morning. It may be occasionally advantageous to defer elective surgery in an asthmatic patient until late in the morning or midday, when bronchomotor tone is optimal.

## What Are the Stimuli for an Asthmatic Attack?

The stimuli that can precipitate an acute episode of bronchial asthma include allergens, exercise, mechanical stimulation, infection, and emotional stress, as well as occupational, environmental, and pharmacologic agents.[2] The patient who is prone to bronchial asthma generally has a genetic predisposition to the disease and responds to an antigenic challenge by developing bronchospasm. The inheritance of bronchial asthma is complex, and our knowledge of it is incomplete. Patients with allergic or atopic (extrinsic) asthma usually have a family history of atopy.

## What Are the Mediators of Bronchial Asthma?

Immunoglobulin E (IgE) secreted by B cells attaches to receptors on mast cells and basophils. Activation of these receptors on mast cells results in the release of potent biologic mediators that trigger an asthmatic attack. The mediators include prostanoids, leukotrienes (LT), bradykinins, eosino-

**TABLE 54–1.** Characteristic Features of Bronchial Asthma, Chronic Bronchitis, and Emphysema

|  | Bronchial Asthma | Chronic Bronchitis | Emphysema |
|---|---|---|---|
| Age of onset | <30 y | >50 y | >60 y |
| History of smoking | No | Yes | Yes |
| Symptoms | Paroxysmal | Chronic | Chronic |
| Chest radiograph | Normal | Increased markings | Hyperinflation |
| $FEV_1$ | Decreased during attack | Decreased | Decreased |
| TLC | Usually normal | Usually normal | Increased |
| RV | Usually normal | Usually normal | Increased |
| $Pao_2$ | Normal | Decreased | Decreased |
| $Paco_2$ | Normal | Elevated | Normal |
| $Dlco$ | Normal | Normal | Decreased |

$Dlco$, diffusing capacity of the lung for carbon monoxide; $FEV_1$, forced expiratory volume in 1 second; $Paco_2$, partial pressure of carbon dioxide, arterial; $Pao_2$, partial pressure of oxygen, arterial; RV, residual volume; TLC, total lung capacity.

**TABLE 54–2.** Mediators of Bronchospasm in Asthma

**Factors That Produce Bronchoconstriction**

Prostanoids ($PGD_2$, $PGF_{2K}$)
Thromboxane $A_2$
Leukotrienes ($LTC_4$, $LTD_4$)
Platelet activating factor
Adenosine
Bradykinin
Substance P
Calcitonin gene-related peptide

**Factors That Produce Increased Capillary Permeability**

Prostanoids (prostacyclin)
Platelet activating factor

**Factors That Produce Increased Secretion of Mucus**

Leukotrienes ($LTC_4$, $LTD_4$)
Platelet activating factor

**Chemotactic Agents That Produce Inflammatory Response (infiltration with neutrophils and eosinophils)**

Leukotrienes ($LTB_4$)
Adenosine
Bradykinin
Eosinophilic chemotactic factor
Lymphocyte chemotactic factor
High molecular weight neutrophils
Chemotactic factor of anaphylaxis

philic chemotactic factors, and others (Table 54–2). The role of LTs in bronchial asthma is being extensively studied, and anti-LT drugs are under evaluation. LTs $B_4$, $C_4$, $D_4$, and $E_4$ are important to vascular permeability and smooth muscle constriction.[5] These mediators are released from mast cells, macrophages, and respiratory epithelial cells of the bronchioles and produce bronchoconstriction and increased capillary permeability with increased airway edema. The end result is bronchoconstriction, inflammation, increased mucus production, and destruction of ciliated epithelium.[6,7]

## What Are the Features of Chronic Bronchitis?

Cough, sputum production, recurrent infection, and airway obstruction are characteristic of chronic bronchitis. Excessive smoking causes hyperplasia of mucus glands in the trachea and large bronchi with production of copious quantities of mucoid secretions. Obstruction to airflow results from changes in small airways, associated emphysematous changes, an increased number of epithelial goblet cells, edema of mucous membranes, and smooth muscle hypertrophy.

The sputum is nonpurulent in the early phases of chronic bronchitis but becomes purulent late due to colonization. The degree of airway obstruction parallels infection of the sputum. Translocation of serum proteins and glycoproteins into the sputum occurs. Tracheal mucus velocity decreases secondary to reduced mucociliary activity. Goblet cells and nonciliated squamous epithelial cells replace normal ciliated epithelium.

## What Are the Features of Emphysema?

Emphysema produces abnormal and permanent enlargement of air spaces distal to the terminal bronchioles. The walls of these air spaces are destroyed, but no fibrosis occurs.[4,8] The

elastic and collagen framework of the lung is destroyed by *elastase,* a proteolytic enzyme that is secreted by neutrophils and other inflammatory cells. Normally, a glycoprotein ($\alpha_1$-antitrypsin) and a macroglobulin ($\alpha_2$-antitrypsin) protect lung elastin.

Smoking produces a low-grade inflammatory reaction and increases the number of neutrophils in the blood and lung tissue; this produces elastolytic injury. Smoking can also alter the inhibitory effects of glycoproteins on elastase. Smokers with $\alpha_1$-antitrypsin deficiency may develop *centrilobular emphysema* by age 40 years. Nonsmokers with this deficiency may develop *panacinar emphysema* by age 60 years.

## What Are the Features of Asthmatic Bronchitis?

The diagnosis of asthmatic bronchitis is applied to patients with airway obstruction, chronic productive cough, and considerable difficulty with episodic bronchospasm. This syndrome may be a result of severe progressive classic asthma or a variant of chronic bronchitis. These patients have frequent and severe recurrences of bronchospasm.

# SIGNS AND SYMPTOMS

## What Are the Signs and Symptoms of Bronchial Asthma?

There are several types of bronchial asthma (Table 54–3). Atopic asthma or extrinsic asthma usually occurs in younger patients (<30 years). A family history of atopy, elevated levels of IgE, positive skin tests for atopy, and positive bronchial challenge tests are diagnostic. Intrinsic asthma manifests in older individuals without a family history of atopy. The blood and sputum of these patients may have an increased number of eosinophils. These patients may have autoantibodies to smooth muscle as well as autoimmune diseases.

Exercise-induced asthma is precipitated by hyperpnea and by heat and water loss from respiratory mucosa. Environmental, infectious, and occupational asthmas are precipitated by a variety of pollutants and infections. The clinical features of an acute attack of bronchial asthma include dyspnea and cough. Physical examination reveals tachypnea, wheezing, and tachycardia. Some patients also exhibit diaphoresis and pulsus paradoxus. Excessive production of mucus causes plugging of bronchioles, which leads to air trapping. Chest radiographs reveal an increase in the anteroposterior diameter of the chest. Mucus secretions and mucus plugs contain eosinophils, ciliated epithelium, Charcot-Leyden crystals (L150 phospholipase), and Curschmann spirals (strands of mucus). As the attack resolves and symptoms abate, the patient develops a productive cough to clear the obstructed airways.

**TABLE 54–3.** Types of Asthma

| | |
|---|---|
| Atopic (extrinsic) | Occupational |
| Intrinsic | Aspirin-induced |
| Exercise-induced | Psychogenic |
| Environmental/infectious | |

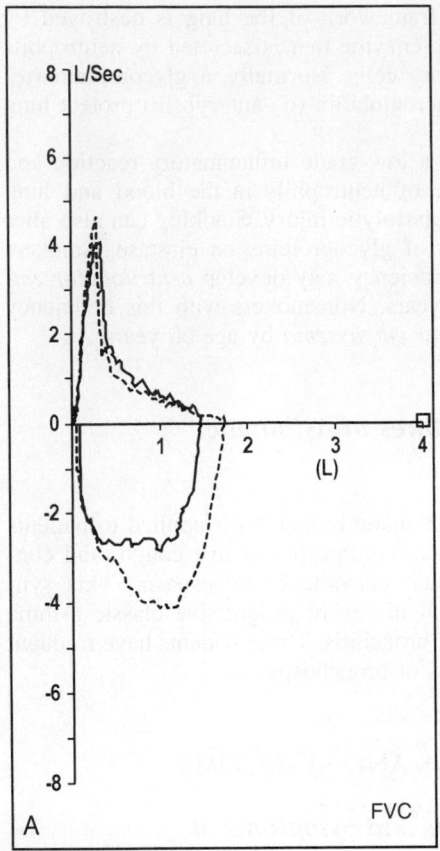

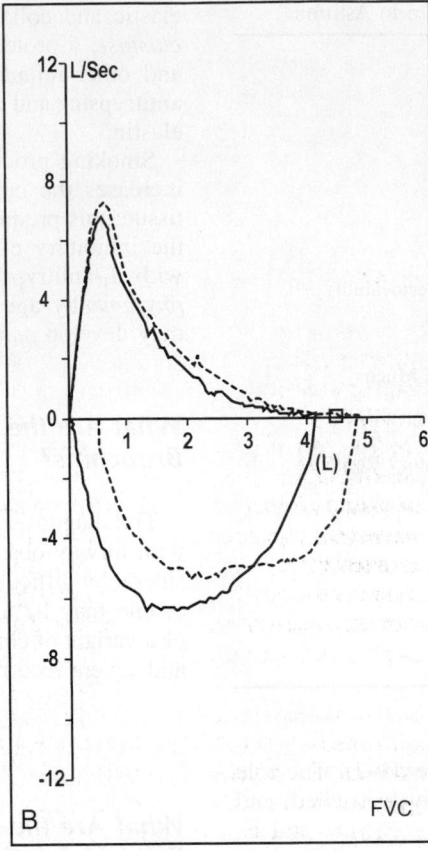

**FIGURE 54–1.** Flow-volume loops in a patient with chronic obstructive pulmonary disease before and after bronchodilator administration. *A,* No appreciable improvement in pulmonary function occurred after the bronchodilator was given. *B,* Flow-volume loop in a patient with bronchial asthma, which shows improvement ($FEV_1 > 15\%$) in pulmonary functions. FVC, forced vital capacity; solid line, pretreatment; dashed line, posttreatment.

## What Are the Signs and Symptoms of Chronic Obstructive Lung Disease?

Patients with a history of cigarette smoking and a family history of COLD are highly likely to have some component of COLD. Symptoms include progressive dyspnea, anorexia, nausea, chest pain, and occasionally hemoptysis.[9,10] Signs include tachypnea, pursed-lip breathing, use of accessory muscles of respiration, tracheal tug, and pulsus paradoxus. Auscultation of the chest usually reveals distant breath sounds, rhonchi, crackles, and wheezing. Progressive chronic hypoxemia results in pulmonary hypertension and cor pulmonale. Presence of cor pulmonale should be considered in patients with hypoxemia, p-pulmonale syndrome on the electrocardiogram (ECG), and right ventricular hypertrophy.

## What Does Pulmonary Function Testing Reveal in Bronchial Asthma?

Pulmonary function tests (PFTs) during an asthmatic attack reveal an increase in total lung capacity (TLC), functional residual capacity (FRC), and residual volume (RV).[7] Decrease in forced vital capacity (FVC), forced expiratory flow during the middle portion of the FVC ($FEF_{25\%-75\%}$), maximum expiratory flow rates (MEFRs), and forced expiratory flow between 200 and 1200 mL of the FVC ($FEF_{200-1200}$) are indicative of airway obstruction.[7,11,12] The response to bronchodilator therapy can be measured as a guide to therapy (Fig. 54–1).

## What Elements of Pulmonary Function Tests Are Effort-Dependent?

FVC is dependent not only on airway obstruction but also on lung elastic properties, absolute volume of air in the lungs, and voluntary patient effort. MEFRs and $FEF_{25\%-75\%}$ are effort-independent (<75% of FVC) and can be used for quantification of airway obstruction. Closing volume is elevated, which leads to premature airway closure.

## What Changes in Pulmonary Function Are Present in Chronic Obstructive Lung Disease?

As a general rule, pulmonary function in COLD patients reveals evidence of airway obstruction and parenchymal hyperinflation (Table 54–4). A reduction in $FEV_1$, $FEF_{25\%-75\%}$,

**TABLE 54–4.** Features of Emphysematous Patients

| Decreased | Increased |
| --- | --- |
| Lung recoil | Residual volume |
| $D_{LCO}$ | Functional residual capacity |
| $FEV_1$ | |
| MEFV | |
| $FEF_{25\%-75\%}$ ± $PaO_2$ | |

$D_{LCO}$, diffusing capacity of the lung for carbon monoxide; $FEF_{25\%-75\%}$, forced expiratory flow, midexpiratory phase; $FEV_1$, forced expiratory volume in 1 second; MEFV, maximum expiratory flow volume.

maximum flow at 75% of vital capacity, midexpiratory flow, and prolonged expiration indicate obstructive airway disease.[13,14]

Increase in residual volume and TLC also occur.[10,14] Specific airway compliance and dynamic compliance are reduced. An increased alveolar-to-arterial oxygen partial pressure gradient occurs secondary to abnormal regional ventilation in the lower lobes from poor compliance.

Emphysematous patients without hypersecretion of mucus exhibit the features listed in Table 54–4. In patients with pure chronic bronchitis, areas of low ventilation-perfusion ($\dot{V}/\dot{Q}$) matching dominate and produce both hypoxemia and hypercarbia. Characteristically, the airway obstruction in patients with COLD does not improve as significantly after the administration of bronchodilators as it does in patients with asthma.

Airway resistance increases and specific conductance decreases during an asthmatic attack. As a result, both resistive and elastic work of breathing increase.[15,16] Development of $\dot{V}/\dot{Q}$ abnormalities leads to hypoxemia and hypercarbia. Hypercarbia during an asthmatic attack indicates a severe episode.

## What Are the Cardiovascular Changes During an Asthmatic Attack?

Acute airway obstruction with air trapping produces deterioration in cardiovascular function. Sinus tachycardia, premature ventricular contractions, p-pulmonale syndrome, right axis deviation, right bundle branch block, clockwise rotation of the heart, right ventricular strain pattern, and ST-T changes are known to occur. ST-T changes can be nonspecific or indicative of myocardial ischemia. Pulsus paradoxus and leftward shift of the interventricular septum with decreased left ventricular stroke volume are manifestations of severe airway obstruction.

## What Conditions Aggravate Bronchial Asthma?

Pregnancy, psychiatric disorders, sinusitis with nasal polyposis, aspirin allergy, obesity, cardiac disease, sleep apnea, and gastroesophageal reflux adversely affect the asthmatic patient. COLD has an obvious negative impact. Sometimes treatment with β-adrenergic agonist drugs can close small and large airways with mucoid impaction, resulting in deterioration of pulmonary function. This occurs because sometimes the primary problem with wheezing is related to excessive secretions rather than bronchospasm. If the bronchi are dilated, and the secretion problem is not addressed, an actual increase in secretions can occur. Then, when the β₂ effect wears off, the patient has a load of secretions that plug the airways.

## What Challenge Tests Are Available for Bronchial Asthma?

A number of tests challenge the reactivity of bronchial airways. Nonantigenic agents such as histamine and methacholine can be used to elicit bronchoconstriction and to evaluate therapy. Inhalation of cold air and voluntary hyperpnea are used to provoke exercise-induced asthma. Inhalation of gases such as sulfur dioxide and ozone, as well as exposure to occupational agents, may provoke bronchospasm in susceptible individuals.

## TREATMENT

### What Are the Goals in the Treatment of Bronchial Asthma?

The primary goals of therapy are reversal of bronchospasm and control of airway inflammatory reaction.[17–19] Airway hypersensitivity and hyperreactivity lead to bronchospasm. Inflammation and inflammatory mediators not only produce edema and cellular infiltration of the airways but also contribute to bronchial hypersensitivity. Inflammation and loss of respiratory epithelium expose autonomic and nonautonomic nerve endings. Stimulation of these nerve endings results in the release of neuropeptides (substance P, neurokinin A, calcitonins, and gene-related peptides) that contribute to airway hyperreactivity. Pharmacologic therapy includes these drug categories:

1. Bronchodilators (β₂ agonists)
2. Anti-inflammatory agents (adrenocorticosteroids)
3. Inhibitors of mediator release (cromolyn sodium)
4. Inhibitors of LTs (mediators) synthesis
5. Anticholinergic agents

### Bronchodilators

The primary drugs for the treatment of bronchial asthma are bronchodilators. Airway smooth muscle contains a large number of β₂-adrenergic receptors. β-Adrenergic compounds increase intracellular adenosine monophosphate, activate protein kinases, inhibit myosin phosphorylation, and lower intracellular calcium levels. All of these effects promote bronchial smooth muscle relaxation and bronchodilation. β-Adrenergic agonists also stabilize mast cells and cholinergic nerve endings and prevent release of mediators.

Several classes of β₂-adrenergic agonists (Table 54–5) can be given in inhalation form.[20–22] Inhaled drugs are effective and tend to be less toxic than parenteral preparations (see Table 54–5). Subcutaneous epinephrine, in particular, is more toxic than inhaled epinephrine when administered to hypoxemic patients. Oral preparations (syrups and tablets) are also available for the resorcinols (terbutaline, metaproterenol) and albuterol.

### Methylxanthines

Methylxanthines are synergistic with β-adrenergic agonists. Theophylline is most frequently used and can be administered orally or parenterally (Table 54–6).[23,24] Although their precise mechanism of action is not clear, methylxanthines increase cyclic adenosine monophosphate by inhibition of phosphodiesterase.

The late response to allergens is also inhibited by an anti-inflammatory action. Theophylline, oxtriphylline, anhydrous theophylline (Elixophyllin), and dyphylline are rapid-acting methylxanthines. Slow-release compounds that contain anhydrous theophylline are available. Intravenous theophylline is

**TABLE 54–5.** Inhaled β-Adrenergic Agonist Bronchodilators

| | | Dose | | |
|---|---|---|---|---|
| | Receptor Activity | Metered-Dose Inhaler* | Aerosol | Activity Duration (h) |
| Catecholamines | | | | |
| Epinephrine | $\alpha_1$, $\beta_1$, $\beta_2$ | 160-250 µg | 1%-2.25% solution, 0.01 mL/kg tid-qid | <1 |
| Isoproterenol | $\beta_1$, $\beta_2$ | 120-130 µg (chloride), 80 µg (sulfate) | 0.5% solution, 0.02 mL/kg qid | <1 |
| Isoetharine | $\beta_2$ | 340 µg | 1% solution, 0.02 mL/kg qid | <1 |
| Resorcinols | | | | |
| Metaproterenol | $\beta_2$ | 650 µg | 5% solution, 0.01-0.03 mL/kg tid-qid | <3 |
| Albuterol | $\beta_2$ | 90 µg | 0.5% solution, 0.01 mL/kg tid-qid | <4 |

*The usual patient dose with a metered-dose inhaler is two puffs.
tid, three times a day; qid, four times a day.

administered with a loading dose of 6 mg/kg over 20 minutes, followed by 0.9 mg/kg/h to maintain a serum level of 10 to 20 µg/mL. Rapid improvement generally occurs within 15 minutes of loading dose administration.[25,26] Side effects include nausea, vomiting, diarrhea, restlessness, insomnia, irritability, headache, seizures, tachycardia, dysrhythmias, hypotension, hypertension, diuresis, flushing, and fever.[25-27] Aminophylline clearance may be decreased by viral infections, cardiac failure, hepatic disease, and drugs such as erythromycin, cimetidine, and troleandomycin, predisposing the patient to aminophylline toxicity. Increased clearance may result from cigarette smoking and hepatic enzyme induction (phenobarbital).

## Adrenocorticosteroids

Corticosteroids are effective for treating bronchial asthma because they suppress inflammation and prevent the release of mediators from mast cells.[28-30] Neither oral nor inhaled preparations are effective for acute attacks of bronchial asthma. Inhaled steroids are useful in maintenance therapy to reduce the systemic effects of orally administered steroids (sodium and chloride retention, gastric hyperacidity, hypertension, psychosis, hypokalemia, increased intraocular pressure, muscle atrophy, diabetes mellitus, poor wound healing, osteoporosis, cataracts, and adrenal suppression). Several preparations of corticosteroids are available (Table 54–7).

## Cromolyn Sodium and Nedocromil Sodium

Cromolyn sodium (Intal) and nedocromil sodium (Tilade) inhibit mast cell degranulation by stabilizing the cell membranes.[31] They block or attenuate bronchoconstriction after the patient has been exposed to allergens or irritants. The protective effect lasts for 3 to 4 hours. They can be administered prophylactically by inhalation in the form of powder or a solution with a metered-dose inhaler (MDI). Side effects include throat irritation, cough, transient skin rashes, and occasional bronchospasm. Nedocromil, in particular, has an unpleasant taste.

## Anticholinergic Agents

Anticholinergics block muscarinic airway receptors, inhibit vagal cholinergic tone, and produce bronchodilation. Ipratropium bromide (administered with an MDI), atropine methylnitrate, and glycopyrrolate methyl bromide (administered as aerosols) are three inhaled bronchodilators that are currently available.[32] The quaternary anticholinergics have fewer side effects because of their low level of systemic absorption. Anticholinergics are particularly useful in conjunction with β-agonists.

## Drugs Acting on Leukotrienes

LTs, derived from lipoxygenases of arachidonic acid metabolism, produce increased mucus, airway wall edema, and bronchoconstriction. Zileuton (Zyflo) and montelukast (Singulair) are LT antagonists. These drugs are useful for treating asthma, particularly as supplemental therapy with β-adrenergic agonists or steroids.[33] In addition, they may increase serum

**TABLE 54–6.** Parenteral Bronchodilators

| | Dose and Route of Administration |
|---|---|
| *Methylxanthines* | |
| Aminophylline | 6 mg/kg IV loading dose |
| | 0.5-0.9 mg/kg/h maintenance |
| *β-Adrenergic Agonists* | |
| Epinephrine | 0.1-0.5 mg SC |
| | 1-4 µg/min IV (10-50 ng/kg/min) |
| Isoproterenol | 0.5-5 µg/min IV |
| Ephedrine | 25-50 mg IM or SC 5-25 mg IV |
| Terbutaline | Maximum of 0.5 mg in 4 h |
| Albuterol | 10 µg/min IV |

IM, intramuscular; IV, intravenous; SC, subcutaneous.

**TABLE 54–7.** Corticosteroid Preparations for Treatment of Asthma

| | Potency Equivalents |
|---|---|
| *Systemic Steroids* | |
| Hydrocortisone | 1 |
| Prednisone | 5 |
| Prednisolone | 4 |
| Methylprednisone | 4 |
| Triamcinolone | 5 |
| Dexamethasone | 30 |
| *Inhaled Steroids* | |
| Beclomethasone dipropionate (Beclovent) 250 µg/puff | 800 µg/d |
| Flunisolide (AeroBid) 250 µg/puff | 1000 µg/d |
| Triamcinolone acetonide (Azmacort) 100 µg/puff | 1000-1600 µg/d |

concentrations of theophylline, warfarin, and propranolol and can induce vasculitis. Further clinical evaluation is needed before these drugs are commonly used.

## How Do You Treat Chronic Obstructive Lung Disease Patients?

Treating COLD patients includes the following principles:

- Patient
  Stop smoking
- Physician
  Treat reversible bronchospasm
  Provide chest physiotherapy
  Treat complications (including hypoxemia, hypercarbia, respiratory tract infection, and cor pulmonale)

## What Drugs Are Useful for Chronic Obstructive Lung Disease Patients?

The use of bronchodilators is the mainstay of treatment in managing reversible bronchospasm or bronchospasm producing airflow limitation. β-Adrenergic agonists, ipratropium bromide, and aminophylline are commonly used.[34] Ipratropium has been found to be much more effective in patients with COLD than in patients with asthma.[35] Corticosteroids are useful in patients with asthmatic bronchitis.

## Do Ancillary Measures Help?

Observation of appropriate bronchial hygiene, cessation of smoking, avoidance of allergens and airway irritants, and use of antibiotic therapy for airway infection result in further improvement of pulmonary function.

### Mobilization of Secretions

Mobilization of airway secretions is a goal of adjunctive therapy for COLD. Adequate systemic hydration, effective cough training, and chest physiotherapy (chest percussion, vibration, postural drainage) all help mobilize airway secretions.

Iodinated glycerol is useful as an expectorant and mucolytic. Other oral mucolytic agents include thioprimine and 2-mercaptoethane. Acetylcysteine is an excellent mucolytic agent that can be administered as an aerosol or by direct instillation into the tracheobronchial tree. Voluntary exercises and training of respiratory muscles, including upper abdominal muscles, is also helpful.

### Oxygen

Hypoxemia should be treated promptly with supplemental oxygen. Patients with pulmonary hypertension, cor pulmonale, polycythemia, exercise intolerance, impaired cognition, nocturnal restlessness, and morning headache benefit considerably.

## PREOPERATIVE MANAGEMENT

## How Do You Evaluate Patients With Bronchial Asthma and Chronic Obstructive Lung Disease Preoperatively?

Patients with a history of bronchial asthma, smoking, COLD, and abnormal PFTs are at increased risk for developing pulmonary complications following surgery.[36,37]

Preanesthetic evaluation for bronchial asthma should include identification of precipitating and seasonal variation, frequency of attacks, time and duration of last attack, and maintenance medications.[38,39] The physical examination should include assessment of respiratory rate, accessory respiratory muscles, heart rate, and blood pressure, in addition to auscultation of the chest for wheezing and rhonchi, elicitation of pulsus paradoxus, and awareness of the possible signs of pulmonary hypertension. The physical examination should focus on the patient's breathing pattern (eg, rate, depth, and accessory muscle use) and chest auscultation. A chest radiograph that demonstrates lung hyperinflation, cardiac enlargement, atelectasis, pneumonia, or pleural effusion is indicative of increased perioperative risk.

Additional information may be obtained from sputum examination, chest roentgenogram, arterial blood gases (ABGs), and PFTs. PFTs assess the type and degree of airway obstruction, evaluate the response to bronchodilators, help determine perioperative risk, and provide guidelines for postoperative care. Measurements of FVC, forced expiratory volume in 1 second ($FEV_1$), and $FEF_{25\%-75\%}$ indicate the severity of airway obstruction. A strong correlation exists among the $FEV_1$, $PaO_2$, and $PaCO_2$: the lower the $FEV_1$, the higher the $PaCO_2$.

Evaluation of the patient with COLD should include medical history (focusing on the presence and severity of dyspnea), smoking history, productive cough, wheezing, and the previous anesthesia effects. The patient's ability to cough and clear secretions is also of considerable importance. Age over 60 years and obesity are other factors that increase perioperative risk.

## What Are the Guidelines for Pulmonary Function Tests?

There are no specific guidelines for performing preoperative PFTs. Depending on the type of surgery, clinical examination of the patient is sufficient to suggest when to take ABG measurement and routine spirometry. Spirometry should include FVC, $FEV_1$, $FEV_1/FVC$, and $FEF_{25\%-75\%}$. The results can be compared with normal predicted values. A typical flow volume loop with spirometric measurements for a patient with COLD is shown in Figure 54–1A.

ABG measurement during room air breathing is an excellent method to determine a patient's ability to exchange oxygen and carbon dioxide at rest. A resting $PaCO_2$ of $\geq 45$ mm Hg is associated with greater postoperative risk. The site of surgical incision markedly affects respiratory function postoperatively. Sophisticated measures of pulmonary function, such as split-lung function testing, may be required for pulmonary resection. Epstein and colleagues developed a cardiopulmonary risk index, which is the sum of a modified Goldman

**TABLE 54–8.** Pulmonary Function Criteria Indicative of Increased Perioperative Risk

| | Predicted Value | |
|---|---|---|
| | *Abdominal Surgery* | *Thoracic Surgery* |
| FVC | <70% | <70% |
| FEV₁ | <70% | <1.0 L |
| FEF$_{25\%-75\%}$ | <50% | <50% |
| MVV | <50% | <50% |
| RV | — | >47% |
| Paco₂ | >45 mm Hg | >45 mm Hg |
| Mean PAP | >45 mm Hg | >22 mm Hg |

FEF$_{25\%-75\%}$, forced expiratory flow, midexpiratory phase; FEV₁, forced expiratory volume in 1 second; FVC, forced vital capacity; MVV, maximum voluntary ventilation; Paco₂, partial pressure of carbon dioxide, arterial; PAP, pulmonary artery pressure; RV, residual volume.

Modified from Gass GD, Olsen GN. Preoperative pulmonary function testing to predict postoperative morbidity and mortality. *Chest.* 1986;89:127.

(cardiac) index and pulmonary risk factors. The pulmonary risk factors include obesity, smoking, productive cough, diffuse wheezing or rhonchi, an FEV₁:FVC ratio <70%, and Paco₂ >45 mm Hg.[39,40]

## What Is the Outcome After Upper Abdominal Surgery in Chronic Obstructive Lung Disease Patients?

An upper abdominal incision is associated with reduced diaphragmatic excursion and reduced effectiveness of cough due to pain. These 2 factors lead to atelectasis, bronchitis, and pneumonia. After upper abdominal surgery, these complications occur in 25% of patients without COLD. Those with COLD and abnormal PFTs have a postoperative complication rate of 42%.

Proper preoperative preparation of patients with COLD can reduce the postoperative complication rate from 60% to 22%.[41] An increased likelihood of postoperative complications can be anticipated if the vital capacity is <75% of predicted, the FEV₁ is <70% of the FVC, the FEF$_{25\%-75\%}$ is <50% of the FVC, and the maximum voluntary ventilation is <50% of predicted values (Table 54–8).

If preoperative preparation does not improve pulmonary function, a high incidence of complications should be anticipated. Each patient with severe dysfunction must be considered on an individual basis, and the risk-benefit ratio of each patient for a given surgical procedure must be determined.

## What Factors Increase the Risks of Thoracic Surgery?

Multiple factors influence the perioperative risk following thoracic surgery (see Table 54–8). Traditional PFTs can predict the perioperative risk. Patients undergoing thoracic surgery for lobectomy or pneumonectomy have an increased postoperative risk with FVC <2 L, FEV₁ <1.2 L, FEV₁/FVC <35%, FEF$_{25\%-75\%}$ <1.6 L, a midexpiratory flow rate <200 L/min, and a maximum voluntary ventilation <50% of the predicted value. Other pulmonary function values indicative of high risk include an increased residual volume, a diffusing

capacity of the lung for carbon monoxide ≤50%, a Paco₂ >45 mm Hg, mean pulmonary artery pressure >22 mm Hg, and pulmonary vascular resistance ≥190 dynes/s/cm⁻⁵.[42] Because the pulmonary tissue intended for resection may be noncontributory to ventilation, split PFTs that employ ¹³³Xe radiospirometry may be useful for predicting the effect of the actual loss of functional pulmonary tissue.

## What Is Lung Volume Reduction Surgery and What Are the Indications?

Lung volume reduction surgery involves resection of 20% to 30% of each lung in severe emphysema. The surgery can be done via a median sternotomy, sequential thoracoscopy, or thoracotomy. The surgery reduces severe hyperinflation, restores elastic recoil in small airways with reduction of airway resistance, restores chest wall elastic recoil, improves $\dot{V}/\dot{Q}$, and reduces residual lung volume. There are criteria established to include or exclude patients from surgery. Inclusion criteria include NYHA class III–IV, evidence of airflow obstruction (FEV₁ <30% of predicted), hyperinflation (FRC or TLC >120% of predicted), reduction of maximum inspired pressure (MIP) or transdiaphragmatic pressure by at least 50%, hyperinflation by chest radiograph or CT scan, and $\dot{V}/\dot{Q}$ mismatch quantitatively evaluated in the planned resection part of the lung. The exclusion criteria include refractory hypoxemia, severe hypercapnia requiring mechanical ventilation, significant cardiovascular disease, severe pulmonary hypertension (mean pulmonary artery pressure ≥50 mm Hg), severely debilitated condition, significant extrapulmonary disease, and psychologic dysfunction.[43–45]

## How Do You Prepare Chronic Obstructive Lung Disease Patients for Anesthesia and Surgery?

A number of therapeutic modalities can be employed preoperatively to improve perioperative outcome (Table 54–9).[46–52] Improved outcome, however, is predicated on the presence of a reversible component of the patient's COLD. Because most treatments require more than overnight preparation, the necessary amount of time must be planned preoperatively for effective therapy. Cessation of smoking for 12 to 24 hours before surgery does not improve pulmonary function but does reduce the effects of nicotine. Reduced carboxyhemoglobin levels decrease the likelihood of erroneous pulse oximeter readings (functional versus fractional saturation). Smoking should be

**TABLE 54–9.** Therapy to Reduce Pulmonary Risk

Cessation of smoking
Treatment of pulmonary infection
Bronchodilator therapy
Nutritional support
Respiratory or chest physiotherapy
Decreased anesthesia or surgical time (risk increased with operations >3 h)
Effective postoperative analgesia (systemic or neuraxial narcotics)
Maximum breathing exercises (incentive spirometry, nasal mask continuous positive airway pressure)
Early postoperative mobilization and ambulation
Heparin prophylaxis in selected cases

**TABLE 54–10.** Risk Reduction Strategies

**Preoperative**

Encourage cessation of cigarette smoking for at least 8 wk.
Treat airflow obstruction in patients with chronic obstructive lung disease or asthma.
Administer antibiotics and delay surgery if respiratory infection is present.
Begin patient education regarding lung expansion maneuvers.

**Intraoperative**

Limit duration of surgery to <3 h.
Use spinal or epidural anesthesia.*
Avoid use of pancuronium.
Use laparoscopic procedures when possible.
Substitute less ambitious procedure for upper abdominal or thoracic surgery when possible.

**Postoperative**

Use deep-breathing exercises or incentive spirometry.
Use continuous positive airway pressure.
Use epidural analgesia.*
Use intercostal nerve block.*

*This strategy is recommended, although variable efficacy has been reported in the literature.
From Smetana GW. Preoperative pulmonary evaluation. *N Engl J Med.* 1999;340:937.

stopped for at least 8 weeks for any improvement in pulmonary function to be optimally realized.[40] Risk reduction strategies that apply to both COLD and asthmatic patients are shown in Table 54–10.

## How Do You Prepare a Patient With Bronchial Asthma for Anesthesia and Surgery?

Preanesthetic preparation with respiratory therapy, cessation of smoking, treatment with bronchodilators, and physical training with deep breathing exercises reduces the incidence of postoperative complications. The asymptomatic patient who does not require maintenance medication can undergo anesthesia and surgery with little risk of postoperative complications. Avoidance of allergens, active or passive smoke, infection, alcohol, and nonsteroidal anti-inflammatory drugs is helpful.[51,52]

## ANESTHETIC MANAGEMENT

### What Factors Are Important in Planning Anesthesia for an Asthmatic Patient?

In planning an anesthetic for the patient with asthma, the anesthesiologist must answer several questions (Table 54–11). Functional recovery from an acute episode of asthma may require several days to a week. Consequently, induction of

**TABLE 54–11.** Planning the Anesthetic Management of Patients With Asthma

When was the last acute episode?
What time of day is best for anesthesia and surgery?
What allergens or irritants precipitate bronchospasm?
What medications are used for treatment of asthma?
What potential drug interactions can occur during anesthesia?

anesthesia soon after an acute episode may provoke another attack.

Airway resistance in the asthmatic patient is generally greatest in the early morning hours. Although few data are available concerning the interaction of this diurnal pattern and anesthesia, delaying anesthesia and surgery until the late morning hours, as previously noted, may be beneficial. Exposure to known irritants and allergens during the perioperative period should be avoided.

Interactions between anesthesia and bronchodilators such as β-adrenergic agonists and aminophylline may result in cardiac dysrhythmias. Changes in aminophylline levels and clearance may also occur during anesthesia.

### Preanesthetic Medications

Patients should continue taking medications for treatment of bronchial asthma such as bronchodilators, corticosteroids, sedatives, and anticholinergic medications. Patients receiving chronic corticosteroid therapy (especially oral) may require supplemental corticosteroids during the perioperative period if they are considered to be at risk for steroid-induced adrenal suppression.

Administration of inhaled bronchodilators in the preoperative holding area may also be beneficial. Auscultation of the chest for wheezing before induction should be performed to determine whether bronchoconstriction has developed since the preoperative evaluation. In patients with a history of atopy, antihistamines (histamine receptor antagonists) may be beneficial. Histamine$_2$ (H$_2$) receptors are necessary for inhibitory feedback for H$_1$ receptors; thus, sodium citrate may be preferable to cimetidine or other drugs in that class if an antacid is used.

Regional anesthesia is preferred by many anesthesiologists for extremity, perineal, and lower abdominal surgeries. It avoids potential bronchoconstrictive stimuli such as tracheal intubation and minimizes potential drug interactions. However, the occurrence of bronchospasm after spinal anesthesia suggests that unopposed vagal effects following sympathetic blockade, as well as depression of adrenal function with decreased levels of endogenous steroids and catecholamines, may not make this the perfect alternative either.

### What Are the Potential Problems With General Anesthesia?

#### Induction Agents and Muscle Relaxants

When general anesthesia is necessary, several considerations merit attention. Thiopental, methohexital, etomidate, and propofol in usual clinical doses have long been thought to have no direct effect on bronchomotor tone and have been used in the asthmatic patient. More recent data are at odds with this impression. They suggest that propofol is the preferred intravenous induction agent. This derives from the observation that in the in vitro human airway rings that were either normal or sensitized with asthmatic serum, neither etomidate nor propofol altered baseline tone, whereas thiopental induced a dose-dependent bronchial contraction.[53] Furthermore, both propofol and etomidate reduced histamine reactivity in both normal and asthma serum-sensitized human bronchial muscle, but this beneficial effect was much greater with propofol.[53] This in vitro observation is supported by a clinical study showing a much greater incidence of wheezing in asymptomatic asthmatic patients following a thiobarbiturate induction (45%) than a propofol induction (0%).[54] This pattern was also observed with nonasthmatic patients where 16% wheezed following thiobarbiturate induction and 3% wheezed following propofol induction.[54]

Bronchospasm that occurs after the administration of these drugs is often secondary to the direct mechanical stimulus of tracheal intubation. Ketamine is a bronchodilator and may be advantageous for the patient with bronchospasm. Nasotracheal intubation should be avoided in patients with an aspirin allergy because of the high incidence of the presence of nasal polyps. A laryngeal mask airway is a good alternative in patients undergoing short procedures under general anesthesia who do not require neuromuscular blockade to avoid tracheal stimulation.

Succinylcholine can be used to relax muscles for tracheal intubation. Although d-tubocurarine, mivacurium, and atracurium are associated with histamine release, clinical experience suggests that they can be safely used. Vecuronium, rocuronium, and cisatracurium can be used without any side effects. Pancuronium can produce tachycardia, especially in the presence of β-adrenergic agonists. Reversal of neuromuscular blockade with neostigmine or pyridostigmine, together with an anticholinergic, has not been shown to produce any adverse effects in asthmatic patients who are *not* actively wheezing.

### Inhalation Agents

Halogenated inhalation anesthetics (halothane, isoflurane, enflurane, desflurane, and sevoflurane) produce bronchodilation and are efficacious for the asthmatic patient. In fact, some of these anesthetics have been used in intensive care units for the treatment of status asthmaticus. Desflurane can sometimes produce airway irritation and is best avoided in an asthmatic patient.

### Lidocaine

Lidocaine decreases bronchomotor tone. However, the direct instillation of lidocaine into the tracheobronchial tree may produce reflex bronchoconstriction. Consequently, use of intravenous lidocaine is preferable.

### Drugs That Promote Bronchospasm

A number of drugs can release histamine, provoke bronchospasm, or produce anaphylactoid reactions (Table 54–12). They must be used with caution or avoided in patients with asthma.

**TABLE 54–12.** Drugs Associated With Histamine Release or Bronchoconstriction

Vancomycin
Histamine$_2$ antagonists
β-Adrenergic blockers (propranolol)
Anticholinesterases without concomitant anticholinergic agents
Radiopaque dyes
Prostaglandins with bronchoconstrictor effects
Protamine

### What Monitoring Is Indicated?

Routine intraoperative monitoring of the asthmatic patient should include ECG, blood pressure, end-tidal $CO_2$ measurement, pulse oximetry, and chest or esophageal stethoscope evaluation. If wheezing is present, insertion of an arterial catheter and periodic measurement of partial pressures of the ABG are highly recommended. If an upward sloping capnogram is observed, an increased arterial-to-end tidal $CO_2$ gradient is to be expected. A technique that can be used to assess this gradient noninvasively is to allow a complete exhalation to occur by turning off the ventilator until the capnogram is seen to plateau or begin its descent (caused by aspiration of fresh gas into the elbow by a sidestream gas monitor). The resulting peak exhaled $CO_2$ should be much closer to the arterial value.

### When Should Tracheal Extubation Be Performed?

Extubation of the trachea during deep levels of anesthesia has the potential advantage of preventing reflex bronchospasm that usually results from tracheal irritation. However, many patients, such as those with gastroesophageal reflux or poor pulmonary function, are not good candidates for "deep extubation." These patients' tracheas must be extubated when protective airway reflexes have returned.

## INTRAOPERATIVE BRONCHOSPASM

Intraoperative bronchospasm can present a significant challenge to the anesthesiologist. Bronchospasm results in air trapping, intrinsic positive end-expiratory pressure (PEEP), decrease in cardiac output, and hypotension, as well as increases in pulmonary arterial, right ventricular, and right atrial pressures.

### How Should It Be Treated?

#### Differential Diagnosis

The hallmark sign of bronchospasm is wheezing. However, a number of causes of intraoperative wheezing are not related to intrinsic bronchoconstriction (Table 54–13). These causes must be considered before treatment is begun. If they have been eliminated and asthmatic bronchoconstriction is suspected, treatment with bronchodilators should be initiated.

#### Inhaled Bronchodilators

Inhaled bronchodilators can be administered with an MDI attached to the tracheal tube or in aerosol form. The inhaled bronchodilator should be administered near the tracheal tube through the inspiratory limb of the breathing circuit or at the junction of the elbow connector and the tracheal tube (Fig. 54–2).

This treatment is best accomplished during manual ventilation, particularly if an MDI is used, so that the respiratory effect can be optimized (ie, by a deep manual inspiration with the drug delivery into the circuit at midinspiration, followed

**TABLE 54–13.** Causes of Intraoperative Wheezing

Light anesthesia
Bronchial asthma
Chronic obstructive lung disease
Fluid overload
Acute left ventricular failure
Mechanical obstruction of the tracheal tube
Endobronchial intubation
Foreign body aspiration
Pulmonary aspiration of gastric acid
Persistent coughing against the tracheal tube
Pulmonary embolism

by an end-inspiratory hold). Metered dose or aerosol administration are equally effective. $\beta_2$-Adrenergic agonists can produce tachycardia and must be cautiously used in patients with ischemic heart disease. MDI delivery is significantly compromised by rainout onto the endotracheal tube. Thus, it is not unusual to need 4 to 10 doses (if no adverse side effects are noted) to achieve good results. Intravenous aminophylline requires more time to onset of action than do inhaled bronchodilators. Adjunctive therapy consists of a slow ventilatory rate and a low ratio of inspiratory to expiratory rate, application of expiratory retard, and adequate preload.

## How Do You Manage Chronic Obstructive Lung Disease Patients Intraoperatively?

Regional anesthesia is advantageous for patients with COLD undergoing surgery on the limbs, lower abdomen, and perineum. Sedation during regional anesthesia may negate the beneficial pulmonary-sparing effects of the regional anesthetic. Spinal or epidural anesthesia at a level higher than T10 may cause an ineffective cough due to abdominal muscle dysfunction. Continuous spinal or epidural anesthesia may have the advantage in allowing better control of the level of anesthesia. Brachial plexus anesthesia or more specific nerve blocks are associated with a low pulmonary morbidity. If an interscalene block is contemplated, it is useful to be reminded

that at least 80% of the time, the ipsilateral phrenic nerve is blocked as well.

## How Is General Anesthesia Used in Chronic Obstructive Lung Disease Patients?

If general anesthesia is required, no specific contraindications relate to commonly used induction agents such as thiopental, methohexital, propofol, etomidate, or ketamine, but propofol is emerging as the drug of choice if there is a reactive airway component associated with the COLD.[53,54] Volatile halogenated agents do not produce bronchoconstriction and are suitable for patients with COLD.[55–57] Intravenous agents such as narcotics and benzodiazepines should be selectively used in these patients because of their generally slower elimination.

Nitrous oxide has been shown to increase pulmonary vascular resistance and pulmonary artery pressure in patients with pulmonary hypertension and should not be used in patients with cor pulmonale. In patients with blebs or bullae, nitrous oxide can produce an increase in their pressure and volume and can potentially increase the risk of pneumothorax.

Muscle relaxation can be produced with succinylcholine or nondepolarizing muscle relaxants. Neuromuscular blockade monitoring is particularly important in these patients to decrease the risk of respiratory failure from residual neuromuscular block.

## What Problems Might Arise Intraoperatively?

### Cardiovascular

Intraoperative cardiovascular changes such as hypertension or supraventricular tachyarrhythmia should not be treated with nonselective $\beta$-adrenergic blockers because these drugs may provoke bronchospasm. Such bronchospasm is unpredictable and can be severe. Cardioselective esmolol and metoprolol have, however, been used to good advantage without worsen-

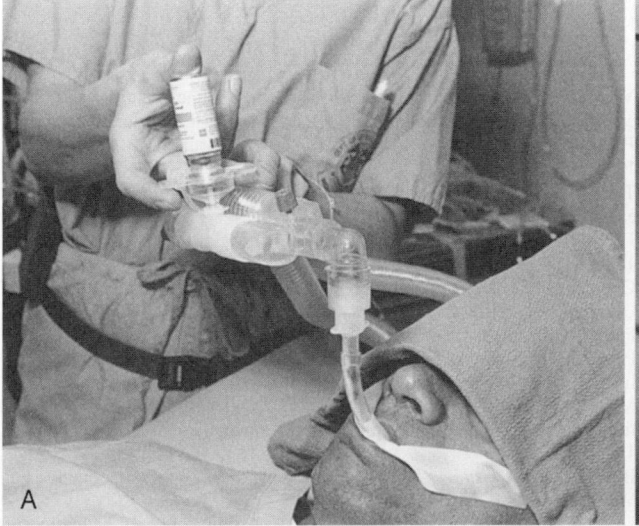
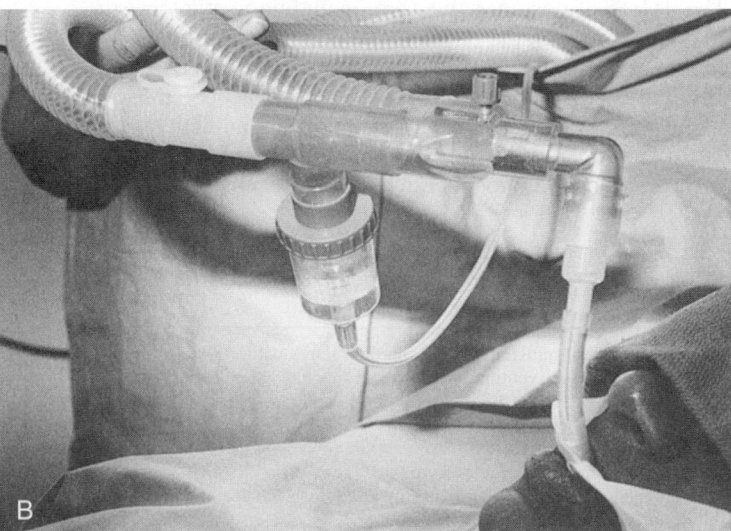

**FIGURE 54–2.** A simple way of administering inhalation bronchodilator at the inspiratory limb of the anesthetic circuit. Metered-dose inhaler (*A*) and aerosol (*B*) can be attached and administered without a special device. A special device does allow them to be attached between the Y-piece and the endotracheal tube.

**TABLE 54–14.** Causes of Acute Increases in Airway Pressure With or Without Hemodynamic Changes During Anesthesia

Inspissated secretions in the tracheobronchial tree
Bronchospasm from bronchial asthma or chronic obstructive lung disease
Pulmonary edema with wheezing
Pulmonary embolism with wheezing
Partial obstruction of tracheal tube
Tension pneumothorax
Endobronchial intubation

ing bronchospasm.[58] Although no significant worsening of pulmonary function is typically noted, it is important to consider that in one series of 50 COLD patients, 6% had asymptomatic decreases in their $FEV_1$ after esmolol infusion.[59] Because there is still some effect on bronchomotor tone, if the asthma is severe, this must be done cautiously. Another option is to treat atrial tachycardia with diltiazem or verapamil.

### Respiratory

A slow respiratory rate with prolonged expiratory time is recommended during controlled ventilation to prevent air trapping. Humidification of inspired anesthetic gases prevents inspissation of secretions.

An increase in airway pressure and systemic hypotension should alert the anesthesiologist to the possibility of air trapping or tension pneumothorax. The causes of increased intraoperative airway pressure are listed in Table 54–14.

A number of causes of intraoperative wheezing must be eliminated before it can be assumed that intrinsic bronchospasm has developed. If bronchospasm is the cause, an inhaled bronchodilator (eg, ipratropium, β-adrenergic agonist, or halogenated inhaled anesthetic) can be administered. Treatment of intraoperative bronchospasm is outlined in Table 54–15.

## POSTOPERATIVE MANAGEMENT

### What Postoperative Care May Be Needed for Intraoperative Bronchospasm?

The degree of postoperative care, including ventilatory support, is dependent on the preoperative status and intraoperative events. For example, the patient with active bronchospasm who requires emergent surgery may require postoperative mechanical ventilation. The asymptomatic patient with an uneventful intraoperative course requires no special postoperative care. Bronchodilator therapy should be continued in all

**TABLE 54–15.** Treatment of Intraoperative Wheezing and Increasing Airway Pressure

Stop nitrous oxide administration and ventilate lungs with 100% oxygen.
Discontinue mechanical ventilation and begin manual ventilation.
Increase expiratory time (ratio of inspiratory to expiratory time >1:3).
Decrease respiratory rate.
Increase depth of anesthesia.
Administer intravenous lidocaine (1 mg/kg).
Administer inhaled bronchodilator (use metered-dose inhaler or aerosol).
Permit spontaneous ventilation, if feasible.
Perform tracheal extubation at a deep level of anesthesia at the conclusion of procedure if not contraindicated.

asthmatic patients. Postoperative analgesia can be provided with neuraxial or parenteral narcotics.

### How Is Postoperative Weaning Accomplished?

The level of postoperative ventilatory care depends on the severity of the COLD and on the surgical site. Patients with severe COLD should be weaned from the ventilatory support and managed with extubation as would any patient with respiratory failure. Measurement of ABG and bedside PFTs may provide useful guidance for tracheal extubation.

Site of surgery (eg, upper abdominal surgery) and residual effects of anesthetics, narcotics, and muscle relaxants must be considered. Postoperative respiratory therapy such as chest physiotherapy or incentive spirometry may be beneficial.

Postoperative pain control with epidural narcotic administration may benefit patients following thoracotomy and upper abdominal surgery. Because COLD patients are often particularly sensitive to the respiratory depressant effects of narcotics, consider an analgesic regimen that includes a narcotic and a nonsteroidal compound (eg, ketorolac).

In conclusion, patients with bronchial asthma and COLD can present interesting and challenging problems during and following anesthesia and surgery. Proper preoperative evaluation, in addition to preoperative, intraoperative, and postoperative management can reduce complications.

### References

1. McFadden ER Jr. Asthma: general features, pathogenesis, and pathophysiology. In: Fishman AP, ed. *Pulmonary Diseases and Disorders.* Vol 2. 2nd ed. New York, NY: McGraw-Hill; 1988:1295.
2. Dawson A, Simon RA. Bronchospastic disorders: an overview. In: Dawson A, Simon RA, eds. *The Practical Management of Asthma.* Orlando, Fla: Grune & Stratton; 1984:3.
3. Petty TL. Definitions in chronic obstructive pulmonary disease. *Clin Chest Med.* 1990;11:363.
4. Pierce JA, Niewoehner DE, Thurlbeck WM, et al. *Standards for the Diagnosis and Care of Patients With Chronic Obstructive Pulmonary Disease (COPD) and Asthma.* New York, NY: American Thoracic Society; 1981:225.
5. Henderson WR Jr. The role of leukotrienes in inflammation. *Ann Intern Med.* 1994;121:684.
6. Kaliner MA, McFadden ER Jr. Bronchial asthma. In: Samter M, Talmage DW, Frank MM, et al, eds. *Immunological Disease.* Vol 2. Boston, Mass: Little, Brown & Co; 1988:1067.
7. McFadden ER Jr. Asthma: airway dynamics, cardiac function, and clinical correlates. In: Middleton E Jr, Reed CE, Ellis EF, et al, eds. *Allergy, Principles, and Practice.* Vol 2. 3rd ed. St Louis, Mo: CV Mosby; 1988:1018.
8. Thurlbeck WM. Pathophysiology of chronic obstructive pulmonary disease. *Clin Chest Med.* 1990;11:389.
9. Flenley DC. Chronic obstructive pulmonary disease. *Dis Mon.* 1988;34:543.
10. Georgopoulous D, Anthonisen NR. Symptoms and signs of COPD. In: Cherniack NS, ed. *Chronic Obstructive Pulmonary Disease.* Philadelphia, Pa: WB Saunders; 1991:357.
11. Peres L, Sybrecht G, Maclem PT. The mechanism of increase in total lung capacity during acute asthma. *Am J Med.* 1976;61:165.
12. McFadden ER Jr, Kiser R, DeGroot WJ. Acute bronchial asthma: relations between clinical and physiologic mechanisms. *N Engl J Med.* 1973;288:221.
13. Bates DV. *Respiratory Function in Disease.* 3rd ed. Philadelphia, Pa: WB Saunders; 1989:152.
14. Hoppin FG Jr. Pulmonary function tests for diagnosis and evaluation of COPD. In: Cherniack NS, ed. *Chronic Obstructive Pulmonary Disease.* Philadelphia, Pa: WB Saunders; 1991:363.

15. Bates DV. *Respiratory Function in Disease.* 3rd ed. Philadelphia, Pa: WB Saunders; 1989:218.
16. Shetter Al, Bailey WC, Bleecker UR, et al. *Guidelines for the Diagnosis and Treatment of Asthma.* Rockville, Md: National Institute of Health, US Dept of Health and Human Services; August 1991:1.
17. McFadden ER Jr. Asthma: acute and chronic therapy. In: Fishman AP, ed. *Pulmonary Diseases and Disorders.* Vol 2. 2nd ed. New York, NY: McGraw-Hill; 1988:1311.
18. Webb-Johnson DC, Andrew JL Jr. I: Bronchodilator therapy. *N Engl J Med.* 1977;297:476.
19. Webb-Johnson DC, Andrew JL Jr. II: Bronchodilator therapy. *N Engl J Med.* 1977;297:758.
20. Summer W, Elston R, Tharp L, et al. Aerosol bronchodilator delivery methods: relative impact on pulmonary function and cost of respiratory care. *Arch Intern Med.* 1989;149:618.
21. Newman SP, Clark SW. The proper use of metered dose inhalers. *Chest.* 1984;86:342.
22. Orgel HA, Kemp JP, Tinkelman DG, et al. Bitolterol and albuterol metered dose aerosols: comparison of two long acting beta-2 adrenergic bronchodilators for treatment of asthma. *J Allergy Clin Immunol.* 1985;75:55.
23. McFadden ER Jr. Methylxanthines in the treatment of asthma: the rise, the fall, and the possible rise again. *Ann Intern Med.* 1991;115:323.
24. Barnes PJ. A new approach to the treatment of asthma. *N Engl J Med.* 1989;321:1517.
25. Piafsky KM, Ogilvie RI. Dosage of theophylline in bronchial asthma. *N Engl J Med.* 1975;292:1218.
26. Hendeles L, Weinberger M. Theophylline: a "state of the art" review. *Pharmacotherapy.* 1983;3:2.
27. Bukowsky M, Nakatsu K, Munt PW. Theophylline reassessed. *Ann Intern Med.* 1984;101:63.
28. Morris HG. Mechanisms of action and therapeutic role of corticosteroids in asthma. *J Allergy Clin Immunol.* 1985;75:1.
29. Spector SL. The use of corticosteroids in treatment of asthma. *Chest.* 1985;87:73S.
30. Fanta CH, Rossing TH, McFadden ER Jr. Glucocorticoids in acute asthma: a critical controlled trial. *Am Rev Respir Dis.* 1982;125:94S.
31. Patalano F, Ruggieri F. Sodium cromoglycate: a review. *Eur Repir J.* 1989;2:556.
32. Gross NJ, Skorodin MS. Anticholinergic, antimuscarinic bronchodilators. *Am Rev Respir Dis.* 1984;129:356.
33. Drazen JM, Israel E, O'Byrne PM. Treatment of asthma with drugs modifying the leukotriene pathway. *N Engl J Med.* 1999;340:197.
34. Ziment I. Pharmacologic therapy of obstructive airway disease. *Clin Chest Med.* 1990;11:461.
35. Wesseling G, Mostert R, Wouters EF. A comparison of the effects of anticholinergic and beta-2 agonist and combination therapy on respiratory impedance in COPD. *Chest.* 1992;101:166.
36. Geiger K, Hedley-White J. Preoperative and postoperative considerations. In: Ewiss EB, Segal MS, Stein M, eds. *Bronchial Asthma.* 2nd ed. Boston, Mass: Little, Brown & Co; 1985:892.
37. Warner DO, Warner MA, Barnes RD, et al. Perioperative respiratory complications in patients with asthma. *Anesthesiology.* 1996;85:460.
38. Harman E, Lillington G. Pulmonary risk factors in surgery. *Med Clin North Am.* 1979;63:1289.
39. Epstein SK, Faling LJ, Daly BD, et al. Predicting complications after pulmonary resection: preoperative exercise testing vs. a multifactorial cardiopulmonary risk index. *Chest.* 1993;104:694.
40. Smetana GW. Preoperative pulmonary evaluation. *N Engl J Med.* 1999;340:937.
41. Gass GD, Olsen GN. Preoperative pulmonary function testing to predict postoperative morbidity and mortality. *Chest.* 1986;89:127.
42. Frost EAM. Preanesthetic assessment of the patient with respiratory disease. *Anesth Clin North Am.* 1990;8:657.
43. Criner GJ, O'Brien G, Furukawa S, et al. Lung volume reduction surgery in ventilator-dependent COPD patients. *Chest.* 1996;110:877.
44. Lefrak SS, Yusen RD, Trulock EP, et al. Recent advances in surgery for emphysema. *Annu Rev Med.* 1997;48:387.
45. Brenner M, Yusen R, McKenna R Jr, Sciurba F, et al. Lung volume reduction surgery for emphysema. *Chest.* 1996;110:205.
46. Rehder K, Sessler AD, Marsh HM. General anesthesia and the lung. *Am Rev Respir Dis.* 1975;112:541.
47. Stein MA. Preoperative pulmonary function evaluation and therapy for surgical patients. *JAMA.* 1970;211:787.
48. Van de Meter JM, Watring WG, Linton LA, et al. Prevention of postoperative pulmonary complications. *Surg Gynecol Obstet.* 1972;135:229.
49. Egan TD, Wong KC. Perioperative smoking cessation and anesthesia: a review. *J Clin Anesth.* 1992;4:63.
50. Nunn JF, Milledge JS, Chen D, et al. Respiratory criteria of fitness for surgery and anaesthesia. *Anaesthesia.* 1988;43:543.
51. Kingston HGG, Hirshman CA. Perioperative management of the patient with asthma. *Anesth Analg.* 1984;63:844.
52. Fung D, Smith NT. Anesthetic considerations in asthmatic patients. In: Gershwin EE, ed. *Bronchial Asthma. Principles of Diagnosis and Treatment.* Orlando, Fla: Grune & Stratton; 1986:525.
53. Ouedraogo N, Roux E, Forestier F, et al. Effects of intravenous anesthetics on normal and passively sensitized human isolated airway smooth muscle. *Anesthesiology.* 1998;88:317.
54. Pizov R, Brown RH, Weiss YS, et al. Wheezing during induction of general anesthesia in patients with and without asthma. A randomized blind trial. *Anesthesiology.* 1995;82:1111.
55. Pasch T, Kamp HD, Petermann H. The effect of halothane, enflurane, and isoflurane on resistance and compliance in patients with asthma or chronic obstructive lung diseases. *Anaesthesist.* 1991;40:65.
56. Pietetak S, Weenig CS, Hickey RF, et al. Anesthetic effects of ventilation in patients with chronic obstructive pulmonary disease. *Anesthesiology.* 1975;42:160.
57. Pasch T, Kamp HD, Grimm H, et al. Effect of isoflurane on respiratory mechanics. *Anasthesiol Intensivther Notfallmed.* 1986;21:1.
58. Tafreshi MJ, Weinacker AB. Beta-adrenergic blocking agents in bronchospastic diseases: a therapeutic dilemma. *Pharmacotherapy.* 1999;19:974.
59. Gold MR, Dec GW, Cocca-Spofford D, et al. Esmolol and ventilatory function in cardiac patients with COPD. *Chest.* 1991;100:1215.

# CHAPTER 55

# Pulmonary Edema

Eran Segal

Azriel Perel

Pulmonary edema is defined as the abnormal accumulation of fluid in the extravascular space of the lung. It is associated with disturbances of lung volumes, lung mechanics, and gas exchange; can be the result of diverse causes (Table 55–1); and always represents a potential threat to life.

In the perioperative period, pulmonary edema is a relatively rare event. Cooperman and Price described 40 cases of pulmonary edema and calculated that its overall incidence is 1:4500.[1] The true incidence is probably higher because many patients have an increase in extravascular lung water (EVLW) without overt alveolar pulmonary edema. In their series of 1004 patients who formed the basis of the cardiac risk index, Goldman and coworkers found 36 patients who developed perioperative pulmonary edema, 58% of whom had no history of congestive heart failure (CHF).[2] The mortality rate in this subgroup was 57%, whereas those patients who developed heart failure without pulmonary edema had a lower overall mortality rate of 15%.

More recently, Arieff described a group of patients who developed postoperative pulmonary edema after a variety of surgical procedures.[3] Common to all patients was an underestimation of fluid administration and weight gain in the first days after surgery. This excess fluid was probably a significant factor in the development of pulmonary edema. Arieff also studied 1 year's surgical procedures in a major tertiary medical center. Among 8195 major operations, 7.6% developed pulmonary edema, with a mortality rate of 11.9%.[3]

**TABLE 55–1.** Some Conditions Associated With Perioperative Pulmonary Edema

| |
|---|
| Congestive heart failure |
| Coronary ischemia |
| Fluid overload |
| Sepsis |
| Aspiration |
| Embolism |
| Neurogenic pulmonary edema |
| Reexpansion pulmonary edema |
| Negative pressure (postobstructive) pulmonary edema |
| Aortic clamping |
| Lung resection |
| Cardiopulmonary bypass |

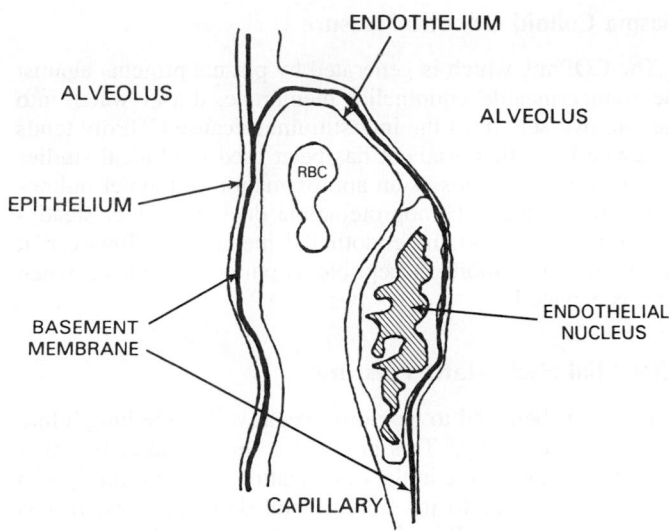

**FIGURE 55–1.** Schematic representation of the alveolocapillary membrane microanatomy. Note the basement membrane, which lies between the endothelial and the epithelial sides of the membrane. RBC, red blood cell.

Because the impact of pulmonary edema on surgical outcome is significant, anesthesiologists must be familiar with its diagnosis and management. Most patients can be treated successfully if diagnosis is made early and appropriate care is promptly initiated.

## PATHOGENESIS

### What Are the Important Anatomic Considerations?

Major structures involved in the pathogenesis of pulmonary edema are the microvascular endothelium, alveolar epithelium, interstitium, and pulmonary lymphatic system (Fig. 55–1).

#### Microvascular Endothelium

The endothelium is composed of a monolayer of cells situated on a basement membrane. Junctions between endothelial cells contain pores that allow the free passage of water and ions. They act as a sieve for protein molecules; of these molecules, only the smaller ones, such as albumin, normally can pass with relative freedom, whereas larger ones, such as globulin and fibrinogen, cannot.

#### Alveolar Epithelium

Alveolar epithelial cells, which are situated on their own basement membrane, are composed of type 1 and type 2 pneumocytes. *Type 1 pneumocytes* are large, flat cells that line the alveoli as a continuous sheet and have tight gaps (pores) in their junctions. Thus, the alveolar wall is much less permeable than is the endothelial wall; this explains the many instances in which pulmonary edema remains in the interstitium without filling the alveoli. *Type 2 pneumocytes* are cuboidal stem cells that produce surfactant.

#### Pulmonary Interstitium

Between the endothelial and alveolar layers lies the thin part of the interstitium; its thicker component surrounds the larger blood vessels and airways. This space is a fibrin and collagen matrix that contains the pulmonary lymphatic vessels that drain the pulmonary microvascular filtrate.

## PATHOPHYSIOLOGY

### How Does Pulmonary Edema Present?

Pulmonary edema can be classified into three stages. The first involves EVLW accumulation in the interstitial space. Cuffs of fluid appear around bronchi and blood vessels, but oxygenation is often not severely impaired. During the second stage, fluid enters the alveoli, and hypoxemia appears owing to increased ventilation-perfusion ($\dot{V}/\dot{Q}$) mismatching. The third and most dramatic stage is that of airway flooding (Fig. 55–2). Because of the reduction in compliance induced by the increased EVLW, there is an increased work of breathing and a smaller functional residual capacity (FRC).

Much of the clinical presentation of pulmonary edema can by ascribed to these pathophysiologic mechanisms. The patient becomes tachypneic, in an attempt to compensate for the reduced tidal volume. There may be signs of an increased inspiratory effort with alae nasi, suprasternal and intercostal retractions, and anxiety.

### What Is the Starling Equation?

The Starling equation incorporates the major forces that take part in transvascular (microvascular [mv] and interstitial [is]) fluid exchange ($\dot{Q}f$) (Fig. 55–3). These include the hydrostatic pressure gradient (Pmv minus Pis), which favors transudation of fluid from the microvessels, and the colloid oncotic pressure gradient (COPmv minus COPis), which normally draws water into the microvessels. The resulting balance, $\dot{Q}f$, is the total amount of fluid that traverses the endothelial membrane. The equation is dominated by Kf, the fluid filtra-

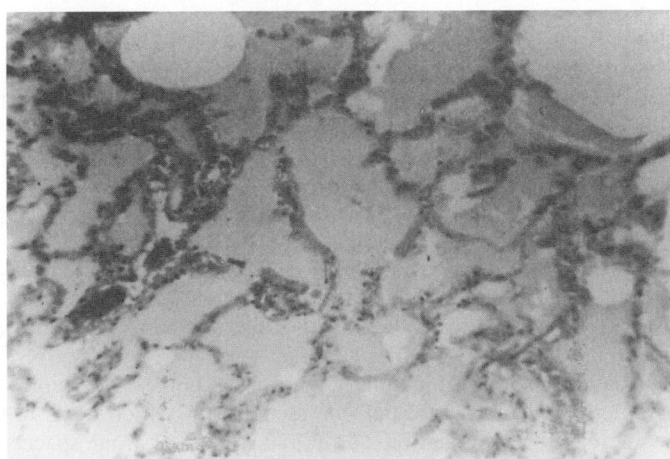

**FIGURE 55–2.** Histologic section of lung from a patient with severe cardiogenic pulmonary edema. Note that the alveolar spaces were almost completely filled with pulmonary edema fluid. (Courtesy of J. Kopolovic, MD, Chair, Department of Pathology, Sheba Medical Center, Tel-Hashomer, Israel.)

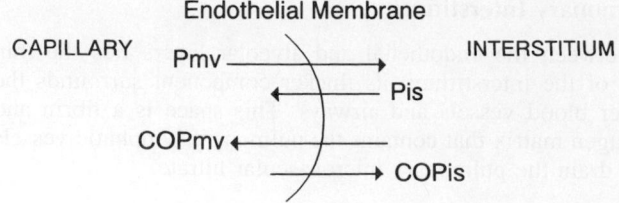

$$\dot{Q}f = Kf\left[(Pmv - Pis) - \sigma(COPmv - COPis)\right]$$

**FIGURE 55–3.** The Starling equation describes the forces involved in transvascular fluid flux. The microvascular hydrostatic (Pmv) and the interstitial oncotic (COPis) pressures act in concert to drive fluid into the interstitium. The interstitial hydrostatic (Pis) and microvascular colloid oncotic (COPmv) pressures oppose this shift. ($\sigma$, reflection coefficient.)

tion coefficient that expresses the number and size of the endothelial membrane pores and the surface area available for fluid exchange.

Pulmonary edema is usually caused either by an increase in the pulmonary Pmv (cardiogenic) or by a change in the permeability characteristics of the microvascular membrane (noncardiogenic). The practical value of the Starling equation is conceptualization of pulmonary edema formation.

## Microvascular Hydrostatic Pressure

The main determinant of filtration across the endothelium is the Pmv. When the left side of the heart fails, its end-diastolic volume increases owing to incomplete ejection. The resultant elevated pressure leads to increased left atrial, pulmonary venous, and pulmonary microvascular pressures.

Other downstream factors that can also affect Pmv include left atrial myxoma, mitral and aortic valve disease, decreased left ventricular compliance, and sudden increases in the peripheral vascular resistance. Clinically, Pmv is often estimated by the pulmonary artery occlusion pressure (PAOP), although it may be more accurately calculated as follows:

$$Pmv = LAP + 0.4\,(PAP - LAP)$$

where PAP and LAP are the mean pulmonary artery and left atrial pressures, respectively. The constant, 0.4, denotes the estimated fraction of pulmonary vascular resistance that is downstream from the exchange vessels.

Pmv is influenced by gravity; in the upright position, it may be as much as 30 cm $H_2O$ higher at the bases than at the apices of the lungs. Because fluid and protein probably cross pulmonary arterioles and venules as well as the capillaries, the operative Pmv within different segments of the pulmonary microvasculature can be quite different. High pulmonary perfusion pressures increase the passage of tracer substances into the interstitium from the intravascular space.

In patients with high capillary pressures, the alveolar capillary membrane may develop "stress failure," which leads to the increased accumulation of fluid in the interstitial space. Situations such as extreme physical activity, neurogenic pulmonary edema, and lung overinflation lead to capillary membrane failure and thus constitute a type of high-pressure pulmonary edema.[4]

## Plasma Colloid Oncotic Pressure

The COPmv, which is generated by plasma proteins against the semipermeable endothelial membrane, draws water into the microvessels from the interstitium. Because COPmv tends to negate Pmv, this gradient has been used in clinical studies of critically ill patients as an approximation of the net pulmonary fluid balance.[5] Hypoproteinemia does not affect steady-state filtration across the endothelial membrane. However, it makes the lungs more susceptible to pulmonary edema when Pmv is elevated.

## Interstitial Hydrostatic Pressure

The Pis is believed to be more "negative" in the lung hilum than in the periphery.[6] This gradient within the interstitium is probably a major force in the mobilization of interstitial lymph from the periphery to its more central drainage sites. It acts in concert with the Pmv in the promotion of filtration from the microvessels into the interstitium and is important in negating the alveolar surface tension force and in keeping the alveoli dry.

## Interstitial Colloid Oncotic Pressure

Data concerning COPis are derived mainly from analysis of lung lymph.[7] The pulmonary lymph, which is normally produced at a rate of 10 mL/h, contains about 60% as much protein as the plasma. Distribution of proteins is determined by their capacity to cross the microvascular barrier. Thus, lymph albumin concentration is about 80% of the serum albumin concentration, but fibrinogen is almost absent in lymph.

The drainage capacity of the pulmonary lymphatic system may be overcome when large amounts of filtrate enter the interstitium from the intravascular space, leading to an increase in EVLW and interstitial edema, with or without overt alveolar edema.

## CLINICAL IMPLICATIONS

### How Are Pressure and Permeability Pulmonary Edema Differentiated?

Elevated left atrial pressure increases both lymph flow and EVLW content.[8] Pulmonary edema associated with an increase in hydrostatic pressure is relatively low in protein content because water primarily leaves the microvessels and passes into the interstitium. During increased permeability edema, the Kf is the primarily deranged variable, so that increased water and protein traverse the endothelial membrane. Because the membrane, in essence, loses its barrier function with respect to the passage of protein molecules, the normal oncotic pressure gradient between the plasma and interstitium may be abolished.

### Etiology

Although the clinical picture of pulmonary edema is quite consistent, important etiologic differences must be distinguished if the response to therapy is to be enhanced. Thus, more than academic interest should spur clinicians to differen-

**TABLE 55–2.** Differentiating High-Pressure and Increased Permeability Pulmonary Edema

|  | High-Pressure Pulmonary Edema | Increased Permeability; Low-Pressure Edema |
|---|---|---|
| Filling pressures | High | Usually normal or low |
| Cardiac output | Often low | Often high |
| Edema fluid protein–to–protein plasma ratio | <0.5 | >0.6 |
| Heart size (on radiograph) | Large | Normal |

tiate between high-pressure edema (as occurs in CHF) and permeability edema (as occurs in the acute respiratory distress syndrome [ARDS]) (Table 55–2). Such distinction is often difficult because patients may present with pulmonary edema owing to increases in both pressure and permeability. In the perioperative period, many patients with heart disease decompensate for various reasons. Thus, high-pressure pulmonary edema is relatively more frequent. At the same time, reasons for ARDS in the perioperative period are numerous, and pulmonary edema due to aspiration, blood transfusion, and sepsis is well recognized.

### Edema Fluid Analysis

When pulmonary edema results in flooding of the airways, its analysis may be helpful in differentiating the cause. With increased pressure, the fluid has a transudate-like quality and a low edema fluid–to–plasma protein ratio. When increased permeability is responsible, the edema fluid–to–plasma protein concentration ratio is usually >0.60.[9] Remember, however, that within 1 to 2 days, resorption of alveolar fluid increases the ratio, even in high-pressure edema. Hence, the usefulness of this test is limited to the initial presentation.[10]

## How Does Pulmonary Edema Affect Lung Volumes and Mechanics?

Accumulation of lung fluid has dramatic effects on volumes and mechanics. The FRC in patients with pulmonary edema is greatly decreased; this leads to increased venous admixture and hypoxemia, even before alveolar flooding occurs. The reduction in FRC also activates stretch receptors that are responsible for the characteristic dyspnea. Finally, the reduced FRC causes markedly reduced lung compliance and a significant increase in the work of breathing.

Patients with pulmonary edema, therefore, revert to a pattern of rapid, shallow breathing and usually develop acute respiratory alkalosis. If the ratio of dead space to tidal volume is increased because of preexisting chronic obstructive pulmonary disease (COPD) or other factors, carbon dioxide ($CO_2$) retention may eventually develop.[11] Increased airway resistance may also contribute to the increased work of breathing.

## How Can Pulmonary Edema Be Recognized?

### Awake Patients

The clinical presentation in awake patients can be quite variable. Initial signs and symptoms may include unexplained agitation, increased blood pressure (BP) and heart rate due to generalized stress, and hypoxemia. Patients are dyspneic and tachypneic because of reduced lung compliance, activation of pulmonary interstitial stretch receptors, and shallow, rapid ventilation. Increased inspiratory effort is associated with intercostal retractions and accessory muscle activation.

When the respiratory rate exceeds 30 breaths per minute, the resistive work of breathing increases significantly, leading to eventual fatigue and ventilatory failure. Inspiratory crackles reflect the sound of gas flowing through the fluid-filled distal airways. If pulmonary edema is mainly interstitial, the auscultatory findings are usually minimal.

### Anesthetized Patients

Recognition of intraoperative pulmonary edema in the anesthetized patient is more difficult than in the awake patient because few of the physical signs and none of the symptoms are present. Pulmonary edema should be suspected whenever an increase in airway pressure is associated with an apparent sudden decrease in compliance. Increased airway resistance also may cause sudden increases in airway pressure and is characterized by a large difference between the peak and plateau airway pressures. This can be assessed by ventilating the patient with a respiratory pattern that includes an end-inspiratory hold. Obviously, other underlying problems may be responsible for an acute decrease in lung compliance, such as pneumothorax, atelectasis, kinking of the endotracheal tube (ETT), or obstruction with secretions.

The most common sign of pulmonary edema in the anesthetized patient is progressive hypoxemia that is relatively unresponsive to an increase in the fraction of inspired oxygen ($FIO_2$). Hypoxemia is not a specific sign of edema. As is the case with reduction in compliance, it may be caused by bronchial intubation, atelectasis, or tube obstruction. Nevertheless, its appearance during anesthesia warrants careful investigation to exclude the possibility of pulmonary edema. In severe cases of pulmonary edema, edema fluid may appear in the ETT. Rarely, filling of the breathing circuit with edema fluid, which is often heard rather than seen, may be the initial presenting sign.

### Oxygenation and Ventilation

#### Hypoxemia

The functional impairment associated with pulmonary edema is usually evaluated on the basis of the degree of hypoxemia relative to the administered $FIO_2$ ($PaO_2/FIO_2$). In normal lungs, or in those in which $\dot{V}/\dot{Q}$ is low but finite (ie, >0, implying that the air spaces are open), the $PaO_2$ rises when the $FIO_2$ is increased, so that $PaO_2/FIO_2$ remains relatively constant. With pulmonary edema, however, right-to-left shunting of blood through nonventilated lung regions often occurs. Therefore, the low $PaO_2$ may not respond appropriately to an increase in $FIO_2$, implying the presence of lung areas with a $\dot{V}/\dot{Q}$ ratio of 0.

Minimal pulmonary edema may be associated with only slight lowering of the $PaO_2$, which can remain unnoticed if the patient is breathing oxygen ($O_2$)-enriched gas; the decrease in the $PaO_2$ may be missed despite monitoring with a pulse oximeter because arterial $O_2$ saturation decreases only when reductions in $PO_2$ of <100 mm Hg occur. Thus, pulse oximetry does not replace periodic measurement of arterial blood gases to examine the response to therapy in the patient who develops intraoperative pulmonary edema.

### Hypercapnia

A gradual increase in $Paco_2$ may signify worsening of edema, diminished alveolar minute ventilation, or both. This change can result from an increase in the anesthesia circuit's gas compression and compliance-related volume caused by the higher airway pressures.

### Lung Mechanics

Other parameters that reflect the functional impairment during pulmonary edema include alterations in lung mechanics—particularly lung compliance and work of breathing—which can be continuously monitored with advanced software (Fig. 55–4). Plateau airway pressure can be readily measured and used in the repeated calculation of static compliance. This parameter provides a good indication of the severity of the edema as well as a means to assess changes in the patient's clinical state.

In recent years, the importance of pressure-volume curves of the lung has been stressed. Using these curves may help in titration of mechanical ventilation particularly with respect to prevention of ventilator-induced lung injury. Obtaining a pressure-volume curve to establish the upper and lower inflection points so as to enable optimization of ventilatory parameters is not readily available clinically, but with the advent of commercial graphic monitors for respiratory mechanics, it is possible to use information from them to direct therapy.

### Chest Radiography

#### High Pressure

In the absence of airway flooding, and because of the often nonspecific clinical picture, chest radiography is a major diagnostic tool.[12] In high-pressure edema, radiographic pro-

**TABLE 55–3.** Commonly Found Radiologic Differences Between High-Pressure and Increased-Permeability Pulmonary Edema

| Radiologic Feature | High-Pressure Pulmonary Edema | Increased-Permeability Pulmonary Edema |
|---|---|---|
| Pleural effusion | Yes | No |
| Butterfly pattern | Yes | No |
| Peripheral distribution | No | Yes |
| Air bronchogram | No | Yes |
| Heart size | Large | Small |

gression is predictable, with increased vascular markings appearing in the upper lung regions when the PAOP is about 15 mm Hg and signs of interstitial edema at a PAOP of 15 to 25 mm Hg. These signs include peribronchial cuffing or thickening of the peribronchial walls and Kerley B lines, which represent thickened interlobular septa.

When the PAOP is >25 mm Hg, alveolar flooding that appears as patchy air-space opacification is usually seen. Such opacification may be most prominent near the mediastinum and take the form of a butterfly, with the peripheral lung fields remaining relatively clear. The butterfly pattern is due to the greater degree of ventilation in the periphery of the lungs, which reduces the presence of fluid in the air spaces. A higher Pmv in the proximal pulmonary vessels may also contribute to this phenomenon. A large heart size is also typical of alveolar flooding of cardiogenic origin (Table 55–3).

#### Increased Permeability

The chest radiograph or a computed tomography scan obtained during permeability edema often shows diffuse inhomogeneous infiltrates (Fig. 55–5). The picture may vary according to the underlying pathology.

### Is Measurement of Extravascular Lung Water Clinically Useful?

Measurement of EVLW is potentially a attractive tool for the management of pulmonary edema. The direct measure-

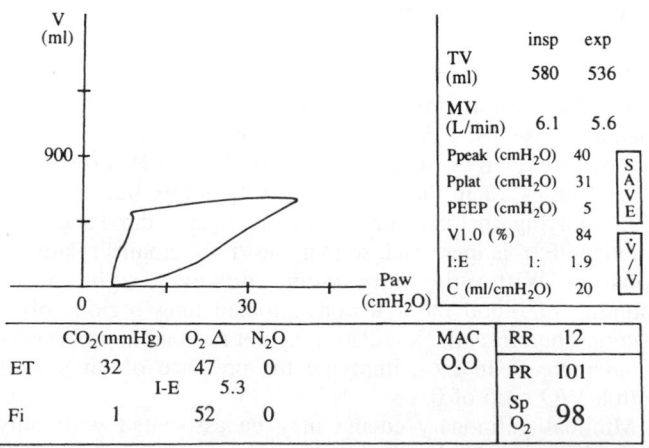

**FIGURE 55–4.** Printout from a lung mechanics monitor. The compliance of the patient's lungs is 20 mL/cm $H_2O$. The resistive component of the patient's lungs can also be appreciated by the large difference between the peak and plateau airway pressures.

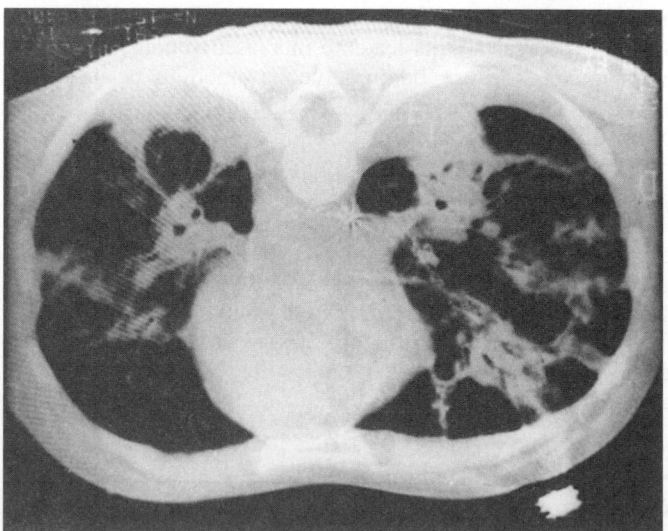

**FIGURE 55–5.** Computed tomography scan of a patient with severe acute respiratory distress syndrome, demonstrating the inhomogeneous type of injury in this disorder. (Photograph courtesy of Professor J.J. Rouby, Department of Anesthesiology, Hôpital Pitie-Salpetrier, Paris, France.)

ment of EVLW can be done with a double dilution technique, using a cold solution with indocyanine green dye. The difference in the volume of distribution of both indicators (temperature and dye) is the volume of the EVLW. This technique requires the use of specially designed catheters and equipment and thus is impractical for routine clinical use.

Another technique for the measurement of EVLW uses a central venous injection site and an intraarterial sensor placed into the femoral or axillary artery to measure the temperature change, from which cardiac output and EVLW can be computed. The technique makes the measurement of EVLW easily available at the bedside. This may lead to increased relevance and use of EVLW as a clinical tool in the diagnosis and management of pulmonary edema.[13]

## PREOPERATIVE TREATMENT

The therapeutic approach to pulmonary edema includes three major elements: (1) normalization of oxygenation and ventilation, (2) reduction of excessive EVLW, and (3) identification and treatment of the underlying disease. Because the major pathophysiology of pulmonary edema is well understood and its response to certain therapeutic maneuvers is well established, treatment should begin immediately, even when the actual cause is still unclear.

$O_2$ therapy, improvement of FRC and lung mechanics by continuous positive airway pressure (CPAP), and, if necessary, intubation and mechanical ventilation constitute the first therapeutic measures. The use of diuretics to achieve rapidly a negative water balance may be indicated if the patient's condition allows a decrease in preload in high-pressure edema. When possible, the cause should be determined. Identification of the causative mechanism may be of utmost importance in assessing the edema's natural course and prognosis and in directing more definitive therapy. When pulmonary edema is suspected or diagnosed, several general supportive measures should be taken (Table 55–4).

### What Is the Role of Positioning?

Patients with pulmonary edema should be placed in a head-up position whenever possible. In this position, the pulmonary Pmv is minimized, and lung mechanics improve through gravitational augmentation of diaphragmatic descent. The head-up position, especially when combined with lowering of the legs, also reduces venous return, a factor of importance in patients with high-pressure edema. Immediate partial relief of dyspnea often follows.

These positional considerations are especially important in surgical patients. Preoxygenation and induction should be

**TABLE 55–4.** Therapeutic Measures for Patients With Pulmonary Edema

| | |
|---|---|
| Positioning | Head-up position |
| Oxygen | High $F_{IO_2}$ |
| Negative fluid balance | When tolerated |
| Positive end-expiratory pressure | With mask or endotracheal tube |
| Drugs | Diuretics, vasodilators, inotropes |

$F_{IO_2}$, fraction of inspired oxygen.

performed with the patient sitting upright until loss of consciousness is achieved. The patient should then be rapidly repositioned and tracheal intubation performed. If insertion of a central catheter is indicated, a modest Trendelenburg position is appropriate for the short duration of the venipuncture. Preparation and draping should be done with the patient in a head-up position.

### How Should Oxygen Be Administered?

Although the hypoxemia that occurs during pulmonary edema characteristically does not respond significantly to $O_2$ therapy because of shunting, $O_2$ administration is still the first therapeutic measure. This is so because elevating the $Pa_{O_2}$ even slightly in hypoxemic patients may significantly increase $O_2$ saturation and delivery. The highest $F_{IO_2}$ possible should be delivered. During anesthesia, the patient must be ventilated with 100% $O_2$ until evidence of adequate oxygenation with a lower $F_{IO_2}$ is demonstrated. Administration of 100% $O_2$ also has direct therapeutic value during the acute phase of pulmonary edema associated with air embolism because it promotes resorption of intravascular nitrogen.

### Why Is Positive Pressure Ventilation of Value?

#### Continuous Positive Airway Pressure

The ultimate supportive measure in pulmonary edema is face mask–administered CPAP in patients who have adequate spontaneous minute ventilation and an intact sensorium. Increasing the FRC by keeping the airway pressure positive at end-expiration is often sufficient to reduce the work of breathing and "flatten" the edema fluid on the walls of the tracheobronchial tree.

Use of the CPAP mask should be considered in the preoperative period, when the patient is prepared for surgery, or in the postoperative period, when pulmonary edema appears after extubation. In the latter instance, the anesthesiologist should be sure that the patient is fully conscious, has adequate pharyngeal reflexes, and shows adequate respiratory drive.

#### Mechanical Ventilation and Positive End-Expiratory Pressure

Intraoperative ventilation in the presence of pulmonary edema should include positive end-expiratory pressure (PEEP) delivered through a breathing circuit that is fitted with one of the various available after-market PEEP valves. Continuous administration of PEEP during transport to the postanesthesia care unit (PACU) is mandatory and should be performed with an appropriate transport ventilator, a PEEP valve attached to the self-inflating bag, or a Mapleson-D circuit with an attached manometer so that PEEP can be continuously provided and monitored.

Although mechanical ventilation and PEEP can be dramatically effective, the attendant reduction of preload must be taken into consideration in hypovolemic patients. Once mechanical ventilation has been instituted, its gradual discontinuation (weaning) should be started when the patient is stabilized and the edema has resolved.

## *How Should Fluid Management Proceed?*

### Positive Balance

Fluid management in cases of pulmonary edema has been the subject of much controversy in critical care medicine. The most common approach is the aggressive reduction of filling pressures (ie, keeping the patient "dry"). This approach, however, may cause hemodynamic instability and dangerously reduce perfusion to other organs, such as the kidneys.

Schuller and associates[14] retrospectively analyzed 89 patients with pulmonary edema in a medical intensive care unit (ICU). They found that survivors had no significant fluid gain or increases in EVLW. Patients with a low fluid gain (<1 L) had a better chance of survival, a shorter duration of mechanical ventilation requirement, and a shorter ICU stay compared with patients with a highly positive fluid balance.

The question to be answered is whether positive fluid balance is a marker or a cause of poor outcome. The investigators concluded that increased fluid administration is partially responsible for some patients' poor outcome, and that if it is hemodynamically tolerated, a strategy of keeping patients dry is appropriate.

Intraoperatively, when active bleeding occurs in the presence of pulmonary edema, adequate fluid resuscitation should be carried out, even at the price of worsening edema. However, short bursts of rapidly administered fluids should be avoided because they may locally increase pulmonary Pmv.

### Colloid Therapy

Another approach is to attempt to increase the COPmv by infusing colloid solutions. This approach has been criticized because of the risk for infused colloid leaking into the interstitium, resulting in delayed edema resolution. Colloid infusions are also more expensive than crystalloid solutions, and no well-controlled study documents their superiority.

Shires and associates[15] examined the difference between EVLW in patients receiving colloid solutions and EVLW in those who were given lactated Ringer's injection intraoperatively. No difference in EVLW occurred between the two groups. Although the patients receiving crystalloid solutions required twice as much fluid to achieve the same hemodynamic goals, this difference had no significance with respect to lung function.

Whatever fluid is chosen, attention should be given to maintaining adequate organ perfusion. Acute postoperative renal failure or critical illness carries grave prognostic implications, whereas worsening of $\dot{V}/\dot{Q}$ mismatch because of increased EVLW can usually be treated adequately with positive pressure ventilation.

## *Which Drugs Are Potentially Beneficial?*

The most useful drugs are diuretics, which can have a strikingly therapeutic effect in some patients. Besides reducing total body water, they may exert a beneficial effect owing to venodilation and increased COPmv.[16] When pulmonary edema is due to CHF, other measures for preload reduction, such as intravenous nitroglycerin administration or regional anesthesia to the lower half of the body, may be of value.

The reduction of pulmonary artery pressure with vasodilators may be of benefit as well and has been suggested to improve outcome in ARDS patients.[17] However, intravenously administered vasodilators can increase the production of lung lymph and may also increase shunt and hypoxemia by blunting hypoxic pulmonary vasoconstriction. Recently, a great deal of attention has been given to use of nitric oxide (NO) in the treatment of hypoxemia and pulmonary hypertension in critically ill patients with pulmonary edema. In a model of pulmonary edema induced in sheep by endotoxin infusion, Bjertnaes and associates[18] showed that inhaled NO could reduce pulmonary lymph flow by reducing microvascular pressures and also reducing permeability.

The clinical significance of inhaled NO on outcome from severe ARDS is, as yet, uncertain.[19] Other useful drugs are those directed at specific problems, such as sepsis, cardiac decompensation, or ischemia. Drugs that directly influence increased microvascular permeability are still considered experimental.

## *How Is the Patient With Cardiac Disease Managed?*

Cardiac disorders, in particular ischemic heart disease, constitute a frequent cause of morbidity and mortality during anesthesia and surgery.[20] In adults undergoing cardiac or noncardiac surgery, perioperative myocardial infarction (MI), CHF, and pulmonary edema are among the most common causes of perioperative mortality.[21] Anesthesiologists, therefore, should carefully assess the patient with suspected heart disease preoperatively so that they may anticipate episodes of cardiac decompensation and optimize therapy.

### History

The patient history is extremely important. Goldman and colleagues[2] showed that a history and physical signs of CHF (an S3 gallop or the presence of jugular venous distention) are the strongest predictors of a cardiac complication in the perioperative period. Information should be sought concerning daily activities and the patient's functional capacity. Because most patients are seen while they are at rest, those with mild to moderate CHF may be comfortable during the preoperative visit but may become dyspneic while walking into the examination room, undressing, or lying flat for a few minutes.

### Physical Examination

Patients with chronic CHF are usually malnourished. They often show evidence of increased adrenergic activity that is reflected by peripheral vasoconstriction; pale, cold extremities; and a rapid but weak peripheral pulse. Examination of the lung fields may reveal fine inspiratory crackles at both lung bases. Ankle or sacral edema, an enlarged liver, and hepatojugular reflux due to right heart failure are often present.

### Diagnostic Studies

The preoperative evaluation is also enhanced by objective measurements of left ventricular function (such as echocardiography) or radionuclide studies (to assess ejection fraction). Echocardiography is probably the better of the two methods because it also shows wall motion abnormalities and valvular function.

## Preoperative Medication

A critical issue in the management of patients with ischemic heart disease concerns preoperative medication. Episodes of ischemia are often unrecognized. The natural preoperative increase in stress can increase the frequency of ischemia. During such ischemic episodes, the associated acute reduction in left ventricular function may bring about an acute episode of pulmonary edema. Thus, patients should be adequately sedated when arriving for surgery. Some patients, however, may not tolerate heavy sedation that compromises respiratory drive and function. Hypoxemia in the preoperative admitting area should be prevented by administering $O_2$ to those patients who are suspected of having heart failure. The development of acute pulmonary edema in the immediate preoperative period is illustrated by the following case history.

### CASE HISTORY 1

A 67-year-old man arrived in the preoperative admitting area for a total hip replacement. The patient's previous medical history included ischemic heart disease and an acute MI 3 years earlier. He was seen the previous evening by an anesthesiologist who decided that he was not in optimal condition for surgery. Therefore, the anesthesiologist postponed the case. Owing to administrative error, the patient was brought to the operating room without having received his regular medications. Upon his arrival in the admitting area, he immediately started to complain of shortness of breath. A chest radiograph revealed pulmonary edema (Fig. 55–6).

Preparation of patients with CHF for surgery includes optimization of cardiac medications. Intravenous nitrates may improve coronary perfusion as well as preload and afterload conditions for the failing left ventricle. Intravenous dopamine or dobutamine may be started even before surgery to improve cardiac contractility.

## Pulmonary Artery Catheterization

Elective surgery must be delayed until CHF is controlled. A pulmonary artery (PA) catheter may be inserted preoperatively

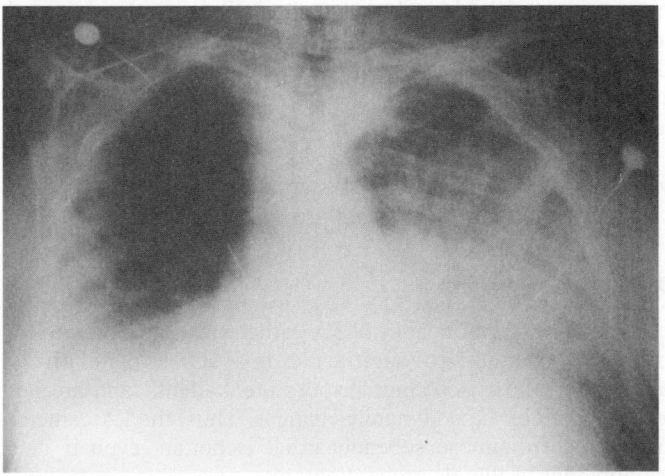

**FIGURE 55–6.** Chest radiograph of a patient who arrived in the operating room without being prepared for surgery. The patient developed chest pain and shortness of breath in the admitting area. The radiograph shows diffuse interstitial and intraalveolar opacifications. Peribronchial cuffing may be seen in the right lung field.

because gross aberrations of hemodynamic function are frequently unrecognized during clinical examination alone.[22] The PA catheter should be used to establish the optimal filling pressures for the failing heart and to titrate drug therapy.

Patients with pulmonary edema should undergo surgery only in an emergency and when a conservative alternative is not available. The minimum possible procedure is the one that should be performed in these instances.

## INTRAOPERATIVE PULMONARY EDEMA

### How Is the Patient With Acute Respiratory Failure Managed?

The patient with pulmonary edema and ARDS who requires surgery usually comes from the ICU or emergency department and may suffer from trauma, sepsis, aspiration, and other life-threatening conditions. Operative procedures may range from aggressive, stressful surgery for trauma or sepsis to "minor" procedures such as tracheotomy. Evaluation of the ICU patient with ARDS includes familiarization with the respiratory status and ventilatory parameters because most patients need similar levels of support during transport and surgery.

### Transport

Transport of the patient from the ICU to the operating room can be a serious challenge. The anesthesiologist should be involved in planning the transport and make sure that an adequate $O_2$ supply is available and that appropriate PEEP levels are provided throughout the transport. Use of a transport ventilator capable of providing CPAP and the required inspiratory pressures and minute ventilation is highly desirable (see Chapter 23).

### Oxygenation

A major problem in many ARDS patients is the maintenance of adequate oxygenation during surgery. Biery and coworkers[23] reviewed 200 surgical procedures in patients who required mechanical ventilation for respiratory failure. The patients were divided into those with ARDS (n = 49), pneumonia (n = 20), atelectasis (n = 65), cardiogenic pulmonary edema (n = 11), and acute ventilatory failure that was due mostly to neurologic dysfunction (n = 55).

Most of the patients who developed intraoperative hypoxemia had ARDS and sepsis and were undergoing laparotomy. However, hypoxemia was usually short-lived, and oxygen levels returned to preoperative values a few hours after surgery. The mortality rate within the first 3 postoperative days was quite low compared with overall in-hospital mortality. Thus, most of even the sickest patients survive the operative procedure.

### Ventilation

The type of ventilator used during anesthesia for patients with pulmonary edema may present an unexpected problem. Schapera and associates[24] studied patients with respiratory failure who were ventilated during surgery with an Ohio anesthesia ventilator (Ohmeda, Madison, Wis) or with a Siemens 900C critical care ventilator (Schaumberg, Ill). Those ventilated with the Siemens 900C did better in terms of oxygenation and reduction of pulmonary shunt intraoperatively.

### Choice of Ventilator

The same investigators conducted a bench study of different anesthesia ventilators and concluded that in situations of reduced compliance, increased resistance, and high minute ventilation, many anesthesia ventilators fail to provide the required ventilation parameters.[25] They recommended that for patients with a preoperative minute ventilation of >15 L and a peak inspiratory pressure of >50 cm $H_2O$, a critical care–type ventilator should be used intraoperatively.

### Choice of Mode

Because patients frequently are given neuromuscular blocking agents during surgery, partial ventilatory support measures, such as synchronized intermittent mandatory ventilation or pressure-support ventilation, must be replaced by controlled mechanical ventilation. Such change may lead to the development of excessive airway pressure as well as an increase in the compressible volume within the anesthetic circuit. A diminution of the patient-delivered tidal volume may result. Ideally, minute volume should be measured at the airway to obviate the effect of gas compression and circuit compliance. An arterial blood gas analysis after stabilization in the operating room is also useful because it is common for ARDS patients to have significant differences between arterial and end-tidal $CO_2$ levels.

The current trend in mechanical ventilation of patients with acute lung injury calls for "lung protective ventilation strategy." The concept involves a minimization of tidal volume and plateau pressures, while at the same time ensuring a PEEP level higher than the lower inflection point on the volume-pressure curve. Such a strategy has been shown to improve outcome in patients with acute lung injury and ARDS in a multicenter study.[26] In an experimental model in rats, the damage of high volumes led to a reduced capacity of the lungs to clear edema fluid.[27]

When providing low tidal volumes and low pressures to the patient with ARDS who is spontaneously breathing, care must be taken that the inspiratory flow of the ventilator satisfies the patient's inspiratory flow demand. Patients who have a high inspiratory flow demand may create excessive negative pressures to a degree that can induce negative pressure pulmonary edema.[28]

### How Should Anesthesia Be Induced and Maintained?

The administration of anesthesia to the patient with pulmonary edema is a major feat. Anesthetic-induced stress reduction from a high adrenergic state, if not immediately accompanied by ventilatory and hemodynamic support, may cause hypotension and a vicious circle that is difficult to control. Induction of anesthesia, therefore, requires agents that, at least in theory, maintain cardiac output (narcotics, ketamine, or etomidate). Care must be taken to prevent further myocardial ischemia in patients with coronary artery disease. In these

patients and in those with mitral stenosis, agents that may cause tachycardia are best avoided.

The maintenance of anesthesia may be complicated by hemodynamic instability and thus requires careful titration of anesthetic and vasoactive drugs. Consideration must be given to the effects of ventilation or different anesthetics on pulmonary vascular resistance and venous admixture because hypercarbia increases pulmonary vascular resistance and because all inhalation agents depress hypoxic pulmonary vasoconstriction.

### How Should the Patient With Pulmonary Edema Be Monitored?

All patients with or at risk for pulmonary edema intraoperatively should be monitored with pulse oximetry, capnography, and an arterial catheter. When cardiac ischemia is the cause of pulmonary edema, automated ST-segment analysis and transesophageal echocardiography should be used when available.

#### Pulmonary Artery Catheterization

The insertion of a PA catheter may be indicated. Measurement of left ventricular filling pressures may be invaluable for both diagnosis and management, especially in patients with CHF undergoing major surgery associated with blood loss and large fluid shifts. At the same time, care should be exercised in inserting the catheter and using the data obtained. In critically ill patients in the ICU, Connors and colleagues[29] have shown that PA catheters may be associated with excess mortality. Because this relationship was not due to complications of the PA catheter insertion, it is possible that the problem lies with the attempt to optimize pressures and cardiac output.

#### Differential Diagnosis

A major reason for performing PA catheterization is to differentiate high-pressure from increased-permeability pulmonary edema. Fein and colleagues[30] reported that in 70 consecutive patients, 40% of those suspected of having cardiogenic pulmonary edema had left ventricular filling pressures that were actually low. In contrast, patients with increased pulmonary microvascular permeability were, for the most part, diagnosed correctly on clinical grounds alone. It has also been shown that using a PA catheter appropriately affects clinical decisions in most patients.[31]

Some studies have shown a definite outcome difference when critically ill and high-risk surgical patients are managed with aggressive monitoring and goal-directed therapy.[32]

#### Detection of Ischemia

Another potential benefit of PA catheterization is its ability to detect ischemia. Although a rise in PAOP is a relatively late marker, most ischemic episodes are "silent" and are not accompanied by hemodynamic changes. Thus, the PA catheter may help to diagnose subendocardial ischemia, even if it is not apparent in the electrocardiogram.

A major problem is that physicians who care for patients with PA catheters on an irregular basis do not have adequate knowledge to make the most of this technique.[33] In addition, PA catheter use is not without risks and complications. In the previously mentioned series described by Fein and colleagues, almost 25% of the patients had a major complication associated with PA catheterization.[30]

## What Is Neurogenic Pulmonary Edema?

After severe injury to the central nervous system (trauma, subarachnoid hemorrhage, stroke, or seizures), an acute form of neurogenic pulmonary edema may occur. The classic explanation for neurogenic pulmonary edema is that the severe damage to the brain induces a "sympathetic storm." The high levels of catecholamine cause a sudden increase in the pulmonary Pmv because of reduced left ventricular compliance and the shift of a large portion of the blood volume from the systemic circulation into the pulmonary circulation. The large increase in perfusion of the pulmonary microvessels is thought to cause pore stretching, which is, in turn, responsible for the high protein content in the edema fluid that is recovered. Thus, neurogenic pulmonary edema results from a combination of high pressure and increased permeability.[34]

This syndrome frequently is short-lived and resolves rapidly with appropriate supportive therapy. However, it carries a grave neurologic prognosis. The reason for rapid clearance of pulmonary edema fluid has been shown to be related to the effect of epinephrine on the alveoli. This effect could be blocked by adrenalectomy, β-blockade, or sodium channel blockade.[35] Clinicians should be aware that the use of PEEP during neurogenic pulmonary edema may compromise cerebral perfusion by reducing cardiac output and impeding cerebral venous return.

## How Does Embolization Produce Pulmonary Edema?

### Air

Air embolism can be encountered during neurosurgical procedures that are carried out with the patient in the sitting position and also during spine, hip, and prostate gland surgery. It is occasionally seen after an inspiratory effort in the presence of a disconnected central venous catheter or after infusion of air through a pressurized fluid bag or as a result of the malfunction of an infusion system.

If a large amount of air suddenly enters the venous circulation, cardiac arrest may ensue owing to arrhythmias, airlock in the right ventricle, or both. However, when air enters at a slower rate, the bubbles reach the pulmonary microvessels, and significant pulmonary edema may develop.

An early diagnosis should prompt an effort to remove as much air as possible through a central venous or right atrial catheter if one is present and if the source is from the upper half of the body.[36] Administration of 100% $O_2$ improves bubble reabsorption and oxygenation. PEEP should be immediately employed because it prevents further entry of air into the venous circulation until the port of entry is identified and sealed. However, in the presence of a probe-patent foramen ovale, paradoxic left-sided embolism may occur. Corticosteroids have been found to be effective in reducing the pulmonary damage only when they are administered before air embolism, and thus they have no role in the therapy of air embolism.[37]

### Fat

The fat embolism syndrome usually appears 24 to 72 hours after long bone fracture and is characterized by mental confusion, thrombocytopenia, and petechiae in addition to respiratory failure. Increased pulmonary microvascular permeability is caused not only by the embolization of fat globules released from the bone marrow (because this is found after every bone fracture) but also by an as yet unidentified factor that causes activation of the complement or coagulation cascade. Moreover, intravenously administered fat globules do not produce the syndrome in experimental animals unless associated massive soft tissue trauma is also present. The release of free fatty acids by the action of lipase on neutral fat may also play a role in this process. The computed tomography scan image of pulmonary edema in fat embolism syndrome has been described recently; the investigators claimed that this syndrome was different from other causes of increased permeability pulmonary edema.[38]

The incidence of severe fat embolism syndrome appears to be decreasing, most likely as a result of better and earlier fixation of fractures, careful administration of fluids, and earlier diagnosis. If a fracture has not been stabilized, it should be stabilized to stop this source of further embolization. Some investigators recommend the use of corticosteroids in the early management of fat embolism syndrome. Otherwise, the treatment is entirely supportive. Development of intraoperative pulmonary edema due to fat embolism during orthopedic surgery is extremely rare.

## POSTOPERATIVE PULMONARY EDEMA

### Why Does It Occur?

Acute pulmonary edema may develop in the immediate postoperative period. Of the 40 cases of perioperative edema studied by Cooperman and Price,[1] most occurred within the first 30 to 60 minutes postoperatively and were usually due to increased BP in patients with previously known, poorly controlled hypertension. The following report illustrates such a case.

### CASE HISTORY 2

A 76-year-old man underwent endoscopic ureterectomy for stricture. His medical history included ischemic heart disease with an MI 4 years earlier and coronary artery bypass graft 1 year later. He did not have symptoms and was not receiving any cardiac medications. During the procedure, which was performed with the patient under general anesthesia, he was stable but had elevated BP (180 to 190/115 mm Hg) even after fentanyl administration. Labetalol was administered in 5-mg increments until BP and pulse rate were well controlled.

The patient was easily aroused at the end of the procedure and, therefore, was extubated and transported to the PACU. His $O_2$ saturation while he breathed room air was 87%. He complained of mild shortness of breath, and a chest radiograph revealed pulmonary edema (Fig. 55–7). The postoperative electrocardiogram was unchanged compared with a preoperative electrocardiogram, and creatine kinase (MB) levels were not elevated. He was treated with 100% $O_2$ and furosemide, and his status improved over a few hours.

As noted previously, Arieff[3] described a number of patients with fatal postoperative pulmonary edema. The most signifi-

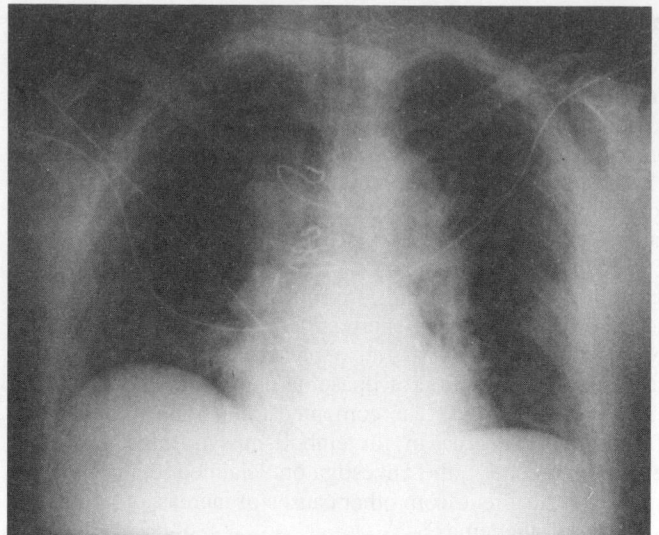

**FIGURE 55–7.** Chest radiograph of a patient with ischemic heart disease and a previous coronary artery bypass graft who developed hypertension and hypoxemia after a urologic procedure. The radiograph demonstrates enlargement of the vascular pedicles with cephalization of the pulmonary vascular markings consistent with cardiogenic pulmonary edema.

cant factor leading to pulmonary edema in these patients was fluid accumulation, which may have been underestimated by the treating clinicians. No laboratory or monitoring system can predict the development of pulmonary edema with any accuracy. Therefore, it remains to the clinician to be alert to the possibility of excessive fluid administration and to treat the patient appropriately.[39] The immediate postoperative period may be the first time that intraoperative pulmonary edema is diagnosed. It should be suspected when the patient exhibits signs and symptoms of respiratory failure after reversal of muscle paralysis and cessation of mechanical ventilation. When respiratory difficulty is encountered, the ETT should be kept in place while further doses of narcotics are administered. A chest radiograph should be obtained as soon as possible. If pulmonary edema is seen, adequate mechanical ventilatory support should be maintained while the cause is sought.

The cause is not always apparent; common problems in the differential diagnosis include overhydration, aspiration, and sympathetic overstimulation. Even when the reason cannot be defined, the prognosis is usually good if general principles of therapy are maintained (ie, negative fluid balance, tailored respiratory support, and cautious weaning).

## Hyperadrenergic State and the Use of Naloxone

Emergence from anesthesia is characterized by significant sympathetic discharge, even in patients whose hemodynamic responses were well controlled during surgery. This sympathetic overstimulation can lead to hypertension and myocardial ischemia in patients with preexisting heart disease. The excess catecholamine flux is further increased by pain, shivering, inadequate reversal of muscle paralysis, and anxiety. Adequate analgesia probably decreases the incidence and severity of these episodes.

Excessive catecholamine discharge has also been implicated as the reason for pulmonary edema after the administration of naloxone at the end of surgery. When naloxone is administered in doses that eliminate analgesia, the sudden, overwhelming

sensation of pain results in a massive discharge of catecholamines, which may cause severe dysrhythmias as well as pulmonary edema. Postoperative respiratory depression, therefore, should be treated with small (20-μg) increments of naloxone to achieve a relatively selective reversal of respiratory depression without elimination of analgesia. Even when obvious signs of distress are not present, pulmonary edema may follow administration of naloxone.[40]

This phenomenon serves as further evidence for the role of catecholamine-induced pulmonary edema, which is probably the result of a severe, nonhomogeneous constriction of segments of the pulmonary microvasculature. The administration of barbiturates and narcotics has been shown to prevent adrenaline-induced pulmonary edema in experimental models.

## Relief of Airway Obstruction (Negative Pressure Pulmonary Edema)

Pulmonary edema that appears after acute or prolonged airway obstruction is an intriguing problem.[41,42] It may appear in patients who develop airway obstruction during induction or emergence, particularly young adults who generate large "negative" (subambient) intrapleural pressures during the period of obstruction. A recent report described a patient who developed negative pressure pulmonary edema during emergence as a result of biting on a laryngeal mask while making a strong inspiratory effort.[43] The relief of such obstruction by intubation or by resolution of laryngospasm can be followed by acute pulmonary edema.[44] In a patient in the decubitus position, negative pressure pulmonary edema may present unilaterally.[45] All patients with laryngospasm during induction or emergence should be watched for at least 2 hours. Pulmonary edema can appear as late as 4 hours after an episode of airway obstruction.[46]

### Etiology

Pulmonary edema that develops after airway obstruction is most probably caused by the large negative pericapillary inspiratory pressures that favor the transudation of fluid from the intravascular to the interstitial and airway spaces of the lung. Other factors also play a role. Among these are the increase in venous return and pulmonary blood volume secondary to the negative intrathoracic pressures as well as the activation of hypoxic pulmonary vasoconstriction, which elevates pulmonary Pmv and promotes the efflux of fluid to the extravascular space.

Increased sympathetic tone during episodes of airway obstruction causes further systemic vasoconstriction and additional increases in pulmonary blood volume. Intraoperative fluid overload has also been implicated, although documented PAOP values in patients with negative pressure pulmonary edema have usually been low.

### Aspiration of Gastric Contents

Aspiration of gastric contents usually occurs during induction and emergence. At these times, patients are prone to aspirate because they are unconscious and do not mobilize their protective airway reflexes. Aspiration during induction usually manifests during surgery. Aspiration during emergence appears in the first minutes or hours postoperatively. Aspira-

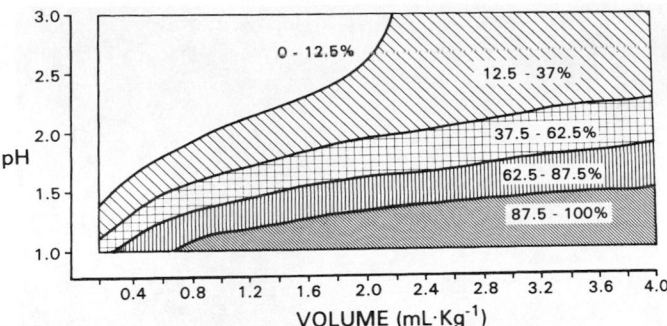

**FIGURE 55–8.** Predicted mortality rates (%) after aspiration. Each *shaded area* represents the mortality rate interval predicted for a specific pH and volume of solution aspirated. (From Janiec CF, Modell JH, Gibbs CP, et al. Pulmonary aspiration: effects of volume and pH in the rat. *Anesth Analg.* 1984;63:667.)

tion is not always accompanied by obvious signs of regurgitation.

The time from aspiration to its clinical presentation and the degree of pulmonary dysfunction depend on the pH and the quantity of the aspirate[47] (Fig. 55–8). An aspirate with a pH of <2.5 and a quantity of >20 mL is thought to cause a clinically significant problem in adult patients based on extrapolation of animal data. Particulate matter in the aspirate also causes serious damage because it can result in airway obstruction or granulomatous pneumonia. Risk factors for aspiration are listed in Table 55–5.

### CASE HISTORY 3

A 34-year-old man underwent emergency appendectomy. His previous medical history included familial Mediterranean fever with recurrent episodes of peritonitis. The patient had not had anything to eat or drink for the previous 8 hours. Induction and surgery were uneventful, and the patient was extubated in the operating room while still somewhat somnolent. Upon arrival in the recovery room, he vomited a large amount of clear, greenish fluid. He was turned on his side and his oropharynx immediately suctioned.

Ten minutes later, he experienced severe respiratory distress. He was intubated and ventilated with an $FIO_2$ of 1.0 and a PEEP

**TABLE 55–5.** Some Conditions Associated With High Risk for Aspiration

| | |
|---|---|
| Full stomach | Trauma |
| Intestinal obstruction | Large intraabdominal mass |
| Pregnancy | Diabetes |

of 10 cm $H_2O$. A chest radiograph revealed pulmonary edema with widespread opacification of both lung fields (Fig. 55–9A). After 12 hours of therapy, a repeat chest radiograph taken during 5 cm $H_2O$ PEEP showed marked improvement (see Fig. 55–9B).

Aspiration is the most important complication to prevent. Elective surgery patients at high risk should receive histamine-2 antagonists preoperatively to reduce gastric acidity. A single dose of metoclopramide (10 mg for a 70-kg patient) increases lower esophageal sphincter tone and improves gastric emptying. We routinely administer 200 mg of cimetidine or 50 mg of ranitidine intravenously, together with 10 mg of metoclopramide, 30 to 45 minutes before induction of high-risk patients. A nonparticulate antacid should be added to this regimen in emergency patients to neutralize what is already in the stomach. Placement of a nasogastric tube preinduction is advocated by some. This measure certainly decreases the gastric volume but does not predictably empty the stomach.

## MISCELLANEOUS CAUSES

### What Is Reexpansion Pulmonary Edema?

Rapid evacuation of the pleural space in cases of pneumothorax or pleural effusion sometimes leads to pulmonary edema in the reexpanded lung. The exact mechanism that causes this entity is unclear but may involve the production of negative interstitial pressures during the reexpansion that lead to a permeability defect.[48] It can occur in a single lung or even a single lobe after evacuation of air or fluid from the pleural space.[49] It is also occasionally seen as a bilateral phenomenon after evacuation of a single lung.

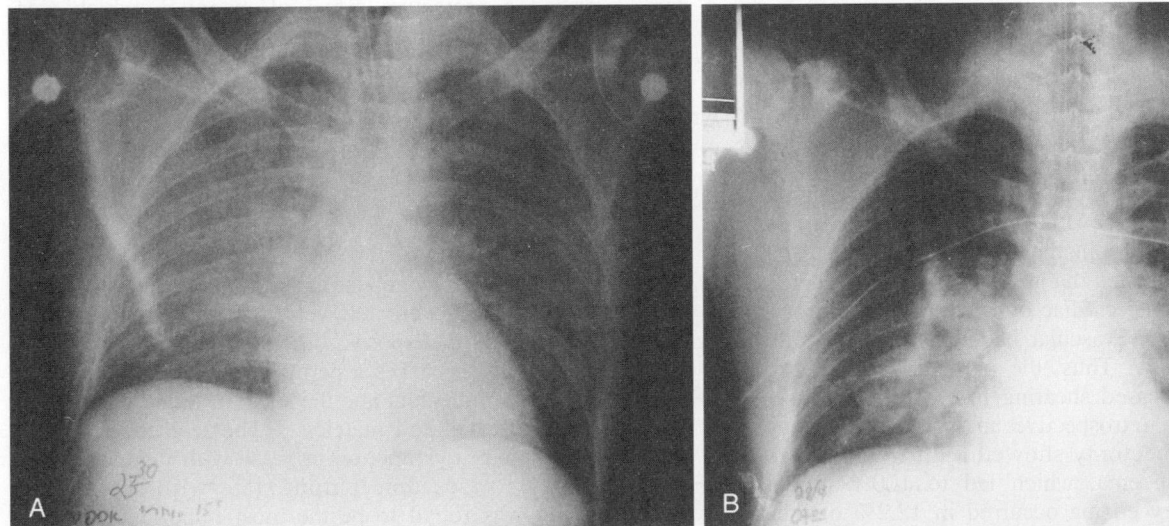

**FIGURE 55–9.** *A*, Chest radiograph of a patient who aspirated in the recovery room. The film was taken 15 minutes after the aspiration and shows widespread interstitial and intraalveolar opacification consistent with acid aspiration. *B*, Radiograph of the same patient taken 12 hours later. Substantial improvement is apparent.

The disorder probably can be prevented by evacuating a long-standing pneumothorax or pleural effusion slowly. When a patient complains of chest pain after insertion of a chest tube (in the situation of long-standing lung collapse), the tube should be intermittently clamped and evacuation accomplished gradually over 10 to 15 minutes.[50]

## Why Does Unilateral Pulmonary Edema Occur?

### Mechanical Causes

A number of causes are possible for unilateral pulmonary edema. Most are mechanical factors and include the aforementioned cases of pulmonary edema after reexpansion and the relief of obstruction to a single lobe (as by laser surgery of an obstructing neoplasm).[51] Mechanical obstruction of the pulmonary veins after open heart surgery for congenital heart disease has been suggested as a cause.[52] Previous sympathectomy, which prevents edema in the denervated side, may result in contralateral manifestations.[53]

### Position

Patients in the lateral decubitus position tend to develop edema in the dependent lung because of increased hydrostatic pressure; this is described in the following case.

### CASE HISTORY 4

A 20-year-old man underwent surgery to remove a plate that had been placed for internal fixation of a fracture of the femur 6 months previously. The procedure was performed with the patient under general anesthesia in the right lateral decubitus position. The surgery lasted 2 hours, and the patient received 2 L of crystalloid solution during surgery. Upon arrival in the PACU, his $O_2$ saturation was low, and he required an $O_2$ mask with an $FIO_2$ of 0.40 to 0.50 to maintain saturation above 90%. His chest radiograph revealed predominantly right-sided edema (Fig. 55–10).

## Why Does Lung Resection Lead to Pulmonary Edema?

Pulmonary edema may appear in the first postoperative hours after lung resection. This entity has been described after both pneumonectomy and lobar resection. Manipulation of the lung, altered hemodynamics, intraoperative fluid overload, and reduced lymphatic capacity play a part in the formation of this disorder. Mathru and coworkers[54] reported on patients in whom the protein fraction in the edema fluid was >0.6 of that in plasma and suggested that this was caused by increased permeability. The normal cardiac output that flows through a much smaller pulmonary vascular bed is associated with increased PAP and PAOP. Thus, the permeability defect can be caused by the increased shearing forces at microvascular junctions. Recently, a retrospective analysis of 197 patients undergoing pneumonectomy showed a 2.5% incidence of manifest pulmonary edema, which led to 100% mortality. Premanifest pulmonary edema occurred in 12.2% of the patients. The administration of fresh-frozen plasma and the use of ventilation with high pressures during surgery were associated with an increased risk for pulmonary edema.[55]

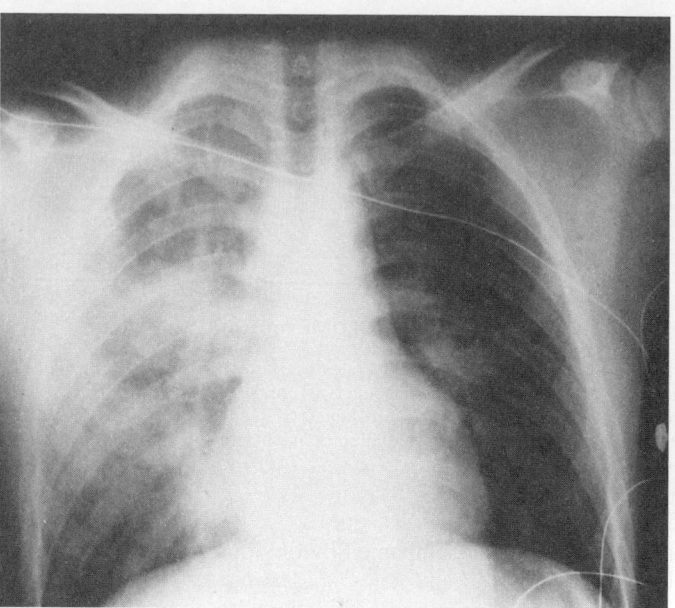

**FIGURE 55–10.** Chest radiograph showing unilateral pulmonary edema in a patient who presented with moderate hypoxemia in the recovery room after a lengthy orthopedic procedure performed in the right lateral decubitus position.

## What Are the Effects of Aortic Cross-Clamping?

In patients who undergo aortic surgery, pulmonary edema may be caused by a number of factors. These patients often have intrinsic heart disease, and cardiac decompensation can follow aortic cross-clamping. In addition, after aortic clamping, the problems of reperfusion may occur. In a number of studies, Hechtman's group[56] showed that ischemia and reperfusion of a large body mass cause production of arachidonic acid metabolites. These metabolites (in particular, thromboxane) cause an elevation of PAP, margination of polymorphonuclear leukocytes in the lung, and an increase in EVLW. Four to 8 hours after clamping, a decrease in oxygenation and an increase in airway pressures and EVLW (as assessed with chest radiography) were noted. The investigators described a protective effect of mannitol, which was ascribed to the free radical scavenging properties of this drug.[57]

## Why Does Pulmonary Edema Follow Open Heart Surgery?

### Cardiopulmonary Bypass

Pulmonary edema may appear in the immediate post-bypass period secondary to severe left ventricular dysfunction. The heart-lung machine predisposes to hemodilution and a reduction of COP and also causes a permeability defect secondary to activation of complement and the sequestration of polymorphonuclear leukocytes and platelets.[58] The incidence and severity of pulmonary dysfunction increase with increasing bypass times. A low cardiac output state with splanchnic hypoperfusion was found to be the most important determinant of ARDS development after cardiac surgery. In this series, ARDS occurred in 1% of the patients and was associated with a high mortality rate of close to 70%.[59]

## Silent Ischemia

Another reason for post–open heart surgery pulmonary edema may be the ischemia that occurs in patients in the first few days after surgery. This ischemia, which is usually silent, has been correlated with adverse cardiac outcome, including pulmonary edema. The efficacy of intensive postoperative analgesia with a continuous infusion of sufentanil to reduce ischemia has been shown.[60] This approach may also reduce the risk for pulmonary edema due to such ischemic episodes.

## References

1. Cooperman LH, Price HL. Pulmonary edema in the operative and postoperative period: a review of 40 cases. *Ann Surg.* 1970;172:883.
2. Goldman L, Caldera DL, Nussbaum SR, et al. Multifactorial index of cardiac risk in noncardiac surgical procedures. *N Engl J Med.* 1977;297:845.
3. Arieff AI. Fatal postoperative pulmonary edema: pathogenesis and literature review. *Chest.* 1999;115:1371.
4. West JB, Mathieu-Costello O. Structure, strength, failure, and remodeling of the pulmonary blood-gas barrier. *Annu Rev Physiol.* 1999;61:543.
5. Rackow EC, Fein IA, Siege J. The relationship of the colloid osmotic pulmonary artery wedge pressure gradient in pulmonary edema and mortality in critically ill patients. *Chest.* 1982;82:433.
6. Guyton AC, Parker JC, Taylor AE, et al. Forces governing water movement in the lung. In: Fishman AP, Renkin EM, eds. *Pulmonary Edema.* Bethesda, Md: American Physiological Society; 1979:65.
7. Staub NC, Flick M, Perel A, et al. Lung lymph as a reflection of interstitial fluid. In: Hargens AR, ed. *Tissue Fluid Pressure and Composition.* Baltimore, Md: Williams & Wilkins; 1981:113.
8. Erdmann AJ III, Vaughn TR Jr, Brigham KL, et al. Effect of increased vascular pressure on lung fluid balance in unanesthetized sheep. *Circ Res.* 1975;37:271.
9. Sprung CL, Long WM, Marcial EH, et al. Distribution of proteins in pulmonary edema: the value of fractional concentrations. *Am Rev Respir Dis.* 1987;136:957.
10. Matthay MA, Wiener-Kronish JP. Intact epithelial barrier function is critical for the resolution of alveolar edema in humans. *Am Rev Respir Dis.* 1990;142:1250.
11. Perel A, Williamson DC, Modell JH. Effectiveness of CPAP by mask for pulmonary edema associated with hypercarbia. *Intensive Care Med.* 1983;9:17.
12. Morgan PW, Goodman LR. Pulmonary edema and adult respiratory distress syndrome. *Radiol Clin North Am.* 1991;29:943.
13. Neumann P. Extravascular lung water and intrathoracic blood volume: double versus single indicator dilution technique. *Intensive Care Med.* 1999;25:216.
14. Schuller D, Mitchell JP, Calandrino FS, et al. Fluid balance during pulmonary edema: is fluid gain a marker or a cause of poor outcome? *Chest.* 1991;100:1068.
15. Shires GT III, Peitzman AB, Albert SA, et al. Response of extravascular lung water to intraoperative fluids. *Ann Surg.* 1983;197:515.
16. Wickerts CJ, Blomqvist H, Berg B, et al. Furosemide, when used in combination with positive end-expiratory pressure, facilitates the resorption of extravascular lung water in experimental hydrostatic pulmonary oedema. *Acta Anesth Scand.* 1991;35:776.
17. Humphrey H, Hall J, Sznajder I, et al. Improved survival in ARDS patients associated with a reduction in pulmonary capillary wedge pressure. *Chest.* 1990;97:1176.
18. Bjertnaes LJ, Koizumi T, Newman JH. Inhaled nitric oxide reduces lung fluid filtration after endotoxin in awake sheep. *Am J Respir Crit Care Med.* 1998;158:1416.
19. Dellinger RP, Zimmerman JL, Taylor RW, et al. Effects of inhaled nitric oxide in patients with acute respiratory distress syndrome: results of a randomized phase II trial. Inhaled Nitric Oxide in ARDS Study Group. *Crit Care Med.* 1998;26:15.
20. Segal E. The preoperative evaluation of the patient with heart disease. *Probl Anesth.* 1992;6:22.
21. Browner WS, Li J, Mangano DT. Study of perioperative ischemia research group: in-hospital and long-term mortality in male veterans following non-cardiac surgery. *JAMA.* 1992;268:228.
22. DelBGuercio LRM, Cohn D. Monitoring operative risk in the elderly. *JAMA.* 1980;243:1350.
23. Biery DR, Marks JD, Schapera A, et al. Factors affecting perioperative pulmonary function in acute respiratory failure. *Chest.* 1990;98:1455.
24. Schapera A, Marks JD, Minagi H, et al. Perioperative pulmonary function in acute respiratory failure: effect of ventilator type and gas mixture. *Anesthesiology.* 1989;71:396.
25. Marks JD, Schapera A, Kraemer ARW. Pressure and flow limitations of anesthesia ventilators. *Anesthesiology.* 1989;71:403.
26. The Acute Respiratory Distress Syndrome Network. Ventilation with lower tidal volumes as compared with traditional tidal volumes for acute lung injury and the acute respiratory distress syndrome. *N Engl J Med.* 2000;342:1301.
27. Lecuona E, Saldias F, Comellas A, et al. Ventilator-associated lung injury decreases lung ability to clear edema in rats. *Am J Respir Crit Care Med.* 1999;159:603.
28. Kallet RH, Alonso JA, Luce JM, et al. Exacerbation of acute pulmonary edema during assisted mechanical ventilation using a low-tidal volume, lung-protective ventilator strategy. *Chest.* 1999;116:1826.
29. Connors AF Jr, Speroff T, Dawson NV, et al. The effectiveness of right heart catheterization in the initial care of critically ill patients. *JAMA.* 1996;276:889.
30. Fein AM, Goldberg SK, Walkenstein MD, et al. Is pulmonary artery catheterization necessary for the diagnosis of pulmonary edema? *Am Rev Respir Dis.* 1984;129:1006.
31. Marinelli WA, Weinert CR, Gross CR, et al. Right heart catheterization in acute lung injury: an observational study. *Am J Respir Crit Care Med.* 1999;160:69.
32. Shoemaker WC, Appel PL, Kram HB, et al. Prospective trial of supranormal values of survivors as therapeutic goals in high-risk surgical patients. *Chest.* 1988;94:1176.
33. Iberti TJ, Fischer EP, Leibowitz AB, et al. Multicenter study of physicians' knowledge of the pulmonary artery catheter. Pulmonary Artery Catheter Study Group. *JAMA.* 1990;264:2928.
34. Smith WS, Matthay MA. Evidence for a hydrostatic mechanism in human neurogenic pulmonary edema. *Chest.* 1997;111:1326.
35. Lane SM, Maender KC, Awender NE, et al. Adrenal epinephrine increases alveolar liquid clearance in a canine model of neurogenic pulmonary edema. *Am J Respir Crit Care Med.* 1998;158:760.
36. Artru A. Venous air embolism in prone dogs positioned with the abdomen hanging freely: percentage of gas retrieved and success rate of resuscitation. *Anesth Analg.* 1992;75:715.
37. Jerome EH, Bonsignore MR, Albertine KH, et al. Timing of corticosteroid treatment: effect on lung lymph dynamics in air embolism lung injury in awake sheep. *Am Rev Respir Dis.* 1990;142:872.
38. Arakawa H, Kurihara Y, Nakajima Y. Pulmonary fat embolism syndrome: CT findings in six patients. *J Comput Assist Tomogr.* 2000;24:24.
39. Kirby RR. Perioperative fluid therapy and postoperative pulmonary edema: cause-effect relationship? *Chest.* 1999;115:1224.
40. Johnson C, Mayer P, Grosz D. Pulmonary edema following naloxone administration in a healthy orthopedic patient. *J Clin Anesth.* 1995;7:356.
41. Kamal RS, Agha S. Acute pulmonary oedema: a complication of upper airway obstruction. *Anaesthesia.* 1984;39:464.
42. Deepika K, Kenaan CA, Barrocas AM, et al. Negative pressure pulmonary edema after acute upper airway obstruction. *J Clin Anesth.* 1997;9:403.
43. Devys JM, Balleau C, Jayr C, et al. Biting the laryngeal mask: an unusual cause of negative pressure pulmonary edema. *Can J Anaesth.* 2000;47:176.
44. Herrick IA, Mahendran B, Penny FJ. Postoperative pulmonary edema following anesthesia. *J Clin Anesth.* 1990;2:116.
45. Sullivan M. Unilateral negative pressure pulmonary edema during anesthesia with a laryngeal mask airway. *Can J Anaesth.* 1999;46:1053.
46. Glasser SA, Siler JN. Delayed onset of laryngospasm-induced pulmonary edema in an adult outpatient. *Anesthesiology.* 1985;62:370.
47. James CF, Modell JH, Gibbs CP, et al. Pulmonary aspiration: effects of volume and pH in the rat. *Anesth Analg.* 1984;63:665.
48. Timby J, Reed C, Zeilender S, et al. "Mechanical" causes of pulmonary edema. *Chest.* 1990;98:973.
49. Vuong TK, Dautheribes C, Robert J, et al. Reexpansion pulmonary edema localized to a lobe. *Chest.* 1988;93:1170.
50. Milano S, Tassi GF. Pneumothorax evacuation. *Chest.* 1988;93:443.
51. Miro AM, Shivaram U, Finch PJP. Noncardiogenic pulmonary edema following laser therapy of a tracheal neoplasm. *Chest.* 1989;96:1430.
52. Schiff GA, Simpson JI. Unilateral pulmonary edema after atrial septal defect repair. *Anesthesiology.* 1991;74:7851.
53. Flick MR, Kanzler GB, Block AJ. Unilateral pulmonary edema with

contralateral thoracic sympathectomy in the adult respiratory distress syndrome. *Chest.* 1975;68:736.

54. Mathru M, Blakeman B, Dries DJ, et al. Permeability pulmonary edema following lung resection. *Chest.* 1990;98:1216.

55. van der Werff YD, van der Houwen HK, Heijmans PJ, et al. Postpneumonectomy pulmonary edema: a retrospective analysis of incidence and possible risk factors. *Chest.* 1997;111:1278.

56. Paterson IS, Klausner JM, Pugatch R, et al. Noncardiogenic pulmonary edema after abdominal aortic aneurysm surgery. *Ann Surg.* 1989;209:231.

57. Paterson IS, Klausner JM, Goldman G, et al. Pulmonary edema after aneurysm surgery is modified by mannitol. *Ann Surg.* 1989;210:796.

58. Klancke KA, Assey ME, Kratz JM, et al. Postoperative pulmonary edema in postcoronary artery bypass graft patients. *Chest.* 1983;84:529.

59. Christenson JT, Aeberhard JM, Badel P, et al. Adult respiratory distress syndrome after cardiac surgery. *Cardiovasc Surg.* 1996;4:15.

60. Mangano DT, Siliciano D, Hollenberg M, et al. Postoperative myocardial ischemia: therapeutic trials using intensive analgesia following surgery. *Anesthesiology.* 1992;76:342.

# The Neonate

Timothy W. Martin
Joanne M. Stoner

## INTRAOPERATIVE MONITORING

*What Are the Basics?*

*What Is the Value of Pulse Oximetry?*

*What Is the Value of Capnometry/Capnography?*

## PYLORIC STENOSIS

*What Are the Primary Concerns?*

*How Is Anesthesia Managed?*

## CONGENITAL ABDOMINAL WALL DEFECTS

*What Are They?*

*What Are Potential Complications?*

*What Are the Major Management Problems?*

*How Is Anesthesia Managed?*

## NECROTIZING ENTEROCOLITIS

*What Is it?*

*What Are the Presenting Signs?*

*What Does Medical and Surgical Management Involve?*

*How Is Anesthesia Managed?*

## PATENT DUCTUS ARTERIOSUS

*What Are the Characteristics?*

*What Are the Clinical Signs?*

*How Is Anesthesia Managed?*

## TRACHEOESOPHAGEAL FISTULA

*What Is It?*

*How Is It Diagnosed?*

*What Should Be Done Before Surgery?*

*How Is Anesthesia Managed?*

## CONGENITAL DIAPHRAGMATIC HERNIA

*What Is It?*

*What Are the Effects?*

*How Is It Diagnosed?*

*How Is It Treated?*

*How Is Anesthesia Managed?*

## NEONATAL RESUSCITATION

*When Is It Necessary?*

*What Is the Basic Approach?*

*What Is the Role of Drug Therapy?*

*How Should Drugs or Fluids Be Administered?*

The special considerations and unique features of pediatric anesthesia (discussed in Chapter 57) are most evident and affect anesthetic care most significantly in neonates. In addition, infants younger than 1 year of age account for more than half of the anesthesia-related pediatric cardiac arrests in the Pediatric Perioperative Cardiac Arrest (POCA) Registry.[1] The differences between anesthesia for neonates and adults may be viewed from several perspectives, as outlined in Table 56–1.

## PAIN AND ITS PERCEPTION

### *Do Neonates Require Anesthesia?*

Since approximately the mid-1980s, a significant volume of research has addressed the issue of neonatal anesthetic

**TABLE 56–1.** Contrasting Areas of Neonatal and Adult Anesthetic Requirements

**Anatomic and Physiologic Features**

Airway and respiratory system
Cardiovascular system
Kidney and body fluid distribution
Thermoregulation

**Preexisting or Chronic Medical Problems**

Infant respiratory distress syndrome
Persistent pulmonary hypertension
Intraventricular hemorrhage
Anemia
Retinopathy of prematurity

**Preanesthetic Preparation**

Fasting requirements
Premedication
Equipment and operating room setup
Intraoperative management

**Airway and Ventilation**

Vascular access
Fluid management
Monitoring

**Surgical Disorders and Procedures**

Pyloric stenosis
Tracheoesophageal fistula
Gastroschisis and omphalocele
Necrotizing enterocolitis
Diaphragmatic hernia
Patent ductus arteriosus

**Postoperative Problems**

Apnea/bradycardia
Pain

**Neonatal Resuscitation**

requirements and the consequences of withholding appropriate anesthesia from surgical patients. Before this time, neonates were subjected to repeated major surgery and painful stimuli without the provision of what could be considered even minimal analgesia. To illustrate this point, in a 1970 discussion of anesthesia for premature neonates, the following statement was made:

*Most of these babies do not need halothane. All they need is a little ventilatory support. They do not need much agent at all. A little bit of adhesive tape holds them down.*[2]

Since that time, we have come to terms with the realization that a great number of neonates born in the era of "modern" anesthesia have been and, in some instances, continue to be, undermedicated; a double standard has existed in our approach to providing anesthesia and analgesia for newborns and adults.

An enlarging body of knowledge in more recent years has demonstrated that neonates are capable of mounting an intense metabolic response to stress that can be ameliorated by the use of analgesics.[3] Research showing that actual outcomes are improved with the use of analgesics has led to dramatic changes in the field of neonatal anesthesia.[4] However, the progress realized in operative anesthesia for newborns and small infants has not been uniformly transferred to related practices, such as the routine use of postoperative analgesics or sedation in the neonatal intensive care unit (NICU).[4]

## How Do Neonates Perceive Pain?

Because pain is generally defined as a subjective phenomenon, strongly influenced by previous emotional and painful experiences, it is difficult to evaluate in neonates. For this reason, the suggestion has been made that nociceptive activity, or the perception of tissue damage, is more appropriately studied in neonates than is the phenomenon of pain.[5]

The inherent inability of neonates to express the subjective component of pain had previously been used to infer that, as a group, they were incapable of experiencing painful stimuli. The current definition of pain implies that the experience is learned through early life experiences. However, one prominent researcher in the field has argued that pain perception is an inherent quality of life itself, and a part of the human condition. Further, it is the subjective experience or verbal description that is learned, rather than the perception of the noxious stimulus itself.[6] Historically, reasons why neonates and sick infants have been provided little or no anesthesia have included poorly understood neonatal requirements for anesthesia, inadequate monitoring, and fear of inducing cardiovascular instability with what previously had been a limited selection of anesthetic agents.[7]

### Neural Development

Investigations in recent years have demonstrated that neonates possess the anatomic, functional, and neurochemical systems necessary for pain perception.[5,8,9] Archaic developmental arguments that had been used to justify the withholding of anesthesia from neonates, including an underdeveloped nervous system, the absence of mature pain receptors, and the incomplete myelinization of neonatal peripheral nerves, have been refuted.

It is now known that the neural pathways that transmit impulses from painful stimuli can be traced from sensory receptors in the skin to the cerebral cortex of newborn infants. The lack of complete myelination of the nervous system at birth has frequently served as an argument that neonates are not capable of pain perception although, even in adults, nociceptive impulses are often transmitted by unmyelinated nerve fibers. The electroencephalographic patterns of premature and term newborns allow distinction between wakefulness and sleep and demonstrate changes in response to tactile stimuli, indicating functional integrity of a neonate's nervous system. In addition, neurochemical systems, including the tachykinins and endogenous opioids (enkephalins and endorphins), are demonstrable in fetuses and neonates.

It is possible that the neonate is more sensitive to pain than older age groups. To summarize the major points of recent work:

- There is a defined physiologic basis for increased pain sensitivity in neonates.
- Prolonged hyperalgesia after acute painful stimuli in preterm neonates may lead to chronic pain states.
- Acute physiologic responses to painful stimuli may cause adverse neurologic outcomes, including intraventricular hemorrhage and periventricular leukomalacia.
- Interventions designed to provide preemptive analgesia may lessen the incidence of adverse neurologic outcomes.
- There appears to be an association of neurobehavioral and developmental sequelae resulting from repetitive painful interventions during a NICU stay.[10]

The gestational timetable for maturation of pain pathways in a human fetus and neonate is illustrated in Figure 56–1.

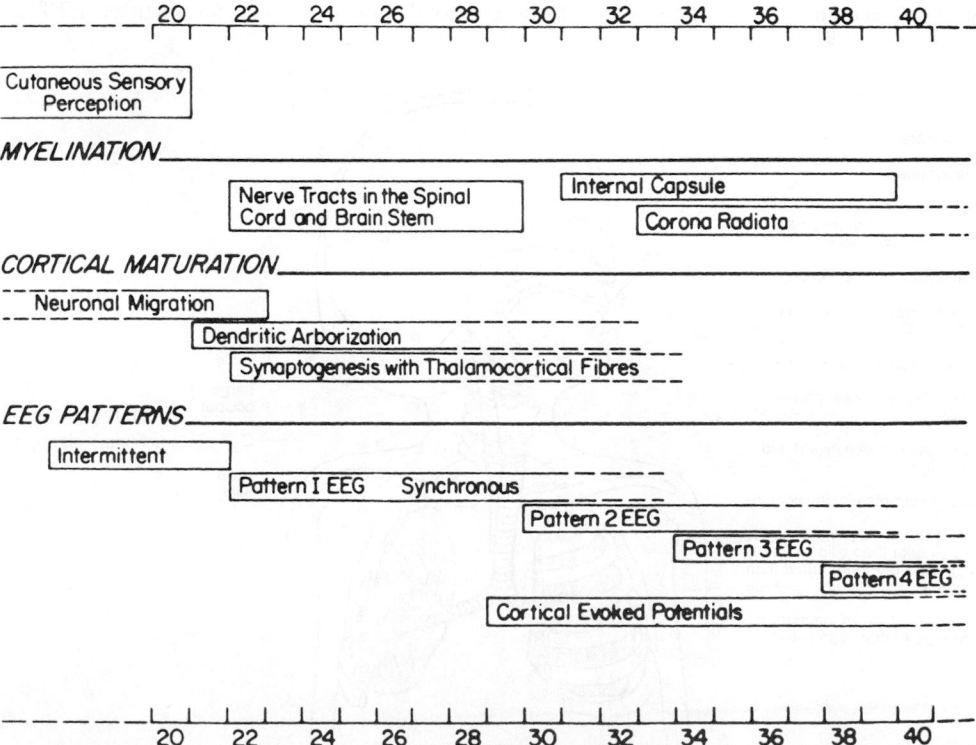

FIGURE 56–1. Schematic diagram of the development of structures and functions necessary for pain perception from weeks 20 to 40 of gestation. (Reprinted from Anand KJS, Hickey PR. Pain and its effects in the human neonate and fetus. *N Engl J Med.* 1987;317:1322.)

### What Are the Responses to Pain?

Physiologic and metabolic responses to pain and surgical stress similar to those observed in children and adults have been documented in neonates.[11] Parameters such as heart rate, blood pressure, and respiratory rate and metabolic indicators such as serum glucose and lactic acid levels increase in the presence of pain or inadequate analgesia. The anatomic and functional requirements for long-term memory (principally the limbic system and diencephalon) are present in neonates; although painful experiences may not be subject to conscious recall, such events probably affect later development and behavior.[5]

The relative plasticity of the neonatal brain suggests that repetitive painful insults may affect neuronal and synaptic organization permanently. On the other hand, exposure of the same developing brain to psychoactive drugs may also lead to unknown changes, the long-term consequences of which are largely unknown. Clearly, much remains to be learned in this field.[10]

## THE RESPIRATORY SYSTEM

A number of features of the neonate's airway and respiratory system have clinical implications. For purposes of discussion, these can be divided into the conductive airway, from the nares to the trachea, and the lower respiratory tract, including not only the lungs but also the chest wall and diaphragm (Fig. 56–2).

### What Should Be Known About the Airway?

#### Nasopharynx

The nares are relatively narrow and, together with the nasal passages, account for nearly two thirds of the total airway resistance.[12] When not crying, neonates are obligate nose breathers. The relationship of the epiglottis to the soft palate allows infants to isolate the breathing and feeding channels effectively and to perform both processes simultaneously. Any anatomic abnormality, disease process, or artificial medical appliance (eg, nasogastric tube) may significantly increase airway resistance and the work of breathing in spontaneously ventilating newborns.

#### Tongue and Epiglottis

The tongue is relatively large compared with the oral cavity and may predispose to airway obstruction and increase the difficulty of laryngoscopy during intubation. Because the epiglottis is integral to simultaneous breathing and swallowing, it is narrower, shorter, and somewhat omega shaped, and it has a tendency to protrude more into the hypopharynx.

#### Larynx

The larynx is located higher in the neck, as demonstrated by the position of the glottis at the level of the third cervical vertebra.[13] In adults, the glottis is at the level of C-5. The more cephalad location of the neonatal glottis creates the *impression* that the larynx is anterior during laryngoscopy, thus occasionally making laryngeal exposure and intubation more difficult. The neonatal cricoid ring is underdeveloped, imparting a funnel shape to the larynx and making this the narrowest segment of the upper airway.

This feature assumes significance in the selection of endotracheal tubes (ETTs) and the development of laryngeal and tracheal edema due to any of various causes. The fit of an ETT at the cricoid cartilage must not be so tight that it induces mucosal ischemia; otherwise, after extubation the short-term problem of increased resistance to airflow and the long-term problem of tracheal stenosis may result. In practice, intubating with an uncuffed ETT of a size that allows a small air leak at

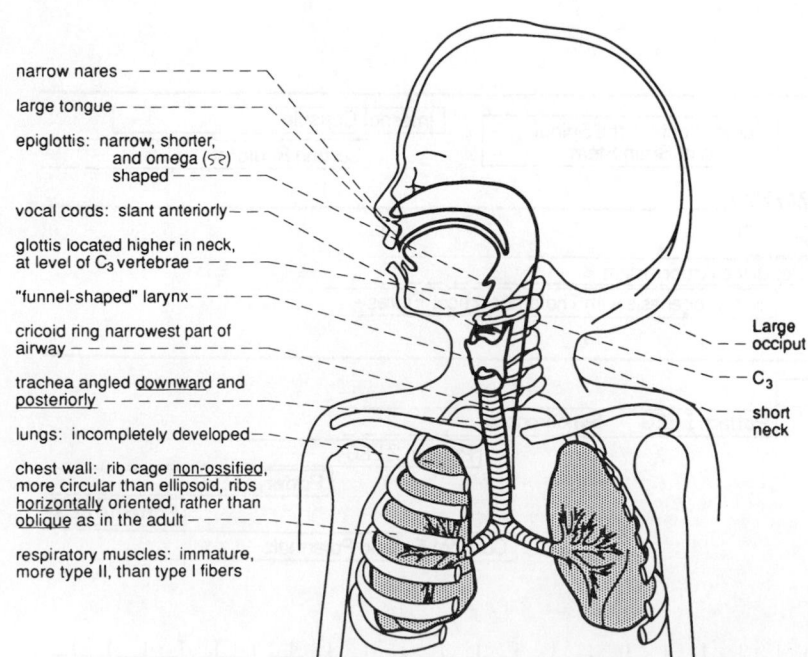

narrow nares

large tongue

epiglottis: narrow, shorter, and omega (ℭ) shaped

vocal cords: slant anteriorly

glottis located higher in neck, at level of $C_3$ vertebrae

"funnel-shaped" larynx

cricoid ring narrowest part of airway

trachea angled <u>downward</u> and <u>posteriorly</u>

lungs: incompletely developed

chest wall: rib cage <u>non-ossified</u>, more circular than ellipsoid, ribs <u>horizontally</u> oriented, rather than <u>oblique</u> as in the adult

respiratory muscles: immature, more type II, than type I fibers

Large occiput

$C_3$

short neck

**FIGURE 56–2.** Diagram depicting the significant features of the neonatal airway and respiratory system that differ from those in adults.

an inflation pressure of 20 to 30 cm $H_2O$ appears to prevent this complication.

### Trachea

A neonate's trachea is angled downward and posteriorly, unlike the straight downward projection in an adult.

### Neck and Occiput

Although not parts of the airway, the occiput and neck of a newborn have features that affect airway management. The large occiput causes the head to be flexed anteriorly, sometimes making effective bag-valve-mask ventilation and laryngoscopy difficult; this problem is compounded if the head is elevated on folded towels or a headrest, as is frequently done before elective intubation in adults. Optimum positioning of the head, neck, and shoulders is achieved by placing a small rolled towel in a transverse position at the level of the shoulders.

## What Should Be Known About the Lungs?

The lungs are incompletely developed at birth and continue to develop through a process of alveolar septation for the first 18 months of life. During this period, there is a significant increase in the capillary and air space volumes of the lungs. Although it had previously been thought that the lungs do not attain their full complement of alveoli until approximately 8 years of age, it now appears that the adult number of alveoli may be attained by age 2 years. Beyond this point, most new growth occurs through an increase in the volume of existing alveoli.[14,15] The alveoli are composed of two types of pneumocytes: predominant type I cells, which provide the structure of the alveolus, and type II cells, which produce surfactant as early as the 24th week of gestation. Surfactant is a mixture of phospholipids and proteins; it reduces surface tension in the alveoli, preventing alveolar collapse as lung volumes are reduced during expiration.

On a weight basis, tidal volume, dead space, the ratio of dead space to tidal volume, and functional residual capacity (FRC) are nearly the same as in adults. Because of a neonate's elevated metabolic rate and an oxygen ($O_2$) consumption that is two to three times an adult's rate of 3 mL/kg/min, alveolar ventilation also is 2 to 3 times an adult's volume.

The ratio of alveolar ventilation to FRC approaches 5:1 in neonates, compared with a ratio of approximately 1.4:1 in adults.[16] This significant difference explains the rapidity of oxyhemoglobin desaturation and hypoxemia after apnea and the increased rate of inhalation anesthetic uptake. Atelectasis and gas trapping can occur because closing volume, the lung volume at which terminal airway closure begins, is higher in infants. Even within the excursion of normal tidal volumes, some airway closure occurs, primarily as a result of underdevelopment of tissues that contribute to the elastic recoil of the lungs.[17]

## What Should Be Known About the Chest Wall and Respiratory Muscles?

The chest wall and muscles of respiration must also mature. The nonossified rib cage is more circular than ellipsoid and is very compliant. The individual ribs are more horizontally oriented than oblique as in adults; hence, the accessory muscles of respiration have a shorter course and generate a less forceful contraction.[18] These features make a newborn essentially a diaphragmatic breather. The respiratory muscles are also different. In neonates, they are composed of a lower percentage of slow-twitch, high-oxidative muscle fibers (type I), which are capable of sustained activity; newborn infants are therefore predisposed to respiratory muscle fatigue.[19]

## THE CARDIOVASCULAR SYSTEM

## What Should Be Known About the Fetal Circulation?

A discussion of the neonatal cardiovascular system begins with an assessment of the fetal circulation (Fig. 56–3). The circulatory system must complete several adaptations to convert from the *parallel* pulmonary and systemic circuits of a fetus to the *series* components of an infant and adult.

### The Ductus Venosus

In utero, unsaturated blood in the descending aorta is carried to the placenta by two umbilical arteries to pick up $O_2$. It then returns to the body through the umbilical vein. There, approximately half of the returning blood enters the ductus venosus, then the inferior vena cava (IVC), effectively bypassing the liver. The other half of the returning oxygenated blood enters the hepatic circulation.[20]

### The Foramen Ovale

Poorly oxygenated blood from the body and oxygenated blood from the placenta and IVC are *partially* mixed in the right atrium. The blood then may pass into the right ventricle or through the foramen ovale into the left atrium, bypassing the pulmonary circulation. Most of the oxygenated blood from the placenta and IVC is shunted through the foramen ovale, to the left atrium and ventricle, then into the ascending aorta, where it is primarily directed to the major arteries of the head and upper extremities.[21] Poorly oxygenated blood from the superior vena cava primarily enters the right ventricle and pulmonary artery.

### The Ductus Arteriosus

Another anatomic shunt, the ductus arteriosus, serves to allow most (90%) of the blood in the pulmonary artery to bypass the lungs (and the high-resistance pulmonary vascular circuit) to enter the aorta.[20] The flow dynamics are such that most of this blood courses into the descending aorta to the arteries of the abdomen and lower extremities or the umbilical arteries and placenta.

## What Changes Occur at Birth?

At birth, the lungs are inflated with the onset of ventilation, and intraalveolar fluid is expelled, resulting in an elevation in arterial partial pressure of $O_2$ ($PaO_2$) and reduction in pulmo-

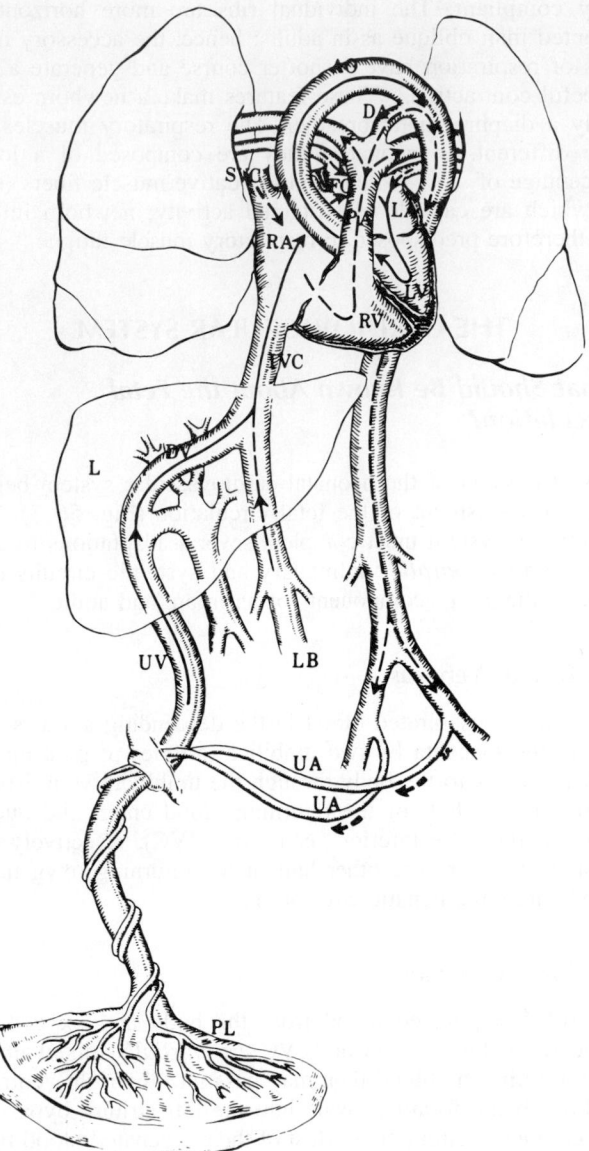

**FIGURE 56–3.** The fetal circulation. The *solid line with arrows* indicates the pathway that oxygenated blood follows from the placenta to the fetal heart. AO, aorta; DA, ductus arteriosus; DV, ductus venosus; FO, foramen ovale; IVC, inferior vena cava; L, liver; LA, left atrium; LB, lower body; LV, left ventricle; PA, pulmonary artery; PL, placenta; RA, right atrium; RV, right ventricle; SVC, superior vena cava; UA, umbilical artery; UV, umbilical vein. (From Rimar S, Urban MK. Newborn physiology and development. In: Bell C, Hughes CW, Oh TH, eds. *The Pediatric Anesthesia Handbook.* St Louis, Mo: CV Mosby; 1991:1.)

nary vascular resistance (PVR). Pulmonary blood flow increases fivefold.[20] Simultaneously, the umbilical cord is clamped, and the placenta is separated from the neonatal body and circulation. Systemic vascular resistance immediately increases. The effect of these profound hemodynamic changes and oxygenation is to promote *functional* closure of the fetal shunts; permanent anatomic closure of the ductus arteriosus and foramen ovale may take several weeks, and in a small number of individuals it never occurs. The rate of probe patency of the foramen ovale in older children and adults has been estimated to be as high as 34%.[22]

## How Does the Neonatal Heart Differ?

Several features of the neonatal heart and its innervation are unlike those of older children and adults.

### Structure

At birth, the right and left ventricles have equivalent muscle masses and wall thicknesses.[23] The fetal and neonatal myocardium has a lower percentage of contractile mass than mature myocardium. Neonatal myocytes have a greater density of nuclei, mitochondria, and endoplasmic reticulum, which support cell growth but do not contribute to mechanical work. These noncontractile elements are gradually replaced with increasingly organized myofibrils in the first several months of extrauterine life as the left ventricle grows to meet the demands of the systemic circulation and becomes the dominant ventricular chamber.

### Innervation

The parasympathetic innervation of the heart is well established at birth, but the sympathetic nervous supply is incomplete.

The clinical implications of these observations are that a neonate's heart is less compliant and possesses a very limited ability to alter myocardial contractility; hence, stroke volume is relatively fixed.[24] Maintenance of the cardiac output primarily depends on sustaining a relatively high normal heart rate, which, coupled with the cited predominance of parasympathetic vagal activity in neonates, explains the abrupt onset of hypotension and poor systemic perfusion observed in response to hypoxemia or noxious stimulation.

### Heart Rate and Rhythm

The heart rate and cardiac output of the newborn (350 mL/kg/min) are considerably higher than in adults to compensate for the elevated $O_2$ consumption, metabolic rate, and limited myocardial contractility of the newborn. Despite the elevated neonatal heart rate and cardiac index, blood pressures of neonates are significantly lower than those of older patients, reflecting reduced systemic vascular resistance.[25] Table 56–2 indicates normally expected vital signs in neonates.

## THE KIDNEYS

### How Do They Differ?

The neonatal kidneys, like the heart and lungs, are functionally immature at birth and must continue to develop through-

**TABLE 56–2.** Normal Neonatal Vital Signs*

| Measurement | Premature | Term |
| --- | --- | --- |
| Heart rate (beats per minute) | 150 ± 30 | 140 ± 30 |
| Mean systolic blood pressure (mm Hg) | 55 ± 10 | 75 ± 10 |
| Mean diastolic blood pressure (mm Hg) | 40 ± 5 | 50 ± 8 |
| Respiratory rate (breaths per minute) | 40-70 | 35-60 |

*Significant variations may exist among and within individual neonates in the first hours and days of life.

out the first year of life to attain adult levels of efficiency. Significant differences are noted in neonatal renal blood flow, glomerular filtration rate (GFR), and tubular function, as reflected in urine concentrating ability. During gestation, the fetal kidneys receive 3% to 7% of the cardiac output. This amount provides growth and developmental needs and the formation of a small amount of urine, which in turn becomes an important constituent of the amniotic fluid.

In contrast, mature kidneys receive approximately 20% of the cardiac output, a level not achieved until 2 years of age. Renal blood flow increases rapidly in the first weeks of life as a result of mechanisms analogous to those in the pulmonary circulation at birth: increased cardiac output and mean arterial pressure and reduced renal vascular resistance.[26]

## Glomerular Development

The adult number of nephrons, and hence glomeruli, is achieved by the 34th week of gestation. For this reason, a neonate's observed GFR of 30% of the healthy adult value is due to reduced glomerular surface area, ultrafiltration pressure, and glomerular capillary permeability.[27] The GFR is 5 mL/min/m$^2$ at 28 weeks' gestational age, 12 mL/min/m$^2$ at 40 weeks, and 25 mL/min/m$^2$ by the end of the second postnatal week.[20] Adult rates of GFR are reached at approximately 1 year of age.

## Renal Tubular Development

The renal tubules, consisting of the proximal and distal convoluted tubules, loops of Henle, and collecting ducts, likewise demonstrate immature function at birth; premature infants at 30 weeks' gestational age can concentrate urine to an osmolarity only slightly greater than that of plasma. By 1 month of age, urine with a maximal osmolarity of 550 to 700 mOsm/L may be produced. Urine concentrating ability is therefore less than half that of the adult.[20] The clinical significance of this limitation is that neonates are more susceptible to dehydration when nonrenal water losses are increased.

Although a neonate's kidneys are widely reported to be obligate sodium losers, this "defect" seems to be present only in premature infants; healthy term infants not subjected to stresses such as hypoxia, hyperbilirubinemia, or intrinsic renal disease are capable of maintaining a positive sodium balance. They may, however, experience difficulty excreting an excessive sodium load.[26] The normally expected levels of serum electrolytes, blood urea nitrogen, and creatinine are listed in Table 56–3.

## HEAT LOSS

### Why Does It Occur?

The problems of maintaining normal body temperature and avoiding hypothermia are pervasive in the care of all neonates, particularly in the operating room and during transport. Although neonates possess central regulatory mechanisms that respond to body and environmental temperature fluctuations, a number of factors predispose to hypothermia. These include an increased ratio of body surface area to mass, increased minute ventilation, poor body insulation, and a limited ability to shiver and generate heat.

**TABLE 56–3.** Normal Neonatal Laboratory Values*

| Determination | Premature | Term |
| --- | --- | --- |
| *Arterial Blood Gases* | | |
| pH | 7.35-7.46 | 7.35-7.45 |
| Po$_2$ (mm Hg) | 45-75 | 50-80 |
| Pco$_2$ (mm Hg) | 27-45 | 30-40 |
| *Blood Chemistry* | | |
| Sodium (mEq/L) | 135-145 | 140-150 |
| Potassium (mEq/L) | 4.5-6.5 | 4.5-6.5 |
| Chloride (mEq/L) | 100-110 | 96-108 |
| Glucose (mg/dL) | 40-80 | 40-100 |
| Blood urea nitrogen (mg/dL) | 5-20 | 5-20 |
| Creatinine (mg/dL) | 0.5-1.5 | 0.3-1.2 |
| *Hematology* | | |
| Hemoglobin (g/dL) | 15-19 | 16-21 |
| Hematocrit (%) | 50-60 | 52-68 |
| Platelets (1000/mm$^3$) | 150-300 | 150-400 |

*Values reflect range of "normal" measurements at approximately 24 hours of life; significant variations may exist, depending on birth weight, source of blood sampled, and age at time of sample.

Heat loss occurs through four mechanisms: radiation, evaporation of water in the respiratory tract or from the skin surface, conduction, and convection. Failure to maintain reasonably normal body temperature often results in depression of organ system function, hypoperfusion acidosis, apnea, and interference with normal metabolic processes. Recommendations for preventing hypothermia are listed in Table 56–4.

### What Is Nonshivering Thermogenesis?

The phenomenon of nonshivering thermogenesis is a neonate's primary means of counteracting body heat loss.[28] This mechanism begins with the liberation of catecholamines (norepinephrine) as skin and mucosal temperatures decline. Norepinephrine induces the metabolism of fatty acids in a newborn's brown fat tissues, with resultant heat production.

## PREEXISTING MEDICAL CONDITIONS

Critically ill neonates often have preexisting medical conditions that may be related to the indication for surgery. To the extent that these processes may affect intraoperative management or, conversely, that anesthetic maneuvers may influence

**TABLE 56–4.** Recommendations for the Prevention of Hypothermia in Neonates During Anesthesia and Surgery

Warmed operating room*
Radiant heat lamp
Warming blanket or mattress
Humidified and warmed inspired gases
Warming of intravenous fluids and blood products
Warming of irrigating solutions
Covering exposed body parts with transparent plastic wrap
Covering acceptable body parts with heated, forced air blanket (eg, Bair Hugger)

*Ideally, the operating room temperature is set as close as possible to the neonate's thermoneutral zone (32°-37°C), the environmental temperature range in which oxygen consumption is minimized.

the course of disease, the anesthesiologist must have an understanding of neonatal medical conditions. Among others, these include persistent pulmonary hypertension of the newborn (PPHN), infant respiratory distress syndrome (IRDS), intraventricular hemorrhage (IVH), and anemia.

## What Is Persistent Pulmonary Hypertension of the Newborn?

In 1969, Gersony recognized a group of term infants with structurally normal hearts who became cyanotic with only mild respiratory distress shortly after birth.[29] These infants had the development or persistence of increased PVR that was equal to or greater than the systemic vascular resistance. Systemic hypoxemia often resulted because of right-to-left shunting of blood across persistent fetal pathways (the foramen ovale and ductus arteriosus). This pattern of shunting was reflected in the condition's original name, *persistent fetal circulation.* This name was subsequently changed to PPHN to describe more accurately the condition's pathophysiologic process and reflect the reality that the fetal circulation, which includes the umbilical vessels and placenta, no longer exists.[30] PPHN usually becomes apparent within the first day of extrauterine life in term or postterm newborns. One multicenter review of PPHN cited a prevalence of 1.9 per 1000 live births. Despite significant variation in treatment practices among centers, there was no significant difference in mortality rates among centers, with an overall mortality rate with PPHN of 11%.[31]

## What Factors Contribute to Neonatal Pulmonary Hypertension?

Several factors that are at least partially under the control of the anesthesiologist in the perioperative period may trigger or sustain the elevation in PVR and the ensuing worsening cycle of increased hypoxemia, right-to-left shunting, and congestive heart failure. They include acidemia, hypoxemia, hypercarbia, hypothermia, polycythemia, hypoglycemia, hypomagnesemia, and hypocalcemia.[32,33] These factors are more important with respect to transiently elevated pulmonary pressures than persistently elevated values.[30]

## What Clinical Disorders Are Associated With Persistent Pulmonary Hypertension of the Newborn?

A large number of clinical disorders or perinatal insults may be associated with PPHN. These can be categorized into three groups according to their presumed cause[30]:

1. Normal pulmonary vascular development with active pulmonary vasoconstriction in response to a stimulus, such as an infectious process or perinatal aspiration syndrome
2. True maldevelopment of the pulmonary vessels, which may be idiopathic or precipitated by factors such as chronic intrauterine asphyxia or the meconium aspiration syndrome
3. Underdevelopment of the lung, with decreased vessel number or reduced pulmonary artery cross-sectional area, as in congenital diaphragmatic hernia (CDH)

## What Are the Physical Findings in Persistent Pulmonary Hypertension of the Newborn?

Physical findings in newborns with PPHN include tachypnea, central cyanosis, prominent right ventricular impulse and loud pulmonary component ($P_2$) of the second heart sound, normal or decreased peripheral pulses, and normal systemic blood pressure until the late stages of congestive heart failure.[34] Diagnosis is made on the basis of the clinical setting; physical examination; demonstration of ductal right-to-left shunting with at least a 10 mm Hg stepdown in $Pao_2$ from the right arm (usually preductal) to the descending aorta or lower extremities (postductal)[35]; echocardiography; and, in a few cases, cardiac catheterization. Echocardiography should be a part of the diagnostic evaluation in all infants suspected of having PPHN to rule out cyanotic congenital heart disease, document right-to-left shunting at the ductus and foramen ovale, and measure systolic time intervals.[30]

## How Is Persistent Pulmonary Hypertension of the Newborn Managed?

Initial therapies for PPHN involve correcting any potentially transient causes or exacerbating factors, while addressing associated disease processes. General goals include lowering the pulmonary arterial pressure, maintenance of systemic blood pressure, reversal of right-to-left shunts, and improved arterial and tissue oxygenation. In general, a target $Pao_2$ of 80 to 100 mm Hg is recommended, with no evidence of improved outcome but the possibility of increased $O_2$ toxicity with $Pao_2$ >100 mm Hg.[36] Conservative medical management of these infants may reduce the need for extracorporeal membrane oxygenation (ECMO) and improve outcome.[37,38]

### Mechanical Ventilation

If conservative measures fail, mechanical ventilation with positive end-expiratory pressure (PEEP) should provide some alveolar recruitment and improve oxygenation.[39] Sedation, usually with opioids, frequently is used to minimize the neonate's sensitivity to external stimuli. The use of muscle relaxants is controversial because they may lead to alveolar collapse in the dependent regions of the lungs and should probably be reserved for infants requiring high inspiratory pressures.[30,39] The next step is to induce respiratory alkalosis. Alternative ventilatory modes such as high-frequency jet ventilation (HFJV) and high-frequency oscillatory ventilation (HFOV) have been used in infants with PPHN. HFJV has been found to lower both $Paco_2$ and ventilatory pressures, but to have no effect on outcome.[40] HFOV was not found to reduce the need for ECMO in these infants.[41] As long as adequate ventilation is ensured, metabolic alkalosis may be induced with a continuous infusion of sodium bicarbonate.[42]

### Drugs

Pharmacologic measures to reduce PVR may be required. Surfactant deficiency plays a role in some of the disease processes that lead to PPHN, and although the application of exogenous surfactant makes empiric sense, its use in PPHN is still considered experimental.[30] The vasodilator tolazoline was historically the most commonly used drug to dilate the pulmonary vascular bed. However, its effects on the vasculature are not specific to the pulmonary circulation, and the agent's systemic effects frequently lead to an unacceptably high incidence of hypotension-related complications. Tolazoline is now rarely used to treat PPHN.[30] Other pharmacologic agents including magnesium, adenosine triphosphate-MgCl$_2$, prostacyclin, and prostaglandin D$_2$, have been tried without proven results in infants with PPHN.[30]

Nitric oxide (NO) has been shown selectively to dilate the pulmonary vasculature and improve oxygenation in infants with PPHN.[43] In a randomized, controlled study of 235 term infants with PPHN, NO did result in a reduction in the need for ECMO. However, its use did not alter the mortality rate, probably because all infants who failed medical management were placed on ECMO.[44] Many patients with PPHN do respond to NO therapy, but the response appears to be variable, with respect both to individual patients and different clinical centers.[45]

## Advanced Therapy

Infants with PPHN and otherwise refractory respiratory failure may be considered for ECMO therapy. Of course ECMO is invasive, costly, and carries its own morbidity. ECMO use is usually considered when the underlying disease process is potentially reversible and has an expected mortality rate of at least 80%.[46] Survival rates in infants treated with ECMO for a variety of underlying disease processes are as follows: meconium aspiration, 93%; sepsis, 76%; idiopathic PPHN, 83%; and CDG, 58%.[47] Surgical ligation of a patent ductus arteriosus (PDA) in PPHN with right-to-left shunting is not indicated and may precipitate acute right ventricular failure.[48]

## What Is Infant Respiratory Distress Syndrome?

IRDS, often referred to as *hyaline membrane disease*, is principally a disorder of premature infants.

### Pathogenesis

IRDS is caused by a deficiency of pulmonary surfactant, which is a mixture of phospholipids (lecithin and sphingomyelin) and proteins produced by type II pneumocytes. Surfactant reduces surface tension at the air-water interface in the alveoli. A deficiency leads to alveolar and small airways collapse at end-expiration, preventing maintenance of the FRC necessary for gas exchange and resulting in hypoxemia and acidemia. With atelectasis and airway collapse, pulmonary compliance is reduced and the work of breathing is increased; the highly compliant neonatal chest wall, described earlier, makes efforts to expand the lungs and maintain FRC even more difficult. Hypoxemia and acidemia lead to pulmonary hypertension and vasoconstriction, which further reduce surfactant production in a circuitous fashion.

### Clinical Presentation

This syndrome is noted in premature infants in the first hours of life, particularly after perinatal asphyxia, maternal diabetes mellitus, or cesarean delivery. The incidence is reduced after "stressful pregnancies" (hypertension, infection), maternal drug addiction, and the administration of corticosteroids to the mother during pregnancy.[20] Physical signs include tachypnea, nasal flaring, grunting, and chest wall retractions. Breath sounds are often reduced.[49] Arterial blood gas analysis reveals hypoxemia and acidemia, which commonly is both respiratory (hypercarbia) and metabolic in origin. Chest radiography demonstrates the classic ground-glass appearance, with scattered air bronchograms throughout both lungs.

### Operating Room Problems

Neonates who have IRDS and who require a surgical procedure typically present with hypoxemia, increased O$_2$ requirement, hypercarbia, and reduced pulmonary compliance. Oxygenation and ventilation represent an added challenge to the usual problems of caring for premature infants, particularly if the ventilator or breathing circuit used is different from that in the NICU. For unstable patients or neonates with advanced ventilatory requirements, consider using the NICU ventilator in the operating room for the surgical procedure or accomplishing the procedure in the NICU if possible.

Infants with IRDS commonly require longer inspiratory times and higher levels of inspiratory pressure and PEEP to achieve optimal oxygenation and ventilation. Each of these maneuvers increases mean airway pressure, which is variable but optimal at approximately 12 to 14 cm H$_2$O in patients with IRDS.[20]

### Exogenous Surfactant

Research has focused on administering exogenous surfactant materials to premature infants, either at birth or with the onset of respiratory distress.[50] Surfactant replacement therapy, which improves oxygenation and pulmonary compliance within minutes, can significantly alter the course of IRDS and may result in a reduction of complications, including barotrauma, bronchopulmonary dysplasia (BPD), and pulmonary interstitial emphysema.

## What Is Intraventricular Hemorrhage?

IVH refers to bleeding that begins around the capillaries of the subependymal germinal matrix and may then extend to the ventricles and brain parenchyma.[51] Neonatal vessels in the brain appear to possess several characteristics and distribution factors that may predispose them to disruption. Parenchymal hemorrhagic necrosis occurring in association with germinal matrix hemorrhage or IVH, once thought to be caused by extension of the intraventricular bleed, may actually result from a separate process of venous infarction in the white matter.[52,53]

IVH occurs most commonly in premature infants but may also develop in severely asphyxiated term infants. Before the advent of computed tomographic scanning and intracranial sonography, the diagnosis of IVH was based on clinical findings of abrupt-onset hypotension, acute anemia, metabolic acidosis, full fontanel, apnea and bradycardia, altered sensorium, and seizures.[52] Noninvasive computed tomographic and ultrasound (US) scanning have demonstrated that many cases are asymptomatic and that as many as 90% of very low-birth-weight infants have IVH at some point in the first hours or days of life.[54,55] On the basis of US examination of the head, IVH may be graded according to the following scheme[20]:

**Grade I.** Hemorrhage in germinal matrix only
**Grade II.** Blood fills lateral ventricle
**Grade III.** Grade II plus ventricle distended
**Grade IV.** Parenchyma involved

### Predisposing Factors

Several factors in addition to prematurity are thought to increase risk. Experimentally, intraventricular hemorrhages have been produced in the wake of reperfusion after induced hypotension and hypovolemia. Autoregulation of cerebral perfusion may also be impaired in neonates, placing them at increased risk of intracerebral bleeds with increases in blood pressure. Other conditions thought to be associated with IVH include increased venous pressure, asphyxia, pneumothorax, and IRDS.

Procedures such as tracheal suctioning, awake intubation, and poorly synchronized mechanical ventilation during spontaneous breathing have been associated with significant intracranial hypertension in premature neonates, and may therefore predispose to the development of IVH.[56,57] Rapid volume expansion and hypercapnia may also increase cerebral blood flow and thereby potentially cause IVH.[52] Not surprisingly, medications that interfere with the blood coagulation cascade may also predispose to IVH. Of interest is a pilot report suggesting that preemptive analgesia with a continuous morphine infusion may reduce the incidence of poor neurologic outcome (including IVH) in preterm neonates.[4]

### Anesthetic Contribution

Anesthesiologists who encounter a neonate with documented IVH or one who is at risk for development of IVH should attempt to use an anesthetic regimen, ventilator therapy, and a fluid management plan that minimizes the potential for abrupt changes in cerebral blood flow and intracranial pressure. Although an open anterior fontanel may help to protect against intracranial pressure elevations, wide fluctuations in arterial blood pressure during light anesthesia or stimulation are apt to be transmitted to the relatively fragile vasculature of the neonatal germinal matrix, with the potential for resulting hemorrhage. Correction of acid-base abnormalities, coagulation defects, and hypothermia is also important.[54]

### *Why Does Anemia Occur?*

Healthy term neonates are born with a mean umbilical cord hemoglobin of 16.8 g/dL, whereas preterm infants younger than 34 weeks' gestational age have somewhat lower mean values, in the range of 15 to 16 g/dL.[58] An occasional healthy neonate is born with a hemoglobin as high as 20 g/dL. With birth and exposure to the $O_2$-rich environment of extrauterine life, erythropoiesis in the neonatal marrow comes to a virtual standstill.

Hemoglobin in term newborns typically reaches a nadir of 9.0 to 11.0 g/dL in the third month of life, whereas premature infants may experience even lower hemoglobin concentrations within a shorter period.[59] In addition to this "physiologic"

anemia, critically ill neonates may become anemic with consequent reductions in $O_2$-carrying capacity as a result of sepsis, hemolytic processes, nutritional deficiencies, and repeated blood sampling for laboratory studies.

### Fetal and Adult Hemoglobin

Normally, the onset of physiologic anemia of early infancy is not accompanied by clinical evidence of tissue $O_2$ deficits because fetal hemoglobin, which has a relatively high $O_2$ affinity ($P_{50} = 19$ mm Hg), is being replaced by adult hemoglobin. Fetal hemoglobin differs from normal adult hemoglobin in that it has two $\alpha$ and two $\gamma$ globin chains, whereas adult hemoglobin has two $\alpha$ and two $\beta$ chains. Fetal hemoglobin comprises 60% to 80% of all hemoglobin at term birth, but by 4 to 5 months of age, constitutes only 3% of newly synthesized hemoglobin.[60] Adult hemoglobin has a lower $O_2$ affinity, as reflected in its $P_{50}$ value of approximately 27 mm Hg, implying that it more readily releases $O_2$ to the tissues (Fig. 56–4). When one or more of the anemia-inducing processes mentioned earlier compounds normal, physiologic anemia, a neonate may manifest the clinical signs and problems of tachypnea, tachycardia, poor weight gain, apnea, bradycardia, pallor, and lethargy.[61]

### The Minimally Acceptable Hemoglobin

Until the 1990s, common practice in NICUs was to maintain hemoglobin values of at least 12 to 13 g/dL. Although some investigations supported the notion that transfusions improve the symptoms of anemia, particularly the incidence of apnea/bradycardia spells, others failed to demonstrate any consistent benefit of red blood cell transfusions.[61,62]

Concerns about the transmission of blood-borne infectious diseases have cast doubt on the wisdom of routinely transfusing neonates to achieve some arbitrary hemoglobin or hemato-

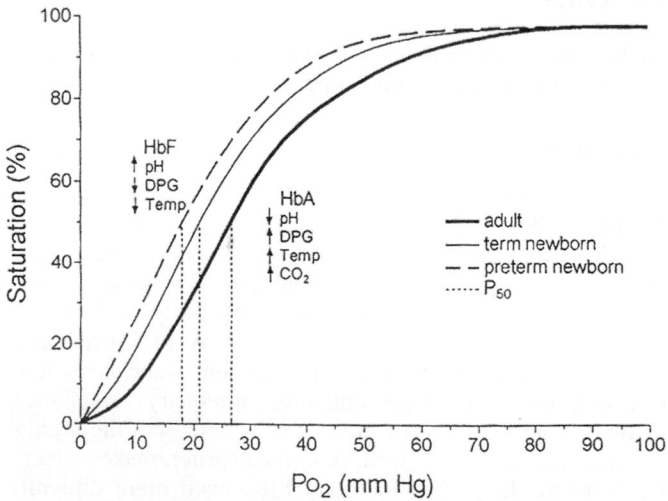

**FIGURE 56–4.** The oxygen dissociation curve of hemoglobin at different stages of development. The approximate $P_{50}$ (ie, oxygen tension at which the hemoglobin is 50% saturated) of adult blood is 27 mm Hg, that of a term newborn infant is 22 mm Hg, and that of a preterm newborn is 18 mm Hg. The heterotropic modifiers of hemoglobin function shown can increase (leftward shift) or decrease (rightward shift) hemoglobin oxygen affinity. (From Bard H. Hemoglobin synthesis and metabolism during the neonatal period. In: Christensen RD, ed. *Hematologic Problems of the Neonate.* Philadelphia, Pa: WB Saunders; 2000:375.)

crit value. The neonatal patient should never be transfused on the basis of hemoglobin concentration alone.[59] However, Welborn and colleagues showed that former preterm infants with hematocrit values of 25% to 30% were much more likely to experience postoperative apnea than those with a hematocrit >30%.[63]

Nevertheless, rigid and arbitrary requirements for preoperative hemoglobin values in neonates seem inappropriate; rather, each case should be approached on an individual basis, considering factors such as an infant's gestational and postconceptual ages, anticipated blood loss, history of apnea/bradycardia spells, and provisions for postoperative monitoring.

## Transfusion Guidelines

In general, severely anemic neonates or former premature infants should be transfused if their preoperative hematocrit is <25%. Above this level, it is reasonable to proceed with minimal blood loss procedures, but all caregivers should be aware that the infant may be more likely to experience postoperative apnea; therefore, appropriate monitoring with pulse oximetry, capnography, and an electrocardiogram (ECG) must be provided. To the extent that surgery in neonates or former premature infants in the first months of life is seldom purely elective, the possibility of postponing surgery is not often a practical option.

## RETINOPATHY OF PREMATURITY

### What Is It?

Retinopathy of prematurity (ROP) was formerly known as *retrolental fibroplasia*, a descriptive term that applies only to a subset of patients with advanced ROP. It is a disorder characterized by abnormal proliferation of small retinal vessels. As its name implies, ROP is almost exclusively a disease of premature infants (<37 weeks' gestational age), although a number of other factors have been associated with it, including low birth weight, $O_2$ therapy, shock, sepsis, poor nutritional status, and ambient light exposure.[64] The incidence and severity of ROP appear to have declined sharply in the 1990s because of factors such as exogenous surfactant use, continuous pulse oximetry, use of maternal antenatal steroids, and improved neonatal nutrition.[65,66]

### How Does It Develop?

Although the exact role of these factors in the pathogenesis of ROP is unclear, the fundamental problem appears to be that at the time of a premature birth, vascularization of the retina is incomplete; a variable area of the peripheral retina is avascular. At some point in early postnatal life, the delicately growing vessels at the margin of vascular development sustain an injury related to the previously mentioned factors. Vascularization of the remaining retina must then be accomplished through a repair response rather than normal angiogenesis (Fig. 56–5). Abnormal vessel proliferation, retinal hemorrhage, scarring, and detachment may result. Possible sequelae of ROP include myopia, strabismus, glaucoma, amblyopia, and blindness.[67]

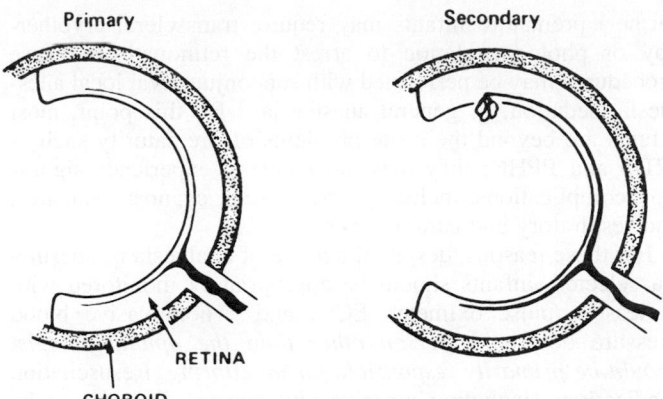

**FIGURE 56–5.** The mechanism of oxygen in retinopathy of prematurity. The primary response of vasoconstriction of the anterior retinal vessels and the later proliferation of remaining vascular components are demonstrated. (From Patz A. Retinopathy of prematurity. In: Tasman WS, Jaeger EA, eds. *Duane's Clinical Ophthalmology*. Vol 3. Philadelphia, Pa: JB Lippincott; 1990:3.)

### What Is the Role of Oxygen Therapy?

An understanding of ROP is essential for anesthesiologists because of the likely influence of $O_2$ therapy (specifically, hyperoxygenation) on the pathogenesis of the disease and because affected infants may require monitoring and sedation or a general anesthetic for retinal cryoablation or laser photocoagulation.

$O_2$ therapy is only one of many contributing factors in ROP, although it is one of the most widely recognized and one of the few that can be controlled. $O_2$ involvement in ROP is confused by the observation that many premature infants who receive it never have the problem, but others, including some term infants never exposed to $O_2$ supplementation, contract the disease.[68] After $O_2$ was first implicated in the early 1950s, therapy was widely restricted, and exposure for premature infants was limited to 40% $O_2$ or less.[69] By the 1960s, although the incidence of ROP had fallen sharply, the problem of brain damage and death among premature infants had become more significant. In fact, for every case of ROP blindness prevented, 16 infants were estimated to have died in the United States.[70]

### What Are Oxygen Administration Guidelines?

Attempts to define a "safe" level or duration of supplemental $O_2$ exposure have been unsuccessful.[71] Under optimal and stable conditions, it has been suggested that $O_2$ and ventilatory therapy should maintain the preductal (right arm) $PaO_2$ between 50 and 80 mm Hg and the pulse oximetric $O_2$ saturation ($SpO_2$) between 85% and 92% until 44 weeks of conceptual age when the retinal vasculature is mature.[72] However, because of rapid changes in the level of arterial oxygenation during surgical procedures, it is reasonable to allow some safety margin with $SpO_2$ values as high as 95%. During periods of airway manipulation (bronchoscopy, intubation) or profound hemodynamic instability, 100% $O_2$ should be provided even if it induces short periods of hyperoxygenation.[57]

### What Are the Anesthetic Implications?

Because 4 to 6 weeks normally must pass for ROP to become evident on ophthalmoscopic examination, older (or former) premature infants may require transscleral cryotherapy or photocoagulation to arrest the retinopathy.[73] These procedures may be performed with subconjunctival local anesthesia, sedation, or general anesthesia.[74] By this point, most infants are beyond the acute problems of prematurity such as IRDS and PPHN; they may, nonetheless, experience significant complications, including bradycardia, cyanosis, seizures, and respiratory and cardiac arrest.[75]

For these reasons, despite the mode of analgesia or anesthesia selected, infants should be appropriately monitored with at least a pulse oximeter, ECG, and a noninvasive blood pressure device. *A person other than the ophthalmologist should be primarily responsible for monitoring.* Resuscitation medications, including atropine and epinephrine, should be readily available in addition to equipment for airway support and positive-pressure ventilation.

## ANESTHETIC PROBLEMS OF FORMER PREMATURE INFANTS

The dramatically increased survival rate of premature neonates since the early 1980s has resulted in greater numbers of former premature infants presenting for surgical procedures. These patients have been demonstrated to be at higher risk of perioperative complications than term infants, and several scoring systems have been proposed to quantitate this risk.[76–78] Table 56–5 outlines the major anesthetic considerations that may apply to former premature infants. Most perioperative complications in this group are related to the airway and respiratory systems and include apnea, atelectasis, and aspiration.

---

**TABLE 56–5.** Anesthetic Considerations in Former Premature Infants

---

**Effects of Chronic Organ System Dysfunction**

*Pulmonary*

Chronic lung disease; bronchopulmonary dysplasia
Recurrent pneumonias
Chronic aspiration (secondary to gastroesophageal reflux)

*Cardiac*

Persistent patent ductus arteriosus
Cardiomyopathy

*Central Nervous System*

Delayed development
Impaired respiratory and cardiovascular reflexes
Apnea
Seizures
Hydrocephalus
Retinopathy of prematurity

**Airway Management Problems**

Subglottic stenosis
Tracheobronchomalacia
Impaired airway reflexes

**Metabolic/Fluid Management Problems**

Poor nutritional status
Tendency toward hypoglycemia
Fragile bones, joints, and tissues
Relative hypovolemia secondary to chronic fluid restriction and diuretics
Difficult venous or arterial access
Increased disposition to hypothermia (reduced amounts of brown fat and subcutaneous tissue)

---

## What Is Bronchopulmonary Dysplasia?

The diagnosis of BPD, as originally described by Northway in 1967, required a history of chronic ventilatory support combined with specific radiologic changes in the chest. The definition of BPD has continued to evolve as more is learned about the disease process. One definition refers to BPD as any respiratory sequelae in an infant who reaches 36 weeks' postconceptual age but remains hospitalized because of continued $O_2$ or mechanical ventilator support or is discharged on such therapy.[79]

The cause of BPD appears to be multifactorial, but implicated factors include $O_2$ toxicity, volutrauma or barotrauma, endotracheal intubation, and sepsis.[80] BPD is thought to result from a disturbed repair process after pulmonary tissue injury, with the likely involvement of chemical mediators in the inflammatory cascade.[81] Infants with BPD may demonstrate hypoxemia, hypercarbia, reactive airways disease, and increased PVR. Treatment includes the use of antenatal steroids in mothers at risk for premature delivery, exogenous surfactant after delivery, assisted ventilation with the lowest possible airway pressures to minimize barotrauma, and judicious fluid management.

Infants with known BPD respond to furosemide, inhaled bronchodilators, and steroids, although the long-term risk-benefit ratio of these therapies remains uncertain.[80] Infants with BPD are particularly sensitive to fluid overload and tend to have an increased incidence of lower respiratory tract infections and airway hyperreactivity. The most severe result of BPD is chronic pulmonary hypertension and cor pulmonale. The overall mortality rate of BPD is 10%.[79]

## What Is the Significance of Postanesthetic Apnea?

Postanesthetic apnea in the former premature infant has been thought to be due to immaturity of central respiratory control, although the distinctions between central, obstructive, and mixed apnea are becoming less obvious as evidence suggesting similar underlying pathophysiologic processes accumulates.[82]

The occurrence of postoperative apnea in infants recovering from general anesthesia for minor procedures was first described in 1982.[76] Since then, a number of studies have attempted to determine the risk factors for postanesthetic apnea and to delineate the age beyond which the risk of apnea should no longer be of concern. Isolated reports of postoperative apnea in otherwise healthy *term* infants have been published.[83,84] Even in the absence of anesthesia and surgery, a baseline incidence of apneic episodes >15 seconds' duration occurs in approximately 60% of premature infants.[85] Recommended postconceptual ages that define the upper limit below which the former premature infant is at increased risk of postanesthetic apnea have ranged from 44 to 60 weeks.[86,87] Siblings of infants who were victims of sudden infant death syndrome are probably not at increased risk of postanesthetic apnea.[88]

Because of the relatively broad range of recommended cutoff ages defining an increased risk of postanesthetic apnea, the selection of an age for a given institution or practitioner is in part arbitrary and must be based on the experience and comfort level of the anesthesiologist and the degree of risk he or she is willing to tolerate. However, as with other anesthetic questions that lack clear, objective answers (eg, minimum fasting intervals before elective surgery), it is frequently necessary for the anesthesiologists in a given department or institution to arrive at some consensus that drives practice and policy.

An important study published in 1995 reported the results of a combined analysis of all patients reported in earlier investigations of postanesthetic apnea in infants. Conclusions of this analysis were as follows:

- The occurrence of apnea is strongly and inversely related to gestational and postconceptual age.
- Apnea continuing at home is an associated risk factor.
- Small-for-gestational age infants appear to be relatively *protected* from apnea compared with larger infants.
- Anemia is a significant additional risk factor, especially in infants >43 weeks' postconceptual age.
- A relationship between postanesthetic apnea and a history of necrotizing enterocolitis (NEC), neonatal apnea, IRDS, BPD, or operative use of opioids or muscle relaxants could not be demonstrated.

This study reported that the risk of apnea in nonanemic infants who are free of apnea in the postanesthesia care unit is not less than 1% (with 95% statistical confidence) until the postconceptual age was 56 weeks with a gestational age of 32 weeks, or a postconceptual age of 54 weeks with a gestational age of 35 weeks.[89]

### Postoperative Apnea Monitoring

Postanesthetic apnea is most likely to appear within the first 12 hours after anesthesia, although it has been reported as late as 48 hours after surgery. Monitoring for at least 12 (preferably 24) hours after anesthesia on an inpatient or "observation" status should be provided for all former premature infants below the predetermined cutoff age; at the authors' institution, the cutoff is 52 weeks' postconceptual age for infants born before 37 weeks' gestation. At a minimum, monitoring should include an apnea/bradycardia monitor and pulse oximeter in a clinical setting with personnel capable of dealing with periodic breathing and overt apnea episodes.

### Prevention

Intravenous caffeine base, 10 mg/kg intraoperatively, appears to stimulate central respiratory control centers and minimize or eliminate the incidence of apnea in patients at risk.[90] Another preparation of caffeine, caffeine benzoate, may be more readily available and is typically administered in a dose of 20 mg/kg. Other agents that have been used to treat or provide prophylaxis against apnea are theophylline and doxapram.[91] Regional anesthesia may lessen the risks of perioperative respiratory complications and shorten the hospital stay, although infants have experienced apnea after regional anesthesia.[92,93] A recent correspondence found no difference in postoperative apnea in infants undergoing either spinal or general anesthesia.[94]

## PREOPERATIVE FASTING GUIDELINES

Many surgical procedures in neonates are performed on an urgent or emergent basis. This fact, in combination with the knowledge that neonatal disease and surgical disorders often interfere with gastric emptying and normal gastrointestinal function, mandates that most neonates be considered to have a full stomach regardless of the time since the last oral intake.

### *What Is the Appropriate NPO Interval?*

There is no set of universally accepted fasting guidelines for neonates in North America, the United Kingdom and Ireland, or, for that matter, the rest of the world.[95] For cases in which surgery is scheduled semielectively or electively, formula administered by mouth or gavage should be withheld for 4 to 6 hours and clear fluids such as dextrose in water solutions for 2 hours before the anticipated time of induction of anesthesia.[57,96] In determining the fasting interval, the anesthesiologist must consider the risk of dehydration and hypoglycemia on the one hand and the possibility of increasing the volume of gastric contents and thereby increasing the potential for regurgitation and aspiration on the other. Because human breast milk passes through the stomach more rapidly than does formula, some practitioners allow breast milk up to 2 to 3 hours before surgery.[97] However, most pediatric anesthesiologists surveyed in recent years require 4 hours of fasting after a breast milk feeding.[98,99]

### Modifying Factors

Neonates with disorders known to delay gastric emptying should be fasted for longer periods if the surgical condition allows. An intravenous infusion of 5% dextrose in quarter normal saline at a rate of 4 mL/kg/h should be instituted to prevent hypoglycemia and the development of an excessive fluid deficit. A similar practice is recommended for any neonatal surgical patient who is not otherwise at increased risk of aspiration and in whom the time of anesthetic induction is not known or delayed.

## PREMEDICATION

Premedication, for practical purposes in the neonate, is limited to anticholinergic agents. The goals of premedication in older children and adults, including anxiolysis, sedation, and preoperative amnesia, appear to have no application in neonates because separation anxiety does not become an issue until approximately 6 to 9 months of age. The stress of separation and invasive procedures may influence later behavior such as feeding patterns and sleep cycles, but no evidence shows that preoperative sedation alters such effects.[100]

### *What Are the Desired Effects?*

The anticholinergics atropine, glycopyrrolate, and scopolamine blunt the vagal cardiovascular responses to laryngoscopy, nasogastric suctioning, the potent inhalation anesthetics, and succinylcholine. Other effects of these drugs include drying of oral secretions, reduced gastric fluid volume and acidity, and sedation (atropine and scopolamine).[101]

Considerable variation exists with respect to the dosage, route of administration, and timing of premedication with these drugs. Although oral administration of atropine has achieved some popularity in older infants and toddlers, in the neonatal period, the anticholinergics are given intramuscularly, subcutaneously, or intravenously.[83] The dose of atropine is 10 to 20 μg/kg intravenously and 20 μg/kg intramuscularly or subcutaneously (minimum total dose of 100 μg, or 0.1 mg). The dose of glycopyrrolate is 5 to 10 μg/kg intravenously and 10 to 15 μg/kg intramuscularly.

## What Side Effects May Occur?

A number of potential drawbacks should be considered. These include the drying of lower respiratory tract secretions and the possibility that an ETT or lower natural airway may become plugged; persistent tachycardia; and elevation of body temperature due to the inhibition of sweating. Historically, the routine preoperative use of anticholinergics was often questioned because their administration could mask hypoxemia with its attendant bradycardia. The widespread use of pulse oximetry today largely has eliminated this concern.

## AIRWAY MANAGEMENT

The techniques of airway management are based on the anatomic and physiologic features discussed previously. In addition to the specifics concerning tracheal intubation, controversial issues include whether all neonates require intubation for general anesthesia and the practice of awake versus anesthetized intubation.

### Should Neonates Be Intubated Routinely?

Numerous justifications are offered for routine intubation of neonates who require general anesthesia. These include assurance of airway patency, reduction of dead space compared with mask ventilation, decreased likelihood of gastric distention and aspiration, and facilitated control of ventilation.

Is mask general anesthesia acceptable for neonates? Nearly every anesthesiologist has been faced with a vigorous, healthy term neonate who requires an anesthetic for a very brief procedure, such as suture removal after cleft lip repair, or probing and dilation of urethral meatal stenosis. In such cases, depending on the skill of the individual practitioner, mask anesthesia is a suitable alternative. Maintenance of spontaneous ventilation with occasional assisted breaths helps to avoid excessively deep anesthesia and the hemodynamic derangements that accompany it. In most cases, however, tracheal intubation carries very low morbidity, and its advantages greatly exceed its disadvantages.[102]

### Should the Trachea Be Intubated Before or After Anesthesia Induction?

In the past, conventional neonatal anesthetic practice dictated that many newborns undergo intubation while awake. This practice has been justified on the basis of immaturity of airway protective reflexes; the rapidity with which oxyhemoglobin desaturation and hemodynamic instability develop in neonates once the airway is lost; and the fear that neonates may tolerate inhalation or intravenous induction poorly before securing the airway.

On the other hand, concern has existed since at least the mid-1980s over additional airway trauma, arterial hypertension, and the potential for intracranial hemorrhage, especially in premature infants, when awake intubation is accomplished.[103,104] Many practitioners also believe that newborns should be afforded the same benefit of anesthesia during this painful and stressful procedure as would older children or adults.[105] There are certainly instances in which "awake" intubation is clearly preferred, as in adults, such as during cardiopulmonary resuscitation, in situations involving profound hemodynamic instability, or when the airway is already compromised and mask ventilation is expected to be difficult or impossible. However, the trend in clinical practice appears to be toward the provision of sedation or anesthesia before elective intubation, such as occurs in the operating room.[106]

### What Techniques and Equipment Are Applicable?

Intubation requires an appropriately sized ETT and laryngoscope; the means to deliver positive-pressure ventilation with $O_2$; suction apparatus; appropriate monitoring devices; medications including atropine, succinylcholine, and an intravenous anesthetic; and, whenever possible, a skilled assistant. So-called deep intubation under inhalation anesthesia without a muscle relaxant is possible in the neonate but requires considerable skill and experience to avoid excessive hypotension or bradycardia or precipitation of laryngospasm during the attempt at ETT insertion.[107]

After intravenous induction, preoxygenation should be provided with 100% $O_2$ and a secure mask fit before intubation. Most practitioners prefer straight laryngoscope blades (usually Miller 0 or 1) because they provide better glottic visibility and occupy less space in the mouth.

#### Endotracheal Tubes

ETTs are commonly made of clear polyvinylchloride and should be nontapered and uncuffed. A selection above and below the anticipated required size should be available. Small premature infants <1000 g frequently require a tube of 2.5 mm inside diameter (ID), but most larger premature and term neonates accommodate 3.0-mm ID tubes. An occasional large term infant may require a 3.5-mm ID tube.

The range of clinically appropriate ETT lengths in neonates is from 7 cm (gum to midtrachea distance) in 1000-g premature infants to 10 cm in term newborns.[108] ETTs typically are considerably longer; shortening them to 2 to 3 cm beyond the anticipated depth at the gum or alveolar ridge reduces the dead space and resistance to gas flow and the tendency for narrow tubes to kink. Making the cut at an oblique angle facilitates reattaching the ETT-breathing circuit adapter.

Conventional anesthetic practice dictates that an audible leak should be detectable at <30 cm $H_2O$ peak airway pressure; otherwise, the tracheal mucosal perfusion pressure is exceeded and tissue ischemia may develop, with the potential for subglottic edema and delayed subglottic stenosis.[109] If the leak is too great (occurring at <10 cm $H_2O$ pressure), effective positive-pressure ventilation may be difficult, necessitating insertion of a larger ETT.

## INTRAOPERATIVE VENTILATION

### Should Manual or Mechanical Techniques Be Used?

How neonatal surgical patients should be ventilated entails the issues of manual versus mechanical support, the various available breathing circuits, the choice of ventilator, and appropriate ventilator settings. In practice, a combination of manual and mechanical ventilation is frequently used, as in older children and adults. Traditionally, manual ventilation in the newborn had been most strongly advocated as the principal means of ventilatory support, and certainly there are specific patients and points during an operative procedure when manual ventilation is required. However, today's improved anesthesia and ICU ventilators have made the effective intraoperative mechanical ventilation of the neonate more achievable and practical, thereby freeing the anesthesiologist's hands for other tasks.

### Manual

The primary justification for this practice is that ventilation by hand allows rapid detection of the acute changes in compliance and resistance encountered during neonatal surgery and compensation for these changes. That manual ventilation or the use of an "educated hand" measures up to this claim and is superior to mechanical ventilation has been questioned.[110,111]

### Mechanical

Mechanical techniques are capable of predictable and constant ventilation over time (although this advantage is never guaranteed) and free the anesthesia practitioner's hands to perform other duties. Of course, if a change in ventilation is detected by the continuous assessment of breath sounds and chest movement or readings of monitoring devices, manual ventilation can be immediately restored.[112]

The important points to recall are that a means of providing manual ventilation must always be available and the limitations of the specific breathing circuit and ventilator in use must be understood. Regardless of whether a neonate is ventilated by manual or mechanical means, changes in lung-thorax compliance can significantly alter the actual tidal volume because of the compliance and compression volume of the breathing circuit as well as the leak around the uncuffed tube.

### How Should Mechanical Ventilation Be Administered?

Several alternatives are available to provide mechanical ventilation in the operating room. In very small premature infants (<1000 g) and patients with significant IRDS or labile oxygenation and ventilation due to any cause, an attractive option is to use the ventilator, mode, and settings that are being used in the NICU. This normally restricts the anesthesiologist to the use of intravenous agents (opioids, barbiturates,

muscle relaxants), which is seldom a problem because most of these patients continue to require mechanical ventilation after surgery. During the procedure, particularly if it involves the thorax or abdomen, ventilatory and $O_2$ requirements may frequently change, and the anesthesiologist should be prepared to provide manual ventilation or changes in mechanical ventilator settings. If the patient has been receiving some form of high-frequency ventilation, particularly HFOV, it is usually necessary temporarily to revert to conventional ventilation during the procedure.

The volume-limited (or preset) ventilators found on most anesthesia machines can also be effectively used in most cases. For neonates, it is necessary to recognize that the set and measured tidal volumes on the anesthesia machine are only rough guides to effective ventilation. The authors' approach is initially to set the excursion volume of the ventilator bellows to its minimum setting. The set tidal volume (or minute ventilation) is then gradually increased as the fresh gas flow and inspiratory-to-expiratory time (I:E) ratio are adjusted to provide adequate tidal volume based on patient observation and monitoring variables. The age and size of the patient and any existing disease processes determine ventilatory rate.

### Settings and Strategy

A large number of variables can be adjusted to optimize oxygenation and ventilation, particularly if one of the newer and highly sophisticated ventilators normally found in the ICU is used. These include peak inspiratory pressure (PIP), inspiratory time, tidal volume, PEEP, rate, pressure support, inspired $O_2$ concentration ($FIO_2$), ventilation mode, and rate. There has been significant attention devoted to minimizing the potentially damaging effects of mechanical ventilation through the implementation of so-called lung-protective strategies. At best, defining lung protective strategies in neonates is difficult because of profound variation in stages of lung development and the characteristics of different disease processes. In general, the trend is toward the use of smaller tidal volumes, more frequent use of PEEP, tolerance of mild to moderate degrees of hypercapnia, and the use of adjuncts such as surfactant and oscillatory ventilation in the effort to reduce pulmonary damage and other multiple organ dysfunction.[113]

Although the ventilator settings are determined by the presence and stage of any cardiopulmonary disease processes, typical initial values include a PIP of 15 to 18 cm $H_2O$, tidal volume of 8 to 10 mL/kg, PEEP of 0 to 3 cm $H_2O$, ventilatory rate of 24 breaths per minute, and an I:E ratio of 1:2. The adequacy of tidal volume is assessed by observation of chest wall movement, breath sounds, and the capnograph and pulse oximeter readings. The $FIO_2$ is adjusted to maintain $SpO_2$ between 93% and 98%. Requirements for the fresh gas flow rate vary depending on the breathing circuit in use and the presence or absence of a carbon dioxide ($CO_2$) absorber. Fresh gas flow rates for common neonatal ventilators are typically 5 to 10 L/min.[114]

### What Circuits Are Available?

#### Nonrebreathing

Historically, and in many institutions today, neonates have been ventilated during anesthesia with any of several "semi-open" nonrebreathing circuits, such as the Bain modification of the Mapleson D system (illustrated in Chapter 57) and the Jackson-Rees modification of the Ayres T-piece.[115] These systems lack unidirectional valves and a $CO_2$ absorber; hence, they eliminate much of the work of spontaneous ventilation and facilitate manual detection of subtle changes in lower airway resistance. $CO_2$ elimination and adequacy of ventilation are determined by fresh gas flow (which must be $\geq 2.5$ L/min and twice minute ventilation during spontaneous ventilation to prevent rebreathing), tidal volume, and respiratory rate.[116,117]

## Circle

Lightweight plastic pediatric circle systems with small-diameter tubing have become increasingly popular for use in infants and neonates and function identically to well-known adult circle systems. By necessity, pediatric circles include one-way valves that must be opened with each breath. Experts usually recommend that neonates not be allowed (or required) to breathe spontaneously without assistance for more than a few minutes.[118]

# VASCULAR ACCESS

## *What Are the Indications?*

Intravenous access is indicated in all anesthetized neonates for the purposes of administering anesthetic drugs, resuscitative medications, fluids, and blood products. When the neonate is critically ill or has a significant thoracoabdominal disease process, intravenous access should be established before the induction of anesthesia.

The size and number of intravenous catheters are determined by the nature of the surgical procedure and the potential for major blood and third space fluid loss. For infants receiving infusions of parenteral hyperalimentation fluid or vasoactive medications, an additional venous access site or lumen of a central venous catheter is recommended for administration of anesthetic agents and bolus fluids. Because access to neonates and infants under surgical drapes and surrounded by members of the surgical team can be difficult and limited, and because of the relatively slow intravenous infusion rates and high intravenous tubing "dead spaces" used in these patients, it is helpful to plug a flushed section of microbore intravenous tubing into an intravenous line near the point of entry of the intravenous catheter. The other end of the microbore flush tubing with mounted syringe is located near the anesthesiologist. This technical point greatly facilitates the prompt administration and effect of medications and special fluids.

## *What Sites Should Be Used?*

Peripheral veins usually are easily seen and may be cannulated with 22- or 24-gauge intravenous catheters. Sequentially larger guidewires (0.18-0.25 mm) and catheters (18-20 gauge) may be placed. Alternatively, access to large central veins can be obtained at the femoral, subclavian, and internal and external jugular veins.[119,120] Common sites of peripheral access are the dorsum of the hand, antecubital fossae, greater saphenous vein on the medial surface of the ankle just anterior to the medial malleolus, and dorsal and lateral surfaces of the foot. Scalp vein needles may be used for administering medications and maintenance fluids but in our experience are not reliable for large-volume fluid infusions and boluses; they should be used only after depletion of sites on the extremities.

## *How Is Insertion Performed?*

### General Considerations

Thorough preparation and planning are essential to secure reliable venous access. A varied selection of appropriate-sized catheters should be available and within reach of the person attempting placement. The extremity should be immobilized by an assistant or padded support. Strict attention to asepsis should be ensured by the use of gloves and topically applied iodine solution or alcohol.

Helpful maneuvers include the following:

1. Nicking the skin at the site of anticipated entry of the catheter-over-the-needle device to prevent catheter drag at the skin surface
2. Removing the plastic cap from the hub of the intravenous needle assembly before venipuncture
3. After placement of the catheter, initially verifying correct intravenous location by hooking up an intravenous fluid-filled syringe attached to a T-connector extension set and injecting a small amount of fluid

If little or no resistance to injection is noted and the site does not become indurated or infiltrated, the intravenous tubing providing fluid administration is attached to the venous catheter.

Because all neonates can be assumed to have anatomic connections or shunts between the left and right sides of the heart, meticulous attention should be given to clearing the intravenous tubing of all bubbles. Microdrip (60 drops/mL) fluid administration sets with calibrated, limited-volume (100-150 mL) fluid chambers are typically used for neonates and infants. An electronic infusion pump may be used to provide more precise control of fluid administration rates.

### Umbilical Catheterization

The umbilical vessels, including one vein and two arteries, provide an alternative source of vascular access in neonates and are typically used by the staff in the NICU before surgery. Umbilical venous catheters may be used to monitor central venous pressure and to administer fluids and medications. Catheters in the umbilical artery are used to monitor arterial pressure and to administer drugs and fluids in emergency situations.

The location of umbilical catheter tips must be verified before surgery to minimize the potential for inward or outward migration of a catheter during surgery; disastrous complications, including visceral artery thrombosis and liver necrosis or cirrhosis, may result from many fluids and medications administered through an incorrectly located umbilical catheter.[121] The tip of an umbilical artery catheter may be either "low" just above the bifurcation of the femoral arteries (L3-L4) or "high" above the diaphragm (T6-T9). The tip of an umbilical venous catheter should rest in the IVC near the junction with the right atrium, beyond the ductus venosus.

## Alternate Arterial Sites

Other sites for arterial cannulation include the radial, dorsalis pedis, posterior tibial, and femoral arteries. Arterial cannulation is indicated for continuous blood pressure monitoring and analysis of blood gases and pH. If possible, the right radial artery should be cannulated because it is representative of preductal blood flow for arterial blood gas measurements.

## FLUID ADMINISTRATION

### *What Are the Basic Requirements?*

Fluid management in neonatal surgical patients includes normal maintenance requirements, replacement of any preexisting deficit, and both third space fluid and acute blood losses. A typical term neonate has a water content of 75% to 80% and a blood volume of 80 to 90 mL/kg.[122] Premature infants may have a blood volume as great as 105 mL/kg.

### Maintenance

The average fluid requirement in a healthy neonate is approximately 100 mL/kg/d, or 4 mL/kg/h.[123] Various processes such as congenital heart disease, BPD, and the use of radiant warmers and phototherapy may increase or decrease this basic fluid requirement. Electrolyte replacement must be accounted for in maintenance fluids; appropriate amounts of sodium and chloride are usually provided by quarter normal saline. Potassium may be added (in the presence of adequate renal function) with 1 to 2 mEq/100 mL of maintenance fluid.

### Preexisting and Intraoperative Losses

Most critically ill neonates receive nothing by mouth and have received intravenous maintenance fluids for some time before surgery or have never taken oral fluids. Fluid deficits may result from incomplete or inadequate volume replacement before surgery. Third space fluid losses are particularly significant in patients with gastroschisis, omphalocele, NEC, and ruptured meningomyelocele.

### *What Fluids Are Indicated?*

### Balanced Electrolyte Solutions

During major operative procedures involving manipulation and exposure of large visceral surfaces, replacement with 2 to 15 mL/kg/h of balanced salt solution (normal saline or Ringer's injection, lactated) is necessary to replenish intravascular fluid volume.[124] Preexisting and intraoperative deficits associated with hypotension, metabolic acidosis, and oliguria require bolus fluid therapy; 10 to 20 mL/kg of balanced salt solution or a colloid volume expander is repeatedly administered over 5 to 10 minutes as blood pressure, heart rate, and urine output are monitored. Large volumes of 100 to 200 mL/kg or greater may be required to restore and maintain normal intravascular volume and hemodynamics.

### Colloids

Colloid preparations, such as 5% albumin, plasma protein fraction, and fresh-frozen plasma, commonly are used in the fluid resuscitation of neonates, perhaps to a greater extent than in adults. The justification for this practice is not well defined but has been based on concerns that neonates are less tolerant of large fluid and salt loads, are perhaps more susceptible to the detrimental effects of interstitial edema, and are frequently experiencing at least a low-grade coagulopathy when critically ill. Colloids do remain in the intravascular compartment longer than crystalloids but are more expensive.[123]

### Glucose and Hyperalimentation Solutions

Limited neonatal glycogen stores, the frequent absence of normal enteral nutrition, and the stress of the disease state and surgery necessitate that glucose be provided in a 5% to 12.5% concentration in the maintenance fluids to meet caloric requirements and prevent hypoglycemia. Critically ill neonates often receive all or a significant portion of their maintenance fluids from parenteral hyperalimentation solutions. Approaches to the management of hyperalimentation fluids vary, with some advocating administration of 10% dextrose in place of the hyperalimentation fluid during surgery to prevent rebound hypoglycemia. In most instances, the hyperalimentation fluid can be continued during surgery. In any case, blood glucose levels should be monitored at least hourly.

### *How Is Blood Loss Replaced?*

Until recent years, hematocrit values were maintained in the minimum range of 35% to 40% because of a neonate's greater $O_2$ consumption and a limited ability to increase $O_2$ delivery by increases in cardiac output. The heightened concern of blood-borne infectious disease transmission has caused "target" hematocrit values in neonates to drift downward, as in older patients.

As blood is lost, intravascular volume replacement initially is provided in the form of isotonic crystalloid or colloid. Crystalloids are normally replaced in a 3:1 ratio to blood loss to compensate for the extravascular shift of fluid. Colloids and blood products should be warmed from their refrigerated temperatures, and are provided in a 1:1 ratio with blood loss after the allowable blood loss has been exceeded. Ten to 20 mL/kg of packed red blood cells is commonly administered by a manual syringe or calibrated infusion pump, after which the clinical situation is reassessed.

Packed erythrocytes have a hematocrit of 65% to 75%; overzealous transfusion may induce a dangerously high hematocrit and hyperviscosity. One solution to this problem is to dilute the packed red blood cells with warm isotonic saline to a hematocrit of 45% to 50% before transfusion. All blood products and bolus crystalloids should be warmed before administration.

## INTRAOPERATIVE MONITORING

### *What Are the Basics?*

Monitoring during anesthesia and surgery includes two distinct but related functions: assessment of homeostasis of the patient's physiologic status and evaluation of equipment performance (breathing systems, ventilator, and intravenous infusion pumps). At a minimum, monitoring should comply with the American Society of Anesthesiologists' Standards for Basic Intra-Operative Monitoring; practically, this approach includes a precordial or esophageal stethoscope, continuous ECG, noninvasive blood pressure measurement, a temperature probe, pulse oximetry, and capnography.[125] Additional measurements that may be required in selected patients include nerve stimulation, continuous invasive blood pressure, and urine output. Selective laboratory studies obtained during anesthesia, including determination of hemoglobin or hematocrit, serum glucose, electrolytes, and blood coagulation parameters, are also a form of monitoring and may be required.

## What Is the Value of Pulse Oximetry?

The most significant monitoring advances in clinical practice since the mid-1980s are pulse oximetry and capnometry. Neonates and infants younger than 6 months are at greatest risk of experiencing at least one major episode such as accidental extubation, esophageal intubation, circuit disconnect, or kinking of the ETT.[126]

Pulse oximetry is relatively simple to use, particularly compared with transcutaneous $O_2$ monitoring.[127] It provides early evidence of impending oxyhemoglobin desaturation before hypoxemia-induced changes in vital signs or clinically apparent cyanosis develops.[128] It may also be used to guide the $FiO_2$ selection and thereby lessen the risk of hyperoxia in premature neonates. This is the one situation in which the high $SpO_2$ alarm setting can be used to advantage. Inferences concerning intravascular volume status, cardiac output, and peripheral vasoconstriction may be made when a well-placed oximeter cannot consistently detect arterial pulsations.[129]

From a practical standpoint, oximeter probes are often placed or wrapped (depending on the design of the probe) around the palm of the hand or the foot in neonates. In determining probe placement, consideration should be given to accessibility, potential for motion, compression, and light interference, as well as the vascular supply of the location (proximal or distal) to the ductus arteriosus.

## What Is the Value of Capnometry/Capnography?

### Indications

Capnometry, the measurement of $CO_2$ partial pressure in a gas mixture, and capnography, the representation of $CO_2$ partial pressure as a waveform over time, provide a large amount of information about a patient and the function of the artificial airway, breathing system, and ventilator. $CO_2$ analysis facilitates the detection of critical incidents, breathing system leaks, and rebreathing, and assists the assessment of ventilation.

### Limitations

Expired gas can be analyzed with a mainstream- or sidestream-type monitor; each has its limitations. Accurate measurements of true end-expired $CO_2$ partial pressure can be difficult with a sidestream analyzer in which the gas to be measured is aspirated from the airway or breathing circuit. This problem is particularly evident in nonrebreathing systems with relatively high fresh gas flows and in the presence of

significant cardiopulmonary disease.[130] Accuracy is also decreased with low sampling flow rates (<100 mL/min).[131] An ETT with a built-in distal sampling port or a mainstream analyzer improves the validity of $CO_2$ readings. A mainstream analyzer "reads" gas in the airway or circuit but is bulky and may lead to kinking or dislodgment of the ETT.

## PYLORIC STENOSIS

Infantile hypertrophic pyloric stenosis is a relatively common gastrointestinal disorder, with an incidence that may approach 1 in 300 live births in some geographic locations.[132] It typically presents as nonbilious projectile vomiting between the second and sixth weeks of life. Boys are approximately four times more likely to be affected than girls.

The cause of pyloric stenosis is unknown, although a number of factors, including genetic inheritance, infection, and pyloric irritation with subsequent edema and obstruction, may play a part.[133] Infants with this disorder have been diagnosed increasingly early in the course of the disease. As a result, the profound metabolic derangement consisting of a hypochloremic, hypokalemic, hyponatremic metabolic alkalosis and hypovolemia is less frequently encountered. Diagnosis is made on the basis of history and physical examination and is confirmed by a barium contrast study of the stomach (Fig. 56–6) or US of the upper abdomen.[134]

## What Are the Primary Concerns?

Pyloric stenosis is a medical emergency first and surgical emergency second. As such, the initial point of management after diagnosis is to correct disturbances in acid-base, fluid, and electrolyte status.

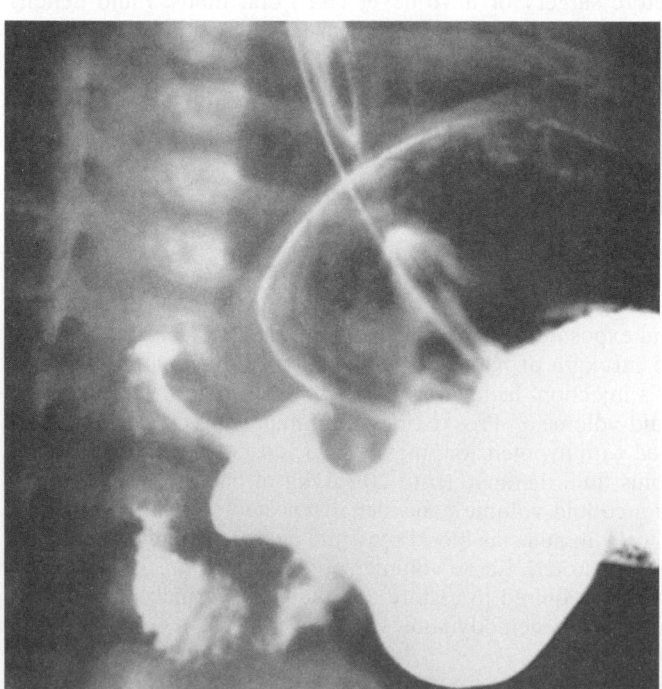

**FIGURE 56–6.** Barium contrast study of the stomach in a patient with pyloric stenosis. The fundus is at the *upper right,* and the area of the pylorus is seen on the *left* overlying the vertebra.

## Fluid Therapy

The exact nature and quantity of intravenous fluid required depend on the severity of these derangements. For mild to moderate hypovolemia (5%-15% loss of body weight), 50 to 100 mL/kg fluid replacement may be provided with normal saline. Half the deficit should be replaced during the first 8 hours, and the remaining half in the next 16 hours.

## Acid-Base Status

For severe hypovolemia and alkalosis ($HCO_3^-$ >42 mEq/L), several boluses of normal saline (20 mL/kg) are required, followed by replacement of the remaining deficit as outlined earlier. Potassium may be added to the intravenous fluid when urine output is adequate (>0.5 mL/kg/h). A urinary chloride concentration >20 mEq/L after fluid resuscitation is proposed as a useful indicator of satisfactory volume replacement.[133]

## *How Is Anesthesia Managed?*

A number of anesthetic considerations are implicit in the care of infants with pyloric stenosis in addition to the standard tenets of neonatal anesthesia. After fluid resuscitation and the correction of acid-base and electrolyte abnormalities, the neonate must be regarded as having a full stomach owing to impaired gastric emptying. Before either awake intubation or rapid-sequence induction and intubation, a *new* orogastric or nasogastric tube should be passed into the stomach and put to suction. A prospective investigation compared the efficacy and complications of three induction and intubation techniques in patients with pyloric stenosis: awake intubation with an $O_2$ insufflating laryngoscope, rapid-sequence induction, and modified rapid-sequence induction with mask ventilation through cricoid pressure. Rapid-sequence induction was identified as the technique of choice, there being no advantages realized by the alternatives.[135]

Muscle relaxants allow a reduction in the dose of inhalation anesthetics, improve surgical exposure, and minimize the risk of perforation of the duodenal mucosa. Some infants with pyloric stenosis may have postanesthetic apnea after surgery, which may reflect uncorrected alkalosis in the blood or cerebrospinal fluid; for this reason, narcotics should be used sparingly (if at all).[136,137] Postoperative analgesia may be provided by infiltration of the surgical wound with bupivacaine and the administration of rectal acetaminophen.[138]

## CONGENITAL ABDOMINAL WALL DEFECTS

## *What Are They?*

Omphalocele and gastroschisis are congenital abdominal wall defects requiring emergent surgical repair. Considerable confusion exists about the terminology for these lesions and the distinction between them, with resultant difficulty in comparing treatments and outcomes in patient series at different locations.

## Omphalocele

Omphalocele (Fig. 56–7) is a herniation of the abdominal viscera that occurs into the base of the umbilical cord through

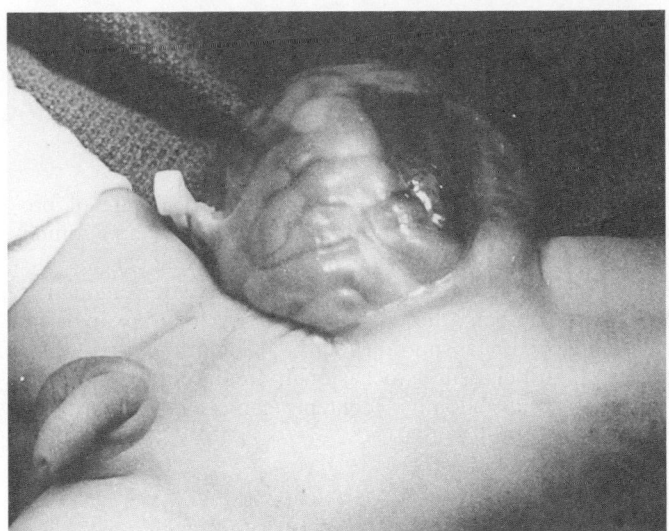

**FIGURE 56–7.** Omphalocele, with herniated abdominal organs covered by a translucent membranous sac.

a central wall defect. Herniated organs are covered by a membranous sac and may include the intestine, stomach, liver, and spleen. Omphalocele has an incidence of 1 in 5000 to 10 000 live births and is frequently associated with other congenital anomalies (76%).[139] Potential coexisting defects include congenital heart disease, chromosomal trisomy, and the Beckwith-Wiedemann syndrome of hypoglycemia, macroglossia, and visceromegaly. Approximately 33% of patients with an omphalocele are premature.

## Gastroschisis

Gastroschisis (Fig. 56–8) is an evisceration of bowel through a full-thickness defect in the abdominal wall, typically to the right of the umbilical cord. No membrane or sac covers the eviscerated organs, which characteristically are thickened and matted together. Fifty percent of patients with this defect

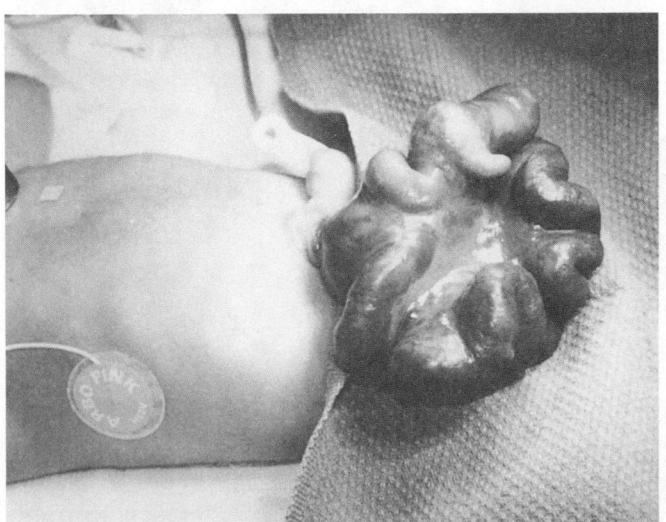

**FIGURE 56–8.** Gastroschisis. Note the lack of a membranous covering and the confluent appearance of the intestine. The herniation has actually occurred to the right of the umbilicus.

are premature, but it is less likely to be associated with other congenital defects.

## What Are Potential Complications?

Patients with gastroschisis are most likely to die of processes related to prematurity or intestinal and wound complications, whereas death in patients with omphalocele is often related to their low birth weight and coexisting anomalies. With both disorders, the abdominal cavity may be small and underdeveloped, causing difficulty at the time of surgical repair. An artificial silo is occasionally required to enclose the viscera until all abdominal contents can later be returned to the abdomen[140] (Fig. 56–9).

## What Are the Major Management Problems?

Problems encountered before surgery persist into the operative period and include difficulty with maintenance of body temperature, significant fluid loss through the exposed viscera, and infection. Placing the exposed viscera into a plastic or gauze wrap before surgery reduces heat and fluid loss. Additional measures such as warming the ambient environment, ventilator gases, and fluids to be infused are crucial.

### Fluid Requirements

Fluid requirements vary depending on the size of the wall defect and the amount of exposed viscera. Parameters that can be monitored to guide fluid resuscitation include systolic blood pressure, heart rate, urine output, base deficit, and hematocrit. Hemoconcentration, as evidenced by increasing hematocrit, may denote hypovolemia. As in other instances of neonatal fluid resuscitation, colloid preparations are used

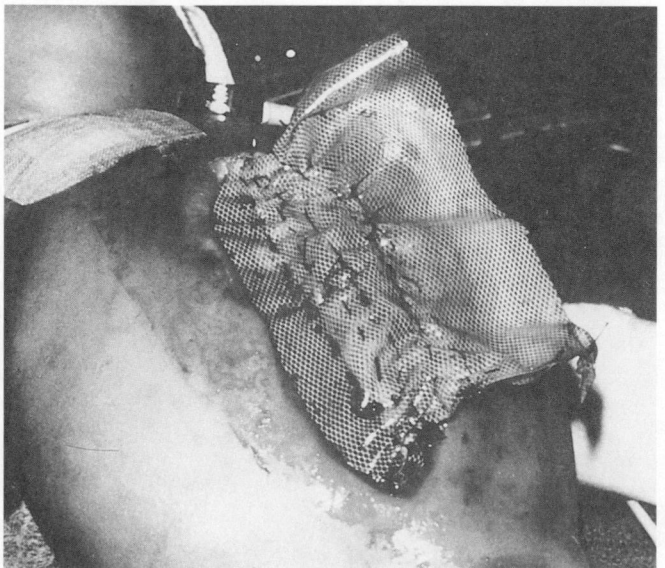

**FIGURE 56–9.** Artificial silo in place to contain abdominal viscera after omphalocele repair. This patient has undergone sequential reduction of the silo contents and is photographed before removal of the silo and closure of the abdominal wall.

frequently in 10 to 20 mL/kg increments.[141] As much as 300 to 400 mL/kg of crystalloid may be needed immediately before surgery and during surgical repair. Significant amounts of blood loss usually are not encountered.

### Airway

If they are not already intubated in the NICU, patients presenting for surgical repair of an abdominal wall defect may be intubated either after rapid intravenous induction of anesthesia or, in the presence of anticipated difficult airway or hemodynamic instability, awake. Nasogastric or orogastric tube decompression of the stomach should precede induction.

## How Is Anesthesia Managed?

Anesthesia is provided by a combination of an opioid (usually fentanyl) and a nondepolarizing muscle relaxant. A potent inhalation anesthetic may be used to supplement the intravenous agents if the patient tolerates it. Nitrous oxide should be avoided in these patients because of the possibility that it may contribute to intestinal distention and interfere with successful closure of the abdomen. It is important that intravenous access in the upper extremities be obtained (if not already present) because return of the viscera to the abdominal cavity may impair venous drainage of the lower extremities.

### Adequacy of Ventilation

As the eviscerated or herniated organs are returned to the abdominal cavity, the PIP, adequacy of ventilation, and hemodynamic stability must be closely monitored. Return of all herniated organs and primary closure of abdominal wall defects may be associated with severe limitation of diaphragmatic excursion and reduction of venous return of blood from the lower extremities and abdomen, with a subsequent reduction in cardiac output and impaired systemic perfusion.

Failure of primary operative repair of omphalocele and gastroschisis was associated with intragastric pressures >20 mm Hg, reductions of cardiac index of ≥0.78 L/min/m², and increases in central venous pressure of ≥4 mm Hg in one report.[142] In the presence of such indices or a PIP significantly >30 cm $H_2O$, an artificial silo may be necessary to cover the eviscerated organs. The hernia may then be gradually reduced over a period of up to 10 days.

### Extubation

The decision to extubate is influenced by the size of the defect, the extent of fluid loss and resuscitation, the residual effects of anesthetic agents, and the presence of other problems such as IRDS and congenital heart disease.

### Monitoring

Monitoring includes all standard parameters. Invasive blood pressure monitoring is optional (but often required) and largely depends on pulmonary status, the size of the lesion, and the extent of existing or anticipated acid-base derangements.

## NECROTIZING ENTEROCOLITIS

### What Is It?

Neonatal NEC is not a congenital anomaly. It is acquired and is primarily a disease of premature low-birth-weight infants; it is seen in 10% of patients with birth weight <1.5 kg.[20] It is rare in term infants, although in some reports up to 10% of patients are term infants.[143] The incidence and mortality rate of NEC vary among institutions, with clusters of "outbreaks" developing at different times.

### Causes

A large number of conditions in addition to prematurity are associated with NEC, including perinatal asphyxia and hypoxemia, umbilical vessel catheterization, episodes of hypotension or shock, PDA, exchange transfusions, polycythemia, and hyperosmolar feedings. The disease appears to involve hypoperfusion of the intestinal mucosa. The result is mucosal inflammation, ischemia, necrosis, bowel wall perforation, and sepsis. Other factors that appear to be important in the etiology of NEC include bacterial colonization of the gut and the presence of a substrate, usually formula feedings, in the gut lumen.[144]

### What Are the Presenting Signs?

Neonates with NEC may present with a number of nonspecific signs, including lethargy, pallor, irritability, temperature instability, apnea, and bradycardia. Abdominal findings include distention (Fig. 56–10), tenderness, gastric retention, gastrointestinal hemorrhage, and erythema of the abdominal wall. Later in the disease, signs of sepsis and disseminated

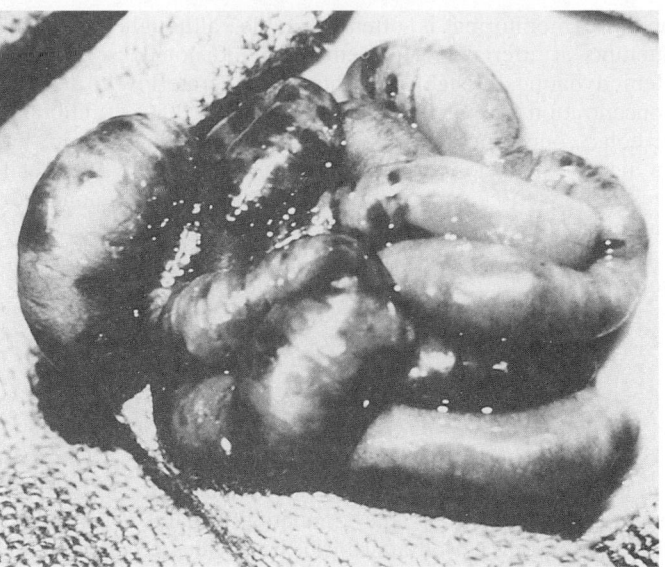

**FIGURE 56–11.** Intestine of a patient with necrotizing enterocolitis during exploratory laparotomy. Note dark patches of intestinal wall necrosis.

intravascular coagulation may appear. Pneumatosis intestinalis (gas in the intestinal wall) is considered pathognomonic of NEC and may be associated with the presence of portal venous gas.

### What Does Medical and Surgical Management Involve?

Medical management of NEC includes discontinuation of enteral feeding, orogastric or nasogastric decompression of the stomach, administration of intravenous fluids, electrolytes, and antibiotics, and institution of parenteral hyperalimentation. Specific blood products, such as packed red blood cells, platelets and fresh-frozen plasma, may be required to correct anemia, thrombocytopenia (platelets <100 000/mm³), and any coagulopathy.

Indications for surgical intervention vary.[145] The only universally accepted criterion is perforation of the bowel wall with pneumoperitoneum. Other possible indications include failed medical management, positive findings on paracentesis, erythema of the abdominal wall, or a fixed abdominal mass. Surgical management consists of exploratory laparotomy, resection of the necrotic segment, and usually external ostomy diversion.[146] Very small infants (<1000 g) may be managed with intraperitoneal drainage as a temporizing measure, but most require subsequent laparotomy.[147] The appearance of the intestine at the time of laparotomy is shown in Figure 56–11.

### How Is Anesthesia Managed?

Anesthetic management includes the same airway concerns and options previously discussed for the abdominal wall defects and pyloric stenosis. Most of these patients are premature; therefore, the usual problems and risks associated with hyperoxia and hypothermia apply. If the disease has evolved to sepsis and peritonitis, third space fluid losses may be large, necessitating vigorous fluid resuscitation. Invasive arterial

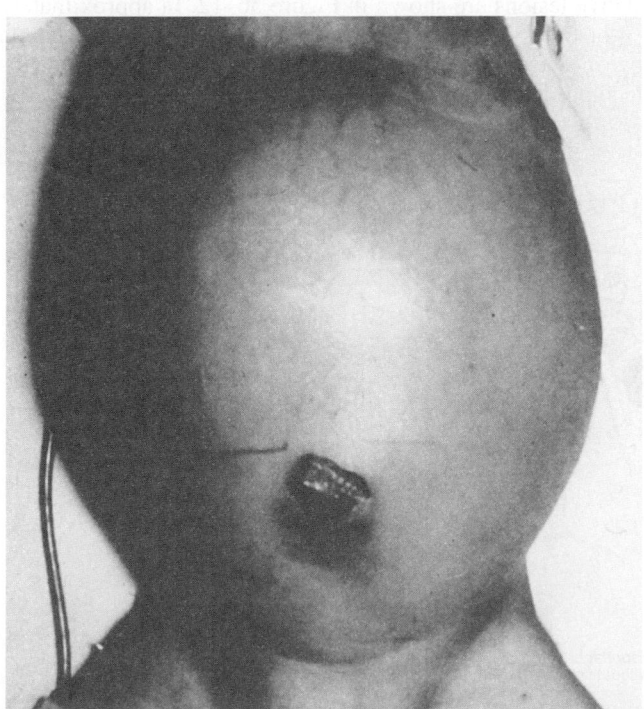

**FIGURE 56–10.** Photograph of chest and distended abdomen of a neonate with necrotizing enterocolitis before exploratory laparotomy.

pressure monitoring is often desirable, although prolonged attempts at arterial line placement should not delay surgery. Hemodynamically stable patients may tolerate low to normal concentrations of potent inhalational agents (0.5-1.3 minimum alveolar concentration [MAC]). Unstable patients require incremental small doses of an opioid such as fentanyl. Skeletal muscle relaxation is maintained in all patients with a nondepolarizing muscle relaxant. Nitrous oxide is not used because it might contribute to intestinal distention and an increase in the volume of intraluminal gas pockets.

## PATENT DUCTUS ARTERIOSUS

### What Are the Characteristics?

The term *patent ductus arteriosus* signifies only that a remnant of the normal fetal circulation remains open for an abnormally long period after birth. It provides no information about the direction of blood flow across the shunt or the underlying pathologic processes that may be responsible for continued patency of the ductus. Normally, the elevated $PaO_2$ after birth promotes functional (and later, anatomic) closure of the ductus within the first days of life.

Infants with a symptomatic PDA typically are premature and have left-to-right shunting of blood across the ductus and various degrees of respiratory distress syndrome and congestive heart failure. PDA occurs in 30% of very low-birth-weight premature infants with IRDS.[20] Infants with certain forms of congenital heart disease (eg, tricuspid or pulmonary atresia) may depend on patency of the ductus to provide pulmonary blood flow. Those with PPHN have increased PVR causing a right-to-left shunt across the ductus. Ligation of a PDA in such patients usually is not indicated and may induce abrupt right ventricular failure.[148] A small number of otherwise healthy term infants also may have PDA, but these cases are thought to be related to a defect in the mucoid endothelial layer and the muscular media.[149,150]

### What Are the Clinical Signs?

Clinical features of PDA with predominant left-to-right shunting include a typical continuous or systolic cardiac murmur, hyperactive precordium, widened pulse pressure (>35 mm Hg), bounding peripheral pulses, and findings of respiratory distress. The heart is enlarged (as seen on a chest radiograph), with evidence of volume overload of the pulmonary vasculature. Diagnosis is confirmed by echocardiography. Initial management includes fluid restriction, diuresis, mechanical ventilation, and treatment with a prostaglandin synthetase inhibitor, such as indomethacin, in appropriate candidates.[151]

### How Is Anesthesia Managed?

Surgical ligation of the PDA is undertaken in patients who have refractory respiratory or cardiac failure and who have failed medical therapy. These neonates are usually critically ill. They frequently are already intubated and receiving conventional support or high-frequency ventilation and continuous infusions of inotropic agents. Patients are placed in the right lateral decubitus position just before the procedure. Monitoring should include a right precordial stethoscope and an arterial line in most instances.

### Fluids

Preoperative fluid restriction and diuretic therapy often induce a hypovolemic state. Many patients benefit from a bolus (10 mL/kg) of crystalloid or colloid before the induction of anesthesia.[152]

### Induction and Maintenance

Induction is typically accomplished with a combination of narcotic (fentanyl, 10-50 μg/kg) and a nondepolarizing muscle relaxant. If the patient has been receiving high-frequency ventilation, it is necessary to convert to conventional ventilation just before the procedure. Means of providing manual ventilation must be readily available. The $FIO_2$ and mean airway pressure normally must be increased when the thoracic cavity is opened and the left lung is compressed. Occlusion of the PDA normally is associated with elevation of the systemic blood pressure and narrowing of the pulse pressure.

Our practice is to monitor $SpO_2$ and peripheral pulses with a pulse oximeter both preductally and postductally in the event that the subclavian artery or aortic arch is occluded or ligated erroneously. The procedure of surgical ligation of the ductus arteriosus usually requires approximately 30 minutes. Mechanical ventilation is continued after the procedure.

## TRACHEOESOPHAGEAL FISTULA

### What Is It?

The anomaly of tracheoesophageal fistula (TEF) and esophageal atresia (EA) includes various anatomic defects; representative lesions are shown in Figure 56–12. In approximately 80% of cases, the defect consists of EA with a distal fistula between the lower trachea and the segment of esophagus extending upward from the stomach.

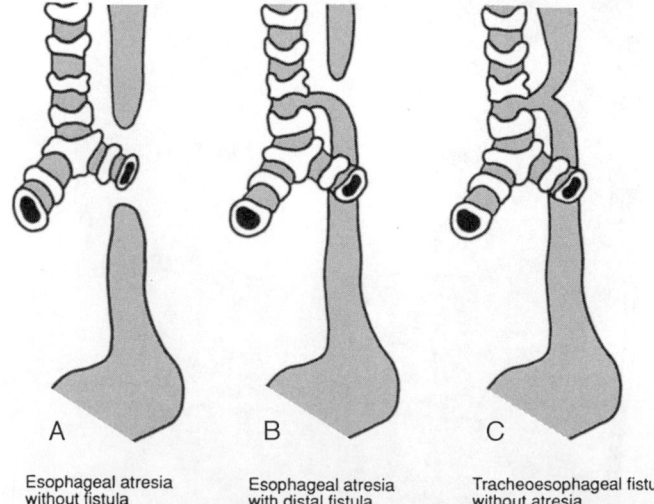

Esophageal atresia without fistula

Esophageal atresia with distal fistula

Tracheoesophageal fistula without atresia

A     B     C

**FIGURE 56–12.** Three configurations of the tracheoesophageal fistula (TEF)/esophageal atresia (EA) complex. *A*, EA without TEF. *B*, The most common variant of EA. *C*, An H-type fistula.

The disorder has an incidence of 1 in 3500 live births and an overall survival rate of 90%.[153] It is associated with other congenital anomalies in 30% to 50% of patients, the most common of these being cardiovascular and other gastrointestinal defects (eg, imperforate anus). A complex of congenital anomalies known as the *VATER association* is found in approximately 10% of patients with TEF. In addition to TEF/EA, this "syndrome" consists of vertebral, anal, renal, and radial bony abnormalities.[154] Approximately one third of newborns with combined TEF/EA and EA alone are premature.

## How Is It Diagnosed?

In most cases, the diagnosis is made shortly after birth when a suction catheter cannot be advanced through the esophagus into the stomach or when respiratory symptoms of coughing, choking, and cyanosis develop after initial feedings. Polyhydramnios is often present with EA during pregnancy. In cases without fistula, no gas is demonstrable in the abdomen.

Preoperative evaluation should include instillation of a small amount of contrast material (barium or metrizamide) into the blind esophageal pouch (Fig. 56–13) to help define the extent of atresia and any proximal fistula (rare). In addition, US evaluation of the renal and cardiac systems is warranted to identify the existence of significant associated lesions.

## What Should Be Done Before Surgery?

Before surgery, the goal of management in patients with TEF/EA is to minimize pulmonary complications through

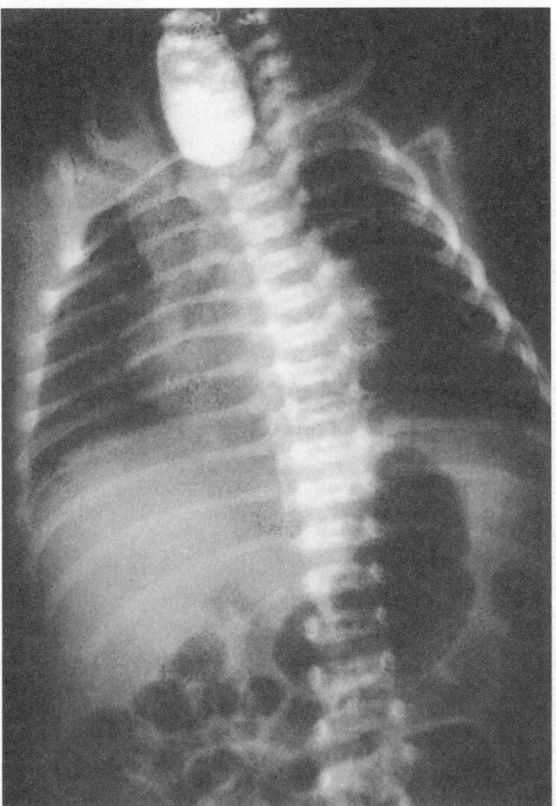

**FIGURE 56–13.** Chest radiograph of a patient with esophageal atresia. The collection of barium in a dilated, blind upper esophageal pouch is demonstrated.

strict observance of NPO status. The patient's head is elevated and continuous suction of the proximal esophageal pouch is carried out, along with provision of supplemental $O_2$ as required. Bronchoscopy is frequently performed to define the existence and location of the TEF (if present) and the presence of any other defects, such as a laryngeal cleft or tracheomalacia.

Spontaneous ventilation should be maintained during bronchoscopy before ligation of the fistula to minimize the passage of gas under positive pressure through the fistula and into the gastrointestinal tract. In the event of a large TEF with significant gastric distention, a small-caliber suction catheter may be passed through the fistula to decompress the stomach, after which a Fogarty balloon catheter is advanced to occlude the fistula until the surgical ligation is performed. After bronchoscopy, the infant is intubated.

## How Is Anesthesia Managed?

### Intubation

When bronchoscopy is not required before the surgical procedure, the anesthesiologist is faced with the question of whether to perform awake intubation or an intravenous induction with or without a muscle relaxant. In light of improved monitoring techniques and the recognition of neonatal anesthetic requirements, we intubate after administering intravenous anesthetics unless airway anomalies make intubation difficult or the patient is moribund. Succinylcholine may be used to allow rapid return of spontaneous ventilation, although the authors have had good success with intubating after administration of thiopental alone; many neonates continue to ventilate spontaneously and maintain satisfactory oxygenation, and do not require positive pressure ventilation until after the TEF has been ligated.

### Endotracheal Tube Position

After intubation, the tip of the tracheal tube should be positioned distal to the fistula but above the carina. It is sometimes helpful to rotate the tube 90% from its usual insertion orientation so that the bevel is angled anteriorly, allowing the distal part of the tube to cover the fistula opening in the posterior tracheal wall.

Another approach is to place the tracheal tube intentionally into either mainstem bronchus and then withdraw it slowly to the point at which bilateral breath sounds are auscultated. This maneuver places the tip of the tube below the level of the fistula in all but the lowest of abnormalities.

### Patient's Position

Patients are typically placed in the left lateral decubitus position, and the procedure of fistula ligation and esophageal anastomosis is effected through a lateral thoracotomy incision, usually with a retropleural approach. It is important that preoperative echocardiograms be used to attempt to identify whether the aortic arch is left- or right-sided because this facilitates optimum positioning and surgical approach.

### Maintenance

Anesthesia is maintained with inhaled anesthetics or intravenous narcotics or both, depending on the infant's condition and whether extubation of the trachea after surgery is anticipated. Spontaneous ventilation, when possible, is ideal in patients with distal TEF in that it minimizes gas entry into the gastrointestinal tract. We have anesthetized a number of neonates with birth weights of 2500 to 3500 g who have tolerated 1.5 MAC inhalation agent (isoflurane) in 100% $O_2$ with spontaneous ventilation and acceptable hemodynamics. Nitrous oxide should be avoided because it may contribute to abdominal distention and often is tolerated poorly during thoracotomy when one lung is compressed and deflated.

### Extubation

The decision to extubate is based on the knowledge of the infant's preoperative pulmonary status, the type of anesthetic administered, and any coexisting medical conditions. The passage of suction catheters into the trachea beyond the level of the fistula or the esophagus should be avoided out of concern that they may disrupt the fistula ligation or esophageal repair.

## CONGENITAL DIAPHRAGMATIC HERNIA

### What Is It?

CDH has an incidence of 1 in 2000 to 5000 live births. It most commonly (70%-85%) involves the herniation of abdominal contents (stomach, spleen, liver, and intestine) through the left posterolateral diaphragm at the site of the Bochdalek foramen. It is thought to occur at approximately the eighth week of gestation as a result of the premature return of the midgut to the abdominal cavity from the umbilical stalk. Separation of the pleural and peritoneal cavities by closure of the diaphragm does not occur until the 9th to 12th week of gestation. In a small percentage of cases, herniation of abdominal organs also can occur through the substernal sinus (Morgagni foramen) or the esophageal hiatus. The disorder is far more than a mere herniation of abdominal contents into the thorax; CDH bears a complex pathophysiology associated with pulmonary hypoplasia and hypertension that remain as problems after operative reduction of the hernia.[155]

### What Are the Effects?

The presence of midgut structures in the thoracic cavity impedes normal lung development, resulting in pulmonary hypoplasia, which is often bilateral but more severe on the ipsilateral side of the hernia. Pulmonary hypoplasia is marked by reduced lung weight, smaller numbers of terminal bronchioles and alveoli, and a significant reduction in the total cross-sectional area of the pulmonary vascular bed.[156] The walls of pulmonary arteries demonstrate thickening of both the adventitia and media.[157] These abnormalities and the propensity to development of pulmonary hypertension, despite operative reduction of the hernia, are responsible for the persistent overall mortality rate of approximately 50%.

### How Is It Diagnosed?

Many cases are now diagnosed prenatally by US. After birth, the diagnosis of CDH is based on the demonstration of

gas-filled loops of bowel in the chest (Fig. 56–14), often with a shift of mediastinal structures to the opposite side. Clinical signs include a scaphoid abdomen, barrel chest, reduced or absent breath sounds on the side of the hernia, and, in a small number of patients, bowel sounds in the chest. Various degrees of respiratory distress may be observed, depending on the amount of herniated viscera and the degree of pulmonary hypoplasia (Fig. 56–15). Other congenital anomalies frequently associated with CDH include malrotation of the intestine (50%), congenital heart disease (23%), and central nervous system and genitourinary disorders (15%-20%).

### How Is It Treated?

CDH historically was one of the true neonatal surgical emergencies requiring operative intervention within the first several hours of extrauterine life. In some cases and institutions, when a patient has severe respiratory distress shortly after birth, this approach is still followed. However, in many centers, delayed surgery after a period of medical stabilization (depending on coexisting congenital problems, the degree of respiratory compromise, and the equipment and technology available to manage this group of critically ill neonates) has become the standard practice.[158] Because of the high mortality rate among these infants, a range of management plans exists. There is no single accepted standard or time for operative intervention.

### Preoperative Stabilization

Infants with respiratory distress cannot be expected to improve significantly without surgical repair of the hernia, but

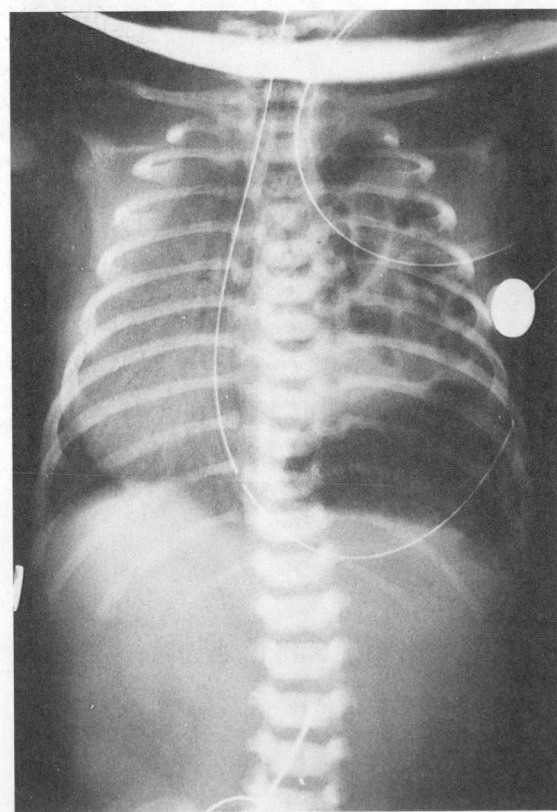

**FIGURE 56–14.** Left-sided congenital diaphragmatic hernia, with loops of intestine in left hemithorax.

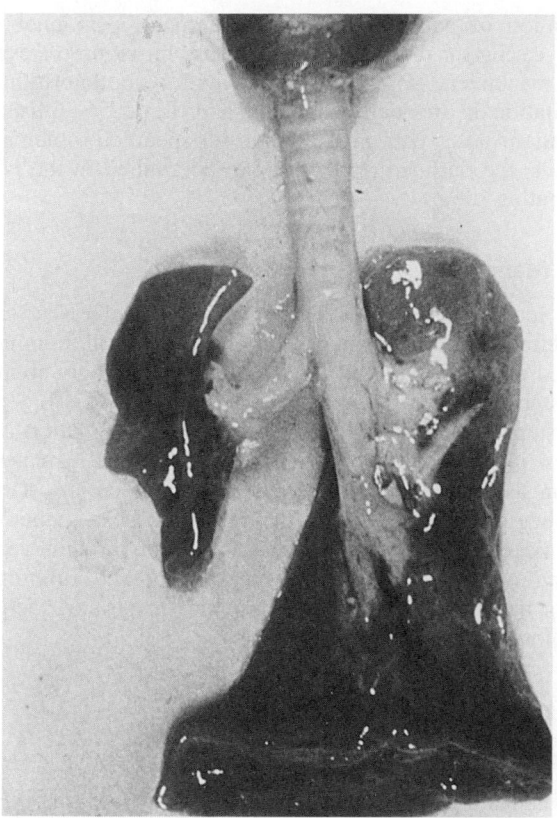

**FIGURE 56–15.** Tracheobronchial structures and lungs in postmortem specimen from a neonate who died from congenital diaphragmatic hernia. Note the marked hypoplasia of the right lung.

surgery alone does not "cure" these patients. Increased reactivity of the pulmonary circulation and pulmonary hypertension may persist or worsen after surgery. For this reason, many neonates with CDH today undergo a period of stabilization and medical evaluation before surgery. If the equipment and appropriate personnel are available, infants may be supported by ECMO before, during, and after surgery.[159] Although still controversial, it appears that ECMO significantly improves survival rates for neonates with CDH and a predictive mortality risk exceeding 80%.[160]

Preoperative treatment includes orogastric or nasogastric tube decompression of the stomach, positioning in a semi-upright manner to minimize compression of lung tissue by abdominal contents, and conservative intravenous fluid therapy to avoid volume overload and exacerbation of pulmonary hypertension. Conditions that induce or contribute to pulmonary vasoconstriction, such as hypothermia, acidosis, hypoxemia, and hypercarbia, must be treated.[161] Infants with early respiratory distress usually require intubation and mechanical ventilation before surgery. There is some evidence that minimizing lung injury through "permissive hypercapnia" and gentle ventilation rather than aggressive hyperventilation may reduce the need for ECMO and improve outcome.[162,163] HFJV and HFOV have had only limited success in the management of infants with CDH.[164,165]

### How Is Anesthesia Managed?

#### Induction

Mask ventilation should be avoided. This technique often forces gas into the gastrointestinal tract and exacerbates pulmonary compression.[139] Intubation may be accomplished either awake or after rapid-sequence intravenous induction in stable patients. After intubation, restriction of the PIP to 20 to 25 cm $H_2O$ minimizes the chance of creating a pneumothorax. The temptation to inflate the atelectatic hypoplastic lung or lungs aggressively must be resisted.

Rapid respiratory rates of 60 to 80 breaths per minute help to compensate for smaller-than-normal tidal volumes and restricted PIPs. This approach may also help to induce a mild state of hypocarbia and respiratory alkalosis, alleviating pulmonary vasoconstriction.

Nonventilatory strategies to reduce PVR include administration of direct vasodilating or α-adrenergic blocking medications, such as sodium nitroprusside, nitroglycerin, prostaglandin $E_1$, tolazoline, or chlorpromazine. These vasodilators often are begun in the presence of poor systemic oxygenation and pulmonary hypertension refractory to nonpharmacologic manipulation. They predispose to systemic hypotension and frequently require simultaneous administration of increased fluid and a combined inotrope/vasopressor such as dopamine.

#### Maintenance

Anesthesia for CDH repair is usually provided with a combination of narcotics and nondepolarizing muscle relaxants. In some cases, anesthesia with a narcotic (fentanyl) or isoflurane may lower PVR and has been maintained after surgery.[166] Most surgeons reduce the hernia and repair the diaphragm through an upper abdominal incision, which allows them to correct malrotation or other associated gastrointestinal anomalies. The abdominal cavity may be underdeveloped, as in omphalocele and gastroschisis.

Tight abdominal closure sometimes contributes to postoperative respiratory compromise and vena caval compression, with concomitant reduction of venous return and cardiac output. During surgery, close attention must be paid to body temperature maintenance, the possibility of pneumothorax with sudden cardiopulmonary compromise (particularly in the hemithorax opposite the hernia), intravascular fluid volume, and acid-base balance.

#### Postoperative Care

Completion of the operative procedure is not the end of the challenge in caring for these patients. The classic "honeymoon period" of improved ventilation and oxygenation observed immediately after surgery is often abruptly terminated by recurrent bouts of pulmonary hypertension, hypercapnia, and hypoxemia. Intensive medical maneuvers to influence PVR are required.

### NEONATAL RESUSCITATION

The subject of neonatal resuscitation encompasses the provision of life support and interventions in the delivery room, NICU, and operating room. Although the underlying disease or impaired physiologic processes leading to cardiorespiratory arrest or profound hemodynamic instability may vary in these settings, the fundamental principles of resuscitation outlined in the final section of this chapter are generally the same.

Six percent of the approximately 3.8 million infants born each year in the United States require life support in the delivery room or nursery; in infants with a birth weight <1500 g, the requirement for resuscitation rises to 80%.[167] In most cases, the need for neonatal resuscitation can be anticipated on the basis of maternal history, antenatal diagnostic techniques, and fetal monitoring. Adequate resuscitation involves the skills of at least two to three health care providers. For these reasons, anesthesiologists must have a sound understanding of neonatal resuscitation techniques.

## When Is It Necessary?

Conditions that place a neonate at increased risk of asphyxia and requiring resuscitation are listed in Table 56–6; these may be divided into maternal, delivery-related, and fetal/neonatal factors.

## Apgar Scoring

The Apgar scoring system remains in nearly universal use to assess a neonate's general condition and degree of compromise after delivery.[168,169] It is based on 5 objective measurements:

1. Heart rate
2. Respiratory effort
3. Muscle tone
4. Reflex irritability
5. Color

A score from 0 to 2 is assigned for each clinical sign, with a maximum possible score of 10, at 1- and 5-minute intervals after birth.

A number of caveats must be remembered in using Apgar scores. First, resuscitation must not be withheld until an Apgar score is obtained; assessment of a patient begins immediately at birth, and appropriate interventions are applied as indicated. Second, the scoring system was not designed for premature infants, in whom several of the measurements can be difficult to apply meaningfully.[170] Third, scores should not be used in an attempt to predict long-term neurologic outcome.[171]

## What Is the Basic Approach?

Successful neonatal resuscitation depends on appropriate anticipation of neonates at increased risk of asphyxia, proper preparation of equipment, the environment, personnel who will be caring for the patient, and prompt initiation of resuscitation maneuvers. Figure 56–16 provides an algorithm for resuscitation in the delivery room and Table 56–7 lists the medications used; with modification for specific problems and therapies, the outlined principles can be applied in the NICU or operating room.

## Initial Maneuvers

The interventions that compose the neonatal resuscitation procedure begin with simple, noninvasive, and commonly required maneuvers and progress to the increasingly sophisticated steps required by smaller numbers of infants.[172] Simple initial steps include placing the neonate in the supine or lateral position under a radiant warmer with the head in a neutral position as drying and suctioning are provided. Most newborns begin spontaneous ventilations with these maneuvers, but if necessary, additional stimulation can be achieved by slapping or flicking the soles of the feet and rubbing an infant's back. Assessment of heart rate, respiratory activity, and color is undertaken at this time.

## Ventilation

### Bag-Mask

If a neonate remains apneic or has a heart rate <100 beats per minute, bag-valve-mask ventilation should be instituted. In newborns known or strongly suspected of having a diaphragmatic hernia, positive-pressure ventilation should be commenced through an ETT. Ventilations should be provided at a rate of 40 breaths per minute; initial lung inflation may require a peak pressure of 30 to 40 cm $H_2O$ or higher, and subsequent breaths should require 15 to 20 cm $H_2O$ pressure. Important is not so much what the airway pressure manometer shows but that gas exchange is accomplished at the lowest feasible inflation pressure.

### Tracheal Intubation

If mask ventilation is difficult, causes including poor mask fit, obstruction of the airway by the tongue, or congenital airway abnormalities must be sought and the airway and head positions reassessed. In some cases, laryngoscopic examina-

**TABLE 56–6.** Conditions That Place Neonates at Increased Risk for Requiring Resuscitation

| Maternal | Delivery | Fetal/Neonatal |
|---|---|---|
| Age >35 y | Cesarean section | Meconium staining of amniotic fluid |
| Diabetes mellitus | Abnormal fetal presentations | Prematurity |
| Toxemia of pregnancy | Prolapsed umbilical cord | Multiple gestations |
| Hypertension | Cord compression | Intrauterine fetal growth retardation |
| Anemia | Maternal hypotension | Polyhydramnios |
| Blood type isoimmunization | Use of forceps (other than low elective) | Oligohydramnios |
| Antepartum hemorrhage (placenta previa or abruptio placentae) | Prolonged rupture of membranes | Immature lecithin-to-sphingomyelin ratio |
| Drug therapy (narcotics, lithium, recreational drugs, magnesium, alcohol) | Difficulty with delivery | Fetal malformation (diaphragmatic hernia, congenital heart disease) |
| Previous fetal or neonatal death | Prolonged labor | Gestation >42 wk |
| Poor or no prenatal care | | Indices of fetal distress during labor (low fetal scalp pH, abnormal fetal monitoring tracing) |
| Maternal infections | | |
| Low estriol levels | | |

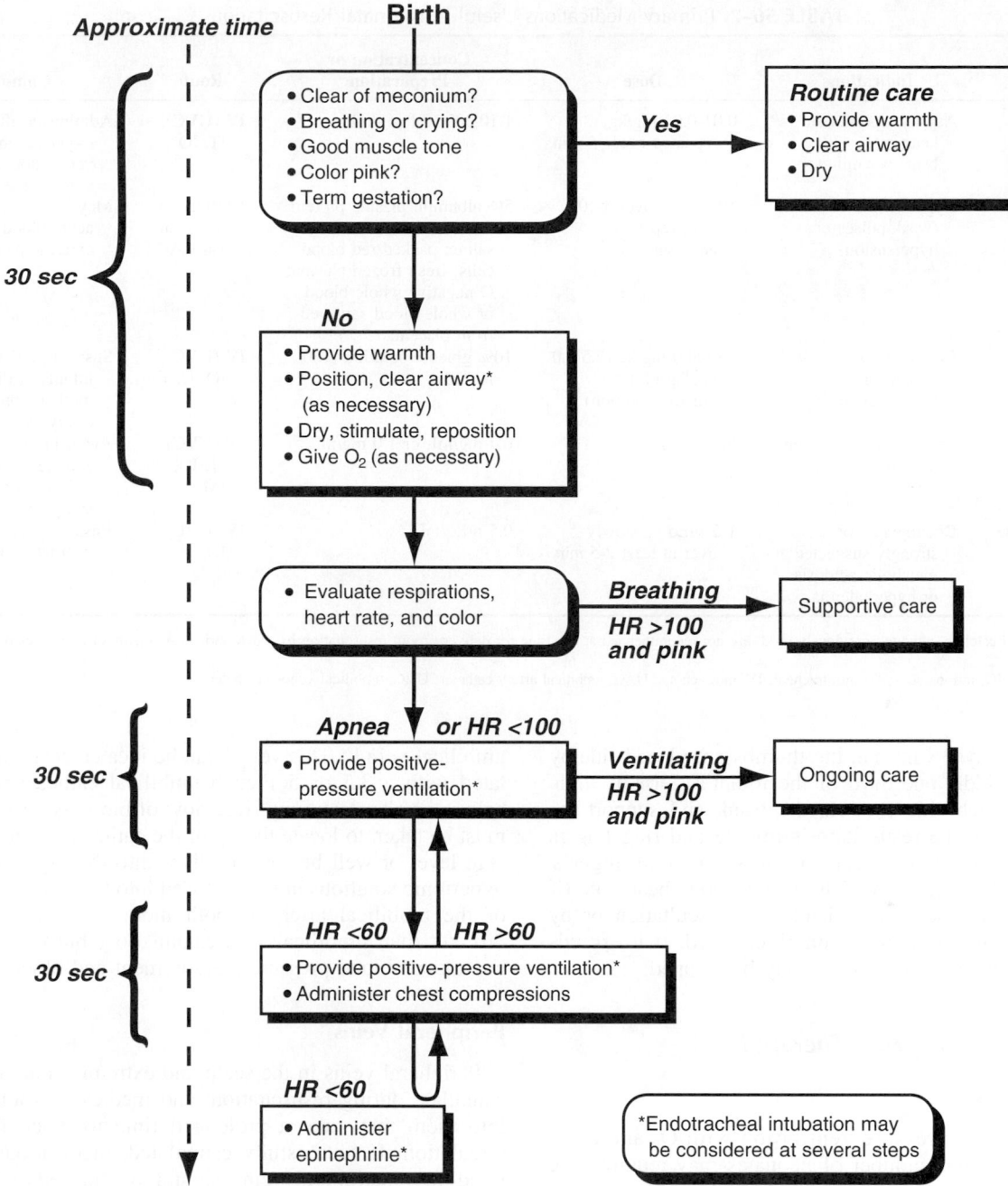

**Approximate time**

**Birth**

- Clear of meconium?
- Breathing or crying?
- Good muscle tone
- Color pink?
- Term gestation?

**Yes** →

**Routine care**
- Provide warmth
- Clear airway
- Dry

**30 sec**

**No**

- Provide warmth
- Position, clear airway*
  (as necessary)
- Dry, stimulate, reposition
- Give O₂ (as necessary)

- Evaluate respirations,
  heart rate, and color

**Breathing**
**HR >100**
**and pink** →

Supportive care

**Apnea    or HR <100**

**30 sec**

- Provide positive-
  pressure ventilation*

**Ventilating**
**HR >100**
**and pink** →

Ongoing care

**HR <60    HR >60**

**30 sec**

- Provide positive-pressure ventilation*
- Administer chest compressions

**HR <60**

- Administer
  epinephrine*

*Endotracheal intubation may
be considered at several steps

**FIGURE 56–16.** Algorithm for resuscitation of the newly born infant. (From Niermeyer S, Kattwinkel J, Van Reempts P, et al. International Guidelines for Neonatal Resuscitation: An Excerpt From the Guidelines 2000 for Cardiopulmonary Resuscitation and Emergency Cardiovascular Care: International Consensus on Science [electronic article]. *Pediatrics.* 2000;106[3]:e29.)

tion of the upper airway and tracheal intubation are required. Other indications for endotracheal intubation include the need for suctioning thick, particulate meconium and prolonged controlled ventilation.

After 15 to 30 seconds of adequate ventilation, the heart rate should be reassessed. Controlled ventilation may be stopped if the heart rate is >100 beats per minute and adequate spontaneous respirations are present. If the pulse is absent or the heart rate is <60 beats per minute, chest compressions should be started. If the heart rate is 60 to 100 beats per minute and rising, assisted ventilation should be continued but chest compressions may be withheld or stopped. In the event that a heart rate is <80 beats per minute and is not rising, both assisted ventilation and chest compressions should be provided.

### Chest Compressions

Chest compressions in neonates should be provided at a rate of ≥120 beats per minute, with the goal of depressing the sternum one half to three fourths of an inch with each stroke. Because of the prime importance of effective ventilations in neonates, chest compressions must be interposed with ventilations in a 3:1 ratio; this may result in the actual provision of 90 compressions and 30 ventilations each minute.[171] Correct finger placement for compressions can be accom-

**TABLE 56–7.** Primary Medications Useful in Neonatal Resuscitation

| Medication | Indications | Dose | Concentration or Preparation | Route | Comments |
|---|---|---|---|---|---|
| Epinephrine | Asystole, persistent heart rate <80 beats per minute | 0.01-0.03 mg/kg, repeated every 5 min | 1:10,000 (0.1 mg/mL) | IV (UVC), IT, IO | Administer after oxygenation, ventilation, chest compressions fail |
| Volume expander | Hypovolemia or shock (weak pulses or hypotension) | 10 mL/kg over 5-10 min; repeat as necessary | 5% albumin; plasma protein fraction; 0.9% (normal) saline; packed red blood cells; fresh frozen plasma; O-negative whole blood or whole blood salvaged from placenta | IV, IO; can be given via UAC | May be required with acute blood loss or extreme pallor |
| Glucose | Confirmed or suspected hypoglycemia | 250-500 mg/kg (2.5-5.0 mL/kg of 10% glucose solution) | 10% glucose solution (100 mg/mL) | IV (UVC), IO, UAC | Suspect particularly in infants of diabetic mothers, preterms, asphyxia |
| Naloxone | Ventilatory depression, narcotic-induced | 0.1 mg/kg | 0.4 mg/mL or 1.0 mg/mL | IV (UVC), IT, IO, IM | Avoid in infants of opiate-addicted mothers—may induce withdrawal symptoms |
| Sodium bicarbonate | Documented or strongly suspected metabolic acidosis or hyperkalemia | 1-2 mEq/kg slowly over at least 2-5 min | 0.5 mEq/mL | IV (UVC), IO | Ensure appropriate ventilation is provided |

*Note:* Atropine and calcium, although previously used, are not recommended at this time for delivery room resuscitation by the American Academy of Pediatrics or the American Heart Association.

IM, intramuscular; IO, intraosseous; IT, intratracheal; IV, intravenous; UAC, umbilical artery catheter; UVC, umbilical venous catheter.

plished in two ways.[173] In one, the thumbs are placed side by side over the middle one third of the infant's sternum while the fingers on each side encircle the trunk and support the back. In the other, the resuscitator's middle and ring fingers are used to provide two-finger compressions one finger's breadth below the nipple line. The spontaneous heart rate (if any) should be checked periodically by auscultation or by lightly grasping the base of the umbilical cord. If it exceeds 80 beats per minute, compressions may be stopped.

## What Is the Role of Drug Therapy?

### Indicated Agents

Despite positive-pressure ventilation with $O_2$ and chest compressions, a small number of neonates may require drug and fluid therapy. Drugs that have a role in the acute phase of neonatal resuscitation include epinephrine, naloxone, glucose, and plasma volume expanders (see Table 56–7). Calcium chloride or calcium gluconate should *not* be used without a specific diagnosis involving hypocalcemia or hyperkalemia. The vagolytic agent atropine, although useful in the initial resuscitation of older infants and children, is not a first-line drug in neonatal resuscitation.[172] Atropine and sodium bicarbonate may have a role in the NICU after definitive therapies have begun.

## How Should Drugs or Fluids Be Administered?

### Umbilical Vein

The preferred route of medication administration in neonatal resuscitation when no vascular access is in place is the umbilical vein.[174] This vessel can be located easily and cannulated with a 3.5 or 5 French umbilical catheter passed just below the skin level until free flow of blood is observed. Care must be taken to locate the tip of the catheter either just below skin level or well beyond the liver into the high IVC so that hypertonic solutions are not infused into the liver. Cannulation of the umbilical artery is both more time consuming and difficult than umbilical vein cannulation, but does allow for continuous blood pressure measurement and blood sampling.

### Peripheral Veins

Peripheral veins in the scalp and extremities are difficult to cannulate during resuscitation, and medications administered into them may take a prolonged time to reach the central circulation. If successfully cannulated, medications administered into peripheral veins should be flushed with several milliliters of normal saline to promote passage into the central circulation.

### Intraosseous

Intraosseous administration of drugs and fluids in neonates has been described, but experience with the technique in the newborn is limited.[175] (See Chapter 57 for a more in-depth discussion of intraosseous infusions.)

### Trachea

The intratracheal route can be used to administer epinephrine, naloxone, atropine, and lidocaine. Recommendations for intratracheal doses range from onefold to fivefold the standard intravenous dose for the drug. The effectiveness of an intratracheal drug can be increased by diluting it with 2 to 3 mL of normal saline and injecting through a suction catheter or feeding tube passed to the tip of the RTT of the intubated patient, and then providing several positive pressure ventilations.

## References

1. Morray JP, Posner K. *POCA Registry Newsletter.* Seattle, Wash: University of Washington Department of Anesthesiology; (10):Winter/Spring 2000.

2. Webb E, Ward RJ, Crawford EW, et al. Anesthetic experience for infants under 2500 grams weight. *Anesth Analg.* 1970;49:767.

3. Anand KJS, Hickey PR. Halothane-morphine compared with high-dose sufentanil for anesthesia and postoperative analgesia in neonatal cardiac surgery. *N Engl J Med.* 1992;326:1.

4. Anand KJS, McIntosh N, Lagercrantz H, et al. Analgesia and sedation in preterm neonates who require ventilatory support. *Arch Pediatr Adolesc Med.* 1999;153:331.

5. Anand KJS, Hickey PR. Pain and its effects in the human neonate and fetus. *N Engl J Med.* 1987;317:1321.

6. Anand KJS. Neonatal analgesia and anesthesia: introduction [review]. *Semin Perinatol.* 1998;225:347.

7. Berry FA, Gregory GA. Do premature infants require anesthesia for surgery? *Anesthesiology.* 1987;67:291.

8. Fitzgerald M. Development of pain pathways and mechanisms. In: Anand KJS, McGrath P, eds. *Pain in Neonates.* 1st ed. Amsterdam, The Netherlands: Elsevier; 1993:19.

9. Abu-Saad HH, Bours GJ, Stevens B, et al. Assessment of pain in the neonate. *Semin Perinatol.* 1998;22:402.

10. Anand KJS. Clinical importance of pain and stress in preterm neonates. *Biol Neonate.* 1998;73:19.

11. Anand KJS, Aynsley-Green A. Measuring the severity of surgical stress in newborn infants. *J Pediatr Surg.* 1988;23:297.

12. Ferris BG, Mead J, Opie LH. Partitioning of respiratory flow resistance in man. *J Appl Physiol.* 1964;19:653.

13. Eckenhoff JE. Some anatomic considerations of the infant larynx influencing endotracheal anesthesia. *Anesthesiology.* 1951;12:401.

14. Haddad GG, Perez-Fontan JJ. Development of the respiratory system. In: Behrman RE, Kliegman RM, Jenson HB, eds. *Nelson Textbook of Pediatrics.* 16th ed. Philadelphia, Pa: WB Saunders; 2000:1235.

15. Reid L. The lung: its growth and remodeling in health and diseases. *AJR Am J Roentgenol.* 1977;129:777.

16. Cook DR, Marcy JH. Pediatric anesthetic pharmacology. In: Cook DR, Marcy JH, eds. *Neonatal Anesthesia.* 1st ed. Pasadena, Calif: Appleton-Davies; 1988:87.

17. Mansell A, Bryan AC, Levison H. Airway closure in children. *J Appl Physiol.* 1972;33:711.

18. Harris TR. Physiological principles. In: Goldsmith JP, Karotkin EH, eds. *Assisted Ventilation of the Neonate.* 2nd ed. Philadelphia, Pa: WB Saunders; 1988:22.

19. Keens TG, Bryan AC, Levison H, et al. Developmental pattern of muscle fiber types in human ventilatory muscles. *J Appl Physiol.* 1978;44:909.

20. Habel A, Scott R. *Notes on Paediatrics: Neonatology.* 1st ed. Oxford, United Kingdom: Butterworth-Heinemann; 1998.

21. Friesen RH. Neonatal physiologic adaptations and their anesthetic implications. In: Diaz JH, ed. *Perinatal Anesthesia and Critical Care.* 1st ed. Philadelphia, Pa: WB Saunders; 1991:263.

22. Hagen PT, Scholz DG, Edwards WD. Incidence and size of patent foramen ovale during the first ten decades. *Mayo Clin Proc.* 1984;59:17.

23. Bernstein D. The fetal to neonatal circulatory transition. In: Behrman RE, Kliegman RM, Jenson HB, eds. *Nelson Textbook of Pediatrics.* 16th ed. Philadelphia, Pa: WB Saunders, 2000:1337.

24. Friedman WF. The intrinsic physiologic properties of the developing heart. *Prog Cardiovasc Dis.* 1972;15:87.

25. Goudsouzian NG. Anatomy and physiology in relation to pediatric anesthesia. In: Katz J, Steward DJ, eds. *Anesthesia and Uncommon Pediatric Diseases.* 1st ed. Philadelphia, Pa: WB Saunders; 1987:1.

26. Shaffer SE, Norman ME. Renal function and renal failure in the newborn. *Clin Perinatol.* 1989;16:199.

27. Larson L, Aperia A, Elinder G. Structural and functional development of the nephron. *Acta Paediatr Scand Suppl.* 1983;305:56.

28. Downes JJ, Heiser MS. Temperature regulation in the pediatric patient. *Semin Anesth.* 1984;3:37.

29. Gersony W, Duc G, Sinclair J. PFC syndrome (persistence of the fetal circulation). *Circulation.* 1969;39(suppl):iii-87.

30. Hansen T, Corbet A. Disorders of the transition. In: Taeusch HW, Ballard RA, eds. *Avery's Diseases of the Newborn.* 7th ed. Philadelphia, Pa: WB Saunders; 1998:602.

31. Walsh-Sukys MC, Tyson JE, Wright LL, et al. Persistent pulmonary hypertension of the newborn in the era before nitric oxide: practice variation and outcomes. *Pediatrics.* 2000;105:14.

32. Borland LM. Persistent pulmonary hypertension of the newborn. In: Cook DR, Marcy JH, eds. *Neonatal Anesthesia.* 1st ed. Pasadena, Calif: Appleton-Davies; 1988:49.

33. Rudolph A. High pulmonary vascular resistance after birth. *Clin Pediatr.* 1980;19:585.

34. Hagedorn MI, Gardner SL, Abman SH. Respiratory diseases. In: Merenstein GB, Gardner SL, eds. *Handbook of Neonatal Intensive Care.* 2nd ed. St Louis, Mo: CV Mosby; 1989:365.

35. Levin DL, Heymann MA, Kitterman JA, et al. Persistent pulmonary hypertension of the newborn infant. *J Pediatr.* 1976;89:626.

36. Hansen T, Gest A. Oxygen toxicity and other ventilatory complications of treatment of infants with persistent pulmonary hypertension. *Clin Perinatol.* 1984;11:653.

37. Dwortez G, Moya F, Sabo B, et al. Survival of infants with persistent pulmonary hypertension without extracorporeal membrane oxygenation. *Pediatrics.* 1989;84:1.

38. Wung WT, James L, James E. Management of infants with severe respiratory failure and persistence of the fetal circulation without hyperventilation. *Pediatrics.* 1985;76:488.

39. Steinhorn R. Persistent pulmonary hypertension of the newborn. *Acta Anaesthesiol Scand Suppl.* 1997;111:135.

40. Carlo W, Beoglos A, Chatburn R, et al. High-frequency jet ventilation in neonatal pulmonary hypertension. *Am J Dis Child.* 1989;143:233.

41. Clark R, Yoder B, Sell M. Prospective, randomized comparison of high-frequency oscillation and conventional ventilation in candidates for extracorporeal membrane oxygenation. *J Pediatr.* 1994;124:447.

42. Ward RM. Persistent pulmonary hypertension. In: Nelson NM, ed. *Current Therapy in Neonatal-Perinatal Medicine.* 2nd ed. Toronto, Ontario, Canada: BC Decker; 1990:331.

43. Roberts J, Fineman J, Morin F, et al. Inhaled nitric oxide and persistent pulmonary hypertension of the newborn. *N Engl J Med.* 1997;336:605.

44. Inhaled nitric oxide in full-term and nearly full-term infants with hypoxic respiratory failure. The Neonatal Inhaled Nitric Oxide Study Group. *N Engl J Med.* 1997;336:597.

45. Abman SH. New developments in the pathogenesis and treatment of neonatal pulmonary hypertension. *Pediatr Pulmonol.* 1999;18(suppl):201.

46. Gomez M, Hansen T, Corbet A. Therapies for intractable respiratory failure. In: Taeusch HW, Ballard RA, eds. *Avery's Diseases of the Newborn.* 7th ed. Philadelphia, Pa: WB Saunders; 1998:595.

47. Kanto W. A decade of experience with neonatal extracorporeal membrane oxygenation. *J Pediatr.* 1994;24:335.

48. Daberkow E, Washington RL. Cardiovascular diseases and surgical interventions. In: Merenstein GB, Gardner SL, eds. *Handbook of Neonatal Intensive Care.* 2nd ed. St Louis, Mo: CV Mosby; 1989:427.

49. Thompson AE, Cook DR. Respiratory care. In: Cook DR, Marcy JH, eds. *Neonatal Anesthesia.* 1st ed. Pasadena, Calif: Appleton-Davies; 1988:203.

50. Merritt TA, Hallman M, Bloom BT, et al. Prophylactic treatment of very premature infants with surfactant. *N Engl J Med.* 1986;315:785.

51. Minarcik CJ, Beachy P. Neurologic disorders. In: Merenstein GB, Gardner SL, eds. *Handbook of Neonatal Intensive Care.* 2nd ed. St Louis, Mo: CV Mosby; 1989:501.

52. Goddard-Finegold J, Mizrahi EM, Lee RT. The newborn nervous system. In: Taeusch HW, Ballard RA, eds. *Avery's Diseases of the Newborn.* 7th ed. Philadelphia, Pa: WB Saunders; 1998:839.

53. Volpe J. Neurologic outcome of prematurity. *Arch Neurol.* 1998;55:297.

54. Hegyi T. Intraventricular hemorrhage. In: Nelson NM, ed. *Current Therapy in Neonatal-Perinatal Medicine.* Toronto, Ontario, Canada: BC Decker; 1990:289.

55. Volpe J. Germinal matrix-intraventricular hemorrhage of the premature infant. In: Volpe J, ed. *Neurology of the Newborn.* 3rd ed. Philadelphia, Pa: WB Saunders; 1995:403.

56. Friesen RH, Honda AT, Thieme RE. Changes in anterior fontanelle pressure in preterm infants during tracheal intubation. *Anesth Analg.* 1987;66:874.

57. Diaz JH. Anesthetic management of premature neonates. In: Diaz JH, ed. *Perinatal Anesthesia and Critical Care.* 1st ed. Philadelphia, Pa: WB Saunders; 1991:281.

58. Christensen RD. Expected hematologic values for neonates. In: Chris-

tensen RD, ed. *Hematologic Problems of the Neonate.* 1st ed. Philadelphia, Pa: WB Saunders; 2000:117.

59. Ohls RK. Evaluation and treatment of anemia in the neonate. In: Christensen RD, ed. *Hematologic Problems of the Neonate.* 1st ed. Philadelphia, Pa: WB Saunders; 2000:137.

60. Bard H. Hemoglobin synthesis and metabolism during the neonatal period. In: Christensen RD, eds. *Hematologic Problems of the Neonate.* 1st ed. Philadelphia, Pa: WB Saunders; 2000:365.

61. Keyes WG, Donohue PK, Spivak JL, et al. Assessing the need for transfusion of premature infants and the role of hematocrit, clinical signs, and erythropoietin levels. *Pediatrics.* 1989;84:412.

62. Joshi ATG, Shandloff P. Blood transfusion effect on the respiratory pattern of preterm infants. *Pediatrics.* 1987;80:79.

63. Welborn LG, Hannallah RS, Luban NLC, et al. Anemia and postoperative apnea in former preterm infants. *Anesthesiology.* 1991;74:1003.

64. Phelps DL. Retinopathy of prematurity. In: Nelson NM, ed. *Current Therapy in Neonatal-Perinatal Medicine.* Toronto, Ontario, Canada: BC Decker; 1990:350.

65. Bullard SR, Donahue SP, Feman SS, et al. The decreasing incidence and severity of retinopathy of prematurity. *J AAPOS.* 1999;3:46.

66. Hussain N, Clive J, Bhandari V. Current incidence of retinopathy of prematurity. *Pediatrics.* 1999;1043:e26.

67. Porat R. Care of the infant with retinopathy of prematurity. *Clin Perinatol.* 1984;11:123.

68. Stafani FH, Ehalt H. Non–oxygen-induced retinitis proliferans and retinal detachment in full-term infants. *Br J Ophthalmol.* 1974;58:490.

69. Flynn JT. Retinopathy of prematurity. *Pediatr Clin North Am.* 1987;34:1487.

70. Cross KW. Cost of preventing retrolental fibroplasia. *Lancet.* 1973;2:954.

71. Olitsky SE, Nelson LB. Disorders of the retina and vitreous. In: Behrman RE, Kliegman R, Jenson HB, eds. *Nelson Textbook of Pediatrics.* 16th ed. Philadelphia, Pa: WB Saunders; 2000:1925.

72. Martyn LJ. Pediatric ophthalmology. In: Behrman RE, Vaughan VC, Nelson WE, eds. *Nelson Textbook of Pediatrics.* 12th ed. Philadelphia, Pa: WB Saunders; 1983:1761.

73. Kalina RE. Update on retinopathy of prematurity. *West J Med.* 1990;153:188.

74. Sternberg P, Lopez PF, Lambert HM, et al. Controversies in the management of retinopathy of prematurity. *Am J Ophthalmol.* 1992;113:198.

75. Brown GC, Tasman WS, Naidoff M, et al. Systemic complications associated with retinal cryoablation for retinopathy of prematurity. *Ophthalmology.* 1990;97:855.

76. Steward DJ. Preterm infants are more prone to complications following minor surgery than are term infants. *Anesthesiology.* 1982;56:304.

77. Welborn LG, Ramirez N, Oh TH, et al. Evaluation of anesthetic risks in premature infants [abstract]. *Anesthesiology.* 1984;61:A417.

78. Mayhew JF, Bourke DL, Guinee WS. Evaluation of the premature infant at risk for premature complications. *Can J Anaesth.* 1987;34:627.

79. Hansen T, Corbet A. Chronic lung disease. In: Taeusch HW, Ballard RA, eds. *Avery's Diseases of the Newborn.* 7th ed. Philadelphia, Pa: WB Saunders; 1998:634.

80. Barrington KJ, Finer NN. Treatment of bronchopulmonary dysplasia. *Clin Perinatol.* 1998;251:177.

81. Groneck P, Speer C. Pulmonary inflammation in the pathogenesis of bronchopulmonary dysplasia. *Pediatr Pulmonol.* 1997;16(suppl):29.

82. Ruggins NR. Pathophysiology of apnea in preterm infants. *Arch Dis Child.* 1991;66:70.

83. Noseworthy J, Duran C, Khine HH. Post-operative apnea in a full-term infant. *Anesthesiology.* 1989;70:879.

84. Tetzlaff JE, Annand DW, Pudimat MA, et al. Postoperative apnea in a full-term infant. *Anesthesiology.* 1988;69:426.

85. Daily WJR, Klaws M, Meyer HBB. Apnea in premature infants: monitoring, incidence, heart rate changes, and an effect of environment temperature. *Pediatrics.* 1969;43:510.

86. Malviya S, Swartz J, Lerman J. Are all preterm infants younger than 60 weeks postconceptual age at risk for postanesthetic apnea? *Anesthesiology.* 1993;78:1076.

87. Kurth CD, LeBard SE. Association of postoperative apnea, airway obstruction, and hypoxemia in former premature infants. *Anesthesiology.* 1991;75:22.

88. Steward DJ. Is there a risk of general anesthesia triggering SIDS? Possibly not! *Anesthesiology.* 1985;63:326.

89. Coté CJ, Zaslavsky A, Downes JJ, et al. Postoperative apnea in former preterm infants after inguinal herniorrhaphy. *Anesthesiology.* 1995;82:809.

90. Welborn LG, Hannallah RS, Fink R. High-dose caffeine suppresses postoperative apnea in former preterm infants. *Anesthesiology.* 1989;71:347.

91. Peliowski A, Finer NN. A blinded, randomized, placebo-controlled trial to compare theophylline and doxapram for the treatment of apnea of prematurity. *J Pediatr.* 1990;116:648.

92. Somri M, Gaitini L, Viada S, et al. Postoperative outcome in high-risk infants undergoing herniorrhaphy: comparison between general and spinal anesthesia. *Anaesthesia.* 1998;53:762.

93. Watcha MF, Thach BT, Gunter JB. Postoperative apnea after caudal anesthesia in an ex-premature infant. *Anesthesiology.* 1989;71:613.

94. Kunst G, Linderkamp O, Holle R, et al. The proportion of high-risk preterm infants with postoperative apnea and bradycardia is the same after general and spinal anesthesia. *Can J Anaesth.* 1998;94.

95. Eriksson LI, Sandin R. Fasting guidelines in different countries. *Acta Anaesthesiol Scand.* 1996;40:971.

96. Blumenthal I, Ebel A, Pildes RS. Effect of posture on the pattern of stomach emptying in the newborn. *Pediatrics.* 1979;63:532.

97. Tomomasa T, Hyman PE, Itoh K, et al. Gastroduodenal motility in neonates: response to human milk compared to cow's milk formula. *Pediatrics.* 1987;80:4343.

98. Emerson BM, Wrigley SR, Newton M. Pre-operative fasting for paediatric anaesthesia: a survey of current practice. *Anaesthesia.* 1998;534:326.

99. Ferrari LR, Rooney FM, Rockoff MA. Preoperative fasting practices in pediatrics. *Anesthesiology.* 1999;90:978.

100. Richards MPM, Bernal JF, Brackbill Y. Early behavioral differences: gender or circumcision? *Dev Psychobiol.* 1976;9:89.

101. Salem MR, Wong AY, Mani M, et al. Premedicant drugs and gastric juice pH and volume in pediatric patients. *Anesthesiology.* 1976;44:216.

102. Marcy JH, Cook DR. Basic neonatal anesthesia and monitoring. In: Cook DR, Marcy JH, eds. *Neonatal Anesthesia.* 1st ed. Pasadena, Calif: Appleton-Davies; 1988:143.

103. Marshall TA, Deeder R, Pai S. Physiologic changes associated with endotracheal intubation in preterm infants. *Crit Care Med.* 1984;12:501.

104. Wells JT, Ment LR. Prevention of intraventricular hemorrhage in preterm infants. *Early Hum Dev.* 1995;42:209.

105. Armstrong TS, Byers GF, Johnston GM. Tracheal intubation in infants [letter]. *Anesth Analg.* 1998;876:1455.

106. Peutrell JM, Wilkins DG. Pyloric stenosis in full term babies: a postal survey of the management by paediatric anaesthetists. *Paediatr Anaesth.* 1994;4:93.

107. Politis GD, Tobin JR, Morell RC, et al. Tracheal intubation of healthy pediatric patients without muscle relaxant: a survey of technique utilization and perceptions of safety. *Anesth Analg.* 1999;88:737.

108. Tochen ML. Orotracheal intubation in the newborn infant. *J Pediatr.* 1979;95:1050.

109. Finholt DA, Henry DB, Raphaely RC. Factors affecting leak around endotracheal tubes in children. *Can Anaesth Soc J.* 1985;32:326.

110. Gregory GA. Anesthesia for premature infants. In: Gregory GA, ed. *Pediatric Anesthesia.* New York, NY: Churchill Livingstone; 1989:803.

111. Spears RS, Yeh A, Fisher DM, et al. The "educated hand": can anesthesiologists assess changes in neonatal pulmonary compliance manually? *Anesthesiology.* 1991;75:693.

112. Steward DJ. Mechanical versus manual ventilation of the lungs of infants in the operating room. *Anesthesiology.* 1992;76:479.

113. Clark RH, Slutsky AS, Gerstmann DR. Lung protective strategies of ventilation in the neonate: what are they? *Pediatrics.* 2000;1051:112.

114. Fox WW, Spitzer AR, Shutack JG. Positive-pressure ventilation: pressure- and time-cycled ventilators. In: Goldsmith JP, Karotkin EH, eds. *Assisted Ventilation of the Neonate.* 2nd ed. Philadelphia, Pa: WB Saunders; 1988:146.

115. Bain JA, Spoerel WE. A streamlined anesthetic system. *Can Anaesth Soc J.* 1972;19:426.

116. Miller DM. Breathing systems for use in anesthesia: evaluation using a physical lung model and classification. *Br J Anaesth.* 1988;60:555.

117. Badgwell JM, Wolf AR, McEvedy BA, et al. Fresh gas formulae do not accurately predict end-tidal $PCO_2$ in paediatric patients. *Can J Anaesth.* 1988;35:581.

118. Coté CJ. Pediatric equipment. In: Coté CJ, Ryan JF, Todres ID, et al, eds. *A Practice of Anesthesia for Infants and Children.* 2nd ed. Philadelphia, Pa: WB Saunders; 1993:483.

119. Metz RI, Lucking SE, Chaten FC, et al. Percutaneous catheterization of the axillary vein in infants and children. *Pediatrics.* 1990;85:531.

120. Coté CJ, Jobes DR, Schwartz AJ, et al. Two approaches to cannulation of a child's internal jugular vein. *Anesthesiology.* 1979;50:371.

121. Roberts JD, Todres ID, Coté CJ. Neonatal emergencies. In: Coté CJ, Ryan JF, Todres ID, et al, eds. *A Practice of Anesthesia for Infants and Children.* 2nd ed. Philadelphia, Pa: WB Saunders; 1993:225.

122. Furman EB, Roman GD, Lemmer LAS, et al. Specific therapy in water, electrolyte, and blood-volume replacement during pediatric surgery. *Anesthesiology.* 1975;42:187.

123. Liu LMP. Fluid management. In: Coté CJ, Ryan JF, Todres ID, et al, eds. *A Practice of Anesthesia for Infants and Children.* 2nd ed. Philadelphia, Pa: WB Saunders; 1993:171.

124. Shires T, Williams J, Brown F. Acute changes in extracellular fluids associated with major surgical procedures. *Ann Surg.* 1961;154:803.

125. American Society of Anesthesiologists. Standards for basic intraoperative monitoring. In: American Society of Anesthesiologists, ed. *Directory of Members.* Park Ridge, Ill: American Society of Anesthesiologists, 2000:477.

126. Coté CJ, Rolf N, Liu LMP, et al. A single-blind study of combined pulse oximetry and capnography in children. *Anesthesiology.* 1991;74:980.

127. Rooth G, Huch A, Huch R. Transcutaneous oxygen monitors are reliable indicators of arterial oxygen tension (if used correctly). *Pediatrics.* 1987;79:283.

128. Coté CJ, Goldstein EA, Coté CJ. A single-blind study of pulse oximetry in children. *Anesthesiology.* 1988;68:184.

129. Partridge BL. Use of pulse oximetry as a non-invasive indicator of intravascular volume status. *J Clin Monit.* 1987;3:263.

130. Badgwell JM, McLeod ME, Lerman J, et al. End-tidal $PCO_2$ measurements sampled at the distal and proximal ends of the endotracheal tube in infants and children. *Anesth Analg.* 1987;66:959.

131. Gravenstein N. Capnometry in infants should not be done at lower sampling flow rates. *J Clin Monit.* 1989;5:63.

132. Katz S, Basel D, Branski D. Prenatal gastric dilatation and infantile hypertrophic pyloric stenosis. *J Pediatr Surg.* 1988;23:1021.

133. Bissonette B, Sullivan P. Pyloric stenosis. *Can J Anaesth.* 1991;38:668.

134. Spicer RD. Infantile pyloric stenosis: a review. *Br J Surg.* 1982;69:128.

135. Cook-Sather SD, Tulloch HV, Cnaan A, et al. A comparison of awake versus paralyzed tracheal intubation for infants with pyloric stenosis. *Anesth Analg.* 1998;86:945.

136. MacDonald NJ, Fitzpatrick GJ, Moore KD, et al. Anaesthesia for congenital hypertrophic pyloric stenosis: a review of 350 patients. *Br J Anaesth.* 1987;59:672.

137. Andropoulos DB, Heard MB, Johnson KL, et al. Postanesthetic apnea in full-term infants after pyloromyotomy. *Anesthesiology.* 1994;80:216.

138. Habre W, Schwab C, Gollow I, et al. An audit of postoperative analgesia after pyloromyotomy. *Paediatr Anaesth.* 1999;9:253.

139. Dierdorf SF, Krishna G. Anesthetic management of neonatal surgical emergencies. *Anesth Analg.* 1981;60:204.

140. Schwartz MZ, Tyson KRT, Milliorn K, et al. Staged reduction using a Silastic sac is the treatment of choice for large congenital abdominal wall defects. *J Pediatr Surg.* 1983;18:713.

141. Philippart AI, Canty TG, Filler RM. Acute fluid volume requirements in infants with anterior abdominal wall defects. *J Pediatr Surg.* 1972;7:553.

142. Yaster M, Buck JR, Dudgeon DL, et al. Hemodynamic effects of primary closure of omphalocele/gastroschisis in human newborns. *Anesthesiology.* 1988;69:84.

143. Marcy JH, Cook DR. Common surgical conditions of the newborn. In: Cook DR, Marcy JH, eds. *Neonatal Anesthesia.* 1st ed. Pasadena, Calif: Appleton-Davies; 1988:159.

144. Kosloske AM, Musemeche CA. Necrotizing enterocolitis of the neonate. *Clin Perinatol.* 1989;16:97.

145. Kliegman RM, Fanaroff AA. Necrotizing enterocolitis. *N Engl J Med.* 1984;310:1093.

146. Stoll BJ, Kliegman RM. Digestive system disorders. In: Behrman RE, Kliegman RM, Jenson HB, eds. *Nelson Textbook of Pediatrics.* 16th ed. Philadelphia, Pa: WB Saunders; 2000:510.

147. Ahmed T, Ein S, Moore A. The role of peritoneal drains in treatment of perforated necrotizing enterocolitis: recommendations from recent experience. *J Pediatr Surg.* 1998;3310:1468.

148. Gersony WM. Patent ductus arteriosus in the neonate. *Pediatr Clin North Am.* 1986;33:545.

149. Gittenberger-de-Groot AC. Persistent ductus arteriosus: most probably a primary congenital malformation. *Br Heart J.* 1977;6:610.

150. Bernstein D. Acyanotic congenital heart disease: the left-to-right shunt lesions. In: Behrman RE, Kliegman RM, Jenson HB, eds. *Nelson Textbook of Pediatrics.* 16th ed. Philadelphia, Pa: WB Saunders; 2000:1365.

151. Gersony WM, Peckham GJ, Ellison RC, et al. Effects of indomethacin in premature infants with patent ductus arteriosus: results of a national collaborative study. *J Pediatr.* 1983;102:895.

152. Robinson S, Gregory G. Fentanyl-air-oxygen anesthesia for ligation of patent ductus arteriosus in preterm infants. *Anesth Analg.* 1981;60.331.

153. Reyes HM, Meller JL, Loef D: Management of esophageal atresia and tracheoesophageal fistula. *Clin Perinatol.* 1989;16:79.

154. Barry JE, Auldist AW. The VATER association: one end of a spectrum of anomalies. *Am J Dis Child.* 1974;128:769.

155. Thebaud B, Mercier JC, Dinh-Xuan AT. Congenital diaphragmatic hernia: a cause of persistent pulmonary hypertension of the newborn which lacks an effective therapy. *Biol Neonate.* 1998;745:323.

156. Kitagawa M, Hislop A, Boyden EA, et al. Lung hypoplasia in congenital diaphragmatic hernia: a quantitative study of airway, artery, and alveolar development. *Br J Surg.* 1971;58:342.

157. Taira Y, Yamataka T, Miyazaki E, et al. Comparison of the pulmonary vasculature in newborns and stillborns with congenital diaphragmatic hernia. *Pediatr Surg Int.* 1998;14:30.

158. Clark RH, Hardin WD, Hirschl RB, et al. Current surgical management of congenital diaphragmatic hernia: a report from the Congenital Diaphragmatic Hernia Study Group. *J Pediatr Surg.* 1998;33:1004.

159. Truog RD, Schena JA, Hershenson MB, et al. Repair of congenital diaphragmatic hernia during extracorporeal membrane oxygenation. *Anesthesiology.* 1990;72:720.

160. The Congenital Diaphragmatic Hernia Study Group. Does extracorporeal membrane oxygenation improve survival in neonates with congenital diaphragmatic hernia? The Congenital Diaphragmatic Hernia Study Group. *J Pediatr Surg.* 1999;345:720.

161. Tiefenbrunn LJ, Riemenschneider TA. Persistent pulmonary hypertension in the newborn. *Am Heart J.* 1986;111:564.

162. Bohn DJ, Pearl R, Irish MS, et al. Postnatal management of congenital diaphragmatic hernia. *Clin Perinatol.* 1996;23:843.

163. Kays DW, Langham MR, Ledbetter DJ, et al. Detrimental effects of standard medical therapy in congenital diaphragmatic hernia. *Ann Surg.* 1999;230:340.

164. Hartman GE. Diaphragmatic hernia. In: Behrman RE, Kliegman RM, Jenson HB, eds. *Nelson Textbook of Pediatrics.* 16th ed. Philadelphia, Pa: WB Saunders; 2000:1231.

165. Kamata S, Usui N, Okuyama H, et al. Prolonged preoperative stabilization using high-frequency oscillatory ventilation does not improve the outcome in neonates with congenital diaphragmatic hernia. *Pediatr Surg Int.* 1998;13:542.

166. Vacanti JP, Crone RK. The pulmonary hemodynamic response to perioperative anesthesia in the treatment of high-risk infants with congenital diaphragmatic hernia. *J Pediatr Surg.* 1984;19:672.

167. Emergency Cardiac Care Committee and Subcommittees, American Heart Association. Guidelines for cardiopulmonary resuscitation and emergency cardiac care, part VII: neonatal resuscitation. *Circulation.* 2000;102(suppl I):I-343–I-357.

168. Apgar V. Proposal for method of evaluation of newborn infant. *Anesth Analg.* 1953;32:260.

169. Casey BM, McIntyre DD, Leveno KJ. The continuing value of the Apgar score for the assessment of newborn infants. *N Engl J Med.* 2001;344:467.

170. Catlin EA, Carpenter MW, Brann BSI, et al. The Apgar score revisited: influence of gestational age. *J Pediatr.* 1986;109:865.

171. Nelson KB, Ellenberg JH. Neonatal signs as predictors of cerebral palsy. *Pediatrics.* 1979;64:225.

172. Subcommittee on Pediatric Resuscitation. Newborn resuscitation. In: Chameides L, Hazinski MF, eds. *Pediatric Advanced Life Support.* Dallas, Tex: American Heart Association; 1997:9-1.

173. Todres ID, Rogers MC. Methods of external cardiac massage in the newborn infant. *J Pediatr.* 1975;86:781.

174. Bloom RS, Copley C. *Textbook of Neonatal Resuscitation.* Dallas, Tex: American Heart Association; 1987.

175. Kelsall AW. Resuscitation with intraosseous lines in neonatal units. *Arch Dis Child.* 1993;68:324.

# CHAPTER
# 57

# The Pediatric Patient

Timothy W. Martin
Joanne M. Stoner

*What Are Maintenance Fluids?*

*What Are Fasting Fluid Deficits?*

*What Constitutes Intraoperative Fluid Loss?*

MONITORING

*What Is Routine?*

*When Should Monitors Be Applied to the Child?*

*What Is the Role of Pulse Oximetry and Capnography?*

*What Common Intraoperative Problems May Be Detected?*

REGIONAL ANESTHESIA

*What Is Its Role?*

POSTANESTHETIC PROBLEMS

*What Are Some Common Problems Encountered After Anesthesia?*

*What Are the Causes of Airway Obstruction in the Postanesthesia Care Unit?*

*How Is Laryngospasm Recognized?*

*What Causes Postintubation Croup, and How Is It Treated?*

*Why Does Hypoxemia Occur?*

*What Are Potential Causes of Delayed Emergence?*

*What Is Emergence Delerium?*

*How Is Postoperative Pain Managed?*

*Why Do Nausea and Vomiting Occur?*

*How Are Postanesthetic Nausea and Vomiting Managed?*

Physicians whose practices encompass both children and adults often must be reminded that pediatric patients are not simply little adults. Within the realm of anesthetic practice, children pose a number of different problems and have requirements that separate them from adults, who are generally the foundation on which instruction and training in anesthesia are based.

Perhaps the most obvious differences between the juvenile and adult patient concern the physical size of the body and its constituent structures. Often related to variations in gross size are differences in physiologic processes and pharmacologic responses that have significant implications for the pediatric anesthesia practice. These differences are of greatest magnitude in the premature and term neonate and gradually diminish at varying rates over the first 10 to 15 years of life as anatomic, physiologic, and metabolic growth and maturation take place. By mid-adolescence, the teenage child may be considered physically (if not socially and psychologically) an adult for anesthetic purposes.

The many differences briefly outlined imply not only that anesthesiologists caring for children should be knowledgeable of pediatric anesthesia but also that there are in fact numerous institutional and "system" requirements for providing appropriate pediatric anesthetic care. Taken together, these features comprise the pediatric perioperative anesthesia environment, details of which have been described and set forth by the American Academy of Pediatrics.[1] The most highly skilled and experienced pediatric anesthesiologist would have great difficulty providing optimum quality care in an environment that lacked the other health care personnel, facilities, and equipment to support the provision of pediatric anesthesia services.

Because anatomic and physiologic differences are most profound in the neonatal and infant periods, they are considered in Chapter 56. This chapter emphasizes the preoperative evaluation and preparation of the pediatric patient and common features of the induction, maintenance, and monitoring of anesthesia in children. Concluding sections discuss the postoperative problems encountered in the treatment of children as well as anesthetic approaches to pediatric laryngoscopy and bronchoscopy, tonsillectomy and pressure-equalizing tube insertion, and sedation for magnetic resonance imaging (MRI) procedures.

## PREANESTHETIC ASSESSMENT: GENERAL CONSIDERATIONS

### What Are Normal Vital Signs and Weights in Children?

Every clinician involved in providing anesthesia care for children should be aware of the actual and age-specific reference body weight and vital signs for each patient. Knowledge of this information provides the basis for a number of different anesthetic assessments and interventions in the preoperative, intraoperative, and postoperative periods. For example, the child's usual or baseline weight, heart rate, and blood pressure (BP) are useful in the evaluation of chronic disease states and fluid volume status during the preanesthetic assessment. Intraoperatively, the same parameters must be considered in determining drug dosages, intravenous fluid requirements, and appropriate hemodynamic responses to anesthesia and surgical stimulation. For these purposes, the data in Table 57–1 are provided as a reference.

### What Information Must Be Exchanged Preoperatively?

The preanesthetic interview provides an opportunity for the anesthesiologist to obtain a great deal of information about the child's medical and surgical history, recent state of health, and general temperament, particularly as it relates to anticipated reactions to separation from the parents and to anesthetic induction (Fig. 57–1). In addition, and as important, the interview serves to allow parents and older children an improved understanding of the anesthetic experience, perioperative period, and potential complications of anesthesia. Nothing substitutes for a frank, unhurried, and appropriately detailed discussion of what the patient and parents can expect on the day of surgery, both in and out of the operating room. To expect that the preoperative encounter should obviate the need for pharmacologic maneuvers to sedate the child before surgery is unrealistic. However, it should significantly allay parental anxieties and fears, which not uncommonly exceed those of the juvenile patient and often influence the anxieties of the child.

#### From the Parents and Child

Important information to be gathered includes current medications; any history of drug intolerance or allergies, including latex products; previous surgical procedures or anesthetics, and the problems experienced with them; and general informa-

**TABLE 57–1.** Weights and Vital Signs for Children

| Age | Resting Heart Rate (per minute) | Resting Blood Pressure (All Values ±10 mm Hg) | | Resting Respiratory Rate (per min) | Weight (kg), 50th Percentile | |
|---|---|---|---|---|---|---|
| | | Boys | Girls | | Boys | Girls |
| Newborn | 120 (±25) | 70/50 | 70/50 | 45 (±15) | 3.4 | 3.2 |
| 6 mo | 140 (±30) | 95/50 | 90/50 | 40 (±10) | 8 | 7 |
| 1 y | 120 (±20) | 95/55 | 95/50 | 35 (±10) | 10 | 9.6 |
| 2 y | 110 (±30) | 95/60 | 95/60 | 35 (±5) | 12.6 | 12 |
| 4 y | 100 (±35) | 90/55 | 90/55 | 25 (±8) | 17 | 16 |
| 6 y | 95 (±25) | 95/60 | 95/60 | 22 (±7) | 21 | 20 |
| 8 y | 90 (±25) | 100/60 | 100/60 | 22 (±7) | 25 | 25 |
| 10 y | 80 (±20) | 100/65 | 100/65 | 22 (±7) | 32 | 33 |
| 12 y | 75 (±20) | 105/65 | 110/70 | 20 (±5) | 40 | 42 |
| 14 y | 70 (±20) | 110/65 | 110/70 | 20 (±5) | 50 | 50 |

Data from Hamill PW, Drizd TA, Johnson CL, et al. NCHS Growth Charts, 1976. Monthly Vital Statistics Report. US Department of Health, Education and Welfare, Washington, DC. Report of the Second Task Force on Blood Pressure Control in Children—1987. *Pediatrics.* 1987;79:1, and Baldwin GA. Vital signs for age. In: Baldwin GA, ed. *Handbook of Pediatric Emergencies.* Boston, Mass: Little, Brown; 1989:46.

tion that focuses on the cardiovascular and respiratory systems. For infants and toddlers, be sure to inquire about the gestational and neonatal periods and about any illnesses or difficulties that may have been encountered. If a chronic disease state or surgical condition with systemic manifestations is present, further specific questioning should be pursued to define the anticipated effect of the disorder on anesthesia and recovery. Postpubertal girls should be specifically questioned for symptoms of anemia and the possibility of pregnancy.

### To the Parents and Child

As indicated previously, information is exchanged bidirectionally during the preoperative interview. Specific points to be explained to the responsible adult or adults caring for the infant or school-aged child include fasting guidelines, plans for premedication, the anticipated induction technique, vascular access and airway adjuncts (particularly if the latter are to remain in place postoperatively), plans for the use of blood products (if applicable), and any regional anesthetic techniques to be applied for anesthetic maintenance or postoperative analgesia. A description of what can be expected in the postanesthesia care unit (PACU) or intensive care unit (ICU) after surgery is also prudent.

## What Pertinent Information Can Be Obtained From the Medical Record?

### Previous Anesthetics

Although in most cases, sufficient information can be obtained in the course of the preanesthetic interview and the physical examination, in some instances, the medical record may provide invaluable data. This observation is perhaps most true with children who previously have experienced anesthesia; in this case, information regarding responses to premedication, ease of parental separation and induction, airway management, tolerance of anesthesia, and complications may be obtained.

### Disease Processes

The records of children with disease processes likely to influence the response to anesthesia, such as cardiac and

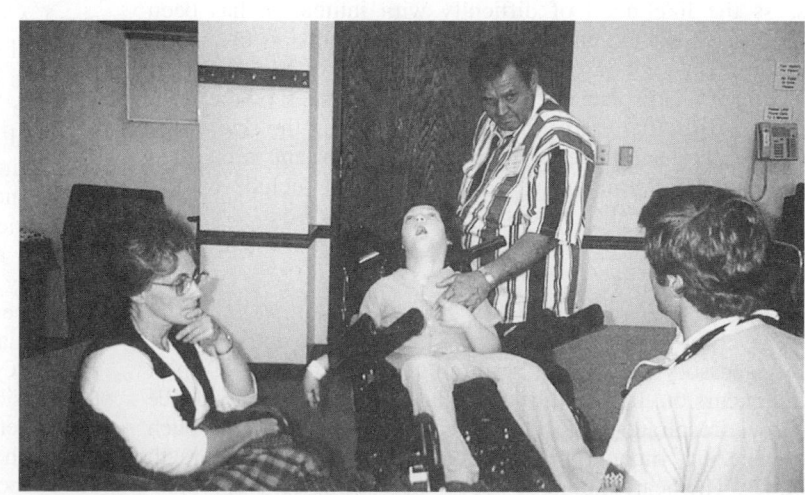

**FIGURE 57–1.** Anesthesiologist conducting the preanesthesia interview of a child and parents.

pulmonary disorders, may contain details unavailable to or unknown by the parents. An example is cardiac catheterization or echocardiographic data in the child with congenital heart disease. Such data may define anatomic abnormalities; the presence, direction, and degree of shunting; the existence of pulmonary hypertension; and an estimate of ventricular function. In children with symptoms of an upper respiratory tract infection (URI), an idea of the frequency and typical course of such infections can be obtained to assist in making the decision about whether to proceed with or to reschedule surgery. The medical record also frequently indicates recent weights and vital signs and may list drug intolerance or allergies as well as any medications being taken.

### Caretakers

The medical record of the child also typically contains information about the responsible caretaker, such as which adult or adults or agencies are legally responsible for the child, how the parent or consent-granting authority can be reached if that individual is not with the child, and how far the caretaker and pediatric outpatient must travel to reach a hospital should complications develop after surgery.

## What Does the Routine Preanesthetic Physical Examination Encompass?

### Upper Airway

As is generally the case in adults, the emphasis of the preoperative examination of the child is on the cardiovascular and respiratory systems. The upper airway should be evaluated for several reasons: (1) to identify any evidence of URI that may place the child at increased risk of airway or pulmonary complications perioperatively; (2) to recognize any features that may make airway management and intubation difficult; and (3) to identify any loose teeth. In the absence of any of the several congenital abnormalities known to be associated with unusual or difficult facial and airway anatomy, such as the Pierre-Robin, Treacher-Collins, or Goldenhar syndromes, pediatric patients rarely are unable to be ventilated by mask and intubated.

In contrast to adults, no systematic classification scheme to assess the likelihood of difficulty with intubation has been developed for children.[2] However, key elements of the airway examination include evaluation of the size of the mandible and potential displacement space for the tissues of the floor of the mouth, the size of the oral aperture, and the size of the tongue. The last of these is particularly important in children with any of several metabolic disorders that include macroglossia as a typical feature.

### Chest

The chest should be physically inspected to detect use of any accessory muscles of respiration or asymmetry of chest wall excursion. It should be auscultated to detect any evidence of lower respiratory infection or reactive airways disease, such as wheezing, rhonchi, crackles, or areas of diminished breath sounds. The heart should be auscultated during several inhalation-exhalation cycles to detect any murmurs.

### Skin and Nail Beds

The skin and nail beds merit examination to detect or evaluate a variety of conditions, including cyanosis, anemia, ecchymoses, hypovolemia, diffuse skin rashes (which may indicate the presence of any of several systemic diseases, such as measles or chicken pox), and the suitability of different sites for venous cannulation.

## What Laboratory Studies Should Be Performed?

Most healthy children who are to undergo elective surgery require no routine laboratory testing, chest radiography, and electrocardiographic (ECG) testing in the absence of specific symptoms, signs, or known disease processes. Preoperative studies in children should largely be determined by the nature of any preexisting disease states and by the type and extent of the anticipated surgery.[3,4] However, a survey of the membership of the Society for Pediatric Anesthesia found that many physicians continue to order routine preoperative laboratory tests.[5]

### Hemoglobin and Hematocrit

Although requirements vary among anesthesiologists and institutions, a strong case can be made for measuring hemoglobin or hematocrit in infants <6 months of age, patients with chronic disease, and postmenarchal girls before all but the most minor of procedures.[5] Infants typically experience the nadir of hemoglobin and hematocrit values at about 3 months of age (physiologic anemia of infancy), whereas adolescent girls are prone to iron-deficiency anemia if nutritional habits and iron intake are suboptimum. In these cases, hemoglobin or hematocrit testing may be considered indicated on the basis of history rather than performed for routine screening purposes.

### Pregnancy Testing in Teenage Girls

There are several justifications for routine preanesthetic pregnancy testing in teenage girls. The rate of teenage pregnancies in many areas of the United States has been increasing, such that these now represent 13% to 23% of all pregnancies.[6] Accurate histories concerning sexual activity and the potential for pregnancy in teenagers may be difficult to obtain, although one investigation in which all pregnancy tests were negative concluded that education of adolescents about the potential risks of anesthetics may result in reliable histories.[7] As in adults, there are significant concerns regarding teratogenicity and the potential for spontaneous abortion should an anesthetic be administered. Pregnancy testing before surgery is often an emotionally charged issue that is strongly influenced by legal, ethical, and religious concerns.

A recent prospective study of 261 ambulatory surgery patients at a tertiary pediatric hospital identified a 1.3% positive pregnancy test rate (3 patients); these three patients denied the possibility of pregnancy and reported that their last menstrual period had been <3 weeks before the scheduled surgery.[8] The Society for Pediatric Anesthesia survey of preoperative laboratory tests in children found that pregnancy testing was required by 43% of respondents.[5] There is significant variation among practitioners who perform routine pregnancy testing as to when testing begins; in some cases, a history of menarche (first menses) triggers the pregnancy test, whereas in others, a designated age cutoff triggers the test. Two studies found no patients with positive pregnancy tests before surgery who were <15 years of age.[8,9]

## What Is Known About Aspiration in Children?

The pulmonary aspiration of gastric contents remains one of the most feared of anesthetic complications. Historically, 26% of anesthesia-related mortality in children was related to the aspiration of blood or vomitus in the perioperative period.[10] A large retrospective review of aspiration during anesthesia confirmed that children are more likely to experience aspiration than adults (8.6 aspirations per 10 000 children aged 1-9 years, in contrast to 2.9 aspirations per 10 000 adults). However, despite the increased incidence and an overall mortality rate following aspiration of 5%, no deaths in pediatric patients were attributable specifically to aspiration.[11]

A large prospective study of anesthetic complications in infants and children revealed a lower aspiration incidence of about 1.2 per 10 000 anesthetics and no mortality attributable to aspiration.[12] Whether owing to increased awareness of the problem of pulmonary aspiration or to improved anesthetic practices and skill on the part of anesthesia practitioners, these data suggest that the incidence of aspiration and the associated mortality have decreased compared with those of previous years.

## What Are Appropriate Fasting Guidelines?

### Historical Approach

The question of what constitutes an adequate preoperative fasting period in children has been the subject of significant research and debate. The principal justification for prohibiting oral intake before surgery since the late 1940s (since the work of Mendelson[13] and Teabeault[14]) has been to minimize the risk for pulmonary aspiration should the patient experience gastroesophageal reflux or vomiting in the perioperative period when airway reflexes may be impaired by anesthetics. Until relatively recently, all oral intake has been treated equally, and the adult fasting standard of nil per os (NPO) after midnight (or 6-8 hours) has been applied to children for elective procedures. The question of pharmacologic prophylaxis against pulmonary aspiration is addressed later in this chapter in the discussion of premedication.

### Gastric Fluid Characteristics

The characteristics of a gastric aspirate that are most closely associated with an increased risk for pulmonary aspiration syndrome are a pH of <2.5, a volume of >0.4 mL/kg, and a high level of particulate matter in the aspirate.[15] Since 1976, a large number of investigators have demonstrated that despite standard preoperative fasts of at least 4 hours (and usually 8-12 hours), a high percentage of children continue to have gastric fluid characteristics that place them at increased risk for pulmonary aspiration syndrome, as shown in Table 57-

2.[16-20] Despite the assumption of this increased risk, a recent prospective study of perioperative aspiration in infants and children found clinically important pulmonary aspiration to be an uncommon event, with a frequency of 1:2632 anesthetics, or 0.04%.[21] Although a priori, the recognition of increased gastric fluid volume as a risk factor for aspiration would seem to make sense, even this supposition has been questioned.[22,23]

### Solid Foods Versus Clear Liquids

A number of studies have recently examined fasting practices and resulting gastric fluid volumes in children presenting for elective procedures.[24-26] These investigations clearly indicate that allowing healthy children to consume clear liquids (water, non–pulp-containing apple juice, fruit punch) until 2 hours before the induction of general anesthesia does not significantly alter gastric residual volumes or pH, nor does it increase the risk for pulmonary aspiration. In fact, because clear liquids facilitate gastric emptying, gastric fluid volumes may actually be lower and pH values higher in patients allowed to consume clear liquids preoperatively. Few would disagree that solid foods (including dairy products and pulp-containing juices) should continue to be withheld for at least 6 to 8 hours, even in children, because these foods require significantly longer gastric emptying times.

The benefits of allowing clear liquids during the fasting period in children include providing a more humane experience for the patient and family, a reduced chance of anesthetic induction in a hypovolemic child, and a possibly reduced risk for intraoperative or postoperative hypoglycemia. The downside of a liberalized clear liquid policy includes the potential for delays in the surgical schedule should the operating room allow for an earlier than anticipated start time. Also, the possibility exists that allowing this exception to the traditional absolute NPO mandate may increase the likelihood that other food substances will be ingested in addition to clear liquids, increasing uncertainty as to the true nature of gastric contents in the individual patient.

### Current Recommendations

At this time, anesthesiologists should continue to withhold solid foods (including dairy products) for 6 hours in children under 3 years of age and for 8 hours in children over 3 years of age before elective surgery, but allow clear fluids to be consumed up to 2 hours before induction. Children known to be at increased risk for having a full stomach should continue to have even clear liquids withheld for the traditional period of at least 6 to 8 hours.

**TABLE 57–2.** Pediatric Patients at Elevated Risk for Aspiration Following Standard Fast (>4 Hours)

| Investigator | pH < 2.5 (%) | Mean Gastric Volume | Combined % at Risk* |
|---|---|---|---|
| Salem et al.[16] | 90 | 0.6 mL/kg | Not applicable |
| Goudsouzian et al.[17] | 100 | 0.53 mL/kg | 64 |
| Cote et al.[18] | 96 | 0.78 mL/kg | 76 |
| Manchikanti et al.[19] | 92 | 0.49 mL/kg | 60 |
| Meakin et al.[20] | 100 | 0.25 mL/kg | 22 |

*Percentage of patients with both a gastric pH < 2.5 and a gastric volume > 0.4 mL/kg.

## UPPER RESPIRATORY TRACT INFECTION

### How Should It Be Assessed?

One of the most commonly encountered problems in the preoperative evaluation of children is the presence of symptoms or signs of a URI. Clinical findings, including a sore or scratchy throat, sneezing, malaise, fever, rhinorrhea, nonproductive cough, and nasal or sinus congestion, may be nonspecific and overlap with manifestations of noninfectious disorders, such as allergies and vasomotor rhinitis. Although laboratory studies and chest radiographs may provide some assistance in clinical decision making, there is no substitute for directly examining and talking with the caretakers (and patient, if applicable) to assess the nature, chronicity, and severity of clinical findings.

### Acuity of Symptoms

The parent or other caretaker should be questioned regarding the presence of not only current URI symptoms but also symptoms that have occurred within the preceding month. A recent, resolving URI is suggested to be associated with the same or an even greater risk for perioperative complications than is an existing infection.[27] When evidence of chronic allergy or URI symptoms is present, parents are frequently able to indicate whether the child's current clinical status is typical for the individual patient or unusual, as in the presence of a higher-than-normal fever, reduced activity level, or change in behavior.

As stated previously, some indications warrant routine preoperative laboratory or radiologic studies. Decisions concerning the management of children with URI symptoms must be based primarily on the clinical impression of whether the patient's condition is likely secondary to an infectious process. The white blood cell count may be depressed, normal, or elevated in the child with a viral URI and is therefore of little help in the decision-making process. Chest radiographs are indicated only when symptoms such as a productive cough or findings on physical examination, including crackles, wheezing, or areas of decreased breath sounds, are present. In these cases, a lower respiratory tract process (pneumonia, asthma) more likely than not is present in addition to the URI.

### Cancellation of Surgery

Because of airway reactivity and secretions, children with a URI are generally thought to be at risk for the complications described in the next section. The issue, once the diagnosis of a URI has been made, is whether to proceed with an elective surgical procedure or to postpone surgery for 4 to 6 weeks to allow resolution.

### Anesthesia and Surgery Should Not Be Canceled

One prospective investigation of 489 pediatric patients undergoing myringotomy under mask general inhalation anesthesia found no significant difference in perioperative complications among children without symptoms of URI, children with symptoms who met predetermined URI criteria, and children with symptoms who failed to meet URI criteria.[27] This study further suggested that the duration of certain URI symptoms, including sore throat, sneezing, and fever, was shorter in patients who underwent anesthesia and surgery than in a control group of patients with symptoms who did not undergo surgery but were evaluated over the course of a 3-week follow-up period. This finding was likely the result of the beneficial effect of myringotomy on upper respiratory tract physiology, although the possibility exists that the anesthetic itself may have exerted a beneficial influence on the course of the viral syndrome.

Other considerations that may argue against the postponement of surgery include the nature of the surgical procedure, the chronic and never-resolving nature of some upper respiratory symptoms, and social issues, including the distance traveled for surgery and the expense and effort undertaken by parents (eg, time away from work, obtaining caretakers for other children) to present their child for surgery. Although the purist might argue that such social considerations should have no place in clinical decision making, the reality is that such concerns are important and do influence medical decisions.

Some practitioners argue that even if complications related to URI develop, they are readily managed with modern medications and airway and respiratory maneuvers. It is at this point that the nature and urgency of the surgical procedure must be considered to assess relative risks and benefits.

### Anesthesia and Surgery Should Be Canceled

Children who undergo elective anesthesia and surgery in the presence of a URI may be at increased risk for a number of complications, including perioperative hypoxemia, bronchospasm, and prolonged oxygen ($O_2$) requirement and intubation postoperatively.[28] One large retrospective review of prospectively gathered information demonstrated that children with a URI were 2 to 7 times more likely than healthy children to experience a respiratory complication in the perioperative period, depending on the specific respiratory event examined.[29] This investigation also demonstrated that tracheal intubation in children with a URI is associated with about twice the number of adverse respiratory events as is endotracheal intubation in the absence of a URI.

### Recommendations

The decision to proceed with elective surgery in the presence of a current or recent URI should be made only after the parents and surgeon understand the potential risks of perioperative respiratory complications. As with most medical judgments, it should be based on a risk-benefit analysis that includes such factors as the age of the patient, nature of the proposed surgery, frequency of URIs, history of previous respiratory complications, and any coexisting medical problems that may further complicate management. If the determination is made to postpone surgery, it should not be rescheduled until 4 to 6 weeks after the resolution of signs and symptoms.

### What Perioperative Problems May Occur?

The child who has experienced a viral URI within the previous month or who currently exhibits evidence of a URI may be at increased risk for a number of perioperative problems and complications, although the data on this subject are frequently conflicting. Perhaps the first association between preexistent respiratory infections and perioperative morbidity was made in 1936, when the following was stated:

*The presence of any respiratory tract infection, even mild pharyngitis or oral sepsis, substantially increases the incidence of postoperative respiratory infections.*[30]

### Airway

Potential problems that may be encountered include laryngospasm, airway obstruction, coughing, breath holding, hemoglobin desaturation, atelectasis, and bronchospasm. A 1984 study of laryngospasm during anesthesia indicated that children with URIs experienced nearly a 10-fold increase in incidence.[31] Inflammatory changes resulting from infection increase secretions, which may obstruct endotracheal tubes (ETTs) or predispose to the development of airway closure with atelectasis and pneumonia. The incidence of bronchospasm in intubated patients is increased in the presence of a URI.[28] Atelectasis and pulmonary dysfunction induced by URI may be manifested by hemoglobin desaturation in the operating room or PACU. One small study showed that 20% of children with a history or current signs and symptoms of URI had hemoglobin saturations below 95% while they breathed room air in the PACU.[32]

### Pulmonary Function

Pulmonary function may be compromised during or after URI, despite the absence of overt evidence of lower respiratory tract involvement. Some changes may be subclinical, as demonstrated by a longitudinal study of spirometric changes experienced by healthy children during periods both with and without a URI. Adjusted mean values of forced vital capacity, 1-second forced expiratory volume, peak expiratory flow, and several other variables all decreased during uncomplicated URIs.[33]

Proposed mechanisms that account for observed spirometric changes and clinical wheezing or airway hyperreactivity are complex and likely interact to create the clinical picture of bronchospasm. They include viral stimulation of immunoglobulin E antibody production with resultant hypersensitivity, enhanced mediator release from basophils and mast cells, diminished β-adrenergic function in bronchial smooth muscle, and epithelial injury with sensitization of airway receptors, which may trigger cholinergic reflex bronchospasm.[34]

## ASTHMA

### *How Is Reactive Airways Disease Assessed and Managed?*

Asthma is a chronic disease of the tracheobronchial tree in which episodic increases in resistance to airflow result from heightened responsiveness to endogenous or exogenous stimuli, or both. It is one of the most common conditions encountered in children, affecting 10% to 15% of boys and 7% to 10% of girls at some time during childhood, and both the prevalence and mortality have been increasing.[35] As a clinical entity, asthma may occur in any of a variety of scenarios, from the older child or young adult with only a remote history of asthma or wheezing as a toddler, to the asymptomatic child

who is well-controlled with bronchodilators, and, finally, to the patient with an exacerbation of asthma and respiratory distress who presents for emergency surgery or requires tracheal intubation in the course of treatment of status asthmaticus. The clinical approach depends primarily on the activity and time course of the disease in the individual patient.

### Classification

Several classification schemes have been proposed that are based on the causes or stimuli that induce bronchospasm. *Extrinsic* asthma is most common in children, in whom an allergy to some external substance and elevated levels of serum immunoglobulin E (IgE) can often be demonstrated. *Intrinsic* asthma, by contrast, has no apparent allergic cause but rather is a respiratory tract infection or some form of chronic lung disease, such as cystic fibrosis or bronchopulmonary dysplasia. It occurs more commonly in adolescents and adults.

Other varieties of asthma include exercise- and aspirin-induced forms, which may overlap or coexist with extrinsic or intrinsic asthma.

### Pathophysiology

The principal pathophysiologic features of asthma include a reduction in the diameter of the airways, thickening of the bronchial mucosa owing to inflammation and edema, and the collection of thick secretions within the tracheobronchial tree. Several potential defects induce these changes, although the relative importance or applicability of a specific abnormality may vary from patient to patient. They include an imbalance of the autonomic nervous system's control of bronchomotor tone; alterations in the properties of the smooth muscle cells within the bronchial walls[36]; or abnormal immune function with increased IgE formation and mast cell degranulation, particularly in the case of extrinsic asthma in children.

The result of these underlying changes is gas trapping, ventilation-perfusion mismatching, atelectasis, and increased dead space ventilation. Pulmonary function studies reveal increased residual volume, functional residual capacity, and total lung volume and reduced expiratory flow rates, vital capacity, expiratory reserve volume, and inspiratory capacity.[37]

### Therapeutic Implications

It is at the level of these defects that our somewhat incomplete understanding of the mechanism of action of the drugs used to treat asthma is found. Because parasympathetic-cholinergic or α-adrenergic stimulation promotes bronchoconstriction either by direct innervation or humoral passage of mediators, substances such as atropine or ipratropium may reverse or block bronchospasm induced by these mechanisms. Likewise, because β₂-adrenergic stimulation promotes bronchodilation, β-agonists such as epinephrine and albuterol may be used therapeutically as bronchodilators.

Theophylline, an agent commonly used as a bronchodilator, may have several different actions. The classic effect of intracellular phosphodiesterase inhibition with resultant elevation of cyclic adenosine monophosphate levels and consequent bronchodilation appears to be of minor importance at clinically useful theophylline concentrations of 10 to 20 μg/mL.[38] Other possible benefits of theophylline include inhibition of adenosine-induced bronchoconstriction and interference with the synthesis or effects of prostaglandins.[39] The use of theophylline to treat asthma in children is now largely obsolete owing to numerous side effects and questionable effects on asthma-related mortality.[40]

Corticosteroids are thought to have a number of actions, including inhibition of the release of mediators of bronchoconstriction and inflammation, reduction of bronchial mucosal edema, and potentiation of β-adrenergic receptors.[41] Inhaled formulations have limited effects on nonpulmonary tissues and the hypothalamic-pituitary-adrenal axis.

## History and Physical Findings

Preoperative evaluation of the child with asthma is centered on determining the current activity of the disease and what is required (if anything) to improve the patient's condition. The history of the disease, which includes the child's age at onset, triggering stimuli, the number of clinic and hospital visits, the number of severe episodes requiring mechanical ventilation, and current medications, should be reviewed. Physical examination should include not only assessment of the chest and a search for wheezing, diminished breath sounds, and delayed expiration but also assessment of vital signs, the use of accessory muscles of respiration, hydration status, cyanosis, and any evidence of URI or pneumonia.

## Laboratory Tests

As with the general preoperative evaluation of all patients, routine laboratory testing has no place; studies must be guided by the patient's condition. The symptom-free patient with normal results on physical examination requires nothing; the child with a fever, focal chest findings, and some degree of respiratory distress may require a chest radiograph, complete blood count with white blood cell differential, and an arterial blood gas analysis. Older children may be able to undergo spirometry. If bronchospasm or symptomatic asthma is found, elective surgery should be postponed while the bronchodilator regimen is adjusted and any infectious process is treated or resolved.

## Anesthetic Implications

Anesthetic management of the asthmatic child also depends on the patient's condition. Use of preoperative bronchodilators (oral or inhaled) should be continued until the time of surgery. If the patient is currently taking or has received systemic steroids within the 6-month period before surgery, "stress" steroid coverage for all but minor surgical procedures should be provided. An acceptable dosage is the equivalent of 2 to 3 mg/kg/d of methylprednisolone perioperatively.[42] Premedication with sedatives as outlined later in this chapter may be beneficial to the extent that anxiety and fear may contribute to the development of bronchospasm.

### Regional Techniques

Asthmatic patients may be provided with either general or regional anesthesia. Regional techniques make it possible to avoid airway instrumentation and intubation, but in the case of moderately high levels of spinal or epidural anesthesia, they may interfere with the patient's ability to cough or use some of the accessory muscles of respiration. The concern that thoracic pharmacologic sympathectomy secondary to spinal or epidural anesthesia may induce a predominance of parasympathetic tone to the tracheobronchial tree and thereby promote bronchospasm appears to be more theoretic than practical.

### General Techniques

**Intravenous Induction Agents.** In considering intravenous induction agents for general anesthesia, sodium thiopental, etomidate, ketamine, and propofol have been successfully used in asthmatic patients, despite the fact that thiopental has been demonstrated to induce histamine release in vitro.[43]

**Inhalation Agents.** Either halothane or sevoflurane may be used for inhalation induction because these drugs have the most tolerable odors and are most agreeable to children. After inhalation or intravenous induction, any of the potent inhalation anesthetics may be administered because isoflurane, enflurane, and halothane possess equivalent bronchodilating properties.[44] However, because of the propensity of halothane to sensitize the myocardium to the effects of catecholamines,[45] it may induce problems with arrhythmia in the asthmatic patient who has received β-agonists and theophylline preparations.

**Narcotics and Muscle Relaxants.** Some narcotics (morphine, meperidine) and muscle relaxants (succinylcholine, the aminosteroid agent rapacuronium, and the benzylisoquinoline agents atracurium, mivacurium, metocurine, and doxacurium) have the potential to cause histamine release, depending on dosage and speed of administration. As with thiopental, these agents have been safely used in patients with asthma, but in view of the wide variety of narcotics and muscle relaxants available today, the use of agents that are not associated with histamine release or exacerbation of bronchospasm is perhaps most prudent. Such drugs include fentanyl and related compounds and most of the steroid muscle relaxants (pancuronium, vecuronium, pipecuronium). Nevertheless, circumstances may occur in which a drug like succinylcholine is indicated despite the presence of asthma, as when rapid muscle relaxation for tracheal intubation is essential.

## How Is Intraoperative Wheezing Managed?

The first step in the management of intraoperative wheezing is to determine the cause; it is dangerous to assume that any intraoperative wheezing in a patient with known asthma is in fact due to the asthma. Other causes of wheezing, including airway secretions, kinking of the ETT, bronchial mainstem intubation, airway foreign body, and pulmonary edema, should be searched for and either treated or excluded. If the wheezing is thought to be due to asthma, the inspired $O_2$ concentration should be increased and the anesthetic level deepened with appropriate intravenous and inhalational agents as hemodynamically tolerated. A $\beta_2$-agonist (usually albuterol) should be given using a metered-dose inhaler and mixing chamber attached to the proximal end of the ETT. Some patients may require treatment with an inhaled (ipratropium) or systemic (atropine) anticholinergic agent. Still fewer patients require treatment with systemic corticosteroids intraoperatively.

## Miscellaneous Considerations

Other maneuvers that are helpful in asthmatic patients include passive or active humidification of inspired gases, administration of intravenous lidocaine before intubation, awake extubation, or tracheal suctioning,[46] and provision of mask anesthesia without intubation or deep extubation of the trachea at the conclusion of surgery in appropriate patients.

## CONGENITAL HEART DISEASE

### *What Are the Implications for Noncardiac Surgery?*

No other group of children, with the possible exception of those with an abnormal or difficult airway, elicit as much anxiety among anesthesiologists as pediatric patients with unrepaired or palliated congenital heart disease. For the most part, definitive surgical management of congenital cardiac lesions is reserved for pediatric centers; the anesthetic considerations in pediatric cardiac surgery are discussed in Chapter 62. However, a fundamental understanding of the nature of congenital cardiac lesions and of implications for anesthetic management of noncardiac surgery is essential.

### Pathophysiologic Flow Characteristics

Various congenital cardiac lesions can be thought of in terms of their pathophysiologic flow characteristics (Table 57–3). In the first two of the categories, blood is shunted through abnormal circulatory connections or pathways as a function of pressure channels and of the relative pulmonary and systemic vascular resistances. In the third category, no shunting of blood occurs in the absence of coexisting lesions, although various cardiac chambers and vascular beds may be affected by the obstruction to forward blood flow.

**TABLE 57–3.** Pathophysiologic Classification of Congenital Cardiac Lesions

**Increased Pulmonary Blood Flow**

Atrial septal defect
Ventricular septal defect
Patent ductus arteriosus
Atrioventricular canal
Anomalous coronary arteries
Transposition of the great vessels*
Anomalous pulmonary venous drainage
Truncus arteriosus*
Single ventricle*

**Decreased Pulmonary Blood Flow**

Tetralogy of Fallot
Pulmonary atresia
Tricuspid atresia
Ebstein's anomaly
Truncus arteriosus*
Transposition of the great vessels*
Single ventricle*

**Obstruction to Blood Flow**

Aortic stenosis
Pulmonary stenosis
Coarctation of the aorta
Asymmetric septal hypertrophy

*Classification as an increased or decreased pulmonary blood flow lesion depends on absence or presence (respectively) of obstruction to pulmonary blood flow and relative pulmonary and systemic vascular resistance.

From Schwartz AJ, Campbell FW. Pathophysiological approach to congenital heart disease in pediatric anesthesia. In: Lake CL, ed. *Pediatric Cardiac Anesthesia.* Norwalk, Conn: Appleton & Lange; 1988:9.

### Preanesthetic Management

The child with congenital heart disease scheduled for non-cardiac surgery should have the same preoperative evaluation as previously discussed in addition to several further investigations. Specifically, the history and physical examination should seek any evidence of cyanosis or congestive heart failure. Cyanosis is typically found in lesions with reduced pulmonary blood flow, pulmonary hypertension, or both, and with predominant right-to-left shunting of blood. Congestive heart failure, conversely, usually results from increased pulmonary blood flow, increased pulmonary venous return, and left ventricular overload.

The nature and extent of previous palliative or corrective surgical procedures should be elucidated together with the child's current functional state as indicated by activity, symptoms, and objective measurements, including echocardiography and cardiac catheterization data. Chronic use of cardiac medications (digoxin, diuretics, antidysrhythmics) should be noted, continued until the time of surgery, and resumed postoperatively in either oral or parenteral form, as required. Patients demonstrating cyanosis are likely to have polycythemia secondary to chronic hypoxemia. An unusually high hematocrit places a child at risk for thrombotic complications. Platelet counts, although frequently elevated, may conceal platelet function abnormalities and potential defects in hemostasis.

### Premedication

No lesion-specific approach to anesthesia and intraoperative management exists for children with congenital heart disease. Rather, the current degree of cardiopulmonary compensation, the anticipated surgical procedure, and the associated stresses dictate the approach. Preanesthetic sedation is usually indicated for the general reasons described later in this chapter and for the specific benefit of alleviating anxiety and sympathetic activation, which may impair cardiovascular function before and during induction.

### *What Are the Anesthetic Effects on Cardiopulmonary Function?*

A number of anesthetic factors influence cardiovascular and pulmonary function perioperatively, any of which may be beneficial or deleterious, depending on the pathophysiology involved.[47]

### Cardiac Output

Forward blood flow (cardiac output) may be enhanced by judiciously increased intravascular volume expansion and increasing heart rate, inotropic agents, and vasodilators (in normovolemia). Inhalation anesthetics and α-adrenergic blockers, which normally are myocardial depressants, may actually improve cardiac output in patients with hypertrophic cardiomyopathy and ventricular outflow obstruction. Cardiac output is reduced by hypervolemia, dysrhythmias, ischemia, and, in the presence of hypovolemia, vasodilators and increased mean airway pressures.

## Systemic and Pulmonary Vascular Resistance

The resistances in the pulmonary and systemic circulations are influenced in numerous ways. Sympathetic stimulation (as in light anesthesia) and α-adrenergic agonists may increase both systemic and pulmonary vascular resistance. Hypoxemia, acidosis, hypercarbia, hypervolemia, and increased airway pressure also increase pulmonary vascular resistance. Both systemic vascular resistance and pulmonary vascular resistance are decreased by inhalation anesthetic agents, vasodilators, and α-adrenergic antagonists. $O_2$, alkalosis, hypocarbia, prostaglandin $E_1$, prostacyclin, and nitric oxide additionally reduce pulmonary vascular resistance.

## What Other Factors Are Critical to Management?

### Endocarditis Prophylaxis

Children with certain congenital heart defects who undergo surgery in which transient bacteremia is possible (dental; ear, nose, and throat; gastrointestinal; and genitourinary procedures) require prophylaxis against bacterial endocarditis. Sources of controversy and confusion in discussions of procedure-related endocarditis include which cardiac defects are associated with increased risk and which surgical procedures are likely to cause bacteremia and therefore merit antibiotic prophylaxis. In 1997, the American Heart Association issued its most recent set of formal recommendations for the prophylaxis and prevention of procedure-related endocarditis (Table 57–4). Six major points relating to the current recommendations are as follows:

1. Most cases of endocarditis cannot be attributed to a specific procedure.
2. Cardiac conditions have been stratified into high, moderate, and negligible risk based on the seriousness of outcome should endocarditis develop.
3. Specific procedures that could lead to bacteremia and thus merit prophylaxis are more clearly specified.
4. An algorithm is presented for patients with mitral valve prolapse to define better which patients require prophylaxis.
5. The initial amoxicillin dose for oral and dental procedures was reduced to 2 g; the follow-up (6-8 hours postprocedure) dose was eliminated; and alternatives other than erythromycin for penicillin-allergic patients are offered.
6. The prophylactic regimens for gastrointestinal and genitourinary procedures are simplified.

The only patients not requiring such prophylaxis are those who are more than 6 months postrepair of a secundum-type atrial septal defect (without patch) or postligation of a patent ductus arteriosus. Importantly, tracheal intubation alone is not an indication for bacterial endocarditis prophylaxis.

### Air Embolization

With all forms of intravenous access, meticulous care should be provided to ensure that air does not enter the tubing or venous system. Once air gains access to the venous circulation, it may pass through a probe-patent foramen ovale or any other abnormal channel between the pulmonary and systemic circulations. A paradoxic air embolus, with resultant central nervous system (CNS) or myocardial ischemia or infarction, can result.

## MALIGNANT HYPERTHERMIA

### What Is Malignant Hyperthermia?

Malignant hyperthermia (MH) is a pharmacokinetic disorder that rarely occurs outside of the administration of certain anesthetic drugs, including depolarizing muscle relaxants (succinylcholine) and the potent inhalation anesthetics (halothane, enflurane, isoflurane, sevoflurane, and desflurane) (Table 57–5). When triggered by a combination of one or more of these agents, it induces a clinical state of hypermetabolism marked by hypercapnia, tachycardia, arrhythmias, metabolic acidosis, skeletal muscle rigidity, rhabdomyolysis, and profound temperature elevation. Before the use of dantrolene, MH carried a mortality rate of at least 64%, but in modern centers with accessible supplies of this drug, the mortality rate is <10%. MH has been said to be more common in children than adults, although as noted by Brandom and Gronert, the disorder is sufficiently rare that it is difficult to estimate its true incidence without selection bias.[48]

An anxiety-provoking and potentially confusing clinical situation arises during the provision of anesthesia for the patient who is susceptible to MH.[49] Confusion is greatest when a personal or family history of MH is questionable or poorly documented. Management is relatively straightforward for patients with a history of a fulminant MH crisis or a positive halothane-caffeine contracture test after muscle biopsy.

### Who Is at Risk?

Patients considered at risk for a reaction include those who have survived an MH episode or who have positive muscle biopsy results; first-degree relatives of such patients; first-degree relatives with known muscle or skeletal abnormalities or chronically elevated creatine kinase levels; and patients who have experienced masseter spasm after administration of halothane and succinylcholine.

### Why Does It Occur?

The fundamental defect in human beings responsible for the development of MH is a malfunction of the ryanodine receptor (RYR1), a large protein molecule that normally regulates the release of calcium from the sarcoplasmic reticulum of skeletal muscle cells. The inciting cellular event is a large increase in the level of intracellular ionized calcium secondary to a drug-induced disturbance or perturbation of membrane function involving the ryanodine receptor. The elevated intracellular calcium then induces skeletal muscle contracture and acceleration of aerobic and anaerobic metabolism. The acute clinical findings in an MH crisis were noted previously in the definition of the disorder. Late manifestations include central nervous system changes of cerebral edema and coma, renal failure, and disseminated intravascular coagulation. Not all of these clinical findings or complications may be evident in each patient.

**TABLE 57–4.** Bacterial Endocarditis Prophylaxis in Children

**A. Cardiac Conditions Associated With Endocarditis**

*Endocarditis Prophylaxis Recommended*

*High Risk*

Prosthetic cardiac valves
Previous bacterial endocarditis
Complex cyanotic congenital heart disease
Surgically constructed systemic pulmonary shunts or conduits

*Moderate Risk*

Most other congenital cardiac malformations (other than above or below)
Acquired valvar dysfunction (eg, rheumatic heart disease)
Hypertrophic cardiomyopathy
Mitral valve prolapse with valvar regurgitation and/or thickened leaflets

*Endocarditis Prophylaxis Not Recommended*

*Negligible Risk*
(no greater risk than the general population)

Isolated secundum atrial septal defect
Surgical repair of atrial or ventricular septal defect or patent ductus
    arteriosus (without residua beyond 6 months)
Previous coronary artery bypass graft surgery
Mitral valve prolapse without valvar regurgitation
Physiologic, functional, or innocent heart murmurs
Previous Kawasaki disease without valvar dysfunction
Previous rheumatic fever without valvar dysfunction
Cardiac pacemakers and implanted defibrillators

**B. Procedures and Endocarditis Prophylaxis**

*Prophylaxis Recommended*

*Invasive Dental Procedures*

Extractions
Periodontal procedures
Dental implant placement
Endodontic surgery
Prophylactic cleaning of teeth when bleeding is anticipated

*Respiratory Tract*

Tonsillectomy and/or adenoidectomy
Surgical operations that involve respiratory mucosa
Rigid bronchoscopy

*Gastrointestinal Tract*

Sclerotherapy of esophageal varices
Esophageal stricture dilation
Endoscopic retrograde cholangiography with biliary obstruction
Biliary tract surgery
Surgical operations that involve intestinal mucosa

*Genitourinary Tract*

Prostatic surgery
Cystoscopy
Urethral dilation

*Prophylaxis Not Recommended*

*Minimally Invasive Dental Procedures*

Restorative dentistry
Local anesthetic injections (nonintraligamentary)
Placement of rubber dams
Postoperative suture removal
Taking of oral impressions
Fluoride treatments

*Respiratory Tract*

Endotracheal intubation
Flexible bronchoscopy with or without biopsy
Tympanostomy tube insertion

*Gastrointestinal Tract*

Transesophageal echocardiography
Endoscopy with or without gastrointestinal biopsy

*Genitourinary Tract*

Vaginal hysterectomy
Vaginal delivery
Cesarean section
In uninfected tissue:
    Urethral catheterization
    Uterine dilation and curettage
    Therapeutic abortion
    Sterilization procedures
    Insertion or removal of intrauterine devices

*Other*

Cardiac catheterization, including balloon angioplasty
Implanted cardiac pacemakers, implanted defibrillators, and stents
Incision or biopsy of surgically scrubbed skin
Circumcision

**C. Prophylactic Regimens**

*Dental, Oral, Respiratory Tract, or Esophageal Procedures*

Standard general prophylaxis: amoxicillin, 50 mg/kg orally to max 2 g 1 h
    before procedure
Unable to take oral medications: ampicillin, 50 mg/kg IM or IV within 30
    min before procedure
Allergic to penicillin: clindamycin *or* 20 mg/kg orally to max 600 mg 1 h
    before procedure
Cephalexin or cefadroxil: 50 mg/kg orally to max 2 g 1 h before procedure
Azithromycin or clarithromycin 15 mg/kg orally to max 500 mg 1 h before
    procedure
Allergic to penicillin and unable to take oral medications:
    Clindamycin, 20 mg/kg IV within 30 min before procedure, *or*
    Cefazolin, 25 mg/kg IM or IV within 30 min before procedure

*Genitourinary and Gastrointestinal Procedures*

High-risk patients: ampicillin plus gentamicin. Ampicillin, 50 mg/kg to max
    2 g IM or IV plus gentamicin 1.5 mg/kg within 30 min of starting the
    procedure; 6 h later, ampicillin, 25 mg/kg IM or IV, or amoxicillin, 25
    mg/kg orally
High-risk patients allergic to amoxicillin: ampicillin, vancomycin plus
    gentamicin. Vancomycin, 20 mg/kg IV over 1–2 h (max, 1 g) plus
    gentamicin 1.5 mg/kg IV/IM; complete infusion within 30 min of starting
    procedure
Moderate-risk patients amoxicillin or ampicillin. Amoxicillin, 50 mg/kg
    orally 1 h before procedure. Or, ampicillin, 50 mg/kg IV/IM within 30
    min of starting the procedure
Moderate-risk patients allergic to ampicillin/amoxicillin: vancomycin plus
    gentamicin. Vancomycin, 20 mg/kg IV over 1–2 h (max, 1 g); complete
    infusion within 30 minutes of starting procedure

From Dajani AS, Taubert KA, Wilson W, et al. Prevention of bacterial endocarditis. *JAMA.* 1997;277:1794.

## How Is Preanesthetic Assessment Carried Out?

### History and Physical Examination

The first priority is to obtain a detailed history, perform a physical examination, and review any available medical and anesthetic records. Parents of known or potentially susceptible children should be counseled regarding the nature, diagnosis, and treatment of MH and how the impending anesthetic will be tailored to avoid triggering an episode. An increasing number of parents of MH-susceptible children are knowledgeable of the disorder and its implications because of improved patient education and the activities of the Malignant Hyperthermia Association of the United States.

A number of other disorders have been associated with

**TABLE 57–5.** Anesthetic Drugs and Malignant Hyperthermia

| Triggering Agents | Nontriggering Agents |
|---|---|
| Succinylcholine | Narcotics |
| Decamethonium | Benzodiazepines |
| Halothane | Barbiturates |
| Enflurane | Propofol |
| Isoflurane | Nitrous oxide |
| Sevoflurane | Etomidate |
| Desflurane | Nondepolarizing muscle relaxants |
| | Anticholinesterases |
| | Ketamine* |
| | Ester-type local anesthetics |
| | Amide-type local anesthetics* |
| | Anticholinergics (atropine) |

*Agents considered to be safe in malignant hyperthermia–susceptible patients, but this belief is controversial.

MH; that is, their presence appears to increase the risk for an MH episode during an anesthetic. Most notable among these are several myopathies, including Duchenne-type muscular dystrophy, King-Denborough syndrome, and central core disease. The latter appears to be the only one in which MH susceptibility should be assumed until proved otherwise.[48] Other conditions with relatively weak associations with MH include strabismus, ptosis, idiopathic kyphoscoliosis, and even inguinal and umbilical hernias. The neuroleptic malignant syndrome (NMS) is a distinct disorder that resembles MH clinically but is triggered by psychiatric drugs that induce dopaminergic blockade. NMS has an onset over hours or days rather than the minutes to fraction of an hour that herald the onset of an MH episode.

### Are Any Laboratory Studies Useful in Assessing Patients Before Surgery?

Noninvasive or minimally invasive studies to evaluate potentially MH-susceptible patients do not exist, although molecular genetic analysis[50] and MRI spectroscopy[51] may have some clinical utility as supplements to the caffeine-halothane contracture test in diagnosing and assessing specific individuals and families. Knowledge of serum levels of creatine kinase is useful in that if they are elevated in a close relative of an individual known to be MH susceptible, that relative may likewise be considered susceptible. However, measurement of serum creatine kinase or other muscle enzymes has no place as an independent screening tool for MH.

Postponement of elective surgery and insistence that a patient who may be MH-susceptible undergo a muscle biopsy and caffeine-halothane contracture testing is impractical. To do so would require the patient to travel to one of the few centers where standardized testing is performed and to undergo a surgical procedure. Such testing can and should be arranged for a later date, if indicated; in the meantime, such a patient may be safely anesthetized with nontriggering agents without the need to apply the label or diagnosis of MH.

### What Are the Anesthetic Considerations?

After evaluation and counseling, anesthesia may proceed with a variety of nontriggering anesthetic techniques. A com-

mon approach is to administer a rectal, oral, or intravenous barbiturate or benzodiazepine and to complete the induction with inhalation of nitrous oxide and $O_2$ administered by mask. Anesthesia is then maintained with a balanced technique that consists of the administration of nitrous oxide, $O_2$, narcotics, propofol,[52] and nondepolarizing muscle relaxants. Depending on the surgical site, it may be reasonable to provide a regional anesthetic (eg, caudal or lumbar epidural or peripheral nerve block) as the primary anesthetic technique or as a part of a combined general and regional anesthetic.

Routine monitors include pulse oximetry and capnography. A "clean" anesthesia machine with a fresh carbon dioxide ($CO_2$) absorber, disposable circuit, and no vaporizers that has been flushed with high-flow $O_2$ for a minimum of 10 to 12 minutes may be used to ventilate the patient.[53,54] If a nontriggering anesthetic technique and appropriately prepared anesthesia machine or breathing circuit are used, dantrolene prophylaxis is not necessary, although it should be readily available.

### How Is a Malignant Hyperthermia Episode Treated?

The cornerstone of treatment of MH is rapid administration of dantrolene. This drug works within skeletal muscle cells at the level of excitation-contraction coupling and is thought to inhibit calcium release from the sarcoplasmic reticulum.[55] It is provided as a lyophilized powder in 20 mg vials that also contain 3 g of mannitol and an amount of sodium hydroxide to maintain the pH at 9 to 10. The powder in each vial must be reconstituted with 60 mL of sterile water before administration in an initial dose of 2.5 mg/kg. The MH episode normally responds to total dantrolene doses of <10 mg/kg. Other steps in the treatment of an MH episode are listed in Table 57–6.

## LATEX SENSITIVITY

### What Is Latex Allergy?

Allergic reactions to natural rubber or latex are an important clinical concern in both pediatric and adult patients. As of August 1997, the US Food and Drug Administration had received >2300 reports of allergic reactions to latex-containing medical products, including 53 cardiac arrests and 17 deaths.[56]

The problem of latex sensitivity appears to be a relatively new phenomenon. The first reports of intraoperative anaphylactic reactions caused by latex sensitization appeared in 1989.[57–59] However, the problem may have been noted at least 5 years earlier.[60] Three types of adverse reaction to latex are known, only two of which are allergic in nature. Irritant contact dermatitis is a nonimmunologic reaction caused by direct skin damage. Contact dermatitis from latex-containing products has been recognized for years. In general, it has been thought that the irritants involved were part of the manufacturing process and not the latex itself.[61] Contact dermatitis can range from mild transient redness to severe swelling with bullae formation. Skin damage induced by irritants may result in increased antigen exposure and enhancement of the likelihood of developing a true allergic reaction.[62]

**TABLE 57–6.** Management of an Acute Malignant Hyperthermia Episode

1. Discontinue all anesthetic agents and request help from additional anesthesia and surgery personnel.
2. Hyperventilate patient with 100% oxygen, preferably from a "clean" anesthesia machine with a fresh $CO_2$ absorber or from a nonrebreathing circuit with maximum oxygen flow.
3. Terminate surgical procedure (if necessary) as soon as feasible.
4. Mix each 20-mg bottle of dantrolene with 60 mL of sterile-water; administer initial intravenous dose of 2.5 mg/kg.
5. Obtain additional intravenous access and an arterial line for continuous measurement of blood pressure and arterial blood gas analysis.
6. Begin surface cooling and lavage of body cavities with iced saline as necessary to reduce body temperature.
7. Administer additional dantrolene in 2 mg/kg increments up to a total of 10 mg/kg every 10–15 min as needed based on resolution of tachycardia, hyperthermia, and muscle rigidity.
8. Treat metabolic acidosis with sodium bicarbonate and persistent dysrhythmias with procainamide, after confirming adequate treatment with intravenous dantrolene.
9. Monitor serum electrolytes, urinary output, and blood coagulation status; treat hyperkalemia with intravenous glucose and insulin, and treat oliguria with intravenous fluids (dantrolene preparation contains 3 g of mannitol per vial) and furosemide.
10. Transfer to intensive care unit and monitor for 1–3 d for late effects of malignant hyperthermia episode. Continue intravenous dantrolene 1–2.5 mg/kg for first 24 h after episode and for reappearance of features of malignant hyperthermia.
11. Counsel family and discuss referral of relatives for muscle biopsy to MHAUS:

MHAUS
(Malignant Hyperthermia Association of the United States)
PO Box 3231
Darien, CT 06820
(203)-655-3007

True allergic reactions to latex are classified as either type I (anaphylactic, mediated by IgE) or type IV (mediated by sensitized T cells). Type I, immediate-hypersensitivity reactions to latex involve latex-specific IgE, the formation of which has been induced by a previous exposure. Cross-linking of IgE by latex allergen on the surface of mast cells and basophils results in the liberation of physiologic mediators, including tryptase, histamine, prostaglandins, eosinophilic chemotactic factor of anaphylaxis, leukotrienes, kinins, and platelet-activating factor. These mediators then induce the manifestations of the allergic response. The spectrum of reactions includes immediate itching and hives in the area of exposure to rhinorrhea, swollen eyes, generalized rash or hives, bronchospasm, and anaphylaxis.[56] Of particular concern to anesthesiologists is that anaphylactic reactions related to latex exposure appear to occur most commonly intraoperatively.[63]

Type IV, delayed-hypersensitivity reactions to latex-containing products are similar in nature to the response caused by poison ivy. A rash that usually appears from 6 to 72 hours after initial contact and may progress from mild erythema to severe skin damage with blister and bullae formation characterizes this type of allergy.[56] The relationship between type I and type IV allergic reactions is not clear, although one investigator found that 79% of patients with a type I response had previously had symptoms suggestive of a type IV response.[64]

### Which Patients Are at Risk?

Four groups of people appear to be at increased risk for latex allergy[56]:

1. Patients who have had multiple surgical procedures
2. Workers, including health care personnel, with frequent occupational latex exposure
3. Atopic individuals with a history of multiple allergies
4. Individuals with specific food allergies (avocados, kiwis, bananas, chestnuts, and stone fruits)

One of the first groups of patients found to be at increased risk for latex reactions was children with spina bifida.[57] Since then, others have suggested that it is the number of surgical procedures rather than spina bifida per se that is related to latex-induced sensitization.[65]

### How Is an Allergic Response to Latex Avoided?

The first step in preventing latex allergy is to minimize repeated exposure. Latex-containing medical devices should be used only when they are superior to alternative nonlatex products. When latex-containing materials are deemed to be necessary, products with low levels of antigens and powder-free gloves should be considered first.[66] In general, powdered gloves contain higher levels of latex antigen than those that are powder free. In addition, the glove allergens may adhere to the powder and become aerosolized when the gloves are donned.[67]

### How Are Intraoperative Reactions to Latex Minimized?

In 1991, because of reports of severe allergic reactions to latex-containing medical products and devices, the US Food and Drug Administration recommended that all patients be questioned about latex sensitivity in the course of obtaining the general history.[68] The preanesthesia evaluation should seek specific information about latex sensitivity and historical risk factors. Individuals who are found to be at elevated risk for latex sensitivity should be provided with a latex-free environment perioperatively. Pharmacologic prophylaxis originally found to be effective in preventing reactions to intravenous contrast materials has not been universally adopted and applied in latex-sensitive patients.[69] Current recommendations in management favor strict latex avoidance over reliance on prophylactic drug therapy with antihistamines and corticosteroids.[61,70]

## PREMEDICATION AND PREPARATION FOR ANESTHESIA

### What Are the Goals?

The approaches to pediatric premedication since the late 1980s are altogether different than the techniques used before that time, largely owing to the introduction of midazolam. However, the primary goals of premedication—or perhaps more appropriately, preinduction of anesthesia[71]—have remained the same: to provide smooth and atraumatic separation of the child from the parents and to facilitate the induction of anesthesia. An additional benefit, although seldom a primary indication, is reduction of intraoperative anesthetic requirements.

### Reduction of Stress

Beyond these objectives, several additional justifications can be suggested for preinduction pharmacologic preparation. These include provision of amnesia for the period of separation and induction of anesthesia; vagolysis and reduction of secretions, as discussed in the section on anticholinergic agents; reduction of physiologic stress, as in patients with congenital heart disease; and provision of analgesia for the preinduction placement of invasive catheters and monitors.

## Which Patients Are or Are Not Candidates?

In determining which children should receive pharmacologic preparation before anesthesia and surgery, it is perhaps easier to identify those patients who are *not* candidates for preoperative sedation. Infants <1 year of age traditionally have been premedicated with an anticholinergic agent alone, although many vigorous and healthy 9- and 10-month-old infants may benefit from a sedative.

Children with abnormal airways, respiratory distress, increased intracranial pressure, and hemodynamic compromise should receive premedication (if at all) only in the continuous presence of a practitioner skilled in airway management and in the presence of appropriate monitoring devices and resuscitative equipment.

Almost all other patients, from late infancy through adolescence, benefit from some form of preinduction medication. With the wide variety of agents and techniques available, little justification can be advanced for a crying, kicking, and screaming child hauled off to the operating room where he or she is laid upon and restrained by two or three assistants while a mask is clamped onto his or her face.

## Should Anticholinergic Agents Be Administered?

A long-standing practice in pediatric anesthesia has been to administer an anticholinergic drug—usually atropine, but occasionally glycopyrrolate—before or at the time of induction. The primary justification for this practice has been to block parasympathetically mediated reductions in heart rate or even asystole that may occur after the administration of intravenous succinylcholine and increasing concentrations of the potent inhalation anesthetics, or after airway manipulation.

The cardiac output of newborns, infants, and small children is highly dependent on maintenance of an adequate heart rate because of a limited ability to compensate with increases in stroke volume and myocardial contractility. Therefore, atropine commonly has been administered either orally, intravenously, intramuscularly, or even rectally to promote hemodynamic stability.

Other benefits of preinduction anticholinergics include drying of oral secretions and a mild degree of sedation, which is observed only after the administration of atropine. Glycopyrrolate, a quaternary ammonium compound, is unable to pass the blood-brain barrier, and thus exerts no CNS effects.

### Risks and Side Effects

The anticholinergic agents, although generally regarded as safe, are not without potential risks and side effects. In some patients, particularly those with congenital cardiac lesions such as aortic stenosis, the relative or absolute tachycardia induced by atropine and glycopyrrolate may reduce effective cardiac output. Atropine diminishes sweat gland activity and may interfere with thermoregulation, resulting in an elevation in body temperature. Newborns and patients with pulmonary disease such as cystic fibrosis may experience drying and impaired clearance of pulmonary secretions, which may promote atelectasis and pneumonia.

Although anticholinergic drugs reduce gastric fluid secretion,[16] they decrease lower esophageal sphincter tone, thereby producing opposing effects on the potential for gastric fluid reflux and pulmonary aspiration. Finally, although the effect is essentially cosmetic, atropine commonly causes flushing of the cheeks, neck, and trunk.

### Indications

The administration of preoperative anticholinergic drugs must frequently be in accord with institutional guidelines and policies regarding the route and timing of dosing and the patients for which they are indicated. To state that any drug, including an anticholinergic, is always required for all infants or all children is too simplistic and is contrary to the concept of individually tailoring an anesthetic for each patient.

A reasonable approach is to provide a preinduction anticholinergic agent to infants and children with increased oral secretions; to newborns and small infants undergoing mask inhalation induction of anesthesia; and to any child undergoing mask induction in whom intravenous access is expected to be difficult. In an effort to avoid awake intramuscular injections, patients who are to receive intravenous succinylcholine or to undergo procedures likely to elicit vagal reflexes (eg, laryngoscopy or bronchoscopy and strabismus surgery) may receive intravenous atropine immediately after intravenous access is obtained.

### Doses

Several points concerning the dosing of anticholinergic agents require mention. Whether atropine or glycopyrrolate is administered before induction, predrawn syringes containing intravenous atropine and those containing intramuscular atropine should be readily available. A low threshold should prevail for administering a dose of atropine once the heart rate begins to decline below the lower acceptable limit. Such therapy may well offset the significantly reduced cardiac output and prolonged circulation time that accompany the onset of bradycardia.[72]

The minimum dose of atropine for an infant or child of any size is 0.1 mg. Smaller doses may induce a paradoxical slowing of the heart rate that is thought to be due to a weak peripheral muscarinic, cholinergic agonist effect.[73] The intravenous dose is 10 to 20 $\mu$g/kg, and the intramuscular dose is 20 $\mu$g/kg. Atropine also effectively dries secretions and attenuates the bradycardic responses to halothane in infants when it is given orally in a dose of 20 to 40 $\mu$g/kg,[41] although many practitioners find the oral route less efficacious than others. Glycopyrrolate is provided in a dose of 5 $\mu$g/kg intravenously or 10 $\mu$g/kg intramuscularly.

**TABLE 57–7.** Current Preinduction Medications

| Agent | Dose | Route | Onset |
|---|---|---|---|
| *Benzodiazepines* | | | |
| Midazolam | 0.5-1.0 mg/kg | PO | 15-30 min |
| | 0.02-0.1 mg/kg | IV | 1-3 min |
| | 0.08-0.25 mg/kg | IM | 5-10 min |
| | 0.2 mg/kg | IN | 10 min |
| | 0.3-1 mg/kg | PR | 10-20 min |
| Diazepam | 0.1-0.5 mg/kg | PO, IM, PR | 60 min |
| *Narcotics* | | | |
| Fentanyl | 15-20 μg/kg | OT | 5-30 min |
| | 0.5-1 μg/kg | IV | 1-3 min |
| | 1-3 μg/kg | IM | 5-15 min |
| Sufentanil | 1.5-4.5 μg/kg | IN | 7-10 min |
| Morphine | 0.05-0.1 mg/kg | IV | 3-10 min |
| | 0.1-0.2 mg/kg | IM | 30-45 min |
| *Barbiturates* | | | |
| Methohexital | 6-10 mg/kg | IM | 3-5 min |
| | 20-35 mg/kg | PR | 5-10 min |
| Thiopental | 25-35 mg/kg | PR | 5-10 min |
| Pentobarbital | 2-4 mg/kg | PO, IM, PR | 45-90 min |
| *Dissociative Anesthetics* | | | |
| Ketamine | 6-10 mg/kg | PO | 10-20 min |
| | 2-6 mg/kg | IM | 30 s to 2 min |
| | 3 mg/kg | IN | 20 min |
| | 10 mg/kg | PR | 10 min |
| *Hypnotics* | | | |
| Chloral hydrate | 50-75 mg/kg | PO | 30-60 min |

IN, intranasally; OT, oral transmucosal; PR, per rectum.

## What Are the Alternatives for Preoperative Sedation?

Table 57–7 lists commonly used premedicant agents and their approximate doses, routes of administration, and onset times. As with most anesthetic drugs, intravenous administration (when appropriate) should be titrated to clinical effect. Because of significant patient variability, particularly among children who are chronically exposed to sedatives and anesthetics, individual requirements may fall below or well above the indicated ranges.

The expected clinical effects and uses of these agents depend on the dosage and route of administration. For example, ketamine in a low intramuscular dose of 2 mg/kg[42] and midazolam in an intravenous dose of 0.05 mg/kg may be regarded as sedatives. In higher doses, ketamine (5 mg/kg intramuscularly) and midazolam (0.3 mg/kg intravenously) may be considered induction agents. The same principle applies for the rectal administration of the short-acting barbiturates methohexital and thiopental, which typically induce sleep and loss of consciousness rather than the anxiolysis, sedation, and euphoria usually observed with the indicated doses of midazolam.

Because of the availability of a variety of administration techniques for agents with relatively rapid onsets of action and short durations of effect, such as midazolam, fentanyl, sufentanil, and ketamine, classic pediatric premedicants, including pentobarbital, secobarbital, and chloral hydrate, are infrequently used in modern anesthetic practice.

## Midazolam

Midazolam administered by the oral, nasal, and rectal routes has achieved great popularity and is probably now the most commonly used pediatric premedication in the United States. It may be given incrementally intravenously with great predictability and control. It may also be given intramuscularly, although the needle stick is undesirable.[74] In the interest of avoiding fear-inducing and painful intramuscular injections, less invasive and more tolerable routes of administration have been popularized, including a needleless injection system that uses carbon dioxide to power the cartridge administering the medication.[75,76]

In some children, midazolam may cause paradoxical excitement and agitation that may not be observed until postoperatively in the PACU. This frustrating adverse response may be reversed with flumazenil in a dose of 0.01 mg/kg intravenously, titrated to effect. Excessive sedation or prolonged emergence due to midazolam may also be reversed with flumazenil, although resedation is possible.[77] Overall, the administration of midazolam is generally thought to provide for a smoother separation from the parents and induction of anesthesia and to lessen the incidence of negative postoperative behaviors.[78,79] However, one study found an increase in adverse postoperative behavior after premedication administration.[80]

### *Oral*

Oral midazolam safely induces a state of tranquillity and euphoria in children, but seldom sleep[81,82] (Fig. 57–2). It has a somewhat narrow window of optimum sedation that lasts from 15 to 45 minutes after administration; after this period, children appear to return to their baseline mental state quite

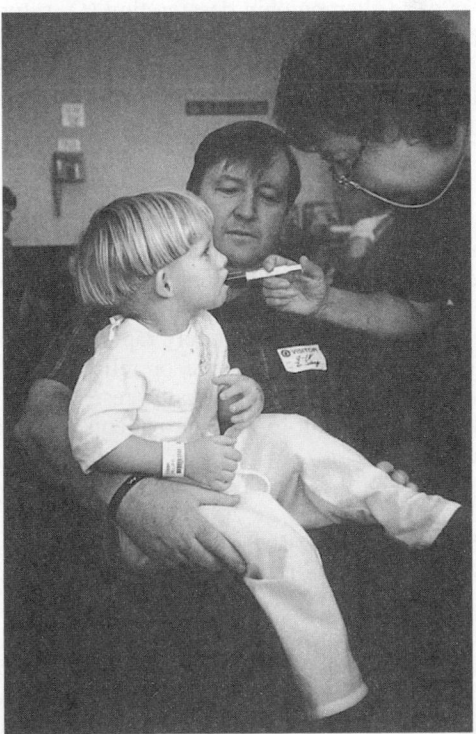

**FIGURE 57–2.** Administration of an oral preinduction medication with a syringe.

rapidly. Oral midazolam is now available in a cherry-flavored syrup from the manufacturer, or the intravenous formulation may be added to a small volume of clear juice or flavoring with added sweetener. Nevertheless, children may find the preparation bitter and refuse, spit, or vomit the mixture.

### Nasal

Midazolam may also be administered intranasally in drops or an aerosol. Intranasal administration has the advantages of greater bioavailability (55%, in contrast to the 18% to 19% for the rectal and oral routes)[83] and, as a consequence, reduced dosage, lower cost, and a somewhat more rapid onset of action. The drawback of intranasal midazolam is that it burns and causes as many as 84% of patients to cry.[84]

### Rectal

Rectal midazolam diluted with normal saline to a volume of 5 mL is perhaps most appropriate for infants and toddlers and for patients in whom an oral preparation is contraindicated.[85] Occasionally, an older child may prefer this route of administration.

## Fentanyl and Sufentanil

Fentanyl, in the form of oralets, which allow oral transmucosal absorption,[86] and intranasally administered sufentanil have also attracted a great deal of interest as pediatric premedicants.[71] These opioid agents have the advantage of providing analgesia for preinduction vascular catheter insertion and postoperative analgesia following short procedures. The downside of opioid premedication includes an increased incidence of nausea and vomiting. Patients may also experience reduced ventilatory compliance ("stiff chest"), pruritus, and mild degrees of oxyhemoglobin desaturation ($O_2$ saturation as measured by pulse oximetry [$SpO_2$] < 95%). Personnel skilled in airway management and appropriate resuscitative equipment must be immediately available after administration of these agents.

## Ketamine

Ketamine, a dissociative anesthetic with sedative and analgesic properties, may be given through a number of alternative orifices in addition to the standard intravenous and intramuscular routes. Although it acts relatively rapidly, in our experience, it has not been as predictable or reliable as similarly administered midazolam. We generally reserve its use for uncooperative and difficult-to-manage patients, in whom it is given intramuscularly.

## Should Pharmacologic Prophylaxis Against Aspiration Be Provided?

The practice of routine pharmacologic prophylaxis against aspiration in pediatric patients has never been widespread. It is usually reserved for patients with known factors placing them at increased risk for passive gastroesophageal reflux or vomiting and then the pulmonary aspiration syndrome. These risk factors include known or suspected gastroesophageal re-

flux, history of esophageal dysfunction, gastrointestinal obstruction or some other acute abdominal process, impaired or absent airway reflexes, recent ingestion of a meal with subsequent trauma or onset of acute illness, and obesity.

## Antacids

Sodium citrate, a clear, nonparticulate antacid, effectively increases the gastric content pH in children when administered in a dose of 0.4 mL/kg.[87] One concern about antacids has been the increase of gastric fluid volume that follows their use; as a result, patients commonly present with significant gastric residual volumes after standard fasts. In addition, impaired gastric emptying may result.[88]

## Histamine-2 Antagonists

The histamine-2 ($H_2$)-receptor antagonists include cimetidine, ranitidine, and famotidine. These drugs reduce the volume and elevate the pH of gastric mucosal secretions and have demonstrated efficacy in children.[17,89] The dose of cimetidine is 5 to 7.5 mg/kg by either the intravenous, intramuscular, or oral routes; that of ranitidine is 0.5 to 1.0 mg/kg intravenously or intramuscularly and 2 mg/kg orally. Intramuscular and intravenous injections must be given at least 1 hour before the anticipated induction of anesthesia (1.5-3 hours for oral doses).

The major drawback of the $H_2$-receptor antagonists is the prolonged time they must be administered before surgery, which is particularly a problem with outpatients. If they are given <2 hours before induction, they should be administered by intramuscular injection or after awake venous catheterization. Such injections may be beneficial and justified in a patient at increased risk for gastroesophageal reflux and pulmonary aspiration but cannot be recommended for routine use in all pediatric surgical patients. Instead, one should focus attention on skillful airway management at the time of anesthetic induction and emergence, nasogastric and orogastric suctioning, and the potential consideration of an alternate anesthetic technique (eg, regional anesthesia) in the child at increased risk for aspiration.

## Metoclopramide

Metoclopramide, which increases the tension of the lower esophageal sphincter and facilitates gastric emptying, likewise may be given in a dose of 0.1 mg/kg intravenously or orally. This drug also exhibits an antiemetic effect. It exerts its effects within minutes of intravenous or intramuscular administration, but must be given at least 1 hour before induction when the oral preparation is used. This medication is contraindicated in patients with known or suspected gastrointestinal obstruction.

## A Practical Approach

If time allows, children with full stomachs should undergo a 6- to 8-hour fast in the interest of maximizing any possible gastric emptying. Infants and small children should receive intravenous fluids during this period. If not contraindicated (eg, metoclopramide in the presence of intestinal obstruction), pharmacologic agents, including sodium citrate, $H_2$-receptor antagonists, and metoclopramide, may be administered to in-

**TABLE 57–8.** Equipment Needs in the Operating Room

| | |
|---|---|
| M | Machine, anesthesia |
| S | Suction |
| M | Monitors |
| A | Airway |
| I | Intravenous |
| D | Drugs |
| S | Special equipment |

crease gastric pH, reduce gastric volume, and facilitate gastric emptying.

Depending on the specific surgical condition, the patient's mental status, and coexisting medical problems, regional anesthetic techniques may be considered. Nasogastric or orogastric suctioning of gastric contents before induction and extubation may be attempted if general anesthesia is provided. However, multiorificed gastric tubes are not capable of removing large food particles, and one should never assume that because the stomach has been suctioned, it is also empty.

## What Are the Essential Equipment Requirements?

In the course of preparing the operating room, a prepared checklist or predetermined routine should be followed so as not to omit any essential element of care. Valuable time and patient safety are jeopardized when appropriate checks and equipment preparation are not performed before the patient's arrival in the operating room.

Although a variety of different preanesthesia checklists have been developed in recent years, one published by the US Food and Drug Administration in 1986 has achieved widespread use.[90] Additionally, it is suggested that the individual practitioner be thoroughly familiar with the manufacturers' recommendations and procedures for the start-up and use of all items. The mnemonic MS MAIDS (Table 57–8) serves as a useful guide to follow in ensuring that all areas of supply and equipment preparation have been considered.

### Suction

Reliable central wall or portable suction must be continuously available in all anesthetizing locations. An appropriate selection of soft suction catheters in sizes 6, 8, and 10 French should be available for use with pediatric-sized ETTs in addition to rigid Yankauer suction instruments for large volumes

of oral secretions. Soft, flexible catheters can be used to suction and decompress the stomach of infants and toddlers, whereas multiorificed tubes specifically designed for nasogastric or orogastric use may be required in older children and adolescents.

### Airway

Airway supplies that must be available in a range of appropriate sizes include masks, oral and nasopharyngeal airways, laryngeal mask airways (LMAs), functional laryngoscope handles with blades, and ETTs with tube stylets. Suggested sizes of different items used in pediatric airway management are summarized in Table 57–9. Clear, see-through masks with an air-filled plastic cushion around the rim are in widespread use; allow visualization of lip color, oral secretions, and emesis; and provide a snug fit for most children.

### *Endotracheal Tubes*

Uncuffed ETTs are commonly used in children up to about 8 years of age; before this age, the narrowest portion of the pediatric airway is in the subglottic region at the level of the cricoid cartilage, and proper placement of a cuffed tube would result in the inflated cuff resting above the narrowest portion of the airway.

Whether a leak is present around the ETT should be ascertained after intubation. Its presence implies that the fit of the tube is not too snug. Significant tracheal mucosal edema and ischemia, which may lead to postintubation croup in the recovery period[91] or acquired subglottic stenosis several weeks or months after the period of intubation, will thus be less likely.

The technique of checking the leak around an ETT should be standardized[92]; the patient should be supine, with the head in a neutral, straight, and forward position, and deeply anesthetized or paralyzed with a muscle relaxant to minimize the effects of regional laryngeal muscle tone on the leak. The ETT should be at an appropriate depth for the age and size of the patient.

With the pop-off valve closed, airway pressure in the circuit is slowly increased as fresh gas enters the circuit or as the anesthesia bag is gently compressed. The anesthetist notes the leak pressure by auscultating over the larynx with a stethoscope or by listening near the patient's mouth while observing the airway pressure manometer. An audible leak should occur within the pressure range of 10 to 30 cm $H_2O$; too great a leak may make controlled ventilation difficult with normal

**TABLE 57–9.** Suggested Sizes of Pediatric Airway Equipment

| Age | Oral Airways | Laryngoscope Blades | Endotracheal Tubes (mm ID) |
|---|---|---|---|
| Preterm neonate | 40-50 | Miller 0 | 2.5-3.0 |
| Term neonate | 50 | Miller 0 | 3.0-3.5 |
| 3-6 mo | 60 | Miller 1 | 3.5 |
| 6-12 mo | 60 | Miller 1 | 4.0 |
| 2 y | 70 | Phillips 1, Miller 1 | 4.5 |
| 4 y | 70 | Phillips 1, Miller 2 | 5.0 |
| 6 y | 70-80 | Phillips 1, Miller 2, MacIntosh 2 | 5.5 |
| 8 y | 80 | Miller 2, MacIntosh 2 | 6.0 |
| 10 y | 80 | Miller 2, MacIntosh 2 | 6.5-7.0 |

fresh gas flows, whereas a leak above 30 cm $H_2O$ or no detectable leak indicates a tight ETT-larynx interface and the potential for tracheal mucosal ischemia.

ETT size (in millimeters of internal diameter [mm ID]) can be estimated by observing the circumference of the child's little finger or by using the following formula:

$$mm\ ID = 16 + Age\ in\ Years \div 4 \qquad \text{(Equation 1)}$$

The appropriate depth of insertion of an ETT in centimeters from the lips is calculated as the internal diameter of the tube multiplied by 3, or 10 plus the patient's age in years.

## Intravenous Supplies

Necessary intravenous supplies include venous catheters in an assortment of sizes from 18 to 24 gauge, alcohol or iodine preparation pads, tourniquets, adhesive tape or clear plastic patches to secure and protect the catheter insertion site, and an infusion set with an appropriate intravenous fluid. For patients who weigh less than about 25 kg, a mini-drip set with a burette or small-volume fluid chamber that delivers 1 mL of fluid for every 60 drops affords more precise control of the fluid administration rate and reduces the maximum flow rate and potential for accidental administration of excessive intravenous fluid. Optional equipment that may be indicated for use with specific patients includes electronic infusion pumps and fluid warmers.

## Temperature Control

Depending on the age and size of the patient and the nature and duration of the surgical procedure, consideration should be given to the use of some combination of techniques or devices to maintain or elevate core body temperature. These include increasing the ambient temperature of the operating room, use of a radiant heat lamp and heating blanket on the operating table, insertion of a humidifier or passive heat and moisture exchanger ("artificial nose") into the breathing circuit, administration of blood and fluids through warming devices, and covering of the patient with plastic wraps or a warmed forced-air blanket.

## INDUCTION OF ANESTHESIA

### Should the Parents Be Present for Anesthetic Induction?

The practice of allowing one or both parents of a pediatric surgical patient to be present at the time of anesthetic induction has become increasingly popular in recent years, particularly at pediatric centers. Psychologists and pediatricians have been aware of the benefit of minimizing the period of parent-child separation for many years.[93] The provision of anesthetic and surgical care on an outpatient basis has focused attention on methods to get the child into the operating room, to induce anesthesia for the procedure, and to prepare the child for discharge with a minimum of premedication and recovery time. Several of the premedication schemes described earlier have resulted from this interest, as has the interest in parental presence for anesthetic induction (PPAI), which may minimize

or alleviate the requirement for premedication and its potential for delayed recovery[94,95] (Fig. 57–3).

An investigation of anxiety in pediatric patients and their parents in which children received either midazolam 0.5 mg/kg, PAP alone without midazolam, or neither intervention revealed that oral midazolam was more effective than PPAI or no intervention in managing children's and parents' anxiety during the perioperative period.[96] Another study examined the frequency of 5% halothane induction for behavioral distress during inhalation induction with the combination of PPAI and oral midazolam compared with PPAI alone. The combination of PPAI and oral midazolam resulted in fewer than 5% rapid halothane inductions than did PPAI alone.[97] In an attempt to define further the patient population that would benefit the most from PPAI, yet another study concluded that children over 4 years of age, those with a parent with low trait anxiety, and those with a low baseline level of activity and temperament benefited from PPAI.[98]

## Options

Allowing a parent to be present for anesthetic induction poses several potential logistic and management problems. Perhaps the most obvious is how to get the parent to the site of anesthetic induction, which is usually within or adjacent to the sterile environment of the operating room. Some operating suites are constructed with adjoining induction rooms into which parents may go dressed in street clothes; after induction, the parents leave, the airway is secured, and intravenous access is obtained (if necessary) either in the induction room or after transfer to the operating room.

An alternative but somewhat more cumbersome approach is to have parents change into regular operating room scrub wear or put on a coverall "bunny suit" for access to the operating room. If bringing the parent to the induction site creates too many problems, the final option is to bring the induction site to the parent in the preoperative clinic or holding area. In this case, nearly any of the premedication techniques discussed previously may be employed with the goal of inducing anxiolysis and a state beyond sedation.

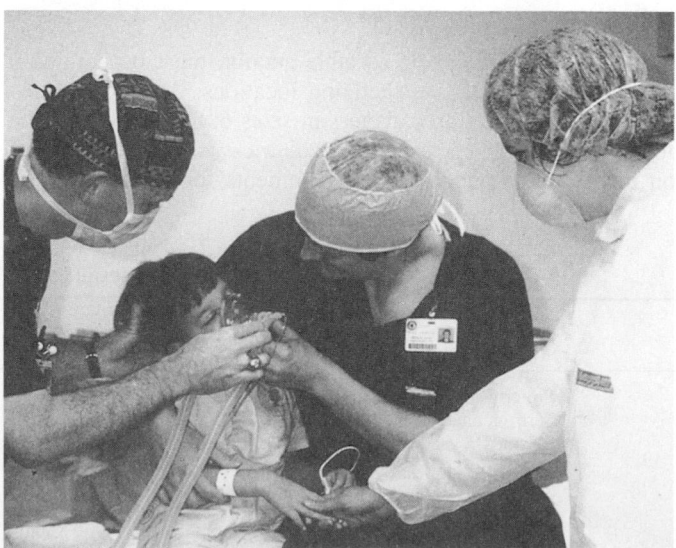

**FIGURE 57–3.** A parent (the mother) present with a child for induction of anesthesia in the operating room.

## Precautions

Several caveats to allowing parental presence for induction of the child merit discussion. Wherever it is to occur, be it in an induction room or a holding area, airway equipment and resuscitative drugs must be readily available. The anesthetist caring for the patient should have an understanding of and be comfortable with parental presence. Provider concerns include fear of the parent watching or being critical during induction, having to divide one's attention between the child and parent, and fear that parental anxiety may make the child more upset.[95] Another potential concern is that of added liability for the anesthesiologist should the parent faint or suffer some other complication in observing the induction.

Finally, parents should be well informed before induction of their child as to what they may expect to see and experience and should be aware that they may be asked to leave the room immediately if a complication or emergency arises. One study demonstrated that a significant number of parents experience anxiety or become upset while observing their child's induction, particularly as the child loses consciousness and becomes limp.[99] However, most felt their presence was beneficial to the child's emotional well-being (88%) and assisted the anesthesiologist (65%).

## What Are the Options for Anesthesia Induction and Airway Management?

The topics of anesthesia induction and airway management are inseparable and go hand-in-hand. Although there is a nearly infinite number of variations in induction techniques, inhalation, intravenous (including rapid-sequence intubation), and intramuscular inductions constitute the principal approaches. Not infrequently, individual patients are induced with a combination of techniques. After anesthesia induction, the airway can be managed and maintained with a face mask, LMA, or ETT, depending on a variety of considerations. Although, strictly speaking, awake intubation represents an approach to airway management with specific indications, it may be regarded as an alternative induction technique in the sense that the airway is secured before the induction of unconsciousness with inhalation or intravenous agents. Airway management approaches are considered first.

## AIRWAY MANAGEMENT

### Which Patients Are Candidates for Mask Anesthesia?

Guidelines for selecting general anesthesia delivered by a mask rather than an ETT are similar to those for adults. In general, patients who are scheduled for elective surgery and have had an appropriate NPO interval, do not appear to have a difficult airway (eg, micrognathia, macroglossia, or tracheal deviation), and are having surgery that does not compromise the airway nor affects pulmonary compliance are candidates for mask inhalation anesthesia. Although the duration of surgery is not an absolute determinant, cases that last longer than 1 hour tend to be more easily managed with a LMA or endotracheal intubation. Classic pediatric mask airway procedures include bilateral myringotomy with pressure equalization tube placement, inguinal hernia repair, circumcision, and short, distal orthopedic procedures (eg, cast changes or wound irrigation).

A variety of congenital or acquired disorders may make mask ventilation or tracheal intubation difficult (Table 57–10). In most cases, the history and physical examination reveal conditions known to be associated with difficult pediatric airway management, and in many cases, it is the airway abnormality for which the patient is undergoing a surgical procedure. Unlike the case with adults, in our experience, truly unanticipated difficult airways in children are unusual. Physical features associated with difficult intubation include micrognathia, macroglossia, microstomia, maxillary hypoplasia, and a short neck with limitation of cervical spine mobility.

### How Is the Laryngeal Mask Airway Used in Children?

The LMA is a device that rests in the hypopharynx forming a low-pressure seal around the laryngeal inlet after either inhalation or intravenous induction of general anesthesia and blind insertion. Notably, the LMA contains no latex and may be reused several hundred times after gentle cleaning and steam autoclaving. In general, any anesthetic for which mask ventilation is acceptable would be suitable for use of the LMA, although the LMA can be used for procedures that might be considered too lengthy for ventilation using the face mask alone. Additionally, the LMA provides the advantage of freeing the anesthesiologist's hands for other tasks. A compar-

**TABLE 57–10.** Conditions Associated With Difficult Pediatric Airway Management

| Congenital | Acquired |
|---|---|
| Choanal atresia | Infections |
| Subglottic stenosis (may be acquired) | Epiglottitis |
| Cystic hygroma | Laryngotracheitis |
| Tumors | Peritonsillar abscess |
| Angiofibroma | Burns |
| Hemangioma | Trauma (facial or cervical) |
| Craniofacial syndromes | Foreign body aspiration |
| Crouzon's syndrome | Tumors (oral cavity, neck, or mediastinum) |
| Apert's syndrome | Papillomatosis |
| Goldenhar's syndrome | Juvenile rheumatoid arthritis |
| Treacher Collins | |
| Pierre Robin | |
| Freeman-Sheldon | |
| Hallermann-Streiff | |
| Inborn errors of metabolism | |
| Hurler syndrome | |
| Pompe's disease | |
| Chromosomal abnormalities | |
| Trisomy-21 (Down's syndrome) | |
| Trisomy-13 | |
| Trisomy-18 | |
| Cri du chat (5p − ) syndrome | |
| Turner's syndrome | |
| Beckwith-Wiedemann syndrome | |
| Mediastinal vascular rings | |

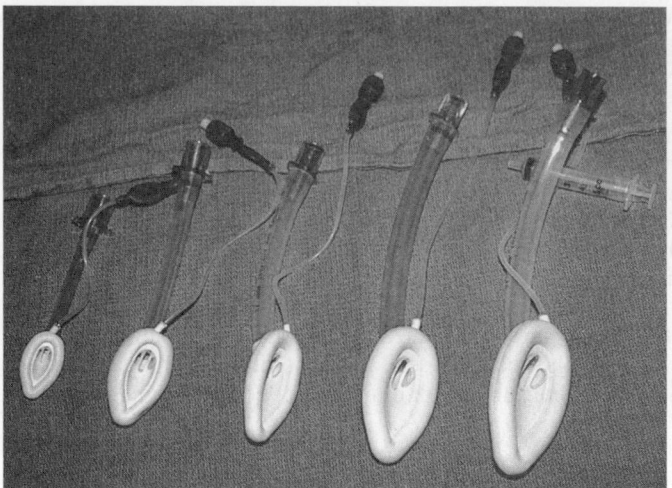

**FIGURE 57–4.** Assortment of laryngeal mask airways in various sizes.

ison of airway management between the LMA and endotracheal intubation in children with URI revealed a higher incidence of bronchospasm and arterial $O_2$ desaturation events in the patients who were intubated, although all respiratory complications in both groups were easily managed.[100]

The LMA is available in a range of sizes for pediatric patients, including size 1 for newborns through small infants weighing 5 kg; the recently released size 1.5 for infants weighing 5 to 10 kg; size 2 for large infants and toddlers weighing 10 to 20 kg; size 2.5 for children weighing 20 to 30 kg; and size 3 for children weighing >30 kg (Fig. 57–4). Some older children and adolescents may require the larger (adult) size 4 or 5 LMA.[101] The technique of LMA insertion is similar to that in adults, and with continued experience, first-time insertion success rates in children improve from about 60% to 98%[102,103] (Figs. 57–5 and 57–6). After insertion and connection to the breathing circuit, either spontaneous or positive pressure assisted ventilation may be employed. In the

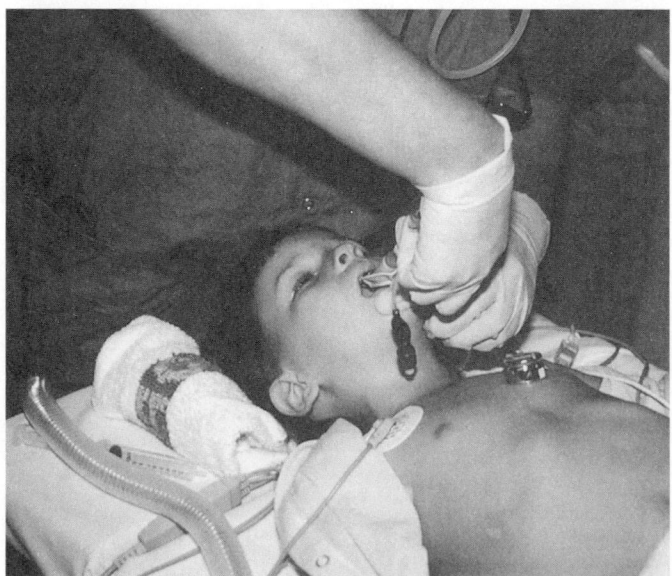

**FIGURE 57–5.** Initial phase of insertion of a laryngeal mask airway into the pharynx of a child. The cuff is deflated, and the device is inserted "blindly" into the mouth along the hard palate.

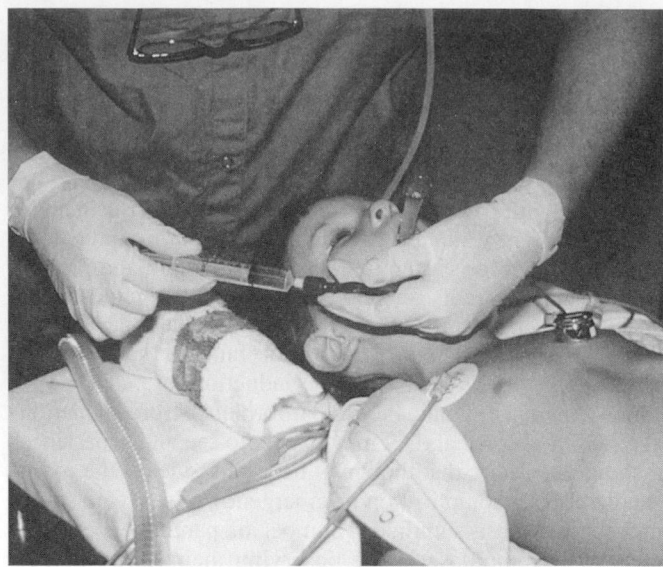

**FIGURE 57–6.** Final phase of laryngeal mass airway insertion. The cuff is inflated before securing the device with tape and inserting a roll of gauze or a "bite block" into the mouth.

latter case, one investigation demonstrated an initial mean leak pressure of 25 cm $H_2O$ after cuff inflation.[104] It is helpful to place rolled gauze between the upper and lower teeth on either side of the LMA to assist with stabilization and to minimize biting of the device upon emergence. Additionally, the breathing circuit should be secured so that it does not cause the LMA to become dislodged.

In addition to routine anesthetic use for elective diagnostic and surgical procedures, the LMA has been successfully used in difficult airway management, as an aid to fiberoptic intubation, and in neonatal resuscitation.[105,106] At the conclusion of the anesthetic, our practice is to remove the LMA when normal airway reflexes have returned and the patient has begun reaching for the LMA, although some practitioners prefer to remove the LMA before emergence and to maintain the patient's airway with a face mask.

## How Is the Trachea Intubated?

Once the child has reached a satisfactory level of anesthesia through the inhalation or intravenous route, direct laryngoscopy is attempted. If the vocal cords and glottis are visualized, the trachea is intubated with an appropriately sized ETT. If the glottis is not visualized, simple maneuvers, including a change in head and neck position, use of a different laryngoscope blade, and application of cricoid pressure, should be considered. If these adjustments fail to allow visualization of the glottis, alternative techniques of intubation, the need for which were anticipated before beginning the induction, are attempted.

At no time should the child receive a muscle relaxant until effective, controlled mask ventilation has been demonstrated. The choice of a muscle relaxant to facilitate difficult intubation is largely a matter of personal preference. For some practitioners, succinylcholine is still the preferred agent for use before securing the difficult airway, although mivacurium[107] or rapacuronium may serve as suitable alternatives for those wishing to avoid the use of succinylcholine in children.

## Failed Attempts

If the patient is unable to be ventilated by mask or develops hemodynamic instability or oxyhemoglobin desaturation, consideration should be given to discontinuing anesthesia and attempting intubation either while the patient is awake or on another day. Alternatively, proceeding to emergency percutaneous needle or surgical cricothyrotomy may be considered. Specific clinical circumstances and the experience of the anesthesiologist determine which of these alternatives is most appropriate. In some cases, awake intubation may be indicated from the start, as in the neonate with an obstructing airway mass or in the unstable trauma victim.

## Alternative Techniques

Alternative techniques of intubation that may be applied in either the awake (with or without airway topicalization) or anesthetized child include the following:

1. Blind nasal intubation, which requires spontaneous ventilation
2. Use of several variations of small-caliber fiberoptic laryngoscopes,[108] some of which employ an LMA as a guide[109]
3. Use of devices such as a lighted stylet (*lightwand*)[110,111] or a Bullard laryngoscope[112]
4. *Retrograde intubation,* in which the ETT is advanced through the nose or mouth and into the trachea over a guidewire that has been passed through an introducer in the cricothyroid membrane and into the upper airway[113] (Fig. 57–7)

## *When Is Awake Intubation Indicated?*

Patients with profound hemodynamic instability or abnormal airways in whom mask ventilation and tracheal intubation are expected to be difficult should be intubated while awake. After denitrogenation with 100% $O_2$ and as tight a mask fit as is practical, intubation may be accomplished blindly by the nasal route, orally or nasally with direct laryngoscopy, or, if time allows, with a pediatric fiberoptic laryngoscope. Insufflation of $O_2$ with a side port on the laryngoscope blade or through the suction channel of the flexible fiberoptic laryngoscope may help to minimize oxyhemoglobin desaturation during the intubation process. Appropriate monitors include a pulse oximeter, ECG testing, automated BP device, and a capnograph to verify proper ETT placement following intubation. Suction equipment and an assistant skilled in applying cricoid pressure (Fig. 57–8) should be available.[114,115]

## *How Is Inhalation Induction Performed?*

Numerous methods are available for induction of general anesthesia; several are extensions of premedication techniques, and each has its own benefits, unique applications, and risks. The choice of technique is influenced by the patient's medical condition and ability to cooperate, the nature and duration of the surgical procedure, and the skill and training of the practitioner. Although mask inhalation of potent vapor agents is the most common means of inducing anesthesia in children younger than about 10 years of age,[116] other

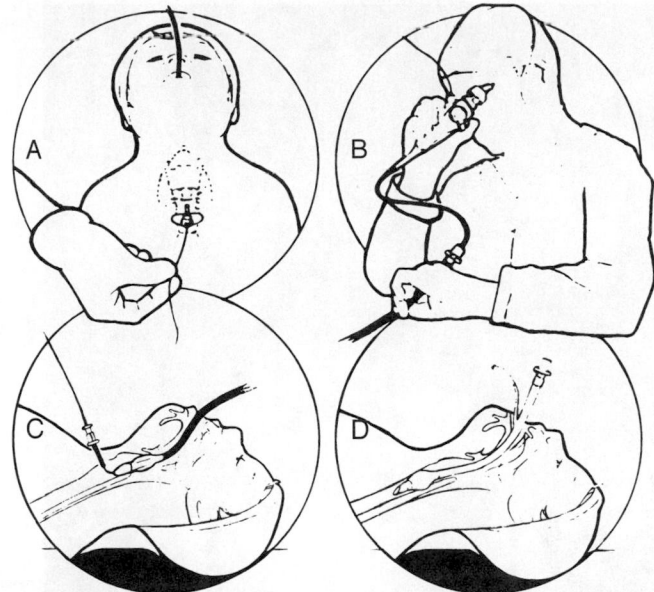

**FIGURE 57–7.** Technique of retrograde intubation in a child, using a fiberoptic laryngoscope. *A,* A flexible guidewire is introduced through a needle or intravenous catheter that has been inserted into the cricothyroid membrane, into the larynx, and up through the vocal cords and mouth. *B,* The guidewire is inserted into the suction channel of a fiberoptic laryngoscope over which an appropriately sized endotracheal tube has been placed. *C,* The fiberoptic laryngoscope is advanced over the guidewire into the larynx and upper trachea. *D,* The endotracheal tube is advanced over the fiberscope into the trachea, with fiberoptic visualization of the endotracheal tube tip within the trachea before removal of the guidewire and fiberscope. (Modified from Lechman MJ, Donahoo JS, MacVaugh H. Endotracheal intubation using percutaneous retrograde guidewire insertion followed by antegrade fiberoptic bronchoscopy. *Crit Care Med.* 1986;14:589.)

techniques include intravenous, intramuscular, and rectal approaches (Fig. 57–9).

## The Classic Approach

A variety of inhalation induction techniques are available, many of which are facilitated by nasal, oral, intramuscular, or rectal premedication. The classic mask induction begins with the administration of a high-flow mixture of nitrous oxide and

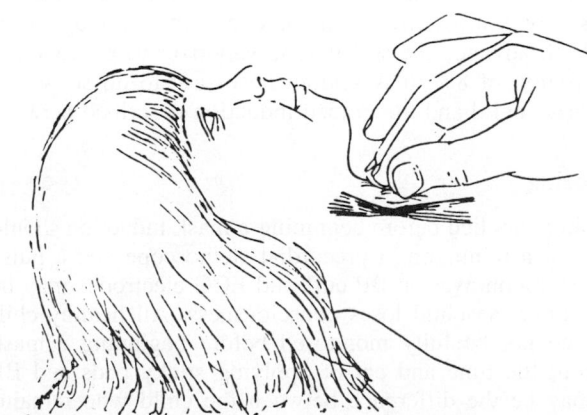

**FIGURE 57–8.** The correct application of cricoid pressure (Sellick maneuver) in a child. (Reprinted by permission of Quadrant HealthCom Inc from Goudsouzian N. Aspiration in children: practical implications. *Anesthesiol Rev.* 1984;11:6, Copyright 2000 by Quadrant HealthCom Inc.)

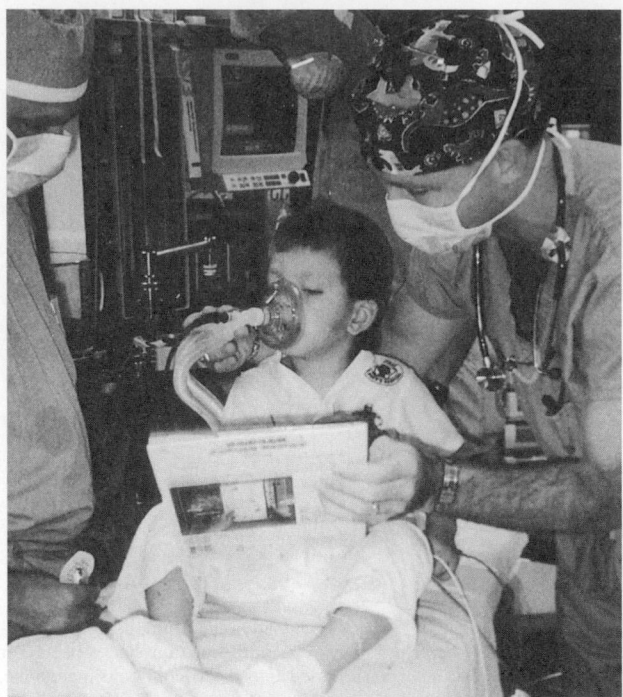

**FIGURE 57–9.** Mask, or inhalation induction of a child.

$O_2$ (60%-70% nitrous oxide) through a cupped hand or loosely applied face mask. As the child becomes stunned or more sedated, the mask can be held snugly to the face, and a potent agent (halothane or sevoflurane) can be added in a low concentration ranging from 0.25% to 0.5%. The concentration of the volatile agent is increased in 0.25% to 0.5% increments with every fourth breath that the child takes.

If the potent agent is advanced too slowly or if the fresh gas flow is too low, the patient may experience a period of prolonged excitement (body movement, breath holding, and agitation) during induction. If the anesthetic concentration is increased too rapidly, the child may likewise withdraw from the mask or develop breath holding or laryngospasm. The maximum indicated vaporizer "dial" concentration of volatile anesthetic administered is dependent on the medical condition and speed of induction of the patient. A healthy toddler or child readily tolerates a 3% to 4% concentration of halothane *with spontaneous ventilation* during induction, whereas an aggressively fluid-restricted infant does not. Although it is possible to advance the sevoflurane vaporizer to a maximum concentration of 8%, it is seldom necessary to do so with a cooperative child and the graded induction described here.

## Monitoring

Monitors applied before beginning a mask induction should include, at a minimum, a precordial stethoscope and a pulse oximeter; a noninvasive BP cuff and ECG electrodes may be applied after the child loses consciousness. All healthy children need not be fully monitored before beginning a mask induction; the time and act of applying sticky pads and BP cuffs may be the difference between the child who remains calm and cooperative and one who decompensates and becomes difficult to manage.

Full preinduction monitoring is reasonable in small infants and any older child with a significant cardiac or pulmonary abnormality that may affect the induction. Only after the child has reached a light plane of surgical anesthesia should an intravenous catheter be placed. After placement, the anesthetic may be maintained by mask, or the patient may be intubated with or without the use of a muscle relaxant.

## Variations in Technique

As indicated previously, variations of the mask inhalation induction exist. These include the omission of nitrous oxide, the use of a potent agent other than halothane or sevoflurane, and the single-breath technique.[117] In addition to some form of premedication, distraction with a story, bubbles (Fig. 57–10), or game (eg, a "blow-up the balloon" contest) or placement of a fruity scent inside of the mask is often helpful.

Many anesthesiologists omit nitrous oxide from their anesthetic regimens because of the wide variety of supplemental short-acting intravenous anesthetics, narcotics, and regional techniques now available; the reduction of inspired $O_2$ and the possibility that this low-potency agent may contribute to postoperative nausea and vomiting (PONV) are two reasons for its omission.[118]

Isoflurane, enflurane, or desflurane may be administered in place of halothane or sevoflurane. However, these agents are more pungent and less well tolerated by awake children and are more potent respiratory depressants than halothane; in our practice, they have no place in inhalation induction.

The single-breath technique, somewhat of a misnomer, requires a cooperative and capable child to take a deep, vital capacity breath from a primed anesthesia circuit containing 5% halothane and 60% to 70% nitrous oxide. The patient must then take several regular breaths before eye closure and loss of the eyelid reflex are attained. Similarly, a high-dose sevoflurane induction technique has been described that is particularly useful in young children and patients in whom a lack of cooperation with induction is anticipated. In this case, the breathing circuit is primed with 8% sevoflurane and a 2:1 mixture of nitrous oxide and $O_2$ at a 6 L/min total fresh gas flow rate for 3 minutes before placing the mask on the child's face. This technique appears to be well tolerated from the

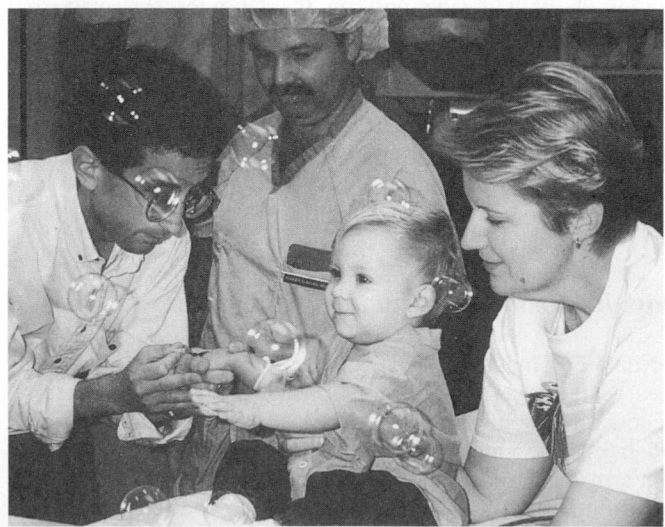

**FIGURE 57–10.** The use of distraction techniques, such as blowing bubbles and a musical storybook, during an intravenous start and induction of anesthesia.

standpoints of patient acceptance, airway management, and hemodynamics.[119]

## How Is Intravenous Induction Performed?

General anesthesia may also be induced by the intravenous route.[120–123] Although it is the standard technique in some pediatric centers, intravenous induction is generally reserved for small neonates and premature infants; for older children who may prefer awake placement of an intravenous catheter rather than a mask induction; for children who are considered at elevated risk for pulmonary aspiration or are hemodynamically unstable; and for patients who already have an intravenous catheter in place for treatment of a medical or surgical condition. It is desirable to attempt denitrogenation of the lungs with 100% inspired mask and as tight a mask fit as possible before intravenous induction, although clearly the age and activity level of the patient may make denitrogenation difficult. Intravenous induction agents provide the most rapid loss of consciousness and can be titrated based on patient response and hemodynamic status. Commonly used agents and doses are indicated in Table 57–11.

## What Is Rapid-Sequence Induction and Intubation?

Rapid-sequence induction and intubation (RSI) is a specific form of intravenous induction in which an induction agent and muscle relaxant are administered in quick succession; after the loss of consciousness and the onset of muscle relaxation, the trachea is intubated. The goal of RSI is to minimize the amount of time between the point of unconsciousness and the point that the airway is secured with a styletted ETT. RSI is typically indicated in patients with normal airways in whom intubation is not expected to be difficult and who are at increased risk for pulmonary aspiration (eg, patients with full stomachs, gastroesophageal reflux, or intestinal obstruction).

RSI should be preceded by denitrogenation of the lungs with 100% $O_2$, and cricoid pressure (Sellick maneuver) should be applied before the loss of consciousness (see Fig. 57–8). Classically, no positive pressure ventilation is provided until the ETT is in place in the trachea. However, in children, it is often necessary to perform a so-called modified RSI with mask ventilation and cricoid pressure, owing to difficulty obtaining effective denitrogenation and the rapidity with which young patients become desaturated after the onset of apnea. Induction agents for RSI include thiopental, propofol, etomidate, and ketamine. Acceptable muscle relaxants include succinylcholine (see later), rocuronium, rapacuronium, and vecuronium. Caution must be exercised when performing the near-simultaneous injection of thiopental and one of these nondepolarizing relaxants into an intravenous line; a precipitate may form, stopping the flow of intravenous fluid and distracting the anesthesiologist from the priority of airway management and intubation. Solutions to this annoying complication include providing a flush of crystalloid solution after the induction drug or administering the medications through different injection ports, possibly in separate intravenous lines. After confirmation of appropriate ETT placement by auscultation and detection of end-tidal $CO_2$, cricoid pressure is released, and the stomach is suctioned.

Although an RSI is the preferred method of inducing general anesthesia in a child with a normal airway and a full stomach, an occasional patient may be encountered in whom attempts at awake peripheral intravenous catheter placement have failed. The options in this case are to insert a percutaneous central line, perform a peripheral venous cutdown, or proceed with an inhalation induction and establish venous access after the child is anesthetized.

## How Are Intramuscular and Rectal Induction Performed?

The intramuscular and rectal routes are extensions of premedication techniques in which lower dosages of medications are used. The distinction between preanesthetic sedation and anesthetic induction with these approaches lies in a gray zone, however. Although they allow induction outside of the operating room in the parents' presence, they have the potential to induce airway obstruction and respiratory depression.

Intramuscular induction agents include methohexital (administration of 8-10 mg/kg of a 5% solution, which is followed by loss of consciousness in 3-5 minutes)[124] and ketamine (administration of 3-10 mg/kg, with loss of consciousness in 1-2 minutes). Rectal induction is usually accomplished with 25 to 35 mg/kg of methohexital or thiopental administered with a well-lubricated, shortened suction catheter affixed to a syringe; loss of consciousness usually occurs within 10 minutes.

Our experience with intramuscular and rectal midazolam is that it provides effective sedation but seldom results in actual loss of consciousness with dosages of 0.3 to 0.5 mg/kg.

## ANESTHETIC MAINTENANCE

### What Breathing Circuit Should Be Used?

Pediatric breathing circuits may be divided into circle systems and variations of the Mapleson classification of semio-

**TABLE 57–11.** Intravenous Induction Agents in Children

| Agent | Concentration | Dose | Comments |
|---|---|---|---|
| Thiopental | 2.5% | 4-6 mg/kg | Rapid, smooth induction with blood pressure reduction similar to propofol<br>Reduce dose in hypovolemic or compromised patients |
| Methohexital | 1.0% | 1-2 mg/kg | May cause seizure activity; shorter elimination half-life than thiopental<br>Frequent excitatory phenomena with induction |
| Ketamine | 1.0% | 1-2 mg/kg | Useful in hypovolemic patients; increases oral secretions<br>May induce dreaming, nystagmus, extremity movement |
| Propofol | 2% | 2-3 mg/kg | Often burns on intravenous administration, less frequently with larger, more proximal veins<br>Probably less nausea and vomiting than with other agents |

pen, nonrebreathing circuits. The work of breathing necessary to overcome the resistance of the one-way valves in an adult circle system by a spontaneously breathing neonate or infant may predispose to fatigue, hypoventilation, and atelectasis. The Bain circuit, a coaxial modification of the Mapleson D circuit (Fig. 57–11), contains no such valves and is therefore associated with less work of breathing. Other advantages include a degree of warming of inspired gases as they flow through tubing within the expiratory limb of the circuit and the rapidity with which change in the concentration of gases delivered to the patient can be achieved.

For most pediatric cases, particularly infants and neonates, ventilation is assisted or controlled. Hence, a pediatric circle system can be used safely in most children. The range of recommended fresh gas flow rates for partial or nonrebreathing circuits is quite wide. However, adequate fresh gas flow is a critical factor to prevent rebreathing of $CO_2$ in any circuit without a $CO_2$ absorber. A minimum fresh gas flow of 2.5 to 3.0 L/min with an additional 100 mL/kg/min is recommended for the Bain circuit.[125] Even higher fresh gas flow rates of 2 to 3 times the minute volume of ventilation also have been recommended, particularly during spontaneous breathing.[126] Capnography should be used to adjust fresh gas flows and minute ventilation after anesthesia induction.

## How Do the Inhalation Agents Compare?

Anesthetic drugs and adjunctive agents such as muscle relaxants used to maintain the state of general anesthesia after one of the induction techniques discussed previously are essentially the same as those employed in adults. However, the dose responses and clinical use of these medications frequently differ in children. Examples of such differences in the case of the commonly used inhalation agent halothane are the higher minimum alveolar concentration (MAC) values in infants and small children[127] and the widespread use of halothane for mask induction of general anesthesia. Sevoflurane has also achieved popularity as a mask induction and maintenance inhalation agent, particularly for relatively brief outpatient procedures. This agent has virtually replaced the use of halothane in Japan.[128]

### General Features

The potent inhalation agents halothane, enflurane, isoflurane, desflurane, and sevoflurane are the only drugs that are individually capable of providing amnesia, analgesia, control of autonomic nervous system reflexes, and muscle relaxation. The potent inhaled agents may be used alone or in combination with adjuvants such as nitrous oxide and narcotics for the maintenance of anesthesia. Given the available agents,

enflurane has no application in pediatric anesthesia because it offers no particular advantages and possesses a number of undesirable features. These include a somewhat pungent, disagreeable odor, low potency (higher MAC) when compared with halothane and isoflurane, profound respiratory depression during spontaneous ventilation, and a small but significant degree of metabolism that results in liberation of potentially nephrotoxic-free fluoride ions during prolonged administration. The major disadvantage of desflurane in pediatrics is the great difficulty with which mask inhalation induction is performed when using this drug; if an intravenous induction is possible, the low solubility of desflurane provides for a relatively rapid emergence that can be associated with agitation and delirium. These emergence features frequently result in the use of sedatives and opioids to control the child, which may negate the benefit of the low solubility and rapid emergence.

The principal inhalation agents employed in children are halothane, sevoflurane, and isoflurane. Halothane has an agreeable odor and is, therefore, associated with less breath holding, coughing, and laryngospasm than is isoflurane. Halothane and isoflurane MAC values (at age 6 months, when MAC peaks) are about 30% to 50% greater than adult values, being 1.1% and 1.7%, respectively. Like halothane, sevoflurane has a pleasant odor and is associated with minimum airway irritation. As with the other potent inhalation anesthetics, the MAC of sevoflurane is increased in infancy to about 3.3%, after which it slowly declines to the 2% value found in adults.

### Hemodynamic Effects

Halothane and isoflurane differ significantly in their hemodynamic effects, a fact that has implications for the anesthetic management of infants, who have limited myocardial contractile reserve, and of children with congenital heart disease. Halothane is a myocardial depressant and tends to reduce heart rate, whereas isoflurane tends to maintain or increase heart rate and to reduce peripheral vascular resistance, thus minimizing reductions in cardiac index. Greater cardiovascular reserve and ability to tolerate intravenous fluid challenges are said to occur with the use of isoflurane.[129]

In general, the hemodynamic effects of sevoflurane are similar to those of isoflurane, and stability of BP and heart rate is retained during the maintenance phase of anesthesia.[130]

### Speed of Induction

Despite isoflurane's lower blood-gas solubility coefficient (1.4), which would be expected to provide more rapid anesthetic induction and recovery than halothane (the blood-gas solubility coefficient of halothane is 2.4), most clinical studies fail to demonstrate a significant difference between the agents. One report suggested shorter induction and elimination times for isoflurane.[131] This observation, in combination with many practitioners' clinical impression that children anesthetized with isoflurane may wake up and recover more rapidly, support the widespread practice of switching from halothane to isoflurane after induction. In general, however, halothane and isoflurane can be used interchangeably with similar results. Inhalation induction with sevoflurane is rapid, owing to its acceptable odor and low solubility (blood-gas partition coefficient of 0.6).

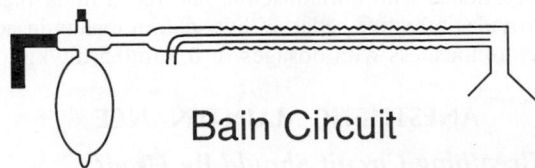

**Bain Circuit**

**FIGURE 57–11.** Schematic diagram of the Bain circuit, demonstrating its coaxial design, with inner inspiratory flow tubing, outer (corrugated) expiratory flow channel, and anesthesia bag.

## Of What Value Are the Opioids?

The opioids, or narcotics, are used both as supplements to inhalation anesthesia and, in higher dosages, as primary anesthetic agents. As adjuvants, doses include morphine, 0.05 to 0.2 mg/kg; meperidine, 0.5 to 1.0 mg/kg; fentanyl, 1 to 3 $\mu$g/kg/h; sufentanil, 0.1 to 0.3 $\mu$g/kg/h; and alfentanil, 10 to 50 $\mu$g/kg/h. Opioids blunt the cardiovascular responses to surgical stimulation, reduce the requirement for inhalation agents, and contribute to postoperative analgesia.

Fentanyl, 10 to 50 $\mu$/kg, and sufentanil, 3 to 15 $\mu$g/kg, are frequently used as primary anesthetics in children with significant cardiovascular instability or in those who are undergoing cardiac surgery.[132] In these settings, these drugs must be used with muscle relaxants. Because the narcotics may not provide adequate amnesia, even with high dosages, they are supplemented with benzodiazepines or low concentrations of the potent inhalation agents.

Remifentanil is a relatively new rapid- and ultrashort-acting opioid that is metabolized by nonspecific esterases in the blood. It is almost always administered by continuous infusion, although it has been given in a bolus dose to blunt the hemodynamic response to endotracheal intubation.[133] It has been used as a supplement to other agents during general anesthesia during a variety of procedures, including microlaryngobronchoscopy, craniotomy, and posterior spinal fusion. It has also been used in conjunction with propofol to provide total intravenous anesthesia.[134] Suggested infusion rates vary considerably, depending on the simultaneous administration of other anesthetic agents, from about 0.05 to 1 $\mu$g/kg/min.[135,136] It is essential that some provision is made for analgesia (regional block or longer acting opioid) after painful procedures and the discontinuation of a remifentanil infusion.

Among the side effects of opioids are respiratory depression, chest wall rigidity, and bradycardia, particularly with rapid intravenous administration of higher dosages. Morphine and meperidine additionally induce histamine release, and meperidine may additionally induce tachycardia. The latter agent is seldom used in pediatric anesthesia.

## When Are Muscle Relaxants Indicated?

Muscle relaxants are used to facilitate tracheal intubation after anesthetic induction and provide neuromuscular blockade throughout some procedures. They may be necessary for improved surgical exposure or to prevent dangerous patient movement should the level of anesthesia become unexpectedly light, although muscle relaxation should rarely be used as a substitute for good anesthesia with inhalation or intravenous anesthetics; emergency cases associated with life-threatening hemodynamic instability are the exception. Differences in the pharmacokinetic and pharmacodynamic responses to muscle relaxants in pediatric and adult patients have received a great deal of attention in the anesthesia literature.[137] Most significant are the altered volumes of distribution of these water-soluble drugs and immaturity of the neuromuscular junction, particularly in the neonatal and early infancy periods.[138]

### Nondepolarizing Agents

The nondepolarizing muscle relaxants are indicated in Table 57–12 along with their effective ($ED_{95}$) and intubating doses.

**TABLE 57–12.** Initial (Intubating) and Maintenance Doses of Nondepolarizing Muscle Relaxants in Children

| Drug | Intubating Dose ($\mu$g/kg) | Maintenance Dose* ($\mu$g/kg) |
|---|---|---|
| *Benzylisoquinolines* | | |
| Atracurium | 500-600 | 100-300 |
| Cisatracurium | 200 | 50-100 |
| Doxacurium | 500 | 30-100 |
| Metocurine | 300 | 100-200 |
| Mivacurium | 200-300 | 100-200 |
| D-Tubocurarine | 600 | 200-400 |
| *Aminosteroids* | | |
| Pancuronium | 100 | 10-50 |
| Pipecuronium | 100 | 20-50 |
| Rapacuronium | 2000 | NR |
| Rocuronium | 600-1200 | 100-500 |
| Vecuronium | 100 | 20-50 |

*Maintenance doses are variable and should be guided by monitors of neuromuscular transmission (eg, train-of-four ratios), coadministration of other anesthetics (especially potent inhalational agents), and time-course of the procedure.

NR, not recommended.

The choice for a specific case is based on the anticipated duration of the procedure and the expected side effects of the agents. Because of significant variability in the individual response to muscle relaxants, monitors of neuromuscular function should be used to guide dosing.

Whether routine reversal of the short- to intermediate-acting nondepolarizing relaxants (atracurium, cisatracurium, vecuronium, rocuronium, rapacuronium) should be employed is controversial. Up to 70% of acetylcholine receptors at the neuromuscular junction may be blocked in the presence of an intact twitch response.[139] Infants and small children with increased $O_2$ consumption and ventilatory requirements may be predisposed to subclinical muscle weakness and respiratory failure. These facts suggest the advisability of reversal. Yet, if an adequate interval has elapsed since the agent was last administered, and if adequate recovery of neuromuscular function can be demonstrated clinically[140] and with neuromuscular transmission (train-of-four) monitoring, the withholding of reversal agents such as edrophonium or neostigmine and close observation are probably satisfactory.[137]

### Succinylcholine

Succinylcholine is the only depolarizing muscle relaxant in clinical use in the United States and remains the shortest acting of all relaxants. It has also been the only agent to be safely and effectively given intramuscularly when muscle relaxation is required but an intravenous route is lacking,[141] although rapacuronium may be the first truly viable alternative to succinylcholine for intramuscular administration.[142]

Succinylcholine is associated with a number of potential side effects or complications that make its use less attractive. These include cardiac dysrhythmias, masseter spasm, rhabdomyolysis, and MH. Additionally, succinylcholine preparations now bear the warning that severe arrhythmias and cardiac arrest may result from administration of the drug to children (usually boys) with occult myopathies. In view of these potential problems, many anesthesiologists who care for children now reserve succinylcholine for use in specific circumstances. These include RSI, treatment of laryngospasm that is refractory to 100% $O_2$ and positive pressure ventilation, and instances in which the longer duration of muscle relaxation provided by the nondepolarizing agents is undesirable. The short- to intermediate-acting nondepolarizing relaxants mivacurium, rapacuronium, and rocuronium are often used as suitable alternatives to succinylcholine, although onset time and duration of action are generally longer than with succinylcholine.[107]

## How Should Ketamine and Propofol Be Used?

The intravenous drugs ketamine and propofol, which are typically used as induction agents, may also be used in incremental boluses or by continuous infusion for the maintenance of general anesthesia. Ketamine is particularly useful in hypovolemic patients and may also be given intramuscularly, but it is associated with several undesirable side effects, including dreaming, vomiting, increased intracranial pressure, and increased production of secretions.

Propofol is noted for the rapidity of recovery from its desired effects and for the low incidence of side effects, such as vomiting, headache, and confusion. It is particularly useful in short-duration procedures on outpatients and in situations when inhalation anesthetics are difficult or impossible to administer, such as when sedation must be provided for MRI procedures and jet ventilation for bronchoscopy or airway surgery.[143,144] The required continuous infusion rate of propofol ranges from 50 to 300 μg/kg/min, depending on the nature of procedural stimulation and any inhalational anesthetics or opioids that are administered simultaneously.

## FLUID THERAPY AND BLOOD TRANSFUSION

### Which Children Require Intravenous Access?

If the question of intravenous access for a particular patient arises, it probably should be used. It should always be provided for a neonate receiving general anesthesia; in children with any metabolic derangement (eg, diabetes mellitus, dehydration, hyponatremia); for cases in which there exists the possibility of significant blood loss; for any procedure that is scheduled to last over 30 minutes; and for any patient in whom postoperative nausea or vomiting, or both, are anticipated. The only cases that do not routinely require intravenous access before the procedure are short, minimally invasive procedures in relatively healthy patients, such as pressure-equalizing tube placement, suture removal, limb cast changes, and some cases of examination under anesthesia. Common sites of catheter placement are shown in Figure 57–12.

### What Are the Available Alternatives to Vascular Access?

#### Central Venous Access

Pediatric vascular access frequently poses a daunting challenge. Along with the usual peripheral access sites, central

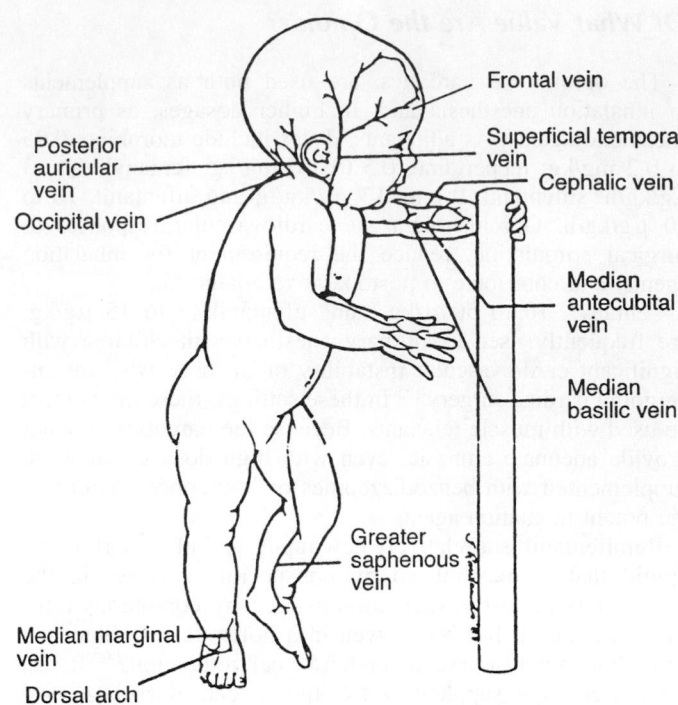

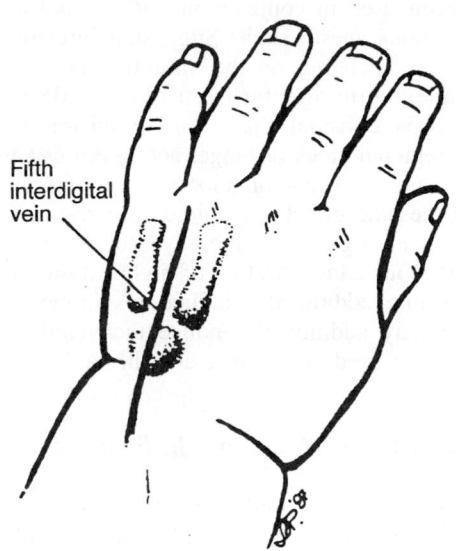

**FIGURE 57–12.** Peripheral intravenous access sites in the child. (From Baldwin GA. *Handbook of Pediatric Emergencies*. Boston, Mass: Little, Brown; 1989:18.)

venous access may be obtained through the external or internal jugular, subclavian, or femoral veins.

#### Intraosseous Access

Should intravenous sites prove inaccessible, fluid resuscitation and the administration of medications may be accomplished through an intraosseous cannula in emergencies. Catecholamines, whole blood, calcium, antibiotics, digitalis, heparin, lidocaine, atropine, and sodium bicarbonate have been infused using this route.[145]

A large (16- to 18-gauge) hypodermic needle, spinal needle with stylet, or bone marrow needle may be placed into the

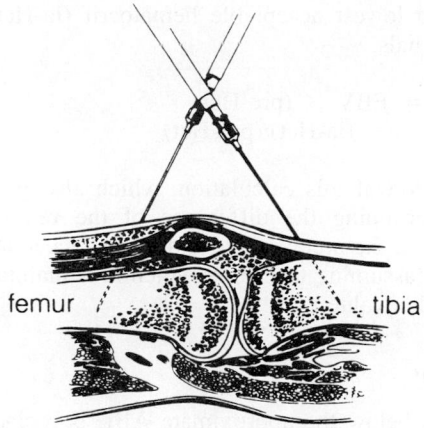

**FIGURE 57–13.** Placement of an intraosseous needle in the distal femur or proximal tibia. Note orientation away from the epiphyseal plate. (From Rosetti VA, Thompson BM, Miller J, et al. Intraosseous infusion: an alternative route of pediatric intravascular access. *Ann Emerg Med.* 1985;14:585.)

marrow cavity of any long bone. Typically, the tibia is chosen as the easiest and least complicated site. The technique is accomplished by placing the needle on the anterior surface of the tibia, 1 to 3 cm inferior to the tibial tuberosity. The needle is positioned perpendicular to the plane of the tibial surface and directed slightly caudad to avoid the epiphyseal plate[146] (Fig. 57–13). When the needle tip is in the bone marrow cavity, bone marrow aspirate should be obtainable, and a free flow of infusate should ensue.

## Endotracheal Access

Some medications may also be administered through the ETT. These include lidocaine, atropine, naloxone, and epinephrine.

## *What Are Maintenance Fluids?*

Comprehensive fluid management includes consideration of maintenance fluid requirements, preexisting water and electrolyte deficits, and intraoperative losses of fluid and blood. Maintenance fluids are those that would normally be consumed orally by the child to provide for the needs of caloric expenditure and metabolism, insensible water loss through the skin and respiratory tract, and measurable water loss through urinary and fecal excretion.

## Infusion Rate

Administration rates may be calculated on the basis of weight, body surface area, or elaborate measures of metabolic rate.[147] For the initial 10 kg of body weight, 100 mL/kg of water is needed for each 24-hour period. For the second 10-kg increment of weight, 50 mL/kg is required per 24-hour period; and for every 1 kg above 20 kg, 25 mL/kg per 24-hour period is needed.

If the 24-hour day is rounded up to 25 hours, the "4-2-1" rule may be applied to determine the hourly basal fluid requirement in any patient. For example, a 30-kg normothermic child in a normal indoor environment would require 70 mL/h of maintenance fluid: 40 mL/h for the initial 10 kg; 20 mL/h for the next 10 kg; and 10 mL/ h for the final 10 kg.

Of course, water alone is not infused because there are additional needs for electrolytes and glucose; the requirement for sodium is 3 mEq, that for potassium is 2 mEq, and that for chloride is 2 mEq per 100 mL of water. Quarter-normal (0.22%) saline with 20 mEq/L added potassium most closely approximates these requirements. Glucose is commonly added as well to meet part of the energy substrate need and to increase the tonicity of the intravenous fluid solution.

### Glucose Requirements

The issue of how much (if any) glucose to provide in the intravenous fluids for a surgical procedure on a child remains controversial, and a wide variation of practice exists among pediatric anesthesiologists. On the one hand, routine administration of a 5% glucose-containing intravenous solution as the sole fluid during surgery frequently results in hyperglycemia.[148] Subsequent osmotic diuresis and the possibility of worsened neurologic outcome should a cerebral ischemic event occur intraoperatively are concerns. On the other hand, administration of glucose-free solutions presents the risk of the patient becoming hypoglycemic while anesthetized, with consequent impairment of function or damage of the nervous[149,150] or other organ systems.

The optimum glucose infusion concentration appears to range between 1.0% and 2.5%.[151,152] That glucose requirements are lower during anesthesia and surgery than during the awake state is a result of the sympathoadrenal stress response to surgery, decreased glucose use, and increased gluconeogenesis.[153]

To insist that every pediatric patient receive intravenous glucose during surgery is unreasonable. Healthy, well-nourished children undergoing short procedures (<1 hour) may receive a glucose-free infusion as long as all caregivers involved understand that a small but real chance exists that the patient may be asymptomatically hypoglycemic before or during surgery. For this reason, performing a finger- or heel-stick blood glucose analysis should be considered after anesthesia induction; if the results indicate a low glucose level, glucose should be added to the intravenous infusion.

Patients at risk for hypoglycemia, as indicated in Table 57–13, should receive supplemental glucose in their intravenous fluids. Ideally, glucose is infused at a constant rate during surgery, preferably by piggybacking the glucose-containing solution into the main intravenous infusion. Alternatively, a dedicated second intravenous catheter can be used.

**TABLE 57–13.** Children at Increased Risk for Hypoglycemia During Anesthesia

| Infants | Children |
|---|---|
| Preterm infants | Patients receiving total parenteral nutrition |
| Infants of diabetic mothers | Malnourished or chronically diseased patients |
| Infants with erythroblastosis fetalis | Patients receiving insulin therapy |
| Infants small for gestational age | Patients who have been nil per os for prolonged periods |
| | Patients with certain glycogen storage diseases |
| | Patients undergoing prolonged surgical procedures |
| | Patients with insulin-secreting tumors |

## What Are Fasting Fluid Deficits?

The subject of preoperative fasting periods and resultant fluid deficits was discussed earlier in this chapter. The fasting fluid deficit is calculated by multiplying the hourly maintenance fluid rate by the number of hours since the patient last ingested oral fluids. One half of this deficit is administered in addition to the maintenance fluid during the first hour of anesthesia; the remaining half is infused during the next 2 hours.[154] The fluid used to make up the fasting deficit is the same as that used for the maintenance infusion.

## What Constitutes Intraoperative Fluid Loss?

Intraoperative fluid losses include so-called third space loss and actual blood loss.

### Third Space Loss

Third space loss is the result of the transfer of isotonic fluid primarily from the extracellular compartment to a nonfunctional interstitial compartment. A number of conditions in addition to surgical tissue trauma may result in significant third space loss, including burns, gastrointestinal tract obstruction, infections, and blunt trauma. These fluid losses are difficult to quantify and must be estimated based on such factors as the size of the incision, the exposure of visceral surfaces, and the degree of inflammation present. Third space loss is replenished with non–glucose-containing isotonic fluid at rates that range from 1 mL/kg/h for minor procedures with minimal tissue injury to as much as 20 mL/kg/h for large abdominal incisions with extensive inflammation or tissue injury.

### Blood Loss

Any intraoperative blood loss exceeding the minimum amount of 1% of estimated blood volume should be replaced in some fashion. The first step in replacement is to determine the allowable blood loss, that is, the volume of lost blood below which replacement will be provided by crystalloid or colloid preparations and above which a blood component such as packed red blood cells will be given. Calculation of the allowable blood loss requires an estimate of the patient's total blood volume, preoperative hematocrit, and the lowest acceptable hematocrit without a blood product transfusion. The total blood volume is about 90 mL/kg in the full-term infant; this value declines to 70 mL/kg by the age of 1 year.

### Lowest Acceptable Hematocrit

The lowest acceptable hematocrit, or so-called transfusion trigger, for all patients has steadily drifted downward because of the heightened concern of exposing patients to blood-borne infectious agents such as HIV and hepatitis viruses.[155] The hematocrit of an otherwise healthy child who is expected to make an uncomplicated recovery from surgery may be allowed to decrease to between 18% and 20% without transfusion. Some patients with chronic disease states may require higher minimum hematocrit values. With these considerations in mind, the allowable blood loss (ABL) is determined by the following relationship, in which the preoperative hematocrit

(pre-Hct) and lowest acceptable hematocrit (la-Hct) are entered as decimals:

$$ABL = EBV \times (pre\text{-}Hct) - (la\text{-}Hct)/(pre\text{-}Hct) \qquad \text{(Equation 2)}$$

An expansion of this calculation, which also yields ABL, involves determining the difference of the red blood cell masses between the preoperative and lowest acceptable hematocrit values (assuming that normovolemia is maintained) and multiplying this value by 3.

### Replacement

Blood loss below the approximate ABL is replaced in the ratio of 2 to 3 mL of isotonic, non–glucose-containing crystalloid per 1 mL of blood loss, or in a 1:1 ratio with a colloidal preparation such as 5% albumin or 5% plasma protein fraction. For patients with a preexisting coagulopathy or a dilutional coagulopathy secondary to massive blood loss and transfusion, fresh frozen plasma may be used as an alternative colloid preparation, although dilutional coagulopathy is most commonly secondary to thrombocytopenia. Once the ABL has been exceeded, packed red blood cells should be administered.

Older children and adolescents may receive an entire unit of blood, not unlike adults. Infants and small children should receive packed red blood cells in 5- to 10-mL/kg increments by syringe or from subdivided units of blood. Serial hematocrit determinations, ongoing blood loss, and the hemodynamic response to the red blood cell infusion determine the speed and amount of transfusion. To the extent possible, a transfusion from a single-donor source should be continued once the child has been exposed to the blood. This approach optimizes the hematocrit and minimizes the chance of the patient requiring a second transfusion from another donor hours or days later. The justification for administration of all blood products should be clearly documented on the anesthetic record.

## MONITORING

It is imperative to recognize that the real monitor of the patient's physiologic status and response to anesthesia is the anesthesiologist or anesthetist who is observing the patient and the array of monitoring devices attached to the patient or anesthesia delivery system. The application of the ASA monitoring standards alone does not guarantee a desirable patient outcome, and individual patient needs and common sense should be considered in devising specific monitoring approaches.[156]

## What Is Routine?

Routine monitoring in pediatric anesthesia includes, at a minimum, measures that satisfy the standards for basic intraoperative monitoring adopted by the American Society of Anesthesiologists.[157] These include the following:

1. The presence of an anesthetist at all times
2. Monitoring of adequate oxygenation, as provided by an $O_2$ analyzer with audible alarm for low fraction of inspired $O_2$, and pulse oximeter

3. Monitoring of adequate ventilation, as provided by assessment of qualitative signs (chest excursion, movement of reservoir breathing bag, auscultation of breath sounds by precordial or esophageal stethoscope), capnography, and a functioning "disconnect" alarm if the patient is being mechanically ventilated

4. A continuous ECG and arterial BP measured at least every 5 minutes

5. Measurement of body temperature when clinically significant changes in body temperature are intended, anticipated, or suspected

To this list may be added monitoring of neuromuscular transmission in children receiving muscle relaxants in the course of anesthesia. Select patients may require monitoring of urine output, central venous pressure, and neurophysiologic functioning.

Detailed discussion of the function and application of monitoring systems is provided elsewhere in this text. In pediatric patients, pertinent issues include the timing of application of monitors at the time of anesthetic induction and the provision of size-adjusted appliances (eg, ECG pads, BP cuffs, pulse oximetry probes) for the same monitoring systems as would be employed in adults.

### When Should Monitors Be Applied to the Child?

The subject of timing of monitor application at induction must consider the patient's anxiety and activity levels and underlying physiologic status. Particularly in the toddler and preschool-aged population, it may be necessary to proceed with the initial phases of induction with only a precordial stethoscope or pulse oximeter in place, and to apply additional modalities (BP, ECG) gradually as the patient loses consciousness. Success with the preinduction placement of monitors in young children is heavily influenced by the effects of any preanesthetic sedative given, the use of distraction techniques (blowing bubbles, playing with stuffed animals or noise books), and the rapport the anesthesiologist has established with the patient.

### What Is the Role of Pulse Oximetry and Capnography?

Pulse oximetry has been shown to reduce the incidence of critical desaturation events in children undergoing general anesthesia.[158] Capnography provides the earliest diagnosis of esophageal intubation, accidental disconnections within the breathing circuit, inadvertent extubation, and ETT obstruction.[159] It may also reflect the onset of problems, including MH, venous air or particulate embolism, and acute changes in cardiac output.

### What Common Intraoperative Problems May Be Detected?

#### Airway Obstruction

Airway obstruction in the narrow sense implies loss of upper airway patency from causes such as posterior displacement of the tongue into the oropharynx. Premature placement of an oral airway, the presence of blood and secretions in proximity to the larynx, and surgical manipulation during light anesthesia may trigger laryngospasm.

Management of upper airway obstruction includes placement of an artificial oral or nasal airway, administration of 100% $O_2$ with low-level continuous positive airway pressure (3-5 cm $H_2O$), and performance of simple maneuvers such as a chin-lift or jaw-thrust. If laryngospasm fails to respond to these measures, a small dose of intravenous succinylcholine (0.2-0.5 mg/kg) induces relaxation of the laryngeal muscles and facilitates assisted or controlled ventilation. Consideration should then be given to intubating the trachea.

In a broader sense, airway obstruction includes ETT occlusion by secretions or tissue; lower airway compromise due to bronchospasm or foreign bodies; and extrinsic compression of the intrathoracic airway by tumors or surgical manipulation.

#### Oxyhemoglobin Desaturation

Oxyhemoglobin desaturation indicated by a decreased $SpO_2$ results from any process that interferes with $O_2$ uptake or transport. Problems may involve the supply of $O_2$ to the breathing circuit, airway obstruction, cardiac dysfunction, and impaired perfusion of specific limbs or tissue beds. When desaturation develops abruptly during anesthesia, apnea, airway obstruction, ETT displacement, or malfunction of the ventilator and breathing circuit is commonly responsible.

The immediate response should be to administer 100% $O_2$ manually by mask or ETT, to assess airway patency, and to begin a sequential check of all elements from the $O_2$ source to the peripheral circulation. Remember that surgical maneuvers may be causative (positioning, packing, and clamping). Only after other possibilities are excluded should the possibility of monitor inaccuracy or artifact be considered. Inaccuracies may result from excessive ambient light, impaired perfusion to the site of the oximeter probe, patient movement, partial probe displacement, and electrical interference.

#### Temperature Fluctuations

Pediatric patients may experience significant reductions or increases in body temperature during surgery. Because of their greater ratio of body surface area to weight, they are at higher risk of significant heat loss and hypothermia in the operating room. However, because this risk is now generally well recognized by anesthesiologists and operating room nursing personnel, hyperthermia due to overzealous measures to maintain body temperature, in our experience, is nearly as common a problem as significant hypothermia. This is particularly the case with procedures involving limb tourniquets, limited patient exposure, or the application of casts that cover a large portion of the patient's body.

MH is distinguished from more common causes of intraoperative temperature elevation on the basis of findings that generally appear earlier, such as hypercarbia and nonrespiratory acidosis.

#### Blood Pressure Fluctuations

BP is usually measured noninvasively at 3- to 5-minute intervals with automated oscillotonometric devices. Other noninvasive techniques that are occasionally employed include ultrasound flow detection with intermittent cuff occlusion over a peripheral artery and the use of a manual sphygmomanometer and stethoscope to auscultate Korotkoff sounds. Invasive arterial BP monitoring may be indicated in patients with significant cardiopulmonary disease and hemodynamic instability or in patients with significant anticipated blood or fluid losses perioperatively. In toddlers and preschool-aged children up to 6 years of age, a 22-gauge catheter is used in nearly any peripheral artery but most commonly the radial and dorsalis pedis arteries. A 20-gauge catheter may be used in older children. The adequacy of collateral arterial supply to the extremity under consideration and the nature and site of the proposed surgery should be assessed in choosing an arterial catheter site.

Intraoperative hypotension is commonly due to bradycardia, hypoxemia, hypovolemia, and relative anesthetic overdose. Myocardial dysfunction, in the absence of a known history of congenital cardiac disease, is an unusual cause. Other causes include inappropriately sized BP cuffs, anaphylaxis, sepsis, and tension pneumothorax.

Hypertension may be secondary to pain or light anesthesia, excessive intravenous fluid administration, hypercarbia, or the use of inappropriately small BP cuffs. A small number of pediatric patients have an organic source that is usually identified preoperatively, such as coarctation of the aorta, chronic renal disease, or a catecholamine-secreting tumor.

## Cardiac Arrhythmias

### Bradycardia

Primary cardiac dysrhythmias are uncommon in the absence of structural heart disease. Sinus or junctional bradycardia or sinus tachycardia may occur in response to a host of acute clinical derangements. Before the popularization of pulse oximetry, the dictum that bradycardia reflects hypoxemia until proven otherwise prevailed. Although hypoxemia remains an important and common cause of bradycardia, it is now easier to exclude, allowing earlier consideration of other possibilities. These include light or inadequate anesthesia with consequent vagal stimulation; any of several neural responses such as the oculocardiac reflex; and drug effects (with the use of potent inhalation anesthetics, narcotics, or cholinesterase inhibitors).

### Sinus Tachycardia

Sinus tachycardia, the diagnosis of which should include consideration of the patient's age and usual heart rate, may occur secondary to hypovolemia, light anesthesia, hypoxemia (early), hypercarbia, temperature elevation, or drug effect.

### Premature Ventricular Contractions

Premature ventricular contractions may appear in the setting of light anesthesia or impaired ventilation and usually resolve spontaneously with correction of these conditions. Halothane-induced sensitization of the heart to dysrhythmias should be considered, especially with concomitant use of epinephrine infiltration at the surgical site; however, children appear to be more resistant to dysrhythmias than adults in this situation.[160]

## REGIONAL ANESTHESIA

### What Is Its Role?

Regional anesthesia has proved to be useful as a primary technique and as an adjunct to general anesthesia. Physiologic considerations in patients 6 months of age or younger include a minimal hemodynamic response to extensive conduction blockade. Hypotension following sympathectomy is rare because cardiac output, BP, and carotid blood flow are well maintained.[161] Myelination of the CNS is not complete until about 18 months of age; hence, effective neural blockade may be achieved with lower concentrations of local anesthetics. Maximum recommended doses for local anesthetics are shown in Table 57–14.

### Caudal Epidural

Caudal analgesia or anesthesia is one of the most useful, commonly administered regional techniques in children. The placement of a caudal epidural needle is illustrated in Figure 57–14. Because the distal end of the dura can be as low as the S-3 level in neonates, care should be taken when advancing the needle into the caudal space to avoid unintended dural puncture. As with most other regional techniques, it is prudent to aspirate the syringe gently before commencing the injection of the local anesthetic mixture to detect the presence of blood, which might indicate intravascular or intraosseous placement of the needle tip. Although the electrocardiogram should be closely monitored during the incremental caudal injection to detect early signs of intravascular local anesthetic injection, several investigations have reported the unreliability of "test

**TABLE 57–14.** Current Use of Local Anesthetics for Regional Anesthesia and Analgesia in Children

| Drug | Use | Concentration Range (%)* | Dose or Volume | Maximum Dose (mg/kg)† |
|------|-----|--------------------------|----------------|------------------------|
| Tetracaine | Spinal (<3 y) | 0.2-0.5 | 0.4-0.8 mg/kg | 2 |
| Bupivacaine | Single-shot caudal/epidural | 0.125-0.5 | 0.5-1.25 mL/kg | 3 |
| | Continuous lumbar epidural | 0.075-0.5 | 0.1-0.2 mL/kg/h | |
| Ropivacaine | Single-shot caudal/epidural | 0.2-0.5 | 0.5-1.25 mL/kg | ? 3–4‡ |
| | Intravenous regional | 0.2 | 0.6-1 mL/kg | |
| Lidocaine | Tissue infiltration | 0.5-1 | As required, up to maximum dose | 5 (up to 10 mg/kg with 1:200 000 epinephrine) |
| | Intravenous regional | 0.5 | 0.6-1 mL/kg | 5 |

*Higher concentrations apply to more dense, "surgical" blocks, whereas lower concentrations are employed for analgesia and pain management.
†These are suggested safe upper limits for a single dose of local anesthetic administration. Accidental intravenous or intraarterial injection of even a fraction of these amounts may result in toxicity.
‡A maximum single dose of ropivacaine is probably 3-4 mg/kg using the caudal route; the drug is less toxic than bupivacaine.

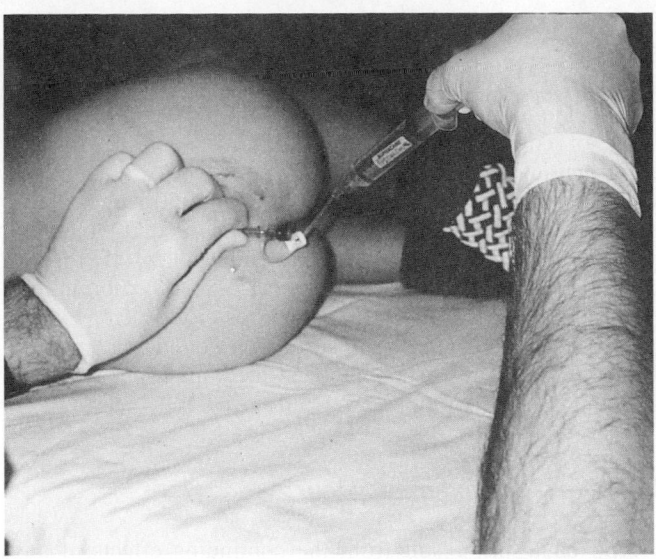

**FIGURE 57–14.** Insertion of a single-shot caudal block needle in a child. The child is in the right lateral decubitus position. After palpation of the sacral hiatus between the sacral cornua, a 22-gauge "B"-bevel needle is placed into the caudal epidural space. After aspiration of a syringe attached to the needle for blood, the local anesthetic mixture is injected.

dosing" with epinephrine-containing local anesthetic solutions.[162,163] When present, ECG changes may include both tachycardia and relative bradycardia, as well as various ST-segment and T-wave changes, particularly a markedly increased amplitude of the T wave.[164] Urinary retention is a possibility following this block, although most children void within 6 to 8 hours. Postoperative voiding, therefore, need not be a criterion for discharge from the PACU in the otherwise comfortable child.

For surgery below the diaphragm, 0.25% bupivacaine (with epinephrine, 1:200 000) in a dosage of 1 mL/kg (maximum, 40 mL) provides good anesthetic conditions for surgery.[165] Postoperative analgesia with minimum motor blockade may be obtained with similar dosing of 0.125% bupivacaine. Analgesia of longer duration (8-24 hours) may be obtained with caudally administered preservative-free morphine in a dose of 0.03 to 0.05 mg/kg diluted in 5 mL of preservative-free normal saline. Ventilatory response to $CO_2$ is attenuated with epidural doses of morphine as low as 0.05 mg/kg; therefore, patients should be monitored for about 24 hours after epidurally administered morphine.[166]

The role of ropivacaine, a relatively new long-acting amide local anesthetic, in pediatric anesthetic practice is currently unclear. This agent is provided as a single enantiomer with properties similar to those of bupivacaine but with a lower potential for CNS and cardiovascular toxic side effects. Ropivacaine also has the potential to cause less motor block than bupivacaine. Although the drug has several theoretic advantages, it is unclear whether its higher cost will offset its benefits in routine clinical practice.[167,168]

## Lumbar and Thoracic Epidural

Lumbar and thoracic epidural anesthesia, provided through catheters placed at these levels or through a catheter threaded cephalad from a caudal insertion site, are becoming more

popular in children. Technical and equipment difficulties with these approaches, as well as the ability to obtain comparable analgesia by using different local anesthetic and opioid agents through the caudal route, may make these approaches less useful for the general anesthesiologist who practices pediatric anesthesia infrequently.

Advantages of these approaches include a reduction in the total volume and dose of local anesthetic required to achieve analgesia, a decrease in the endocrine stress response to surgery, and the ability to use a continuous infusion of a lipophilic opioid, such as fentanyl, that is prone to less migration within the cerebrospinal fluid.[169] For lumbar epidural administration, 0.75 mL/kg of 0.25% bupivacaine with 1:200 000 epinephrine provides good surgical analgesia; incremental dosing with 0.125% bupivacaine, with or without fentanyl, 1 to 2 μg/kg, provides satisfactory postoperative analgesia. With continuous or prolonged infusions, the total dose of bupivacaine should not exceed 0.4 mg/kg/h in older infants and children and 0.2 mg/kg/h in younger infants.[170,171]

## Spinal

Intrathecal anesthesia is an option for high-risk formerly premature infants undergoing infraumbilical procedures (primarily inguinal hernia repair). Spinal anesthesia without supplemental sedation in these infants can reduce the incidence of apnea that occurs after general anesthesia.[172,173] Nevertheless, studies indicate that apnea monitoring is required for all high-risk infants postoperatively, regardless of anesthetic technique.[174] Tetracaine in a dose of 0.4 to 0.8 mg/kg with or without epinephrine generally provides adequate anesthesia. It is important to realize that the time to return of motor function after intrathecal hyperbaric tetracaine is about 80% shorter in children; hence, this technique requires a relatively quick surgeon.[175]

## Peripheral Nerve Blocks

Specific individual nerve blocks may be useful in pediatric practice. Block of the dorsal nerve of the penis is easily performed with 0.8 mL of 1.0% plain lidocaine in the newborn and with 1 to 3 mL of 0.25% bupivacaine in older children. This nerve's major anterior and minor posterior divisions supply all but the base of the penis, which is innervated by branches from the genitofemoral and ilioinguinal nerves. Dorsal nerve block provides good anesthesia for circumcision and postoperative analgesia for hypospadias repair. The ilioinguinal and iliohypogastric nerves are also easily blocked by simple infiltration of the abdominal wall medial to the anterosuperior iliac spine.[175] This block can provide excellent analgesia for inguinal hernia repair and orchiopexy.

## Intravenous Regional

Intravenous regional anesthesia (Bier block) is useful to provide extremity anesthesia for procedures of limited duration in cooperative patients. After limb exsanguination, the tourniquet should be inflated to about 50 mm Hg above the measured systolic BP. Lidocaine in a dosage range of 2.5 to 5.0 mg/kg in a concentration of 0.5% is generally the agent of choice.[165,175]

## POSTANESTHETIC PROBLEMS

### What Are Some Common Problems Encountered After Anesthesia?

A number of different problems may be encountered after anesthesia in the PACU or ICU. Although some of these are common to both adult and pediatric patients, approaches to assessment and management may vary. Common problems include airway obstruction (postintubation croup and stridor), hypoxemia, delayed emergence, delirium, pain, and nausea and vomiting.

### What Are the Causes of Airway Obstruction in the Postanesthesia Care Unit?

Airway obstruction may occur at any point from the time of extubation in the operating room or PACU until hours after surgery on the ward or in the ICU. A major cause is resedation from the effects of residual anesthetic agents or analgesics given in the operating room or PACU, with resulting decreased muscle tone and relaxation of the muscles of the floor of the mouth and pharynx. Another cause is laryngospasm (see later). Large amounts of secretions and foreign bodies (eg, emesis, throat packs) may also lead to airway obstruction. Airway infringement can also result from the effects of anatomic distortions due to disease processes and surgical procedures, as in laryngeal papillomatosis and cervical hematomas.

Most cases of postanesthetic airway obstruction resolve with simple maneuvers such as opening the mouth and providing a chin-lift or jaw-thrust, or placing the child on his or her side. Some patients may require placement of a size-appropriate oral nasopharyngeal airway, depending on level of consciousness. Infrequently, reintubation or direct surgical intervention, as in the case of posttonsillectomy hemorrhage or expanding cervical hematoma, may be required.

### How Is Laryngospasm Recognized?

Laryngospasm is recognized by the presence of a paradoxic rocking motion of the abdominal and chest walls with ventilatory effort and sternal and intercostal retractions. High-pitched squeaky (partial obstruction) or absent (complete obstruction) breath sounds can result, leading to oxyhemoglobin desaturation and hypoxemia. Light anesthesia, pain, and the presence of secretions on, or irritation of, the vocal cords may cause it. Treatment consists of administering 100% $O_2$ and continuous positive airway pressure through a tight-fitting mask. If the laryngospasm does not abate, succinylcholine, 0.1 to 0.2 mg/kg intravenously, often relieves it without necessitating reintubation.

### What Causes Postintubation Croup, and How Is It Treated?

Postintubation croup and stridor denote a specific subset of children with airway obstruction that is thought to be due to swelling or edema in the larynx, usually at the level of the cricoid ring. The incidence is about 1% of pediatric anesthe-

tics.[91] As the name implies, endotracheal intubation, usually with a tight-fitting tube that failed to provide a leak below 30-cm $H_2O$ pressure, is implicated. Other contributing factors may include frequent changes in head and tube position, the effects of cold and dry medical gases, and URI. It may develop at any time in the first 24 hours after extubation but usually occurs within the first several hours. Treatment consists of the progressive application of humidified $O_2$, administration of nebulized racemic epinephrine (0.25-0.5 mL of 2.25% racemic epinephrine solution in 2.5-5 mL normal saline), and perhaps an intravenous corticosteroid such as dexamethasone (0.25-0.5 mg/kg).[176] Rarely, a child may require reintubation for severe postintubation croup associated with oxygenation and ventilation difficulties.

### Why Does Hypoxemia Occur?

Hypoxemia may result from the continuing effects of any preexisting disease processes that impair oxygenation, or it may be a complication of the anesthetic or surgical procedure. At first, it is essential to ensure that the patient is receiving supplemental $O_2$ in the desired concentration and through an appropriate airway adjunct. As the patient is examined, evidence that the clinical findings (eg, presence or absence of airway obstruction or respiratory distress, cyanosis) corroborate the pulse oximeter readings should be sought. Specific anesthetic- and surgery-related causes of hypoxemia include airway obstruction; profound hypoventilation or apnea; reduction of functional residual capacity owing to anesthetic or surgical effects; bronchospasm; pneumothorax; pulmonary embolic events; and congestive heart failure resulting from fluid volume overload or the negative inotropic effects of anesthetics. Therapy is directed at the likely cause of hypoxemia.

### What Are Potential Causes of Delayed Emergence?

Delayed emergence may be said to exist whenever it appears that a patient is not awakening or emerging from the effects of administered anesthetics within the anticipated time period. The anesthesiologist who cares for infants and children must be able to assess and manage delayed emergence in an organized fashion. First, the "ABCs" should be checked to ensure that the patient has a patent and stable airway and that there are no significant problems with ventilation or oxygenation as assessed by observation of the patient and the trends of vital sign and monitoring parameters, chiefly the oxyhemoglobin saturation and end-tidal carbon dioxide (if applicable). The fluid and perfusion status of the patient should be reviewed. Second, the anesthesia and PACU records should be reviewed with an eye toward the combination, dosing, and timing of administration of preanesthetic sedatives and intraoperative anesthetics and opioids. Depending on the clinical situation, it may be appropriate to attempt pharmacologic reversal with specific antagonists, including cholinesterase inhibitors for the nondepolarizing muscle relaxants, flumazenil for the benzodiazepines, and naloxone for the opioids. Third, metabolic or electrolyte derangements due to preexisting disease processes or the effects of the surgical procedure should be sought and managed; examples include hypoglycemia and hyponatremia. Fourth, pathologic CNS events such as intracranial hemorrhage or increased intracranial pressure due to some other cause should be excluded.

## What Is Emergence Delirium?

Another relatively common PACU problem in children is severe disorientation or emergence delirium. Preoperative and intraoperative use of anticholinergics (mainly atropine), benzodiazepines, ketamine, and the sole use of the potent inhalation anesthetics are associated with this phenomenon. Although not always easy, emergence delirium must be differentiated from abnormal behavior due to hypoxemia or pain. Paradoxical reaction to midazolam occurs in about 1% of patients and manifests as inconsolable crying, combativeness, disorientation, dysphoria, tachycardia, agitation, and restlessness.[177] Older children have described hallucinations as a part of this symptom complex.

After ensuring that the ABCs are intact and reviewing the anesthetic record and nature of the operative procedure, it is usually prudent to treat the delirious child as if he or she is experiencing pain. If, after applying appropriate analgesics that may include local anesthetics, nonsteroidal nonopioid analgesics, or opioids, the child is still "out-of-sorts," it may be appropriate to attempt to reverse the effects of any previously administered benzodiazepines or anticholinergics. Flumazenil in an initial dose of 0.01 mg/kg may be administered to reverse midazolam and diazepam.[177,178] Although not frequently used, the tertiary amine anticholinesterase physostigmine may also be given in an initial dose of 0.01 mg/kg to treat the central anticholinergic syndrome. In selected cases, it is remarkably effective.

## How Is Postoperative Pain Managed?

Pain is the most common problem seen in any patient population after surgery, although pediatric patients, particularly infants, have historically received fewer analgesics intraoperatively and postoperatively. It is essential that age- and cognitive development–appropriate pain assessment methods be employed and that not all instances of crying and tachycardia be automatically assumed to be secondary to pain.

Pain can be attenuated prophylactically in the operating room with adjunctive regional techniques (caudal, epidural, or intrathecal use of local anesthetics or narcotics, or both) or the parenteral administration of analgesic medications. Acetaminophen administered orally before the procedure in a dose of 10 mg/kg with or without midazolam is useful for brief procedures for which no intravenous line is placed. Alternatively, acetaminophen may be given rectally in a dose of 20 to 30 mg/kg while the patient is anesthetized or soon after entry into the PACU. Ketorolac, a nonsteroidal antiinflammatory drug, is effective in alleviating postsurgical pain by the intravenous (0.5-1 mg/kg, maximum 30 mg) administration of a bolus dose or a continuous infusion of 0.17 mg/kg/h.[179] Ketorolac is generally avoided in cases such as tonsillectomy in which rebleeding is a serious concern. Intravenous morphine (0.025-0.1 mg/kg) or fentanyl (0.5-1 μg/kg) is titrated to effect in ameliorating moderate to severe acute pain. If the patient is to be hospitalized after the surgical procedure, consideration should be given to providing an opioid by means of a patient-controlled analgesia (PCA) device. Ideally, the PCA pump is prepared and available for the patient and parent to use in the PACU before transfer to a ward.

## Why Do Nausea and Vomiting Occur?

PONV occurs commonly in pediatric surgical patients. Certain procedures, such as repair of strabismus, middle and inner ear surgery, and tonsillectomy are associated with a high incidence of nausea and vomiting (approaching 80% of patients) if no antiemetic therapy is provided. Other contributing factors include a longer duration of anesthesia and surgery, a history of motion sickness, and a previous history of PONV. Although nausea or vomiting is not a serious complication in the sense that some other PACU complications are, it may lead to hypovolemia and electrolyte disturbances that necessitate costly hospital admission immediately or several days after outpatient surgery. Nausea and vomiting are among the most distressing and commonly cited complaints in surgical patients.[180]

## How Are Postanesthetic Nausea and Vomiting Managed?

The proper approach to managing PONV begins with anticipating its development and instituting appropriate prophylactic measures in the operating room. Decompression of the stomach with an orogastric tube during surgery and immediately before emergence and extubation relieves gaseous distention and the accumulation of fluids and secretions that can promote nausea and vomiting. Attention should be devoted to ensuring appropriate intravenous fluid replacement intraoperatively. As always, consideration should be given to providing effective relief of pain and anxiety postoperatively because these may be associated with PONV. Clinical data are conflicting as to whether nitrous oxide actually promotes nausea and vomiting, although in practice, many clinicians attempting to reduce PONV to the lowest possible incidence omit its use. Use of propofol is associated with a reduced incidence of nausea and vomiting.[181] In procedures known to be associated with a high risk for PONV, or when opioids have been used, it is appropriate to administer an antiemetic prophylactically.

A large number of antiemetic agents have been employed prophylactically and after the fact in managing PONV. The fact that so many drugs are used implies that there is no panacea, including the serotonin receptor antagonists ondansetron, dolasetron, and gravisetron, that is 100% effective in alleviating this frustrating complication of what is frequently an otherwise perfect anesthetic. In addition to not being uniformly effective, many antiemetics possess significant side effects, including excessive sedation and extrapyramidal reactions. Commonly used medications include metoclopramide (0.1-0.15 mg/kg intravenously),[182] droperidol (25-75 μg/kg intravenously), and the serotonin antagonists ondansetron (0.05-0.1 mg/kg, maximum 4 mg intravenously)[183] and dolasetron (12.5 mg).[184]

### References

1. American Academy of Pediatrics, Section on Anesthesiology. Guidelines for the pediatric perioperative anesthesia environment. *Pediatrics*. 1999;1032:512.

2. Riazi J. The difficult pediatric airway. In: Benumof JL, ed. *Airway Management: Principles and Practice*. St Louis, Mo: CV Mosby; 1996:585.

3. O'Connor ME, Drasner K. Preoperative laboratory testing of children undergoing elective surgery. *Anesth Analg*. 1990;70:176.

4. Hannalah RS. Preoperative investigations. *Paediatr Anaesth*. 1995;5:325.

5. Patel RI, DeWitt L, Hannallah RS. Preoperative laboratory testing in children undergoing elective surgery: analysis of current practice. *J Clin Anesth*. 1997;9:569.

6. Stevens-Simon C, White MM. Adolescent pregnancy. *Pediatr Ann*. 1991;20:322.

7. Malviya S, D'Errico C, Reynolds P, et al. Should pregnancy testing be routine in adolescent patients prior to surgery? *Anesth Analg*. 1996;82:854.

8. Wheeler M, Coté CJ. Preoperative pregnancy testing in a tertiary care children's hospital: a medico-legal conundrum. *J Clin Anesth*. 1999;111:56.

9. Azzam FJ, Padda GS, DeBoard JW, et al. Preoperative pregnancy testing in adolescents. *Anesth Analg*. 1996;82:4.

10. Graff TD, Phillips OC, Benson DW, et al. Baltimore anesthesia study committee: factors in pediatric anesthesia mortality. *Anesth Analg*. 1964;43:407.

11. Olsson GL, Hallen B, Hambraeus-Jonzon K. Aspiration during anesthesia: a computer-aided study of 185,358 anaesthetics. *Acta Anaesthesiol Scand*. 1986;30:84.

12. Tiret L, Nivoche Y, Hatton F, et al. Complications related to anesthesia in infants and children. *Br J Anaesth*. 1988;61:263.

13. Mendelson CL. The aspiration of stomach contents into the lungs during obstetrical anesthesia. *Am J Obstet Gynecol*. 1946;52:191.

14. Teabeault JR. Aspiration of gastric contents: an experimental study. *Am J Pathol*. 1952;28:51.

15. Roberts RB, Shirley MA. Reducing the risk of acid aspiration during Cesarean section. *Anesth Analg*. 1974;53:859.

16. Salem MR, Wong AY, Mani M, et al. Premedicant drugs and gastric juice pH and volume in pediatric patients. *Anesthesiology*. 1976;44:216.

17. Goudsouzian N, Coté CJ, Liu LMP, et al. The dose-response effects of cimetidine on gastric pH and volume in children. *Anesthesiology*. 1981;55:553.

18. Coté CJ, Goudsouzian NG, Liu LMP, et al. Assessment of risk factors related to the acid-aspiration syndrome: gastric pH and residual volume. *Anesthesiology*. 1982;56:70.

19. Manchikanti L, Colliver JA, Marrero TC, et al. Assessment of age-related acid aspiration risk factors in pediatric, adult, and geriatric patients. *Anesth Analg*. 1985;64:11.

20. Meakin G, Dingwall AE, Addison GM. Effects of fasting and oral premedication on the pH and volume of gastric aspirate in children. *Br J Anaesth*. 1987;59:678.

21. Warner MA, Warner ME, Warner DO, et al. Perioperative pulmonary aspiration in infants and children. *Anesthesiology*. 1999;90:66.

22. Schreiner MS. Gastric fluid volume: is it really a risk factor for pulmonary aspiration. *Anesth Analg*. 1998;87:754.

23. Schwartz DL, Connelly NR, Theroux CA, et al. Gastric contents in children presenting for upper endoscopy. *Anesth Analg*. 1998;87:757.

24. Nicolson S, Dorsey A, Schreiner M. Shortened preanesthetic fasting interval in pediatric cardiac surgical patients. *Anesth Analg*. 1992;74:694.

25. Splinter WM, Stewart JA, Muir JG. Large volumes of apple juice preoperatively do not affect gastric pH and volume in children. *Can J Anaesth*. 1990;37:36.

26. Schreiner MS, Triebwasser A, Keon TP. Ingestion of liquids compared with preoperative fasting in pediatric outpatients. *Anesthesiology*. 1990;72:593.

27. Tait AR, Knight PR. The effects of general anesthesia on upper respiratory tract infections in children. *Anesthesiology*. 1987;67:930.

28. Rolf N, Coté CJ. Frequency and severity of desaturation events during general anesthesia in children with and without upper respiratory infections. *J Clin Anesth*. 1992;4:200.

29. Cohen MM, Cameron CB. Should you cancel the operation when a child has an upper respiratory tract infection? *Anesth Analg*. 1991;72:282.

30. Rovenstine EA, Taylor IB. Postoperative respiratory complications: occurrence following 7874 anesthesias. *Am J Med Sci*. 1936;191:807.

31. Olsson GL, Hallen B. Laryngospasm during anesthesia: a computer-aided incidence study in 136,929 patients. *Acta Anaesthesiol Scand*. 1984;28:567.

32. DeSoto H, Patel RI, Soliman IE, et al. Changes in oxygen saturation following general anesthesia in children with upper respiratory infection signs and symptoms undergoing otolaryngological procedures. *Anesthesiology*. 1988;68:276.

33. Collier AM, Pimmel RL, Hasselblad V, et al. Spirometric changes in normal children with upper respiratory infections. *Am Rev Respir Dis*. 1978;117:47.

34. Busse WW. Respiratory infections: their role in airway responsiveness and the pathogenesis of asthma. *J Allergy Clin Immunol*. 1990;85:671.

35. Sly M. Asthma. In: Behrman RE, Kliegman RM, Jenson HB, eds. *Nelson Textbook of Pediatrics*. Philadelphia, Pa: WB Saunders; 2000:664.

36. Takiyawa T, Thurlbeck WM. Muscle and mucous gland size in the major bronchi of patients with chronic bronchitis, asthma, and asthmatic bronchitis. *Am Rev Respir Dis*. 1971;104:331.

37. Woolcock AJ, Read J. Lung volumes in exacerbations of asthma. *Am J Med*. 1966;41:259.

38. Goldberg P, Leffert F, Gonzalez M, et al. Intravenous aminophylline therapy for asthma: a comparison of two methods of administration in children. *Am J Dis Child*. 1980;134:596.

39. Horobin DF, Manku MS, Franks DJ, et al. Methylxanthine phosphodiesterase inhibitors behave as prostaglandin antagonists in a perfused rat mesenteric artery preparation. *Prostaglandins*. 1977;13:33.

40. Wilson JD, Sutherland DC, Thomas AC. Has the change to beta agonist combined with oral theophylline increased cases of fatal asthma? *Lancet*. 1981;1:1235.

41. Burrows FA, Lerman J. Immune and allergic disorders. In: Katz J, Steward DJ, eds. *Anesthesia and Uncommon Pediatric Diseases*. Philadelphia, Pa: WB Saunders; 1987:429.

42. Wilson DF. Asthma. In: Berry FA, eds. *Anesthetic Management of Difficult and Routine Pediatric Patients*. New York, NY: Churchill Livingstone; 1990:285.

43. Hirshman CA, Edelstein RA, Ebertz JM, et al. Thiobarbiturate-induced histamine release in human skin mast cells. *Anesthesiology*. 1985;63:353.

44. Hirshman CA, Edelstein G, Peetz S, et al. Mechanism of action of inhalational anesthesia on airways. *Anesthesiology*. 1982;56:107.

45. Munson ES, Tucker WK. Doses of epinephrine causing arrhythmias during enflurane, methoxyflurane, and halothane anesthesia in dogs. *Can Anaesth Soc J*. 1975;22:495.

46. Downes H, Gerber N, Hirshman CA. IV lignocaine in reflex and allergic bronchoconstriction. *Br J Anaesth*. 1980;52:873.

47. Schwartz AJ, Campbell FW. Pathophysiological approach to congenital heart disease. In: Lake CL, ed. *Pediatric Cardiac Anesthesia*. Norwalk, Conn: Appleton & Lange; 1988:9.

48. Brandom BW, Gronert GA. Malignant hyperthermia. In: Motoyama EK, Davis PJ, eds. *Smith's Anesthesia for Infants and Children*. St Louis, Mo: CV Mosby; 1996:809.

49. Britt BA, Kwong IHF, Endrenyi L, et al, eds. *Malignant Hyperthermia: Current Concepts*. New York, NY: Appleon-Century-Crofts; 1979.

50. Levitt RC. Prospects for the diagnosis of malignant hyperthermia susceptibility using molecular genetic approaches. *Anesthesiology*. 1992;76:1039.

51. Olgin J, Argor Z, Rosenberg H, et al. Non-invasive evaluation of malignant hyperthermia susceptibility with phosphorus nuclear magnetic resonance spectroscopy. *Anesthesiology*. 1988;68:507.

52. Verburg MP, DeGrood PM. Safety of propofol in malignant hyperthermia (preliminary results). *Anesthesia*. 1988;43(suppl):121.

53. Beebe JJ, Sessler DI. Preparation of anesthesia machines for patients susceptible to malignant hyperthermia. *Anesthesiology*. 1988;69:395.

54. McGraw TT, Keon TP. Malignant hyperthermia and the clean machine. *Can Anaesth Soc J*. 1989;36:530.

55. Morgan KG, Bryant SH. The mechanism of action of dantrolene sodium. *J Pharmacol Exp Ther*. 1977;201:138.

56. Task Force on Latex Sensitivity of the ASA Committee on Occupational Health of Operating Room Personnel. *Natural Rubber Latex Allergy: Considerations for Anesthesiologists*. Park Ridge, Ill: American Society of Anesthesiologists; 1999:1.

57. Slater J. Rubber anaphylaxis. *N Engl J Med*. 1989;320:1126.

58. Leynadier F, Pecquet C, Dry J. Anaphylaxis to latex during surgery. *Anaesthesia*. 1989;44:547.

59. Gerber A, Jorg W, Zbinden S, et al. Severe intraoperative anaphylaxis to surgical gloves: latex allergy, an unfamiliar condition. *Anesthesiology*. 1989;71:800.

60. Hirshman CA. Latex anaphylaxis [editorial]. *Anesthesiology*. 1992;77:223.

61. Holzman RS. Latex allergy: an emerging operating room problem. *Anesth Analg*. 1993;76:635.

62. Beers MA, Berkow R, eds. *The Merck Manual of Diagnosis and Therapy.* Whitehouse Station, NJ: Merck Research Laboratories; 1999.

63. Sussman G, Tarlo S, Dolovitch J. The spectrum of IgE-mediated responses to latex. *JAMA.* 1991;265:2844.

64. Charous B, Hamilton R, Yungiger J. Occupational latex exposure: characteristics of contact and systemic reactions in 47 workers. *J Allergy Clin Immunol.* 1994;84:12.

65. Porri F, Pradal M, Lemiere C, et al. Association between latex sensitization and repeated latex exposure in children. *Anesthesiology.* 1997;86:599.

66. DHHS (NIOSH) Publication No. 97-135. NIOSH Alert: preventing allergic reactions to natural rubber latex in the workplace. US Department of Health and Human Services; 1997. Available at: http://www.cdc.gov/niosh/latexalt.html. Accessed March 2001.

67. Yunginger JW, Jones RT, Fransway AF, et al. Extractable latex allergens and proteins in disposable medical gloves and other rubber products. *J Allergy Clin Immunol.* 1994;93:836.

68. Food and Drug Administration. FDA medical alert: allergic reactions to latex-containing medical devices. Rockville, Md: Food and Drug Administration; 1991.

69. Lasser EC, Berry CC, Talner LB, et al. Pretreatment with corticosteroids to alleviate reactions to intravenous contrast materials. *N Engl J Med.* 1987;317:845.

70. Holzman R. Clinical management of latex-allergic children. *Anesth Analg.* 1997;85:529.

71. Henderson JM, Brodsky DA, Fisher DM, et al. Preinduction of anesthesia in pediatric patients with nasally administered sufentanil. *Anesthesiology.* 1988;68:671.

72. Zimmerman G, Steward DJ. Bradycardia delays the onset of action of intravenous atropine in infants. *Anesthesiology.* 1986;65:320.

73. Stoelting RK. Anticholinergic drugs. In: Stoelting RK, eds. *Pharmacology and Physiology in Anesthetic Practice.* Philadelphia, Pa: JB Lippincott; 1987:232.

74. Rita L, Seleny FL, Mazurek A, et al. Intramuscular midazolam for pediatric preanesthetic sedation: a double-blind controlled study with morphine. *Anesthesiology.* 1985;63:528.

75. Greenberg R, Maxwell L, Zahural M, et al. Preanesthetic medication of children with midazolam using the biojector jet injector. *Anesthesiology.* 1995;83:264.

76. Polillo AM, Kiley J. Does a needleless injection system reduce anxiety in children receiving intramuscular injections? *Pediatr Nurs.* 1997;231:47.

77. Cook DR, Davis PJ, Lerman J. Pharmacology of pediatric anesthesia. In: Motoyama EK, Davis PJ, eds. *Smith's Anesthesia for Infants and Children.* St Louis, Mo: CV Mosby; 1996:159.

78. Kain ZN, Mayes L, Wang SM, et al. Postoperative behavioral outcomes in children. *Anesthesiology.* 1999;90:758.

79. Holm-Knudsen R, Carlin J, Mckenzie I. Distress at induction of anesthesia in children: a survey of incidence, associated factors and recovery characteristics. *Paediatr Anaesth.* 1998;8:383.

80. Mcgraw T, Kendrisk A. Oral midazolam premedication and postoperative behavior in children. *Paediatr Anaesth.* 1998;8:117.

81. Spahr-Schopfer IA, McMillan C, Sikich N, et al. Safety of oral midazolam premedication for use in children [abstract]. *Anesthesiology.* 1991;75:A921.

82. Feld LH, Negus JB, White PF. Oral midazolam preanesthetic medication in pediatric outpatients. *Anesthesiology.* 1990;73:831.

83. Delaunay L, Murat I, Rey E, et al. Pharmacokinetics of intranasal and intravenous midazolam in young children [abstract]. *Anesthesiology.* 1991;75:A923.

84. Karl HW, Keifer AT, Rosenberger JL, et al. Comparison of the safety and efficacy of intranasal midazolam or sufentanil for preinduction of anesthesia in pediatric patients. *Anesthesiology.* 1992;76:209.

85. Spear RM, Yaster M, Berkowitz ID, et al. Preinduction of anesthesia in children with rectally administered midazolam. *Anesthesiology.* 1991;74:670.

86. Conard PL, Rosenblum M, Weisman SJ, et al. Safety and efficacy of oral transmucosal fentanyl citrate (OTFC) for procedures in children [abstract]. *Anesthesiology.* 1991;75:A954.

87. Henderson IM, Spence DG, Clarke WN, et al. Sodium citrate in pediatric outpatients. *Can J Anaesth.* 1987;34:560.

88. Salem MR, Wong AY, Collins VJ. The pediatric patient with a full stomach. *Anesthesiology.* 1973;39:435.

89. Sandhar BK, Goresky GV, Maltby JR, et al. Effect of oral liquids and ranitidine on gastric fluid volume and pH in children undergoing outpatient surgery. *Anesthesiology.* 1989;71:327.

90. Food and Drug Administration. Anesthesia apparatus checkout recommendations, 1993. Available at: http://www.fda.gov/cdrh/humfac/ancsckot/html. Accessed March 2001.

91. Koka BV, Jeon IS, Andre JM, et al. Postintubation croup in children. *Anesth Analg.* 1977;56:501.

92. Finholt DA, Henry DB, Raphaely RC. Factors affecting leak around endotracheal tubes in children. *Can Anaesth Soc J.* 1985;32:326.

93. Vernon D, Schulman J, Foley JM. Changes in children's behavior after hospitalization. *Am J Dis Child.* 1966;111:581.

94. Schulman J, Foley JM, Vernon D, et al. A study of the effect of the mother's presence during anesthesia induction. *Pediatrics.* 1967;39:111.

95. Hannallah RS, Rosales JK. Experience with parents' presence during anesthesia induction in children. *Can Anaesth Soc J.* 1983;30:286.

96. Kain ZN, Mayes LC, Wang SM, et al. Parental presence during induction of anesthesia versus sedative premedication: which intervention is more effective? *Anesthesiology.* 1998;89:1147.

97. Gillerman RG, Hinkle AJ, Green HM, et al. Parental presence plus oral midazolam decreases frequency of 5% halothane inductions in children. *J Clin Anesth.* 1996;8:480.

98. Kain ZN, Mayes LC, Caramico LA, et al. Parental presence during induction of anesthesia: a randomized controlled trial. *Anesthesiology.* 1996;85:1212.

99. Honig J, Maguire E, Hannallah RS. Parents' response to observing anesthesia induction in their children [abstract]. *Anesthesiology.* 1991;75:A1051.

100. Tait AR, Pandit UA, Voepel-Lewis T, et al. Use of the laryngeal mask airway in children with upper respiratory tract infections: a comparison with endotracheal intubation. *Anesth Analg.* 1998;86:706.

101. Brimacombe JR, Brain AIJ, Berry AM. *The Laryngeal Mask Airway: A Review and Practical Guide.* London, United Kingdom: WB Saunders; 1997.

102. Johnston DF, Wrigley SR, Robb PJ, et al. The laryngeal mask airway in paediatric anaesthesia. *Anaesthesia.* 1990;45:924.

103. Lopez-Gil M, Brimacombe J, Cebrian J, et al. The laryngeal mask airway in pediatric practice: a prospective study of skill acquisition by resident anesthesiologists. *Anesthesiology.* 1996;84:807.

104. Epstein RH, Ferouz F, Jenkins MA. Airway sealing pressures of the laryngeal mask airway in pediatric patients. *J Clin Anesth.* 1996;8:93.

105. Barnes SD. Emergent intubation of the difficult pediatric airway using the laryngeal mask airway. *Am J Crit Care.* 1996;55:376.

106. Brimacombe JR, Berry AM. The laryngeal mask airway: a consideration for the NRP guidelines? *Can J Anaesth.* 1995;42:88.

107. Goudsouzian NG, Alifimoff JK, Eberly C, et al. Neuromuscular and cardiovascular effects of mivacurium in children. *Anesthesiology.* 1989;70:237.

108. Berthelsen P, Prytz S, Jacobsen E. Two-stage fiberoptic nasotracheal intubation in infants: a new approach to difficult pediatric intubation. *Anesthesiology.* 1985;63:457.

109. Maekawa N, Mikawa K, Obara H. The laryngeal mask may be a useful device for fiberoptic airway endoscopy in pediatric anesthesia. *Anesthesiology.* 1991;75:169.

110. Holzman RS, Nargozian CD, Florence FB. Lightwand intubation in children with abnormal upper airways. *Anesthesiology.* 1988;69:784.

111. Rehman MA, Schreiner MS. Oral and nasotracheal light wand guided intubation after failed fiberoptic bronchoscopy. *Paediatr Anaesth.* 1997;7:349.

112. Borland LM, Casselbrand M. The Bullard laryngoscope: a new indirect oral laryngoscope (pediatric version). *Anesth Analg.* 1990;70:105.

113. Audenaert SM, Montgomery CL, Stone B, et al. Retrograde-assisted fiberoptic tracheal intubation in children with difficult airways. *Anesth Analg.* 1990;73:660.

114. Sellick BA. Cricoid pressure to control regurgitation of stomach contents during induction of anesthesia. *Lancet.* 1961;1961:2:404.

115. Salem MR, Wong AY, Fizzolti GF. Efficacy of cricoid pressure in preventing aspiration of gastric contents in pediatric patients. *Br J Anaesth.* 1972;44:401.

116. Gregory GA. Induction of anesthesia. In: Gregory GA, eds. *Pediatric Anesthesia.* New York, NY: Churchill Livingstone; 1989:539.

117. Liu LMP, Ryan JF. Modified single breath induction of anesthesia in children with and without nitrous oxide [abstract]. *Anesthesiology.* 1989;71:A1008.

118. Alexander GD, Skupski JN, Brown EM. The role of nitrous oxide in postoperative nausea and vomiting. *Anesth Analg.* 1984;63:175.

119. Epstein RH, Stein AL, Marr AT, et al. High concentrations versus incremental induction of anesthesia with sevoflurane in children: a comparison of induction times, vital signs, and complications. *J Clin Anesth.* 1998;10:41.

120. Brett CM, Fisher DM. Thiopental dose-response relations in unpremedicated infants, children, and adults. *Anesth Analg.* 1987;66:1024.

121. Liu LMP, Coté CJ, Goudsouzian NG, et al. Response to intravenous induction doses of methohexital in children. *Anesthesiology.* 1981;55:A330.

122. Hannallah RS, Baker SB, Casey W, et al. Propofol: effective dose and induction characteristics in unpremedicated children. *Anesthesiology.* 1991;74:217.

123. Sevel PS, Lowdon JS. Propofol: a new intravenous anesthetic. *Anesthesiology.* 1989;71:260.

124. Varner PD, Ebert JP, McKay RD, et al. Methohexital sedation of children undergoing CT scan. *Anesth Analg.* 1985;64:643.

125. Bain JA, Spoerel WE. A streamlined anesthetic system. *Can Anaesth Soc J.* 1972;19:426.

126. Miller DM. Breathing systems for use in anesthesia: evaluation using a physical lung model and classification. *Br J Anaesth.* 1988;60:555.

127. Lerman J, Robinson S, Willis MM, et al. Anesthetic requirements for halothane in young children 0-1 and 1-6 months of age. *Anesthesiology.* 1983;59:421.

128. Cohen IT, Motoyama EK. Intraoperative and postoperative management. In: Motoyama EK, Davis PJ, eds. *Smith's Anesthesia for Infants and Children.* St Louis, Mo: Mosby–Year Book; 1996:313.

129. Murray D, Vandewalker G, Metherne GP, et al. Pulsed Doppler and two-dimensional echocardiography: comparison of halothane and isoflurane on cardiac function in infants and small children. *Anesthesiology.* 1987;67:211.

130. Sarner JB, Levine M, Davis PJ, et al. Clinical characteristics of sevoflurane in children: a comparison with halothane. *Anesthesiology.* 1995;82:38.

131. Wren WS, McShane AJ, McCarthy JG, et al. Isoflurane in pediatric anesthesia: induction and recovery from anesthesia. *Anaesthesia.* 1985;40:315.

132. Davis PJ, Cook DR, Stiller RL, et al. Pharmacodynamics and pharmacokinetics of high-dose sufentanil in infants and children undergoing cardiac surgery. *Anesth Analg.* 1987;66:203.

133. Robinson DN, O'Brien K, Kumar R, et al. Tracheal intubation without neuromuscular blockade in children: a comparison of propofol combined either with alfentanil or remifentanil. *Paediatr Anaesth.* 1998;8:467.

134. Morton NS. Total intravenous anesthesia (TIVA) in paediatrics: advantages and disadvantages. *Paediatr Anaesth.* 1999;93:279.

135. Davis PJ, Lerman J, Suresh S, et al. A randomized multicenter study of remifentanil compared with alfentanil, isoflurane, or propofol in anesthetized pediatric patients undergoing elective strabismus surgery. *Anesth Analg.* 1997;84:982.

136. Glass PSA, Gan TJ, Howell S. A review of the pharmacokinetics and pharmacodynamics of remifentanil. *Anesth Analg.* 1999;894S:S7.

137. Goudsouzian NG. Neuromuscular blocking agents in children. *Paediatr Anaesth.* 1991;1:75.

138. Goudsouzian NG. The infant and the myoneural junction. *Anesth Analg.* 1986;65:1208.

139. Waud BE, Waud DR. The relation between the response to "train-of-four" stimulation and receptor occlusion during competitive neuromuscular block. *Anesthesiology.* 1972;37:413.

140. Mason LJ, Betts EK. Leg lift and maximum inspiratory force: clinical signs of neuromuscular blockade reversal in neonates and infants. *Anesthesiology.* 1980;52:441.

141. Liu LMP, DeCook TH, Gousouzian NG, et al. Dose response to intramuscular succinylcholine in children. *Anesthesiology.* 1981;55:599.

142. Reynolds LM, Infosino A, Brown R, et al. Intramuscular rapacuronium in infants and children: dose-ranging and tracheal intubating conditions. *Anesthesiology.* 1999;91:1285.

143. Morton NS, Johnston G, White M, et al. Propofol in paediatric anaesthesia. *Paediatr Anaesth.* 1992;2:89.

144. Borgeat A, Popovic V, Meier D, et al. Comparison of propofol and thiopental/halothane for short-duration ENT surgical procedures in children. *Anesth Analg.* 1990;71:511.

145. Glaeseer PW, Losek JD. Emergency intraosseous infusions in children. *Am J Emerg Med.* 1986;4:36.

146. Rosetti VA, Thompson BM, Miller J, et al. An alternative route of pediatric intravascular access. *Ann Emerg Med.* 1985;14:885.

147. Lindahl SGE. Energy expenditure and fluid and electrolyte requirements in anesthetized infants and children. *Anesthesiology.* 1988;69:377.

148. Hongnat JM, Murat I, St Maurice C. Evaluation of current paediatric guidelines for fluid therapy using two different dextrose hydrating solutions. *Paediatr Anaesth.* 1991;1:95.

149. Sieber FE, Smith DS, Traystman RJ, et al. Glucose: a reevaluation of its intraoperative use. *Anesthesiology.* 1987;67:72.

150. Lanier WL, Stangland KJ, Scheithauer BW, et al. The effects of dextrose infusion and head position on neurologic outcome after complete cerebral ischemia in primates: examination of a model. *Anesthesiology.* 1987;66:39.

151. Welborn LG, Hannallah RS, McGill WA, et al. Glucose concentrations for routine intravenous infusion in pediatric outpatient surgery. *Anesthesiology.* 1987;67:427.

152. DuBois MC, Gouyet L, Murat I, et al. Lactated Ringer's with 1% dextrose: an appropriate solution for perioperative fluid therapy in children. *Paediatr Anaesth.* 1992;2:99.

153. Welborn LG, McGill WA, Hannallah RS, et al. Perioperative blood glucose concentrations in pediatric outpatients. *Anesthesiology.* 1986;65:543.

154. Furman EB, Roman GD, Lemmer LAS, et al. Specific therapy in water, electrolyte, and blood-volume replacement during pediatric surgery. *Anesthesiology.* 1975;42:187.

155. Ward JW, Holmberg SD, Allen JR, et al. Transmission of human immunodeficiency virus (HIV) by blood transfusion screened as negative for HIV antibody. *N Engl J Med.* 1988;318:473.

156. Brodsky JB. What intraoperative monitoring makes sense? *Chest.* 1999;1155:101S.

157. American Society of Anesthesiologists. Standards for basic intraoperative monitoring. In: *Directory of Members.* Park Ridge, Ill: American Society of Anesthesiologists; 2000:477.

158. Coté CJ, Goldstein EA, Coté MA. A single-blind study of pulse oximetry in children. *Anesthesiology.* 1988;68:184.

159. Coté CJ, Rolf N, Liu LMP, et al. A single-blind study of combined pulse oximetry and capnography in children. *Anesthesiology.* 1991;74:980.

160. Karl HW, Swedlow DB, Lee KW, et al. Epinephrine-halothane interactions in children. *Anesthesiology.* 1983;58:142.

161. Payen D, Ecoffey C, Carli C, et al. Pulsed Doppler ascending aortic, carotid, brachial, and femoral artery blood flows during caudal anesthesia in infants. *Anesthesiology.* 1987;67:681.

162. Desparmet J, Mateo J, Ecoffey C, et al. Efficacy of an epidural test dose in children anesthetized with halothane. *Anesthesiology.* 1990;72:249.

163. Brendel JK, Yemen TA, Berry FA. Intravenous injection of local anesthetic: identification with isoproterenol and epinephrine in children during halothane anesthesia. *Reg Anesth.* 1993;18:49.

164. Fried EB, Bailey AG, Valley RD. Electrocardiographic and hemodynamic changes associated with unintentional intravascular injection of bupivacaine with epinephrine in infants. *Anesthesiology.* 1993;79:394.

165. Yaster M, Maxwell LG. Pediatric regional anesthesia. *Anesthesiology.* 1989;65:590.

166. Attis J, Ecoffey C, Sandouk P, et al. Epidural morphine in children: pharmacokinetics and $CO_2$ sensitivity. *Anesthesiology.* 1986;65:590.

167. DaConceicao MJ, Cohelo L, Khalil M. Ropivacaine 0.25% compared with bupivacaine 0.25% by the caudal route. *Paediatr Anaesth.* 1999;9:229.

168. Bosenberg AT, Ivani G. Regional anaesthesia: children are different [editorial]. *Paediatr Anaesth.* 1998;8:447.

169. Murat I, Walker J, Esteve C, et al. Effect of lumbar epidural anesthesia on plasma cortisol levels in children. *Can J Anaesth.* 1988;35:20.

170. Berde C. Toxicity of local anesthetics in infants and children. *J Pediatr.* 1993;1225:S14.

171. Berde C. Convulsions associated with pediatric regional anesthesia. *Anesth Analg.* 1992;75:164.

172. Abajian CJ, Mellish RWP, Browne AF, et al. Spinal anesthesia for surgery in the high-risk infant. *Anesth Analg.* 1984;63:359.

173. Sartorelli KH, Abajian JC, Kreutz JM, et al. Improved outcome utilizing spinal anesthesia in high-risk infants. *J Pediatr Surg.* 1992;278:1022.

174. Welborn LG, Broadman LM, Rice LJ, et al. Postoperative apnea in former preterm infants: prospective comparison of spinal and general anesthesia. *Anesthesiology.* 1990;72:838.

175. Rice JL. Regional anesthesia and analgesia. In: Motoyama EK, Davis PJ, eds. *Smith's Anesthesia for Infants and Children.* St Louis, Mo: CV Mosby; 1996:403.

176. Kuusela A, Vesikari T. A randomized double-blind, placebo-controlled trial of dexamethasone and racemic epinephrine in the treatment of croup. *Acta Paediatr Scand.* 1988;77:99.

177. Massanari M, Novitsky J, Reinstein LJ. Paradoxical reactions in children associated with midazolam use during endoscopy. *Clin Pediatr.* 1997;3612:681.

178. Thakker P, Gallagher TM. Flumazenil reverses paradoxical reaction to midazolam in a child. *Anaesth Intensive Care.* 1996;244:505.

179. Forrest JB, Heitlinger EL, Revell S. Ketorolac for postoperative pain management in children. *Drug Saf*. 1997;165:309.

180. Watcha MF, White PF. Postoperative nausea and vomiting: its etiology, treatment, and prevention. *Anesthesiology*. 1992;77:162.

181. Martin TM, Nicholson SC, Bargas MS. Propofol anesthesia reduces emesis and airway obstruction in pediatric outpatients. *Anesth Analg*. 1993;76:144.

182. Ferrari LD, Donlon JV. Metoclopramide reduces the incidence of nausea and vomiting after tonsillectomy in children. *Anesth Analg*. 1992;75:351.

183. Watcha MF, Bras PJ, Cieslak GD, et al. The dose-response relationship of ondansetron in preventing postoperative emesis in pediatric patients undergoing ambulatory surgery. *Anesthesiology*. 1995;82:47.

184. Kovac AL, Scuderi PE, Boerner TF, et al. Treatment of postoperative nausea and vomiting with single intravenous doses of dolasetron mesylate: a multicenter trial. *Anesth Analg*. 1997;85:546.

CHAPTER

58

# The Geriatric Patient

Ray Roy

## DEMOGRAPHICS

*What Is Geriatric Anesthesia?*

*What Is the Difference Between Life Expectancy and Life Span?*

*What Percentage of Elderly Will Become Surgical Patients?*

## MORBIDITY AND MORTALITY

*Does Advancing Age Affect the American Society of Anesthesiologists Physical Status?*

*What Is the Effect of Advanced Age on Perioperative Morbidity and Mortality?*

*What Are Perioperative Mortality and Morbidity Rates for Elderly Patients?*

*When Do Anesthesia-Related Complications Occur?*

*When Do Perioperative Myocardial Infarctions Occur?*

## CARDIOVASCULAR SYSTEM

*Should All Elderly Patients Receive β-Adrenergic Receptor Blocking Agents Perioperatively?*

*Should All Elderly Patients Receive α2-Agonists Perioperatively?*

*What Are the Definitions of Intraoperative Hypotension and Hypertension?*

*What Is the Significance of New T-Wave Inversions Following Anesthesia?*

*Do Patients With Bundle Branch Blocks Require Preoperative Prophylactic Placement of Pacemakers?*

*Does Prophylactic Percutaneous Transluminal Coronary Angioplasty Reduce the Incidence of Adverse Cardiac Outcomes After Noncardiac Surgery?*

## AIRWAY AND PULMONARY SYSTEM

*Should Elderly Smokers Be Permitted to Smoke Preoperatively?*

*Does Airway Obstruction Determined by Preoperative Spirometry Predict Perioperative Complications in Smokers?*

*What Is the Best Way to Preoxygenate Elderly Patients?*

*Are Elderly Patients More Likely to Be Difficult to Ventilate by Mask?*

*Does a Laryngeal Mask Airway Cause Less Airway Irritation Than an Endotracheal Tube?*

*What Percentage of Oxygen Should Be Administered to Elderly Patients Intraoperatively?*

*Should Elderly Patients Automatically Receive Supplemental Oxygen in the Postoperative Period After Major Surgery, Even If $SpO_2$ Is >95%?*

## INHALATIONAL AGENTS

*What Is the Effect of Advancing Age on Inhalational Anesthesia Endpoints?*

*Does End-Tidal Gas Concentration Accurately Reflect Brain Concentration of Inhalational Agents?*

*Do Electroencephalographic Markers of Anesthetic Endpoints Need to Be Adjusted for Age?*

*Are Mask Inductions Easier in Older Patients Than in Younger Ones?*

*Does Changing From Isoflurane to Desflurane Near the End of the Procedure Accelerate Recovery?*

*Does Spinal or Epidural Anesthesia Reduce Minimum Alveolar Concentration and MACawake of Potent Inhalational Agents?*

*Do Inhalational Agents Affect How Hypovolemia Manifests Itself in Elderly Patients?*

*What Is the Role of Nitrous Oxide?*

## INTRAVENOUS AGENTS

*How Does Advancing Age Affect Doses of Intravenous Agents?*

*What Is the Optimum Duration of Injection for Propofol?*

## SEDATIVES

*Does Sedation Affect Hypoxic Control of Cardiorespiratory Responses?*

*Is There a Sedative That Does Not Potentiate the Effects of Intravenous Opioids?*

*Does Spinal or Epidural Anesthesia Increase Sensitivity to Intravenous Sedation?*

## NEUROMUSCULAR BLOCKING AGENTS

*Does Advancing Age Change the Onset Time for Neuromuscular Blocking Agents?*

*What Is the Effect of Advancing Age on the Duration of Action of Neuromuscular Blocking Agents?*

*Should Long-Acting Neuromuscular Blocking Agents Be Administered to Elderly Patients Whose Tracheas Are to Be Extubated at the End of the Surgical Procedure?*

## POSTOPERATIVE ANALGESIA

*Does Regional Analgesia Affect Outcome?*

REGIONAL VERSUS GENERAL ANESTHESIA

*Are There Theoretical Reasons to Prefer Regional Anesthesia?*

*Is Regional Anesthesia Safer Than General Anesthesia?*

*Is There a Difference Between Regional and General Anesthesia?*

GUIDING PRINCIPLES

*How Do You Approach Patients With the Choice Between Regional and General Anesthesia?*

*What Are the Ten Commandments for Anesthetizing Elderly Patients?*

## DEMOGRAPHICS

### What Is Geriatric Anesthesia?

*Geriatrics* may be defined as the health and social care of the *elderly,* who are traditionally defined by demographers, insurers, and employers as individuals over the age of 65 years. *Geriatric medicine* is the subdiscipline within geriatrics that is devoted to the medical care of the elderly. Geriatric medicine is recognized as a distinct specialty, and 75 years is often used as the defining age. Although *geriatric anesthesia* is the term generally applied to the perioperative medical care of older surgical patients, Muravchick coined *geroanesthesia* as a synonym.[1] Three texts devoted to geriatric anesthesia that cover information not found in this chapter are recommended to the reader.[1-3]

Anesthesiologists tend to have two extreme views of older patients. The optimistic "cup-is-more-than-half-full" lens is the one through which Roizen peers in his bestseller, *Real-Age.*[4] He describes lifestyle changes that aging anesthesiologists can make to delay the onset and lessen the impact of chronic disease and, in so doing, maximize their own life expectancy and quality of life.

The pessimistic "cup-is-less-than-half-empty" lens is the one through which most anesthesiologists see their elderly patients. Although this chapter concentrates more on age-related changes than on the consequences of chronic disease, the two areas are intertwined and clinically less important for the clinician to separate when actually administering anesthesia.

In "younger" elderly patients, chronic disease is a stronger factor than the natural aging process when it comes to the erosion of organ reserve. This chapter asks questions addressed in articles that have appeared in the anesthesia literature since 1997 and are pertinent to the care of the reasonably healthy geriatric patient.

### What Is the Difference Between Life Expectancy and Life Span?

On longevity:

*I enjoy it because I have my health and I can do things.*
*—SARAH KNAUSS*[5]

Sarah Knauss made the above comment when she was interviewed at age 115 years. According to the 1999 *Guinness Book of Records,* the oldest authenticated age for a woman is 122 years and 164 days, and the oldest authenticated age for a man is 120 years and 237 days.[6] Until recently the oldest person to undergo major surgery was 111 years and 105 days.[6] A woman from the United Kingdom holds the current record. Her fractured right femoral shaft was repaired when she was 113 years old. General anesthesia was administered. She was discharged from the hospital on postoperative day (POD) 23, lived an additional 9 months, and celebrated her 114th birthday.[7]

But life span is not defined as the longest age anyone has ever attained. Rather, it is the average age of all those who died of natural causes, that is, death in the absence of disease and trauma. *Life expectancy* at birth is defined as the average age that members of a population are expected to attain when premature causes of death are taken into account. In 1980, Fries suggested that human life span was approximately 85 years. He proposed that the "ideal" human mortality curve, a plot of the number of patients dying versus their age at death, described a normal distribution centered at 85 years, with an SD of 4 years.[8] He hypothesized that if all premature causes of death could be eliminated, 95% of all mortality would be compressed between 2 SD of 85 years, which was thought to be the average life span. The age range for natural death would be between 77 and 93 years. Health care planning based on this optimistic preventive health care model predicts fewer elderly individuals presenting for surgery. However, newer data suggest that life span may be longer than 85 years, perhaps as old as 100 years. Also, the rate at which life expectancy in the United States is approaching life span is slowing down. The most current life expectancy data for men and women in the United States are presented in Table 58–1.[9] Thus, morbidity and mortality, instead of being compressed within fewer years, now appear to be distributed over an increased number of years. Health care planning based on this model predicts more infirm elderly presenting for surgery. Elective surgery in this population, such as total hip and knee replacements, has the potential to actually improve longevity by improving physical function and independence.[10]

### What Percentage of Elderly Will Become Surgical Patients?

By 2010, the number of people aged 65 years or older is projected to exceed one fifth (20%) of the population in Japan, Italy, Germany, Greece, Belgium, Spain, the United Kingdom, France, the Netherlands, and the Czech Republic. The number will exceed 15% in Australia, Canada, the United States,

**TABLE 58–1.** Life Expectancy at Birth in the United States in 1997

|  | Age (y) |
|---|---|
| **Women** | |
| White | 79.9 |
| Black | 74.7 |
| **Men** | |
| White | 74.3 |
| Black | 67.2 |

From Centers for Disease Control and Prevention. Mortality patterns—United States, 1997. *MMWR.* 1999;48:664.

**TABLE 58–2.** Age-Related Annual Rate (per 100 Population) of Anesthetic Administrations in France in 1996*

| Ages (y) | Male | Female |
|---|---|---|
| 35-44 | 8.9 | 13.2 |
| 55-64 | 17.7 | 14.6 |
| 75-84 | 30.2 | 23.5 |

*Anesthetics include general anesthesia or intravenous sedation (77%), regional anesthesia with and without intravenous sedation (21%), and combined regional plus general anesthesia (2%) for surgery, endoscopy, and radiology or other diagnostic or therapeutic nonsurgical procedures.

Adapted from Clergue F, Auroy Y, Pequignot F, et al. French survey of anesthesia in 1996. *Anesthesiology.* 1999;91:1509.

**TABLE 58–4.** Age Distribution of Surgical Procedures in France in 1996

| Specialty | Percentage Within Age Range (y) | | | |
|---|---|---|---|---|
| | *15-54* | *55-74* | *75-84* | *>84* |
| Orthopedics | 29.1 | 26.3 | 23.9 | 35.8 |
| Ophthalmology | 2.1 | 12.8 | 29.8 | 27.5 |
| General Surgery (GI) | 11.8 | 15.9 | 13.4 | 12.6 |
| Urology | 4.0 | 11.5 | 10.9 | 7.6 |
| Vascular | 4.4 | 7.6 | 5.3 | 4.1 |
| Gynecology | 17.0 | 6.2 | 3.0 | 2.0 |

GI, gastrointestinal.

Adapted from Clergue F, Auroy Y, Pequignot F, et al. French survey of anesthesia in 1996. *Anesthesiology.* 1999;91:1509.

Poland, Russia, Argentina, and Taiwan. It will exceed 10% in South Korea, Chile, Thailand, China, Turkey, Brazil, Venezuela, Peru, South Africa, Colombia, Mexico, India, and Malaysia.[11]

When the 1980 and 1996 data were compared in France,[12] the annual rate of procedures requiring anesthesia increased from 6.6 to 13.5 per 100 global population. For men aged 75 to 84 years, the 1996 rate was 30.2 per 100 population. The rates for specific age groups are presented in Table 58–2. In 1996, one third of all procedures were performed on patients older than 60 years and 3% on patients older than 84 years. For patients over 60 years of age, the increase in the number of procedures was 196% from 1980 to 1996. As expected with advancing age, there was a progressive decrease in the percentage of patients who were American Society of Anesthesiologists (ASA) physical status (PS) I and a progressive increase in the percentage who were ASA PS II through IV (Table 58–3). Orthopedic, ophthalmologic, gastrointestinal, and urologic surgery accounted for 75% to 85% of all procedures on patients 75 years of age and older (Table 58–4).

## MORBIDITY AND MORTALITY

### Does Advancing Age Affect the American Society of Anesthesiologists Physical Status?

The ASA PS traditionally has been viewed as independent of age. However, if chronic disease reduces organ reserve enough to raise PS, then it stands to reason that aging, even in the absence of disease, will, by itself, eventually also reduce organ reserve sufficiently to be associated with a higher PS. I

**TABLE 58–3.** Distribution of American Society of Anesthesiologists Physical Status of Patients Requiring Surgery in France in 1996

| Ages (y) | ASA PS (%) | | | |
|---|---|---|---|---|
| | *1* | *2* | *3* | *4 + 5* |
| 35-44 | 77 | 18 | 4 | 1 |
| 45-54 | 62 | 30 | 7 | 1 |
| 55-64 | 40 | 44 | 14 | 2 |
| 65-74 | 22 | 53 | 22 | 3 |
| 75-84 | 12 | 54 | 30 | 4 |
| >84 | 5 | 45 | 42 | 8 |

ASA, American Society of Anesthesiologists; PS, physical status.

Data from Clergue F, Auroy Y, Pequignot F, et al. French survey of anesthesia in 1996. *Anesthesiology.* 1999;91:1509.

propose that those people who live long enough to enter the age distribution associated with natural death should have an increased PS, even if they have been fortunate enough to avoid significant chronic disease. White women in the United States aged 80 years and older and white men aged 75 years and older—those whose ages now are greater than the life expectancy at birth for their gender (see Table 58–1)—perhaps should be classified as PS III, regardless of their apparent health. Any patient age 85 years and older—that is, older than the life span initially accepted by Fries[8]—perhaps should be classified as PS IV. Many of these patients maintain homeostasis well and appear very fit, but all have organ reserve sufficiently reduced to make restoration of homeostasis more difficult when it is distorted by surgical disease, surgical procedure, or an anesthetic than when they were younger. This view is not the one that was applied to the data presented in Table 58–3. Perhaps the best argument against modifying the ASA PS based on age-only information is hidden in the clever question attributed to Satchel Paige, "How old would you be if you didn't know how old you were?" As yet, there are no absolute accepted markers of human age, but PS can be determined from the level of maximal activity at which a patient is capable of performing regardless of age.

### What Is the Effect of Advanced Age on Perioperative Morbidity and Mortality?

Perioperative mortality and morbidity increase with advancing age.[13,14] In an analysis of the 1991–1992 Medicare Claims database, Fleisher and associates demonstrated increasing mortality with increasing age in patients who had undergone elective major vascular surgery.[14]

Perioperative mortality and morbidity also increase with increasing ASA PS. Is age the significant risk factor, or is age an indirect marker for increasing severity of chronic disease states? The question is relevant because chronologic age cannot be altered, but disease may be prevented or treated.[4] In the Fleisher study, preoperative stress testing was associated with decreased mortality presumably because it (1) identified those patients who subsequently benefited from coronary artery bypass grafting or percutaneous transluminal angioplasty before their vascular surgery, (2) provided information that influenced perioperative management, or (3) meant that the procedure was performed at an institution with a good support system and sufficient numbers to suggest experienced providers. The consensus opinion is that erosion of organ reserve or acute disruption of homeostasis is more likely to occur from disease than from age-related changes, at least until the age range associated with natural death is reached.

## What Are Perioperative Mortality and Morbidity Rates for Elderly Patients?

The total perioperative risk (TPR) can be expressed *conceptually* by the following equation[15]:

$$TPR = M + S + MS + [A + (AM + AS + AMS)]$$

where M is the risk due to a coexisting medical condition independent of surgery and anesthesia, S is the surgery risk due to surgery independent of the coexisting medical condition and anesthesia, MS is the risk resulting from the interaction of surgery and the medical condition, A is the risk due to anesthesia independent of any coexisting medical disease and surgery, AM is the anesthesia-related medical risk (eg, postoperative myocardial dysrhythmia or infarction associated with intraoperative hypothermia),[16] AS is the anesthesia-related surgical risk (eg, increased postoperative surgical infection associated with intraoperative hypothermia,[17] or normoxic rather than hyperoxic oxygen administration intraoperatively and during recovery),[18] and AMS is the risk resulting from the interaction of anesthesia, surgery, and the medical condition (eg, postoperative pulmonary edema).[19] The term (AM + AS + AMS) is the anesthesia-related risk, and [A + (AM + AS + AMS)] is the total anesthesia risk.

Early studies focused only on A, which included the death from loss of the airway and cardiac arrest during anesthesia unrelated to the surgical problem. With death as the outcome marker, A is approximately 1:250 000 for all patients regardless of age, coexisting medical condition, surgical illness, surgical procedure, ASA PS, or anesthetic technique; [A + (AM + AS + AMS)] is approximately 1:13 000[20]; and TPR is approximately 1:500 in a typical surgical tertiary care population.[21] Because the anesthesia-related death rate is so low, studies using it as the only outcome marker would require prohibitively large numbers of patients. Thus, death cannot be the only endpoint in studies designed to establish the superiority of a particular anesthetic agent, technique, or provider.

If major morbidity is added to the mortality outcomes examined in the aforementioned tertiary care population, the risk encompassed by the anesthesia-related terms ranges between 1:125 and 1:1500.[21] Outcome studies now are feasible but require several hundred to several thousand patients. Many studies will have to be multicentered or a meta-analysis of multiple, identically designed, single-centered studies. Studies with smaller numbers of patients are typically performed with surrogate outcome markers that occur more frequently, for example, tachycardia rather than myocardial ischemia or myocardial ischemia rather than myocardial infarction (MI), or even tachycardia rather than MI, although the validity of drawing conclusions using surrogate outcome markers is frequently and rightfully questioned. Also, the larger a study must be to demonstrate clinical significance the less significant the answer to the clinical question becomes.

This discussion focuses on how the clinician should look at the literature and develop evidence-based anesthetic administration and management. But how does it help answer the patient who asks what are his or her risks? First, patients tend to be more concerned about total perioperative risk than anesthesia risk isolated from surgical risk because they are aware that anesthesia is required if surgery is to be performed. To quote the same risk of death from both anesthesia-only causes as 1:250 000 and from anesthesia-related causes as 1:13 000 to a bedridden, 75-year-old patient presenting for coronary artery surgery with unstable angina and to a vigorous 75-year-old patient presenting for cataract surgery is a misuse of statistics.

Second, as yet, there are few studies of anesthesia-related complications whose results provide specific numeric risks that are appropriate for quoting to individual elderly patients with specific disease states presenting for specific operations. However, it is well established that 40% of Medicare patients undergoing noncardiac surgery suffer perioperative complications.[22] There is ample evidence to state that there are (1) factors associated with increased risk; (2) approaches to reduce, but not eliminate, the occurrence rate of untoward events; and (3) techniques to minimize the adverse impact of these untoward events when they do occur.

Finally, although much anesthesia training and practice is directed toward anticipating, monitoring for, and preventing "need-to-rescue" situations, the frequency with which these situations occur correlates more tightly with severity of illness than quality of care. A high outlier, the "failure-to-rescue" rate, is a stronger indicator of substandard care than a high outlier, "need-to-rescue" rate, but it is still hard not to believe that the greater the frequency of need-to-rescue events, the greater the likelihood of making an error when responding to these urgent or emergent conditions.

## When Do Anesthesia-Related Complications Occur?

Anesthesia complications that occur intraoperatively are often linked to poor preoperative preparation of the patient. One of four aggressive therapies is frequently required in elderly patients before the induction of anesthesia: (1) volume administration to restore normal intravascular volume in patients who are hypovolemic because of dehydration, bowel preparation, sepsis, ascites, or blood loss; (2) diuresis or dialysis to restore normal intravascular volume in patients who are hypervolemic because of congestive heart failure (CHF) or renal dysfunction; (3) administration of β-adrenergic receptor antagonists to normalize blood pressure (BP) and heart rate in patients with hypertension and heart rates >80 beats per minute (bpm); or (4) hydration of patients who received radiographic contrast dye injections or nonsteroidal antiinflammatory drug administrations within 24 hours of the scheduled surgery. Epidural or spinal anesthesia is contraindicated in hypovolemic patients but either one is an excellent choice in hypervolemic patients.

Most perioperative complications in elderly patients manifest themselves postoperatively. An untoward event that is triggered postoperatively is less likely to be *anesthesia*-related, but it still may be *analgesia*-related. An untoward event that is triggered intraoperatively but only manifests postoperatively is likely to be anesthesia-related. Most anesthesia-related complications manifest themselves beyond the postanesthesia care unit (PACU) on PODs 1 through 5, well after the direct effects of anesthetic agents are gone. The median day of occurrence for MI is either the day of surgery or POD 1, depending on diagnostic criteria; for CHF, pulmonary edema, pneumonia, and atelectasis, it is POD 2; and for cerebral vascular accident and pulmonary embolism, POD 3.[23] Examples of anesthesia-related complications triggered intraoperatively and manifested postoperatively include the following:

1. Postoperative atelectasis and pneumonia occurring more frequently in patients receiving long-acting neuromuscular blocking agents than in patients receiving intermediate-acting ones[24]
2. Wound infection, ileus, and postoperative cardiac events occurring more frequently in patients who develop mild hypothermia compared with those who are maintained normothermic[17]
3. Postoperative ileus lasting longer in patients who have not received intravenous lidocaine infusions[25] or who have not had local anesthetics added to the epidural opioid infusions[26]
4. Wound infection appearing more frequently in patients to whom 30% oxygen is administered in the operating and recovery rooms than in those to whom 80% oxygen is administered[18]
5. Postoperative myocardial ischemia occurring more frequently in patients who do not receive β-blockers.[27–31]

## When Do Perioperative Myocardial Infarctions Occur?

In a prospective study that evaluated 323 noncardiac surgery patients with ischemic heart disease, Badner and colleagues determined that 18 MIs (5.6%) were diagnosed in the postoperative period: 8 on the day of surgery, 6 on POD 1, 3 on POD 2, and 1 on POD 4.[32] An analysis of these 18 perioperative MIs reveals that 17% were fatal, 83% were not associated with angina, 39% had only chemical evidence of infarction, and 56% developed clinical findings: atrial fibrillation in 2 patients, hypotension in 4, and pulmonary edema in 4. Although the study was not designed to determine the relative safety of regional versus general anesthesia, the infarction rate was 9.5% (4 of 42) with regional anesthesia and 5.0% (14 of 281) with general anesthesia. Echocardiographic criteria or increased serum levels of creatine kinase isoenzymes or troponin were used to establish the diagnosis.

Zaugg and associates found that if the serum level of cardiac troponin I is used as a surrogate marker for cardiac injury, 8 of 19 noncardiac surgery patients not receiving β-blockade and 9 of 40 receiving atenolol had peak troponin levels associated with myocardial damage during noncardiac surgery.[29] One third of the serum elevations occurred intraoperatively. In the 19 patients not receiving atenolol, 3 of the 8 with elevated cardiac troponin I had levels normally associated with MI. Intraoperative ST-segment analysis did not reveal evidence of myocardial ischemia, and postoperative electrocardiographs (ECGs) did not meet criteria for diagnosis of MI.

The large majority of perioperative MIs diagnosed by chemical criteria are not associated with angina, hemodynamic instability, Q-waves, and ventricular failure. Mangano pointed out that validation studies have yet to be performed to determine the best criteria for diagnosing perioperative MI. In summary, most perioperative MIs occur within the first 2 days

of surgery, with the greatest frequency during or within 24 hours of the surgery. But the clinical significance of asymptomatic non–Q-wave infarctions remains to be established.[33]

## CARDIOVASCULAR SYSTEM

### Should All Elderly Patients Receive β-Adrenergic Receptor Blocking Agents Perioperatively?

In a 1998 editorial entitled "β-Adrenergic-Blocking Drugs. Incredibly Useful, Incredibly Underutilized," Warltier stated that "the evidence is overwhelming that patients at risk for coronary artery disease (CAD) will dramatically benefit from administration of these drugs. Unfortunately, the β-blockers are underused for reasons that are not clear."[27] Three studies using the long-acting, $\beta_1$-selective adrenergic agonists, atenolol (Tenormin) and bisoprolol (Zebeta), have appeared supporting Warltier's contention.

Poldermans and associates[28] screened 1351 patients presenting for elective abdominal aortic or infrainguinal arterial reconstruction. From the 846 who were determined to possess one or more cardiac risk factors, 173 had positive dobutamine echocardiographic studies. Of these, 61 were excluded: 53 who were already receiving β-blockers and 8 who already had very severe wall motion abnormalities at rest or during stress testing. The remaining 112 were randomized into two groups: 59 received bisoprolol and 53 received customary therapy. The study was designed to be twice as large but was stopped at the halfway point for ethical reasons because statistical and clinical significance was achieved in favor of β-blocker administration (Table 58–5).

Zaugg and colleagues demonstrated that patients receiving atenolol showed improved hemodynamic stability during emergence and in the postoperative period.[29] They also observed a trend toward lower cardiac troponin I release in the atenolol groups, but the groups were not large enough for the differences to achieve statistical significance. Interestingly the β-blockade did not reduce the neuroendocrine stress response to surgery but did appear to reduce postoperative analgesic requirements and allow faster recovery from anesthesia. This study supported an earlier one by Wallace and colleagues that demonstrated decreased incidence of postoperative myocardial ischemia in at-risk patients who received atenolol versus placebo starting in the immediate preinduction period and continued for 7 days postoperatively.[30]

Although many well-constructed clinical studies have demonstrated that β-blockade, established preoperatively and maintained intraoperatively and postoperatively, reduces the incidence of myocardial ischemia and infarction, most anesthesiologists tend not to establish and maintain β-blockade. Instead, they administer short-acting β-blockers, such as esmolol, metoprolol, or labetalol, intravenously and intermit-

**TABLE 58–5.** Effects of Bisoprolol on Perioperative Morbidity

| Group | Cardiac Death | Nonfatal Myocardial Infarction | Total |
|---|---|---|---|
| Bisoprolol | 2/59 (3.4%) | 0 | 2/59 (3.4%) |
| Standard care | 9/53 (17%) | 9/53 (17%) | 18/53 (34%) |

tently (eg, before intubation and during emergence). This practice helps to reduce the incidence of myocardial ischemia intraoperatively, but no study has yet demonstrated the effectiveness or ineffectiveness of this approach in reducing the incidence of perioperative MI. Postoperative myocardial ischemia is reduced when β-blockers are prophylactically administered postoperatively to maintain a heart rate <80 bpm.[31]

Most studies demonstrating the benefits of perioperative β-blockade actually only demonstrate the benefits of acute β-blockade initiated in the perioperative period (ie, immediately before being enrolled in their respective studies, the patients were not receiving β-blockers). Thus, the effects of fresh β-blockade were compared with no β-blockade. A different but related question is whether maintenance of chronic β-blockade established >30 days before surgery and continued throughout the perioperative period improves outcome.

This issue was addressed by Sear and colleagues, who retrospectively examined perioperative ambulatory ECGs from 453 noncardiac surgery patients enrolled in four previously reported studies.[34] The 70 patients who were receiving chronic β-adrenergic blocking agents had the same incidence of postoperative silent myocardial ischemia as the other 385 patients (including some who were receiving chronic calcium channel entry blockers). By far, the best predictor of postoperative silent myocardial ischemia was ECG evidence of preoperative silent ischemia. Other significant risk factors included chronic calcium channel blockade, arterial hypertension, and vascular surgery. In this relatively small, general surgical population, 45% of whom were older than 70 years, age >70 years did not achieve statistical significance as a risk factor. In conclusion, supplementing chronic β-blockade with additional β-blockers may not reduce the incidence of postoperative silent ischemia, but it is better than withdrawing β-blockers or treating intraoperative hypertension or tachycardia with calcium channel blockers.

### Should All Elderly Patients Receive α₂-Agonists Perioperatively?

Clonidine, dexmedetomidine, and mivazerol are three $\alpha_2$-agonists that have been studied in clinical trials as anesthesia adjuvants that may reduce perioperative myocardial ischemia and infarction. In a 1999 editorial, Ebert suggested that clonidine may help limit cardiac mortality and morbidity by aiding anesthesiologists in "gaining control of the autonomic nervous system."[35] In elderly patients, sympathovagal balance may be improved by decreasing sympathetic tone and increasing vagal control. Clonidine restores, and perhaps increases, vagally mediated reflex activity that is typically depressed in the postoperative period and decreases resting sympathetic tone centrally. The hemodynamic stability associated with clonidine actually refers to lesser variability in BP and heart rate throughout the perioperative period around a setpoint of a lower basal BP. Clonidine does not impair the ability of the baroreflex to increase sympathetic outflow during hypotension.[36] Clonidine does increase the sensitivity to bolus injections of α-agonists such as phenylephrine but not to vasodilators like sodium nitroprusside.[37]

However, unlike the favorable conclusions on routine β-blocker administration, the role for $\alpha_2$-agonists still remains to be established. In 1897 patients with established CAD undergoing surgery, mivazerol administration did not alter the rates of MI or death. But in the vascular surgery subgroup of 904 patients, there was a trend toward fewer MIs and a significant reduction in the number of other primary cardiac endpoints.[38] From an anesthetic perspective, the upside of clonidine administration is that patients experience fewer episodes of hypertension and tachycardia, a hemodynamic combination that increases the incidence of myocardial ischemia. The downside of clonidine administration is the more frequent occurrence of hypotension during anesthesia that may lead to increased infusion of fluid, vasopressors, or inotropes.

### What Are the Definitions of Intraoperative Hypotension and Hypertension?

Keeping systolic pressure within 20% of baseline systolic pressure is a commonly taught rule-of-thumb that has not been proven in well-designed clinical outcome studies. According to this dictum, a patient whose systolic BPs normally range between 180 and 200 mm Hg should be managed such that his or her systolic BPs are maintained between 144 and 160 mm Hg. However, with the exception of patients with critical left main coronary lesions (or their equivalent), tight aortic stenosis, and very significant left ventricular hypertrophy, systolic BPs between 90 and 120 mm Hg are well tolerated. Systolic BPs between 160 and 180 are well tolerated if heart rates are maintained in the 50 to 70 bpm range. However, lower BPs and faster heart rates are necessary to maximize the forward stroke volume and cardiac output of patients with mitral or aortic regurgitation. Deliberate hypotension with mean arterial pressures in the 45 to 55 mm Hg range is also well tolerated in normovolemic patients during epidural anesthesia if cardiac output is maintained by administering low dose inotropic infusions.[39]

The coronary perfusion pressure necessary to prevent ischemia varies with anesthetic technique. It is higher with opioid-based techniques and lower with potent inhalational anesthetics. Less ischemia occurs during inhalational anesthesia if BP is maintained with lower alveolar concentrations than with higher alveolar concentrations and phenylephrine infusion.[40]

Another rule-of-thumb for maintaining adequate coronary perfusion pressure and minimizing myocardial ischemia is to keep the rate-pressure product below that which causes angina during exercise testing. (The rate-pressure product is the heart rate in beats per minute multiplied by mean arterial pressure in mm Hg.) However, hypertension and tachycardia during exercise is different hemodynamically than hypertension and tachycardia during anesthesia and after surgery. These data are not always available preoperatively.

Perhaps a better rule-of-thumb may be to keep the pressure/rate quotient >1. The pressure rate quotient is the mean arterial pressure in mm Hg divided by the heart rate in bpm. Myocardial ischemia, in a dog model at least, was minimized if the mean arterial pressure was greater than the heart rate. But BPs and heart rates must not be extremely high or low.[41] In simpler terms, tachycardia is not good for patients with ischemic heart disease, and the combination of hypotension and tachycardia is even worse.

Raby and colleagues used Holter monitoring in the 24 hours preceding vascular surgery to identify patients with preoperative silent myocardial ischemia. They determined for each patient the minimal heart rate at which these ischemic events occurred and defined this rate as the ischemic threshold for that patient. They then used esmolol infusions postoperatively to keep the heart rate below the ischemic threshold. Postoperative myocardial ischemia was markedly reduced in the patient population most likely to experience postoperative ischemia.[42]

In summary, if one accepts functional definitions for hypotension, hypertension, bradycardia, and tachycardia as those limits above or below which significant threat to organ function occurs, then the numbers associated with these limits are dependent on patient factors, severity of disease, acute surgical requirements, and anesthetic technique. In the absence of limits applicable to elderly patients, monitoring emerges as a crucial component for effective care, although, even here, there is reason to question the accuracy of automated devices that are used to measure BP.[43]

### What Is the Significance of New T-Wave Inversions Following Anesthesia?

The incidence of new T-wave changes after anesthesia observed in the PACU and not associated with other signs or symptoms of myocardial ischemia is approximately 18%. This observation holds true after regional or general anesthesia regardless of age. In a prospective study of 394 consecutive patients who were not undergoing cardiac or neurosurgical procedures, a flattening of T waves was seen in 46 and inversion was seen in 25.[44] In another prospective study, 21% of 206 men undergoing transurethral prostate resection developed ECG changes postoperatively (mostly T wave changes), but none experienced cardiac symptoms or developed sustained creatine kinase MB elevations.[45] In the elderly, new T-wave inversions create a problem. It is not cost effective to work up each occurrence if it is not associated with clinical signs and symptoms of cardiovascular dysfunction. But the elderly do not always present with textbook signs and symptoms of myocardial ischemia. The threshold to rule out an MI should be low if there are other "soft" signs of cardiovascular dysfunction.[46,47]

### Do Patients With Bundle Branch Blocks Require Preoperative Prophylactic Placement of Pacemakers?

Chronic bifascicular block will progress to complete heart block within 5 years in 5% to 10% of patients. Anesthesia and surgery do not affect this conversion rate. In nine retrospective studies involving a total of 341 patients with asymptomatic chronic bifascicular block or left bundle branch block, the incidence of serious block progression was <1%. Prophylactic insertion of temporary transvenous pacemakers is no longer recommended in these patients. This consensus opinion was supported by a prospective study of 106 asymptomatic patients with this degree of conduction block using Holter monitoring for 24 hours before the induction of anesthesia.[48] The patients received general, spinal, or epidural anesthesia. Block progression, not to complete heart block but to second-degree atrioventricular block Mobitz type I without hemodynamic impairment, occurred in 2 patients, both of whom started with right bundle branch block and left anterior fascicular block with normal P-R intervals (1 intraoperatively and another 2 hours postoperatively). A third patient developed second-de-

gree atrioventricular block with subsequent cardiac arrest 3 days postoperatively during an infusion of neostigmine for stimulation of bowel function. Bradycardia that responded quickly to pharmacologic therapy occurred in a total of 9 patients: intraoperatively in 7 and postoperatively in 2. The incidence of bradyarrhythmias with or without hypotension was no different in patients with prolonged P-R intervals than in those with normal P-R intervals. In conclusion, although the routine insertion of prophylactic pacemakers in these patients is not necessary, they are prone to bradyarrhythmias, which anesthesiologists must be prepared to treat. The precautionary availability of a working transcutaneous pacing system for immediate application is recommended.

### Does Prophylactic Percutaneous Transluminal Coronary Angioplasty Reduce the Incidence of Adverse Cardiac Outcomes After Noncardiac Surgery?

In a retrospective study of cardiac complications after noncardiac surgery, percutaneous transluminal coronary angioplasty (PTCA) did not reduce the incidence of postoperative MI or death.[49] In this study, 686 patients who had undergone PTCA were compared with 686 matched patients with CAD who had not undergone PTCA and with 2155 normal controls. PTCA did reduce the incidence of postoperative myocardial ischemia and CHF by 50%.

## AIRWAY AND PULMONARY SYSTEM

### Should Elderly Smokers Be Permitted to Smoke Preoperatively?

In a study using exhaled carbon monoxide (CO) concentrations as evidence of acute smoking, Woehlck and coworkers demonstrated that many patients who smoke cigarettes either deny being smokers or continue to smoke cigarettes on the day of surgery.[50] In a setting in which the preoperative instructions are clearly given not to smoke, 0.9% of patients who claimed to be nonsmokers, 4.3% who claimed to have been prior smokers, and 24.5% who were acknowledged smokers admitted violating these instructions when confronted with biochemical evidence that they had done so.

Smoking involves inhalation of CO. CO causes problems in at least four ways:

1. CO binds to hemoglobin to produce carboxyhemoglobin (COHb), which reduces oxygen carrying capacity.
2. CO impairs release of nitric oxide from hemoglobin and limits the ability of red blood cells to autoregulate local blood flow.
3. CO binds to myoglobin and impairs cardiac muscle function.
4. Pulse oximetry overestimates oxygen saturation in the presence of COHb.

Patients with CAD, whose COHb concentration is 2% to 6% of their total hemoglobin concentration, the range typically seen in cigarette smokers, experience more myocardial ischemia during exercise than when only trace COHb is present.

When cigarette smoke is the source of CO, greater myocardial ischemia is observed in patients at the same concentration of COHb that is obtained when a pure source of CO is inhaled. This observation suggests that cigarette smoke contains additional toxins which impair myocardial oxygen utilization. In their study of 740 patients under the age of 65 years with no history or symptoms of ischemic heart disease or peripheral vascular disease, Woehlck and colleagues also demonstrated that the probability of intraoperative ST depression increased with increased exhaled CO concentrations. Their patient population was not anemic and was presenting for elective noncardiac, non–major vascular surgery. The probability of preoperative smoking-induced myocardial ischemia is increased in anemic patients, in patients with known CAD, and in patients presenting for vascular or cardiac surgery.

Having stated the detriments of preoperative cigarette smoking one must also note that acute cessation of smoking may also lead to problems. Cigarette smoke is an airway irritant that leads to coughing. Smokers need to cough because of increased sputum production. With acute cessation, sputum production continues, but cough itself is inhibited by analgesic and sedative drugs, and cough effectiveness is depressed by splinting from pain. Smokers retain secretions that can cause bronchospasm or obstruct airways and lead to atelectasis and pneumonia. It takes at least 2 months for sufficient improvement of ciliary and small airway function and decrease in sputum production to decrease postoperative respiratory morbidity to below that found in active smokers.[51] Postoperative pulmonary complications occur 3 times more frequently in patients with lung disease when they are compared with patients without lung disease.[52] In summary, acute cessation of smoking does not reduce intraoperative or postoperative pulmonary events or complications but will decrease the likelihood of myocardial ischemia.

### Does Airway Obstruction Determined by Preoperative Spirometry Predict Perioperative Complications in Smokers?

Because postoperative pulmonary complications occur more frequently in patients with chronic obstructive lung disease, it stands to reason that the severity of airway obstruction, as measured by forced expiratory flow volume in 1 second ($FEV_1$), should predict these complications. In fact, Warner and colleagues determined that $FEV_1$ predicts the occurrence of perioperative bronchospasm but does not predict the need for prolonged endotracheal intubation or prolonged intensive care admission after abdominal surgery.[52] Optimized preoperative pulmonary therapy, effective treatment of bronchospasm, and current standards of anesthetic and postoperative care probably contributed positively to this "negative" finding.

### What Is the Best Way to Preoxygenate Elderly Patients?

Although four deep breaths of 100% oxygen within 30 seconds may be an acceptable technique to preoxygenate healthy younger patients, it is not as satisfactory a technique in elderly patients because it does not provide maximal preoxygenation.

**TABLE 58–6.** Times to Desaturation After Three Different Techniques for Preoxygenation

| Type of Patient | Definition of Desaturation* | Preoxygenation Technique | | |
|---|---|---|---|---|
| | | 4DB/30S | TV/3 min | 8DB/60s |
| Elderly | $SaO_2$ >90% | 212 | 408 | |
| Elderly | $SaO_2$ >93% | 222 | 324 | |
| CABG | $SpO_2$ >95% | 167 | 224 | 313 |

*Desaturation situation: apnea with open airway exposed to room air.

CABG, coronary artery bypass graft; 4DB/30s, 4 deep breaths of 100% oxygen within 30 seconds at oxygen flows of 10 L/min; TV/3min, tidal volume breathing of 100% oxygen for 3 minutes at oxygen flows of 5 L/min; 8DB/60s, 8 deep breaths of 100% oxygen within 60 seconds at oxygen flows of 10 L/min.

Data from Benumof JL. Preoxygenation: best method for both efficacy and efficiency? *Anesthesiology.* 1999;91:603 *and* Baraka A, Taha SK, Aouad MT, et al. Preoxygenation: comparison of maximal breathing and tidal volume breathing techniques. *Anesthesiology.* 1999;91:612.

Maximal preoxygenation is needed in elderly patients for at least three reasons.

1. Desaturation occurs faster in older patients than in younger adults for any given oxygenation technique.
2. The time to peak relaxation from succinylcholine or non-depolarizing neuromuscular blocking agents is delayed in proportion to age during a rapid sequence induction (Table 58–6).
3. The elderly are more likely than younger patients to suffer a cardiac event from desaturation because of the higher incidence of ischemic heart disease.

Maximal preoxygenation, as described by Benumof, is achieved when not only the alveolar and arterial compartments are filled with oxygen but also the tissue and venous compartments.[53] Practically, the technique providing maximal preoxygenation should be defined as the one that produces the longest time before desaturation and not the one that produces the highest $PaO_2$ (see Table 58–6). A technique that seems to provide maximal oxygenation in the shortest period of time is one in which eight deep breaths of 100% oxygen are taken within 60 seconds with an oxygen flow of 10 L/min.[54] With deep breathing techniques, the higher oxygen flow rates lead to higher $PaO_2$.

### Are Elderly Patients More Likely to Be Difficult to Ventilate by Mask?

Difficulty in mask ventilation was encountered in 5% of patients (75 of 1502) who were prospectively studied for this specific event.[55] It was predicted at the time of the preoperative assessment in only 17% of these 75 patients. This 5% incidence is higher than the 0.07% to 1.4% reported in prospective studies more focused on difficult intubation and less than the 15% reported in retrospective studies. Five elements emerged as independent variables:

1. Age older than 55 years
2. Body mass index >26 kg/m²
3. Presence of a beard
4. Lack of teeth
5. History of snoring

The presence of two of these factors indicated a high likelihood of difficult mask ventilation but did not correlate with difficulty in endotracheal intubation. Shaving a beard and retaining lower dentures are actions that may be taken to improve mask ventilation, but neither action has been studied prospectively to determine efficacy in older patients.

## Does a Laryngeal Mask Airway Cause Less Airway Irritation Than an Endotracheal Tube?

Two studies focused on this question. In the Kim and Bishop study, respiratory system resistance was higher in patients immediately after endotracheal intubation but decreased to the level measured in patients with laryngeal mask airways (LMAs) within 10 minutes.[56] In these patients, anesthesia was induced with thiopental and fentanyl and intubation or LMA placement facilitated with succinylcholine. Measurements were made immediately after LMA placement or intubation and after 10 minutes of isoflurane inhalation.

In the study by Berry and coworkers, patients were randomized to either LMA or endotracheal tube (ETT) groups and were anesthetized with propofol, fentanyl, isoflurane, nitrous oxide, and vecuronium.[57] Measurements were made at tidal volumes of 5, 10, and 15 mL/kg.

Peak inspiratory pressure, mean airway resistance, and pulmonary airway resistance were all lower in the LMA group. Clearly avoiding the highly innervated larynx and trachea reduces reflex bronchoconstriction. Using an LMA may avoid triggering bronchospasm in patients with reactive airway disease; however, an LMA does not permit adequate controlled ventilation of patients with active severe bronchospasm.

In both studies, neuromuscular blocking agents and controlled ventilation were used with LMAs. This practice is contrary to teaching in some training centers in the United States where LMAs are predominantly used with spontaneous ventilation. If controlled ventilation through an LMA is contemplated, minute ventilation must be provided with higher respiratory rates and lower tidal volumes than typically used through an ETT. I frequently use controlled ventilation through an LMA, but I demand that two conditions be met in patients with bronchospastic disease. First, patients must not be actively wheezing before LMA insertion. Second, the patients must remain supine throughout the surgery so that the LMA may be exchanged for an ETT should bronchospasm develop.

## What Percentage of Oxygen Should Be Administered to Elderly Patients Intraoperatively?

There are now many recognized advantages to higher inhaled oxygen concentrations (80% oxygen), even when the arterial oxygen saturation is 100% at lower inhaled concentrations. Use of high inhaled intraoperative and postoperative oxygen concentrations has lead to decreased postoperative nausea and vomiting (PONV),[58] decreased postoperative tachycardia, and possibly decreased myocardial ischemia,[59] in addition to possibly improved wound healing, less dehiscence, and decreased surgical infections because of increased tissue oxygenation.[60]

A presumed disadvantage of higher oxygen concentration is increased atelectasis. However, Akca and associates determined that the incidence and severity of postoperative atelectasis was the same when patients inhaled 80% oxygen and 20% nitrogen as when they inhaled 30% oxygen and 70% nitrogen[60] during anesthesia for colon resection. I feel that the evidence is mounting for all elderly patients to receive 50% to 80% oxygen during general anesthesia and in the recovery room.

## Should Elderly Patients Automatically Receive Supplemental Oxygen in the Postoperative Period After Major Surgery, Even If $SpO_2$ Is >95%?

Higher inspired oxygen concentrations may decrease PONV. Grief and colleagues studied the effect of inhaled oxygen concentration, 30% versus 80%, intraoperatively and postoperatively on the incidence of PONV in 231 patients after colon resection.[58] The average age was 60 years, and no patients received nitrous oxide or prophylactic antiemetics. Their data are presented in Table 58-7. Even though $SpO_2$ was maintained above 95% in both groups, the higher oxygen group experienced less PONV. The authors theorized that patients undergoing colon resection probably suffered some regional intestinal ischemia, which caused the release of serotonin, a potent trigger of nausea and vomiting. Ischemia was less likely in the 80% oxygen group. Hyperoxia also produces a vagally mediated bradycardia. It is possible that there is concomitant vagal release of acetylcholine, which also produces intestinal vasodilation, improves oxygenation, and reduces serotonin release.

## INHALATIONAL AGENTS

### What Is the Effect of Advancing Age on Inhalational Anesthesia Endpoints?

Human studies demonstrate that the MAC of any inhalational agent associated with the absence of physical signs of withdrawal from the surgical incision in 50% of patients is reduced with advancing age. The average decrease in MAC is approximately 6% per decade for all agents.[61] For isoflurane, MAC is 1.49% at 1 year of age, 1.17% at 40 years of

**TABLE 58–7.** Effect of Supplemental Oxygen on Postoperative Nausea and Vomiting After Colon Resection

|  | 30% O₂ (n = 119) | 80% O₂ (n = 112) | p |
|---|---|---|---|
| **0-6 h After Surgery** | | | |
| Nausea (%) | 15 | 8 | |
| Vomiting (%) | 2 | 0 | |
| **Total (%)** | **15** | **8** | **0.141** |
| **6-24 h After Surgery** | | | |
| Nausea (%) | 22 | 10 | |
| Vomiting (%) | 6 | 2 | |
| **Total (%)** | **22** | **10** | **0.045** |

Modified from Grief R, Laciny S, Rapf B, et al. Supplemental oxygen reduces the incidence of postoperative nausea and vomiting. *Anesthesiology.* 1999;91:1246.

age, and 0.91% at 80 years of age. No similar study in human beings has been performed for nitrous oxide, but in laboratory rats in hyperbaric chambers, the MAC for nitrous oxide also decreased with advancing age. When burst-suppression in the electroencephalogram (EEG) is used as an endpoint, elderly patients anesthetized with 1.7% end-tidal isoflurane experience a greater frequency of burst-suppression events and spend a greater proportion of time with a burst-suppression EEG pattern with each event than younger patients.[62] MAC is dramatically reduced by the concomitant administration of benzodiazepines and opioids and by spinal or epidural anesthesia.

MACawake, the minimum alveolar concentration of an inhalational agent associated with failure to respond to "Open your eyes" command, also decreases with advancing age.[63] MACawake can be determined in the absence of surgery or at the end of surgery and with or without airway appliances. MACawake is less if it is determined when anesthesia is administered by mask without other airway appliances and in the absence of surgery (preoperative MACawake) than when it is determined postoperatively with an ETT or LMA in place (postoperative MACawake). Aging reduces postoperative MACawake more than it reduces preoperative MACawake. This observation is reasonable because somatic and visceral pain thresholds increase with advancing age. A potentially painful stimulus of fixed intensity is less likely to awaken an older patient than a younger one. Aging also reduces MAC more than it reduces the postoperative MACawake. Thus, theoretically, if the end-tidal inhalational agent concentration is adjusted so that it is equi-MAC (as opposed to equi–end-tidal) for younger and older patients, older patients should actually awaken earlier than younger ones. In practice, however, most anesthesiologists overestimate how much inhalational agent an elderly patient requires, especially when BP is used as the primary guide for anesthetic depth. Also, inhalational agents are rarely given alone. Concomitantly administered intravenous agents markedly decrease MAC and MACawake.[64] Thus, older patients tend to take longer to awaken than younger ones.

### Does End-Tidal Gas Concentration Accurately Reflect Brain Concentration of Inhalational Agents?

During the maintenance phase of anesthesia, the end-tidal gas concentration parallels brain concentration; however, end-tidal gas monitoring significantly overestimates brain concentration during anesthesia induction and underestimates brain concentration during emergence.[65] This hysteresis effect is more dramatic with a more soluble agent, such as isoflurane, and less dramatic with a less soluble agent, such as desflurane. Failure to take this effect into account leads to prolonged emergence times. Patients are amnestic for a variable period of time in the recovery room after inhalational anesthesia with halothane, enflurane, isoflurane, and sevoflurane. The rate at which the brain concentration ratio approaches zero is indicated in Table 58–8 and compared with the rate at which the alveolar concentration ratio decreases. Because of this hysteresis effect, MACawake determined when the vaporizer is immediately turned off is lower than MACawake determined when the vaporizer is turned down in small stepwise decrements every 10 to 15 minutes before *off* is reached: 0.34

**TABLE 58–8.** Comparison of Cerebral and Alveolar Elimination for Isoflurane

| Time (min) | Concentration Ratio | |
| --- | --- | --- |
| | *Cerebral* | *Alveolar* |
| 0-6 | 0.686 | 0.242 |
| 6-12 | 0.337 | 0.102 |
| 12-18 | 0.236 | 0.072 |
| 18-24 | 0.136 | 0.056 |
| 24-30 | 0.101 | 0.047 |
| 90-120 | 0.048 | 0.017 |

Modified from Lockhart SH, Cohen Y, Yasuda N, et al. Cerebral uptake and elimination of desflurane, isoflurane, and halothane from rabbit brain: an in vivo NMR study. *Anesthesiology.* 1991;74:575.

MAC versus 0.22 MAC for isoflurane and sevoflurane.[66] The most common clinical reason why anesthesiologists are reluctant to turn down the anesthetic agent toward the end of surgery is that the older patient tends to become hypertensive, which is interpreted as light anesthesia. Emergence is then prolonged with inhaled agents other than desflurane. The administration of antihypertensives, such as labetalol or hydralazine, as inhalational agents are being withdrawn, helps avoid this problem and promotes hemodynamic stability during emergence, extubation, and recovery.

### Do Electroencephalographic Markers of Anesthetic Endpoints Need to Be Adjusted for Age?

It is well established that increasing age reduces potent inhalational agent requirements and endpoints such as MAC and MACawake. Until recently, it had not been established whether the bispectral indices or spectral edge frequencies associated with these endpoints require correction for the age of the patient. Fortunately, there is no age-adjustment required. Increasing age reduced the end-tidal sevoflurane concentrations required to suppress responses to a verbal command but did not change the bispectral index and 95% spectral edge frequency associated with this endpoint. During sevoflurane anesthesia, the best-to-worst predictor of a response to a verbal command is the bispectral index (BIS) > end-tidal sevoflurane concentration > the 95% spectral edge frequency > BP and/or heart rate.[63]

### Are Mask Inductions Easier in Older Patients Than in Younger Ones?

Mask induction of anesthesia is faster in elderly patients than in younger patients for several reasons. First is the previously described lower MAC. Second, decreased airway reflex activity in older patients limits breath-holding, which commonly delays induction in younger ones. Third, lower cardiac outputs, more likely in older patients than in younger ones, enhance the rate of induction. Although the resting cardiac output in healthy elderly patients is generally the same as that seen in younger patients, elderly patients who have hypertension or who are taking β-blockers do have lower resting cardiac outputs. All inhalational agents are myocardial depressants. If the myocardial depressant effects of inhalational agents are not offset by vasodilation, as they tend to be with isoflurane, then their inhalation will speed induction. There is also less tachycardia in elderly patients during induction and therefore less compensation for the reduced stroke volume. Older patients are more likely to become hypertensive, and their cardiac output decreases with minimal stimulus. The increase in cardiac output in response to stimulation is less with advancing age. Opposing the tendency toward more rapid induction is a slight increase in solubility of inhalational agents with advancing age. Also, mask inductions are slightly prolonged when patients have chronic obstructive lung disease.

## Does Changing From Isoflurane to Desflurane Near the End of the Procedure Accelerate Recovery?

The answer is no. This question was addressed in a brilliant clinical study, and this practice should be discouraged as costly and ineffective.[67] The results of this study should not be interpreted to mean that desflurane should be avoided completely. In fact, with its rapid emergence profile, it is an ideal agent in the elderly if it used for the entire anesthetic with low flows.

## Does Spinal or Epidural Anesthesia Reduce Minimum Alveolar Concentration and MACawake of Potent Inhalational Agents?

Two patients are to undergo a colon resection. One will receive a combined epidural-general anesthesia. The other will be given just a general anesthesia. Will both patients require the same amount of inhalational agent to achieve the same depth of anesthesia before the surgical incision if stimulated in a dermatome not anesthetized by the epidural?

This question was directly answered in two recent clinical studies. The minimum alveolar concentration (MAC) for sevoflurane was determined in 3 groups of patients: group E, T2 epidural lidocaine; group C, epidural saline (control); and group I, epidural saline with intravenous lidocaine (lidocaine infusion rate was chosen to produce plasma levels equivalent to those seen from systemic absorption of lidocaine after epidural injection).[68] The MAC stimulus was a 10-second burst of 50 Hz, 60 mA tetanic electrical stimulus in the C5 dermatome seeking purposeful movement of the head. The MAC of sevoflurane was 0.52% in Group E, 1.04 in Group I, and 1.18% in Group C. T2 epidural anesthesia reduced MAC by 50%. In an earlier study, MACawake for isoflurane was determined to be 0.28% to 0.31% ($\approx$25% of MAC) with varying plasma levels of lidocaine and 0.18% (approximately 15% of MAC) with epidural lidocaine.[69] The reductions in MAC and MACawake were not due to systemic absorption of epidurally administered lidocaine.

Lower levels of inhalational agents during combined epidural-general anesthesia are required for ETT tolerance and to prevent intraoperative awareness as compared with general anesthesia without a functioning epidural. Emergence is prolonged if the same alveolar concentration of inhalational agent is maintained during combined epidural-general anesthesia as during general anesthesia without an epidural.

## Do Inhalational Agents Affect How Hypovolemia Manifests Itself in Elderly Patients?

Unanesthetized patients develop tachycardia before they become hypotensive as hypovolemia evolves. Inhalational agents interfere with baroreceptor function. Therefore, hypovolemia during inhalational anesthesia tends to manifest itself more with hypotension than with tachycardia. Systolic arterial pressure decreases during the inspiratory phase of positive pressure ventilation. The magnitude of this variability increases with hypovolemia.[70] Other parameters that affect this variability include positive end-expiratory pressure, lung and chest wall compliance, mode of ventilation, and inspiratory:expiratory ratio. There are two components to this change in systolic pressure: a contribution above baseline and one below. An increase in the down component reflects a decrease in venous return and hypovolemia. An increase in the up component reflects an augmentation of cardiac output with increased preload during left ventricular ejection in the expiratory phase. The up component may increase significantly in left ventricular failure because of the afterload reducing effect of increased intrathoracic pressure. A normal variation in systolic pressure is about 8 to 10 mm Hg, with the down component being 6 to 8 mm Hg. Greater variations suggest hypovolemia as a likely cause. Similar variations have been reported in pulse oximetry traces and with the Finapres noninvasive, beat-to-beat BP device.

## What Is the Role of Nitrous Oxide?

Two major benefits of nitrous oxide are (1) reduction of MAC of more potent and more soluble inhalational agents, which enables faster emergence from inhalational anesthesia; and (2) less cardiovascular depression when nitrous oxide is administered with isoflurane versus isoflurane administered alone at equi-MAC concentrations. When 1.05% isoflurane in oxygen was compared with 0.55% isoflurane and 50% nitrous oxide in 70-year-old patients, heart rate was lower, cardiac index and stroke volume were higher, and systolic and diastolic BP and systemic vascular resistance essentially were unchanged in the nitrous oxide group.[71] Nitrous oxide behaved like an "inhalational opioid." I consider 50% to 70% nitrous oxide to be equivalent to approximately 5 $\mu$g/kg of fentanyl.

The use of nitrous oxide in the elderly is decreasing for several reasons. First, elderly patients require a higher inspired oxygen concentration than younger patients to maintain the same intraoperative $PaO_2$ or $SpO_2$, so that less nitrous oxide can be given. Second, there are significant benefits now being ascribed to higher inspired oxygen concentrations (eg, 80%), including reduced nausea and infection rates, less postoperative tachycardia and perhaps myocardial ischemia, and less bowel distention, which facilitates closure with less demand for muscle relaxation and minimizes ileus. Thus, given a choice between nitrous oxide and the described potential benefits, more anesthesiologists are against using nitrous oxide. Third, nitrous oxide reduces movement by reducing MAC, but it does not produce muscle relaxation. Higher concentrations of potent inhalational agents reduce the dose requirements for neuromuscular blocking agents. Residual concentrations of neuromuscular blocking agents have been implicated in postoperative pulmonary complications. Fourth, MAC and

MACawake are reduced to a greater extent in the elderly than popularly appreciated, especially if intravenous drugs are also administered, so that nitrous oxide is a less important contributor to depth of anesthesia than in younger patients or older anesthetic techniques. Fifth, less soluble potent inhalational agents, sevoflurane and especially desflurane, are now available so that emergence times are diminished. Sixth, opioids do what nitrous oxide does intraoperatively but in addition residual opioid effects smooth out emergence in ways that nitrous oxide cannot.

## INTRAVENOUS AGENTS

### How Does Advancing Age Affect Doses of Intravenous Agents?

*Elderly patients require smaller doses of intravenous anesthetic drugs than younger patients.*

—*STEVEN SHAFER*[72]

Shafer begins and ends an elegant chapter with this sentence and supports it with 118 references.[72] This statement is certainly valid when comparing a population of older patients with a population of younger patients. However, the dose that produces a specific endpoint in a randomly selected individual elderly patient may be greater than, the same as, but usually less than the dose for a randomly selected individual young patient. For any given drug, the dose-response curve becomes broader and shifts to the left for a population of older patients, but it still overlaps with the taller, more narrow curve for a population of younger patients. The dose that is required to achieve but not exceed a particular endpoint is more difficult to determine in older patients than in younger patients. Elderly individuals demonstrate considerable variability in effect of aging on organ function; in severity of chronic disease; in social habits that affect drug disposition, such as cigarette smoking and alcohol consumption; and of additive or synergistic effects associated with polypharmacy.

The mechanisms for decreased dose requirements are pharmacokinetic changes associated with aging and disease, pharmacodynamic changes associated with aging, or a combination of the two. Using EEG endpoints as the principal measure of drug effect, a pharmacokinetic explanation has been determined to be the primary one that explains decreased requirements for thiopental and etomidate in older patients. The steady-state plasma concentrations reflect fixed effect-site (brain) concentrations associated with various endpoints that are independent of age for these drugs. A decreased volume of distribution is usually measured. Thus, for any given bolus dose, the plasma concentration is higher in elderly patients than in younger ones. A carefully chosen smaller bolus dose in the elderly will produce the same brain concentration seen with a larger bolus dose in young patients and have the same effect.

A pharmacodynamic explanation for a decreased dose has been determined for midazolam, alfentanil, and fentanyl. Only small pharmacokinetic differences are noted between older and younger patients for these drugs, but the steady-state plasma concentration, and therefore the effect-site (brain) concentration, is lower for any given anesthesia endpoint.

More complex age-related effects are seen with propofol and remifentanil. Remifentanil simulations based on an EEG model suggest that age is an important variable in calculating bolus doses (elderly doses one half that of young) and infusion rates (elderly doses one third of young).[73,74] For propofol, at any given infusion rate, the resulting plasma concentrations are higher in older patients. To achieve the same target level, the infusion rates must be higher in younger patients than in older patients. When the propofol infusion is discontinued, the plasma concentrations of propofol fall faster in older patients. Despite several rigorous attempts to determine whether an age-related pharmacodynamic effect exists for propofol, to me it is unclear whether one exists, and if it does, whether it is clinically significant.[75,76]

### What Is the Optimum Duration of Injection for Propofol?

It has been suggested that the optimum duration of injection for propofol is 2 minutes if the goal is to administer the minimum amount of drug to achieve loss of consciousness with minimum hemodynamic side effects. Faster injection increases peak arterial concentration, but the arterial peak is too transient to permit maximum loading of the brain because of a relatively long blood-brain equilibration time for propofol (4.32 minutes versus 1.22 minutes for thiopental). For injections slower than 2 minutes, drug lost to redistribution limits brain concentrations to less than those seen with 2 minute injections. Hemodynamic side effects correlate better with arterial concentrations than with brain concentrations.[77,78] Thus, propofol is not a good drug for rapid sequence inductions and intubations. For thiopental, the maximum brain concentration occurs 1.5 minutes after a bolus injection. Thus, it is more suitable for faster administration rates and for rapid sequence inductions than propofol. Wakeling and colleagues hold a contrary opinion.[79] They suggest that when the target is the effect compartment concentration rather than the plasma concentration, induction occurs more rapidly without significant hemodynamic changes.

## SEDATIVES

### Does Sedation Affect Hypoxic Control of Cardiorespiratory Responses?

Hypoxia triggers a biphasic response with regard to ventilation. In the absence of medication, hypoxemia lasting $<5$ minutes stimulates the peripheral chemoreceptors of the carotid bodies. Hypoxemia lasting $>5$ minutes depresses the respiratory center of the brain. The acute hypoxic response hence is hyperventilation followed within 3 to 5 minutes by a gradual diminution in minute ventilation to a lower steady-state minute ventilation after 15 to 20 minutes. With oxygen saturation in the 80% to 90% range, there is release and accumulation of inhibitory neurotransmitters such as γ-aminobutyric acid (GABA), which may contribute to the central depression. Because many sedatives bind to GABA receptors, they may inhibit this hypoxic ventilatory response. When healthy volunteers were challenged with hypoxia to a $PaO_2$ of 50 mm Hg, propofol infusions to a BIS index of 76 caused a 50% reduction in the ventilatory response to acute hypoxia.[80] Coadministration of fentanyl, alfentanil, diltiazem, antimycotics, and macrolide antibiotics inhibits the clearance of metabolism of midazolam by hepatic microsomal cytochrome P4503A (CYP3A)[81] and may contribute to the frequent hypoxemia and apnea seen after sedation with midazolam and opioids.[82]

### Is There a Sedative That Does Not Potentiate the Effects of Intravenous Opioids?

Diphenhydramine is commonly administered as a sedative, an antipruritic, and an antiemetic. Administered alone, it modestly stimulates ventilation by augmenting the interaction of hypoxic and hypercarbic drives. When diphenhydramine is administered in combination with a systemic opioid such as alfentanil to healthy 23- to 38-year-old patients, it counteracted the decrease in the slope of the ventilatory response to carbon dioxide by alfentanil. It also counteracted the alfentanil-induced decrease in minute ventilation when the end-tidal carbon dioxide tension was 54 mm Hg. Diphenhydramine neither counteracted nor worsened the effect of alfentanil on response to hypoxia. Thus, diphenhydramine is a sedative that does not appear to potentiate the effect of opioids on ventilatory responses to hypoxia and hypercarbia.[83]

### Does Spinal or Epidural Anesthesia Increase Sensitivity to Intravenous Sedation?

Two patients request sedation for a urologic procedure. One has just received a T4-6 spinal anesthetic. The other requests monitored anesthesia care. Will both patients require the same amount of midazolam or propofol to achieve loss of consciousness?

This question was directly answered in four recent clinical studies and one animal study. The ED50 for loss of consciousness for intravenous midazolam was 75% less during T8 spinal bupivacaine anesthesia[84] and 80% less during T8 epidural bupivacaine anesthesia when compared to monitored anesthesia care.[85] Intramuscular bupivacaine also reduced the ED50, but not to the same extent. When midazolam is administered at a rate of 1 mg every 30 seconds to healthy women about to undergo gynecologic procedures, the women in the spinal group required only 7.6 mg to achieve loss of consciousness *versus* 14.7 mg in the monitored anesthesia care group.[86] (This study can be criticized for too rapid administration of midazolam since its peak effect occurs at 3-5 minutes. Had the midazolam been administered at a dose of 1 mg every 3-5 minutes, the doses in both groups would have been less.) When morphine was added to the spinal and propofol substituted for midazolam and infused at a rate of 20 mg/kg/h, loss of consciousness was achieved sooner (4.7 versus 6.0 minutes) in the spinal group.[87] In a relevant rat study, spinal bupivacaine reduced the dose of intraperitoneal thiopental associated with blocking the corneal reflex by one third. The brain concentration of thiopental in the bupivacaine spinal group associated with an absent corneal reflex was also one third the concentration in the saline spinal group.[88] Thus, both spinal and epidural anesthesia dramatically reduce sedative requirements for midazolam and propofol.

This question has also been indirectly addressed in several other studies. The BIS50 is the BIS index below which 50%

of patients experience loss of consciousness. When the BIS50 for midazolam was determined in healthy volunteers in one study of monitored anesthesia care[89] and compared with the BIS50 determined during spinal or epidural anesthesia,[90] it was higher in the regional anesthesia study (79 versus 70). Thus, the BIS50 for loss of consciousness is not a constant. Regional anesthesia attenuates sensory input to the brain and shifts the BIS50 to a higher index. A higher BIS50 and a lower midazolam dose are associated with loss of consciousness during spinal or epidural anesthesia than during monitored anesthesia care. Similarly, 0.5 mg of midazolam was predictably associated with apnea in elderly patients during spinal anesthesia in one study,[91] but in another, it produced only mild sedation in 16 of 29 patients (and no apparent sedation in 13 of 29) at 7 minutes during monitored anesthesia care.[92] However, at 15 minutes during monitored anesthesia care, 3 of 29 became moderately sedated and 1 of 29 deeply sedated after 0.5 mg.

Spinal and epidural anesthesia reduce sedative requirements, presumably by decreasing afferent input to the brain. This observation may be the new mechanism Keats[93] was looking for to explain the cardiac arrests during spinal anesthesia reported in the closed claims study,[94] especially in view of the effects of sedatives and opioids on hypoxic control of the cardiorespiratory responses discussed previously.

## NEUROMUSCULAR BLOCKING AGENTS

### Does Advancing Age Change the Onset Time for Neuromuscular Blocking Agents?

The onset time for neuromuscular blocking agents is prolonged in the elderly. The onset times for succinylcholine, 1 mg/kg, and for vecuronium, 0.1 mg/kg, average 71 seconds and 222 seconds, respectively, for 20- to 40-year-olds and 95 seconds and 295 seconds, respectively, for 60- to 80-year-olds.[95] Priming or defasciculating doses of nondepolarizing muscle agents markedly impair oxygen saturation and pulmonary function in elderly patients.[96] Defasciculating doses also delay the onset time for succinylcholine. This information is important during the performance of rapid sequence inductions. I no longer administer defasciculating doses before injection of succinylcholine in elderly patients.

### What Is the Effect of Advancing Age on the Duration of Action of Neuromuscular Blocking Agents?

The same initial dose of nondepolarizing muscle agents is required for older patients as for younger patients, but the duration of action is prolonged for pancuronium, vecuronium, and rocuronium.[97] The recovery profile for cisatracurium and laudanosine concentrations is unaffected by age.[98] Mild intraoperative hypothermia to 34.7°C doubles the duration of action of neuromuscular blocking agents and prolongs the time to recovery after neostigmine.[99] Thus, intermediate-acting muscle relaxants can become long-acting muscle relaxants in cold elderly patients.

### Should Long-Acting Neuromuscular Blocking Agents Be Administered to Elderly Patients Whose Tracheas Are to Be Extubated at the End of the Surgical Procedure?

There is considerable economic pressure to use pancuronium for longer surgeries. However, accumulating evidence shows that long-acting neuromuscular blocking agents are associated with longer recovery room stays[100] and an increased incidence of postoperative pulmonary complications, such as atelectasis and pneumonia.[24] The likelihood of postoperative pulmonary complications with long-acting muscle relaxants increases with advanced age, increased duration of surgery, decreased body temperature, and increased density of neuromuscular blockade required for laparotomies compared with orthopedic procedures. There is also evidence to suggest that a sizable percentage of patients who satisfy rigorous extubation criteria in the operating room after reversal of their neuromuscular blockade deteriorate in the recovery.[24,101] I recommend that short- to intermediate-acting muscle relaxants be used in all elderly patients for whom extubation is planned at the end of the surgical procedure.

## POSTOPERATIVE ANALGESIA

### Does Regional Analgesia Affect Outcome?

In 1987, Yeager and colleagues demonstrated that the incidence of postoperative complications in high risk patients was greater after general anesthesia with parenteral opioid analgesia than after combined epidural-general anesthesia followed by epidural analgesia.[19] When the study was repeated for a single operation, that is, surgery on the abdominal aorta, and when postoperative analgesia was standardized (both groups received postoperative epidural analgesia), there was no difference in the outcomes between regional and general anesthesia.[102] Thus, it is possible that the results in the first study, interpreted as favoring combined epidural-general anesthesia, may actually have demonstrated the positive impact of postoperative epidural analgesia.[103] Liu and colleagues determined that after colon surgery, if postoperative analgesia was provided with epidural local anesthetic agents combined with morphine, there were fewer side effects and much shorter times to reach discharge criteria than if postoperative analgesia was provided by either intravenous morphine or epidural morphine.[26] Clearly, different postoperative analgesic regimens affect outcome. Patients are more likely to receive epidural postoperatively if epidural anesthesia is used for the surgery either with intravenous sedation or combined with general anesthesia. However, Gwirtz and colleagues reported on the successful provision of postoperative analgesia with intrathecal opioids in 5969 adults.[104] For 98%, the spinal administration took place at the end of surgery while the patient was still receiving a general anesthetic.

## REGIONAL VERSUS GENERAL ANESTHESIA

### Are There Theoretical Reasons to Prefer Regional Anesthesia?

Regional anesthesia and analgesia completely block the stress response associated with surgery if normothermia and nutrition are maintained perioperatively. Carli and Halliday compared two anesthetic techniques in patients who were undergoing elective colorectal surgery: combined epidural-general anesthesia with postoperative epidural analgesia and general anesthesia and parenteral analgesia.[105] They used an increase in muscle protein degradation and a decrease in muscle protein synthesis as their markers for surgical stress. Their patients were continuously nourished and kept normothermic for 48 hours. In the continuous epidural anesthesia and analgesia group, there was no change in the rates of muscle protein degradation and synthesis in the perioperative period. In the general anesthesia with traditional analgesia group, the typical changes in protein metabolism were observed.

Regional anesthesia also prevents central sensitization, or spinal cord "wind-up," and in doing so provides preemptive analgesia (ie, analgesic requirements are diminished postoperatively if regional anesthesia is established before surgical incision is made). Both Shir[106] and Gottschalk and associates[107] demonstrated this phenomenon in patients undergoing radical prostatectomy. Shir divided patients into three groups, epidural-only anesthesia, combined epidural-general anesthesia, and general anesthesia. The epidural-only group received significantly more local anesthesia via the epidural than the combined epidural-general group. In all patients, postoperative analgesia was provided with epidural patient-controlled analgesia (PCA). The epidural PCA demand was significantly less in the epidural-only group compared with both general anesthesia groups. Gottschalk and colleagues divided their patients into three intraoperative groups: epidural local anesthetic, epidural opioid, and no epidural medication. All patients received a general anesthetic, and all patients received epidural PCA for postoperative analgesia. Significantly less epidural PCA was required in the epidural local anesthetic group compared with the control group than in the epidural fentanyl group versus control group. Overall, the preemptive analgesia groups experienced 33% less pain while hospitalized. At 9½ weeks, 86% of the preemptive analgesia groups were pain-free and more active compared with 47% in the control group. If less pain medication is required, the side effects of opioid medications, such as respiratory depression, ileus, and urinary retention, which prolong length of stay,[26] may be reduced.

### Is Regional Anesthesia Safer Than General Anesthesia?

In outcome studies in the late 1970s and 1980s, there was a strong perception that regional anesthesia was safer than general anesthesia. A widely cited study at that time by McLaren suggested that the 28-day mortality rate in elderly hip surgery patients for general anesthesia was 4 times that found for those who had spinal anesthesia: 28% versus 7%, respectively.[108] Advocates of regional anesthesia also pointed to a retrospective study that suggested a greater incidence of dehiscence of large bowel anastomoses after general anesthesia than when general anesthesia was combined with a high spinal block.[109] The results of later studies, much better designed, forced a reevaluation of this debate. When the large bowel anastomosis study was repeated prospectively in 1988, the dehiscence rate was 17% regardless of anesthetic technique.[110] The findings of McLaren were contradicted in multiple larger prospective studies that subsequently found no difference in 28-day mortality rates for regional versus general anesthesia, 6% to 7% versus 6% to 8%, respectively, for hip surgery.[111,112] In a recent retrospective cohort study of 9425 consecutive patients who were 60 years of age or older (mean, 80.3 years) and who required repairs of fractured hips, the 7-day mortality rates were 1.3% for regional anesthesia and 1.6% for general anesthesia. The 30-day mortality rates were 4.4% and 5.4%, respectively.[113] Finally, there was no difference in the incidence of postoperative cardiovascular or cerebrovascular complications or cognitive dysfunction after elective total knee replacement in a study of 262 elderly patients who received either general anesthesia with PCA or epidural anesthesia and analgesia.[114]

When perioperative hemodynamics are well monitored and tightly controlled and equivalent postoperative analgesia is provided, no difference in cardiac morbidity or mortality is reported in patients undergoing lower extremity vascular surgery with general, spinal, or epidural anesthesia.[115,116] New or unstable angina appeared postoperatively in several patients in studies in which the epidural analgesia was discontinued. Two observations from these studies are particularly relevant. First, a greater effort on the part of the anesthesia care team was required to keep BPs and heart rates within protocol limits during and after general anesthesia (eg, with the administration of β-adrenergic blocking agents or nitroglycerin, vasoconstrictor, or inotropic agent infusions).[117,118] Second, patients who had an inadequate regional anesthetic were significantly more likely to die during their hospitalization than patients who had received a general anesthetic or a successful regional anesthetic.[115] Thus, well-managed general anesthetics, although more demanding from a hemodynamic control perspective, yield outcomes equivalent to successful regional anesthetic blocks, and inadequate regional anesthetic blocks yield outcomes worse than those observed after general anesthesia. Although clinical perceptions and theoretical considerations suggest that regional anesthesia should be safer than general anesthesia, there appears to be no difference between the two in mortality and major cardiovascular morbidity in most patient populations.

## Is There a Difference Between Regional and General Anesthesia?

There is common clinical perception among anesthesiologists that regional anesthesia is safer than general anesthesia. Although earlier clinical studies tended to support this perception, more recent ones have not. There are four major differences between past and current anesthesia studies:

1. More aggressive use of β-adrenergic blocking agents
2. The maintenance of intraoperative normothermia
3. More timely administration of antibiotic prophylaxis
4. The acceptance of lower hematocrits before transfusion is deemed necessary

Preoperative withdrawal of β-blockers is associated with an increase in silent myocardial ischemia. The addition of β-blockers is associated with a decreased incidence of untoward cardiovascular outcomes in patients with CAD undergoing noncardiac surgery. Because patients are more likely to be hypertensive and to develop tachycardia after general anesthesia than after regional anesthesia, the argument could be made that administration of β-blockers improves outcomes more after general anesthesia than after regional anesthesia. Similarly, some of the stress of surgery and subsequent hemodynamic lability is not really due to the surgery but to the stress of recovery from mild hypothermia.

Maintenance of intraoperative hypothermia may reduce the complications associated with general anesthesia greater than those associated with regional anesthesia. If there is a difference in morbidity and mortality between the two anesthetic approaches, administration of β-blockers and maintenance of normothermia may reduce the frequency of complications so that many more patients may need to be in a study in order to achieve statistical significance. One of the advantages of regional anesthesia consistently reported is reduced blood loss. However, this reduced blood loss has not necessarily translated into reduced blood transfusion because of the acceptance of a lower hematocrit before a transfusion is triggered.

There have been significant improvements in general anesthetic techniques since 1990. The introduction of the LMA and anesthetic agents with faster, more pleasant recovery profiles have reduced the stress of general anesthesia and shortened length of stay in the PACU and ambulatory surgery units to less than that seen with lidocaine spinal anesthesia. Although pain scores are slightly higher after general anesthesia than after spinal anesthesia, propofol-desflurane-fentanyl combinations are now being recommended over spinal anesthesia in these settings in elderly patients.[119]

There is a growing body of evidence that spinal and epidural anesthesia are commonly managed in ways that remove some of their advantages and narrow any possible difference between regional and general anesthesia. This controversial assertion refers to two practices. The first is a dictum that the systolic BP during spinal and epidural anesthesia should be maintained within 20% of baseline. In fact, cardiac function is improved in most elderly patients with CHF if the systolic BP is allowed to settle between 90 and 100 mm Hg during spinal and epidural anesthesia.[120,121] The second practice is the intravenous administration of 8 to 15 mL/kg of crystalloid solution before the administration of the spinal or epidural in hopes of preventing hypotension. The amount of volume administered has not been demonstrated to reduce the incidence of hypotension.[122] This prehydration frequently becomes a problem postoperatively when the block resolves. The hypervolemic state that results increases the risk of urinary retention, myocardial ischemia, and pulmonary edema. I recommend fluid restriction of the normovolemic elderly patient presenting for spinal and epidural anesthesia, viewing fluid administration like a drug that is administered judiciously, and treatment of hypotension unrelated to blood loss with inotropes or vasopressors.

## GUIDING PRINCIPLES

### How Do You Approach Patients With the Choice Between Regional and General Anesthesia?

It is difficult to ignore clinical perceptions. Death and major morbidity are only minimum outcome markers to which anesthesiologists respond. Additional endpoints may be more important in the selection process. Anesthesiologists remember the ease of administration. They remember patient satisfaction. Elderly patients tend to look better in recovery after regional anesthesia than after general. "Which is safer?" the patient asks. Every anesthesiologist must anticipate this question and be prepared with an answer. The patient wants a 1-word answer: regional or general. As usual, the question is simple and direct, but the answer is much more complex. I answer in either of two ways. "Both are safe. But I am particularly concerned about certain medical problems that you have. For this operation and with your medical problems I think that regional (or general) is preferred because . . . ." Or "Both are safe. Each has its advantages and disadvantages. Because you are most concerned about . . . . I would suggest . . . ." For any anesthesia provider, the answer takes into account his or her comfort level with the various possible anesthetic techniques, interpretation of the medical literature, opinions of expert colleagues, ability of medical personnel who may be assisting with the administration of the anesthetic, pressure of the clinical situation, concerns of the surgeon, and perception of what the patient really prefers but may be reluctant to state.

### What Are the Ten Commandments for Anesthetizing Elderly Patients?

1. Choose drug doses carefully. Elderly patients have variable, most likely decreased requirements. Take into account the additive and synergistic effects of drug combinations.
2. Think regional anesthesia but be prepared to resuscitate or administer a general anesthetic.
3. Administer β-blockers.
4. Give antibiotics in a timely fashion.
5. Avoid hypothermia.
6. Be prepared for greater hemodynamic instability intraoperatively and postoperatively.
7. Plan postoperative analgesia carefully.
8. Monitor for subclinical events. Remember that signs and symptoms of untoward events are often nonspecific in the elderly.
9. Allow the elderly more time to respond to questions, requests, and drugs, and time to emerge from anesthesia and achieve extubation criteria.
10. Remember that bad outcomes occasionally occur despite good care.

### References

1. Muravchik S. *Geroanesthesia.* St Louis, Mo: Mosby-Year Book; 1997.
2. McLeskey C, ed. *Geriatric Anesthesiology.* Baltimore, Md: Williams & Wilkins; 1997.
3. Silverstein JH, ed. Geriatric anesthesia. *Anesthesiol Clin North Am.* 2000;18 (special issue).
4. Roizen MF. *RealAge.* New York, NY: HarperCollins, 1999.
5. Oldest person in the world dies at 119 after quiet life. *Winston-Salem Journal.* December 31, 1999:A2.
6. *The Guinness Book of Records 1999.* London, United Kingdom: Guinness Publishing; 1999:162, 170.
7. Oliver CD, White SA, Platt MW. Surgery for a fractured femur and elective ICU admission at 113 yr of age. *Br J Anaesth.* 2000;84:260.
8. Fries JF. Aging, natural death, and the compression of morbidity. *N Engl J Med.* 1980;303:130.
9. Centers for Disease Control and Prevention. Mortality patterns—United States, 1997. *MMWR.* 1999;48:664.
10. Raja SN, Haythornthwaite JA. Anesthetic management of the elderly. *Anesthesiology.* 1999;91:909.
11. Emerging-Market Indicators. *The Economist.* March 4, 2000:108.
12. Clergue F, Auroy Y, Pequignot F, et al. French survey of anesthesia in 1996. *Anesthesiology.* 1999;91:1509.
13. Klopfenstein CE, Herrmann FR, Michel JP, et al. The influence of an aging surgical population on the anesthesia workload: a ten-year surgery. *Anesth Analg.* 1998;86:1165.
14. Fleisher LA, Eagle KA, Shaffer T, et al. Perioperative and long-term mortality rates after major vascular surgery: the relationship to preoperative testing in the Medicare population. *Anesth Analg.* 1999;89:849.
15. Roy RC, Overdyk FJ. The adult patient. In: Morell RC, Eichhorn JH, eds. *Patient Safety in Anesthetic Practice.* New York, NY: Churchill Livingstone; 1997:160.
16. Frank SM, Fleisher LA, Breslow MJ, et al. Perioperative maintenance of normothermia reduces the incidence of morbid cardiac events. *JAMA.* 1997;277:1127.
17. Leslie K, Sesler DI. The implications of hypothermia for early tracheal extubation following cardiac surgery. *J Cardiothorac Vasc Anesth.* 1998;12(6 suppl 2):30.
18. Greif R, Akca O, Horn E-P, et al. Supplemental perioperative oxygen to reduce the incidence of surgical wound infection. *N Engl J Med.* 2000;342:161.
19. Yeager MP, Glass DD, Neff RK, et al. Epidural anesthesia and analgesia in high-risk surgical patients. *Anesthesiology.* 1987;66:729.
20. Legasse RS. Defining anesthesia-related mortality [abstract]. *Anesthesiology.* 1998;89:A1215.
21. Legasse RS, Steinberg ES, Katz RI, et al. Defining quality of perioperative care by statistical process control of adverse outcomes. *Anesthesiology.* 1995;82:1181.
22. Silber JH, Kennedy SK, Even-Shoshan O, et al. Anesthesiologist direction and patient outcomes. *Anesthesiology.* 2000;93:152.
23. Johannessen NW, Jensen PF, Moller JT. When do postoperative complications occur? A prospective study of 20,802 patients [abstract]. *Anesthesiology.* 1991;75:A863.
24. Berg H, Roed J, Viby-Mogensen J, et al. Residual neuromuscular block is a risk factor for postoperative pulmonary complications. *Acta Anesthesiol Scand.* 1997;41:1095.
25. Groudine SB, Fisher HA, Kaufman RP Jr, et al. Intravenous lidocaine speeds the return of bowel function, decreases postoperative pain, and shortens hospital stay in patients undergoing radical retropubic prostatectomy. *Anesth Analg.* 1998;86:235.
26. Liu SS, Carpenter RL, Mackey DC, et al. Effects of perioperative analgesic technique on rate of recovery after colon surgery. *Anesthesiology.* 1995;83:757.
27. Warltier DC. β-adrenergic blocking drugs. Incredibly useful, incredibly underutilized. *Anesthesiology.* 1998;88:2.
28. Poldermans D, Boersma E, Bax JJ, et al. The effect of bisoprolol on perioperative mortality and myocardial infarction in high-risk patients undergoing vascular surgery. *N Engl J Med.* 1999;341:1789.
29. Zaugg M, Tagliente T, Lucchinetti E, et al. Beneficial effects from β-adrenergic blockade in elderly patients undergoing non-cardiac surgery. *Anesthesiology.* 1999;91:1674.
30. Wallace A, Layug B, Tateo I, et al. Prophylactic atenolol reduces postoperative myocardial ischemia. *Anesthesiology.* 1998;88:7.
31. Urban MK, Markowitz SM, Gordon MA, et al. Postoperative prophylactic administration of β-adrenergic blockers to patients at risk of myocardial ischemia. *Anesth Analg.* 2000;90:1257.
32. Badner NH, Knill RL, Brown JE, et al. Myocardial infarction after non-cardiac surgery. *Anesthesiology.* 1998;88:572.
33. Mangano DT. Adverse outcome after surgery in the year 2001—a continuing odyssey. *Anesthesiology.* 1998;88:561.
34. Sear JW, Foex P, Howell SJ. Effect of chronic intercurrent medication

with β-adrenoceptor blockade or calcium entry blockade on postoperative silent myocardial ischemia. *Br J Anaesth.* 2000;84:311.

35. Ebert TJ. Is gaining control of the autonomic nervous system important to our specialty? *Anesthesiology.* 1999;90:651.

36. Parlow JL, Begou G, Sagnard P, et al. Cardiac baroreflex during the postoperative period in patients with hypertension. Effect of clonidine. *Anesthesiology.* 1999;90:651.

37. Parlow JL, Sagnard P, Begou G, et al. The effects of clonidine on sensitivity to phenylephrine and nitroprusside in patients with essential hypertension recovering from surgery. *Anesth Analg.* 1999;88:1239.

38. Oliver MF, Goldman L, Julian DG, et al. Effect of mivazerol on perioperative cardiac complications during non-cardiac surgery in patients with coronary heart disease. The European mivazerol trial (EMIT). *Anesthesiology.* 1999;91:951.

39. Williams-Russo P, Sharrock NE, Mattis S, et al. Randomized trial of hypotensive epidural anesthesia in older adults. *Anesthesiology.* 1999;91:926.

40. Smith JS, Roizen MF, Cahalan MK, et al. Does anesthetic technique make a difference? Augmentation of systolic blood pressure during carotid endarterectomy: effects of phenylephrine versus light anesthesia and of isoflurane versus halothane on the incidence of myocardial ischemia. *Anesthesiology.* 1988;69:846.

41. Buffington CW. Hemodynamic determinants of ischemic myocardial dysfunction in the presence of coronary stenosis in dogs. *Anesthesiology.* 1985;63:651.

42. Raby KE, Brull SJ, Timimi F, et al. The effect of heart rate control on myocardial ischemia among high-risk patients after vascular surgery. *Anesth Analg.* 1999;88:477.

43. Shuler CL, Allison N, Holcomb S, et al. Accuracy of an automated blood pressure device in stable inpatients: optimum vs routine use. *Arch Intern Med.* 1998;158:714.

44. Breslow MJ, Miller CF, Parker SD, et al. Changes in T-wave morphology following anesthesia and surgery: a common recovery-room phenomenon. *Anesthesiology.* 1986;64:398.

45. Ashton CM, Thomas J, Wray NP, et al. The frequency and significance of ECTG changes after transurethral prostate resection. *J Am Geriatr Soc.* 1991;39:575.

46. Sharkey SW, Sear W, Hodges M, et al. Reversible myocardial contraction abnormalities in patients with acute noncardiac illness. *Chest.* 1998;114:98.

47. Okada M, Yotsukura M, Shimada T, et al. Clinical implications of isolated T wave inversion in adults: electrocardiographic differentiation of the underlying causes. *J Am Coll Cardiol.* 1994;24:739.

48. Gauss A, Hubner C, Radermacher P, et al. Perioperative risk of bradyarrhythmias in patients with asymptomatic chronic bifascicular block or left bundle branch block. *Anesthesiology.* 1998;88:679.

49. Posner KL, Van Norman GA, Chan V. Adverse cardiac outcomes after noncardiac surgery in patients with prior percutaneous transluminal coronary angioplasty. *Anesth Analg.* 1999;89:553.

50. Woehlck HJ, Connolly LA, Cinquegrani MP, et al. Acute smoking increases ST depression in humans during general anesthesia. *Anesth Analg.* 1999;89:856.

51. Warner MA, Offord KP, Warner ME, et al. Role of preoperative cessation of smoking and other factors in postoperative pulmonary complications: blinded prospective study of coronary artery bypass patients. *Mayo Clin Proc.* 1989;64:609.

52. Warner DO, Warner MA, Offord KP, et al. Airway obstruction and perioperative complications in smokers undergoing abdominal surgery. *Anesthesiology.* 1999;90:372.

53. Benumof JL. Preoxygenation. Best method for both efficacy and efficiency? *Anesthesiology.* 1999;91:603.

54. Baraka A, Taha SK, Aouad MT, et al. Preoxygenation. Comparison of maximal breathing and tidal volume breathing techniques. *Anesthesiology.* 1999;91:612.

55. Langeron O, Masso E, Huraux C, et al. Prediction of difficult mask ventilation. *Anesthesiology.* 2000;92:1229.

56. Kim ES, Bishop MJ. Endotracheal intubation, but not laryngeal mask airway insertion, produces reversible bronchoconstriction. *Anesthesiology.* 1999;90:391.

57. Berry A, Brimacombe J, Keller C, et al. Pulmonary airway resistance with the endotracheal tube versus laryngeal mask airway in paralyzed anesthetized adult patients. *Anesthesiology.* 1999;90:395.

58. Grief R, Laciny S, Rapf B, et al. Supplemental oxygen reduces the incidence of postoperative nausea and vomiting. *Anesthesiology.* 1999;91:1246.

59. Rosenberg-Adamsen S, Lie C, Bernhard A, et al. Effect of oxygen treatment on heart rate after abdominal surgery. *Anesthesiology.* 1999;90:380.

60. Akca O, Podolsky A, Eisenhuber E, et al. Comparable postoperative pulmonary atelectasis in patients given 30% or 80% oxygen during and 2 hours after colon resection. *Anesthesiology.* 1999;91:991.

61. Mapleson WW. Effect of age on MAC in humans: a meta-analysis. *Br J Anaesth.* 1996;76:179.

62. Schwartz AE, Tuttle RH, Poppers PJ. Electroencephalographic burst suppression in elderly and young patients anesthetized with isoflurane. *Anesth Analg.* 1989;68:9.

63. Katoh T, Bito H, Sata S. Influence of age on hypnotic requirement, bispectral index, and 95% spectral edge frequency associated with sedation induced by sevoflurane. *Anesthesiology.* 2000;92:55.

64. Katoh T, Ikeda K. The effects of fentanyl on sevoflurane requirements for loss of consciousness and skin incision. *Anesthesiology.* 1998;88:18.

65. Lockhart SH, Cohen Y, Yasuda N, et al. Cerebral uptake and elimination of desflurane, isoflurane, and halothane from rabbit brain: an *in vivo* NMR study. *Anesthesiology.* 1991;74:575.

66. Katoh T, Suguro Y, Kimura T, et al. Cerebral awakening concentration of sevoflurane and isoflurane predicted during slow and fast alveolar washout. *Anesth Analg.* 1993;77:1012.

67. Neuman MR, Weiskopf RB, Gong DH, et al. Changing from isoflurane to desflurane toward the end of anesthesia does not accelerate recovery in humans. *Anesthesiology.* 1998;88:914.

68. Hodgson PS, Liu SS, Gras TW. Does epidural anesthesia have general anesthetic effects? A prospective, randomized, double-blinded, placebo-controlled trial. *Anesthesiology.* 1999;91:1687.

69. Inagaki Y, Mashimo T, Kuzukama A, et al. Epidural lidocaine delays arousal from isoflurane anesthesia. *Anesth Analg.* 1994;79:368.

70. Stoneham MD. Less is more . . . using systolic pressure variation to assess hypovolemia. *Br J Anaesth.* 1999;83:550.

71. McKinney MS, Fee JPH. Cardiovascular effects of 50% nitrous oxide in older adult patients anaesthetized with isoflurane or halothane. *Br J Anaesth.* 1998;80:169.

72. Shafer SL. Pharmacokinetics and pharmacodynamics of the elderly. In: McLeskey CH, ed. *Geriatric Anesthesiology.* Baltimore, Md: Williams & Wilkins; 1997:123.

73. Minto CF, Schnider TW, Egan TD, et al. Influence of age and gender on the pharmacokinetics and pharmacodynamics of remifentanil. *Anesthesiology.* 1997;86:10.

74. Minto CF, Schnider TW, Shafer SL. Pharmacokinetics and pharmacodynamics of remifentanil. *Anesthesiology.* 1997;86:24.

75. Schnider TW, Minto CF, Shafer SL, et al. The influence of age on propofol pharmacodynamics. *Anesthesiology.* 1999;90:1502.

76. Kazama T, Ikeda K, Morita K, et al. Comparison of the effect-site $k_{e0}$s of propofol for blood pressure and EEG bispectral index in elderly and younger patients. *Anesthesiology.* 1999;90:1517.

77. Zheng D, Upton RN, Martinez AM, et al. The influence of the bolus injection rate of propofol on its cardiovascular effects and peak blood concentrations in sheep. *Anesth Analg.* 1998;86:1109.

78. Ludbrook GL, Upton RN, Grant C, et al. The effect of rate of administration on brain concentrations of propofol in sheep. *Anesth Analg.* 1998;86:1301.

79. Wakeling HG, Zimmerman JB, Howell S, et al. Targeting effect compartment or central compartment concentration of propofol. *Anesthesiology.* 1999;90:92.

80. Nieuwenhuijs D, Sarton E, Teppema L, et al. Propofol for monitored anesthesia care. Implications on hypoxic control of cardiorespiratory responses. *Anesthesiology.* 2000;92:46.

81. Oda Y, Mizutani K, Hase I, et al. Fentanyl inhibits metabolism of midazolam: competitive inhibition of CVP3A4 *in vitro. Br J Anaesth.* 1999;82:900.

82. Bailey PL, Pace NL, Ashburn MA, et al. Frequent hypoxemia and apnea after sedation with midazolam and fentanyl. *Anesthesiology.* 1990;73:826.

83. Babenco HD, Blouin RT, Conard PF, et al. Diphenhydramine increases ventilatory drive during alfentanil infusion. *Anesthesiology.* 1998;89:642.

84. Tversky M, Shagal M, Finger J, et al. Subarachnoid bupivacaine blockade decreases midazolam and thiopental hypnotic requirements. *J Clin Anesth.* 1994;6:487.

85. Tversky M, Shifrin V, Finger J, et al. Effect of epidural bupivacaine block on midazolam hypnotic requirements. *Reg Anesth.* 1996;21:209.

86. Ben-David B, Vaida S, Gaitini L. The influence of high spinal anesthesia on sensitivity to midazolam sedation. *Anesth Analg.* 1995;81:525.

87. Kurata J, Sugahara M, Mukaida K, et al. High spinal anesthesia in-

creases the sensitivity to the soporific effects of propofol in humans. *Anesth Analg.* 1998;86;S282.

88. Eappen S, Kissin I. Effect of subarachnoid bupivacaine block on anesthetic requirements for thiopental in rats. *Anesthesiology.* 1998;88:1036.

89. Glass PS, Bloom M, Kearse L, et al. Bispectral analysis measures sedation and memory effects of propofol, midazolam, isoflurane, and alfentanil in healthy volunteers. *Anesthesiology.* 1997;86:836.

90. Liu J, Singh H, White PF. Electroencephalogram bispectral analysis predicts the depth of midazolam-induced sedation. *Anesthesiology.* 1996;84:64.

91. Inada E, Mizumoto K, Fujioka S, et al. A low dose of midazolam causes apnea in geriatric patients under spinal anesthesia. *Anesthesiology.* 1998;89:A822.

92. Fredman B, Lahav M, Zohar E, et al. The effect of midazolam premedication on mental and psychomotor recovery in geriatric patients undergoing brief surgical procedures. *Anesth Analg.* 1999;89:1161.

93. Keats AS. Anesthesia mortality—a new mechanism. *Anesthesiology.* 1988;68:2.

94. Caplan RA, Ward RJ, Posner K, et al. Unexpected cardiac arrest during spinal anesthesia: a closed claims analysis of predisposing factors. *Anesthesiology.* 1988;68:5.

95. Koscielniak-Nelson ZJ, Bevan JC, Popovic V, et al. Onset of maximum neuromuscular block following succinylcholine or vecuronium in four age groups. *Anesthesiology.* 1993;79:229.

96. Aziz L, Jahangir SM, Choudhury SN, et al. The effect of priming with vecuronium and rocuronium on young and elderly patients. *Anesth Analg.* 1997;85:663.

97. Bevan DR, Fiset P, Balendran P, et al. Pharmacodynamic behaviour of rocuronium in the elderly. *Can J Anaesth.* 1993;40:127.

98. Ornstein E, Lien CA, Matteo RS, et al. Pharmacodynamics and pharmacokinetics of cisatracurium in geriatric surgical patients. *Anesthesiology.* 1996;84:520.

99. Leslie K, Sessler DI, Bjorksten AR, et al. Mild hypothermia alters propofol pharmacokinetics and increases the duration of action of atracurium. *Anesth Analg.* 1995;80:1007.

100. Ballantyne JC, Chang Y. The impact of choice of muscle relaxant on postoperative recovery time: a retrospective study. *Anesth Analg.* 1997;86:65.

101. Kopman AF, Yee PS, Neuman GG. Relationship of the train-of-four fade ratio to clinical signs and symptoms of residual paralysis in awake volunteers. *Anesthesiology.* 1997;86:65.

102. Baron JF, Bertrand M, Barre E, et al. Combined epidural and general anesthesia versus general anesthesia for abdominal aortic surgery. *Anesthesiology.* 1991;75:611.

103. Liu S, Carpenter RL, Neal JM. Epidural anesthesia and analgesia. *Anesthesiology.* 1995;82:1474.

104. Gwirtz KH, Young JV, Byers RS, et al. The safety and efficacy of intrathecal opioid analgesia for acute postoperative pain: seven years experience with 5969 surgical patients at Indiana University Hospital. *Anesth Analg.* 1999;88:599.

105. Carli F, Halliday D. Continuous epidural blockade arrests the postoperative decrease in muscle protein fractional synthetic rate in surgical patients. *Anesthesiology.* 1997;86:1033.

106. Shir Y. The effect of epidural versus general anesthesia on postoperative pain and analgesic requirement in patients undergoing radical prostatectomy. *Anesthesiology.* 1994;89:49.

107. Gottschalk A, Smith DS, Jobes DR, et al. Preemptive epidural analgesia and recovery from radical prostatectomy: a randomized controlled trial. *JAMA.* 1998;279:1076.

108. McLaren AD. Mortality studies. *Reg Anesth.* 1982;7:S172.

109. Aitkenhead AR, Wishart HY, Brown DA, et al. High spinal nerve block for large bowel anastomosis. *Br J Anaesth.* 1978;50:177.

110. Worsley MH, Wishart HY, Peebles-Brown DH, et al. High spinal nerve block for large bowel anastomosis. *Br J Anaesth.* 1988;60:836.

111. Davis FM, Woolner DF, Frampton C, et al. Prospective, multi-centre trial of mortality following general or spinal anesthesia for hip fracture surgery in the elderly. *Br J Anaesth.* 1987;59:1080.

112. Valentin N, Lomholt B, Jensen JS, et al. Spinal or general anesthesia for surgery of the fractured hip. A prospective study of mortality in 578 patients. *Br J Anaesth.* 1986;58:284.

113. O'Hara DA, Duff A, Berlin JA, et al. The effect of anesthetic technique on postoperative outcomes in hip fracture repair. *Anesthesiology.* 2000;92:947.

114. Williams-Russo P, Sharrock NE, Mattis S, et al. Cognitive effects after epidural vs general anesthesia in older patients. *JAMA.* 1995;274:44.

115. Bode RH Jr, Lewis KP, Zarich SW, et al. Cardiac outcome after peripheral vascular surgery. A comparison of general and regional anesthesia. *Anesthesiology.* 1996;84:3.

116. Christopherson R, Beattie C, Frank SM, et al. Perioperative morbidity in patients randomized to epidural or general anesthesia for lower extremity vascular surgery. *Anesthesiology.* 1993;79:422.

117. Crowley H. More beta blockers are required to control tachycardia in general than epidural anesthesia. *Anesth Analg.* 1990;70:S74.

118. Glavan JJ. Association of hypertension and heart rate lability with intraoperative myocardial ischemia. *Anesth Analg.* 1995;80:SCA105.

119. Fredman B, Zahar E, Philipov A, et al. The induction, maintenance, and recovery characteristics of spinal versus general anesthesia in elderly patients. *J Clin Anesth.* 1998;10:623.

120. Baron J-F, Corlat P, Mundler D, et al. Left ventricular global and regional function during lumbar epidural anesthesia in patients with and without angina pectoris. *Anesthesiology.* 1987;66:621.

121. Sharrock NE, Mineo R, Urquhart B, et al. Haemodynamic effects and outcome analysis of hypotensive extradural anesthesia in controlled hypertensive patients undergoing total hip arthoplasty. *Br J Anaesth.* 1991;67:17.

122. Buggy D, Higgins P, Moran C, et al. Prevention of spinal anesthesia-induced hypotension in the elderly: comparison between preanesthetic administration of crystalloids, colloids, or no prehydration. *Anesth Analg.* 1997;84:106.

# CHAPTER

# 59

# The Obstetric Patient

Tammy Y. Euliano
Donald Caton

Obstetric anesthesia presents exceptional challenges and opportunities. The privilege of caring for patients during such an extraordinary time and the opportunity to optimize their delivery can be one of the most rewarding experiences in medicine. Yet, events on the labor and delivery ward can be some of the most terrifying for anesthesiologists. Although these events cannot be eliminated, knowledge of the factors that make obstetric anesthesia different from other subspecialty areas is vital to providing optimal care.

First, the patient population is unique: physically, physiologically, and in response to drugs and techniques.

Second, anesthesia affects two individuals, and the effects of anesthetic interventions on the fetus are thus a substantial concern.

Third, despite the appearance on many wards, the process of labor and delivery is normal and natural. The vast majority of deliveries proceed to completion with a good outcome independent of our involvement. This fact puts on us the onus of demonstrating that our efforts to relieve pain leave both the patient and her child no worse off than if we had done nothing at all.

Fourth, the analgesic goal is often only the control of pain, rather than complete relief.

Finally, and perhaps most important, the delivery of a child, including the pain associated with it, has different social and personal implications from the pain associated with a surgical procedure such as an appendectomy. For a brief period, the anesthesiologist enters an intimate and emotional time in the life of the patient and her family. We must therefore be especially sensitive to their psychologic and physical needs and be ready to work with them.

The principles and standards of good anesthesia care apply to every patient, regardless of the location within the institution or the clinical situation. We must adapt these general rules to the circumstances of obstetric patients, to their physiology or pathophysiology, and to the surgical requirements. Such considerations help us to develop a special set of guidelines for this subspecialty (Table 59–1). These guidelines do not nullify general principles of good care but merely modify them.

We must occasionally ignore elements of the guidelines specific for obstetric anesthesia and revert to principles of general operating room (OR) care. This situation usually occurs when a patient has a concurrent medical or surgical problem—severe cardiac or pulmonary disease, for example—that overshadows the obstetric considerations. Similarly, the presence of an obscure medical problem for which there is no specific information to guide us in her obstetric anesthetic management, as with Marfan syndrome or a rare metabolic disorder, requires reference to the large body of information gained from our work in the OR.

## NORMAL CHANGES IN PREGNANCY

Pregnancy involves significant changes in virtually every maternal tissue and function. These changes form the basis for many aspects of our care of obstetric patients.

### *What Cardiovascular Changes Occur?*

Virtually every segment of the maternal cardiovascular system adapts to support the fetus and minimize the impact of aortocaval compression (Table 59–2). Increased blood volume and cardiac output are accompanied by decreased systemic vascular resistance and increased venous capacity; thus, at term, blood pressure (BP) and central venous pressure are approximately normal. By about 20 weeks' gestation, the uterus is of sufficient size to compress the vena cava or aorta when the patient is supine. Ten percent of parturients become symptomatic in this position, and 5% experience severe hypotension and bradycardia (*supine hypotensive syndrome*). Even in asymptomatic parturients, uterine blood flow falls by an average of 20%.[1] Thus, all pregnant patients should be maintained in a left tilted position of at least 15° when they are supine.

The sympathetic response to labor pain induces additional

**TABLE 59–1.** Guidelines for Obstetric Anesthesia

**Goals of Obstetric Anesthesia**

Alleviate the pain of labor.
Provide optimum conditions for operative obstetrics.
   Cesarean section
   Vaginal delivery
   Application of forceps
   Repair of lacerations and episiotomy
   Relaxation of the uterus

**Constraints Governing Obstetric Anesthesia**

Interfere as little as possible with the progress of labor and delivery.
Minimize the effects of drugs on the infant.
Maintain fetal homeostasis, including reflexes involved in the adaptation to
   extrauterine life.

**TABLE 59–2.** Physiologic Changes at Term Pregnancy

| Variable | Change |
|---|---|
| Total blood volume | ↑ 45% |
| Plasma volume | ↑ 55% |
| Red blood cell volume | ↑ 30% |
| Stroke volume | ↑ 25% |
| Heart rate | ↑ 20% |
| Cardiac output | ↑ 50% |
| Systemic vascular resistance | ↓ 30% |
| Pulmonary vascular resistance | ↓ 50% |
| Venous capacitance | ↑ 50% |
| Minute ventilation | ↑ 35% |
| Alveolar ventilation | ↑ 75% |
| Tidal volume | ↑ 30% |
| Respiratory rate | ↑ 5% |
| Functional residual capacity | ↓ 20% |
| Oxygen consumption | ↑ 50% |

stresses on the cardiovascular system, which may be at least partially abated with adequate analgesia. After delivery, autotransfusion from contraction of the uterus and improved venous return from relief of aortocaval compression further increase cardiac output up to 75%[2] (Fig. 59–1). These changes are of particular concern and possible consequence in patients with preexisting cardiac disease (eg, mitral stenosis).

### *What Pulmonary Changes Occur?*

Early in pregnancy, progesterone increases the sensitivity of the central respiratory center to carbon dioxide ($CO_2$).[3] This reduction in the $CO_2$ set-point causes an increase in minute

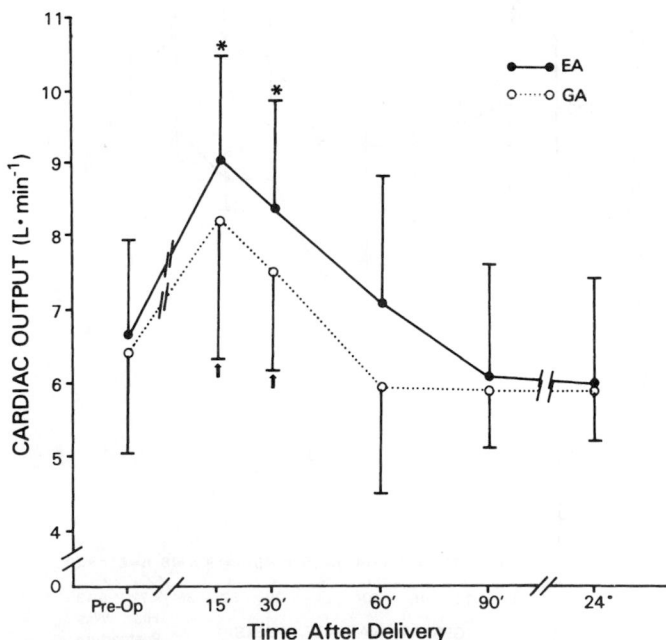

**FIGURE 59–1.** Cardiac output with cesarean section. The data illustrate the rise that occurs immediately following, several minutes after, and 1 day after delivery. The type of anesthesia used had no significant effect on the magnitude or pattern of response. (From James CF, Banner T, Caton D. Cardiac output in women undergoing cesarean section with epidural or general anesthesia. *Am J Obstet Gynecol.* 1989;160:1178.)

ventilation and a compensated respiratory alkalosis. A typical arterial blood gas at term would be as follows:

| pH | $PaCO_2$ | $PaO_2$ | $HCO_3^-$ |
|-----|-----|-----|-----|
| 7.44 | 30 | 103 | 20 |

Oxygen ($O_2$) consumption (and $CO_2$ production) progressively increases during gestation (Fig. 59–2). Surprisingly, the increased minute ventilation is achieved primarily through increased tidal volume (see Table 59–2).[4] Increased chest circumference through flaring of the rib cage maintains most lung volumes in spite of the enlarged uterus. A notable exception is the 20% reduction in functional residual capacity.

The pulmonary metabolic changes of decreased functional residual capacity with increased $O_2$ consumption combine to incite rapid desaturation during periods of apnea (Fig. 59–3). In addition, the relative hypocapnia must be considered during controlled ventilation. Although acidosis should be avoided, hyperventilation reduces venous return and causes a leftward shift of the oxyhemoglobin dissociation curve, potentially resulting in decreased fetal $PaO_2$. Increased cardiac output reduces alveolar dead space, abolishing the usual difference between arterial and end-tidal $CO_2$.[5] Thus, the end-tidal $CO_2$ during controlled ventilation should be maintained at 30 to 32 mm Hg.

During the peripartum period, most smooth muscle becomes highly reactive. Bronchospasm among asthmatics and smokers may become a significant problem when tracheal intubation is required.[6]

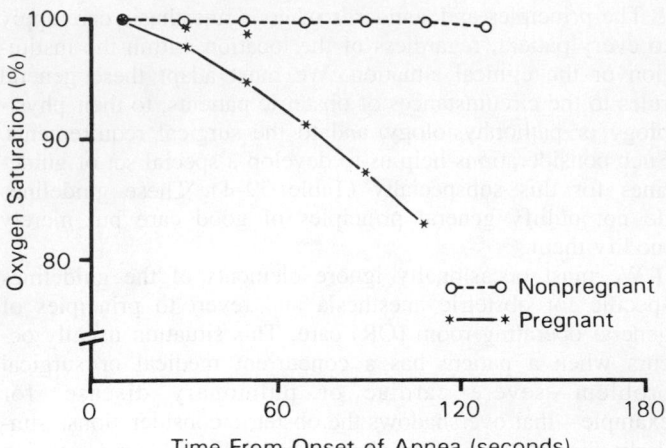

**FIGURE 59–3.** Oxygen saturation measured by pulse oximetry of a pregnant and nonpregnant patient. The pregnant patient was also obese. The rapid decline in saturation was caused by the decreased functional residual capacity and the increased metabolic rate.

## Why Are Parturients Always Considered a "Full Stomach"?

Most pregnant women experience heartburn induced by changes in the gastrointestinal system including (1) increased intragastric pressure due to the enlarged uterus; (2) decreased lower esophageal sphincter tone due to an upward shift of the stomach and esophagus, as well as hormone-induced lower esophageal sphincter relaxation; and (3) increased gastric acid secretion, in part due to placental secretion of gastrin. Gastric emptying, although normal during pregnancy, is slowed during labor due to anxiety, pain, and opioids.[7] These factors, along with recent oral intake, place parturients at a markedly increased risk for pulmonary aspiration of gastric contents with impaired consciousness (eg, general anesthesia, seizure).

### Acid Aspiration Prophylaxis

Acid aspiration remains the single most common cause of maternal mortality from anesthesia in the United States.[8] Some have advocated a nil per os (NPO) status for laboring women, citing the historic risk factors for acid aspiration: gastric fluid pH <2.5 and volume >25 mL (although data for the latter are weak,[9] and twice the volume is probably safe[10]). The current American Society of Anesthesiologists Practice Guidelines[11] recommend "modest amounts of clear liquids . . . for uncomplicated laboring patients," but they recommend against any solid food ingestion.

For cesarean section, oral administration of 15 to 30 mL 0.3 M sodium citrate (nonparticulate antacid) no more than 30 minutes before delivery is recommended. Additional measures that have proven effective include histamine$_2$ receptor antagonists (even 30 minutes before induction if administered intravenously[12]), omeprazole, and metoclopramide. Cricoid pressure is essential during rapid-sequence induction of general anesthesia.

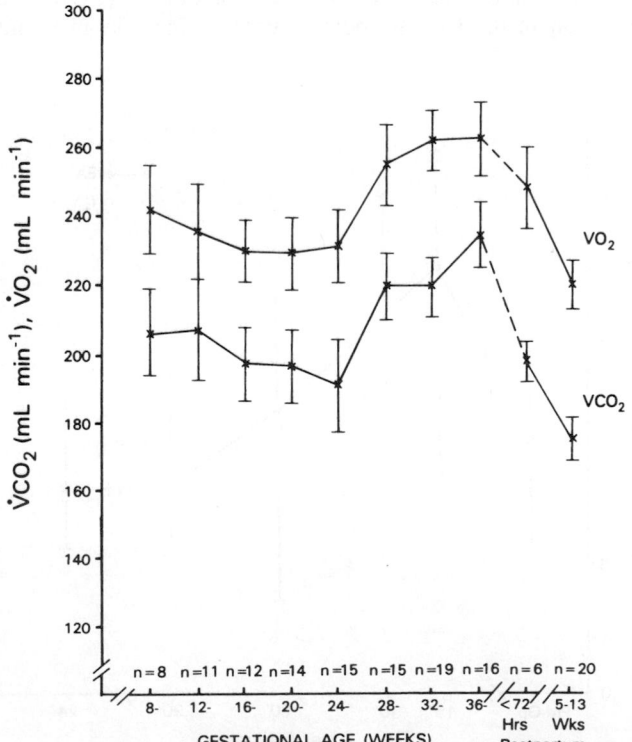

**FIGURE 59–2.** Oxygen consumption and carbon dioxide production of normal patients during pregnancy. Most of the increase during the third trimester reflects the high metabolic activity of the fetal, placental, and uterine tissues. (From Rees GB, Broughton Pipkin F, et al. A longitudinal study of respiratory changes in normal human pregnancy with cross-sectional data on subjects with pregnancy-induced hypertension. *Am J Obstet Gynecol.* 1990;162:826.)

## What Renal and Hepatic Changes Occur?

Increased renal plasma flow of 75% to 80% and increased glomerular filtration rate of 50% result in mild glucosuria.

Serum urea nitrogen and creatinine fall slightly (8-9 mg/dL and 0.5-0.6 mg/dL, respectively).

Liver transaminase levels increase to the upper limits of normal, and bile stasis predisposes to the formation of gallstones. Albumin levels fall primarily due to dilution, resulting in decreased protein binding of many medications (eg, local anesthetics, thiopental).

## What Uterine Changes Occur?

The uterus must enlarge to accommodate the growing fetus. The fetus depends on uterine blood flow for exchange of $O_2$, nutrients, $CO_2$, and heat with the maternal circulation. Uterine blood flow at term is approximately 700 mL/min (12% of maternal cardiac output) and depends on maintenance of adequate perfusion pressure (Fig. 59–4). Although there are no vasodilators selective for the uterine vasculature, nor vasopressors that exclude it, ephedrine appears to increase maternal BP with the least increase in uterine vascular resistance (UVR). Phenylephrine increases UVR, but this effect may be offset by an increase in perfusion pressure, maintaining uterine blood flow.[13] Most practitioners choose to avoid using it, however.

## What Hematologic Changes Occur?

Plasma volume increases more than red blood cell mass (see Table 59–2), resulting in a dilutional anemia with a normal hematocrit of approximately 35%. At term, parturients are in a hypercoagulable state due to increases in several clotting factors. Increased platelet turnover is countered by increased production, netting a normal or slightly decreased platelet count. However, 8% of healthy parturients will have a platelet count of $<150\ 000/\mu L$, and almost 1% will be $<100\ 000/\mu L$.[14] Although a diagnosis of exclusion that is best made retrospectively, gestational thrombocytopenia is a benign condition and requires only careful surveillance as long as the platelet count is $>50\ 000/\mu L$.[15]

### Transfusion

The average blood loss during an uncomplicated, singleton vaginal delivery ranges from 400 to 600 mL. With twins or an uncomplicated cesarean section, this number is doubled. Transfusion is extremely rare for several reasons: (1) despite the relatively large volume of blood loss, it contains fewer red cells because of the dilutional anemia; (2) immediately after delivery, central blood volume is increased approximately 500 mL due to improved venous return from the periphery and uterine contraction; and (3) within 2 weeks of delivery, the maternal blood volume approximates prepartum levels resulting in hemoconcentration. Transfusion is reserved for symptomatic patients or those with preexisting conditions (cardiac disease in particular) in whom the reduction in $O_2$-carrying capacity is not tolerated. If substantial blood loss is anticipated, and transfusion is not an option (eg, patient is a Jehovah's Witness), intraoperative autologous blood collection and autotransfusion (Cell Saver) should be considered.[16]

## Should Coagulation Be Assessed Before Regional Anesthesia?

The answer is a simple "yes," and usually a history directed at discerning a bleeding predisposition is adequate. Although used since the early 1900s, the bleeding time does not predict risk of hemorrhage.[17,18] In fact, no single test is entirely suitable. Despite the 1% risk of significant gestational thrombocytopenia, some recommend against routine assessment of platelet count, citing the potential for increased morbidity from unnecessarily invasive obstetric management.[19]

Because preeclamptic patients are at risk for developing HELLP (*h*emolysis, *e*levated *l*iver enzymes, *l*ow *p*latelets) syndrome, their platelet count should be determined. Determination of a partial thromboplastin time (PTT) and prothrombin time (PT) are necessary in preeclampsia only if the platelet count or lactate dehydrogenase level is abnormal.[20] Coagulation studies should also be performed in parturients with moderate to severe placental abruption or prolonged fetal death in utero.[21]

The minimum safe platelet count for regional anesthesia is a matter of debate. Beilin and colleagues[22] found no reported neurologic complications in 30 patients who underwent epidural placement with platelets $<100\ 000/\mu L$ (69 000-98 000). It is our practice to withhold epidural analgesia for a platelet count $<80\ 000/\mu L$. For those with $<100\ 000$ platelets/$\mu L$ or with evidence of a declining platelet count, we use a low concentration of local anesthetic, supplemented with opioids. This technique allows a greater chance of detecting an evolving epidural hematoma because motor weakness would not be expected from the anesthetic alone.

## What Physical Changes Occur?

In addition to an enlarged abdomen, the rib cage expands and the breasts increase in volume, sometimes to the point of interfering with placement of the laryngoscope blade (a short handle or straight blade are helpful). Swelling of mucous membranes is common, causing many women to complain of a "stuffy nose," as well as recurrent epistaxis. This may complicate nasotracheal intubation or nasogastric tube placement. In preeclamptic patients, generalized edema may involve the vocal cords and should be suspected in the presence of hoarseness. Elsewhere in the body, relaxin hormone affects ligaments, resulting in complaints of backache (particularly in the sacroiliac joint) and joint injuries. Effects of relaxin are evident during placement of neuraxial anesthesia, with re-

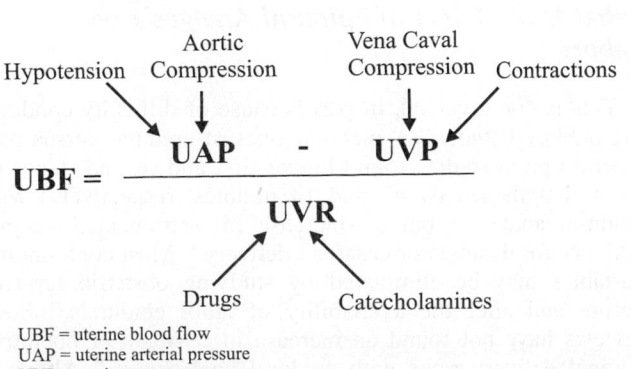

$$UBF = \frac{UAP - UVP}{UVR}$$

with labels: Hypotension, Aortic Compression, Vena Caval Compression, Contractions pointing to UAP and UVP; Drugs, Catecholamines pointing to UVR.

UBF = uterine blood flow
UAP = uterine arterial pressure
UVP = uterine venous pressure
UVR = uterine vascular resistance

**FIGURE 59–4.** Uterine blood flow determinants.

duced resistance and a different feel to needle insertion, increasing the risk of dural puncture.

## LABOR

### What Are the Stages of Labor?

The first stage of labor begins with the onset of regular uterine contractions sufficient to cause cervical change and ends with complete cervical dilation. During this phase, pain is mediated by sympathetic fibers that enter the spinal cord at T10-12 (Fig. 59–5). Patients may complain of back pain, particularly with an abnormal fetal presentation (eg, occiput posterior).

The first stage of labor may be subdivided into a *latent phase* of slow cervical dilation and a more rapid *active phase* (>1.2 cm/h nullipara, >1.5 cm/h multipara). Most women enter the active phase between 3 and 5 cm dilation. The second stage begins with complete cervical dilation and ends with delivery of the infant. Pain during this stage is primarily somatic sacral in origin (S2-4) due to distention of the vagina, vulva, and perineum. The third stage is from the delivery of the infant to the delivery of the placenta.

### What Are the Analgesic Options?

Prepared childbirth reduces labor pain scores in primiparas[23] but may not reduce their desire for analgesia. Inhalation analgesia with nitrous oxide is used occasionally at our institution, and successful use of desflurane has been reported.[24] Although formerly popular, the "Penthrane whistle" (a low-tech method for patient-controlled delivery of methoxyflurane) has fallen out of favor due to concerns over loss of airway reflexes, amnesia, and delivery room pollution.

### Parenteral Opioids

Opioids such as meperidine or an agonist-antagonist such as butorphanol or nalbuphine are frequently offered. The latter are growing in popularity due to the "ceiling effect" on respiratory depression,[25] although no maternal or neonatal benefit has been documented. Patient-controlled intravenous opioid analgesia with meperidine or fentanyl has met with variable success.

### Regional Analgesia

Various nerve blocks have been used for labor analgesia. Although it provides pain relief for the first stage, the *paracervical block* is not popular in the United States due to a high rate of fetal complications, particularly bradycardia.[26] In Scandinavian countries, however, a low-dose superficial paracervical block technique is commonly used.[27] *Pudendal block* is effective for the second stage of labor; complications are primarily related to failure of the block and local anesthetic toxicity from multiple attempts. *Lumbar sympathetic block* at the L2 level provides excellent first-stage analgesia without motor block and has been reported to both shorten the duration of labor and improve a dysfunctional labor pattern.[28,29] Although complications are rare, the technique has not become popular, in part because it is unfamiliar and requires multiple injections.

Epidural analgesia is most commonly employed. A thorough meta-analysis of randomized controlled trials comparing epidural analgesia with parenteral opioids for labor[30] found improved patient satisfaction with the former. *Continuous spinal* analgesia has not regained popularity since the microcatheter was removed from the US market. The risk of spinal headache is too great in this population to use the 18- or 20-gauge epidural catheters available.

The choice of analgesic technique should be based on coexisting medical conditions, patient preferences, and clinical resources, as well as the availability, experience, and skill level of the obstetrician and anesthetist.

### What Is the Effect of Epidural Analgesia on Labor?

This is controversial, in part because of difficulty conducting unbiased studies. A meta-analysis of epidural versus parenteral opioid studies found longer first and second stages of labor (lengthened by 42 and 14 minutes, respectively) with epidural analgesia but no increase in instrumented vaginal delivery for dystocia or cesarean delivery.[30] Most confounding variables may be eliminated by studying obstetric services before and after the availability of labor epidurals.[31] Such reviews have not found an increase in cesarean or operative vaginal delivery rates with epidural analgesia.[32–34] Although more controversial, early (3-5 cm dilation) administration of epidural analgesia does not prolong labor, increase the use of

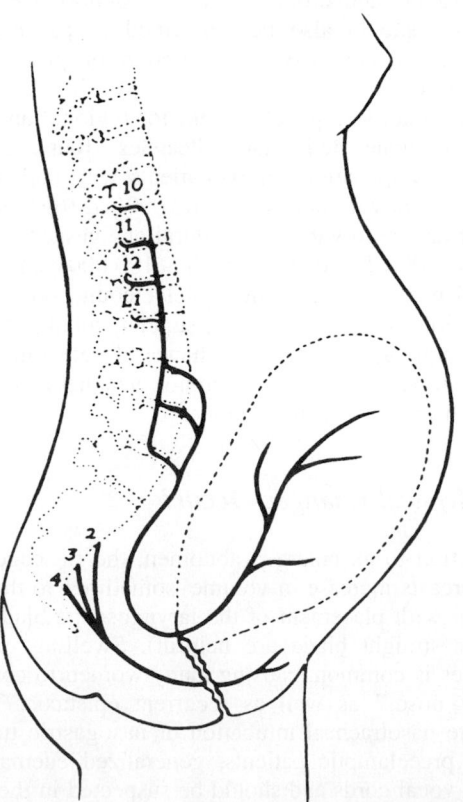

**FIGURE 59–5.** Pain pathways of labor. Stage 1: Sympathetic fibers that travel through Frankenhauser's plexus at the cervix, then with the hypogastric nerves to the paravertebral sympathetic chain at L2-3, then through the dorsal root ganglia of T10-L1. Stage 2: Somatic to S2-4 via the pudendal nerve.

oxytocin, or increase the incidence of operative delivery in nulliparous patients.[35]

## What Is the Effect of Analgesia on the Fetus and Newborn?

Drug transfer across the placenta is similar to that across the blood-brain barrier. That is, low molecular weight, highly lipid soluble agents that are not highly protein bound readily traverse into the fetal circulation. Timing of drug administration is also important; for example, meperidine levels in the neonate are highest 2 to 3 hours after intravenous maternal administration[36] due to ion trapping of metabolites.

With neuraxial analgesia, the maternal blood levels of most agents are minimized. In fact, the meta-analysis by Halpern and colleagues found improved neonatal outcomes with epidural analgesia versus parenteral opioids (fewer Apgar scores <7 at 1 and 5 minutes, less use of naloxone, and fewer newborns with low pH).[30]

Maternal opioids may cause neonatal respiratory depression and delayed sucking ability, perhaps interfering with early breastfeeding. Intrapartum, even small doses of opioids affect the fetal heart rate (FHR) tracing. The decreased short-term beat-to-beat variability may obscure interpretation. No similar effect has been reported with the local anesthetics employed for epidural analgesia.

## What Technique Should Be Used for Neuraxial Analgesia?

### Epidural

Table 59–3 is a sample technique employed at our institution. Several points deserve further comment. The choice of loss of resistance fluid is controversial. Although some advocate air, severe headache and neurologic deficits have been attributed to pneumocephalus and cord compression.[37] We prefer saline with a small air bubble. Lack of compression of the bubble is an excellent sign of proper location and is particularly useful when observing placement by a trainee.

The test dose has also been a matter of debate. Use of epinephrine as an intravascular marker is hampered by baseline maternal heart rate variability, coupled with pain-induced

---

**TABLE 59–3.** Sample Technique for Initiation of Labor Epidural Analgesia

1. Fluid bolus: 10 mL/kg of balanced salt solution or hetastarch, preferably warmed
2. Sitting or lateral decubitus position based on patient preference with blood pressure and continuous heart rate monitoring of both mother and fetus
3. Location of epidural space by LOR to saline technique with needle bevel aligned parallel to long-axis of spine
4. Test dose: 3 mL 1.5% to 2% lidocaine with epinephrine 1:200 000
5. Catheter threaded approximately 5 cm into epidural space
6. Patient allowed to straighten back, followed by catheter taping
7. After negative aspiration, catheter bolused with 5 to 10 mL low-concentration local ± opioid
8. PCEA initiated at 6 to 10 mL/h; 4 to 5 mL demand bolus with 15-min lockout and 20 to 30 mL/h maximum

LOR, loss of resistance; PCEA, patient-controlled epidural analgesia.

---

tachycardia during contractions. In addition, intravascular epinephrine increases UVR and may dramatically increase BP in preeclamptic patients. Some contend that negative aspiration alone is sufficient,[38] but others disagree.[39] We recommend the use of 15 µg epinephrine in 1.5% to 2% lidocaine (3 mL of local anesthetic containing epinephrine at a concentration of 1:200 000) injected immediately after a contraction, with continuous maternal and FHR monitoring. An increase in maternal heart rate of >10 beats/minute is 100% sensitive and 73% specific for intravascular placement.[40]

Overthreading of the catheter may adversely affect the quality of the block; 5 cm appears to be the optimal distance.[41] Taping of the catheter should not occur until the patient straightens her back, as the distance from the skin to the ligamentum flavum changes significantly, particularly in obese patients.[42]

### Combined Spinal-Epidural

It was hoped that combined spinal-epidural (CSE) analgesia would overcome some of the purported drawbacks of conventional epidural analgesia (delayed onset of analgesia, motor blockade, prolonged first stage of labor, increased risk of dystocia), in part by allowing patients to ambulate. In fact, CSE may result in more rapid cervical dilation when compared with conventional epidural analgesia,[43] but this effect is unrelated to ambulation.[44] There is no decrease in the incidence of cesarean section,[45] but the combined technique does provide a more rapid onset of analgesia, resulting in improved patient satisfaction after 20 minutes.[44] The major drawback is the 40% to 50% incidence of moderate to severe intrathecal opioid-induced pruritus,[46] although this is usually self-limited.

Several techniques for CSE have been proposed, but the needle-through-needle technique is most popular. When the epidural space is located by loss of resistance, the fluid used for identification is not injected because this may push the dura out of reach of the spinal needle, which only protrudes 10 to 15 mm beyond the epidural needle tip. A 25- or 27-gauge pencil point spinal needle is advanced through the epidural needle until cerebrospinal fluid is obtained. Bupivacaine, 2.5 mg (1 mL of 0.25%) with 10 µg sufentanil (0.2 mL) is commonly injected, resulting in analgesia within 5 minutes and minimal motor blockade. Care must be taken with the administration of epidural fluid (either local or saline) to avoid cephalad spread of the intrathecal drugs due to compression of the intrathecal space.[47] Before clearing for ambulation, examination should include motor assessment: straight leg raises, partial deep knee bends, and assessment for orthostatic hypotension.

It appears that some practitioners use CSE exclusively, whereas others are less impressed with its benefits over standard epidural analgesia. Patients for whom we prefer this technique include the following:

1. Women very early in labor
2. Those who wish to ambulate
3. Patients in late stages of labor (need rapid onset with minimal motor weakness)

However, if Tsen and colleagues' study[43] demonstrating more rapid cervical dilation is successfully replicated, we will reconsider this position.

## How Should a Labor Epidural Be Dosed?

Continuous infusion is superior to intermittent bolusing because it reduces the potential for tachyphylaxis. Patient-controlled epidural analgesia (PCEA) (basal infusion rate supplemented by on-demand boluses) provides the patient some control and has become the method of choice at our institution (Table 59–4). The neurologic and cardiovascular toxicity profiles of both ropivacaine[48] and levobupivacaine[49] are more favorable than that of bupivacaine. Early reports of reduced motor blockade from ropivacaine did not recognize its significantly lower potency.[50] In our practice, using fractionated dosing for boluses and PCEA for labor, the improved toxicity profile probably does not outweigh the increased cost of either new drug.

## What Should Be Done About an Inadvertent Dural Puncture?

Ideally, the needle or catheter is removed and replaced at a different interspace. If, however, an experienced anesthetist punctured the dura after a prolonged attempt at epidural placement, and if the anesthesia care team will not change during the expected time to delivery, consider placing the epidural catheter into the subarachnoid space. Although not supported by a controlled study,[51] some have found a reduced risk of postdural puncture headache (PDPH) with this management[52] (and personal experience). Use of an intrathecal catheter during labor can provide superior analgesia but must be accompanied by extreme caution. The patient and the entire care team, particularly the nursing staff, should be aware. Bupivacaine, 2.5 mg, with or without fentanyl 10 μg on patient request (approximately every 1-2 hours, in our experience) provides effective analgesia with minimal motor weakness.

Although some recommend prophylactic epidural blood patch (EBP), we do not. Depending on bevel orientation, 30% to 70% of patients will not develop PDPH and, of those who do, up to 70% may be treated with caffeine alone. Thus, most EBP patients would receive an unnecessary invasive procedure.

## How Can Inadequate Epidural Analgesia Be Improved?

Pain may recur via several mechanisms:

1. Catheter location outside the epidural space, either through migration or failure of original placement

2. Progression of labor with descent of the fetal head (ie, a change in the pain pattern)
3. Fetal malposition, particularly occiput-posterior with persistent maternal back pain
4. Bladder distention
5. Rarely, abruption or uterine rupture.

The first step in assessing such pain is to ascertain whether the epidural is working. If there is any question, an unequivocal test dose should be administered (eg, 5 mL of 1.5%-2% lidocaine with 1:200 000 epinephrine). Such a dose would be expected to cause recognizable motor weakness, the lack of which identifies placement outside the epidural space. If failure of the catheter is not recognized until complete cervical dilation, pudendal block or intrathecal injection of bupivacaine ± opioid should be considered.

If the epidural has clearly been functioning, the analgesia level should be determined and the patient questioned about the character and location of the pain. Although its etiology is unclear,[53] management options for unilateral epidural anesthesia include withdrawing the catheter 1 to 2 cm (depending on the original depth of insertion), bolusing the catheter with the patient's unblocked side down, or replacing the catheter. Back pain may indicate an abnormal fetal presentation (eg, occiput-posterior) and is often difficult if not impossible to eradicate. Addition of opioid to the infusion may be helpful. Presence of other "hot spots" is similarly treated with opioids.

## What Monitoring and Recordkeeping Are Appropriate?

The American Society of Anesthesiologists' Guidelines for Regional Anesthesia in Obstetrics state only that vital signs and FHR must be monitored and documented by a qualified individual.[54] Our practice is to record vital signs for at least 20 minutes after institution of labor analgesia and after any manual re-doses. In the interim, the BP cycles at 15-minute intervals with appropriate alarm settings and is recorded at 30-minute intervals by the nursing staff. There are standing orders for the nursing staff in the event of altered consciousness, respiratory distress, or hemodynamic instability.

## What Are the Complications of Neuraxial Analgesia and How Should They Be Managed?

### Hypotension

Due to the sympathectomy induced by neuraxial anesthesia, hypotension is the most common side effect. Volume expan-

**TABLE 59–4.** Suggested Labor Epidural Dosing Regimen

| Procedure | Medication | Concentration (%) | Opioid | Volume |
|---|---|---|---|---|
| Test dose | Lidocaine + epinephrine 1:200 000 | 1.5–2 | | 3 mL |
| Initial bolus | Bupivacaine/levobupivacaine | 0.0625–0.125 | Fentanyl 2.5–10 μg/mL | 5–10 mL |
| | Ropivacaine | 0.1–0.2 | Fentanyl 2.5–10 μg/mL | 5–10 mL |
| Infusion | Bupivacaine/levobupivacaine | 0.0625*–0.125 | Fentanyl 2.5 μg/mL | 6–10 mL/h + 4 mL q15m NTE 25 mL/h |
| | Ropivacaine | 0.1*–0.2 | Fentanyl 2.5 μg/mL | 6–10 mL/h + 4 mL q15m NTE 25 mL/h |
| Top up | Lidocaine | 0.5–1 | | 10–15 mL |
| | Bupivacaine/levobupivacaine | 0.1 | | 10–15 mL |
| | Ropivacaine | 0.15 | | 10–15 mL |

*The lowest concentrations usually require opioids, frequently unnecessary at the higher concentrations.
NTE, not to exceed.

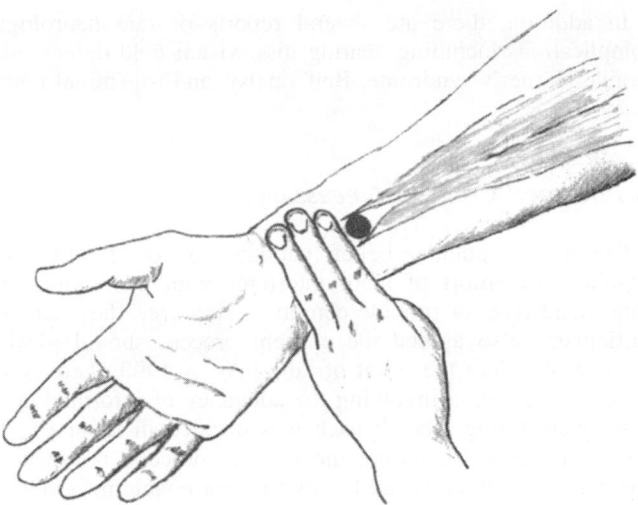

FIGURE 59–6. Location of the P-6 antinausea acupressure point.

sion (10 mL/kg lactated Ringer's or 1 L hetastarch 6% given immediately before the block)[55,56] and avoidance of aortocaval compression can minimize the decline in BP. Although hetastarch is a better prophylactic, it is not commonly used for this application. When necessary, ephedrine is the vasopressor of choice because it restores uterine blood flow.[57] Prophylactic ephedrine infusion may be superior to bolus administration.[58] Despite its effects on UVR, phenylephrine is an acceptable vasopressor in the face of refractory hypotension.[13]

## Pruritus

Neuraxial (particularly intrathecal) opioids may cause itching in a dose-dependent manner.[59] Treatment options include diphenhydramine, nalbuphine, naloxone, and ondansetron.[60] Patients should be warned to avoid traumatic scratching while under sensory blockade.

## Nausea and Vomiting

Nausea occurring immediately after neuraxial dosing should be assumed secondary to hypotension and treated with intravenous fluids, uterine displacement, and ephedrine. Delayed onset is primarily due to use of neuraxial opioids. Management options include standard nonsedating antiemetic medications such as metoclopramide and ondansetron, as well as dexamethasone[61,62] and acupressure.[63] The latter is achieved by applying pressure to the P-6 acupoint located about three of the patient's fingerbreadths proximal to the transverse crease of the wrist, between the tendons of the flexor carpi radialis and palmaris longus. Mild discomfort is elicited with deep pressure at this location (Fig. 59–6).

## Pyrexia

Although the mechanism is unclear, epidural analgesia is an independent risk factor for the development of maternal fever, particularly in nulliparous patients with prolonged labor.[64] In a flawed but highly publicized study,[65] epidural analgesia was linked to neonatal sepsis evaluations, even in the absence of maternal fever. A subsequent study countered this finding.[64] Protocols for neonatal sepsis evaluation should take

into consideration the expected increase in maternal temperature with prolonged epidural analgesia (>5 hours).[66]

## Shivering

Predelivery shivering occurs in about 20% of laboring patients without an epidural[67,68] and in up to 33% with epidural analgesia. Much of this shivering is nonthermoregulatory and is not relieved by use of warming blankets.[69] Although warmed intravenous fluids,[70] warmed injectate, and use of fentanyl[71] may reduce the incidence of shivering, intravenous κ-receptor agonists (eg, meperidine 12.5-25 mg, nalbuphine 5-10 mg) and intravenous clonidine (0.15 mg)[72] are effective treatments.

## Postdural Puncture Headache

Because the risk factors for PDPH include female gender, age range 20 to 40 years, history of PDPH or migraine headaches, and possibly pregnancy itself, it is particularly common in the obstetric population. The technique-related risk factors include needle size and shape, bevel direction, and number of dural punctures. Using 25- to 27-gauge pencil point (Whitacre or Sprotte) needles for spinal anesthesia and inserting epidural needles with the bevel parallel to the long axis of the spine[73] minimize the risk. Occasionally, there is difficulty threading the epidural catheter with this needle orientation. Threading can be facilitated by expanding the epidural space by injecting either anesthetic or saline, or by rotating the needle 90°. The latter is performed with backward traction on the needle to avoid dural scoring or coring, followed by reassessment for lack of resistance to injection and careful assessment to verify that the catheter was not threaded intrathecally. Some have advocated always rotating the needle cephalad, finding a lower incidence of one-sided blocks and improved analgesic spread.[74]

Although the majority of PDPHs resolve spontaneously, the circumstances of new motherhood necessitate early treatment. The first step is confirming the diagnosis (Table 59–5). Usually, the clinical presentation is sufficient, but if in doubt, additional studies may be indicated. Mild PDPH can often be satisfactorily managed with analgesics alone. Although dehydration may exacerbate the headache, vigorous hydration is of no benefit. For a severe headache, intravenous caffeine sodium benzoate (500 mg) is effective in most patients and curative (sometimes requiring two doses) in about 70%.[75] In fact, for patients who recognize PDPH only after discharge, oral caffeine[76] (or theophylline[77]) may be effective. A single study has shown the effectiveness of subcutaneous sumatrip-

**TABLE 59–5.** Differential Diagnosis of Postpartum Headache

Tension headache
Postdural puncture headache
Migraine
Hypertension
Sinusitis
Pneumocephalus
Caffeine withdrawal
Meningitis
Subarachnoid hemorrhage
Cortical vein thrombosis
Subdural hematoma
Brain tumor or arteriovenous malformation

tan as well.[78] EBP—placement of 10 to 20 mL autologous blood in the epidural space—remains the definitive therapy, with an initial success rate of 90% or more but recurrence occurring in up to 30%.[79] EBP may be repeated one time. Because the injected blood spreads primarily cephalad,[80] injection should be performed at or below the site of the original dural puncture. Risks of EBP include repeat dural puncture, back pain, transient neurologic deficits, and possibly inadequate analgesia with a subsequent epidural.[81]

## Local Anesthetic Toxicity

Accidental intravascular injection or systemic absorption of local anesthetic may result in toxic blood levels. Initial symptoms include perioral numbness and tinnitus, with progression to convulsions, and respiratory and cardiac arrest. Aspiration before each local anesthetic bolus and fractionated dosing can virtually eliminate this complication. Treatment of toxicity includes supplemental $O_2$ and thiopental (50-75 mg), or benzodiazepine for treatment or prophylaxis of seizures. In the event of cardiac arrest, prompt delivery of the fetus may improve maternal survival. If bupivacaine cardiac toxicity is suspected, prolonged cardiopulmonary resuscitation is indicated, and bretylium, rather than lidocaine, should be used to treat ventricular arrhythmias.

## Neurologic Complications

It is exceedingly rare to cause direct nerve damage while placing a neuraxial anesthetic in an awake patient. The etiology of nerve damage is more likely fetal compression of nerves in the pelvis or excessive flexion of the hip during maternal pushing. The latter may become more likely when symptoms are blocked by epidural analgesia. The majority of these nerve injuries resolve in a matter of months. Epidural hematoma is a potentially catastrophic complication, but is thankfully rare in a patient with normal hemostasis.

Remember to remind labor assistants during stage 2 pushing to deflex the patient's hips between contractions to avoid femoral nerve damage from prolonged femoral nerve compression.

## Total Spinal Anesthesia

A total spinal may result from inadvertent intrathecal injection of an epidural dose of local anesthetic, injection of intrathecal medications after dilation of the epidural space, or injection of epidural volume after placement of local anesthetic in the intrathecal space. Treatment is supportive, including airway or ventilatory management and cardiovascular support. If the intrathecal solution is hyperbaric, reverse Trendelenburg position may be helpful, but hemodynamic instability may require a head-down position. Delayed onset of an unexpectedly high anesthetic level following epidural dosing may be due to a subdural catheter location.[82]

## Backache

In the only prospective study to date, epidural analgesia did not affect the incidence of postpartum backache.[83] Those who have reported an increased incidence of backache after epidural for labor find that it is primarily postural and not severe.[84]

In addition, there are several reports of rare neurologic complications including hearing loss, visual field defects, diplopia, Horner's syndrome, Bell's palsy, and trigeminal nerve palsy.[85]

## Is Informed Consent Necessary?

Contrary to popular belief, patients do not feel that the ongoing discomfort of labor interferes with their ability to understand risks or provide consent.[86] However, these survey participants also agreed the consent process should ideally occur well before the onset of labor. As of 1990, there were three closed claims involving the adequacy of informed consent given during labor[87]; each was decided in favor of the anesthesiologist. Regarding the consent process, no specific documentation was required, only that reasonable information be given, including general acknowledgment of serious risks with an approximate probability of occurrence and an opportunity for the patient to ask questions. Although some recommend only a note on the chart to this effect,[87] others suggest a full written consent.[86]

# CESAREAN SECTION

## What Are the Anesthetic Options?

Anesthetic options for cesarean section are largely dependent on the indication for the procedure. Elective operations are almost exclusively performed under regional anesthesia for several reasons, including patient preference, ability to have a companion present in the OR, reduced neonatal depression, and improved postoperative pain control with long-acting neuraxial opioids. The case-fatality risk ratio of general versus regional anesthesia was reported at 16.7[8] and was determined through analysis of anesthesia-related maternal deaths. Much of the increased risk is probably due to the circumstances requiring general anesthesia (eg, emergency surgery, morbid obesity, coagulopathy) rather than the anesthetic technique itself.[8] It is our practice to encourage regional anesthesia but not to force it on an unwilling patient.

For laboring patients in whom the risk of general anesthesia may be increased (those with morbid obesity or a difficult airway), we discuss with the obstetricians the need to avoid emergency cesarean section (ie, consider cesarean earlier with a nonreassuring FHR tracing) and encourage the early placement of an epidural catheter, perhaps without dosing.

## Regional Techniques

A T4 level is required for cesarean section, although the procedure may be better tolerated with a T2 level, with reduced nausea and vomiting, particularly if the surgeon exteriorizes the uterus.

### Epidural

After intravascular volume loading of the patient, epidural anesthesia is achieved with 10 to 30 mL of local anesthetic (lidocaine 2% with epinephrine, bupivacaine 0.5%, 2-chloroprocaine [2-CP] 3%, ropivacaine 1%). Onset time may be reduced by alkalinization (lidocaine, 2-CP), perhaps by use of warmed local anesthetics,[88] injection in the lateral decubitus position,[89] and injection through the needle before placement of the catheter. Addition of fentanyl to the local anesthetic may improve the quality of the block and reduce maternal discomfort. If administered at least 10 minutes after epinephrine-containing local anesthetics, maternal blood levels of fentanyl are insignificant due to local vasoconstriction and decreased uptake. After delivery of the infant, preservative-free morphine, 2 to 3 mg, is administered through the epidural catheter, providing 12 to 24 hours of postoperative pain relief. Use of 2-CP reduces the analgesic efficacy of epidural morphine,[90] necessitating more liberal supplemental postpartum analgesia.

In the presence of a labor epidural, there appears to be little decrease in the local anesthetic volume required to attain a T4 surgical level. In those instances in which such a level cannot be obtained despite adequate dosing, removal of the catheter and placement of a spinal anesthetic may be considered. Although reduction of the spinal dose may result in a continued inadequate block, the risk of high spinal in this setting may be as high as 11%, perhaps due to compression of the intrathecal space by the volume in the epidural space.[91] Having witnessed this complication on three occasions, one of which required emergency intubation, we recommend early assessment of the epidural's function before administering a large dose of local anesthetic. In fact, if a labor epidural was providing only a "spotty" block, it is removed and a spinal placed instead.

### Spinal

The most common drug for spinal anesthesia is hyperbaric bupivacaine 0.75%. Addition of epinephrine may delay the onset of the block[92] and does not substantially increase the duration, although it may increase the intensity. Fentanyl, 10 to 20 μg, may improve the quality of the block, and morphine sulfate (Duramorph) 0.1 mg is effective for postoperative pain relief.[59]

### Combined Spinal-Epidural

A combined spinal-epidural may offer the advantages of both modalities: the onset speed of a spinal anesthetic coupled with the reduced hypotension and duration flexibility of an epidural.[93,94]

### General Anesthesia

Because the depressant effects of anesthetic agents on the fetus depend on the induction to delivery interval (preferably <8 minutes),[95] general anesthesia is not induced until the obstetricians are ready for incision. After placing the patient supine with left lateral tilt (or a left hip wedge), monitors are applied while the patient is prepped and draped. Following preoxygenation, a rapid-sequence induction is performed with an induction agent (usually thiopental), succinylcholine, and cricoid pressure. Fasciculations may not occur and thus are not a reliable indicator of adequate intubating conditions. The endotracheal tube should be one-half size smaller than usual due to the frequent presence of airway edema. A short-handled laryngoscope may be useful due to mammomegaly. Because volatile anesthetic agents may cause uterine relaxation and increased blood loss, their concentration must be minimized.

Once correct endotracheal tube placement is confirmed, nitrous oxide 50% in $O_2$ is provided, with a low concentration of volatile anesthetic (one-half minimum alveolar concentration [MAC] or less). This regimen is tolerated because MAC is reduced 40% at term. Minute ventilation should be titrated to an end-tidal $CO_2$ pressure of 30 to 32 mm Hg to maintain normal maternal pH. Following delivery, nitrous oxide concentration is increased to 70%, and intravenous opioids may be added. Due to laxity of the abdominal musculature, addition of nondepolarizing muscle relaxants is rarely required and should be particularly avoided for patients on magnesium.

Although recall is rare, awareness under general anesthesia is common. In fact, in one study, 97% of patients were aware at skin incision, with 80% sensing pain. After 2 minutes, 20% were still aware, with 7% experiencing pain.[96] Therefore, we advocate speaking to the patient immediately after intubation, acknowledging that they can hear and assuring them that they will be more deeply asleep soon.

## How Should the Difficult Airway Be Managed?

The first goal is advance recognition of the difficult airway (Table 59–6). Management of the patient with an anticipated difficult airway is controversial. Total spinal or intravascular local anesthetic toxicity may necessitate emergency airway management; thus, some consider the difficult airway a contraindication to regional anesthesia. Probably the most conservative management is awake intubation of these patients. A slowly dosed epidural is a safe alternative. In fact, when parturients with a difficult airway are identified early in labor, the obstetrician should be notified that emergency cesarean section under general anesthesia is not a safe option. This may encourage early placement of a labor epidural for future dosing and an earlier obstetric decision regarding cesarean section.

Although recognition of potential airway problems and advanced planning are optimal, two thirds of patients in whom intubation was difficult were unexpected, even on retrospective examination.[97] It is imperative that all anesthetists have a plan and appropriate equipment for this scenario (see Chapter 53). Although anesthesiologists are trained to manage such a situation in the main operating suite, there are additional considerations in obstetrics:

1. Maternal status. In a "can't intubate, can't ventilate" scenario leading to hemodynamic instability, resuscitation of

**TABLE 59–6.** Difficult Intubation Relative Risk Factors

| Risk Factor | Relative Risk |
| --- | --- |
| Mallampati class | |
| II | 3.23 |
| III | 7.58 |
| IV | 11.30 |
| Short neck | 5.01 |
| Receding mandible | 9.71 |
| Protruding maxillary incisors | 8.0 |

Adapted from Rocke DA, Murray WB, Rout CC, et al. Relative risk analysis of factors associated with difficult intubation in obstetric anesthesia. *Anesthesiology.* 1992;77:71.

the mother may be enhanced by delivery of the fetus, improving venous return.
2. Status of the fetus. Although FHR monitoring is a poor predictor of compromise, there are clearly emergent conditions (eg, cord prolapse, abruption, uterine rupture) in which rapid delivery of the fetus is essential. This, of course, must be balanced with maternal risk.
3. Risk of aspiration. Unlike the general OR population, mask ventilation or use of a laryngeal mask airway (LMA) are suboptimal solutions.

Because of the comfort level of many anesthesiologists with LMAs, they are often the first device used in the "can't intubate" setting. Placement of the LMA may improve ventilation, but endotracheal intubation through the mask is probably indicated for airway protection. An alternative is the esophageal-tracheal Combitube with the aid of a laryngoscope.[98] The tube reduces the risk of aspiration and can be used for ventilation whether it is located in the esophagus or trachea. Like the LMA, the Combitube (in the more common esophageal position) will not overcome ventilation problems due to laryngospasm. The obstetric suite should be equipped with a readily accessible difficult airway box, including the capability for percutaneous tracheal insufflation and ventilation.

## How Should Postoperative Pain Be Managed?

One of the advantages of regional anesthesia for cesarean section is the excellent pain control provided by neuraxial opioids. Intrathecal morphine, 0.1[59,99] to 0.3 mg,[100] or epidural morphine, 3 mg,[101] provides 12 to 24 hours of analgesia with tolerable side effects including nausea and vomiting (20% intrathecal,[59] 40% epidural[101]), pruritus (51% intrathecal,[59] 58% epidural[101]), and urinary retention. Due to delayed onset of neuraxially administered opioids, breakthrough pain in the postanesthesia care unit is common. In the postpartum period, intravenous ketorolac (even in breastfeeding women, due to minimal excretion into breast milk[102]) or opioids are effective treatments.

## FETAL MONITORING

## How Is the Fetus Monitored During Late Pregnancy?

Although maternal recognition of fetal movement is sufficient in the low-risk patient, several tools (Table 59–7) are used to evaluate fetal well-being for those in high-risk categories (eg, coexisting medical diseases, gestation >42 weeks, suspected intrauterine growth retardation). The results of these tests may indicate a need for early delivery. Typically, delivery before 37 weeks' gestation is preceded by amniocentesis to document fetal lung maturity (fetal lung maturity >55 or lecithin/sphingomyelin ratio >2.0). A negative result may prompt a 48-hour course of maternal steroids followed by delivery.

**TABLE 59–7.** Prenatal Fetal Assessment

| Assessment Tool | Data Obtained | Comments |
|---|---|---|
| Ultrasound | EFW, AFI | Rule out IUGR, macrosomia<br>Rule out oligo- or polyhydramnios |
| Nonstress test | FHR pattern over 30 min | Follow-up score <9 with CST |
| Contraction stress test | FHR response to contractions induced by oxytocin or nipple stimulation | Negative test good indicator of fetal well-being, 25% false-positive |
| Biophysical profile | Fetal breathing, movement, tone, AFI, NST | Normal: 8-10; suspect: 4-6 → repeat in several hours; critical: 0-2 |
| Doppler velocimetry | Systolic/diastolic flow ratio in umbilical artery | Absent or reversed diastolic flow suggests increased placental vascular resistance |
| Amniocentesis | FLM, L/S ratio | Test of fetal lung maturity |

AFI, amniotic fluid index; CST, contraction stress test; EFW, estimated fetal weight; FHR, fetal heart rate; FLM, fetal lung maturity; IUGR, intrauterine growth retardation; L/S, lecithin/sphingomyelin; NST, nonstress test.

## How Is Fetal Well-Being Assessed During Labor?

There is currently no optimal tool for intrapartum fetal assessment. Because the fetus responds to hypoxia with a change in heart rate, FHR monitoring (either continuous electronic or intermittent auscultation) is the standard of care (Tables 59–7 and 59–8). The predictive value of continuous electronic FHR monitoring is unclear, and its specificity is poor, contributing to increased operative delivery rates.[103]

Fetal scalp blood pH determinations may be used to confirm fetal acidosis with a nonreassuring FHR tracing. A pH <7.20 on more than one sample encourages expeditious delivery. Unfortunately, the laboratory requirements for such measurements have eliminated the procedure from most small hospitals. Alternatively, the presence of accelerations in response to fetal scalp stimulation suggests a pH of at least 7.19.[104] A similar response is seen with vibroacoustic stimulation (application of an artificial larynx to the maternal abdomen).

**TABLE 59–8.** Fetal Heart Rate Monitoring

| Feature | Characteristics | Affected by |
|---|---|---|
| Baseline fetal heart rate | Normal: 120-160 bpm at term | Gestational age, hypoxia, maternal fever, intrauterine infection, medications, fetal cardiac anomaly |
| Long-/short-term variability (see Fig. 59–7) | | Hypoxia, atropine, opioids |
| Early deceleration (Fig. 59–8) | Onset and offset coincide with contraction | Head compression with vagal response |
| Variable deceleration (see Fig. 59–8) | Often abrupt | Umbilical cord compression |
| Late deceleration (see Fig. 59–8) | Begin 10-30 s after start of contraction, and end similarly; smooth and repetitive | Hypoxia |

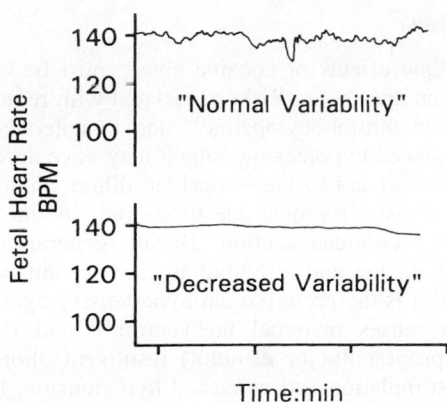

**FIGURE 59–7.** Fetal heart rate variability. Illustration of normal and abnormal beat-to-beat variability. Loss of variability has been attributed to fetal brain injury, hypoxia, and drugs. At present, no accepted methods exist to measure variability or to establish limits of normal or abnormal change.

Fetal scalp pulse oximetry and monitoring of fetal cerebral oxygenation with near-infrared spectroscopy remain experimental.

## What Determines an Urgent or Emergency Cesarean Section?

Due to the poor predictive value of FHR monitoring, the time frame for delivery of an infant is a frequent area of

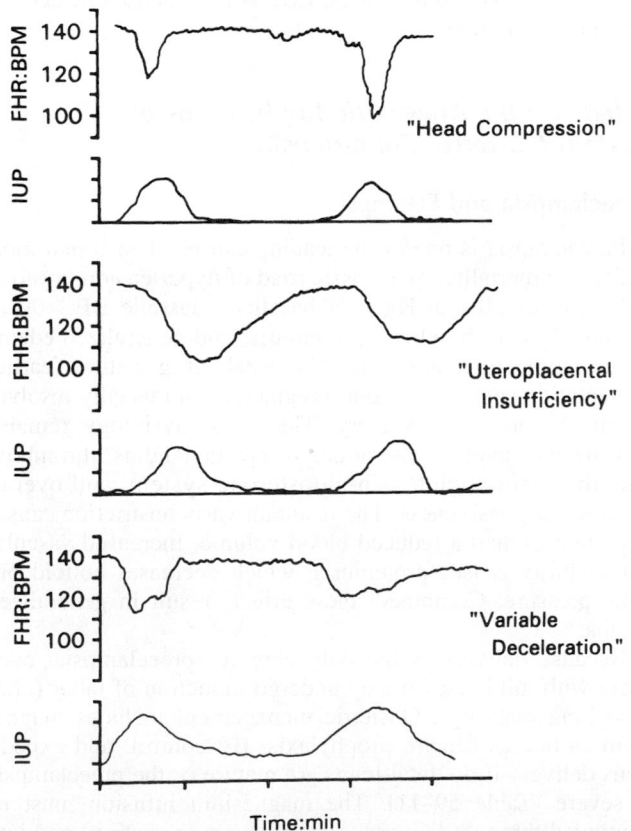

**FIGURE 59–8.** Abnormal fetal heart rate tracings. Three patterns of abnormal response of fetal heart rate tracings in relation to uterine contractions.

**TABLE 59–9.** Apgar Scoring

| Sign | 0 | 1 | 2 |
|---|---|---|---|
| Heart rate | Absent | <100/min | >100/min |
| Respiratory effort | Absent | Gasping/irregular; weak cry | Good; strong cry |
| Muscle tone | Flaccid, limp | Some flexion | Normal |
| Reflex irritability | No response | Grimace/minimal reaction | Cry, cough, sneeze |
| Color | Pale; blue | Acrocyanosis | Pink |

contention between obstetricians and anesthesiologists. The only published guideline is the ability to start an emergency cesarean delivery "within 30 minutes of the decision to operate."[105]

## NEONATAL RESUSCITATION

### What Is the Anesthesiologist's Responsibility?

Although our primary responsibility is to our patient, the mother, it is in her best interests to have a healthy child. Therefore, if the mother is stable, a nurse should be assigned (temporary transfer of care) to watch the patient's vital signs while the anesthesiologist assists with the resuscitation of a distressed neonate.[54]

### How Is the Newborn Assessed?

Apgar scores (Table 59–9) are assigned 1 and 5 minutes after delivery. Although useful for assessing the need for resuscitation, the score has not proven predictive of long-term outcome.[106] Umbilical cord blood gases are often obtained. A pH of 7.20 has traditionally been considered the lower limit of normal, although this may be overly conservative. Only a pH <7.00 has been associated with an increased incidence of neonatal death.[107]

### What Are the Current Guidelines for Resuscitation?

A brief overview is provided in Table 59–10, but frequent review of current neonatal resuscitation practices is recommended. Recall that neonatal distress is most often caused

**TABLE 59–10.** Neonatal Resuscitation Overview

1. Administer supplemental oxygen and stimulate the baby.
2. If meconium is present, intubate and suction before positive-pressure ventilation.
3. With ineffective spontaneous respiration or heart rate <100 bpm, begin bag-valve-mask ventilation. Use minimum inflation pressure required to effect chest movement, usually <35 cm $H_2O$.
4. If heart rate <60 bpm after 30 s of adequate ventilation, begin chest compressions.
5. If heart rate remains <60 bpm after 30 s, administer epinephrine IV or via ETT.

ETT, endotracheal tube; IV, intravenous.

by hypoxia; therefore, improving oxygenation is the primary treatment goal.

# HIGH-RISK OBSTETRICS

## How Do Common Medical Conditions Impact Anesthetic Management?

### Asthma

Approximately 10% of asthmatic women will have symptoms of asthma during labor.[108] Epidural analgesia is useful for labor in these patients, particularly in those with stress- or exercise-induced asthma. For operative delivery, the risk of respiratory distress from intercostal muscle paralysis during regional anesthesia must be balanced against the substantial risk of bronchospasm from endotracheal intubation. Topical anesthesia of the airway should be considered, and ketamine, 2 mg/kg, may be the preferred induction agent due to its bronchodilating properties. The bronchodilatory effects of volatile agents may not be evident at the low concentrations used to minimize their uterine relaxant effects. The pharmacologic treatment of postpartum hemorrhage is limited due to the bronchospastic side effects of both 15-methylprostaglandin $F_{2\alpha}$ (carboprost tromethamine [Hemabate]) and the ergot alkaloids (methylergonovine). β-Blockers in the management of hypertension must be used with caution.

### Cardiovascular Disease

Severe preexisting cardiac disease, particularly pulmonary hypertension, may portend a disastrous course. Fetal growth is a good marker of cardiac reserve; that is, a fetus that is normal size for gestational age is unlikely if maternal cardiac function is severely impaired. Appropriate monitoring is essential, particularly in the early postpartum period when cardiac demands are greatest.

### Prior Back Surgery

Epidural analgesia should not necessarily be withheld from patients with prior back operations, including laminectomy or Harrington rod placement.[109] The patient should be informed, however, of the increased chance of dural puncture, inadequate analgesia, and difficult placement requiring multiple attempts, as well as the risk of back pain for several days after delivery. Review of a prior spine film may identify an area without instrumentation or bony fusion; if none exists, consider the caudal route, lumbar sympathetic blocks, or other analgesic alternatives.

### Diabetes

Pregnancy affects insulin sensitivity and increases the risk of ketoacidosis. There is an increased risk of fetal anomalies, and macrosomia is common and may necessitate cesarean delivery. Although no anesthetic technique is contraindicated, the accelerated atherosclerosis of diabetes may affect the placenta; therefore, uterine perfusion must be maintained and anesthesia-induced hypotension avoided. Because insulin crosses the placenta readily, the neonate is at risk for hypoglycemia.

### Cocaine Abuse

The multiple effects of cocaine abuse must be considered in planning an anesthetic. Risks associated with regional anesthesia include thrombocytopenia[110] and exaggerated sympathectomy-induced hypotension, which may have an unpredictable response to ephedrine—consider dilute phenylephrine. Despite these risks, regional anesthesia remains the preferred anesthetic for cesarean section. During general anesthesia, severe hypertension and arrhythmias may accompany intubation. Labetalol is the preferred antihypertensive agent because hydralazine causes maternal tachycardia[111] and β-blockade alone (eg, propranolol or esmolol) results in unopposed α-adrenergic stimulation and worsened hypertension. Halothane and ketamine are avoided to limit catecholamine-induced arrhythmias, and volatile anesthetics should be carefully titrated because MAC may be increased (acute cocaine) or decreased (chronic cocaine) depending on the timing of the last cocaine use.

### HIV

Obstetric management of HIV-infected patients remains a matter of intense research. Some evidence suggests that elective cesarean section reduces vertical transmission by 50%,[112] although it appears that vaginal delivery is safe with adequate antiviral therapy and a low viral titer. From an anesthetic perspective, we must consider the often coexisting conditions of substance abuse, hepatitis B, and other venereal diseases (particularly syphilis). Regional anesthesia is not contraindicated in HIV-infected patients, although thrombocytopenia is common and may be severe in 1.5% of these patients.[113] Failing conservative measures, EBP is not contraindicated for treatment of PDPH.[114]

## What Are the Anesthetic Implications of Certain Obstetric Conditions?

### Preeclampsia and Eclampsia

Preeclampsia is one of the leading causes of maternal morbidity and mortality. The classic triad of hypertension (systolic BP >140 or 30 mm Hg over baseline, diastolic BP >90 or 15 mm Hg over baseline), proteinuria, and generalized edema occurs some time after the 20th week of gestation (earlier presentation suggests a molar pregnancy) and usually resolves within 48 hours of delivery. The pathophysiology remains obscure but involves alterations in prostaglandins, thromboxane, the renin-angiotensin-aldosterone system, and overall vascular responsiveness. The resultant vasoconstriction causes hypertension and a reduced blood volume. Increased vascular permeability causes proteinuria, which decreases colloid oncotic pressure. Combined, these effects result in generalized edema.

Because delivery is the only cure for preeclampsia, even those with mild disease may undergo induction of labor (after fetal lung maturity). Obstetric management includes magnesium sulfate as seizure prophylaxis, BP control, and expeditious delivery if the fetal lungs are mature or the preeclampsia is severe (Table 59–11). The magnesium infusion must be continued through delivery (even if cesarean section) and into the postpartum period. Magnesium toxicity (Table 59–12) is treated with intravenous calcium.

**TABLE 59–11.** Diagnostic Features of Severe Preeclampsia

Blood pressure: SBP >160, DBP >110
Proteinuria: >5 g/24 h
Oliguria: <500 mL/24 h
CNS symptoms: headache, visual disturbance
Pulmonary edema or cyanosis
Right upper quadrant pain: from hepatic swelling → stretch of the hepatic capsule
HELLP syndrome: *h*emolysis, *e*levated *l*iver enzymes, *l*ow *p*latelets

CNS, central nervous system; DBP, diastolic blood pressure; SBP, systolic blood pressure.

## Labor

A platelet count should be obtained on all patients with preeclampsia. If there is no bleeding history and >100 000 platelets/μL, further assessment of coagulation is unnecessary. Many advocate placement of the epidural catheter early in labor to aid in BP control and for use during potential cesarean (a frequent sequela due to failed induction and/or uteroplacental insufficiency). In addition, if placed before development of HELLP syndrome-induced coagulopathy, the epidural may be used safely and removed after the platelet count rebounds (48 hours after delivery). With severe preeclampsia refractory to labetalol and hydralazine, invasive arterial BP monitoring may be indicated, particularly if nitroglycerin or nitroprusside infusions are considered. With oliguria or pulmonary edema, central monitoring may be useful; a pulmonary artery catheter may provide more reliable insight into left-sided filling pressures than a central venous catheter.[115]

## Cesarean Section

For cesarean section in a preeclamptic patient, a slowly dosed epidural is preferable to a spinal anesthetic due to the patient's depressed volume status. Hypotension should be managed with careful volume loading and small doses of ephedrine (2.5-5 mg) due to hypersensitivity to vasopressors. If general anesthesia is required, BP should be controlled before induction with labetalol or vasodilator infusion (nitroglycerin or nitroprusside). The latter may require invasive arterial pressure monitoring. An opioid such as fentanyl is useful at induction to blunt the hypertensive response to laryngoscopy. The pediatricians should be warned that neonatal ventilatory depression might occur as a result. Intraoperatively, BP should be maintained within 30% of the desired preoperative levels. Cerebral autoregulation can shift after a relatively short period of hypertension (days); therefore, hypotension may be poorly tolerated. If nondepolarizing muscle relaxants are administered, they must be used cautiously

**TABLE 59–12.** Magnesium Effects

| Level (mg/dL) | Effects |
|---|---|
| 4–8 | Therapeutic range; warmth, flushing, tocolysis, anticonvulsant, mild vasodilation |
| 5–10 | ECG changes: PR prolongation, QRS widening |
| 10–12 | Loss of deep tendon reflexes |
| 12–15 | Respiratory depression, SA and AV nodal block |
| 25–30 | Cardiac arrest |

AV, atrioventricular; ECG, electrocardiogram; SA, sinoatrial.

with frequent monitoring because of the dramatic prolongation of their effect caused by magnesium.

## Abnormal Presentation

Mode of delivery in breech presentation is an area of continued debate. Some advocate elective cesarean delivery, whereas others recommend an individualized approach based on obstetric history, estimated fetal weight (avoid if <1500 g or >4000 g), and possibly radiographic pelvimetry. Vaginal delivery usually entails delay of maternal expulsive efforts until the breech has reached the perineum and then allowing delivery to at least the level of the fetal umbilicus before providing obstetric assistance. Piper forceps may be applied to extract the fetal head. Epidural analgesia may help reduce the urge to push early, relax the pelvic floor for delivery, allow placement of forceps, and provide a method for rapid anesthesia in the event of emergency cesarean section. Fetal head entrapment may require cervical or perineal relaxation. Uterine (and some cervical) relaxation may be provided by emergency rapid sequence induction with a high concentration (2-3 MAC) of volatile agent or by intravenous or sublingual administration of nitroglycerin.[116] Perineal entrapment may require profound epidural anesthesia or general anesthesia with neuromuscular blockade.

## Multiple Gestation

Multiple gestation results in exaggerated cardiopulmonary changes and an increased risk of aortocaval compression. Epidural anesthesia should be encouraged in these patients due to the high rate of cesarean section and the potential for emergency cesarean even after delivery of the first twin. Epidural analgesia may also help with attempts at internal or external version of the second twin.

## What Antepartum Hemorrhage Etiologies Are of Concern?

Vaginal bleeding may occur from many sources including vaginal or cervical irritation, but three etiologies merit special attention.

## Placenta Previa

Placenta previa typically presents as painless vaginal bleeding from a placental implantation in advance of the fetal presenting part. Cesarean section is usually required but may be delayed for fetal lung maturity if the bleeding is minimal. Perinatal mortality is 2.3%.[117] There is a likelihood of substantial blood loss because (1) the placenta may be cut during incision, (2) the lower uterine segment does not contract as well as the normal fundal implantation site, and (3) there is an increased chance of placenta accreta, potentially requiring an emergency cesarean hysterectomy. Patients with placenta previa may require additional intravenous access, and availability of blood products should be considered.

## Abruption

Premature separation of the placenta from the decidua results in bleeding, much of which may be retroplacental and unrecognized even with ultrasound. Unlike placenta previa, these patients usually experience pain and uterine tenderness. Perinatal mortality may be as high as 36%.[118] Anesthetic management for labor or cesarean requires consideration of the volume status. Ketamine may be the preferred induction agent and volume resuscitation is essential.

### Uterine Rupture

A typical presentation is hypotension, cessation of labor, and fetal distress in a parturient with a history of uterine surgery. Pain is not a reliable finding; therefore, epidural analgesia is safe and unlikely to mask uterine rupture in patients undergoing vaginal birth after cesarean.[119] Anesthetic management frequently involves general anesthesia due to the uncertain blood volume and potential for hysterectomy.

## What Types of Embolism Are Common in the Pregnant Patient?

### Pulmonary Thromboembolism

Pulmonary thromboembolism occurs with increased frequency in pregnancy due to venous stasis and hypercoagulability.

### Venous Air Embolism

Venous air embolism may occur in 50% of patients during cesarean delivery.[120] Reverse Trendelenburg position probably does not reduce the incidence,[121] but exteriorization of the uterus may increase it.[122]

### Amniotic Fluid Embolism

Although fortunately a rare event, amniotic fluid embolism has devastating consequences with 61% mortality and neurologically intact survival in only 15%.[123] In the most comprehensive review to date (46 cases[123]), 70% occurred during labor, 11% after vaginal delivery, and 19% during cesarean section after delivery of the infant. Of the 13 patients who experienced amniotic fluid embolism after delivery, the mean time to onset of symptoms was 8 minutes. The etiology is not entirely clear but probably involves an anaphylactoid reaction to some component of amniotic fluid, resulting in pulmonary hypertension and bronchoconstriction. The resultant profound hypoxia causes biventricular dysfunction and cardiovascular collapse.[124] Only the latter stage has been observed in human beings, probably due to the lack of invasive monitoring during the initial insult. Clinically, the most common presenting features are dyspnea and cyanosis, fetal bradycardia (if undelivered), and seizures. Those patients who survive the first several hours may go on to develop disseminated intravascular coagulation (DIC). Treatment is supportive and should include high concentrations of supplemental $O_2$ and intense cardiovascular monitoring.

### Postpartum Hemorrhage

The most common etiology of hemorrhage is uterine atony. Oxytocin infusion reduces the incidence and, coupled with external uterine massage, is effective therapy in most cases.

The second line of therapy is the ergot alkaloids, ergonovine and methylergonovine. These are usually administered subcutaneously (0.2 mg) and can cause significant cardiovascular effects including pulmonary and coronary vasoconstriction, as well as bronchospasm. Several prostaglandins have also proven valuable: the most common is 15-methylprostaglandin $F_{2\alpha}$ (carboprost tromethamine) dosed 250 μg intramuscularly or intramyometrially every 15 to 30 minutes. Side effects include bronchospasm and hypoxemia from increased intrapulmonary shunting.[125]

Other causes of postpartum hemorrhage include coagulopathy, DIC, retained placenta, placenta accreta, and uterine inversion. After correction of coagulopathies, management of continued bleeding may include angiography with embolization of the supplying arteries, surgical ligation of those vessels, or emergency hysterectomy with an average blood loss of more than 2 L.[126]

## OTHER PROCEDURES IN LABOR AND DELIVERY

## What Are the Anesthetic Considerations for Other Procedures?

### Postpartum Bilateral Tubal Interruption

The proximity of the fallopian tubes to the abdominal wall in the postpartum period enables access through a small infraumbilical incision. Conversely, an interval bilateral tubal interruption (BTI), performed at least 6 weeks postpartum, requires general anesthesia and laparoscopy with all the attendant risks. Postpartum BTI is typically performed under regional anesthesia. Reactivation of an existing labor epidural should be successful (>90%) if less than 24 hours have elapsed since delivery, but this probability declines with a longer interval.[127] Removal of the epidural and use of spinal anesthesia may reduce overall costs.[128] Failed reactivation of an epidural catheter followed by subarachnoid block with the potential for a high spinal are strong reasons to place a new spinal anesthetic in a patient who is amenable. Because gastric emptying is delayed during labor, the ASA Practice Guidelines[11] recommend that any patient planning an elective postpartum BTI within 8 hours of delivery should have no oral intake of solid foods during labor and postpartum. Although slowed at 12 hours postpartum,[129] gastric emptying returns to nonpregnant rates 18 hours after an uncomplicated vaginal delivery.[7]

### Cerclage

Patients with cervical dilation early in pregnancy often require placement of a cervical pursestring suture. The required T8-10 level is typically achieved with a spinal. Sedation must consider the stage of pregnancy, although the small amounts required are unlikely to affect the developing fetus.

### Version

Conversion of a breech presentation to vertex may avert the need for cesarean section. External cephalic version requires application of significant force to the maternal abdomen. Traditionally, maternal discomfort has limited the force applied, presumably reducing the risk of fetal injury or uterine rupture. Ultrasound, electronic FHR monitoring, and the ability to perform immediate cesarean delivery have increased the safety of this procedure, and the success rate may be safely increased when performed under epidural anesthesia (T6 level with 2% lidocaine with epinephrine).[130]

## References

1. Kauppila A, Koskinen M, Puolakka J, et al. Decreased intervillous and unchanged myometrial blood flow in supine recumbency. *Obstet Gynecol.* 1980;55:203.
2. Ueland K, Hansen JM. Maternal cardiovascular dynamics. 3. Labor and delivery under local and caudal analgesia. *Am J Obstet Gynecol.* 1969;103:8.
3. Lyons HA, Antonio R. The sensitivity of the respiratory center in pregnancy and after the administration of progesterone. *Trans Assoc Am Phys.* 1959;72:173.
4. Spätling L, Fallenstein F, Huch A, et al. The variability of cardiopulmonary adaptation to pregnancy at rest and during exercise. *Br J Obstet Gynaecol.* 1992;99(suppl 8):1.
5. Shankar KB, Moseley H, Kumar Y, et al. Arterial to end tidal carbon dioxide tension difference during caesarean section anaesthesia. *Anaesthesia.* 1986;41:698.
6. Turner ES, Greenberger PA, Patterson R. Management of the pregnant asthmatic patient. *Ann Intern Med.* 1980;93:905.
7. Whitehead EM, Smith M, Dean Y, et al. An evaluation of gastric emptying times in pregnancy and the puerperium. *Anaesthesia.* 1993;48:53.
8. Hawkins JL, Koonin LM, Palmer SK, et al. Anesthesia-related deaths during obstetric delivery in the United States, 1979–1990. *Anesthesiology.* 1997;86:277.
9. Schreiner MS. Gastric fluid volume: is it really a risk factor for pulmonary aspiration? [editorial]. *Anesth Analg.* 1998;87:754.
10. Raidoo DM, Rocke DA, Brock-Utne JG, et al. Critical volume for pulmonary acid aspiration: reappraisal in a primate model. *Br J Anaesth.* 1990;65:248.
11. American Society of Anesthesiologists. Practice guidelines for obstetrical anesthesia: a report by the American Society of Anesthesiologists Task Force on Obstetrical Anesthesia. *Anesthesiology.* 1999;90:600.
12. Rout CC, Rocke DA, Gouws E. Intravenous ranitidine reduces the risk of acid aspiration of gastric contents at emergency cesarean section. *Anesth Analg.* 1993;76:156.
13. Thomas DG, Robson SC, Redfern N, et al. Randomized trial of bolus phenylephrine or ephedrine for maintenance of arterial pressure during spinal anaesthesia for Caesarean section. *Br J Anaesth.* 1996;76:61.
14. Burrows RF, Kelton JG. Thrombocytopenia at delivery: a prospective survey of 6715 deliveries. *Am J Obstet Gynecol.* 1990;162:731.
15. Anteby E, Shalev O. Clinical relevance of gestational thrombocytopenia of <100,000/microliters. *Am J Hematol.* 1994;47:118.
16. Rebarber A, Lonser R, Jackson S, et al. The safety of intraoperative autologous blood collection and autotransfusion during cesarean section. *Am J Obstet Gynecol.* 1998;179:715.
17. Lind SE. The bleeding time does not predict surgical bleeding. *Blood.* 1991;77:2547.
18. Rodgers RP, Levin J. A critical reappraisal of the bleeding time. *Semin Thromb Hemost.* 1990;16:1.
19. Rouse DJ, Owen J, Goldenberg RL. Routine maternal platelet count: an assessment of a technologically driven screening practice. *Am J Obstet Gynecol.* 1998;179:573.
20. Barron WM, Heckerling P, Hibbard JU, et al. Reducing unnecessary coagulation testing in hypertensive disorders of pregnancy. *Obstet Gynecol.* 1999;94:364.
21. Basu SN, Constantine G, Bareford D. The rational use of coagulation studies in obstetrics: an audit. *Br J Obstet Gynaecol.* 1990;97:452.
22. Beilin Y, Zahn J, Comerford M. Safe epidural analgesia in thirty parturients with platelet counts between 69,000 and 98,000 mm(-3). *Anesth Analg.* 1997;85:385.
23. Melzack R, Taenzer P, Feldman P, et al. Labour is still painful after prepared childbirth training. *Can Med Assoc J.* 1981;125:357.
24. Abboud TK, Swart F, Zhu J, et al. Desflurane analgesia for vaginal delivery. *Acta Anaesthesiol Scand.* 1995;39:259.
25. Gal TJ, DiFazio CA, Moscicki J. Analgesic and respiratory depressant activity of nalbuphine: a comparison with morphine. *Anesthesiology.* 1982;57:367.
26. Puolakka J, Jouppila R, Jouppila P, et al. Maternal and fetal effects of low-dosage bupivacaine paracervical block. *J Perinat Med.* 1984;12:75.
27. Ranta P, Jouppila P, Spalding M, et al. Paracervical block—a viable alternative for labor pain relief? *Acta Obstet Gynecol Scand.* 1995;74:122.
28. Hunter CA. Uterine motility studies during labor: observations on bilateral sympathetic nerve block in the normal and abnormal first stage of labor. *Am J Obstet Gynecol.* 1963;85:681.
29. Leighton BL, Halpern SH, Wilson DB. Lumbar sympathetic blocks speed early and second stage induced labor in nulliparous women. *Anesthesiology.* 1999;90:1039.
30. Halpern SH, Leighton BL, Ohlsson A, et al. Effect of epidural vs parenteral opioid analgesia on the progress of labor: a meta-analysis. *JAMA.* 1998;280:2105.
31. Zhang J, Klebanoff MA, DerSimonian R. Epidural analgesia in association with duration of labor and mode of delivery: a quantitative review. *Am J Obstet Gynecol.* 1999;180:970.
32. Lyon DS, Knuckles G, Whitaker E, et al. The effect of instituting an elective labor epidural program on the operative delivery rate. *Obstet Gynecol.* 1997;90:135.
33. Yancey MK, Pierce B, Schweitzer D, et al. Observations on labor epidural analgesia and operative delivery rates. *Am J Obstet Gynecol.* 1999;180:353.
34. Impey L, MacQuillan K, Robson M. Epidural analgesia need not increase operative delivery rates. *Am J Obstet Gynecol.* 2000;182:358.
35. Chestnut DH, McGrath JM, Vincent RDJ, et al. Does early administration of epidural analgesia affect obstetric outcome in nulliparous women who are in spontaneous labor? *Anesthesiology.* 1994;80:1201.
36. Kuhnert BR, Kuhnert PM, Tu AS, et al. Meperidine and normeperidine levels following meperidine administration during labor, II: fetus and neonate. *Am J Obstet Gynecol.* 1979;133:909.
37. Saberski LR, Kondamuri S, Osinubi OY. Identification of the epidural space: is loss of resistance to air a safe technique? A review of the complications related to the use of air. *Reg Anesth.* 1997;22:3.
38. Norris MC, Ferrenbach D, Dalman H, et al. Does epinephrine improve the diagnostic accuracy of aspiration during labor epidural analgesia? *Anesth Analg.* 1999;88:1073.
39. Birnbach DJ, Chestnut DH. The epidural test dose in obstetric patients: has it outlived its usefulness? [editorial]. *Anesth Analg.* 1999;88:971.
40. Colonna-Romano P, Lingaraju N, Godfrey SD, et al. Epidural test dose and intravascular injection in obstetrics: sensitivity, specificity, and lowest effective dose. *Anesth Analg.* 1992;75:372.
41. Beilin Y, Bernstein HH, Zucker-Pinchoff B. The optimal distance that a multiorifice epidural catheter should be threaded into the epidural space. *Anesth Analg.* 1995;81:301.
42. Hamilton CL, Riley ET, Cohen SE. Changes in the position of epidural catheters associated with patient movement. *Anesthesiology.* 1997;86:778.
43. Tsen LC, Thue B, Datta S, et al. Is combined spinal-epidural analgesia associated with more rapid cervical dilation in nulliparous patients when compared with conventional epidural analgesia? *Anesthesiology.* 1999;91:920.
44. Collis RE, Harding SA, Morgan BM. Effect of maternal ambulation on labour with low-dose combined spinal-epidural analgesia. *Anaesthesia.* 1999;54:535.
45. Nageotte MP, Larson D, Rumney PJ, et al. Epidural analgesia compared with combined spinal-epidural analgesia during labor in nulliparous women. *N Engl J Med.* 1997;337:1715.
46. Dunn SM, Connelly NR, Steinberg RB, et al. Intrathecal sufentanil versus epidural lidocaine with epinephrine and sufentanil for early labor analgesia. *Anesth Analg.* 1998;87:331.
47. Takiguchi T, Okano T, Egawa H, et al. The effect of epidural saline injection on analgesic level during combined spinal and epidural anesthesia assessed clinically and myelographically. *Anesth Analg.* 1997;85:1097.
48. Santos AC, Arthur GR, Wlody D, et al. Comparative systemic toxicity of ropivacaine and bupivacaine in nonpregnant and pregnant ewes. *Anesthesiology.* 1995;82:734.
49. Huang YF, Pryor ME, Mather LE, et al. Cardiovascular and central nervous system effects of intravenous levobupivacaine and bupivacaine in sheep. *Anesth Analg.* 1998;86:797.
50. Polley LS, Columb MO, Naughton NN, et al. Relative analgesic potencies of ropivacaine and bupivacaine for epidural analgesia in labor: implications for therapeutic indexes. *Anesthesiology.* 1999;90:944.
51. Norris MC, Leighton BL. Continuous spinal anesthesia after unintentional dural puncture in parturients. *Reg Anesth.* 1990;15:285.
52. Dennehy KC, Rosaeg OP. Intrathecal catheter insertion during labour

reduces the risk of post-dural puncture headache. *Can J Anaesth.* 1998;45:42.

53. Asato F, Hirakawa N, Oda M, et al. A median epidural septum is not a common cause of unilateral epidural blockade. *Anesth Analg.* 1990;71:427.

54. Guidelines for Regional Anesthesia in Obstetrics. (Approved by ASA House of Delegates on October 12, 1988 and last amended on October 18, 2000.) In: *American Society of Anesthesiologists Directory of Members 2001.* Park Ridge, Ill: ASA; 2001:504.

55. Park GE, Hauch MA, Curlin F, et al. The effects of varying volumes of crystalloid administration before cesarean delivery on maternal hemodynamics and colloid osmotic pressure. *Anesth Analg.* 1996;83:299.

56. Ueyama H, He Y, Tanigami H, et al. Effects of crystalloid and colloid preload on blood volume in the parturient undergoing spinal anesthesia for elective cesarean section. *Anesthesiology.* 1999;91:1571.

57. James FM, Greiss FCJ, Kemp RA. An evaluation of vasopressor therapy for maternal hypotension during spinal anesthesia. *Anesthesiology.* 1970;33:25.

58. Kang YG, Abouleish E, Caritis S. Prophylactic intravenous ephedrine infusion during spinal anesthesia for cesarean section. *Anesth Analg.* 1982;61:839.

59. Dahl JB, Jeppesen IS, Jorgensen H, et al. Intraoperative and postoperative analgesic efficacy and adverse effects of intrathecal opioids in patients undergoing cesarean section with spinal anesthesia. *Anesthesiology.* 1999;91:1919.

60. Borgeat A, Stirnemann HR. Ondansetron is effective to treat spinal or epidural morphine-induced pruritus. *Anesthesiology.* 1999;90:432.

61. Fujii Y, Saitoh Y, Tanaka H, et al. Granisetron/dexamethasone combination for reducing nausea and vomiting during and after spinal anesthesia for cesarean section. *Anesth Analg.* 1999;88:1346.

62. Goedhals L, Heron JF, Kleisbauer JP, et al. Control of delayed nausea and vomiting with granisetron plus dexamethasone or dexamethasone alone in patients receiving highly emetogenic chemotherapy: a double-blind, placebo-controlled, comparative study. *Ann Oncol.* 1998;9:661.

63. Ho CM, Hseu SS, Tsai SK, et al. Effect of P-6 acupressure on prevention of nausea and vomiting after epidural morphine for post-cesarean section pain relief. *Acta Anaesthesiol Scand.* 1996;40:372.

64. Philip J, Alexander JM, Sharma SK, et al. Epidural analgesia during labor and maternal fever. *Anesthesiology.* 1999;90:1271.

65. Lieberman E, Lang JM, Frigoletto F Jr, et al. Epidural analgesia, intrapartum fever, and neonatal sepsis evaluation. *Pediatrics.* 1997;99:415.

66. Camann WR, Hortvet LA, Hughes N, et al. Maternal temperature regulation during extradural analgesia for labour. *Br J Anaesth.* 1991;67:565.

67. Jaameri KE, Jahkola A, Perttu J. On shivering in association with normal delivery. *Acta Obstet Gynecol Scand.* 1966;45:383.

68. Panzer O, Ghazanfari N, Sessler DI, et al. Shivering and shivering-like tremor during labor with and without epidural analgesia. *Anesthesiology.* 1999;90:1609.

69. Buggy D, Gardiner J. The space blanket and shivering during extradural analgesia in labour. *Acta Anaesthesiol Scand.* 1995;39:551.

70. Workhoven MN. Intravenous fluid temperature, shivering, and the parturient. *Anesth Analg.* 1986;65:496.

71. Shehabi Y, Gatt S, Buckman T, et al. Effect of adrenaline, fentanyl and warming of injectate on shivering following extradural analgesia in labour. *Anaesth Intensive Care.* 1990;18:31.

72. Mercadante S, De Michele P, Letterio G, et al. Effect of clonidine on postpartum shivering after epidural analgesia: a randomized, controlled, double-blind study. *J Pain Symptom Manage.* 1994;9:294.

73. Norris MC, Leighton BL, DeSimone CA. Needle bevel direction and headache after inadvertent dural puncture. *Anesthesiology.* 1989;70:729.

74. Huffnagle SL, Norris MC, Arkoosh VA, et al. The influence of epidural needle bevel orientation on spread of sensory blockade in the laboring parturient. *Anesth Analg.* 1998;87:326.

75. Sechzer PH, Abel L. Post-spinal anesthesia headache treated with caffeine. *Curr Ther Res.* 1978;24:307.

76. Camann WR, Murray RS, Mushlin PS, et al. Effects of oral caffeine on postdural puncture headache. A double-blind, placebo-controlled trial. *Anesth Analg.* 1990;70:181.

77. Feuerstein TJ, Zeides A. Theophylline relieves headache following lumbar puncture. Placebo-controlled, double-blind pilot study. *Klin Wochenschr.* 1986;64:216.

78. Carp H, Singh PJ, Vadhera R, et al. Effects of the serotonin-receptor agonist sumatriptan on postdural puncture headache: report of six cases. *Anesth Analg.* 1994;79:180.

79. Taivainen T, Pitkanen M, Tuominen M, et al. Efficacy of epidural

blood patch for postdural puncture headache. *Acta Anaesthesiol Scand.* 1993;37:702.

80. Beards SC, Jackson A, Griffiths AG, et al. Magnetic resonance imaging of extradural blood patches: appearances from 30 min to 18 h. *Br J Anaesth.* 1993;71:182.

81. Crawford JS. Epidural blood patch [letter]. *Anaesthesia.* 1985;40:381.

82. Reynolds F, Speedy HM. The subdural space: the third place to go astray. *Anaesthesia.* 1990;45:120.

83. Russell R, Dundas R, Reynolds F. Long term backache after childbirth: prospective search for causative factors. *BMJ.* 1996;312:1384.

84. Russell R, Groves P, Taub N, et al. Assessing long term backache after childbirth. *BMJ.* 1993;306:1299.

85. Day CJ, Shutt LE. Auditory, ocular, and facial complications of central neural block. A review of possible mechanisms. *Reg Anesth.* 1996;21:197.

86. Pattee C, Ballantyne M, Milne B. Epidural analgesia for labour and delivery: informed consent issues. *Can J Anaesth.* 1997;44:918.

87. Knapp RM. Legal view of informed consent for anesthesia during labor. *Anesthesiology.* 1990;72:211.

88. Clark V, McGrady E, Sugden C, et al. Speed of onset of sensory block for elective extradural caesarean section: choice of agent and temperature of injectate. *Br J Anaesth.* 1994;72:221.

89. Reid JA, Thorburn J. Extradural bupivacaine or lignocaine anaesthesia for elective caesarean section: the role of maternal posture. *Br J Anaesth.* 1988;61:149.

90. Karambelkar DJ, Ramanathan S. 2-Chloroprocaine antagonism of epidural morphine analgesia. *Acta Anaesthesiol Scand.* 1997;41:774.

91. Furst SR, Reisner LS. Risk of high spinal anesthesia following failed epidural block for cesarean delivery. *J Clin Anesth.* 1995;7:71.

92. Moore CH, Wilhite A, Pan PH, et al. The addition of epinephrine to subarachnoid administered hyperbaric bupivacaine with fentanyl for cesarean delivery: the effect on onset time. *Reg Anesth.* 1992;17:202.

93. Fan SZ, Susetio L, Wang YP, et al. Low dose of intrathecal hyperbaric bupivacaine combined with epidural lidocaine for cesarean section—a balance block technique. *Anesth Analg.* 1994;78:474.

94. Davies SJ, Paech MJ, Welch H, et al. Maternal experience during epidural or combined spinal-epidural anesthesia for cesarean section: a prospective, randomized trial. *Anesth Analg.* 1997;85:607.

95. Datta S, Ostheimer GW, Weiss JB, et al. Neonatal effect of prolonged anesthetic induction for cesarean section. *Obstet Gynecol.* 1981;58:331.

96. King H, Ashley S, Brathwaite D, et al. Adequacy of general anesthesia for cesarean section. *Anesth Analg.* 1993;77:84.

97. Hawthorne L, Wilson R, Lyons G, et al. Failed intubation revisited: 17-yr experience in a teaching maternity unit. *Br J Anaesth.* 1996;76:680.

98. Bishop MJ, Kharasch ED. Is the Combitube a useful emergency airway device for anesthesiologists? *Anesth Analg.* 1998;86:1141.

99. Palmer CM, Emerson S, Volgoropolous D, et al. Dose-response relationship of intrathecal morphine for postcesarean analgesia. *Anesthesiology.* 1999;90:437.

100. Skilton RWH, Kinsella SM, Smith A, et al. Dose response study of subarachnoid diamorphine for analgesia after elective caesarean section. *Int J Obstet Anesth.* 1999;8:231.

101. Fuller JG, McMorland GH, Douglas MJ, et al. Epidural morphine for analgesia after caesarean section: a report of 4880 patients. *Can J Anaesth.* 1990;37:636.

102. Brocks DR, Jamali F. Clinical pharmacokinetics of ketorolac tromethamine. *Clin Pharmacokinet.* 1992;23:415.

103. Thacker SB. The efficacy of intrapartum electronic fetal monitoring. *Am J Obstet Gynecol.* 1987;156:24.

104. Clark SL, Gimovsky ML, Miller FC. The scalp stimulation test: a clinical alternative to fetal scalp blood sampling. *Am J Obstet Gynecol.* 1984;148:274.

105. American Academy of Pediatrics and The American College of Obstetricians and Gynecologists. *Guidelines for Perinatal Care.* 4th ed. 1997:112.

106. Seidman DS, Paz I, Laor A, et al. Apgar scores and cognitive performance at 17 years of age. *Obstet Gynecol.* 1991;77:875.

107. Goldaber KG, Gilstrap LC, Leveno KJ, et al. Pathologic fetal acidemia. *Obstet Gynecol.* 1991;78:1103.

108. Schatz M, Harden K, Forsythe A, et al. The course of asthma during pregnancy, post partum, and with successive pregnancies: a prospective analysis. *J Allergy Clin Immunol.* 1988;81:509.

109. Daley MD, Rolbin SH, Hew EM, et al. Epidural anesthesia for obstetrics after spinal surgery. *Reg Anesth.* 1990;15:280.

110. Kain ZN, Mayes LC, Pakes J, et al. Thrombocytopenia in pregnant women who use cocaine. *Am J Obstet Gynecol.* 1995;173:885.

111. Vertommen JD, Hughes SC, Rosen MA, et al. Hydralazine does not

restore uterine blood flow during cocaine-induced hypertension in the pregnant ewe. *Anesthesiology.* 1992;76:580.

112. The Inernational Perinatal HIV Group. The mode of delivery and the risk of vertical transmission of human immunodeficiency virus type 1—a meta-analysis of 15 prospective cohort studies. The International Perinatal HIV Group. *N Engl J Med.* 1999;340:977.

113. Louache F, Vainchenker W. Thrombocytopenia in HIV infection. *Curr Opin Hematol.* 1994;1:369.

114. Tom DJ, Gulevich SJ, Shapiro HM, et al. Epidural blood patch in the HIV-positive patient. Review of clinical experience. San Diego HIV Neurobehavioral Research Center. *Anesthesiology.* 1992;76:943.

115. Newsome LR, Bramwell RS, Curling PE. Severe preeclampsia: hemodynamic effects of lumbar epidural anesthesia. *Anesth Analg.* 1986;65:31.

116. O'Grady JP, Parker RK, Patel SS. Nitroglycerin for rapid tocolysis: development of a protocol and a literature review. *J Perinatol.* 2000;1:27.

117. Crane JM, van den Hof MC, Dodds L, et al. Neonatal outcomes with placenta previa. *Obstet Gynecol.* 1999;93:541.

118. Nielson EC, Varner MW, Scott JR. The outcome of pregnancies complicated by bleeding during the second trimester. *Surg Gynecol Obstet.* 1991;173:371.

119. ACOG Practice Bulletin. Vaginal birth after previous cesarean delivery. *Int J Gynecol Obstet.* 1999;66:197.

120. Vartikar JV, Johnson MD, Datta S. Precordial Doppler monitoring and pulse oximetry during cesarean delivery: detection of venous air embolism. *Reg Anesth.* 1989;14:145.

121. Lew TW, Tay DH, Thomas E. Venous air embolism during cesarean section: more common than previously thought. *Anesth Analg.* 1993;77:448.

122. Handler JS, Bromage PR. Venous air embolism during cesarean delivery. *Reg Anesth.* 1990;15:170.

123. Clark SL, Hankins GD, Dudley DA, et al. Amniotic fluid embolism: analysis of the national registry. *Am J Obstet Gynecol.* 1995;172:1158.

124. Hankins GD, Snyder RR, Clark SL, et al. Acute hemodynamic and respiratory effects of amniotic fluid embolism in the pregnant goat model. *Am J Obstet Gynecol.* 1993;168:1113.

125. Hankins GD, Berryman GK, Scott RTJ, et al. Maternal arterial desaturation with 15-methyl prostaglandin F2 alpha for uterine atony. *Obstet Gynecol.* 1988;72:367.

126. Chestnut DH, Dewan DM, Redick LF, et al. Anesthetic management for obstetric hysterectomy: a multi-institutional study. *Anesthesiology.* 1989;70:607.

127. Goodman EJ, Dumas SD. The rate of successful reactivation of labor epidural catheters for postpartum tubal ligation surgery. *Reg Anesth Pain Med.* 1998;23:258.

128. Viscomi CM, Rathmell JP. Labor epidural catheter reactivation or spinal anesthesia for delayed postpartum tubal ligation: a cost comparison. *J Clin Anesth.* 1995;7:380.

129. Jayaram A, Bowen MP, Deshpande S, et al. Ultrasound examination of the stomach contents of women in the postpartum period. *Anesth Analg.* 1997;84:522.

130. Carlan SJ, Dent JM, Huckaby T, et al. The effect of epidural anesthesia on safety and success of external cephalic version at term. *Anesth Analg.* 1994;79:525.

CHAPTER

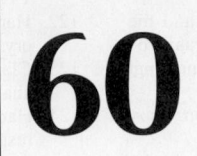

# 60

# Nonobstetric Surgery in the Pregnant Patient

Michael A. Frölich

Thomas W. Lebert II

Christopher F. James

## SUMMARY

Not uncommonly, pregnant patients have to undergo surgery for nonobstetric reasons; in the United States, about 50 000 to 70 000 women per year undergo surgery while pregnant, an incidence of 0.75% to 2%.[1,2] Appendectomy is the most common nonobstetric operation during pregnancy, closely followed by cholecystectomy and ovarian cystectomy. Many different procedures have been performed successfully during pregnancy, including open heart procedures,[3] neurosurgical procedures requiring hypotensive techniques and hypothermia,[4] and liver transplantation.[5] Some of the more common reasons for surgical intervention are listed in Table 60–1. The prevalence of trauma during pregnancy is also increasing. In some areas of the United States, especially the inner cities, trauma is the leading cause of maternal mortality.

## MATERNAL CONSIDERATIONS

### *What Are the Major Concerns?*

To provide safe anesthesia to the pregnant patient, one must consider not only the physiologic changes but also at what point they occur during gestation and how they affect the administration of anesthesia. Fetal concerns include the possible teratogenic effects of anesthetic agents, avoidance of intrauterine fetal asphyxia, and prevention of premature labor. Maternal considerations result from the physiologic changes of pregnancy, which are summarized in this chapter. A more detailed discussion is presented in Chapter 59.

The cardiovascular system undergoes significant alteration under the influence of the hormonal milieu of pregnancy. Changes include increased oxygen ($O_2$) consumption, increased heart rate, and increasing cardiac output, with a peak effect at 28 to 32 weeks of gestation.[6] Blood pressure (BP) falls during the second trimester, with a greater decrease in the diastolic pressure, resulting in an increase in pulse pressure. The increase in blood volume occurs to a greater extent in the plasma component than in the red blood cell mass, resulting in physiologic anemia even though the actual red blood cell mass is increased.

Aortocaval compression, which results from the impingement of the weight of the uterus on the aorta and vena cava, can occur as early as the 18th week of gestation. Usually, however, it is not significant until after the 24th week. Aortic compression may lead to decreased uterine perfusion with normal maternal upper extremity BP measurements; thus, BP measurement in the lower extremities may be prudent in the third trimester, especially if the procedure must be performed in the supine position.

Other physiologic adjustments that occur during pregnancy are altered glucose homeostasis and maternal respiratory alkalosis. The compensated maternal respiratory alkalosis is probably due to hyperventilation, which begins early in pregnancy and is thought to result from increased progesterone as well as sensitivity of the central nervous system. After the fifth month of pregnancy, the functional residual capacity, expiratory reserve volume, and lung residual volume are decreased by 20% because of the gravid uterus pushing on the diaphragm.

Table 60–2 and Figure 60–1 summarize some of the physiologic alterations in pregnancy.

## Do Pregnant Patients Have Reduced Anesthetic Requirements?

Gestation is associated with a decrease in drug requirement for both general and regional anesthesia. The reduction in minimum alveolar concentration (MAC) for both halothane and isoflurane may be as great as 25% to 40%.[7] This change has been attributed to the sedative effects of high progesterone levels and, more recently, to increased levels of endogenous endorphins.[8]

Progesterone and other biochemical factors may also be responsible for an enhancement in membrane sensitivity to local anesthetics, thereby reducing requirements for these

**TABLE 60–2.** Anesthetic Implicatons of the Physiologic Changes in Pregnancy

| Change | Implication |
|---|---|
| *Gastrointestinal* | |
| Increased gastric volume, volume acidity, relaxed LES | Drug modification of gastric contents |
| Respiratory | |
| Increased $O_2$ consumption | Protect airway, early intubation |
| Decreased FRC | Apnea leads to rapid hypoxemia |
| Lowered $Paco_2$/serum bicarbonate | Preoxygenation, denitrogenation |
| | Decreased tolerance of acidosis |
| | Interpretation of ABG results |
| *Cardiac* | |
| Increased CO | Decreased UBF if CO not maintained |
| Aortocaval compression | Maintenance of uterine displacement |
| Increased plasma volume | Volume status to maintain UBF |
| | Interpretation of CVP and PAOP |
| *Hematologic* | |
| Dilutional anemia | Interpretation of CBC and coagulation panel |
| Leukocytosis | |
| Hypercoagulability | Prophylaxis for DVT |
| *Central Nervous System* | |
| Decreased MAC | Vigilance with sedation (especially non–operating room locations) |
| | Sensitivity to analgesics or anesthetics |
| *Renal* | |
| Increased RBF, GFR ureteral compression | Interpretation of BUN creatinine levels |
| | Vigilance toward development of UTI |

ABG, arterial blood gas; BUN, blood urea nitrogen; CBC, complete blood count; CO, cardiac output; CVP, central venous pressure; DVT, deep vein thrombosis; FRC, functional residual capacity; GFR, glomerular filtration rate; LES, lower esophageal sphincter; MAC, minimum alveolar concentration; PAOP, pulmonary artery occlusion pressure; RBF, renal blood flow; UBF, uterine blood flow; UTI, urinary tract infection.

drugs as early as the first trimester.[9] Decreases in the total dose requirement for spinal or epidural anesthesia occur with increasing duration of gestation. These decreases are probably related to the decreased volume of the epidural space and cerebrospinal fluid that is brought about by epidural venous engorgement and the previously mentioned hormonal effects.[10–12]

The increase in vascularity increases the incidence of unintended epidural intravascular injection of local anesthetics to as much as 10%. Along with the increased sensitivity of local anesthetics in pregnancy is their increased systemic toxicity, which may be due in part to the increased free fraction of highly protein-bound drugs such as bupivacaine.[13]

**TABLE 60–1.** Reasons for Surgical Intervention During Pregnancy

**Abdominal**
Appendectomy
Ovarian surgery (cyst, torsion)
Cholecystectomy (laparoscopic)

**Nonabdominal**
Breast surgery
Thyroidectomy
Parathyroidectomy
Cardiac surgery
Neurosurgery

**Trauma**
Blunt (motor vehicle accident)
Penetrating (gunshot wound, stabbing)

**Pregnancy-Related**
Cervical cerclage
Fetal surgery

## FETAL CONSIDERATIONS

### What Are the Primary Fetal Physiologic Concerns?

Whenever a pregnant patient undergoes surgery, two patients are placed at risk. Fetal hazards can be minimized by an understanding of the fetal effects of maternal drug administration and of the operation. The most important acute fetal risk related to maternal surgery and anesthesia is intrauterine asphyxia. Therefore, the anesthesiologist's primary concerns are the perioperative maintenance of maternal $O_2$-carrying capacity, $O_2$ affinity, $Pao_2$, and uteroplacental blood flow. Maintenance of normal maternal $Pao_2$, $Paco_2$, maternal

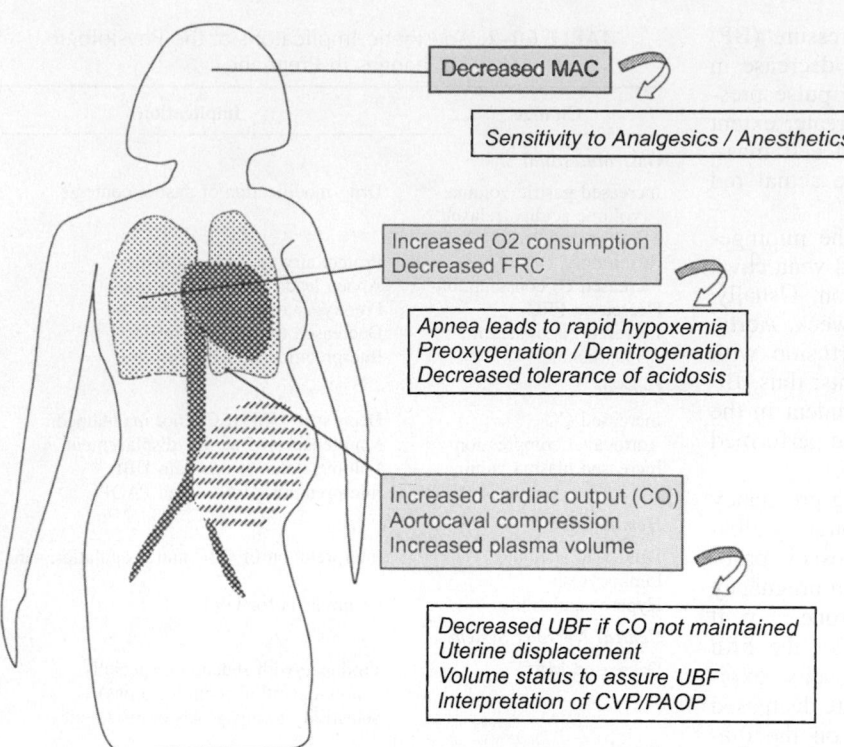

**FIGURE 60–1.** Anesthetic implications of the physiologic changes in pregnancy. The changes outlined in *shaded boxes* necessitate a modification in the anesthetic management (outlined in *clear boxes*). CVP, central venous pressure; FRC, functional residual capacity; MAC, minimal alveolar concentration; PAOP, pulmonary artery occlusion pressure; UBF, uterine blood flow.

BP, and uterine vascular resistance is of paramount importance.[14]

## Uteroplacental Perfusion

Uterine blood flow is described by the following equation that is based on Ohm's law:

$$UBF = \frac{UAP - UVP}{UAR}$$

where UBF is uterine blood flow, UAP is uterine artery pressure, UVP is uterine venous pressure, and UAR is uterine artery resistance.

Normally, 10% of a pregnant patient's cardiac output goes to the uterus; this value is 1% in the nonpregnant patient. The placenta accounts for about 80% of this blood flow; the balance supplies the uterine smooth muscle. Autoregulation of uterine vessels does not occur; thus, flow is directly proportional to maternal mean arterial pressure. Interventions that increase uterine venous pressure or uterine artery resistance decrease uterine blood flow and may lead to placental hypoperfusion and fetal asphyxia (Table 60–3).

## Uterine Vasoconstriction

The uterine vasculature normally functions in a state of near-maximum vasodilation, and a significant reserve for vasoconstriction is present should maternal needs require it. Maternal hyperventilation leads to vasoconstriction and reduces placental perfusion. The rise in maternal pH associated with hyperventilation increases the affinity of maternal hemoglobin for $O_2$, thereby further reducing $O_2$ delivery to the fetoplacental unit.

Administration of direct-acting vasoconstrictors such as phenylephrine—if given in large doses—reduces uterine perfusion by direct vasoconstriction; therefore, indirectly acting agents, such as ephedrine, which has fewer α-adrenergic receptor effects, are the drugs of choice.[15,16] Hypoventilation and maternal hypercapnia lead to fetal respiratory acidosis, which in turn, if severe, can lead to fetal myocardial depression and hypotension. Hyperventilation can result in umbilical artery constriction, and uterine blood flow can also be reduced by positive pressure ventilation. Maternal hypoxemia, from a myriad of factors (eg, pulmonary aspiration, difficulty in tracheal intubation, total spinal block) results in fetal hypoxemia. Maternal hyperoxia, however, presents no fetal risk of retinopathy of prematurity or of premature closure of the ductus arteriosus because, even in the presence of a maternal $PaO_2$ of 600 mm Hg, the fetal $PaO_2$ does not exceed 50 to 60 mm Hg.[17]

Maternal hypotension should be avoided when possible, and if it occurs, the patient must be treated aggressively with intravenous fluids, lateral positioning, decreased levels of anesthesia, and aggressive use of ephedrine. If these measures fail, low-dose phenylephrine and epinephrine may be indicated. Despite preblock hydration and positioning, the

---

**TABLE 60–3.** Factors That Decrease Uteroplacental Perfusion

**Decreased Uterine Arterial Pressure**

Hypotension
Hypovolemia

**Increased Uterine Venous Pressure**

Inferior vena cava compression
Increased uterine tone (hypercarbia, oxytocin, ergots, ketamine)

**Increased Uterine Artery Resistance**

α-Adrenergic vasopressors
Endogenous catecholamines
Ketamine (>1 mg/kg first trimester)

incidence of hypotension in the term pregnant patient under regional anesthesia is as high as 80%.[18]

Fetal risks may be presented by an acute, single anesthetic exposure for a surgical procedure or by subacute or chronic low-dose occupational anesthetic exposure of a parent who works in an operating room. Numerous studies have been published, but conclusions are limited by these studies' retrospective nature, by inherent variables such as maternal health and multiple drug exposures, by the lack of needed control groups, and by the limited sample sizes.

## What Is the Risk of Chronic Low-Dose Anesthetic Exposure?

### Spontaneous Abortion

Although multiple reports have been published regarding an increased risk of both spontaneous abortion and congenital anomalies among operating room personnel, a causal relationship has never been demonstrated. The American Society of Anesthesiologists (ASA) conducted an extensive nationwide survey in 1974 that appeared to demonstrate an increased rate of spontaneous abortion among female operating room personnel compared with their non–operating room hospital personnel counterparts.[19] Among female dentists who used inhalation agents in their practice, a reportedly higher incidence of spontaneous abortion existed than among those who limited their practice to the use of local anesthetics.[20]

### Congenital Anomalies

Although multiple studies have alluded to a correlation between the occupational exposure of women to subanesthetic concentrations of inhalation anesthetics and an increased occurrence of spontaneous abortion, a correlation of such exposure with increased risk of congenital abnormalities has not been documented. Many factors, such as maternal health, work-related stress differences, and the level and frequency of exposure to trace anesthetics, could not be controlled. Furthermore, the efficient scavenging systems used today limit the relevance of these data in the current work environment.

## What Is the Risk of Acute Anesthetic Exposure?

### Organogenesis

In general, the most critical stage of development is thought to be during the period of organogenesis, which in human beings occurs roughly from postconception days 15 to 56. Because the genitourinary system and the central nervous system continue to develop throughout the course of gestation, even into the neonatal period, extended periods of sensitivity are present throughout the course of pregnancy. Nevertheless, organogenesis represents the most critical period.[21]

### Congenital Abnormalities

In a more recent review of a Swedish registry of 5405 cases, no increase in congenital malformations or stillbirths was noted in the offspring of patients having surgery, and no specific type of anesthesia or surgery was associated with adverse outcome. However, the incidence of low-birth-weight infants and neonatal deaths within the first 7 days of life was increased.[22] In these and other studies, an increased risk for congenital anomalies could not be demonstrated.[23]

### Teratogenicity

Several premedicants and anesthetic drugs have been demonstrated to be teratogenic in some animal models under particular conditions.[24] Furthermore, certain physiologic risks associated with the administration of an anesthetic, such as hypoxia, hypotension, and hypercapnia, may be teratogenic in some animals. Multiple factors are involved in determining whether a particular drug or agent will be teratogenic in human beings (Table 60–4). Drugs that have been shown to cause particular defects in animal models may have no such effect in human beings. In addition, duration and dose of exposure play a significant role. Teratogens that have been documented are listed in Table 60–5.

Although teratogenesis may occur after exposure to very high doses or prolonged chronic exposure to low doses, one cannot conclude that a single short exposure during the course of an anesthetic case will cause the same defect. The fetal gestational age is also a critical element. Susceptibility or enhanced sensitivity from exposure to a particular agent during one stage of fetal or embryonic development occurs rarely or not at all at a different stage.[23]

## What Are the Risks of Specific Agents and Other Factors?

### Nitrous Oxide

Among the commonly used anesthetic agents, nitrous oxide use during pregnancy has been the subject of the greatest controversy. Concerns stem from (1) uterine vascular vasoconstriction and decreased uterine blood flow in animal studies and (2) the potentially toxic effect that nitrous oxide may pose relative to its ability to inactivate the enzyme methionine synthetase.[25] This enzyme is responsible for the production of methionine and tetrahydrofolate, which are important elements in the process of myelination. Hence, the potential for central nervous system aberration subsequent to the exposure to nitrous oxide is an important consideration.

The inactivation of methionine synthetase by nitrous oxide appears to last for several days. However, its effect has not been demonstrated to be clinically significant in human studies. Some investigators have advocated the administration of methionine, folinic acid, and vitamin $B_{12}$ to patients undergoing anesthesia with nitrous oxide during pregnancy as a "rescue" technique because of the theoretic toxicity. Although this problem has not been proved to be clinically significant,

**TABLE 60–4.** Some Factors That Affect the Teratogenicity of Drugs

Dose of drug or agent
Duration of patient exposure
Embryonic or fetal stage at time of exposure
Genetic susceptibility to individual drug effects

**TABLE 60–5.** Drugs Known to Be Teratogens

| Agents | Effects |
| --- | --- |
| Angiotensin-converting enzyme inhibitors | Fetal renal tubular dysplasia, neonatal renal failure, lack of cranial ossification |
| Alcohol | Growth restriction, mental retardation, microcephaly, midfacial hypoplasia, renal and cardiac defects |
| Androgens | Virilization of female, advanced genital development in male |
| Carbamazepine | Neural tube defects, minor craniofacial defects, fingernail hypoplasia, microcephaly |
| Chemotherapy agents | Increased risk for spontaneous abortions, various anomalies |
| Cocaine | Bowel atresias; malformations of heart, limbs, face and genitourinary tract; microcephaly; cerebral infarcts |
| Coumadin | Nasal hypoplasia, stippled bone epiphyses, broad short hands with shortened phalanges |
| Diethylstilbestrol | Clear-cell adenocarcinoma of the vagina or cervix, vaginal adenosis, abnormalities of the cervix and uterus, and testes |
| Kanamycin and streptomycin | Hearing loss, 8th nerve damage |
| Lead | Increased abortion rates, stillbirths |
| Lithium | Congenital heart disease, especially Ebstein's anomaly |
| Mercury | Cerebral atrophy, microcephaly, mental retardation, spasticity, seizures, blindness |
| Phenytoin | Mental retardation, microcephaly, dysmorphic craniofacial features, cardiac defects, hypoplastic nails and distal phalanges |
| Tetracycline | Hypoplasia of tooth enamel, permanent discoloration of deciduous teeth |
| Trimethadione and paramethadione | Cleft lip or palate, cardiac defects, microcephaly, mental retardation, facial abnormalities, ophthalmologic, limb and genitourinary tract abnormalities |
| Valproic acid | Neural tube defects, especially spinal bifida; minor facial defects |
| Vitamin A and derivatives | Increased abortion rate, micrognathia, central nervous system defects, thymic agenesis, craniofacial dysmorphism, microphthalmia, cleft lip and palate, mental retardation |

Adapted from American College of Obstetricians and Gynecologists (ACOG). *ACOG Educational Bulletin # 236.* Washington, DC: ACOG; April 1997.

most anesthesiologists in obstetrics advocate the avoidance of nitrous oxide for pregnant patients whenever possible but especially during the first trimester.

## Potent Inhalation Agents

No major structural abnormalities could be found among rats exposed to 0.75 of the MAC of halothane, enflurane, or isoflurane.[26] Single exposure for brief periods appears highly unlikely to produce fetal abnormalities. A second, somewhat serendipitous advantage to the use of these agents during pregnancy is the fact that all the potent inhalation agents, including the newer ones, sevoflurane and desflurane, are known to reduce uterine contractility and, therefore, may provide some benefit to reduce the risk for intraoperative premature uterine contractility. On the other hand, higher MAC concentrations (approaching 2 MAC levels) of inhalation agents can indirectly decrease uterine blood flow by decreasing maternal cardiac output.

## Sodium Thiopental and Other Sedative Drugs

An increase in the incidence of congenital abnormalities after sodium thiopental use has been shown in some animal species. However, the administration of sodium thiopental to 152 women in their first trimester and undergoing cervical cerclage was not associated with an increase in the occurrence of fetal anomalies.[27]

Such has not been the case with the use of benzodiazepines. These drugs are among the most frequently administered medications in the United States. Although investigations of fetal outcome after in utero exposure have led to discrepant results, two separate retrospective studies have shown an association between high-dose maternal diazepam use and fetal cleft lip or cleft palate.[28,29] No such linkage has been established in prospective studies with other benzodiazepines or sedative agents.[30]

## Narcotics

The effects of in vitro and in vivo narcotics have been evaluated extensively. Chronic administration of morphine to pregnant rats did not lead to increased incidence of congenital anomalies, but it was found to be associated with decreased fetal and maternal weight gain, decreased litter counts, and an increased number of term stillbirths.[31] Parallel results have also been observed in human narcotic addicts and in those taking methadone.[32]

Animal studies involving the chronic administration of newer synthetic agents such as fentanyl have failed to demonstrate impairment in reproductive capability or in the occurrence of fetal anomalies.[33] Little, if any, evidence shows that the short, single exposure of pregnant women to narcotic agents in routine doses is associated with adverse fetal outcome.

Codeine-containing compounds have been shown to be teratogenic when used in the first trimester. Compounds containing codeine may be used in the second and third trimesters for short intervals with little fetal risk.[34,35] Nonsteroidal antiinflammatory agents block prostaglandin synthesis and may lead to in utero premature closure of the ductus arteriosus. Cases of fatal neonatal pulmonary hypertension have been reported with use of these agents near term.[36] Short courses of indomethacin have been used in the early third trimester as a tocolytic agent for preterm labor with little reported fetal morbidity. In most cases, however, nonsteroidal antiinflammatory agents are to be avoided in the pregnant patient.

## Muscle Relaxants

Despite the presence of skeletal abnormalities in chick embryos exposed to D-tubocurarine, no evidence suggests adverse fetal effects in pregnant human beings exposed to the usual range of clinically used muscle relaxants. Developmental abnormalities did not occur in cultured rat embryos until much greater than usual (30 times) clinical doses of D-tubocurarine, pancuronium, atracurium, and vecuronium were administered.[37]

Reversal of neuromuscular blockade at the end of a case can be avoided in certain circumstances, especially with judicious use of the shorter-acting nondepolarizing neuromuscular blockers, such as mivacurium, rocuronium, and rapacuronium. When reversal of muscle relaxation is indicated, it should be performed with caution and the usual coadministration of an anticholinergic to avoid acute increases in acetylcholine that may promote uterine contractions.

## Local Anesthetics

Although local anesthetics, even in very low concentrations, have been shown in vitro to reversibly reduce cell division, studies have failed to demonstrate an increased rate of fetal malformation with exposure to amides or esters.[38] Cardiac and neural sensitivity to local anesthetics is increased in pregnancy.[39]

## Hypoxia and Hyperoxia

Hypoxia is teratogenic in several animal species.[40] Complications that can lead to maternal and fetal hypoxemia must be prevented with deliberate and careful anesthetic management. The fears of uterine and placental vasoconstriction in the face of maternal hyperoxia are unfounded.

No studies demonstrate fetal hypoxia in the face of maternal hyperoxia. Furthermore, as was noted earlier, increasing maternal $PaO_2$ to as high as 600 mm Hg cannot produce a fetal $PaO_2$ of $>60$ mm Hg because of the high metabolic activity of the placenta and the lack of autoregulation between the maternal and placental circulations.[41] Hyperbaric $O_2$, however, does increase the incidence of fetal anomalies, although these effects appear to be more related to the high-pressure state than to maternal hyperoxia.[42]

## Hypocarbia and Hypercarbia

Hypocarbia interferes not only with maternal and fetal acid-base balance (see Uteroplacental Perfusion) but also with fetal development. Hypercarbia, manifested by exposing rats to elevated inhaled tensions of carbon dioxide ($CO_2$) for periods of 24 hours, results in a high incidence of fetal cardiac anomalies.[43] Whether these effects are mediated in relation to direct exposure to higher levels of $CO_2$ or, more likely, as a result of the physiologic aberration that occurs in the face of hypercarbia (acidosis, vasoconstriction of uterine vessels, change in hemoglobin affinity for $O_2$, and direct fetal myocardial depression) has not been determined.

In summary, although surgery during pregnancy is associated with an increased incidence of spontaneous abortion and fetal demise, these outcomes cannot be attributed to the anesthetic. Rather, the increased risk appears to be related to the procedure itself, the site of maternal surgery, and the mother's underlying medical condition that may have precipitated the need for surgical intervention.

Obviously, hypoxia, hypercarbia, and hypotension have multiple deleterious effects, and careful anesthetic management of these factors is critical. No clinical evidence shows that any particular anesthetic type or technique is associated with improved fetal outcome.

## What Is the Risk of Maternal Diagnostic Irradiation?

Indicated diagnostic radiologic procedures may be undertaken with care in the pregnant patient. Adverse fetal effects are unlikely with adequate technique but have been reported. Direct fetal irradiation of 10 cGy (10 000 millirad [mrd], 1 cGy = 1 mrd) has been shown to produce fetal defects.[44–46] Microcephaly is the single most common defect observed. Intrauterine growth retardation and poor fetal development have also been described. Doses of direct irradiation to the fetus of 1 cGy or less have not been shown to produce fetal defects.[47]

Concern exists that any in utero radiation exposure increases the risk for neonatal and childhood neoplasms, and thus any radiation exposure during gestation should be undertaken with care.[48,49] If a significant alteration in clinical management is to be undertaken because of findings obtained from a radiologic procedure, the potential risk to the fetus is warranted. The estimated fetal radiation exposure associated with several radiodiagnostic procedures is shown in Table 60–6.

Radionuclide procedures may also be performed if patient management decisions depend on their results. Radiation doses to the fetus are generally low with most investigational radionuclide procedures. Most of these agents are cleared renally, and it is important to place an indwelling bladder catheter to reduce total radiation doses to the fetus because urine is retained in the maternal bladder and the fetus may be exposed to larger radiation doses.

In summary, irradiation during pregnancy should be avoided whenever possible. Diagnostic irradiation during pregnancy for medically indicated procedures should not be withheld if it is deemed necessary. Exposure of low-dose radiation ($<5$ Gy) to the fetus should not form the basis for termination of pregnancy. Fortunately, ultrasonography often can replace radiographic procedures.

## What Is the Risk of Preterm Labor?

Premature labor is a rare complication of nonobstetric surgery. With the exception of lower abdominal and pelvic procedures, there is little risk of precipitating labor.[50] Maternal hypotension with a resultant decrement in uterine perfusion may lead to premature uterine contraction activity. The prophylactic use of β-adrenergic tocolytic drugs is not recommended because their potential complications of vasodilation and tachycardia are not outweighed by any clinical benefits.[51] Procedures of the lower abdomen or pelvis requiring manipu-

**TABLE 60–6.** Estimated Radiation Exposure to the Shielded Fetus From Commonly Ordered Radiographs

| Examination | Mean (mGy) | Maximum (mGy) |
|---|---|---|
| ***Conventional Radiographic Examinations*** | | |
| Abdomen | 1.4 | 4.2 |
| Chest | <0.01 | <0.01 |
| Intravenous urogram | 1.7 | 10 |
| Lumbar spine | 1.7 | 10 |
| Pelvis | 1.1 | 4 |
| Skull | <0.01 | <0.01 |
| Thoracic spine | <0.01 | <0.01 |
| ***Fluoroscopic Examinations*** | | |
| Barium meal (UGI) | 1.1 | 5.8 |
| Barium enema | 6.8 | 24 |
| ***Computed Tomography*** | | |
| Abdomen | 8.0 | 49 |
| Chest | 0.06 | 0.96 |
| Head | <0.005 | <0.005 |
| Lumbar spine | 2.4 | 8.6 |
| Pelvis | 25 | 79 |

UGI, upper gastrointestinal series.
From Pregnancy and medical radiation. *Ann ICRP.* 2000;30(1):1.

lation of the uterus may stimulate uterine contractions. When there is extensive uterine manipulation in the second and third trimester and premature contractions ensue, tocolytic therapy with β-adrenergic agents may be used. A single subcutaneous or intravascular dose of terbutaline sulfate, 0.25 mg, or intravenous (100-200 μg) or sublingual nitroglycerin is often sufficient to arrest contractions. Occasionally, if frank labor ensues and the risks for fetal prematurity are significant (<32 weeks' gestation), intravenous magnesium sulfate may be given if there are no maternal contraindications. An initial loading dose of 4 to 6 g of a 20% solution of magnesium sulfate is given over 20 to 30 minutes, followed by a maintenance dose of 2 to 4 g/h. Magnesium sulfate carries a risk for respiratory depression or arrest and cardiac arrhythmias. Toxic side effects may be reversed with calcium given intravenously (1 g of a 10% solution of calcium gluconate).

First-trimester or early second-trimester uterine cramping may be treated with progesterone to attempt uterine quiescence. Data justifying these endeavors have shown some clinical effect, although minimal. Hydroxyprogesterone is given as an intramuscular dose of 250 mg.[52]

In most clinical conditions that require surgery (eg, acute appendicitis or acute cholecystitis), the severity of the maternal disease outweighs the potential consequences of not performing surgery, and the resulting fetal risks are much greater than the small potential for premature labor with surgery.

## PREPARING THE PATIENT FOR SURGERY

### What Are the Major Concerns?

Five major concerns must be addressed before anesthesia is administered to a pregnant surgical patient (Table 60–7). Elective surgery should be postponed until after parturition. When surgery is deemed necessary, it should be avoided during the first trimester, if at all possible, so long as the mother's health is not in jeopardy. Early second-trimester surgery also may be more appropriate if the peaks in blood volume, cardiac output, and aortocaval compression that occur in the third trimester are to be avoided. As was noted previously, procedures within the pelvic cavity pose the greatest risk for preterm labor.

### Preoperative Management

A thorough preoperative evaluation is extremely important. In addition to the obviously important gathering of information, it allows the anesthesiologist to explain the relative risks involved and to reassure the patient that a safe and effective anesthetic can be provided for the mother and fetus.

Anxiety and pain should be allayed with narcotics alone or in combination with a major tranquilizer. Diazepam and possi-

bly other benzodiazepines should be avoided during organogenesis.

The preoperative administration of histamine$_2$ antagonists, metoclopramide, or both may be well advised to decrease the risk for pneumonitis should aspiration occur. A clear, nonparticulate antacid such as sodium citrate is useful to neutralize preexisting gastric secretions. Uterine displacement is advisable from the second trimester onward during transport, anesthesia, surgery, and recovery to avoid aortocaval compression.

### Monitoring

In addition to basic intraoperative monitoring, as set forth in the guidelines of the ASA, more serious conditions may dictate the need for invasive maternal monitors. The fetal heart rate should also be recorded continuously whenever possible. If the surgical field makes this an impossible task, presence of the fetal heart rate should be documented preoperatively and after induction of anesthesia with the surgeon or obstetrician present; subsequent continuous monitoring should be initiated at the end of surgery. During intraabdominal cases, periodic fetal heart rate monitoring with a sterile ultrasonic transducer may be prudent.

The fetal heart rate can be detected as early as the 16th week of gestation with ultrasound. It is obviously a good indicator of uteroplacental function. Variability after the 25th week of gestation is a good indicator of fetal well-being. However, this variability is commonly lost after the administration of parenteral narcotics, barbiturates, sedative-hypnotics, and potent inhalation agents; regional anesthetic techniques do not usually affect variability.[53]

Intraoperatively, beat-to-beat variability is therefore of little diagnostic value. The clinician should use the basal fetal heart rate for the assessment of fetal well-being. The normal fetal heart rate ranges from 120 to 160 beats/min and is usually low-normal during sleep cycles of the fetus. Lower heart rates during sleep cycles (in the 110 beats/min range) can be observed in pregnancies close to term.

Whenever possible intraoperatively, and in all patients postoperatively, monitoring of uterine contractility with a tocodynamometer is advised for up to 24 hours. This technique is also most useful in assessing the need for tocolytic therapy. Aggressive treatment of preterm labor is advised, as was mentioned previously.

### Trauma and Pregnancy

Trauma during pregnancy is a frequent event complicating about 1 in every 12 pregnancies.[54] Because trauma and other forms of violence are the leading causes of death in the reproductive age group, it is not surprising that trauma is the leading cause of nonobstetric maternal death.[55] One particular concern is the effect of trauma itself on the pregnancy. Abruptio placentae has been well documented after trauma during pregnancy,[56–59] and its clinical manifestations and deleterious effects on the pregnancy have recently become better understood. Additionally, there appears to be substantial risk for fetal maternal hemorrhage after trauma during pregnancy.[60]

### What Are the Specific Concerns of Trauma in Pregnancy?

The uterus and its contents are themselves subject to serious, even catastrophic, injury, which constitutes one of the

**TABLE 60–7.** Key Anesthetic Concerns for the Administration of Anesthesia During Pregnancy

Maternal safety
Fetal well-being
Avoidance or prevention of preterm labor
Fetal and uterine monitoring
Maintenance of uteroplacental perfusion

major reasons that trauma during pregnancy is such a unique event.

***Abruptio placentae*** complicates between 1% and 5% of minor injuries, compared with 40% to 50% of major (ie, life-threatening) injuries.[61] In the trauma patient who is beyond 20 weeks' gestation, cardiotocodynamometry appears to be particularly sensitive in identifying patients with abruptio placentae.[62]

***Uterine rupture*** is an infrequent but potentially life-threatening complication of trauma, involving only 0.6% of all injuries during pregnancy. It tends to occur only when there is direct abdominal impact associated with substantial traumatic force.

***Direct fetal injury*** is also an infrequent but potentially serious event-complicating trauma during pregnancy. Numerous cases of direct fetal injury have been reported, but because it is such an uncommon event, the incidence is uncertain.

***Penetrating abdominal trauma*** during pregnancy has remarkably disparate prognosis for the fetus and the gravida. Visceral injuries to the mother complicate only 19% of gunshot wounds to the uterus, whereas the fetus is injured nearly two thirds of the time.[63] Subsequent perinatal mortality rates vary from 41% to 71%.

## Is Cardiopulmonary Resuscitation Different in the Pregnant Patient?

The advanced cardiac life support guidelines for pharmacologic and electroshock interventions should be followed as in nonpregnant patients, remembering the importance of manual uterine displacement to enhance cardiac return.[64] Closed chest compressions can restore about one third of the cardiac output of a nonpregnant arrest victim. Chest compression forces decrease by about 20% when the mother is tilted.[65] In the face of maternal cardiac arrest, consideration must be given to perimortem cesarean delivery if initial resuscitation efforts are unsuccessful. Initialization of a perimortem cesarean delivery within 4 minutes of maternal cardiac arrest maximizes maternal and fetal survival. Neonatal outcome after 15 minutes of maternal cardiac arrest is poor.[66]

## What Are the General Principles of Trauma Management in the Pregnant Patient?

Management of the penetrating trauma begins with completely undressing the patient, followed by careful inspection of all entrance and exit wounds because victims are occasionally shot or stabbed multiple times. Radiographs of the area in two projections are often helpful to localize a bullet if an exit wound is not seen. Fortunately, the uterus and its contents can often stop the progression of a projectile, limiting the extent of maternal injury to the abdominal wall and the uterus.

Unfortunately, signs of peritoneal irritation are less reliable during pregnancy, and changes in vital signs due to blood loss may occur relatively late owing to an increase in blood volume. These latter observations mandate a relatively aggressive approach to exploratory laparotomy for gunshot wounds to the abdomen during pregnancy. The indications for tetanus

prophylaxis are not changed because of pregnancy and should be administered to appropriate candidates.

The use of cardiotocographic monitoring in pregnant victims of trauma beyond 20 weeks' gestation appears to predict reliably those patients who will develop abruptio placentae. Because abruptio placentae usually becomes manifest shortly after injury, monitoring should be initiated after the woman is stabilized. The duration of monitoring is controversial. However, a minimum of 4 hours of monitoring should allow identification of patients who subsequently develop abruptio placentae or preterm delivery.

# ANESTHETIC ADMINISTRATION

## What Techniques Are Useful?

The choice of anesthesia should be based on the mother's condition, the mother's choice, and the extent of the planned surgery.

### Subarachnoid Block

A subarachnoid block is our preferred method for those procedures that lend themselves to this technique. Spinal anesthesia is preferred because maternal and fetal drug exposure is limited to a very small dose of local anesthetic. The risk for hypotension is, of course, a major consideration and makes prehydration and aggressive treatment essential.

### Lumbar Epidural and Caudal Epidural Block

Lumbar epidural or caudal anesthesia provides the same advantages as spinal anesthesia. However, more local anesthetic agent (5-7 times the spinal dose) is necessary, increasing the risk for systemic local anesthetic toxicity. The increased risk for local anesthetic toxicity is also compounded by the increased epidural vein engorgement, especially later in gestation, making epidural vein cannulation more common.[11,67] The incidence and degree of hypotension with an epidural block may be less than with spinal anesthesia, owing to a slower onset of action. Other regional blocks should be used when possible, such as in upper extremity surgery.

### Combined Spinal Epidural Anesthesia

The combined spinal epidural technique has been used successfully for labor analgesia and cesarean sections and in patients undergoing urologic, gynecologic, and general surgery of the lower abdomen and orthopedic procedures.[68] Theoretical advantages of this technique for surgery in the pregnant patient include (1) a lower total dose of local anesthetic compared with a conventional epidural technique, (2) avoidance of a high spinal block that results in hypotension and so forth by using a smaller spinal dose with the combined technique as compared with a conventional single-shot spinal technique, and (3) the flexibility of a prolonged block, if needed, with the epidural component.[66-69]

### General Anesthesia

General anesthesia is necessary when the operative procedure involves the head, neck, or thorax or when medical circumstances dictate its use. The common induction agents—thiopental, propofol, etomidate, and ketamine—have all been found safe when used judiciously. However, high doses of thiopental (6-8 mg/kg) and ketamine (2 mg/kg) have produced neonatal depression.[70,71] Ketamine at higher doses of 2.0 mg/kg has been shown to decrease uterine blood flow by increasing uterine tone when administered in the first half of pregnancy.[72] Propofol compares favorably with thiopental for induction of anesthesia; however, there have been rare case reports and animal studies that have demonstrated severe maternal bradycardia following propofol and succinylcholine combinations for rapid-sequence inductions.[73] Etomidate has been used sparingly in the pregnant patient, secondary to involuntary muscle movements and neonatal cortisol suppression.[74]

Maintenance of anesthesia with potent inhalation agents has the advantage of decreasing uterine tone, producing uterine artery vasodilation, and increasing uterine blood flow at 1.0 MAC. However, at higher doses (1.5-2.0 MAC), decreases in maternal cardiac output result and lead to decreased uterine blood flow. With the lower solubilities of the newer inhalation agents sevoflurane and desflurane, theoretical advantages include a more rapid recovery from anesthesia. Both sevoflurane and desflurane have demonstrated similar maternal and fetal effects and outcome when compared with isoflurane, enflurane, and spinal anesthesia in patients undergoing cesarean section.[75,76]

A combined epidural and general anesthetic offers several advantages. It provides loss of consciousness with a lower concentration of volatile anesthetic, thereby reducing fetal exposure. It further affords the opportunity to administer less systemic medication and avoids the use of nitrous oxide. Finally, it provides an ideal approach to postoperative pain control through the use of neuraxial narcotics.

Table 60–8 lists recommended guidelines for the administration of these anesthetics to a pregnant patient.

## Can Hypotensive Anesthesia Be Provided Safely?

### Inhalation Agents

Hypotensive anesthesia reportedly has been performed successfully, although some cases of its use have resulted in fetal

**TABLE 60–8.** Guidelines for Administration of Anesthetics to Pregnant Patients

| Spinal Epidural | General |
| --- | --- |
| Avoid premedicants if possible | Avoid premedicants if possible |
| 30 mL of 0.3 M sodium citrate preoperatively | 30 mL of 0.3 M sodium citrate preoperatively |
| | Left uterine displacement |
| Fetal and uterine monitoring (with obstetrician present) | Preoxygenation |
| Treat hypotension aggressively | |
| Left uterine displacement | Fetal and uterine monitoring (with obstetrician present) |
| | Rapid sequence with cricoid pressure |
| Supplemental O$_2$ | |
| Upper and lower extremity blood pressure monitoring | Upper and lower extremity blood pressure monitor |

M, molarity.

distress and even death.[77,78] Among the drugs commonly used for this purpose, the halogenated agents probably are contraindicated because of the myocardial depression and reduced cardiac output that result from the need for the administration of high concentrations.

### Antihypertensive Agents (Nitroprusside, Nitroglycerin, Trimethophan)

Although sodium nitroprusside has the potential for cyanide toxicity in the fetus, as demonstrated by animal studies with supraclinical doses, it has been used successfully without ill effects for induced hypotension in pregnancy at low doses and for short intervals.[79] Nitroglycerin is essentially nontoxic and has been demonstrated to be effective in clinical trials and, thus, has been more commonly used over nitroprusside in pregnancy.[80] However, its onset is slower and may not be effective for a severe hypertensive crisis. Note that both nitroprusside and nitroglycerin are potent cerebral vasodilators and should be used with caution in patients with intracranial mass lesions and increased intracranial pressure.

Trimethophan, a short-acting, ganglionic-blocking drug with a high molecular weight, minimally crosses the blood-brain barrier and placenta. Thus, it has minor effects on maternal intracranial pressure (except in severe cases) and limited fetal involvement. Control of hypertension with this agent may not be adequate, owing to the risk for tachyphylaxis. Its side effects include pupillary dilation and pseudocholinesterase inhibition.

### β-Adrenergic Blocking Agents

Labetalol has been used for acute management of hypertension in pregnant patients and has been shown to be safe and efficacious. β-Adrenergic blocking agents have also been used in conjunction with nitroprusside, nitroglycerin, and hydralazine to limit the resultant reflex tachycardia with these agents. Labetalol, a mixed α- and β-adrenergic blocking agent, and esmolol, a short-acting β-adrenergic blocking agent, do not decrease uterine blood flow. In a gravid ewe model, acute intravenous administration of labetalol did not produce appreciable fetal β-adrenergic blockade, whereas esmolol resulted in fetal β-adrenergic blockade and fetal hypoxemia.[81,82] Chronic use of β-blockers has resulted in intrauterine growth restriction and fetal β-adrenergic blockade. Most of those studies were older and involved the use of propranolol, and whether intrauterine growth retardation was the result of the β-adrenergic blocker, the underlying disease state, or a combination of both is not entirely clear.

### Monitoring

When induced hypotension is required, the reduction in maternal BP should be limited in extent and duration. Direct arterial pressure monitoring of the mother is advocated, and frequent assessment of maternal acid-base regulation is essential if fetal acidosis is to be avoided. The fetal heart rate must be monitored throughout the case. Lower extremity BP monitoring may be particularly helpful during induced hypotension because the effects of aortocaval compression will be proportionately greater.

## Is Laparoscopic Surgery Advisable During Pregnancy?

The most common intraabdominal problems—acute appendicitis, cholecystitis, and ovarian lesions—have been managed successfully with open techniques. Numerous clinical accounts of successful laparoscopic cholecystectomy,[83] laparoscopic appendectomy,[84] and ovarian cystectomy[85] led many to feel that laparoscopic surgery in nonobstetric conditions would also be safe for both mother and unborn child. Despite a report of seven cases describing two patients with intrauterine fetal death and another two with incomplete abortions, recent data from the Swedish Health Registry have demonstrated the efficacy and safety of laparoscopic surgery during pregnancy.[72,86]

## Physiologic Alterations Associated With Laparoscopic Surgery

Several studies of $CO_2$ pneumoperitoneum in animal models have demonstrated physiologic alterations in fetal BP and pulse rate (both tachycardia and bradycardia); maternal and fetal hypoxemia, acidosis, and hypercarbia have been noted in sheep and baboons during insufflation with $CO_2$.[87–89]

Standard recommendations for instituting $CO_2$ pneumoperitoneum include hyperventilating the mother with close monitoring of end-tidal $CO_2$ ($ET_{CO_2}$) to prevent fetal acidosis.[90] In some patients, arterial $Pa_{CO_2}$ values during insufflation may be underestimated by $ET_{CO_2}$ measurements. $ET_{CO_2}$ significantly underestimated maternal $Pa_{CO_2}$ by 15 mm Hg and lagged behind it in the studies of Hunter and colleagues.[87] In experimental animals, hyperventilation has not been sufficient to prevent hypercarbia and acidosis.[72–75]

Although laparoscopic cholecystectomy, appendectomy, and ovarian cystectomy have been performed successfully in pregnancy, caution should be taken, with emphasis on maintenance of low intraabdominal insufflation pressure, limitation of insufflation time, and even laparoscopic surgery without any insufflating gas at all. The typical precautions for surgery in a pregnant patient also pertain to laparoscopy, including uterine displacement, lead shielding of the fetus and fetal monitoring when appropriate, and, more specifically, an open technique for trocar placement to avoid uterine injury.

## Are Osmotic Diuretics Safe to Use During Pregnancy?

Osmotic diuretics such as mannitol are frequently used in neurosurgical procedures to optimize surgical exposure and reduce cerebral edema. Unfortunately, the use of these drugs leads to a net loss of water from the fetus to the mother through renal excretion and can result in severe fetal dehydration.[91] Hence, they should be used only when absolutely necessary and preferably in low doses.

## Is Hypothermia Safe?

Hypothermia is used during certain cardiac and neurosurgical procedures in an attempt to reduce metabolic $O_2$ requirements. Reports have indicated successful use of moderate

hypothermia (30°C) during pregnancy.[92] Although placental blood flow decreases secondary to increased uterine vascular resistance, $O_2$ transport remains unaffected. The fetus becomes hypothermic, and metabolic requirements drop. Provided that maternal blood gases and acid-base status are optimized, the fetus appears to tolerate moderate hypothermia. Some evidence suggests that hypothermia during pregnancy may induce a fetal adrenocortical response. This effect has been suggested to be an inciting factor in the onset of labor in a normal-term pregnancy.[93] Therefore, the possibility of preterm labor may also be greater in these patients.

## How Should Hyperventilation Be Provided?

As described previously, extreme hyperventilation causes decreases in uterine blood flow and placental $O_2$ delivery, which can potentially lead to fetal hypoxemia and acidosis. Mild hyperventilation (decreases in maternal $Pa_{CO_2}$ of 5-7 mm Hg) may be well tolerated. This technique should be undertaken only with a fetal heart rate monitor in place and with the surgeon's understanding that ventilation will be returned to normal as soon as possible or when any sign of fetal distress is observed. Hyperventilation should be reserved for cases in which it is considered essential (ie, in the presence of maternal cerebral edema and increased intracranial pressure).

## How Is Cardiopulmonary Bypass Performed?

The incidence of cardiac disease during pregnancy is <2%. However, the problems of this disease are significant in pregnancy because the cardiovascular demands are markedly increased. Although successful procedures with good outcomes have been performed on pregnant patients who require cardiopulmonary bypass, fetal mortality can be high. Whenever possible, these operations should be performed early in the second trimester, after organogenesis, and before the period of risk for premature labor and hemodynamic alterations that peaks in the third trimester.

High pump flows, upper-limit pressures, and normothermic perfusion are recommended. Recall that the cardiac output of a pregnant patient increases with increasing gestational age. Although moderate hypothermia (32°C) is probably safe, more profound hypothermia may lead to fetal dysrhythmias and death. Moreover, despite adequate mean arterial pressure during cardiopulmonary bypass, increased uterine tone may decrease placental perfusion.

Fetal bradycardia often occurs with the onset of cardiopulmonary bypass and may continue throughout the pump run despite high flow rates, adequate pressures, and homeostatic control of acid-base balance. Frequently, a compensatory fetal tachycardia occurs after cardiopulmonary bypass. Uterine and fetal monitoring should be continued into the postbypass and postoperative periods.

## FETAL SURGERY

Fetal surgery has been performed in human beings since the 1980s. A select group of disorders amenable to potential improvement by fetal treatment has been identified and includes fetal urinary tract obstruction, fetal diaphragmatic hernia, fetal congenital cystic adenomatoid malformation, and fetal sacrococcygeal teratoma.

## What Type of Monitoring Is Recommended for Fetal Surgery?

Intraoperatively, mothers are monitored with ASA standard monitors. A central venous and radial arterial catheter may be helpful to follow hemodynamics closely throughout the perioperative course. The average maternal blood loss ranges from 200 to 1000 mL.

In a fetal surgical operation, the mother is supine, with her right side slightly elevated to prevent aortocaval compression by the gravid uterus. Fetal monitoring is maintained with a radiotelemetric device for electrocardiogram, a temperature monitor, and an intrauterine pressure monitor, which is affixed to the fetal chest or back.[94] A miniaturized pulse oximeter is wrapped around the fetal hand. The fetus receives intramuscular pancuronium (0.2 mg/kg). The fetus may also receive intramuscular fentanyl (50 µg/kg) before the hysterotomy to help ablate the fetal stress response if maternal plasma fentanyl levels are not maintained at a high level.

Postoperatively, obstetric ultrasound and fetal echocardiography, which substitute for a fetal physical examination, are performed daily. An obstetric ultrasound is performed weekly thereafter. Care in the first 48 hours after surgery is provided in an intensive care unit with a designated fetal ultrasound machine and fetal monitors. The patient is then transferred to the obstetric ward, with limited ambulation beginning on postoperative day 3 to 5 and discharge from the hospital averaging 8 days postsurgery. The fetus is delivered by cesarean section at a tertiary center when either the membranes rupture or labor cannot be controlled, which usually occurs before 36 weeks' gestation.

## What Are the Potential Complications of Fetal Surgery?

Preterm labor remains the main impediment to fetal surgery. The incidence of preterm labor is about 70%. Other complica-

**TABLE 60–9.** Guide Chart to Drug Use in Breast-Feeding Women Requiring Anesthesia

| Drug Groups | Individual Drugs | | |
| --- | --- | --- | --- |
| | *Indicated* | *Controversial or Contraindicated* | *Comments and Effects on Infant* |
| Opioids | Morphine | | |
| | | Meperidine | Neurobehavioral depression |
| | Codeine | | |
| | Fentanyl | | |
| | Sufentanil | | |
| | Alfentanil | | |
| Nonopioid analgesics | Paracetamol | | |
| | | Aspirin | Risks of Reye's syndrome, platelet dysfunction, hypoprothrombinemia, metabolic acidosis, kernicterus |
| | Ibuprofen | | The short-term use of ibuprofen (800–1600 mg/d) can be considered safe |
| | Flubiprofen | | |
| | Indomethacin | | Monitor; convulsions reported in one infant |
| | Diclofenac | | |
| | Ketorolac | | Single doses appear to be safe |
| Intravenous induction agents | Thiopental | | |
| | Propofol | | |
| Inhalational agents | All | | |
| Muscle relaxants | | | Theoretically safe |
| Anticholinergics | Atropine | | Possible risk for antimuscarinic effects |
| | | Hysine | Possible risk for antimuscarinic effects |
| | Glycopyrrolate | | Theoretically safe |
| Anticholinesterases | Neostigmine | | |
| | Pyridostigmine | | |
| Local anesthetics | Lidocaine | | |
| | Bupivacaine | | |
| | Cocaine | | |
| Benzodiazepines | | Diazepam | Lethargy, weight loss, sedation |
| | Lorazepam | | |
| | Midazolam | | |
| | Temazepam | | |
| Histamine₂ antagonists | Cimetidine | | Caution: significant amount of drugs excreted in breast milk |
| | Ranitidine | | |
| | Famotidine | | |
| | Nizatidine | | |
| Antiemetics and neuroleptics | | Metoclopramide | Caution with repeated administration: animal studies suggest possible adverse effects on infant's nervous system |
| | | Domperidone | |
| | | Chlorpromazine | |
| | | Haloperidol | |
| | | (Ondansetron) | Lack of clinical experience |
| | | (Dolasetron) | |

tions may include amniotic fluid leak (requiring reoperation and closure), pulmonary edema (secondary to tocolysis), and the development of the maternal mirror syndrome[95] as well as maternal and fetal infections. The prevention and treatment of preterm labor includes the use of volatile anesthetics and the administration of rectal indomethacin, magnesium sulfate, and intravenous nitroglycerin. Postoperatively, the patient can be weaned from nitroglycerin and magnesium sulfate by substituting subcutaneous terbutaline.

## ANESTHESIA AND BREAST FEEDING

### Are There Special Precautions for the Breast-Feeding Mother?

The principal physicochemical properties of a drug that determine the extent of drug transfer into breast milk are the $pK_a$ partition coefficient (relative solubilities in fat and water) and molecular weight. Human milk has a mean pH of 7.09, which is lower than that of the plasma.[96] This results in different drug dissociation and unequal total concentrations of drugs in the two media. As a general rule, weak acids achieve a lower concentration in milk than in plasma (M/P ratio <1.0), whereas weak bases achieve a higher M/P ratio (>1.0); nonionized (lipid-soluble) drugs enter the breast milk from maternal plasma by passive diffusion down a concentration gradient.

Provided the drugs are chosen with care, elective surgery should not be postponed, and breast feeding should be continued in the immediate postoperative period. Table 60–9 provides a brief review of indicated and contraindicated drugs during lactation.

**Premedication.** Therapeutic doses of temazepam may be used. Lorazepam, midazolam, opioids, and glycopyrrolate may be used safely. Histamine$_2$ receptor antagonists and antiemetics (eg, metoclopramide) should not be used routinely but rather only if strongly indicated.

**Induction.** Only thiopental (induction doses) and propofol (induction and maintenance doses) have been shown to be safe.

**Muscle Relaxants and Maintenance of Anesthesia.** On the basis of their pharmacokinetic profiles, the use of muscle relaxants and halothane, enflurane, and isoflurane for maintenance of anesthesia appears to be safe despite the lack of complete supporting data. Analgesia may be supplemented by opioids.

**Postoperative Analgesia.** Therapeutic doses of opioids may be used. Nonsteroidal antiinflammatory drugs, such as diclofenac and ibuprofen, and regional techniques using local anesthetics and opioids may be used. When opioids are required, it is preferable to avoid the use of meperidine because decreased fetal neurobehavioral scores are associated with this drug. Opioids should be used with caution in mothers nursing infants with respiratory problems. Aspirin is contraindicated because of its association with Reye's syndrome in children.

## SUMMARY

A number of concerns must be addressed when providing anesthetic care for the pregnant surgical patient. Basic consid-

**TABLE 60–10.** Basic Concerns During Anesthesia for Pregnant Patients

The physiologic changes of pregnancy must be understood, and the anesthetic implications must be taken into account.

Maternal blood pressure and uteroplacental perfusion must be maintained. Hypotension and aortocaval compression must be avoided; however, should they occur, aggressive treatment must be initiated promptly.

Anesthetic techniques that limit the exposure of both mother and fetus should be chosen. Agents should be chosen that have a proven record of safety. Regional anesthesia should be used whenever possible.

The implications of surgery and anesthesia during pregnancy, including our current knowledge regarding the lack of known teratogenicity among the commonly used anesthetic agents, should be discussed with the patient.

Finally, fetal heart rate and uterine activity should be monitored intraoperatively and postoperatively, depending on the gestation. If changes are noted, appropriate action should be taken; this may include tocolysis for premature labor; alteration of anesthetic or surgical techniques, hemodynamics, or oxygenation for fetal distress; and cesarean delivery if fetal demise occurs.

erations common to all such cases are summarized in Table 60–10. With these considerations in mind, safe, efficient, and uneventful anesthesia can be provided.

### References

1. Brodsky JB, Cohen EN, Brown BW Jr, et al. Surgery during pregnancy and fetal outcome. *Am J Obstet Gynecol.* 1980;138:1165.
2. Mazze RI, Kallen B. Reproductive outcome after anesthesia and operation during pregnancy: a registry study of 5405 cases. *Am J Obstet Gynecol.* 1989;161:1178.
3. Strickland RA. Oliver WC Jr, Chantigian RC, et al. Anesthesia, cardiopulmonary bypass, and the pregnant patient. *Mayo Clin Proc.* 1991;66:411.
4. Donchin Y, Anzirav B, Sahar A, et al. Sodium nitroprusside for aneurysm surgery in pregnancy, report of a case. *Br J Anaesth.* 1978;50:849.
5. Merritt WT, Dickstein R. Beattie C, et al. Liver transplantation during pregnancy: anesthesia for two procedures in the same patient with successful outcome of pregnancy. *Transplant Proc.* 1991;23:1996.
6. Ueland K, Novy M, Peterson EN, et al. Maternal cardiovascular dynamics. *Am J Obstet Gynecol.* 1969;104:856.
7. Palahniuk RJ, Shnider SM, Eger EI II. Pregnancy decreases the requirements for inhaled anesthetic agents. *Anesthesiology.* 1974;41:81.
8. Csontos K, Rust M, Holt V, et al. Elevated plasma beta-endorphin levels in pregnant women and their neonates. *Life Sci.* 1979;25:835.
9. Fagraeus L, Urban BJ, Bromage PR. Spread of epidural analgesia in early pregnancy. *Anesthesiology.* 1983;58:184.
10. Marx GF, Oka Y, Orkin LR. Cerebrospinal fluid pressures during labor. *Am J Obstet Gynecol.* 1967;84:213.
11. Igarashi T, Hirabayashi Y, Shimizu R, et al. The fiberscopic findings of the epidural space in pregnant women. *Anesthesiology.* 2000;92:1631.
12. Morishima HO, Pedersen H, Finster M, et al. Bupivacaine toxicity in pregnant and nonpregnant ewes. *Anesthesiology.* 1985;63:134.
13. Tsen LC, Tarshis J, Denson DD, et al. Measurements of maternal protein binding of bupivacaine throughout pregnancy. *Anesth Analg.* 1999;89:965.
14. Konieczko KM, Chapple JC, Nunn JF. Fetotoxic potential of general anesthesia in relation to pregnancy. *Br J Anaesth.* 1987;59:449.
15. Adamsons K, Mueller-Heubach E, Myers RE. Production of fetal asphyxia in rhesus monkeys by administration of catecholamines to the mother. *Am J Obstet Gynecol.* 1971;109:248.
16. James FM III, Griess FC Jr, Kemp RA. An evaluation of vasopressor therapy for maternal hypotension during spinal anesthesia. *Anesthesiology.* 1970;33:25.
17. Khazin AF, Hon EH, Hahre FW. Effects of maternal hyperoxia on the fetus, I: oxygen tension. *Am J Obstet Gynecol.* 1971;109:628.
18. Webb AA, Shipton EA. Re-evaluation of i.m. ephedrine as prophylaxis against hypotension associated with spinal anaesthesia for caesarean section. *Can J Anaesth.* 1998;45:367.
19. American Society of Anesthesiologists Ad Hoc Committee on the Effect of Trace Anesthetics on the Health of Operating Room Personnel. Occu-

pational disease among operating room personnel. *Anesthesiology.* 1974;41:321.

20. Cohen EN, Brown BW, Wu ML, et al. Occupational disease in dentistry and chronic exposure to trace anesthetic gases. *J Am Dent Assoc.* 1980;101:21.

21. Tuchmann-Duplessis H. The effects of teratogenic drugs. In: Phillip EE, Barnes J, Newton M, eds. *Scientific Foundations of Obstetrics and Gynecology.* London, United Kingdom: Heinemann; 1970:636.

22. Mazze RI, Kallen B. Reproductive outcome after anesthesia and operation during pregnancy: a registry study of 5,405 cases. *Am J Obstet Gynecol.* 1989;161:1178.

23. Brodsky JB, Cohen EN, Brown BW, et al. Surgery during pregnancy and fetal outcome. *Am J Obstet Gynecol.* 1980;138:1165.

24. Wilson JG. Experimental studies on congenital malformations. *J Chron Dis.* 1959;10:111.

25. Nunn JF, Chanarin I. Nitrous oxide inactivates methionine synthetase. In: Eger EI II, ed. *Nitrous Oxide/N₂O.* New York, NY: Elsevier; 1985:211.

26. Mazze RI, Funinaga M, Rice SA, et al. Reproduction and teratogenic effects of nitrous oxide, halothane, isoflurane, and enflurane in Sprague-Dawley rats. *Anesthesiology.* 1986;64:334.

27. Heinnen OP, Slone D, Shapiro S. *Birth Defects and Drugs in Pregnancy.* Littleton, Mass: Publishing Sciences Group; 1977.

28. Safra M, Oakley GP. Association between cleft lip with or without cleft palate and prenatal exposure to diazepam. *Lancet.* 1975;2:478.

29. Saxen I, Saxen L. Association between maternal intake of diazepam and oral clefts. *Lancet.* 1975;2:498.

30. Hartz SC, Heinnen OP, Shapiro S, et al. Antenatal exposure to meprobamate and chlordiazepoxide in relation to malformation, mental development and childhood mortality. *N Engl J Med.* 1975;292:726.

31. Zagon IS, McLaughlin PJ. Effects of chronic morphine administration on pregnant rats and their offspring. *Pharmacology.* 1977;15:302.

32. Naeye RL, Blanc W, LeBlanc W, et al. Fetal complications of maternal heroin addiction: abnormal growth, infection and episodes of stress. *J Pediatr.* 1973;83:1055.

33. Fujinaga M, Mazze RI, Jackson EC, et al. Reproductive and teratogenic effects of sufentanil and alfentanil in Sprague-Dawley rats. *Anesth Analg.* 1988;67:166.

34. Briggs GG, Bodendorfer TW, Freeman RK, et al. *Drugs in Pregnancy and Lactation: A Reference Guide to Fetal and Neonatal Risk.* Baltimore, Md: Williams & Wilkins; 1994.

35. Pedersen H, Finster M. Anesthetic risk in the pregnant surgical patient. *Anesthesiology.* 1979;51:439.

36. Shepard TF. Human teratogenicity. *Adv Pediatr.* 1986;33:225.

37. Fujinaga M, Badden JM, Mazze RI. Developmental toxicity of nondepolarizing muscle relaxants in cultured rat embryos. *Anesthesiology.* 1992;76:999.

38. Heinnen OP, Slone D, Shapiro S. *Birth Defects and Drugs in Pregnancy.* Littleton, Mass: Publishing Sciences Group; 1977:337.

39. Moller RA, Datta S, Fox J, et al. Effect of progesterone on the cardiac electrophysiologic action of bupivacaine and lidocaine. *Anesthesiology.* 1992;76:604.

40. Grabowski CT. The teratogenic effects of graded doses of hypoxia on the chicken embryo. *Am J Anat.* 1958;103:313.

41. Khazin AF, Hon EH, Hahre FW. Effects of maternal hyperoxia on the fetus, I: oxygen tension. *Am J Obstet Gynecol.* 1971;109:628.

42. Fern BH. Teratogenic effects of hyperbaric oxygen. *Proc Soc Exp Biol Med.* 1964;116:975.

43. Haring OM. Cardiac malformations in rats induced by exposure of the mother to carbon dioxide during pregnancy. *Circ Res.* 1960;8:1218.

44. Brent RL. The effects of embryonic and fetal exposure to x-ray, microwaves, and ultrasound. *Clin Obstet Gynecol.* 1983;26:484.

45. Houston CS. Diagnostic irradiation of women during the reproductive period. *Can Med Assoc J.* 1977;117:648.

46. Mossman KL, Hill LT. Radiation risks in pregnancy. *Obstet Gynecol.* 1982;60:237.

47. Pentel RL, Brown ML. Genetically significant dose to the United States population from diagnostic medical roentgenology. *Radiology.* 1968;90:209.

48. Stewart A, Kneale GW. Radiation dose effects in relation to obstetric x-rays and childhood cancers. *Lancet.* 1970;1:1185.

49. Totter JR, MacPherson HS. Do childhood cancers result from prenatal x-rays? *Health Phys.* 1981;40:511.

50. Hunt MG, Martin JN Jr, Martin RW, et al. Perinatal aspects of abdominal surgery for nonobstetric disease. *Am J Perinatol.* 1989;6:412.

51. Kammerer WD. Non-obstetric surgery in pregnancy. *Med Clin North Am.* 1987;71:551.

52. Hill LM, Johnson CE, Lee RA. Prophylactic use of hydroxyprogesterone caproate in abdominal surgery during pregnancy: a retrospective evaluation. *Obstet Gynecol.* 1975;46:287.

53. Liu P, Warren TM, Ostheimer GW, et al. Foetal monitoring in parturients undergoing surgery unrelated to pregnancy. *Can Anaesth Soc J.* 1985;32:525.

54. Peckham CH, King RW. A study of intercurrent conditions observed during pregnancy. *Am J Obstet Gynecol.* 1963;87:609.

55. Varner MW. Maternal mortality in Iowa from 1952 to 1986. *Surg Obstet Gynecol.* 1989;168:555.

56. Crosby WM, Costiloe JP. Safety of lap-belt restraint for pregnant victims of automobile collisions. *N Engl J Med.* 1971;284:632.

57. Goodwin TM, Breen MT. Pregnancy outcome and fetomaternal hemorrhage of noncatastrophic trauma. *Am J Obstet Gynecol.* 1990;162:665.

58. Pearlman MD, Tintinalli JE, Lorenz RP. A prospective controlled study of outcome after trauma during pregnancy. *Am J Obstet Gynecol.* 1990;162:1502.

59. Rothenberger D, Quattlebaum FW, Perry JF, et al. Blunt maternal trauma: a review of 103 cases. *J Trauma.* 1978;18:173.

60. Rose PG, Strohm PL, Zuspan FP. Fetomaternal hemorrhage following trauma. *Am J Obstet Gynecol.* 1985;153:844.

61. Elliott M. Vehicular accidents and pregnancy. *Aust N Z J Obstet Gynaecol.* 1966;6:279.

62. Perlman MD, Tintinalli JE, Lorenz RP. A prospective controlled study of outcome after trauma during pregnancy. *Am J Obstet Gynecol.* 1990;162:1502.

63. Buchsbaum HJ. Penetrating injury of the abdomen. In: Buchsbaum HJ, ed. *Trauma in Pregnancy.* 1st ed. Philadelphia, Pa: WB Saunders; 1979:82.

64. American Heart Association: Cardiac arrest associated with pregnancy. Guidelines 2000 for cardiopulmonary resuscitation and emergency cardiovascular care. International Consensus on Science. *Circulation.* 2000;102(suppl I):I-247.

65. Rees GAD, Willis BA. Resuscitation in late pregnancy. *Anaesthesia.* 1988;43:347.

66. Katz VL, Dotters DJ, Droegemueller E. Perimortem cesarean delivery. *Obstet Gynecol.* 1986;27:408.

67. Morishima HO, Pedersen H, Finster M, et al. Bupivacaine toxicity in pregnant and nonpregnant ewes. *Anesthesiology.* 1985;63:134.

68. Rawal N, Van Zundert A, Holmstrom B, et al. Combined spinal-epidural technique. *Reg Anesth.* 1997;22:406.

69. Fan SZ, Susetio L, Wang YP, et al. Low dose of intrathecal hyperbaric bupivacaine combined with epidural lidocaine for cesarean section: a balance block technique. *Anesth Analg.* 1994;78:474.

70. Kosaka Y, Takahashi T, Mark LC. Intravenous thiobarbiturate anesthesia for cesarean section. *Anesthesiology.* 1969;31:489.

71. Janeczko GF, El-Etr AA, Younes S. Low-dose ketamine anesthesia for obstetrical delivery. *Anesth Analg.* 1974;53:828.

72. Oats JN, Vasey DP, Waldron BA. Effects of ketamine on the pregnant uterus. *Br J Anaesth.* 1979;51:1163.

73. Baraka A. Severe bradycardia following propofol-suxamethonium sequence. *Br J Anaesth.* 1988;61:482.

74. Reddy BK, Pizer B, Bull PT. Neonatal serum cortisol suppression by etomidate compared with thiopentone for elective caesarean section. *Eur J Anaesth.* 1988;5:171.

75. Gambling DR, Sharma SK, White PF, et al. Use of sevoflurane during elective cesarean birth: a comparison with isoflurane and spinal anesthesia. *Anesth Analg.* 1995;81:90.

76. Abboud TK, Zhu J, Richardson M, et al. Desflurane: a new volatile anesthetic for cesarean section: maternal and neonatal effects. *Acta Anaesthesiol Scand.* 1995;39:723.

77. Minielly R, Yupze AA, Drake CG. Subarachnoid hemorrhage secondary to ruptured cerebral aneurysm in pregnancy. *Obstet Gynecol.* 1979;53:64.

78. Robinson JL, Chir B, Hall CJ, et al. Subarachnoid hemorrhage in pregnancy. *J Neurosurg.* 1972;37:27.

79. Donchin Y, Amirav B. Sodium nitroprusside for aneurysm surgery in pregnancy. *Br J Anaesth.* 1978;50:849.

80. Wheeler AS, James FM III, Meis PJ, et al. Effects of nitroglycerin and nitroprusside on the uterine vasculature of gravid ewes. *Anesthesiology.* 1980;52:390.

81. Eisenach JC, Castro MI. Maternally administered esmolol produces fetal beta-adrenergic blockade and hypoxemia in sheep. *Anesthesiology.* 1989;71:718.

82. Eisenach JC, Mandell G, Dewan DM. Maternal and fetal effects of labetolol in pregnant ewes. *Anesthesiology.* 1991;74:292.

83. Schorr RT. Laparoscopic colecystectomy and pregnancy. *J Laparoendosc Surg.* 1993;3:291.

84. Schreiber JH. Laparoscopic appendectomy in pregnancy. *Surg Laparosc Endosc.* 1990;4:100.

85. Reedy MB, Kallen B, Kuehl TJ. Laparoscopy during pregnancy: a study of five fetal outcome parameters with the use of the Swedish Health Registry. *Am J Obstet Gynecol.* 1997;177:673.

86. Amos DJ, Schorr SJ, Norman PF, et al. Laparoscopic surgery during pregnancy. *Am J Surg.* 1996;171:435.

87. Hunter J. Swanson L, Thornburgh K. Carbon dioxide pneumoperitoneum induces fetal acidosis in a pregnant ewe model. *Surg Endosc.* 1995; 9:272.

88. Reedy MB, Galan HL, Bean-Lijewski JD, et al. Maternal and fetal effects of laparoscopic insufflation in the gravid baboon. *J Am Assoc Gynecol Laparosc.* 1995;4:399.

89. Cruz AM, Southerland LC, Duke T, et al. Intraabdominal carbon dioxide insufflation in the pregnant ewe: uterine blood flow, intraamniotic pressure, and cardiopulmonary effects. *Anesthesiology.* 1996;85:1395.

90. Soper NJ. Effect of nonbiliary problems on laparoscopic cholecystectomy. *Am J Surg.* 1993;165:522.

91. Bruns PD, Linder RO, Brose VE, et al. The placental transfer of water from fetus to mother following intravenous administration of hypertonic mannitol to the maternal rabbit. *Am J Obstet Gynecol.* 1963;86:160.

92. Stange K, Halldin M. Hypothermia in pregnancy. *Anesthesiology.* 1983;58:460.

93. Levy DL, Warriner RA, Burges GE. Fetal response to cardiopulmonary bypass. *Obstet Gynecol.* 1980;56:112.

94. Jennings RW, Adzick NS, Longaker MT. Radio-telemetric fetal monitoring during and after open fetal surgery. *Surg Obstet Gynecol.* 1993;176:59.

95. van Selm M, Kanhai HH, Gravenhorst JB. Maternal hydrops syndrome: a review. *Obstet Gynecol Surv.* 1991;46:785.

96. Ansell C, Moore A, Barrie H. Electrolyte and pH changes in human milk. *Pediatr Res.* 1977;11:1177.

CHAPTER

# 61

# Abdominal Surgery

Sergio Gregoretti

# THE ABDOMINAL WALL

## Why Does It Get Tight?

Muscle relaxation is essential in abdominal surgery to allow exposure of abdominal contents and minimize motion in the surgical field. The "tight" abdomen about which surgeons often complain is the result of a spinal polysynaptic reflex. It is evoked by painful stimuli applied to the abdominal wall and peritoneum and by traction on the intraabdominal viscera.[1] Afferent pathways include the intercostal and splanchnic nerves, whereas efferent impulses travel through the intercostal and, if the stimulus is strong enough, the phrenic nerves, causing contraction of the abdominal wall muscles and diaphragm.[2]

This reflex is particularly noticeable during skin incision, peritoneal opening, placement of retractors, and intraabdominal exploration. It tends to fatigue, becoming less effective with time despite continuous stimulation. This fact may explain why during surgery, once exposure is achieved, the need for additional relaxation is decreased.

Contraction of the abdominal wall can still be elicited late during an operation either by a strong sudden stimulus, such as traction on the mesentery, or when the viscera are repositioned in the abdomen and the peritoneum closed. Because a tight abdomen results from a spinal reflex, it can still be observed in patients with a spinal cord injury at T5 and higher despite complete loss of abdominal wall sensation. It also can occur in brain-dead subjects during organ procurement for transplantation.

## How Is It Relaxed?

Abdominal relaxation can be obtained by interrupting the spinal reflex at different sites. Regional techniques (intercostal nerve blocks combined with celiac plexus block, as well as spinal or epidural anesthesia) provide relaxation mainly by preventing afferent stimuli from reaching the spinal cord.[3] All inhaled and intravenous anesthetics, with the exception of the opioids and ketamine, provide some degree of relaxation by depressing the reflex pathways at the spinal cord level.[4]

Muscle relaxants act on the efferent side of the reflex,

blocking motor impulses to the muscles. The intense degree of relaxation required during abdominal surgery can be obtained only by muscle relaxants or regional anesthesia techniques. The degree of relaxation that modern inhaled anesthetics provide is usually inadequate for operations in the abdomen, but enhances the relaxation provided by other drugs.

## GENERAL ANESTHESIA

General anesthesia is most common for abdominal operations. Induction is usually achieved with an intravenous agent, followed by tracheal intubation facilitated by a muscle relaxant. Tracheal intubation is mandatory because of the high incidence of regurgitation of gastrointestinal (GI) contents during manipulation of the stomach, biliary tract, and other abdominal contents.

### Is Hyperventilation Helpful?

Hyperventilation has been widely used during abdominal surgery because of empiric evidence that it enhances muscle relaxation and improves operating conditions. The mechanisms by which it affects muscle relaxation are largely unknown.[5] Hypocapnia, however, decreases cardiac output and blood flow to several organs, including the liver and intestines.[6,7] Because intraabdominal surgical manipulations and the anesthetic agents significantly decrease splanchnic blood flow,[8] it is perhaps preferable to maintain carbon dioxide ($CO_2$) tension within normal limits. Normocarbia also allows more rapid restoration of spontaneous breathing at the end of the procedure, particularly when opioids have been used.[9,10]

### What Are the Options?

Anesthesia can be maintained by intermittent doses or continuous infusions of intravenous agents such as thiopental, propofol, and opioids, usually combined with nitrous oxide. However, the inhaled halogenated anesthetics (isoflurane, desflurane, sevoflurane) probably are the most commonly used drugs. They reliably control hemodynamic reflex responses elicited by the intense stimuli encountered during abdominal surgery, and their concentrations can be easily decreased when the stimuli are less intense or absent. In addition, they exhibit predictable pharmacokinetic activity and, even after very long procedures, patients can be awakened within minutes after these agents have been discontinued.

Halogenated anesthetics also potentiate the effects of muscle relaxants.[4] Therefore, when a halogenated agent is used, less relaxant is required for adequate surgical conditions, and reversal of the residual block at the end of the procedure is easier. Furthermore, in the presence of a halogenated agent, recovery from neuromuscular blockade tends to be more gradual, more time is available to recognize the need for additional relaxant, and abrupt motion of the surgical field is avoided.

### Which Inhaled Agent Is Best?

Any of the available inhaled agents can be satisfactory for abdominal surgery. Few would argue that the pharmacologic differences among anesthetics are much less important for a good outcome than the skill, clinical acumen, and vigilance of the anesthesia provider. However, isoflurane seems to maintain liver and intestinal blood flow better than other inhaled agents during abdominal procedures.[11-14] Thus, a case can be made in favor of this agent when a decrease in splanchnic blood flow may be particularly detrimental. These circumstances include patients with liver disease, in whom further deterioration of liver function may result in overt failure, and patients undergoing major liver resections, in whom damage to the residual liver may jeopardize survival. There is some evidence that desflurane preserves hepatic and intestinal blood flow as well as isoflurane.[15]

### What Is the Role of Nitrous Oxide?

Although halogenated agents combined with a muscle relaxant can provide excellent anesthetic conditions during abdominal operations, they are often used in combination with nitrous oxide and opioids. Features that make nitrous oxide attractive are fast uptake and elimination, minimal cardiovascular effects, its additive anesthetic effects to those of the halogenated agents, and low cost.

Nitrous oxide can be used at the beginning of the procedure to ensure maintenance of the anesthetic state while the effects of the intravenous induction agents are dissipating. The halogenated agent may then be gradually introduced and titrated according to blood pressure changes. Nitrous oxide reduces the required concentration of the halogenated agent by approximately 50%. Therefore, hypotension is less likely, particularly during periods of little surgical stimulation. Toward the end of the procedure, the potent agent can be discontinued well ahead of completion. Anesthesia is maintained with nitrous oxide, thus allowing more rapid awakening.

### What Are the Roles of Opioids?

Opioids are used because of their "sparing" effect on the requirements for halogenated agents and their minimal cardiovascular effects. These drugs are particularly useful at the beginning of the procedure when the most intense surgical stimulation occurs. Toward the end of the operation, the anesthesiologist should rely more on the inhaled agents than the opioid to control hemodynamics, thus avoiding excessive, opioid-induced depression of the respiratory center. At the end of surgery, opioids used intraoperatively facilitate a smoother emergence from anesthesia and provide some residual analgesia.

## MUSCLE RELAXANTS

Muscle relaxation during abdominal surgery is commonly obtained with nondepolarizing agents. If succinylcholine is used to facilitate tracheal intubation, the maintenance nondepolarizing agent should be administered after the patient shows some signs of recovery from the succinylcholine. This approach rules out the possibility of a genetically abnormal pseudocholinesterase and provides useful information about anesthetic depth (ie, lack of movement during this period of negligible muscle relaxant effect suggests an adequate anesthetic level).

## How Is the Muscle Relaxant Chosen?

The factors pertinent to abdominal surgery that influence the choice of a muscle relaxant are the duration of the procedure and preexisting diseases that affect relaxant pharmacokinetics. Short procedures such as an appendectomy, which may be completed in 30 minutes, or an exploratory laparotomy that may be rapidly aborted call for the use of a short- or intermediate-acting agent. For short procedures, an infusion of succinylcholine is also appropriate; should the procedure become more complex and extended, a switch to a nondepolarizing agent is easily accomplished.

Long-acting agents are appropriate for procedures lasting ≥2 hours. However, even when they are used in procedures of several hours' duration, the long-acting agents are associated with a significantly higher postoperative incidence of residual neuromuscular blockade than are the intermediate-acting agents.[16,17] A case can be made, therefore, for the use of intermediate-acting agents in lengthy procedures.

## What Factors Affect the Duration of Muscle Relaxation?

Situations that commonly affect relaxant pharmacokinetics during abdominal surgery include obstructive jaundice (cholestasis) and cirrhosis of the liver.

### Obstructive Jaundice

Obstructive jaundice prolongs the elimination half-life but does not affect the volume of distribution of pancuronium[18] and vecuronium.[19] Although this issue has not been specifically addressed, obstructive jaundice probably begins to affect the pharmacokinetics of these relaxants only when the bilirubin level is >5 mg/dL.[19] In practice, the initial dose of pancuronium and vecuronium in patients with severe jaundice does not need to be adjusted, but the duration of the block is approximately 50% longer than normal.[18,19] To avoid an excessive dose, the maintenance doses need to be smaller than usual and administered only when signs of recovery from the block are noted. Apart from gallamine, the kinetics of which are not altered in obstructive jaundice and which is no longer in use,[20] the pharmacokinetics of no other relaxant have been studied in patients with cholestasis. Clinical experience indicates that atracurium and cisatracurium administered to these patients do not have a prolonged effect.

### Cirrhosis

Cirrhosis and other severe liver diseases may prolong the duration of succinylcholine block because of the associated decrease in plasma pseudocholinesterase activity. In practice, succinylcholine use in the presence of liver disease does not pose any problem because the increase in duration of the block amounts to a few minutes at most.[21]

A common clinical impression is that the initial dose of nondepolarizing relaxants needs to be larger than usual in patients with cirrhosis to achieve a given degree of block. The need for additional doses is decreased for pancuronium,[22] whereas for vecuronium and rocuronium this phenomenon becomes evident only after prolonged administration (ie, after the third or fourth "top-up" dose).[23–26] The maintenance doses for atracurium and cisatracurium are unchanged in cirrhosis or other liver diseases.[27,28]

In patients with cholestasis and severe liver disease, any relaxant can be safely used if it is titrated to effect. Atracurium and cisatracurium are excellent choices because of their unique elimination that does not depend on liver or kidney function.

## How Should Muscle Relaxants Be Given?

The relaxants should be given in doses adequate to provide favorable surgical conditions, while at the same time avoiding an overdose (ie, excessive duration) and consequently a block difficult to reverse at the end of the procedure. The first dose of the nondepolarizing relaxant is given according to the known pharmacology of the drug. Subsequent doses, usually one third to one fifth of the initial one, are administered when evidence of block dissipation is noted. Neuromuscular block is best assessed by a peripheral nerve stimulator. Clinical criteria are also useful.

## How Should the Nerve Stimulator Be Used?

The use of a peripheral nerve stimulator may be associated with several pitfalls that lead the clinician to judge a block to be adequate, whereas in reality it is not. To avoid these pitfalls, the following factors are important.

First, a strong control twitch must be obtained before any relaxant is given. This response is used as a control against which to compare the twitches elicited during the onset, maintenance, and recovery of the block.

Second, although the motor responses evoked by peripheral nerve stimulation can be recorded on paper and examined very precisely, in clinical practice the evaluation is visual or tactile and, by nature, very imprecise. If the ulnar nerve is stimulated, as is most commonly done, tactile evaluation of the contraction of the adductor pollicis is preferred. The best results are obtained if slight tension is applied to the thumb before the stimulus. Contractions of the fourth and fifth fingers are sometimes present while the thumb is completely paralyzed. These contractions probably occur because the hypothenar muscles are slightly more resistant to the relaxant than the adductor pollicis, and should be disregarded when a train-of-four count assessment of the block is made.[29] If the facial nerve is stimulated, the contractions of the orbicularis oculi muscle are evaluated visually.

Third, when the neuromuscular block is monitored at the adductor pollicis, care should be taken to prevent cooling of the arm and hand being examined. Cooling of the limb out of proportion to the rest of the body may cause a persistent block of the thumb at a time when the muscles in other parts of the body have recovered from the block.

Different muscles respond differently to muscle relaxants; therefore, the results obtained for one muscle cannot automatically be extrapolated to other muscles. The muscle usually monitored is the adductor pollicis, whereas in abdominal surgery the diaphragm and the abdominal muscles are of most concern. After a bolus dose of relaxant, the block of the diaphragmatic and abdominal muscles is probably as intense as that of the adductor pollicis.[30,31] However, both diaphragm and abdominal muscles recover from the block much faster than does the adductor pollicis (Fig. 61–1). This fact explains the frequent clinical situation in which contractions of the abdomen occur despite minimum or absent motor response of the thumb to ulnar nerve stimulation.[32] The orbicularis oculi muscle shows the same response to relaxants as does the diaphragm (see Fig. 61–1). Monitoring of this muscle may therefore be preferable to monitoring the adductor pollicis when intense diaphragmatic paralysis is important.

### How Are Clinical Criteria Used?

Slight limb movements, small contractions of the abdominal wall or diaphragm, hiccups, and the surgeon's comments on the quality of the relaxation form the basis for clinical evaluation. Experience shows that other useful signs that the block is dissipating and will soon be inadequate are a sudden increase in heart rate and blood pressure during what otherwise appears to be a perfectly adequate anesthetic. That these hemodynamic changes are related to inadequate relaxation is confirmed by the fact that an additional dose of relaxant rapidly returns these parameters to the prior status quo. Validation of this clinical observation is left to the reader. Bucking on the endotracheal tube and elevated peak airway pressures are signs of grossly inadequate relaxation.

Movements of the facial muscles (grimacing, winking, or wrinkling of the forehead), in view of the great resistance of these muscles to relaxants, are more likely signs of inadequate anesthesia than inadequate relaxation and are best treated by verbal reassurance to the patient, accompanied by a small dose of thiopental or opioid and by increasing the concentration of the inhaled agent.

Finally, even when the peripheral nerve stimulator is used, the practitioner should look at the patient and surgical field and integrate the clinical observations with the information provided by the nerve stimulator. Should an apparent disparity arise, defer to the clinical observations.

### When Is the Need for Relaxation Greatest?

The requirement for muscle relaxation encompasses the entire length of the operation. The need is greatest at the beginning when the peritoneum is opened and the surgical area exposed and at the end when the peritoneum is closed. At the beginning of a laparotomy, adequate relaxation is present when no twitch of the thumb is detected in response to a train-of-four stimulation of the ulnar nerve. Later in the case, less intense relaxation is needed. Some recovery of neuromuscular function is allowed until 1 or 2 twitches in response to train-of-four stimulation are detected. At this point, an additional dose of relaxant should be given. However, as noted previously, even when no response of the thumb to ulnar nerve stimulation is present, diaphragmatic contractions can occur in response to intense surgical stimuli. If ulnar nerve stimulation is used to ensure diaphragmatic inactivity when the train-of-four count at the thumb is zero, the posttetanic count method may be used.[33] If only 2 or 3 twitches are detected after the tetanic stimulus, even the strongest surgical stimulation does not evoke diaphragmatic activity.[34] Alternatively, the orbicularis oculi muscle, which responds to relaxants similarly to the diaphragm, can be monitored and sufficient relaxant given to suppress any response to facial nerve stimulation.[31]

### Hiccups: A Minor Nuisance?

Hiccups are an intermittent spasm of the diaphragm of reflex origin.[35] The afferent limb of the reflex is composed of the vagus and phrenic nerves, with the "hiccup center" located in the spinal cord between the third and fifth cervical segments. The efferent limb is the phrenic nerve. Hiccups usually occur during procedures in the upper abdomen and are caused by visceral stimulation or irritation of the diaphragm. Hiccups signal that the diaphragm is not fully paralyzed and require treatment only if they are interfering with the surgeon's work. Although several pharmacologic treatments for hiccups have been suggested,[36] the best treatment is to block the reflex pathway concerned by giving a further dose of muscle relaxant or by deepening the level of anesthesia with

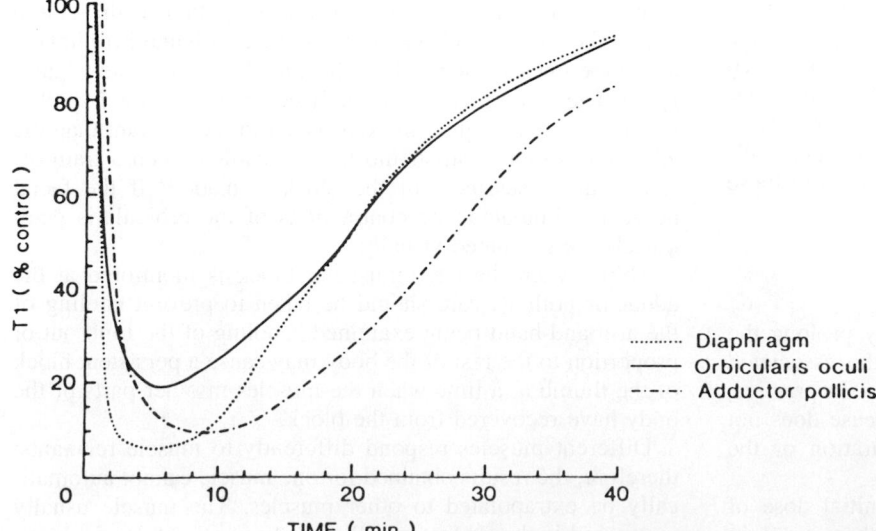

Legend:
.......... Diaphragm
—— Orbicularis oculi
–··–··– Adductor pollicis

**FIGURE 61–1.** Intensity and time course of neuromuscular block at the diaphragm, orbicularis oculi, and adductor pollicis after administration of vecuronium, 0.07 mg/kg. The block is expressed as amplitude of the first twitch to train-of-four stimulation (T1) relative to control. The diaphragm recovers from the block much more quickly than does the adductor pollicis. The block at the orbicularis oculi is nearly identical to that at the diaphragm. The clinical implications of these observations are explained in the text. (From Donati F, Meistelman C, Plaud B. Vecuronium neuromuscular blockade at the diaphragm, the orbicularis oculi, and adductor pollicis muscles. *Anesthesiology.* 1990;73:870.)

a small dose of thiopental or a higher concentration of inhaled agent.

## How Can Inadequate Relaxation During Peritoneal Closure Be Handled?

Inadequate relaxation is occasionally present during peritoneal closure, when only 15 to 20 more minutes of anesthesia are needed. Several avenues can be followed to solve the dilemma of satisfying operative demands while at the same time avoiding a dose of anesthetic or relaxant that makes awakening unduly prolonged or reversal of the block difficult. A small intravenous dose of thiopental or lidocaine and an increase in the concentration of the inhaled agents sometimes are enough to solve the problem. Manual hyperventilation is also helpful. If the abdominal contractions are powerful, however, only an additional dose of relaxant will bring the situation under control. When intermediate-acting agents such as vecuronium or atracurium have been used throughout the procedure, a small dose of the same relaxant is appropriate.

### Succinylcholine

When a long-acting relaxant has been used, an additional dose of the same drug would probably produce a block too long in duration for the remaining procedure and cause difficulty with reversal. In this situation, succinylcholine is a tempting but controversial choice. Some authorities object to the use of succinylcholine when the effect of a nondepolarizing block is dissipating because the block induced is somewhat variable and accompanied by a transient reversal of the residual nondepolarizing block.[37,38] In addition, when neostigmine or a similar drug is administered to reverse the residual nondepolarizing block, it may potentiate the effect of the previous dose of succinylcholine. Finally, there is a remote possibility that succinylcholine administration may be followed by a long-lasting block, should the patient have atypical plasma pseudocholinesterase.

Others argue that the brief antagonism of the nondepolarizing block is of little relevance and, provided a large enough dose of succinylcholine is administered (ie, 1 mg/kg), adequate relaxation can be consistently obtained for the few minutes needed.[38] Any succinylcholine/neostigmine interaction can be easily avoided if neostigmine is not administered until at least 15 minutes has elapsed after the administration of succinylcholine.[38] If a peripheral nerve stimulator is used, the residual nondepolarizing block is reversed only when the twitch has recovered to the level present before the administration of succinylcholine.

### Intermediate-Duration Relaxants

To avoid the succinylcholine controversy, the use of a shorter-acting nondepolarizing agent may seem an attractive choice. Unfortunately, shorter-acting agents administered during the recovery phase of a neuromuscular block established with long-acting agents usually cause a prolonged block far exceeding the 15 to 20 minutes required. For instance, vecuronium in a dose of 1 mg given during the recovery phase of a metocurine, pancuronium, or pipecuronium block causes a profound block that lasts 30 to 60 minutes.[39–41] Atracurium in a dose of 5 mg administered after pancuronium provides a

block of the same duration as 1 mg pancuronium.[42] A dose of 50 to 70 µg/kg of mivacurium given after pancuronium causes a block lasting approximately 60 minutes.[43,44] The problem can be circumvented by using very small doses of the shorter-acting agent. For instance, vecuronium 0.25 mg and atracurium 2 mg provide a block lasting approximately 15 minutes when administered after tubocurarine.[45] Mivacurium 10 µg/kg prolongs a pancuronium block by 20 to 25 minutes.[43] Because mivacurium is metabolized by plasma cholinesterase, there is the remote possibility of a prolonged block even after such a low dose in patients with atypical plasma pseudocholinesterase.[46]

## Does Neostigmine Affect Bowel Anastomosis?

Neostigmine is an anticholinesterase agent commonly used to reverse the effects of nondepolarizing muscle relaxants. In addition to its action on the skeletal muscle, it also causes forceful contractions of the bowel that persist for several minutes.[47] These contractions are unaffected by the concomitantly administered anticholinergic drug,[48,49] but are completely prevented by inhaled agents.[49] The effects of edrophonium and pyridostigmine, the other common reversal agents, have not been investigated.

In patients undergoing bowel resection and anastomosis, the hyperperistalsis induced by neostigmine has been postulated to disrupt the newly constructed anastomosis by putting excessive traction on the suture line.[50] The suggestion that inhaled agents completely inhibit neostigmine-induced contractions was discounted on the grounds that these agents are usually discontinued before neostigmine administration and therefore cannot be relied on to prevent the hyperperistalsis caused by neostigmine. Several subsequent studies have failed to link the use of neostigmine to an increased incidence of anastomotic breakdown,[51,52] leading to the current opinion that neostigmine is an unlikely cause of anastomotic complications.

## Can Muscle Relaxation Be Reestablished Shortly After Reversal?

Shortly after a neuromuscular block has been reversed with an anticholinesterase agent, unexpected circumstances such as an incorrect sponge count may require prompt reexploration of the abdomen with a short period of intense muscle relaxation. In this situation, the anesthesiologist may be reluctant to use succinylcholine because the inhibition of plasma pseudocholinesterase by the anticholinesterase agent may result in an excessively prolonged block. This concern, however, is unfounded. If edrophonium was the anticholinesterase agent used, it has no effect on plasma pseudocholinesterase and, accordingly, on the duration of a dose of succinylcholine subsequently administered.[53] A block caused by 1 mg/kg succinylcholine administered immediately after neostigmine or pyridostigmine (ie, when pseudocholinesterase activity is maximally inhibited) lasts approximately 30 minutes.[54] A smaller dose (eg, 0.5 mg/kg) provides approximately 15 minutes of relaxation. Should the block wear off before surgery is completed, additional doses of succinylcholine can be safely administered.

The inhibitory effect of neostigmine or pyridostigmine on

plasma pseudocholinesterase lasts approximately 60 minutes.[55] Therefore, no prolongation of succinylcholine block occurs when an hour or more has elapsed since the last dose of anticholinesterase.

## SPINAL AND EPIDURAL ANESTHESIA

### What Level of Sensory Block Is Needed for Upper Abdominal Procedures?

Upper abdominal procedures require an intense sensory block up to a T4 level. In actuality, however, a sensory level at T1 to T2 is needed, because analgesia at the upper level of the block tends to be tenuous, and only a sensory block up to T1 to T2 ensures a "surgical" block at the lower level T4. This high a level of anesthesia can be safely obtained only by a continuous epidural technique. Because an excessive dose of local anesthetic may be required if the injection is given at the lumbar level, the epidural puncture should be performed at a midthoracic level.

### Is Regional Anesthesia as the Sole Anesthetic Adequate for Upper Abdominal Surgery?

Despite an adequate sensory level, upper abdominal surgery under regional anesthesia is often marred by pain, nausea, and vomiting when the surgeon manipulates the viscera and by difficulty with respiration when retractors and packs are in place. In addition, relaxation of the abdominal muscles is not always satisfactory. For these reasons, regional anesthesia for an upper abdominal procedure is virtually always combined with endotracheal general anesthesia that eliminates patient discomfort, ensures adequate ventilation, and allows the use of relaxants if the surgical field is unsatisfactory.

### What Level of Sensory Block Is Needed for Lower Abdominal Procedures?

Surgery below the umbilicus requires a sensory block at T4 to T5 for both patient and surgeon satisfaction. This sensory level can be obtained equally well by spinal or epidural anesthesia. If the operating time is estimated to be less than 2 hours, a spinal or a single-shot epidural anesthetic can be used. However, because the duration of operations cannot always be predicted reliably, a case can be made for routine placement of an epidural catheter that allows prolongation of the block if needed. Obviously, a continuous epidural technique is chosen if postoperative analgesia is to be provided by the epidural route. Continuous spinal anesthesia has several appealing features, but concerns about serious neurologic complications have limited the widespread use of the technique.

### Is Regional Anesthesia Alone Adequate for Lower Abdominal Procedures?

Although regional anesthesia can provide satisfactory conditions for lower abdominal surgery, it also is often combined with general anesthesia to improve patient comfort. The combination prevents pain and nausea or the discomfort caused by a head-down position or by lying on the operating table for several hours. General anesthesia also allows administration of muscle relaxants should the abdominal relaxation provided by the regional block be inadequate.

### Technique for Combined Regional and General Anesthesia

A single-shot spinal or epidural block should be performed before the induction of general anesthesia to detect paresthesias or radicular pain during lumbar puncture and injection of the local anesthetic. If a continuous epidural technique is used, once the epidural catheter has been placed and the test dose administered, induction of general anesthesia first is expedient to allow placement of the urethral catheter and sterile preparation of the field without waiting for the block to be fully developed.

General anesthesia is induced with the intravenous agent of choice, followed by tracheal intubation. Topical anesthesia of the larynx and trachea with 4% lidocaine enhances tolerance of the endotracheal tube. Light anesthesia is maintained with nitrous oxide supplemented as needed by minimal concentrations of a halogenated agent or small doses of intravenous agents.

Ventilation can be spontaneous[56] or controlled. Controlled ventilation is mandatory when muscle relaxants are used but can also be easily established without muscle relaxants after a small dose of fentanyl and moderate hyperventilation (end-tidal $CO_2$ of approximately 30 mm Hg). During such "light" anesthesia, insertion of a nasogastric tube invariably is associated with the patient straining and bucking. This sequence can be avoided by inserting the nasogastric tube immediately after the endotracheal tube when the intubating level of muscle relaxant and induction agent is still present.

### How Is Hypotension Treated?

The combination of general and regional anesthesia is associated with a much greater decrease in blood pressure than when either technique is used alone. This hypotension responds poorly to fluid administration and is preferably treated with ephedrine or phenylephrine.[57–59]

### Is Regional Anesthesia Better Than General Anesthesia?

Numerous studies have addressed the question as to whether regional anesthesia offers any significant advantage over general anesthesia in abdominal surgery. The techniques have been compared in relation to several intraoperative and postoperative factors, including blood loss and the need for transfusion,[60,61] postoperative lung function and respiratory complications,[60,62] wound dehiscence,[60] anastomotic breakdown after bowel resection,[61] incidence of deep venous thrombosis,[60,63,64] postoperative weight loss and nitrogen balance,[65] duration of postoperative ileus, and postoperative mental dysfunctioning.[66] No clinically important differences in these areas have been demonstrated, and no convincing evidence favors one technique over the other for abdominal procedures.

In skillful hands, either is acceptable; once again, a successful outcome is related more to careful monitoring and control of physiologic variables than to the method of anesthesia.

## HYPOTENSION RELATED TO SURGICAL MANEUVERS

### Why Does It Occur?

Surgical maneuvers, particularly during procedures in the upper abdomen, may cause hypotension that can be explained by mechanical, reflex, or humoral mechanisms.

### Mechanical Causes

Placement of packs, retractors, or other instruments in the right upper abdominal quadrant or displacement of the liver can cause a drop in blood pressure by compression of the inferior vena cava and impedance to venous blood return. If invasive monitoring is used, the decrease in venous return is indicated by a rapid fall in filling pressures. Mechanical obstruction of the inferior vena cava should be promptly identified and relieved; treatment with fluids and vasopressors is seldom needed.

### Reflex Mechanisms

Hypotension may follow traction and manipulation of the biliary tract, colon, uterus and ovaries, and parietal peritoneum.[67] If a patient is conscious during regional anesthesia, such maneuvers can also cause discomfort, nausea, and vomiting. The decrease in blood pressure caused by manipulation of intraabdominal structures is associated with bradycardia in approximately 50% of patients.[67] Bradycardia is sometimes severe and appears to be the primary event that causes the reduction in blood pressure.[68]

These hemodynamic changes are usually ascribed to a reflex mechanism (Fig. 61–2). Impulses conducted by visceral and somatic pathways are postulated to increase parasympathetic tone or inhibit sympathetic activity. The ensuing hypotension is secondary to a decrease in heart rate or vasodilation in the splanchnic area, with blood pooling and decreased venous return. Severe reflex bradycardia during intraabdominal procedures seems to occur more commonly than in the past, particularly in younger patients with a greater vagal tone.[69] This observation probably is explained by the fact that in modern anesthesia practice, drugs with vagolytic activity (atropine, gallamine, pancuronium) are less frequently used,

whereas opioids with vagotonic effects are commonly administered. As a consequence, the effects on the heart by the vagal reflexes elicited during surgery are not only unopposed but facilitated.

### Humoral Mechanisms

Hypotension caused by systemic vasodilation and associated with a compensatory increase in heart rate and cardiac output characteristically follows traction on the small bowel mesentery.[70] These changes are commonly observed in patients undergoing aortic surgery when the small bowel is exteriorized to expose the abdominal aorta (Table 61–1). In addition to the hemodynamic changes, marked flushing of the skin in the head and neck areas develops in approximately two thirds of patients. The greatest changes in blood pressure and heart rate occur 5 to 10 minutes after mesenteric traction and persist 30 to 45 minutes. Pretreatment with aspirin and ibuprofen is effective in preventing these hemodynamic changes, supporting the hypothesis that they are mediated by intestinal release of prostacyclin.[71,72]

### How Is It Treated?

When serious hemodynamic changes of reflex origin occur, any surgical maneuver should stop promptly. Treatment of severe bradycardia with intravenous atropine is preferable to glycopyrrolate because of its more rapid rate of onset.[73] If the heart rate is normal, ephedrine effectively restores blood

**TABLE 61–1.** Hemodynamic Measurements and Derived Data Before and After Mesenteric Traction in 20 Patients Undergoing Aortic Surgery*

| Hemodynamic Parameters | Premesenteric Traction† | Postmesenteric Traction† |
|---|---|---|
| Heart rate (beats per minute) | 67 ± 13 | 77 ± 17 |
| Mean arterial pressure (mm Hg) | 105 ± 20 | 81 ± 19 |
| Cardiac output (L/min) | 5.8 ± 1.9 | 7.7 ± 2.3 |
| Stroke volume (mL) | 88 ± 25 | 100 ± 22 |
| Central venous pressure (mm Hg) | 11 ± 5 | 10 ± 5 |
| Pulmonary artery occlusion pressure (mm Hg) | 18 ± 6 | 16 ± 6 |
| Systemic vascular resistance (dynes/s/cm$^{-5}$) | 1423 ± 504 | 839 ± 405 |

*All changes were statistically significant.
†Values are expressed as mean ± standard error of the mean.
Modified from Seltzer JL, Ritter DE, Starsnic MA, et al. The hemodynamic response to traction on the abdominal mesentery. *Anesthesiology.* 1985;63:96.

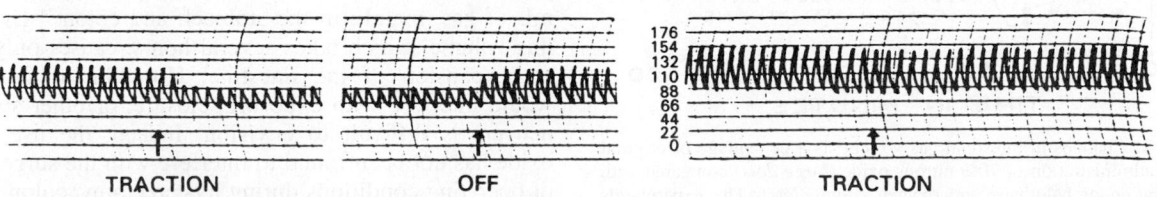

TRACTION          OFF          TRACTION

**FIGURE 61–2.** Continuous arterial pressure recordings (measured in millimeters of mercury) during traction on the transverse colon. Traction produced an immediate fall in blood pressure from 122/66 to 87/57, but the heart rate remained unchanged *(left tracing).* Note the prompt return to the control blood pressure on release of traction *(middle tracing).* The *third tracing* illustrates the effect of similar traction after separation of the colon from its mesentery. The rapid changes in blood pressure when the stimulus was applied and released and the unchanged blood pressure after the mesentery was severed strongly suggest a reflex mechanism. (From Eather KF, Peterson LH, Dripps RD. Studies of circulation of anesthetized patients by new method for recording arterial pressure and pressure pulser contours. *Anesthesiology.* 1949;10:125.)

pressure. Hypotension and tachycardia due to mesenteric traction may require fluid and phenylephrine administration.

## NITROUS OXIDE AND BOWEL DISTENTION

### Why Does It Occur?

The bowel contains variable proportions of nitrogen, hydrogen, and methane.[74] These gases are much less soluble in the blood than is nitrous oxide. When nitrous oxide is respired, it can enter the intestinal lumen far more readily than nitrogen and the other gases can be removed from it. As a result, the bowel, having highly compliant walls, increases its volume.

### Concentration and Duration of Administration

The change in bowel volume depends on the nitrous oxide concentration and duration of administration. When 70% nitrous oxide is administered, a twofold increase in intestinal gas volume occurs in 2 hours, and up to a threefold increase occurs by 4 hours (Fig. 61–3). Bowel volume progressively increases until equilibrium is reached between the concentra-

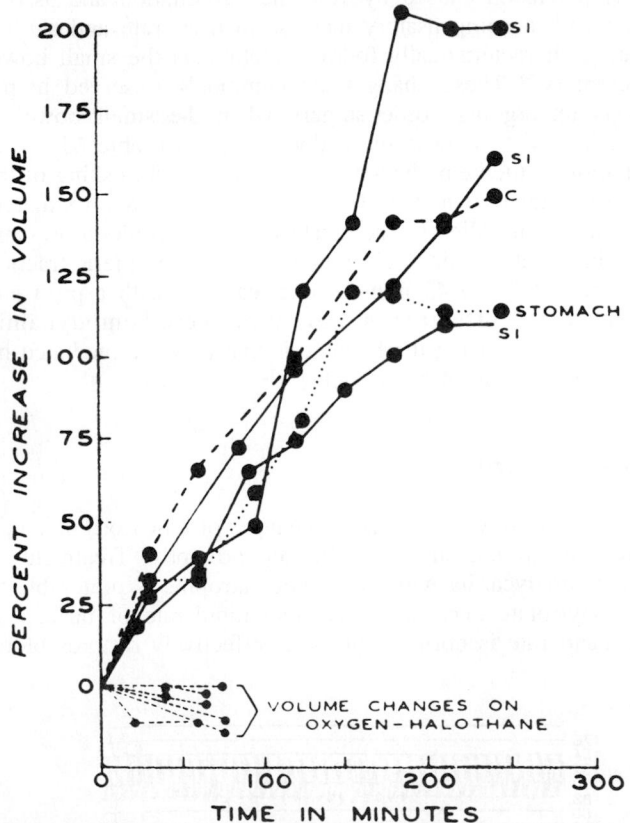

**FIGURE 61–3.** Changes in intestinal gas volume as a percentage of original volume with administration of 70% nitrous oxide *(large dots)* compared with the administration of halothane and oxygen *(small dots)*. The experiments were performed in isolated segments of animal stomach, small bowel (SI), and colon (C) into which a measured volume of air was injected. The animals were then given nitrous oxide to breathe. The volume changes in the bowel were then measured at intervals. (From Eger EI, Saidman LJ. Hazards of nitrous oxide anesthesia in bowel obstruction and pneumothorax. *Anesthesiology.* 1965;26:61.)

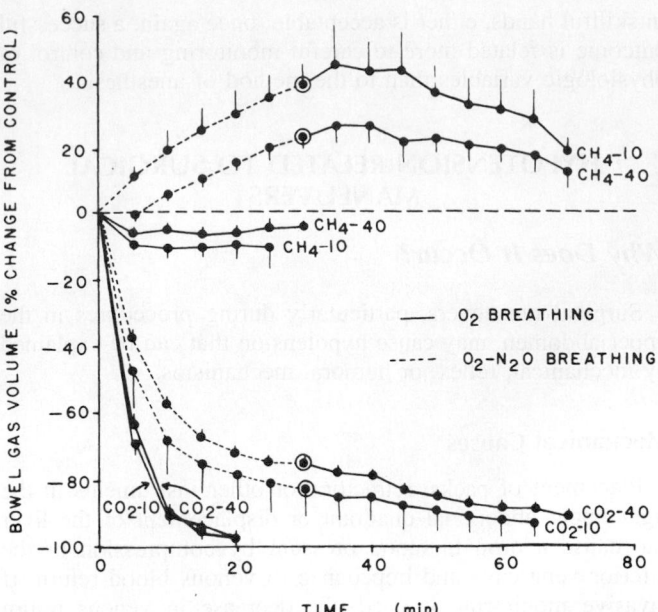

**FIGURE 61–4.** Effect of 100% $O_2$ or 21% $O_2$-balanced $N_2O$ ($O_2$-$N_2O$) administration on bowel gas volume. Four bowel segments are represented, each of which was initially injected with 10 mL (ambient temperature and pressure, dry) or 40 mL of methane ($CH_4$-10, $CH_4$-40) or carbon dioxide ($CO_2$-10, $CO_2$-40). The changeover from $O_2$-$N_2O$ to $O_2$ breathing at 30 minutes is indicated by a *circle*. The means $\pm$ standard error of the mean of the results from four dogs are given. (From Steffey EP, Johnson BH, Eger EI II, et al. Nitrous oxide: effect on accumulation rate and uptake of bowel gases. *Anesth Analg.* 1979;58:407.)

tion of nitrous oxide in the blood and bowel lumen, a process that takes 5 to 6 hours. Should the administration of 70% nitrous oxide continue until equilibrium is reached, the bowel volume would at most increase fourfold.[75]

When nitrous oxide concentration is limited to 50%, the increase in volume is less. Should nitrous oxide administration continue until equilibrium, the volume of intestinal gas doubles at most. Discontinuation of nitrous oxide reverses the gas expansion, but bowel deflation takes place slowly[76] (Fig. 61–4).

### Is It a Problem in Normal Patients?

Surgeons sometimes express concern that during abdominal procedures, nitrous oxide, by distending the bowel, might interfere with surgical conditions. This concern is not supported by theoretical considerations or empiric data. The potential for intestinal distention with nitrous oxide in normal people is very limited. The intestine usually contains <200 mL of gas, mainly in the stomach and colon.[74] Even tripling this volume, which takes several hours, causes only a moderate expansion of the intestine. How this modest increase would interfere with exposure, closure, or other surgical maneuvers is difficult to envision. Indeed, the use of nitrous oxide has not been found to interfere with the surgeon's rating of operating conditions during hysterectomy, colon surgery, or laparoscopic procedures.[77–79] In practice, however, a distended bowel is occasionally noted when the abdomen is opened. In such patients, the anesthesiologist may consider limiting nitrous oxide concentration to 50% or discontinuing the agent altogether.

A distended stomach should be decompressed by inserting a nasogastric tube and does not pose a contraindication to the use of nitrous oxide.

### Can Nitrous Oxide Be Used With Intestinal Obstruction?

Nitrous oxide administration to patients with intestinal obstruction is more problematic. Further dilation of an already distended intestine carries several risks and should be avoided. Nitrous oxide, however, expands the bowel slowly, and the dilation observed during the first hour of administration is probably of little clinical relevance (see Fig. 61–4). According to Eger and Saidman, "it would seem prudent to consider bowel obstruction as a relative contraindication to nitrous oxide at inspired concentration exceeding 50%, particularly if it is anticipated that anesthesia will be prolonged."[75]

Nitrous oxide, therefore, is still acceptable in a patient with bowel obstruction, provided it is administered for a short time (ie, until the abdomen is open), the cause of the intestinal obstruction has been determined, and a plan has been made to relieve it. In most cases of severe abdominal obstruction, the surgeon effects some kind of decompression of the intestine (long intestinal tube or enterotomy) before proceeding to the rest of the operation. If the planned procedure is of long duration, options for nitrous oxide use are complete avoidance, use in a concentration not exceeding 50%, or use only as an aid during induction and emergence.

## NARCOTIC ADMINISTRATION AND BILIARY SPASM

Opioid analgesics such as morphine, meperidine, and fentanyl are known to cause contraction of the choledochoduodenal sphincter (sphincter of Oddi) and an increase in intrabiliary pressure. This effect, also present during anesthesia with potent inhaled agents, is promptly reversed by naloxone.[80] The agonist-antagonist agents, butorphanol and nalbuphine, have only negligible effects on the sphincter of Oddi.[80–82]

### Is It a Problem?

Most surgeons operating on the biliary tract routinely perform intraoperative cholangiography to detect stones in the common bile duct and verify its patency. Narcotics are considered by many to be contraindicated during biliary tract surgery because they may cause an intense contraction of the sphincter of Oddi. The resulting interference with the passage of contrast from the common bile duct into the duodenum can thereby simulate a mechanical obstruction, potentially leading to an unnecessary exploration of the biliary tract.

This concern seems unfounded. Surgeons are well aware that the contrast material may fail to enter the duodenum because of a spasm of the sphincter. This event is characterized radiologically by a smoothly tapered distal sphincter and a bile duct of normal diameter.[83] Failure of the dye to enter the duodenum as an isolated finding does not represent an indication for surgical exploration of the biliary tract. It must be associated with stones or other signs of long-standing

mechanical obstruction such as a dilated common bile duct. Narcotics obviously do not have anything to do with these latter pathologic findings.

### Are Other Factors Responsible?

The incidence of spasm of the sphincter of Oddi during operative cholangiography is low. Even when a fentanyl-based anesthetic was used, a spasm was detected in only approximately 3% of the patients.[84] The cause of this spasm is not clear. In addition to narcotics, surgical manipulation and the irritant effect of the contrast dye have been cited. When spasm of the sphincter of Oddi is suspected, administration of glucagon or cholecystokinin is invariably followed by relaxation and flow of contrast medium into the duodenum.[83] Naloxone and nalbuphine[85] may be used if spasm is thought to be related to a previously administered opioid; they do not resolve spasm induced by other factors.

## NASOGASTRIC TUBES

### What Types Are Available?

#### Single Lumen

Nasogastric tubes are used to decompress the stomach by removing fluid and gas. A Levin tube is a single-lumen tube, the major drawback of which is that suction can be applied only intermittently. If continuous suction is applied, once the stomach is empty, the gastric mucosa is sucked into the distal orifice and occludes it. As a consequence, fluid or air that reaccumulates in the stomach cannot be removed.

#### Double Lumen

More popular, but not necessarily more effective, are nasogastric tubes designed to be used with continuous suction.[86] These tubes have a double lumen: one for suction and one, the "sump," that is left open to ambient air. When continuous suction is applied and the stomach is empty, the sump lumen allows air to enter the stomach, preventing the gastric mucosa from obstructing the tube. A sucking sound around the proximal port of the sump lumen signals that the tube is properly functioning. Should fluid reaccumulate, air entrainment stops until the fluid has been suctioned out.

In elective abdominal surgery, the nasogastric tube is usually placed after induction of anesthesia for patient comfort, whereas in emergency procedures, the patient arrives in the operating room with a nasogastric tube already in place. Only the placement of gastric tubes in tracheally intubated and anesthetized patients is discussed in this chapter.

### When Is the Tube Inserted Through the Mouth?

A gastric tube is usually placed through the nose, but if it is to be removed at the end of surgery, the oral route is preferred to avoid epistaxis. The oral route is also indicated in the presence of basal skull fractures to prevent accidental intracranial introduction[87] or when nasal deformities or facial fractures make transit through the nose impossible.

### Is It Contraindicated in Patients With Esophageal Varices?

Placement of a gastric tube in patients with portal hypertension and esophageal varices is often considered to be contraindicated because of fear of variceal bleeding. Recent data indicate that this fear is largely unfounded, and patients with esophageal varices should not be denied the benefits of a nasogastric tube.[88]

### How Is It Inserted?

Before insertion, a deep level of anesthesia or, preferably, intense neuromuscular block should be present to prevent straining and bucking. When succinylcholine is used during induction of anesthesia, the nasogastric tube should be inserted either immediately after the endotracheal tube has been secured or delayed until neuromuscular block from the maintenance nondepolarizing agent is well established. If the gastric tube is placed later, deep neuromuscular block (ie, no more than 1 twitch using a train-of-four count) keeps the patient from moving in response to this stimulus.

### Technique

A properly lubricated nasogastric tube is inserted through the larger naris and advanced parallel to the floor of the nasal cavity in an anteroposterior direction. Resistance is sometimes met in the posterior pharynx because the tube does not negotiate the sharp angle between the nasopharynx and oropharynx. If the resistance is not overcome by gentle manipulation, the tip of the tube can be retrieved by the operator's index finger in proximity to the soft palate and directed into the oropharynx.

Most of the time, the tube advances easily into the stomach. Proper position is confirmed by return of gastric juice with aspiration or by gastric palpation when the abdomen is open. The tube is then secured by a mesentery or umbilical bridge, thereby avoiding any pressure on the nostrils (Fig. 61–5).

### Why Does the Ventilator Sometimes Alarm?

Manipulation of a gastric tube in the esophagus of a mechanically ventilated patient may cause (1) gas volume occasionally to be lost from the breathing circuit; (2) the low-pressure alarm of the ventilator to sound; or (3) the bellows actually to collapse, especially when the tube is attached to suction. These problems occur when the gastric tube accidentally enters the trachea, causing air leak both around the endotracheal tube cuff and through the tube itself. Removal and repositioning solves the problem.

### What Can the Anesthesiologist Do if the Tube Will Not Pass?

Should the tube fail to enter the esophagus, several maneuvers may be attempted. If an esophageal stethoscope or other

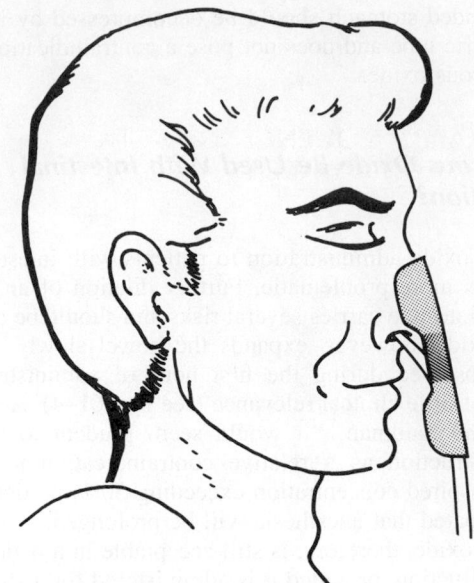

**FIGURE 61–5.** Umbilical bridge. Pinching the midsection of a strip of 1-inch tape so that it sticks to itself creates an umbilical bridge that allows the practitioner to secure a nasogastric tube to the nose without applying pressure to the tip of the nose. (From Guyton DC. Oral, nasopharyngeal, and gastrointestinal systems. In: Gravenstein N, ed. *Manual of Complications During Anesthesia.* Philadelphia, Pa: JB Lippincott; 1991:632.)

probe is already in place, it should be removed and replaced after the nasogastric tube has been inserted or reinserted simultaneously. These tubes are sufficiently flexible that if their plastic surface contacts that of another, they stick and coil rather than advance.

A patient's head can also be turned to the side, or the thyroid cartilage can be grasped between the thumb and index finger and lifted anteriorly while the gastric tube is advanced. These maneuvers open an esophagus that is normally collapsed by gravity.[89] Should they fail, a laryngoscope is inserted into the oropharynx, the esophageal opening is visualized, and the tube is pushed in, possibly with the help of Magill forceps.

Another technique uses a nasoesophageally placed endotracheal tube.[90] A 7.5-mm internal diameter endotracheal tube with the connector removed is cut lengthwise along one side and inserted through the nose into the esophagus. A lubricated 18 French nasogastric tube is then passed through the lumen of the endotracheal tube into the stomach. The endotracheal tube is removed from the nose and, having been previously split, peeled away from the nasogastric tube.

### How Is a Long Tube Passed?

A surgeon may sometimes wish to decompress a greatly distended bowel at the beginning of the procedure. Decompression can be accomplished by advancing a long tube from the stomach along the entire length of the small bowel to the ileocecal valve while suction is continuously applied. The tube, approximately 120 inches long, is introduced into the stomach through the nose or mouth, depending on whether it is to be left in position. One, or sometimes two, balloons are present at the distal end and are inflated with air or water once the tube is in the stomach. This process enables the surgeon to grasp the tube and advance it past the pylorus into the small bowel. Once the tube is in place, the balloons must be deflated.

## RAPID-SEQUENCE INDUCTION IN EMERGENCY ABDOMINAL SURGERY

Patients requiring emergency abdominal surgery have a "full stomach" and therefore are at risk for pulmonary aspiration should regurgitation or vomiting occur during induction of anesthesia. These patients, however, seldom have food in the stomach because vomiting usually has already occurred before their admission. Gastric contents usually represent GI secretions, fecaloid fluid when bowel obstruction is present, or blood.

In these patients, a rapid-sequence induction technique[91] combined with cricoid pressure is indicated.[92] However, before initiating a rapid-sequence induction, the anesthesiologist should assess a patient's anatomy by conventional laryngoscopy to verify that tracheal intubation is feasible. If uncertainty exists, awake intubation with local anesthesia may be the safest method to secure the airway.

### Should the Patient Be Ventilated?

During rapid-sequence induction, mask ventilation before tracheal intubation is believed to be contraindicated by many anesthesiologists because positive-pressure ventilation may cause gastric insufflation and increases the chance of regurgitation. In addition, it is feared that should regurgitation occur, mask ventilation can "push" the regurgitated material into the airways. However, properly applied cricoid pressure completely occludes the esophagus, and thereby prevents passive fluid regurgitation and keeps air from being pushed into the stomach.[92-94] In this circumstance, gentle mask ventilation does not seem contraindicated.[92,95]

Some patients, despite protracted preoxygenation, very rapidly develop hypoxemia when apneic during a conventional rapid-sequence induction.[96] Obesity, lung disease, and abdominal distention due to bowel obstruction or ascites greatly decrease the functional residual capacity (FRC) and hence the amount of oxygen ($O_2$) available when ventilation is discontinued. To avoid hypoxemia, these patients may require a "modified" rapid-sequence induction, in which mask ventilation with $O_2$ is given before intubation while cricoid pressure is continuously applied.

### What Is Done When a Nasogastric Tube Is in Place?

When a nasogastric tube is in place, it should be suctioned before induction. The tube is then left open to ambient air or connected to continuous suction, if it is a sump type. This procedure does not guarantee that the stomach is empty.

Whether a nasogastric tube should be removed before induction is controversial. A gastric tube does not interfere with an adequate esophageal seal when cricoid pressure is applied.[93] In addition, it can act as a pop-off valve should intragastric pressure suddenly increase while cricoid pressure is applied[93] (Fig. 61–6). A gastric tube, however, makes an

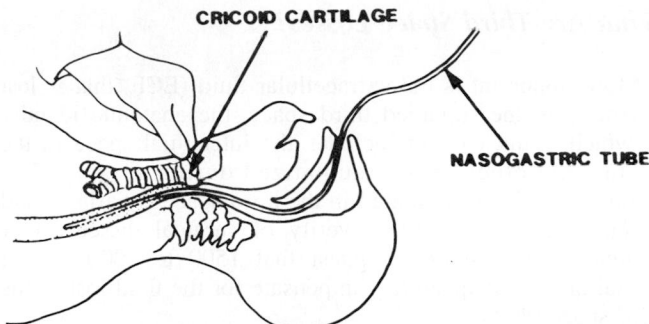

**FIGURE 61–6.** Firmly applied cricoid pressure is effective in sealing the esophagus around an esophageal tube against an intraesophageal pressure of up to 100 cm $H_2O$. (Modified from Salem MR, Joseph NJ, Heyman HJ, et al. Cricoid compression is effective in obliterating the esophageal lumen in the presence of a nasogastric tube. *Anesthesiology.* 1985;63:444.)

airtight mask fit difficult and therefore may interfere with adequate mask ventilation. Hence, removal may be preferable when the need for mask ventilation is likely because of low $O_2$ reserve (decreased FRC), high $O_2$ consumption (sepsis), or potentially difficult intubation.

### Should Cricoid Pressure Be Released if the Patient Vomits?

Cricoid pressure should immediately be released if a patient actively vomits, lest esophageal rupture occur.[92,97] Vomiting, which requires powerful abdominal contractions, should rarely, if ever, occur during rapid-sequence induction if succinylcholine is administered through a freely running intravenous catheter immediately after the intravenous induction agent.[92]

## INTRAOPERATIVE FLUID MANAGEMENT

### What Is the Preoperative Deficit and Basal Fluid Requirement?

The amount of fluid administered intraoperatively depends on the basal requirements, replacement of deficits incurred before anesthesia, and replacement of intraoperative losses. In adults, basal fluid requirements amount to 75 to 100 mL/h and represent the water needed for urine production and to replace that evaporated through the skin and lungs.[98] Preexisting fluid deficits in patients undergoing elective surgery are caused by the 8 to 10 hours of preoperative fasting and total 500 to 1000 mL.[99] Preoperative fluid deficits encountered in patients with acute intraabdominal disease are often significantly larger and should be replaced as much as possible before surgery.

### What Is the Intraoperative Fluid Deficit?

Intraoperative water losses result from evaporation through the exposed surface of the bowel and humidification of dry respiratory gases. These losses usually are negligible. Additional loss that can be easily measured is represented by the fluid drained through the nasogastric tube.

## What Are Third Space Losses?

More important is the extracellular fluid (ECF) that is lost internally in the so-called third space, the anatomic identity of which is unclear but includes the interstitial space in the wound and other areas traumatized during surgery. The amount of fluid accumulated in the third space is variable and depends, in part, on the severity of surgical dissection or trauma.[100] Most studies suggest that 1500 to 2000 mL of crystalloids is adequate to compensate for the fluid lost in the third space.[101–104]

## How Are Fluids Replaced?

The total amount of fluids required for most abdominal procedures, in the absence of significant blood loss, is 2000 to 3000 mL, usually supplied as lactated Ringer's solution. Deficits due to fasting are quickly replaced just before or during anesthesia induction, and the rest is infused at a rate of 8 to 10 mL/kg/h of surgery. In addition, 2 or 3 mL of lactated Ringer's is infused for each milliliter of blood lost, until the blood loss has reached 800 to 1000 mL (15%-20% of the circulatory volume). Should blood loss continue, packed red blood cells, additional crystalloids, or colloids need to be administered. These guidelines are general; the amount and type of fluid administered may vary considerably according to specific clinical situations. The goal of fluid administration is to maintain stable hemodynamic function with adequate organ perfusion.

Limiting the volume of intraoperative fluids to what really is needed is based on two considerations. First, excess fluid is retained and accumulates as edema in the skin and other organs such as the intestine and skeletal muscle.[105] A growing consensus suggests that such edema may not be completely benign.[106,107] Second, retained fluids are mobilized on the second to third postoperative day and returned to the vascular compartment. Although mobilized fluids are well handled by patients with a normal heart and kidneys, pulmonary edema may occur should the cardiovascular system be unable to tolerate the increase in intravascular volume or the kidneys unable to increase urine output.

### Useful Rules of Thumb

To maintain hemodynamic function and organ perfusion without excessive expansion of the ECF compartment, the following considerations may be useful:

1. If the procedure lasts several hours, not because of its inherent complexity but because, for example, the surgeon is particularly slow or the report on a specimen sent for tissue diagnosis is greatly delayed, the hourly fluid rate should be decreased.
2. Low blood pressure during periods of minimal surgical stimulation probably is better treated by lightening the anesthetic or administering a vasopressor than by administering a fluid bolus.
3. If large amounts of crystalloids (>4000 mL) have been given in the absence of significant blood loss and the circulation is still unstable, colloids should be considered to minimize tissue edema.[108]

4. Colloids are useful to replace blood loss in elderly patients and in patients with cardiac diseases to decrease the fluid load and thus the risk of postoperative edema.
5. An hourly urinary output of >1 mL/kg suggests that the fluid rate can be decreased.
6. Intraoperative oliguria (ie, urinary output <0.5 mL/kg/h) does not always mean that the fluid rate needs to be increased. The first step is to rule out compression or kinking of the urine collecting system. A sudden drop in urine output can often be observed when a patient is placed in a steep head-down position. As a result, the bladder neck is moved uppermost, and urine pools at the bottom of the bladder rather than flowing through the urinary catheter into the collecting system. This situation does not require treatment; brisk flow of urine is observed when a patient's position is returned to horizontal.
7. In evaluating fluid replacement, observe the hemodynamic changes that occur over time (ie, the trend rather than the absolute values) and resist the temptation to treat "the numbers" instead of the patient. For instance, a central venous pressure (CVP) of 3 mm Hg that has not changed in a patient with normal blood pressure and pulse rate and adequate urinary output does not require treatment. Conversely, a drop in CVP from 9 to 6 mm Hg associated with sudden blood loss requires prompt intervention even if the blood pressure and heart rate have not changed significantly.

## What Is Normovolemic Oliguria?

Intraoperative oliguria is often caused by hypovolemia but sometimes occurs in patients with normal kidneys, hemodynamics, and blood volume.[109] This "normovolemic" oliguria is a benign phenomenon that does not indicate poor kidney perfusion, nor is it associated with postoperative renal failure.[109,110]

Low urinary output in the presence of normal kidney perfusion and adequate hydration probably is a consequence of the combined effects of the anesthetic agents and the neurohumoral changes set in motion by surgical trauma. Normal urinary output resumes soon after completion of anesthesia.

If the volume status is uncertain, a bolus of 500 mL of crystalloid is administered over 5 to 10 minutes. Should urine output increase, the diagnosis of hypovolemia is confirmed and additional fluid may be required.[109] If the urine output remains scanty after the fluid bolus and all else seems stable, normovolemic oliguria is likely. The clinician may then do nothing, or a small dose (5-10 mg) of furosemide can be administered intravenously. Urine production usually increases within 15 to 20 minutes.

## What Is the Effect of Preoperative Bowel Preparation?

In patients undergoing colon and rectal surgery, preoperative cleansing of the bowel of fecal material is important to decrease septic complications. The bowel can be effectively cleansed by oral administration of balanced electrolyte solutions to which osmotically active substances such as mannitol or polyethylene glycol are added. These solutions promptly cause watery diarrhea and are usually administered over several hours in large volumes until the rectal effluent is clear.

## Fluid Deficits and Excesses

Depending on the composition of the solution, a positive or a negative fluid balance may result due to the translocation of water and electrolytes through the intestinal mucosa.[111] Neither event is desirable; fluid absorption may result in hypervolemia and pulmonary edema, whereas fluid loss may cause hypovolemia and hypotension.

An electrolyte solution containing polyethylene glycol (Go-Lytely) has gained popularity because it leaves the fluid balance virtually unaffected. Water and electrolytes are neither absorbed nor secreted from the bowel.[112] Patients treated with this solution usually do not manifest hypovolemia or hemodynamic instability during induction of anesthesia.

## How Is Management Changed by an Acute Intraabdominal Pathologic Process?

Patients with an acute intraabdominal pathologic process often present with significant ECF deficits and electrolyte imbalance. External losses are secondary to vomiting, prolonged nasogastric suction, diarrhea, and intestinal fistulas. If the fluid lost is predominantly gastric juice, the result is hypochloremic, hypokalemic metabolic alkalosis. Potassium is present in the gastric juice, but the main reason for hypokalemia in vomiting is renal excretion as $H^+$ ions are conserved. The loss of intestinal and pancreatic juices, which contain bicarbonate, tends to produce metabolic acidosis.

## Where Does the Fluid Go?

Internal fluid losses occur in bowel obstruction, peritonitis, and acute pancreatitis. Bowel obstruction fluid, which is similar to plasma in protein and electrolyte content, accumulates in the intestinal lumen above the obstruction and in the walls of the involved bowel. Peritonitis is associated with the loss of plasma-like fluid as edema of the parietal and visceral peritoneum and as exudate into the peritoneal cavity. Additional fluid loss occurs into the atonic bowel that invariably accompanies peritonitis. When the vascular supply to the bowel is compromised because of strangulation or thromboembolism of the intestinal vessels, a significant amount of blood can extravasate into the wall and lumen of the necrotic bowel, further decreasing the circulating volume.

In acute pancreatitis, large amounts of fluid are sequestered in the retroperitoneal space and in the inflamed peritoneal cavity. In the hemorrhagic form of pancreatitis, a large amount of blood is also lost internally.

Fluid loss through the GI tract causes ECF contraction, the magnitude of which depends on the underlying disease process and its duration. Volume depletion is particularly severe in extensive peritonitis and pancreatitis because of the large areas involved in the inflammatory process and in bowel obstruction because of both external and internal losses. Small bowel obstruction in this respect is more serious than large bowel obstruction because fluid losses are larger and progress more rapidly. The ECF volume reduction may eventually lead to shock with hypotension, tachycardia, and oliguria. Obvious signs of hypovolemia indicate an ECF deficit in excess of 20% to 25%.

## Replacement

Fluid deficits secondary to GI disease are replaced with lactated Ringer's solution or, if gastric juice loss is prominent, normal saline because of its high chloride content. Potassium chloride is added when adequate urinary output is established.

## Estimation of Deficit

The ECF deficit and, therefore, the volume of fluid replacement is difficult to estimate. A decrease in body weight represents external fluid losses but obviously does not provide information about the amount of internal fluid sequestration. Also, the body weight before dehydration took place frequently is unknown. In the absence of hemorrhage, the hematocrit increases in proportion to the ECF deficit. If the hematocrit before and after the fluid loss is known, calculation of the deficit is possible.[113]

Plasma electrolyte determinations give an idea of alterations in composition but not of the ECF volume deficit. In practice, according to the severity of the illness, several liters of crystalloids are rapidly infused after placement of a central catheter for pressure monitoring.

## Adequacy of Replacement

Fluids are administered until the blood pressure, heart rate, heart filling pressures, and hourly urinary output have reached satisfactory values. Reestablishment of adequate perfusion is also indicated by warm, dry skin, brisk capillary refill, improvement of metabolic acidosis, and an increase in cardiac output and mixed venous $O_2$ saturation. Blood pressure, heart rate, and heart filling pressures can be normal despite a considerable volume depletion.[114] Fluids are administered until the CVP and pulmonary artery occlusion pressures (PAOP) are 10 to 12 mm Hg and 15 to 18 mm Hg, respectively, and further 250-mL fluid boluses cause an excessive increase in filling pressures.

Another method to assess the adequacy of the circulatory volume is to measure blood pressure and heart rate changes in response to postural stress.[115] When a patient arises from a supine to a sitting position, with both legs horizontal and the chest at an angle of 45°, an increase in heart rate of 10 beats per minute associated with a fall in blood pressure $\geq 15$ mm Hg indicates a persistent volume deficit. Additional fluids are administered until the hemodynamic changes with alterations in posture are minimal.

## Colloid Administration

Patients with peritonitis, ischemic bowel, or protracted bowel obstruction suffer large losses of protein-rich fluids. If they remain unstable despite large volumes of crystalloids, colloids such as 6% hetastarch or 5% albumin may be beneficial.

A combination of crystalloids and colloids should also be considered for elderly patients, in whom more rapid replenishment of the circulatory volume and reestablishment of adequate organ perfusion may be desirable. This combination also may be useful for patients with preexisting cardiac disease to limit fluid volume requirements. With correction of the fluid deficit and plasma volume, the hematocrit may drop significantly, revealing preexistent anemia or blood sequestration. Blood transfusion may then be indicated.

### Timing of Replacement

Patients who have incurred large fluid and plasma losses must be resuscitated as adequately as possible before induction of anesthesia. Otherwise, a dramatic fall in blood pressure will be associated with the loss of sympathetic tone and vasodilatation. The induction of anesthesia for emergency surgery should be delayed while crystalloids or colloids, or both, are rapidly infused. This preinduction volume resuscitation can usually be accomplished in less than 15 minutes. Although surgery is urgent, the extra time invested in stabilizing a patient before anesthesia may avert a disaster.

## ACUTE GASTROINTESTINAL BLEEDING

Patients with GI bleeding require emergency surgery when they manifest persistent or recurrent bleeding despite conservative treatment, including endoscopic electrocoagulation or laser coagulation, selective intraarterial vasopressin infusion, and transcatheter arterial embolization. These patients are almost invariably hypovolemic, often hypotensive or in frank shock, and require intravascular volume resuscitation before anesthesia can be safely induced.

### What Should Be Done Before Induction?

The first step in the management of hemorrhagic patients is to establish adequate venous access, preferably by placing two large-bore cannulas. The second step is to estimate the severity of blood loss and resuscitation needs based on blood pressure, heart rate, mental status, capillary refill, and urinary output. Hemoglobin concentration is of no use in assessing blood volume status in patients who are acutely bleeding or in those who have been bleeding intermittently for 24 to 48 hours and have received multiple transfusions.

Patients with hypotension, tachycardia, apprehension, or clouding of consciousness have lost at least 30% of their circulating blood volume and require prompt resuscitation with crystalloids or colloids and blood.[116] Usually, 2 L of crystalloid is rapidly infused, followed by 2 units of blood. The situation is then reevaluated, and additional fluids or blood is administered until a satisfactory blood pressure and heart rate are obtained. Colloids are also recommended because they allow more rapid and sustained restoration of blood volume, cardiac output, and organ perfusion.

Patients with less hemodynamic compromise are initially resuscitated with crystalloids or colloids; blood administration is less urgent. While volume resuscitation takes place, arterial and central venous catheters are placed for pressure monitoring and acid-base evaluation. After the blood volume has been restored, hemoglobin or hematocrit is measured to assess the need for additional blood transfusion.

### How Should Anesthesia Be Induced?

Once adequate hemodynamics have been obtained, anesthesia is carefully induced with the agent of choice (eg, etomi-

date, ketamine, or thiopental). The latter drug is used in a reduced dose, while the blood pressure is closely watched and additional fluids are promptly administered should it decrease. A rapid-sequence induction is mandatory.

Patients with acute GI bleeding sometimes arrive in the operating room with normal blood pressure and heart rate. By no means should this observation be considered proof of normovolemia. Younger patients in particular can compensate surprisingly well for a loss of up to 20% of their blood volume.[117] Induction of anesthesia in patients with compensated contraction of blood volume may be followed by a dramatic decline in blood pressure. A prudent approach is to expand the circulatory volume by infusing rapidly 1 L of crystalloid just before induction of anesthesia to compensate for any hidden volume deficit. Anesthesia is then induced following the same precautions previously outlined.

### What Should Be Done Intraoperatively?

Fluid resuscitation continues intraoperatively according to blood pressure, heart filling pressures, urinary output, and other clinical signs. These patients commonly have concurrent medical problems such as cirrhosis, sepsis, and renal failure that may compound the coagulopathy associated with massive blood loss. A coagulation profile should therefore be obtained at the earliest opportunity and fresh frozen plasma (FFP) and platelets administered as needed.

## SPLENECTOMY

Most elective splenectomies are performed for hematologic diseases. Conditions in which splenectomy may be beneficial include hemolytic anemias, idiopathic thrombocytopenic purpura, hypersplenism, and leukemias. In Hodgkin's disease, a staging laparotomy is performed, including splenectomy, liver biopsy, and abdominal lymph node sampling.

Patients scheduled for splenectomy, depending on the underlying disease, may have anemia, thrombocytopenia, and other coagulation disorders. Close cooperation with the surgeon and the hematologist is essential to make them ready for surgery. These patients also may have received recent chemotherapy, the implications of which should be recognized.

Removal of a spleen of normal size is usually an uncomplicated procedure. If the spleen is large, particularly in the presence of portal hypertension, intraoperative bleeding may be significant; venous access adequate for rapid volume replacement and transfusion is required.

### When Should Platelet Transfusion Occur?

Patients presenting for splenectomy may be extremely thrombocytopenic. Thus, a preoperative platelet transfusion would seem advantageous. However, because the spleen is normally the cause of thrombocytopenia, platelet administration before ligation of the splenic artery is futile. If the platelet count is <20 000/mm³, or bleeding is thought to be related to a platelet deficiency, infusion of platelets is reasonable after splenic artery ligation. The infused platelets have a clinical effect within minutes of administration and, because the spleen has been removed, have a normal lifespan of approximately 10 days.

## OBSTRUCTIVE JAUNDICE

Patients with obstructive jaundice (cholestasis) present three problems:

1. Vitamin K malabsorption leads to coagulopathy with an increased prothrombin time secondary to a deficit of vitamin K-dependent clotting factors. Patients with obstructive jaundice are routinely treated for 2 to 3 days before surgery with intramuscular vitamin K to normalize the prothrombin time. FFP should be used only in those patients who do not respond to vitamin K treatment.
2. Cholestasis modifies the pharmacokinetics of pancuronium, vecuronium, and probably rocuronium because the latter drug is eliminated predominantly by the liver and excreted unmodified in the bile.[26] Atracurium and cisatracurium, because of their peculiar metabolism, are popular muscle relaxants in these patients.
3. Patients with obstructive jaundice are at increased risk of postoperative renal failure. Acute renal failure occurs in 5% to 10% of patients undergoing surgery for relief of obstructive jaundice and is associated with a 75% mortality rate.[118,119]

### Why Does Renal Failure Occur?

A number of studies have examined the effects of jaundice on renal function.[120,121] Overall, renal function and renal blood flow do not seem significantly altered by obstructive jaundice, per se. The mechanisms leading to kidney failure after surgery for obstructive jaundice remain uncertain. A decrease in the ECF volume,[122] increased sensitivity of the kidneys to an ischemic insult,[123] and endotoxemia[118] have been suggested.

### How Is Postoperative Renal Failure Prevented/Improved?

Anesthetic management of patients with jaundice requires liberal preoperative and intraoperative fluid administration,[123,124] guided preferably by assessment of urinary output and CVP. Hypotension should be avoided to prevent kidney hypoperfusion. Jaundiced patients seem to be unusually sensitive to a blood volume deficit. A moderate blood loss, usually well tolerated by normal subjects, may be followed in these patients by an exaggerated fall in blood pressure.[118] Accordingly, any blood loss needs to be carefully replaced, and early use of colloids and blood is recommended.

Mannitol administration has long been recommended to prevent renal failure in jaundiced patients.[125] One study, however, did not show any effect of this agent with respect to an increase in creatinine clearance or decrease in the incidence of postoperative renal failure.[126] Mannitol perhaps should be reserved for those patients in whom urine output is inadequate despite normal blood pressure and normal or slightly increased heart filling pressures. Should mannitol fail to improve urine output, dopamine, or fenoldopam in small doses are reason-

able choices, although no data are available to prove that such therapy is of any benefit in jaundiced patients.

## HEPATIC RESECTION

Indications for hepatic resection include primary or metastatic carcinoma of the liver and a variety of benign lesions (eg, cysts, granulomas, vascular malformations).

### What Factors Determine Surgical Risk?

Preoperative liver function has a fundamental role in determining the risk of this type of surgery, the outcome of which largely depends on the ability of the residual liver to undergo compensatory regeneration. Up to 75% of a normal liver can be resected safely without postoperative liver failure. After a resection of this magnitude, the residual liver regenerates fairly rapidly to reach approximately 75% of the preoperative size within 1 year.[127]

Patients with concomitant chronic liver disease are usually considered poor candidates for major liver resection because of increased risk of postoperative liver failure. This is of considerable practical relevance because approximately 40% of patients with primary malignancy of the liver have cirrhosis or chronic hepatitis. Data indicate, however, that selected patients with underlying chronic liver disease can undergo a major liver resection with an acceptable mortality rate. Criteria for selection include good hepatic functional reserve—as suggested by serum bilirubin <2 mg/dL, prothrombin time <4 seconds above normal, serum albumin >3 g/dL—and no clinical evidence of portal hypertension (ie, ascites, splenomegaly, and varices). The measurement of the clearance of indocyanine green has also been reported to be of some use in determining patient tolerance of major liver resection.[128–130]

### What Are the Common Liver Resections?

From a surgical standpoint, the liver is divided into two parts: a right and left liver, each with its own portal and arterial vascular supply and biliary drainage. The demarcation line between the two livers, called the *main portal scissura,* runs on the surface of the liver from the medial margin of the gallbladder anteriorly to the vena cava posteriorly. There is no external visible mark that permits the identification of the two livers, but the division becomes apparent if the blood supply to one liver is interrupted: the ischemic liver darkens, thus creating a clear demarcation between the two sides. The right and left livers are further divided into four segments each. The right liver comprises segments V to VIII and the left liver segments I to IV (Fig. 61–7). Segment I is the caudate lobe. A major resection involves the removal of three or more segments. Removal of one or two segments is called *segmentectomy.*

There are four common types of major liver resections (because there are two nomenclatures used to identify liver resections, both are reported here): (1) right hepatectomy, that is, removal of segments V, VI, VII, and VIII (alternative: right hepatic lobectomy); (2) left hepatectomy, that is, removal of segments I, II, III, and IV (left hepatic lobectomy); (3) right lobectomy, that is, removal of segments IV, V, VI, VII, and

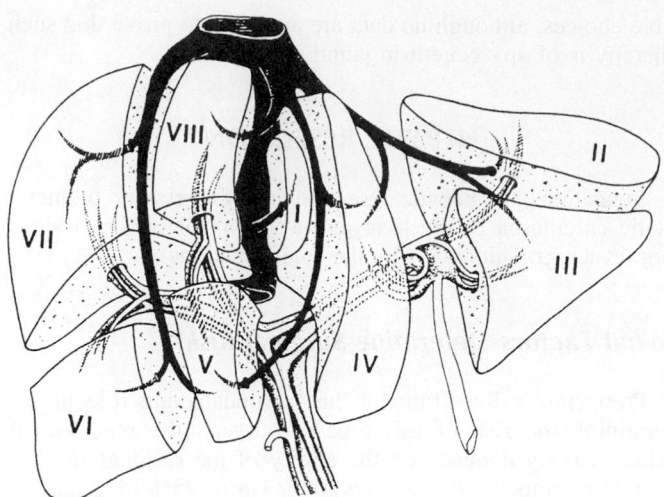

**FIGURE 61–7.** View of the segments of the liver. The right liver includes segments V to VIII. The left liver includes segments I to IV. Each segment is independent with regard to the portal and arterial vascularization and biliary drainage. (From Bismuth H. Surgical anatomy and anatomical surgery of the liver. *World J Surg.* 1982;6:3.)

VIII (extended right hepatic lobectomy); and (4) left lobectomy, that is, removal of segments I, II, and III (left lateral segmentectomy; Fig. 61–8).

## What Are the Technical Steps of a Liver Resection?

A liver resection essentially consists of three steps: control of the afferent vessels (portal and arterial), parenchymal transection, and control of the efferent vessels (hepatic veins). How vascular control is obtained and the sequence of these

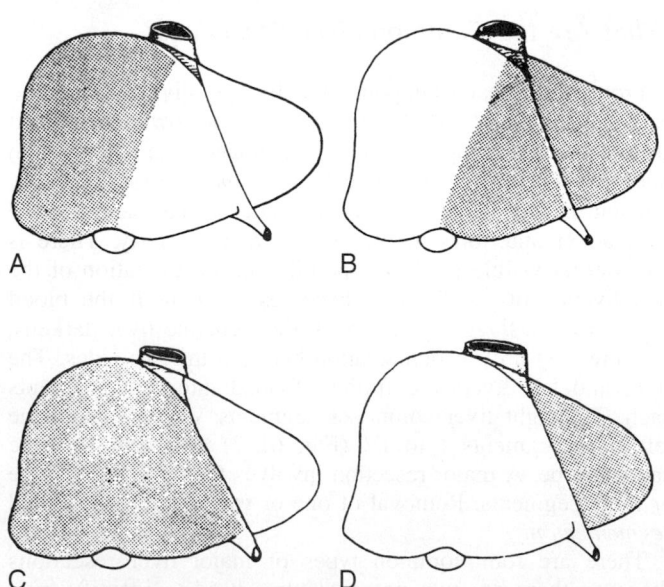

**FIGURE 61–8.** The four common major liver resections. The shaded areas represent the part of liver to be resected. *A and B,* Right and left hepatectomy. The line of transection is the main portal scissura. *C and D,* Right and left lobectomy. The line of transection is the umbilical scissura. (From Bismuth H. Surgical anatomy and anatomical surgery of the liver. *World J Surg.* 1982;6:3.)

steps may vary considerably depending on several factors, not the least of which is the surgeon's personal preference. It is, therefore, advisable for the anesthesiologist to discuss the planned technique with the surgeon before surgery.

In general, control of the afferent vessels relevant to the area to be resected is obtained first. These vessels are divided usually just outside of the liver substance at the hilus. The parenchyma is then transected along the line of demarcation that separates the devascularized liver from the perfused one. The efferent hepatic veins are ligated and divided from within the liver substance as the parenchymal transection progresses toward the vena cava. Eventually the main hepatic vein draining the area to be resected is divided and the specimen removed. Alternatively, extrahepatic control of the hepatic veins is obtained before starting parenchymal dissection.

After mobilization of the right or left side of the liver, depending on the type of resection, an extensive dissection is performed along the retrohepatic vena cava until the confluence of the hepatic vein of interest and the vena cava is reached. Once the hepatic vein is isolated, it may either be temporarily occluded by using a tourniquet and divided at the end of parenchymal transection or immediately divided and the parenchyma transected.

During parenchymal transection, significant portal and arterial bleeding may occur from the perfused side of the liver. An effective way of controlling this bleeding is temporarily to clamp the main portal vein and hepatic artery, thus interrupting the blood flow to the whole liver (total inflow occlusion). This maneuver is called *portal triad clamping (PTC),* or the *Pringle maneuver* after the surgeon who first described it.[131]

## What Are the Hemodynamic Consequences of Portal Triad Clamping?

PTC is followed by modest hemodynamic changes. Heart filling pressures and cardiac output decrease by 10% to 20%, while arterial blood pressure remains at, or may slightly increase above, preclamping levels because of an increase in systemic vascular resistance (SVR).[132] Clamping of the portal vein is well tolerated, probably because of effective portosystemic shunts through which the splanchnic blood can return to the caval system.

Hemodynamic changes during PTC usually do not require treatment and the small decrease in CVP that is often observed during PTC may actually be beneficial in decreasing backbleeding from the hepatic veins (see following section). Unclamping of the portal triad is followed by a decrease in blood pressure that may persist several minutes, particularly when clamping time was protracted.

## Is a Low Central Venous Pressure Useful During Hepatic Resections?

Low CVP may reduce blood loss during parenchymal transection and facilitate the surgeon's work during the dissection of the vena cava and hepatic veins. During parenchymal transection, even when total inflow occlusion is used, significant hepatic venous back-bleeding may occur. Low pressure in the hepatic veins minimizes back-bleeding and makes control of intraparenchymal hepatic venous bleeding easier.[133-135]

Dissection of the vena cava or hepatic veins is easier in the presence of low venous pressure because the walls of these veins are lax. Also, should a venous injury occur, low pressure in the vessel allows easier control of the bleeding. Although a CVP <6 mm Hg has been advocated, an alternative approach consists in a judicious fluid administration titrated to maintain the CVP close to the value measured at the beginning of surgery. If during the procedure the surgeon finds the veins too distended or the back-bleeding excessive, the CVP can be easily decreased with an infusion of nitroglycerin. The low CVP is then maintained until the specimen is removed and hemostasis is completed. Thereafter, fluids can be liberally administered to correct any volume deficit. The disadvantage of a low CVP is a potentially increased risk of venous air embolism (see next section) but, in practice, this has not been found to be the case.[133]

## What Is Hepatic Total Vascular Exclusion and When Is It Used?

Hepatic total vascular exclusion (TVE) combines portal triad clamping (total inflow occlusion) with the clamping of the infrahepatic and suprahepatic vena cava (total outflow occlusion). TVE is used to resect large, centrally located tumors, and tumors close to the hepatic veins or infiltrating the vena cava. The major risk associated with the resection of such tumors is laceration of the vena cava or hepatic veins, resulting in massive hemorrhage and possibly air embolism. Vascular inflow occlusion alone does not prevent bleeding either from the vena cava or the hepatic veins, or air embolism. Addition of infrahepatic and suprahepatic vena caval clamping allows total vascular exclusion of the liver, thereby obviating these risks and providing a virtually bloodless field.

Once TVE is established, the liver is transected and the major vascular structures are secured from within the parenchyma with minimal blood loss. Most of the bleeding occurs from the raw surface of the remaining liver when the clamps are released and blood flow is restored to vessels that were transected while the liver was ischemic.

## What Are the Hemodynamic Consequences of Total Vascular Exclusion?

When clamps are sequentially applied to the portal triad and the infrahepatic and suprahepatic vena cava, the sudden decrease in venous return causes a 40% to 60% drop in cardiac output and a 20% decrease in pulmonary artery diastolic and wedge pressures. The decrease in cardiac output is due to a decrease in stroke volume. Heart rate is usually increased. Arterial pressure may be unchanged or decreased depending on the ability of the patient to increase SVR to compensate for the decreased cardiac output.[136] These changes are partially prevented by fluid loading to a target CVP of 12 to 15 mm Hg or pulmonary artery diastolic pressure of 15 to 17 mm Hg before clamping.[137] Occasionally, vasopressors are needed in addition to fluids to maintain an adequate blood pressure. Caval clamping causes renal venous congestion, which may be detrimental to the kidney. To prevent renal damage, some recommend an infusion of low-dose dopamine and the administration of mannitol before caval clamping.

It is common practice to perform a trial clamping lasting 3 to 5 minutes to determine if the patient tolerates the maneuver. Sometimes, an improvement in blood pressure and cardiac output occurs after a few minutes of clamping. It is unusual for an initially well-tolerated vascular exclusion to become poorly tolerated thereafter.

At the end of the hepatectomy, the caval clamps are released first to reestablish venous return from the lower body and stabilize the hemodynamics before the liver is reperfused. On clamp release, blood pressure and cardiac output increase to preclamp values, heart rate decreases, and a brief period of pulmonary hypertension lasting 5 to 10 minutes is common.[137] Also common is a mixed (respiratory and metabolic) acidosis, which does not require treatment and disappears over 30 minutes.

In spite of optimal treatment, 10% to 15% of patients do not tolerate vascular exclusion because of unacceptable low blood pressure or cardiac output. One option is clamping the aorta above the celiac artery before the inferior vena cava clamps are applied. Clamping of the aorta allows adequate blood pressure during TVE,[136,138] but has the disadvantage of causing renal and spinal cord ischemia with possible renal failure and paraplegia. Another option is to use a TVE technique whereby total outflow occlusion is obtained by clamping the major hepatic veins but not the vena cava.[139,140] This technique preserves the caval blood flow, and its hemodynamic effects are limited to those caused by portal triad clamping.[141]

## What Are the Potential Hazards of Hepatic Vascular Inflow Occlusion?

Whereas hepatic inflow occlusion used on its own or as part of a TVE technique is very effective in decreasing bleeding, it may cause ischemic damage to the remnant liver, and postoperative liver failure is thus a major concern.[142] A normal liver can tolerate a warm ischemia time of 1 hour; there is evidence that this time may be extended to 90 minutes.[143,144] A cirrhotic or otherwise diseased liver does not tolerate ischemia as well. The safe period of ischemia for an abnormal liver is not well established, but ischemic time should be kept to <1 hour.[145]

To avoid the risk of ischemia associated with uninterrupted clamping of the portal triad maintained for the 30 to 45 minutes necessary to complete the liver transection, intermittent clamping has been advocated (clamping periods of 15-20 minutes followed by 5 minutes of reperfusion). Intermittent clamping may allow cumulative ischemic times of 2 hours and seems particularly beneficial when the liver is cirrhotic.[146-148] A minor drawback to intermittent clamping is bleeding from the transected surface when the clamp is released. When TVE is used, the hemodynamic changes caused by clamping and unclamping of the vena cava make intermittent clamping impossible. However, during TVE with selective occlusion of the hepatic veins and preservation of caval flow, intermittent clamping has been successfully used.[141]

## What Is the Anesthetic Management?

The main problem encountered during surgery is blood loss. Large-bore venous catheters and arterial and central venous catheters for pressure monitoring are therefore recommended, as well as the use of devices that allow the rapid infusion of warm fluids or blood. Pulmonary artery catheters, at least in patients with good heart function, are not particularly useful during routine hepatic resections but may be helpful when a TVE technique is used with inferior vena caval clamping.

General anesthesia with low-dose isoflurane combined with an opioid is a popular technique because it preserves liver blood flow. However, the extent of hepatic resection, blood loss, and associated periods of hemodynamic instability, as well as damage to the residual liver during vascular occlusion are far more important than any anesthetic agent in determining postoperative hepatic function. The use of nitrous oxide, which, per se, does not impair liver function,[149] is optional; some prefer to avoid it because of the slight risk of air embolism during surgery.

Should a large blood loss occur requiring volume resuscitation and blood or blood product administration, three points are relevant: first, patients undergoing live resection tolerate well hematocrit values of 30%. Such moderate hemodilution has no adverse effects on postoperative liver function, even in the presence of chronic liver disease.[150,151] Second, various factors such as reduction in liver parenchyma, underlying liver disease, and temporary liver ischemia may impair citrate metabolism. As a consequence, citrate toxicity and hypocalcemia may occur after rapid administration of blood and FFP. Treatment with calcium chloride, preferably guided by measurements of serum ionized calcium, may be needed. Third, after surgery there is temporary impairment of liver function. As a consequence, prothrombin time invariably increases by an average of 4 seconds above normal, and levels of coagulation factors V and II decrease by approximately 50%. These changes are maximal on the first postoperative day and normalize in approximately 1 week. Serum albumin concentration is also markedly decreased and slowly rises toward normal in 2 to 3 weeks.[152,153] Accordingly, 5% albumin and FFP may be preferred over crystalloids for volume replacement in these patients, considering that albumin and clotting factors lost during surgery are not replaced by the liver as promptly as usual. FFP is usually administered when the prothrombin time is >2 seconds above normal.

Venous air embolism is a well-recognized intraoperative hazard associated with operations on the liver. It may occur during transection of the liver parenchyma or other surgical maneuvers involving the main hepatic veins or the vena cava. Occlusion of the portal vein and hepatic artery during liver resection does not prevent air embolism, which occurs through open hepatic veins. When total vascular occlusion is used, and the suprahepatic vena cava or the main hepatic veins are clamped, air embolism is prevented during the resection phase but may occur when venous outflow is reestablished and air trapped in the veins is mobilized. Placing the patient in a head-down position seems to prevent (counterintuitively) venous air embolism. In a series of approximately 500 liver resections performed using a head-down tilt, the incidence of clinically significant air embolism was 0.4%.[133]

## PATIENTS WITH ASCITES

Patients with ascites who require intraabdominal surgery pose several problems. When the ascites is large, impairment of ventilation mandates tracheal intubation followed by me-

chanical ventilation. Ventilatory encroachment is sometimes so great that patients do not tolerate the supine position even for a short time, making induction of anesthesia problematic. This problem can be prevented by performing paracentesis before surgery to remove enough fluid to allow patients to assume the supine position.

Another way to overcome the problem is to position patients on the operating table in a semisitting position as tolerated, preoxygenate, administer the intravenous induction agent, and then rapidly change the operating table position to allow mask ventilation and intubation. A rapid-sequence induction is advisable because of the increased intragastric pressure. Because of the distended abdomen, a rapid fall in $O_2$ saturation can occur during induction using a conventional rapid-sequence technique. A modified technique in which mask ventilation is used before intubation may therefore be considered.

### What Happens When Ascitic Fluid Is Acutely Drained?

When the procedure requires a laparotomy, ascites is removed at the beginning of surgery through a small skin incision. Studies have investigated the immediate and delayed hemodynamic effects of removal of large volumes (5 L) of ascitic fluid.[154] Most of the data have been obtained in patients with cirrhosis, but they apply equally to patients with malignancy-induced ascites.[155]

Ascitic fluid drainage is followed by an increase in cardiac output, mainly because of an increase in stroke volume, but the arterial blood pressure does not change because the SVR decreases[156] (Fig. 61–9). The CVP and PAOP are unchanged or slightly decreased.[154–156] Renal function and urinary output remain unchanged or may improve[154,156,157] (Fig. 61–10). The circulatory blood volume is unchanged immediately and up to 48 hours after paracentesis.[158,159]

These results indicate that a large peritoneal effusion and the concomitant increase in intraperitoneal pressure are detrimental because they compress the inferior vena cava and possibly the portal vein, thereby decreasing venous return to the heart. The decrease in cardiac output elicits a compensatory SVR increase to maintain normal blood pressure.

The data do not lend support to a commonly held belief that the removal of ascitic fluid is hazardous because of sudden hypotension or cardiovascular collapse. The sporadic reports of these untoward hemodynamic events date back to more than 30 years, when paracentesis was performed with patients in the sitting position. The very infrequent episodes of collapse observed during paracentesis likely were syncopal (vasovagal) episodes.[154]

Despite the absence of hemodynamic compromise after paracentesis, some evidence suggests that patients with advanced liver disease may occasionally experience a delayed deterioration of kidney function with oliguria and avid sodium retention. The renal dysfunction that may follow paracentesis in cirrhotic patients can be adequately prevented by administration of albumin or synthetic colloids such as dextran 70 and hetastarch, in a dose of 8 g/L of ascitic fluid removed.[157,160] It seems, therefore, prudent to administer an appropriate dose of 25% albumin or synthetic colloid to patients with a large ascites removed at the beginning of surgery.

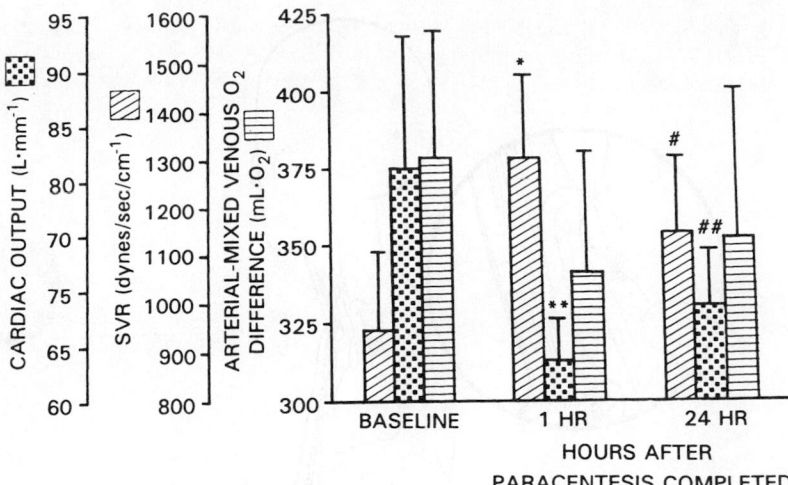

**FIGURE 61–9.** Changes in cardiac output, systemic vascular resistance (SVR), and the difference in arterial-mixed venous oxygen content observed 1 hour and 24 hours after large-volume paracentesis (range, 4-15 L) in patients (n = 10) with cirrhotic ascites. (From Simon DM, McCain JR, Bonkovsky HL, et al. Effects of therapeutic paracentesis on systemic and hepatic hemodynamics and on renal and hormonal function. *Hepatology.* 1987;7:423.)

## PERITONEOVENOUS SHUNTING

Peritoneovenous (PV) shunting is rarely used, the main indication being treatment of refractory ascites secondary to cirrhosis or malignancy.

### *How Is It Performed?*

The most common PV shunt in use today was developed by Le Veen and associates.[161] This shunt consists of one limb

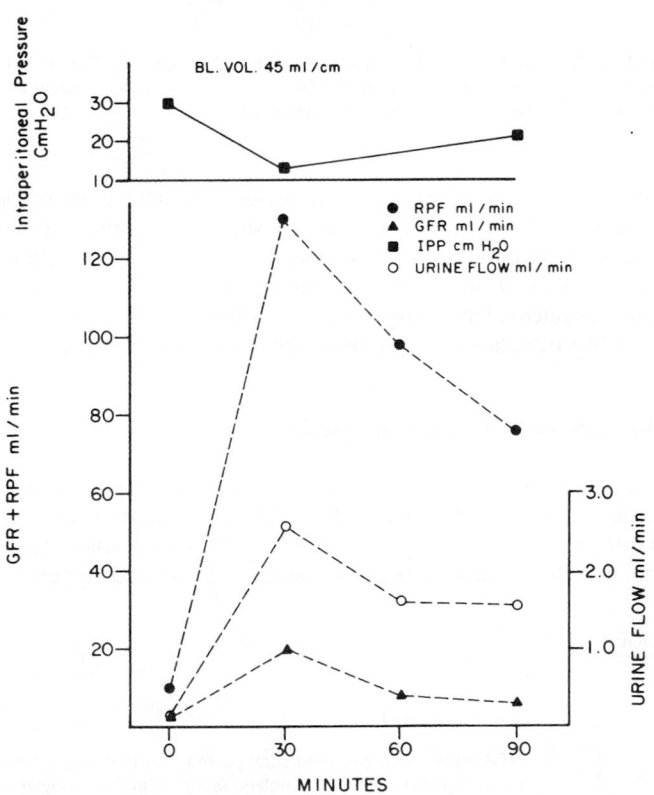

**FIGURE 61–10.** Change in intraperitoneal pressure, renal plasma flow (RPF), glomerular filtration rate (GFR), and urine flow in a representative patient with cirrhosis after a 2000-mL paracentesis. The deterioration in RPF and urine flow at 90 minutes is probably secondary to the reduction in circulatory volume caused by the continuous formation of ascitic fluid. (From Cade R, Wagemaker H, Vogel S, et al. Hepatorenal syndrome: studies of the effect of vascular volume and intraperitoneal pressure on renal and hepatic function. *Am J Med.* 1987;82:427.)

that is inserted through a small abdominal incision to lie free in the peritoneal cavity. The peritoneal limb is connected to a one-way valve placed extraperitoneally but underneath the abdominal wall muscles. A long tunneling instrument is used to pass the venous limb subcutaneously from the abdominal wound to the neck, where it is inserted into the internal jugular vein and positioned at the junction of superior vena cava and right atrium (Fig. 61–11). The one-way valve opens when a pressure gradient >3 cm $H_2O$ is established between the peritoneal cavity and the venous system; ascitic fluid then flows into the systemic circulation. Effective decompression of the peritoneal cavity is obtained without the ensuing vascular volume depletion that often complicates paracentesis.

### *How Should Anesthesia Be Administered?*

Patients undergoing PV shunt placement, besides having large ascites, are often in poor physical condition because of the underlying neoplastic or liver disease and are sometimes in kidney failure. The procedure can be performed under local anesthesia with sedation[161] or under general anesthesia. If the latter technique is chosen, rapid-sequence induction and tracheal intubation are mandatory, followed by mechanical ventilation. The ascitic fluid is drained at the beginning of the procedure so that patients can breathe more easily after surgery.

### *What Complications Follow Peritoneovenous Shunting?*

The placement of a PV shunt is followed by a wide array of complications. Serious, albeit rare, complications occurring perioperatively include pneumothorax due to damage to the pleura when the tunneling instrument is pushed subcutaneously up the chest wall, trauma to the recurrent laryngeal nerve, air embolism, pulmonary edema, and disseminated intravascular coagulation.[162] The latter is ascribed to substances present in the ascitic fluid that interfere with coagulation when they are infused into the systemic circulation. The precise triggering mechanisms, however, are unknown.

Postshunt coagulopathy can be effectively prevented by removing the ascites during surgery. Replacement of discarded

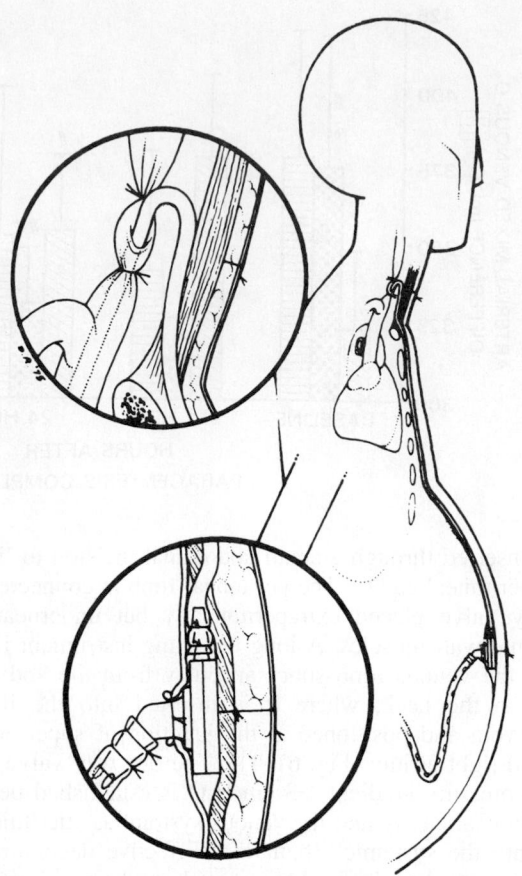

**FIGURE 61–11.** Schematic drawing of the LeVeen shunt after placement. Ascites is drained into the internal jugular vein through the intraperitoneal tubing. The one-way valve lies extraperitoneally and deep to the abdominal muscles *(lower enlarged view)*. The venous collecting tube traverses the subcutaneous tissue of the chest wall into the neck, where it enters the internal jugular vein *(upper enlarged view)*. (From LeVeen HH, Wapnick S, Grosberg S, et al. Further experience with peritoneo-venous shunt for ascites. *Ann Surg.* 1976;184:574.)

ascitic fluid with normal saline infused into the peritoneal cavity before opening the shunt has been advocated to decrease further the incidence and severity of coagulopathy[163] (Fig. 61–12). Treatment of the coagulopathy includes FFP, platelets, and possibly antifibrinolytic agents (eg, aminocaproic or tranexamic acid).[162]

## PORTOSYSTEMIC SHUNTS

Portosystemic shunts are usually performed to decompress the portal system in cirrhotic patients with bleeding esopha-

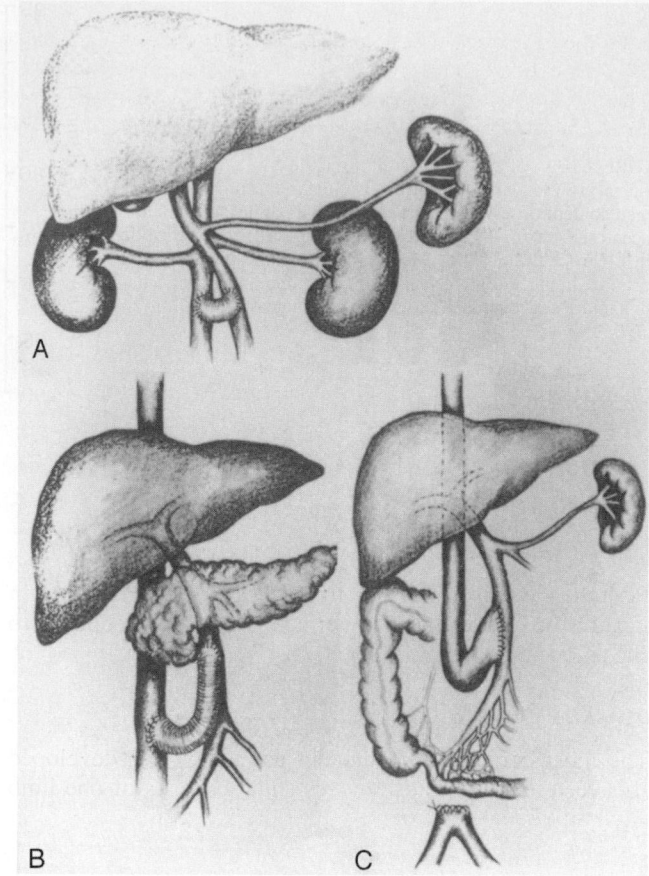

**FIGURE 61–13.** Portacaval shunts. *A*, End-to-side shunt. *B*, Side-to-side shunt. *C*, H-graft. (From Terblanche J. The surgeon's role in the management of portal hypertension. *Ann Surg.* 1989;209:381.)

geal varices caused by portal hypertension. The number of these procedures has decreased significantly because of the success in treating variceal bleeding by transesophageal sclerotherapy, a much less invasive and costly technique.[164] Emergency portacaval shunting, which is complicated by very high mortality rate, has in many institutions become obsolete.

### *What Shunts Are Performed?*

Several variants of portosystemic shunts have been described (Figs. 61–13 to 61–15). The most common are the end-to-side or side-to-side portacaval and distal splenorenal shunts. Often, patients requiring surgery for portal hyperten-

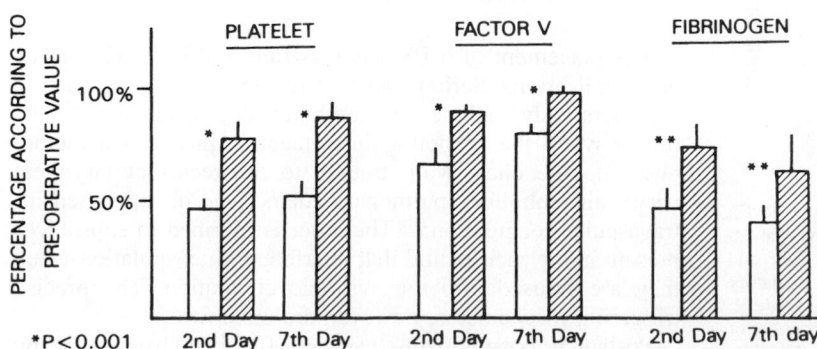

**FIGURE 61–12.** Mean percentage and standard error of the mean of the decrease of platelets, factor V, and fibrinogen in patients of group 1 (without replacement of ascitic fluids; *open bars*) and of group 2 (with replacement of ascitic fluids with normal saline solution; *shaded bars*) on the second and seventh postoperative days.

sion are potential candidates for liver transplantation. Interest in mesocaval and other shunts that interfere the least anatomically with a subsequent liver transplant is therefore growing.

The hemodynamic effects of portosystemic shunts have been studied extensively, particularly in reference to liver blood flow.[165,166] Of practical importance is that usually minimum systemic hemodynamic changes are observed intraoperatively when a newly fashioned portacaval shunt is opened. In general, the type of shunt chosen by the surgeon is irrelevant to the anesthetic management.

## What Factors Predict Postoperative Outcome?

Surgical outcome largely depends on preoperative liver function. The risk assessment for cirrhotic patients undergoing

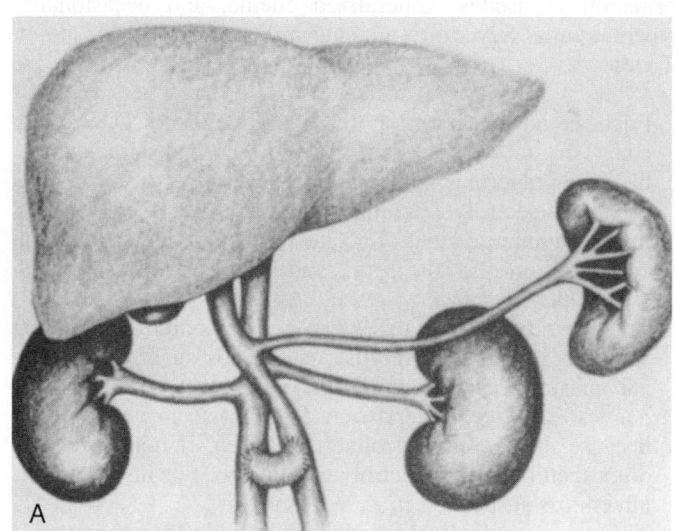

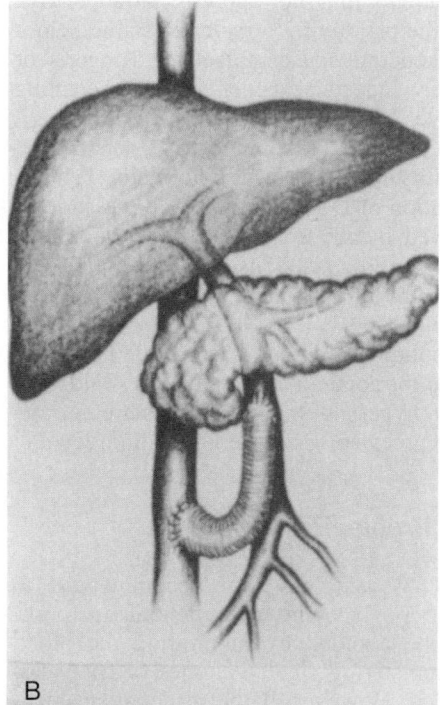

**FIGURE 61–14.** Mesocaval shunts. *A,* H-graft. *B,* C-graft. (From Terblanche J. The surgeon's role in the management of portal hypertension. *Ann Surg.* 1989;209:381.)

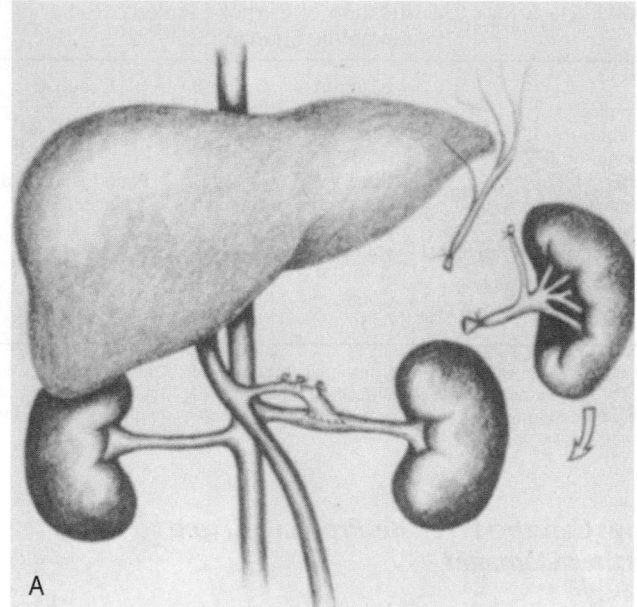

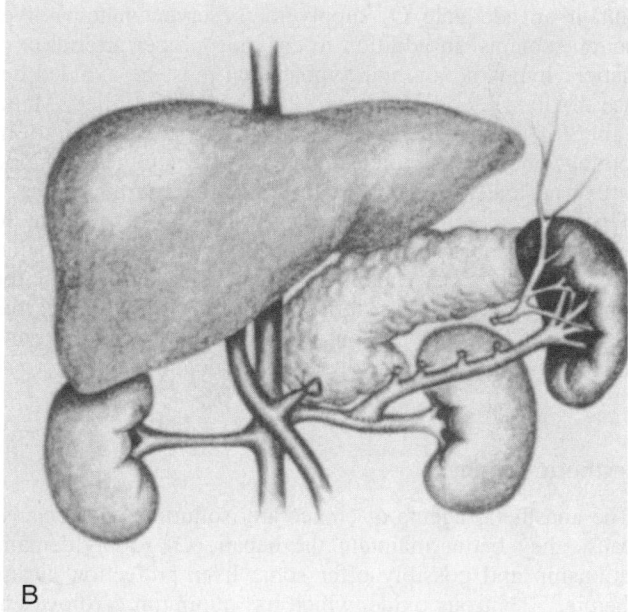

**FIGURE 61–15.** Splenorenal shunts. *A,* Central splenorenal shunt. *B,* Selective distal splenorenal shunt. (From Terblanche J. The surgeon's role in the management of portal hypertension. *Ann Surg.* 1989;209:381.)

portosystemic shunts is usually based on a slightly revised version of Child's classification[167,168] (Table 61–2). Patients in group A with good liver function usually fare well, whereas patients in groups B and C with poor liver function have a grimmer outcome.

## Can the Usual Drugs Be Used?

Hepatic cirrhosis significantly affects the pharmacodynamics and pharmacokinetics of a large number of drugs. In practice, however, any commonly used anesthetic drug can safely be used in these patients, provided it is titrated to the desired effect. The use of relaxants in patients with liver disease was discussed previously.

**TABLE 61–2.** Risk Classification of Cirrhotic Patients Requiring Portosystemic Shunting

| | Group A | Group B | Group C |
|---|---|---|---|
| Bilirubin (mg/dL) | <2.0 | 2.0–3.0 | >3 |
| Albumin (g/dL) | >3.5 | 3.0–3.5 | <3 |
| Ascites | None | Controlled | Poorly controlled |
| Encephalopathy | None | Minimum | Advanced |
| Nutrition | Excellent | Good | Poor |
| Prothrombin time (seconds above control) | <4 | 4–6 | >6 |
| Surgical risk | Good (<5%) | Moderate (10%) | Poor (50%) |

Data from Child CG. Major problems in clinical surgery. In: Child CG, Coon WW, eds. *The Liver and Portal Hypertension.* Philadelphia, Pa: WB Saunders; 1964:50; and Pugh RNH, Murray-Lyon IM, Dawson JL, et al. Transection of the esophagus for bleeding varices. *Br J Surg.* 1973;60:646.

## How Can the Liver Be Protected From Further Damage?

A specific goal during anesthesia in cirrhotic patients is to maintain an adequate $O_2$ supply to preserve whatever liver function remains. In addition to ensuring proper arterial oxygenation, hypovolemia and hypotension must be avoided because the liver blood supply will be severely curtailed. Maintenance of a normal circulatory volume is of paramount importance because hypotension results after a moderate blood loss that normally would not cause blood pressure changes.

This poor tolerance to hypovolemia probably is due to impaired vasoconstriction in response to sympathetic stimulation,[169] as well as an inability to mobilize blood from the splanchnic pool into the systemic circulation.[170] Arterial partial pressure of $CO_2$ ($Paco_2$) should be maintained within normal limits because liver blood flow is best maintained with normocarbia.[7]

### Anesthetic Choice

The anesthetic agents of choice are isoflurane and fentanyl because they better maintain the hepatic $O_2$ supply-demand relationship and possibly offer some liver protection during ischemia.[11,12] Nitrous oxide, which has minimum cardiovascular depressant effects, is a useful addition because patients with cirrhosis are prone to hypotension and often do not tolerate isoflurane except at very low concentrations that may be inadequate to provide unconsciousness.

### Monitoring

The main intraoperative problem is hemorrhage due to venous congestion of the splanchnic area. The risk of profuse bleeding, combined with the need for maintaining the blood pressure and blood volume as close to normal as possible, mandates adequate venous access and placement of an arterial catheter for continuous pressure monitoring.

Whether a central venous or pulmonary artery catheter should be placed is controversial. My preference is to use a pulmonary artery catheter in patients in Child groups B and C based on the assumption that aggressive hemodynamic management may help to preserve liver and kidney function and improve outcome.

If a pulmonary artery catheter is used and cardiac output is measured, cirrhotic patients often have a hyperdynamic circulation characterized by high cardiac output, low-normal systemic blood pressure, low SVR, and a narrow arteriovenous $O_2$ content difference because of a high mixed venous $O_2$ saturation. This hemodynamic pattern is characteristic of cirrhosis and does not require intervention.

## What Are the Requirements for Fluid Management?

Intraoperative fluid management of cirrhotic patients is also somewhat controversial. Solutions of 5% dextrose in water ($D_5W$) are sometimes recommended instead of sodium-containing solutions based on the premise that these patients retain sodium and that the sodium retention is responsible for formation of ascites, generalized edema, and occasionally hypernatremia. Several arguments militate against this point of view:

1. First, the advocates of the intraoperative use of $D_5W$ often equate crystalloid solutions with 0.9% normal saline, which has a supranormal sodium concentration of 156 mEq/L. Balanced electrolyte solutions currently used have a much lower sodium content. Lactated Ringer's has a sodium concentration of 130 mEq/L, and its use is not associated with hypernatremia.
2. Those who argue against the use of sodium-containing solutions recommend the use of colloids such as albumin and plasma to maintain adequate intraoperative hemodynamics. This recommendation does not seem very logical because these colloids contain as much, if not more, sodium than balanced electrolyte solutions. For instance, 5% albumin is suspended in normal saline.
3. Therapeutic considerations that are valid in long-term treatment of cirrhotic patients may not apply to intraoperative management when the priority is to maintain stable hemodynamics. The intraoperative use of lactated Ringer's or similar solutions may indeed be beneficial by preventing hypovolemia and liver hypoperfusion.
4. Cirrhotic patients are particularly prone to hyponatremia, owing to their inability to excrete water normally.[171] Intraoperative administration of $D_5W$ solutions to these patients may thus be followed by severe hyponatremia. A serum sodium level <130 mEq/L is considered an important cause of encephalopathy in cirrhotic patients.[172]

In my opinion, a solution to this controversy is to use lactated Ringer's as the intraoperative maintenance fluid. The solution causes neither hypernatremia nor hyponatremia and may partially correct a preexisting low serum sodium level.

## Is Hypoglycemia a Problem?

Administration of $D_5W$ also has been recommended to prevent intraoperative hypoglycemia. This phenomenon probably is rare and can be avoided by monitoring the blood glucose level and administering small volumes of 25% glucose solutions as needed. However, if the reader is not convinced by the position presented and chooses to infuse $D_5W$, it is necessary to monitor the serum sodium concentration closely. Should the sodium level decrease to 130 mEq/dL, the

$D_5W$ is discontinued and replaced with lactated Ringer's solution.

### How Is Oliguria Managed?

Urinary output should be monitored and maintained at $>0.5$ mL/kg/h. Oliguria is best prevented by careful replacement of intraoperative losses. Poor urinary output is primarily due to inadequate volume replacement and needs to be treated as such.

Oliguria occasionally persists despite normal cardiac output and filling pressures. The approach to this condition consists in further expanding the circulatory volume, preferably with albumin or FFP,[154] until a CVP or PAOP of 18 to 20 mm Hg is reached. Oliguria refractory to volume expansion is very difficult to reverse. Low-dose dopamine, or fenoldopam, as well as diuretics such as furosemide and mannitol, may be tried, but the results are often disappointing.

### Why Does Coagulopathy Occur?

Surgical bleeding may be compounded by coagulopathy associated with the underlying liver disease and the dilutional coagulopathy that follows resuscitation for large blood losses. During surgery, repeated assessments of the prothrombin time and platelet count may be needed to guide replacement therapy. After surgery, these patients should be admitted to an intensive care unit because of significant continued fluid translocation and complications of bleeding, liver failure, encephalopathy, and kidney failure.

## EFFECTS OF ABDOMINAL SURGERY ON PULMONARY FUNCTION

Pulmonary dysfunction is invariably present after laparotomy. The primary changes occur in lung mechanics, which in turn are responsible for impaired gas exchange.

### What Abnormalities Occur?

Pulmonary abnormalities are characterized by a restrictive pattern, with a decrease in forced vital capacity (FVC) and FRC.[173,174] The forced expired volume in 1 second ($FEV_1$) is also decreased, but the ratio of $FEV_1$ to FVC remains at preoperative values.[175]

The magnitude and duration of the postoperative lung abnormality depend on the site of surgical incision. The closer the incision to the diaphragm, the greater and more prolonged the reduction in postoperative lung volumes. After upper abdominal surgery, the FVC may decrease by $\geq50\%$ and the FRC by 20% to 25% (Fig. 61–16). The largest lung volume changes occur on the first postoperative day. Thereafter, they begin to recover, with a gradual return to normal by the seventh postoperative day. The changes in FVC and FRC observed after lower abdominal surgery are smaller and resolve more rapidly (Fig. 61–17). Whether lung function is better preserved after laparotomies performed with a transverse rather than vertical incision remains controversial.[176–178]

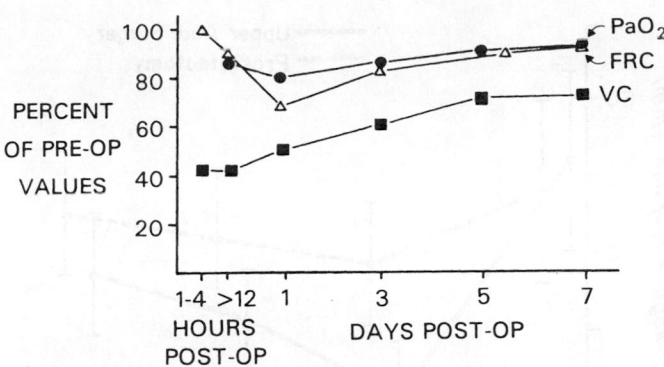

**FIGURE 61–16.** Postoperative vital capacity (VC), functional residual capacity (FRC), and partial pressure of arterial oxygen ($PaO_2$ while breathing room air) as percentages of preoperative values after upper abdominal surgery. (From Craig DB. Postoperative recovery of pulmonary function. *Anesth Analg.* 1981;60:46.)

### What Causes the Restrictive Defect?

The restrictive defect after abdominal surgery primarily results from a decreased diaphragmatic activity, best evidenced by the marked decrease in diaphragm excursion during maximum inspiration[179–181] (Fig. 61–18). Abnormal contraction of the abdominal and low intercostal muscles during expiration also plays a role.[182,183] The reduced diaphragm activity is probably secondary to a reflex inhibition of the phrenic nerve output mediated by stimuli originating in the abdominal cavity.

General anesthesia consistently decreases the FRC. However, this effect is transitory, and the FRC rapidly returns to preoperative values shortly after a patient has regained consciousness.[174] Therefore, anesthesia is unlikely to have a role in causing the low FRC that persists for many days after abdominal surgery.

### Does Pain Influence Postoperative Lung Function?

Pain has only a small contributory role in causing postoperative lung dysfunction. Even with complete pain relief obtained by epidural administration of local anesthetics, FVC is only partially restored and FRC is virtually unchanged[184,185]

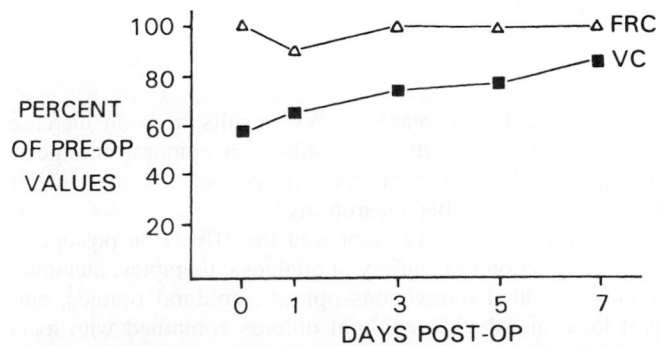

**FIGURE 61–17.** Postoperative vital capacity (VC) and functional residual capacity (FRC) as percentages of preoperative values after lower abdominal surgery. (From Craig DB. Postoperative recovery of pulmonary function. *Anesth Analg.* 1981;60:46.)

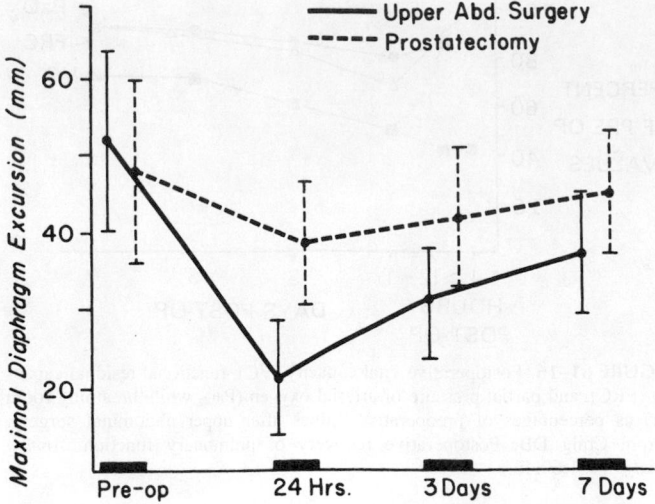

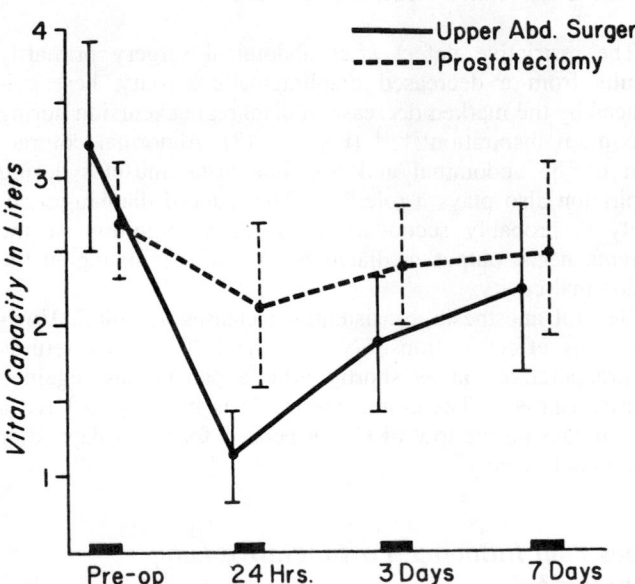

FIGURE 61–18. Mean changes in maximum diaphragmatic excursion (A) and vital capacity (B) after upper or lower (prostatectomy) abdominal surgery. The diaphragmatic excursion measured by fluoroscopy during maximum respiratory efforts was greatly decreased after upper abdominal surgery and correlated well with the decrease in vital capacity. The changes in diaphragmatic excursion and vital capacity were much less important after lower abdominal surgery. (From Tahir AH, George RB, Weil H, et al. Effects of abdominal surgery upon diaphragmatic function and regional ventilation. *Int Surg.* 1973;58:337.)

(Table 61–3). The increase in FVC results from an increase in diaphragmatic activity, suggesting that epidural anesthesia interrupts, at least in part, the afferent stimuli that inhibit diaphragm activity after laparotomy.[186]

Several studies[187] have compared the effects on postoperative lung function of a variety of analgesic therapies, including patient-controlled intravenous opioids, epidural opioids, epidural local anesthetics, epidural opioids combined with local anesthetics, intrapleural local anesthetic, and intercostal nerve block. No technique has been found superior in terms of improvement of postoperative lung volumes.

## What Is the Effect of Laparotomy on Oxygenation?

After abdominal surgery, arterial partial pressure of $O_2$ (Pa$O_2$) is consistently lower than before the operation. The average decrease in Pa$O_2$ is accentuated more after upper than lower abdominal operations (15 and 6 mm Hg, respectively) in patients breathing room air.[188,189] The decrease in Pa$O_2$ is slightly greater in elderly patients.[189] Pa$O_2$ is lowest the first 24 to 48 hours after surgery, then recovers in parallel with the recovery of lung mechanics (see Fig. 61–16). The decrease in Pa$O_2$ is not improved by postoperative pain relief.[190] The defect in arterial oxygenation after abdominal operations is a consequence of reduced FRC and is due to ventilation ($\dot{V}$) and perfusion ($\dot{Q}$) mismatch, with an increase in lung zones with a zero (true shunt) or low $\dot{V}/\dot{Q}$ ratio.[174]

True right-to-left shunt probably is due to the development of small atelectases in the dependent lung regions.[191] Regions with low $\dot{V}/\dot{Q}$ develop when the closing capacity (ie, the lung volume at which airway closure starts to occur) exceeds the FRC, resulting in small airway closure during normal tidal breathing.[173,174] The relative contributions of shunting and low $\dot{V}/\dot{Q}$ to postoperative hypoxemia vary from patient to patient in an unpredictable fashion.

This fact may explain the seemingly paradoxical observation that changing a patient position from supine to sitting in the early postoperative period improves the FRC[192] but does not consistently improve the Pa$O_2$, which in some patients may actually deteriorate.[193-195] It has been postulated that when the main cause of impaired oxygenation is an unfavorable relation of FRC to closing capacity, change in position is followed by an increase in Pa$O_2$ because the FRC becomes larger and the $\dot{V}/\dot{Q}$ mismatch due to airway closure is reduced. Conversely, when the main cause of hypoxemia is a true shunt, the sitting position is associated with a decrease in Pa$O_2$ because of a 10% decrease in cardiac output, which magnifies the effects of shunt on Pa$O_2$.[195]

The deficit in oxygenation that follows abdominal surgery usually is modest and well tolerated; most patients have no need for supplemental $O_2$, apart from perhaps the brief period of recovery from the anesthetic. Patients with low preoperative

**TABLE 61–3.** Lung Dysfunction and Postoperative Pain*

| | Before Surgery (Control) | After Surgery | |
| --- | --- | --- | --- |
| | | Before Epidural Injection | 1 h After Epidural Injection |
| Forced vital capacity (mL) | 3300 ± 208 | 1308‡ ± 115 | 1930‡ ± 144§ |
| Functional residual capacity (mL) | 2500 ± 104 | 2208‡ ± 127 | 2220‡ ± 130 |
| Pa$O_2$ (mm Hg) | 74 ± 3 | 64† ± 3 | 67 ± 2 |
| Pa$CO_2$ (mm Hg) | 39 ± 1 | 39 ± 1 | 38 ± 2 |

Pa$O_2$, partial pressure of arterial oxygen; Pa$CO_2$, partial pressure of arterial carbon dioxide.

*Values are expressed as mean ± standard error of the mean.
†P < .05.
‡P < .01 versus control.
§P < .01 versus before epidural injection.
Modified from Mankikian B, Cantineau JP, Bertrand M, et al. Improvement of diaphragmatic function by a thoracic extradural block after upper abdominal surgery. *Anesthesiology.* 1988;68:379.

$PaO_2$, such as the elderly or those with significant lung disease, may show unacceptably low postoperative $PaO_2$ values, with $O_2$ saturation <90%. They require $O_2$ therapy for a few days, usually at moderate concentrations of 30% to 35%, until gas exchange improves. Pulse oximetry during the recovery period in the postanesthesia care unit identifies patients who still require supplemental $O_2$ after discharge to the ward.

## PULMONARY COMPLICATIONS

Pulmonary complications after abdominal surgery can be divided into two categories: acute ventilatory failure and atelectasis/pneumonia. Anesthesiologists are more directly involved with the former; the latter complications are often in the domain of other physicians and are briefly discussed in this chapter.

### Who Is at Risk for Acute Ventilatory Failure and Why Does It Occur?

Acute ventilatory failure occurs immediately or shortly after surgery in patients with severe underlying pulmonary disease who cannot tolerate the further impairment in lung function brought about by the surgical procedure. The respiratory muscles, already chronically stressed, rapidly fatigue in the presence of the increased workload imposed by the acute reduction in lung volume that follows surgery. Ventilatory failure then ensues, followed by hypercapnia and hypoxemia.

Patients with an FVC or $FEV_1$ <50% of predicted normal or $FEV_1$/FVC <50% are usually considered at risk for ventilatory failure, particularly after upper abdominal procedures that most affect lung function.[196] This risk, however, seems to be low (5%-10%); even patients with grossly abnormal spirometry (ie, $FEV_1$ as low as 15% of normal, $FEV_1$/FVC as low as 26%) can undergo abdominal surgery without necessarily needing postoperative mechanical ventilation.[197–199]

### What Is the Anesthetic Approach to Patients at Risk for Ventilatory Failure?

These patients require vigorous preoperative care to optimize their residual lung function. Physiotherapy, antibiotics, and bronchodilators are indicated to clear purulent sputum and relieve airway obstruction.

The anesthetic technique (general versus regional), as discussed previously, has no influence on postoperative lung function. When general anesthesia is used, the anesthetic should be planned to have the patient awake and able to breathe spontaneously as soon as possible after surgery is completed. High-dose opioid techniques should be limited to cases in which postoperative ventilatory support is planned electively. Care has to be exercised to ensure complete reversal of the neuromuscular block at the end of surgery, particularly if a long-acting agent has been used.

On emergence from anesthesia, patients who do not meet criteria for extubation are ventilated in the postanesthesia care unit until the effects of residual anesthesia dissipate, hypothermia and hemodynamic instability are corrected, and adequate pain relief has been obtained.

Most of the patients who require ventilatory support immediately after surgery improve their respiratory function within a few hours, allowing rapid weaning and extubation. If the patient cannot be extubated or rapidly deteriorates after surgery, requiring reintubation, ventilatory support is usually needed only for a few days because the effects of surgery on the lungs are temporary and reversible. Patients with poor lung function are sometimes ventilated "prophylactically" for 18 to 24 hours. However, no evidence shows that prophylactic ventilation offers any advantage over a policy of extubating patients as soon as feasible. Postoperative ventilatory failure in patients with poor lung function undergoing abdominal surgery is associated with a very low mortality rate.[197,198] "Prohibitive" lung function that contraindicates abdominal surgery because of excessive mortality due to respiratory causes apparently does not exist. Patients should not be denied the benefits of an operation on the grounds of poor respiratory function.

### What Are the Incidence and Risk Factors of Atelectasis/Pneumonia After Abdominal Surgery?

Atelectasis and pneumonia are very common after abdominal surgery. The acute restrictive defect that follows abdominal surgery is associated with a decreased ability to breathe deeply and cough efficiently. Poor lung expansion and plugging of the bronchi by retained sputum eventually cause parenchymal collapse or infection. The reported incidence of these pulmonary complications varies widely, mainly because of large differences in the diagnostic criteria used. If only clinically important complications are considered (ie, requiring therapy or prolonging hospital stay), their incidence after upper abdominal surgery in healthy, nonsmoking patients is approximately 7%.[200] After lower abdominal surgery, the incidence is half of that. The risk of atelectasis/pneumonia is moderately increased in the elderly and in patients in poor physical condition or those who are obese.[201] Smoking, chronic bronchitis with mucus hypersecretion, and chronic obstructive pulmonary disease increase the incidence of these complications to 50% to 75%.[200]

It has been reported that patients who received pancuronium during anesthesia and in whom residual neuromuscular block was detectable in the recovery room were at increased risk for postoperative pulmonary complications. In contrast, postoperative residual block after the use of intermediate-duration relaxants, such as vecuronium and atracurium, did not increase the pulmonary risk.[202] The practical consequences of this study are, in my opinion, as follows: if a long-acting relaxant is chosen during an abdominal procedure in a patient at high risk for pulmonary complications, utmost care has to be used to ensure a complete recovery from the neuromuscular block. Alternatively, a case can be made for the use in these patients of intermediate-duration muscle relaxants. Pulmonary complications after abdominal surgery, even in patients with severe pulmonary disease, are associated with a very low mortality rate.[197,198]

### What Can Be Done to Prevent Postoperative Atelectasis/Pneumonia?

Respiratory maneuvers aimed to reexpand lung volumes and clear secretions are very effective in decreasing postoperative lung complications. The simplest maneuver is to position patients in a semisitting position, thus increasing the expiratory reserve volume and greatly improving the ability to cough.[203] Other techniques include intermittent positive-pressure breathing, continuous positive airway pressure delivered at intervals by mask, and deep-breathing exercises with or without the aid of an incentive spirometer.

All these techniques are equally effective in decreasing the incidence of pulmonary complications, but none enhances the restoration of normal lung volumes or Pao$_2$.[204,205] Accordingly, techniques such as intermittent positive-pressure breathing or continuous positive airway pressure that require expensive apparatus can hardly be justified. Patients without risk factors for postoperative pulmonary complications do not require more than frequent deep breathing exercises supervised by a nurse or respiratory therapist.[206,207] High-risk patients may benefit by the addition of incentive spirometry to their physical therapy.[208]

### Does Postoperative Analgesia Influence Pulmonary Outcome?

It is widely assumed that adequate pain relief after abdominal surgery decreases the incidence of pulmonary complications because it allows deeper breathing and improves lung expansion, enhances coughing, improves patient compliance to physiotherapy, and facilitates early ambulation. Although epidurally administered opioids and, particularly, the combination of opioids and local anesthetics provide excellent analgesia after abdominal surgery,[209] it is not established whether these techniques decrease the incidence of postoperative pulmonary complications compared with systemic opioids.[187] My bias is to recommend the use of epidural opioid-local anesthetic combinations to provide analgesia after abdominal surgery in patients at high risk for pulmonary complications.

### What Are the Pulmonary Effects of Laparoscopic Procedures?

After laparoscopic procedures, the decrease in lung volumes (FVC, FRC) and Pao$_2$ is less and of shorter duration than after similar open procedures. For instance, 24 hours after laparoscopic cholecystectomy, FEV$_1$ and FVC are approximately 70% to 80% of preoperative values, whereas they are 50% to 60% of preoperative values after open cholecystectomy. Lung volumes return to preoperative values in 3 days after laparoscopic cholecystectomy (ie, 4-5 days earlier than after open cholecystectomy).[210,211] Laparoscopic procedures in the upper abdomen (eg, cholecystectomy) affect lung volumes more and for a longer time than laparoscopic procedures in the lower abdomen (eg, inguinal hernia repair, myomectomy).[212,213] Diagnostic laparoscopy or laparoscopy with minimal visceral involvement such as tubal ligation has no effect on postoperative lung function.[212,214]

Lung function changes after laparoscopic surgery are attributed to the same mechanisms responsible for the changes observed after laparotomy (ie, abnormal function/activity of the respiratory muscles caused by reflexes originating from traumatized intraabdominal organs).[213,215] Because laparoscopic surgery only modestly affects lung function, it is not surprising that the incidence of pulmonary complications after laparoscopies is dramatically lower than that after laparotomies. In one large study, the incidence of postoperative pulmonary complications after laparoscopic cholecystectomy was 0.3%.[216]

## POSTOPERATIVE INTESTINAL MOTILITY

Operations in the abdominal cavity are followed by a period of decreased GI motility, referred to as *postoperative ileus* and characterized by ineffective peristalsis and atony. Stomach and small bowel motor activity returns within 24 hours after surgery. The colon shows a more profound inhibition that persists at least 48 hours. Decreased motility of the colon contributes most significantly to the duration of postoperative ileus.

### What Causes Ileus?

The etiology of postoperative ileus remains largely unknown. The most accepted hypothesis is that postoperative ileus is due to spinal reflexes originating from the abdomen and involving sympathetic efferent nerves to the gut; however, other factors have a role as well, such as manipulation of the bowel, electrolyte imbalances, and reduced plasma concentrations of the intestinal hormone motilin.[217] The duration of ileus does not correlate with the degree of operative handling of the bowel, nor with the extent of dissection or duration of surgery.[218]

#### Anesthetic Effects

Inhaled anesthetic agents greatly depress bowel motility, but this effect is promptly reversed when they are withdrawn. Therefore, they do not seem to have any role in causing long-lasting postoperative ileus.[219] Concerns that intraoperative use of nitrous oxide might delay the recovery of bowel function after intestinal surgery[220] have not been substantiated by recent studies.[78,221,222] It is difficult to envision how nitrous oxide, which in itself does not affect bowel motility[219] and is completely reabsorbed from the intestinal lumen in a few hours, would influence the duration of postoperative ileus.

#### Opioids

Opioids have a well-known depressant effect on bowel motility.[223] Because they are widely used to provide analgesia after abdominal surgery, separation of their effects on bowel function from those of the surgical procedure is difficult. Although comparisons are lacking, no clinically significant difference is thought to exist between the various opioids in terms of duration of postoperative ileus. The route of administration also seems unimportant because the duration of ileus is the same after epidural or parenteral opioids.[224] The agonist-antagonist opioids (pentazocine, nalbuphine, and others) apparently exert a depressant effect on bowel motility similar to that of the pure agonists; therefore, their use does not seem to offer any advantage.

#### Epidural Anesthesia and Analgesia

Epidural anesthesia used during abdominal surgery has no effect on the duration of postoperative ileus. It is as yet unclear whether postoperative epidural analgesia with local anesthetics, alone or in combination with opioids, shortens the duration of postoperative ileus compared with conventional analgesia with parenteral opioids. Several investigators found a faster recovery of bowel function with epidural analgesia, but others were unable to confirm this finding.[225] The best results in terms of recovery of bowel function after abdominal surgery have been obtained when the epidural catheter was placed at thoracic level and epidural analgesia maintained for 2 to 3 days.[226]

### Propofol

An in vitro study has shown that clinically relevant concentrations of propofol inhibit spontaneous contractile activity at the gastric and colonic smooth muscle.[227] Possible implications for propofol-sedated patients in the intensive care unit are obvious.

### Is Ileus Treatable?

There is no specific therapy for postoperative ileus. Its treatment is merely supportive, consisting of nasogastric decompression, intravenous fluid administration, and correction of existing metabolic abnormalities. Early ambulation does not enhance the restoration of normal bowel function after laparotomy.[228]

Several pharmacologic agents have been tried in the treatment of postoperative ileus, including metoclopramide, erythromycin (a motilin agonist), and cisapride. The results have been disappointing, and the patients often have been troubled by side effects.[229] At present, it is unclear whether faster recovery of bowel function after surgery is advantageous, or whether postoperative ileus is a useful biologic response that "puts the bowel to rest" and enhances the healing process. For instance, in an animal model, the administration of metoclopramide in the early postoperative period was associated with an increased incidence of dehiscence in colonic anastomoses.[230] Until this controversy is resolved, the value of pharmacologic interventions directed to shorten the duration of postoperative ileus remains speculative.

## SURGERY OF THE ABDOMINAL WALL AND ABDOMINAL WALL HERNIAS

### Which Anesthetics Are Appropriate?

#### Ventral Hernias

Ventral hernias (umbilical, epigastric, and postincisional) can be repaired under general anesthesia or, if the incision is at or below the umbilicus, regional anesthesia. If regional anesthesia is chosen, a sensory block to T5 is recommended to prevent pain when the peritoneum is opened. The repair of a giant ventral hernia may cause postoperative ventilatory problems that necessitate mechanical ventilation.

#### Inguinal and Femoral Hernias

Inguinal and femoral hernias can be operated on under local,[231] general, spinal, or epidural anesthesia. The degree of muscle relaxation required is usually moderate, and muscle relaxants can be used sparingly or avoided altogether. If regional anesthesia is used, a sensory block to T5 is preferred to prevent pain when traction is applied to the spermatic cord or the peritoneum. Laparoscopic repair of inguinal hernias also has gained some popularity. A laparoscopic approach usually requires general anesthesia.[232]

Hernia repairs performed under general or spinal anesthesia are followed by the same incidence of postoperative urinary retention, backache, and respiratory complications.[233,234] The main difference is that the incidence of nausea, vomiting, and sore throat (if tracheal intubation has been performed) is greater after general anesthesia. Postspinal headache and other minor neurologic problems (temporary paresthesias or radicular pain) may complicate spinal anesthesia.

### Choice of Local Anesthetic

If hernia repair is performed under regional anesthesia, prompt recovery of motor and bladder function is desirable; therefore, short-acting local anesthetics are preferred. Hyperbaric 5% lidocaine provides excellent surgical conditions and quick recovery. Unfortunately, the spinal use of this anesthetic, even at lower concentrations of 1% to 2%, has been associated with transient postoperative neurologic symptoms consisting of backache and pain in the buttocks or legs.[235] The incidence of this complication varies with the type of surgery and is approximately 5% after inguinal hernia repair.[236] Hyperbaric bupivacaine, very rarely associated with transient neurologic symptoms, is a suitable alternative for spinal anesthesia, but the slow recovery of motor and bladder function makes this agent less desirable in an outpatient setting.[237,238]

Lidocaine, 2%, and chloroprocaine, 3%, both with 1:200 000 epinephrine, are the agents of choice for epidural anesthesia.[239] Very effective and long-lasting postoperative analgesia can be obtained by infiltrating the surgical area with 30 to 40 mL of 0.25% bupivacaine.[240] This method of pain relief is particularly attractive for outpatients.[241]

### Strangulated Hernias

Spinal anesthesia may be particularly advantageous for patients with strangulated hernias, provided the circulatory volume is normal and no other specific contraindications are present. This technique obviates the significant risk of pulmonary aspiration during the induction of general anesthesia in these patients.

During induction of anesthesia for repair of an incarcerated hernia, the bowel may retreat into the peritoneal cavity before the surgeon can confirm its viability. Under such circumstances, abdominal exploration may be indicated to examine the incarcerated segment.

Whether the untimely reduction of an incarcerated hernia is more likely during general or spinal anesthesia apparently never has been investigated. No data validate maneuvers sometimes used to prevent this event from occurring, such as inducing anesthesia with a patient in the head-up position or having the surgeon or an assistant hold the hernia during induction until the incision can be made.

## INTRAABDOMINAL HYPERTENSION AND THE ABDOMINAL COMPARTMENT SYNDROME

An acute increase in intraabdominal pressure (IAP), which normally in a recumbent subject is close to atmospheric pressure, has profound effects on several organ systems. The level at which IAP becomes intraabdominal hypertension (IAH) and begins to exert detrimental effects is not certainly defined, but it is probably approximately 15 mm Hg.[242,243] The severity of these deleterious effects is roughly proportional to the pressure developed in the abdomen. The most severe cases of IAH, if left untreated, lead uniformly to organ failure and death. The term *abdominal compartment syndrome* has been proposed to describe all the pathophysiologic derangements caused by IAH.

## What Is the Physiopathology of Intraabdominal Hypertension?

The most important adverse effects of IAH are on the cardiovascular system, lungs, kidneys, and intracranial pressure.[244] These effects are purely mechanical in origin, caused by direct compression of intraabdominal vessels or organs and by the cephalad displacement of the diaphragm with a concomitant increase in intrathoracic pressure. Prompt decompression of the abdomen reverses all the derangements caused by IAH.

### Cardiovascular Effects

An increase in IAP invariably decreases the cardiac output, while blood pressure is maintained within normal range by a compensatory increase in SVR. The decrease in cardiac output is mainly due to a decrease in stroke volume, which results from a decreased venous return from the inferior and superior vena cava and direct compression of the heart. Inferior caval flow is decreased because of compression of the inferior vena cava and the portal vein. The increased intrapleural pressure that accompanies IAH decreases superior caval flow and compresses the heart, thus decreasing end-diastolic ventricular volumes. Also, the increased intrapleural pressure is transmitted to the intrathoracic vessels, leading to spuriously elevated central venous, pulmonary arterial, and pulmonary wedge pressures.[245] If the measured pleural pressure is subtracted from these, the "true" pressures may be normal or lower than normal. Because cardiac contractility is usually preserved, the decrease in cardiac output caused by an increased IAP can be corrected by circulating volume expansion with crystalloids, blood, and the like[245] (Figs. 61–19 to 61–21).

Because in the presence of IAH, central venous and pulmonary wedge pressures become unreliable indicators of heart preload (unless intrapleural pressure is measured as well), volume administration is best guided by repeated measurements of cardiac output and mixed venous oxygen saturation. Normalization of cardiac output with volume expansion is often only a temporizing measure because the detrimental effects of IAH on the lung and the kidney persist unabated.

### Pulmonary Effects

Elevated IAP displaces the diaphragm cephalad, causing a marked reduction in lung volumes and lung compliance. If the patient is breathing spontaneously, respiratory failure quickly follows, requiring intubation and mechanical ventilation. Because of the low lung compliance, high peak inspiratory pressures (PIPs) are needed to maintain adequate tidal volume. Positive end-expiratory pressure is invariably applied to main-

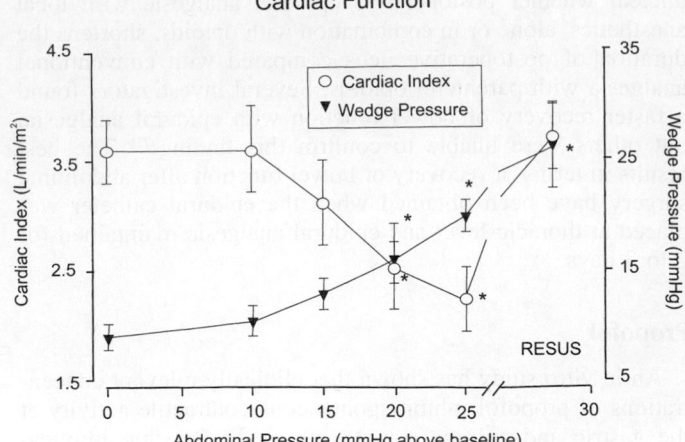

**FIGURE 61–19.** Effects of intraabdominal pressure on cardiac index and pulmonary wedge pressure in an animal model. When abdominal pressure was 25 mm Hg, intravascular volume was expanded with an infusion of saline (RESUS). *$P < .05$ versus baseline. (From Ridings PC, Bloomfield GL, Blocher CR, et al. Cardiopulmonary effects of raised intra-abdominal pressure before and after intravascular volume expansion. *J Trauma.* 1995;39:1071.)

tain oxygenation. In the most severe cases of IAH, mechanical ventilation of the lungs becomes difficult and hypoxia and hypercarbia ensue.

### Renal Effects

Renal dysfunction caused by IAH is characterized by oliguria progressing to anuria and azotemia. Oliguria can be observed at IAP of 15 to 20 mm Hg, whereas at pressures of 25 to 30 mm Hg, urine flow stops altogether.[246] Normalization of cardiac output with volume expansion, dopamine, and diuret-

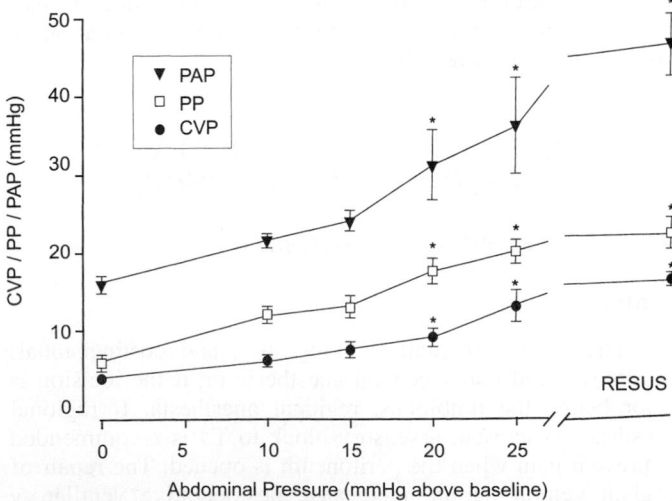

**FIGURE 61–20.** Effects of intraabdominal pressure on pulmonary artery pressure (PAP), central venous pressure (CVP), and pleural pressure (PP) in an animal model. When abdominal pressure was 25 mm Hg, intravascular volume was expanded with an infusion of saline (RESUS). *$P < .05$ versus baseline. (From Ridings PC, Bloomfield GL, Blocher CR, et al. Cardiopulmonary effects of raised intra-abdominal pressure before and after intravascular volume expansion. *J Trauma.* 1995;39:1071.)

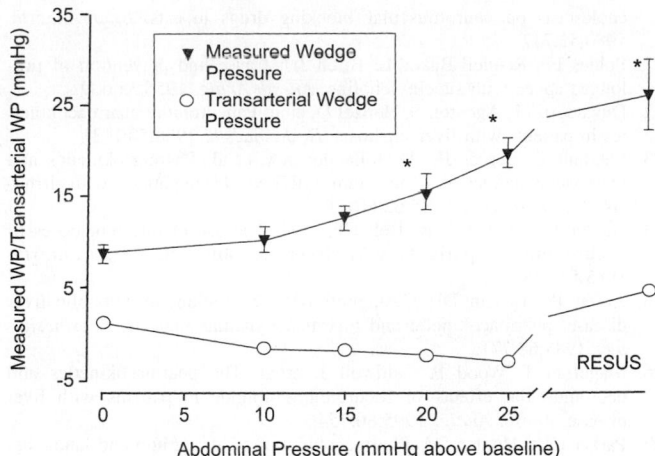

**FIGURE 61–21.** Effects of intraabdominal pressure on the measured wedge pressure and transarterial wedge pressure (measured wedge pressure − pleural pressure) in an animal model. When abdominal pressure was 25 mm Hg, intravascular volume was expanded with an infusion of saline (RESUS). *P < .05 versus baseline. (From Ridings PC, Bloomfield GL, Blocher CR, et al. Cardiopulmonary effects of raised intra-abdominal pressure before and after intravascular volume expansion. *J Trauma.* 1995;39:1071).

ics is ineffective in improving urinary output and renal function. Oliguria or anuria in patients with IAH are late and ominous events, invariably preceded by cardiac and pulmonary compromise. Renal dysfunction is probably caused by direct compression of renal parenchyma and renal veins with markedly decreased renal blood flow and glomerular filtration rate.[247] Ureteral compression has no role in causing renal failure in the presence of IAH.

### Intracranial Effects

IAH may cause an increase in intracranial pressure, probably by increasing intrathoracic pressure and CVP with consequent obstruction of the cerebral venous outflow. The notion that in the presence of coexisting intracranial hypertension, IAH can further increase intracranial pressure, has obvious important therapeutic implications.[248]

## What Causes an Increase in Intraabdominal Pressure?

Because the abdominal cavity is enclosed by walls with limited compliance, an increase in volume of its contents eventually causes an increase in pressure in the cavity itself. The more rapid the increase in volume, the higher is the increase in pressure, because little adaptive stretching of the abdominal walls occurs. Because of the anatomic relation between the abdominal cavity and retroperitoneal space, an increase in volume of the latter also increases IAP. Common causes of increased IAP include intraperitoneal hemorrhage, distention or edema of the bowel, ascites, pancreatitis, and retroperitoneal hemorrhage or edema. In surgical practice, IAH is most frequently seen after surgery for major abdominal trauma, but it may complicate any abdominal surgery.

## How Is Intraabdominal Pressure Measured?

IAP can be measured directly by connecting an intraperitoneal catheter to a water manometer or pressure transducer or,

more commonly, by measuring the pressure inside the urinary bladder.[246] The bladder is an intraabdominal, extraperitoneal organ with a thin, compliant wall. When the bladder is empty or moderately distended (≤50 mL), intravesical pressure has been shown closely to parallel IAP up to 70 mm Hg. Bladder pressure is easily measured using the Foley catheter already in place in virtually every patient at risk for IAH. With the patient supine, the tubing to the urine collecting bag is clamped just past the sampling port, and 50 mL of saline is instilled into the bladder through the sampling port with a needle. The needle is then connected to a water manometer or a pressure transducer, and bladder pressure is measured using the pubic symphysis as the zero reference point. The tubing and Foley should be free of air.

## How Is Intraabdominal Hypertension Diagnosed?

The diagnosis of IAH is primarily clinical and should be suspected in every critically ill patient with a *distended, tense abdomen,* who requires mechanical ventilation with high PIP. Hemodynamic measurements indicate a low cardiac output, which usually improves with fluid administration in spite of high heart filling pressures. Urinary output may be poor or absent. IAP, measured with the urethral catheter, is markedly elevated, with values at times in excess of 30 mm Hg.

## What Is the Treatment for Intraabdominal Hypertension?

The only treatment of IAH is surgical decompression of the abdomen (decompressive laparotomy). The decision as to whether to proceed with surgery should be based on a careful evaluation of the patient's condition. If active bleeding is suspected, prompt exploration of the abdomen is often indicated. If IAH is secondary to factors such as visceral edema, retroperitoneal hematoma, abdominal packing, and so forth, abdominal decompression should be decided on the basis of concomitant deterioration of cardiovascular, pulmonary, and renal function. Oliguria and difficult mechanical ventilation with progressive hypercarbia are strong indications for decompression.

Some authors have recommended the measurement of IAP to guide the treatment of patients with IAH. In general, at IAP <20 mm Hg, a temporizing attitude may be appropriate, with the treatment aimed at maintaining cardiac output and organ perfusion with fluid/drug administration. At IAP between 20 and 25 mm Hg, abdominal decompression should be seriously considered, and is mandatory at IAP >25 mm Hg.[249] Patients, however, do not respond uniformly to the same levels of IAP. For this reason, the measurement of IAP is less important than clinical assessment of overall patient conditions in deciding the appropriate therapy.

## What Happens When Intraabdominal Hypertension Is Relieved?

Abdominal decompression is followed by an almost immediate decrease in PIP. Lung gas exchange rapidly improves with a decrease in $Paco_2$ and an increase in $Pao_2$. Renal dysfunction is also promptly reversed, as indicated by an increase, at times brisk, in diuresis. Sudden and severe hypotension, sometimes leading to cardiac arrest, has been reported immediately after abdominal decompression.[250] A possible explanation of this hemodynamic instability is a sudden decrease in SVR from resumption of flow in the decompressed splanchnic bed.[251] Hypotension after abdominal decompression is treated with potent $\alpha$-adrenoreceptor agonists such as epinephrine or norepinephrine[252] and fluid administration.[251] The latter should be guided by hemodynamic measurements, lest the fluid overload commonly present in these patients be worsened. A decrease in applied positive end-expiratory pressure may also be beneficial in ameliorating hemodynamic instability after abdominal decompression.

## References

1. Downman CBB. Skeletal muscle reflexes of splanchnic and intercostal nerve origin in acute spinal and decerebrate cats. *J Neurophysiol.* 1955;18:217.
2. Kugelberg E, Hagbarth KE. Spinal mechanism of the abdominal and erector spine skin reflexes. *Brain.* 1958;81:290.
3. Albano JP, Garnier L. Bulbo-spinal respiratory effects originating from the splanchnic afferents. *Respir Physiol.* 1983;51:229.
4. Ngai SH. Action of general anesthetics in producing muscle relaxation: interaction of anesthetics with relaxants. In: Katz RL, ed. *Muscle Relaxants.* Amsterdam, The Netherlands: North-Holland; 1975:279.
5. Downes H. Hyperventilation and abdominal reflex inhibition. *Anesthesiology.* 1963;24:617.
6. Foex P. Effects of carbon dioxide on the systemic circulation. In: Prys-Roberts C, ed. *The Circulation in Anaesthesia.* London, United Kingdom: Blackwell Scientific Publications; 1980:295.
7. Gelman S. Carbon dioxide and hepatic circulation. *Anesth Analg.* 1989;69:149.
8. Gelman S. Disturbances in hepatic blood flow during anesthesia and surgery. *Arch Surg.* 1976;111:881.
9. Cartwright P, Prys-Roberts C, Gill K, et al. Ventilatory depression related to plasma fentanyl concentrations during and after anesthesia in humans. *Anesth Analg.* 1983;62:966.
10. Schwartz AE, Matteo RS, Ornstein E, et al. Pharmacokinetics of sufentanil in neurosurgical patients undergoing hyperventilation. *Br J Anaesth.* 1989;63:385.
11. Nagano K, Gelman S, Parks DA, et al. Hepatic oxygen supply-uptake relationship and metabolism during anesthesia in miniature pigs. *Anesthesiology.* 1990;72:902.
12. Nagano K, Gelman S, Parks D, et al. Hepatic circulation and oxygen supply-uptake relationships after hepatic ischemic insult during anesthesia with volatile anesthetics and fentanyl in miniature pigs. *Anesth Analg.* 1990;70:53.
13. Goldfarb G, Debaene B, Ang ET, et al. Hepatic blood flow in humans during isoflurane-$N_2O$ and halothane-$N_2O$ anesthesia. *Anesth Analg.* 1990;71:349.
14. Noldge GFE, Priebe HJ, Kopp KH, et al. Differences in effects of isoflurane and enflurane on splanchnic oxygenation and hepatic metabolism in the pig. *Anesth Analg.* 1990;71:258.
15. O'Riordan J, O'Beirne HA, Young Y, et al. Effects of desflurane on splanchnic microcirculation during major surgery. *Br J Anaesth.* 1997;78:95.
16. Andersen BN, Madsen JV, Schurizek BA, et al. Residual curarization: a comparative study of atracurium and pancuronium. *Acta Anaesthesiol Scand.* 1988;32:79.
17. Bevan DR, Smith CE, Donati F. Postoperative neuromuscular blockade: a comparison between atracurium, vecuronium, and pancuronium. *Anesthesiology.* 1988;69:272.
18. Somogyi AA, Shanks CA, Triggs EJ. Disposition kinetics of pancuronium bromide in patients with total biliary obstruction. *Br J Anaesth.* 1977;49:1103.
19. Lebrault C, Duvaldestin P, Henzel D, et al. Pharmacokinetics and pharmacodynamics of vecuronium in patients with cholestasis. *Br J Anaesth.* 1986;58:983.
20. Westra P, Houwertjes MC, DeLange AR, et al. Effect of experimental cholestasis on neuromuscular blocking drugs in cats. *Br J Anaesth.* 1980;52:747.
21. Foldes FF, Rendell-Baker L, Birch JH. Cause and prevention of prolonged apnea with succinylcholine. *Anesth Analg.* 1956;35:609.
22. Duvaldestin P, Agoston S, Henzel D, et al. Pancuronium pharmacokinetics in patients with liver cirrhosis. *Br J Anaesth.* 1978;50:1131.
23. Lebrault C, Berger JL, D'Hollander AA, et al. Pharmacokinetics and pharmacodynamics of vecuronium (ORG NC 45) in patients with cirrhosis. *Anesthesiology.* 1985;62:601.
24. Hunter JM, Parker CJR, Bell CF, et al. The use of different doses of vecuronium in patients with liver dysfunction. *Br J Anaesth.* 1985;57:758.
25. Arden JR, Lynam DP, Castagnoli KP. Vecuronium in alcoholic liver disease: pharmacokinetic and pharmacodynamic analysis. *Anesthesiology.* 1988;68:771.
26. Magorian T, Wood P, Caldwell J, et al. The pharmacokinetics and neuromuscular effects of rocuronium bromide in patients with liver disease. *Anesth Analg.* 1995;80:754.
27. Parker CJR, Hunter JM. Pharmacokinetics of atracurium and laudanosine in patients with hepatic cirrhosis. *Br J Anaesth.* 1989;62:177.
28. De Wolf AM, Freeman JA, Scott VL, et al. Pharmacokinetics and pharmacodynamics of cisatracurium in patients with end-stage liver disease undergoing liver transplantation. *Br J Anaesth.* 1999;76:624.
29. Lee C. Train-of-4 quantitation of competitive neuromuscular block. *Anesth Analg.* 1975;54:649.
30. Derrington MC, Hindocha N. Comparison of neuromuscular block in the diaphragm and hand after administration of tubocurarine, pancuronium, and alcuronium. *Br J Anaesth.* 1990;64:294.
31. Donati F, Meistelman C, Plaud B. Vecuronium neuromuscular blockade at the diaphragm, the orbicularis oculi, and adductor pollicis muscles. *Anesthesiology.* 1990;73:870.
32. Saddler JM, Marks LF, Norman J. Comparison of atracurium-induced neuromuscular block in rectus abdominis and hand muscles of man. *Br J Anaesth.* 1992;69:26.
33. Viby-Mogensen J, Howardy-Hansen P, Chraemmer-Jorgensen B, et al. Posttetanic count (PTC): a new method of evaluating an intense nondepolarizing neuromuscular block. *Anesthesiology.* 1981;59:1089.
34. Fernando PUE, Viby-Mogensen J, Bonsu AK, et al. Relationship between posttetanic count and response to carinal stimulation during vecuronium-induced neuromuscular blockade. *Acta Anaesthesiol Scand.* 1987;31:593.
35. Lewis JH. Hiccups: causes and cures. *J Clin Gastroenterol.* 1985;7:539.
36. Bannon MG. Termination of hiccups occurring under anesthesia. *Anesthesiology.* 1991;74:385.
37. Rouse JM, Bevan DR. Mixed neuromuscular block. *Anesthesia.* 1979;34:608.
38. Feldman SA. Rational use of muscle relaxants and anticholinesterase in clinical practice. In: Hamilton WK, ed. *Muscle Relaxants.* 2nd ed. Philadelphia, Pa: WB Saunders; 1979:221.
39. Rashkovsky OM, Agoston S, Ket JM. Interaction between pancuronium bromide and vecuronium bromide. *Br J Anaesth.* 1985;57:1063.
40. Ornstein E, Matteo RS, Weinstein JA, et al. The effect of maintenance dose vecuronium on preestablished metocurine- or vecuronium-induced neuromuscular blockade. *Anesthesiology.* 1988;69:954.
41. Smith I, White PF. Pipecuronium-induced prolongation of vecuronium neuromuscular block. *Br J Anaesth.* 1993;70:446.
42. Whalley DG, Lewis B, Bedocs NM. Recovery of neuromuscular function after atracurium and pancuronium maintenance of pancuronium block. *Can J Anaesth.* 1994;41:31.
43. Erkola O, Rautoma P, Meretoja OA. Mivacurium when preceded by pancuronium becomes a long-acting muscle relaxant. *Anesthesiology.* 1996;84:562.
44. Kim KS, Shim JC, Kim DW. Interactions between mivacurium and pancuronium. *Br J Anaesth.* 1997;79:19.
45. Middleton CM, Pollard BJ, Healy TEJ, et al. Use of atracurium or vecuronium to prolong the action of tubocurarine. *Br J Anaesth.* 1989;62:659.
46. Ostergaard D, Jensen E, Jensen FS, et al. The duration of action of mivacurium-induced neuromuscular block in patients homozygous for the atypical plasma cholinesterase gene. *Anesthesiology.* 1991;75:A774.
47. Yellin AE, Newman J, Donovan AJ. Neostigmine-induced hyperperistalsis. *Arch Surg.* 1973;106:779.
48. Child CS. Prevention of neostigmine-induced colonic activity. *Anesthesia.* 1984;39:1083.
49. Wilkins JL, Hardcastle JD, Mann CV, et al. Effects of neostigmine and atropine on motor activity of ileum, colon, and rectum of anaesthetized subject. *BMJ.* 1970;1:793.

50. Bell CMA, Lewis CB. Effect of neostigmine on integrity of ileorectal anastomoses. *BMJ.* 1968;3:587.

51. Brown EN, Daughety MJ, Petty WC. Integrity of intestinal anastomoses following muscle relaxant reversal with neostigmine. *Anesth Analg.* 1973;52:118.

52. Morisot P, Loygue J, Guilmet EC. Effets de la décurarisation postopératoire par la néostigmine sur les anastomoses digestives. *Can Anaesth Soc J.* 1975;22:144.

53. McCoy EP, Mirakhur RK. Comparison of the effects of neostigmine and edrophonium on the duration of action of suxamethonium. *Acta Anaesthesiol Scand.* 1995;39:744.

54. Sunew KY, Hicks RG. Effects of neostigmine and pyridostigmine on duration of succinylcholine action and pseudocholinesterase activity. *Anesthesiology.* 1978;49:188.

55. Baraka A, Wakid N, Mansour R, et al. Effect of neostigmine and pyridostigmine on the plasma cholinesterase activity. *Br J Anaesth.* 1981;53:849.

56. Morgan M, Norman G. The effect of extradural analgesia combined with light general anaesthesia and spontaneous ventilation on arterial blood gases and physiological dead space. *Br J Anaesth.* 1975;47:955.

57. Stephen GW, Lees MM, Scott DB. Cardiovascular effects of epidural block combined with general anesthesia. *Br J Anaesth.* 1969;41:933.

58. Germann PAS, Roberts JG, Prys-Roberts C. The combination of general anaesthesia and epidural block, I: the effects of sequence of induction on haemodynamic variables and blood gas measurements in healthy patients. *Anaesth Intensive Care.* 1979;7:229.

59. Wright PMC, Fee JPH. Cardiovascular support during combined extradural and general anaesthesia. *Br J Anaesth.* 1992;68:585.

60. Hjortso NC, Neumann P, Frosig F, et al. A controlled study on the effect of epidural analgesia with local anaesthetics and morphine on morbidity after abdominal surgery. *Acta Anaesthesiol Scand.* 1985;29:790.

61. Worsley MH, Wishart HY, Brown P, et al. High spinal nerve block for large bowel anastomosis: a prospective study. *Br J Anaesth.* 1988;60:836.

62. Ravin MB. Comparison of spinal and general anesthesia for lower abdominal surgery in patients with chronic obstructive pulmonary disease. *Anesthesiology.* 1971;35:319.

63. Hendolin H, Tuppurainen T, Lahtinen J. Thoracic epidural analgesia and deep vein thrombosis in cholecystectomized patients. *Acta Chir Scand.* 1982;148:405.

64. Mellbring G, Dahlgren S, Reiz S, et al. Thromboembolic complications after major abdominal surgery: effects of thoracic epidural analgesia. *Acta Chir Scand.* 1983;149:263.

65. Kehlet H. Effect of pain-relieving techniques on postoperative protein economy. *Br J Clin Pract.* 1988;63:121.

66. Jones MJT. The influence of anesthetic methods on mental functioning. *Acta Chir Scand Suppl.* 1988;555:169.

67. Rocco AG, Vandam LD. Changes in circulation consequent to manipulation during abdominal surgery. *JAMA.* 1957;16:14.

68. Doyle DJ, Mark PWS. Reflex bradycardia during surgery. *Can J Anaesth.* 1990;37:219.

69. Coventry DM, McMenemin I, Lawrie S. Bradycardia during intraabdominal surgery. *Anaesthesia.* 1987;42:835.

70. Seltzer JL, Ritter DE, Starsnic MA, et al. The hemodynamic response to traction on the abdominal mesentery. *Anesthesiology.* 1985;63:96.

71. Gottlieb A, Skrinska VA, O'Hara P, et al. The role of prostacyclin in the mesenteric traction syndrome during anesthesia for abdominal aortic reconstructive surgery. *Ann Surg.* 1989;209:363.

72. Hudson JC, Wurm WH, O'Donnell TF Jr, et al. Ibuprofen pretreatment inhibits prostacyclin release during abdominal exploration in aortic surgery. *Anesthesiology.* 1990;72:443.

73. Mirakhur RK, Jones CJ, Dundee JW. Effects of intravenous administration of glycopyrrolate and atropine in anaesthetized patients. *Anaesthesia.* 1981;36:277.

74. Levitt MD, Bond JH. Intestinal gas. In: Sleisenger MH, Fordtran JS, eds. *Gastrointestinal Disease.* 4th ed. Philadelphia, Pa: WB Saunders; 1989:257.

75. Eger EI II, Saidman LJ. Hazards of nitrous oxide anesthesia in bowel obstruction and pneumothorax. *Anesthesiology.* 1965;26:61.

76. Steffey EP, Johnson BH, Eger EI II, et al. Nitrous oxide: effect on accumulation rate and uptake of bowel gases. *Anesth Analg.* 1979;58:405.

77. Karlsten R, Kristensen JD. Nitrous oxide does not influence the surgeon's rating of operating conditions in lower abdominal surgery. *Eur J Anaesthiol.* 1993;10:215.

78. Krogh B, Jernjensen P, Henneberg SW, et al. Nitrous oxide does not influence operating conditions or postoperative course in colonic surgery. *Br J Anaesth.* 1994;72:55.

79. Taylor E, Feinstein R, White PF, et al. Anesthesia for laparoscopic cholecystectomy: is nitrous oxide contraindicated? *Anesthesiology.* 1992;76:541.

80. Radnay PA, Duncalf D, Novakovic M, et al. Common bile duct pressure changes after fentanyl, morphine, meperidine, butorphanol, and naloxone. *Anesth Analg.* 1984;63:441.

81. McCammon RL, Stoelting RK, Madura JA. Effects of butorphanol, nalbuphine, and fentanyl on intrabiliary tract dynamics. *Anesth Analg.* 1984;63:139.

82. Vatashsky E, Haskel Y. Effect of nalbuphine on intrabiliary pressure in the early postoperative period. *Can Anaesth Soc J.* 1986;33:433.

83. Carey LC, Ellison CE. Cholecystostomy, cholecystectomy, and intraoperative evaluation of the biliary tree. In: Nyhus LM, Baker RJ, eds. *Mastery of Surgery.* Vol 1. 2nd ed. Boston, Mass: Little, Brown & Co; 1992:873.

84. Jones RM, Fiddian-Green R, Knight PR. Narcotic-induced choledochoduodenal sphincter spasm reversed by glucagon. *Anesth Analg.* 1980;59:946.

85. Humphreys HK, Fleming NW. Opioid-induced spasm of the sphincter of Oddi apparently reversed by nalbuphine. *Anesth Analg.* 1992;74:308.

86. Ikard RW, Federspiel CF. A comparison of Levin and sump nasogastric tubes for postoperative gastrointestinal decompression. *Am Surg.* 1987;53:50.

87. Galloway DC, Grundis J. Inadvertent intracranial placement of nasogastric tube through a basilar skull fracture. *South Med J.* 1979;72:240.

88. Ritter DM, Rettke ST, Hughes RW, et al. Placement of nasogastric tubes and esophageal stethoscopes in patients with documented esophageal varices. *Anesth Analg.* 1988;67:283.

89. Mundy DA. Another technique for insertion of nasogastric tubes. *Anesthesiology.* 1979;50:374.

90. Siegel IB, Kahn RC. Insertion of difficult nasogastric tubes through a nasoesophageally placed endotracheal tube. *Crit Care Med.* 1987;15:876.

91. Stept WJ, Safar P. Rapid induction/intubation for prevention of gastric content aspiration. *Anesth Analg.* 1979;49:633.

92. Sellick BA. Cricoid pressure to control regurgitation of stomach contents during induction of anaesthesia. *Lancet.* 1961;2:404.

93. Salem MR, Joseph NJ, Heyman JH, et al. Cricoid compression is effective in obliterating the esophageal lumen in the presence of a nasogastric tube. *Anesthesiology.* 1985;64:443.

94. Salem MR, Wong AY, Mani M, et al. Efficacy of cricoid pressure in preventing gastric inflation during bag-mask ventilation in pediatric patients. *Anesthesiology.* 1974;40:96.

95. Lawes EG, Campbell I, Mercer D. Inflation pressure, gastric insufflation, and rapid sequence induction. *Br J Anaesth.* 1987;59:315.

96. Jense HG, Dubin SA, Silverstein P, et al. Effect of obesity on safe duration of apnea in anesthetized humans. *Anesth Analg.* 1991;72:89.

97. Ralph SJ, Wareham CA. Rupture of the esophagus during cricoid pressure. *Anaesthesia.* 1991;46:40.

98. Hayes MA, Goldenberg MD. Renal effects of anesthesia and operation mediated by endocrines. *Anesthesiology.* 1963;24:487.

99. Albert SN, Shibuya J, Economooulous B, et al. Simultaneous measurement of erythrocyte, plasma, and extracellular fluid volumes with radioactive tracers. *Anesthesiology.* 1968;29:908.

100. Shires T, Williams J, Brown F. Acute change in extracellular fluids associated with major surgical procedures. *Ann Surg.* 1961;154:803.

101. Shires T, Jackson DE. Postoperative salt tolerance. *Arch Surg.* 1962;84:703.

102. Roberts JP, Roberts JD, Skinner C, et al. Extracellular fluid deficit following operation and its correction with Ringer's lactate. *Ann Surg.* 1984;202:1.

103. Irvin TT, Hayter CJ, Modgill VK, et al. Plasma-volume deficits and salt and water excretion after surgery. *Lancet.* 1972;2:1159.

104. Shizgal HM, Solomon S, Gutelius JR. Body water distribution after operation. *Surg Gynecol Obstet.* 1977;144:35.

105. Pappova E, Bachmeier W, Crevoisier J-L, et al. Acute hypoproteinemic fluid overload: its determinants, distribution, and treatment with concentrated albumin and diuretics. *Vox Sang.* 1977;33:307.

106. Chan STF, Kapadia DR, Johnson AW, et al. Extracellular fluid volume expansion and third space sequestration at the site of small bowel anastomoses. *Br J Surg.* 1983;70:35.

107. Lowell JA, Schifferoecker C, Driscoll CF, et al. Postoperative fluid overload: not a benign problem. *Crit Care Med.* 1990;18:728.

108. Nielsen OM, Engell HC. The importance of plasma colloid osmotic

pressure for interstitial fluid volume and fluid balance after elective abdominal vascular surgery. *Ann Surg.* 1986;203:25.

109. Zaloga GP, Hughes SS. Oliguria in patients with normal renal function. *Anesthesiology.* 1990;72:598.

110. Mackenzie AI, Donald JR. Urine output and fluid therapy during anaesthesia and surgery. *BMJ.* 1969;3:619.

111. Ambrose NS, Keighley MRB. Physiological consequences of orthograde lavage bowel preparation for elective colorectal surgery: a review. *J R Soc Med.* 1983;76:767.

112. Davis GR, Santa Ana CA, Morawski SG, et al. Development of a lavage solution associated with minimal water and electrolyte absorption or secretion. *Gastroenterology.* 1980;78:991.

113. Skillmann JJ, Critchlow JF. Postoperative hemorrhage and volume depletion. In: Nyhus LM, Baker RJ, eds. *Mastery of Surgery.* 2nd ed. Boston, Mass: Little, Brown & Co; 1992:48.

114. Shippy CR, Appel PL, Shoemaker WC. Reliability of clinical monitoring to assess blood volume in critically ill patients. *Crit Care Med.* 1984;12:107.

115. Amoroso P, Greenwood RN. Posture and central venous pressure measurements in circulatory volume depletion. *Lancet.* 1989;2:258.

116. Stene JK, Grande CM, Giesecke A. Shock resuscitation. In: Stene JK, Grande CM, eds. *Trauma Anesthesia.* Baltimore, Md: Williams & Wilkins; 1991:100.

117. Shenkin HA, Cheney RH, Govons SR, et al. On the diagnosis of hemorrhage in man: a study of volunteers bled large amounts. *Am J Med Sci.* 1944;208:421.

118. Wait RB, Kahng KU. Renal failure complicating obstructive jaundice. *Am J Surg.* 1989;157:256.

119. Greig JD, Kurkowski ZH, Matheson NA. Surgical morbidity and mortality in one hundred and twenty-nine patients with obstructive jaundice. *Br J Surg.* 1988;75:216.

120. Green J, Beyar R, Bomzon L, et al. Jaundice, the circulation, and the kidney. *Nephron.* 1984;37:145.

121. Sitprija V, Kashemsant U, Sriratanaban A, et al. Renal function in obstructive jaundice in man: cholangiocarcinoma model. *Kidney Int.* 1990;38:945.

122. Martinez-Rodenas F, Oms L, Carulla X, et al. Measurements of body water compartments after ligation of the common bile duct in the rabbit. *Br J Surg.* 1989;76:461.

123. Dawson JL. Jaundice and anoxic renal damage: protective effect of mannitol. *BMJ.* 1964;1:810.

124. McPherson GA, Benjamin IS, Blumgart LH. Improving renal function in obstructive jaundice without preoperative drainage [letter]. *Lancet.* 1984;1:511.

125. Dawson JL. Postoperative function in obstructive jaundice: effect of mannitol diuresis. *BMJ.* 1965;1:32.

126. Gubern JM, Sancho JJ, Simo J, et al. A randomized trial on the effect of mannitol on postoperative renal function in patients with obstructive jaundice. *Surgery.* 1988;103:39.

127. Miyagawa S, Kawasaki S, Noike T, et al. Liver regeneration after extended right hemihepatectomy in patients with hilar or diffuse bile duct carcinoma. *Hepatogastroenterology.* 1999;46:364.

128. Matsumata T, Higashi H, Shimada M, et al. Indications for major hepatectomy in cirrhotic liver. *Hepatogastroenterology.* 1994;41:165.

129. Fan ST, Lai EC, Lo CM, et al. Hospital mortality of major hepatectomy for hepatocellular carcinoma associated with cirrhosis. *Arch Surg.* 1995;130:198.

130. Farges O, Malassagne B, Flejou JF, et al. Risk of major liver resection in patients with underlying chronic liver disease: a reappraisal. *Ann Surg.* 1999;229:210.

131. Pringle JH. Notes on the arrest of hepatic hemorrhage due to trauma. *Ann Surg.* 1908;48:541.

132. Delva E, Camus Y, Paugam C, et al. Hemodynamic effects of portal triad clamping in humans. *Anesth Analg.* 1987;66:864.

133. Mendelez JA, Arslan V, Fischer ME, et al. Perioperative outcomes of major hepatic resections under low central venous pressure anesthesia: blood loss, blood transfusion, and the risk of postoperative renal dysfunction. *J Am Coll Surg.* 1998;187:620.

134. Johnson M, Mannar R, Wu AVO. Correlation between blood loss and inferior vena cava pressure during liver resection. *Br J Surg.* 1998;85:188.

135. Jones R, Moulton CE, Hardy KJ. Central venous pressure and its effects on blood loss during liver resection. *Br J Surg.* 1998;85:1058.

136. Delva E, Barberousse JP, Nordlinger B, et al. Hemodynamic and biochemical monitoring during major liver resection with use of hepatic vascular exclusion. *Surgery.* 1984;95:309.

137. Emont JC, Kelley SD, Heffron TG, et al. Surgical and anesthetic management of patients undergoing major hepatectomy using total vascular exclusion. *Liver Transpl Surg.* 1996;2:91.

138. Stephen MS, Gallagher PJ, Sheil AG, et al. Hepatic resection with vascular isolation and routine supraceliac aortic clamping. *Am J Surg.* 1996;171:351.

139. Elias D, Lasser P, Debaene B, et al. Intermittent vascular exclusion of the liver (without vena cava clamping) during major hepatectomy. *Br J Surg.* 1995;82:1535.

140. Elias D, Dube P, Bonvalot S, et al. Intermittent complete vascular exclusion of the liver during hepatectomy: technique and indications. *Hepatogastroenterology.* 1998;45:389.

141. Cherqui D, Malassagne B, Colau PI, et al. Hepatic vascular exclusion with preservation of the caval flow for liver resection. *Ann Surg.* 1999;230:24.

142. Arnoletti JP, Brodsky J. Reduction of transfusion requirements during major hepatic resection for metastatic disease. *Surgery.* 1999;125:166.

143. Quan D, Wall WJ. The safety of continuous hepatic inflow occlusion during major liver resection. *Liver Transpl Surg.* 1996;2:99.

144. Evans PM, Vogt DP, Mayes JT, et al. Liver resection using total vascular exclusion. *Surgery.* 1998;124:807.

145. Huguet C, Gavelli A, Bona S. Hepatic resection with ischemia of the liver exceeding one hour. *J Am Coll Surg.* 1994;178:454.

146. Wu CC, Hwang CR, Liu TJ, et al. Effects and limitations of prolonged intermittent ischemia for hepatic resection of the cirrhotic liver. *Br J Surg.* 1996;83:121.

147. Man K, Fan S, Ng I, et al. Tolerance of the liver to intermittent Pringle maneuver in hepatectomy for liver tumors. *Arch Surg.* 1999;134:533.

148. Belghiti J, Noun R, Malafosse R, et al. Continuous versus intermittent portal triad clamping for liver resection: a controlled study. *Ann Surg.* 1999;229:369.

149. Lampe GH, Wauk LZ, Whitendale P, et al. Nitrous oxide does not impair hepatic function in young or old surgical patients. *Anesth Analg.* 1990;71:606.

150. Makuuchi M, Takayama T, Gunven P, et al. Restrictive versus liberal blood transfusion policy for hepatectomies in cirrhotic patients. *World J Surg.* 1989;13:644.

151. Sejourne P, Poirier A, Meakins JL, et al. Effect of haemodilution on transfusion requirements in liver resection. *Lancet.* 1989;9:1380.

152. Suc B, Panis Y, Belghiti J, et al. "Natural history" of hepatectomy. *Br J Surg.* 1992;79:39.

153. Pelton JJ, Hoffman JP, Eisenber BI. Comparison of liver function tests after hepatic lobectomy and hepatic wedge resection. *Am Surg.* 1998;64:408.

154. Arroyo V, Gines P, Planas R, et al. Paracentesis in the management of cirrhotics with ascites. In: Epstein M, ed. *The Kidney in Liver Disease.* 3rd ed. Baltimore, Md: Williams & Wilkins; 1989:578.

155. Cruikshank DP, Buchsbaum HJ. Effects of rapid paracentesis: cardiovascular dynamics and body fluid composition. *JAMA.* 1973;225:1361.

156. Simon DM, McCain JR, Bonkovsky HL, et al. Effects of therapeutic paracentesis on systemic and hepatic hemodynamics and on renal and hormonal function. *Hepatology.* 1987;7:423.

157. Cade R, Wagemaker H, Vogel S, et al. Hepatorenal syndrome: studies of the effect of vascular volume and intraperitoneal pressure on renal and hepatic function. *Am J Med.* 1987;82:427.

158. Kao HW, Rakov NE, Savage E, et al. The effect of large volume paracentesis on plasma volume: a cause of hypovolemia? *Hepatology.* 1985;5:403.

159. Pinto P, Amerian J, Reynolds TB. Large-volume paracentesis in nonedematous patients with tense ascites: its effects on intravascular volume. *Hepatology.* 1988;8:207.

160. Planas R, Gines P, Arroyo V, et al. Dextran 70 versus albumin as plasma expanders in cirrhotic patients with tense ascites treated with total paracentesis. *Gastroenterology.* 1990;99:1736.

161. LeVeen HH, Christoudias G, Moon JP, et al. Peritoneo-venous shunting for ascites. *Ann Surg.* 1974;180:580.

162. LeVeen HH, Ip M, Ahmed N, et al. Coagulopathy post peritoneovenous shunt. *Ann Surg.* 1987;205:305.

163. Biagini JR, Belghiti J, Fekete F. Prevention of coagulopathy after placement of peritoneovenous shunt with replacement of ascitic fluid by normal saline solution. *Surg Gynecol Obstet.* 1986;163:315.

164. Cello JP, Grendell JH, Crass RA, et al. Endoscopic sclerotherapy versus portocaval shunt in patients with severe cirrhosis and acute variceal hemorrhage. *N Engl J Med.* 1987;316:11.

165. Reichel FA, Owen OE. Hemodynamic parameters in human hepatic cirrhosis. *Ann Surg.* 1979;190:523.

166. Steegmuller KW, Markin HM, Hollis HW Jr. Intraoperative hemodynamic investigations during portacaval shunt. *Arch Surg.* 1984;119:269.

167. Child CG. Major problems in clinical surgery. In: Child CG, Coon WW, eds. *The Liver and Portal Hypertension*. Philadelphia, Pa: WB Saunders, 1964:50.

168. Pugh RNH, Murray-Lyon IM, Dawson JL, et al. Transection of the esophagus for bleeding varices. *Br J Surg*. 1973;60:646.

169. Lunzer MR, Newman S, Bernard AG, et al. Impaired cardiovascular responsiveness in liver disease. *Lancet*. 1975;2:382.

170. Greenway CV. Role of splanchnic venous system in overall cardiovascular homeostasis. *Fed Proc*. 1983;42:1678.

171. Vaamonde CA. Renal water handling in liver disease. In: Epstein M, ed. *The Kidney in Liver Disease*. 3rd ed. Baltimore, Md: Williams & Wilkins; 1989:31.

172. Arieff A. Hyponatremia and hypernatremia in liver disease. In: Epstein M, ed. *The Kidney in Liver Disease*. 3rd ed. Baltimore, Md: Williams & Wilkins; 1989:73.

173. Craig DB. Postoperative recovery of pulmonary function. *Anesth Analg*. 1981;60:46.

174. Wahba RWM. Perioperative functional residual capacity. *Can J Anaesth*. 1991;38:384.

175. Latimer RG, Dickman M, Day WC, et al. Ventilatory patterns and pulmonary complications after upper abdominal surgery determined by preoperative and postoperative computerized spirometry and blood gas analysis. *Am J Surg*. 1971;122:622.

176. Ali J, Khan TA. The comparative effects of muscle transection and median upper abdominal incisions on postoperative pulmonary function. *Surg Gynecol Obstet*. 1979;148:863.

177. Garcia-Valdecasas JC, Almenara R, Cabrer C, et al. Subcostal incision versus midline laparotomy in gallstone surgery: a prospective and randomized trial. *Br J Surg*. 1988;75:473.

178. Becquemin JP, Piquet J, Becquemin MH, et al. Pulmonary function after transverse or midline incision in patients with obstructive pulmonary disease. *Intensive Care Med*. 1985;11:247.

179. Tahir AH, George RB, Weil H, et al. Effects of abdominal surgery upon diaphragmatic function and regional ventilation. *Int Surg*. 1973;58:337.

180. Ford GT, Whitelaw WA, Rosenal TW, et al. Diaphragm function after upper abdominal surgery in humans. *Am Rev Respir Dis*. 1983;127:431.

181. Simmonneau G, Vivien A, Sartene R, et al. Diaphragm dysfunction induced by upper abdominal surgery. *Am Rev Respir Dis*. 1983;128:899.

182. Dureuil B, Cantineau JP, Desmonts JM. Effects of upper or lower abdominal surgery on diaphragmatic function. *Br J Anaesth*. 1987;59:1230.

183. Duggan JE, Drummond GB. Abdominal muscle activity and intraabdominal pressure after upper abdominal surgery. *Anesth Analg*. 1989;69:598.

184. Mankikian B, Cantineau JP, Bertrand M, et al. Improvement of diaphragmatic function by a thoracic extradural block after upper abdominal surgery. *Anesthesiology*. 1988;68:379.

185. Scott NB, Mogensen T, Bigler D, et al. Continuous thoracic extradural 0.5% bupivacaine with or without morphine: effect on quality of blockade, lung function, and the surgical stress response. *Br J Anaesth*. 1989;62:253.

186. Pansard JL, Mankikian B, Bertrand M, et al. Effects of thoracic extradural block on diaphragmatic electrical activity and contractility after upper abdominal surgery. *Anesthesiology*. 1993;78:63.

187. Ballantyne JC, Carr DB, deFerranti S, et al. The comparative effects of postoperative analgesic therapies on pulmonary outcome: cumulative meta-analysis of randomized, controlled trials. *Anesth Analg*. 1998;86:598.

188. Kitamura H, Sawa T, Ikezono E. Postoperative hypoxemia: the contribution of age to the maldistribution of ventilation. *Anesthesiology*. 1972;36:244.

189. Diament ML, Palmer KNV. Postoperative changes in gas tensions of arterial blood and in ventilatory function. *Lancet*. 1966;2:180.

190. Whealthy R, Somerville I, Sapford D, et al. Postoperative hypoxemia: comparison of extradural, I.M., and patient-controlled analgesia. *Br J Anaesth*. 1990;64:267.

191. Strandberg A, Tokics L, Brismar B, et al. Atelectasis during anaesthesia and in the postoperative period. *Acta Anaesthesiol Scand*. 1986;30:154.

192. Hsu HO, Hickey RF. Effect of posture on functional residual capacity postoperatively. *Anesthesiology*. 1976;44:520.

193. Vaughan RW, Wise L. Postoperative arterial blood gas measurement in obese patients: effect of position on gas exchange. *Ann Surg*. 1975;182:705.

194. Russell WJ. Position of patient and respiratory function in immediate postoperative period. *BMJ*. 1981;283:1079.

195. Bonnet F, Bourgain JL, Mtamis D, et al. The influence of position on ventilation-perfusion distribution after abdominal surgery. *Acta Anaesthesiol Scand*. 1988;32:585.

196. Glass GD, Olsen GN. Preoperative pulmonary function testing to predict postoperative morbidity and mortality. *Chest*. 1986;89:127.

197. Kroenke K, Lawrence VA, Theroux JF, et al. Operative risk in patients with severe obstructive pulmonary disease. *Arch Intern Med*. 1992;152:967.

198. Warner DO, Warner MA, Offord K, et al. Airway obstruction and perioperative complications in smoker undergoing abdominal surgery. *Anesthesiology*. 1999;90:372.

199. Nunn JF, Milledge JS, Chen D, et al. Respiratory criteria of fitness for surgery and anaesthesia. *Anaesthesia*. 1988;43:543.

200. Dilworth JP, White RJ. Postoperative chest infection after upper abdominal surgery: an important problem for smokers. *Respir Med*. 1992;86:205.

201. Pasulka PS, Bistrian BR, Benotti PN, et al. The risk of surgery in obese patients. *Ann Intern Med*. 1986;104:540.

202. Berg H, Viby-Mogensen J, Roed J, et al. Residual neuromuscular block is a risk factor for postoperative pulmonary complications: a prospective, randomized, and blinded study of postoperative pulmonary complications after atracurium, vecuronium and pancuronium. *Acta Anaesthesiol Scand*. 1997;41:1095.

203. Wiren JE, Lindell SE, Hellekant C. Pre- and post-operative lung function in sitting and supine position related to postoperative chest x-ray abnormalities and arterial hypoxemia. *Clin Physiol*. 1983;3:257.

204. Christensen EF, Schultz P, Jensen OV, et al. Postoperative pulmonary complications and lung function in high-risk patients: a comparison of three physiotherapy regimens after upper abdominal surgery. *Acta Anaesthesiol Scand*. 1991;35:97.

205. Thomas JA, McIntosh JM. Are incentive spirometry, intermittent positive pressure breathing, and deep breathing exercises effective in the prevention of postoperative pulmonary complications after upper abdominal surgery? *Phys Ther*. 1994;74:3.

206. Roukema JA, Carol EJ, Prins JG. The prevention of pulmonary complications after upper abdominal surgery in patients with noncompromised pulmonary status. *Arch Surg*. 1988;123:30.

207. Schwieger I, Gamulin Z, Forster A, et al. Absence of benefit of incentive spirometry in low-risk patients undergoing elective cholecystectomy: a controlled randomized study. *Chest*. 1986;89:652.

208. Hall JC, Tarala RA, Tapper J, et al. Prevention of respiratory complications after abdominal surgery: a randomized clinical trial. *BMJ*. 1996;312:148.

209. Dahl JB, Rosenber J, Hansen BL, et al. Differential analgesic effects of low dose epidural morphine and morphine-bupivacaine at rest and during mobilization after major abdominal surgery. *Anesth Analg*. 1992;74:362.

210. Putensen-Himmer G, Putensen C, Lammer H, et al. Comparison of postoperative respiratory function after laparoscopy or open laparotomy for cholecystectomy. *Anesthesiology*. 1992;77:675.

211. Schauer PR, Luna J, Ghiatas AA, et al. Pulmonary function after laparoscopic cholecystectomy. *Surgery*. 1993;114:389.

212. Joris J, Kaba A, Lamy M. Postoperative spirometry after laparoscopy for lower abdominal or upper abdominal surgical procedures. *Br J Anaesth*. 1997;79:422.

213. Erice F, Fox GS, Salib YM, et al. Diaphragmatic function before and after laparoscopic cholecystectomy. *Anesthesiology*. 1993;79:966.

214. Benhamu D, Simmoneau G, Poynard T, et al. Diaphragm function is not impaired by pneumoperitoneum after laparoscopy. *Arch Surg*. 1993;128:430.

215. Couture JG, Chartrand D, Gagner M, et al. Diaphragmatic and abdominal muscle activity after endoscopic cholecystectomy. *Anesth Analg*. 1994;78:733.

216. The Southern Surgeons Club. A prospective analysis of 1518 laparoscopic cholecystectomies. *N Engl J Med*. 1991;324:1073.

217. Rennie JA, Christofides ND, Mitchenere P, et al. Neural and humoral factors in postoperative ileus. *Br J Surg*. 1980;67:694.

218. Graber JN, Schulte WJ, Condon RE, et al. Relationship of duration of postoperative ileus to extent and site of operative dissection. *Surgery*. 1982;92:87.

219. Condon RE, Cowles V, Ekbom GA, et al. Effects of halothane, enflurane, and nitrous oxide on colon motility. *Surgery*. 1987;101:81.

220. Scheinin B, Lindgren L, Scheinin TM. Preoperative nitrous oxide delays bowel function after colonic surgery. *Br J Anaesth*. 1990;64:154.

221. Giuffre M, Gross JB. The effects of nitrous oxide on postoperative bowel motility. *Anesthesiology*. 1986;65:699.

222. Jensen AJ, Kalman SH, Nystrom P, et al. Anaesthetic technique does

not influence postoperative bowel function: a comparison of propofol, nitrous oxide and isoflurane. *Can J Anaesth.* 1992;39:938.

223. Wilson JP. Postoperative motility of the large intestine in man. *Gut.* 1975;16:689.

224. Scheinin B, Asantila R, Orko R. The effect of bupivacaine and morphine on pain and bowel function after colonic surgery. *Acta Anaesthesiol Scand.* 1987;31:161.

225. Liu SS, Carpenter RL, Mackey DC, et al. Effects of perioperative analgesic technique on rate of recovery after colon surgery. *Anesthesiology.* 1995;83:757.

226. Steinbrok RA. Epidural anesthesia and gastrointestinal motility. *Anesth Analg.* 1998;86:830.

227. Lee TL, Ang SBL, Dambisya YM, et al. The effect of propofol on human gastric and colonic muscle contractions. *Anesth Analg.* 1999;89:1246.

228. Waldenhausen JHT, Schirmer BD. The effect of ambulation on recovery from postoperative ileus. *Ann Surg.* 1990;212:671.

229. Resnick J, Greewald DA, Brandt LJH. Delayed gastric emptying and postoperative ileus after nongastric abdominal surgery: part II. *Am J Gastroenterol.* 1997;92:934.

230. Garcia-Olmo D, Paya J, Lucas FJ, et al. The effects of the pharmacological manipulation of postoperative intestinal motility on colonic anastomoses: an experimental study in a rat model. *Int J Colorect Dis.* 1997;12:73.

231. Von Bahr V. Local anesthesia for inguinal herniorraphy. In: Eriksson E, ed. *Illustrated Handbook in Local Anaesthesia.* 2nd ed. Philadelphia, Pa: WB Saunders; 1979:52.

232. Rudkin GE, Maddern GJ. Peri-operative outcome for day-case laparoscopic and open inguinal hernia repair. *Anaesthesia.* 1995;50:586.

233. Urbach KF, Lee WR, Sheely LL, et al. Spinal or general anesthesia for inguinal hernia repair? *JAMA.* 1964;190:137.

234. Petros JG, Rimm EB, Robillard RJ, et al. Factors influencing postoperative urinary retention in patients undergoing elective inguinal herniorrhaphy. *Am J Surg.* 1991;161:431.

235. Pollock JE, Liu SS, Neal JM, et al. Dilution of spinal lidocaine does not alter the incidence of transient neurologic symptoms. *Anesthesiology.* 1999;90:445.

236. Pollock JE, Neal JM, Stephenson CA, et al. Prospective study of the incidence of transient radicular irritation in patients undergoing spinal anesthesia. *Anesthesiology.* 1996;84:1361.

237. Hiller A, Rosenberg P. Transient neurological symptoms after spinal anesthesia with 4% mepivacaine and 0.5% bupivacaine. *Br J Anaesth.* 1997;79:301.

238. Hampl KF, Heinzmann-Wiedmer S, Luginbuehol I, et al. Transient neurologic symptoms after spinal anesthesia. *Anesthesiology.* 1998;88:629.

239. Kopacz DJ, Mulroy MF. Chloroprocaine and lidocaine decrease hospital stay and admission rate after outpatient epidural anesthesia. *Reg Anesth.* 1990;15:19.

240. Tverskoy M, Cozacov C, Ayache M, et al. Postoperative pain after inguinal herniorrhaphy with different types of anesthesia. *Anesth Analg.* 1990;70:29.

241. Ryan JA Jr, Adye BA, Jolly PC, et al. Outpatient inguinal herniorrhaphy with both regional and local anesthesia. *Am J Surg.* 1984;148:313.

242. Ivatury RR, Diebel L, Porter JM, et al. Intra-abdominal hypertension and the abdominal compartment syndrome. *Surg Clin North Am.* 1997;77:783.

243. Fietsam R, Villalba M, Glover JL, et al. Intra-abdominal compartment syndrome as a complication of ruptured abdominal aortic aneurysm repair. *Am Surg.* 1989;55:396.

244. Saggi BH, Sugerman HJ, Ivatury RR, et al. Abdominal compartment syndrome. *J Trauma.* 1998;45:597.

245. Ridings PC, Bloomfield GL, Blocher CR, et al. Cardiopulmonary effects of raised intra-abdominal pressure before and after intravascular volume expansion. *J Trauma.* 1995;39:1071.

246. Kron IL, Harman PK, Nolan SP. The measurement of intra-abdominal pressure as a criterion for abdominal re-exploration. *Ann Surg.* 1984;199:28.

247. Harman PK, Kron IL, McLachlan HD, et al. Elevated intra-abdominal pressure and renal function. *Ann Surg.* 1982;196:594.

248. Bloomfield GL, Dalton JM, Sugerman HJ, et al. Treatment of increasing intracranial pressure secondary to the acute abdominal compartment syndrome in a patient with combined abdominal and head trauma. *J Trauma.* 1995;39:1168.

249. Burch JM, Moore EE, Moore FA, et al. The abdominal compartment syndrome. *Surg Clin North Am.* 1996;76:833.

250. Morris JA, Eddy VA, Blinman TA, et al. The staged celiotomy for trauma: issues in unpacking and reconstruction. *Ann Surg.* 1993;217:5763.

251. Shelly MP, Robinson AA, Hesford JW, et al. Haemodynamic effects following surgical release of increased intra-abdominal pressure. *Br J Anaesth.* 1987;59:800.

# 62

# Anesthesia for Pediatric Cardiovascular Surgery

## Laurie K. Davies

The care of children undergoing cardiovascular surgery provides a remarkable challenge to the anesthesiologist. In the 1960s, only a small fraction of patients with congenital heart disease (CHD) were offered surgical repair or palliation. Those who were offered repair or palliation experienced significant mortality and morbidity. Since the early 1970s, however, improvements in diagnostic capability, cardiopulmonary bypass (CPB) techniques, monitoring, and perioperative care have permitted more complicated procedures to be performed on smaller, sicker children with remarkable success. Even today, operative procedures and technology are being constantly modified in an effort to further improve the safety and outcome for these special children.

Each child presents a unique set of circumstances and pathophysiologic concerns. Much of the knowledge regarding appropriate management for adults undergoing cardiac surgery will not apply to these children. Anesthesiologists caring for these patients must be flexible and innovative. Rigid protocols rarely are appropriate; instead, an individualized plan for each patient is mandatory. Team effort and good communication are essential to the success of a pediatric cardiovascular surgical program. Being a part of a successful team and caring for these patients are among the most exciting and rewarding experiences in medicine today.

## MAJOR CONGENITAL HEART LESIONS

### *What Are Their Characteristics?*

#### Incidence

CHD is relatively uncommon. It is estimated to occur in somewhat fewer than 1% of all live births (Table 62–1).[1] The true incidence is probably quite a bit higher. Much fetal wastage is thought to occur because of the presence of congenital heart defects that are incompatible with life. Also, some heart lesions (eg, bicuspid aortic valve and patent ductus arteriosus [PDA]) may be relatively asymptomatic early in life. Thus, the true incidence of CHD is unknown.

Available studies have tried to estimate CHD prevalence in selected populations.[2,3] Certain lesions are more likely to become manifest early in life than are others. Thus, the prevalence of these symptomatic lesions is falsely elevated. With these caveats in mind, the lesions most likely to be encountered in the first year of life are ventricular septal defect (VSD), transposition of the great vessel (TGV), Tetralogy of Fallot, coarctation of the aorta, and hypoplastic left heart syndrome.[2]

Different reference populations may demonstrate different patterns of CHD. For instance, infants who are premature and small for their gestational ages have an increased prevalence of CHD (especially VSD and PDA) compared with full-term newborns.[4] Congenital heart defects are more common among infants of diabetic mothers than among those of nondiabetic mothers.[5] Infants with abnormal chromosomes have an increased frequency of congenital heart defects. About 23% to

**TABLE 62–1.** Reported Estimate of Prevalence per 1000 Live Births for Specific Congenital Heart Defects

| Defect | Prevalence |
| --- | --- |
| Ventricular septal defect | 0.38 |
| Transposition | 0.21 |
| Tetralogy of Fallot | 0.21 |
| Coarctation of aorta | 0.18 |
| Hypoplastic left-sided heart syndrome | 0.16 |
| Patent ductus arteriosus | 0.14 |
| Atrioventricular septal defect | 0.12 |
| Pulmonary stenosis | 0.19 |
| Pulmonary atresia | 0.07 |
| Secundum atrial septal defect | 0.07 |
| Total anomalous pulmonary venous drainage | 0.06 |
| Tricuspid atresia | 0.06 |
| Aortic stenosis | 0.04 |
| Double-outlet right ventricle | 0.03 |
| Truncus arteriosus | 0.03 |
| Other | 0.18 |

Modified from Daniels SR. Epidemiology. In: Long WA, ed. *Fetal and Neonatal Cardiology*. Philadelphia, Pa: WB Saunders; 1990:430.

56% of children with trisomy 21 have CHD.[6] The most common defects in children with Down syndrome appear to be VSD, atrial septal defect (ASD), PDA, and atrioventricular canal defects.[7]

#### Severity

Patients with CHD present a broad spectrum of severity of illness. Some patients may be asymptomatic and found only incidentally to have an ASD or PDA. Others may be moribund with congestive heart failure (CHF), cyanosis, or a combination of the two. Keith studied 10 535 cases of cardiac defects at the Hospital for Sick Children in Toronto from 1950 to 1970.[8] Twenty-seven percent of the patients died during the period of observation, and 34% died during the first month of life.

#### Prognosis

The outlook for these children today has improved considerably over that of previous years. A better understanding of the pathophysiology of individual lesions allows a rational treatment care plan to be developed. Earlier complete repairs of CHD are being performed successfully, often resulting in avoidance of the long-term sequelae of unrepaired CHD. Cardiac transplantation also has become a viable option for some children whose lesions cannot be surgically repaired. For any of these options to be successful, the patient's care must be thoughtfully individualized with vigilance, anticipation, and meticulous attention to detail.

## PHYSIOLOGIC CONSIDERATIONS

### *What Is the Difference Between Fetal and Adult Circulation?*

In order to develop an understanding of the clinical and anesthetic implications of CHD, one must be familiar with fetal and adult circulations. Three important channels characteristic of the circulation in utero allow preferential shunting of blood: ductus venosus, foramen ovale, and ductus arteriosus (Fig. 62–1).

#### Ductus Venosus

Well-oxygenated blood from the placenta, with a $Po_2$ of about 33 mm Hg, travels through the umbilical vein to enter the liver.[9] The ductus venosus allows about one half of this blood to be shunted from the liver directly into the inferior vena cava.

#### Foramen Ovale

About one third of the blood entering the right atrium from the inferior vena cava is preferentially shunted across the foramen ovale into the left atrium. On the other hand, superior vena cava blood (which is poorly oxygenated) primarily enters the right ventricle, with 2% to 3% crossing the foramen ovale.

#### Ductus Arteriosus

Right ventricular blood is largely shunted across the ductus arteriosus into the descending aorta (rather than perfusing the high-resistance pulmonary circulation).

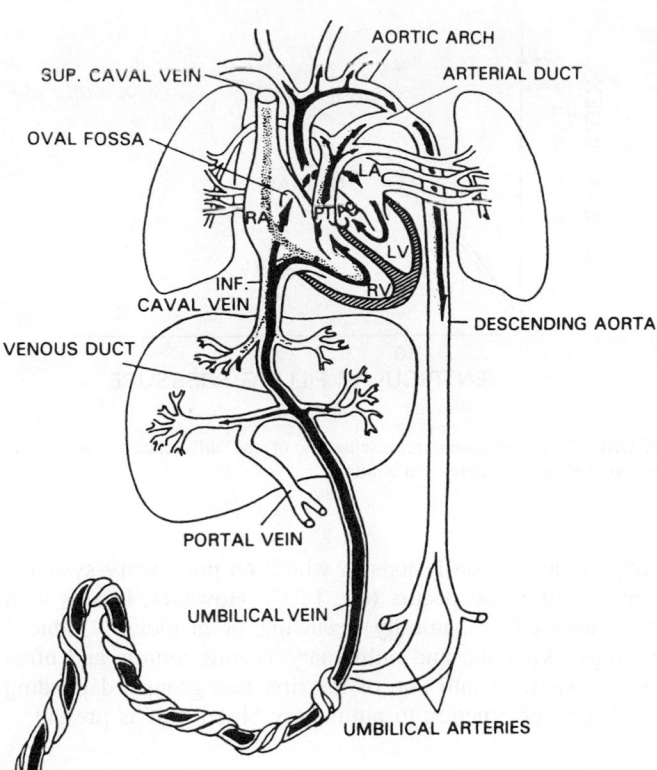

**FIGURE 62–1.** Diagram of the course of the fetal circulation. (From Ho SY, Angelini A, Moscoso G. Developmental cardiac anatomy. In: Long WA, ed. *Fetal and Neonatal Cardiology.* 1st ed. Philadelphia, Pa: WB Saunders; 1990:4.)

## Implications

The structure of the fetal circulation allows the well-oxygenated blood (which has a high glucose content) from the inferior vena cava to preferentially perfuse the brain, coronary circulation, and upper extremities. The lower portion of the body receives blood with a low oxygen content from the ductus arteriosus.[10] Hence, the systemic and pulmonary circulations in the fetus function in parallel, with each ventricle receiving only a portion of the systemic cardiac output.[11] The adult situation, in contrast, requires the two circulations to work in series, each processing the entire cardiac output.

## *What Is the Transitional Circulation?*

At birth, remarkable changes occur rapidly in the circulation that allow the infant to adapt to the stresses of extrauterine life.[12] A period of transition in the neonatal circulation occurs before permanent adaptation to the normal adult pattern takes place. This transitional stage is unstable and may exist for a few hours or for many weeks, depending on the stresses imposed. Factors contributing to the instability of the transitional circulation are the state of the ductus arteriosus, foramen ovale, and pulmonary vascular bed, as well as the immaturity of the neonatal heart. Conditions that may prolong the transitional circulation include hypoxia, hypothermia, acidosis, hypercarbia, sepsis, and CHD.[13]

### Closure of the Ductus Arteriosus

Functional closure of the ductus arteriosus usually occurs within a few hours of birth, but anatomic closure may not occur for several weeks.[14] During this period, the resistance to ductus arteriosus blood flow is responsive to changes in $PaO_2$; that is, increased $PaO_2$ increases duct resistance, and decreased $PaO_2$ decreases resistance. Prostaglandin $E_1$ ($PGE_1$) infusion relaxes the ductal musculature and increases ductal flow, which may be left-to-right, right-to-left, or bidirectional.[15] Maintenance of ductal patency may be important for the infant with cyanotic heart disease until repair or palliative surgery can be performed.

### Closure of the Foramen Ovale and Ductus Venosus

The foramen ovale functionally closes when left atrial pressure exceeds right atrial pressure; this usually occurs within a few hours after birth. Anatomic closure does not occur for many months, and about 30% of adults demonstrate probe patency of the foramen ovale.[16] Right-to-left intracardiac shunting may occur across this area with coughing or the Valsalva maneuver or if pulmonary hypertension develops. Umbilical arteries and veins close shortly after birth, as does the ductus venosus. The latter forms the ligamentum venosum.

### Pulmonary Vascular Resistance

Pulmonary vascular resistance is high in utero, but it declines rapidly after birth. Usually, it is lower than systemic levels within 24 hours of birth. Thereafter, it falls at a moderate rate for 5 to 6 weeks and then more gradually for the next 2 to 3 years.[17,18] During this period, a child's pulmonary vascular bed is more reactive than an adult's, and a rise in pulmonary artery (PA) pressure can easily be produced by hypoxemia, hypercarbia, acidosis, or bronchospasm. If this reaction occurs shortly after birth, it may result in shunting across the ductus arteriosus or foramen ovale or another cardiac defect. Later in life, usually only a patent foramen ovale or cardiac defect remains as a possible shunt site.

## *How Is a Child's Heart Structurally Different Than That of an Adult?*

### Size

At birth, both ventricles are approximately equal in size and wall thickness. With the change-over from the fetal circulation, the left ventricle must accommodate a greater pressure and volume workload; conversely, the pressure load of the right ventricle is reduced, and its volume work is only slightly increased. The left ventricle hypertrophies in response to the increased workload and becomes roughly twice as heavy as the right ventricle by about 6 months of age.[19]

### Ultrastructure

The neonate's heart is ultrastructurally immature. Myofibrils are arranged in a disorderly fashion and have a smaller percentage of contractile proteins than do those in the adult (30% versus 60%).[20] Autonomic innervation is also incomplete at birth. The sympathetic innervation to the heart is decreased as are cardiac catecholamine stores.[21] In contrast, the parasympathetic innervation of the neonatal heart is comparable with that of the adult heart.[22] These observations are often cited to explain the frequent vagal predominance that occurs in infants compared with adults.

Sympathetic innervation also is immature in the peripheral vasculature. Therefore, control of vascular tone and myocardial contractility in infants depends largely on adrenal function and circulating or exogenously administered catecholamines. There are also differences in myocardial calcium metabolism.[23] In the mature myocardium, the sarcoplasmic reticulum is the predominant source of calcium ion for excitation-contraction coupling, but the sarcoplasmic reticulum is poorly developed in the immature heart. Because the neonatal myocardial cell is deficient in T-tubules that, in the mature myocardium, provide electrical coupling between the cell membrane and the sarcoplasmic reticulum, it is incapable of internal release and reuptake of calcium for contraction and instead depends on transmembrane calcium transport for the development of tension. These differences in calcium handling by the cell provide some explanation for the clinical observation that newborns require greater serum ionized calcium levels for optimal myocardial contractility.

## Compliance

The immature heart has a functionally decreased compliance when compared with the adult heart. This difference, in part, reflects the ultrastructure of the heart and the increased volume load that each ventricle must handle with the transition from a parallel fetal to an adult series circulation.[13] The right and left ventricles are more intimately interrelated as a result of this decreased compliance and similarity in size. Dysfunction of one ventricle quickly leads to biventricular failure. Reduced compliance also means that the immature heart is more sensitive to volume overload. A neonate's ventricular function curve is shifted to the right and downward compared with that of an adult. Over the physiologic range of ventricular filling pressures, stroke volume changes are, in fact, small.

This relatively fixed stroke volume makes a neonate highly dependent on heart rate and sinus rhythm for optimal cardiac output. In comparison, the adult heart is much more responsive to changes in preload to effect a change in stroke volume and thereby change cardiac output. Increases in pressure work are poorly tolerated by both the right and left sides of the immature heart. The neonate, therefore, responds poorly to either volume or pressure loading because resting cardiac function is on or near the plateau of the cardiac function curve (Fig. 62–2).

## *How Are Congenital Cardiac Lesions Meaningfully Characterized?*

### Flow Pattern

Patients with congenital heart defects are a diverse group. Rather than memorize an approach to each lesion, one should group the many anatomic varieties into a few understandable categories (Table 62–2). Most defects can be assigned to one of three groups:

1. Those resulting in increased pulmonary blood flow
2. Those resulting in decreased pulmonary blood flow
3. Those resulting in obstruction to blood flow

The first two groups feature an abnormal shunt pathway, whereas the third group has no shunting of blood. A fourth

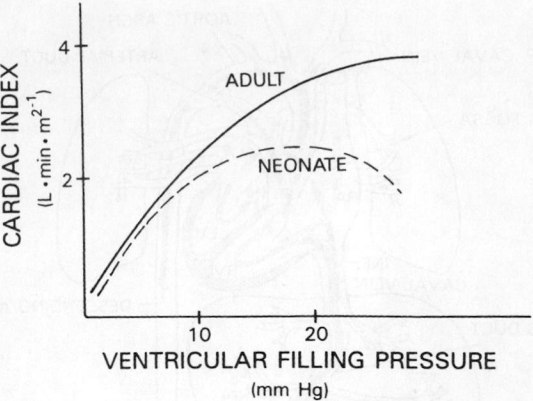

**FIGURE 62–2.** Schematic representation of the difference in ventricular function between neonates and adults.

group could include lesions in which no pulmonary-systemic exchange of blood occurs (eg, TGV). However, infants with TGV have either naturally occurring or artificially induced mixing of systemic and pulmonary venous returns and often can be classified into one of the first two groups, depending on whether obstruction to pulmonary blood flow is present.

## Cyanosis Versus Heart Failure

Cyanosis and CHF are the major manifestations of CHD. Thus, the pathophysiologic classification must be related to the clinical status. Cyanosis occurs most commonly with lesions in which pulmonary blood flow is anatomically de-

**TABLE 62–2.** Flow Characteristics of Various Congenital Cardiac Lesions

**Increased Pulmonary Blood Flow Lesions**

Atrial septal defect
Ventricular septal defect
Patent ductus arteriosus
Endocardial cushion defect (atrioventricular canal abnormality)
Anomalous origin of coronary arteries
Transposition of the great arteries*
Anomalous pulmonary venous drainage*
Truncus arteriosus*
Single ventricle*

**Decreased Pulmonary Blood Flow Lesions**

Tetralogy of Fallot
Pulmonary atresia
Tricuspid atresia
Ebstein anomaly
Truncus arteriosus*
Transposition of the great arteries*
Single ventricle*

**Obstructive Lesions**

Aortic stenosis
Pulmonary stenosis
Coarctation of the aorta
Asymmetric septal hypertrophy

*Systemic hypoxemia occurs as a result of the mixing of systemic and pulmonary venous returns. Classification as an increased or decreased pulmonary blood flow lesion depends on the absence or presence within the anatomic variation of obstruction to pulmonary blood flow.

Modified from Schwartz AJ, Campbell FW. Pathophysiological approach to congenital heart disease. In: Lake CL, ed. *Pediatric Cardiac Anesthesia.* Norwalk, Conn: Appleton & Lange; 1988:9.

creased or functionally decreased as mixing of systemic and pulmonary venous blood occurs.

CHF occurs most commonly in shunt lesions with excessively increased pulmonary blood flow or obstructive lesions that stress the ventricle beyond its capacity to pump effectively.[24] Note that a child can be cyanotic but still fall into the category of having a lesion with increased pulmonary blood flow and may even manifest CHF. An example of such a situation is an infant with TGV and a large VSD. Even the most complex lesions usually fall into one of the three categories, even if they are characterized by mixed features (see Table 62–2).[24]

## When and Why Do Patients Become Symptomatic?

Many types of CHD may not be detected immediately after birth. The age at which heart defects become manifest obviously depends on the type of lesion, its severity, and the state of the infant's transitional circulation. Increased pulmonary blood flow lesions typically become symptomatic as pulmonary vascular resistance decreases and shunt flow to the lungs increases. These changes may take days to weeks to occur. Also, if the defect is small, it may remain asymptomatic.

Decreased pulmonary blood flow lesions often are detected earlier, usually because they result in significant cyanosis. If obstruction to pulmonary blood flow is severe, patients with such lesions may be dependent on left-to-right flow across their PDA. As the PDA closes in the first few days of life, hypoxemia becomes even more pronounced and may be incompatible with survival.

Infants with TGV and an inadequate intracardiac communication become extremely cyanotic as their PDA closes. On the other hand, if a large VSD or PDA is present, these patients develop excessive pulmonary blood flow as the pulmonary vascular resistance decreases during the first few weeks of extrauterine life. Left untreated, hypertrophic vascular changes and pulmonary hypertension will occur.

Left-sided obstructive lesions cause pulmonary congestion without pulmonary volume overload. They impede flow from the pulmonary venous system to the systemic arterial system and can precipitate CHF. The symptomatology and age at presentation depend on the severity of the lesion. If the ductus arteriosus is patent, it allows right-to-left shunting of blood around the lesion, improving systemic perfusion but causing cyanosis.

## PREOPERATIVE ASSESSMENT

## What Should the Anesthesiologist Look for?

In developing an anesthetic plan for these children, be sure to understand the pathophysiology of the individual lesion and to appreciate the degree of clinical symptomatology. As in any other assessment, taking of a careful history and the physical examination are probably the most important parts of the preoperative evaluation. Remember that the infant cannot tell you the symptoms experienced, and the parents often fail to understand the significance of some of their observations.

### Age at Presentation

The age at presentation often provides a clue to the severity of the lesion. Infants with decreased pulmonary blood flow or inadequate mixing may be persistently cyanotic or may have intermittent episodes that are often associated with agitation, crying, or exercise. If a child is older, cyanotic episodes may be associated with "squatting" (which increases systemic vascular resistance and promotes increased pulmonary blood flow). Particularly severe episodes can result in loss of consciousness or seizures.

### Frequency of Episodes

The frequency of these episodes also suggests the severity of the lesion. Knowledge that cyanotic episodes are intermittent confirms the dynamic nature of the shunt and should alert one to the fact that the same scenario is probable during anesthesia and surgical manipulations. Alterations in systemic and pulmonary vascular resistance may result in profound changes in the magnitude of the right-to-left shunt.

### Cyanosis

During the physical examination, an important consideration is that clinical cyanosis depends on the absolute concentration of deoxygenated hemoglobin in the blood rather than on the oxygen saturation. More than 3 g/dL of deoxygenated arterial blood hemoglobin should make central cyanosis recognizable.[25] The oxyhemoglobin saturation at which central cyanosis becomes clinically apparent varies from about 62% when hemoglobin level is 8 g/dL to about 88% in the polycythemic infant whose hemoglobin level is 24 g/dL. Thus, cyanosis is more easily detected when the infant's hematocrit (Hct) is elevated. However, recognition of cyanosis is more difficult if a newborn has a significant proportion of fetal hemoglobin because it is more highly saturated at a given $Po_2$ (Fig. 62–3).[25] Therefore, the newborn with a high proportion of fetal hemoglobin may require a large reduction in $Pao_2$ before central cyanosis is clinically apparent.[25]

### Respiration

Infants with cyanotic heart disease often have an increased tidal volume. Clubbing of the fingers may also occur but may not be evident early in life. Children with decreased pulmonary blood flow usually have exercise intolerance. Progressive polycythemia is characteristic of lesions with inadequate pulmonary blood flow. Infants with preductal coarctation of the aorta may demonstrate cyanosis that is restricted to the lower half of the body if the right ventricle supplies the descending aorta with deoxygenated blood via a PDA.

### Congestive Heart Failure

Infants with too much pulmonary blood flow present with CHF early in infancy when the pulmonary vascular resistance decreases. A history of feeding difficulties and failure to thrive are characteristic of CHF in infancy. Other features include tachypnea, tachycardia, inappropriate sweating (often with feeding), nasal flaring, sternal and intercostal retractions, cardiomegaly, and hepatomegaly. A history of wheezing, frequent respiratory infections, and pneumonia is common. The distinc-

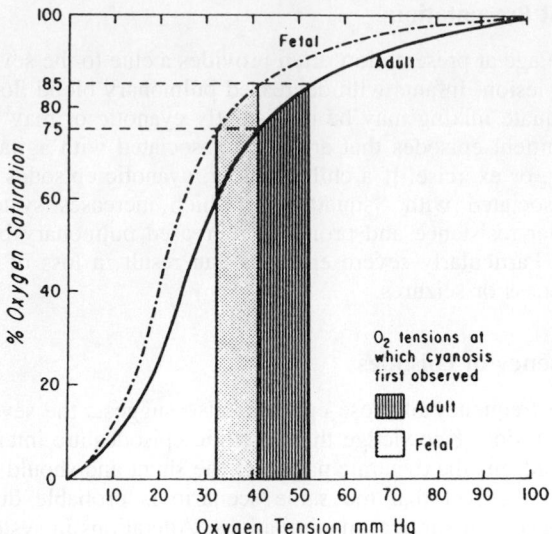

**FIGURE 62–3.** Hemoglobin-oxygen dissociation curves for fetal and adult hemoglobin. Note that an infant with a high proportion of fetal hemoglobin will have a very low PaO$_2$ (33-42 mm Hg) before cyanosis is observed. (From Lees MH, King DH. Heart disease in the newborn. In: Adams FH, Emmanouilides GC, Riemenschneider TA, eds. *Heart Disease in Infants, Children and Adolescents.* Baltimore, Md: Williams & Wilkins; 1989:844.)

tion between left-sided and right-sided heart failure in the newborn is less obvious than in the adult. Peripheral edema and râles are rarely present in the infant. Systemic perfusion may be compromised as evidenced by decreased pulses, pallor, and poor capillary refill. A severely compromised infant may be apathetic and have a weak cry and little spontaneous movement.

Left-sided obstructive lesions may also cause CHF with clinical manifestations that are similar to those of pulmonary volume overload. Note, however, that the symptoms are a result of pulmonary venous congestion without abnormal shunting. If the lesion is located so that left ventricular *outflow* is obstructed, left ventricular hypertrophy will develop; if the site of obstruction involves the *inflow* to the left ventricle, left ventricular hypertrophy does not occur and left ventricular end-diastolic pressure is normal.

### Associated Anomalies

Look carefully for associated congenital anomalies because they are common in newborns with cardiac disease. Other problems unique to the newborn or premature infant include difficulty with temperature regulation, impaired nutrition, susceptibility to dehydration and hypoglycemia, respiratory difficulties, coagulation abnormalities, and central nervous system (CNS) disorders.

### *What Preoperative Laboratory Studies Are Helpful?*

Laboratory studies of particular interest include Hct, white blood cell count, coagulation profile, and electrolyte and serum glucose determinations. Sickle cell screening and measurement of digoxin level should be included when applicable.

### Hematocrit

The hematocrit progressively rises as hypoxemia becomes more profound. In fact, periodic checks of the hematocrit provide a simple method to follow the patient's level of hypoxemia. Increasing hematocrit may serve as a cue for the appropriate timing of surgery for patients with complex cyanotic lesions. A high hematocrit can result in increased blood viscosity, which can lead to spontaneous thrombosis and resultant cerebral, renal, or pulmonary infarctions. This process may be aggravated by the relative dehydration produced by a long period without oral intake. If the polycythemia is sufficiently severe (ie, hematocrit is >60%-65%), phlebotomy may be required. Patients with cyanotic CHD are prone to develop coagulopathies because of platelet dysfunction and hypofibrinogenemia.[26,27] These patients also have a blunted ventilatory response to hypoxia.[28]

### White Blood Cell Count

Elevations in white blood cell count and a white blood cell shift in the differential should raise the suspicion of a systemic infection. Fever and upper respiratory infection must be ruled out. Children with elevated white blood cell counts should not be electively anesthetized because immunologic function is compromised by CPB. Also, prosthetic material is frequently used in the surgical repair; if this material is inadvertently seeded by a bacteremia, the consequences may be disastrous.

### Coagulation Studies

Results of coagulation studies must be normal before CPB can be performed. A family history of bleeding tendencies should be sought. Unsuspected factor deficiencies have manifested and caused uncontrollable bleeding following surgery, when it may be difficult to identify the source of the problem. It may be particularly difficult to accurately test for a coagulopathy in patients who are polycythemic. The testing matrix for a protime or partial thromboplastin time assumes that a certain amount of plasma is present. If a patient's hematocrit is exceptionally high, he or she will have a proportionately lesser amount of plasma for the reagents. Thus, the results may be spuriously elevated even when the patient does not have a factor deficiency or an inhibitor. If the concern exists, one may wish to perform a 1:1 dilution with normal plasma. If the test result normalizes, this is suggestive that the patient's coagulation status is acceptable.

### Electrolytes

Electrolyte problems may be present in the newborn, especially if the child is receiving medication or total parenteral nutrition. Hypokalemia, hypomagnesemia, hypocalcemia, and hypoglycemia should be ruled out. Hypocalcemia is common in children with DiGeorge syndrome (a congenital disorder of the third and fourth branchial arches that is associated with thymic hypoplasia and congenital heart defects, especially aortic arch abnormalities).

### Glucose

Hypoglycemia is especially common in infants with hypoplastic left-sided heart syndrome. The newborn's myocardium has an increased glucose dependence compared with the adult myocardium; thus, hypoglycemia may aggravate myocardial failure.[29] Hypoglycemia can occur because of reduced synthetic function, decreased glycogen stores, or reduced systemic perfusion resulting in compromised hepatic function. Under anesthesia, hypoglycemia will be masked and may be missed unless the anesthesiologist looks for it. Conversely, these children often come to the operating room with concentrated dextrose in their hyperalimentation solution. Steroids are commonly administered on CPB and when combined with dextrose, can result in significant hyperglycemia. Substantial literature exists showing the detrimental effects of hyperglycemia during complete, incomplete, and focal cerebral ischemia in animals and adult people.[30–33] Specific data are lacking in children, although Steward and colleagues[34] suggested a worsened neurologic outcome with hyperglycemia in a retrospective review of 34 children undergoing deep hypothermic circulatory arrest (DHCA). In contrast, the Boston Circulatory Arrest Study suggested that normal blood glucose levels during reperfusion were associated with poorer neurologic outcome, whereas hyperglycemic levels appeared associated with better outcome.[35] It has been speculated that in the immature brain, substrate deficiency may be an issue and that normal blood glucose levels during the reperfusion period after cerebral ischemia in infants may be insufficient for complete cerebral recovery.

### Digoxin

Many children scheduled for heart surgery are receiving digoxin. Following CPB, both a rebound increase in digoxin level and an increased sensitivity to the drug have been reported.[36] Perioperative dysrhythmias are common and may be related to digoxin toxicity; other factors may play a role in this enhanced toxicity, including hypokalemia, calcium fluxes, hypomagnesemia, and decreased creatinine clearance. Therefore, verify that the digoxin level is within the normal range and withhold digoxin preoperatively.

### Sickling Test

A sickling test should be performed in appropriate children. Hypothermia, acidosis, and anemia—as induced by CPB—as well as decreased perfusion enhance sickling if hemoglobin S is present. If the sickling test result is positive, hemoglobin electrophoresis should be performed to delineate the type of hemoglobinopathy. Depending on the type of defect, exchange transfusion may be indicated before CPB.

### Electrocardiography

The electrocardiogram (ECG) shows great variability, especially during the first 24 hours of life. In some instances, the ECG is diagnostically helpful. For example, extreme left or right axis deviation with counterclockwise frontal vector and right ventricular hypertrophy suggests a form of endocardial cushion defect.

### Echocardiography and Cardiac Catheterization

Two-dimensional echocardiography with quantitative Doppler and color flow mapping has revolutionized the diagnosis of CHD. In many institutions, the technology has become so

refined that most surgical procedures are performed on the basis of this study alone. Cardiac catheterization is used to confirm the diagnosis and to provide information concerning vascular resistance, the magnitude of shunts, and coronary anatomy.

### Chest Radiography

Chest radiography serves to evaluate the type and severity of heart disease. It is also used to identify simulators of heart disease (eg, meconium aspiration, mediastinal masses, pneumothorax, hyaline membrane disease, and diaphragmatic hernia) and to rule out significant pulmonary pathology.

## What Should the Anesthesiologist Tell the Family About Risk?

### Anesthetic Risk

A comprehensive evaluation of anesthetic complications and outcome in 500 consecutive patients undergoing CHD operations has been performed.[37] Several anesthetic agents were used, including thiopental, ketamine, narcotics, and inhalation agents. No apparent differences in outcome were detected with these different agents. During hospitalization, a perioperative mortality of 6.3% occurred; no death was directly attributable to anesthesia. Anesthetic complications (major and minor) occurred in 2% of cases.

A 1991 abstract examined risk in patients with CHD undergoing noncardiac surgery.[38] A total of 135 anesthetic procedures in 110 patients were analyzed. Almost one half of the patients (47%) experienced an *adverse event,* which was broadly defined as any unexpected event that was not part of a routine, uncomplicated anesthetic case (Table 62–3). Not all adverse events resulted in perioperative complications. Uncompensated CHF, cyanosis, and uncorrected heart disease were associated with a higher risk of adverse events. Patients with tetralogy of Fallot had the highest incidence of adverse events (9 of 13 patients); the most common complication involved airway difficulties. Thus, patients with CHD represent a challenge in both cardiac and noncardiac surgery.

### Neurologic Sequelae

Morbidity and mortality vary, depending on the lesion being repaired or palliated and the institution involved. Ironically,

**TABLE 62–3.** 135 Operations (Noncardiac Surgery) With Perioperative Complications in Patients With Congenital Heart Disease

| Adverse Event | No. of Patients |
| --- | --- |
| Airway emergency | 22 |
| Bronchospasm | 4 |
| Dysrhythmias | 17 |
| Circulatory instability | 16 |
| Acidosis | 2 |
| Hypoglycemia | 1 |
| Delayed emergence | 4 |
| Nausea/emesis | 5 |

From Strafford MA, Henderson KH. Anesthetic morbidity in congenital heart disease patients undergoing noncardiac surgery. *Anesthesiology.* 1991;75:A1056.

as mortality has decreased, important morbidities have become more prominent. Neurologic sequelae remains one of the most common and potentially devastating complications of CHD and its repair. Early postoperative neurologic dysfunction may occur in as many as 25% of these children, with seizures occurring in approximately 20% of neonates following CPB.[39,40] The seizures are generally self-limited, with some early series reporting no long-term adverse sequelae.[41,42] However, the group from Boston was the first to prospectively study a relatively homogeneous group of infants with TGV undergoing repair using either a predominantly low-flow CPB or DHCA strategy. They demonstrated that seizures are an important prognostic indicator of neurodevelopmental outcome.[43] The study also showed that there was a significantly higher incidence of seizures among infants randomized to circulatory arrest compared with those randomized to low-flow bypass. Follow-up of these children has shown a continued significant association between postoperative seizures and outcome, with a considerable decrement in cognitive and verbal skills assessments as well as motor skills.[44] Avoidance of circulatory arrest is not the entire solution to the problem, however; the Boston group showed that even when continuous bypass was used, a risk of seizures and suboptimal neurodevelopmental outcome existed.

Multiple factors contribute to the risk for neurodevelopmental sequelae. A complex interaction of preoperative, perioperative, and postoperative events can conspire to produce brain injury. Many children with CHD have pre-existing brain malformations.[45] Multiple chromosomal anomalies with combined cardiac and neurologic features have been described, the best known being Down syndrome (trisomy 21) and the Catch-22 spectrum of conditions that is associated with microdeletions in the 22q11 region of chromosome 22.[46] Neurologic manifestations of the Catch-22 spectrum may be subtle early in life but become more apparent over time. The potential impact of this chromosomal anomaly is enormous because monosomy 22q11 has an estimated prevalence of 5% to 10% in the population of children with CHD. Brain injury may also be acquired in the preoperative period. Abnormal cardiovascular function may be associated with poor brain growth, embolic infarction, cerebrovascular thrombosis, and abscess formation. Hopefully, earlier diagnosis and repair of CHD in children will limit this mechanism of brain injury. Hypoxic-ischemic-reperfusion injury is thought to be the principal mechanism of brain injury occurring in the intraoperative period.[47] Injury can also occur in the postoperative period during which unstable hemodynamics and increased cerebral energy needs may result in a mismatch of oxygen supply and demand to the brain. Intensive research is ongoing in this area of brain injury to try to prevent this important problem.

### When Should Oral Intake Stop?

Nil per os guidelines used for other infants and children can generally be used in patients with CHD. Evidence suggests that clear liquids can be continued until 2 to 4 hours before surgery.[48] In children with cyanotic heart disease, meticulous attention must be paid to the patient's state of hydration. Specifically, orders are written to awaken the child 2 hours before surgery to offer clear liquids. If uncertainty exists concerning the precise time of surgery, place an intravenous catheter and begin an infusion to prevent dehydration in patients with cyanotic heart disease.

### What Sedation Is Appropriate?

The need for sedation must be individualized, but certain guidelines can be offered. A thorough explanation to the patient and family is in order because the parents' anxiety is often transmitted to the child. Neonates and infants under the age of 6 months rarely require any sedation because separation anxiety is not an issue. In older children, if intravenous access is already established and the child's parents are allowed to accompany him or her to the preoperative holding area, additional sedation may be unnecessary because incremental intravenous agents can be titrated before transfer to the operating room.

Children between the ages of 1 and 5 years benefit most from judicious sedation. A variety of agents and routes can be used. I prefer to avoid intramuscular injections and use either intravenous or oral midazolam. If given intravenously, I titrate in 0.1- to 0.25-mg increments, whereas if given orally, I give 0.5 mg/kg. Patient acceptance is improved if the drug is offered in sweetened apple juice. An oral dose of 0.5 mg/kg typically results in easy separation from the parents at 10 to 20 minutes. If given intranasally, 0.2 mg/kg will be effective at about 10 to 15 minutes. These patients must be monitored when sedation is given. Pulse oximetry and careful observation are mandatory because the hemodynamic status may be adversely and unpredictably affected if hypercarbia or hypoxemia occur.

Some physicians routinely administer anticholinergics preoperatively. Others give atropine in the operating room only if clinically necessary. Keep in mind that slow heart rates are often not tolerated in infants whose stroke volume is relatively fixed.

### When Does the Patient Need Intravenous Access?

Children requiring vasoactive infusions preoperatively come to the operating room with such access already available. For others, the timing of intravenous access is strictly up to the anesthesiologist involved. For many cases, a gentle inhalation induction with subsequent expeditious venous catheter placement before intubation is appropriate. Again, if the timing of surgery is uncertain, preoperative intravenous catheter placement is desirable to avoid dehydration, especially in children with cyanotic heart disease.

### When Is Prostaglandin E₁ Indicated?

$PGE_1$ is indicated whenever it is thought that maintaining, reopening, or enlarging an existing ductus arteriosus will benefit the neonate. Common situations in which it is used include the presence of (1) lesions with decreased pulmonary blood flow, (2) TGV, and (3) left-sided heart outflow obstruction.

With TGV, the response to $PGE_1$ is variable, but in some infants, mixing of systemic and pulmonary circulation improves sufficiently to reduce hypoxemia slightly and to relieve acidosis. With left-sided heart outflow obstruction (eg, hypoplastic left-sided heart syndrome, coarctation) $PGE_1$ will open the ductus and allow right-to-left flow across it, thereby improving systemic perfusion and perhaps even coronary blood flow. It also may dilate the pulmonary vascular bed.

Stabilization of the infant before surgical intervention with $PGE_1$ infusion often results in improved outcome. Side effects include apneic spells, seizures, systemic hypotension, inhibition of platelet aggregation, peripheral edema, and unexplained fever. Cortical proliferation in long bones can occur with chronic use. Because $PGE_1$ is rapidly metabolized, it must be continuously infused, usually at a dose of 0.05 to 0.1 μg/kg/min. As much as 80% of circulating $PGE_1$ is metabolized in one pass through the lungs; thus, the ductal response diminishes within minutes after its discontinuation.

# EQUIPMENT AND INFUSIONS

## What Is Required?

Care for an infant undergoing heart surgery demands meticulous attention to detail and extreme vigilance. A well thought-out plan should be developed before induction so that all equipment needed is available and in working order (Table 62–4).

### Anesthetic and Surgical Considerations

The anesthesia machine and circuit should be checked as for all procedures. Multiple sizes of endotracheal tubes (ETTs), masks, and laryngoscope blades must be available. Appropriate equipment to keep the infant warm may be needed, including a heating-cooling blanket, radiant warming lights, a fluid warmer, and a heated humidifier. A working operating room table that allows optimal positioning to facilitate surgical exposure is required. A defibrillator with both nonsterile (external) and sterile (internal) paddles, a dual-chamber pacemaker generator, a cardiac output computer, and a coagulation analyzer must be operational. A fibrillator is frequently also needed intraoperatively to induce ventricular fibrillation during open chamber procedures.

### Monitoring

Equipment needed to monitor the patient includes a pulse oximeter, a hemodynamic monitor, appropriate catheters for arterial and venous cannulation, transducers (zeroed and calibrated to mercury), a blood pressure cuff, a stethoscope, thermistors, and a mixed venous oxygen saturation monitor. Equipment used to monitor CNS function may include electroencephalography (EEG), transcranial Doppler (TCD), jugular venous saturation monitors, and near-infrared spectroscopy. Transesophageal echocardiography has become an extraordinarily valuable tool for both diagnostic purposes (eg, confirmation and delineation of anatomy, detection of unsuspected defects or residual defects postrepair) and ventricular function and volume monitoring.

### Intravenous Fluids

Two intravenous fluid sets should be prepared, and all air bubbles should be removed from the tubing. This task is made easier if one begins with warm fluid; microbubble formation seems to occur less frequently than if cold fluid is allowed to warm when the room temperature is raised. All intravenous and monitoring tubing must be bubble-free whenever a potential shunt is present because intracardiac shunts can be bidirectional and may become right-to-left during surgery. Air filters can be used but should not be relied on to trap all air; thus, every effort must be expended to remove air from intravenous tubing. Another drawback to air filters is that they slow down intravenous infusions significantly and may make it difficult to keep up with volume replacement.

A method to carefully control and limit intravenous fluid intake is important because many patients have barely compensated excess pulmonary blood flow and volume. Infusion using a limited amount in a burette chamber and a minidripper, use of infusion pumps with set volumes, or administration of fluid via syringe in bolus increments are methods that can be used to limit intake. At least three infusion pumps that allow accurate titration of vasoactive drugs should be available.

### Preparation of Infusions

Appropriate intravenous solutions for mixing infusions (eg, normal saline and 5% dextrose in water) and cassettes for the pumps should be on hand. Common infusions to have available on short notice include sodium nitroprusside, epinephrine, dopamine, and amrinone or milrinone.

Some thought should be given to the appropriate concentrations for the patient's body size so that fluid overload can be minimized. In general, I find it useful to mix the infusions so that a starting dose infuses at about 2 to 3 mL/h. In the following example for sodium nitroprusside, I solve for concentration so that my infusion pump rate is approximately 2 to 3 mL/h:

$$\text{Rate} \atop (2\text{-}3 \text{ mL/h}) = \frac{\text{μg/kg/min} \times \text{Weight (kg)} \times 60 \text{ min/h}}{\text{Concentration (μg/mL)}}$$

If the patient weighs 10 kg and a starting dose of 1 μg/kg/min is desired, the formula follows:

$$3 \text{ mL/h} = \frac{1 \text{ μg/kg/min} \times 10 \text{ kg} \times 60 \text{ min/h}}{200 \text{ μg/mL}}$$

Therefore, I would mix 50 mg of sodium nitroprusside in 250 mL of diluent for a final concentration of 200 μg/mL and begin my infusion at 3 mL/h. Table 62–5 lists commonly used drugs and bolus doses or initial infusion rates.

In general, infusions are not prepared unless they are needed. Instead, commonly needed drugs are mixed in syrin-

**TABLE 62–4.** Equipment Used During Pediatric Cardiac Surgery

| | |
|---|---|
| Heating/Cooling blanket | Pacemaker generator |
| Radiant warming lights | Coagulation analyzer |
| Fluid warmer | Fibrillator |
| Heated humidifier | Infusion pumps |
| Defibrillator (external, internal) | Transesophageal echocardiography |

**TABLE 62–5.** Nonanesthetic Drugs and Dosages*

| | Drug | Dose |
|---|---|---|
| Inotropic infusions | Epinephrine | 0.01-0.1 μg/kg/min |
| | Isoproterenol | 0.01-0.1 μg/kg/min |
| | Norepinephrine | 0.01-0.1 μg/kg/min |
| | Dopamine | 2-10 μg/kg/min |
| | Dobutamine | 2-10 μg/kg/min |
| | Amrinone† | 2-2.5 mg/kg bolus divided over 30-60 min, followed by 5-20 μg/kg/min infusion |
| | Milrinone | 50 μg/kg bolus, followed by 0.4-0.8 μg/kg/min infusion |
| Vasodilator infusions | Nitroglycerin | 1-2 μg/kg/min |
| | Nitroprusside | 1-5 μg/kg/min |
| | Aminophylline | 0.5 mg/kg slowly, followed by 0.5-1 mg/kg/h infusion‡ |
| | Prostaglandin E₁ | 0.05-0.1 μg/kg/min |
| | Labetalol | 10-100 mg/h |
| Antiarrhythmic drugs | Lidocaine | 1-mg/kg bolus 0.03 mg/kg/min infusion |
| | Adenosine | 0.15 mg/kg bolus |
| | Procainamide | 2 mg/kg over 5 min |
| | Dilantin | 2-4 mg/kg over 5 min |
| | Bretylium | 5 mg/kg bolus |
| | Amiodarone | 5 mg/kg over 1 h, then 5 mg/kg over 12 h (repeat as needed) |
| β-blocking drugs | Propranolol | 0.01-0.1 mg/kg |
| | Esmolol | 0.5-1 mg/kg bolus 100-300 μg/kg/min infusion |
| Others | Calcium chloride | 10-20 mg/kg |
| | Sodium bicarbonate | 1 mEq/kg (or as determined by base deficit) |
| | Phenylephrine | 1-10 μg/kg |
| | Ephedrine | 0.05-0.2 mg/kg |
| | Heparin | ≥3 mg/kg (300 U/kg) |
| | Protamine | ≥3 mg/kg |

*The dose of each drug varies with the clinical context.
†Cannot be mixed in dextrose-containing solutions.
‡Maintenance rate determined by plasma levels.

ges so that a small bolus can be given if required. If needed repetitively, an infusion is mixed. Table 62–6 shows drugs that should be imminently available in syringes at the beginning of each pediatric cardiac surgical case. A narcotic, a benzodiazepine, and a muscle relaxant are also on hand for ready use.

## Blood and Blood Products

Blood products appropriate to the particular procedure and patient size should also be readied in advance. Preparation may range from typing and screening for simple procedures to typing and cross-matching of multiple units of blood or platelets (or both) and fresh frozen plasma for complex pump cases. At the University of Florida, infants younger than 4 months of age undergo typing and screening and then preferentially receive type O blood without a cross-match because the risk of transfusion reaction is low.

Transfusion-acquired cytomegalovirus infection is generally a benign entity in immunocompetent patients who receive blood. However, immunologically immature patients (especially low-birth-weight infants) can become symptomatic if infected. Therefore, our routine is to use cytomegalovirus-negative blood products in infants younger than 4 months of age. For infants with aortic arch abnormalities, blood products

should be irradiated because these cardiac lesions may be associated with DiGeorge syndrome. Such patients may have an absent thymus and are susceptible to graft versus host disease following transfusion.

## ANESTHETIC INDUCTION AND MAINTENANCE

### What Monitors Are Needed Before Induction?

No absolute rule exists for determining the amount of monitoring necessary before induction. In some patients, particularly if a "steal" induction is ideal, anesthesia can be started with just a pulse oximeter and a precordial stethoscope. Then, as the patient is induced, ECG and blood pressure monitoring can be quickly established. In others, it may be preferable to begin with all monitors (even invasive ones) in place. Generally, arterial and central venous catheters are placed postinduction.

### When Does a Patient Need Intravenous Access Preinduction?

The timing of intravenous access, as noted previously, is often a matter of personal preference. However, polycythemic patients must be well hydrated either by mouth or intravenously. Children with extremely poor cardiac function and who require inotropes may not tolerate an inhalation induction; thus, an intravenous induction is preferred. Most other pediatric patients tolerate a judicious inhalation induction with subsequent placement of intravenous catheters.

If myocardial reserve is impaired, a high-dose inhalation technique cannot be used for long; once catheters are placed, a transition is made to either a completely intravenous narcotic technique or to a combination of intravenous and inhalation techniques. If the anesthesiologist is uncertain about his or her ability to place an intravenous catheter rapidly during an inhalation induction, it should be inserted before induction.

**TABLE 62–6.** Bolus Drugs Available in Syringes

| Drug | Syringe Concentrations | Bolus Dose |
|---|---|---|
| Calcium chloride | 100 mg/mL | 10-20 mg/kg |
| Epinephrine | 10 μg/mL | 0.2-1 μg/kg (inotropy) |
| | 100 μg/mL | 10-100 μg/kg (cardiac arrest) |
| Isoproterenol | 20 μg/mL | 1-10 μg |
| Phenylephrine | 100 μg/mL | 1-10 μg/kg |
| Lidocaine | 20 mg/mL | 1 mg/kg |
| Esmolol* | 10 mg/mL | 0.5-1 mg/kg |
| Heparin | 1000 U/mL | 300 U/kg (cardiopulmonary bypass) |
| | | 100 U/kg (vascular nonpump) |
| Atropine | 0.4 mg/mL | 0.01-0.02 mg/kg |
| Succinylcholine | 20 mg/mL | 1-2 mg/kg |
| Ephedrine | 5 mg/mL | 0.05-0.2 mg/kg |
| Sodium thiopental | 25 mg/mL | 3-5 mg/kg |
| Pancuronium | 1 mg/mL | 0.1-0.15 mg/kg (intubation) |

*Available for treatment of hypercyanotic spells in patients with tetralogy of Fallot.

## How Does Cardiac Disease Affect the Rate of Induction?

### Inhalation Agents

Intracardiac shunting can alter the uptake of inhalation anesthetics.[49] The final effect on rate of induction depends on the size and direction of the shunt and the patient's cardiac output. A right-to-left intracardiac shunt prolongs induction due to the slow uptake of anesthetic into the blood. If high concentrations of agents are used to speed induction and a relative anesthetic overdose occurs, it is difficult to remedy because the inhalation agents are also slow to be eliminated. A left-to-right shunt generally has a negligible effect on the speed of induction if the systemic perfusion is preserved at a normal level. A left-to-right shunt may speed induction when it coexists with a large right-to-left shunt.

### Intravenous Agents

Response to intravenously administered drugs is faster with a right-to-left shunt because the dilution effect and the pulmonary transit time are reduced in proportion to the magnitude of the shunt. A left-to-right shunt has a minimal effect on the response to intravenous drugs if systemic perfusion is preserved.

## What Problems Are Likely to Occur During Induction?

Any number of untoward events can occur during induction of anesthesia in pediatric patients with heart disease.

### Airway Obstruction

Airway obstruction is poorly tolerated in these patients, especially small infants or those with cyanotic heart disease. The margin for error is extremely small because minor problems can quickly become life-threatening. Airway obstruction that causes hypoxemia or hypercarbia increases pulmonary vascular resistance. A reversal of a left-to-right intracardiac shunt or aggravation of a right-to-left shunt may result, exacerbating the problem and creating a vicious cycle.

### Dysrhythmias

The patient may become bradycardic or develop a nodal rhythm with induction. Because stroke volume is relatively fixed, cardiac output suffers in this context. Acidosis can occur quickly when perfusion is marginal; this further depresses myocardial contractility, increasing pulmonary and decreasing systemic vascular resistances.

Dysrhythmias can result from many causes, including light anesthesia, hypoxemia, hypercarbia, drugs, and electrolyte abnormalities.

Significant potential problems may occur during central venous access acquisition. The drapes or patient position may serve to kink the ETT as it warms to body temperature. Dysrhythmias during this phase are generally induced mechanically from the catheter or guidewire. Familiarity with the lengths of the catheter kit components makes insertion to excessive depth less likely. Mechanically induced dysrhythmias respond better to removal of the stimulus than to pharmacologic therapy.

## What Anesthetic Technique Should the Anesthesiologist Use?

The choice of drug or drugs is not as important as is an understanding of the lesion's pathophysiology. Of help is the development of hemodynamic goals for each patient in terms of heart rate, contractility, preload, systemic vascular resistance, and pulmonary vascular resistance (Table 62–7).[50] In several lesions, overriding considerations dominate. An appropriate approach for a patient with aortic insufficiency may be totally different than that for a patient with Tetralogy of Fallot. Once the goals are defined, appropriate agents, dosages, and routes of administration can be selected. Many agents can be used as long as they are administered in a thoughtful fashion.

## How Should the Patient Be Positioned?

Data are scarce regarding the safest way to position a patient for heart surgery. The major issues are prevention of brachial plexus injury and optimal surgical access. I find it useful to place the patient in a supine position on a heating blanket covered with a thin sheet and to abduct the upper arms 90° with the hands above the head to allow easy access to and inspection of arterial and venous cannulation sites. The shoulders and elbows are supported at an angle of about 30° above the table by a "wedge" cushion in order to lessen the danger of any stretch on the brachial plexus. A study[51] suggested that bilateral somatosensory evoked potential monitoring of the median and ulnar nerves may be useful to predict (and perhaps to help prevent) such injuries during cardiac surgery. The applicability of this technique to children is unknown at this time.

Access to the patient's head is crucial for visual inspection to rule out superior vena cava syndrome, for pupil evaluation, and for airway manipulation. A piece of egg crate foam can

**TABLE 62–7.** Cardiac Grid for Common Congenital Heart Diseases (Desired Hemodynamic Changes)

| | Preload | PVR | SVR | HR | Contractility |
|---|---|---|---|---|---|
| ASD | ↑ | ↑ | ↓ | N | N |
| VSD (right-to-left) | N | ↓ | ↑ | N | N |
| VSD (left-to-right) | ↑ | ↑ | ↓ | N | N |
| Idiopathic hypertrophic subaortic stenosis | ↑ | N | N − ↑ | *↓ | *↓ |
| PDA | ↑ | ↑ | ↓ | N | N |
| Coarctation | ↑ | N | ↓ | N | N |
| Valvular pulmonic stenosis | ↑ | ↓ | N | ↓ | ↑ |
| Infundibular pulmonary stenosis | ↑ | ↓ | N | ↓ | *↓ |
| Aortic stenosis | ↑ | N | *↑ | *↓ | N − ↑ |
| Mitral stenosis | ↑ | N − ↓ | N | *↓ | N − ↑ |
| Aortic regurgitation | ↑ | N | ↓ | N − ↑ | N − ↑ |
| Mitral regurgitation | ↑ | N − ↓ | ↓ | N − ↑ | N − ↑ |

*An overriding consideration.

HR, heart rate; N, normal or no change; PVR, pulmonary vascular resistance; SVR, systemic vascular resistance.

From Moore RA. Anesthesia for the pediatric congenital heart patient for noncardiac surgery. *Anesthesiol Rev.* 1981;8:27.

**TABLE 62–8.** Monitors and Infusions

| Cardiac Lesion | ART | Multilumen CVP* | PA* | LA | Foley | Drug Infusions Anticipated |
|---|---|---|---|---|---|---|
| ASD | + | + | | | + | None |
| VSD | + | | + | + | + | SNP, ± Epi, Isuprel, Amrinone |
| Transposition (Jatene) | + | + | ± | + | + | NTG, SNP, ± Epi |
| Tetralogy of Fallot | + | | + | ± | + | SNP, ± Epi |
| Atrioventricular canal | + | | + | + | + | SNP, Epi, ± Isuprel, Amrinone |
| Total anomalous pulmonary venous return | + | + | + | + | + | SNP, ± Epi, Isuprel, Amrinone |
| Aortic stenosis | + | + | | + | + | NTG, ± Dopamine, Epi |
| Truncus arteriosus | + | + | + | + | + | SNP, Epi, Isuprel, Amrinone |
| Tricuspid atresia (Fontan) | + | + | | + | + | SNP, Epi, Isuprel |
| Patent ductus arteriosus | | | | | | None |
| Coarctation | + (right radial) | + | | | ± | SNP, Labetalol |
| Blalock-Taussig shunt | + † | + | | | ± | None |

*Choice of CVP versus PA line is often made on basis of patient size.
†Arterial line must be opposite to the surgical site.
ART, arterial catheter; CVP, central venous pressure (catheter); Epi, epinephrine; LA, left atrial catheter; NTG, nitroglycerine; PA, pulmonary artery catheter; SNP, sodium nitroprusside.

be placed under the patient's head to minimize the chance of pressure necrosis; many heart surgery cases are lengthy, and low perfusion pressure occurs during CPB. Because infants have such large occiputs, elevation of the head in this way may occasionally result in encroachment on the surgical field. Placing a small bolster underneath the patient's shoulders is helpful to bring the patient's chin off the chest.

## MONITORING

Anesthetic induction generally proceeds with noninvasive monitors. A 5-lead ECG is used to facilitate detection of rhythm disturbances and myocardial ischemia. An esophageal lead can also be used to more easily diagnose dysrhythmias, especially when tachycardia is present.[52] Lead $V_5$ can be placed in its normal position and covered with an adhesive drape to protect it from the surgical scrub solutions. The monitor mode of the ECG will minimize baseline drift, whereas the diagnostic mode allows better resolution of the P and T waves and ST segments.

### When Is an Arterial Catheter Indicated?

An indwelling arterial catheter is required whenever continuous monitoring of arterial pressure or frequent blood sampling is necessary. All procedures using CPB require placement of an arterial catheter because noninvasive methods are not useful if no pulsatile flow is present. Most closed-heart procedures also benefit from beat-to-beat monitoring of arterial pressure.

The arterial catheter is placed after intubation, preferably percutaneously in the nondominant radial artery. Other sites commonly used include the dorsalis pedis, posterior tibial, femoral, and, rarely, temporal arteries. A surgical cutdown is used only as a last resort because of the disproportionately high incidence of thrombosis and infection. For coarctation repairs, the arterial catheter must be placed in the right radial artery; if this is unsuccessful, the catheter can be placed in a temporal artery. In patients with a Blalock-Taussig shunt, the catheter must be placed on the side opposite the Blalock-

Taussig shunt or in a lower extremity artery (Table 62–8). A 22- or 24-gauge catheter is used, depending on the child's size.

## When Is Central Venous Access Needed?

### Central Venous Catheters

Central venous access is established routinely when a knowledge of right-sided heart filling pressure trends is desired or the need to administer vasoactive drugs rapidly exists. Access to the central circulation also allows placement of PA or pacing catheters. The decision as to which type and size of catheter should be used depends on the type of operation performed and on the size and clinical status of the patient.

A central venous catheter is routine in patients undergoing CPB. Monitoring superior vena caval pressure during extracorporeal circulation is useful in assessing adequacy of venous drainage, particularly when two venous cannulas are used. A central catheter with at least two lumens allows drug and fluid delivery via one lumen and uninterrupted central venous pressure (CVP) measurements via the other.

My guidelines for catheter length and size are shown in Table 62–9. Follow-up verification of appropriate catheter position occurs on review of the postoperative chest film.

**TABLE 62–9.** Guidelines for Central Venous Pressure Catheter Size and Length in Relationship to Patient Size

| Patient Weight | Internal Jugular Catheter Size* | Central Venous Pressure Catheter Length |
|---|---|---|
| <2.5 kg | 3 Fr SL or 4 Fr DL | 5 cm |
| 2.5-5.0 kg | 4 Fr DL or 5 Fr DL | 5 cm |
| 5-10 kg | 5 Fr DL or 5 Fr introducer | 8 cm |
| 10-20 kg | 5 Fr DL or 6 Fr introducer | 8–12 cm |
| >20 kg | 5-7 Fr DL or 6 Fr introducer | 12–15 cm |

*Catheter size is also influenced by operative procedure. If significant blood loss is anticipated and peripheral venous access is limited, a larger size CVP catheter may be preferred.
DL, double-lumen; Fr, French; SL, single-lumen.

## Pulmonary Artery Catheters

Monitoring of PA pressure is helpful when pulmonary vascular resistance is problematic. Placement of the PA catheter can be accomplished percutaneously or by the surgeon using a direct transthoracic approach. If the patient is too small to accept a balloon flotation catheter, a combined percutaneous and direct intraoperative approach can be employed. In this scenario, the catheter is placed through a sterility sheath into the introducer and advanced into the superior vena cava. When the chest and heart are open, the surgeon can then advance it into the proximal PA. In complex cardiac anomalies with shunts, the surgeon generally will thread the percutaneously placed PA catheter into position at the end of the surgical procedure because the catheter is often in the field of repair.

Continuous mixed venous oximetry is also available with selected catheters and may be helpful in titrating vasoactive infusions, in providing an early warning of deteriorating cardiac output, and in assessing residual shunts. The patient's size must be large enough to accommodate a 5 to 6 French introducer to facilitate percutaneous placement of such a PA catheter.

Smaller infants requiring PA pressure monitoring will have transthoracic PA catheters placed at the close of surgery. The PA catheter is also useful postoperatively to assess pressure gradients by carefully measuring pull-back pressures during removal. Some PA catheters allow measurement of cardiac output by thermodilution; however, this method is not often used in small children because of the significant fluid load it imposes on the patient.

## Left Atrial Catheters

Left atrial pressure monitoring is commonly used in patients with CHD because disparities in left- and right-sided heart function are often present. This catheter is inserted by the surgeon at the end of repair, usually via the right superior pulmonary vein. One must be careful in its use; because the catheter is in the left side of the heart, the risk of systemic embolization of clot or air is real. A risk of bleeding and cardiac tamponade is present when it is removed.

## *Where Should Temperature Be Measured?*

The optimal site for temperature monitoring during cardiac cases is controversial; remember that gradients exist between various sites (Fig. 62–4).[53] Commonly used are the esophagus, nasopharynx, rectum, tympanic membrane, blood, and bladder. Temperature monitoring is important because the rate of cooling and rewarming appears to have significant influence on brain injury. Wide gradients (>10°C) between body and perfusate temperature in dogs correlated with brain cell necrosis and death.[54] Monitoring in at least two sites is advisable to ensure that the temperature gradient between inflow (blood temperature) and core (bladder or rectal temperature) does not exceed 10°C and that uniform cooling and warming has occurred.

## *How Do End-Tidal and Arterial Carbon Dioxide Pressures Correlate?*

Monitoring of end-tidal carbon dioxide partial pressure ($P_{ET}CO_2$) is used to corroborate tracheal intubation. The arte-

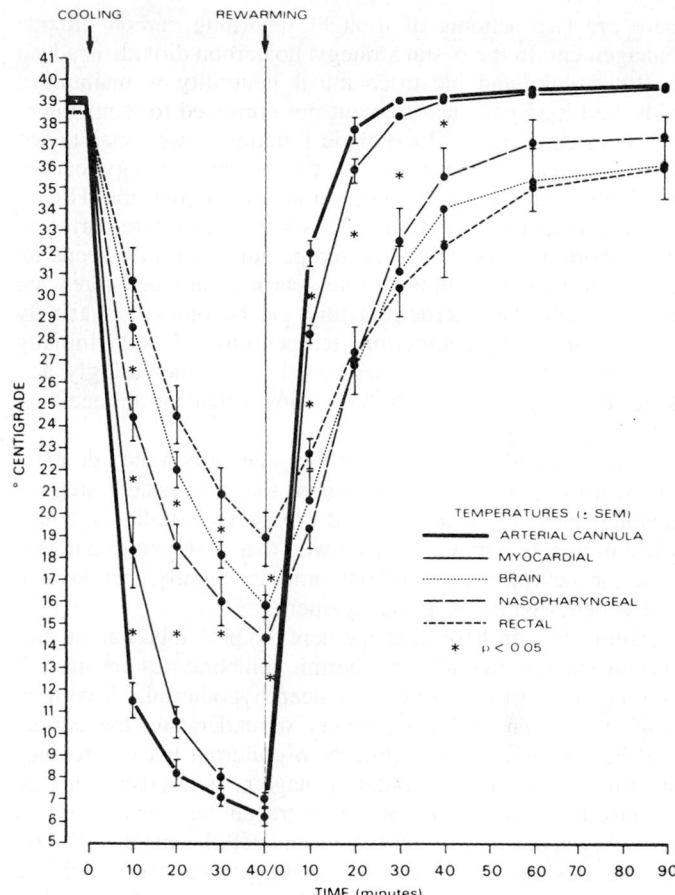

**FIGURE 62–4.** Average temperature ($\pm$ SEM) of arterial cannula, myocardium, cerebral cortex, nasopharynx, and rectum during 40 minutes of cooling and 90 minutes of rewarming during cardiopulmonary bypass in 6 pigs. (From Stefaniszyn HJ, Novick RJ, Keith FM, et al. Is the brain adequately cooled during deep hypothermic cardiopulmonary bypass? *Curr Surg.* 1983;40:294.)

rial to end-tidal carbon dioxide partial pressure difference ($P[a-ET]CO_2$) can be increased in patients with cardiopulmonary disease. It also may be increased in small children, depending on the sampling site and ventilatory pattern. Patients with CHD have altered ventilation-perfusion ratios; this produces abnormalities of both the physiologic dead space to tidal volume ratio ($V_{DS}/V_T$) and venous admixture ($\dot{Q}s/\dot{Q}t$).

In patients with cyanotic heart disease, in whom $\dot{Q}s/\dot{Q}t$ can be large, $P_{ET}CO_2$ significantly underestimates $PaCO_2$.[55] Because intracardiac shunting is often dynamic, the $P(a-ET)CO_2$ is ever-changing; thus, even $P_{ET}CO_2$ trends are not reliable in these patients. Periodic measurement of $PaCO_2$ is necessary to document adequate ventilation. $P_{ET}CO_2$ monitoring during PA banding reflects the decrease in pulmonary blood flow. As the band is tightened, the $P(a-ET)CO_2$ gradient increases.

## *How Should Blood Gases Be Managed During Cardiopulmonary Bypass?*

The strategy for management of the pH has received considerable attention over the past few years. Blood gas management strategy may be more important in children because greater degrees of hypothermia are used, resulting in more profound differences in blood carbon dioxide levels. Briefly, there are two schools of thought regarding carbon dioxide management. In the α-stat strategy, no carbon dioxide is added to the circuit, and electrochemical neutrality is maintained with the blood gas measurement not corrected to temperature (ie, reported at 37°C). Enzymatic function is well maintained in this milieu. In contrast, with the pH-stat strategy, carbon dioxide is added to the system to maintain a constant pH over varying temperatures. Blood gases are temperature-corrected and reported at actual body temperature. In this scenario, hydrogen ions accumulate, total carbon dioxide stores are elevated, and the microcirculatory pH becomes increasingly acidotic at deep hypothermic temperatures. It was initially believed that intracellular pH also became increasingly acidotic, but more recent data have shown that the intracellular pH changes only slightly.[56]

In adults, evidence suggests either that carbon dioxide management on CPB does not matter or that an α-stat strategy is advantageous. Three randomized prospective studies of adults using moderate hypothermia showed that postoperative neurologic or neuropsychologic outcome is slightly, but consistently, better with α-stat management.[57–59]

Although acid-base management is probably not as important when moderate hypothermic temperatures are used, it may be critical in the setting of deep hypothermia. Investigations have been performed to try to understand the correct acid-base management approach in children, but controversy remains. Theoretically, α-stat management has some appeal because maintenance of constant intracellular electrochemical neutrality appears essential for normal cellular function.[60] Animal studies suggest that α-stat management is beneficial in terms of myocardial protection and contractility.[61,62] The electrical stability of the heart is improved (less spontaneous ventricular fibrillation) using α-stat pH regulation compared with pH-stat.[63] During anoxic perfusion, there is a decrease in the extent and magnitude of brain lesions when the perfusate has a higher pH, whereas an acidic perfusate enhances the extent of the lesions.[64] The cerebral blood flow (CBF) during pH-stat hypothermia actually is far in excess of metabolic need.

On one hand, proponents of the α-stat method suggest that these unnecessarily high blood flows with pH-stat may place the brain at risk for damage due to microemboli, cerebral edema, or high intracranial pressure, or it may actually predispose to an adverse redistribution of blood flow ("steal") away from marginally perfused areas in patients with cerebrovascular disease. On the other hand, proponents of the pH-stat strategy suggest that enhanced CBF may be helpful in improving cerebral cooling before the initiation of circulatory arrest. In fact, total CBF is increased, global cerebral cooling is enhanced, and a redistribution of brain blood flow occurs during pH-stat management. An increased proportion of CBF is distributed to deep brain structures (thalamus, brainstem, and cerebellum) when pH-stat management is used.[65]

However, other data suggest that cerebral metabolic recovery after circulatory arrest may be better with the α-stat method than the pH-stat mode. This variation in results has led some authors to advocate a cross-over strategy; that is, using a pH-stat approach during the first 10 minutes of cooling to provide maximal cerebral metabolic suppression, followed by a change to α-stat strategy to remove the severe acidosis that accumulates during profound hypothermia with the use of pH-stat. This approach appears to offer maximal metabolic recovery in animals[66] (Fig. 62–5).

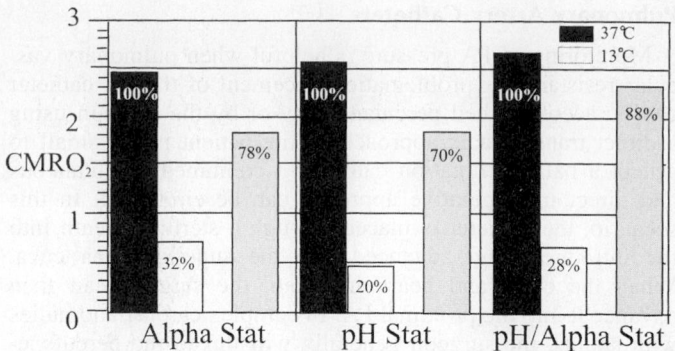

**FIGURE 62–5.** The effects of three different cooling strategies (α-stat, pH-stat, and a cross-over of pH-stat followed by α-stat) on cerebral metabolic suppression before deep hypothermia and circulatory arrest (DHCA) and the recovery of cerebral metabolism after DHCA. The pH-stat strategy provides better cerebral metabolic suppression before DHCA than α-stat, but cerebral metabolic recovery after DHCA is poor. Initial cooling with a pH-stat strategy followed by conversion to α-stat before DHCA results in the greatest cerebral metabolic recovery after DHCA. *Solid black bar*, 37°C; *white bar*, 13°C; *gray bar*, after DHCA. DHCA, deep hypothermic circulatory arrest. (From Kern FH, Greeley WJ. pH-Stat management of blood gases is not preferable to α-stat in patients undergoing brain cooling for cardiac surgery. *J Cardiothorac Vasc Anesth.* 1995;9:215.)

Choice of acid-base management may be particularly important in the subgroup of patients with aortopulmonary collaterals where cerebral cooling is problematic. It appears that the addition of carbon dioxide during cooling enhances cerebral perfusion and improves cerebral metabolic recovery.[67] Kurth and colleagues demonstrated, in a piglet model, two mechanisms by which pH-stat management may be beneficial to the brain.[68] They showed that pH-stat increases the rate of brain cooling and that the rate of brain oxygen depletion during DHCA is considerably slower with pH-stat management than with α-stat management. A recent randomized, single-center trial in infants younger than 9 months of age found that infants managed with a pH-stat strategy generally had better outcomes than those managed with an α-stat strategy.[69] The pH-stat infants had a significantly shorter recovery time to first EEG activity and a tendency to fewer EEG-manifested seizures. In the subset of transposition babies, those assigned to pH-stat tended to have a higher cardiac index despite a lower requirement for inotropic agents, less frequent acidosis and hypotension, and a shorter duration of mechanical ventilation and intensive care unit stay. Although the numbers are small, this study challenges the concept that α-stat management is more physiologic and protective during deep hypothermia in infants. The data suggest that pH-stat management may actually enhance systemic and cerebral protection in this group of patients.

### Why the Apparent Difference in Outcome Between Adults and Children Relative to pH Management?

It may relate to differences in mechanism of brain injury during CPB. In adults, emboli appear to play a prominent role in adverse neurologic outcome.[70] It is thus postulated that the decrease in CBF associated with α-stat management might be protective by limiting cerebral microemboli. On the other hand, the mechanism of injury in children may relate more to hypoperfusion or activation of excitotoxic pathways.[71] If a pII-stat strategy is employed, the increase in CBF may be beneficial in ensuring complete brain cooling and slowing oxygen consumption, thus increasing the brain's tolerance for DHCA.

## How Should the Central Nervous System Be Monitored?

CNS insults associated with cardiac surgery remain an unsolved problem. Brain damage can occur as a result of global hypoxia-ischemia or focal emboli. EEG has been used to try to provide a measure of cerebral electrical activity and function during cardiac surgery. Unfortunately, the EEG may not be reliable in predicting or preventing brain ischemia during CPB because of the effects of hypothermia and anesthetic agents and because of the likelihood of focal embolic injury. Newer computerized, processed EEG monitors are less cumbersome and allow easier recognition of trends and abrupt changes. The advantage of EEG is that it can be obtained in patients of any age or size with no risk and may be effective in detecting catastrophic events that cause global ischemia. EEG can also be useful in assessing adequacy of cerebral cooling by ensuring electrocerebral silence before circulatory arrest.

CBF has been measured using the Fick principle and [133]xenon clearance.[72] Unfortunately, this technique does not provide continuous measurement of CBF and is more applicable to the research setting rather than clinical care. TCD sonography uses the Doppler principle to detect shifts in frequency of reflected signals from blood in motion to calculate flow velocity.[73] Because it is thought that the diameters of the large cerebral arteries insonated are relatively constant, trends in flow velocity should pattern those of CBF. Thus, even though quantitative measurement of CBF cannot be made from TCD sonography, qualitative inferences may be appropriate. TCD can also provide an indirect measure of cerebral vascular resistance (which is increased with elevated intracranial pressure or markedly elevated CVP). TCD can be helpful in detecting suboptimally placed cannulas, which can distort the superior vena cava and impede cerebral venous drainage. It is also useful in detecting cerebral emboli. At present, the technology does not allow determination of emboli type (air versus particulate) or size.

Cerebral metabolism has been estimated by monitoring jugular venous bulb saturation, the cerebral equivalent of "mixed venous" blood.[74] A low saturation suggests an elevation in cerebral metabolism, outstripping the cerebral oxygen provided. However, this blood is the effluent from many areas of the brain, and regional areas of cerebral hypoperfusion can easily be missed. Near-infrared spectroscopy is a noninvasive method of monitoring brain oxygen saturation (cerebral oximetry).[75] Its noninvasiveness is appealing, but it also suffers from the drawback that it only reflects global perfusion.

A retrospective study suggested that neurologic monitoring and appropriate interventions may make a difference in outcome for these patients.[76] The researchers used a multimodal approach to monitoring: EEG, TCD, and cerebral oximetry. An interventional algorithm was used to detect and correct specific deficiencies in cerebral perfusion or oxygenation or to increase cerebral tolerance to ischemia or hypoxia. They observed significant changes in 70% of patients, and intervention was deemed appropriate in 74% of these patients with neurophysiologic changes. Obvious neurologic sequelae (eg, seizure, movement, vision or speech disorder) occurred in 7% of patients without noteworthy change, 6% of patients with intervention, and 26% of patients without intervention ($P = 0.001$). The researchers also noted a significant cost savings with appropriate intervention: the length of stay was increased in the patients with neurologic injury. This retrospective study is certainly encouraging, and, hopefully, the results can be reproduced in other clinical centers.

Because neurologic morbidity is an issue, I believe neurologic monitoring will become more prevalent, and techniques will be refined over the next decade. Anesthesiologists will become more skilled in "pattern recognition" of scenarios that require intervention.

## What Is the Role of Echocardiography?

Perioperative echocardiography is increasingly used in many centers for pediatric cardiac surgery. Both epicardial and, more recently, transesophageal echocardiography studies have been performed to better define cardiac anatomy and assess surgical repair. Technologic improvements allow better imaging, smaller probe size, and multiplane capability, thereby substantially increasing the information provided by this modality. The ultimate role of echocardiography in the operating room and intensive care unit is still evolving and will hinge on demonstration of improved outcome in these patients.

In one study of congenital heart repairs, epicardial echocardiographic Doppler color flow imaging demonstrated previously unappreciated anatomic details in 18% of patients before bypass.[77] After repair, the color flow imaging proved to be a much more sensitive method to assess quality of repair than was the surgeon's subjective impression. In 15% of cases in which the surgeon was satisfied, epicardial echocardiography after repair revealed persistent problems that required attention. If the unacceptable result determined by color flow imaging was not successfully revised before the patients left the operating room, only 21% had favorable outcomes compared with 83% of those whose results were successfully revised. When ventricular dysfunction was indicated, an unfavorable outcome was also predictable.

# CARDIOPULMONARY BYPASS

## How Does It Differ in Children?

The physiology of extracorporeal circulation is similar in adults and children. The details of CPB are covered in Chapter 17 and are not repeated here. However, significant differences in technique are applied to infants and small children (Table 62–10).[78] Smaller cannulas are used in children; however, proportionally, they may be so large that they obstruct venous drainage into the heart or arterial outflow from it before institution of bypass or after its discontinuation. Most cardiac repairs in children necessitate the use of dual venous cannulas so that all venous blood can be diverted to the bypass circuit and the heart can be opened to allow repair of the intracardiac defect.

**TABLE 62–10.** Differences in Adult Versus Pediatric Cardiopulmonary Bypass

| Parameter | Adult | Pediatrics |
|---|---|---|
| Hypothermic temperature | Rarely below 25°-32°C | Commonly 15°-20°C |
| Use of total circulatory arrest | Rare | Common |
| Pump prime | | |
|   Dilution effects on blood volume | 25%-33% | 200%-300% |
|   Additional additives in pediatric primes | | Blood, albumin |
| Perfusion pressures | Typically 50-80 mm Hg | 20-50 mm Hg |
| Influence of pH management strategy | Minimal at moderate hypothermia | Marked at deep hypothermia |
| Measured PaCO₂ differences | 30-45 mm Hg | 20-80 mm Hg |
| Glucose regulation | | |
|   Hypoglycemia | Rare; requires significant hepatic injury | Common; reduced hepatic glycogen stores |
|   Hyperglycemia | Frequent; generally easily controlled with insulin | Less common; rebound hypoglycemia may occur |

Modified from Kern FH, Schulman SR, Lawson DS, et al. Extracorporeal circulation and circulatory assist devices in the pediatric patient. In: Lake C, ed. *Pediatric Cardiac Anesthesia.* 3rd ed. Stamford, Conn: Appleton & Lange; 1998:219.

## Profound Hypothermia and Total Circulatory Arrest

An alternative method employed in small children with complex heart disease is profound hypothermia and total circulatory arrest. This technique employs a single venous drainage cannula during the period of cooling. When a core temperature of about 15° to 20°C is reached, the pump is stopped and the venous cannula removed. The major advantage of this technique is that it provides excellent exposure without cannulas or blood in the operative field. Deep hypothermia also enhances myocardial protection, decreases CPB time, and decreases blood trauma. As previously mentioned, the Boston Circulatory Arrest study showed that the use of circulatory arrest is associated with a higher risk of seizures. There was a strong correlation between duration of circulatory arrest and occurrence of seizures. Seizures in the perioperative period significantly increased the risk of both lower IQ scores and neurologic abnormalities.[79] On the basis of this study, most centers have minimized the use of DHCA. When it must be used, make every effort to limit its duration to <35 to 40 minutes.

## Venous Drainage

Venous drainage problems are more common in children than in adults. The inferior vena cava is short, and inadvertent cannulation of the hepatic veins is possible. If this occurs, marked engorgement of the splanchnic vessels can result in mesenteric ischemia. Problems with superior vena cava drainage are also possible, especially if a left superior vena cava is present. Occlusion of this vessel causes significant venous hypertension; it must be cannulated or cerebral ischemia may result. Careful attention should be paid to superior vena cava pressure by frequent inspection of the head and CVP reading.

The upper venous cannula can easily be kinked or drainage otherwise impaired with retraction of the heart.

### Systemic-to-Pulmonary Artery Shunt Occlusion

When CPB is first initiated, the surgeon must quickly occlude any systemic-to-PA shunts (eg, PDA or Blalock-Taussig shunt). Otherwise, continued perfusion of these shunts will lead to underperfusion of the systemic circulation, possible hemorrhagic edema of the lungs, and continued pulmonary venous return with possible overdistention of the left side of the heart.

### Perfusion Flow and Pressure

CPB flow rates are proportionately higher in infants and children than in adults, ranging from 80 to 150 mL/kg/min. Adult rates usually range from about 1.8 to 2.2 L/min/m², or about 50 mL/kg/min. Perfusion pressures associated with adequate oxygenation and perfusion tend to be lower in children (20-50 mm Hg). The optimal pressure or flow is unclear, and significant interinstitutional variation exists.

### Moderate Hypothermia and Ventricular Fibrillation

Moderate hypothermia combined with ventricular fibrillation is used often in pediatric cardiac repair. With this technique, the patient is cooled to about 28° to 30°C, and the heart is fibrillated but continues to be perfused because an aortic cross-clamp is not placed. The surgeon can then open the cardiac chambers without risking the entrainment of air into the left side of the heart and subsequent ejection into the arterial circulation.

Deliberate fibrillation is often used during work on the right side of the heart or for relatively simple repairs such as ASD closure. The advantages of deliberate fibrillation with moderate hypothermia include a favorable myocardial supply-demand ratio, decreased risk of air embolus to the brain, and avoidance of aortic cross-clamping and cardioplegia. However, surgical exposure is limited because of the significant amount of blood in and continued motion of the heart. Therefore, aortic cross-clamping and cardioplegic protection of the heart are necessary for more complex intracardiac repairs, especially in small children.

### Bypass Circuit Volume

The bypass circuit volume is large relative to the blood volume in infants. In pediatric CPB circuits, the priming volume is about 700 mL, whereas the estimated blood volume of a 3-kg neonate is 250 to 300 mL. The hematocrit, accordingly, is reduced by approximately 70%. In contrast, an adult CPB circuit is primed with 1500 mL for a patient with an estimated blood volume of 5 L; a <25% drop in hematocrit results. Small infants undergoing complex repairs often require transfusion of red blood cells, platelets, and fresh frozen plasma to offset the dilutional reduction of hematocrit and clotting factors.

### *When Should Blood Be Added to the Bypass Circuit?*

In general, hemodilution during bypass is desirable and tolerated because microcirculatory perfusion is improved and metabolic needs are reduced by hypothermia. However, if the hematocrit is lowered too far, oxygen-carrying capacity is diminished, and anaerobic metabolism results. The ideal hematocrit during CPB is unknown. However, for most complex repairs, a hematocrit of 20% to 25% during CPB is used.

The CPB circuit must be primed. Each circuit has an obligatory volume that is required to fill the tubing, filters, and oxygenator. Even in small infants, who require the smallest tubing possible, the obligatory prime, as has already been mentioned, is about 700 to 750 mL. Therefore, red blood cells are commonly added to the priming solution to reach the desired hematocrit. Calculation of the hematocrit on bypass is simple:

1. Determine the patient's estimated blood volume.
2. Multiply the estimated blood volume by the measured hematocrit (Hct) to yield the patient's red blood cell mass (RBCM).
3. Ask the perfusionist what the circuit priming volume is.
4. Add the estimated blood volume to the priming volume to obtain the total volume on bypass (CPBV).
5. Predicted hematocrit on bypass is RBCM/CPBV.
6. If the predicted hematocrit on bypass is less than desired, the quantity of red blood cells that must be added is calculated as follows:

$$CPBV \times Desired\ Hct = Required\ RBCM$$

$$\frac{Required}{RBCM} - \frac{Patient's}{RBCM} = RBCM\ to\ Be\ Added$$

### How Is Anticoagulation Managed?

Heparin is given to prevent initiation of the coagulation cascade by contact of blood with the bypass circuit. A dose of 300 U/kg is generally sufficient, although 400 U/kg are sometimes recommended for neonates. This dose is given through a central catheter after aspiration to verify blood return.

### Activated Clotting Time

Documentation of heparin effect can be made by measuring activated clotting time about 3 to 5 minutes later. A value of 300 to 400 seconds appears adequate to prevent clotting on bypass.

Activated clotting time is relatively simple to determine and is reasonable to monitor because an occasional patient does exhibit marked heparin resistance. The activated clotting time can also signal a potentially catastrophic drug administration error when a substance other than heparin is injected. If the patient remains normothermic, the activated clotting time is generally rechecked every 20 to 30 minutes. With significant hypothermia, heparin effect is prolonged.

### Should Antifibrinolytics Be Used?

In an effort to minimize transfusion requirements, many groups have focused on preservation of platelet function and prevention of fibrinolysis, using drugs such as ε-aminocaproic acid and aprotinin. Although the data that support the de-

creased transfusion requirement in redo operations in adults are fairly convincing, it is not as clearcut in infants. Some groups have reported dramatic decreases in blood loss, whereas others have shown no difference in donor exposures to banked blood.[80-82] Many of the studies performed on aprotinin usage in children are difficult to interpret due to wide variations in dosage regimens, patient age, type of operation, and other factors. When aprotinin is dosed according to patient weight or body surface area, much lower plasma concentrations than those found in the adult population result.[83] It appears that the large volume of the pump prime relative to the patient's small blood volume leads to a greater dilution of the drug during bypass. In order to compensate for the hemodilution, additional aprotinin may need to be added to the prime to achieve plasma levels sufficient to inhibit activation of the coagulation cascade.

### How Are Patients Weaned?

Success in weaning from bypass is critically dependent on the surgeon's ability to completely repair the defect. Residual shunts, obstruction, or valvular dysfunction are tolerated poorly following bypass.

### Preparation

Be certain the patient is optimally prepared before attempting discontinuation of bypass (Table 62–11). Near the end of the surgical repair, gradual rewarming is begun. Temperature gradients are common; be sure that the patient is thoroughly and evenly rewarmed. The speed and method of rewarming may be critical. Postischemia hyperthermia is particularly deleterious in the setting of altered cerebral energy metabolism.[84] Mild degrees of hypothermia have been shown to be protective. Infusion of afterload-reducing agents, such as sodium nitroprusside, during rewarming may be helpful to dilate the vascular bed and promote uniform rewarming. Allowing time for reperfusion of the heart after the cross-clamp is removed makes possible dissipation of "evil humors" (*cardioplegia*) and re-establishment of aerobic metabolism.

### Heart Rate and Rhythm

Sinus rhythm is essential because ventricular function is typically impaired following bypass and ischemia. Optimal heart rate is also important in improving cardiac output because stroke volume may be less than ideal. A heart rate of 120 to 160 beats per minute (bpm) is desirable. The atrium may be paced if the patient has a slower sinus rate, or

---

**TABLE 62–11.** Checklist for Discontinuation of Bypass

1. Complete rewarming (core temperature ≥35°C).
2. Complete reperfusion of heart after cardioplegia.
3. Sinus rhythm with appropriate heart rate.
4. Evaluate ST changes.
5. Check electrolytes, blood gases, and hematocrit.
6. Optimize pulmonary function.
7. Check hemodynamic monitors.
8. Prepare vasodilator or inotropic drugs, if indicated.
9. Prepare platelets and fresh frozen plasma, if indicated.

sequential atrioventricular pacing may be required if a rhythm other than sinus exists. New ECG ST changes may indicate the presence of air in the coronary arteries or ongoing myocardial ischemia. A transient increase in coronary perfusion pressure (as occurs with application of a partial occlusion clamp to the aorta distal to the aortic cannula) promotes clearance of this air.

### Other Monitored Parameters

Hemodynamic monitors should be rechecked and transducers rezeroed. The surgeon may elect to insert a left atrial pressure catheter to assess ventricular filling and function. Laboratory values, including hematocrit, potassium, ionized calcium, arterial blood gas partial pressures, and pH, should be rechecked after aortic cross-clamp release and before discontinuation of bypass is attempted.

### Vasoactive Drugs

Vasodilator and inotropic drugs should be available for infusion by calibrated pumps, especially after intracardiac repair. Significant hemodynamic compromise may result from hypoxic-ischemic reperfusion injury superimposed on marginal baseline ventricular function. Ventricular performance usually is readily improved by inotrope or combined inotrope and vasodilator support. Impaired postoperative cardiac performance is clearly associated with higher morbidity and mortality. In one study, acute cardiac failure accounted for over 59% of postoperative deaths in children younger than 2 years of age.[85]

### Cardiovascular Changes

Arterial pressure may be normal or above normal when cardiac output is high, normal, or low; thus, knowledge of it is not helpful with regard to diagnosis of cardiac dysfunction (Fig. 62–6).[86] Following CPB, systemic vascular resistance is generally high in both adults and children because of circulating catecholamines and antidiuretic hormone, as well as other influences.[87] In the neonate, this response may be amplified,

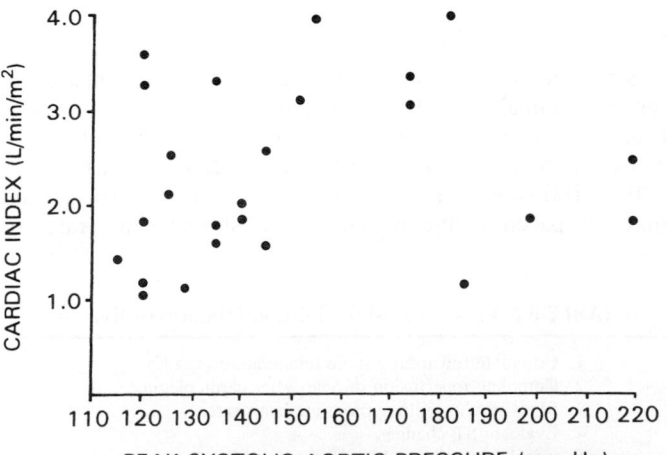

**FIGURE 62–6.** Comparison of cardiac index and peak systolic pressure in 25 adult patients during the first 4 hours after open intracardiac operations. (From Kouchoukos NT, Karp RB. Management of the postoperative cardiovascular surgical patient. *Am Heart J.* 1976;92:517.)

leading to uninhibited vasoconstriction and a marked disparity between aortic or femoral and radial artery blood pressures.

### Afterload Reduction

Children tolerate an increased pressure workload poorly. Therefore, afterload reduction (generally with sodium nitroprusside) may be useful to improve cardiac output. Cardiac index increased 20% after infusion of sodium nitroprusside in 16 infants after intracardiac surgery.[88] A further 20% increase was achieved by restoration of left atrial pressure to baseline values. When cardiac output is still impaired after vasodilator therapy, a combination of afterload reduction, volume expansion, and inotropic support is warranted.

### *Measurement of Blood Pressure*

If the blood pressure is low during attempted weaning from bypass, another method of blood pressure measurement must be available to check the accuracy of the peripheral data. The surgeon can easily place an exploring needle into the ascending aorta (often at the site of the previous cardioplegia infusion) and connect it to a pressure transducer. A noninvasive (cuff) blood pressure measurement also can be obtained.

In small children, a significant difference in blood pressure measurements is often present between central aortic and peripheral arterial sites. The reason for this discrepancy is not clear, but it usually resolves over time. Before starting administration of inotropes or vasopressors, be certain that the pressure measurement is accurate. If the discrepancy persists, placement of a femoral arterial catheter helps to guide therapy.

## How Is Increased Pulmonary Vascular Resistance Managed?

Pulmonary function must be optimized before discontinuation of bypass is attempted. Increased pulmonary vascular resistance results from increased lung water, complement activation, catecholamines, and atelectasis.

### Lung Expansion and Oxygenation

The lungs must be vigorously re-expanded to increase functional residual capacity (Fig. 62–7).[89] The ETT is not routinely suctioned because suctioning may precipitate bleeding in anticoagulated patients. Any wheezing is vigorously treated with inhaled bronchodilators. I prefer albuterol, 2.5 mg, administered via a nebulizer attached between the ETT and the circle system. If secretions prevent appropriate deflation of the lungs, careful suctioning with a soft red rubber catheter is indicated.

Vigorous hyperventilation without positive end-expiratory pressure is one of the most powerful tools available to decrease pulmonary vascular resistance.[90] The pulmonary vascular responsiveness to hypercarbia is accentuated in the postbypass period; thus, even small increases in $PaCO_2$ are associated with significant increases in resistance. High inspired oxygen concentrations should be used, and metabolic acidosis should be avoided.

### Pharmacologic Interventions

$\alpha$-Stimulation causes pulmonary vasoconstriction, whereas $\beta$-stimulation causes vasodilation. Many pharmacologic

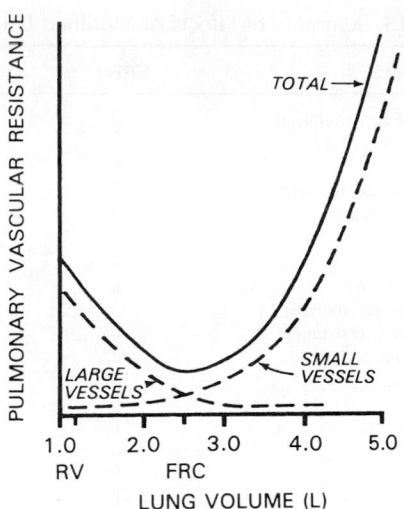

**FIGURE 62–7.** An asymmetric U-shaped curve relates total pulmonary vascular resistance to lung volume. The trough of the curve occurs when lung volume equals functional residual capacity (FRC). Total pulmonary resistance is the sum of resistance in small vessels (increased by increasing lung volume) and in large vessels (increased by decreasing lung volume). RV, residual volume. (From Benumof JL. Respiratory physiology and respiratory function during anesthesia. In: Miller RD, ed. *Anesthesia.* 2nd ed. New York, NY: Churchill Livingstone; 1986:1122.)

agents have been used with only marginal success in the attempt to selectively decrease pulmonary vascular resistance. The ones most commonly used include sodium nitroprusside, nitroglycerin, isoproterenol, aminophylline, amrinone, milrinone, PGE$_1$, and perhaps adenosine. Inhaled nitric oxide offers promise as a truly selective pulmonary vasodilator but has only recently been made commercially available.[91]

Factors that increase or decrease pulmonary vascular resistance are summarized in Table 62–12.

## POSTBYPASS ISSUES

### What Is Modified Ultrafiltration and When Is It Used?

The inflammatory response on bypass is significant and may be responsible for much of the morbidity seen in these

**TABLE 62–12.** Alteration of Pulmonary Vascular Resistance

| Increase Resistance | Decrease Resistance |
| --- | --- |
| Hypoxia | Oxygen |
| Hypercarbia | Hypocarbia |
| Acidosis | Alkalosis |
| Hyperinflation | Normal functional residual capacity |
| Atelectasis | Blocking sympathetic stimulation |
| Sympathetic stimulation | Low hematocrit |
| Surgical constriction | Modified ultrafiltration |
| High hematocrit | Nitric oxide |
| | Phosphodiesterase inhibitors |

Modified from Hickey PR, Wessel DL: Anesthesia for treatment of congenital heart disease. In: Kaplan JA, ed. *Cardiac Anesthesia.* 2nd ed. Orlando, Fla: Grune & Stratton; 1987:656.

children. Endothelial injury can cause an increase in total body water and increased capillary permeability, with resultant multiorgan failure. Conventional ultrafiltration on CPB has been used to try to prevent tissue edema but is limited. It is difficult to remove much water during bypass and still maintain a safe acceptable reservoir volume. In 1993, Naik and Elliott described a technique of modified ultrafiltration (MUF) that is performed in the immediate postbypass period.[92,93] The aortic cannula is left in place and approximately 10 to 30 mL/kg/min of blood is siphoned from the aorta, pumped through a hemoconcentrator (dialysis membrane), and returned to the right atrium (Fig. 62–8). Volume is infused from the reservoir as necessary to maintain hemodynamic stability. Multiple studies have documented the effectiveness of MUF in ameliorating many of the adverse effects of CPB. MUF improves hemodynamics, reduces total body water (Fig. 62–9), and decreases the need for blood transfusions compared with nonfiltered controls.[94] It is associated with significant increases in hematocrit, fibrinogen, and total plasma protein levels, but no change in platelet count.[95] MUF has been shown to improve intrinsic left ventricular systolic function, improve diastolic compliance, increase blood pressure, and decrease inotropic drug use in the early postoperative period.[96] It has been shown to decrease levels of the lung vasoconstrictor, endothelin-1, significantly decrease the pulmonary-systemic pressure ratio after CPB, and it may help prevent pulmonary hypertensive crises.[97] It improves lung compliance, reduces cytokine levels,

**FIGURE 62–8.** A diagram of a modified ultrafiltration system. After CPB, modified ultrafiltration proceeds using the blood cardioplegia roller pump from the CPB circuit. Blood is pumped from the aortic cannula through the ultrafilter and heat exchanger and is reinfused into the patient through the venous cannula. CPB, cardiopulmonary bypass. (From Kern FH, Shulman SR, Lawson DS, et al. Extracorporeal circulation and circulatory assist devices in the pediatric patient. In: Lake CL, ed. *Pediatric Cardiac Anesthesia.* 3rd ed. Stamford, Conn: Appleton & Lange; 1998:219. Reproduced with permission of The McGraw-Hill Companies.)

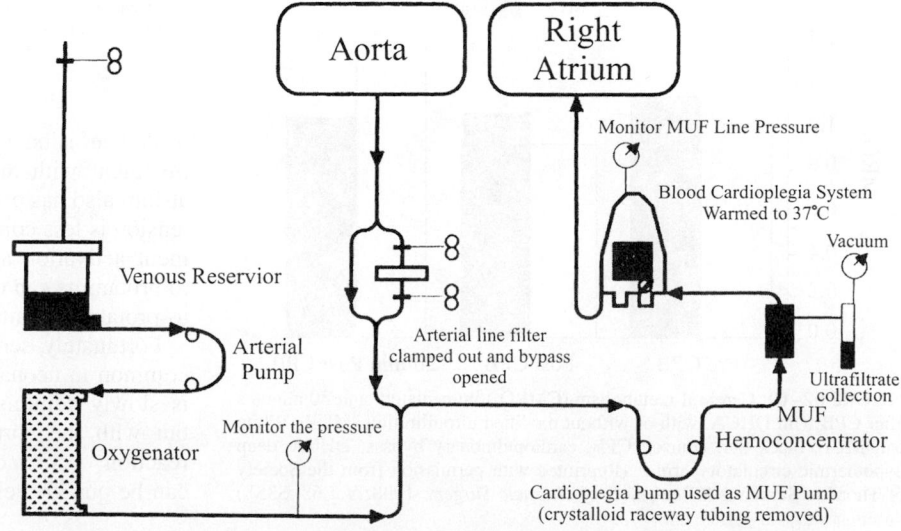

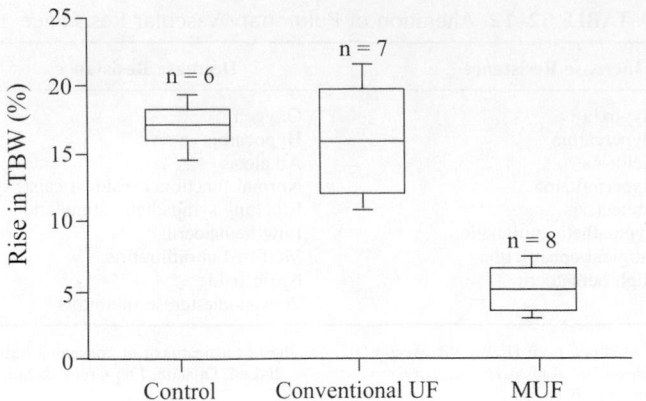

**FIGURE 62–9.** Percentage increase in total body water (TBW) with conventional ultrafiltration (UF), modified ultrafiltration (MUF), and on filtration. (Reprinted with permission from the Society of Thoracic Surgeons [*The Annals of Thoracic Surgery,* 1998, Vol 6S, S35].)

**TABLE 62–13.** Summary of Effects of Modified Ultrafiltration

| Feature | Effect | References |
|---|---|---|
| Total body water accumulation | ⇓ | A |
| Hematocrit | ⇑ | A, B, C |
| Blood loss | ⇓ | A, C, D |
| Blood transfusion requirement | ⇓ | A, C, D |
| Colloid osmotic pressure | ⇑ | B, E |
| Cardiac output | ⇑ | A, F |
| Heart rate | ⇓ | F |
| Arterial blood pressure | ⇑ | A, F |
| Systemic vascular resistance | ⇔ | G |
| Pulmonary vascular resistance | ⇓ | G, H |
| Diastolic compliance | ⇑ | F |
| Inotropic drug use | ⇓ | F |
| Renal function | ⇔ | A |
| Cerebral recovery from DHCA | ⇑ | B, I |
| Plasma endothelin-1 | ⇓ | H |
| Lung compliance | ⇑ | J |
| Cytokine levels | ⇓ | K |
| Activated complement levels | ⇓ | L |
| Heparin concentration | ⇑ | M |

Modified from Elliott MJ. Recent advances in paediatric cardiopulmonary bypass. *Perfusion.* 1999;14:237.

ᴬNaik SK, Knight A, Elliott MJ. A prospective randomized study of a modified technique of ultrafiltration during pediatric open-heart surgery. *Circulation.* 1991;84:III422.

ᴮDaggett CW, Lodge AJ, Scarborough JE, et al. Modified ultrafiltration versus conventional ultrafiltration: a randomized prospective study in neonatal piglets. *J Thorac Cardiovasc Surg.* 1998;115:336.

ᶜDraaisma AM, Hazekamp MG, Frank M, et al. Modified ultrafiltration after cardiopulmonary bypass in pediatric cardiac surgery. *Ann Thorac Surg.* 1997;64:521.

ᴰFriesen RH, Campbell DN, Clarke DR, et al. Modified ultrafiltration attenuates dilutional coagulopathy in pediatric open heart operations. *Ann Thorac Surg.* 1997;64:1787.

ᴱAd N, Snir E, Katz J, et al. Use of the modified technique of ultrafiltration in pediatric open-heart surgery: a prospective study. *Isr J Med Sci.* 1996;32:1326.

ᶠDavies MJ, Nguyen K, Gaynor JW, et al. Modified ultrafiltration improves left ventricular systolic function in infants after cardiopulmonary bypass. *J Thorac Cardiovasc Surg.* 1998;115:361.

ᴳNaik SK, Balaji S, Elliott MJ. Modified ultrafiltration improves haemodynamics after cardiopulmonary bypass in children. *J Am Coll Cardiol.* 1992;19:37A.

ᴴBando K, Vijay P, Turrentine MW, et al. Dilutional and modified ultrafiltration reduces pulmonary hypertension after operations for congenital heart disease: a prospective randomized study. *J Thorac Cardiovasc Surg.* 1998;115:517.

ᴵSkaryak LA, Kirshbom P, DiBernardo LR, et al. Modified ultrafiltration improves cerebral metabolic recovery after circulatory arrest. *J Thorac Cardiovasc Surg.* 1995;109:744.

ᴶMeliones JN, Gaynor JW, Wilson BG, et al. Modified ultrafiltration reduces airway pressure and improves lung compliance after congenital heart surgery. *J Am Coll Cardiol.* 1995;25:271A.

ᴷMillar AB, Armstrong L, van der Linden J, et al. Cytokine production and hemofiltration in children undergoing cardiopulmonary bypass. *Ann Thorac Surg.* 1993;56:1499.

ᴸAndreasson S, Gothberg S, Berggren H, et al. Hemofiltration modifies complement activation after extracorporeal circulation in infants. Ann Thorac Surg. 1993;56:1515.

ᴹWilliams GD, Ramamoorthy C, Totzek FR, et al. Comparison of the effects of red cell separation and ultrafiltration on heparin concentration during pediatric cardiac surgery. *J Cardiothorac Vasc Anesth.* 1997;11:840.

and removes activated complement (C3a and C5a).[98–100] After DHCA, MUF also improves the brain's ability to use oxygen[101] (Fig. 62–10). The data summarizing its beneficial effects are shown in Table 62–13.

## How Should Protamine Be Administered?

Protamine is given following termination of CPB to neutralize the effects of heparin. It is not administered until MUF is complete and the venous cannula has been removed. Generally, a dose of 3 to 4.5 mg/kg (1-1.5 mg for every 100 U of heparin) is given. Satisfactory reversal of heparin is suggested by return of the activated clotting time to baseline value. Protamine can cause serious adverse reactions in some patients. These reactions include systemic hypotension, pulmonary hypertension, and allergic reactions. The mechanism for these events is not entirely clear but may involve antibody-mediated immune responses, complement activation, and histamine release.

Histamine release is provoked by rapid administration of large doses of protamine. Slow administration with a con-

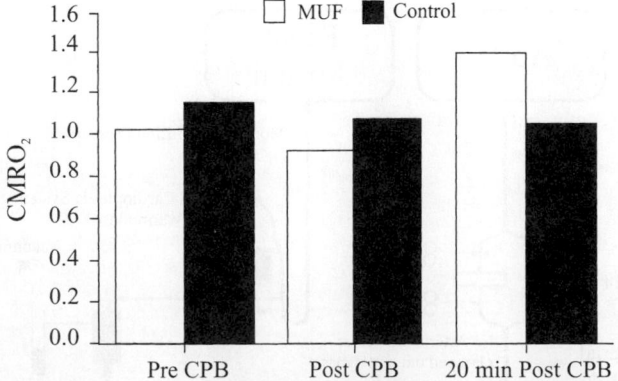

**FIGURE 62–10.** Cerebral metabolism (CMRO$_2$) immediately and 30 minutes after CPB with DHCA, with or without modified ultrafiltration (MUF). White bar, MUF; black bar, control. CPB, cardiopulmonary bypass; DHCA, deep hypothermic circulatory arrest. (Reprinted with permission from the Society of Thoracic Surgeons [*The Annals of Thoracic Surgery,* 1998, Vol 6S, S35].)

trolled infusion is effective in limiting this side effect. Pretreatment with antihistamine or administration into the left atrium also has been proposed. Catastrophic pulmonary hypertension is less common and probably occurs owing to complement activation and thromboxane release. Allergic reactions to protamine can occur, usually in patients with prior exposure to protamine-containing insulin preparations.

Fortunately, serious reactions to protamine appear to be less common in neonates and children than in adults. If protamine is slowly administered after removal of the venous cannula but with the aortic cannula still in place, should a severe reaction occur, additional heparin is administered, and CPB can be quickly reinstituted.

## What Are the Causes of Low Cardiac Output?

Low cardiac output can have many causes but is categorized according to its major determinants: heart rate, rhythm, contractility, preload, and afterload.

### Heart Rate

Infants and children have a relatively fixed cardiac stroke volume and therefore modify cardiac output by heart rate changes. Thus, cardiac output is considered to be rate-dependent. Heart rates ≥120 bpm should be the goal in an effort to optimize cardiac output. A lower heart rate should be treated either pharmacologically or by pacing.

### Dysrhythmias

Dysrhythmias following CPB are often tolerated poorly and may require electrical conversion. Sinus rhythm at a reasonable rate is crucial to maximize cardiac output. Do not hesitate to use electrical pacing to optimize myocardial performance. Unfortunately, arrhythmias that are caused by abnormal automaticity may occur and may be difficult to treat. Junctional ectopic tachycardia (JET) is an uncommon but life-threatening arrhythmia seen almost exclusively in neonates and infants following congenital heart surgery.[102] JET is of special significance for the anesthesiologist because it usually manifests intraoperatively or in the immediate postoperative period. JET remains among the more difficult tachycardias to control, leading to severe hemodynamic instability and death. It is thought to result from abnormal automaticity with the focus of active discharge located at the AV node or the proximal bundle of His and yet the atrial tissue is not directly involved in the arrhythmia mechanism. Therefore, an important characteristic of this tachyarrhythmia is a lack of response to cardioversion, overdrive pacing, and conventional medications.

JET is classically recognized as a narrow QRS tachycardia with AV dissociation, and an atrial rate that is slower than the ventricular rate. Typically, peak JET rates range from 170 to 300 bpm. Retrograde conduction and retrograde P-waves can be seen on the ECG. Interestingly, a wide QRS may be seen if there is an associated bundle branch block that occurs either as a rate-dependent aberration or as a fixed abnormality due to surgical damage of the bundle branch.

Postoperatively, JET has been generally refractory to most of the conventional antiarrhythmic drugs. Remarkably, it usually resolves on its own within the first 3 days of presentation. Therapy should be directed toward decreasing the junctional rate to allow atrial pacing with atrioventricular synchrony to reestablish hemodynamic stability.

### Decreased Contractility

Poor contractility can occur due to surgical trauma (as from a ventriculotomy incision), pre-existing volume or pressure overload condition, injury to or air in a coronary artery, residual effects of myocardial ischemia and reperfusion, metabolic and acid-base derangements, hypoxemia, and drug effects.

### Decreased Preload

Decreased preload may occur from hypovolemia, cardiac tamponade, positive airway pressure, and increased pulmonary vascular resistance that causes diminished return to the left side of the heart.

### Increased Afterload

Increased afterload can be a major problem for both the left and right sides of the heart. Many congenital lesions are associated with pulmonary vascular changes and pulmonary hypertension. Thus, control of right ventricular function and afterload is crucial to maintain adequate cardiac output.

## What Are the Causes of and Treatments for Excessive Bleeding?

### Causes

Most commonly, patients bleed postoperatively as a result of inadequate surgical hemostasis. Inadequate heparin neutralization can also be a factor. Thrombocytopenia or platelet dysfunction is the next most common cause. Platelets are sequestered in the bypass circuit and become dysfunctional because of surface exposure and hypothermia.

Patients with cyanotic heart disease and significant polycythemia have a baseline abnormality of platelet function and clotting factors. They often demonstrate a decrease in factors II, V, VII, VIII, and IX; hypofibrinogenemia; and an increase of fibrin split products, all of which may lead to excessive bleeding.[103] Although the use of positive end-expiratory pressure to "tamponade" the bleeding and decrease mediastinal drainage has been recommended,[104] another study failed to confirm this effect.[105]

### Treatment

While a source of bleeding is sought, the patient must be aggressively treated with volume replacement. Crystalloid solutions are the mainstay of therapy, but their administration should be tempered by the knowledge that a total body inflammatory response after bypass leads to problems with increased vascular permeability and edema. Decreased colloid oncotic pressure can be a problem following CPB because of hemodilution and destruction of serum proteins; judicious use of albumin-containing solutions may be warranted.

If continuing red blood cell loss is a problem, packed red blood cell transfusion is indicated. Typically, a hematocrit of 25% to 30% in acyanotic and 30% to 40% in cyanotic children seems reasonable. In children with good cardiac reserve following simple repairs, an even lower hematocrit of 18% to 20% may be well tolerated. If no surgical source is found and the activated clotting time is normal, an empiric platelet transfusion is often used. Only following prolonged, deep hypothermic cases in small infants should transfusion with cryoprecipitate or fresh frozen plasma be necessary.

## What Metabolic Problems Are Likely?

### Potassium Disorders

Metabolic derangements are relatively common. Hyperkalemia and hypokalemia are the most common electrolyte abnormalities. Hyperkalemia is commonly seen immediately after the cross-clamp is removed if large amounts of cardioplegic solution have been used. If cardiac output is poor, hyperkalemia may remain problematic. Typically, hypokalemia evolves because patients exhibit a marked kaliuresis after bypass. Unless the serum potassium value is $\geq 4.5$ mEq/ L or renal function is impaired, I almost routinely begin a potassium chloride infusion of 1 to 4 mEq/h following CPB. Remember that dysrhythmias associated with digitalis toxicity are enhanced by hypokalemia.

## Calcium Abnormalities

Hypocalcemia occurs frequently, especially following rapid transfusion of blood products. A decrease in the ionized fraction can lead to decreased myocardial contractility and decreased vascular smooth muscle tone.

## Miscellaneous Problems

Hypomagnesemia can occur and can enhance ventricular irritability. Hyperglycemia is common following CPB and is relatively resistant to treatment with insulin. Sodium changes typically do not present a major problem after bypass, although hypernatremia can occur if large quantities of sodium bicarbonate have been given.

## When Is the Patient Extubated?

Most patients undergoing complex repairs remain intubated and mechanically ventilated for several hours to days after surgery. This approach allows heavy sedation, recovery of myocardial function, and stabilization of hemodynamic status. For simple repairs (eg, ASD, simple VSD, and coarctation), extubation may be considered at the end of the procedure if the patient is stable and awake and if bleeding is controlled. Obviously, all normal criteria for extubation, including reversal of muscle relaxation, normothermia, good spontaneous ventilation, and the ability to maintain and protect the airway, should be present.

## References

1. Daniels SR. Epidemiology. In: Long WA, ed. *Fetal and Neonatal Cardiology*. Philadelphia, Pa: WB Saunders; 1990:425.
2. Fyler DC. Report of the New England Regional Cardiac Program. *Pediatrics*. 1980;65(suppl):375.
3. Ferencz C, Rubin JD, McCarter RJ, et al. Congenital heart disease: prevalence at livebirth: the Washington-Baltimore Infant Study. *Am J Epidemiol*. 1985;121:31.
4. Levy RJ, Rosenthal A, Fyler DC, et al. Birth weight of infants with congenital heart disease. *Am J Dis Child*. 1978;132:249.
5. Rowland TW, Hubbell JP, Nadas AS. Congenital heart disease in infants of diabetic mothers. *J Pediatr*. 1973;83:815.
6. Hoffman JIE. Incidence of congenital heart disease, I: postnatal incidence. *Pediatr Cardiol*. 1995;16:103.
7. Warkany J, Passarge E, Smith LB. Congenital malformations in autosomal trisomy syndromes. *Am J Dis Child*. 1966;112:502.
8. Keith JD. Prevalence, incidence and epidemiology. In: Keith JD, Rowe RD, Vlad P, eds. *Heart Disease in Infancy and Childhood*. New York, NY: Macmillan; 1978:3.
9. Rudolph AM. The changes in the circulation after birth. *Circulation*. 1970;41:343.
10. Lake CL. Cardiac embryology, growth and development. In: Lake CL, ed. *Pediatric Cardiac Anesthesia*. Norwalk, Conn: Appleton & Lange; 1988:27.
11. Ho SY, Angelini A, Moscoso G. Developmental cardiac anatomy. In:

Long WA, ed. *Fetal and Neonatal Cardiology*. Philadelphia, Pa: WB Saunders; 1990:3.
12. Davies LK, Davis RF. Cardiothoracic anesthesia. In: Brown DL, ed. *Risk and Outcome in Anesthesia*. Philadelphia, Pa: WB Saunders; 1992:258.
13. Hickey PR, Crone RK. Cardiovascular physiology and pharmacology in children: normal and diseased pediatric cardiovascular systems. In: Ryan JF, Todres ID, Cote CJ, et al, eds. *A Practice of Anesthesia for Infants and Children*. Orlando, Fla: Grune & Stratton; 1986:176.
14. Gessner IH, Klovetz LJ, Hensen RW, et al. Hemodynamic adaptations in the newborn infant. *Pediatrics*. 1965;36:752.
15. Clyman RI, Heymann MA, Rudolph AM. Ductus arteriosus responses to prostaglandin $E_1$ at high and low oxygen concentrations. *Prostaglandins*. 1977;13:219.
16. Hagen PT, Scholz DG, Edwards WD. Incidence and size of patent foramen ovale during the first ten decades: a necropsy study of 965 normal hearts. *Mayo Clin Proc*. 1984;59:17.
17. Emmanouilides GC, Moss AJ, Duffie ER, et al. Pulmonary arterial pressure changes in human newborn infants from birth to three days of age. *J Pediatr*. 1964;65:327.
18. Rudolph AM. *Congenital Disease of the Heart: Clinical-Physiologic Considerations in Diagnosis and Management*. Chicago, Ill: Yearbook Medical; 1974:29.
19. Keen EN. The postnatal development of the human cardiac ventricles. *J Anat*. 1955;89:484.
20. Friedman WF. Intrinsic physiological properties of the developing heart. *Prog Cardiovasc Dis*. 1972;15:87.
21. Friedman WF, Pool PE, Jacobowitz D, et al. Sympathetic innervation of the developing rabbit heart: biochemical and histochemical comparisons of fetal, neonatal, and adult myocardium. *Circ Res*. 1968;23:25.
22. Sinha SN, Armour JA, Randall WC. Development of autonomic innervation of the heart. *Circulation*. 1973;48(suppl 4):37.
23. Klitzner TS. Maturational changes in excitation-contraction coupling in mammalian myocardium. *J Am Coll Cardiol*. 1991;17:218.
24. Schwartz AJ, Campbell FW. Pathophysiological approach to congenital heart disease. In: Lake CL, ed. *Pediatric Cardiac Anesthesia*. Norwalk, Conn: Appleton & Lange; 1988:7.
25. Lees MH, King DH. Heart disease in the newborn. In: Adams FH, Emmanouilides GC, Riemenschneider TA, eds. *Heart Disease in Infants, Children and Adolescents*. Baltimore, Md: Williams & Wilkins; 1989:842.
26. Paul MH, Currimbhoy Z, Miller RA, et al. Thrombocytopenia in cyanotic congenital heart disease. *Circulation*. 1961;24:1013.
27. Kontras SB, Sirak HD, Newton WA Jr. Hematologic abnormalities in children with congenital heart disease. *JAMA*. 1966;195:611.
28. Edelman NH, Lahiri S, Braudol L, et al. The blunted ventilatory response to hypoxia in cyanotic congenital heart disease. *N Engl J Med*. 1970;282:405.
29. Amatayakul O, Cumming GR, Haworth JC. Association of hypoglycemia with cardiac enlargement and heart failure in newborn infants. *Arch Dis Child*. 1970;45:717.
30. Lanier WL, Stangland KJ, Scheithauer BW, et al. The effects of dextrose infusion and head position on neurologic outcome after complete cerebral ischemia in primates: examination of a model. *Anesthesiology*. 1987;66:39.
31. Pulsinelli WA, Waldman S, Rawlinson D, et al. Moderate hyperglycemia augments ischemic brain damage: a neuropathologic study in the rat. *Neurology*. 1982;32:1239.
32. Pulsinelli WA, Levy DE, Sigsbee B, et al. Increased damage after ischemic stroke in patients with hyperglycemia with or without established diabetes mellitus. *Am J Med*. 1983;74:540.
33. Nakakimura K, Fleischer JE, Drummond JC, et al. Glucose administration before cardiac arrest worsens neurologic outcome in cats. *Anesthesiology*. 1990;72:1005.
34. Steward DJ, DaSilva CA, Flegel T. Elevated glucose levels may increase the danger of neurologic deficit following profoundly hypothermic cardiac arrest. *Anesthesiology*. 1988;68:653.
35. Burrows FA. Neurologic protection in pediatric cardiac surgery. Workshop at: Society of Cardiovascular Anesthesiologists 20th Annual Meeting; April 25-29, 1998; Seattle, Wash.
36. Morrison J, Killip T. Serum digitalis and arrhythmia in patients undergoing cardiopulmonary bypass. *Circulation*. 1973;47:341.
37. Hickey PR, Hansen DD, Norwood WI, et al. Anesthetic complications in surgery for congenital heart disease. *Anesth Analg*. 1984;63:657.
38. Strafford MA, Henderson KH. Anesthetic morbidity in congenital heart disease patients undergoing noncardiac surgery [abstract]. *Anesthesiology*. 1991;75:A1056.

39. Ferry P. Neurologic sequelae of cardiac surgery in children. *Am J Dis Child.* 1987;141:309.

40. Helmers SL, Wypij D, Constantinou JE, et al. Perioperative electroencephalographic seizures in infants undergoing repair of complex congenital cardiac defects. *Electroencephalogr Clin Neurophysiol.* 1997;102:27.

41. Ehyai A, Fenichel GM, Bender HW Jr. Incidence and prognosis of seizures in infants after cardiac surgery with profound hypothermia and circulatory arrest. *JAMA.* 1984;252:3165.

42. O'Dougherty M, Wright FS, Garmezy N, et al. Later competence and adaptation in infants who survive severe heart defects. *Child Dev.* 1983;54:129.

43. Newburger JW, Jonas RA, Wernovsky G, et al. A comparison of the perioperative neurologic effects of hypothermic circulatory arrest versus low flow cardiopulmonary bypass in infant heart surgery. *N Engl J Med.* 1993;329:1057.

44. Bellinger DC, Wypij D, Kuban KCK, et al. Developmental and neurological status of children at 4 years of age after heart surgery with hypothermic circulatory arrest or low-flow cardiopulmonary bypass. *Circulation.* 1999;100:526.

45. Miller G, Vogel H. Structural evidence of injury or malformation in the brains of children with congenital heart disease. *Semin Pediatr Neurol.* 1999;6:20.

46. Strauss A, Johnson M. The genetic basis of pediatric cardiovascular disease. *Semin Perinatol.* 1996;20:564.

47. DuPlessis AJ. Mechanisms of brain injury during infant cardiac surgery. *Semin Pediatr Neurol.* 1999;6:32.

48. Nicolson SC, Dorsey AT, Schreiner MS. Shortened preanesthetic fasting interval in pediatric cardiac surgical patients. *Anesth Analg.* 1992;74:694.

49. Tanner GE, Angers DG, Barash PG, et al. Effect of left-to-right, mixed left-to-right, and right-to-left shunts on inhalational anesthetic induction in children: a computer model. *Anesth Analg.* 1985;64:101.

50. Moore RA. Anesthesia for the pediatric congenital heart patient for noncardiac surgery. *Anesthesiol Rev.* 1981;8:23.

51. Hickey C, Gugino LD, Aglio LS, et al. Intraoperative somatosensory evoked potential monitoring predicts peripheral nerve injury during cardiac surgery. *Anesthesiology.* 1993;78:29.

52. Greeley WJ, Kates RA, Bushman GA, et al. Intraoperative esophageal electrocardiography for dysrhythmia analysis and therapy in pediatric cardiac surgical patients. *Anesthesiology.* 1986;65:669.

53. Stefaniszyn HJ, Novick RJ, Keith FM, et al. Is the brain adequately cooled during deep hypothermic cardiopulmonary bypass? *Curr Surg.* 1983;40:294.

54. Almond CH, Jones JC, Snyder HM, et al. Cooling gradients and brain damage with deep hypothermia. *J Thoracic Cardiovasc Surg.* 1964;48:890.

55. Burrows FA. Physiologic dead space, venous admixture, and the arterial to end-tidal carbon dioxide difference in infants and children undergoing cardiac surgery. *Anesthesiology.* 1989;70:219.

56. Swain JA, McDonald TJ, Robbins RC, et al. Relationship of cerebral and myocardial intracellular pH to blood pH during hypothermia. *Am J Physiol.* 1991;260:H1640.

57. Stephan H, Weyland A, Kazmaier S, et al. Acid-base management during hypothermic cardiopulmonary bypass does not affect cerebral metabolism but does affect blood flow and neurological outcome. *Br J Anaesth.* 1992;69:51.

58. Patel RL, Turtle MR, Chambers DJ, et al. Alpha-stat acid-base regulation during cardiopulmonary bypass improves neuropsychologic outcome in patients undergoing coronary artery bypass grafting. *J Thorac Cardiovasc Surg.* 1996;111:1267.

59. Murkin JM, Martzke JS, Buchan AM, et al. A randomized study of the influence of perfusion technique and pH management strategy in 316 patients undergoing coronary artery bypass surgery, II: neurologic and cognitive outcomes. *J Thorac Cardiovasc Surg.* 1995;110:349.

60. Hickey PR, Hansen DD. Temperature and blood gases: the clinical dilemma of acid-base management for hypothermic cardiopulmonary bypass. In: Tinker J, ed. *Cardiopulmonary Bypass: Current Concepts and Controversies.* Philadelphia, Pa: WB Saunders; 1989:1.

61. McConnell DH, White F, Nelson RL, et al. Importance of alkalosis in maintenance of "ideal" blood pH during hypothermia. *Surg Forum.* 1975;26:263.

62. Poole-Wilson PA, Langer GA. Effect of pH on ionic exchange and function in rat and rabbit myocardium. *Am J Physiol.* 1975;229:570.

63. Swain JA, White FN, Peters RM. The effect of pH on the hypothermic ventricular fibrillation threshold. *J Thoracic Cardiovasc Surg.* 1984;87:445.

64. Norwood WI, Norwood CR, Castaneda AR. Cerebral anoxia: effect of deep hypothermia and pH. *Surgery.* 1979;86:203.

65. Aoki M, Nomura F, Stromski ME, et al. Effects of pH on brain energetics after hypothermic circulatory arrest. *Ann Thorac Surg.* 1993;55:1093.

66. Skaryak LA, Chai PJ, Kern FH, et al. Blood gas management and degree of cooling: Effects on cerebral metabolism before and after circulatory arrest. *J Thorac Cardiovasc Surg.* 1995;110:1649.

67. Kirshbom PM, Skaryak LA, DiBernardo LR, et al. pH-stat cooling improves cerebral metabolic recovery after circulatory arrest in a piglet model of aorto-pulmonary collaterals. *J Thorac Cardiovasc Surg.* 1996;111:147.

68. Kurth CD, O'Rourke MM, O'Hara IB. Comparison of pH-stat and alpha-stat cardiopulmonary bypass on cerebral oxygenation and blood flow in relation to hypothermic circulatory arrest in piglets. *Anesthesiology.* 1998;89:110.

69. DuPlessis AJ, Jonas RA, Wypij D, et al. Perioperative effects of alpha-stat versus pH-stat strategies for deep hypothermic cardiopulmonary bypass in infants. *J Thorac Cardiovasc Surg.* 1997;114:990.

70. Hammon JW, Stump DA, Kon ND, et al. Risk factors and solutions for the development of neurobehavioral changes after coronary artery bypass grafting. *Ann Thorac Surg.* 1997;63:1613.

71. Vannucci RC. Mechanisms of perinatal ischemic brain damage. In: Jonas RA, Newburger JW, Volpe JJ, eds. *Brain Injury and Pediatric Cardiac Surgery.* Boston, Mass: Butterworth-Heinemann; 1996:201.

72. Kern FH, Greeley WJ, Ungerleider RM. The assessment of cerebral function during paediatric cardiopulmonary bypass. *Perfusion.* 1993;8:63.

73. Van der Linden J, Priddy R, Ekroth R, et al. Cerebral perfusion and metabolism during profound hypothermia in children. A study of middle cerebral artery ultrasonic variables and cerebral extraction of oxygen. *J Thorac Cardiovasc Surg.* 1991;102:103.

74. Goetting MG, Preston G. Jugular bulb catheterization: experience with 123 patients. *Crit Care Med.* 1990;18:1220.

75. Daubeney PE, Pilkington SN, Janke E, et al. Cerebral oxygenation measured by near-infrared spectroscopy: comparison with jugular bulb oximetry. *Ann Thorac Surg.* 1996;61:930.

76. Austin EH III, Edmonds HL Jr, Auden SM, et al. Benefit of neurophysiologic monitoring for pediatric cardiac surgery. *J Thorac Cardiovasc Surg.* 1997;114:707.

77. Ungerleider RM, Greeley WJ, Sheikh KH, et al. Routine use of intraoperative epicardial echocardiography and Doppler color flow imaging to guide and evaluate repair of congenital heart lesions. *J Thorac Cardiovasc Surg.* 1990;100:297.

78. Lake CL, Schwartz AJ, Campbell FW. Extracorporeal circulation. In: Lake CL, ed. *Pediatric Cardiac Anesthesia.* Norwalk, Conn: Appleton & Lange; 1988:155.

79. Jonas R. Neurological protection during cardiopulmonary bypass/deep hypothermia. *Pediatr Cardiol.* 1998;19:321.

80. Royston D. High dose aprotinin therapy: a review of the first five years' experience. *J Cardiothorac Vasc Anesth.* 1992;6:76.

81. Boldt J, Knothe C, Zickmann B, et al. Comparison of two aprotinin dosage regimens in pediatric patients having cardiac operations: influence on platelet function and blood loss. *J Thorac Cardiovasc Surg.* 1993;105:705.

82. D'Errico CC, Shayevitz JR, Martindale SJ, et al. The efficacy and cost of aprotinin in children undergoing reoperative open heart surgery. *Anesth Analg.* 1996;83:1193.

83. Mossinger H, Dietrich W. Activation of hemostasis during cardiopulmonary bypass and pediatric aprotinin dosage. *Ann Thorac Surg.* 1998;65:S45.

84. Buss MI, McLean RF, Wong BI, et al. Cardiopulmonary bypass, rewarming, and central nervous system dysfunction. *Ann Thorac Surg.* 1996;61:1423.

85. Parr CVS, Blackstone EH, Kirklin JW. Cardiac performance and mortality early after intracardiac surgery in infants and young children. *Circulation.* 1975;51:867.

86. Kouchoukos NT, Karp RB. Management of the postoperative cardiovascular surgical patient. *Am Heart J.* 1976;92:513.

87. Gall WE, Clarke WR, Doty DB. Vasomotor dynamics associated with cardiac operations. *J Thorac Cardiovasc Surg.* 1982;83:724.

88. Appelbaum A, Blackstone EH, Kouchoukos NT, et al. Effect of afterload reduction on cardiac output in infants after intracardiac surgery [abstract]. *Circulation.* 1975;51, 52(suppl II):II151.

89. Benumof JL. Respiratory physiology and respiratory function during anesthesia. In: Miller RD, ed. *Anesthesia.* 2nd ed. New York, NY: Churchill Livingstone; 1986:1122.

90. Hickey PR, Wessel DL. Anesthesia for treatment of congenital heart disease. In: Kaplan JA, ed. *Cardiac Anesthesia.* 2nd ed. Orlando, Fla: Grune & Stratton; 1987:635.

91. Miller OI, Celermajer DS, Deanfield JE, et al. Very low-dose inhaled nitric oxide: a selective pulmonary vasodilator after operations for congenital heart disease. *J Thorac Cardiovasc Surg.* 1994;108:487.

92. Naik SK, Elliott MJ. Ultrafiltration and paediatric cardiopulmonary bypass. *Perfusion.* 1993;8:101.

93. Elliott MJ. Ultrafiltration and modified ultrafiltration in pediatric open-heart operations. *Ann Thorac Surg.* 1993;56:1518.

94. Naik SK, Knight A, Elliott MJ. A prospective randomized study of a modified technique of ultrafiltration during pediatric open-heart surgery. *Circulation.* 1991;84:III422.

95. Friesen RH, Campbell DN, Clarke DR, et al. Modified ultrafiltration attenuates dilutional coagulopathy in pediatric open-heart operations. *Ann Thorac Surg.* 1997;64:1787.

96. Davies MJ, Nguyen K, Gaynor JW, et al. Modified ultrafiltration improves left ventricular systolic function in infants after cardiopulmonary bypass. *J Thorac Cardiovasc Surg.* 1998;115:361.

97. Bando K, Vijay P, Turrentine MW, et al. Dilutional and modified ultrafiltration reduces pulmonary hypertension after operations for congenital heart disease: a prospective randomized study. *J Thorac Cardiovasc Surg.* 1998;115:517.

98. Meliones JN, Gaynor JW, Wilson BG, et al. Modified ultrafiltration reduces airway pressure and improves lung compliance after congenital heart surgery. *J Am Coll Cardiol.* 1995;25:271A.

99. Millar AB, Armstrong L, van der Linden J, et al. Cytokine production and hemofiltration in children undergoing cardiopulmonary bypass. *Ann Thorac Surg.* 1993;56:1499.

100. Andreasson S, Gothberg S, Berggren H, et al. Hemofiltration modifies complement activation after extracorporeal circulation in infants. *Ann Thorac Surg.* 1993;56:1515.

101. Skaryak LA, Kirshbom P, DiBernardo LR, et al. Modified ultrafiltration improves cerebral metabolic recovery after circulatory arrest. *J Thorac Cardiovasc Surg.* 1995;109:744.

102. Botero M, Davies LK. Diagnosis and management of arrhythmias in children after surgery. *Semin Cardiothorac Vasc Anes.* 2001;5:122.

103. Ekert H, Gilchrist GS, Stanton R, et al. Hemostasis in cyanotic heart disease. *J Pediatr.* 1970;76:221.

104. Hoffman WS, Tomasello DN, MacVaugh H. Control of postcardiotomy bleeding with PEEP. *Ann Thorac Surg.* 1982;34:71.

105. Murphy DA, Finlayson DC, Craver JM, et al. Effect of positive end-expiratory pressure on excessive mediastinal bleeding after cardiac operations: controlled study. *J Thorac Cardiovasc Surg.* 1983;85:864.

CHAPTER

# 63

# Anesthesia for Adult Cardiovascular Surgery

Gregory M. Janelle

Monica Botero

Emilio B. Lobato

Today, over one half million cardiac surgery procedures are carried out annually in the United States, with absolute numbers doubling every 5 years. The population of adult patients undergoing cardiac surgery in the 21st century has evolved to one of increasing age and extensive medical therapy, often with a previous history of angioplasty or revascularization. Perioperative care for patients undergoing cardiac surgery involves some of the greatest challenges in our specialty. The combination of complicated preoperative pathophysiologic states and the invasive nature of the operative procedures carried out under largely nonphysiologic conditions has led to technologic and pharmacologic advances in anesthesia for cardiac procedures that are unparalleled in anesthesia for other types of surgery.

## PREOPERATIVE EVALUATION

Only through a meticulous understanding of a patient's pathophysiology and severity of illness can a specific anesthetic plan be made. Technologically advanced invasive and noninvasive tests can delineate much about the extent of cardiovascular disease processes. However, the patient's history of clinical signs and symptoms of cardiovascular disease can often provide a wealth of information about the manner and degree to which a patient is affected and should never lose its emphasis.

### *What Are the Goals of the Preoperative Assessment?*

#### Duke Activity Status Index

The Duke Activity Status Index provides a standard for assessing patients' baseline liveliness and reserve (metabolic equivalent test [MET])[1]:

#### 1 MET

- Can you take care of yourself?
- Eat, dress, or use the toilet?
- Walk indoors around the house?
- Walk a block or two on level ground at 2 to 3 mph?

#### 4 to 10 METs

- Do light work around the house like dusting or washing dishes?
- Climb a flight of stairs or walk up a hill?
- Walk on level ground at 4 mph?
- Run a short distance?

- Do heavy work around the house like scrubbing floors or lifting or moving heavy furniture?
- Participate in moderate recreational activities like golf, bowling, dancing, doubles tennis, or throwing a baseball or football?

**10 METs**

- Participate in strenuous sports like swimming, singles tennis, football, basketball, or skiing?

## What Are the Clinical Signs and Symptoms of Myocardial Ischemia?

### Angina Pectoris

#### Categorization

Angina is commonly categorized according to the Canadian Cardiovascular Society grading scale[2]:

**Class I.** Angina occurs only with strenuous or protracted physical activity.
**Class II.** Slight limitation of vigorous physical activity such as walking up a hill briskly.
**Class III.** Marked limitation of physical activity, with symptoms occurring during the activities of daily living.
**Class IV.** Symptoms occur at rest, with inability to perform the activities of daily living.

Angina that has a predictable and reproducible pattern for longer than 3 months is labeled *stable angina*. Any change in the pattern, intensity, or duration, as well as the occurrence of angina at rest, defines *unstable angina*. The classification proposed by Braunwald[3] (Table 63–1) defines unstable angina according to the intensity and precipitating factors and the temporal association with a myocardial infarction (MI). It is simple to use and has been found to correlate with the pathophysiology and predict outcome.[4]

Although angina is the single most common symptom of myocardial ischemia, it is important to note that anginal symptoms usually occur as a late consequence of a cascade of events. In fact, some patients (eg, diabetics) may not complain of angina but rather exhibit "anginal" equivalents such as shortness of breath, palpitations, or dizziness. Earlier manifestations of acute ischemia include abnormalities in diastolic and systolic left ventricular (LV) function, followed by abnormal myocardial lactate metabolism, electrocardiographic (ECG) changes, and eventually anginal symptoms.[5,6] However, the vast majority (>75%) of ischemic episodes by ECG criteria in patients with chronic stable angina may occur in the absence of angina.[5] The incidence of silent ischemia is even higher in the diabetic population because of the neuropathy that develops as a consequence of microvascular disease in the diabetic patient's cardiac pain fibers. It is also important to note that myocardial dysfunction may exist for 60 to 120 minutes following resolution of angina or ischemia-induced ECG changes, as a result of myocardial stunning.[7]

## What Are the Clinical Signs and Symptoms of Congestive Heart Failure?

### Dyspnea

#### New York Heart Association Activity Scale

Dyspnea is commonly quantified by a patient's functional reserve as described previously. Patients with congestive heart failure (CHF) are often categorized according to the New York Heart Association (NYHA) according to their functional status as follows[8]:

**Class I.** No limitation of physical activity.
**Class II.** Mild limitation of physical activity. Ordinary physical activity may result in fatigue, dyspnea, or angina.
**Class III.** Marked limitation in physical activity. Symptoms occur with less than ordinary physical exertion.
**Class IV.** Symptoms occur at rest. Unable to perform any physical activity without discomfort.

### Orthopnea and Paroxysmal Nocturnal Dyspnea

The process by which orthopnea and paroxysmal nocturnal dyspnea (PND) occur is similar and one that the failing heart cannot tolerate. Subsequently, pulmonary edema (PE) develops and may be associated with coughing, wheezing, diaphoresis, and even overt cyanosis. Patients often avoid or ameliorate PND by elevating their heads during sleep. Therefore, the number of pillows on which one sleeps can be used as a gross means of quantifying the severity of PND. In fact, it is not uncommon to find patients with severely decompensated CHF who sleep in a reclining chair or inclined hospital bed.

### Edema and Nocturia

Patients should be questioned about ankle edema that worsens throughout the day. Also, nocturia may be caused by

---

TABLE 63–1. Classification of Unstable Angina

| Severity | Clinical Circumstances | | |
| | A. Presence of Extracardiac Condition (Secondary UA) | B. Absence of Extracardiac Condition (Primary UA) | C. Develops Within 2 Weeks After AMI (Postinfarction UA) |
| --- | --- | --- | --- |
| I. New onset of severe angina or accelerated angina; no rest pain | IA | IB | IC |
| II. Angina at rest within past month but not within preceding 48 h (subacute UA) | IIA | IIB | IIIB |
| III. Angina at rest within 48 h (acute UA) | IIIA | IIIB | IIIC |

AMI, acute myocardial infarction; UA, unstable angina.
From Braunwald E. Unstable angina: a classification. *Circulation.* 1989;80:410.

position-dependent redistribution of peripheral edema fluid to the intravascular volume and subsequent renal excretion of excess water.

## Syncope and Palpitations

Cardiac syncope is typically characterized by a sudden loss of consciousness without prodrome. Patients lose consciousness as a consequence of inadequate brain perfusion due to a variety of causes, including arrhythmias (eg, ventricular tachycardia, ventricular fibrillation, atrial fibrillation with rapid ventricular response, high-degree atrioventricular nodal block, asystole); LV outflow obstruction (eg, aortic stenosis [AS], hypertrophic obstructive cardiomyopathy); or simply low output states (eg, vasovagal syncope). When syncope is due to arrhythmias, patients may experience palpitations, an unpleasant awareness of the heartbeat often described as "skipping," "jumping," or "racing" in nature.

## How Can Patients With a Normal Ejection Fraction Have Congestive Heart Failure?

The syndrome of CHF is characterized predominantly by symptoms of organ congestion due to elevated venous pressures. Most commonly, these are the result of the inability of the myocardium to eject an adequate stroke volume due to depressed contractility (systolic dysfunction), which leads to an increase in end-diastolic volume and filling pressure (diastolic dysfunction) and results in PE (LV failure) or peripheral edema (right ventricular failure). In some patients, the predominant abnormality is either ventricular relaxation or increased wall stiffness despite adequate systolic function. Therefore, higher filling pressures are required to maintain stroke volume. In this circumstance, any increase in heart rate or exaggerated fluid infusion will result in a steep increase in filling pressure, thus leading to symptoms of CHF.

## How Is the Preoperative Electrocardiogram Helpful?

The heart rate (HR) and rhythm may indicate the adequacy of therapy with antidysrhythmic and rate-controlling agents (eg, digoxin, β-adrenergic blockers). Measurement of the PR, QRS, and QT intervals provides information about the conduction system. The ECG may show evidence of ischemia or previous MI. The lead tracings in which evidence of infarction is seen may provide information about the location of coronary artery stenosis (Table 63–2). The ECG frequently appears normal, even in the presence of severe coronary artery disease (CAD).[9]

## How Is the Chest Radiograph Helpful?

Radiographic signs of CHF are correlated with poor ventricular function. Specifically, four radiographic indices are important indicators[10]:

1. The cardiothoracic ratio
2. Total heart volume
3. LV volume
4. Signs of CHF

The latter are specific indicators of abnormal ejection fraction, end-systolic volume, cardiac index, stroke work index, end-diastolic volume, and end-diastolic pressure. The chest radiograph can also appear normal in patients with significant ventricular dysfunction.

## What Is the Role of Noninvasive Cardiac Studies?

Patients who present with new-onset angina or who undergo cardiac evaluation before noncardiac surgery may undergo various noninvasive cardiac studies.

**TABLE 63–2.** Relationship Between Electrocardiographic Findings Relecting Myocardial Ischemia and Area of Myocardium Involved

| Electrocardiogram Lead | Coronary Artery Responsible for Myocardial Ischemia | Area of Myocardium That May Be Involved |
|---|---|---|
| II, III, aVF | Right coronary artery | Right atrium<br>Interatrial septum<br>Right ventricle<br>Sinoatrial node<br>Atrioventricular node<br>Posterior fascicle of left bundle<br>Posterior one third of interventricular septum<br>Posterior papillary muscle |
| $V_3$–$V_5$ | Left anterior descending coronary artery | Anterolateral aspects of left ventricle<br>Right bundle branch<br>Anterior fascicle of left bundle<br>Posterior fascicle of left bundle<br>Anterior two thirds of interventricular septum<br>Anterior papillary muscle<br>Posterior papillary muscle |
| I, aVL | Left circumflex coronary artery | Lateral aspects of left ventricle<br>Sinoatrial node<br>Atrioventricular node<br>Posterior fascicle of left bundle |

From McCammon RL. Coronary artery disease. In: Stoelting RK, Dierdorf SF, McCammon RL, eds. *Anesthesia and Coexisting Disease.* 2nd ed. New York, NY: Churchill Livingstone; 1988:1.

## Exercise Treadmill Testing

Exercise treadmill testing provides an important assessment of functional capabilities. Patients are progressively exercised to a target heart rate. They are monitored for symptomatic and ECG evidence of myocardial ischemia (Fig. 63–1). This test is particularly helpful in that it can suggest which lead to monitor for intraoperative ischemia detection.

## Thallium-201 Perfusion Scan

A thallium-201 perfusion study may be performed in conjunction with exercise treadmill testing. Thallium-201 is a radioactive potassium analogue that is taken up by areas of myocardium that are perfused. It is injected during peak exercise, and areas of ischemia or previous infarction appear as cold spots on the imaging. After 2 to 4 hours of rest following exercise, imaging is repeated. Areas that were ischemic but still viable become perfused, and the defect on the image disappears (reversible defect). Areas of previous infarction remain as cold spots (fixed defect).

## Dipyridamole-Thallium Imaging

Dipyridamole-thallium imaging can be performed in patients who cannot exercise (owing to musculoskeletal disorders, claudication, other reasons). Dipyridamole simulates exercise by inducing dilation of coronary arteries. Stenotic vessels cannot dilate normally; therefore, less thallium is taken up in areas supplied by them than in areas supplied by normal coronary arteries. On images taken later, thallium redistributes into these areas of relative ischemia.

## Echocardiography

Echocardiography can be used preoperatively to assess regional wall motion, ventricular systolic and diastolic function, chamber pressures, valvular areas, interchamber gradients, in-

ECG PATTERNS INDICATIVE OF MYOCARDIAL ISCHEMIA

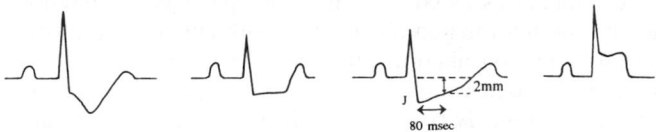

ECG PATTERNS NOT INDICATIVE OF MYOCARDIAL ISCHEMIA

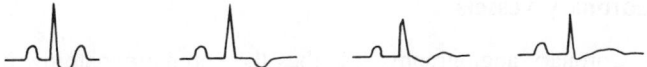

**FIGURE 63–1.** Electrocardiographic criteria for myocardial ischemia during exercise treadmill testing: at least 1 mm of J point depression with downsloping or horizontal ST segments; slowly upsloping ST segment depression with 2 mm of ST segment depression measured at 80 ms after the J point; and ST segment elevation. ST segment depression usually indicates nontransmural ischemia, whereas ST segment elevation connotes transmural injury. Downsloping S depression more often indicates severe two- and three-vessel coronary artery disease than does horizontal or slowly upsloping ST segment depression. ST segment elevation indicates high-grade, usually proximal coronary artery stenosis in patients without previous myocardial infarction. (Reproduced with permission from Goldschlager N. Use of the treadmill test in the diagnosis of coronary artery disease in patients with chest pain. *Ann Intern Med.* 1982;97:383.)

tracardiac and extracardiac masses, valvular function, and the presence of intracardiac shunts. Although echocardiography may be a useful test to diagnose ventricular dysfunction, a resting echocardiogram tells little about the potential for developing ischemia in a patient with severe CAD without history of MI. The echocardiographic detection of new wall motion abnormalities after peak exercise correlates well with the severity of coronary artery stenoses found on angiography.[11] The use of contrast echocardiography to identify coronary stenoses and successful revascularization may play a more significant role in the future as the technology evolves.

## Stress Echocardiography

Stress echocardiography can be used to determine both the area of myocardium at risk and the potential for improvement following revascularization. Patients exercise on a treadmill until target heart rates are achieved and then rapidly undergo echocardiography examinations. Comparisons are made among baseline, peak exercise, and recovery examinations to determine areas of myocardium at risk for ischemia. Patients who are not candidates for exercise treadmill testing are given incrementally increased doses of dobutamine (DSE), often with the addition of atropine, to pharmacologically increase heart rate to at least 85% of their maximum predicted value. Echocardiographic views are obtained between doses and following discontinuation of drug therapy in order to determine the areas (if any) at risk for developing *demand ischemia,* which is ischemia that occurs due to increased metabolic requirements. High concordance rates exist between cardiac catheterization data and DSE findings.

## Radionuclide Studies

Radionuclide angiography plays a less important role now than in the past. It measures ejection fraction and provides an assessment of wall motion. Thus, it can be used to evaluate ventricular function and the impact of CAD.

## Fluorodeoxyglucose Studies

Patients with severely depressed ventricular function due to ischemic cardiomyopathy may not be considered candidates for surgical revascularization. However, in certain cases, areas of myocardium may be "stunned" due to an antecedent MI, but not irreversibly infarcted. Uptake of fluorodeoxyglucose (FDG) in these areas of myocardial stunning provides evidence for potential myocardial recovery and improvement in function following successful revascularization. Combined metabolic single photon emission computed tomography (CT) imaging with FDG and β-methyl-iodophenyl-pentadecanoic acid (BMIPP) can further reveal areas of high metabolic mismatch (FDG/BMIPP) and has been shown to have potential for more efficient therapeutic revascularization.[12]

## *How Are Cardiac Catheterization Data Used?*

Most patients presenting for cardiac surgery have undergone diagnostic cardiac catheterization. Cardiac catheterization provides the most precise information about the location and severity of coronary stenoses, ventricular function, pulmonary

**TABLE 63–3.** Normal Hemodynamic Values Measured at Cardiac Catheterization

|  |  | a Wave | v Wave | Systolic | End-Diastolic | Mean |
|---|---|---|---|---|---|---|
| Pressures (mm Hg) | Right atrium | 2–10 | 2–10 |  |  | 0–8 |
|  | Right ventricle |  |  | 15–30 | 0–8 |  |
|  | Pulmonary artery |  |  | 15–30 | 3–12 | 9–16 |
|  | Pulmonary capillary wedge | 3–15 | 3–12 |  |  | 1–10 |
|  | Left atrium | 3–15 | 3–12 |  |  | 1–10 |
|  | Left ventricle |  |  |  |  |  |
|  | Aorta |  |  | 100–140 | 3–12 |  |
|  |  |  |  | 100–140 | 60–90 | 70–105 |
| Oxygen consumption index (mL/min/m²) |  | 110–150 |  |  |  |  |
| Arteriovenous $O_2$ difference (mL/dL) |  | 3–5 |  |  |  |  |
| Cardiac index (L/min/m²) |  | 2.6–4.2 |  |  |  |  |

From Grossman W. Cardiac catheterization. In: Braunwald E, ed. *Heart Disease: A Textbook of Cardiovascular Medicine.* 4th ed. Philadelphia, Pa: WB Saunders; 1992:180.

and systemic vascular resistance (PVR and SVR), and valvular function, and the presence of intracardiac shunts.

Although the hemodynamic data obtained at cardiac catheterization can be extremely helpful in understanding the pathophysiology in a particular patient, keep in mind that these data are dependent on multiple factors such as filling conditions, the presence or absence of ischemia, autonomic activity, and so on. Thus, it is not surprising that sometimes the data at catheterization and preinduction do not correlate.

## Pressure Measurement

The reported hemodynamic measurements should include baseline data such as the patient's HR, rhythm, and blood pressure (BP). Chamber pressures are reported as systolic and end-diastolic pressures for the ventricles and as mean pressure for the atria. Normal values are shown in Table 63–3. Pressure measurements are also used to calculate SVR and PVR. If stenotic valves are present, valve areas and pressure gradients are reported. The orifice areas of stenotic valves are calculated from the pressure gradient and flow across a valve by Gorlin's formulas (Table 63–4).

## Cardiac Output

Cardiac output (CO) can be determined by Fick's oxygen ($O_2$) method or by an indicator dilution technique (dye dilution or thermodilution). There is generally good correlation between the two techniques. Fick's $O_2$ method requires estima-

tion of $O_2$ consumption by collection of expired air during a 3-minute period. CO is then calculated as follows:

$$\text{Cardiac Output (L/min)} = \frac{O_2 \text{ Consumption (mL/min)}}{C\,(a - \bar{v})\,O_2 \text{ (mL/L)}}$$

(Equation 1)

Thermodilution CO is considerably easier to perform, but Fick's method is more accurate in patients with low CO, regurgitant valvular lesions, and intracardiac shunts.

## Ventricular Function

The angiography portion of the cardiac catheterization report provides information about ventricular function, coronary anatomy, and the presence of regurgitant valvular lesions. The ventriculogram may be omitted in patients with poor ventricular function for fear that they may decompensate with injection of a large bolus of contrast material. It may also be omitted in patients with significant renal dysfunction. The report of ventriculography contains information about global LV function, as assessed by wall motion and ejection fraction, and specific information about areas with abnormal wall motion. Wall motion abnormalities may be described as *hypokinesis* (decreased contractility), *akinesis* (no contractile motion), or *dyskinesis* (outward wall motion). A ventricular aneurysm or thrombus may be noted as well.

## Coronary Vessels

Coronary angiography describes the coronary anatomy, including details about the sizes of vessels, the location of any anatomic variations, and the presence of calcifications and stenoses. Stenoses are characterized according to their length, the degree of diameter narrowing, and the presence of collateral filling. Narrowing of luminal diameter by 50% corresponds to a 75% reduction in cross-sectional area, and this is regarded as hemodynamically significant. The incidence of coronary spasm may be noted by including ergonovine in the study to stimulate spasm or the use of nitroglycerin (NTG) to relieve it. Normal coronary artery anatomy is depicted in Figure 63–2.

**TABLE 63–4.** Gorlin's Formulas for Calculation of Stenotic Valve Areas

$$\text{Aortic valve area (cm}^2\text{)} = \frac{F}{44.5\sqrt{\Delta}}$$

$$\text{Mitral valve area (cm}^2\text{)} = \frac{F}{38.0\sqrt{\Delta P}}$$

$$\text{Flow (mL/s)} = \frac{\text{Cardiac output (mL/min)}}{\text{DFP (s/min) or SEP (s/min}^2\text{)}}$$

DFP, diastolic filling period; SEP, systolic ejection period. These are calculated by measuring the diastolic filling time or systolic ejection time per beat and multiplying by heart rate. F, flow across the valve (mL/s); $\Delta P$, mean pressure gradient across the valve (mm Hg).

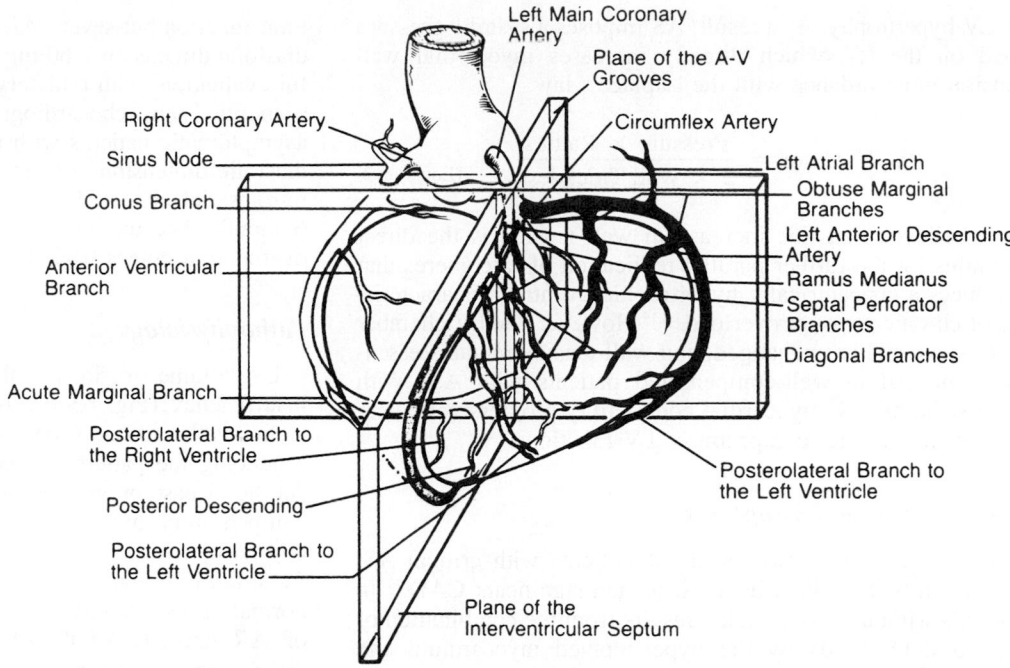

**FIGURE 63–2.** Normal anatomy of the coronary arteries. The right coronary artery and the left circumflex coronary artery lie in the same plane, whereas the left anterior descending coronary artery travels perpendicular to that plane. Each gives rise to branches as shown. The left circumflex artery is shown in black, the left anterior descending artery in gray, and the right coronary artery in white. (From Bashore TM, Chapman MJ. Basic anatomy and physiology of the heart. In: Bashore TM, ed. *Invasive Cardiology: Principles and Techniques.* 1st ed. Toronto, Ontario, Canada: BC Decker; 1990:79.)

## What Are the Considerations for the Patient With Valvular Disease?

### Aortic Stenosis

#### Natural History

Valvular AS is more common in men and is usually congenital or degenerative in origin.[13] Isolated, acquired disease usually results from calcification or degeneration of a congenitally bicuspid or previously normal tricuspid valve.[14] In the natural history of AS, there is a long latent period during which there is gradually increasing obstruction and pressure load on the myocardium while the patient remains asymptomatic; yet morbidity and mortality are low.[15] Cardiac catheterization and Doppler studies indicate that some patients show a decrease in valve area of 0.1 to 0.3 $cm^2$ per year and an increase in the systolic pressure gradient across the valve of 10 to 15 mm Hg per year. It appears that progression of AS is more rapid in patients with degenerative calcific disease than in those with congenital disease; still, the rate of progression of AS in an individual patient is uncertain.[15]

When the classic symptoms of angina, syncope, and heart failure develop, the prognosis changes dramatically. Survival curves show that the interval from the onset of symptoms to the time of death is 2 years in patients with heart failure, 3 years in those with syncope, and 5 years in those with angina.[16,17] Sudden death is known to occur in patients with severe AS but it is an uncommon event in asymptomatic patients, occurring probably <1% per year.[15]

An optimal schedule for repeated medical examination in patients with AS has not been defined yet. Current understanding of the natural history of AS and indications for surgical intervention do not support the use of annual echocardiographic studies to assess changes in valve area in asymptomatic patients. However, serial echocardiograms are helpful to assess changes in LV hypertrophy and function. Therefore, in patients with severe AS, a yearly echocardiogram may be appropriate. In patients with moderate AS, serial studies every

2 years are satisfactory, and in patients with mild AS, serial studies can be performed every 5 years. Echocardiography should be performed more frequently if there is a change in clinical findings.[15]

#### Pathophysiology

The normal aortic valve area is 2.6 to 3.5 $cm^2$. Symptoms generally occur when the valve area has narrowed to one fourth its normal size (ie, 0.5 $cm^2/m^2$), and the peak systolic gradient across the valve exceeds 50 mm Hg in the presence of a normal CO.

Stenosis at the level of the aortic valve results in a pressure gradient from the LV to the aorta (Fig. 63–3). In adults with AS, this obstruction usually increases gradually over a prolonged period, and LV output is maintained by the presence

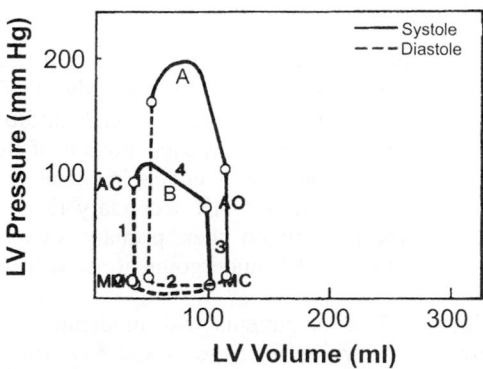

**FIGURE 63–3.** Comparison of left ventricular pressure-volume loops: moderate aortic stenosis (A) showing markedly elevated left ventricular systolic pressure, elevated end-systolic and end-diastolic volume, and increased diastolic pressure versus normal ventricle (B). AC, aortic valve closure; AO, aortic valve opening; MC, mitral valve closure; MO, mitral valve opening. (Redrawn from Moore RA, Martin DE. Anesthetic management for the treatment of valvular heart disease. In: Hensley FA Jr, Martin DE, eds. *A Practical Approach to Cardiac Anesthesia.* 2nd ed. Boston, Mass: Little, Brown and Co; 1995:298,300.)

of LV hypertrophy. As a result, AS imposes a systolic pressure load on the LV, which directly increases myocardial wall tension in accordance with the Laplace's law:

$$\text{Wall Tension} = \frac{\text{Pressure} \times \text{Radius}}{2 \times \text{Wall Thickness}} \qquad \text{(Equation 2)}$$

It is believed that this increase in wall tension is the direct stimulus for the further parallel replication of sarcomeres that produces a concentrically hypertrophied ventricle characteristic of chronic pressure overload.[18,19] However, the LV chamber size is essentially unchanged, and wall tension remains essentially normal in well-compensated patients with AS. With long-standing AS, myocardial contractility progressively deteriorates and further compromises LV function.

### Clinical Signs and Symptoms

Angina occurs in two thirds of patients with critical AS, and about half of them have associated significant CAD.[19] In patients without CAD, angina results from the combination of increased $O_2$ needs by the hypertrophied myocardium and reduced $O_2$ delivery secondary to the excessive compression of coronary vessels.[13]

Syncope is most commonly due to the reduced cerebral perfusion that occurs during exertion when arterial pressure declines as a result of systemic vasodilation in the presence of fixed CO. Syncope at rest may occur as a result of transient atrial fibrillation resulting in decreased ventricular filling and decreased CO or transient ventricular block due to extension of the calcification of the valve into the conduction system.

Exertional dyspnea with orthopnea and PE result in pulmonary venous hypertension and are relatively late symptoms in AS.[13]

The most common sign of AS is a systolic ejection murmur radiating to the neck and best heard in the aortic area. In mild AS, the murmur usually peaks early in systole. As the severity of the AS increases, the murmur peaks progressively later in systole and may become softer as CO decreases.[20]

## Aortic Regurgitation

### Natural History

Aortic regurgitation (AR) is usually acquired. It may occur as a result of an abnormality of the aortic valve leaflets due to rheumatic heart disease or bacterial endocarditis or in association with any disease that causes dilation of the aortic root, preventing leaflet coaptation such as in connective tissue disorders or aortic dissection.[21] AR secondary to aortic root disease is now more common than primary valve disease among patients with pure AR undergoing aortic valve replacement.[22]

Approximately 75% of patients with moderately severe to severe chronic AR survive for 5 years and 50% for 10 years after diagnosis.[13,23] Without surgical treatment, death usually occurs within 4 years after the development of angina and within 2 years after the onset of heart failure.[13]

Asymptomatic patients with mild AR, little or no LV dilation, and normal LV systolic function can be evaluated on a yearly basis. If there is no clinical evidence that regurgitation has worsened, routine echocardiography can be performed every 2 to 3 years. Asymptomatic patients with normal sys-

tolic function but severe AR and significant LV dilation (end-diastolic dimension >60 mm) require more frequent and careful evaluation, with a history and physical examination every 6 months and echocardiography every 6 to 12 months. In asymptomatic patients with more advanced LV dilation (end-diastolic dimension >70 mm or end-systolic dimension >50 mm), serial echocardiograms should be obtained every 4 to 6 months because the risk of developing symptoms or LV dysfunction ranges from 10% to 20% per year.[15]

### Pathophysiology

LV volume overload is the characteristic feature of aortic insufficiency (Fig. 63–4). As a result of increased end-diastolic wall tension, serial replication of sarcomeres occurs, producing the pattern of eccentric ventricular hypertrophy.[18] As the disease progresses, recruitment of preload reserve and compensatory hypertrophy allow the ventricle to maintain normal ejection performance despite the elevated afterload.[15] *LV systolic dysfunction,* defined as an ejection fraction below normal at rest, is initially reversible. However, as the amount of AR exceeds >60% of stroke volume, progressive LV dilation and hypertrophy occur, leading to irreversible myocardial damage.[24]

### Clinical Signs and Symptoms

Acute AR causes a sudden increase in LV filling pressures and PE. Patients develop sudden manifestations of cardiovascular collapse with severe dyspnea and hypotension.

In patients with chronic AR, exertional dyspnea, orthopnea, and PND are the characteristic complaints. Although the typical diastolic blowing murmur heard along the left sternal border is the usual sign of AR, the peripheral signs of hyperdynamic circulation indicates that the disease is severe. Some of these signs include *Corrigan pulse* (a bounding, full carotid pulse with a rapid downstroke), *Musset's sign* (head bobbing), *Quincke pulse* (systolic plethora and diastolic blanching in the nail bed when gentle pressure is placed on it), and *Hill sign* (SBP in the leg at least 30 mm Hg higher than that in the

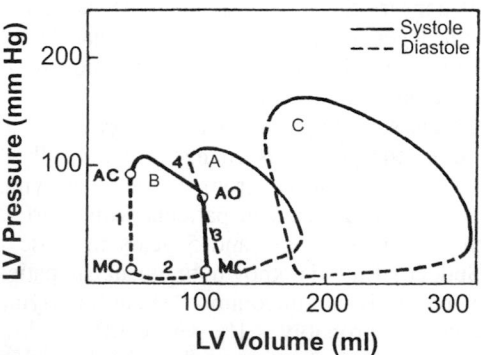

**FIGURE 63–4.** Comparison of left ventricular pressure-volume loops: acute aortic insufficiency (A), showing elevated left ventricular systolic and diastolic volumes, as well as a high left ventricular end-diastolic pressure; chronic aortic insufficiency (C) showing markedly increased systolic and diastolic volumes and a lower end-diastolic pressure versus normal ventricle (B). AC, aortic valve closure; AO, aortic valve opening; MC, mitral valve closure; MO, mitral valve opening. (Redrawn from Moore RA, Martin DE. Anesthetic management for the treatment of valvular heart disease. In: Hensley FA Jr, Martin DE, eds. *A Practical Approach to Cardiac Anesthesia.* 2nd ed. Boston, Mass: Little, Brown & Co; 1995:298,304.)

arm).[20] In addition to the typical murmur of AR, a mid- and late-diastolic apical rumble, the *Austin Flint murmur*, is common in severe AR and may occur in the presence of a normal mitral valve. This murmur appears to be created as the aortic jet impinges on the mitral valve, causing it to vibrate; and also by rapid antegrade flow across a mitral orifice that is narrowed by the rapidly rising LV diastolic pressure, producing physiologic stenosis.[13,20]

## Mitral Stenosis

### Natural History

Mitral stenosis (MS) is typically rheumatic in origin and primarily affects women.[23] Only 25% of patients have isolated MS, whereas 40% have combined MS and MR.[25,26] Other rare causes include systemic lupus erythematosus and carcinoid and rheumatoid arthritis. Methysergide is an uncommon but documented cause of MS.[27] Although calcification of the mitral annulus usually causes mitral regurgitation (MR), when subvalvular or intravalvular extension is extensive, MS may result.[13]

In developed countries, there is a long latent period of 20 to 40 years from the occurrence of rheumatic fever to onset of symptoms.[15] It then takes approximately 3 years for most patients to progress from mild disability (ie, early class II) to severe disability (ie, class III or IV).[13] However, when significant limiting symptoms occur, the 10-year survival rate is only 0% to 15%; when there is severe pulmonary hypertension, mean survival drops to <3 years.[15]

In the asymptomatic patient, yearly reevaluation is recommended; at this time, a history, physical examination, chest radiograph, and ECG should be obtained. A yearly echocardiogram is not recommended unless there is a change in clinical status.[15]

### Pathophysiology

The normal mitral valve area is 4.0 to 6.0 cm$^2$. Narrowing of the valve area to <2.5 cm$^2$ must occur before development of symptoms.[15] With a valve area <1 cm$^2$, a significant left atrioventricular pressure gradient is required to maintain a normal CO at rest (Fig. 63–5). In turn, the elevated left atrial pressure increases pulmonary capillary pressures, resulting in exertional dyspnea.[13]

## Clinical Signs and Symptoms

The symptoms of MS stem from increased left atrial pressure and reduced CO, primarily caused by mechanical obstruction of filling of the ventricle. In patients with markedly elevated PVR, right ventricular function is often impaired. Patients with MS usually have symptoms typical of left-sided heart failure: dyspnea on exertion, orthopnea, and PND. Less frequently, they have hemoptysis, hoarseness, and symptoms of right-sided heart failure.[20] Physical examination findings include a diastolic low-pitched rumbling murmur, best heard at the apex, that may radiate to the axilla or lower left sternal area. Although the intensity of the murmur is not strictly related to the severity of stenosis, the duration of the murmur is a guide to the severity of mitral narrowing.[13] The opening snap that precedes the classic rumble appears to be caused by the sudden tensing of the valve leaflets after the valve cusps have completed their opening excursion and occurs when the sudden movement of the mitral dome into the LV suddenly stops.[28] The presence of a loud P2, right ventricular lift, elevated neck veins, ascites, and edema indicates that pulmonary hypertension producing right ventricular overload has developed. This is a dismal sign in the progression of MS because pulmonary hypertension increases the risk associated with surgery.[20,29]

## Mitral Regurgitation

### Natural History

Mitral regurgitation (MR) occurs from defects of any of the structures of the mitral valve apparatus, which include the valve leaflets per se, the mitral annulus, the chordae tendineae, and the papillary muscles.[13,30] MR due to abnormalities of the valve leaflets not only may follow rheumatic heart disease, an increasingly uncommon cause, but also may occur as a result of infective endocarditis.[25] The mitral annulus is a soft and flexible structure that measures approximately 10 cm in circumference in the adult and constricts during LV systolic contraction, playing an important role in valve closure. Any condition that causes severe dilation of the LV, especially dilated ischemic cardiomyopathy or severe degenerative calcification, can cause MR.[13,31] The chordae may be congenitally abnormal or may rupture due to trauma, endocarditis, or rheumatic fever; however, in most cases, no cause for this rupture is apparent, other than increased mechanical strain.[13] The papillary muscles, perfused by the terminal portion of the coronary vascular bed, are particularly at risk for ischemia, and its dysfunction results in transient or permanent incomplete leaflet coaptation.

The natural history of MR is variable and depends largely on the cause of the underlying disorder. Symptoms usually do not develop in patients with chronic MR until the LV fails. The time interval between the initial attack of rheumatic fever and the development of symptoms tends to exceed two decades.[13,24] Once significant symptoms occur, the 5-year survival rate may be only 45%.[32]

Asymptomatic patients with mild MR and no evidence of LV enlargement or dysfunction or pulmonary hypertension can be followed up on a yearly basis. Annual echocardiography is

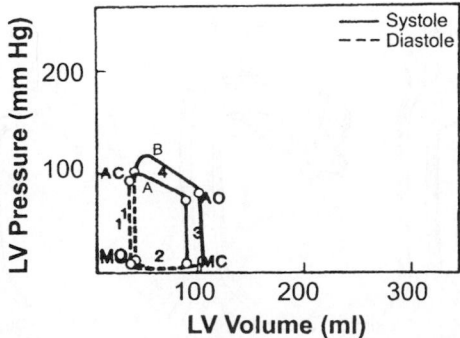

**FIGURE 63–5.** Comparison of left ventricular pressure-volume loops: mitral stenosis (A), showing decreased left ventricular systolic and diastolic volumes, and decreased systolic and end-diastolic pressures versus normal ventricle (B). AC, aortic valve closure; AO, aortic valve opening; MC, mitral valve closure; MO, mitral valve opening. (Redrawn from Moore RA, Martin DE. Anesthetic management for the treatment of valvular heart disease. In: Hensley FA Jr, Martin DE, eds. *A Practical Approach to Cardiac Anesthesia.* 2nd ed. Boston, Mass: Little, Brown & Co; 1995:298,307.)

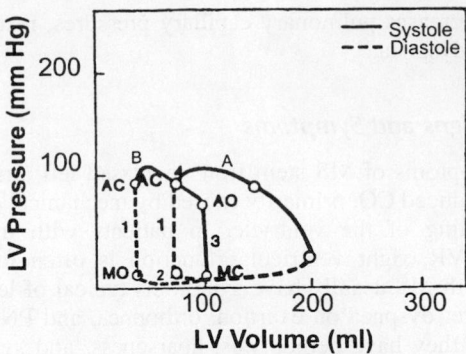

**FIGURE 63–6.** Comparison of left ventricular pressure-volume loops: moderate mitral insufficiency (A), showing increased left ventricular end-systolic and end-diastolic volumes with some increase in left ventricular end-diastolic pressure versus normal ventricle (B). AC, aortic valve closure; AO, aortic valve opening; MC, mitral valve closure; MO, mitral valve opening. (Redrawn from Moore RA, Martin DE. Anesthetic management for the treatment of valvular heart disease. In: Hensley FA Jr, Martin DE, eds. *A Practical Approach to Cardiac Anesthesia.* 2nd ed. Boston, Mass: Little, Brown & Co; 1995:298,312.)

recommended for patients with moderate MR or if there is clinical evidence that regurgitation has worsened. Asymptomatic patients with severe MR should be evaluated with a history, physical examination, and echocardiography every 6 to 12 months to assess the transition to LV dysfunction. Exercise testing is especially important if a good history of the patient's exercise capacity cannot be obtained.[15]

### Pathophysiology

In acute MR, the volume overload increases preload sarcomere length, which results in an increase of LV end-diastolic volume (LVEDV) from 150 mL to 170 mL (Fig. 63–6). Although the ejection fraction increases acutely, the forward stroke volume is reduced because part of the stroke volume is regurgitated into the left atrium. Initially, chronic MR is compensated by the development of eccentric cardiac hypertrophy, which allows for an increase in total stroke volume as well as forward stroke volume. Accordingly, enlargement of the left atrium allows the volume overload to generate lower filling pressures. In this phase of compensated MR, the patient may be entirely asymptomatic, even during vigorous exercise. The transition to chronic decompensated MR is characterized by LV dysfunction. In this phase, end-systolic volume is increased, and forward stroke volume is decreased, resulting in increased LV filling pressure and pulmonary congestion.[13,20,33]

### Clinical Signs and Symptoms

Acute, severe mitral regurgitation causes a sudden increase in left atrial pressure, leading to severe PE and symptoms of acute LV failure. Unless such patients are treated aggressively, a fatal outcome is almost certain.

Physical examination of patients with MR demonstrates a displacement of the LV apical impulse due to cardiac enlargement. A third heart sound, caused by rapid filling of the LV, does not necessarily indicate heart failure. Although the most prominent physical finding is the high-pitched holosystolic murmur, best heard at the apex, with radiation to the axilla and left infrascapular area, little correlation has been established between the intensity of the murmur and the severity of MR.[34]

## *What Information Should Be Obtained From Patients With Thoracic Aortic Disease?*

### Aortic Aneurysm

Aneurysms of the thoracic aorta can be classified according to their size, shape (saccular, fusiform), location, and etiology. Most are caused by either atherosclerosis or cystic medial necrosis, but less frequently they can occur as a result of an inflammatory process (syphilitic aortitis). Patients may exhibit symptoms such as pain, hoarseness from involvement of the recurrent laryngeal nerve, or recurrent pneumonitis from left bronchial compression. Findings consistent with AR may accompany ascending aneurysms due to dilation of the aortic valve. Transverse arch aneurysms are usually not associated with cerebral ischemia unless concomitant dissection is present. Descending aneurysms may produce midscapular pain due to bony erosion of the thoracic spine (see Chapter 65).

The diagnosis is made either by chest radiograph or CT scan. However, angiography delineates the extent of the aneurysm and also other important information such as the coronary anatomy and the presence of AR.

### Dissection

Dissection is one of the most common problems of the thoracic aorta. It occurs as a result of a tear in the intimal layer, which then becomes separated from the media by an expanding hematoma. The anatomic classifications of thoracic aortic dissections have been described (Fig. 63–7). DeBakey's classification (types I, II, III) considers the site of the tear on the extent of aortic involvement. Dailey's (Stanford's) classification categorizes dissections into types A (ascending aorta) and B (distal to the left subclavian), regardless of the site of the tear. The latter classification has important prognostic values: type A dissections are always considered a surgical disease, whereas in selected patients, type B dissections may be managed medically.

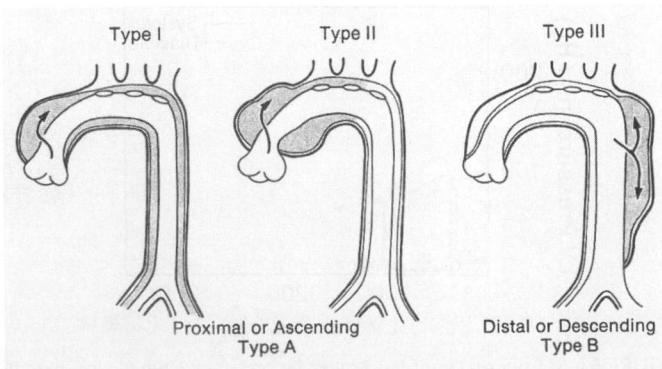

**FIGURE 63–7.** The anatomic classification of thoracic aortic dissections. DeBakey types I and II and Stanford type A involve the ascending aorta and arch. DeBakey type III and Stanford type B originate distal to the left subclavian artery. (From Benumof JL. Anesthesia for emergency thoracic surgery. In: Benumof JL, ed. *Anesthesia for Thoracic Surgery.* 1st ed. Philadelphia, Pa: WB Saunders; 1987:375.)

A common symptom associated with type A dissections is severe chest pain that is "tearing" in character. Dissections involving the aortic root are frequently accompanied by AR or myocardial ischemia. Shock may result from hemopericardium, MI, or acute LV failure. Involvement of the arch vessels may be associated with diminished pulse on the upper extremities and symptoms of cerebral ischemia. Chest radiograph findings include a wide mediastinum and loss of the aortic knob. The diagnosis can be established with high sensitivity and specificity by CT scanning, magnetic resonance imaging, or transesophageal echocardiography (TEE). However, aortography still remains as the confirmatory test. Because of the rapidity of diagnosis with TEE, it has become the initial test of choice in many centers. In addition, TEE allows for the diagnosis of aortic insufficiency, tamponade, and myocardial ischemia.

### Rupture

Aortic rupture is most commonly occurs in the descending aorta and is frequently associated with multiple injuries. Occasionally, the ascending aorta can be involved. Death usually occurs from a massive hemothorax or hemomediastinum.

## What Electrophysiologic Disorders Are Important?

Patients with reentry atrial and ventricular tachydysrhythmias are commonly treated using catheter ablation techniques in the cardiac catheterization laboratory,[35] but some still require ablation of reentry pathways or ventricular aneurysmectomy. Others with a history of recurrent ventricular tachycardia or ventricular fibrillation undergo placement of an automatic internal cardioverter-defibrillator (AICD).

The nature of the dysrhythmias and their associated symptoms, the status of antidysrhythmic therapy, and the apparent success or lack of success in controlling the problem should be determined by history, Holter monitoring, and electrophysiologic studies. Ventricular dysfunction and CHF should be ascertained if present. Patients with precipitation atrial reentrant tachydysrhythmias, such as the Wolff-Parkinson-White syndrome, may have normal ventricular function and be in otherwise good health. Others may have severe ventricular dysfunction due to ischemic cardiomyopathy or idiopathic cardiomyopathy.

### Pulmonary Function

Preoperative pulmonary function tests should be considered in patients scheduled for AICD implantation. Patients treated with amiodarone may develop interstitial lung fibrosis as a toxic side effect of the drug. They tend to have reduced total lung capacity and diffusion capacity.[36] Chronic obstructive lung disease should also be ruled out.

Depending on the surgical approach, one-lung ventilation may be used intraoperatively; thus, optimization of pulmonary function is especially important. If a patient may not be able to tolerate such an approach, an alternative (eg, subxiphoid or median sternotomy) can be suggested.

## THE PREOPERATIVE PERIOD

After preoperative evaluation, the anesthetic plan is constructed. It involves decisions about continuation of long-term medications, administration of preoperative sedation, choice of monitors, and intraoperative anesthetic management.

## What Medications Should Be Continued in Patients With Coronary Artery Disease?

Patients with CAD are usually treated with one or more antianginal agents, including nitrates, β-adrenergic blockers, and calcium channel blockers. Antihypertensive medications, such as angiotensin-converting enzyme inhibitors, angiotensin II inhibitors, or the centrally acting α-adrenergic agonist clonidine may also be part of the long-term treatment regimen. Other commonly prescribed medications include diuretics, antiarrhythmics, digoxin, potassium supplements, insulin, oral hypoglycemic agents, heparin, and aspirin.

### Nitrates

Oral, sublingual, or topical nitrates (eg, NTG, isosorbide dinitrate, isosorbide mononitrate) exert antianginal effects primarily by their systemic vasodilating effects.[37] They reduce preload by dilating capacitance veins, thereby decreasing myocardial oxygen consumption ($M\dot{V}O_2$) via decreasing LV end-diastolic diameter and wall tension. They also reduce afterload by dilating systemic arteries and arterioles, further decreasing $M\dot{V}O_2$. Direct vasodilation in the coronary circulation primarily involves large conductive vessels.[38]

Because nitrate therapy may contribute to stable hemodynamic function and help to prevent myocardial ischemia, it should be continued in the perioperative period. If a patient uses sublingual NTG for episodes of chest pain, the anesthesiologist should include a preoperative order that it be sent to the operating room (OR) for use as needed. Patients receiving intravenous NTG should continue to receive it during transport to the OR.

### β-Blockers

Patients receiving β-adrenergic blockers should continue to receive them perioperatively. These agents have beneficial effects in ischemic heart disease, primarily through reduction in HR, decrease in force of contraction, platelet aggregation, and decreased renin production. The cardiac effects of β-adrenergic blockade are more marked under conditions of increased myocardial demand and increased sympathetic tone, such as during exercise. For this reason, β-blockers are particularly effective in patients with exercise-induced angina. This fact may also explain their benefit in the perioperative period because they may blunt the tachycardiac, hypertensive response to tracheal intubation and surgical stimuli. Tachycardia is the hemodynamic response most commonly associated with perioperative ischemia that is attributed to a change in hemodynamics.[39,40]

In the past, discontinuation of β-adrenergic blockade was recommended before surgery for fear of dangerous interaction with general anesthetic agents.[41] This concern is unfounded.[42,43] Hemodynamic management is not complicated by the continuation of β-blockers. Discontinuation of β-adrenergic blockade not only deprives patients of its beneficial effects but also may lead to rebound phenomena. Nervousness, sweating, and tachycardia may be followed by life-threatening hypertension, myocardial ischemia, and infarction.[44]

One possible exception involves a long-acting β-blocker, nadolol, which some investigators suggest should be converted to a shorter acting drug on the day of surgery to avoid prolonged bradycardia and myocardial depression after cardiopulmonary bypass (CPB).

## Calcium Channel Blockers

Calcium channel blockers are a common part of the therapy of ischemic heart disease. The various agents exert different hemodynamic effects, including systemic vasodilation, slowing of atrioventricular conduction, depression of myocardial contractility, and prevention of coronary spasm. Interestingly, evidence that calcium channel blockers have a significant role in preventing perioperative myocardial ischemia is lacking.[45,46]

Potential adverse side effects of continuing calcium channel blockers in cardiac surgical patients include decreased SVR, myocardial depression, and atrioventricular conduction block. However, these side effects can be overcome with vasoconstrictors, inotropes, and atrioventricular sequential pacing. Because calcium channel blockers in particular patients may play a part in control of hypertension, prevention of supraventricular tachydysrhythmias, and relief of Prinzmetal angina, logic suggests they provide similar benefit in the perioperative period and should therefore be continued.

## Clonidine

Clonidine is an $\alpha_2$-adrenergic agonist commonly used to treat hypertension. Clonidine must be continued perioperatively to avoid the rebound hypertensive crisis associated with withdrawal as early as 8 hours after the last dose. Alternate routes of administration should be considered either preoperatively or in the early postoperative period before patients are able to receive it orally. The transdermal route is an option that must be anticipated in that it requires 24 to 48 hours to reach peak effect. Rectal administration requires 45 minutes.[47]

## Aspirin

Prophylactic aspirin should be discontinued 1 week before scheduled cardiac surgery. Continuation of aspirin in the preoperative period significantly increases blood loss and transfusion requirements.[48]

## Should Antidysrhythmics Be Continued for Implantation of an Automatic Internal Cardioverter-Defibrillator?

The cardiologist who treats a patient preoperatively and postoperatively should make the decision about continuation of antidysrhythmic medications. However, the anesthesiologist and surgeon should be aware of the decision and understand its implications because the issue is somewhat controversial.

Some antiarrhythmic medications affect the testing and function of an AICD. The defibrillation threshold may be elevated by antidysrhythmic medications.[49] Class I antiarrhythmic agents would be expected to increase defibrillation threshold by depression of sodium conductance, and class III

agents would be expected to lower depolarization threshold by decreasing potassium conductance.[50] In doses used clinically, however, this is not necessarily true. Class IC agents, such as encainide and flecainide, reliably increase the defibrillation threshold in animal models.[51,52] Chronic oral administration of amiodarone has been shown to raise energy requirements for defibrillation in patients at the time of AICD implantation.[53–55] Other antidysrhythmic agents appear to be clinically less significant in altering the defibrillation threshold. Slowing of conduction by class I agents and amiodarone may also cause slowing of ventricular tachycardia and may interfere with tachycardia detection by the AICD.

The best solution is to maintain patients on a stable antidysrhythmic regimen through the perioperative period. If a patient will not be maintained on such medications postoperatively, they should be stopped 1 to 2 days before surgery and the patient kept on continuous ECG monitoring.[56] A much longer period is necessary for amiodarone because it has a mean elimination half-life of 52 days.[57]

If a patient is to be maintained on antidysrhythmic medications postoperatively, they should be continued perioperatively so that the AICD can be tested under the same pharmacologic conditions that will be present thereafter.

## How Should Preoperative Sedation Be Managed Before Cardiac Surgery?

### General Considerations

Preoperative medication should help to alleviate a patient's anxiety, suppress the pain that may be associated with the placement of intravascular catheters, and induce amnesia. The preoperative discussion should make clear to patients that you are sensitive to their concerns and should provide enough information so that none of the invasive procedures are complete surprises.

Anxiolytic treatment helps to reduce the chance that ischemia may result from a patient's sympathetic response to apprehension. Appropriate use of local anesthesia limits the pain associated with placement of invasive monitors but does not completely prevent it. Preoperative medications that provide amnesia are important for two reasons: most patients do not want to remember the immediate preoperative period, and preoperative medication may also prevent awareness and recall of intraoperative events, particularly when the planned anesthetic is primarily opioid-based.

### Functional Status

Although all of these characteristics are desirable, the dosing of preoperative medication should be based on a patient's functional status. Not all patients want or need preoperative sedation. Many times, all that is needed is to compassionately reassure patients and allow them the choice to receive such medication at any time if they feel that it might be helpful.

If sedation is required, doses of most sedatives are judiciously reduced in (1) elderly patients, (2) those with poor ventricular function, (3) patients who appear to be especially susceptible to soft tissue airway obstruction, and (4) with known or suspected pulmonary hypertension (especially patients with valvular disease). Such patients are more safely managed by the administration of a small dose of a benzodiazepine before transfer to the OR. Additional sedation with intravenously administered opioids or benzodiazepines can be titrated for placement of intravascular catheters in the OR, where closer observation and monitoring can be performed. Patients who are anticoagulated receive either orally or intravenously administered premedications only.

All cardiac surgery patients who have received a sedative premedication should be transported to the OR with supplemental $O_2$ readily available to provide a margin of safety. This practice is especially important for patients with pulmonary hypertension that may be significantly worsened by hypoxemia. No matter what degree of sedation is chosen, patients about to undergo cardiac surgery should not be left unattended for long periods after receiving preoperative medication. Ideally, they should be observed in a preoperative holding area. Pulse oximetry may provide added safety by identifying desaturation and extremes of HR. Table 63–5 lists some suggested preoperative medication regimens.

## Should Sedation Be Administered Before Undergoing Thoracic Aortic Surgery?

The decision to administer sedation to patients undergoing thoracic aortic surgery will depend on whether the patient is in a chronic stable condition or has an acute evolving process and is hemodynamically unstable. Sedation in stable patients should be done judiciously because a patient who is rendered stuporous will be impossible to monitor for neurologic findings as an indication of progression of the disease. Patients with a dissection must be alert enough to describe the location and quality of pain, which may indicate progression of the process. If a patient is hemodynamically stable, careful administration of analgesics can be beneficial by preventing pain-induced tachycardia and hypertension, which may exacerbate the disease process.

## What Monitors Are Required?

The basic intraoperative monitors for any anesthetic as outlined by the American Society of Anesthesiologists apply to cardiac anesthesia as well. They include an inspired $O_2$ analyzer, pulse oximeter, ECG machine, and BP cuff, as well as qualified anesthesia personnel in the room throughout the procedure. Beyond these basic monitors, cardiac anesthesia requires additional devices or techniques that should be considered standard because of the severity of illness of the patients and the invasive nature of the surgical procedure.

**TABLE 63–5.** Suggested Preoperative Medications

| Good LV function | Diazepam, 0.1–0.15 mg/kg PO<br>Morphine, 0.1 mg/kg IM<br>Scopolamine, 0.005 mg/kg IM |
|---|---|
| Good LV function, anticoagulated | Diazepam, 0.1–0.15 mg/kg PO<br>Methadone, 0.1 mg/kg PO |
| Poor LV function, advanced age | Diazepam, 0.07–0.1 mg/kg PO, or midazolam, 0.02–0.04 IM<br>Morphine 0.05 mg/kg IM |
| Poor LV function, pulmonary hypertension | Diazepam, 0.07–0.1 mg/kg PO, or midazolam, 0.02–0.04 mg/kg IM |

IM, intramuscularly; LV, left ventricular; PO, orally.

## Electrocardiogram

ECG is an important monitor of HR and rhythm, atrioventricular conduction, and myocardial ischemia. Changes occur suddenly in cardiac procedures. Conduction disturbances commonly result from anesthetic agents, electrolyte and temperature changes, ventricular irritability from intravascular wires and catheters, manual manipulation of the heart and intrathoracic structures, and surgically induced disruption of conduction pathways. The preferred leads are lead II, which provides the best P-wave morphology as well as right coronary artery (RCA) distribution in most patients, and $V_5$, which provides information that correlates with left coronary artery (LCA) distribution.

## Blood Pressure

Arterial BP must be monitored by an intra-arterial catheter in addition to a BP cuff. Intra-arterial pressure monitoring provides continuous beat-to-beat measurement. BP is subject to sudden and dramatic change during cardiac surgery, owing to the patient's cardiovascular disease, changes in heart rhythm, effects of anesthetic agents and airway manipulation, surgical stimulation, and direct manipulation of the heart and great vessels. During CPB, only an intra-arterial catheter can reliably measure the nonpulsatile arterial pressure.

### Catheter Location

The specific location of the catheter is determined by the preference of the anesthesiologist and the requirements of the procedure. Aortic arch pressure is the measurement that is most closely related to LV stroke volume, LV contractility, and SVR.[4,58] Direct arterial BP measurement is obtained at more distal sites, with consequent attenuation of the aortic pressure waveform. Although mean arterial pressure (MAP) may be fairly consistent throughout the arterial tree, systolic pressure, flow, and waveform characteristics in peripheral arteries are often divergent from those of the aorta (Fig. 63–8). Radial or femoral arterial catheters are most commonly used for cardiac surgery because of their easy accessibility and relative safety.

Following CPB, it is not uncommon to experience dramatically lower pressures recorded from radial arteries compared with simultaneously recorded central arterial pressures (aortic or femoral). This may be due to either damping from temperature-induced vasoconstriction or the presence of peripheral arteriovenous shunting, which may occur following CPB. Whichever the case, the phenomenon often resolves with time, during which direct aortic pressure may be measured by the pressure in the aortic cannula (if still present), by passing sterile tubing connected to a needle placed in the field, or by placing a femoral arterial line.

During coronary artery bypass graft (CABG) surgery in which a left internal mammary artery (IMA) graft is used, traction of the Favoloro retractor on the sternum and left chest wall may cause "tenting" of the left subclavian artery. This might lead to damping or loss of a left radial arterial pressure tracing. As many anesthesiologists prefer placing radial artery catheters in patients' nondominant wrists, left radial catheters may be the preferred site in some institutions when not otherwise contraindicated. If so, it may prove useful to monitor BP with a noninvasive cuff on the right arm. This method can be

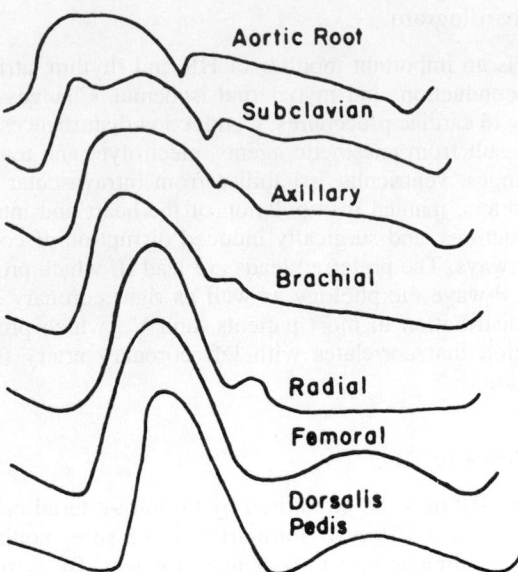

**FIGURE 63–8.** The arterial pressure wave undergoes considerable attenuation as it passes from the aorta to distal arterial sites. Although the measured mean pressure is fairly constant, there is considerable disparity among systolic pressures measured at various sites. (From Bedford RF. Invasive blood pressure monitoring. In: Blitt CD, ed. *Monitoring in Anesthesia and Critical Care Medicine.* 2nd ed. New York, NY: Churchill Livingstone; 1990:93.)

accomplished safely because the period of dissection of the IMA is not particularly stimulating and tends to be associated with hemodynamic stability.

Insertion of a second intraarterial catheter may be necessary for thoracic aortic aneurysm repair. The locations of the catheters are determined by the type of aneurysm and the planned location of aortic cross-clamps and are discussed later.

### Assessment of Intravascular Volume

Intravascular volume is indirectly assessed by central venous pressure (CVP), pulmonary artery pressure (PAP), and pulmonary artery occlusion pressure (PAOP), or by measurement of left atrial pressure (LAP) through a catheter placed by the surgeon. Such assessment is essential to maintain hemodynamic stability in cardiac surgery patients. It is especially important during weaning from CPB when intravascular volume (preload) is optimized by delivering blood from the CPB circuit reservoir.

In estimating preload, it is necessary to keep in mind that the actual value a clinician is attempting to ascertain in order to maximize myocardial performance along the Starling curve is the LVEDV. Use of intravascular catheters necessarily implies that pressure measurements are directly related to volume status. Although this assumption is generally true, many things must be kept in mind.

Not all patients have "normal" systolic or diastolic function. An LAP of 8 mm Hg might indicate an adequate LVEDV, whereas for a patient with long-standing AS and LVH, the same value might represent gross underfilling of a noncompliant ventricle. Additionally, due to risks inherent to cardiac surgery, such as ischemia from prolonged cross-clamp time, inadequate myocardial preservation or revascularization, or reperfusion injury, the same patient may have extraordinarily different loading conditions with the same LAP before and after CPB.

Furthermore, it is important to remember the anatomic locations of the catheters from which one extrapolates pressure measurements to volumetric assumptions. If one is attempting to ascertain LVEDV, then certainly the LV end-diastolic pressure (LVEDP) provides the closest measurement. In the absence of functional MS, the LAP during diastole should equal the LVEDP. In the absence of intrinsic lung disease or pulmonary hypertension, the PAOP should approximate the LAP. Likewise, with normal lung compliance and a competent pulmonic valve, the PA diastolic pressure closely approximates the PAOP. The right ventricular (RV) systolic pressure equals the pulmonary artery (PA) systolic pressure in the absence of pulmonic or infundibular stenosis. Likewise, the RV diastolic pressure is the same as the right atrial pressure (RAP) during diastole in the absence of tricuspid stenosis, which is equal to the CVP. Relationships become more complicated in the presence of intracardiac shunts.

### Central Venous Catheter

As discussed, the CVP indicates RAP. During CPB, CVP should also be monitored to assess the adequacy of superior vena caval drainage and, indirectly, cerebral venous drainage. In some cases, the CVP may be the only intravascular volume monitor necessary, for example, atrial septal defect repair or CABG surgery in a patient with well-preserved ventricular function.

### Pulmonary Artery Catheter

**Pressure Monitoring.** A PA catheter is commonly used during cardiac surgery to measure CVP, PAP, and PAOP. In addition to providing valuable hemodynamic information, it can also help to detect myocardial ischemia.

Frequent indications for use of a PA catheter are outlined in Table 63–6. Although the use of a PA catheter with aggressive treatment of hemodynamic aberrations in patients with CAD may decrease perioperative MI and mortality,[59,60] a prospective study has shown no difference in outcome whether a PA catheter or CVP catheter was used.[61] The decision about which to use should be based on the severity of cardiac disease, the nature of the procedure, and the anesthesiologist's and sur-

**TABLE 63–6.** Indications for Use of a Pulmonary Artery Catheter During Cardiac Surgery

Patients for CABG surgery with
  Poor LV function (EF <0.4 or LVEDP >18 mm Hg)
  LV wall motion abnormalities
  Recent MI (<6 mo)
  Complications of recent MI (acute mitral insufficiency, ventricular septal rupture, ventricular aneurysm)
  Unstable angina requiring intravenous nitroglycerin or intraaortic balloon counterpulsation
Valvular disease
Combined coronary and valvular disease
Pulmonary hypertension
Complex cardiac lesions
Thoracic aortic surgery requiring cross-clamping
Patients with significant systemic disease (eg, renal, hepatic)

CABG, coronary artery bypass graft; EF, ejection fraction; LV, left ventricular; LVEDP, left ventricular end-diastolic pressure; MI, myocardial infarction.
Modified from Kaplan JA. Hemodynamic monitoring. In: Kaplan JA, ed. *Cardiac Anesthesia.* 2nd ed. Orlando, Fla: Grune & Stratton; 1987:179.

**TABLE 63–7.** Derived Hemodynamic Parameters From Pulmonary Artery Catheter Data

| Formula | Units | Normal Range |
|---|---|---|
| $CI = \dfrac{CO}{BSA}$ | L/min/m$^2$ | 2–5 |
| $SV = \dfrac{CO}{HR}$ | mL/beat | 60–90 |
| $SI = \dfrac{SV}{BSA}$ | mL/beat/m$^2$ | 40–60 |
| $LVSWI = \dfrac{1.36\,(MAP - PCWP)}{100} \times SI$ | g/m/m$^2$ | 45–60 |
| $RVSWI = \dfrac{1.36\,(PAP - CVP)}{100} \times SI$ | g/m/m$^2$ | 5–10 |
| $SVR = \dfrac{(MAP - CVP)}{CO} \times 80$ | dynes/s/cm$^5$ | 900–1500 |

BSA, body surface area; CI, cardiac index; CO, cardiac output; CVP, central venous pressure; HR, heart rate; LVSWL, left ventricular stroke work index; PAP, mean pulmonary artery pressure; PCWP, pulmonary capillary wedge pressure; PVR, pulmonary vascular resistance; RVSWI, right ventricular stroke work index; SI, stroke index; SV, stroke volume; SVR, systemic vascular resistance.

From Kaplan JA. Hemodynamic monitoring. In: Kaplan JA, ed. *Cardiac Anesthesia*. 2nd ed. Orlando, Fla: Grune & Stratton; 1987:179.

geon's preferences for completeness of hemodynamic information.

**Cardiac Output.** Measurement of CO is a more reliable means to assess cardiac performance than is BP. In order to standardize for body size differences, it is often expressed as cardiac index (Table 63–7). CO is most easily measured using a thermodilution PA catheter. The injectate is a crystalloid solution at a temperature lower than the patient's blood temperature. Iced injectate is not necessary for accuracy or reproducibility,[62] and the solution may be saline, 5% dextrose, or lactated Ringer's, all of which have similar specific gravity and specific heat.[63] The injection should be made in triplicate at the same time in the respiratory cycle, typically at end-expiration.

CO measurements can be erroneous in patients with intracardiac shunts or right-sided valvular lesions. Thermodilution techniques measure right-sided CO, which normally is the same as left-sided output. Left-to-right blood flow across an atrial septal or ventricular septal defect, however, causes the measured CO to be greater than actual left-sided CO and is of little or no value. Similarly, regurgitation through or stenosis of either the tricuspid valve or pulmonic valve leads to erroneous CO measurements because of the altered blood flow and, therefore, thermodilution. Hence, although a PA catheter may still provide useful information about PAP, PAOP, and CVP, it should not be placed for the purpose of measuring CO in patients with intracardiac shunts or right-sided valvular lesions.

Once the CO and filling pressures have been measured, other hemodynamic variables can be calculated (see Table 63–7). Although these parameters can aid in the understanding of a patient's hemodynamic status, undue emphasis should not be placed on them. They are derived rather than directly measured values like HR, CO, and BP. Consequently, they are affected by small changes in each of the measured parameters, as well as by technical inaccuracies in measurement.

As an example, SVR is the parameter most commonly used in the clinical setting to assess LV afterload, that is, the force opposing ventricular fiber shortening during LV ejection. However, during the pharmacologic manipulations commonly required for cardiac anesthesia, the SVR does not reflect true

LV afterload, which depends on a multitude of factors both internal and external to the myocardium.[64] These factors include the myocardial contractile state, intraventricular pressure, geometric characteristics of the LV, elasticity and geometry of blood vessels, inertial properties of blood, and viscosity of blood.

**Continuous Mixed Venous Oxygen Saturation.** Continuous mixed venous $O_2$ saturation ($S\bar{v}O_2$) can be monitored with specially designed PA catheters. The $S\bar{v}O_2$ should reflect the global adequacy of body tissue perfusion (ie, the balance between tissue $O_2$ demand and delivery). When the patient's temperature is relatively stable, a decrease in $S\bar{v}O_2$ most likely indicates decreased $O_2$ delivery to the tissues. CO, arterial $O_2$ saturation ($SaO_2$), and hematocrit are assessed to determine the cause, if it is unclear, and appropriate treatment is begun. Several factors can be responsible for changes in $S\bar{v}O_2$ (Table 63–8).

### Left Atrial Pressure

LAP can be measured directly with a catheter placed by the surgeon. This procedure minimizes the effect of airway pressure, pulmonary compliance, and pulmonary hypertension that may alter PAOP accuracy, but it does not accurately indicate LVEDP in the presence of mitral valvular disease. An LA catheter also introduces the risk of bleeding and air or thrombus embolization directly into the left-sided vasculature.

**TABLE 63–8.** Factors That Influence $S\bar{v}O_2$

**Causes of Decreased $S\bar{v}O_2$**

Decreasing or low cardiac output
Low $SaO_2$
Anemia
Increased oxygen consumption (hyperthermia, shivering)

**Causes of Increased $S\bar{v}O_2$**

High cardiac output (sepsis, liver failure)
Decreased oxygen consumption (hypothermia, sepsis, liver failure)
Cyanide toxicity
Falsely elevated $S\bar{v}O_2$ by wedging of the catheter in a pulmonary capillary bed

## Transesophageal Echocardiography

TEE enables experienced clinicians to continually assess regional wall motion, preload, ventricular systolic and diastolic function, chamber pressures, degree of valvular stenoses or regurgitant lesions, function of valvular prostheses, interchamber gradients, intracardiac and extracardiac masses, congenital and other undiagnosed structural abnormalities, disease of the ascending and descending aorta, pulmonary emboli, and the presence and severity of intracardiac shunts. TEE enables post-CPB assessment of adequacy of revascularization, success of valvular repair, and function of prosthetic valves, and diagnosis of surgically created complications. TEE frequently allows one to identify pathology not diagnosed preoperatively. It also influences changes in both surgical and anesthetic management. At our institution, all cardiac surgery patients are monitored with intraoperative TEE.

## Urine Output

Urine output is routinely monitored during cardiac surgery. It provides a "soft" indication of the adequacy of renal perfusion and function. Renal perfusion may be altered by inadequate intravascular volume as a result of diuretic and vasodilator therapy, inadequate perfusion pressure as a result of poor CO or vasodilator therapy, impairment of renal blood flow by vasoconstrictors and CPB, changes in neurohumoral levels, and various other factors.

Renal function during cardiac surgery must be maintained to prevent acute renal failure. This goal is best accomplished by ensuring adequate intravascular volume and CO before and after CPB and adequate perfusion during CPB. Hemoglobinuria may be seen during cardiac surgery, most commonly as a result of hemolysis but occasionally from a transfusion reaction during CPB. Treatment with diuretics such as mannitol or furosemide is frequently recommended but remains controversial.

## Temperature

Temperature must be monitored to ensure adequate, even cooling and rewarming during CPB. It can be measured at various sites. Tympanic membrane temperature is the best indication of brain temperature but its measurement has been associated with traumatic perforation.[65] Temperatures at other sites are compared with tympanic membrane temperature as a standard, with rectal, bladder, esophageal, and nasopharyngeal temperatures correlating most closely.[66]

Core cooling during CPB, however, induces significant differences in temperature measured at various sites (Fig. 63–9). Esophageal and nasopharyngeal temperatures decrease most rapidly with cooling and increase most rapidly with rewarming.[67] Conversely, temperature changes most slowly in the rectum. Bladder temperature is intermediate in rate of cooling and rewarming,[67] but at the conclusion of bypass, it most closely indicates the temperature afterdrop that occurs postoperatively.[68]

## Coagulation

Intraoperative coagulation monitoring is essential for management of the anticoagulation necessary for CPB and for assessment of post-CPB coagulation. The activated clotting

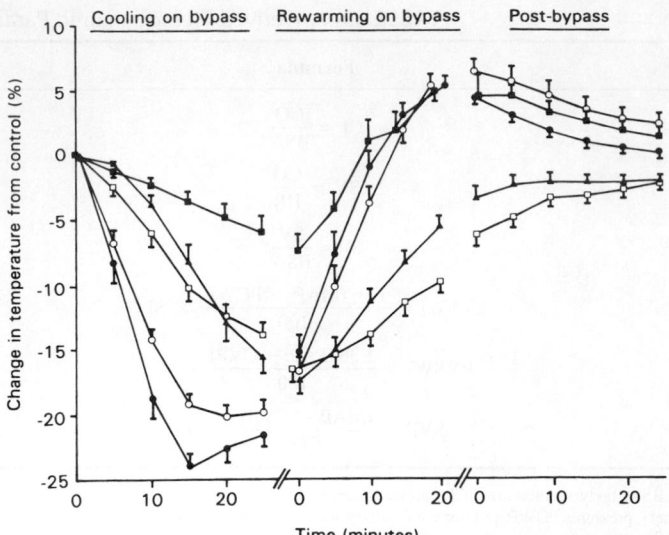

**FIGURE 63–9.** Changes in temperature measured at various sites during active cooling on cardiopulmonary bypass, rewarming on bypass, and postbypass. The changes are expressed as percentage change from control. Sites are esophageal (*solid circles*), nasopharyngeal (*open circles*), bladder (*solid triangles*), rectal (*open squares*), and thumb (*solid squares*). *Bars* indicate SEM. (From Bone ME, Feneck RO. Bladder temperature as an estimate of body temperature during cardiopulmonary bypass. *Anaesthesia.* 1988;43:181.)

time (ACT) is a simple but useful test of heparin activity. Measurement of heparin concentration may also be of value. Thromboelastography monitors the viscoelastic coagulation, and Sonoclot (Scienco Inc, Morrison, Colo.), although perhaps not routine in this setting, offers additional help in diagnosing and targeting treatment of post-CPB coagulation problems.

## Electroencephalogram

Electroencephalography (EEG) offers potential benefits in cardiac anesthesia. The depth of anesthesia during high-dose opioid anesthesia with muscle relaxation is difficult to assess clinically. Induction of anesthesia with opioids produces progressive slowing of EEG activity. Processed EEG monitoring montages, such as the bispectral index, have made assessment more manageable in the OR.[69] Whether EEG improves anesthetic management by indicating the need for additional agents is beyond the scope of this chapter and is discussed in detail in Chapter 21.

The EEG is useful to assess adequate dosing of barbiturates to induce electrical silence during CPB or deep hypothermic circulatory arrest. Simply monitoring two-channel bipolar leads can provide small reassurance with bihemispheric perfusion, although the small particulate matter and air emboli purported to cause adverse neurologic sequelae following CPB are often missed by the large expanse of cortical areas covered with this practice, resulting in a high false-negative rate. However, observation of asymmetric activity has led to the timely discovery of inadvertent aortic cannula malposition and obstructed carotid flow, as well as global hemispheric embolic events.

## Regional Cerebral Oximetry

Cerebral oximetry applies the basic principles of near-infrared spectroscopy (NIRS) to determine the regional mixed venous $O_2$ saturation of brain tissue, providing a quantitative measurement of the relationship of $O_2$ supply and demand. As monitors are routinely placed over the forehead bilaterally, its limitations include the relatively large sample areas (resulting in falsely normal values for discrete areas of frontal perfusion) and lack of information for areas perfused by the middle cerebral arteries and posterior circulation. In addition, NIRS values can also change due to extracerebral factors (eg, decrease in skin temperature) without reflecting any changes in intracerebral oxygenation.

NIRS can be useful to assess successful engagement of retrograde cerebral perfusion during cases of deep hypothermic circulatory arrest, as well as determining whether hemispheric blood flow is symmetric. Saturation values <40%, may be required to increase cerebral $O_2$ delivery (eg, increased hematocrit or fraction of inspired $O_2$ [$FIO_2$], CO-pump flow or adding $CO_2$ to increase cerebral blood flow [CBF]) or decrease cerebral $O_2$ consumption (eg, through hypothermia or administration of barbiturates); however, compelling evidence associating use of regional cerebral oximetry with improved neurologic outcome is still lacking.[70] Recently, Yao and colleagues showed that any single cerebral oximeter reading <45% in patients undergoing cardiac surgery significantly correlated with prolonged intensive care unit (ICU) and hospital stay.[71]

## Transcranial Doppler

Transcranial Doppler (TCD) devices allow clinicians to ascertain CBF velocities continuously through the use of ultrasound probes applied to the head and typically focused on either the middle cerebral or anterior cerebral artery. Continuous flow can also be readily documented during CPB. This allows for rapid recognition of asymmetric blood flow following surgical maneuvers and institution of CPB in the areas studied. Because the detection of CBF requires three-dimensional manipulation of the probe in order to find target vessels, and because minute changes of probe positions can result in complete loss of signals, the technique is exceedingly more difficult than simple application of two-channel EEG or cerebral oximetry sensor. Subjective experience has shown that certain patient populations, such as postmenopausal women and black patients, often have inadequate "windows" to obtain Doppler signals, perhaps due to increased ossification. TCD also allows for quantification of high-intensity transient signals (HITS) indicative of microemboli from either gaseous or particulate matter.

As yet, the number of HITS has not been shown to correlate with postoperative neurologic dysfunction in cardiac surgical procedures. However, in a recent report, the incidence of cerebral dysfunction (evidenced by antisaccadic eye movement error) showed a significant correlation with the number of HITS, which was higher following coronary bypass on-pump than with off-pump bypass surgery.[72]

## Which Monitors Are Used to Detect Intraoperative Myocardial Ischemia?

One of the most important goals in the management of patients undergoing cardiac surgery, particularly CABG surgery, is the prevention or timely detection of myocardial ischemia. If all ischemia were related to hemodynamic aberrations such as tachycardia, hypertension, or hypotension, so-

phisticated ischemia monitoring might not be necessary. Despite maintenance of stable hemodynamic parameters, however, ischemia still occurs.[39] Therefore, detection is extremely important to allow treatment to be initiated before harmful consequences occur.

## Electrocardiogram

### Lead Selection

The ECG continues to be the mainstay of intraoperative ischemia monitoring. Most commonly, leads II and $V_5$ are monitored in the OR. Lead II is important for dysrhythmia detection, and $V_5$ is the single most sensitive (75%) lead for intraoperative ischemia detection.[73] The combination of leads II and $V_5$ is 80% sensitive in the detection of myocardial ischemia.[73] The combinations of $V_4/V_5$ and $II/V_4/V_5$ are 90% and 96% sensitive, respectively.[73] These two-lead combinations are not readily available on most conventional OR ECG monitors.

Particularly in the cardiac surgical OR, the capability of recording the ECG on paper should be available. This allows comparison of tracings from different times during the procedure. Automated ST analysis has also improved the anesthesiologist's ability to detect and treat ischemic changes that might otherwise be overlooked.

### Limitations

Although the ECG remains the most commonly used ischemia monitor in the OR, questions have arisen about its sensitivity and specificity. ECG evidence of myocardial ischemia exists as one point along a continuum of manifestations of the imbalance between myocardial $O_2$ supply and demand. Earlier manifestations include regional lactate production, decrease in LV compliance, and development of regional wall motion abnormalities (RWMAs).

Myocardial lactate production cannot be readily measured in the clinical setting, but changes in LV compliance may be reflected in the PAP and PAOP tracings. RWMAs can be detected by echocardiography, a monitoring modality that is finding widespread application in cardiac anesthesia. A study of patients undergoing percutaneous transluminal coronary angioplasty has demonstrated the time course of ischemic manifestations in awake patients[74] (Table 63–9).

Ischemia is difficult to diagnose in patients who have LV hypertrophy or who are receiving digoxin therapy because of abnormal ST segments that are present even without ischemia. Ischemic changes cannot be diagnosed in patients with left bundle branch block or a paced rhythm. Subendocardial ische-

**TABLE 63–9.** Time Course of Ischemic Manifestations in Patients Undergoing Percutaneous Transluminal Coronary Angioplasty

| Ischemic Manifestation | Time to Onset |
|---|---|
| Regional wall motion abnormalities | 19 ± 8 s |
| Electrocardiographic ST segment changes | 30 ± 5 s |
| Angina pectoris | 39 ± 10 s |

From Hauser AM, Gangadharan V, Ramos RG, et al. Sequence of mechanical, electrocardiographic, and clinical effects of repeated coronary artery occlusion in human beings: echocardiographic observations during coronary angioplasty. *J Am Coll Cardiol.* 1985;5:193.

**TABLE 63–10.** Conditions Associated With ST Segment Depression

| | |
|---|---|
| Myocardial ischemia | Athletic heart syndrome |
| Digitalis treatment | Prolonged QT syndromes |
| Quinidine treatment | Mitral valve prolapse |
| Left bundle branch block | Increased intracranial pressure |
| Ventricular pacing | Pheochromocytoma |
| Acute cor pulmonale (eg, pulmonary embolism) | |

mia does not always cause ECG changes. Finally, even when ST changes are present on an ECG, they are not always specific for ischemia but may be caused by other conditions (Table 63–10).

## Pulmonary Artery Catheter

PA catheters initially were thought to play a role in ischemia monitoring. Kaplan and Wells reported that an increase in PAOP and the development of abnormal a-c and v waves preceding ECG changes was suggestive of ischemia.[75] This finding may reflect increased LV diastolic wall tension and reduced LV compliance as a result of the development of subendocardial ischemia.

Subsequent studies comparing changes in PAOP with RWMAs suggest that PAOP changes are less sensitive.[76,77] Although such changes can be associated with ischemia, it appears that neither they nor the development of abnormal waveforms is a sensitive or reliable early indicator of myocardial ischemia. It has also been demonstrated that PAOP following CPB becomes a much less reliable measure of preload, especially in patients with pre-CPB systolic dysfunction. Due to the increased risk of the potentially fatal complication of PA rupture, the balloon of the PA catheter should not be wedged under full systemic heparinization necessitated by CPB. In addition, the presence of hypothermia renders the PA more susceptible to rupture. At our institution, the PA catheter is pulled back several centimeters at the initiation of CPB, and the balloon is not inflated again, even after the administration of protamine.

## Transesophageal Echocardiography

TEE appears to be a sensitive monitor of myocardial ischemia. Smith and colleagues studied 50 patients undergoing myocardial revascularization or other vascular surgery.[78] New-onset RWMAs detected by TEE were seen more frequently than ST segment changes. No patients developed new ECG changes without new RWMAs. In patients who developed both RWMAs and ST segment changes, the RWMAs tended to occur earlier. Of four patients who suffered perioperative MI, one had persistent RWMAs and ST segment changes, two had persistent RWMAs without ST segment changes, and one had only transient RWMAs without ST segment changes.

Leung and colleagues studied 50 patients undergoing myocardial revascularization.[79] Similarly, RWMAs were detected more frequently than ST segment changes, and echocardiographic evidence of postbypass ischemia was correlated with adverse cardiac outcome. Of the ischemic episodes, 73% were not associated with even a 20% change in HR, BP, or PA pressure.

TEE appears to be a sensitive monitor for ischemia, even in patients with left bundle branch block, paced rhythm, LV hypertrophy, digoxin therapy, or subendocardial ischemia. The ECG is considerably less sensitive under these circumstances.

In both of the previously quoted studies, many patients with new RWMAs did not have adverse cardiac outcomes. Thus, the specificity of TEE as a monitor of ischemia has been questioned. Causes of RWMAs other than myocardial ischemia or infarction may include nonuniform contractility in various regions of the LV,[80] myocardial stunning,[81] altered loading conditions, tethering of normally perfused myocardium adjacent to ischemic tissue,[82] or abnormal sequence of septal depolarization (left bundle branch block, ventricular pacing). In a more recent study, however, Comunale and associates argued that TEE remains twice as predictive as ECG in identifying patients who have an MI.[83] Despite questions about its specificity, TEE appears to be a valuable monitor of myocardial ischemia.

## ANESTHETIC MANAGEMENT BEFORE CARDIOPULMONARY BYPASS

Before induction of anesthesia, appropriate hemodynamic goals should be determined for each patient, depending on the particular cardiovascular pathophysiology. The anesthetic plan can then be tailored with specific objectives in mind, and responses to deviations from planned limits in hemodynamic parameters can be logically implemented as they occur.

## What Are the Hemodynamic Goals in Anesthetic Management in Coronary Artery Disease?

The prevention of myocardial ischemia depends on balancing myocardial $O_2$ supply and demand. Hemodynamic goals should be chosen with this goal in mind. Myocardial $O_2$ supply is determined by the arterial $O_2$ content ($CaO_2$) of blood and coronary blood flow. Myocardial $O_2$ demand is determined by heart rate, contractility, preload, and afterload (Table 63–11).

## Myocardial Oxygen Supply

### Arterial Oxygen Content

$CaO_2$ can be calculated from the following equation:

$$CaO_2 \text{ (mL/dL)} = (1.39) \text{ (Hb) (\% saturation)} + (0.003) \text{ (PO}_2)$$

(Equation 3)

**TABLE 63–11.** Determinants of Myocardial Oxygen Balance

| Myocardial $O_2$ Supply | Myocardial $O_2$ Demand |
|---|---|
| Arterial $O_2$ content | Heart rate |
| Coronary blood flow | Myocardial contractility |
| Perfusion pressure | Wall tension |
| Mechanical effects | Afterload |
| Neural effects | Preload |
| Stenoses | |
| Collaterals | |

The lowest safe hemoglobin concentration for any particular patient with CAD is difficult to determine but probably lies in the range of 8 to 10 g/100 mL. Patients should receive an $FIO_2$ that maintains the $SaO_2$ >95%. Any leftward shift of the oxyhemoglobin dissociation curve (hypothermia, alkalosis, or decreased concentration of 2,3-diphosphoglycerate) can contribute to decreased availability of $O_2$ at the tissues.

### Coronary Blood Flow

Coronary blood flow is determined by a number of mechanical, metabolic, hormonal, and anatomic factors. The coronary arteries arise from the root of the aorta and give rise to numerous branches over the epicardial surface (see Fig. 63–2). These vessels subdivide into additional branches that course through the myocardium to form a subendocardial plexus.

Isovolemic contraction of the LV generates high tension within the myocardium, causing abrupt cessation in blood flow of the intramyocardial distribution of the left coronary artery (Fig. 63–10). Left coronary flow begins to rise gradually during systole but occurs primarily during diastole. Approximately 85% of coronary blood flow to the LV occurs during diastole. The 15% that occurs during systole is primarily epicardial. Intracavitary systolic pressures of the RV are much lower, allowing for significant coronary blood flow to the RV during systole and diastole.

When coronary autoregulation is normal, diastolic flow to the subendocardium is augmented by vasodilation and the presence of an anatomically greater density of subendocardial vasculature compared with the subepicardium. Nevertheless, the subendocardium is particularly susceptible to ischemia during tachycardia because it is primarily the diastolic portion of the cardiac cycle that is shortened by increasing heart rate.

### Coronary Perfusion Pressure

Perfusion pressure of most organs is calculated from the MAP minus the venous pressure of the organ. The driving pressure for blood perfusing the subendocardium is the aortic diastolic pressure. Because most of the subendocardial venous drainage is via the thebesian veins into the LV cavity, the venous pressure for subendocardial perfusion is the LVEDP. Thus, the equation that determines coronary perfusion pressure (CPP) is as follows:

$$CPP = \text{Diastolic BP} - \text{LVEDP} \qquad \text{(Equation 4)}$$

For this reason, any increase in LVEDP places the subendocardium at risk of ischemia (ie, CHF due to fluid overload, or decreased ventricular compliance due to long-standing LVH from AS or the onset of myocardial ischemia).

### Metabolic Factors

Metabolic factors have an important regulatory role in coronary blood flow, which is closely coupled to $M\dot{V}O_2$. Coronary vascular resistance (CVR) is varied on a beat-to-beat basis. Factors of importance in mediating this control of vascular resistance include adenosine, hydrogen ion, carbon dioxide, lactic acid, nitric oxide, and possibly other compounds.

### Autonomic Innervation

Coronary arteries have sympathetic adrenergic and muscarinic cholinergic receptors. Their roles in determining coronary blood flow are unclear, but they appear to be less important than metabolic factors.

### Anatomic Characteristics

The anatomic characteristics of CAD influence coronary blood flow. Stenoses decrease blood flow by increasing resistance. In atherosclerotic CAD, the stenoses are fixed. In Prinzmetal angina, they are dynamic as a result of vasospasm. The degree of stenosis and the compensatory development of collateral vessels determine the susceptibility of the myocardium to ischemia.

### Myocardial Oxygen Demand

Increased HR increases $M\dot{V}O_2$. The increase is related not only to the increased work of more beats per minute but also to an associated increase in contractility with increasing heart rate (the Treppe phenomenon). At the same time, tachycardia decreases myocardial $O_2$ supply, especially to the LV, by shortening the diastolic perfusion time. An increase in contractility also increases the work of the heart and therefore increases $M\dot{V}O_2$.

The $M\dot{V}O_2$ is closely related to ventricular wall tension. Wall tension is determined by both intracavitary pressure and volume, as was noted previously, by Laplace's law (see Equation 2).

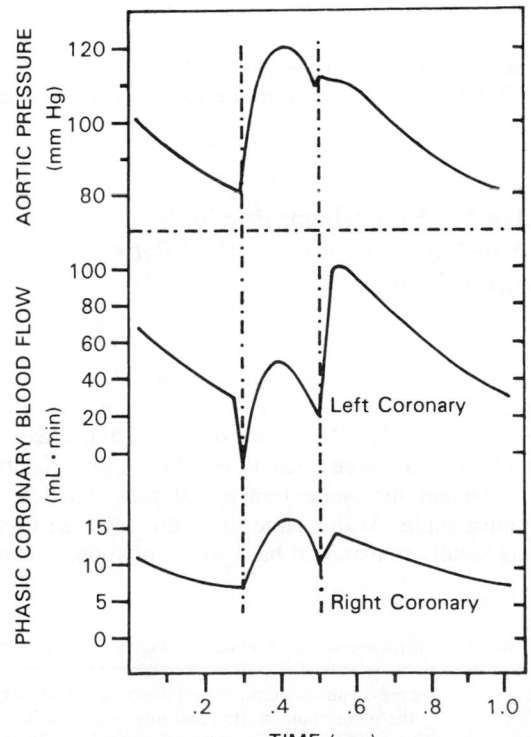

**FIGURE 63–10.** Comparison of phasic coronary blood flow in the left and right coronary arteries in relation to aortic pressure. Left coronary artery blood flow peaks during diastole. Right coronary artery blood flow peaks during systole. (From Berne RM, Levy MD. *Cardiovascular Physiology.* 2nd ed. St Louis, Mo: CV Mosby; 1972.)

Increased intraventricular pressure at the end of systole (afterload) and increased intraventricular volume at the end of diastole (preload) increase both wall tension and $M\dot{V}O_2$. Increased wall thickness, as occurs in LV hypertrophy, tends to decrease wall tension and $M\dot{V}O_2$ for a given area of the heart, but the increase in myocardial mass increases overall myocardial $O_2$ demand.

The hemodynamic goals for patients with CAD are outlined in Table 63–12. Avoidance of tachycardia appears to be the most important goal. Although most ischemia is not associated with hemodynamic abnormalities, they constitute the most easily prevented subset. Even with close adherence to these hemodynamic goals, careful ischemia monitoring should be carried out and treatment of ischemia planned.

### Is Routine Use of Intravenous Nitroglycerin Effective?

Prophylactic intraoperative use of NTG infusion has been suggested as potentially beneficial therapy for patients with CAD.[84] NTG might prevent ischemia by decreasing $M\dot{V}O_2$ via decreases in preload and afterload. It may also improve myocardial perfusion by direct effects on coronary arteries. However, a controlled study using a prophylactic infusion of 0.5 μg/kg/min demonstrated no more efficacy in the prevention of myocardial ischemia than did placebo.[85] Higher doses of 1 μg/kg/min also have not been shown to change outcome.

A potential adverse effect of prophylactic NTG infusion is unnecessary venodilation, leading to increased fluid requirements. Although this therapy may have no deleterious hemodynamic effect, it can lead to hemodilution and increased blood product transfusion requirements later in the procedure.[85] A more prudent approach may be to use NTG when it is specifically indicated by hypertension, increased filling pressures, or any sign of myocardial ischemia.

### What Are the Hemodynamic Goals in the Anesthetic Management of Patients With Aortic Stenosis?

Avoidance of any decrease in systemic vascular resistance is of paramount importance in the anesthetic management of patients with AS. Vasodilation will not reduce the work of the LV, but it will reduce CPP, leading to life-threatening ischemia.

Avoidance of bradycardia and maintenance of sinus rhythm and normal intravascular volume are also important. The hypertrophied and noncompliant LV requires a coordinated atrial

**TABLE 63–12.** Hemodynamic Goals for Coronary Artery Disease

| Heart rate | <70 to control $M\dot{V}O_2$ and allow time for diastolic coronary perfusion |
| --- | --- |
| Rhythm | Sinus is preferred |
| Preload | Decrease in order to decrease wall tension and increase coronary perfusion pressure |
| Afterload | Decrease slightly to decrease wall tension, but maintain adequate pressure for coronary perfusion |
| Contractility | Decrease to reduce $M\dot{V}O_2$ as long as adequate cardiac output is maintained |

**TABLE 63–13.** Hemodynamic Goals for Aortic Stenosis

| Heart rate | Low heart rate (50–70 bpm) is best to control $M\dot{V}O_2$ and prevent ischemia. Severe bradycardia is associated with decreased cardiac output because stroke volume is relatively fixed. |
| --- | --- |
| Rhythm | Sinus rhythm is very important. |
| Preload | Must be maintained or increased to maintain ventricular filling in a poorly compliant ventricle in order to maintain cardiac output. |
| Afterload | Must be maintained or increased to avoid reductions in coronary perfusion pressure. |
| Contractility | Maintain. |

contraction to provide adequate LV filling; otherwise, a sudden fall in CO may cause severe hypotension. Likewise, atrial fibrillation with rapid ventricular response may cause ischemia and should be treated aggressively. Bradycardia is also poorly tolerated because of the inability of the LV to generate a compensatory response to maintain CO by increasing stroke volume (Table 63–13).

### What Are the Hemodynamic Goals in the Anesthetic Management of Patients With Aortic Regurgitation?

Maintenance of normal intravascular volume and normal or decreased systemic vascular resistance is crucial because the primary mechanism for the regurgitant flow is an increase in stroke volume. However, overzealous fluid replacement can result in PE, and excessive decreases in afterload may result in myocardial ischemia because the aortic diastolic pressure is already low.

Avoidance of bradycardia is beneficial because the increased diastolic time will exacerbate regurgitation (Table 63–14).

### What Are the Hemodynamic Goals in the Anesthetic Management of Patients With Mitral Stenosis?

Maintenance of sinus rhythm and avoidance of tachycardia are extremely important. In patients with MS, the gradient across the mitral valve is critically dependent on HR. For instance, doubling the HR from 60 to 120 decreases the duration of diastole more than threefold.[14] Consequently, in order to maintain the same transmitral flow, the left atrial pressure must triple. At the same time, this increase in filling pressure is rapidly transmitted back to the pulmonary capillar-

**TABLE 63–14.** Hemodynamic Goals for Aortic Insufficiency

| Heart rate | Increase causes shortening of diastolic, which decreases the regurgitant fraction and increases cardiac output. |
| --- | --- |
| Rhythm | Sinus is preferred but less important than in other valvular lesions. |
| Preload | Increase to maximize forward cardiac output. |
| Afterload | It is very important to decrease afterload to favor forward cardiac output. |
| Contractility | Maintain. |

**TABLE 63–15.** Hemodynamic Goals for Mitral Stenosis

| | |
|---|---|
| Heart rate | Slow to allow more diastolic time for flow across mitral valve. |
| Rhythm | Sinus rhythm is very important. If atrial fibrillation is present, control ventricular rate. |
| Preload | Must be maintained or slightly increased to provide adequate flow across the mitral valve for left ventricular filling. Excessive preload may cause pulmonary edema. |
| Afterload | Systemic vascular resistance should be maintained. Decreases do not improve cardiac output. Increases in pulmonary vascular resistance should be avoided. |
| Contractility | Maintain to provide adequate cardiac output. |

ies, which may result in PE and RV failure. Moreover, the inability to maintain LV filling may result in hypotension.

On one hand, systemic vascular resistance must be maintained because stroke volume is unlikely to increase with afterload reduction. On the other hand, vasodilation may induce RV ischemia by decreasing the aortic diastolic pressure necessary for adequate perfusion of the right ventricle (Table 63–15).

## What Are the Hemodynamic Goals in the Anesthetic Management of Patients With Mitral Regurgitation?

Decreased SVR is the primary hemodynamic goal in the anesthetic care of patients with MR, for the increased afterload worsens the regurgitant fraction. In addition, faster than normal HRs are beneficial because bradycardia can increase the regurgitant volume by increasing LVEDV and mitral annular distention.[14]

Preload reduction may be beneficial, as long as it is not excessive, because adequate volume to maintain adequate forward stroke volume is essential. Similarly, excessive volume expansion can also worsen the regurgitation by increasing the radius of the LV (Table 63–16).

## When Did "Fast-Track" Cardiac Anesthesia Begin?

Anesthesia for adult cardiovascular surgery has undergone radical changes in its most fundamental approach. In the 1970s and 1980s, the basic anesthetic management for CABG patients consisted of a high-dose narcotic technique, such as morphine sulfate (often 0.5-3.0 mg/kg or more) combined

**TABLE 63–16.** Hemodynamic Goals for Mitral Regurgitation

| | |
|---|---|
| Heart rate | Maintain or increase. Bradycardia worsens regurgitant flow. |
| Rhythm | Sinus is preferred, although it is less crucial than in mitral stenosis. |
| Preload | Maintain or slightly increase. Avoid extremes of high (increases regurgitant flow) or low (inadequate cardiac output) preload conditions. |
| Afterload | Decrease to improve forward cardiac output. |
| Contractility | Maintain or increase to decrease left ventricular volume. |

with droperidol, the "neuroleptic" regimen. Subsequently, it was the norm for patients to remain endotracheally intubated for up to several days postoperatively. As nearly all anesthetics other than narcotics typically have been associated with negative inotropic effects, this approach was thought to be the safest for the patient. In fact, some anesthetics that we commonly use today were considered relatively contraindicated for cardiac anesthesia; isoflurane, for example, was avoided for years by many clinicians because of the theoretic risk of coronary steal in the patient with CAD. Consequently, with sole anesthetic regimens often consisting of narcotics, droperidol, and muscle relaxants, the incidence of intraoperative recall was reportedly as high as 28%. With the advent of the synthetic opioids, fentanyl and sufentanil became popular substitutions for morphine and were not accompanied by histamine release and its associated complications. However, the dose ranges used by most clinicians for cardiac procedures were still astronomical by today's standards, with doses often exceeding 100 to 150 $\mu$g/kg and 15 to 30 $\mu$g/kg for fentanyl and sufentanil, respectively.

As cardiac anesthesia moved toward the 21st century, these regimens underwent drastic changes. As early as 1973, early extubation following CPB was thought to have potential benefits. Klineberg and coworkers reported 31 patients studied during this time frame who were allowed to wake passively.[86] Of these patients, 16% were extubated within 15 hours of ICU admission and 45% were extubated 15 to 20 hours post-ICU admission. The same group then studied 72 patients from 1975 to 1976 and actively reversed muscle relaxants and somnolence, allowing for 62.5% of patients to be extubated within 5 hours of ICU admission and 91% within 20 hours of ICU admission. This aggressive regimen allowed for 46% of patients to be discharged from the ICU within 24 hours and 73% within 48 hours. This study also introduced the strict *fast-track* pathway, allowing for early extubation only if certain criteria were met. These were estimated blood loss (EBL) <100 mL/h, urine output >80 mL/h, tolerate CVP with minimal vasopressors, absence of dangerous arrhythmias, and a $Pao_2$ >100 mm Hg on 50% $Fio_2$. Muscle relaxants were reversed with neostigmine or atropine, somnolence reversed with physostigmine, and patients were placed on 60% T-piece for 1 hour. Following this period, arterial blood gases, forced vital capacity (FVC), and minute ventilation ($\dot{V}E$) were measured. If the vital capacity (VC) >10 mL/kg, VC/2 × 30 > $Pco_2$ × $\dot{V}E$/40, and patients were awake and cooperative, then extubation was performed.

No patients in either part of the study were reintubated. In the subsequent study, three patients in the early extubation limb were readmitted to ICU: two with supraventricular tachycardia (SVT), and one with ventricular tachycardia (VT). No mortality was reported.

Despite these observations, early extubation following cardiac surgical procedures did not gain general acceptance until the late 1990s. Despite the fact that the patient population presenting for cardiac surgery includes that of increasing age, more concomitant diseases, higher incidence of redo procedures, and frequently severely depressed cardiac function, recent improvements have made early extubation a safe alternative. With improvements in surgical techniques, myocardial protection, CPB perfusion techniques, anesthetic agents, hemostatic drugs ($\epsilon$-aminocaproic acid [EACA], tranexamic acid, aprotinin), intraoperative monitoring techniques (PA catheters, TEE), and antiarrhythmic drugs (sotalol, amiodarone), early extubation has become the norm rather than the exception in many centers.

## What Is a Fast-Track Anesthetic Regimen?

*Fast-tracking* refers to early tracheal extubation following cardiac surgery, typically within the first 8 hours postoperatively. Regimens vary from institution to institution, but the overall focus is that of "balanced" anesthesia. Multiple combinations of narcotics, benzodiazepines, propofol, and inhalational agents have been successfully reported, with an emphasis on much lower narcotic doses than previously administered in order to facilitate early emergence from anesthesia, early return to spontaneous ventilation, early extubation, early mobilization, earlier ICU discharge, shorter hospital length of stay (LOS), and consequently lower total hospital costs.

## What Anesthetic Agents Can Be Safely Used for Cardiovascular Anesthesia?

Since the advent of cardiac anesthesia, the goals of anesthetic regimens have been geared toward cardiovascular stability with an emphasis on avoiding drugs that have negative inotropic effects. As previously described, this goal originally limited the tailored cardiac anesthetic to a heavily narcotic-based technique.

Despite these findings, early cardiac anesthetic techniques commonly consisted of high-dose opioids, resulting in prolonged somnolence, long-term postoperative ventilatory requirements, and prolonged ICU stays.

For years, it had been assumed that the patient at risk for ischemia would necessarily have less intraoperative ischemic events if kept under strict hemodynamic control. Hemodynamic goals toward reducing "demand ischemia" included keeping patients' rate pressure product (RPP) (HR × systolic BP [SBP]) <12 000 or the pressure rate quotient (MAP/HR) >1 in order to optimize the ratio of myocardial $O_2$ supply to demand, with some evidence implicating an association between abnormalities in these measurements with myocardial irritability.[87] With this in mind, along with the advent of fast-track cardiac anesthetic concerns, anesthetic regimens were revisited in the 1990s in order to determine whether the hemodynamic stability provided by narcotic-based techniques actually created less morbidity and mortality. During this period, it was suggested by one study, which found that <30% of intraoperative ECG changes or segmental wall motion abnormalties (SWMAs) noted on TEE were preceded by acute changes in any hemodynamic parameter, that perhaps $O_2$ supply was the more important determinant of intraoperative ischemia.[88] In fact, neither PA catheter pressure measurements nor the specialized indices of ischemia susceptibility (RPP and MAP/HR) appeared to be useful in predicting TEE episodes. For this reason, agents that had previously been avoided except in small doses were reconsidered. Several techniques are discussed, with accompanying advantages and disadvantages noted.

## ANESTHETIC TECHNIQUES

## Why Are High-Dose Opioids Used?

Narcotics have long been regarded as the gold standard of cardiac anesthetic agents because of their profound analgesic properties, smooth hemodynamic profile, and lack of negative inotropy and their ability to blunt the response to circulating catecholamines associated with laryngoscopy and sternotomy. Although high doses of narcotics are commonly known to attenuate the hemodynamic response to surgical stimulation, it has been shown that even astronomic doses of narcotics by today's standards (50-100 µg/kg fentanyl, 10-30 µg/kg sufentanil) are unable to completely abolish the sympathetic responses to laryngoscopy and sternotomy, as defined by a 15% or more increase in SBP from control and a hormonal response of 50% or more increase over control (renin, aldosterone, cortisol, and catecholamines).[89] In fact, induction and intubation has been shown to be attainable with equal hemodynamic stability with 15 or 60 µg/kg of fentanyl.

## What Are the Disadvantages of High-Dose Opioid Anesthesia?

### Inadequate Amnesia

As narcotics provide only analgesia and, less reliably, hypnosis, adjuncts to the narcotic-based techniques often consisted of premedication with scopolamine or benzodiazepines along with intraoperative administration of benzodiazepines or droperidol for amnesia. Unfortunately, these techniques, when coupled with the added uncertainty of amnestic periods during hypothermia and CPB, produce amnesia less reliably than the inhalation-based anesthetic regimens often used in noncardiac surgery. As a result, cardiac anesthesia has shared the dubious distinction with obstetric (7%-28%) and trauma anesthesia (up to 43%) of up to a 28% incidence of explicit intraoperative awareness[90] as opposed to 0.2% during general surgery.[91–93]

### Chest Wall Rigidity

Induction of anesthesia with high doses of opioids, particularly fentanyl, sufentanil, and alfentanil, may be associated with chest wall rigidity. This decrease in compliance makes ventilation difficult or impossible. The resultant increase in arterial partial pressure of carbon dioxide (Paco$_2$) leads to an increase in circulating catecholamines that may cause systemic and pulmonary hypertension, tachycardia, and myocardial ischemia.

Many pharmacologic adjuncts have been suggested to prevent this rigidity, including benzodiazepines, $\alpha_2$-adrenergic agonists, serotonin antagonists, and dopaminergic agonists. The most effective preventive measure—and the most effective treatment once chest wall rigidity occurs—is muscle relaxation. A small dose of nondepolarizing muscle relaxant before induction is not as effective as administration of a paralyzing dose simultaneously with the opioid[94] (Fig. 63–11).

### Respiratory Depression

High-dose opioid anesthesia produces prolonged respiratory depression. Patients require mechanical ventilation for several hours postoperatively and may not be extubated until the day after surgery. Although this may not adversely affect a patient's outcome, it does prolong the stay in the ICU and increases the cost of hospitalization.

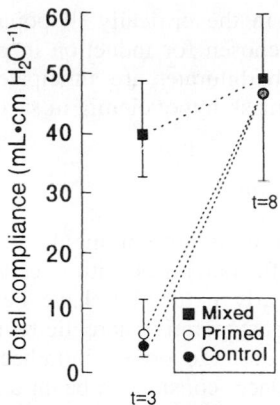

**FIGURE 63–11.** Ventilatory compliance during three different induction sequences. The control group received a placebo at time 0; followed by a 2-minute infusion of sufentanil, 3 μg/kg, from 1 to 3 minutes; followed by pancuronium, 0.1 mg/kg, at 4 minutes. The primed group received 1 mg of pancuronium at time 0; a 2-minute infusion of sufentanil, 3 μg/kg, at 1 to 3 minutes; and the balance of pancuronium, 0.1 mg/kg, at 4 minutes. The mixed group received a placebo at time 0; a 2-minute infusion of sufentanil, 3 μg/kg, and pancuronium, 0.1 mg/kg, from 1 to 3 minutes; and a placebo at 4 minutes. Ventilatory compliance was significantly greater for the mixed group at 3 minutes compared with the control and primed groups. At 8 minutes, there was no difference in ventilatory compliance among the 3 groups. (From Horrow JC, Abrams JT, Van Riper DF, et al. Ventilatory compliance after three sufentanil-pancuronium induction sequences. *Anesthesiology.* 1991;75:969.)

## Volatile Inhalational Anesthetics

Inhalational agents are known to be negative inotropes that can beneficially decrease $M\dot{V}O_2$ and cause coronary vasodilation at the expense of decreasing CPP and increasing HR. Isoflurane, in particular, has been commonly avoided because of the theoretic risk of coronary steal, a phenomenon thought to occur in patients with "steal-prone" anatomy. Patients with total occlusion of one coronary artery that is supplied distally by collateral flow from another coronary artery with a ≥50% stenosis are thought to be particularly at risk.

More recent human experimental evidence has contradicted these findings. Leung and colleagues used TEE and continuous Holter ECG to study the relative risk of myocardial ischemia in high-risk patients undergoing elective CABG surgery using isoflurane or sufentanil anesthesia under strict control of hemodynamics and found that the duration and severity of TEE episodes were not significantly different between the two groups.[95] TEE ischemic episodes and isoflurane concentrations did not have any correlation, and the duration and severity of ECG ischemic episodes did not differ in patients receiving either isoflurane or sufentanil. In a later study, the incidence of ischemia was similar among patients with and without steal-prone coronary anatomy in those who received isoflurane or sufentanil anesthesia.[96] A related study found minimal direct effects of halothane and isoflurane on CVR, diastolic coronary pressure, and collateral myocardial blood flow, suggesting that neither agent is likely to cause myocardial ischemia by a coronary steal mechanism.[97] Other studies have similarly shown neither a difference in outcome in regimens consisting of isoflurane, halothane, and enflurane in patients with steal-prone anatomy,[98] nor a difference in mortality rates or duration of hospitalization when using a primary opioid versus an inhalational agent.

One clinical study suggested that isoflurane may even offer protection against ischemia. Patients with CAD were observed for signs and symptoms of ischemia at rest, during rapid atrial pacing while they were awake, and during rapid atrial pacing with isoflurane–nitrous oxide anesthesia. The rate at which signs of ischemia (ST segment changes, angina in awake patients, increases in PAOP, or onset of v waves) developed was lower during isoflurane anesthesia than in awake patients.[99]

### Clinical Significance

Analysis of angiographic data from the Coronary Artery Surgery Study registry revealed that 23% of patients in the registry have "steal-prone" coronary anatomy.[100] However, isoflurane is commonly used in patients with CAD with few apparent signs of myocardial ischemia. It has been suggested that isoflurane does not often cause ischemia despite its vasodilating properties because, unlike a pure vasodilator such as adenosine, it also possesses a negative inotropic effect.[101] It may decrease $M\dot{V}O_2$ enough by depressing the contractility to such a degree that coronary blood flow redistribution is less harmful than expected. Isoflurane's ability to decrease BP by decreasing SVR and depressing myocardial contractility enables CO to be maintained, which is an attractive feature in the management of CAD. For many anesthesiologists, the clinical significance of isoflurane-induced coronary steal is not convincing, and therefore, it is still commonly used in this setting.

### Benzodiazepines

Induction of anesthesia with a benzodiazepine is associated with relative hemodynamic stability and profound amnesia. Additional anesthesia with opioids, inhalation agents, or other intravenous agents is necessary to blunt the response to noxious stimuli. The interaction of a benzodiazepine and a potent opioid administered within minutes of each other may lead to significant hypotension due to a decrease in SVR.[102,103] Diazepam may provide smoother hemodynamic conditions than midazolam by causing a smaller increase in HR and a smaller decrease in MAP.[104]

However, when used judiciously, no adverse effects on overall outcome have been shown. Instead, midazolam usage has been shown to reduce opioid use and facilitate early extubation.[105] It is the practice of our institution to titrate benzodiazepine doses to provide hemodynamic stability and reliable amnesia.

### Ketamine

Ketamine, when administered alone, often produces unwanted increases in HR and BP. When it is administered with a benzodiazepine or an opioid, however, these detrimental effects generally are not encountered, and hemodynamic stability is maintained.[106–109] When ketamine is used in combination with opioids, benzodiazepines, or other sedatives, hallucinations and emergence delirium are unlikely.

It is uncertain whether ketamine-induced increases in CBF and intracranial pressure increase the risk of neurologic complications during cardiac surgery. However, ketamine-based techniques compare favorably with various other anesthetic regimens in outcome studies of patients undergoing cardiac surgery.[110,111] In addition, ketamine and diazepam were shown to be associated with lower fluid requirements and shorter postoperative stays in ICUs than noted for a high-dose opioid technique.[111]

## Propofol

The literature also provides support for the safe use of propofol with narcotics in cardiac anesthesia when compared with enflurane-opioid, or pure opioid-based techniques.[112,113] Typically, HR and CO increase following intubation, whereas SVR decreases after intubation and then returns to baseline during surgery. Stroke index changes were similar between groups and were directly related to changes in SVR. Regional and global coronary blood flow, $M\dot{V}O_2$, and lactate extraction ratio were constant. The use of a propofol infusion plus fentanyl, 15 $\mu$g/kg, has been shown to result in lower HR pre-CPB and facilitate earlier awakening and extubation when compared with midazolam, 3 to 6 mg, and fentanyl, 60 $\mu$g/kg, without significant differences in thermodilution assessment of right heart function.

## Clonidine

Clonidine as an adjunct to other anesthetics in the cardiac surgical population has been associated with reduced opioid and anesthetic requirements, shortened periods of postoperative ventilation, reduced plasma catecholamine levels, and decreased myocardial ischemia.[114,115] Unfortunately, its use has also been associated with increased requirements for pacemaker use and unstable hemodynamics (severe hypotension and vasodilation), precluding its use from routine practice.[115,116]

## Barbiturates

Barbiturates, including primarily sodium thiopental and methohexital, are commonly administered as induction agents along with the agents previously discussed. Doses of 5 mg/kg of thiopental or 1 mg/kg of methohexital caused a decrease in stroke volume and arterial pressure mainly attributable to venous pooling and not to a primary negative inotropic effect. Myocardial $O_2$ consumption decreases with the accompanying changes in hemodynamics[117]; however, a compensatory tachycardia may offset these potential benefits. Gunaydin and Babacan suggested that barbiturate induction with continued administration of 3 mg/kg/h during CPB may convey a lower incidence of postoperative cerebral hypoperfusion, and therefore a decreased risk of postoperative delirium when compared with high-dose fentanyl anesthesia in cardiac surgery.[118]

Patients with ventricular dysfunction, pressure-dependent CAD, or valvular disease may not tolerate the decreased stroke volume or BP resulting from barbiturate administration, especially when magnified by coadministration of other agents for induction (narcotics, benzodiazepines). For this reason, induction doses are typically reduced to produce hypnosis without the undesired hemodynamic consequences.

## Etomidate

Etomidate is an anesthetic that induces only minor cardiovascular changes; its influence on the endocrine system, however, has reduced its clinical indication. It use has been associated with a dose-dependent adrenal suppression, which may be more profound in the critically ill population. Although etomidate is often chosen for induction in patients when the adverse effects of barbiturates are anticipated to be ill-tolerated, it can still unmask hypovolemia in susceptible patients.

## Intrathecal Morphine

Intrathecal morphine is not commonly administered at our institution. Successful outcomes with excellent postoperative pain control and early extubation have been reported.[119,120] Despite decreased postoperative narcotic requirements associated with the use of large doses, intrathecal morphine has what many practitioners consider to be an unsatisfactory risk-benefit ratio.

Intrathecal morphine in smaller doses than originally investigated was associated in a randomized, prospective study with a significantly increased incidence of respiratory depression without significantly reducing postoperative narcotic requirements.[121,122] Its use does not reliably attenuate the stress response during and after cardiac surgery, as originally hypothesized, and bloody taps result in either cancellation of surgery or an intraoperative delay in systemic heparinization due to the potentially increased risk of the rare development of subarachnoid or epidural hematoma.[123]

## Thoracic Epidural Anesthesia

Thoracic epidural anesthesia (TEA) is thought by some proponents to have potential benefits in patients undergoing CABG surgery by producing superior perioperative analgesia, stress response attenuation, and cardiac sympatholysis.[124] Unlike intrathecal morphine analgesic supplementation, TEA combined with general anesthesia has been shown to attenuate the myocardial sympathetic response to CPB in association with decreased myocardial injury.[125] TEA can reduce respirator time and the need for parenteral analgesics after CABG without significant differences in ventilation-perfusion ($\dot{V}/\dot{Q}$) matching, oxygenation, or atelectasis formation.[126] However, TEA continues to have a questionable risk-benefit ratio. Many patients actually relate higher pain scores localized in the region of the leg incision for vein harvest than to the sternal incision site. Moreover, despite the fact that there has never been a case of thoracolumbar epidural hematoma formation following CPB with central neuraxial blockade, it is the current recommendation of the American Society of Regional Anesthesia[127] that surgery involving CPB be delayed following a bloody tap for either intrathecal narcotic administration or epidural analgesia.[128] For this reason, many institutions either place epidurals on the evening before surgery, limiting the technique to those not presenting for same-day procedures, or do not commonly administer TEA for patients undergoing CPB.

## Opioid Antagonists

The practice of facilitating early somnolence or reversing it with opioid antagonists has many potential complications. This practice has been associated with ventricular irritability, acute PE, hypertension, increased requirements for postoperative analgesics, renarcotization, and unacceptable increases in pain.[129–132]

## Does the Choice of Anesthetic Influence Outcome?

The fact that so many different anesthetic techniques are used in cardiac anesthesia makes one wonder if the specific method chosen really makes a difference. Primary anesthetic techniques for CABG surgery have been examined in two studies, each with more than 1000 patients.[110,133] Compared with patients receiving sufentanil, those receiving halothane, enflurane, or isoflurane were more likely to have episodes of intraoperative hypotension, were less likely to have hypertension both intraoperatively and postoperatively, and required a shorter period of tracheal intubation.[133] The incidences of ischemia, tachycardia, and adverse outcome did not differ among the various techniques. A comparison of high-dose fentanyl, moderate-dose fentanyl, sufentanil, diazepam-ketamine, and halothane likewise showed no difference in morbidity or mortality.[110] Diazepam-ketamine–anesthetized patients had a lower incidence of hypotensive episodes.

### Physiologic Effects

Hemodynamic and other physiologic effects differ greatly among anesthetic agents. The different effects do not, however, correlate well with outcome variables. Other factors, including preoperative cardiac status, perioperative hemodynamic stability, incidence of perioperative myocardial ischemia, and technical quality of coronary bypass grafts, are more important than the choice of anesthetic agents. As long as an anesthesiologist is fully aware of a patient's pathophysiology and the pharmacology of the agents chosen and promptly treats hemodynamic aberrations and myocardial ischemia, the anesthetic agents themselves are of secondary importance.

### Balanced Anesthesia

The selection of a combination of agents, each with a desired effect, allows the provision of a more complete anesthetic, which is chosen based on a particular patient's pathophysiology. Because interactions may occur between various anesthetic agents, vasoactive agents must be immediately available to increase or decrease HR, BP, and myocardial contractility. These combinations may decrease the total doses of anesthetic agents and their duration of action.

Some suggested combinations of anesthetic agents are listed in Table 63–17. They are not meant to serve as a cookbook but to provide guidelines in dosing that are then adjusted according to a patient's response. Other combinations not listed may also be efficacious. Extensive reviews of the hemodynamic effects of anesthetic agents in patients undergoing cardiac surgery have been published.[134–136]

### What Are the Benefits of Fast-Track Cardiac Surgery?

Quasha and associates noted in 1980 that pulmonary complications were markedly diminished when patients were extubated early, possibly due to better return of mucociliary function, decreased atelectasis, and decreased perioperative pneumonia.[137] In addition to the potential pulmonary benefits, elimination of positive pressure ventilation has also been shown to improve diastolic compliance[138] and intrapulmonary shunt fraction, in addition to allowing earlier chest tube removal, mobilization, food intake, and ICU and hospital discharge.[139]

One of the major advantages to early extubation is the overall cost of hospital stay. Complications in the perioperative period are the main determinants of aberrancy from average costs following CABG. Although reexploration for postoperative bleeding or atrial arrhythmias can increase costs by 30% to 40%, stroke or IABP support can increase perioperative hospital costs by three- to fivefold. Fast-tracking does not appear to increase complications. Several studies have demonstrated no increase in rate or cost of complications with early extubation anesthesia (EEA), and in fact reveal total cost savings >20%. Significant differences are realized primarily in costs incurred while in the ICU (almost 40% less in the EEA group) and appear related to ICU nursing costs, supplies (51.4%), respiratory therapy and ventilator management (29.4%), and physician fees (16.8%). Unchanged variables include total preoperative costs, anesthetic drug costs, and OR costs.[140,141]

### How Are Patients Determined to Be Candidates for Early Extubation?

There have been several criteria proposed for selection of patients to a fast-track protocol. They are similar in that a preoperative determination of the overall physical status of the patient seems to play a role in the postoperative course from not only a cardiovascular stability standpoint but also a multiorgan system approach. Tables 63–18 and 63–19 present some guidelines for selection.

### Has Fast-Tracking Increased the Incidence of Awareness With Cardiac Surgery?

A recent study reported a 0.3% incidence of awareness during fast-track cardiac anesthesia, which is the lowest ever reported to date during cardiac surgery. The balanced anesthetic technique used in this report consisted of continuous administration of volatile (isoflurane) or intravenous (propofol) anesthetic agents before, during, and after CPB.[142]

## MANAGEMENT OF SURGICAL EVENTS IN CARDIAC SURGERY

Certain surgical events are of particular importance to anesthesiologists, either because of their physiologic impact or because of the participatory role an anesthesiologist must have.

### What Should Be Anticipated After Induction and Intubation?

After these events follows a period of minimum stimulation, during which antiseptic preparation and draping take place. Raising the legs to scrub for saphenous vein dissection leads to an increase in drainage from lower extremity veins, produc-

**TABLE 63–17.** Suggested Cardiac Anesthesia Techniques

| | Induction | Maintenance | Comments |
|---|---|---|---|
| High-dose opioid | Fentanyl, 50–100 µg/kg<br><br>Sufentanil, 10–25 µg/kg | Additional boluses or infusion:<br>Fentanyl, 1–5 µg/kg/h<br><br>Sufentanil, 0.3–2 µg/kg/h | Benzodiazepine or volatile agent for amnesia.<br>Volatile agent or vasoactive agent for breakthrough tachycardia and hypertension.<br>Preferred technique in patients with poor ventricular function. |
| Moderate-dose opioid | Fentanyl, 10–50 µg/kg<br>Sufentanil, 3–10 µg/kg | Benzodiazepine, volatile agent, and additional opioid boluses or infusion:<br>Fentanyl, 0.2–2 µg/kg/h<br>Sufentanil, 0.1–1 µg/kg/h | Well tolerated by patients with preserved ventricular function who can benefit from decreased contractility associated with higher concentrations of volatile agents. |
| Opioid-benzodiazepine | Sufentanil, 1–2.5 µg/kg<br>Midazolam, 0.1 mg/kg | Volatile agent or infusion:<br>Sufentanil, 0.7–1.5 µg/kg/h<br>Midazolam, 0.07–0.15 mg/kg/h | Give induction doses over at least 5 min.<br>Treat breakthrough by increasing the infusion rate, adding volatile agent or vasoactive agent. |
| Opioid-propofol | Propofol, 1–2 mg/kg<br>Remifentanil, 1–2 mg/kg | Propofol, 100–200 µg/kg/min<br>Remifentanil, 0.5–2 mg/kg/min | Fast emergence. May require longer acting narcotics for pain control postoperatively.<br>Expensive. |
| Benzodiazepine | Diazepam, 0.2–0.6 mg/kg<br>Midazolam, 0.1–0.3 mg/kg | Opioids and volatile agents | Induction produces mild hypotension. Other anesthetic agents are necessary to prevent tachycardia and hypertension in response to noxious stimuli. Opioids must be carefully and slowly titrated to prevent hypotensive interaction. (Avoid large doses of benzodiazepines in elderly patients and patients with hepatic dysfunction.) |
| Diazepam-ketamine | Diazepam, 0.3–0.4 mg/kg<br>Ketamine, 2 mg/kg | Volatile agent, opioids, or an infusion of ketamine, 1 mg/kg/h | Minimal hemodynamic effects, even with poor ventricular function. |
| Midazolam-ketamine | Midazolam, 0.5 mg/kg<br>Ketamine, 2 mg/kg | Volatile agent, opioids, or vasoactive agents and an infusion of midazolam, 0.04 mg/kg/h, ketamine, 1 mg/kg/h | Minimal hemodynamic effects, even with poor ventricular function. |
| Opioid-ketamine | Ketamine, 1–2 mg/kg and fentanyl, 10 µg/kg or sufentanil, 1–2 µg/kg | Volatile agent, opioid, or vasoactive agent and an infusion of ketamine, 1 mg/kg/h, and fentanyl, 0.5–2 µg/kg/h, or sufentanil, 0.2–1 µg/kg/h | Minimal hemodynamic effects, even with poor ventricular function. |

ing an increase in filling and systemic pressures. These changes revert when the legs are returned to table level. During this period, the anesthesiologist records postinduction hemodynamic data, places the TEE probe if one is used, ensures that the patient is safely positioned with all intravenous catheters and invasive monitors functioning, and prepares for the next noxious stimuli—incision and sternotomy. The depth of anesthesia should be increased in anticipation of these events to treat hypertensive or tachycardiac breakthrough and myocardial ischemia. When intraoperative ischemia occurs, it is most commonly associated with induction, intubation, skin incision, sternotomy, and cannulation for CPB.[38]

### Sternotomy

At the time of sternotomy, a patient's lungs should be deflated to decrease the risk of laceration of the pleura or lung

**TABLE 63–18.** Selecting Patients for EEA:
Preoperative Severity Scoring

| | |
|---|---|
| Emergency | 6 |
| Serum Cr >1.9 | 4 |
| Serum Cr 1.6–1.8 | 1 |
| Severe LV dysfunction | 3 |
| Redo sternotomy | 3 |
| MR | 3 |
| Age >75 y | 2 |
| Prior vascular surgery | 2 |
| COPD on medication | 2 |
| Hct <34% | 2 |
| AS | 1 |
| Weight ≤65 kg | 1 |
| Diabetes on medication | 1 |
| Cerebrovascular Dz | 1 |
| Age 65–74 y | 1 |

AS, aortic stenosis; COPD, chronic obstructive pulmonary disease; Cr, creatinine; Dz, disease; EEA, early extubation anesthesia; Hct, hematocrit; LV, left ventricular; MR, mitral regurgitation.
From Higgins TL. Safety issues regarding early extubation after coronary artery bypass surgery. *J Cardiothorac Vasc Anesth.* 1995;95(suppl 1):24.

**TABLE 63–19.** Postoperative Criteria for Early Extubation

Awake and responsive to commands
Adequate gag reflex
Able to maintain pH >7.35 on CPAP
Hemodynamically stable without arrhythmias
Mediastinal bleeding <100 mL/h × 2 h
Fully rewarmed (T >36°C), no shivering
Well-perfused with adequate urine output

From Verrier ED, Wright IH, Cochran RP, et al: Changes in cardiovascular surgical approaches to achieve early extubation. *J Cardiothorac Vasc Anesth.* 1995; 95(suppl):10.

parenchyma by the sternal saw. The lungs may be immediately substernal during full inflation. Deflation is most reliably accomplished by detaching one limb of the breathing circuit until sternotomy is complete.

In a patient who has previously undergone cardiac surgery, close attention during sternotomy is especially important. The heart or coronary bypass grafts may be adherent to the sternum. An oscillating saw, which resembles a cast cutter, is used to cut through the sternum. Ventilation may be continued when sternotomy is complete. Blood should be available in the OR and already cross-checked with the patient's identification so that it can be rapidly transfused if the heart or great vessels are injured, especially for redo procedures when scarring may cause adherence of the heart or great vessels to the sternum.

The surgeon should prepare the femoral area for potential femoral artery cannulation. In emergency situations requiring urgent initiation of CPB, the cardiotomy suction can be placed in the chest following systemic heparinization to serve as a venous return line, and the aortic line can be attached to the femoral arterial cannula to initiate "sucker bypass." Alternatively, femoral artery–femoral vein bypass can be established before sternotomy or in the event of major bleeding or cardiovascular collapse.

### Should Autologous Blood Be Drawn Before and Infused After Cardiopulmonary Bypass?

Intraoperative withdrawal of blood before CPB for infusion afterward is done in many institutions as a blood conservation measure. The theoretic benefit is that fresh autologous whole blood that has not been exposed to the adverse effects of CPB on platelets is then available for transfusion after discontinuation of CPB.

Blood is withdrawn through an arterial or venous catheter and collected in a bag containing heparin or citrate. Alternatively, the perfusionist can withdraw blood through the venous cannula after heparinization. This should provide a safe source of red blood cells, coagulation factors, and platelets.

#### Risks

Potential risks exist. An equal volume of colloid or three times the volume of blood in crystalloid must be infused during collection to preserve hemodynamic stability. Patients with a preoperative hematocrit <33% to 35% probably do not benefit much because after withdrawal of blood, the initiation of CPB may cause hemodilution to a hematocrit <20%. Withdrawal of blood through an arterial or intravenous catheter can be time-consuming and distracting to the anesthesiologist. Inadequate mixing of the blood with an anticoagulant or blood withdrawal in excess of the citrate anticoagulation capacity ($\approx$450 mL) can allow coagulation. Strict aseptic technique is another consideration because the withdrawn blood is a perfect culture medium and is usually stored at room temperature.

#### Outcome Analysis

The most important questions are whether or not intraoperative blood harvesting plus reinfusion improves coagulation, decreases post-CPB bleeding, and ultimately decreases trans-

fusion requirement. Unfortunately, the literature does not provide clear answers. Some reviews suggest equivocal results.[143,144] Other factors related to surgical technique (intraoperative blood salvage from the surgical site, limitation of pre-CPB fluid administration, collection and autotransfusion of chest tube drainage, and a willingness to accept normovolemic anemia) are probably more important in determining perioperative blood use.[143] Withdrawal of heparinized blood through the venous cannula is simpler, less time-consuming, and less distracting than withdrawal of nonheparinized blood through an arterial or venous catheter if this approach is chosen.[144]

### What Are the Concerns During Internal Mammary Artery Dissection?

If the IMA is to be used as a bypass graft, the surgeon dissects it out after sternotomy. The left IMA is usually grafted to the left anterior descending coronary artery. In patients with previous saphenous vein grafting or vein stripping procedures, the right IMA may also be used.

The IMA lies along the anterior chest wall posterior to the cartilages of the first six ribs, about 1.25 cm from the lateral margin of the sternum. A Favoloro retractor is placed to lift the sternum, and the operating table is tilted away from the surgeon. While tilting the table, the anesthesiologist should ensure that tension on the endotracheal tube does not displace it. The effect of this position change on the transducers' zero reference levels must also be considered. If a radial arterial catheter has been placed on the side to which the table is tilted, the tracing may be lost, as discussed earlier. Alternative BP monitoring must be available. Finally, the arm may be compressed between the patient's chest and the retractor post, causing neurologic damage (particularly by compression of the radial nerve in the spiral groove of the humerus) or ischemia to the hand.

Mechanical ventilation of the lungs during IMA dissection may obscure the surgical field. Reduction of tidal volume and increase of respiratory rate to maintain constant alveolar ventilation are often helpful.

The surgeon may occasionally use papaverine or another vasodilator to maximally dilate the IMA. It may be injected into the IMA and tissue surrounding it, or a sponge soaked with the vasodilator may be applied. Transient systemic hypotension may ensue.

### How Is Heparin Administered in Preparation for Cardiopulmonary Bypass?

Heparin is administered before the initiation of CPB. Contact between blood and the materials of the CPB circuit activates the coagulation and the fibrinolytic systems; enough heparin must be administered to prevent gross and microscopic coagulation. Its effect is most commonly monitored by assessing the ACT.

At the beginning of the procedure, preferably after skin incision, a blood sample is withdrawn to determine a baseline ACT. Before cannulation of the aorta and right atrium, heparin is administered in a dose of 300 to 400 units/kg. The ACT is measured again before initiation of CPB. An ACT >400 seconds is the minimum safe degree of anticoagulation for CPB.[145] If the priming solution contains 5000 to 10 000 units of heparin, CPB may be initiated when the ACT, after the dose of heparin, is close to 400 seconds. The ACT should again be measured immediately after the initiation of CPB, and typically at routine intervals (30-60 minutes) during prolonged bypass runs.

Heparin should be administered through a central venous catheter after aspiration to ensure blood return. Some surgeons prefer to inject heparin directly into the RA to be certain that it is delivered to the central circulation.

### Heparin Resistance

Adequate anticoagulation after a standard dose of heparin cannot be assumed. If the ACT is inadequate for CPB, additional heparin should be given in doses of 5000 to 10 000 units. If additional doses do not result in an adequate ACT, reasons for heparin resistance should be considered (Table 63–20).

One cause of heparin resistance that does not respond well to even large doses of heparin is antithrombin III deficiency. Antithrombin III is a plasma protein that acts as an inhibitor of thrombin and the serine proteases. Heparin acts by binding to antithrombin III, speeding up the relatively slow inhibitory action of antithrombin III on thrombin. Patients with antithrombin III deficiency have a tendency toward thrombosis and a resistance to the anticoagulant effect of heparin. Transfusion of two units of fresh-frozen plasma provides enough antithrombin III to overcome heparin resistance.

### What Are the Concerns During Cannulation for Cardiopulmonary Bypass?

After the pericardium is opened, the surgeon prepares for aortic and RA cannulation. The aorta is cannulated first so that if a problem develops with atrial cannulation, such as significant dysrhythmia or hemorrhage, bypass can be immediately instituted or volume infusion from the CPB pump through the aortic cannula can be established, respectively. If

**TABLE 63–20.** Conditions and Situations Causing Real or Apparent Heparin Resistance

**Technical Reasons**

Mislabeled heparin syringe
Heparin not injected intravascularly (extravasation, tubing disconnected, other)

**Heparin Resistance**

Previous or ongoing administration of heparin
Heparin-induced thrombocytopenia
Pregnancy
Use of oral contraceptives
Intraaortic balloon counterpulsation
Shock
Previous administration of streptokinase
Antithrombin III deficiency
Low-grade disseminated intravascular coagulation
Infective endocarditis
Presence of a clot within the body (intracardiac thrombus)
Increased platelet count

Data from Anderson EF. Heparin resistance prior to cardiopulmonary bypass. *Anesthesiology.* 1986;64:504; and Romanoff ME, Rung GW. Anesthetic management in the precardiopulmonary bypass period. In: Hensley FA Jr, Martin DE, eds. *The Practice of Cardiac Anesthesia.* Boston, Little, Brown & Co; 1990:202.

difficulty is encountered with atrial cannulation and hemodynamic instability results, CPB can be initiated by sucker bypass, in which the cardiotomy suckers substitute for the atrial cannula.

### Aortic Cannulation

In preparation for aortic cannulation, the SBP should be reduced to about 100 mm Hg to decrease the risk of aortic dissection. Aortic cannulation frequently is associated with a hypertensive response despite deep anesthesia because it is more stimulating than the events preceding it or because of direct stimulation of sympathetic nerves in the aortic arch.

BP control may be achieved by increasing the concentration of the volatile agent or by administering short-acting vasoactive agents such as NTG, sodium nitroprusside (SNP), or esmolol. After the aortic cannula is placed and the CPB tubing is connected, the surgeon and anesthesiologist should visually inspect the tubing and cannula for the presence of air bubbles before any volume is infused to the patient. Following inspection, the perfusionist is frequently asked to test the cannula by infusing a volume of pump prime while inspecting the pressure to determine if the cannula is indeed intraluminal. Pressures >300 mm Hg may indicate inappropriate location of the cannula, either between the muscular layers of the aorta or in a manner that obstructs forward flow. It is imperative to document intraluminal placement in the event that sudden initiation of CPB becomes necessary due to complications in placing subsequent cannulae.

### Atrial Cannulation

RA cannulation may involve a single two-stage cannula or two separate cannulas to drain the superior vena cava (SVC) and inferior vena cava (IVC). A two-stage cannula is used most often for CABG and aortic valve procedures. RA cannulation may be complicated by supraventricular dysrhythmias, including atrial fibrillation, which may lead to decreased CO and hypotension. This problem is particularly troublesome in a patient with a poorly compliant LV whose filling and CO are dependent on the atrial kick. Cardioversion is the treatment of choice in this situation. If it is unsuccessful and hemodynamic instability results, expedient initiation of CPB may be necessary.

For procedures involving right atriotomy, such as ASD repairs, tricuspid surgery, and a trans–right atrial approach to the mitral valve, two separate cannulas are placed to ensure drainage from both the SVC and IVC. With either approach, it is important to monitor CVP continuously during CPB. Perfusionists may note a decrease in venous return in the event of an obstructed cannula; however, adequate return may exist when partial obstruction occurs due to improper placement, surgical manipulation, or cannula orifice obstruction caused by position against a venous or atrial wall. As cerebral perfusion pressure during bypass is most accurately determined by MAP (CPB perfusion pressure) − CVP (in the absence of intracranial hypertension), occlusion of SVC return (as evidenced by a rising CVP) can cause catastrophic cerebral hypoperfusion or cerebral edema due to venous congestion.

### Cardioplegia Catheters

The surgeon also places one or more cardioplegia catheters for anterograde, retrograde, or both types of cardioplegia delivery. Anterograde cardioplegia is delivered either via a needle placed in the ascending aorta proximal to the aortic cannula or directly into the coronary arteries following application of the aortic cross-clamp and open aortotomy, as in aortic valve replacement or aortic root-arch replacement. Insertion of the former cardioplegia needle is usually hemodynamically insignificant; however, as with aortic cannulation, the SBP should remain around 100 mm Hg to reduce the risk of dissection.

Retrograde cardioplegia is routinely administered through a catheter that is placed through the right atrium and into the coronary sinus. Because manual guidance is typically required to ensure that the catheter lies in an appropriate position, surgical compression of right-sided heart structures is often accompanied by hypotension due to a decrease in venous return. This decreased preload can often be overcome by volume resuscitation from the aortic cannula or temporarily compensated for by administration of short-acting vasoconstrictors. In some patients who are less tolerant, it may be necessary to wait until CPB is instituted to properly position the retrograde cardioplegia cannula.

Oftentimes, a sterile pressure tubing is passed over the drapes to the anesthesiologist. Once the tubing is attached to the retrograde cannula, the pressure may be transduced. On administration of retrograde cardioplegia, a typical waveform can be used to confirm appropriate placement in the coronary sinus, and the perfusionist may limit flow so that maximum pressures of 30 to 35 mm Hg limit the amount of myocardial edema that may develop with excessive coronary venous pressures.

### How Must the Anesthesiologist Prepare for Cardiopulmonary Bypass?

Before the initiation of CPB, anticoagulation must be adequate as assessed by an ACT >400 seconds. The intravenous infusions may be turned off except for one central venous catheter, into which medications may be administered and through which the CVP is monitored.

### Physical Examination

The patient's neck and eyes should be examined before and immediately after initiation of CPB in order to detect improper placement of aortic and venous cannulas. Sudden distention of the jugular veins and development of facial edema may indicate obstruction to cerebral venous drainage. Palpation of a thrill on one side of the neck or a temperature difference between left and right sides of the neck suggests misplacement of the aortic cannula such that the majority of flow is being directed to only half of the cerebral circulation. The pupils should be small and equal before CPB. A sudden change may occur with a misplaced aortic or venous cannula.

### Monitors

On initiation of CPB, changes in cerebral monitoring devices, as discussed previously, can indicate cannula malposition, and thus arterial pressure and CVP should be continuously monitored.

Elevated PA pressures may be indicative of ventricular distention. This may occur due to aortic insufficiency following electrical silence or fibrillation, when perfusion from the aortic cannula drains into a nonpumping LV across an incompetent aortic valve. It may also occur gradually due to continued return of blood to the LV or left atrium via the thebesian veins, bronchiolar circulation, or an intracardiac shunt. Whatever the case, due to increased wall tension, myocardial $O_2$ consumption is higher in a distended ventricle, whereas coronary perfusion pressure is lower than that in an appropriately decompressed ventricle; it may be necessary to place an LV vent (typically through the right superior pulmonary vein). In some cases, as with severe aortic insufficiency, the surgeon may prefer to place the LV vent before institution of CPB in anticipation of overdistention. Continued LV ejection usually prevents distention from occurring; however, it is often prudent to advise the surgeon when fibrillation or ventricular asystole occurs because his or her attention may be focused on other matters.

### Hemodilution and Drug Concentrations

With the initiation of CPB, significant hemodilution occurs, with resultant decreases in the plasma concentrations of most drugs. Consideration should be given to the administration of additional opioids and amnestic agents around the time of initiation of CPB to counteract this effect.

### Blood Pressure Control

BP commonly drops with the initiation of CPB. This observation has been attributed to one or more causes. Hemodilution reduces the hematocrit and concentrations of plasma proteins, thus reducing the viscosity of blood. Vasodilation may occur in response to hemodilution or to the loss of pulsatile flow. Acute dilution of circulating catecholamines may also produce vasodilation. This sudden decrease in MAP may not be clinically important if a patient's temperature is rapidly lowered with the initiation of CPB. If normothermia is maintained, however, restoration of perfusion pressure (50-80 mm Hg) is more important. Therefore, phenylephrine should be immediately available for bolus injection (40-200 μg doses) or continuous infusion.

### Aortic Dissection

Hypotension associated with markedly elevated aortic line pressure from the CPB pump and decreased venous drainage to the reservoir can occur with an aortic dissection at the cannulation site. A hematoma may be seen within the wall of the aorta. This finding necessitates discontinuation of CPB to reposition the aortic cannula and repair the dissection.

### Pulmonary Artery Catheter Positioning

The PA catheter should be withdrawn to the main PA (usually ≈5 cm) during CPB to decrease the risk of PA rupture. The catheter becomes stiff when the patient is cooled, and emptying and manipulating the heart cause it to advance as well. With rewarming, the catheter length may straighten out, also causing the tip to advance. The PA pressure tracing should be observed throughout CPB and should be 15 mm Hg or less. Higher pressures may be a sign that the catheter is "overwedging," and it should be withdrawn farther. With adequate venous drainage, the RA should be relatively empty and the CVP should be <5 mm Hg. Similarly, elevated PA pressures may be indicative of ventricular distention. This may occur due to aortic insufficiency following electrical silence or fibrillation, when perfusion from the aortic cannula drains into a nonpumping LV across an incompetent aortic valve. It may also occur gradually due to continued return of blood to the LV or left atrium via the thebesian veins, bronchiolar circulation, or an intracardiac shunt. Whatever the case, due to increased wall tension, myocardial $O_2$ consumption is higher in a distended ventricle, whereas coronary perfusion pressure is lower than an appropriately decompressed ventricle, and it may be necessary to place an LV vent (typically through the right superior pulmonary vein). In some cases, as with severe aortic insufficiency, the surgeon may prefer to place the LV vent before institution of CPB in anticipation of overdistention. As mentioned, continued LV ejection usually prevents distention from occurring; however, it is often prudent to advise the surgeon when fibrillation or ventricular asystole occurs because his or her attention may be focused on other matters.

## "Inspired" Gas

Once adequate CPB flow is reached, the inspired gas mixture is changed to air, the anesthetic vaporizer is turned off, and the ventilator may be turned off. This switch to air is thought to decrease the degree of post-CPB intrapulmonary shunt by decreasing both the direct toxic effects of a high $FIO_2$ and absorption atelectasis. No advantage in regard to postoperative pulmonary function results from continuing ventilation. The pulse oximeter and gas analyzer (or capnograph, if separate) may also be turned off because they do not provide useful information during CPB.

## What Is a "Snorkel"?

It has become the practice of many cardiac anesthesiologists and perfusionists in our institution to continuously monitor gases from the exhaust tubing of the membrane oxygenator on the CPB machine by extending monitoring tubing from this site to the gas analyzer, a practice we refer to as *snorkeling*. Snorkeling provides continuous measurements of end-tidal $O_2$, $CO_2$, and volatile agent concentrations, therefore enabling the perfusionist and anesthesiologist to monitor oxygenation, ventilation, and anesthetic delivery during CPB. Because of the increased solubility of gases in solution during hypothermia, significant gradients are often observed in $CO_2$ concentrations during cooling, whereas reverse gradients are evident on rewarming when compared with concomitant arterial blood gas (ABG) measurements.

Snorkeling allows for confirmation of adequate oxygenation of the perfusate more rapidly than ABG measurements can be made, and has successfully identified at least one potentially catastrophic event in which an $O_2$ flow meter delivered an inadequate $FIO_2$ to the membrane oxygenator. Snorkeling also enables the anesthesiologist to determine more timely redosing of intravenous anesthetic agents on rewarming because end-tidal agent concentrations are readily measured, allowing for administration of drugs based on anesthetic thresholds rather than on temperature thresholds. Although a study has not yet been performed to determine changes in outcome, drug utilization, or incidence of intraoperative recall using this device, it is extremely cheap, easy to perform, and offers absolutely no risk to patients.

## WEANING AND SEPARATION FROM CARDIOPULMONARY BYPASS

The process of weaning and separation from CPB is the climax of cardiac surgical procedures. It tests the success of surgical interventions and provides a challenge to the anesthesiologist to optimize hemodynamic variables through this important transitional period.

## What Preparations Should Be Made During Cardiopulmonary Bypass?

Toward the end of CPB, the anesthesiologist formulates a plan for hemodynamic management based on an assessment of ventricular function. This assessment is drawn from preoperative information (history and physical examination, cardiac catheterization data); pre-CPB information (eg, response to anesthetic and surgical manipulations, hemodynamic parameters, TEE); the apparent status of ventricular function during CPB as seen on visual inspection and TEE; and the surgeon's impression of the adequacy of the surgery (quality of coronary bypass grafts, valve replacement and repair, and so on).

Depending on this assessment, inotropes, vasodilators, and vasoconstrictors are selected and prepared. NTG, SNP, and an inotrope such as dopamine, dobutamine, or epinephrine should be available in all procedures. If it is believed that an inotrope will be necessary, the infusion should be started at least 5 minutes before weaning to allow time for the drug to circulate, reach steady state, and begin to exert its effects. Starting an inotrope earlier than necessary may worsen ischemic injury and reperfusion injury by raising $MVO_2$.[146,147]

### Venting of Air

After an open cardiac procedure, air remains in the left side of the heart. Before weaning from CPB and before the heart is allowed to eject blood, efforts must be made to remove the air to avoid embolization to the coronary and cerebral vasculature. With the head lowered (Trendelenburg position), the patient is manually ventilated to force air and blood back to the left side of the heart from the pulmonary vasculature. While the heart is tilted back and forth, air is aspirated through a needle at the apex or through an aortic root vent. TEE can be used to assess the presence of residual intracardiac air. The surgeon may insert a 25-gauge needle into the coronary grafts to allow air and blood to exit. This procedure also confirms blood flow in the grafts.

### Cardiac Pacing

A pacemaker must be available. Function of the pacemaker may be confirmed during CPB after the surgeon places epicardial leads. Pacing facilitates weaning from CPB by optimizing heart rate (70-100 bpm) and providing synchronous atrioventricular contraction (atrial pacing or atrioventricular sequential pacing).

## Rewarming

Patients must be adequately rewarmed. Although esophageal and nasopharyngeal temperatures rise rapidly with rewarming, the temperature of peripheral tissues rises more slowly. Rectal temperature should be at least 35°C before separation from CPB. Otherwise, the SVR may remain high, and hypothermia will recur. It has been shown that rewarming with concurrent administration of nitrosodilators increases peripheral rewarming, reduces the degree of post-CPB temperature afterdrop, and reduces time to extubation.[148]

## Metabolic Status

Electrolyte concentrations and acid-base status should be investigated. Potassium concentration may be slightly elevated at the end of CPB owing to absorption of cardioplegia solution, but it usually decreases soon afterward as long as renal function is adequate. Severe hyperkalemia may induce conduction disturbances and depress contractility. Hypokalemia in this setting ($K^+$ <4 mEq/L) predisposes to ventricular irritability and should be corrected before weaning from CPB. Mild hypocalcemia at the end of CPB is common and probably does not warrant treatment while on CPB. Severe hypocalcemia may develop, particularly in patients who require transfusion of citrate-preserved blood products during CPB, and may induce myocardial depression and systemic vasodilation.[149] Severe hypocalcemia (<0.80 mmol/L) should be treated with calcium salts after separation from CPB (see later discussion).

## Fluids and Blood

Intravenous fluids should be available for infusion after weaning from CPB. Thresholds for transfusion of packed red blood cells before weaning vary from institution to institution and from patient to patient but are generally around a hemoglobin concentration of <7.0 g/100 mL if it is suspected that $O_2$ delivery after CPB may be marginal owing to low CO. Otherwise, crystalloid solutions and colloids such as hydroxyethyl starch, purified protein fraction, or albumin should be available.

## Anesthetic Requirements

During the rewarming phase of CPB, metabolism of drugs increases and cerebral function increases. Therefore, anesthetic requirements likewise increase. At this time, additional opioids, amnestic agents, and muscle relaxants may be required. Some prefer not to administer additional muscle relaxants because they are not necessary for completion of the operation, and their use prevents patients' movements indicating awareness.

Choice of a "landmark" temperature at which additional anesthetic is administered may help an anesthesiologist to develop a routine so that this factor is not overlooked. For example, at a blood (not rectal) temperature of 35°C, additional intravenous agents may be given and any inhaled agent being administered into the pump may be discontinued. This process allows adequate time for inhaled anesthetics to wash out, so that residual myocardial depressant effects will be dissipated at the time of weaning from CPB. Greater than 90% washout of inhaled anesthetics requires approximately 15 minutes[150] (Fig. 63–12).

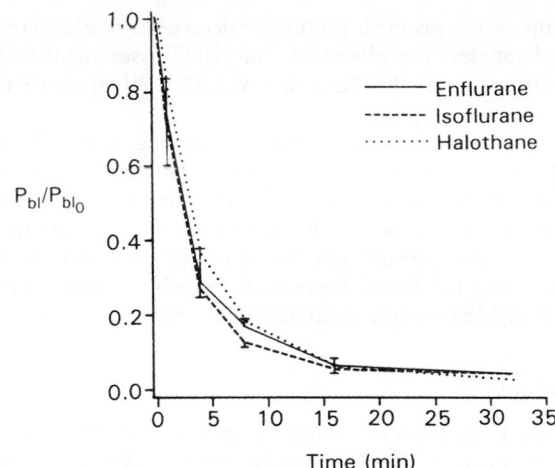

**FIGURE 63–12.** Washout of inhaled anesthetics using an in vitro model of cardiopulmonary bypass at 24° to 26°C. The partial pressures of anesthetics are expressed as the ratio of the partial pressure of anesthetic in blood at a given time, divided by the partial pressure of anesthetic in blood just prior to discontinuation of administration. Washout of anesthetics during rewarming may be more rapid because of decreased solubility of gases in blood with increasing temperatures. (From Nussmeier NA, Moskowitz GJ, Weiskopf RB, et al. In vitro anesthetic washing and washout via bubble oxygenators: influence of anesthetic solubility and rates of carrier gas inflow and pump blood flow. *Anesth Analg.* 1988;67:982.)

As mentioned previously, snorkeling may be useful as a guide to administering additional anesthetics, rather than simply gross temperature thresholds.

## Monitoring and Ventilation

The pressure transducers must be recalibrated and the other monitors (pulse oximeter, gas analyzers, and so on) turned on before weaning from CPB. The lungs are gently reexpanded by manually delivering first a few small-volume and then a few large-volume breaths and sustaining airway pressure at approximately 20 cm $H_2O$ for a few seconds in order to reexpand atelectatic segments. Then mechanical ventilation is resumed with 100% $O_2$. Administration of a few small breaths first is especially important after the left IMA has been used as a graft because the inflated lung may apply tension on it. If this occurs, the surgeon can revise the IMA path.

When all of these preparations have been made and there is agreement among the surgeon, anesthesiologist, and perfusionist that conditions are optimum, the patient is weaned from CPB.

## How Are Weaning and Separation Accomplished?

### Technique

Weaning from CPB involves a gradual transition from complete support of perfusion and oxygenation by the CPB pump to resumption of these functions by the heart and lungs. The venous line is partially occluded by the surgeon or perfusionist to allow gradual filling of the right side of the heart, ejection into the pulmonary vasculature, and return of blood to the left side of the heart for distribution to the systemic vasculature. As this process increases left-sided preload, the inflow from the pump to the aorta is gradually decreased while hemodynamic parameters are observed and visual assessment of ventricular function in the field and via TEE (if present) takes place.

With partial occlusion of the venous line, some blood is still returned to the pump while the remainder returns to the right side of the heart. Preload is adjusted according to the hemodynamic response by altering the amount of venous line occlusion to provide enough blood for adequate CO without overdistending the heart. Distention must be avoided because it increases $M\dot{V}O_2$ while reducing CPP.

## Assessment

Preload is estimated by the appearance of the heart, the measurements of CVP, PA diastolic pressure, PAOP, LA pressure (as available), and the TEE assessment of LV volume. LV compliance may change significantly compared with pre-CPB values, so pressure readings can be misleading. The gradient between PA diastolic pressure and PAOP also may change significantly.[151] Thus, if PA diastolic pressure is chosen as a measure of preload, a correlation between it and PAOP should be measured after CPB (following the administration of protamine and reassurance that the PA catheter has not migrated). This change in compliance persists for at least the first few hours postoperatively.[152] The PA diastolic pressure and PAOP, therefore, may need to be higher than before CPB to obtain a similar filling volume.

As pump flow is decreased to approximately 1 L/min, if the heart is able to generate adequate systemic pressure (>90 mm Hg systolic) at the desired preload, CPB may be terminated. Pump flow is stopped, and both the venous and aortic lines are clamped, but connections are left intact while the hemodynamic status is monitored. Preload may still be augmented by transfusing volume from the CPB through the aortic cannula in increments of 50 to 100 mL.

This sequence of events may be accomplished quickly in patients with adequate ventricular function. Patients with poor ventricular function, at higher risk for ventricular distention and failure, may benefit from slower weaning with more careful adjustment of preload and inotropic support.

## *What Are the Hemodynamic Goals?*

The hemodynamic goals for all post-CPB patients are similar unless residual valvular lesions are present. The means of attaining those goals differ according to a patient's ventricular function and afterload condition (Table 63–21).

### Heart Rate

The HR must be adequate to provide sufficient CO (usually 70-100 bpm). In many patients, lower HRs may be inadequate because of the altered ventricular compliance discussed earlier. Higher HRs also may be detrimental by shortening the diastolic period, decreasing stroke volume through insufficient diastolic filling, and decreasing coronary perfusion. At the same time, increased HR increases $M\dot{V}O_2$. Bradycardia is most easily overcome by pacing. The treatment options for tachycardia are discussed later.

Heart rhythm should be sinus rhythm. Atrioventricular sequential pacing may be used to overcome heart block. Dys-

**TABLE 63–21.** Hemodynamic Goals After Cardiopulmonary Bypass

| | |
|---|---|
| Heart rate | Moderate heart rate (70–90 bpm) is best to maintain adequate cardiac output without increasing $M\dot{V}O_2$ excessively. |
| Rhythm | Sinus rhythm is preferred. Atrioventricular sequential pacing is equally beneficial. |
| Preload | Preload must be enough to support adequate cardiac output without overdistending. |
| Afterload | Reduced afterload decreases wall tension and $M\dot{V}O_2$ and increases cardiac output. Afterload must be high enough to allow adequate systemic and coronary perfusion pressures. |
| Contractility | Contractility should be increased to maintain adequate cardiac output without excessively increasing $M\dot{V}O_2$ and inducing ischemia. |

rhythmias should be treated pharmacologically and electrically as indicated.

### Preload

Preload should be optimized as outlined previously. Additional volume may be transfused from the CPB reservoir via the aortic cannula, or volume may be infused intravenously. It is most convenient to administer volume from the reservoir until the time of aortic decannulation. This process takes full advantage of a patient's autologous blood contained in the pump before transfusing homologous blood or infusing crystalloids and colloids, which lead to further hemodilution. Excessive preload may be relieved by infusion of intravenous NTG or administration of a diuretic. Severe overload can be relieved by reopening the venous line or atriotomy site and phlebotomizing blood to the CPB reservoir.

### Afterload

Reduction of afterload is advantageous to a post-CPB heart. Decreased wall stress lowers $M\dot{V}O_2$, which lessens the risk of ischemia. Afterload reduction favors forward flow from the LV. This relationship is especially important in patients with mild residual mitral regurgitation and in patients with a poorly compliant LV. In patients who are post-CPB after mitral valve replacement for either mitral insufficiency or MS, afterload reduction is also essential.

### Contractility

Myocardial contractility should be optimized in order to maintain an adequate CO. Contractility may be assessed by TEE or visual inspection. It can also be inferred indirectly in relationship to other hemodynamic parameters. The choice of inotropic support depends on the severity of ventricular dysfunction, loading conditions, HR, and personal preference. Currently available inotropes are listed in Table 63–22.

The efficacy of the inotrope chosen must be reassessed frequently so additional drugs be added or alternatives sought. If aggressive inotropic support fails to improve hemodynamic status, a return to CPB may be indicated to "unload" the heart. Then, correctable causes of ventricular dysfunction are identified and corrected. Not uncommonly, combinations of inotropes (ie, phosphodiesterase type III [PDEIII] inhibitors

**TABLE 63–22.** Inotropic Medications

| Drug | Dosing | | Benefits | Risks |
|---|---|---|---|---|
| | *Bolus* | *Infusion* | | |
| Dopamine | — | 2–20 µg/kg/min | Increased renal blood flow at low doses<br>Mild vasoconstriction at moderate doses | Tachycardia<br>Dysrhythmias<br>Vasoconstriction at high doses |
| Dobutamine | — | 2–20 µg/kg/min | Vasodilation<br>Little tachycardia at low doses | Tachycardia at high doses<br>Dysrhythmias at high doses<br>Nonselective vasodilator |
| Epinephrine | 5–10 µg | 0.02–0.50 µg/kg/min | Most potent inotrope<br>Bronchodilation | Tachycardia<br>Dysrhythmias<br>Vasoconstriction |
| Norepinephrine | — | 0.03–0.30 µg/kg/min | Most potent vasoconstrictor | Vasoconstriction<br>Tachycardia<br>Dysrhythmias |
| Isoproterenol | — | 0.02–0.50 µg/kg/min | Most potent $\beta_1$- and $\beta_2$-agonist<br>Bronchodilation<br>Increases heart rate<br>Vasodilator | Tachycardia<br>Dysrhythmias<br>Hypotension |
| Amrinone | 0.75–3.0 mg/kg (over 10 min) | 5–20 µg/kg/min | Inodilator, less tachycardia | Hypotension with rapid bolus<br>Thrombocytopenia with prolonged infusion (>48 h) |
| Milrinone | 50 µg/kg over 10 min | 0.5–0.75 µg/kg/min | Inodilator, less tachycardia, improved coronary flow | Hypotension with rapid bolus |

+ β-adrenergic receptor agonists) are required and consideration is given to mechanical support.

## PROBLEMS AFTER BYPASS

After separation from CPB, close monitoring of patients continues because this period may be fraught with various complicating circumstances (Table 63–23).

### What Are the Causes and Treatment of Left Ventricular Failure?

LV failure after CPB has many causes (Table 63–24). Rapid identification is important to determine therapy. If the cause is surgically correctable, the patient is returned to CPB and the repair is made. Otherwise, LV failure may be treated by pharmacologic means, by intravenous fluid administration, and by ensuring adequate ventilation and oxygenation.

### Ischemia

Myocardial ischemia is treated by administration of NTG to decrease preload and improve coronary collateral blood flow. CPP is raised by improving CO with inotropes, adminis-

**TABLE 63–23.** Postcardiotomy Bypass Problems

| | |
|---|---|
| Left ventricular failure | Coagulopathy |
| Right ventricular failure | Acid-base abnormalities |
| Myocardial ischemia | Electrolyte abnormalities |
| Dysrhythmias | Bronchospasm |
| Pulmonary hypertension | Pulmonary edema |
| Prosthetic valve failure | Hypothermia |
| Protamine reactions | Pacemaker failure |

tering fluids to increase preload if necessary, and administering phenylephrine to increase peripheral vascular tone. If a patient is anemic, blood transfusion may improve ischemia by raising $O_2$ delivery. Tachycardia may be controlled by administering additional anesthetic agents, a β-blocker, digoxin, or a calcium channel blocker.

The choice of inotrope may also influence the occurrence of myocardial ischemia. Whereas β-agonists such as epinephrine improve contractility, they may do so at the expense of increased $M\dot{V}O_2$. PDEIII inhibitors not only increase contractility but also myocardial blood flow[153]; thus $M\dot{V}O_2$ remains relatively unchanged or slightly increased. Blas and colleagues recently demonstrated fewer episodes of post-CPB ischemia in patients receiving milrinone compared to those receiving epinephrine.[154] Also, it has been shown that milrinone increases grafted IMA flow as well as nitroglycerin and may protect against graft vasoconstriction during phenylephrine administration.[155]

### Myocardial Stunning

Ventricular dysfunction that is not related to ongoing ischemia but rather is a result of reperfusion injury is treated with inotropes and, as long as perfusion pressure is adequate, vasodilators. Dopamine, dobutamine, phosphodiesterase inhibitors, and epinephrine are most commonly used. Although both β-receptor agonists and PDEIII inhibitors produce a similar increase in cardiac index, the inodilator properties of the latter may offer some potential advantages, such as (1) less increase in $M\dot{V}O_2$, (2) native coronary and graft vasodilation,[156] (3) increased LV compliance,[157] and (4) decreased SVR and PVR.

### Acid-Base Status

Acid-base and electrolyte abnormalities must be promptly identified and corrected to avoid dysrhythmias and to allow maximum benefits of inotropes.

**TABLE 63–24.** Causes of Left Ventricular Failure

| | | |
|---|---|---|
| Ischemia | Coronary graft failure | Thrombosis |
| | | Constriction by suture at proximal or distal anastomosis |
| | | Kinking of graft |
| | | Air in graft |
| | | Vein graft sewn in backward (no flow across valves) |
| | Inadequate internal mammary artery graft flow | Inadequate coronary blood flow |
| | | Incomplete revascularization |
| | | Inadequate coronary perfusion pressure |
| | | Coronary embolism (air, clot, plaque) |
| | | Coronary spasm |
| | Ischemic myocardial damage | Tachycardia (shortening of diastole) |
| | | Increased myocardial $O_2$ demand |
| | | Incomplete myocardial protection during cardiopulmonary bypass |
| | | Myocardial infarction |
| Valve failure | Prosthetic valve | Sewn in backward |
| | | Perivalvular leak |
| | | Mechanical failure (immobile disk) |
| | Native valve | Ischemic papillary muscle dysfunction or rupture |
| Gas exchange problems | Hypoxemia | Inadequate $F_{IO_2}$ |
| | | Mechanical ventilator failure |
| | | Bronchospasm |
| | | Pulmonary edema |
| Inadequate preload | Hypoventilation | |
| Volume overload | | |
| Reperfusion injury | | |
| Miscellaneous causes of decreased contractility | Preexisting left ventricular failure | |
| | Medications | Blockade |
| | |   Calcium channel blockers |
| | |   Inhalation anesthetics |
| | |   Antiarrhythmics |
| | Acidemia | |
| | Electrolyte abnormalities | Hypocalcemia |
| | | Hyperkalemia |

From Romanoff ME, Larach DR. Weaning from cardiopulmonary bypass. In: Hensley FA Jr, Martin DE, eds. *The Practice of Cardiac Anesthesia.* Boston, Mass: Little, Brown & Co; 1990:252.

## Artifact

Monitoring artifacts should also be considered. The arterial pressure measured in a radial artery after CPB is often significantly lower than the aortic pressure either because of decreased forearm vascular resistance with rewarming[158] or because of hypovolemia and vasoconstriction.[159] If doubt exists concerning the accuracy of pressure measured from a radial arterial catheter after CPB, a more central arterial pressure should be measured (BP cuff, aortic cannula, needle placed in the aortic root, femoral arterial catheter).

When these measures are unsuccessful, mechanical support (intraaortic balloon pump or LV assist device) may become necessary.

## What Are the Causes and Treatment of Right Ventricular Failure?

Many of the factors responsible for LV failure also may cause RV failure. Additional possibilities are listed in Table 63–25. The RV, because of its thinner wall, is affected more by increases in afterload. Therefore, any factors that result in increased PVR place a patient at risk for RV failure.

## Ischemia

Ischemic RV failure is treated similarly to ischemic LV failure. Although the emphasis has been placed on the LV in consideration of myocardial ischemia, the RV is also susceptible to ischemia, and the effects are detrimental to overall cardiac function. Also, ischemia may develop secondarily in right-sided heart failure. In response to pulmonary hypertension, the cavitary diameter of the RV increases, thereby increasing wall stress and restricting subendocardial blood flow, which in turn leads to depression of RV contractility.[160]

**TABLE 63–25.** Causes of Right Ventricular Failure

Right ventricular ischemia or infarction
Preexisting pulmonary hypertension
  Chronic mitral stenosis or insufficiency
  Septal defect (atrial or ventricular)
Respiratory disease
  Chronic obstructive lung disease
  Adult respiratory distress syndrome
Effects of mechanical ventilation
  Positive pressure ventilation
  Positive end-expiratory pressure
Protamine reaction (pulmonary vasoconstriction)
Pulmonary embolism (air, thrombus)

## Control of Preload

Maintaining preload is important to provide adequate RV stroke volume and LV function. When RV failure is caused solely by pump failure (eg, RV infarction), simply augmenting preload may be sufficient to overcome the poor contractility and low CO. However, excessive RV preload can induce a leftward septal shift and thereby impair LV diastolic filling. Inotropic support in this situation may be more beneficial.[161]

## Pulmonary Vascular Resistance

Simple maneuvers such as hyperventilation, elimination hypoxia, administration of nitrosodilators, or administration of β-agonists by either parenteral or inhalational routes may sufficiently reduce PVR to acceptable levels. However, other maneuvers may become necessary. Several approaches are described.

### Prostaglandin E₁ and Norepinephrine

When RV failure is caused more by high afterload than pump failure alone, the combination of inotropic support and pulmonary vasodilation, along with augmentation of preload, may be most effective. One successful technique that has been described is the administration of prostaglandin E₁ (PGE₁) and norepinephrine through RA and LA catheters, respectively.[162]

PGE₁ is a potent pulmonary vasodilator that is metabolized in the pulmonary vasculature. Incomplete metabolism and shunting to the systemic circulation lead to systemic vasodilation as well. Norepinephrine infusion via an LA catheter provides some compensatory systemic vasoconstriction and inotropic stimulation. Central venous infusions of ultra–short-lived substances such as adenosine ultimately may be useful to provide selective pulmonary vasodilation.

### Nitric Oxide

Inhaled nitric oxide is a powerful pulmonary vasodilator.[163] It is devoid of systemic hypotensive effects because it is rapidly inactivated by binding to hemoglobin in the pulmonary vasculature. It selectively dilates pulmonary vasculature only in areas that are being ventilated, allowing for a reduction in PVR and a potential improvement in $\dot{V}/\dot{Q}$ mismatching. At present, it is only approved as an investigational drug but in the future it may become widely available.

### Inhibition of Phosphodiesterase Type III

The combined inotropic and vasodilating effects of the phosphodiesterase type III (PDEIII) inhibitors amrinone and milrinone may prove beneficial in RV failure. PDEIII inhibition has been shown to be effective in this situation, more by reduction of RV afterload than by direct inotropic effects.[164] Milrinone is preferred in many institutions due to thrombocytopenia that may develop in association with prolonged administration of amrinone.

## What Mechanical Devices Can Be Used?

When pharmacologic treatment is inadequate for a patient with post-CPB heart failure, mechanical assist devices may become necessary. They include the IABP, ventricular assist devices (VADs), and the total artificial heart.

## Intraaortic Balloon Pump

The IABP is the most commonly used circulatory assist device. The indications for IABP use are (1) intractable cardiac failure after CPB, (2) preoperative stabilization of refractory angina or LV failure, and (3) complications of MI refractory to pharmacologic therapy.[165] It functionally increases coronary artery perfusion and decreases LV afterload.

### Mechanism of Action

The IABP is placed percutaneously or by surgical cutdown via a femoral artery or the aorta. It is advanced to the descending aorta so that the balloon lies distal to the left subclavian artery and proximal to the renal arteries (Fig. 63–13). The balloon inflates at the beginning of diastole (closure of the aortic valve), forcing blood into the coronary ostia, thereby augmenting coronary artery perfusion. With the beginning of systole, it deflates, causing a sudden decrease in afterload and favoring increased ejection of blood from the LV. The IABP is triggered automatically by either the ECG or arterial pressure waveform. The timing of inflation and deflation is critical to provide maximum benefit.

### Effectiveness

The IABP is effective only if a patient has some ventricular function and a fairly regular rhythm. It is meant to assist LV output and is ineffective in the presence of extremely severe ventricular dysfunction, asystole, severe ventricular dysrhyth-

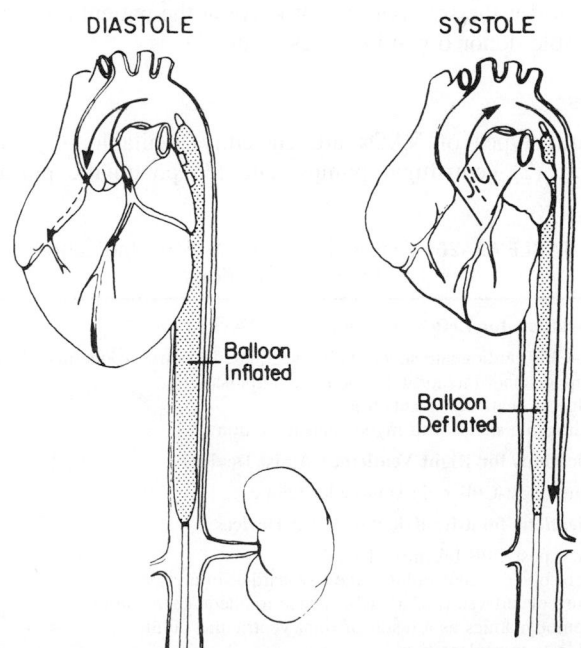

**FIGURE 63–13.** Proper positioning of the intraaortic balloon pump below the left subclavian artery and above the renal arteries. The balloon inflates during diastole, forcing blood into the coronary arteries. It deflates during systole, creating a void that decreases impedance to left ventricular ejection. (From Maccioli GA, Lucas WJ, Norfleet EA. The intraaortic balloon pump: a review. *J Cardiothorac Anesth.* 1988;2:365.)

mias, and rapid or irregular atrial or ventricular rhythms. Irregular rhythms make IABP timing difficult. Rapid rates allow insufficient time for ventricular filling. If these problems cannot be corrected by pharmacologic means or pacing, a VAD may be more appropriate.

### Contraindications

The IABP is contraindicated in patients with significant aortic insufficiency. Diastolic inflation increases regurgitant flow and worsens LV failure. Femoral placement may be difficult or impossible in patients with peripheral vascular disease, although occasionally, devices may be surgically placed directly into the descending aorta. The device is relatively contraindicated in patients with thoracic or abdominal aortic aneurysms.

## Ventricular Assist Devices

VADs may be used to augment LV or RV function and for short or extended periods in the ICU. Indications and contraindications are listed in Table 63–26.

An LVAD takes over the work of the LV. The ventricle is unloaded through an LA or LV cannula, and blood is returned to the aorta via the LVAD. When the LVAD is placed only temporarily, LA access is preferred. When isolated RV failure is present or when an LVAD cannot function properly, a RVAD may be implanted. The RV is unloaded with a cannula placed in the RA appendage, and blood is returned to the PA.

The goal of mechanical circulatory assistance is to decrease $M\dot{V}O_2$ while allowing time for metabolic recovery of the myocardium. If sufficient ventricular recovery to allow weaning from mechanical assistance does not occur, consideration is given to the use of such a device as a bridge to transplantation. In many institutions, VADs are being placed prophylactically in prospective transplant recipients with deteriorating function for the sole purpose of keeping the patient alive until a suitable donor organ becomes available.

### Types

Three types of VADs are currently available: (1) roller pumps, (2) centrifugal pumps, and (3) pneumatic pulsatile

**TABLE 63–26.** Ventricular Assist Devices: Indications and Contraindications

**Indications for Left Ventricular Assist Devices**

Post-CPB cardiogenic shock with inadequate response to pharmacologic support and intraaortic balloon counterpulsation
Bridge to heart transplantation
Cardiogenic shock with myocardial infarction

**Indications for Right Ventricular Assist Devices**

Isolated post-CPB right ventricular failure

**Indications for Biventricular Assist Devices**

Severe post-CPB biventricular failure
Severe biventricular failure after myocardial infarction
Failure of left ventricular assist device to adequately improve hemodynamics as a result of right ventricular failure
Bridge to transplantation

**Contraindications to Ventricular Assist Devices**

No reasonable expectation of ventricular recovery in a patient not considered a candidate for heart transplantation
Sepsis

CPB, cardiopulmonary bypass.

pumps. Roller pumps are readily available, simple, and inexpensive, but they require systemic anticoagulation, produce nonpulsatile flow, and induce significant blood trauma.

The advantages of centrifugal pumps are that they are readily available, simple, and relatively inexpensive. They do not require full heparinization, but if no heparin is used, the pump head must be changed every 48 to 72 hours.[166]

Pneumatic assist pumps provide pulsatile flow. They are designed to minimize blood trauma and to operate without systemic heparinization, so complete reversal of heparin may be accomplished. Newer pneumatic VADs are much more portable and enable patient ambulation; however, the devices still require an extensive system of external tubing and an external power source.

VAD technology is a field constantly in flux. The large, bulky, nonportable machines of the past are rapidly being replaced with smaller, more efficient, less hematologically destructive models that enable patients to survive for weeks and months while awaiting transplantation. Some models even enable patients to ambulate with the working devices. A recent innovative pump is actually implanted endovascularly, where it functions as a centrifugal pump without external wires, extracorporeal flow, or external power sources. With promising early European outcome studies, it appears this VAD will be increasingly used in the early 21st century.

### Management Goals

The management goal of VAD therapy is to maintain adequate perfusion to all tissues. Assessment includes evaluation of acid-base status, arterial and venous $O_2$ saturation, and urine output. Appropriate hemodynamic goals are to maintain a cerebral perfusion pressure >50 mm Hg, an LA pressure of about 10 mm Hg, and a cardiac index of 2.4 L/min/m².[167] The unassisted ventricle may benefit from inotropes or vasodilators. Most patients require 3 to 7 days of support with a VAD and can then be successfully weaned to pharmacologic support. Ventricular recovery and successful discharge from the hospital have been reported in as many as 40% of patients who require VAD support for cardiogenic shock following cardiac surgery.[167] Without VAD support, these patients would die.

### Total Artificial Heart

In a few centers, a total artificial heart is available as a bridge to heart transplantation. Disadvantages include its irreversibility and a high incidence of complications including bleeding, thrombosis, and multiple organ failure.

## What Are the Causes and Treatment of Dysrhythmias?

### Ventricular Dysrhythmias

Dysrhythmias in post-CPB patients are common (Table 63–27). Rapid search for the cause and prompt treatment are essential. Ventricular tachycardia and ventricular fibrillation should be immediately treated with internal defibrillation. Table 63–28 lists agents used in the treatment of ventricular tachydysrhythmias.

**TABLE 63–27.** Causes of Dysrhythmias After Cardiopulmonary Bypass

| | | |
|---|---|---|
| Cardiac dysfunction | Impaired myocardial $O_2$ supply | Low $Pao_2$ |
| | | Low blood $O_2$-carrying capacity |
| | | Impaired coronary perfusion (residual coronary stenoses, emboli, low perfusion pressure) |
| | | Impaired cellular $O_2$ use (nitroprusside-induced cyanide toxicity) |
| | Cell death, trauma | Myocardial infarction |
| | | Inadequate myocardial protection during cardiopulmonary bypass |
| | | Reperfusion injury |
| | | Surgical trauma |
| | Specific cardiac abnormalities | Congenital |
| | | Valvular disease (mitral valve prolapse, mitral insufficiency related to papillary muscle dysfunction or rupture) |
| | | Cardiomyopathy |
| | | Long QT syndrome (congenital; electrolyte, metabolic, or drug induced) |
| Acid-base and electrolyte disorders | Hyperkalemia | Renal dysfunction, residual cardioplegia, rapid transfusion of stored blood, rapid administration of potassium chloride |
| | Hypokalemia | |
| | Hypermagnesemia, hypomagnesemia | |
| | Hypercalcemia, hypocalcemia | |
| | Acidosis, alkalosis | |
| | Hypercarbia, hypocarbia | |
| Electromechanical cardiac stimulation | Surgical manipulation | |
| | Intravascular catheter or wire (pulmonary artery catheter, pacing wire) | |
| | Overdistention of atrium or ventricle | |
| | Macroshock, microshock | |
| | Pacemaker induced | Malfunction |
| | | Inappropriate discharge |
| | | Inappropriate settings |
| | R-on-T phenomena | |
| Autonomic imbalance | Inadequate anesthesia for surgical stimulation | |
| | Reflex activation with hypotension | |
| | Myocardial ischemia | |
| Drugs | Drug overdose | |
| | Idiosyncratic or allergic drug reaction | |
| | Pharmacokinetic or pharmacodynamic drug interactions | |
| | Specific drugs | Anesthetics and muscle relaxants |
| | | Proarrhythmic effects of antiarrhythmics (long QT) |
| | | Digitalis toxicity |
| | | Catecholamines or sympathomimetics |
| | | Calcium channel blockers |
| | | Beta-blockers |
| | | Cholinergic or anticholinergic drugs |
| | | Respiratory drugs (aminophylline, β-agonists) |
| | Hypothermia | Incorrect electrocardiogram interpretation |
| | Pseudodysrhythmias | Electrocardiographic artifacts (extracardiac electrical signals, electrical interference) |

Modified from Springman SR, Atlee JL. The etiology of intraoperative arrhythmias. *Anesth Clin North Am.* 1989;7:293.

**TABLE 63–28.** Antiarrhythmic Drugs Used in the Treatment of Ventricular Tachydysrhythmias

| Drug | Intravenous Loading Dose | Infusion |
|---|---|---|
| Lidocaine | 1.5 mg/kg × 2 doses | 1–4 mg/min (15–50 μg/kg/min) |
| Procainamide | 20–50 mg/min up to 1000 mg, control of dysrhythmia, hypotension, or >50% increase in QRS duration | 2 mg/kg/h |
| Bretylium | 5–10 mg/kg over 10 min | 5–10 mg/kg over 10 min every 6 h or 1–2 mg/min |
| Amiodarone | 150 mg over 10 min | 360 mg over 6 h (1 mg/min) followed by 540 mg over 18 h (0.5 mg/min) |
| Esmolol | 0.5 mg/kg | 50 μg/kg/min |
| Magnesium | 2 g over 6 min | 1–2 g/h for 5 h |

## Supraventricular Dysrhythmias

Supraventricular tachydysrhythmias, such as atrial fibrillation and tachycardia, should be treated with synchronized internal cardioversion. Although arterial blood is drawn for evaluation of blood gases, acid-base status, and electrolyte concentrations, efforts should be made to optimize preload and afterload. Because ischemia is such an important cause of post-CPB dysrhythmias, its presence should be assumed and coronary perfusion optimized by raising perfusion pressure and administering NTG. Antidysrhythmic therapy should then be added as indicated.

Supraventricular tachycardia can be difficult to treat. Various medications are available, but each has undesirable side effects (Table 63–29). Digitalis is unlikely to be effective acutely and carries the risk of inducing toxic ventricular and supraventricular dysrhythmias. Verapamil, procainamide, and β-blockers all may cause myocardial depression. Procainamide may induce a long QT interval and predispose to ventricular dysrhythmias.

Edrophonium may exert undesirable cholinergic side effects, most notably bronchospasm, and also requires additional dosing of muscle relaxants to prevent patients' movement. Adenosine can be used, but early experience in post-CPB patients with CAD indicates that it may cause ischemia by inducing coronary steal.[168]

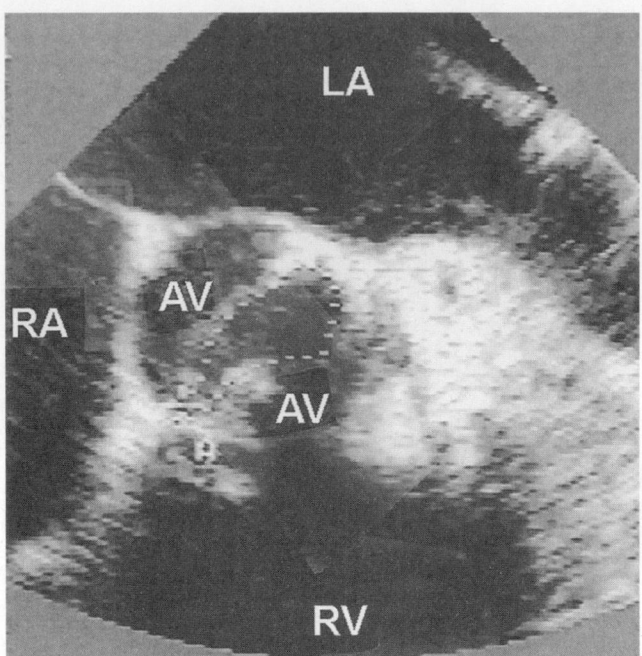

**FIGURE 63–14.** Two-dimensional transesophageal echocardiogram of a patient with bicuspid aortic valve showing the stenotic valve area (dotted line). AV, aortic valve; LA, left atrium; RA, right atrium; RV, right ventricle.

## How Is Valvular Function Assessed?

Until the introduction of TEE, assessment of valvular function after CPB was based on observation of overall cardiac function and observation of the PAP, PAOP, and CVP waveforms. TEE has made evaluation of valvular function much more straightforward (Fig. 63–14 and color plates 63–1 through 63–4).

The mitral and aortic valves, in particular, are well visualized with TEE. Mitral regurgitation after mitral valve repair or replacement or due to ischemic dysfunction of papillary muscles can be assessed during weaning from CPB. In patients undergoing mitral or aortic valve replacement, detection of valvular dysfunction and residual gradients after CPB may prompt a return to CPB for correction and is predictive of postoperative cardiac morbidity and mortality if left uncorrected.[169] Similarly, pathologic perivalvular leaks are readily identified.

Even in centers in which TEE is not available for all procedures, it is often brought to the OR and used for assessment of valve function after mitral valve replacement. The development of omniplane probes, which allow rotation of the piezoelectric crystals in planes that enable three-dimensional examination, has enabled clinicians to glean an extraordinary amount of information semi-invasively that previously was not possible.

## How Is the Dose of Protamine Determined?

### Standard Doses

The proper dose of protamine depends on the remaining heparin activity after CPB. It may be given as a standard dose based on the original dose of heparin or the total dose of heparin during CPB (eg, 1 mg protamine per 100 units of heparin).

### Heparin Versus Activated Clotting Time Dose-Response Curve

The protamine dose may also be determined from the dose-response curve of heparin dose versus ACT constructed before CPB (Fig. 63–15). This curve is easily generated using a graph in which ACT is on the x-axis and heparin dose (in milligrams per kilogram) on the y-axis. The baseline ACT determines the point corresponding to no heparin, and the postheparin ACT, the second point corresponding to the administered heparin dose. Because the relationship is linear, these two points are all that is needed.

The ACT after bypass is then plotted on the line, the effective remaining heparin dose is read off the axis, and the appropriate protamine dose (1 mg per 100 units of remaining heparin activity) is then based on the heparin dose predicted to give that ACT value.[170]

**TABLE 63–29.** Antiarrhythmic Drugs Used in the Treatment of Supraventricular Tachycardia After Cardiopulmonary Bypass

| Drug/Treatment | Intravenous Dose |
| --- | --- |
| Synchronized internal cardioversion | Start at 10–20 J |
| Overdrive pacing | |
| Digoxin | 0.5–1.0 mg |
| Esmolol | 0.5 mg/kg (if effective, consider infusion) |
| Verapamil | 0.075–0.15 mg/kg |
| Edrophonium | 5–10 mg |
| Procainamide | 20–50 mg/min to effect, up to 1000 mg or toxic effect (hypotension, QRS prolonged by 50%) |
| Adenosine | 6–12 mg |

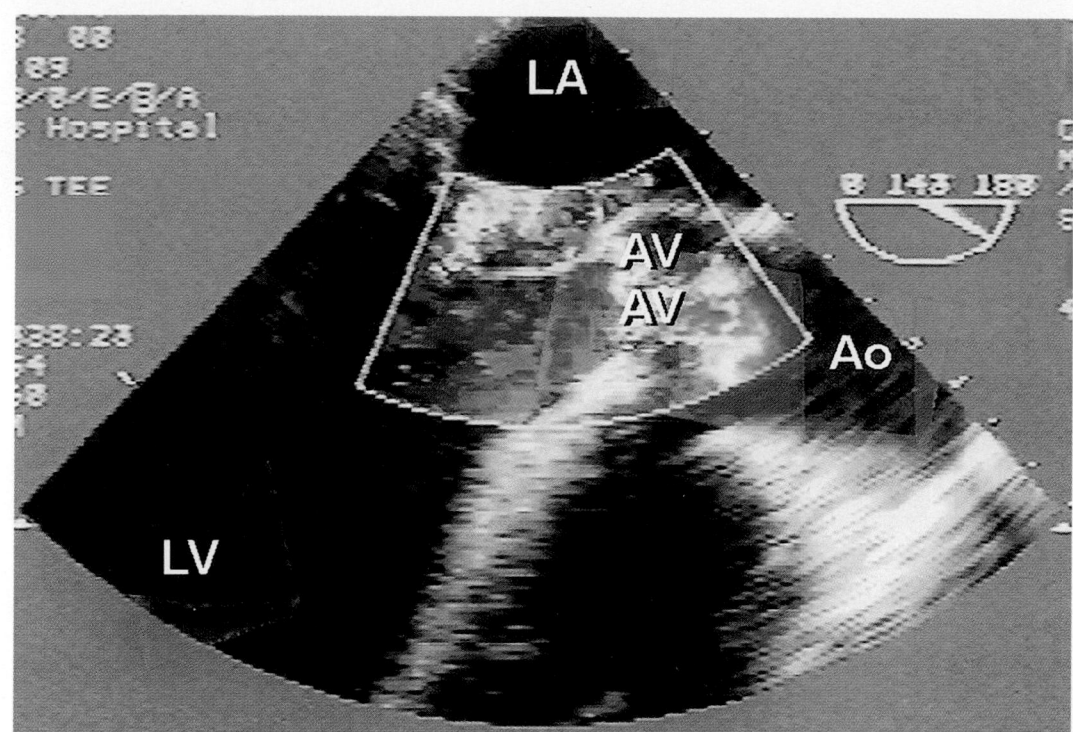

**COLOR PLATE 63–1.** Color flow imaging of the left ventricular outflow tract in a patient wiht aortic stenosis demonstrating turbulent flow through the stenotic orifice. Ao, aorta; AV, aortic valve; LA, left atrium; LV, left ventricle.

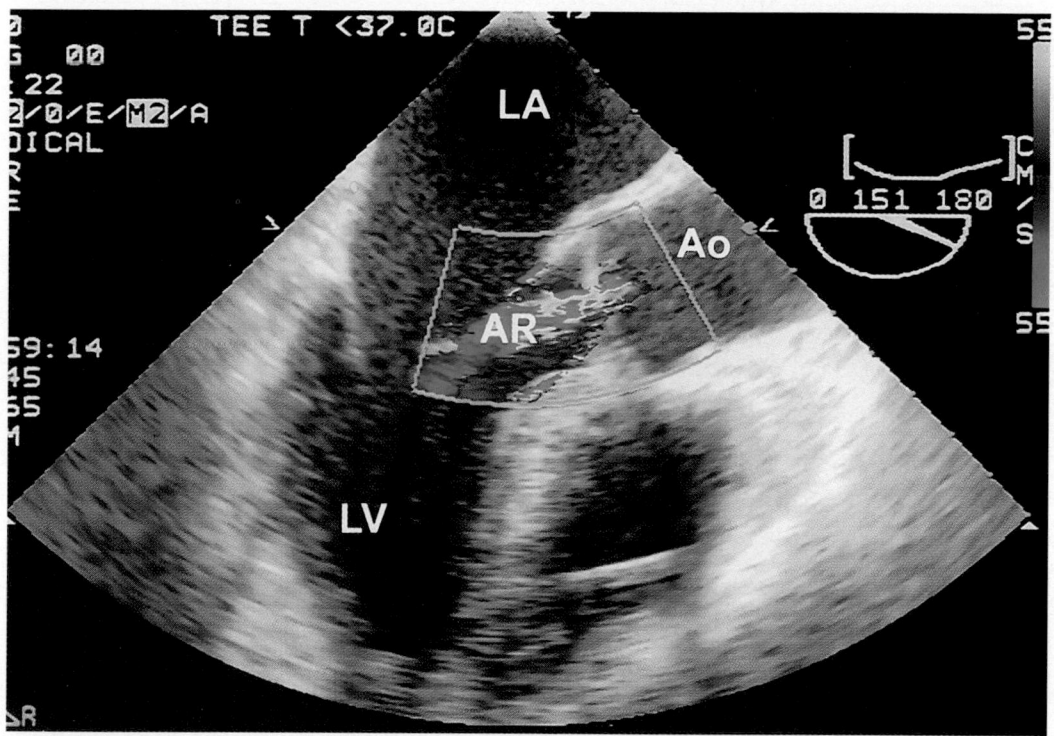

**COLOR PLATE 63–2.** Transesophageal color flow echocardiogram of a patient with aortic insufficiency. The regurgitant jet is seen as a multicolored display protruding into the left ventricle. Ao, aorta; AV, aortic valve; LA, left atrium; LV, left ventricle.

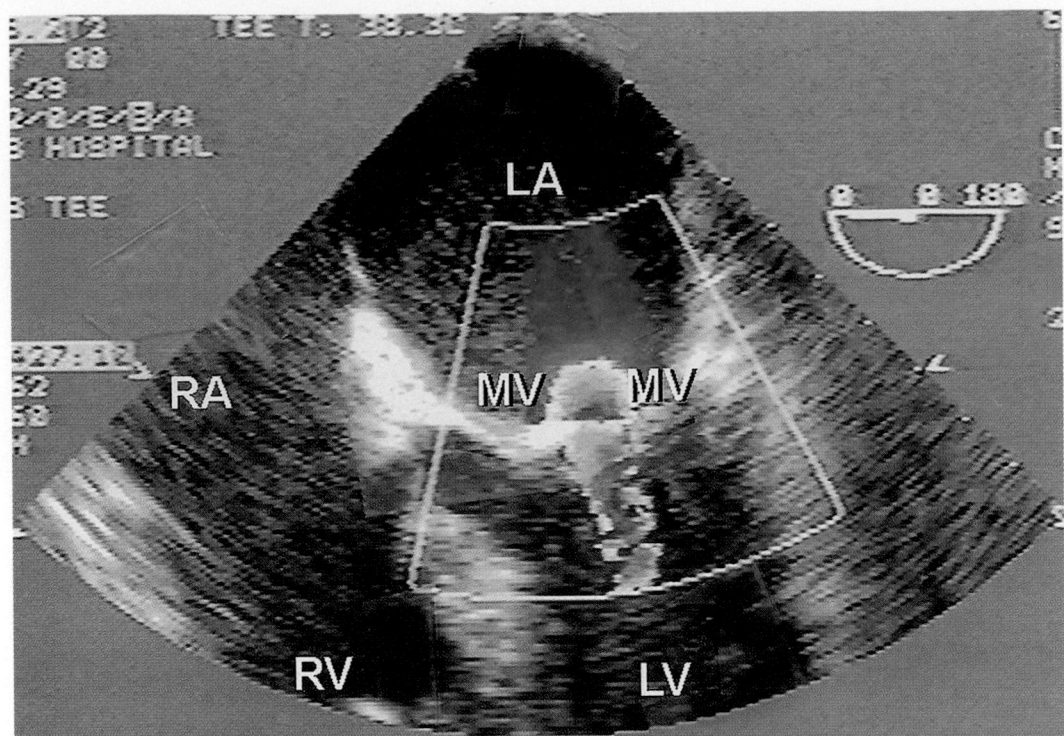

**COLOR PLATE 63–3.** Transesophageal color flow echocardiogram of a patient with mitral stenosis demonstrating the turbulent jet. The domed mitral valve can be seen between the left atrium and the left ventricle. LA, left atrium; LV, left ventricle; MV, mitral valve; RA, right atrium; RV, right ventricle.

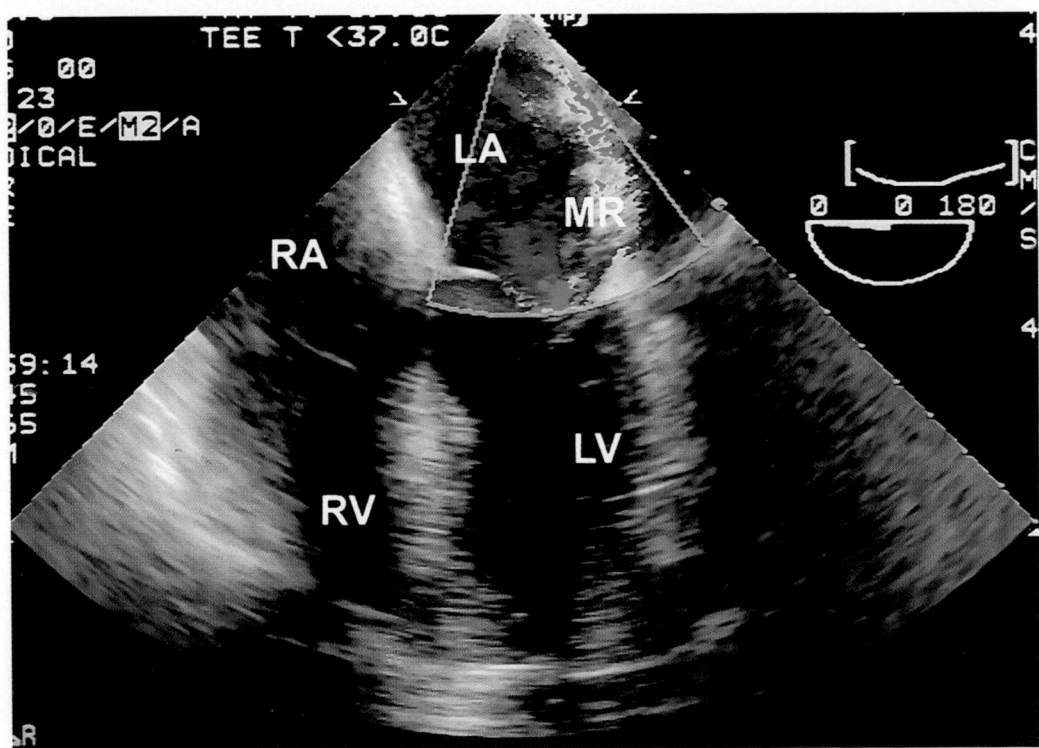

**COLOR PLATE 63–4.** Transesophageal color flow echocardiogram of a patient with mitral insufficiency. The regurgitant jet is seen as a multicolored display protruding into the left atrium. LA, left atrium; LV, left ventricle; MR, mitral regurgitant jet; RA, right atrium; RV, right ventricle.

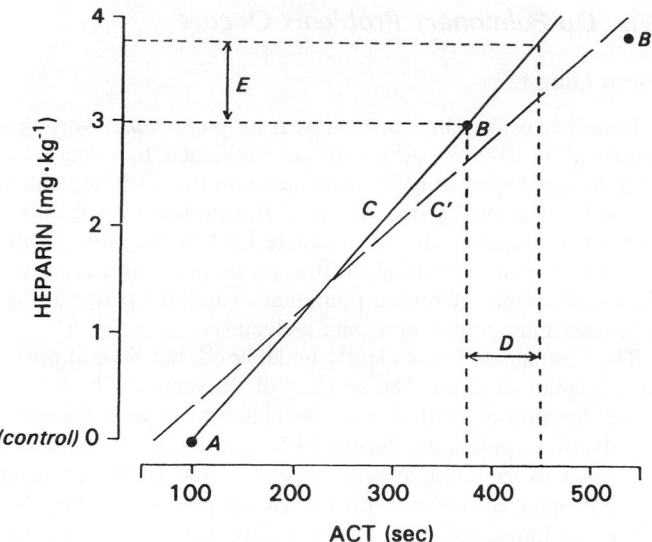

**FIGURE 63–15.** Construction and use of the heparin dose-activated coagulation time (ACT) response curve. A, plot ACT control versus no heparin; B, plot ACT response versus initial heparin dose; C, draw dose-response curve; D, locate desired ACT increase; E, locate corresponding change in circulating heparin and administer this dose. B', plot new ACT response versus expected circulating heparin. C', revise dose-response curve. Repeat D-C' as needed. (From Cohen JA. Activated coagulation time method for control of heparin is reliable during cardiopulmonary bypass. *Anesthesiology.* 1984;60:122.)

## Protamine Titration

A third technique for determining the appropriate dose of protamine is the protamine titration technique. It may be accomplished manually by adding variable amounts of protamine to tubes of blood, determining which clots first, and then calculating a proportional dose of protamine based on the patient's estimated blood volume. Protamine titration may also be performed mechanically with an automated heparin-protamine titration system.

## Heparin Concentration

Heparin and protamine management may also be carried out based on measurement of heparin concentration. One study demonstrated that when anticoagulation was based on heparin concentration rather than ACT, higher heparin concentrations were maintained during CPB with less activation of the coagulation system but with greater post-CPB blood loss.[171] The same investigators found that heparin rebound after CPB was more common when management was based on heparin concentration rather than on ACT.[172] As long as patients were closely monitored postoperatively by measuring ACT and treating with additional doses of protamine, heparin rebound did not lead to excessive postoperative bleeding. The additional measurement of heparin concentration appears to be neither detrimental nor beneficial. Its clinical role has yet to be fully elucidated.

Whatever technique is chosen to determine protamine dose, the ACT should be measured 5 to 10 minutes after protamine administration. Additional protamine may be given to return the ACT to the baseline range or, if the patient was receiving heparin preoperatively, to the normal range ($\approx$100-160 seconds).

## What Are the Manifestations and Risks of Protamine Toxicity?

Protamine is known to cause various degrees of adverse cardiovascular responses, some of which are predictable and some of which are not. Protamine reactions have been classified into three types.[173]

### Hypotensive (Type I) Reaction

Transient hypotension with rapid injection is a predictable adverse effect, so protamine should be administered slowly (eg, through a minidripper diluted in 100 mL saline). The calculated dose should be given over 10 minutes or more. Injection through a peripheral rather than central venous catheter may be preferable to allow more dilution of protamine before its delivery to the pulmonary vasculature. Administration of protamine via the left atrium or aorta does not appear to offer any advantage over peripheral administration. The hypotension associated with rapid injection results from systemic vasodilation and may be treated with a vasoconstrictor such as phenylephrine and volume as needed.

### Anaphylactic and Anaphylactoid (Type II) Reactions

An adverse response to protamine may be a true allergic reaction (anaphylaxis) or a reaction due to the release of vasoactive mediators or the activation of complement (anaphylactoid reaction).

Patients who are allergic to fish may develop an allergic reaction to protamine because it is prepared from salmon gonads. Patients who have had a vasectomy commonly develop an antibody to their own sperm, which theoretically may cross-react with protamine. However, the clinical significance of this relationship is doubtful.

Diabetic patients who have been treated with NPH insulin or PZI insulin commonly develop antibodies to protamine, which is an ingredient in these preparations. However, no prospective data document an increased incidence of these reactions in diabetic compared with nondiabetic patients.

### Catastrophic Pulmonary Vasoconstriction (Type III) Reaction

This reaction is characterized by systemic hypotension in the presence of severe pulmonary vasoconstriction and elevated PAP. (A type I or type II reaction is characterized by systemic hypotension and decreased PAP.) The postulated mechanism involves activation of the complement system in the pulmonary vasculature by heparin-protamine complexes. Release of lysosomal enzymes causes additional activation of the arachidonic acid pathways to form thromboxane, a potent vasoconstrictor.[174] This type of reaction may result in RV failure and must be treated as such.

## Should Calcium Salts Be Administered Routinely?

Once thought to be valuable inotropes, calcium salts have now been recognized as potentially harmful medications. Calcium plays an important part in ischemia and reperfusion injury.[174]

## Ionized Hypocalcemia

Serum ionized calcium is commonly measured during cardiac surgery. Mild ionized hypocalcemia (0.80-1.00 mmol/L) is common during CPB. Animal studies have demonstrated that administration of calcium to treat severe hypocalcemia (<0.60 mmol/L) results in significant improvement in ventricular function, but administration of calcium at a normal baseline calcium concentration causes little improvement.[175] Although BP may increase after administration of calcium under normocalcemic conditions, it is a result of increased SVR and is not associated with increases in CO or stroke volume.[176]

To test the efficacy of calcium administration in post-CPB patients with mild hypocalcemia, a randomized, controlled study was conducted.[177] Calcium chloride or a placebo was administered on separation from CPB. Although administration of calcium raised ionized calcium concentration and MAP significantly, no difference in cardiac index was detected between the calcium and placebo groups in the first few minutes after separation. Increased MAP without an increase in CO results from an increase in afterload, which implies increased $M\dot{V}O_2$.

Although administration of calcium salts may be indicated in patients with significant hypocalcemia, it does not appear to be beneficial in patients with the slightly decreased ionized calcium concentrations commonly noted during cardiac surgery. Furthermore, ionized calcium concentration returns to normal levels in the post-CPB period even without administration of calcium salts.[178]

## Detrimental Effects

The potential detrimental effects of calcium on the post-CPB heart relate to the role of intracellular calcium in ischemic damage. During reperfusion of ischemic myocardium, large amounts of intracellular calcium accumulate.[179–181] An increase in intracellular calcium activates various enzymes (phospholipases, proteases, and nucleases) that may contribute to ischemic damage. Activation of calcium-adenosine triphosphatase may increase the use of adenosine triphosphate, which is already in short supply in the ischemic cells. Mitochondrial oxidative phosphorylation may become uncoupled.[182] Other potential problems include coronary spasm and dysrhythmias[183] and an increased risk of pancreatitis.[184] A recent study demonstrated that routine administration of bolus doses of calcium chloride reduced grafted IMA flow despite significantly increased CPP.[185]

## Indications

Despite these concerns, the issue of calcium administration after CPB remains controversial because of its widespread use and apparent safety, at least when measured ionized calcium concentration is low.[186] Also, the relationship of intracellular to extracellular concentrations of calcium after its administration remains unknown. Situations in which administration of calcium is clearly indicated include treatment of severe hypocalcemia associated with transfusion of citrate-containing blood products and treatment of severe hyperkalemia.

## *Why Do Pulmonary Problems Occur?*

### Pump Lung

Postreperfusion lung, also known as *pump lung,* was first described in 1960.[187] Although its incidence has decreased with the development of improvements in the CPB apparatus, it is still occasionally encountered. The problem represents a form of noncardiogenic PE, characterized by hypoxemia due to intrapulmonary shunting, diffuse pulmonary infiltrates on a chest radiograph, increased pulmonary capillary permeability, decreased lung compliance, and atelectasis.

The mechanism is not clearly understood, but several possible explanations exist. The severity of PE seems to be related to the duration of CPB. It may be related to hypoperfusion of the alveolar epithelium during CPB, depletion of surfactant, activation of the complement system by the CPB circuit, or by neutrophil activation with release of proteolytic enzymes within the lungs during CPB. It has also been reported following protamine administration.[188]

### Bronchospasm

Post-CPB bronchospasm may occur, particularly in patients with COPD. Observation of the chest reveals that the lungs expand with inspiration but fail to empty with expiration. The treatment of bronchospasm after CPB may be complicated by the dysrhythmogenic potential of the available treatments in patients already at risk for dysrhythmias.

Treatment with a nebulized $\beta_2$-adrenergic agonist should be attempted first and is quite effective in many patients. When bronchospasm is extremely severe; however, nebulized medications may not be effectively delivered to areas of air trapping. Other treatments that may be considered include intravenous lidocaine, glycopyrrolate, epinephrine, and aminophylline. If ventricular function is adequate, inhaled anesthetics may provide some bronchodilation. The use of mechanical expiratory retardation, similar to that used in COPD, may also be effective.[189]

## *Why Does Coagulopathy Occur?*

Coagulopathy after CPB may have many causes (Table 63–30). Preexisting coagulation problems should be carefully sought in the preoperative evaluation. Adequate surgical hemostasis is extremely important. The sites most likely to be responsible for postoperative bleeding are the IMA harvest site and its coronary anastomosis, the proximal and distal anastomoses of vein grafts, side branches of vein grafts, sites of cannulation (especially aortic cannulation), and the sternum.

### Heparin and Protamine

Inadequate reversal of heparin should be diagnosed by measuring the ACT. Postoperatively, heparin rebound may occur. This is a return of heparin effect despite initially adequate reversal. If suspected, the blood should be tested for prolongation of the ACT. Excess protamine weakens clot structure and has been associated with a dose-related anticoagulant effect mediated by a reduction in ADP-induced platelet aggregation, which may significantly prolong the ACT, partial

**TABLE 63–30.** Causes of Postcardiopulmonary Bypass Coagulopathy

Inadequate surgical hemostasis
Residual heparin effect
Inadequate reversal with protamine
Heparin rebound
Thrombocytopenia
Platelet dysfunction
    Aspirin induced
    Related to activation during cardiopulmonary bypass
    Hypothermia induced
Pre-existing coagulopathy
    Congenital
    Acquired disorders (liver disease, uremia, hematologic diseases)
    Induced by medications (warfarin, heparin, antiplatelet drugs, tissue
        plasminogen activator, streptokinase)
Decreased coagulation factors
Primary fibrinolysis
Disseminated intravascular coagulation

thromboplastin time (PTT), platelet count, and platelet aggregation. This is especially true if platelet numbers were already decreased and protamine-to-heparin ratios are ≥1.3 mg/100 units.[190] Administration of a small excess of protamine appears unlikely to induce a clinically recognizable coagulopathy.[191,192]

### Platelets and Platelet Function

The most common causes of abnormal coagulation caused by CPB are thrombocytopenia and qualitative platelet dysfunction. Thrombocytopenia not only is due in part to hemodilution but also results from destruction at blood-gas interfaces, such as in the cardiotomy suction and bubble oxygenator. Williams and associates determined that among laboratory tests including hematocrit, prothrombin time (PT), PTT, platelet count, fibrinogen concentration, and thromboelastography, platelet count during CPB was the variable most significantly associated with intraoperative blood loss and 12-hour chest tube output.[193]

Qualitative platelet dysfunction may be more important and occurs whether a membrane oxygenator or bubble oxygenator is used. One potential cause of platelet dysfunction after CPB and in the postoperative period is hypothermia.[194] Contact between platelets and the artificial surfaces of the CPB circuit also leads to platelet activation, manifested by release of α-granules, platelet factor 4, and α-thromboglobulin.[195,196] These activated platelets continue to circulate and exhibit abnormal aggregation and adhesion.[196,197] Platelet function improves over a few hours after CPB.

### Coagulation Factors

Concentrations of coagulation factors decrease during CPB by up to 50% owing to hemodilution, but abnormal coagulation should not be noted until concentrations of coagulation factors are reduced to 30% or less of normal (10%-15% for Factor V).[195] These decreases may occur in procedures requiring unusually large amounts of fluids, including transfusion of packed red blood cells and washed blood.

### Fibrinolysis

Although anticoagulation with heparin also limits fibrinolytic activity, fibrinolysis is known to occur during CPB.[198]

Fibrinolytic activity seems to return to baseline rapidly after CPB, so the significance of this phenomenon is uncertain. Inhibition of fibrinolysis by antifibrinolytic agents during CPB may reduce blood loss, however, as discussed later.

### Disseminated Intravascular Coagulation

Disseminated intravascular coagulation may occur during cardiac surgery, but as in other surgical settings, it is extremely rare. When coagulation studies demonstrate thrombocytopenia, prolonged PT and PTT, hypofibrinogenemia, and the presence of fibrin degradation products, the coagulopathy is more likely a result of severe hemodilution, and the fibrin degradation products are related to low-grade fibrinolysis during CPB. However, disseminated intravascular coagulation can be noted in the presence of sepsis, hemolytic transfusion reactions, and allergic reactions.

## How Are Coagulation Problems Diagnosed and Treated?

The diagnosis of post-CPB coagulopathy is problematic. If pre-existing coagulation problems are known, therapy may be guided by preoperative plans. If residual heparin activity is the only problem, it should be readily diagnosed by measuring the ACT (and perhaps the heparin concentration) and treating with additional protamine. Diagnosis and treatment of other coagulation problems depend on three possible approaches: (1) empirical treatment, (2) standard coagulation tests, or (3) viscoelastic coagulation testing.

### Empiric Treatment

Empirical treatment is often used to treat "nonsurgical bleeding" because standard coagulation tests may take too long to be helpful in a patient with clinically significant bleeding. Because platelet dysfunction is the most likely coagulation defect, treatment with desmopressin (DDAVP) or transfusion of platelets may be indicated while awaiting results of standard coagulation tests.

If these measures do not correct the apparent coagulopathy, no other cause is identified, and test results have not yet returned, transfusion of fresh-frozen plasma may be the next logical step. Although this approach is not particularly scientific, the wide range of transfusion practice in the United States suggests that some variation of this approach is commonly used.[199] However, prophylactic transfusion of platelets or fresh-frozen plasma, even in patients with preoperative risk factors for platelet dysfunction, has not proven to be beneficial.[200,201]

### Standard Coagulation Tests

In some centers, results are returned rapidly from the coagulation laboratory. Standard coagulation tests are also helpful in the postoperative period. Blood products must be transfused only to treat documented bleeding and should not be used merely to correct abnormal laboratory results. This admonition is illustrated by the finding in one study that 80% of patients had a prolonged PT that was a poor predictor of postoperative bleeding.[202]

If bleeding is present, useful goals of therapy include platelet count >100 000/mm³, PT and PTT <1.2 times the control value, and fibrinogen >100 mg/dL. A postoperative bleeding time <10 minutes precludes platelet dysfunction. Unfortunately, the bleeding time is not generally available intraoperatively because it requires time and attention, access to an extremity, and standardization of the technique.

## Viscoelastic Tests

Viscoelastic coagulation monitors, namely thromboelastography (TEG) and Sonoclot, may also be beneficial in guiding coagulation therapy. The advantages of these techniques follow:

1. They require small specimens of blood.
2. They can be performed in the OR without sending specimens to a laboratory.
3. Results are usually obtained more rapidly than with standard coagulation tests.
4. They provide more information about qualitative platelet function, clot formation, and fibrinolysis than can be obtained with standard coagulation tests.

Both techniques are better predictors of post-CPB bleeding than standard coagulation tests.[203,204] In vitro incubation of TEG samples with heparinase allows TEG monitoring during CPB, despite heparin anticoagulation. Although a decrease in the speed of clot formation has been shown under hypothermic conditions, a temperature-induced absolute deterioration in clot quality is not observed.[205] In a direct comparison study, TEG provided higher sensitivity, specificity, and accuracy and lower false-positive and false-negative rates than Sonoclot measurements.[206]

## Is Desmopressin Efficacious After Cardiopulmonary Bypass?

Initial experience with DDAVP suggested that it may decrease blood loss in complex cardiac procedures.[207,208] The mechanism of action of DDAVP appears to be a release of von Willebrand factor, which is involved in the interaction of platelets with subendothelial tissue. Subsequent studies have not confirmed significant benefits of DDAVP after CPB.[209,210]

DDAVP may improve platelet function in some patients (eg, patients with uremia or patients taking antiplatelet drugs preoperatively), but its routine use does not appear warranted. When administered, the intravenous dose is 0.3 µg/kg over 15 to 20 minutes to avoid hypotension.

## Do Antifibrinolytic Agents Reduce Blood Loss?

Three antifibrinolytic agents have been studied in the setting of cardiac surgery to determine whether clinically significant reductions in blood loss and transfusion requirements may be obtained. The agents studied are EACA, tranexamic acid, and aprotinin.

## ε-Aminocaproic Acid

Randomized trials of EACA have been shown to decrease blood loss by about 10% to 20% without apparent increased risk of thrombotic complications.[211,212] EACA exerts its effects by binding to the platelet lysine binding site to inhibit plasmin-induced platelet aggregation.[213] TEG analysis has shown that patients who receive EACA injection have a better coagulation profile, and the qualitative platelet function is also better after CPB.[214]

Dosage recommendations in adults include a 100 mg/kg loading dose before CPB and a 10 mg/kg/h maintenance infusion continued for 4 hours during and after CPB; however, clinicians frequently administer a loading dose of 5 g followed by a continuing infusion at the rate of 1 g/h. Often, an additional 5 g load is placed in the pump prime to compensate for the additional circulating blood volume encountered when instituting CPB. Renal excretion is the primary route of elimination, prompting recommendations for alteration of the dosing regimen in patients with renal failure to an EACA loading dose of 50 mg/kg and a maintenance infusion of 25 mg/kg/h.[215]

## Tranexamic Acid

Randomized trials of tranexamic acid have also been shown to decrease blood loss by about 10% to 20% without apparent increased risk of thrombotic complications[216,217] Tranexamic acid is a synthetic derivative of the amino acid lysine, which exerts its antifibrinolytic effect through the reversible blockade of lysine binding sites on plasminogen molecules.[218] As such, tranexamic acid inhibits plasmin's catalytic activity in a similar fashion to that of EACA, decreasing the frequency of the presence of fibrin split products and increasing the platelet dense granule content of adenosine diphosphate. This inhibition of plasmin-induced partial platelet activation during CPB preserves qualitative platelet function.[219]

Pinosky and coworkers compared tranexamic acid and EACA and found that although intraoperative blood loss between the two groups was similar, tranexamic acid was more effective in reducing blood loss postoperatively following CABG.[220]

Dosing regimens for tranexamic acid in adults most commonly include a loading dose of 10 mg/kg followed by an infusion of 1 mg/kg/h. As with EACA, elimination is largely via renal excretion, that smaller doses may be enough to maintain therapeutic levels in patients with renal insufficiency.[221]

## Aprotinin

Aprotinin has been extensively studied and is in widespread use outside the United States. Its efficacy in markedly reducing blood loss and transfusion requirements in cardiac surgery has been well documented.[222,223] Aprotinin is a broad-spectrum protease inhibitor that modulates the systemic inflammatory response associated with CPB surgery. Its mechanism of action has not been completely determined but may include inhibition of kallikrein-activated fibrinolysis, inhibition of fibrinogenolysis, and inhibition of release of endothelial plasminogen activator. Aprotinin exerts its antiinflammatory response by inhibiting proinflammatory cytokine release, reducing glycoprotein loss in platelets, and preventing the expression of proinflammatory adhesive glycoproteins in granulocytes.

In prospective, randomized studies, there have been conflicting reports regarding potential advantages of aprotinin over EACA and tranexamic acid. Menichetti and associates reported significantly decreased transfusion requirements in an aprotinin test group compared with groups receiving either EACA or tranexamic acid[224]; however, Trinh-Duc and coworkers reported no difference in a comparison of aprotinin and EACA.[225] Although use of aprotinin has been safely documented in cases involving deep hypothermic circulatory arrest, there currently remains much controversy on the subject.

Aprotinin prolongs ACT measurements, and fatal thrombosis has been noted with its use.[226] It has been observed that kaolin-based ACTs are not increased to the same degree by aprotinin as are celite ACTs. Although protocols vary, a minimal celite ACT of 750 seconds or kaolin ACT of 480 seconds is recommended in the presence of aprotinin.[227] Many clinicians routinely administer heparin doses of 400 units/kg rather than the more conventional 300 units/kg dose when concomitantly administering aprotinin.

There are two main dosing regimens for aprotinin. The high-dose or full-dose regimen consists of a loading dose of 2 million kallikrein-inhibiting units (KIU), 2 million KIU into the pump prime volume, and 500 000 KIU/h of operation as a continuous intravenous infusion. The low-dose or half-dose regimen consists of one half of the preceding values. Although the high-dose regimen has not been shown to convey significantly decreased blood transfusion requirements and may carry an increased risk of perioperative renal insufficiency, a progressive benefit toward reducing adverse perioperative neurologic sequelae has been reported.[228]

Anaphylactic and anaphylactoid reactions have been reported following aprotinin administration, but the overall incidence of these potentially catastrophic events is reportedly <1%. However, special concerns are warranted among patients who have been previously exposed to aprotinin, in whom the incidence of hypersensitivity or anaphylactic reactions is 2.7%. The incidence of a hypersensitivity or anaphylactic reaction following reexposure is increased when the reexposure occurs within 6 months of the initial administration (5.0% for reexposure within 6 months; 0.9% for re-exposure >6 months). For this reason, it is considered prudent to delay aprotinin administration until surgical exposure allows for rapid cannulation and institution of CPB. Many clinicians do this as a routine precaution even among primary exposures. It is the norm in our institution to administer a test dose of 1 mL before giving a full loading dose and to delay loading the pump prime until safe administration has been established.

Because of the associated risks conveyed by the use of aprotinin and the additional cost of the drug compared with either EACA or tranexamic acid, aprotinin use is often reserved for patients undergoing redo-sternotomy procedures and in cases in which massive transfusion requirements are anticipated, such as those requiring prolonged CPB times or deep hypothermic circulatory arrest.

## OTHER APPROACHES TO CARDIAC SURGERY

### What Are Some Other Approaches to Conventional Coronary Artery Bypass Grafting Using Cardiopulmonary Bypass?

The 1990s brought many technologic changes to cardiac surgery. Along with emerging technologies, novel approaches

to performing cardiac surgery and previously attempted approaches were technically modified in order to be performed with improved safety. Among the most popular approaches are off-pump coronary artery bypass (OPCAB) grafting; minimally invasive, direct vision coronary artery bypass (MIDCAB) grafting, port-access heart surgery, and transmyocardial laser revascularization (TMLR).

### What Is Off-Pump Coronary Artery Bypass Grafting?

This surgical technique, as with conventional CABG surgery, entails a median sternotomy approach; however, in OPCAB surgery, the bypass grafts are anastomosed without the aid of CPB. Hence, the usual surgical steps undertaken to prepare for CPB (including aortic cannulation, venoatrial cannulation, and so on) are omitted. Instead, the grafts are anastomosed under conditions of normothermia and moderate anticoagulation (typically heparin doses of 100 U/kg) on an actively beating heart. Relative bradycardia is often preferred by surgeons to facilitate the procedure and can be accomplished with an esmolol infusion (50-150 µg/kg/min) titrated to effect. Occasionally, bolus doses of adenosine may be administered for particularly difficult stitches in order to cause a brief period of sinus arrest. However, with the advent of newer and more effective stabilization devices, the surgical field is often fixed in a relatively stable position regardless of the heart rate.

Although this approach obviates the need for cooling, rewarming, hemodilution, and additional risks of CPB (cannulation, cross-clamping, nonpulsatile flow, platelet dysfunction, and so on), it carries its own risks and difficulties. It does not preclude the use of partial aortic occlusion, which is still performed for proximal vein graft anastomoses. Perhaps the most difficult hemodynamic insults occur during distal anastomoses while the target vessel is occluded. During this period, distal myocardium, which was perhaps already receiving a paucity of blood flow, becomes reliably ischemic. Wall motion on TEE typically progresses from baseline to hypokinesis to akinesis and often dyskinesis. CO often suffers, producing systemic hypotension. Arrhythmias occur despite prophylaxis with lidocaine, especially during RCA-distribution anastomoses, often requiring pacing or defibrillation.

In addition to the surgically induced ischemia, the location of anastomoses often requires nonphysiologic heart positions, ranging from multiple laparotomy pads placed behind the heart to physical retraction of the heart, and resulting in both decreased filling and abnormal geometric cardiac deformations that are not conducive to normal ejection.

Added to the conditions of decreased venous return, ischemia, hypotension, and an overall low CO state often herald the need for NTG for coronary and graft vasodilation and β-blockade for a relative bradycardia to facilitate the anastomosis. This combination often results in the seemingly self-defeating need for fluid administration, inotropic support, or administration of vasoconstrictors. Reperfusion following restoration of normal coronary blood flow does not necessarily solve the antecedent problems; the myocardium may remain stunned without a return to baseline performance, may have completed actual infarction with even relatively short occlusion times, and often actually precipitates further arrhythmias as the accumulated products of anaerobic metabolism are suddenly washed out.

In 10% to 25% of cases, due to either the impossibility of complete revascularization off bypass, physiologic intolerance of cardiac retraction or coronary occlusion, or graft malfunction, it is necessary to convert to CPB.[229] Despite these hemodynamic insults, patients are often successfully extubated in the OR following completion of surgery, and if not, they are frequently successfully fast-tracked.

## What Does Minimally Invasive, Direct Vision Coronary Artery Bypass Grafting Entail?

The major difference between MIDCAB and OPCAB is the surgical incision. Rather than a median sternotomy, the MIDCAB incision is a left parasternal minithoracotomy incision. This incision is smaller than a full sternotomy and more aesthetically pleasing to many patients; however, consequent to the limited incision, surgical exposure is logically limited as well. It is usually applicable only for patients with simple single vessel disease of the LAD coronary artery or proximal disease of the circumflex coronary artery; however, RCA anastomoses via this approach have been reported as well. One-lung ventilation is frequently necessary to facilitate surgical exposure. The minimally invasive approach has also been used for intracardiac congenital lesions, using a left parasternal minithoracotomy for VSD repairs and a right submammary incision for ASD repairs.[230]

Anastomoses are performed as with OPCAB on the beating heart, and, consequently, disadvantages include the technical challenge of less exposure and more difficulty with cardiac motion. Early reports have yielded variable patency rates and unique complications such as stenosis at the retractor site.[231] A major disadvantage of this approach to OPCAB is the lack of access for conventional cannulation should a catastrophic complication occur, necessitating urgent conversion to CPB. Femoral cannulation can be successfully used should this need arise.

## Does the Surgical Approach Change Perioperative Outcome?

One would anticipate that the omission of CPB and its associated complications would provide overwhelming advantages of OPCAB and MIDCAB to conventional CABG; however, evidence remains unclear. Although CBP has complications related to clotting factor destruction, hemodilution, particulate embolization, and others, CPB does ensure at least constant CO. Although nonpulsatile blood flow is nonphysiologic and may change distal perfusion, end-organ perfusion may be better in some patients than in those with low CO of OPCAB due to intraoperative cardiac positioning and ischemia. Additionally, hypothermia is often performed with CPB, offering some end-organ advantages in that $O_2$ consumption is decreased regardless of supply conditions. Cardioplegia may offer benefits regarding myocardial $O_2$ supply, consumption, and reperfusion injuries that do not exist with OPCAB. Similarly, patency rates of OPCAB grafts do not appear as good as with conventional CABG, perhaps due to the difficulty of operating on a moving surgical field as well as from proximal

postoperative coronary stenoses that have been implicated from the stabilization devices.

One recent study compared patients undergoing fast-track CABG with conventional CPB (group A) versus MIDCAB (group B) versus OPCAB (group C). Group A had more vessels revascularized with no significant difference in morbidity, mortality, or postoperative LOS. Group B tended to be younger patients with single vessel disease, whereas group C had significant differences in preoperative cardiovascular status and comorbid conditions (more LV dysfunction, CHF, and symptomatic PVD) compared with group A but had fewer vessels bypassed. Group C patients had reduced postoperative LOS without increasing mortality or readmission rate, regardless of age, sex, or associated comorbidity.[232]

Hence, at this time, there exists a need for more randomized, controlled, prospective trials examining this dilemma, which will likely produce different advantages of alternative surgical approaches based on preoperative cardiovascular status, comorbid conditions, and number and location of grafts to be performed.

## To What Does Port-Access Cardiac Surgery Refer?

Port access surgery was developed to improve exposure of the target vessels in a quiet operating field while still limiting the incision, with improved cosmetic results, reduced pain, shorter hospital stays, and an earlier return to normal activity.[233] It combines the limited paramedian thoracotomy incision (left or right, depending on the surgical procedure) with CPB. Because the surgical field is limited and access to the anatomic structures for cannulation is often impossible, port-access surgery involves percutaneous placement of a femoral to IVC/RA venous drainage cannula, an endoaortic balloon clamp via the femoral artery, an endopulmonary vent, an endosinus catheter, and a contralateral endoarterial return cannula. Once the often time-consuming process of placing these cannulas is completed, systemic heparinization is accomplished and the operation is carried out in a bloodless, motionless surgical field under CPB.

Complications of port-access surgery include endoaortic balloon occluder malposition, stroke, coronary sinus rupture, wound infections, vascular insufficiency, pulmonary complications, early recurrent ischemia caused by anastomotic restenosis, sinus node dysfunction, and low CO.

## What Is Transmyocardial Laser Revascularization?

TMLR is a process of increasing regional myocardial perfusion by actually boring multiple holes through the ventricular wall with the use of a holmium:YAG, argon, or $CO_2$ laser. The theory for TLMR was based on the existence of naturally occurring sinusoids connecting myocardial arterioles that was originally described in 1933 by Wearn and colleagues.[234] This discovery led to initial trials with transmyocardial revascularization with needle punctures as early as 1965.[235] Laser technology was first used to create these channels in 1982[236]; however, the approach has only recently been promoted as a nonexperimental approach for treatment of patients with refractory class III-IV angina not amenable to percutaneous transluminal coronary angioplasty (PTCA) or CABG. The procedure is typically performed through a left anterolateral thoracotomy incision. Confirmation of completion of each attempt can be provided with concurrent use of TEE; vaporization plumes are readily identified when the laser penetrates the full thickness of the myocardium and comes into contact with blood. Depending on the area of myocardium to be treated, multiple channels (often 10-40) are made in a gridlike pattern over the myocardial surface. Contrast echocardiography can be used to document regional improvements in blood flow intraoperatively.[237]

Experience with this technique remains somewhat limited; however, TMLR has been shown to reduce angina by an average of two classes in patients with angina resistant to medical treatment and otherwise untreatable by either PTCA or CABG. Although long-term improvements in regional blood flow have been shown by positron emission tomography studies,[238] there are conflicting reports regarding long-term patency.[239–242] Cardiologists have begun performing catheter-based TMLR in which channels are created from the endocardial surface using holmium:YAG and Xe:Cl lasers.

It is unknown whether the increased perfusion resulting from TMLR is a result of direct blood flow from the "lased" channels or neoangiogenesis caused by the laser-induced myocardial injury. Survivors of TLMR surgery have reliably reduced angina scores, reduced doses of antianginal medications, reduced hospital admissions per year, and improved exercise tolerance.[243] However, despite some evidence that short-term and long-term functional performance and symptomatology are improved following TMLR,[241] early mortality rates for TMLR are often high. Additionally, despite documentation that blood flow is increased, no studies have demonstrated a significant improvement in ejection fraction. This has led to the hypothesis that symptomatic improvement results not from a lack of ischemia due to increased blood flow, but rather from permanent laser-induced injury to afferent cardiac nerve fibers.[244]

### What Is "Volume Reduction Surgery"?

Surgical alternatives to medical therapy have been sought due to the 50% 3-year mortality of patients with end-stage cardiac failure. These include cardiac transplantation (see Chapter 73) and LV volume reduction surgery. The pioneering work on this type of surgery was performed by Batista and associates[245]; hence, the procedure is often referred to as the *Batista procedure*. The procedure is performed on the subset of patients suffering from end-stage dilated cardiomyopathies, who primarily suffer from forward pump failure due to a chronic physiologic aberrancy resulting from the increased radius of the ventricle as described by the law of Laplace:

$$Pressure = 2 \times Wall\ Tension\ Radius$$

Therefore, wall tension must increase twofold for each corresponding increase in ventricular radius in order to generate the same ventricular pressure. LV volume reduction surgery involves either an inter- or extrapapillary resection of the LV wall in order to decrease the ventricular radius, thereby improving myocardial contractility. Initial reports describe an approximate 10% increase in ejection fraction with functional improvement in 80% of patients to NYHA class I or II[245,246];

however, early failures have been unpredictable, and the incidence of the use of mechanical support as rescue therapy has led to a need for extremely careful patient selection.

### Are There Any Other Recent Innovations Pertaining to Anesthesia for Adult Cardiac Surgery?

Robotically assisted microsurgery for endoscopic CABG has been successful and reported.[247] Using this technique, the operator actually performs anastomoses at a remote site from the patient, using computer virtual reality technology to control a robotic arm that provides the physical interface between surgeon and patient.

## SURGERY USING DEEP HYPOTHERMIA

### When Is Deep Hypothermia Indicated?

Patients undergoing operations of the thoracic aorta, although a small subset of the population undergoing heart surgery, constitute a formidable challenge for the cardiothoracic team today. The main challenge is to provide the patient with adequate cerebral protection from prolonged ischemia and emboli during the surgical procedure. Clearly, the single most important advance in the area of cerebral protection has been the institution of deep hypothermia (temperatures of 18°-20°C).[248] In adults, the use of deep hypothermic circulatory arrest (DHCA) is traditionally instituted for those with aortic arch involvement in order to provide a dry and motionless field. Recently, DHCA has been described as an alternative to aortic cannulation in the presence of extensive atheromatous disease of the ascending aorta, as well as during thoracoabdominal aneurysm repairs.

The cerebral protection that hypothermia provides is mainly due to a temperature-related reduction of cerebral metabolic rate of $O_2$ ($CMRO_2$), which reduces the need for $O_2$ delivery and blood flow requirements proportionally. This relationship between $CMRO_2$ and temperature is exponential and expressed as a temperature coefficient or Q10 (the difference in $CMRO_2$ at two temperatures differing by 10°C). The cerebral protective effect of hypothermia probably involves more than a reduction in $CMRO_2$ and most likely includes the prevention of release of excitatory neurotransmitters and delay of the onset of biochemical reactions that eventually lead to cell death.

### What Is the Safe Limit for Deep Hypothermic Circulatory Arrest?

It is important to recognize that DHCA does not *eliminate* the possibility of cerebral ischemia, but only *delays* it. Metabolic and enzymatic reactions persist, although at a lower speed. Mezrow and colleagues demonstrated that 39% of baseline metabolic activity and significant EEG slow wave activity persists at 18°C in some patients.[249] Studies suggest that the "safe" period of DHCA at a temperature around 20°C is approximately 40 to 45 minutes.[250,251] Longer DHCA periods are associated with an increased incidence of neurologic ischemic insults with accompanying morbidity. The duration of DHCA should be kept as short as possible to minimize the possibility of cerebral ischemia

## What Are the Alternatives to Deep Hypothermic Circulatory Arrest?

Besides the fact that DHCA does not provide unlimited cerebral protection, other disadvantages include the prolonged period of CPB time required to cool and rewarm the patients, coagulation abnormalities resulting in excessive bleeding, and the increased risk of organ dysfunction. Because some operations may exceed the limits for DHCA, alternative methods have been described.

### Selective Antegrade Cerebral Perfusion

This technique involves distal clamping of the aorta, along with cannulation of the innominate, left common carotid, and subclavian arteries. These vessels are then perfused in an antegrade fashion to ensure a constant supply of $O_2$ to the brain with preservation of autoregulation, thus allowing for more complex and time-consuming procedures to take place. Another advantage is that surgery can be performed under moderate hypothermia (24°-27°C), thus decreasing the severity of coagulopathy and organ failure. Disadvantages include a more complicated technique, multiple cannulation sites, distortion of the aorta, and the increased risk of cerebral embolization and stroke due to dislodgment of atheromatous debris.

### Retrograde Cerebral Perfusion

This simpler technique for ensuing cerebral protection is actually utilized as an adjunct to DHCA. Retrograde cerebral perfusion (RCP) uses a continuous flow through the superior vena cava, cerebral vasculature, and arch vessels during DHCA. Initially used to treat massive cerebral air embolism, RCP effectively flushes out microemboli that occur during CPB. In addition, it allows for the brain to be cooled at a lower temperature than the rest of the body. The amount of retrograde flow that actually reaches the brain is uncertain because some of the flow is diverted through the azygous and extracranial veins. Although protection against cerebral ischemia occurs, elevated RCP pressures may result in cerebral edema.[251] Studies in animals suggest that RCP pressures (measured at the level of the internal jugular vein) between 20 to 25 mm Hg will supply the lowest perfusion pressure that provides effective CBF without increasing cerebral water content.[252,253] The value of RCP to extend the protective effect of DHCA is controversial. RCP lasting <30 minutes appears to be safe, whereas RCP periods >60 to 100 minutes have been associated with significant neurologic dysfunction.[254]

## What Are Some of the Adjuvant Measures for Cerebral Protection?

### Barbiturates

The administration of barbiturates in the presence of hypothermia-induced isoelectric EEG seems to add little to cerebral protection. The consequence is a slow emergence with potential delays in diagnosis of neurologic injury. However, if EEG activity is present despite deep hypothermia, the administration of sodium thiopental (3-10 mg/kg) titrated to isoelectricity is indicated.

### Corticosteroids

The use of steroids to minimize cerebral edema associated with DHCA is advocated by some but their benefits are unproved. Methylprednisolone in large doses has been administered before DHCA.

### Mannitol

Mannitol in doses of 0.5 g to 1 g/kg is given to produce osmotic diuresis and minimize intracranial pressure.

### Glucose Control

Although management of blood sugar during CPB is controversial, there is a general agreement that brain damage due to ischemia is exacerbated in the presence of hyperglycemia. Serum blood glucose should be obtained at frequent intervals in order to adjust insulin dosage.

### Local Cooling

Ice packs placed around the head to provide topical cooling of the brain may provide additional protection.

## OTHER PROCEDURES NOT REQUIRING CARDIOPULMONARY BYPASS: PACEMAKER IMPLANTATION

### What Are the Anesthetic Considerations?

Implantation of a permanent transvenous pacemaker may be carried out in a cardiac catheterization laboratory or an OR. Most commonly, access to a subclavian vein is obtained, and pacemaker leads are inserted under fluoroscopic guidance. A subcutaneous pocket is then created for the pulse generator.

A permanent pacemaker is indicated for conduction defects or bradydysrhythmias that result in symptoms of inadequate CO, such as lightheadedness, syncope, or CHF. Pacemakers may also be used to suppress ventricular and supraventricular tachydysrhythmias.

Some patients will already have a temporary transvenous pacemaker, external pacemaker, or esophageal pacemaker in place. If not, alternative pacing equipment must be available. A transcutaneous pacemaker provides rapid, noninvasive pacing capability if the need arises. The equipment necessary to insert a transvenous pacing wire via the right or left internal jugular vein should be available. Esophageal pacers, because of the proximity of the esophagus to the left atrium, reliably capture and pace the atrium and are especially useful in patients with symptomatic bradycardia, sick sinus syndrome, and occasionally for asystole; however, for ventricular capture to occur, the intrinsic atrioventricular nodal conduction system must remain intact. For this reason, esophageal pacing is ineffective for advanced second-degree or third-degree atrioventricular block. Resuscitation drugs such as atropine, isoproterenol, and epinephrine should be available to treat bradycardia. Stimulation of the endocardium with a pacemaker electrode can induce dysrhythmias. These most often resolve spontaneously with removal of the mechanical stimulus, but antidysrhythmic agents should be readily available as well.

### Local Infiltration and Regional Block

Pacemaker implantation can be performed with infiltration of local anesthesia if at all possible. Intravenous sedation should be administered judiciously. To provide adequate anesthesia without oversedation of patients who are often critically ill, a technique of regional anesthesia has been described.[255] The technique involves the combination of a cervical plexus block and blocks of the second, third, and fourth intercostal nerves. An interscalene cervical plexus block is performed with 15 mL of a local anesthetic mixture consisting of 1% mepivacaine, 0.2% tetracaine, and 1:200 000 epinephrine. Blocks of T2, T3, and T4 are performed with 3 mL for each nerve. Safe and effective anesthesia is obtained without the need for supplemental analgesics.

### General Anesthesia

If general anesthesia is required, temporary pacing with a transcutaneous or transvenous pacemaker should be established before induction. The specific technique should be chosen with consideration of a patient's ventricular function. Otherwise, no specific anesthetic agents are contraindicated for pacemaker implantation.

## AUTOMATIC INTERNAL CARDIOVERTER-DEFIBRILLATOR IMPLANTATION

### *What Are the Indications?*

Indications for AICD implantation are listed in Table 63–31. An AICD improves survival of patients at high risk for sudden death. Pharmacologic treatment of recurrent ventricular tachydysrhythmias has been disappointing.[256,257] Patients who meet the criteria in Table 63–31 are considered for AICD implantation if the dysrhythmia is life threatening, causing sudden death, syncope, or severe hemodynamic compromise. It must not be related to acute MI, myocardial ischemia, electrolyte abnormalities, or drug toxicity. The device is contraindicated in incessant ventricular tachycardia or fibrillation (ie, one or more episodes daily) because the AICD battery would be rapidly depleted.

### *What Are the Components?*

An AICD device consists of two defibrillating electrodes, one or two rate-sensing electrodes, and a pulse generator (Figs. 63–16 and 63–17). The first defibrillating electrode is either an intravascular spring electrode placed in the superior vena cava near the RA or a wire mesh patch sewn to the RA or RV. The second defibrillating electrode is a wire mesh patch sewn to the apex of the LV.

The rate-sensing electrode system is either a pair of screw-in electrodes placed in normal epicardium or a single transvenous electrode attached to the RV endocardium like a pace-

**TABLE 63–31.** Indications for Implantation of Automatic Internal Cardioverter-Defibrillator

**Conditions for Which There Is General Agreement**

One or more documented episodes of hemodynamically significant ventricular tachycardia or ventricular fibrillation in a patient in whom electrophysiologic testing and ambulatory monitoring cannot be used to accurately predict efficacy of therapy.

One or more documented episodes of hemodynamically significant ventricular tachycardia or ventricular fibrillation in a patient in whom no drug was found to be effective or no drug currently available and appropriate was tolerated.

Continued inducibility at electrophysiologic study of hemodynamically significant ventricular tachycardia or ventricular fibrillation despite the best available drug therapy or despite surgery or catheter ablation if drug therapy has failed.

**Conditions for Which Use Is Frequent but There Is Divergence of Opinion About Their Necessity**

One or more documented episodes of hemodynamically significant ventricular tachycardia or ventricular fibrillation in a patient in whom drug efficacy testing is possible.

Recurrent syncope of undetermined origin in a patient with hemodynamically significant ventricular tachycardia or ventricular fibrillation induced at electrophysiologic study in whom no effective or no tolerated drug is available or appropriate.

Modified from Guidelines for implantation of cardiac pacemakers and antiarrhythmia devices: a report of the American College of Cardiology/American Heart Association Task Force on Assessment of Diagnostic and Therapeutic Cardiovascular Procedures (Committee on Pacemaker Implantation). *J Am Coll Cardiol.* 1991;18:1.

maker lead. The ends of the electrodes are tunneled subcutaneously to a left upper quadrant pouch, where the pulse generator is placed.

### *How Does the Device Function?*

The sensing electrode system of an AICD determines HR and characteristics of the ECG waveform. Specifically, a probability density function analyzes the amount of time the QRS complex spends away from the isoelectric baseline. During ventricular tachycardia or coarse ventricular fibrillation, the waveform deviates from the isoelectric baseline much more

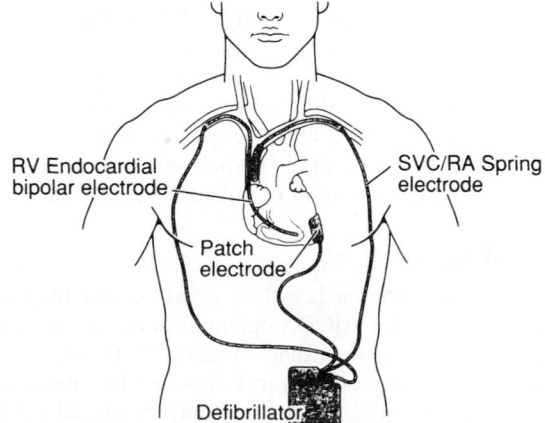

**FIGURE 63–16.** Automatic internal cardioverter-defibrillator with an electrode configuration consisting of a transvenous rate-sensing bipolar electrode, a transvenous defibrillating spring electrode, and a single epicardial defibrillating patch electrode. (From Deutsch N, Hantler CB, Morady F, et al. Perioperative management of the patient undergoing automatic internal cardioverter-defibrillator implantation. *J Cardiothorac Anesth.* 1990;4:236.)

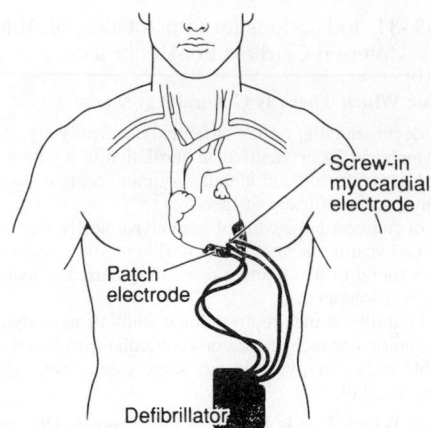

**FIGURE 63–17.** Automatic internal cardioverter-defibrillator with electrode configuration consisting of a screw-in rate-sensing electrode and two epicardial defibrillating patch electrodes. (From Deutsch N, Hantler CB, Morady F, et al. Perioperative management of the patient undergoing automatic internal cardioverter-defibrillator implantation. *J Cardiothorac Anesth.* 1990;4:236.)

than during sinus rhythm. The sensing of rapid HR or a rapid HR and altered ECG morphology leads to activation of the countershock sequence.

Five to 15 seconds are required for the AICD to determine that a malignant dysrhythmia is in progress. An additional 5 to 15 seconds is required to charge the energy-storage capacitors. A 25-J pulse is then delivered. The sensing and charging cycles are repeated, if necessary, and up to three more shocks of 30 J each may be delivered.

## What Is the Surgical Approach?

The possible surgical approaches for AICD implantation are median sternotomy, left subxiphoid, left subcostal, and left anterior thoracotomy. More recently, AICDs have become more portable and have been placed transvenously with generator placement in the infraclavicular location as with other pacemaker devices.

### Median Sternotomy

If a patient is undergoing a concurrent cardiac surgical procedure, the AICD is placed via median sternotomy at the completion of the primary procedure. Some surgeons prefer this approach even if a patient is not undergoing another cardiac operation. It affords the best exposure for placement of the AICD components, allows rapid cannulation for CPB if complications develop, and is associated with less postoperative pain than a thoracotomy or subcostal approach.[258,259]

### Subxiphoid Approach

The subxiphoid approach is less invasive and may be the preferred technique for AICD implantation in patients without previous or concurrent cardiac surgery.[260] Through a subxiphoid incision, the pericardium is opened for placement of electrodes. Alternatively, the patches may be placed extrapericardially.

### Anterior Thoracotomy

Anterior thoracotomy is most useful in patients with previous median sternotomy. This approach minimizes the dissection required for placement of patches and decreases the risk of injury to bypass grafts. A subcostal approach has also been used. In all of these approaches, a subcutaneous pocket is created in the left upper quadrant or left paraumbilical area in order to house the pulse generator.

## What Are the Intraoperative Anesthetic Considerations?

### Monitoring

Patients undergoing AICD implantation should be monitored according to the degree of myocardial dysfunction. All patients should have intraarterial BP monitoring. A PA catheter is frequently placed to assist in the intraoperative and postoperative hemodynamic management. Alternatively, a CVP catheter may be sufficient if ventricular function is well preserved.

### Dysrhythmia Control

An external defibrillator should be immediately available at all times in case ventricular tachycardia or ventricular fibrillation develops. Such dysrhythmias preferably should not be treated with antidysrhythmics before AICD implantation, because they are unlikely to be successful and may alter fibrillation and defibrillation thresholds during testing. If external defibrillation alone does not halt malignant ventricular dysrhythmias, however, the combination of external defibrillation with lidocaine, procainamide, and bretylium may be necessary in a life-threatening situation.

Other emergency medications to have immediately available include ephedrine, atropine, and epinephrine (in both 100 μg/mL and 4-10 μg/mL concentrations). Isoproterenol is sometimes used to facilitate dysrhythmia induction.

### General Anesthesia

A general anesthetic technique is used. Consideration should be given to epidural or intrathecal narcotics for postoperative pain management, particularly when a thoracotomy or subcostal approach is used. The choice of anesthetic agents depends on a patient's ventricular function and whether or not a concurrent cardiac surgical procedure is planned. For isolated AICD implantation, extubation at the end of the procedure or in the early postoperative period is usually possible. Placement of a double-lumen tube for one-lung ventilation facilitates surgical exposure and may protect against trauma to the lung when the thoracotomy approach is used.

Intraoperatively, after placement of the electrodes, a series of tests are performed to ensure that the sensing and defibrillating components function adequately. Testing involves induction of ventricular tachycardia and ventricular fibrillation several times to determine adequate sensing and the defibrillation threshold for each dysrhythmia. Hypotension develops as the dysrhythmia is induced but resolves after each defibrillation. In some patients, treatment with ephedrine, 5 mg, or epinephrine, 10 μg, may be necessary to assist recovery of BP and contractility.

External defibrillator pads or paddles must be in place, and internal paddles must be available in case defibrillation is unsuccessful with the AICD electrodes. Despite the fact that many of these patients have marginal myocardial function, electrophysiologic testing both intraoperatively and postoperatively has not been shown to further depress LV function.[261,262]

## PERICARDIOTOMY

### *What Are the Indications?*

Pericardiotomy is used to drain a pericardial effusion or to relieve pericardial tamponade. It is performed emergently after cardiac surgery, thoracic surgery, or chest trauma when hemodynamic measurements suggest pericardial tamponade. Semielective pericardiotomy is indicated in patients with chronic pericardial effusions due to malignancy, renal disease, connective tissue disorders, and so on. When pericardial tamponade develops as a result of nonsurgical, nontraumatic etiologies, immediate pericardiocentesis is the treatment of choice.

### *What Are the Signs and Symptoms of Pericardial Tamponade?*

Fluid accumulation in the pericardial space causes increased intrapericardial pressure and impairment of venous return, and it ultimately leads to decreased stroke volume and CO. Reflex tachycardia and vasoconstriction develop to maintain CO and BP. Systemic hypotension results as filling pressures (mean RA and LA, PAOP, and LV and RV diastolic pressures) tend to equalize.[263] Other clinical findings include jugular venous distention, pulsus paradoxus, and muffled heart sounds. The chest radiograph may show mediastinal widening. Echocardiography demonstrates location and size of effusion, and ultrasound may be used to aid in guiding pericardiocentesis. Although not all effusions cause tamponade, echocardiographic evidence of RA collapse and RV diastolic collapse are indicative of hemodynamically significant fluid accumulation. Similarly, Doppler interrogation of transmitral flow, pulmonary venous flow, transtricuspid flow, and hepatic venous flow can be used to document typical respiratory variations seen with hemodynamically significant effusions in experienced hands.

It is important to note that especially following cardiac surgery, fluid collections and blood clots may be well localized, and compression of discrete areas may result in tamponade. Diagnosis of this "single chamber" tamponade can be delineated with echocardiography, and frequently requires surgical exploration, as the location and nature of the clot preclude successful pericardiocentesis.

### *What Are the Anesthetic Considerations?*

#### Pericardial Tamponade

The hemodynamic goals in a patient with tamponade physiology are to prevent decreases in preload, afterload, HR, and contractility in order to maximize CO. Monitoring should include an arterial catheter and, in most cases, a central venous catheter.

For a patient who develops pericardial tamponade in the early postoperative period after cardiac or thoracic surgery while still intubated, administration of an opioid and a muscle relaxant may provide sufficient anesthesia. In other patients

who are hemodynamically unstable, pericardiocentesis or subxiphoid pericardiotomy should be performed with local anesthesia only. If a patient is stable enough to receive sedation, small doses of ketamine are a good choice.[264] If general anesthesia is an absolute necessity, as in cases of single chamber tamponade not amenable to pericardiocentesis, induction should be accomplished in a manner that allows for continuous spontaneous ventilation. Institution of positive-pressure ventilation in these critically ill patients results in positive intrathoracic pressure, which frequently proves deleterious to blood return to a ventricle which is already unable to fill, resulting in profound hypotension and possibly precipitating sudden death.

#### Chronic Pericardial Effusion

Patients with chronic pericardial effusions may be well compensated enough to receive a general anesthetic, but the same hemodynamic goals as for pericardial tamponade should be kept in mind until pericardial fluid has been removed. Until that has been accomplished, spontaneous ventilation, perhaps including awake intubation, should be maintained to avoid reductions in venous return due to positive-pressure ventilation.

### *How Can Spinal Cord Electrical Stimulation Be Used for Patients With Intractable Angina?*

There has been recent multidisciplinary interest in the treatment of patients with refractory chest pain with inoperable coronary anatomy through the use of spinal cord electrical stimulation (SCES). The principle of SCES can be applied to these patients in much the same fashion as for other sufferers of chronic pain due to somatic origins. SCES has been shown to improve or abolish the time to angina of patients paced at or above previous angina-inducing threshold heart rates.[265] Although mortality in these patients does not appear to be affected, use of SCES in this select patient population has the potential to improve quality of life.

### References

1. Hlakty MA, Boineau RE, Higgenbotham MB, et al. A brief self-administered questionnaire to determine functional capacity [the Duke Activity Status Index]. *Am J Cardiol.* 1989;64:651.
2. Campeau L. Grading of angina pectoris. *Circulation.* 1975;54:522.
3. Braunwald E. Unstable angina: a classification. *Circulation.* 1989;80:410.
4. Van Mittenburg-Van Zijl AJ, Simoons ML, Veerhoek RJ, et al. Incidence and follow-up of Braunwald subgroups in unstable angina pectoris. *J Am Coll Cardiol.* 1995;25:1286.
5. Parker JO, Chiong MA, West RO, et al. Sequential alterations in myocardial lactate metabolism, ST segments, and left ventricular function during angina induced by atrial pacing. *Circulation.* 1969;40:113.
6. Upton MT, Rerych SK, Newman GE, et al. Detecting abnormalities in left ventricular function during exercise before angina and ST-segment depression. *Circulation.* 1980;62:341.
7. Ambrosio G, Betocchi S, Pace L, et al. Prolonged impairment of regional contractile function after resolution of exercise induced angina. *Circulation.* 1996;94:2455.
8. Goldman L, Cook EF, Loscalzo A. Comparative reproducibility and validity of systems for assessing cardiovascular functional class: advantages of a new specific activity scale. *Circulation.* 1981;64:1227.
9. Benchimol A, Harris CL, Desser KB, et al. Resting electrocardiogram in major coronary artery disease. *JAMA.* 1973;224:1489.

10. Mangano DT. Preoperative assessment of the patient with ischemic heart disease. In: Mangano DT, ed. *Preoperative Cardiac Assessment.* Philadelphia, Pa: JB Lippincott; 1990:1.

11. Sheikh KH, Bengston JR, Helmy S, et al. Relation of quantitative coronary lesion measurements to the development of exercise-induced ischemia assessed by exercise echocardiography. *J Am Coll Cardiol.* 1990;15:1043.

12. Sato H, Iwasaki T, Toyama T, et al. Prediction of functional recovery after revascularization in coronary artery disease using (18)F-FDG and (123)I-BMIPP SPECT. *Chest.* 2000;117:65.

13. Braunwald E. Valvular heart disease. In: Braunwald E, ed. *Heart Disease: A Textbook of Cardiovascular Medicine.* 5th ed. Philadelphia, Pa: WB Saunders; 1997:1007.

14. Cahalan MK. Anesthesia for cardiac valvular surgery. International Anesthesia Research Society 2000 review course lectures. *Anesth Analg.* 2000;(suppl IARS):1.

15. ACC/AHA Practice Guidelines. *Executive Summary. Guidelines for the Management of Patients With Valvular Heart Disease. A Report of the American College of Cardiology/American Heart Association Task Force on Practice Guidelines. Committee on Management of Patients With Valvular Heart Disease. Circulation.* 1998;98:1949.

16. Ross J, Braunwald E. The influence of corrective operations on the natural history of aortic stenosis. *Circulation.* 1968;37(suppl 5):61.

17. Frank S, Johnson A, Ross J Jr. Natural history of valvular aortic stenosis. *Br Heart J.* 1973;35:41.

18. Jackson JM, Thomas SJ. Valvular heart disease. In: Kaplan JA, ed. *Cardiac Anesthesia.* 4th ed. Philadelphia, Pa: WB Saunders; 1999:727.

19. Hakki AH, Kimbiris D, Iskandrian AS, et al. Angina pectoris and coronary artery disease in patients with severe aortic valvular disease. *Am Heart J.* 1980;100:441.

20. Carabello BA, Crawford FA Jr. Valvular heart disease. *N Engl J Med.* 1997;337:32.

21. Hartman GS, Thomas SJ. Valvular heart disease. In: Yao J, Fun-Sun F, eds. *Yao & Artusio's Anesthesiology: Problem-Oriented Patient Management.* 4th ed. Philadelphia, Pa: JB Lippincott; 1998:194.

22. Dare AJ, Veinot JP, Edwards WD, et al. New observations on the etiology of aortic valve disease. *Human Pathol.* 1993;24:1330.

23. Olson, L, Subramanian R, Ackermann DM. Surgical pathology of the mitral valve: a study of 712 cases spanning 21 years. *Mayo Clin Proc.* 1987;62:22.

24. Moore RA, Martin DE. Anesthetic Management for the treatment of valvular heart disease. In: Hensley FA Jr, Martin DE, eds. *A Practical Approach to Cardiac Anesthesia.* 2nd ed. Boston, Mass: Little, Brown & Co; 1995:311.

25. Kumar A, Sinha M, Sinha DNP. Chronic rheumatic heart diseases in Ranchi. *Angiology.* 1982;33:141.

26. Delahaye F, Delahaye J, Ecochard R, et al. Influence of associated valvular lesions on long-term prognosis of mitral stenosis: a 20-year follow-up of 202 patients. *Eur Heart J.* 1991;12(suppl B):77.

27. Misch, KA. Development of heart valve lesions during methysergide therapy. *BMJ.* 1974;2:365.

28. Barrington WW, Boudoulas J, Bashore T, et al. Mitral stenosis: mitral dome excursion and M1 and the mitral opening snap—the concept of reciprocal heart sounds. *Am Heart J.* 1988;115:1280.

29. Waed C, Hancockk BW. Extreme pulmonary hypertension caused by mitral valve disease: natural history and results of surgery. *Br Heart J.* 1975;37:74.

30. Carabello BA. Mitral regurgitation. In: Rahimtoola SH, ed. *Valvular Heart Disease and Endocarditis. Atlas of Heart Diseases.* Vol 11. St Louis, Mo: Mosby; 1997;9.1.

31. Boltwood CM, Tei C, Wong M, et al. Quantitative echocardiography of the mitral complex in dilated cardiomyopathy: the mechanism of functional mitral regurgitation. *Circulation.* 1983;68:498.

32. Munoz S, Gallardo J, Diaz-Gorrin JR. et al. Influence of surgery on the natural history of rheumatic mitral and aortic valve disease. *Am J Cardiol.* 1975;35:234.

33. Carabello BA. Mitral regurgitation: basic pathophysiologic principles. *Mod Concepts Cardiovasc Dis.* 1988;57:53.

34. Schreiber TL, Fisher J, Mangla A, et al. Severe "silent" mitral regurgitation: a potentially reversible cause of refractory heart failure. *Chest.* 1989;96:242.

35. Grossman W, Barry B. Cardiac catheterization. In: Heart Disease: Braunwald E, ed. *A Textbook of Cardiovascular Medicine.* 3rd ed. Philadelphia, WB Saunders, 1988;250.

36. Kudenchuk PJ, Pierson DJ, Greene HL, et al. Prospective evaluation of amiodarone pulmonary toxicity. *Chest.* 1984;86:541.

37. Parker JO. Nitrate therapy in stable angina pectoris. *N Engl J Med.* 1987;316:1635.

38. Fam WM, McGregor M. Effect of coronary dilator drugs on retrograde flow in areas of myocardial ischemia. *Circ Res.* 1964;15:355.

39. Slogoff S, Keats AS. Does perioperative myocardial ischemia lead to postoperative myocardial infarction? *Anesthesiology.* 1985;62:107.

40. Slogoff S, Keats AS. Further observations on perioperative myocardial ischemia. *Anesthesiology.* 1986;65:539.

41. Viljoen JF, Estafanous FG, Kellner GA. Propranolol and cardiac surgery. *J Thorac Cardiovasc Surg.* 1972;64:826.

42. Slogoff S, Keats AS, Hibbs CW, et al. Failure of general anesthesia to potentiate propranolol activity. *Anesthesiology.* 1977;47:504.

43. Kopriva CJ, Brown ACD, Pappas G. Hemodynamics during general anesthesia in patients receiving propranolol. *Anesthesiology.* 1978;48:28.

44. Weiner N. Drugs that inhibit adrenergic nerves and block adrenergic receptors. In: Gilman AG, Goodman LS, Rall TW, et al, eds. *Goodman and Gilman's The Pharmacological Basis of Therapeutics.* 7th ed. New York, NY: Macmillan; 1985:181.

45. Slogoff S, Keats AS. Does chronic treatment with calcium entry blocking drugs reduce perioperative myocardial ischemia? *Anesthesiology.* 1988;68:676.

46. Chung F, Houston PL, Cheng DCH, et al. Calcium channel blockade does not offer adequate protection from perioperative myocardial ischemia. *Anesthesiology.* 1988;69:343.

47. Berge KH, Lanier WL. Myocardial infarction accompanying acute clonidine withdrawal in a patient without history of ischemic coronary artery disease. *Anesth Analg.* 1991;72:259.

48. Taggart DP, Siddiqui A, Wheatley DJ. Low-dose preoperative aspirin therapy, postoperative blood loss, and transfusion requirements. *Ann Thorac Surg.* 1990;50:425.

49. Babbs CF. Alteration of defibrillation threshold by antiarrhythmic drugs: a theoretical framework. *Crit Care Med.* 1981;9:362.

50. Gottlieb CG, Horowitz LN. Potential interactions between antiarrhythmic medication and the automatic implantable cardioverter defibrillator. *PACE.* 1991;14:898.

51. Fain ES, Dorian P, Davy J-M, et al. Effects of encainide and its metabolites on energy requirements for defibrillation. *Circulation.* 1986; 73:1334.

52. Reiffel JA, Coromilas JM, Zimmerman JM. Drug-device interactions: clinical considerations. *PACE.* 1985;8:369.

53. Fogoros RN. Amiodarone-induced refractoriness to cardioversion. *Ann Intern Med.* 1984;100:699.

54. Troup PJ, Chapman PD, Olinger GN, et al. The implanted defibrillator: relation of defibrillating lead configuration and clinical variables to defibrillation threshold. *J Am Coll Cardiol.* 1985;6:1315.

55. Guarnieri T, Levine JH, Veltri EP, et al. Success of chronic defibrillation and the role of antiarrhythmic drugs with the automatic implantable cardioverter/defibrillator. *Am J Cardiol.* 1987;60:1061.

56. Gaba DM, Wyner J, Fish KJ. Anesthesia and the automatic implantable cardioverter/defibrillator. *Anesthesiology.* 1985;62:786.

57. Holt DW, Tucker GT, Jackson PR, et al. Amiodarone pharmacokinetics. *Am Heart J.* 1983;106:840.

58. Bedford RF. Invasive blood pressure monitoring. In: Blitt CD, ed. *Monitoring in Anesthesia and Critical Care Medicine.* 2nd ed. New York, NY: Churchill Livingstone; 1990:93.

59. Moore CH, Lombardo TR, Allums JA, et al. Left main coronary artery stenosis: hemodynamic monitoring to reduce mortality. *Ann Thorac Surg.* 1978;26:445.

60. Rao TLK, Jacobs KH, El-Etr AA. Reinfarction following anesthesia in patients with myocardial infarction. *Anesthesiology.* 1983;59:499.

61. Tuman KJ, McCarthy RJ, Spiess BD, et al. Effect of pulmonary artery catheterization on outcome in patients undergoing coronary artery surgery. *Anesthesiology.* 1989;70:199.

62. Nelson LD, Anderson HB. Patient selection for iced versus room temperature injectate for thermodilution cardiac output determination. *Crit Care Med.* 1986;13:182.

63. Wolman RL, Shah J, Shapiro JH. Does the type of injectate solution alter the result of thermodilution cardiac output measurements? Paper presented at: Annual Meeting of the Society of Cardiovascular Anesthesiologists; May 5–8, 1991; San Antonio, Tex.

64. Lang RM, Borow KM, Neumann A, et al. Systemic vascular resistance: an unreliable index of left ventricular afterload. *Circulation.* 1986;74:1114.

65. Wallace CT, Marks WE, Adkins WY, et al. Perforation of the tympanic membrane: a complication of tympanic thermometry during anesthesia. *Anesthesiology.* 1974;41:290.

66. Cork RC, Vaughan RW, Humphrey LS. Precision and accuracy of intraoperative temperature monitoring. *Anesth Analg.* 1983;62:211.

67. Bone ME, Feneck RO. Bladder temperature as an estimate of body temperature during cardiopulmonary bypass. *Anaesthesia.* 1988;3:181.

68. Ramsay JG, Ralley FE, Whalley DG, et al. Site of temperature monitoring and prediction of afterdrop after open heart surgery. *Can Anaesth Soc J.* 1985;32:607.

69. Scott JC, Ponganis KV, Stanski DR. EEG quantitation of narcotic effect: the comparative pharmacodynamics of fentanyl and sufentanil. *Anesthesiology.* 1985;62:234.

70. Cook DJ, Oliver WC Jr, Orszulak TA, et al. A prospective, randomized comparison of cerebral venous oxygen saturation during normothermic and hypothermic cardiopulmonary bypass. *J Thorac Cardiovasc Surg.* 1994;107:1020.

71. Yao FF, Tseng C, Braverman JM, et al. Cerebral oxygen desaturation is associated with prolonged lengths of stay in the intensive care unit and hospital [abstract]. *Anesthesiology.* 1999;91:A123.

72. Bhaskerao B, VanHimbergen D, Edmonds HL Jr, et al. Evidence for improved cerebral function after minimally invasive bypass surgery. *J Card Surg.* 1998;13:27

73. London MJ, Hollenberg M, Wong MG, et al. Intraoperative myocardial ischemia: localization by continuous 12-lead electrocardiography. *Anesthesiology.* 1988;69:232.

74. Hauser AM, Gangadharan V, Ramos RG, et al. Sequence of mechanical, electrocardiographic and clinical effects of repeated coronary artery occlusion in human beings: echocardiographic observations during coronary angioplasty. *J Am Coll Cardiol.* 1985;5:193.

75. Kaplan JA, Wells PH. Early diagnosis of myocardial ischemia using the pulmonary artery catheter. *Anesth Analg.* 1981;60:789.

76. Haggmark S, Hohner P, Ostman M, et al. Comparison of hemodynamic, electrocardiographic, mechanical, and metabolic indicators of intraoperative myocardial ischemia in vascular surgical patients with coronary artery disease. *Anesthesiology.* 1989;70:19.

77. van Daele MERM, Sutherland GR, Mitchell MM, et al. Do changes in pulmonary capillary wedge pressure adequately reflect myocardial ischemia during anesthesia? A correlative preoperative hemodynamic, electrocardiographic, and transesophageal echocardiographic study. *Circulation.* 1990;81:865.

78. Smith JS, Cahalan MK, Benefiel DJ, et al. Intraoperative detection of myocardial ischemia in high-risk patients: electrocardiography versus two-dimensional transesophageal echocardiography. *Circulation.* 1985;72:1015.

79. Leung JM, O'Kelly B, Browner WS, et al. Prognostic importance of postbypass regional wall-motion abnormalities in patients undergoing coronary artery bypass graft surgery. *Anesthesiology.* 1989;71:16.

80. Haendchen RV, Wyatt HL, Maurer J, et al. Quantitation of regional cardiac function by two-dimensional echocardiography, I: patterns of contraction in the normal left ventricle. *Circulation.* 1983;67:1234.

81. Braunwald E, Kloner RA. The stunned myocardium: prolonged postischemic ventricular dysfunction. *Circulation.* 1982;66:1146.

82. Force T, Kemper A, Perkins L, et al. Overestimation of infarct size by quantitative two-dimensional echocardiography: the role of tethering and of analytic procedures. *Circulation.* 1986;73:1360.

83. Comunale ME, Body SC, Ley C, et al. The concordance of intraoperative left ventricular wall-motion abnormalities and electrocardiographic S-T segment changes: association with outcome after coronary revascularization. Multicenter Study of Perioperative Ischemia (McSPI) Research Group. *Anesthesiology.* 1998;88:945.

84. Coriat P, Daloz M, Bousseau D, et al. Prevention of intraoperative myocardial ischemia during noncardiac surgery with intravenous nitroglycerin. *Anesthesiology.* 1984;61:193.

85. Lowenstein E, Hallowell P, Levine FH, et al. Cardiovascular response to large doses of intravenous morphine in man. *N Engl J Med.* 1969;28:1389.

86. Klineberg PL, Geer RT, Hirsh RA, et al. Early extubation after coronary artery bypass graft surgery. *Crit Care Med.* 1977;5:272.

87. Campbell RL, Langston WG, Ross GA. A comparison of cardiac rate-pressure product and pressure-rate quotient with Holter monitoring in patients with hypertension and cardiovascular disease: a follow-up report. *Oral Surg Oral Med Oral Pathol Oral Radiol Endod.* 1997;84:125.

88. Leung JM, O'Kelly BF, Mangano DT. Relationship of regional wall motion abnormalities to hemodynamic indices of myocardial oxygen supply and demand in patients undergoing CABG surgery. *Anesthesiology.* 1990;73:802.

89. Philbin DM, Rosow CE, Schneider RC, et al. Fentanyl and sufentanil anesthesia revisited: how much is enough? *Anesthesiology.* 1990;73:5.

90. Choneim MM, Block RI. Learning and consciousness during general anesthesia. *Anesthesiology.* 1992;76:279.

91. Schwender D, Klasing S, Daunderer M, et al. Awareness during general anesthesia. Definition, incidence, clinical relevance, causes, avoidance and medicolegal aspects. *Anaesthesist.* 1995;44:743.

92. Liu WHD, Thorp TAS, Graham SG, et al. Incidence of awareness with recall during general anaesthesia. *Anaesthesia.* 1991;46:435.

93. Jordening H, Pedersen T. The incidence of conscious awareness in a general population of anesthetized patients. *Anesthesiology.* 1991; 75:A1055.

94. Horrow JC, Abrams JT, Van Riper DF, et al. Ventilatory compliance after three sufentanil-pancuronium induction sequences. *Anesthesiology.* 1991;75:969.

95. Leung JM, Goehner P, O'Kelly BF, et al. Isoflurane anesthesia and myocardial ischemia: comparative risk versus sufentanil anesthesia in patients undergoing coronary artery bypass graft surgery. The SPI (Study of Perioperative Ischemia) Research Group. *Anesthesiology.* 1991;74:838.

96. Leung JM, Hollenberg M, O'Kelly BF, et al. Effects of steal-prone anatomy on intraoperative myocardial ischemia. The SPI Research Group. *J Am Coll Cardiol.* 1992;20:1205.

97. Cason BA, Verrier ED, London MJ, et al. Effects of isoflurane and halothane on coronary vascular resistance and collateral myocardial blood flow: their capacity to induce coronary steal. *Anesthesiology.* 1987;67:665.

98. Slogoff S, Keats AS, Dear WE, et al. Steal-prone coronary anatomy and myocardial ischemia associated with four primary anesthetic agents in humans. *Anesth Analg.* 1991;72:22.

99. Tarnow J, Markschies-Hornung A, Schulte-Sasse U. Isoflurane improves the tolerance to pacing-induced myocardial ischemia. *Anesthesiology.* 1986;64:147.

100. Buffington CW, Davis KB, Gillespie S, et al. The prevalence of steal-prone coronary anatomy in patients with coronary artery disease: an analysis of the Coronary Artery Surgery Study registry. *Anesthesiology.* 1988;69:721.

101. Lillehaug SL, Tinker JH. Why do "pure" vasodilators cause coronary steal when anesthetics don't (or seldom do)? *Anesth Analg.* 1991;73:681.

102. Tomicheck RC, Rosow CE, Philbin DM, et al. Diazepam-fentanyl interaction—hemodynamic and hormonal effects in coronary artery surgery. *Anesth Analg.* 1983;62:881.

103. Roekaerts P, de Lange S. Con: midazolam is not the sedative of choice to supplement narcotic anesthesia. *J Cardiothorac Vasc Anesth.* 1993;7:620.

104. Samuelson PN, Reves JG, Kouchoukos NT, et al. Hemodynamic responses to anesthetic induction with midazolam or diazepam in patients with ischemic heart disease. *Anesth Analg.* 1981;60:802.

105. Newman M, Reves JG. Pro: midazolam is the sedative of choice to supplement narcotic anesthesia. *J Cardiothorac Vasc Anesth.* 1993;7:76.

106. Kumar SM, Kothary SP, Zsigmond EK. Plasma free norepinephrine and epinephrine concentrations following diazepam-ketamine induction in patients undergoing cardiac surgery. *Acta Anaesthesiol Scand.* 1978;22:593.

107. Jackson APF, Dhadphale PR, Callaghan ML, et al. Haemodynamic studies during induction of anaesthesia for open-heart surgery using diazepam and ketamine. *Br J Anaesth.* 1978;50:375.

108. Tuman KJ, McCarthy RJ, Ivankovich AD. Perioperative hemodynamics using midazolam-ketamine for cardiac surgery [abstract]. *Anesth Analg.* 1988;67:S238.

109. Newsome LR, Moldenhauer CC, Hug CC Jr, et al. Hemodynamic interactions of moderate doses of fentanyl with etomidate and ketamine. *Anesth Analg.* 1985;64:260.

110. Tuman KJ, McCarthy RJ, Spiess BD, et al. Does choice of anesthetic agent significantly affect outcome after coronary artery surgery? *Anesthesiology.* 1989;70:189.

111. Tuman KJ, Keane DM, Spiess BD, et al. Effects of high-dose fentanyl on fluid and vasopressor requirements after cardiac surgery. *J Cardiothorac Anesth.* 1988;2:419.

112. Vermeyen KM, De Hert SG, Erpels FA, et al. Myocardial metabolism during anaesthesia with propofol—low dose fentanyl for coronary artery bypass surgery. *Br J Anaesth.* 1991;66:504.

113. Manara AR, Monk CR, Bolsin SN, et al. Total i.v. anaesthesia with propofol and alfentanil for coronary artery bypass grafting. *Br J Anaesth.* 1991;66:716.

114. Flacke JW, Bloor BC, Flacke WE, et al. Reduced narcotic requirement by clonidine with improved hemodynamic and adrenergic stability in patients undergoing coronary bypass surgery. *Anesthesiology.* 1987;67:11.

115. Dorman BH, Zucker JR, Verrier ED, et al. Clonidine improves perioperative myocardial ischemia, reduces anesthetic requirement, and alters hemodynamic parameters in patients undergoing coronary artery bypass surgery. *J Cardiothorac Vasc Anesth.* 1993;7:386.

116. Abi-Jaoude F, Brusset A, Ceddaha A, et al. Clonidine premedication for coronary artery bypass grafting under high-dose alfentanil anesthesia: intraoperative and postoperative hemodynamic study. *J Cardiothorac Vasc Anesth.* 1993;7:35.

117. Schaps DK. Effect of barbiturates on myocardial metabolism and hemodynamics. *Fortschr Med.* 1982;100:1404.

118. Gunaydin B, Babacan A. Cerebral hypoperfusion after cardiac surgery and anesthetic strategies: a comparative study with high dose fentanyl and barbiturate anesthesia. *Ann Thorac Cardiovasc Surg.* 1998;4:12.

119. Aun C, Thomas D, St John-Jones L, et al. Intrathecal morphine in cardiac surgery. *Eur J Anaesthesiol.* 1985;2:419.

120. Swenson JD, Hullander RM, Wingler K, et al. Early extubation after cardiac surgery using combined intrathecal sufentanil and morphine. *J Cardiothorac Vasc Anesth.* 1994;8:509.

121. Chaney MA, Nikolov MP, Blakeman BP, et al. Intrathecal morphine for coronary artery bypass graft procedure and early extubation revisited. *J Cardiothorac Vasc Anesth.* 1999;13:574.

122. Chaney MA, Furry PA, Fluder EM, et al. Intrathecal morphine for coronary artery bypass grafting and early extubation. *Anesth Analg.* 1997;84:241.

123. Chaney MA, Smith KR, Barclay JC, et al. Large-dose intrathecal morphine for coronary artery bypass grafting. *Anesth Analg.* 1996;83:215.

124. Riedel BJ, Wright IG. Epidural anesthesia in coronary artery bypass grafting surgery. *Curr Opin Cardiol.* 1997;12:515.

125. Loick HM, Schmidt C, Van Aken H, et al. High thoracic epidural anesthesia, but not clonidine, attenuates the perioperative stress response via sympatholysis and reduces the release of troponin T in patients undergoing coronary artery bypass grafting. *Anesth Analg.* 1999;88:701.

126. Tenling A, Joachimsson PO, Tyden H, et al. Thoracic epidural anesthesia as an adjunct to general anesthesia for cardiac surgery: effects on ventilation-perfusion relationships. *J Cardiothorac Vasc Anesth.* 1999;13:258.

127. Kaplan R. ASRA consensus statements for anticoagulated patients. American Society of Regional Anesthesia. *Reg Anesth Pain Med.* 1999;24:477.

128. Ho AM, Chung DC, Joynt GM. Neuraxial blockade and hematoma in cardiac surgery: estimating the risk of a rare adverse event that has not (yet) occurred. *Chest.* 2000;117:551.

129. Michaelis LL, Hickey PR, Clark TA, et al. Ventricular irritability associated with the use of naloxone hydrochloride. Two case reports and laboratory assessment of the effect of the drug on cardiac excitability. *Ann Thorac Surg.* 1974;18:608.

130. Flacke JW, Flacke WE, Williams GD. Acute pulmonary edema following naloxone reversal of high-dose morphine anesthesia. *Anesthesiology.* 1977;47:376.

131. Bailey PL, Clark NJ, Pace NL, et al. Antagonism of postoperative opioid-induced respiratory depression: nalbuphine versus naloxone. *Anesth Analg.* 1987;66:1109.

132. Ramsay JG, Higgs BD, Wynands JE, et al. Early extubation after high-dose fentanyl anaesthesia for aortocoronary bypass surgery: reversal of respiratory depression with low-dose nalbuphine. *Can Anaesth Soc J.* 1985;32:597.

133. Slogoff S, Keats AS. Randomized trial of primary anesthetic agents on outcome of coronary artery bypass operations. *Anesthesiology.* 1989;70:179.

134. Sebel PS, Bovill JG. Opioid analgesics in cardiac anesthesia. In: Kaplan JA, ed. *Cardiac Anesthesia.* 2nd ed. Orlando, Fla: Grune & Stratton; 1987:67.

135. Reves JG, Flezzani P, Kissin I. Pharmacology of intravenous anesthetic induction drugs. In: Kaplan JA, ed. *Cardiac Anesthesia.* 2nd ed. Orlando, Fla: Grune & Stratton; 1987:125.

136. Lowenstein E, Reiz S. Effects of inhalation anesthetics on systemic hemodynamics and the coronary circulation. In: Kaplan JA, ed. *Cardiac Anesthesia.* 2nd ed. Orlando, Fla: Grune & Stratton; 1987:3.

137. Quasha AL, Loeber N, Feeley TW, et al. Postoperative respiratory care: a controlled trial of early and late extubation following coronary-artery bypass grafting. *Anesthesiology.* 1980;52:135.

138. Jardin F, Farcot JC, Boisante L, et al. Influence of positive end-expiratory pressure on left ventricular performance. *N Engl J Med.* 1981;304:387.

139. Cheng DC, Karski J, Peniston C, et al. Early tracheal extubation after coronary artery bypass graft surgery reduces costs and improves re-

source use. A prospective, randomized, controlled trial. *Anesthesiology.* 1996;85:1300.

140. Cheng DC. Impact of early tracheal extubation on hospital discharge. *J Cardiothorac Vasc Anesth.* 1998;12(6 suppl 2):35.

141. Cheng DC. Fast track cardiac surgery pathways: early extubation, process of care, and cost containment. *Anesthesiology.* 1998;88:1429.

142. Dowd NP, Cheng DC, Karski JM, et al. An intraoperative awareness in fast-track cardiac anesthesia. *Anesthesiology.* 1998;89:1068.

143. Robblee JA. Pro: blood should be harvested immediately before cardiopulmonary bypass and infused after protamine reversal to decrease blood loss following cardiopulmonary bypass. *J Cardiothorac Anesth.* 1990;4:519.

144. Starr NJ. Con: blood should not be harvested immediately before cardiopulmonary bypass and infused after protamine reversal to decrease blood loss following cardiopulmonary bypass. *J Cardiothorac Anesth.* 1990;4:522.

145. Young JA, Kisker CT, Doty DB. Adequate anticoagulation during cardiopulmonary bypass determined by activated clotting time and the appearance of fibrin monomer. *Ann Thorac Surg.* 1978;26:231.

146. Ward HB, Einzig S, Wang T, et al. Comparison of catecholamine effects on canine myocardial metabolism and regional blood flow during and after cardiopulmonary bypass. *J Thorac Cardiovasc Surg.* 1984;87:452.

147. Lazar HL, Buckberg GD, Foglia RP, et al. Detrimental effects of premature use of inotropic drugs to discontinue cardiopulmonary bypass. *J Thorac Cardiovasc Surg.* 1981;82:18.

148. Deakin CD, Petley GW, Smith D. Pharmacological vasodilatation improves efficiency of rewarming from hypothermic cardiopulmonary bypass. *Br J Anaesth.* 1998;81:147.

149. Drop LJ. Ionized calcium, the heart, and hemodynamic function. *Anesth Analg.* 1985;64:432.

150. Nussmeier NA, Moskowitz GJ, Weiskopf RB, et al. In vitro anesthetic washin and washout via bubble oxygenators: influence of anesthetic solubility and rates of carrier gas inflow and pump blood flow. *Anesth Analg.* 1988;67:982.

151. Heinonen J, Salmanpera M, Takkunen O. Increased pulmonary artery diastolic–pulmonary wedge pressure gradient after cardiopulmonary bypass. *Can Anaesth Soc J.* 1985;32:165.

152. Hansen RM, Viquerat CE, Matthay MA, et al. Poor correlation between pulmonary arterial wedge pressure and left ventricular end-diastolic volume after coronary artery bypass graft surgery. *Anesthesiology.* 1986;64:764.

153. Lobato EB, Beaver T, Martin TD: Comparison of milrinone and low dose epinephrine on grafted left internal mammary artery flow after cardiopulmonary bypass. *Anesth Analg.* 1997;84:SCA46.

154. Blas ML, Janelle GM, Urdaneta F, et al. Myocardial ischemia/infarction following cardiopulmonary bypass during coronary artery bypass grafting: does the inotrope matter? *Anesthesiology.* 2000;93;A259.

155. Urdaneta F, Janelle GM, Rayburn TA, et al. Effects of nitroglycerin versus milrinone, alone and in combination, on grafted internal mammary artery flow: abstracted. *Anesth Analg.* 1999;88:SCA45.

156. Lobato EB, Urdaneta F, Martin TD, et al. Effects of milrinone versus epinephrine on grafted internal mammary artery flow after cardiopulmonary bypass. *J Cardiothorac Vasc Anesth.* 2000;14:9.

157. Lobato EB, Martin TD, Gravenstein N. Milrinone, not epinephrine, improves left ventricular compliance. *J Cardiothorac Vasc Anesth.* 2000;14:473.

158. Stern DH, Gerson GI, Allen FB, et al. Can we trust the direct radial artery pressure immediately following cardiopulmonary bypass? *Anesthesiology.* 1985;62:557.

159. Mohr R, Lavee J, Goor DA. Inaccuracy of radial artery pressure measurement after cardiac operations. *J Thorac Cardiovasc Surg.* 1987;94:286.

160. Lavr MB, Strauss HW, Pohost GM. Right and left ventricular geometry: adjustments during acute respiratory failure. *Crit Care Med.* 1979;7:509.

161. Swerdlow CD, Winkle RA, Mason JW. Determinants of survival in patients with ventricular tachyarrhythmias. *N Engl J Med.* 1983;308:1436.

162. Wilber DJ, Garan H, Finkelstein D, et al. Out-of-hospital cardiac arrest: use of electrophysiologic testing in the prediction of long-term outcome. *N Engl J Med.* 1988;318:19.

163. Blakeman BM, Wilber D, Pifarre R. Median sternotomy for implantable cardioverter/defibrillator. *Arch Surg.* 1989;124:1065.

164. Gartman DM, Bardy GH, Allen MD, et al. Short-term morbidity and mortality of implantation of automatic implantable cardioverter-defibrillator. *J Thorac Cardiovasc Surg.* 1990;100:353.

165. Watkins L Jr, Taylor E Jr. The surgical aspects of automatic implantable cardioverter-defibrillator implantation. *PACE.* 1991;14:953.

166. Antunes ML, Spotnitz HM, Livelli FD Jr, et al. Effect of electrophysiological testing on ejection fraction during cardioverter/defibrillator implantation. *Ann Thorac Surg.* 1988;45:315.

167. Stoddard MF, Redd RR, Buckingham TA, et al. Effects of electrophysiologic testing of the automatic implantable cardioverter-defibrillator on left ventricular systolic function and diastolic function. *Am Heart J.* 1991;122:714.

168. Reddy S, Curtiss EI, O'Toole JD, et al. Cardiac tamponade: hemodynamic observations in man. *Circulation.* 1978;58:265.

169. Kaplan JA, Bland JW Jr, Dunbar RW. The perioperative management of pericardial tamponade. *South Med J.* 1976;69:417.

170. Bull BS, Huse WM, Brauer FS, et al. Heparin therapy during extracorporeal circulation, II: the use of a dose-response curve to individualize heparin and protamine dosage. *J Thorac Cardiovasc Surg.* 1975;69:685.

171. Gravlee GP, Haddon WS, Rothberger HK, et al. Heparin dosing and monitoring for cardiopulmonary bypass: a comparison of techniques with measurement of subclinical plasma coagulation. *J Thorac Cardiovasc Surg.* 1990;99:518.

172. Gravlee GP, Rogers AT, Dudas LM, et al. Heparin management protocol for cardiopulmonary bypass influences postoperative heparin rebound but not bleeding. *Anesthesiology.* 1992;76:393.

173. Horrow JC. Protamine allergy. *J Cardiothorac Anesth.* 1988;2:225.

174. Cheung JY, Bonventre JV, Malis CD, et al. Calcium and ischemic injury. *N Engl J Med.* 1986;314:1670.

175. Drop LJ, Geffin GA, O'Keefe DD, et al. Relation between ionized calcium concentration and ventricular pump performance in the dog under hemodynamically controlled conditions. *Am J Cardiol.* 1981;47:1041.

176. Drop LJ, Scheidegger D. Plasma ionized calcium concentration: important determination of the hemodynamic response to calcium infusion. *J Thorac Cardiovasc Surg.* 1980;79:425.

177. Royster RL, Butterworth JF IV, Prelipp RC, et al. A randomized, blinded, placebo-controlled evaluation of calcium chloride and epinephrine for inotropic support after emergence from cardiopulmonary bypass. *Anesth Analg.* 1992;74:3.

178. Robertie PG, Butterworth JF IV, Royster RL, et al. Normal parathyroid hormone responses to hypocalcemia during cardiopulmonary bypass. *Anesthesiology.* 1991;75:43.

179. Zimmerman ANE, Daems W, Hulsmann WC, et al. Morphologic changes of heart muscle caused by successive perfusion with calcium-free and calcium-containing solutions (calcium paradox). *Cardiovasc Res.* 1967;1:201.

180. Shen AC, Jennings RB. Myocardial calcium and magnesium in acute ischemic injury. *Am J Pathol.* 1972;67:417.

181. Henry PD, Schuchlieb R, Davis J, et al. Myocardial contracture and accumulation of mitochondrial calcium in ischemic rabbit heart. *Am J Physiol.* 1977;233:H677.

182. Jennings RB, Ganote CE. Mitochondrial structure and function in acute myocardial ischemic injury. *Circ Res.* 1976;38:(Suppl 1):I80.

183. Moffit EA, Sethna DH, Gray RJ, et al. Effects of calcium on the coronary and systemic circulation in patients after coronary surgery. *Can Anaesth Soc J.* 1982;29:313.

184. Fernandez-Del Castillo C, Harringer W, Warshaw AL, et al. Risk factors for pancreatic cellular injury after cardiopulmonary bypass. *N Engl J Med.* 1991;325:382.

185. Janelle GM, Urdaneta F, Martin TD, et al. Effects of calcium chloride on grafted internal mammary artery flow after cardiopulmonary bypass. *J Cardiothorac Vasc Anesth.* 2000;14:4.

186. Koski G. Con: calcium salts are contraindicated in weaning of patients from cardiopulmonary bypass after coronary artery surgery. *J Cardiothorac Anesth.* 1988;2:570.

187. Baer DM, Osborn JJ. The post perfusion pulmonary congestion syndrome. *Am J Clin Pathol.* 1960;34:442.

188. Urdaneta F, Lobato EB, Kirby RR, et al. Noncardiogenic pulmonary edema associated with protamine administration during coronary artery bypass graft surgery. *J Clin Anesth.* 1999;11:675.

189. Weng JT, Smith D, Graybar G, et al. Hypotension secondary to air trapping treated with expiratory flow retard. *Anesthesiology.* 1984;60:82.

190. Mochizuki T, Olson PJ, Szlam F, et al. Protamine reversal of heparin affects platelet aggregation and activated clotting time after cardiopulmonary bypass. *Anesth Analg.* 1998;87:781.

191. Kresowik TF, Wakefield TW, Fessler RD 2d, et al. Anticoagulant effects of protamine sulfate in a canine model. *J Surg Res.* 1988;45:8.

192. Ellison N, Ominsky AJ, Wollman H. Is protamine a clinically important anticoagulant? a negative answer. *Anesthesiology.* 1971;35:621.

193. Williams GD, Bratton SL, Riley EC, et al. Coagulation tests during cardiopulmonary bypass correlate with blood loss in children undergoing cardiac surgery. *J Cardiothorac Vasc Anesth.* 1999;13:398.

194. Valeri ACR, Cassidy G, Khuri S, et al. Hypothermia-induced reversible platelet dysfunction. *Ann Surg.* 1987;205:175.

195. Harker LA, Malpass TW, Branson HE, et al. Mechanism of abnormal bleeding in patients undergoing cardiopulmonary bypass: acquired transient platelet dysfunction associated with selective α-granule release. *Blood.* 1980;56:824.

196. Rinder CS, Bohnert J, Rinder HM, et al. Platelet activation and aggregation during cardiopulmonary bypass. *Anesthesiology.* 1991;75:388.

197. Rinder CS, Mathew JP, Rinder HM, et al. Modulation of platelet surface adhesion receptors during cardiopulmonary bypass. *Anesthesiology.* 1991;75:563.

198. Kucuk O, Kwaan HC, Frederickson J, et al. Increased fibrinolytic activity in patients undergoing cardiopulmonary bypass operation. *Am J Hematol.* 1986;23:223.

199. Goodnough LT, Johnston MFM, Toy PTCY. The variability of transfusion practice in coronary artery bypass surgery. *JAMA.* 1991;265:86.

200. National Institutes of Health Consensus Conference. Platelet transfusion therapy. *JAMA.* 1987;257:1777.

201. National Institutes of Health Consensus Conference. Fresh-frozen plasma: indications and risks. *JAMA.* 1985;253:551.

202. Bachmann F, McKenna R, Cole ER, et al. The hemostatic mechanism after open-heart surgery, I: studies on plasma coagulation factors and fibrinolysis in 512 patients after extracorporeal circulation. *J Thorac Cardiovasc Surg.* 1975;70:76.

203. Spiess BD, Tuman KJ, McCarthy AJ, et al. Thromboelastography as an indicator of postcardiopulmonary bypass coagulopathies. *J Clin Monit.* 1987;3:25.

204. Tuman KJ, Spiess BD, McCarthy RJ, et al. Comparison of viscoelastic measures of coagulation after cardiopulmonary bypass. *Anesth Analg.* 1989;69:69.

205. Kettner SC, Kozek SA, Groetzner JP, et al. Effects of hypothermia on thromboelastography in patients undergoing cardiopulmonary bypass. *Br J Anaesth.* 1998;80:313.

206. Shih RL, Cherng YG, Chao A, et al. Prediction of bleeding diathesis in patients undergoing cardiopulmonary bypass during cardiac surgery: viscoelastic measures versus routine coagulation test. *Acta Anaesthesiol Sin.* 1997;35:133.

207. Salzman EW, Weinstein MJ, Weintraub RM, et al. Treatment with desmopressin acetate to reduce blood loss after cardiac surgery: a double-blind randomized trial. *N Engl J Med.* 1986;314:1402.

208. Czer LSC, Bateman ATM, Gray RJ, et al. Treatment of severe platelet dysfunction and hemorrhage after cardiopulmonary bypass: reduction in blood product usage with desmopressin. *J Am Coll Cardiol.* 1987;9:1139.

209. Rocha E, Llorens R, Paramo JA, et al. Does desmopressin acetate reduce blood loss after surgery in patients on cardiopulmonary bypass? *Circulation.* 1988;77:1319.

210. Hackmann T, Gascoyne RD, Naiman SC, et al. A trial of desmopressin (1-desamino-8-D-arginine vasopressin) to reduce blood loss in uncomplicated cardiac surgery. *N Engl J Med.* 1989;321:1437.

211. Vander Salm TJ, Ansell JE, Okike ON, et al. The role of epsilon-aminocaproic acid in reducing bleeding after cardiac operation: a double-blind randomized study. *J Thorac Cardiovasc Surg.* 1988;95:538.

212. Montesano RM, Gustafson PA, Palanzo DA, et al. The effect of low-dose epsilon-aminocaproic acid on patients following coronary artery bypass surgery. *Perfusion.* 1996;11:53.

213. Watabe A, Ohta M, Matsuyama N, et al. Characterization of plasmin-induced platelet aggregation. *Res Commun Mol Pathol Pharmacol.* 1997;96:341.

214. Liu YC, Tsai TP. The effect of coagulation protection with combination of epsilon aminocaproic acid and plasma saver in open-heart surgery. *Acta Anaesthesiol Sin.* 1998;36:149.

215. Butterworth J, James RL, Lin Y, et al. Pharmacokinetics of epsilon-aminocaproic acid in patients undergoing aortocoronary bypass surgery. *Anesthesiology.* 1999;90:1624.

216. Horrow JC, Hlaavacek J, Strong MD, et al. Prophylactic tranexamic acid decreases bleeding after cardiac operations. *J Thorac Cardiovasc Surg.* 1990;99:70.

217. Brown RS, Thwaites BK, Mongan PD. Tranexamic acid is effective in decreasing postoperative bleeding and transfusions in primary coronary artery bypass operations: a double-blind, randomized, placebo-controlled trial. *Anesth Analg.* 1997;85:963.

218. Dunn CJ, Goa KL. Tranexamic acid: a review of its use in surgery and other indications. *Drugs.* 1999;57:1005.

219. Soslau G, Horrow J, Brodsky I. Effect of tranexamic acid on platelet ADP during extracorporeal circulation. *Am J Hematol.* 1991;38:113.

220. Pinosky ML, Kennedy DJ, Fishman RL, et al. Tranexamic acid reduces bleeding after cardiopulmonary bypass when compared to epsilon aminocaproic acid and placebo. *J Card Surg.* 1997;12:330.

221. Andersson L, Eriksson O, Hedlund PO, et al. Special considerations with regard to the dosage of tranexamic acid in patients with chronic renal diseases. *Urol Res.* 1978;6:83.

222. Royston D, Bidstrup BP, Taylor KM, et al. Effect of aprotinin on need for blood transfusion after repeat open-heart surgery. *Lancet.* 1987;2:1289.

223. Bidstrup BP, Royston D, Sapsford RN, et al. Reduction in blood loss and blood use after cardiopulmonary bypass with high dose aprotinin (Trasylol). *J Thorac Cardiovasc Surg.* 1989;97:364.

224. Menichetti A, Tritapepe L, Ruvolo G, et al. Changes in coagulation patterns, blood loss and blood use after cardiopulmonary bypass: aprotinin vs tranexamic acid vs epsilon aminocaproic acid. *J Cardiovasc Surg.* 1996;37:401.

225. Trinh-Duc P, Wintrebert P, Boulfroy D, et al. Comparison of the effects of epsilon-aminocaproic acid and aprotinin on intra- and postoperative bleeding in heart surgery. *Ann Chir.* 1992;46:677.

226. Alvarez JM, Goldstein J, Mezzatesta J, et al. Fatal intraoperative pulmonary thrombosis after graft replacement of an aneurysm of the arch and descending aorta in association with deep hypothermic circulatory arrest and aprotinin therapy. *J Thorac Cardiovasc Surg.* 1998;115:723.

227. Dietrich W, Dilthey G, Spannagl M, et al. Influence of high-dose aprotinin on anticoagulation, heparin requirement, and celite- and kaolin-activated clotting time in heparin-pretreated patients undergoing open-heart surgery. A double-blind, placebo-controlled study. *Anesthesiology.* 1995;83:679.

228. Levy JH, Pifarre R, Schaff HV, et al. A multicenter, double-blind, placebo-controlled trial of aprotinin for reducing blood loss and the requirement for donor-blood transfusion in patients undergoing repeat coronary artery bypass grafting. *Circulation.* 1995;92:2236.

229. Soltoski P, Salerno T, Levinsky L, et al. Conversion to cardiopulmonary bypass in off-pump coronary artery bypass grafting: its effect on outcome. *J Card Surg.* 1998;13:328.

230. Wu YC, Chang CH, Lin PJ, et al. Minimally invasive cardiac surgery for intracardiac congenital lesions. *Eur J Cardiothorac Surg.* 1998;14(suppl I):S154.

231. Pagni S, Qaqish N, Senior DG, et al. Anastomotic complications in minimally invasive coronary bypass grafting. *Ann Thorac Surg.* 1997;63:S64.

232. Ott RA, Gutfinger DE, Steedman R, et al. Initial experience with beating heart surgery: comparison with fast-track methods. *Am Surg.* 1999;65:1018.

233. Navia J, Cosgrove D. Minimally invasive mitral valve operations. *Ann Thorac Surg.* 1996;63(suppl):S35.

234. Wearn JT, Mettier SR, Klumpp TG, et al. The nature of the vascular communications between the coronary arteries and the chambers of the heart. *Am Heart J.* 1933;9:143.

235. Sen PK, Udwadia TE, Kinare SG, et al. Transmyocardial acupuncture: a new approach to myocardial revascularization. *J Thorac Cardiovasc Surg.* 1965;50:181.

236. Mirhoseine M, Muckerheide M, Cayton MM. Transventricular revascularization by laser. *Lasers Surg Med.* 1982;2:187.

237. Choo SJ, Shah PM, Oury JH, et al. Contrast echocardiography as an intraoperative method to determine the area of myocardium perfused by transmyocardial laser channels: an experimental study. *J Card Surg.* 1998;13:484.

238. Frazier OH, Cooley DA, Kadipasaoglu KA, et al. Myocardial revascularization with a laser: preliminary results. *Circulation.* 1995;92(suppl):1158.

239. Hardy RI, Bove KE, James FW, et al. A histologic study of laser-induced transmyocardial channels. *Lasers Surg Med.* 1987;6:563.

240. Cooley DA, Frazier OH, Kadipasaoglu KA, et al. Transmyocardial laser revascularization. Anatomic evidence of long-term channel patency. *Tex Heart Inst J.* 1994;21:220.

241. Horvath KA, Smith WJ, Laurence RG, et al. Recovery and viability of an acute myocardial infarct after transmyocardial laser revascularization. *J Am Coll Cardiol.* 1995;25:258.

242. Kohmoto T, Fisher PE, Gu A, et al. Does blood flow through holmium:YAG transmyocardial laser channels? *Ann Thorac Surg.* 1996;61:861.

243. Horvath KA, Cohn LH, Cooley DA, et al. Transmyocardial laser revascularization: results of a multicenter trial with transmyocardial laser revascularization used as sole therapy for end-stage coronary artery disease. *J Thorac Cardiovasc Surg.* 1997;113:645.

244. Kwong KF, Kanellopoulos GK, Nickols JC, et al. Transmyocardial laser treatment denervates canine myocardium. *J Thorac Cardiovasc Surg.* 1997;114:883.

245. Batista RJ, Santos JL, Takeshita N, et al. Partial left ventriculectomy to improve left ventricular function in end-stage heart disease. *J Card Surg.* 1996;11:96.

246. McCarthy JF, McCarthy PM, Starling RC, et al. Partial left ventriculectomy and mitral valve repair for end-stage congestive heart failure. *Eur J Cardiothorac Surg.* 1998;13:337.

247. Stephensen ER, Sankholkar S, Ducko CT, et al. Robotically assisted microsurgery for endoscopic coronary artery bypass grafting. *Ann Thorac Surg.* 1998;66:1065.

248. Griepp RB, Sunson EB, Hollingsworth JF, et al. Prosthetic replacement of the aortic arch. *J Cardiovasc Surg.* 1975;70:1051.

249. Mezrow CK, Midiulla PS, Sadeghi AM, et al. Evaluation of cerebral metabolism and quantitative electroencephalography after hypothermic circulatory arrest and low flow cardiopulmonary bypass at different temperatures. *J Thorac Cardiovasc Surg.* 1994;107:1006.

250. Svensson LG, Crawford S, Hess KR, et al. Deep hypothermia with circulatory arrest: determinants of stroke and early mortality in 656 patients. *J Thorac Cardiovasc Surg.* 1993;106:19.

251. Ergin MA, Griepp EB, Lansman SL, et al. Hypothermic circulatory arrest and other methods of cerebral protection during operations of the thoracic aorta. *J Card Surg.* 1994;9:525.

252. Nojima T, Magara T, Nakajima Y, et al. Optimum perfusion pressure for experimental retrograde perfusion. *J Cardiovasc Surg.* 1994;107:548.

253. Usui A, Oohara K, Liu TL, et al. Determination of the optimum retrograde cerebral perfusion conditions. *J Thorac Cardiovasc Surg.* 1994;107:300.

254. Usui A, Abe T, Murase M. Early clinical results of retrograde cerebral perfusion for aortic arch operations in Japan. *Ann Thorac Surg.* 1996;62:94.

255. Raza SM, Vasireddy AR, Candido KD, et al. A complete regional anesthesia technique for cardiac pacemaker insertion. *J Cardiothorac Vasc Anesth.* 1991;5:54.

256. Swerdlow CD, Winkle RA, Mason JW. Determinants of survival in patients with ventricular tachyarrhythmias. *N Engl J Med.* 1983;308:1436.

257. Wilber DJ, Garan H, Finkelstein D, et al. Out-of-hospital cardiac arrest: use of electrophysiologic testing in the prediction of long-term outcome. *N Engl J Med.* 1988;318:19.

258. Blakeman BM, Wilber D, Pifarre R. Median sternotomy for implantable cardioverter/defibrillator. *Arch Surg.* 1989;124:1065.

259. Gartmann DM, Bardy GH, Allen MD, et al. Short-term morbidity and mortality of implantation of automatic implantable cardioverter-defibrillator. *J Thorac Cardiovasc Surg.* 1990;100:353.

260. Watkins L Jr, Taylor E Jr. The surgical aspects of automatic implantable cardioverter-defibrillator implantation. *PACE.* 1991;14:953.

261. Antunes ML, Spotnitz HM, Livelli FD Jr, et al. Effect of electrophysiological testing on ejection fraction during cardioverter/defibrillator implantation. *Ann Thorac Surg.* 1988;45:315.

262. Stoddard MF, Redd RR, Buckingham TA, et al. Effects of electrophysiologic testing of the automatic implantable cardioverter-defibrillator on left ventricular systolic function and diastolic function. *Am Heart J.* 1991;122:714.

263. Reddy S, Curtiss EI, O'Toole JD, et al. Cardiac tamponade: hemodynamic observations in man. *Circulation.* 1978;58:265.

264. Kaplan JA, Bland JW Jr, Dunbar RW. The perioperative management of pericardial tamponade. *South Med J.* 1976;69:417.

265. Bagger JP, Jensen BS, Johannsen G. Long-term outcome of spinal cord electrical stimulation in patients with refractory chest pain. *Clin Cardiol.* 1998;21:286.

CHAPTER

# 64

# Anesthetic Considerations for Thoracic Surgery

William C. Wilson

PART **I**

# SPECIAL CONCEPTS OF THORACIC SURGERY

Modern anesthetic management of thoracic surgery patients requires expeditious preoperative evaluation and preparation, specialized intraoperative monitoring techniques, and efficacious postoperative analgesia. However, separation of the lungs is what differentiates thoracic anesthesia from other subspecialties in anesthesiology. Accordingly, this chapter focuses on the mechanics of one-lung ventilation (1LV) and the anesthetic considerations relevant to procedures requiring 1LV.

Thoracic operations requiring 1LV have numerous disease- and procedure-specific anesthetic considerations. For example, anatomic derangements (eg, stenotic left mainstem bronchus, aberrant supracarinal origin of the right mainstem bronchus) have specific anesthetic considerations during lung separation. Additionally, thoracic anesthesiologists need to be aware of the various types of benign and malignant tumors that can be treated by surgery (versus radiation therapy), as well as the side effects of radiation or chemotherapy. This chapter provides the information required to care for classic thoracotomy patients. In addition, other frequently encountered thoracic surgical procedures, such as mediastinoscopy and bronchoscopy, and care of thoracic trauma are reviewed here in separate sections. Finally, newer procedures in thoracic surgery with specific anesthetic considerations, such as lung volume reduction surgery (LVRS) and video-assisted thoracic surgery (VATS) are also covered. Other thoracic surgery subjects addressed elsewhere in this book (eg, thoracic aortic aneurysm resection, esophageal surgery) are not reviewed here.

## PREOPERATIVE EVALUATION FOR PULMONARY RESECTION

Numerous specific preoperative issues must be evaluated in the thoracic surgery patient. However, because the vast majority of thoracic surgical procedures (noncardiac, noncardiopulmonary bypass) involve resection or repair of lung or bronchial tissue, preoperative evaluation of a patient requiring pulmonary resection should address the following three questions:

1. What is the tissue type (ie, is it treatable by surgery)?
2. Has the tumor spread too far for surgical excision (ie, what is the stage)?
3. Is the patient likely to tolerate the planned surgery (ie, is he or she fit for surgery)?

## Which Pathologic Processes, Presenting as a Mass in the Lung, Are Surgical Lesions?

Both benign and malignant processes can present as a lung mass. Benign pulmonary masses include hemangiomas, carcinoid tumors, sequestrations, nonmycobacterial granulomatous disease (eg, Wegener's granulomatosis), and infectious processes (including bacterial pneumonias, tuberculosis, fungal mycetoma, hydatid cyst). Viral and mycoplasma pneumonias typically present as diffuse patchy alveolar infiltrates on chest radiographs and are not treated by resection. Several of the aforementioned benign infiltrative processes do have specific anesthetic considerations (detailed later in chapter).

The vast majority of pulmonary resections are performed for removal of malignant tissue. Accordingly, preoperative evaluation considerations should focus on issues relevant to the care of patients presenting with lung cancer.

Currently, lung cancer is the second most common type of cancer in the United States (15% of all cancer) and accounts for the greatest number of deaths in both men and women (28% of all cancer deaths).[1] Historically, lung cancer was a disease predominantly afflicting men. By 1965, the male-female ratio peaked at 7:1; however, by 1975, the ratio had slipped to 4:1, and by 1993, the ratio had evened out at 1.2:1.0.[2]

*Bronchogenic carcinoma* is a term commonly used to describe most lung cancers, but it is imprecise because not all arise from the bronchi. Peripheral adenocarcinomas typically arise from bronchioli. Lung cancer is most logically divided into two major categories: small cell (oat cell, small cell lung cancer [SCLC]), which accounts for 20% to 25% of all primary lung cancer, and non–small cell lung cancer (NSCLC), which accounts for the remaining 75% of cases.

### Small Cell Lung Cancers Are Rarely Operable Lesions

Prognosis in SCLC is usually poor, with average survival being 3 months following diagnosis for untreated patients. Therapy for SCLC rarely involves surgery because these patients usually present with disseminated disease, with metastasis to bone (35%), liver (25%), central nervous system, lymph nodes, subcutaneous tissue, or pleura (10%).[3] However, in some early stage patients (T1-T2 N0 M0), surgical treatment followed by chemotherapy has been successful.[4] The only prospective, randomized phase 3 trial of SCLC found similar survival rates for patients receiving induction chemotherapy and radiation followed by surgery or observation.[5] Therefore, surgical resection cannot currently be recommended as standard treatment. Rather, surgery is reserved for a small group

of selected patients with early stage disease, such as those who are found to have SCLC at thoracotomy (Table 64–1). Regardless of the diagnostic setting, whenever lung biopsy reveals SCLC, these patients should be referred for chemotherapy within 1 week, and they should start chemotherapy within 2 weeks of diagnosis.[6]

### Special Anesthetic Considerations for Patients With Small Cell Lung Cancer

Endocrinologic abnormalities and neurologic paraneoplastic syndromes are extremely common with SCLC. Forty percent of patients with SCLC manifest the syndrome of inappropriate antidiuretic hormone production (SIADH). The enhanced secretion of atrial natruretic hormone in these patients may further exacerbate this tendency toward hyponatremia, intravascular hypovolemia, and hypotension (particularly during induction of general anesthesia). Additionally, patients with SCLC may express the Eaton-Lambert myasthenic syndrome due to cross-reactivity between tumor associated antigens and calcium-gated ion channels. These patients are at increased risk for prolonged neuromuscular blockade.[7]

## Surgery Should Be Considered for All Cases of Non–Small Cell Lung Cancer

Non–small cell cancers are divided into 6 main types:

1. Epidermoid or squamous cell ($\pm 45\%$)
2. Adenocarcinoma ($\pm 20\%$)
3. Large cell anaplastic ($\pm 10\%$)
4. Bronchial carcinoid ($<5\%$)
5. Alveolar cell carcinoma ($<3\%$)
6. Sarcoma ($<1\%$)

Although prognosis is variable depending on the type of NSCLC and stage at diagnosis (see Table 64–1), all NCLCs respond to therapy in a similar way. Surgery is currently the only curative treatment for NSCLC and should be considered in all patients. However, $<20\%$ of NSCLC patients present at a stage that is amenable to surgical excision.[8] Furthermore, of those patients with NSCLC who undergo surgery, $<50\%$ survive 5 years.[9]

### Special Systemic Manifestations of Non–Small Cell Lung Cancer

Although cough, hemoptosis, weight loss, chest pain, and dyspnea are the usual presenting symptoms for lung cancer, endocrinologic and paraneoplastic syndromes are occasionally the presenting complaint. Although tumors secreting adrenocorticotropic hormone (Cushing syndrome) and antidiuretic hormone (hyponatremia and SIADH) are more common with SCLS (oat cell), secretion of parathormone (and consequent hypercalcemia) is more common with squamous cell carcinoma.[10,11] Bronchial carcinoids can cause carcinoid syndrome (although this is more common with gastrointestinal carcinoids that have metastasized to the liver). Other systemic manifestations of bronchial carcinomas include myopathies, neuropathies, and skin lesions (eg, acanthosis nigricans).[12] Additionally, apical lung cancers in the superior sulcus (known as Pancoast tumors) can invade the cervical sympa-

**TABLE 64–1.** Histologic Types of Primary Lung Cancers, Their Incidence, and the Utility of Surgical Resection

| Histologic Type of Lung Cancer | % of all Lung Cancer | Is Surgical Resection Indicated? | Comments (smoking association., prognosis) |
|---|---|---|---|
| Squamous cell (epidermoid) | 45* | Yes, providing stage < $T_3 N_2 M_0$ Tends to metastasize locally, and later than other bronchogenic carcinomas. | Growth rate is more rapid than other NSCLCs. Is associated with smoking. Prognosis is fair, good if caught early. |
| Small cell (oat cell) | 20%–25% | Rarely, in early-stage ($T_1$-$T_2 N_0 M_0$) in combination with postoperative chemotherapy. 80% respond to chemotherapy but most relapse and die within 2 years. Radiation therapy is used for local control. | Usually disseminated at diagnosis. SIADH and other endocrine or paraneoplastic syndromes common. Cigarette smoking accounts for >90% of cases. Prognosis is very poor. |
| Adenocarcinoma (most common: bronchial origin, uncommon: bronchioloalveolar) | 15%–25%* | Yes, providing stage < $T_3 N_2 M_0$ | Tend to be peripheral, slower growing, sometimes associated with areas of scarring, less closely associated with smoking. Prognosis is usually good. |
| Large cell anaplastic | 10% | Yes, providing stage < $T_3 N_2 M_0$ May represent SCCA or adenocarcinomas too undifferentiated to identify cell type. | Rapid growth rate and undifferentiated cell type. Is associated with smoking. Prognosis is poor. |
| Bronchial carcinoid (bronchial adenoma) | <5% | Yes, providing stage < $T_3 N_2 M_0$ Slowly growing, but locally invasive. | Usually age <40 years, occasionally metastasize. Prognosis is good. |
| Alveolar cell (bronchiolar) | <3% | Yes, providing stage < $T_3 N_2 M_0$ behaves more like a benign expanding lesion because it rarely invades. | Native septal wall architecture preserved. Occurs in patients of all ages. Prognosis is usually good. |
| Sarcoma | <1% | Yes, providing stage < $T_3 N_2 M_0$ | Arise from the connective tissue framework of lung. Prognosis varies. |

TNM relates to the international non–small cell lung carcinoma primary size of tumor (T); nodal involvement (N); distant metastasis (M) staging system (see text for details). Prognosis stated takes into consideration the stage of the disease at presentation (ie, early versus late stage).
*The incidence of squamous cell carcinoma of the lung is on the decrease, and the incidence of adenocarcinoma of the lung is on the increase.
SIADH, syndrome of inappropriate antidiuretic hormone production.
The incidences in this table taken in part from Landis SH, Murray T, Bolden S, et al. Cancer statistics, 1988. *CA Cancer J Clin.* 1998;48:6; Humphrey WS, Smart CR, Winchester DP. National survey of the pattern of care for carcinoma of the lung. *J Thorac Cardiovasc Surg.* 1990;100:837; and Galofre M, et al. Pathologic classification and surgical treatment of bronchogenic carcinoma. *Surg Gynecol Obstet.* 1964;119:51.

thetic plexus (causing pain in the distribution of the ulnar nerve) or the subclavian vein (causing a superior vena cava syndrome [SVCS]) or cause a Horner syndrome (ipsilateral ptosis, miosis, exophthalmos, and anhidrosis).

## What Is the International Staging System for Non–Small Cell Lung Cancer

Staging—the quantitative determination of the extent of tumor spread—for lung cancer uses the international TNM classification first agreed on in 1986, revised in 1992, and revised again in 1997.[13] The TNM classification requires determination of the tumor size (T), the extent of nodal involvement (N), and the presence or absence of metastasis (M), and is summarized in Table 64–2.

Briefly, a T1 tumor is <3 cm in its greatest dimension and is completely surrounded by lung or visceral pleura with no bronchoscopic evidence of invasion in any main bronchus. T2 indicates that the tumor is >3 cm in diameter, or invades the visceral pleura or main bronchi (but >2 cm from the carina), or is associated with obstructive atelectasis or pneumonia. Tumors that invade the parietal pleura, extend closer to the carina than 2 cm, or are associated with collapse of an entire lung are labeled T3. T4 tumors are those associated with a malignant pleural effusion or invasion of generally unresect-

able structures such as the heart, great vessels, trachea, vertebral body, carina, or esophagus. N0 indicates no nodal involvement; N1 indicates ipsilateral peribronchial or hilar nodal involvement within visceral pleura; N2 indicates involvement of ipsilateral mediastinal or subcrinal nodes; and N3 indicates contralateral mediastinal or hilar, supraclavicular, or interscalene nodes. M0 indicates no evidence of distant metastasis and M1 means distant metastasis present.

When each TNM value is summarized for a patient, a stage grouping can be assigned that correlates with prognosis and dictates operability. The stage groupings are also summarized in Table 64–2. Operations are usually indicated for stage I–IIIa and not for IIIb–IV. However, controversy exists regarding the proper staging of satellite lesions in the ipsilateral lobe of the primary lesion. In the 1992 criteria, this would be a high *grade T* designation; however, according to the 1997 revision, this is categorized as *metastatic disease*. Okada and colleagues have recently reported data that indicate ipsilateral satellite lesions should be reclassified according to the 1992 standards because this would categorize the lesion as operable, and thus improve survival.[14]

Despite significant advances, the diagnosis of lung cancer continues to portend a dismal overall prognosis. Of every 100 patients with lung cancer, 65 will be inoperable at presentation. Of the 35 who receive operations, only 20 will have resectable disease. Of those 20 patients, 8 will be alive in 5 years, and only 4 will be alive at 10 years.

**TABLE 64–2.** International TNM Staging for Non-Small Cell Lung Cancer*

| Category | Class | Criteria Required for Classification |
|---|---|---|
| Primary Size of Tumor (T) | $T_0$ | No evidence of primary tumor by cytology, bronchoscopy, or radiographic evaluation |
| | $T_1$ | Tumor is 3 cm or less in its greatest dimension, but completely surrounded by tissue |
| | $T_2$ | Tumor >3 cm in diameter, or invades the visceral pleura, or has postobstructive atelectasis or pneumonia, but does not extend within 2 cm of carina |
| | $T_3$ | Tumor invades the parietal pleura, associated with total lung collapse, extends within 2 cm of (but does not involve) carina |
| | $T_4$ | Tumor associated with a malignant pleural effusion or invades generally unresectable structures (heart, great vessels, trachea or carina, vertebral bodies, esophagus) |
| Extent of Nodal Involvement (N) | $N_0$ | No nodal involvement |
| | $N_1$ | Involvement within visceral pleura |
| | $N_2$ | Involvement of nodes on ipsilateral mediastinum |
| | $N_3$ | Contralateral mediastinal hilar, supraclavicular, or interscalene nodes |
| Evidence of Metastasis (M) | $M_0$ | No evidence of distant metastasis |
| | $M_1$ | Distant metastasis present |
| Stage Groupings† | Stage I | $T_{<3} N_0 M_0 \rightarrow$ Surgery indicated |
| | Stage II | $T_{<3} N_{<2} M_0 \rightarrow$ Surgery indicated |
| | Stage IIIa | $T_{<4} N_{<3} M_0 \rightarrow$ Surgery indicated |
| | Stage IIIb | $T_{0-4} N_{0-3} M_0 \rightarrow$ No surgical benefit |
| | Stage IV | $T_{1-4} N_{0-3} M_1 \rightarrow$ No surgical benefit |

*Staging criteria from Mountain CF. A new international staging system for lung cancer. *Chest.* 1986;89(suppl 4):225S.

†Controversy exists as to whether ipsilateral satellite lesions represent disease more akin to direct extension (higher T score) or metastasis (see text for explanation).

## Is Your Patient Fit for Surgery?

### History, General Risk Factors, and Physical Examination

History is mainly focused on the airways, exercise tolerance, dyspnea symptoms, oxygen ($O_2$) use, sputum production, and bronchodilator use. Additionally, several demographic factors are associated with survival from lung cancer. Women survive longer than men following lung cancer excision for all grades and stages of NSCLC.[15] Age >60 years has been shown to correlate with a worse prognosis,[16,17] as does malnutrition and low serum protein.[18] Prior radiation therapy, which may have airway implications, and chemotherapy (eg, bleomycin), which may cause pulmonary pathology, are important elements of a patient's history. Additionally, four easily rectified deleterious aspects of the patient's condition should be sought out and eliminated if present: smoking, bronchospasm, copious secretions, purulent secretions. These conditions—and their specific impacts and treatments—are discussed further in the section on preoperative preparation. It also bears mentioning here that cessation from smoking, even for a few days, may have a significant positive impact on postoperative outcome (Table 64–3).

**TABLE 64–3.** Beneficial Effects of Smoking Cessation and Time Course

| Time Course | Beneficial Effects |
|---|---|
| 12–24 h | Decreased CO and nicotine levels |
| 48–72 h | CO-Hb levels normalized, ciliary function improves |
| 1–2 wk | Decreased sputum production |
| 4–6 wk | PFTs improve |
| 6–8 wk | Immune function and metabolism normalizes |
| 8–12 wk | Decreased overall postoperative morbidity and mortality |

CO, carbon monoxide; CO-Hb, carboxyhemoglobin; PFTs, pulmonary function tests.

Although spirometric and other quantitative tests are more predictive, physical examination findings may identify respiratory problems that relate to increased perioperative risk. Inspection may reveal a barrel-shaped thorax, suggestive of chronic obstructive lung disease (COLD), kyphoscoliosis, obesity, pectus excavation, prior mastectomy, radiation therapy, or a burn scar suggestive of restrictive physiology. Scars from tracheotomy may indicate tracheomalacia or tracheal stenosis and consequent difficulty in placing double-lumen tubes (DLTs). Scars from prior chest tube or thoracotomy indicate significant pulmonary surgical history—expect more bleeding during the case.

Additional peripheral signs of disease include cyanosis, clubbing, and nicotine-stained fingers. Pursed-lip exhalation suggests obstructive disease. Accessory muscle use suggests lung disease or impaired diaphragm function. The patient's back should be inspected for lesions that would contraindicate placement of a thoracic epidural. Palpation identifies asymmetric chest excursion and accessory muscle use. Percussion of the posterior chest measures diaphragm excursion, abnormal pleural fluid, or consolidation. A receding diaphragm during inspiration suggests phrenic nerve dysfunction. Auscultation frequently demonstrates distant faint breath sounds in COLD patients. Focally decreased breath sounds may occur with atelectasis, pulmonary infiltrates, empyema, or effusion. Rales may indicate congestive heart failure. All of these abnormal findings require chest radiographic evaluation. The ability to take a deep breath and cough vigorously is a basic indicator of the ability to clear secretions and prevent atelectasis.

### Bronchoscopic Airway Examination for Staging

The bronchoscopic examination is critical for staging (determining resectability), planning operative therapy, and deciding on the method of lung separation. Deviations from normal anatomy has clear implications for preoperative planning; thus, the anesthesiologist must understand normal and abnormal airway anatomy.

## Normal Airway Anatomy and Important Bronchoscopic Landmarks

The airway begins at the mouth and nares and extends through the oropharynx or nasopharynx into the supraglottic area, through the vocal cords, and into the trachea. The main function of the upper airway is to humidify air and to provide a passageway to the trachea.

The trachea begins at the level of the sixth cervical vertebrae in adults (Fig. 64–1). It is 10 to 15 cm long and ends at the carina (bifurcation of right and left mainstem bronchi) at about the fourth thoracic vertebrae in adults. The diameter of the trachea ranges from 1.5 to 2.5 cm. It is flattened posteriorly, rounded anteriorly, and supported by 15 to 20 horseshoe-shaped cartilaginous "rings." The flat posterior wall of the trachea is comprised of longitudinal smooth muscle fibers that continue their course down the right and left mainstem bronchi, and hence are used for determining right from left during fiberoptic bronchoscopic (FOB) examination. The anterior horseshoe-shaped cartilages continue as well.

The length of the right mainstem bronchus is about 2 to 2.5 cm; the left mainstem bronchus is 4.5 to 5 cm long in most adults. Rarely, the right mainstem bronchus has its take-off from the trachea just above the carina (as is common in dogs). In this situation, right-sided DLTs are contraindicated.

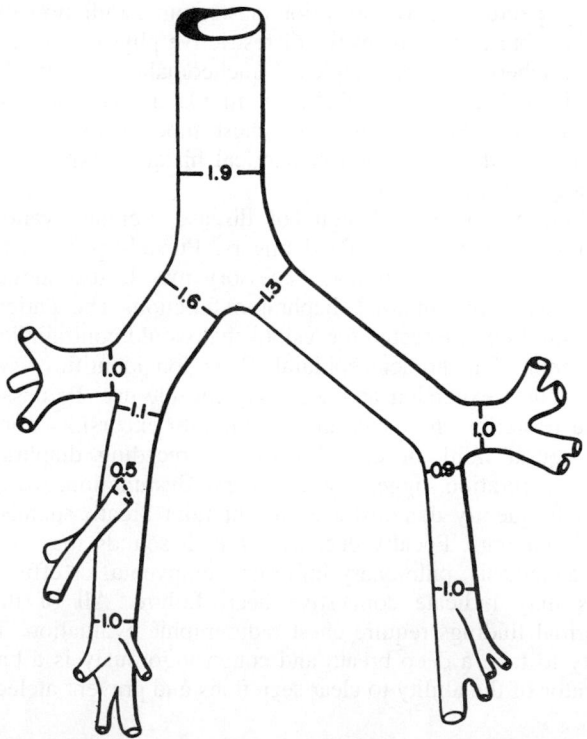

**FIGURE 64–1.** Mean tracheobronchial tree diameter (in cm) Note the right main stem bronchus is 1.5 to 2.0 cm in length. Whereas, the left main stem bronchus is 4.5 to 5.0 cm in length. Also note that the superior segments of both the right and left lower lobes are not depicted in this figure (see Fig. 64–2). (From Merendino KA, Keriluk LB. Human measurements involved in tracheobronchial resection and reconstruction procedures. *Surgery.* 1954;35:590.)

A left-sided DLT should be used for right-sided surgery, and a left-sided bronchial blocker (BB) should be considered for left-sided surgery. Occasionally, the left mainstem bronchus is stenotic, hindering placement of a left-sided DLT (see discussion section). The surgeon should tell the anesthesiologist these details preoperatively.

## Deferring the Staging Bronchoscopic Examination to the Operating Room

Bronchoscopy should be performed during the staging workup of any patient with a lung mass. However, for cost-saving reasons, certain patients with radiographically discrete lung lesions may have fiberoptic airway examination deferred to the operating room (OR).

The down side of the deferred FOB examination is that an intrabronchial lesion may be found, requiring biopsy, and may obviate surgical resection. When the FOB study is performed at this time, the patient submits himself or herself to significant additional risks and discomfort (placement of an arterial line, thoracic epidural, induction of general anesthesia). As mentioned previously, preoperative knowledge of any abnormal anatomy is critical for planning lung separation techniques. For these reasons, we believe that FOB examination should be performed by the pulmonologists in advance of surgery.

## Whole-Lung Pulmonary Function Tests Should Be Obtained on All Patients Scheduled for Pulmonary Resection

Approximately 30% of thoracotomy patients experience postoperative pulmonary complications.[19] These complications are related to both the removal of lung tissue and alterations in chest wall mechanics.[20] Several pulmonary function tests (PFTs) have definite direct predictive value in selecting candidates for pulmonary resection, including spirometry, determination of diffusion capacity of lung for carbon monoxide ($DL_{CO_2}$), room air arterial blood gas (ABG) values, among others. Furthermore, PFTs are useful for determining the risk of postoperative pulmonary complications (Table 64–4).[21]

### Spirometry

Spirometry is a simple, reliable, and inexpensive test with postoperative predictive value. The spirometer provides multiple lung volume measurements, including vital capacity (VC) and tidal volume ($V_T$). To measure VC, the patient inhales to total lung capacity, then exhales, either slowly (slow VC) or forcibly (forced VC) to residual volume. Figure 64–1 shows a spirogram for a normal individual. The normal VC is approximately 70 mL/kg; in a lean, healthy 70-kg adult, this would equal 5,000 mL. Table 64–4 displays minimal pulmonary function criteria for various sized pulmonary resections.

Additionally, spirometry provides information regarding dynamic airway disease. The forced expiratory volume in 1 second ($FEV_1$) is inversely correlated with the degree of obstructive airways disease. Patients without significant obstructive disease will exhale >80% of their VC in 1 second. The maximum midexpiratory flow rate is measured in the middle of the timed expiratory spirogram, also abbreviated as $FEV_{25\%-75\%}$. The $FEV_{25\%-75\%}$ provides the best measure of obstructive airways disease because it eliminates from consid-

**TABLE 64–4.** Minimal Preoperative Measurements or Predictions (of Postoperative Pulmonary Function) for Various Sized Pulmonary Resections

| Pulmonary Function Test | Units and Designation (Preoperative Value Versus Postoperative Prediction) | Normal | Pneumonectomy | Lobectomy | Wedge or Segmental Resection |
|---|---|---|---|---|---|
| $FEV_1$ | Liters (measured preoperatively) | >4.0 | >2.1–1.7 | >1.2–1.0 | >0.6–.9 |
| | Percentage (measured preoperatively) | >80% FVC | >50% FVC | >40% FVC | >40% FVC |
| | Liters (predicted postoperatively) | N/A | >0.9–0.8 | >1 | >0.6–.9 |
| $FEV_{25-75\%}$ | Liters (measured preoperatively) | >2 | >1.6 | 0.6–1.6 | >0.6 |
| FVC | Liters | >5.0 | >2.0 | — | — |
| MVV | Liters/minute (measured for 1 minute preoperatively) | 100 | >50 | >40 | >25 |
| | % predicted (measured preoperatively) | 100% | >50% | >40% | 25% |
| $DL_{CO}$ | % predicted (measured preoperatively) | 100% | >60% | — | — |
| | % (predicted postoperatively) | NA | >40% | — | — |
| Exercise Testing | Stair climbing (measured preop) | >10 flights | >5 flights | >3 flights | >2 flights |
| | $VO_2$max (L/min) | 2.8 | >1 | >1 | >1 |
| | Oxy-Hb sat drop with exercise | None | <3% | <5% | <5% |
| $PaO_2$ | mm Hg (whole lung measured preoperatively) | >90 | >80 | >70 | >60 |
| $PaCO_2$ | mm Hg (whole lung measured preoperatively) | 40 | <45 | <50 | <55 |

Volume and $VO_{2max}$ values based upon a 70 kg adult.

$DL_{CO}$, diffusing capacity; $FEV_1$, volume of gas exhaled in the first second; FVC, forced vital capacity; MVV, maximum voluntary ventilation; PFT, pulmonary function testing; sat, saturation; $VO_2$max, maximum oxygen consumption.

Data from Benumof JL. *Anesthesia for Thoracic Surgery.* 2nd ed. Philadelphia, Pa: WB Saunders; 1995:234; Gass GD, Olsen GN. Clinical significance of pulmonary function tests. Preoperative pulmonary function testing to predict postoperative morbidity and mortality. *Chest.* 1986;89:127; Crapo RO. Pulmonary function testing: current concepts. *N Engl J Med.* 1994;331:25; Thomas SD, Berry PD, Russel GN. Is this patient fit for thoracotomy and resection of lung tissue? *Postgrad Med J.* 1995;71:331.

eration the initial highly effort-dependent portion of the timed expiratory spirogram. If either the $FEV_1$ or the $FEV_{25\%-75\%}$ is less than acceptable for the planned resection (see Table 64–4), the test should be repeated after bronchodilator therapy. If the values remain low (eg, $FEV_1$ <2 L in a patient scheduled for pneumonectomy), split function tests should be performed.[22] Spirometry values do not return to baseline until 6 to 8 weeks postoperatively.[23]

### Flow-Volume Loops

Recording the inspiratory and expiratory flow versus volume (as opposed to time, as in spirometry) creates a semicircular loop with diagnostic power for separating obstructive from restrictive diseases. Flow-volume loops are also capable of separating variable intrathoracic (eg, tracheomalacia) from extrathoracic (eg, vocal cord paralysis) obstructive lesions. However, no prospective trials have shown flow-volume loops to be in any way superior to spirometry in predicting postoperative morbidity or mortality in patients undergoing thoracic surgery.

### Maximum Voluntary Ventilation

The *maximum voluntary ventilation,* also known as the maximum breathing capacity, is the maximum volume in liters that a patient can breathe over a 1 minute interval. The maximum voluntary ventilation provides a measure of pulmonary reserve. However, it is an extremely effort dependent PFT. The best results occur with a motivated patient and an encouraging physician who can coach the patient to properly perform the test.

### Diffusing Capacity

$DL_{CO2}$ relates the ability of gas to be transferred between the alveolar epithelium and the capillary membrane. Carbon monoxide (CO) is the gas used to study diffusion, as these results extrapolate well to diffusion of $O_2$. Decreased $DL_{CO2}$ is observed in cases of increased cardiac output, low hemoglobin concentration, ventilation-perfusion ($\dot{V}/\dot{Q}$) abnormalities, decreased surface area of the alveolar capillary membrane (eg, emphysema, bronchiectasis) or thickened membranes (eg, interstitial lung disease). One of the latter two explanations is deduced in patients with relatively normal cardiac outputs and hemoglobin values.

In one study of 38 preoperative and operative risk factors, $DL_{CO2}$ was the most important predictor of postoperative death and pulmonary complications.[24] A postresection value of >40% of normal is considered acceptable. Because of the measurement technique (single VC breath beginning at residual volume, breathing a mixture of helium and 0.03% CO), patients who have been smoking heavily before study (high residual CO values) may have falsely abnormal values.

### Exercise Testing

Exercise testing is a time proven, clinically useful, preoperative test of pulmonary fitness for surgical resection. However, exercise testing in impaired patients is a nonspecific predictor of suitability for lung resection because these tests are effort-dependent and involve more than just the pulmonary system (ie, they require adequate cardiovascular and skeletal-muscular function). Despite these shortcomings, several simple tests such as stair climbing or stationary bike riding continue to be used.

Patients should be able to walk >300 meters in 6 minutes (3 km/h) and should not suffer a decrease of >5% in arterial saturation to be considered for pulmonary resection. A more precise method to determine exercise tolerance is to formally measure maximum $O_2$ consumption ($\dot{V}O_2$max) in an exercise laboratory. A $\dot{V}O_2$max of 40 mL/kg/min (2.8 L/min in a 70 kg adult) is normal, whereas a $\dot{V}O_2$max <15 mL/kg/min (<1 L/

min in a 70 kg adult) is associated with an increased risk of postoperative pulmonary complications.[25]

### Room Air Arterial Blood Gas Studies

Room air hypercarbia ($PaCO_2$ >45 mm Hg) has been identified as a significant predictor of postoperative respiratory failure and death for several decades.[26,27] However, hypercapnia may result from reversible processes such as bronchospasm or a treatable infection. Therefore, attempts should be made to correct all potentially reversible conditions before obtaining the baseline ABG measurement. Persistent hypercarbia indicates high-risk for lung resection and is an indication to perform further testing, including split function lung studies.

Room air hypoxemia is an additional criterion for increased risk. However, changes in $PaO_2$ following thoracotomy and lung resection are variable. Indeed, some tumors may have already completely occluded both a bronchus and the blood supply to the corresponding lung segments. These patients have already undergone a functional autoresection by the tumor, and removal of the diseased portion of the lung should not yield any further decrement in $PaO_2$. Other patients may show an actual improvement in $PaO_2$ following thoracotomy and lung resection.[28] This occurs because a tumor may be obstructing the bronchus, resulting in atelectasis and infection, with some continued blood flow to the corresponding lung segment (shunt). Removal of that lung segment, with the concomitant ligation of its pulmonary blood flow, will eliminate the physiologic shunt, resulting in an increased $PaO_2$. Some patients with compromised respiratory reserve who undergo resection of a lobe for a small peripheral lung tumor that is not already causing $\dot{V}/\dot{Q}$ mismatch may have a decrease in their $PaO_2$ after the resection. However, aside from the above considerations, a room air saturation <90% or a change of >5% during exercise is associated with increased operative risk. On one hand, patients capable of performing PFTs and exercising at the levels indicated earlier (see Table 64–4) should be considered for pulmonary resection. On the other hand, patients incapable of producing the cutoff values shown in Table 64–4 have >75% chance of postoperative pulmonary complications.

### Split Function Lung Studies Are Reserved for Patients With Marginal Baseline Pulmonary Function Tests

Whenever patients fail to achieve any of the minimal values shown in Table 64–4, and pulmonary resection is required, right-left (individual lung) split function tests are indicated. The goal of split function lung testing is to estimate preoperatively the relative contribution of the diseased lung relative to the overall existing lung function. If the remaining lung tissue is inadequate, severe hypoxemia and cor pulmonale may result, leading to disability or death. Split function lung studies can be obtained via bronchospirometry, the lateral position test,[29, 30] $\dot{V}/\dot{Q}$ lung scanning, and balloon occlusion studies.[31]

Bronchospirometry, an early method of measuring split function, is the most direct technique.[32] An awake patient is prepared with topical anesthetics, a DLT is passed into the patient's airway, and spirometry measurements are taken from each side of the lung. Because of the invasive nature and patient discomfort associated with bronchospirometry, radioisotopic $\dot{V}/\dot{Q}$ scanning has replaced this test in most centers.

The lateral position test is a method of obtaining spirometric measurements in first the supine position, followed by both lateral positions, and back to supine. In most patients, the functional residual capacity (FRC) increases in the lateral position compared with the supine. The relative increase in FRC from each lung correlates with $O_2$ consumption and minute ventilation derived via bronchospirometric techniques.[33] However, radioisotopic $\dot{V}/\dot{Q}$ scanning correlates better with postoperative function when lung pathology is assymetric.[34]

### Ventilation-Perfusion Scans

$\dot{V}/\dot{Q}$ scans have replaced the extremely uncomfortable bronchospirometry studies. $\dot{V}/\dot{Q}$ scans use inhaled radioactive tracers, xenon ($^{133}$Xe), technetium ($^{99}$Tc)-labeled aerosol (for determining ventilation), and intravenous radioactive tracers such as $^{99}$Tc-labeled albumin microspheres (for perfusion measurements). This technique of radiospirometry yields accurate predictions of postoperative lung function.[35–37]

Radioactive scanning yields data on regional perfusion, regional ventilation, and regional lung volumes, from which one can estimate the percentage of lung function contributed by the lung segment to be removed. The perfusion scan alone is as accurate as the combined $\dot{V}/\dot{Q}$ scans in predicting postoperative pulmonary function. Preoperative prediction of pulmonary function after pneumonectomy is calculated as follows:

$$\text{Predicted Postoperative FEV}_1 = \text{Preoperative FEV}_1 \times \text{Perfusion (\%) to Remaining Lung}$$

For example, if the preoperative $FEV_1$ is 2 L and the perfusion to the lung that is to remain after resection is 45%, the predicted postoperative $FEV_1$ is 900 mL.

In the absence of adequate resolution of the $\dot{V}/\dot{Q}$ scans (especially at the lobar level), calculation of predicted pulmonary function after segmentectomy can be calculated by knowing the number of segments in each lobe. Using the nomenclature of Jackson and Huber[38] the distribution of the 19 segments (Fig. 64–2) is as follows:

Right upper lobe = 3
Right middle lobe = 2
Right lower lobe = 5
Left upper lobe (LUL) = 4
Left lower lobe = 5

Some texts consider the LUL to have 5 segments because the left apico-posterior segment branches into 2 subsegments. Loss of function due to segmental resection is calculated as follows:

$$\text{Preoperative FEV}_1 \times \text{Number of Functional Segments to Be Resected/Total Number of Segments in Both Lungs}^{39}$$

Most references support a lower limit of 800 mL as the minimal predicted postoperative $FEV_1$ that will be tolerated by the patient. This is based both on the observation that

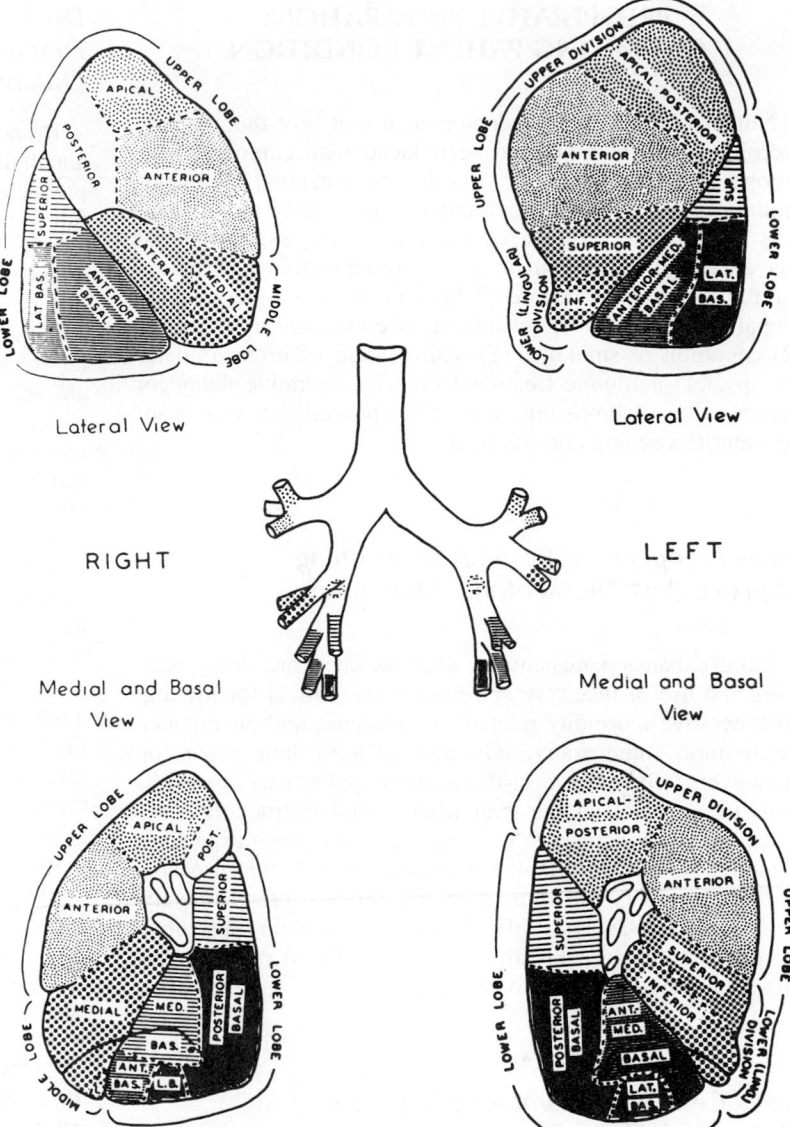

**FIGURE 64–2.** Tracheobronchial branching correlated with subdivision of the lungs. Each bronchus is marked the same as the segment it branches out to supply, and should be designated by the same name. The terminology used is that suggested by Jackson and Huber. (Modified from Jackson CL, Huber JF. Correlated anatomy of the bronchial tree and lungs with a system of nomenclature. *Dis Chest.* 1943;9:319.)

patients with COLD and an $FEV_1$ <800 mL have significant reduction in their level of daily function[40] and on a study suggesting that patients with COLD begin retaining carbon dioxide ($CO_2$) and develop hypercapnia when their $FEV_1$ value is <800 mL.[41]

### Unilateral Pulmonary Artery Occlusion

The pulmonary arteries (PAs) of normal patients are thin, distensible structures that passively dilate in response to increased cardiac output. However, patients with PA hypertension have less compliant PAs that cannot dilate to accommodate the increased flow. Forcing all of the blood to flow through only one PA in a pulmonary hypertensive patient (as would occur with a pneumonectomy) can lead to severe pulmonary hypertension in the remaining artery and consequent acute right heart failure.

The distensibility and compliance of the PA that will remain following pneumonectomy can be tested preoperatively by passing a balloon-fitted catheter (similar to a Swan-Ganz cath-

eter) into the main PA scheduled for resection (under fluoroscopic guidance). The 5-mL balloon is inflated, halting pulmonary blood flow through the diseased side, thus forcing all of the blood to travel through the side that would remain postpneumonectomy.

This test is somewhat unphysiologic in terms of ventilation, as the occluded side represents entirely dead space ventilation and the nonoccluded side has an increased transpulmonary shunt due to the increased blood flow from the occluded side. Regardless of these shortcomings, reproducible benchmark findings have been published. If the mean PA pressure exceeds 40 mm Hg (some authors use 35 mm Hg), the $PaCO_2$ exceeds 60 mm Hg, or the $PaO_2$ decreases below 45 mm Hg, with temporary occlusion of one PA, the patient is unlikely to tolerate pneumonectomy without developing cor pulmonale and right ventricular failure.[42,43] Regardless of the preoperative PFT or PA pressure data, temporary intraoperative PA occlusion testing (vascular clamp on PA proposed for resection) should always proceed pneumonectomy in order to verify that the patient can indeed tolerate the condition.

## PREOPERATIVE PREPARATION: OPTIMIZING PATIENT CONDITION

Numerous studies have documented that post-thoracotomy morbidity and mortality can be reduced with comprehensive preoperative preparation.[44-46] Besides, optimization of nonpulmonary systems (eg, cardiovascular, renal, and so on), maneuvers designed to promote postoperative lung expansion and gas exchange are the mainstay of preoperative preparation for thoracotomy procedures.[47] Specific areas of preoperative preparation include (1) rehabilitation education and training, (2) cessation of smoking, (3) optimization of bronchodilator therapy, (4) antibiotic treatment or brief operative delay for exacerbation of bronchitis, and (5) improved secretion management (loosening and removal).

### Does Preoperative Respiratory Training Improve Post-Thoracotomy Outcome?

Lung expansion maneuvers, such as deep breathing exercises and use of incentive spirometry, are critical for limiting postoperative morbidity related to atelectasis and pneumonia. Furthermore, preoperative education in these lung expansion maneuvers will reduce post-thoracotomy pulmonary complications to a greater degree than when initial instruction is delayed until after surgery.[48] The specific type of lung expanding maneuver is not important; the critical factor is that it occurs and that patients are trained in the process preoperatively. A recent meta-analysis of 14 studies comparing incentive spirometry and deep breathing exercises found no statistical difference between the two modalities.[49]

### Does Cessation of Smoking Improve Outcome in Thoracic Surgery?

Smoking has been a known risk factor for postoperative pulmonary complications since 1944.[50] Unfortunately, mortality and overall morbidity do not decrease significantly until 8 weeks of smoking abstinence has elapsed.[51,52] Despite this, smoking cessation for 12 to 48 hours preoperatively does convey several significant benefits by decreasing the concentration of carboxyhemoglobin (CO-Hb) and nicotine levels and improving ciliary function.[53,54] Indeed, cessation from smoking for 8 to 12 hours will decrease carboxyhemoglobin from nearly 8% to <4%. Decreasing the carboxyhemoglobin levels in blood increases the $O_2$-carrying capacity and shifts the oxyhemoglobin disassociation curve back to the right (improves $O_2$ delivery to tissues).[55] Other benefits of smoking cessation before surgery include improvement in PFTs, ciliary activity, immunity, and sputum clearance, as well as a decreased stimulus for bronchoconstriction.[56]

Additionally, abstinence from smoking will decrease myocardial ischemic events as well. Smokers have a 12-fold higher incidence of ischemic episodes (by Holter monitor) compared with nonsmokers with the same degree of clinical and angiographically proven coronary artery disease.[57] The benefits of smoking cessation are summarized in Table 64–3.

### Do Bronchodilators Improve Pulmonary Function Tests or Post-Thoracotomy Outcome?

Bronchodilation with a combination of inhaled $\beta_2$-agonist, anticholinergics, and steroids are the mainstay of modern preoperative preparation for COLD patients scheduled for thoracotomy.

Stimulation of $\beta_2$-adrenergic receptors with selective $\beta_2$-agonists such as albuterol leads to activation of adenylate cyclase followed by increased formation of cyclic adenosine monophosphate (cAMP). The increased amount of intracellular cAMP results in bronchodilation. Selective $\beta_2$-agonists are administered as inhaled aerosols, either via nebulizer or metered-dose inhaler (MDI). Selective $\beta_2$-agonists are the preferred drugs in the treatment of acute bronchospasm because of their rapid onset (initial benefit in seconds, peak effect in 15 minutes, lasting 4-6 hours), low systemic absorption, and less severe cardiovascular side effects compared with theophylline (ie, less tachycardia and dysrhythmias).

Anticholinergic drugs inhibit parasympathetic vagal innervation of the tracheobronchial tree, resulting in a decrease in the intracellular level of cyclic guanylic acid monophosphate, which mediates bronchoconstriction. Marini and coworkers discovered that inhaled atropine alone improved $FEV_1$ in 85% of patients with COLD.[58] When atropine was given together with terbutaline, the $FEV_1$ improved in 93% of the patients, whereas terbutaline alone improved $FEV_1$ in only 56% of patients.

Ipratropium bromide (Atrovent) is a quaternary ammonium derivative of atropine, available as an aerosol (nebulizer or MDI), that shares atropine's bronchodilator properties. However, ipratropium bromide is poorly absorbed from the tracheobronchial tree and does not easily cross the blood-brain barrier. Thus, ipratropium's therapeutic margin of safety is wide compared with atropine's, and severe side effects such as tachycardia, blurred vision, dry mouth, and hesitancy of micturition are rare. Compared with $\beta_2$-agonists, ipratropium's onset is slower (75% effect achieved in 15 minutes, complete effect in 1 hour, lasting 6-8 hours). Ipratropium's major clinical role is in the treatment of patients with chronic lung disease, in whom this drug usually is at least as potent a bronchodilator as the $\beta_2$-adrenergic agents.[59,60] Ipratropium should be considered first line therapy for COLD patients because they have increased baseline cholinergic tone compared with normal patients.[61] Both ipratroprium and a $\beta_2$-agonist (eg, albuterol) should be co-administered to COLD patients before lung resection because there is an additive bronchodilating effect that occurs with these drugs.[62]

Inhaled steroids do not directly relax bronchial smooth muscle; however, they do promote bronchodilation and inhibit bronchial hyperresponsivness. Inhaled steroids are the best known compounds to decrease mucosal edema and suppress inflammation in the tracheobronchial tree.[63] Inhaled steroids are slow to act, and some patients will tend to omit their use because they do not notice the more dramatic effects that result from $\beta_2$-agonists and ipratropium.

Systemic corticosteroids should be considered preoperatively for patients who have required steroid therapy in the past and are not at their baseline status before surgery.[64] A short course of perioperative corticosteroids does not increase the incidence of perioperative infections or other complications in patients with asthma.[65] It is likely, but unproved, that this favorable risk-benefit ratio also pertains to COLD patients and immunosuppressed lung cancer patients.

Cromolyn sodium stabilizes mast cell membranes, preventing their degranulation and release of chemical mediators responsible for bronchospasm, edema, and inflammation. This drug is useful in the prevention of bronchospastic attacks (especially in asthmatics) but has no role in the treatment of an acute attack and, in general, is less useful in older patients with COLD.

Methylxanthines, such as theophylline and aminophylline, are phosphodiesterase inhibitors that directly promote the accumulation of intracellular cAMP by inhibition of its enzymatic breakdown. The increased cAMP promotes bronchial smooth muscle relaxation. Additionally, aminophylline improves diaphragmatic contractility and the patient's resistance to fatigue.[66] Aminophylline has been shown to improve function in end-stage COLD patients with severe "fixed" obstruction (FEV >30%, unresponsive to $\beta_2$-agonists) due to the increasing strength of respiratory muscles.[67,68] Unfortunately, aminophylline has a narrow therapeutic window, with multiple significant side effects. Nausea, vomiting, dizziness, restlessness, tachycardia, dysrhythmias, and myocardial ischemia are common at serum levels above the therapeutic range (5-20 $\mu$g/mL). Additionally, seizures are seen in toxic states.

Despite these significant shortcomings, a selected few high-risk patients may merit the addition of aminophylline to the standard preoperative regimen of inhaled $\beta_2$-agonists, ipratropium, and inhaled steroids.[69] However, aminophylline blood levels must be closely monitored in these high-risk patients to avoid toxicity.

### Do Preoperative Antibiotics Improve Outcome?

Antibiotic therapy should be reserved for patients with a diagnosed acute or chronic infection because indiscriminate use only selects out more virulent organisms. A change in the color or quantity of sputum produced by a COLD patient may indicate infection. Amoxicillin, or another antibiotic effective against *Haemophilus influenzae* and pneumococci (the pathogens usually found in these patients' respiratory tracts), should be used until results of a Gram stain or culture and sensitivity tests indicate an alternate pathogen. An older prospective study found a lower incidence of postoperative pulmonary complications and even a lower mortality rate in the group of patients treated with prophylactic antibiotics before lung surgery.[70] However, no recent prospective studies have demonstrated any benefit of prophylactic antibiotics preceding the resection of noninfected lung tissue.

### Which Maneuvers Help Loosen and Remove Pulmonary Secretions?

Systemic hypovolemia and electrolyte imbalance should be corrected before surgery. This helps decrease the viscosity of bronchial secretions and facilitates their removal from the bronchial tree by increasing the tracheal transport velocity.[71] Humidification of bronchial secretions can be accomplished by use of an ultrasonic nebulizer or a respiratory humidifier.

Use of mucolytic agents such as acetylcysteine (Mucomyst) or an oral expectorant such as potassium iodide can benefit patients with viscous secretions. These mucolytic drugs decrease viscosity by depolymerizing mucopolysaccharides.[72] Unfortunately, these drugs are also irritating to the airways and can cause bronchospasm in sensitive patients.

Mobilization of secretions is achieved by a combination of deep breathing, vigorous coughing, postural drainage, and chest percussion.[73] Coughing alone in weak and debilitated patients is insufficient to clear peripheral airways because they are unable to generate a high enough air flow rate to sheer the secretions away from the airway wall. Weak and debilitated patients with inefficient cough capabilities benefit most from chest physical therapy.

### Do Patients With Gastroesophageal Reflux Disease Merit Specific Preoperative Preparation?

Since Kennedy first reported the association between pulmonary symptoms and gastroesophageal reflux disease (GERD) almost 4 decades ago,[74] numerous papers have reported improvement of asthma symptoms with antireflux medication[75] and surgery.[76] Likewise, GERD has been increasingly appreciated as a risk factor for perioperative aspiration. These patients are presumed to chronically aspirate greater quantities of gastric contents than normal patients during sleep. Many of these patients have reactive airway symptoms due to airway irritation. However, some investigators believe the asthma-like symptoms are due to a vagally mediated esophagobronchial reflex.[77] Antireflux therapy alleviates asthma symptoms but may not quantitatively improve PFTs.[78] Yet, one study demonstrated that antireflux surgery improves GERD symptoms and asthma symptoms, decreases asthma medication use, and improves pulmonary function in 90%, 79%, 88%, and 27% respectively.[79]

In my practice, I have found that some GERD patients may have chronic scarring of the epiglottis and an abnormal airway that can contribute to difficult intubation. These patients should receive preoperative nonparticulate antacids (Bicitra) and gastropropulsive medications such as metoclopramide. However, caution should be observed in administering $H_2$-receptor blockers (famotidine, ranitidine) due to the possibility of provoking bronchospasm. Histamine mediates bronchoconstriction via the $H_1$ receptor, whereas the $H_2$ receptor mediates bronchial dilation. Indiscriminate use of $H_2$ blockade could provoke unopposed bronchospasm via $H_1$. Thus, in cases involving COLD or asthmatic patients, where $H_2$ blockers are considered important, co-administration of $H_1$ blockade (Benadryl) should occur.

## INTRAOPERATIVE MONITORING

The intraoperative monitoring requirements of patients undergoing thoracic surgery is dictated by the degree of underlying respiratory and cardiac disease, the magnitude of the planned surgery, and in some cases by the proficiency of the surgeon. (Also see Chapters 18-20.) This approach has been termed a *tiered monitoring system*,[80] in which patients are stratified according to their physiologic condition and the anticipated demands of surgery so that increasing levels of monitoring sophistication are used for increasingly sick patients or complex surgeries (Table 64–5).

**TABLE 64–5.** Tiered Monitoring System for Thoracic Surgery Based on the Amount of Pre-existing Lung Disease, General Physical Condition, and Planned Operation

| Tiered System | Patient Category | Gas Exchange | Airway Mechanics | Endotracheal Tube Position | PA Pressures | Cardiovascular Status |
|---|---|---|---|---|---|---|
| *Tier I* Essential monitors used in all patients* | Routine healthy patients without special intraop conditions. | Color of tissues and shed blood $SpO_2$ $PETCO_2$ | Feel of breathing bag, stethoscope, PIP, $PETCO_2$ | EBBS (except ipsilateral tube clamp - > ipsilateral breath sounds disappear). Ballotable balloon in SSN, FOB after patient placed in lateral decubitus position | Not measured | NIBP, pulse oximeter waveform, ECG, $PETCO_2$, esophageal stethoscope, ± CVP ± invasive arterial pressure monitoring. |
| *Tier II* Special intermittent or continuous monitoring needs | Healthy patients with special procedures, or sick patients with routine procedures | As above plus frequent ABG studies | As above plus spirometry. Individual and whole lung compliance | FOB to verify tube position while in supine position, as well as in lateral decubitus position | Measure $P_{PA}$ if lobectomy or lung resection | As above, plus invasive arterial pressure monitoring, + CVP, + PA catheter (if poor EF, PA, HTN) ± TEE |
| *Tier III* Advanced monitoring | Sick patients with special intraoperative conditions. | As above plus $Q_s/Q_t$, $VD/VT$ frequent VBGs | As above plus airway resistance | As above plus frequent re-checks to verify position | Measure PA, CO, PVR, SVR, a-vDO$_2$ | As above plus PA + TEE |

*Presumes complete machine, ventilator, suction check, and routine monitors are in use including inspired $O_2$, precordial and/or esophageal stethoscope, capnography, $PETCO_2$, pulse oximeter ($SpO_2$), ECG, noninvasive arterial blood pressure, neuromuscular blockade (twitch) monitor, temperature probe. Each successive tier includes all of the monitoring modalities used in the lower numbered tier in addition to the ones listed in each successive tier.

ABG, arterial blood gas; a-vDO$_2$, arterial venous content difference (the amount consumed by tissue metabolism); CO, cardiac output; CVP, central venous pressure; EBBS, equal bilateral breath sounds; ECG, electrocardiogram; EF, ejection fraction; FOB, fiberoptic bronchoscope; HTN, hypertension; NIBP, noninvasive blood pressure; PA, pulmonary artery; Ppa, pulmonary arterial pressure; $PETCO_2$, partial pressure of end-tidal $CO_2$; PIP, peak inspiratory pressure; PVR, pulmonary vascular resistance; $Q_s/Q_t$, right to left transpulmonary shunt; $SpO_2$, saturation of oxygen measured by pulse oximetry; SSN, suprasternal notch; SVR, systemic vascular resistance; TEE, transesophageal echocardiography; VBGs, mixed venous blood gases; $VD/VT$, dead space to tidal volume ratio.

Various monitors used in general anesthesia have specific considerations for thoracic procedures and will be briefly reviewed in this section using an organ systems approach. The greatest emphasis is placed on neurologic considerations, pulmonary function, and cardiovascular monitoring because these systems are at great risk of injury (brain, spinal cord) or significant interference (heart and lungs) during thoracic anesthesia.

## What Are the Important Neurologic Monitoring Considerations for Thoracic Surgery?

The patient's neurologic status is tested and documented before placing a thoracic epidural or invasive lines and monitors. Thoracic epidurals provide excellent postoperative analgesia but should only be placed and tested preoperatively in awake teenage through adult patients. Placing thoracic epidurals in anesthetized, teenage through adult patients exposes them to significant neurologic risk that may not be apparent until the patient wakes up with paraplegia.[81] Pediatric patients may have thoracic epidurals placed via the caudal technique while asleep.[82] The patient's neurologic status is tested and documented again at the end of all thoracic cases because certain procedures (eg, thoracic aorta surgery, tumor excisions extending into the mediastinum) are associated with spinal cord injury.[83] Any postoperative impairment of neurologic status must be immediately evaluated. Specific neurologic monitoring for thoracic aortic surgery (somatosensory-evoked potentials, motor-evoked potentials) has been reviewed,[84] and is more thoroughly discussed in Chapter 21.

## Neurologic Monitoring Considerations Related to the Lateral Decubitus Position

The lateral decubitus position provides ample opportunities for neck and brachial plexus injuries. Be sure to maintain the neck in-line with the thoracic vertebra by resting the head on a doughnut-shaped sponge pillow supported by folded towels or blankets as necessary. In-line axial spine immobilization is particularly important in the trauma patient who is undergoing an emergency thoracotomy for repair of an aortic rupture.

An axillary roll is placed under the dependent chest up toward, but not entirely within, the axilla (proper placement of the axillary roll allows insertion of an arm between the patient's axilla and the axillary roll). The character of the patient's dependent arm pulse should be unchanged after moving from the supine to the lateral decubitus position (the anesthesiologist should specifically look for and verify this).

## Temperature Measurement and Neurologic Protection

Neuroprotection with mild hypothermia has been demonstrated in multiple animal models.[85,86] Additionally, several clinical studies involving human subjects have shown some improvement in neurologic outcome following treatment of traumatic brain injury with moderate hypothermia.[87] Despite these favorable data, the risk-benefit ratio for moderate hypothermia has not yet been completely elucidated. Yet, it is likely that neurologic outcomes will be improved using mild hypothermia (35°C) in patients undergoing procedures with a high risk of neurologic injury (eg, thoracotomy for thoracic spine surgery). When central nervous system protection is being considered, brain temperature should be closely monitored. Tympanic or nasopharyngeal temperatures correlate most closely with brain temperature.[88] The Swan-Ganz catheter thermistor provides a good measure of both core and brain temperature for patients not on cardiopulmonary bypass (CPB).

### Spinal Cord and Cerebral Perfusion Pressure

Cerebral perfusion pressure (CPP), calculated as (CPP = mean arterial pressure [MAP] − intracranial pressure [ICP]), normally measures >70 mm Hg. Certain thoracic procedures (eg, thoracic aortic surgery) require close vigilance of these concepts because increased ICP may impair spinal cord perfusion. In situations in which an ICP monitor is not indicated, high ICPs may still be interpolated from high central venous pressure (CVP) measurements. Because jugular venous blood drains into the central venous circulation, high CVP (>20-30 mm Hg) will increase ICP (decreasing the perfusion pressure to brain and spinal cord). If this occurs during thoracic aortic surgery in the setting of a low MAP, the CPP will be dangerously low, and spinal cord blood flow will be dangerously impaired.

## What Are the Important Respiratory System Monitoring Considerations During Thoracic Surgery?

Monitoring of respiratory function during thoracic surgery must minimally include auscultation of the breath sounds with an esophageal stethoscope and observation of the depth and rate of ventilation. During the procedure, after the patient has been prepped and draped, a stethoscope can usually be passed into either axilla to monitor baseline ventilation and spot check critical events. Once the chest is open, operative lung ventilation can be directly observed, but nondependent lung ventilation is best monitored by a stethoscope placed in the dependent axilla. Monitoring breath sounds gives valuable information about respiratory depth and rate, presence of wheezing, rales, or rhonchi; and occurrence and duration of apnea.

### Fraction of Inspired Oxygen Monitoring

An $O_2$ analyzer should be used during all anesthetics to confirm the fraction of inspired $O_2$ ($FIO_2$) administered. Most thoracic surgery patients should receive 100% $O_2$ during 1LV. Lung transplant recipients are a notable exception. Other exceptions include patients previously exposed to pulmonary toxic chemotherapeutic drugs (eg, bleomycin). These patients should have their $FIO_2$ decreased as low as possible, providing the patient is able to maintain an $SpO_2$ >95%.

### Oxygen Saturation Monitoring

Pulse oximetry has become a standard essential monitor over the last decade and is particularly accurate in the range of 85% to 100% saturation. During thoracic surgery, oximetry may fail to register during periods of hypotension. Hypotension occurs due to significant intrinsic postive end-expiratory pressure (PEEP). This can be mitigated by using a slower respiratory rate and a relatively long exhalation time, allowing permissive hypercapnia. Another frequent contributor to loss of the pulse oximetry signal is volume depletion from hemorrhage, circulatory shock, or iatrogenic causes of under repletion. Thoracotomy patients are typically managed "on the dry side," with minimal volume replacement and perioperative diuresis.

### Arterial Blood Gas Monitoring

ABG monitoring is an essential component of thoracotomy management. Intra-arterial catheters should be used in all patients undergoing 1LV. A baseline ABG, followed by frequent subsequent samples, should be monitored in debilitated patients. Healthy patients may not require a baseline intraoperative blood gas evaluation but must have free access available should an emergency occur. If the pulse oximeter falters, and the chest is open, visualization of healthy pink flesh in the operative field is comforting, and the patient's well being can be further confirmed with an ABG. If the chest is closed, quickly pulling back on a syringe connected to the arterial line can quickly reveal oxygenation status: bright red arterial blood ("all is well") or chocolate brown ("arrest impending"). In either case, confirmation is established by evaluating the ABG.

### Ventilation Monitoring

Adequacy of ventilation must be continuously monitored using multiple modalities such as a stethoscope, either precordial or esophageal, and the spirometer on the anesthesia machine (which measures the exhaled $V_T$). Airway pressures provide valuable information about changes in lung compliance, alterations in airway resistance (bronchospasm, secretions, blood, pus), or changes in the patency of DLT (eg, kink) or position change (eg, migration). Airway pressures are frequently altered when changing between 1LV and two-lung ventilation (2LV) and with migration of DLT within the airways.

### End-Tidal Carbon Dioxide Monitoring

Monitoring of end-tidal $CO_2$ ($PETCO_2$) is essential during thoracic anesthesia. During 2LV in the supine position, there is usually a good correlation between the $PETCO_2$ and the $PaCO_2$, with the $PETCO_2$ being 2 to 4 mm Hg less than the $PaCO_2$ due to alveolar dead space ventilation ($VD_{alveolar}$).[87,88] However, COLD patients have a wider gap between the $PETCO_2$ and the $PaCO_2$ because of their vastly increased $VD_{alveolar}$.[89] The $VD_{alveolar}$ increases further with placement in the lateral decubitus position and further still during 1LV in the lateral decubitus position[92]; the amounts must be determined by ABG. Werner and colleagues noted almost no gradient in exhalate from the dependent lung (almost all West's zone 2 and 3), and a gradient of 11 mm Hg for the exhalate from the nondependent lung (mainly zone 1, high $\dot{V}/\dot{Q}$, increased $VD_{alveolar}$).[93]

Continuous breath-by-breath display of the $PETCO_2$ waveform should be monitored for evidence of bronchospasm. COLD patients classically exhibit a continuous upslope of end-tidal trace. This should be evaluated in COLD patients and the results following bronchodilator therapy should be noted. Additionally, alarms on the capnography machine are engineered to alert the anesthesiologist to any episodes of apnea or airway disconnects; which frequently occur in these cases. Capnography can also be used as a reflection of cardiac output changes once a stable $P_{ETCO_2}$–$Pa_{CO_2}$ gradient has been established. Furthermore, in experienced hands, capnography can be used to detect proper placement of DLTs. In one study, authors simultaneously sampled gas from the bronchial and tracheal lumens of a DLT, displaying them on two separate capnographs. The $P_{ETCO_2}$ values and waveforms were compared to determine proper positioning of the DLT.[94]

## What Are the Important Cardiovascular Monitoring Considerations for Thoracic Surgery?

The heart rate and blood pressure (BP) are the most basic cardiovascular parameters which require monitoring during thoracic surgery. Heart rate and rhythm should be monitored via several modalities: esophageal stethoscope, (precordial for esophageal cases), pulse oximetry, electrocardiograph (ECG), and arterial line. For patients requiring more advanced monitoring, the heart rate and rhythm are assessed by reviewing the ECG and central line wave forms (CVP or PA catheter) and the picture obtained via transesophageal echocardiography (TEE). All thoracotomy patients should be monitored with an invasive arterial monitor. The specific cardiovascular monitoring considerations imposed by thoracic surgery will be enumerated for each of these monitoring modalities.

### Electrocardiogram

Dysrhythmias are common with thoracic surgical procedures. An ECG is essential for monitoring rhythm abnormalities and for detecting myocardial ischemia. An ECG monitor that can display 2 channels simultaneously is optimal. Lead II is superior for monitoring the cardiac rhythm because of the clarity and size of the P wave. However, the precordial leads are the most sensitive for detecting significant myocardial ischemia. Indeed, London and associates studied a large cohort of patients with known coronary artery disease undergoing noncardiac, mainly vascular surgery and found that $V_5$ was most sensitive, detecting 75% of ischemic events.[95] Simultaneously monitoring both leads $V_4$ and $V_5$ increased sensitivity to 90%, whereas the standard II and $V_5$ array was only 80% sensitive (Fig. 64–3). Because lead II is most sensitive for P wave evaluation and detects inferior wall ischemia, simultaneous monitoring of lead II and $V_5$ is recommended. The $V_5$ lead is classically placed over the left fifth intercostal space. However, I frequently modify this location to accommodate the surgical field.

### Invasive Arterial Blood Pressure Monitoring

Invasive arterial BP monitoring is required of all patients undergoing thoracotomy. It may be placed after induction of anesthesia in otherwise healthy thoracotomy patients. However, the arterial catheter should be placed preoperatively (before induction) on all systemically ill patients at high risk for hemodynamic deterioration during induction. An arterial line serves the dual purpose of providing access for repetitive ABG samples and continuous beat-to-beat measurement of

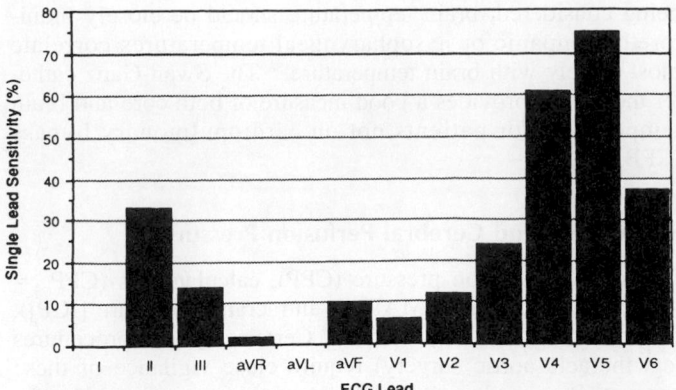

**FIGURE 64–3.** Single-lead sensitivity for detection of myocardial ischemia during noncardiac surgery. (From London MJ, Hollenberg M, Wong MG, et al. Intraoperative myocardial ischemia: localization by continuous 12-lead electrocardiography. *Anesthesiology.* 1988;69:232.)

arterial BP throughout the case, beginning with placement of the thoracic epidural catheter and induction of anesthesia.

### Thoracic Surgery Events That May Impair Intra-Arterial Pressure Measurement

Continuous BP monitoring is critical for most thoracic surgery cases because intrinsic PEEP, surgical manipulations, and intravascular volume shifts can cause acute, profound changes in arterial BP. Not only do the absolute systolic, diastolic, and mean pressures have important clinical relevance, but the information contained in the arterial pressure waveform has important hemodynamic information (including rate, rhythm, preload, afterload, and contractility).[96–98]

### Considerations for Selecting the Optimum Site for Arterial Cannulation

Any large peripheral artery can be used for catheterization. Sites commonly used during thoracic anesthesia include the radial, femoral, and ulnar arteries. During thoracotomy, the radial arterial catheter can be placed in either arm. Some authors prefer the dependent arm, arguing it is easier to stabilize and care for the catheter in that location. As long as the axillary roll is inserted properly (as detailed previously), the dependent arm usually provides an accurate waveform. For mediastinoscopy, it is useful to place the catheter in the right arm and use it to monitor the magnitude and duration of innominate artery compression by the mediastinoscope (see later discussion).[99]

The dorsalis pedis, brachial, axillary, and posterior tibial arteries are less favorable due to the higher risk of ischemia. In neonates, the umbilical artery is an excellent source of pressure monitoring and blood sample acquisition, providing no coarctation or patent ductus exists.

Choosing the site for arterial cannulation includes consideration of many factors. Typically, the radial artery of the nondominant hand is used. When this site is unsuitable, alternate sites are chosen based on four criteria:

1. The artery should be large enough to accurately reflect systemic BP.
2. The chosen site should be free of cellulitis or nearby infected or devitalized tissue.

3. There should be sufficient collateral flow to prevent distal ischemia (dorsalis pedis is a poor choice in the elderly diabetic patient with peripheral vascular disease).

4. The artery should be proximal to any anatomic aberrations (ie, use the right arm for patients with aortic coarct or patent ductus arteriosus).

Table 64–6 lists arterial line positioning considerations for various thoracic procedures.

### Risks of Arterial Cannulation and the Impact of Thoracic Surgery

The risk of radial artery cannulation with a 20 g Teflon catheter is extremely low in adults.[100] This risk may be further decreased by using the Allen test.[101] The Allen test verifies the patency of the ulnar artery, which supplies the majority of the blood flow to the hand.[102] The Allen test is performed by exsanguinating the hand (clenched fist), then occluding both the ulnar and radial arteries. The hand is then opened loosely

---

**TABLE 64–6.** Procedure-Driven Arterial Catheter Site Selection for Thoracic Anesthesia

**Aortic Coarctation Repair**

Right radial artery monitoring is advocated for three reasons: (1) in a preductal coarct, the left radial pressure will be less than the right; (2) the left subclavian flow may be impaired during placement of the aortic X-clamp; and (3) the left subclavian artery may be incorporated into the repair.

**Blalock-Taussig Shunt**

Monitor the contralateral radial artery in patients who are scheduled to undergo, or already have one of these subclavian-to-pulmonary artery shunts.

**Internal Mammary Artery Grafting**

Monitor the contralateral radial artery in patients scheduled to undergo internal mammary artery (IMA) grafting because the sternal and rib cage retraction caused by the Favaloro retractor can distort the ipsilateral subclavian artery. The left side is usually retracted for a left IMA; use the right radial artery in these patients.

**Mediastinoscopy**

Mediastinoscopy tends to obstruct the innominate artery, thus impairing the right radial pulse and right carotid artery inflow. Decisions regarding optimum catheter placement are based on that information and the following reasoning. If time of innominate artery obstruction is considered most important (eg, left carotid obstruction, flow dependent on right carotid artery that branches off the innominate), then monitor with the right radial artery. Monitor with the left radial artery if uninterrupted arterial pressure wave form is essential (carotids fine, tight left main).

**Patent Ductus Arteriosus**

Monitor the right radial artery because femoral or umbilical arteries (postductal) register pressures significantly lower than at the ascending aortic arch.

**Postcardiopulmonary Bypass**

After cardiopulmonary bypass, especially following circulatory arrest, there is frequently a disparity between the peripheral and the central intra-arterial blood pressures. The peripheral (radial) pressure is lower than the central (aortic, femoral, subclavian) due to a decreased hand and forearm arteriolar (and/or capillary) resistance relative to arterial resistance in the upper limb.

**Thoracic Aortic Aneurysm Repair**

If *ascending*, use left radial. For *arch portion*, use right radial (usually need circulatory arrest). If *descending*, use right radial. If a Gott shunt or fem-fem bypass is used, one should concomitantly measure the right radial artery and one of the femoral arteries to verify adequacy of distal perfusion and pressure.

---

(palm up), and ulnar artery compression is released. If the hand pinks up within 3 to 5 seconds, a normal test is declared. Pale digits for >5 seconds following ulnar release is distinctly abnormal. Some have impuned the Allen test because small numbers of patients have been able to tolerate catheterization despite an abnormal test,[103] and others have recognized devastating arterial injury despite an entirely normal test.[104] Although the predictive value of the Allen test is imperfect, its use should still be considered the standard of care. An abnormal Allen test should initiate a search for an alternate site (eg, contralateral radial, femoral, and so on). If no other site is available, then the abnormal artery must be used with the knowledge that there is an ill-defined increased ischemic risk. Furthermore, the patient should be made aware of this fact preoperatively.

In certain situations (severe vasoconstriction or severe vasodilation), the femoral arterial catheter will more closely reflect the aortic pressure than the radial catheter.[105] Relevant conditions in thoracic anesthesia include the cystic fibrosis patient undergoing lung transplant and patients requiring deep hypothermic circulatory arrest (DHCA) such as thoracic aortic aneurysm surgery and PA thromboendarterectomy surgery.[106] These patients are frequently unstable hemodynamically, and the femoral artery will provide a systolic, diastolic, and MAP reading that are significantly greater (both statistically and clinically) than the radial artery pressures.[107] Additionally, certain procedures (eg, thoracic aortic aneurysm repair) are best managed with pressure measurements obtained above (right radial) and below (either femoral artery) the lesions.[108] The complication rate from percutaneous cannulation of the femoral artery is no greater than that of the radial artery.[109,110]

### Is Measurement of Urine Output Helpful in Thoracic Patients?

The Foley catheter provides an acceptable reflection of intravascular volume in patients with normal renal function and normal serum osmolality (absence of hyperglycemia, alcohol intoxication, mannitol therapy) and in the absence of other diuretics (eg, caffeine, furosemide). However, urine output is not responsive enough to reflect intravascular volume on a beat-to-beat or even minute-to-minute basis. Rather, urine output is most useful in determining adequacy of renal perfusion on a hourly basis. Accordingly, during acute events common to thoracic surgery (massive exsanguination, clamping of major vascular structures, severe intrinsic PEEP), more direct and rapidly responsive measures of intravascular volume and organ perfusion are needed (eg, arterial line, CVP, PA catheter, TEE).

### Which Thoracic Surgery Patients Benefit From Central Venous Pressure Monitoring?

CVP monitoring is considered a second tier monitoring device (recommended if the patient has significant systemic disease, ie, chronic renal failure or is undergoing a high-risk procedure). CVP reflects the relationship between the patient's blood volume, venous tone, and right ventricular performance. In patients without significant cardiac disease or pulmonary hypertension, the CVP also provides a useful reflection of right (and left) ventricular preload. Additionally, it provides a port for the administration of cardiovascular drugs and the insertion of a PA catheter or transvenous pacemaker.

### Central Venous Access Considerations for Thoracic Surgery

The central line catheter can be placed via a subclavian, internal jugular (IJ), external jugular, femoral, or antecubital vein route. The external jugular access is discouraged during thoracotomy because the catheter often kinks when the head is rotated back toward the midline (as is customary for placing the neck in a neutral position during the lateral decubitus position). If a subclavian technique is chosen, one should cannulate the vein on the same side as the thoracotomy. This avoids the development of a pneumothorax on the dependent side, which could lead to severe (life-threatening) hypoxemia when 1LV is subsequently instituted. Antecubital sites are preferred for neurology cases in which access to the head is difficult but are a relatively poor choice for thoracic surgery. This is because the long arm catheters have a propensity for migration into the right ventricle and the subsequent triggering of dysrhythmias. Such migration frequently occurs with arm extension (such as that required for the lateral decubitus position). The right IJ vein is recommended for central access during thoracotomy cases because the success rate is highest,[111] and major complications are fewest.[112] A left IJ catheter may occasionally be selected as the best first choice in patients undergoing a left thoracotomy who have significant baseline disease in the right lung (eg, left single lung transplant).

### *Which Thoracic Surgery Patients Benefit From Pulmonary Artery Catheterization?*

PA catheterization is a second or third tier monitor reserved for patients in whom the CVP poorly reflects intravascular volume status (impaired LV function, severe coronary artery disease, known PA hypertension, mitral or tricuspid valve pathology). Additionally, PA catheters are indicated for high-risk procedures (thoracic aorta cross-clamping) or when significant pulmonary vascular flow diversion is anticipated (lobectomy or pneumonectomy) and to detect the need for CPB (to temporarily bypass the pulmonary vasculature) during lung transplantation.

Information available from PA catheters includes left-sided filling pressures, measurement of cardiac output, sampling mixed venous blood, calculation of systemic and pulmonary vascular resistances, and PA and wedge pressure waveform analysis. The PA catheter provides estimates of left ventricular (LV) preload (ie, LV end-diastolic volume [LVEDV]) by measuring LV end-diastolic pressure (LVEDP). This LVEDP/LVEDV relationship is altered by changes in LV compliance (eg, myocardial ischemia, tissue edema). Many investigators have demonstrated a poor correlation between pulmonary capillary wedge pressure (PCWP) and LVEDV in acutely ill patients.[113] In situations where assessment of LVEDV is critical (eg, hypotension, low cardiac output, normal or high filling pressures by CVP and PCWP in COLD patients undergoing major lung resection or lung transplant), using a TEE provides the most accurate direct view of LV preload and contractility.[114] However, pneumonectomy or lung transplantation in patients with pulmonary hypertension also requires a test clamp of the PA to be resected.

### Right-Left Heart Interactions May Impair Pulmonary Artery Catheter Measurements

Another factor influencing the measurements obtained by a PA catheter is the interdependence of right ventricle and LV. Ventricular interdependence can be misleading when the interventricular septum encroaches on the LV cavity, leading to elevated PCWP measurements. In this situation, the elevated PCWP associated with the decreased cardiac output can be interpreted as LV failure when, in fact, a decrease rather than an increase may have occurred in LVEDV. This situation most commonly occurs with large tidal volumes or high levels of PEEP[115] and is particularly problematic in COLD patients undergoing 1LV. The TEE is a better monitor of LV volume in this situation as well.

### Lateral Decubitus Position and One-Lung Ventilation Effects on the Pulmonary Artery Catheter

Several important points must be considered when interpreting PA catheter data obtained from thoracotomy patients in lateral decubitus position. First, >90% of PA catheters float to and locate in the right lung.[116] This right-sided propensity is only partly due to the increased right-sided blood flow and pathway curvature. It is possible to increase the incidence of left-sided PA catheter positioning to 50% when advanced with the patient in the right lateral decubitus position (implying the importance of balloon flotation vertically upward as well).[117]

Second, during a right thoracotomy with the patient in the left lateral decubitus position, the PA catheter will likely be in the operative, nondependent lung. This "up" lung is either collapsed if 1LV is employed or mainly functioning as West zone 1 or 2 if ventilated. When the PA catheter is in zone 1 or 2 of the lung, the pressure recorded during catheter wedging is more reflective of the airway pressure than left atrial pressure, especially if a large tidal volume, PEEP, or continuous positive airway pressure (CPAP) is applied to the up lung. Furthermore, hypovolemia, hypotension, and decreased cardiac output all decrease perfusion to the nondependent lung and further exacerbate this condition, leading to near or total collapse of the pulmonary veins.

Third, Cohen and coworkers reported that during right thoracostomies with the PA catheter in the right, nondependent lung, cardiac output measurements will be underestimated.[118]

Conversely, during left thoracotomy (right lateral decubitus position), when the PA catheter is located in the right dependent lung (which is well perfused and functioning as a zone 3), measurement of wedge pressure and cardiac output more accurately reflects both left atrial pressure and true flow. The reason for the disparity in cardiac output measurements is partially due to decreased flow through the nondependent lung for physiologic reasons (gravity, hypoxic pulmonary hypertension [HPV]), and partly due to distorted anatomy and stagnant blood flow. In the same study, Cohen and colleagues found that mixed venous saturation ($S\bar{v}o_2$) is lower during right thoracostomies compared with left when the catheter is in the right lung, probably due to stagnant blood flow. Furthermore, alterations from surgical manipulation can yield additional unpredictable artifacts.

However, when the nondependent up lung is ventilated with varying levels of PEEP, no difference in cardiac output or $S\bar{v}o_2$ can be detected when simultaneously measured from PA catheters located in the dependent or the nondependent lungs.[119] Furthermore, Landais and colleagues measured cardiac output by the thermodilution method during left thoracotomy in the right lateral decubitus position in dogs with both lungs being ventilated via a single-lumen endotracheal tube (ETT). That study concluded that no difference occurred in cardiac output measured whether the thermistor was located in the main trunk of the PA or in either the right or the left branches of the dependent or nondependent lung.[120] Additionally, Feinglass and associates found no difference in a sheep unilateral lung injury model regardless of whether the catheter was in the injured lung or uninjured lung side.[121] Finally, Gunther and coworkers found no difference in critically ill adults between decubitus or supine positioning.[122]

The mode of ventilation (controlled versus spontaneous) and the degree of lung compliance have important influences on PEEP/CPAP-induced discrepancies between PAWP and LAP. During spontaneous ventilation in compliant lungs with the patient in the lateral decubitus position, even when the PA catheter was located in zone 1 or 2 (ie, in the up lung above the level of the left atrium), the PAWP remained an accurate reflection of LAP, even with CPAP as high as 20 mm Hg.[123] However, if the patient was on controlled ventilation (as is the usual case during thoracotomy), large PEEP-induced discrepancies occurred between PAWP and LAP. The noncompliant lung does not transmit PEEP as readily to the pulmonary vasculature, and therefore the noncompliant lung PAWP more accurately reflects LAP. The difference between PAWP and LAP with the PA catheter in the up lung was significantly less in noncompliant lungs than in compliant lungs, with PEEP values >10 mm Hg.

In summary, when the PA catheter is in the nondependent lung, which is either collapsed or ventilated with large tidal volumes, PEEP, or CPAP, the PA wedge pressure (PAWP) may not reflect left atrial pressure (LAP). When the PA catheter is in the dependent lung and presumably in the zone 3 region, PAWP should accurately reflect LAP, even when PEEP is applied to the dependent lung. During 2LV in the lateral decubitus position, the cardiac output will be accurately measured regardless of which side the PA catheter resides. However, during 1LV, the cardiac output is underestimated when the PA catheter is in the nondependent operative side.

Finally, these differences are greatest during positive pressure ventilation versus spontaneous ventilation and in compliant (COLD) lungs versus noncompliant stiff (ARDS) lungs.

### Avoidance of Pulmonary Artery Rupture During Thoracic Surgery

A comprehensive discourse on the complications of central venous and PA catheterization is beyond the scope of this chapter. These have been exhaustively tabulated by Shah and colleagues in 1984,[124] and by Zion and associates in 1990,[125] and are thoroughly reviewed in Chapter 20 and elsewhere.[126] However, the rare but catastrophic complication of PA catheterization, PA rupture, has particular relevance to thoracic anesthesia and justifies discussion.

The risk factors associated with PA rupture include overaggressive advancement of catheter, pulmonary hypertension, mitral stenosis, female gender (twice as common as in males), advanced age, hypothermia, and anticoagulation. Inflation of the PA catheter balloon in the distal vessels is probably the

most important factor due to the high pressures generated by the balloon.[127]

Mortality from PA rupture is approximately 46% but in the setting of anticoagulation soars to 70%.[128] The most frequent sign of PA rupture is hemoptysis. Manipulation of the heart and mediastinum during thoracic surgery can predispose to perforation of the PA because the PA catheter's tip may be propelled into a more distal position in the pulmonary circulation. Always avoid advancing the PA catheter to the periphery of the PA tree and always look for evidence of its distal migration during a procedure (wedge trace displayed on monitor when the balloon is deflated). Most importantly, during pulmonary resections (especially on the right side), the PA catheter must be pulled back before test clamp and resection because PA catheters have been sewn into various structures with lethal results.

### What Is the Role of Transesophageal Echocardiography in Thoracic Anesthesia?

TEE is an established monitoring and diagnostic tool for the cardiothoracic anesthesiologist. Techniques for insertion, interpretation, and complications have been comprehensively reviewed elsewhere.[129] The main benefit of TEE lies in the fact that direct visualization of both ventricular and atrial chambers provides instantaneous information on preload. Contractility is also directly visualized using the short axis view.[130] Monitoring for ischemia and wall motion abnormalities is excellent with TEE, and automated real-time technologies are emerging.[131] Valvular function can be assessed using color-labeled directional flow and Doppler techniques. Abnormal holes can be detected via direct view or administration of agitated saline. Pericardial effusions and their effect on atrial and ventricular function are well visualized. Of particular relevance to thoracic surgery is observation of the effect of right-left heart interactions and increased pulmonary vascular resistance in COLD patients on PA catheter readings. See Chapter 20 for more details on cardiovascular monitoring.

## LUNG SEPARATION

### What Are the Absolute and Relative Indications for Lung Separation?

The indications for separation of the two lungs have historically been absolute and relative. Some believe this distinction is arbitrary because any relative indication may progress to an absolute indication at any moment. Indeed, there is a continuum from strong to weak indications. However, the anesthesiologist must be able to recognize when the lungs absolutely need separation (absolute indication) and when the separation is being accomplished mainly for convenience of the surgeon (relative indication).

#### Absolute Need for Lung Separation

There are four absolute indications for lung separation (Table 64–7).

1. The separation of one lung from the other is needed to prevent the spillage of blood or pus from the affected to the nonaffected lung.

**TABLE 64–7.** Indications for Lung Separation and or One-Lung Ventilation

**ABSOLUTE**

*Isolation of One Lung From the Other to Prevent Spillage or Contamination*

Infection
Massive hemorrhage

*Control of Ventilation Distribution*

Bronchopleural fistula
Bronchopleural cutaneous fistula
Tracheobronchial tree disruption (penetrating or blunt trauma)
Surgical opening of a major conducting airway
Giant unilateral lung bulla or cyst
Life-threatening hypoxemia due to unilateral lung disease

*Unilateral Bronchopulmonary Lavage*

*Bilateral Sequential Lung Transplantation (Without Cardiopulmonary Bypass)*

**RELATIVE**

*Surgical Exposure: Highest priority*

Thoracic aortic aneurysm
Pneumonectomy
Upper lobectomy
Mediastinal exposure
Thoracoscopy

*Surgical Exposure: Lower Priority*

Middle and lower lobectomies
Esophageal resection
Anterior thoracic spine procedures
Minimally invasive coronary artery surgery
Internal mammary artery harvest for noninvasive surgery

*Control of Ventilation Distribution*

Severe (but not life-threatening) hypoxemia due to unilateral lung disease
Post cardiopulmonary bypass for pulmonary thromboendarterectomy with reperfusion pulmonary edema

2. Many unilateral lung problems require lung separation and differential ventilation: (a) large bronchopleural or bronchocutaneous fistula where the low resistance to air flow causes inhalation flow delivered via positive pressure ventilation to exit the airways with little transmitted to the contralateral normal lung; (b) tracheobronchial tree disruption as may occur following penetrating or blunt trauma; (c) severe life-threatening unilateral lung disease requiring differential ventilation[132]; and (d) following single lung transplantation for primary pulmonary hypertension (excess blood flow to the newly transplanted lung) or following single lung transplantation for emphysema (excessive ventilation of the nontransplanted lung).
3. Performance of unilateral pulmonary alveolar lavage for pulmonary alveolar proteinosis.
4. Bilateral single lung transplantation for diseases not requiring CPB cannot be expeditiously and safely accomplished without lung separation. When CPB is planned at the start of the case, a single-lumen tube may be used.

### Relative Indications for Lung Separation

The relative indications for lung separation surround the needs of facilitating surgical exposure (see Table 64–7). Although most of the procedures listed as a relative indication for lung separation could be accomplished without lung separation, generally it would take much more time, be less safe, and put the patient at risk for excessive secondary lung injury

from retraction of the lung. The secondary traction-induced lung injury can significantly impair gas exchange both intraoperatively,[133] and postoperatively.[134] The highest priority is for thoracic aortic aneurysm repair and pneumonectomy. The descending aorta runs through most of the left hemithorax, and pneumonectomy requires dissection of the structures in the lung hilum. Similarly, an upper lobectomy is more difficult to perform without lung separation than either a middle lobectomy or a lower lobectomy and is categorized accordingly. Severe unilateral lung disease is another relative indication. However, if the condition becomes life-threatening, then it becomes an absolute indication for lung separation and differential ventilation.

## What Techniques Are Used for Separating the Lungs?

The lungs can be separated by use of either a DLT or a BB. Correct positioning of DLTs and BBs is often the most important determinant as to whether thoracic surgery (in particular 1LV cases) and differential lung ventilation in the intensive care unit proceed smoothly. If the method of lung separation is correct, the operative nondependent lung will collapse completely and easily, the surgeon will be able to work efficiently with less damage to the operative lung, and the nonoperative lung will remain unobstructed and easy to ventilate.

### Double-Lumen Tubes

#### History of the Development of the Modern (Robertshaw) Double-Lumen Tube

The concept of lung separation began in the late 1880s with physiologic experimentation on dogs. However, throughout the 1920s, patients continued to receive mask ventilation for most thoracic procedures such as drainage of tuberculous empyema in the prone position. The first documented account of true 1LV was published by Waters and Gale of Madison, Wisconsin, in 1932.[135] Their tube had one lumen, a distal curvature, and one large cuff that both sealed the trachea and blocked the bronchus contralateral to the intubated bronchus. Magill developed a similar tube in London in 1935, although his tube had a wire-reinforced bronchial tip. Crafoord, a Swedish surgeon, accomplished lung separation by stuffing a ribbon gauze pack down a bronchus ("tampon" technique) using a rigid bronchoscope in 1938. Jacobaeus and Frenckner invented the first double lumen apparatus, but it was a crude rigid metal device used for bronchospirometry.[136]

The first flexible DLT was invented by Carlens in Sweden in 1949.[137] This DLT had a carinal hook that allowed blind placement. However, problems with the carinal hook included laryngeal trauma during insertion, amputation of the hook during passage, malposition of the tube caused by the hook, and physical interference of closing the bronchial stump during pneumonectomy.[138] For these reasons, some anesthesiologists adopted a practice of cutting off the hook before use. This tube is still available in four sizes (41, 39, 37, and 35 French).

Several additional modifications of right- and left-sided Carlens tubes were developed. However, not until the late 1950s, when Robertshaw came to Manchester to work as a thoracic anesthesiologist, was a better tube invented. Robertshaw developed his tube with the close cooperation of the Leyland and Birmingham Rubber Company of Lancashire, England. He molded two D-shaped tubes back to back to increase the airway chambers, thus allowing passage of larger suction catheters and lower airway resistance than the Carlens tube. Robertshaw produced the final prototype in 1962, and his is now by far the most commonly used type of DLT.[139] For a more thorough discourse on the history of 1LV, readers are referred to the delightful review by Lee.[140]

### Double-Lumen Tube Types and Sizes Available for Adults

There are seven sizes of commonly available adult Robertshaw DLTs (26, 28, 32, 35, 37, 39, and 41 French).

In general, the largest DLT that fits should be used to minimize airway resistance and increase ease of FOB and suction catheter passage. The height of the patient correlates better than the weight in selecting a DLT size. Short patients (4'6-5'5") should use a 35 to 37 French left-sided DLT; for medium height patients (5'5"-5'10"), a 37 to 39 French left-sided DLT is recommended; and for tall patients (5'11"-6'4"), a 39 to 41 French left-sided DLT is optimum.[141] In my experience, airways tend to be larger than would be predicted by height alone in chronic smokers and in patients with bronchiectasis or chronic pulmonary infections (eg, cystic fibrosis). Therefore, these patients can tolerate larger DLTs than would be predicted by their height. Additionally, men tend to have larger airways than women of the same height due, in part, to men tending to have longer torsos than women.

### Double-Lumen Tube Selection for Right Versus Left Thoracostomies

When surgery is performed on the right lung, a left-sided DLT is used (Fig. 64–4A). When surgery of the left lung is performed, either a left- or right-sided DLT is used (see Fig. 64–4B). However, because the margin of safety in positioning a right-sided DLT is much less than for a left-sided DLT (because the length of the right mainstem bronchus— approximately 1.5-2.0 cm—is much shorter than the length of the left mainstem bronchus—approximately 5.0-5.5 cm),[142] use of a right-sided DLT for left lung surgery increases the risk of either blockade of the right upper lobe (right-sided DLT in too far; endobronchial cuff blocks right upper lobe)

or the left lung (right-sided DLT out too far;, endobronchial cuff blocks carinal area and left lung). To avoid these complications, a left-sided DLT can be used for most cases requiring 1LV. If clamping of the left mainstem bronchus is necessary, the DLT can be withdrawn at that time (after deflating the cuffs) into the trachea and then used as a single-lumen tube (deflate only the left lumen cuff and use both of the lumens to ventilate the right lung) (see Fig. 64–4C).

### Indications for a Right-Sided Double-Lumen Tube

A right-sided DLT is indicated only when a left-sided DLT is contraindicated. Relative contraindications to using a left-sided DLT include the following conditions: (1) a large exophytic lesion in the left mainstem bronchus; (2) the left mainstem bronchus is critically stenotic; (3) the left mainstem bronchus is distorted by either a left lower lobe or LUL tumor, causing the left mainstem bronchus to take off from the trachea at a sharp angle. Under these circumstances, it may not be possible to insert the left endobronchial lumen into the left mainstem bronchus (even when using an FOB as a stylet).

### Airway Equipment Required to Be Present Before Attempting Double-Lumen Tube Placement

Selection and preparation of DLT airway equipment ahead of time is essential, especially for practitioners who infrequently place DLTs. Of particular importance for thoracic anesthesia is to preoperatively select the DLT, testing both the tracheal and bronchial cuffs, and locating and test fitting the 15-mm airway adapter hookups. Additionally, the anesthesiologist should secure a large rubber-shod Kelly clamp for sequential 1LV testing. Finally, verification of proper function and immediate availability of a pediatric FOB is essential because it will be required for confirmation of correct DLT positioning.

### Conventional Method for Double-Lumen Tube Insertion

The conventional method of DLT insertion, using rigid direct laryngoscopy, begins with placing the patient in a standard sniffing position. Adequate preoxygenation is accomplished followed by induction of general anesthesia. The abil-

**FIGURE 64–4.** Use of left-sided and right-sided double-lumen tubes for left- and right-lung surgery (as indicated by the clamp). When surgery is going to be performed on the right lung, a left-sided double-lumen tube should be used (A). When surgery is going to be performed on the left lung, a right-sided double-lumen tube can be used (B). However, because of uncertainty as to the alignment of the right upper lobe ventilation slot to the right upper lobe orifice, a left-sided double-lumen tube can also be used for left lung surgery (C). If the left-lung surgery requires a clamp to be placed high on the left mainstem bronchus, the left endobronchial cuff should be deflated, the left-sided double-lumen tube pulled back into the trachea, and the right lung ventilated through both of the lumens (ie, use the double-lumen tube as a single-lumen tube). (From Benumof JL. *Anesthesia for Thoracic Surgery.* 2nd ed. Philadelphia, Pa: WB Saunders; 1995:341.)

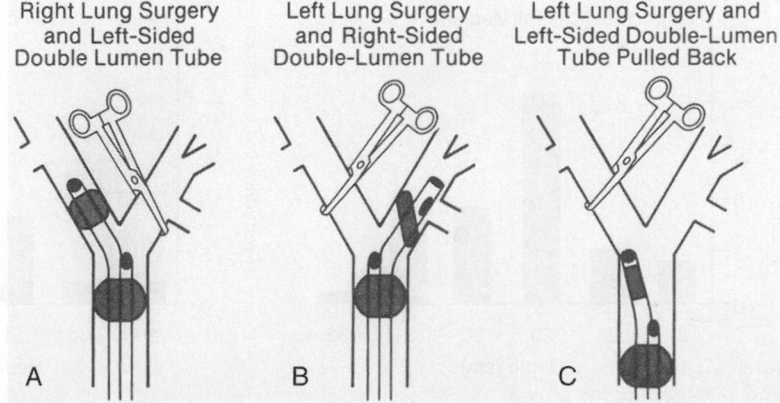

Right Lung Surgery and Left-Sided Double Lumen Tube

Left Lung Surgery and Right-Sided Double-Lumen Tube

Left Lung Surgery and Left-Sided Double-Lumen Tube Pulled Back

A  B  C

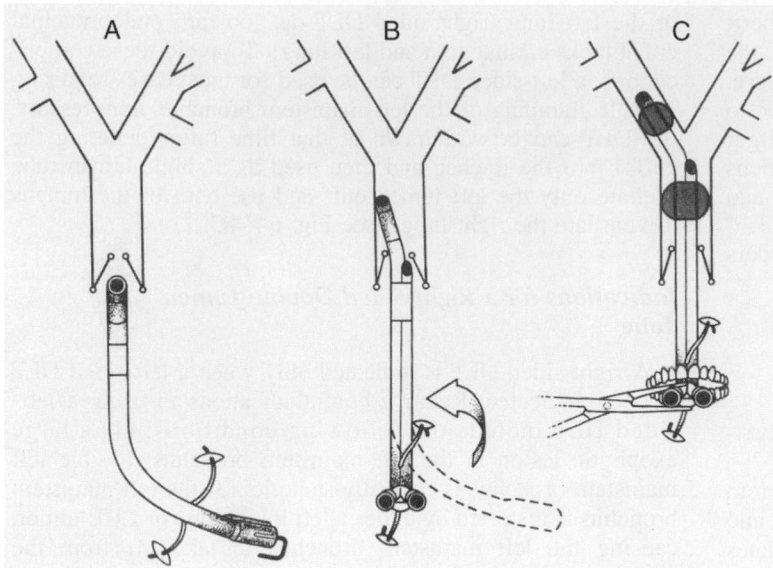

**FIGURE 64–5.** This schematic diagram depicts the passage of the left-sided double-lumen tube in a supine patient. *A,* The tube is held with the distal curvature concave anteriorly and the proximal curve concave to the right and in a plane parallel to the floor. The tube is then inserted through the vocal cords until the left cuff passes the vocal cords. The stylet is then removed. *B,* The tube is rotated 90° counterclockwise so that the distal curvature is concave to the left and in a plane parallel to the floor, whereas, the proximal curvature is concave anteriorly. *C,* The tube is inserted until either a moderate resistance to further passage is encountered or the end of the common molding of the two lumens is at the teeth. Both cuffs are then inflated, and both lungs are ventilated. Finally, one side is clamped while the other side is ventilated and vice versa (see text for further explanation). (From Benumof JL. *Anesthesia for Thoracic Surgery.* 2nd ed. Philadelphia, Pa: WB Saunders; 1995: 343.)

ity to mask ventilate is demonstrated, and neuromuscular blockade is administered. Intermittent mask ventilation is provided until optimum intubating conditions are demonstrated by neuromuscular blockade twitch monitor. Next, direct laryngoscopy is performed, the DLT tip is passed through the glottic chink under direct vision, and the tube is rotated 90° (leftward for a left DLT or rightward for a right DLT) so that the proximal curve is concave anteriorly and the distal curvature points toward the bronchus intended for cannulation (Fig.

64–5). The tube is then pushed in until moderate resistance to further passage is encountered (on average, 29 ± 2 cm at the upper incisors). Just like selection of DLT size, the optimum depth of insertion correlates with the height of the patient (Fig. 64–6). For patients 4′6″ to 5′5″, 27 ± 2 cm at the upper incisors is the optimum depth of insertion; for patients 5′5″ to 5′10″, 29 ± 2 cm is optimum; and for patients 5′10″ to 6′4″, 31 ± 2 cm is the optimum depth. Final depth of insertion is determined by clinical examination and FOB (discussion follows).

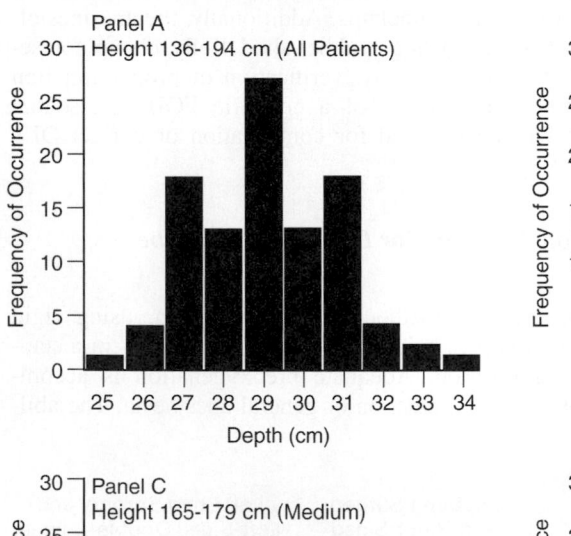

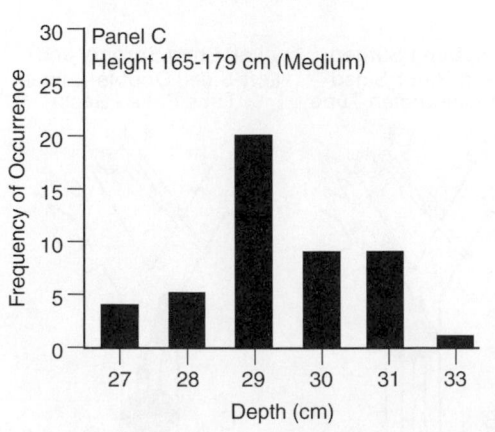

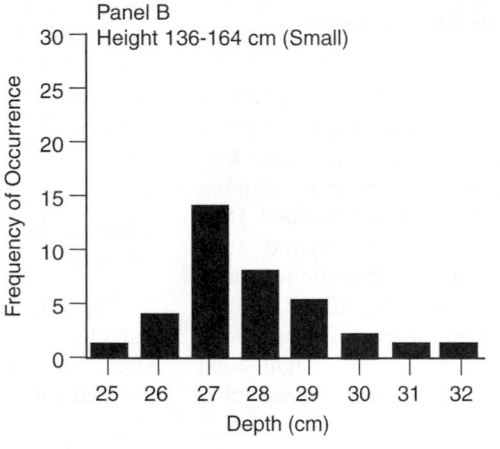

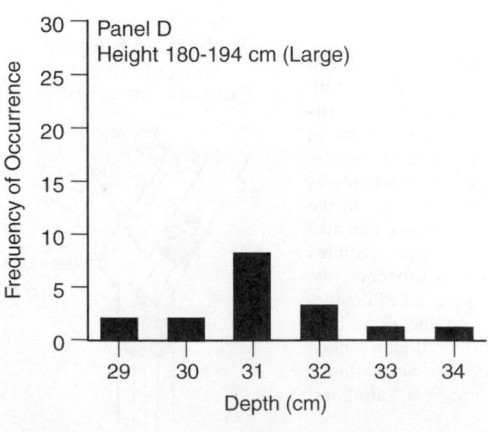

**FIGURE 64–6.** The depth of insertion for left double-lumen tubes for all patients and for three grouped intervals based on patient height. The average depth of insertion is 29 cm. Tall patients averaged 31 cm, whereas short patients averaged 27-cm depth of insertion. At each grouped interval, the depth of insertion was normally distributed. (From Brodsky JB, Benumof JL, Ehrenwerth J, et al. Depth of placement of left double-lumen endobronchial tubes. *Anesth Analg.* 1991;73:570.)

### Fiberoptic Bronchoscopic Guided Initial Insertion of the Double-Lumen Tube

Routine insertion of the bronchial lumen of a DLT into the appropriate mainstem bronchus is usually successfully accomplished blindly. However, when difficulty is encountered, bronchial placement may be guided by FOB (Fig. 64–7). The DLT is first placed in the trachea in a conventional manner (laryngoscopy, manual tube insertion) until the tracheal cuff just passes the vocal cords; the tracheal cuff is inflated, and both lungs are ventilated through both lumens (use the DLT as if it were a single-lumen tube). A pediatric FOB can then be inserted into the bronchial lumen through a self-sealing diaphragm incorporated in the elbow connector to the bronchial lumen (which permits continued positive-pressure ventilation through that lumen around the FOB), and passed into the appropriate mainstem bronchus. The tracheal cuff is then deflated, and the bronchial lumen is guided over the FOB stylet into the appropriate mainstem bronchus. The FOB is then withdrawn from the bronchial lumen and passed down the tracheal lumen to determine the precise DLT position (fine-adjust the depth of insertion so that the blue endobronchial cuff is just below the tracheal carina—see next section).

### Direct and Indirect Methods for Verification of Double-Lumen Tube Position

FOB (a direct measure) should be used to verify DLT position in all patients after final positioning and before surgery and should also be used whenever positioning is unclear. However, there are four indirect cardinal observations that the anesthesiologist should be able to make after initial passage of a properly placed DLT using unilateral clamping:

1. The breath sounds should only be heard on the side contralateral to the clamp, and the breath sounds should disappear on the ipsilateral (clamped) side.
2. The contralateral (nonclamped) lung should feel reasonably compliant.
3. Only the contralateral chest should rise and fall with ventilation, giving the chest a rocking boat motion.
4. The respiratory gas moisture should disappear on inhalation and reappear on exhalation on the ventilated side, and the respiratory gas moisture should be stationary on the clamped side.

### Common Double-Lumen Tube Malpositions and Their Diagnoses Using Indirect Methodology

There are three gross malpositions for a DLT (Fig. 64–8). The DLT can be in too far in the left or the right mainstem bronchus, or it may be inserted not far enough, so that both lumens are in the trachea. In each malposition, the left cuff, when inflated, blocks the right lumen; this situation can be taken advantage of to diagnose the DLT malposition. When the left cuff is inflated and the left lumen is clamped (ventilation is only through the right lumen), the left cuff will block the right lumen in all three malpositions, and the breath sounds are either absent or diminished. When the left cuff is then deflated, breath sounds are heard on the left side when the DLT is in too far on the left; breath sounds are heard on both sides when the DLT is out too far; and breath sounds are only heard in the right lung when the DLT is in too far on the right.

### Why Indirect Methods for Double-Lumen Tube Position Verification Are Unreliable

Reasons for the failure of the indirect methods for DLT position verification follow: (1) once the patient is prepared and draped, the chest is less available for auscultation (to improve auscultation, listen in the axilla, which is typically available throughout the case); (2) use of breath sounds as an endpoint is often insensitive because of pre-existing lung disease and loud ORs; (3) the tube may migrate during the case (surgical traction, patient coughing, patient turning); (4) the tube may be just barely malpositioned; and (5) a combination of all of the above.

### Final Double-Lumen Tube Position Should Always Be Verified Using a Fiberoptic Bronchoscope

The FOB should be used in every case to verify final DLT placement because indirect methods are imprecise. Initially, routine use of the FOB provides practice and preparation so that quick remedies can be made using the FOB during malposition emergencies. Furthermore, whenever there is any doubt as to the precise location of the DLT (which includes the initial insertion), it may be resolved by the use of an FOB. The FOB should remain in the OR for subsequent use throughout the case until the DLT is removed.

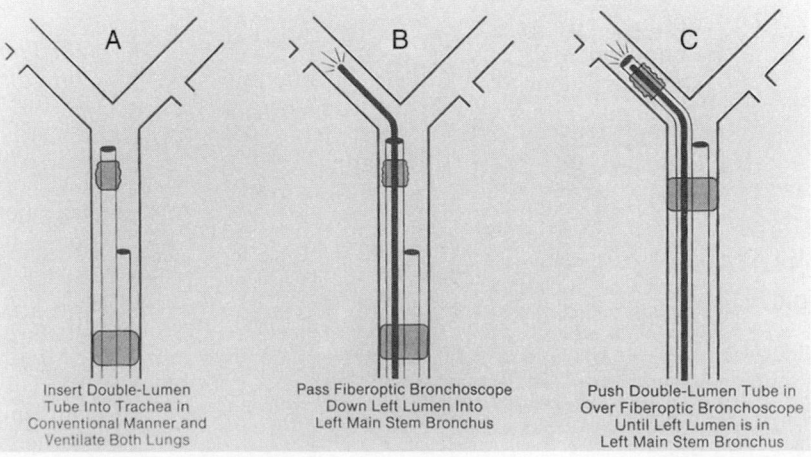

**FIGURE 64–7.** This schematic diagram portrays use of the fiberoptic bronchoscope (FOB) to insert a left-sided double-lumen tube (DLT). The DLT can be put into the trachea in a conventional manner, and both lungs can be ventilated by both lumens (A). The FOB may be inserted into the left lumen of the DLT through a self-sealing diaphragm in the elbow connector to the left lumen; this allows continued positive-pressure ventilation of both lungs through the right lumen without creating a leak. After the FOB has been passed into the left mainstem bronchus (B), it is used as a stylet for the after coming left lumen of the DLT (C). The FOB is then withdrawn. Final precise positioning of the DLT is performed with the FOB by ensuring that the left lumen of the DLT lies proximal to the take off of the left upper lobe bronchus. Next, the right (Tracheal) lumen of the DLT is cannulated with the FOB to ensure that the left bronchial balloon does not herniate over the carina and obstruct the right main stem bronchial lumen (see Fig. 64–9). (From Benumof JL. *Anesthesia for Thoracic Surgery.* 2nd ed. Philadelphia, Pa: WB Saunders; 1995:350.)

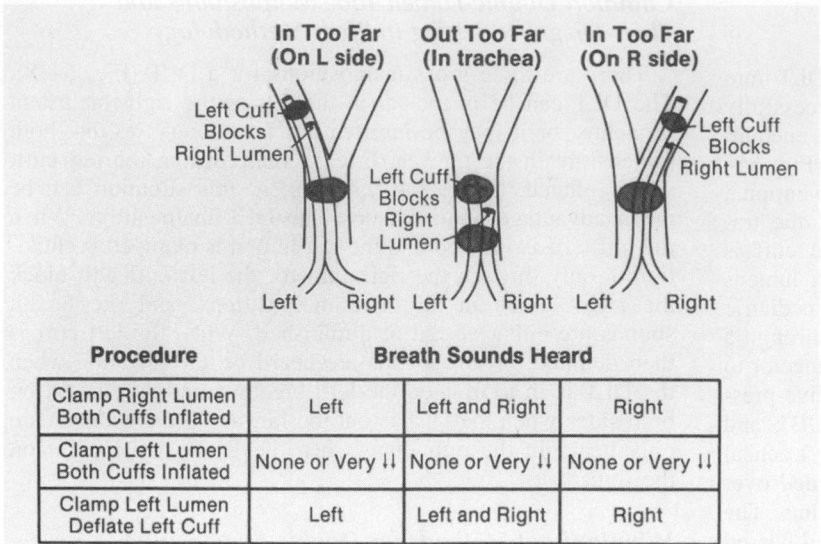

| Procedure | Breath Sounds Heard | | |
|---|---|---|---|
| Clamp Right Lumen<br>Both Cuffs Inflated | Left | Left and Right | Right |
| Clamp Left Lumen<br>Both Cuffs Inflated | None or Very ↓↓ | None or Very ↓↓ | None or Very ↓↓ |
| Clamp Left Lumen<br>Deflate Left Cuff | Left | Left and Right | Right |

**FIGURE 64–8.** There are three major (involving a whole lung) malpositions of a left-sided double-lumen endotracheal tube. The tube can be in too far on the left (both lumens are in the left mainstem bronchus), out too far (both lumens are in the trachea), or down the right mainstem bronchus (at least the left lumen is in the right mainstem bronchus). In each of these three malpositions, the left cuff, when fully inflated, can completely block the right lumen. Inflation and deflation of the left cuff while the left lumen is clamped creates a breath sound differential diagnosis of tube malposition. (See text for full explanation.) L, left; R, right; ↓, decreased. (From Benumof JL. *Anesthesia for Thoracic Surgery.* 2nd ed. Philadelphia, Pa: WB Saunders; 1995:347.)

Large bronchoscopes that are easily passed down adult-sized 7.0 to 8.0 ETTs are too large to use in DLTs. However, a pediatric FOB (outside diameter <4.0 mm) can be passed down the lumens of all sized (35, 37, 39, 41 French) DLTs. A 4.9-mm outside diameter FOB will not pass down the 35 French and is a tight squeeze through a 37 French tube.

The simplest way to determine DLT position is to pass the FOB down the right lumen, much as one might pass a suction catheter. Looking down the right lumen, the endoscopist should see a clear straight-ahead view of the tracheal carina, the left lumen going off the left side and the upper surface of the blue left endobronchial cuff just below the tracheal carina (Fig. 64–9). Looking down the right lumen, the endoscopist should not see the left cuff herniating over the carina or the carina pushed over to the right and compromising the right mainstem bronchial orifice.

### Left-Sided Double-Lumen Tubes Are Safer Because of Their Greater Margin of Error

The outermost acceptable position of a left-sided DLT occurs when the left endobronchial cuff is just below the tracheal

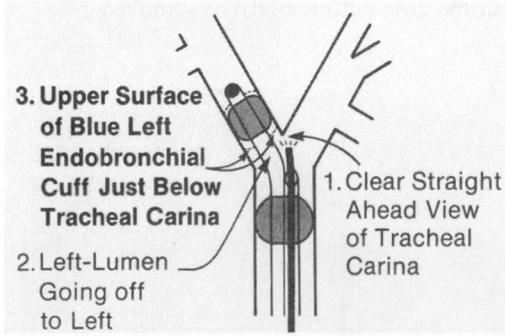

**FIGURE 64–9.** This schematic diagram portrays use of the fiberoptic bronchoscope down the right (tracheal) lumen of the left-sided double-lumen tube (DLT) to verify precise positioning. The endoscopist should see a clear straight-ahead view of the tracheal carina, the left lumen of the DLT going off into the left mainstem bronchus, and, most importantly, the upper surface of the blue left endobronchial cuff just below the tracheal carina. No portion of the blue balloon should herniate over the carina, as this could obstruct the right side of the lung. (From Benumof JL. *Anesthesia for Thoracic Surgery.* 2nd ed. Philadelphia, Pa: WB Saunders; 1995:352.)

carina. If a left-sided DLT is pulled out any further, the left endobronchial cuff will obstruct the trachea and the right mainstem bronchus. The innermost acceptable position occurs when the distal tip of the left lumen is at the LUL bronchus because further insertion could obstruct the LUL. The distance between the right and left lumen tip for a left-sided DLT is approximately 70 to 75 mm, which is longer than the length of the left mainstem bronchus (50-55 mm in both men and women). Thus, it is possible for the right (tracheal) lumen to be above the tracheal carina while the left (bronchial) lumen tip obstructs the LUL. The distance between the upper surface of the left endobronchial balloon and the tip of the left lumen is 25 mm (which is shorter than the shortest left mainstem bronchus). Thus, when the upper surface of the left endobronchial balloon is just below the tracheal carina, it is virtually impossible for the left tip to obstruct the LUL.

Confirmation of correct right-sided DLT position is similar to correct verification of left-sided DLT position, except that it is also necessary to pass the FOB down the bronchial lumen and confirm that the right upper lobe ventilation slot is opposite the right upper lobe bronchial orifice (Fig. 64–10). The margin of error for a right-sided DLT is far less than that for a left-sided tube because the length of the right mainstem bronchus is much shorter than the left (see Figs. 64–1 and 64–2). Additionally, the right-sided anatomy is more variable than the left.

### DLT Placement Considerations for Patients With Difficult Airways

Patients with difficult airways identified during the preoperative evaluation should have their tracheas intubated while they are awake using an FOB with a pre-ensleeved DLT. Indications for FOB-guided DLT placement include (1) situations where alignment of the oral, pharyngeal, and laryngeal axes are difficult or ill-advised (eg, cervical spine injury or neck fixed in a halo brace), and (2) situations in which difficult direct laryngoscopy are predicted (ie, hyomental distance [HMD] <6 cm, Mallampati class III or IV) (Table 64–8), especially in patients with a small mouth opening and those with temporomandibular joint (TMJ) disease.

After completely anesthetizing the patient's airway with

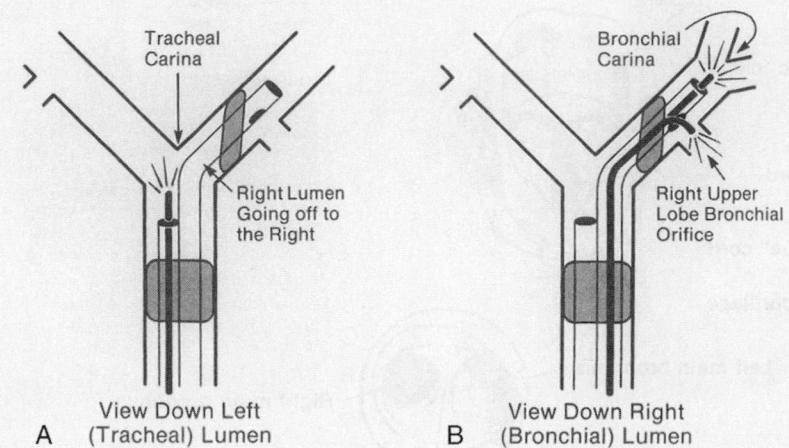

**FIGURE 64–10.** This schematic diagram portrays use of a fiberoptic bronchoscope (FOB) to verify precise right-sided double-lumen tube (DLT) position. A) When the FOB is passed down the left (tracheal) lumen, the endoscopist should see a clear straight-ahead view of the tracheal carina and the right lumen of the DLT going off into the right mainstem bronchus. B) When the FOB is passed down the right (bronchial) lumen, the endoscopist should see the bronchial carina off in the distance; when the FOB is flexed laterally and cephalad and passed through the right upper lobe ventilation slot, the right upper lobe bronchial orifice should be visualized. The classic view of the three segmental bronchi (anterior, posterior, and apical) of the right upper lobe is similar to the image of a Mercedes Benz logo. (From Benumof JL. *Anesthesia for Thoracic Surgery*. 2nd ed. Philadelphia, Pa: WB Saunders; 1995:353.)

topical anesthetics (and nerve blocks, if necessary), the FOB is placed through the bronchial lumen of the DLT. The FOB is then advanced into the airway under direction vision until the epiglottis or the laryngeal aperture is identified. Once the glottic opening or the epiglottis is in view (Fig. 64–11), the FOB is maneuvered through the vocal cords and into the trachea. The FOB is then advanced further down the trachea to a position just above the carina. At this point, the DLT is threaded over the FOB through the larynx and into the trachea. If the ETT does not advance easily, it may be hung up at the

**TABLE 64–8.** Anatomic Predictors of Difficult Intubation: Minimal Acceptable Values and Significance of Airway Examination

| Airway Evaluation Measurements | Minimal Acceptable Value | Significance of Examination |
|---|---|---|
| *QUANTITATIVE* | | |
| *Interincisor Gap* Space between upper and lower incisors measured in centimeters | >3 cm | A positive result (>3 cm) means a 2-cm deep flange on a MacIntosh or Miller blade can be easily inserted without hitting teeth. |
| *Oropharyngeal Class* Obtained with patient sitting to maximize predictability. In patients with a known or suspected C-spine injury, examine patient supine, with neck neutral. | ≤ Class II (see text for definition of Mallampati classes) | A positive result (≤ Class II) means the tongue is reasonably small in relation to the size of the oropharyngeal cavity and should be relatively easy to retract out of the line of site. |
| *Mandibular Space Length (hyomental or thyromental distance)* If C-spine injury, use method of Rocke et al. (head in neutral position) rather than that of Frerk (head fully extended) | ≥6 cm (hyomental distance) or ≥7 cm (thyromental distance) or 3 ordinary sized finger breadths | A positive result means that the larynx is reasonably posterior relative to the other upper airway structures resulting in a favorable line of site. |
| *Range of Motion of Head and Neck* Unable to test in patient with possible C-spine injury | Neck flexed on chest 35° and head extended on neck 80° (sniffing position) | The sniffing position aligns the oral, pharyngeal and laryngeal axis creating a favorable line of site. |
| *QUALITATIVE* | | |
| *Length of Neck* | A qualitative evaluation. A quantitative index has not been determined. | A short fat neck is a known confounder in intubation. However, no specific values have been prospectively tested. |
| *Thickness of Neck* | Qualitative/relative | A thick neck decreases the ability to align the upper airway axes. |
| *Length of Incisors* | Qualitative/relative | Long incisors increase the difficulty of aligning the oral and pharyngeal axes (creates a sharper angle between the two axes). |
| *Buck Teeth* Involuntary anterior overriding of maxillary teeth on the mandibular teeth | Absence of overriding of maxillary teeth upon mandibular teeth | The significance of buck teeth is impairment of glottic visualization; similar to the obstruction caused by long incisors. |
| *Mandibular Translation* Voluntary protrusion of the mandibular teeth anterior to maxillary teeth | Ability to protrude mandibular teeth anterior to maxillary teeth | Test of temporomandibular function. A positive result predicts that a good view of the larynx with conventional laryngoscopy is likely. |
| *Palate Configuration* | Should not appear very narrow or highly arched | A narrow palate decreases the oropharyngeal volume and ability to visualize the larynx when both the laryngoscope and endotracheal tube are in the mouth. |

Modified from Wilson WC, Benumof JL. Pathophysiology, evaluation, and treatment of the difficult airway. *Anesth Clin North Am.* 1998;16:29.

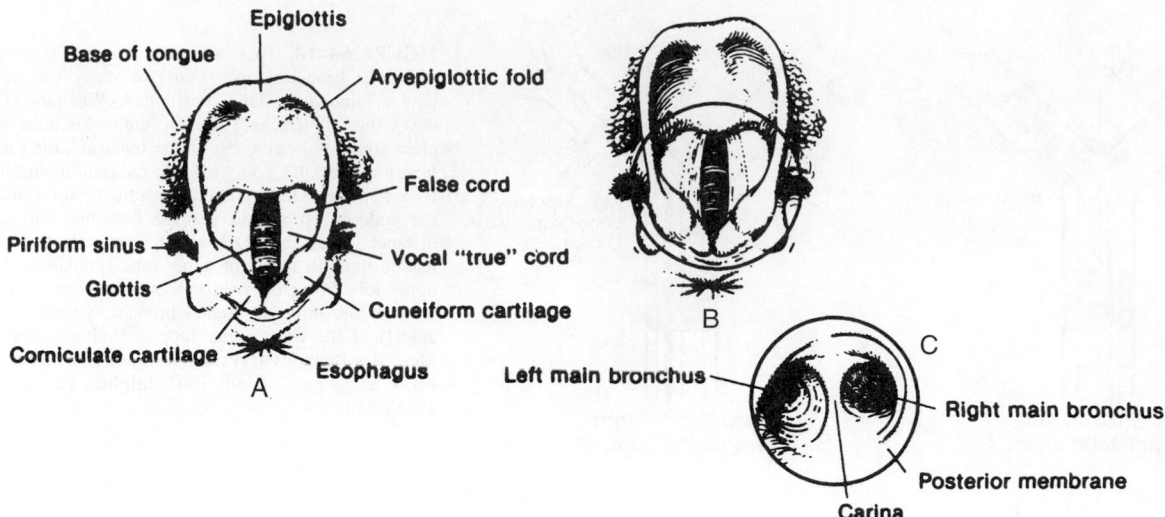

**FIGURE 64–11.** View of the larynx and carina via a fiberoptic bronchoscope. *A,* The normal anatomy of the larynx. *B,* View obtained from a fiberoptic bronchoscope positioned just above the laryngeal inlet. *C,* After passage of the FOB through the vocal cords and down the trachea, the carina comes into view. The tracheal cartilages are C-shaped and are joined posteriorly with a membrane. This anatomy allows for identification of the various portions of the tracheal bronchial tree. (From Zuppan J. Fiberoptic bronchoscopy in anesthesia and critical care. In: Benumof JL, ed. *Clinical Procedures in Anesthesia and Intensive Care.* Philadelphia, Pa: JB Lippincott; 1992:260.)

arytenoids or at the laryngeal aperture. This can either be due to a size discrepancy between the DLT and the FOB or because the DLT is too large in general. If hang up occurs, it is appropriate to rotate the DLT 90° to 180° to facilitate passage of the DLT past the obstruction. If the DLT still will not pass with these maneuvers, the DLT and FOB should be left in place and a laryngoscope gently placed to provide exposure (nerve blocks are usually required for patients to tolerate awake placement of a rigid direct laryngoscope). The laryngoscopist tries to visualize the hang up. This maneuver can also be of assistance if the bronchoscopist has trouble cannulating the glottis. In this case, the laryngoscopist can place the FOB through the cords, or near enough to the cords so the bronchoscopist can steer the FOB through the cords. While still retaining laryngoscopic view, the DLT is advanced into the midtracheal position. If none of these maneuvers allow passage into the trachea, the FOB and DLT are removed together as a unit and a smaller DLT used.

After placing the DLT into the midtrachea, a period of rest and ventilation of both lungs with the DLT in the midtrachea can now take place, and the patient can be put to sleep (deferring bronchial placement till the patient is deeply asleep). Alternatively, providing excellent distal topicalization with good patient cooperation and high $O_2$ saturation, the FOB can be steered into the appropriate bronchus and the DLT advanced over it into the final position. Similarly, the FOB can be used to guide DLT placement in apneic or anesthetized patients. These patients should be preoxygenated and laryngoscopy used to expose the glottis, while the bronchoscopist steers the FOB and DLT into the trachea.

### Bronchial Blockers

BBs are balloon-tipped luminal catheters (eg, Fogarty embolectomy catheter) that can be placed under FOB guidance into a mainstem bronchus, thereby inhibiting ventilation beyond the blockage and facilitating 1LV. BBs now are commercially available as a structurally combined apparatus, joined to a single-lumen tube, marketed as the Univent Tube (Fugi

Systems Corp, Tokyo, Japan). Additionally, free standing BBs continue to be used.

### Pros and Cons of Bronchial Blockers Compared With Double-Lumen Tubes

The advantage of using a BB for lung separation is that the single-lumen ETT can be used before and after lung separation without the need for exchanging the DLT for a single-lumen tube. This is particularly advantageous in patients with difficult airways preoperatively, or in those who will be edematous postoperatively (long duration thoracic, spine case performed in the prone position).

However, the disadvantages of the BBs compared with DLT lung separation include the inability to extensively suction or ventilate the lung distal to the blocker (while inflated). Also, there is increased placement time using BBs compared with a DLT (less significant when using the Univent tube). Additionally, there is a propensity for the BB to back out of the bronchus into the trachea, loosing the seal separating the two lungs, which can lead to two catastrophic complications. First, if the BB was being used to seal off a fluid (blood or pus) in one lung, then both lungs may become contaminated with the fluid. Second, the trachea will be at least partially obstructed by the blocker, and ventilation will be greatly impaired. The Univent tube has been re-engineered and is much more stable in the bronchus than earlier designs but still not as stable as a DLT. A new system (Arndt Endobronchial Blocker, see later) has a lower pressure, larger volume cuff, which makes it about as stable as the Univent tube. Regardless of the device, bronchial blockage requires that the anesthesiologist continuously and intensively monitor the compliance and breath sounds of the ventilated lung and have a bronchoscope in the room throughout the case.

### Indications and Placement Considerations for Bronchial Blockers

In general, BBs are most suitable for nonpulmonary procedures requiring 1LV, rather than lung operations requiring

1LV, because of the inability to ventilate or suction debris from the blocked lung and because of the more frequent incidence of BB migration compared with DLT. BBs are best placed in the left mainstem bronchus for left-sided surgery (greater margin of error). For right lower or middle lung surgery, the BB can be placed in the right-sided bronchus intermedius (providing the surgeon does not mind that this allows ventilation of the right upper lobe). For right upper lobe surgery, the BB can be placed either in the right mainstem bronchus (prone to migration with surgical manipulation) or at the orifice of the right upper lobe). This tends to be more stationary; however, air can leak around the BB in this position due to the disparity between diameter of the right mainstem bronchus (1.6 cm), the right upper lobe bronchus (1.0 cm), and the bronchus intermedius (1.1 cm) (see Fig. 64–1).

### The Univent Bronchial Blocker Tube

The Univent tube is a single-lumen tube (adult sizes 7.0 and 8.0 mm ID) that has a small lumen along the anterior concave side of the tube (Fig. 64–12). This lumen contains a small hollow lumen catheter (~17 gauge) with a cuff at the end of the tube. This secondary moveable, small lumen, cuffed catheter serves as a BB when the catheter is advanced into either mainstem bronchus and the cuff is inflated.

**Insertion Technique for the Univent Tube.** The Univent tube is inserted in the following manner. First, the single-lumen tube, along with the BB, is inserted as a unit into the trachea (Fig. 64–13). The cuff on the main ETT lumen is inflated, and the patient is ventilated and oxygenated. An FOB is inserted through a self-sealing diaphragm in the elbow connector to the single-lumen tube while ventilation is maintained around the FOB (but within the single-lumen tube). The right and left mainstem bronchi are identified by noting

the relationship of the mainstem bronchi to the posterior membrane and the anterior cartilaginous rings. The tube of the BB is located by moving the BB in and out just beyond the end of its own and the main lumens of the Univent tube. Next, the main single-lumen tube is turned so that the concavity of the tube is facing the side to be blocked. The BB is then advanced into the mainstem bronchus under direct vision, the balloon is inflated just so the cephalad surface of the balloon is just below the tracheal carina, and the FOB is then withdrawn.

### Independent Bronchial Blockers

Besides the commercially available Univent tube, BBs can also be passed independently of the single-lumen tube. The independent BB most often used for adults is a Fogarty occlusion (embolectomy catheter with balloons, which range from 3-6 mL).[143] The Fogarty embolectomy catheter comes with a stylet in place so that it is possible to place a curvature at the distal tip (like a hockey stick) to facilitate entry into the larynx and either mainstem bronchus (by twirling the proximal end).

**Insertion Technique for Independent Bronchial Blockers.** If no ETT is in place, the operator exposes the larynx and places a single-lumen tube with a high-volume cuff in the trachea. The Fogarty catheter is then placed either inside or alongside the single-lumen tube. Placement of the Fogarty catheter inside the single-lumen tube can be greatly facilitated by use of two elbow connectors with self-sealing diaphragms that are connected in series with the anesthesia circuit attached to the proximal end of the connectors.[144] The distal end of the elbow connectors is attached to the patient's single-lumen ETT. The Fogarty catheter can be easily introduced through the diaphragm of one of the elbow connectors while the other diaphragm allows insertion of an FOB to verify correct placement of the catheter in the mainstem bronchus. In either case, an FOB is passed down to the end of the single-lumen tube through a self-sealing diaphragm in the elbow connector (which permits continued positive-pressure ventilation around the FOB), and the Fogarty catheter is visualized below the tip of the single-lumen tube. The proximal end of the BB is then twirled in the fingertips until the hockey stick–shaped distal tip locates in the desired mainstem bronchus. The catheter balloon is then inflated under direct visualization, and the FOB is withdrawn through the self-sealing diaphragm. The self-sealing diaphragm in the elbow connector containing the BB should be made airtight. The BB within the single-lumen tube technique may also be used with a tracheotomy.[145] Placing the BB outside the lumen of the single-lumen tube has the advantage of increased stability during suctioning and bronchoscopy.

**Arndt Endobronchial Blocker Set.** Most independent BBs have the disadvantage of being difficult to properly place, even with the help of an FOB. Indeed, sometimes placement of an independent BB requires rigid bronchoscopy for placement. However, the new Arndt Endobronchial Blocker (Cook Critical Care, Bloomington, Ind) incorporates a novel snare-guided BB that makes positioning far easier (Fig. 64–14). The Arndt Endobronchial Set works with any standard ETT. After intubation, the Arndt multiport airway adapter is connected between the ETT and the ventilation circuit using standard 15 mm connectors. Additionally, specific ports exist for insertion of the FOB and the special snare-tipped endobronchial cathe-

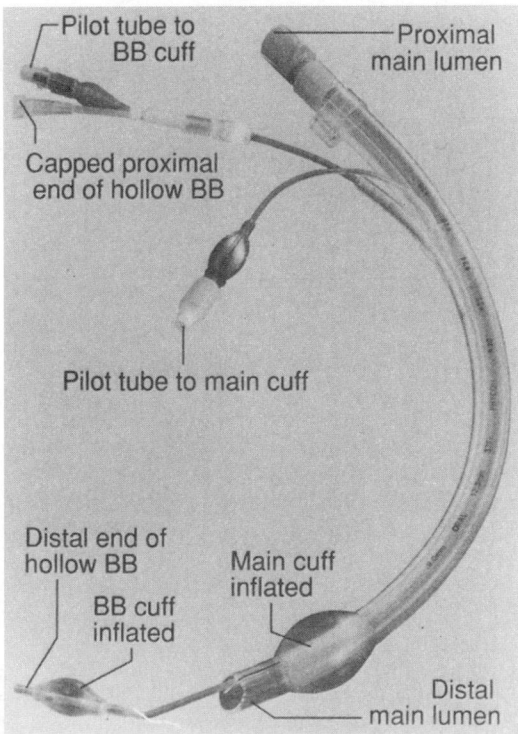

**FIGURE 64–12.** The Univent single-lumen tube bronchial blocker system.

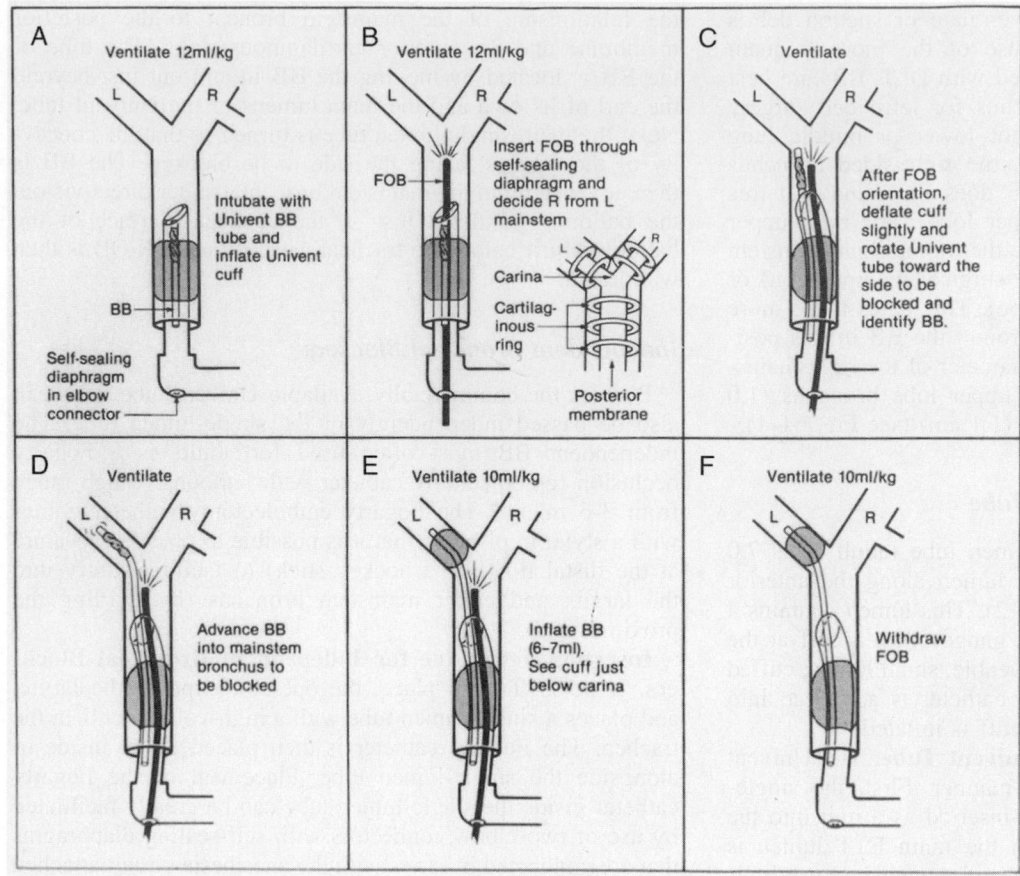

**FIGURE 64–13.** The sequential steps of the fiberoptic-aided method of inserting and positioning the Univent bronchial blocker in the left mainstem bronchus are illustrated. One- and two-lung ventilation is achieved by simply inflating and deflating, respectively, the bronchial blocker balloon. FOB, fiberoptic bronchoscope. (From Benumof JL. *Anesthesia for Thoracic Surgery.* 2nd ed. Philadelphia, Pa: WB Saunders; 1995:372.)

ter. The FOB is passed through the loop of the endobronchial catheter snare. The snare-guided bronchial blocker is slid along the FOB to the desired spot. Alternatively, the snare can be tightened gently around the distal tip of the FOB. The endobronchial catheter can then be guided into the desired bronchus under direct vision by the ensnared FOB. Once positioning is verified by the FOB, the string may be removed and the resulting 1.8-mm lumen may be used for suctioning (not great) or for insufflation of $O_2$ or application of operative lung CPAP. Two minor drawbacks to this device are its high

cost and the inability to reinsert the string (once removed) to facilitate redirection of the endobronchial blocker if necessary.

### Pediatric-Sized Double-Lumen Tubes, Bronchial Blockers, and Other Lung Separation Devices

Young teenagers (ages 13-14 years) can frequently use an adult-sized 35 French DLT. The smallest left-sided DLTs made by Mallinckrodt are 32, 28, and 26 French; these can be used by 12-, 10-, and 8-year-old children, respectively. The smallest

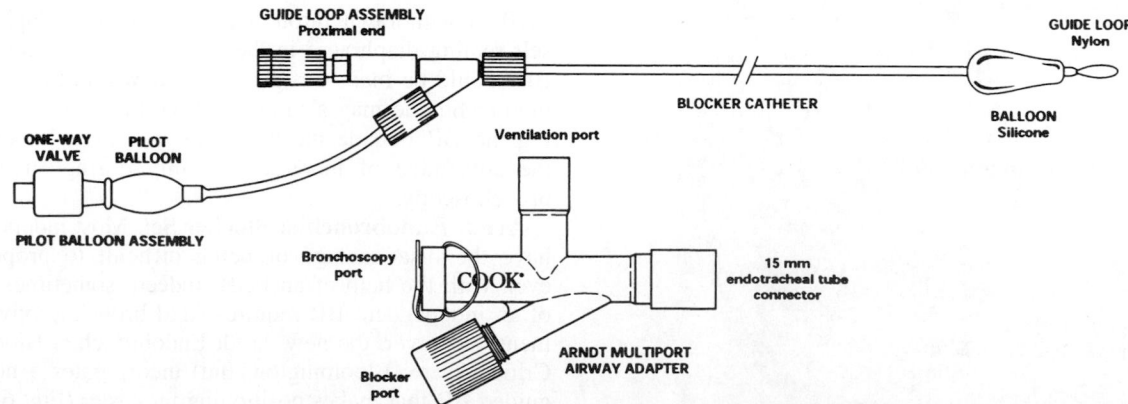

**FIGURE 64–14.** The Arndt Endobronchial Blocker System. This system consists of an endobronchial blocker catheter and an Arndt multiport airway adapter. The airway adapter has a specific bronchoscopy port and bronchial blocker port, as well as two standard 15-mm airway connectors to connect the ventilator system to the patient's endotracheal tube. The endobronchial blocker has a novel snare (nylon loop) at the distal tip. The endobronchial blocker is placed through the blocker port of the airway adapter and into the patient's endotracheal tube. Next, the fiberoptic bronchoscope (FOB) is passed through the bronchoscopy port of the airway adapter, and the tip of the FOB is placed within the snare of the endobronchial blocker. The snare loop is tightened, and then the FOB can guide the endobronchial blocker into the appropriate bronchus. See text for further explanation.

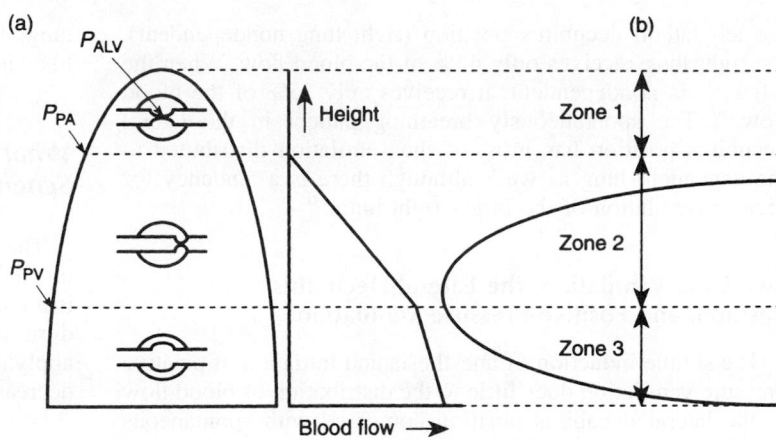

**FIGURE 64–15.** The three-zone model of the lung showing how the distribution of blood flow from top to bottom of the lung (center) is determined by the alveolar (Palv), pulmonary artery (Ppa) and pulmonary venous (Ppv) pressures. Zone 1, which may be present in the erect lung (a), is not present in the supine position (b) because the vertical height of the lung is less than Ppa, however, some Zone 1 would be present in the lateral decubitus position (see Fig. 64–16). (From Sykes K. Pulmonary physiology during one-lung ventilation. In: Gosh S, Latimer RD, eds. *Thoracic Anaesthesia.* Oxford, United Kingdom: Butterworth-Heinemann; 1999:25. Reprinted by permission of Butterworth-Heinemann, a division of Reed Educational & Professional Ltd.)

right-sided tube is the 32 French; the 28 and 26 French currently come only as a left-sided DLT. Leyland Rubber has made some special order right- and left-sided DLTs for 6- to 8-year-old children, largely for bronchopulmonary lavage of alveolar proteinosis. For smaller children, BBs or mainstem intubation are techniques typically used when lung separation is necessary. There are 3.5 and 4.5 Univent tubes available for 6- to 10-year-old children. For bronchial blockade in small children (19 kg or less), a Fogarty embolectomy catheter with a balloon capacity of 0.5 mL or a Swan-Ganz catheter (1-mL balloon) should be used.[146] Naturally, these catheters have to be positioned under direct vision; an FOB method is perfectly acceptable, except the FOB outside diameter must be approximately 2 mm to fit inside the ETT. Otherwise, the BB must be situated with a rigid bronchoscope. Pediatric patients of intermediate size will require intermediate-sized occlusion catheters and appropriate judgment on the mode of placement (ie, rigid versus FOB). Additionally, Marraro bilumen uncuffed tubes have been used in neonates weighing as low as 1500 g to 5 year olds.[147]

## MANAGEMENT OF ONE-LUNG VENTILATION

### How Is Ventilation-Perfusion Normally Distributed?

The pulmonary circulation is a low pressure, low resistance system under normal conditions. Therefore, the distribution of flow is primarily determined by gravity, with the majority of perfusion occurring in the dependent portion of the lung. Ventilation is also affected by gravity with the top of the lung having more negative pleural pressure than the bottom of the lung. Given that the lung is about one quarter as dense as water, there is approximately 7.5 cm $H_2O$ pressure gradient from the top to the bottom of a 30 cm tall lung.[148] In 1964, West and coworkers described the distribution of blood flow in relation to vascular and alveolar pressures.[149] Since then, three classical "zones of West" have been recognized in the upright chest: zone 1 (top of the lung) has relatively high $\dot{V}/\dot{Q}$ (PA > Ppa > Ppv); zone 2 (middle of the lung) has relatively matched $\dot{V}/\dot{Q}$ (Ppa > PA > Ppv); zone 3 (bottom of the lung) has relatively low $\dot{V}/\dot{Q}$ (Ppa > Ppv > PA). (PA, alveolar pressure; Ppa, pulmonary artery pressure; and Ppv, pulmonary venous pressure.) In the supine position, little zone

1 exists because the vertical height of the lung is less than the Ppa (Fig. 64–15).

### What Are the Ventilation-Perfusion Relationship Changes That Occur in the Lateral Decubitus Position During Two-Versus One-Lung Ventilation (Spontaneous Versus Positive Pressure Ventilation)?

#### Two-Lung Ventilation, Lateral Decubitus Position, and the Spontaneously Breathing Patient

In the lateral decubitus position, the nondependent lung is comprised of mainly zone 1 and zone 2, whereas the dependent lung is comprised of zone 2 and zone 3 (Fig. 64–16). In the upright position, the right lung receives approximately 55% of the blood flow, with 45% going to the left lung. In

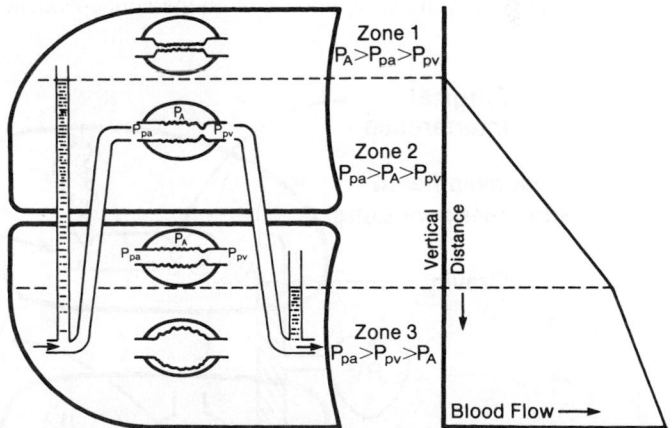

**FIGURE 64–16.** Schematic representation of the effects of gravity on the distribution of pulmonary blood flow in the lateral decubitus position. The vertical gradient in the lateral decubitus position is less than that in the upright position, but more than the supine position (see Fig. 64–15). Consequently, there is less zone 1 and more zone 2 and zone 3 blood flow in the lateral decubitus position compared with the upright position. Nevertheless, pulmonary blood flow increases with lung dependency and is greater in the dependent lung compared with the nondependent lung. PA, alveolar pressure; Ppa, pulmonary artery pressure; Ppv, pulmonary venous pressure. (Modified from Benumof JL. Physiology of the open chest and one-lung ventilation. In: Kaplan JA, ed. *Thoracic Anesthesia.* New York, NY: Churchill Livingstone; 1983.)

the left lateral decubitus position (right lung nondependent), the right lung receives only 45% of the blood flow. When the left lung is nondependent, it receives only 35% of the blood flow.[149] The spontaneously breathing patient in the lateral decubitus position has most of the ventilation distributed to the dependent lung as well, although there is a tendency for greater ventilation of the larger right lung.[151]

### Two-Lung Ventilation, the Lateral Decubitus Position, and Positive-Pressure Ventilation

The simple induction of anesthesia and initiation of positive pressure ventilation does little to the distribution of blood flow in the lateral decubitus position compared with spontaneous ventilation. However, the distribution of ventilation between the two lungs is dramatically altered, as the majority of ventilation is switched from the dependent lung to the nondependent lung. Indeed, the nondependent lung receives about 55% of the positive pressure ventilation.[152] Similar findings are observed in children.[153] When the chest is open, there is an even greater disparity between ventilation (greater in the nondependent lung) and perfusion (greater in the dependent lung).

### One-Lung Ventilation, the Lateral Decubitus Position, and Positive Pressure Ventilation

When 1LV is employed, the nondependent lung is the nonventilated and collapsed (atelectatic) lung. Switching from 2LV to 1LV dramatically improves the $\dot{V}/\dot{Q}$ matching to the dependent (ventilated) lung. However, there will still be some blood traveling through the nondependent lung. This blood represents an obligate right-to-left transpulmonary shunt. Anything that increases the blood flow to the nondependent lung decreases the blood flow to the dependent lung and worsens shunt. Figure 64–17 summarizes the influences on pulmonary blood flow. Vasodilators and high-dose general anesthetics will inhibit HPV and increase blood flow to the nondependent lung. Excessive tidal volume or dependent lung PEEP will likewise force more blood to the nondependent lung.

### What Is the Optimum Initial Management Scheme for One-Lung Ventilation?

The optimum initial management scheme for 1LV is based on the $\dot{V}/\dot{Q}$ issues reviewed previously. Systemic hypoxemia is a constant threat and must be avoided by optimizing dependent lung ventilation and quickly re-expanding and or applying CPAP to the nondependent lung when saturations decrease.

### Optimization of Fraction of Inspired Oxygen

Although $O_2$ toxicity and absorption atelectasis are bonafide concerns, the benefit of supplying 100% $O_2$ exceeds the risks when applied for short periods in all patients except those who have received certain chemotherapy drugs (see later discussion). A high $F_{IO_2}$ in the ventilated lung has the benefit of maintaining the $PaO_2$ at higher safer levels rather than hypoxemic levels, which may threaten myocardial and cerebral vitality. Additionally, a high dependent lung $F_{IO_2}$ promotes vasodilation and increases the ability to accommodate the increased blood flow redistribution due to nondependent lung HPV.[154,155]

For considerations of absorption atelectasis, an optimum $F_{IO_2}$ is 0.8 to 0.9 because increasing the $F_{I}N_2$ to the 0.1 to 0.2 range greatly diminishes the possibility of absorption atelectasis (by allowing some nitrogen to splint open low $\dot{V}/\dot{Q}$ regions).[156] At the same time, the diminution in $PaO_2$ should be trivial in most patients.

### *Oxygen-Induced Pulmonary Toxicity*

Molecular $O_2$ is a powerful oxidizing agent, and multiple reactive $O_2$ species occur. Superoxide, hydrogen peroxide

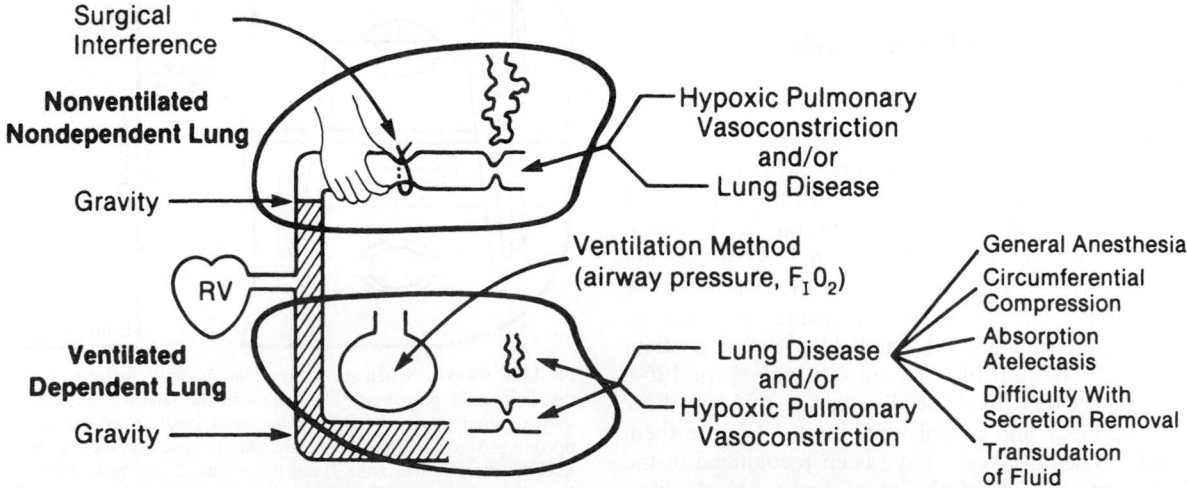

**FIGURE 64–17.** This schematic diagram shows the major determinants of blood flow distribution during one-lung ventilation. Blood flow to the nonventilated, nondependent lung is reduced by the force of gravity, surgical interference (compression, tying off of vessels), hypoxic pulmonary vasoconstriction, or lung disease (vascular obliteration, thrombosis). Blood flow to the ventilated, dependent lung is increased by gravity; however, dependent lung blood flow and vascular resistance may be altered in either direction depending on the method of ventilation (amount of airway pressure, $F_{IO_2}$, and the amount of dependent lung disease and/or hypoxic pulmonary vasoconstriction). Factors that may increase the amount of dependent lung disease intraoperatively are listed on the extreme right of the figure (see Fig. 64–18). (From Benumof JL. *Anesthesia for Thoracic Surgery.* 2nd ed. Philadephia, Pa: WB Saunders; 1995:408.)

($H_2O_2$), and the hydroxyl radicals are some the best understood toxic, reactive intermediates. Superoxide ($O_2^-$) is formed when one electron is added to molecular $O_2$. Superoxide then undergoes a dismutation reaction (catalyzed by superoxide dismutase) to yield $H_2O_2$. The $H_2O_2$ formed is further reduced via either another dismutase reaction (catalyzed by catalase) or directly by glutathione (catalyzed by glutathione peroxidase) to form $H_2O$.[157]

In the mammalian species, almost all respired $O_2$ is reduced via a series of linked electron-carrying enzymes in mitochondria, producing water without discharging harmful intermediates.[158] However, some reactive $O_2$ species are invariably produced.[159–161] Normally, an elaborate array of extracellular and cytoplasmic antioxidant defense mechanisms protect the cell from oxidant injury (including catalase, superoxide dismutase, glutathione, and peroxidase). However, when production of toxic $O_2$ species exceeds clearance, cellular damage occurs.

Considerable evidence has accumulated implicating oxidant-mediated cell injury in the pathophysiology of pulmonary $O_2$ toxicity,[162,163] endotoxic lung injury,[164,165] emphysema, immune-complex alveolitis,[166] aspiration pneumonia,[167] interstitial lung disease,[168, 169] and ischemia-reperfusion mediated lung injury.[170–175]

The dose toxicity curve for human beings is only approximate because it varies according to barometric pressure, $F_{IO_2}$, level of antioxidant exposure (ie, drugs such as bleomycin), integrity of the normal endogenous antioxidant defense system, as well as whether or not reperfusion is occurring following an anoxic period. $O_2$ toxicity begins with >6 hours of exposure to 200% to 500% $O_2$ (2-5 atmospheres), or >12 hours of exposure at 100% $O_2$, or >24 hours of exposure at 80% $O_2$, or >36 hours exposure at 60% $O_2$.[176]

### Chemotherapeutics That Promote Oxygen Toxicity

Multiple chemotherapeutic drugs may cause pulmonary toxicity. However, four classes of drugs deserve major focus because these have been documented to clearly increase the propensity for pulmonary toxicity, especially in conjunction with increased $F_{IO_2}$.

**Cyclophosphamide (Nitrogen Mustard).** Nitrogen mustards comprise a group of toxic vesicating alkylating drugs that were synthesized in 1854 and used during World War I (WWI) for the vesicant action on the eyes, skin, and lungs.[177] In the interval between WWI and WWII, the nitrogen mustards were extensively but secretly studied. After WWII, these data were declassified and efforts toward using these drugs as antineoplastics began.

Cyclophosphamide, a nitrogen mustard, promotes three major forms of pulmonary toxicity: (1) an acute, IgE-mediated hypersensitivity reaction similar to that seen with methotrexate, bleomycin, and procarbazine[178]; (2) noncardiogenic pulmonary edema (rare)[179]; and (3) pulmonary fibrosis (most common form of toxicity). In these cases, cyclophosphamide depletes the body store of antioxidants,[180] and the unchallenged reactive oxidant species injure cellular membranes.[181] Exposure to high concentrations of $O_2$ has been demonstrated to result in an increased risk of damage in animals.[182]

**Carmustine (Nitrosourea).** Carmustine, also known as BCNU, is associated with pulmonary toxicity that is heralded by a decrease in diffusion capacity and has an average incidence of 25%. At doses higher than 1500 mg/m², the incidence may be as high as 30% to 50%.[183] Preexisting lung disease, concomitant exposure to cyclophosphamide, and tobacco use increase the risk of pulmonary toxicity from BCNU (Table 64–9).[184,185] The long-term pulmonary effects of BCNU exposure are particularly striking. O'Driscoll and colleagues report that in children with brain tumors treated with carmustine and radiation, there was a 35% fatality rate from pulmonary fibrosis, with two thirds of these patients dying of progressive fibrosis. Fibrosis may be encountered up to 17 years after cessation of the drug.[186] Rare case reports of carmustine-associated acute pulmonary venous vasculitis have been cited, similar to that seen with mitomycin and bleomycin.[187]

**Bleomycin (Antibiotic).** Bleomycin is an antibiotic product of a *Streptomyces* species, which is a mixture of several sulfur-containing glycopeptides. They function principally by binding to DNA, with resulting strand damage and ultimate inhibition of DNA synthesis.

Pulmonary toxicity occurs in three forms. The first is an acute IgE-mediated hypersensitivity reaction, similar to that seen with cyclophosphamide.[188,189] A second form of toxicity is an acute pulmonary venous vasculitis with resultant pulmonary hypertension. A third and most worrisome pulmonary toxicity is dose-dependent chronic pneumonitis, with or without progressive fibrosis. Bleomycin results in direct injury to the pulmonary capillary endothelium, followed by injury to the type I and type II pneumocytes, with progressive fibrosis of the alveolar-capillary membrane and a decreased diffusion capacity and restrictive lung pattern.[190] Toxicity is at least partially caused by free radical formation, explaining the tendency of $O_2$ therapy to worsen the effect of bleomycin toxicity.[191] The role of radiation in stimulating free radical formation further potentiates bleomycin toxicity.[192]

The risk of toxicity is approximately 5% at doses up to 400 units but increases exponentially at higher doses.[193] Toxicity has been noted at doses as low as 100 units, although the presence of other risk factors is considered to have contributed to these cases.[194] Other risk factors include advanced age; combination therapy with other toxins, including cyclophosphamide; chest irradiation (doses >3300 rads); and smoking.[195]

Reports of postoperative complications, including death among patients exposed to bleomycin, first appeared in 1978.[196,197] The prominent risk factor was initially thought to be $O_2$ therapy and excessive crystalloid administration, although subsequent studies have implicated only the former.[198–200] A few poorly controlled studies questioned the role of $O_2$ therapy in the pathogenesis of bleomycin toxicity; because these experiments did not control the bleomycin dose and degree of exposure, they should not be used as evidence to disregard $F_{IO_2}$ levels.[201,202] Given the current information, $O_2$ exposure must be carefully limited to patients with a history of exposure to bleomycin. This may be challenging in the case of selective 1LV (eg, excision of lung cancer after bleomycin chemotherapy). A useful means of providing precisely controlled $O_2$ concentrations was described by Hughes and Benumof.[203]

**Mitomycin C (Antibiotic).** Mitomycin C is an antibiotic produced by a Streptomyces species and could also be classified as an alkylating agent. Mitomycin forms covalent bonds with DNA, creating cross-links that inhibit DNA synthesis. Additionally, Mitomycin C promotes an elaboration of $O_2$-free radicals. The mechanism of mitomycin-induced pneumo-

**TABLE 64–9.** Pulmonary Toxicity of Antineoplastic Drugs

| Drug | Incidence and Injury Type | Dose-Related Toxicity | Does $O_2$ Worsen? | Other Risk Factors |
|---|---|---|---|---|
| **Alkylating Agents** | | | | |
| Cyclophosphamide | <1% pulmonary fibrosis*† | No | Yes | None |
| Ifosfamide | Rare interstitial pneumonitis† | No | Unknown | None |
| Chlorambucil | Rare interstitial pneumonitis | 2000 mg over 6 months | Unknown | None |
| Melphalan | Rare interstitial pneumonitis | ? | Unknown | None |
| Busulfan | 4% pulmonary fibrosis | ? doses >500 mg | No | Advanced age, prolonged or combined treatment with radiation therapy |
| **Nitrosureas‡** | | | | |
| Carmustine | 25% pulmonary fibrosis§ | Yes, doses >1500 mg/m² | Yes | Prior lung disease, tobacco use, cyclophosphamide |
| **Antimetabolities** | | | | |
| Methotrexate | 8% incidence of hypersensitivity pneumonitis* | Rare at dose 20 mg/wk | No | None |
| Ara-C | Rare noncardiogenic pulmonary edema | High dose only | No | None |
| **Plant Derivatives** | | | | |
| Vincristine | Rare pulmonary infiltrates with fibrosis | Only with mitomycin | No | Mitomycin coadministration |
| **Antineoplastic Antibiotics** | | | | |
| Bleomycin | 5%–40% incidence of chronic pulmonary fibrosis*§ | Yes, dose >100 units | Yes | Cyclophosphamide, advanced age, radiation therapy, tobacco use |
| Mitomycin | 3%–12% incidence of interstitial pneumonitis§ | No | Yes | Radiation therapy |
| Procarbazine | Hypersensitivity, pneumonitis | No | No | None |

*Hypersensitivity pneumonitis rarely seen.
†Noncardiogenic pulmonary edema rarely seen.
†All nitrosureas have been associated with pulmonary disease.
§Acute pulmonary venous vasculitis rarely seen.

nitis is not fully understood, but is thought to be similar to the mechanism responsible for bleomycin-related pulmonary fibrosis (see above).[204] The incidence of pulmonary fibrosis does not appear to be dose-related, although $O_2$ therapy and thoracic irradiation are probably contributory.[205,206] The incidence of fibrosis approaches 12% with a 50% mortality.[207,208] Rare cases of mitomycin-associated pulmonary venous vasculitis have also been noted, similar to that seen with carmustine and bleomycin.[209]

### Optimization of the Initial Ventilation Scheme for One-Lung Ventilation

The dependent lung should be ventilated with approximately 8 to 10 mL/kg. Larger tidal volumes increase dependent lung alveolar pressures and vascular resistance,[210] thereby forcing more blood upward to the nondependent lung, impairing HPV and increasing shunt.[211,212] Similarly, little or no dependent lung PEEP should be used initially.

The respiratory rate should be adjusted so that the $Paco_2$ remains at 40 mm Hg. The dependent lung $V_T$ of 10 mL/kg represents a decrease of approximately 20% from the usual two-lung $V_T$ of 10 to 15 mL/kg. Thus, the respiratory rate usually needs to be increased approximately 30% because there is slightly increased dead space ventilation in the 1LV condition compared with 2LV.[213] Hypocapnia is avoided be-

cause the increased mean airway pressure required to achieve it can increase nondependent lung blood flow (blunting HPV),[214] and systemic hypocapnia can inhibit nondependent lung HPV.[215] Conversely, hypercapnia is avoided because it can increase the dependent lung vascular resistance and force more blood flow up to the nondependent lung and increase shunt (Fig. 64–18).

### What Are the Options for Treatment of Hypoxemia During One-Lung Ventilation?

If $O_2$ saturation begins to diminish, (1) ensure that the patient is being ventilated with 100% $O_2$; (2) verify that hemodynamic status is adequate; (3) use an FOB to ensure proper positioning of the lung separation apparatus (DLT or BB) and to ensure that secretions or blood are not occluding ventilated bronchi; (4) use differential lung ventilation techniques (intermittent re-inflation of the nondependent lung, nondependent lung CPAP, followed by dependent lung PEEP); and (5) if hypoxemia persists, consider clamping the operative (nondependent) lung. Additionally, in patients with pulmonary vascular hypertension, inhaled nitric oxide (iNO) may be beneficial. The following sections detail the effects of differential lung ventilation techniques.

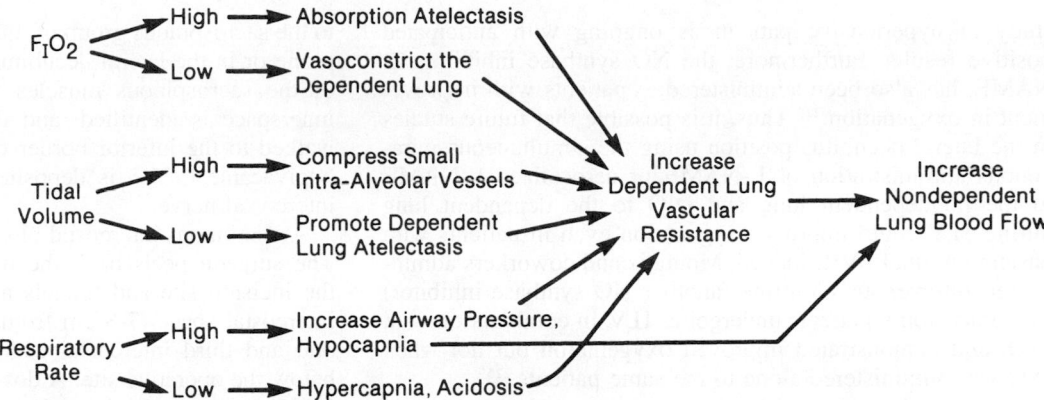

**FIGURE 64–18.** The method of ventilation of the dependent lung during one-lung ventilation can be a major determinant of the amount of nondependent lung blood flow. (From Benumof JL. *Anesthesia for Thoracic Surgery.* 2nd ed. Philadephia, Pa: WB Saunders; 1995:409.)

## Limitations of Intermittent Operative Lung Re-Inflation for Improving PaO₂

Intermittent re-inflation of the collapsed operative (nondependent) lung during 1LV usually results in an immediate significant increase in PaO₂. Indeed, Malmkvist demonstrated that intermittent lung re-expansion, occurring every 5 minutes, resulted in a PaO₂ that was twice the value obtained in a control group that did not receive intermittent re-inflation.[216] The problem with intermittent re-inflation of the operative lung is that it is impractical and bothersome to the surgeon and may not be compatible with surgery in certain situations.

## Operative (Nondependent) Lung Continuous Positive Airway Pressure Dramatically Improves PaO₂

Hypoxemia during 1LV (in patients with properly positioned DLT or BBs) is mainly due to shunt occurring in the nondependent lung. Therefore, it is surprising that manipulations of the V̇/Q̇ of the nondependent lung have the greatest effect on PaO₂. Completely occluding blood flow to the nondependent (operative) lung will eliminate this source of shunting. However, clamping the delicate PAs can only be done after they have been dissected out, and should only be reserved for emergency situations unless the entire operative lung is planned for resection (ie, pneumonectomy or transplant situation). Conversely, manipulation of the ventilation to the operative, nondependent lung can dramatically improve oxygenation with little disruption of the surgical field.

Low levels of operative lung CPAP maintain the patency of the nondependent lung airways, allowing gas exchange between O₂-filled alveoli and the capillary blood flow.[217] In essentially all human clinical studies of nondependent lung, CPAP (in the 5-10 cm H₂O range) has led to significant reproducible improvement in PaO₂.[218] Furthermore, nondependent lung CPAP is better tolerated by the surgeons than intermittent re-inflation because the surgical field is minimally disturbed.

## Nonoperative (Dependent) Lung Positive End-Expiratory Pressure Sometimes Decrease Oxygenation Rather Than Improve It

Application of PEEP to the nonoperative (dependent), ventilated lung results in two separate countervailing effects. The beneficial effect is that the administration of pressure to the alveoli and distal airways at end-exhalation tends to recruit

lung volume, increase FRC, and keep alveoli open that would otherwise become atelectatic and thus decrease shunt in the dependent lung. The nonbeneficial effect of dependent lung PEEP is that the increased airway pressure will tend to divert blood away from the dependent ventilated lung up to the nondependent, nonventilated lung and increase shunt through that lung, thus decreasing PaO₂. Accordingly, it is not surprising that dependent lung PEEP studies have demonstrated variable results, with some patients decreasing and others increasing their oxygenation.[219–221] Overall, the variable results and countervailing effects of dependent lung PEEP argues against using it as a primary therapy. Rather, dependent lung PEEP should only be employed after nondependent lung CPAP has been administered (Fig. 64–19).

## Role of Inhaled Nitric Oxide in Improving Oxygenation During One-Lung Ventilation in the Lateral Decubitus Position

Nitric oxide (NO) is a potent vasodilator of vascular smooth muscle. iNO provides selective pulmonary vasodilation to segments of the lung that are well ventilated, thus improving V̇/Q̇ matching. Rich and colleagues administered iNO to cardiac patients undergoing 2LV and demonstrated a significant reduction in pulmonary vascular resistance (PVR).[222] Subsequently, the same investigators administered iNO to supine patients undergoing 1LV with a BB and noted a decrease in PVR again (mainly in those with elevated PVRs).[223] In 1997, Wilson and coworkers hypothesized that administration of iNO to the dependent ventilated lung in patients undergoing 1LV in the lateral decubitus position would vasodilate the dependent ventilated lung and thus decrease the amount of blood forced to transit the nondependent lung.[224] However, they studied patients with normal PVR and consequently did not demonstrate any reduction in PVR or shunt. A follow-up

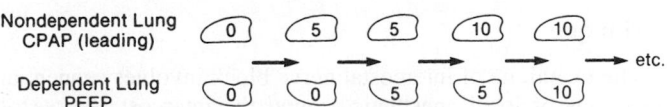

**FIGURE 64–19.** A search for optimal nondependent-lung continuous positive airway pressure (CPAP) and dependent-lung positive end-expiratory pressure (PEEP) is performed by leading with nondependent-lung CPAP and following with dependent-lung PEEP. Leading with nondependent-lung CPAP removes the deleterious arterial oxygenation blood flow diversion effects of dependent lung PEEP. (From Benumof JL. *Anesthesia for Thoracic Surgery.* 2nd ed. Philadelphia, Pa: WB Saunders; 1995:427.)

study in hypertensive patients is ongoing with anticipated positive results. Furthermore, the NO synthase inhibitor, L-NAME, has also been administered to patients with improvement in oxygenation.[225] Thus, it is possible that future studies in the lateral decubitus position using the simultaneous intravenous administration of L-NAME or aerosolized L-NAME to the nondependent lung and iNO to the dependent lung during 1LV could improve oxygenation even in patients with baseline normal PVR. Indeed, Moutafis and coworkers administered intravenous almitrine (another NO synthase inhibitor) to thoracostomy patients undergoing 1LV, in combination with iNO, and demonstrated improved oxygenation but not when iNO was administered alone to the same patients.[226]

## POST-THORACOTOMY ANALGESIA

The evolution of efficacious postoperative analgesic techniques has allowed thoracic anesthesia to mature into the well developed specialty it is today. The muscle sparing thoracotomy has resulted in improved muscle strength and spirometry values and less postoperative pain than the standard posterolateral thoracotomy.[227] However, effective analgesia is still particularly critical in the first 48 hours postoperatively.[228] Indeed, many of the complications following thoracic surgery are directly attributable to postoperative pain (splinting, poor pulmonary function) or the direct side effects of analgesic techniques (hypotension, respiratory depression, increased fluid requirements).

A thoracotomy incision is one of the most painful insults caused by surgery. This is partly due to the extensive innervation of the structures that are damaged during surgery, the continuous motion of the operative site and surrounding structures, and the various chest tubes and drains that irritate the pleura. Most thoracotomy incisions are made at the T5 innerspace, but the pain extends 2 to 3 dermatomes on either side of the incision. Additionally, the shoulder may be positioned in an uncomfortable orientation, the lung can become contused during operation, and the pleura irritated, and intercostal nerves can become trapped within sutures. Besides the intercostal nerves, pain signals can travel down the phrenic (diaphragmatic pleura), vagus (lung and mediastinal pleura), and cervical spinal nerves (shoulder and arm). Sympathetic nerves which innervate the lung may also play a role. Besides patient-controlled analgesia (reviewed in Chapters 13 and 14), five analgesic techniques are of particular importance in thoracic surgery: intercostal nerve blocks, epidural analgesia, cryoanalgesia, intrapleural catheters, and paravertebral blocks.

### What Is the Role of an Intercostal Block for Post-Thoracotomy Analgesia?

#### Technique

The technique of intercostal nerve block involves sequential injections of local anesthetic around the intercostal nerve of the thoracotomy site, as well as two to three levels above and below the operative site. This can be accomplished directly by the surgeon while performing an open thoracotomy (or during thoracoscopy) or can be done percutaneously by the anesthesiologist at the end of the procedure. The conventional percutaneous approach is accomplished posteriorly, just lateral

to the sacrospinous group of muscles. The patient is positioned prone or in the lateral decubitus position, and the lateral edge of the sacrospinous muscles is identified. The rib at each innerspace is identified, and the 22-g short bevel needle is walked to the inferior border of the rib, where 3 to 5 mL of bupivacaine 0.25% is deposited. This is continued for each intercostal nerve.

A continuous intercostal block can be performed in the OR. The surgeon peels back the parietal pleura from the ribs at the incision site and tunnels an 18-g Tuohy to the posterior intercostal space (7-8 cm from the posterior midline). A second and third intercostal catheter can be placed above and below the operative site. A dose of 3 to 10 mL of bupivacaine 0.25% can be administered to each catheter (total dose not to exceed 15 mL/h).

#### Advantages

The advantage of the continuous intercostal over the intrapleural catheter is that there is no diffusion barrier to overcome for the intercostal catheter, and the local anesthetic is delivered directly to the site of action without being diluted in the pleural space with blood or fluids or evacuated out the chest tubes.

#### Disadvantages

The disadvantage compared with a paravertebral block is that the intercostal block frequently misses the posterior rami of the intercostal nerve. The disadvantage compared with intrapleural catheters is that the intercostal block frequently misses the diaphragmatic pleura and diaphragmatic structures. Common complications of intercostal nerve blocks—when performed for procedures other than thoracotomy—include pneumothorax[229] and hemothorax.[230] These complications can be minimized with meticulous technique. Furthermore, when performed on the operative side for a thoracotomy, a chest tube should already be in place to evacuate blood and air.

### Is Thoracic Epidural Analgesia the Current Gold Standard for Post-Thoracotomy Pain?

Thoracic epidural analgesia is the current gold standard for post-thoracotomy analgesia because most believe there is subjectively better analgesia with this technique than with any other. However, no randomized trials have documented a benefit of a thoracic epidural over other regional anesthetic techniques, and most show no difference between a lumbar placed epidural and a thoracic epidural when quantitative measurements are taken.[231] Furthermore, the high block necessary for adequate analgesia when using local anesthetics is associated with systemic hypotension, bradycardia, and decreased cardiac output due to the consequent sympathectomy.[232]

Some prefer epidural opioids because there is less hypotension. However, these have their own set of side effects including respiratory depression, nausea, puritis, and urinary retention. Most acknowledge that a combined opiate and dilute local anesthetic diminishes the major toxicity of each drug type and maximizes the therapeutic benefit.[233] I successfully administer a combination of low dose hydromorphone HCl (Dilaudid) and dilute bupivacaine to achieve excellent postoperative analgesia, with rare local anesthetic or opioid induced side effects. However, there is still the issue of neurologic risk during placement, which is catastrophic when it occurs, even though it is rare. Because of this devastating complication, thoracic epidural catheters should only be placed in awake patients. Pediatric patients can have their epidural placed via the sacral hiatus and advanced to the thoracic level under anesthesia (but placement should be verified by radiograph).

## Placement Tips

The following thoracic epidural catheter placement tips are provided in an effort to share my University of California, San Diego (UCSD) experience and, hopefully, make your patient's experience more comfortable.

1. Both the midline and paramedian approaches are feasible. However, I recommend that epidurals be placed using the paramedian approach when inexperienced in this technique because the midline approach is notorious for false loss of resistance when advancing the needle.
2. Catheters are placed above T8 to ensure coverage of the operative site. The epidural catheter is threaded a minimum of 3 cm, preferably 5 cm.
3. A test dose of 3 to 6 mL of 2% lidocaine with epinephrine 1:200 000 should be administered to rule out intravenous catheter positioning and to demonstrate a band of anesthesia before inducing anesthesia.
4. When inexperienced physicians are encountering difficulty placing thoracic epidurals, they should acknowledge their need for expert assistance sooner rather than later. Accordingly, a more experienced colleague or faculty member should be sought for assistance. In some centers, an anesthesiologist pain specialist may be the most experienced individual and asked to place the epidural preoperatively.
5. Once the catheter is in place, 3 mL of 0.25% to 0.5% bupivacaine plus morphine sulfate (Duramorph) (see dosing recommendations) should be administered followed by 3 mL 0.25% to 0.5% bupivacaine every 20 to 30 minutes throughout the case.

   Initial Thoracic Duramorph Bolus Dosing Recommendations
   >65 years of age: 1 mg
   <65 years of age: 2-3 mg
6. Postoperative epidural orders should be written in the OR and sent to the pharmacy at the beginning of the case so they will be available to the patient as soon as the patient leaves the OR to enter the PACU or SICU.

   Standard Orders Follow
   Bupivacaine 1/16% with hydromorphone 20 μg/mL
   Continuous infusion: 6 to 10 mL/h
   Patient-controlled epidural analgesia (PCEA) bolus dose: 3 mL
   Lockout: 30 minutes
   Clinician activated boluses: up to 6 mL every 30 minutes
7. If the patient is not receiving adequate analgesia, immediately postoperatively, the catheter position must be reconfirmed and rebolused; if it is still not functional, a new catheter should be placed de novo or another analgesic technique employed.

## What Is Cryoanalgesia, and How Does It Provide Analgesia?

Direct application of a cryoprobe on the thoracic intercostal nerve can provide long-lasting analgesia along the dermatome of the nerves treated. Nelson and colleagues published the technique in 1974[234]; however, it was Katz who popularized the procedure among anesthesiologists and pain physicians beginning in 1980.[235] The biophysiology of cryoanalgesia was described in 1981 by Myers and associates. They demonstrated that direct application of the ice ball to the nerve caused axonal degeneration without damage to the supporting structures (the neurolemma).[236] Preservation of the intraneural and perineural connective tissues allows regenerating axons, Schwann cells, and their capillaries to grow along the existing scaffolding, thus reinnervating the temporarily ablated dermatome. Approximately 1 to 3 months following cryoanalgesia, full restoration of nerve structure and function is accomplished, without neuritis or neuroma formation.

### Efficacy of Cryoanalgesia for Post-Thoracotomy Pain Control

Cryoanalgesia has been shown to dramatically decrease narcotic requirements and improve postoperative pulmonary function.[237,238] Cryoanalgesia patients may have some minimal to moderate pain following the procedure. However, the pain is rarely due to incisional discomfort but rather represents shoulder or arm pain due to chest tube irritation of the pleura or shoulder pain due to positioning in the lateral decubitus position. I have had excellent results with supplemental ketorolac tromethamine (Toradol), 30 mg intravenous, administered in the OR just before extubation with diminution in these minor complaints. Others have correctly observed that analgesia is improved when the chest tubes exit from dermatomes blocked by cryoanalgesia and that once the chest tubes are removed, most patients are almost pain-free.[239]

### Cryoanalgesia Apparatus

I have successfully used a Frigitronics model CCS-100 (Shelton, Conn) device, which uses nitrous oxide gas to cool a 5 mm diameter probe in a controlled temperature range from +10°C to -60°C. Nitrous oxide gas is one of a number of gases used to obtain sub-zero temperatures. In this case, the nitrous oxide is delivered under high pressure (700 psi) to the tip of the cryoprobe. Internally, at the tip, the gas is throttled through a tiny nozzle, with a resulting drop in pressure. This rapid gas expansion, combined with the pressure drop, results in a significant temperature decrease. This phenomenon is called the *Joule-Thomson effect*. The actual temperature at the cryoprobe tip is controlled by changing the pressure differential. By adjusting the back pressure of the exhaust gas, the pressure differential at the nozzle is regulated, and a specific temperature other than the minimum (−60°C) temperature can be monitored and controlled. For cryoanalgesia, I use −60°C. However, because a minute amount of fluid surrounds the nerve tissue, an ice ball forms on the nerve, and the nerve tissue itself is approximately −20°C.

### Cryoprobe Application Technique During Thoracotomy

The nerve is gently dissected out in the intercostal space posteriorly approximately 1 to 2 cm from the costovertebral ligament. The cryoprobe is then applied to the exposed nerve and an ice ball is formed. Some use two 30-second freeze cycles separated by a 5-second thaw. However, experience with a single 30 second freeze resulted in no loss of analgesia but did show a significant reduction in the period of numbness (from 3.0-1.2 months).[241] Despite this finding, surgeons at UCSD have been performing a 3-minute freeze directly on the dissected nerve with excellent postoperative analgesia. The numbness in patients begins to remit in 3 to 6 weeks.

### Complications of Cryoanalgesia

The numbness that occurs during the ablative period is generally well tolerated. However, some young women have reported distress at having lost sensation in the nipple area. Because most surgeons make their incision at the fifth intercostal space and freeze nerves between T3 and T7, temporary numbness of the nipple is a universal occurrence with efficacious cryoanalgesia.

Other postoperative complications in patients followed for up to 6 months include dysesthesias and intercostal muscle paralysis.[241] However, it is impossible to distinguish whether these nerve injuries are due to cryoablation or surgical manipulation of the tissues.[242] Indeed, up to 44% of post-thoracotomy patients had persistent pain in one study.[243] The only drawback I see is the time required to perform the blocks (approximately 4-5 minutes per level).

### *Why Are Intrapleural Catheters an Unpredictable Mode of Post-Thoracotomy Analgesia?*

Intrapleural analgesia typically uses a percutaneously placed catheter (sometimes placed under direct vision by the surgeon) in the space between the parietal and visceral pleura. A posterior intercostal space between the 4th and 8th ribs is usually chosen. Most reports use 0.5% to 0.25% bupivacaine in volumes of 20 to 40 mL. Typically, analgesia is inadequate after 3 to 4 hours. Also, the block can be unpredictable due to the loss of local anesthetic via the chest tubes, and the drug does not spread well to the intercostal space or alleviate the chest wall discomfort from the chest tubes. Most authors recommend clamping the chest tubes for 30 minutes after each bolus (which are needed every 4-6 hours). Patients with large bronchopleural fistulas may not tolerate chest tube clamping. Additionally, blood levels of bupivacaine as low as 2.3 μg/kg have been associated with seizure activity,[244] and values above this range are not uncommon using this technique.[245] Because intrapleural analgesia is unpredictable (variable loss of drug out of chest drains, binding with blood in the pleural space, and rapid systemic absorption), intrapleural block is only recommended where other choices are unavailable.

### *How Are Paravertebral Blocks Employed?*

Paravertebral blocks are placed posteriorly, just lateral to the vertebral bodies, and can be performed as single shot injections at multiple levels, or several catheters can be inserted for continuous infusion of local anesthetic. Both posterior and anterior rami of the intercostal nerve at the level are usually anesthetized.

Although thoracic epidural is the current gold standard, newer more efficacious techniques await development (eg, intraoperative intercostal nerve blockade with slow release bupivacaine and morphine—released from microspheres).

## PART II

# SPECIAL PROCEDURES AND CONDITIONS

### MEDIASTINOSCOPY

### *How Was Mediastinoscopy Developed and How Is It Performed Today?*

The concept of mediastinal exploration for tissue diagnosis was first reported by Harkens and coworkers in 1954.[246] However, Carlens introduced the mediastinoscope as a method of tissue acquisition in 1959.[247] Pearson refined the operative technique that remains in use today.[248] The procedure, most accurately described as *cervical mediastinoscopy,* is carried out in the following manner. A small incision is made across the suprasternal notch. Blunt dissection of the pretracheal fascia is carried out (ultimately between the trachea and the aortic arch) into the mediastinum. A tunnel is created along the anterior and lateral walls of the trachea, behind the aortic arch, and down to the carina (Fig. 64–20). The mediastinoscope is used to create the shore up the walls and illuminate the tunnel created by blunt dissection using the surgeon's finger, suction, cautery apparatus, and gauze-tipped forceps (among other instruments).

### *What Are the Indications for Mediastinoscopy?*

Mediastinoscopy is used to obtain the diagnosis of mediastinal masses and for the staging of known lung cancers with computed tomography (CT) or chest radiograph evidence of mediastinal adenopathy.[249] The benefits of mediastinal tissue diagnosis is clearly seen in differentiating the tissue response to therapy between lymphomas (respond to radiation therapy) and thymomas (require resection). Mediastinoscopy may be scheduled as a solitary procedure (eg, diagnosis of a solitary mediastinal mass) or in conjunction with bronchoscopy and preceding a thoracotomy (when staging for lung cancer).

### *Which Structures Can Be Sampled by Cervical Mediastinoscopy?*

The mediastinoscope positioning allows sampling of the lymph nodes located in the anterior and lateral paramainstem bronchi, anterior subcarina and anterior and lateral paratracheal areas. Left-sided apical and central lesions are not well sampled with cervical mediastinoscopy. For these lesions, a

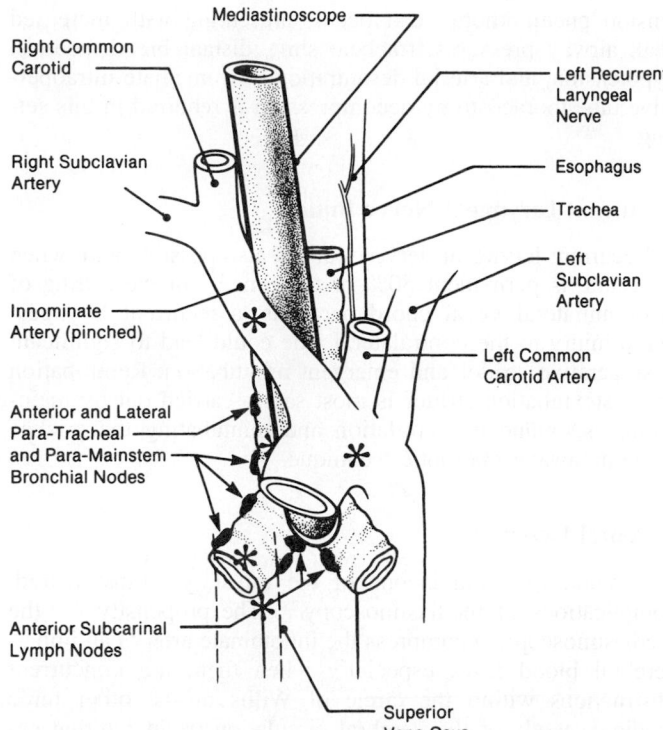

**FIGURE 64–20.** This schematic diagram shows the placement of a mediastinoscope into the superior mediastinum. The mediastinoscope passes in front of the trachea but behind the thoracic aorta. This location of the mediastinoscope allows for sampling of anterior and lateral para-mainstem bronchial lymph nodes, anterior subcarinal lymph nodes, and anterior and lateral paratracheal lymph nodes. Anatomic structures that can be compressed by the mediastinoscope (see areas marked by an *) and that can cause major complications are the thoracic aorta (rupture, reflex bradycardia), innominate artery (decreased right carotid blood flow can cause cerebral vascular symptoms, and decreased right subclavian flow can cause loss of right radial pulse), trachea (inability to ventilate), and vena cava (risk of hemorrhage and superior vena cava syndrome). (From Benumof JL. *Anesthesia for Thoracic Surgery.* 2nd ed. Philadelphia, Pa: WB Saunders; 1995:505.)

left anterior mediastinotomy is preferred (second rib interspace, just lateral to the sternum). A mediastinoscope is often used with this approach; it gives excellent access to left-sided centrally located and apical pathology as well as access to the thymus and structures in the anterior mediastinum.

## What Are the Anesthetic Considerations for Mediastinoscopy?

Most of the anesthetic considerations for mediastinoscopy revolve around preparing for complications and limiting those that may occur. Large bore venous access is a must (patient may be put to sleep with a small intravenous needle; however, a large bore intravenous needle must be in place before starting the case because of the ever-present threat of acute massive hemorrhage). In the case of SVCS, large bore access should be secured in a tributary of the inferior vena cava (IVC.) Arterial line monitoring is not absolutely required but, when indicated, should usually be placed in the right radial artery so as to detect the duration of compression of the innominate, right subclavian (inconsequential) or carotid arteries. Otherwise, keep the right arm free for analysis of the pulse and place a BP cuff on the left arm for accurate sequential BP

measurements. Other monitoring standards should be observed without special precautions.

The patient's hematocrit should be known and a type and crossmatch sent to the blood bank before initiating the mediastinoscopy. Because the surgical procedure is relatively brief, short-acting drugs are preferable. Just as in other elective situations, if the patient's airway appears to be difficult to intubate, it should be intubated using an awake technique (preferably FOB). If the laryngoscopy and mask ventilation appear to be easy yet the patient has a large mediastinal mass and airway stridor symptoms in the supine position, a spontaneous ventilation technique for induction is indicated.

For most cases, a total intravenous anesthetic using fentanyl 2 to 5 μg/kg or alfentanil 30 to 50 μg/kg along with propofol 2 mg/kg for induction, followed by an infusion of atracurium, 0.5 mg/kg, works well. In lieu of the propofol infusion, inhaled sevoflurane is appropriate. With both of these techniques, the patient has excellent anesthesia during the vigorous dissection and mediastinal lymph node biopsy portion and has decreasing levels of narcotic and muscle relaxation at the end of the case, when the surgeon and anesthesiologist are awaiting return of frozen samples from pathology.

A double-lumen ETT is not required for mediastinoscopy; rather, a single-lumen ETT is generally used. An armored or nonkinking ETT is advisable for situations in which tracheomalacia is anticipated or in a rare re-do mediastinoscopy (relative contraindication) in which supraordinary pressure may be exerted on the trachea and increase the risk of ETT compression.

## Does the Anesthetic Technique Differ When Planning for a Solitary Mediastinoscopy Versus a Planned Consecutive Mediastinoscopy Followed by Thoracotomy?

When there is a low probability of positive lymph nodes in a consecutive procedure (mediastinoscopy followed by thoracotomy), my practice is to prepare for a thoracotomy including the placement of a thoracic epidural before the patient goes to sleep (in order to verify positioning in an awake patient) and placement of an arterial catheter (before or after induction). However, my practice is to initially intubate the trachea with a single lumen ETT, and if biopsies come back negative, I convert to a DLT while the patient is still asleep.

If there is a high probability of positive lymph nodes and low likelihood that the case will proceed to an open thoracotomy, I prepare the patient in the same fashion as for a known solitary mediastinoscopy. If the lymph nodes are negative, I proceed in one of two ways: (1) the patient is allowed to wake up fully before placement of a thoracic epidural and then proceeds to a DLT intubation in the standard fashion; or (2) I proceed to a DLT while the patient is anesthetized and employ a technique other than thoracic epidural for postoperative analgesia. I do not endorse placing a thoracic epidural in any adult patient unless that patient is fully conscious, able to participate in the procedure, and able to report any untoward signs and symptoms of improper catheter placement. Needless to say, thorough and clear discussion must occur between the surgeon and anesthesiologist for these cases in order to avoid conflicts.

## What Are the Complications of Mediastinoscopy and Their Appropriate Anesthetic Management?

Table 64–10 shows the most common complications seen in patients who undergo mediastinoscopy. Most of these complications require specific immediate therapy.

### Hemorrhage

Hemorrhage is the most common serious complication from mediastinoscopy and the most difficult to manage acutely, especially when sudden and massive. Patients with SVCS are at somewhat higher risk for venous bleeding due to the higher venous pressures present. However, the importance of obtaining an accurate tissue diagnosis and employing appropriate therapy does not preclude mediastinoscopy in this setting.[250] The appropriate anesthetic response is as follows:

1. Begin rapid volume infusion via an already placed large bore intravenous needle. If the tear is from a tributary of the superior vena cava (SVC), infusion should go via the tributary of IVC (saphenous vein intravenous or femoral vein).
2. Send for blood that was typed and crossed before procedure.
3. Support circulation pharmacologically (phenylephrine, ephedrine, dopamine, epinephrine, atropine as appropriate) while volume repletion is ongoing and the surgeon is gaining control (emergency median sternotomy for right-sided lesions, left thoracotomy for left-sided lesions).
4. Ensure adequate oxygenation and ventilation.
5. Turn off all anesthetic drugs until the patient is resuscitated and stable vital signs are achieved.

### Pneumothorax

Pneumothorax is the next most common serious complication from mediastinoscopy. Both cervical mediastinoscopy and anterior mediastinotomy are mainly extrapleural. However, a small tear in the pleura can occur. Accordingly, an early postoperative chest radiograph is advisable, although the majority of these patients do not require treatment. Intraoperative

tension pneumothorax can occur, presenting with increased peak airway pressures, tracheal shift, distant breath sounds, hypotension, and arterial desaturation.[251] Immediate intraoperative tube thoracostomy decompression is required in this setting.

### Recurrent Laryngeal Nerve Injury

Recurrent laryngeal nerve injury is also possible and, when it occurs, is permanent 50% of the time.[252] In the setting of prior unilateral vocal chord paralysis, a recurrent laryngeal nerve injury to the contralateral side could lead to significant postoperative stridor and emergent reintubation. Reintubation for postextubation stridor is most safely carried out by maintaining spontaneous ventilation and reintubating the trachea using an awake fiberoptic technique.

### Cerebral Ischemia

Cerebral ischemia is one of the rarest, yet most feared, complications of mediastinoscopy.[253] The propensity for the mediastinoscope to compress the innominate artery can impair cerebral blood flow, especially when there are concurrent obstructions within the circle of Willis or the other three feeding vessels of the cerebral circulation (right internal carotid, and the right and left vertebral arteries). Other problems related to innominate artery compression include reflex bradycardia (treat with atropine or halt compression) and diminished right subclavian and right radial pulse (less risk of tissue damage than the inconvenience to BP monitoring from the right extremity).

### Venous Air Embolism

Venous air embolism is a constant threat when venous vessels are torn or during blunt dissection or biopsy acquisition. Positive pressure ventilation in the supine or Trendelenburg position will limit this complication, whereas spontaneous ventilation and slight head elevation (sometimes requested to decrease venous engorgement) will increase the risk of venous air embolism.

## THORACOSCOPY AND VIDEO-ASSISTED THORACIC SURGERY

### How Has Thoracoscopy Developed Into Video-Assisted Thoracic Surgery?

Thorascopy was first described in 1910 by Jacobeus, a Swedish physician who used a cystoscope to inspect the pleura and lyse adhesions between the lung and chest wall of tuberculosis patients. This technique was widely used until the discovery of streptomycin in 1945, after which thoracoscopy was relegated almost solely as a diagnostic tool. This trend changed dramatically in the early 1990s when a wide array of instruments, originally used for laparoscopy (graspers, retractors, lasers, cryoprobes), began to be used above the diaphragm. Furthermore, the advent of new devices engineered specifically for thoracoscopy (eg, lung stapling devices) and the development of high resolution endoscopic video equipment propelled thorascopy toward the current

**TABLE 64–10.** Major Complications of Mediastinoscopy

| Complication | Emergency Anesthetic Treatment |
|---|---|
| Hemorrhage | Rapid volume repletion; use a tributary of the inferior vena cava if venous hemorrhage (volume repletion through a tributary of the superior vena cava will likely be lost at the site of injury). |
| Tracheal compression | Monitor airway pressures, use armored tube. |
| Pneumothorax | Maintain vigilance, administer 100% $O_2$, place chest tube. |
| Recurrent laryngeal nerve injury | Emergent re-intubation if stridor severe or associated with desaturation. |
| Cerebral ischemia | Devastating if occurs, but rare. Limit innominate artery compression. |
| Bradycardia | Reflex bradycardia may be seen with compression of the innominate artery. Therapy is atropine and cessation of compression. |

widely used modality for operations involving thoracic lesions.[254]

## What Are the Benefits of Video-Assisted Thoracic Surgery Over Thoracoscopy?

Significant advances in videoscopic technology during the 1990s caused VATS to supersede thoracoscopy as the operative technique of choice. The benefits of VATS over thoracoscopy include (1) the visualization is of superior quality; (2) the surgeon's hands are free to operate (with the specialized instruments); (3) others in the OR can follow the case progress (scrub nurse and assistants can anticipate surgical needs, anesthesiologists can predict physiologic permutations, and track case progress); and (4) there is increased ability to maintain sterility in the operative field.

## What Are the Diagnostic and Therapeutic Indications for Video-Assisted Thoracic Surgery?

The most common diagnostic indications for VATS include evaluation of pleural pathology, determining the cause of pleural effusions, staging of lung cancer, evaluation of mediastinal pathology, and staging of esophageal pathology. Because 5% to 10% of patients with lung cancer present with an ipsilateral pleural effusion, VATS-assisted pleuroscopy should always proceed thoracotomy in patients with a cytologically negative pleural effusion.[255]

The therapeutic role of VATS has expanded to include wedge resection of solitary lung lesions,[256] lobectomy,[257] resection of emphysematous blebs, LVRS, treatment of pericardial disease (including creation of a pericardial window), and minimally invasive coronary surgery (including harvesting of internal mammary artery) among others.

## What Are the Benefits of Video-Assisted Thoracic Surgery Compared With Thoracotomy?

The main benefits of VATS over formal thoracotomy involve decreased thoracic wall tissue injury and subsequent pain leading to improved postoperative pulmonary function.[258] Indeed, VATS patients tend to be more active earlier, with less atelectasis and a lower incidence of postoperative pneumonia.

Some disadvantages to VATS still remain compared with open thoracotomy, including limitations in instrumentation, difficulty in assessment and control of hemorrhage, decreased tactile discrimination (palpation occurs by probing with an instrument, rather than with fingers and hands), lack of 3-dimensional view, increased equipment expense, and increased learning curve.

## What Is the Surgical Technique for Video-Assisted Thoracic Surgery?

The typical VATS procedure is performed in the lateral decubitus position, facilitated by lung separation using a DLT

(if general anesthesia and positive pressure ventilation are used—as discussed below). Although there is significant variability, depending on the procedure, a minimum of three incisions are typically required (Fig. 64–21). One incision is required for the scope, the others for various instruments. Most insertion points occur at intercostal spaces located between the third and eighth ribs.

## What Are the Anesthetic Techniques Used for Video-Assisted Thoracic Surgery?

VATS can be performed with a local field block, regional epidural, or general anesthesia. Surgeons and anesthesiologists must work together to orchestrate a safe operative plan. VATS should be regarded as a major operation, and the anesthesiologist must always be prepared to convert to a formal thoracotomy if trouble is encountered (eg, major hemorrhage, other technical difficulty, failure to locate the lesion, tight pleural adhesions, and so on). Regardless of the anesthetic technique used, 100% $O_2$ is recommended for all thoracotomy procedures, unless contraindicated due to sensitivity to $O_2$ toxicity (eg, lung transplantation, prior exposure to drugs, increasing free radical production, or decreasing their clearance) as described in this chapter.

Local anesthesia field block at the various ports is simple, yet usually associated with some discomfort to the patient even if the pleural space is infiltrated with local anesthesia. Intercostal nerve blocks at the level of each port and one interspace above and below provides slightly better surgical anesthesia; if block is placed posteriorly, it anesthetizes parietal pleural sensation as well. These techniques are most

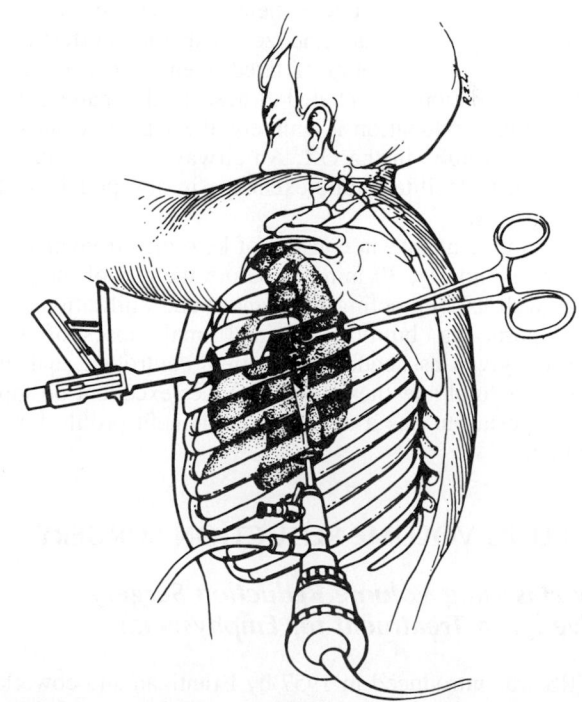

**FIGURE 64–21.** Incisions for thoracoscope and instruments. The instruments may consist of staplers, lasers, cautery, cryoprobe, retractors, and graspers. (Reprinted with permission from the Society of Thoracic Surgeons [*The Annals of Thoracic Surgery* 1992, Vol 54, page 421.])

suitable for pleural evaluation, drainage, and biopsy.[259] Thoracic epidural anesthesia provides a similar level of anesthesia but may need supplementation if a port outside of the band of anesthesia is required. Providing spontaneous ventilation continues, a DLT is unnecessary because some spontaneous collapse of the operated lung will occur as soon as air enters the pleural space. However, the operative lung will paradoxically contract with inhalation and expand with exhalation during spontaneous ventilation with an iatrogenic pneumothorax. Thus, some lung retraction will be required in order to maintain adequate visualization. Additionally, some surgeons will insufflate $CO_2$ to improve visualization. Although this practice was previously thought to be unnecessary and dangerous, pressures up to 10 cm $H_2O$ are well tolerated in normovolemic patients.[260]

General anesthesia is the most frequently used anesthetic technique for VATS at my institution and is most suitable for major therapeutic thoracoscopies.[261] Monitoring includes an arterial line and other standard monitors. Large bore access is required before surgery commences but may be placed after induction of anesthesia. The need for CVP and PA catheterization is patient- and procedure-specific (see Intraoperative Monitoring). Induction and maintenance drugs with rapid elimination or redistribution are best suited to VATS (eg, propofol, sevoflurane, desflurane). Neuromuscular blockade facilitates placement of a left-sided DLT and the application of positive pressure ventilation, and provides stable operating conditions. Accordingly, short- to moderate-acting drugs (eg, atracurium, vecuronium) are optimal.

### What Are the Postoperative Considerations for Video-Assisted Thoracic Surgery?

The majority of patients undergoing VATS may have their tracheas extubated in the OR. Patients with severe preexisting lung disease should be anesthetized with the shortest-acting drugs available, a minimum of fixed agent, and a minimum or total elimination of inhaled drugs. If the patient is so debilitated that extubation is unlikely, the DLT is changed to a single-lumen tube in the OR. An airway exchange catheter can be used to facilitate tube exchange in any patient with a difficult airway.

Postoperative analgesia consists of ketorolac tromethamine, 30 mg intravenously, 30 minutes before the end of the procedure, as well as long-acting local anesthetic infiltration of the surgical ports (eg, bupivacaine) and small doses of opiate analgesics, given as needed, via patient-controlled analgesia. Thoracic epidural anesthesia also provides excellent postoperative analgesia but has a negative risk-benefit profile for this procedure.

## LUNG VOLUME REDUCTION SURGERY

### How Has Lung Volume Reduction Surgery Evolved as a Treatment for Emphysema?

LVRS was introduced in 1957 by Brantigan and coworkers as a method of treating nonbullous emphysema.[262] In this initial article, the surgical rationale was much as it is today. They wrote: "It is an operation directed at restoration of a physiologic principle. It is not concerned with removal of pathologic tissue." However well intentioned, their technique was soon abandoned due to the high morbidity (persistent air-leaks) and high mortality. The concept was reintroduced by Cooper and colleagues in 1995 using a similar technique they termed *reduction pneumonectomy*.[263] They used a median sternotomy approach and an automatic stapler to excise the most severely diseased portions of the lung (20%-30% of the lung volume). The 20 patients with severe emphysema used in this study demonstrated significant improvement at 3 months following surgery in $FEV_1$, indices of dyspnea, and health related quality of life, as well as decreased use of $O_2$ and corticosteroids. Demand for the LVRS skyrocketed in the late 1990s as others showed similar favorable results.[264]

### What Is the Mortality From Lung Volume Reduction Surgery?

It has been difficult to compare the mortality from LVRS with nonoperative therapy because no long-term randomized trials have yet been completed. However, it is known that patients with severe emphysema awaiting lung transplantation have an annual mortality rate of approximately 8%,[265] whereas the perioperative (usually 30 days) mortality for LVRS ranges between 0 and 19%.[266]

Despite the high perioperative mortality, short-term results from LVRS are generally good with increased $FEV_1$ of 25% to 58% measured 3 to 6 months postoperatively. The duration of benefit has been variable, but most reports show significant improvement for as long as 2 to 3 years before patients deteriorate back toward their preoperative status. Interestingly, bilateral VATS as the technique for LVRS seems to have better survival than bilateral LVRS using an open sternotomy technique.[267]

### Does Medicare Cover the Costs of Lung Volume Reduction Surgery?

A National Institutes of Health workshop in September 1995 declared that LVRS was being performed with insufficient evaluation in many patients, and in December 1996, the Health Care Financing Administration (HCFA) declared that LVRS would not be covered by Medicare until it was scientifically proven to be defensible regarding the risks and benefits.[268] Subsequently, HCFA joined with the National Heart, Lung, and Blood Institute to sponsor a randomized trial comparing LVRS with optimal medical therapy. This high profile study is called the National Emphysema Treatment Trial and has attracted several prominent institutions, including ours at UCSD. Enrollment began in 1997, and all participants in the trial receive intensive medical therapy and rehabilitation. Half of these patients are also randomly selected to undergo LVRS. However, enrollment has been slow because most patients recognize that participation in the study means they have only a 50% chance of receiving the operation. Others withdraw from the study if they are allocated to the nonoperative arm of the study and find ways to pay for their LVRS at private centers.

### What Are the Anesthetic Considerations for Lung Volume Reduction Surgery?

The surgical approach (median sternotomy, bilateral thoracotomy versus bilateral VATS) affects the anesthetic technique employed. The specific details of management of 1LV and considerations for thoracotomy or VATS have been discussed elsewhere. However, the overall goals remain the same:

1. Avoid high airway pressures (prone to rupturing emphysematous bullae).
2. Allow long exhalation time (prone to air trapping with consequent hemodynamic deterioration).
3. Limit any fixed agent at the end of the case so that the trachea can be extubated in the OR (this limits postoperative bronchopulmonary fistula and decreases the propensity for $CO_2$ retention, a frequent postoperative problem.
4. Provide optimum postoperative analgesia via ketorolac and thoracic epidural to improve patient comfort and pulmonary toilet.

Monitoring includes an arterial line for beat-to-beat evaluation of BP. Intraoperative hypotension is a frequent occurrence in these cases, sometimes requiring significant augmentation with inotropes or pressors following thoracic epidural induced vasodilation or transient removal of the ETT from the ventilator to allow exhalation and venous return in cases of severe air trapping. The patient is then reconnected to the ventilator with a longer exhalation time. The arterial line is also invaluable in following the degree of postoperative $CO_2$ retention, which usually occurs for the first 24 hours postoperatively. I have found that a continuous ABG monitor has been invaluable in these patients. Additionally, central venous monitoring along with TEE for evaluation of myocardial performance or a PA catheter is often helpful.

A thoracic epidural is placed with the patient awake before the induction of anesthesia. Before induction, ipratropium bromide and albuterol inhalers are administered. Anesthesia is induced with short-acting agents (propofol, 2 mg/kg) or etomidate if hemodynamically unstable. Systemic opiates are avoided, and small doses of opiates combined with dilute bupivacaine are administered via the thoracic epidural. Nondepolarizing neuromuscular blocking drugs are used to facilitate DLT intubation. Placement of the left DLT is confirmed by FOB. Maintenance of anesthesia is best accomplished with intravenous propofol infusion, thus eliminating dependence on the lungs for elimination of potent vapors via exhalation. Furthermore, because propofol is a bronchodilator, there is no benefit attributable to inhaled drugs for this procedure.[269] Intermediate-acting neuromuscular blockade is used and monitored quantitatively to ensure reversibility at the end of the case.

Management of ventilation is a critical component of anesthetic management. There are four goals of ventilatory management:

1. Avoidance of hypoxia
2. Avoidance of hyperinflation, due to air trapping and consequent hypotension
3. Avoidance of high airway pressures and consequent barotrauma
4. Maintenance of optimum DLT position to facilitate lung separation for operative exposure.

These goals are continually reevaluated during the case. Avoidance of hypoxia is facilitated by use of 100% $O_2$, and frequent suctioning is guided by FOB to ensure airway patency and DLT positioning. Maneuvers aimed at avoiding hypoxia places greater emphasis on nondependent lung CPAP over dependent lung PEEP for this population of patients.

Initial maneuvers to limit hyperinflation begin with reduced tidal volumes (ie, 7 mL/kg), decreased I:E ratio (1:4-1:5) and decreased respiratory rate, further increasing the exhalation time. Some consequent permissive hypercapnia (during the case) is well tolerated. Intermittent disconnection from the ventilator to prevent excessive gas trapping should be routinely performed and emergently pursued in the face of increasing airway pressures and decreasing BP. An acute tension pneumothorax on the nonoperative side is a constant threat that must be considered early in the differential and treated promptly in the setting of hypotension, deteriorating $O_2$ saturation, and increasing airway pressures.

The goal is to have the patient's trachea extubated in the OR because of concern that positive pressure ventilation can potentiate barotrauma and may worsen any preexisting bronchopulmonary fistulas. Also, there is concern of bucking and coughing postoperatively. Accordingly, only small doses of fixed agents are used. At UCSD, I have extubated the trachea while the patient is still under deep anesthesia, and I maintain mask ventilation until the patient regains airway reflexes. Occasionally, I have replaced the ETT with a laryngeal mask airway. I also prophylax against nausea and vomiting with odansetron and metoclopramide HCl (Reglan). The vast majority of these patients retain $CO_2$ postoperatively; thus, only small doses or no intravenous narcotics are used.[270] Occasionally, small doses of naloxone are used postoperatively to promote increased minute ventilation.

Because of poor baseline pulmonary function, many of these patients will have suboptimal weaning and extubation criteria. This, coupled with perioperative pulmonary edema, residual anesthetics, chest tube air leaks, and excessive pain, can make extubation difficult. If immediate postoperative extubation is not possible, the DLT is exchanged for a single lumen ETT, and the patient should be maintained on the minimum pressure support necessary to maintain an adequate minute ventilation.

## PERCUTANEOUS IMAGE-GUIDED THORACIC PROCEDURES

### What Are the Anesthetic Considerations for Drainage of Pleural Effusions and Pulmonary Fluid Collections?

Percutaneous catheter drainage of intrathoracic collections has evolved as an extension of similar interventional radiologic procedures in the abdomen. The advent of CT and sonography, which allow detection and characterization of pleural and parenchymal collections, combined with advances in drainage catheter design and interventional techniques, have made imaging-guided management of intrathoracic collections a safe and effective alternative to traditional surgical and thoracoscopic drainage modalities.[271] Image-guided management is ideal for extremely ill patients and for those who have undergone multiple thoracic operations.

Anesthetic need for percutaneous fluid drainage is minimal, typically requiring only local anesthesia at the skin and monitored anesthetic care. However, critically ill patients require extensive aggressive monitoring, sometimes making CT-guided procedures less attractive due to the need for transport.

Thus, for these patients, parenchymal disease manipulation may not be feasible, whereas bedside ultrasound-guided placement of intrapleural drainage catheters is more easily accomplished.

### What Is the Role of Radiofrequency Ablation in the Treatment of Lung Cancer?

Radiofrequency (RF) ablation for malignant lung lesions is a new technology just beginning to emerge in the United States. However, anesthesiologists have extensive experience with RF ablation of liver tumors.[272] Additionally, >500 cases of RF ablation for lung tumors have been performed in China, >100 at the University of Mississippi, several at Providence, RI, and a few at UCSD (S. Rose, personal communication, January 2001). Because of the extreme likelihood that RF ablation technology for unresectable lung cancer will expand in the next 2 years, some discussion is warranted.

### Radiofrequency Ablation Theory and Technique

A multi-tine RF ablation probe (Radiotherapeutics Corp, Sunnyvale, Calif) is placed into the middle of the target tumor under CT guidance. (Figs. 64–22 and 64–23). High-frequency energy (30-40 W for lung tissue) is transmitted to the tips of the ablation probe (which is otherwise shielded). The current model generator is capable of transmitting up to 90 W of power, so careful attention to the energy setting is important.[273] RF-induced temperature elevation results when the high frequency alternating current (~460 MHz) flows from the tip of an electrode through the surrounding tissue. Ionic agitation is produced as the ions attempt to follow the change in direction of the alternating current around the electrode tip. This ionic agitation creates frictional heating and coagulation of the targeted tissue around the electrode.[274] Energy via the RF ablation probe is delivered until a complete rise in the tissue impedance occurs, indicating complete coagulation of tis-

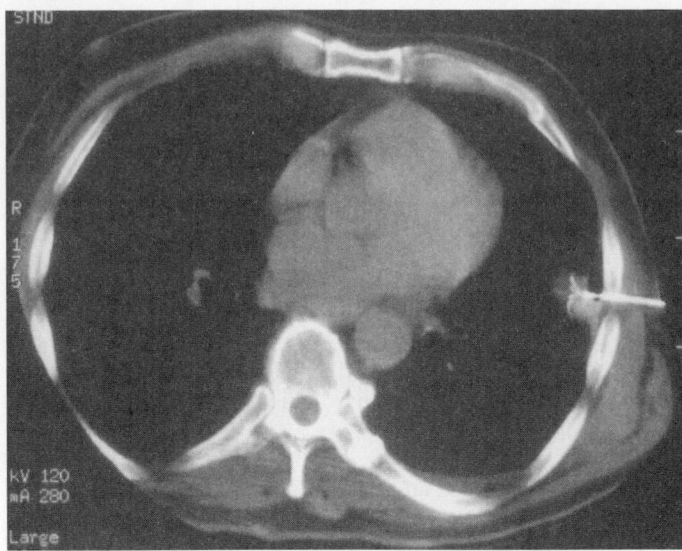

**FIGURE 64–23.** Computed tomography of chest demonstrating a multi-tine needle electrode (Radiotherapeutics Corp, Sunnyvale, Calif) deployed into the target (non–small cell lung cancer) tissue. (Courtesy of Patrick E. Sewell, MD, University of Mississippi Medical Center, Jackson, Mississippi.)

sue.[275] Some RF ablation probes deliver energy until a target temperature is reached indicating tumor coagulation.

### Indications for RF Ablation of Pulmonary Lesions

Indications for RF ablation are still evolving. Although RF ablation has been reported in animals,[276] and as combination therapy for bronchial malignancies,[277] only one group has reported results in human beings to date.[278]

Currently, the application of RF ablation to address lung cancer is under study and tends to be relegated to palliative therapy. Appropriate patients are those with otherwise unresectable pulmonary lesions not invading the major pulmonary vessels or mediastinum, and who are not candidates for radiation therapy or are either not candidates for or who have failed systemic chemotherapy. Currently, the maximum tumor size amenable to RF ablation is approximately 4 cm. Tumors >2.5 cm diameter may require multiple catheter placements (S. Rose, personal communication, January 2001).

### Anesthetic Considerations for Radiofrequency Ablation

I have just begun to perform this procedure at UCSD. I use standard monitoring, 5-lead ECG, arterial line and two large-bore intravenous needles (due to the risk of hemorrhage). A single lumen ETT is employed, and I use an intravenous infusion of propofol, opiates, nerve muscular blocker (NMB), and occasionally low dose Sevoflurane for maintenance. During most of the procedure, the anesthetic requirement is low, requiring <1 MAC anesthetic. However, during the actual RF ablation periods, there is a significant increase in anesthetic requirements. The trachea is extubated immediately postprocedure, unless there is a preexisting contraindication.

Currently, these cases take 4 to 8 hours, depending on the number and size of tumors (multiple scans and rescans to ensure proper probe positioning during ablation). Because of

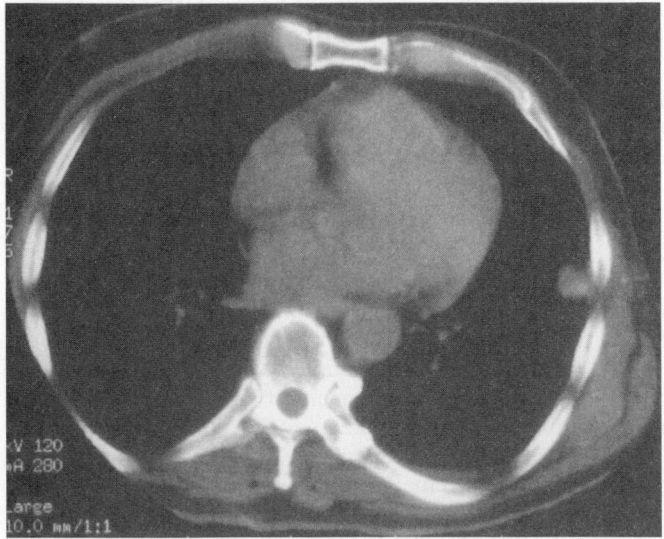

**FIGURE 64–22.** Computed tomography of chest in patient with non-small cell lung cancer, before radiofrequency ablation. Note target tissue approximately 1.5 cm × 1.5 cm adjacent to the left chest wall. (Courtesy of Patrick E. Sewell, MD, University of Mississippi Medical Center, Jackson, Mississippi.)

the long duration of these procedures, patients must be padded far more substantially than is normally required for a CT scan of the chest. This may require bringing in a thicker mattress than is usually used for CT scans to decrease the possibility of decubitus ulcers and positioning injuries. It is anticipated that the procedure time will decrease to 1 to 2 hours when refined. At that time, it is likely that local anesthesia with monitored anesthesia care will be appropriate. Cases are performed in the CT scan suite, and all of the equipment required for anesthesia in a main OR is taken to the anesthetizing location.

## Common Complications of Radiofrequency Ablation

All patients demonstrate radiographic evidence of postoperative focal pulmonary edema in the surrounding tissue due to the local thermal injury (Fig. 64–24). All patients develop at least a small pleural effusion, but like the tissue edema, it typically resolves in 2 to 3 weeks (Fig. 64–25). The immediate postoperative pneumothorax rate is approximately 20% to 30%. These small pneumothoraces are typically treated with immediate aspiration under radiographic guidance, and rarely require a tube thoracostomy. By 2 to 3 days, the residual pneumothorax rate is down to the 5% range. Some patients complain of dyspnea postoperatively; this occurs more frequently in patients with poor baseline pulmonary function. Additionally, many of the patients will manifest blood-tinged sputum, but frank hemoptysis is rare.

RF ablation for pulmonary lesions may be associated with

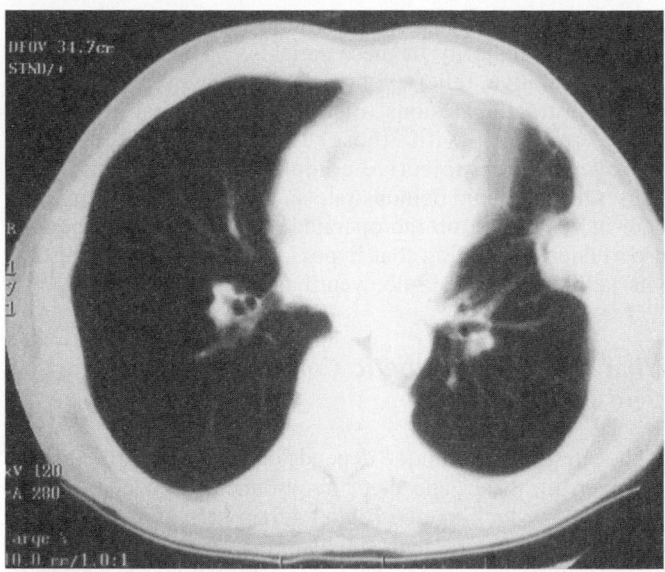

**FIGURE 64–25.** Computed tomography of chest in patient one month following radiofrequency ablation of lesion (non-small cell lung cancer). Note the thermal lesion is still substantially larger than the initial tumor (but biopsy is negative for viable malignant cells). Additionally, the rim of edematous tissue has regressed. Finally, the pneumothorax has resolved. (Courtesy of Patrick E. Sewell, MD, University of Mississippi Medical Center, Jackson, Mississippi.)

an increased risk of neurologic impairment resulting from air emboli released into the arterial circulation. It is known, from the liver ablation experience, that numerous microbubbles are evacuated via the surrounding blood vessels (some are likely nitrogen bubble emboli produced from the tissue heating). In the liver, the hepatic veins drain blood to the IVC and then to the lungs, which should filter out most emboli. However, when RF ablation is carried out in the lungs, pulmonary venous emboli may go directly to the left atrium, out the LV, and subsequently to the coronary (thus the need for an arterial line and 5-lead ECG) and cerebral circulation. At UCSD, Dr Steven Rose has performed simultaneous carotid duplex ultrasonography during RF ablation of pulmonary tumors to document this phenomena of microbubble embolization to the brain. So far, no cases of postoperative neurologic deficits have been reported in association with RF ablation of pulmonary lesions. Finally, due to the constant possibility of major hemorrhage and hemoptysis, a DLT and FOB should be immediately available throughout the case.

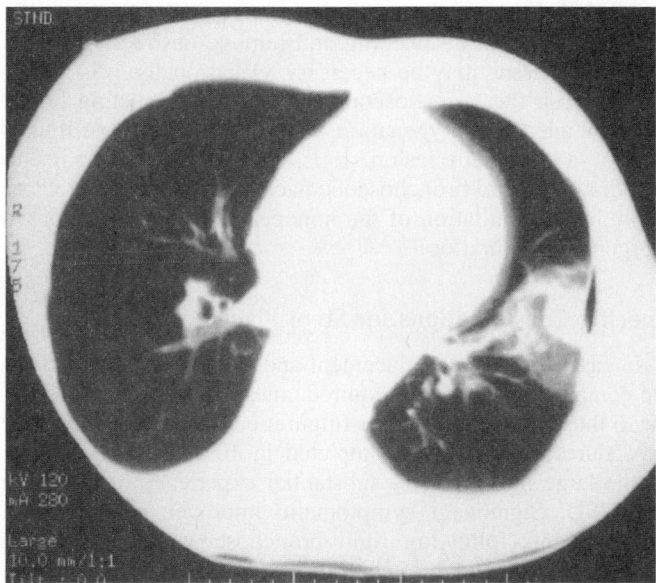

**FIGURE 64–24.** Computed tomography of chest in patient immediately following radiofrequency ablation of lesion (non–small cell lung cancer). Note the thermal lesion is substantially larger than the initial tumor (the goal is to create a margin of thermally ablated normal tissue around the target lesion which is essentially similar to what the surgical margins would be). There is also a rim of edematous tissue surrounding the thermal lesion; this typically dissipates by 2 to 3 days postablation. A small pneumothorax is noted just lateral to the thermal lesion. Immediately following radiofrequency ablation, 20% to 30% of patients will have a small pneumothorax. These are typically treated with syringe evacuation, without thoracostomy. By 48 hours, only approximately 7% of patients will have CT evidence of a pneumothorax. (Courtesy of Patrick E. Sewell, MD, University of Mississippi Medical Center, Jackson, Mississippi.)

## RIGID BRONCHOSCOPY FOR LASER AND STENT PLACEMENT

### Which Lesions Are Amenable to Laser Fulguration or Stent Placement?

There are many causes of tracheal and bronchial narrowing. Those lesions, which are inside the tracheal or bronchial wall (bronchogenic cancer, carcinoids, bronchogenic papillomas), are extremely amenable to laser fulguration, with marked improvement in symptoms of stridor and dyspnea. Conversely, laser therapy is contraindicated for stridor emanating from an extrinsic lesion.[279] These cases are treated with rigid stents placed under direct vision using a rigid bronchoscope, as are patients with tracheomalacia.

The greatest benefit occurs in partially obstructing lesions, with the vast majority of these patients experiencing immediate postoperative relief of symptoms. However, even completely obstructing lesions (of brief duration) can be significantly relieved with these techniques, resulting in improvement in subjective complaints and objective $\dot{V}/\dot{Q}$ scans. One study did demonstrate an average of 50% improvement in ventilation on the operated side and an 25% increase in perfusion, indicating that hypoxic pulmonary vasoconstriction had been relieved once ventilation was restored.[280]

## What Are the Anesthetic Considerations for Rigid Bronchoscopy?

The anesthetic technique depends on the procedure planned. However, the basic anesthetic requirements needed for rigid bronchoscopy facilitate both laser fulguration and stent placement. These requirements include complete immobility of the patient, maintenance of adequate $O_2$ saturation, ability to ventilate, and ability to suction blood, tumor fragments, and other debris from the major airways. Because of these requirements, local anesthetic techniques, although possible, are dangerous and uncomfortable for the patient. At UCSD, general anesthetic techniques are used, typically with controlled mechanical ventilation (though one surgeon still prefers spontaneous ventilation). Spontaneous ventilation does provide the theoretical benefit of decreased propensity to debris blown into distal airways (during a positive pressure breath). However, the ability to maintain an adequate plane of anesthesia, which allows spontaneous ventilation in a patient, yet simultaneously prevents major gross body movements during rigid bronchoscopy for laser surgery and stent placement, is almost impossible.

## What Is the University of California, San Diego, Anesthetic Technique for Rigid Bronchoscopy?

Patients are evaluated thoroughly by the anesthesiologist and discussed in a preoperative conference with the rigid bronchoscopist (usually a pulmonologist). In this conference, the patient's chest radiograph, CT scan, and other relevant data are displayed, as are images of the airway from prior bronchoscopies (if it is a repeat patient, which is common). The operative goals are discussed, potential problems are identified, and a team strategy is developed. Once all information is considered, an anesthetic plan emerges.

The typical anesthetic plan involves preoperative administration of inhaled steroids, ipratropium bromide, albuterol, intravenous methyl-prednisolone sodium succinate (Solu-Medrol) (125 mg). In the OR, standard monitors are placed. After careful preoxygenation for 3 to 5 minutes, intravenous induction is accomplished with 2 to 3 mg/kg of propofol and 20 to 50 µg/kg of alfentanil (depending on anticipated procedure duration [1 µg/kg/minute of anesthesia-works for cases up to 45 min. in duration]). The ability to ventilate is established; succinylcholine, 1 to 2 mg/kg, is administered for short duration cases; and atracurium for cases >20 minutes is occasionally used. After the neuromuscular blockade takes effect, direct laryngoscopy is performed, and the tracheobronchial tree is sprayed with lidocaine using a laryngotracheal

kit. At this time, the airway is turned over to the rigid bronchoscopist, and anesthesia is maintained with a propofol infusion of 100 to 300 µg/kg/min, and a syringe of propofol is placed in the stopcock of the intravenous line in case the patient moves.

A rubberized mouth guard is placed over the upper incisors, and the rigid bronchoscope is inserted through the cords and into the upper trachea under direct vision. Immediately after insertion of the rigid bronchoscope, the anesthesia ventilation system is attached to the 15-mm airway adapter side arm of the rigid bronchoscope. I use a coaxial Mapelson D circuit (Bain circuit) because it is lightweight and less bulky than the standard circle system. Next, the mouth is packed with saline-wetted gauze, which is tucked into the folds around the glottis with McGill forceps. This is done to decrease the air leak occurring between the glottic chink and the rigid bronchoscope; occasionally, I pack the nose with petroleum jelly gauze as well. Positive pressure ventilation is maintained by hand because there are frequent exchanges of equipment pieces, which are inserted through the self-sealing diaphragm on the end of the rigid bronchoscope (Fig. 64–26). Whenever this seal is broken, ventilation is withheld because anesthetic gases and the patient's debris can be exhaled into the surgeon's face.

### Specific Considerations for Laser Fulguration

If the surgeon decides to use laser fulguration, all OR personnel are required to put on protective eyeware, and the $F_{IO_2}$ is decreased <40% in balance nitrogen (no $N_2O$). If any desaturation <90% occurs, laser fulguration ceases, and ventilation with 40% $O_2$ is used, with rapid escalation to 100% as needed to return the saturation above 90%. Additionally, suctioning to control bleeding and remove obstructing pieces of necrotic tissue may be necessary. Occasionally, it is necessary to push the bronchoscope tip past an obstructing lesion to allow adequate oxygenation. Alternatively, during fulguration of a mainstem lesion, it is occasionally necessary to withdraw the rigid bronchoscope back into the main trachea to allow better ventilation of the nonoperative side and improve oxygenation saturation.

### Specific Considerations for Stent Placement

In cases where stent placement and or dilation of an extrinsic compressing lesion is required, anesthetic techniques similar to those outlined for laser fulguration are employed. These procedures are typically completed in 10 to 15 minutes due to the large numbers and substantial experience of the team at UCSD. Significant symptomatic improvement occurs in most patients following rigid bronchoscopy for both stent placement and laser bronchoscopy. Accordingly, every effort is made to extubate the trachea of these patients in the OR.

## UNILATERAL BRONCHOPULMONARY LAVAGE FOR PULMONARY ALVEOLAR PROTEINOSIS

Unilateral bronchopulmonary lavage is used to remove the lipoproteinaceous material that accumulates in the airways of patients with pulmonary alveolar proteinosis. The phospholipoproteinaceous material is derived from surfactant which

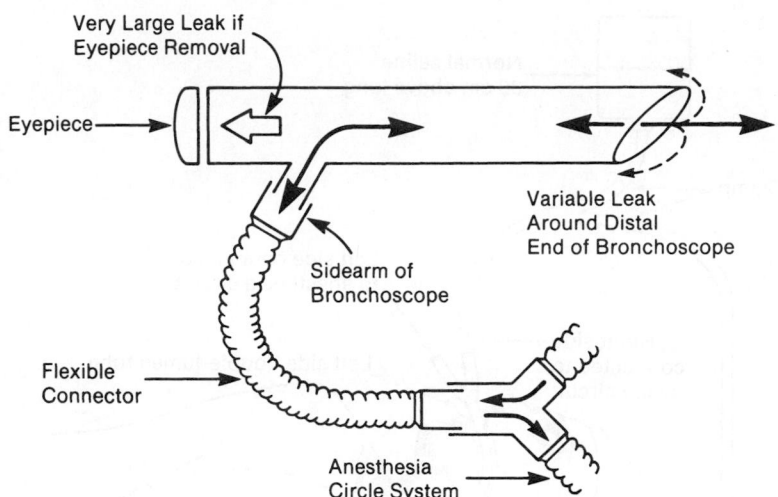

**FIGURE 64–26.** This schematic diagram shows a rigid ventilating bronchoscope system, which consists of the anesthesia circle system attached to a flexible connector that is attached to the sidearm of the bronchoscope. I recommend use of the Mapelson D (Bain circuit) because of the light weight and decreased dead space compared to the system depicted here. With the proximal eyepiece in place, most of the inspired gas goes into the patient. However, since the bronchoscope cannot fully fill the area of the trachea, there is a variable leak around the distal end of the bronchoscope. Exhaled gases are evacuated through the anesthesia circle system (or exhalation limb of the Bain circuit—if used). When the eyepiece is removed, there is a very large leak out the proximal end of the bronchoscope. The anesthesiologist remains vigilant so as not to ventilate at this time, otherwise the surgeon may be splashed with debris that emerges out of the eyepiece. (From Benumof JL. *Anesthesia for Thoracic Surgery.* 2nd ed. Philadelphia, Pa: WB Saunders; 1995:502.)

builds up due to abnormal clearance mechanisms, rather than increased production.[281] There are at least two congenital forms of the disease, as well as secondary forms that result from chemical exposure.[282]

### How Is the Diagnosis of Pulmonary Alveolar Proteinosis Made?

Patients present with progressive hypoxemia and dyspnea (first with exertion, later at rest). PFTs demonstrate a restrictive process, with significant, progressive right-to-left shunt. The classic chest radiographic picture consists of patchy airspace consolidation in a "bat wing" or "butterfly" distribution.[283] CT scans more clearly define the extent of disease and help differentiate pulmonary alveolar proteinosis from other diagnostic entities (ie, sarcoidosis, extrinsic allergic alveolitis, pulmonary fibrosis, and tuberculosis). The definitive diagnosis is based on histologic samples obtained via biopsy (via transbronchial, percutaneous, or open thoracotomy techniques).[284]

### What Are the Indications for Unilateral Bronchopulmonary Lavage?

The threshold symptoms requiring unilateral bronchopulmonary lavage vary with the patient's lifestyle and general constitution. Generally, a room air $PaO_2$ <60 at rest or $O_2$ dependency for normal activities are threshold indications.

### What Is the Technique for Unilateral Bronchopulmonary Lavage?

Unilateral bronchopulmonary lavage is carried out under general anesthesia using a left-sided DLT. The most severe side is lavaged first, and after a few days' rest, the contralateral side is lavaged (Fig. 64–27). The procedure takes several hours to lavage 10 to 20 L of warmed isotonic saline in 500- to 1000-mL aliquots. The lavaged effluent is initially dark brown in color. The material removed appears like grains of sand, which settle to the bottom of the collection bottle. When the lavage effluent clears, the lavage is complete.

### What Are the Anesthetic Considerations for Unilateral Bronchopulmonary Lavage?

Standard monitoring for a thoracotomy is used, including an arterial line and central venous monitoring. After preoxygenation, general anesthesia is induced, and a nondepolarizing neuromuscular blockade administered. The largest left-sided DLT that will fit is inserted; this facilitates drainage during lavage removal and suctioning at the end of the case (when the lung must be as clear of fluid as possible). Final positioning of the left DLT is verified with an FOB, and an underwater cuff seal test is used to verify that tracheal and bronchial cuffs will hold against 50 cm $H_2O$ pressure. The patient is maintained in the supine position, which balances blood flow and spillage to the contralateral lung (Table 64–11).

The patient's anesthesia is maintained with propofol infusion or an inhaled agent (isoflurane, sevoflurane, or desflurane). Neuromuscular blockade is maintained to minimize the risk of movement associated with DLT migration. After baseline pulmonary compliance is measured for each lung, lavage begins.

Warmed isotonic saline is infused by gravity at a height of 30 cm above the midaxillary line. When flow ceases, the lung is assumed to be full, and drainage is allowed (by gravity) to a collection bottle held 20 cm below the midaxillary line.

**TABLE 64–11.** Unilateral Lung Lavage Effect on Patient Positioning

| Position | Advantages | Disadvantages |
|---|---|---|
| Lateral decubitus (nondependent, lavaged lung) | Minimizes blood flow to the nonventilated lung | Maximizes the possibility of spillage into dependent lung |
| Lateral decubitus (dependent, lavaged lung) | Minimizes the possibility of spillage into dependent lung | Maximizes blood flow to the nonventilated lung |
| Supine | Balances spillage and blood flow | |

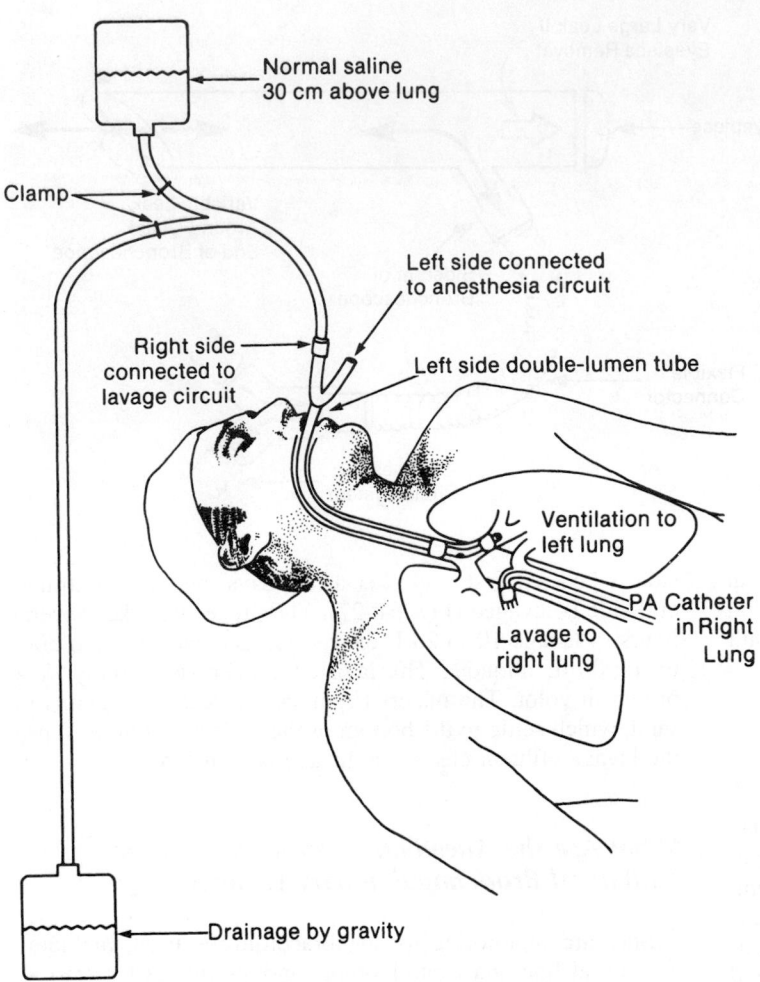

**FIGURE 64–27.** Technique for providing unilateral pulmonary lavage. A left sided double-lumen endotracheal tube allows ventilation to the left lung during lavage of the right lung (and vice versa). Normal saline is infused and drained by gravity; clamps on the connection tubes determine direction of fluid flow. PA, pulmonary artery. (From Benumof JL. *Anesthesia for Thoracic Surgery.* 2nd ed. Philadelphia, Pa: WB Saunders; 1995:549.)

Systemic arterial oxygenation will predictably improve with infusion of saline because more blood flow is diverted to the ventilated lung and deteriorates with drainage of the effluent.[285] Conversely, cardiac output decreases slightly during infusion of the saline (due to the increased pulmonary vascular resistance)[286] and returns to baseline after drainage of the effluent.

After the last effluent becomes clear, the lavage portion of the procedure is terminated, and the recovery portion begins. The recovery period consists of chest wall percussion and suctioning with postural drainage along with intermittent large tidal volumes. When the compliance of the lavage returns to the prelavage value, neuromuscular blockade is reversed, and the patient is allowed to emerge from general anesthesia in the usual fashion. Weaning and extubation criteria are the same as with any thoracic surgery patient. If the patient is not a candidate for extubation, the DLT is changed to a single-lumen ETT, and the patient is ventilated conventionally with some PEEP.

Postextubation, the patient is encouraged to cough and deep breathe, get out of bed and ambulate, and use an incentive spirometer. After 3 to 5 days' recovery, the patient's oxygenation, exercise tolerance, and general condition is usually markedly improved from the preprocedure condition. At this time, lavage of the contralateral lung may commence. The anesthetic considerations are the same as for the first lung except that oxygenation problems are usually much less severe than the first procedure because now a nearly normal lung will

be used to support oxygenation. Bilateral sequential lavage performed on the same day is risky but is practiced at some centers.[287]

## PULMONARY THROMBOENDARTERECTOMY

### What Is Chronic Thromboembolic Pulmonary Hypertension? What Is a Pulmonary Thromboendarterectomy?

Pulmonary thromboendarterectomy (PTE) is a potentially curative procedure for chronic thromboembolic pulmonary hypertension (CTEPH). PTE is currently the only curative treatment for CTEPH. Medical management provides only limited improvement in symptoms, and the only reasonable alternative is lung transplantation. Compared with lung transplantation, PTE has a lower surgical mortality, better long-term survival, shorter waiting period before surgery, and fewer long-term complications. Because PTE is gaining popularity worldwide, anesthesiologists must make themselves aware of the procedure and its associated perioperative considerations.

### Which Patients Develop Chronic Thromboembolic Pulmonary Hypertension?

CTEPH is a progressive debilitating disease resulting from incompletely resolved pulmonary emboli (PE). Most patients experience a major deep venous thrombosis (DVT) and subsequent PE, although the initial event may go undetected in many. The embolus undergoes incomplete resolution, and the patient experiences a "honeymoon" period followed months to years later by insidious and unremitting cardiopulmonary deterioration. In the United States, approximately 600 000 patients develop PE annually.[288] Approximately 150 000 of these patients die leaving 450 000 survivors. The vast majority of survivors enjoy complete dissolution of their emboli following therapy with heparin and warfarin sodium (Coumadin). However, 0.5% of the survivors have unresolved PE. It is these 2500 or more patients who develop CTEPH annually in the United States alone.

### How Has the Pulmonary Thromboendarterectomy Technique Evolved Into Today's Procedure?

It was not until the late 1960s that CTEPH was recognized widely as a distinct diagnostic entity and the need to perform a complete endarterectomy (not merely a thrombectomy) became understood. In 1973, the first PTE was performed at UCSD.[289] After this case, the use of median sternotomy (rather than thoracotomy) and need for CPB gained popularity. In the 1980s and 1990s, innovations in surgical and anesthetic techniques led to improvements in outcome.

### What Is the Diagnostic Workup for Chronic Thromboembolic Pulmonary Hypertension?

Once CTEPH is suspected, the diagnostic goals are to (1) confirm the presence of thromboembolic disease, (2) quantify the degree of pulmonary hypertension, and (3) search for the etiology or contributing factors (such as hypercoagulability).

Most CTEPH patients present with progressive dyspnea on exertion. This finding in young individuals is particularly significant because it is otherwise rare. Exercise-induced syncope may be present in late stages of the disease. A documented history of PE is helpful but not absolutely necessary.

Physical examination typically demonstrates evidence of right heart failure. Precordial examination reveals a right ventricular heave, and a unique murmur is heard on auscultation of the lung fields.[290] This systolic sound results from turbulent flow through partially obstructed or recannalized pulmonary vessels.

The hematocrit is frequently elevated due to secondary polycythemia, with values in the 45% to 55% range being common. Liver function tests may be abnormal in a nonspecific pattern, reflecting hepatic congestion. Prothrombin time (PT) and partial thromboplastin time (PTT) are usually normal. No clear dysfunction in the fibrinolytic system has yet been identified.[291] Furthermore, antithrombin III (ATIII), protein C, and protein S are abnormal in <1% of patients with CTEPH.[292] The only prothrombotic factor yet identified in this patient population is the lupus anticoagulant (present in approximately 10% of patients with CTEPH).[293]

The ECG shows evidence of right ventricular hypertrophy. PFT reveals a decreased carbon monoxide (CO) diffusing capacity and a moderate restrictive defect. The decreased CO diffusion capacity is a combination of both decreased membrane diffusion and decreased capillary blood volume.[294]

ABG analysis universally reveals an increased alveolar-arterial (A-a) $O_2$ gradient which markedly widens with exercise. Dead space ventilation is increased, leading to a compensatory increase in minute ventilation. As dead space ventilation increases with exercise, hypercarbia may result.[295] When multiple inert gas elimination technique (MIGET) is performed, moderate-to-large $\dot{V}/\dot{Q}$ mismatches are documented; this distinguishes the disease from primary pulmonary hypertension or COLD, where small patchy inequalities are present. $\dot{V}/\dot{Q}$ scans, however, often dramatically underestimate central pulmonary vascular obstruction in patients with CTEPH.

Chest radiography (Fig. 64–28) typically demonstrates clear airway spaces, with relative oligemia in the affected lobes of the lungs, reflecting the diminished pulmonary blood flow. Additionally, evidence of right ventricular enlargement is present. Finally, the greater diameter of the left main PA (seen on the radiograph as the shadow above the left main stem bronchus) compared with that of the aorta is a subtle finding invariably seen with CTEPH.[296] Occasionally, pulmonary infarcts are seen, but these are rare.

Recently, spiral computerized tomography (CT) scanning and magnetic resonance imaging (MRI) have shown utility in the evaluation of CTEPH.[297] The CT scan shows a characteristic mosaic appearance due to variable regional pulmonary blood flow (Fig. 64–29).

Right heart catheterization demonstrates the severity of pulmonary hypertension. The echocardiogram demonstrates function and severity of disease. A classic end stage CTEPH

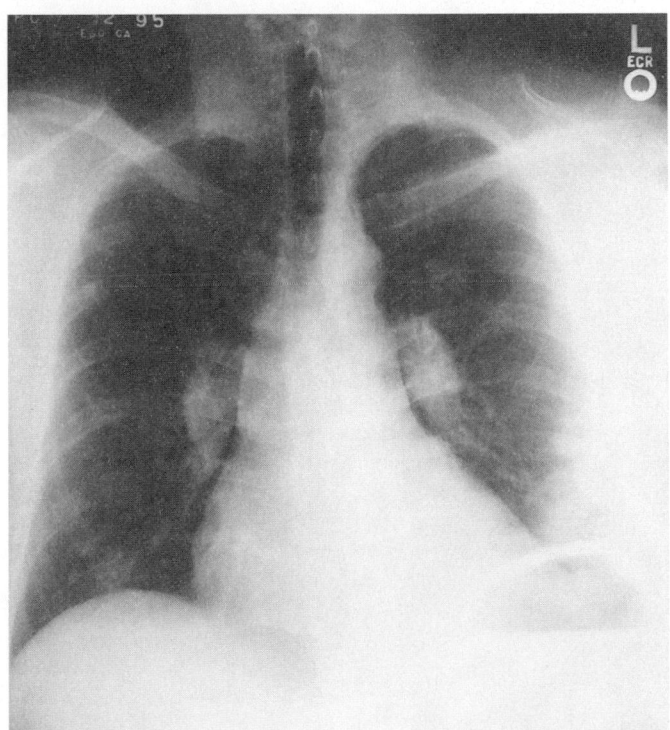

**FIGURE 64–28.** The chest radiograph of a patient with chronic thromboembolic pulmonary hypertension (CTEPH). This patient had a left sided pulmonary infarct, which is rare (pleural based, slightly underpenetrated—just above the gastric air bubble). Note the bilaterally prominent hilar pulmonary arteries which abruptly cut off. There is a paucity of any pulmonary vessels superiorly, and only a few in the lower lobes. The left pulmonary artery is actually larger than the aorta in this radiograph (an almost universal feature in CTEPH).

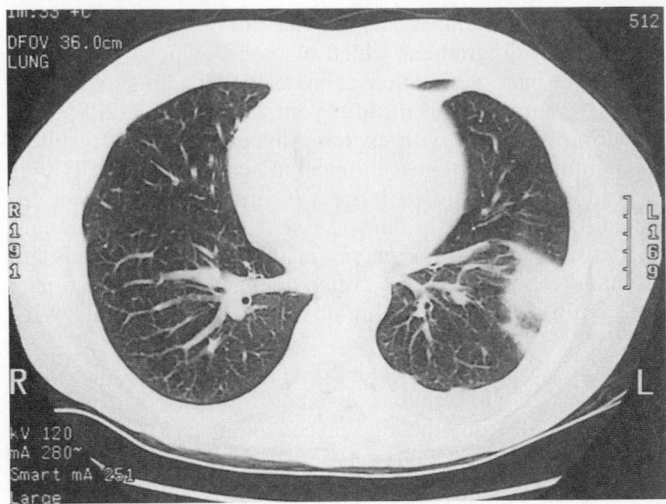

**FIGURE 64–29.** A chest CT scan of the same patient whose chest x-ray is shown in Figure 64–28. The characteristic mosaic appearance of the lung, due to the variable regional perfusion, is demonstrated. The left sided pulmonary infarct, is well seen. A small left sided effusion is also noted.

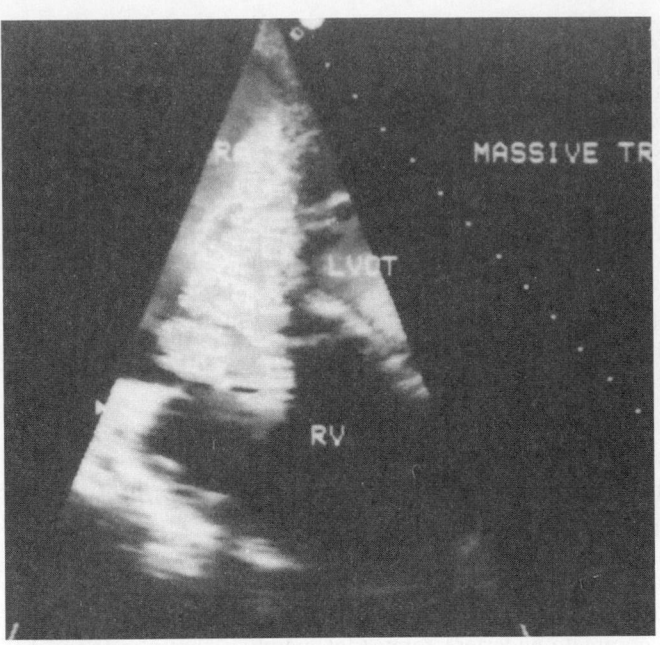

**FIGURE 64–31.** A transesophageal echocardiogram during systole of the same patient shown in Figure 64–30. Note the massive tricuspid regurgitant (TR) jet created by the turbulent backflow of blood out of the leaky tricuspid valve. This tricuspid regurgitation resolved postoperatively, following removal of the obstructing PTE lesion. LVOT, left ventricular outflow tract; RA, right atrium, RV, right ventricle.

patient will demonstrate massive right atrial and right ventricular enlargement (Fig. 64–30). Typically, the LV is relatively small due to impingement from the hypertrophic right ventricle and diminished left-sided preload.[298] Tricuspid regurgitation is frequently found using Doppler color-flow measurements (Fig. 64–31). Occasionally, thrombi are noted in the right atrium, and obstructive material is frequently found in the PAs (Fig. 64–32).

Pulmonary arteriography has been an invaluable diagnostic modality providing characteristic patterns, including (1) irregular arterial contours, (2) abrupt cut-off or narrowing of vessels, (3) PA webs and bands, (4) pouch defects, and (5) obstruction of lobar or segmental arteries at their point of origin (Fig. 64–33).[299] CT and MRI are adding important information. However, the, pulmonary arteriogram remains the gold standard for evaluating pulmonary vascular obstruction in these patients. Although an invasive test, >600 pulmonary angiograms have been completed with non-ionic contrast at UCSD without a single fatality.

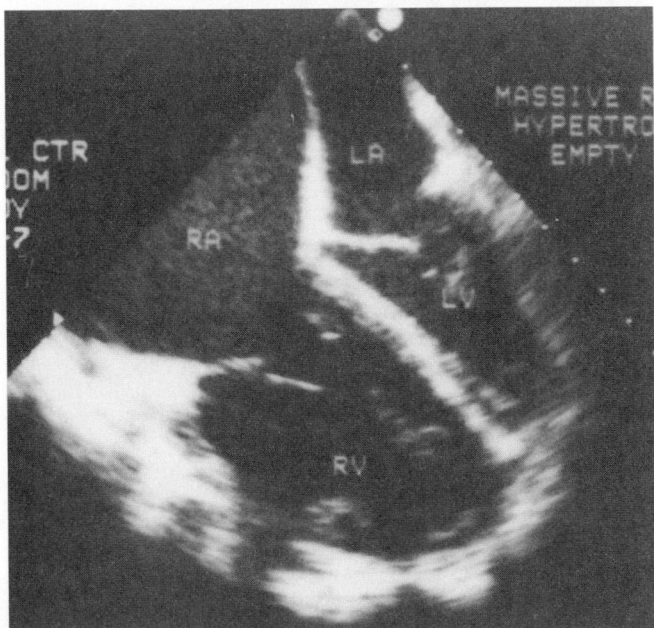

**FIGURE 64–30.** A four chamber view transesophageal echocardiogram of a patient with chronic thromboembolic pulmonary hypertension (CTEPH). The right atrium (RA) is massively dilated, the right ventricle (RV) is hypertropic and distended. The interventricular septum is bulging in toward the diminutive empty left ventricle (LV). Both the left atrium (LA) and LV are small and empty.

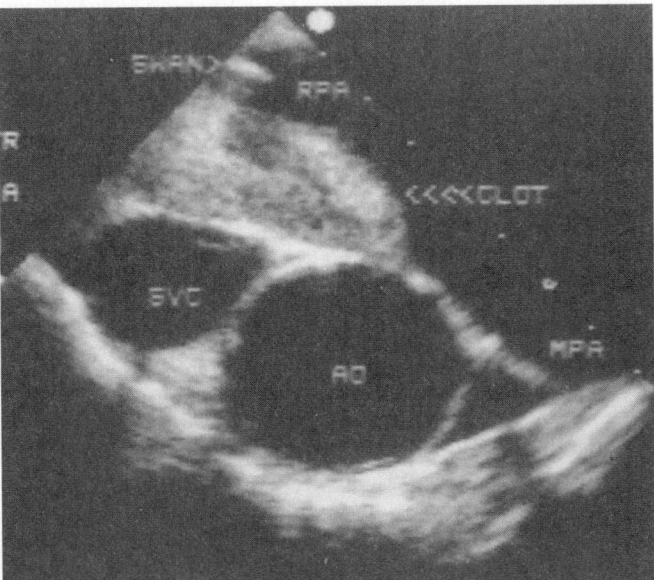

**FIGURE 64–32.** A transesophageal echocardiogram demonstrating a thrombus in the right pulmonary artery (RPA) of a patient with CTEPH. Note the small shadow caused by the pulmonary artery catheter seen in the superior vena cava (SVC) and RPA (marked SWAN). AO, aorta; <<<< Clot, thrombus; MPA, main pulmonary artery.

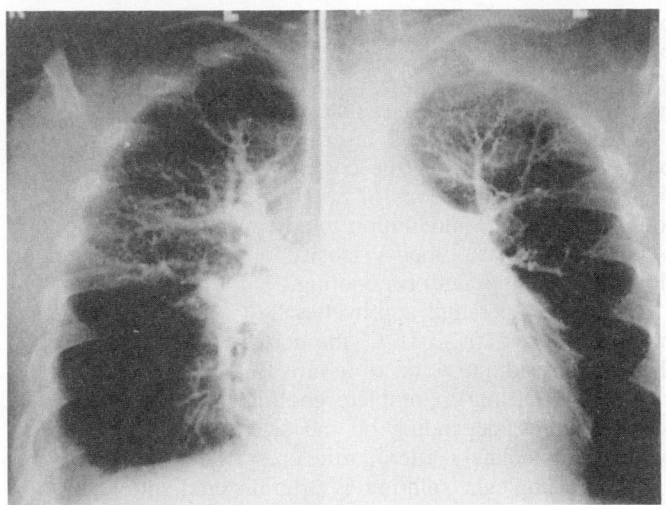

**FIGURE 64–33.** Right and left pulmonary arteriograms demonstrate lack of filling to the periphery. The specimen removed from this patient is shown in Figure 64–34. (From Jamieson SW, Kapelanski DP. Pulmonary endarterectomy. *Curr Probl Surg.* 2000;37:165.)

## What Are the Criteria for Surgery Selection?

The majority of patients have pulmonary vascular resistance (PVR) >300 dynes/sec/cm$^{-5}$. It is not uncommon to encounter values >1000 dynes/sec/cm$^{-5}$ and suprasystemic PA pressures. Important in the process is the patient's willingness to accept the mortality rate of the procedure, which, at UCSD, is 5% to 7%.[3] There are no levels of right-sided heart dysfunction, extent of disease, functional impairment, or pulmonary vascular resistance that contraindicate this operation. The UCSD selection criteria for PTE are shown in Table 64–12.

## What Are the Important Anesthetic Management Principles for the Pulmonary Thromboendarterectomy Patient?

### Hemodynamic Considerations for Induction and the Precardiopulmonary Bypass Period

Although a small percentage of patients with CTEPH presenting for PTE have associated LV pathology (<10%), the vast majority do not. Accordingly, hemodynamic assessment and decision making considerations are centered on optimiza-

tion of right ventricular function, and are outlined in Table 64–13. The right ventricle is hypertrophic and dilated, as is the right atrium. Because of the high right-sided pressures, the coronary blood supply to the right ventricle is constantly at risk. Maintenance of adequate systemic vascular resistance (SVR), preserving the inotropic state and maintaining normal sinus rhythm tends to preserve systemic hemodynamics as well as right coronary perfusion. The preoperative cardiac catheterization data—including cardiac output, pulmonary vascular resistance (PVR), patency of coronary arteries, and right ventricular end-diastolic pressure (RVEDP)—are particularly useful in planning the induction sequence. Elevated RVEDP (>14 mm Hg), moderate to severe tricuspid regurgitation, and preoperative PVR >1000 dynes/sec/cm$^{-5}$ are signs of impending decompensation. In such cases, institution of inotropic (eg, dopamine or epinephrine) and pressor support (eg, phenylephrine) should be considered for the induction and prebypass period.

### Induction

Induction is targeted at maintenance of hemodynamic stability. Moderate doses of etomidate (0.1-0.2 mg/kg) or midazolam (0.1 mg/kg) in conjunction with fentanyl 5 to 50 μg/kg are given in divided doses while hemodynamic response is assessed. Phenylephrine (50-100 μg) is frequently necessary to maintain right coronary artery (RCA) perfusion pressure; MAP in the 75 to 85 mm Hg range is usually sufficient.

**TABLE 64–12.** University of California, San Diego, Criteria for Pulmonary Thromboendarterectomy Surgery

Hemodynamically significant pulmonary vascular obstruction (PVR >300 dynes/sec/cm$^{-5}$)
Significant functional impairment
  Dyspnea and fatigue exacerbation with exertion
  Oxygen dependence, or oxygen and nitric oxide dependence
Proximal location of pulmonary thrombi (surgical access possible)
Absence of significant coexisting disease (eg, liver failure, renal failure, malignancy, psychiatric illness)
Patient must desire surgery based on dissatisfaction with cardiopulmonary status or prognosis
Patients and family must be willing to accept the morbidity and mortality of the procedure (current 5%-7%)

PVR, pulmonary vascular resistance.

**TABLE 64–13.** Hemodynamic Considerations for Chronic Thromboembolic Pulmonary Hypertension Patients Undergoing Pulmonary Thromboendarterectomy for Induction and During the Precardiopulmonary Bypass Period

**Pathophysiology: RV Hypertrophy**

The RV hypertrophy seen in CTEPH patients is a right-sided equivalent of the hypertrophic LV seen in patients with aortic stenosis. Because the RV did not evolve as a high pressure ventricle, at end stage, the RV becomes dilated, weak, and begins to fail.

**Hemodynamic Goals**

| | |
|---|---|
| HR | Slow (60–80 bpm) |
| Rhythm | Sinus |
| RV Preload | Maintain the elevated CVP |
| LV Preload | Cannot easily manipulate (LV is typically dry) |
| SVR | Keep normal or elevated |
| PVR | Do not exacerbate (avoid hypoxia, hypercarbia, acidosis, anxiety). |
| Contractility | Maintain. Do not allow myocardial depression. |

**Induction Considerations**

Maintain right coronary artery perfusion pressure
Avoid drugs or maneuvers that decrease SVR
Avoid myocardial depressants
Etomidate is a good induction drug for patients in failure (ie, RVEDP > 12–14 range)
If concerned, start dopamine pre-induction
Treat hypotension with phenylephrine
Be prepared to immediately cardiovert if AF or VF occurs (CPR will likely be futile)
Use TEE (postinduction) to guide volume of the LV (which is typically healthy but empty).

AF, atrial fibrillation; CPB, cardiopulmonary bypass; CPR, cardiopulmonary resuscitation; CTEPH, chronic thromboembolic pulmonary hypertension; HR, heart rate; LV, left ventricle; PTE, pulmonary thromboendarterectomy; PVR, pulmonary vascular resistance; RV, right ventricle; RVEDP, right ventricular end-diastolic pressure; SVR, systemic vascular resistance; TEE, transesophageal echocardiography; VF, ventricular fibrillation.

The benefit of phenylephrine therapy for patients with severe pulmonary hypertension was documented by Rich and associates, who showed increased right ventricular performance (increased MAP and coronary artery perfusion pressure and maintenance of cardiac output) with phenylephrine administration.[300] When anesthetic depth and muscle relaxation are deemed to be adequate, the trachea is intubated with a single-lumen ETT.

## Placement of Additional Monitoring Postinduction and Before Cardiopulmonary Bypass

In addition to standard monitors and radial arterial catheter placed pre-induction, other hemodynamic monitors are inserted with the patient anesthetized in order to minimize discomfort. The PA catheter is placed in the right IJ vein but flotation through the tricuspid valve may be difficult because of tricuspid regurgitation. If it cannot be placed in the PA (rarely), it is left in the SVC (~15 cm), and an attempt is made later under echocardiographic guidance.

Next, a femoral arterial catheter is placed. This is because the systemic arterial pressure is significantly underestimated by the radial artery catheter in the post-CPB period. The mechanism for this involves peripheral vasodilation.[301] A TEE probe is then inserted. I have found the TEE to be an extremely valuable monitor for assessing cardiac function, ventricular filling during PTE. Additionally, I perform an agitated saline study to determine the presence of an atrial septal defect.[302] Electroencephalogram (EEG) electrodes are placed and the processed EEG is monitored throughout the procedure. The patient's head is then wrapped in a circulating cold water cooling blanket.

Other monitors include a urinary catheter with temperature monitoring capabilities, a rectal temperature probe, and tympanic membrane temperature probe which provides a fairly reliable estimation of brain temperature.[303] The rectal and bladder probes estimate core temperature, thus helping quantitate thermal gradients. The PA catheter measures the blood temperature, which is allowed to differ no >10°C from the core temperature during cooling and warming.

The fluid warmers are turned off in preparation for cooling, and additional fentanyl or midazolam is administered as necessary before chest incision. Potent inhalational agents such as isoflurane are used sparingly, if at all. When the hematocrit and hemodynamics permit, 1 to 2 units of autologous blood are harvested for reinfusion after CPB.

## Median Sternotomy and Deep Hypothermic Circulatory Arrest

The surgical approach involves a median sternotomy and CPB. Although used in the past, a lateral thoracotomy is suboptimal.[304] A median sternotomy allows treatment of both PAs, which is necessary in almost all cases. The use of CPB with periods of complete DHCA provides the bloodless operative field necessary for complete meticulous lobar and segmental dissections.[305]

Following median sternotomy, CPB is established with ascending aortic cannulation, and two caval cannulae are inserted for venous return to the bypass pump. Cooling begins immediately using CPB temperature adjustment and cooling blankets, which are placed under the patient and around the head. A gradient of 10°C is maintained between the arterial blood and the bladder/rectal temperature. A temporary PA vent is inserted. When the temperature descends to approximately 26° to 27°C, the heart slows or begins to fibrillate. At this time, an LV vent is inserted through the right upper pulmonary vein. During the cooling phase venous $O_2$ saturation increases. Saturations of 80% are typical at 25°C, rising to 90% at 20°C. Hemodilution to a hematocrit of 18% to 25% is used to decrease blood viscosity, optimize capillary blood flow, and promote uniform cooling.

As core temperature approaches 20°C, and brain temperature approaches 16° to 18°C, the aorta is cross-clamped, and thiopental is administered to assure EEG isoelectricity (typically 500-1000 mg). Complete cooling typically requires 45 to 60 minutes, depending on the size and perfusion of the patient. Immediately after aortic cross-clamping, cold crystalloid cardioplegia solution is administered into the aortic root. Additional myocardial protection is afforded by a cooling jacket around the heart.

## Surgical Technique for Pulmonary Thromboembolism

The right PA endarterectomy plane is established and dissection continues until bronchial artery back-bleeding impairs good visualization. At this point, circulatory arrest is imperative. Bronchial artery backflow in these patients is frequently substantial and without circulatory arrest, and complete endarterectomy cannot be accomplished. It has been suggested that the procedure be referred to as *pulmonary endarterectomy* rather than PTE because it is the endarterectomy that is critical to the success of the operation. Figure 64–34 shows the specimen obtained from a successful pulmonary endarterectomy. The corresponding pulmonary arteriogram (from the same patient) is shown in Figure 64–33.

Circulatory arrest is limited to 20 minute periods to prevent neurologic damage. An experienced surgeon can usually accomplish the entire unilateral endarterectomy within this time period. If additional arrest time is necessary, reperfusion is carried out at 18°C core temperature for a minimum of 10

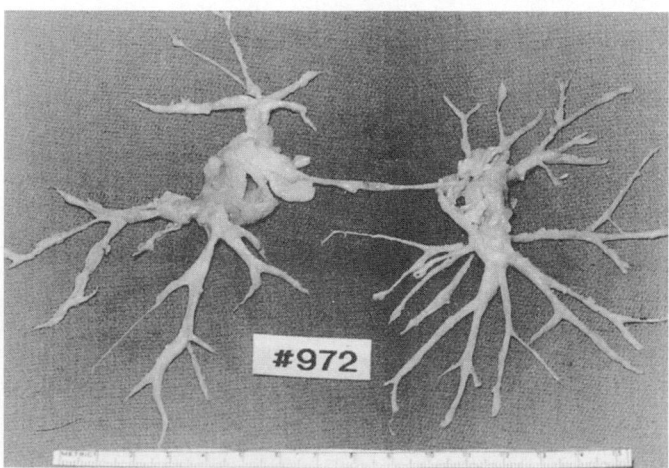

**FIGURE 64–34.** Operative specimen removed from patient whose pulmonary arteriogram is shown in Figure 64–33. The ruler measures 15 cm. It is not uncommon to remove more material at operation than would be suggested by the arteriograms. (From Jamieson SW, Kapelanski DP. Pulmonary endarterectomy. *Curr Probl Surg.* 2000;37:165.)

minutes. At the completion of the endarterectomy, perfusion is reestablished while the PA incision is closed.

Next, the left PA is incised and an endarterectomy is performed as described above. Following completion of the left endarterectomy, the right atrium is explored for the presence of an ASD, which is repaired if present. Any additional procedures such as coronary artery bypass grafting (CABG) or valve replacement can be performed during the rewarming period.

## Anesthetic Considerations During Deep Hypothermic Circulatory Arrest

The anesthetic considerations immediately before and during DHCA are summarized in Table 64–14. Immediately before DHCA arrest, the lungs are gently ventilated with unwarmed room air (not $O_2$). The purpose of this is to empty remaining blood from the pulmonary veins and bronchial vessels, providing a bloodless surgical field. Room air is preferred for this maneuver because of the theoretical concern that 100% $O_2$ during circulatory arrest may lead to bronchial or alveolar injury (involving $O_2$ derived free radical mediated mechanisms).

During DHCA, the anesthesiologist ensures that the head cooling blanket is functioning properly, the EEG is isoelectric, and all stopcocks and intravenous solutions are turned to the *off* position. This decreases the risk of entraining air into the vasculature during exsanguination. Furthermore, flushing of arterial or venous lines during DHCA is strictly avoided as this may allow air, debris, or warm saline to be infused into the cerebral circulation

## Anesthetic Considerations During Post–Deep Hypothermic Circulatory Arrest (Rewarming Period)

On rewarming, the head cooling blanket is removed, and additional anesthetic (eg, benzodiazepine or propofol infusion, muscle relaxant) is administered. The aortic cross-clamp is removed, and full perfusion is restored. The myocardial cooling jacket is removed, and methylprednisolone, 500 mg (stabilizes cellular membranes and decreases reperfusion pulmonary edema), and mannitol, 12.5 g (to promote diuresis and free radical scavenging), are administered. Research is ongoing at

**TABLE 64–14.** Anesthetic Considerations Immediately Before and During Deep Hypothermic Circulatory Arrest

Ensure ice is applied to head, or ice water bath ($\pm$ 4°C) is circulating through and cooling water blanket applied to the patient's head.

Ensure patient's core temperature is 18°C or lower.

Be sure all fluid warmers are shut off (these should remain off from the start of the case until the perfusionist is instructed to begin active rewarming).

Turn off all stopcocks toward the patient.

Do not allow any flushing of arterial or venous lines during DHCA. (Otherwise air, debris, or room temperature saline may perfuse the cerebral blood vessels and increase the risk of neurologic complications).

Ensure patient's EEG is isoelectric. (If not, 500–1000 mg STP administered).

Immediately prior to DHCA, several large tidal volume breaths are delivered to the patient with unwarmed room air.

DHCA, deep hypothermic circulatory arrest; STP, sodium thiopental.

UCSD to assess the benefit of these theoretically advantageous maneuvers. A 10°C gradient between blood and bladder/rectal temperature is maintained but not exceeded during rewarming. Warming more quickly (>10°C gradient) promotes systemic gas bubble formation and uneven warming. Rewarming times are variably related to the patient's weight and systemic perfusion; 90 to 120 minutes are usually required to achieve a core temperature of 36.5°C. The heart generally begins to beat spontaneously with a bradycardiac rhythm as the blood temperature approaches 25° to 30°C; defibrillation is occasionally necessary.

## Anesthetic Considerations During Separation From Cardiopulmonary Bypass

Preparation for separation from CPB occurs as for most cardiac cases. However, for PTE patients, we use a generous $V_T$ (12-15 mL/kg) to provide adequate lung expansion and 5 cm of PEEP. End-tidal $CO_2$ ($ETCO_2$) is a poor measure of ventilation adequacy in these patients both pre- and post-CPB because dead space ventilation is an integral part of the disease process. After successful surgery, however, the arterial-$ETCO_2$ gradient is decreased compared with preoperative values.

While still on CPB, the TEE is used to detect intracavitary air as well as to evaluate left and right ventricular function. The femoral artery pressure is monitored as it is a more accurate measure of aortic pressure than the radial artery pressure at this time (for reasons described previously). The anesthesiologist checks the airway for frothy sputum or bleeding due to the risk of reperfusion pulmonary edema and airway bleeding, two of the most dreaded complications of this procedure which may manifest at this time.

Separation from CPB occurs as the venous return line is clamped and the heart is allowed to fill. I typically separate from CPB with the CVP in the 10 to 16 mm Hg range and use TEE for assessing the function and volume of the ventricles. Generally, the CVP is the best postoperative filling pressure correlate (in successful operations); recall that the LV is typically normal preoperatively, just empty and starving for blood.

I routinely use a dopamine infusion (3-5 μg/kg/min) both for its mild inotropic activity and renal dopaminergic effect. In patients with particularly poor ventricular function, epinephrine, 0.4 to 1.5 μg/kg/min, is added. If the surgery has been successful, the TEE reveals immediate post-PTE improvements in the left- and right-sided geometry.[306] The distention of the right atrium and right ventricle is greatly decreased, resulting in improvement of function of both ventricles. Tricuspid regurgitation, if it was present before the endarterectomy, has greatly decreased or resolved; it is for this reason that tricuspid valve repair is generally not performed as part of this operation. Significant improvement in hemodynamic status is noted, including a doubling of the cardiac index, dramatic decrease in PA pressures, and a drop in the PVR to 25% of the preoperative value.

## Anesthetic Considerations During and Following Cardiopulmonary Bypass

If autologous blood was harvested before CPB, it is now reinfused. Frothy sputum, if present, likely indicates the onset of reperfusion pulmonary edema. In this case, the ETT is quickly suctioned and increasing amounts of PEEP are applied beginning with 5 cm $H_2O$, escalating to 7.5, and up to 10 cm $H_2O$. If frank blood is returning from the ETT, surgical bleeding is the probable culprit. Although it may not be of much benefit, PEEP is increased and aggressive suctioning of the blood ensues. If severe bleeding persists, FOB is used to evaluate the source of bleeding, and lung isolation maneuvers (BBs, double-lumen ETT) are considered.

Following heparin reversal, the pericardium and thoracic cavity is inspected for bleeding sources. The anesthesiologist verifies heparin reversal with an activated clotting time (ACT). A cell-saver is used to recover shed blood and process blood remaining in the bypass circuit. Mediastinal tubes are placed, and the chest is closed. Bleeding diathesis is rare, and transfusion requirements are usually minimal.

### What Concerns Unique to Pulmonary Thromboembolism Complicate Postoperative Management?

Postoperative management of the PTE patient is similar to that following most other types of CPB. The patient tends to awaken in 6 to 12 hours following PTE. We typically extubate the trachea on postoperative day number one. However, two major postoperative complications unique to PTE (reperfusion pulmonary edema and PA steal) can delay weaning and extubation for prolonged periods. Reperfusion pulmonary edema is a localized form of high permeability (noncardiogenic) lung injury—a form of adult respiratory distress syndrome (ARDS)—localized to the area of lung in which the endarterectomy *was performed*. It usually occurs within the first 24 hours but may appear up to 72 hours following PTE.[307] In most cases, it is mild; reperfusion edema resulting in clinically significant morbidity occurs in only 10% of cases. In its most severe form, it begins immediately post-CPB in the OR as described previously. These patients are often extremely ill, requiring aggressive intensive care and ventilator management. Pressure control, PEEP, and inverse ratio ventilation are used judicially in an effort to improve $\dot{V}/\dot{Q}$ matching and minimize further pulmonary injury.

PA steal represents a postoperative redistribution of PA blood away from the previously well perfused segments into the newly endarterectomized segments.[308] Whether the cause is failure of autoregulation in the newly endarterectomized segments or secondary small vessel changes in the previously open segments has not been clarified. However, long-term follow-up has documented a decrease in pulmonary vascular steal in the majority of patients, suggesting a remodeling process in the pulmonary vascular bed.[309]

### What Is the Long-Term Outcome Following Pulmonary Thromboembolism?

The long-term hemodynamic and systematic outcomes have been equally encouraging. Systematic improvement has been documented for as long as 12 months following the surgery with every indication that the improvements are essentially permanent. A study of UCSD patients having received pulmonary endarterectomy between 1970 and 1995 indicates that most patients experience a sustained improvement in functional status indefinitely.[310] The majority of patients who were initially NYHA class III and IV status returned to NYHA

class I and II and are able to resume normal activities. In addition, resolution of hypertensive changes within the pulmonary vascular bed occur and remodeling of the right ventricle continues over weeks to months.

All patients are maintained on life-long anticoagulation therapy with warfarin. Although thromboembolic recurrence has been detected in a few patients in whom anticoagulation therapy was discontinued or allowed to fall below therapeutic levels, there have been no documented occurrences of recurrent thromboembolic events in patients who have been maintained on adequate anticoagulation. The neurologic outcome is generally good, although occasionally patients exhibit neuropsychiatric changes which can include paranoia, euphoria, and, rarely, focal deficits. There has been a decrease in the frequency and magnitude of neurologic deficits in the last 10 years at UCSD. This improvement has been attributed to decreased circulatory arrest times and improved cerebral protection.

## THORACIC TRAUMA

### What Are the Indications for Thoracotomy Following Thoracic Trauma?

Emergency department thoracotomy (single-lumen ETT used) is indicated for patients with penetrating thoracic injuries with signs of life in the field who do not respond to fluids and begin to lose their vital signs in the resuscitation area.[311] Survival rates following emergency thoracotomy are low for patients with abdominal hemorrhage, a blunt mechanism of injury, and those without signs of life in the field. For these patients, significant judgment is required.

Urgent thoracotomy with planned lung separation (DLT) following thoracic trauma is reserved for patients with (1) massive thoracic bleeding (>1000 mL initially following thoracostomy and >200 mL/h for several hours); (2) massive air leak (especially with known tracheo-bronchial injury); and (3) diaphragmatic rupture. Delayed thoracotomy (also requiring a DLT) is indicated following resuscitation and stabilization for repair of thoracic spine lesions, esophageal injuries, clotted hemothorax, and delayed empyema. However, with the advent of VATS, open thoracotomy is less frequently used in many of the less emergent conditions.[312]

The majority of patients who have sustained thoracic trauma (90% blunt and 75%-80% penetrating) are treated nonoperatively with tube thoracostomy and endotracheal intubation. Therefore, most thoracic trauma patients are seen initially by the anesthesiologist for airway management in the emergency room.

### What Is the Major Cause of Death Following Thoracic Trauma?

Exsanguinating hemorrhage is the most common acute cause of death following thoracic trauma.[313,314] Anesthesiologists caring for trauma victims must always consider airway management concurrently with circulatory support during trauma resuscitation. However, immediate large bore vascular access and aggressive volume administration are the most important initial maneuvers for massive hemorrhage.

At least two large bore peripheral intravenous needles must

be established and secured early. IJ venous catheters can be placed if cervical spine injury is cleared (allowing the head to be turned). Similarly, subclavian or femoral venous access can also be obtained.

## Does the Site of Injury Dictate Optimum Location of Intravenous Access?

The site of injury dictates optimum anatomic location for peripheral intravenous catheter placement. However, in extremis, access is established wherever possible. Following thoracic injuries, at least one large bore line should enter a tributary of the IVC. If an IJ or subclavian central line is placed, it should be inserted ipsilateral to any hemothorax or pneumothorax. In the absence of major abdominal or lower extremity injuries, femoral vein access is equally acceptable and provides reliable CVP trending (even though the wave form variation is opposite that seen from lines placed in the SCV during spontaneous ventilation).

## Is Catheter Size Important in Trauma?

The largest bore catheters available should be inserted during resuscitation of the hemorrhaging trauma patient. According to Poiseuille's law, the rate of fluid flow is directly proportional to the fourth power of the catheter radius and the pressure gradient across the catheter, and is inversely proportional to the length of the catheter and fluid viscosity:

$$Q = \pi r^4 (\Delta P)/8\ nL$$

where $Q$ = flow, $\pi$ = pi, $r$ = radius, $\Delta P$ = pressure gradient, $n$ = viscosity of fluid, and $L$ = length. Doubling the internal diameter of the venous catheter increases the flow through the catheter 16-fold. Flow through a 14-gauge, 2.5-inch catheter is about twice the flow through a 16-gauge, 12 inch catheter.[315] Flow through a 14-gauge catheter with a pressure infusion cuff at 200 mm Hg provides a flow about 400 mL/min.[316] An 8 French catheter introducer provides about twice the flow as a 14-gauge catheter.[317]

## What Is the Minimum Monitoring Required for Thoracic Trauma?

Minimum monitoring for the hemorrhaging trauma patient includes pulse oximeter, end-tidal $CO_2$, ECG, automated BP cuff, temperature probe, and esophageal or precordial stethoscope. For assessment of intravascular volume, blood replacement, and systemic perfusion, an arterial line and CVP should be placed in all severely traumatized patients as soon as more life-threatening concerns are addressed (ABCs of cardiopulmonary resuscitation).

## How Are Advanced Monitoring Modalities Affected by Thoracic Trauma?

An arterial catheter is preferably inserted in an upper extremity (right upper optimal). The femoral artery is a second-

ary choice because it is "down stream" in the event of temporary aortic cross-clamping (which may be required during emergency thoracotomy). A CVP catheter can be used therapeutically for volume and vasopressor administration as well as diagnostically for volume assessment and aids in the diagnosis of pericardial tamponade or tension pneumothorax.

A PA catheter is not usually required initially. However, in patients with persistent hypotension not explained by hypovolemia, a PA catheter is helpful in determining if the problem is poor contractility (myocardial contusion, ischemia) versus systemic vasodilation versus other causes (pericardial tamponade, and so on).

A transesophageal echocardiogram (TEE) probe can be placed following induction and provides the best assessment of intravascular volume, myocardial dysfunction (contusion, tamponade, ischemia, intracardiac air), and can also be used as a monitor for pericardial tamponade, aortic injury, and PE.[318]

A Foley catheter should be placed in all patients with severe trauma either transuretherally or via a suprapubic tube if the patient has urethral trauma. The urine quantity and concentration is a good measure of perfusion to the kidneys.

## Which Specific Thoracic Injuries Pose an Immediate Threat to Life?

### Flail Chest

#### Definition/Presentation

Classically, a flail chest involves three or more adjacent ribs fractured in two or more places (Fig. 64–35). When the fractured ribs occur in one hemithorax, the nonaffected hemithorax expands properly with inhalation, whereas the

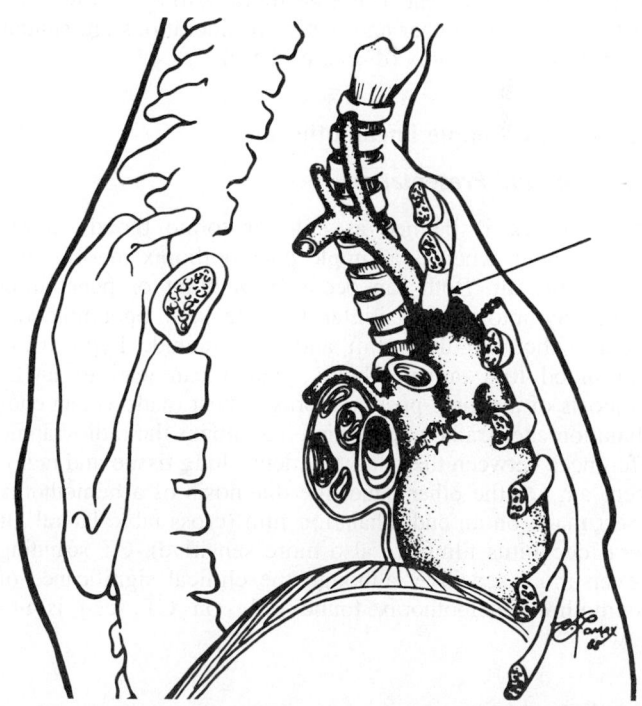

**FIGURE 64–35.** Drawing demonstrating a constellation of thoracic injuries that might be sustained following massive trauma; including a flail chest equivalent. The drawing shows rupture of the trachea and avulsion of the innominate artery by a fractured manubrium. (From Pate JW. Tracheobronchial and esophageal injuries. *Surg Clin North Am.* 1989;69:111.)

affected "flail segment" paradoxically contracts toward the nonaffected side, making ventilation inefficient. A flail chest involves any chest wall injury severe enough to cause ventilatory failure. Additionally, patients with multiple rib fractures are at high risk for developing a pneumo- or hemothorax. Furthermore, positive pressure ventilation further increases the risk of tension pneumothorax.

### Anesthetic Management

Intubation and mechanical ventilation is frequently required for a flail chest. Tube thoracostomy is also frequently required if there is associated hemothorax or pneumothorax.

Analgesia is important. Patients with rib fractures with little or no underlying pulmonary contusion benefit greatly from a thoracic epidural. However, patients suffering a major pulmonary contusion will likely require several days of intubation and mechanical ventilation. Accordingly, these patients benefit less from a thoracic epidural, as systemic analgesia is satisfactory.

## Tension Pneumothorax

### Definition and Presentation

A tension pneumothorax is defined as extra-anatomic air (in the pleural space) under pressure. The patient typically presents with decreased breath sounds, shifted heart sounds, dyspnea, trachea shift from midline, hyperresonance on percussion, distended neck veins, hypotension, and pulseless electrical activity (PEA).

### Anesthetic Management

Chest tube placement or needle thoracostomy followed by chest tube is used. Other anesthetic considerations are similar to simple pneumothorax (discussed later).

## Hemothorax: Simple Pneumothorax

### Definition and Presentation

Hemothorax is defined as extra-anatomic blood (in the pleural space), whereas a simple pneumothorax involves extra-anatomic air. Both can occur from blunt or penetrating trauma. Symptoms are similar to a tension pneumothorax except without midline shift and may include hypotension from blood loss in hemothorax, which can lead to EMD. Diagnosis of a simple pneumothorax is best made via an end-exhalation chest radiograph which maximizes the radiographic differences between the relatively dense lung tissue and radiolucent air. On the other hand, the diagnosis of a hemothorax is best made on an end-inhalation film (cross table lateral, or lateral decubitus films are also more sensitive). CT scanning is even more sensitive, although the clinical significance of pneumothorax-hemothorax found only on CT scan is unknown.

### Anesthetic Management

Chest tube placement is the primary management. Some recommend placing a chest tube simply for rib fractures in patients requiring positive-pressure ventilation. I do not endorse this approach. Nitrous oxide is generally avoided due to its propensity to expand the volume of noncommunicating gas-filled structures. Additionally, patients scheduled for air transport should have chest tubes placed in even the smallest pneumothorax that might otherwise be treated with observation.

## Cardiac Tamponade

### Definition/Presentation

Cardiac tamponade is defined as accumulation of fluid (in trauma blood) in the pericardial space. The pathophysiology involves sudden cardiovascular collapse once a critical volume is reached. The pressure/volume curve of the pericardial space is flat initially; once a critical volume is achieved, the compliance decreases sharply, impairing filling of both atrium and right ventricle initially. Subsequently, the LV becomes empty, and cardiac output is impaired as there is a normalization of all central pressures. The patient classically presents with Beck's triad (jugular venous distention, muffled heart sounds, hypotension). Additionally, pulsus paradoxus will be significant. If the systolic pressure variation between inhalation and end exhalation is >10 mm Hg, "pulsus paradoxus" is present. Echocardiography is an excellent tool for verification of tamponade; however, intraoperative TEE is best.

### Anesthetic Management

Rapid fluid repletion, occasional inotropic supplementation, and pericardiocentesis are the usual immediate therapeutic goals. The anesthetic goals are to maintain spontaneous ventilation and avoid myocardial depression or any drugs that might decrease heart rate. (Tachycardia is the normal physiologic compensation required to maintain cardiac output in the setting of diminished stroke volume).

Local anesthesia, in the awake spontaneously ventilating patient, should be used to temporarily facilitate temporary decompression via pericardiocentesis. Frequently after modest fluid removal, hemodynamic status will temporarily improve. This emergency (temporary) decompression will frequently allow the patient to tolerate a general anesthetic, and a more complete tamponade decompression (via a pericardial window). Median sternotomy for repair of cardiac injury is occasionally required. Indeed, a prepped anterior thorax and gowned and gloved surgeons is the best approach for any severe case.

## Myocardial Contusion

### Definition/Presentation

Blunt trauma to the anterior chest wall (steering wheel, baseball, and hockey puck) can cause a myocardial contusion. Many will have a normal rhythm; however, most patients with significant trauma of this type will have some rhythm disturbance, as well as sudden ventricular fibrillation.[139] The myocardial contusion can progress with impaired pump function. Patients with myocardial contusion will be less able to tolerate pericardial tamponade than a normal heart and more rapidly progress to EMD. The best diagnostic test is echocardiography.

## Anesthetic Management

Patients with known or suspected myocardial contusion (fractured sternum) must be monitored in a telemetry unit until cardiac ectopy abates. Specific intervention is seldom needed, and the stable patient does not require diagnostic imaging studies to "prove" the presence of cardiac contusion unless there is significant ectopy or hemodynamic instability. These patients can experience an acute decrease in pump function and deteriorate to EMD or cardiac rupture and EMD.

## Aortic Rupture

### Definition/Presentation

The definition of aortic rupture is tear of all 3 layers of the aorta (intima, media, adventitia). This is in contrast to a thoracic aortic dissection, which occurs typically in patients with atherosclerotic aortic disease or other medical causes (ie, syphilitic aortitis, Marfan, and so on). Aortic rupture classically occurs in deceleration trauma (fall from height, high speed motor vehicle accident). 85% of aortic rupture patients expire at the scene or en route to the hospital. Most ruptures occur at the ligamentum arteriosum. Chest radiograph reveals a widened mediastinum, blurred and enlarged aortic knob, esophageal deviation to the right (look at NG tube), and apical cap (blood collected at the upper apex of the lungs). The patient will frequently have other evidence of significant deceleration impact (first and second rib fractures, and so on). Definitive diagnosis can be made by angiogram or CT. More recently, TEE has been used with success.

### Anesthetic Management

BP is controlled in the low normal range with a combination of esmolol, to prevent shear forces (high dp/dt), and nitroprusside, to provide rapid minute-to-minute titration. After the placement of two large bore intravenous needles and a right radial arterial line, these patients need an expeditious workup. Occasionally this is best accomplished in the OR. Indeed, the longer the time from the accident to arrival in the OR, the greater the chance of hypotension, EMD, and cardiac arrest. In the OR, after induction, a DLT is placed in preparation for lung separation during the left thoracotomy and aortic repair. Patients are usually placed on fem-fem bypass via the left femoral artery. The right femoral artery should be monitored via an invasive catheter so that the anesthesiologist can monitor perfusion pressure above (right radial arterial line) and below (femoral arterial line) the lesion.

## Tracheobronchial Disruptions

### Definition/Presentation

A tracheobronchial disruption is defined as any interruption of the airway integrity occurring below the glottis due to either blunt or penetrating trauma. A tracheobronchial injury should be suspected in any patient who has sustained blunt or penetrating trauma to the neck or chest. The vast majority of these patients will present with evidence of extra-anatomic air seen on the chest radiograph, and many will have subcutaneous air. The trachea and bronchi can be involved at any level. However, following blunt trauma, >80% occur within 2.5 cm of the carina.[320]

## Anesthetic Management

The literature provides little guidance for emergency airway management of patients with airway disruption because these injuries are relatively uncommon (occurring in only 14% of cases of penetrating neck trauma),[42] and most studies are retrospective.[3] Additionally, the diversity of concomitant injuries and hemodynamic status at presentation makes broad recommendations difficult. Shearer and Giesecke recently reviewed their experience with 107 patients with penetrating neck trauma requiring definitive airway management at Parkland Memorial Hospital, finding that neither the zone of injury nor the mechanism correlated with degree of intubation difficulty or the primary choice of surgical airway.[145]

At UCSD, we have established the following guidelines: If the airway injury is large, an awake technique using direct vision is indicated (surgical airway or FOB intubation). If the disruption is small, then the technique chosen is less critical. However, whatever technique is selected, one must avoid applying positive pressure ventilation proximal to the injury, as this could convert a relatively small tear into a large or complete airway disruption or cause mediastinal air.

Awake intubation with spontaneous ventilation is indicated for a major airway tear because this avoids exposing the disruption to positive pressure ventilation (which may cause airway and mediastinal emphysema). Furthermore, the airway may be held together by muscle tone in the strap muscles along the airway, and this tone could be lost using a rapid sequence technique involving muscle paralysis. Fiberoptic intubation is the awake technique of choice because it allows for visualization of airway disruption (diagnosis) as well as assured placement of the ETT cuff distal to the disruption (treatment). A DLT can be placed as well using an awake technique under fiberoptic guidance if necessary.

In general, intubation by conventional laryngoscopy should not be the primary technique for a subglottic disruption because the ETT could pass out the disruption into the mediastinum, thereby worsening or completing it. Ideally, one would like to maintain a view of the airway (FOB, surgical airway). An FOB may not be an option if the airway is grossly bloody, full of emesis, or if there is a stat situation (eg, concomitant severe closed head injury [GCS<9], full arrest) or the patient is uncooperative. One should always consider inserting a DLT via any intubation route/entry point if a distal unilateral tear is highly suspected. Furthermore, a complex distal tear may require cardiopulmonary support or bypass for resuscitation or definitive treatment if concomitant vascular injury is present,[150] whereas disruptions limited primarily to the airway can usually be repaired using a DLT.

## References

1. Landis SH, Murray T, Bolden S, et al. Cancer Statistics, 1998. *CA Cancer J Clin.* 1998;48:6.
2. Cook RM, Miller YE, Bunn PA. Small cell lung cancer: etiology, biology, clinical features, staging, and treatment. *Curr Probl Cancer.* 1993;17:69.
3. Mackay B, Lukeman JM, Ordonez NG. *Tumors of the Lung.* Philadelphia, Pa: WB Saunders; 1991.
4. Shepherd FA. Role of surgery in the management of small cell lung cancer. In: Aisner J, Arriagada R, Green MR, et al, eds. *Comprehensive Textbook of Thoracic Oncology.* Baltimore, Md: Williams & Wilkins; 1996:439.
5. Lad T, Piantadosi S, Thomas P, et al. A prospective randomized trial to determine the benefit of surgical resection of residual disease following

response of small cell lung cancer to combination chemotherapy. *Chest.* 1994;106(suppl 6):320S.

6. Adjei AA, Marks RS, Bonner JA. Current guidelines for the management of small cell lung cancer. *Mayo Clin Proc.* 1999;74:809.

7. Hunter JM, Bell CF, Florence AM, et al. Vecuronium in the myasthenic patient. *Anesthesia.* 1985;40:848.

8. Simmonds P. Managing patients with lung cancer. New guidelines should improve standards of care [editorial]. *BMJ.* 1999;319:527.

9. Mountain CF. A new international staging system for lung cancer. *Chest.* 1986;89(suppl 4):225S.

10. Tishler AS, Dichter MA, Biales B, et al. Neuroendocrine neoplasms and their cells of orgin. *N Engl J Med.* 1977;296:919.

11. Yesner R. Spectrum of lung cancer and ectopic hormones. *Pathol Annu.* 1978;13:217.

12. Brown J, Winklemann KK. Acanthosis nigricans—a study of 90 cases. *Medicine.* 1968;47:33.

13. Mountain CF. Revisions in the international system for staging lung cancer. *Chest.* 1997;111:1710.

14. Okada M, Tsubota N, Yoshimura M, et al. Evaluation of TNM classification for lung carcinoma with ipsilateral intrapulmonary metastasis. *Ann Thorac Surg.* 1999;68:326.

15. Mitsudomi T, Tateishi M, Oka T, et al. Longer survival after resection of non–small cell lung cancer in Japanese women. *Ann Thorac Surg.* 1989;48:639.

16. Keagy BA, Lores ME, Starek PJK, et al. Elective pulmonary lobectomy: factors asociated with morbidity and operative mortality. *Ann Thorac Surg.* 1985;40:349.

17. Khoman LJ, Meyer JA, Ikins PM, et al. Random versus predictable risks of mortality after thoracotomy for lung cancer. *J Thorac Cardiovasc Surg.* 1986;91:51.

18. Windsor JA, Hill GL. Risk factors for postoperative pneumonia. *Ann Surg.* 1988;208:209.

19. Ferguson MK. Preoperative assessment of pulmonary risk. *Chest.* 1999;115:58S.

20. Busch E, Verazin G, Antkowiak JG, et al. Pulmonary complications in patients undergoing thoracotomy for lung carcinoma. *Chest.* 1994;105:760.

21. Gass GD, Olsen GN. Clinical significance of pulmonary function tests. Preoperative pulmonary function testing to predict postoperative morbidity and mortality. *Chest.* 1986;89:127.

22. Boysen PG, Block AJ, Olsen GN, et al. Prospective evaluation for pneumonectomy using the technetium quantitative perfusion lung scan. *Chest.* 1977;72:422.

23. Bastin R, Moraine J-J, Bardocsky G, et al. Incentive spirometry performance. *Chest.* 1997;111:559.

24. Fergguson MK, Little L, Rizzo L, et al. Diffusion capacity predicts morbidity and mortality after pulmonary resection. *J Thoracic Cardiovasc Surg.* 1988;96:894.

25. Neuberg GW, Friedman SH, Weiss MD, et al. Cardiopulmonary exercise testing: the clinical value of gas exchange data. *Arch Intern Med.* 1988;148:2221.

26. Milledge JS, Nunn JF. Criteria of fitness for anesthesia in patients with chronic obstructive lung disease. *BMJ.* 1975;3:670.

27. Stein M, Koota GM, Simon M, et al. Pulmonary evaluation of surgical patients. *JAMA.* 1962;181:765.

28. Kristersson S, Lindell SE, Svanberg L. Prediction of pulmonary function loss due to pneumonectomy using $^{133}$Xe-radiospirometry. *Chest.* 1972;62:694.

29. Schoonover GA, Olsen GN, Habibian MR, et al. Lateral position test and quantitative lung scan in the preoperative evaluation for lung resection. *Chest.* 1984;86:854.

30. Marion JM, Alderson PO, Lefrak SS, et al. Unilateral lung function: comparison of the lateral position test with radionuclide ventilation-perfusion studies. *Chest.* 1976;69:5.

31. Carlens E, Hanson HE, Nordenstrom B. Temporary unilateral occlusion of the pulmonary artery. *J Thorac Surg.* 1951;22:527.

32. Neuhaus H, Cherniak NS. A bronchospirometric method of estimating the effect of pneumonectomy on the maximum breathing capacity. *J Thorac Cardiovasc Surg.* 1968;55:144.

33. Hazlett DR, Watson RL. Lateral position test: a simple, inexpensive, yet accurate method of studying the separate functions of the lungs. *Chest.* 1970;59:276.

34. Schoonover JA, Olsen GN, McLain WC. Lateral position test and quantitative lung scan in the preoperative evaluation for lung resection. *Chest.* 1984;86:854.

35. Boysen PG, Harris JO, Block AJ, et al. Prospective evaluation for pneumonectomy using perfusion scanning. *Chest.* 1981;80:163.

36. Crapo RO. Pulmonary function testing. Current concepts. *N Engl J Med.* 1994;331:25.

37. Olsen GN, Weiman DS, Bolton JW, et al. Submaximal invasive exercise testing and quantitative lung scanning in the evaluation for tolerance of lung resection. *Chest.* 1989;95:267.

38. Jackson CL, Huber JF. Correlated anatomy of the bronchial tree and lungs with a system of nomenclature. *Dis Chest.* 1943;9:319.

39. Wernly JA, DeMeester TR, Kirchner PT, et al. Clinical value of quantitative ventilation-perfusion lung scans in the surgical management of bronchogenic carcinoma. *J Thorac Cardiovasc Surg.* 1980;80:535.

40. Olsen GN, Block AJ, Swenson EW, et al. Pulmonary function evaluation of the lung resection candidate: a prospective study. *Am Rev Respir Dis.* 1975;111:379.

41. Segall JJ, Butterworth BA. Ventilatory capacity in chronic bronchitis in relation to carbon dioxide reduction. *Scand J Respir Dis.* 1966;47:215.

42. Laros CD, Swierenga J. Temporary unilateral pulmonary artery occlusion in the preoperative evaluation of patients with bronchial carcinoma. *Med Thorac.* 1967;24:269.

43. Tisi GM. Preoperative evaluation of pulmonary function. *Am Rev Respir Dis.* 1979;119:293.

44. Gracey DR, Divertie MB, Didier EP. Preoperative pulmonary preparation of patients with chronic obstructive pulmonary disease. *Chest.* 1979;76:123.

45. Olsen GN. Perioperative respiratory care. *Clin Chest Med.* 1993;14:205.

46. Thomas SD, Berry PD, Russell GN. Is this patient fit for thoracotomy and resection of lung tissue? *Postgrad Med J.* 1995;71:331.

47. Brooks-Brunn JA. Postoperative atelectasis and pneumonia. *Heart Lung.* 1995;24:94.

48. Castillo R, Haas A. Chest physical therapy: comparative efficacy of preoperative and postoperative in the elderly. *Arch Phys Med Rehabil.* 1985;66:376.

49. Thomas JA, McIntosh JM. Are incentive spirometry, intermittent positive pressure breathing, and deep breathing exercises effective in the prevention of postoperative pulmonary complications after upper abdominal surgery? A systematic overview and meta-analysis. *Phys Ther.* 1994;74:3.

50. Morton HJV. Tobacco smoking and pulmonary complications after surgery. *Lancet.* 1944;1:368.0

51. Pearce AC, Jones RM. Smoking and anesthesia: preoperative abstinence and perioperative morbidity. *Anesthesiology.* 1984;61:576.

52. Warner MA, Tinker JH, Divertie MB. Preoperative cessation of smoking and pulmonary complications in pulmonary dysfunction. *Anesthesiology.* 1983;59:A60.

53. Kambam JR, Chen LH, Hyman SA. Effect of short-term smoking halt on carboxyhemoglobin and P50 values. *Anesth Analg.* 1986;65:1186.

54. Benowitz NL. Pharmacologic aspects of cigarette smoking and nicotine addiction. *N Engl J Med.* 1988;319:1318.

55. Davies JM, Latto IP, Jones JG, et al. Effects of stopping smoking for 48 hours on oxygen availability from the blood: a study on pregnant women. *BMJ.* 1979;2:355.

56. Jones RM. Smoking before surgery: the case for stopping smoking. *BMJ.* 1985;290:1763.

57. Barry J, Meade K, Nabel EG, et al. Effect of smoking on the activity of ischemic heart disease. *JAMA.* 1989;261:398.

58. Marini JJ, Lakshmimara Y, Kradyan WA. Atropine and terbutaline aerosols in chronic bronchitis. *Chest.* 1981;80:285.

59. Gross NJ. Ipratropium bromide. *N Engl J Med.* 1988;319:486.

60. Crompton GK. A comparison of responses to bronchodilator drugs in chronic bronchitis and chronic asthma. *Thorax.* 1968;23:46.

61. Gross NJ, Co E, Skorodin MS. Cholinergic bronchomotor tone in COPD: estimates of its amount in comparison with that of normal subjects. *Chest.* 1989;96:984.

62. The COMBIVENT Inhalation Aerosol Study Group. In chronic obstructive pulmonary disease, a combination of ipratropium and albuterol is more effective than either agent alone: an 85-day multicenter trial. *Chest.* 1994;105:1411.

63. Lam A, Newhouse MT. Management of acute asthma and chronic airflow limitation: are methylxanthines obsolete? *Chest.* 1990;98:44.

64. Mendella LA. Manfreda J, Warren CP, et al. Steroid response in stable chronic obstructive pulmonary disease. *Ann Intern Med.* 1982;96:17.

65. Kabalin CS, Yarnold PR, Grammer LC. Low complication rate of corticosteroid-treated asthmatics undergoing surgical procedures. *Arch Intern Med.* 1995;155:1379.

66. Aubier M, De Troyer A, Sampson M, et al. Aminophylline improves diaphragmatic contractility. *N Engl J Med.* 1981;305:249.

67. Drazen JM, Gerard C. Reversing the irreversible. *N Engl J Med.* 1989;320:1555.

68. Murciano D, Auclair MH, Pariente R, et al. A randomized, controlled trial of theophylline in patients with severe chronic obstructive pulmonary disease. *N Engl J Med.* 1989;320:1521.

69. Vaz Fragoso CA, Miller MA. Review of the clinical efficacy of theophyllin in the treatment of chronic obstructive pulmonary disease. *Am Rev Respir Dis.* 1993;147:S40.

70. Cooper DKL. The incidence of postoperative infection and the role of antibiotic prophylaxis in pulmonary surgery: a review of 221 consecutive patients undergoing thoracotomy. *Br J Dis Chest.* 1981;75:154.

71. Chopra SK, Taplin GV, Simmons DH. Effects of hydration and physical therapy on tracheal transport velocity. *Am Rev Respir Dis.* 1977;115:1009.

72. Scheffiner AC. The mucolytic activity and mechanism of action and metabolism of acetylcysteine. *Pharmacol Ther.* 1964;1:47.

73. May DB, Munt PW. Physiologic effects of chest percussion and postural drainage in patients with stable chronic bronchitis. *Chest.* 1979;75:29.

74. Kennedy JH. "Silent" gastroesophageal reflux: an important but little known cause of pulmonary complications. *Dis Chest.* 1962;42:42.

75. Ekstrom T, Lindgren BR, Tibbling L. Effects of ranitidine treatment on patients with asthma and a history of gastroesophageal reflux: a double blind crossover study. *Thorax.* 1989;44:19.

76. Overholt RH, Voorhees RJ. Esophageal reflux as a trigger in asthma. *Dis Chest.* 1966;49:464.

77. Castell DO, Schnatz PF. Gastroesophageal reflux disease and asthma: reflux or reflex? *Chest.* 1995;108:1186.

78. Field SK. A critical review of the studies of the effects of simulated or real gastroesophageal reflux on pulmonary function in asthmatic adults. *Chest.* 1999;115:848.

79. Field SK, Gelfand GAJ, McFadden SD. The effects of antireflux surgery on asthmatics with gastroesophageal reflux. *Chest.* 1999;116:766.

80. Benumof JL. *Anesthesia for Thoracic Surgery.* 2nd ed. Philadelphia, Pa: WB Saunders; 1995:234.

81. Bromage PR, Benumof JL: Paraplegia following intracord injection during attempted epidural anesthesia under general anesthesia. *Reg Anesth Pain Med.* 1998;23:104.

82. Krane EJ, Dalens BJ, Murat J, et al: The safety of epidurals placed during general anesthesia. *Reg Anesth Pain Med.* 1998;23:433.

83. Lovstad RZ, Steen PA, Forsman M. Paraplegia after thoracotomy—not caused by the epidural catheter. *Acta Anaesthesiol Scand.* 1999;43:230.

84. de Haan P, Kalkman CJ, Jacobs MJ. Spinal cord monitoring with myogenic motor evoked potentials: early detection of spinal cord ischemia as an integral part of spinal cord protective strategies during thoracoabdominal aneurysm surgery. *Semin Thorac Cardiovasc Surg.* 1998;10:19.

85. Clifton GL, Jiang JY, Lyeth BG, et al. Marked protection by moderate hypothermia after experimental traumatic brain injury. *J Cereb Blood Flow Metab.* 1991;11:114.

86. Bustow R, Dietrich WD, Globus MYT, et al. Small differences in intraischemic brain temperature critically determine the extent of ischemic neuronal injury. *J Cereb Blood Flow Metab.* 1987;7:729.

87. Marion DW, Penrod LE, Kelsey SF, et al. Treatment of traumatic brain injury with moderate hypothermia. *N Engl J Med.* 1997;336:540.

88. Schuhmann MU, Suhr DF, Gosseln HH, et al. Local brain surface temperature compared to temperatures measured at standard extracranial monitoring sites during posterior fossa surgery. *J Neurosurg Anesthesiol.* 1999;11:90.

89. Fletcher R, Jonson B. Deadspace and the single breath test for carbon dioxide during anesthesia and artifical ventilation. *Br J Anesth.* 1984;56:109.

90. Fletcher R. The arterial endtidal-$CO_2$ difference during cardiothoracic surgery. *J Cardiothorac Anesthesiol.* 1990;4:105.

91. Yamanaka MK, Sue DY. Comparison of arterial–end-tidal $CO_2$ difference and dead space/tidal volume ratio in respiratory failure. *Chest.* 1987;92:832.

92. Nunn JF. The distribution of inspired gas during thoracic surgery. *Ann R Coll Surg.* 1961;28:223.

93. Werner O, Malmkvist G, Beckman A, et al. Carbon dioxide elimination from each lung during endobronchial anesthesia. *Br J Anaesth.* 1984;56:995.

94. Shankar KB, Moseley HS, Kumar AY. Dual end-tidal $CO_2$ monitoring and double lumen tubes. *Can J Anaesth.* 1992;39:100.

95. London MJ, Hollenberg M, Wong MG, et al. Intraoperative myocardial ischemia: localization by continuous 12 lead-electrocardiography. *Anesthesiology.* 1988;69:232.

96. Young C, Mark J, White W, et al. Clinical evaluation of continuous noninvasive blood pressure monitoring: accuracy and tracking capabilities. *J Clin Monit.* 1995;11:245.

97. Weissman C, Ornstein E, Young W. Arterial pulse contour analysis trending of cardiac output: hemodynamic manipulations during cerebral arteriovenous malformation resection. *J Clin Monit.* 1993;9:347.

98. Coriat P, Vrillon M, Perel A, et al. A comparison of systolic blood pressure variations and echocardiographic estimates of end-systolic left ventricular size in patients after aortic surgery. *Anesth Analg.* 1994;78:56.

99. Petty C. Right radial artery pressure during mediastinoscopy. *Anesth Analg.* 1979;58:428.

100. Bedford RF, Wollman H. Complications of percutaneous radial artery cannulation: an objective prospective evaluation in man. *Anesthesiology.* 1973;38:228.

101. Allen EV. Thromboangiitis obliterans: methods of diagnosis of chronic occlusive arterial lesions distal to the wrist with illustrated cases. *Am J Med Sci.* 1929;178:237.

102. Mozersky DJ, Buckley CJ, Hagood C, et al. Ultrasonic evaluation of the palmer circulation. *Am J Surg.* 1973;126:810.

103. Slogoff S, Keats AS, Arlund C. On the safety of radial artery cannulation. *Anesthesiology.* 1983;59:42.

104. Mangano DT, Hickey RF. Ischemic injury following uncomplicated radial artery catheterization. *Anesth Analg.* 1979;58:55.

105. Rulf ENR, Mitchell MM, Prakash O, et al. Measurement of arterial pressure after cardiopulmonary bypass with long radial artery catheters. *J Cardiothoracic Anesth.* 1990;4:19.

106. Wilson WC. Anaesthesia for pulmonary thromboendarterectomy. In: Ghosh S, Latimer RD, eds. *Thoracic Anaesthesia.* Oxford, United Kingdom: Butterworth Heinemann; 1999:223.

107. Urzua J. Aortic-to-radial arterial pressure gradient after bypass [letter]. *Anesthesiology.* 1990;73:191.

108. Kopman E, Ferguson TB. Intraoperative monitoring of femoral artery pressure during replacement of aneurysm of descending thoracic aorta. *Anesth Analg.* 1977;56:603.

109. Russell JA, Joel M, Hudson RJ, et al. Prospective evaluation of radial and femoral artery catheterization sites in critically ill patients. *Crit Care Med.* 1983;11:936.

110. Gurman GM, Kriemerman S. Cannulation of big arteries in critically ill patients. *Crit Care Med.* 1985;13:217.

111. Verweis J, Kester A, Stroes W, et al. Comparison of 3 methods for measuring central venous pressure. *Crit Care Med.* 1986;14:288.

112. Sznajder JI, Kester A, Stroes W, et al. Central vein catheterization: failure and complication rates by 3 percutaneous approaches. *Arch Intern Med.* 1986;146:259.

113. Raper R, Sibbald WJ. Misled by the wedge. *Chest.* 1986;89:427.

114. Cheung AT, Savino JS, Weiss, et al. Echocardiographic and hemodynamic indexes of left ventricular preload in patients with normal and abnormal ventricular function. *Anesthesiology.* 1994;81:376.

115. Jardin F, Farcot JC, Boisante L, et al. Influence of PEEP on left ventricular performance. *N Engl J Med.* 1981;304:387.

116. Benumof JL. Where pulmonary arterial catheters go: intrathoracic distribution. *Anesthesiology.* 1977;46:336.

117. Parlow JL, Milne B, Cervenko FW. Balloon floatation is more important than flow direction in determining the position of flow-directed pulmonary artery catheters. *J Cardiothoracic Vasc Anesthesiol.* 1992;6:20.

118. Cohen E, Eisenkraft JB, Thys D, et al. Hemodynamics and oxygenation during one lung anesthesia: right vs left [abstract]. *Anesthesiology.* 1985;63:3A, A566.

119. Hasan FM, Malanga A, Corrao WM, et al. Effect of catheter position on thermodilution cardiac output during continuous positive-pressure ventilation. *Crit Care Med.* 1984;12:387.

120. Landais A, Morin JP, Roche A, et al. Measurement of cardiac output by the thermodilution method during left thoracotomy in the lateral position in the dog. *Acta Anaesthesiol Scand.* 1990;34:158.

121. Feinglass NG, Lucas S, Gallenger TJ. Pulmonary artery measurements during unilateral lung injury in sheep. *Anesth Analg.* 1989;68:S82.

122. Guenther NR, Kay J, Chenag EY, et al. Comparing pulmonary artery catheter measurements in the supine, prone, and lateral decubitus positions. *Crit Care Med.* 1987;15:383.

123. Berryhill RE, Benumof JL. PEEP-induced discrepancy between pulmonary arterial wedge pressure and left atrial pressure: the influence of controlled vs. spontaneous ventilation and compliant vs. noncompliant lungs in the dog. *Anesthesiology.* 1979;46:303.

124. Shah KB, Rao TLK, Laughlin S, et al. A review of pulmonary artery catheterization in 6245 patients. *Anesthesiology.* 1984;61:271.

125. Zion MM, Balkin J, Rosemann D, et al. Use of pulmonary artery

catheters in patients with acute myocardial infarction: analysis of experience in 5,841 patients in the SPRINT registry. *Chest.* 1990;98:1331.

126. Ehrenwerth J, Urban MK. Monitoring during thoracic surgery. *Probl Anesth.* 1990;4:306.

127. Durbin CG. The range of pulmonary artery catheter balloon inflation pressures. *J Cardiothorac Anesth.* 1990;4:39.

128. Hannan AT, Brown M, Bigman O. Pulmonary artery catheter induced hemorrhage. *Chest.* 1984;85:128.

129. Kahn RA, Konstadt SN, Louie EK, et al. Intraoperative echocardiography. In: Kaplan JA, Reich DL, Konstadt SN, eds. *Cardiac Anesthesia.* 4th ed. Philadelphia, Pa: WB Saunders; 1999:401.

130. Clements FM, Harpole DH, Quill T, et al. Estimation of left ventricular volume and ejection fraction by two-dimensional transesophageal echocardiography: comparison of short axis imaging and simultaneous radionucleotide angiography. *Br J Anaesth.* 1990;64:331.

131. Cahalan MK, Ionescu P, Melton HJ, et al. Automated real time analysis of intraoperative transesophageal echocardiograms. *Anesthesiology.* 1993;78:477.

132. Kvetan V, Carlon GC, Howland WS. Acute pulmonary failure in asymmetric lung disease: approach to management. *Crit Care Med.* 1982;10:114.

133. Anderson HW, Benumof JL. Intrapulmonary shunting during one-lung ventilation and surgical manipulation. *Anesthesiology.* 1981;55:A377.

134. Boysen PG. Pulmonary resection and postoperative pulmonary function. *Chest.* 1980;77:718.

135. Gale JW, Waters RM. Closed endobronchial anesthesia in thoracic surgery. *J Thorac Surg.* 1932;1:432.

136. Jacobaeus HC, Frenckner P, Bjorkman S. Some attempts at determining the volume and function of each lung separately. *Acta Medica Scand.* 1932;79:174.

137. Carlens E. A new flexible double lumen catheter for bronchospirometry. *J Thoracic Surg.* 1949;18:742.

138. Newman RW, Finer GE, Downs JE. Routine use of the Carlens double-lumen endobronchial catheter: an experimental and clinical study. *J Thorac Cardiovasc Surg.* 1961;42:327.

139. Robertshaw FL. Low resistance double-lumen endobronchial tubes. *Br J Anaesth.* 1962;34:76.

140. Lee G. History and equipment: the evolution of endobronchial apparatus for one-lung ventilation and anesthesia. In: Ghosh S, Latimer RD, eds. *Thoracic Anaesthesia.* Oxford, United Kingdom: Butterworth Heinemann; 1999:1.

141. Brodsky J, Benumof JL, Ehrenwerth J. Depth of placement of left double-lumen endobronchial tubes. *Anesth Analg.* 1991;73:570.

142. Benumof JL, Partridge B, Salvatierra C, et al. Margin of safety in positioning modern double-lumen tubes. *Anesthesiology.* 1987;67:729.

143. Ginsberg RJ. New technique for one lung anesthesia using an endobronchial blocker. *J Thorac Cardiovasc Surg.* 1981;82:542.

144. Larson CE, Gaisor TA. A device for endobronchial blocker placement during one-lung anesthesia. *Anesth Analg.* 1990;71:311.

145. Ziberstein M, Katz RI, Levy A, et al. An improved method for introducing an endobronchial blocker. *J Cardiothorac Anesth.* 1990;4:481.

146. Veil R. Selective bronchial blocking in a small child. *Br J Anaesth.* 1969;41:453.

147. Nicoll SJB, Bingham R. Paediatric thoracic anaesthesia. In: Ghosh S, Latimer RD, eds. *Thoracic Anaesthesia.* Oxford, United Kingdom: Butterworth Heinemann; 1999:189.

148. Hoppin FG, Green ID, Mead J. Distribution of pleural surface pressure. *J Appl Physiol.* 1969;27:863.

149. West JB, Dollery CT, Naimark A. Distribution of blood flow in isolated lung: relation to vascular and alveolar pressures. *J Appl Physiol.* 1964;19:713.

150. Wulff KE, Aulin I. The regional lung function in the lateral decubitus position during anesthesia and operation. *Acta Anesthesiol Scand.* 1972;16:195.

151. Svanberg L. Influence of posture on lung volumes, ventilation and circulation in normals. *Scand J Clin Lab Invest.* 1957;9(suppl 25):1.

152. Larson A, Malmkvist G, Werner O. Variations in lung volume and compliance during pulmonary surgery. *Br J Anaesth.* 1987;59:585.

153. Larson A, Jonmarker C, Jogi P, et al. Ventilatory consequences of the lateral position and thoracotomy in children. *Can J Anaesth.* 1987;34:141.

154. Johansen I, Benumof JL. Flow distribution in abnormal lung as a function of FIO₂ [abstract]. *Anesthesiology.* 1979;51:369.

155. Scanlon TS, Benumof JL, Wahrenbrock EA, et al. Hypoxic pulmonary vasoconstriction and the ratio of hypoxic lung to perfused normoxic lung. *Anesthesiology.* 1978;49:177.

156. Dantzker DR, Wagner PD, West JB. Instability of lung units with low V̇/Q̇ ratios during O₂ breathing. *J Appl Physiol.* 1975;38:886.

157. Risberg B, Smith L, Ortenwall P. Oxygen radicals and lung injury. *Acta Anaesthesiol Scand.* 1991;35:106.

158. Fridovich I, Freeman B. Antioxidant defenses in the lung. *Ann Rev Physiol.* 1986;48:693.

159. Heffner JE, Repine JE. Pulmonary stratagies of antioxidant defense. *Am Rev Respir Dis.* 1989;140:531.

160. Phan SH, Gannon DE, Varani J, et al. Xanthine oxidase activity in rat pulmonary artery endothelial cells and its alteration by activated neutrophils. *Am J Pathol.* 1989;134:1201.

161. Lucchesi BR, Werns SW, Fantone JC. The role of the neutrophil and free radicals in ischemic myocardial injury. *J Mol Cell Cardiol.* 1989;21:1241.

162. Martin WJ II, Gadek JE. Oxidant injury of lung parenchymal cells. *J Clin Invest.* 1981;68:1277.

163. Ryan SF. Acute alveolar injury: experimental models. In: Gill J, ed. *Models of Lung Disease: Microscopy and Structural Methods.* New York, NY: Marcel Dekker; 1990;641.

164. Demling R, Lalonde C, Seekamp A, et al. Endotoxin causes hydrogen peroxide-induced lung lipid peroxidation and prostanoid production. *Arch Surg.* 1988;123:1337.

165. Milligan SA, Hoeffel JM, Goldstein IM. Effect of catalase on endotoxin-induced acute lung injury in unanesthetized sheep. *Am Rev Respir Dis.* 1988;137:420.

166. Warren JS, Johnson KJ, Ward PA. Consequences of oxidant injury. In: Crystal RG, West JB, ed. *The Lung: Scientific Foundations.* Vol 2. New York, NY: Raven Press; 1991:1829.

167. Stothert JC Jr, Basadre JO, Herndon D, et al. Conjugated diene production after airway acid aspiration. *Prog Clin Bio Res.* 1989;299:69.

168. Clement A, Chandelat K, Masliah J, et al. A controlled study of oxygen metabolite release by alveolar macrophages from children with interstitial lung disease. *Am Rev Respir Dis.* 1987;136:1424.

169. Kaelin RM, Lapance Y, Tschoop JM. Diffuse interstitial lung disease associated with hydrogen peroxide inhalation in a dairy worker. *Am Rev Respir Dis.* 1988;137:1233.

170. Allison RC, Kyle J, Adkins KW, et al. Effect of ischemia reperfusion or hypoxia reoxygenation on lung vascular permeability and resistance. *J Appl Physiol.* 1990;69:597.

171. Lynch MJ, Grum CM, Gallagher KP, et al. Xanthine oxidase inhibition attenuates ishcemic-reperfusion lung injury. *J Surg Res.* 1988;44:538.

172. Klausner JM, Paterson IS, Kobzik L, et al. Oxygen free radicals mediate ischemia-induced lung injury. *Surgery.* 1989;105:192.

173. Detterbeck FC, Keagy BA, Paull DE, et al. Oxygen free radical scavengers decrease reperfusion injury in lung transplantation. *Ann Thorac Surg.* 1990;50:204.

174. Horgan MJ, Lum H, Malik AB. Pulmonary edema after pulmonary artery occlusion and reperfusion. *Am Rev Respir Dis.* 1989;140:1421.

175. Kennedy TP, Rao NV, Hopkins C, et al. Role of reactive oxygen species in reperfusion injury of the rabbit lung. *J Clin Invest.* 1989;83:1326.

176. Clark JM. Pulmonary limits of oxygen tolerance in man. *Exp Lung Res.* 1988;14:897.

177. Calabresi P, Chabner BA. Antineoplastic agents. In: Gilman AG, Rall TW, Nies AS, et al, eds. *Goodman and Gilman's The Pharmacological Basis of Therapeutics.* 8th ed. New York, NY: Pergamon Press; 1990.

178. Weiss RB. Hypersensitivity reaction to cancer chemotherapy. *Semin Oncol.* 1982;9:5.

179. Cooper JA Jr, White DA, Matthay RA. Drug-induced pulmonary disease, part 1: cytotoxic drugs. *Am Rev Respir Dis.* 1986;133:321.

180. Smith AC, Boyd MR. Preferential effects of 1,3-bis(2-chloroethyl)-1-nitrosourea (BCNU) on pulmonary glutathione reductase and glutathione/glutathione disulfide ratios: possible implications for lung toxicity. *J Pharmacol Exp Ther.* 1984;229:658.

181. Freeman BA, Crapo JD. Biology of disease: free radicals and tissue injury. *Lab Invest.* 1982;47:412.

182. Hakkinen PJ, Whiteley JW, Witschi HR. Hyperoxia, but not thoracic X-irradiation, potentiates bleomycin- and cyclophosphamide-induced lung damage in mice. *Am Rev Resp Dis.* 1982;126:281.

183. Weinstein AS, Diener-West M, Nelson DF, et al. Pulmonary toxicity of carmustine in patients treated for malignant glioma. *Cancer Treat Rep.* 1986;70:943.

184. Aronin PA, Mahaley MS Jr, Rudnick SA, et al. Prediction of BCNU pulmonary toxicity in patients with malignant gliomas: an assessment of risk factors. *N Engl J Med.* 1980;303:183.

185. Weiss RB, Muggia FM. Pulmonary effects of carmustine (bischloroethylnitrosourea, BCNU) [letter]. *Ann Intern Med.* 1979;91:131.

186. O'Driscoll BR, Hasleton PS, Taylor PM, et al. Active lung fibrosis up

to 17 years after chemotherapy with carmustine (BCNU) in childhood. *N Engl J Med.* 1990;323:378.

187. Doll DC, Ringenberg QS, Yarbro JW. Vascular toxicity associated with antineoplastic agents. *J Clin Oncol.* 1986;4:1405.

188. DeVita VT Jr. Principles of chemotherapy. In: Divita VT, Hellman S, Rosenberg SA, eds. *Cancer: Principles and Practice of Oncology.* Philadelphia, Pa: Lippincott; 1981:132–155.

189. Cooper JA, Zitnik R, Matthay RA. Mechanisms of drug-induced pulmonary disease. *Annu Rev Med.* 1988;39:395.

190. Cooper JA Jr, White DA, Matthay RA. Drug-induced pulmonary disease, part 1: cytotoxic drugs. *Am Rev Respir Dis.* 1986;133:321.

191. Oberley LW, Buettner GR. The production of hydroxyl radical by bleomycin and iron (II). *Fed Exp Biol Soc.* 1979;97:47.

192. Gross NJ. The pathogenesis of radiation-induced lung damage. *Lung.* 1981;159:115.

193. Ginsberg SJ, Comis RL. The pulmonary toxicity of antineoplastic agents. *Semin Oncol.* 1982;9:34.

194. Iacovino JR, Leitner J, Abbas AK, et al. Fatal pulmonary reaction from low doses of bleomycin. An idiosyncratic tissue response. *JAMA.* 1976;235:1253.

195. Waid-Jones MI, Coursin DB. Perioperative considerations for patients treated with bleomycin. *Chest.* 1991;99:993.

196. Goldiner PL, Carlon GC, Cvitkovic E, et al. Factors influencing postoperative morbidity and mortality in patients treated with bleomycin. *BMJ.* 1978;1:1664.

197. Allen SC, Riddell GS, Butchart EG. Bleomycin therapy and anaesthesia. The possible hazards of oxygen administration to patients after treatment with bleomycin. *Anaesthesia.* 1981;36:60.

198. Toledo CH, Ross WE, Hood CT, et al. Potentiation of bleomycin toxicity by oxygen. *Cancer Treat Rep.* 1982;66:359.

199. Tryka AF, Skornik WA, Godleski JJ, et al. Potentiation of bleomycin-induced lung by exposure to 70% oxygen: morphologic assessment. *Am Rev Respir Dis.* 1982;126:1074.

200. Tryka AF, Godleski JJ, Brain JD. Differences in effects of immediate and delayed hyperoxia exposure on bleomycin-induced pulmonary injury. *Cancer Treat Rep.* 1984;68:759.

201. Douglas MJ, Coppin CM. Bleomycin and subsequent anaesthesia: a retrospective study at Vancouver General Hospital. *Can Anaesth Soc J.* 1980;27:449.

202. LaMantia KR, Glick JH, Marshall BE. Supplemental oxygen does not cause respiratory failure in bleomycin-treated surgical patients. *Anesthesiology.* 1984;60:65.

203. Hughes SA, Benumof JL. Operative lung continuous positive airway pressure to minimize FIo₂ during one-lung ventilation. *Anesth Analg.* 1990;71:92.

204. McDonald S, Missaillidou D, Rubin P. Pulmonary complications. In: Abeloff MD, Armitage JO, Lichter AS, et al, eds. *Clinical Oncology.* New York, NY: Churchill Livingstone; 1995.

205. Orwoll ES, Kiessling PJ, Patterson JR. Interstitial pneumonia from mitomycin. *Ann Intern Med.* 1978;89:352.

206. Desidero D, Alegesan R, Fischer M, et al. Intraoperative FIo₂ and the development of mitomycin-induced post-operative interstitial pneumonitis. *Anesthesiology.* 1990;73:A1177.

207. Gunstream SR, Seidenfeld JJ, Sobonya RE, et al. Mitomycin-associated lung disease. *Cancer Treat Rep.* 1983;67:301.

208. Stover DE. Adverse effects of treatment. In: DeVita VT, Hellman S, Rosenberg SA, eds. *Cancer: Principles and Practice of Oncology.* 3rd ed. Philadelphia, Pa: JB Lippincott; 1989:2166.

209. Doll DC, Ringenberg QS, Yarbro JW. Vascular toxicity associated with antineoplastic agents. *J Clin Oncol.* 1986;4:1405.

210. Kerr JH. Physiological aspects of one lung (endobronchial) anesthesia. *Int Anesthesiol Clin.* 1972;10:61.

211. Finley TN, Hill TR, Bonica JJ. Effect of intrapleural pressure on pulmonary shunt to atelectatic dog lung. *Am J Physiol.* 1963;205:1187.

212. Benumof JL, Rogers SN, Moyce PR, et al. Hypoxic pulmonary vasoconstriction and whole lung PEEP in the dog. *Anesthesiology.* 1979;51:503.

213. Baker RW, Burki NK. Alterations in ventilatory pattern and ratio of dead-space to tidal volume. *Chest.* 1987;92:1013.

214. Benumof JL, Wahrenbrock EA. Blunted hypoxic pulmonary vasoconstriction by increased lung vascular pressures. *J Appl Physiol.* 1975;38:846.

215. Benumof JL, Mathers JM, Wahrenbrock EA. Cyclic hypoxic pulmonary vasoconstriction induced by concomitant carbon dioxide changes. *J Appl Physiol.* 1976;41:466.

216. Malmkvist G. Maintenance of oxygenation during one-lung ventilation: effect of intermittent reinflation of the collapsed lung with oxygen. *Anesth Analg.* 1989;68:763.

217. Hogue CW. Effectiveness of low levels of non-ventilated lung continuous positive airway pressure in improving arterial oxygenation during one-lung ventilation. *Anesth Analg.* 1994;79:364.

218. Benumof JL, Gaughan S, Ozaki GT. Operative lung constant positive airway pressure with the Univent bronchial blocker tube. *Anaesth Analg.* 1992;74:406.

219. Capan LM, Turndorf H, Chandrakant P, et al. Optimization of oxygenation during one lung anesthesia. *Anesth Analg.* 1980;59:847.

220. Katz JA, Laverne RG, Fairley HB, et al. Pulmonary oxygen exchange during endobronchial anesthesia: effects of tidal volume and PEEP. *Anesthesiology.* 1982;56:164.

221. Cohen E, Salter O, Ali J. Effect of incremental PEEP on PaO₂ and SvO₂ during OLV. *Anesth Analg.* 1991;72:S43.

222. Rich GF, Lowson SM, Johns RA, et al. Inhaled nitric oxide selectively decreases pulmonary vascular resistance without impairing oxygenation in patients undergoing cardiac surgery. *Anesthesiology.* 1993;78:57.

223. Rich GF, Lowson SM, Johns RA, et al. Inhaled nitric oxide selectively decreases pulmonary vascular resistance without impairing oxygenation during one lung ventilation in patients undergoing cardiac surgery. *Anesthesiology.* 1994;80:57.

224. Wilson WC, Kapelanski DP, Benumof JL, et al. Inhaled nitric oxide (40 ppm) during one-lung ventilation, in the lateral decubitus position, does not decrease pulmonary vascular resistance or improve oxygenation in normal patients. *J Cardiothorac Vasc Anesth.* 1997;11:172.

225. Freden F, Berglund JE, Reber A, et al. Inhalation of nitric oxide synthase inhibitor to a hypoxic or collapsed lung lobe in anesthetized pigs: effects on pulmonary blood flow distribution. *Br J Anaesth.* 1996;77:414.

226. Moutafis M, Liu N, Dalibon N, et al. The effects of inhaled nitric oxide and its combination with intravenous almitrine on PaO₂ during one-lung ventilation in patients undergoing thoracoscopic procedures. *Anaesth Analg.* 1997;85:1130.

227. Hazelrigg SR, Landreneau RJ, Boley TM, et al. The effect of muscle sparing versus standard posterolateral thoracotomy on pulmonary function, muscle strength, and postoperative pain. *J Thorac Cardiovasc Surg.* 1991;101:394.

228. Kavanagh BP, Katz J, Sandler AN. Pain control after thoracic surgery. A review of current techniques. *Anesthesiology.* 1994;81:737.

229. Holzer A, Kapral S, Hellwagner K, et al. Severe pneumothorax after intercostal nerve blockade. A case report. *Acta Anaesthesiol Scand.* 1998;42:1124.

230. Dangoisse M, Collins S, Glynn CJ. Haemothorax after attempted intercostal catheterisation. *Anaesthesia.* 1994;49:961.

231. Bouchard F, Drolet P. Thoracic versus lumbar administration of fentanyl using patient-controlled epidural after thoracotomy. *Reg Anesth.* 1995;20:385.

232. Etches RC, Gammer TL, Cornish R. Patient-controlled epidural analgesia after thoracotomy: a comparison of meperidine with and without bupivacaine. *Anesth Analg.* 1996;83:81.

233. Burgess FW, Anderson DM, Colonna D, et al. Thoracic epidural analgesia with bupivacaine and fentanyl for postoperative thoracotomy pain. *J Cardiothorac Vasc Anesth.* 1994;8:420.

234. Nelson KM, Vincent RG, Bourke RS, et al. Intraoperative intercostal nerve freezing to prevent post-thoracotomy pain. *Ann Thorac Surg.* 1974;18:280.

235. Katz J, Nelson W, Forest R, et al. Cryoanalgesia for postthoracotomy pain. *Lancet.* 1980;1:512.

236. Myers RR, Powell HC, Heckman HM, et al. Biophysical and pathological effects of cryogenic nerve lesion. *Ann Neurol.* 1981;10:478.

237. Gough JD, Williams AB, Vaughan RS, et al. The control of post-thoracotomy pain. A comparative evaluation of thoracic epidural fentanyl infusions and cryoanalgesia. *Anaesthesia.* 1988;43:780.

238. Rooney S, Jain S, McCormack P, et al. A comparison of pulmonary function tests for post-thoracotomy pain using cryoanalgesia and transcutaneous nerve stimulation. *Ann Thorac Surg.* 1986;41:204.

239. Roxburgh JC, Markland CG, Ross BA, et al. Role of cryoanalgesia in the control of pain after thoracotomy. *Thorax.* 1987;42:292.

240. Maiwand MO, Makey AR, Rees A. Cryoanalgesia after thoracotomy. Improvement of technique and review of 600 cases. *J Thorac Cardiovasc Surg.* 1986;92:291.

241. Muller LC, Salzer GM, Ransmayr G, et al. Interoperative cryoanalgesia for post-thoracotomy pain relief. *Ann Thorac Surg.* 1989;48:15.

242. Katz J. Cryoanalgesia for postthoracotomy pain. *Ann Thorac Surg.* 1989;48:5.

243. Kalas E, Perttunen K, Kaasinen S. Pain after thoracic surgery. *Acta Anaesthesiol Scand.* 1992;36:96.

244. Ryan DW. Accidental intravenous injection of bupivacaine: a complication of obstetrical epidural anesthesia. *Br J Anaesth.* 1983;45:907.

245. Seltzer JL, Larijani GE, Goldberg ME, et al. Intrapleural bupivacaine—a kinetic and dynamic evaluation. *Anesthesiology.* 1987;67:798.

246. Harkens DE, Black H, Clauss R, et al. A single cervical mediastinal exploration for tissue diagnosis of intrathoracic disease. *N Engl J Med.* 1954;251:1041.

247. Carlens EL. Mediastinoscopy: a method for inspection and tissue biopsy in the superior mediastinum. *Dis Chest.* 1959;36:343.

248. Pearson FG. Mediastinoscopy: a method of biopsy in the superior mediastinum. *J Thorac Cardiovasc Surg.* 1965;49:11.

249. Hammond ZT, Anderson RC, Myers BF, et al. The current role of mediastinoscopy in the evaluation of thoracic disease. *J Thorac Cardiovasc Surg.* 1999;118:894.

250. Mineo TC, Ambrogi V, Nofroni I, et al. Mediastinoscopy in superior vena cava obstruction: analysis of 80 consecutive patients. *Ann Thorac Surg.* 1999;68:223.

251. Furgang FA, Saidman LJ. Bilateral tension pneumothorax associated with mediastinoscopy. *J Thorac Cardiovasc Surg.* 1972;63:329.

252. Ashbaugh DG. Mediastinoscopy. *Arch Surg.* 1970;100:568.

253. Mackie AM, Watson CB. Anaesthesia and mediastinal masses. *Anaesthesia.* 1984;39:899.

254. Lewis RJ, Caccavale RJ, Sisler GE, et al. One hundred consecutive patients undergoing video-assisted thoracic operations. *Ann Thorac Surg.* 1992;54:421.

255. Kaiser LR. Diagnostic and therapeutic uses of pleuroscopy (thoracoscopy) in lung cancer. *Surg Clin North Am.* 1989;67:1081.

256. Miller DL, Allen MS, Trastek VF, et al. Video thoracoscopic wedge excision of the lung. *Ann Thorac Surg.* 1992;54:410.

257. McKenna RJ, Wolf RK, Brenner M, et al. Is lobectomy by video-assisted thoracic surgery an adequate cancer operation? *Ann Thorac Surg.* 1998;66:1903.

258. Landreneau RJ, Hazelrigg SR, Mack MJ. Post-operative pain related morbidity. Video-assisted thoracic surgery versus thoracotomy. *Ann Thorac Surg.* 1993;56:800.

259. Bonniot JPA, Homasson JPD, Roden SL. Pleural and lung cryobiopsies during thoracoscopy. *Chest.* 1989;95:492.

260. Toashiya O, Imanaka K, Endoh M. Hemodynamic effects of carbon dioxide insufflation under single-lung ventilation during thoracoscopy. *Ann Thorac Surg.* 1999;68:29.

261. Plummer S, Hartley M, Vaughan RS. Anaesthesia for telescopic procedures in the thorax. *Br J Anaesth.* 1998;80:223.

262. Brantigan OC, Mueller E, Kress M. A surgical approach to pulmonary emphysema. *Am Rev Respir Dis.* 1959;80:194.

263. Cooper JD, Trulock EP, Triantafillou AN, et al. Bilateral pneumonectomy (volume reduction) for chronic obstructive pulmonary disease. *J Thorac Cardiovasc Surg.* 1995;109:106.

264. Sciurba FC, Rogers RM, Kennen RJ, et al. Improvement in pulmonary function and elastic recoil after lung reduction surgery for diffuse emphysema. *N Engl J Med.* 1996;334:1095.

265. Hosenpud JD, Bennett LE, Keck BM. Effect of diagnosis on survival benefit of lung transplantation for end-stage lung disease. *Lancet.* 1998;351:24.

266. Fessler HE, Wise RA. Lung volume reduction surgery: is less really more? *Am J Respir Crit Care Med.* 1999;159:1031.

267. Brenner M, McKenna RJ, Chen JC. Survival following bilateral staple lung volume reduction surgery for emphysema. *Chest.* 1999;115:390.

268. National Institutes of Health News Advisory. December 20, 1996. Available at: http://www.nih.gov/news/pr/dec96/nhlbi-20.htm. Accessed September 10, 1999.

269. DeSouza G, deLisser EA, Turry P. Comparison of propofol with isoflurane for maintenance of anesthesia in patients with chronic obstructive pulmonary disease. *J Cardiothoracic Vasc Anaesth.* 1995;9:24.

270. Triantafillou AN. Anesthetic management of bilateral volume reduction surgery. *Sem Thorac Cardiovasc Surg.* 1996;8:94.

271. Klein JS, Schultz S, Heffner JE. Interventional radiology of the chest: image-guided percutaneous drainage of pleural effusions, lung abscess, and pneumothorax. *AJR Am J Roentgenol.* 1995;164:581.

272. Pearson AS, Izzo F, Fleming RV, et al. Intraoperative radiofrequency ablation or cryoablation for hepatic malignancies. *Am J Surg.* 1999;178:592.

273. Putnam JB, Thomsen SL, Siegenthaler M. Therapeutic implications of heat-induced lung injury. In: Ryan TP, ed. *Matching the Energy Source to the Clinical Need.* Bellingham, Wash. SPIE Optical Engineering Press; 2000:139.

274. McGahan JP, Brock JM, Tesluk H, et al. Hepatic ablation with use of radio-frequency electrocautery in the animal model. *JVIR.* 1992;3:291.

275. Curley SA, Izzo F, Delrio P, et al. Radiofrequency ablation of unresectable primary and metastatic hepatic malignancies. *Ann Surg.* 1999;230:1.

276. Goldberg SN, Gazelle GS, Compton SS, et al. Radiofrequency tissue ablation in the rabbit lung: efficacy and complications. *Acad Radiol.* 1995;2:776.

277. Marasso A, Bernardi V, Gai R, et al. Radiofrequency resection of bronchial tumors in combination with cryotherapy: evaluation of a new technique. *Thorax.* 1998;53:106.

278. Dupuy DE, Zagoria RJ, Akerley W. Percutaneous radiofrequency ablation of malignancies in the Lung. *AJR Am J Roentgenol.* 2000;174:57.

279. Jacobson MJ, Lo Cicero J. Endobronchial treatment of lung carcinoma. *Chest.* 1991;100:837.

280. George PJM, Clark G, Tolfree S, et al. Changes in regional ventilation and perfusion of the lung after endoscopic laser treatment. *Thorax.* 1990;45:248.

281. Ramirez J, Harlan WJ Jr. Pulmonary alveolar proteinosis. Nature and origin of alveolar lipid. *Am J Med.* 1968;45:502.

282. Shah PL, Hansell D, Lawson PR. Pulmonary alveolar proteinosis: clinical aspects and current concepts on pathogenesis. *Thorax.* 2000;55:67.

283. Rameriz J. Pulmonary alveolar proteinosis. A roentgenologic analysis. *AJR Am J Roentgenol.* 1964;92:571.

284. Rubenstein I, Mullen BM, Hoffstein V. Morphologic diagnosis of idiopathic pulmonary alveolar proteinosis. *Arch Intern Med.* 1988;148:813.

285. Cohen E, Eisenkraft JB. Bronchopulmonary lavage: effects on oxygenation and hemodynamics. *J Cardiothoracic Anesth.* 1990;4:609.

286. Alfery DD, Zamost BG, Benumof JL. Unilateral lung lavage: blood flow manipulation by ipsilateral pulmonary artery balloon inflation. *Anesthesiology.* 1981;55:376.

287. Shah PL, Hansell D, Lawson PR, et al. Pulmonary alveolar proteinosis: clinical aspects and current concepts on pathogenesis. *Thorax.* 2000;55:67.

288. Dalen JE, Alpert JS. Natural history of pulmonary embolism. *Prog Cardiovasc Dis.* 1975;17:257.

289. Moser KM, Braunwald NS. Successful surgical intervention in severe chronic thromboembolic pulmonary hypertension. *Chest.* 1973;64:29.

290. Auger WR, Moser KM. Pulmonary flow murmurs: a distinctive physical sign found in chronic pulmonary thromboembolic disease. *Clin Res.* 1989;37:145A.

291. Olman MA, Marsh JJ, Lang IM, et al. Endogenous fibrinolytic system in chronic large-vessel thromboembolic pulmonary hypertension. *Circulation.* 1992;86:1241.

292. Fedullo PF, Auger WR, Channick RN, et al. Chronic thromboembolic pulmonary hypertension. *Clin Chest Med.* 1995;16:353.

293. Auger WR, Permpikul P, Moser KM. Lupus anticoagulant, heparin use, and thrombocytopenia in patients with chronic thromboembolic pulmonary hypertension: a preliminary report. *Am J Med.* 1995;99:392.

294. Bernstein RJ, Ford RL, Clausen JL, et al. Membrane diffusion and capillary blood volume in chronic thromboembolic pulmonary hypertension. *Chest.* 1996;110:1430.

295. Kapitan KS, Buchbinder M, Wagner PD, et al. Mechanisms of hypoxemia in chronic thromboembolic pulmonary hypertension. *Am Rev Respir Dis.* 1989;139:1149.

296. Bergin CJ. Chronic thromboembolic pulmonary hypertension: the disease, the diagnosis, and the treatment. *Semin Ultrasound CT MR.* 1997;18:383.

297. Bergin CJ, Sirlin CB, Hauschildt JP, et al. Chronic thromboembolism: diagnosis with helical CT and MR imaging with angiographic and surgical correlation [see comments]. *Radiology.* 1997;204:695.

298. Dittrich HC, Chow LC, Nicod PH. Early improvement in left ventricular diastolic function after relief of chronic right ventricular pressure overload. *Circulation.* 1989;80:823.

299. Auger WR, Fedullo PF, Moser KM, et al. Chronic major-vessel thromboembolic pulmonary artery obstruction: appearance at angiography. *Radiology.* 1992;182:393.

300. Rich S, Gubin S, Hart K. The effects of phenylephrine on right ventricular performance in patients with pulmonary hypertension [see comments]. *Chest.* 1990;98:1102.

301. Urzua J. Aortic-to-radial arterial pressure gradient after bypass [letter]. *Anesthesiology.* 1990;73:191.

302. Dittrich HC, McCann HA, Wilson WC. Identification of interatrial communication in patients with elevated right atrial pressure using surface and transesophageal contrast echocardiography. *J Am Coll Cardiol.* 1993;21(suppl):135A.

303. Schuhmann MU, Suhr DF, v Gosseln HH, et al. Local brain surface temperature compared to temperatures measured at standard extracranial monitoring sites during posterior fossa surgery. *J Neurosurg Anesthesiol.* 1999;11:90.

304. Jamieson SW. Pulmonary thromboendarterectomy [editorial]. *Heart.* 1998;79:118.

305. Jamieson SW, Auger WR, Fedullo PF, et al. Experience and results

with 150 pulmonary thromboendarterectomy operations over a 29-month period. *J Thorac Cardiovasc Surg.* 1993;106:116; discussion, 26.

306. Dittrich HC, Nicod PH, Chow LC, et al. Early changes of right heart geometry after pulmonary thromboendarterectomy. *J Am Coll Cardiol.* 1988;11:937.

307. Levinson RM, Shure D, Moser KM. Reperfusion pulmonary edema after pulmonary artery thromboendarterectomy. *Am Rev Respir Dis.* 1986;134:1241.

308. Olman MA, Auger WR, Fedullo PF, et al. Pulmonary vascular steal in chronic thromboembolic pulmonary hypertension. *Chest.* 1990;98:1430.

309. Moser KM, Metersky ML, Auger WR, et al. Resolution of vascular steal after pulmonary thromboendarterectomy. *Chest.* 1993;104:1441.

310. Archibald CJ, Auger WR, Fedullo PF, et al. Long-term outcome after pulmonary thromboendarterectomy. *Am J Respir Crit Care Med.* 1999;160:523.

311. Rhee PM, Acosta J, Bridgeman A, et al. Survival after emergency department thoracotomy: review of published data from the past 25 years. *J Am Coll Surg.* 2000;190:288.

312. Mineo TC, Ambrogi V, Cristino B, et al. Changing indications for thoracotomy in blunt chest trauma after the advent of videothoracoscopy. *J Trauma.* 1999;47:1088.

313. Feliciano DV, Rozycki, GS. Advances in the diagnosis and treatment of thoracic trauma. *Surg Clin North Am.* 1999;79:1417.

314. Hardman JG, Mahajan RP. Anaesthetic management of the severely injured patient: chest injury. *Br J Hosp Med.* 1997;58:157.

315. Millikan JS, Cain TL, Hansbrough J, et al. Rapid volume replacement for hypovolemic shock: a comparison of techniques and equipment. *J Trauma.* 1984;24:428.

316. Mateer JR, Thompson BM, Aprahamian C, et al. Rapid fluid resuscitation with central venous catheters. *Ann Emerg Med.* 1983;12:149.

317. Dutky PA, Stevens SL, Maull KI, et al. Factors affecting rapid fluid resuscitation with large bore introducer catheters. *J Trauma.* 1989;29:856.

318. Wilson WC, Frankville DD, Maxwell W, et al. Massive intraoperative pulmonary embolus diagnosed by transesophageal echocardiography. *Anesthesiology.* 1994;81:504.

319. Maron B, Poliac L, Kaplan J, et al. Blunt impact to the chest leading to sudden death from cardiac arrest during sports activities. *N Engl J Med.* 1995;333:337.

320. Jones WS, Mavroudis C, Richardson JD, et al. Management of tracheobronchial tree disruption resulting from blunt trauma. *Surgery.* 1984;95:319.

CHAPTER

# 65

# Surgery of the Descending Thoracic Aorta

Stuart J. Weiss

John G. Augoustides

## AORTIC DISEASE

*What Is the Normal Anatomy of the Aorta?*

*What Are the Physiologic Factors That Influence Aortic Wall Stress?*

*What Differentiates Aneurysms From Pseudoaneurysms?*

*How Are Aneurysms Characterized and Managed?*

*How Are Dissections Characterized and Managed?*

*What Are Transections, and How Are They Managed?*

*What Characterizes Congenital Coarctation, and How Is It Managed?*

*What Are the Diagnostic Imaging Methods for Major Aortic Pathology?*

*What Are the Most Common Coexisting Diseases and Their Implications for the Anesthesiologist?*

## ANESTHETIC INDUCTION AND MAINTENANCE AND POSTOPERATIVE ISSUES

*What Are the Preoperative Anesthetic Considerations?*

*What Are the Goals and Strategies for the Conduction of Intraoperative Anesthesia?*

*What Are the Considerations for Ventilatory Management?*

*Is There a Role for Epidural Anesthesia?*

*What Are the Issues of Circulatory Management During the Period of Aortic Clamping?*

*What Therapeutic Interventions Can Be Used to Decrease the Risk for Postoperative Renal Failure?*

*Why Does Paraplegia Occur, and What Can Be Done to Prevent It?*

*What Are the Techniques and Strategies to Enhance Distal Spinal Cord Perfusion?*

*Does Paraplegia Occur in Patients Having Abdominal Aortic Surgery?*

*What Are the Management Strategies for Coagulation and Transfusion Therapies?*

*Should Patients Be Extubated in the Operating Room?*

*Is There a Role for the Anesthesiologist in Postoperative Care?*

## CONCLUSION

Patients undergoing operation on the aorta and its major branches present a formidable anesthetic challenge. The high incidence of severe coexisting disease and advanced age, combined with the abrupt and severe physiologic impact of the operations, impose a significant burden on these patients. Perhaps in no other area of surgery have anesthesiologists made such key contributions during the past 30 years. In the mid-1960s, the 6-day mortality rate for undergoing major aortic reconstruction was 25% to 30%. At present, the rate has decreased to <3%.

Several factors have played an important role in enhancing perioperative care and reducing the death rate: better preoperative assessment, improved monitoring techniques, new anesthetics, and refined surgical techniques and graft materials.[1] In addition, an improved understanding of the pathologic homeostatic mechanisms that are operative in patients suffering from vascular disease has been critical. The discussion in this chapter is limited to those issues directly related to the basic pathophysiology of the major aortic lesions and the perioperative management of patients undergoing major aortic operations.

## AORTIC DISEASE

### What Is the Normal Anatomy of the Aorta?

The aorta is the major conduit for the transport of blood throughout the body and sustains tremendous shearing forces with each left ventricular systolic ejection. It is a compliant elastic structure that absorbs and converts some of the kinetic energy of left ventricular ejection into potential energy that is stored in the wall of the aorta. During diastole, the elastic recoil of the vessel wall converts the stored energy to a kinetic force that serves to augment blood flow.

The normal aorta ranges from 2.5 to 3 cm in diameter and is composed of three layers: (1) a thin inner layer, the tunica intima; (2) a thick middle layer, the tunica media; and (3) a thin outer layer, the tunica adventitia (Fig. 65–1). The tunica intima is lined with endothelial cells. The tunica media adds

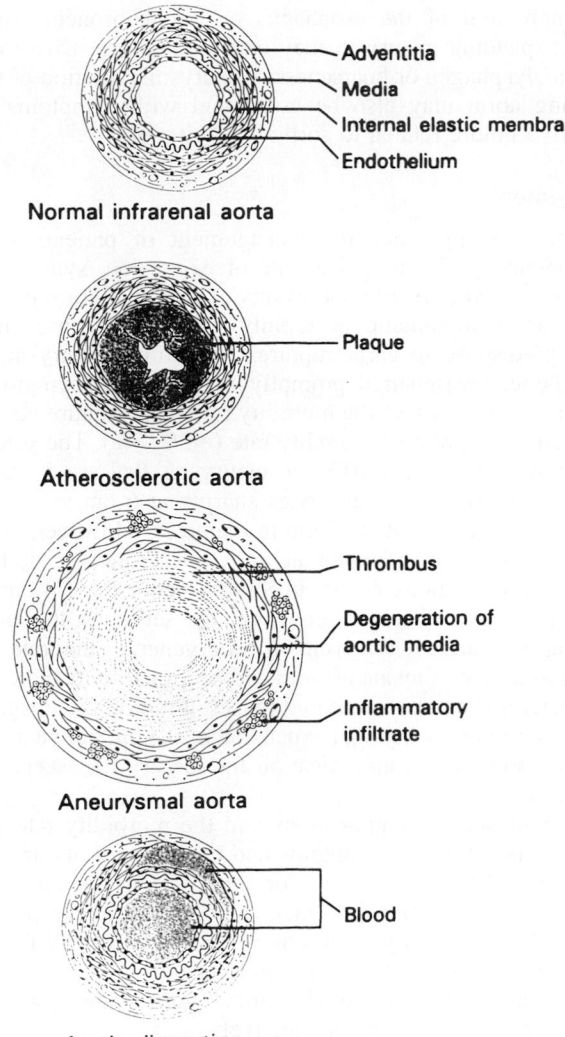

Adventitia
Media
Internal elastic membrane
Endothelium

**Normal infrarenal aorta**

Plaque

**Atherosclerotic aorta**

Thrombus

Degeneration of
aortic media

Inflammatory
infiltrate

**Aneurysmal aorta**

Blood

**Aortic dissection**

**FIGURE 65–1.** Schematic representation of the normal aorta with its three distinct layers: the intima, the media, and the adventitia. Atherosclerosis results in intimal thickening secondary to the formation of plaque. An aneurysm is a dilation of an artery with degeneration of the media. The inner lining is a layer of thrombus. Aortic dissection results from an intimal tear and a consequent plane of blood cleaving the media. (From Tilson MD III, Brophy CM. Pathogenesis of aneurysms. In: Greenfield J, ed. *Surgery: Scientific Principles and Practice.* Philadelphia, Pa: JB Lippincott; 1993:1676.)

tensile strength to the vessel wall and is composed of laminated and intertwining sheets of elastic tissue arranged in a spiral manner. Medial degeneration is the major pathophysiologic process that leads to weakening of the aortic wall. This structural weakness predisposes to dissection and aneurysm formation. The third layer, the tunica adventitia, contains the vasa vasorum and lymphatics that nourish the vessel.

## What Are the Physiologic Factors That Influence Aortic Wall Stress?

The physiologic attributes that influence the development of aortic pathology are described by Laplace's law, which relates tension of the aortic wall to internal pressure and radius according to the following equation:

$$T = P \times R/\delta$$

(Equation 1)

where T denotes the circumferential wall tension, P the internal pressure, R the internal radius, and δ the wall thickness. Rupture occurs when the circumferential wall tension exceeds the wall tensile strength. Increases in arterial blood pressure or vessel diameter result in an increase in wall tension with a concomitant risk for rupture. Thinning of the aortic wall, as caused by aneurysmal dilation or dissection, significantly increases wall tension and the likelihood of rupture. The relationships described in Equation 1 have been confirmed by clinical findings, thereby implicating hypertension and large aneurysms as significant risk factors for rupture.[2]

## What Differentiates Aneurysms From Pseudoaneurysms?

A true aortic aneurysm is defined as a >50% increase in the diameter of the normal aorta.[3] The most common etiologies of aortic aneurysms are mycotic processes, atherosclerosis, collagen vascular disease (Marfan and Ehlers-Danlos syndromes), and congenital deficits (coarctation, bicuspid aortic valves). Mycotic aneurysm formation was the major cause of aortic aneurysms in the first half of the 20th century; syphilis was the most common infectious agent. Syphilitic aortitis predominantly affects the ascending aorta and typically develops 10 to 20 years after the acute infection. Antibiotic therapy arrests infection but does not reverse the damage.

At present, the most common predisposing factors that lead to medial degeneration and structural weakening of the aorta are hypertension, infiltration of atheroma associated with atherosclerosis, and smoking.[4] Another common etiology that predisposes to aneurysm formation is chronic aortic dissection. Destruction and disruption of the elastin fibers of the media cause further dilation and weakening in the vessel wall, thereby directly increasing wall tension (Laplace's law). As the aneurysm progressively enlarges, the wall tension correspondingly increases, and encroachment on adjacent structures and rupture become more likely.

Pseudoaneurysms represent focal defects in the integrity of the vessel wall. In contrast to an aneurysm, which contains all three layers of the vessel wall, a pseudoaneurysm lacks one or more layers of the aortic wall. Pseudoaneurysms form at sites of local weakening of the vessel wall; these areas can develop after infection, after trauma, or at cannulation sites from previous surgeries.

## How Are Aneurysms Characterized and Managed?

### Location

Seventy-five percent of all aortic aneurysms are located in the infrarenal abdominal aorta (Fig. 65–2). Of the remaining, 25% are located in the ascending aorta, 30% in the aortic arch, and 45% in the descending thoracic aorta.[5] Although less common, thoracoabdominal aneurysms pose greater challenges for intraoperative management of the circulation and neuroprotection.

### Shape

The morphology of an aneurysm is related to the risk for rupture and choice of management strategies. There are two

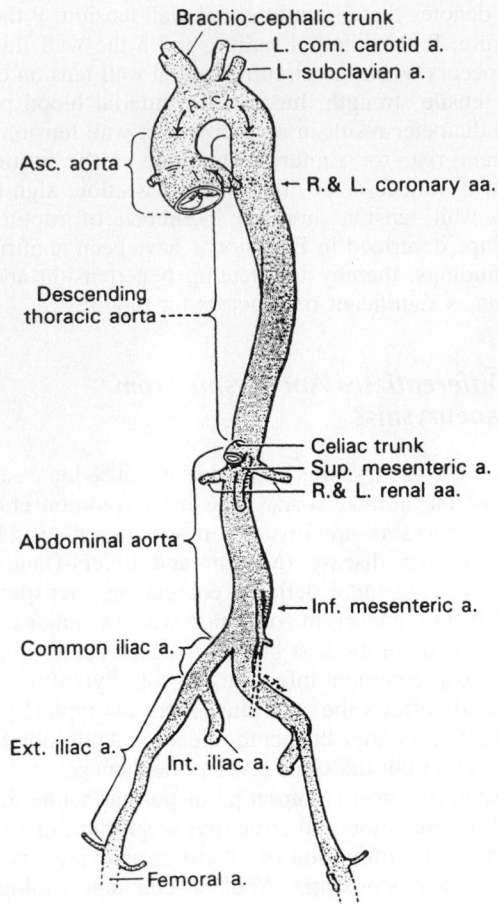

**FIGURE 65–2.** Anatomy of the aorta.

basic types. A *fusiform aneurysm* is a spindle-shaped dilation that symmetrically encompasses the circumference of the aorta. Most aneurysms, particularly abdominal aortic aneurysms caused by atherosclerosis, are fusiform. A *saccular aneurysm* is a pouchlike dilation that begins at a narrow neck. Saccular aneurysms have a higher rate of rupture and may be treated surgically regardless of size. However, many aneurysms cannot be strictly characterized as examples of either type but may demonstrate characteristics of both.

## Classification

Thoracoabdominal aneurysms may involve the entire thoracic and abdominal aorta. The classification scheme that was developed by Crawford is widely used to characterize the extent of aortic pathology. It is used to determine the surgical approach, conduct of the operation, and operative risk (Fig. 65–3). Type I aneurysms are limited to the area distal to the left subclavian and proximal to the renal arteries. Type II aneurysms extend from the left subclavian artery to below the renal arteries. Type III involve less than half the thoracic aorta and substantial portions of the abdominal aorta. Type IV aneurysms involve the upper abdominal aorta.

## Symptoms

Thoracic aortic aneurysms may produce symptoms described as a throbbing or aching sensation in the chest. Extrin-

sic compression of the esophagus or tracheobronchial tree by the expanding aneurysm may cause coughing, wheezing, dyspnea, dysphagia, or hoarseness. Aneurysmal dilation of the ascending aorta may also be associated with symptoms of congestive failure related to aortic regurgitation.

## Management

Factors that influence the management of patients with aortic aneurysms include size, rate of expansion, symptoms, location, and type. Aortic aneurysms of any size are repaired if they are symptomatic or rapidly growing because such factors predispose to early rupture. Ascending aneurysms 5 cm or larger are repaired promptly regardless of symptoms because at this diameter, the mortality rate from rupture equals or exceeds the operative mortality rate ($\approx$3%-5%). The yearly risk for rupture is about 10% for aneurysms that are 5 cm in diameter. The rate of rupture rises sharply at 6 cm to almost 40% for aneurysms that are 7 cm in diameter.[6] However, even small aneurysms can rupture at any time. Autopsy studies have noted that rupture occurs in 8% of aneurysms <4 cm in diameter. Hence, diameter alone cannot serve as the only criterion for surgical intervention.[7] In general, the rate of expansion in size of an aneurysm is proportional to its increase in diameter and can be monitored by serial radiologic imaging studies. A rate of aneurysmal expansion of 0.4 cm per year has also been proposed as an indication for surgery for ascending thoracic aneurysms.[2]

The incidence of complications and the morbidity rate are related to the acuity of symptoms and the urgency of surgical intervention. The mortality rate for elective aortic aneurysmal resection is about 3%[8]; for emergency repair of a ruptured abdominal aortic aneurysm, it ranges from 15% to 78% (average, $\approx$50%).[9] The most common judgmental error associated with mortality of ruptured abdominal aortic aneurysms is failure to repair the aneurysm electively.

In the past, elective repair of aortic aneurysms in high-risk patients with multiple severe comorbidities represented a population with a prohibitive perioperative risk. Aneurysm resection was delayed unless the predicted life expectancy exceeded 2 years. The technology of using deployment of aortic intravascular stents may provide a new therapeutic option for these patients.

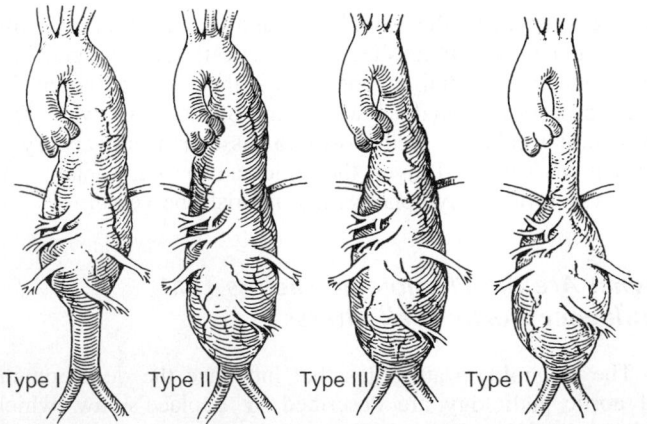

**FIGURE 65–3.** Crawford's classification of aortic aneurysms: types I, II, III, and IV. (From Naslund TC, Hollier LH. Thoracoabdominal aneurysm. In: Cameron JL, ed. *Current Surgical Therapy.* 4th ed. St Louis, Mo: Mosby–Year Book; 1992:674.)

## How Are Dissections Characterized and Managed?

### Pathology and Pathophysiology

Dissections of the thoracic portion of the aorta are frequently lethal aortic catastrophes, occurring twice as often as ruptured abdominal aortic aneurysms. Unlike aortic aneurysm formation, which is a chronic process unless rupture or leakage occurs, aortic dissection is an acute event. Acute dissections of the ascending aorta are true emergencies, with a mortality rate of 1% to 2% per hour during the first 48 hours. Dissections can involve any portions of the aorta or its branch vessels. Factors that predispose to ascending aortic dissection include atherosclerosis, systemic hypertension, and collagen vascular diseases, such as Marfan and Ehlers-Danlos syndromes, which cause medial necrosis. Atherosclerosis is the most common cause of aortic disease and is the primary etiology of dissections confined to the descending aorta. The presence of systemic hypertension causes degeneration of the vasa vasorum and compromises the nutritional supply to the tunica media. Episodes of hypertension, which increase intraluminal pressure, and disruption of vessel wall integrity caused by dissection markedly increase the risk for acute rupture.

Aortic dissections originate from a transverse defect or tear in the intima of the aorta. This defect produces an intimal flap that redirects the pulsatile flow of blood into the tunica media, producing a false lumen. Once blood has dissected into the tunica media, the pressure within the false lumen can propagate the dissection either proximally or distally. Blood flow within the false lumen can also cause further intimal tears and rupture back into the true lumen, creating secondary communications between the two lumens. Dissections that span aortic branch vessels may cause malperfusion syndromes that result from occlusion of the branch vessel, extension of the dissection into the branch vessel, or the reduced blood flow from the false lumen supplying the branch vessel.

### Symptoms

Aortic dissection is more common in men than women, with a ratio of about 2:1, and most often occurs between the ages of 40 and 70 years. Most aortic intimal tears are located in the thoracic aorta and have an incidence of 70% in the ascending aorta, 8% in the aortic arch, 21% in the aortic isthmus and descending thoracic aorta, and 1% in the abdominal aorta.[10] The most common presenting symptom of aortic dissection is severe unremitting chest pain that is often described as "tearing," "ripping," or "stabbing." Rarely is the dissection painless. The location of pain may indicate the location of the dissection. Pain in the anterior thorax, neck, throat, jaw, or teeth suggests ascending aorta or arch dissections. Pain in the back or abdomen suggests dissection in the descending thoracic aorta. Other presenting symptoms may include vasovagal manifestations such as sweating, apprehension, nausea and vomiting, and near syncope. Less common presenting symptoms include congestive heart failure, confusion, and stroke. Acute mental status changes or focal neurologic deficits may indicate malperfusion of branch vessels in the aortic arch.

Aortic dissections can rupture in one of several ways. External rupture into the mediastinum or pleural space often

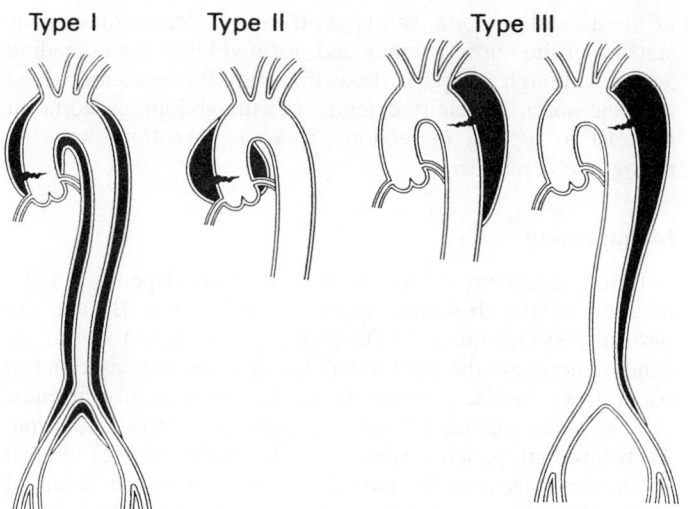

**FIGURE 65–4.** DeBakey's classification of aortic dissections. (Adapted from DeBakey ME, McCollum CH, Crawford ES, et al. Dissection and dissecting aneurysms of the aorta: twenty-year follow-up of five hundred twenty-seven patients treated surgically. *Surgery.* 1982;92:1118.)

results in exsanguination with acute hemodynamic collapse. If the rupture thromboses, it may develop into a mediastinal hematoma or pleural effusion, more often in the left pleura. Alternatively, an acute pericardial effusion with tamponade physiology can also rapidly lead to hemodynamic collapse. Obviously, the presence of any amount of pericardial fluid in a patient with aortic dissection is an alarming sign and should signal rapid intervention.

### Classifications Schemes

Multiple classifications systems based on the location of the dissection have been proposed; DeBakey's[11] (Fig. 65–4) and Dailey's (or Stanford's)[12] (Fig. 65–5) classifications are the most commonly used. Involvement of the ascending aorta is the single most important predictor of clinical outcome. Neither the origin of intimal dissection nor the extent of distal extension of the dissection significantly influences subsequent clinical presentation. Types I, II, and A indicate involvement

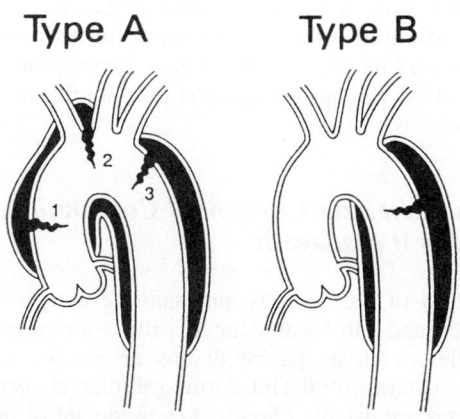

**FIGURE 65–5.** Dailey's (Stanford's) classification of aortic dissections. Numbers indicate potential locations of the site of primary intimal tear. (Adapted with permission from Miller DC, Stinson EB, Oyer PE, et al. Operative treatment of aortic dissections: experience with 125 patients over a sixteen-year period. *J Thorac Cardiovasc Surg.* 1979;78:365.)

of the ascending aorta, and types III and B denote dissections starting at the aortic isthmus and not involving the ascending aorta. Although a type B dissection may be restricted to the thoracic aorta, it usually extends into the abdominal aorta. In contrast to type A dissections, type B dissections have no retrograde component.

## Management

Initial treatment of an acute dissection depends on the location of the dissection (type A versus type B) and the patient's symptoms.[13–15] Dissections that begin in the ascending aorta are the most lethal. Cardiac decompensation can occur from cardiac tamponade, aortic valvular insufficiency, rupture with exsanguination, or coronary artery occlusion. Therefore, all patients with type A dissection are surgical candidates. Because the mortality rate for surgical repair of uncomplicated type B dissections is greater than that associated with medical therapy, surgical intervention should be deferred unless extenuating circumstances arise. Evidence of vascular obstruction, compromise of a major aortic branch, or failure of intensive medical therapy is an indication for more aggressive intervention.

## What Are Transections, and How Are They Managed?

An aortic transection is often the result of a sudden deceleration injury sustained from a motor vehicle accident. Acute traumatic aortic rupture or transection is a dehiscence of all or part of the aortic wall resulting from intense deceleration of the body that produces strain between fixed and mobile structures. The forward displacement of the heart, proximal aorta, and lungs creates a shearing and torsion effect on the upper thoracic aorta that is relatively fixed to the posterior thorax by adhesions and intercostal arteries. The most common location is at the insertion of the ligamentum arteriosum (formally the ductus arteriosum) below the left subclavian. Other reported locations of aortic transection are the arch and ascending aorta.

Within the first hour, 80% of patients die from acute rupture and exsanguination. Initially, bleeding may be contained by the mediastinal pleura, but may rupture into the pleural space with minimal perturbation of position or hemodynamics. An untreated aortic transection progresses to formation of a pseudoaneurysm and retains a high risk for acute rupture. Survival is dependent on prompt recognition and appropriate surgical intervention.

## What Characterizes Congenital Coarctation, and How Is It Managed?

Coarctation of the aorta is an anatomic narrowing of the aortic lumen and can be associated with other cardiovascular abnormalities, such as patent ductus arteriosus, ventricular septal defect, and mitral and aortic valvular abnormalities.[16] These lesions are usually classified as preductal or postductal, according to the location of the stricture in relation to the ductus. The incidence of occurrence is higher in males than females.[16] Although most patients with coarctation are diagnosed in infancy, others are diagnosed as an adult. Aortic coarctation increases afterload to the left ventricle, causing myocardial hypertrophy. Patients may also develop systemic hypoperfusion below the area of coarctation or congestive heart failure from left ventricular overload or intracardiac shunting.

The timing and choice of surgical intervention are dependent on the patient's age, symptoms, location of coarctation, and presence of associated cardiovascular abnormalities. In contrast to that in patients undergoing thoracic aneurysm repair, the incidence of spinal cord paraplegia or paraparesis is relatively low: 0.14% to 0.41%.[17–19] The lesser incidence of spinal cord complication is most likely attributable to the development of extensive collateral vascularity.

## What Are the Diagnostic Imaging Methods for Major Aortic Pathology?

### Chest Radiograph

Chest radiographs are useful screening examinations; findings are abnormal in 80% of patients with dissection of the thoracic aorta.[20] Although widely available, they have a low sensitivity and specificity for detecting and characterizing aortic pathology. The elderly population has a high prevalence of focal intimal calcification that can be observed by radiography. Separation of this intimal calcification from the adventitial border >1 cm is referred to as the *calcium sign* and indicates aortic dissection. Apical capping, widened mediastinum, lateral displacement of the left mainstem bronchus, and obliteration of the usual clear space between the aortic knob and left pulmonary artery are evidence of aortic dilation. Aneurysms may also appear as localized dilations of the aorta but are difficult to distinguish from other mediastinal masses unless the vessel lumen is outlined by calcification in the vessel wall.

### Angiography

Although aortography has long been considered the gold standard for diagnosing aortic dissection, newer diagnostic modalities have replaced its routine use.[21] Radiographic contrast media injected into the aorta permits visualization of the lumen of the aorta and blood flow in the aortic branch vessels, including the coronary arteries. Aortography can identify visceral artery obstruction or stenosis. Angiographic diagnosis of aortic dissection is based on demonstrating an intimal flap that separates the true and false lumens. However, false-negative results may occur if both the true and false lumens of the aorta simultaneously opacify during injection of the contrast agent. Aortography is less valuable for defining aneurysms because it shows only the size of the lumen and cannot detect the presence of mural thrombus or the overall size.

### Computed Tomography

Computed tomography with intravenous injection of contrast material has been used with success in the diagnosis and subsequent long-term follow-up of aortic disease.[22,23] This method is most reliable for defining the location and size of aortic aneurysms. Its specificity for the diagnosis of type A aortic dissections is limited by its ability to differentiate intimal flaps from artifacts. It is anticipated that the sensitivity and specificity will increase with improvements in technology.

## Magnetic Resonance Imaging

Magnetic resonance imaging and magnetic resonance angiography are currently the best technologies for imaging the entire aorta and its branch vessels in the transverse axis, sagittal, or frontal imaging planes. Both technologies can provide an accurate measure of aortic dimensions and detect blood flow in true and false lumens, thrombus, intimal flaps, and aortic regurgitation. For these reasons, they are considered the most specific tests for the diagnosis and classification of aortic dissection.[22,24,25] The availability, expense, and time required for image acquisition, however, limit its use in the hemodynamically unstable patient.

## Transesophageal Echocardiography

Echocardiography often is the diagnostic modality of choice. It is particularly valuable for the timely and accurate diagnosis of major vascular pathology of the aortic root. Transesophageal echocardiography (TEE) is portable, can be used in the operating room, and can be performed in <30 minutes, making it ideal for use in emergencies or when the patient's condition is unstable.[21] TEE can image the ascending and descending thoracic aorta in detail but provides limited imaging of the distal ascending aorta and aortic arch because the trachea and left mainstem bronchus limit the acoustic window.[26] Despite the limited imaging planes, clinical studies have demonstrated a >95% sensitivity and specificity for the diagnosis of aortic dissection and traumatic injury with TEE.[21,22,27,28] TEE can accurately measure the diameter of the ascending aorta, the sinotubular junction, and the aortic valve annulus. It also provides assessment of cardiac function and detection of pericardial effusions, aortic valvular insufficiency, and regional wall motion abnormalities.

## *What Are the Most Common Coexisting Diseases and Their Implications for the Anesthesiologist?*

### Atherosclerosis

Atherosclerosis is one of the most common cardiovascular diseases and is a significant factor leading to aortic dilation, aneurysm formation, or dissection. In addition, the presence of atheroma may be important as a marker for coexisting coronary artery disease and as a potential source of embolic cerebrovascular events. Risk factors that have been strongly associated with severe atherosclerotic disease of the aorta include advanced age, peripheral vascular disease, coronary artery disease, and carotid stenosis. The presence of significant arterial atherosclerosis can complicate certain technical aspects of surgery and increase the risk for postoperative stroke, renal failure, and ischemia that results from embolization after manipulation of the friable aorta.

### Coronary Artery Disease

The dominant risk factor for perioperative morbidity and mortality in patients scheduled for abdominal aortic aneurysmectomy is found to be cardiac (47%), followed by pulmonary (31%), age older than 85 years (17%), renal failure (2%), retroperitoneal fibrosis (2%), and cirrhosis with ascites (1%)[8]

(Table 65–1). Hertzer and colleagues showed that only 8% of patients undergoing vascular surgery had normal coronary arteries as determined by angiography.[29] Thirty-one percent (25% correctable and 6% inoperable) had severe coronary artery disease. The presence of coronary stenosis may increase a patient's vulnerability to ischemia or infarction caused by hemodynamic instability, transient hypotension, anemia, postoperative hypercoagulability, or ruptured atherosclerotic plaques. Various interventions have been proposed to improve the outcome for these high-risk patients. A recent randomized multicenter study found that administration of a β-adrenergic receptor antagonist significantly reduced the incidence of death related to cardiac causes and nonfatal infarction in high-risk vascular patients.[30] This study and others strongly support the perioperative administration of a β-adrenergic receptor antagonist in high-risk patients undergoing major surgery to decrease the risk for cardiac-related morbidity and mortality.[30,31]

All patients having vascular surgery should undergo some cardiac evaluation. Poor exercise tolerance, the history of angina, or an abnormal electrocardiogram (ECG) mandates further evaluation. Myocardial stress testing (treadmill, Persantine thallium myocardial imaging, or stress echocardiography) is a common study used to select those patients at highest risk for ischemia. Patients having a positive test that is consistent with coronary artery disease often receive left heart catheterization. Confirmation of significant coronary artery disease by angiography may lead to angioplasty, stenting, or coronary artery bypass grafting either before or at the time of surgical intervention.

Aortocoronary bypass before aortic resection lowers perioperative mortality.[32] In the case of an emergency, most cardiac evaluations are often aborted, and intraoperative ECG and TEE are used to diagnose ischemia and guide therapy. Even in the absence of documented coronary artery disease, all patients undergoing aortic surgery should be considered at risk for myocardial ischemia. Risk factors such as myocardial hypertrophy and a history of hypertension lability of blood pressure and heart rate render these patients at increased risk for myocardial ischemia.[33] Therefore, the goals of perioperative management should include optimizing the balance of myocardial oxygen ($O_2$) supply by ensuring adequate perfusion while limiting metabolic demands.

### Hypertension

Hypertension is the most common cardiovascular disease and an important factor contributing to the development of

**TABLE 65–1.** Prevalence of Coexisting Disease in Patients Scheduled for Vascular Surgery

| Coexisting Disease | Prevalence (%) |
|---|---|
| Hypertension | 40–60 |
| Heart disease | 50–70 |
| Angina | 10–20 |
| Previous myocardial infarction | 40–60 |
| Congestive heart failure | 5–15 |
| Diabetes mellitus | 8–12 |
| Chronic obstructive lung disease | 25–50 |
| Renal disease | 5–25 |

Adapted from Clark NJ, Stanley TH. Anesthesia for vascular surgery. In: Miller RD, ed. *Anesthesia.* 3rd ed. New York, NY: Churchill Livingstone; 1990:1694.

aortic and cardiac pathology. Although the diagnosis of left ventricular hypertrophy may be suggested by ECG criteria, echocardiography is considered the best diagnostic tool.[34] A history of chronic hypertension and major sequelae of left ventricular myocardial hypertrophy have significant implications for perioperative hemodynamic management. Chronic hypertension shifts circulatory autoregulation of various organs, such as the brain and kidney, rendering them susceptible to ischemia. Left ventricular hypertrophy places the patient at increased risk for myocardial ischemia, even in the absence of discrete significant coronary stenosis. An imbalance of myocardial supply and demand can trigger transient myocardial ischemia and dysfunction. Patients with a history of chronic hypertension often demonstrate labile blood pressure and are, therefore, at increased risk for aortic rupture or dissection. Such patients may require aggressive hemodynamic control that often necessitates an infusion of vasodilators (sodium nitroprusside, nitroglycerin, and nicardipine) and a β-adrenergic antagonist (esmolol).

### Pulmonary Disease

A history of pulmonary disease poses a number of perioperative management challenges for the anesthesiologist. For example, an acute exacerbation of reactive pulmonary disease illustrates one such problem. Sympathomimetic bronchodilators are associated with hypertension and tachycardia and, therefore, are relatively contraindicated in hypertensive patients with unstable aortic disease. The presence of reactive airway disease may also be a relative contraindication to the use of β-adrenergic antagonists, which are used to control hemodynamics. One of the most challenging intraoperative problems is that of maintaining adequate respiratory function during surgery of the descending thoracic aorta.

Single-lung isolation is a common technique to facilitate surgical exposure of the descending thoracic aorta. Aneurysmal dilation of the aorta may distort the trachea or mainstem bronchus, making single-lung isolation difficult. Even after appropriate placement of the endotracheal tube (ETT), the presence of significant lung disease may compromise the anesthesiologist's ability to ventilate and oxygenate adequately during single-lung isolation. Postoperatively, these patients may experience a further decrement of lung function, thus jeopardizing their ability to wean from mechanical ventilation. Trauma to the diaphragm or phrenic nerve significantly increases the postoperative difficulties of weaning and maintaining adequate pulmonary toilet after extubation. A preoperative evaluation (pulmonary function tests and arterial blood gas) for patients with significant pulmonary disease may help guide perioperative management.

### Renal Disease

Patients with preexisting renal disease pose specific challenges to the anesthesiologist by complicating issues of hemostasis, drug administration, and fluid management. The qualitative platelet dysfunction associated with end-stage renal disease may be attenuated by preoperative hemodialysis or the administration of desmopressin (1-deamino-8-D-arginine-vasopressin, DDAVP). The choice of drugs and dosing regimen of all pharmacologic agents must take into consideration the presence and severity of renal disease. The problems of fluid management may require intraoperative ultrafiltration

during cardiopulmonary bypass (CPB) or the use of aggressive diuretic therapy. As expected, patients with a history of renal disease are also at high risk for further decrement in postoperative renal function. Specific intraoperative management issues associated with risk for renal ischemia and prophylaxis are discussed later (see What Therapeutic Interventions Can Be Used to Decrease the Risk for Postoperative Renal Failure?).

## ANESTHETIC INDUCTION AND MAINTENANCE AND POSTOPERATIVE ISSUES

### What Are the Preoperative Anesthetic Considerations?

The presence of coexisting disease and acuity of the patient's presentation guide the preoperative evaluation (Table 65–2). At a minimum, the preoperative cardiovascular examination should include a 12-lead ECG to assess for myocardial ischemia and a chest radiograph. Coronary arteriography is usually performed in patients undergoing elective aortic aneurysm repair because of the high incidence of associated coronary artery disease. In more urgent circumstances, preoperative echocardiography is frequently performed to evaluate ventricular and valvular function. A neurologic examination should assess mental status, motor strength, and sensory function to differentiate a preexisting neurologic deficit from a new postoperative deficit. The preoperative detection of new carotid bruits or asymmetric blood pressures obtained in the upper extremities may indicate the need for modifying circulatory management.

### Preoperative Stabilization of Hemodynamics

Patients with acute aortic dissection or large symptomatic aortic aneurysms are typically admitted to an intensive care unit for medical control of blood pressure. Because hypertension increases the risk for aortic rupture or propagation of a dissection, pharmacologic therapy is initiated to reduce systolic blood pressure and decrease the velocity of left ventricular ejection. Systolic blood pressure is typically decreased to a range of 100 to 120 mm Hg, or the lowest blood pressure

**TABLE 65–2.** Issues of Preoperative Management

| | |
|---|---|
| Sequelae of aortic disease | Peripheral vascular insufficiency, hemothorax, hypertension, hypotension, pulseless extremities, tracheal deviation |
| Cardiopulmonary examination | Auscultation of heart and lungs, jugular venous distention, murmurs, pulse pressure, electrocardiogram, echocardiogram |
| Neurologic examination | Mental status, motor and sensory deficits of the lower extremities |
| Vascular examination | Vascular (pulses and blood pressure of upper and lower extremities), malperfusion (bowel, neurologic, renal, extremities) |
| Presence of morbidities | Coronary artery disease, hypertension, renal disease, pulmonary disease |
| Hemodynamic concerns | Set target blood pressure and heart rate and achieve goals by titration of analgesics, vasodilators, and β-blockers. |
| Blood products | Type and cross-match for red blood cell count. |

that permits adequate end-organ perfusion. In patients with aortic regurgitation, decreasing the systemic vascular resistance improves cardiac performance by increasing cardiac output. Blood pressure control is usually achieved with a combination of narcotic analgesics to relieve pain, vasodilators to decrease arterial pressure, and β-adrenergic receptor antagonists to decrease heart rate and the force of ventricular ejection.

Alternatively, patients who present with sustained hypotension need fluid resuscitation and evaluation for emergent surgical intervention. Causes of this hypotension include aortic rupture, malperfusion syndromes, cardiac tamponade, severe aortic valvular regurgitation, myocardial ischemia or infarction, and heart block. Resuscitative efforts are directed at hemodynamic stabilization, the support of vital organ function, and preparing the patient for surgery.

## What Are the Goals and Strategies for the Conduction of Intraoperative Anesthesia?

The goals of anesthesia for surgery of the aorta are similar to those for any procedure: to minimize patient morbidity and to maximize patient benefit while providing acceptable surgical conditions (Table 65–3). During transport, patients should receive adequate preoperative sedation, and antihypertensive therapy should be continued. Antibiotic prophylaxis with cefazolin, 1 g, or vancomycin, 1 g, intravenously, is administered at least 30 minutes before skin incision. Because the potential for blood loss during the operation is substantial, 4 to 6 units of packed red blood cells should be typed and cross-matched for immediate availability. Typically, two large gauge (>16 gauge) peripheral intravenous catheters are placed for intraoperative volume resuscitation. Alternatively, an 8.5 French catheter can be placed in a central vein for rapid volume resuscitation.

### Monitors

#### Hemodynamic

Most hemodynamic monitors are placed before the induction of general anesthesia. In addition to the routine monitors, invasive monitoring of systemic and cardiac pressures is crucial in guiding perioperative hemodynamic management (Table 65–4). Arterial catheters allow for continuous blood pressure monitoring and serial blood sampling for blood gases, acid-base status, and glucose metabolism. The arterial catheter is usually placed in the right upper extremity when the left subclavian is close to the operative site. Central venous or

**TABLE 65–3.** Major Anesthetic Goals During Vascular Surgery

Maintain adequate level of analgesia, sedation, amnesia, and muscle relaxation.
Maintain stable cardiac function and hemodynamics using invasive hemodynamic monitoring to administer vasoactive drugs judiciously.
Maintain adequate urine output by hydration and the use of mannitol and/or dopamine (particularly suprarenal aortic cross-clamping).
Maintain adequate oxygen-carrying capacity by using volume replacement and blood products.
Maintain adequate body temperature.
Maintain acid-base status.

**TABLE 65–4.** Issues of Intraoperative Management

| | |
|---|---|
| Antibiotics | Cefazolin, 1 g, or vancomycin, 1 g |
| Intravenous access | Minimum 16 gauge (×2); preference for right upper extremity when left brachiocephalic vein is at risk of being ligated |
| | *Optional: Rapid infuser with high-flow-capacity tubing* |
| Monitors | Radial arterial cannula (right side if left subclavian line is to be clamped); a second arterial line from surgical field to monitor distal aortic pressure during bypass; pulmonary artery catheter; urine output; temperature (bladder, nasopharyngeal); CSF pressure |
| | *Optional: SSEP, EEG, MEP, TEE* |
| Temperature control | Fluid warmers, raise room temperature, forced air blankets, bypass |
| Induction of anesthesia | If emergent: rapid-sequence blockers, metoclopramide, sodium citrate; control hypertensive episodes |
| Tracheal intubation | Double-lumen tube or bronchial blocker (placement may be difficult because of tracheal deviation or collapse of the mainstem bronchus related to aortic pathology. After surgery, the double-lumen tube is replaced with single-lumen tube) |
| Maintenance of anesthesia | Balanced anesthetic techique that permits assessment of neurologic status within 6 h postoperatively |
| Antifibrinolytic therapies | Epsilon aminocaproic acid (Amicar); aprotinin |
| Position | Right lateral decubitus with groins exposed |
| Pressure points | Check eyes, nose, elbows, arms, ears, lower extremities |
| Gastric tube | Nasogastric tube in place before transfer to the ICU |
| Surgical approach | Left lateral thoracotomy, with possible retroperitoneal incision |
| Techniques of circulatory management | Simple clamp-and-sew; passive shunt (variable distal pressure); active shunt (left atrial to femoral artery bypass), distal MAP >60 mm Hg |
| Neurologic protection | Control blood sugar, 90–200 mg/dL |
| | *Optional: Solu-Medrol, mannitol, 0.25–0.5 kg 30–45 min before cross-clamping, MSO₄ before cross-clamp ischemia* |
| | CSF drain placed in lower lumbar region after induction, zeroed at the level of the lower thoracic spine, and CSF pressure maintained at 10 mm Hg; hypothermic circulatory arrest (T, 18°C); mild hypothermia (T, 33°C) |
| Renal protection | *Optional: shunt, dopamine, fenoldopam, and mannitol infusions* |

CPB, cardiopulmonary bypass; CSF, cerebrospinal fluid; EEG, electroencephalogram; ICU, intensive care unit; MAP, mean arterial pressure; MEP, motor evoked potentials; SSEP, somatosensory evoked potentials; TEE, transesophageal echocardiogram.

pulmonary artery catheters are used to assess volume status and to guide fluid replacement therapy and titration of vasoactive drugs. Although slightly more difficult to place, cannulation of the nondependent side (left side) for cases requiring right lateral decubitus positioning allows for easier access during surgery. In addition, placement of TEE may be indicated in cases of significant cardiac dysfunction or refractory intraoperative hypotension.

#### Temperature

Monitoring body temperature is necessary to ensure adequate cooling for neural protection and rewarming after the operative procedure. Body temperature is monitored from several locations. A temperature probe in the bladder or rectum provides an estimate of core body temperature; a probe in the nasopharynx provides an estimate of central nervous system temperature; and the temperature probe built into the pulmonary artery catheter provides an estimate of the blood temperature.

## Neurologic

Neurologic monitoring is useful for intraoperative clinical management and as a research tool for cases involving a significantly increased risk for central nervous system ischemia. The electroencephalogram (EEG) is commonly used to determine the timing of deep hypothermic circulatory arrest and diagnose the cerebral ischemia. The EEG may also prove useful as a guide for blood pressure management when flow-related changes in the EEG activity are noted intraoperatively.

For surgery of the descending thoracic aorta in which ischemic paraplegia is a concern, somatosensory evoked potentials (SSEP) have been used to monitor the integrity of the spinal cord and effect changes in intraoperative management.[35–41] However, the prognostic value of SSEP in determining the risk for spinal cord ischemia remains controversial.

Postoperative paraplegia is possible, even with normal SSEP tracings.[37,42] SSEP monitors electrical neural activity of the dorsal spinal columns (sensory nerve tracks of vibration and proprioception) but does not monitor the crucial ventral motor tracks, which are at highest risk for ischemia. A relatively new and promising monitoring technique records spinal cord function using motor evoked potentials (MEPs). Transcranial magnetic stimulation of upper motor neurons is used to detect global spinal cord ischemia in the area of the ventral motor neurons that is supplied by the crucial anterior spinal artery. Several investigators have successfully used this technique to prospectively reverse ischemic changes in MEPs by increasing distal and proximal blood pressures.[43] Availability of neurologic monitoring and personnel is an important limiting factor for the routine use of these techniques in many institutions.

## Cerebrospinal Fluid

Another commonly used monitoring technique and therapeutic modality for spinal cord preservation during surgery of the descending thoracic aorta is that of draining cerebrospinal fluid (CSF). The rationale for CSF drainage is to augment spinal cord blood flow by minimizing intraspinal pressure, thus increasing perfusion pressure to the spinal cord.[35,44] The CSF drain is placed at the level of the lumbar vertebra after the induction of anesthesia while the patient is positioned in the lateral decubitus position. The drain is connected to a closed drainage system and the pressure transduced using manometry or an electronic transducer (heparin and flush bag are eliminated). At our institution, CSF pressures are continuously monitored and fluid drained to maintain a pressure of <10 mm Hg.

## Renal Function

During all major vascular operations, the quantity of urine produced is closely monitored. The rationale is that urine production, presumably, is an index of the adequacy of renal blood flow and reflects intravascular volume status. The kidneys are resilient to ischemia and, in general, even if suprarenal and infrarenal aortic cross-clamp times are kept to 40 minutes or less, no impairment of renal function (eg, rise in creatinine levels) occurs postoperatively.[45] A more detailed discussion about perioperative renal dysfunction and prophylactic strategies is presented later in this chapter.

## General Anesthesia

### Induction

The induction of anesthesia must be tailored with concern to the patient's preoperative cardiopulmonary status, volume status, and the extent and acuity of aortic pathology. In the hemodynamically stable patient with good cardiac function and adequate volume status, the choice of an induction agent is of less concern than in the unstable patient. The administration of incremental doses of a narcotic analgesic (fentanyl or sufentanil), in combination with sedative-hypnotic agents, typically produces predictable and favorable hemodynamic responses. Midazolam is a good choice as an adjunct for induction to produce anxiolysis and amnesia, in addition to reducing the incidence of narcotic-induced chest wall rigidity. In cases of hypovolemia, intravascular volume expansion is suggested, and the administration of drugs that depress myocardial function or further dilate the vasculature should be avoided.

General anesthesia is typically maintained with a combination of sedative-hypnotics, potent inhalation anesthetic agents, narcotics, and muscle relaxants. A long-acting nondepolarizing muscle relaxant such as pancuronium is used if renal function is adequate for the elimination of the drug. In the case of renal insufficiency, a more logical choice is a muscle relaxant such as atracurium or cisatracurium, which do not rely on renal metabolism.

A major concern during the induction of general anesthesia is the presence of sequelae that would markedly affect the hemodynamics. Hemopericardium can compromise the hemodynamics by decreasing cardiac preload, thereby causing tamponade-like physiologic effects. The classic strategy of "fast and full" can be achieved by administration of volume and sympathomimetic agents to increase heart rate and contractility. The use of induction agents such as etomidate and ketamine is consistent with the maintenance of previously stated goals of minimal change in the hemodynamics. Surgeons should be available should the pericardial effusion need to be drained emergently. Another potential complicating factor in patients with a type A dissection and aneurysm of the ascending aorta is the presence of aortic insufficiency. The anesthetic management of these patients is best accomplished by decreasing afterload and maintaining a slightly increased heart rate to minimize the retrograde flow into the left ventricle. Most patients undergoing aortic surgery are at increased risk for myocardial ischemia related to coronary artery disease, left ventricular hypertrophy, or compromised blood flow related to aortocoronary dissection or malperfusion. The anesthesiologist should monitor the ECG tracing for changes consistent with ischemia and adjust hemodynamics to minimize $O_2$ consumption while providing adequate coronary perfusion.

It is often challenging to minimize such fluctuations in blood pressure. The occurrence of hypertension associated with laryngoscopy and intubation markedly increases the risk for aortic rupture. Narcotics alone are often not effective in attenuating the hypertension and tachycardia associated with major vascular surgery. Such episodes of hypertension can be attenuated by increasing the depth of anesthesia with inhalation agents that can be quickly eliminated as the blood pressure decreases and with a titration of short-acting agents such as esmolol or vasoactive agents such as sodium nitroprusside or nitroglycerin.

**TABLE 65–5.** Comparison of Management Issues Between Surgery of the Ascending Arch and the Descending Thoracic Aorta

| Management | Ascending to Arch of Aorta | Descending Thoracic Aorta | Intravascular Stents |
|---|---|---|---|
| Patient position | Supine | Right lateral decubitus | Supine (fluoroscopy table) |
| Incision | Median sternotomy | Left thoracotomy | Femoral |
| Special circulatory management | *Cardiopulmonary bypass option: deep hypothermic circulatory arrest* | 1. Simple clamp-and-sew<br>2. Passive shunt<br>3. Active shunt (partial bypass)<br>4. *Cardiopulmonary bypass option: deep hypothermic circulatory arrest* | |
| Ventilatory management | Single-lumen endotracheal tube | One-lung ventilation (double-lumen tube or bronchial blocker) | Single-lumen endotracheal tube |
| Hematologic management | | | |
|   Blood loss | + | + + + | + |
|   Transfusion | ± | + + + | − |
| Antifibrinolytic | ± | + + | − |
| Ischemic risks | Cerebral | Spinal cord, renal, splanchnic | Spinal cord, renal, splanchnic |
| Anesthetic techniques | General anesthesia | General anesthesia, ± epidural | General anesthesia |

### Maintenance

The major goal is to produce stable hemodynamics with agents that preserve cardiac performance. The most commonly used strategy is that of a narcotic-based, balanced anesthetic technique that is supplemented by inhalation agents. Inhalation anesthetic agents are commonly used as adjuncts to provide amnesia, analgesia, and intraoperative hypotension. These agents have the added advantage of being administered during CPB and eliminated soon after the completion of surgery. The use of volatile anesthetics should be limited, however, when using EEG or SSEP monitoring to prevent interference.[46] Devising an anesthetic plan that would allow for emergence and extubation in the operating room is not a problem. Most patients are permitted to emerge from anesthesia and sedation in the intensive care unit after they are adequately rewarmed and hemodynamically stable.

### What Are the Considerations for Ventilatory Management?

Surgical and anesthetic considerations for the descending thoracic aorta differ from those of the ascending aorta and are presented in Table 65–5. Surgery of the ascending aorta and arch is approached by median sternotomy using the standard CPB circuit with cannulation of the ascending aorta; surgery of the descending thoracic aorta, on the other hand, employs alternative techniques of circulatory management, patient positioning, and ventilatory management. The surgical approach is through a left thoracotomy with the patient in a modified right lateral decubitus position to provide vascular access to the femoral vessels for institution of partial circulatory bypass. In addition, exposure of the descending thoracic aorta requires selective ventilation of the dependent right lung and collapse of the nondependent left lung.

Selective right lung ventilation with collapse of the left lung is achieved by placement of a double-lumen ETT or bronchial blocker (Univent, Fuji Systems Corp, Tokyo, Japan). Because this aneurysm often encroaches on the left mainstem bronchus, great care must be exercised not to rupture it during endobronchial tube placement. Preoperative diagnostic imaging studies can be of great assistance in alerting the clinician to potential difficulties. Placement of a double-lumen ETT is

the most common and dependable technique used to enable selective lung ventilation. Alternatively, a bronchial blocker can be used to provide one-lung anesthesia. Although bronchial blockers require more experience and expertise to position correctly, they offer the advantages of eliminating the exchange to a single-lumen ETT at the completion of surgery, quick reinstitution of selective ventilation if surgical reexploration is required, and better access for fiberoptic bronchoscopy to maintain pulmonary toilet.

The ability to establish selective ventilation should be verified by bronchoscopy in both the supine and lateral decubitus positions (Table 65–6). Because the left mainstem bronchus lies inferior to the aorta, compression by aortic pathology may distort or compress the anatomy and therefore complicate the ability to secure selective lung ventilation. Selective one-lung ventilation usually results in periods of relative or severe $O_2$ desaturation. The most commonly used management strategies include the use of continuous positive airway pressure, use of positive end-expiratory pressure, institution of $O_2$ flow, and temporary reinstitution of two-lung ventilation (Table 65–7). More discussion about the pathophysiology and ventilation strategies of selective one-lung ventilation is presented in Chapter 68.

### Is There a Role for Epidural Anesthesia?

The use of epidural anesthesia as an adjunct during major vascular surgery in the descending thoracic aorta involves many tradeoffs that may affect circulatory management and

**TABLE 65–6.** Basic Strategies for Management of One-Lung Ventilation

1. Assess adequacy of oxygenation and ventilation by monitoring pulse oximetry, capnography, and arterial blood gases.
2. Delay initiation of single-lung ventilation until patient positioning is completed.
3. Confirm correct lung isolation by auscultation or more definitively by visualization using fiberoptic bronchoscopy.
4. Increase inspired oxygen concentration to decrease the risk for systemic hypoxia.
5. Adjust ventilation to maintain normocapnia and avoid atelectasis in the dependent, ventilated lung.

**TABLE 65–7.** Strategies for Management of Hypoxemia During One-Lung Ventilation

1. Increase inspired concentration of $O_2$ to 100%; increase tidal volume.
2. Confirm position of the double-lumen tube or bronchial blocker using fiberoptic bronchoscopy.
3. Add CPAP at 5 cm $H_2O$ to nondependent lung.
4. Add PEEP at 5 cm $H_2O$ to dependent lung.
5. Institute intermittent positive pressure ventilation of the nondependent lung with 100% $O_2$.
6. Repeat steps 3 and 4, increasing CPAP and PEEP to 10 cm $H_2O$.
7. Consider asking the surgeon to clamp the pulmonary artery supplying the nondependent lung.
8. *If none of the previous 5 maneuvers is successful, resume two-lung ventilation.*

CPAP, continuous positive airway pressure; PEEP, positive end-expiratory pressure.

complicate the detection of a new neurologic deficit after surgery. Some investigators have reported significant complications with this technique in the setting of major vascular surgery. However, others have touted its many benefits.[6,47–54]

Epidural anesthesia has been shown to decrease the incidence of myocardial ischemia, provide excellent muscle relaxation, and improve distal vascular graft perfusion and postoperative ventilatory mechanics. However, one of the most feared complications is the development of an epidural hematoma with subsequent neurologic deficit.[47] Many of the patients with vascular disease come to the operating room with heparin infusions or are subsequently administered heparin, or they develop coagulopathies during the course of the operation. Massive volume shifts and dilutional thrombocytopenia commonly occur and may render patients especially susceptible to an epidural hematoma. The authors acknowledge that this same argument may be used for patients who receive an intrathecal catheter for CSF drainage. However, placement of an elective epidural catheter preoperatively doubles the theoretic risk of hematoma formation. As of this time, there have been no studies demonstrating that these patients are at increased risk by placing the epidural several hours before heparinization.

Rao and El-Etr placed epidural catheters in patients scheduled for aortic coronary bypass.[48] They found that epidural catheters in the setting of full heparinization did not increase the rate of complications. However, in their study, if blood was observed in the epidural needle during placement of the catheter, surgery was delayed for 24 hours to allow for adequate clot formation.

The postponement of surgery is not an attractive option in today's economic climate or for patients undergoing emergent procedures. Even if the epidural is placed preoperatively, at least 1 hour before heparinization, one should be cautioned against using it until the patient is awake and a baseline neurologic assessment obtained. Administration of any drug volume into the epidural space will theoretically increase the pressure within the vertebral canal, thus essentially antagonizing the putative benefit of CSF drainage to increase spinal cord perfusion pressure (SCPP). Additionally, the risk for paraplegia associated with this type of surgery necessitates adequate documentation without the confounding variable of residual postoperative motor weakness resulting from local anesthetic activity.

## What Are the Issues of Circulatory Management During the Period of Aortic Clamping?

Circulatory management during complex aortic reconstruction can be categorized into two groups (see Table 65–5). Surgery involving the ascending aorta or arch necessitates full CPB with the option of using special techniques in the case of deep hypothermic circulatory arrest. Alternatively, circulatory management during surgery involving the descending thoracic aorta may incorporate one of several techniques: simple clamp and sew, passive shunting, partial bypass, or routine CPB.

Regardless of the technique chosen, all patients require some degree of anticoagulation during the period of aortic cross-clamping. The techniques of simple clamping and passive shunting require a minimal amount of anticoagulation. The partial bypass circuit that includes a centripetal pump, a reservoir, and a temperature coil requires more than the former techniques but less than routine CPB because it lacks an oxygenator. The use of a complete CPB circuit requires full anticoagulation. However, the previous guidelines for heparin administration are being revised because of the more common use of heparin-coated circuits and oxygenators. At some institutions, a full bypass circuit may be set up with the exclusion of certain parts, such as the oxygenator or cardiotomy reservoir. The guidelines for anticoagulation are institution and surgeon specific.

Regardless of the technique of circulatory management, an anesthesiologist should strive to achieve two major therapeutic goals during the period of cross-clamping: (1) the prevention of hypertensive injury to those organs located proximal to the cross-clamp (heart and brain); and (2) the prevention of hypotensive injury to those organs distal to the cross-clamp (segments of the spinal cord, kidneys, and gut). Although these goals are easily promulgated, their achievement is often difficult.

### Simple Aortic Cross-Clamping

The technique of simple aortic cross-clamping was introduced by Crawford.[55] The major advantage of this technique is that it requires no special equipment and thus is readily applicable at most medical centers, especially for emergencies such as an impending rupture or a leaking aneurysm. Two of the major limitations of this technique that predispose to increasing the risk for complications are the duration of ischemia distal to the aortic cross-clamp and the time constraints that may limit reimplantation of potentially important segmental arteries.

Clamping of the proximal descending thoracic aorta results in acute hemodynamic perturbations that can trigger cardiac failure (Table 65–8). The sudden increase in left ventricular afterload may cause myocardial ischemia or volume overload in the presence of valvular insufficiency. Although coronary blood flow may increase after aortic cross-clamping, any potential benefit may be undermined by the increased metabolic demands associated with the increased wall tension and decreased coronary perfusion pressure related to the increased left ventricular end-diastolic pressure.[56] Intraoperative myocardial ischemia may persist despite aggressive administration of inotropes and nitroglycerin. However, Roizen and colleagues found that despite a 93% incidence of ischemic changes diag-

**TABLE 65–8.** Effect of Aortic Cross-Clamp Level on Myocardial Variables (Percentage Change From Baseline Values)

| Cardiovascular Parameter | Supraceliac | Suprarenal and Infrarenal | Infrarenal |
|---|---|---|---|
| Mean arterial pressure (mm Hg) | 54 | 5* | 2* |
| Pulmonary capillary wedge pressure (mm Hg) | 38 | 10* | 0* |
| End-diastolic area (cm²) | 28 | 2* | 9* |
| End-systolic area (cm²) | 69 | 10* | 11* |
| Ejection fraction (%) | −38 | 10* | 3* |
| Abnormal motion of wall (% of patients) | 92 | 33* | 0* |
| New myocardial infarctions (% of patients) | 8 | 0* | 0* |

*Statistically different from group undergoing supraceliac aortic occlusion ($P < 0.05$). Adapted from Roizen JF, Beaupre PN, Alpert RA, et al. Monitoring with two-dimensional transesophageal echocardiography: comparison of myocardial function in patients undergoing supraceliac, suprarenal-infraceliac, or infrarenal aortic occlusion. *J Vasc Surg.* 1984;1:300.

nosed by TEE, only 8% of these patients were actually shown to have a perioperative myocardial infarction.[57] In addition to TEE, acute ventricular dysfunction may be detected by the pulmonary artery catheter as an increased pulmonary artery occlusion pressure or by ECG as ST segment changes or acute hypotension.

Anticipation and appreciation of the pathophysiology of aortic cross-clamping is essential to avert a hypertensive crisis. The proximal pressure should be allowed to remain elevated in hopes of improving distal blood flow through collateral circulation. However, the specific target blood pressure range should be individualized so as not to jeopardize cardiac function. In preparation for cross-clamping, the adequacy of anticoagulation should be confirmed, the preload decreased, and depth of anesthesia increased. Vasodilators such as nitroglycerin, anesthetics, and calcium channel antagonists should be titrated to achieve a low-normal blood pressure immediately before clamping. After the aorta is clamped, the infusions of vasodilators should be increased to maintain the systemic vascular resistance in the low-normal range. The choice of vasodilator is controversial because distal aortic and spinal cord perfusion will also decrease. The reader is cautioned against the use of sodium nitroprusside, because of its association with poor neurologic outcomes. The overly aggressive control of proximal aortic pressure with any vasodilator may inadvertently compromise distal spinal cord perfusion.

Unclamping of the thoracic aorta often results in a sudden marked increase in systemic vascular resistance that may precipitate acute cardiovascular collapse. This decrease in cardiac afterload and preload may be related to ischemic metabolites, hypovolemia, left ventricular dysfunction, and redistribution of blood.[58,59] Disastrous consequences can be averted by anticipation and preparation. The surgical and anesthesia teams should maintain good communication to provide adequate warning before the release of the aortic cross-clamp and subsequent reperfusion. The process of releasing the cross-clamp should be slow and deliberate, gradually increasing flow as the blood pressure tolerates. Blood products and vasopressors should be readily available to treat the decrease in blood pressure. Before unclamping, the anesthesiologist should discontinue any vasodilators, decrease anesthetic agents, initiate volume resuscitation to increase preload, and consider administration of a vasopressor immediately before release of the clamp. If hypotension is refractory to bolus administration of vasopressors and volume, the surgeon should temporarily reclamp the aorta to restore pressure. Immediately after cross-clamp release, patients exhibit a combined metabolic and respiratory acidosis and some degree of hyperkalemia. The acidosis resolves with increased ventilation and bicarbonate administration. However, unless a patient is significantly acidemic (pH <7.25), sodium bicarbonate is not administered. Rather than administer bicarbonate empirically, the repletion of bicarbonate should be guided by the following equation:

$$\text{Dose (mEq)} = 0.2 \text{ BW (kg)} \times \text{BE (mEq/kg)}$$

(Equation 2)

where BW and BE denote body weight and base deficit, respectively. One half the calculated dose of bicarbonate can be administered as a bolus and then acid-base status rechecked. Saleh and colleagues showed that sodium bicarbonate infusion at a rate of 0.05 mEq/kg/min was not associated with sudden shifts in pH, $P_{CO_2}$, potassium, or serious cardiac dysrhythmias.[60] In contrast to its requirement in thoracoabdominal aortic surgery, sodium bicarbonate is rarely needed during repair of abdominal aortic aneurysms. Because of the risk for malignant arrhythmias, significant hyperkalemia should be aggressively managed with sodium bicarbonate, calcium, and the administration of insulin and dextrose.

### Passive Shunting

The technique of passively shunting blood from the proximal aorta distally was introduced in an effort to provide distal perfusion and reduce the dramatic hemodynamic changes and complications associated with clamping and unclamping. Passive shunting does provide some distal perfusion but may not ensure adequate distal aortic perfusion.[61,62] Distal aortic perfusion is dependent on shunt diameter and length as well as left ventricular function. Another technical limitation of this strategy is that it does not allow for active temperature control to cool or rewarm the patient. Verdant and associates reported that the use of passive shunt in 380 patients was associated with a low incidence (0.4%) of paraplegia.[61] The same authors described 40 cases with the use of a centrifugal pump (Medtronic, Biomedicus Inc, Eden Prairie, Minn) and reported that partial bypass significantly increased distal flow and pressure. Although previously proponents of passive shunting, they recognized that partial bypass provided superior physiologic conditions and altered their routine surgical practice.

The hemodynamic challenges posed by clamping and unclamping of the thoracic aorta are significantly attenuated by passive shunting as compared with the simple clamp-and-sew technique. However, the anesthesiologist must still be prepared to treat any acute changes in blood pressure and heart rate. In skilled hands, there appears to be a role for passive shunting because it provides good results while being inexpensive and readily available.

### Partial Bypass

Active shunting using partial bypass reliably offers several advantages beyond passive shunting or simple cross-clamping (see later discussion about strategies for spinal cord protection). Partial bypass provides better distal aortic perfusion, allows for control of systemic cooling and warming, and provides for rapid volume transfusion in the event of major hemorrhage. Oxygenated blood is removed from the proximal cannulation site in the left atrium or left pulmonary vein and infused into the distal aorta or femoral artery. Anticoagulation is required, but heparin administration may be reduced when using heparin-coated circuits or excluding the oxygenator and cardiotomy reservoir from the bypass circuit. The typical partial bypass flows of 25 to 40 mL/kg/min provide adequate distal flow and decompression of the heart.

The proximal and distal perfusion is a balance of left ventricular preload, venous drainage to the bypass circuit, and vascular tone. The precise management of these variables requires clear communication and cooperation between the anesthesiologist and perfusionist. The mean proximal pressure, as monitored from the right radial artery, should be maintained at least 60 to 70 mm Hg to guarantee adequate cerebral and coronary perfusion. This proximal pressure can be increased by volume administration or decreasing the rate of bypass flow. Decreased venous drainage for the bypass circuit increases left ventricular preload and thereby increases proximal systemic pressure. The distal mean arterial pressure, as monitored from a femoral artery or distal aorta, should be maintained at >60 mm Hg to provide adequate distal perfusion.[62] The distal aortic pressure can be increased by increasing flow of the centripetal pump or augmenting vascular tone by administration of phenylephrine.

## Cardiopulmonary Bypass

The choice of full CPB is an option for patients with severe pulmonary or cardiac dysfunction or when the aortic pathology involves the distal arch and proximal descending thoracic aorta. This technique offers the advantages of maintaining total control of respiratory function for patients who are unable to tolerate single-lung ventilation and of preventing cardiac decompensation related to acute changes in afterload. Use of CPB dissociates the hemodynamic control from cardiac function, allowing for deep hypothermic circulatory arrest in cases that require proximal anastomosis at the aortic arch. For a more in-depth discussion of the management issues of CPB and circulatory arrest, see Chapter 17.

## The Future Is Here: Intraaortic Stents

A new and increasingly popular technology is that of implantation of endovascular stents to treat diseases of the thoracic[63-69] and abdominal aorta.[70-73] This emerging technology typifies the general movement in medicine toward less invasive procedures, which we hope will result in a lower rate of complications and shorter recuperative period. The intravascular stent is a compressed wire cage covered with a woven fabric sheath that is deployed into position by inflation of an intraaortic balloon (Fig. 65–6). As the stent decreases in length, the aortic diameter increases, and the stent is anchored into the wall of the aorta by hooks.

The implantation of endovascular prostheses has been used to treat aortic aneurysms, pseudoaneurysms,[66,70] traumatic transections,[74] congenital coarctation,[75] dissections, mycotic aneurysms,[69] aortoesophageal fistula,[68] and aortopulmonary fistulas.[76] The 30-day mortality rate was about 9% to 15%.[77-79]

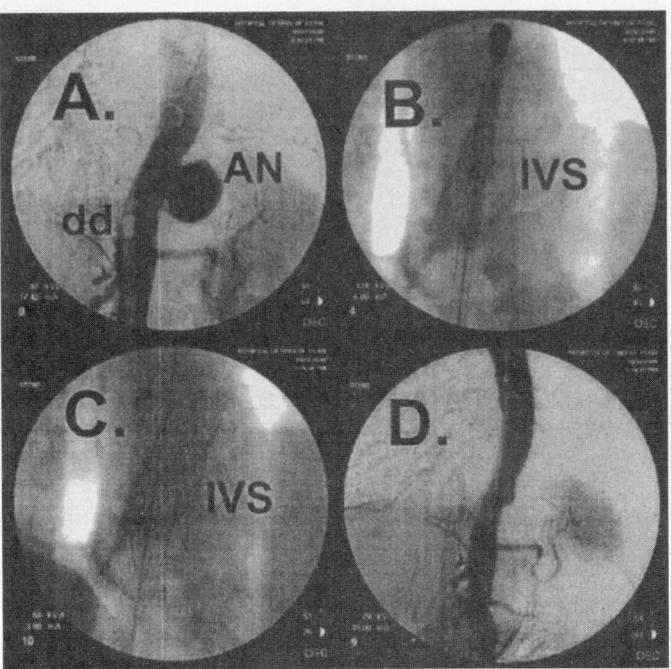

**FIGURE 65–6.** Deployment of intravascular stent to thoracic pseudoaneurysm. *A*, A 71-year-old patient with severe lung disease and a leaking thoracic pseudoaneurysm (AN) is visualized by angiography. The intravascular deployment device (dd) can be seen below the lesion. *B*, Deployment of the first intravascular stent (IVS) across the opening of the pseudoaneurysm and a second stent being positioned proximal to the lesion. *C*, The netlike appearance of the 3 stents across the aortic defect is visualized by fluoroscopy. *D*, The efficacy of the intravascular stent to exclude the pseudoaneurysm is demonstrated by angiography.

In addition, other acute and long-term complications include repositioning of the stent, perforation with rupture or leak, emboli, renal insufficiency, stroke, and paralysis.[80,81] The leakage of blood at the graft site is a potentially lethal complication. It most commonly occurs at the site of distal or proximal attachment and presents either asymptomatically as an incidental finding on follow-up computed tomography scan or clinically as cardiovascular distress from an expanding hematoma or frank exsanguination. However, the incidence of such complications should decrease with the increasing experience of the operator and improvements in technology.

Preoperative evaluation should be the same as for any patient having major vascular surgery (see previous section, What Are the Most Common Coexisting Diseases and Their Implications for the Anesthesiologist?). Management of anesthesia for endovascular stenting is dependent on multiple factors such as experience of the surgical team, location and pathology of the aortic disease, and anticipation of an inflammatory response with increased fluid requirement postoperatively. Most patients undergoing intraaortic stenting have general anesthesia, but alternative techniques such as epidural and local anesthesia with sedation have been also used successfully. Choice of monitors should include placement of arterial cannula and strong consideration of central venous access for close intraoperative and postoperative monitoring. In addition, TEE has been used to confirm aortic pathology and placement of the stent, in addition to providing hemodynamic assessment.[82] However, application of TEE for these procedures at our institution is infrequent because most of the information that it provides is redundant, and the availability of TEE is limited. Although the procedure is noninvasive, all patients having deployment of an intravascular stent are at risk for sudden conversion to an open repair of the aortic pathology. Conversion may occur because of failure to position the intravascular stent appropriately, acute aortic dissection, or perforation of the aorta that may present either as a small extravasation of contrast dye with formation of a hematoma or as acute hypotension resulting from frank rupture. The incidence of conversion ranges from 2% to 8%.[66,77] Because of postoperative fluid requirements and the risk for acutely converting to an open procedure, we routinely place at least one large intravenous catheter.

A less invasive surgical procedure does not mean a benign postoperative course. These patients undergo an inflammatory reaction, which seems similar to that experienced for an open procedure.[83] These patients are at risk for increased alveolar-to-arterial gradients, large fluid shifts, hyperpyrexia, and arrhythmias and require titration of $O_2$ supplementation and fluid replacement in a closely monitored setting.

### What Therapeutic Interventions Can Be Used to Decrease the Risk for Postoperative Renal Failure?

One of the most common complications after aortic surgery is that of renal failure.[84] The reported incidence of postoperative renal failure is between 3% and 18% in thoracoabdominal operations[85,86] and 40% after ruptured abdominal aortal aneurysms, with intermediate numbers for elective procedures.[87] In many of the same studies, the mortality rate for postoperative renal failure in patients with ruptured aortic aneurysms has been reported to be as high as 90%. Although the main culprit for acute renal failure is decreased perfusion during the perioperative period, there are other factors that may place additional risk. These include a history of preoperative renal dysfunction, hypotension, diabetes, and associated atherosclerotic disease. In addition, the administration of intravenous contrast for angiography may worsen preexisting renal dysfunction. Intraoperative factors such as general anesthetics, intraoperative hypotension, atheromatous embolization, surgical trauma, reperfusion injury secondary to free radicals (reactive hyperemia), and an increase in plasma renin activity also contribute to perioperative impairment of renal function.[88-90] Five basic approaches to decrease the incidence of renal failure are presented in Table 65–9.

Many management strategies have attempted to improve outcome but, in general, the documented benefit has been controversial. Strategies to preserve renal function entail mod-

**TABLE 65–9.** Methods to Prevent Renal Failure During the Perioperative Period

Optimize intravascular volume status, avoiding hypovolemia.
Avoid or adjust dose of nephrotoxic medications.
Ensure adequate recovery of renal function after contrast dye administration.
Maintain good indices of cardiac performance and perfusion pressures.
Avoid use of vasopressor medications that decrease renal blood flow.
Limit use of diuretic therapy that would cause hypovolemia.
Institute drug therapy: mannitol, dopamine (efficacy unproven).
Minimize duration of suprarenal aortic cross-clamping.
Use distal shunts to increase renal blood flow.
Use hypothermia during aortic cross-clamping.

ifying preoperative, intraoperative, and postoperative management. Patients should be adequately hydrated before and after receiving intravenous contrast, and surgery should be postponed until renal function returns to baseline.[8] Another important strategy for renal protection is the avoidance of potentially nephrotoxic drugs. Some drugs such as nonsteroidal inflammatory drugs (ie, ketorolac) have deleterious effects on renal blood flow and should be avoided. In addition, other drugs such as some antibiotics can be nephrotoxic and should therefore be avoided or dosed by level.

The risk for intraoperative renal failure is multifactorial and reflects ischemia from the transient interruption of vascular supply, embolic injury, reperfusion injury, and relative hypoperfusion associated with hypovolemia. Surgery on the descending aorta often involves a period of renal ischemia or hypoperfusion until blood flow can be reestablished. The use of vascular shunts during prolonged ischemic periods has been shown to decrease the risk for postoperative renal failure. Alternatively, the administration of renoplegia with cold crystalloid does not decrease the risk for postoperative renal dysfunction.[91] In addition to ischemia-hypoperfusion and emboli, humoral mediators released during a systemic inflammatory response may exacerbate preexisting renal dysfunction due to vasoconstriction, redistribution of blood flow, and changes in vascular permeability.

Hypovolemia is perhaps one of the more common factors precipitating postoperative renal dysfunction. Maintenance of adequate intravascular volume may be difficult in these patients because of third spacing and fear of the pulmonary consequences of volume overload. In addition, diuretics are commonly administered as prophylactic agents before aortic cross-clamping of renal flow. It is unclear whether there is any prophylactic benefit to using diuretics for renal preservation. Administration of diuretics to increase urine output can exacerbate renal dysfunction by turning latent hypovolemia into prerenal azotemia. Moreover, the administration of diuretics intraoperatively to protect renal function may mask intravascular hypovolemia and cause further depletion.

Mannitol (0.25-0.5 g/kg) is commonly administered intraoperatively to increase urine output and protect renal function. Its protective effects are through two mechanisms: (1) scavenging of free radicals and thus attenuating reperfusion injury, and (2) a tendency to reverse cortical ischemia.[92,93] Renal injury is associated with a shift of blood flow from the cortical to juxtamedullary nephrons. The net result is salt retention and a reduction in urine output. Mannitol can reverse this shift by inciting an osmotic diuresis and preventing cortical ischemia. However, these putative clinical benefits have not been conclusively proven to improve outcome. In addition to the postulated renal benefits, mannitol may protect the spinal cord from ischemia by decreasing CSF pressure and thereby increasing the distal cord perfusion pressure.

The administration of renal-dose dopamine (1-3 μg/kg/min) is widely practiced but has not been shown to provide effective renal protection. Although dopamine increases urine output, increased urine output is not necessarily associated with improved creatinine clearance and outcome. Duke and colleagues compared the renal effects of dopamine and dobutamine in postoperative critically ill patients.[94] Dobutamine improved creatinine clearance but did not increase urine output. The true role of dopamine may lie in its ability not only to produce natriuresis but also to maintain supernormal hemodynamics and provide prophylaxis against mesenteric hypoperfusion. Perhaps a more receptor-specific DA-1 receptor agonist such as fenoldopam will improve outcome. Fenoldopam may be advantageous by increasing renal blood flow and producing a natriuresis while decreasing systemic and splanchnic vascular resistance.[95,96]

The most important therapeutic strategy to protect the kidneys is that of optimizing the hemodynamics or maintaining $O_2$ delivery. One should increase cardiac output with the goal of slightly increasing preload and contractility. It is advisable to avoid vasoconstrictors such as phenylephrine or norepinephrine, which tend to elevate the blood pressure but may compromise renal perfusion.

## Why Does Paraplegia Occur, and What Can Be Done to Prevent It?

### Anterior Spinal Artery Syndrome

The most devastating complication following surgery of the descending aorta is paraplegia, with an incidence that ranges from 1% to 40%.[97–99] The clinical presentation resembles the anterior spinal artery syndrome, which results from occlusion of the artery radicularis magna (artery of Adamkiewicz) that supplies the anterior portion of the spinal cord. The associated neurologic deficit is localized to the anterior aspect of the spinal cord and characterized by loss of motor function and pinprick sensation (Fig. 65–7). The vibratory and position sensations that travel in the posterior column are supplied by the posterior spinal arteries and remain intact.

### Perfusion

Susceptibility to spinal cord ischemia is related to perfusion of the spinal cord. Aortic cross-clamping during surgery com-

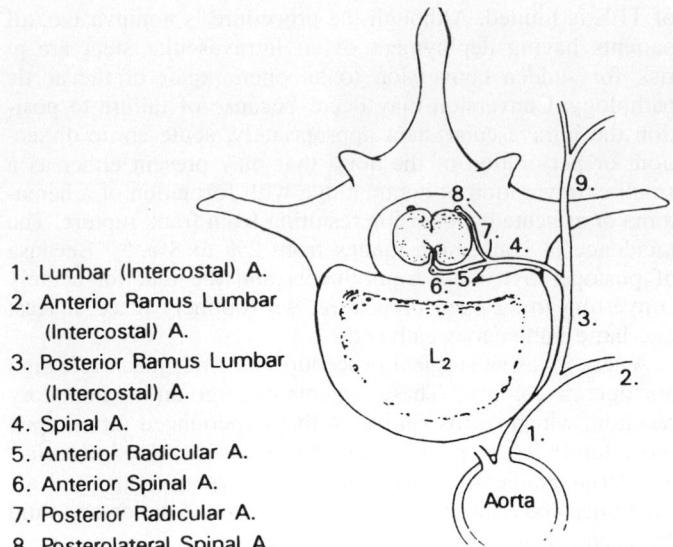

1. Lumbar (Intercostal) A.
2. Anterior Ramus Lumbar (Intercostal) A.
3. Posterior Ramus Lumbar (Intercostal) A.
4. Spinal A.
5. Anterior Radicular A.
6. Anterior Spinal A.
7. Posterior Radicular A.
8. Posterolateral Spinal A.
9. Muscular Branches

**FIGURE 65–8.** Spinal cord blood supply. (Adapted from Szilagyi DE, Hageman JH, Smith RF, et al. Spinal cord damage in surgery of the abdominal aorta. *Surgery.* 1978;83:38.)

promises regional blood flow, rendering perfusion of the anterior spinal cord tenuous (Fig. 65–8). Unlike the posterior third of the spinal cord, which is supplied by two posterior spinal arteries, the anterior two thirds of the cord is supplied by a single anterior spinal artery that has poor collateral blood flow, particularly at the midthoracic level (see Fig. 65–7). The posterior spinal artery, which has a well-developed collateral flow, is less dependent on the integrity of individual radicular vessels and is thus more resistant to ischemia. In addition, the posterior spinal artery is continuous through the length of the spinal cord. However, the anterior spinal artery generally lacks this vertical continuity and relies on radicular branches for its blood supply.

At the level of the cervical spinal cord, the anterior spinal artery is primarily supplied by branches of the vertebral artery and remains relatively well perfused during thoracic aortic cross-clamping. At the level of the lumbar sacral cord, the anterior spinal artery is supplied by several branches of the internal iliac arteries. Because of relative luxury perfusion, clamping of the aorta during a repair of an abdominal aortic aneurysm is rarely associated with paraplegia.[100,101] However, the anterior artery spinal cord perfusion of the middle and lower thoracic region is more tenuous because it is supplied only by a few radicular arteries (branches of intercostal arteries), the largest of which is the artery of Adamkiewicz. Multiple levels of the thoracic cord do not have individual radicular branches and depend on the artery radicularis magna. The absence of luxury perfusion at the thoracic level results in watershed areas of the spinal cord that are susceptible to ischemic injury during aortic cross-clamping. Conventional opinion states that there is only one artery radicularis magna. However, the belief of a single dominant supply of blood may need to be appended. The critical blood supply of the spinal cord may depend on several vessels.[43,102]

### Risk Factors

The risk for paraplegia is related to three major risk factors: acuity of surgery, extent of aortic pathology, and duration of

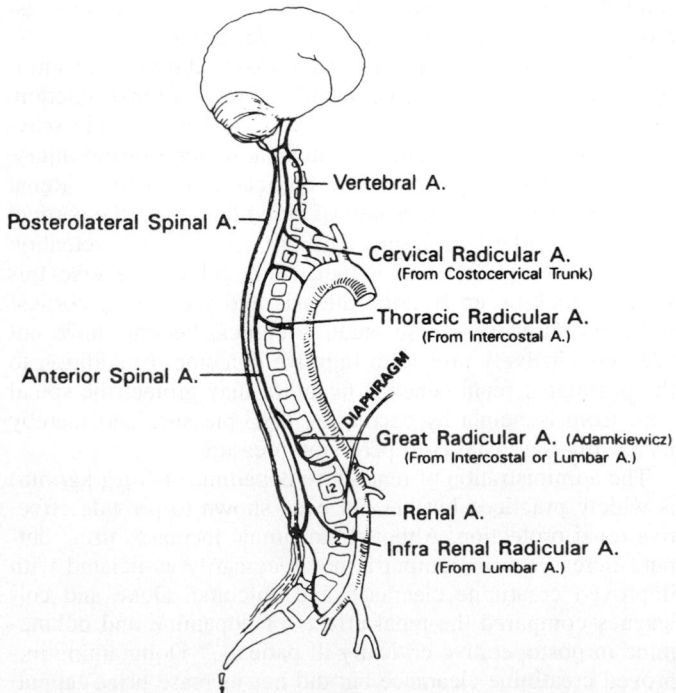

Vertebral A.
Posterolateral Spinal A.
Cervical Radicular A. (From Costocervical Trunk)
Thoracic Radicular A. (From Intercostal A.)
Anterior Spinal A.
DIAPHRAGM
Great Radicular A. (Adamkiewicz) (From Intercostal or Lumbar A.)
Renal A.
Infra Renal Radicular A. (From Lumbar A.)

**FIGURE 65–7.** Spinal cord blood supply. (Adapted from Szilagyi DE, Hageman JH, Smith RF, et al. Spinal cord damage in surgery of the abdominal aorta. *Surgery.* 1978;83:38.)

aortic cross-clamping. Emergency aortic surgery is associated with a higher risk for neurologic complications than is an elective procedure. Patients with chronic aortic disease are believed to develop collateral circulation, making them more resistant to temporary interruption than to aortic cross-clamping.[103] The incidence of paraplegia is related to the location, extent of aortic pathology, and origins of the vascular supply. Neurologic deficits are most commonly associated with type II aneurysms, followed by type I and, least commonly, type III and type IV aneurysms.[104] This distribution reflects the origin of the artery of Adamkiewicz, which is variable but usually arises between the levels of T5 and L3. Its origin is between T5 and T8 in 15% of patients, between T9 and T12 in 60%, and at L1 in 14% of patients, with the remainder arising from either L2 or L3.[101,105]

Ischemic periods of >30 minutes, as defined by the duration of aortic cross-clamping, markedly increase the risk for postoperative paralysis.[106-108] The duration of aortic cross-clamping is not the only period in which the patient is in jeopardy. The patient remains at significant risk for new neurologic deficits within the first 3 postoperative days. Reperfusion hyperemia and edema from intraoperative ischemia make the cord especially vulnerable in patients who have marginal circulation because of pressure-dependent collateral blood flow. Other possible mechanisms of postoperative neurologic injury include hypercoagulable states, spinal cord edema, hypotension, and vascular spasm of a vessel that supplies an already tenuous circulation.

## What Are the Techniques and Strategies to Enhance Distal Spinal Cord Perfusion?

Our current understanding of spinal cord ischemia following thoracoabdominal aortic repair has evolved from animal research and clinical experience. A number of surgical, pharmacologic, and circulatory strategies have developed over the years to reduce the incidence of cord ischemia, yet a great deal of controversy still exists with regard to the optimal protective strategy. The multiplicity of strategies and adjuncts attests to the view that no single method has been totally effective universally. Rather, individual surgeons and institutions have adopted methods that have proven effective in reducing spinal cord injury when compared with historical controls. The major paradigm is that a decreased $O_2$ demand and an increased supply of blood and $O_2$ result in a decreased risk for spinal cord ischemia.

### Circulatory Management

The risk for postoperative paraplegia rises rapidly after 30 minutes of thoracic aortic cross-clamp time.[106-108] Mauney and associates reported that their experience with the clamp-and-sew technique without use of adjunct therapies (1987-1994) was associated with a 10% incidence of spinal cord injury.[109] Distal aortic perfusion is often performed to preserve spinal cord, mesenteric, and renal blood flow to regulate body temperature and eliminate the physiologic consequences of clamping and releasing the aortic cross-clamp. The need and benefit for implementing shunts during cross-clamp times of <30 minutes is controversial.[99,110]

Aortic bypass is accomplished by either implantation of an extraluminal "passive shunt" (ie, Gott shunt: a heparin-bonded shunt from the apex of the left ventricle to the femoral artery) or institution of active bypass from the left atrium to the femoral artery using a centrifugal pump. Passive shunt techniques do not consistently provide adequate bypass because of inherent limitations of device design and the inability to monitor and control flow accurately. More important, passive distal shunting may not prevent the deleterious decrease in SCPP that follows aortic cross-clamping.[111] Active shunting using the left atrium–to–femoral artery technique is superior to passive shunts in effecting proximal unloading by allowing for precise adjustment of blood flow to equilibrate proximal and distal aortic pressures. The adequacy of distal perfusion is monitored by measuring the distal aortic pressure and assessing the affect on neurophysiologic monitoring. The blood pressure distal to the aortic cross-clamp is commonly monitored with a femoral arterial catheter or a cannula inserted into the aorta by the surgeon. Jacobs and colleagues found that the mean distal aortic pressure that was required to maintain adequate cord perfusion was 66 mm Hg, but varied widely among individuals, ranging from 48 to 110 mm Hg.[62] Although these bypass techniques require heparinization, which may increase blood loss, the risk for such interventions is outweighed by their potential benefit during surgical repair of the thoracic aorta.

### Surgical Technique

The application of therapeutic interventions to protect the cord from intraoperative ischemia will fail if the vascular supply is sacrificed. Most surgeons attempt to reimplant intercostal arteries, especially in the region of thoracic aorta at T9 to T12.[112] Few surgeons localize the artery of Adamkiewicz preoperatively, whereas some use intraoperative SSEP or MEP to ascertain an island of segmental intercostal arteries to reattach. Preoperative localization of the artery of Adamkiewicz by angiography, which has a success rate of only 65%, is time-consuming and may increase the risk for renal injury related to dye injection.[113] Although the artery of Adamkiewicz is important, other segmental arteries may also be important contributors to spinal cord supply in circumstances of decreased spinal cord perfusion.[43,102]

The thoracic radicular and iliolumbar arteries may achieve greater importance under perioperative circumstances. In contrast to these segmental arteries, the artery of Adamkiewicz has a hairpin downward bend that preferentially directs the flow of blood distally in the caudal direction. Because of this, many investigators have recommended that the posterior wall of the aorta be preserved and reattached as a pedicle of the prosthetic graft to revascularize the thoracic spinal cord. The size of this vascular pedicle is determined by the extent of back-bleeding when the aorta is opened. The practice of vascular reanastomosis is supported by clinical observations of Griepp and colleagues, who found that neurologic deficits were encountered only when >10 segmental arteries were sacrificed.[102]

### Drainage of Cerebrospinal Fluid

A major strategy to prevent spinal cord ischemia is to maintain adequate spinal cord blood flow (SCBF) and SCPP. Although perfusion pressures that protect the spinal cord against ischemic injury have been determined in a dog model during supraceliac aortic cross-clamping, no corresponding critical level has been established in human beings. Differences in the anatomic spinal cord blood supply between human beings and dogs probably make comparisons between the two species inappropriate.

The spinal cord and associated structures are contained in a nondistensible bony vertebral channel. Because the spinal cord is susceptible to "compartment syndrome," any intervention that affects either SCBF or spinal cord fluid pressure (SCFP) affects SCPP. SCPP is defined as the difference between distal mean arterial pressure (MAP) and SCFP:

$$SCPP = Distal\ MAP - SCFP \qquad \text{(Equation 3)}$$

Cross-clamping the thoracic aorta in dogs and human beings increases the SCFP and therefore decreases SCPP.[114] This decrease in SCPP may be exacerbated by the use of sodium nitroprusside to control proximal hypertension because it increases SCFP and decreases distal aortic pressure (see The Use of Vasodilators). The price paid for overly aggressive treatment of proximal hypertension may be postoperative paraplegia.

Equation 3 provides the rationale for various therapeutic interventions (Table 65–10). The most notable is that withdrawal of CSF increases SCPP and blood flow to the spinal cord. Most studies in human beings that reported beneficial

**TABLE 65–10.** Strategies to Decrease the Risk for Spinal Cord Deficits

**Increase Spinal Cord Perfusion Pressure**

*Increase distal aortic pressure*

Proximal hypertension during simple clamp-and-sew technique
Passive shunt (eg, Gott shunt)
Partial bypass (ie, left atrium to femoral artery)
Cardiopulmonary bypass
Restricted use of vasodilators that decrease distal spinal cord perfusion

*Decrease CSF pressure*

CSF drainage

**Decrease Spinal Cord Vascular Resistance**

Intrathecal papaverine (dilates anterior spinal artery)

**Decrease Metabolic Rate**

General hypothermia (mild, deep hypothermic circulatory arrest)
Selective hypothermia (infusion in epidural space)

**Pharmacologic Therapies**

Steroids
Magnesium
Mannitol

*Therapies With Some Efficacy in Animal Studies*

NMDA antagonists
Calcium-channel blockers
Allopurinol
Superoxide dismutase
Naloxone
Barbiturates, propofol
Desferoxamine
Aprotinin
Prostaglandin $E_1$

**Other Strategies**

Aggressive control of blood glucose (avoid hyperglycemia)
Reimplantation of segmental arteries
Monitoring (SSEP, MEP, CSF pressure, distal aortic pressure)

CSF, cerebrospinal fluid; MEP, motor evoked potentials; NMDA, *N*-methyl-D-arginine; SSEP, somatosensory evoked potentials.

effects of CSF drainage are limited because they employed a multimodality approach and retrospective controls.[35,39,44,112,115] Safi and colleagues reported that the incidence of paraplegia in type II repairs using a simple clamp-and-sew technique was appreciably lowered from 29.6% to 8.1% when CSF drainage was combined with distal aortic perfusion.[112] However, in the only randomized prospective study in human beings that examined the role of CSF drainage, postoperative paraplegia or paresis was not prevented.[116] Failure to observe a significantly improved outcome may have been related to the study design, which limited the amount of CSF drainage to 50 mL.

Although the effectiveness of CSF drainage in human beings remains debatable, it is a relatively safe procedure and may prolong the period of ischemia before irreversible neurologic damage occurs. At our institution, CSF is drained to maintain a pressure rise of 10 mm Hg or less. Monitoring and draining of CSF pressure should extend into the postoperative period as well. The potential benefits of CSF drainage are believed to outweigh the risk for side effects, which include headache and, rarely, intrathecal hemorrhage or transtentorial herniation.

## Monitoring

The monitoring of spinal cord function during surgery of the thoracic aorta affords the anesthesiologist and surgeon the opportunity to detect neurologic ischemia in order to alter intraoperative management in the hope of improving outcome (see Table 65–10). SSEP and MEP have been presented in a previous section and receive more comprehensive discussion in Chapter 21. The early detection of spinal cord ischemia may allow for the timely institution of protective measures (distal aortic perfusion, sequential aortic clamping, and selective segmental artery reattachment) that are aimed at restoring adequate spinal cord blood supply. Faberowski and colleagues found that the incidence of intraoperative interventions was 26.4% and that no patient had sustained a neurologic deficit.[41] Although the frequency of their interventions was higher than expected, such monitoring has a definite role in the current practice of this high-risk surgery.

## The Use of Vasodilators

Vasodilators play an important role in controlling hypertension, preventing aortic rupture, and decreasing afterload on the heart, especially during aortic cross-clamping in the absence of distal bypass or during the postoperative period. The choice of vasodilator may affect outcome by deleteriously decreasing spinal cord perfusion, thereby increasing the risk for ischemia. The most commonly used vasoactive agents, nitroglycerin and sodium nitroprusside, differ in regard to their effects on CSF dynamics and the risk for postoperative paraplegia. Sodium nitroprusside decreases SCPP by decreasing blood pressure distal to the aortic cross-clamp and increasing CSF pressure.[117,118] This effect cannot be prevented by drainage of CSF. Nitroglycerin has a better profile with a lower risk for neurologic injury. Although it also decreases SCPP, its effects on CSF dynamics can be counteracted by drainage of CSF.

However, use of any vasodilator that decreases distal perfusion pressure may compromise SCBF. A recent study showed that animals undergoing phlebotomy to lower proximal arterial pressure had significantly better distal aortic pressure, SCPP, and postoperative motor function when compared with those receiving nitroprusside or nitroglycerin.[119]

Intraoperative hypertension can be treated by adjusting left atrial–to–femoral artery bypass and administering more narcotic analgesic or by temporarily increasing the inhalational agent. The reader should be cautioned that inhalational agents used to control proximal hypertension could also reduce SCPP.[120] Other vasoactive agents, such as calcium channel blockers, may be associated with an improved safety profile by decreasing the risk for reperfusion vasospasm that would compromise SCPP.

## Mechanisms of Cell Injury

Spinal cord injury induced by ischemia is a consequence of an initial insult and subsequent reperfusion injury processes that involve various pathochemical events, leading to progressive tissue death and apoptosis. It is these latter processes that are the targets of pharmacologic interventional treatment. Mechanisms of cellular injury involve multiple deleterious processes that include release of excitatory neurotransmitters and generation of free radicals.[121,122] The levels of excitatory amino acids—glutamate and aspartate—significantly increase in response to spinal cord ischemia and reperfusion.[123–126] In various animal models, NMDA receptor antagonists decreased the incidence of paraplegia and extent of histologic damage.[127,128] Activated neutrophils have also been implicated in the damage of endothelial cells by releasing inflammatory mediators, such as neutrophil elastase and $O_2$ free radicals, which perpetuate the cascade of edema and cell injury.[129]

## Pharmacologic Intervention

A major thrust of pharmacologic therapy is to protect against the initial ischemic insult and antagonize the cascade of deleterious reactions that characterize the reperfusion injury. Many investigators have attempted to modulate these reactions with free radical scavengers, antioxidants, excitatory neurotransmitter antagonists, and calcium channel blockers (see Table 65–10).

Steroids are commonly used during thoracic aortic surgery for spinal cord protection. The rationale for their use is not based on prospective trials of spinal cord ischemia but on acute spinal cord trauma. The National Acute Spinal Cord Injury Study was a multicenter prospective randomized placebo-controlled trial that evaluated the efficacy of methylprednisolone or naloxone to attenuate the injury from acute spinal cord trauma and to improve outcome.[130] Patients received either a 30 mg/kg dose of methylprednisolone, followed by an infusion of 5.4 mg/kg/h for the next 23 hours; 5.4 mg/kg of naloxone, followed by an infusion of 4 mg/kg/h for the next 23 hours; or placebo. Significant improvement in both motor and sensory function at 6 weeks, 6 months, and 1 year occurred with incomplete and complete spinal cord lesions in patients receiving methylprednisolone; no benefit was found with naloxone.[130]

Possible complications of steroid administration include immunosuppression and hyperglycemia-induced infection and neurologic injury. Other pharmacologic adjuncts include mannitol as a free radical scavenger and magnesium as a calcium antagonist and membrane stabilizer.[131] The protease inhibitor, aprotinin, may improve neurologic function as well as coagu-

lation status. Recently, aprotinin was found to reduce spinal cord injury in a model of transient spinal cord ischemia in rabbits.[132] At best, many pharmacologic agents to attenuate the ischemia-induced cascade of cell injury and death have been investigated in animals, but few have advanced to clinical trials. As yet, the clinical application of NMDA inhibitors, free radical scavengers, and calcium channel antagonists remains an area of active research. A list of suggested pharmacologic adjunct therapies is presented in Table 65–10.

Pharmacologic adjuncts have also been used to improve spinal cord perfusion. Intrathecal papaverine and intravenous prostaglandin $E_1$ have been demonstrated to improve neurologic outcome in animal studies and have been incorporated clinically in a multifaceted approach with other therapies.[115,133–136]

## Hypothermia

By far, the most effective strategy to increase ischemic tolerance is hypothermia. Along with lowering the metabolic rate, hypothermia reduces the loss of intracellular adenosine triphosphate, with resolution of lactate accumulation, and decreases the release of the excitatory neurotransmitter glutamate.[124–126] The technique of hypothermia has proved successful when applied to selective cooling of the spinal cord or the whole body.[137–139]

The institution of mild to moderate hypothermia is common for routine cardiac operations. This technique has been extended recently to provide brain protection in cases of prolonged circulation arrest. Several investigators have successfully used profound hypothermia for circulatory arrest in patients undergoing extensive thoracoabdominal aneurysmectomy.[140–142] These investigators advocate the use of this technique for surgery involving the proximal descending thoracic aorta when control of the proximal aorta may be difficult or when the risk for cerebral embolism is high. Even a slight reduction in body temperature of 3°C doubled the duration of ischemia that could be reversibly sustained in rabbits.[131] Many surgeons employ mild hypothermia (33°-34°C), by positioning a heat exchanger in the bypass circuit to cool and rewarm patients efficiently.

Several investigators advocate the use of selective cooling of the spinal cord. Cambria and associates reported that regional cooling of the spinal cord using the clamp-and-sew technique without bypass provided results comparable to those cases managed with active bypass.[138] They infused iced saline (4°C) into the epidural space 30 minutes before cross-clamping to lower the temperature of the spinal cord to 26°C. Any intervention, whether pharmacologic or mechanical, that affects SCFP ultimately affects SCBF. Although any volume infused into the epidural space increases SCFP and decreases SCPP, the authors reported that the incidence of paraplegia decreased from 23% to 2.9%.[138] It is unlikely that this technique will achieve widespread implementation because of the inability to control intrathecal pressures and the common availability of distal bypass.

## Ischemic Preconditioning

The strategy of ischemic preconditioning for neural protection has recently gained interest. Brief periods of ischemia with subsequent perfusion are theorized to render tissues more resistant to subsequent, more prolonged ischemic insults. Several animal studies have demonstrated that the induction of a short period of spinal cord ischemia provides a protective benefit and improves neurologic outcome.[143–146] The putative mechanism of ischemic tolerance induced by preconditioning may involve formation of new proteins, such as heat-shock proteins, or modification of existing molecules.[146] The clinical application of this strategy to thoracic aortic surgery has not been reported. Practical factors, such as timing of ischemic conditioning, the interval required to produce its putative protective benefit, and clinical efficacy, are unknown. The risk for embolization and rupture associated with manipulation of the aorta renders the widespread application of this strategy unlikely.

## Does Paraplegia Occur in Patients Having Abdominal Aortic Surgery?

The incidence of spinal cord damage following abdominal aortic surgery is low: 0.25% in a series of 3164 patients.[101] All cases of paraplegia occurred after aneurysmal aortic surgery; none followed surgery for occlusive aortic disease. The incidence of postoperative paraplegia in patients having emergency surgery for ruptured abdominal aortic aneurysm was 10 times higher than in patients having surgery for unruptured aneurysms. The probability of spinal cord ischemia would be markedly increased if the aorta is cross-clamped proximal to the takeoff of the artery of Adamkiewicz in patients who do not have extensive, well-developed infrarenal lumbar radicular arteries.[100] In addition, other secondary factors that were mentioned in the previous sections are probably crucial to the development of postoperative paraplegia following abdominal aortic cross-clamping.

## What Are the Management Strategies for Coagulation and Transfusion Therapies?

The approach to blood component transfusion should be rational and timely. The first principle is to employ perioperative blood conservation whenever possible. Preoperative autologous donation is indicated when possible, especially in patients with a rare blood phenotype or multiple red blood cell antibodies. The American Association of Blood Banks recommends autologous donation in patients having a hemoglobin concentration >11 g/dL.[147] Contraindications to autologous blood donation include severe aortic stenosis, unstable angina, or left main coronary artery disease.

In cases of elective surgery, preoperative red blood cell mass may be increased by iron supplementation or erythropoietin therapy. Intraoperatively, red blood cell salvage using cell-saver technology should be routine, but its implementation in the presence of infection should be arrested. Another commonly used intraoperative strategy is acute isovolemic hemodilution in patients with a hematocrit of >30%. The harvested whole blood is administered after surgical blood loss or CPB to avoid bypass-induced platelet dysfunction. Use of these strategies may avoid or limit allogeneic red blood cell transfusion, which is especially important for the perioperative care of Jehovah's Witnesses.

In general, a single hemoglobin concentration should not be used as a transfusion threshold for all patients. The decision to transfuse red blood cells is multifactorial. Red blood cell transfusion is almost always indicated with a hemoglobin concentration of <6 g/dL and is rarely indicated with a hemoglobin concentration of >10 g/dL.[148] The threshold to transfuse is lower for this surgical population of patients because of the prevalence of concomitant coronary artery disease, impaired ventricular function, and chronic obstructive pulmonary disease than for younger patients without coincident disease. Transfusion of red blood cells is not the only therapy that increases $O_2$ delivery to the tissues. For example, an increase in hemoglobin content from 9 to 10 g/dL elevates $O_2$ delivery by 11%. However, increasing cardiac performance from a cardiac index of 2.0 to 2.5 increases $O_2$ delivery by 25%.

Intraoperative blood loss may be significant and lead to a quantitative decrease of coagulation factors and platelets and to a qualitative dysfunction of platelets. The rationale for transfusion of component therapy should be based on laboratory data and experience. Often, this type of testing is unavailable within the operating room, and obtaining test results in a timely manner is problematic. Some institutions have the availability of a thromboelastography, which analyzes the coagulation changes. Thromboelastography can assess platelet and clotting factor function and diagnose bleeding dyscrasias as well as hypercoagulable states that can occur after aortic surgery.[149]

The timely assessment of platelet quantity and function is often unavailable. The decision for platelet transfusion proceeds most often on clinical impression and the presence of microvascular bleeding. Platelet transfusion is usually indicated for microvascular bleeding with a platelet count of $<50 \times 10^9$. Platelet therapy for platelet counts between 50 and $100 \times 10^9$ should consider anticipated blood loss, presence of microvascular bleeding, or qualitative platelet dysfunction from aspirin administration, uremia, or CPB. The qualitative platelet dysfunction related to aspirin therapy or bypass cannot be reversed pharmacologically. However, uremia-induced platelet dysfunction can be reversed with the administration of DDAVP.[150] Any putative beneficial effect of DDAVP for a coagulopathy caused by cirrhosis or aspirin is, as yet, unproved. DDAVP, at a dosage of 0.3 µg/kg, should be slowly administered intravenously to avoid the occurrence of hypotension. The onset of action is about 30 minutes. The necessity for repeat administration should be determined by the presence of clinical bleeding and laboratory testing. Tachyphylaxis is observed with repeated administration.

A coagulopathy may also result from factor deficiencies related to hemodilution and consumption. Administration of fresh frozen plasma is indicated for microvascular bleeding with either an activated partial thromboplastin time or a prothrombin time >1.5 times normal.[148] Fresh frozen plasma dosed at 10 to 15 mL/kg usually achieves a minimum of 30% of plasma factor concentrations, which, in most instances, is adequate for effective hemostasis. In addition, fresh frozen plasma administration acutely reverses a warfarin sodium (Coumadin)-induced coagulopathy.[148] In elective situations, parenteral administration of vitamin K produces the same effect within 12 hours.

Blood loss and transfusion requirements may be reduced by administration of antifibrinolytic agents (ε-aminocaproic acid, tranexamic acid, and aprotinin), which have proved efficacious in cardiac surgery.[151–153] ε-Aminocaproic acid and tranexamic acid inhibit plasmin-induced fibrinolysis. Both of these agents are widely available, are inexpensive, and have a wide therapeutic index with a good safety profile.

Aprotinin is a protease inhibitor that is isolated from bovine lung. It has a variety of effects on the coagulation pathway and inflammatory response. It prevents fibrinolysis by inhibition of plasmin and kallikrein and protects platelets by preserving adhesive glycoproteins, making them resistant to damage.[154] Aprotinin also attenuates the inflammatory response and has been implicated as a neuroprotective agent. Although aprotinin has been shown to be more efficacious for minimizing blood loss and transfusion, it has a number of potential detractors, such as cost, concerns of thrombosis, and risk for allergic reaction with subsequent exposures.[132,155]

## Should Patients Be Extubated in the Operating Room?

All patients remain intubated after major thoracic aortic surgery. If a double-lumen ETT is used, it is usually changed to a large single-lumen ETT (>8 mm) to perform pulmonary toilet adequately and to facilitate weaning from mechanical ventilation. Excessive left-lung manipulation during surgery may result in alveolar trauma and bronchial hemorrhage that may be exacerbated by heparinization during bypass. Any secretions and blood clots can partially obstruct the airway causing ventilation-perfusion ($\dot{V}/\dot{Q}$) mismatching and clinically significant alveolar-arterial $O_2$ gradients. In addition, patients may remain intubated for a prolonged time because of compromised respiratory mechanics related to pain, phrenic nerve paralysis, and diaphragmatic dysfunction. The timing for extubation depends on factors such as adequate rewarming, pain control, respiratory pattern, respiratory mechanics, neurologic status, hemostasis, and hemodynamics.

The exchange of a double-lumen for a single-lumen ETT may be performed by direct laryngoscopy. If the vocal cords cannot be visualized and the airway appears edematous, tube exchange may be facilitated by using an ETT changer or by fiberoptic laryngoscopy. However, if the tube exchange is judged to place the patient at increased risk, the double-lumen ETT can be changed later in the intensive care unit after airway swelling has receded. As discussed previously, the newer ETTs (Univent, Arndt) that contain a bronchial blocker obviate changing the tube at the end of the procedure.

## Is There a Role for the Anesthesiologist in Postoperative Care?

There is a definite role for the anesthesiologist as an intensivist or as a consultant in the postoperative period. Anesthesiologists are often institutional experts in airway management, mechanical ventilation with double-lumen ETTs, titration of muscle relaxants and sedatives, and administration of postoperative analgesia. Anesthesiologists also have expertise in invasive hemodynamic monitoring, use of vasoactive agents, and TEE. As a profession, we should embrace these challenges to improve patient care while educating the medical staff of our diverse role in providing perioperative care.

At the time of transfer to the intensive care unit, the patient should be hemodynamically stable and adequately sedated. A high priority should be given to maintaining tight management of blood pressure to avoid untoward stress on the new suture

lines (Table 65–11). The target mean arterial blood pressure typically ranges from 65 to 75 mm Hg but is adjusted accordingly in the presence of carotid artery or coronary artery disease. These goals are best achieved by the infusion of a vasodilator (nitroglycerin, sodium nitroprusside, or nicardipine) and sedation, with careful titration of small doses of a narcotic or benzodiazepine. Alternatively, the degree of sedation may be better controlled with an infusion of propofol or, in the future, with other agents, such as central $\alpha_2$-adrenergic receptor agonists, and dexmedetomidine.[156] Postoperative sedation should continue until the patients are adequately rewarmed, at which time it should be titrated to permit smooth emergence with minimal hypertension and tachycardia.

Patients are often hypothermic after major aortic surgery because of the heat loss from the pericardial, pleural, and peritoneal cavities. Postoperative hypothermia increases the risk for coagulopathy, bleeding, infection, and myocardial ischemia. The use of forced warmed air blankets should be initiated early to normalize body temperature.

Any episodes of hypotension should be aggressively treated to avoid further ischemic insult to the spinal cord or kidney that may contribute to poor neurologic outcome. Maintaining tight hemodynamic control during the initial postoperative period is important to permit recovery from any ischemic and perfusion injuries that occurred during the intraoperative period. The anesthetic technique should permit an adequate neurologic evaluation within several hours after surgery. Although the classic anterior spinal artery occlusion syndrome affects bilateral motor function, a common clinical presentation is unilateral motor weakness. Detection of a new neurologic deficit should be aggressively pursued by increasing mean arterial pressure and draining more CSF in an attempt to increase SCPP. In addition, specific diagnostic imaging studies may detect potentially correctable lesions, such as an epidural hematoma. Because of the risk for adverse outcome related to intraoperative management, the epidural catheter should not be injected with local anesthetic until a neurologic examination has been performed.

### Postoperative Analgesia

Postoperative analgesia is always indicated. The route of analgesic delivery is either epidural or parenteral. Epidural catheter placement may proceed before surgery at the time of

**TABLE 65–11.** Issues of Postoperative Management

| | |
|---|---|
| Hemodynamic | Maintain BP within target range by titration of vasodilators or vasopressors; aggressively avoid episodes of hypotension. |
| Electrolytes | Maintain K$^+$ ≥ 4 mEq/L, Mg$^{2+}$ ≥ 2.5 mEq/L |
| Excessive bleeding | Correct coagulopathy, increase PEEP, rewarm. Consider decreasing target BP. |
| Renal function | Maintain euvolemia; avoid vasopressors or therapies that would decrease renal blood flow. |
| Neurologic | Neurologic examination within 4–6 h. Drain CSF to maintain CSF pressure 10–15 mm Hg; retain drain 48–72 h. |
| Postoperative analgesia | Epidural after neurologic examination; PCEA, PCA, narcotic administration as needed. |
| Pulmonary dysfunction | Phrenic nerve or diaphragm dysfunction, pain, mucus plugging. |

BP, blood pressure; CSF, cerebrospinal fluid; K$^+$, potassium; Mg$^+$, magnesium; PCA, patient-controlled analgesia; PCEA, patient-controlled epidural analgesia; PEEP, positive end-expiratory pressure.

catheter insertion for CSF drainage. Alternatively, the epidural catheter may be placed after surgery in the intensive care unit. To minimize the risk for complications, placement is contraindicated in patients with coagulopathy or paraspinal infection, or in whom an adequate neurologic examination has not been performed. The initial dosing of the epidural catheter should proceed cautiously, so as not to precipitate a sympathectomy-induced episode of hypotension. The drop in blood pressure can be attenuated by a bolus of intravenous fluid or the administration of a vasopressor. The drug concentration and infusion rate of the epidural should be titrated so that it does not produce a significant neurologic deficit that would compromise postoperative neurologic examination. At our institution, the epidural infusion of 0.05% bupivacaine and a narcotic (0.001% fentanyl or 0.01% morphine) is started on postoperative day 1 at a rate of 5 to 10 mL/h. Parenteral narcotics can be administered by patient-controlled analgesia or by the medical staff as required. Narcotic analgesia is titrated to patient comfort, respiratory rate, and mean arterial pressure.

## Postoperative Respiratory Function

Patients with advanced aortic disease are typically at increased risk for postoperative pulmonary complications as a consequence of their age and, oftentimes, a history of tobacco use. Large aortic aneurysms can impinge against the trachea or left mainstem bronchus, resulting in bronchomalacia. This leads to dynamic airway obstruction that persists postoperatively. Large aneurysms can also cause narrowing of the airway as a consequence of direct external mechanical compression, or deviation of the trachea and left mainstem bronchus. In addition, patients may experience a significant decrease in respiratory function postoperatively that is related to disturbances in ventilatory function or lung injury. Phrenic nerve dysfunction may result from traction or surgical manipulation; diaphragmatic dysfunction can be caused by surgical dissection at the site of the thoracoabdominal aneurysm. Clinically, these patients exhibit poor parameters of ventilatory function (decreased vital capacity, tidal volume, and negative expiratory force) and have difficulty weaning from mechanical ventilation. Radiographically, the left hemidiaphragm is elevated and may be associated with persistent lower-lobe atelectasis. Confirmation of diaphragmatic dysfunction can be achieved by performing the "sniff test." The patient attempts a quick forceful inspiration while the diaphragmatic motion is evaluated by fluoroscopy. Normally, the diaphragm moves down with inspiration, and thus the absence of movement or upward diaphragmatic movement suggests injury to the diaphragm or the phrenic nerve. Postoperative respiratory insufficiency may also be caused by pulmonary contusions incurred by surgical traction, infection, or edema. These patients have an increased $O_2$ requirement and a significant alveolar-arterial gradient. A diagnostic and therapeutic bronchoscopy should be performed to maximize pulmonary toilet to remove any blood clots and secretions and obtain a sample for culture.

## CONCLUSION

Providing anesthesia for patients undergoing surgical repair of the descending thoracic aorta can be one of the most challenging, yet rewarding, endeavors. The anesthesia care team can play a vital role in organizing and coordinating the efforts of other participating hospital services, such as the intensive care unit, preoperative evaluation, operating room personnel, perfusionists, intraoperative echocardiography, intraoperative neurophysiologic monitoring, and blood bank.

The pace of the preoperative preparations and the ability to provide perioperative patient care are dictated by the acuity of the patient. In the case of an emergency, the preoperative evaluation must be prioritized, focusing on defining the extent of aortic pathology and evaluating cardiorespiratory status. Patients undergoing surgical repair of the descending thoracic aorta require special considerations for the perioperative ventilatory and circulatory management.

Intubation with either a double-lumen ETT or bronchial blocker significantly improves surgical exposure by allowing single-lung ventilation of the dependent lung and deflation of the nondependent left lung. After intubation, patients are placed in the right lateral decubitus position to maximize surgical exposure and to obtain access to the femoral vessels. Circulatory management during periods of induction and aortic cross-clamping can have profound effects on the risk for aneurysm rupture, cardiac function, hemodynamic lability, and incidence of postoperative neurologic deficits. The aggressive control of blood pressure is required to prevent hypertension-induced rupture of the aorta and hypotension-induced ischemia of the spinal cord. During the period of aortic cross-clamping, the simple technique of clamp-and-sew has been successfully applied to cases with a short cross-clamp duration of <30 minutes. However, the alternative techniques, which involve perfusion of the aorta distal to the cross-clamp, are generally accepted to reduce hemodynamic lability, cardiac stress, and improve neurologic outcome during most cross-clamp durations of longer than 30 minutes.

One of the most feared complications of aortic surgery is paraplegia. Clamping of the thoracic aorta may compromise blood flow to the anterior spinal cord, rendering the patient at risk for postoperative paraplegia. The multiple intraoperative strategies used for spinal cord preservation employ several anesthetic, surgical, and pharmacologic interventions. The major goals of management seek to maximize spinal cord perfusion and minimize the risk for ischemic injury. Spinal cord perfusion may be improved by increasing perfusion of the areas distal to the aortic cross-clamp with partial bypass or by decreasing SCFP by draining spinal fluid. By far, the most effective strategy to increase ischemic tolerance is hypothermia. Along with lowering the metabolic rate, hypothermia reduces the loss of intracellular adenosine triphosphate and decreases the release of excitatory neurotransmitters. The technique of hypothermia has proved successful when applied to selective cooling of the spinal cord or the whole body. A number of pharmacologic adjunct interventions have been suggested, but confirmation of improved clinical outcome in human beings is debatable.

Intraoperative blood loss may be significant and can lead both to a quantitative decrease of platelets and coagulation factors and to a qualitative decrease of platelet function. The anesthesiologist is ultimately responsible for confirming the availability and directing the transfusion of blood products. Ideally, the rationale for the transfusion of component therapy should be based on laboratory data and experience. However, the inability to obtain test results in a timely manner often necessitates that the decisions for transfusion therapy proceed on clinical impression and the presence of microvascular bleeding.

The role of the anesthesiologist has expanded beyond that of the operating room into the critical care unit. Often, anesthesiologists are the institutional experts for airway management, mechanical ventilation, hemodynamic monitoring, and postoperative pain control. The intraoperative anesthetic technique should permit an adequate neurologic evaluation within several hours after surgery. Detection of a new neurologic deficit should be aggressively pursued by increasing mean arterial pressure, draining CSF in an attempt to increase SCPP, and obtaining further diagnostic studies. As the patient emerges from anesthesia, plans for postoperative analgesia should be implemented. The most common routes of analgesic delivery are either epidural or parenteral. Epidural catheter placement may proceed before surgery or after surgery in the intensive care unit. To minimize the risk for complications, placement is contraindicated in patients with a coagulopathy, or in whom an adequate neurologic examination has not been performed.

## References

1. Crawford ES, Saleh SA, Babb JWI, et al. Infrarenal abdominal aortic aneurysm: factors influencing survival after operation performed over a 25-year period. *Ann Surg.* 1981;193:699.
2. Cronenwett JL, Sargent SK, Wall MH, et al. Variables that affect the expansion rate and outcome of small abdominal aortic aneurysms. *J Vasc Surg.* 1990;11:260.
3. Johnston KW, Rutherford RB, Tilson MD, et al. Standards for reporting on arterial aneurysms. Subcommittee on Reporting Standards for Arterial Aneurysms Ad Hoc Committee on Reporting Standards, Society for Vascular Surgery. *J Vasc Surg.* 1991;13:452.
4. Ross R. Pathophysiology of atherosclerosis. In: Wilson SF, Hobson RW, eds. *Vascular Surgery Principles and Practice.* New York, NY: McGraw-Hill; 1987:11.
5. Joyce JW, Fairburn JFI, Kincaid OW, et al. Aneurysms of the thoracic aorta, a clinical study with special reference to prognosis. *Circulation.* 1964;29:176.
6. Rutherford RB. Infrarenal aortic aneurysms. In: Rutherford R, ed. *Vascular Surgery.* Philadelphia, Pa: WB Saunders; 1984:755.
7. Darling RC, Messina CR, Brewster DC, et al. Autopsy study of unoperated abdominal aortic aneurysms: the case for early resection. *Cardiovasc Surg.* 1977;56:161.
8. Hollier LH. Surgical management of abdominal aortic aneurysms in the high risk patient. *Surg Clin North Am.* 1986;66:269.
9. Wakefield TW, Whitehouse TWJ, Wu SC, et al. Abdominal aortic aneurysm rupture: statistical analysis of factors affecting outcome of surgical treatment. *Surgery.* 1982;91:586.
10. Roberts WC. Aortic dissection: anatomy, consequences, and causes. *Am Heart J.* 1981;101:195.
11. DeBakey ME, Cooley DA, Creech OJ. Surgical considerations of dissecting aneurysms of the aorta. *Ann Surg.* 1955;142:586.
12. Dailey PO, Trueblood HN, Stinson EB, et al. Management of acute aortic dissections. *Ann Thorac Surg.* 1970;10:237.
13. Ergin MA, Galla JD, Lansman S, et al. Acute dissections of the aorta: current surgical treatment. *Surg Clin North Am.* 1985;65:721.
14. Miller DC, Mitchell RS, Oyer PE, et al. Independent determinants of operative mortality for patients with aortic dissection. *Circulation.* 1984;70:1153.
15. Wolfe WG, Moran JF. The evolution of medical and surgical management of acute aortic dissection. *Circulation.* 1977;56:503.
16. Campbell M. Natural history of coarctation of the aorta. *Br Heart J.* 1970;32:633.
17. Keen G. Spinal cord damage and operations for coarctation of the aorta: aetiology, practice, and prospects. *Thorax.* 1987;42:11.
18. Crawford FA Jr, Sade RM. Spinal cord injury associated with hyperthermia during aortic coarctation repair. *J Thorac Cardiovasc Surg.* 1984;87:616.
19. Brewer LAD, Fosburg RG, Mulder GA, et al. Spinal cord complications following surgery for coarctation of the aorta: a study of 66 cases. *J Thorac Cardiovasc Surg.* 1972;64:368.
20. Itzchak Y, Rosenthal T, Adar R, et al. Dissecting aneurysm of the thoracic aorta: reappraisal of radiologic diagnosis. *AJR Am J Roentgenol.* 1975;125:559.
21. Kearney PA, Smith DW, Johnson SB, et al. Use of transesophageal echocardiography in the evaluation of traumatic aortic injury. *J Trauma.* 1993;34:696.
22. Nienaber CA, von Kodolitsch Y, Nicolas V, et al. The diagnosis of thoracic aortic dissection by noninvasive imaging procedures. *N Engl J Med.* 1993;328:1.
23. Sommer T, Fehske W, Holzknecht N, et al. Aortic dissection: a comparative study of diagnosis with spiral CT, multiplanar transesophageal echocardiography, and MR imaging. *Radiology.* 1996;199:347.
24. Nienaber CA, Spielmann RP, von Kodolitsch Y, et al. Diagnosis of thoracic aortic dissection: magnetic resonance imaging versus transesophageal echocardiography. *Circulation.* 1992;85:434.
25. Nienaber CA, von Kodolitsch Y, Brockhoff CJ, et al. Comparison of conventional and transesophageal echocardiography with magnetic resonance imaging for anatomical mapping of thoracic aortic dissection. A dual noninvasive imaging study with anatomical and/or angiographic validation. *Int J Card Imaging.* 1994;10:1.
26. Rennollet R, Engberding R, Visser CA, et al. Transesophageal imaging of the thoracic aorta in aortic dissection. In: Erbel RKB, Brennecke R, eds. *Transesophageal Echocardiography: A New Window to the Heart.* Berlin, Germany: Springer-Verlag; 1989:140.
27. Buckmaster MJ, Kearney PA, Johnson SB, et al. Further experience with transesophageal echocardiography in the evaluation of thoracic aortic injury. *J Trauma.* 1994;37:989.
28. Laissy JP, Blanc F, Soyer P, et al. Thoracic aortic dissection: diagnosis with transesophageal echocardiography versus MR imaging. *Radiology.* 1995;194:331.
29. Hertzer NR, Beven EG, Young JR, et al. Coronary artery disease in peripheral vascular patients. *Ann Surg.* 1984;199:223.
30. Poldermans D, Boersma E, Bax JJ, et al. The effect of bisoprolol on perioperative mortality and myocardial infarction in high-risk patients undergoing vascular surgery. Dutch Echocardiographic Cardiac Risk Evaluation Applying Stress Echocardiography Study Group. *N Engl J Med.* 1999;341:1789.
31. Wallace A, Layug B, Tateo I, et al. Prophylactic atenolol reduces postoperative myocardial ischemia. McSPI Research Group. *Anesthesiology.* 1998;88:7.
32. Hertzer NR, Young JR, Kramer JR, et al. Routine coronary angiography prior to elective aortic reconstruction: results of selective myocardial revascularization in patients with peripheral vascular disease. *Arch Surg.* 1979;114:1336.
33. Hollenberg M, Mangano DT, Browner WS, et al. Predictors of postoperative myocardial ischemia in patients undergoing noncardiac surgery. The Study of Perioperative Ischemia Research Group. *JAMA.* 1992;268:205.
34. Devereux RB, Alonso DR, Lutas EM, et al. Echocardiographic assessment of left ventricular hypertrophy: comparison to necropsy findings. *Am J Cardiol.* 1986;57:450.
35. Grubbs P, Marini CP, Toporoff B, et al. Somatosensory evoked potentials and spinal cord perfusion pressure are significant predictors of postoperative neurologic dysfunction. *Surgery.* 1988;104:216.
36. Cunningham JNJ, Laschinger JC, Merkin HA, et al. Measurement of spinal cord ischemia during operations upon the thoracic aorta. *Ann Surg.* 1982;196:285.
37. Ginsburg HH, Shetter AG, Raudzens PA. Postoperative paraplegia with preserved intraoperative somatosensory evoked potentials: case report. *J Neurosurg.* 1985;63:296.
38. Kaplan BJ, Friedman WA, Alexander JA, et al. Somatosensory evoked potential monitoring of spinal cord ischemia during aortic operations. *Neurosurgery.* 1986;19:82.
39. Shahin GM, Hamerlijnck RP, Schepens MA, et al. Upper and lower extremity somatosensory evoked potential recording during surgery for aneurysms of the descending thoracic aorta. *Eur J Cardiothorac Surg.* 1996;10:299.
40. Grabitz K, Sandmann W, Stuhmeier K, et al. The risk of ischemic spinal cord injury in patients undergoing graft replacement for thoracoabdominal aortic aneurysms. *J Vasc Surg.* 1996;23:230.
41. Faberowski LW, Black S, Trankina MF, et al. Somatosensory-evoked potentials during aortic coarctation repair. *J Cardiothorac Vasc Anesth.* 1999;13:538.
42. Takaki O, Okumura F. Application and limitation of somatosensory evoked potential monitoring during thoracic aortic aneurysm surgery: a case report. *Anesthesiology.* 1985;63:700.
43. de Haan P, Kalkman CJ, Meylaerts SA, et al. Development of spinal

cord ischemia after clamping of noncritical segmental arteries in the pig. *Ann Thorac Surg.* 1999;68:1278.

44. McCullough JL, Hollier LH, Nugent M. Paraplegia after thoracic aortic occlusion: influence of cerebrospinal fluid drainage. *J Vasc Surg.* 1988;7:153.

45. Alpert RA, Roizen MF, Hamilton WK, et al. Intraoperative urinary output does not predict postoperative renal function in patients undergoing abdominal aortic revascularization. *Surgery.* 1984;95:707.

46. Schindler E, Muller M, Zickmann B, et al. Modulation of somatosensory evoked potentials under various concentrations of desflurane with and without nitrous oxide. *J Neurosurg Anesth.* 1998;10:218.

47. Spurny OM, Rubin S, Wolf JW, et al. Spinal epidural hematoma during anticoagulant therapy: report of two cases. *Arch Intern Med.* 1964;114:103.

48. Rao TLK, El-Etr AA. Anticoagulation following placement of epidural and subarachnoid catheters: an evaluation of neurological sequelae. *Anesthesiology.* 1981;55:618.

49. Barron HC, LaRaja RD, Rossi G, et al. Continuous epidural analgesia in the heparinized vascular surgical patient: a retrospective review of 912 patients. *J Vasc Surg.* 1987;6:144.

50. Baron JF, Bertrand M, Barre E, et al. Combined epidural and general anesthesia versus general anesthesia for abdominal aortic surgery. *Anesthesiology.* 1991;75:611.

51. Tuman KJ, McCarthy RJ, March RJ, et al. Effects of epidural anesthesia and analgesia on coagulation and outcome after major vascular surgery. *Anesth Analg.* 1991;71:696.

52. Yeager MP, Glass DD, Neff RK, et al. Epidural anesthesia and analgesia in high-risk patients. *Anesthesiology.* 1987;66:729.

53. Bunt TJ, Manczuk M, Varley K. Continuous epidural anesthesia for aortic surgery: thoughts on peer review and safety. *Surgery.* 1987;101:706.

54. Mason RA, Newton GB, Cassel W. Combined epidural and general anesthesia in aortic surgery. *J Cardiovasc Surg.* 1989;31:442.

55. Crawford ES. Thoracoabdominal and abdominal aortic aneurysms involving renal, superior mesenteric and celiac arteries. *Ann Surg.* 1974;179:763.

56. Roberts AJ, Nora JD, Hughes WA, et al. Cardiac and renal responses to cross-clamping the descending thoracic aorta. *J Thorac Cardiovasc Surg.* 1983;86:732.

57. Roizen MF, Beaupre PN, Alpert RA, et al. Monitoring with two-dimensional transesophageal echocardiography. *J Vasc Surg.* 1984;1:300.

58. O'Connor C, Rothenberg DM. Anesthetic considerations for descending thoracic aortic surgery: part II. *J Cardiothorac Vasc Anesth.* 1995;9:734.

59. O'Connor C, Rothenberg DM. Anesthetic considerations for descending thoracic aortic surgery: part 1. *J Cardiothorac Vasc Anesth.* 1995;9:581.

60. Saleh SA, Crawford ES, Bomberger RA, et al. Intraoperative acid-base management for the resection of thoracoabdominal aneurysms: a comparison of continuous infusion of sodium bicarbonate versus the bolus. *Anesth Analg.* 1982;61:213.

61. Verdant A, Page A, Cossette R, et al. Development of circulatory support during 420 aneurysm resections of the descending thoracic aorta. *Ann Chir.* 1996;50:619.

62. Jacobs M, Meylaerts SA, de Haan P, et al. Strategies to prevent neurologic deficit based on motor-evoked potentials in type I and II thoracoabdominal aortic aneurysm repair. *J Vasc Surg.* 1999;29:48.

63. Deshpande A, Mossop P, Gurry J, et al. Treatment of traumatic false aneurysm of the thoracic aorta with endoluminal grafts. *J Endovasc Surg.* 1998;5:120.

64. Ishimaru S, Kawaguchi S, Koizumi N, et al. Preliminary report on prediction of spinal cord ischemia in endovascular stent graft repair of thoracic aortic aneurysm by retrievable stent graft. *J Thorac Cardiovasc Surg.* 1998;115:811.

65. Kato M, Kaneko M, Kuratani T, et al. New operative method for distal aortic arch aneurysm: combined cervical branch bypass and endovascular stent-graft implantation. *J Thorac Cardiovasc Surg.* 1999;117:832.

66. Mitchell RS, Dake MD, Sembra CP, et al. Endovascular stent-graft repair of thoracic aortic aneurysms. *J Thorac Cardiovasc Surg.* 1996;111:1054.

67. Murgo S, Dussaussois L, Golzarian J, et al. Penetrating atherosclerotic ulcer of the descending thoracic aorta: treatment by endovascular stent-graft. *Cardiovasc Interv Radiol.* 1998;21:454.

68. Oliva VL, Bui BT, Leclerc G, et al. Aortoesophageal fistula: repair with transluminal placement of a thoracic aortic stent-graft. *J Vasc Interv Radiol.* 1997;8:35.

69. Semba CP, Sakai T, Slonim SM, et al. Mycotic aneurysms of the thoracic aorta: repair with use of endovascular stent-grafts. *J Vasc Interv Radiol.* 1998;9:33.

70. Cutry AF, Whitley D, Patterson RB. Midaortic pseudoaneurysm complicating extensive endovascular stenting of aortic disease. *J Vasc Surg.* 1997;26:958.

71. Duda SH, Raygrotzki S, Wiskirchen J, et al. Abdominal aortic aneurysms: treatment with juxtarenal placement of covered stent-grafts. *Radiology.* 1998;206:195.

72. Marin ML, Parsons RE, Hollier LH, et al. Impact of transrenal aortic endograft placement on endovascular graft repair of abdominal aortic aneurysms. *J Vasc Surg.* 1998;28:638.

73. Takolander R. Conservative treatment, stent grafting or open repair of abdominal aortic aneurysms. *Ann Chir Gynaecol.* 1998;87:167.

74. Rousseau H, Soula P, Perreault P, et al. Delayed treatment of traumatic rupture of the thoracic aorta with endoluminal covered stent. *Circulation.* 1999;99:498.

75. Suarez de Lezo J, Pan M, Romero M, et al. Immediate and follow-up findings after stent treatment for severe coarctation of aorta. *Am J Cardiol.* 1999;83:400.

76. Miyata T, Ohara N, Shigematsu H, et al. Endovascular stent graft repair of aortopulmonary fistula. *J Vasc Surg.* 1999;29:557.

77. Heilberger P, Ritter W, Schunn C, et al. Results and complications after endovascular reconstruction of aortic aneurysms. *Zentralbl Chir.* 1997;122:762.

78. Mitchell RS, Miller DC, Dake MD. Stent-graft repair of thoracic aortic aneurysms. *Semin Vasc Surg.* 1997;10:257.

79. Jacobowitz GR, Lee AM, Riles TS. Immediate and late explantation of endovascular aortic grafts: the endovascular technologies experience. *J Vasc Surg.* 1999;29:309.

80. Dake MD, Miller DC, Mitchell RS, et al. The "first generation" of endovascular stent-grafts for patients with aneurysms of the descending thoracic aorta. *J Thorac Cardiovasc Surg.* 1998;116:689.

81. Lindholt JS, Sandermann J, Bruun-Petersen J, et al. Fatal late multiple emboli after endovascular treatment of abdominal aortic aneurysm: case report. *Int Angiol.* 1998;17:241.

82. Moskowitz DM, Kahn RA, Konstadt SN, et al. Intraoperative transoesophageal echocardiography as an adjuvant to fluoroscopy during endovascular thoracic aortic repair. *Eur J Vasc Endovasc Surg.* 1999;17:22.

83. Eberle B, Weiler N, Duber C, et al. Anesthesia in endovascular treatment of aortic aneurysm: results and perioperative risks. *Anaesthetist.* 1996;45:931.

84. Martin LF, Atnip RG, Holmes PA, et al. Prediction of postoperative complications after elective aortic surgery using stepwise logistic regression analysis. *Am Surg.* 1994;60:163.

85. Torsello G, Kutkuhn B, Kniemeyer H, et al. Prevention of acute renal failure in suprarenal aortic surgery: results of a pilot study. *Zentralbl Chir.* 1993;118:390.

86. Svensson LG, Crawford ES, Hess KR, et al. Experience with 1509 patients undergoing thoracoabdominal aortic operations. *J Vasc Surg.* 1993;17:357.

87. Chawla SK, Najafi H, Ing TS, et al. Acute renal failure complicating ruptured abdominal aortic aneurysm. *Arch Surg.* 1975;110:521.

88. Bush HL. Renal failure following abdominal aortic reconstruction. *Surgery.* 1983;93:107.

89. Myers BD, Miller DC, Mehigan JT, et al. Nature of the renal injury following total renal ischemia in man. *J Clin Invest.* 1984;73:329.

90. Miller DC, Myers BD. Pathophysiology and prevention of acute renal failure associated with thoracoabdominal or abdominal aortic surgery. *J Vasc Surg.* 1987;5:518.

91. Svensson LG, Coselli JS, Safi HJ, et al. Appraisal of adjuncts to prevent acute renal failure after surgery on the thoracic or thoracoabdominal aorta. *J Vasc Surg.* 1989;10:230.

92. Abbott WM, Austen WG. The reversal of renal cortical ischemia during aortic occlusion by mannitol. *J Surg Res.* 1974;16:482.

93. Barry KG, Cohen A, Knochel JP. Mannitol infusion, II: the prevention of acute functional renal failure during resection of an aneurysm of the abdominal aorta. *N Engl J Med.* 1961;264:967.

94. Duke GJ, Briedis JH, Weaver RA. Renal support in critically ill patients: low-dose dopamine or low-dose dobutamine? *Crit Care Med.* 1994;22:1919.

95. Schiffer ER, Schwieger IM, Gosteli P, et al. Systemic and splanchnic oxygen supply-demand relationship with fenoldopam, dopamine and noradrenaline in sheep. *Eur J Pharmacol.* 1995;286:49.

96. Mathur VS, Swan SK, Lambrecht LJ, et al. The effects of fenoldopam, a selective dopamine receptor agonist, on systemic and renal hemodynamics in normotensive subjects. *Crit Care Med.* 1999;27:1832.

97. Crawford ES, Fenstermacher JM, Richardson W, et al. Reappraisal of

adjuncts to avoid ischemia in the treatment of thoracic aortic aneurysms. *Surgery.* 1970;67:182.

98. Najafi H, Javid H, Hunter J, Serry C, et al. Descending aortic aneurysmectomy without adjuncts to avoid ischemia. *Ann Thorac Surg.* 1980;30:326.

99. Crawford ES, Crawford JL, Safi HJ, et al. Thoracoabdominal aortic aneurysms: preoperative and intraoperative factors determining immediate and long-term results of operations in 605 patients. *J Vasc Surg.* 1986;3:389.

100. Rosenthal D. Spinal cord ischemia after abdominal aortic operation: is it preventable? *J Vasc Surg.* 1999;30:391.

101. Szilagyi DE, Hageman JH, Smith RF, et al. Spinal cord damage in surgery of the abdominal aorta. *Surgery.* 1978;83:38.

102. Griepp RB, Ergin MA, Galla JD, et al. Looking for the artery of Adamkiewicz: a quest to minimize paraplegia after operations for aneurysms of the descending thoracic and thoracoabdominal aorta. *J Thorac Cardiovasc Surg.* 1996;112:1202.

103. Williams GM, Perler BA, Burdick JF, et al. Angiographic localization of spinal cord blood supply and its relationship to postoperative paraplegia. *J Vasc Surg.* 1991;13:23.

104. Crawford ES, Coselli JS. Thoracoabdominal aneurysm surgery. *Semin Thorac Cardiovasc Surg.* 1991;3:300.

105. Wadouh F, Lindemann E, Arndt CF, et al. The arteria radicularis magna anterior as a decisive factor influencing spinal cord damage during aortic occlusion. *J Thorac Cardiovasc Surg.* 1984;88:1.

106. Livesay JJ, Cooley DA, Ventemiglia RA, et al. Surgical experience in descending thoracic aneurysmectomy with and without adjuncts to avoid ischemia. *Ann Thorac Surg.* 1985;39:37.

107. Katz NW, Blackstone EH, Kirklin JW, et al. Incremental risk factors for spinal cord injury following operation for acute traumatic aortic transection. *J Thorac Cardiovasc Surg.* 1981;81:669.

108. Diehl JT, Cali RF, Hertzer NR, et al. Complications of abdominal aortic reconstruction: an analysis of perioperative risk factors in 557 patients. *Ann Surg.* 1983;197:49.

109. Mauney MC, Tribble CG, Cope JT, et al. Is clamp and sew still viable for thoracic aortic resection? *Ann Surg.* 1996;223:534.

110. Crawford ES, Walker HS, Saleh SA, et al. Graft replacement of aneurysm in descending thoracic aorta: results without bypass or shunting. *Surgery.* 1981;89:73.

111. Kaplan DK, Atsumi N, D'Ambra MN, et al. Distal circulatory support for thoracic aortic operations: effects on intracranial pressure. *Ann Thorac Surg.* 1995;59:448.

112. Safi HJ, Miller CC 3rd. Spinal cord protection in descending thoracic and thoracoabdominal aortic repair. *Ann Thorac Surg.* 1999;67:1937.

113. Heinemann MK, Brassel F, Herzog T, et al. The role of spinal angiography in operations on the thoracic aorta: myth or reality? *Ann Thorac Surg.* 1998;65:346.

114. Marini CP, Grubbs P, Toporoff B, et al. Effect of sodium nitroprusside on spinal cord perfusion pressure and paraplegia during aortic cross-clamping. *Ann Thorac Surg.* 1989;47:379.

115. Robertazzi RR, Cunningham JN Jr. Intraoperative adjuncts of spinal cord protection. *Semin Thorac Cardiovasc Surg.* 1998;10:29.

116. Crawford ES, Svensson LG, Hess K, et al. A prospective randomized study of cerebrospinal fluid drainage to prevent paraplegia after high-risk surgery on the thoracoabdominal aorta. *J Vasc Surg.* 1991;13:36.

117. Marini CP, Levison J, Caliendo F, et al. Control of proximal hypertension during aortic cross-clamping: its effect on cerebrospinal fluid dynamics and spinal cord perfusion pressure. *Semin Thorac Cardiovasc Surg.* 1998;10:51.

118. Marini CP, Nathan IM, Efron J, et al. Effect of nitroglycerin and cerebrospinal fluid drainage on spinal cord perfusion pressure and paraplegia during aortic cross-clamping. *J Surg Res.* 1997;70:61.

119. Simpson JI, Eide TR, Schiff GA, et al. Effect of nitroglycerin on spinal cord ischemia after thoracic aortic cross-clamping. *Ann Thorac Surg.* 1996;61:113.

120. Grum DF, Svensson LG. Changes in cerebrospinal fluid pressure and spinal cord perfusion pressure prior to cross-clamping of the thoracic aorta in humans. *J Cardiothorac Vasc Anesth.* 1991;5:331.

121. Ilhan A, Koltuksuz U, Ozen S, et al. The effects of caffeic acid phenethyl ester (CAPE) on spinal cord ischemia/reperfusion injury in rabbits. *Eur J Cardiothorac Surg.* 1999;16:458.

122. Lombardi V, Valko L, Stolc S, et al. Free radicals in rabbit spinal cord ischemia: electron spin resonance spectroscopy and correlation with SOD activity. *Cell Molec Neurobiol.* 1998;18:399.

123. Brock MV, Redmond JM, Ishiwa S, et al. Clinical markers in CSF for determining neurologic deficits after thoracoabdominal aortic aneurysm repairs. *Ann Thorac Surg.* 1997;64:999.

124. Farooque M, Hillered L, Holtz A, et al. Effects of moderate hypothermia on extracellular lactic acid and amino acids after severe compression injury of rat spinal cord. *J Neurotrauma.* 1997;14:63.

125. Ishikawa T, Marsala M. Hypothermia prevents biphasic glutamate release and corresponding neuronal degeneration after transient spinal cord ischemia in the rat. *Cell Molec Neurobiol.* 1999;19:199.

126. Wakamatsu H, Matsumoto M, Nakakimura K, et al. The effects of moderate hypothermia and intrathecal tetracaine on glutamate concentrations of intrathecal dialysate and neurologic and histopathologic outcome in transient spinal cord ischemia in rabbits. *Anesth Analg.* 1999;88:56.

127. Nakamichi T, Kawada S. Glutamate neurotoxicity during spinal cord ischemia: development of a delayed-onset paraplegia model. *Nippon Kyobu Geka Gakkai Zasshi.* 1997;45:1667.

128. Danielisova V, Chavko M. Comparative effects of the N-methyl-D-aspartate antagonist MK-801 and the calcium channel blocker KB-2796 on neurologic and metabolic recovery after spinal cord ischemia. *Exp Neurol.* 1998;149:203.

129. Taoka Y, Okajima K. Spinal cord injury in the rat. *Prog Neurobiol.* 1998;56:341.

130. Bracken MB, Shepard MJ, Collins WF, et al. A randomized, controlled trial of methylprednisolone or naloxone in the treatment of acute spinal-cord injury. *N Engl J Med.* 1990;322:1405.

131. Vacanti FX, Ames A. Mild hypothermia and $Mg^{++}$ protect against irreversible damage during CNS ischemia. *Stroke.* 1984;15:695.

132. Sirin BH, Yilik L, Ortac R, et al. Aprotinin reduces injury of the spinal cord in transient ischemia. *Eur J Cardiothoracic Surg.* 1997;12:913.

133. Ohtake H, Urayama H, Katada S, et al. Prevention of spinal cord ischemia by selective intercostal arterial infusion of prostaglandin E1. *J Vasc Surg.* 1998;28:301.

134. Sun J, Hirsch D, Svensson G. Spinal cord protection by papaverine and intrathecal cooling during aortic crossclamping. *J Cardiovasc Surg.* 1998;39:839.

135. Svensson LG, Grum DF, Bednarski M. Appraisal of CSF alterations during aortic surgery with intrathecal papaverine administration and CSF drainage. *J Vasc Surg.* 1990;11:423.

136. Svensson LG, Stewart RW, Cosgrove DM, et al. Intrathecal papaverine for the prevention of paraplegia after operation on the thoracic or thoracoabdominal aorta. *J Thorac Cardiovasc Surg.* 1988;96:823.

137. Marsala M VI, Galik J, Radonak J, et al. Panmyelic epidural cooling protects against ischemic spinal cord damage. *J Surg Res.* 1993;55:21.

138. Cambria RP, Davison JK, Zannetti S, et al. Clinical experience with epidural cooling for spinal cord protection during thoracic and thoracoabdominal aneurysm repair. *J Vasc Surg.* 1997;25:234.

139. Cambria RP. Thoracoabdominal aortic aneurysm repair: how I do it. *Cardiovasc Surg.* 1999;7:597.

140. Kieffer E, Koskas F, Walden R, et al. Hypothermic circulatory arrest for thoracic aneurysmectomy through left-sided thoracotomy. *J Vasc Surg.* 1994;19:457.

141. Rokkas CK, Cronin CS, Nitta T, et al. Profound systemic hypothermia inhibits the release of neurotransmitter amino acids in spinal cord ischemia. *J Thorac Cardiovasc Surg.* 1995;110:27.

142. Kouchoukos NT, Daily BB, Rokkas CK, et al. Hypothermic bypass and circulatory arrest for operations on the descending thoracic and thoracoabdominal aorta. *Ann Thorac Surg.* 1995;60:67.

143. Fan T, Wang CC, Wang FM, et al. Experimental study of the protection of ischemic preconditioning to spinal cord ischemia. *Surg Neurol.* 1999;52:299.

144. Lukacova N, Marsala M, Halat G, et al. Neuroprotective effect of graded postischemic reoxygenation in spinal cord ischemia in the rabbit. *Brain Res Bull.* 1997;43:457.

145. Matsuyama K, Chiba Y, Ihaya A, et al. Effect of spinal cord preconditioning on paraplegia during cross-clamping of the thoracic aorta. *Ann Thorac Surg.* 1997;63:1315.

146. Zvara DA, Colonna DM, Deal DD, et al. Ischemic preconditioning reduces neurologic injury in a rat model of spinal cord ischemia. *Ann Thorac Surg.* 1999;68:874.

147. American Association of Blood Banks. *Blood Transfusion Therapy: A Physician's Handbook.* 5th ed. Bethesda, Md: American Association of Blood Banks; 1996.

148. American Society of Anesthesiologists. Practice guidelines for blood component therapy: A report by the American Society of Anesthesiologists Task Force on Blood Component Therapy. *Anesthesiology.* 1996;84:732.

149. Gibbs NM, Crawford GPM, Michalopoulos N. Thromboelastographic patterns following abdominal aortic surgery. *Anesth Int Care.* 1994;22:534.

150. Manucci PM, Remuzzi G, Pusineri F, et al. Desamino-8-d-arginine vasopressin shortens the bleeding time in uremia. *N Engl J Med.* 1983;308:8.

151. Hardy JF, Desroches J. Natural and synthetic antifibrinolytics in cardiac surgery. *Can J Anaesth.* 1992;39:353.

152. Horrow JC, Hlavacek J, Strong MD, et al. Prophylactic tranexamic acid decreases bleeding after cardiac operations. *J Thorac Cardiovasc Surg.* 1990;99:70.

153. Jordan D, Delphin E, Rose E. Prophylactic epsilon-aminocaproic acid (EACA) administration minimizes blood replacement therapy during cardiac surgery. *Anesth Analg.* 1995;80:827.

154. Van Oeveren W, Harder MP, Roozendal KJ, et al. Aprotinin protects platelets against the initial effect of cardiopulmonary bypass. *J Thor Cardiovasc Surg.* 1990;99:788.

155. Godet G, Bertrand M, Samama CM, et al. Aprotinin to decrease bleeding and intraoperative blood transfusion requirements during descending thoracic and thoracoabdominal aortic aneurysmectomy using cardiopulmonary bypass. *Ann Vasc Surg.* 1994;8:452.

156. Talke P, Li J, Jain U, Leung J, et al. Effects of perioperative dexmedetomidine infusion in patients undergoing vascular surgery. The Study of Perioperative Ischemia Research Group. *Anesthesiology.* 1995;82:620.

# 66

# Genitourinary Surgery

Jerry J. Berger

Genitourinary (GU) surgery encompasses renal, ureteral, bladder, and prostate procedures. Although these procedures can be performed under general anesthesia, the neuronal innervation of these GU structures allows regional anesthesia and local anesthesia to be considered in many cases. Many of the anesthetic considerations that relate to abdominal surgery are applicable to urogenital surgery as well. In addition, special problems occur in selected operations such as transurethral resection of the prostate (TURP) and laser surgery. These problems are emphasized in this chapter. Anesthetic considerations for renal transplantation are discussed in Chapter 76.

## ANATOMIC CONSIDERATIONS

### What Is the Celiac Plexus?

The celiac plexus comprises visceral afferent and efferent fibers from T5 to T12[1] and parasympathetic fibers that originate in the cranial and sacral areas. It innervates the kidneys, ureters, and adrenal glands. Innervation of the kidneys is thoracolumbar in origin (T12-L2).

## Splanchnic Nerves

All three splanchnic nerves, which are preganglionic, synapse in the celiac plexus. The postganglionic fibers travel to the aortic, renal, and hypogastric plexuses that provide innervation to the viscera. The lumbar sympathetic ganglia lie at the anterolateral border of the vertebral bodies. The lumbar sympathetic chain innervates the urogenital organs, colon, and rectum.[2]

Celiac plexus and lumbar sympathetic blocks are not used alone for surgical procedures because they provide exclusively autonomic blockade. Thus, they must be combined with other somatic nerve blocks. Because of their relative technical ease, epidural or spinal anesthetics (*neuraxial blockade*) that block both autonomic and somatic nerves usually are chosen when a regional anesthetic technique is desired.

## What Is the Lumbar Plexus?

The lumbar plexus (Fig. 66–1) derives its innervation from the L1, L2, L3, L4, and L5 somatic nerve roots. Together with the T11 and T12 somatic nerve roots, it innervates the inguinal region and canal, including the spermatic cord. After traveling between the transverse and internal oblique muscles, the 11th and 12th thoracic nerves pass through the rectus sheath. Their roots innervate the rectus muscle and sheath and the internal, external, and transverse oblique muscles.

## Ilioinguinal and Iliohypogastric Nerves

The T12 and L1 roots form the ilioinguinal and iliohypogastric nerves, which are retroperitoneal until they penetrate the transverse oblique muscle. The internal oblique muscle is penetrated more medially, and the nerves enter the inguinal canal on the anterior surface of the spermatic cord.

## Genitofemoral Nerve

The genitofemoral nerve is derived from the L1 and L2 nerve roots and is located on the posterior surface of the spermatic cord. The genital branch supplies sensation to the cremaster muscle and the scrotum. The femoral branch innervates the Scarpa fascia and a small area on the anterior thigh.[3]

## Pudendal Nerves

The pudendal nerves are derived from the somatic roots of S2, S3, and S4 from the sacral plexus. The nerves branch under the pubic bone to produce the left and right dorsal nerves of the penis; the nerves supply all innervation to the penis.[4]

## Regional Anesthesia of the Inguinal Region

Regional anesthesia of the inguinal region may be advantageous for several reasons. Earlier ambulation, earlier discharge, and lower morbidity occur in patients receiving this anesthetic compared with those who are administered a general anesthetic. It may be the technique of choice in patients with severe systemic illnesses, especially those that involve the pulmonary and cardiac systems.[4] Regional blockade of

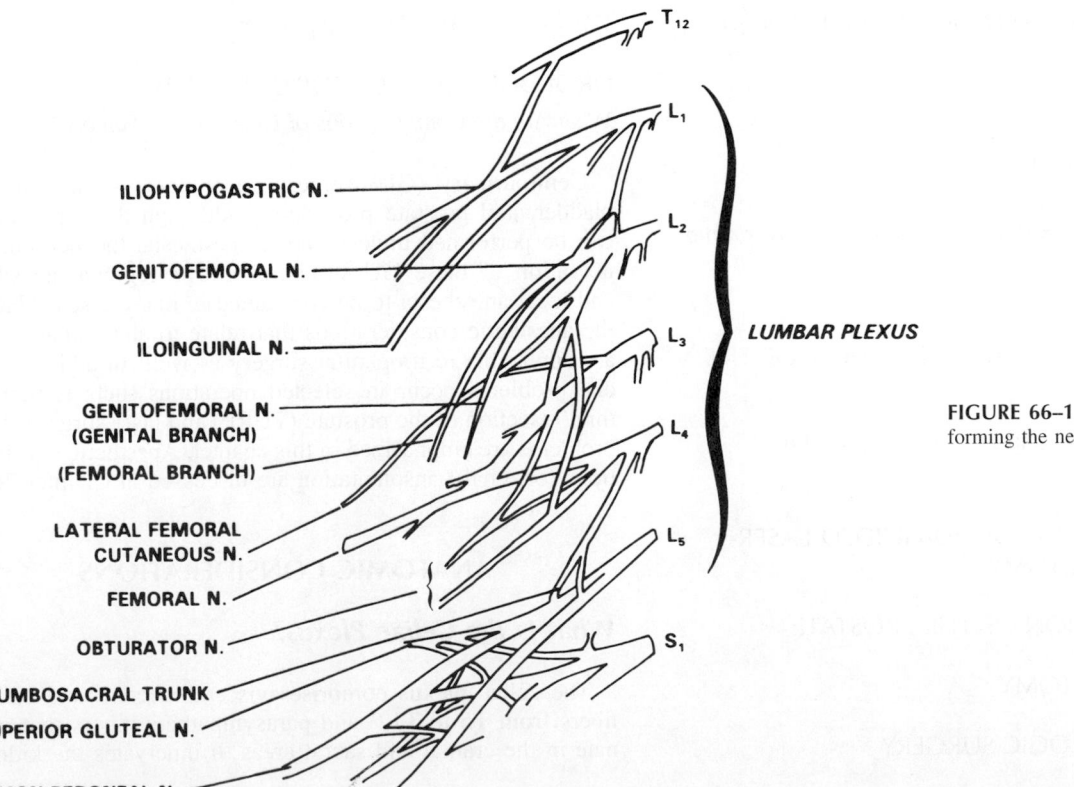

**FIGURE 66–1.** View of the lumbar plexus forming the nerves of the inguinal region.

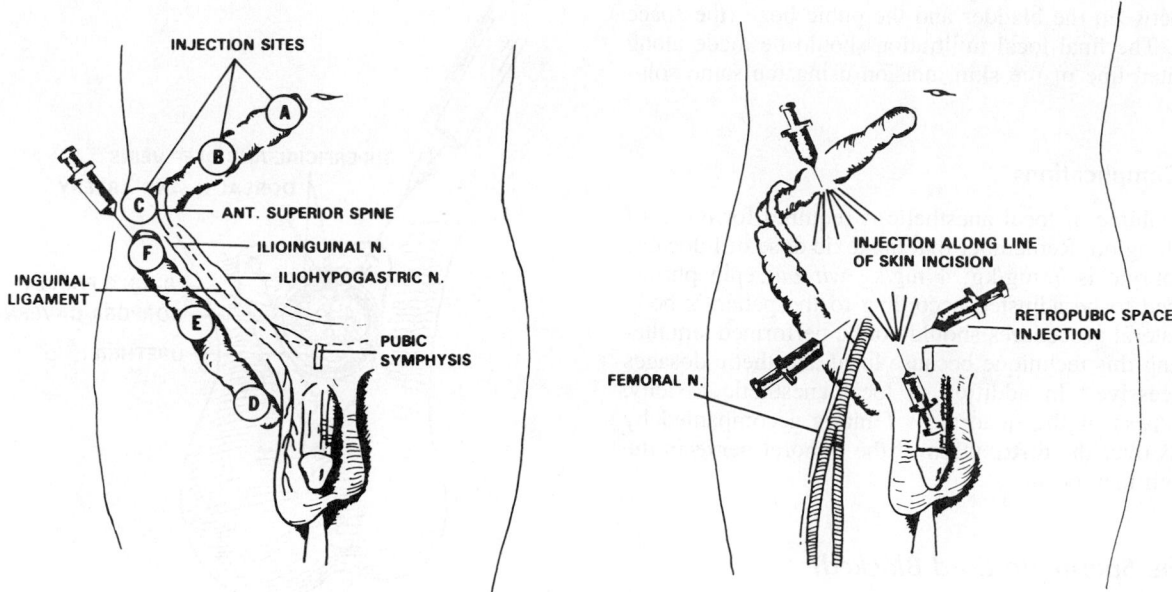

**FIGURE 66–2.** Overall view of the injection sites for complete ilioinguinal anesthesia.

this area should provide significant postoperative analgesia in patients undergoing surgical manipulation of the inguinal canal, spermatic cord, and testes.

## What Is the Technique?

Blockade of the inguinal region requires several injections. Landmark identification is imperative (Fig. 66–2). A line is drawn from the anterosuperior iliac spine to the umbilicus. A second line is drawn from the anterosuperior iliac spine to the pubic tubercle along the course of the inguinal ligament. The initial injection is performed along the first line, 1 inch from the anterosuperior iliac spine, and anesthetizes the ilioinguinal and iliohypogastric nerves. A 22- or 25-gauge 1½- or 2-inch needle is inserted through a skin wheal and advanced downward and lateral to the iliac crest. Five to 10 mL of 1%

lidocaine with epinephrine (1:200 000) are injected along the medial aspect of the iliac bone. The needle is then withdrawn and reinserted slightly more medially so that the infiltration is fanned out, and another 4 to 5 mL of the solution are injected deep into the transversalis fascia. The injection is continued as the needle is withdrawn. The procedure is repeated several times as the needle is advanced more medially (Fig. 66–3).

Twenty milliliters of a 0.5% lidocaine solution with epinephrine (1:200 000) are injected subcutaneously along the two lines that were drawn previously. The index finger should palpate the femoral artery during injection to prevent puncture and intravascular injections. After infiltration, the needle is inserted perpendicular to the skin above and lateral to the superior ramus of the pubic bone. Additional injections of the same solution (15 mL total) are made on each side of the spermatic cord, into the rectus muscle attachments to the pubis, along the superior ramus of the pubic bone, and into

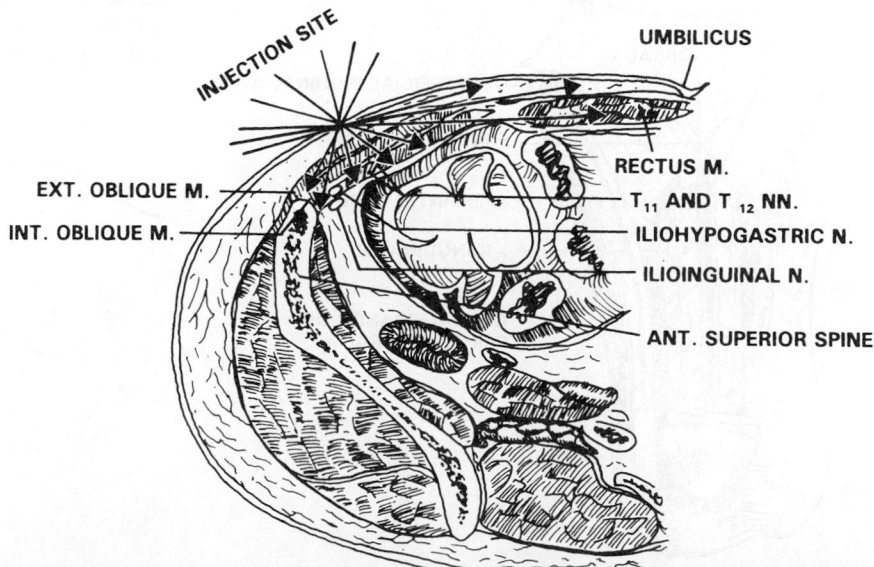

**FIGURE 66–3.** Sagittal view of the abdominal wall at the level of the umbilicus. Injection of local anesthetic and the fanning technique are shown.

the space between the bladder and the pubic bone (the space of Retzius). The final local infiltration should be made along the anticipated line of the skin incision using the same solution.[3]

## Potential Complications

A large volume of local anesthetic is required for block of the inguinal region. Remember that the toxic dose of lidocaine with epinephrine is 7 mg/kg; 4 mg/kg *without* epinephrine. Dosages need to be adjusted according to the patient's body weight. Bilateral procedures should not be performed simultaneously using this technique because local anesthetic dosages will be excessive.[4] In addition to local anesthetic toxicity, motor weakness of the quadriceps femoris accompanied by sensory loss over the distribution of the femoral nerve in the anterior thigh may occur.

## How Is the Spermatic Cord Blocked?

Regional nerve block involving the spermatic cord may be used for surgical procedures of the scrotum, including orchiectomy, vasovasostomy, spermatocelectomy, and hydrocelectomy.[5,6] A 25-gauge 1½-inch needle must be used to inject 10 mL of 1% lidocaine (*without* epinephrine) into each spermatic cord just below the superficial inguinal ring. The entire cross-sectional area of the cord is infiltrated, with special care being taken in the region of the vas deferens.[4] Another injection is made along the anterior scrotal skin, where the incision is to be made. Care should be taken to prevent a hematoma in this sensitive area (Fig. 66–4).

## How Is a Penile Block Performed?

### Innervation

Regional anesthesia may be used for operations on the penis and all of its structures, including the prepuce, urethra,

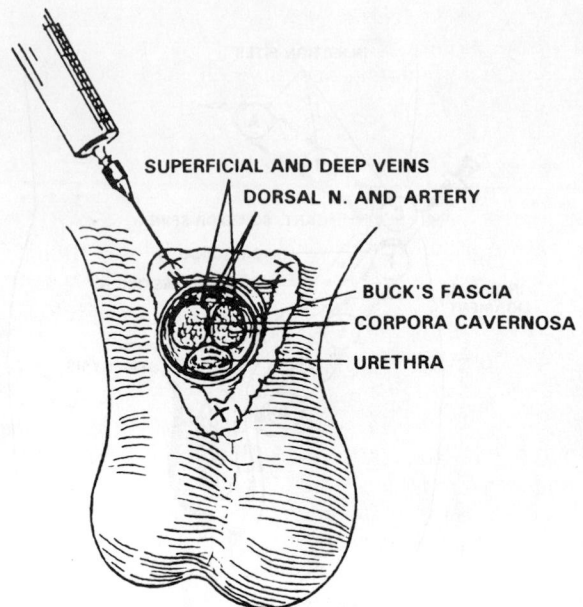

**FIGURE 66–5.** Injection points for penile block.

glans, and corpora cavernosa. Although the most frequent indication is circumcision, placement of penile prostheses and manipulation of the urethra can also be performed satisfactorily. The left and right dorsal nerves of the penis, which are branches of the pudendal nerves, are formed by the S2, S3, and S4 roots. The dorsal nerve of the penis branches into anterior and posterior components after it passes underneath the pubic bone. The anterior branches supply sensation to the dorsum of the penis and the glans. The smaller posterior branches innervate the underside of the penis and frenulum. Skin at the base of the penis is innervated by the ilioinguinal nerve and, occasionally, a branch of the genitofemoral nerve (see Fig. 66–4).[3]

### Technique

Block of the penis is performed using a 25- or 27-gauge ¾-inch needle. Intradermal skin wheals are raised ½ inch caudal and ½ inch medial to each pubic tubercle (Figs. 66–5 and 66–6). The intradermal wheals are connected by intradermal and subcutaneous infiltration of 10 mL of 1% lidocaine,

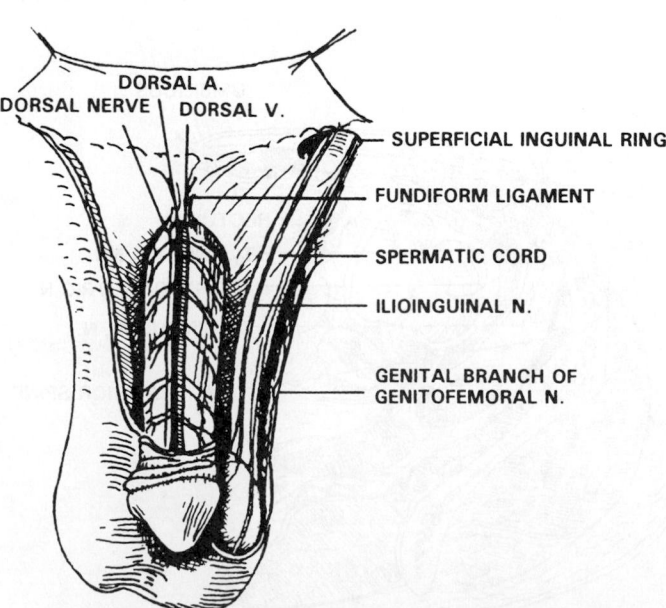

**FIGURE 66–4.** Relevant neuroanatomy of the penis.

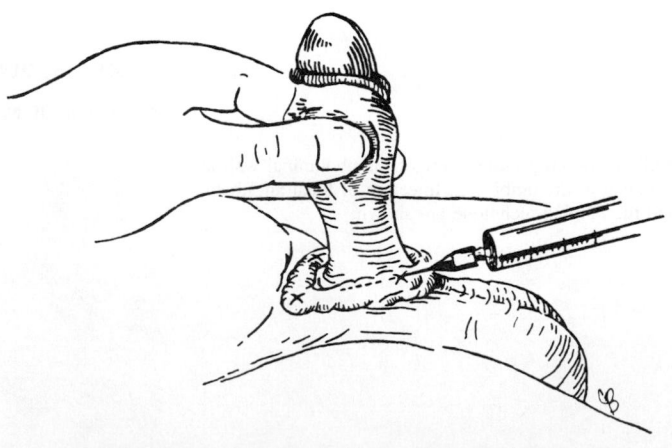

**FIGURE 66–6.** Intradermal skin wheals for penile block.

with or without epinephrine (1:200 000). A skin wheal also is raised on the median raphe of the scrotum at the base of the penis, and the intradermal and subcutaneous infiltrations are extended bilaterally to this point; 20 mL of the anesthetic solution is used.[3] Care must be taken not to inject intravascularly.

Duration of analgesia is 1 to 3 hours; the longer duration follows injection of epinephrine-containing solutions. Impotence following penile block apparently has followed placement of the local anesthetic under the penile fascia.

## INTERPLEURAL ANESTHESIA

Interpleural anesthesia has been advocated for patients undergoing a variety of procedures from cholecystectomies to renal surgery. Trivedi and coworkers described interpleural block with 30 mL of 0.5% bupivacaine for patients undergoing percutaneous nephrostomy and nephrolithotomy.[7] The ultimate role of interpleural block in regional anesthesia remains to be defined, but advantages over segmental epidural or subarachnoid block are not obvious.

### How Is It Performed?

Interpleural catheters are placed using 16- or 18-gauge Tuohy needles that are inserted along the superior border of the eighth rib, 8 to 10 cm from the posterior midline. The needle is advanced using either a loss of resistance technique with a glass syringe or a hanging drop method. When the pleural cavity is identified, a catheter is placed 5 to 6 cm past the end of the needle. A 3 mL test dose of 0.5% bupivacaine with epinephrine (1:200 000) is injected; this is followed by a loading dose of 20 to 30 mL.

Advocates of this block point to its maintenance of hemodynamic stability as a distinct advantage. The duration of effect is claimed to be 9 to 10 hours.[8] Reverse diffusion of local anesthetic from the parietal pleura to the intercostal muscles and also to the intercostal nerves is thought to provide analgesia.

### What Problems May Occur?

#### Local Anesthetic Toxicity

Questions arise as to whether local anesthetic toxicity is a major concern when using this route of injection.[9] Vascular absorption of local anesthetics from this region is high and may lead to toxicity. Seltzer and colleagues measured blood levels at different time intervals following administration of a 30-mL dose of 0.5% bupivacaine with epinephrine (1:100 000) and found absorption from the pleural space is similar to that in other areas of the body. Maximum bupivacaine plasma concentrations were reached between 10 and 30 minutes and ranged from 1.1 to 3.3 μg/mL.[10] Plasma levels of bupivacaine, 4 μg/mL, are associated with central nervous system toxicity. The toxic dose of bupivacaine is 3 mg/kg. Lower concentrations of bupivacaine in the injectate were correlated with poor pain relief.[10] Although no studies have been done using ropivacaine 0.5% for interpleural anesthesia, it may be a better choice in this location with its relatively

lower rate of cardiotoxicity (safe cumulative dose of 770 mg over a 24-hour period in adults).

### Other Complications

Possible complications include pneumothorax, hemothorax, empyema, systemic local anesthetic toxicity, intravascular injection, and Horner's syndrome. Contraindications to interpleural block include pleural fibrosis, pleural effusion, pleural infections, pneumothorax, and severely compromised cardiorespiratory function.[7]

## PROSTATIC SURGERY

Benign prostatic hyperplasia generally begins in the fourth decade of life. When hyperplasia becomes symptomatic, patients usually require surgery to alleviate its symptoms. If a prostate cancer occurs, it may be treated with either radiation therapy or surgical excision.

### What Is the Purpose of Balloon Dilation?

Balloon dilation of the prostate initially was used as an alternative to more invasive TURP surgery in high-risk patients. The procedure involves dilation of the prostatic urethra with a balloon catheter of up to size 90 French that is inflated for 10 minutes.[11] The incidence of complications from the procedure is extremely low, and it now is offered to an increasing number of patients with symptomatic benign prostatic hyperplasia.[12]

#### Anesthesia

Initially, the procedure was performed using general or regional anesthesia because dilation is painful. This approach necessitated long postanesthesia care unit (PACU) stays for monitoring. It is now increasingly performed with local anesthesia or with a combination of local anesthesia and intravenous sedation.

### Technique

The technique involves placement of the patient in a dorsal lithotomy position. Reddy anesthetized the perineum using a 25-gauge needle to infiltrate 1% lidocaine bilaterally into the skin 1 cm above and lateral to the anal orifice.[11] While a finger is placed in the rectum, a 20-gauge, 5-inch spinal needle is advanced, and 5 mL of 1% lidocaine is infiltrated along the left lateral border of the prostate to the junction of the prostate and left seminal vesicle. Ten to 15 mL of 1% lidocaine is deposited in this area. The same procedure is then performed on the right side. If the needle is placed too far anteriorly or laterally, it will hit the pubic ramus and must be redirected. The dilation can then be performed, usually without any additional sedative or analgesic supplement.

### Sedoanalgesia

Alternatively, local anesthetic instillation or infiltration techniques have been used. The urethra can be anesthetized by instillation of 2% lidocaine jelly. Concurrent intravenous sedation is achieved with short-acting narcotics, alone or combined with a benzodiazepine, such as midazolam, or with a propofol infusion, 30 to 50 µg/kg/min titrated to effect. The combination of local anesthesia and sedation is referred to as *sedoanalgesia* and has been used with great success in urology.[13] Advantages of these local techniques are shorter stays in PACUs and improved outpatient performance on discharge.

## How Is Prostatic Resection Accomplished?

The prostate gland can be excised by transurethral resection or an open approach. Large prostate glands (>80 g) are generally best resected by open prostatectomy. Prostate procedures are most often performed with the patient in a lithotomy position and with the operating table adjusted to some degree of the Trendelenburg tilt. Padding under the hips to provide better exposure of the prostate also is often used. The prostate is a vascular structure; thus, bleeding may be significant and at times difficult to control, regardless of the surgical approach employed.

### Open Prostatectomy

This procedure can be safely and effectively accomplished using a general, regional, or combined anesthetic technique. The head-down position, the use of retractors, and the length of the procedure normally dictate the need for a general anesthetic, either alone or in combination with epidural anesthesia. Benefits of regional and combination techniques include decreased intraoperative blood loss (37%), lowered incidence of pelvic deep vein thrombosis (DVT) (77%), and the ability to provide postoperative analgesia with epidural narcotics.[14]

A lowered mean arterial pressure (inflow) and decreased venous tone (outflow) are the mechanisms likely to influence the beneficial effect on blood loss and thrombosis. Placement of and dosing through the epidural catheter before induction of general anesthesia avoid most hemodynamic changes and allow the patient to identify a paresthesia should one occur. Use of a central venous catheter is also frequently recommended because the bladder is open during the procedure; thus urine output is not available to help guide fluid management and substantial bleeding can occur.

## Does Venous Air Embolism Occur?

Venous air embolism is a possibility, and its occurrence in this setting has been described.[15] The actual incidence of this complication during open prostatectomy is unknown. However, the hydrostatic pressure gradient between the prostatic fossa and the right side of the heart when the patient is in a head-down position, the extensive venous plexus, the use of retractors, and significant blood loss in combination predispose patients to such embolism. This complication merits inclusion in the differential diagnosis of intraoperative hypotension.

### Transurethral Resection

TURP still is the primary method used to relieve bladder outlet obstruction from prostatic hyperplasia. In a cooperative study that evaluated 3885 patients, Mebust and associates reviewed patient demographics. The average patient age was 69 years; 81% of patients were white, 10% were black, 5% were Hispanic, and 0.3% were Asian (the ethnic affiliation of 3% of patients was not recorded). The age distribution of patients was as follows: 15% were younger than 60 years; 38% were aged from 60 to 69 years; 35% were aged from 70 to 79 years; and 12% were older than 80 years.[16] Only 24.3% had no other recorded medical problems (Table 66–1).

### Anesthesia

In the study of Mebust and associates, 77% of surgeries were performed with spinal anesthesia, 20% were performed with general anesthesia, and the remaining 3% used either epidural or local anesthesia.[16]

### Spinal Anesthesia and Transurethral Resection

It is commonly believed that a subarachnoid sensory block to the T10 dermatome is required for adequate anesthesia during TURP.[17] Evans, in a study of 350 patients, concluded that a block to the upper level of L3 was sufficient for anesthesia in all cases of TURP, although he failed to objectively evaluate the perception of the patient's pain.[18] Beers and colleagues looked at the adequacy of an L3 block in relationship to pain scores that were defined as a visual analogue scale of <5.[19] They concluded that a block of L1 or greater provided adequate anesthesia for patients undergoing TURP. However, 38% of patients with a block of L3 or less had an inadequate block. Dubuisson stated that innervation of the muscles and deep structures does not strictly conform to the overlying dermatomes and that the deep segmental innervation of the pubic arch is supplied by L2, L3, and L4 roots.[20] Beers and associates said that a subarachnoid block to a level of between T12 and L1 might be reasonable in patients in whom adverse pulmonary effects may occur with a higher level.

### Local Anesthetics for Subarachnoid Block

#### Lidocaine

Jones and coworkers studied the dose of lidocaine (75 mg or 100 mg) necessary to provide adequate anesthesia for cystoscopy.[21] No difference was found in the onset of the drug

**TABLE 66–1.** Transurethral Resection of the Prostate and Coexisting Disease

| Disease | Percentage |
|---|---|
| Pulmonary | 14.1 |
| Gastrointestinal | 13.2 |
| Hypertension | 43 |
| Previous myocardial infarction | 12.3 |
| Dysrhythmias | 12.4 |
| Renal insufficiency | 9.8 |
| Diabetes | 9.8 |

From Mebust WK, Holtgrewe HL, Cockett ATK, et al. Transurethral prostatectomy: immediate and postoperative complications: a cooperative study of 13 participating institutions evaluating 3885 patients. *J Urol.* 1989;14:243.

based on dose, but recovery of motor function occurred at 95.5 + 7.38 minutes after the 75-mg dose when compared with 129 + 9.5 minutes with the 100-mg dose. The time difference between onset of motor recovery and full motor recovery was 22 minutes sooner in the 75-mg lidocaine group (7.2 + 1.2 minutes versus 29.5 minutes). They concluded that the larger dose did not confer any clinical advantage.

Although subarachnoid hyperbaric lidocaine has been studied in patients undergoing cystoscopy or TURP, the incidence of transient neurologic deficit symptoms that can occur afterward limit its use. Prospective studies with spinal lidocaine have shown incidence of transient radicular irritation (TRI) to be 10% to 37%.[22–24] Procedures done with the patient in a flexed knee or flexed hip position, as in GU procedures, appear predisposed to TRI. Patients with TRI present with central pain (burning, electrical quality, hypersensitivity, or decreased sensation). Normally, this is self-limited, resolving over a few days. Pandadero and associates reported a case of a patient with pain in the hips, buttocks, and legs.[25]

Alternative spinal anesthetics may include meperidine (pethidine). Sia and colleagues injected either 2 mL of 0.5% bupivacaine or 40 mg of meperidine intrathecally in patients undergoing TURP and found no significant difference in the degree of hypotension.[26] Meperidine had a significantly greater reduction in heart rate, less motor block, and a shorter period of postoperative analgesia, but it had a higher incidence of nausea and vomiting. Although intrathecal meperidine can be used as an alternative agent for local anesthetics in subarachnoid block, it does not offer any advantage to the hemodynamic side effects of local anesthetics and has an increased incidence of other side effects that were disconcerting to patients.

In some areas, local anesthesia with sedation is growing in popularity; for example, small glands can be resected using this approach.[13] Regional anesthesia is the preferred method for patients undergoing TURP because it facilitates early recognition of complications (Table 66–2).

## Complications

**Morbidity and Mortality.** Uchida and coworkers reviewed 1931 patients who underwent TURP from 1971–1985 and noted a total of 516 complications in 465 patients (an overall complication rate of 13.4%). Blood transfusions were necessary in 13.1% of patients.[27] Morbidity and blood transfusion rates were 9.5% and 6.1%, respectively, in patients who had surgery during the later period; the earlier period group had

**TABLE 66–2.** Signs and Symptoms of Complications of Transurethral Resection of the Prostate

| Complication | Signs and Symptoms |
|---|---|
| Fluid overload | Tachypnea; ↓ SpO₂ |
| Hyponatremia | Restlessness, confusion, nausea, seizures |
| Glycine toxicity | Encephalopathy; transient blindness (rarely) |
| Bladder perforation | |
| | *Extraperitoneal* |
| | Decreased irrigating fluid return, abdominal pain and distention, nausea, sweating |
| | *Intraperitoneal* |
| | Rapid onset of extraperitoneal symptoms as well as shoulder pain |

an incidence of 17.2% and 20.2%, respectively. Extravasation of irrigant was the most common intraoperative complication (3.5%). Acute epididymitis, urethral strictures, and a second TURP resulting from postoperative contracture of the bladder neck were observed in 1.6%, 1.5%, and 0.7% of patients. TURP syndrome occurred in 0.4% of patients. Mebust and associates noted 9 postoperative deaths (0.23%). In patients with benign disease, mortality was 0.1%.[16] A *postoperative death* was defined as one that occurred during the postoperative hospital period or within 30 days of surgery regardless of the cause. This is a decrease in mortality rate from the 2.5% rate in the 1960s.

Causes of death were sepsis in 5 patients, myocardial infarction (MI) in 1 patient, and other nonspecific conditions in 3 patients. No intraoperative deaths occurred. A total of 272 complications (6.9%) occurred intraoperatively.[16]

**Myocardial Ischemia.** Roos and colleagues noted patients who undergo TURP have an average mortality between 1% and 1.5%, related most commonly to cardiovascular disease.[28] Wong and associates studied 39 patients undergoing TURP to determine the incidence of perioperative ischemia.[29] There was an 18% incidence of ST segment changes consistent with myocardial ischemia. Patients who had more prostatic tissue resected and larger blood losses were more likely to have an episode of ST segment changes that was consistent with myocardial ischemia. These ischemic episodes were often accompanied by changes in heart rate, blood pressure (BP), or operative events. Edwards and coworkers monitored 100 patients undergoing TURP with either general or spinal anesthesia for myocardial ischemia.[30] The incidence of ischemia was between 18% and 26% and occurred more often in patients with known ischemic heart disease. There was an increase in both the incidence and the duration of myocardial ischemia postoperatively after anesthesia but no significant difference between general and spinal anesthesia. Factors that increased the incidence of myocardial ischemia follow:

1. Previous ischemic heart disease
2. Hypertension
3. Vascular disease
4. Diabetes
5. Abnormal preoperative electrocardiograph (ECG)

Hahn and colleagues found that the risk of MI after TURP correlated with the absorption of irrigating fluid.[31] The relative risk associated with absorption of 500 mL or more of irrigating solution was 1.6 (95% confidence interval [CI] for a first time MI after TURP and 6.1 (95% CI) for a reinfarction associated with the procedure. A blood loss of 375 mL or more without a 500-mL fluid absorption was associated with a decreased relative risk of first time MI (0.4 relative risk). A blood loss of 275 mL or less during TURP, but associated with an absorption of more than 500 mL of irrigating fluid, led the patient to have a 4.4 times greater risk for developing an acute MI.

In another study, Hahn and coworkers concluded that a moderately reduced hemoglobin level before TURP (10.0-12.9 g/dL) doubled (2.0 relative risk) the risk of acute MI.[32]

**Bleeding.** Blood loss during TURP can be significant. Mebust and associates reported an intraoperative transfusion rate of 2.5% and a postoperative transfusion rate of 3.9% of two units or greater with TURP.[33] The most common complication was bleeding sufficient to require transfusion in 2.5% of patients. When resection time is >90 minutes, the incidence of intraoperative bleeding is 7.3% (compared with 0.9% when resection time is <90 minutes).[16] The near constant flow of irrigating solution makes assessment of blood loss difficult. Additionally, the infusion of irrigating solution through the opened prostatic venous channels, combined with the absorption of fluid from retroperitoneal and perivesical spaces, masks the usual hemodynamic changes associated with blood loss.

## Intravascular Volume Loss

Perioperative hypotension is frequently preceded by blood loss. It may at times be explained by hyponatremia and hypertension that lead to a net water flux along osmotic and hydrostatic pressure gradients out of the intravascular space and into the lungs. This triggers pulmonary edema and hypovolemic shock.[34,35] Sympathectomy secondary to regional anesthesia may compound the TURP syndrome.

Transurethral resection of larger glands (ie, >50 g) and procedures that are of long duration (ie, >1 hour) are associated with increased blood loss. A useful rule-of-thumb is that blood loss of 15 mL per gram of resected tissue should be anticipated.[36,37] Kirollos and Campbell studied whether regional anesthesia reduced blood loss in comparison to general anesthesia.[38] There was a tendency for less blood loss with regional, but it was not statistically significant. Madsen and Madsen, however, showed a significant advantage of spinal anesthesia in preventing blood loss compared with general anesthesia.[39] The amount of prostate tissue resected is the only consistent variable in determining blood loss. Abrams and colleagues and Smyth and associates found that when resected tissue weight exceeded 35 g, blood loss was in excess of the linear correlation shown with the weight of resected prostatic tissue.[40,41]

Aspirin has been used as an antithrombotic agent in the prevention of thromboembolus after surgery and was thought to pose an increased risk of bleeding in patients undergoing TURP.[42] Ala-Opas and Gronlund studied 82 patients receiving 250 mg of aspirin daily who underwent TURP and concluded that blood loss was not enhanced by aspirin.[43] Avoidance of aspirin before TURP appears unnecessary.

Resections of prostate glands weighing >45 g have a statistically greater incidence of intraoperative bleeding (10%) than smaller glands (0.9%) and require a greater amount of time to perform. The incidence of the TURP syndrome is also higher (1.5% compared with 0.8% for smaller glands).

## Coagulopathies and Transurethral Resection of the Prostate

Smyth and coworkers studied patients receiving either general or spinal anesthesia for TURP and found that blood loss in TURP patients was independent of the anesthetic technique.[41] The type of anesthesia used to prevent blood loss was thought to be a matter of personal choice. Six percent of patients developed subclinical intravascular coagulopathies, correlating with the resected prostate tissue mass. Immediate and postsurgical bleeding is the most frequent complication during TURP. Nielsen and associates studied whether the activation of the extrinsic tissue plasminogen activator (TPA)-related fibrinolysis is implicated in the blood loss during TURP.[44] After studying 24 patients, they concluded that although the fibrinolytic system is activated during and after TURP, the increased activity is not of pathophysiologic importance for blood loss.

Bell and associates used the thromboelastograph (TEG) to assess the changes in overall coagulation status and define the degree of systemic fibrinolysis occurring in patients undergoing TURP.[45] There was no evidence by TEG of fibrinolysis in patients during the perioperative period; however, noteworthy was that from 3 hours to 10 to 14 days postoperatively, the TEG variables showed a hypercoagulable state. It was concluded that there was no role of *systemic* fibrinolysis in primary and secondary hemorrhage following TURP. However, Nielsen and coworkers investigated in situ fibrinolysis as a cause of bleeding after TURP.[44] Concentrations of the urokinase and TPA-related fibrinolysis were measured in the urine of 24 men who underwent TURP to determine if the changes were related to postoperative blood loss. Blood loss after TURP was correlated with the increase of urinary fibrinolytic activity, most likely caused by TPA. These findings may support the notion that blood loss after TURP can be significantly reduced after the administration of antifibrinolytic drugs, especially if given locally such as with bladder instillation. Routine use of antifibrinolytic drugs was, however, not recommended.

## Hypothermia and Irrigant Temperature

Hypothermia results from reduced temperatures in the operating room and the use of room temperature irrigating solutions. Routine use of irrigating solutions that are warmed to body temperature prevents this complication. If room temperature irrigating fluids are used, the average decrease in body temperature is 1.8°C for a 70-minute TURP.[46] Pit and associates studied patients undergoing TURP comparing isothermic solutions with room temperature solutions and found a statistically significant difference in core temperatures between the two groups.[47] The isothermic group had a decrease of only 0.74°C, whereas the room temperature group had a 1.71°C drop in temperature after a resection time of only 30 minutes.

## Sepsis

Sudden cardiovascular collapse, rigors, or tachycardia suggest the presence of bacteremia. Treatment is symptomatic and includes broad-spectrum antibiotic coverage. Procedures on the vascular GU system predispose the patient to intravascular inoculation and bacteremia if an infection is present. Thus, prostate or urinary tract infections should be ruled out and, if present, treated preoperatively.

## Obturator Nerve Stimulation

Stimulation of the obturator nerve by the electric resectoscope sometimes occurs. The obturator nerve traverses the pelvis adjacent to the inferolateral wall of the bladder, the bladder neck, and the lateral prostatic urethra. It is a branch of the lumbar plexus (L2-4). As it emerges from the obturator canal, it divides into the superficial and profunda branches. The superficial branch innervates the short, long, and gracilis adductor muscles. The profunda branch innervates the adductor magnus and internus muscles.

Adductor contraction results from direct stimulation of the

motor neurons within the obturator nerve by the electrical current from the resectoscope.[48] Jerking of the legs may be so violent that it causes inadvertent bladder perforation or makes the urologist unable to resect the prostate adequately. Neuromuscular blocking agents prevent adductor contraction; a spinal or epidural anesthetic, however, does not.[49] Although nondepolarizing and depolarizing agents accomplish neuromuscular blockade, direct muscle stimulation from the current can best be prevented by using a depolarizing agent. If repetitive adductor muscle contraction is a problem during general anesthesia, a succinylcholine infusion should be considered.

The obturator nerve can be blocked. In one series, an obturator block obtained with 30 mL of 2% lidocaine with epinephrine produced complete ablation of adductor spasm in 11 of 13 patients; the remaining 2 patients had 80% reduction of the spasm.[50]

To perform the block, the adductor longus tendon is palpated where it inserts into the pubic tubercle. A 22-gauge spinal needle is placed 2 cm lateral and caudad to the pubic tubercle (Fig. 66–7). The needle is aimed at an angle slightly lateral (15°-20°) and cephalad (10°-30°) and is advanced to the superior pubic ramus. It is then *walked* off the inferior margin of the superior pubic ramus and advanced 1.5 to 2 cm in a posterior, superior, and lateral direction (Fig. 66–8). One half of the volume is injected, the needle is withdrawn and repositioned 1 cm laterally, and one half of the remaining lidocaine is injected. The needle is again repositioned 1 cm medial to the original site, and the remainder of the anesthetic is injected (Fig. 66–9).[50]

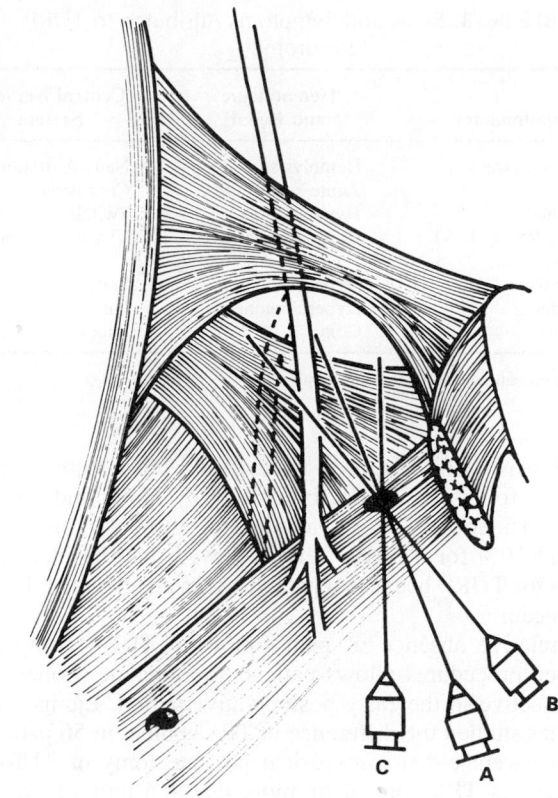

**FIGURE 66–8.** Site of local anesthetic infiltration for obturator nerve block. *A*, Midobturator canal. *B*, One centimeter lateral. *C*, One centimeter medial.

### Venous Thrombosis

A potentially devastating complication after prostatic surgery is DVT with resultant pulmonary embolus. Nicolaides and coworkers studied 50 patients who underwent TURP or retropubic prostatic resection.[51] They found that the incidence

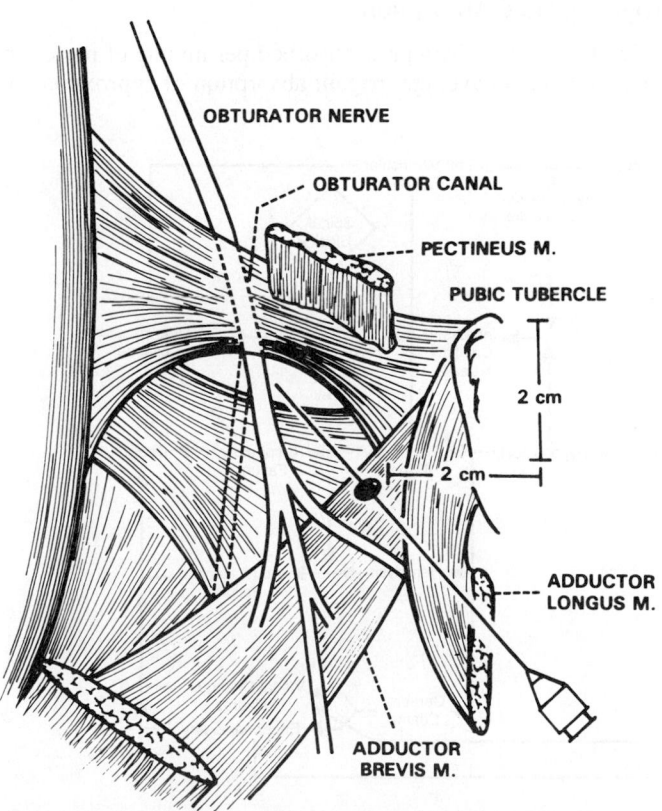

**FIGURE 66-7.** View of the obturator nerve as it passes through the obturator canal. (Redrawn from Augspurger RR, Donohue RE. Prevention of obturator nerve stimulation during transurethral surgery. *J Urol.* 1980;123:170.)

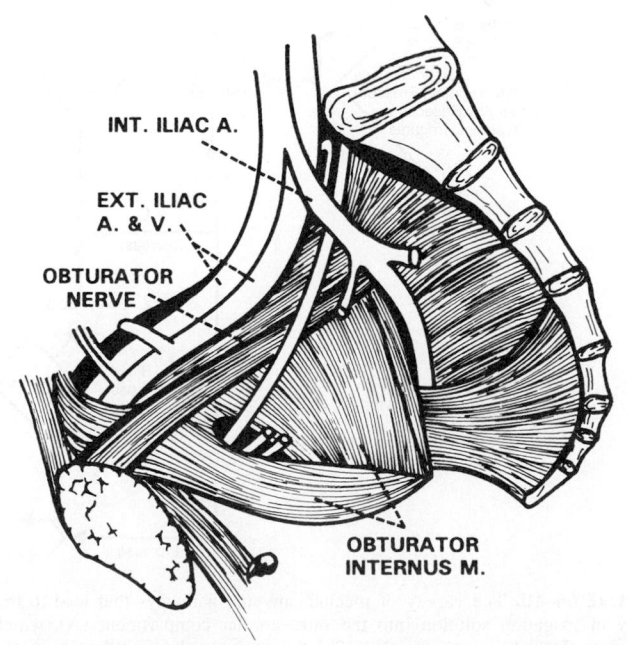

**FIGURE 66-9.** View of the obturator nerve as it passes through the pelvis.

**TABLE 66–3.** Signs and Symptoms Attributed to TURP Syndrome

| Cardiopulmonary | Hematologic and Renal | Central Nervous System |
|---|---|---|
| Respiratory distress | Hemolysis | Nausea/vomiting |
| Cyanosis | Acute renal failure | Confusion |
| Hypertension | Hyponatremia | Twitches |
| Widened QRS or ↑ ST segment | Hypo-osmolality | Visual disturbance |
| Dysrhythmia | Hyperglycinemia | Seizures |
| Bradycardia | Hyperammonemia | Paralysis |
| Hypotension | Coma | Shock |

TURP, transurethral resection of the prostate.

of DVT was 47.6% following retropubic prostatectomy and only 6.8% following TURP. In a study by Mayo and associates, the incidence of DVT was 51% for retropubic prostatectomy and 10% for TURP.[52] They believed that the incidence was less for TURP because a patient's legs are elevated during this procedure.

The relative absence of pain following TURP compared with open procedures allows patients to ambulate sooner and be more active in the early postoperative period. Ljunger and colleagues studied the difference in TPA content in 56 patients who underwent either transvesical prostatectomy or TURP.[53] A decrease in TPA content by more than 0.5 unit was found in 75% of the patients who had transvesical surgery compared with only 30% of the patients in the TURP group on the first postoperative day. No difference in the activity decrease was noted between general and regional anesthesia patients. These authors concluded that the TPA difference may in part be responsible for the increased incidence of DVT following open versus TURP.

## THE TRANSURETHRAL RESECTION OF THE PROSTATE SYNDROME

### What Is It?

The *TURP syndrome* is a complication that can occur during or after TURP in up to 10% of patients.[54] A disproportionately higher mortality is noted in those patients who develop it compared with those who do not. Acute intravascular volume shifts and acute changes in plasma solute concentrations are responsible. The latter include hyponatremia, decreased serum osmolarity, and increased glycine and ammonia concentrations. Manifestations of this syndrome as well as the systems that are affected are varied (Table 66–3).

### What Causes It?

The mechanisms and pathways that lead to TURP are illustrated in Figure 66–10.

### Osmolality Changes

The most serious derangement in the TURP syndrome is not hyponatremia, per se, but rather the acute hypo-osmolality that it causes; this hypo-osmolality, in turn, results in cerebral and pulmonary edema.[35,54] Serum sodium determination is not always a reliable indicator of serum osmolality or of the TURP syndrome; however, it is the most quickly determined surrogate for osmolality.

### Irrigating Fluid Absorption

Ten to 30 mL of irrigant is absorbed per minute of resection time, yielding an average irrigant absorption of approximately

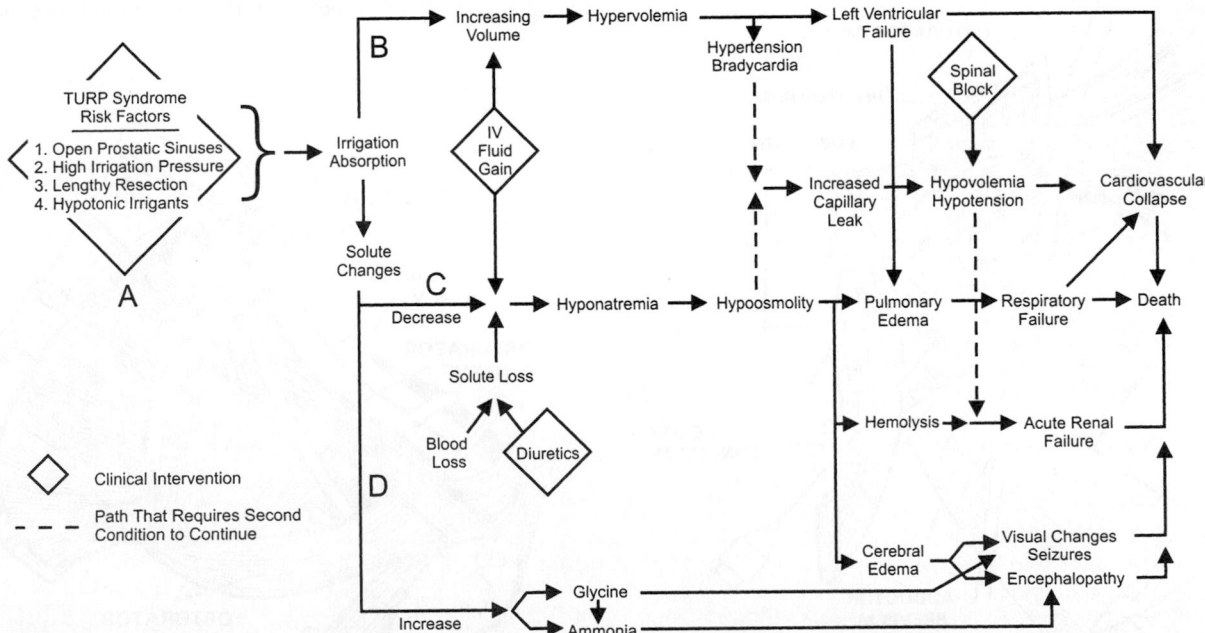

**FIGURE 66–10.** The variety of mechanisms and pathways that lead to transurethral resection of the prostate (TURP) syndrome. The triggering event is the entry of irrigation solution into the intravascular compartment (A), which increases intravascular volume (B) with its sequelae and decreases (C) and/or increases (D) solute concentration. The figure shows the complex interactions that need to be considered when the TURP syndrome unfolds. IV, intravenous. (From Gravenstein D. Transurethral resection of the prostate [TURP] syndrome: a review of the pathophysiology and management. *Anesth Analg.* 1997; 84:438.)

1000 mL in the course of an operation.[55] Absorption of irrigant during TURP can lead to rapid volume expansion and lead to hypertension and reflex bradycardia. In extreme cases, absorption can approach 200 mL/min of volume.[56] The rate of irrigating fluid absorption is also related to the height of the irrigating fluid reservoir above the bladder. Ideally, the fluid reservoir irrigating pressure should not exceed venous pressure, but it should be sufficiently great to maintain visibility and to wash away blood and tissue.

If the intravesical pressure is kept <15 cm $H_2O$, irrigant absorption usually stops. The most commonly used system is one in which the resectoscope simultaneously irrigates and drains irrigating fluid. This method keeps the irrigating fluid pressure relatively low unless the hydrostatic pressure of the fluid reservoir exceeds the low resistance drainage capacity of the resectoscope or unless the drainage channel becomes obstructed.

Van Renen and Reymann studied the effect of height on the absorption of irrigating solutions at 70 cm and 150 cm and concluded that the height of the solution is not important in developing the hyponatremia and hypo-osmolality associated with TURP.[57] Careful attention to surgical technique, by avoiding overdistention of the bladder and opening of major venous sinuses, is a more important factor. This is in contrast to Madsen and Naber, who found that intravesicular pressure >30 mm Hg increased irrigant absorption and recommended limiting the height of the irrigant to 40 cm or using a continuous irrigating resectoscope or suprapubic trocar to minimize it.[58] If the intravesicular pressure is limited to 15 mm Hg or less, irrigant absorption is negligible.[59]

### What Irrigating Fluids Are Available?

A TURP requires a solution that does not conduct electricity and that provides a clear visual field. It has evolved from plain water in the past to 1.5% glycine and Cytal (2.7% sorbitol and 0.54% mannitol). Plain water irrigation has been virtually abandoned because it causes unacceptable degrees of hemolysis, hyponatremia, and renal failure.

Nonelectrolyte 1.5% glycine solution is slightly hypo-osmolar (230 mOsm), but it is inexpensive when compared with Cytal, which is isotonic. An additional consequence is that glycine has ammonia as a metabolic byproduct and, thus, predisposes the patient to sequelae of hyperglycemia and hyperammonemia, which can lead to encephalopathy and transient blindness. Solutions of 1.2% glycine, 2.5% glycine, 5% mannitol, and 5% sorbitol are also used. Three percent sorbitol has an osmolality of 178 mOsm/kg. Other sorbitol solutions may be formulated to be isotonic. Osmolarity calculations for irrigation solutions are based on no interaction between solute particles. Particles do, however, interact in solution; thus, the calculated osmolarity values are slightly greater (10-20 mOsm/kg) than the measured osmolality of the solution.[35]

Hahn and colleagues found no clear advantage to lowering the concentration of glycine from 1.5% to 1% in irrigating solutions because the type of solution had no effect on the total incidence of symptoms.[60] Akan and associates looked at three different irrigating solutions for patients undergoing TURP: 1.5% glycine, 5% mannitol, and 2.7% sorbitol.[61] Mannitol was believed to cause more hypervolemia, although it was not clinically significant. Glycine has the potential to

**TABLE 66–4.** Acute Changes in Serum Sodium

| Serum Sodium | Electrocardiographic Changes | Irritability |
|---|---|---|
| 120 mEq/L | May see widened QRS | Restlessness; confusion |
| 115 mEq/L | Widened QRS; ↑ ST | Nausea; vomiting; semicoma |
| 100 mEq/L | Ventricular tachycardia or fibrillation | Seizures |

From Berger JJ. Transurethral resection of the prostate. Lesson 20. *Curr Rev Clin Anesth.* 1981;1:165.

cause hyperammonemia. Sorbitol has none of these adverse effects.

### How Is It Diagnosed?

The occurrence of any of the signs or symptoms listed in Table 66–3, the presence of any of the ECG changes listed in Table 66–4, or a resection that lasts longer than 60 minutes suggests the urgent need for serum sodium measurement and, if available, a serum osmolality determination. One percent ethanol in the irrigating solution has also been used as a marker for early detection of both irrigating fluid absorption and hyponatremia (Figs. 66–11 and 66–12).[62] This assessment is an alternative to repetitive serum sodium and osmolality determinations and measures the ethanol content of the expired breath with a Breathalyzer. Ethanol 1% in glycine 1.5% is currently marketed in the United Kingdom and Scandinavia for monitoring irrigant absorption during TURP. Physicians in Switzerland have reduced the concentration of ethanol down

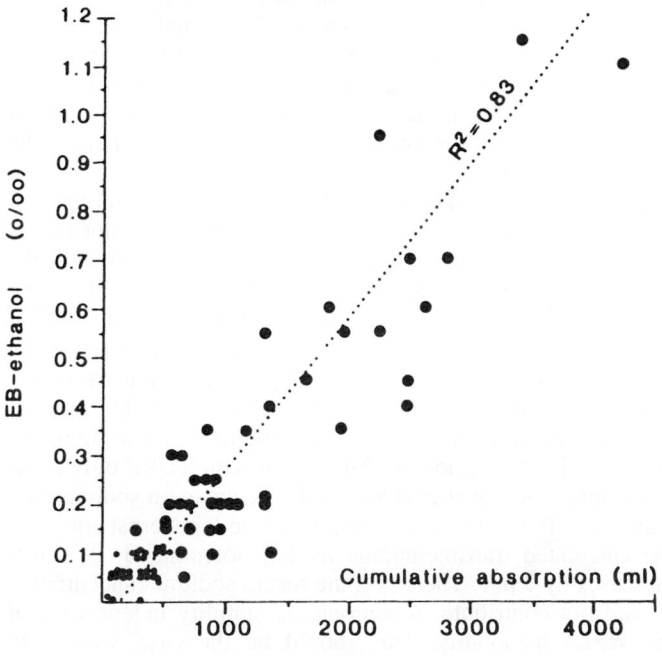

**FIGURE 66–11.** The relationship between the ethanol concentration in the expired breath (EB-ethanol) and the cumulative absorption of irrigant measured for 10-minute periods during transurethral resection. (From Hahn RG. Early detection of the TUR syndrome by marking the irrigating fluid with 1% ethanol. *Acta Anaesthesiol Scand.* 1989;33:147.)

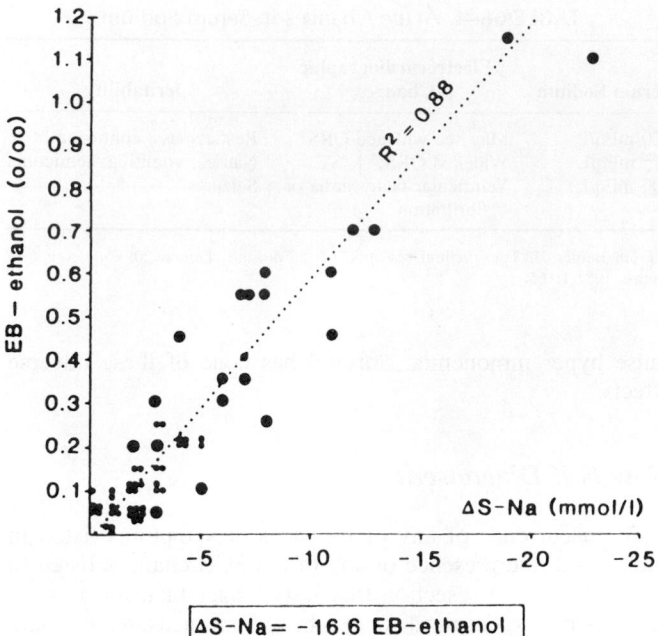

$$\Delta S\text{-}Na = -16.6 \ EB\text{-}ethanol$$

**FIGURE 66–12.** The relationship between the ethanol concentration in the expired breath (EB-ethanol) and the change in the serum sodium concentration since the commencement of the operation. The data relate to the end of the 10-minute period during resections when the EB-ethanol concentration indicated that irrigant was being absorbed. (From Hahn RG. Early detection of the TUR syndrome by marking the irrigating fluid with 1% ethanol. *Acta Anaesthesiol Scand.* 1989;33:147.)

to 0.5% but with an associated lower sensitivity than the 1% concentration.[63] Hahn, however, pointed out that except for the above countries, virtually no one in the United States is using this method.[64] Part of the problem may be that the incidence of the TURP syndrome in the United States is low, calculated to be between 0.5 and 2 cases per year in any given surgical department. Proponents of the ethanol detection system point out that studies show that irrigant absorption of >1000 mL occurs in between 5% to 10% of patients who undergo TURP.[65–67]

Patients with marked hyponatremia may show no signs of water intoxication[67]; therefore, hyponatremia may not be the sole or primary cause of the neurologic manifestations of the TURP syndrome. Acute hypo-osmolality is more likely the cause of the central nervous system malfunction in the TURP syndrome. This can be anticipated because the blood-brain barrier's pore size of 8 Å is essentially impermeable to sodium but freely permeable to water.[35] The Nernst equation predicts that the decrease in extracellular sodium concentration that accompanies the hypo-osmolality seen with TURP only minimally alters neuronal excitability. By replacing a sodium (Na) value of 140 mmol/L with 100 mmol/L in the Nernst equation, the calculated transmembrane resting potential of −60 mV increases by 9 mV. Therefore, the serum sodium concentration should not contribute to neuronal excitability independent of the serum osmolality. This should be the case, even with the serum sodium changes typically associated with TURP syndrome.

The brain quickly reacts within seconds to minutes by decreasing intracellular Na, K, Cl. In conjunction, idiogenic osmoles act to decrease intracellular osmolality and prevent swelling.[68] These compensatory mechanisms may not work fast enough, allowing cerebral edema from hypo-osmolality

to occur. This edema is caused by decreased osmolality and not by decreased serum colloid oncotic pressure.

## When Is the Transurethral Resection of the Prostate Syndrome Treated?

The TURP syndrome probably should be treated only if it is symptomatic, that is, a patient should not be treated just because his serum sodium level is decreased.[69] If TURP syndrome occurs intraoperatively, the operation should be concluded as quickly as possible using the minimum acceptable irrigating fluid pressure. The acute treatment endpoint should be resolution of symptoms rather than complete correction of hyponatremia.[69]

This conservative approach minimizes the risk of central pontine myelinolysis from overly rapid correction of hyponatremia (hypo-osmolality).[35,70] Myelinolysis is rare and is more commonly seen in cases of chronic hypo-osmolality. Its association with hyponatremia is unclear.[71]

### Central Pontine Myelinolysis

When treatment is instituted too slowly for symptomatic hyponatremia (<0.7 mmol/L/h) in order to avoid central pontine myelinolysis, a higher morbidity and mortality occurs than if too rapid correction is done (>1.0 mmol/L/h).[72] Correction rates of 1.5 to 2.0 mmol/L/h have been reported safe (to prevent CPM) even though they do not take into account changes in osmolality.[73,74] Some scientists state that osmotic changes are more detrimental to patients with a correction of chronic hyponatremia than those with acute hyponatremia correction.[75,76] Patient symptoms from hyponatremia may be the most important factor in determining treatment and the associated morbidity and mortality. In the absence of symptoms, instituting therapy may risk too rapid a correction. The correction rate is frequently difficult to control. Serum osmolality should therefore be monitored. Correction of osmolality should only be aggressive until patient symptoms resolve and then be continued slowly at a rate of <1.5 mmol/L/h.

## How Is It Treated?

In addition to rapid conclusion of the procedure, treatment of symptomatic TURP syndrome may necessitate administration of 3% saline. Seizures are treated with thiopental or a benzodiazepine, whereas fluid overload is treated with diuresis. The diuresis should be initiated with furosemide, 20 to 40 mg intravenously, because the aberration is free water excess rather than an absolute sodium deficiency. The amount of sodium necessary to correct the deficit can be calculated using the following equation:

mEq of Sodium Deficit = Desired Sodium (mEq/L)
(usually not more than 130 mEq/L) −
[Measured (Current) Sodium (mEq/L) × TBW (L)]

(Equation 1)

in which TBW is total body water.

Because 3% saline contains 513 mEq/L of sodium, the volume required is calculated as follows:

$$\text{mL Required} = \text{mEq of Sodium Deficit}/513 \text{ mEq/L} \times 100$$

(Equation 2)

(For 5% saline, substitute 855 mEq/L for 513 mEq/L.)

## Treatment of Hyponatremia and Hypo-Osmolality

Pretreatment with hypertonic saline may decrease the degree of dilutional hyponatremia[77] and the incidence of hypo-osmolality–related TURP syndrome. It may, however, aggravate the incidence and severity of the hypervolemia symptoms. Serum sodium levels do not reflect serum osmolality. The serum sodium should be measured alone and the irrigant osmolality reported if the irrigant contains osmotically active solutes such as glycine, mannitol, and sorbitol. If the irrigant's osmolality is near normal, no intervention should take place to correct the serum sodium in asymptomatic patients with low serum sodium concentrations.[35]

Only one quarter to one half of the calculated deficit correcting fluid volume should be administered unless symptoms resolve earlier; if this occurs, administration is stopped. Serum sodium measurement is repeated after fluid administration based on this partial deficit correction. Measurement of serum sodium, osmolality, or both, is a key factor in the early diagnosis and treatment of TURP syndrome. Some clinicians determine these values as often as every 15 to 30 minutes. Be sure that the baseline and subsequent determinations are made with the same analyzer because significant differences can occur when using different analyzers.

## Hyperammonemia

Prophylactic administration of intravenous L-arginine markedly moderates the increase in blood ammonia concentration in fasting patients receiving intravenous glycine. Infusion of L-arginine during or at the end of glycine administration prevents further increases in blood ammonia concentration and accelerates the return to normal levels.[78] Doses of L-arginine 4 g (20 mmol) infused over 3 minutes or 38 g (180 mmol) infused over 120 minutes have been recommended. No toxicity was noted with either regimen. The cost of a 300-mL bottle of preservative-free L-arginine with an osmolality of 950 mOsm/kg is approximately US$85.

## Hyperglycinemia

Glycine may be involved in TURP-related encephalopathy and seizure activity by its action on the *N*-methyl-D-aspartate (NMDA) receptor system.[79,80] Seizures associated with hyponatremia and hypo-osmolality are resistant to benzodiazepine and anticonvulsant therapy. This treatment may lead to apnea. NMDA receptor antagonists or glycine antagonists are better choices to stop these seizures.[80] In addition, magnesium exerts a negative control on the NMDA receptor. Serum magnesium levels in TURP syndrome may be lowered by dilution and increase seizure activity. Magnesium therapy for seizures in patients undergoing TURP with a glycine irrigant may deserve consideration.

## Diuretics for Treatment of the Transurethral Resection of the Prostate Syndrome

A study by Tsao and colleagues compared the use of 30 mg intravenous furosemide to 0.5 g/kg intravenous glycerol for treating TURP syndrome.[81] Although glycerol produced significantly less urine 1 hour after the operation, it has the potential to be superior in protecting against water intoxication because it produces higher plasma osmolality and less rebound cerebral edema.

# TRANSURETHRAL ELECTROVAPORIZATION OF THE PROSTATE

Newer techniques have been developed for resection of benign prostatic hypertrophy (BPH) other than the classic TURP using a resectoscope and irrigant. They range from transurethral electrovaporization of the prostate (TUVP), transurethral ultrasound-guided laser-induced prostatectomy (TULIP), visual laser ablation of the prostate (VLAP), and transurethral needle ablation (TUNA).

TUVP of the prostate is a new technique for treatment of benign hypertrophy of the prostate.[82] Electrosurgery uses electrical energy to heat tissue. If the application of the electrical energy is slow or only in small amounts, cells will only heat and dehydrate. However, if the energy applied is great enough, the heat produced will vaporize the cellular contents and cause the cell to explode. TUVP is accomplished using a rolling electrode that is grooved and spiky. It concentrates the electrosurgical current at the ridges of the grooved surface that are in direct contact with the tissue.[82] An area of high current density is provided where it contacts the tissues, resulting in a thermal reaction that raises the tissue temperature to the point of vaporization (>100°C). The procedure is performed under irrigation to prevent desiccation of the tissues and facilitate the vaporization process. The coagulation depth increases with higher power and multiple passes of the vaporizing electrode but does not exceed 2 to 3 mm beyond the vaporized cavity. The irrigant fluid removes most of the heat.

Several studies have compared TURP and TUVP under continuous glycine irrigation.[82,83] They find that the two techniques are equivalent in relieving the patient's symptoms. TUVP, however, permitted shorter hospital stays with a reduction in cost. The decrease in Na, hemoglobin, and hematocrit were significantly lower with TUVP than with TURP. TUVP was found to cause only minimal absorption of the irrigant. With TUVP, there is a lower incidence of bleeding, a decreased need for transfusion, and a significantly lower drop in hematocrit compared with TURP, and less irrigant absorption. The need for postoperative irrigation following TUVP has been abandoned due to the lack of bleeding.

Kupeli and associates noted that decreases in serum sodium were insignificant in TURP and TUVP but the drop was less in the TUVP group.[84] Talic modified the TUVP electrode into a winged tip.[85] He noted no significant drop in hematocrit in most patients. However, a perforation of the prostatic capsule did occur in one patient in whom the device was used in the coagulation mode to stop a bleeding vessel. This patient developed a TURP syndrome, requiring treatment with hypertonic saline for 24 hours. Therefore, it is key the surgeon and anesthesiologist communicate because TURP syndrome may occur even with TUVP if perforation takes place.

Ekengren and Hahn studied 26 patients undergoing TUVP and 100 undergoing TURP monitoring to evaluate blood loss, fluid absorption by ethanol method, and hemodynamic stability.[86] Results showed that blood loss with TUVP was lower per minute. The volume of irrigant tended to be smaller with TUVP. Fluid absorption was detected in most patients during TUVP, although only small volumes were absorbed. Most absorption could not be detected by measuring serum sodium but by the ethanol breath analysis method.

The advantages of TUVP versus TURP are listed in Table 66–5. Remember that the TURP syndrome, although much less likely, may still occur with TUVP, especially if the prostatic capsule is perforated.

## TRANSURETHRAL NEEDLE ABLATION OF THE PROSTATE

TUNA is an outpatient method of coagulating prostate tissue using interstitial low-level radiofrequency current. TUNA generates prostatic tissue temperatures in excess of 100°C by using radiofrequency (RF) energy.[87] The result is irreversible damage and tissue necrosis after 3 to 5 minutes of exposure. The urethra is cooled by injection of cold saline through the catheter irrigating port, but continuous bladder irrigation is unnecessary. The active electrode (needle) has a small surface area and delivers the RF current into the target tissue. The prostate cells resist the passage of the electrical current, generating thermal energy by inductive heating of water molecules and friction. This process eventually leads to tissue heating and ablation by coagulation necrosis. The thermal lesions occur only in the localized area of RF current near the active electrode. The lesion size is proportional to the amount of tissue in contact with the exposed needle length and the magnitude of the energy delivered. The second electrode is the indifferent electrode applied externally to the patient. It acts as a ground and, therefore, does not cause any tissue damage.

### Procedure

The patient is placed in the dorsal lithotomy position. Lidocaine jelly 2% is injected intraurethrally at least 10 minutes before the start of the procedure. Frequently, local anesthesia is supplemented with intravenous sedation. General or spinal anesthesia is not usually required. Kahn and associates studied patients undergoing TUNA and found that 57% of the surgeries were performed under local anesthesia with 2% lidocaine gel and intravenous midazolam 1.25 to 5 mg.[88] Two of the patients <65 years, under local anesthesia, had to have the procedure aborted because of excessive pain and the procedures were subsequently performed under general anesthesia. Fourteen patients were <65 years: 10 received general anes-

**TABLE 66–5.** Advantages of TUVP Versus TURP

| | |
|---|---|
| Shorter hospital stay | Less blood loss |
| Less irrigant absorption | Less incidence of blood transfusion |
| Less decrease in serum sodium | No postoperative irrigation necessary |

TURP, transurethral resection of the prostate; TUVP, transurethral electrovaporization of the prostate.

**TABLE 66–6.** Advantages of TUNA Versus TURP

| |
|---|
| Less blood loss |
| Less irrigant absorption |
| Extremely low incidence of transfusion |

TUNA, transurethral needle ablation; TURP, transurethral resection of the prostate.

thesia, 2 had epidurals, and 2 had spinal anesthesia. No patient required a blood transfusion nor manifested signs of fluid absorption. Narayan and colleagues concluded that in a large majority of patients (57%), TUNA could be performed under local anesthesia with intravenous supplementation.[89]

The advantages of TUNA versus TURP are listed in Table 66–6.

## TRANSURETHRAL ULTRASOUND-GUIDED LASER-INDUCED PROSTATECTOMY

Transurethral ultrasound (US) has been added to the laser induced prostatectomy (TULIP) to show the depth and configuration of the benign prostatic hypertrophied tissue in the path of the laser beam.[90] The TULIP system was developed to optimize laser prostatectomy. It consists of a transurethral probe and a US imager. The 20-French probe incorporates a side firing laser window and split US transducer. The TULIP probe is enclosed in a sleeve filled with sterile water. The US imager displays a real time 90° sector scan image from the transducer. Tissue depth up to 4 cm below the surface of the urethra can be imaged, allowing the urologist to determine the specific areas of the prostate requiring laser treatment. The TULIP system can be coupled to most Nd:YAG lasers. The laser energy penetrates beneath the surface of the tissue and causes coagulation necrosis along the length of the passage. Constant laser beam standoff is maintained; tissue is not ablated, vaporized, or acutely removed; and bleeding, therefore, does not occur. Minimal irrigation fluid is required and the procedure is essentially bloodless while visualized under US imaging and not by cystoscopy. McCullough studied 150 patients using the TULIP procedure to relieve bladder outlet obstruction secondary to benign prostatic hypertrophy.[90] Anesthesia consisted of spinal (67%), general (22%), regional block (6%), and local (5%) anesthesia. Ninety-five percent of the cases were estimated to have blood loss <50 mL. The other 5% were estimated to have blood loss between 50 mL and 200 mL. No blood transfusions were required. The average amount of irrigant used was only 1.7 L.

## VISUAL LASER ABLATION OF THE PROSTATE

VLAP, a right angle delivery system coupled to a Nd:YAG laser, has several potential advantages over traditional TURP including the use of local anesthesia alone, a lower incidence of hemorrhage, and fewer complications. Anson and colleagues studied 166 patients undergoing either VLAP or TURP and noted only a significant decrease in hematocrit at 24 hours with TURP.[91] No patient in the VLAP group received a transfusion; the incidence of transfusion with TURP was 12%. The serum sodium decreased significantly in both groups postoperatively but none were in a problematic range. Complications of VLAP include delay in spontaneous voiding. To circumvent this problem, Anson and associates recommended that urethral catheters be left in place for 5 days postoperatively.

Narayan and coworkers found that 33% of patients required catheterization for >3 days after laser therapy, and 11% required >5 days of catheterization.[89] Dysuria was higher in the VLAP patients. Costello and associates studied the changes in hemoglobin and serum sodium in patients undergoing TURP versus laser prostatectomy.[92] The laser group had a slight fall in hemoglobin in the recovery room that did not last 24 hours. Serum sodium demonstrated no difference between preoperative levels and levels in the recovery room. The TURP group showed statistically significant drops in both hemoglobin and serum sodium levels in the recovery room and 24 hours later. They concluded that VLAP provided greater safety than TURP, with an absence of bleeding and absence of irrigant absorption, thus minimizing electrolyte alterations that would reduce the morbidity and mortality seen with conventional TURP. Cummings and colleagues, in a study that monitored irrigant absorption by ethanol levels, found minimal to no irrigant absorbed with the laser technique.[93]

The advantages and disadvantages of using VLAP over TURP are listed in Table 66–7.

### Local Anesthesia for Laser Prostatectomy

Leach studied 46 men undergoing visual laser-assisted prostatectomy (VLAP) using local anesthesia with a periprostatic block.[94] The procedure involved infiltration of a 50:50 mixture of 1% plain lidocaine and 0.5% bupivacaine. A total of 10 mL was injected perineally just lateral to the urethra on each side, using a 21-gauge spinal needle inserted at the base of the prostate. Infiltration was continued while the needle was withdrawn distally to the prostatic apex under digital rectal control. Intravascular injection was avoided. Additional anesthetic effect was obtained with intraurethral 1% lidocaine jelly. Intravenous mild sedation was provided with midazolam. No effort was made to analyze the adequacy of the anesthetic or patient acceptance (Fig. 66–13). Akalin and associates used an 18-gauge spinal needle to perform a similar block with 2% lidocaine and supplemented the infiltration with a topical gel that contained 2% lidocaine and 0.05 g chlorhexidine hydrochloride given by the transurethral route.[95] Pain scores on a scale of 0 to 4 were obtained. Eight of 12 patients had grade 0 pain (none), and 4 of 12 felt grade 1. All 12 patients responded that they would choose this type of anesthesia again.

Karlsen and Lund provided anesthesia for VLAP with 20 mg/mL of lidocaine gel intraurethrally for a total dose of 40

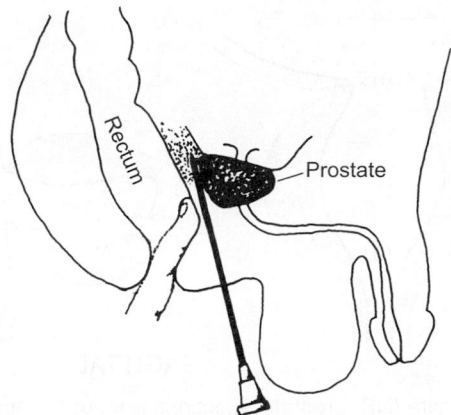

**FIGURE 66–13.** Periprostatic transperineal local anesthetic injection under digital rectal control. (Reprinted from *Urology,* Vol 43, Leach GE, Sirls L, Ganabathi K, et al. Outpatient visual laser-assisted prostatectomy under local anesthesia. Page 149, Copyright 1994, with permission from Elsevier Science.)

mL and kept it in place with a distal penile clamp for 10 minutes.[96] Intravenous sedation was given with midazolam or diazepam and fentanyl. All patients received anti-inflammatory medication with 500 mg of naproxen preoperatively. All cases were completed with this anesthetic technique. Mean dosage of sedation was accomplished with midazolam, 3.5 mg and fentanyl, 0.15 mg. Patient acceptance was good, and no patient expressed pain to the anesthesiologist or surgeon. Karlsen and Lund noted that the threshold level for pain differs among individuals and cultures and concluded that any patient who felt comfortable with a diagnostic cystoscopy performed using intraurethral lidocaine gel anesthesia will find this technique satisfactory for laser coagulation of the prostate.

Birch and coworkers described a technique for TURP performed under local anesthesia with sedation (sedoanalgesia) in 100 patients.[97] The size of the prostate to be resected was limited to those <40 g. Sedation was provided by intravenous midazolam, and 20 g of 2% lidocaine gel was applied locally to the urethra and clamped in place. Injection of 1% lidocaine was delivered beneath the trigone of the bladder, just lateral and medial to the ureteral orifices. One percent lidocaine with epinephrine 1:200 000 (5 mL) was infiltrated into the bladder neck at the 5-, 7-, 2-, and 10-o'clock positions and into the prostate at the 3- and 9-o'clock positions. Visual analogue scale averaged 10 on a scale of 0 to 100 for the prostatic resection. Birch and coworkers concluded that sedoanalgesia preserved detrusor function and sphincter coordination, while allowing immediate ambulation with resumption of normal diet (Fig. 66–14).[97]

## RADICAL PROSTATECTOMY

Radical prostatectomy is performed by an open surgical technique for patients who are suffering from cancer of the prostate. Although treatments are available for minimally invasive prostate cancers (eg, radiation, localized excision), radical prostatectomy with or without nerve sparing is the most common technique.

### Choice of Anesthetic

Neuraxial blockade as the anesthetic for surgery of the lower abdomen and lower limbs has been shown to positively

**TABLE 66–7.** VLAP Versus TURP

| Advantages | Disadvantages |
| --- | --- |
| Lower incidence of bleeding | Higher incidence of dysuria |
| Lower incidence of transfusion | |
| Lower incidence of irrigant absorption | Longer duration of urethral catheterization |
| Anesthesia may be provided solely by local anesthetics or in combination with IV sedation | |

TURP, transurethral resection of the prostate; VLAP, visual laser ablation of the prostate.

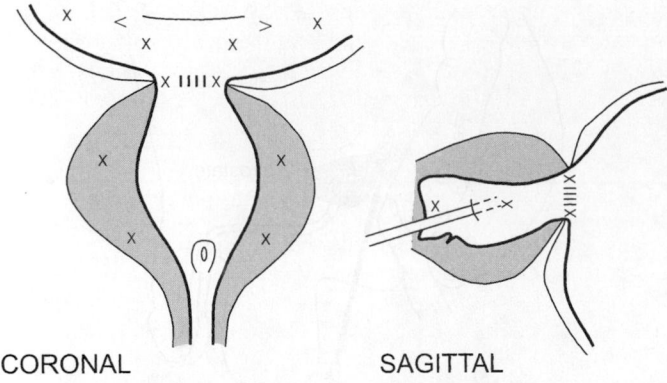

CORONAL                    SAGITTAL

x: Injection site (NB: prostatic injections are out to capsule)

**FIGURE 66–14.** Local anesthetic injection sites. Injection sites in trigone, bladder neck, and prostate. (Reprinted from *Urology*, Vol 38, Birch BR, Gelister JS, Parker CJ, et al. Transurethral resection of prostate under sedation and local anesthesia [sedoanalgesia]. Experience in 100 patients. Page 113, Copyright 1991, with permission from Elsevier Science.)

affect the perioperative neuroendocrine and metabolic responses as compared with general anesthesia. It remains controversial whether neuraxial blockade improves the postoperative morbidity in radical prostatectomy patients when compared with general anesthesia. Shir and associates compared patients receiving either epidural anesthesia, combined epidural and general anesthesia, and general anesthesia alone for the incidence of postoperative pain, bleeding, urine output, fever, length of paralytic ileus, and length of hospitalization.[98] There were no major differences in perioperative complications during radical prostatectomy with any of the anesthetic techniques. However, intraoperative and postoperative epidural analgesia should be considered separately when studying the effects on perioperative morbidity.

Stevens and coworkers randomized prostatectomy patients into two groups to note the recovery time of bowel function: one undergoing general anesthesia and intravenous morphine PCA and one using thoracic epidural anesthesia and "light" general anesthesia, followed by epidural morphine analgesia.[99] Although patients undergoing light general anesthesia have significantly less (mean, 34%) intraoperative blood loss compared with the general group, return of bowel function and postoperative pain scores were equal 1 day postoperatively, regardless of treatment type. The epidural group did show significantly shorter times to first flatus and bowel movement, although there were no differences between the groups to first bowel sounds, first oral and solid intake, and the time of discharge from the hospital.

In contrast, there has been a trend by urologists to forego the use of epidural analgesia secondary to the trend in reduction of postoperative stays for patients treated with radical prostatectomy.[100,101] This direction by urologists has, in part, been accomplished by avoiding narcotic analgesics and using parenteral ketorolac. They feel that epidural analgesia may contribute to longer anesthetic times and increased postoperative costs. Most of the patients given ketorolac did not receive adequate analgesia and required supplemental intravenous opioids. Gottschalk and colleagues studied the effects of preemptive analgesia with epidural fentanyl or bupivacaine on postoperative pain scores in a total of 100 men undergoing radical prostatectomy.[102] Those who received preemptive analgesia were more active at 3.5 weeks after surgery and experienced 33% less pain during hospitalization than those not receiving it.

## Indigo Carmine

Indigo carmine is often used during urologic procedures as a dye to localize ureteral orifices and identify severed ureters and fistulous connections.[103] It is used during radical prostatectomy. In most patients, its usual effect is hypertension and bradycardia immediately after injection. Several cases of severe hypotension, bradycardia, vomiting, and bronchoconstriction have been also reported.[104–106] The most probable cause of these symptoms includes an anaphylactoid reaction or reaction similar to 5-hydroxytryptamine (5-HT) because indigo carmine has a molecular structure that resembles two molecules of 5-HT.

**Treatment.** Treatment includes all medications used in anaphylactoid reactions: specifically, the rapid infusion of crystalloid solution; antihistamines such as diphenhydramine HCl (Benadryl), ephedrine, or epinephrine, depending on the severity of the reaction; and atropine for bradycardia.

## PRIAPISM AND UROLOGIC SURGERY

Penile tumescence is a well-known complication that may occur during any urologic surgery that involves manipulation of the penis such as cystoscopy and TURP. Development of priapism during these procedures can make it technically difficult to continue surgery.

Quinney and Lomas noted in a case report the four options available to cause detumescence of the patient under regional anesthesia[107]:

1. Abandon the operation
2. Convert from a spinal anesthetic to a general anesthetic
3. Surgically decompress the erect penis
4. Pharmacologically induce penile detumescence

Pharmacologic manipulation is the usual preferred means of achieving a flaccid penis, with a variety of drugs being used. Both α- and β-agonists have become the drugs of choice to accomplish this goal. Because α-antagonists can be used in the treatment of impotence, metaraminol, an α-agonist, was first used by Brindley to treat priapism.[108] Metaraminol has both direct and indirect actions and overall effects similar to norepinephrine. Its α-adrenergic stimulatory effect predominates, raising both systolic and diastolic pressures.[109] Lue reported three deaths secondary to the systemic absorption of metaraminol after intraoperative intracavernosal injection.[110] Adrenaline at doses as low as 10 μg/mL injected into the corpora cavernosa also has been effective in treating priapism.[111] Phenylephrine and ephedrine have also been injected intracavernosally with success.[112,113]

β-Receptors are known to be present in the corpora cavernosa, although in fewer numbers than α-receptors. Shantha and coworkers intravenously injected terbutaline to cause detumescence.[114] Terbutaline may be a safer alternative to α-agonists because it has more $\beta_2$ activity than $\beta_1$ and is less likely to increase peripheral vascular tone and left ventricular wall tension. Terbutaline may, however, cause marked tachycardia. Ketamine has also been reported to relieve priapism during general anesthesia.[115] The topical application of ethyl chloride sprayed directly on the erect penis was shown by Miller and Galizia to have varying degrees of success in treatment.[116]

A summary of the pharmacologic methods for achieving detumescence is listed in Table 66–8. Detumescence can also be accomplished by draining the corpora cavernosa with a needle, but this can lead to long-term fibrosis and penile damage. If surgically feasible, the procedure is usually discontinued if detumescence is not accomplished.

## NEPHRECTOMY

This procedure is performed on the donor for living-related kidney transplantation and is the operation of choice for the treatment of renal cell carcinoma. Depending on the surgeon's preference and on the extent of the tumor (eg, possible invasion of inferior vena cava), the affected kidney may be removed via a transabdominal flank or thoracoabdominal incision. In all cases, the operating table is adjusted to provide maximum exposure of the kidney, which is otherwise partially obscured by the lower rib cage. One or two ribs may be removed.

### How Should Anesthesia Be Administered?

Intraoperative management of a patient includes placement of intra-arterial and central venous catheters. If the tumor extends into the inferior vena cava or the right atrium, transesophageal echocardiography is helpful to identify tumor embolus if it occurs and provides another monitor of cardiac function and volume status.

#### Preemptive and Postoperative Analgesia

A combined technique using epidural and general anesthesia not only facilitates muscle relaxation and decreases the requirement for volatile anesthetics and narcotics but also provides a route for pre-emptive and postoperative analgesia. The average length of hospitalization was almost 2 days shorter for donor nephrectomy patients who received postoperative pain management by epidural fentanyl infusion compared with those who received morphine with a patient-controlled analgesia device.[117]

### What Problems Should Be Anticipated?

#### Pneumothorax

Because the kidney lies in the posterior upper abdomen adjacent to the posterior diaphragmatic attachment, the possibility of an intraoperative pneumothorax exists. This complication may first manifest as unexplained hypotension on closure of the abdomen. When it occurs, it is ipsilateral to the surgery and is readily treated by simple aspiration and tube thoracostomy.

#### Inferior Vena Caval Obstruction and Bleeding

A second possible complication is inferior vena caval obstruction from retractor placement. This problem is most likely to occur during right nephrectomy and radical nephrectomy for tumor. Similarly, the right renal vein is shorter than the left, and thus caval injury and bleeding is also more likely during a right radial nephrectomy. The diagnosis of both pneumothorax and inferior vena caval obstruction is facilitated by the presence of an intra-arterial catheter.

## CYSTECTOMY

Total cystectomy is performed on patients with deeply infiltrating cancer of the bladder. It requires removal of the bladder and its replacement with an ileal conduit. Bladder extirpation with the prostatic urethra and, frequently, the pelvic lymph nodes, is associated with a great deal of blood loss. The ileal conduit urinary diversion portion of the procedure usually incurs little additional blood loss.

### How Should Anesthesia Be Administered?

Ryan compared two anesthetic regimens for this procedure: epidural anesthesia utilizing bupivacaine, 0.5% plain, supplemented with nitrous oxide–oxygen–enflurane versus general anesthetic-relaxant using nitrous oxide–oxygen–fentanyl and pancuronium.[118] The epidural group had a significantly lower average (taken at 5-minute intervals) systolic BP (80 mm Hg versus 115 mm Hg) and a markedly lower mean blood loss. A wide variation in blood loss occurred within each group. All patients had similar cardiovascular changes during the first 12 hours postoperatively.

#### Controlled Hypotension

Ahlering and coworkers studied controlled hypotension to reduce blood loss during radical cystectomy.[119] Hypotension was induced with enflurane or trimethaphan to maintain BP at 90/60 mm Hg. The mean operative blood loss was reduced significantly in the hypotensive group compared with the normotensive group (740 ± 14 mL versus 821 ± 78 mL, respectively). Ninety percent of the normotensive patients received blood transfusions compared with only 69% of the hypotensive patients. Controlled hypotension, particularly in combination with substantial blood loss, is not without risks that include myocardial ischemia, infarction, stroke, and ischemic optic neuropathy.

#### Radical Cystectomy and Blood Transfusion

Radical cystectomy is frequently associated with a large volume of blood loss that necessitates blood transfusion. Alternative means to controlled hypotension have been sought to decrease the incidence of homologous blood transfusion.

**TABLE 66–8.** Pharmacologic Methods for Detumescence

| Application | Drug | | |
| | β-Agonist | α-Agonist | Anesthetics |
| --- | --- | --- | --- |
| Systemically administered | Terbutaline | | Ketamine |
| Direct penile injection | Ephedrine Epinephrine (10 μg/mL) | Metaraminol Phenylephrine (0.5 mg/9 mL) | |
| Topical | | | Ethyl chloride spray |

An alternative to homologous transfusion is autologous transfusion. Three ways of performing autologous transfusion are phlebotomy of the patient several weeks to months before the operation and hemodilution with intraoperative phlebotomy. This method of banking a patient's own blood preoperatively, in combination with recombinant erythropoietin, is effective in reducing the need for homologous blood transfusion during radical cystectomy.[120,121] Advanced phlebotomy will delay surgery for several weeks while the red cell mass increases during this period. An alternative method, the hemodilution technique, requires that the blood be collected immediately before the surgical procedure while being replaced with a sufficient volume of crystalloid and colloid solution. Atallah and colleagues studied 20 patients who underwent hemodilution postinduction of anesthesia, and 10 patients who underwent hemodilution while awake.[122] Hemodynamic variables and hematologic and coagulation factors were monitored. Acute hemodilution in awake or anesthetized patients did not result in significant hemodynamic disruption in patients undergoing radical cystectomy.

The Shands Hospital at the University of Florida has developed a protocol for acute normovolemic hemodilution (ANH) for surgery.[123]

## What Is Acute Normovolemic Hemodilution?

ANH is a method to minimize the red cell loss during surgery. Blood is collected from the patient before any surgical blood loss takes place and is stored in citrate anticoagulant-containing plastic bags while the patient's blood volume is maintained by infusion of colloid and/or crystalloid solutions. The patient's red cell level is diluted to the allowable minimum based on medical considerations and maintained at that level by reinfusion of the collected blood and non-red cell containing solutions until surgical loss is complete. This ensures that all surgically lost blood contains the minimum red cell level deemed acceptable to the patient. The materials required to achieve ANH are listed in Table 66–9.

## Procedure

### Preoperative Preparation
1. Document initial red blood cell level. If the hematocrit is <36% or hemoglobin is <12.0 g/dL, ANH will not be sufficient to warrant its use.
2. Calculate the quantity of blood that can be collected. For patients without coronary or other significant cardiac disease, a postcollection target of hemoglobin, 9.0 g/dL, is appropriate.

**TABLE 66–9.** Materials Required to Achieve Acute Normovolemic Hemodilution

Baxter Fenwal autologous blood collection kit with Luer connector 4R5012
6-inch extension set with wide bore stopcock: Medex MX7306
HemoCue Analyzer
Sebra Model 1040 digital blood shaker
Blood warmer
Pressure infusion bags

Calculation of the amount of blood to be collected (using 70 mL/kg as ideal body weight):

$$V = EBV \times [Ho - Hf]/Hav$$

where V is the volume of blood (mL) that may be removed; EBV is the estimated blood volume (mL); Ho is the initial hemoglobin; Hf is the target hemoglobin after collection (9 g/dL); Hav is the average hemoglobin (Ho + Hf)/2. (H variables may be hematocrit or hemoglobin so long as use is consistent.)

3. Open the Fenwal Blood Collection kit and foil pouch, discarding the red blood band in the kit so that it does not become co-mingled with the identification bands associated with existing blood bank orders. The product collected should not leave the operating room unless it is infusing into the patient.
4. Attach each blood-pack unit in the foil to a Y-type connector set with Luer lock and close both blue clamps. There will a spike on each setup.
5. Set up a blood warmer flushed with hetastarch (Hespan).

### Intraoperative Collection
6. Induce anesthesia. Start a large intravenous catheter (12-gauge or larger) in the arm opposite the established infusion and cap with a 6-inch extension set.
7. Measure the initial hemoglobin level with the HemoCue.
8. Connect the Luer fitting of the first bag Luer connector system to the 6-inch extension stopcock, making sure the tubing is clamped or the stopcock is closed.
9. Begin replacement fluid infusion. For a four-unit collection, two 500-mL bags of hetastarch followed by a 500 mL bag of 3% NaCl, followed by isotonic crystalloid solutions is suggested. For larger collections, add another 500 mL bag of 3% NaCl.
10. Use the Sebra to collect blood so that it is immediately mixed with the citrate anticoagulant. Set the quantity to be collected at 425 mL to prevent overfilling the bags and associated inadequate anticoagulation. The red and green lights and digital volume display allow easy monitoring to confirm adequate flow. Make sure the tubing is mechanically clamped before removing it from the Sebra electronic clamp. Label the unit as to the order of the draw.
11. Recheck the patient's hemoglobin level after each unit is collected.

### Intraoperative Reinfusion
12. The end of blood collection is presumed to be the lowest point in the hemoglobin level that is allowable; therefore, reinfusing the last (most dilute) collected unit should begin when more than a negligible amount of blood loss begins. Use the HemoCue often to determine if you are under- or overtransfusing back to the patient. Reinfuse the units in reverse order of their collection.
13. Toward the end of the surgical procedure, the rate of reinfusion can increase so that the postsurgical hemoglobin is well above the target and all units are infused or infusing when the patient leaves the operating room.

### Caution

Clotting of the collected blood unit destroys the efficacy of ANH. Do not cool the units so that platelet function is optimally preserved. The anticoagulant solution is theoretically sufficient for 450 mL of blood. Because the product is not cooled, it is suggested that no more than 425 mL of blood is drawn or else there is a possibility of clotting. As hematocrit falls, the acellular volume that contains the ionized calcium that the citrate must chelate increases as a percentage of the total volume collected. Therefore, it is recommended to reduce the volume of subsequent collected units, and by the fourth and fifth bag, collect only 375 mL. A turgid bag can hold 600 mL and will clot. If the patient has high calcium or calcium is administered intravenously, the citrate in the bag may be insufficient to prevent clotting.[122]

Intraoperative autotransfusion is the process of reinfusing the patient's blood that is recovered during the operation itself. Intraoperative autotransfusion is not widely accepted in cancer surgery because of the risk that the blood might be contaminated with cancer cells. Pisters and Wajsman reported a 5-year study at the University of Florida using intraoperative autotransfusion in radical cystectomy and prostatectomy patients.[124] No adverse effects on malignancy recurrence or survival rates were reported. Yamada and coworkers, in a retrospective study of 71 patients who underwent radical prostatectomy under controlled hypotensive anesthesia, examined the impact of preoperative autologous blood collection on perioperative blood requirements.[125] They found that 21 of 37 patients were anemic at hospitalization secondary to autologous blood donation. In addition, the data suggested that 2 weeks' time was insufficient to stimulate the bone marrow erythropoiesis by natural means. Efforts to increase the erythropoietin response preoperatively by administering erythropoietin were suggested. The need for homologous blood transfusion was noted to have decreased from 21% to 8% in patients undergoing radical prostatectomy with autologous blood transfusion. Park and associates studied 10 patients undergoing radical cystectomy using intraoperative autologous transfusion (IAT) in order to evaluate its efficacy in blood replacement.[126] IAT was successful in reducing the need for autologous blood but did not eliminate it unless it was in combination with predeposited autologous blood.

## NONCHROMAFFIN PARAGANGLIOMAS

Nonchromaffin paragangliomas of the bladder do occur, but most are inactive. A tumor that released catecholamines has been reported.[127] Such a tumor occasionally is malignant. A patient may present with the classic symptoms of a pheochromocytoma (hypertension, tremulousness, anxiety, and a pounding sensation in the head and chest).

### How Should Anesthesia Be Managed?

Preoperative treatment should be similar to that for patients with pheochromocytomas. α-Blockers followed by β-blockers, calcium channel blockers, and inhibitors of catecholamine synthesis are administered with magnesium sulfate as needed. In the reported case, prazosin and propranolol were used. Additional nifedipine was added to control BP.[128]

Several anesthetic techniques have been used during resection of catecholamine-producing tumors, and no one method was proven to be superior. A continuous infusion of sodium nitroprusside titrated to effect, as well as bolus doses of

phentolamine, may be necessary to maintain an acceptable BP.[128]

## LASER SURGERY FOR NONPROSTATIC SURGERY

### What Are the Applications?

In addition to radical surgery for bladder carcinomas, laser treatment in outpatient settings is used for these tumors and for genital condylomata. Carbon dioxide ($CO_2$), argon, and Nd:YAG lasers are most frequently used in urologic surgery.

#### Carbon Dioxide Laser

The $CO_2$ laser can be used in relatively inaccessible areas. Its advantage is that it can cut and coagulate tissue while maintaining a bloodless field. A major disadvantage is that it cannot penetrate a quantity of water >0.1 mm in depth; therefore, it cannot be used in water or urine-filled organs. Its role in urology is in the treatment of cutaneous lesions such as condylomata acuminata and of premalignant and malignant cutaneous lesions of the penis.

#### Argon Laser

The argon laser can be used with a fiberoptic guide. Water does not prevent its penetration; thus, it can be used to treat lesions within the bladder. Argon laser use, combined with concomitant administration of intravenous hematoporphyrin derivatives, produces tumoricidal effects on bladder cancer. Urethral strictures also can be removed. With increasing power settings, large defects in the tissue occur that can lead to bladder perforation. Therefore, the argon laser is limited to the treatment of superficial bladder cancers.

#### ND:YAG Laser

The Nd:YAG laser is most useful for urologic surgery. Its tissue-penetrating ability is the most potent of the three available lasers. It can be used in water or urine without loss of power and can be adapted to a fiberoptic light source. Bloodless destruction of cancer cells and a minimal risk of bladder perforation are its advantages. Contraindications to its use are the presence of large or extensive tumors that require increased photoradiation. Patients with potential bladder outlet obstruction must be observed for urinary retention postoperatively.

### How Is Anesthesia Administered?

#### Bladder Cancer

Male and female patients with bladder cancer can undergo Nd:YAG laser surgery with intravenous sedation and an instillation of 2% lidocaine hydrochloride jelly into the urethra. If extensive or numerous tumors are present, the patient may require a general or regional anesthetic. The PACU stay may be prolonged following a regional anesthetic case. Evaluation of the abdomen to assess for rigidity or tenderness is done before discharge to verify that no laser-induced intraperitoneal perforations have occurred.

## Condylomata Acuminata

When the laser is used for the treatment of condylomata acuminata, >90% of patients receive local anesthesia. One percent lidocaine is infiltrated at the base of each lesion. If the warts involve the penis, a penile block is performed. For urethral condylomata, a general or regional anesthetic is usually administered because local anesthetic alone is not sufficient to prevent pain caused by the laser phototherapy.[127]

## NONINVASIVE UROLOGIC SURGERY

Since the early 1980s, a large proportion of traditionally open urologic surgical procedures have been eliminated by technology that allows intervention with minimally invasive techniques. Percutaneous nephrostomy and urethroscopy enable 90% of procedures that involve calculi of the upper urinary tract to be performed endoscopically. Patients who previously had to stay in the hospital 1 to 2 weeks after an open surgical procedure and could not go back to work for weeks can now be discharged within 24 hours and can return to work within a few days. Virtually the only remaining indication for open surgery is the combination of a stone and stenosis at the ureteropelvic junction.

### *What Are the Anesthetic Requirements?*

Because nephrostomy and urethroscopy are performed without a scalpel, minimal tissue trauma occurs; thus, the need for general anesthesia is greatly reduced. For elderly or high-risk patients who require urologic procedures, a local anesthetic frequently is the technique of choice.

## UROLOGIC LAPAROSCOPIC SURGERY

The number of urologic surgeries performed using a laparoscope has increased over the last several years, including laparoscopic nephrectomy, varicocelectomy, pelvic lymph node dissection, and evaluation for cryptorchidism.[129] Future urologic procedures that may be performed by this method include intra-abdominal orchiectomy, isolated partial cystectomy, ureterolysis, treatment of intractable lymphoceles, biopsy of intrapelvic or abdominal masses, bladder suspension, and repair of inguinal hernia.

Laparoscopic surgery has risks and complications that are inherent not only with the technique but also from anesthesia. Overall mortality rate in a large series of gynecologic surgeries was reported to be 0.03%. Researchers reported a minor complication rate of 4% with laparoscopic surgery.[129–131] Major complication rates for laparoscopic surgery were 0.6%.[132]

### *What Are the Complications of Laparoscopic Surgery?*

Laparoscopic complications[129–133] and their treatment are listed in Table 66–10.

### Pulmonary

Positioning during laparoscopic surgery may place the patient in several positions that affect pulmonary dynamics

**TABLE 66–10.** Laparoscopic Complications and Treatment

**Complications**

Related to the onset of pneumoperitoneum
Emphysema: subcutaneous, properitoneal, omental
Tension pneumoperitoneum
Gas embolism
    Diagnosis: marked drop in end-tidal $CO_2$
    Windmill murmur by auscultation
    Sudden decrease in oxygen saturation
    Decrease in blood pressure
Trocar insertion: bleeding, visceral injury
Burns, tissue dissection injury, failed surgical attempt
Postoperatively unrecognized bowel injury, other visceral injury, shoulder
    tip pain and deep vein thrombosis

**Treatment**

Stop gas insufflation
Place patient in a steep left lateral Trendelenberg position to possibly
    minimize the gas obstruction of the right ventricular outflow tract
Attempt to aspirate the gas from a central venous catheter if present
Place a central venous catheter at the junction of the right atrium and
    superior vena cava if resuscitation efforts are difficult
Use cardiopulmonary resuscitation guidelines for general resuscitation with
    any cardiac arrest

(Trendelenburg position, lateral decubitus position). Fahy and associates studied the effects of the lateral decubitus position and split torso positioning on respiratory mechanics in patients undergoing laparoscopic donor nephrectomy and found that respiratory mechanics during laparoscopic nephrectomy differ from other laparoscopic procedures.[134] The position for the procedure was responsible for an increase in lung compliance, a decrease in chest wall compliance, and an increase in chest wall resistance. Compliance of the chest wall decreased more with abdominal insufflation than with other procedures.

With split torso positioning, the muscle and connective tissue of the rib cage and abdominal wall are most likely stretched, causing the decreases in chest wall compliance. Lung elastance decreases as a result of an increase in functional residual capacity. Although these changes in respiratory mechanics did little clinically to the healthy patients undergoing laparoscopic nephrectomy, Fahy and colleagues cautioned that patients with underlying cardiopulmonary disease may have significant changes in respiratory mechanics with this procedure and recommended some type of monitoring. (Although not mentioned, peak inspiratory pressure monitoring would be the most accessible means.)

The Trendelenburg position causes the weight of the abdominal contents to press on the diaphragm.[135] The head-down position decreases lung volumes and may cause atelectasis.[136] In combination with the pressure exerted by insufflation of the abdomen during laparoscopy, further restriction of the diaphragm and decreases in pulmonary compliance occur.[137] Pneumomediastinum, pneumothorax, and pneumopericardium may also develop. A pneumothorax, if sufficiently large, may require decompression with a chest tube.[138,139]

### Cardiac Complications

Cardiac dysrhythmias are a frequent complication of laparoscopic surgery. Bradyarrhythmias have been reported to occur between 25% and 47%, with Myles reporting 30% with insufflation or traction on pelvic structures.[140,141] Insufflated $CO_2$ is systemically absorbed via the large peritoneal surface area and can lead to hypercarbia. Increased blood $CO_2$ levels can cause tachycardia and premature ventricular contractions. Increased ventilation is commonly necessary to normalize $CO_2$ levels. An increase in intra-abdominal pressure and vena cava compression may lead to decreased venous return and resulting hypotension, as well as a decrease in circulating volume and cardiac output. For this reason, insufflation pressure should not exceed 15 mm Hg.

## General Anesthesia

General anesthesia is most frequently the method of choice for intra-abdominal urologic procedures. The major advantage of general anesthesia for laparoscopic surgery is controlled patient ventilation and complete amnesia and analgesia. Although not always present, muscle paralysis during general anesthesia avoids the likelihood that the patient will strain with trocar placement. This could result in bowel or vascular damage. The patient under general anesthesia will not detect the discomfort and referred shoulder pain associated with pneumoperitoneum.[130] Many agents have been investigated in search of the ideal general anesthetic for laparoscopic surgery. DeGrood and associates compared four anesthetic techniques, including propofol, etomidate, thiopental, and isoflurane, and found that a total intravenous technique with propofol caused less nausea and a faster recovery than that of an inhalational technique with isoflurane.[142] Most general anesthetic techniques are suitable for laparoscopic surgery.

The only controversial anesthetic is nitrous oxide. Nitrous oxide causes little diaphragmatic irritation but supports combustion in the presence of oxygen and electrocautery. It is considered to be contraindicated by some.[132] The disadvantages of using nitrous oxide are (1) increased incidence of postoperative nausea; (2) increase in gas volume (as much as 100% after 2 hours of use); and (3) rapid expansion of a pneumothorax.[143,144]

## Regional Anesthesia

Regional anesthesia (spinal and epidural) is not frequently used for laparoscopic surgery because the $CO_2$ pneumoperitoneum will limit diaphragmatic movement and the patient's ability to breathe. Gas irritation of the diaphragm may also lead to considerable discomfort and shoulder pain if the patient is awake. Several studies have, however, shown regional anesthesia to be a safe alternative to general anesthesia in laparoscopic procedures of short duration.[145,146] Advantages may include a lower incidence of postoperative nausea and vomiting and a shorter postoperative recovery time.

## Local Anesthesia

Infiltrative techniques with local anesthetics have been tried in combination with sedation. The most commonly used local anesthetics that are infiltrated subcutaneously are 0.5% bupivacaine and 1% lidocaine.[147] Topical anesthetic cream (lidocaine; prilocaine [EMLA]) has also been used. Sedoanalgesia is usually provided intravenously with opioids and midazolam. Although local anesthesia avoids the risks associated with general or regional anesthesia, the patient may suffer from abdominal or referred shoulder pain, in addition to intraoperative anxiety and respiratory compromise from gas insufflation. Local anesthesia should only be considered for laparoscopic procedures of extremely short duration in a cooperative patient.

## Sedoanalgesia

Many urologic procedures, both endoscopic and open, can be performed following local or regional anesthesia. Owing to the patient's embarrassment or anxiety, or due to the extent of the procedure, local anesthesia may not provide an acceptable alternative. If it is anxiety, administration of an anxiolytic agent can improve the conditions of surgery considerably. If the limiting factor is the extent of the procedure, regional or general anesthesia is performed. Sedoanalgesia, as was noted earlier, places equal emphasis on sedation and analgesia.

Birch and colleagues reported the results of this technique for 1020 patients. The short-acting benzodiazepine, midazolam, provided the hypnosedation and amnesia, whereas intramuscular meperidine and topical lidocaine gel provided the analgesia.[97] Midazolam was administered 20 to 30 minutes before surgery in a dose of 0.1 to 0.12 mg/kg intramuscularly. In elderly, unfit patients, the dosage was reduced 30% to 60%. The urethra was anesthetized with 2% lidocaine gel 10 to 15 minutes after premedication was given. Monitoring included ECG, automatic BP measurement, and pulse oximetry.

If a patient was still anxious before the procedure began, midazolam was titrated intravenously in 1-mg increments. Cystoscopies required no further anesthetic supplementation. However, for biopsies, diathermy, and incisions, 1% lidocaine with epinephrine (1:200 000) was injected into the area. The investigators concluded that sedoanalgesia greatly increased the efficiency of outpatient surgeries. Eighty percent of their patients were fit for discharge 1 hour postoperatively.[97,148]

## References

1. Thompson G, Moore D. Celiac plexus intercostal and minor peripheral blocks. In: Cousins MJ, Bridenbaugh PO, eds. *Clinical Anesthesia and Management of Pain*. 2nd ed. Philadelphia, Pa: JB Lippincott; 1988:503.
2. Lofstrom JB, Cousins M. Sympathetic neural blockade of upper and lower extremities. In: Cousins MJ, Bridenbaugh PO, eds. *Clinical Anesthesia and Management of Pain*. 2nd ed. Philadelphia, Pa: JB Lippincott; 1988:483.
3. Moore D. Block of the inguinal region. In: Moore D, ed. *Regional Blockade*. 4th ed. Springfield, Ill: Charles C Thomas; 1981:167.
4. Cassady JJI. Regional anesthesia for urologic procedures. *Urol Clin North Am.* 1987;14:43.
5. Fuchs GF. Cord block anesthesia for scrotal surgery. *J Urol.* 1982;128:718.
6. Kaye KW, Lange PH, Fraley EE. Spermatic cord block in urologic surgery. *J Urol.* 1982;128:720.
7. Trivedi NS, Robalino J, Shevde K. Intrapleural block: a new technique for regional anesthesia during percutaneous nephrostomy and nephrolithotomy. *Can J Anaesth.* 1990;37:479.
8. Perestad F, Stromskag KE. Interpleural catheter in the management of postoperative pain: a preliminary report. *Reg Anesth.* 1986;11:89.
9. Covino BG. Interpleural regional analgesia [editorial]. *Anesth Analg.* 1988;67:427.
10. Seltzer JL, Larijani GE, Goldberg ME, et al. Intrapleural bupivacaine: a kinetic and dynamic evaluation. *Anesthesiology.* 1987;67:798.
11. Reddy PK. New technique to anesthetize the prostate for transurethral balloon dilation. *Urol Clin North Am.* 1990;17:55.
12. Reddy PK, Wasserman W, Castaneda F, et al. Balloon dilatation of the prostate for treatment of benign hyperplasia. *Urol Clin North Am.* 1988;15:529.
13. Birch BRP, Anson KM, Miller RA. Sedoanalgesia in urology: a safe, cost-effective alternative to general anesthesia: a review of 1020 cases. *Br J Urol.* 1990;66:342.
14. Hendolin H, Mattila MAK, Poikolainen E. The effect of lumbar epidural

analgesia on the development of deep vein thrombosis of the legs after open prostatectomy. *Acta Chir Scand.* 1981;147:425.

15. Albin MS, Ritter RR, Reinhart R, et al. Venous air embolism during radical retropubic prostatectomy. *Anesth Analg.* 1992;74:191.

16. Mebust WK, Holtgrewe HL, Cockett ATK, et al. Transurethral prostatectomy: immediate and postoperative complications: a cooperative study of 13 participating institutions evaluating 3,885 patients. *J Urol.* 1989;14:243.

17. Raj PP, Gesund P, Phero J, et al. Rational choice for surgical procedures. In: Raj PP, ed. *Clinical Practice of Regional Anesthesia.* New York, NY: Churchill-Livingstone; 1991:231.

18. Evans TI. Regional anesthesia for transurethral resection of the prostate—which method and which segments? *Anaesth Intensive Care.* 1974;2:240.

19. Beers RA, Kane PB, Nsouli I, et al. Does a mid-lumbar block level provide adequate anesthesia for transurethral prostatectomy? *Can J Anaesth.* 1994;9:807.

20. Dubuisson D. Nerve root damage and arachnoiditis. In: Wall PD, Melzak R, eds. *Textbook of Pain.* 3rd ed. Edinburgh, United Kingdom: Churchill-Livingstone; 1994:711.

21. Jones RDM, Rushmer J, Chan SSC. Pharmacodynamics of subarachnoid hyperbaric 5% lignocaine. *Acta Anaesthesiol Scand.* 1996;40:350.

22. Pollack JE, Neal JM, Stephenson CA, et al. Prospective study of the incidence of transient radicular irritation in patients undergoing spinal anesthesia. *Anesthesiology.* 1996;84:1361.

23. Hampl KF, Schneider MC, Ummenhofer W, et al. Transient neurologic symptoms after spinal anesthesia. *Anesth Analg.* 1995;81:1148.

24. Tarkkila P, Huhtala J, Tuominen M. Transient radicular irritation after spinal anaesthesia with hyperbaric 5% lignocaine. *Br J Anaesth.* 1995;74:328.

25. Pandadero A, Monedero P, Fernandez-Liesa I, et al. Repeated transient neurological symptoms after spinal anesthesia with hyperbaric 5% lidocaine. *Br J Anaesth.* 1998;81:471.

26. Sia AT, Chow MY, Koay CK, et al. Intrathecal pethidine: an alternative anaesthetic for transurethral resection of prostate? *Anaesth Intensive Care.* 1997;25:650.

27. Uchida T, Ohori M, Soh S, et al. Factors influencing morbidity in patients undergoing transurethral resection of the prostate. *Urology.* 1999;53:98.

28. Roos NP, Wennberg JE, Malenka DJ, et al. Mortality and reoperation after open and transurethral resection of the prostate for benign prostatic hyperplasia. *N Engl J Med.* 1989;320:1120.

29. Wong DH, Hagar JM, Christiano M, et al. Incidence of perioperative myocardial ischemia in TURP patients. *J Clin Anesth.* 1996;8:627.

30. Edwards ND, Callaghan LC, White T, et al. Perioperative myocardial ischemia in patients undergoing transurethral surgery: a pilot study comparing general with spinal anesthesia. *Br J Anaesth.* 1995;74:368.

31. Hahn RG, Nelsson S, Farahmand Y, et al. Operative factors and the long term incidence of acute myocardial infarction after transurethral resection of the prostate. *Epidemiology.* 1996;7:93.

32. Hahn RG, Nilsson A, Farahmand BY, et al. Blood hemoglobin and the long term incidence of acute myocardial infarction after transurethral resection of the prostate. *Eur Urol.* 1997;31:199.

33. Mebust WK, Holtgrewe HL, Cockett ATK, et al. Transurethral prostatectomy: immediate and postoperative complications. A cooperative study of 13 participating institutions evaluating 3885 patients. *J Urol.* 1989;141:243.

34. Ceccarelli EE, Mantell TK. Studies of fluid and electrolyte alterations during transurethral prostatectomy. *J Urol.* 1961;85:75.

35. Gravenstein D. Transurethral resection of the prostate (TURP) syndrome: a review of the pathophysiology and management. *Anesth Analg.* 1997;84:438.

36. Levin K, Nyren O, Pompeius R. Blood loss, tissue weight, and operating time in transurethral prostatectomy. *Scand J Urol Nephrol.* 1981;15:197.

37. Nielson KK, Andersen K, Asbjorn VF, et al. Blood loss in transurethral prostatectomy: epidural vs. general anesthesia. *Int Urol Nephrol.* 1987;19:287.

38. Kirollos MM, Campbell N. Factors influencing blood loss in transurethral resection of the prostate (TURP): auditing TURP. *Br J Urol.* 1997;80:111.

39. Madsen RE, Madsen PO. Influence of anesthesia form on blood loss in transurethral prostatectomy. *Anesth Analg.* 1967;46:330.

40. Abrams PH, Shah PJR, Bryning K, et al. Forum: blood loss during transurethral resection of the prostate. *Anaesthesia.* 1982;37:71.

41. Smyth R, Cheng D, Asokumar B, et al. Coagulopathies in patients after transurethral resection of the prostate: spinal versus general anesthesia. *Anesth Analg.* 1995;81:680.

42. Watson CJE, Deane AM, Doyle PT, et al. Identifiable factors in post-prostatectomy hemorrhage: the role of aspirin. *Br J Urol.* 1990;66:85.

43. Ala-Opas MY, Gronlund SS. Blood loss in long term aspirin users undergoing transurethral prostatectomy. *Scand J Urol Nephrol.* 1996;30:203.

44. Nielsen JD, Gram J, Holm-Nielsen A, et al. Postoperative blood loss after transurethral prostatectomy is dependent on in situ fibrinolysis. *Br J Urol.* 1997;80:889.

45. Bell CRW, Cox DJA, Murdock PJ, et al. Thromboelastographic evaluation of coagulation in transurethral prostatectomy. *Br J Urol.* 1996;78:737.

46. Rabke HB, Jenicek JA, Khouri E. Hypothermia associated with transurethral resection of the prostate. *J Urol.* 1962;87:447.

47. Pit MJ, Tegelaar RJ, Venema PL. Isothermic irrigation during transurethral resection of the prostate: effects on perioperative hypothermia, blood loss, resection time and patient satisfaction. *Br J Urol.* 1996;78:99.

48. Augspurger RR, Donohue RE. Prevention of obturator nerve stimulation during transurethral surgery. *J Urol.* 1980;123:170.

49. Narins L, Lief PA. Abolition of mass femoral muscular contractions during transurethral resection. *J Mt Sinai Hosp.* 1957;24:23.

50. Hradec E, Soukup F, Novah J, et al. The obturator nerve block: preventing damage of the bladder wall during transurethral surgery. *Int Urol Nephrol.* 1983;15:149.

51. Nicolaides AN, Field ES, Kakkar VV, et al. Prostatectomy and deep vein thrombosis. *Br J Surg.* 1972;59:487.

52. Mayo ME, Halil T, Browse NL. The incidence of deep vein thrombosis after prostatectomy. *Br J Urol.* 1971;43:738.

53. Ljunger H, Bergquist D, Isacson S. Plasminogen activator activity in patients undergoing transvesical and transurethral prostatectomy. *Eur Urol.* 1983;9:24.

54. Ghanem AN, Ward JP. Osmotic and metabolic sequelae of volumetric overload in relation to the TUR syndrome. *Br J Urol.* 1990;66:71.

55. Hahn RG. Relations between irrigant absorption rate and hyponatremia during transurethral resection of the prostate. *Acta Anaesthesiol Scand.* 1987;32:53.

56. Hahn RG, Ekengren JC. Patterns of irrigating fluid absorption during transurethral resection of the prostate as indicated by ethanol. *J Urol.* 1993;149:502.

57. Van Renen RG, Reymann U. Comparison of the effect of two heights of glycine irrigation solution on serum sodium and osmolality during transurethral resection of the prostate. *Aust N Z J Surg.* 1997;67:874.

58. Madsen PO, Naber KC. The importance of the pressure in the prostatic fossa and absorption of irrigating fluid during the transurethral resection of the prostate. *J Urol.* 1973;109:446.

59. Hjertberg H, Petterson B. The use of bladder pressure warning device during transurethral prostatic resection decreases absorption of irrigating fluid. *Br J Urol.* 1992;69:56.

60. Hahn RG, Nilsson A, Farahmand BY, et al. Operative factors and the long term incidence of acute myocardial infarction after transurethral resection of the prostate. *Epidemiology.* 1996;7:93.

61. Akan H, Sargin S, Turkseven F, et al. Comparison of three different irrigation fluids used in transurethral prostatectomy based on plasma volume expansion and metabolic effects. *Br J Urol.* 1996;78:224.

62. Hahn RG. Early detection of the TUR syndrome by marking the irrigating fluid with 1% ethanol. *Acta Anaesthesiol Scand.* 1989;33:149.

63. Konrad C, Gerber HR, Schiepfer G, et al. Transurethral resection syndrome: effect of the introduction into clinical practice of a new method for monitoring fluid absorption. *J Clin Anesth.* 1998;10:360.

64. Hahn RG. Ethanol monitoring of fluid absorption in anesthesiology practice. *J Clin Anesth.* 1998;10:357.

65. Hahn RG, Ekengren JC. Patterns of irrigation fluid absorption during transurethral resection of the prostate as indicated by ethanol. *J Urol.* 1993;149:502.

66. Checketts MR, Duthie WH. Expired breath ethanol measurement to calculate irrigating fluid absorption during transurethral resection of the prostate: experience in a district general hospital. *Br J Urol.* 1996;77:198.

67. Norlen H, Allgen LG, Vinnars E, et al. Glycine solution as an irrigating agent during transurethral prostatic resection. *Scand J Urol Nephrol.* 1986;20:19.

68. Andrew RD. Seizure and acute osmotic change: clinical and neurophysiological aspects. *J Neurol Sci.* 1991;101:7.

69. Norenberg MD, Papendick RE. Chronicity of hyponatremia as a factor in experimental myelinolysis. *Ann Neurol.* 1984;15:544.

70. Brunner JE, Redmond AM, Haggar AM, et al. Central pontine myeli-

nolysis and pontine lesions after rapid correction of hyponatremia: a prospective magnetic resonance imaging study. *Ann Neurol.* 1990;27:61.

71. Layon AJ, Bernards WC, Kirby RR. Fluids and electrolytes in the critically ill. In: Civetta JM, Kirby RR, Taylor RW, eds. *Critical Care.* 2nd ed. Philadelphia, Pa: JB Lippincott; 1992:457.

72. Arieff AI, Ayus JC, Fraser CL. Hyponatremia and death or permanent brain damage in healthy children. *BMJ.* 1992;304:1218.

73. Ayus JC, Krothapalli RK, Arieff AI. Treatment of symptomatic hyponatremia and its relation to brain damage: a prospective study. *N Engl J Med.* 1987;317:1190.

74. Cheng J, Zikos D, Skopicki HA, et al. Long-term neurologic outcome in psychogenic water drinkers with severe symptomatic hyponatremia—the effect of rapid correction. *Am J Med.* 1990;88:561.

75. McManus ML, Churchwell KB, Strange K. Regulation of cell volume in health and disease. *N Engl J Med.* 1995;333:1260.

76. Lien YH, Shapiro JI, Chan L. Study of brain electrolytes and organic osmolytes during correction of chronic hyponatremia. *J Clin Invest.* 1991;88:303.

77. Russell D. Painless loss of vision after transurethral resection of the prostate. *Anaesthesia.* 1990;45:218.

78. Fahey JL. Toxicity and blood ammonia rise resulting from intravenous amino-acid administration in man: the protective effect of L-arginine. *J Clin Invest.* 1957;36:1647.

79. Kish SJ, Dixon LM, Burnham WM, et al. Brain neurotransmitters in glycine encephalopathy. *Ann Neurol.* 1988;24:458.

80. Schwarcz R, Meldrum B. Excitatory amino acid antagonists provide a therapeutic approach to neurological disorders. *Lancet.* 1985;2:140.

81. Tsao CM, Lui PW, Jang JH, et al. Comparison of diuretic effects of glycerol with furosemide after transurethral prostatectomy. *Acta Anaesthesiol Sin.* 1996;34:184.

82. Shokeir AA, Al-Sisi YM, Farage MA, et al. Transurethral prostatectomy: a prospective randomized study of conventional resection and electrovaporization in benign hyperplasia. *Br J Urol.* 1997;80:570.

83. Hammadeh MY, Fowlis GA, Singh M, et al. Transurethral electrovaporization of the prostate—a possible alternative to transurethral resection: a one-year follow-up of a prospective randomized trial. *Br J Urol.* 1998;81:721.

84. Kupeli S, Baltaci S, Soygur T, et al. A prospective randomized study of transurethral resection of the prostate and transurethral vaporization of the prostate as a therapeutic alternative in the management of men with BPH. *Eur Urol.* 1998;34:15.

85. Talic RF. Transurethral electrovaporization—resection of the prostate using the "wing" cutting electrode: preliminary results of safety and efficacy in the treatment of men with prostatic outflow obstruction. *Urology.* 1999;53:106.

86. Ekengren J, Hahn RG. Complications during transurethral vaporization of the prostate. *Urology.* 1996;48:424.

87. Beduschi MC, Oesterling JE. Transurethral needle ablation of the prostate: a minimally invasive treatment for symptomatic benign prostatic hyperplasia. *Mayo Clin Proc.* 1998;73:696.

88. Kahn SA, Alphonse P, Tewari A, et al. An open study of the efficacy and safety of transurethral needle ablation of the prostate in treating symptomatic benign prostatic hyperplasia: the University of Florida experience. *J Urol.* 1998;160:1695.

89. Narayan P, Fournier G, Indudhara R, et al. Transurethral evaporation of prostate (TUEP) with Nd:YAG laser using a contact free beam technique: results in 61 patients with benign prostatic hyperplasia. *Urology.* 1994;43:813.

90. McCullough DL, Roth RA, Babayan RK, et al. Transurethral ultrasound-guided laser-induced prostatectomy: National Human Cooperative Study results. *J Urol.* 1993;150:1607.

91. Anson K, Nawrocki J, Buckley J, et al. A multicenter randomized prospective study of endoscopic laser ablation versus transurethral resection of the prostate. *Urology.* 1995;46:305.

92. Costello TG, Crowe H, Costello AJ. Laser prostatectomy versus transurethral resection of the prostate for benign prostatic hypertrophy: comparative changes in haemoglobin and serum sodium. *Anaesth Intensive Care.* 1997;25:493.

93. Cummings JM, Parra RO, Bouiller JS, et al. Evaluation of fluid absorption during laser prostatectomy by breath ethanol techniques. *J Urol.* 1995;154:2080.

94. Leach GE, Sirls L, Ganabathi K, et al. Outpatient visual laser assisted prostatectomy under local anesthesia. *Urology.* 1994;43:149.

95. Akalin Z, Mungan NA, Basar H, et al. Transurethral resection of the prostate and laser prostatectomy under local anesthesia. *Eur Urol.* 1998;33:202.

96. Karlsen SJ, Lund M. Visual laser coagulation of the prostate using

97. Birch BR, Gelister JS, Parker CJ, et al. Transurethral resection of prostate under sedation and local anesthesia (sedoanalgesia). *Urology.* 1991;38:113.

98. Shir Y, Frank SM, Brendler CB, et al. Postoperative morbidity is similar in patients anesthetized with epidural and general anesthesia for radical prostatectomy. *Urology.* 1994;44:232.

99. Stevens RA, Mikat-Stevens M, Flanigan R, et al. Does the choice of anesthetic technique affect the recovery of bowel function after radical prostatectomy. *Urology.* 1998;52:213.

100. See WA, Fuller JR, Toner ML. An outcome study of patient-controlled morphine analgesia, with or without ketorolac, following radical retropubic prostatectomy. *J Urol.* 1995;154:1429.

101. Koch MO, Smith JA Jr, Hodge EM, et al. Prospective development of a cost-effective program for radical retropubic prostatectomy. *Urology.* 1994;44:311.

102. Gottschalk A, Smith DS, Jobes DR, et al. Preemptive epidural analgesia and recovery from radical prostatectomy: a randomized controlled trial. *JAMA.* 1998;279:1076.

103. Eisenkop SM, Richman R, Platt LD, et al. Urinary tract injury during cesarean section. *Obstet Gynecol.* 1982;112:591.

104. Shir Y, Raja SN. Indigo carmine-induced severe hypotension in patients undergoing radical prostatectomy. *Anesthesiology.* 1993;79:378.

105. Erickson JC, Widmer BA. The vasopressor effect of indigo carmine. *Anesthesiology.* 1968;29:188.

106. Jeffords DL, Lange PH, Dewolf WC. Severe hypertensive reaction to indigo carmine. *Urology.* 1977;9:180.

107. Quinney N, Lomas I. Treatment of priapism during transurethral resection of the prostate. *Br J Hosp Med.* 1995;54:393.

108. Brindley GS. New treatment for priapism [letter]. *Lancet.* 1984;2 (8396):220.

109. Wong KC. Sympathomimetic drugs. In: Smith NT, Miller RD, Corbascio AN, eds. *Drug Interactions in Anesthesia.* Philadelphia, Pa: Lea & Febiger; 1981:74.

110. Lue FT. Functional evaluation of penile hemodynamics [editorial comments]. *J Urol.* 1988;139:737.

111. Zappala SM, Howard PJ, Hopkins TB, et al. Management of intraoperative penile erections with diluted epinephrine solutions. *Urology.* 1992;40:76.

112. Walther PJ, Meyer AF, Woodworth BC. Intraoperative management of penile erection with intracorporeal phenylephrine during endoscopic surgery. *J Urol.* 1987;137:738.

113. Walther PJ, Meyer AF, Woodworth BE. Intraoperative management of penile erection with intracorporeal phenylephrine during endoscopic surgery. *J Urol.* 1987;137:738.

114. Shantha TR, Finnerty DP, Rodriguez AP. Treatment of persistent penile erection and priapism using terbutaline. *J Urol.* 1989;141:1427.

115. Gale AS. Ketamine prevention of penile turgescence. *JAMA.* 1972;219:1629.

116. Miller PD, Galizia EJ. Management of erections during transurethral surgery using ethyl chloride spray. *Br J Urol.* 1993;71:105.

117. Dixon CL, Sefton W, Gravenstein N. Epidural analgesia after donor nephrectomy decreases duration of hospitalization [abstract]. *Reg Anesth.* 1992;17:75.

118. Ryan DW. Anaesthesia for cystectomy: a comparison of two anaesthetic techniques. *Anaesthesia.* 1982;37:554.

119. Ahlering TE, Henderson JB, Skinner DG. Controlled hypotensive anesthesia to reduce blood loss in radical cystectomy for bladder cancer. *J Urol.* 1983;129:953.

120. Goodnough LT, Riddell J, Kursh E, et al. Utilization and efficacy of autologous blood predeposit in radical prostatectomy and lymphadectomy: implications for blood conservation and physician education program. *Urology.* 1992;40:201.

121. Faris PM, Ritter MA, Abels RI. The effects of recombinant human erythropoietin in perioperative transfusion requirements in patients having a major orthopedic operation. *J Bone Joint Surg Am.* 1996;78:62.

122. Atallah MM, Banoub SM, Saied MM. Does timing of hemodilution influence the stress response and overall outcome? *Anesth Analg.* 1993;76:113.

123. Bjoraker, DB. Protocol for autologous blood transfusion for radical cystectomy. Shands Hospital at the University of Florida, Gainesville, Florida.

124. Pisters LL, Wajsman Z. Use of predeposit autologous blood and intraoperative autotransfusion in urologic cancer surgery. *Urology.* 1992;40:211.

125. Yamada AH, Lieskovsky G, Skinner DG, et al. Impact of autologous

blood transfusions on patients undergoing radical prostatectomy using hypotensive anesthesia. *J Urol.* 1993;149:73.

126. Park KI, Kojima O, Tomoyoshi T. Intra-operative autotransfusion in radical cystectomy. *Br J Urol.* 1997;79:717.

127. Malloy TR, Wein AJ. Laser treatment of bladder carcinoma and genital condylomata. *Outpatient Urol Surg.* 1987;14:121.

128. Splinter WM, Milne B, Nickel C, et al. Perioperative management for resection of a malignant nonchromaffin paraganglioma of the bladder. *Can J Anaesth.* 1989;36:215.

129. Winfield HN, Donovan JF, See WA, Loening SA, et al. Urological laparoscopic surgery. *J Urol.* 1991;146:941.

130. Monk TG, Weldon C. Anesthetic considerations for laparoscopic surgery. *J Endourol.* 1992;6:89.

131. Cuschieri A, Berci G, McSherry CK. Laparoscopic cholecystectomy. *Am J Surg.* 1990;159:273.

132. Borten M. Complications of pneumoperitoneum. In: Ponsky JL, ed. *Laparoscopic Complications: Prevention and Management.* Philadelphia, Pa: BC Decker; 1986:265.

133. Borten M. Instrumentation. In: Ponsky JL, ed. *Laparoscopic Complications: Prevention and Management.* Philadelphia, Pa: BC Decker; 1986:9.

134. Fahy BG, Barnas GM, Flowers JL, et al. Effects of split torso positioning and laparoscopic surgery for donor nephrectomy on respiratory mechanics. *J Clin Anesth.* 1998;10:103.

135. Inglis JM, Brooke BN. Trendelenburg tilt—an obsolete position. *BMJ.* 1956;2:343.

136. Wilcox S, Vandam LD. Alas poor Trendelenburg and his position. *Anesth Analg.* 1988;67:574.

137. Scott DB. Some effects of peritoneal insufflation of carbon dioxide at laparoscopy. *Anaesthesia.* 1970;25:590.

138. Kalhan SB, Reaney JA, Collins RL. Pneumomediastinum and subcutaneous emphysema during laparoscopy. *Cleve Clin J Med.* 1990;57:639.

139. Pascual JB, Baranda MM, Tarrero MT, et al. Subcutaneous emphysema, pneumomediastinum, bilateral pneumothorax and pneumopericardium after laparoscopy. *Endoscopy.* 1990;22:59.

140. Myles PS. Arrhythmias during laparoscopy. *Br J Anaesth.* 1989;63:365.

141. Harris MNE, Plantevin OM, Crowler A. Cardiac arrhythmias during anesthesia for laparoscopy. *Br J Anaesth.* 1984;56:1213.

142. DeGrood PM, Harbers JB, van Egmond J, et al. Anaesthesia for laparoscopy: a comparison of five techniques including propofol, etomidate, thiopentone and isoflurane. *Anaesthesia.* 1987;42:815.

143. Eger EI, Saidman LJ. Hazards of nitrous oxide anesthesia in bowel obstruction and pneumothorax. *Anesthesiology.* 1965;26:61.

144. Lonie DS, Harper NJN. Nitrous oxide anesthesia and vomiting. *Anaesthesia.* 1986;41:703.

145. Bridenbaugh LD, Soderstrom RM. Lumbar epidural block anesthesia for outpatient laparoscopy. *J Reprod Med.* 1979;23:85.

146. Ciofolo MJ, Clergue F, Seebacher J, et al. Ventilatory effects of laparoscopy under epidural anesthesia. *Anesth Analg.* 1990;70:357.

147. Alexander GD, Goldruth M, Brown EM, et al. Outpatient laparoscopic sterilization under local anesthesia. *Am J Obstet Gynecol.* 1973;116:1065.

148. Miller RA, Birch BRP, Anson KU, et al. The impact of minimally invasive surgery and sedoanalgesia on urological practice. *Postgrad Med.* 1990;66(suppl):572.

CHAPTER

# 67

# Anesthesia for Orthopedic Surgery

F. Kayser Enneking

Mark T. Scarborough

Walter W. Virkus

## DEEP VENOUS THROMBOSIS AND PULMONARY EMBOLISM

*What Factors Place Patients at Risk?*

*What Is the Appropriate Drug Therapy for Deep Venous Thrombosis Prophylaxis?*

*How Does Anesthesia Influence Postoperative Thromboembolism?*

## INFECTION

*When Are Prophylactic Antibiotics Indicated?*

*Which Antibiotics Are Most Effective?*

*Why Is Antibiotic Coverage Crucial?*

## ORTHOPEDIC TRAUMA

*What Factors Are Important in Evaluation?*

*What Is the Significance of an Open Fracture in Multiple Trauma?*

*How Much Bleeding Can Occur From Femur and Pelvic Fractures?*

*When Should Military Antishock Trousers Be Released?*

*What Studies Should Be Performed to Evaluate the Cervical Spine?*

*Why Do Closed Femur Fractures Require Early Stabilization?*

*Which Orthopedic Injuries Require Emergent or Urgent Surgery?*

*What Is the Prognosis for Elderly Patients Who Sustain Hip Fractures?*

## TOTAL JOINT REPLACEMENT

*What Are the Fluid Requirements?*

*What Is the Anticipated Blood Loss During Various Arthroplasties?*

*What Are Other Unique Complications?*

*When Should Invasive Monitors Be Used?*

*Why Does Hypotension Occur During Lower Extremity Joint Replacement?*

*Why Are Some Total Joints Placed Without Cement?*

*Why Is Muscle Relaxation Necessary During Total Hip Replacement?*

## RHEUMATOID ARTHRITIS

*Why Do These Patients Have Difficult Airways?*

*What Other Systemic Involvement Is Important?*

*Is Regional Anesthesia Advantageous?*

## ORTHOPEDIC ONCOLOGY

*Why Should Impending Pathologic Fractures Be Stabilized?*

*What Is an Osteoid Osteoma, and How Is It Treated?*

*What Problems Are Common to Patients With Bone Cancers?*

*Which Procedures Have a Potential for Massive Blood Loss?*

## SCOLIOSIS

*Does the Underlying Cause of Scoliosis Have Anesthetic Implications?*

*What Are the Respiratory Effects?*

*Why Do Curves >65° Need to Be Corrected?*

*How Is Spinal Cord Function Monitored Intraoperatively?*

*When Are Anterior Approaches to the Spine Used?*

*What Is Important About Instrumentation for Spinal Surgery?*

## AMPUTATIONS AND PHANTOM LIMB PAIN

*What Causes Phantom Limb Pain?*

*How Can Phantom Limb Pain Be Prevented?*

## AMBULATORY ORTHOPEDIC SURGERY

*What Are the Causes of Pain During Arthroscopic Procedures?*

*What Can You Do to Improve Arthroscopic Visualization?*

## REGIONAL ANESTHESIA

*What Are the Important Factors in Upper Extremity Blocks?*

*What Are the Important Considerations in Lower Extremity Blocks?*

*Does Regional Anesthesia Reduce Morbidity or Mortality for Hip Fractures?*

*What Are the Advantages of Regional Anesthesia?*

## BLOOD LOSS

*What Measures Should Be Taken Preoperatively for Projected Blood Loss?*

*How Can Intraoperative Blood Loss Be Decreased?*

## POSITIONING

*Why Are Chest Rolls Used in the Prone Position?*

*What Is the Correct Position for Longitudinal Chest Rolls?*

*What Are Important Considerations When Using the Beach-Chair Position?*

*What Are Potential Complications of the Lateral Decubitus Position?*

*What Are Potential Complications of the Lateral Decubitus Position?*

*What Are the Potential Complications?*

*What Is the Optimal Tourniquet Inflation and Release Scheme?*

*Why Are Surgeons Reluctant to Deflate a Tourniquet Intraoperatively?*

*What Is the Optimal Tourniquet Pressure?*

*What Causes Bleeding Distal to an Inflated Tourniquet?*

*What Is Tourniquet Pain?*

*What Physiologic Effects Occur With Tourniquet Deflation?*

## SPLINTING

*Why Is the Timing of the Wake-Up Important in Orthopedic Cases?*

*What Are the Dangers Associated With Plaster Splints?*

Orthopedic surgery encompasses a broad spectrum of procedures, from simple closed reduction of a dislocated joint to complicated removal and reconstruction of a failed total joint arthroplasty. Patients of all ages undergo orthopedic procedures and have a wide range of associated illnesses. Anesthesiologists should be aware of the spectrum of disease states and the specific perioperative considerations frequently encountered during orthopedic procedures. This chapter approaches this broad topic by category, addressing both specific and general problems encountered in the care of orthopedic patients.

## DEEP VENOUS THROMBOSIS AND PULMONARY EMBOLISM

### What Factors Place Patients at Risk?

Orthopedic patients are at higher risk for deep venous thrombosis (DVT) and subsequent pulmonary embolus (PE) than most other surgical patients. Decreased mobility after joint surgery, trauma, or spine injury is a contributing factor to the development of DVT in this patient population. Furthermore, many operative procedures involve direct manipulation of major vessels, or involve manipulation of the extremity leading to temporary kinking of the vessels. DVT and PE occur most often following hip and knee surgery. The incidence in some trauma patients has been reported to be as high as 80%.[1] Fatal PE is reported in 1% to 3% of patients who did not receive prophylaxis against thrombosis after total hip replacement.[2] With prophylaxis, the incidence of DVT can be reduced to as low as 20% and fatal PE can be nearly eliminated.[3,4]

The cited incidence of DVT depends on the mechanism for documentation of embolism (ie, venography, pulmonary angiography, Doppler, or ultrasonographic [US] studies). In the orthopedic population, risk factors include hip surgery, advanced age, female gender, previous thromboembolic disease, malignancy, and prolonged bed rest.

Many investigations have been performed to examine the incidence of DVT and PE and identify the ideal method of prophylaxis. Venous thrombosis prophylaxis can be divided into mechanical and pharmacologic methods. Mechanical methods include compression stockings, sequential compression devices, and plantar foot pumps. Pharmacologic agents include dextran, aspirin, fractionated and unfractionated heparin, and warfarin. Mechanical methods alone are not thought to be adequate prophylaxis and should be used in concert with a pharmacologic agent.

### What Is the Appropriate Drug Therapy for Deep Venous Thrombosis Prophylaxis?

The ideal drug therapy for DVT prophylaxis is still a matter of debate. Dextran is not used due to its cost and its side effects of volume overload and hypersensitivity. A minority of surgeons use aspirin, in conjunction with mechanical methods. However, studies have indicated that its effectiveness is questionable.[5,6] For routine DVT prophylaxis after arthroplasty surgery, the majority of surgeons use either warfarin or fractionated low molecular weight heparin (LMWH) in conjunction with mechanical methods. No study has shown one to be definitively superior. Some studies have shown that the DVT/PE incidence is lower with LMWH but with a higher bleeding complication rate.[5,7] Other studies have shown no significant differences between the two therapies.[8] Both regimens will likely continue to be used until a study shows a clear difference.

In the trauma patient, the issue of DVT prophylaxis is more difficult. Although these patients are clearly at risk, their compromised medical condition can make pharmacologic anticoagulation dangerous. These patients frequently require repeated surgical procedures, making continuous anticoagulation impossible. There are a number of ongoing studies reviewing this problem, but current practice is typically low-dose subcutaneous heparin or LMWH, depending on the patient's potential for bleeding complications, along with diligent use of mechanical methods.

### How Does Anesthesia Influence Postoperative Thromboembolism?

The influence of regional anesthesia on the incidence of postoperative thromboembolism is real but perhaps less important today than it was in the past. Evidence suggests a lower incidence of DVT in patients undergoing total hip replacement with epidural anesthesia than with general anesthesia.[9,10] However, when the patients in the general anesthetic group were given antithrombotic prophylaxis, no difference occured.[11,12] Because new techniques have been developed to prevent DVT (low-dose sodium warfarin, LMWH, and the routine use of pneumatic intermittent compression stockings), the advantage of the intraoperative technique may be less important.[13]

## INFECTION

### When Are Prophylactic Antibiotics Indicated?

Prophylactic antibiotics are indicated for all clean orthopedic operative procedures that involve implantation of foreign materials, including prostheses, plates, and screws, or the transplantation of tissues (whether autologous or allograft). Appropriate antibiotic prophylaxis for soft tissue procedures, particularly those of short duration, is less clear.

The timing of the administration of the antibiotics is critical and should be done at least 5 minutes before the inflation of a tourniquet or before the incision so that prophylactic soft tissue and bone antibiotic drug levels are achieved at the operative site. The recommended duration of prophylactic antibiotic administration is 24 to 48 hours postoperatively (eg, cefazolin, 1 g intravenously every 8 hours for 24-48 hours in a healthy adult).

The routine preoperative culturing of open fractures is no longer considered to be beneficial; antibiotic administration should not be delayed for this practice.

### Which Antibiotics Are Most Effective?

Cefazolin (Kefzol or Ancef) is the most commonly used prophylactic antibiotic. This antibiotic has good bone penetration characteristics, provides broad-spectrum microbial coverage of the most commonly encountered orthopedic pathogens (staphylococci and streptococci), is relatively inexpensive, and has been used successfully for many years.

In penicillin-allergic patients, vancomycin is most frequently used as an alternative prophylactic antibiotic agent. However, vancomycin requires approximately 1 hour for its complete administration if the "red man syndrome" is to be avoided; furthermore, this drug is expensive. Most importantly, its use leads to the formation of vancomycin-resistant organisms, which are becoming an increasingly important medical issue. Clindamycin can also be used as an alternative for penicillin-allergic patients. It can be given as a bolus, has relatively few side effects, and is inexpensive.

### Why Is Antibiotic Coverage Crucial?

Many orthopedic procedures involve implantation of synthetic materials such as rods, prostheses, plates, and allografts. Some bacteria readily bind to such materials by elaborating glycocalyx. Once bound, infection can be established by proliferation of implant-bound bacteria. Prophylactic antibiotic therapy dramatically reduces the incidence of infection in hip replacement surgery from 2% to 3% to less than 1% in

most series.[14] Patzakis and coworkers reported a decrease in infection rate for open fractures from 13% to 2.3% when prophylactic antibiotics were administered.[14]

The potential for wound contamination is high in orthopedic procedures for several reasons. Many procedures are relatively long and frequently performed under ischemic conditions. If antibiotics have not been administered before tourniquet inflation, the wound provides an ideal medium for bacterial growth. Also, preparation of the bone for implantation by drilling and reaming causes local bone necrosis and thus provides another site for bacterial proliferation and glycocalyx production.

Once the presence of a bone infection has been established, it is difficult to eradicate. Frequently, extensive bone débridement and prolonged antibiotic therapy are required. Reconstruction can only take place after the infection is cleared and is often technically difficult. Because of the potential risk of blood-borne microorganisms seeding implanted synthetic material, some physicians recommend the use of prophylactic antibiotics for any procedure that might lead to bacteremia. The recommendations are similar to those for subacute bacterial endocarditis prophylaxis.

## ORTHOPEDIC TRAUMA

### What Factors Are Important in Evaluation?

#### Patient Profiles

Although trauma can occur in any age group, it frequently involves patients under the age of 30 years. Alcohol and illegal drug use are common in trauma patients. Blood and urine samples for toxicology screening should be obtained as part of the preoperative work-up. Acute intoxication might change the anesthetic management by altering the patient's responses to certain drug therapies, by rendering the patient unable to cooperate for a regional technique, or by slowing arousal following general anesthesia. Intoxicated patients are potentially dangerous to themselves and others. Universal precautions should be observed in all trauma settings because the risk of exposure to a variety of body fluids is high.

### What Is the Significance of an Open Fracture in Multiple Trauma?

Multiple trauma resulting from a high-velocity motor vehicle accident is one of the most common causes of orthopedic injuries (Table 67–1). Patients may have dramatic and obvious extremity trauma without other readily apparent injury. Mechanism of injury is an important factor in guiding patient care. High-energy injuries must raise suspicion for multisystem injury. The magnitude of force required to cause an open fracture is such that the patient must be systematically evaluated for other less apparent associated injuries to the chest, abdomen, and neurologic axis, as well as the musculoskeletal system. Enormous external forces are required to disrupt the pelvis; consequently, associated injuries are common. Blood loss can be >20 units in some cases. The reported mortality rate is 5% to 20%, and each patient has an average of 2.7 other associated major injuries.[15]

**TABLE 67–1.** Common Orthopedic Injuries

| Injury | Imaging | Treatment | Emergent Fixation Required |
|---|---|---|---|
| Cervical spine | Cross-table lateral radiograph; cervical spine series; CT; MRI | Halo cast versus cervical instrumentation versus cervical fusion | Not unless progressive neurologic compromise occurs |
| Thoracic spine; lumbar spine | AP, lateral radiograph; CT | Cast versus instrumentation and fusion | Not unless progressive neurologic compromise occurs |
| Pelvic fracture | CT; AP radiograph | ORIF versus external fixation | If patient hemodynamically stable, wait at least 72 h; if patient hemodynamically unstable, fixation ASAP |
| Femur fractures | AP; lateral radiograph | ORIF versus external fixation | Yes, within 24 h |
| Open fracture | Radiograph | Irrigation and débridement; ORIF versus external fixation | Yes, within 6-8 h |
| Open fracture with arterial injury | Radiograph; angiography | Irrigation and dériderment; arterial repair ORIF versus amputation | Yes, ASAP |
| Knee dislocation | Radiograph; angiography | Repair ligaments and popliteal vessels | Yes, ASAP |
| Hip dislocation | Radiograph; CT | May require muscle relaxation for closed reduction versus open reduction | Yes, ASAP |
| Shoulder dislocation | Radiograph | May require muscle relaxation for closed reduction versus open reduction | Yes, ASAP |
| Supracondylar elbow fracture; no vascular compromise; if vascular/neuro compromise | Radiograph | Closed reduction percutaneous pinning versus ORIF | Yes, within 6-8 h<br><br>Yes, ASAP |
| Compartment syndromes | Compartment pressure measurement | Fasciotomy | Yes, ASAP |
| Hip fracture | Radiograph; CT; MRI | IF versus hip replacement | Yes, within 24 h<br>Yes, within 48 h |
| Septic joint | Joint aspiration | Irrigation and débridement | Yes, ASAP |
| Other closed fractures | Radiograph; CT | Closed reduction versus percutaneous pinning versus ORIF | Yes, within 24 h or 2-5 d later, when swelling has reduced |

AP, anteroposterior; ASAP, as soon as possible; CT, computed tomography; IF, internal fixation; MRI, magnetic resonance imaging; Neuro, neurologic; ORIF, open reduction.

## Associated Injuries

Typical injuries resulting from rapid acceleration and deceleration include flexion and extension injuries to the spine; pulmonary and cardiac contusions caused by the seatbelt or steering wheel; shearing of organ pedicles that are anatomically fixed, including the ascending aorta and mesentery; femoral and acetabular fractures; ligamentous knee injuries; and hip dislocations.

Airbag deployment in motor vehicles has improved the chance of surviving high-impact motor vehicle accidents, particularly for unrestrained drivers. However, airbag deployment can cause injuries even in low-impact collisions, including chemical burns, ocular trauma, upper limb fractures, lacerations, and fatal cervical spine disarticulation.[16]

If the patient is ejected from a vehicle or sustains a fall from a height, the injury pattern differs. A systematic evaluation from head to toe should be undertaken according to ATLS protocols. Closed head injuries and cervical spine trauma should be suspected, especially in victims of motorcycle accidents, pedestrians struck by a motor vehicle, and occupants ejected from cars. Flail chest, hemothorax, and pneumothorax are common thoracic injuries in these patients. Laparotomy is frequently required for abdominal injuries, following evaluation by computed tomography (CT) scan or diagnostic peritoneal lavage.

Urethral and bladder injuries require early urologic consultation. Catheterization of the bladder with a Foley catheter should be performed when the patient arrives at the hospital. Blood at the urethral meatus requires a retrograde urethrogram before urinary catheter insertion to avoid exacerbating a urethral injury. Suprapubic catheters can contaminate future ab-dominal and pelvic surgical approaches and should only be used as a last resort. Rectal or vaginal lacerations and small- and large-bowel perforations are commonly associated with pelvic fractures. These injuries require primary repair, a diverting colostomy, or both.

Neurologic injury can be secondary to spinal cord injury or can occur from traction injury to the lumbosacral plexus. Although spinal cord injuries secondary to vertebral column fractures are treated by stabilizing the bony injury, no treatment exists for injuries to the lumbosacral plexus. Injury to the conus medullaris at L1 or the sacral nerve roots may lead to bowel or bladder incontinence and sexual dysfunction.

## How Much Bleeding Can Occur From Femur and Pelvic Fractures?

Closed femoral fractures cause damage to the thigh musculature that can result in the sequestered loss of up to 4 to 6 units of blood into the thigh before tamponade occurs. Compartment syndromes of the thigh have been reported in association with this type of injury, but they are uncommon.[17]

Pelvic fractures may result in uncontrollable retroperitoneal bleeding. Patients with such fractures that disrupt the pubic symphysis (open book-type fractures) are at high risk for massive blood loss. The average blood loss associated with closed fractures of the pelvis is 6 units, in contrast to 18 units for open pelvic fractures.

Methods to control blood loss associated with pelvic fractures include external fixation, angiographic embolization, wound packing, military antishock trouser placement, ligation of ruptured vessels, and, rarely, hemipelvectomy. The most desirable approach is pelvic external fixation, which involves placing metal pins in both iliac wings and connecting the pins with an external frame. The iliac wings are then compressed, and the fixator is tightened; this stabilizes the pelvis. External fixation is a quick, reliable method to control hemorrhage and does not interfere with general surgical or urologic access to the patient for other procedures.

## When Should Military Antishock Trousers Be Released?

Military antishock trousers may be applied by paramedical personnel before hospital transfer to support blood pressure (BP) and stabilize lower extremity fractures. They are being taken out of use in an increasing number of major cities because of complications associated with their use. If they are placed for BP support, they should be released incrementally as soon as possible after hemodynamic stability has been achieved with concurrent volume replacement. If they are placed only for fracture stabilization and the patient is hemodynamically stable, they should be removed immediately on arrival to the emergency department. Multiple case reports describe compartment syndromes that develop when military antishock trousers are inflated for longer than 120 minutes.[18–20]

## What Studies Should Be Performed to Evaluate the Cervical Spine?

If the patient arrives in extremis, intubation with direct visualization by the anesthesiologist (with the assistance of the surgeon who holds the head and neck in rigid traction) should be performed without delay. The neck must be held firmly in the neutral position until the cervical spine has been examined radiographically.

Screening lateral radiographs of the cervical spine from the occiput to the first thoracic vertebra must be obtained in any patient admitted with a history of major skeletal trauma, a fall, head or facial injury, neurologic symptoms, or loss of consciousness. The bone architecture and alignment of the cervical spine should be evaluated and the adjacent soft tissues examined for swelling. Cervical neutrality should be maintained in patients with a possible cervical neck injury (those with neck pain, paresthesias, or momentary paralysis at the scene) until a formal orthopedic or neurosurgical evaluation has been performed, even if findings on screening cross-table lateral radiography are negative. Remember that the cervical spine cannot be cleared with radiographs alone, and either a clinical examination or magnetic resonance imaging must also be performed to rule out a ligamentous injury. Almost all patients who need emergent or semi-emergent surgical intervention for trauma will not have a cleared cervical spine before surgery. A patient demonstrating diffuse extremity numbness or weakness, suggestive of a spinal cord injury, is usually also given intravenous steroids based on the 1998 findings of the Third National Acute Spinal Cord Injury study.[21] The dose for this treatment is a 30 mg/kg bolus of methylprednisolone, followed by a continuous infusion of 5.4/mg/kg/h for 23 hours. For patients in whom methylprednisolone therapy is initiated within 3 hours of injury, 24-hour maintenance is appropriate. Patients starting therapy 3 to 8

hours after injury should be maintained on the regimen for 48 hours unless there are complicating medical factors.[22] This therapy must be instituted within 8 hours of injury for any beneficial effect to be expected.

## Why Do Closed Femur Fractures Require Early Stabilization?

Early stabilization of femur fractures in multiple trauma patients decreases the incidence of complications.[23] Rigid internal fixation allows early mobility and improved respiratory care. The result is a decrease in the incidence of acute respiratory failure, fat emboli, and pneumonia. When fracture stabilization is delayed for >24 hours, the length of the intensive care unit stay and the overall duration of hospitalization are increased. Hospital costs are nearly 50% greater for these patients than for patients whose fractures are stabilized.[24]

The greatest improvement in outcome has been shown in patients with the highest injury severity scores.[25] Such patients should be brought to the operating room (OR) as soon as their diagnostic work-up is completed. Patients with closed head injury and elevated intracranial pressure must be assessed on an individual basis. Early fracture fixation can cause an elevation of intracranial pressure, which may have an adverse effect on the neurologic outcome of these patients. Communication among the anesthetist, neurosurgeon, and orthopedic surgeon is vital in these cases.

Multitrauma patients with femur fractures must be carefully monitored during manipulation of the femoral canal. Studies using echocardiography have shown that large amounts of medullary fat and debris are introduced into the venous system during reaming of the femoral canal.[26] In patients with preexisting traumatic lung injury, such embolization may increase the risk of progressive lung dysfunction. Episodes of hypoxemia or increased pulmonary vascular resistance may occur during these cases and should be treated aggressively.

## Which Orthopedic Injuries Require Emergent or Urgent Surgery?

Table 67–1 outlines the urgency of many common orthopedic injuries. In general, emergent surgery (ie, in the next available OR) should be carried out whenever a limb is at risk for disruption of its blood supply. This scenario may result from direct trauma to the vessels or from joint dislocation. Open fractures require urgent irrigation and débridement within a maximum of 6 to 8 hours from the time of injury to prevent deep-seated bone infections.

Closed fractures requiring open repair need surgical attention before the development of skin breakdown from edema formation (fracture blisters). These blisters can develop within 12 hours if the extremity is not properly elevated. Any surgical reduction of a fracture is facilitated by muscular paralysis, which can be accomplished with general or regional anesthesia. Dislocations of the hip should be relocated within 6 hours to restore blood supply to the femoral head and prevent avascular necrosis. Unlike dislocations occurring in total hip arthroplasties (THAs), traumatic dislocations in normal hips should ideally be reduced in a setting of complete muscular paralysis to minimize further injury to the femoral head during relocation. This can be accomplished with both general anes-

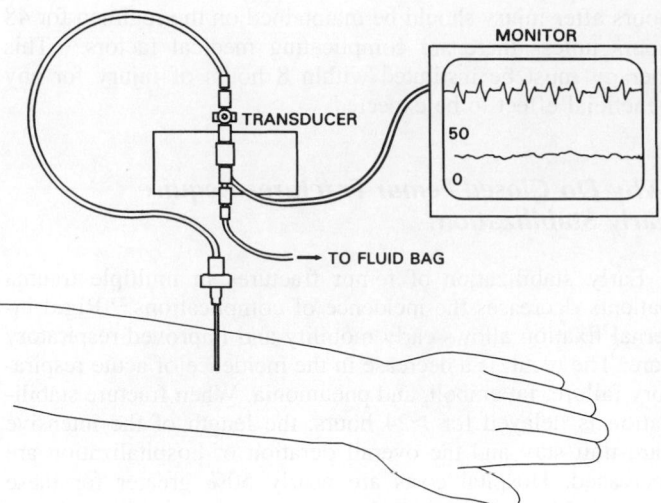

**FIGURE 67–1.** Measurement of tissue (compartment) pressure following orthopedic extremity trauma.

thesia and neuromuscular blocking agents or with regional anesthesia and dense motor blockade. Knee dislocations require urgent operative intervention because they are frequently associated with vascular injury.

Compartment syndromes are diagnosed by measuring pressures within an anatomic compartment, such as the volar aspect of the forearm (Fig. 67–1). The technique is as simple as taking a calibrated pressure transducer and attaching a needle where you would normally attach the catheter. The needle is then aseptically inserted into the compartment in question. If the pressure fluctuates when the adjacent tissue is compressed, the system should be functioning properly.

The extremity is usually tense, and capillary refill may be delayed. The quality of the pulse is not a reliable indicator of compartment pressures. Compartment syndromes of soft tissue or from bone injuries can develop intraoperatively if vascular access catheters infiltrate or in the presence of poor extremity positioning.[27] The problem should be brought to the immediate attention of the surgical team. Treatment of compartment syndromes includes emergent surgical fasciotomy. Whether regional anesthesia in the postoperative period masks compartment syndrome is controversial. Although reports of missed compartment syndrome in the presence of regional anesthesia and epidural analgesia exist, most authors do recognize a change in pain level with the development of the compartment syndrome.[28,29]

### What Is the Prognosis for Elderly Patients Who Sustain Hip Fractures?

The mortality rate for the American Society of Anesthesiologists class 3 and 4 patients is 6-fold that for age-matched controls during the first year following hip fracture.[30] Many studies have attempted to assess the cause of the high rates of morbidity and mortality in the elderly population. The single best predictor of mortality is preoperative mental status.[31]

## TOTAL JOINT REPLACEMENT

Replacement of diseased joints with implantable prosthetic devices is a major advance in orthopedic surgery since the

early 1960s. The vast majority of patients who undergo replacement surgery are >60 years of age and are generally in good health. Of concern, however, are the patients with arthritis who may not report symptoms of cardiac or respiratory insufficiency because they have made adaptive changes in their lifestyle that severely restrict their activity level. Younger patients who require joint replacement fall into one of three categories: those with congenital anomalies, those with trauma to the joint, and those with severe systemic disease frequently requiring steroid therapy.

### What Are the Fluid Requirements?

Primary total joint replacements usually do not involve tremendous fluid shifts. A transient decrease in BP occurs at predictable times during THA (cementing) and total knee arthroplasty (TKA) (tourniquet release) and should be anticipated with an appropriate volume replacement strategy. Fluids should be administered based on preoperative deficit, maintenance requirements, estimated blood loss, and third space losses. The fluid replacement requirement for primary THA is approximately 5 mL/kg/h and that for total knee and shoulder replacements is approximately 4 mL/kg/h.

### What Is the Anticipated Blood Loss During Various Arthroplasties?

#### Total Hip Arthroplasty

Intraoperative blood loss during an uncomplicated primary THA for arthritis is usually between 400 and 800 mL when cemented prostheses are placed. If a noncemented prosthesis is placed, higher blood losses can be expected both intraoperatively and postoperatively.

Anticipated blood loss during THA for congenital deformities, malignant bone lesions, or revision of a previous joint replacement is much less predictable. Frequently, these operations are technically difficult to perform, and blood loss of more than 1500 mL is not uncommon (Table 67–2).

#### Total Knee Replacement

Because a total knee replacement is performed below the point where the tourniquet is placed, blood loss does not begin until the tourniquet is deflated. Some orthopedists close the wound and apply the dressing before they release the tourniquet, thereby minimizing intraoperative blood loss. However, this strategy does not reduce total blood loss, which averages 200 to 600 mL regardless of when the tourniquet is deflated.

**TABLE 67–2.** Procedures Likely to Have an Estimated Blood Loss of >1 Liter

| |
|---|
| Revision total hip arthroplasty |
| Arthroplasty for congenital hip deformity |
| Removal of infected prosthesis |
| Intramedullary rodding of a femur fracture |
| Resection and reconstruction of bone lesions |
| Bilateral total knee arthroplasties |
| Biopsy of any sacral lesion |
| Spinal fusion at >3 levels |

## Total Shoulder Replacement

The most common diagnoses for patients requiring total shoulder arthroplasty (TSA) are rheumatoid arthritis and osteoarthritis. These operations are frequently technically difficult, and average blood losses vary from 300 to 1000 mL.

## What Are Other Unique Complications?

Brachial plexus injury is a significant risk following TSA. Lynch and colleagues[32] reported a 4% incidence of brachial plexus injury following TSA in 417 operations. The presumed mechanism of injury was stretching of the upper and middle cords of the plexus during operation. They reported a high correlation with a particular surgical approach (the long deltopectoral approach) and with a short operating time.

## Removal of an Infected, Loose, or Broken Prosthesis

During removal of an infected prosthesis, major blood loss can be anticipated as the surgeon attempts a deep débridement. Frequently, these procedures last several hours and a slow steady venous ooze from the bone occurs while the surgeon removes contaminated cement and tissue. If there is evidence of active infection, use of a cell saver is contraindicated.

## When Should Invasive Monitors Be Used?

The decision to place invasive monitors should always be made on a case by case basis, depending on the patient's physical status and on the type of operation to be performed. Certain procedures present the potential for tremendous blood loss. Patients who are to have such procedures should undergo invasive monitoring of their arterial and central venous pressures.

Intraoperative transesophageal echocardiography (TEE) has become the gold standard for emboli detection during joint arthroplasties and fracture fixation operations. Sulek and associates[33] reported on patients having both TEE and transcranial Doppler monitoring during routine TKA. They found more than half of the patients had evidence of echogenic microemboli as detected by TEE following tourniquet release. All the patients with TEE evidence of emboli had evidence of cerebral microemboli by transcranial Doppler. Although there were no neurologic deficits attributed to the cerebral microembolisms detected in this study, other investigators have reported evidence of long-term cognitive dysfunction in up to 5% of patients undergoing TKA.[34]

## Why Does Hypotension Occur During Lower Extremity Joint Replacement?

Immediately after the femoral prosthesis has been cemented, the majority of patients who undergo hip replacement surgery experience a decrease in BP for several minutes. Two mechanisms probably are responsible. First, emboli of fat, marrow, and air are extruded from the femoral canal into the pulmonary circulation, resulting in transient pulmonary arteriolar obstruction. Second, direct vasodilation is caused by the methylmethacrylate monomer.

If a tourniquet is not used for a total knee replacement, hypotension from the same mechanism may occur when the femoral component is seated. The degree of hypotension is usually not as great as that associated with tourniquet use, probably because a smaller volume of marrow is displaced. However, TKA is usually performed with a tourniquet, and hypotension is most likely to occur immediately after tourniquet release. Although hypotension is thought to be related to the presence of small emboli, other factors related to ischemia of the extremity, including reactive hyperemia and the release of adenosine, might also play a role.

## Why Are Some Total Joints Placed Without Cement?

Fixation of total joint prosthesis can be accomplished with acrylic cement or using a "press fit" technique. The indications for choosing one technique over another are controversial among orthopedic surgeons. In theory, uncemented joints should have increased longevity because the prosthesis becomes biologically incorporated into the native bone. Uncemented prostheses are usually placed in young patients and in more active older patients.

Whether uncemented prostheses actually last longer than cemented ones is debatable. The uncemented joints require a prolonged period of nonweight-bearing ambulation and thus are not recommended in debilitated patients. Press fit prostheses are easier to revise than are cemented ones; this feature is a distinct advantage in young patients who can anticipate revision every 5 to 10 years, depending on their activity level.

## Why Is Muscle Relaxation Necessary During Total Hip Replacement?

During THA, the head of the femur is dislocated from its position in the acetabulum. This maneuver does not require flaccid paralysis; however, the powerful quadriceps and hip flexor muscles will hamper this action if some degree of muscle relaxation is not used. Application of regional techniques or administration of a muscle relaxant during general anesthesia is suitable. The combination of muscle relaxation and surgical manipulation results in postoperative lower back discomfort in almost all hip replacement patients, regardless of the anesthetic technique chosen.

## RHEUMATOID ARTHRITIS

Rheumatoid arthritis is an autoimmune system–mediated inflammatory process that affects connective tissue. Joint instability and destruction are the primary manifestations of this disease. Typically, patients have morning stiffness, pain on motion, swelling, and tenderness of multiple joints. The incidence of rheumatoid arthritis is about 0.5%, and the disease occurs most frequently in women between the ages of 30 and 60 years. Exacerbations and remissions over a patient's lifetime characterize the natural history of the disease. Patients frequently require multiple orthopedic interventions.

## Why Do These Patients Have Difficult Airways?

Cervical instability, micrognathia, and limited mobility of the temporomandibular joints and cervical spine are common findings. Radiographic evidence of cervical spine involvement can be found in ≤90% of patients.[35] The most common form involving the cervical spine is atlantoaxial instability. This condition allows excessive motion between C1 and C2 and can result in cervical spinal cord impingement. Cervical spine flexion-extension radiographs should be obtained preoperatively in all rheumatoid patients in whom intubation is required.

A subset of patients develop triplanar deviation of the larynx in which the larynx is displaced caudally, deviated to the left, rotated to the right, and anteriorly angulated (Fig. 67–2).[30,36] Involvement of the cricoarytenoid joints decreases the diameter of the airway such that smaller than anticipated endotracheal tubes must be used for intubation.

A detailed airway examination should be performed to assess for possible paresthesias or dizziness with neck motion in all planes, tracheal deviation, and hoarseness. Physical examination and flexion-extension lateral cervical spine films usually identify those patients who require awake fiberoptic intubation and positioning.

## What Other Systemic Involvement Is Important?

The incidence of heart disease is increased in patients with rheumatoid arthritis compared with age-matched controls.[37]

Coronary arteritis, conduction defects, valvular heart disease, and pericarditis have been attributed to rheumatoid disease and should be sought. Extrinsic and intrinsic restrictive lung disease can occur. Pulmonary function tests should be performed preoperatively if the rheumatoid patient has complaints of dyspnea. Anemia is frequently present as well.

Review of the drug history is essential. These patients frequently take large doses of nonsteroidal anti-inflammatory drugs. Platelet dysfunction and renal impairment as a result of this therapy should be evaluated preoperatively. Steroid therapy is commonly employed clinically during exacerbation of the disease. Perioperative stress steroid coverage is most commonly achieved by administering a large dose of a corticosteroid drug (ie, 100 mg of hydrocortisone) before, during, and after the operation if the patient has received exogenous steroids within the previous 6 months. No controlled studies have confirmed the necessity for these large doses.

Gold salts, hydroxychloroquine sulfate (Plaquenil Sulfate), penicillamine, and methotrexate are used to treat rheumatoid arthritis. The most common adverse side effect of these drugs is suppression of the hematopoietic system, but renal and hepatic damage can also occur. In addition, gold salts rarely can cause interstitial lung disease.

## Is Regional Anesthesia Advantageous?

Patients with severe disease often have progression of joint dysfunction and airway involvement throughout their lifetimes. Intubation can be a harrowing experience for the patient and the anesthesiologist. Severe hypoxia may occur during a difficult intubation, even in the conscious but sedated patient, during fiberoptic bronchoscopy.

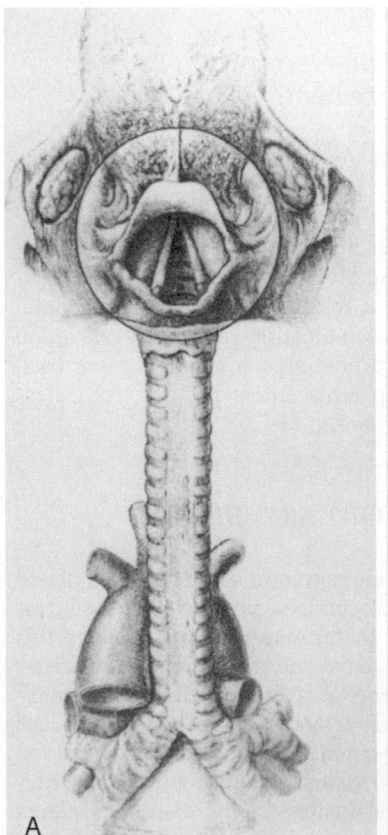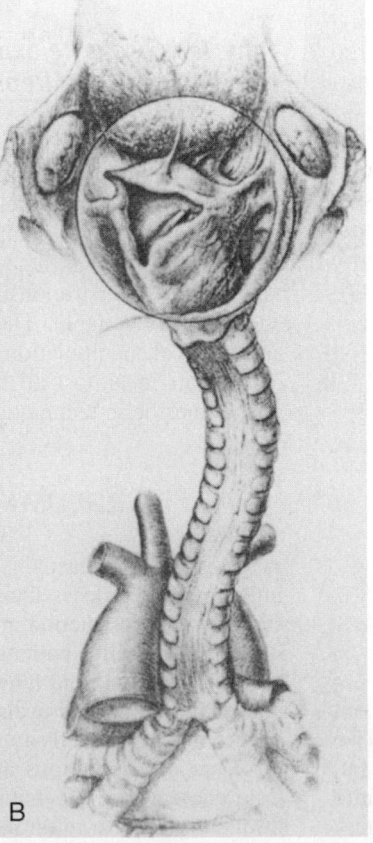

**FIGURE 67–2.** *A,* Normal position of the trachea and larynx. Circled area represents view through a fiberoptic bronchoscope. *B,* Deviated position of the trachea and larynx associated with severe rheumatoid arthritis. Note the triaxial deviation of the airway and the small glottic opening. (From Keenen MA, Siles CM, Kaufman RL. Acquired laryngeal deviation associated with the cervical spine disease in erosive polyarticular arthritis. *Anesthesiology.* 1983;58:441.)

Extubation may also be problematic. Airway edema, especially after a traumatic intubation, causes critical narrowing of an already compromised airway and thus makes extubation unwise. Thus, selecting a regional technique that avoids airway manipulation may be prudent. However, it must be conducted with recognition that emergency intubation may not be possible.

Positioning during a regional anesthetic procedure is almost an art form. Rheumatoid arthritis patients often have other joint involvement that makes it difficult for them to be maintained in the same position for many hours regardless of how well padded they are. Finally, these patients will return to the OR for future surgery; therefore, frank discussion of their disease and anesthetic options is essential to gain their cooperation and understanding. Unless they are exceptionally motivated, no significant advantage is gained with regional anesthesia during major joint replacement procedures.

## ORTHOPEDIC ONCOLOGY

Orthopedic oncology encompasses a wide range of diagnostic, therapeutic, and reconstructive procedures in patients of all age groups. Although primary bone tumors are exceedingly rare, soft tissue sarcomas and metastatic bone disease are frequently encountered. Anesthesiologists should be aware of specific concerns that are applicable to almost any oncology patient.

### Why Should Impending Pathologic Fractures Be Stabilized?

Patients treated prophylactically for impending fractures have a lower surgical mortality, fewer complications, fewer stabilization failures, and more successful rehabilitation than those who suffer pathologic fractures.[38] All pathologic fractures should undergo stabilization if the patient's quality of life will be improved by the procedure (ie, if the procedure will provide pain relief or improved mobility).

### What Is an Osteoid Osteoma, and How Is It Treated?

An osteoid osteoma is a painful small benign bone lesion that usually occurs in children and young adults and is located most often in the femur and tibia. In the past, these were treated with surgical excision. Recently, these lesions have been effectively treated with CT-directed radiofrequency ablation. This technique involves putting a needle into the nidus of the lesion under CT guidance. The lesion is then heated to 90°C for several minutes. Because the procedure is painful, it is done under either regional or general anesthesia. This noninvasive technique can be performed on an ambulatory basis.

### What Problems Are Common to Patients With Bone Cancers?

#### Pain

Bone lesions frequently are painful. Patients commonly take large doses of analgesics and may have a tolerance to narcotics and other sedatives. An accurate drug history is necessary to anticipate and plan for their postoperative needs. Oral narcotic doses should be converted to an equivalent parenteral dose that is administered while the patient remains in nil per os status. Stress doses of steroids are *not* indicated if steroids were used for chemotherapeutic purposes only.

#### Chemotherapy

Frequently, oncology patients receive chemotherapy that results in anemia, granulocytopenia, thrombocytopenia, or any combination of these. The introduction of granulocyte-stimulating factors and recombinant erythropoietin lessens the severity of bone marrow suppression that results from chemotherapy. Hypercalcemia may occur in cancer patients, especially those with metastatic disease, and should be checked before any surgical procedure. Specific inquiry should be made regarding the use of doxorubicin (Adriamycin), vincristine, and bleomycin in any chemotherapy regimen.

#### Doxorubicin

Doxorubicin can cause immediate and cumulative dose-dependent cardiomyopathy. The lifetime maximum dose of doxorubicin is 450 mg/m² of body surface area. Toxic effects are dose related and are potentiated by radiation therapy of the mediastinum. If a patient has received doxorubicin at any time, a preoperative assessment for cardiac symptoms should be sought; if they are present, the patient should, at a minimum, be evaluated with echocardiography.

#### Vincristine

Vincristine can be neurotoxic; any neurologic defects should be documented preoperatively, especially before a regional technique is used.

#### Bleomycin

Bleomycin causes pulmonary fibrosis in 10% of patients who receive a full course of this drug (300 U). The extent of involvement can be followed with measurements of carbon monoxide–diffusing capacity. Because the severity of fibrosis can possibly be potentiated by the administration of oxygen ($O_2$-enriched gases), any patient with a decreased carbon monoxide diffusing capacity should not receive >30% of inspired $O_2$, if possible.

#### Metastatic Disease

Tumors metastatic to bone commonly have associated pulmonary involvement; conversely, the lungs are the most common site of metastatic primary sarcomas. Therefore, bone cancer patients require a preoperative chest radiograph that can be used to search for pulmonary metastases and malignant pleural effusions.

### Which Procedures Have a Potential for Massive Blood Loss?

#### Large Resections

The most common orthopedic oncology procedures that result in large volumes of blood loss are large bone tumor resections in the spine, pelvis, sacrum, proximal femur, and shoulder girdle (see Table 67–2). Surgery in these areas precludes use of a tourniquet, and control of bleeding may be difficult. Sacral tumor resections are renowned for massive blood loss. The rich sacral venous plexus is often violated, and blood loss is difficult to control. Entire blood volume losses are not uncommon.

In cases in which the tumor is in such a location that a tourniquet can be used, resection is usually done with the tourniquet inflated. Blood loss in these cases follows deflation of the tourniquet during the complex bone reconstruction. Often, the blood loss is a slow ooze that is difficult to quantify but can exceed 1000 mL.

## Biopsies

Biopsies of musculoskeletal tumors sometimes result in massive blood loss. Sacral tumors, metastatic renal cell carcinoma, and some other primary bone tumors may result in blood loss of >1 L from a small biopsy incision. After tissue is obtained, bleeding from the biopsy site can be controlled by packing the bone defect with bone cement.

Preoperative communication between the anesthesiologist and the surgeon about the procedure, the positioning, and the potential for blood loss is essential to anticipate each patient's needs. Venous access must be established at the beginning of these procedures because the blood loss that occurs frequently is fast and furious.

## SCOLIOSIS

Surgical correction of scoliosis is considered in patients with spinal curves that exceed 45° or those patients with smaller curves that have been observed to progress on sequential radiographs. Other indications include trunk deformity, pain, decreasing cardiopulmonary status, familial history of severe scoliosis, and loss of function. Risk factors for spinal cord injury during repair of kyphoscoliosis include severe deformity, congenital scoliosis, kyphosis, neurofibromatosis, and prior neurologic deficit.[39]

### Does the Underlying Cause of Scoliosis Have Anesthetic Implications?

Idiopathic scoliosis accounts for approximately 70% of all cases. Patients are most commonly adolescent girls who have no other systemic diseases. Congenital scoliosis can result from vertebral anomalies (eg, spina bifida) and may be associated with neurologic deficits. These patients commonly have tethered spinal cords, which increase the risk of neurologic damage and paraplegia during corrective surgery.[40] In addition, a high incidence of cardiovascular, gastrointestinal, and urologic anomalies is associated with congenital scoliosis (VATER syndrome [*v*ertebral defects, imperforate *a*nus, *tr*acheo*e*sophageal fistula, and *r*adial and *r*enal dysplasia]).

Neuromuscular scoliosis can be classified as neuropathic or myopathic. With the eradication of polio, neuropathic scoliosis is most commonly the result of cerebral palsy. The muscular dystrophies are the cause of most myopathic scoliosis. Curvature worsens as muscular weakness progresses. Respiratory impairment from muscular weakness can be a significant problem for these patients postoperatively; thus, screening pulmonary function tests are essential.[41] Neurofibromatosis is another common cause of neuromuscular scoliosis. Anesthetic considerations associated with neurofibromatosis include paying strict attention to the possibility of airway neurofibromas.

### What Are the Respiratory Effects?

Patients with idiopathic scoliosis have a restrictive lung defect that is the result of rib cage deformity. This deformity impairs development of the number of vascular units per volume of lung.[42] The lungs, being compressed by the rib cage deformity, have reduced compliance and abnormal ventilation-perfusion characteristics. These create increases in the ratio of dead space–to–tidal volume and the alveolar-arterial $O_2$ partial pressure difference. Hypercapnia, arterial hypoxemia, and pulmonary hypertension often result. The severity of these derangements is directly related to the degree of curvature. The vital capacity is not severely impaired until the curve progresses to >60° (Fig. 67–3).

The rib cage abnormality in idiopathic scoliosis is usually not as severe as it is in patients with neuromuscular scoliosis, but the same mechanisms of respiratory impairment can be present. In addition, these patients have muscle weakness that impairs their ability to sigh and cough. Frequently, they have abnormal airway reflexes and are therefore prone to aspiration.

### Why Do Curves Greater Than 65° Need to Be Corrected?

If the spinal deformity is <65°, lung function can be considered normal.[43] Patients with greater curves should be thoroughly evaluated for pulmonary and cardiac dysfunction preoperatively. Surgical correction will not restore normal pulmonary function, but it will arrest further progression and preserve a patient's mobility.

### How Is Spinal Cord Function Monitored Intraoperatively?

#### Wake-Up Test

The *wake-up test*, as the name implies, involves discontinuation of the anesthetic and reversal of neuromuscular blockade after distraction of the spine. Patients are asked to move an arm to confirm cooperation; then, they are asked to move their legs to confirm motor function. The anesthetic is then readministered, and the operation is continued.

A narcotic-based anesthetic is most often administered because it can be reversed with a narcotic antagonist. An intravenous technique using propofol or an inhalation technique using isoflurane with nitrous oxide have also been used. Regardless of the technique, few patients have any recall of the test. If they are informed about the test preoperatively, emergence is smoother and usually more rapid. The major limitation of the wake-up test is that it only gives information at a single moment during the operation.

#### Somatosensory Evoked Potentials

Somatosensory evoked potentials (SSEPs) provide a continuous monitor of neural integrity. They are widely accepted as

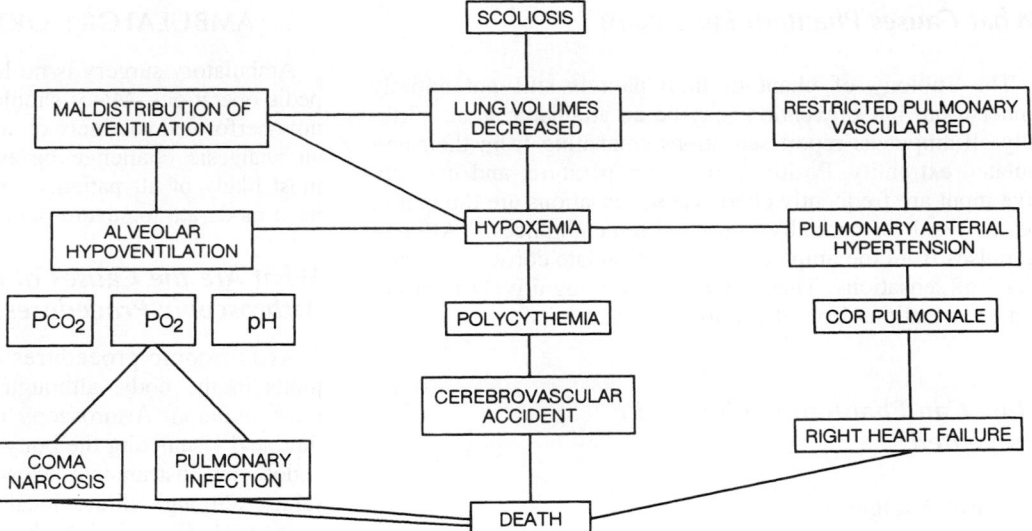

**FIGURE 67–3.** Pathophysiology of severe scoliosis. (Courtesy of Dr Henry Levison.)

the standard of care for any procedure in which spinal cord integrity might be compromised. SSEPs are gathered using electroencephalographic (EEG) monitoring during the presentation of a repetitive peripheral electrical stimulus. Neural impulses travel from the site of stimulus to the brain. Because these impulses are not discernible in the raw EEG data, the stimulus is repeated thousands of times. When these impulses are collated, random impulses in the raw EEG are canceled, and a distinctive series of waves emerges.

Baseline tracings are recorded for continuous comparison throughout the perioperative period. If a significant change in the *amplitude* (height) or *latency* (time from impulse to detection at the brain) from baseline occurs, neural integrity must be verified, and a wake-up test should be performed.

No *true false-negative results* (abnormal sensory function with no change in the SSEP observed) have occurred with properly conducted SSEP monitoring. This technique does not monitor motor function; however, in scoliosis surgery, SSEP changes correlate reliably with motor changes. *False-positive results* (normal sensory function with a significant change in SSEP) can occur for a variety of reasons. Abrupt changes in temperature, BP, and depth of anesthesia produce dramatic changes. Anesthetic techniques also influence the SSEP trace quality. A continuous infusion of narcotics complemented with low dose isoflurane and avoidance of nitrous oxide is the preferred technique to maximize the quality of SSEP monitoring during spine surgery.

### When Are Anterior Approaches to the Spine Used?

Anterior approaches are used when the anterior elements of the spine must be accessed for soft tissue release, tumor removal, bone grafting, or internal fixation. These approaches typically are used for severe forms of scoliosis, some cases of congenital scoliosis, spinal trauma, infection, tumors, or severe kyphotic deformities. Due to the proximity of the aorta, vena cava, and segmental vertebral vessels, large blood losses are possible during these procedures.

### What Is Important About Instrumentation for Spinal Surgery?

The range of instrumentation used in spinal surgery has grown over the past decade from a few simple rod and hook components to innumerable complex systems (eg, the Harrington, Cotrel-Dubousset, Scottish-Rite, and Luque systems). The system is not as important as the technique used for securing the hardware to the spinal column and the susceptibility of the spinal cord tissue to injury. Traction, compression, or direct trauma to the spinal cord can cause neural injury. When the instrumentation system is distracted or compressed, neural injury can occur. Following such cord manipulation, evaluation of neural function is critical.[44]

Sublaminar wires are used with a variety of instrumentation systems for rigid spinal fixation (eg, Luque rods, Cotrel-Dubousset, and, occasionally, Harrington rods). They require the passage of a wire beneath the lamina immediately adjacent to the neural elements, exposing the neural structures to the potential for direct injury. In up to 25% of cases in which sublaminar wires are used, slight changes in the monitored SSEP have been reported.[45,46]

Blindness resulting from ischemic optic neuropathy following spine surgery has been recognized as a more frequent complication than previously appreciated. Potential culprits cited were induced hypotension, decreased intraoperative hemoglobin, positioning, or some combination thereof. A survey conducted by the Scoliosis Research Society documented 37 cases of blindness following spine surgery.[47] In these cases, 92% were for complex instrumented fusions.

### AMPUTATIONS AND PHANTOM LIMB PAIN

Unfortunately, amputations are neither uncommon nor are they likely to become obsolete in the near future. The most common indications are ischemia, infection, trauma, and cancer. Frequently, these operations are the best option to restore a patient's mobility and function (provided that he or she will be free of pain).

## What Causes Phantom Limb Pain?

The etiology of phantom limb pain is still not entirely understood, but prevention may be an attainable goal. Virtually all amputees report sensations emanating from their amputated extremity. Position, touch, temperature, and nociceptive input are frequently cited. These sensations are thought to be the result of centrally imprinted remembrances.[48] Afferent impulses from the amputated nerve stimulate cortical "memories" of sensations. These memories are cognitively interpreted as sensations from the amputated extremity.

## How Can Phantom Limb Pain Be Prevented?

### Epidural Analgesia

In a study of 24 patients undergoing lower extremity amputation, epidural anesthesia with local anesthetic, narcotic, and clonidine decreased the incidence of phantom limb pain from 73% in controls to 8% in the study group at 1 year.[49] In another small study of 11 patients with painful extremities that required amputation, epidural analgesia was provided for 3 days preoperatively to render the extremity pain-free before amputation. Postoperative pain was managed with intravenous and oral narcotics. At the 12-month follow-up examination, none of these patients developed phantom limb pain. In the control group of 15 patients whose preoperative pain was controlled with intravenous and oral narcotics only, a 27% incidence of phantom pain was present at 1 year.[50] Together, these small studies imply that the use of epidural anesthesia preoperatively—to control or eradicate pain—may decrease the incidence of phantom limb pain after amputation.

### Local Anesthetic Bathing

Another technique for providing analgesia following amputation is infusion of local anesthetics through catheters placed intraoperatively directly along the nerve sheaths. The technique is relatively simple and easily managed. Six reports have been published about this technique.[51–56] Favorable results from four of these studies suggest a reduction in postoperative narcotic requirements and a decrease in the incidence of phantom limb pain. Two of the studies found no significant differences from control groups. A major difference between the positive and negative studies is the volume of local anesthetic used (Table 67–3).

**TABLE 67–3.** Results of Continuous Local Anesthetic Perfusion of Amputated Nerves

| | Nerve Sheath Catheters | | |
|---|---|---|---|
| | Bupivacaine Dosage | Narcotic Sparing Effect | Inhibition of Phantom Limb Pain |
| Malawar et al[52] | NS | + | + |
| Fisher and Meller[51] | 25 mg/h | + | + |
| Elizaga et al[53] | 7.8 mg/h | − | − |
| Pinzur et al[55] | 5 mg/h | − | − |
| Enneking et al[56] | 15 mg/h | + | + |

## AMBULATORY ORTHOPEDIC SURGERY

Ambulatory surgery is no longer used just for minor orthopedic operations. Major shoulder and knee reconstructions are now performed routinely on an outpatient basis. This presents an analgesic challenge because orthopedic patients are the most likely of all patients undergoing ambulatory surgery to have moderate to severe pain postoperatively.[57]

## What Are the Causes of Pain During Arthroscopic Procedures?

Arthroscopic procedures are performed on virtually all joints in the body, although knee arthroscopy remains the most common. Arthroscopy involves distending a joint with fluid and visualizing the bony and ligamentous structures with endoscopic instruments. Most commonly, the fluid is normal saline, although dilute local anesthetic solutions have also been used. Pain during the procedure usually results from distention of the capsule that surrounds the joint and during the introduction of instruments through the capsule. Irrigant is infused to keep the joint distended and to wash away blood and debris. Again, the irrigant can be saline or dilute local anesthetic. If local anesthetic is used as the distending fluid, most knee arthroscopies can be done with minimal analgesics.[58] This technique has also been described for ankle arthroscopy but is not commonly employed for other procedures yet.

At the conclusion of most arthroscopic procedures, local anesthetic is injected intraarticularly for postoperative pain relief. This practice has recently been examined in a systematic review of double-blind, randomized, controlled trials.[59] The review concludes that a small improvement in postknee arthroscopy pain scores, which is short lived, can be demonstrated following intraarticular instillation of bupivacaine. This effect is probably dose dependent because the positive studies correlated with higher mean bupivacaine doses.

The use of intraarticular narcotics is even more controversial than use of intraarticular local anesthetics. There is clear animal data to suggest that intraarticular injection of narcotics does suppress pain in a model of induced inflammation.[60] Clinically, the degree of synovial inflammation may be an important factor in response to intraarticular narcotic injection.

### Intraarticular Local Anesthetic Techniques

Intraarticular injection of local anesthetic has become a popular method of providing anesthesia for knee arthroscopy in busy ambulatory practices. The portal sites are injected superficially and a local anesthetic is injected intraarticularly. The technique works best if the intraarticular injection is performed 20 to 30 minutes preoperatively. Supplemental intravenous sedation is often required intraoperatively during the insertion of the trocars through the capsule. This technique requires an able surgeon and willing patient; with that combination, it is extraordinarily successful.[58]

## What Can You Do to Improve Arthroscopic Visualization?

Bleeding from synovial vessels can obscure the arthroscopic surgical field. There are four options to improve visualization:

1. A tourniquet can be inflated for all procedures except shoulder arthroscopy.

2. If tourniquet inflation is not an option, the inflow pressure of irrigant can be increased. This will lead to greater extravasation of irrigant into the surrounding tissues.
3. Many surgeons will request a reduction in the systolic BP to <100 mm Hg. There have been no formal studies correlating systolic BP with improved visualization during shoulder arthroscopy.
4. The addition of epinephrine to the irrigant solution (1 mg epinephrine to each 3-L bag) is also an option. This must be done before the initiation of the bleeding or the epinephrine may increase the patient's BP as it is systemically absorbed.

None of these techniques have been formally compared, but the options should be discussed with the surgeon.

## Monitoring

In the beach-chair or semirecumbent position, air embolism is a theoretic risk because the operative field is above the heart. Two cases of air embolism during shoulder arthroscopy have been reported.[61,62] However, in one case, air was injected to distend the joint before irrigant administration. Monitoring of end-tidal $CO_2$ is probably sufficient to provide data in the event of this unlikely occurrence.

Electrocardiographic leads require unique placement during shoulder arthroscopy. The arm lead for the operative side should be placed medial to the scapula on that side so that it is out of the surgical field. If the patient is at risk for ischemia, a $V_5$ or $V_4$ lead is readily preserved. If BP is to be measured noninvasively, the lower extremity should be used so as not to interfere with pulse oximetry monitoring and vascular access. However, one should remember to compensate for the hydrostatic effect of measuring BP at a point significantly below the level of the head and the heart.

## Nerve Damage

The entire brachial plexus can be stretched during shoulder surgery if the upper extremity is not supported adequately. This complication can occur if the patient is pulled off the edge of the operating table to promote exposure of both sides of the shoulder. In addition, the axillary and radial nerves may be compressed during dissection of the shoulder. The incidence of brachial plexus injury during TSA has been reported to be as high as 4%.[32] During shoulder arthroscopy, cutaneous branches of the axillary nerve are particularly at risk with portal placement.[63]

## REGIONAL ANESTHESIA

By virtue of its concentration on the extremities, orthopedic surgery lends itself to the use of regional anesthetics. Whether a real advantage accrues with such techniques is a constant source of debate among anesthesiologists worldwide. Conflicting studies have attempted to distinguish a difference in outcome for orthopedic patients as a result of the anesthetic techniques employed. Only recently have rehabilitation strategies to exploit the improved pain management offered by continuous regional anesthesia been employed. Several studies have now shown improvement in rehabilitation with continuous peripheral nerve blocks compared with patient-controlled intravenous narcotics.[64–66] As a result, new emphasis and enthusiasm are being placed on refining techniques, drugs, and equipment.

## What Are the Important Factors in Upper Extremity Blocks?

As in real estate, the most important consideration is "location, location, location." After location, one must consider the potential complications as well as the unique advantages of each block.

### Intravenous Regional Techniques

Intravenous regional blocks of the upper extremity are technical "no-brainers" that require an intravenous catheter, an Esmarch bandage, and a tourniquet. This simplicity has allowed surgeons to perform these blocks in emergency department settings for years without much guidance from anesthesiologists. They have a reliable, rapid onset and are safe when used with the proper equipment and drugs. They are most effective for distal procedures of short duration.

A double-cuff tourniquet is most commonly used. However, if a single cuff is a better fit because of the shape of an arm, then that should be used. The tourniquet should be checked and calibrated before placement on the patient. Tourniquet failure is the most common cause of complications.

Many agents and additives have been used over the years. Lidocaine, prilocaine, and preservative-free chloroprocaine are the safest agents available because of their rapid clearance and low toxicity. Bupivacaine should not be used for an intravenous regional anesthetic because of potentially high levels with tourniquet release. In volunteers, ropivacaine caused fewer central nervous system side effects than lidocaine following tourniquet release.[67] The authors speculated that delayed washout of the ropivacaine, because of increased tissue binding, led to lower peak levels of ropivacaine compared to lidocaine. There are few reports of ropivacaine for intravenous regional anesthesia at this time.

Several studies have examined the role of additives in improving patient comfort with intravenous regional anesthesia. Clonidine in doses of 1 μg/kg improved intraoperative tourniquet tolerance and increased the length of time to first request for pain medication with minimal side effects.[68,69] Ketorolac has also been shown to extend the duration of pain relief following intravenous regional anesthesia with lidocaine when used in doses as small as 15 mg.[70]

### Brachial Plexus Blocks

Axillary and interscalene blocks are the most commonly used brachial plexus blocks. Both of these approaches are relatively simple to master, provide consistent blockade, and have few complications with appropriate patient selection.

#### Axillary

Axillary blocks are safe and have a low risk of complications. The incidence of postoperative paresthesias is no different with the transarterial approach than it is with the eliciting of paresthesias.[71] The highest reported success rate for axillary block has been with a transarterial approach and comes close to 99% in experienced hands. With a transarterial approach, one must be ever vigilant for signs and symptoms of local anesthetic toxicity because of the possibility of intravascular injection. The axillary artery is the most consistent landmark for the axillary approach to the brachial plexus. If the artery is not palpable, a Doppler or US probe can be used to direct the needle to the neurovascular bundle block. Because this block has relatively simple landmarks, it is often the easiest brachial plexus block to perform. With the use of large volumes of local anesthetic, 40 to 50 mL, adequate anesthesia above the elbow can be achieved with an axillary approach.[72] Supplementation with separate musculocutaneous and intercostal brachialis injections improves the success of this block in most patients.

### Interscalene

For shoulder surgery, an interscalene block is the only technique that predictably provides shoulder relaxation.[73] However, it does not reliably provide a complete sensory block of the hand and is a poor choice for hand surgery and particularly for any surgery that involves the sensory distribution of the ulnar nerve.

Complications of interscalene blocks are higher than with any other approach to the brachial plexus. Complications of interscalene blocks include vertebral artery and subarachnoid injection and the spread of the local anesthetic solution into the epidural space, which results in a high cervical epidural blockade. One should always also expect a phrenic nerve paralysis from blockade of C3, C4, and C5 fibers. Bilateral interscalene blocks should never be performed, and the performance of these blocks in patients with limited respiratory reserve should be carefully considered.

The interscalene block is unique in its ability to provide shoulder relaxation. Traditionally, a paresthesia below the elbow is required for reliable brachial plexus blockade. Roch and colleagues reported the use of shoulder paresthesia for patients who had an interscalene brachial plexus block for shoulder surgery.[73] In 45% of these patients, the initial elicited paresthesia was to the shoulder, whereas in 55% of patients, a paresthesia was distal to the shoulder. All of the patients developed a brachial plexus block adequate for shoulder surgery.

### Continuous Brachial Plexus Blocks

There are several approaches to the brachial plexus for continuous catheter placement including axillary, infraclavicular, interscalene, and intersternocleidomastoid (interSCM) techniques. In a study of analgesic techniques in patients undergoing major shoulder surgery, continuous interscalene blocks were compared with intravenous patient-controlled analgesics and found to decrease narcotic related side effects and improve rehabilitation scores.[64] Interestingly, patients in the continuous interscalene block group had a much higher satisfaction rating as well.

Consideration for continuous techniques includes the ease of catheter introduction, the reliable development of anesthesia, and the stability of the catheter once placed. In our experience, the interSCM approach has best met these criteria. This technique, described by Pham and associates,[74] uses the two heads of the sternocleidomastoid as landmarks. An insulated needle is directed at a 45° angle to the skin and stimulated. When the appropriate muscle twitch is achieved, a dose of local anesthetic is administered through the needle and then the catheter is introduced. The interSCM provides the rapid, reliable development of dense surgical anesthesia and can provide analgesia for the entire upper extremity depending on which trunk is stimulated.

### Continuous Local Anesthetic Infusions

Continuous infusions of local anesthetics through catheters placed in the wound or directly on nerve sheaths has been used to control postoperative pain with great success.[64–66,75–77] Significant reductions in postoperative narcotic use occurred in patients who required iliac bone graft harvesting. A continuous infusion of 0.25 bupivacaine at 5 mL/h was used to bathe the harvest site as long as a drain remained in place.[76]

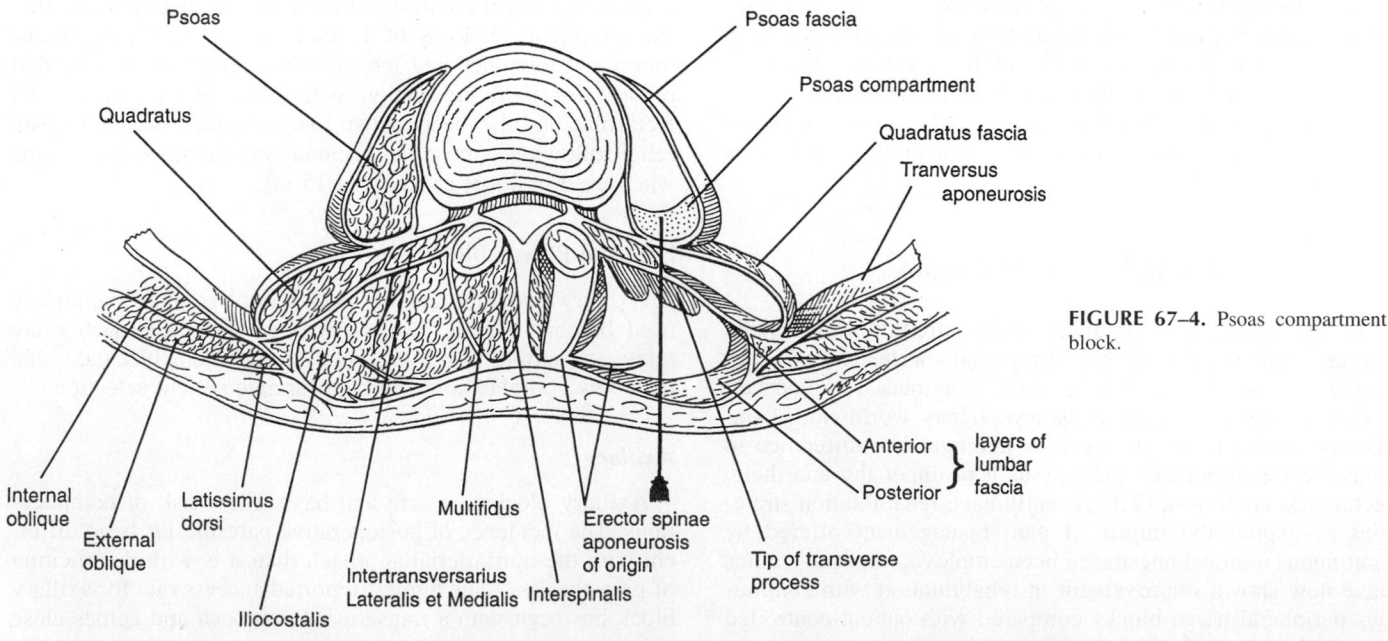

**FIGURE 67–4.** Psoas compartment block.

In our experience, we have found dilute solutions of local anesthetic, most commonly bupivacaine 0.125% to 0.25% or ropivacaine 0.2%, to provide excellent analgesia when infused at a small, constant rate with additional patient-controlled boluses available. The addition of the patient-controlled boluses allows a lower constant infusion rate to be used. Singelyn and Van der Elst found lower local anesthetic consumption, improved pain scores with motion, and higher patient satisfaction when patient-controlled lumbar plexus block was compared to continuous-rate lumbar plexus block after THA.[75]

Rawal and colleagues used the technique of wound perfusion to provide at-home analgesia for ambulatory surgery patients.[77] In this report of 60 patients, excellent analgesia was reported with no side effects or complications in a wide variety of patients including orthopedic patients. Continuous local anesthetic perfusion of peripheral nerves and wounds has been done on a limited basis in the United States and is currently under investigation.

## What Are the Important Considerations in Lower Extremity Blocks?

Many factors must be considered when choosing an appropriate lower extremity regional technique for anesthesia or extended analgesia. These factors include surgical incision site, patient's desired mobility, and anticoagulation status.

Subarachnoid block provides adequate anesthesia for all operations of the lower extremity. Epidural blockade, however, is occasionally inadequate for operations on the foot or ankle because of sacral sparing. This can be overcome with increased volume of local anesthetic and low siting (ie, L4-5 placement) of the catheter. Femoral sciatic block provides excellent anesthesia for procedures on the distal extremity but is associated with a higher rate of tourniquet pain than neuraxial techniques. Intravenous regional blocks in the lower extremity frequently are limited to foot and ankle surgery. Ankle blocks work well for anesthesia of the foot if placed 20 to 40 minutes before surgery and if an Esmarch tourniquet is used at the ankle. However, if a thigh tourniquet is used, pain from its application will rapidly make the patient uncomfortable. Sciatic nerve block at the popliteal fossae is an excellent choice for foot and ankle surgery; however, if surgery enters the territory of the saphenous nerve, the sciatic nerve block must be supplemented.

Postoperative mobility is important for rehabilitation following major lower extremity surgery and, hence, the popularity of epidural analgesia following major lower extremity orthopedic operations. Epidural analgesia has several common limitations: bilateral blockade, sympathetic blockade leading to orthostatic hypotension, and urinary retention. Potentially severe respiratory depression, the association of spinal hematoma with epidural analgesia, and the use of LMWH also limit its application (Table 67-4).

Because of these considerations, interest in the use of continuous lumbar plexus blockade is increasing. There are several approaches to the lumbar plexus, but we have found the psoas compartment block the easiest and most reliable technique for continuous catheter placement. Landmarks for this technique are the iliac crest and the L4 spinous process (Figs. 67-4 and 67-5). A mark 3-cm lateral and 5-cm caudal is made. A 6-inch stimulating needle is directed slightly medial

**TABLE 67-4.** Comparison of Techniques for Continuous Postoperative Pain

|  | Epidural | Peripheral Nerve Block |
|---|---|---|
| Unilateral blockade | No | Yes |
| Urinary retention | Yes | No |
| Respiratory monitoring requirement | Yes | No |
| Spinal hematoma risk with low molecular weight heparin | Yes | No |
| Technically difficult to place | No | No, lower extremity |
| Additional sedatives ad lib | No | Yes |

and cephalad until the L5 transverse process is struck. The needle is walked off the transverse process and introduced until a twitch is perceived in the quadriceps. A bolus of local anesthetic is administered, and a catheter is threaded into the potential space of the psoas compartment. This will provide anesthesia in the distribution of the lumbar plexus and that of the femoral, lateral femoral cutaneous, and obturator nerves. It will not block the gluteal nerves or the sciatic nerve. Thus, this block must be supplemented with additional nerve blocks or general anesthesia for many common lower extremity procedures. It does provide excellent analgesia for many of these procedures including THA and TKA and anterior cruciate ligament reconstruction.[65,66,75]

Orthopedic surgeons have a variety of anticoagulation strategies for postoperative patients including both pharmacologic and mechanical options.

The most common pharmacologic agents used following orthopedic surgery are warfarin and LMWH. Warfarin has

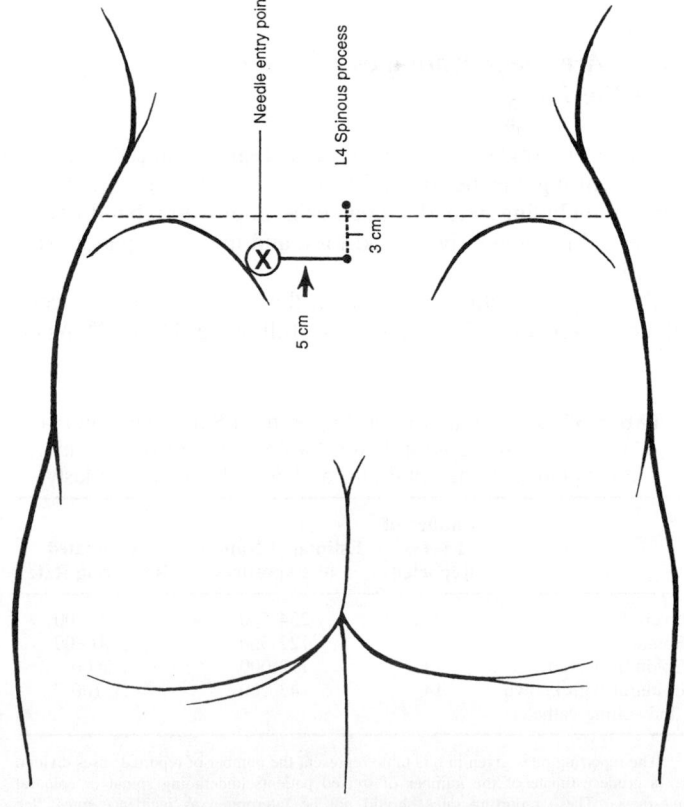

**FIGURE 67-5.** Psoas compartment block landmarks.

been used safely in conjunction with continuous epidural analgesia for many years. There are only two case reports of patients developing a spinal hematoma while receiving epidural analgesia and perioperative low dose warfarin prophylaxis.[78,79] In contrast, in the 5 years that LMWH was available before April 1998, approximately 40 reports of spinal hematoma associated with epidural analgesia and LMWH therapy were reported to the US Food and Drug Administration.[80] These numbers have led statisticians to estimate the risk of spinal hematoma in patients receiving LMWH and continuous epidural analgesia to be approximately 1 in 3100[80] (Table 67–5). This prompted the American Society for Regional Anesthesia and Pain Management to convene a consensus conference on regional anesthesia and anticoagulation. The conference recommendations have been published and can be used as a guide in the decision-making process regarding neuraxial anesthesia and analgesia in the presence of various anticoagulation therapies.[81–90]

### Does Regional Anesthesia Reduce Morbidity or Mortality for Hip Fractures?

McKenzie and associates reported on mortality at 2 weeks following hip fracture repair in a comparison of spinal and general anesthesia. Patients in the spinal group had a mortality of 5% compared with 15% for those who received general anesthesia.[91] However, at 2 months, the cumulative mortality in each group reportedly was the same. Sorenson and Pace combined 13 studies that compared regional anesthesia with general anesthesia for surgical repair of femoral neck fractures.[92] With a database that included 2000 patients, they found the difference in mortality to be insignificant (2.7% less following regional anesthesia).

### What Are the Advantages of Regional Anesthesia?

There are several advantages that regional anesthesia can confer during the perioperative period following orthopedic surgery including extended analgesia, improved rehabilitation, decreased intraoperative blood loss, and improved patient satisfaction.

Recently, two studies examined the role of analgesic technique on rehabilitation parameters following TKA.[65,66] When

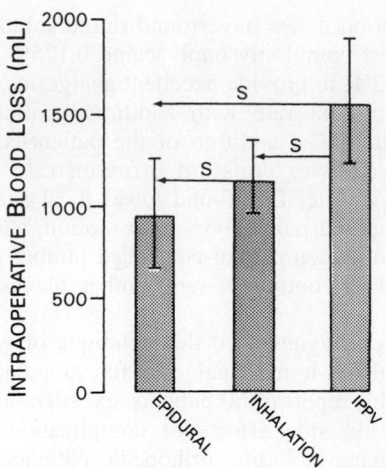

**FIGURE 67–6.** Intraoperative blood loss during total hip arthroplasty. Epidural, spontaneous ventilation without intubation; inhalation, general endotracheal anesthesia (GETA) with spontaneous ventilation; IPPV, GETA with controlled intermittent positive-pressure ventilation; S, significant difference. (From Modig J. Regional anesthesia and blood loss. *Acta Anaesthesiol Scand.* 1988;32:45.)

compared with intravenous PCA narcotic therapy, both continuous epidural and continuous lumbar plexus block were found to provide equivalent and superior outcome scores including percentage of physical therapy goals achieved, degree of knee flexion immediately and during late follow-up, and decreased hospital stays.

Modig showed a clear reduction in blood loss during total hip replacement procedures performed under epidural anesthesia compared with those performed under general anesthesia.[93] This difference extends into the postoperative period and should be considered a real advantage (Fig. 67–6). The mechanism is thought to be related to decreases in venous pressures. Allowing the patient to ventilate spontaneously reduces transmitted thoracic pressure caused by positive-pressure ventilation. This effect, coupled with reduced venous tone from the sympathectomy, makes a difference in the amount of oozing that occurs from open bone interstices.

Patient satisfaction is one of the more important patient outcomes. Continuous peripheral nerve blocks have been shown to have higher patient satisfaction ratings when compared with intravenous narcotic therapy in several studies for both upper and lower extremity surgery.[64,65,75] The satisfaction seems to be related to the ability to participate in physical therapy with greater facility.

## BLOOD LOSS

The unique anatomy of bone, which is characterized by movement of the blood supply through solid interstices, often impairs hemostasis during operative procedures. No vessels can be ligated on raw bone surfaces. Bone wax is effective at plugging bleeding surfaces, but it inhibits bone union and therefore is infrequently used by orthopedic surgeons. Thus, patients undergoing orthopedic surgery are predisposed to continuous blood loss intraoperatively and often into the postoperative period. Any mechanism to decrease the mass of red blood cell loss intraoperatively should be aggressively pursued.

**TABLE 67–5.** Estimated Reporting Rate of Spinal Hematoma After Spinal and Epidural Anesthesia With Enoxaparin in Patients Undergoing Total Hip and Total Knee Arthroplasty

| | Number of Events Reported | Estimated Number of Exposures | Estimated Reporting Rate* |
|---|---|---|---|
| Overall | 22 | 234 500 | 1:10 700 |
| Spinal | 3 | 122 500 | 1:40 800 |
| Epidural overall | 17 | 112 000 | 1:6600 |
| Epidural with known indwelling catheter | 14 | 43 200 | 1:3100 |

*The reporting rates given in this table represent the number of reported cases divided by a crude estimate of the number of treated patients undergoing spinal or epidural anesthesia. These reporting rates should not be interpreted as incidence rates. See reference 80 for more details.

## What Measures Should Be Taken Preoperatively for Projected Blood Loss?

### Preoperative Autologous Blood Donation

Preoperative autologous blood donation is the gold standard for blood conservation in most orthopedic practices. For procedures associated with predictable large estimated blood losses, preoperative autologous blood donation lowers homologous blood transfusions. Erythropoietin therapy can facilitate the donation of blood preoperatively.[94,95] This effect is particularly useful in female patients.[95]

### Hemodilution

Intraoperative hemodilution should be considered for patients who arrive in the OR with a hemoglobin level of 12 g/dL or greater and in whom the blood loss can be projected to be at least 1 L. Acute normovolemic hemodilution (ANH) is an excellent alternative to preoperative autologous blood donation for orthopedic surgery.[96–98] The cost of ANH is substantially less than preoperative autologous blood donation, there is no room for clerical errors in its administration, and ANH is equivalent to preoperative autologous blood donation in terms of reduction in homologous blood requirements.[99] It can also be used in conjunction with autologous blood donation. In a study of ANH in conjunction with autologous blood donation and intraoperative blood scavenging, Oisha and colleagues[100] found a lower mean autologous blood transfusion requirement when compared with a control group without ANH.

### Blood Salvage

Blood salvaging devices have been used for many years with great success. Few contraindications to the reinfusion of wasted scavenged blood exist (among them are sickled red blood cells, active infection, and cancerous contamination). These devices are cost effective for procedures in which the blood loss can be predicted to be >500 mL.

## How Can Intraoperative Blood Loss Be Decreased?

### Induced Hypotension

Hypotensive anesthesia decreases blood loss in hip replacement surgery, spinal surgery, and orthognathic surgery.[96–98] Hypotension has been accomplished with a variety of agents and techniques, including the use of sodium nitroprusside, trimethaphan, deep inhalation anesthesia, and regional anesthesia.

Because most blood loss during orthopedic procedures comes from continual bone oozing, any technique that decreases peripheral venous pressure might be expected to decrease intraoperative blood loss (Fig. 67–7). A direct correlation exists between peripheral venous pressure measured in the wound and intraoperative blood loss.[93] Therefore, spontaneous ventilation, regional anesthesia, and vasodilator-induced hypotension with a drug such as nitroglycerin should decrease intraoperative blood loss.

Another benefit of induced hypotension is the vast improve-

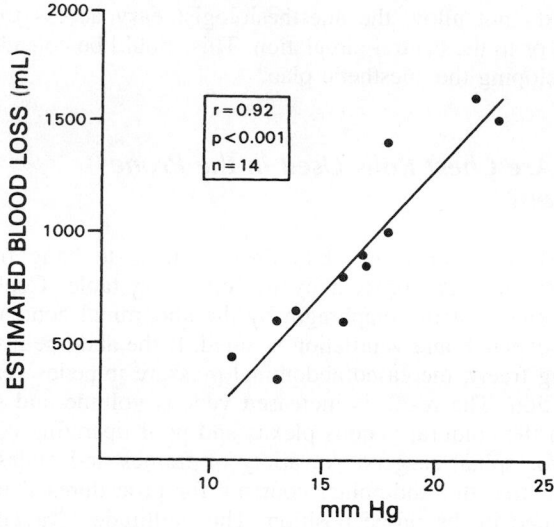

**FIGURE 67–7.** Relationship between mean venous pressure and intraoperative blood loss during total hip arthroplasty. (From Modig J. Regional anesthesia and blood loss. *Acta Anaesthesiol Scand.* 1988;32:46.)

ment it brings about in the quality of the operating field. Even modest reductions in mean arterial pressure provide a clearer, drier operating field. Lessard and associates documented this improvement using a 5-point scale to rate the quality of the operative field (Fig. 67–8) during induced hypotension.[98]

Factors that should be considered before induced hypotension include severe systemic hypertension, severe coronary artery disease, and history of cerebrovascular accident. There is concern that induced hypotension may be a factor in the development of postoperative cortical blindness following complex spinal surgery.[47] This association is of concern and should be discussed with your surgical colleagues.

## POSITIONING

The most important goals of positioning for any operation are patient safety and optimal surgical conditions. In order to meet these goals during orthopedic procedures, the desired positioning should be discussed preoperatively. Many of the positions commonly used (prone, lateral decubitus, and beach-

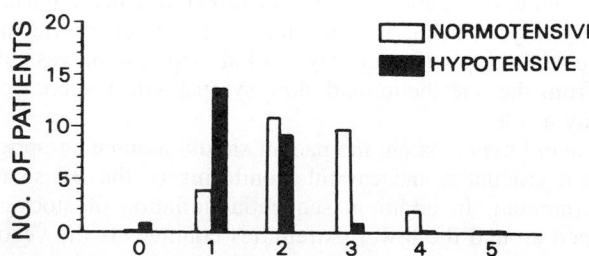

**FIGURE 67–8.** Quality of surgical field in normotensive and hypotensive conditions. 0, No bleeding, virtually bloodless field; 1, bleeding so mild that it is not a surgical nuisance; 2, moderate bleeding that is a nuisance but that does not interfere with accurate dissection; 3, moderate bleeding that moderately compromises surgical dissection; 4, heavy but controllable bleeding that significantly interferes with dissection; 5, massive uncontrollable bleeding. (Graph from Lessard MR, Trepanier CA, Baribault JP, et al. Isoflurane-induced hypotension in orthognathic surgery. *Anesth Analg.* 1989;69:379. Scale from Fromme GA, MacKenzie RA, Gould AB, et al. Controlled hypotension for orthognathic surgery. *Anesth Analg.* 1986;42:356.)

chair) do not allow the anesthesiologist easy access to the airway or to the central circulation. This should be considered in developing the anesthetic plan.

### Why Are Chest Rolls Used in the Prone Position?

Chest rolls allow the abdominal contents to hang freely without being compressed by the operating table. Cephalic displacement of the diaphragm by the abdominal contents is thus prevented, and ventilation is aided. If the abdomen is not hanging freely, increased abdominal pressure impedes venous circulation. The result is increased venous volume and pressure in the epidural venous plexus and poor operating conditions for spinal surgery. A variety of frames and tables are used to free the abdominal contents for procedures that are performed in the prone position. The multitude of available devices attests to the difficulty associated with achieving the ideal prone position.

### What Is the Correct Position for Longitudinal Chest Rolls?

The cephalad end of longitudinal chest rolls should extend to just below the clavicle so that they avoid clavicular impingement on the brachial plexus. The breasts should be directed medially, if possible; they should not be brought out laterally. Nipples should not be compressed by the chest rolls. The abdomen should hang freely between the rolls, which should extend to the iliac crests. Male genitalia should be in a neutral position and free of compression. The knees should be padded and the feet supported by pillows. The arms should be carefully padded and tucked or abducted, but not by >90° from the sides and anterior to the plane of the thorax.

### What Are Important Considerations When Using the Beach-Chair Position?

When using the upright, semirecumbent, beach-chair position, several important considerations must be kept in mind. As the patient is changing position from supine to partially seated and upright, attention must be directed to hemodynamic stability. Hypotension is frequently encountered during this maneuver.[98] Hypovolemia, myocardial depression, vasodilation from the anesthetic, and slow sympathetic response can all play a role.[101]

To avoid hypotension, the patient should assume an upright position gradually, and careful monitoring of the BP should be paramount. In addition, sequential inflation of stockings wrapped around the lower extremities counteracts the venous pooling that occurs when the patient is in this position.

If the anesthetic plan calls for intubation, the endotracheal tube should be secured on the side opposite the operative site. The head must be firmly secured to the frame of the bed in a forward-facing direction. This prevents the head from turning opposite to the surgical field and stretching the brachial plexus. It also helps to prevent accidental extubation during exuberant surgical manipulation of the extremity.

### What Are Potential Complications of the Lateral Decubitus Position?

Careful attention must be directed toward the dependent extremities when the patient is positioned in the lateral decubitus position. Compression of the neurovascular bundle in the axilla can occur if a chest roll does not support the weight of the torso. This problem may result in nerve palsies, compartment syndromes, or both.

Complications in the dependent leg during hip surgery performed in the lateral decubitus position rarely occur. Lachiewicz and Latimer reported six cases of swelling of the gluteal muscle compartments, rhabdomyolysis, myoglobinuria, and sciatic nerve palsy.[102] Risk factors for these complications included obesity, prolonged operating time, and lateral decubitus position. Complications ranging from nerve palsies to ischemia of the dependent leg that resulted in acute renal failure and death have been reported during THA.[103] Careful padding and gentle flexion of the hip, buttocks, and knee of the dependent extremity also can minimize these problems. Figure 67–9 demonstrates the correct placement of the buttock support for the lateral decubitus position.

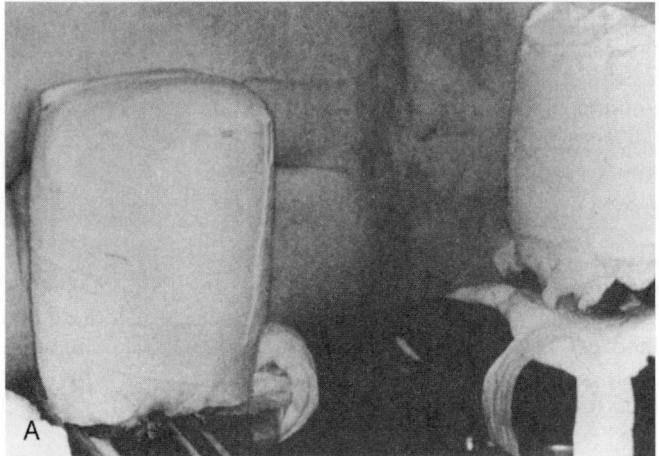

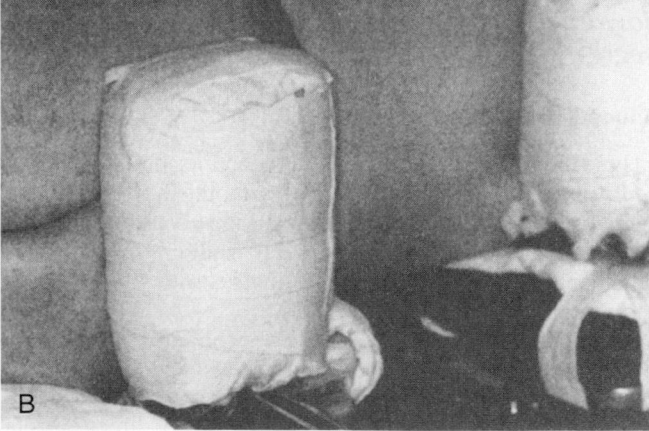

**FIGURE 67–9.** Placement of buttock supports for the lateral decubitus position. *A*, Incorrect placement of the posterior pad on the gluteal muscles can cause gluteal crush injury. *B*, Correct placement of the posterior pad on the sacrum frees the gluteal muscles. (From Lachiewicz PF, Latimer HA. Rhabdomyolysis following total hip arthroplasty. *J Bone Joint Surg [Br]*. 1991;73:578.)

# TOURNIQUETS

Tourniquets are frequently applied during extremity surgery to limit blood loss, to provide a bloodless surgical field, and to perform intravenous regional blockade. Anesthesiologists and surgeons are jointly responsible for their proper application and use in the OR.

## What Are the Potential Complications?

Neural damage, muscle necrosis, arterial thrombosis, DVT, and skin injury are reported complications of tourniquet use. The incidence of complications is low when properly calibrated equipment is used and a schedule of inflation-deflation times is followed. In 21 of 25 cases in which the tourniquet was checked after a tourniquet-induced injury occurred, patients had been exposed to excessive pressure caused by tourniquet malfunction.[95] Proper tourniquet calibration should be verified before each use.

### Nerve Damage

Nerve damage is the result of direct axonal compression of the nerve, usually at the edge of the cuff. Excessive cuff pressure appears to be the major factor leading to nerve injury, with duration of application as a secondary influence.[104] Symptoms of tourniquet-induced nerve injury range from transient mild paresthesias to permanent paralysis of the nerves involved. The radial nerve is most frequently involved in tourniquet-induced palsies. Being located adjacent to the humerus allows it to be easily compressed against the bone by the tourniquet. Lower extremity nerve injuries are much less common because their greater muscle mass protects the nerves and because in the lower extremity, the peroneal nerve is the only nerve located close to a bone.

### Muscle Damage

Muscle damage from tourniquet-induced ischemia is less dramatic than nerve damage in its presentation but probably occurs with greater frequency. Saunders and associates reported on 48 patients who underwent knee surgery with the use of a thigh tourniquet. Eighty-five percent of the patients with thigh tourniquets inflated for 60 minutes or longer demonstrated abnormal electromyographic data and muscle weakness. The incidence of abnormal electromyograms in this study directly correlated with the length of tourniquet inflation (Table 67–6). In all patients, the electromyographic abnormali-

**TABLE 67–6.** Effect of Tourniquet Time on Quadriceps Function After Knee Arthroscopy*

| No. of Patients | Tourniquet Time (min) | Abnormal Electromyogram No. (%) |
| --- | --- | --- |
| 13 | ≥60 | 11 (85) |
| 14 | 30–60 | 10 (71) |
| 12 | 15–30 | 7 (58) |
| 9 | <15 | 2 (22) |

*Tourniquet inflation may cause significant electromyographic abnormalities postoperatively.

From Saunders KC, Louis DL, Weingarden SI, et al. Effect on tourniquet time on postoperative quadriceps function. *Clin Orthop.* 1979;143:194.

ties resolved over varying amounts of time up to 5 months postoperatively.[105]

Edema associated with reperfusion hyperemia develops immediately on tourniquet deflation. Tissue edema, pallor, stiffness, weakness without paralysis, and subjective numbness of the extremity characterize the post-tourniquet syndrome. This syndrome is probably the result of the edema compressing on the vessels, joint capsules, and nerve endings. The symptoms usually resolve within a week of the insult, although the edema may take longer to disappear.

## What Is the Optimal Tourniquet Inflation and Release Scheme?

Sapega and colleagues performed histologic canine muscle studies following a variety of inflation-deflation schemes.[106] They demonstrated a direct relationship between the time of continuous tourniquet inflation and the extent of muscle damage. By limiting the initial period of ischemia to 90 minutes, they found that recovery before reinflation of the tourniquet could be achieved in 5 minutes.[107] Thus, for procedures likely to exceed 2 hours, surgeons should be encouraged to deflate the tourniquet after 90 minutes to allow a 5-minute reperfusion period.

## Why Are Surgeons Reluctant to Deflate a Tourniquet Intraoperatively?

Edema formation begins immediately when the tourniquet is deflated. Visualization of anatomic structures is often difficult after even short periods of tourniquet inflation, not because blood is present in the field but because edema occludes the structures. If the tourniquet is released after the application of dressings and splinting devices, many surgeons believe the amount of edema formation is reduced. In addition, they believe that blood loss is decreased if a pressure dressing is applied before tourniquet release. Therefore, if an entire procedure is anticipated to be accomplished in <150 minutes, most surgeons prefer not to deflate the tourniquet for reperfusion.

In defense of this practice, data from human studies have demonstrated that the rate of metabolite accumulation and high-energy phosphate depletion decreased with increasing tourniquet time.[107] This is thought to be the result of decreased metabolic needs that occur with cooling of the unperfused extremity. However, surgeons should be informed (which should be charted) of the amount of ischemic time that has elapsed at hourly intervals for the first 2 hours, again at 2.5 hours, and at 15-minute intervals thereafter.

## What Is the Optimal Tourniquet Pressure?

Tourniquet inflation pressure frequently is chosen arbitrarily to be 250 mm Hg for the upper extremities and 350 mm Hg for the lower extremities. These values may be satisfactory for normally shaped extremities in nonhypertensive patients who require short periods of tourniquet inflation. In patients requiring long tourniquet inflation times, in hypertensive patients, and in extremely thin or obese patients, a more scientific approach should be used.

The inflation pressure required to eliminate the pulse detected by a US Doppler flow meter can be determined before tourniquet inflation. For upper extremity operations, 50 mm Hg should be added to the Doppler occlusion pressure; for lower extremity operations, 75 mm Hg should be added. Using this scheme, Reid and coworkers achieved adequate hemostasis in a series of 84 patients with tourniquet inflation pressures of 135 to 255 mm Hg for the upper extremities and 175 to 305 mm Hg for the lower extremities.[108]

The width of the tourniquet is another important factor to consider in choosing a tourniquet inflation pressure. Standard 8.5-cm pneumatic tourniquets exert the highest pressure at the midcuff subcutaneous level. The pressure diminishes at deeper tissue planes and toward the cuff edges. Moore and colleagues demonstrated Doppler occlusion pressures that were lower than systolic BPs using a tourniquet 15-cm in width. They theorized that "an accumulation of frictional resistance along the compressed length" of the cuff accounted for the subsystolic pressures required to stop detectable flow.[109] Perhaps 15-cm cuffs should always be used when possible.

## What Causes Bleeding Distal to an Inflated Tourniquet?

Inadequate extremity exsanguination is the most common cause of bleeding distal to a tourniquet. This problem requires release of the tourniquet and re-exsanguination of the extremity. During an intravenous regional anesthetic case, this approach is unacceptable. Thus, one must be meticulous in exsanguination during preparation for this block.

Insufficient hemostasis from inadequate inflation pressure is most likely to occur in hypertensive patients. Wide swings in BP may allow arterial breakthrough, a fact that should be considered when choosing an inflation pressure for hypertensive patients. Arterial breakthrough can be treated by increasing the tourniquet inflation pressure, as long as the extremity does not require re-exsanguination.

Tourniquet "ooze" is due to the entry of blood into the bone medulla through nutrient arteries proximal to the tourniquet. This problem cannot be treated by increasing the tourniquet inflation pressure.[104]

## What Is Tourniquet Pain?

### Characteristics

Tourniquet pain is an ill-defined, dull, aching pain as described by patients who undergo operations that require tourniquet inflation. It usually occurs 45 to 60 minutes after inflation of the tourniquet, even when otherwise adequate surgical levels of general and regional anesthesia are provided. During general anesthesia, it is manifested by hypertension, which has been reported to occur in as many as 66% of patients. During regional anesthesia, the patient may complain of an annoying ache that is accompanied by restlessness and agitation.[110] In either case, release of the tourniquet provides instant relief. With reinflation, the pain usually occurs after a shorter interval than it did initially.

### Cause

The pathologic basis of tourniquet pain is not entirely understood. Because unmyelinated C fibers transmit impulses associated with dull, persistent, poorly localized pain, it is these fibers that are probably responsible.[111–113] In an in vitro model, Gissen and coworkers showed that C fibers are more resistant to local anesthetic-induced conduction blockade than are the larger A fibers.[112] In addition, they found that as tetracaine concentrations decreased, C fiber action potential amplitudes returned to normal levels, whereas A fiber action potentials were still suppressed. Bupivacaine did not exhibit this differential effect to the same extent.

This theory of tourniquet pain is well supported by the findings of Concepcion and associates, who reported significantly less tourniquet pain in patients anesthetized with intrathecal bupivacaine than in those given tetracaine for lower extremity procedures, despite the presence of longer tourniquet times in the bupivacaine group.[111]

## What Physiologic Effects Occur With Tourniquet Deflation?

Following deflation of a lower extremity tourniquet, the most obvious clinical effects are hypotension, a transient increase in end-tidal carbon dioxide tension, and a small decrease in patient temperature. These changes can also be seen with deflation of upper extremity tourniquets, but the degree of change usually is not as significant. Presumably, postischemic reactive hyperemia induced by tissue anoxia and reperfusion of a cooled extremity are responsible.

The exact mediators of postischemic reactive hyperemia have not been identified, but clinicians frequently refer to them as "evil humors." Leading candidates are bradykinin, lactate, adenosine, and inorganic phosphate. After tourniquet deflation, increased blood flow to the extremity rapidly washes out the products of anaerobic metabolism. End-tidal carbon dioxide may increase as much as 18 mm Hg during this washout phase.[114]

Transient temperature decreases of as much as 1.5°C may be seen at this time. Significant convective heat loss can occur in the unperfused extremity during prolonged tourniquet inflation. The vasodilation associated with postischemic reactive hyperemia make it difficult to regain the pretourniquet deflation temperature.

Hypotension frequently occurs in the immediate postdeflation period and probably has a variety of causes. Central blood volume is acutely decreased as blood returns to the postischemic vasodilated extremity. This factor, coupled with the dramatic relief of tourniquet pain, may result in transient moderate systolic hypotension. Adequate volume replacement before tourniquet deflation attenuates this effect.

# SPLINTING

## Why Is the Timing of the Wake-Up Important in Orthopedic Cases?

Orthopedic cases that involve reduction and fixation of fractures, ligament repair, or other fixation of anatomic structures require postoperative immobilization for adequate healing. The first step in postoperative immobilization is the application of a splint that provides rigid immobilization and accommodates postoperative swelling. In such cases, the patient must remain immobile. Splints using plaster of Paris require roughly 10 minutes to become rigid following application. Premature cessation of the anesthetic can have dire consequences, including loss of fracture reduction or failure of the repair. Some splints are placed for patient comfort and do not require patient immobility during application. Querying the surgeon as to the appropriate time for patient wake-up is appreciated and recommended.

### What Are the Dangers Associated With Plaster Splints?

Plaster of Paris splinting material hardens with an exothermic chemical reaction. Burns can result from this reaction. Adequate ventilation of the plaster material is important to prevent excessive heat accumulation. The splint should not be covered with blankets or be in contact with plastic-covered pillows during the exothermic phase (in the operative setting, this phase usually lasts until after the patient reaches the postanesthesia care unit).

## CONCLUSION

Orthopedic surgery and orthopedic anesthesia continue to evolve and innovate. There are several foreseeable trends. The use of LMWHs will continue to expand. As anesthesiologists, we must acknowledge this fact and develop schemes for anesthesia and analgesia that accommodate this evolving practice. The trend toward more complicated surgeries being performed on an outpatient basis will continue to grow. Again, we must expand our role as perioperative physicians to become outpatient "analgesiologists" and patient advocates. As the data accumulate in regard to improved rehabilitation scores in the presence of continuous peripheral nerve blockade, we must expand our knowledge base of these techniques both on a clinical and basic science level. These are but some of the challenges that await us.

### References

1. Geerts WH, Code KI, Jay RM, et al. A prospective study of venous thromboembolism after major trauma. *N Engl J Med.* 1994;331:1601.
2. Collins R, Scrimgeour A, Yusef S, et al. Reduction in fatal pulmonary embolism and venous thrombosis by perioperative administration of subcutaneous heparin. *N Engl J Med.* 1988;318:1162.
3. Kaempffe FA, Lifeso RM, Meinking C. Intermittent pneumatic compression versus Coumadin: prevention of deep venous thrombosis in lower extremity total joint arthroplasty. *Clin Orthop.* 1991;269:89.
4. Hull RD, Raskob GE, Gent M, et al. Effectiveness of intermittent pneumatic leg compression for preventing deep vein thrombosis after total hip replacement. *JAMA.* 1990;263:2313.
5. Imperiale TF, Speroff T. A meta-analysis of methods to prevent venous thromboembolism following total hip replacement. *JAMA.* 1994;271:1780.
6. Haas B, Insall JN, Scuderi GR, et al. Pneumatic sequential-compression boots compared with aspirin prophylaxis of deep-vein thrombosis after total knee arthroplasty. *J Bone Joint Surg [Am].* 1990;72:27.
7. Hull R, Raskob G, Pineo G, et al. A comparison of subcutaneous low-molecular-weight heparin with warfarin sodium for prophylaxis against deep-vein thrombosis after hip or knee implantation. *N Engl J Med.* 1993;329:1370.
8. Leclerc JR, Geerts WH, Desjardins L, et al. Prevention of venous thromboembolism after knee arthroplasty. A randomized, double-blind trial comparing enoxaparin with warfarin. *Ann Intern Med.* 1996;124:619.
9. Modig J, Borg T, Karlstrom G, et al. Thromboembolism after total hip replacement: role of epidural and general anesthesia. *Anesth Analg.* 1983;62:174.
10. Sharrock NE, Haas SB, Hargett MJ, et al. Effects of epidural anesthesia on the incidence of deep-vein thrombosis after total knee arthroplasty. *J Bone Joint Surg [Am].* 1991;73:502.
11. Francis CW, Pellegrini VD, Marder VJ, et al. Comparison of warfarin and external pneumatic compression in prevention of venous thrombosis after total hip replacement. *JAMA.* 1992;267:2911.
12. Vresilovic EJ, Hozack WJ, Booth RE, et al. Incidence of pulmonary embolism after total knee arthroplasty with low-dose Coumadin prophylaxis. *Clin Orthop.* 1993;286:27.
13. Hodge WA. Prevention of deep vein thrombosis after total knee arthroplasty: Coumadin versus pneumatic calf compression. *Clin Orthop.* 1991;271:101.
14. Patzakis MJ, Harvey JP Jr, Ivler D. The role of antibiotics in the management of open fractures. *J Bone Joint Surg [Am].* 1974;56:532.
15. Perry JF. Pelvic open fractures. *Clin Orthop.* 1980;151:41.
16. Mohamed AA, Banerjee A. Patterns of injury associated with automobile airbag use. *Postgrad Med J.* 1998;74:455.
17. Viegas S, Rimoldi R, Scarborough M, et al. Acute compartment syndrome in the thigh: a case report and review of the literature. *Clin Orthop.* 1988;234:232.
18. Taylor DC, Salvian AJ, Shackleton CR. Crush syndrome complicating pneumatic antishock garment (PASG) use. *Injury.* 1988;19:43.
19. Bass RR, Allison EJ, Reines HD, et al. Thigh compartment syndrome without lower extremity trauma following application of pneumatic antishock trousers. *Ann Emerg Med.* 1983;12:382.
20. Johnson BE. Anterior tibial compartment syndrome following use of MAST suit. *Ann Emerg Med.* 1981;10:209.
21. Bracken MB, Shepard MJ, Holford TR, et al. Methylprednisolone or tirilazad mesylate administration after acute spinal cord injury: 1-year follow up. Results of the Third National Acute Spinal Cord Injury randomized controlled trial. *J Neurosurg.* 1998;89:699.
22. Bracken MB, Shepard MJ, Collins WF Jr, et al. Methylprednisolone or naloxone treatment after acute spinal cord injury: 1-year follow-up data. Results of the second National Acute Spinal Cord Injury Study. *J Neurosurg.* 1992;76:23.
23. Seibel R, LaDuca J, Hassett JM, et al. Blunt multiple trauma (ISS 36), femur traction, and the pulmonary failure-septic state. *Ann Surg.* 1985;202:283.
24. Bone LB, Johnson KD, Weigelt J, et al. Early versus delayed stabilization of femoral fractures: a prospective randomized study. *J Bone Joint Surg [Am].* 1989;71:336.
25. Johnson KD, Cadambi A, Seibert GB. Incidence of adult respiratory distress syndrome in patients with multiple musculoskeletal injuries: effect of early operative stabilization of fractures. *J Trauma.* 1985;25:375.
26. Morawa LG, Manley MT, Edidin AA, et al. Transesophageal echocardiographic monitored events during total knee arthroplasty. *Clin Orthop.* 1996;331:192.
27. Willsey DB, Peterfreund RA. Compartment syndrome of the upper arm after pressurized infiltration of intravenous fluid. *J Clin Anesth.* 1997;9:428.
28. Eyres KS, Hill G, Magides A. Compartment syndrome in tibial shaft fracture missed because of a local nerve block [letter]. *J Bone Joint Surg [Br].* 1996;78:996.
29. Dunwoody JM, Reichert CC, Brown KL. Compartment syndrome associated with bupivacaine and fentanyl epidural analgesia in pediatric orthopaedics. *J Pediatr Orthop.* 1997:17:285.
30. White BL, Fisher WD, Laurin CA. Rate of mortality for elderly patients after fracture of the hip in the 1980s. *J Bone Joint Surg [Am].* 1987;69:1335.
31. Ions GK, Stevens J. Prediction of survival in patients with femoral neck fractures. *J Bone Joint Surg [Br].* 1987;69:384.
32. Lynch NM, Cofield RH, Silbert PL, et al. Neurologic complications after total shoulder arthroplasty. *J Shoulder Elbow Surg.* 1996;5:1:53.
33. Sulek CA, Davies LK, Enneking FK, et al. Cerebral microembolism diagnosed by transcranial Doppler during total knee arthroplasty: correlation with transesophageal echocardiography. *Anesthesiology.* 1999;91:672.
34. Williams-Russo P, Sharrock NE, Mattis S, et al. Cognitive effects after epidural versus general anesthesia in older patients. *JAMA.* 1995;274:44.
35. Pellicci PM, Ranawat CS, Tsairis P. A prospective study of the progression of rheumatoid arthritis of the cervical spine. *J Bone Joint Surg [Am].* 1981;63:342.
36. Keenen MA, Siles CM, Kaufman RL. Acquired laryngeal deviation

associated with the cervical spine disease in erosive polyarticular arthritis. *Anesthesiology.* 1983;58:441.

37. Cathcart ES, Spodick DH. Rheumatoid heart disease: a study of the incidence and nature of cardiac lesions in rheumatoid arthritis. *N Engl J Med.* 1962;266:959.

38. Zuckerman JD, ed. *Orthopedic Knowledge Update 3: Hip Trauma.* Park Ridge, Ill: American Academy of Orthopedic Surgeons; 1990:499.

39. Byerly SI. Complications of spinal surgery. In: John Atlee, ed. *Complications in Anesthesia.* Philadelphia, Pa: WB Saunders; 1999:902.

40. MacEwen GD, Bunnell WP, Sriram K. Acute neurological complications in the treatment of scoliosis: a report of the Scoliosis Research Society. *J Bone Joint Surg [Am].* 1975;57:404.

41. Millne B, Rosales JK. Anesthetic consideration in patients with muscular dystrophy undergoing spinal fusion and Harrington rod instrumentation. *Can Anaesth Soc J.* 1982;29:750.

42. Kafer ER. Idiopathic scoliosis: mechanical properties of the respiratory system and the ventilatory response to carbon dioxide. *J Clin Invest.* 1975;55:1153.

43. Holtby HM, Relton JES. Orthopedic diseases. In: Katz J, ed. *Orthopedic Diseases.* Philadelphia, Pa: WB Saunders; 1987:370.

44. Bieber E, Tolo V, Uematsu S. Spinal cord monitoring during posterior spinal instrumentation and fusion. *Clin Orthop.* 1988;229:121.

45. Luque ER. Sequential spinal instrumentation of the lumbar spine. *Clin Orthop.* 1986;203:126.

46. Rossier AB, Cochran TP. The treatment of spinal fusion with Harrington compression rods and sequential sublaminar wiring: a dangerous combination. *Spine.* 1984;9:796.

47. Myers MA, Hamilton SR, Bogosian AJ, et al. Visual loss as a complication of spine surgery: a review of 37 cases. *Spine.* 1997;22:1325.

48. Katz J, Melzack R. Pain "memories" in phantom limbs: review and clinical observations. *Pain.* 1990;43:319.

49. Jahangiri M, Jayatunga AP, Bradley JW, et al. Prevention of phantom pain after major lower limb amputation by epidural infusion of diamorphine, clonidine and bupivacaine. *Ann R Coll Surg Engl.* 1994;76:324.

50. Bach S, Noreng MF, Tjelden NU. Phantom limb pain in amputees during the first 12 months following limb amputation, after preoperative lumbar epidural blockade. *Pain.* 1988;33:297.

51. Fisher A, Meller Y. Continuous postoperative regional analgesia by nerve sheath block for amputation surgery: a pilot study. *Anesth Analg.* 1991;72:300.

52. Malawer MM, Buch R, Khurana JS, et al. Postoperative infusional continuous regional analgesia: a technique for relief of postoperative pain following major extremity surgery. *Clin Orthop.* 1991;266:227.

53. Elizaga AM, Smith DG, Sharar SR, et al. Continuous regional analgesia by intraneural block: effect on postoperative opioid requirements and phantom limb pain following amputation. *J Rehabil Res Dev.* 1994;31:179.

54. Pavy TJ, Doyle DL. Prevention of phantom limb pain by infusion of local anaesthetic into the sciatic nerve. *Anesth Intensive Care.* 1996;24:599.

55. Pinzur MS, Garla PG, Pluth T, et al. Continuous postoperative infusion of a regional anesthetic after an amputation of the lower extremity. A randomized clinical trial. *J Bone Joint Surg [Am].* 1996;78:1501.

56. Enneking FK, Scarborough MT, Radson EA. Local anesthetic infusion through nerve sheath catheters for analgesia following upper extremity amputation: clinical report. *Reg Anesth.* 1997;22:351.

57. Chung F, Ritchie ED, Su J. Postoperative pain in ambulatory surgery. *Anesth Analg.* 1997;8:816.

58. Lintner S, Shawen S, Lohnes J, et al. Local anesthesia in outpatient knee arthroscopy: a comparison of efficacy and cost. *Arthroscopy.* 1996;12:482.

59. Møiniche S, Mikkelsen S, Wetterslev J, et al. A systematic review of intra-articular local anesthetic for postoperative pain relief after arthroscopic knee surgery. *Reg Anesth Pain Med.* 1999;24:430.

60. Nagasaka H, Awad H, Yaksh TL. Peripheral and spinal actions of opioids in the blockade of the autonomic response evoked by compression of the inflamed knee joint. *Anesthesiology.* 1996;85:808.

61. Habeggar R, Siebenmann R, Kieser CH. Lethal air embolism during arthroscopy. A case report. *J Bone Joint Surg [Br].* 1989;71:314.

62. Faure EA, Cook RI, Miles D. Air embolism during anesthesia for shoulder arthroscopy. *Anesthesiology.* 1998;89:805.

63. Segmuller HE, Alfred SP, Zilio G, et al. Cutaneous nerve lesions of the shoulder and arm after arthroscopic shoulder surgery. *J Shoulder Elbow Surg.* 1995;4:254.

64. Borgeat A, Shappi B, Biasca N, et al. Patient-controlled analgesia after major shoulder surgery. *Anesthesiology.* 1997;87:1343.

65. Singelyn FJ, Deyaert M, Joris D, et al. Effects of intravenous patient-controlled analgesia with morphine, continuous epidural analgesia, and continuous three-in-one block on postoperative pain and knee rehabilitation after unilateral total knee arthroplasty. *Anesth Analg.* 1998; 87:88.

66. Capdevila X, Barthelet Y, Biboulet P, et al. Effects of perioperative analgesic technique on the surgical outcome and duration of rehabilitation after major knee surgery. *Anesthesiology.* 1999;91;8.

67. Hartsmannsgruber MWB, Silverman DG, Halaszynski TM, et al. Correlation of side effects and plasma levels following ropivacaine and lidocaine for IVRA. *Anesthesiology.* 1999;91:A853.

68. Gentili M, Bernard JM, Bonnet F. Adding clonidine to lidocaine for intravenous regional anesthesia prevents tourniquet pain. *Anesth Analg.* 1999;88:1327.

69. Reuben SS, Steinberg RB, Klatt JL, et al. Intravenous regional anesthesia using lidocaine and clonidine. *Anesthesiology.* 1999;91:654.

70. Reuben SS, Steinberg RB, Kreitzer JM, et al. Intravenous regional anesthesia using lidocaine and ketorolac. *Anesth Analg.* 1995;81:110.

71. Goldberg ME, Gregg C, Larijan GE, et al. A comparison of three methods of axillary approach to brachial plexus blockade for upper extremity surgery. *Anesthesiology.* 1987;66:814.

72. Schroeder LE, Horlocker TT, Schroeder DR. The efficacy of axillary block for surgical procedures about the elbow. *Anesth Analg.* 1996;83:747.

73. Roch JJ, Sharrock NE, Neudachin L. Interscalene brachial plexus block for shoulder surgery: a proximal paresthesia is effective. *Anesth Analg.* 1992;75:386.

74. Pham DC, Gunst JP, Gouin F, et al. A novel supraclavicular approach to brachial plexus block. *Anesth Analg.* 1997;85:111.

75. Singelyn FJ, Van der Elst P. Continuous "3-in-1" block after total hip replacement continuous or patient-controlled infusion? *Anesth Analg.* 1998;86:S315.

76. Brull SJ, Lieoponis JV, Murphy MJ, et al. Acute and long-term benefits of iliac crest donor site perfusion with local anesthetics. *Anesth Analg.* 1992;74:145.

77. Rawal N, Axelsson K, Hylander J, et al. Postoperative patient-controlled local anesthetic administration at home. *Anesth Analg.* 1998;86:86.

78. Badenhorst CH. Epidural hematoma after epidural pain control and concomitant postoperative anticoagulation [letter]. *Reg Anesth.* 1996;21:272.

79. Woolson ST, Robinson RK, Khan NQ, et al. Deep venous thrombosis prophylaxis for knee replacement: warfarin and pneumatic compression. *Am J Orthop.* 1998;27:299.

80. Schroeder DR. Statistics: detecting a rare adverse drug reaction using spontaneous reports. *Reg Anesth Pain Med.* 1998;23(suppl 2):183.

81. Horlocker TT, Wedel DJ. Anticoagulation and neuraxial block: historical perspective, anesthetic implications, and risk management. *Reg Anesth Pain Med.* 1998;23(Suppl 2):129.

82. Heit JA. Low-molecular-weight heparin: biochemistry, pharmacology, and concurrent drug precautions. *Reg Anesth Pain Med.* 1998;23(suppl 2):135.

83. Enneking FK, Benzon H. Oral anticoagulants and regional anesthesia: a perspective. *Reg Anesth Pain Med.* 1998;23(suppl 2):140.

84. Urmey WF, Rowlingson J. Do antiplatelet agents contribute to the development of perioperative spinal hematoma? *Reg Anesth Pain Med.* 1998;23(suppl 2):146.

85. Rosenquist RW, Brown DL. Neuraxial bleeding: fibrinolytics/thrombolytics. *Reg Anesth Pain Med.* 1998;23(suppl 2):152.

86. Liu SS, Mulroy MF. Neuraxial anesthesia and analgesia in the presence of standard heparin. *Reg Anesth Pain Med.* 1998;23(suppl 2):157.

87. Horlocker TT, Wedel DJ. Neuraxial block and low-molecular-weight heparin: balancing perioperative analgesia and thromboprophylaxis. *Reg Anesth Pain Med.* 1998;23(suppl 2):164.

88. Tryba M. European practice guidelines: thromboembolism prophylaxis and regional anesthesia. *Reg Anesth Pain Med.* 1998;23(suppl 2):178.

89. Schroeder DR. Statistics: detecting a rare adverse drug reaction using spontaneous reports. *Reg Anesth Pain Med.* 1998;23(suppl 2):183.

90. Landow L. Monitoring adverse drug events: the Food and Drug Administration Medwatch reporting system. *Reg Anesth Pain Med.* 1998;23(suppl 2):190.

91. McKenzie PJ, Wishart HY, Smith G. Long-term outcome after repair of fractured neck of femur: comparison of subarachnoid and general anesthesia. *Br J Anaesth.* 1984;56:581.

92. Sorenson RM, Pace NL. Anesthetic techniques during surgical repair of femoral neck fractures: a meta-analysis. *Anesthesiology.* 1992; 77:1095.

93. Modig J. Regional anaesthesia and blood loss. *Acta Anaesth Scand Suppl.* 1988;89:44.

94. Goodnough LT, Rudnick S, Price TH, et al. Increased preoperative collection of autologous blood with recombinant human erythropoietin therapy. *N Engl J Med.* 1989;17:1163.

95. Tyrba M. Epoetin alfa plus autologous blood donation and normovolemic hemodilution in patients scheduled for orthopedic and vascular surgery. *Semin Hematol.* 1997;33(2 Suppl 2):34.

96. McNeil TW, DeWald RL, Kuo KN, et al. Controlled hypotensive anesthesia in scoliosis surgery. *J Bone Joint Surg [Am].* 1974;56:1167.

97. Barbier-Bohm G, Desmonts JM, Couderc E, et al. Comparative effects of induced hypotension and normovolaemic hemodilution on blood loss in total hip arthroplasty. *Br J Anaesth.* 1980;52:1039.

98. Lessard MR, Trepanier CA, Baribault JP, et al. Isoflurane-induced hypotension in orthognathic surgery. *Anesth Analg.* 1989;69:379.

99. Monk TG, Goodnough LT. Acute normovolemic hemodilution. *Clin Orthop.* 1998;357:74.

100. Oishi CS, D'Lima DD, Morris BA, et al. Hemodilution with other blood reinfusion techniques in total hip arthroplasty. *Clin Orthop.* 1997;June(339):132.

101. Elliott BA. Positioning and monitoring. In: Wedel DJ, ed. *Orthopedic Anesthesia.* New York, NY: Churchill Livingstone; 1993:101.

102. Lachiewicz PF, Latimer HA. Rhabdomyolysis following total hip arthroplasty. *J Bone Joint Surg [Br].* 1991;73:576.

103. Smith JW, Pellicci PM, Sharrock NE. Complications after total hip replacement. *J Bone Joint Surg [Am].* 1989;71:528.

104. Monroe MC. The arterial tourniquet. In: Gravenstein N, ed. *Manual of Complications During Anesthesia.* Philadelphia, Pa: JB Lippincott; 1991:683.

105. Saunders KC, Louis DL, Weingarden SI, et al. Effect of tourniquet time on postoperative quadriceps function. *Clin Orthop.* 1979;143:194.

106. Sapega AA, Heppenstall RB, Chance B, et al. Optimizing tourniquet application and release times in extremity surgery: a biochemical and ultrastructural study. *J Bone Joint Surg [Am].* 1985;67:303.

107. Haljamae H, Enger E. Human skeletal muscle energy metabolism during and after complete tourniquet ischemia. *Ann Surg.* 1975;182:9.

108. Reid HS, Camp RA, Jacob WH. Tourniquet hemostasis: a clinical study. *Clin Orthop.* 1983;177:230.

109. Moore MR, Garfin SR, Hargens AR. Wide tourniquets eliminate blood flow at low inflation pressures. *J Hand Surg.* 1987;12A:1006.

110. Valli H, Rosenberg DH, Kytta J, et al. Arterial hypertension associated with the use of a tourniquet with either general or regional anesthesia. *Acta Anaesth Scand.* 1987;31:279.

111. Concepcion MA, Lambert DH, Welch KA, et al. Tourniquet pain during spinal anesthesia: a comparison of plain solutions of tetracaine and bupivacaine. *Anesth Analg.* 1988;67:828.

112. Gissen AJ, Covino BG, Gregus J. Differential sensitivities of mammalian nerve fibers to local anesthetic agents. *Anesthesiology.* 1980;53:467.

113. Stewart A, Lambert DH, Concepcion MA. Decreased incidence of tourniquet pain during spinal anesthesia with bupivacaine: a possible explanation. *Anesth Analg.* 1988;67:833.

114. Dickson M, White H, Kinney W, et al. Extremity tourniquet deflation increases end-tidal $P_{CO_2}$. *Anesth Analg.* 1990;70:457.

C H A P T E R

# 68

# Otolaryngologic and Maxillofacial Surgery

Alexander W. Gotta

Lynne Ferrari

Colleen A. Sullivan

## LASER SURGERY

*What Is the Laser and Why Is It Used?*

*What Are the Risks of Laser Surgery?*

*What Techniques Are Used to Provide Anesthesia for Laser Surgery of the Airway?*

## AIRWAY EMERGENCIES

*Who Aspirates Foreign Bodies?*

*How Should the Child Who Has Aspirated a Foreign Body Be Anesthetized?*

*What Are the Intraoperative Complications to Avoid?*

## DENTAL REPAIRS IN RETARDED AND UNCOOPERATIVE PATIENTS

*What Problems Should Be Anticipated?*

*How Is Anesthesia Managed?*

## CRANIOFACIAL TRAUMA

*What Anatomic Structures Determine the Sites of Fracture?*

*When Do Mandibular Fractures Occur?*

*How Are Facial Fractures Classified?*

*How Do Le Fort Fractures Influence Anesthetic Management?*

*What Are the Effects and Implications of Temporomandibular Joint Injuries?*

*What Are the Most Frequent Associated Injuries?*

## AWAKE TRACHEAL INTUBATION

*What General Concepts Are Applicable?*

*How Is the Patient Prepared?*

*What Is the Sensory Innervation of the Larynx?*

*How Is the Superior Laryngeal Nerve Blocked?*

*Why Not Block the Recurrent Laryngeal Nerves?*

*How Is Translaryngeal Analgesia Obtained?*

*Can the Airway Be Anesthetized by Inhalation of Local Anesthetic?*

*Is There a Risk of Local Anesthetic Overdose?*

## ALTERNATIVE TECHNIQUES TO SECURE THE AIRWAY

*What Is a Bimandibular Fracture?*

*What Problems Are Associated With Emergency Airway Management?*

*When Are Fiberoptic Techniques Indicated?*

*Why Not Take an Awake Look?*

*What Is the Role of the Laryngeal Mask Airway in Head and Neck Surgery?*

*What Are the Indications for Tracheotomy?*

*How Should a Patient Whose Jaw Is Wired Be Extubated?*

Anesthetic management for surgery of the head and neck presents a series of challenges to the anesthesiologist. The airway may be obstructed by tumor, abscess, or trauma. The patient, struggling for every breath, may be difficult to intubate, and use of an anesthetic that impairs respiratory drive is fraught with peril. The art of nasotracheal intubation must be mastered, as well as the use of fiberoptic intubating techniques. Awake intubation is often an unpleasant necessity, and the role of the laryngeal mask airway is yet to be defined. The creation of a surgical airway by tracheostomy or crico-

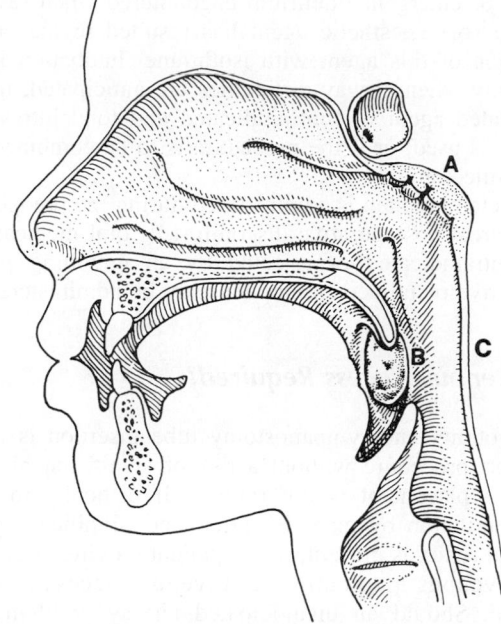

**FIGURE 68–1.** Sagittal view of the relevant anatomic relationships of the upper airway. A, adenoids; B, palatine tonsil; C, posterior wall of pharynx.

thyrotomy must be considered, as well as jet ventilation. Both surgeon and anesthesiologist are competing for the same space (Fig. 68–1) and must learn to cooperate and share, but never compromise the patient's safety. We consider here the variety of anesthetic challenges and plans for clinical management. Finally, the indications for and the time and place of extubation maximally test clinical judgment.

## MYRINGOTOMY

### What Are the Indications?

Chronic or recurrent otitis media is a highly prevalent pediatric disorder. Untreated, this condition may lead to middle ear damage and permanent hearing impairment. Consequently, elective myringotomy with insertion of tympanotomy tubes is among the most commonly performed pediatric surgical procedures. Nonpurulent effusions appear to be related to abnormal eustachian tube function, which results in impaired venting of the middle ear. Bacterial infection is frequently superimposed and is treated with appropriate antibiotics before myringotomy.

### Which Technique Is Preferred?

Bilateral myringotomy with tube insertion is typically a very short operation. Sedative premedication may outlast the procedure and usually is not necessary. Parental presence during induction of general anesthesia is often as effective, if not better, than pharmacologic premedication. Mask induction and maintenance of anesthesia using oxygen ($O_2$), nitrous oxide ($N_2O$), and a volatile agent are routine. Although halothane had been the inhalation agent of choice, sevoflurane is now the preferred volatile agent for induction of anesthesia, followed by isoflurane for anesthetic maintenance. The high incidence of emergence delirium encountered when sevoflurane is the sole anesthetic agent has resulted in the popular combination of this agent with isoflurane. Intubation is performed only when airway difficulties are anticipated, the use of an inhaled agent is contraindicated and total intravenous anesthesia is used, or if the procedure is to be combined with adenotonsillectomy.

Oral acetaminophen is administered during the preoperative period to treat postoperative discomfort. If oral medication is either contraindicated or rejected by an unwilling patient, intraoperative rectal acetaminophen may be administered.

### Is Intravenous Access Required?

Myringotomy and tympanostomy tube insertion is a relatively short procedure without a risk of significant bleeding, and fluid replacement is not routine. If difficulty in maintaining ventilation by mask is anticipated, significant gastroesophageal reflux is present, or the patient requires intraoperative intravenous medication, intravenous access might be considered. Should an unanticipated airway problem arise, intramuscular succinylcholine may be used at a dose of 1 to 4 mg/kg.[1,2] In infants and children, 2 to 3 mg/kg of succinylcholine intramuscularly usually provides effective treatment of laryngospasm, and should be combined with atropine 0.02 mg/kg to prevent bradycardia. Intramuscular administration of succinylcholine results in a delayed onset and longer duration of action than with the intravenous route.

## ADENOTONSILLECTOMY

### What Are the Indications?

Indications for adenotonsillectomy as well as timing and risks versus benefits are topics of considerable debate among pediatricians and otolaryngologists.[3] Absolute indications include unilateral enlargement (suggesting neoplasm), airway obstruction, or sleep apnea. Chronic or recurrent tonsillitis and obstructive tonsillar hyperplasia are the major indications for surgical removal, although other indications do exist[4,5] (Table 68–1). Tonsillectomy is required when tonsillitis recurs despite adequate medical therapy and when it is associated with peritonsillar abscess or acute airway obstruction. Halitosis, persistent pharyngitis, and cervical adenitis may accompany chronic tonsillitis.

Patients with obstructive sleep apnea (OSA) often experience some relief of symptoms after tonsillectomy. The severity of the disease is not always related to the degree of tonsillar hypertrophy, and patients with the most severe sleep apnea do not necessarily have the largest tonsils. Children with OSA

**TABLE 68–1.** Indications for Adenotonsillectomy

Recurrent tonsillitis or adenoiditis
Acute tonsillitis or adenoiditis
Peritonsillar abscess
Airway obstruction/sleep apnea*
Failure to thrive
Cor pulmonale
Unilateral enlargement/tonsillar or adenoidal mass*

*Absolute indications.

are usually between the ages of 2 and 6 years and have one or more of the following: snoring, daytime somnolence, failure to thrive, developmental delay, recurrent respiratory tract infections, craniofacial dysmorphism, cor pulmonale, and cardiac dysrhythmias. OSA in children may occur in association with congenital neuromuscular or craniofacial anomalies such as Pierre Robin and Treacher Collins syndromes, which may make airway management extremely difficult. Two thirds of children and adults with OSA are obese.[6] Many of the effects of OSA are reversed after tonsillectomy.

### How Are Patients Assessed?

Because of the high frequency of associated respiratory problems in children undergoing adenotonsillectomy, the presence of a recent upper respiratory infection or tonsillitis and current use of antibiotics, antihistamines, or other medicines should be sought. Because many over-the-counter medications contain aspirin or aspirinlike compounds, which might interfere with coagulation, the use of these compounds must be specifically identified. A history of abnormal bleeding should also be selectively elicited because postoperative bleeding is one of the most serious complications of this surgery. If there is a history of recent aspirin or nonsteroidal antiinflammatory drug (NSAID) use or if there is a coagulation abnormality, a coagulation screening profile and evaluation of platelet function should be included in the preoperative assessment. Without a specific indication, the value of routine coagulation testing has been debated.[7,8]

Parents should be questioned for the presence of OSA and, if it is present, the results of the polysomnogram should be reviewed and recorded. The diagnosis of sleep apnea syndrome is confirmed by the presence of one or more of the following findings during graphic recordings of respiration during a period of natural sleep: apnea determined by complete cessation of airflow on auscultation; $O_2$ desaturation (measured by pulse oximetry) to <90%; obstructive apnea determined by the absence of respiration for a minimum of 10 seconds, accompanied by paradoxical movement of the rib cage and abdomen; and nasopharyngoscopy- or cinefluoroscopy-documented upper airway obstruction.[9]

The physical examination should begin with observation of the patient, especially noting the presence of audible respiration, mouth breathing, nasal quality of the speech, and chest retractions. These children are often mouth breathers and have long faces, retrognathic mandibles, and high-arched palates, the result of chronic nasopharyngeal obstruction.[10] The oropharynx should be inspected to determine the degree of tonsillar hypertrophy because tonsils that occupy >50% of the hypopharynx may be associated with difficulty in mask ventilation. Although mask ventilation may be difficult, laryngoscopy and tracheal intubation should not be because the tonsils are supraglottic structures. Wheezing, rales, or stridor heard on chest auscultation may indicate upper airway obstruction resulting from hypertrophied tonsils and adenoids or inflammation of the lower airway.

The importance of laboratory examination is constantly being reevaluated. Routine measurement of hemoglobin is unnecessary in otherwise healthy children because the incidence of isolated anemia in pediatric surgical patients is only 2%.[11–13] Patients in whom there is a high likelihood of anemia, such as infants younger than 1 year of age and those with a history of prematurity or chronic illness, should have a hemoglobin measurement. The large number of false-positive laboratory tests combined with the relatively low incidence of inherited and acquired coagulopathies raises doubts about the value of routine coagulation screening before adenotonsillectomy.[14,15] Chest radiography and electrocardiography are not required unless a specific history of abnormalities in these areas is elicited, such as recent pneumonia, bronchitis, upper respiratory infection, or history consistent with OSA or cor pulmonale. In patients with severe OSA, a preoperative arterial blood gas measurement and echocardiogram may be indicated.[16]

## How Is Anesthesia Managed?

### Induction

Pediatric patients without airway obstruction may be premedicated if necessary. However, preoperative premedication may interfere with ventilatory function in the postoperative period, so it is best used cautiously. Patients with OSA should not receive premedication because they are at risk for postoperative apnea simply as a result of their disease and sedative premedication may further impair respiratory function. The presence of a parent in the operating room for the induction of anesthesia in children is very effective and is usually better accepted than a pharmacologic agent. After mask induction using $O_2$, $N_2O$, and a volatile agent, intravenous access is obtained. In the older child and adult, intravenous induction of general anesthesia is accomplished with propofol, 2 to 3 mg/kg. The most frequently used agent for mask induction is sevoflurane, but some practitioners still prefer to use halothane. Intubation is then performed using a nondepolarizing muscle relaxant. An oral RAE tube commonly is chosen, although a conventional endotracheal tube is acceptable. There is a great deal of controversy surrounding the use of cuffed or uncuffed endotracheal tubes. For pediatric patients, most practitioners still favor the use of an uncuffed endotracheal tube with a leak at 20 to 30 cm $H_2O$ pressure. If a cuffed endotracheal tube is chosen, the same conditions for a leak apply; otherwise, the risk of postextubation croup is high.[17] The tube is taped to the midline of the lower lip, where it is secured by the tongue blade of a mouth gag. Continuous capnography and auscultation of breath sounds are essential because kinking, extubation, or bronchial intubation may occur.

### Maintenance

Many techniques are suitable for anesthetic maintenance. A volatile agent in combination with narcotic is a standard approach, either with or without muscle relaxant. Total intravenous anesthesia also is effective in all age groups, using a short-acting opioid such as remifentanil combined with propofol, $N_2O$, and a muscle relaxant. Ketorolac and other NSAIDs are contraindicated in tonsillectomy patients because of the increased risk of bleeding.[18] Alternatively, local anesthetic (eg, bupivacaine 0.25%) may be instilled into the tonsillar fossa at the conclusion of the procedure.[19] Postoperative nausea and vomiting is very common after adenotonsillectomy, and an antiemetic should be administered prophylactically. Intraoperative fluid should be given in an amount to compensate for

the NPO losses as well as intraoperative blood loss because it is common for patients not to drink in the first 12 hours after surgery.

### Emergence and Extubation

After completion of surgery, the pharynx is gently cleared using a soft catheter. Suctioning of the stomach is also performed to remove any gas that may contribute to postoperative nausea and vomiting rather than to remove blood, which is rarely present. On verification of hemostasis, anesthesia is discontinued and muscle relaxants are reversed, if they have been used. Lidocaine, 1.5 mg/kg intravenously, reduces the incidence of postextubation laryngospasm in adult patients. The trachea is extubated either with the patient awake and responsive or "deeply" to prevent coughing and bucking on the endotracheal tube. Either method is acceptable. The patient is placed in the lateral "tonsil" position during recovery, so that blood and secretions drain out, thus avoiding laryngospasm.

Although adenoidectomy is customarily an ambulatory procedure, in many centers posttonsillectomy patients are admitted for overnight observation. Selection of patients for ambulatory tonsillectomy is individualized and based on the needs of the patient, family, and referring physician.[20] Ambulatory patients should be observed for 6 to 8 hours before leaving the hospital. Discharged patients are instructed to return to the hospital in case of bleeding, vomiting, lightheadedness or dizziness, palpitations, or mental status changes. Patients who are younger than 3 years of age or have abnormalities in the coagulation profile, multisystem medical problems, or craniofacial abnormalities, or who live beyond a reasonable distance to the hospital, are not candidates for outpatient tonsillectomy.[21]

## How Is Posttonsillectomy Bleeding Managed?

Postoperative hemorrhage occurs at a frequency of 0.1% to 8.1%; 75% of cases occur within 6 hours of surgery and the remaining 25% may be observed as late as the sixth postoperative day. The tonsillar fossa is the site in 67% of cases of postoperative bleeding; 27% occur in the nasopharynx, and bleeding occurs in both locations in the remaining 7%. Control of bleeding can be achieved using pharyngeal packs and cautery. If this approach fails, patients must return to the operating room for exploration and surgical hemostasis. Large volumes of blood originating from the tonsillar bed may be swallowed and this is often not appreciated by the patient, parent, or surgeon. All patients with posttonsillectomy hemorrhage must therefore be considered to have a full stomach, and anesthetic precautions must be taken. A rapid-sequence induction, accompanied by cricoid pressure and a styletted endotracheal tube, are suggested. Before anesthetic induction, it is essential that the blood pressure be checked in both the erect and supine positions ("tilt test"), looking for orthostatic changes resulting from decreases in intravascular volume. In addition, intravenous access must be established, volume replacement initiated, hematocrit measured, and a blood sample for type and crossmatch sent before induction. Various laryngoscope blades, handles, and endotracheal tubes must be available. Suction apparatus should be prepared in duplicate because blood in the airway may impair visualization of the vocal cords and cause plugging of the endotracheal tube or suction apparatus; if one suction apparatus becomes blocked with a blood clot, another should be readily available.

Both intravenous- and inhalation-based anesthetic techniques are appropriate. However, patients should be responsive at the conclusion of surgery and be extubated awake. These surgical procedures usually are very brief, so the anesthetic should be planned accordingly. Criteria for having discharged patients return to the hospital for evaluation of post-tonsillectomy bleeding are listed in Table 68–2.

## How Is Postoperative Pulmonary Edema Detected and Treated?

Acute postoperative negative pressure pulmonary edema (NPPE) is an infrequently recognized but potentially life-threatening complication encountered when airway obstruction is suddenly relieved. One proposed mechanism is that during inspiration before adenotonsillectomy, the *negative* (subambient) intrapleural pressure that is generated causes an increase in venous return, enhancing pulmonary blood volume. In the healthy child without airway obstruction, pleural pressure ranges between $-2.5$ and $-10$ cm $H_2O$ during inspiration. Intrapleural pressure generated in the child with airway obstruction can be as low as $-30$ cm $H_2O$, which, when transmitted to the interstitial peribronchial and perivascular spaces, causes disruption of the capillary walls of the pulmonary microvasculature. Concurrent with a negative transpulmonary gradient is an increase in venous return to the right side of the heart, thus increasing preload. In the setting of "leaky capillaries," transudation of fluid into the alveolar space is facilitated.[22] Counterbalancing this sequence, positive intrapleural and alveolar pressure is generated during exhalation, thereby decreasing venous return and pulmonary blood volume. This sequence is similar to an expiratory "grunt" mechanism in which the transpleural pressures generated are similar to those present during a Valsalva maneuver. The rapid relief of airway obstruction results in decreased airway pressure, an increase in venous return, an increase in pulmonary hydrostatic pressure, hyperemia, and, finally, pulmonary edema. The all-important counterbalance of the expiratory "grunt" in limiting pulmonary venous return is lost when the obstruction is relieved. Contributing factors are the increased volume load on both ventricles and the inability of the pulmonary lymphatic system acutely to remove large amounts of fluid. Prevention of this situation may be attempted during induction of anesthesia by applying moderate amounts of continuous positive pressure to the airway, thus allowing time for circulatory adaptation to take place. This physiologic sequence is similar to that seen in patients with severe acute airway obstruction secondary to epiglottitis or laryngospasm.[23] The presentation of NPPE is the appearance of frothy pink fluid in the endotracheal tube of an intubated patient or the presence of a decreased $O_2$ saturation, wheezing, dyspnea, and increased respiratory rate in the immediate postoperative period in a previously extubated patient. In mild cases the patient may present with minimal symptoms.

The differential diagnosis of NPPE includes aspiration of gastric contents, adult respiratory distress syndrome, congestive heart failure, intravascular volume overload, and anaphylaxis. A chest radiograph showing diffuse, usually bilateral interstitial pulmonary infiltrates combined with an appropriate clinical history confirms the diagnosis. Treatment is usually supportive with maintenance of a patent airway, $O_2$ administration, and diuretic therapy in some cases. Tracheal intubation and mechanical ventilation with positive end-expiratory pressure may be necessary in severe cases. Resolution is usually rapid and may occur within hours of surgery. Most cases resolve without treatment within 24 hours. No method reliably predicts which children will experience this clinical syndrome after their airway obstruction has been resolved.

## How Are Postoperative Pain, Nausea, and Vomiting Addressed?

Pain is minimal after adenoidectomy but severe after tonsillectomy. Significant differences in the degree of postoperative pain are related to the method of tonsil removal. An increase in pain medication requirement, otalgia, and patient irritability have been noted in patients who have undergone tonsillectomy by means of electrocautery and laser excision compared with a technique of sharp dissection. Intraoperative administration of corticosteroids may decrease edema formation and subsequent patient discomfort. Infiltration of the peritonsillar space with local anesthetic and epinephrine is effective in reducing intraoperative blood loss in addition to decreasing postoperative pain.[24] Each tonsillar pillar is infiltrated with 3 to 5 mL of 0.25% bupivacaine containing a 1:200 000 dilution of epinephrine. This approach substantially diminishes immediate postoperative as well as long-term posttonsillectomy pain. An explanation for the long-term pain relief may be that neural blockade prevents nociceptive stimulus impulses from entering the central nervous system during and immediately after surgery, thus suppressing the formation of a sustained, hyperexcitable state that is responsible for the maintenance of postoperative pain. The anesthesiologist must remember, however, that intravascular, especially intraarterial, injection of local anesthetic can be lethal. Pain may be treated by administration of small repeated doses of narcotic. NSAIDs should be avoided because the potential interference with coagulation can prove disastrous.

Inadequate management of pain predisposes children to an increased incidence of postoperative nausea and vomiting. The combined effects of irritant blood in the stomach, interference with the gag reflex by edema, and stimulation of receptors in the chemoreceptor trigger zone contribute to the cause of vomiting, which can occur in up to 60% of tonsillectomy patients. Vigorous use of antiemetic agents, gastric decompression with an orogastric tube (remember never to insert a nasogastric tube in the postadenoidectomy patient), adequate treatment of pain, and quiet emergence from anesthesia are interventions that can help to diminish the rate of posttonsillectomy vomiting. NSAIDs are avoided. Antiemetic agents such as droperidol, 50 to 75 mg/kg, metoclopramide, 0.15 mg/kg, and ondansetron, 0.1 mg/kg, often are effective in

**TABLE 68–2.** Condition of Patients Who Should Remain in or Return to the Hospital After Tonsillectomy

| | |
|---|---|
| Prolonged postoperative vomiting | Agitation |
| Tachycardia | Orthostatic hypotension |
| Obtundation | Excessive distance from the hospital |

controlling postoperative emesis in pediatric patients. Dehydration from poor oral intake after tonsillectomy occurs at a frequency of 1% and should be offset by intravenous hydration to restore intravascular volume during surgery. If children cannot tolerate oral fluid administration secondary to pain or if vomiting is severe despite antiemetic administration, admission to the hospital or other inpatient facility is warranted.

## MIDDLE EAR SURGERY

### What Are the Implications of Patient Positioning?

Typically, the table is turned 90° from the induction position, with the patient's head turned toward the anesthetic machine. Three likely problems can occur: (1) circuit disconnection under the drapes; (2) mainstem intubation resulting from caudal movement of the tube when the head is turned or if the neck is flexed; and (3) inadvertent extubation due to either traction on the endotracheal tube or extension of the neck with rostral movement of the endotracheal tube.

The risk of disconnection is minimized by removing strain from all of the slip-fit connections, by the use of a long breathing circuit, and by the use of a tube holder. Mainstem intubation is not so much avoided as it is identified by auscultation of both hemithoraces after the bed and patient are in their final position. However, particularly in children, auscultation of the chest often is unreliable as an indication of appropriate endotracheal tube positioning. Accidental extubation is guarded against in similar fashion to disconnection. Ventilation must be continuously monitored during surgery using a stethoscope and capnometry so that any problems can be immediately identified and corrected.

### Is Nitrous Oxide Contraindicated?

$N_2O$ diffuses into air-filled spaces much faster than nitrogen diffuses out. An increased gaseous pressure or volume, or both, occurs within the space, depending on its compliance. The intact middle ear is a noncompliant air-filled space that is intermittently vented to the oropharynx through the eustachian tube. This venting occurs both actively (as during swallowing) and passively (when middle ear pressure [MEP] exceeds 20-40 cm $H_2O$ in normal people).[25]

MEP rises at a rate of approximately 1 cm $H_2O$/min under 67% $N_2O$ anesthesia. Hence, MEP peaks and is passively vented after 30 to 40 minutes in normal patients. However, passive or even active venting may be impaired in the presence of sinusitis, pharyngitis, or otitis, and after adenoidectomy.[26] Tympanic membrane rupture has occurred under such conditions and is generally a risk when MEP exceeds 100 cm $H_2O$.[27]

### Discontinuation

Tympanic membrane perforation or mastoidectomy opens the middle ear cavity; hence, MEP equilibrates with atmospheric pressure. When the cavity is then closed, as in placement of a tympanic membrane graft, blood-borne $N_2O$ diffuses into the space and increases MEP. If it cannot be vented through the eustachian tube, the graft is often dislodged.

Discontinuation of $N_2O$ has the opposite effect: diffusion out of the space causes reductions in pressure. Preanesthetic levels of MEP are usually reached within an hour after discontinuation, and in some cases, considerable subatmospheric pressure may result. Because the eustachian tube functions as a one-way valve, passive venting of negative MEP does not normally occur. When equilibration is not achieved by active measures such as yawning or swallowing, negative MEP may result in nausea, vomiting, serous otitis media, hemotympanum, and stapes disarticulation with resultant hearing loss.[28,29]

Obviously, the use of $N_2O$ should be restricted not only in middle ear surgery but in all patients with a history of otolaryngologic disease. Recommendations include limiting concentrations and discontinuing the agent before middle ear closure. However, increasing MEPs have been observed even 10 to 20 minutes after discontinuation.[28,29] Based on the foregoing considerations, we prefer to avoid $N_2O$, particularly because anesthesia can easily be maintained with other agents, such as propofol by infusion and volatile anesthetic agents.

## OTOLOGIC AND PAROTID SURGERY

### Should Muscle Relaxants Be Used?

The facial nerve courses through a periosteal sheath in the medial wall of the tympanic cavity. After it emerges from the stylohyoid foramen, ramifications of the nerve traverse and envelop the substance of the parotid gland (Fig. 68–2). Thus, it is susceptible to injury during otologic and parotid surgery. Direct electrical stimulation is used to facilitate nerve identification and thereby prevent facial nerve palsy. Although considerable degrees of neuromuscular blockage allow response to direct stimulation, many surgeons prefer that nondepolarizing muscle relaxants be completely avoided.

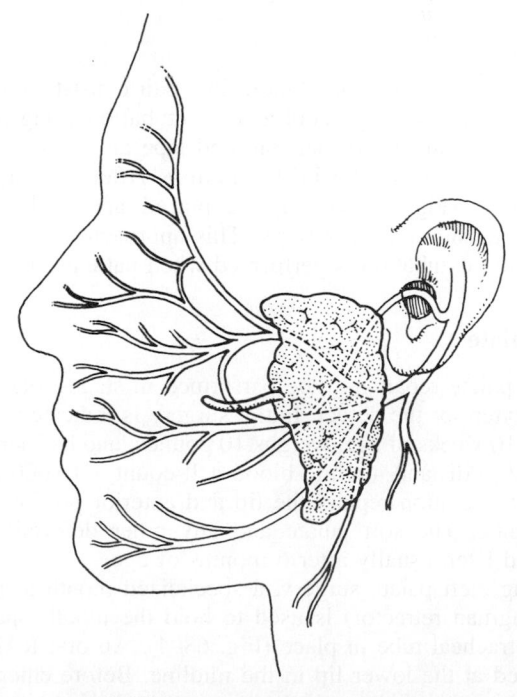

**FIGURE 68–2.** Facial nerve distribution.

Intermediate-acting drugs are acceptable, provided that careful monitoring of the neuromuscular junction is maintained and precisely documented. Communication with the surgeon allows spontaneous recovery of neuromuscular transmission when use of the nerve stimulator is anticipated. A long-acting relaxant should not be used for intubation or anesthetic management. Surgeons who disclaim the need for a nerve stimulator often change their minds during surgery, thus necessitating a change in the anesthetic plan, which may be difficult to carry out. Because neuromuscular blockade is not otherwise necessary for this surgery, we believe that these drugs are best avoided whenever possible. If they have been used, recovery of neuromuscular function should be documented in the record.

### Is Induced Hypotension Useful?

Successful use of an operating microscope requires a virtually bloodless surgical field. In the past, some have advocated profound degrees of deliberate hypotension to achieve these results.[30] In fact, one blinded study found no correlation between blood pressure and the surgeon's assessment of operative conditions.[31] Although most patients tolerate modest reductions in blood pressure, the safety and benefit of extreme levels of hypotension are not documented. In most instances, a modest[32] head-up position, topical and injected vasoconstrictors, and systolic blood pressure reduction to 75% of awake level are satisfactory.

In summary, during otologic surgery, general anesthesia using a potent volatile agent allows avoidance of $N_2O$, avoidance of longer-acting muscle relaxants, and easy titration to the desired blood pressure.

## CLEFT LIP AND PALATE

### How Is the Airway Secured?

#### Cleft Lip

Management of unilateral cleft lip repair consists of routine induction, followed by endotracheal intubation using an oral RAE tube.[33] Tincture of benzoin and tape are used to secure the tube to the lower lip in the midline. After the surgery, a Logan bow (Fig. 68–3) may be placed across the lip to decrease tension on the sutures. This approach impairs mask ventilation; extubation is performed when patients are awake.

#### Cleft Palate

Cleft palate repair may be performed in stages, depending on the extent of the defect. Initial surgery is indicated when a child is 10 weeks of age, weighs 10 pounds, and has hemoglobin of 10 g/dL and a white blood cell count <10 000/mm[3].[34] The first operation repairs the lip and anterior portion of the hard palate. The soft palate and any other deformities are corrected later, usually after 6 months of age.

During cleft palate surgery, a specialized mouth gag (Millard-Dingman retractor) is used to hold the mouth open and an endotracheal tube in place (Fig. 68–4). An oral RAE tube is secured at the lower lip in the midline. Before emergence, a suture is placed through the tongue to eliminate the need

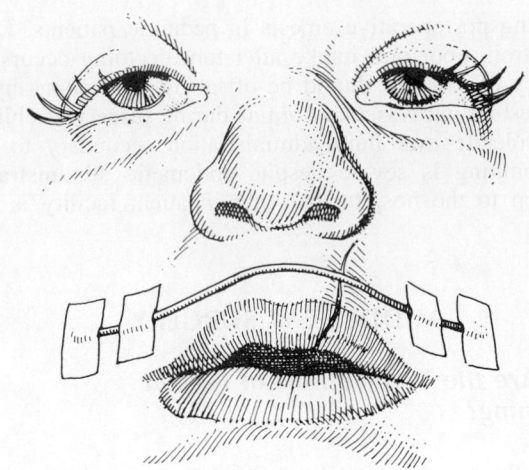

**FIGURE 68–3.** Logan bow.

for an oral airway, because the latter risks damaging the palatal repair. If soft tissue–related obstruction occurs during emergence or recovery, traction on the suture usually alleviates the problem.

## CALDWELL-LUC PROCEDURE

### What Are the Indications?

The Caldwell-Luc procedure is performed to gain access to the maxillary sinus. The operation consists of an incision and osteotomy above the ipsilateral premolars. Usually indicated for the drainage of chronic infection, the approach is also used for biopsies and for reduction and fixation of inferior orbital fractures.

### What Are the Anesthetic Concerns?

Although an antrostomy can be performed using local anesthesia, general anesthesia is usually chosen and is often necessary for additional work in the antrum. Orotracheal intubation

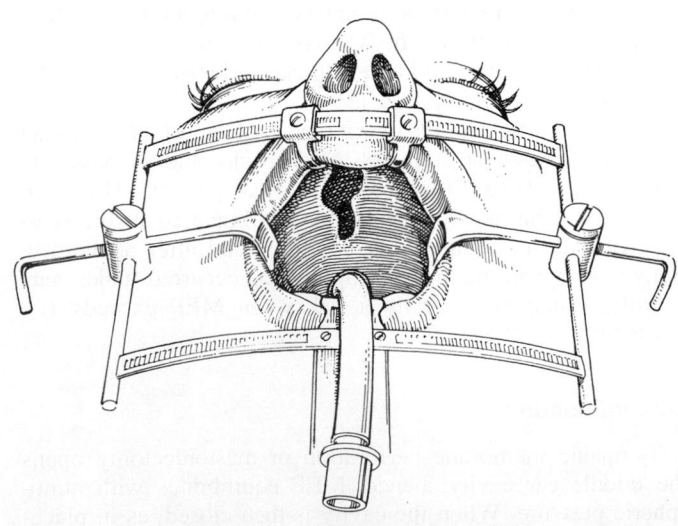

**FIGURE 68–4.** Millard-Dingman retractor.

**TABLE 68–3.** Minimizing Epinephrine-Induced Ventricular Irritability Using General Anesthesia*

| Agent (1.25 MAC) | Maximum Recommended Dose (in 0.5% lidocaine) |
|---|---|
| Halothane | 2.1 µg/kg |
| Enflurane | 3.4 µg/kg |
| Isoflurane | 6.7 µg/kg |

Incidence of arrhythmias is not related to dose of inhaled agent.
Nitrous oxide does not enhance epinephrine-induced irritability.
Use of lidocaine as a vehicle increases the arrhythmogenic dose of epinephrine.
Epinephrine concentrations stronger than 1:100 000 increase risk of ectopy without increasing hemostasis.
In adults, do not exceed 10 mL in 10 min or 30 mL in 1 h using epinephrine 1:100 000.
Avoid hypoxia, hypercarbia, and light anesthesia.
Presence of sympathetic-modifying drugs increases the risk of arrhythmias (eg, β-agonists, tricyclic antidepressants, monoamine oxidase inhibitors, methyldopa, cocaine, aminophylline, reserpine, and guanethidine).
Ephedrine (1:1000) or phenylephrine (1:10 000) may be substituted for infiltration; both are far less arrhythmogenic.
Intravenous lidocaine, β-blockers, or both are effective agents when treatment is necessary.

*Isoflurane is the potent volatile agent of choice when epinephrine injection is anticipated.
MAC, minimum alveolar concentration.

and fixation of the tube in the contralateral corner of the mouth are routine.

Injection of epinephrine-containing solutions is common, and concomitant use of halogenated anesthetics increases the risk of ventricular arrhythmias. The anesthesiologist is obliged to monitor the dose of epinephrine injected and to observe for any systemic signs of absorption. Arrhythmias may occur in the absence of hypertension. Limitation of epinephrine dose, provision of adequate anesthetic depth, and avoidance of hypoxia, hypercarbia, and halothane minimize the risk of ventricular ectopy[35,36] (Table 68–3).

## PHARYNGEAL ABSCESS

### What Is It?

The site and size of the collection affect the decision about how to secure the airway. Abscess formation tends to occur either adjacent to an infected tonsil, where it is called *quinsy*, or in the posterior pharyngeal wall. Quinsy causes severe pain and trismus, and it occasionally may obstruct the airway. Risks of general anesthesia include difficult intubation and aspiration. In particular, right-sided quinsy may interfere with glottic visualization; therefore, drainage under local anesthesia is preferred when possible. In most cases, however, the high and lateral location does not impair glottic visualization. Nevertheless, retropharyngeal collections may obliterate the hypopharynx and must be managed with extreme caution. Preoperative discussion with the surgeon is thus important to identify the abscess site because of the obvious implications for airway management.

### How Is the Airway Secured?

#### Awake Intubation

A large or tense and fluctuant abscess presents a formidable dilemma. Rupture after induction can result in disastrous aspi-

ration of purulent material. Severe infections are accompanied by generalized edema and hyperemia of all pharyngeal mucosa that may further complicate both ventilation and laryngoscopy. Hence, drainage using local anesthesia or awake intubation may be attempted.

#### Tracheotomy

These approaches usually require sedation, which, when combined with topical and local anesthesia, impairs protective reflexes. In some cases, tracheotomy may be necessary either to relieve airway obstruction or to protect the trachea from purulent drainage, because the infection is surgically drained into the pharynx. A plan for airway management must be discussed and agreed on with the surgeon before the operation.

## TEMPOROMANDIBULAR JOINT PROCEDURES

### What Are the Indications for Arthroscopy of the Temporomandibular Joint?

The most common diagnoses leading to arthroscopic study of the temporomandibular joint (TMJ) in an extensive multicenter study of 3200 patients and 4800 joints are summarized in Table 68–4.[37]

### What Problems Should Be Anticipated in Tracheal Intubation?

Because of anatomic changes in the joint, there may be decreased mobility of the jaw. This immobility may limit or prevent visualization of the larynx and intubation under direct vision. The anesthesiologist must examine the pertinent radiographs and consult with the surgeon to determine the advisability of awake intubation.

### What Other Problems Might Exist?

Psychological disorders are a major concomitant or even causative factor of TMJ dysfunction. There is a 74% incidence of major depression and somatoform disorders.[38]

### How Is the Anesthetic Managed?

General anesthesia with nasotracheal intubation gives the surgeon appropriate access and exposure.

**TABLE 68–4.** Most Common Diagnoses Leading to Arthroscopic Examination of the Temporomandibular Joint

| Condition | Incidence |
|---|---|
| Internal joint derangement with closed lock | 28.3% |
| Internal joint derangement with painful clicking | 16.1% |
| Osteoarthritis | 11.5% |
| Hypermobility | 3.0% |
| Fibrous ankylosis | 2.4% |
| Arthralgia | 2.1% |

## When Should the Patient Be Extubated?

Before extubation, the oropharynx must be examined carefully, and the area of the TMJ internally and externally must be searched, for any evidence of swelling. If irrigation fluid escapes the capsule of the TMJ, it may dissect under the mucosa of the oropharynx and close the airway either partially or completely. Mild swelling is usually progressive, and the patient must not be extubated until the turgor has disappeared completely, usually within 4 to 6 hours.[39]

## THYROID

### What Airway Management Problem Should Be Anticipated in a Patient With a Large Goiter?

An enlarged thyroid may wrap itself around the trachea and even extend into the thorax. The trachea may be narrowed or deviated to one side. Computed tomography (CT), magnetic resonance imaging (MRI), and radiographs of the tracheal air column (not soft tissue) help to determine the extent of anatomic distortion.

### How Should a Patient With a Large Goiter Be Intubated?

If marked anatomic distortion is present, the patient should be intubated awake. A long (uncut), soft (eg, warmed heat-labile) endotracheal tube should be passed through the vocal cords and the stylet quickly removed. The tube should be gently threaded into the trachea until it reaches the carina, and then pulled back slightly. Breath sounds must be auscultated on both sides of the chest. Because the tube now acts as a stent in the trachea, the surgeon cannot compress the trachea distal to the tube as he or she manipulates an intrathoracic goiter.

### What Problems Might Arise at Extubation?

With long-standing goiters, there may be erosion of the tracheal rings and the development of tracheomalacia. After removal of the thyroid and before closure of the wound, the surgeon should be asked to palpate the trachea to determine if it is softer than normal. If there is any doubt, the tube should be removed over a ventilating tube changer. With extensive resection of the thyroid, the recurrent laryngeal nerves are in danger and vocal cord paralysis may occur.

## LUDWIG'S ANGINA

### What Is It?

Ludwig's angina is a cellulitis of the floor of the mouth caused by bacterial infection of the sublingual and submandibular spaces.[40,41] Brawny induration of the neck is present, and the tongue is usually pushed upward into the oral cavity, obstructing the airway. An ominous sign is an edematous

**TABLE 68–5.** Characteristics of Ludwig's Angina

| |
|---|
| Induration of the neck |
| Trismus |
| Dysphonia |
| Drooling |
| Edema and elevation of the tongue |
| Dyspnea |
| Stridor |

tongue extending out of the mouth. Often, little or no pus is present. The cause is usually infection at the root of a second or third lower molar. These roots lie below the mylohyoid ridge; thus, infection spreads easily by continuity through the spaces. Antibiotic therapy should be instituted but may be of little value because of a mixed flora. Surgical treatment consists of airway decompression and drainage of pus if present (Table 68–5).

### How Is the Airway Secured?

Although some have advocated inhalation induction and intubation without tracheotomy,[42,43] our experience is that awake, preliminary tracheotomy is preferable. Fiberoptic intubation, either oral or nasal, is extremely difficult because of anatomic distortion, erythema, and edema. The patient in obvious respiratory distress and with airway obstruction should not be anesthetized before securing the airway.[44]

## AIRWAY NEOPLASIA

### How Is the Airway Evaluated?

Neoplasia can so distort the anatomy of the airway that tracheal intubation is difficult, if not impossible.

#### Historical Facts

Any intraoral mass can become so large that it makes direct visualization of the larynx impossible. Lesions in the airway may lead to hypoventilation and even asphyxiation if neglected. Prior treatment of an airway lesion often causes significant problems. Radiation therapy can stiffen normally pliable tissues and make laryngoscopy difficult. If one or both TMJs have been included in the radiation field, the mouth may be impossible to open. Friable or vascular lesions may bleed quite severely if manipulated during intubation. Prior surgery, especially mandibulectomy (partial or complete), may also distort the anatomy and make intubation impossible. When evaluating the patient, the clinician should specifically seek a history of respiratory distress. Dysphagia indicates an expanding mass growing out of the airway and impinging on the esophagus.

#### Physical Findings

The patient's ability to open his or her mouth must be evaluated. If the intraoral lesion is readily apparent, it must be evaluated for size and texture (using a gloved finger). Is the tongue mobile? Is the lesion friable? Does it bleed on gentle manipulation? Direct or mirror laryngoscopy may also aid in evaluating the tumor and will have been performed by the surgeon before surgery. The surgeon's findings should be reviewed or discussed before anesthetizing a patient.

### Radiographic and Laboratory Studies

Advanced radiographic techniques such as CT scanning or MRI can give a very clear assessment of tumor location, size, invasion of adjacent tissue, degree of encroachment, and airway compromise. Measurements made during review of these studies can also identify if a smaller endotracheal tube than usual is needed. Pulmonary function tests may help to determine the extent of airway obstruction. Arterial blood gas values may assist in assessing total ventilatory adequacy.

## How Is Intubation Performed?

If there is any doubt about the ability to intubate an anesthetized patient, awake intubation is mandated. Fiberoptic intubation may be unsuccessful in the presence of a severely altered airway and risks serious hemorrhage if a friable tumor is traumatized by the bronchoscope. Above all, a compromised airway must not be put at greater risk by attempting to intubate a paralyzed patient because a surgeon gives assurance that he or she can rapidly perform a tracheotomy. Even in the best circumstances, a tracheotomy requires more than 5 minutes to complete.

## RADICAL HEAD AND NECK SURGERY

The most important and vulnerable nerves during radical head and neck surgery are the recurrent laryngeal, superior laryngeal, and phrenic. Damage may occur to any or all of these structures. The resulting functional loss may be complete or incomplete and permanent or temporary, depending on whether the nerve is completely or partially severed or is trapped by surrounding edematous tissue in a closed fascial plane.

## What Are the Effects of Recurrent Laryngeal Nerve Damage?

If both recurrent laryngeal nerves are partially damaged, the glottis closes when the endotracheal tube is removed (Fig. 68–5, Part III). This situation is obviously an acute emergency and demands immediate recognition and reintubation. After total section of both nerves, the vocal cords are fixed in midposition (see Fig. 68–5, Part III).

The problem is much more difficult to recognize if only one recurrent laryngeal nerve has been sectioned because the glottis does not close completely and the vocal cord on the injured side is drawn (adducted) immobile to the center of the glottic chink (see Fig. 68–5). The diagnosis is suggested by postoperative hoarseness and confirmed by laryngoscopy.

Attempts to visualize the larynx directly at the time of extubation or immediately afterward to determine mobility of both cords are usually unavailing and prone to giving a false sense of security. The denervated cord often moves passively in the turbulent air stream passing through the larynx.

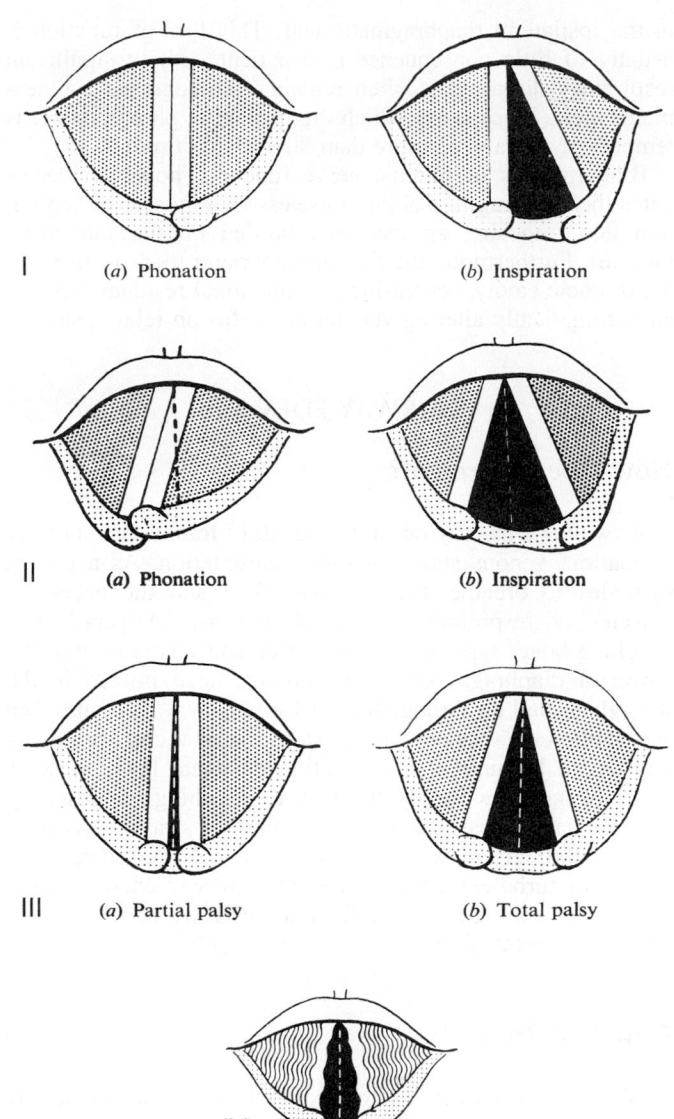

**FIGURE 68–5.** *I,* Pure abductor palsy. *II,* Abductor and adductor palsy. *III,* Bilateral damage to the recurrent laryngeal nerves. *IV,* Bilateral palsy of the recurrent laryngeal nerves with palsy of the external branch of the superior laryngeal nerve.

## What Are the Effects of Superior Laryngeal Nerve Damage?

Section of the superior laryngeal nerve denervates the cricothyroid muscle, a tensor of the vocal cords. Permanent loss of function of this nerve does not close the larynx, but the patient may not be able to vocalize high-pitched tones. More important, loss of function of the internal branch of the superior laryngeal nerve causes loss of sensation in the larynx. The laryngeal protective reflexes are thus ablated, making the patient vulnerable to aspiration of oral secretions and food.

## What Are the Effects of Phrenic Nerve Damage?

The phrenic nerve lies deep within the neck and is well protected. Section of this nerve leads to loss of motor activity in the ipsilateral diaphragmatic leaf. This loss of function is usually of little consequence in a patient without significant respiratory disease and often remains unrecognized (witness interscalene block, after which the ipsilateral phrenic nerve is temporarily paralyzed more than 80% of the time).

Bilateral loss of phrenic nerve function, however, denervates the diaphragm, making it useless as a muscle of ventilation and imposing an increased burden on the intercostal muscles. Furthermore, the flaccid diaphragm tends to rise into the thoracic cavity, decreasing the functional residual capacity and dramatically altering ventilation-perfusion relationships.

## AIRWAY EDEMA

### How Does It Present?

Airway edema may occur as a result of trauma or traumatic intubation, venous stasis, or fluid resuscitation. As a patient struggles to breathe, the alae nasi flare and the accessory muscles of respiration are called into use. A paradoxical "rocking boat" type of respiration frequently is present as the powerful diaphragm sucks the thoracic cage inward in the struggle to pull air through the narrowed airway. Patients often are diaphoretic, cyanotic, and anxious. Normal conversation is impossible because of the resulting dyspnea. If the process develops more insidiously, the work of breathing progressively increases and is associated with inspiratory stridor. Auscultation of the larynx with a stethoscope helps to detect the sounds of turbulent airflow. Subglottic airway edema related to tracheal intubation typically manifests within the first 4 hours after extubation.

### How Is It Treated?

With severe airway edema, restoration of the airway by tracheal intubation, translaryngeal ventilation, or tracheotomy is indicated, the route determined by clinical assessment and relative immediacy of the problem. Steroid administration (eg, dexamethasone, 4 to 12 mg intravenously), either as prophylaxis or treatment, is common, but with little scientific evidence of efficacy. Humidified air/$O_2$ while the patient is kept in a head-elevated position is adequate therapy in mild cases. Racemic epinephrine (0.5-1 mL of a 2% solution diluted to a volume of 3-5 mL) nebulized through a face mask or mouthpiece, acting as a topical vasoconstrictor, has been efficacious in treating upper airway edema.[45]

## AIRWAY OBSTRUCTION IN CHILDREN

### How Is Stridor Evaluated in Infants and Children?

Breathing during turbulent airflow secondary to an obstructed airway results in stridor. Obstruction of the upper airway is identified as inspiratory stridor; stridor during exhalation is due to obstruction of the lower airway. Obstructive lesions of the midtrachea cause biphasic stridor. The age of the patient at the time of presentation may aid in determining the etiology because vocal cord paralysis is often present at

birth, whereas laryngotracheomalacia develops early in infancy, and cysts or masses of the vocal cords usually develop later in childhood. Symptomatic improvement may occur in specific positions and these should be sought in the history, both to elucidate the etiology and for use during anesthetic induction to decrease the effects of obstruction on the airway. The general condition of the child and the degree of airway compromise should be noted. Identification of lesions impinging on the trachea may be aided by chest radiograph and upper gastrointestinal series. CT, MRI, and pulmonary function testing (including flow volume loops) are helpful, if available, but are not routinely obtained in the pediatric population. The intervention that is routinely recommended in the evaluation of stridor is laryngoscopy and bronchoscopy under general anesthesia.

### How Are Laryngoscopy and Bronchoscopy Performed in Infants and Small Children?

Anesthetic induction is best accomplished by inhalation of volatile agents by mask, after which the examination of the airway begins. Small infants may be brought into the operating room unpremedicated. However, if premedication is necessary in the older child, caution should be used because respiratory depression and worsening of airway obstruction may occur. After placement of appropriate monitors, pulse oximeter probe, blood pressure cuff, electrocardiographic electrodes, and precordial stethoscope, inhalation induction by mask is accomplished with 100% $O_2$ and increasing concentrations of a nonirritating volatile agent (halothane or sevoflurane). Patients should be placed in a position that facilitates ventilation (often sitting). After sufficient depth of anesthesia has been obtained, intravenous access should be secured. An antisialagogue is often administered to decrease secretions, which may interfere with visualization of the airway.

If the surgeon wishes to view the vocal cord movement, paralysis is omitted, the vocal cords are sprayed with 2% lidocaine, and the surgeon performs laryngoscopy. Subsequently, a short- or intermediate-acting muscle relaxant is administered, and when paralysis is confirmed, the rigid bronchoscope is passed through the vocal cords and the lower airway is examined. Ventilation may be continued through the side arm of the rigid bronchoscope. It is unwise to pass the rigid bronchoscope through unparalyzed vocal cords because coughing and bucking may lead to tracheal tears, dislocation of the arytenoid cartilage, or laryngospasm. If paralysis has not worn off or been reversed, the patient is intubated and allowed to emerge from anesthesia. If the patient is no longer paralyzed at the conclusion of the procedure, emergence from anesthesia can be supported by mask ventilation of 100% $O_2$.

## LARYNGOTRACHEAL RECONSTRUCTION

### Who Requires Laryngotracheal Reconstruction?

Children who have significant tracheal stenosis may benefit from reconstructive surgery. In the pediatric population, the overwhelming majority of patients are those in whom airway compromise is a result of prolonged intubation. Often, these children were born prematurely and required tracheal intuba-

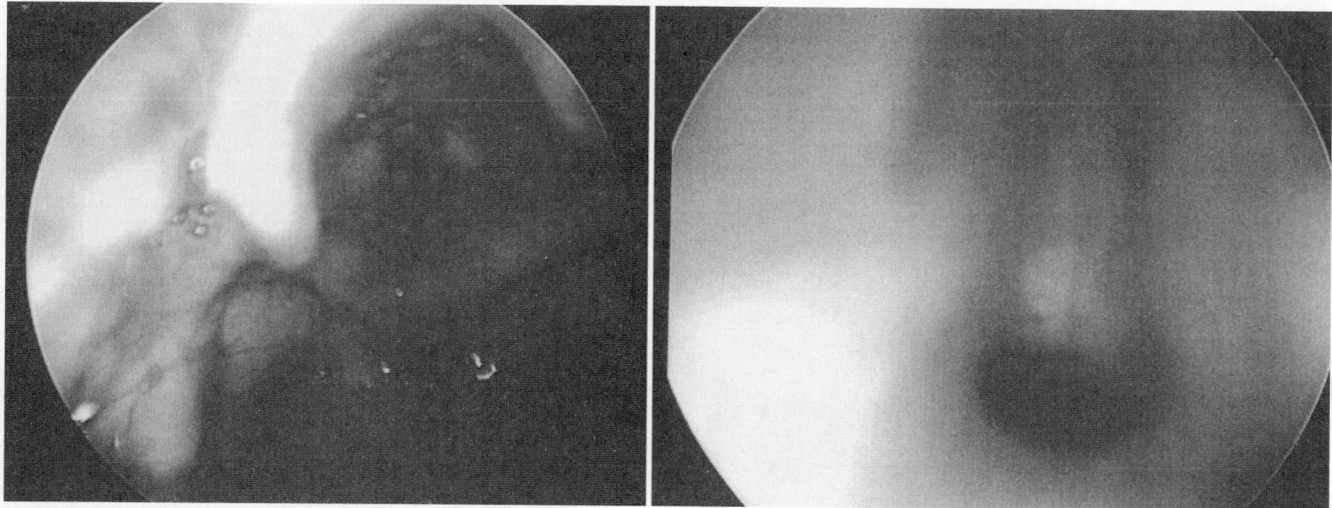

**FIGURE 68–6.** Vocal cords and immediate subglottic trachea in a 4-year-old boy with severe tracheal stenosis secondary to prolonged neonatal intubation.

tion and mechanical ventilation during the neonatal period (Fig. 68–6). In these patients, other problems associated with prematurity (eg, a patent ductus arteriosus, intraventricular hemorrhage) should be explored during the preoperative evaluation. The incidence of tracheal stenosis is between 1% and 8%.[46,47] Mild cases of subglottic stenosis can be managed without tracheotomy. However, in the more severely affected patients, tracheotomy is required to stabilize the airway until the child is ready for reconstructive surgery. Most children with symptomatic subglottic stenosis do not outgrow their stenosis.

## What Is the Best Anesthetic Plan for This Surgical Procedure?

Because most patients have already undergone tracheostomy, anesthetic induction is best accomplished by inhalation of volatile agents through the tracheostomy tube. $N_2O$, $O_2$, and sevoflurane are the most widely used agents for this purpose. Once the patient is anesthetized, a long-acting muscle relaxant is administered and the tracheostomy tube is removed and replaced with a reinforced flexible endotracheal tube that is sutured to the chest wall (Figs. 68–7 and 68–8). If an uncuffed endotracheal tube is chosen, it should be placed in the right mainstem bronchus and then withdrawn until bilateral breath sounds are heard. If a cuffed endotracheal tube is used, it should be inserted into the tracheostomy stoma, inflated, and pulled back until the cuff is just below the stoma. General anesthesia should be maintained with a narcotic-based technique and minimal volatile agent (Fig. 68–9).

Once the posterior wall of the trachea has been augmented with rib graft cartilage, the flexible endotracheal tube is removed and the patient is intubated from above through the vocal cords. In this way, the anterior surface of the trachea can be augmented and the tracheostomy stoma closed. Laryngotracheal reconstruction patients usually remain intubated in the intensive care unit for 3 to 5 days while primary healing of the tracheal suture line around the endotracheal tube stent takes place.

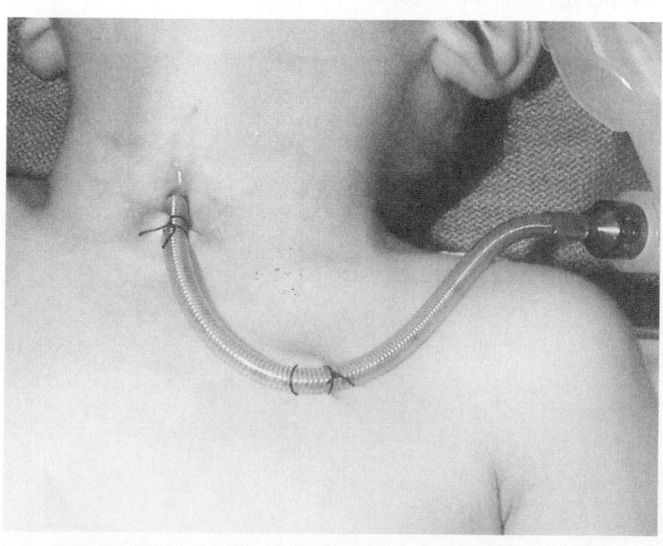

**FIGURE 68–7.** Flexible endotracheal tube sutured to chest wall.

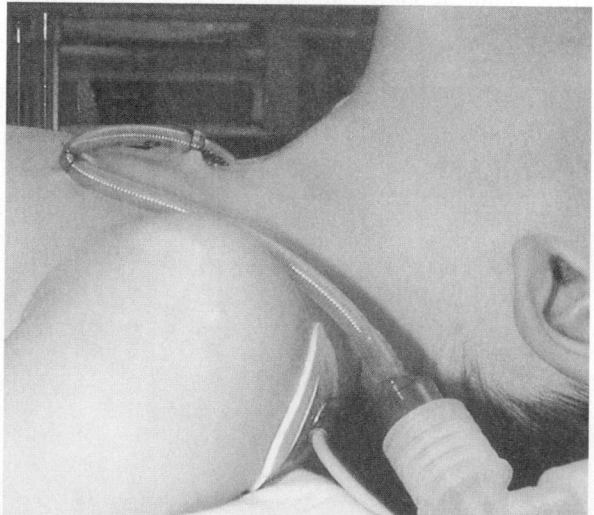

**FIGURE 68–8.** Lateral view of chest wall with endotracheal tube sutured. Note that the tube is secured to one side of the chest to allow a surgical field to be created to harvest rib cartilage for grafting onto the trachea.

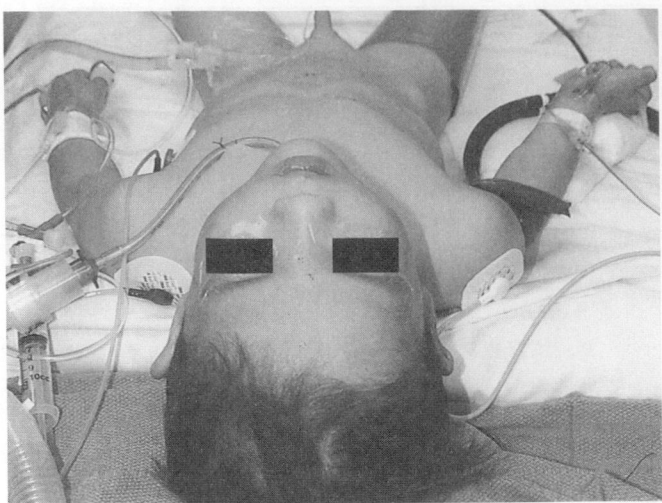

**FIGURE 68–9.** View of fully monitored patient.

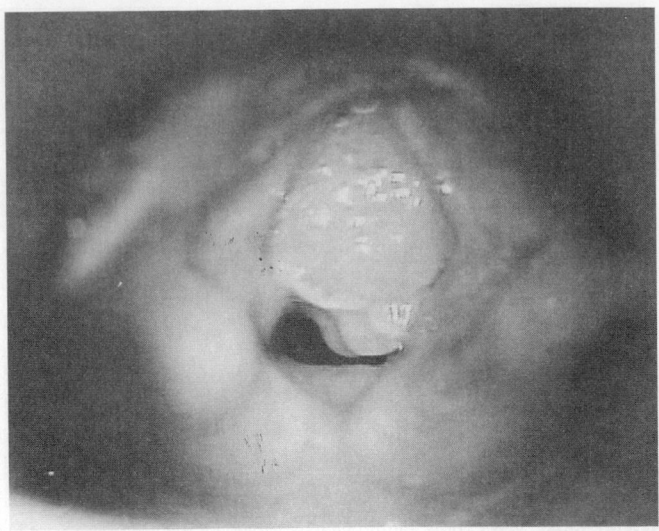

**FIGURE 68–11.** Preoperative view of an untreated laryngeal papilloma in a child.

## What Are the Postoperative Considerations?

Patients remain intubated for several days. Therefore, they should be transported to the intensive care unit after surgery. Coughing and bucking on the endotracheal tube are to be avoided at all costs because the fresh tracheal suture line may be damaged. Patients may be maintained on assisted ventilation with or without paralysis.

The patient returns to the operating room after the fifth postoperative day for a trial extubation. All sedatives, narcotics, and muscle relaxants should be discontinued before arrival in the operating room. General anesthesia is best accomplished with topical administration of 2% lidocaine to the vocal cords and propofol administered by infusion. Avoidance of volatile anesthetic agents is recommended to prevent coughing and agitation during emergence in the newly extubated patient (Fig. 68–10).

## LASER SURGERY

### What Is the Laser and Why Is It Used?

*L*ight *a*mplification by *s*timulated *e*mission of *r*adiation (laser) has been one of the most important modalities in changing the surgical approach to the compromised airway. The laser provides precision in targeting lesions with minimal bleeding and edema, as well as preservation of surrounding structures and rapid healing. It consists of a tube with reflective mirrors at either end and an amplifying medium between them to generate electron activity that results in the production of light. The $CO_2$ laser is the most widely used in medical practice, having particular application in the treatment of laryngeal or vocal cord papillomas, laryngeal webs, resection of redundant subglottic tissue, and coagulation of hemangiomas (Figs. 68–11 and 68–12). Lasers are an especially useful modality for the surgeon because the invisible beam of light provides an unobstructed view of the lesion during resection. The energy emitted by a $CO_2$ laser is absorbed by water, including the water contained in blood and tissues. Human tissue is approximately 80% water, and laser energy absorbed by tissue water rapidly increases the temperature, denaturing protein and causing vaporization of the target tissue. The thermal energy of the laser beam cauterizes capillaries as it vaporizes tissues; therefore, bleeding is minimal and little postoperative edema occurs.[48–50]

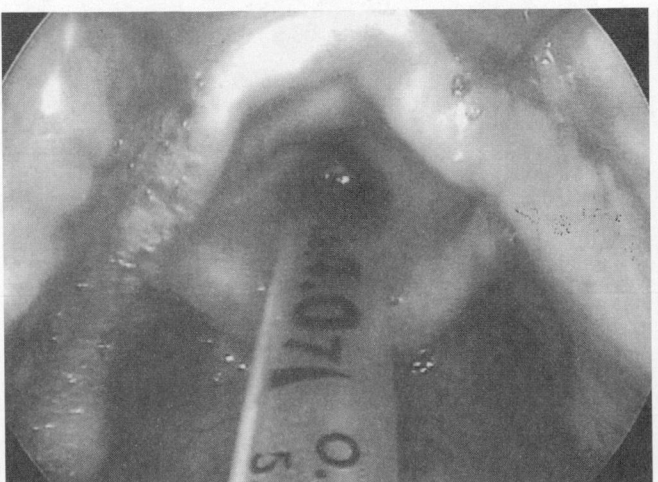
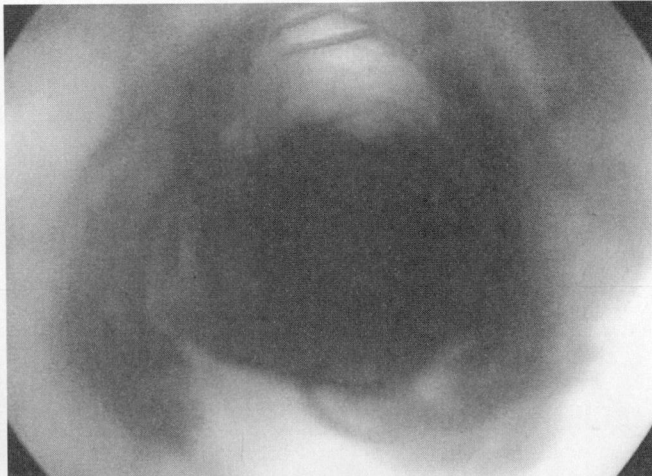

**FIGURE 68–10.** Vocal cords 5 days after surgery with endotracheal tube in place. Note the widened subglottic trachea immediately after extubation.

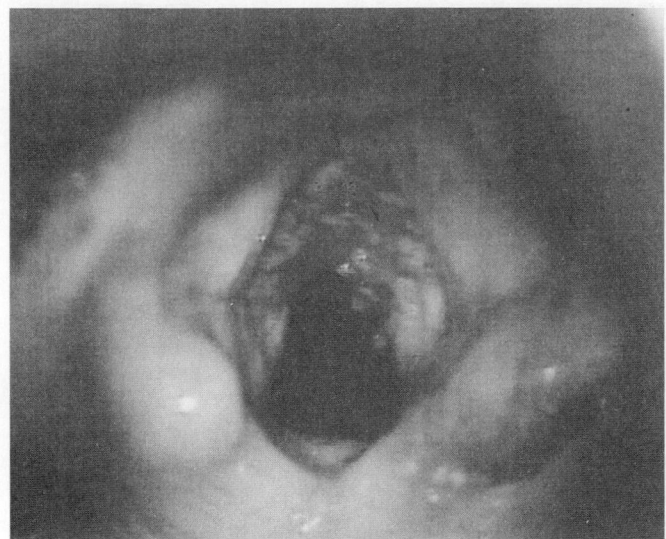

**FIGURE 68–12.** View of the larynx after laser resection of the papilloma seen in Figure 68–11.

## What Are the Risks of Laser Surgery?

A misdirected laser beam may cause injury to a patient or to unprotected operating room personnel. The eyes are especially vulnerable to laser injury, and all operating room personnel should wear laser-specific eye goggles with side protectors to prevent injury. Because of the limited penetration of the $CO_2$ laser, it may cause injury only to the cornea. Other lasers, such as the Nd:YAG, have a deeper penetration and may cause retinal injury and scarring. The eyes of a patient undergoing laser treatment must be protected by taping them shut, followed by the application of wet gauze pads to the eyelids and covering with a metal shield. Any stray beam is absorbed by the wet gauze, preventing penetration of the eyes. Laser radiation increases the temperature of absorbent material, and flammable objects such as surgical drapes must be kept away from the path of the laser beam. Wet towels should be applied to exposed skin of the face and neck when laser is being used in the airway to avoid cutaneous burns from deflected beams. Laser smoke plumes may cause damage to the lungs. The use of specially designed surgical masks for filtering of laser smoke is recommended.

## What Techniques Are Used to Provide Anesthesia for Laser Surgery of the Airway?

Most anesthetic techniques are suitable for laser surgery provided that patients are immobile and the laser beam can be directed at a target that is entirely still and in full view. Because both $N_2O$ and $O_2$ support combustion, the primary gas for anesthetic maintenance should consist of blended air and $O_2$ or helium and $O_2$. A pulse oximeter should be used at all times.[51]

The airway may be managed with an endotracheal tube or without. The choice of endotracheal tube used during laser surgery can affect the safety of the technique. All standard polyvinyl chloride (PVC) endotracheal tubes are flammable and can ignite and vaporize when in contact with the laser beam. Specially manufactured laser-protective endotracheal

tubes should be used, and cuffed endotracheal tubes should be inflated with sterile saline to which methylene blue has been added so that if a laser spark strikes the cuff and burns a hole, it will be readily be detected by the blue dye and extinguished by the saline.[52] The outer diameter of each size of laser-specific endotracheal tube is considerably greater than the PVC counterpart, especially in the small sizes used for pediatric anesthesia. Therefore, other ways of supporting the airway are used.

When the apneic technique is chosen, the child is anesthetized and rendered immobile by the use of a muscle relaxant or deep inhalation of a volatile agent. The trachea is not intubated and the airway is given over to the surgeon, who uses the laser for very brief periods. In between laser applications, the patient is ventilated by mask or intubated briefly. Because apnea is a component of this technique, it is prudent for the patient to be ventilated with 100% $O_2$. There is a potential for debris and resected material to enter the trachea as well as an increased risk of tracheal injury resulting from repeated intubation.

The jet ventilation technique involves the delivery of $O_2$ under pressure through a variable reducing valve.[53] Additional room air is entrained, and the patient is ventilated with this combination of gas. The advantage of this technique is a quiet surgical field because large chest excursions of the diaphragm are eliminated and ventilation of the patient is uninterrupted. In morbidly obese patients and those with severe small airway disease, effective ventilation is not accomplished with this technique and an alternate technique should be used.

Spontaneous ventilation is also possible when a surgical laryngoscope fitted with an $O_2$ insufflation port is inserted into the larynx. The volatile anesthetic gas is mixed with $O_2$ and administered through the side port. Anesthesia is maintained without muscle relaxant in the spontaneously breathing patient in this manner. Infusion of propofol may be supplemented to decrease the concentration of inhaled volatile agent and the vocal cords may be sprayed with 4% lidocaine to decrease reactivity.[54] This technique is advantageous in that long periods of uninterrupted laser application may be provided. Disadvantages include the absence of complete control of the airway, no protection from laryngospasm, and no protection from debris entering the airway. Motion of the vocal cords also is present, and adequate scavenging is difficult.

## AIRWAY EMERGENCIES

### Who Aspirates Foreign Bodies?

The aspiration of a foreign body in the airway is a major cause of accidental death in pediatric patients younger than 1 year of age. A history of coughing or choking while eating should suggest the possibility of foreign body aspiration in a child with a new onset of wheezing (Fig. 68–13). Physical findings include decreased breath sounds, tachypnea, stridor, wheezing, and fever. Few foreign bodies are identifiable on radiologic examination because 90% are radiolucent. However, air trapping, mediastinal shift, and atelectasis may be noted (Fig. 68–14). The most common site of foreign body aspiration is the mainstem bronchus, right more frequently than left.

### How Should the Child Who Has Aspirated a Foreign Body Be Anesthetized?

All aspirated foreign bodies in the airway should be removed in the operating room. The procedure should be considered to be an emergency. No sedation should be administered before removal of the foreign body. If the child has recently eaten, and the airway is severely compromised, full stomach precautions must be taken and anesthesia should be induced intravenously (topical EMLA [eutectic mixture of local anesthetics] cream may be applied to the skin before intravenous insertion in small children) by rapid sequence and gentle cricoid pressure maintained during intubation. If the child has adequate ventilation and oxygenation, anesthesia may be induced by inhalation of 100% $O_2$ and a volatile anesthetic agent by mask. The most commonly used agents are sevoflurane and halothane. Inhalation induction can be prolonged secondary to obstruction of the airway, and $N_2O$ should be avoided to reduce air trapping distal to the obstruction. The surgeon inserts a rigid bronchoscope and removes the aspirated object. Spontaneous ventilation should be preserved until the location and nature of the foreign body have been determined.

Once the foreign body has been removed, examination of the entire tracheobronchial tree is carried out to detect any additional objects or fragments. Often vigorous irrigation and suctioning distal to the obstruction are required to remove

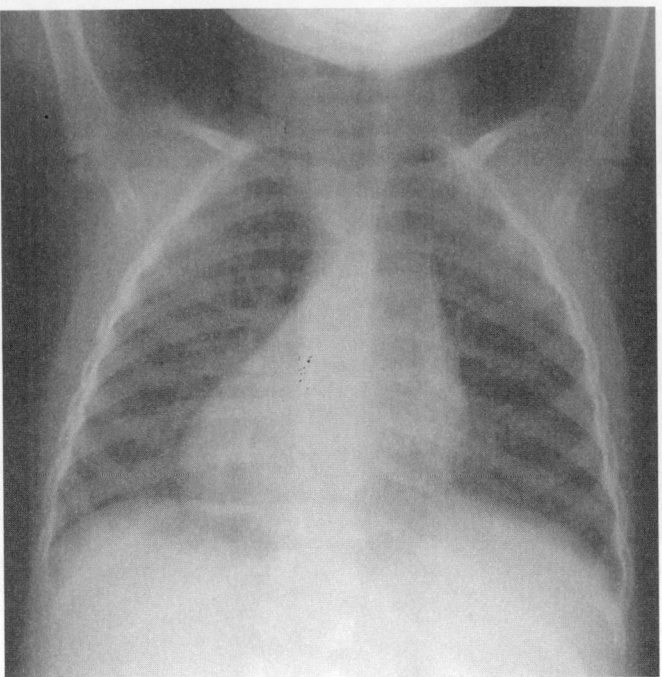

**FIGURE 68–14.** Chest radiograph of the 2-year-old patient seen in Figure 68–13 after aspiration of a peanut fragment. Note the hyperinflation of the right lung and shift of the mediastinum to the left.

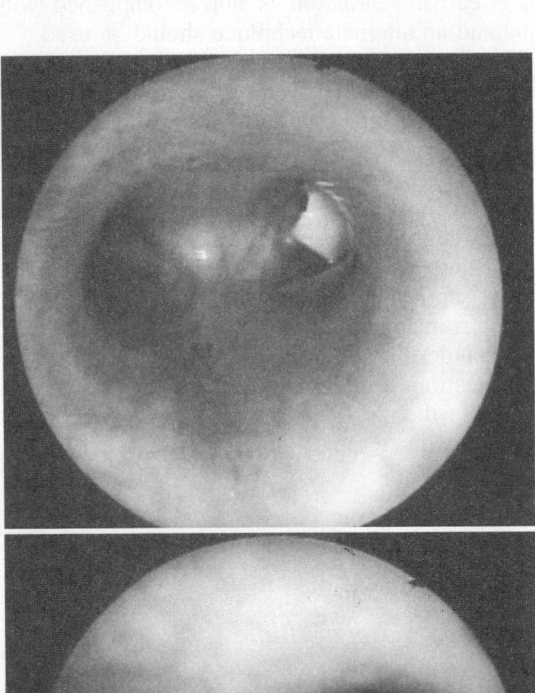

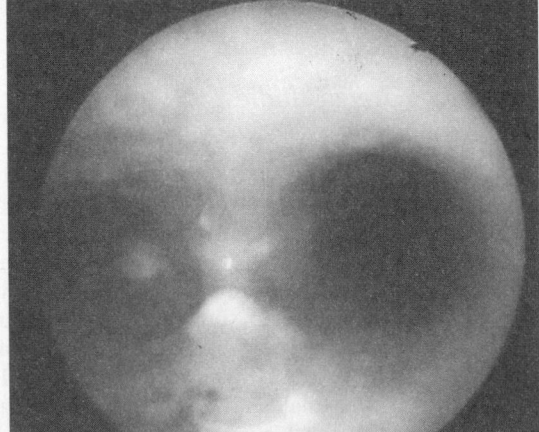

**FIGURE 68–13.** Aspirated peanut fragment in the right mainstem bronchus of a 2-year-old girl. Note the view after bronchoscopic removal of the fragment.

accumulated secretions and prevent the possibility of postobstructive pneumonia. Steroids are administered if inflammation of the airway mucosa is observed. Close postoperative observation of the patient is required so that intervention may be early in the event of respiratory compromise secondary to airway edema or infection, which may ensue.[55]

### What Are the Intraoperative Complications to Avoid?

Hypoxia and hypercarbia due to inadequate ventilation are caused by an excessively large leak around the bronchoscope or, more commonly, by inability to provide adequate gas exchange through a narrow-lumen bronchoscope fitted with an internal telescope. These conditions are remedied by frequent removal of the telescope and withdrawal of the bronchoscope to the midtrachea, allowing effective ventilation to resume. Bronchospasm may occur during examination of the respiratory tract and should be treated with increasing depths of anesthesia, nebulized albuterol, or intravenous bronchodilators. Although rare, pneumothorax should be suspected if acute deterioration during the procedure occurs. Close communication with the surgeon is essential.

## DENTAL REPAIRS IN RETARDED AND UNCOOPERATIVE PATIENTS

### What Problems Should Be Anticipated?

Because of the care and attention needed to maintain good dental hygiene, retarded patients, both children and adults, often have marked deterioration in tooth and gum health and require operative dental repair. Patients may have significant congenital malformations not as readily apparent as the retardation and, of course, may have acquired any disease common to their more fortunate peers. Because retarded patients usually cannot give a satisfactory history, discovery and evaluation of significant alterations in cardiac or pulmonary function that may affect anesthetic management can be difficult and challenging.

### How Is Anesthesia Managed?

If the patient is placid, anesthetic management does not differ markedly from that of a normal child or adult. Unfortunately, retarded patients may be disruptive and even violent, representing a potential danger to themselves and to those who care for them. The sedative medication that a patient takes regularly must be continued into the perioperative period and started again as soon as possible after anesthesia and surgery are completed.

Retarded patients frequently develop a close personal relationship with a parent, friend, or health care worker. This personal associate should be allowed to accompany the patient to the operating room, where his or her presence may have a calming effect that transforms a potentially stormy induction into a more pleasant entry to the anesthetized state.

### Induction Technique

Whenever possible, an intravenous infusion should be initiated before any attempts at anesthetic induction because intravenous agents are usually much better tolerated than attempts at mask induction. The anesthesiologist should not adhere rigidly to definite drugs and dosages for premedication because patients vary considerably in their states of agitation, maintenance medication, and increased metabolic activity secondary to enzyme induction.

Rectal instillation of a barbiturate (eg, thiopental) or short-acting benzodiazepine (eg, midazolam) may have superficial appeal. However, inserting a tube in the rectum is often more difficult and presents greater hazards to the physician or nurse than starting an intravenous infusion.

Oral midazolam is very effective to sedate retarded children. We use 0.5 mg/kg orally in apple juice in the preoperative holding area. Patients are continuously observed and monitored with a pulse oximeter after this premedication.

A further cautionary note is to be aware of gingival hyperplasia. Many of these patients receive phenytoin (Dilantin) to control seizures. Because the gingiva is highly vascular, surgical manipulation may lead to greater than anticipated blood loss.

## CRANIOFACIAL TRAUMA

The facial skeleton is in contact with the cranial skeleton. Because great forces are generated in the mouth during the normal process of mastication, bony buttresses and arches prevent displacement of one skeleton against the other.[56] Horizontal posterior displacement is limited by the zygomatic process of the temporal bone; oblique posterior displacement, by the pterygoid process of the sphenoid bone; and vertical posterior displacement, by the greater wing of the sphenoid

bone. Upward displacement is checked by the zygomatic process of the frontal bone, the nasal part of the frontal bone, and the roof of the mandibular fossa. In addition to the bony buttresses, a series of arches is present in the craniofacial skeleton. The arch created by the zygomatic process of the temporal bone extends through the zygoma to the zygomaticomaxillary suture. Another extends between the head and neck of the mandibular condyle, to the coronoid process.

### What Anatomic Structures Determine the Sites of Fracture?

#### Dispersal of Forces

The buttresses and arches of the craniofacial skeleton redistribute and disperse the forces generated in the oral cavity during chewing and protect the skeleton from displacement or fracture by these forces. A normal vector of force dispersion redistributes physiologic forces and forces resulting from a blow to the face. A blow to the mandible may fracture the jaw at the point of impact or at other points in the bone. The fracture very rarely extends into the cranium because the force follows a normal dispersion vector and is redistributed (Fig. 68–15).

A blow to the face from the front, however, and especially from the front and above, does not follow a normal vector of force dispersion. An abnormal shearing force that may be generated tends to tear the facial skeleton away from the cranium and may extend a fracture into the base of the skull (see Fig. 68–15). The possibility of basilar skull fracture, therefore, must always be considered in the patient with severe midface trauma.[57–62]

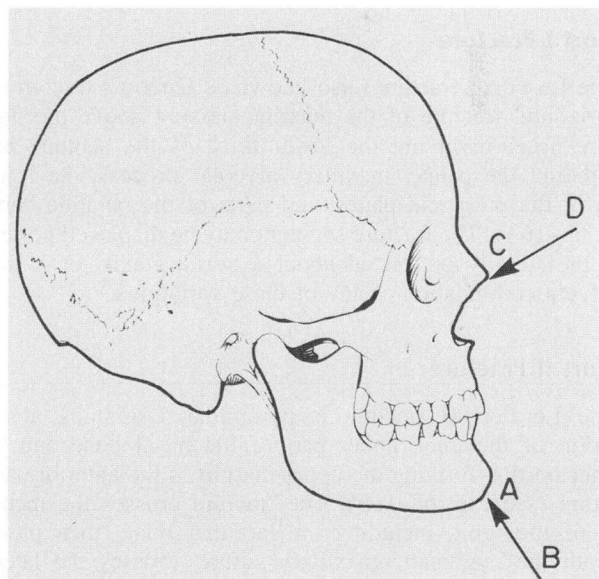

**FIGURE 68–15.** Dispersion of forces in craniofacial trauma. A blow along the line *AB* follows a normal vector of force dispersion and distribution. The mandible may be fractured, but the fracture line does not extend into the skull. A blow along the line *CD* does not follow a normal vector of force dispersion and distribution and generates an abnormal shearing force that may tear the facial skeleton and cranial skeleton. (Reproduced from Gotta AW. Maxillofacial trauma: anesthetic considerations. *ASA Refresh Courses Anesthesiol.* 1987;15:39, with permission.)

## *When Do Mandibular Fractures Occur?*

The mandible is a tubular bone and derives its strength from the bony cortex.[58] It is strongest and least vulnerable to fracture at its anteroinferior border, where the cortex is thickest. The cortex thins, and vulnerability to fracture increases posteriorly. Thus, most fractures of the mandible occur in the ramus. Another common site of fracture is in the body of the mandible at the level of the first or second molar.

The site of fracture is determined to some extent by the nature of the traumatic blow. High-velocity and high-impact types of injuries, such as those produced in an automobile accident, create a high incidence of condylar, subcondylar, and angle of the ramus fractures. Low-velocity, low-impact forces, such as a blow by a fist or fall, tend to produce symphyseal, parasymphyseal, and body fractures. Because of the mandible's unique horseshoe shape, any blow creates shearing forces that tend to fracture it at its weakest points, no matter where the point of impact may be.

## *How Are Facial Fractures Classified?*

Early in the preceding century, Rene Le Fort of Lille, France, published the results of a series of interesting and even bizarre experiments on cadavers and cadaver skulls.[63] Intact cadavers were dropped from a height onto a stone floor, or severed heads were compressed in a vise. The soft tissue was then carefully dissected away to reveal underlying structural damage. Le Fort had two goals: (1) to determine the relationship between soft tissue trauma and fractures of the facial bones, and (2) to ascertain the common lines of fracture of the midface. He noted no pathognomonic soft tissue representation of facial features and delineated the midfacial fractures that bear his name Le Fort I, Le Fort II, and Le Fort III.

### Le Fort I Fracture

The Le Fort I fracture (also known as Guérin's fracture) is a horizontal fracture of the maxilla, passing above the floor of the nose, involving the lower third of the septum, and mobilizing the palate, maxillary alveolar process, the lower third of the pterygoid plates, and parts of the palatine bones (Fig. 68–16*A*). The fracture segment may be displaced posteriorly or laterally or rotated about a vertical axis, or it may involve a combination of any of these variations.

### Le Fort II Fracture

The Le Fort II fracture is pyramidal, beginning at the junction of the thick upper part of the nasal bone and the thinner portion forming the upper margin of the anterior nasal aperture (see Fig. 68–16*B*). The fracture crosses the medial wall of the orbit, including the lacrimal bone, then passes beneath the zygomaticomaxillary suture, crosses the lateral wall of the antrum, and traverses posteriorly through the pterygoid plates.

### Le Fort III Fracture

In a Le Fort III fracture, the midface is separated from the cranium (see Fig. 68–16*C*). The fracture line extends through

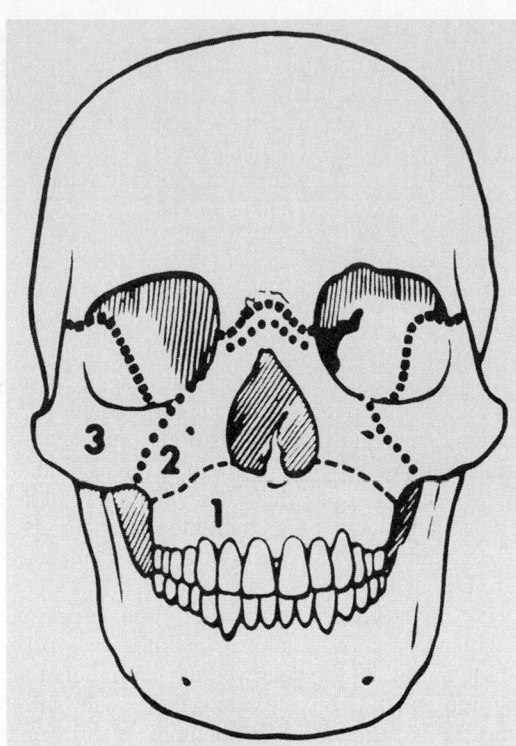

**FIGURE 68–16.** A Le Fort I fracture (1) is a horizontal fracture of the maxilla. A Le Fort II fracture (2) is a pyramidal fracture of the midface, whereas a Le Fort III fracture (3) separates the facial and cranial skeletons. (Reproduced from Gotta AW. Maxillofacial trauma: anesthetic considerations. *ASA Refresh Courses Anesthesiol.* 1987;15:39, with permission.)

the base of the nose and the ethmoid in its depth and through the orbital plates in proximity to the cribriform plate, which may also be fractured. It crosses the lesser wing of the sphenoid and then passes downward to the pterygomaxillary fissure and sphenopalatine fossa. From the base of the inferior orbital fissure, it extends laterally and upward to the frontozygomatic suture and downward and backward to the root of the pterygoid plates. The zygomatic arch of the temporal bone is usually fractured bilaterally.

## *How Do Le Fort Fractures Influence Anesthetic Management?*

### Le Fort I

A Le Fort I fracture usually affords little difficulty for an anesthesiologist. Patients may be intubated orally or nasally, and the airway usually is secured without problem.

### Le Fort II

A Le Fort II fracture involves fracture of the nose and is thus a relative but not absolute contraindication to nasal intubation. Because the force of the blow to the midface necessary to create this type of fracture is substantial, the clinician must always consider the possibility of a concomitant fracture of the base of the skull. Unless this possibility is definitively ruled out by a radiograph or CT scan, nasal intubation of any type should be avoided.

## Le Fort III

Basilar skull fracture is much more likely with a Le Fort III fracture because the ethmoid bone is involved in the fracture line. Although fracture of the cribriform plate of the ethmoid is not *per se* part of the definition of a Le Fort III fracture, it *may* be involved. In such cases, the intracranial subarachnoid space may be open and communicating with the nasal cavity, rendering it vulnerable to false passage of a nasally placed tube (endotracheal or gastric) and infection.

Attempted nasotracheal intubation of a patient with a basilar skull fracture involves the very serious risks of introducing the tube into the skull, dragging contaminated foreign material into the subarachnoid space and causing meningitis. The tube may also inflict severe damage to the brain itself. Even positive-pressure ventilation with bag and mask predisposes to introduction of foreign material into the subarachnoid space.[64]

Clinical signs and findings suggestive of basilar skull fracture are listed in Table 68–6. Whenever a basilar skull fracture is suspected or is confirmed radiologically, nasal intubation is contraindicated.

## What Are the Effects and Implications of Temporomandibular Joint Injuries?

The temporomandibular articulation is a ginglymoarthrodial joint, with a hingelike action allowing flexion and extension in only one plane. Two articulations are present: one is between the condyle and articular disk, and the other is between the disk and the mandibular fossa. Motion of the joint takes place in both parts. As the joint opens, the condyle glides forward (translation of the mandible).

### Technique of Intubation

Patients with maxillofacial trauma may be unable to open their mouths, thus presenting special problems for an anesthesiologist who must intubate the trachea. The most common causes of jaw immobility are pain, trismus, and edema. Pain responds to anesthetics and muscle relaxants and presents no serious problem. Trismus is spasm of the masseter muscles; it also responds similarly. However, the time of fracture, duration of trismus, and prior imposed immobility deserve consideration. If the fracture is more than 2 weeks old, fibrosis is present in the masseter muscles; fibrotic muscles do *not* respond to an anesthetic and muscle relaxant. Edema is rarely so severe that it presents a major challenge. However, awake intubation *must* be considered.

### Functional Impairment

Several fractures may directly cause impairment of the TMJ. Mechanical dysfunction of the joint does not respond to anesthetics and relaxants, and proven or suspected mechanical

**TABLE 68–6.** Clinical Signs and Findings Suggestive of Basilar Skull Fracture

| |
|---|
| Blood behind a tympanic membrane |
| Periocular ecchymosis ("raccoon eyes") |
| Predisposing facial fracture (Le Fort II or III) |

**TABLE 68–7.** Incidence of Other Injuries Associated With Maxillofacial Trauma

| Injury | High Velocity (Vehicular) | Low Velocity (Personal) |
|---|---|---|
| Major (life-threatening) | 32% | 4% |
| Minor | 31% | 10.5% |

From Luce EA. Review of 1,000 major facial fractures and associated injuries. *Plast Reconstruct Surg.* 1979;63:26.

impairment necessitates awake intubation. If the condyle is fractured, TMJ function may be disrupted by bony fragments in the joint. A fracture of the zygomatic arch of the temporal bone drives fractured segments onto the coronoid process, limiting translation of the mandible. The zygomatic arch is well protected by the temporalis fascia, which splits into two leaves, lateral and medial, thus enveloping the arch. However, a blow to the side of the head from above may be powerful enough to rupture this membrane and fracture the bone. TMJ dysfunction must be considered in any displaced fracture of the zygomatic arch.

## What Are the Most Frequent Associated Injuries?

The nature and incidence of associated injuries in patients with maxillofacial trauma depend on the nature of the inciting force. In one study that compared high-velocity, high-impact forces with low-velocity, low-impact forces, both major and minor associated injuries were significantly higher in high-velocity injuries (Table 68–7).

### Cervical Spine

Perhaps most vexing to anesthesiologists is trauma to the cervical spine that injures the spinal cord or puts it at risk during the perioperative period. Radiographs of the cervical spine are indicated for any suspicion of cervical spine injury (pain or tenderness in the neck, loss of consciousness, or neurologic signs and symptoms indicative of spinal injury). Practitioners should always err on the conservative side and order too many "negative" radiographs rather than miss a cervical spine injury.

Tracheal intubation of patients with cervical spine injury risks further and often irreparable damage to the spinal cord. In one study of 2555 patients with facial skeletal trauma, 32 patients (1.3%) sustained cervical spine injury. Of these, 11 (34%) were unstable.[65] In patients with mandibular fracture, associated injuries were varied[66] (Table 68–8).

## AWAKE TRACHEAL INTUBATION

### What General Concepts Are Applicable?

Nasotracheal intubation is relatively (but not absolutely) contraindicated in patients with a nasal fracture. The greater the degree of deformity, the greater is the contraindication. Basilar skull fracture is a contraindication to nasotracheal intubation. In instances of severe fracture-deformity of the

**TABLE 68–8.** Mandibular Fractures: Associated Injuries

| Type of Injury | Number | Percentage |
| --- | --- | --- |
| Facial fracture | 70 | 35 |
| Intracranial | 30 | 15 |
| Cervical spine (fracture-dislocation) | 12 | 6 |
| Extremity | 42 | 21 |
| Chest | 27 | 14 |
| Abdominal | 6 | 3 |
| Airway problem | 13 | 6 |

From Busuito MJ, Smith DJ, Robson MC. Mandibular fractures in an urban trauma center. *J Trauma*. 1986;26:826. © Williams & Wilkins, 1986.

nose or basilar skull fracture, the route of choice is oral intubation or, if this approach is not feasible, tracheotomy.

Nasotracheal intubation is the preferred technique with mandibular fractures requiring internal fixation because the fixation apparatus cannot be closed over an oral tube. If nasal intubation is not feasible and tracheotomy is undesirable, it may be possible for the fixation apparatus to be placed, but not closed with wires, until the patient is awake and the oral tube is removed.

## How Is the Patient Prepared?

Placement of a rather large plastic endotracheal tube into an awake patient's airway is a formidable and unpleasant task. The larynx is designed to prevent entry of foreign material, and the protective reflexes are acute and potent.

### Topical Anesthesia

The nose, mouth, and oropharynx can be anesthetized with topically applied local anesthetics. The first step is to administer atropine or glycopyrrolate. If the oropharyngeal mucosa is not relatively dry, topical anesthesia is impaired by dilution and diffusion across the saliva to the tissues. Inhalation of vaporized lidocaine has been recommended as an effective technique to anesthetize the airway. Our experience suggests that this method is neither as dependable nor as effective as direct topical application coupled with bilateral superior laryngeal nerve block.

### Cocaine

Local anesthetics may be applied by anesthetic-soaked cotton pledgets in the nose. Cocaine is an especially useful agent because it is a potent topical anesthetic and the only one that, in conventional concentrations (2%-4%), is also a vasoconstrictor.[67] However, cocaine has an illicit value that makes its storage hazardous. Also, cocaine is toxic. Although the toxic dose is usually calculated at approximately 200 mg in an adult, serious toxicity has resulted from as little as 50 mg.

### Lidocaine

We favor lidocaine, 2% to 4%, to which is added a few drops of phenylephrine hydrochloride (0.25%) or oxymetazoline (0.05%) for vasoconstriction. This combination of drugs has neither the street value nor the toxicity of cocaine. Atomizers are unreliable and do not produce a uniform dose. We

suggest drawing the anesthetic into a syringe and squirting it into the nose and mouth. Anesthesiologists commonly forgo application of local anesthetic in the mouth, especially if the jaw is wired shut, but local anesthetic can be injected past the wires through an intravenous catheter without difficulty.

## What Is the Sensory Innervation of the Larynx?

Innervation of the larynx is provided by the superior laryngeal nerve, a branch of the vagus nerve derived from the nodose ganglion. It travels with the main trunk of the nerve to the level of the larynx, where it angles forward and terminates in internal (sensory) and external (motor) branches.[68] The external branch penetrates and innervates the cricothyroid muscle, a tensor of the vocal cords. The internal branch penetrates the thyrohyoid membrane and ramifies immediately, providing sensory innervation from the base of the tongue to the vocal cords. After penetrating the thyrohyoid membrane, the nerve rests in a closed space bounded superiorly by the inferior surface of the hyoid bone, inferiorly by the superior edge of the thyroid cartilage, medially by the laryngeal mucosa, and laterally by the thyrohyoid membrane (Fig. 68–17).

## How Is the Superior Laryngeal Nerve Blocked?

The nerve can be blocked by placing a needle in the closed space and depositing a local anesthetic.[69] The landmarks are

1. The hyoid bone, a freely movable bone in the upper neck that articulates with no other bone (see Fig. 68–17)
2. The thyroid cartilage
3. The thyrohyoid membrane, which binds the two together

A patient's head should be extended to maximize the distance between the hyoid and thyroid cartilages. A 22- or 23-gauge needle attached to a syringe containing 2 mL of 2% lidocaine is directed at the hyoid, parallel to the coronal plane. When the needle strikes the bone, a characteristic gritty feeling may be appreciated. The sensation is like that felt

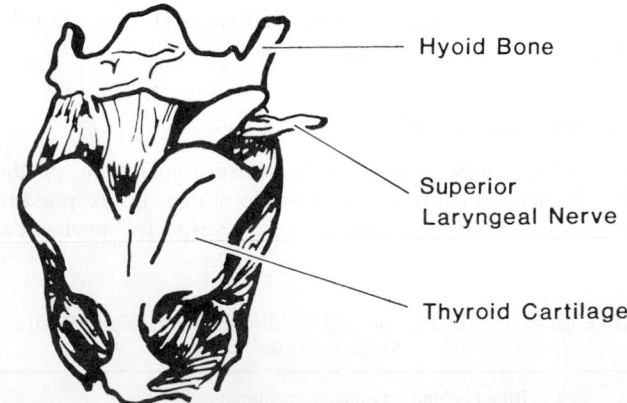

**FIGURE 68–17.** Anatomic relationships of the superior laryngeal nerve, hyoid bone, and thyroid cartilage.

during an intercostal block when the rib is struck. The needle is then "walked" caudad, until it slips off the bone and through the thyrohyoid membrane. Aspiration should yield nothing, at which point the anesthetic may be injected and the block repeated on the opposite side. If air is aspirated, the needle is in the larynx; blood indicates penetration of a blood vessel, such as one of the major structures in the carotid sheath, the carotid artery, or the internal jugular vein. The superior laryngeal artery is also close by.

### Contraindications

Contraindications to a superior laryngeal nerve block include (1) a full stomach because the block will ablate protective laryngeal reflexes, (2) infection at the site of the block, and (3) tumor at the site of the block. We consider these to be relative, not absolute, contraindications that necessitate careful, individual, case-by-case assessment of risk versus benefit. With a full stomach, if there is trained help, good suction, and a mobile table, benefit often exceeds risk.

### Complications

Complications of the block include intravascular injection of local anesthetic with subsequent seizure. The only other complication we have personally witnessed is one instance of a small, easily contained hematoma.

### Why Not Block the Recurrent Laryngeal Nerves?

Sensory innervation of the trachea is provided by the recurrent laryngeal nerves. Because these nerves also provide motor innervation of the intrinsic muscle of the larynx, their block risks acute airway closure and is contraindicated.

### How Is Translaryngeal Analgesia Obtained?

Sensory analgesia can be provided by translaryngeal application of local anesthetic. The cricothyroid membrane is identified in the midline. Major neural or vascular structures are absent in this area, and penetration of the membrane entails no great risk. A 22-gauge needle attached to a syringe containing 4 mL of 2% lidocaine is thrust through the membrane until air is freely aspirated. The patient is instructed to inhale deeply and then exhale maximally. At the end of expiration, the lidocaine is rapidly injected, and the needle removed from the neck. Local anesthetic striking the carina stimulates a vigorous cough that sprays droplets along the trachea and the inferior surface of the vocal cords. The procedure should be done using both hands to steady the syringe and needle. When the inevitable cough occurs, the needle can be rapidly withdrawn so that it does not lacerate or puncture the posterior tracheal wall.

### Can the Airway Be Anesthetized by Inhalation of Local Anesthetic?

As a supplement to, but not as an alternative, superior laryngeal and translaryngeal block, the patient may inhale nebulized local anesthetic. This technique requires the patient's cooperation because the agent must be inhaled for at least 20 minutes, with deep breaths to allow precipitation of the anesthetic into the deeper recesses of the airway. Pain may limit cooperation.

### Is There a Risk of Local Anesthetic Overdose?

The amount of local anesthetic causing toxicity is controversial and the limits applied are arbitrary and unscientific.[70] Toxic reaction is less likely due to overdose than to intravascular injection. The anesthesiologist has the option of choosing that dose he or she thinks toxic and then manipulating the drug concentration and amount to keep within this arbitrary limit.

## ALTERNATIVE TECHNIQUES TO SECURE THE AIRWAY

Occasionally, the airway must be secured quickly, often under suboptimal conditions. This situation is most likely to occur with severe crush injury of the face or massive destruction such as that caused by a shotgun blast.

### What Is a Bimandibular Fracture?

Particularly dangerous is a bimandibular fracture, in which the body of the mandible has been fractured on both sides.[71] If the distal fracture segment is mobilized, it may be distracted posteroinferiorly by the muscles of the floor of the mouth (genioglossus, mylohyoid, and digastric). As the fracture segment is distracted, it brings with it the tongue and paraglottic soft tissues, pushing them into the upper airway and causing severe and even complete airway obstruction.

Because of the characteristic foreshortening of the mandible associated with this injury, it is sometimes known as an *Andy Gump fracture* after the popular comic strip character with a hypoplastic mandible. If the airway is stable, awake intubation may be attempted. But, if the airway is compromised, awake intubation may prove unsuccessful and a surgical airway (tracheostomy or cricothyroidotomy) must be secured. If surgical help is not readily available, gentle, but forceful, anterior traction on the mandible may reduce the fracture and reestablish a patent airway.

### What Problems Are Associated With Emergency Airway Management?

In any instance of acute upper airway closure, when oral or nasal intubation is either contraindicated or has failed, the airway must be secured by tracheotomy, cricothyroidotomy, or translaryngeal ventilation. Emergency tracheotomy in a patient struggling furiously for every breath is harrowing, difficult, and sometimes impossible. Operative or percutaneous cricothyroidotomy through the cricothyroid membrane may be performed more quickly but should be converted to a tracheotomy within 24 to 48 hours.

## When Are Fiberoptic Techniques Indicated?

Fiberoptic intubation techniques should be considered whenever a patient must be intubated awake. The indication is relative, not absolute, because awake intubation may be effected under direct vision or even blindly. However, fiberoptic techniques are difficult after failed attempts at awake blind nasal intubation because of nasopharyngeal trauma, coupled with epistaxis, erythema, edema, and secretions.

If serious doubt exists about the feasibility of awake intubation under direct vision, fiberoptic visualization and intubation are indicated and should be tried first. Awake intubation is mandated with dysfunction of the TMJ that locks the jaw shut, fibrosis of the masseter muscles after prolonged trismus, or immobilization of the jaw. Extensive facial trauma with anatomic distortion, hemorrhage, erythema, and edema often makes fiberoptic techniques impossible.

Failed fiberoptic techniques should never be followed by administration of anesthetic agents and muscle relaxants in an attempt to visualize the airway. To do so entails the very serious risk of failure to intubate and ventilate. Failed fiberoptic techniques mandate awake intubation under direct visualization, if possible, or tracheotomy, if necessary.

## Why Not Take an Awake Look?

Visualizing the larynx of an awake patient in an attempt to determine if it is safe to anesthetize and intubate the patient is a technique fraught with peril. The muscle tone and respiration of the awake patient may help to identify the larynx, but these aids are lost in the anesthetized patient. If a difficult intubation is anticipated and the awake look visualizes the larynx, an endotracheal tube should be placed immediately.

## What Is the Role of the Laryngeal Mask Airway in Head and Neck Surgery?

In an emergency situation—cannot intubate, cannot ventilate—any technique that may secure the airway must be used. In a nonemergency situation, the currently available laryngeal mask airway modes are of limited utility. They have been used successfully in tonsillectomy and may be useful in myringotomy, but radical surgery or trauma surgery demands a well-protected airway secure from the entrance of blood or pus. This goal can be obtained only by oral or nasotracheal intubation with a cuffed tube or by a surgical airway. The laryngeal mask airway often provides inadequate seal and protection of the lower airway.[72,73]

## What Are the Indications for Tracheotomy?

Tracheotomy is occasionally necessary in cases of severe maxillofacial trauma. In most instances of Le Fort III fractures, tracheotomy is performed. Indications include (1) severe anatomic distortion that makes oral or nasotracheal intubation impossible, (2) airway obstruction when oral or nasotracheal intubation is impossible, and (3) basilar skull fracture when oral intubation is not feasible because of the surgical technique or approach. Basilar skull fracture is a contraindication to nasotracheal intubation. If, in the presence of basilar skull fracture, the surgeon cannot work with an oral tube in place, tracheotomy is the most prudent choice.

## How Should a Patient Whose Jaw Is Wired Be Extubated?

Extubation of a patient whose jaw is wired demands judgment about timing, available equipment, and a suitable plan for reintubation or securing the airway in another manner, on an emergent basis. An oral surgeon or otolaryngologist should be immediately available to cut the wires if necessary. In addition, equipment to perform translaryngeal jet ventilation should be at the bedside. A tracheotomy set should also be readily available.

If extensive edema is present, particularly near the angle of the jaw, extubation should be deferred for at least 24 hours. One useful technique is to insert a fiberoptic bronchoscope through the endotracheal tube and then to remove the tube over the bronchoscope, leaving the bronchoscope in the larynx and trachea. Should intubation become necessary, the bronchoscope is already in place and the tube can be reinserted expeditiously. This technique should be used only with nasotracheal extubation so that the patient cannot bite and damage the fiberoptic bronchoscope. An alternative approach, which must be used with orotracheal intubation, is to extubate the patient over a ventilating tube changer. Before extubation, it is necessary to ensure that patients are awake, reactive, and responsive to verbal commands and that they meet all criteria for removal of ventilatory support.

## References

1. Liu L, DeCook C, Goudsouzian N, et al. Dose response to intramuscular succinylcholine in children. *Anesthesiology.* 1981;55:599.
2. Goudsouzian N. Relaxants in pediatric anesthesia. *Clin Anesthesiol.* 1985;3:539.
3. McGoldrick K. Anesthesia for elective ENT surgery. In: McGoldrick K, ed. *Anesthesia for Ophthalmic and Otolaryngologic Surgery.* Philadelphia, Pa: WB Saunders; 1992:97.
4. Berkowitz R, Zalzal G. Tonsillectomy in children under 3 years of age. *Arch Otolaryngol Head Neck Surg.* 1990;116:685.
5. Deutsch ES. Tonsillectomy and adenoidectomy: changing indications. *Pediatr Clin North Am.* 1996;43:1319.
6. Guilleminault C. Obstructive sleep apnea: the clinical syndrome and historical perspective. *Med Clin North Am.* 1985;69:1187.
7. Eisenberg J, Clarke J, Sussman S. Prothrombin and partial thromboplastin times as preoperative screening tests. *Arch Surg.* 1982;117:48.
8. Rohrer J, Michelotti M, Nahrwold D. Prospective evaluation of the efficacy of preoperative coagulation testing. *Ann Surg.* 1988;208:554.
9. Chaban R, Cole P, Hoffstein V. Site of upper airway obstruction in patients with idiopathic obstructive sleep apnea. *Laryngoscope.* 1988;98:641.
10. Smith R, Gonzalez C. The relationship between nasal obstruction and craniofacial growth. *Pediatr Clin North Am.* 1989;36:1423.
11. O'Connor M, Drasner K. Preoperative laboratory testing of children undergoing elective surgery. *Anesth Analg.* 1990;70:176.
12. Baron M, Gunter J, White P. Is the pediatric preoperative hematocrit determination necessary? *South Med J.* 1992;85:1187.
13. Berry F. Preoperative assessment and general management of outpatients. *Int Anesthesiol Clin.* 1982;20:3.
14. Burk C, Miller L, Handler S, et al. Preoperative history and coagulation screening in children undergoing tonsillectomy. *Pediatrics.* 1992;89:691.
15. Gabriel P, Eccofey P, Mazoit X. Relationship between clinical history, coagulation tests and bleeding during tonsillectomy in children. *Anesthesiology.* 1996;69:A1281.
16. Brown O, Manning S, Ridenour B. Cor pulmonale secondary to tonsillar

and adenoidal hypertrophy: management considerations. *Int J Pediatr Otorhinolaryngol.* 1988;16:138.

17. Khine H, Corddry D, Kettrick R, et al. Comparison of cuffed and uncuffed endotracheal tubes in young children during general anesthesia. *Anesthesiology.* 1997;86:627.

18. Judkins J, Dray T, Hubbell R. Intraoperative ketorolac and posttonsillectomy bleeding. *Arch Otolaryngol Head Neck Surg.* 1996;122:932.

19. Goldsher M, Podoshin L, Fradis M, et al. Effects of peritonsillar infiltration on posttonsillectomy pain. *Ann Otol Rhinol Laryngol.* 1996;105:868.

20. Guida R, Mattucci K. Tonsillectomy and adenoidectomy: an inpatient or outpatient procedure? *Laryngoscope.* 1990;100:491.

21. Brown O, Cunningham M. Tonsillectomy and adenoidectomy inpatient guidelines: recommendations of the AAO-HNS Pediatric Otolaryngology Committee. *Am Acad Otolaryngol Head Neck Surg Bull.* September 1996:36.

22. Feinberg A, Shabino C. Acute pulmonary edema complicating tonsillectomy and adenoidectomy. *Pediatrics.* 1985;75:112.

23. Galvis A, Stool S, Bluestone C. Pulmonary edema following relief of acute upper airway obstruction. *Ann Otol.* 1980;89:124.

24. Jebeles J, Reilly J, Gutierrez J, et al. Tonsillectomy and adenoidectomy pain reduction by local bupivacaine infiltration in children. *Int J Pediatr Otorhinolaryngol.* 1993;25:149.

25. Davis I, Moore J, Lahiri S. Nitrous oxide and the middle ear. *Anaesthesia.* 1978;34:147.

26. Owens W, Gustave F, Sclaroff A. Tympanic membrane rupture with nitrous oxide anesthesia. *Anesth Analg.* 1978;57:283.

27. Armstrong H, Hein J. The effect of flight on the middle ear. *JAMA.* 1937;109:417.

28. Patterson M, Bartlett P. Hearing impairment caused by intratympanic pressure changes during general anesthesia. *Laryngoscope.* 1976;86:399.

29. Waun N, Sweitzer R, Hamilton W. Effect of nitrous oxide on middle ear mechanics and hearing acuity. *Anesthesiology.* 1967;28:846.

30. Kerr A. Anesthesia with profound hypotension for middle ear surgery. *Br J Anaesth.* 1977;49:477.

31. Eltringham R, Young P, Fairburn M, et al. Hypotensive anesthesia for microsurgery of the middle ear: a comparison between enflurane and halothane. *Anaesthesia.* 1982;37:1028.

32. Crysdale W, Russell D. Complications of tonsillectomy and adenoidectomy in 9409 children observed overnight. *CMAJ.* 1986;135:1139.

33. Chaing T, Sukis A, Ross D. Tonsillectomy performed on an outpatient basis: report of a series of 40,000 bases without a death. *Acta Otolaryngol.* 1968;88:105.

34. Goudsouzian N, Miler V. Anesthesia for plastic surgery in children. In: Abadir A, Humayun S, eds. *Anesthesia for Plastic and Reconstructive Surgery.* St Louis, Mo: Mosby–Year Book; 1991:211.

35. Johnston R, Eger E, Wilson C. A comparative interaction of epinephrine with enflurane, isoflurane and halothane in man. *Anesth Analg.* 1976;55:709.

36. Tucker W, Packstein A, Munson E. Comparison of arrhythmic doses of adrenaline, metaraminol, ephedrine, and phenylephrine during isoflurane and halothane anesthesia in dogs. *Br J Anaesth.* 1974;46:392.

37. McCain JP, Sander B, Koslin MG, et al. Temporomandible joint arthroscopy: a 6 year multicenter retrospective study of 4,831 joints. *J Oral Maxillofac Surg.* 1992;15:926.

38. Kinney RK, Gatchel RJ, Ellis E, et al. Major psychological disorders in chronic TMD patients. *J Am Dent Assoc.* 1992;123:49.

39. Hendler BH, Levin LM. Postobstructive pulmonary edema as a sequela of temporomandibular joint arthroscopy: a case report. *J Oral Maxillofac Surg.* 1993;51:315.

40. Burke J. Angina ludovici: a translation, together with a biography of Wilhelm Frederick von Ludwig. *Bull Hist Med.* 1939;7:1115.

41. Patterson HC, Kelly JH, Strome M. Ludwig's angina: an update. *Laryngoscope.* 1982;92:370.

42. Loughnan TE, Allen DE. Ludwig's angina. The anesthetic management of nine cases. *Anaesthesia.* 1985;40:295.

43. Allen D, Loughman TE, Ord RA. A re-evaluation of the role of tracheostomy in Ludwig's angina. *J Oral Maxillofac Surg.* 1985;43:436.

44. Har-El G, Aroesty JH, Shaha A, et al. Changing trends in deep neck abscess: a retrospective study of 110 patients. *Oral Surg Oral Med Oral Pathol.* 1994;77:446.

45. Jordan W, Graves C, Elwyn R. A new therapy for postintubation laryngeal edema and tracheitis (croup) in children. *JAMA.* 1970;212:585.

46. Marshak G, Grundfast K. Subglottic stenosis. *Pediatr Clin North Am.* 1982;28:941.

47. Ratner I, Whitfield J. Acquired subglottic stenosis in the very low birthweight infant. *Am J Dis Child.* 1983;137:40.

48. Lu J. Lasers in medicine: implications for the anesthesiologist. In: Lake C, ed. *Advances in Anesthesiology.* St louis, Mo: Mosby; 1994:113.

49. Ferrari L, Vasallo S. Anesthesia for otorhinolaryngology procedures. In: Cote C, Ryan J, Todres I, et al, eds. *A Practice of Anesthesia for Infants and Children.* Philadelphia, Pa: WB Saunders; 1992:318.

50. Hermens J, Bennett M, Hirshman C. Anesthesia for laser surgery. *Anesth Analg.* 1983;62:218.

51. McLeskey C. Anesthetic management of patients undergoing laser surgery. In: *IARS Review Course Lectures.* Cleveland, Ohio: International Anesthesia Research Society; 1988;135.

52. Sosis M, Dillon F. Saline-filled cuffs help prevent laser-induced polyvinylchloride endotracheal tube fires. *Anesth Analg.* 1991;72:187.

53. Weeks D. Laboratory and clinical description of the use of jet-Venturi ventilator during laser microsurgery of the glottis and subglottis. *Anesth Rev.* 1985;12:32.

54. Quintal M, Ferrari L, Cunningham M. Tubeless spontaneous respiration technique for pediatric microlaryngeal surgery. *Arch Otolaryngol Head Neck Surg.* 1997;123:209.

55. Ferrari L. Anesthesia for pediatric ENT surgery, routine and emergent. *ASA Refresh Course Lect.* 1996;24:57.

56. Gotta AW. Maxillofacial trauma: anesthetic considerations. *ASA Refresh Courses Anesthesiol.* 1987;15:39.

57. Gotta AW. Management of the traumatized airway. *ASA Refresh Courses Anesthesiol.* 1995;23:103.

58. Haskell R. Applied surgical anatomy. In: Rowe NL, Williams JL, eds. *Maxillofacial Injuries.* Edinburgh, United Kingdom: Churchill Livingstone; 1985:3.

59. Huelke DF. Mechanics in the production of mandibular fractures: a study of the "stress coat" technique, I: symphyseal impacts. *J Dent Res.* 1961;40:1042.

60. Huelke DF, Patrick LM. Mechanics in the production of mandibular fractures: strain-gauge measurements of impacts to the chin. *J Dent Res.* 1964;43:437.

61. Halazonetis JA. The weak regions of the mandible. *Br J Oral Surg.* 1968;6:37.

62. Hahum AM. The biomechanics of facial bone fracture. *Laryngoscope.* 1975;85:140.

63. Le Fort R. Etude experimentale sur les fractures de la machoire superieure. *Rev Chir.* 1901;23:208, 360, 479.

64. Kitahata L, Collins W. Meningitis as a complication of anesthesia in a patient with a basal skull fracture. *Anesthesiology.* 1970;32:282.

65. Davidson J, Birdsell D. Cervical spine injury in patients with facial skeletal trauma. *J Trauma.* 1989;29:1276.

66. Busuito M, Smith D, Robson M. Mandibular fractures in an urban trauma center. *J Trauma.* 1986;26:826.

67. Ritchie J, Cohen P. Cocaine, procaine and other synthetic local anesthetics. In: Goodman L, Gilman A, eds. *The Pharmacological Basis of Therapeutics.* New York, NY: Macmillan; 1975:338.

68. Durhan CF, Harrison TS. The surgical anatomy of the superior laryngeal nerve. *Surg Gynecol Obstet.* 1964;118:38.

69. Gotta AW, Sullivan CA. Superior laryngeal nerve block: an aid to intubating the patient with fractured mandible. *J Trauma.* 1984;24:83.

70. Scott DB. Maximum recommended dose of local anaesthetic drugs. *Br J Anaesth.* 1989;63:373.

71. Seshul MB, Sinn DP, Gerlock AJ. The Andy Gump fracture of the mandible: a cause of respiratory obstruction or distress. *J Trauma.* 1978;18:611.

72. Bailey P, Brimacombe JR, Keller C. The flexible LMA: literature consideration and practical guide. *Int Anesthesiol Clin.* 1998;36:111.

73. Ferson DZ, Brimacombe J, Brain AIJ, et al. The intubating laryngeal mask airway. *Int Anesthesiol Clin.* 1998;36:183.

# 69

# Neurologic Surgery

Michael E. Mahla

In neuroanesthesia, unlike other subspecialties of anesthesiology, the organ system involved with the surgical procedure is also the primary site of action of the hypnotic, analgesic, and amnestic effects of anesthetic drugs. This distinction is important for two reasons. First, anesthetic drugs have profound effects on central nervous system (CNS) function and may alter homeostatic mechanisms such as autoregulation or the vascular response to carbon dioxide ($CO_2$). In addition, measurable parameters, such as cerebral blood flow (CBF), cerebral blood volume (CBV), and cerebral metabolism

(CMRo$_2$), may be changed. Because of these effects, anesthetic drugs have the potential to alter unfavorably blood flow and intracranial pressure (ICP). If CNS pathology already has altered ICP and CBF, further drug-induced changes or even drug-induced vital sign changes may cause permanent damage independently of the surgical procedure.

Second, the normal effects of drugs that we use may be difficult to distinguish from the signs and symptoms produced by many different types of CNS pathology. For example, distinguishing between unresponsiveness produced by residual levels or isoflurane, fentanyl, and pancuronium and the unresponsiveness produced by inadvertent interruption of the middle cerebral artery following aneurysm clipping can be difficult but is vitally important. The effects of anesthetic drugs eventually dissipate without harm. Loss of blood supply to the frontal, parietal, and temporal lobes, however, has long-term devastating effects that often are not reversible. Thus, an important goal of neuroanesthesia is that the hypnotic effects of anesthetic drugs should dissipate rapidly at the conclusion of the operation to allow early assessment of neurologic function and rapid detection of potentially reversible surgical problems.

## NEUROPHYSIOLOGY AND NEUROPHARMACOLOGY

### Do Anesthetics or Adjunctive Drugs and Techniques Influence Outcome?

No prospective randomized or retrospective study in neurosurgical patients has shown a superior patient outcome with one anesthetic technique compared with another. Clinicians are presented with a wide array of frequently conflicting laboratory and clinical data from studies that elucidate the primary CNS properties and side effects of most anesthetic and adjunctive therapeutic drugs (eg, vasodilators and vasopressors). Major conclusions regarding the appropriateness of these drugs during neurologic surgery are often reached without any evidence that they affect ultimate outcome or influence intraoperative surgical conditions.[1-3] Authors of these studies emphasize, however, that clinicians must be aware of the CNS effects of the drugs they use in order to use each drug *appropriately*. For example, a drug that increases CBV is inappropriate for a patient with increased ICP unless some therapeutic intervention, such as hyperventilation or mannitol diuresis, is employed to prevent a further rise in ICP.

The clinician should be aware that many of the techniques thought to be very important in the management of the neurosurgical patient are now being called into question. Two important examples of this phenomenon are the routine use of hyperventilation and ICP-based management of the neurosurgical patient. Many authors now advise against the routine use of hyperventilation; some go so far as to say that hyperventilation should never be used without a method that simultaneously measures the effects of hyperventilation on CBF. Other authors now emphasize that maintenance of cerebral perfusion pressure (CPP) is much more important, per se, than reduction of intracranial pressure. These authors recommend the use of vasopressors and volume to increase cardiac output and blood pressure and thereby maintain CPP. They believe that previously recommended methods of reducing ICP, including hyperventilation and fluid restriction, actually cause

cerebral damage by reducing the delivery of oxygen to tissues. As is the case with anesthetic drugs, definitive outcome studies either proving or disproving these statements are still lacking; nonetheless, several smaller studies suggest that these concepts have some merit.[4-12]

### What Homeostatic Mechanisms Are Important During Neurologic Surgery?

Both anesthetic and adjunctive medications affect normal CNS function and important homeostatic regulatory mechanisms. Many of these parameters are measurable, including autoregulation of blood flow, vascular responsiveness to CO$_2$, CMRo$_2$, CBF, CBV, and ICP.

#### Autoregulation of Cerebral or Spinal Cord Blood Flow

If an organ is able to autoregulate, blood flow is maintained at a constant value over a range of perfusion pressures. CBF is constant and normal at mean perfusion pressures that range from 50 to 130 mm Hg (Fig. 69–1A). If a pathologic condition or drug causes loss of autoregulation, blood flow varies directly with perfusion pressure (see Fig. 69–1B). Perfusion pressures that would produce normal blood flows with intact autoregulation often produce abnormal flows when autoregulation is impaired. Low flows may produce ischemia, and high flows may cause edema and hemorrhage. Thus, more rigid control of blood pressure to maintain normal CBF appears to be important in such patients whether autoregulation is impaired by drugs or by pathologic change.

#### Responsiveness to Carbon Dioxide

Carbon dioxide is a potent cerebral vasodilator. Decreases in CO$_2$ cause cerebral vasoconstriction and reduction in CBF and CBV. This normal cerebrovascular response enables the clinician to reduce brain bulk during surgery by hyperventilating the patient and is the basis of one treatment for reduction

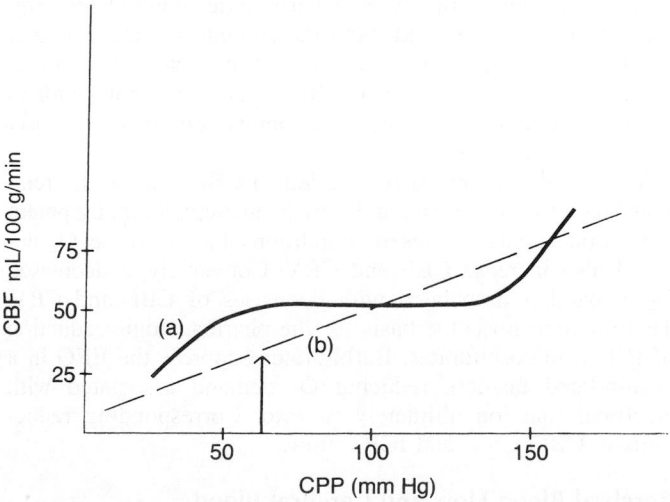

**FIGURE 69–1.** Normal autoregulation (a) and failure of autoregulation (b). *Arrow* shows a mean cerebral perfusion pressure that would produce a normal cerebral blood flow (CBF) if autoregulation were intact and a low CBF if autoregulation had failed.

of elevated ICP. This method of lowering ICP, although effective, may in fact be harmful in some circumstances and should be used only circumspectly and when other methods have failed (discussion follows). If vascular responsiveness to $CO_2$ is impaired or lost, however, hyperventilation no longer is effective in reducing brain bulk or in lowering ICP. Because hyperventilation may have undesirable effects, such as reduction of perfusion to other organs or elevation of mean airway pressures (MAPs) with decreased venous return to the heart, the loss of vascular responsiveness to $CO_2$ is important to ascertain.

## Cerebral Oxygen Demand

Oxygen ($O_2$) is used equally by the brain to maintain both function and cellular integrity. As the $O_2$ supply decreases, the brain first sacrifices function and devotes all available $O_2$ to the maintenance of cellular integrity. Further reduction in $O_2$ may result in cell damage or cell death. When the $O_2$ supply is restored, function returns to normal, provided that cellular damage has not occurred. The $CMRO_2$ is important for several reasons. It may determine the relative risk to the brain of an ischemic insult. Further, the relationship between $CMRO_2$ and CBF forms the basis of pharmacologically induced reduction of ICP.

## Brain Tolerance to Ischemic Insults

Until recently, most clinicians believed that reduction of $CMRO_2$ was the most important factor during attempts to increase brain tolerance to an ischemic insult. Therefore, drugs that lowered $CMRO_2$ were thought to protect the brain from intraoperative ischemia. However, studies have suggested that reduction of $CMRO_2$ is not always associated with ischemic cerebral protection. In addition, some drugs that do not decrease $CMRO_2$ appear to be protective in animal experiments.[13-15] Another previous supposition was that to obtain maximal cerebral protection from barbiturates, a burst suppression pattern on the electroencephalogram (EEG) indicating maximal reduction in $CMRO_2$ is needed. At least in the rat model, burst suppression does *not* appear to be necessary for maximal protection from transient focal ischemia.[16] This observation has potentially enormous implications for anesthetic management. If the dose of barbiturate required for cerebral protection is reduced, both the associated cardiovascular depression and prolonged wake-up time may be reduced. Available data suggest that $CMRO_2$ is an important factor in determining CNS tolerance to ischemia, but this is clearly only part of the story.

The $CMRO_2$ is normally coupled to CBF. Unless the relationship between demand and flow is uncoupled (eg, by potent inhalation agents), drugs or conditions that increase $O_2$ demand also increase CBF and CBV. Conversely, a decreased $O_2$ demand is associated with decreases of CBF and CBV. This relationship is the basis for the pharmacologic reduction of ICP with barbiturates. Barbiturates suppress the EEG in a dose-related fashion, reducing $O_2$ demand associated with electrical function ultimately to zero. Corresponding reductions in CBF, CBV, and ICP follow.

## Cerebral Blood Flow and Cerebral Blood Volume

CBF provides the brain with $O_2$ for function and maintenance of cellular integrity. Reductions in CBF to less than 10 to 20 mL/100 g per minute under anesthesia are associated with a loss of function; reductions to less than 5 to 10 mL/100 g per minute result in loss of cellular integrity and death.[17,18]

Changes in CBV are normally directly related to changes in CBF. How much CBV changes with a change in CBF is unknown and probably depends on the mechanism by which the change occurs. CBV may also change without a change in CBF as, for example, during a change in head position from elevated to supine. Changes in CBV are normally not clinically significant. However, in patients with poor intracranial elastance (ie, in patients whom large changes in ICP occur with small changes in intracranial volume), increases or decreases in CBV can produce similar changes in ICP.

## Intracranial Pressure

The ICP is important for two reasons. First, it is a primary determinant of CPP, which is defined as MAP minus ICP or central venous pressure (CVP), whichever is greater:

$$CPP = MAP - ICP \text{ (or CVP)} \qquad \text{(Equation 1)}$$

If MAP remains constant and ICP increases, CPP decreases. This decrease becomes important once CPP falls below the lower limits for cerebral autoregulation. In patients with impaired autoregulation, blood flow may fall substantially with increases in ICP that do not cause CPP to drop below the lower limits for autoregulation (see Fig. 69–1). If the fall in blood flow is significant enough, loss of function and cellular death may ensue.

The numeric value of the ICP is less important than that of the CPP. Moderate elevations in ICP may actually be beneficial. After subarachnoid hemorrhage (SAH), an increase in ICP (while CPP is still within the autoregulatory range) reduces the transmural wall pressure of the aneurysm and the risk for rebleeding without reducing CBF. Indeed, some authors now recommend a CPP-based management protocol, particularly in head-injured patients. They do not use traditional methods of lowering ICP (eg, including barbiturates, hyperventilation, and hypothermia) but, instead, depend on vascular volume expansion and vasopressors to raise blood pressure and also on cerebrospinal fluid drainage *in addition to* judicious use of mannitol to reduce ICP, thus producing a resultant CPP of 70 mm Hg or greater.[19-23]

ICP may vary between the cerebral and spinal compartments. Significant regional elevations in pressure can produce a pressure gradient sufficient to cause herniation of the contents of one compartment into another. This finding is fairly common when significant elevation of supratentorial ICP causes the temporal lobe or lobes to herniated through the tentorium cerebri. The resulting compromise of blood flow to the herniated brain tissue causes loss of function and cell death.

## *What Drug Effects Are Important?*

Table 69–1 summarizes much of the animal and human data available on many drugs that are commonly used during anesthesia for craniotomies.[14,24-96] The effects shown represent a synthesis of frequently conflicting animal and human studies as well as my opinion regarding the clinical importance of the

**TABLE 69–1.** Anesthetic Effects on Physiologic Variables

| Drug or Drug Class* | CMRo$_2$ | CBF | CBF/CMRo$_2$ | CBV | AR | CO$_2$ | BP | ICP | CPP |
|---|---|---|---|---|---|---|---|---|---|
| Barbiturates (includes etomidate) | ↓ | ↓ | 0 | ↓ | N | ↓ | ↓ | ↓ | ↑, ↓, 0* |
| Propofol | ↓ | ↓ | 0, ? ↓ | ↓ | N | N | ↓ | ↓ | ↑, ↓, 0 |
| Benzodiazepines | ↓ | ↓ | 0 | ↓ | N | N | ↓ | ↓ | ↑, ↓, 0* |
| Opiates, including remifentanil | 0 | ↓, ? ↑ | 0 | 0 | N | N | 0, ↓ | 0, ? ↑ | 0, ↓ |
| Ketamine | ↑ | ↑ | 0, ↑ | ↑ | ? | N | ↑ | ↑ | ↑, ↓, 0* |
| Nitrous oxide† | ↑ | ↑ | 0 | ↑ | N | N | 0, ↓ | 0, ↑ | 0, ↓ |
| Halothane | ↓ D | ↑ | ↑ | ↑ | ↓ D | ↓ D | ↓ | 0, ↑ | ↓ |
| Enflurane | ↓ D, ↑ ‡ | ↑ | ↑ | ↑ | ↓ D | N | ↓ | 0, ↑ | ↓ |
| Isoflurane, desflurane | ↓ D | ↑ | ↑ | ↑ | ↓ D | N | ↓ | 0, ↑ | ↓ |
| Sevoflurane§ | ↓ | ↑ | ↑ | ↑ | ↓ | N | ↓ | 0, ↑ | ↓ |
| Succinylcholine | 0 | 0, ↑ | 0, ↑ | 0, ↑ | N | N | 0 | 0, ↑ | 0, ↓ |
| Pancuronium | 0 | 0 | 0 | 0 | N | N | 0, ↑ | 0 | 0 |
| Doxacurium, pipecuronium, vecuronium, rocuronium, rapacuronium (not studied yet) | 0 | 0 | 0 | 0 | N | N | 0 | 0 | 0 |
| Atracurium | 0 | 0 | 0 | 0 | N | N | 0, ↓ | 0, ↑ | 0, ↓ |
| Cisatracurium | 0 | 0 | 0 | 0 | N | N | 0 | 0 | 0 |
| α- and β-Blocking agents | 0 | 0 | 0 | 0 | N | N | ↓ | 0 | ↓ |
| Sodium nitroprusside | 0 | ↑ | ↑ | ↑ | ↓ | ↓ | ↓ | ↑ | ↓ |
| Nitroglycerin | 0 | ↑ | ↑ | ↑ | ↓ | ↓ | ↓ | ↑ | ↓ |
| Trimethaphan | 0 | 0 | 0 | 0 | N | ↓ | ↓ | 0 | ↓ |
| Calcium channel blocking agents | 0 | ↑ | ↑ | N, ↓ | N | ↓ | 0 | 0 | |
| Phenylephrine | 0 | 0, ↑ | 0, ↑ | | N | N | ↑ | 0, ↑ | 0, ↑ |
| Ephedrine | 0, ↑ | 0, ↑ | 0, ↑ | | N | N | ↑ | 0, ↑ | 0, ↑ |

*Overall effect depends on what changes more—blood pressure or ICP.

†In anesthetized patients or animals (ie, when N$_2$O is added to another agent, such as a barbiturate, the value will not exceed that in an awake subject).

‡High dose, during seizure.

§Some studies suggest that effects seen with sevoflurane are less both in magnitude and in clinical significance than with the other inhaled agents.

AR, cerebral autoregulation; BP, blood pressure; CO$_2$, vascular response to carbon dioxide; CPP, cerebral perfusion pressure; D, dose-related effect; N, preserves normal function in usual anesthetic dose range; 0, no clinically important effect; ↑, increases parameter; ↓, decreases parameter.

If more than one effect is shown, effect varies, depending on patient pathology or if unresolved controversy exists.

Data from references 14 and 24–96.

reported effects. Thus, the table shows no important effect of a given drug—even when the literature reports an effect—if in my opinion, the effect is not *clinically* important.

When planning to use any during neurologic surgery, the anesthesiologist needs to consider its effects on CPP, CBF, and CBV. Provided that each of these interdependent values can be kept within acceptable limits, use of a particular drug or drug combination is unlikely to affect outcome in any fashion that can be currently measured.

The importance of each of these parameters varies from operation to operation (Table 69–2). Sodium nitroprusside administered to reduce blood pressure in a patient with a large intracranial mass may increase ICP because of its effects on CBV. This drug, therefore, is generally not chosen to lower blood pressure in such patients. On the other hand, because sodium nitroprusside increases CBF, it is a drug of choice for the relatively unusual times that induced hypotension is used during aneurysm clippings because CBF is preserved even at low CPP.

Clearly, an understanding of the pathophysiology of the disease state involved and the nature of the planned operation is necessary before anesthetic or associated drugs are chosen for use during surgery. Drugs and adjunctive measures (such as hyperventilation or mannitol administration) can be chosen

**TABLE 69–2.** Examples of the Changing Relative Importance of Physiologic Parameters With Different Types of Neurosurgical Operations

| Type of Operation | CBF | CBV | CPP | Rationale |
|---|---|---|---|---|
| Craniotomy for large intracranial mass | 3 | 3 | 3 | Increased CBF increases CBV, which in turn increases ICP and decreases CPP. |
| Craniotomy for clipping of intracranial aneurysm | 3 | 2 | 3 | Preservation of CBF is very important. ICP is usually not elevated to dangerous levels. Hyperventilation may lower CBF, CBV, and ICP and increase the risk for rebleeding. |
| Craniotomy following head trauma | 3 | 3 | 3 | Maintenance of CPP is critical to survival. |
| Transsphenoidal resection of pituitary mass | 1 | 1 | 1 | Poor intracranial elastance is rare. Hyperventilation-induced decreases in ICP may impair tumor delivery through the sphenoid sinus. |
| Vertebrectomy and posterior spinal fusion | 3 | 1 | 3 | Preservation of cerebral and spinal cord blood flow during induced hypotension is important. |
| Ventriculoperitoneal shunt | 3 | 3 | 3 | Intracranial elastance is often poor. Same considerations apply as for craniotomy for mass. |
| Microvascular decompression of cranial nerves V or VIII | 1 | 1 | 1 | Patient has a normal brain. Technique should help minimize retraction. |

CBF, cerebral blood flow; CBV, cerebral blood volume; CPP, central perfusion pressure; ICP, intracranial pressure. 1, parameters may vary greatly without changing operating conditions; 2, moderately important to large changes may produce significant changes in operating conditions; 3, critically important to small changes in these parameters may greatly change operating conditions.

that minimally affect, or even improve, preexisting physiologic disturbances.

## POSITIONING

The most common patient positions during neurosurgical procedures are the supine, prone, three-quarter prone, and sitting positions. Table 69–3 lists those positions used during specific types of neurosurgical procedures.

### Why Do Neurosurgeons Choose One Position Over Another?

#### General Considerations

Perhaps the most important reason for choosing a surgical position is familiarity. Surgeons trained to perform acoustic tumor resections or cervical decompression laminectomies with patients in the sitting position are likely to continue using that position in practice. Next is a desire to provide optimum operating conditions. Intracranial neurosurgical procedures generally involve removal of a neoplasm or require retraction of brain in order to gain access to a neoplasm, blood vessel, or cranial nerve. Neoplasms may elevate ICP, reduce intracranial elastance, or both. Correct positioning can lessen ICP or reduce the amount of retractor pressure necessary for exposure by facilitating venous drainage (head-up position) and by reducing CBV. Incorrect positioning (eg, with the head down or turned so far as to occlude jugular venous drainage) can increase ICP or the need for retraction because of increased brain bulk. Similar positioning considerations apply for spinal surgery. Table 69–4 identifies common positioning errors that affect directly the surgical procedure and their consequences.

**TABLE 69–3.** Most Common Positions for Neurosurgical Procedures

| Operation | Position |
|---|---|
| Lumbar laminectomy or disk surgery, thoracic or lumbar spinal cord surgery | Prone, lateral decubitus |
| Cervical laminectomy, disk, or spinal cord surgery | Supine (anterior approach)<br>Sitting (posterior approach)<br>Prone (posterior approach) |
| Craniotomy for aneurysm | *Anterior circulaton:* supine with head turned<br>*Basilar apex:* supine with head turned, or lateral decubitus<br>*Posterior circulation:* three-quarter prone or prone |
| Craniotomy for mass resection | *Frontal:* supine<br>*Temporal:* supine with head turned, or lateral decubitus<br>*Parietal:* supine with head turned, or lateral decubitus<br>*Occipital:* three-quarter prone, prone, or sitting<br>*Posterior fossa:* three-quarter prone, prone, or sitting |
| Transsphenoidal resection | Supine, head elevated (beach-chair) |
| Microvascular decompression | Three-quarter prone, or sitting |

**TABLE 69–4.** Common Positioning Errors in Neuroanesthesia

| Error | Consequence |
|---|---|
| Head rotated too far | Venous drainage obstructed<br>Increased CBV<br>Increased CSF (decreased reabsorption and increased production)<br>Increased ICP or increased brain bulk |
| Head flexed too far | Decreased upper cervical spinal cord and medullary blood flow → quadriplegia |
| Head not elevated | Decreased venous drainage<br>Increased CBV<br>Increased ICP or increased brain bulk |
| Abdomen not free in prone position | Increased venous bleeding<br>Increased difficulty with ventilation |

### Gravitational Effects

Positioning may help to improve exposure by taking advantage of gravitational effects. When a patient is in the three-quarter prone position, the cerebellum may be positioned so that the amount of retraction necessary to move it out of the way during microvascular decompression of the 5th or 7th cranial nerve is decreased. The sitting position allows blood and cerebrospinal fluid (CSF) to drain out of the incision without the need for constant suctioning and thereby improves visibility. Finally, proper positioning places the surgical field in a location that makes the surgeon maximally comfortable during these frequently protracted operations.

### How Is Anesthesia Affected by Surgical Position?

#### Venous Air Embolism

Positioning may create special monitoring needs. Any time the incision is above the level of the heart, the patient is at risk for venous air embolism. The distance of the incision above the heart and size of the incision are also important. For example, a posterior fossa exploration with a patient in the sitting position is associated with a much higher incidence of venous air embolism than is a posterior cervical laminectomy with a patient in the same position. Air embolism has also been reported during spine surgery where the incision is not very far above the level of the heart but is very long with a large exposed surface area.[97]

My practice is to monitor all patients with head-elevated positions for venous air embolism. If the risk is significant (eg, as with posterior fossa explorations in the sitting position), a right atrial catheter is placed at the superior vena cava–right atrial junction for aspiration of large, hemodynamically significant air emboli.[98–100] Air embolism can occur in any neurosurgical procedure. Table 69–5 lists the procedures that I consider to be associated with the highest risk.

**TABLE 69–5.** Neurosurgical Procedures in Which Air Embolism Risk is Greatest

Sitting posterior fossa exploration
Sitting cervical laminectomies
Craniofacial reconstructions, especially for cranial synostosis

## IMPACT OF NEUROLOGIC DISEASE ON ANESTHETIC MANAGEMENT

### What Aspects Are Important?

Eight specific areas should be addressed (Table 69–6). I consider relevant neuroanatomy, physiology, pathology, and the nature of the planned surgical procedure to be particularly important.

### Neuroanatomy, Physiology, and Pathology

In planning the anesthetic for a patient with a large brain tumor, such as a glioblastoma multiforme, the size of the mass and whether significant mass effect and surrounding edema are present must be known. In patients with large mass effect, small changes in CBV likely will produce a marked rise in ICP. In addition, large areas of the brain may not autoregulate blood flow normally; increases or decreases in blood pressure that normally would not cause concern may have disastrous consequences.

In contrast, when planning the anesthetic for a patient undergoing a microvascular decompression of the 5th cranial nerve for trigeminal neuralgia, factors such as ICP, autoregulation, and anatomy are expected to be entirely normal. No special planning is needed except that imposed by coexisting diseases, such as heart disease, hypertension, lung disease, or hepatic enzyme induction produced by the medications being used to treat the trigeminal neuralgia.

### Surgical Procedure

The nature of the surgical procedure often has a major impact on management. Resection of a large tumor in the posterior fossa that involves multiple cranial nerves makes intraoperative bradycardic episodes more likely. It may also seriously impair postoperative airway reflexes, thus necessitating prolonged tracheal intubation. If temporary occlusion of major cerebral vessels during aneurysm clipping is planned, preoperative anticipation of moderate hypothermia and possible barbiturate cerebral protection is helpful. The nature of the procedure and the location of the lesion also allow planning of the intraoperative position. Close communication with the surgeon is essential to allow the anesthesiologist to plan optimally for any given operation.

### Functional Status

Functional status of the nervous system is a major concern. Patients with preexisting neurologic compromise likely will suffer at least transient worsening of neurologic function after surgery. This finding is particularly true of patients with depressed mental status. Transient neurologic deterioration may necessitate at least brief postoperative retention of the endotracheal tube. For example, I rarely extubate a patient with a grade III SAH after aneurysm clipping. Whether a postoperative deficit was, in fact, also present preoperatively is essential to know. If a deficit was *not* present before surgery, its presence after surgery may represent a complication of the surgical procedure that is partially or fully correctable if it is recognized promptly.

### Coexisting Disease

Neurosurgical procedures are often conducted on patients with other systemic illnesses. These illnesses sometimes make special techniques or even something as basic as positioning very risky. For a patient with severe chronic obstructive lung disease and a large posterior fossa brain tumor, the prone position can make deliberate hyperventilation difficult or impossible. If the same patient instead requires surgery for removal of a thoracic vertebral body, deliberate hypotension to reduce blood loss may cause severe hypoxemia because of vasodilator-induced loss of hypoxic pulmonary vasoconstriction.

### Premedication

Because the target organ is the CNS, premedication is sometimes hazardous in patients with neurologic disease. The effect of a benzodiazepine may be greatly exaggerated and lead to coma in a patient with a frontal mass. Respiratory depression associated with many premedicants can increase $PaCO_2$, CBF, CBV, and ICP. Premedications should *never* be given routinely. The risks for hypoventilation, an exaggerated preoperative effect, and persistent postoperative influence must be carefully balanced against the anticipated benefits of reduced patient anxiety and blood pressure and of increased patient comfort.

When no special risk factors are present, as for a patient about to undergo lumbar disk surgery or transsphenoidal resection of a small pituitary tumor, premedication may be given as needed or desired. When significant risk is involved (eg, a patient with a large intracranial mass and elevated ICP), but premedication is thought to be necessary, the premedication should be given only in carefully monitored environments with pulse oximetry available and individuals skilled in emergency airway management immediately at hand.

### Monitoring

Intraoperative monitoring during neurosurgical procedures is determined by multiple factors, including the anticipated blood loss; special techniques, such as induced hypotension or barbiturate coma; positioning; the nature of the planned procedure; and the patient's overall medical condition.

Consider a microvascular decompression of the trigeminal nerve. In this procedure, a sponge is placed between the trigeminal nerve and a nearby blood vessel that is compressing the nerve. The procedure is generally not associated with a large blood loss and does not require special anesthetic techniques. It is usually conducted with the patient in the three-quarter prone position, which does not create special

**TABLE 69–6.** Approach to the Neurosurgical Patient

| Special Areas for Consideration |
| --- |
| Neuroanatomy, physiology, and pathology related to the disease process and the planned surgical procedure |
| Nature of the planned surgical procedure |
| Preoperative functional level of the nervous system |
| Other systemic illnesses |
| Premedication |
| Intraoperative monitoring |
| Induction and maintenance of anesthesia (special techniques) |
| Emergence from anesthesia |

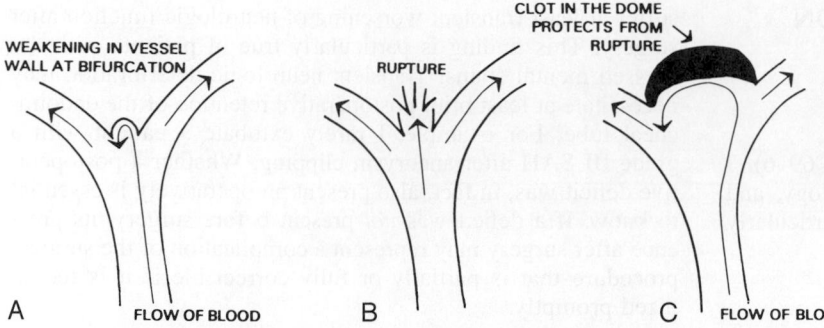

**FIGURE 69–2.** Schematic representation of aneurysm development. *A*, Asymptomatic small intracranial aneurysm. *B*, Aneurysmal rupture. *C*, Formation of giant aneurysm with wall reinforced by clot that may be calcified.

monitoring needs. However, the cerebellum must be retracted medially, and this stretches the 8th cranial nerve. Large blood pressure variations during the time of sponge placement, as well as postdecompression hypertension that requires vasodilator treatment, are common.

Assuming the patient is otherwise healthy, monitoring consists of continuous electrocardiography; blood pressure monitoring with the cuff on the *nondependent* arm so that the patient does not lie on the cuff during the case; pulse oximetry using the *dependent* hand to assess grossly perfusion of the dependent arm as well as oxyhemoglobin saturation; end-tidal $CO_2$ monitoring to assess the adequacy of hyperventilation; intraarterial catheter placement after induction to assist with blood pressure management; and recording of auditory evoked potentials (not usually performed by the anesthesiologist) to help detect damage to the 8th cranial nerve caused by cerebellar retraction (see Chapter 21).

## Induction and Maintenance

Induction and maintenance techniques are most likely selected based on familiarity. Many laboratory studies show *theoretic* advantages or disadvantages to various anesthetic and adjunctive drugs. The data in Table 69–1 combined with the relative goals in Table 69–2 allow development of a strategy for most neurosurgical procedures. Preoperative planning for special anesthetic and adjunctive procedures, such as induced hypotension or barbiturate cerebral protection, obviously is of great importance.

## Emergence

Finally, as has been stated previously, the target organ of both the operation and the anesthetic is the same. Anesthetic drugs routinely cause impairment of CNS function that often is indistinguishable from surgically induced damage. Anesthetic-induced problems improve as drug levels fall; surgical problems do not. A very short time may be available before potentially reversible problems become irreversible. Thus, the effects of anesthetic drugs must be minimized at the conclusion of surgery so that the neurosurgeon can assess the level of function and be reasonably sure that any problems detected are not induced by the anesthetic. Preoperative planning to ensure reversibility is thus an important goal for all neurologic surgery. Sometimes, of course, such reversibility is impossible, as in the case of the patient who is given large doses of sodium thiopental during surgery for cerebral protection.

# NEUROVASCULAR SURGERY

## What Is an Intracranial Aneurysm?

### Pathogenesis

An intracranial aneurysm is produced by a weakening in the wall of a blood vessel, usually at a bifurcation (Fig. 69–2). Turbulent flow of blood at the bifurcation predisposes that area to aneurysmal dilation. As the aneurysm enlarges, the elastance of the wall decreases. Wall tension rises, and the risk for rupture and SAH increases. If the aneurysm does not rupture, it may continue to grow and become a giant aneurysm (ie, >2 cm in diameter). Table 69–7 shows those anatomic and physiologic characteristics of a patient's intracranial aneurysm and SAH that likely affect anesthetic management.

### Morbidity and Mortality

About 11 of 100 000 individuals experience SAH. About 28 000 patients with aneurysmal hemorrhages reach hospitals for treatment annually in the United States. Despite improvements in the surgical, anesthetic, and medical management of these patients, the overall mortality rate remains about 50%.

The most common causes of mortality include rebleeding and vasospasm (delayed ischemic encephalopathy). Of those who survive the initial hemorrhage, 19% of those whose aneurysms are not surgically clipped rebleed in the first 2 weeks; half of these patients die.[101] Roughly 60% of patients with SAH, whether clipped or unclipped, develop vasospasm. About half of these patients have symptoms, with signs ranging from focal neurologic deficit to massive stroke and death.[102] Many neurosurgeons now believe that vasospasm following SAH produces more morbidity than rebleeding.

## When Should Surgery Be Performed After Hemorrhage?

Aneurysmal SAH is a condition that requires surgical repair to prevent rebleeding. No reliably effective medical manage-

**TABLE 69–7.** Important Anatomic and Physiologic Factors for Patients Undergoing Aneurysm Surgery

| | |
|---|---|
| Location | Vasospasm? |
| Size | Systemic manifestations |
| Rupture? | Preexisting medical illness |

ment is available. Timing of aneurysm surgery after SAH, however, remains controversial. Because SAH may produce cerebral edema, aneurysm exposure during surgery early after SAH is sometimes technically more difficult and associated with increased need for brain retraction to expose the aneurysm. This retraction subjects the neural tissue to increased pressures at a time when it may already be ischemic. On the other hand, early operation limits further morbidity and mortality from aneurysm rebleeding. Finally, early clipping of the aneurysm increases the safety of hypervolemic, hypertensive therapy, a promising approach to the treatment and prevention of vasospasm.

A multicenter, prospective, international cooperative study on the timing of aneurysm surgery demonstrated that many patients whose surgery was delayed had major complications or died before surgery.[103–105] However, patients who survived had better postoperative results if surgery was delayed until the second week after SAH. Overall morbidity and mortality were nearly identical for both the early and delayed surgery groups. There has been little change in opinion regarding timing, per se, since this study. Many investigators have begun to question whether subgroups of patients could be identified who could benefit from early aggressive surgical treatment versus those whose outcome would unlikely be improved by early surgical management.[106–108] In addition, the availability of endovascular approaches for treatment of symptomatic and asymptomatic intracranial aneurysm may substantially alter the management options for some patients with intracranial aneurysms. Investigations into the normal course of patients with unruptured cerebral aneurysms have improved our understanding of when patients with grade 0 (unruptured) aneurysms should have their aneurysms obliterated either surgically or by an endovascular approach.[109,110]

Surprisingly, neither advanced age nor high grade of hemorrhage reliably predicts a poor functional outcome, and patients cannot be readily shunted to medical or expectant management based on high grade or age alone.[106–108] Indeed, one study recommended early surgical management for elderly patients with low-grade hemorrhage and no other organ failure.[107] A large international study of patients with unruptured cerebral aneurysms demonstrated a very low risk for rupture (<0.05% per year) provided the aneurysm was less than 10 mm in size. Patients with aneurysms 10 mm or larger had a higher rate of rupture, but it was still less than 1% per year unless the aneurysm was a giant aneurysm (2.5 cm or larger), in which case the risk was 6% in the first year. Patients who had previously bled from another aneurysm were at substantially higher risk for rupture (0.5% per year). Considering the morbidity and mortality associated with clipping a grade 0 aneurysm, the risk for morbidity and mortality related to surgery exceeded the 7.5-year risk for rupture in patients with an aneurysm smaller than 10 mm without previous history of rupture of another aneurysm.[109]

## Why Is Location of the Aneurysm Important?

### Positioning

The location of the aneurysm determines the patient's position. In general, anterior circulation aneurysms may be approached with the patient supine and the head slightly turned. Basilar aneurysms are approached with the patient either in the full lateral position or supine and the head turned to a greater extent. Posterior fossa aneurysms are usually approached with the patient in the three-quarter prone or prone position.

### Treatment of Catastrophic Rupture

The location of the aneurysm also affects planning for intraoperative catastrophic rupture. Hemorrhage from aneurysms located at bifurcations of terminal arteries (such as the middle cerebral artery) may be readily controlled with a temporary clip on the parent vessel (Fig. 69–3). Those located on vessels with multiple points of inflow and outflow are more problematic. For example, an aneurysm on the anterior communicating artery may require temporary clips on both anterior cerebral arteries to control intraoperative hemorrhage. Although good intravenous access is needed in all cases, even better access is needed in cases in which hemorrhage cannot be as easily controlled. The only patients I have seen who died from uncontrolled hemorrhage during surgery had basilar apex aneurysms.

## How Does Aneurysm Size Affect Anesthetic Management?

The size of an aneurysm may create special problems. As an aneurysm enlarges, major outflow vessels and perforating

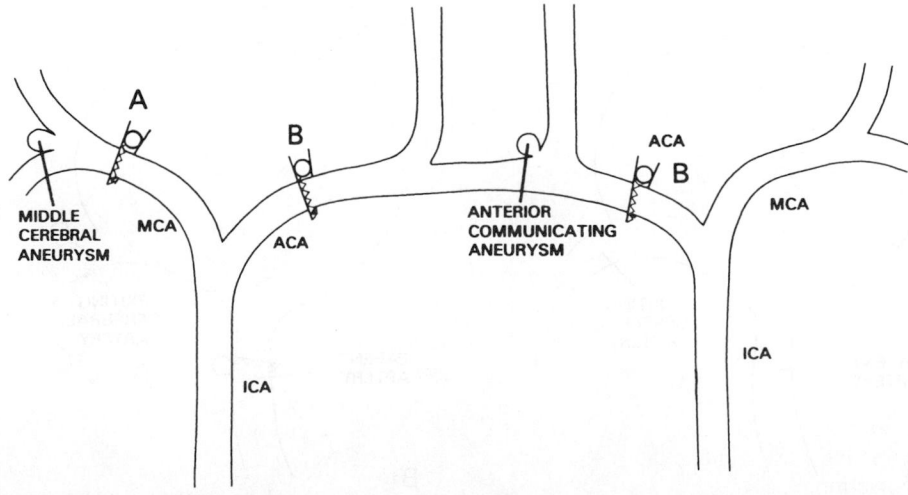

**FIGURE 69–3.** Planning for rupture. A, A temporary clip on the middle cerebral artery (MCA) that stops bleeding from a ruptured MCA aneurysm. B, Rupture of an anterior communicating artery aneurysm may require clips on both anterior cerebral arteries (ACA) to control intraoperative hemorrhage. ICA, internal carotid artery.

vessels are more likely to be involved in the aneurysm's dome (Fig. 69–4). Repair sometimes necessitates temporary occlusion of the vessels supplying the aneurysm (see Fig. 69–4). In such a case, tolerance to focal ischemia may be increased by lowering the $CMRO_2$ with barbiturates or, perhaps even more importantly, by decreasing the patient's temperature. Review of the angiogram and discussion with the surgeon preoperatively can help the anesthesiologist to anticipate the need for such therapy. I routinely reduce the patient's temperature to 33°C in the event that the surgeon unexpectedly and temporarily must place a clip on a major cerebral vessel. A pilot trial (larger study now underway) suggests that mild hypothermia may, indeed, be helpful.[111]

## Why Does Aneurysm Rupture Matter?

Ruptured aneurysms are at high risk for rebleeding. This risk can be minimized by careful control of blood pressure. Preoperative insertion of invasive arterial monitoring catheters facilitates this control, but insertion must be as painless as possible because noxious stimuli may cause hypertension. Patients with preoperative hypertension who need sodium nitroprusside for control of blood pressure *require* invasive monitoring. Patients who are normotensive and stable may have the arterial catheter placed after induction but preferably before strong stimuli such as laryngoscopy occur.

A study conducted in human beings undergoing aneurysm clipping showed that the pressure inside the aneurysm lumen and the artery supplying it are equal unless the aneurysm is thrombosed.[112] Aneurysmal wall tension is related directly to the radius of the aneurysm, which in turn is related to the pressure inside the aneurysmal lumen. Sudden increases or decreases in blood pressure, unless the aneurysm is partially thrombosed, are fully transmitted to the aneurysm wall, alter wall tension, and may cause rupture.

### Increased Intracranial Pressure

Aneurysmal rupture causes a rapid increase in ICP immediately after SAH. This increase in ICP helps to tamponade the aneurysm and stop bleeding. The ICP usually returns to mildly elevated levels in a matter of minutes to hours. However,

blood in the CSF interferes with CSF reabsorption and may cause hydrocephalus. In addition, hemorrhage into the parenchyma of the brain produces an intracerebral hematoma. In either of these cases, ICP may remain elevated at the time the patient arrives in the operating room.

For patients with altered mental status and hydrocephalus, a ventriculostomy catheter is often inserted preoperatively. CSF pressure is then very gradually reduced over several hours to improve cerebral perfusion (but generally is not reduced to <20 mm Hg). Sometimes, dramatic improvements in neurologic status may be seen after this intervention. Although a decrease in ICP improves cerebral perfusion and CBF, aneurysmal transmural wall pressure increases and makes rebleeding more likely. Any reduction in CSF pressure, therefore, must be very gradual. When patients with ruptured intracranial aneurysm who have a ventriculostomy in place are transported anywhere, either to the operating room or for diagnostic studies, the ventriculostomy should be turned *off* for transport. Inadvertently dropping the CSF collection bag to the floor while moving the patient could result in rapid drainage of CSF and a catastrophic lowering of ICP, leading to rebleeding of the aneurysm. After the patient arrives at the new site, the ventriculostomy drainage system can be reset to provide drainage at the proper ICP.

### Loss of Cerebral Autoregulation

Aneurysmal rupture can result in loss of cerebral autoregulation, which may be diffuse or restricted mainly to the vascular bed involved with the hemorrhage. Reductions in blood pressure that normally do not cause a decrease in CBF may cause marked decreases in such cases (see Fig. 69–1). When induced hypotension is deemed necessary, the adequacy of cerebral perfusion should be monitored with an electroencephalogram or somatosensory evoked potentials (SSEPs), if possible (see Chapter 21).

## Why Does Cerebral Vasospasm Follow Aneurysmal Rupture?

Vasospasm is a potentially devastating physiologic disturbance that occurs in some patients 72 hours or more after

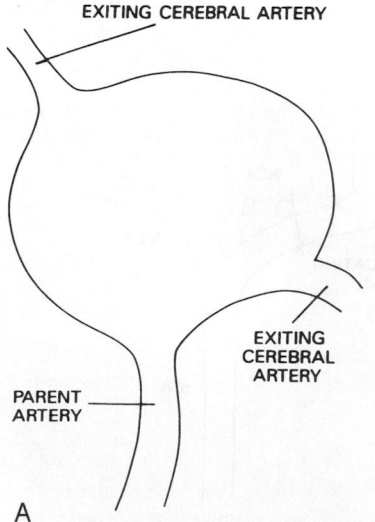

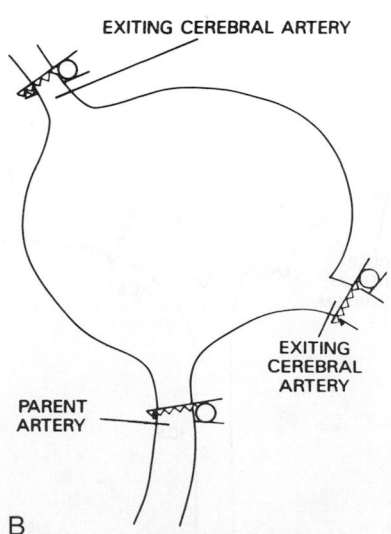

**FIGURE 69–4.** Schematic representation of giant aneurysms. *A,* As aneurysms enlarge, they may involve other vessels in addition to the parent vessel. Shown here, an aneurysm enlarges to involve two exiting cerebral arteries. *B,* Operative repair (if possible) may involve temporary or permanent occlusion of major cerebral vessels.

SAH. It is not seen in a patient with aneurysms that have not ruptured and, interestingly, is not commonly seen in patients with SAH from causes other than an aneurysm. Manifestations are highly variable, ranging from an asymptomatic condition seen only on cerebral angiography to severe cerebral ischemia with focal or global neurologic deficits and massive stroke.

## Pathophysiology and Diagnosis

Vasospasm is thought to be caused by the breakdown of red blood cells in CSF; the risk increases with increased amounts of blood (Fischer grade on the computed tomography [CT] scan). The exact mechanism for vasospasm remains unclear, but recent studies suggest that the answers will likely be found in the realm of molecular biology.[113–115] The condition is initially diagnosed by a typically gradual deterioration of the level of consciousness and the development of focal neurologic findings. Headache is common, and blood pressure frequently increases. These clinical findings can also be caused by other treatable lesions, such as rebleeding, hematoma, hydrocephalus, or metabolic abnormalities (commonly hyponatremia). After these other lesions are excluded, the diagnosis of vasospasm may be confirmed angiographically. Noninvasive transcranial Doppler ultrasound measurements of blood flow velocities in the basal arteries of the brain can also detect and document the severity of vasospasm (see Chapter 21).

## Clinical Implications

Detection of vasospasm is critical because patients are at particular risk if they become hypotensive. Vessels distal to the vasospastic site are no longer able to autoregulate, and critical reductions in CBF may occur with decreases in blood pressure even to the "normal" range (see Fig. 69–1). In the awake patient, such a reduction in flow is usually detectable by the onset of a focal or global neurologic deficit.

While the patient is anesthetized, the neurologic examination is unavailable; electrophysiologic brain monitoring may be used to determine the lower limits of blood pressure tolerated in areas supplied by the vasospastic vessels. With such monitoring, the clinician may properly balance the need for decreased blood pressure to prevent aneurysm rupture and to facilitate clipping against the requirement for higher blood pressure to ensure adequate perfusion through vasospastic vessels.

## Treatment

### Hypervolemic, Hypertensive Therapy

No reliably effective treatment exists for vasospasm, even as we enter the 21st century. Hypervolemic, hypertensive, hemodilution therapy, although still controversial, remains the mainstay of management of cerebral vasospasm.[116,117] Increases of cardiac output and MAP are thought to overcome the vessel narrowing produced by vasospasm and to restore normal blood flow. A prospective study examining the effects of prophylactic hypervolemic hypertensive therapy (HHT) demonstrated a marked reduction in morbidity and mortality in patients with post-SAH vasospasm[33] (Table 69–8). Treatment of established vasospasm with HHT was also shown to be effective in a series of 118 consecutive SAH patients.[118]

**TABLE 69–8.** Hypervolemic Hypertensive Therapy for Cerebral Vasospasm

Mean arterial pressure, >110 mm Hg
Pulmonary capillary wedge pressure, 18–20 mm Hg
Hematocrit, 30–33%
Cardiac index, >3.0 (use inotrope if increased filling pressures are not enough to accomplish this)

Overall, the rate of death and major neurologic deficit in this series was an impressively low 7%.

HHT produces a hyperdynamic circulation and may increase the risk for aneurysm rupture if it is initiated before clipping. Early aneurysm clipping allows HHT to be undertaken without fear of rupture or cerebral swelling, which would impede surgical aneurysm exposure. Further studies involving larger numbers of patients are needed before this therapy becomes a standard of care. Many patients, unfortunately, do not benefit from this therapy for reasons that are not clear. Regardless of whether patients benefit from therapy, HHT is associated with serious cardiac and pulmonary complications in some patients and is usually performed with the guidance of pulmonary catheter monitoring. Despite these drawbacks, this therapeutic modality has found widespread clinical use, both alone and in combination with other therapies.

### Calcium Channel Blockers

Calcium channel blocker therapy for prophylaxis and treatment of established vasospasm appears promising and can be used safely whether or not the aneurysm is clipped.[119,120] Enterally administered nimodipine is most commonly used. Unfortunately, as with HHT, not all patients benefit. Use of nimodipine, as well as some of the other calcium entry blockers, appears to be associated with the need for increased volume therapy intraoperatively to maintain blood pressure.

### Clot Removal

Because the risk for cerebral vasospasm increases with the amount of blood in the subarachnoid space, removal of clot theoretically might lessen vasospasm. Early trials using surgical irrigation to remove blood had promising results, but clot removal takes time, may be difficult, and may itself produce brain damage. A phase I trial using recombinant tissue plasminogen activator instilled by ventriculostomy to facilitate clot removal was completed.[121] Ten patients with grade 3 or 4 SAH were enrolled in the study. Six of these patients showed good outcome 3 months after SAH. These results, although promising, must be duplicated in trials with larger numbers of patients.

### Cerebral Angioplasty

Patients who fail medical treatment may respond to cerebral angioplasty. An initial study involving a small number of patients reported good results after forced balloon dilation of vasospastic vessels following aneurysm clipping.[122] A subsequent larger study confirmed these results.[123] However, such therapy requires trained neuroradiologists or neurosurgeons, who are only available at a limited number of centers. A risk for arterial rupture or dissection follows this procedure; therefore, it is used only on patients with severely narrowed vessels who are not responsive to medical management.

### 21-Aminosteroid Treatment

Studies with the 21-aminosteroid compound, tirilazad mesylate, have suggested that this compound may also be helpful in the treatment of vasospasm.[124,125] Initial studies revealed a beneficial effect only in men. Later studies, however, also demonstrated a beneficial effect in women, although with significantly higher doses. This drug, however, is clearly not as effective as investigators had initially hoped, and it is not clear that treatment with tirilazad is superior to more traditional HHT-based therapy.

### Other Treatment Modalities

Other treatment modalities being examined and showing some promise include intrathecal nitroprusside[126,127] and the use of antioxidants to block the generation of reactive oxygen intermediates in the CSF by oxyhemoglobin.[128]

### Does Preoperative Vasospasm Treatment Affect Anesthetic Management?

When HHT is used preoperatively, the patient must be examined carefully for evidence of pulmonary edema. Increased concentrations of $O_2$ and expiratory positive airway pressure may be needed intraoperatively to obtain adequate oxygenation. Some of the calcium channel antagonists, particularly nimodipine, may reduce systemic vascular resistance. If calcium channel blockers are used preoperatively, this effect may necessitate greater amounts of intravenous fluids, vasopressors, or both to maintain adequate blood pressure while the patient is anesthetized.

### How Does Aneurysm Clipping Differ From Other Neurosurgical Operations?

Aneurysms are rarely superficial, and access to them can generally be obtained only by spreading anatomic fissures or by retraction on a lobe of the brain (Fig. 69–5). Anterior circulation aneurysms are usually approached by a pterional craniotomy. The sylvian fissure is split, and the frontal and temporal lobes are retracted to reveal the aneurysm. Basilar apex aneurysms usually require a temporal craniotomy and retraction of the temporal lobe superiorly.

Retractor pressure reduces perfusion to the underlying brain and may produce neurologic damage, particularly if perfusion is already reduced by vasospasm or induced hypotension. Therapy directed at decreasing brain bulk is useful in decreasing the amount of retractor pressure necessary to expose the aneurysm (Table 69–9). Methods of reducing brain bulk include mannitol infusion, CSF removal by spinal drain or ventriculostomy, and hyperventilation.

Hyperventilation may be deleterious. A rapid lowering of ICP, as has been discussed previously, can increase transmural aneurysmal pressure, predisposing to rupture. It may also produce further reduction in blood flow to areas of the brain

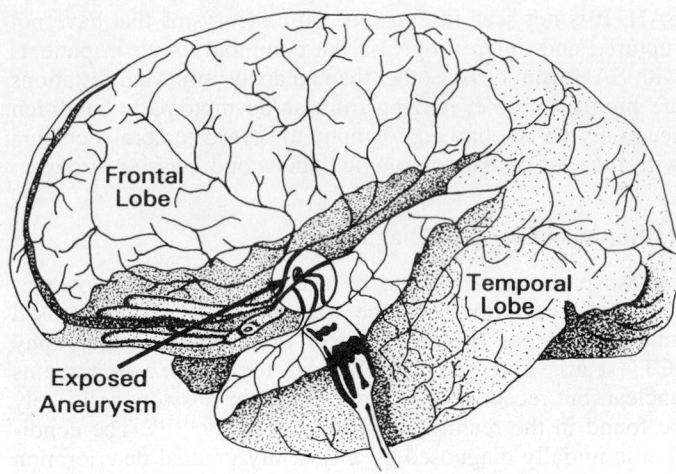

**FIGURE 69–5.** Aneurysms are generally accessible only by retracting brain tissue. In this case, the sylvian fissure is split and retracted, revealing a middle cerebral artery aneurysm.

already at risk for ischemia. Hyperventilation may be necessary to reduce retractor pressure if the other methods are inadequate. It should only be instituted after dural opening unless ICP is very high and then only if absolutely necessary.

### What Is the Impact of Preoperative Central Nervous System Function?

Central nervous system function after SAH is usually determined by four primary factors: brain injury produced by the subarachnoid hemorrhage; cerebral vasospasm; loss of cerebral autoregulation; and hydrocephalus. Patients with focal or global alterations of CNS function and high-grade SAH (Table 69–10) are likely to have a problem in at least one of these areas. Maintenance of adequate cerebral perfusion during surgery is particularly important in these patients, who have lost the ability to maintain and control CBF.

### How Does Subarachnoid Hemorrhage Alter Other Organ Systems?

Marked abnormalities can occur in other organ systems after SAH. The most overt problems are cardiopulmonary in origin.

#### Cardiovascular

New-onset hypertension or exacerbation of previously existing hypertension is common and frequently requires administration of intravenous antihypertensives, such as nitroprus-

**TABLE 69–9.** Methods to Minimize Retractor Pressure Needed for Exposure

Hyperventilation
Mannitol infusion
Cerebrospinal fluid drainage (spinal drain, ventriculostomy)
Pharmacologic
Positioning (enhanced venous drainage)

**TABLE 69–10.** Classification System for Aneurysmal Subarachnoid Hemorrhage

| Grade | Description |
|-------|-------------|
| 0 | Asymptomatic, never ruptured |
| 1 | Headache only, no other symptoms |
| 2 | Severe headache, nuchal rigidity, cranial nerve deficit |
| 3 | Global alteration of consciousness, major focal neurologic deficit (eg, hemiparesis) |
| 4 | Deep coma |
| 5 | Moribund |

side, nitroglycerin, esmolol, or labetalol. Cardiac ischemia may also be produced. Numerous case reports describe electrocardiographic changes with SAH. Early articles suggested that these changes did not correlate with significant myocardial damage or dysfunction.[129,130] One study supports the view that true myocardial dysfunction after SAH may occur and should be investigated in patients who show significant electrocardiographic abnormalities.[131] The exact mechanism that produces cardiac damage is not clear. One recent animal study suggests that myocardial ischemia may *not* be the important mechanism producing left ventricular dysfunction because the dysfunction was not associated with evidence of coronary vasospasm or of global or regional myocardial blood flow disturbances. Also unclear is how often cardiac dysfunction occurs after SAH and how it should affect management. A retrospective review of 72 patients with aneurysmal subarachnoid hemorrhage classified cardiac involvement based on peak elevation of the CK-MB band.[132] The study revealed no significant cardiac problems in 36 patients (CK-MB, <1%), mild problems in 21 (CK-MB, 1–2%), moderate problems in 6 (CK-MB, >2%), and severe problems in 9 (CK-MB, >2% with wall cardiac motion abnormalities). In this study, the most severe myocardial involvement appeared only in patients with the highest CK-MB levels, poor neurologic grade, and female gender. Usually, electrocardiographic changes and wall-motion abnormalities resolve within a few days after SAH.[131] Because these myocardial problems nearly always improve significantly in a few days, it would seem prudent to delay surgery in the most severely affected individuals (left ventricular function severely impaired), particularly if interventions such as temporary vessel occlusion with barbiturate coma and induced hypertension are planned. There are no data to suggest that individuals with milder involvement are at increased risk for perioperative myocardial complications, and delay of surgery does not appear to be warranted.

### Pulmonary

Cardiogenic and noncardiogenic pulmonary edema has also been reported after SAH. Treatment with increased inspired $O_2$, positive pressure ventilation, or continuous positive airway pressure may be required perioperatively. Hypervolemic hypertensive therapy frequently makes this problem worse and may necessitate prolonged intubation and ventilatory support.

### How Does Preexisting Disease Affect Anesthetic Management?

As just noted, SAH has the potential to cause ischemic myocardial damage in patients without coronary disease. The impact of such damage may be even greater on patients with preexisting ischemic cardiac disease. Reductions in diastolic blood pressure and increases in heart rate accompanying induced hypotension needed for aneurysm clipping may not be tolerated. Patients with preexisting pulmonary disease sometimes experience marked decreases in $PaO_2$ if induced hypotension is required because the associated inhibition of hypoxic pulmonary vasoconstriction leads to worsening of intrapulmonary shunt. Worsening of renal function after induced hypotension may occur in patients with preexisting disease. Mannitol administration may obscure decreases in urine output that would otherwise occur.

### Should Preoperative Medication Be Used?

#### Sedatives

Patients undergoing cerebral aneurysm clipping after SAH are often heavily premedicated to prevent anxiety- or pain-induced fluctuations in blood pressure. The preoperative neurologic condition of the patient, however, makes *unmonitored* premedication dangerous. Increased ICP from hydrocephalus or intracranial hematoma worsens with respiratory depression and increased $PaCO_2$. Preoperative global depression of mental status caused by the hemorrhage or by subsequent vasospasm often leads to inordinate sensitivity from any premedication.

Premedication may result in somnolence, which can simulate neurologic changes that could occur with rebleeding or worsening vasospasm. Rebleeding and vasospasm may preclude operation; therefore, the ability to distinguish between premedication effects and rebleeding is vitally important. My practice is to avoid any CNS-active premedicants until I can be with the patient continuously.

Patients presenting for elective aneurysm clipping (ie, patients who have had no recent SAH), who do not have a giant aneurysm that causes significant mass effect, may be safely premedicated. Short-acting agents should be used so that *postoperative* somnolence does not result. Somnolence could also result from clip misplacement, retraction, or a postsurgical hematoma. A long-acting premedicant drug might create difficulties in the differential diagnosis of postoperative somnolence.

#### Anticonvulsants

Patients with SAH are at high risk for seizures. They are usually given phenytoin (Dilantin) or phenobarbital on admission to the hospital. Anticonvulsant blood levels should be checked if possible, and the anticonvulsant should be continued preoperatively and throughout surgery into the postoperative period.

### What Monitoring Should Be Used?

#### Urgent or Emergent Clipping

Invasive arterial blood pressure monitoring should be started before induction, if possible, for any hypertensive patient with SAH. Many patients with SAH require intravenous antihypertensive agents and already have an arterial catheter in place. Normotensive, otherwise healthy patients with SAH may have the arterial catheter placed after induction but before such a potent stimulus as intubation.

Some patients with SAH who are thought to be at high risk for vasospasm may already have a pulmonary artery or central venous catheter in place to monitor HHT therapy before surgery. Patients with significant symptomatic coronary artery disease or SAH-induced cardiovascular dysfunction may benefit from continuous ST-segment analysis, pulmonary artery pressure monitoring, two-dimensional transesophageal echocardiography, or all three. These monitors improve the detection of myocardial ischemia or left ventricular failure induced by HHT or by special techniques, such as deliberate hypotension or barbiturate cerebral protection. If these techniques cause serious cardiovascular compromise, appropriate therapy (eg, volume therapy, inotropic agent administration, or β-blockade) is instituted.

### Elective Clipping

Patients undergoing elective aneurysm clipping may have invasive monitors placed after induction. I also place a central venous catheter for the administration of vasoactive drugs when an immediate effect is desired (such as rapidly induced hypotension following inadvertent rupture). I routinely employ a long-arm catheter; this approach avoids the potential complications of pneumothorax or carotid puncture. More invasive monitoring is used if preexisting disease or special techniques, such as barbiturate cerebral protection, are anticipated.

### Electrophysiologic Monitoring

Cortical SSEPs may be used to monitor cerebral function during aneurysm clippings.[133,134] The best results are seen with anterior circulation aneurysms. If blood flow through the anterior or middle cerebral arteries is reduced, the SSEPs are attenuated or lost. Because most aneurysms are proximally located, all sections of cortex supplied by the artery are equally affected; hence, loss of SSEPs correlates with loss of motor functions as well.

The posterior circulation provides blood through perforating vessels to the somatosensory pathway as it ascends through the brainstem to the thalamus. However, this circulation also supplies blood to large portions of the brainstem that are not involved with the somatosensory pathway. Thus, damage can occur to motor pathways and to the reticular formation, resulting in motor deficit or global depression of consciousness, or both, without any change in SSEPs.[135]

In summary, anterior circulation aneurysms should be monitored with SSEPs whenever possible. Evoked potentials are particularly useful for determining the adequacy of CBF during vasospasm; induced hypotension or hyperventilation; after placement of the aneurysm clip; and during temporary occlusion of major cerebral vessels, even if barbiturates are given. Evoked potentials may also be useful for monitoring the brain during clipping of posterior circulation aneurysms. However, correlation with outcome in this area is not as good.

### How Is Anesthesia Managed?

Multiple anesthetic regimens can be used for aneurysm clipping. Common goals of these techniques are listed in Table 69–11. Which drug regimen is used is not particularly important provided that it meets as many of the goals as possible. After induction of anesthesia, good intravenous access should be obtained. Particular care should be taken with patient positioning because these operations are usually very long. Padding of pressure points is even more important if induced hypotension is planned because perfusion of compressed tissue is further reduced.

### Control of Intracranial Pressure

Patients with SAH rarely have very high ICPs. However, as was discussed previously, therapy directed at decreasing brain bulk is useful to reduce the amount of retractor pressure necessary to expose the aneurysm (see Table 69–9). If possible, anesthetic and adjunctive therapeutic drugs that do not increase brain bulk significantly should be chosen (see Table 69–1). Such choices are not always possible, but the therapeutic maneuvers listed in Table 69–9 often compensate for anesthetic drug-induced increases in brain bulk.

Normocapnia, as determined by preoperative blood gas partial pressure measurements, is maintained throughout surgery. The need and risk for hyperventilation have been discussed in detail previously. Mannitol should be withheld until just before the removal of the bone flap. This regimen produces a maximum decrease in brain bulk at a time when retraction is needed to expose the aneurysm. Spinal fluid drainage through a ventriculostomy or by a spinal drain may be used during some aneurysm clippings. No more than 25 mL of fluid should be drained slowly at one time over 10 to 20 minutes. Fluid should *never* be aspirated. Rapid drainage of CSF produces hypertension, a sharp decrease in ICP, and a predisposition to aneurysmal rupture.

### Fluid Therapy

The patient should be kept at least normovolemic during surgery to maintain adequate blood pressure and cardiac output and to minimize the effects of preexisting vasospasm on CBF. Hypervolemia associated with HHT may increase cerebral edema and the degree of retractor pressure needed for exposure. I do not recommend instituting hypervolemia until after the aneurysm is clipped. After clipping, particularly if the patient is at risk for vasospasm, moderate hypervolemia is indicated.

The type of fluid used for this therapy is somewhat controversial. Most clinicians employ a mixture of crystalloid, colloid, and blood to produce hypervolemia and maintain a hematocrit at about 30%.[136] Maintenance of at least normal

---

**TABLE 69–11.** Anesthetic Goals During Aneurysm Surgery

1. Prevention of rapid changes in blood pressure
2. Prevention of rapid changes in intracranial pressure
3. Reduction of brain oxygen consumption
4. Maintenance of adequate cerebral blood flow
5. Reduction in brain bulk to minimize retraction needed just before removal of bone flap
6. Minimal suppression of evoked potentials and electroencephalogram, if employed (see Tables 21–13 and 21–14)
7. Prevention of position-related injuries in these lengthy operations
8. Rapid emergence

plasma osmolality appears to be very important in the prevention of postoperative cerebral edema.

Animal data suggest that glucose-containing fluids worsen outcome after global cerebral ischemia. In the absence of documented hypoglycemia, such fluids should be avoided because these patients are at significant risk for intraoperative cerebral ischemia.

## Induced Hypotension

Pressure inside an aneurysm is about the same as arterial pressure.[32] The radius of the aneurysm changes in direct proportion to this pressure, and aneurysmal wall tension changes proportionately to the aneurysmal radius. Induced hypotension, therefore, greatly decreases wall tension and the risk for intraoperative rupture. It also decreases aneurysmal bulk, thereby facilitating placement of a clip on the neck of the aneurysm, which otherwise would be obscured by its dome.

### Risks

Induced hypotension is associated with substantial risk. CBF may be critically reduced, resulting in ischemia. This problem is most common in the patient with preexisting vasospasm, long-standing arterial hypertension, or both. Hypotension should be used only with caution in these patients. EEG analysis or cortical SSEP is helpful to determine the limits of hypotension when it is needed. Hypotension may also be harmful to other organ systems, as has been discussed previously. Many neurosurgeons request hypotension only when catastrophic rupture is imminent or has occurred.

A recent retrospective study has confirmed the risk for even limited induced hypotension during surgery. A retrospective review of 84 consecutive patients demonstrated that any intraoperative use (even of very short duration) had a significantly negative effect on the long-term outcome of subarachnoid hemorrhage. Intraoperatively induced hypotension was also associated with more frequent and more severe manifestations of vasospasm postoperatively.[137]

### Agents

Certain hypotensive drugs preserve CBF better than do others. Sodium nitroprusside and isoflurane appear to be the current agents of choice. The former agent is easy to titrate and preserves adequate CBF even in the face of severe hypotension (MAP, 40 mm Hg).[138] Thus, sodium nitroprusside is useful if intraoperative rupture of the aneurysm occurs.

Rapid adjustments of blood pressure are more difficult with isoflurane. However, this drug has a potential advantage over sodium nitroprusside because it maintains CBF *and* reduces brain $O_2$ consumption.[139] Unfortunately, isoflurane, in the high concentrations sometimes necessary for hypotension, suppresses both the EEG values and cortical evoked potentials. Thus, although CBF may supply the brain with sufficient $O_2$, documentation of the adequacy of perfusion is not possible. In addition, evidence suggests that despite reductions of $CMRO_2$, isoflurane may not protect the brain from focal ischemia.[13]

### Hyperventilation

Because hyperventilation normally reduces CBF, it should be employed with caution when induced hypotension (which may also reduce CBF) is used. One study[140] demonstrated that moderate hypocarbia (arterial partial pressure of $CO_2$, 30 mm Hg) and induced hypotension within the autoregulatory range (MAP, $>50$ mm Hg) are usually associated with adequate CBF. Other studies have shown that vasodilators used to induce hypotension impair the brain's vascular response to $CO_2$. Monitoring with EEG or SSEP may be helpful to guide therapy. I do not recommend use of hyperventilation unless other methods to control brain bulk have been unsuccessful.

## Cerebral Protection

### Hypothermia

The only widely accepted method of producing brain protection is reduction in $CMRO_2$. This reduction may be accomplished by active or passive cooling. Cerebral $O_2$ demand is reduced by about 7% per 1°C decrease in temperature.[141] The temperature should be kept above 33°C because the incidence of serious ventricular dysrhythmias begins to increase below this level. A recent pilot study leading to an ongoing trial of intraoperative hypothermia during aneurysm clipping suggested that routine use of mild to moderate hypothermia is helpful.[111]

### Electroencephalographic Suppression

The $O_2$ consumed during generation of the cortical spontaneous EEG may be reduced by several drugs, including barbiturates, etomidate, propofol, and isoflurane (see Table 69–1). The only drugs that nearly all experts agree produce protection from focal ischemia are the barbiturates. Complete suppression of the spontaneous EEG with barbiturates reduces brain $O_2$ requirements by about 50%.[142]

This level of suppression may require large doses of barbiturate (eg, a loading dose of 15 mg/kg of thiopental followed by an infusion of 10-30 mg/kg/h). Additional barbiturate produces no further reduction in cerebral $O_2$ demand. Because high-dose barbiturate administration is accompanied by marked cardiovascular depression, inotropic support is often required. Phenylephrine, dopamine, dobutamine, epinephrine, and other inotropes have been used successfully in this setting. Interestingly, cortical SSEPs may still be monitored even with total barbiturate suppression of the EEG. Recent studies in animals have suggested that this high dose of barbiturates may not be needed and that lower doses (still showing significant EEG activity) may still provide maximal protection.[16]

## What Factors Are Important During Emergence?

Most patients who were not neurologically impaired preoperatively may be extubated immediately postoperatively after normal neurologic function has been documented. Patients who do not promptly return to normal function should remain intubated until a cause is determined. Usually, a CT scan or angiography is needed. Blood pressure should be maintained at normal to moderately elevated levels. This approach is particularly important in patients with vasospasm.

Patients who were obtunded preoperatively usually do not improve in the immediate postoperative period. They should not be extubated, nor should those with vasospasm undergoing vigorous HHT who may need continued postoperative positive pressure ventilation. When postoperative maintenance of intubation is planned, frequent assessment of the patient's neurologic status is critical. After initial neurologic assessment, a propofol infusion may be useful. Rapid return to normal mental status occurs after the infusion is discontinued, even if it has been used for a prolonged period.[143]

### What About Endovascular Therapy?

Endovascular therapy, primarily involving the electrolytically detachable platinum coils (the Guglielmi Detachable Coil system, or GDC coiling [Boston Scientific-Target Therapeutics, Natick, Mass]) has recently become a viable option for the treatment of some intracranial aneurysms. Selection of candidates is based on aneurysm-specific *and* patient-specific considerations. Although discussion of the characteristics that make a given aneurysm suitable for GDC coiling is beyond the scope of this chapter, consideration of patient characteristics is entirely appropriate (see Chapter 52). GDC coiling is conducted either in the neuroradiology suite or in the operating room in combination with a surgical procedure. When used alone as treatment for an aneurysm, this procedure involves considerably less stress for the patient with severe medical risk factors. The procedure may require general anesthesia in most patients because absolute immobility is needed at many points during the procedure. Although case reports and series exist in which local anesthesia with sedation is used, this technique is only possible with very cooperative patients with either unruptured aneurysms or low-grade (I or II) SAH.[144–148] In cases in which general anesthesia is necessary (most, in my experience), all of the considerations discussed previously apply equally well.

### What Is an Arteriovenous Malformation?

Cerebral arteriovenous malformations (AVMs) are composed of thin-walled vessels that provide varying degrees of direct arteriovenous shunt, depending on their size and flow. These malformations cause preoperative symptoms by a number of mechanisms, including hemorrhage, mass effect, and "steal" of blood flow from the surrounding normal brain. Common presenting symptoms include seizures and headaches of varying severity. Hemorrhage produces symptoms similar to those following aneurysmal hemorrhage.

Most AVMs are now treated preoperatively by neuroradiologic embolization. Thrombogenic material is injected into the major arterial feeders of the malformation. It then lodges in the smaller vessels and reduces flow through the malformation. This technique helps to reduce intraoperative blood loss and the likelihood of "breakthrough" bleeding or edema after the arterial inflow to a high-flow AVM is occluded.

AVMs should not be confused with cavernous malformations or venous malformations, which are also associated commonly with seizures and headache. Unlike AVMs, these lesions only rarely present with hemorrhage; because they lack an arterial component, significant intraoperative bleeding is rare.

#### Breakthrough Bleeding and Edema

If flow through an AVM is sufficiently high, the surrounding normal brain receives inadequate blood flow. In response, the vessels supplying the normal brain dilate to better "compete" with the AVM for blood flow. When the arterial inflow to a high-flow AVM is abruptly stopped during surgery, the surrounding brain receives a much higher blood flow than it did before AVM interruption. Vessels leading to the surrounding brain that have been chronically vasodilated are initially unable to constrict to reduce flow. The resultant very high blood flow can lead to cerebral edema and frank hemorrhage in the normal brain.

Although the previous explanation is generally accepted, newer data suggest that, as with many other aspects of therapy in neurosurgical patients, the mechanism is not so simple. Data from several carefully conducted studies suggest that pressure autoregulation is actually intact in the brain surrounding an AVM but is shifted to the left in a fashion analogous to the shift to the right occurring in hypertensive patients. These studies also demonstrated no association between preoperative regional arterial hypotension surrounding the AVM and the postoperative breakthrough bleeding phenomenon.[149–152]

The phenomenon of breakthrough bleeding does occur, however, and when it does, it may be very difficult to manage and involves massive hemorrhage. After AVM inflow occlusion, I routinely lower blood pressure to a mean of 50 to 60 mm Hg in patients with high-flow AVMs provided that other organ systems will tolerate hypotension. Even if intraoperative breakthrough bleeding or edema appears to be absent during surgery, either condition may develop after dural closure. This reduction in blood pressure is sometimes necessary for several days before restoration of normal autoregulation occurs. In extreme cases not controlled by these measures, high-dose barbiturates can be used to reduce blood flow and cerebral edema.

## SPINAL COLUMN AND SPINAL CORD SURGERY

### What Are the Indications?

Generally, patients undergo surgery on the spinal cord or spinal column because they have symptoms related to compression of neural tissue. Common etiologic factors include congenital abnormalities, trauma, degenerative disease, and neoplasms—both intrinsic and extrinsic to the CNS.

Mechanisms of neural compression are shown in Table 69–12 and Figure 69–6. Herniation of disk tissue or abnormal bone compression posterolaterally compresses nerve roots at their exit from the spinal column and produces radiculopathy at the involved level (Table 69–13). Above L1 to L2, such changes may compress the spinal cord and produce myelopathy (see Table 69–13). Stenosis of the spinal canal can also produce radiculopathy or myelopathy. More commonly, stenosis worsens the degree of neural compression produced by disk herniation or bone prominences.

Instability that results from trauma, degenerative diseases (eg, rheumatoid arthritis), or congenital abnormalities (eg, trisomy 21, Klippel-Feil syndrome) can also produce radiculopathy or myelopathy. Associated neural compression is variable in severity, depending on a patient's position or motion. Symptoms and signs of radiculopathy or myelopathy (see Table 69–13) may be severe under baseline conditions or occur only at extremes of rotation, flexion, or extension.

**TABLE 69–12.** Common Mechanisms of Neural Compression in Patients With Disease of the Spinal Column or Spinal Cord*

| Pathology | | Symptoms |
|---|---|---|
| Disk herniation (D, T) | Posterolateral† | Radicular pain, paresthesias, weakness (radiculopathy) |
| | Posterior† | Pain, paresthesias or weakness in spinal cord (or cauda equina distribution caudal to disk herniation [myelopathy]) |
| Bone compression (D, T) | Lateral† | Radicular pain, paresthesias |
| | Anterior† | Pain, paresthesias, or weakness in spinal cord, or cauda equina distribution caudal to bone compression |
| | Spinal canal stenosis | Radiculopathy or myelopathy, or both, depending on where stenosis occurs and whether there is concomitant disk or bone compression |
| Instability (C, D, T) | | Radiculopathy, myelopathy, or both, depending on where the instability produces compression |
| Neoplasm | Intramedullary | Sensory, motor, or cerebellar symptoms in distribution of spinal cord distal to lesion |
| | Extramedullary | Radiculopathy, myelopathy, or both |
| Syrinx (intramedullary fluid collection) | | Sensory, motor, or cerebellar symptoms in distribution of spinal cord distal to lesion |

*See also Figure 69–7.
†Denotes direction of herniation or location of bone compression. C, congenital; D, degenerative; T, trauma-induced.

Patients may not have symptoms, as is frequently the case with patients who have rheumatoid arthritis and atlantoaxial instability.[153]

Nerve root neoplasms can produce radiculopathy in the associated dermatome as the nerve root is progressively stretched by the growing tumor. This neoplasm can also compress the adjacent spinal cord by encroaching on the limited confines of the spinal column. Intramedullary tumors (arising from the spinal cord) produce myelopathy by stretching white-matter pathways and displacing gray matter. Metastatic tumors may involve the bone support structures of the spinal cord and invade the epidural space. Radiculopathy, myelopathy, or both, often result.

Finally, when the normal circulation of CSF is disrupted by tumor or trauma, dissection of fluid into the spinal cord may occur. An intramedullary fluid collection, known as a *syrinx*, displaces and stretches white matter pathways and compresses gray matter.

### Why Are Radiculopathy and Myelopathy Important?

These syndromes have significance in four main areas: the method of intubation, positioning, the choice of muscle relaxants during surgery (if used), and blood pressure control.

### Intubation and Postioning

#### Cervical Radiculopathy

Intubation and positioning are particularly important in patients with cervical spine pathology because the cervical spine is considerably more mobile than is the thoracic or lumbar spine. Thus, positioning changes are more likely to cause exacerbations of preexisting neural compression.

Patients with cervical radiculopathy have one or more compressed nerve roots. Changes in neck alignment associated with intubation are unlikely to cause nerve root damage because the roots are relatively resistant to brief periods of worsened compression or ischemia. Most patients with cervical radiculopathy can be intubated after induction of general anesthesia unless the preoperative cervical range of motion is also severely compromised.

Prolonged nerve root compression associated with positioning, however, can produce permanent damage. Patients with radiculopathy can be tested preoperatively for the development of symptoms by placing them in the planned surgical position for at least 5 minutes. A 5-minute test is used because such symptoms may take time to develop; shorter exposure of a patient to a surgical position may not demonstrate more slowly developing symptoms.

#### Cervical Myelopathy

Patients with cervical myelopathy have spinal cord compression at one or more levels. The spinal cord is more sensitive to ischemic damage from compression than are the nerve roots. Position changes that result from intubation may cause increased spinal cord compression. More importantly,

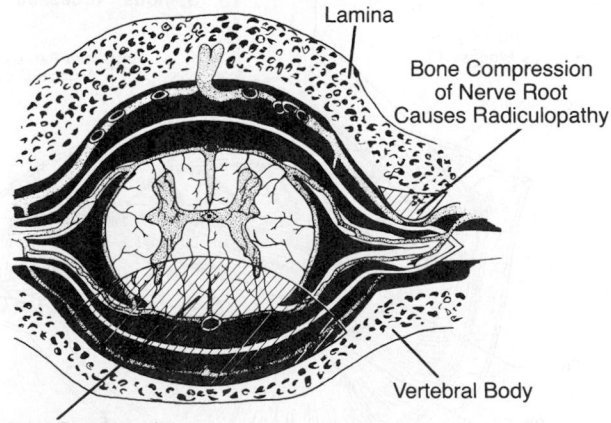

**FIGURE 69–6.** Schematic of myelopathy versus radiculopathy. Compression of the nerve root produces radiculopathy. Compression of the spinal cord produces myelopathy.

**TABLE 69–13.** Radiculopathy Versus Myelopathy

| Syndrome | Motor Function | Sensory Function | Reflexes |
|---|---|---|---|
| Radiculopathy (signs and symptoms restricted to dermatome) | Normal or weak | Pain or numbness | Decreased |
| Myelopathy (signs and symptoms caudal to lesion) | Normal or weak; spasticity common | Pain or numbness | Increased |

worsened compression can result from surgical positioning. Extreme care must be taken with intubation and positioning.

I recommend awake intubation and positioning for any patient with cervical myelopathy so that the patient can warn the anesthesiologist when symptoms are produced by neck movement. In the absence of instability, permanent neurologic damage from intubation and positioning is unlikely to occur in patients with cervical myelopathy. Nevertheless, the consequences of damage to the cervical spinal cord are so great that I consider awake intubation and positioning worthwhile. The actual injury rate is unknown, but isolated cases of sudden, unexpected perioperative death of myelopathic patients have been reported.[154]

### Thoracic and Lumbar Radiculopathy and Myelopathy

Radiculopathy and myelopathy in the thoracic or lumbar spine are unlikely to be affected by intubation and positioning. Only in patients with gross instability does positioning cause worsening of spinal cord compression in these areas. In these rare cases, awake intubation and awake positioning may be helpful.

### Muscle Relaxants

Patients with myelopathy and even radiculopathy are at increased risk for hyperkalemia after succinylcholine administration.[155] In almost all cases, the deficit that results from the radiculopathy and myelopathy is not stable or long-term (ie, unchanged for 6 months or longer). Thus, succinylcholine use should generally be avoided in such patients.

### Blood Pressure Control

Blood pressure control is critically important in myelopathic patients. Spinal cord perfusion pressure is defined as MAP minus CSF pressure. In patients with spinal cord compression, however, the perfusion pressure is actually MAP minus the compression pressure. Decreases in blood pressure that would normally cause no concern may cause spinal cord ischemia. Electrophysiologic monitoring may be helpful to decide what level of hypotension needs to be treated (see Chapter 21). In the absence of such monitoring, however, blood pressure should be maintained at or above the patient's normal range, and although induced hypotension may be requested by the surgeon to reduce blood loss, induced hypotension should *never* be used in myelopathic patients unless a worsened neurologic deficit is an acceptable postoperative outcome.

### What Operations Are Performed to Relieve Neural Compression?

### Diskectomy

Diskectomy is the procedure of choice for disk herniations. In the lumbar spine, this procedure is usually performed through a small, posterior laminotomy. The herniated disk is removed, often with the aid of an operating microscope. In the thoracic spine, a herniated disk may be removed using a posterior approach similar to that used for lumbar surgery or, in some cases, anteriorly through a lateral thoracotomy. In the

latter situation, the lung is retracted or deflated (one-lung ventilation).

A lateral extracavitary approach may largely replace thoracotomy to approach disks that cannot be removed posteriorly.[156] With this technique, a small segment of the proximal portion of several ribs is removed. The lung is retracted laterally, exposing the vertebral bodies and the intervertebral disk (Fig. 69–7).

In the cervical spine, disk herniations are most commonly removed using an anterior approach. A small transverse incision is made adjacent to the trachea. Vascular structures are retracted laterally (the trachea may be retracted medially), exposing the vertebral column, and the disk is removed.

New, relatively noninvasive endoscopic procedures are now available and have been used to treat disk herniations in the lumbar, thoracic, and cervical spine (discussion follows).

### Decompression

### Laminectomy, Foraminotomy

In cases of bony compression, the approach depends on whether the compression is caused by posterior, lateral, or anterior elements or by a combination of spinal column components. Global compression is usually treated with laminectomy. If bony decompression of nerve roots is necessary, the nerve root foramen may be widened (foraminotomy). Anterior compression is more difficult to treat. Sometimes, it may be relieved by widening the spinal canal with a posterior laminectomy.

### Vertebrectomy

Alternatively, anterior compression is relieved by removing all or a portion of the vertebral body. In the lumbar region, vertebrectomy may be performed using a lateral extracavitary approach while the patient is in a prone position or using a retroperitoneal, thoracoabdominal approach while the patient is in a lateral position. Thoracic vertebrectomy may also be done in the lateral position with a thoracotomy or in the prone

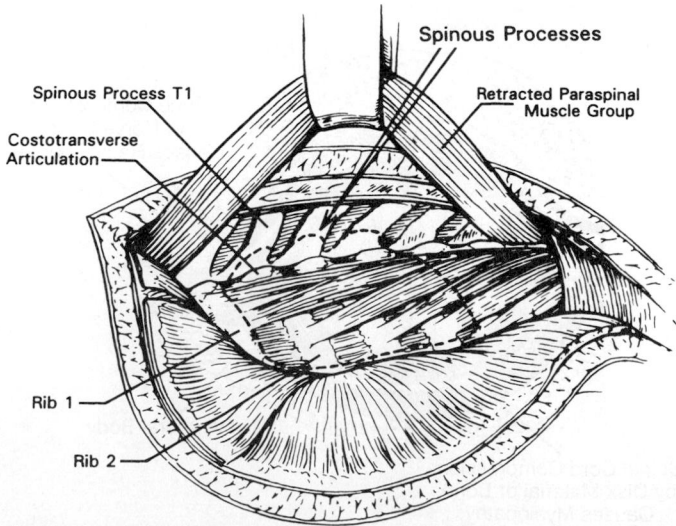

**FIGURE 69–7.** Schematic of lateral extracavitary approach to the thoracic spine. Removal of the proximal portion of two ribs and retraction of the lung allows access to the spinal column.

position through a lateral extracavitary approach (see Fig. 69–7). In the cervical region, vertebrectomy is performed in the supine position from an anterior approach with retraction on the trachea and vascular structures (as for diskectomy). As with diskectomy, less invasive procedures have again surfaced as an alternative therapy at all levels of the spine.

### Stabilizations and Fusions

Instability may be congenital or result from trauma, other spine surgery (eg, vertebrectomy), or degenerative disease. It is usually corrected with some form of posterior spinal fusion. Most commonly, fusion is accomplished with both hardware and autologous or homologous bone grafting.

### Tumor Excision

The surgical approach to intrinsic spinal neoplasms or spinal cord syrinx is usually posterior laminectomy, the extent of which is determined by the size of the lesion. Extrinsic or metastatic neoplasms that involve the vertebral bodies are approached in the same fashion as anterior bone compression. Those in the epidural space are usually approached posteriorly.

## Why Is Preoperative Functional Status Important?

### Acute Versus Chronic Changes

Patients with rapidly deteriorating neurologic function must have expedient correction of neural compression if return of function is to occur. If these patients have coexisting disease that can have a potential impact on anesthetic management, work-up and treatment must occur quickly before CNS deterioration becomes irreversible. The outcome of patients with acute traumatic myelopathy may be improved by the administration of high-dose methylprednisolone given within 8 hours of the injury (30-mg/kg bolus followed by a 23-hour infusion at 5.4 mg/kg per hour).[157,158]

Patients with chronic loss of function or pain may be treated more electively; coexisting disease can be adequately evaluated and appropriate treatment started. Knowledge of the level of neurologic function helps to determine whether radiculopathy or myelopathy will affect the methods of intubation and positioning, blood pressure control, and the choice of relaxants.

### Blood Pressure Aberrations

Autonomic control of blood pressure is often deranged in acutely or chronically myelopathic patients. Acute, high spinal cord injury may produce spinal shock. The patient loses sympathetic control of heart rate and blood pressure and becomes hypotensive and bradycardic. Compensation for anesthetic-induced cardiovascular depression or hemorrhage with increases in heart rate and peripheral vascular resistance cannot occur. Direct-acting vasopressors and positive chronotropic agents are often necessary to prevent further spinal cord injury from hypotension. Patients with chronic injury may show a similar failure of autonomic dysfunction but, in addition, can develop autonomic hyperreflexia.

### Autonomic Hyperreflexia

When noxious sensations reach the spinal cord, a normal, sympathetically induced spinal reflex causes vasoconstriction in the region of the injury. Generalized vasoconstriction is modulated or prevented by supraspinal sympathetic control. Patients with chronic myelopathy from any mechanism, but most commonly after complete spinal cord injury, permanently lose supraspinal control of the sympathetic nervous system. Thus, local vasoconstriction following noxious stimuli may become generalized. If the level of spinal cord injury is at T6 or higher, vasodilation above the lesion is insufficient to compensate for generalized vasoconstriction below the lesion. Severe hypertension frequently results. This syndrome is known as *autonomic hyperreflexia*. It should be anticipated and prevented with spinal blockade or deep anesthesia or be rapidly treated with vasodilators.

## How Does Preexisting Disease Affect Anesthetic Management?

Operative trauma associated with spine surgery varies greatly among the different procedures. A lumbar diskectomy does not usually involve major blood loss or fluid shifts. A thoracic vertebrectomy, however, may be associated with major retraction on the lung as well as large blood loss and third space fluid requirements. The impact of preexisting disease increases with operative trauma.

### Cardiovascular Function

Preexisting cardiac disease presents problems in any of these operations but has a larger impact during procedures associated with large blood loss or significant third space fluid requirements. In addition, these operations are often conducted with a patient in the prone position. Patients with poor ventricular function may not tolerate the decreased venous return that sometimes occurs. Because these operations are frequently associated with large blood loss, induced hypotension is often used. Reductions in diastolic pressure and increases in heart rate may be poorly tolerated.

Some neurosurgeons prefer that patients undergoing certain spinal operations not be given muscle relaxants so that inadvertent manipulation of neural tissue can be detected by patient movement. An amount of anesthetic agent sufficient to ensure immobility of a patient with poor ventricular function may result in significant undesired hypotension, particularly during periods of reduced stimulation. These patients usually require at least partial neuromuscular blockade to prevent movement-induced injury during microsurgery or pin fixation of the head.

### Pulmonary Fixation

Patients with preexisting pulmonary disease often experience marked decreases in $Pao_2$ during induced hypotension. Vasodilator-induced inhibition of hypoxic pulmonary vasoconstriction is in large part responsible, as has been discussed previously. The weight of the body on the thorax and cephalic movement of the diaphragm, which are associated with the prone position, reduce functional residual capacity and worsen shunt.

## Should Patients Be Premedicated?

Unlike patients undergoing some intracranial procedures, patients scheduled for spine surgery are not at increased risk for premedication compared with the general population unless they have a high cervical lesion and impaired ventilation. Premedication generally may be given as indicated.

## What Monitoring Is Needed?

### General Considerations

Monitoring for spine surgery should be determined by the factors shown in Table 69–14. Otherwise, healthy patients having disk surgery for radiculopathy can be monitored noninvasively. Those undergoing major spine operations associated with significant blood loss and fluid shifts benefit from invasive arterial blood pressure monitoring, particularly if induced hypotension is planned. Invasive arterial monitoring also facilitates frequent blood gas and laboratory analyses. Central venous pressure monitoring may also be helpful to guide fluid management. Whenever possible, SSEPs should be monitored during operations that jeopardize the spinal cord or its perfusion through distraction or induced hypotension.

### Preoperative Neurologic Function and Coexisting Disease

Patients undergoing spine operations who are myelopathic require close monitoring of blood pressure to prevent hypotension-induced worsening of neurologic function. Even minor reductions in blood pressure from baseline should be quickly corrected. Patients with serious cardiopulmonary disease may benefit from invasive monitoring even for relatively minor spine procedures.

## How Is Anesthesia Induced and Maintained?

Many reasonable anesthetic regimens can be used for patients undergoing spine operations, the common goals of which are listed in Table 69–15. Provided that the regimen chosen meets as many of these goals as possible, the choice

**TABLE 69–14.** Factors Determining Monitoring During Spine Operations

**Nature of the Operation**

Anticipated blood loss
Use of special techniques, such as induced hypotension, one-lung ventilation
Spinal cord blood flow or neural structures at risk from surgery
Positioning of patient

**Preoperative Level of Neurologic Function**

Patient with myelopathy at risk for aggravation of neurologic deficit by hypotension
Patient with complete spinal cord injury at T6 or higher at risk for autonomic hyperreflexia

**Coexisting Disease**

Preexisting cardiac, pulmonary, or renal disease

**TABLE 69–15.** Anesthetic Goals During Spine Surgery

1 Preserve spinal cord perfusion
2 Protect patient from position-related injury
3 Minimize blood loss
4 Provide good exposure for surgeons
5 Minimal effect on electrophysiologic monitoring if used (see Chapter 21)
6 Rapidly reversible to assess neurologic examination

of drug or drugs is relatively unimportant. Positioning, however, is extremely important.

### Positioning

With the exception of some cervical operations, these procedures are conducted with patients in the prone or lateral position. Careful positioning that avoids stretching or compression of nerves helps to prevent injury during these frequently lengthy operations. Meticulous padding helps to prevent skin breakdown. The prone patient should be placed on chest rolls or a frame that allows the abdomen to be suspended above the table; this minimizes intraabdominal pressure. Increases in intraabdominal pressure are also undesirable from a pulmonary standpoint because higher airway pressures will be necessary for ventilation, the functional residual capacity will decrease, and ventilation-perfusion mismatch will increase. Intraabdominal pressure increases also impede inferior vena caval venous return to the heart, diverting blood to the epidural venous plexus and the azygos system. Distention of these veins increases surgical bleeding.

### Head Position in Lumbar and Thoracic Spine Operations

In lumbar and lower thoracic operations, head position is unimportant to the surgeon. The head is neutral or turned to the side and placed on a padded "donut" (Fig. 69–8A). The dependent eye and ear must be absolutely free of pressure to prevent blindness and external ear necrosis, respectively. Turning the head to the side, however, may impede cerebral venous drainage. Because large amounts of intravenous fluids are frequently needed during these operations, severe swelling of the face, tongue, pharynx, and larynx often occurs.

Several foam headrests are available that allow the patient to be positioned face-down with the head in the neutral position (see Fig. 69–8B). This position allows unimpeded venous drainage from the head and minimizes soft tissue swelling. These headrests also have cutout sections that prevent pressure on the eyes. Even with the best precautions, however, pressure-related injury to the head may occur during these very lengthy operations. The only reliable way to prevent pressure-related injury to the head is to attach a pinion that suspends the head (see Fig. 69–8C).

### Head Position in Cervical Spine Operations

During operations on the cervical spine, the head *must* be kept midline, with the amount of flexion or extension adjustable, depending on the type and level of the operation. Most surgeons use a head pinion to hold the head absolutely immobile. If head flexion is desired, I limit the amount so that at least two fingerbreadths of space remains between the mentum

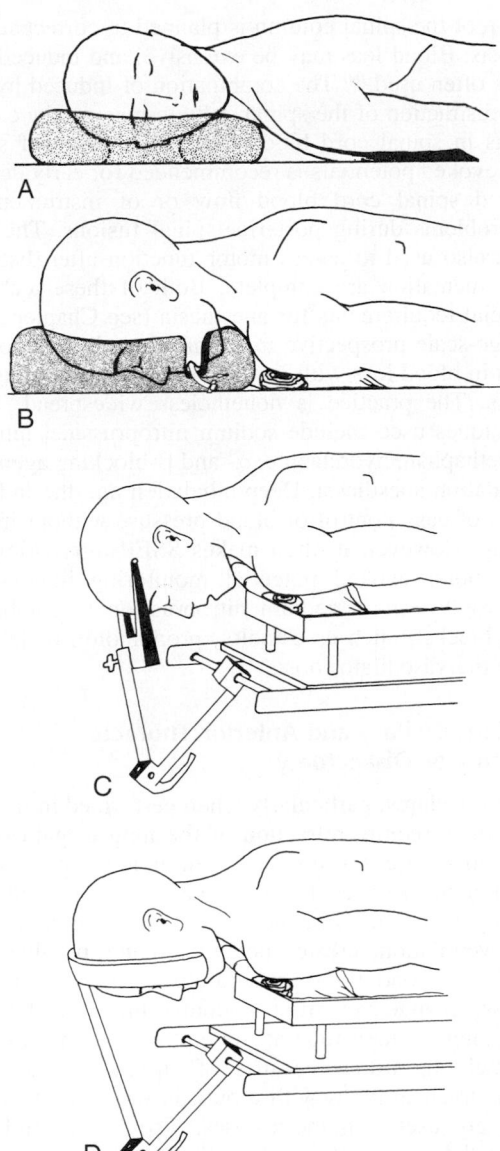

of the endotracheal tube if the patient's mouth clamps shut during periods of light anesthesia. This complication is much more difficult to treat in the prone position. Oral airways commonly have been used for this purpose. With head flexion, however, this airway may compress the hard and soft palates, producing mucosal necrosis.[159] In addition, it may impair venous drainage from the tongue, resulting in swelling. Because of these problems, I use a hard plastic sleeve that fits over the endotracheal tube and prevents bite occlusion (Fig. 69–9). These sleeves are frequently used for intubated intensive care unit patients. They do not impair venous drainage of the tongue, and the potential for palatal pressure injury is minimal.

### Fluid Therapy

No data show that one fluid strategy is superior to another during spine surgery. Most clinicians use a mixture of crystalloid and colloid solutions. Blood products are given based on intraoperative losses and the presence of coexisting diseases. I have found that an infusion of up to 1 L of 3% saline solution substantially reduces the total intravenous fluid requirements and appears to reduce postoperative peripheral edema. Although glucose-containing solutions administered during spinal cord ischemia have not been studied in an

**FIGURE 69–8.** Positioning the head in the prone position. *A*, The head is rotated to the side and placed on a soft foam "donut." Eyes and ears are free of pressure. *B*, The head in the neutral position. The head rests on a foam cushion with a cutout for eyes, nose, and endotracheal tube. *C*, The head in the neutral position. The head is supported by a pinion and is suspended. *D*, The head in the neutral position. The head rests on a horseshoe-shaped headrest that leaves the eyes and nose free of pressure.

and manubrium. A head pinion allows great flexibility in flexing or extending the neck during initial positioning.

Alternatively, the patient may be placed on a foam horseshoe-shaped headrest. The eyes, nose, and mouth are in the open area of the horseshoe, and the forehead and malar eminence are in contact with the foam (see Fig. 69–8D). In my opinion, this headrest should be used only for operations expected to last less than 3 hours. Despite the best precautions, it may cause pressure injuries to the forehead and cheeks if surgery is prolonged or if induced hypotension is used.

### Bite Block Insertion

Some type of bite block should be used in all patients undergoing surgery in the prone position to prevent occlusion

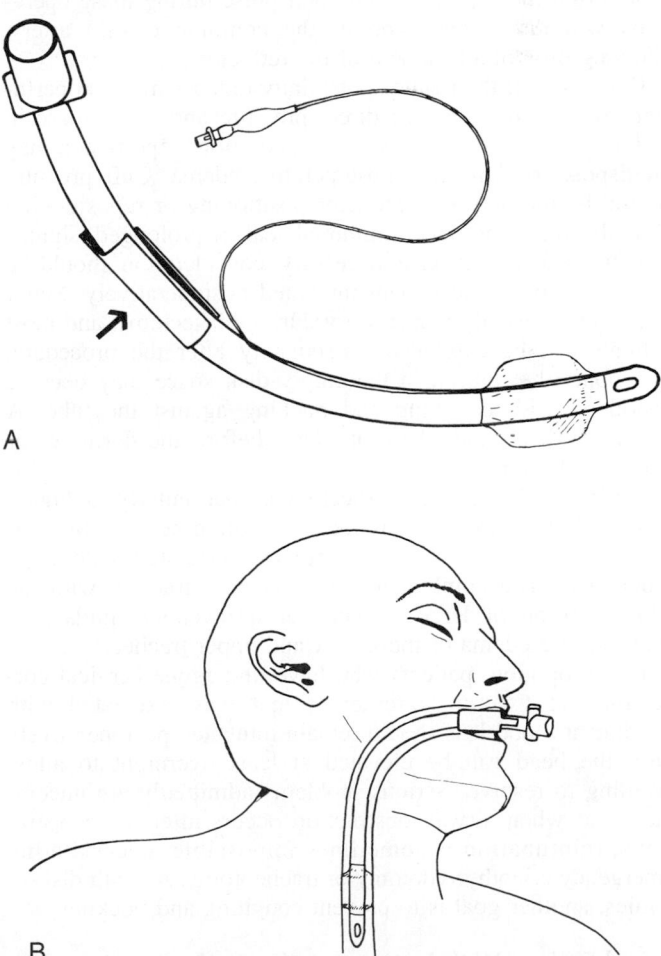

**FIGURE 69–9.** Bite block protection of the endotracheal tube. *A*, A hard plastic sleeve around the endotracheal tube fits between the teeth. *B*, There is no pressure on the palate, and venous drainage from the tongue is not impaired.

animal model, I do not use them unless hypoglycemia is documented.

## Do Anesthetic Considerations Vary With the Operation?

### Lumbar Microdiskectomy

Lumbar microdiskectomy is usually not associated with major blood loss. However, the aortic bifurcation and iliac arteries are just ventral to the anterior longitudinal ligament in the lumbosacral area; inadvertent laceration of a major artery may occur with resultant massive blood loss. This loss is usually occult because the retroperitoneal hemorrhage does not escape through the small hole in the anterior longitudinal ligament. The diagnosis should be considered early if unexplained, intractable hypotension occurs during lumbar disk surgery. Failure to diagnose and treat usually results almost immediately in a lethal outcome.

### Anterior Cervical Diskectomy, Corpectomy, or Fusion

Exposure during these operations is obtained by lateral retraction of vascular structures and medial retraction of the trachea. The former action may cause compression of the common carotid artery and cerebral ischemia in some patients. Monitoring the superficial temporal pulse during these operations will detect occlusion of the common carotid artery, allowing prompt adjustment of the retractor.

Retraction of the trachea potentially reduces mucosal perfusion by two mechanisms: direct pressure and an increase in endotracheal tube cuff pressure. Restoration of perfusion may predispose to significant postoperative edema. Cuff pressure should be retested after retractor positioning or repositioning and adjusted to produce a minimal seal. If prolonged, significant tracheal retraction is necessary, consideration should be given to leaving the patient intubated postoperatively. Major retraction is usually unnecessary during diskectomy, and most patients can be extubated immediately after the procedure. The bone plug placed in the empty disk space may become dislodged with coughing and bucking against the tube. A technique that avoids these problems before and during extubation is desirable.

During multiple-level corpectomies, particularly at higher levels (C3-C5), extensive retraction is often needed. In addition, these operations are sometimes associated with large blood loss. The combination of tracheal retraction with the administration of large amounts of intravenous fluids may cause severe edema of the larynx and upper trachea.

In my opinion, patients who have undergone cervical corpectomy at two or more levels that was associated with significant blood loss should remain intubated postoperatively until the head can be elevated at least overnight to allow swelling to resolve. Serious problems admittedly are uncommon, but when airway obstruction occurs after these operations, reintubation is sometimes impossible, necessitating emergency cricothyroidotomy or tracheotomy. As with diskectomies, another goal is to prevent coughing and bucking.

### Spinal Fusions With Instrumentation and Distraction

Many forms of spinal instrumentation place neural tissue at risk, particularly if instruments invade the spinal canal or if distraction of the spinal column is planned to correct scoliosis or kyphosis. Blood loss may be extensive, and induced hypotension is often used.[160] The combination of induced hypotension and distraction of the spinal column may produce critical reductions in spinal cord blood flow. Monitoring of sensory or motor evoked potentials is recommended for early detection of reduced spinal cord blood flow or of instrumentation-related problems during posterior spinal fusions. The wake-up test is also used to assess motor function after distraction and instrumentation are complete. Both of these techniques have special requirements for anesthesia (see Chapter 21).

No large-scale prospective randomized studies demonstrate reduction in blood loss with induced hypotension during these operations. The practice is nonetheless widespread. Agents and techniques used include sodium nitroprusside, nitroglycerin, trimethaphan, hydralazine, α- and β-blocking agents, and deep inhalation anesthesia. Deep inhalation anesthesia has the advantage of easy control of blood pressure without invasive monitoring. However, it often makes SSEP monitoring difficult and motor evoked potential monitoring impossible. I prefer nitroglycerin or sodium nitroprusside in combination with a β-blocker, such as esmolol, propranolol, or labetalol, to reduce the vasodilator dose.

### Lateral Extracavitary and Anterior Thoracic Corpectomy or Diskectomy

These procedures, particularly when performed in the upper thoracic spine, require retraction of the lung to gain optimal exposure. In such cases, one-lung ventilation may be helpful to the surgeon. Two cautionary notes are important. First, induced hypotension to reduce blood loss, combined with one-lung ventilation, creates potential major problems with oxygenation. Second, if the procedure is associated with major blood loss, changeover from a double-lumen endotracheal tube to a single-lumen tube at the end of the operation may be extremely hazardous because of airway edema. I have found endotracheal tubes with a built-in bronchial blocker to be extremely useful in these cases. The bronchial blocker may be withdrawn at the end of the operation, making an endotracheal tube exchange unnecessary.

### Neoplasms

Spinal neoplasms necessitate special anesthetic considerations because of the potential for bleeding and because of the need to monitor spinal cord function. The greatest blood loss may be expected from tumors that involve the skeleton. Control of hemorrhage from these lesions is difficult until resection is complete, and the potential for massive blood loss is high. Preoperative embolization of the tumor may help to reduce intraoperative blood loss.

Patients with neoplasms frequently have myelopathy. Thus, avoiding even minor degrees of hypotension is a major goal. Induced hypotension to reduce blood loss should not be used, in my opinion, despite the risks associated with transfusion. If myelopathy is not present, deliberate hypotension may be useful.

### Trauma

Spine trauma creates special anesthetic considerations because of instability, spinal cord injury, the potential for bleeding, and the need to monitor spinal cord function.

## Instability

The impact of spinal instability is greatest in the cervical region. Movement of the head and neck during intubation and positioning may cause injury or exacerbate preexisting injury. Patients with an unstable cervical spine should be intubated and positioned while awake, if possible, so that the neurologic function can be carefully monitored. Alternatively, if a patient cannot tolerate awake intubation and positioning, SSEPs may be monitored and then continued during the stabilization procedure. Such monitoring helps to ensure that proper spinal alignment is maintained and that the instrumentation used for stabilization does not injure the spinal cord.

Because of support from surrounding tissues, movement has much less impact on thoracic and lumbar spinal alignment. Most patients with instability in these regions can be intubated and positioned after induction of anesthesia with little risk for damage to the spinal cord. However, if the patient has severe instability with bone or disk material in the spinal canal, I recommend awake positioning or, if asleep, SSEP monitoring.

## Injury

Spinal cord injury associated with trauma affect four areas of anesthetic management: sympathetic nervous system function; choice of muscle relaxants; control of blood pressure; and use of steroids to improve outcome.

**Sympathetic Dysfunction.** As was discussed earlier, both acute and chronic spinal cord injury may affect sympathetic nervous system function. Spinal shock often occurs in the acute setting and produces hypotension and bradycardia; autonomic hyperreflexia may occur in the chronically injured patient. The latter condition does not occur until after spinal shock has resolved. Direct-acting vasopressors and vasodilators should be readily available to control blood pressure in both the acute and chronically injured patient.

**Succinylcholine-induced Hyperkalemia.** After loss of innervation following nerve, spinal cord, or brain injury, rapid up-regulation of acetylcholine receptors on the muscle membranes occurs and becomes significant 48 hours after the injury. After that time, succinylcholine administration may produce a massive release of potassium, particularly if the denervated muscle mass is large. Thus, succinylcholine may be used safely if needed for an acute injury situation but should be avoided if the injury is more than 48 hours old. Chronically denervated muscle will atrophy, and succinylcholine is unlikely to produce hyperkalemia if stable denervation injuries are older than 6 months. However, I still avoid this drug, even in chronically denervated patients, unless a rapid-sequence induction is absolutely necessary.

**High-Dose Methylprednisolone.** High-dose methylprednisolone, begun within 8 hours of the spinal cord injury with a bolus dose of 30 mg/kg, followed by a 23-hour infusion of 5.4 mg/kg per hour, significantly improved outcome in a prospective, randomized, placebo-controlled study.[157,158] This therapy should be initiated in any patient presenting for surgery acutely following spinal cord injury or when spinal cord injury occurs or is suspected intraoperatively.

**Blood Pressure Control.** Blood pressure control is important for patients with spinal cord injury. Spinal cord blood flow decreases after injury when the injured spinal cord cannot autoregulate its blood flow. Decreases in blood pressure reduce blood flow and potentially aggravate the injury. Induced hypotension, as noted previously, should not be used to reduce blood loss.

## How Do the Newer Noninvasive Approaches Change Anesthetic Management?

The basic concepts regarding blood pressure, fluid management, and anesthetic choice are not significantly affected if an endoscopic technique is planned. Endoscopic techniques have become popular because major spine operations can be conducted through small incisions that are thought to be associated with quicker recovery, less pain, and overall less morbidity than traditional approaches (there is a significant lack of comparative outcome studies, however).[161–171]

In the lumbar spine, both posterior diskectomy and anterior vertebral surgery may be approached through the endoscope. Anesthetic considerations are similar to other lumbar posterior procedures or anterior laparoscopic procedures. Some authors have reported using monitored anesthesia care (MAC) techniques for the posterior lumbar microscopic endoscopic diskectomies. I have found that technique very unsatisfactory, usually resulting in an oversedated patient in the prone position with an unprotected airway.

The greatest anesthetic considerations, and perhaps the greatest patient benefit, come from thoracoscopic approaches to thoracic disks and anterior fusions. Instead of recovering from a large lateral thoracotomy and rib resection, these patients recover only from four or five small incisions and chest tube placement. Instrumentation is being developed and used that would allow a solely thoracoscopic correction of thoracic scoliosis. In these thoracoscopic cases, one-lung ventilation is absolutely essential for the success of the operation.

There are several choices for one-lung ventilation, including double-lumen endotracheal tubes and the newer single-lumen tubes that allow easy placement of a built-in bronchial blocker. These newer tubes offer two significant advantages. First, they are relatively easy to place. The initial placement is identical to that of a regular endotracheal tube. The bronchial blocker is then placed in the correct bronchus with the help of a bronchoscope. Second, at the end of the operation, if the patient needs to remain mechanically ventilated for a period of time, the bronchial blocker can be completely withdrawn, and the patient can readily tolerate the remaining normal, single-lumen tube. I have not, however, found these tubes to be useful in these operations for two reasons. Should oxygen desaturation occur with one-lung ventilation, therapeutic options are limited with this tube. For example, it is not possible to apply continuous positive airway pressure to the deflated lung to improve oxygenation. Second, lung deflation has not been as complete or rapid. Because near-complete deflation is needed for exposure to the spine, significant delays have occurred while waiting for the lung to deflate. More experience from multiple institutions and clinicians is needed before a clear decision regarding choice of tube used for single-lung ventilation can be made.

An additional consideration introduced by this operation involves often prolonged deflation of a lung. In several cases at the University of Florida, the lung has been deflated for more than 8 hours. Experience with such a prolonged intraoperative period of unilateral lung deflation is limited. Patients with chronic deflation of a lung secondary to a pleural effusion or pneumothorax have experienced significant pulmonary edema as a result of reexpansion. Although I have not yet observed this phenomenon in a patient undergoing thoracoscopic spine surgery, these patients should be observed closely for a prolonged period (at least overnight) in an intensive care unit or recovery area until more experience with prolonged lung deflation is gained.

Posterior cervical procedures are also possible using the microscopic endoscopic technique. At our institution, the few cases that have been done have all been done in the sitting position. This position was chosen to allow for better drainage of blood from the incision and for surgeon comfort. Because the incision is above the level of the heart, air embolism is clearly possible, although we have not yet seen any significant air emboli.

## INTRACRANIAL NEOPLASM

### What Are Intracranial Neoplasms?

Intracranial neoplasms may arise from any intracranial tissue or may be metastatic. An estimated 24 000 primary brain tumors and an equal number of metastatic brain tumors are diagnosed each year in the United States, resulting in an overall incidence of 8 to 10 per 100 000 population.[172] Tumors that arise from glial cells are the most common, followed by those that arise from the meninges. Characteristics vary according to the type of neoplasm. Those that are important to anesthetic management are listed in Table 69–16, whereas some of the more common types of intracranial tumors and their important characteristics are categorized in Table 69–17.

### Why Are Tumor Size and Rate of Growth Important?

Size of a tumor would seem, a priori, to be the most important factor determining ICP. The ICP–volume curve (Fig. 69–10) demonstrates that pressure changes very little until a *significant* volume is added. Most figures similar to this one do not specify numeric values on the *X* axis because the point at which ICP increases varies with the rate at which the volume is added. For example, a rapidly growing mass, such as an epidural hematoma (which expands over minutes) or a glioblastoma multiforme (Fig. 69–11*A*) with edema (which expands over weeks or months), produces a much higher ICP than a very slowly growing meningioma (which expands over years) (see Fig. 69–11*B*) that is actually twice as large.

As a rapidly growing tumor or hematoma increases in size, compensatory mechanisms act immediately to prevent rises in

**TABLE 69–16.** What Properties of Brain Tumors Are Important?

Size
Growth rate → intracranial pressure and cerebral elastance
Location
Surrounding edema
Vascularity
Effects on neurologic function
Seizures?

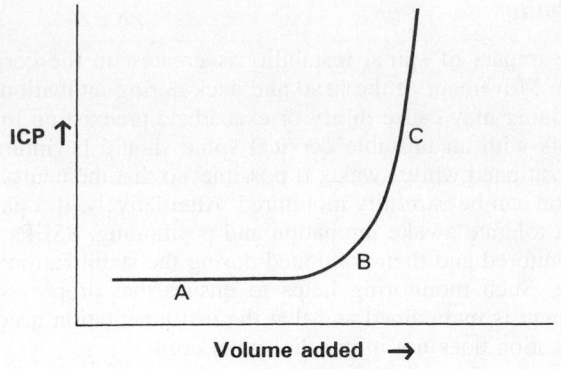

**FIGURE 69–10.** Intracranial elastance curve. A, Normal elastance. B, Reduced elastance (small intracranial pressure [ICP] increase with increasing intracranial volume). C, Poor elastance (large ICP increase with minimal increase in cerebral volume).

ICP: CSF is displaced to spinal levels, and CBV (mainly venous) is decreased. Neural tissue, however, is not acutely compressible; once CSF and blood mechanisms have been exhausted, pressure begins to rise rapidly (see Fig. 69–10B and C). A global rise in ICP is accompanied by direct pressure of the expanding mass on adjacent neural tissue; this causes loss of function.

Chronic, gradual compression of neural tissue can also occur. The slowly growing tumor may reach a very large size, producing slow displacement and compression of neural tissue without any increase in ICP. Displacement of CSF or blood may not even occur, and structures such as the falx cerebri or the ventricles may not show any shift from normal position (see Fig. 69–11*B*). CT and magnetic resonance imaging (MRI) may provide clues as to whether a mass has caused an increase in ICP (Table 69–18). These signs are by no means quantitative and do not substitute for pressure measurements. Thus, size and rate of growth must be considered together when one tries to determine whether a patient has elevated ICP, decreased intracranial elastance, or both.

### Why Is Treatment of Cerebral Edema Important?

Some tumors cause the surrounding brain to develop edema (see Table 69–17). Brain edema surrounding a tumor is indicative of the failure of normal capillary endothelial blood–brain barrier function. Sodium, which normally does not cross the blood–brain barrier, crosses freely and brings water with it, producing cerebral edema located mainly in the white-matter extracellular space. This edema is termed *vasogenic edema*. When edema is limited to a small area or is mild in degree, it is of little clinical significance. When more generalized or severe, however, edema leads to loss of neural function. The increase in brain water surrounding a mass further aggravates any increase in ICP caused by tumor size and rate of growth. Reduction of this edema with preoperative steroid treatment often substantially lowers ICP and improves cerebral elastance. Steroids are thought to restore normal capillary permeability. Their effect is rapid, with improvement of symptoms noted in hours.

**TABLE 69–17.** Important Properties of Common Intracranial Neoplasms

**Skull**

ICP rarely elevated
May be very vascular

**Meninges (meningioma)**

Cause symptoms by compressing neural tissue
Slow growth, may attain very large size with relatively few symptoms
ICP varies, but in general is not frank elevated because of slow growth; elastance may be poor
Supratentorial or infratentorial in location
Often hypervascular; blood loss may be great
Variable edema
Seizures common

**Glial Cells (glioma, oligodendroglioma, optic nerve glioma, medulloblastoma, ependymoma)**

Cause symptoms by compressing neural tissue
Highly malignant gliomas grow rapidly, whereas less malignant gliomas grow slowly
ICP varies, may be very high with rapid growing tumors
Supratentorial or infratentorial in location
Variable vascularity, frequently hypovascular
Variable edema
Seizures common

**Pituitary Gland (pituitary adenoma)**

Cause symptoms secondary to endocrine dysfunction and compression of surrounding tissue (optic nerve, cranial nerves III, IV,
    and VI, hypothalamus)
Growth slow
ICP usually normal
Usually not hypervascular
Edema uncommon

**Hypophyseal Duct (craniopharyngioma)**

Cause symptoms by compressing pituitary gland (panhypopituitarism, diabetes insipidus) and optic chiasm
Growth rate slow
ICP may be elevated, especially if tumor invades third ventricle and causes hydrocephalus
Not hypervascular
Edema uncommon

**Blood Vessel (hemangioblastoma)**

Cause symptoms by cerebellar compression
Growth rate variable
Posterior fossa hypertension possible
Occurs only in posterior fossa or spinal cord; most commonly in cerebellum, occasionally arise from brainstem
Brainstem compression possible
Very hypervascular, massive hemorrhage possible
Hematocrit frequently high on presentation

**Cranial Nerve (acoustic schwannoma, other cranial nerve schwannomas rare)**

Cause symptoms by stretching 8th cranial nerve (deafness, tinnitus), adjacent cranial nerves (VII, V, IX, X), and with large tumors,
    compression of cerebellum (ataxia), brainstem, and fourth ventricle (hydrocephalus)
Growth rate slow
Posterior fossa hypertension with large tumors; supratentorial ICP elevated when hydrocephalus occurs
Involvement of 9th and 10th cranial nerves may depress airway reflexes
Vascularity variable
Edema uncommon

**Metastatic (lung, melanoma, breast, renal, gastrointestinal)**

Cause symptoms by compressing neural tissue
Growth rate variable, but usually rapid
ICP varies, may be very high with rapidly growing tumors
Supratentorial or infratentorial in location
Variable vascularity
Variable edema
Seizures common

ICP, intracranial pressure.

## How Does Tumor Location Influence Management?

### Positioning

Location of a tumor affects many aspects of anesthetic management. First, it determines the position chosen for surgery. In general, all positions used for craniotomy have some degree of head elevation, the details of which were discussed earlier.

### Retraction and Brain Bulk Reduction

Location also determines the need for surgical retraction and affects the requirement for brain bulk reduction (hyperventilation, mannitol, spinal fluid drainage). If the tumor is

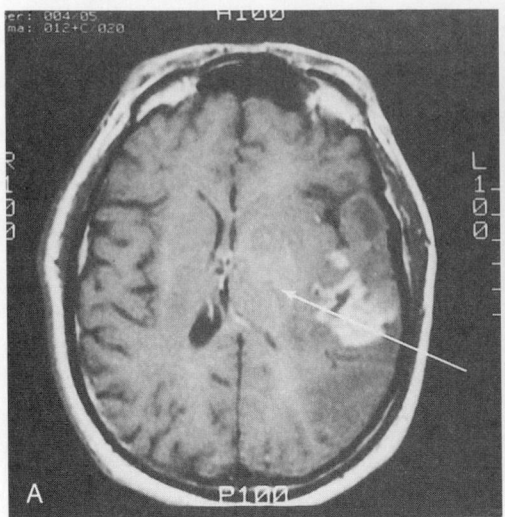 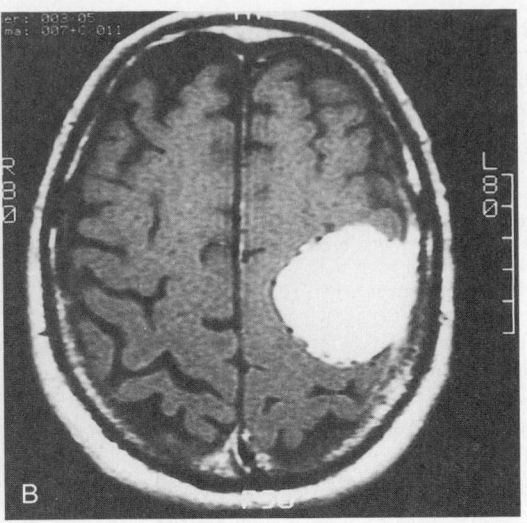

**FIGURE 69–11.** *A,* Magnetic resonance image of a patient with rapidly growing glioblastoma multiforme. Note the shift of structures *(arrow)* and loss of cortical folds. *B,* Magnetic resonance image of a patient with a slow-growing meningioma. Note the absence of shift in structures and the preservation of cortical folds despite the presence of a very large tumor.

located on the cortical surface, retraction is minimal. In this case, if ICP is not elevated, mannitol and hyperventilation are usually unnecessary and sometimes deleterious. For example, if mannitol is given during resection of a small, superficial meningioma, the distance between the dura and cortical surface at the conclusion of surgery can be increased greatly, allowing a postoperative collection of blood and CSF. On the other hand, if this same small meningioma is located on the sphenoid wing, retraction of the frontal and temporal lobes is needed to reach the tumor. Mannitol and perhaps hyperventilation in this case are beneficial because these reduce the amount of retractor pressure necessary for tumor exposure. Again, however, there is increased concern about the effects of hyperventilation on cerebral blood flow, and many clinicians would recommend its use only when other measures, such as mannitol, positioning, and anesthetic technique, have been optimized to reduce brain bulk.

### Nearby Structures

Tumor location near or involving important intracranial structures can be a critical factor. A large sphenoid wing meningioma frequently envelops the carotid artery, middle cerebral artery, or both. In this case, large-bore venous access is needed in the event that major hemorrhage occurs. Electrophysiologic monitoring and barbiturate cerebral protection are useful if temporary vessel occlusion is necessary for tumor resection.

### Why Is Vascularity Important?

Tumors have widely varying vascularity (see Table 69–17). Meningiomas, hemangioblastomas, and some metastatic le-

**TABLE 69–18.** Computed Tomographic and Magnetic Resonance Imaging Signs of Increased Intracranial Pressure*

Shift of structures from normal anatomic position
Small or absent ventricles
Loss of cortical folds
Loss of cerebrospinal fluid in prepontine and mesencephalic cisterns
Cerebral edema (white matter)
Hydrocephalus with loss of cortical folds

*See also Figure 69–11A.

sions carry a significant risk for serious intraoperative hemorrhage. These tumors may be embolized preoperatively to help reduce intraoperative blood loss. Resection of vascular tumors necessitates large-bore intravenous access. Measurement of central venous or pulmonary artery pressures helps to guide fluid replacement.

## What Operations Are Performed?

### Craniotomy

Surgical procedures for intracranial neoplasms are performed for several reasons, including definitive, curative removal, debulking of tumor mass in nonsurgically curable lesions, and tissue biopsy for pathologic diagnosis. For curative removal and debulking operations, a formal craniotomy is performed, and the lesion is completely removed. Lesions in the frontal, temporal, parietal, and occipital regions are approached by removing a plate of bone (ie, craniotomy), opening the dura, and excising the tumor.

If the tumor is not on the surface, retraction of neural tissue or an incision in the cortex is necessary to gain access for tumor removal or debulking. The bone plate is usually replaced after surgery. Because of the thickness of the bone in the suboccipital region, craniotomy with removal of a bone plate is often not possible. Instead, burr holes are made and then widened by removing small bites of bone at a time (craniectomy). This bone is usually not replaced.

### Stereotactic Surgery

### Local Anesthetics

For patients in whom surgical cure is either impossible or associated with major morbidity, tissue diagnosis may be obtained using stereotactic neurosurgical techniques performed with local anesthetics. These techniques greatly decrease surgical trauma and hospital stay. Before stereotactic neurosurgery, the patient's head is secured in a radiopaque frame using local anesthesia for pin fixation. CT or MRI is then made (Fig. 69–12A). The radiopaque frame places reference points on the CT scan. Using these reference points, computer calculations are made to localize the tumor with reference to the frame.

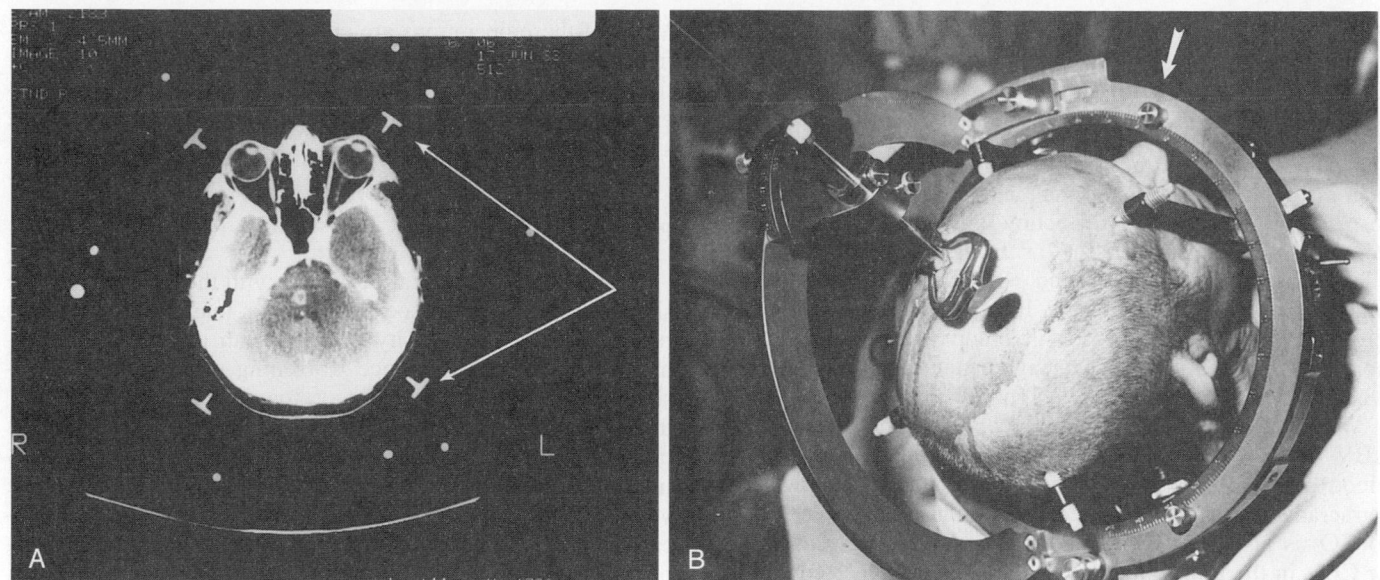

**FIGURE 69–12.** *A,* Computed tomography scan of a patient with a stereotactic frame in place. Note the coordinates placed by the frame on the scan *(arrow).* *B,* A patient in the operating room with a stereotactic frame in place. Note that this frame interferes with access to the airway *(arrow).*

Upon completion, the patient is taken to the operating room, and the scalp is prepared. A sterile operating frame is attached to the stereotactic frame (see Fig. 69–12*B*). Using coordinates determined from CT or MRI, the surgeon drills a small burr hole using local anesthesia. A biopsy needle is placed to a calculated depth, and the tissue sample is sent to the lab. Once the adequacy of the sample is confirmed by frozen section, the incision is closed, and CT is again used to make certain that hemorrhage has not occurred. The patient is discharged home the next day.

### General Anesthesia

When the patient is not cooperative, stereotactic biopsy may also be done under general anesthesia. If the stereotactic frame is placed on the patient's head before the induction of anesthesia, airway management may be extremely difficult because the inferior portion of the frame crosses in front of the mouth and nose and interferes with both mask ventilation and intubation (see Fig. 69–12). If possible, the patient should be anesthetized and intubated before placement of the frame.

Alternatively, the frame may be placed under local anesthesia in the CT scanner as was described previously. The patient is then taken to the operating room, and an awake, fiberoptic tracheal intubation is performed. When the airway is secured, induction of general anesthesia follows. Some newer stereotactic devices allow removal of the portion of the frame in front of the airway, thus avoiding these problems.

Finally, and perhaps the best alternative, stereotactic frames are presently available for both CT and MRI that have a removable front piece, allowing essentially normal access to the airway. However, options for the patient's head position remain severely limited, and patients with marginal or difficult airway anatomy may not be able to be intubated with the usual instrumentation. I have found the low profile Bullard (Circon ACMI, Stamford, Conn) or Upsher (Upsher Laryngoscope Corp, Foster City, Calif) instrumentation very helpful in this circumstance.

## How Does Preoperative Neurologic Function Influence Management?

### General Considerations

Tumors have a variety of effects on preoperative neurologic function. Faster growing tumors with surrounding edema and tumors located near eloquent areas of the brain (ie, areas whose function may be tested by clinical examination) have the greatest effects. Vasogenic edema may also produce loss of function. In contrast, slowly growing tumors may reach a large size without changing neurologic function at all.

### Seizures

New onset of seizures is a common presentation of an intracranial mass. Seizures can occur with tumors of any size. They are most common with those located in the cerebral cortex. Tumors in subcortical regions or in the posterior fossa are not usually accompanied by seizure activity. Therapeutic anticonvulsant levels should be attained preoperatively in patients with seizures. Unless intraoperative electrocorticography for seizure localization is planned, therapy should be continued during surgery, and levels should be checked again postoperatively.

Patients with cortical tumors who do not have seizures are usually started on prophylactic anticonvulsants either preoperatively or during surgery. This therapy helps to prevent postoperative seizures, which are common after manipulation of the cerebral cortex. Patients with subcortical tumors (eg, pituitary adenoma) or with tumors in the posterior fossa (eg, acoustic neuroma) do not usually require seizure prophylaxis.

Many anticonvulsants induce hepatic microsomal enzymes. Thus, another consequence of anticonvulsant therapy is that hepatically metabolized anesthetic drugs (eg, muscle relaxants and narcotics) can have a remarkably reduced duration of clinical effect.

## Homeostatic Mechanisms

Laboratory studies of experimental brain tumors and clinical data suggest that autoregulation and $CO_2$ responses are impaired or absent.[173,174] Tumors may also influence homeostatic mechanisms in the surrounding brain. If function of an area of the brain remains normal, autoregulation and response to $CO_2$ are likely intact. If function is lost, either from direct compression of neural tissue or from the development of edema, both autoregulation and response to $CO_2$ are likely impaired or lost in that region. If autoregulation is lost (see Fig. 69–1B), slight decreases in blood pressure within the normal range may produce a significant reduction in CBF, whereas increases augment CBF and CBV.

When intracranial elastance is poor, even small changes in CBV produce large changes in ICP. Thus, careful control of blood pressure is extremely important in the patient with an intracranial mass and impaired autoregulation. If the response to $CO_2$ is also lost, hyperventilation does not decrease CBF or CBV in the affected area. Other methods of ICP control or brain bulk reduction, such as mannitol infusion and drainage of CSF through a ventriculostomy catheter, must be used in these patients.

### Rapidity of Deterioration

Patients with intracranial mass, severe headache, and rapidly deteriorating level of consciousness likely have significantly elevated ICP and may be close to herniation. When coexisting disease affects anesthetic management, work-up and treatment must take place quickly. No medical conditions take priority over surgical decompression of a patient with impending cerebral herniation.

Patients with preoperative *focal* abnormalities may also need urgent surgery. A large pituitary tumor may be associated with rapidly deteriorating vision. Urgent optic nerve decompression is needed to prevent permanent blindness. Preoperative communication with the neurosurgeon helps to determine the urgency of an individual operation.

## How Does Preexisting Disease Affect Anesthetic Management?

Operative trauma associated with intracranial tumor resection varies greatly. Removal of a small, superficial, low-grade glioma does not usually involve major blood loss or fluid shifts. Mannitol is unnecessary to reduce ICP. Removal of a large meningioma or glioblastoma multiforme, however, may be associated with a significant blood loss. In this situation, mannitol may be necessary to reduce brain bulk and lower ICP.

### Cardiovascular Function

Preexisting cardiac disease may present problems in any of these operations but has a greater impact during procedures that are associated with large blood loss or that require mannitol administration to lower ICP. Acutely, mannitol increases preload and may precipitate congestive heart failure. Later, mannitol-induced reduction of ventricular preload is not well tolerated by patients with poor ventricular function and can result in significant hypotension unless preload is maintained.

Many of these operations are conducted with patients in positions other than the supine. Patients with poor ventricular function, as has been noted repeatedly, may not tolerate decreased venous return that is sometimes associated with the sitting, prone, or three-quarter prone positions.

### Pulmonary Function

Nearly all neurosurgical positions, with the exception of the sitting position, are associated with a marked reduction in functional residual capacity. Patients with preexisting pulmonary disease may experience worsening of ventilation-perfusion mismatch after positioning, particularly in the prone, three-quarter prone, or lateral position. Unless the patient is obese, the sitting position is generally well tolerated. In addition, patients with significant bronchospastic disease may be very difficult to hyperventilate when this technique is indicated. Hyperventilation may result in air-trapping and lung overdistention secondary to failure of the lungs to deflate.

## Can Patients With Intracranial Masses Be Safely Premedicated?

Patients with intracranial masses may be sensitive to premedication for two reasons. First, many premedications produce respiratory depression. Increases in $PaCO_2$ cause increases in CBF, and CBV and may result in a dangerous increase in ICP. Second, some brain tumors, particularly those located in the frontal lobes or in the posterior fossa, appear to cause increased sensitivity to the sedating and respiratory depressant properties of premedicant drugs.

Therefore, the simplest and safest answer to the question posed by this section is "no." However, many of these patients are appropriately anxious and benefit from anxiolysis. Patients with intracranial masses but normal intracranial elastance readily tolerate mild to moderate respiratory depression and exhibit normal sensitivity to premedication. Several sedative medications, such as diphenhydramine and hydroxyzine, are not associated with respiratory depression. Some premedications, such as barbiturates, although producing respiratory depression, may be associated with a smaller increase in CBV because of their own cerebral vasoconstricting properties.

My premedication practice for these patients is shown in Table 69–19. This policy clearly is very conservative. However, because most of these patients are admitted to the hospital *after* surgery, no other method is both feasible *and* safe.

---

**TABLE 69–19.** Premedication for Patients With Intracranial Masses

---

After the preoperative interview, if the patient appears calm, a premedication is usually not needed.

If the patient appears very anxious, the patient is brought to the preoperative holding area, and premedication is given. Pulse oximetry with the patient breathing room air is monitored to facilitate early detection of respiratory depression. Neurologic function is monitored by the preoperative nursing personnel.

Do not give premedication or sleeping medications to patients with brain tumors who are in unmonitored environments.

---

**TABLE 69–20.** Factors Influencing Monitoring for Removal of an Intracranial Mass

**Nature of the Operation**
Limited procedure for tissue diagnosis versus definitive removal
Anticipated blood loss
Location of the lesion, adjacent neural structures at risk from surgery
Sudden vital sign changes likely during manipulation of neural structures
Positioning of the patient
**Preoperative Intracranial Elastance and Intracranial Pressure**
**Coexisting Disease**
Preexisting cardiac, pulmonary, or renal disease

## What Monitoring Is Necessary?

Monitoring needs for intracranial mass resections are determined by several factors (Table 69–20). As with other neurosurgical procedures, coexisting cardiac, pulmonary, or renal disease may impose requirements independent of the operation.

### Type of Operation

The first consideration, obviously, is the nature of the operation. A limited stereotactic procedure conducted under local anesthesia needs only routine, noninvasive monitoring. Definitive resection of a highly vascular large meningioma that may involve major blood loss necessitates invasive arterial pressure monitoring.

Resection of mass lesions located next to eloquent CNS structures may require special monitoring to prevent neurologic damage. Consider the patient with a left temporal lobe mass located near the speech center. To localize the speech center precisely and thus prevent inadvertent resection of eloquent tissue, resection is best performed using local anesthesia. The function of the neural tissue can then be tested while the patient is awake and can talk (see Chapter 21).

Localization within the motor cortex is possible by using direct intraoperative electrical stimulation of the cortex and by observing a peripheral motor response. In similar fashion, the sensory cortex may be localized by electrical stimulation of peripheral nerves and by recording the response directly from the cortex.

Occasionally, tumors are located near or involve structures that, when manipulated, may cause large changes in blood pressure or heart rate. For example, some posterior fossa tumors involve the vagus nerve. Resection of these tumors may be associated with sudden severe bradycardia or asystole. Central venous access in these cases is helpful to administer drugs for correction of life-threatening, surgically induced hemodynamic instability.

### Positioning

Resections, particularly when tumors are located in the posterior fossa, may be conducted with the patient in the sitting position. As discussed previously, the precordial Doppler and central venous catheter are helpful in the diagnosis and treatment of venous air embolism. Many posterior fossa explorations are conducted with the patient in the three-quarter prone position; they are also associated with a significant incidence of air embolism.[175] In my experience, craniofacial repairs in children and bifrontal craniotomies in adults are also associated with a high incidence of venous air emboli. Precordial Doppler monitoring is noninvasive and inexpensive. I use it routinely when the head is elevated more than 20°.

### Increased Intracranial Pressure and Decreased Elastance

Preoperative intracranial elastance and ICP also influence monitoring. Patients with high ICP or poor intracranial elastance are at high risk for hypotension-related decreases in cerebral perfusion. If possible, invasive arterial monitoring should be started before induction of anesthesia to enable rapid detection and correction of hypotension.

## How Should Anesthesia Be Managed?

Anesthetic planning for removal of intracranial masses centers on three factors: the type of operation, the type of tumor (see Table 69–17), and the patient's position (see Tables 69–3 and 69–4). Multiple anesthetic regimens can be used (see Table 69–1). Common goals are listed in Table 69–21. As always, provided that the anesthetic regimen chosen meets as many of these goals as possible, the choice of drug and technique is relatively unimportant to the operation's success. Outcome studies examining intraoperative conditions and postoperative parameters, such as rapidity of emergence and use of antihypertensive agents, fail to demonstrate a difference between drug regimens when all drugs are used appropriately.[1–3]

### Positioning

Careful positioning that avoids nerve stretching, and compression and application of padding to avoid pressure on the skin help to avoid position-related injury in these frequently lengthy operations.

#### Head Position

Elevation of the head above the level of the heart facilitates venous drainage and minimizes the effect of intracranial venous blood volume on intracranial elastance and ICP. A balance assessment between the beneficial ICP and elastance effects of head elevation and the harmful risk for air embolism must be made.

No studies determining the degree of head elevation that produces an ideal balance have been performed. The normal CVP of most patients is between 5 and 15 cm $H_2O$. I speculate

**TABLE 69–21.** Anesthetic Goals During Intracranial Tumor Surgery

1. Prevention of decreases in cerebral perfusion and cerebral blood flow; prevent decreases in blood pressure; prevent increases in ICP
2. Reduction in brain bulk *if needed* to decrease intracranial pressure and minimize retraction needed for tumor exposure
3. Protection of patient from position-related injury, including air embolism
4. Rapid emergence to allow neurologic assessment at the conclusion of surgery

that for a normovolemic patient, a head elevation of 20° or less is probably not associated with greatly subatmospheric cerebral venous pressures and high risk for venous air embolism. This degree of elevation still provides excellent venous drainage and minimizes venous blood volume. Rotation of the head away from midline may impede venous drainage and increase cerebral venous blood volume. Significant rotation may also impede vertebral artery flow.[176]

If surgical exposure requires a head rotation of more than 30°, I turn the body until neck rotation is less than 30° while keeping the head fixed in position. This goal may require that the patient be placed nearly lateral, lateral, or even beyond lateral into the three-quarter prone or prone position. When the surgeon requests head flexion, I limit it so that at least 2 fingerbreadths of distance remain between the mentum and the manubrium.

### Bite Block Insertion

Some type of bite block is desirable to prevent occlusion of the endotracheal tube if the patient's mouth clamps shut during periods of light anesthesia. Because craniotomies are frequently associated with some degree of head flexion, the oral airway, as discussed previously, may compress the hard and soft palates, producing mucosal necrosis.[159] A hard plastic sleeve that is fitted over the endotracheal tube effectively prevents bite occlusion (see Fig. 69–9) without causing oropharyngeal injury.

## How Should Ventilation Be Managed?

As discussed previously, use of hyperventilation to lower ICP has become controversial, especially in patients with significant head trauma. In one study involving patients undergoing resection of a brain tumor, hyperventilation caused evidence of cerebral hypoperfusion as measured by jugular venous oxygen desaturation in a significant number (>50%) of patients anesthetized with a combination of propofol and fentanyl.[177] In my practice, I do not currently use hyperventilation during brain tumor surgery unless it is clearly known that the patient has poor elastance and elevated ICP. In those cases, I will use mild hyperventilation ($Paco_2$, 30–35 mm Hg) both before induction and during surgery until I can see the dura and assess intradural pressure. If there is good brain relaxation obtained from careful positioning, appropriate use of anesthetic agents, mannitol, and fluid management, I gradually restore normocapnia over the next 30 minutes. If intradural pressure appears to be high when the bone flap is removed, I use moderate hyperventilation ($Paco_2$, 25–30 mm Hg) until the surgeon is able to open the dura and obtain decompression by removal of CSF and the tumor itself. At that point, I gradually adjust ventilation to return the patient to normocapnia as soon as possible.

Although it is not clear what the best management of $CO_2$ during craniotomy for tumor actually is, available evidence would suggest that routine prophylactic hyperventilation is not warranted; although hyperventilation may be needed to control intracranial hypertension before dural opening, it should not be the first and only technique used. There is now also substantiation that even during prolonged surgery, the end-tidal $CO_2$-to–$Paco_2$ gradient remains stable over time.[178] Once the gradient's magnitude has been established, end-tidal $CO_2$ may be used in lieu of blood gas analysis to determine the degree of hyperventilation actually being used unless major changes in pulmonary status occur during surgery (eg, massive blood loss requiring major fluid resuscitation, development of bronchospasm).

## How Should Fluids Be Managed?

Classic teaching recommends that patients undergoing resection of an intracranial tumor should be kept relatively hypovolemic to prevent edema-related increases in brain bulk and ICP. As our understanding of the blood–brain barrier has improved, several investigators have questioned the wisdom of this management. Three concepts—osmolality, tissue elastance, and colloid oncotic pressure—must be understood.

### Plasma Osmolality

Osmolality is the number of osmotically active particles per kilogram of solvent (Osm/kg). Osmolality is determined by a measurement technique known as *freezing-point depression*. A solution with more osmotically active particles than another shows greater depression of its freezing point. Solution osmolality (a measured parameter) may be roughly estimated by calculation of its osmolarity. The calculation assumes that all dissolved molecules completely dissociate in solution. For example, normal saline has a sodium chloride concentration of 154 mmol/L. Completely dissociated, this solution would have a concentration of 154 mEq/L of sodium and 154 mEq/L of chloride. The calculated osmolarity is 154 × 2 = 308 mOsm/L. Sodium chloride molecules, however, are not completely dissociated in solution. This observation is important because a nondissociated molecule of sodium chloride is only one osmotically active particle, whereas a dissociated molecule generates two osmotically active particles. Thus, fewer than predicted osmotically active particles are present, and normal saline has a measured osmolality of only 280 mOsm/kg. See Table 69–22 for the osmolarities and osmolalities of other intravenous fluids.

Osmotically active particles draw water across a semipermeable biologic membrane (such as the capillary wall or cell membrane) until the same osmolality is present on both sides of the membrane. Osmotic activity may also be described

**TABLE 69–22.** Osmolarity and Osmolality of Common Intravenous Fluids

| Fluid | Osmolarity (mOsm/L) | Osmolality (mOsm/kg) |
|---|---|---|
| Water | 0 | 0 |
| $D_5W$ | 252 | 259 |
| $D_5$ .2NS | 325 | 321 |
| NS | 308 | 282 |
| LR | 273 | 250 |
| $D_5LR$ | 525 | 524 |
| 3% Saline | 1027 | 921 |
| 6% Hetastarch | 310 | 307 |
| 20% Mannitol | 1098 | 1280 |
| Plasma protein fraction | — | 261 |

$D_5$ .2NS, 5% dextrose in 0.2 normal saline; $D_5LR$, 5% dextrose in lactated Ringer's solution; $D_5NS$, 5% dextrose in normal saline; $D_5W$, 5% dextrose in water.

in terms of osmotic pressure, estimated by the following equation:

$$\text{Osmotic Pressure (mm Hg)} = 19.3 \times \text{Osmolality (mOsm/kg solution)}$$

(Equation 2)

For plasma with a normal osmolality of 280 mOsm/kg, the osmotic pressure is more than 5400 mm Hg. Sodium chloride accounts for most of the plasma osmolality and, thus, osmotic pressure. Plasma proteins account for slightly more than 1 mOsm/kg or 24 mm Hg of osmotic pressure.

### Hypoosmotic Fluids

If hypoosmotic intravenous fluids are given (eg, 5% dextrose in water, 0.45% sodium chloride, or lactated Ringer's solution <280 mOsm/kg), plasma osmolality falls. Osmotic pressure changes cause water to pass from the capillaries into the interstitial space throughout the body, including the brain. As an example, an acute drop in plasma osmolarity of 20 mOsm/L (decrease in sodium from 140 to 130 mEq/L) results in a net osmotic pressure change of nearly 400 mm Hg, drives water into the interstitium, and produces edema.

### The Blood-Brain Barrier

Outside the CNS, sodium normally crosses the capillary endothelial barrier into the interstitial space, drawing water with it. Administration of a large isosmotic fluid load that causes an increase in capillary hydrostatic pressure, therefore, may produce peripheral edema even in a normal patient until lymphatic and excretory mechanisms eliminate the excess solute and water. However, the blood-brain barrier does not normally allow sodium to cross. Administration of a large isosmotic fluid load does *not* produce interstitial cerebral edema, even though edema may occur elsewhere. Most experts now agree that the *osmolality* of administered fluid has a much greater impact on cerebral edema formation than does the absolute *amount* of intravenous fluid.

### Tissue Elastance

Tissue elastance is defined as the change in interstitial pressure per milliliter of volume added. It can be considered a measure of the tendency of a tissue to develop edema. A highly elastic tissue, such as the bowel wall, readily forms edema. Interstitial hydrostatic pressure does not increase until a very large amount of edema is present. The brain, however, with its dense network of glial cells, is inelastic. Interstitial hydrostatic pressure begins to rise rapidly even with minimal edema. Thus, usual capillary hydrostatic pressure changes are insufficient to cause significant edema. A drop in serum osmolality, however, produces a significant driving force for edema formation in the brain and the rest of the body.

### Colloid Oncotic Pressures

The osmotic (oncotic) pressure exerted by plasma proteins (24 mm Hg) is very small when compared with the total osmotic pressure (>5400 mm Hg). However, osmotic pressure exerted by sodium chloride is nearly the same on both sides of the capillary membrane, whereas proteins are predominantly intravascular. The colloid oncotic pressure, therefore, plays an important role in helping to keep fluids intravascular.

Because the colloid oncotic pressure is normally only about 24 mm Hg, a fall in this value cannot produce much interstitial edema. That which forms is primarily in elastic tissues, such as the bowel wall or the lungs, that can increase water content without immediately increasing tissue hydrostatic pressure. In the inelastic brain, however, an increase in brain water caused by decreased colloic oncotic pressure results in an immediate increase in tissue hydrostatic pressure that opposes further edema formation. Even large decreases in colloid oncotic pressure are unlikely to cause significant cerebral edema.

### The Bottom Line

The preceding discussion is somewhat theoretic and assumes normal blood-brain barrier function. In many patients with brain tumors, however, this normal function is lost, and sodium may readily cross into the interstitial space. However, at least in brain trauma, experimental evidence suggests that increases in cerebral edema associated with decreases in plasma osmolality occur primarily in areas of normal brain (ie, the blood-brain barrier is intact). In my opinion, the most important goals of intraoperative fluid management during surgery for removal of brain tumors (and in fact for all intracranial neurologic surgery) are maintenance of at least normal plasma osmolality, adequate cardiac output, and cerebral perfusion.

### Fluids of Choice

Maintenance of normal (290 mOsm/kg) osmolality can be readily accomplished using isosmotic fluids. I generally use 0.9% sodium chloride solution. Lactated Ringer's solution, although generally thought to be isosmotic, actually has an osmolality of only 250 mOsm/kg and should, in my opinion, not be used during intracranial surgery. I avoid the administration of dextrose during intracranial surgery unless hypoglycemia is documented.

### Syndrome of Inappropriate Antidiuretic Hormone Secretion

Some patients with intracranial masses develop the syndrome of inappropriate antidiuretic hormone secretion and come to the operating room with an already decreased serum osmolality. In these patients, I gradually return the sodium level to normal values at a rate of 1 to 2 mEq/L per hour using mannitol (free water diuresis) and isotonic 0.9% sodium chloride. Occasionally, a slow infusion of hypertonic saline is needed.

### Summary

Prevention of cerebral edema by fluid restriction makes no sense if this goal is accomplished at the cost of decreased cardiac output, blood pressure, and CBF. If the patient has excellent cardiovascular function and maintains blood pressure and cardiac output even with decreased preload, fluid restriction may not be harmful. A patient with poor ventricular function, however, may require restoration of normal preload after mannitol administration if hypotension develops. I emphasize again that the amount of fluid administered is a much less important factor driving the formation of cerebral edema than is the plasma osmolality.

## What Factors Are Particularly Important During Emergence?

### Blood Pressure Control

Control of blood pressure during emergence is very important. Bleeding may readily occur from incompletely resected tumors or from the tumor bed. I aggressively treat elevations of more than 20% above the blood pressure just before dural closure and prefer short-acting drugs such as sodium nitroprusside and esmolol during this very labile period. After extubation and transport to the intensive care unit have been completed, the magnitude of blood pressure changes usually decreases. In this more stable period, weaning from sodium nitroprusside with substitution of longer-acting drugs such as labetalol as needed is appropriate.

### Neurologic Assessment

Quick emergence from anesthesia at the conclusion of the operation is needed to allow assessment of neurologic status. If the patient does not promptly return to baseline status, a CT scan is needed to exclude a postoperative hematoma.

### Continued Intubation and Ventilation

Patients with preoperative severe global neurologic impairment should remain intubated at the conclusion of surgery. Continued intubation allows careful control of arterial partial pressures of $O_2$ and $CO_2$ during this critical period. Muscle relaxation and sedation should be minimized.

## CONCLUSIONS

Neuroanesthetic management, including choice of drugs, special techniques, positioning, and fluid management, directly affects normal and pathologic neurologic function. Unlike many other organ systems, neural tissue has only a limited capacity for repair or regeneration. Surgically induced or anesthetic-induced damage thus may produce permanent change in function. As our understanding of anesthetic effects has improved and new monitoring techniques have become available, appropriate anesthetic management has made major contributions to the ease and success of increasingly complex neurosurgical procedures.

This chapter provides a framework to organize large amounts of data concerning anesthetic drugs and special techniques, neurophysiology and neuroanatomy, neuropathology, and neurosurgical procedures into a coherent, logical approach to the neurosurgical patient. Although the scope is necessarily limited, the approaches discussed for vascular neurosurgery, spine surgery, and tumor surgery are equally applicable to patients with any neurosurgical problem.

### References

1. Grundy BL, Pashayan AG, Mahla ME, et al. Three balanced anesthetic techniques for neuroanesthesia: infusion of thiopental sodium with su-

fentanil or fentanyl compared with inhalation of isoflurane. *J Clin Anesth.* 1992;4:372.
2. From RP, Warner DS, Todd MM, et al. Anesthesia for craniotomy: a double-blind comparison of alfentanil, fentanyl and sufentanil. *Anesthesiology.* 1990;73:896.
3. Todd MM, Warner DS, Sokoll M, et al. A prospective, comparative trial of three anesthetics for elective supratentorial craniotomy: propofol/fentanyl, isoflurane/nitrous oxide, and fentanyl/nitrous oxide. *Anesthesiology.* 1993;78:1005.
4. Schierhout G, Roberts I. Hyperventilation therapy for acute traumatic brain injury. *Cochrane Database Syst Rev.* 2000;2:CD000566.
5. Marion DW, Spiegel TP. Changes in the management of severe traumatic brain injury: 1991–1997. *Crit Care Med.* 2000;28:16.
6. Robertson CS, Valadka AB, Hannay HJ, et al. Prevention of secondary ischemic insults after severe head injury. *Crit Care Med.* 1999;27:2086.
7. Roberts I, Schierhout G, Alderson P. Absence of evidence for the effectiveness of five interventions routinely used in the intensive care management of severe head injury: a systemic review. *J Neurol Neurosurg Psychiatry.* 1998;65:729.
8. Schneider GH, Sarrafzadeh AS, Kiening KL, et al. Influence of hyperventilation on brain tissue—$PO_2$, $PCO_2$, and pH in patients with intracranial hypertension. *Acta Neurochir Suppl (Wien).* 1998;71:62.
9. Thiagarajan A, Goverdhan PD, Chari P, et al. The effect of hyperventilation and hyperoxia on cerebral venous oxygen saturation in patients with traumatic brain injury. *Anesth Analg.* 1998;87:850.
10. Allen CH, Ward JD. An evidence-based approach to management of increased intracranial pressure. *Crit Care Clin.* 1998;14:485.
11. Rosner MJ. Rosner SD, Johnson AH. Cerebral perfusion pressure: management protocol and clinical results. *J Neurosurg.* 1995;83:949.
12. Fortune JB, Feustel PJ, Graca L, et al. Effect of hyperventilation, mannitol, and ventriculostomy drainage on cerebral blood flow after head injury. *J Trauma.* 1995;39:1091.
13. Nehls DG, Todd MM, Spetzler RF, et al. A comparison of the cerebral protective effects of isoflurane and barbiturates during temporary focal ischemia in primates. *Anesthesiology.* 1987;66:453.
14. Hoffman WE, Pelligrino D, Werner C, et al. Ketamine decreases plasma catecholamines and improves outcome from incomplete cerebral ischemia in rats. *Anesthesiology.* 1992;76:755.
15. Miura Y, Grocott HP, Bart RD, et al. Differential effects of anesthetic agents on outcome from near-complete but not incomplete global ischemia in the rat. *Anesthesiology.* 1998;89:391.
16. Schmid-Elsaesser R, Schroder M, Zausinger S, et al. EEG burst suppression is not necessary for maximum barbiturate protection in transient focal cerebral ischemia in the rat. *J Neurol Sci.* 1999;162:14.
17. Messick JM, Casement B, Sharbrough FW, et al. Correlation of regional cerebral blood flow (rCBF) with EEG changes during isoflurane anesthesia for carotid endarterectomy: critical rCBF. *Anesthesiology.* 1987;66:344.
18. Sundt TW, Sharbrough FW, Piepgras DG, et al. Correlation of cerebral blood flow and electroencephalographic changes during carotid endarterectomy: with results of surgery and hemodynamics of cerebral ischemia. *Mayo Clin Proc.* 1981;56:533.
19. Procaccio F, Stocchetti N, Citerio G, et al. Guidelines for the treatment of adults with severe head trauma (part I). Initial assessment; evaluation and pre-hospital treatment; current criteria for hospital admission; systemic and cerebral monitoring. *J Neurosurg Sci.* 44:1.
20. Procaccio F, Stocchetti N, Citerio G, et al. Guidelines for the treatment of adults with severe head trauma (part II). Criteria for medical treatment. *J Neurosurg Sci.* 2000;44:11.
21. Manley GT, Hemphill JC, Morabito D, et al. Cerebral oxygenation during hemorrhagic shock: perils of hyperventilation and the therapeutic potential of hypoventilation. *J Trauma.* 2000;48:1025.
22. Rosner MJ. Introduction to cerebral perfusion pressure management. *Neurosurg Clin North Am.* 1995;6:761.
23. Cruz J. The first decade of continuous monitoring of jugular bulb oxyhemoglobin saturation: management strategies and clinical outcome. *Crit Care Med.* 1998;26:344
24. Kassel NF, Hitchon PW, Gerk MK, et al. Influence of changes in arterial $pCO_2$ on cerebral blood flow and metabolism during high-dose barbiturate therapy in dogs. *J Neurosurg.* 1981;54:615.
25. Cold GE, Eskesen V, Eriksen H, et al. CBF and $CMRO_2$ during continuous etomidate infusion supplemented with $N_2O$ and fentanyl in patients with supratentorial tumour: a dose response study. *Acta Anaesthesiol Scand.* 1985;29:490.
26. Pinaud M, Lelausque JN, Chetanneau A, et al. Effects of propofol on cerebral hemodynamics and metabolism in patients with brain trauma. *Anesthesiology.* 1990;73:404.

27. Weinstabl C, Mayer N, Jammerle AF, et al. The effects of propofol bolus administration on the intracranial pressure in craniocerebral trauma. *Anaesthetist.* 1990;39:521.
28. Eng C, Lam AM, Mayberg TS, et al. The influence of propofol with and without nitrous oxide on cerebral blood flow velocity and $CO_2$ reactivity in humans. *Anesthesiology.* 1992;77:872.
29. Fox J, Gelb AW, Enns J, et al. The responsiveness of cerebral blood flow to changes in arterial carbon dioxide is maintained during propofol-nitrous oxide anesthesia in humans. *Anesthesiology.* 1992;77:453.
30. Van Hemelrijck J, Fitch W, Mattheussen M, et al. Effect of propofol on cerebral circulation in the baboon. *Anesth Analg.* 1990;71:49.
31. Larsen R, Hilfiker O, Radke J, et al. The effects of midazolam on the general circulation, cerebral blood flow and cerebral oxygen consumption in man. *Anaesthetist.* 1981;30:18.
32. Forster A, Juge O, Morel D. Effects of midazolam on cerebral hemodynamics and cerebral vasomotor responsiveness to carbon dioxide. *J Cereb Blood Flow Metab.* 1983;3:246.
33. Forster A, Juge O, Morel D. Effects of midazolam on cerebral blood flow in human volunteers. *Anesthesiology.* 1982;56:453.
34. Jobes DR, Kennell E, Bitner R, et al. Effects of morphine-nitrous oxide anesthesia on cerebral autoregulation. *Anesthesiology.* 1975;42:30.
35. McPherson RW, Traystman RJ. Fentanyl and cerebral vascular responsivity in dogs. *Anesthesiology.* 1984;60:180.
36. McPherson RW, Krempansanka E, Eimerl D. Effects of alfentanil on cerebral vascular reactivity in dogs. *Br J Anaesth.* 1985;57:1232.
37. Sperry RJ, Bailey PL, Reichman MV, et al. Fentanyl and sufentanil increase intracranial pressure in head trauma patients. *Anesthesiology.* 1992;77:416.
38. Weinstabl C, Mayer N, Richling B, et al. Effect of sufentanil on intracranial pressure in neurosurgical patients. *Anaesthesia.* 1991;46:837.
39. Shupak RC, Harp JR. Comparison between high-dose sufentanil-oxygen and high-dose fentanyl-oxygen for neuroanesthesia. *Br J Anaesth.* 1985;57:375.
40. Marx W, Shah N, Long C, et al. Sufentanil, alfentanil and fentanyl: impact on cerebrospinal fluid pressure in patients with brain tumors. *J Neurosurg Anesthesiol.* 1989;1:3.
41. Turner DM, Kassell NF, Sasaki T, et al. Cerebral and systemic vascular effects of naloxone in pentobarbital-anesthetized normal dogs. *Neurosurgery.* 1984;14:276.
42. Thiel A, Adams HA, Fengler G, et al. Studies using S (+) ketamine on probands: computerized EEG-analysis and transcranial Doppler ultrasonography. *Anaesthetist.* 1992;41:604.
43. Cavazzuti M, Porro CA, Biral GP, et al. Ketamine effects on local cerebral blood flow and metabolism in the rat. *J Cereb Blood Flow Metab.* 1987;7:806.
44. Young WL, Prohovnik I, Correll JW, et al. Cerebral blood flow and metabolism in patients undergoing anesthesia for carotid endarterectomy: a comparison of isoflurane, halothane, and fentanyl. *Anesth Analg.* 1989;68:712.
45. Miletich DJ, Ivankovich AD, Albrecht RF, et al. Absence of autoregulation of cerebral blood flow during halothane and enflurane anesthesia. *Anesth Analg.* 1976;55:100.
46. Algotsson L, Messeter K, Nordstrom CH, et al. Cerebral blood flow and oxygen consumption during isoflurane and halothane anesthesia in man. *Acta Anaesthesiol Scand.* 1988;32:15.
47. Madsen JB, Cold GE, Hansen ES, et al. The effect of isoflurane on cerebral blood flow and metabolism in humans during craniotomy for small supratentorial cerebral tumors. *Anesthesiology.* 1987;66:332.
48. Madsen JB, Cold GE, Eriksen HO, et al. CBF and $CMRO_2$ during craniotomy for small supratentorial cerebral tumours in enflurane anesthesia: a dose-response study. *Acta Anaesthesiol Scand.* 1986;30:633.
49. Muzzi D, Losasso T, Dietz N, et al. The effect of desflurane and isoflurane on cerebrospinal fluid pressure in humans with supratentorial mass lesions. *Anesthesiology.* 1992;76:720.
50. Archer DP, Labrecque P, Tyler JL, et al. Cerebral blood volume is increased in dogs during administration of nitrous oxide or isoflurane. *Anesthesiology.* 1987;67:642.
51. Algotsson L, Messeter K, Rosen I, et al. Effects of nitrous oxide on cerebral haemodynamics and metabolism during isoflurane anaesthesia in man. *Acta Anaesthesiol Scand.* 1992;36:46.
52. Roald OK, Forsman M, Heier MS, et al. Cerebral effects of nitrous oxide when added to low and high concentrations of isoflurane in the dog. *Anesth Analg.* 1991;72:75.
53. Baughman VL, Hoffman WE, Miletich DH, et al. Cerebrovascular and cerebral metabolic effects of $N_2O$ in unrestrained rats. *Anesthesiology.* 1990;73:269.
54. Kaieda R, Todd MM, Warner DS. The effects of anesthetics and $PaCO_2$ on the cerebrovascular, metabolic, and electroencephalographic responses to nitrous oxide in the rabbit. *Anesth Analg.* 1989;68:135.
55. Baughman VL, Hoffman WE, Thomas C, et al. The interaction of nitrous oxide and isoflurane with incomplete cerebral ischemia in the rat. *Anesthesiology.* 1989;70:767.
56. McPherson RW, Briar JE, Traystman RJ. Cerebrovascular responsiveness to carbon dioxide in dogs with 1.4% and 2.8% isoflurane. *Anesthesiology.* 1989;70:843.
57. Archer DP, Labrecque P, Tyler JL, et al. Measurement of cerebral blood flow and volume with positron emission tomography during isoflurane administration in the hypocapnic baboon. *Anesthesiology.* 1990;72:1031.
58. Artru AA. Partial preservation of cerebral vascular responsiveness to hypocapnia during isoflurane-induced hypotension in dogs. *Anesth Analg.* 1986;65:660.
59. McPherson RW, Traystman RJ. Effects of isoflurane on cerebral autoregulation in dogs. *Anesthesiology.* 1988;69:493.
60. Young WL, Prohovnik I, Correll JW, et al. A comparison of cerebral blood flow reactivity to $CO_2$ during halothane versus isoflurane anesthesia for carotid endarterectomy. *Anesth Analg.* 1991;73:416.
61. Leon LE, Bissonette B. Cerebrovascular responses to carbon dioxide in children anesthetized with halothane and isoflurane. *Can J Anaesth.* 1991;38:817.
62. Lutz LJ, Milde JH, Milde LN. The response of the canine cerebral circulation to hyperventilation during anesthesia with desflurane. *Anesthesiology.* 1991;74:504.
63. Lanier WL, Milde JH, Michenfelder JD. Cerebral stimulation following succinylcholine in dogs. *Anesthesiology.* 1986;64:551.
64. Lanier WL, Milde JH, Michenfelder JD. The cerebral effects of pancuronium and atracurium in halothane-anesthetized dogs. *Anesthesiology.* 1985;63:589.
65. Grubb RL, Raichle ME. Effects of hemorrhagic and pharmacologic hypotension on cerebral oxygen utilization and blood flow. *Anesthesiology.* 1982;56:3.
66. Larsen R, Drobnik L, Teichmann J, et al. The effects of halothane-, nitroprusside-, and trimethaphan-induced hypotension on cerebral blood flow and intracranial pressure. *Anaesthetist.* 1979;28:494.
67. Weiss MH, Spence J, Apuzzo ML, et al. Influence of nitroprusside on cerebral pressure autoregulation. *Neurosurgery.* 1979;4:56.
68. Stange K, Lagerkranser M, Sollevi A. Nitroprusside-induced hypotension and cerebrovascular autoregulation in the anesthetized pig. *Anesth Analg.* 1991;73:745.
69. Candia GJ, Heros RC, Lavyne MH, et al. Effect of intravenous sodium nitroprusside on cerebral blood flow and intracranial pressure. *Neurosurgery.* 1978;3:50.
70. Artru AA. Cerebral vascular responses to hypocapnia during nitroglycerine-induced hypotension. *Neurosurgery.* 1985;16:468.
71. Burt DE, Verniquet AJ, Homi J. The response of the canine intracranial pressure to systemic hypotension induced with nitroglycerine. *Br J Anaesth.* 1982;54:665.
72. Ishikawa T, Funatsu N, Okamoto K, et al. Cerebral and systemic effects of hypotension induced by trimethaphan or nitroprusside in dogs. *Acta Anaesthesiol Scand.* 1982;26:643.
73. Ulrich K, Kuschinsky W. In vivo effects of alpha-adrenoreceptor agonists and antagonists on pial veins of cats. *Stroke.* 1985;16:880.
74. Davis DH, Sundt TM Jr. Relationship of cerebral blood flow to cardiac output, mean arterial pressure, blood volume and alpha and beta blockade in cats. *J Neurosurg.* 1980;52:745.
75. Madsen PL, Vorstrup S, Schmidt JF, et al. Effect of acute and prolonged treatment with propranolol on cerebral blood flow and cerebral oxygen metabolism in healthy volunteers. *Eur J Clin Pharmacol.* 1990;39:295.
76. Dahlgren N, Ingvar M, Siesjo BK. Effect of propranolol on local cerebral blood flow under normocapnic and hypercapnic conditions. *J Cereb Blood Flow Metab.* 1981;1:429.
77. Gaab MR, Hollerhage HG, Walter GF, et al. Brain edema, autoregulation, and calcium antagonism: an experimental study with nimodipine. *Adv Neurol.* 1990;52:391.
78. Hill AC, Schecter WP, Mori H, et al. The effect of verapamil on cerebral cortical and spinal cord blood flow during proximal descending aortic occlusion. *J Trauma.* 1988;28:1214.
79. Pearce WJ, Bevan JA. Diltiazem and autoregulation of canine cerebral blood flow. *J Pharmacol Exp Ther.* 1987;242:812.
80. Brooks DJ, Redmond S, Mathias CJ, et al. The effect of orthostatic hypotension on cerebral blood flow and middle cerebral artery velocity in autonomic failure, with observations on the action of ephedrine. *J Neurol Neurosurg Psychiatry.* 1989;52:962.
81. Bundgaard H, von Oettingen G, Larsen KM, et al. Effects of sevoflurane

on intracranial pressure, cerebral blood flow, and cerebral metabolism: a dose-response study in patients subjected to craniotomy for cerebral tumours. *Acta Anaesthesiol Scand.* 1998;42:621.

82. Duffy CM, Matta BF. Sevoflurane and anesthesia for neurosurgery: a review. *J Neurosurg Anesthesiol.* 2000;12:128.

83. Artru AA, Lam AM, Johnson JO, et al. Intracranial pressure, middle cerebral artery flow velocity, and plasma inorganic fluoride concentrations in neurosurgical patients receiving sevoflurane or isoflurane. *Anesth Analg.* 1997;85:587.

84. Baker KZ. Desflurane and sevoflurane are valuable additions to the practice of neuroanesthesiology: pro. *J Neurosurg Anesthesiol.* 1997;9:66.

85. Tempelhoff R. The new inhalational anesthetics desflurane and sevoflurane are valuable additions to the practice of neuroanesthesia: con. *J Neurosurg Anesthesiol.* 1997;9:69.

86. Bedforth NM, Hardman JG, Nathanson MH. Cerebral hemodynamic response to the introduction of desflurane: a comparison with sevoflurane. *Anesth Analg.* 2000;91:152.

87. Bedforth NM, Girling KJ, Harrison JM, et al. The effects of sevoflurane and nitrous oxide on middle cerebral artery blood flow velocity and transient hyperemic response. *Anesth Analg.* 1999;89:170.

88. Summors AC, Gupta AK, Matta BF. Dyamic cerebral autoregulatioin during sevoflurane anesthesia: a comparison with isoflurane. *Anesth Analg.* 1999;88:341.

89. Warner DS. Experience with remifentanil in neurosurgical patients. *Anesth Analg.* 1999;89(4 suppl):S33.

90. Guy J, Hindman BJ, Baker KZ, et al. Comparison of remifentanil and fentanyl in patients undergoing craniotomy for supratentorial space-occupying lesions. *Anesthesiology.* 1997;86:514.

91. Tipps LB, Coplin WM, Murry KR, et al. Safety and feasibility of continuous infusion of remifentanil in the neurosurgical intensive care unit. *Neurosurgery.* 2000;46:596.

92. Albanese J, Viviand X, Potie F, et al. Sufentanil, fentanyl, and alfentanil in head trauma patients: a study on cerebral hemodynamics. *Crit Care Med.* 1999;27:407.

93. Lauer KK, Connolly LA, Schmelling WT. Opioid sedation does not alter intracranial pressure in head injured patients. *Can J Anaesth.* 1997;44:929.

94. Schramm WM, Strasser K, Bartunek A, et al. Effects of rocuronium and vecuronium on intracranial pressure, mean arterial pressure, and heart rate in neurosurgical patients. *Br J Anaesth.* 1996;77:607.

95. Schramm WM, Papousek A, Michalek-Sauberer A, et al. The cerebral and cardiovascular effects of cisatracurium and atracurium in neurosurgical patients. *Anesth Analg.* 1998;86:123.

96. Kovarik WD, Mayberg TS, Lam AM, et al. Succinylcholine does not change intracranial pressure, cerebral blood flow velocity, or the electroencephalogram in patients with neurologic injury. *Anesth Analg.* 1994;78:469.

97. Albin MS, Ritter RR, Pruett CE, et al. Venous air embolism during lumbar laminectomy in the prone position: report of three cases. *Anesth Analg.* 1992;75:152.

98. Bunegin L, Albin MS, Helsel PE, et al. Positioning the right atrial catheter: a model for reappraisal. *Anesthesiology.* 1981;55:343.

99. Hanna PG, Gravenstein N, Pashayan AG. In vitro comparison of central venous catheters for aspiration of air embolism: effect of catheter type, catheter tip position, and cardiac inclination. *J Clin Anesth.* 1991;3:290.

100. Colley PS, Artru AA. Bunegin-Albin catheter improves air retrieval and resuscitation from lethal venous air embolism in upright dogs. *Anesth Analg.* 1989;68:298.

101. Philips LH, Whisnant JP, O'Fallon WM, et al. The unchanging pattern of subarachnoid hemorrhage in a community. *Neurology.* 1980;30:1034.

102. Weir B. Medical aspects of the preoperative management of aneurysms: a review. *Can J Neurol Sci.* 1981;8:21.

103. Flamm ES. The timing of aneurysm surgery. *Clin Neurosurg.* 1986;33:147.

104. Adams HP. Early management of the patient with recent aneurysmal subarachnoid hemorrhage. *Stroke.* 1986;17:1068.

105. Disney L, Weir B, Petruk K. Effect on management and mortality of a deliberate policy of early operation on supratentorial aneurysms. *Neurosurgery.* 1987;20:695.

106. Versafi PP, Talamonti G, D'Aliberti G, et al. Surgical treatment of poor-grade aneurysm patients. *J Neurosurg Sci.* 1998;42(1 suppl 1):43.

107. Lan Q, Ikeda H, Jimbo H, et al. Considerations on surgical treatment for elderly patients with intracranial aneurysms. *Surg Neurol.* 2000;53:231.

108. Duke BJ, Kindt GW, Breeze RE. Outcome after urgent surgery for grade IV subarachnoid hemorrhage. *Surg Neurol.* 1998;50:169.

109. International Study of Unruptured Intracranial Aneurysms Investigators. Unruptured intracranial aneurysms—risk of rupture and risks of surgical intervention. [Published erratum appears in *N Engl J Med.* 1999;340:744]. *N Engl J Med.* 1998;339:1725.

110. Juvela S, Porras M, Poussa K. Natural history of unruptured intracranial aneurysms: probability of and risk factors for aneurysm rupture. *J Neurosurg.* 2000;93:379.

111. Hindman BJ, Todd MM, Gelb AW, et al. Mild hypothermia as a protective therapy during intracranial aneurysm surgery: a randomized prospective pilot trial. *Neurosurgery.* 1999;44:23.

112. Ferguson GG. Direct measurement of mean and pulsatile blood pressure at operation in human intracranial saccular aneurysms. *J Neurosurg.* 1972;36:560.

113. Dietrich HH, Dacey RG Jr. Molecular keys to the problems of cerebral vasospasm. *Neurosurgery.* 2000;46:517.

114. Pasqualin A. Epidemiology and pathophysiology of cerebral vasospasm following subarachnoid hemorrhage. *J Neurosurg Sci.* 1998;42(1 suppl 1):15.

115. Mayberg MR. Cerebral vasospasm. *Neurosurg Clin North Am.* 1998;9:615.

116. Ullman JS, Bederson JB. Hypertensive, hypervolemic, hemodilutional therapy for aneurysmal subarachnoid hemorrhage. *Crit Care Clin.* 1996;12:697.

117. Oropello JM, Weiner L, Benjamin E. Hypertensive, hypervolemic, hemodilutional therapy for aneurysmal subarachnoid hemorrhage: is it efficacious? No. *Crit Care Clin.* 1996;12:709.

118. Awad IA. Clinical vasospasm after subarachnoid hemorrhage: response to hypervolemic hemodilution and arterial hypertension. *Stroke.* 1987;18:365.

119. Tettenborn D, Porto L, Ryman T, et al. Survey of clinical experience with nimodipine in patients with subarachnoid hemorrhage. *Neurosurg Rev.* 1987;10:77.

120. Allen GS, Ahn HS, Preziosi TJ, et al. Cerebral arterial spasm: a controlled trial of nimodipine in patients with subarachnoid hemorrhage. *N Engl J Med.* 1983;309:308.

121. Zabramski JM, Spetzler RF, Lee KS, et al. Phase I trial of tissue plasminogen activator for the prevention of vasospasm in patients with subarachnoid hemorrhage. *J Neurosurg.* 1991;75:189.

122. Zubrov YLN, Nikiforov BM, Shustin VA. Balloon catheter techniques for dilation of constricted cerebral arteries after aneurysmal subarachnoid hemorrhage. *Acta Neurochir.* 1984;70:65.

123. Bejjani GK, Bank WO, Olan WJ, et al. The efficacy and safety of angioplasty for cerebral vasospasm after subarachnoid hemorrhage. *Neurosurgery.* 1998;42:979.

124. Haley EC Jr, Kassell NF, Apperson-Hansen C, et al. A randomized, double-blind, vehicle-controlled trial of tirilazad mesylate in patients with aneurysmal subarachnoid hemorrhage: a cooperative study in North America. *J Neurosurg.* 1997;86:467.

125. Lanzino G, Kassell NF. Double-blind, randomized, vehicle-controlled study of high-dose tirilazad mesylate in women with aneurysmal subarachnoid hemorrhage. Part II. A cooperative study in North America. *J Neurosurg.* 1999;90:1018.

126. Thomas JE, Rosenwasser RH, Armonda RA, et al. Safety of intrathecal sodium nitroprusside for the treatment and prevention of refractory cerebral vasospasm and ischemia in humans. *Stroke.* 1999;30:1409.

127. Thomas JE, Rosenwasser RH. Reversal of severe cerebral vasospasm in three patients after aneurysmal subarachnoid hemorrhage: initial observations regarding the use of intraventricular sodium nitroprusside in humans. *Neurosurgery.* 1999;44:48.

128. Asano T, Natsui T. Antioxidant therapy against cerebral vasospasm following aneurysmal subarachnoid hemorrhage. *Cell Mol Neurobiol.* 1999;19:31.

129. Beard EF, Robertson JW, Robertson RCL. Spontaneous subarachnoid hemorrhage simulating acute myocardial infarction. *Am Heart J.* 1959;58:755.

130. Diamond T, Segal F. Subarachnoid hemorrhage masquerading electrocardiographically as acute myocardial infarction. *Heart Lung.* 1984;13:451.

131. Pollick C, Cujec B, Parker S, et al. Left ventricular wall motion abnormalities in subarachnoid hemorrhage: an echocardiographic study. *J Am Coll Cardiol.* 1988;12:600.

132. Mayer SA, Lin J, Homma S, et al. Myocardial injury and left ventricular performance after subarachnoid hemorrhage. *Stroke.* 1999;30:780.

133. Friedman WA, Chadwick GM, Verhoeven FJS, et al. Monitoring of somatosensory evoked potentials during surgery for middle cerebral artery aneurysms. *Neurosurgery.* 1991;29:83.

134. Friedman WA, Kaplan BL, Day AL, et al. Evoked potential monitoring

during aneurysm operation: observations after fifty cases. *Neurosurgery.* 1987;20:678.

135. Little JR, Lesser RP, Lüders H. Electrophysiologic monitoring during basilar aneurysm operation. *Neurosurgery.* 1987;20:421.

136. Solomon RA, Fink M, Lennihan L. Early aneurysm surgery and prophylactic hypervolemic hypertensive therapy for the treatment of subarachnoid hemorrhage. *Neurosurgery.* 1988;23:699

137. Chang HS, Hongo K, Nakagawa H. Adverse effects of limited hypotensive anesthesia on the outcome of patients with subarachnoid hemorrhage. *J Neurosurg.* 2000;92:971.

138. Pinaud M, Souron R, Lelausque JN, et al. Cerebral blood flow and oxygen consumption during nitroprusside-induced hypotension to less than 50 mm Hg. *Anesthesiology.* 1989;70:255.

139. Newberg LA, Milde JH, Michenfelder JD. The cerebral metabolic effects of isoflurane at and above concentrations that suppress cortical electrical activity. *Anesthesiology.* 1983;59:23.

140. Artru AA, Katz RA, Colley PS. Autoregulation of cerebral blood flow during normocapnia and hypocapnia in dogs. *Anesthesiology.* 1989;70:288.

141. Michenfelder JD, Theye RA. Hypothermia: effect on canine brain and whole body metabolism. *Anesthesiology.* 1968;29:1107.

142. Michenfelder JD. The in vivo effects of massive concentrations of anesthetics on canine cerebral metabolism. In: Fink BR, ed. *Molecular Mechanisms of Anesthesia.* New York, NY: Raven Press; 1975:537.

143. Carrasco G, Molina R, Costa J. Propofol versus midazolam in short-, medium-, and long-term sedation of critically ill patients. *Chest.* 1993;103:557.

144. Debrun GM, Aletich VA, Kehrli P, et al. Selection of cerebral aneurysms for treatment using Guglielmi detachable coils: the preliminary University of Ilinois at Chicago experience. *Neurosurgery.* 1998;43:1281.

145. Raftopoulos C, Mathurin P, Boscherini D, et al. Prospective analysis of aneurysm treatment in a series of 103 consecutive patients when endovascular embolization is considered the first option. *J Neurosurg.* 2000;93:175.

146. Johnston SC, Wilson CB, Halbach VV, et al. Endovascular and surgical treatment of unruptured cerebral aneurysms: comparison of risks. *Ann Neurol.* 2000;48:11.

147. Vespa PM, Gobin YP. Endovascular treatment and neurointensive care of ruptured aneurysms. *Crit Care Clin.* 1999;15:667.

148. Thomas JE, Armonda RA, Rosenwasser RH. Endosaccular thrombosis of cerebral aneurysms: strategy, indications, and technique. *Neurosurg Clin North Am.* 2000;11:101.

149. Kader A, Young WL. The effects of intracranial arteriovenous malformations on cerebral hemodynamics. *Neurosurg Clin North Am.* 1996;7:767.

150. Young WL, Kader A, Ornstein E, et al. Cerebral hyperemia after arteriovenous malformation resection is related to "breakthrough" complications but not to feeding artery pressure. The Columbia University Arteriovenous Malformation Study Project. *Neurosurgery.* 1996;38:1085.

151. Young WL, Pile-Spellman J, Prohovnik I, et al. Evidence for adaptive autoregulatory displacement in hypotensive cortical territories adjacent to arteriovenous malformations. Columbia University AVM Study Project. *Neurosurgery.* 1994;34:601.

152. Young WL, Kader A, Prohovnik I, et al. Pressure autoregulation is intact after arteriovenous malformation resection. *Neurosurgery.* 1993;32:491.

153. Halla JT, Hardin JG, Vitek J, et al. Involvement of the cervical spine in rheumatoid arthritis (Review). *Arthritis Rheum.* 1989;32:652.

154. Yaszemski MJ, Shepler TR. Sudden death from cord compression associated with atlanto-axial instability in rheumatoid arthritis. *Spine.* 1990;15:338.

155. Kay NH, Blogg CE. Rises in serum potassium after suxamethonium following a brachial plexus injury. *Anaesthesia.* 1982;37:1217.

156. Fessler RG, Dietze DD Jr, MacMillan MM, et al. Lateral parascapular extrapleural approach to the upper thoracic spine. *J Neurosurg.* 1991;75:349.

157. Bracken MB, Shepard MJ, Collins WF, et al. A randomized, controlled trial of methylprednisolone or naloxone in the treatment of acute spinal-cord injury: results of the Second National Acute Spinal Cord Injury Study. *N Engl J Med.* 1990;322:1405.

158. Bracken MB, Shepard MJ, Collins WF Jr, et al. Methylprednisolone or naloxone treatment after acute spinal cord injury: 1-year follow-up data. Results of the second national acute spinal cord injury study. *J Neurosurg.* 1992;76:23.

159. Stauffer JL, Petty TL. Cleft tongue and ulceration of hard palate: complications of oral intubation. *Chest.* 1978;74:317.

160. Lennon RL, Hosking MP, Gray JR, et al. The effects of intraoperative blood salvage and induced hypotension on transfusion requirements during spinal surgical procedures. *Mayo Clin Proc.* 1987;62:1090.

161. Burgos J, Rapariz JM, Gonzalez-Herranz P. Anterior endoscopic approach to the thoracolumbar spine. *Spine.* 1998;23:2427.

162. Huang TJ, Hsu RW, Liu HP, et al. Video-assisted thorascopic surgery to the upper thoracic spine. *Surg Endosc.* 1999;13:123.

163. Arlet V. Anterior thoracoscopic spine release in deformity surgery: a meta-analysis and review. *Eur Spine J.* 2000;9(suppl 1):S17.

164. Newton PO, Shea KG, Granlund KF. Defining the pediatric spinal thoracoscopy learning curve: sixty-five consecutive cases. *Spine.* 2000;25:1028.

165. Rothenberg S, Erickson M, Eilert R, et al. Thoracoscopic anterior spinal procedures in children. *J Pediatr Surg.* 1998;33:1168.

166. Lische V, Westphal K, Behne M, et al. Thoraocoscopic microsurgical technique for vertebral surgery: anesthetic considerations. *Acta Anasthesiol Scand.* 1998;42:1199.

167. Slotman BJ, Stein SC. Laminectomy compared with laparoscopic diskectomy and outpatient laparoscopic diskectomy for herniated L5-S1 intervertebral disks. *J Laparoendosc Adv Surg Tech A.* 1998;8:261.

168. Ditsworth DA. Endoscopic transforaminal lumbar discectomy and reconfiguration: a posterio-lateral approach into the spinal canal. *Surg Neurol.* 1998;49:588.

169. Brayda-Bruno M, Cinnella P. Posterior endoscopic discectomy (and other procedures). *Eur Spine J.* 2000;9(suppl 1):S24.

170. Lieberman IH, Willsher PC, Litwin DE, et al. Transperitoneal laparoscopic exposure for lumbar interbody fusion. *Spine.* 2000;25:509.

171. O'Dowd JK. Laparoscopic lumbar spine surgery. *Eur Spine J.* 2000;9(Suppl 1):S3.

172. Walker AE, Robins M, Weinfeld FD. Epidemiology of brain tumors: the national survey of intracranial neoplasms. *Neurology* 1985;35:219.

173. Kato A, Sako K, Diksic M, et al. Regional glucose utilization and blood flow in experimental brain tumors studied by double tracer autoradiography. *J Neurooncol.* 1985;3:271.

174. Panther LA, Baumbach GL, Bigner DD, et al. Vasoactive drugs produce selective changes in flow to experimental brain tumors. *Ann Neurol.* 1985;18:712.

175. Black S, Ockert DB, Oliver WC, et al. Outcome following posterior fossa craniectomy in patients in the sitting or horizontal positions. *Anesthesiology.* 1988;69:49.

176. Hanakita J, Miyake H, Nagayasu S, et al. Angiographic examination and surgical treatment for bow hunter's stroke. *Neurosurgery.* 1988;23:228.

177. Jansen GF, van Praagh BH, Kedaria MB, et al. Jugular bulb oxygen saturation during propofol and isofurane/nitrous oxide anesthesia in patients undergoing brain tumor surgery. *Anesth Analg.* 1999;89:358.

178. Sharma SK, McGuire GP, Cruise CJ. Stability of the arterial to endtidal carbon dioxide difference during anaesthesia for prolonged neurosurgical procedures. *Can J Anaesth.* 1995;42:498.

CHAPTER

# 70

# Outpatient Anesthesia

Ian Smith

Terri G. Monk

## PAIN MANAGEMENT
*What Role Do Nonopioid Analgesics Play in Pain Management?*
*What Is Multimodal Analgesia?*

## UNANTICIPATED ADMISSION, READMISSION, AND FOLLOW-UP

## OFFICE-BASED ANESTHESIA
*Are the Standards of Care Different in an Office-Based Practice?*
*What Is the Mortality Rate in Office-Based Surgery?*

## CONCLUSION

If growth and diversity are measures of success, then ambulatory surgery must clearly be a success. From its initial beginnings, generally in a hospital-based setting, the number of cases involving elective surgery performed on an ambulatory basis (Fig. 70–1) and the range of patients and procedures deemed suitable for this approach have grown rapidly. During the early expansion, freestanding ambulatory surgical centers began to develop. These centers offered patients the convenience of minor operations in more accessible locations, away from the hospital environment. At first, the selection criteria, both medical and surgical, for freestanding units were more stringent than were those in hospital-affiliated centers. However, as experience has grown, so too has the range of activities. In the latest evolution, there is a move to shift the more minor procedures away from even freestanding units and into the surgeon's office—the so-called office-based anesthesia. Initially, office-based procedures were limited to surgical procedures that could be performed with local anesthesia (often supplemented with sedation), but increasingly general anesthesia is also being used in the office setting.

The expansion of day surgery has not been solely an American phenomenon. Ambulatory surgery is becoming increasingly popular in many other parts of the world. Countries such as Canada, Great Britain, and Australia are among the leading exponents outside of the United States, but ambulatory surgery is beginning to develop in many parts of Europe, Latin America, and the Far East. At present, freestanding and office-based practices are still comparatively uncommon outside of North America; however, based on recent history, this is likely to change in the future.

What has fueled this massive expansion in ambulatory surgery? The major driving forces have been financial and political concerns. In a privately (or insurance-) funded system, ambulatory surgery is simply less expensive than a comparable procedure performed on an inpatient basis. Similarly, the costs in freestanding units are generally lower than are those found in hospital-affiliated centers, and the cost in office-based practice is even less expensive. Such are the pressures to cut health care costs that many insurance companies will no longer fund the full cost of inpatient treatment for many procedures, even when there are strong medical contraindications to ambulatory surgery. Presumably, similar pressures may in due course come to bear on hospital-based and even freestanding ambulatory centers.

Ambulatory surgery is also attractive to other health care systems. In a publicly funded system, ambulatory surgery permits more to be achieved with the same limited resources. The inherent efficiency of ambulatory surgery may also reduce waiting times for elective surgery. There is a danger, however, that the increased accessibility afforded by a move to ambulatory surgery may significantly increase public demand, so that total costs remain unchanged or may even rise. Nevertheless, the end result has been to achieve more with the funds available.

Despite the political and financial forces driving ambulatory surgery, the practice does have considerable benefits. Patients appreciate the convenience of surgery on a "same day" basis, and most would prefer to recover in the familiar surroundings of their own homes, provided that they are comfortable. Because ambulatory surgery is dependent on rapid recovery and control of pain and postoperative sickness for its success, the focus of care in these settings is to provide patients with a pleasant postoperative experience. Where inpatient care is planned, there is a temptation to pay less attention to pain and side effects because these "can always be treated later." In practice, such treatment may be delayed and patients suffer. Ambulatory surgery is often more efficient than in-hospital surgery, with less potential for delays and cancellations. With

**FIGURE 70–1.** Total number of elective operations performed annually in the United States (*dotted line*) and the percentage of that total performed on hospital inpatients, on outpatients within a hospital, in a freestanding ambulatory surgery center, and in a surgeon's office. The total percentage of outpatient procedures is also shown. Data for 2001 are projected values. (Data from SMG Marketing Group, Chicago, Ill, 1996.)

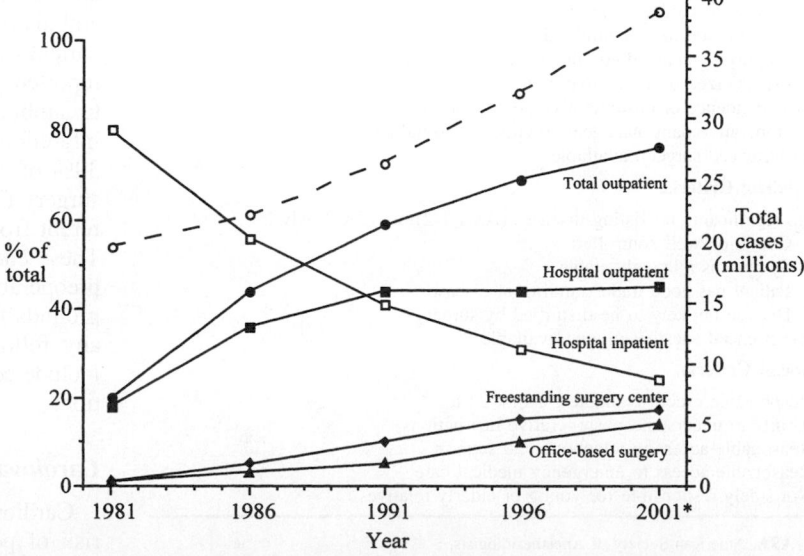

a guaranteed date (and often time) for surgery, there is also less likelihood of cancellation or "no-show" by the patient.

With ambulatory surgery, there is also often a shift of emphasis from treating the disease to the care of the whole person undergoing a (relatively) minor procedure. Because the whole process is "active," with a high ratio of nursing staff to patients and a focus on details of care that can influence recovery, the patient usually feels well taken care of. This improved quality of care with ambulatory surgery has often been an unexpected bonus in countries that have adopted the practice for purely financial reasons.

## PREOPERATIVE PATIENT SELECTION

Despite the expansion in ambulatory surgery, the technique will never be suitable for all patients and surgical procedures. Patients should be selected based on surgical, medical, and social criteria (Table 70–1). It has often been suggested that the duration of surgery should be reasonably short. Various time limits have been proposed, but these limits are often revised. The magnitude of the surgical trauma is undoubtedly more important than the actual duration, and with minimally invasive surgical techniques, more extended procedures are often performed on an ambulatory basis. Recovery from anesthesia (and sedation) will take longer after more prolonged procedures, but this effect is less marked with modern hypnotic agents than with older drugs. Nevertheless, postoperative adverse events are still found to be substantially more common with longer procedures.[1] Unanticipated postoperative hospital admission (ie, failed ambulatory surgery) is also more likely after prolonged or extensive surgery.[2,3] Even when patients are successfully discharged, their functional state may be substantially depressed for several days.[4]

Currently, one of the major factors that determines the suitability of a given procedure for ambulatory surgery is the associated level of postoperative pain. Improvements in analgesic regimens and surgical techniques that reduce postoperative pain are constantly allowing the boundaries of ambulatory surgery to be advanced.

## What Factors Should Be Considered When Determining the Patient's Feasibility for Ambulatory Surgery?

### Age

Age as such is not a contraindication to ambulatory surgery, although elderly patients are more likely to have adverse medical or social factors and may require a greater degree of postdischarge supervision. Adverse intraoperative events (primarily cardiovascular) were more common with increasing age, whereas postoperative events (mostly related to pain, nausea, and vomiting) decreased with advancing years.[1]

For most children, ambulatory surgery offers major benefits, including less time away from the home and family. Ex-premature babies are at increased risk of postoperative apnea, a phenomenon that can occur up to 60 weeks' postconceptional age.[5,6] Earlier than this age, surgery should probably be confined to major life- or sight-threatening conditions, such as hernia repair and congenital cataract correction. With the increasing specialist management of children, such patients would, hopefully, present to dedicated pediatric ambulatory surgery centers or inpatient facilities for their surgery.

### Medical Criteria

The preexisting medical condition of the patient is important, but with the reluctance of insurance companies and health maintenance organizations (HMOs) to pay for inpatient care for a procedure commonly accepted as ambulatory, increasingly unhealthy patients are presenting for ambulatory surgery. Intraoperative complications are associated with various preexisting medical conditions, especially hypertension, obesity, smoking, respiratory and cardiovascular diseases, and diabetes.[1,7,8] Most of these perioperative problems occur during the operation itself or during the early recovery phase. Nevertheless, patients with more extensive disease (eg, American Society of Anesthesiologists [ASA] class 3) have been shown to more likely require overnight admission after planned ambulatory procedures.[2,3] Despite increased perioperative problems, major morbidity and mortality associated with ambulatory surgery appear to be low. In a review of 38 598 patients attending the Mayo clinic, Warner and colleagues reported 31 major complications (with two deaths) related to ambulatory surgery.[9] The two deaths (from myocardial infarction) occurred more than 7 days after surgery. Likewise, 39% of all complications occurred more than 48 hours after surgery (Table 70–2). The overall morbidity appeared no different from a comparable section of the relevant population.[9] These encouraging results should be regarded as evidence of preoperative selection and patient preparation, rather than as grounds for complacency. They also serve as a reminder that any follow-up of the success of ambulatory surgery should include contact with patients at least 1 week after their operation.

### Cardiovascular Disease

Cardiovascular disease is common and can increase the risk of perioperative complications. Excellent guidelines for

---

**TABLE 70–1.** Outline of the Major Selection Criteria for Ambulatory Surgery

**Surgical Criteria**

Operation of moderate duration
Minimal blood loss or fluid shifts
No highly specialized equipment required
No specialized postoperative care
Low incidence of postoperative complications
Postoperative pain manageable without hospital care
Experienced surgeon available

**Medical Criteria**

No significant preexisting diseases (ASA 1-2) or ASA 3 only if
    Condition well controlled
    Symptoms relatively stable
    Patient has good understanding of disease
    Disease unlikely to be disturbed by surgery
Experienced anesthesiologist available

**Social Criteria**

Responsible escort available for first 24 h
Ability to understand postoperative instructions
Reasonable access to telephone and support
Reasonable access to emergency medical care
Not solely responsible for young or elderly relatives

ASA, American Society of Anesthesiologists.

**TABLE 70–2.** Major Morbidity and Mortality in the 30 Days After Ambulatory Surgery in 38 598 Patients Attending the Mayo Clinic From 1988 to 1990

| Event | Total | Within 48 Hours |
| --- | --- | --- |
| Myocardial infarction | 14 (0.036%)* | 9 |
| Central nervous system defect | 7 (0.018%) | 5 |
| Pulmonary embolus | 5 (0.013%) | 2 |
| Respiratory failure | 5 (0.013%) | 3 |
| **Overall** | **31 (0.08%)†** | **19** |

*Two patients died on the seventh postoperative day; symptoms appeared intraoperatively and on the fourth day, respectively.

†An additional two patients died as passengers in automobile accidents that were unrelated to surgery.

Values are number (percentage) of occurrences.

Data from Warner MA, Shields SE, Chute CG. Major morbidity and mortality within 1 month of ambulatory surgery and anesthesia. *JAMA.* 1993;270:1437.

evaluating patients undergoing noncardiac surgery have been issued by the American College of Cardiology and the American Heart Association Task Force.[10] These guidelines give advice on detecting and treating cardiac disease and provide guidance on various risk factors. Most cardiac symptoms should be detected during a routine history and physical examination. Exercise tolerance is a particularly helpful guide. The patient's ability to climb a flight of stairs[11] is a useful cutoff. Patients who fail this basic screening test will require further investigation in order to determine their fitness and to guide therapy.

### Hypertension

Hypertension is a common and significant risk factor for ambulatory surgery.[1,7,8] Hypertension is a major predictor of perioperative myocardial ischemia,[12] and even labile hypertension is associated with left ventricular dysfunction.[13] Patients with existing hypertension should have their treatment optimized and should continue to take their medication on the day of surgery. Newly diagnosed hypertension should be treated before surgery, which should be delayed until the patient is stabilized on medication.

### Respiratory Disease

The most commonly encountered respiratory diseases are asthma, chronic obstructive pulmonary disease (COPD), and respiratory tract infections.

**Asthma.** Asthma should be well controlled by monitoring peak expiratory airflow. Surgery should be avoided during an acute exacerbation (a history of recent systemic steroids may indicate recent poor function). Inhaled bronchodilators should probably be given preoperatively, even if these are usually taken on an "as needed" basis. Most inhaled anesthetics are bronchodilators and may be beneficial. Care should be taken to avoid inadequate levels of anesthesia that may trigger oversensitive airway reflexes.

Nonsteroidal antiinflammatory drugs (NSAIDs) may exacerbate asthma in a few patients (5%-10%). A history of previous NSAID consumption (these drugs are readily available) and their effect, if any, on the patient's asthma should always be taken to guide subsequent pain therapy (discussed later).

**Chronic Obstructive Pulmonary Disease.** COPD is typi-

fied by acute exacerbations against a background of impaired respiratory function. As with asthma, acute exacerbations should be avoided. COPD is less responsive to bronchodilators, but antibiotics may be indicated for associated chest infections. Expiratory flow and exercise tolerance are excellent indicators of disease severity. Local or regional anesthesia is well tolerated, when appropriate.

**Upper Respiratory Tract Infection.** Upper respiratory tract infections (URTIs) are a common source of concern, especially in children. URTIs are associated with increased airway reactivity, which can persist up to 6 weeks,[14] producing bronchospasm, laryngospasm, and arterial oxygen desaturation. Nevertheless, several investigators have found relatively few, generally mild perioperative complications in patients with URTIs.[14] Surgery should certainly be delayed (for 4-6 weeks) if the patient is febrile or has an obvious chest infection, but in other cases can probably proceed safely.[15] More caution may be required if the operation involves the airway. Avoiding instrumentation of the larynx (by the use of a face mask or laryngeal mask) also appears to reduce intraoperative problems.[14,16]

### Obesity

Many other countries practicing ambulatory surgery impose limits on weight. These are usually based on body mass index (BMI), which is calculated by dividing the patient's weight (in kg) by the square of their height (in m). Cutoff values of 30 to 35 $kg/m^2$ are commonly used. Weight has seldom been a contraindication to ambulatory surgery in the United States, perhaps because obesity (and morbid obesity) are so common in this population. Obesity is clearly associated with an increase in perioperative respiratory problems,[1,5,17] but these appear to be early events, and overnight admission is not obviously increased.[3,8] Obesity also increases the difficulty of surgery and provides practical problems for the anesthesiologist. Venous access, block placement, and tracheal intubation are all more difficult. Personal injury to medical personnel during patient positioning is also a major risk.

The management of obese patients is problematic. Advice to lose weight often produces the opposite effect. Obese patients actually benefit from a short-acting anesthetic, avoidance of long-acting opioids, and effective nonopioid analgesia—common features of ambulatory practice. Interestingly, obese patients are more likely to experience significant postoperative pain.[18] The laryngeal mask is generally effective and avoids difficult intubation. Intraoperative reflux is less common than was once thought,[19] although symptoms should be sought, especially in the morbidly obese. In most cases, these patients do well with ambulatory surgery, and it is difficult to see how their management would be improved by pre- or postoperative hospital admission. However, because of the perioperative problems in their care, such patients may be less suitable for office-based anesthesia.

### Diabetes

Non–insulin-dependent diabetic patients usually tolerate ambulatory surgery well. Food and oral hypoglycemic agents are omitted before surgery, and the patient's blood glucose is monitored. Insulin-dependent diabetic patients can also be managed on an ambulatory basis, but their care is more complex. The effects of perioperative stress and preoperative fasting can have conflicting and unpredictable effects on blood sugar.

All patients with diabetes should be carefully evaluated for coexisting cardiovascular disease, the symptoms of which may often be obscured by diabetic neuropathy. With all diabetic patients, local and regional anesthetic techniques should be considered, because these produce less disturbance to the patient's dietary/hypoglycemic regimen.

### Other Diseases

A detailed description of the significance of a wide range of coexisting diseases to the suitability for ambulatory surgery is beyond the scope of this short chapter. The reader is referred to larger textbooks. In general, most underlying conditions are acceptable, provided that they are stable and their management is unlikely to be significantly compromised by the proposed procedure. In many cases, the rapid return to normality permitted by ambulatory anesthesia is beneficial. The basic test to apply in all cases is to consider how much the patient's management would be improved by the following: (1) preoperative hospitalization, or (2) an overnight (or longer) inpatient stay. If no obvious benefit would result from either choice 1 or 2, then the patient is likely to be suitable for ambulatory surgery.

### Specific Anesthetic Problems

Problems with previous anesthetics are not necessarily a contraindication to ambulatory surgery, provided that the problem is known and a solution is obvious. For example, a deficiency in pseudocholinesterase is not a problem if succinylcholine and mivacurium are avoided. There are numerous acceptable alternatives (including spontaneous ventilation with the laryngeal mask) for most patients. Even malignant hyperpyrexia does not need to be a problem if a trigger-free anesthetic from a trigger-free anesthetic machine can be guaranteed. Local anesthesia or monitored anesthesia care (MAC) would probably guarantee this. Facilities for the diagnosis and treatment of malignant hyperpyrexia should nevertheless be available. Difficult tracheal intubation, if known, can usually also be managed. Strategies include avoidance of intubation (by local or regional anesthesia or laryngeal mask airway [LMA]) or awake fiberoptic intubation.

### Social Criteria

Social factors are also important in successful patient selection. Most anesthetics impair cognitive function for some time (perhaps up to 24 hours), and patients should be accompanied home by a responsible escort. A suitable person should also be available to take care of the patient during the first night after surgery and be able to obtain assistance in the (rare) event of major complications. Care of children or elderly family members should also be delegated to the escort during the first 24 hours. Candidates for ambulatory surgery should always have reasonable access to a telephone or other reliable means of reaching medical assistance. The provision of an extended care facility (or hospital hotel) may further extend the scope of ambulatory surgery.

### PREOPERATIVE ASSESSMENT

Failure to select patients well will result in cancellations (through unsuitability), increase perioperative risks and com-

plications, and cause unnecessary admissions and readmissions. Early evaluation allows problems to be detected in time for special investigations to be planned and preexisting medical conditions to be treated. Patients may then be presented for ambulatory surgery in optimum condition or else electively referred for inpatient treatment. The alternative—discovering adverse patient factors on the planned day of operation—inevitably results in expensive delays and cancellations.

### What Procedures Are Used for Preoperative Assessment?

### Preoperative Assessment Clinic

It is common practice to evaluate patients in a preoperative assessment clinic. These are often managed by anesthesiology residents, although physicians, nursing staff, and various other multidisciplinary personnel are increasingly involved.[20,21] These units appear to be highly effective and can significantly reduce costs through fewer cancellations and a reduction in unnecessary preoperative tests.[20] The preoperative clinic provides an opportunity for a full history and physical examination and also allows for the ordering of blood tests and other consultations where indicated. In order to allow adequate time to correct preoperative abnormalities without disrupting scheduled surgery, the assessment should ideally be performed 1 to 2 weeks before the anticipated date of operation. Any evaluation performed earlier than 2 weeks allows too much time for the patient's condition to deteriorate. In reality, preoperative assessment is often performed the day before surgery, resulting in last-minute cancellations and partially defeating the purpose of preoperative screening.

Although the preoperative assessment clinic offers several advantages, there are also some problems. First, such a clinic requires a great deal of resources, including space and personnel, not anticipated in any budget. Second, attending a preoperative clinic requires the patient to make an additional visit to the surgical center, partially negating one of the major advantages of ambulatory surgery. Finally, although the patient may well be seen by an anesthesiologist, this will rarely be the person who will actually administer the anesthetic. Although this may be unimportant for many patients, the opportunity to establish rapport and to discuss the details of the anesthetic technique will be lost. Differences in opinion may also still result in changes being made on the day of surgery, again invalidating the preassessment process.

### Questionnaires

In some areas, alternatives to a preoperative assessment clinic are used to good effect. Once agreed selection criteria are in place, it is relatively easy to screen patients using a series of structured questions. These can be presented in the form of a questionnaire (Fig. 70–2), which can be completed by patients themselves, filled in during an interview with nursing staff or ancillary personnel, or even conducted by telephone.[22] A well-designed form (see Fig. 70–2) has responses aligned, such that potentially adverse factors are easily noticed. The completed questionnaires (and the medical notes, if necessary) can be reviewed by the ambulatory nursing staff 1 to 2 weeks before the planned date of operation.

Will you:-                                    PLEASE TICK THE CORRECT BOX

be able to be driven home by private car?.. | YES | NO |
have someone to take you home?.. | YES | NO |
have a telephone at home?.. | YES | NO |
have easy access to a lavatory?.. | YES | NO |
have someone at home to look after you for 24 hours?.. | YES | NO |

Have you ever suffered from any of the following?:-

| | | | |
|---|---|---|
| heart attack.. | YES | NO |
| angina (chest pain on exercise, at rest or at night).. | YES | NO |
| breathlessness (shortage of breath).. | YES | NO |
| asthma.. | YES | NO |
| bronchitis.. | YES | NO |
| high blood pressure.. | YES | NO |
| heart murmur.. | YES | NO |
| rheumatic fever.. | YES | NO |
| fainting easily.. | YES | NO |
| convulsions or fits.. | YES | NO |
| jaundice (yellowness).. | YES | NO |
| indigestion or heartburn.. | YES | NO |
| kidney or urinary trouble.. | YES | NO |
| anaemia or other blood problem.. | YES | NO |
| excessive bleeding or bruising.. | YES | NO |
| arthritis.. | YES | NO |
| muscle disease or progressive weakness.. | YES | NO |
| diabetes.. | YES | NO |
| deep vein thrombosis.. | YES | NO |
| swollen ankles.. | YES | NO |

If yes, answer the following:
a. do you feel breathless:

at rest.. | YES | NO |
on lying flat.. | YES | NO |
on exertion.. | YES | NO |
on climbing stairs.. | YES | NO |

b. how far can you walk
before breathlessness
stops you?          [ yards ]

Do you:

take any regular medicines
(tablets, patches, injections, inhalers)?.. | YES | NO |   ...If yes please list    1...............................
                                                           2...............................
                                                           3...............................
smoke (cigarettes/pipe)?.. | YES | NO |                    4...............................
                                                           5...............................
drink more than 1½ pints of beer
or 3 shots a day?.. | YES | NO |

|  |  | TYPE OF ANAESTHETIC USED |
|---|---|---|
| What operations have you had before if any? (please list) | 1............................. | GA / SPINAL / LOCAL |
| | 2............................. | GA / SPINAL / LOCAL |
| | 3............................. | GA / SPINAL / LOCAL |
| | 4............................. | GA / SPINAL / LOCAL |
| | 5............................. | GA / SPINAL / LOCAL |

Did you have any anaesthetic or surgical complications? (please list)...   1..........................................
                                                                          2..........................................

**FIGURE 70–2.** Example of a preoperative patient questionnaire. (Simplified version, based on the questionnaire used at North Staffordshire Hospital, Stoke-on-Trent, England.)

Using agreed selection criteria, most patients can be triaged into those who are suitable or unsuitable candidates for ambulatory surgery, with a small third group who require further evaluation by the surgeon or anesthesiologist before a final decision is made. At North Staffordshire Hospital (UK), where such a system has been used for several years,[23] all patients are reviewed on the day of surgery by their surgeon and anesthesiologist in order to detect any new (or overlooked) problems. This system minimizes time spent at the hospital by the patient and has been achieved without the need for additional resources. Its success is reflected by the small number of patients ($<0.5\%$) who are canceled or admitted for reasons that should have been identified previously.

### Laboratory Screening Tests

It is tempting to submit potential ambulatory patients to a series of screening laboratory tests. However, experience suggests that this is unnecessary and wasteful of both time and resources. When laboratory tests are applied to basically healthy patients, most positive results will actually be false-positive. The likely outcome of such findings will be to repeat the test (causing further cost, discomfort, and delay) or ignore the result.[24] If the result is to be ignored, there is clearly little point in performing the test in the first place. One study suggested that at least 60% of preoperative tests were clinically unnecessary and that potentially useful information was obtained in less than 0.2% of cases.[25] Another study in patients of average age of 46 years found at least one abnormal result from screening tests in 84% of patients.[24] In 96% of cases, these abnormalities were simply ignored; repeat testing was ordered in the remainder. Despite these findings, perioperative complications occurred in only 0.6% of patients, and testing was thought to have been helpful in less than 1% of all cases.[24] Preoperative testing may appear more worthwhile for conditions that are difficult to detect clinically, such as anemia. However, it has previously been shown that most patients whose anemia was detected by screening underwent ambulatory anesthesia (without correction of the red blood cell count) without problems.[26] The available evidence suggests that laboratory tests should only be used to further evaluate clinically detected disease and assess its response to therapy.

### Other Screening Tests

Similar comments may be applied to other screening tests. A preoperative electrocardiogram (ECG) is commonly requested to detect asymptomatic cardiac disease. Nevertheless, one study detected no ECG abnormalities in asymptomatic elective surgical patients less than 50 years old, although ECG abnormalities in the group over 50 years of age were almost exclusively found in patients with known cardiovascular risk factors.[27] In the absence of clinical symptoms or risk factors, the ECG is generally not helpful. The preoperative chest radiograph is relatively useless as a screening tool. Any abnormality severe enough to show up in a chest radiograph is likely to have been detected by the history and physical examination. In addition to the expense and inconvenience, a chest radiograph also poses a small health risk to the patient and should not be ordered without good reason.

Many ambulatory centers now require no routine preoperative screening tests, reserving investigation for patients in whom these tests may help to determine the extent or severity of known disease and assess the response to treatment. In some cases, this has required alterations to state laws and local institutional regulations. Such formal policies should not be regarded as a fixed, permanent medicolegal obligation but rather should be revised regularly and modified in light of current evidence.

## PATIENT PREPARATION

### What Information Do Patients Need to Know Before Reporting for Surgery?

After careful selection, ambulatory patients require further preparation in order to make their management safer and more acceptable for everyone involved. Patients need reliable information regarding the effects of surgery on their daily lives. Although pain may be manageable at home, it may be some time before normal activities can be resumed.[4] This will have implications for time away from work and family commitments, thus patients should plan appropriately. Patients must be informed that they cannot drive for 24 to 48 hours after anesthesia so that transport can be arranged. The requirement for an escort and responsible postoperative supervision must also be made clear to patients well before their operation.

Patients also require information on where to report on the day of surgery, when to arrive, where to park, and what to bring with them. They should be supplied with a contact telephone number to use in the event of last minute delays or problems. Patients also need appropriate instructions regarding fasting and whether or not to take their regular medications. Provision of adequate support and information should help to reduce preoperative anxiety.

The admission process should also begin to prepare patients for postoperative pain with the preoperative administration of analgesia and, in high-risk groups, postoperative nausea with selective use of prophylactic antiemetic agents. Important postoperative instructions may also be given, and these instructions should be reinforced in writing and, when possible, repeated to the patient's escort at the time of discharge.

### What Are the Fasting Guidelines?

Patients undergoing general anesthesia should have fasted to minimize the risk of aspiration of stomach contents. Solid food should be avoided for at least 6 hours before surgery, but patients may safely be allowed to drink clear liquids up to 2 hours before induction of anesthesia.[28] Other fluids such as pulp-free fruit juice, tea, and coffee (with small amounts of milk) are also safe. Milk-based drinks (eg, cappuccino) are not appropriate, because milk tends to curdle and form solids that delay gastric emptying. The ASA established a task force to consider all of the available evidence on preoperative fasting and has published its guidelines[29] (Table 70–3). In order to avoid any possible misunderstanding over milk, these guidelines suggest clear tea or black coffee but also permit a range of alternative fluids. Breast milk may safely be given up to 4 hours before anesthesia, but other forms of milk and

**TABLE 70–3.** Summary of The American Society of Anesthesiologists' Guidelines on Preoperative Fasting for Patients Undergoing Elective Surgery*

| Ingested Material | Minimum Fasting Period† (h) |
| --- | --- |
| Clear liquids‡ | 2 |
| Breast milk | 4 |
| Infant formula | 6 |
| Nonhuman milk§ | 6 |
| Light meal‖ | 6 |

*Excludes women in labor.
†Applies to all ages.
‡Clear liquids include water, fruit juices without pulp, carbonated beverages, black tea, and coffee.
§Nonhuman milk is similar to solids, therefore the amount ingested must be considered when determining a safe fasting interval.
‖A light meal consists of toast and clear fluids. Fried or fatty foods or meat may prolong gastric emptying. The amount and type of food ingested must be considered when determining a safe fasting interval.
Modified from American Society of Anesthesiologists Task Force on Preoperative Fasting. Practice guidelines for preoperative fasting and the use of pharmacologic agents to reduce the risk of pulmonary aspiration: application to healthy patients undergoing elective procedures. *Anesthesiology.* 1999;90:896.

all solids should be withheld for at least 6 hours (see Table 70–3). Allowing fluids improves patient satisfaction and also makes medication easier to take. Most regular medications, except for oral hypoglycemic agents, should be taken before ambulatory surgery. In order to benefit from these new guidelines and to reduce preoperative dehydration, patients should probably be advised to drink clear liquids before leaving home.

## What Measures Can Be Taken to Relieve Anxiety?

### Direct Communication

Anxiety is common in patients before all operations. Ambulatory patients have the usual concerns of intraoperative "awareness" and death[30] but are also anxious about postoperative pain, nausea, and vomiting. The anesthetic interview may help these concerns.[31] Fear of death is surprisingly common among ambulatory patients; 30% to 50% of patients report this concern when they are specifically questioned.[30] This fear is dramatically out of proportion to the actual risk of death, which is reported to be in the order of 1 in 11 000.[9] It would be more logical and kinder to offer ambulatory patients strong reassurance that they *will not die* during surgery, rather than recite a long list of rare, medicolegally inspired complications, including death, which will only reinforce irrational beliefs. The patient should also be relieved to know that postoperative pain and nausea are usually manageable and by no means inevitable.

### Premedications

Anxiolytic premedication may be used in exceptional cases but should not be required routinely. Short-acting benzodiazepines (eg, midazolam, temazepam) do not produce a clinically significant delay in recovery times,[32] although these drugs may impair the quality of recovery. This may be more important when "fast-track" recovery is intended (discussed in this chapter). When oral premedication is given, the time available between the patient's arrival and the start of the operation may be too short for the onset of anxiolytic effect, thus paradoxically increasing anxiety. Administration of intravenous benzodiazepines immediately before induction of anesthesia may reduce the hypnotic dose and minimize hypotensive effects (coinduction) but will do little to reduce anxiety at this late stage.

Premedication may be more beneficial in children, who find separation from their parents and induction of anesthesia stressful. Oral midazolam, 0.5 to 0.7 mg/kg is an effective premedication that can facilitate separation from parents and result in a smoother induction.[33] The parenteral preparation of midazolam may be used for oral administration. This has an extremely bitter taste, although it may be masked to some extent by fruit juice or by mixing with a flavored analgesic preparation (eg, acetaminophen or ibuprofen). A commercial oral preparation is available but is expensive. Midazolam may also be administered nasally, resulting in rapid onset of action.[34] Many patients find this route to be especially unpleasant, however.

A good vehicle for preoperative drug administration in children is Oralet, a sucrose matrix–containing drug presented in the form of a lollipop. At present, the only drug available in this format is fentanyl. A dose of 15 to 20 µg/kg is rapidly absorbed through the oral mucosa to reduce agitation, produce sedation, and reduce the requirement for postoperative analgesia.[35,36] However, its use is associated with respiratory depression, a high incidence of pruritus and nausea, and a delay in tolerating oral fluids, resulting in delayed discharge.[35] These disadvantages are all a consequence of the opioid drug rather than the method of delivery. The delivery system probably deserves further investigation with other compounds (eg, benzodiazepines).

### Other Preoperative Drug Administration

In addition to relief of anxiety, there may be benefits from other forms of preoperative drug administration. When postoperative pain and nausea are likely, it is generally desirable to provide prophylactic analgesia and antiemetics. Although these drugs may be given intraoperatively, preoperative oral administration is a useful alternative, especially for analgesia (discussed later). Use of the oral route is inexpensive, and early administration also ensures that an adequate effect has been achieved by the end of surgery.

### *Aspiration Prophylaxis*

Aspiration is rare in ambulatory surgery patients and, when it does occur, rarely causes serious problems.[37,38] Other than routine fasting, there is no evidence to support the need for antacid therapy, histamine$_2$ blockers, or gastropropulsive medications in most ambulatory patients. These medications are not recommended by the ASA task force[29]; however, patients with *significant* acid reflux (which is present when fasted) may require additional measures.

### *Needle Phobia*

In patients who are needle phobic (most children and some adults), it will be desirable to reduce the pain of intravenous cannulation by provision of topical analgesia. Various preparations are available, including lidocaine/prilocaine (EMLA) and amethocaine. Iontophoretic application of local anesthesia is also effective but requires special equipment. These techniques can all reduce the pain of cannulation, provided that they are applied at an appropriate time, although they will have no effect on the actual fear of the procedure. Distraction techniques and a gentle approach are equally important in ensuring an acceptable experience for the patient. Increasingly, inhalation induction with sevoflurane is a realistic alternative for patients with a needle phobia.

### *Regular Medications*

The patient's own regular medication should not be neglected under the heading of preoperative medication. Most regular medications should be continued throughout the perioperative period. This is especially important for antihypertensive drugs and other cardiovascular medications.

## What Are the Final Preparations Before the Patient Goes Into Surgery?

Despite thorough preoperative screening, patients should still meet the anesthesiologist before the operation. This provides an opportunity to check that no important information has been overlooked and that no changes have occurred since the assessment process. This meeting allows the physical examination to be completed, the anesthesia plan to be discussed further or finalized, and a relationship to be established between the patient and the anesthesiologist. The surgeon may also wish to review the patient at this stage to ensure that the operation is still required and that the pathology has not changed dramatically. This also allows an opportunity to identify and mark, if necessary, the operative site.

Once all of these preparations have been made, the patient is ready for anesthesia.

## CHOICE OF ANESTHETIC

Not all anesthetic techniques will be appropriate for all patients and all procedures. Nevertheless, in most cases it will be possible to provide anesthesia with either a general anesthetic or a local or regional technique, in the latter case often supplemented by sedative or analgesic medications. The exact choice depends on the specific nature of the operation, the medical condition and preferences of the patient, and the experience of the anesthesiologist. The relative advantages and disadvantages of each approach must be considered in all cases.

## LOCAL AND REGIONAL ANESTHESIA

### What Are the Advantages and Disadvantages of Local and Regional Anesthesia?

Local and regional anesthesia have the advantage that only that part (or area) of the body undergoing surgery requires anesthesia. Most of the disadvantages (and risks) of general anesthesia are avoided, and the provision of effective intraoperative analgesia usually also ensures adequate postoperative pain relief. Some procedures may be performed by simple local anesthetic infiltration, although a wider range are possible with various regional or central nerve blocks.

There are also disadvantages to local and regional anesthesia. Some techniques may take longer to establish than general anesthesia, although the time is reduced with experience. This additional preoperative time must also be balanced against the ability to take a fully conscious patient out of the operating room immediately after the operation is completed.

Most blocks are painful to some extent; intraoperative discomfort is not universally prevented; and there is a definite failure rate. These factors, as well as the desire to not be "awake" during surgery, can make local anesthetic techniques unpopular with patients. Many of these problems can be reduced, although not completely avoided, by the use of supplemental sedation and systemic analgesia (see the section on MAC).

Regional techniques carry the remote risk of nerve damage. More commonly, there will be the hemodynamic consequences of sympathetic nerve block. Prolonged impairment of motor function, leading to delay in ambulation and urinary retention, is common with some techniques, whereas local anesthetic toxicity and systemic adverse effects are possible with others. These relative disadvantages have to be considered alongside the considerable advantages of local anesthesia.

### What Techniques Are Used for Lower Body Procedures?

#### Spinal and Epidural Anesthesia

These techniques are appropriate for a wide range of lower body procedures. The spinal block is very quick to perform and establish but may be complicated by hypotension and postdural puncture headache (PDPH). The former complication is generally manageable with volume preloading and vasoconstrictors. The incidence of PDPH can be greatly reduced by using fine-gauge (25-27) pencil-point (eg, Whitacre) needles but it is still not eliminated. An epidural block can also reduce these complications, although this advantage must be weighed against a much slower onset time and risk of toxicity if the much larger drug dose is injected into an inappropriate site (eg, subarachnoid or intravascular). The major advantage of the epidural approach is that it allows the placement of a catheter in order to extend the block in the case of prolonged surgery.

#### Choice of Drug

Although prolonged postoperative analgesia is a desirable feature, prolonged motor and sympathetic block are not. For this reason, bupivacaine and tetracaine are too long-lasting for routine ambulatory use. Lidocaine has a more appropriate duration, but reports of neurologic sequelae, including permanent nerve damage, associated with delivering 5% hyperbaric lidocaine through spinal microcatheters[39] have limited its use. This recent uncertainty with regard to the safety of hyperbaric lidocaine has prompted an evaluation of low-dose diluted bupivacaine. Reducing the dose of bupivacaine from 15 to 7.5 mg (diluted up to 3 mL with saline) had no effect on the onset time but reduced discharge time from 471 to 202 minutes.[40] Similar results could be obtained by further reducing the dose to 5 mg (1 mL of 0.5% hyperbaric bupivacaine plus 2 mL saline) and adding 10 µg fentanyl, with the advantage of a slightly more intense intraoperative block.[41] This technique still permitted maximum block (to T8) to be achieved within 10 minutes and may be suitable for ambulatory procedures. Nevertheless, postoperative problems can still occur, and delay in voiding for up to 12 hours has been reported with as little as 5 mg intrathecal bupivacaine.[42]

### What Techniques Are Used for Upper Limb Procedures?

Interscalene block may be used for shoulder or upper arm surgery, but this block is accompanied predictably by hemiparesis of the ipsilateral diaphragm and often by Horner syndrome. Most operations on the arm from the elbow downward may be achieved with an axillary brachial plexus block. Various techniques are described, although all have a modest failure rate and involve relatively large doses of local anesthetic with a consequent risk of toxicity. Lidocaine is a good choice of anesthetic for most procedures, although bupivacaine or ropivacaine may be substituted when prolonged postoperative analgesia is required.

## Intravenous Regional Anesthesia

A simpler approach for hand and forearm surgery is intravenous regional anesthesia. This technique is easily mastered by most anesthesiologists. Because the technique involves deliberate intravascular injection of local anesthetic drug, its safety is totally dependent upon a correctly functioning tourniquet and careful attention to detail. It is vital that the tourniquet is inflated well above the patient's arterial pressure and that tourniquet inflation is maintained for at least 15 to 20 minutes. Patient comfort may be improved with a double cuff, wherein the distal cuff is inflated and the proximal cuff is then released after the onset of pain caused by the tourniquet. To minimize toxicity, lidocaine or, preferably, prilocaine should be used.

### What Are Other Useful Blocks?

Although most lower body procedures can be performed under spinal anesthesia, more localized blocks may reduce complications. Inguinal hernia repairs may be conducted under block of the ilioinguinal and iliohypogastric nerves, combined with infiltration of the line of incision. Various lower limb procedures may be performed with femoral nerve block, sciatic nerve block, three-in-one block, popliteal block, and ankle block. The latter in particular involves several injections of local anesthetic and may be quite painful to perform. The administration of systemic analgesia before performing some of these blocks is recommended.

## MONITORED ANESTHESIA CARE

### What Is Monitored Anesthesia Care?

MAC describes the presence of an anesthesiologist in a monitoring and supportive capacity during procedures performed under local or regional anesthesia or no anesthesia at all. Increasingly, MAC involves the administration of various anxiolytic, hypnotic, amnestic, and analgesic adjuvants to supplement a variety of local anesthetic-based techniques.[43] This may improve patient acceptability and comfort and may also permit more extensive surgery under local anesthesia.[43] These sedative medications can also facilitate various investigative procedures (eg, endoscopy, colonoscopy) that do not require formal anesthesia.

A wide variety of operations may be performed with local infiltration, central nerve blocks, or regional nerve blocks. For some patients, this type of anesthesia may be quite acceptable. Many other patients may experience pain on local anesthetic injection, anxiety about various aspects of surgery, concerns about being awake, boredom or restlessness during the prolonged immobility required by the procedure, or discomfort from various aspects of the operation. These problems may be overcome (or reduced) by the provision of supplemental analgesia, anxiolysis, and hypnosis. The amount of supplemental medication that is required will vary between individuals, operations, and over time during any particular operation.[44] Ideally, each of these different components should be provided by individual drugs, titrated to effect, with short-acting agents so that recovery will be rapid. The currently available drugs come close to making this ideal a reality.

### What Are the Benefits of Monitored Anesthesia Care?

The major benefit of MAC is that it allows many of the disadvantages of general anesthesia to be avoided. Recovery will be faster; protective reflexes will be better preserved; and postoperative nausea and vomiting (PONV) are substantially reduced. Because local anesthesia is used to provide intraoperative analgesia, pain relief will also be good in the early postoperative period. MAC may also be more cost-effective, although there are limited data to confirm this widely held belief.[43] Despite the considerable advantages of MAC, the potential for problems still exists. The ASA recommends that exactly the same standards of care should apply to MAC as for general anesthesia—from the preanesthesia evaluation through patient recovery.[45]

### How Are the Patient's Requirements Assessed During Monitored Anesthesia Care?

Monitoring may be divided into two components: (1) assessing the patient's requirement for supplemental medication and (2) assessing the effect of those drugs on the patient. Monitoring the patient's requirements is best achieved by talking to the patient. This has the additional benefit that the communication itself will usually have a reassuring effect, reducing the need for sedation, whereas the ability to communicate indicates that the patient is not excessively sedated. Various scoring systems can add a degree of objectivity when assessing the patient. Such scores may be useful research tools but lack the other advantages of simple communication. The bispectral index (BSI) may yield further information about the patient's sedation level, although there is considerable interindividual variation[46] that diminishes its usefulness (see detailed discussion in this chapter).

In monitoring the effects of supplemental medications on the patient, it is a fundamental principle that the patient should remain conscious (MAC is often still called *conscious sedation* in other countries). The patient should be calm and relaxed, often (but not always) sleepy, but still responsive to commands. On this basis, MAC is safe; however, keep in mind that many of the drugs used are simply anesthetics at a low dose. It is all too easy to make the transition from sedation to anesthesia, especially because there is considerable overlap between the sedative and anesthetic doses for different individuals. As an uncontrolled (ie, unintended) general anesthetic, MAC can be very dangerous. The necessary drugs and equipment for managing such an eventuality (and a practitioner skilled in their use) must always be available during MAC.[45]

The standard of monitoring should be essentially the same as for general anesthesia, although, in practice, the oxygen saturation and respiratory rate will be of the greatest practical value. Supplemental oxygen is routinely given by many whenever sedative medications are administered. An intravenous cannula attached to a capnograph sample line and inserted into a face mask or nasal cannula (or a commercially available system) can provide a useful respiratory waveform. Again, talking to the patient is an excellent monitor of cerebral oxygenation and perfusion.

## What Type of Sedative-Hypnotics Are Used During Monitored Anesthesia Care?

A variety of sedative-hypnotics can and have been used during MAC. These include various benzodiazepines, barbiturate anesthetics, ketamine, and propofol. Most of these drugs result in slow recovery, poor control, unacceptable side effects, or a combination of these problems. By far the most commonly used sedative-hypnotic agents are midazolam and propofol.

### Midazolam

Midazolam is a water-soluble, nonirritant rapid- and short-acting benzodiazepine that has largely replaced diazepam for MAC. Midazolam has no active metabolites and does not undergo enterohepatic recirculation, resulting in rapid recovery after brief procedures. Increasing age and coexisting medical conditions may enhance the patient's sensitivity to midazolam and increase the variability in response among patients.

Like other benzodiazepines, midazolam produces anxiolysis, combined with varying degrees of amnesia and sedation. The anxiolysis is especially useful, because the fear of being awake during surgery (under local anesthesia) is often much worse than the actual experience. Midazolam also produces some amnesia. This has been considered advantageous in association with unpleasant procedures, although the ethics of this approach are questionable.[47] Many patients find a period of amnesia disturbing; they may wonder who performed the operation[48] and may forget important information and instructions.

Although midazolam lasts for a shorter time than does diazepam, recovery may still be slow after relatively large doses and, especially, after repeated administration of midazolam. Therefore, during more extensive operations, or when more profound sedation is required, it is preferable to use a drug like propofol, which is less likely to accumulate.

### Propofol

Low doses of various anesthetic agents are capable of providing controlled intraoperative sedation. Recovery from the sedative effects of most of these may be prolonged. In contrast, propofol is rapidly distributed and permits rapid recovery after a single bolus or short-term infusion. This rapid recovery also provides excellent response to changes in the rate of continuous infusion and may reduce the incidence of oversedation compared with the use of longer-lasting drugs, such as midazolam.[49]

Infusions of propofol generally provide acceptable sedation.[50] Recovery from sedation is generally faster and more complete after propofol compared with midazolam. For example, comparable sedation was achieved with midazolam, 0.27 mg/kg/h or propofol, 3.7 mg/kg/h, but awakening occurred within 2 minutes of discontinuing propofol compared with 9 minutes after midazolam therapy.[51] Furthermore, psychomotor function was depressed for up to 2 hours after sedation using midazolam but was relatively unchanged after propofol. Several other investigators have found that patients have recovered rapidly and returned to the preoperative state after treatment with propofol compared with recovery times of at least 2 hours after infusions of midazolam.[49,52]

In sedative doses, propofol is also relatively devoid of perioperative side effects. In particular, propofol produces little cardiovascular or respiratory depression and minimal involuntary movements or excitatory effects; this drug has a low incidence of postoperative nausea. Propofol also produces relatively little amnesia for intraoperative events unless patients are rendered unconscious.[50] This may be advantageous, allowing patients to recall important instructions and to be relatively awake during their operation, if they so choose. In situations where intraoperative amnesia is desirable (or requested), it may be achieved by cosedation with midazolam and propofol.

### Sedative Combinations

Propofol offers the benefits of satisfactory and highly controllable sedation during MAC, followed by rapid recovery. Propofol produces relatively little anxiolysis and amnesia. In contrast, midazolam provides excellent anxiolysis and intraoperative amnesia but produces more prolonged and less controllable sedation. The desirable properties of both agents may be combined by using small doses of midazolam (1-2 mg) titrated in conjunction with propofol. Patient anxiety was significantly reduced; sedation scores were increased; and amnesia for early intraoperative events was enhanced by preceding an infusion of propofol with midazolam, 2 mg.[53] This small dose of midazolam had no discernible effect on postoperative sedation, amnesia, or recovery times.[53] Other investigators have also reported benefits from combining propofol with opioids to enhance analgesia during more painful procedures.[54,55]

## When Is Supplemental Anesthesia Necessary During Monitored Anesthesia Care?

During MAC, the analgesic component is provided primarily by the local anesthetic. Supplemental analgesia may be required during the initial local anesthetic injection to prevent pain from pressure and traction on deep tissue planes and other structures outside the area of the local anesthetic block, to reduce discomfort from lying on a hard surface, and to minimize the ache caused by tourniquets. Short-acting opioid analgesics (eg, fentanyl, alfentanil, remifentanil) are the most commonly used adjuvants. Combinations of opioid analgesics and sedative-hypnotics enhance the degree of sedation and can produce highly satisfactory surgical conditions.

Unfortunately, such mixtures can significantly increase the incidence of undesirable side effects. In particular, opioids increase the incidence of nausea and vomiting and are potent respiratory depressants. There is a synergistic interaction between opioids and benzodiazepines to produce even more profound respiratory depression.[56] Great care must be taken when such combinations are used, because fatalities have occurred. In contrast to midazolam, combinations of propofol with opioid analgesics may not exacerbate respiratory depression to the same extent. For example, the incidence of hypoxemia with a propofol-fentanyl combination was one half that experienced with a mixture of midazolam and alfentanil.[54]

### Remifentanil

Remifentanil, the esterase-metabolized, ultra–short-acting opioid, is a μ opioid agonist and has all of the effects and side effects of such drugs. Its extremely short duration of action may enhance the controllability of the desirable effects and may limit the consequences of undesirable ones. Remifentanil, at an infusion of 0.05 to 0.1 μg/kg/min, may provide a useful degree of background analgesia. Remifentanil alone provides no sedation or anxiolysis and thus will usually need to be combined with other sedatives such as midazolam. As with other opioids, interactions with midazolam may occur, although the severity of respiratory depression is usually acceptable, provided that no more than 2 mg of midazolam is used.[57] If respiratory depression occurs with remifentanil, it will rapidly resolve upon reducing or discontinuing the opioid infusion. Because of the intermittent nature of pain during MAC, it may be more desirable to administer remifentanil in small bolus doses (eg, 25 μg) rather than as an infusion. This approach may be more effective, although it may not result in any greater respiratory depression compared with the use of a continuous infusion.[58]

## What Are the Effects of Antagonist Drugs During Monitored Anesthesia Care?

All the effects of opioid analgesics may be antagonized with naloxone, whereas flumazenil will reverse benzodiazepine sedation. The availability of such antagonist drugs represents a useful "escape path" in the event of inadvertent oversedation or respiratory depression. The routine use of these drugs should be strongly discouraged, however, because it introduces two major problems. Reliance on antagonists for rapid recovery encourages the use of excessive sedation; better and more careful titration to effect is a more appropriate strategy. Second, the duration of action of both flumazenil and naloxone is considerably shorter than that of their corresponding agonist drugs (except remifentanil). There is, therefore, the real possibility of a recurrence of excessive sedation or ventilatory depression, which could potentially occur after the patient has been sent home. It is our opinion that antagonist drugs should, therefore, be reserved for emergencies, and patients should be carefully observed for some time if such drugs are required. In the case of remifentanil, stopping the infusion should improve respiratory function before a dose of naloxone can even be prepared. Naloxone is only likely to be required in the case of a massive overdose of remifentanil (ie, a serious drug error).

## What Role Do Inhaled Sedatives Play in Monitored Anesthesia Care?

Inhaled anesthetics can also be used for sedation. This approach has the advantage of being less invasive, and the lungs provide a route for rapid drug elimination. Nitrous oxide ($N_2O$) has been a popular inhaled sedative for many years, especially in dentistry. Various volatile anesthetics have also been used. Of these, sevoflurane is the most pleasant to breathe and has the additional advantage that appropriate sedation is rapidly achieved because of low solubility. Sevoflurane appears to be an effective sedative,[59] with good control of sedation and rapid recovery. One disadvantage of inhaled sedatives is that the risk of unintended transition to general anesthesia may be even higher than with intravenous sedatives. In the absence of a tightly fitting mask, leaks may be considerable, producing pollution of the operating room environment and requiring compensatory high fresh gas flows at increased cost. Unfortunately, tightly fitting masks are often poorly tolerated by the sedated patient who is still conscious. Inhaled sedation may be useful, but practical difficulties limit the widespread adoption of this interesting method of sedation.

## What Are the Future Developments in Monitored Anesthesia Care?

### Benzodiazepines

Ro 48-6791 is a new water-soluble benzodiazepine that is currently under development. This drug is more potent and its effect lasts for a shorter time compared with midazolam therapy. The shorter duration of the medication has allowed patients undergoing endoscopy to return to their awake state, walk unaided, and walk toe-to-heel along a straight line significantly earlier after the last dose of sedative compared with patients who had midazolam therapy.[60] Ro 48-6791 is so shortacting that additional doses (or an infusion) are likely to be required during most procedures. This will not be a problem for anesthesiologists but may be less convenient for nonanesthesiologists, such as endoscopists. Whether Ro 48-6791 will offer clinically significant advantages over midazolam, propofol, or combinations of both drugs is currently unknown, but further evaluation is being undertaken.

### Patient-Maintained Analgesia

There has been considerable interest in allowing patients to adjust their own sedative level in a way similar to patient-controlled analgesia (PCA). Several investigative groups have studied this concept, predominantly using propofol. The basic concept appears sound, with patients being able to self-administer sedation with high levels of satisfaction.[61–63] The potential risk of oversedation remains, however, and patients still require full supervision. A more recent approach is to use an infusion pump programmed with propofol pharmacokinetics to adjust the infusion rate to maintain a constant calculated propofol plasma concentration. Such an approach—target-controlled infusion (TCI)—has been available for general anesthesia for some time in Europe and Australia. For sedation, the computer software is modified such that the plasma concentration gradually declines (to encourage awakening) in the absence of patient input, whereas successful patient demand increases the plasma concentration slightly.[64] This system, known as patient-maintained sedation, is still being developed, and no TCI system (for anesthesia or sedation) currently has regulatory approval in the United States. Although safer in principle than simple PCA, the safety margin between beneficial and harmful effects is generally smaller for sedative-hypnotic drugs than it is for analgesics; therefore, such systems are unlikely to be suitable for patient use without direct supervision. Their only obvious advantage is to give the patient a degree of control; however, this benefit can probably be achieved at lower cost and with reduced drug use by better communication between patients and their anesthesiologists.

## GENERAL ANESTHESIA

General anesthesia can be used for almost any ambulatory procedure; for some procedures such as laparoscopy, there is no good alternative. General anesthesia remains popular with many patients and surgeons. For ambulatory surgery, general anesthesia requires a rapid and smooth onset, good intraoperative conditions with rapid control of anesthetic depth, fast emergence and recovery independent of the duration of anesthesia, and a low incidence of side effects. Of the latter, PONV is probably the most important to minimize.

### Why Is Propofol the Most Commonly Used Intravenous Anesthetic for Ambulatory Surgery?

Propofol is the most commonly used intravenous anesthetic for ambulatory surgery.[65] It provides a smooth induction with good relaxation of pharyngeal muscles, allowing early insertion of an airway or LMA. Pain on injection is common but can be minimized by coadministration of lidocaine. As an induction agent, propofol appears to result in improved early recovery and a modest reduction in PONV compared with alternative intravenous drugs.[65]

Apparent benefits from propofol as an induction agent led to its evaluation for anesthetic maintenance. Initial comparisons of propofol with thiopentone-volatile anesthetic combinations suggested significantly faster recovery after propofol, although this was more related to the change of induction agent than to the elimination of inhaled anesthetics.[65] When propofol is used for induction, recovery times are generally similar, irrespective of whether anesthesia is subsequently maintained with propofol or a halogenated ether.[65]

Nevertheless, propofol has become a popular maintenance anesthetic for ambulatory anesthesia. The most common method of administration is to give an initial bolus for induction, followed by a variable rate infusion for maintenance. Initially, a high infusion rate is administered to compensate for the rapid early distribution of propofol. The infusion rate can be reduced somewhat as the rate of redistribution slows. Further changes to the infusion rate will also be required if the patient demonstrates clinical signs of excessive or inadequate anesthesia. Some of the complexity of propofol administration may be eliminated by using a computer, programmed with population pharmacokinetics, to calculate the necessary infusion rate to achieve and maintain a particular plasma concentration. Such a TCI is generally preferred to a manual infusion scheme[66] and can make it easier to rapidly change the depth of anesthesia.[67]

The beneficial reduction in PONV seen after induction of anesthesia with propofol is more pronounced when propofol is used for maintenance.[68] Although this is still a relatively weak effect, it remains a prominent reason for choosing propofol. Propofol also has an advantage over volatile anesthetics in that it is safe in patients at risk for malignant hyperpyrexia.

One major disadvantage of propofol is its high direct cost. The low cost of anesthesia in relation to surgery and its indirect effect in reducing PONV are often cited in justification of greater expense.[69] Nevertheless, the increased cost of propofol is considerable, even when compared with the newest inhalational agents.[70,71] In particular, significant amounts of propofol often remain to be wasted at the end of each case, a cost that is not experienced with inhaled anesthetics. The recent loss of patent protection for propofol and the advent of generic forms has already substantially reduced the cost.

Propofol is also associated with a high incidence of apnea on induction of anesthesia. This can easily be managed by manual ventilation but can be inconvenient if a spontaneously breathing technique is intended. Unlike inhaled anesthetics, propofol can still be delivered if the patient is hypoventilating. Propofol also commonly induces hypotension on induction. This effect is short-lived, but can be quite profound. Both apnea and hypotension can be reduced by the coadministration of midazolam and/or an opioid analgesic. These drugs significantly reduce the induction dose of propofol and limit the severity of side effects. The TCI system may also reduce side effects by way of a slightly slower, more controlled induction of anesthesia.

### What Other Intravenous Agents Are Used for the Induction of Anesthesia?

IV anesthetics are commonly used for the induction of anesthesia. Methohexitone was popular in the past, but involuntary movements are common and recovery is delayed, especially after shorter-acting maintenance drugs. Etomidate was also evaluated for ambulatory anesthesia but resulted in an unacceptable incidence of PONV. Various steroid anesthetics have been investigated over the years. Although the steroids have some useful benefits, practical problems with solubility and a high incidence of allergic reactions have prevented their practical application. At present, propofol is the intravenous anesthetic of choice.

### What Agents Are Used for Inhalational Anesthesia?

Despite the enthusiasm for propofol, inhaled halogenated ethers remain popular maintenance anesthetics. This is partly related to our familiarity with these drugs and the predictable responses to their administration. The widespread availability of end-expired agent monitoring helps in their clinical delivery but also ensures that drug is being delivered to the patient, potentially reducing the risk of awareness. The use of low-flow anesthesia can make inhaled anesthesia very inexpensive, even with the newer inhaled drugs.[71] In general, the speed and quality of recovery is similar after inhaled anesthetics (when anesthesia is induced with propofol) to that achieved with propofol,[65] provided that PONV is kept under control.

There are various inhaled anesthetics to choose from. Slow recovery and the potential for serious side effects have effectively eliminated halothane, whereas enflurane is now seldom used. Although isoflurane is still popular, interest has recently been focused on the low-solubility agents, desflurane and sevoflurane.

### Desflurane

Desflurane is the least soluble of the available inhaled anesthetics. It is also the most irritating to the airway, thus preventing its safe use as an induction agent. There was initially some concern that this irritation might also pose problems during spontaneous ventilation, although these fears appear groundless.[72] Desflurane is the most stable volatile anesthetic, which may limit its toxic potential. This is probably of limited importance in ambulatory anesthesia. Desflurane can cause harm through production of carbon monoxide in the presence of dry soda lime.

The low solubility of desflurane should ensure rapid recovery. Although some investigations have shown slightly earlier awakening, the majority of evidence suggests that differences in recovery times between desflurane and isoflurane or propofol are only of minor clinical importance.[73] Rapid awakening may be disadvantageous in children, where emergence delirium may occur.[74] In addition, desflurane may be more likely to produce PONV than isoflurane.[75]

With the advent of fast-track recovery (discussed in further detail in this chapter), earlier awakening may become more important. Desflurane anesthesia resulted in a higher proportion of "fast-track eligible" patients than either sevoflurane or propofol.[76] Desflurane may also be more useful after longer ambulatory procedures, because recovery from its effects is less dependent on the duration of administration than it is for other volatile anesthetics.

### Sevoflurane

Sevoflurane is also relatively insoluble, although less so than desflurane. Sevoflurane is also minimally irritating to the airway, thus making it suitable for induction of anesthesia and permitting the abrupt delivery of high inspired concentrations in order to rapidly deepen anesthesia. Sevoflurane is metabolized in vivo and degraded by soda lime to a much greater extent than desflurane. Although there were initially valid concerns as to the production of potentially toxic byproducts, sevoflurane has proved to be very safe in clinical practice. Despite this excellent safety profile, concerns over the risk of nephrotoxicity have prompted the Food and Drug Administration in the United States to warn against the prolonged administration of sevoflurane at relatively low fresh gas flow rates (<1 L/min). Flow rate restrictions have, therefore, been imposed in the United States, and these restrictions have prevented the most economical use of sevoflurane. In the numerous other countries that have no such limitations, sevoflurane is commonly delivered at or below gas flows of 1 L/min, yet clinically relevant toxicity has not been observed.

Like desflurane, the rapid emergence from sevoflurane may cause transient problems in children.[74] Provision of effective analgesia may reduce (but not eliminate) this problem. In adults, sevoflurane also facilitates fast-track recovery better than does propofol.[76] As a maintenance anesthetic, sevoflurane appears to cause less PONV than isoflurane.[77]

### Inhaled Induction

Inhaled induction of anesthesia has always been popular with children. Until relatively recently, halothane was the preferred choice. Sevoflurane, which is less soluble and less irritating, permits faster and smoother induction than halothane, with fewer cardiac dysrhythmias. Sevoflurane has now largely displaced halothane for this indication, despite its significantly higher cost.

Sevoflurane is also such an effective inhaled induction agent that it can be used for that purpose in adults. When 8% sevoflurane is delivered in a tidal breathing technique, induction is smooth, but slightly slower than that achieved with propofol.[78] When a vital capacity technique is used, sevoflurane induction can actually be faster than intravenous induction.[79] This technique has the advantage of maintaining spontaneous ventilation and hemodynamic stability and is acceptable to most patients. It may be especially beneficial to the significant minority of adults who are needle phobic.

### What Is the Volatile Induction and Maintenance of Anesthesia Concept?

Volatile induction and maintenance of anesthesia (VIMA) results from the successful use of sevoflurane as an induction agent in adults. Use of the same anesthetic throughout surgery may reduce complications during the transition from "traditional" intravenous induction to inhaled maintenance and may also permit more rapid awakening after very short procedures.[78] Rapid uptake of anesthetic during the induction phase can permit an earlier adoption of low fresh gas flows and reduces the consumption (and cost) of sevoflurane during maintenance of anesthesia compared with its use after an intravenous induction.[70]

Although one study suggested comparable rates of PONV after either sevoflurane VIMA or propofol anesthesia,[80] other investigations suggest that PONV is more common after VIMA,[67,70] and that the VIMA concept increases PONV with sevoflurane compared with its use solely for maintenance.[70] However, one advantage of the VIMA technique is that it provides excellent control over the depth of anesthesia. This means that intraoperative opioids are rarely needed (provided that adequate nonopioid postoperative analgesia is provided), and the elimination of these drugs reduces PONV to more acceptable levels. VIMA may not be suitable for all patients, perhaps including those at higher than normal risk of PONV, but is a useful and interesting new technique.

### What Are Commonly Used Adjuncts to General Anesthesia?

#### Nitrous Oxide

$N_2O$ is the most commonly used anesthetic adjunct. It has a useful anesthetic-sparing effect and provides a significant degree of intraoperative analgesia. $N_2O$ remains popular, although there are concerns about its environmental effects, the potential for chronic toxicity (for patients and staff), diffusion hypoxia, and a modest increase in PONV. $N_2O$ is not an essential component of anesthesia and can be eliminated from both intravenous and inhaled techniques. It will generally be necessary to use a higher concentration of the hypnotic agent with the addition of an alternative analgesic, usually an opioid if $N_2O$ is avoided. It is more common (but not universal) to deliver intravenous anesthetics without $N_2O$, perhaps because opioid infusions are more commonly used during these techniques.

#### Opioid Analgesics

Opioid analgesics are another common anesthetic adjunct. It is common practice to accompany intravenous induction with propofol with a small bolus of either fentanyl or alfentanil. This approach may smooth induction, reduce the induction dose, and may facilitate LMA insertion or tracheal intubation. However, a bolus dose of a short-acting opioid will provide little, if any, postoperative analgesia and may contribute to PONV.[81,82] These drugs can generally be eliminated from routine practice with little detriment.

If propofol is used for anesthetic maintenance, intraoperative opioid supplements are more likely to be required. Propofol provides no analgesia, and quite high concentrations will be required to prevent intraoperative movement, even in the presence of N$_2$O. Opioid analgesics can significantly reduce the propofol dose requirements while ensuring good intraoperative conditions. Better conditions tend to result from delivering short-acting opioids by continuous infusion, rather than as bolus doses that can induce apnea and hypotension.

## Remifentanil

Alfentanil was previously a popular choice of opioid, but accumulation resulted in delayed recovery of respiratory function or the delivery of a suboptimal dose in compensation for the respiratory depressant effects. The availability of remifentanil allows a more appropriate intraoperative dose to be used while still ensuring a rapid recovery, which can result in improved intraoperative hemodynamic stability.[83] By providing effective intraoperative analgesia with remifentanil, the dose of propofol may be reduced, and recovery may be hastened.

Although respiratory function returns rapidly when remifentanil is discontinued, it is profoundly depressed during infusions of remifentanil, thus making it difficult to maintain spontaneous ventilation during remifentanil-propofol anesthesia.[84] Although ventilation can be assisted without difficulty, the respiratory rate and pattern are lost as indicators of anesthetic depth. Remifentanil may also mask other signs of inadequate anesthesia, and awareness remains a possibility if the propofol dose is reduced too much.[85] Remifentanil may also be used to supplement inhalation anesthesia. Compared with alfentanil, remifentanil prevented intraoperative stress responses to a greater degree and resulted in improved intermediate recovery.[86] Like other opioids, remifentanil may produce PONV. The short duration of remifentanil may limit this effect, but PONV is still likely to be more common than when opioids are avoided.

## How Do You Choose Between Intravenous and Inhaled Anesthetics?

Both intravenous and inhaled anesthetics have a number of relative advantages and disadvantages (Table 70–4). There may be a few cases where an intravenous technique is particularly desirable. Such cases will mainly involve operations around the airway, where inhaled delivery of anesthesia may be difficult. When general anesthesia is required in a patient at risk for malignant hyperpyrexia, propofol is the logical choice. This drug is also likely to be chosen as part of a technique in patients at very high risk of PONV and bronchospasm. In contrast, inhalation anesthetics, at least for induction, are more likely to be chosen for severe needle phobics, especially children. Halogenated ethers may be especially useful if relaxation of muscles is required but neuromuscular block is undesirable. For most cases, a good argument can be made in favor of either form of anesthesia. The ultimate choice invariably comes down to individual preference, and there is no doubt that it is possible to give a very high quality

**TABLE 70–4.** Relative Advantages and Disadvantages of Intravenous and Inhaled Anesthetics for Ambulatory Surgery

**Intravenous Anesthesia**

| *Advantages* | *Disadvantages* |
|---|---|
| Rapid recovery | No measure of actual drug delivery |
| Reduction in PONV (propofol) | |
| Control of anesthesia independent of ventilation | Difficulty in controlling anesthesia (reduced by target-controlled infusion) |
| Ability to provide hypnotic, analgesic, and muscle relaxant components separately | High direct cost |
| Safe in malignant hyperpyrexia (propofol) | Requires infusion pump and disposable equipment |
| Limit airway reactivity (propofol) | Potential for environmental pollution (from disposable items) |

**Inhaled Anesthesia**

| | |
|---|---|
| Rapid recovery | Small increase in PONV (worse in the presence of opioids) |
| End-expired concentration guides *and confirms* drug delivery | Some potentially toxic products (clinical toxicity is rare) |
| Easy to control anesthesia | Require calibrated vaporizer |
| Hypnotic, analgesic, and muscle-relaxant components that are all provided by one drug | Potential for environmental pollution |
| Good bronchodilators | |
| Low direct costs, especially with low flows | |
| Simplicity | |

PONV, postoperative nausea and vomiting.

ambulatory anesthetic with either intravenous or inhaled agents.

## CONDUCTION OF GENERAL ANESTHESIA

### What Are the Advantages and Disadvantages of Tracheal Intubation?

In recent years, it has been common to maintain the patient's airway using a tracheal tube. In the ambulatory setting (and indeed for many other patients), tracheal intubation may have many disadvantages, some of which are listed in Table 70–5. It is a commonly held belief that tracheal intubation is mandatory to protect the patient against pulmonary aspiration of gastric contents. In reality, the incidence of aspiration in fasted, elective ambulatory patients is exceedingly low.[38,87–90] When aspiration does occur, its consequences are generally also mild. For example, in a series of 11 910 patients managed with the LMA, only one case of aspiration was recorded, and the patient did not require admission to an intensive care unit.[89] In a survey of all cases of pulmonary aspiration—elective and emergency—over a 6-year period, the incidence of pulmonary aspiration in elective ASA 1 and 2 patients was approximately 1 in 8000; the morbidity was approximately 1 in 40 000.[38]

Tracheal intubation will not protect against pulmonary aspiration unless a rapid sequence technique is used. Neuromuscular blocking drugs render the larynx incompetent, and the airway is at increased risk until the tracheal tube is in place. Malins and Cooper[90] reported just such a case in a patient about to undergo gynecologic laparoscopy, whereas Warner and colleagues reported that a third of all cases of pulmonary aspiration occurred during laryngoscopy and tracheal intuba-

**TABLE 70–5.** Disadvantages of Tracheal Intubation for Ambulatory Surgical Patients

**Laryngoscopy Required**

Trauma to teeth
Increased HR and BP
Possibility of failure
Risk of awareness during laryngoscopy

**Irritant to the Larynx and Airway**

Postoperative sore throat
Voice abnormalities (eg, in professional singers)
Requires greater depth of anesthesia (slower recovery)
Post-extubation laryngospasm
Increased airway reactivity with recent respiratory tract infection

**Likely to Require a Neuromuscular Block**

Risk of intraoperative awareness
Loss of respiratory rate and pattern as monitors of anesthetic depth
Risk of breathing circuit disconnection
Possibility of inadequate reversal
Possibility of cardiovascular disturbance and increased PONV from "reversal" drugs
Muscle aches with succinylcholine
Increased drug costs

**Airway Protection**

Risk of aspiration before and immediately after intubation
Pharyngeal blood may bypass tracheal cuff

---

BP, blood pressure; HR, heart rate; PONV, postoperative nausea and vomiting.

tion.[38] In addition, tracheal extubation often renders the larynx incompetent for some time,[91] and aspiration can occur after the tracheal tube is removed.[38]

## What Alternatives Are Available for Tracheal Intubation?

There are a number of alternatives to tracheal tubes. The simplest is to use a face mask, but this becomes very tiring for the anesthesia provider during longer procedures. Face masks also result in variable airway quality and intermittent leaks, which may interfere with the ability to use low fresh gas flows. These problems are highly dependent on the skill and vigilance of the anesthesiologist. Holding the face mask in place prevents the anesthesiologist from performing other tasks, such as drug administration or record keeping. A supportive harness can overcome this problem, but trauma to facial nerves is a risk.[92] Pressure on the patient's eye is also a risk when using face masks.[93]

### Laryngeal Mask Airway

A more practical alternative is the LMA, which provides a superior airway to the face mask.[94] The LMA is easily inserted following induction of anesthesia with either propofol or sevoflurane and requires neither laryngoscopy nor neuromuscular block. Once in place, the LMA is well tolerated, requiring a level of anesthesia appropriate to the surgical procedure rather than the deeper levels required with tracheal tubes.[95] This helps to facilitate more rapid recovery (through lower anesthetic drug use) and also provides a clear airway in the emerging patient, the LMA being removed upon awakening.

The LMA is so well tolerated because it occupies an area in the pharynx developmentally adapted to the presence of foreign bodies (in the form of food boluses). In contrast, the tracheal tube crosses the vocal cords, one function of which is to close off in response to direct contact in order to protect the lungs. The LMA leaves these laryngeal reflexes intact (if neuromuscular blocking drugs are not used), which may be one reason why significant aspiration is so uncommon.[89,90] Because it sits over the larynx like an umbrella, the LMA also affords excellent protection against blood and other debris coming from above. In this way, tracheal soiling with blood and subsequent airway-related complications were significantly lower when anesthesia for tonsillectomy was maintained using the LMA compared with the use of a tracheal tube.[96]

### Intubating Laryngeal Mask Airway

Whereas the LMA can provide an excellent airway for numerous ambulatory procedures, there are still situations in which surgical access or the risk of intraoperative aspiration makes tracheal intubation desirable. An alternative to direct laryngoscopy is the intubating LMA (ILMA). The ILMA is modified from the standard LMA by having a shorter, more rigid, and larger diameter tube with a metal handle attached. These differences from the LMA allow the ILMA to be manipulated to provide optimal ventilation and permit the passage of up to a size 8 tracheal tube.[97] The short length of the ILMA reduces the chance of the tracheal tube cuff lying at the level of the vocal cords. The ILMA can be inserted in much the same way as a standard LMA[98] and can be used to provide oxygenation and anesthesia. Once a clear airway is established, the tracheal tube is passed blindly (and carefully) after establishing neuromuscular block. Initial reports suggest successful tracheal intubation in 99.3% of patients with the ILMA,[98] although only 50% were successful first time and 31% required more than two attempts. Regular tracheal tubes may be excessively curved after passing through the ILMA, and thus a dedicated straight latex tube has been produced. The commercially available version has had its tip modified in light of previous experience,[98] and in this form achieved almost 80% first time intubation, with 96.2% intubated within three attempts.[99] Tracheal intubation through the ILMA may be less stimulating, which may be a benefit in the cardiovascularly compromised patient. Although there was a statistically significant increase in heart rate and blood pressure after blind intubation, this increase (3 beats per minute and 9 mm Hg, respectively) was of no clinical significance.[99] It must be remembered that tracheal intubation, however performed, is somewhat traumatic, and there has been at least one case of esophageal perforation by a tube passed through an ILMA; the patient subsequently died.[100]

In the future, continuing modifications to the LMA, including a second cuff to increase glottic seal pressure and a second tube for esophageal drainage, may further reduce the indications for tracheal intubation. A prototype has recently been shown to increase seal pressure and to prevent gastric insufflation during positive pressure ventilation up to 40 cm $H_2O$, while still being easy to insert in children.[101]

### Cuffed Oropharyngeal Airway

A more recent airway management device is the cuffed oropharyngeal airway (COPA). The COPA is a "reinvention" of earlier pharyngeal bulb-type airways. It consists of a Guedel-shaped airway with an inflatable cuff to displace the tongue and help retain the device in position and a 15-mm connection at the other end to attach to a breathing circuit. The COPA is initially inserted like a conventional oral airway. Next, it is held in place with an elasticized strap, and finally the cuff is inflated, using 25 to 40 mL of air. The COPA is available in various sizes: 8, 9, 10, and 11. These sizes refer to the length (in centimeters) of the airway device. The airways are also color coded to facilitate correct selection. The choice of size is determined by estimating the distance between the incisor teeth and the angle of the mandible. The manufacturer recommends choosing a size equal to this distance plus 1 cm, although independent investigators have found a higher first time success rate using mandible-incisor distance plus 2 cm.[102]

There have been a number of comparisons of the COPA with the LMA.[102–105] These have generally demonstrated that (1) the COPA is no less invasive than the LMA[105]; (2) determining the correct size is difficult; and (3) the airway quality is inferior to that achieved with the LMA. In a multicenter evaluation which included the developer's institution,[104] the COPA had a lower first time insertion success rate, required a far higher level of airway support and manipulation, and was much less likely to achieve an excellent airway (Table 70–6). Further investigation by experienced LMA users demonstrated that the COPA was associated with a higher first-time failure rate of 45% compared with 3% with the LMA. In addition, there was a frequent (27%) need for a change of airway size that increased the time needed to establish an effective airway from 49 to 188 seconds.[103]

The COPA is a single-use disposable item, in contrast to the LMA, which is designed to be resterilized (by autoclaving) and reused up to 40 times. Despite the COPA's theoretical advantage of single patient use, no reports of patient-to-patient contamination have appeared with the LMA in over 10 years of use. In reality, the disposable nature of the COPA simply adds to costs (especially if an alternative-sized device has to be used) and contributes to environmental pollution. At the present time, it is difficult to see any obvious place for the COPA in routine ambulatory practice.

**TABLE 70–6.** Comparison of the Cuffed Oropharyngeal Airway With the Laryngeal Mask Airway

|  | LMA | COPA |
| --- | --- | --- |
| Number randomized | 151 | 302 |
| First-time successful insertion | 89% | 81%* |
| Failure of device | 3.4% | 5.4% |
| Time to effective airway(s) | 106 | 150* |
| Airway manipulations: | 4% | 71%* |
| 1–2 Interventions | 4% | 35%* |
| >2 Interventions | 0 | 36%* |
| Head tilt | 3.3% | 54.2%* |
| Chin lift | 1.3% | 42.8%* |
| Jaw thrust | 0.7% | 4.7%* |
| Continuous chin support | 0 | 29.8%* |
| "Excellent" airway | 76.7% | 25.6%* |

*$P < .05$, from the LMA group.
Values are a percentage of patients (%) or the median.
COPA, comparison of the cuffed oropharyngeal airway; LMA, laryngeal mask airway.
Data from Greenberg RS, Brimacombe J, Berry A, et al. A randomized controlled trial comparing the cuffed oropharyngeal airway and the laryngeal mask airway in spontaneously breathing anesthetized adults. *Anesthesiology.* 1998;88:970.

## How Are Neuromuscular Blocks Used in Outpatient Anesthesia?

There is no absolute contraindication to the use of neuromuscular block in ambulatory anesthesia, although the residual effects of these drugs must be thoroughly reversed at the end of anesthesia. Adequate reversal is more likely to be achieved with drugs of intermediate-to-short duration. In single doses, atracurium, vecuronium, and rocuronium are unlikely to present significant problems in the ambulatory setting, but full spontaneous recovery is unlikely except after relatively longer operations. Rocuronium offers a significantly faster onset of action compared with other nondepolarizing alternatives and also appears to have the shortest duration of the intermediate agents.[106] There is some evidence that the use of neostigmine to reverse residual neuromuscular block may contribute to an increase in PONV, although the effect, if any, is weak.[107] Nevertheless, there is some interest in using drugs of sufficiently brief duration that reversal will not be required. The most obvious choice is the depolarizing drug, succinylcholine. This old agent has many unfavorable properties, however, including various cardiac dysrhythmias and occasional reports of cardiac arrest.[108,109] In the ambulatory setting, it is the unacceptably high incidence of myalgia, resulting from muscle fasciculations, that most limits its use.

### Mivacurium

An alternative neuromuscular blocking agent is mivacurium, the cholinesterase-metabolized, nondepolarizing neuromuscular blocking drug. The short duration of action of mivacurium makes spontaneous recovery possible after all but the briefest of procedures.[110,111] Use of mivacurium is not without its difficulties, however. Histamine release may produce hypotension after larger doses, whereas smaller doses result in a delayed onset and variable effect. The duration of action of mivacurium will also be considerably prolonged in the presence of atypical pseudocholinesterase.

### Rapacuronium

Rapacuronium (Raplon; previously ORG 9487) has received its license for clinical use and may become a useful neuromuscular blocking drug for ambulatory use. It was initially believed that this rapid-onset, brief duration agent would be a true nondepolarizing replacement for succinylcholine. In practice, the duration of rapacuronium is likely to be closer to that of mivacurium, but its onset is more rapid. After a dose of 1.5 mg/kg or more, tracheal intubation conditions were excellent or good in >75% of subjects within 90 seconds.[112] The requirement for a rapid-sequence induction is relatively rare in ambulatory patients. In patients with abnormal gastric emptying or significant reflux, succinylcholine may still be the drug of choice. At 50 seconds, tracheal intubating conditions were clinically acceptable in 97.4% of patients receiving succinylcholine, 1 mg/kg, compared with only 89.4% of patients with rapacuronium, 1.5 mg/kg ($P = .004$).[113]

Doses of rapacuronium, 2 mg/kg or less, had a clinical duration of action of no more than 20 minutes, although spontaneous recovery to a train-of-four ratio (TOF) of 70% or more (consistent with safe tracheal extubation) took 30 to 45 minutes.[112] These recovery times are likely to be even longer in the presence of volatile anesthetic agents. As with all nondepolarizing neuromuscular blocking drugs, recovery from rapacuronium may be shortened with reversal agents. Very early administration of reversal drugs (2 minutes after rapacuronium administration) has been reported to substantially shorten recovery, with a TOF ratio of 70% being achieved within 11.6 minutes.[114] This feature may be beneficial with surgical procedures of unpredictable duration or after a failed intubation.

At present, there is relatively limited experience with rapacuronium and few comparisons with established nondepolarizing agents, especially mivacurium and rocuronium. The relative safety of rapacuronium is also unknown and, although unusual for a steroid neuromuscular blocking drug, adverse events probably related to histamine release have been reported.[112,113] Moderate increases in heart rate ($\approx 20\%$) have also been observed after intubating doses of rapacuronium.

## What Alternatives Are Available for Neuromuscular Blocks?

Apart from the alternatives to tracheal intubation discussed above, the patient's trachea may also be intubated under deep anesthesia. This may be facilitated by intravenous or inhalational means. Clinically acceptable conditions may be obtained in most adult patients using combinations of propofol or etomidate with alfentanil,[115] or propofol with remifentanil[116] or sevoflurane.[117] Both propofol-alfentanil[118] and sevoflurane[119] are also effective in children, providing tracheal intubating conditions comparable to those achieved with succinylcholine.

## How Is Anesthetic Depth Monitored?

It has long been a "Holy Grail" of anesthesia to have a reliable method of preventing intraoperative awareness. Much interest has focused on the electroencephalogram (EEG), but previous measures have been hindered by differences in the EEG effects of various anesthetics, the mass of raw EEG data, and a lack of reproducibility with various processed parameters.

### Bispectral Index

The BSI was designed to generate a numeric value that could discriminate between the awake and unconscious states. Validation of the BSI has been difficult, given the absence of a gold standard for detecting awareness and the ethical unacceptability of designing studies with a high likelihood of awareness. Despite these limitations, there is reasonable evidence that most patients will be reliably unaware if the BSI is 60 or below,[46,120] although individual variability remains a possibility. A commercial BSI monitor (Aspect Medical) has been available for a few years.

### Titration

Because of the relative rarity of awareness and the high cost (initial purchase and dedicated disposables) of BSI, there has been considerable financial pressure to use BSI to reduce drug use and speed recovery. In the absence of a reliable anesthetic depth monitor, there has been a tendency to "err on the side of caution," with many patients being excessively anesthetized. By titrating anesthesia to BSI, it has been shown that it is possible to reduce anesthetic consumption, thus reducing costs and recovery times. For example, titrating propofol anesthesia to a BSI value of 45 to 60 (increased to 60-75 near the end of anesthesia) reduced propofol requirements and produced faster early recovery compared with clinical drug delivery.[121] Staff savings are likely from such improved recovery times, although mathematical modeling suggests savings of only $1.50 to $5 per patient, substantially less than the cost of the BSI-dedicated disposables.[122]

When inhalation anesthesia was adjusted to produce a BSI value of approximately 60 throughout, anesthetic consumption was cut by 31% to 38%, and awakening times were shortened by 20% to 50% compared with anesthesia delivery using standard clinical signs.[123] The "deeper" anesthesia produced by this standard approach was reflected in BSI values of approximately 42.[123] The BSI-titrated groups had an increased requirement for neuromuscular blocking drugs; this may have been due to less potentiation from reduced volatile anesthetic dose, but the possibility that it reflected increased movement, possibly indicating inadequate anesthesia, must be considered. The BSI does not appear to reliably predict intraoperative movement.[124] There seems to be a fundamental difference between using BSI as an additional precaution against awareness and using it to intentionally place patients right "on the line" that separates consciousness from wakefulness. Such an approach may be acceptable, but only if we can be *certain* that we know precisely where that line is. In the authors' opinion, the location of the line is not yet sufficiently defined to safely target such BSI values in the presence of neuromuscular block.

### Other Anesthesia Depth Monitors

Although most recent attention has been focused on BSI, there are other potential monitors of anesthetic depth. One promising approach is to use auditory evoked potentials to evaluate patient responses. To simplify the process, an auditory evoked potential index (AEPI) has been developed[125] to derive a single numeric value similar in concept to BSI. Preliminary studies have shown that the AEPI is more reliable than BSI at distinguishing the transition from consciousness to unconsciousness,[126] at least with propofol anesthesia. Further development (including independent validation) of the AEPI is clearly warranted.

Although sophisticated monitors may help to detect awareness, undetected wakefulness remains unlikely in the absence of neuromuscular block. Increased use of the LMA, which is well tolerated without neuromuscular block, may help in this respect.

## RECOVERY

### What Are the Different Stages of Recovery?

Recovery from anesthesia may conveniently be divided into three phases. Early recovery involves the initial awakening from anesthesia (emergence), restoration of protective reflexes, and a degree of hemodynamic stability. Early recovery traditionally occurs in the phase I recovery room or postoperative anesthesia care unit (PACU), where patients are intensively nursed and monitored. With modern, short-acting anesthetics, early recovery is increasingly occurring in the operating room, leading to the concept of fast-track recovery (discussed later). Intermediate recovery occurs in the phase II or step-down unit and continues until the patient can be safely discharged home. Treatment of pain or PONV may be required during the intermediate recovery period, while the wound may be checked and mobilization encouraged. Late recovery continues after discharge until the patient returns to his or her preoperative state. The duration of this phase varies, depending on the length and nature of the surgical procedure and also the age and preexisting condition of the patient. Pain, PONV, and other postoperative complications may still occur during the late recovery period, but these will have to be managed by the patient, his or her family physician, an emergency room, or by readmission. Follow-up of patients should aim to identify particular circumstances that are associated with high complication rates, so that practices may be altered to prevent or reduce their occurrence.

### First Stage of Recovery

The first stage of recovery occurs in the PACU, which should be equipped for full patient monitoring to national standards.[127] In ambulatory units affiliated with inpatient surgical services, a shared PACU facility may be the most efficient arrangement. Isolated or freestanding units will require their own PACU. Such a unit should still be capable of managing all major postoperative complications, although the frequency with which such interventions are required should be low. If the freestanding PACU is used solely for ambulatory surgery, the provision of emergency drugs and equipment may be inefficient because of the rare incidence of major complications. Provision for their management must, nevertheless, be in place. In contrast, a shared PACU facility may be more likely to keep ambulatory patients for an unnecessarily long time and inappropriately administer long-acting drugs (eg, morphine).

The PACU should ideally be situated close to the operating rooms. This may be less important in a shared facility, where an anesthesiologist may be allocated to the PACU but is more important for isolated units where the operative anesthesiologist may also have to manage postoperative complications.

As with inpatients, patients should be adequately transferred to the care of the PACU nursing staff. In particular, pre- and perioperative problems should be mentioned, and any necessary postoperative instructions should be conveyed. The patient's clinical condition and the nature of the surgical procedure will dictate the duration and intensity of monitoring in the PACU. Traditionally, oxygen is administered, but this may be unnecessary according to Gift and colleagues.[128] A series of 293 postoperative patients were randomized to receive oxygen supplementation by various methods, deep breathing exercises but no additional oxygen, or simple room air ventilation. There were no significant differences between the groups in either their admission $SpO_2$ values or in the incidence of oxygen desaturation during the subsequent recovery period. A total of 11 patients experienced oxygen desaturations <90%, all but one of whom already had $SpO_2$ values of 92% or less on admission.[128] Furthermore, admission $SpO_2$ predicted hypoxia in the PACU. Only 8 of 282 patients who

did not experience hypoxia had $SpO_2$ values of 92% or less on arrival to the PACU.[128] On the basis of this evidence, routine supplemental oxygen therapy would only appear to be justified if the $SpO_2$ value is 92% or less when the patient arrives. This relative rarity of postoperative hypoxemia after outpatient surgery is probably a consequence of short duration surgery, rapidly eliminated anesthetic drugs, and a period of high-flow oxygen therapy in the operating room at the end of the surgical procedure.

Traditionally, the PACU has been an ideal environment in which to manage the unconscious patient and to provide airway support. With improvements in ambulatory anesthesia techniques, patients are increasingly likely to be awake when they arrive in the PACU. The PACU also provides an ideal location in which to administer potent intravenous drugs to treat the patient's pain and PONV. Formal assessments of pain and PONV (eg, using visual analog or verbal rating scales) can help in this process.

### Second Stage of Recovery

During the second stage of recovery, the patient is prepared for leaving the ambulatory unit and taking over his or her own care. The patient is gradually mobilized; the use of reclining chairs, rather than beds, may assist in this process. Patients should not be too sleepy; pain and PONV must be controlled; cardiovascular stability must be maintained (including when standing); and the wound must remain problem-free. The motor and autonomic effects of any nerve block should also have worn off, especially in the case of central nerve blocks. During this recovery period, the patient may be given postoperative instructions concerning aftercare, return to normal activities, and any requirement for follow-up. Take-home medication may be supplied if prolonged pain is anticipated. The patient's escort should arrive, and home circumstances should be checked before the patient is discharged.

### *What Is Fast-Track Recovery?*

Because of MAC and the advent of the increasing use of shorter-acting sedative-hypnotics after general anesthesia, patients may already meet all of the PACU discharge criteria when they arrive. On this basis, it would seem logical for such patients to proceed directly to the phase II recovery or step-down unit, thus bypassing the PACU. This fast-track recovery process has several potential benefits (Table 70–7).

The fast-track approach may shorten the recovery process in several ways. First, less time will be lost in handovers and

**TABLE 70–7.** Potential Benefits of Fast-Track Recovery

Awake patients spared the potentially alarming "hi-tech" atmosphere of the PACU
Reduction in workload for PACU staff
Reduction in bureaucracy, paperwork, and logistic delays
Less congestion in the PACU; unit free for major cases
Less opportunity for inappropriate interventions (eg, long-acting opioid analgesia)
May shorten the entire recovery process
Freestanding units need smaller PACU facility
Savings in staff costs

PACU, postanesthetic care unit.

completion of paperwork. Second, pain is more likely to be treated with short-acting, minimally sedating drugs. Finally, there is some evidence that patients may stay a similar length of time in phase II recovery, irrespective of whether or not they have passed through the PACU. Discharge can, therefore, potentially be shortened by the amount of time typically spent in phase I, which is often 30 minutes or more.

Despite these benefits to the patient, the main force driving the use of fast-track recovery, as always, is financial. By requiring fewer PACU staff or by allowing staff to work shorter hours, savings in resources are likely. The magnitude of this savings is quite variable, however, and depends greatly on the nature of the staff contract (eg, part-time, hourly paid, salaried, with or without overtime), the size of the ambulatory population, and the percentage of patients eligible for fast-track recovery.[122] Savings are likely to be greatest with salaried staff and range from $5 to $20 per patient, although there may be no savings at all unless at least the equivalent of one whole job can be saved. In contrast, there will always be savings with staff who are paid on an hourly basis, but these savings are smaller—typically $1 to $5 per patient.[122]

The number of patients eligible for fast-track recovery varies but may increase as experience is gained with the technique. MAC inevitably facilitates fast-track recovery, while the choice of drug can influence the outcome of general anesthesia. For example, after gynecologic laparoscopy, 90% of the women receiving desflurane and 75% of those receiving sevoflurane were eligible for fast-track recovery compared with only 26% who received a continuous infusion of propofol.[76] New monitoring techniques, such as BSI monitoring, may help to hasten recovery,[123] thus facilitating fast-tracking.

Pain and PONV may be more common when the patient awakens from general anesthesia compared with MAC. Although these symptoms may be treated in the step-down unit, their optimum management may be easier (and faster) in the PACU. Because the modified Aldrete score does not consider pain or PONV, some patients may be inappropriately fast-tracked by this measure. A specific fast-track score (Table 70-8) has been devised[129] in the hope of improving the patient's experience by not rushing the patient through the system too quickly. Use of such a score reduces the proportion of fast-track eligible patients and increases the average time required to achieve fast-track eligibility but still shows a benefit of insoluble inhaled anesthetics over propofol.[130] As expected, the revised score appears to significantly reduce the number of patients who require intravenous analgesic or antiemetic medication in the step-down recovery unit.

### What Are the Criteria for Discharge From the Postanesthesia Care Unit?

Patients are usually discharged from the PACU when they are awake and oriented, able to maintain their own airway with a satisfactory breathing pattern and adequate oxygenation, are cardiovascularly stable, and acceptably warm. Any immediate problems, such as pain and PONV, should have been treated, whereas bleeding from the site of operation should be minimal.

### Scoring Systems

Although these various clinical judgments can be made by any competent PACU nurse, it is common to use simple

**TABLE 70–8.** Criteria for Fast-Tracking After Ambulatory Surgery With General Anesthesia

| | | Score |
|---|---|---|
| Level of consciousness | Awake and oriented | 2 |
| | Arousable with minimal stimulation | 1 |
| | Responsive only to tactile stimulation | 0 |
| Physical activity | Able to move all extremities on command | 2 |
| | Some weakness in movement of extremities | 1 |
| | Unable to voluntarily move extremities | 0 |
| Hemodynamic stability | BP ± 15% of baseline | 2 |
| | BP ± 30% of baseline | 1 |
| | BP ± 50% of baseline | 0 |
| Respiratory stability | Respiratory rate 10–20 breaths/min; able to breathe deeply | 2 |
| | Tachypnea with good cough | 1 |
| | Dyspneic with weak cough | 0 |
| Oxygen saturation status | Maintains value >90% on room air | 2 |
| | Needs supplemental oxygen to maintain saturation >90% | 1 |
| | Saturation <90% with supplemental oxygen | 0 |
| Postoperative pain assessment | No or mild discomfort | 2 |
| | Moderate-to-severe pain controlled with IV analgesics | 1 |
| | Persistent moderate-to-severe pain | 0 |
| Postoperative emetic symptoms | No or mild nausea with no active vomiting | 2 |
| | Transient vomiting or retching, controlled with IV antiemetics | 1 |
| | Persistent moderate-to-severe nausea and vomiting | 0 |

The total possible score is 14. Patients who score ≥12 (with no score <1 in any individual category) are eligible for fast-tracking.
BP, blood pressure; IV, intravenous.
From White PF, Song D. New criteria for fast-tracking after outpatient anesthesia: a comparison with the modified Aldrete's scoring system. *Anesth Analg.* 1999;88:1069.

scoring systems in order to standardize the process. Various scoring systems have been advocated. One of the first was proposed by Aldrete and Kroulik in 1970.[131] This simple score assigns points on the basis of activity, breathing, blood pressure, consciousness, and oxygenation. The latter parameter was assessed initially by color; however, with the advent of pulse oximetry, the scoring system was modified[132] and is still widely used in this revised form (Table 70-9).

Discharge criteria have traditionally been clinical. More sophisticated psychomotor tests have little practical benefit in routine care and are reserved for research purposes (where they are also often relatively unhelpful!). Again, discharge criteria are amenable to being incorporated into a scoring system, the most recent of which is the postanesthesia discharge scoring system (PADSS) developed in Toronto[133] (Table 70-10). This scoring system has been shown to predict discharge times that correlate well with traditional criteria.

### Voiding

Previously, patients were always required to be able to tolerate oral fluids and be able to pass urine before they were allowed home. Forcing oral fluids on unwilling patients does not appear to improve subsequent outcome after discharge,[134,135] and may actually increase the risk of PONV.[134] Waiting for the patient to pass urine may significantly delay discharge (especially if the patient has not had liquids) without modifying the occurrence of urinary retention at home.[136] Urinary retention may be more likely in patients with a spinal or epidural block (including caudals) or after inguinal, pelvic, or urologic surgery. In these patients who are at higher risk, it may be advisable to have them void before they are discharged. Alternatively, very specific instructions must be given to seek medical attention if voiding has not occurred within a given time scale.

## What Problems Can Be Expected During Recovery?

A variety of problems may be expected throughout the recovery period, but pain and PONV are the most common. The occurrence of these symptoms is variable, although both are predictable to some extent. For procedures expected to produce postoperative pain, prophylactic analgesia should be given during, or even before surgery. Pain relief should generally be multimodal, using NSAIDs, local anesthesia, and opioids if necessary. Similarly for patients and procedures at high risk of PONV, a "low-risk" anesthetic technique should be used and prophylactic antiemetics should be considered.

## POSTOPERATIVE NAUSEA AND VOMITING

### How Do Postoperative Nausea and Vomiting Affect Recovery?

The occurrence of PONV is unpleasant for patients, delays recovery, and increases cost. PONV is relatively common and, despite improvements in our understanding of its etiology and the availability of effective antiemetics, remains a significant problem in ambulatory anesthesia.[137] PONV is multifactorial,[138] and many of its causes remain outside the control of the anesthesiologist. Some of the more common causes of PONV are listed in Table 70–11.

As well as being unpleasant for the patient, PONV may be a significant cause of unanticipated hospital admissions.[3] PONV often delays recovery even if the patient is subsequently

**TABLE 70–9.** Modified Aldrete Recovery Score

| | | Score |
|---|---|---|
| Activity | Able to move four extremities voluntarily or on command | 2 |
| | Able to move two extremities voluntarily or on command | 1 |
| | Unable to move extremities voluntarily or on command | 0 |
| Respiration | Able to breathe deeply and cough freely | 2 |
| | Dyspnea or limited breathing | 1 |
| | Apneic | 0 |
| Circulation | BP ± 20% of preanesthetic level | 2 |
| | BP ± 20–49% of preanesthetic level | 1 |
| | BP ± 50% of preanesthetic level | 0 |
| Consciousness | Fully awake | 2 |
| | Arousable on calling | 1 |
| | Nonresponsive | 0 |
| Oxygenation | Able to maintain saturation >92% on room air | 2 |
| | Needs oxygen to maintain saturation >90% | 1 |
| | Saturation <90% even with oxygen | 0 |

The total possible score is 10. Patients who score ≥9 are fit for discharge from phase 1 recovery. BP, blood pressure.

From Aldrete JA. The post-anesthesia recovery score revisited [letter]. *J Clin Anesth.* 1995;7:89.

**TABLE 70–10.** Modified Postanesthesia Discharge Scoring System (PADSS)

| | | Score |
|---|---|---|
| Vital signs | *Vital signs must be stable and consistent with age and the preoperative baseline.* | |
| | BP and pulse within 20% of the preoperative baseline | 2 |
| | BP and pulse within 20–40% of the preoperative baseline | 1 |
| | BP and pulse >40% from the preoperative baseline | 0 |
| Activity level | *The patient must be able to ambulate at the preoperative level* | |
| | Steady gait, no dizziness (or meets the preoperative level) | 2 |
| | Requires assistance | 1 |
| | Unable to ambulate | 0 |
| Nausea and vomiting | *The patient should have minimal nausea and vomiting before discharge.* | |
| | Minimal: treated successfully with oral medication | 2 |
| | Moderate: treated successfully with intramuscular medication | 1 |
| | Severe: continues after repeated treatment | 0 |
| Pain | *The patient should have minimal or no pain before discharge.* | |
| | *The level of pain that the patient has should be acceptable to the patient.* | |
| | *Pain should be controllable by oral analgesics.* | |
| | *The location, type, and intensity of pain should be consistent with anticipated postoperative discomfort.* | |
| | Acceptability: yes | 2 |
| | no | 0 |
| Surgical bleeding | *Postoperative bleeding should be consistent with the expected blood loss for the procedure.* | |
| | Minimal: does not require dressing change | 2 |
| | Moderate: up to two dressing changes required | 1 |
| | Severe: more than three dressing changes required | 0 |

The total possible score is 10. Patients who score ≥9 are fit for discharge. BP, blood pressure.

From Marshall S, Chung F. Assessment of "home readiness": discharge criteria and postdischarge complications. *Curr Opin Anesthesiol.* 1997;10:445–450.

discharged, and this delay, combined with the treatment of PONV, is expensive.

The incidence of PONV varies. A substantial proportion of cases do not start until after the patient has been discharged home.[139] The true incidence of PONV may, therefore, be missed and the benefit of preventative measures overestimated if patients are not adequately monitored after discharge.

### What Anesthetic Factors Influence the Incidence of Postoperative Nausea and Vomiting?

Various anesthetic factors may influence the incidence of PONV. Differences appear to exist between the inhaled anesthetics, with desflurane producing more PONV than isoflurane,[75] which in turn produces more nausea than does sevoflurane.[77] Use of sevoflurane for induction and maintenance appears to produce more PONV than when it is used solely for maintenance.[70] $N_2O$ has long been suspected of increasing the incidence of PONV. Meta-analysis of many smaller studies has demonstrated a small increase in vomiting associated with

**TABLE 70–11.** Common Risk Factors for Postoperative Nausea and Vomiting

| Patient factors | Female gender |
|---|---|
| | Nonsmoker |
| | Young age (18–45 years) |
| | Premenstrual |
| | Previous history of PONV |
| | Previous history of motion sickness |
| Surgical factors | Laparoscopy |
| | Other gynecologic procedures |
| | Strabismus surgery |
| | Breast operations |
| | Otolaryngology |
| | Long procedures |
| Anesthetic factors | Opioid analgesics |
| | Etomidate (lipid formulation may be better) |
| | Ketamine |
| | Nitrous oxide |

PONV, postoperative nausea and vomiting.

$N_2O$, but the benefit from its omission is relatively small and probably of little clinical significance.[140] Amongst the intravenous anesthetics, etomidate and ketamine are associated with the highest rates of PONV.

## Propofol

Propofol, as an induction or maintenance agent, is generally associated with lower rates of PONV compared with alternative techniques. Propofol anesthesia can produce a substantial reduction in early PONV.[68] Propofol is a short-acting drug, however, and PONV may recur at a later stage. The number of cases of PONV that can be totally prevented by propofol anesthesia is probably clinically insignificant.[140] Nevertheless, most practitioners would include propofol anesthesia as part of their technique for managing patients at especially high risk for PONV.

## Opioids and Other Drugs

The opioid analgesics are potent causes of PONV. Long-acting drugs, such as morphine, are generally worse than shorter-acting ones like fentanyl.[141] Nevertheless, even modest doses of fentanyl can significantly increase the incidence of PONV associated with either propofol[82] or volatile-based anesthesia.[81]

Some studies have shown that reversal of residual neuromuscular block with neostigmine increases PONV, although this finding is inconsistent. There is probably a very weak benefit from omitting neostigmine, although this must be balanced against the greater risk of residual paralysis.[107] Limiting the use of neuromuscular blocking drugs or using ones which degrade spontaneously is the safest approach.

## What Type of Antiemetic Therapy Is Used for Postoperative Nausea and Vomiting?

Because PONV is common and cannot always be avoided, antiemetic drugs are important. Various antiemetic drugs are available, ranging from anticholinergics and antihistamines to dopamine antagonists, phenothiazine derivatives, and selective antagonists of the 5-hydroxytryptamine type 3 (5-HT$_3$) receptor. The anticholinergic and antihistamine drugs generally have limited efficacy, although they may be more useful in patients with a history of motion sickness. They often cause sedation, which is an undesirable side effect. Metoclopramide is a central dopamine receptor antagonist that is often used as an antiemetic. Unfortunately, metoclopramide is really no more effective than a placebo, which renders it a very cost-ineffective choice despite its low price.[142]

## Droperidol

Droperidol, like the phenothiazines, produces a wide range of effects, although most of its antiemetic activity probably occurs through antagonism at the dopamine receptor level. Droperidol is an effective antiemetic but is associated with frequent side effects, including dizziness, fatigue, sedation, and psychometric effects. Although these effects are more likely at higher doses ($\geq 1$ mg), distressing effects such as akathisia (or restlessness) may occur even with doses of 0.5 mg.[143] Such late symptoms are easily missed because their relation to treatment is often not realized by patients unless specifically questioned, and thus a degree of underreporting is likely. Nevertheless, droperidol is a widely used and cost-effective antiemetic.[144]

## Ondansetron

Selective antagonists of the 5-HT$_3$ receptor were developed to treat emesis resulting from chemotherapy and radiotherapy but are also effective against PONV. Ondansetron was the first of these drugs, but several others (eg, dolasetron, granisetron, tropisetron) have been developed since then. Ondansetron appeared initially to be much more effective than conventional treatments and to be almost devoid of side effects. Although ondansetron does not produce extrapyramidal side effects, headaches and elevated liver enzymes are sometimes seen.

The apparently greater efficacy of ondansetron was partly due to the large number of early trials comparing it with a placebo (or occasionally metoclopramide). Early evaluation of these trials concluded that ondansetron was more effective than droperidol, but its cost rendered it less cost-effective.[144]

A more recent meta-analysis concluded that when PONV was very likely (60%-80% without treatment), 8 mg of ondansetron would prevent vomiting in one of every five patients treated.[145] Three out of every hundred patients treated would develop raised liver enzymes, and a further three would develop a headache. At the more commonly used dose of 4 mg, ondansetron was still effective, although six patients would have to be treated to prevent one case of vomiting compared with five patients at the 8-mg dose.

More recently, ondansetron was compared with low doses of droperidol (0.625 and 1.25 mg) in a large study in high-risk patients. Ondansetron fared no better than did either droperidol dose in achieving a "complete response" (no emesis or antiemetic therapy in 24 hours), whereas 1.25 mg of droperidol was more effective than 4 mg of ondansetron or droperidol, 0.625 mg, in completely preventing nausea.[146]

## Other 5-HT$_3$ Antagonists

Many other 5-HT$_3$ antagonists have now been developed for cancer-induced sickness, and several have been used to treat PONV. As with the early ondansetron studies, most comparisons have been against placebo, a total waste of time given the known efficacy of this drug class. There are few comparative trials with ondansetron, but extrapolation of the placebo work suggests that they will not be significantly better.[147] It is possible that there will be small differences in side effects and most likely large differences in cost.

### How Does the Clinician Decide on Treatment Versus Prophylaxis?

When the likelihood of PONV is high, it is more humane (and often more cost-effective) to give antiemetics prophylactically to prevent symptoms. Because no prophylactic antiemetic is completely effective, some patients will, however, still experience PONV. Others will experience side effects of the antiemetics. Some patients may experience these side effects instead of PONV; others who would not have experienced sickness are exposed to adverse events, whereas some patients may experience both PONV and antiemetic side effects! The balance of desirable and undesirable effects of prophylaxis varies, depending on the drug chosen and the underlying risk of PONV. When the risks of PONV are low, the use of prophylaxis will mainly increase costs and side effects.

Irrespective of whether or not prophylaxis is used, the anesthetic technique should avoid as many potential causes of PONV as possible. When PONV does occur, it should be treated effectively. Some cases of early vomiting may be self-limiting but where symptoms persist, they should be treated promptly. The choice of treatment drug is similar to that used for prevention, although an agent in a different therapeutic class should be used if prophylaxis has failed. The treatment of established PONV appears to be just as effective as its prevention.

### What Other Measures Can Be Taken to Reduce Postoperative Nausea and Vomiting?

As with analgesia, a multimodal approach to antiemesis may be more effective than single drug therapy. For example, combinations of ondansetron with droperidol[148] or steroids[149] are more effective than ondansetron on its own. Steroids may be a useful additional form of antiemetic therapy, because they also appear to reduce postoperative pain.[150]

Simple measures such as adequate intraoperative hydration with 20 mL/kg clear fluid can significantly reduce postoperative nausea during the first 24 hours, with the additional bonus that postoperative drowsiness and dizziness are also improved.[151]

The future will no doubt see further 5-HT$_3$ receptor antagonists, but novel antiemetics may also be developed. Antagonists of the neurokinin$_1$ (NK$_1$) receptor appear to be antiemetics, and prototype drugs are undergoing early trials. While better than placebo, like other antiemetics, they do not prevent PONV. Whether NK$_1$ antagonists will be more effective in combination remains to be seen although, like steroids, these drugs also have analgesic properties.

## PAIN MANAGEMENT

Pain can be expected after every operation, but its incidence and severity vary depending on several factors. Young male patients of ASA class 1 appear to be especially likely to experience severe pain, although this may be a consequence of the type of surgeries that this age group experiences.[18] Severe pain is more likely to occur after certain types of surgery (Table 70–12), as well as after longer operations. Overweight patients are also more likely to experience severe pain, perhaps as a result of relative underdosing with analgesics.[18]

Opioid analgesics are the traditional mainstay of pain management. In the ambulatory setting, these drugs have serious drawbacks (eg, sedation and PONV). Although the degree of sedation produced by modern synthetic opioids seems less than that of older drugs such as morphine, all opioids appear equally likely to produce PONV. Alternatives to opioid analgesics are, therefore, highly desirable to prevent opioid side effects. As more extensive surgery is performed on an ambulatory basis, nonopioid analgesics alone may be insufficient to treat postoperative pain, especially in the early stages. It is, nevertheless, important to use these other drugs as part of a balanced approach to reduce opioid doses.

When opioid analgesics are required, the dose should be titrated to effect to ensure that the lowest dose possible is used. Logic suggests that this process would be easier using drugs with a rapid onset of action (eg, fentanyl rather than morphine). In practice, equipotent doses of fentanyl and morphine were similarly effective and equally rapid in treating postoperative pain.[141] The shorter duration of action of fentanyl resulted in more patients requiring further analgesia later in the recovery process, whereas morphine was associated with an increased incidence of PONV after the patient was discharged.[141]

### What Role Do Nonopioid Analgesics Play in Pain Management?

Various analgesics, such as local anesthetic drugs, NSAIDs, simple analgesics, and tramadol, can be used alone or in combination to reduce or eliminate the use of opioids.

**TABLE 70–12.** Surgical Specialties and Operations Associated With Relatively High or Relatively Low Incidence and Intensity of Pain*

| Surgical Specialty | Pain Likely | Pain Unlikely |
|---|---|---|
| Orthopedic | Shoulder operations | Knee arthroscopy |
| | Removal of hardware | Carpal tunnel |
| | Elbow endoscopy | |
| Urology | Orchiectomy | Cystoscopy |
| | Hydrocele repair | |
| | Circumcision | |
| General Surgery | Hernia repair | Breast biopsy |
| | Varicose vein stripping | |
| Plastic Surgery | Liposuction | Facial surgery |
| | Breast augmentation | |
| Gynecology | Laparoscopic sterilization | Dilation and curettage |
| | Diagnostic laparoscopy | Termination of pregnancy |
| Ophthalmology | Cryopexy | Most other procedures |

*Specialties are listed in order of pain likelihood. Within specialties, more painful procedures are listed first.

Data from Chung F, Ritchie E, Su J. Postoperative pain in ambulatory surgery. *Anesth Analg.* 1997;85:808–816.

## Local Anesthetics

Aside from their use for intraoperative analgesia, local anesthetics are important for postoperative analgesia. Various techniques are appropriate, ranging from regional nerve block to simple wound infiltration or topical application. Applying local anesthesia at the start of the operation will usually produce an anesthetic-sparing effect, although application after surgery appears to provide just as effective postoperative analgesia. The latter approach will definitely not mask tissue planes, distort the anatomy, or spread infection or cancer cells, all of which are objections surgeons sometimes raise to preincisional local anesthetic injection.

There is increasing evidence that simple local anesthetic techniques are as effective as more complex ones. For example, after circumcision in children, pain relief is often provided with a caudal epidural block. This is a relatively simple technique, although it has a small failure rate and occasionally causes urinary retention and leg weakness. Block of the dorsal nerve of the penis has been shown to provide comparable analgesia, without the delay in micturition and ambulation associated with caudal analgesia.[152] Simple topical application of lidocaine jelly is even more simple and less invasive and yet provides equally effective analgesia to a dorsal nerve block.[153] Furthermore, topical anesthesia can be reapplied later for prolonged pain relief, which is a distinct advantage over more invasive blocks.

Similarly, for inguinal hernia repair simple wound infiltration provides as effective analgesia as a more invasive nerve block.[154] For wound infiltration to be effective, however, the local anesthetic probably has to be instilled at least at the subfascial layer.[155] The greatest disadvantage of local anesthetic wound infiltration is that it provides relatively short-lasting analgesia, although this feature is common to all local anesthetic techniques. Nevertheless, local anesthesia provides a useful degree of analgesia in the early postoperative period.

Regional techniques such as caudal blocks may still be useful for bilateral operations or procedures in which the size of the wounds in children would risk exceeding the toxic dose with infiltration anesthesia.

## Nonsteroidal Antiinflammatory Drugs

These drugs are very effective in acute pain[156] and are important in the management of ambulatory patients. There are a wide variety of NSAIDs. These differ considerably in their potency (dose required for a given effect), but there is no evidence that their efficacy differs significantly if an adequate dose is used. Increased potency is not invariably associated with reduced side effects; indeed, the most potent NSAID (ketorolac) also has one of the least favorable side effect profiles.[157] The older drugs, ibuprofen and diclofenac, are among the safest. NSAIDs may be given by various routes, but the oral route is as effective as any and is simple and cheap.[158] There is no particular advantage to the intravenous route in most ambulatory patients.

The NSAIDs work through enzyme inhibition and, therefore, take some time to achieve an analgesic effect (even when given intravenously). Adequate postoperative analgesia is best ensured by preoperative administration. This is most conveniently achieved via the oral route compared with intravenous or rectal administration. Oral NSAIDs are well tolerated, even in fasted patients, and the drug will have been eliminated from the stomach within 1 hour. Sustained release preparations reduce the gastric side effects further, while conferring the additional advantage of prolonged (up to 24 hours) analgesia. When oral administration is impossible (or forgotten), rectal or intravenous administration are viable alternatives, although only a few NSAIDs are available in suitable preparations. Intramuscular administration is best avoided; it is painful and may cause sterile abscesses.

Ketorolac, in particular, has been associated with several reports of serious adverse events. These may be partially related to the drug itself, to the use of too high a dose (the recommended dose has been reduced to 10 mg in many countries), or to indiscriminate use.[156] Despite these effects, most NSAIDs are generally well tolerated. Gastric side effects may occur, but these are uncommon unless administration is continued for more than a few days. Platelet function may be impaired, thus increasing bleeding, although rarely to a clinically significant degree. Renal function may be impaired with high doses; this is a greater problem in the elderly, in combination with other nephrotoxic drugs or when renal function is already compromised. NSAIDs can exacerbate asthma, and at least one such death has been reported.[159] It is estimated that up to 10% of asthmatics are at risk[160] for exacerbation of asthmatic symptoms, but the effect is usually mild. Because NSAIDs are so widely available, most asthmatics will have taken them previously and will be able to provide a negative history of significant exacerbation of airflow obstruction. In the absence of such reassurance, NSAIDs are best avoided in severe asthmatics, in asthmatics with nasal polyps (often associated with aspirin sensitivity), or during an acute exacerbation of asthma.[160] In most patients, the benefits of NSAIDs considerably outweigh their disadvantages. NSAIDs are also very safe and effective in children.

### Selective COX-2 Inhibitors

Cyclooxygenase is now known to exist in two forms.[161] Type 1 is widely present throughout the body and has a predominantly protective role. In particular, it is associated with gastric mucosal integrity and platelet aggregation. The type 2 enzyme is inducible and is primarily associated with inflammation, although it is also found at various other sites, including the juxtaglomerular apparatus of the kidney.[161]

Selective inhibitors of cyclooxygenase type 2 (COX-2) are now available. These drugs (eg, celecoxib, rofecoxib) offer the potential for NSAID analgesia with reduced side effects. They are currently licensed for various forms of arthritis, where they appear to be effective. Gastritis and ulceration are reduced (but not eliminated), and there is no alteration in the bleeding time. Rofecoxib (but not celecoxib) is also licensed for acute pain in adults. These selective COX-2 inhibitors are being evaluated for postoperative pain, but the data are currently limited. Whether these drugs will have an important role in ambulatory anesthesia is currently unknown. Brief use of nonselective NSAIDs is generally well tolerated, except in patients with severe preexisting gastric symptoms. Although an increase in perioperative bleeding is detectable, this is rarely of clinical significance. The selective COX-2 inhibitors may be beneficial in patients at particularly high risk for these problems or in whom even moderately increased bleeding would be dangerous.

It is currently unknown whether selective COX-2 inhibitors will be less inclined to exacerbate severe asthma, but this is unlikely. The potential for renal dysfunction is also unknown but may actually be increased as COX-2 plays a part in renal homeostasis.[161] Finally, it is believed, but by no means proven, that these new drugs will be as effective as other NSAIDs. Nonselective NSAIDs are generally believed to exert their analgesic effect through COX-2 inhibition, yet some effective agents have only minimal COX-2 activity.[161] Inhibition of COX-1 must therefore play some part in acute analgesia. The selective COX-2 inhibitors cost considerably more than their predecessors and are, therefore, unlikely to be used routinely unless a clear advantage can be demonstrated.

## Alternatives to Nonsteroidal Antiinflammatory Drugs

Although NSAIDs are generally safe, they may be best avoided in some patents. Acetaminophen may be an adequate alternative for mild pain but will be inadequate after more major procedures. Codeine, either alone or combined with acetaminophen, is often effective but may increase the incidence of PONV.

### Tramadol

Tramadol is available in several countries. It is an opioid but also produces analgesia by interference with central monoamine pathways. This dual mode of action can provide opioid-like analgesia but with fewer adverse effects, especially respiratory depression. The efficacy of tramadol varies and it may be more useful when pain is moderate rather than severe.[162] Few comparisons between tramadol and NSAIDs have been published, yet the NSAIDs are known to be valuable analgesics for moderate pain. In addition, tramadol does have opioid actions and is thus still associated with significant PONV.[163]

### What Is Multimodal Analgesia?

For most patients, pain relief is inadequate or too short lasting with a single treatment. More effective pain relief may be provided using a multimodal or "balanced" approach.[164] For some patients, this may involve the combination of local anesthetic block or infiltration and an NSAID, but for many others it will also include opioid analgesics. For example, after laparoscopic cholecystectomy, multimodal analgesia with opioid, NSAID, and local anesthesia significantly reduced the incidence and intensity of pain, reduced PONV, and facilitated earlier ambulation and discharge compared with providing no prophylactic analgesia.[165]

Multimodal analgesia may also use other adjuvants as well as different routes of administration. The addition of a single dose of glucocorticoid (eg, betamethasone, 12 mg) after ambulatory surgery may reduce both PONV and postoperative pain.[150] In some cases of chronic inflammation, opioid receptors may be expressed in the periphery. This may explain the variable success of intraarticular morphine in relieving pain after some arthroscopic procedures.[164] There is currently some controversy over whether or not NSAIDs are more effective when administered to the peripheral site of injury. At present, the evidence suggests there is, at best, a very weak effect.

## UNANTICIPATED ADMISSION, READMISSION, AND FOLLOW-UP

The overall rate of unanticipated hospital admission is approximately 1%,[3,136,166] although this figure is likely to rise with more complex procedures being performed. The most common causes of admission, pain and bleeding, are related to the surgical procedure[3,166] although PONV is another significant cause.

After discharge, at least 3% of patients return to[142] or contact[167] the ambulatory surgical unit. About half of these cases are caused by complications; surgical problems such as rebleeding are common.[142] A slightly higher proportion of patients contact their family physician or community nurse,[167] often because of inadequate pain control.

In order to detect potential problems and to improve patient satisfaction, it is desirable to contact patients after their discharge. This type of follow-up can usually be made by telephone. The timing of the call may have to vary with the type of operation. Calling too early may miss numerous late complications,[9] whereas a late call will miss patients who have returned to work. After some procedures, patients may experience distressing symptoms for up to 1 week.[4] Follow-up calls may help detect a trend of certain surgical procedures that are especially associated with postoperative problems,[142] which may modify management of these cases in the future. Simple measures such as providing effective take-home analgesia for procedures associated with significant or prolonged postoperative pain may be beneficial. Detecting late complications is important, because patient dissatisfaction increases with adverse postoperative symptoms.[168,169]

## OFFICE-BASED ANESTHESIA

Despite the fact that office-based anesthesia has gained widespread popularity in the United States in the past few years, it is not a new endeavor. Ralph Waters, MD, an anesthesiologist in Sioux City, Iowa, opened an office-based anesthesia practice for dental surgery in 1915.[170] Office-based surgery continued to grow slowly over the years, but during the 1990s, economic considerations made it the fastest growing locus of surgery (see Fig. 70–1). In 1994, approximately 8.5% of all surgical procedures were performed in the office, and this number was expected to have increased to 14% by 2001.[171]

### Are the Standards of Care Different in an Office-Based Practice?

Office-based anesthesia is a form of outpatient anesthesia and, thus, most of the patient care and anesthetic principles discussed earlier in this chapter apply. At the present time, the majority of operations performed in an office setting are self-pay plastic surgery (70%) and dental procedures, although gynecology, podiatry, ophthalmology, orthopedic, and dermatology procedures are also common.[172] Anesthesia is administered by various providers in the office setting. Surgeons and surgical assistants often administer intravenous sedation themselves,[173] but most office anesthetics in the United States are probably provided by nurse anesthetists under the direction of the attending surgeon or functioning as solo practitioners. The quality of care should be the same whether the anesthetic is performed in a hospital or office setting, and the ASA's Standards for Basic Anesthetic Monitoring and Guidelines for Ambulatory Anesthesia and Surgery should be followed.[174,175] At a minimum, these standards state the following: (1) qualified anesthesia personnel should be present in the room throughout the conduct of all general anesthetics, regional anesthetics, and monitored care procedures; and (2) a patient's oxygenation, ventilation, circulation, and temperature should be continuously evaluated during all anesthetics.[175] However, there is evidence that monitoring standards are substandard in some office practices. A review of monitoring practices by surgeons during aesthetic surgery revealed that 5% of respondents did not measure blood pressure, 7% failed to use pulse oximetry, and 11% did not monitor with an ECG.[173]

## What Is the Mortality Rate in Office-Based Surgery?

Concern over the safety of office-based surgery exists, and a recent report indicates that the mortality rate for some surgical procedures may be exorbitantly high when performed in the office. The overall mortality rate for surgery performed in accredited plastic surgery offices is reported to be 1:57 000.[176] However, the mortality rate after liposuction procedures performed by board-certified plastic surgeons was found to be approximately 1:5000 with most of these deaths occurring the first night after discharge home.[177] These findings have focused media attention on the safety of office-based surgery and will, no doubt, lead to increased government regulation of office procedures in the future.

## CONCLUSION

There is little doubt that moving increasingly complex procedures and less healthy patients from inpatient to ambulatory facilities or offices has shifted much of the cost from hospital and insurance company to the patient and the community.[4] Although this situation is unlikely to be reversed in the near future, good follow-up provides support and reassurance to patients and their caregivers. As even more extensive procedures are contemplated, the provision of some form of postoperative care will become necessary. Patients who stay overnight in hospital after their operation but are discharged within 24 hours (the 23-hour admit) are already classified as "ambulatory" in many centers. Other forms of postoperative care, including hotellike recovery services, may be able to provide some supportive assistance at lower cost than that of full nursing care. Nursing procedures may also be carried out in the community, but the cost of such care may be greater than that of inpatient care if many visits are required.

The future will undoubtedly see further expansion of ambulatory and office-based surgery, but further developments must evaluate the quality and safety of care in these facilities. Increased standards and regulations may also be necessary to prevent outpatient surgery from becoming too aggressive or overambitious.

### References

1. Chung F, Mezei G, Tong D. Pre-existing medical conditions as predictors of adverse events in day-case surgery. *Br J Anaesth.* 1999;83:262.

2. Fortier J, Chung F, Su J. Unanticipated admission after ambulatory surgery: a prospective study. *Can J Anaesth.* 1998;45:612.

3. Gold BS, Kitz DS, Lecky JH, et al. Unanticipated admission to the hospital following ambulatory surgery. *JAMA.* 1989;262:3008.

4. Swan BA, Maislin G, Traber KB. Symptom distress and functional status changes during the first seven days after ambulatory surgery. *Anesth Analg.* 1998;86:739.

5. Malviya S, Swartz J, Lerman J. Are all preterm infants younger than 60 weeks postconceptual age at risk for postanesthetic apnea? *Anesthesiology.* 1993;78:1076.

6. Welborn LG, Ramirez N, Oh TH, et al. Postanesthetic apnea and periodic breathing in infants. *Anesthesiology.* 1986;65:658.

7. Duncan PG, Cohen MM, Tweed WA, et al. The Canadian four-centre study of anaesthetic outcomes, III: are anaesthetic complications predictable in day surgical practice? *Can J Anaesth.* 1992;39:440.

8. Federated Ambulatory Surgery Association. Special Study 1 FASA, Alexandria, Va: FASA; 1986.

9. Warner MA, Shields SE, Chute CG. Major morbidity and mortality within 1 month of ambulatory surgery and anesthesia. *JAMA.* 1993;270:1437.

10. Eagle KA, Brundage BH, Chaitman BR, et al. Guidelines for perioperative cardiovascular evaluation for noncardiac surgery. Report of the American College of Cardiology/American Heart Association Task Force on Practice Guidelines. Committee on Perioperative Cardiovascular Evaluation for Noncardiac Surgery. *Circulation.* 1996;93:1278.

11. Fletcher GF, Balady G, Froelicher VF, et al. Exercise standards. A statement for health care professionals from the American Heart Association. Writing Group. *Circulation.* 1995;91:580.

12. Howell SJ, Hemming AE, Allman KG, et al. Predictors of postoperative myocardial ischaemia. The role of intercurrent arterial hypertension and other cardiovascular risk factors. *Anaesthesia.* 1997;52:107.

13. Glen SK, Elliott HL, Curzio JL, et al. White-coat hypertension as a cause of cardiovascular dysfunction. *Lancet.* 1996;348:654.

14. Jacoby DB, Hirshman CA. General anesthesia in patients with viral respiratory infections: an unsound sleep? *Anesthesiology.* 1991;74:969.

15. Fennelly ME, Hall GM. Anaesthesia and upper respiratory tract infection: a non-existent hazard? [editorial]. *Br J Anaesth.* 1990;64:535.

16. Tait AR, Pandit UA, Voepel-Lewis T, et al. Use of the laryngeal mask airway in children with upper respiratory tract infections: a comparison with endotracheal intubation. *Anesth Analg.* 1998;86:706.

17. Rose DK, Cohen MM, Wigglesworth DF, et al. Critical respiratory events in the postanesthesia care unit: patient, surgical, and anesthetic factors. *Anesthesiology.* 1994;81:410.

18. Chung F, Ritchie E, Su J. Postoperative pain in ambulatory surgery. *Anesth Analg.* 1997;85:808.

19. Illing L, Duncan PG, Yip R. Gastroesophageal reflux during anesthesia. *Can J Anaesth.* 1992;39:466.

20. Pollard JB, Zboray AL, Mazze RI. Economic benefits attributed to opening a preoperative evaluation clinic for outpatients. *Anesth Analg.* 1996;83:407.

21. Kitts JB. The preoperative assessment: who is responsible? *Can J Anaesth.* 1997;44:1232.

22. Patel RI, Hannallah RS. Preoperative screening for pediatric ambulatory surgery: evaluation of a telephone questionnaire method. *Anesth Analg.* 1992;75:258.

23. Claxton AR, Lindsay SA, Watts JC, et al. Ambulatory anesthesia practices in the United Kingdom. *Semin Anesth.* 1997;16:178.

24. Golub R, Cantu R, Sorrento JJ, et al. Efficacy of preadmission testing in ambulatory surgical patients. *Am J Surg.* 1992;163:565.

25. Kaplan EB, Sheiner LB, Boeckmann AJ, et al. The usefulness of preoperative laboratory screening. *JAMA.* 1985;253:3576.

26. Hackmann T, Steward DJ, Sheps SB. Anemia in pediatric day-surgery patients: prevalence and detection. *Anesthesiology.* 1991;75:27.

27. Callaghan LC, Edwards ND, Reilly CS. Utilisation of the pre-operative ECG. *Anaesthesia.* 1995;50:488.

28. Maltby JR, Sutherland AD, Sale JP, et al. Preoperative oral fluids: Is a five-hour fast justified prior to elective surgery? *Anesth Analg.* 1986;65:1112.

29. American Society of Anesthesiologists Task Force on Preoperative Fasting. Practice guidelines for preoperative fasting and the use of pharmacologic agents to reduce the risk of pulmonary aspiration: application to healthy patients undergoing elective procedures. *Anesthesiology.* 1999;90:896.

30. Klafta JM, Roizen MF. Current understanding of patients' attitudes toward and preparation for anesthesia: a review. *Anesth Analg.* 1996;83:1314.

31. Leigh JM, Walker J, Janaganathan P. Effect of preoperative anaesthetic visit on anxiety. *BMJ.* 1977;2:987.

32. Turner GA, Paech M. A comparison of oral midazolam solution with temazepam as a day case premedicant. *Anaesth Intensive Care.* 1991;19:365.

33. Feld LH, Negus JB, White PF. Oral midazolam preanesthetic medication in pediatric outpatients. *Anesthesiology.* 1990;73:831.

34. Wilton NCT, Leigh J, Rosen DR, et al. Preanesthetic sedation of preschool children using intranasal midazolam. *Anesthesiology.* 1988;69:972.

35. Ashburn MA, Streisand JB, Tarver SD, et al. Oral transmucosal fentanyl citrate for premedication in paediatric outpatients. *Can J Anaesth.* 1990;37:857.

36. Feld LH, Champeau MW, Van Steennis CA, et al. Preanesthetic medication in children: a comparison of oral transmucosal fentanyl citrate versus placebo. *Anesthesiology.* 1989;71:374.

37. Kallar SK, Everett LL. Potential risks and preventive measures for pulmonary aspiration: new concepts in preoperative fasting guidelines. *Anesth Analg.* 1993;77:171.

38. Warner MA, Warner ME, Weber JG. Clinical significance of pulmonary aspiration during the perioperative period. *Anesthesiology.* 1993;78:56.

39. Denny NM, Selander DE. Continuous spinal anaesthesia [review]. *Br J Anaesth.* 1998;81:590.

40. Ben-David B, Levin H, Solomon E, et al. Spinal bupivacaine in ambulatory surgery: the effect of saline dilution. *Anesth Analg.* 1996;83:716.

41. Ben-David B, Solomon E, Levin H, et al. Intrathecal fentanyl with small-dose dilute bupivacaine: better anesthesia without prolonging recovery. *Anesth Analg.* 1997;85:560.

42. Tarkkila P, Huhtala J, Tuominen M. Home-readiness after spinal anaesthesia with small doses of hyperbaric 0.5% bupivacaine. *Anaesthesia.* 1997;52:1157.

43. Sá Rêgo MM, Watcha MF, White PF. The changing role of monitored anesthesia care in the ambulatory setting. *Anesth Analg.* 1997;85:1020.

44. Smith I. Monitored anesthesia care: how much sedation, how much analgesia? *J Clin Anesth.* 1996;8:76S.

45. American Society of Anesthesiologists. Standards for basic intraoperative monitoring. In: *ASA Directory of Members.* Park Ridge, Ill: American Society of Anesthesiologists; 1994:735.

46. Liu J, Singh H, White PF. Electroencephalographic bispectral index correlates with intraoperative recall and depth of propofol-induced sedation. *Anesth Analg.* 1997;84:185.

47. Truog RD, Waisel D. Amnesia instead of anesthesia: not always a question of consent. *J Clin Ethics.* 1994;5:153.

48. Philip BK. Hazards of amnesia after midazolam in ambulatory surgical patients [letter]. *Anesth Analg.* 1987;66:97.

49. White PF, Negus JB. Sedative infusions during local and regional anesthesia: a comparison of midazolam and propofol. *J Clin Anesth.* 1991;3:32.

50. Smith I, Monk TG, White PF, et al. Propofol infusion during regional anesthesia: sedative, amnestic and anxiolytic properties. *Anesth Analg.* 1994;79:313.

51. Wilson E, Mackenzie N, Grant IS. A comparison of propofol and midazolam by infusion to provide sedation in patients who receive spinal anaesthesia. *Anaesthesia.* 1988;43(suppl):91.

52. Fanard L, Van Steenberge A, Demeire X, et al. Comparison between propofol and midazolam as sedative agents for surgery under regional anaesthesia. *Anaesthesia.* 1988;43(suppl):87.

53. Taylor E, Ghouri AF, White PF. Midazolam in combination with propofol for sedation during local anesthesia. *J Clin Anesth.* 1992;4:213.

54. Monk TG, Bouré B, White PF, et al. Comparison of intravenous sedative-analgesic techniques for outpatient immersion lithotripsy. *Anesth Analg.* 1991;72:616.

55. Sherry E. Admixture of propofol and alfentanil: use for intravenous sedation and analgesia during transvaginal oocyte retrieval. *Anaesthesia.* 1992;47:477.

56. Bailey PL, Pace NL, Ashburn MA, et al. Frequent hypoxemia and apnea after sedation with midazolam and fentanyl. *Anesthesiology.* 1990;73:826.

57. Avramov M, Smith I, White PF. Interactions between midazolam and remifentanil during monitored anesthesia care. *Anesthesiology.* 1996;85:1283.

58. Sá Rêgo MM, Inagaki Y, White PF. Remifentanil administration during monitored anesthesia care: are intermittent boluses an effective alternative to a continuous infusion? *Anesth Analg.* 1999;88:518.

59. Hartmann T, Hoerauf K, Zavrski A, et al. Light to moderate sedation with sevoflurane during spinal anesthesia. *Acta Anaesthesiol Scand.* 1998;42(suppl 112):221.

60. Tang J, Wang B, White PF, et al. Comparison of the sedation and recovery profiles of Ro 48-6791, a new benzodiazepine, and midazolam in combination with meperidine for outpatient endoscopic procedures. *Anesth Analg.* 1999;89:893.

61. Rudkin GE, Osborne GA, Curtis NJ. Intra-operative patient-controlled sedation. *Anaesthesia.* 1991;46:90.

62. Osborne GA, Rudkin GE, Curtis NJ, et al. Intra-operative patient-controlled sedation: comparison of patient-controlled propofol with anaesthetist-administered midazolam and fentanyl. *Anaesthesia.* 1991;46:553.

63. Ghouri AF, Taylor E, White PF. Patient-controlled drug administration during local anesthesia: a comparison of midazolam, propofol, and alfentanil. *J Clin Anesth.* 1992;4:476.

64. Irwin MG, Thompson N, Kenny GNC. Patient-maintained propofol sedation. Assessment of a target-controlled infusion system. *Anaesthesia.* 1997;52:525.

65. Smith I, White PF, Nathanson M, et al. Propofol: an update on its clinical use. *Anesthesiology.* 1994;81:1005.

66. Russell D, Wilkes MP, Hunter SC, et al. Manual compared with target-controlled infusion of propofol. *Br J Anaesth.* 1995;75:562.

67. Smith I, Thwaites AJ. Target-controlled propofol *vs.* sevoflurane: A double-blind, randomised comparison in day-case anaesthesia. *Anaesthesia.* 1999;54:745.

68. Tramèr M, Moore A, McQuay H. Propofol anaesthesia and postoperative nausea and vomiting: quantitative systematic review of randomized controlled studies. *Br J Anaesth.* 1997;78:247.

69. Rowe WL. Economics and anaesthesia. *Anaesthesia.* 1998;53:782.

70. Smith I, Terhoeve PA, Hennart D, et al. A multicentre comparison of the costs of anaesthesia with sevoflurane or propofol. *Br J Anaesth.* 1999;83:564.

71. Boldt J, Jaun N, Kumle B, et al. Economic considerations of the use of new anesthetics: a comparison of propofol, sevoflurane, desflurane, and isoflurane. *Anesth Analg.* 1998;86:504.

72. Ashworth J, Smith I. Comparison of desflurane with isoflurane or propofol in spontaneously breathing ambulatory patients. *Anesth Analg.* 1998;87:312.

73. Dexter F, Tinker JH. Comparisons between desflurane and isoflurane or propofol on time to following commands and time to discharge: a meta-analysis. *Anesthesiology.* 1995;83:77.

74. Welborn LG, Hannallah RS, Norden JM, et al. Comparison of emergence and recovery characteristics of sevoflurane, desflurane, and halothane in pediatric ambulatory patients. *Anesth Analg.* 1996;83:917.

75. Hough MB, Sweeney B. Postoperative nausea and vomiting in arthroscopic day-case surgery: a comparison between desflurane and isoflurane. *Anaesthesia.* 1998;53:910.

76. Song D, Joshi GP, White PF. Fast-track eligibility after ambulatory anesthesia: a comparison of desflurane, sevoflurane, and propofol. *Anesth Analg.* 1998;86:267.

77. Philip BK, Kallar SK, Bogetz MS, et al. Sevoflurane Multicenter Ambulatory Group: a multicenter comparison of maintenance and recovery with sevoflurane or isoflurane for adult ambulatory anesthesia. *Anesth Analg.* 1996;83:314.

78. Thwaites A, Edmends S, Smith I. Inhalation induction with sevoflurane: a double-blind comparison with propofol. *Br J Anaesth.* 1997;78:356.

79. Philip BK, Lombard LL, Roaf ER, et al. Comparison of vital capacity induction with sevoflurane to intravenous induction with propofol for adult ambulatory anesthesia. *Anesth Analg.* 1999;89:623.

80. Jellish WS, Lien CA, Fontenot HJ, et al. The comparative effects of sevoflurane versus propofol in the induction and maintenance of anesthesia in adult patients. *Anesth Analg.* 1996;82:479.

81. Shakir AAK, Ramachandra V, Hasan MA. Day surgery postoperative nausea and vomiting at home related to perioperative fentanyl. *J One-Day Surg.* 1997;6:10.

82. Sukhani R, Vazquez J, Pappas AL, et al. Recovery after propofol with and without intraoperative fentanyl in patients undergoing ambulatory gynecologic laparoscopy. *Anesth Analg.* 1996;83:975.

83. Philip BK, Scuderi PE, Chung F, et al. Remifentanil compared with alfentanil for ambulatory surgery using total intravenous anesthesia. *Anesth Analg.* 1997;84:515.

84. Peacock JE, Luntley JB, O'Connor B, et al. Remifentanil in combination with propofol for spontaneous ventilation anaesthesia. *Br J Anaesth.* 1998;80:509.

85. Ogilvy AJ. Awareness during total intravenous anaesthesia with propofol and remifentanil [letter]. *Anaesthesia.* 1998;53:308.

86. Cartwright DP, Kvalsvik O, Cassuto J, et al. A randomized, blind comparison of remifentanil and alfentanil during anesthesia for outpatient surgery. *Anesth Analg.* 1997;85:1014.

87. Tiret L, Desmonts JM, Hatton F, et al. Complications associated with anaesthesia: a prospective survey in France. *Can Anaesth Soc J.* 1986;33:336.

88. Kallar SK. Aspiration pneumonitis: fact or fiction? *Probl Anesth.* 1988;2:29.

89. Verghese C, Brimacombe JR. Survey of laryngeal mask airway usage in 11, 910 patients: safety and efficacy for conventional and nonconventional usage. *Anesth Analg.* 1996;82:129.

90. Malins AF, Cooper GM. Laparoscopy and the laryngeal mask airway [letter]. *Br J Anaesth.* 1994;73:121.

91. Burgess GE, Cooper JR, Marino RJ, et al. Laryngeal competence after tracheal extubation. *Anesthesiology.* 1979;51:73.

92. Glauber DT. Facial paralysis after general anesthesia. *Anesthesiology.* 1986;65:516.

93. Munn KA, Williams RT, Shafto CM. Transient unilateral blindness following general anesthesia: case report. *Can Anaesth Soc J.* 1978;25:433.

94. Smith I, White PF. Use of the laryngeal mask airway as an alternative to a face mask during outpatient arthroscopy. *Anesthesiology.* 1992;77:850.

95. Wilkins CJ, Cramp PGW, Staples J. Comparison of the anesthetic requirement for tolerance of laryngeal mask airway and endotracheal tube. *Anesth Analg.* 1992;75:794.

96. Williams PJ, Bailey PM. Comparison of the reinforced laryngeal mask airway and tracheal intubation for adenotonsillectomy. *Br J Anaesth.* 1993;70:30.

97. Brain AI, Verghese C, Addy EV, et al. The intubating laryngeal mask, I: Development of a new device for intubation of the trachea. *Br J Anaesth.* 1997;79:699.

98. Brain AI, Verghese C, Addy EV, et al. The intubating laryngeal mask, II: a preliminary clinical report of a new means of intubating the trachea. *Br J Anaesth.* 1997;79:704.

99. Baskett PJ, Parr MJ, Nolan JP. The intubating laryngeal mask. Results of a multicentre trial with experience of 500 cases. *Anaesthesia.* 1998;53:1174.

100. Branthwaite MA. An unexpected complication of the intubating laryngeal mask. *Anaesthesia.* 1999;54:166.

101. Lopez-Gil M, Brimacombe J, Brain AI. Preliminary evaluation of a new prototype laryngeal mask in children. *Br J Anaesth.* 1999;82:132.

102. Asai T, Koga K, Jones RM, et al. The cuffed oropharyngeal airway. Its clinical use in 100 patients. *Anaesthesia.* 1998;53:817.

103. Brimacombe JR, Brimacombe JC, Berry AM, et al. A comparison of the laryngeal mask airway and cuffed oropharyngeal airway in anesthetized adult patients. *Anesth Analg.* 1998;87:147.

104. Greenberg RS, Brimacombe J, Berry A, et al. A randomized controlled trial comparing the cuffed oropharyngeal airway and the laryngeal mask airway in spontaneously breathing anesthetized adults. *Anesthesiology.* 1998;88:970.

105. Versichelen L, Struys M, Crombez E, et al. Haemodynamic and electro-encephalographic response to insertion of a cuffed oropharyngeal airway: comparison with the laryngeal mask airway. *Br J Anaesth.* 1998;81:393.

106. Chetty MS, Pollard BL, Wilson A, et al. Rocuronium bromide in dental day case anaesthesia: a comparison with atracurium and vecuronium. *Anaesth Intensive Care.* 1996;24:37.

107. Tramèr MR, Fuchs-Buder T. Omitting antagonism of neuromuscular block: effect on postoperative nausea and vomiting and risk of residual paralysis: a systematic review. *Br J Anaesth.* 1999;82:379.

108. Delphin E, Jackson D, Rothstein P. Use of succinylcholine during elective pediatric anesthesia should be reevaluated. *Anesth Analg.* 1987;66:1190.

109. Rosenberg H, Gronert G. Intractable cardiac arrest in children given succinylcholine [letter]. *Anesthesiology.* 1992;77:1054.

110. Tang J, Joshi GP, White PF. Comparison of rocuronium and mivacurium to succinylcholine during outpatient laparoscopic surgery. *Anesth Analg.* 1996;82:994.

111. Ding Y, Fredman B, White PF. Use of mivacurium during laparoscopic surgery: effect of reversal drugs on postoperative recovery. *Anesth Analg.* 1994;78:450.

112. Kahwaji R, Bevan DR, Bikhazi G, et al. Dose-ranging study in younger adult and elderly patients of Org 9487: a new, rapid-onset, short-duration muscle relaxant. *Anesth Analg.* 1997;84:1011.

113. Sparr HJ, Mellinghoff H, Blobner M, et al. Comparison of intubating conditions after rapacuronium (Org 9487) and succinylcholine following rapid sequence induction in adult patients. *Br J Anaesth.* 1999;82:537.

114. Wierda JMKH, van den Broek L, Proost JH, et al. Time course of action and endotracheal intubating conditions of Org 9487, a new short-acting steroidal muscle relaxant: a comparison with succinylcholine. *Anesth Analg.* 1993;77:579.

115. Stevens JB, Vescovo MV, Harris KC, et al. Tracheal intubation using alfentanil and no muscle relaxant: is the choice of hypnotic important? *Anesth Analg.* 1997;84:1222.

116. Stevens JB, Wheatley L. Tracheal intubation in ambulatory surgery patients: using remifentanil and propofol without muscle relaxants. *Anesth Analg.* 1998;86:45.

117. Thwaites AJ, Smith I. A double blind comparison of sevoflurane *versus* propofol and mivacurium for tracheal intubation in day case wisdom tooth extraction [abstract]. *Br J Anaesth.* 1998;80:A36.

118. Steyn MP, Quinn AM, Gillespie JA, et al. Tracheal intubation without neuromuscular block in children. *Br J Anaesth.* 1994;72:403.

119. Thwaites AJ, Edmends S, Tomlinson AA, et al. A double-blind comparison of sevoflurane *vs* propofol and succinylcholine for tracheal intubation in children. *Br J Anaesth.* 1999;83:410.

120. Leslie K, Sessler DI, Schroeder M, et al. Propofol blood concentration and the bispectral index predict suppression of learning during propofol/epidural anesthesia in volunteers. *Anesth Analg.* 1995;81:1269.

121. Gan TJ, Glass PS, Windsor A, et al. Bispectral index monitoring allows faster emergence and improved recovery from propofol, alfentanil, and nitrous oxide anesthesia. *Anesthesiology.* 1997;87:808.

122. Dexter F, Macario A, Manberg PJ, et al. Computer simulation to determine how rapid anesthetic recovery protocols to decrease the time for emergence or increase the phase I postanesthesia care unit bypass rate affect staffing of an ambulatory surgery center. *Anesth Analg.* 1999;88:1053.

123. Song D, Joshi GP, White PF. Titration of volatile anesthetics using bispectral index facilitates recovery after ambulatory anesthesia. *Anesthesiology.* 1997;87:842.

124. Thwaites AJ, Smith I. BIS during TCI propofol or sevoflurane anesthesia [abstract]. *Anesthesiology.* 1998;89:A899.

125. Mantzaridis H, Kenny GNC. Auditory evoked potential index: a quantitative measure of changes in auditory evoked potentials during general anaesthesia. *Anaesthesia.* 1997;52:1030.

126. Gajraj RJ, Doi M, Mantzaridis H, et al. Analysis of the EEG bispectrum, auditory evoked potentials and the EEG power spectrum during repeated transitions from consciousness to unconsciousness. *Br J Anaesth.* 1998;80:46.

127. American Society of Anesthesiologists. *Standards for Postanesthesia Care.* Park Ridge, Ill: American Society of Anesthesiologists; 1994.

128. Gift AG, Stanik J, Karpenick J, et al. Oxygen saturation in postoperative patients at low risk for hypoxemia: is oxygen therapy needed? *Anesth Analg.* 1995;80:368.

129. White PF. Criteria for fast-tracking outpatients after ambulatory surgery [letter]. *J Clin Anesth.* 1998;11:78.

130. White PF, Song D. New criteria for fast-tracking after outpatient anesthesia: a comparison with the modified Aldrete's scoring system. *Anesth Analg.* 1999;88:1069.

131. Aldrete JA, Kroulik D. A postanesthetic recovery score. *Anesth Analg.* 1970;49:924.

132. Aldrete JA. The post-anesthesia recovery score revisited [letter]. *J Clin Anesth.* 1995;7:89.

133. Chung F, Chan VWS, Ong D. A post-anesthetic discharge scoring system for home readiness after ambulatory surgery. *J Clin Anesth.* 1995;7:500.

134. Schreiner MS, Nicolson SC, Martin T, et al. Should children drink before discharge from day surgery? *Anesthesiology.* 1992;76:528.

135. Jin F, Chung F, Norris A, et al. Should adult patients drink before discharge from the ambulatory surgery unit? [abstract]. *Can J Anaesth.* 1998;45(suppl):A25-B.

136. Marshall SI, Chung F. Discharge criteria and complications after ambulatory surgery. *Anesth Analg.* 1999;88:508.

137. Fisher DM. The "big little problem" of postoperative nausea and vomiting. Do we know the answer yet? [editorial] *Anesthesiology.* 1997;87:1271.

138. Watcha MF, White PF. Postoperative nausea and vomiting: its etiology, treatment, and prevention. *Anesthesiology.* 1992;77:162.

139. Carroll NV, Miederhoff P, Cox FM, et al. Postoperative nausea and vomiting after discharge from outpatient surgery centers. *Anesth Analg.* 1995;80:903.

140. Tramèr M, Moore A, McQuay H. Meta-analytic comparison of prophylactic antiemetic efficacy for postoperative nausea and vomiting: propofol anaesthesia *vs* omitting nitrous oxide *vs* total i.v. anaesthesia with propofol. *Br J Anaesth.* 1997;78:256.

141. Claxton AR, McGuire G, Chung F, et al. Evaluation of morphine

versus fentanyl for postoperative analgesia after ambulatory surgical procedures. *Anesth Analg.* 1997;84:509.

142. Twersky R, Fishman D, Homel P. What happens after discharge? Return hospital visits after ambulatory surgery. *Anesth Analg.* 1997;84:319.

143. Foster PN, Stickle BR, Laurence AS. Akathisia following low-dose droperidol for antiemesis in day-case patients. *Anaesthesia.* 1996;51:491.

144. Watcha MF, Smith I. Cost-effectiveness analysis of antiemetic therapy for ambulatory surgery. *J Clin Anesth.* 1994;6:370.

145. Tramèr MR, Reynolds JM, Moore RA, et al. Efficacy, dose-response, and safety of ondansetron in prevention of postoperative nausea and vomiting: a quantitative systematic review of randomized placebo-controlled trials. *Anesthesiology.* 1997;87:1277.

146. Fortney JT, Gan TJ, Graczyk S, et al. A comparison of the efficacy, safety, and patient satisfaction of ondansetron versus droperidol as antiemetics for elective outpatient surgical procedures. *Anesth Analg.* 1998;86:731.

147. Thwaites AJ, Smith I. Novel drugs and anaesthetic techniques for ambulatory (day-case) anaesthesia. *Curr Opin Anaesthesiol.* 1997; 10:421.

148. McKenzie R, Lim NT, Riley TJ, et al. Droperidol/ondansetron combination controls nausea and vomiting after tubal banding. *Anesth Analg.* 1996;83:1218.

149. McKenzie R, Tantisira B, Karambelkar DJ, et al. Comparison of ondansetron with ondansetron plus dexamethasone in the prevention of postoperative nausea and vomiting. *Anesth Analg.* 1994;79:961.

150. Aasboe V, Ræder JC, Groegaard B. Betamethasone reduces postoperative pain and nausea after ambulatory surgery. *Anesth Analg.* 1998;87:319.

151. Yogendran S, Asokumar B, Cheng DCH, et al. A prospective randomized double-blind study of the effect of intravenous fluid therapy on adverse outcomes on outpatient surgery. *Anesth Analg.* 1995;80:682.

152. Vater M, Wandless J. Caudal or dorsal nerve block? A comparison of two local anaesthetic techniques for postoperative analgesia following day case circumcision. *Acta Anaesthesiol Scand.* 1985;29:175.

153. Tree-Trakarn T, Pirayavaraporn S. Postoperative pain relief for circumcision in children: comparison among morphine, nerve block, and topical analgesia. *Anesthesiology.* 1985;62:519.

154. Casey WF, Rice LJ, Hannallah RS, et al. A comparison between bupivacaine instillation versus ilioinguinal/iliohypogastric nerve block for postoperative analgesia following inguinal herniorrhaphy in children. *Anesthesiology.* 1990;72:637.

155. Yndgaard S, Holst P, Bjerre-Jepsen K, et al. Subcutaneously versus subfascially administered lidocaine in pain treatment after inguinal herniotomy. *Anesth Analg.* 1994;79:324.

156. Ballantyne JC, Dershwitz M. The pharmacology of non-steroidal anti-inflammatory drugs for acute pain. *Curr Opin Anaesthesiol.* 1995;8:461.

157. Dordoni PL, Della Ventura M, Stefanelli A, et al. Effect of ketorolac, ketoprofen and nefopam on platelet function. *Anaesthesia.* 1994;49:1046.

158. Tramèr MR, Williams JE, Carroll D, et al. Comparing analgesic efficacy of non-steroidal anti-inflammatory drugs given by different routes in acute and chronic pain: a qualitative systematic review. *Acta Anaesthesiol Scand.* 1998;42:71.

159. Ayres JG, Fleming DM, Whittington RM. Asthma death due to ibuprofen [letter]. *Lancet.* 1987;1:1082.

160. Power I. Aspirin-induced asthma [editorial]. *Br J Anaesth.* 1993;71:619.

161. Hawkey CJ. COX-2 inhibitors. *Lancet.* 1999;353:307.

162. Houmes RJM, Voets MA, Verkaaik A, et al. Efficacy and safety of tramadol versus morphine for moderate and severe postoperative pain with special regard to respiratory depression. *Anesth Analg.* 1992;74:510.

163. Broome IJ, Robb HM, Raj N, et al. The use of tramadol following day-case oral surgery. *Anaesthesia.* 1999;54:289.

164. Kehlet H, Dahl JB. The value of "multimodal" or "balanced analgesia" in postoperative pain treatment [review]. *Anesth Analg.* 1993;77:1048.

165. Michaloliakou C, Chung F, Sharma S. Preoperative multimodal analgesia facilitates recovery after ambulatory laparoscopic cholecystectomy. *Anesth Analg.* 1996;82:44.

166. Greenburg AG, Greenburg JP, Tewel A, et al. Hospital admission following ambulatory surgery. *Am J Surg.* 1996;172:21.

167. Ghosh S, Sallam S. Patient satisfaction and postoperative demands on hospital and community services after day surgery. *Br J Surg.* 1994;81:1635.

168. Tong D, Chung F, Wong D. Predictive factors in global and anesthesia satisfaction in ambulatory surgical patients. *Anesthesiology.* 1997;87:856.

169. Marshall S, Chung F. Assessment of 'home readiness': discharge criteria and postdischarge complications. *Curr Opin Anaesthesiol.* 1997;10:445.

170. Waters RM. The downtown anesthesia clinic. *Am J Surg.* 1919; 33(suppl):71.

171. SMG Marketing Group. *SMG Forecast of Surgical Volume in Hospital/Ambulatory Setting: 1994–2001.* Chicago, Ill: SMG Marketing Group; 1996.

172. Twersky RS. Anaesthetic and management dilemmas in office-based surgery. *Ambulatory Surg.* 1998;6:79.

173. Courtiss EH, Goldwyn RM, Joffe JM, et al. Anesthetic practices in ambulatory surgery. *Plast Reconstr Surg.* 1994;93:792.

174. American Society of Anesthesiologists. *ASA Guidelines for Ambulatory Anesthesia and Surgery, Nonoperating Room Anesthetizing Locations, and Office-Based Anesthesi*a. Park Ridge, Ill: American Society of Anesthesiologists; 1999.

175. American Society of Anesthesiologists. *ASA Standards for Basic Anesthetic Monitoring, Postanesthesia Care.* Park Ridge, Ill: American Society of Anesthesiologists; 1999.

176. Morello DC, Colon GA, Fredricks S, et al. Patient safety in accredited office surgical facilities. *Plast Reconstr Surg.* 1997;99:1496.

177. Grazer FM, de Jong RH. Fatal outcomes from liposuction: census survey of cosmetic surgeons. *Plast Reconstr Surg.* 2000;105:436.

# 71

# Sedation and Analgesia

Antoni M. Nejman

SEDATION
*What Are the Goals?*
*What Are the Indications?*
*What Is the Role for Benzodiazepines?*
*How Are Benzodiazepines Reversed?*
*What Is the Role for Sedative-Hypnotic Anesthetics?*
*What Are the Cost Implications?*

ANALGESIA
*What Are the Effects of Pain?*
*How Should Pain Be Approached Therapeutically?*
*What Is the Role for Narcotics?*
*What Is the Most Effective Delivery Route for Analgesic Medications?*

SUMMARY

## SEDATION

### What Are the Goals?

Sedation is the act of calming,[1] the process of allaying nervous excitement, or a state of being calm.[2] With or without analgesia, it is a condition that potentially results in the loss of protective reflexes for a significant group of patients.[3] This condition is termed *deep sedation*. It may be deliberate, to allow the performance of certain diagnostic or therapeutic interventions (a desirable goal), or inadvertent, as a result of drug overdose, improper monitoring, or both.

Conscious sedation for anesthesia and critical care is a mental state, created by medication or other means, in which the patient is calm and relaxed and is able to maintain his or her airway and protective reflexes while tolerating mild noxious stimuli. As sedation becomes more profound, the patient moves into the zone of light anesthesia and then into general anesthesia.

The aim of sedation should be patient comfort and relaxation and maintenance of the clinician's ability to evaluate neurologic and pulmonary status without compromising the protective reflexes. Adequate analgesia must be considered when a patient is evaluated for sedative requirements. A sedating drug should calm the patient and suppress alertness, arousal, and responses to stimuli. Narcotics are useful for analgesia and for their secondary sedative effects. Hypnotic and anxiolytic drugs are also used for their sedative properties and often are classified as sedatives. The sedative-hypnotic drugs promote drowsiness and facilitate the onset of sleep, but this sleep seldom is identical to normal, physiologic sleep.

Anxiety, fear, distress, hallucinations, disorientation, confusion, agitation, and loss of personal control are frequently part of the hospital experience. We need to identify the neurobehavioral disturbance to select the appropriate management techniques for treatment of the patient. Sedation must not be inappropriately used to mask agitation caused by an underlying undiagnosed or unrecognized pathologic process such as hypercarbia, hypoxia, or increased intracranial pressure.

### What Are the Indications?

Commonly accepted indications are listed in Table 71–1. A point of reference such as the Ramsay Scale[4] is useful when monitoring sedated patients (Table 71–2). Outward calm and tranquility should not always be construed as such; they may reflect paralysis. In a study by Loper and colleagues,[5] 5% of house staff physicians and 10% of intensive care unit (ICU) nurses believed that pancuronium relieved anxiety, leading to a relaxed and passive patient. While striving to reduce the patient's anxiety and pain, we should seek to produce a patient who is calm but able to cooperate. Diagnosis of the behavioral disturbance makes the choice of a pharmacologic agent somewhat easier.

#### Behavioral Disturbances

##### Anxiety

As defined in the *American Psychiatric Association's Psychiatric Glossary,* anxiety is "apprehension, tension, or uneasiness from anticipation of danger, the source of which is largely unknown or unrecognized" (Table 71–3). Most patients in the operating room and the critical care setting experience this emotion.

**TABLE 71–1.** Indications for Sedation

Invasive procedures
  Minor operative procedures
  Wound débridement
  Dressing changes
  Physical therapy
  Central line insertion
  Tracheostomy
  Tube thoracostomy
  Diagnostic laparoscopy/endoscopy
Mechanical ventilation
  Intubated or noninvasive
  With modes that require paralysis
  With modes that control the patient's respiratory mechanics
Acute events
  Resuscitation
  Intubation
  Cardioversion
Decreasing $O_2$ requirements
Prevention of self-harm in the agitated, confused patient
During any kind of therapeutic paralysis
Supplementation of analgesia
Terminal care
Control of physiologic parameters
Management of all patients who are chemically paralyzed

## Delirium

*Delirium* is "the clouding of consciousness with reduced capacity to focus, and sustain attention to environmental stimuli." It tends to develop over a short time (hours to days) and tends to fluctuate over the course of the day. Two of the following characteristics must be present:

1. Perceptual disturbances, including misinterpretations, illusions or hallucinations
2. Speech that is at times incoherent
3. Disturbances of sleep-wakefulness cycles
4. Increased or decreased psychomotor activity

Disorientation and memory impairment are also included in the diagnostic criteria.[6]

## Psychosis

Included are multiple categories of neurobehavioral abnormalities that are manifested as delusions, hallucinations, incoherence, marked loosening of associations, poverty of content of thought, and bizarre behavior.

## Agitation

*Agitation* is "excessive motor activity that is usually nonpurposeful and associated with internal tension." Examples

**TABLE 71–2.** The Ramsay Scale for Assessment of Sedation

| Level | Clinical Description |
|-------|----------------------|
| 1 | Anxious and agitated |
| 2 | Cooperative, oriented, tranquil |
| 3 | Responds only to verbal commands |
| 4 | Asleep; brisk response to light stimulation |
| 5 | Asleep; sluggish response to stimulation |
| 6 | Asleep; no response to stimulation |

**TABLE 71–3.** Behavioral Disturbances and Their Pharmacologic Treatment

| Behavioral Disturbance | Medication |
|------------------------|------------|
| Pain | Analgesics |
| Anxiety | Benzodiazepines |
| Agitation | Sedative-hypnotics |
| Delusions | Neuroleptics |
| Hallucinations | Neuroleptics |
| Delirium | Neuroleptics |
| Withdrawal | Benzodiazepines |

include inability to sit still, fidgeting, pacing, wringing of hands, or pulling of clothes. This condition refers only to the motor manifestations, and not the psychological state. The term *agitation* is often used incorrectly in the critical care setting to categorize more serious disturbances such as delirium or psychosis.

Treatment includes reassurance, elimination of those compounding factors that may be contributing, and, if needed, administration of the appropriate anxiolytic agent.

## What Is the Role for Benzodiazepines?

Benzodiazepines are the agents of choice, but they are also useful for insomnia, irritability, seizures, ethanol withdrawal, and adjustment disorders. Benzodiazepines prevent memory consolidation, thus providing amnesia. They are also effective, to a degree, as skeletal muscle relaxants. They act in the cerebral cortex, substantia nigra, hippocampus, cerebellum, and spinal cord. The benzodiazepine receptor is a complex described as a benzodiazepine/gamma-aminobutyric acid (GABA)/chloride ionophore. In the presence of benzodiazepines, the receptor has an increased affinity for GABA, which, when also present, increases the flow of chloride into the cell.[7] The resultant hyperpolarization decreases overall neuronal excitation in the areas of the brain that modulate anxiety, arousal, and behavioral inhibitions.

Benzodiazepines are safe agents that can be titrated predictably for a range of effects that include anxiolysis, amnesia, anticonvulsive activity, and decreased reaction time and psychomotor activity, and they can be used as a supplement to general anesthesia. The major side effects are cardiovascular and respiratory depression. When benzodiazepines are used in concert with opioids, the decrease in blood pressure is greater than with benzodiazepines alone. Opioids and benzodiazepines used together are synergistic with respect to respiratory depression.

Benzodiazepines are effective at equipotent dosages, so switching from one to another for an improved response is not helpful. The pharmacokinetic profiles and elimination pathways differ and, as such, may influence the choice of agent. Approximately 30 benzodiazepines are available worldwide, but only three are available in the United States for parenteral use (Table 71–4). These three drugs are highly protein bound (96%-98%) and have volumes of distribution ranging from 0.8 to 1.5 L/kg. Alterations in protein binding during sepsis may change the apparent volume of distribution and may necessitate a larger dose of the drug, thus explaining the variability of the drug response in critically ill patients.

**TABLE 71–4.** Benzodiazepines in Brief

| Agent | Metabolism | Half-Life Elimination (h) | Dosing Equivalence (mg/kg IV) | Average Bolus Dose in Adults | Infusion Dose | Comment |
|-------|-----------|--------------------------|-------------------------------|------------------------------|---------------|---------|
| Diazepam | Hepatic oxidation | 21–37 | 0.3–0.5 | 2–20 mg IV/IM, IM absorption unreliable | | Increased effect in aged Delayed clearance with $H_2$ block |
| Midazolam | Hepatic oxidation | 1–4 | 0.15–0.3 | 1–5 mg IV, 30% less with narcotics | 0.05–0.15 mg/kg/h | $H_2$ receptor antagonist does not interefere with metabolism |
| Lorazepam | Conjugation | 10–20 | 0.05 | 1–4 mg IV | 0.01–0.1 mg/kg/h | Less affected by hepatic failure, age, or cimetidine |

IM, intramuscular; IV, intravenous.

Onset of action after bolus injection depends on the rate at which uptake occurs in the brain. Using electroencephalographic (EEG) analysis under identical clinical conditions, maximal effects were measured for an intravenous (IV) bolus injection technique. Maximal diazepam effects were seen by the time the injection was ending; midazolam peaked approximately 5 minutes after the injection; lorazepam took 30 minutes to reach peak activity.[8,9] These facts are important to remember when the need arises for an immediate effect or when the drugs are titrated to effect.

Comparisons in the ICU indicate that midazolam may be better for short-term infusions, whereas lorazepam is appropriate for long-term use. Patients with infusions over 3 to 4.5 days experienced a return to baseline after discontinuation of lorazepam within 4.5 hours, whereas the midazolam comparison group took up to 30 hours,[10] probably because midazolam is more fat soluble. However, requirements for benzodiazepines fluctuate through the course of an ICU stay; a standard infusion for all patients is inappropriate.

## Drug Choices

### Diazepam

Diazepam is insoluble in water and therefore must be dissolved in propylene glycol, ethyl alcohol, benzyl alcohol, and sodium benzoate. In solution, it has a pH of 6.6 to 6.9, and IV or intramuscular (IM) injection may be painful. IM absorption is variable and unpredictable.

Diazepam is metabolized by hepatic microsomal enzymes through oxidative N-demethylation to desmethyldiazepam and oxazepam. Desmethyldiazepam (with an elimination half-life [$t_{1/2}$] of 48-96 hours) is only slightly less potent than diazepam and is probably responsible for the secondary drowsiness seen with diazepam. Oxazepam, although also active, is significant only after repeat doses of diazepam because the levels of the metabolite are clinically minor after a single dose of the parent drug.

As a rough guide, the $t_{1/2}$ of diazepam in hours is equivalent to the patient's age in years, so prudence must be exercised in the older population. The prolonged elimination $t_{1/2}$ in combination with an active metabolite that also has a long $t_{1/2}$ (36-90 hours) may make diazepam an inappropriate choice for infusions. Respiratory depression with increases in $PaCO_2$ is seen with varying doses depending on the patient's physiologic status. Doses of 0.5 to 1.0 mg/kg IV produce minimal reductions in blood pressure but may interfere with compensatory responses in hypovolemic patients. Administration of diazepam followed by IV opioid is associated with decreases in systemic vascular resistance and blood pressure greater than those seen with the opioid alone.

Skeletal muscle relaxation is mediated by diminution of the spinal gamma neuron output, thereby decreasing skeletal muscle tone. Finally, the anticonvulsant properties of diazepam may be effected through the stimulation of GABA, which acts as an inhibitory neurotransmitter.

### Midazolam

Midazolam is mixed in sodium chloride solution, disodium ethylenediaminetetraacetic acid, and benzyl alcohol and adjusted to a pH of 3. Its effects are similar to those of diazepam, with a slightly slower onset. It is two to four times as potent as diazepam but has an elimination $t_{1/2}$ of 1 to 4 hours. It is extremely fat soluble in vivo. Midazolam is metabolized by a hepatic microsomal oxidative mechanism to 1-hydroxymidazolam and 4-hydroxymidazolam. Both of these metabolites are active, but their contribution to clinical effects is still being evaluated.[11] Renal failure does not alter the clearance elimination half-time or volume of distribution of midazolam.[12] Ventilatory depression is similar to that with diazepam, with apnea the result of rapid IV injection of doses in the 0.15-mg/kg range. Midazolam seems to produce greater decreases in blood pressure than does diazepam, especially in the face of hypovolemia.

Midazolam does not prevent the heart rate and blood pressure increases seen with tracheal intubation.

### Lorazepam

Lorazepam is a more potent amnestic than diazepam. Its elimination $t_{1/2}$ is 10 to 12 hours, but its onset is slower. Effects on ventilation and cardiovascular function are similar. It is conjugated with glucuronic acid to form inactive metabolites. Its metabolism is not entirely dependent on hepatic microsomal enzymes, so it is less likely to be affected by hepatic function, age, or interfering drugs such as cimetidine. Many benzodiazepines are available orally (Table 71–5).

## How Are Benzodiazepines Reversed?

Flumazenil is a specific competitive antagonist of all the benzodiazepine effects. When it is administered intravenously, the onset of reversal is usually evident in 1 to 2 minutes, with peak effects at 6 to 10 minutes. The duration of effect is related to the plasma level of flumazenil as well as the dose of benzodiazepine initially administered. Dosing should be

**TABLE 71–5.** Oral Benzodiazepines

| Drug | Initial Dose (mg) | Dosing Interval (h) |
| --- | --- | --- |
| Alprazolam | 0.25–0.5 | 8 |
| Chlordiazepoxide | 5–25 | 6–8 |
| Clonazepam | 0.5 | 8 |
| Diazepam | 2–10 | 6–8 |
| Flurazepam | 15–30 | 3–4 |
| Lorazepam | 1–3 | 24 |
| Oxazepam | 10–15 | 4–6 |
| Prazepam | 10–15 | 6–8 |
| Quazepam* | 7.5–15 | 24 |
| Temazepam* | 15–30 | 24 |
| Triazolam* | 0.125–0.25 | 24 |

*Used primarily for insomnia.

started at 0.2 mg and titrated to a total of 1 mg, keeping in mind that administration of flumazenil may expose benzodiazepine dependence and possibly produce seizure activity. The duration of antagonism is short and resedation remains a concern, especially in cases in which a longer acting benzodiazepine has been given in large quantities. A second course of 1 mg in 0.2-mg increments is appropriate 30 minutes after the initial dosing.

Flumazenil is hepatically metabolized through glucuronide conjugation and not significantly affected by sex, age, or renal failure, or by hemodialysis started 1 hour after the drug is given.

## What Is the Role for Sedative-Hypnotic Anesthetics?

### Barbiturates

Barbiturates often are used to control intracranial hypertension and seizures. Hypotension in the hypovolemic patient is caused by direct myocardial depression. These drugs are potent hepatic enzyme inducers; patients may develop tachyphylaxis, have poor amnestic effects, and have frequent infectious complications. The ultrashort-acting barbiturates, although useful for the rapid induction of unconsciousness and the termination of seizures, are redistributed to fat stores if continued for long periods. This prolongs their effect and can result in coma that lasts for weeks after several days of thiopental infusion.

### Etomidate

Etomidate is a nonbarbiturate, carboxylated, imidazole-containing compound. It is associated with relative cardiovascular stability as an agent for the induction of unconsciousness, but is not appropriate as an infusion sedative because of its suppression of adrenocortical function.[13,14]

### Ketamine

This phencyclidine derivative creates a state of EEG dissociation between the thalamocortical and limbic systems. The patient may appear awake but is noncommunicative. The patient is amnestic, and analgesia is intense. Ketamine stimulates the hepatic enzymes responsible for the breakdown of the drug, thus explaining the frequent development of tolerance to its analgesic effects. Cardiovascular responses resemble those seen with sympathetic nervous system stimulation, with increases in systemic and pulmonary blood pressure, heart rate, and cardiac output. In the patient who is catecholamine depleted and sympathetically exhausted, the direct myocardial depressant effects of ketamine may be unmasked, with an unanticipated drop in blood pressure and cardiac output.

Ketamine does not significantly depress respiration or upper airway skeletal muscle tone. Although airway reflexes are relatively maintained, the patient still must be protected from aspiration. Salivary and tracheobronchial mucous gland secretions are increased, so an antisialagogue may be needed when using ketamine.

Emergence delirium is a common problem (5%-30%)[15] for up to 24 hours after ketamine administration. Patients often complain of vivid, morbid hallucinations and dreams. Benzodiazepines given before ketamine are effective for prevention of this delirium, as is recovery in a quiet, undisturbed environment.

## Propofol

A substituted isopropylphenol, propofol is administered as a 1% solution in an aqueous solution of 10% soybean oil, 2.25% glycerol, and 1.2% purified egg phosphatide. It was initially introduced as an agent that induced unconsciousness in 30 seconds when administered in doses of 2 to 2.5 mg/kg IV. Its elimination $t_{1/2}$ is short (0.5-1.5 hours), its elimination is not affected by cirrhosis, and its clearance is not influenced by renal failure. It has a modest cumulative effect, especially in the elderly. Propofol has become very popular because of its rapid onset and prompt recovery.

The drug also is used frequently for sedation in the ICU. It is extremely useful in those patients who remain severely agitated, despite no apparent underlying or uncorrected etiology (eg, pain, hypoxia), and who are not responding to adequate doses of other sedatives or antipsychotics. It is important for the patient's airway to be controlled because propofol is a profound respiratory depressant, especially when used in concert with narcotics and other sedatives.

Administration should be started slowly to minimize hypotension and overdose. Although a range of 5 to 50 μg/kg/min is usually adequate, higher doses may be required. The infusion should be started at 5 μg/kg/min and increased in increments of 5 to 10 μg/kg/min, waiting 5 to 10 minutes between increases to achieve peak drug effect.

A number of precautions need to be observed when using propofol:

1. Airway control and monitoring for early cardiovascular depression are necessary.
2. It is not an analgesic, so adequate narcotic supplementation is required.
3. 1.0 mL of propofol emulsion contains 1.1 kcal as 0.1 g of fat. Elevation of serum triglycerides may occur with prolonged administration.
4. The emulsion is an ideal culture medium, requiring strict asepsis when handling the vials, syringes, and administration tubing.
5. It should be avoided in patients with soybean or egg allergies.

**TABLE 71–6.** Sedative-Hypnotic Drugs and Doses

| Drug | GA Induction Dose (mg/kg) | Bolus Sedation Dose (mg/kg) | Infusion Dose (mg/kg/m) |
|------|---------------------------|------------------------------|--------------------------|
| Pentothal | 2–5 | 0.5–2 | Not recommended |
| Methohexital | 1–2 | 0.25–1 | Not recommended |
| Etomidate | 0.2–0.4 | 0.05–1 | Not recommended |
| Ketamine | 2–4 | 0.2–1 | 0.01–0.1 |
| Propofol | 2–2.5 | 0.05–0.4 | 0.01–0.2 |

GA, geneal anesthesia.

6. Central venous access is preferred to avoid the transient pain often associated with administration through a peripheral IV line.
7. Quinol metabolites have been known to cause a red-brown or green discoloration of the urine.
8. Wake up and assessment of central nervous system (CNS) function should be carried out daily to determine the minimum necessary dose for sedation.
9. A new brand of propofol with sodium metabisulfite as the preservative has recently been introduced to the market. This formulation should be avoided in patients with bisulfite allergy.

## Sedative-Hypnotics

Characteristics of these substances are outlined in Table 71–6.

### Diphenhydramine

This commonly used ethanolamine antihistamine is chosen not only for its histamine type 1 ($H_1$) receptor blocking properties but also for its side effect profile, including sedation. Doses are 10 to 50 mg IV or deep IM, with a daily maximum of 400 mg.

### Inhalational Anesthetics

These agents occasionally are used outside the operating room, but delivery is by specially calibrated vaporizers, making day-to-day administration in the ICU possible but logistically difficult.

### Haloperidol

Haloperidol (Haldol) is a butyrophenone neuroleptic/antipsychotic that acts in the CNS to block dopaminergic transmission at postsynaptic receptor sites. It may also inhibit central catecholamine reuptake and has α-blocking properties that may cause hypotension. Its $t_{1/2}$ of 12 to 38 hours can result in accumulation. With reference to neuroleptic drugs, Delay and Deniker stated in 1952[16]:

*The apparent indifference or the slowing of responses to external stimuli, the diminution of initiative and anxiety without a change in the state of waking and consciousness or of intellectual faculties constitute the psychological syndrome attributable to the drug.*

This comment very aptly describes the effects seen with haloperidol. The patient appears more calm, is more capable of appropriate response, and is without major respiratory depression. The drug has been used intravenously for over 20 years to manage delirium.[17] Large doses have been used in critically ill patients without harmful side effects.[18–20] Riker and colleagues have described the use of haloperidol in the agitated patient to facilitate weaning from ventilator support.[21] Nevertheless, haloperidol is not approved by the U.S. Food and Drug Administration for IV use.

**Dose.** The recommended dose depends on the level of agitation. Mild cases typically require a dose of 0.5 to 2.0 mg IV; moderate cases, 2 to 5 mg; and severe cases, 5 to 10 mg. Other issues that can modify the dose include the following:

1. Eliminate potential underlying causes of agitation.
2. Use lower doses initially in the elderly.
3. Allow 20 to 30 minutes between doses.
4. After 3 doses, add 0.5 to 1 mg of lorazepam IV concurrently or every other dose.
5. Once the patient is controlled, add the total dose of haloperidol and administer that amount over the next 24 hours.
6. If the patient remains calm, reduce the dose by 50% each 24 hours.
7. The oral dose is twice the IV dose.

If after control is achieved the patient cannot be maintained on an every-4-hour dosing schedule, a continuous infusion of haloperidol should be considered. The infusion should be started at 10 mg/h and titrated by 1 mg/h every 20 minutes to effect control. If agitation continues, repeat boluses of 5 to 10 mg IV are appropriate. Weaning needs to be addressed early so that the patient's degree of agitation/delirium/recovery may be ascertained. It has been demonstrated that in difficult patients, an infusion can decrease the rate of dosing from 23 doses/24 h using intermittent boluses to 7 dosing adjustments/24 h using an infusion.[21]

Side effects include cardiac arrhythmias; hypotension as a result of its α-blocking properties; hypoglycemia; and extrapyramidal syndrome with increased muscle tone in 16%,[22] and more frequently in cocaine abusers.[23] Side effects seem to be decreased with IV administration.[24] Less common side effects include cholestatic jaundice, photosensitivity, rash, weight gain, convulsions, and neurotoxicity in hyperthyroid patients.

**Torsade de Pointes.** Of the cardiac arrhythmias, the most worrisome associated with high-dose haloperidol are ventricular tachyarrhythmias, specifically torsade de pointes (polymorphic ventricular tachycardia). It is often self-terminating, but may degenerate into ventricular fibrillation. The rhythm is frequently heralded by a QT segment prolongation. Although such a prolongation usually is congenital, a number of drugs and abnormalities also cause it. Causes are listed in Table 71–7.

Treatment must be directed at the cause. Discontinuation of

**TABLE 71–7.** Causes of Torsade de Pointes

| | |
|---|---|
| Quinidine | Ingestion of liquid protein |
| Procainamide | Acute ischemia |
| Disopyramide | Bradycardia |
| Phenothiazines | Amyloidosis |
| Tricyclic antidepressants | Acute myocarditis |
| Hypokalemia | Mitral valve prolapse |
| Hypomagnesemia | Central nervous system disease |
| Hypocalcemia | |

the drug, correction of electrolyte abnormalities, and administration of magnesium sulfate as a 2-g bolus are effective.[25] Another reasonable antiarrhythmic drug is bretylium. Although cardioversion does not always prevent repeat bouts of the dysrhythmia, the definitive treatment seems to be atrial overdrive pacing with initial rates of 110 to 150 beats/min.[26]

Rarely (0.5%-1%), patients treated with antipsychotics experience neuroleptic malignant syndrome (NMS). NMS develops over 24 to 72 hours after administration of haloperidol or other potent neuroleptics. The syndrome is characterized by hyperthermia, generalized skeletal muscle hypertonicity, tachycardia and arrhythmias, fluctuating levels of consciousness, increased creatine kinase and liver enzyme levels, autonomic dysfunction (tachycardia, labile blood pressure, and profuse sweating), dyspnea, and incontinence.

The mortality rate is 20% to 30%. Treatment is symptomatic, including discontinuation of the drug, airway control, IV fluids for hypotension, body cooling, and sodium dantrolene, 2 mg/kg IV, repeated every 5 to 10 minutes to a maximum dose of 10 mg/kg.

Acute dyskinesias and dystonias are treated with diphenhydramine, 25 to 50 mg IV every 6 hours. More chronic treatment is provided by anticholinergic drugs such as benztropine, 1 to 2 mg orally or IV; trihexyphenidyl, 2 to 5 mg orally; and procyclidine, 2.5 mg orally 3 times daily. Akathisia (intense feeling of restlessness) is a common extrapyramidal effect that may respond to propranolol if the anticholinergics are not effective.

### Droperidol

Droperidol, another neuroleptic, has a half-life of 2.5 hours, but is much more sedating than haloperidol. Butyrophenone is also used but in smaller dosage ranges.

## What Are the Cost Implications?

In these times of cost constraints it is important to be aware of the overall and individual item costs. These expenses can mount quickly if not monitored. Cost comparisons are shown in Table 71–8. Significant cost minimization can result when these agents are used in combination.

The choice of agent needs to be based on the underlying abnormalities that allow for appropriate use of multiple agents.

Combinations of narcotic analgesics, benzodiazepines, and other sedatives in appropriate doses usually result in a tranquil, pain-free patient.

If all the psychological and sedative approaches have been exhausted and the patient is still at risk, induction of paralysis with the appropriate adjunctive agents may be the only recourse. This happens on occasion, but must be considered a last-ditch measure.

## ANALGESIA

Plato and Aristotle described pain as an emotion or a "passion of the soul." More recent scientists may have described it better as perception of a noxious sensation. A more suitable description might be that pain is an unpleasant experience, both sensory and emotional, that is often perceived in times of physical damage or injury, either actual or anticipated. The physicomechanical aspects and pathways of pain have been well described, but it is important to remember that the emotional state and past experiences play a significant role in how pain is perceived.

## What Are the Effects of Pain?

Nociceptive activity as initiated by a noxious stimulus is not pain until the neural message has been detected, transmitted to the brain, and acted on by numerous neural networks and chemicals. Although many of the neurotransmitters and neural pathways have been elucidated, higher cognitive and emotional processes still are not totally understood.

Pain and nociception are a part of the stress that contributes to the release of catecholamines and other hormones. The distress of pain and anxiety affects the immune system and wound healing.[27,28] The administration of analgesics and sedatives may improve morbidity and mortality rates by decreasing levels of endogenous endorphins that have been implicated in alteration of the immune response.[29]

### Pathophysiology

To look briefly at the pathophysiology of pain, we must start at the initial stimulus. This is usually a mechanical, thermal, chemical, or ischemic insult that causes tissue dam-

**TABLE 71–8.** Cost Comparison of Some Common Agents

| Drug | Cost per Bottle | Milligrams per Bottle | Cost per Milligram | Average Dose/h, 70-kg Man | Daily Infusion Cost |
|---|---|---|---|---|---|
| Propofol | $28.15 | 500 | $0.06 | 210 | $283.75 |
| Ketamine* | $8.63 | 500 | $0.02 | | |
| Haldol | $6.18 | 5 | $1.24 | 5 | $148.32 |
| Meperidine* | $0.14 | 50 | $0.00 | 50 | $3.36 |
| Morphine | $0.48 | 10 | $0.05 | 5 | $5.76 |
| Alfentanil* | $11.55 | 2.5 | $4.62 | 1 | $110.88 |
| Sufentanil* | $16.59 | 0.25 | $66.36 | 0.015 | $23.89 |
| Fentanyl | $0.744 | 0.5 | $1.49 | 0.1 | $3.57 |
| Versed | $8.47 | 5 | $1.69 | 2 | $81.31 |
| Lorazepam* | $11.12 | 40 | $0.28 | 0.25 | $1.67 |
| Diazepam* | $0.278 | 10 | $0.03 | 2 | $1.33 |

These are wholesale costs for a large teaching institution.
*Not often used as infusions in intensive care unit.

**TABLE 71–9.** Nerve Fiber Characteristics

| Nerve Fiber Classification | Diameter (μm) | Myelin | Function | Conduction Velocity (m/sec) |
|---|---|---|---|---|
| A alpha | 12–20 | Yes | Motor | 70–120 |
| A beta | 5–12 | Yes | Pressure/touch | 30–70 |
| A gamma | 5–12 | Yes | Proprioception | 30–70 |
| A delta | 1–4 | Yes | Pain/temperature | 12–30 |
| B | 1–3 | Yes | Preganglionic sympathetic | 14 |
| C sC | 0.3–1.3 | No | Postganglionic sympathetic | 0.7–1.3 |
| C drC | 0.4–1.4 | No | Pain/temperature/ touch | 0.1–2.0 |

age. The activation of nociceptive nerve endings (receptors) or the release of chemical mediators, or both, sends signals to the spinal cord along the primary afferent neurons (Table 71–9). A number of substances sensitize these nerve endings locally and are released in the face of the tissue trauma. Substances that sensitize the neurons to further noxious stimuli and act as mediators of inflammation include $H^+$, $K^+$, lactic acid, histamine, substance P, serotonin, bradykinin, and prostaglandins ($PGE_1 > PGE_2 > PGF_2$).

The cell bodies of these primary afferent neurons reside in the dorsal root ganglia and have projections to the dorsal horn lamina and other areas of the spinal cord, where they synapse with second-order afferent neurons and a series of regulatory neurons. The afferent nociceptive neurons release a number of neurotransmitter substances that activate wide-dynamic-range neurons in the substantia gelatinosa. These substances in the dorsal horn, along with spinal reflexes, act to modulate efferent impulses back to the peripheral nociceptive field, further aggravating the pain receptors[30,31] (Table 71–10). Inhibitory substances also play a role in the regulation of afferent nociceptive impulses at the dorsal horn.

Release of norepinephrine in response to sympathetic reflexes produces smooth muscle spasm, vasoconstriction, and changes in the microcirculation. The resulting ischemia and variation in the chemical environment of the wound augment pain and inflammation at the site of the insult.

The pain message is transmitted through the spinothalamic

**TABLE 71–10.** Substances That Modulate the Synaptic Transmission of Nociceptive Impulses

| Excitatory | Inhibitory |
|---|---|
| L-Glutamate | Enkephalins |
| Aspartate | γ-Aminobutyric acid |
| Vasoactive intestinal peptide | β-Endorphins |
| Cholecystokinin | Norepinephrine |
| Gastrin-releasing peptide | Serotonin |
| Calcitonin gene–related peptide | Somatostatin† |
| Angiotensin II | |
| Substance P* | |
| Dynorphin | |
| Leu-enkephalin | |
| Somatostatin | |
| Sympathetic reflex | |
| Release of norepinephrine | |

*In the synaptic vesicles of unmyelinated C fibers.
†Found in cell without substance P.

and spinoreticular tracts to the thalamus and sensory cortex. CNS brainstem reflexes cause an increase in sympathetic outflow, increased secretion of stress hormones, catabolism, tissue breakdown, and inflammation.

Our concern for the elimination or attenuation of pain stems from more than just an obligation to preserve the patient's peace of mind. Pain impairs ventilatory function, increases intracranial pressures, elevates metabolic rate, raises oxygen consumption, suppresses immune function, and activates a host of endocrine functions. It is impossible to separate totally the surgical stress response from the stress response due to pain because they occur simultaneously and are clearly linked by common pathways.

## How Should Pain Be Approached Therapeutically?

The complexity of the response and a limited understanding of it may help us in our approach to pain control. Ideally, initiation of some kind of afferent blockade preinjury would be effective in reducing stress hormone release. Preemptive analgesia also plays a major role in reduction of the memory of pain.[32] This option is not always available, so we must approach the problem after the insult/surgery.

Where we attempt to interrupt the pain pathway depends on the pharmacologic agents we wish to use (Fig. 71–1).

### Nonsteroidal Antiinflammatory Drugs

The nonsteroidal antiinflammatory drugs (NSAIDs) (Table 71–11) inhibit the prostaglandin-mediated sensitization and amplification of the nociceptive sensory pathways, probably by inhibiting the action of cyclooxygenase (COX) early in the conversion of arachidonic acid to prostaglandin. Ketorolac, the only NSAID available in both oral and parenteral forms, has been proved useful in many situations (60 mg = 100 mg meperidine = 12 mg morphine).

NSAIDs have a ceiling effect for their analgesic properties—that is, beyond a certain dose, the analgesic effect is not increased, but the side effect profile worsens (Fig. 71–2).

Arachidonic acid and its metabolites contribute to the inflammatory response and the modulation of pain. In simple terms, arachidonic acid is formed from cell membrane phospholipids in the presence of chemically or mechanically activated phospholipase $A_2$. Lipoxygenase pathways produce leukotrienes, whereas another pathway is catalyzed by COX-1 or COX-2. COX-2 is induced by cytokines, growth factor, and endotoxin, mainly at the site of inflammation.

COX catalyzes the addition of oxygen to arachidonic acid, which is the first step in a series of reactions involved in the synthesis of prostaglandins, prostacyclins, and thromboxanes, many of which are involved in the inflammatory process. Conventional NSAIDs affect COX-1 and COX-2. COX-1 is expressed in most tissues and is thought to protect the gastric mucosa.[33] The effects of the NSAIDs, which include antiinflammatory activity, antipyresis, and analgesia, result primarily from the inhibition of prostaglandin formation. NSAIDs modify COX-1 and COX-2 activity and the conversion of arachidonic acid to prostaglandin. Selective COX-2 inhibitors have shown antiinflammatory effects with improved

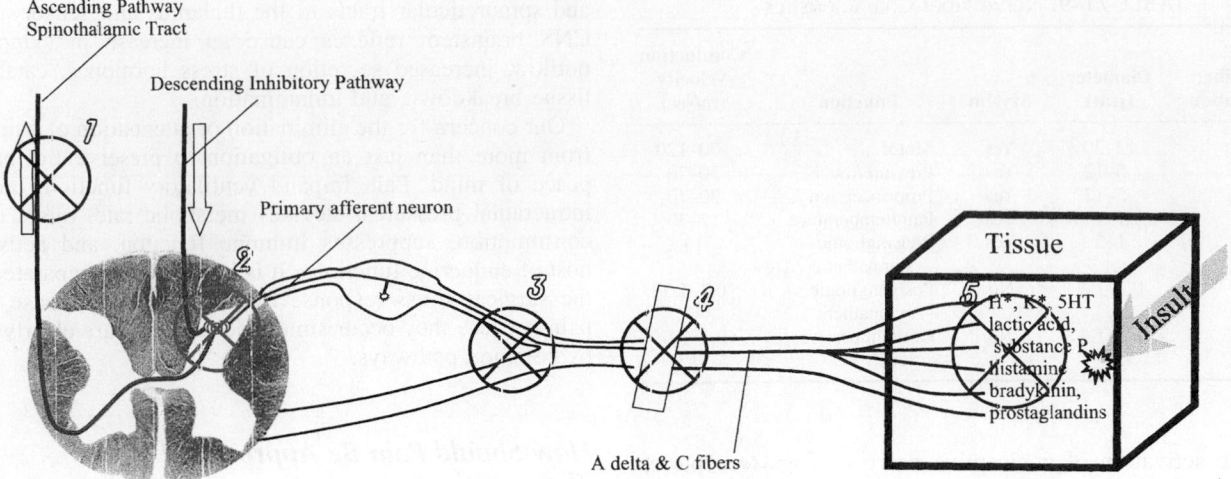

**FIGURE 71–1.** Simplified schematic representation of the pain pathway and sites for modification of stimulus perception.

gastrointestinal tolerance by avoiding effects on COX-1. Rofecoxib inhibits COX-2 but not COX-1.[34]

Aspirin covalently and irreversibly binds to COX-1 and COX-2. In platelets, which have minimal capacity for manufacturing new protein (ie, COX), a single dose of aspirin inhibits COX for the life of the platelets. In contrast, most other NSAIDs are reversible competitive inhibitors of COX activity, and inhibition is determined by their serum levels.

Side effects of NSAIDs include inhibition of platelet function, gastrointestinal ulceration and bleeding, inhibition of uterine motility, inhibition of prostaglandin-mediated renal function, and allergic reactions.

## What Is the Role for Narcotics?

*Papaver somniferum* is the source of the only significant naturally occurring narcotics. Morphine, codeine, and papaverine are all obtained from opium, which is the dried, powdered residue of the juice obtained from the unripe seed capsules of the poppy plant. The semisynthetic narcotics are derived from morphine through chemically induced changes in its structure. Synthetic narcotics resemble morphine but are entirely synthesized.

A group of descending inhibitory nerve fibers originating in the nucleus raphe magnus[4] interface with the first-order afferent neurons to modulate the transmission of afferent impulses. These inhibitory neurons contain β-endorphins (endogenous morphine) and enkephalins that, when released, hyperpolarize the Ad and C fibers, thereby blocking neurotransmitter release presynaptically. Opioids have also been shown to act postsynaptically when applied exogenously[5] and at higher centers, where they modify not only the response to but the perception of and reaction to pain. Morphine and its agonists/antagonists produce their biologic effects by interacting with stereoselective and saturable membrane-bound receptors distributed throughout the CNS. The highest concentration of these receptors is in the limbic system, thalamus, corpus striatum, hypothalamus, midbrain, and spinal cord.

## Mechanism of Action

Opiate receptors include μ (mu), κ (kappa), and δ (delta), which have been reclassified by an International Union of Pharmacology subcommittee as OP1 (δ), OP2 (κ), and OP3 (μ). These receptors are coupled with G-protein (guanine nucleotide-binding protein) receptors and function as modulators, both positive and negative, of synaptic transmission through G-proteins that activate effector proteins[35] (Table 71–12).

Opiates do not alter the pain threshold of afferent nerve endings to noxious stimuli, nor do they affect the conductance of impulses along peripheral nerves. Analgesia is mediated through changes in the perception of pain at the spinal cord

**TABLE 71–11.** Nonsteroidal Antiinflammatory Drugs

| Generic Name | Trade Name | Route | Type | Dosage |
|---|---|---|---|---|
| Indomethacin | Indocin | PO, PR | A, B, C | 25 mg q4h |
| Ketorolac | Toradol | PO, IM, IV, nasal, ophthalmologic | C, A, B | **IV:** 30 mg q6h<br>**IM:** 60 mg q6h (max 120 mg/d)<br>**PO:** 20 mg initial, then 10 mg q6h (max 40 mg/d) |
| Ibuprofen | Motrin, Advil | PO | C, A, B | 400 mg qid |
| Naproxen | Naprosyn | PO | C, A, B | 275–550 mg bid |
| Ketoprofen | Orudis | PO | C, A, B | 150–300 mg qid |
| Celecoxib | Celebrex | PO | B, A, C | 100 mg bid |
| Rofecoxib | Vioxx | PO | B, A, C | 12.5–50 mg/d (max 5 days if 50 mg/d given) |

This is a small sampling of the available NSAIDs.
A, antiinflammatory; B, antipyretic; C, analgesic; IM, intramuscular; IV, intravenous; PO, oral; PR, rectal.

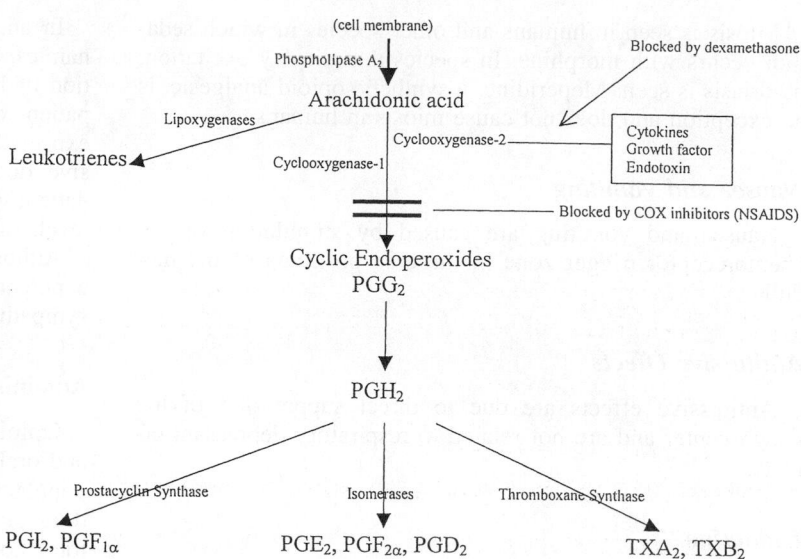

Essential Fatty Acids ⟶ Esterified acid in cell lipid

**FIGURE 71–2.** Cell membrane phospholipid is hydrolyzed by phospholipase $A_2$, releasing arachidonate. Arachidonic acid can then be involved in two pathways. If it is acted on by lipoxygenases, the result is the formation of the precursors of the leukotrienes. The other major pathway involves cyclooxygenases and the formation of the the cyclic endoperoxides, $PGG_2$ and subsequently $PGH_2$, the precursors of the prostaglandins and thromboxanes. Cyclooxygenase-1 (COX-1) is constitutively expressed, while cyclooxygenase-2 (COX-2) is induced by cytokines, growth factors, and endotoxin, an effect blocked by glucocorticoids. COX, cyclooygenase; PG, prostaglandin; PGG and PGH, cyclic endoperoxides; TX, thromboxane. (From Gilman AG, Hardman JG, Limbird LE, et al. In Molinoff PB, Ruddon RW, eds. *Goodman and Gilman's The Pharmacological Basis of Therapeutics.* 9th ed. New York: McGraw-Hill; 1996:1905.)

($\mu_2$-, δ-, κ-receptors) and higher levels in the CNS ($\mu_1$- and $\kappa_3$-receptors). There is no ceiling effect of analgesia for opiates, although the emotional response to pain is altered.

Opioids close voltage-gated calcium channels (κ-receptor agonist) and open calcium-dependent, inwardly rectifying potassium channels (μ- and δ-receptor agonist), resulting in hyperpolarization and reduced neuronal excitability. Binding of the opiate stimulates the exchange of guanosine triphosphate (GTP) for guanosine diphosphate on the G-protein complex. Binding of GTP leads to a release of the G-protein subunit, which acts on the effector system. In the case of opioid-induced analgesia, the effector system consists of adenylate cyclase and cyclic adenosine monophosphate (cAMP) located on the inner surface of the plasma membrane.[36] Thus, opioids decrease intracellular cAMP by inhibiting the adenylate cyclase that modulates the release of nociceptive neurotransmitters such as substance P, GABA, dopamine, acetylcholine, and norepinephrine. Opioids also modulate the endocrine and immune systems. Opioids inhibit the release of vasopressin, somatostatin, insulin, and glucagon.

The stimulatory effects of opioids are the result of "disinhibition" because the release of inhibitory neurotransmitters such as GABA and acetylcholine is blocked, although the exact mechanism for this is unknown.

## Side Effects

### Respiratory Depression

Opioids decrease the respiratory drive by lowering sensitivity to $CO_2$, with subsequent consequences for serum levels, pH, somnolence, and cerebral vasodilation.

### Mood Changes

Opioids produce a clouded sensorium and a feeling of detachment. This is interpreted as pleasant and euphoric by some or unpleasant and alarming by others.

### Sedation

The amount of sedation depends on the opioid, the dose, protein binding, and metabolism. Not all equianalgesic doses of opioids cause an equal level of sedation. Some opioids are excitatory and may cause convulsions.

### Excitation

Low doses of morphine have been known to cause restlessness in some patients, whereas higher doses have caused convulsions.

**TABLE 71–12.** Pharmacology of Opioid Receptors

| | Receptor | | | | |
|---|---|---|---|---|---|
| Action | $\mu_1$ | $\mu_2$ | δ | κ | σ |
| Analgesia | Supraspinal | — | Spinal | Spinal | — |
| Respiration | — | Depresses | Depresses | — | Tachypnea |
| Gastrointestinal | Nausea and vomiting | Constipation | Nausea and vomiting | — | — |
| Genitourinary | Retention | — | Retention | Diuresis | — |
| Mentation | Euphoria | Sedation | — | Sedation | Dyspho |
| Pupil | Miosis | — | — | Miosis | Myd |
| Tolerance | Yes | — | Yes, and dependence | Little | |
| Other | Pruritus | — | Pruritus | | |

## Miosis

Miosis is seen in humans and other species in which sedation occurs with morphine. In species that display excitation, mydriasis is seen. Meperidine, a synthetic opioid analgesic, is an exception and does not cause miosis in humans.

## Nausea and Vomiting

Nausea and vomiting are caused by stimulation of the chemoreceptor trigger zone in the area postrema of the medulla.

## Antitussive Effects

Antitussive effects are due to direct suppression of the cough center and are not related to respiratory depressant effects.

## Endocrine

Endocrine effects associated with opioid administration include elevation of serum prolactin levels, inhibition of vasopressin, and decreased levels of luteinizing hormone, follicle-stimulating hormone, and testosterone.

## Histamine Release

Many opioids cause histamine release with vasodilation. Subsequent hypotension and cutaneous flushing may result in loss of body heat.

## Gastrointestinal System

Small and large bowel tone is increased, but propulsion is slowed, leading to constipation. Increased common bile duct pressure (fentanyl > morphine > meperidine > butorphanol) is reversed by nitroglycerin, atropine, glucagon, and naloxone.

## Cardiovascular

In analgesic doses, morphine has little effect on hemodynamics, but as the dose is increased, vasodilation and inhibition of baroreflexes occur. Sympatholytic vasodilation in the patient with elevated sympathetic tone can cause greater than expected drops in blood pressure with normally nonhypotensive doses. Therefore, caution should be exercised in the patient with serious trauma or cardiovascular disease and high levels of circulating catecholamines.

Although opioids do not suppress the myocardium, there is a potential for dose-dependent bradycardia caused by parasympathomimetic and sympatholytic mechanisms.

## Administration

Opioids are administered intravenously, intramuscularly, and orally. Patient-controlled analgesia (PCA) is increasingly popular, allowing the administration of small IV boluses of drug along with the ability to control the lockout interval, total hourly dose, and underlying basal infusion rate. PCA results in a more uniform level of analgesia and allows the patient latitude in his or her dosing regimen.

The most commonly administered drugs outside the operating room are morphine and meperidine. IV dosing guidelines are summarized in Table 71–13.

During surgery, alfentanil, fentanyl, remifentanil, and sufentanil are preferred. The dosing ranges for these drugs vary depending on the type of anesthetic given, the surgical procedure, and the desired duration of analgesia (Table 71–14).

## Synthetic Opioids

The extent of action of these drugs changes as the duration of the infusion is prolonged. The context-sensitive half-time concept as defined by Hughes and colleagues[37] is the time required for a drug concentration in the central compartment (plasma) to decrease by 50%.

**TABLE 71–13.** Dosing Guidelines for Narcotics Used Outside the Operating Room

| Generic Name | Trade Name | Route | Dosage (mg) | Onset | Peak | Duration | Relative Potency |
|---|---|---|---|---|---|---|---|
| *Natural Alkaloids* | | | | | | | |
| Morphine | | PO | 30–60 | 20–60 min | 60 min | 3–7 h | 0.2 |
| | | IM | 10–15 | 20 min | 30–90 min | 3–4 h | 1 |
| | | IV | 2–10 | 60 sec | 5–10 min | 2–4 h | 1.5 |
| Codeine | | PO | 15–60 | 10–30 min | 1–5 h | 4–6 h | 0.05 |
| | | IM | 15–60 | 15–60 min | 0.5–2 h | 4–6 h | 0.1 |
| *Semisynthetic Derivatives* | | | | | | | |
| Hydromorphone | Dilaudid | IM | 1–4 | 20–30 min | 1 h | 2–3 h | 5 |
| | | PO | 1–4 | 30–60 min | 2 h | 3–4 h | 1.5 |
| Hydrocodone | Vicodin | PO | 5–7.5 | 10–30 min | 30–60 min | 4–6 h | 0.3 |
| Oxycodone | Percodan | PO | 5 | 30 min | 1–2 h | 3–6 h | 0.2 |
| Oxymorphone | Numorphan | IM | 1–1.5 | 30 min | 1 h | 2–3 h | 10 |
| *Synthetics* | | | | | | | |
| Meperidine | Demerol | PO, SC, IM | 25–100 | 10–15 min | 1 h | 3–4 h | 0.1 |
| | | IV | 25–50 | | | | 0.2 |
| Methadone | | IM | 2.5–10 | 15 min | 30–60 min | 4–6 h | 1.2 |
| | | PO | 2.5–10 | 30–60 min | 1.5–2 h | 4–8 h | 1.2 |
| Propoxyphene HCl | Darvon | PO | 65 | 20–60 min | 2–3 h | 3–6 h | 0.25 |
| Levorphanol | Levordromoran | IM | 2–3 | 1 h | 2 h | 4–6 h | 5 |
| | | PO | 2–4 | 1.5 h | 2 h | 4–6 h | 2.5 |
| Tramadol | | PO | 50–100 | | | 4–6 h | 0.1 |

IM, intramuscular; IV, intravenous; PO, oral; SC, subcutaneous.

**TABLE 71–14.** Dosing Guidelines for Intraoperative Narcotics

| Generic Name | Trade Name | Primary Dosing Route | Low Dose | High Dose | Infusion Range | Peak | Relative Potency |
|---|---|---|---|---|---|---|---|
| Alfentanil | Alfenta | IV | 5–10 μg/kg | 150–300 μg/kg | 25–150 μg/kg/h | 1.4 min | 10 |
| Fentanyl | Sublimaze | IV | 1–2 μg/kg | 50–150 μg/kg | 1–4 μg/kg/h | 6.8 min | 75–125 |
| Remifentanil | Ultiva | IV | 0.25–0.5 μg/kg | 1.5–3 μg/kg | 0.025–0.5 μg/kg/min | 1.1 min | 150–200 |
| Sufentanil | Sufenta | IV | 0.1–0.4 μg/kg | 10–30 μg/kg | 0.5–2 μg/kg/h | 6.2 min | 2000–4000 |

IV, intravenous.

Figure 71–3 shows the context-sensitive half-times for the four common synthetic opioids as plotted by a computer simulation. Note that remifentanil's elimination time remains steady regardless of the duration of the infusion. This is a result of its hydrolysis by nonspecific esterases and its lack of dependence on any organ-specific degradation. Remifentanil's context-sensitive half-time of 3 to 4 minutes is ideal for termination of the opioid-based anesthetic and its side effect profile. Termination of the remifentanil infusion requires a supplemental analgesic before discontinuation, or the patient may awaken abruptly without the benefit of any pain control.

Epidural opioids have the advantage of a smaller overall dose and a lower side effect profile, especially when administered by continuous infusion. Placement of the catheter at or near the level of injury or surgery allows smaller doses of narcotics to be administered, whereas more distant placement requires either larger volumes or a less lipophilic drug. Morphine spreads the most and sufentanil (Sufenta) the least. The combination of PCA and epidural infusion, or PCEA (patient-controlled epidural analgesia), seems to result in a lower total dose of drug (Table 71–15).

## Local Anesthetics

Regional anesthesia has been used for many years for deafferentation of the surgical site. It is still in extensive use, alone and in combination with other medications.

Intercostal blocks—intermittent and with indwelling catheters—have been used for analgesia in rib fractures and thoracic surgery, but interpleural catheters may be taking their place. Their ease of placement and the ability to administer the anesthetic in a continuous infusion make them less labor-intensive than repetitive intercostal blocks.

Considerations for interpleural catheters include

1. Placement of the catheter: percutaneous or through chest tube
2. Bolus dosing or continuous infusion
3. Toxicity in the face of mental status changes (is it the medication or not?)
4. Alterations in the interpleural environment: blood, purulence, effusion
5. Pneumothorax rate with the technique

Upper extremity pain often responds well to indwelling interscalene and axillary catheters, which provide good analgesia and sympathectomy and facilitate mobilization by providing muscle relaxation.[38] Lower extremity blocks are used for both analgesia and relaxation during and after surgery. Epidurals with low concentrations of local anesthetics in combination with narcotics have been used to advantage in many situations where one or the other alone does not provide adequate relief.

## α-Adrenergic Receptors

These receptors have been subdivided into $\alpha_1$ and $\alpha_2$ based on selective pharmacologic inhibition (Table 71–16). $\alpha_1$ Receptors are antagonized by prazosin, whereas $\alpha_2$ receptors are antagonized by yohimbine. $\alpha_2$-Adrenoceptors are further subdivided based on pharmacologic or molecular genetic studies into $\alpha_{2A}$, $\alpha_{2B}$, and $\alpha_{2C}$. $\alpha_2$-Adrenoceptors, when activated, initiate their responses through a transmembrane G-protein that inhibits adenyl cyclase, resulting in lower levels of cAMP, decreased phosphorylation of regulatory proteins, and changes in potassium and calcium channels. The resultant efflux of potassium and suppression of calcium entry results in a hyperpolarization of the nerve and decreased release of the stored neurotransmitter.

$\alpha_2$-Adrenoceptors are found in the CNS neurons of the spinal cord lamina, peripheral nerves (somatic and autonomic), primary afferent terminals, in several brainstem nuclei,[39] autonomic ganglia tissues innervated by the sympathetic nervous system, and in postsynaptic effector organs (ie, vascular smooth muscle).

Activation of $\alpha_2$ receptors produces a variety of responses. Presynaptic $\alpha_2$ receptors in sympathetic nerve endings inhibit the release of norepinephrine.[40] Postsynaptic receptor activation in the CNS inhibits sympathetic activity with lowering of blood pressure ($\alpha_{2A}$ receptors), decreased heart rate, and sedation. Spinal cord $\alpha_2$ receptor activation produces analgesia.[41] Peripheral $\alpha_2$ receptor agonism in blood vessels can produce a transient rise in blood pressure ($\alpha_{2B}$ receptors)

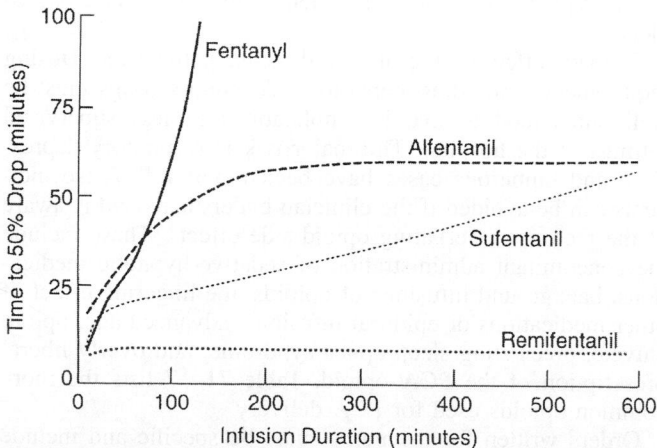

**FIGURE 71–3.** Context-sensitive half-times for the four common synthetic opioids as plotted by a computer simulation.

**TABLE 71–15.** Lipid Solubility and Dosing Guidelines for Epidural Narcotics

| Opioid | Relative Lipid Solubility | Epidural Bolus Dose | Onset Time (min) | Duration (h) | Infusion Concentration (mg/mL) | Infusion Rate (mL/h) |
|---|---|---|---|---|---|---|
| Morphine | 1.4 | 2.5–10 mg* | 45–60 | 8–24 | 0.1 | 4–6 |
| Meperidine | 38.8 | 30–100 mg† | 15–30 | 4–6 | 5–10 | 1–4 |
| Alfentanil | 136 | 15 μg/kg | 15 | 1–1.5 | Seldom used | Seldom used |
| Fentanyl | 813 | 50–100 μg/kg | 15–30 | 2–5 | 4–10 μg/mL | 5–15 mL/h |
| Sufentanil | 1,778 | 10–50 μg/kg | 15 | 4–6 | 0.5–1 μg/mL | 5–10 mL/h |

Note: All dosing must be individualized and the patients closely monitored; these are only guidelines and must be individualized.
*Preservative-free morphine.
†Preservative-free meperidine.

Other $\alpha_2$ receptor stimulation throughout the body results in a reduction in anesthetic requirements during surgery; antisialagogue effects; diuresis (inhibition of antidiuretic hormone); vagally mediated antiarrhythmic effects (significant bradycardia is rare); increased secretion of growth hormone (short lived)[42]; and slight inhibition of insulin release.

The best known of the $\alpha_2$ receptor agonists is clonidine, which was introduced as an antihypertensive in the early 1970s. Clonidine has been administered by oral, epidural, spinal, IV, IM, and transdermal routes. It is a selective partial agonist of $\alpha_2$-adrenoceptors with an $\alpha_2:\alpha_1$ selectivity ratio of 220:1. Dexmedetomidine, a more highly selective $\alpha_2$ agonist with an $\alpha_2:\alpha_1$ selectivity ratio of 1620:1, is still undergoing North American trials. Trials in Europe suggest that IV infusions of dexmedetomidine provide analgesia and reduce anesthetic requirements.

Current uses for clonidine are multiple, but in anesthesia it is primarily used as an oral preoperative medication dosed at 1 to 2 μg/kg. The patient must be warned about potential orthostatic hypotension, and appropriate precautions should be taken.

Intrathecal and epidural clonidine has been used in numerous studies, either alone or in combination with local anesthetics,[43] narcotics,[44,45] or both.[46] The results have shown decreased analgesic requirements for both narcotic and local anesthetic, but as the dose of clonidine increases, so also does sedation and hypotension.

IV dexmedetomidine produces postoperative analgesia and sedation but causes hypotension and bradycardia similar to clonidine. Further studies are ongoing.

## What Is the Most Effective Delivery Route for Analgesic Medications?

The route of medication delivery depends not only on the pharmacology of the medications but also on the support available to administer the drug. An ambulatory patient at home 6 hours after surgery is best treated with oral medication, whereas a patient in the ICU can be appropriately administered IV or neuraxial medication. Most people probably would agree that neuraxial (epidural/spinal) narcotics provide better pain relief with less total drug dosing. Epidural infusions of narcotics and extensive experience with indwelling catheters make this the preferred route.

Local anesthetics in combination with narcotics allow decreased opioid dosing and side effects while providing a decrease in the overall stress response. Local anesthetics in excess result in hypotension, numbness, and loss of motor function, whereas the side effect profile of narcotics includes respiratory depression, pruritus, nausea and vomiting, and urinary retention.

IM analgesic administration is cheap and effective but is very labor intensive for the nursing staff. Staffing and response times to patient requests inevitably result in fluctuating analgesic serum levels with periods of inadequate analgesia followed by excess opioid effect. Intermittent IV opioid dosing results in similar swings, but this can be improved by administration through pumps left in the patient's control.

### Patient-Controlled Analgesia

Patient-controlled IV delivery of opioids is an increasingly popular alternative for the control of postoperative pain. The patient is able to administer analgesic drugs as they are required, but the dosing is limited by the lockout intervals and total dose setting. This mode of administration gives the patient a sense of control and provides consistent serum analgesic levels. PCA requires some patient education but, from the viewpoint of labor and patient satisfaction, is close to ideal.

The side effect profile of opioids remains the same. Dosing requirements and adjustments to PCA pump settings must be well understood to avoid complications in less supervised settings of the hospital. The major risk is respiratory depression, and numerous cases have been reported.[47] These incidents can be avoided if the clinician understands and is aware of the factors exacerbating opioid side effects. These include the concomitant administration of sedative-hypnotic medications, background infusions of opioids, the lingering effect of other medications or epidural infusions, advanced age, opioid naiveté, preexisting sleep apnea syndrome, and overly liberal prescription of the PCA opioid. Table 71–17 lists the more common opioids used for PCA delivery.

Orders written for the pump must be specific and include the drug, the bolus dose, the lockout time between doses, the total dose allowed per unit time, medications for side effects,

**TABLE 71–16.** $\alpha_2$-Agonist Specificity

Relative Agonist Selectivity

*Dexmedetomidine (1620:1)
Guanabenz
Guanfacine
Clonidine (220:1)
*Xylazine (160:1)
Dopamine
Epinephrine
Norepinephrine
Phenylephrine
Methoxamine

$\alpha_2$ ↑

↓ $\alpha_1$

*Not available for clinical use; ( ) indicate $\alpha_2:\alpha_1$ ratio.

**TABLE 71–17.** Patient-Controlled Analgesia Dosing Guidelines for the More Commonly Used Opioids

| Drug | Bolus Dose (mg) | Lockout Interval (min) | 1-h Limit (mg) | Continuous Infusion (mg/h) |
|---|---|---|---|---|
| Fentanyl | 0.015–0.05 | 4–10 | 0.05–0.10 | 0.02–0.075 |
| Hydromorphone | 0.1–0.4 | 10–15 | 0.8–1.5 | |
| Meperidine | 5–15 | 5–15 | 50–75 | 150–250 |
| Morphine | 0.5–2 | 6–20 | 4–10 | 0.1–1 |
| Sufentanil | 0.003–0.015 | 3–10 | 0.01–0.02 | |

exclusion of other sedative hypnotics, the frequency of pain evaluations, the frequency of vital signs, and a contact number for the Pain Service.

## SUMMARY

Analgesia may be approached at a number of locations, from the origin of the stimulus, along the afferent pathway and to the spinal cord, and supraspinally. Blockade of receptor input by the application of local anesthetics or modification of the inflammatory response with NSAIDs has been effective. Epidural and subarachnoid local anesthetics and opioids have proved to be useful with smaller total doses, at least in the case of local anesthetics. Systemic opioids have long been the mainstay of medical pain control despite their well-known side effects. As more information about receptor specificities and the modulation of neurotransmission is developed, specific agonists and antagonists will allow us selectively to block or modify the pain pathways and the perception of this unpleasant sensation.

Although the goal of analgesia is patient comfort, blockade of the stress response is also of paramount importance in the overall treatment of the patient. Selection of the appropriate modality should aim to obtund both of these effects.

## References

1. *Stedman's Medical Dictionary.* 26th ed. Baltimore, Md: Williams & Wilkins; 1995.
2. *Tabers Cyclopedic Medical Dictionary.* 18th ed. Philadelphia, Pa: FA Davis; 1997.
3. *Joint Commission Accreditation Manual for Hospitals.* Oakbrook Terrace, IL; 2000.
4. Ramsay MA, Savege TM, Simpson BR, et al. Controlled sedation with alphaxalone/alphadolone. *BMJ.* 1974;2:256.
5. Loper KA, Butler S, Nessly M. Paralyzed with pain: the need for education. *Pain.* 1989;37:315.
6. American Psychiatric Association. *Quick Reference to the Diagnostic Criteria from DSM III.* Washington, DC: American Psychiatric Association; 1980.
7. Mohler H, Richards JG. The benzodiazepine receptor: a pharmacological control element of brain function. *Eur J Anaesthesiol.* 1988;15:24.
8. Greenblatt DJ, Ehrenberg BL, Gunderman J, et al. Pharmacokinetic and electroencephalographic study of intravenous diazepam, midazolam, and placebo. *Clin J Pharmacol Ther.* 1989;45:356.
9. Greenblatt DJ, Ehrenberg BL, Gunderman J, et al. Kinetic and dynamic study of intravenous lorazepam: Comparison with intravenous diazepam. *J Pharmacol Exp Ther.* 1989;250:134.
10. Pohlman AS, Simpson KP, Hall JB. Continuous intravenous infusion of lorazepam versus midazolam for sedation during mechanical ventilatory support: a prospective randomized study. *Crit Care Med.* 1994;22:1241.
11. Reeves JG, Fragen RJ, Vinik HR, et al. Midazolam: pharmacology and uses. *Anesthesiology.* 1985;62:310.
12. Vinik HR, Reves JG, Greenblatt DJ, et al. The pharmacokinetics of midazolam in chronic renal failure patients. *Anesthesiology.* 1983;59:390.
13. Wagner RL, White PF, Kan PB, et al. Inhibition of adrenal steroidogenesis by the anesthetic etomidate. *N Engl J Med.* 1984;310:1415.
14. Fragen RJ, Shanks CA, Molteni A, et al. Effects of etomidate on hormonal responses to surgical stress. *Anesthesiology.* 1984;61:652.
15. White PF, Way WL, Trevor AJ. Ketamine: its pharmacology and therapeutic uses. *Anesthesiology.* 1982;56:119.
16. Delay J, Deniker P. Trente-huit cas de psychoses traitées par la cure prolongée et continué de. 4560 RP Le Congrès des Al; Et Neurol; De Langue Fr. In Compte Rendu du Congres Masson et Cie. Paris; 1952.
17. Settle EC, Ayd FJ. Haloperidol: a quarter century of experience. *J Clin Psychiatr.* 1983;44:440.
18. Tesar GE, Murray GB, Cassem NH. Use of high dose Haldol in the treatment of agitated cardiac patients. *J Clin Psychopharmacol.* 1985;5:344.
19. Sos J, Cassem NH. Managing postoperative agitation. *Drug Ther.* 1980;10:103.
20. Menza MA, Murray GB, Holmes VF. Decreased extrapyramidal symptoms with intravenous haloperidol. *J Clin Psychiatry.* 1987;48:278.
21. Riker RR, Fraser GL, Cox PM. Continuous infusion of haloperidol controls agitation in critically ill patients. *Crit Care Med.* 1994;22:433.
22. Swett MP. Drug-induced dystonia. *Am J Psychiatry.* 1975;132:532.
23. Kumor K, Sherer M, Jaffe J. Haloperidol-induced dystonia in cocaine addicts. *Lancet.* 1986;2:1341.
24. Dubin WR, Feld JA. Rapid tranquilization of the violent patient. *Am J Emerg Med.* 1989;7:313.
25. Tzivoni D, Keren A. Suppression of ventricular arrhythmias by magnesium. *Am J Cardiol.* 1990;65:1397.
26. Smith WM, Gallagher JJ. "Les torsades de pointes": an unusual ventricular arrhythmia. *Ann Intern Med.* 1980;93:578.
27. Riley V. Psychoneuroendocrine influences on immunocompetence and neoplasia. *Science.* 1981;212:1100.
28. Watkins J, Glynn LE. Symposium on trauma, stress, and immunity at Bath. *Anesthesia.* 1981;36:647.
29. Demling RH. What are the functions of endorphins following thermal injury? [discussion]. *J Trauma.* 1984;24S:172.
30. Jessel TM, Mudge AW, Leeman SE. Release of substance P and somatostatin in vivo from primary different terminals in mammalian spinal cord. *Neurol Sci Abstracts.* 1979;5:611.
31. Henry JL. Effects of substance P on functionally identified units in cat spinal cord. *Brain Res.* 1976;114:439.
32. McQuay HJ. Preemptive analgesia. *Br J Anaesth.* 1992;69:1.
33. Wolfe MM, Lichtenstein DR, Singh G. Gastrointestinal toxicity of nonsteroidal antiinflammatory drugs. *N Engl J Med.* 1999;340:1988.
34. Ehrich EW, Dallob A, De Lepeleire I, et al. Characterization of rofecoxib as a cyclooxygenase-2 isoform inhibitor and demonstration of analgesia in the dental pain model. *Clin Pharmacol Ther.* 1999;65:336.
35. Harrison C, Smart D, Lambert DG. Stimulatory effects of opioids. *Br J Anaesth.* 1998;81:20.
36. Weinstein SM. New pharmacological strategies in the management of cancer pain. *Cancer Invest.* 1998;16:94.
37. Hughes MA, Glass PSA, Jacobs JR. Context-sensitive half-time in multicompartment pharmacokinetic models for intravenous anesthetic drugs. *Anesthesiology.* 1992;76:334.
38. Neimkin RJ, May JWJ, Roberts J. Continuous axillary block through an indwelling Teflon catheter. *J Hand Surg [Am].* 1984;9:830.
39. Unnerstall JR, Kopajtic TA, Kuhar MJ. Distribution of alpha 2 agonist binding sites in the rat and human central nervous system: analysis of some functional, anatomic correlates of the pharmacologic effects of clonidine and related adrenergic agents. *Brain Res Rev.* 1984;7:69.
40. Hyashi Y, Maze M. Alpha 2-adrenoceptor agonists and anaesthesia. *Br J Anaesth.* 1993;71:108.
41. Eisenach J, Detweiler D, Hood D. Hemodynamic and analgesic actions of epidurally administered clonidine. *Anesthesiology.* 1993;78:277.
42. De Kock M, Merello L, Pendeville P, et al. Does intraoperative clonidine administration promote the secretion of growth hormone in the perioperative period? *Acta Anaesthesiol Belg.* 1995;45:175.
43. Carabine UA, Milligan KR, Moore J. Extradural clonidine and bupivacaine for postoperative analgesia. *Br J Anaesth.* 1992;68:132.
44. Van Essen EJ, Bovill JG, Ploeger EJ. Epidural clonidine does not potentiate analgesia produced by extradural morphine after meniscectomy. *Br J Anaesth.* 1991;66:237.
45. Motsch J, Graber E, Ludwig K. Addition of clonidine enhances postoperative analgesia from epidural morphine: a double-blind study. *Anesthesiology.* 1990;73:1067.
46. Mogensen T, Eliasen K, Ejlersen E, et al. Epidural clonidine enhances postoperative analgesia from a combined low-dose epidural bupivacaine and morphine regimen. *Anesth Analg.* 1992;75:607.
47. Etches RC. Respiratory depression associated with patient-controlled analgesia: a review of eight cases. *Can J Anaesth.* 1994;41:125.

CHAPTER

# 72

# Laparoscopic Procedures

Timothy E. Morey
Donn H. Dennis

## GENERAL CONSIDERATIONS
*What Is a Laparoscopic Procedure?*
*Why Is Carbon Dioxide Selected to Distend the Abdomen?*
*What Are the Physiologic Consequences of Carbon Dioxide Pneumoperitoneum?*

## MANAGEMENT OF ANESTHESIA
*What Are the Preoperative Considerations?*

## INTRAOPERATIVE CONSIDERATIONS
*Is General Anesthesia Required for Laparoscopic Surgery?*
*How Is General Anesthesia Conducted?*
*Is a Laryngeal Mask Airway Appropriate?*

## UNIQUE PATIENT POPULATIONS
*Are There Special Differences for Pediatric Patients?*
*Do Laparoscopic Procedures Cause Less Morbidity and Mortality in Sick Patients?*

## COMPLICATIONS
*What Properties of Laparoscopic Procedures Lead to Significant Complications?*

## ECONOMIC, SOCIAL, AND LEGAL ISSUES
*Are Laparoscopic Procedures More Economical?*
*Do Laparoscopic Procedures Require More Operative Time?*
*What Are the Benefits to Society?*
*Does Caring for Patients Undergoing Laparoscopy Represent a Unique Legal Risk to Anesthesiologists?*

Laparoscopy for abdominal and pelvic procedures has been used since the 1960s. Gynecologists pioneered its widespread use for surgery of pelvic organs in the 1970s. More recently, general surgeons have embraced laparoscopy for many surgeries, and this method is now commonly employed not only in large urban medical centers but also in smaller community hospitals. The popularity of the procedure has expanded to include a diverse spectrum of procedures in several surgical subspecialties (Table 72–1). In fact, about 11% of all operations performed by general surgeons use laparoscopy.[1]

In part, migration to laparoscopic techniques is the result of significant postoperative benefits accruing from fewer complications associated with similar open procedures that require larger skin incisions and, more importantly, surgical division of muscle. Furthermore, shorter hospital stays for patients after laparoscopy compared with similar open surgery reap

**TABLE 72–1.** Representative Types of Operations That Can Be Performed Using Laparoscopic Technology

| Surgical Subspecialty | Laparoscopic Procedure |
|---|---|
| General surgery | Adrenalectomy |
| | Appendectomy |
| | Cholecystectomy |
| | Colectomy |
| | Diagnostic laparoscopy |
| | Gastric bypass |
| | Inguinal herniorrhaphy |
| | Jejunostomy |
| | Lysis of adhesions |
| | Liver biopsy |
| | Nissen fundoplication |
| | Pheochromocytoma resection |
| Gynecologic surgery | Bilateral tubal interruption |
| | Diagnostic laparoscopy |
| | Endometriosis ablation |
| | Lysis of adhesions |
| | Oophorectomy and removal of ovarian cysts |
| | Pronuclear-stage transfer of embryos |
| | Salpingectomy |
| | Vaginal hysterectomy |
| Neurologic surgery | Ventriculoperitoneal shunt revision |
| Pediatric surgery | Appendectomy |
| | Colectomy |
| | Diagnostic laparoscopy |
| | Enteroscopy |
| | Gastropexy |
| | Intussusception resection |
| | Meckel's diverticulum resection |
| | Neovaginal construction |
| | Nephrectomy |
| | Ovarian tubal torsion resection |
| | Removal of foreign body in intestines |
| | Removal of teratoma |
| Urologic surgery | Nephrectomy |
| | Penile revascularization |

financial benefits for patients, their employers, and health care financing organizations. Because laparoscopy is now offered by many general, gynecologic, pediatric, and urologic surgeons, anesthesiologists caring for patients undergoing these types of operations should be knowledgeable of the specific benefits of laparoscopy, recognize the unique physiologic changes caused by insufflation, and anticipate the special hazards associated with this surgical technique.

## GENERAL CONSIDERATIONS

### What Is a Laparoscopic Procedure?

Laparoscopy is a surgical technique whereby organs, vessels, and other structures of the abdomen and pelvis are visualized and dissected by deploying a small video camera and surgical instruments through trocars inserted through small skin incisions in the abdominal wall. A trocar is a sharply pointed instrument with a large central lumen for passage of gas, instruments, organs, and other tissues (Figs. 72–1 and 72–2). The image is displayed on a high-resolution video monitor and allows the surgeon to navigate within these cavities and to dissect organs and tissues using blunt and sharp instruments, electrocautery, and lasers (Fig. 72–3). Because the organs and tissues of the abdomen and pelvis are tightly packed, insufflation of this cavity with carbon dioxide during laparoscopy is usually required to elevate the anterior abdominal wall in order to allow adequate visualization of abdominal contents before examination and dissection. To introduce carbon dioxide, a Veress needle is placed blindly through the abdominal wall, usually at the umbilicus. Alternatively, surgeons may perform a minilaparotomy to insert a trocar under direct vision and thereby mitigate the risk for

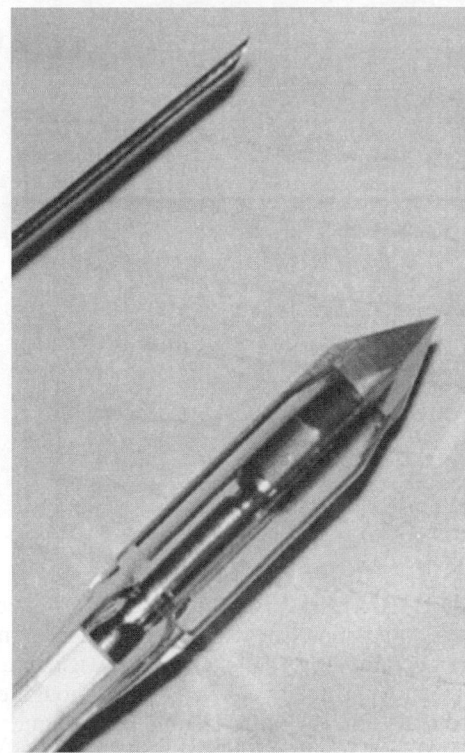

**FIGURE 72–2.** A detailed view of the sharp, Quicke-like point of the Veress needle (*uppermost*) and the pyramidal, sharp end of a 12-mm trocar (*lowermost*). Even a small laceration (1-2 mm) of a vessel may provide a conduit for carbon dioxide entry into the venous vasculature, whereas a large puncture by a trocar may cause massive hemorrhage necessitating rapid conversion to laparotomy to control life-threatening bleeding.

visceral or vascular puncture. Thereafter, an insufflator designed specifically for laparoscopic operations pumps carbon dioxide until an intraabdominal pressure of 8 to 12 mm Hg is achieved at about 4 L of total gas volume (Fig. 72–4).

After the abdomen is ballooned, a camera trocar of 10- to 12-mm diameter is inserted, followed by two or more smaller trocars (5-mm diameter), to allow passage of surgical instruments. Usually, the smaller trocars pass through the abdominal wall under the surgeon's direct vision by use of the video camera. Under good conditions, excellent visualization and color fidelity of abdominal contents are displayed on video monitors. Given the additional bulky equipment required to perform laparoscopy compared with open procedures, proper placement of the equipment requires careful thought to ensure sterility, to provide adequate lines of sight between surgeons and video monitors, to allow foot traffic in the operating room in the event of emergency, and to prevent positional injuries to patients.

### Why Is Carbon Dioxide Selected to Distend the Abdomen?

The ideal gas for abdominal insufflation would be physiologically inert, nonflammable, inexpensive, easily acquired, relatively absorbable by abdominal tissue, and soluble in blood so that it allows rapid pulmonary excretion and thereby minimizes potentially life-threatening effects if embolized into the venous vasculature.[2] Several different gases have been proposed for laparoscopy, including carbon dioxide, nitrous

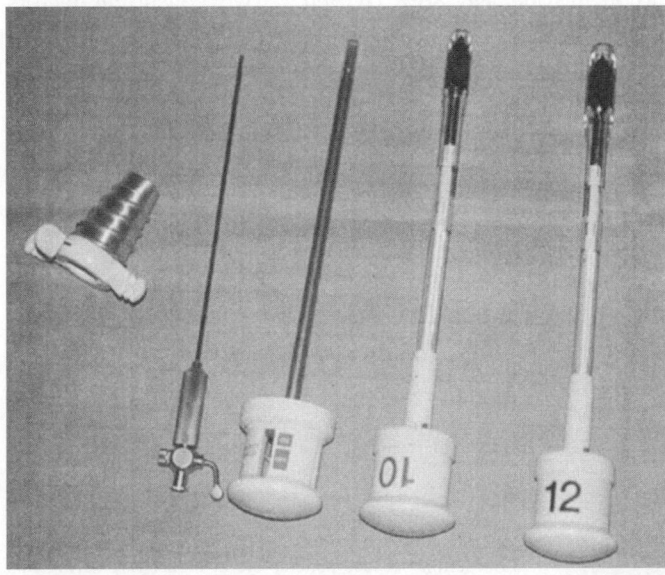

**FIGURE 72–1.** From left to right are shown examples of a screwlike insertion device, a Veress needle, and trocars of various sizes used for carbon dioxide insufflation or passage of a video camera and instruments through the abdominal wall. Note that the Veress needle and trocars of 5-, 10-, and 12-mm diameters are sharp instruments that may be inserted blindly and thereby potentially damage internal organs and blood vessels. Alternatively, some surgeons may wish to use the screwlike port introducer after a minilaparotomy to obviate possible damage from trocar insertion.

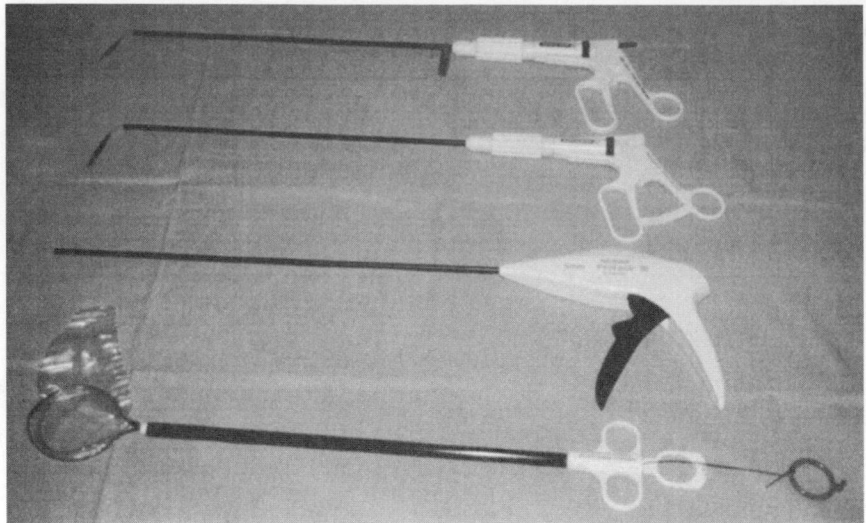

**FIGURE 72–3.** Shown are examples of several surgical instruments used for dissection and manipulation of abdominal contents during laparoscopic procedures. These tools pass through the abdominal wall by means of a 5-mm or larger laparoscopic port. From top to bottom, these instruments are minishears with unipolar electrocautery, a grasping instrument, an endoscopic suturing device, and an endoscopic disposable specimen pouch used to deliver specimens (eg, gall bladder) from the abdominal cavity to the external surgical field.

oxide, argon, and helium. Rarely, pneumoperitoneum may be avoided for operations in which constant suctioning and irrigation is required (eg, hemorrhage) by using a special surgical retractor to lift the abdominal wall, although exposure is inferior to that achieved with pneumoperitoneum.[3–8]

Carbon dioxide is used routinely for abdominal insufflation because it fulfills many of the qualifications previously specified. The primary drawbacks of carbon dioxide are its rapid absorption by abdominal viscera and tissue in conjunction with the possibility of poor pulmonary exchange with resultant adverse physiologic effects, such as hypercarbia (see further discussion later). Nitrous oxide has several desirable qualities for laparoscopy, including relative physiologic inertness, minimal cost, widespread availability, and possibly superior postoperative analgesia.[9,10] Unfortunately, nitrous oxide is an oxidizing agent and may contribute to intraabdominal combustion in the presence of a spark (eg, laser or electrocautery) and a fuel source (eg, methane).[11]

Neuman and colleagues studied the flammability of two endogenously produced bowel gases, hydrogen and methane, in a mixture of nitrous oxide and carbon dioxide and determined that concentrations of nitrous oxide as low as 29% could support combustion of hydrogen[11] (Fig. 72–5). Indeed, several cases of fatal explosions during laparoscopy have been documented and attributed to ignition of native gases in the oxidizing presence of nitrous oxide.[12–15] Helium and argon are noble gases that do not support combustion and cause less physiologic aberrations (eg, hypotension, respiratory acidosis) than does carbon dioxide during abdominal insufflation. When compared with carbon dioxide, however, helium and argon not only induce greater hemodynamic depression if embolized into venous vasculature but also cause death at much smaller volumes than does carbon dioxide[2,16,17] (Fig. 72–6). For these reasons, carbon dioxide remains the most commonly used, safest agent for abdominal insufflation during laparoscopy.

Anesthesiologists, however, should be certain that carbon dioxide is indeed encased in the gas tank linked to the insufflator. Greilich and associates described an intraabdominal explosion in a patient undergoing laparoscopic cholecystectomy after mistaken insufflation with a gas mixture of 14% carbon dioxide and 86% oxygen.[18] Two concurrent factors accounted for this identification error. First, a metal collar obscured the small section of the gas tank painted green (ie, designating the presence of oxygen), so that only the gray portion (ie, designating presence of carbon dioxide) was observable (Fig. 72–7). More disturbingly, the pin index configuration for any gas tank containing greater than 7% carbon dioxide is identical irrespective of the fraction and type

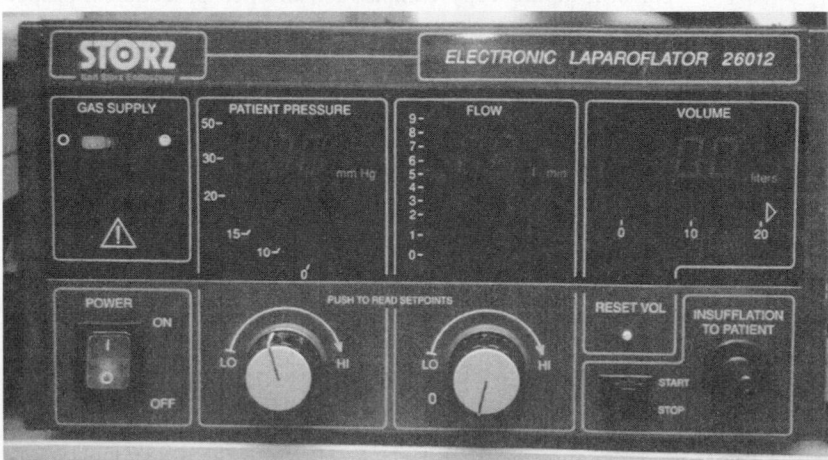

**FIGURE 72–4.** Laparoscopic procedures necessitate additional equipment in the operating room, including a cart holding an insufflating device with a carbon dioxide source. On this "laparoflator," note the prominent display of abdominal pressure, flow rate, and total volume of carbon dioxide delivered. Anesthesiologists may wish to observe the pressures, gas flow, and pressure during the initial insufflation because patients are at higher risk during this setup phase and because abnormally high values may indicate a misplaced Veress needle in a vessel, organ, or subcutaneous tissue.

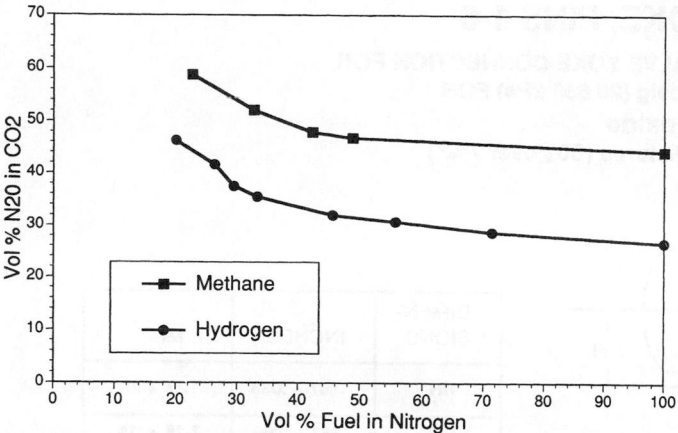

**FIGURE 72–5.** Flammability curves of methane and hydrogen, two gases native to the abdomen, are shown. The percentage of nitrous oxide in carbon dioxide is plotted against the percentage of fuel in nitrogen that supported combustion. Therefore, for a given fuel, the combinations of fuel and oxidizer that lie above and to the right of the curve are capable of supporting combustion. For example, the concentration of nitrous oxide necessary to support 50% hydrogen is about 32%. If nitrous oxide were used for insufflation, concentrations of methane and hydrogen needed to produce combustion would be as small as 20%. (Reprinted with permission from Neuman GG, Sidebotham G, Negoianu E, et al. Laparoscopy explosion hazards with nitrous oxide. *Anesthesiology.* 1993;78:877.)

of the balancing gas, 86% oxygen in this particular case (Fig. 72–8).

### What Are the Physiologic Consequences of Carbon Dioxide Pneumoperitoneum?

Creation of a carbon dioxide pneumoperitoneum causes important physiologic changes in several organ systems not only because of the physical pressure created in the abdomen but also because this gas is readily absorbed by the peritoneum. Although pulmonary and cardiovascular changes are of primary interest, manifestations in the liver, kidneys, central nervous system, and endocrine axis are also important.

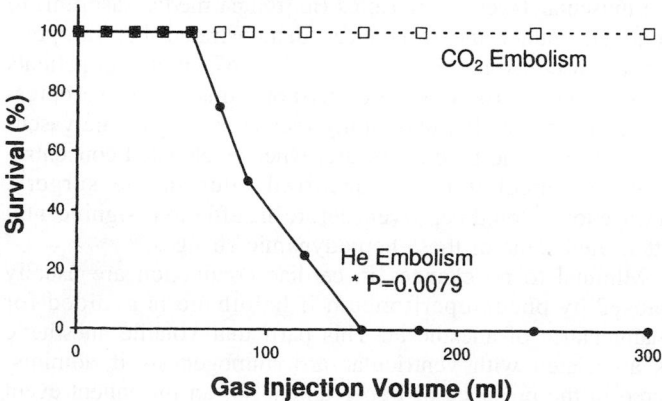

**FIGURE 72–6.** Survival curves for swine subjected to carbon dioxide or helium injected at various rates into the venous vasculature. The lethality of helium was uniform because no animal survived beyond a 120-mL injection compared with carbon dioxide embolism. (Reprinted with permission from Rudston-Brown B, Draper PN, Warriner B, et al. Venous gas embolism: a comparison of carbon dioxide and helium in pigs. *Can J Anaesth.* 1997;44:1104.)

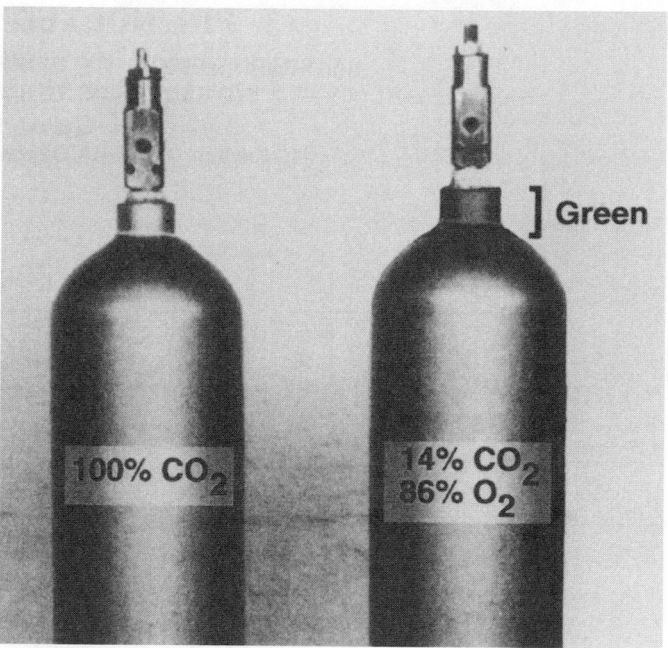

**FIGURE 72–7.** Comparison of 100% carbon dioxide tank (*left*) and 14% carbon dioxide tank (*right*) with a balance of 86% oxygen. Note the green band at the top of the cylinder on the right that denoted the presence of oxygen was covered by a metal collar during the operation. (From Greilich PE, Greilich NB, Froelich EG. Intraabdominal fire during laparoscopic cholecystectomy. *Anesthesiology.* 1995;83:871.)

### Pulmonary

Characteristically, end-tidal carbon dioxide (ie, arterial carbon dioxide tension) rises during pneumoperitoneum. This phenomenon is both time dependent, with plateau values achieved after 15 to 20 minutes, and a function of the patient's American Society of Anesthesiologists (ASA) physical status categorization. That is, the arterial carbon dioxide pressure in ASA II and III patients increased about 3-fold more than that determined in ASA I patients after carbon dioxide insufflation. Although not completely understood, the rapid rise in arterial and end-tidal carbon dioxide after creation of pneumoperitoneum is accounted for by at least two factors: (1) changes in pulmonary dynamics, and (2) absorption of carbon dioxide from the abdomen into the blood.

The increased intraabdominal pressure causes several important changes in the lungs of patients undergoing laparoscopy. Insufflation forces the diaphragm cephalad, compromises inferior pulmonary excursion, and thereby reduces both static and dynamic pulmonary compliance and increases dead space ventilation. If ventilation is not controlled, these changes are primarily mitigated by a more frequent respiratory rate, but end-tidal carbon dioxide concentrations still rise. If controlled ventilation is employed, an increase in minute volume is required to maintain a constant end-tidal carbon dioxide concentration and prevent occurrence of a respiratory acidosis (pH ≈ 7.30) that would otherwise occur. In addition, the displacement of the diaphragm may cause an endotracheal tube previously in the trachea to be forced into a mainstem bronchus[19] (Fig. 72–9).

### Cardiovascular

The cardiac and systemic hemodynamic consequences of abdominal insufflation have been well described, although the

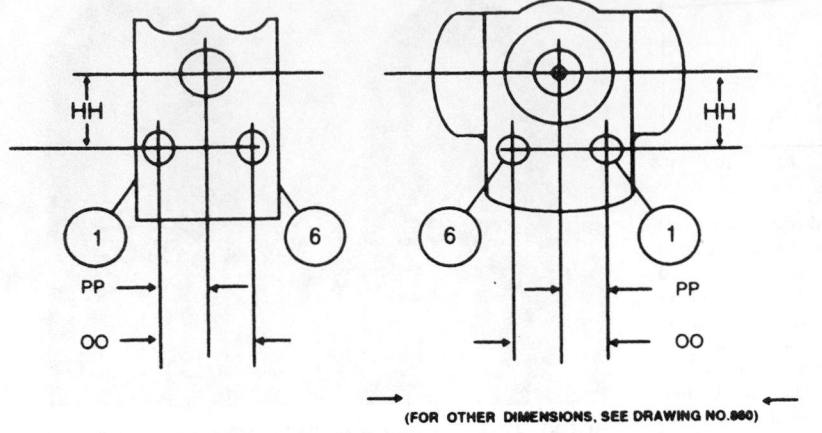

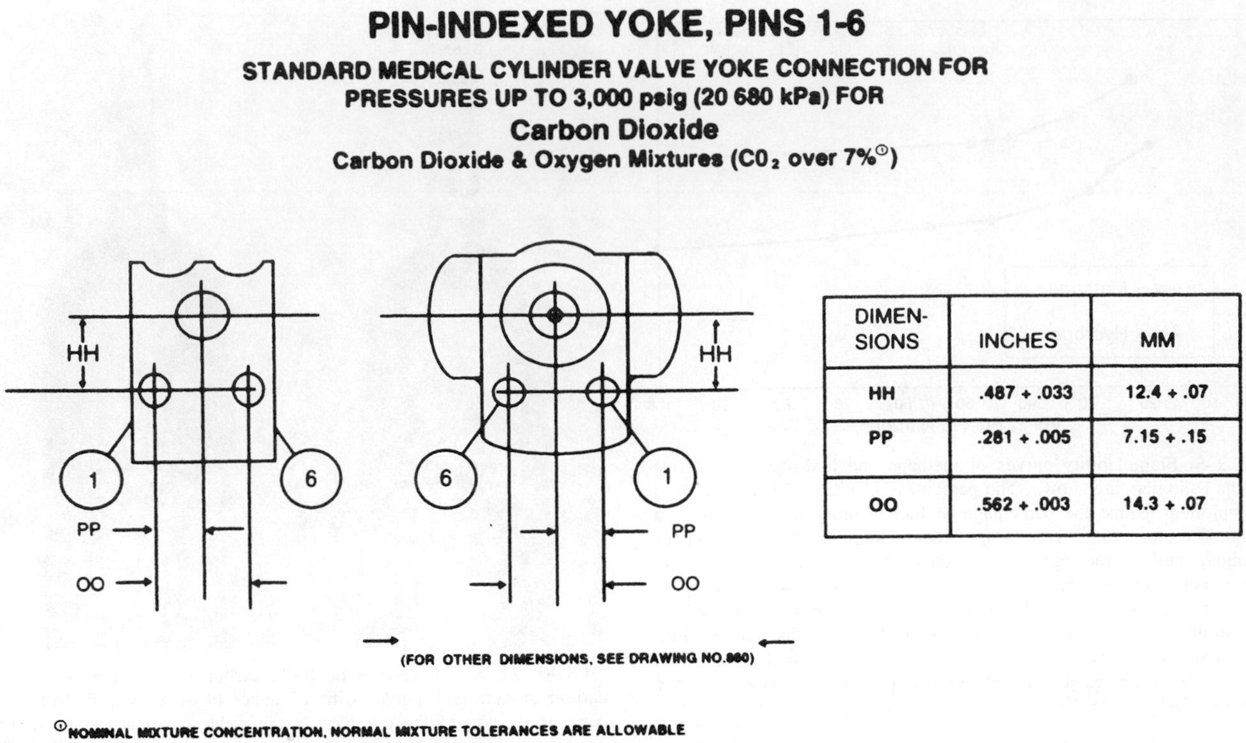

## PIN-INDEXED YOKE, PINS 1-6
### STANDARD MEDICAL CYLINDER VALVE YOKE CONNECTION FOR
### PRESSURES UP TO 3,000 psig (20 680 kPa) FOR
### Carbon Dioxide
### Carbon Dioxide & Oxygen Mixtures (CO₂ over 7%ⓞ)

| DIMEN-SIONS | INCHES | MM |
|---|---|---|
| HH | .487 + .033 | 12.4 + .07 |
| PP | .281 + .005 | 7.15 + .15 |
| OO | .562 + .003 | 14.3 + .07 |

(FOR OTHER DIMENSIONS, SEE DRAWING NO.860)

ⓞNOMINAL MIXTURE CONCENTRATION, NORMAL MIXTURE TOLERANCES ARE ALLOWABLE

**FIGURE 72–8.** Diagram of the Compressed Gas Association (CGA) specifications for tanks containing greater than 7% carbon dioxide (CGA 940). The diagram on the right specifies the dimensions of the inlet valve located on the carbon dioxide collar. The diagram on the left specifies the dimensions of the outlet valve located on the carbon dioxide cylinder yolk. (From Greilich PE, Greilich NB, Froelich EG. Intraabdominal fire during laparoscopic cholecystectomy. *Anesthesiology.* 1995;83:871.)

exact mechanisms whereby these events occur are not clearly understood. As shown by Joris and others, pneumoperitoneum increases systemic blood pressure (≈35%) and systemic vascular resistance (≈65%), but significantly decreases cardiac index (≈20%).[20] Furthermore, the magnitude of change is directly proportional to degree of insufflation pressure used to expand the abdomen. Whereas venous return diminishes during creation of pneumoperitoneum, atrial and ventricular filling pressures increase. This seemingly paradoxical observation may reflect increased intrathoracic pressure secondary to abdominal insufflation. Regardless, pressure data from central venous or pulmonary artery catheters to assess left ventricular loading volumes indirectly should be interpreted cautiously in patients undergoing laparoscopy.

The mechanism by which laparoscopy causes these cardiovascular effects is not clearly delineated but depends partly on elevated concentrations of vasopressin, an endogenous hormone released by the posterior lobe of the pituitary gland. Also called antidiuretic hormone (ADH), this substance causes the muscular layer of arterioles (ie, tunica media vasorum) to contract. Walder and Aitkenhead demonstrated that vasopressin increased from 1.5 ± 0.5 to 123 ± 47 pmol/L in patients undergoing laparoscopy.[21] Furthermore, this rise in vasopressin tended to parallel temporally increases in systemic vascular resistance and blood pressure, whereas elevated concentrations of catecholamines occurred later in the surgery. Intravenous clonidine, given before insufflation, significantly attenuated some of these hemodynamic changes.[20]

Minimal to no changes in cardiac conduction are usually caused by pneumoperitoneum if halothane is avoided for maintenance of anesthesia. This particular volatile anesthetic is associated with ventricular arrhythmogenesis if administered in the presence of hypercapnia, not an infrequent event during carbon dioxide insufflation (Fig. 72–10). Although rare, traction on peritoneal tissue can enhance efferent vagal traffic to the sinus node and slow or abolish spontaneous rhythm. Little data are available regarding the effects of pneumoperitoneum on other indices of cardiac conduction, such as dromotropism and repolarization.

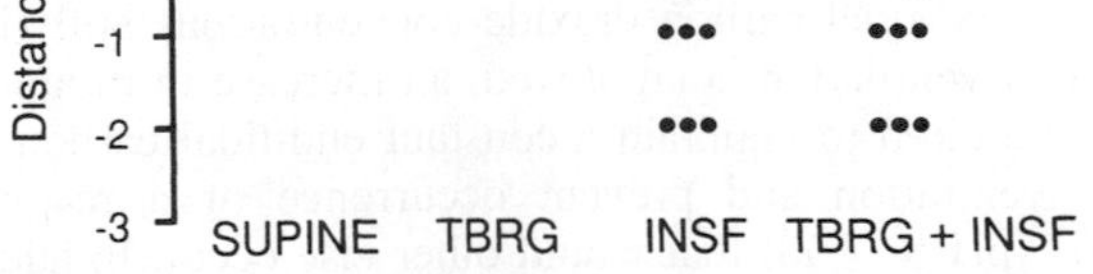

**FIGURE 72–9.** Effects of insufflation and positional changes on the distance from the endotracheal tube to the carina. *Closed circles* represent individual measurements. *Horizontal bars* represent mean values. Negative values indicate endotracheal tube migration into a primary bronchus (ie, mainstem intubation). ETT, endotracheal tube; INSF, postabdominal insufflation of carbon dioxide; TBRG, Trendelenburg position. (From Lobato EB, Paige GB, Brown MM, et al. Pneumoperitoneum as a risk factor for endobronchial intubation during laparoscopic gynecologic surgery. *Anesth Analg.* 1998;86:302.)

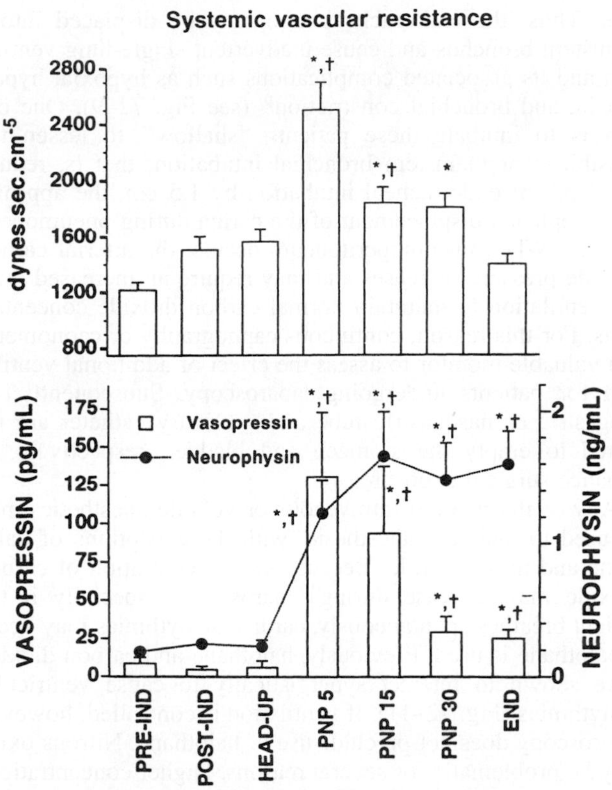

## Systemic vascular resistance

**FIGURE 72–10.** Increased concentrations of vasopressin and neurophysin accompany changes in systemic vascular resistance measured during laparoscopic procedures. PRE-IND, prior to anesthetic induction; POST-IND, 10 min after anesthetic induction; HEAD-UP, 10 min after tilting patient into a 10 head-up position; PNP5, PNP15, and PNP30, 5, 15, and 30 min, respectively, after initiation of abdominal insufflation; END, 30 min after exsufflation. Each point is mean ± SEM of 20 patients undergoing elective laparoscopic cholecystectomy and receiving isoflurane anesthesia. (Reprinted with permission from the American College of Cardiology [*Journal of the American College of Cardiology*, 1998, Vol 32, 1389].)

### Abdominal and Retroperitoneal Organs

The pressure generated by the pneumoperitoneum diminishes blood flow to a number of intraabdominal and retroperitoneal organs, including the kidneys, liver, and gut. In part, the physical pressure of the pneumoperitoneum may compress capillaries in these organs. In addition, humoral mediators, such as renin, could contribute to diminished renal perfusion. The functional consequence of this diminished blood flow to the kidneys resulted in a urinary output of only $0.01 \pm 0.03$ mL/kg/h, compared with $0.85 \pm 0.4$ mL/kg/h in patients undergoing laparoscopic surgery using carbon dioxide pneumoperitoneum or an abdominal wall lift retractor, respectively. Likewise, Koivusalo and colleagues found a significantly greater concentration of $N$-acetyl-β-D-glucosaminidase, an indicator of acute necrosis of the proximal renal tubules, in the patients randomized to the pneumoperitoneum limb of the study.[22] Similar types of findings were observed for organs perfused by other vascular beds, including hepatic, gastric, and mesenteric vessels. One must consider the findings of these studies, however, in the context of clinical care and the absence or paucity of reports detailing renal, hepatic, or intestinal failure after a laparoscopic procedure despite a rapid growth in the frequency of this surgical technique.

### Central Nervous System

Laparoscopy causes increased intracranial pressure.[23] Two mechanisms have been proposed to account for this rise in intracranial pressure: (1) impaired venous return of the lumbar venous plexus and head caused by increased intraabdominal pressure and Trendelenburg positioning, respectively; and (2) increased intracranial flow due to elevated arterial carbon dioxide tensions after abdominal insufflation. For example, intracranial pressure increased from $14 \pm 2$ to $39 \pm 4$ mm Hg when swine were subjected to both 15-mm Hg abdominal pressure during insufflation with carbon dioxide and Trendelenburg position.[24] Probably, both mechanisms account for this rise in intracranial pressure because either insufflation with helium[25] or variation in minute ventilation to keep arterial carbon dioxide pressures constant[26] only partly attenuates increases in intracranial pressure. Notwithstanding these laboratory findings, laparoscopy has been used to assist placement of the peritoneal end of ventriculoperitoneal shunts in patients with preexisting elevated intracranial pressure.[27] Similarly, laparoscopy is used as a screening tool for abdominal injuries in patients suffering trauma who may also have concurrent intracranial injuries.[28] Given the reported safety of procedures in these two patient groups, elevated intracranial pressure does not preclude use of laparoscopy, although more detailed human studies would be useful to delineate this issue further.

## MANAGEMENT OF ANESTHESIA

### What Are the Preoperative Considerations?

As with all patients receiving an anesthetic, a thoughtful preoperative evaluation facilitates delivery of a safe, uneventful anesthetic and prevents or mitigates perioperative medical complications. Given the physiologic effects of carbon dioxide pneumoperitoneum, this evaluation should consider those special factors that contribute to morbidity and mortality in patients undergoing laparoscopy. Specifically, several factors influence the risk that a vessel or organ will be punctured during insertion of the Veress needle or larger trocar that encases the video camera. That is, patients with distorted abdominal anatomy (eg, obesity, prior abdominal surgery with adhesions) are at higher risk for experiencing this complication. In addition, the experience and skill of the surgeon significantly influences this risk. For patients at higher risk for vascular damage, we insert an additional 16-gauge intravenous cannula after induction of anesthesia to provide large-bore access for blood transfusion in the event of vascular perforation.

### INTRAOPERATIVE CONSIDERATIONS

### Is General Anesthesia Required for Laparoscopic Surgery?

Although others have used local or regional techniques, general anesthesia is preferred to anesthetize patients undergoing laparoscopic surgery at my institution for multiple reasons. First, carbon dioxide insufflates the entire abdomen, including the inferior aspect of the diaphragms, and may cause significant discomfort or pain. Because the phrenic nerves originate from the nerve roots of the third, fourth, and fifth cervical vertebrae, diaphragmatic pain is difficult to treat with local or regional anesthesia. Likewise, anesthesia for manipulation of abdominal organs and peritoneal traction may be difficult to achieve using local or regional anesthesia. Centrally acting intravenous agents (eg, narcotics, propofol) may provide mild-to-moderate analgesia but also will desensitize the respiratory drive centers of the medulla oblongata to the effects of increasing carbon dioxide concentrations that occur during laparoscopy and may impede spontaneous ventilation. Second, increased intraabdominal pressure and Trendelenburg positioning hinders spontaneous breathing and may compromise respiratory exchange. Third, muscular relaxation and an immobile operative field aid surgeons to perform a rapid, safe procedure without coughing, retching, or movement by the patient. Fourth, surgeons typically require that an orogastric or nasogastric tube and urinary catheter be inserted to empty the stomach or bladder, respectively, to obtain optimal exposure of abdominal organs. Although patients routinely accept these gastric and bladder catheters in emergency rooms and hospital wards, placement is an additional discomfort that may be avoided by general anesthesia.

Finally, university-based hospitals are postgraduate training facilities for neophyte surgeons who may not yet have acquired the skill and efficiency necessary to complete a laparoscopic procedure in the timely manner necessary for patients experiencing laparoscopy under local or regional anesthesia. For these reasons, nearly all the laparoscopic procedures conducted at our institution are performed under general anesthesia. Laparoscopic gastrostomy, jejunostomy, herniorrhaphy, and other minimal procedures, however, have been satisfactorily performed using local or regional anesthesia combined with intravenous sedation, although these patients may aspirate gastric contents more frequently than patients under general anesthesia.[29–31] Likewise, many gynecologic and other pelvic laparoscopic surgeries have been performed under spinal or epidural blockade with adverse effects when compared with cases done with general anesthesia.

## How Is General Anesthesia Conducted?

Anesthesiologists may safely select from a number of induction agents and neuromuscular antagonists provided these drugs are appropriate for concurrent patient disease and duration of surgery. Endotracheal intubation is the preferred technique to manage oxygenation and ventilation (see subsequent discussion of laryngeal mask airway). During laparoscopy, the diaphragm is displaced cephalad, whereas the endotracheal tube remains immobile owing to its fixation to the skin of the face. Thus, the endotracheal tube may be displaced into a mainstem bronchus and cause inadvertent single-lung ventilation and its associated complications such as hypoxia, hypercapnia, and bronchial constriction[19] (see Fig. 72–9). One option is to intubate these patients "shallow" to lessen the possibility of mainstem bronchial intubation; that is, reduce the depth of endotracheal intubation by 1.5 cm, the approximate cephalad displacement of the carina during pneumoperitoneum. When pneumoperitoneum occurs, the arterial carbon dioxide pressure increases and may require an increased minute ventilation to maintain normal carbon dioxide concentrations. For this reason, continuous capnography or capnometry is a valuable monitor to assess the effect of additional ventilation for patients undergoing laparoscopy. Subsequently, an orogastric or nasogastric tube and a urinary catheter are inserted to empty the stomach and bladder, respectively, to enhance surgical exposure.

Any of the modern intravenous or volatile anesthetics may be used to maintain anesthesia, with the exceptions of halothane and nitrous oxide. Because the concentration of carbon dioxide may increase during laparoscopy, especially if the patient breathes spontaneously, cardiac arrhythmias may occur if halothane is used. Previously, halothane and carbon dioxide were shown to interact synergistically to cause ventricular arrhythmias (Fig. 72–11). If ventilation is controlled, however, laparoscopy does not preclude use of halothane. Nitrous oxide may be problematic for several reasons. Higher concentrations of inspired nitrous oxide act as an oxidizing agent to fuel sources in the abdomen and may contribute to intraabdominal fire. Second, nitrous oxide may further exacerbate the incidence of postoperative nausea and vomiting after laparoscopy. Third, the propensity of nitrous oxide to diffuse into gas-filled cavities may cause the small bowel to increase in size and obscure surgical exposure and to expand any carbon dioxide that may have embolized into the venous vasculature. Fourth, both sevoflurane and desflurane possess blood-gas solubility constants similar to nitrous oxide and are useful alternative agents. For these reasons, avoidance of halothane and nitrous oxide seems prudent when anesthetizing patients for laparoscopic surgery. In addition, propofol should perhaps be avoided when anesthetizing women for pronuclear-stage transfer of embryos because this anesthetic results in a lower ongoing pregnancy rate (29%) when compared with isoflurane use (54%).[32]

## Is a Laryngeal Mask Airway Appropriate?

Use of laryngeal mask airways (LMA) during laparoscopic surgery remains controversial for two reasons. First, aspiration has been observed in patients in whom an LMA was used to

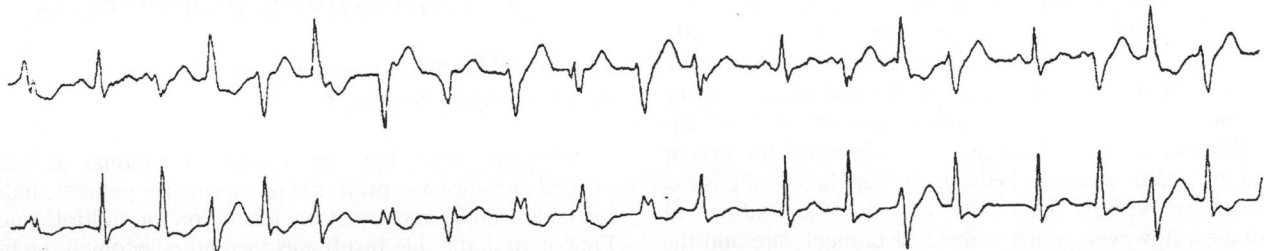

**FIGURE 72–11.** Two-channel electrocardiogram recorded from a patient receiving 1.3 MAC halothane and spontaneously breathing with an end-tidal carbon dioxide pressure of 56-61 mm Hg. Note the frequent ventricular contractions evident on this tracing. Conversion to controlled ventilation by means of an endotracheal tube with a reduction in carbon dioxide pressure to 32-34 mm Hg caused conversion to sinus tachycardia (data not shown).

control the airway.[33,34] Because the LMA does not partition the trachea from the esophagus as a cuffed endotracheal tube does, gastric contents may be more likely to be aspirated. In addition, peritoneal insufflation and Trendelenburg positioning may compress the stomach and thereby cause gastric contents to be expelled into the esophagus, with possible migration into the trachea. The possibility of tracheal aspiration, however, is mitigated by placement in the Trendelenburg position that allows dependent drainage of gastric contents. Second, if spontaneous ventilation is required, the LMA limits the maximum positive pressure to that pressure created by the seal in the posterior pharynx, about 20 mm Hg. Given the displacement of the diaphragm caused by intraabdominal pressure, 8 to 12 mm Hg, positive pressure ventilation may be compromised.

Notwithstanding these objections, several studies have addressed this issue, with varying conclusions regarding use of the LMA during laparoscopic procedures (Table 72–2). In the largest study, Verghese and Brimacombe surveyed medical records from two hospitals and determined that, during laparoscopic cholecystectomy (65 patients) or laparoscopic gynecologic procedures (1469 patients) under general anesthesia with an LMA, less than 0.14% of patients suffered a "critical event," defined to include airway regurgitation, vomiting, and aspiration of gastric contents.[35] Moreover, 44% of these patients were ventilated using positive pressure. Likewise, Bapat and Verghese investigated staining of LMAs placed in 100 patients who ingested methylene blue capsules before receiving general anesthesia for laparoscopic gynecologic operations.[36] Blue stains were noted in only one LMA removed from a patient who had regurgitated on induction, but before LMA placement. No complications were noted in other smaller studies of 15 to 60 patients, although the power of these investigations to detect infrequent complications is low.[37] Given these findings, use of an LMA may not be precluded by abdominal insufflation in the absence of other contraindications to LMA insertion.[38–41]

## UNIQUE PATIENT POPULATIONS

### Are There Special Differences for Pediatric Patients?

Pediatric surgeons have adopted laparoscopy to treat many conditions included in Table 72–1 plus some unique disorders

of childhood, such as intestinal intussusception. Compared with many investigations detailing anesthetic management of adult patients undergoing laparoscopic surgery,[42] few data are available for children beyond case presentations, including reports for patients younger than 12 months of age. Hsing and colleagues, however, did observe that end-tidal carbon dioxide pressure rises more rapidly and achieves plateau values sooner in younger (11-24 months of age) versus older (5-14 years of age) children during carbon dioxide insufflation.[43] Tobias and coauthors described the largest experience managing the anesthetic care of children for brief laparoscopic inspection (<15 min) of the peritoneum and noted small changes in end-tidal carbon dioxide tension ($32 \pm 3$ to $35 \pm 5$ mm Hg) and peak inflating pressures ($20 \pm 3$ to $23 \pm 3$ cm $H_2O$) after insufflation. Their findings regarding changes in blood pressure, heart rate, respiratory rate, and tidal volume are not always consistent but appear to be at least qualitatively similar to those in adult patients. For some of these children, face mask (20 patients) or laryngeal mask (15 patients) ventilation was used without apparent complication. Minimal to no data have been published regarding anesthetic management of patients undergoing longer laparoscopic procedures, except for one study that noted that the end-tidal carbon dioxide concentration overestimates the arterial carbon dioxide pressure.[44] As the horizons of laparoscopy expand to include routine use in children at community hospitals, more detailed consideration will be merited to achieve optimal care for our youngest patients.

### Do Laparoscopic Procedures Cause Less Morbidity and Mortality in Sick Patients?

Laparoscopic procedures clearly improve perioperative outcome for procedures such as cholecystectomy, donor nephrectomy, and other operations compared with open surgery. The primary advantages are less postoperative pain, preservation of diaphragmatic function, a lower frequency of postoperative ileus, shorter hospital stays, and others.[45] These benefits, however, have been observed in a largely healthy patient population (ie, ASA physical classification I and II). Sometimes, surgeons submit more ill patients (ASA III and IV) for operations with poorly justified assurances to patients and anesthesiologists that using a laparoscopic technique mitigates the adverse effects of surgery and anesthesia. Few data and mini-

**TABLE 72–2.** Detection of Esophageal Regurgitation or Tracheal Aspiration of Gastric Contents in Patients Undergoing Laparoscopic Surgery With a Laryngeal Mask Airway

| Investigators | Patient Type (#) | Surgery Type | End Points (Number Detected/Number Observed) |
|---|---|---|---|
| Verghese and Brimacombe, 1996[35] | Adults (1534) | Gynecologic Cholecystectomy | Airway regurgitation, vomiting, or aspiration of gastric contents ($\leq$7/1534) |
| Bapat and Verghese, 1997[36] | Women (100) | Gynecologic | Methylene blue staining of LMA (1/100); methylene blue staining of trachea by visualization with fiberoptic bronchoscopy (0/30); esophageal pH < 4.0 (0/91) |
| Swann et al, 1993[38] | Women (30) | Gynecologic | Regurgitation (0/30) |
| Goodwin et al, 1992[39] | Women (40) | Day stay | Clinical aspiration (0/40) |
| Ho et al, 1998[40] | Women (30) | Day stay | Esophageal pH < 4.0 (0/15) |
| Skinner et al, 1998[39] | Women (30) | Day stay | Esophageal pH < 4.0 (4/30); 3 mechanically and 1 spontaneously ventilated |
| Tobias et al, 1996[37] | Children (15) | Brief, diagnostic laparoscopy | (0/15) |

*Verghese and Brimacombe[34] reported 7 cases of regurgitation, vomiting, and aspiration in 11 910 patients managed with a laryngeal mask airway but did not categorize these adverse events into laparoscopic or open procedures.

mal to no prospective, randomized, outcome-based trials are available comparing laparoscopic and open procedures in this more seriously ill patient population. These limited studies of 13 to 22 patients indicate that those who are ASA class III and IV have hemodynamic and respiratory changes caused by pneumoperitoneum similar to those observed in healthier patients and that laparoscopic procedures can be safely performed for the sicker patients. As with other interventions, such as drug administration and fluid administration, anesthesiologists might be prudent to mitigate the effects of interventions by reducing the rate of abdominal insufflation with carbon dioxide and restricting the maximum angle of Trendelenburg position.

## COMPLICATIONS

### What Properties of Laparoscopic Procedures Lead to Significant Complications?

#### Morbidity and Mortality

A number of surveys have been conducted to determine the complications that may occur as a result of laparoscopic procedures (Table 72–3). Large national registries in Finland (32 205 patients),[46] France (22 966 patients),[47] and The Netherlands (25 764 patients)[48] are the most informative reports owing to their statistical power, and detail overall complication rates of 4.0 to 5.7 per 1000 laparoscopic procedures, a morbidity rate similar to that described for open procedures such as cholecystectomy. The complication rate is higher for operative (12.6 per 1000 cases) than for diagnostic (0.6 per 1000 procedures) laparoscopy.[46] Furthermore, laparoscopic hysterectomy entailed the greatest relative risk for injury to the ureter (risk ratio, 29.0; 95% confidence interval [CI], 23.3, 63.0), bladder (risk ratio, 13.0; CI 6.0, 28.2), and intestines (risk ratio, 1.3; CI 0.6, 2.5).[46] In addition, previous abdominal surgery and lack of surgical experience are independent pre-

dictors of an intraoperative complication requiring conversion to laparotomy.[48]

Overall, many complications are overlooked during laparoscopic operations and become apparent only in the postoperative period. For example, 28.6% (36 of 139 patients) of complications in the French registry were noted after laparoscopy and included urologic, vascular, and bowel injuries. Because anesthesiologists frequently continue caring for patients in the postanesthesia care unit, they should maintain a high degree of suspicion for inadvertent, unrecognized injury in these patients when constructing differential diagnosis of postoperative problems. Although infrequent, two dreaded complications listed in Table 72–3 lead to rapid deterioration and possibly death in patients undergoing laparoscopic procedures. For this reason, the diagnosis and treatment of carbon dioxide venous embolism and hemorrhage are detailed subsequently.

### Carbon Dioxide Venous Embolus

Embolism of gas into the venous vasculature during laparoscopic procedures was first reported in 1951.[49] Although embolism is a rare event, occurring on the order of 15 per 113 253 cases,[50] rapid physiologic decompensation and death may occur unless both the surgeon and anesthesiologist quickly intercede not only to eliminate further embolism but also to treat the cardiovascular collapse caused by the carbon dioxide embolus. Similar to entrainment of air into veins, embolization of carbon dioxide requires the concurrent presence of two conditions: (1) an opening in a vein, and (2) a pressure gradient to drive the gas from the intraabdominal cavity into the venous vasculature.

Laceration of veins occurs during introduction of the pneumoperitoneum needle, during subsequent trocar placement, or later during sharp dissection or electrocautery. The blood vessels most commonly injured during laparoscopic procedures include the distal aorta and its immediate ramifications and associated veins (eg, common iliac vessels) as well as the epigastric, mesenteric, and hepatic vessels.[51,52] Risk factors associated with an increased incidence of vascular injury include patient characteristics that complicate primary cannula insertion (eg, obesity, prior abdominal surgery, distorted anatomy)[53,54] and a surgeon with limited experience (ie, fewer than 100 cases) performing laparoscopic procedures.[55] Of note, the physical dimension of the vasculature opening required to introduce a lethal volume of carbon dioxide may be minimal ($\approx$0.1 cm).[56] That is, a simple perforation of a vein with a Veress needle may produce a sufficiently large conduit for carbon dioxide to egress from the abdomen into the vasculature. In addition, if the patient is placed in Trendelenburg position and the veins are partially compressed owing to abdominal insufflation, a small perforation may not be recognized until frank symptoms of carbon dioxide embolus occur.

Because pressure is required to pump carbon dioxide into the abdomen and lift the anterior abdominal wall to facilitate visualization of organs, the pressure gradient needed for gas embolization is always present during laparoscopy. The recommended pressure used to insufflate the abdomen is 5 to 15 mm Hg. In swine, higher gas pressures (eg, 25-30 mm Hg) and flow rates enhance the possibility that a venous embolism will occur.[57] Although vessel laceration may occur during needle or trocar insertion, carbon dioxide embolus may occur

**TABLE 72–3.** Possible Perioperative Complications Caused by the Requirement for Pneumoperitoneum in Laparoscopic Surgery

| Causative Action | Complication |
| --- | --- |
| Carbon dioxide insufflation | Acid-base disorders from hypercarbia |
| | Cardiovascular abnormalities (eg, hypertension, arrhythmias, diminished cardiac output) |
| | Extraperitoneal insufflation (eg, subcutaneous emphysema, pneumomediastinum, pneumopericardium, pneumothorax, pneumoscrotum) |
| | Mainstem bronchial intubation |
| | Venous gas embolus |
| Needle and trocar insertion | Incisional hernia |
| | Infection |
| | Tumor seeding of peritoneum |
| | Vascular perforation (eg, terminal aorta and its branches, epigastric vessels) |
| | Visceral damage (eg, bile duct laceration, intestinal perforation, uterine injury) |
| Miscellaneous | Retention of foreign body due to limited visualization |
| | Positioning injuries (eg, sciatic neuropraxis) |

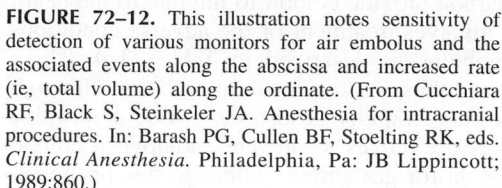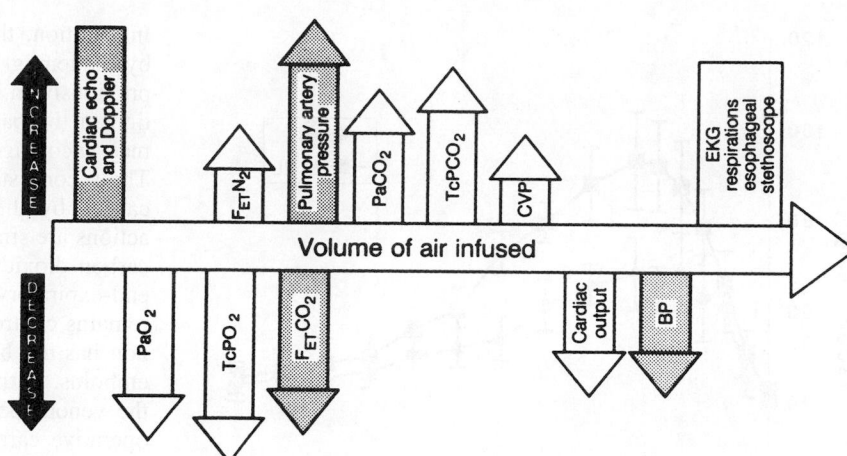

**FIGURE 72–12.** This illustration notes sensitivity of detection of various monitors for air embolus and the associated events along the abscissa and increased rate (ie, total volume) along the ordinate. (From Cucchiara RF, Black S, Steinkeler JA. Anesthesia for intracranial procedures. In: Barash PG, Cullen BF, Stoelting RK, eds. *Clinical Anesthesia*. Philadelphia, Pa: JB Lippincott; 1989:860.)

any time during the operation. Sharp dissection and electrocautery may also cause venous perforation, although the surgeon may be more likely to observe these events because dissection is performed under direct vision, in contrast to blind insertion of the Veress needle. Carbon dioxide emboli occurring after cessation of surgery may be observed as a result of occult accumulation of the gas in the portal circulation and subsequent migration to the heart with a positional change at the conclusion of surgery.[58]

Similar to other types of emboli, a carbon dioxide embolus may progress into the central circulation and cause significant hemodynamic aberrations, cardiovascular collapse, and death.[56,59] The physical findings used to diagnose carbon dioxide embolism are similar to those employed to detect venous embolism of air or thrombus (Fig. 72–12). Doppler techniques are by far the most sensitive indicators of embolic phenomena. Transesophageal echocardiography is an extremely sensitive monitor to detect material embolized into the right heart and can identify essentially all carbon dioxide emboli, even those with volumes as small as 0.1 mL/kg.[60] In fact, Derouin and colleagues observed carbon dioxide embolus in 11 of 16 patients undergoing laparoscopic cholecystectomy, although no concurrent cardiovascular compromise was noted.[61] Although transesophageal echocardiography is probably not indicated in the absence of other coexisting diseases (eg, congestive heart failure), precordial Doppler monitoring is a simpler and far less expensive method that may achieve a similar degree of sensitivity. In clinical practice, however, neither Doppler monitoring technique is routinely used given the low incidence of hemodynamically significant carbon dioxide embolism, the expense of equipment, and the requisite time needed to position monitors correctly while completing busy operating room schedules. Therefore, anesthesiologists must be prepared to confront late signs of carbon dioxide embolism that are caused by hemodynamic compromise and that may progress to cardiovascular collapse if untreated.

All of the late signs of carbon dioxide embolus are similar to those that occur with air embolus, a phenomenon more extensively studied. That is, anesthesiologists may observe (in increasing order of severity) rapid changes in end-tidal carbon dioxide concentrations, increased pulmonary artery pressures, decreased systemic blood pressure, a mill wheel murmur, hypoxia, cardiac arrhythmias, and death. Perhaps the only major distinguishing feature between carbon dioxide and air embolus is the change in end-tidal carbon dioxide. Whereas

this variable always decreases during venous air or thrombotic embolism, some controversy exists regarding its change during carbon dioxide embolism. Clinical evidence exists that demonstrates that end-tidal carbon dioxide concentrations increase during the early stages of carbon dioxide embolus but then decrease as more pulmonary dead space is created.[62,63] Shulman and Aronson observed an increase of end-tidal carbon dioxide from 3.8% to 4.2% in the early phase of embolus[63] (Fig. 72–13). If end-tidal carbon dioxide concentrations do rise during carbon dioxide embolus, this characteristic might serve as a diagnostic feature to distinguish this event from embolic events due to other material (eg, air or thrombus) or hemorrhage when determining the fundamental cause of any severe hypotension and shock that might occur in patients undergoing laparoscopic procedures. Great increases in carbon dioxide (eg, to 60-100 mm Hg) concentrations, however, are more likely caused by injection of the gas into subcutaneous tissue[64] (Fig. 72–14).

In contrast, other reports and some experimental data indicate that end-tidal carbon dioxide concentrations immediately decrease with carbon dioxide embolism even in the early phase of this event. That is, the carbon dioxide emboli exist as gaseous bubbles in blood. In this state, the carbon dioxide is not available for gaseous exchange in the lung. Therefore, the carbon dioxide embolus obstructs pulmonary blood flow

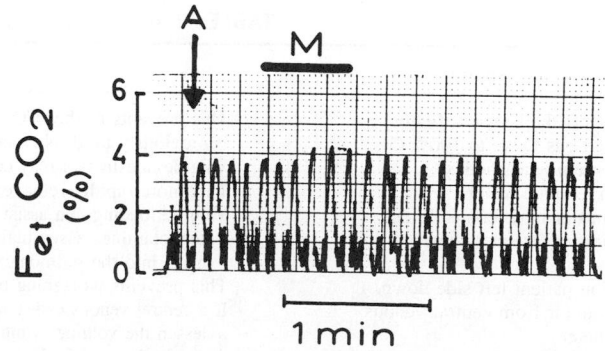

**FIGURE 72–13.** Illustration of an increase in end-tidal carbon dioxide concentration in a woman undergoing diagnostic laparoscopy. Fractional end-tidal carbon dioxide (percentage) versus time is shown. Insufflation of carbon dioxide started at the point denoted as *A*. A cardiac murmur was heard, and insufflation discontinued at the time indicated by *M*. (From Shulman D, Aronson HB. Capnography in the early diagnosis of carbon dioxide embolism during laparoscopy. *Can Anesth Soc J.* 1984;31:455.)

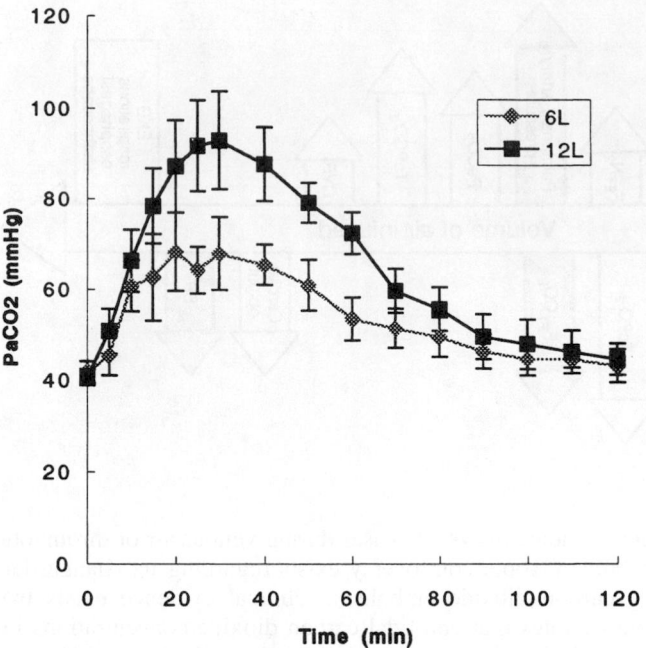

**FIGURE 72–14.** Effect of subcutaneous carbon dioxide insufflation on $Pa_{CO_2}$ measured in swine. From baseline $Pa_{CO_2}$ values of $41.8 \pm 2.3$ mm Hg, $Pa_{CO_2}$ peaked at $68.3 \pm 8.6$ and $92.9 \pm 10.7$ mm Hg for the 6- and 12-L volumes, respectively, 20 to 25 min after insufflation. (Reprinted from *American Journal of Surgery*, Vol 171, Rudston-Brown BC, MacLennan D, Warriner CB, et al. Effect of subcutaneous carbon dioxide insufflation on arterial $PCO_2$, 461, Copyright 1996, with permission from Excerpta Medica Inc.)

similar to embolic events owing to other substances, increases pulmonary dead space, and causes end-tidal carbon dioxide concentrations to decrease. Irrespective of the direction of changes in end-tidal carbon dioxide concentrations, further progression to cardiovascular collapse is similar to air or thrombotic embolism.

Once diagnosed, carbon dioxide embolism requires rapid treatment. The first step is to notify the surgeon and prevent further carbon dioxide entrance into the venous vasculature by abolishing the pressure gradient driving the gas. Therefore, the flow of carbon dioxide pumped by the insufflating device should be reduced to 0 L/min or powered to the off position.

In addition, the pressure gradient can be further diminished by flattening the operating room table if the patient was previously in Trendelenburg position, although further elevation of the patient's head and torso above a horizontal plane may encourage carbon dioxide emboli to migrate to the heart. The second step involves treatment of the adverse conditions caused by the embolus as described in Table 72–4. These actions are similar to those used to treat air embolus, although carbon dioxide is more rapidly absorbed.[62,65] Use of positive end-expiratory pressure valves to prevent paradoxical emboli remains controversial for gas emboli, although this phenomenon has not been specifically investigated for carbon dioxide embolus. If the patient survives the acute embolic event and the venous perforation is surgically corrected, attentive postoperative care in the surgical intensive care unit will be required.

## Hemorrhage

Major vascular injury is a serious complication feared by both surgeons and anesthesiologists because of the mortal danger to the patient's life, the requisite rapidity of diagnosis and treatment to prevent mortality, the associated morbidity such as conversion to an open operation, the high probability for transfusion of blood products, and the possibility of admission to the intensive care unit as well as a longer hospital stay. Fortunately, the frequency of these events is relatively low, with rates of 0.14 per 1000 patients in the United States,[66] and 0.1 to 0.4 per 1000 cases in large Finnish and French national registries that included 103 852 cases and 390 000 trocar insertions.[46,47,67] Vessels reportedly damaged during laparoscopy include the aorta, inferior vena cava, iliac vessels, portal vein, hypogastric artery, mesenteric vessels, and others.[52,68–70] Insertion of the Veress needle and trocars are, however, likely events during which vascular laceration may occur. For example, 76.5% of all injuries reported in the French registry occurred during the setup phase of laparoscopy when the insufflating needle and trocars were placed.[68] For this reason, alternative approaches to create a pneumoperitoneum have been advocated to decrease the incidence of vascular damage. Bonjer and associates used an open technique with a blunt needle to reduce the incidence of perforation from 0.075% of 489 335 patients to zero incidents in 12 444 pa-

**TABLE 72–4.** Treatment of Venous Carbon Dioxide Embolism

| Action | Justification |
| --- | --- |
| Power off the $CO_2$ insufflator. | This prevents further $CO_2$ from entering veins by abolishing the abdomen-to-vein pressure gradient. |
| Convert gas flows to 100% $O_2$. | If previously used, $N_2O$ can rapidly expand gaseous bubbles. Hypoxia is a late symptom of $CO_2$ embolism. |
| Discontinue anesthetics. | Volatile anesthetics may contribute to hypotension and paradoxical emboli. |
| Hyperventilate patient. | This more rapidly removes any $CO_2$ that dissolves into the blood. |
| Administer intravenous fluids. | Volume loading can assist ejection of gas from the heart into the lungs. |
| Administer catecholamines. | Catecholamines assist maintenance of peripheral blood pressure and may force embolized gas from the right heart into the pulmonary vessels. |
| Position patient left side down. | This prevents worsening of "gas lock" in the right ventricular outflow tract. |
| Aspirate air from central venous catheter. | If a central venous catheter near the right atrium is present, aspiration of foam will confirm the diagnosis and may lessen the volume of intravascular $CO_2$ embolus. Alternatively, consider inserting a central venous catheter. |
| Begin cardiopulmonary resuscitation. | Arrhythmias and prolonged hypotension compel anesthesiologists to begin advanced cardiac life support techniques. |
| Consider initiation of cardiopulmonary bypass. | If the resources are present, cardiopulmonary bypass may be useful to resuscitate patients recalcitrant to other treatments. Previously, Diakun successfully resuscitated a patient with a right atrial "gas lock" who otherwise would have died.[62] |
| Consider hyperbaric $O_2$ therapy. | If a hyperbaric chamber is available, high-pressure $O_2$ therapy may be useful to ameliorate any long-term neurologic dysfunction caused by paradoxical $CO_2$ emboli.[65] |

tients undergoing laparoscopic surgery.[71] Vascular injury is not limited to the Veress needle or trocar insertion, however, because subsequent use of scissors, probes, electrocautery, and lasers can also perforate vessels.[72] Although the surgeon is primarily responsible for preventing vascular damage, both anesthesiologists and surgeons must be vigilant to acknowledge these injuries rapidly if these mishaps do occur.

The key feature to saving patients with major vascular injury is early recognition by the operating room team. Whereas hemorrhage may be obvious if the field is flooded with blood, occult retroperitoneal bleeding may be insidious and is apparent only after significant hemodynamic decompensation or at autopsy. Unexplained hypotension unresponsive to fluid and mild vasopressor therapy (eg, ephedrine) is especially concerning during laparoscopy and may be an indication for termination of the procedure or conversion to laparotomy.[73] Other causes of hypotension during laparoscopy, however, must be considered in the differential diagnosis, such as pneumothorax, gas embolism, reverse Trendelenburg position, anesthetic overdose, and others.[45,73] For example, 12.9% of patients undergoing laparoscopic cholecystectomy developed intraoperative hypotension, defined as systolic blood pressure of less than 80 mm Hg for greater than 5 minutes or requiring fluid or vasopressor therapy.[74] The condition of the patient, index of suspicion for vascular damage, and other individual factors dictate the medical judgment made on a case-by-case basis regarding the proper course of action.

Although vessel laceration or puncture may be managed without conversion to open laparotomy, the occurrence of severe hypotension compels the team to locate and repair the site of damage quickly. While the surgeon explores the abdomen and pelvis, the anesthesiologist must act to restore intravascular volume and oxygen delivery with therapy similar to that used for patients with other types of penetrating trauma. Actions may include decreasing the depth of anesthesia, establishment of additional intravenous access, infusion of warmed fluid or packed red blood cells, and prevention of hypothermia. Early recognition and prompt treatment improves the probability of a favorable outcome.

## ECONOMIC, SOCIAL, AND LEGAL ISSUES

Anesthesiologists' responsibilities extend beyond providing direct medical care to patients and include participation on committees of hospitals and professional societies that assess the value, need, and expense of new technology. For this reason, understanding the economic and social issues associated with laparoscopy enhances not only our skill in caring for patients but also our discipline's standing in the medical community and society at large.

### Are Laparoscopic Procedures More Economical?

Notwithstanding any changes in morbidity and mortality owing to laparoscopic techniques, economic issues compel anesthesiologists and surgeons to consider the expenses associated with these techniques compared with traditional, open surgeries. Literature detailing the cost-effectiveness of laparoscopic operations compared with open surgeries mainly encompasses common procedures, such as cholecystectomy and

hysterectomy. The financial impact of laparoscopy on the costs of newer or more complicated operations (eg, colectomy) is not well studied.

The principal cost savings associated with laparoscopic procedures, in terms of open surgeries, is largely attributable to a reduced length of hospital stay and shorter convalescence. Although the reduced inpatient tenure of patients mitigates the additional costs of operative time during laparoscopic procedures (see later discussion) and expenditures for laparoscopic equipment (eg, insufflation devices, video monitors, disposable supplies), the overall savings due to laparoscopy are modest.[75,76] Cost estimates of open versus laparoscopic cholecystectomy vary by surgeon, institution, and region but are approximately equivalent or slightly less with a laparoscopic technique.[77–82] If bile duct injury occurs or intraoperative cholangiography is required, however, the potential financial advantages of laparoscopy are significantly reduced.[79,80,83,84]

The main financial beneficiaries of laparoscopic operations are patients and their employers because of a significantly reduced duration of inpatient care and quicker recovery of patients having laparoscopic procedures.[81–90] For example, the average duration of hospitalization after open and laparoscopic cholecystectomy procedures was 3.7 and 1.3 days, respectively.[78] Likewise, the number of days required before complete resumption of occupational duties or normal activity after cholecystectomy was reduced from 32.4 ± 3.6 to 8.6 ± 9.0 days using laparoscopic techniques.[77] Similar results from other types of surgeries (eg, hysterectomy) have been noted. In children, however, more expedient recovery clearly leads to cost-effectiveness for laparoscopic procedures. For example, the decreased hospital stay for children undergoing laparoscopic appendectomy, fundoplication, cholecystectomy, or splenectomy netted a mean overall savings of $2370, $5391, $1161, $859, respectively, per patient, although operating costs were significantly greater ($442, $634, $848, $1551, respectively) than those determined for similar open surgeries.[91] Recognizing the principal financial beneficiaries of laparoscopy, at least one author has noted that given the fiscal investment required of hospitals to facilitate laparoscopic surgery, it seems somewhat unjust that these institutions appear to receive minimal to no financial gain.[87]

### Do Laparoscopic Procedures Require More Operative Time?

Laparoscopic procedures require a longer duration of operative time to perform than do open procedures.[85,92] For example, the mean surgical time for open or laparoscopic cholecystectomy was determined to be 72 and 107 minutes, respectively, at one hospital.[85] However, this time difference is remarkably tempered by a decrease in operative time duration as the surgeon's experience and skill increases. At one institution, the operative time for laparoscopic cholecystectomy fell from 180 to 45 minutes after 145 patients had undergone this procedure.[93] In addition to operative time, the requirement for additional equipment preparation and need for extra disposable supplies add to the total operating room use required to complete a laparoscopic surgery.

### What Are the Benefits to Society?

The benefits of laparoscopic surgery have been noted by the lay public and have generated political controversy. Patients rapidly learned of the potential postoperative medical benefits of laparoscopic procedures and prompted hospitals to supply necessary equipment and surgeons to expand their operative repertoire to include laparoscopy. Similar to the trend toward ambulatory surgery caused by health care finance organizations and patient desire, the demand for laparoscopic surgery is also consumer driven. This rapid change to laparoscopic techniques precluded large, prospective studies regarding the safety and benefits of open versus laparoscopic procedures. As noted, the overall morbidity and mortality rates are slightly lower for laparoscopy than for open procedures, although the nature of the complications differs slightly. This benefit, however, is significantly mitigated by the increased rate of surgery that accompanied the widespread use of laparoscopy, so that the total number of complications probably has remained almost constant. For example, the annual rate of cholecystectomy in Maryland increased 28% from 1989 to 1992.[94] In one health maintenance organization, the increased rate of cholecystectomy from 1988 to 1992 caused the total economic cost of gallbladder disease to rise 11.4% despite a 25.1% decrease in physician and hospital costs. Notwithstanding these observations, the perception of economic savings and improved outcome for laparoscopy compared with open procedures has forced the medical community to adopt laparoscopy.

As with other valuable services, these benefits have led some observers to study the use of laparoscopy as an index of equal distribution of medical resources, a derivative of the fundamental ethical principle of justice. For example, Arozullah and colleagues determined that from 1992 to 1995, African-American veterans of the Armed Forces of the United States of America had a significantly lower likelihood (relative risk ratio, 0.68; 95% CI, 0.55-0.84) of receiving a laparoscopic cholecystectomy (versus an open procedure) when compared with clinically similar white patients in nationwide Veterans Administration Medical Centers[95] (Fig. 72–15). Likewise, residents of Maryland undergoing laparoscopy tended to be younger, to be white, and to have private health insurance compared with a similar cohort receiving an open procedure.[94] Patients in this more affluent group, however, were less likely

to have acute cholecystitis or a common-duct stone. In view of these observations, anesthesiologists should recognize that our work is scrutinized by colleagues and the public at large for compliance with esteemed social values that prohibit racial, economic, and age discrimination when making medical decisions.

### Does Caring for Patients Undergoing Laparoscopy Represent a Unique Legal Risk to Anesthesiologists?

Given the previously described risks that are unique to laparoscopy, anesthesiologists might consider the possibility that providing care for patients undergoing this type of surgery may represent a specific legal hazard to their practice. To date, the best method to scrutinize damage to patients beyond case reports and anecdotes is analysis of alleged injury caused by professional negligence by anesthesiologists. The Closed Claims Project of the ASA encompasses a large database that includes information on patients that received anesthesia, including patients undergoing laparoscopy. A query revealed that claims (n = 113) involving laparoscopic procedures were mostly filed by young (35 ± 12 years of age), healthy (92% ASA physical classification I or II), female (94%) patients receiving a general anesthetic (97%) (F.W. Cheney, written communication, November 5, 1999).

The nature of the injuries in patients undergoing laparoscopy was similar to those in patients undergoing other types of surgery, with respiratory events (24%) being the most frequent, followed by equipment (15%) and cardiovascular (9%) damaging events. Nerve injury, airway injury, and awareness were slightly more common in laparoscopic claims, whereas brain damage was less common than in claims for patients undergoing other types of surgery. Payments were generally awarded at a similar rate and were lower in claims for laparoscopic procedures with a median amount of $55 000 (range $75 to $14 700 000) compared to $100 000 (range $15 to $23 200 000) for other types of cases. These data may exclude certain adverse advents (eg, retroperitoneal hemorrhage), however, wherein legal action may be primarily pursued against the surgeon instead of the anesthesiologist. Regardless, given the widespread use of laparoscopy for gynecologic cases in women of childbearing age and the relative similarities of damaging events and financial awards between laparoscopic and other types of surgery, these data do not currently justify the claim that laparoscopic cases represent a unique risk for malpractice actions against anesthesiologists.

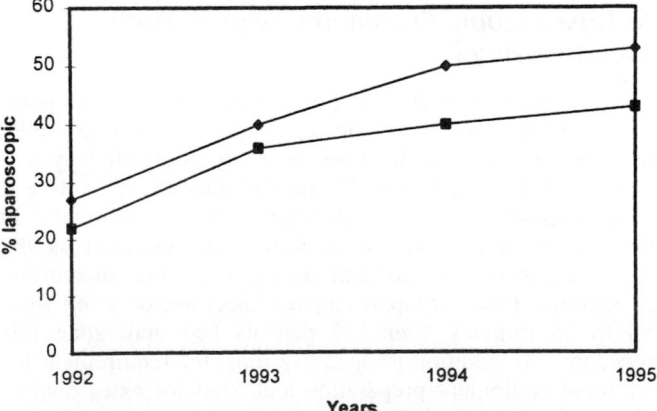

**FIGURE 72–15.** Percentage of cholecystectomy operations performed in 1932 African-American (*squares*) and 14 249 white (*diamonds*) veterans of the Armed Forces of the United States of America for the years 1992–1995 at nationwide Veterans' Administration Medical Centers. (From Arozullah AM, Ferreira MR, Bennett RL, et al. Racial variation in the use of laparoscopic cholecystectomy in the Department of Veterans Affairs medical system. *J Am Coll Surg.* 1999;188:604.)

### References

1. Ritchie WPJ, Rhodes RS, Biester TW. Work loads and practice patterns of general surgeons in the United States, 1995–1997: a report from the American Board of Surgery. *Ann Surg.* 1999;230:533.
2. Rudston-Brown B, Draper PN, Warriner B, et al. Venous gas embolism: a comparison of carbon dioxide and helium in pigs. *Can J Anaesth.* 1997;44:1102.
3. Luks FI, Peers KH, Deprest JA, et al. Gasless laparoscopy in infants: the rabbit model. *J Pediatr Surg.* 1995;30:1206.
4. Rademaker BM, Meyer DW, Bannenberg JJ, et al. Laparoscopy without pneumoperitoneum: effects of abdominal wall retraction versus carbon dioxide insufflation on hemodynamics and gas exchange in pigs. *Surg Endosc.* 1995;9:797.
5. Thoelke MH, Merkelbach D, Ehmann T, et al. The abdominal lift: is

there any advantage for the critically ill patient? *Endosc Surg Allied Technol.* 1995;3:180.

6. Goldberg JM, Maurer WG. A randomized comparison of gasless laparoscopy and $CO_2$ pneumoperitoneum. *Obstet Gynecol.* 1997;90:416.

7. Viani MP, Intra M, Pinto A, et al. Gasless laparoscopic treatment of perforated duodenal ulcer: a case report. *J Laparoendosc Adv Surg Tech A.* 1997;7:249.

8. Paolucci V, Gutt CN, Schaeff B, et al. Gasless laparoscopy in abdominal surgery. *Surg Endosc.* 1995;9:497.

9. Aitola P, Airo I, Kaukinen S, et al. Comparison of $N_2O$ and $CO_2$ pneumoperitoneums during laparoscopic cholecystectomy with special reference to postoperative pain. *Surg Laparosc Endosc.* 1998;8:140.

10. Lipscomb GH, Summitt RLJ, McCord ML, et al. The effect of nitrous oxide and carbon dioxide pneumoperitoneum on operative and postoperative pain during laparoscopic sterilization under local anesthesia. *J Am Assoc Gynecol Laparosc.* 1994;2:57.

11. Neuman GG, Sidebotham G, Negoianu E, et al. Laparoscopy explosion hazards with nitrous oxide. *Anesthesiology.* 1993;78:875.

12. Gunatilake DE. Case report: fatal intraperitoneal explosion during electrocoagulation via laparoscopy. *Int J Gynaecol Obstet.* 1978;15:353.

13. El-Kady AA, Abd-El-Razek M. Intraperitoneal explosion during female sterilization by laparoscopic electrocoagulation: a case report. *Int J Gynaecol Obstet.* 1976;14:487.

14. Drummond GB, Scott DB. Laparoscopy explosion hazards with nitrous oxide [letter]. *BMJ.* 1976;1:586.

15. Khunda S, Ghanima KY. Laparoscopy explosion hazards with nitrous oxide [letter]. *BMJ.* 1976;1:1147.

16. Fleming RY, Dougherty TB, Feig BW. The safety of helium for abdominal insufflation. *Surg Endosc.* 1997;11:230.

17. Mann C, Boccara G, Grevy V, et al. Argon pneumoperitoneum is more dangerous than $CO_2$ pneumoperitoneum during venous gas embolism. *Anesth Analg.* 1997;85:1367.

18. Greilich PE, Greilich NB, Froelich EG. Intraabdominal fire during laparoscopic cholecystectomy. *Anesthesiology.* 1995;83:871.

19. Lobato EB, Paige GB, Brown MM, et al. Pneumoperitoneum as a risk factor for endobronchial intubation during laparoscopic gynecologic surgery. *Anesth Analg.* 1998;86:301.

20. Joris JL, Chiche JD, Canivet JL, et al. Hemodynamic changes induced by laparoscopy and their endocrine correlates: effects of clonidine. *J Am Coll Cardiol.* 1998;32:1389.

21. Walder AD, Aitkenhead AR. Role of vasopressin in the haemodynamic response to laparoscopic cholecystectomy. *Br J Anaesth.* 1997;78:264.

22. Koivusalo AM, Kellokumpu I, Ristkari S, et al. Splanchnic and renal deterioration during and after laparoscopic cholecystectomy: a comparison of the carbon dioxide pneumoperitoneum and the abdominal wall lift method. *Anesth Analg.* 1997;85:886.

23. Moncure M, Salem R, Moncure K, et al. Central nervous system metabolic and physiologic effects of laparoscopy. *Am Surg.* 1999;65:168.

24. Halverson A, Buchanan R, Jacobs L, et al. Evaluation of mechanism of increased intracranial pressure with insufflation. *Surg Endosc.* 1998;12:266.

25. Schob OM, Allen DC, Benzel E, et al. A comparison of the pathophysiologic effects of carbon dioxide, nitrous oxide, and helium pneumoperitoneum on intracranial pressure. *Am J Surg.* 1996;172:248.

26. Rosenthal RJ, Friedman RL, Chidambaram A, et al. Effects of hyperventilation and hypoventilation on $Paco_2$ and intracranial pressure during acute elevations of intraabdominal pressure with $CO_2$ pneumoperitoneum: large animal observations. *J Am Coll Surg.* 1998;187:32.

27. Collure DW, Bumpers HL, Luchette FA, et al. Laparoscopic cholecystectomy in patients with ventriculoperitoneal (VP) shunts. *Surg Endosc.* 1995;9:409.

28. Villavicencio RT, Aucar JA. Analysis of laparoscopy in trauma. *J Am Coll Surg.* 1999;189:11.

29. Duh QY, Senokozlieff-Englehart AL, Choe YS, et al. Laparoscopic gastrostomy and jejunostomy: safety and cost with local vs general anesthesia. *Arch Surg.* 1999;134:151.

30. Ferzli G, Sayad P, Vasisht B. The feasibility of laparoscopic extraperitoneal hernia repair under local anesthesia. *Surg Endosc.* 1999;13:588.

31. Almeida ODJ, Val-Gallas JM. Office microlaparoscopy under local anesthesia in the diagnosis and treatment of chronic pelvic pain. *J Am Assoc Gynecol Laparosc.* 1998;5:407.

32. Vincent RDJ, Syrop CH, Van Voorhis BJ, et al. An evaluation of the effect of anesthetic technique on reproductive success after laparoscopic pronuclear stage transfer: propofol/nitrous oxide versus isoflurane/nitrous oxide. *Anesthesiology.* 1995;82:352.

33. Barker P, Langton JA, Murphy PJ, et al. Regurgitation of gastric contents during general anaesthesia using the laryngeal mask airway. *Br J Anaesth.* 1992;69:314.

34. el Mikatti N, Luthra AD, Healy TE, et al. Gastric regurgitation during general anaesthesia in different positions with the laryngeal mask airway. *Anaesthesia.* 1995;50:1053.

35. Verghese C, Brimacombe JR. Survey of laryngeal mask airway usage in 11,910 patients: safety and efficacy for conventional and nonconventional usage. *Anesth Analg.* 1996;82:129.

36. Bapat PP, Verghese C. Laryngeal mask airway and the incidence of regurgitation during gynecological laparoscopies. *Anesth Analg.* 1997;85:139.

37. Tobias JD, Holcomb GW, Rasmussen GE, et al. General anesthesia using the laryngeal mask airway during brief, laparoscopic inspection of the peritoneum in children. *J Laparoendosc Surg.* 1996;6:175.

38. Swann DG, Spens H, Edwards SA, et al. Anaesthesia for gynaecological laparoscopy: a comparison between the laryngeal mask airway and tracheal intubation. *Anaesthesia.* 1993;48:431.

39. Skinner HJ, Ho BY, Mahajan RP. Gastro-oesophageal reflux with the laryngeal mask during day-case gynaecological laparoscopy. *Br J Anaesth.* 1998;80:675.

40. Ho BY, Skinner HJ, Mahajan RP. Gastro-oesophageal reflux during day case gynaecological laparoscopy under positive pressure ventilation: laryngeal mask vs. tracheal intubation. *Anaesthesia.* 1998;53:921.

41. Goodwin AP, Rowe WL, Ogg TW. Day case laparoscopy: a comparison of two anaesthetic techniques using the laryngeal mask during spontaneous breathing. *Anaesthesia.* 1992;47:892.

42. Joris JL. Anesthetic management of laparoscopy: new developments. In: Miller RD, ed. *Anesthesia.* 4th ed. Issue 2. New York, NY: Churchill Livingstone; 1995:4.

43. Hsing CH, Hseu SS, Tsai SK, et al. The physiological effect of $CO_2$ pneumoperitoneum in pediatric laparoscopy. *Acta Anaesthesiol Sin.* 1995;33:1.

44. Laffon M, Gouchet A, Sitbon P, et al. Difference between arterial and end-tidal carbon dioxide pressures during laparoscopy in paediatric patients. *Can J Anaesth.* 1998;45:561.

45. Cunningham AJ, Brull SJ. Laparoscopic cholecystectomy: anesthetic implications. *Anesth Analg.* 1993;76:1120.

46. Harkki-Siren P, Sjoberg J, Kurki T. Major complications of laparoscopy: a follow-up Finnish study. *Obstet Gynecol.* 1999;94:94.

47. Chapron C, Querleu D, Bruhat MA, et al. Surgical complications of diagnostic and operative gynaecological laparoscopy: a series of 29,966 cases. *Hum Reprod.* 1998;13:867.

48. Jansen FW, Kapiteyn K, Trimbos-Kemper T, et al. Complications of laparoscopy: a prospective multicentre observational study. *Br J Obstet Gynaecol.* 1997;104:595.

49. Jernstrom P. Air embolism during peritoneoscopy. *Am J Clin Pathol.* 1951;21:573.

50. Yacoub OF, Cardona IJ, Coveler LA, et al. Carbon dioxide embolism during laparoscopy. *Anesthesiology.* 1982;57:533.

51. Cottin V, Delafosse B, Viale JP. Gas embolism during laparoscopy: a report of seven cases in patients with previous abdominal surgical history. *Surg Endosc.* 1996;10:166.

52. Nordestgaard AG, Bodily KC, Osborne RWJ, et al. Major vascular injuries during laparoscopic procedures. *Am J Surg.* 1995;169:543.

53. Corson SL, Brooks PG, Soderstrom RM. Gynecologic endoscopic gas embolism. *Fertil Steril.* 1996;65:529.

54. Mlyncek M, Truska A, Garay J. Laparoscopy without use of the Veress needle: results in a series of 1,600 procedures. *Mayo Clin Proc.* 1994;69:1146.

55. Fahlenkamp D, Rassweiler J, Fornara P, et al. Complications of laparoscopic procedures in urology: experience with 2,407 procedures at 4 German centers. *J Urol.* 1999;162:765.

56. Lantz PE, Smith JD. Fatal carbon dioxide embolism complicating attempted laparoscopic cholecystectomy: case report and literature review. *J Forensic Sci.* 1994;39:1468.

57. Bazin JE, Gillart T, Rasson P, et al. Haemodynamic conditions enhancing gas embolism after venous injury during laparoscopy: a study in pigs. *Br J Anaesth.* 1997;78:570.

58. Root B, Levy MN, Pollack S, et al. Gas embolism death after laparoscopy delayed by "trapping" in portal circulation. *Anesth Analg.* 1978;57:232.

59. Beck DH, McQuillan PJ. Fatal carbon dioxide embolism and severe haemorrhage during laparoscopic salpingectomy. *Br J Anaesth.* 1994;72:243.

60. Mann C, Boccara G, Fabre JM, et al. The detection of carbon dioxide embolism during laparoscopy in pigs: a comparison of transesophageal Doppler and end-tidal carbon dioxide monitoring. *Acta Anaesthesiol Scand.* 1997;41:281.

61. Derouin M, Couture P, Boudreault D, et al. Detection of gas embolism by transesophageal echocardiography during laparoscopic cholecystectomy. *Anesth Analg.* 1996;82:119.

62. Diakun TA. Carbon dioxide embolism: successful resuscitation with cardiopulmonary bypass. *Anesthesiology.* 1991;74:1151.

63. Shulman D, Aronson HB. Capnography in the early diagnosis of carbon dioxide embolism during laparoscopy. *Can Anaesth Soc J.* 1984;31:455.

64. Rudston-Brown BC, MacLennan D, Warriner CB, et al. Effect of subcutaneous carbon dioxide insufflation on arterial pCO₂. *Am J Surg.* 1996;171:460.

65. McGrath BJ, Zimmerman JE, Williams JF, et al. Carbon dioxide embolism treated with hyperbaric oxygen. *Can J Anaesth.* 1989;36:586.

66. Geers J, Holden C. Major vascular injury as a complication of laparoscopic surgery: a report of three cases and review of the literature. *Am Surg.* 1996;62:377.

67. Champault G, Cazacu F, Taffinder N. Serious trocar accidents in laparoscopic surgery: a French survey of 103,852 operations. *Surg Laparosc Endosc.* 1996;6:367.

68. Chapron CM, Pierre F, Lacroix S, et al. Major vascular injuries during gynecologic laparoscopy. J Am Coll Surg. 1997;185:461.

69. Usal H, Sayad P, Hayek N, et al. Major vascular injuries during laparoscopic cholecystectomy: an institutional review of experience with 2589 procedures and literature review. *Surg Endosc.* 1998;12:960.

70. Nezhat CR, Childers J, Borhan S. Major vessel injury during advanced laparoscopic surgery. *J Am Assoc Gynecol Laparosc.* 1996;3:S33.

71. Bonjer HJ, Hazebroek EJ, Kazemier G, et al. Open versus closed establishment of pneumoperitoneum in laparoscopic surgery. *Br J Surg.* 1997;84:599.

72. Nezhat C, Childers J, Nezhat F, et al. Major retroperitoneal vascular injury during laparoscopic surgery. *Hum Reprod.* 1997;12:480.

73. Tabboush ZS. When hypotension during laparoscopic cholecystectomy indicates termination of the laparoscopy. *Anesth Analg.* 1994;79:195.

74. Rose DK, Cohen MM, Soutter DI. Laparoscopic cholecystectomy: the anaesthetist's point of view. *Can J Anaesth.* 1992;39:809.

75. Strahm P, Tompkins L, Younes RP. Laparoscopic cholecystectomy: a new technology cost analysis. *HMO Pract.* 1994;8:84.

76. Fullarton GM, Darling K, Williams J, et al. Evaluation of the cost of laparoscopic and open cholecystectomy. *Br J Surg.* 1994;81:124.

77. Schirmer BD, Edge SB, Dix J, et al. Laparoscopic cholecystectomy: treatment of choice for symptomatic cholelithiasis. *Ann Surg.* 1991;213:665.

78. Kelley JE, Burrus RG, Burns RP, et al. Safety, efficacy, cost, and morbidity of laparoscopic versus open cholecystectomy: a prospective analysis of 228 consecutive patients. *Am Surg.* 1993;59:23.

79. Bass EB, Pitt HA, Lillemoe KD. Cost-effectiveness of laparoscopic cholecystectomy versus open cholecystectomy. *Am J Surg.* 1993;165:466.

80. Mowschenson PM. Improving the cost-effectiveness of laparoscopic cholecystectomy. *J Laparoendosc Surg.* 1993;3:113.

81. Berggren U, Zethraeus N, Arvidsson D, et al. A cost-minimization analysis of laparoscopic cholecystectomy versus open cholecystectomy. *Am J Surg.* 1996;172:305.

82. Stoker ME, Vose J, O'Mara P, et al. Laparoscopic cholecystectomy: a clinical and financial analysis of 280 operations. *Arch Surg.* 1992;127:589.

83. McKellar DP, Johnson RM, Dutro JA, et al. Cost-effectiveness of laparoscopic cholecystectomy. *Surg Endosc.* 1995;9:158.

84. Jawad AJ, Kurban K, el-Bakry A, et al. Laparoscopic cholecystectomy for cholelithiasis during infancy and childhood: cost analysis and review of current indications. *World J Surg.* 1998;22:69.

85. McIntyre RCJ, Zoeter MA, Weil KC, et al. A comparison of outcome and cost of open vs. laparoscopic cholecystectomy. *J Laparoendosc Surg.* 1992;2:143.

86. Glinatsis MT, Griffith JP, McMahon MJ. Open versus laparoscopic cholecystectomy: a retrospective comparative study. *J Laparoendosc Surg.* 1992;2:81.

87. Stevens HP, van de Berg M, Ruseler CH, et al. Clinical and financial aspects of cholecystectomy: laparoscopic versus open technique. *World J Surg.* 1997;21:91.

88. Cuschieri A. Day-case (ambulatory) laparoscopic surgery. Let us sing from the same hymn sheet. *Surg Endosc.* 1997;11:1143.

89. Anderson RE, Hunter JG. Laparoscopic cholecystectomy is less expensive than open cholecystectomy. *Surg Laparosc Endosc.* 1991;1:82.

90. Wenner J, Graffner H, Lindell G. A financial analysis of laparoscopic and open cholecystectomy. *Surg Endosc.* 1995;9:702.

91. Luks FI, Logan J, Breuer CK, et al. Cost-effectiveness of laparoscopy in children. *Arch Pediatr Adolesc Med.* 1999;153:965.

92. Fisher KS, Reddick EJ, Olsen DO. Laparoscopic cholecystectomy: cost analysis. *Surg Laparosc Endosc.* 1991;1:77.

93. Woisetschlager R, Wayand W. Laparoscopic cholecystectomy: how does it work and how long does it take? *Surg Endosc.* 1991;5:109.

94. Steiner CA, Bass EB, Talamini MA, et al. Surgical rates and operative mortality for open and laparoscopic cholecystectomy in Maryland. *N Engl J Med.* 1994;330:403.

95. Arozullah AM, Ferreira MR, Bennett RL, et al. Racial variation in the use of laparoscopic cholecystectomy in the Department of Veterans Affairs medical system. *J Am Coll Surg.* 1999;188:604.

# Transplantation

CHAPTER

# 73

# Heart and Lung Transplantation

Mark L. Blas

Emilio B. Lobato

Recent advances in recipient selection, immunosuppressive therapy, and immune surveillance have helped to significantly increase survival following heart and lung transplantation in

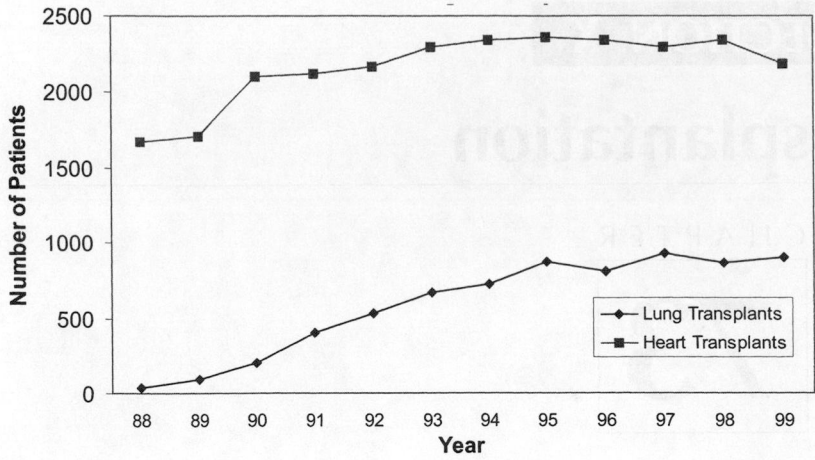

**FIGURE 73–1.** Rise in number of heart and lung transplants, per year, between 1988 and 1999. (Data from UNOS website. Available at: www.unos.org. Accessed 2001.)

the United States. The current 5-year survival rate after heart transplantation is >70%, and the 1-year survival rate after lung transplantation is approximately 75%.[1] In addition, the quality of posttransplantation life has improved. After heart transplantation, 90% of recipients resume a New York Heart Association Class I lifestyle,[2] whereas 80% of lung transplant patients have no exercise limitation at the end of the first year.[3,4] These improvements in lifestyle are in sharp contrast to the 40% to 50% mortality rate of patients with New York Heart Association Class IV heart disease and the severe exercise and lifestyle-limiting debilitation of end-stage lung disease.[5]

As a result of these improvements in both survival and quality of life, there has been an exponential growth in the number of heart and lung transplants since the 1980s. The number of heart transplants increased from 1676 in 1988 to 2185 in 1999, whereas the number of lung transplants increased from 33 in 1988 to 899 in 1999[1] (Fig. 73–1). Along with this growth in the number of transplants, there has also been a proportional growth in the number of transplant centers in the United States. As of 1999, there were at least 242 centers in the United States that perform heart and lung transplantation.[1]

This significant increase in the number of heart and lung transplants has consequently created a relative shortage of organs available for transplant. The number of patients awaiting heart transplantation in the United States increased from 1030 in 1988 to 4290 in 1999.[1] In a similar fashion, the

number of patients awaiting lung transplantation in the United States increased from 69 in 1988 to 3350 in 1999[1] (Fig. 73–2). As a result of this organ shortage, proper selection and stratification of recipients, with "bridge" therapies such as hospitalizations with inotropic support or ventricular assist devices have become integral components in the continuum of modern day heart and lung transplantation. Some cardiac patients may benefit sufficiently from implantation of a left ventricular assist device that its subsequent removal is possible after a period of support.[6]

Important to all anesthesiologists is the fact that with improvements in posttransplant survival, many transplant recipients undergo further operations subsequent to their transplant procedures. As many as one in three heart transplant recipients will present subsequently for a noncardiac operation.[7–15] Although the anesthesiologist providing anesthetic care for the transplant procedure is most likely a specialist in the area, subsequent noncardiac or nonpulmonary surgical procedures may involve any anesthesiologist in practice. As such, a basic understanding of the posttransplant physiology is mandatory for every practicing anesthesiologist.

## HEART AND LUNG TRANSPLANTATION

### Why Are Selection Criteria Critical?

Because the number of potential transplant recipients exceeds the number of organs available for transplantation, care-

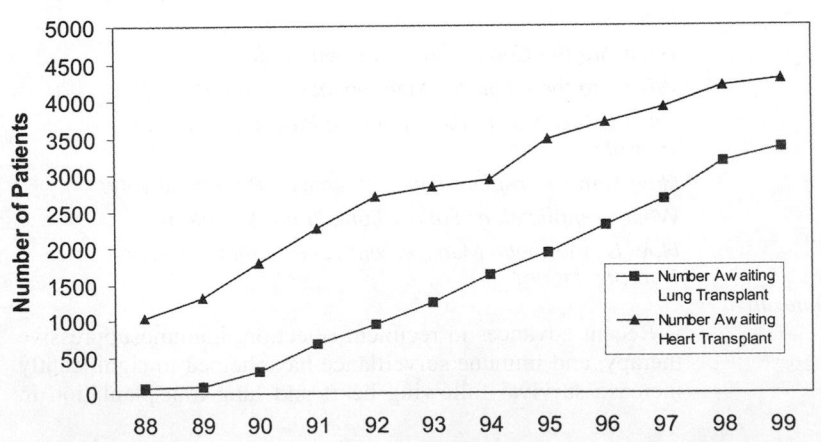

**FIGURE 73–2.** Number of patients awaiting heart or lung transplantation, per year, between 1988 and 1999. (Data from UNOS website. Available at: www.unos.org. Accessed 2001.)

**TABLE 73–1.** Indications for Cardiac Transplantation

End-stage heart disease refractory to other medical or surgical intervention
Prognosis for 1 y survival <75%
New York Heart Association Class III-IV symptoms with maximum medical therapy
Age <60 y (exceptions occur)
Patient emotionally stable, well motivated, and medically compliant
Supportive family

**TABLE 73–3.** Contraindications for Cardiac Transplantation

Elevated pulmonary vascular resistance refractory to vasodilator therapy (>6-8 Wood's units)
Major systemic disease that would independently limit survival (ie, cirrhosis, malignancy, severe cerebrovascular or peripheral vascular disease)
Active systemic infection
Unresolved pulmonary embolism, infarction, or both
Active substance abuse
History of medical noncompliance

ful selection criteria are important to ensure the highest probability of survival for both the recipient and the transplanted organ. Most cardiac and lung transplantation programs have established specific recipient selection criteria for this purpose. These criteria[3,16–21] are summarized in Tables 73–1 and 73–2.

## Heart

Indications for heart transplantation include end-stage organ disease refractory to medical management, likelihood of 1-year survival <75%, and exhaustion of other surgical options.

## Lung

Indications for lung transplantation include advanced pulmonary, vascular, fibrotic, or obstructive disease, with a likelihood of survival <2 years, severe functional limitation, and lack of success of alternative treatment modalities.

### What Are the Contraindications to Heart and Lung Transplantation?

Contraindications to transplantation are typically divided into two categories: strict and relative. *Strict contraindications* for heart or lung transplantation include systemic diseases (including infection and malignancy), severe irreversible pulmonary hypertension (>4–6 Wood's units), history of ongoing substance abuse, and inability to comply with medical regimens.[16,17] Relative contraindications include poorly controlled chronic medical conditions, active collagen vascular disease, and steroid dependence (>20 mg prednisone/d).[3] Contraindications specific for heart transplantation and lung transplantation are summarized in Tables 73–3 and 73–4, respectively.

Notably, one element of the contraindications for heart and lung transplantation has shifted during the past several years. The determination of a "reversible" component of pulmonary hypertension (ie, using a sodium nitroprusside challenge) versus a "fixed" pulmonary vascular resistance (PVR) can aid in the inclusion of patients with high pulmonary artery (PA) pressure onto the transplant roster. Patients with a reversible

component often do as well as patients without elevated PA pressures.[22]

## COMBINED HEART-LUNG TRANSPLANTATION

Historically, combined heart-lung transplantation was the treatment of choice for patients with irreversible pulmonary hypertension. Currently, because many of these patients can be treated with single-lung transplantation, combined transplantation is decreasing in frequency. Combined heart-lung transplantation, however, continues to be the treatment of choice in patients with irreversible pulmonary hypertension, unrepairable congenital defects, and left ventricular failure.

As more and more patients exist in a borderline state while awaiting transplantation, meticulous pretransplant medical management strategies are essential.

### Is Management of Anesthesia Similar to Heart Transplantation?

The anesthetic management for heart-lung transplantation is similar to that of heart transplantation with similar bicaval and aortic cannulations.[23] The airway anastomoses may be either two bibronchial or a single tracheal anastomosis.

### What Types of Complications Occur?

Complications are the same as those found in heart and lung transplantation including reperfusion injury, pulmonary edema, ventricular failure, infection, and rejection.

**TABLE 73–4.** Contraindications for Lung Transplantation

Acute medical illness
Active cancer or malignancy (excepting squamous and basal carcinoma of the skin)
End-stage organ disease from other medical diseases
Active smoking
Severe malnutrition or morbid obesity
History of noncompliance or ongoing substance abuse
Relative: poorly controlled medical conditions, active collagen vascular disease, colonization with pan-resistant bacteria

**TABLE 73–2.** Indications for Lung Transplantation

Advanced obstructive, pulmonary, vascular, or fibrotic disease
Lack of continued success of other treatment modalities
Life expectancy <2 y
Age 65 y or less (single-lung transplant)
Age 60 y or less (double-lung transplant)

Adapted, by permission, from the *New England Journal of Medicine* (Vol 340, page 1081, 1999).

Adapted, by permission, from the *New England Journal of Medicine* (Vol 340, page 1081, 1999).

## HEART TRANSPLANTATION

### What Factors Should Be Considered in End-Stage Heart Disease?

Optimal management of the heart transplant patient requires a thorough understanding of the pathophysiology of end-stage congestive heart failure (CHF). Once this pathophysiology is understood, appropriate management principles become easier to understand and implement.

### Pathophysiology

Impaired contractile function secondary to any of a number of disorders is the common starting point in the progression toward symptomatic heart failure. The loss of contractile function leads to deterioration in the systolic pump function of the heart, which, in turn, leads to CHF and use of compensatory mechanisms by the heart to maintain cardiac output.[24–26] CHF results in increased interstitial lung water, reduced pulmonary compliance, and, in the preterminal stages, pulmonary hypertension.

As cardiac output falls, tissue oxygen delivery becomes inadequate, and vital organ function is compromised. At this stage, the left ventricle functions with worsening contractility, greater preload dependence, and greater afterload sensitivity.[27] Patients with dilated cardiomyopathies are also at risk for myocardial ischemia and infarction.[28]

It is important to recognize that, although the heart is primarily affected in end-stage heart disease, CHF is a multisystem disease. The kidneys, splanchnic organs, and central nervous system (CNS) are all commonly affected by left ventricular dysfunction.

### Anesthetic Implications

Three main cardiovascular abnormalities exist in all patients with end-stage heart disease: impaired myocardial contractility, preload dependence, and afterload sensitivity.

### Abnormal Contractility

The heart with *severely impaired contractility* demonstrates poor tolerance for negative inotropic agents and for agents that decrease heart rate. In this condition, cardiac output is maintained by heart rate because the stroke volume is relatively fixed; this is in contrast to the normal heart, in which stroke volume changes as a function of preload and contractility. If the impaired heart is unable to increase contractility, it will be unable to maintain or increase cardiac output in response to surgical stresses that increase afterload.

A hypertensive response to light anesthesia probably will not occur. In fact, the heart may respond to stress with rapid decompensation.[27] Impaired contractility is associated with a decrease in myocardial catecholamines and in myocardial β-receptor density.[29] This deficit has important implications for anesthetic management. One can expect decreased effectiveness of inotropic agents that act via β-receptor stimulation. This response is particularly common in intensive care unit (ICU) patients who require inotropic support preoperatively. Much higher doses of inotropic agents may be required during anesthesia and surgery. Alternatively, inotropes that bypass the β-receptor (such as phosphodiesterase inhibitors) may be useful.

### Preload Dependence

As heart failure progresses, the principal compensatory mechanism is an increase in left ventricular end-diastolic volume *(preload)*. The heart functions on the flat portion of the Starling curve and requires a higher than normal preload to maintain cardiac output and systemic perfusion.[27] A sudden decreased preload can result in decompensation and circulatory collapse. Significantly, intravascular volume augmentation (increased preload) does not predictably increase stroke volume and can lead to decreased cardiac output.

A number of important factors occur during the course of surgery and should be remembered. Anesthetic agents can result in venodilation and decreased preload; surgery results in volume loss through multiple mechanisms; positive-pressure ventilation can impede venous return to the heart. The importance of closely monitoring intravascular volume status and careful volume replacement cannot be overemphasized.

### Afterload Sensitivity

The third abnormality of importance in understanding the delicate cardiovascular state of these patients is afterload sensitivity. Any increase in afterload or systemic vascular resistance without a corresponding increase in myocardial contractility may result in a rapid decrease in stroke volume, cardiac output, and systemic perfusion.[27] Small decreases in afterload are associated with significant increases in stroke volume. However, large decreases in afterload are also poorly tolerated and may result in hypotension and decreased organ perfusion.

### Summary

The cardiovascular state of the heart transplant patient is usually that of marginal compensation at best. It should be remembered that multiple organ system dysfunction can exist as a result of the chronic low-perfusion state and that any physiologic insult such as sudden change in loading condition, drug-induced myocardial depression, or decreased heart rate can easily and rapidly result in cardiovascular decompensation or collapse.

### How Is a Transplant Candidate Evaluated Preoperatively?

A candidate patient must undergo extensive evaluation by transplant surgeons, cardiologists, and other specialists in order to be listed as a potential recipient.[30,31] This information is typically up-to-date and readily available in the patient's chart or from the transplant coordinator and can help facilitate the preanesthetic evaluation.

The major anesthetic considerations of heart transplantation deal with administering an anesthetic to a patient with a severely compromised ventricle and the multiorgan system sequelae that occur as a result of the chronic low-perfusion state.

### Coexisting Disease

The heart transplant candidate will often have manifestations of severe cardiac failure and usually some reversible components of renal, hepatic, or pulmonary compromise. Evidence of organ dysfunction in the presence of heart failure can be detected in >50% of patients. In one series, 42% of patients were orthopneic on the day of surgery, 27% had peripheral edema, 12% were receiving inotropic support, 2% had an intraaortic balloon pump in place, 41% had renal dysfunction, 52% had liver dysfunction, and 12% had cardiac dysrhythmias.[32]

### History

Emphasis should be placed on previous anesthetic administrations, current medications, a brief review of systems, and drug allergies. In addition, the most recent estimates of cardiac function including electrocardiogram (ECG), echocardiography, and heart catheterization should be available and thoroughly reviewed.

### Physical Examination

The physical examination should concentrate on a patient's vital signs and weight, airway status, neurologic function, and cardiopulmonary system. Simple observation provides the answers to obvious and important questions:

Is the patient ambulatory and thus stable or reasonably compensated, or moribund in the ICU and dependent on mechanical circulatory support?
What catheters are in place and do any need to be replaced to minimize the risk of infection?

Examination of the cardiopulmonary system helps to estimate if the Trendelenburg position will be tolerated for central venous catheter insertion and also to anticipate the cardiovascular response to anesthetic induction.

As with any anesthetic, a thorough examination of the airway should be performed. Anticipation of a difficult airway may necessitate fiberoptic intubation. If this is anticipated, it should be communicated to the transplant coordinator and the patient brought to the operating room (OR) slightly earlier than previously planned.

### Laboratory Tests

It is not uncommon for transplant candidates to be systemically anticoagulated. In addition, hepatic and renal functions are often compromised by the low-perfusion state. Thus, in addition to serum electrolytes and blood counts, coagulation studies and renal function tests are important. The chest radiograph should be examined for signs of CHF such as cardiomegaly and vascular prominence. The ECG should be examined for evidence of ischemia or dysrhythmias.

### Should Transplant Patients Be Treated as a "Full Stomach"?

Several factors are involved in this decision. Because transplant recipients rarely know more than several hours in advance of their impending surgery, it is unusual for them to have been fasting for more than 6 to 8 hours. In addition, the excitement and anticipation toward the surgery may decrease normal gastric emptying. For these reasons, patients are routinely premedicated with histamine$_2$ (H$_2$) blockers and metoclopramide (Reglan) to aid in the gastric emptying process.

Some heart transplantation immunosuppression protocols include the oral administration of cyclosporin A preoperatively, usually with milk or orange juice, neither of which is a clear liquid. For this reason, premedication to minimize the risk of serious aspiration is also appropriate. Metoclopramide, histamine blockers, a nonparticulate antacid, or a combination of these can be used. If a nasogastric tube is placed, it should not be drained lest the immunosuppressant drug be removed.

### Does Anesthesia Equipment Differ From That for Other Open Heart Procedures?

Preparation of anesthetic equipment for heart transplantation is similar to that for other open heart cases, with emphasis on the requirement for maximum sterility. The anesthesia machine should be set up with a sterile, disposable anesthesia bag and circuit.[18,27,33,34] In addition, some centers routinely use bacterial filters on the breathing circuit, although this practice is not universal.[18] In some centers, a sterile intubation tray is also employed.

### What Equipment and Monitors Are Routinely Used?

#### Anesthesia Equipment

Noninvasive monitors include a pulse oximeter, noninvasive blood pressure (BP) cuff, multilead ECG, capnograph, esophageal stethoscope, and temperature probes (esophageal and bladder).[32,35–37] In addition, a Foley catheter with a urometer is placed following induction. Invasive monitors include a radial arterial line, a central venous pulmonary (CVP) or PA catheter, and a transesophageal echocardiography (TEE) probe.

#### Pulmonary Artery Catheters

Whether PA catheterization should be performed in heart transplantation is a subject of controversy. A survey of heart transplantation centers in North America indicated that 32% used the PA catheter before bypass, and 44% used it after bypass.[38,39] Advocates claim that rational anesthetic management is possible only with such monitoring.[38] Others claim that PA catheters are unnecessary for patients who do not have pulmonary hypertension; their use increases the risk of infection, and they must be pulled back into the sterility sheath before removal of the recipient's heart.[19,32,34,35] Still others claim that PA catheters are altogether contraindicated.[36]

A reasonable approach is to use a CVP catheter in patients without pulmonary hypertension. A multilumen polyurethane catheter permits simultaneous drug infusion and CVP monitoring and also minimizes the risk of superior vena caval or right atrial perforation.[40,41] A PA catheter is most useful in patients with pulmonary hypertension. It allows for the titration of inhaled nitric oxide and other pulmonary vasodilators and their effects on PVR. Initially, it is advanced only 15 to 20 cm and used to measure CVP, with the sterility sheath fully extended over the catheter. It can then be advanced into the PA after separation from cardiopulmonary bypass (CPB).

It is important to remember that with the catheter only partially inserted, the CVP port and possibly the venous infusion port may be outside the introducer; therefore, medications given via these routes do not reach the circulation.

Several factors can make placement of a PA catheter difficult in heart transplantation patients, including cardiac dysrhythmias, a large dilated heart with poor ejection fraction, tricuspid regurgitation, and poor tolerance of the head-down position by awake patients.

### Internal Jugular Vein Access

Historically, the use of the right internal jugular vein for central venous access was not recommended due to the need for routine myocardial biopsies postoperatively. This concern has not proven to be valid. The left-sided internal jugular vein can also safely be used but may be more difficult to access and has an increased risk of inadvertent vascular perforation (SVC) by the catheter tip once placed.[40,41] The catheter must be long enough for its tip to reach beyond the junction of the brachiocephalic vein and superior vena cava. Polyurethane or, preferably, "pig-tail" catheters are recommended, as they are less likely to perforate the vessel wall.[41] At our institution, we typically use the right internal jugular vein for central venous access. Use of a transcutaneous ultrasound (US) imaging probe can facilitate central venous cannulation.

### Transesophageal Echocardiography

Due to its low risk of complications, TEE is routinely used to assess fluid status and ventricular and valvular function, as well as to aid in the intracardiac "de-airing" process before separation from CPB.

### Should Premedication Be Given?

The benefits of premedication, including anxiolysis, must be weighed against the possibility of depressed consciousness, hypoxemia, and hemodynamic compromise. We do not typically administer anxiolytics before arrival in the OR. In patients with severe anxiety, small amounts of benzodiazepine can be carefully titrated before transport to the OR.

### What Preparations Should Take Place During the Preinduction Period?

#### Blood

At least two units of packed red blood cells should be present in the OR at the time of incision. In the case of chest reoperation, at least four units should be available.

The immunosuppressed heart transplantation patient is at risk for cytomegalovirus (CMV) sepsis; thus, the blood bank should obtain CMV-free blood products for those patients who lack CMV antibodies.

#### Drugs

Because transplant patients have poor baseline ventricular function, a variety of inotropic and vasoactive agents should be premixed and made immediately available during induc-

tion; direct-acting agents such as dobutamine, epinephrine, phenylephrine, isoproterenol, and sodium nitroprusside are most useful. If available, nitric oxide should also be readily accessible, especially for patients with known pulmonary hypertension.

### Placement of Monitoring Devices

Transplant patients who have previously undergone cardiac surgery are likely to require more time for placement of invasive monitors, chest opening, and cannulation for CPB than other patients. This factor must be considered preoperatively so that donor organ ischemic times are not prolonged unnecessarily. Intravenous catheters and invasive monitors can be placed conveniently under local anesthesia in the ICU before transport to the OR. However, this approach is inherently less sterile. Alternatively, the patient can be transported to the OR early enough to allow sufficient time for catheter insertion under more aseptic conditions.

### Transportation to the Operating Room

Depending on the severity of illness, transportation to the OR may require physician transport. Physicians typically transport patients on vasoactive infusions and mechanical cardiac support, in addition to those requiring telemetry. Patients who have been at home preoperatively and are well compensated can usually be transported safely by nonphysician OR staff. At our institution, patients are typically transported by the anesthesiology service to help monitor and expedite the transportation process.

### Timing of Induction

The transplant coordinator should primarily coordinate the timing of induction. Ideally, timing should balance the anesthesia staff and surgical staff time requirements, while limiting the duration of donor heart ischemic time. Frequent communication between transplant coordinator, anesthesiology, and surgical services is necessary to achieve this goal.

### Infection Control

Infection is a leading cause of morbidity and mortality in heart transplant recipients.[20,42] Thus, all invasive catheters must be placed with sterile technique. For intravenous catheters, the site should be prepped with povidone-iodine and draped with sterile towels; sterile gloves and gown should be worn during insertion. Although suprapubic catheters sometimes are used to minimize the risk of bladder infection, this problem has not proved to be significant; most centers use Foley catheters. Prophylactic antibiotics are given before surgical incision.

### Immunosuppressant Therapy

Intravenous cyclosporin A is started preoperatively. Corticosteroids are typically administered at the time of aortic cross-clamp removal. Other immunosuppressant therapies exist, including tacrolimus, anti-T cell, and azathioprine-based regimens; these are administered according to preestablished protocols.

## What Are Important Considerations During Anesthetic Induction?

Induction of anesthesia is perhaps the most critical period of anesthetic care. In a patient with little or no cardiac reserve, the combination of negative inotropic anesthetic agents, ablation of sympathetic tone, venous dilation, decreases in heart rate, and positive pressure ventilation can result in sudden cardiovascular collapse. The primary goals are to monitor hemodynamic function closely, minimize the administration of negative inotropic agents, maintain heart rate and intravascular volume, avoid arterial and venous dilation, and minimize the risk of aspiration.

### Techniques

Anesthetic techniques used for other cardiac surgical patients who have poor ventricular function are appropriate for the transplant recipient, and many have been used successfully.[18,27,32,33,36–38,43,44] The risk of aspiration must be considered before induction. In the anesthetic management survey of Hensley and associates, aspiration precautions were taken in 88% of cases.[38] Rapid-sequence induction was employed in 11 of 30, and modified rapid-sequence induction, with ventilation through cricoid pressure, was used in 15 of 30 cases. Other studies in which the preoperative administration of oral cyclosporin A was performed did not consider the small amount immunosuppressant to be an indication for a rapid-sequence induction.[33] Generally, one of three approaches is taken.

### Routine Induction

Some authorities prefer a slow, titrated anesthetic induction technique.[19,36] The agents most often used are the potent synthetic narcotics—fentanyl or sufentanil—along with benzodiazepines, low-dose inhaled agents, or scopolamine. These drugs can be titrated slowly or administered by slow infusion.

Care must be taken when inducing anesthesia with high-dose potent synthetic narcotics (especially sufentanil) to avoid slowing of the heart rate from central narcotic-induced vagotonia. Hemodynamic decompensation can be precipitated in patients with rate-dependent cardiac output. This problem usually can be minimized by the simultaneous administration of incremental doses of pancuronium. This drug's vagolytic effects minimize slowing of heart rate.

### Rapid-Sequence Induction

A classic rapid-sequence induction of anesthesia with cricoid pressure is frequently recommended.[32,37,38] The induction agents most commonly used for this technique are ketamine and etomidate. Ketamine is traditionally associated with maintenance of BP due to released catecholamines. However, its indirect sympathomimetic effects may not manifest in these catecholamine-depleted patients, and its direct negative inotropic effects may result in significant hypotension.

Etomidate is a good alternative as it is not associated with significant hemodynamic alterations.

### Modified Rapid Sequence Induction

A third commonly used approach is a modified rapid-sequence induction in which potent synthetic narcotics, muscle relaxants, and benzodiazepines or low-dose inhaled agents are administered slowly with continuous application of cricoid pressure and controlled ventilation.[33] One must realize that this approach does not necessarily guarantee the absence of regurgitation or aspiration.

### Sterile Intubation

Although the trachea cannot be intubated in a sterile fashion, anesthesiologists should attempt to perform the intubation in as sanitary a manner as possible in order to minimize the risk of pulmonary infection. A sterile intubation tray can be used. A designated intubator (second anesthesiologist) drapes the patient's face with sterile towels and performs the intubation with a sterile laryngoscope and endotracheal tube (ETT).[19,34] A nasal intubation should be avoided if at all possible because it predisposes the patient to bacteremia and subsequent sinus infection.

### Summary

For patients coming from home for transplantation who have compensated ventricular function and a full stomach, premedication with $H_2$ blockers and metoclopramide, and a rapid-sequence induction with etomidate or ketamine plus succinylcholine are reasonable. Potent narcotics can be titrated slowly before and after induction, as needed.

For the hospitalized patient who is uncompensated, receiving inotropic support, and in nil per os status (except for oral cyclosporine administration), a slower, modified rapid-sequence induction technique with cricoid pressure is reasonable.

The goals of anesthetic technique should include hemodynamic stability and amnesia and allow for prompt neurologic assessment following the procedure. The ability of the patient to follow simple commands soon after arrival to the ICU is reassuring to both staff and family.

No matter what induction technique is used, the hemodynamic status must be monitored closely; fluids, anesthetics, and vasoactive agents are administered as clinically indicated.

## How Is Maintenance of Anesthesia Accomplished?

### Agent Choice

A variety of anesthetic agents have been used successfully for anesthetic maintenance, and no correlation can be found between anesthetic techniques and operative outcome.[32] A survey of anesthesia practices at 34 centers indicated that narcotic-based anesthesia, which causes minimal cardiac depression, was used in the majority of 1273 heart transplantations, and potent inhaled agents were rarely used as the primary maintenance anesthetic for heart transplantation.[38] Their use has been complicated by hypotension; however, they are used to supplement narcotic-based techniques.[32,44]

### Precautions

The success with which a variety of agents have been used for maintenance of anesthesia during cardiac transplantation suggests that the skill and care with which the anesthetic is administered is probably of greater importance than the particular agent. However, a few points merit discussion.

Benzodiazepines are often used to supplement narcotic anesthesia for heart transplantation. These agents can lower systemic vascular resistance and produce myocardial depression when combined with narcotic agents. Nitrous oxide is not recommended because it can further depress myocardial contractility and may exacerbate the consequences of air emboli.

## Goals

Regardless of the technique used, one must remember several anesthetic goals. Before CPB, maintenance of the patient's baseline hemodynamic state is a primary consideration. Efforts to make a stable patient "better" before CPB are as likely to create more problems as they are to prevent them. Be prepared to administer pharmacologic cardiovascular support. Inotropic support was increased postinduction in 44% of cases according to a 1986 survey.[38] During mobilization and exposure of the heart, hemodynamic instability and cardiac dysrhythmias are common, especially with dissection of adhesions and placement of the vena cava–encircling snares. Constant vigilance and interaction with the surgical team is essential.

Following exposure of the heart, heparin is administered in preparation for cannulation of the great vessels. After adequate anticoagulation is verified and the great vessels are cannulated, if timing has been appropriate, the donor heart arrives, and CPB is initiated.

## What Are the Anesthesiologist's Responsibilities During Cardiopulmonary Bypass?

During CPB, the anesthesiologist should be anticipating the strategy for separation from CPB. Excessive doses of narcotics should be avoided when possible because prolonged mechanical ventilatory support increases the risk of pulmonary infection postoperatively.

### Transplantation and Other Cardiac Procedures

Most anesthesiologists treat CPB similarly in transplantation and other cardiac procedures; however, several considerations are different for heart transplantation. If a PA catheter is in place, it is withdrawn into the proximal superior vena cava before sealing off the vena cava around the venous cannula. Early in the CPB procedure, blood gas measurements often reveal metabolic acidosis; this reflects the large oxygen deficit in the peripheral tissues of patients with severe heart failure. The anesthesiologist and perfusionist should ensure that these abnormalities are corrected before attempting separation from CPB. During reperfusion, the pulmonary circulation is exposed to cytokines and other ischemic neurohumoral metabolites, resulting in free radical injury that can produce a significantly increased PVR. Metabolic acidosis, hypoxemia, and hypercapnia may also exacerbate pulmonary hypertension.

### Agents for Weaning

During CPB, the appropriate inotropic agents must be available for weaning from CPB. These include isoproterenol or

dobutamine, nitroglycerin, and phosphodiesterase type III inhibitors. Prostaglandin $E_1$ ($PGE_1$) should also be readily available because it has been demonstrated to be useful in managing pulmonary hypertension during separation from CPB. Nitric oxide should also be accessible because it allows decreasing PVR without decreasing systemic BP, unlike other vasodilators. Be prepared to administer immunosuppressive agents before removal of the aortic cross-clamp and during reperfusion of the transplanted heart. As with other cardiac procedures performed under CPB, additional narcotics, anesthetics, muscle relaxants, or benzodiazepines are administered during rewarming, as clinically indicated.

## What Is Involved in the Operative Procedure?

### Technical Aspects

#### Donor Heart

A brief description of the transplantation procedure helps one to understand the unique cardiac physiology and pharmacology.[45] The donor heart is resected so that the posterior atrial walls (including the sinoatrial node), pulmonary veins, and vena cava are intact. The great vessels are divided above the semilunar valves. The heart typically receives cardioplegia with preservative solution, and then it is stored in an ice water solution during transport.

#### Recipient Heart

The recipient's heart is exposed using midline sternotomy. Ideally, CPB is initiated just before arrival of the donor heart. The aorta is cross-clamped, and *after* the donor heart is in the room and is determined to be suitable, the recipient's heart is resected. The atria are transected above the atrioventricular grooves, leaving the posterior atrial walls and the sinoatrial node intact. The great vessels are divided above the valves.

#### Anastomoses

The operation requires the completion of 4 major anastomoses. First, the left and right atrial anastomoses are completed, and then the aortic and PA anastomoses are performed. Subsequently, air is evacuated, a second dose of steroid is administered, the cross-clamp is removed, and rewarming is completed. The result is an implanted heart that is totally devoid of autonomic innervation and one that contains two sinoatrial nodes.

The patient is weaned from CPB in the usual manner, except that an infusion of β-agonist (eg, isoproterenol) is used to maintain the heart rate at about 100 beats per minute (bpm). Temporary pacing wires are also placed.

## How Does Denervated Heart Function Affect Anesthetic Management?

The transplanted heart is excluded from all normal autonomic innervation. Thus, its physiologic and pharmacologic response to drugs is altered. These alterations affect postbypass anesthetic management.

It is important to note that, although denervation does not impair the heart's intrinsic impulse formation and conduction system, the heart rate is controlled by the donor sinoatrial node, which does not respond to direct autonomic nervous system stimulation. Thus, the basal heart rate is usually 90 to 100 bpm, the intrinsic rate of a denervated heart.[46]

## Physiologic Alterations

### Exercise

Studies of heart transplantation patients demonstrate that they have an altered hemodynamic response to stress and exercise.[47–52] The rate response of the denervated heart is delayed, gradual, and reduced.[48,49,51] Increase in cardiac output induced by exercise or stress is almost entirely mediated through an increase in stroke volume, as a result of greater venous return and the Frank-Starling mechanism.[44,49] Thus, cardiac output is preload-dependent.

With more progressive and sustained exercise, heart rate and contractility increase in response to circulating catecholamines, the result of which is a greater cardiac output.[49] With cessation of exercise or stress, a more gradual return to baseline hemodynamic values than in normal subjects occurs. This gradual return to baseline correlates with decreasing circulating catecholamine levels.[49]

### Reflex Changes

Denervation also removes the heart from the physiologic control loops that require intact autonomic innervation. Thus, reflex increases in heart rate to augment cardiac output cannot occur immediately in response to vasodilation or sudden blood loss. Also, the heart rate will not respond immediately to inadequate anesthesia; any response in heart rate that results will lag in onset, be minor in magnitude, and lag in termination.

## Pharmacologic Responses

The second major consequence of cardiac denervation is the altered response to various cardiovascular drugs. Because the heart is denervated, medications that act via the autonomic nervous system do not elicit the expected response. For example, atropine normally accelerates heart rate by blocking vagal tone. This effect is not seen in the denervated heart; thus, atropine is totally ineffective in treating bradycardia or conduction system defects.

Although adrenergic neurotransmission has been permanently disrupted, the adrenergic receptors are intact, and the response of the denervated heart to the *direct adrenergic agonists*—isoproterenol, epinephrine, dobutamine, norepinephrine, and phenylephrine—is preserved and can be increased.[53,54] Bradydysrhythmias can be treated with direct β-adrenergic stimulating agents. However, reflex changes associated with direct-acting agents are absent. For example, the reflex bradycardia normally seen in response to phenylephrine hydrochloride administration does not occur.

Drugs that act both directly and indirectly (dopamine) have diminished effects. Although these drugs have not been carefully studied, several reports indicate that they may be useful in cardiac transplant patients.[35–38]

### Antidysrhythmic Agents

**Digoxin.** Digoxin produces little acute change in sinus node activity and atrioventricular conduction because these functions are primarily indirect and autonomically mediated. It has positive inotropic action (direct effect) in heart transplant patients.[46,55,56] Thus, digoxin is not useful for acute control of the ventricular rate in atrial fibrillation. Chronic oral administration, however, effectively depresses atrioventricular conduction, making digoxin useful for long-term rate control in atrial fibrillation.[57]

**β-Blockers.** As expected, β-blockers decrease heart rate in the denervated heart.[58,59] Few studies concerning the effects of β-blockers on cardiac output, ejection fraction, or any other measure of ventricular systolic function have been performed. However, studies have demonstrated that β-blockers can significantly reduce exercise tolerance in these patients.[52,60] As noted earlier, the denervated heart's peak cardiac output is highly dependent on elevated catecholamine levels. Heart transplant patients should be considered *extremely* sensitive to the effects of β-blockers.

**Verapamil.** Verapamil is effective in its direct action on the calcium channels of the transplanted heart and decreases atrial rate and atrioventricular conduction. Thus, it can be used in supraventricular tachydysrhythmias.[61]

**Quinidine and Procainamide.** The electrophysiologic effects of quinidine and procainamide are similar in that they exert both direct and autonomically mediated effects on the heart. The increase in heart rate is due to an atropinelike effect on the sinoatrial and atrioventricular nodes and is absent in the denervated heart.[62] The direct effects of these agents, suppression of the sinoatrial and atrioventricular nodes and of the His-Purkinje conduction, are present, and they appear to be useful to suppress supraventricular dysrhythmias in the denervated heart.[62]

**Lidocaine.** The effects of lidocaine are almost completely independent of the autonomic nervous system (ANS). Thus, lidocaine is useful for control of ventricular dysrhythmias in these patients.

## How Does Separation From Cardiopulmonary Bypass Differ in the Transplant Patient?

### Before Separation From Bypass

The postbypass period of cardiac transplantation presents the obvious requirement for maintenance of anesthesia and management of the acutely denervated and transplanted heart. The newly transplanted heart does not function normally as a result of the typically more prolonged ischemia (often ≥2.5 hours) and cardioplegia that occur during donor cardiectomy and recipient implantation. Additionally, donor brain death may induce myocardial dysfunction before harvest.

### Inotropic Support

Contractility and stroke volume are often decreased, and cardiac output becomes volume-dependent and rate-dependent. Therefore, use of an isoproterenol infusion is common. Left atrial or PA occlusion pressure helps gauge volume status. In the recipient with normal PVR, CVP measurement often suffices. TEE plays a role here as well. It allows verification that therapeutic interventions are adequate and provides a direct, objective assessment of left ventricular volume. This benefit is particularly relevant when left ventricular compliance is decreased because left atrial pressure and PA occlusion pressure do not provide an accurate assessment of volume status or compliance.

### After Release of the Aortic Cross-Clamp

After release of the aortic cross-clamp, a sinus or slow junctional rhythm usually develops. If spontaneous defibrillation has not occurred when core temperature reaches 34°C to 36°C, electrical defibrillation should be undertaken. The intrinsic rate of the denervated heart initially may be quite slow.

### Maintenance of Heart Rate and Contractility

To ensure an adequate heart rate and to enhance contractility, an infusion of isoproterenol, 0.005 to 0.05 μg/kg/min, is begun during the final stages of CPB and is titrated to achieve a heart rate of 90 to 100 bpm. Isoproterenol also decreases PVR, enhances diastolic relaxation, and improves cardiac filling. Dobutamine, which has similar effects to isoproterenol, is used at some sites.[19] Epicardial pacing is occasionally required. Low-dose dopamine is also frequently employed to augment urine output. Dopamine may also produce a slight increase in systemic vascular resistance, offsetting peripheral "isoproterenol-induced" vasodilation.

### Volume Sensitivity

The newly transplanted ischemic heart is volume-sensitive and usually functions best when CVP is 10 to 15 cm $H_2O$. Higher filling pressures are required in cases of graft dysfunction. With adequate heart rate and preload, weaning from CPB is usually straightforward. Occasionally, high doses of isoproterenol or dobutamine and epinephrine, norepinephrine, or amrinone are necessary. This requirement occurs in the setting of pulmonary hypertension and prolonged ischemic times. Only rarely is an intraaortic balloon pump or ventricular assist device support required. Hensley and coworkers reported the use of an intraaortic balloon pump to separate patients from CPB in only 2% of cases.[38]

### After Separation From Bypass

After separation from bypass, anesthetic management is similar to that for most open-heart procedures with a few special considerations. Postoperative function of the graft is substandard for several days.[63] For this reason, most people recommend that isoproterenol not be completely discontinued in the operative and immediate postoperative periods, even if the heart appears to be functioning well.[36]

Transplanted patients typically do well and are good candidates for early extubation. Because prolonged intubation may present a significant infectious disease risk, anesthetic management (narcotic dosing) should be tailored to allow early extubation, if possible. Also, blood products should be avoided, if possible, in these immunocompromised patients to minimize the risk of transmission of unscreened viral agents.

## What Are the Options When Failure to Wean From Bypass Occurs?

In approximately 1% of cases, the donor heart does not function adequately despite aggressive inotropic and intraaortic balloon pump support.[38] The most common cause for failure to wean (45%) is right ventricular dysfunction. Postischemic ventricular dysfunction and, rarely, acute rejection are other causes. In the event of the occurrence of these phenomena, only retransplantation, with temporary mechanical support using a ventricular assist device or total artificial heart as a bridge, will suffice until a suitable donor for retransplantation can be located.

### Right Ventricular Failure and Pulmonary Hypertension

If right ventricular failure from pulmonary hypertension is the reason for inability to wean, retransplantation is *unlikely* to be a cure, and mechanical support with further aggressive pharmacologic and respiratory therapy is recommended.

In the setting of cardiac transplantation, right ventricular failure is almost always secondary to excessive right ventricular afterload; it is imminent when the mean PA pressure exceeds 30 mm Hg.[63] Patients with preexisting pulmonary hypertension are at the greatest risk. Even with mild preexisting disease, severe acute pulmonary hypertension can be seen after CPB. Treatment modalities are summarized in Table 73–5. The most effective treatments are pulmonary vasodilation and inotropic support, along with maintenance of normocarbia or hypocarbia.

Phosphodiesterase inhibitors (milrinone, amrinone) and inhaled nitric oxide have become recent additions in the medical treatment of pulmonary hypertension.

### Prostaglandin E₁

$PGE_1$ in doses of 30 to 150 ng/kg/min, usually lowers PVR when other agents have failed.[64,65] Because of its systemic vasodilating effects, it is typically administered directly into

**TABLE 73–5.** Treatment Modalities for Elevated Pulmonary Artery Pressures and Right Ventricular Failure

**Primary Treatment Modalities**

Correct acidosis/provide alkalosis
Institute hyperventilation
Adjust dose of anesthesia
Minimize positive end-expiratory pressure/continuous positive airway pressure

**Secondary Treatment Modalities**

*Intravenous Vasodilator*

Nitroglycerin, sodium nitroprusside
Phosphodiesterase inhibitor (amrinone, milrinone)
Prostaglandin E₁
Prostacyclin
Inhaled nitric oxide

*Inotropic Support*

Isuprel, epinephrine, dobutamine
Amrinone, milrinone

*Mechanical Support*

Ventricular assist device

the right atrium. In cases where systemic vasodilation becomes a problem, a left atrial infusion of norepinephrine can be helpful.[66]

### Nitric Oxide

Nitric oxide is becoming an integral part of the armamentarium as a selective PA vasodilator. Its selective effects on PVR and lack of systemic vasodilatory effects make it an excellent choice in the treatment of pulmonary hypertension. Numerous studies have been performed showing nitrous oxide's corrective effect on ventilation-perfusion ($\dot{V}/\dot{Q}$) mismatch[67,68] and reduction in mean PA pressure with improvement in cardiac index.[69,70] Typical therapeutic dosages are 20 to 40 ppm inhaled nitrous oxide.

### Inotropic Support

Inotropic agents with vasodilatory properties, such as isoproterenol, milrinone, and dobutamine, should be the primary agents selected. Typically, these are used in combination with a selective PA vasodilator. If the measures discussed fail, institution of mechanical right ventricular support may be the only way to avoid a fatal outcome.

### Hyperventilation

Hyperventilation with minimal positive end-expiratory pressure and correction of acidosis are also important measures to minimize pulmonary vasoconstriction. The effect of hypoventilation or hyperventilation on PVR should not be underestimated. An increase in arterial carbon dioxide partial pressure from only 38 to 49 mm Hg has been shown to cause a 54% increase in PVR, a 34% increase in PAP, and an increase in right ventricular volume.[71]

### How Common Are Cardiac Dysrhythmias?

The denervated heart often exhibits sinus bradycardia or low-grade atrioventricular block in the early postbypass period and thus requires the institution of either chronotropic or pacemaker support. Approximately 5% to 10% of transplant patients have persistence of bradydysrhythmias and require placement of a permanent pacemaker. Patients can develop any of the wide variety of dysrhythmias seen in other cardiac surgical patients; these dysrhythmias may be more common in the denervated heart.[49,72] When treating them, remember that antidysrhythmic and chronotropic agents that act via the ANS will not be effective.

### How Common Is Bleeding?

Bleeding is more likely to be a problem after cardiac transplantation than in the average open-heart surgery patient and is multifactorial in origin (Table 73–6). Many potential cardiac transplantation patients are chronically anticoagulated with warfarin to reduce the risk of thrombotic complications associated with low cardiac output. Some cardiac transplantation patients have decreased levels of coagulation factors secondary to preoperative liver dysfunction. Although efforts are usually made to correct the coagulopathy preoperatively,

**TABLE 73–6.** Potential Causes of Bleeding in the Cardiac Transplantation Patient

| |
|---|
| Anticoagulation therapy |
| Coagulation factor deficiency from hepatic dysfunction |
| Dilutional coagulopathy |
| Thrombocytopenia |
|    Secondary to preoperative heparin therapy |
|    Dilutional |
|    Damage secondary to cardiopulmonary bypass |
| Suture line |

most patients are still anticoagulated to some degree at the time of transplantation.

### Treatment of Coagulopathy

Vitamin K administered before surgery is not effective for at least 24 to 48 hours. In addition, because most transplantation patients have some degree of impaired hepatic function, and because vitamin K effects depend on the hepatic synthesis of water-soluble factors, vitamin K should not be expected to have maximum effectiveness in these patients.

Correction of the coagulopathy preoperatively is not without risk; 2 units of fresh-frozen plasma (FFP) may be enough to precipitate acute heart failure. If correction is necessary preoperatively, careful monitoring and even concomitant administration of a diuretic should be considered. Most patients need FFP or platelets, or both, to correct their bleeding diathesis. This need should be anticipated well in advance so that CMV-free and irradiated blood products can be procured. Do not forget surgical causes of bleeding that are related to the four major anastomoses between the donor heart and the recipient.

### When Is Additional Surgery Necessary After Cardiac Transplantation?

As noted previously, up to 30% of heart transplantation recipients require surgery at a later date. Surgery may be necessary as a result of complications of the transplantation procedure, progression of an underlying disease process, complications of immunosuppressive therapy, or reasons completely unrelated to the transplantation procedure (Table 73–7). These patients provide an anesthetic challenge because the additional surgery often is emergent; patients often are seriously ill, their hearts remain denervated, and severe complications may have developed. A complete preanesthetic evaluation with emphasis on selected areas identifies the significant problems (Table 73–8).

### What Significant Problems Must Be Addressed in the Posttransplant Patient?

#### Infection

Infection is still the number one cause of death in transplant patients. Pulmonary infections are most common (65%), the most serious of which are bacterial and fungal.[20] Optimization of preoperative pulmonary function, extubation as early as

**TABLE 73–7.** Common Surgical Procedures Performed After Cardiac Transplantation

Emergency exploration for mediastinal bleeding
Thoracotomy for repair of perforated endomyocardial biopsy site
Retransplantation
Complications caused by infection
    Laparotomy
    Craniotomy
    Bronchoscopy
    Mediastinoscopy or thoracostomy
    Extremity abscess drainage
Complications caused by steroid treatment
    Repair of hip fracture/total hip replacement
    Laparotomy for perforated viscous cataract excision
Vascular surgery
    Aortic
    Peripheral
    Amputations
Cardioversion
Other procedures
    Elective
    Trauma
    Obstetric

possible, and plans for aggressive postoperative respiratory therapy should be made. Meticulous aseptic technique is mandatory in the management of transplant patients.

## Rejection

### Acute

Acute rejection is the second most common cause of death in the first 2 years after transplantation. Clinical signs of acute rejection include tachycardia, fever, dysrhythmias, and heart failure.[73] The undertaking of surgery and anesthesia during a period of acute rejection places the patient at high risk for morbidity and mortality. In many centers, cardiac catheterization and endomyocardial biopsy are recommended before elective surgery.

The immunologist managing the patient should be consulted so that the appropriate plans are made for perioperative immunosuppressive therapy. Patients continue to receive appropriate immunosuppressive therapy. Elective surgery is generally postponed until after the first year following transplantation, at which time immunosuppressant use will have been reduced to maintenance doses, and acute rejection becomes unlikely.

### Chronic

Chronic rejection, which is manifested as diffuse coronary arteritis, is a complication of heart transplantation. Its prevalence rises progressively with time: 18% at 1 year, 27% at 2

**TABLE 73–8.** Important Anesthetic Considerations in Patients Who Are to Undergo Surgery After Cardiac Transplantation

Physiology and pharmacology of the denervated heart
Risk of infection
Common complications
    Acute rejection
    Chronic rejection/graft arteritis (vasculitis)
    Complications of immunosuppressive therapy
Perioperative maintenance of immunosuppression
Perioperative steroid coverage

years, and 44% at 3 years after transplantation.[74,75] This arteritis tends to be much different from atherosclerosis in that it is diffuse, concentric, and obliterative. Thus, little collateral vessel flow is present, and the lesion is not amenable to angioplasty. Clinical manifestations of chronic rejection do not include angina because the heart is denervated. Instead, the patient usually presents with angina equivalents such as dysrhythmias, heart failure, or sudden death.

## Altered Cardiovascular Function

Although heart transplant patients may be functioning well, they do not have a normal cardiovascular system. As was discussed earlier, they have altered cardiovascular physiologic and pharmacologic responses. In addition, left ventricular dysfunction secondary to chronic rejection, graft arteritis and vasculitis, or both, may be present.

## Chronic Immunosuppression

Chronic immunosuppression is necessary for survival of heart transplantation patients; however, many side effects and complications may result (Table 73–9). The anesthesiologist should review the immunosuppressive regimen and look for the development of these complications, especially renal insufficiency and hypertension. Serum creatinine typically is >2 mg/dL. The implications for drugs that undergo renal clearance are obvious. Patients usually are treated with chronic administration of corticosteroids; thus, supplemental steroids should be considered.

## Miscellaneous Considerations

Because most of these patients have been previously exposed to blood products, they will be more difficult to crossmatch. The need for blood products must be considered preoperatively. CMV infection is devastating in the immunosuppressed patient; therefore, CMV-negative blood should be requested.

Direct-acting vasoactive agents used during cardiac transplantation should also be prepared before the induction of anesthesia. A transvenous or transcutaneous pacemaker should

**TABLE 73–9.** Complications of Immunosuppressive Therapy

| General | Infection | |
| --- | --- | --- |
| | Malignancy | |
| | Pancytopenia | |
| **Agent-Specific** | Cyclosporin A | Renal insufficiency |
| | | Hypertension |
| | Prednisone | Adrenal suppression |
| | | Glucose intolerance |
| | | Hypertension |
| | | Osteoporosis |
| | | Aseptic necrosis |
| | | Gastrointestinal bleeding |
| | | Electrolyte disturbances |
| | | Fragile skin |
| | Azathioprine | Pancytopenia |
| | | Liver dysfunction |
| | T-Cell Agents | Hypotension |
| | | Nausea and vomiting |
| | | Pulmonary edema |
| | | Serum sickness–like syndrome |
| | | Aseptic meningitis |

be readily available for the treatment of bradydysrhythmias if pharmacologic agents are ineffective.

## Does the Anesthetic Technique for a Posttransplant Patient Undergoing Surgery Matter?

A multitude of reports have recommended a variety of anesthetic agents and techniques; general and regional methods have been used without significant problems.[76–82] No evidence shows that regional anesthesia is safer than general anesthesia. Recommendation for a specific technique to the exclusion of others cannot and should not be made. As long as the pharmacologic and physiologic changes discussed earlier are appreciated, the anesthetic technique selected does not appear to be critical.[83]

Several points deserve special emphasis (Table 73–10). Avoid any maneuver that rapidly reduces filling pressures, heart rate, or systemic vascular resistance because transplant patients cannot immediately compensate for these physiologic stresses. They function best with high-normal filling pressures. This admonition is especially important to keep in mind if spinal or epidural anesthesia is used. Changes in heart rate are poor indicators of the adequacy of anesthesia and intravascular volume. Again, drugs that stimulate receptors directly have the most reliable effect in the denervated heart.

## LUNG TRANSPLANTATION

Because of the improved success of lung transplantation, there have been increases in both the number of indications and number of patients presenting for transplantation. Unfortunately, the growth in recipient pool has outpaced the relatively constant and limited supply of donors. As a result, the median waiting time for a lung transplant has increased to approximately 18 months.[1] Common indications for lung transplantation include chronic obstructive pulmonary disease (45%), emphysema, cystic fibrosis, primary pulmonary hypertension, Eisenmenger syndrome, and idiopathic pulmonary fibrosis.[3,4]

Although this chapter is directed toward specific aspects of performing lung transplant anesthesia, Chapter 64 is a good source for a more detailed discussion of anesthetic implications, management, and special techniques for pulmonary and thoracic surgery.

## What Are the Criteria for Recipient Selection and Screening?

Ideally, recipient candidates are referred when their life expectancy is anticipated to be less than 2 years. This period

**TABLE 73–10.** Anesthetic Considerations for the Patient With a Transplanted Heart

| |
|---|
| Avoid |
|   Rapid decreases in filling pressure |
|   Rapid fall in heart rate |
|   Significant decrease in systemic vascular resistance |
| Maintain high-normal filling pressures |
| Use direct-acting vasoactive drugs |
| Perioperative steroid/immunosuppressant coverage |
| Strict aseptic technique |

allows transplantation to infer an increase in overall life expectancy.[3] These patients are typically functionally impaired. However, they must be free from other systemic diseases. A list of indications and contraindications has been given (see Tables 73–2 and 73–4).

Organs are typically allocated to recipients on the basis of waiting time, regardless of illness severity.[84] This is in contrast to heart and liver transplantation in which allocation is prioritized according to illness severity.

Patients with severe pulmonary hypertension may undergo a sodium nitroprusside challenge to determine the "reversibility" of elevated PVR.[22] Patients with a reversible component of pulmonary hypertension can do as well as patients with normal pulmonary pressures.

## What Are the Criteria for Donor Selection and Screening?

A number of factors are important in determining the suitability of cadaveric donors.[3] Early endotracheal intubation limits the possibility of aspiration and subsequent pneumonia before explantation. There must be no evidence of aspiration by history, examination, or bronchoscopy. The donor must have had minimal fluid resuscitation and no known history of pleural disease. Finally, the absence of previous chest tubes or tracheotomy is also desired.

Unfortunately, less than 20% of cadaveric donor lungs are suitable for transplantation secondary to damage from excessive fluid administration, aspiration, and ventilator-assisted pneumonia.[1]

## What Testing Is Performed on the Donor Before Lung Harvest?

Donors should have a clear chest radiograph. Arterial blood gas values should be normal on appropriate ventilator settings. Sputum cultures are taken, and Gram stain should not reveal unusual findings. Last, bronchoscopy is performed before explantation to rule out the presence of masses or infection not seen on chest radiograph.

## What Are the Objectives for Donor-Host Matching?

The two primary objectives in lung transplantation compatibility matching are ABO and size matching.[85] The donor's height should be within ± 20% of the recipient's. The length of the lungs (anteroposterior), as determined by chest radiograph, may also be considered because oversized lungs can result in atelectasis.

## What Anesthesia Equipment and Monitors Are Used in Lung Transplantation?

### Anesthetic Equipment

Noninvasive monitors used during lung transplantation include pulse oximetry and 5-lead ECG, as well as noninvasive BP monitoring and expired gas analysis. Invasive monitors used are radial artery and PA catheters. These patients typically have chronic hypercapnia with elevated PA pressures.

### Pulmonary Artery Catheters

Because of the incidence of pulmonary hypertension, PA monitoring can be extremely useful in the evaluation of changes in PVR. Increases in PA pressure imply an increased load on the right ventricle, which, in severe cases, can progress to right ventricular failure. Responsiveness to pulmonary vasodilators, nitric oxide, or inotropes can be better evaluated with a PA catheter.

### Transesophageal Echocardiography

TEE has become an important monitor during lung transplantation. Evaluation of right and left ventricular function is facilitated, as is volume status. In the absence of a PA catheter, the PA pressure can be estimated if even small amounts of pulmonary or tricuspid valve insufficiency are present. Another important function is to rule out a patent foramen ovale (PFO), as the presence of a PFO may change the surgical technique.

### How Is Infection Control Managed?

The anesthesiologist plays an important role in infection control. Aseptic technique is absolutely critical. Preoperative broad-spectrum antibiotics are also typically given. In addition, the surgeon plays an important role in infection control because the surgical technique chosen for removal of the recipient's native lung may help avoid transfer of sputum and infectious secretions into the contralateral lung or mediastinum.

### When Are Lung Isolation Techniques Necessary?

Depending on the planned procedure, single-lung isolation may or may not be needed. Patients who undergo CPB will not typically need single-lung isolation. However, it is important to remember that while performing transplantation on CPB, individual lung isolation may be requested by the surgeon to test bronchial suture lines before coming off bypass.

Lung isolation can be performed with a double-lumen ETT or with a bronchial blocker. Postoperatively, a double-lumen ETT offers the advantage of selective ventilation of each lung independently, if needed.

### What Factors Should Be Considered During the Preinduction Period?

#### Blood

Typically 2 units of PRBCs are present in the OR at the time of induction. Four units may be needed when chests require reoperation or when CPB is anticipated. CMV-negative blood is used when available.

#### Drugs

Besides the medications typically used for thoracic or pulmonary surgery, other drugs should be available to correct changes in PVR. These include nitroglycerin and nitroprusside, B$_2$-agonists, phosphodiesterase inhibitors, and inhaled nitric oxide.

### Transport and Timing of Induction

As with cardiac transplantation, the transplant coordinator plays the key role in coordinating lung harvest and recipient induction. If placement of a preoperative epidural catheter is anticipated, additional time should be allotted for this procedure, as well as for other problems such as difficult intubation or difficulty obtaining intravenous access.

It is wisest to avoid preoperative sedation before arriving in the OR because these patients are chronically hypoxic and hypercapnic. Acute decompensation can occur with even small doses of sedatives or anxiolytics.

### What Are the Choices for Anesthetic Induction?

As with cardiac transplantation, any of three basic techniques—rapid, modified-rapid (ventilation through cricoid pressure), or controlled induction—can be successfully used. The risks and benefits are similar to other transplant patients, with an even greater emphasis placed on avoiding increases in right ventricular afterload. As with other transplant patients, these patients may not be nil per os and pose a risk for aspiration. Also, many of these patients cannot lie flat because of their respiratory status. (This can be overcome by preoxygenating in the inclined or sitting position and then flattening the OR table after the patient is unconscious.) The key elements to induction are to safely secure the airway with as little myocardial depression as possible.

A gradual, modified rapid-sequence induction with a short-acting hypnotic such as etomidate, a small amount of narcotic, and a nondepolarizing muscle relaxant may help avoid increases in right ventricular afterload.

Finally, regardless of the induction technique, it must be remembered that these patients are typically borderline hypovolemic; therefore, histamine-releasing anesthetic agents and negative inotropic agents should be avoided.

### What Are the Goals for Maintenance of Anesthesia?

The goals of anesthesia for lung transplantation are the same as for other anesthetic procedures: the maintenance of acceptable arterial oxygen saturation and hemodynamic parameters while rendering the patient unconscious for the surgical procedure. The transition from preoperative "spontaneous" ventilation to positive-pressure ventilation to one-lung ventilation poses several challenges to the anesthesiologist. Hyperinflation of the lungs can cause hemodynamic compromise by impeding RV preload. Some patients, with significant right ventricular failure, may not tolerate even moderate amounts of an inhalation anesthetic agent. In such cases, a balanced technique with higher doses of narcotic must be used. One-lung ventilation produces changes in oxygenation and may lead to hypoxemia, whereas changes in CO$_2$ may increase PVR and produce or worsen right ventricular failure.

## Pulmonary Hypertension and Right Ventricular Failure

Right ventricular failure is a common occurrence in patients undergoing lung transplantation with preexisting pulmonary hypertension. Before implementing any pharmacologic treatment, basic parameters including appropriate hyperventilation, maintenance of a slight metabolic alkalosis, maintenance of adequate depth of anesthesia, and minimization of intrathoracic pressure (ie, PEEP and auto-PEEP) should be geared toward lowering PA pressure.

Management is similar to treatment of elevated PA pressures and right ventricular failure, as discussed previously, in the cardiac transplantation portion of this chapter. The approach should be initially directed toward lowering PVR with any of the medications discussed. Addition of an inotrope can be helpful in cases of right ventricular failure. Addition of an α-agent (neosynephrine, epinephrine) can help preserve systemic and coronary perfusion pressures.

## What Is Involved in the Operative Procedure for Lung Transplantation?

Single-lung, double-lung, lobar, and heart-lung transplantations have all been performed. Single-lung transplantation is most frequently performed, as it is technically easier and allows for donation to two recipients. In general, complications from the surgical technique have been greatly reduced since the mid-1980s due to improved anastomotic technique.[86] A bibronchial technique, as opposed to tracheobronchial technique, is used because it reduces ischemic and stenotic complications. Revascularization of the bronchial arteries is controversial but may reduce or slow the development of bronchiolitis obliterans (BO).[87]

### Single-Lung Transplant

Single-lung transplantation is most commonly employed due to its technical ease and because it allows for transplantation of two recipients, as just mentioned. It is typically performed in the lateral decubitus position, and the surgical approach uses a lateral thoracotomy.

The choice of which lung to transplant is based on multiple factors, including a preference for removing the recipient lung with the worst $\dot{V}/\dot{Q}$ mismatching. For technical reasons, the left lung is preferred.

The bronchial anastomosis is performed first, followed by PA anastomosis, with the pulmonary vein anastomosis done last. Glucocorticoids are administered before de-airing and declamping of the vessels.

### Double-Lung Transplant

In double-lung transplantation, supine positioning is used for a transverse sternotomy. Double-lung transplantation typically requires more perioperative transfusions than single-lung transplantation and is more likely to require CPB.[88] The procedure can be performed either on or off CPB.

Bilateral sequential transplantation can be performed in patients when hypoxemia and PA pressures can be controlled and do not severely change with placement of the PA cross-clamp.

Simultaneous transplantation, using CPB, occurs in patients with severely elevated PA pressures or when single-lung oxygenation is difficult. Coagulopathy following bypass is common.

Patients with cystic fibrosis typically have extensive pleural scarring. Surgical exposure can be significantly enhanced by CPB under cardioplegic cardiac arrest.

### Lobar Transplantation

Lobar transplantation has become one therapeutic option in emergent or life-threatening situations where respiratory decompensation has begun or in urgent situations such as in infants with bronchopulmonary dysplasia on extracorporeal membrane oxygenation.[89] In cases where donor shortage would prevent transplantation and result in death, living-related or cadaveric lobar transplantation can be performed. This procedure is not routinely performed at most lung transplantation centers in the United States.

## How Is the Transplant Patient Managed Postoperatively?

### Extubation

Ideally, the lung transplant recipient is extubated on the first or second day following transplantation. This can only be done if judicious fluid management, adequate pain control, and ongoing immunosurveillance are provided.

### Respiratory Support

Postoperatively, positive pressure ventilation is continued. A normal tidal volume (8-12 mL/kg) with 5 to 10 cm of PEEP is appropriate for initial ventilator settings.

Following single-lung transplantation, hyperinflation of a more compliant (ie, COPD) native lung, with hypoventilation of the transplanted lung, may result in hemodynamic compromise from mediastinal shift. In these cases, independent lung ventilation with hypoventilation of the native lung can be helpful.

### Pain Management

Thoracic or lumbar epidural catheters allow for maximum pain relief while minimizing exposure to systemic narcotics. Ideally, this can allow for earlier extubation and ambulation. Timing of placement of these catheters is a source of controversy.

Placement before anticipated CPB and systemic heparinization is avoided. In patients not anticipated to receive systemic heparinization, an attempt should be made to place the catheter in the awake preoperative patient. This allows documentation as to the ease of placement and lack of adverse sequelae such as radicular pain. Often, however, the preoperative period from donor lung visualization to recipient incision is limited. There may not be ample time to allow placement in the awake patient. In these patients, placement following the procedure while the patient continues in the lateral decubitus position may be performed.

## Immunosuppression

Rejection may be seen as early as several days postoperatively. Fever, infiltrates on chest radiograph, and worsening arterial blood gas values all point to rejection. Bronchoscopy is typically performed for tissue diagnosis. Treatment includes pulse steroids and can include changing the immunosuppression regimen.

## Intravenous Fluid Therapy

Fluid therapy is usually restricted postoperatively and, depending on the degree of reperfusion pulmonary edema, a diuresis may be indicated. Systemic BP may be augmented with an alpha or mixed agent (eg, neosynephrine, epinephrine) if necessary.

## What Complications Follow Lung Transplantation?

In general, complications including pneumothorax, hemorrhage, and coagulopathy can be identified and treated as in other thoracic or cardiopulmonary cases. Excessive chest tube drainage, hemoptysis, hemodynamic instability, or abnormal coagulation studies help identify the origin of the problem. As mentioned previously, patients who have undergone CPB are at greater risk for postoperative bleeding. Residual heparin effect can be identified by coagulation studies. Discussion of some of the more significant complications to lung transplantation follows.

### Suture Dehiscence

Although not as much of a concern today, because of improved anastomotic techniques, dehiscence of the bronchial anastomoses can produce life-threatening consequences unless recognized and treated quickly. Acute hemoptysis, changes in ventilatory parameters including peak inspiratory pressure, and sudden changes in the ability to oxygenate should increase suspicion.

### Primary Graft Failure

Although the occurrence of transient, mild pulmonary edema following lung transplantation is common in a small number of patients, it may progress to moderate or severe acute respiratory distress syndrome (ARDS). The development of ARDS in this manner is termed *primary graft failure*. Clinical findings include infiltrates on chest radiograph, hypoxemia, decrease in lung compliance, and worsening pulmonary hypertension. A number of factors that may contribute are ischemia-reperfusion injury, surgical trauma, and lymphatic disruption. Treatment is supportive, including continued mechanical ventilation, inhaled nitric oxide, and independent lung ventilation.[90] Mortality rates may approach 60%.

### Infection

The fact that the allograft is exposed to the external environment is thought to be the reason why lung transplant patients have the highest rate of infection of all organ transplantation. Broad-spectrum antibiotic coverage is usually continued postoperatively and is aimed at nosocomial and aspiration sources until a specific agent can be isolated.

## Rejection

To aid in the detection of rejection, most transplant centers perform some form of surveillance bronchoscopy following transplantation.[91] Although a randomized trial has not yet been performed to assess the clinical impact of these procedures, complications are rare and minimal.

### Acute

Acute rejection is typically seen in the first several days following transplantation. Clinically, acute rejection is seen as new pulmonary infiltrates and new or worsening hypoxemia. Diagnosis is by transbronchial biopsy. Treatment consists of pulse steroids and increasing or changing of the immunosuppression regimen.

### Chronic

Chronic rejection is seen as BO, a syndrome consisting of progressive dyspnea, small airway obstruction, and pulmonary infiltrates. BO is thought to be multifactorial with chronic ischemia as one etiologic factor. Treatment consists of increasing the immunosuppression regimen. Revascularization of the bronchial arteries may improve the prevention of this syndrome.[87]

## How Is Anesthetic Management Carried Out Post–Lung Transplantation?

As with cardiac and other organ transplants, the possibility of further surgical intervention exists. Whether for posttransplant complications (ie, bleeding or wound dehiscence) or for nontransplant-related surgery, the status and function of the transplanted lung must be evaluated, and the surgical plan must incorporate the safest course for the organ and patient. Traditionally, it has been thought that avoidance of a general anesthetic, where the surgical procedure permits, and use of a regional technique is preferable.

## References

1. United Network for Organ Sharing website. Available at: www.unos.org. Accessed 2001.
2. Heck CF, Shumway SJ, Kaye MP. The Registry of the International Society for Heart Transplantation: sixth official report—1989. *J Heart Transplant.* 1989;8:271.
3. Arcasoy SM, Kotloff MD. Lung transplantation. *N Engl J Med.* 1999;340:1081.
4. Hosenpud JD, Bennett LE, Keck BM, et al. The Registry of the International Society for Heart and Lung Transplantation: fifteenth report—1998. *J Heart Lung Transplant.* 1998;17:656.
5. Dargie HJ, McMurray JJ, McDonagh TA. Heart failure—implications of the true size of the problem. *J Intern Med.* 1996;239:309.
6. Hetzer R, Muller J, Weng Y, et al. Cardiac recovery in dilated cardiomyopathy by unloading with left ventricular assist device. *Ann Thorac Surg.* 1999;68:742.
7. Shaw IH, Kirk AJ, Conacher ID. Anesthesia for patients with transplanted hearts and lungs undergoing non-cardiac surgery. *Br J Anaesth.* 1991;67:772.
8. Jones MT, Menkis AH, Kostuk WJ, et al. Management of general surgical problems after cardiac transplantation. *Can J Surg.* 1988;31:259.

9. Isono SS, Woolson ST, Schurman DJ. Total joint arthroplasty for steroid-induced osteonecrosis in cardiac transplant patients. *Clin Orthop.* 1987;217:201.

10. Merrel SW, Ames SA, Nelson EW, et al. Major abdominal complications following cardiac transplantation. *Arch Surg.* 1989;124:889.

11. Disea VJ, Kirkman RL, Tilney NL, et al. Management of general surgical complications following cardiac transplantation. *Arch Surg.* 1989;124:539.

12. Steed DL, Brown B, Reilly JJ, et al. General surgical complications in heart and heart-lung transplantation. *Surgery.* 1985;98:739.

13. Colon R, Frazier OH, Kahan BD, et al. Complications in cardiac transplant patients requiring general surgery. *Surgery.* 1988;103:32.

14. Burton DS, Mochizuki RM, Halpern AA. Total hip arthroplasty in the cardiac transplant patient. *Clin Orthop.* 1978;130:186.

15. Reitz BA, Baumgartner WA, Oyer PE, et al. Abdominal aortic aneurysmectomy in long-term cardiac transplant survivors. *Arch Surg.* 1977;112:1057.

16. Renlund DG, Bristow MR, Lee HR, et al. Medical aspects of cardiac transplantation. *J Cardiothorac Anesth.* 1988;2:500.

17. Copeland JG, Emery RW, Levinson MM, et al. Selection of patients for cardiac transplantation. *Circulation.* 1987;75:2.

18. Firestone L. Heart transplantation. *Int Anesthesiol Clin.* 1991;29:41.

19. Gallo JA, Cork RC. Anesthesia for cardiac transplantation. *Contemp Anesth Pract.* 1987;10:47.

20. Pennock JL, Oyer PE, Reitz BA, et al. Cardiac transplantation in perspective for the future: survival, complications, rehabilitation, and cost. *J Cardiovasc Surg.* 1982;83:168.

21. Achuff SC. Clinical evaluation of potential heart transplantation recipients. In: Baumgartner WA, Reitz BA, Achuff SC, eds. *Heart and Heart-Lung Transplantation.* Philadelphia, Pa: WB Saunders; 1990:51.

22. Costard-Jackle A, Fowler MB. Influence of preoperative pulmonary artery pressure on mortality after heart transplantation: testing of potential reversibility of pulmonary hypertension with nitroprusside is useful in defining a high risk group. *J Am Coll Cardiol.* 1992;19:48.

23. McCarthy PM, Kirby TJ, White RD, et al. Lung and heart-lung transplantation: the state of the art. *Cleve Clin J Med.* 1992;59:307.

24. Weber KT, Janicki JS, Maskin CS. Pathophysiology of cardiac failure. *Am J Cardiol.* 1985;56:3B.

25. Parmley WW. Pathophysiology of congestive heart failure. *Am J Cardiol.* 1985;56:7A.

26. Braunwald E. Heart failure: pathophysiology and treatment. *Am Heart J.* 1981;102:486.

27. Clark NJ, Martin RD. Anesthetic considerations for patients undergoing cardiac transplantation. *J Cardiothorac Anesth.* 1988;2:519.

28. Van de Heuvel AF, Van Veldhuisen DJ, Van der Wall EE, et al. Regional myocardial blood flow reserve impairment and metabolic changes suggesting myocardial ischemia in patients with dilated cardiomyopathy. *J Am Coll Cardiol.* 2000;35:19.

29. Fowler MB, Laser JA, Hopkins GL, et al. Assessment of the β-adrenergic receptor pathway in the intact failing human heart: progressive receptor down-regulation and subsensitivity to agonist response. *Circulation.* 1986;74:1290.

30. Davis FD. Coordination of cardiac transplantation: patient processing and donor organ procurement. *Circulation.* 1987;75:29.

31. Baumgartner WA, Borkon AM, Achuff SC, et al. Organization, development and early results of a heart transplant program: the Johns Hopkins experience. *Chest.* 1986;89:836.

32. Demas K, Wyner J, Mihm FG, et al. Anesthesia for heart transplantation: a retrospective study and review. *Br J Anaesth.* 1986;58:1357.

33. Baum VC. Anesthesia for heart transplantation recipients. *Semin Anesth.* 1990;9:298.

34. Humphrey LS, Blanck TJ. Anesthetic management of the heart or heart-lung transplant patient. In: Baumgartner WA, Reitz BA, Achuff SC, eds. *Heart and Heart-Lung Transplantation.* Philadelphia, Pa: WB Saunders; 1990:103.

35. Grebenik CR, Robinson PN. Cardiac transplantation at Harefield: a review from the anesthetist's standpoint. *Anaesthesia.* 1985;40:131.

36. Ream AK, Fowles RE, Jamieson S. Cardiac transplantation. In: Kaplan JA, ed. *Cardiac Anesthesia.* Vol 2. Philadelphia, Pa: WB Saunders; 1987:881.

37. Wyner J, Finch E. Heart and heart lung transplantation. In: Gelman S, ed. *Anesthesia and Organ Transplantation.* Philadelphia, Pa: WB Saunders; 1987:111.

38. Hensley FA, Martin DE, Larach DR, et al. Anesthetic management for cardiac transplantation in North America—1986 survey. *J Cardiothorac Anesth.* 1987;1:429.

39. Curling PE, Zaidan JR, Murphy DA, et al. Treatment of pulmonary hypertension after human orthotopic heart transplantation. *Anesth Analg.* 1987;66:S37.

40. Ellis L. Hydrothorax as a late complication of central venous indwelling catheters. *Surgery.* 1983;94:842.

41. Gravenstein N, Blackshear RH. In vitro evaluation of relative perforating potential of central venous catheters: comparison of materials, selected models, number of lumens, and angles of incidence to simulated membrane. *J Clin Monit.* 1991;7:1.

42. Kaye MP. The Registry of the International Society for Heart Transplantation: fourth official report—1987. *J Heart Transplant.* 1987;6:63.

43. Berberich JJ, Fabian JA. A retrospective analysis of fentanyl and sufentanil for cardiac transplantation. *J Cardiothorac Anesth.* 1987;1:200.

44. Keats AS, Strong MJ, Girgis KZ, et al. Observations during anesthesia for cardiac homotransplantation in ten patients. *Anesthesiology.* 1969;30:192.

45. Gay WA. Cardiac transplantation: a surgical perspective. *J Cardiothorac Anesth.* 1988;2:513.

46. Mason JW, Stinson EB, Harrison DC. Autonomic nervous system and arrhythmias: studies in the transplanted denervated human heart. *Cardiology.* 1976;61:75.

47. Verani MS, George SE, Leon CA, et al. Performance at rest and during exercise in heart transplant recipients. *J Heart Transplant.* 1988;7:145.

48. Stinson EB, Griepp RB, Schroeder JS, et al. Hemodynamic observations one and two years after cardiac transplantation in man. *Circulation.* 1972;45:1183.

49. Pope SE, Stinson EB, Daughters GT, et al. Exercise response of the denervated heart in long-term cardiac transplant recipients. *Am J Cardiol.* 1980;46:213.

50. McLauglin PR, Klieman JH, Martin RP, et al. The effect of exercise and atrial pacing on left ventricular volume and contractility in patients with innervated and denervated hearts. *Circulation.* 1978;58:476.

51. Pflugfelder PW, Purves PD, McKenzie FN, et al. Cardiac dynamics during supine exercise in cyclosporine-treated orthotopic heart transplant recipients: assessment by radionuclide angiography. *J Am Coll Cardiol.* 1987;10:336.

52. Wielhorski WA, Paiement B, Dyrda I, et al. The performance of nine human hearts before, during, and after transplantation. *Can Anaesth Soc J.* 1970;17:97.

53. Cannom DS, Rider AK, Stinson EB, et al. Electrophysiologic studies in the denervated human heart, II: response to norepinephrine, isoproterenol and propranolol. *Am J Cardiol.* 1975;36:859.

54. Borow KM, Neumann A, Arensman PW, et al. Left ventricular contractility and contractile reserve in humans after cardiac transplantation. *Circulation.* 1985;71:866.

55. Leachman RD, Cokkinos DV, Cabrera R, et al. Response of the transplanted, denervated human heart to cardiovascular drugs. *Am J Cardiol.* 1971;27:272.

56. Goodman DJ, Rossen RM, Ingham R, et al. Sinus node function in the denervated heart: effect of digitalis. *Br Heart J.* 1975;37:612.

57. Ricci DR, Orlick AE, Reitz BA, et al. Depressant effect of digoxin on atrioventricular conduction in man. *Circulation.* 1978;57:898.

58. Bexton RS, Milne JR, Cory-Pearce R, et al. Effect of beta blockade on exercise response after cardiac transplantation. *Br Heart J.* 1983;49:584.

59. Yusuf S, Theodoropoulus S, Dhalla N, et al. Effect of beta blockade on dynamic exercise in human heart transplant recipients. *J Heart Transplant.* 1985;4:312.

60. Cannom DS, Graham AF, Harrison DC. Electrophysiologic studies in the denervated transplanted human heart: response to atrial pacing and atropine. *Circ Res.* 1973;32:268.

61. Bexton RS, Cory-Pearce R, Spurrel RA, et al. Electrophysiologic effects of nifedipine and verapamil in the transplanted human heart. *J Heart Transplant.* 1984;3:97.

62. Mason JW, Winkle RA, Rider AK, et al. The electrophysiological effects of quinidine in the transplanted human heart. *J Clin Invest.* 1977;59:481.

63. Sibbald WJ, Driedger AA. Right ventricular function in acute disease states: pathophysiologic considerations. *Crit Care Med.* 1983;11:339.

64. Armitage JM, Hardesty RL, Griffith BP. Prostaglandin E1: an effective treatment of right heart failure after orthotopic heart transplantation. *J Heart Transplant.* 1987;6:348.

65. Fonger JD, Borkon AM, Baumgartner WA, et al. Acute right heart failure following heart transplantation: improvement with prostaglandin E1 and right ventricular assist. *J Heart Transplant.* 1986;5:317.

66. Schmid ER, Burke C, Engel MH, et al. Inhaled nitric oxide versus intravenous vasodilators in severe pulmonary hypertension after cardiac surgery. *Anesth Analg.* 1999;89:1108.

67. Hermle G, Schutte H, Walmrath D, et al. Ventilation-perfusion mismatch after lung-ischemia-reperfusion. Protective effect of nitric oxide. *Am J Respir Crit Care Med.* 1999;60:1179.

68. Della-Rocca G, Coccia C, Pugliese F, et al. Inhaled nitric oxide in patients with cystic fibrosis during preoperative evaluation and during anesthesia for lung transplantation. *Eur J Pediatr Surg.* 1998;8:262.

69. Moraes D, Loscalzo J. Pulmonary hypertension: newer concepts in diagnosis and management. *Clin Cardiol.* 1997;20:676.

70. Beck JR, Mongero LB, Kroslowitz RM, et al. Inhaled nitric oxide improves hemodynamics in patients with acute pulmonary hypertension after high-risk cardiac surgery. *Perfusion.* 1999;14:37.

71. Vijtanen A, Salmenperä M, Heinonen J. Right ventricular response to hypercarbia after cardiac surgery. *Anesthesiology.* 1990;73:393.

72. Stinson EB, Caves PK, Griepp RB, et al. Hemodynamic observations in the early period after human heart transplantation. *J Thorac Cardiovasc Surg.* 1975;69:264.

73. Schroeder JS, Berke DK, Graham AF, et al. Arrhythmias after cardiac transplantation. *Am J Cardiol.* 1974;33:604.

74. Uretsky BF, Murali S, Reddy S, et al. Development of coronary artery disease in cardiac transplant patients receiving immunosuppressive therapy with cyclosporine and prednisone. *Circulation.* 1987;76:827.

75. Chomette G, Auriol M, Cabrol C. Chronic rejection in human heart transplantation. *J Heart Transplant.* 1988;7:292.

76. Camann WR, Goldman GA, Johnson MD, et al. Caesarean delivery in a patient with a transplanted heart. *Anesthesiology.* 1989;71:618.

77. Eisenkraft JB, Dimich I, Sachdev VP. Anesthesia for major noncardiac surgery in a patient with a transplanted heart. *Mt Sinai J Med.* 1981;48:116.

78. Bricker SRW, Sugden JC. Anesthesia for surgery in a patient with a transplanted heart. *Br J Anaesth.* 1985;40:210.

79. Samuels SI, Wyner J. Anesthesia for surgery in a patient with a transplanted heart. *Br J Anaesth.* 1986;58:1199.

80. McKeown DW, Armstrong IR. Anesthesia for surgery in a patient with a transplanted heart. *Br J Anaesth.* 1986;58:1200.

81. Kanter SF, Samuels SI. Anesthesia for major operations on patients who have transplanted hearts: a review of 29 cases. *Anesthesiology.* 1977;46:65.

82. Cooper DKC, Becerra EA, Novitsky D, et al. Surgery in patients with heart transplants: anesthetic and operative considerations. *S Afr Med J.* 1986;70:137.

83. Samuels SI, Kanter SF. Anesthesia for major surgery in a patient with a transplanted heart. *Br J Anaesth.* 1977;49:265.

84. Hauptman PJ, O'Connor KJ. Procurement and allocation of solid organs for transplantation. *N Engl J Med.* 1997;336:422.

85. Daly RC, McGregor CG. Surgical issues in lung transplantation: options, donor selection, graft preservation, and airway healing. *Mayo Clin Proc.* 1997;72:79.

86. Griffith BP, Magee MJ, Gonzalez IF, et al. Anastomotic pitfalls in lung transplantation. *J Thorac Cardiovasc Surg.* 1994;107:743.

87. Norgaard MA, Olsen PS, Svendsen UG, et al. Revascularization of the bronchial arteries in lung transplantation: an overview. *Ann Thorac Surg.* 1996;62:1215.

88. Triulzi DJ, Griffith BP. Blood usage in lung transplantation. *Transfusion.* 1998;38:12.

89. Vaughn AS, Barr ML, Cohen RG. Lobar transplantation: indications, technique, and outcome. *Thorac Cardiovasc Surg.* 1994;108:403.

90. Date H, Triantafillou AN, Trulock EP, et al. Inhaled nitric oxide reduced human allograft dysfunction. *J Thorac Cardiovasc Surg.* 1996;111:913.

91. Kukafka DS, O'Brien GM, Furukawa S, et al. Surveillance bronchoscopy in lung transplant recipients. *Chest.* 1997;111:377.

# Orthotopic Liver Transplantation

Avner Sidi

Orthotopic liver transplantation (OLT) is the most common liver transplantation procedure and is performed by transplanting the donor liver to the same site after hepatectomy (Fig. 74–1). In heterotopic (auxiliary) liver transplantation, the donor liver is placed in the paravertebral gutter or in the pelvis without removal of the diseased liver.[1] The latter technique is frequently complicated by atrophy of the grafted liver (because of low portal and hepatic arterial blood flow). Therefore, it is recommended only for high-risk surgical patients or those who have reversible liver disease.

## GENERAL CONSIDERATIONS

### What Is the Impact of Timing?

Timing of transplantation is crucial; poor timing may convert an otherwise acceptable candidate for OLT into an unacceptable one because a patient's general neurologic condition, coagulopathy, acidosis, sepsis, and cardiovascular instability are important prognostic determinants (discussed later). Although preoperative severe hypoxemia may be a contraindication to OLT, the adult respiratory distress syndrome associated with hepatic failure improves dramatically with liver transplantation.

Pulmonary infection must be treated before surgery, as must other sources of infection and sepsis. The semiemergent nature of this surgery allows time for the treating physician to correct preoperative abnormalities indicated by a patient's laboratory values. When a patient has grade 4 encephalopathy (discussed later) and depends on mechanical ventilation, it may be too late for OLT.[2] However, to allow a patient's condition to deteriorate to a point that necessitates use of life-support systems before consideration of the transplantation option is unacceptable. The status definition of an OLT recipient—reflecting the urgency for OLT and general condition of the patient—was changed in 1997 (Fig. 74–2). The medical urgency status codes for liver allocation were categorized from 1 (intensive care unit [ICU]-bound) to 3 or 4 (requires continuous care/at home). In the late 1990s, a higher percentage of recipients who required continuous, but not acute, care (status 3) received OLT. On the other hand, a lower percentage of ICU-bound (status 1) patients or those in good general condition at home (status 4) received OLT (see Fig. 74–2).

### Are There Any Contraindications to Orthotopic Liver Transplantation?

Only a few years ago, OLT for fulminant hepatic failure (FHF) was considered ineffective by the time patients reached grade 4 encephalopathy,[2] and a high risk in potentially unstable cardiovascular patients.[3] However, in the 1990s, involvement of the central nervous system (CNS) or cardiovascular system has proven not to be a contraindication to OLT.[4,5] For patients with chronic liver disease and a poor prognosis because of CNS involvement,[6] OLT may be the definitive treatment,[7] especially when appropriate perioperative monitoring and treatment are used.[8] OLT in patients with severe coronary or valvular cardiac disease exposes these patients to the risk of myocardial ischemia, perioperative bleeding, further hepatic damage, renal dysfunction, and neurologic damage.[9] However, there are numerous reports of a successful two-stage surgical procedure (one or two separate sessions) when cardiac surgery preceded[9–12] or followed OLT[5] in which risk factors and survival were carefully estimated when prioritizing surgical and anesthetic therapies.

In fact, OLT had received broader application for patients with not only end-stage hepatic disease, but other organ-specific or systemic diseases.[13] In the setting of OLT and immunosuppression, cardiovascular disease and infection are the two major causes of mortality.[14] Diabetes mellitus has thus been considered to be a major risk factor in renal, cardiac,[15] and liver transplantation.[16] However, OLT (with or without pancreatic transplantation) patient and graft survival was shown not to be affected in diabetes and can be performed safely in carefully selected diabetic patients. Therefore, at present, the only contraindications to OLT may be hepatic cancer and HIV infection.

### Who Are Adult Candidates?

OLT is considered a last resort for virtually every patient with lethal hepatic disease.[2] The list of liver diseases is long (Table 74–1), and selection of appropriate recipients from such a large pool requires individual assessment. In 1982, the annual need for OLT was estimated at 15 per million population.[17] Today's need is even greater because of fewer restrictions on candidacy.

#### Nonmalignant End-Stage Liver Disease

From a purely medical standpoint, the requirement for OLT is relatively clear: nonmalignant end-stage liver disease that will not recur in the hepatic graft. There is little debate over this rationale for transplantation.

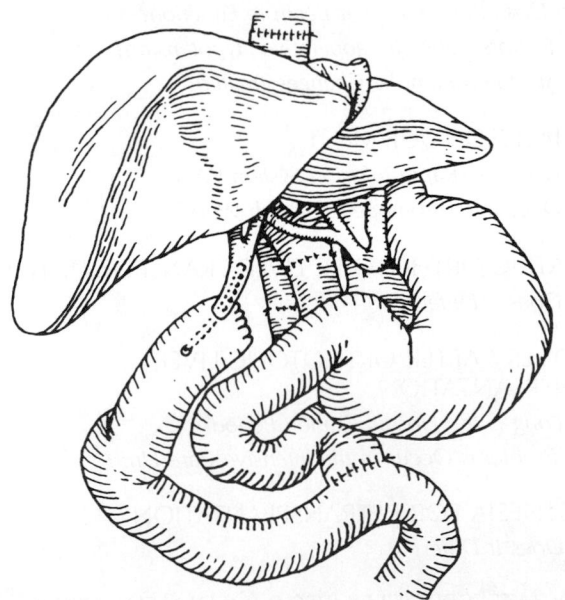

**FIGURE 74–1.** Orthotopic liver transplantation. (Modified from Starzl TE, Demetris AJ, Van Thiel D. Liver transplantation [first of two parts]. *N Engl J Med.* 1989;321:1014, by permission of the *New England Journal of Medicine.*)

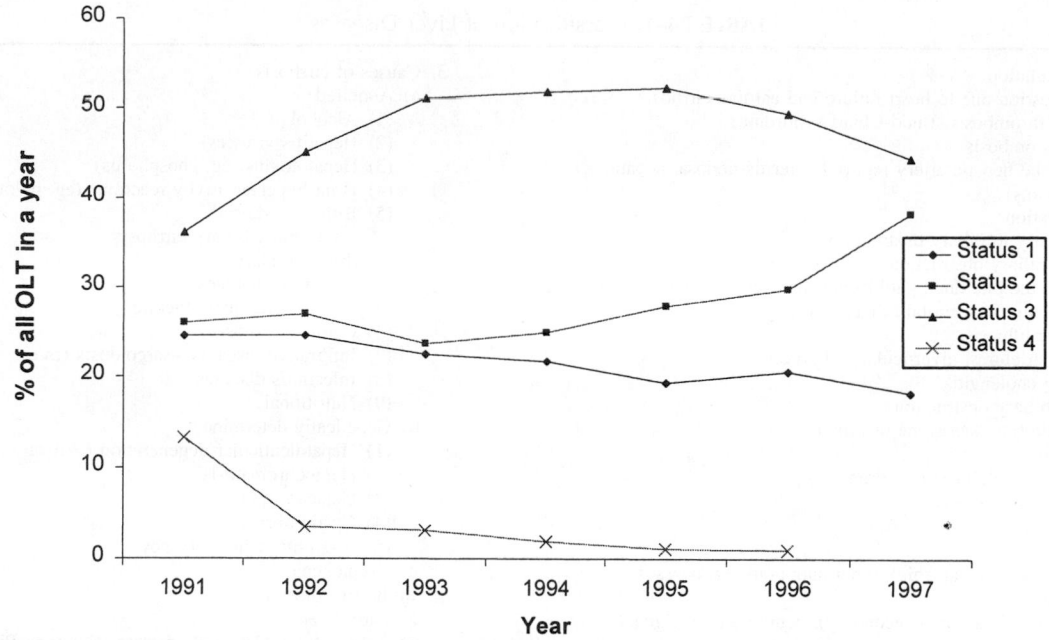

**FIGURE 74–2.** Transplant recipient characteristics: the percentage of all orthotopic liver transplant recipients, in each year during 1991–1997, in each one of the Medical Urgency Status Codes. Created after United Network for Organ Sharing (UNOS) Report 88. Percentages are based on totals excluding unknown cases. The Medical Urgency Status Codes for liver allocation are: (1) acute liver failure, or pediatric transplant candidate <18 years of age in intensive care unit because of acute or chronic liver failure, with a life expectancy of <7 days; (2) hospitalized in an acute care bed for at least 5 days, or intensive care bound; (2A) with a life expectancy without a transplant of <7 days; (3) require continuous care; (4) at home. (Data from United Network for Organ Sharing. Transplant Recipient Characteristics—1988 to 1997. UNOS Scientific Registry, September 8, 1998. United Network for Organ Sharing [UNOS] and the Organ Procurement and Transplantation Network Data Base, Richmond, Virginia.)

## Other Causes of End-Stage Liver Disease

Any other cause of end-stage liver disease is not considered to be a complete contraindication. The most common diagnoses are chronic active hepatitis, cryptogenic cirrhosis, primary biliary cirrhosis, and inborn errors of metabolism.[2,18] A prime example is alcoholic cirrhosis. With multidisciplinary care for substance abuse in properly selected cases, the results of transplantation for Laennec's alcoholic cirrhosis are as good as those for other diseases.

Even patients with hepatitis B cirrhosis, in whom the recurrence of viral infection cannot be reliably prevented, have benefited from transplantation. In addition to disease states that at one time would have ruled out OLT, inflexible age limits have been eliminated, as have many technical or mechanical obstacles such as extensive thrombosis of the portal-mesenteric-splenic veins and scarring due to multiple abdominal operations (ie, for portosystemic shunts).

The inborn errors of metabolism that result partially or completely from known deficiencies of specific liver enzymes or from abnormal products of hepatic synthesis have been treated with the most predictable results. With other, less well-understood disorders, OLT helps to clarify the pathogenesis, either by correcting the inborn error or by failing to do so.

More than 60 distinct liver diseases have been treated with OLT, including 16 in the broad category of inborn errors of metabolism and 14 in the category of cholestatic disease.

## Hepatic Cancer and Human Immunodeficiency Virus Infection

The major controversial issues are whether patients with hepatic cancer and those with antibodies for HIV should be excluded from candidacy. The percentage of patients with a tumor in large transplantation programs ranges from 4% to 34%[2,19]; a crucial requirement for candidacy in this group is that the tumor not have spread beyond the liver. A relatively high percentage of patients can have prolonged benefit from OLT despite a positive HIV test result.[2]

## Who Are Pediatric Candidates?

Half of the pediatric recipients have biliary atresia, making it the leading reason for OLT in this age group[2,18,19] and accounting for 17% of all OLT recipients. Inborn errors of metabolism are a distant second (Tables 74–2 and 74–3). Cholestatic (obstructive) diseases, including biliary atresia, account for 55% of all pediatric recipients (see Table 74–3). Pediatric recipients used to comprise approximately 50% of all transplanted patients in the 1980s; this percentage has decreased to only 20% of total OLT patients in the 1990s[20] (Fig. 74–3).

## Is the Severity of Liver Disease Important to the Prognosis?

The cause of the disease may in itself be an important prognostic determinant.[21] Features that even before surgery predict imminent death include relentless progression, grade 3 or 4 encephalopathy, severe coagulopathy, rapid shrinkage of the liver, metabolic acidosis, cardiovascular instability, and sepsis.[2] Pulmonary infection contraindicates surgery because of the high incidence of life-threatening postoperative pneumonia in immunosuppressed patients.

**TABLE 74–1.** Classification of Liver Diseases

I. Disorders of circulation
  A. Passive congestion due to heart failure and cardiac cirrhosis
  B. Hepatic vein thrombosis (Budd-Chiari syndrome)
  C. Portal vein thrombosis
  D. Disorders of the hepatic artery (eg, polyarteritis nodosa, hepatic artery aneurysms)
  E. Hepatic infarction
II. Disorders secondary to biliary obstruction
  A. Extrahepatic biliary obstruction
    1. Tumors of the bile duct, gallbladder, pancreas, ampulla of Vater, and duodenum, congenital biliary atresia
    2. Choledocholithiasis
    3. Bile duct strictures, diverticula, and so on
    4. Sclerosing cholangitis
  B. Intrahepatic biliary obstruction
    1. Intrahepatic bile duct stone or tumor
    2. Cholangitis
    3. Intrahepatic cholestasis (eg, drugs)
    4. Primary biliary cirrhosis
III. Parenchymal disorders
  A. Focal liver disease
    1. Abscess (pyogenic, amebic); other suppurative processes (eg, actinomycosis)
    2. Neoplasms (primary and secondary), benign and malignant
    3. Cysts (eg, echinococcal, congenital), gummas
    4. Granulomas (sarcoidosis, tuberculosis, berylliosis, histoplasmosis, other)
  B. Diffuse liver disorders
    1. Inborn errors of bilirubin metabolism
      a) Gilbert's syndrome
      b) Dubin-Johnson and Rotor's syndromes
    2. Hepatitis
      a) Viral (Epstein-Barr virus, cytomegalovirus, herpesvirus), hepatitis A, hepatitis B, and hepatitis C viruses
      b) Parasitic leptospirosis
      c) Bacterial
      d) Drug-induced hepatitis
      e) Chronic active hepatitis

    3. Causes of cirrhosis
      a) Acquired
        (1) Alcohol
        (2) Hepatitis virus(es)
        (3) Hepatotoxins (eg, phosphorus)
        (4) Drug hypersensitivity reactions (eg, halothane)
        (5) Biliary cirrhosis
          (a) Primary biliary cirrhosis
          (b) Secondary
            i) Gallstones
            ii) Bile duct stricture
        (6) Cardiac cirrhosis
        (7) Infiltrative diseases—sarcoidosis (rare)
        (8) Infectious diseases
        (9) Nutritional
      b) Genetically determined
        (1) Hepatolenticular degeneration (Wilson's disease)
        (2) Hemochromatosis
        (3) Galactosemia
        (4) Cystic fibrosis
        (5) $\alpha_1$-Antitrypsin deficiency
      c) Cryptogenic
    4. Infiltrative diseases
      a) Fatty liver
      b) Amyloidosis, Gaucher's disease, Neimann-Pick disease
      c) Leukemia, lymphoma
    5. Metabolic
      a) $\alpha_1$-Antitrypsin deficiency
      b) Fibrocystic disease
      c) Fatty liver of pregnancy
      d) Reye's syndrome
IV. Traumatic
  A. Penetrating
  B. Nonpenetrating

Modified from Maddrey W, section ed. Disease of the liver (Section 10). In: Harvey AM, Johns RJ, Owens AH Jr, et al, eds. *The Principles and Practice of Medicine.* 19th ed. New York, NY: Appleton-Century-Crofts; 1979:865, with permission of The McGraw-Hill Companies.

Any surgical procedure poses a risk proportional to the severity of hepatic disease, but the magnitude of surgery also contributes to the outcome and influences it. When reviewing the risk factors in cirrhotic patients (Table 74–4), the clinician should note that (1) only five variables are considered before the surgical procedure; (2) aminotransferases are not included;

and (3) prothrombin time (PT) represents an extremely valuable laboratory test for prognosis and surgical risk assessment.

## What Is the Expected Survival Rate?

Patients requiring <30 units of red blood cells (RBCs) have a survival rate >75%, whereas for those needing >70 units, the survival rate is <15%.[22]

The overall survival rate in different series of patients after introduction of the new immunosuppressive drugs is 70% to 80% (Figs. 74–4 and 74–5). Survival rates remain unchanged for 12 to 18 months after OLT and vary from 75% to 85% according to clinical severity at the time of transplantation.

Increased donor age decreases the successful outcome of liver transplantation from approximately 80% in donors younger than 50 years to 70% in donors over 50 years of age (Fig. 74–6). The graft survival rate also changes according to the recipient's age, and declines after 5 years post-OLT to <60% in recipients older than 65 years or younger than 1 year of age (Fig. 74–7). In the meantime, the 5-year patient survival rate remains at <60% for those older than 65 years and approximately 75% for those younger than 1 year of age. The survival rate after OLT for hepatocellular carcinoma beyond 2 years after surgery declines from approximately 80% to 60%.[23]

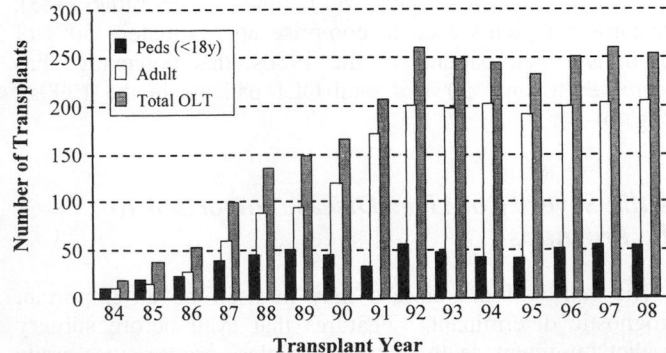

**FIGURE 74–3.** University of California, Los Angeles liver transplantation volume by year (1984–1998). (From Amersi F, Farmer DG, Busuttil RW. Fifteen-year experience with adult and pediatric liver transplantation at the University of California, Los Angeles. In: Ceckos JM, Teraski PI, eds. *Clinical Transplantation 1998.* Los Angeles, Calif: UCLA Tissue Typing Laboratory; 1998:255.)

**TABLE 74–2.** Native Liver Disease in 400 Pediatric and 858 Adult Recipients of Liver Transplants at the University of Pittsburgh, 1981–1988

| Disease | Number of Cases | Percentage |
|---|---|---|
| **Parenchymal** | 522 | 41.5 |
| Postnecrotic cirrhosis | 348 | 27.7 |
| Alcoholic cirrhosis | 76 | |
| Acute liver failure | 54 | |
| Budd-Chiari syndrome | 18 | |
| Congenital hepatic fibrosis | 9 | |
| Cystic fibrosis | 6 | |
| Neonatal hepatitis | 8 | |
| Hepatic trauma | 3 | |
| **Cholestatic** | 544 | 43.2 |
| Biliary atresia | 217 | 17.2 |
| Primary biliary cirrhosis | 186 | |
| Sclerosing cholangitis | 100 | |
| Secondary biliary cirrhosis | 25 | |
| Familial cholestasis | 16 | |
| **Inborn errors of metabolism** | 114 | 9.0 |
| **Tumors** | 78 | 6.2 |
| Primary malignant | 60 | 4.8 |
| Benign | 10 | |
| Metastatic | 8 | |
| **Total** | 1258 | 100 |

Modified from Starzl TE, Demetris AJ, Van Thiel D. Liver transplantation (first of two parts). *N Engl J Med.* 1989;321:1014, by permission of the *New England Journal of Medicine.*

## Fulminant Hepatic Failure

When patients with FHF (with or without brain edema) were selected for OLT according to an established plan or treatment model[24] and aggressively treated according to continuous perioperative measurement of intracranial pressure (ICP), survival rates in the early series ranged from 54% to 75%.[8,22,25–27] However, considering the fact that survival rates in nontransplanted patients with FHF and encephalopathy range from 12% to 67%, depending on the disease origin,[28] there is an advantage to OLT in these patients. The principal cause of death in patients with FHF is cerebral edema,[29] so ICP monitoring is crucial to outcome (see What Kind of

**TABLE 74–3.** Indications for Liver Transplantation in 216 Pediatric Patients

| Obstructive | Number of Cases | % |
|---|---|---|
| **Obstructive** | | |
| Biliary atresia | 106 | 49 |
| $\alpha_1$-Antitrypsin deficiency | 29 | |
| Alagilles' syndrome | 16 | |
| Byler's disease | 2 | |
| *Total* | 153 | 71 |
| **Miscellaneous** | | |
| End-stage liver failure | 30 | 14 |
| Chronic active hepatitis | 6 | |
| Wilson's disease | 5 | |
| Neonatal hepatitis | 5 | |
| Glycogen storage disease | 5 | |
| Familial cholestasis | 5 | |
| Tyrosinemia | 4 | |
| Hepatic tumor | 3 | |
| *Total* | 63 | 29 |
| **Total** | 216 | 100 |

Modified from Borland LM, Martin DJ. Anesthesia consideration for orthotopic liver transplantation. *Contemp Anesth Pract.* 1987;10:157.

**TABLE 74–4.** Surgical Risk Factors in Cirrhotic Patients

| Variable | Points | | |
| | *1* | *2* | *3* |
|---|---|---|---|
| Ascites | None | Moderate | Severe |
| Encephalopathy grade | None | 1-2 | >2 |
| Bilirubin (mg/dL) | 1.5 | 1.5-2.0 | >2.0 |
| Albumin (mg/dL) | 3.5 | 2.0-3.5 | <2.0 |
| Prothrombin time (seconds of control) | 1-4 | 4-6 | >6 |

Good risk (5% mortality): 5-6 points
Moderate risk (10%-20% mortality): 7-9 points
Poor risk (>50% mortality): >10 points
Data from Pugh RNH, Murray-Lyon M, Dawson JL, et al. Transection of the esophagus for bleeding varices. *Br J Surg.* 1973;60:646.

Monitoring Is Used to Evaluate Brain Function in Fulminant Hepatic Failure?, later).

## PREANESTHETIC EVALUATION

### How Does It Differ?

Preoperative evaluation is performed in two stages. In the "early" first stage, all OLT candidates are examined by anesthesiologists. This assessment is to rule out any condition contraindicating surgery and to determine physical aspects that can be improved or tests that should be performed to prepare patients optimally. Similar evaluations by hepatologists, surgeons, intensivists, and nurses can take place in a parallel manner or in a joint meeting with the anesthesiologists. The patient and the family are briefed, and the preoperative care and possible risks explained. A later, second-stage evaluation is performed immediately before surgery.

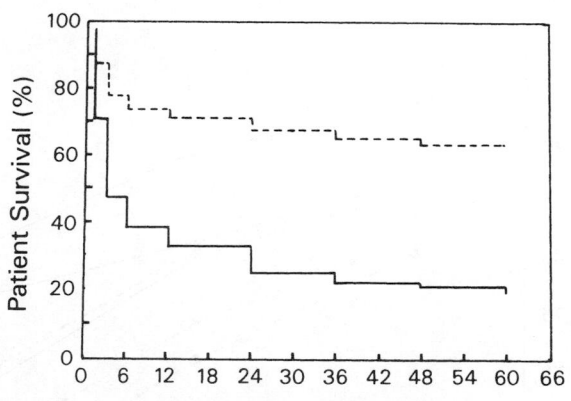

**FIGURE 74–4.** Survival of 170 liver transplant recipients treated before cyclosporin became available (1963–1979) compared with the survival of 1258 recipients treated between 1980 and mid-1988. The patients were treated by a single team at the University of Colorado through 1980 and at the University of Pittsburgh thereafter. The *solid line* denotes patients who received azathioprine (n = 170), and the *broken line* indicates those who received cyclosporin (n = 1258). Survival is calculated by use of the life-table method. (Reprinted from Starzl TE, Demetris AJ, Van Thiel D. Liver transplantation [second of two parts]. *N Engl J Med.* 1989;321:1092, by permission of the *New England Journal of Medicine.*)

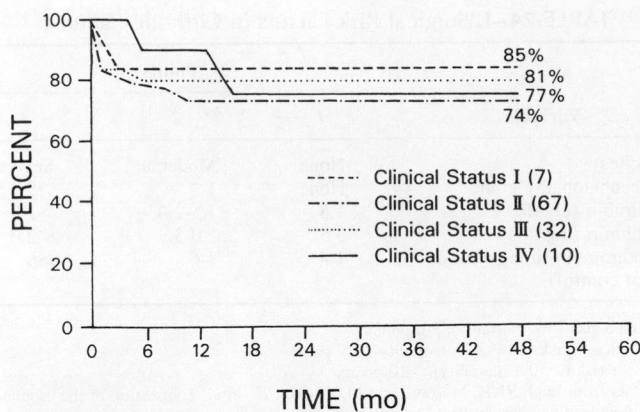

**FIGURE 74–5.** Survival of pediatric patients undergoing liver transplantation. Patients were grouped by clinical status at the time of transplantation. Group I, children who received no medical therapy for liver disease or its complications; group II, children living at home and receiving outpatient medical management; group III, children with accelerating decompensation of their disease; and group IV, children confined to the intensive care unit because of their liver disease or complications. (From Davis PJ, Cook DR. Anesthetic problems in pediatric liver transplantation. *Transplant Proc.* 1989;21:3493. © 1989. Reprinted by permission of Appleton & Lange.)

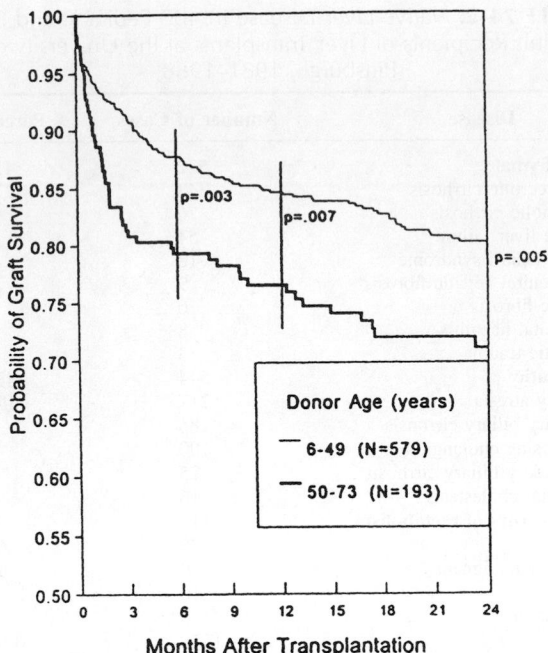

**FIGURE 74–6.** Graft survival by donor age among 772 adults receiving a single-organ liver transplantation at three medical centers between April 15, 1979 and June 30, 1994. (From Hoofnagle JH, Lombardero M, Zetterman RK, et al. Donor age and outcome of liver transplantation. *Hepatology.* 1996;24:89.)

## What Are the Signs and Symptoms of Hepatic Failure?

Failure of hepatic cell function produces generalized manifestations that are constitutional, cutaneous, endocrine, and hematologic (Table 74–5). They reflect the liver's central role in metabolism and homeostasis. The more dramatic include jaundice, ascites, bleeding from varices due to portal hypertension, and mental changes associated with hepatic encephalopathy. Hypoxemia, anemia, and coagulopathy often accompany hepatic disease. Encephalopathy, renal dysfunction, and ascites are also common.

For clinical purposes, patients with liver diseases can be divided into two main groups:

1. Parenchymal disease is usually associated with a hyperdynamic circulatory state. It is characterized by decreased vascular resistance (peripheral vasodilation, increased arteriovenous shunting); increased circulating blood volume

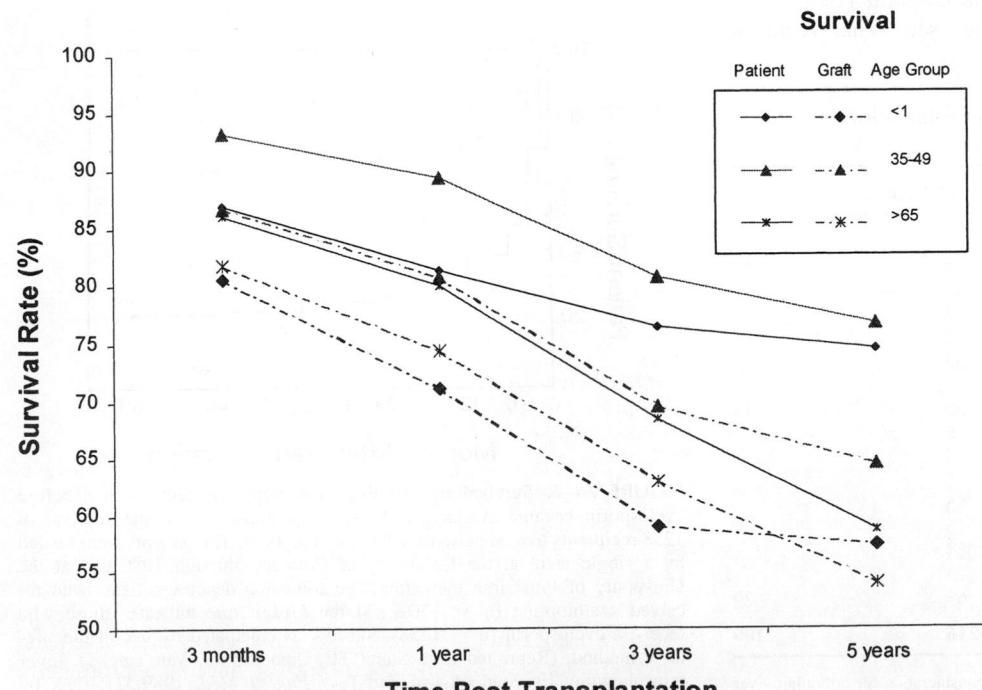

**FIGURE 74–7.** Patient and graft survival rates, in three age groups, at 3 months to 5 years after liver transplantation. Created after United Network for Organ Sharing (UNOS) Report 88. (Data from United Network for Organ Sharing. Patient Survival Rates at Three Months and at One, Three and Five Years. UNOS Scientific Registry Data, as of September 8, 1998. United Network for Organ sharing [UNOS] and the Organ Procurement and Transplantation Network Data Base, Richmond, Virginia.)

TABLE 74–5. Systemic Signs and Symptoms in Hepatic Disease

| Manifestation | Possible Mechanisms |
| --- | --- |
| **Constitutional** | |
| Anorexia | Overall hepatic failure |
| Weight loss | |
| Weakness, fatigue | |
| Nausea | Splanchnic congestion |
| | Ascites |
| Flatulence | Hepatic inflammation |
| Fever | Reduced resistance to infection |
| Fetor hepaticus | Abnormal methionine metabolism |
| **Cardiovascular** | |
| Hyperdynamic circulation | Hormone-induced general vasodilation |
| Bounding pulses–wide pulse pressure | |
| Increased cardiac output | |
| Tachycardia | |
| Increased plasma volume | Associated with portal hypertension |
| Cyanosis | Arteriovenous anastomoses (lung, liver, systemic) |
| Clubbing | Arterial oxygen saturation |
| **Cutaneous and endocrine** | |
| Spider telangiectases | Abnormal metabolism of estrogens and androgens |
| Palmar erythema | |
| Menstrual irregularities | |
| Impotence | |
| Gynecomastia | |
| **Hematologic** | |
| Petechiae | Decreased platelet count often associated with leukopenia and anemia |
| Ecchymoses | Impaired production of coagulation proteins |
| Generalized bleeding tendency | Both of above |

Modified from Maddrey W, section ed. Disease of the liver (Section 10). In: Harvey AM, Johns RJ, Owens AH Jr, et al, eds. *The Principles and Practice of Medicine.* 19th ed. New York, NY: Appleton-Century-Crofts; 1979:865.

and cardiac output; and increased splanchnic (except the liver), pulmonary, and skin blood flow. Systemic and cardiac filling pressures, heart rate, hepatic arterial (but not portal) blood flow, and renal blood flow are maintained.

2. In patients with cholestasis, jaundice is the primary manifestation.

## What Associated Problems May Be Present?

### Cardiovascular

The *hyperkinetic circulation* observed in patients with chronic liver disease is thought to be caused by pulmonary and portosystemic shunts and circulating vasoactive substances (eg, glucagon, ferritin, atrial natriuretic factor, vasodilating prostaglandin E₁, vasoactive intestinal polypeptide) that have not been detoxified in these cirrhotic patients. Plasma volume expansion is probably not a major factor.

A vasodilation-induced decrease in systemic pressure and stimulation of baroreceptors provoke a subsequent increase in sympathetic tone and an increase in arginine vasopressin and renin release. A high cardiac output results, as do splanchnic vasoconstriction and increased preload.

Paradoxically, many cirrhotic patients have impaired contractile function and cardiomyopathy. The production of false neurotransmitters with norepinephrine depletion and low myocardial β-adrenergic receptor density correlates with catechol-

amine hyposensitivity. Overall, a cirrhotic patient's heart has a very limited ability to respond to stress.

### Pulmonary

*Hypoxemia* is often associated with severe hepatic disease and results from ventilation/perfusion abnormalities, including impaired hypoxic pulmonary vasoconstriction; rightward shift of the oxyhemoglobin dissociation curve; hypoventilation due to ascites; decreased pulmonary diffusing capacity resulting from an increase in extracellular fluid; and right-to-left shunts across the lungs. The latter are due to pulmonary spider angiomas, portopulmonary communications, and humoral factors. Tidal volume, vital capacity, and functional residual capacity are decreased, yet compensatory tachypnea can result in respiratory alkalosis. Acute respiratory failure sometimes develops in patients with severe hepatocellular dysfunction, possibly secondary to the decreased hepatic clearance of endotoxin.

### Hematologic

*Anemia,* which may be hypochromic, microcytic, or macrocytic, invariably develops in cirrhotic patients as a result of malabsorption of iron and folic acid, frequent variceal bleeding, and hypersplenism. Furthermore, changes in lipid metabolism of cell membranes shorten RBC survival. In severe hepatocellular disease, a coagulopathy is also evident.

### Central Nervous System

Patients may exhibit minimal confusion (stage 1 encephalopathy), gross mental confusion (stage 2), somnolence and stupor (stage 3), or deep coma with response only to pain (stage 4). Hepatic encephalopathy is considered to be associated with increased blood ammonia levels and accumulations of other substances (eg, mercaptans, short-chain fatty acids, false neurotransmitter, and γ-aminobutyric acid). Several factors may worsen encephalopathy, including diuretics, gastrointestinal bleeding, infection, and further hepatic damage. Brain edema formation appears with FHF, and intracranial hemorrhage may develop with severe coagulopathy.

### Renal Fluids and Electrolytes

Three types of *renal dysfunction* are encountered: (1) hepatorenal syndrome, characterized by low urine sodium ($U_{Na^+}$ <10 mEq/L); (2) tubular necrosis, characterized by high $U_{Na^+}$ excretion with casts; and (3) prerenal azotemia with low $U_{Na^+}$ (Table 74–6). Patients may recover from the last two complications, but hepatorenal syndrome is frequently lethal. It may improve after transplantation.[1]

Differentiation of the syndrome from other renal diseases is very difficult because of the frequent use of complex diuretic therapy. Kidney dysfunction is associated with enhanced renin-angiotensin activity, hyperaldosteronism, increased sympathetic tone, increased antidiuretic hormone activity, increased conjugated bilirubin levels, and altered activity of the renal prostaglandins or kallikrein-kinin systems. Inadequate intravascular volume and cyclosporin-induced nephrotoxicity further impair renal function.

**TABLE 74–6.** Urinary Composition in Oliguria

| Component | Hepatorenal Syndrome | Prerenal Failure | Acute Tubular Necrosis | Hepatorenal Failure |
|---|---|---|---|---|
| Urinary sodium | <10 mEq/L | <25 mEq/L | >25 mEq/L | <10-20 mEq/L |
| Urinary specific gravity | >1.024 | >1.015 | 1.010-1.015 | >1.015 |
| Urinary:plasma osmolality | >2.5:1 | >1.8:1 | ≤1.1:1 | >1.2:1 |
| Urinary:plasma urea | >100:1 | >20:1 | 3:1, rarely >10:1 | >10:1 |
| Urinary:plasma creatinine | >60:1 | >30:1, rarely <10:1 | <10:1 | >40:1 |

Compiled from Mazze RI. Critical care of the patient with acute renal failure. *Anesthesiology.* 1977;47:138; and Miller TR, Anderson RJ, Linas SL, et al. Urinary diagnostic indices in acute renal failure: a prospective study. *Ann Intern Med.* 1978;89:47.

## Blood Volume

Blood volume increases by 10% to 20% above normal levels. However, intravascular volume can be depleted owing to continuous formation of ascites or diuretic therapy to treat ascites. Caution must be exercised during repletion because rapid administration of volume, including blood and its products, may cause intravascular overloading, especially if myocardial dysfunction is evident.

## Hyponatremia

Hyponatremia is a common finding because of water retention due to antidiuretic hormone activity, impaired renal water excretion, or true sodium deficiency (therapeutically produced). This multifactorial combination may explain why preoperative correction of hyponatremia is very difficult and therefore is best accomplished with the aid of hemodynamic and laboratory monitoring.

## Hypokalemia

Hypokalemia is a chronic finding because depletion of total body potassium frequently follows diuretic therapy, inadequate intake, and continuous loss (vomiting and diarrhea). Aggressive and complete correction of acute hypokalemia should be avoided because of the preoperative difficulties in treatment and because the situation usually reverses to hyperkalemia after reperfusion of the new liver (discussed later). Hyperkalemia may be observed in patients with moderate to severe renal dysfunction.

## Acid-Base Derangements

*Metabolic alkalosis* in patients with chronic liver disease is associated with hyperaldosteronism, vomiting, and diarrhea. It is frequently complicated by hypoxia-induced respiratory alkalosis. On the other hand, metabolic acidosis often is found in patients with acute fulminant hepatitis, rapidly progressive hepatic failure, or unrecognized infection.

## What Kind of Monitoring Is Used to Evaluate Brain Function in Fulminant Hepatic Failure?

The etiology of encephalopathy and coma in patients with FHF has been attributed to a vasogenic (extravasation) and cytotoxic (intracellular) type of brain edema[7] due to accumulations of toxins of gut origin (mostly nitrogenous products) that bypass the liver and reach the brain. During OLT, patients may be even more susceptible to sudden changes in ICP because of frequent changes in fluid balance and intravascular volume (blood loss, edema), venous pressures (clamping and unclamping of major vessels), overall hemodynamic stability (low contractility and peripheral vasodilation), and potential intracerebral bleeding (clotting abnormalities). Management of brain edema in patients with FHF depends on objective measurements (eg, ICP monitoring), and the goal is to maintain a cerebral perfusion pressure (CPP) value of >40 mm Hg and ICP measurement <30 mm Hg[7,27] no matter what the cause of the edema. This is no different from the guidelines and goals used in the treatment of brain edema due to head trauma.[29] Thus, preoperative and intraoperative management of patients with FHF and encephalopathy is directed toward decreasing intracranial edema and pressure to control and maintain adequate brain perfusion. When conditions to support cerebral perfusion are optimized,[7] OLT should be considered early for those patients in the poor prognosis group.[24] Variables to consider in the treatment of these patients may be static (eg, age, etiology, jaundice) or dynamic (eg, bilirubin, PT). When patients with FHF were selected for OLT according to an established plan[24] and aggressively treated in response to ICP and CPP monitoring, the survival rate was 54% to 75%[8,25–27]—higher than without monitoring or transplantation (12%-67%).[28] The survival rate was lower than in patients who underwent OLT without FHF (70%-80%).[3]

During surgery, the goals and methods for controlling and maintaining adequate brain perfusion stay the same. Hemodynamic instability is a problem during OLT[1] and can decrease brain perfusion. Additional ways of promoting hemodynamic stability should be used and include vasopressor catecholamines (epinephrine, ephedrine, phenylephrine) for pressure; noncatecholamines (calcium, amrinone) for myocardial contractility; and colloids and noncolloids (crystalloids, plasma, blood) for volume. In our experience, hemodynamic instability can also decrease CPP. In fact, when other means for decreasing ICP are (1) ineffective (eg, due to a nonfunctioning kidney); (2) potentially harmful and causing hemodynamic instability (eg, barbiturates, hyperventilation, furosemide); or (3) already exhausted (eg, mannitol, hyperventilation), the only way then of increasing CPP may be to increase systemic perfusion by pharmacologic agents or volume administration. Hemodynamic instability during OLT also commonly occurs at the time of reperfusion because of metabolic factors, volume overload, air embolism, uncontrolled bleeding, or a combination of these problems.[1] However, treatment (phenylephrine, calcium chloride, epinephrine, and rapid blood administration) at this time may be problematic because the effect may combine with preexisting causes for high ICP and result in a dramatic increase in ICP in those patients with decreased intracranial compliance.[8,26] Therefore, monitoring ICP, CPP, or brain perfusion on a continuous basis is indicated during OLT, and treatment should be judged only according to its ability to improve cerebral perfusion.

Anesthetic management has to be reconsidered and adjusted in specific cases of liver failure with neurologic disease and potential hemodynamic and cardiovascular instability. Barbiturates have traditionally been advocated in cases of elevated ICP, but can potentially cause hemodynamic instability. Isoflurane produces comparatively less cerebral vasodilation than other halogenated inhalational agents, but high doses may still increase ICP.[8] Systemic hypertension (eg, during arterial occlusion) can be treated with nitroprusside, and β-adrenergic receptor blocking agents (esmolol, labetalol) may be indicated.[8] Continuous monitoring of CPP may indicate or contraindicate certain agents, and because there is no single optimum approach, agents and techniques must be tailored to each individual patient using continuous ICP/CPP monitoring.

Intracranial bleeding is a potential and fatal hazard of ICP monitoring and causes death in 5% to 22% of patients.[8,25] Placement of the ICP catheter is a highly invasive procedure and requires expert surgical technique, especially in those patients with coagulopathy. Blood product therapy should be given as needed based on coagulation studies before ICP catheter insertion. There are a variety of different ICP monitoring techniques, including subdural,[8] extradural,[25] and intraventricular[30] monitoring systems. The intraventricular catheter is the most invasive. The extradural—which has the lowest bleeding and complication rate—is probably the least reliable method to measure ICP and does not permit cerebrospinal fluid drainage to treat high ICP. When intracranial bleeding occurs after ICP catheter insertion, the mortality rate can rise as high as 60% in these patients.[8] This is a good reason for seeking alternate, noninvasive techniques such as transcranial Doppler (TCD) and establishing their role as perioperative monitors of CPP in patients with FHF, brain edema, and coagulopathy. TCD monitoring, used extensively in head injury and cerebral circulatory arrest, has also been used in patients with FHF, but failed to show any abnormal flow velocity in cerebral vessels before surgery.[31]

We found that TCD can provide adequate information when CPP is low, and that the information thus obtained regarding low perfusion or high cerebrovascular resistance (pulsatility difference) has a good correlation with CPP and increases dramatically when CPP is <50 to 60 mm Hg. In those instances, the diastolic component of the TCD recording (TCD-D) decreased to near 0, which warned of decreased CPP. In all cases of seriously decreased CPP, TCD-D decreased <10 cm/s.[4]

In conclusion, the outcome of patients with FHF and grade 4 encephalopathy is greatly improved by CPP monitoring. The use of TCD monitoring in addition to or as a replacement for ICP monitoring is effective, especially in patients with coagulopathy. However, further animal and human studies are indicated to show the quantitative relationship between brain perfusion (monitored by TCD) and intracranial pressures (ICP, CPP).

## Why Does Coagulopathy Occur in Chronic Liver Disease?

Coagulopathy in hepatic disease results from the following processes:

1. Malabsorption of substrates
2. Thrombocytopenia, which occurs in 70% of cases owing to hypersplenism
3. Impaired platelet function resulting from small, hypofunctional platelets
4. Increased fibrinolytic activity, with decreased production of antiplasmin and inadequate clearance of tissue plasminogen activators
5. Decreased hepatic synthesis of plasma clotting factors. Levels of all coagulation factors decrease except for fibrinogen and factor VIII (the latter mostly produced in vascular endothelium). Dysfibrinogenemia may follow the formation of abnormally structured fibrinogen.
6. Shortened half-lives of plasma clotting factors due to defective hepatic synthetic function
7. Formation of abnormal coagulation products

## How Much Bleeding Is Expected in Orthotopic Liver Transplantation?

The amount of bleeding expected during OLT is highly variable, ranging in different series from 1 to >100 units of RBCs and fresh-frozen plasma (FFP).[1,19,22] Estimated blood loss ranges from 10 to 1000 mL/kg, with an average of >100 mL/kg.[32] The clinical significance of coagulopathy is confirmed by the correlation between its preoperative severity and intraoperative blood product requirements. Patients with hepatocellular disease and a poor preoperative coagulation profile require more blood products.[22]

### Type of Liver Disease

Statistically significant differences for RBC replacement according to diagnostic group have been reported. Patients with chronic active hepatitis tend to require more blood and blood products than do patients with perisclerosing cholangitis (Table 74–7), although the latter tend to require more blood than those with primary biliary cirrhosis. Patients in the last two categories are usually diagnosed earlier, treated earlier, and sustain less parenchymal damage with less severe subsequent clotting abnormalities.

When patients are classified into risk categories for likelihood of bleeding, according to age, weight, diagnosis, coagulation status, previous operation, and so on (similar to Table 74–4), a significant difference has been noted between high-risk and low-risk cases in adults (Table 74–8). The *median* requirement for RBCs and FFP by those classified as high-risk cases was almost twice that needed in low-risk cases, although the *average* use was similar. This observation probably reflects that a few low-risk patients had substantial bleeding that necessitated a large number of blood units.

A more specific isolation of the relationship between blood and blood components consumed intraoperatively and the extent of liver disease was found with elevated PT (>15.0 seconds) and presence of ascites (Tables 74–9 and 74–10). Pediatric patients have a tendency toward a lower estimated blood loss (see Table 74–8), but mean loss in milliliters per kilogram is similar.[32]

**TABLE 74–7.** Intraoperative Blood and Blood Component Use (in Units) for 66 First-Transplant Patients, Shown by Major Diagnostic Group

| Type of Transfusion | CAH (n = 24) | | PSC (n = 22) | | PBC (n = 20) | | P* |
| --- | --- | --- | --- | --- | --- | --- | --- |
| | *Mean* | *Median* | *Mean* | *Median* | *Mean* | *Median* | |
| Packed red blood cells | 23.7 | 16.9 | 20.7 | 13.7 | 13.5 | 9.4 | .17 |
| Fresh-frozen plasma | 18.3 | 15.0 | 12.4 | 7.5 | 10.3 | 8.5 | .04 |
| Cryoprecipitate | 23.3 | 20.0 | 15.3 | 10.0 | 10.1 | 10.0 | .02 |
| Platelets | 21.9 | 14.5 | 17.0 | 12.0 | 10.7 | 12.0 | .02 |

*Kruskal-Wallis one-way analysis of variance of ranks of median usage for three groups.
CAH, chronic active hepatitis; PSC, primary sclerosing cholangitis; PBC, primary biliary cirrhosis; 17 patients had other diagnoses.
From Motschman TL, Taswell HF, Brecher ME, et al. Intraoperative blood loss and patient and graft survival in orthotopic liver transplantation: their relationship to clinical and laboratory data. *Mayo Clin Proc.* 1989;64:346. By permission.

## What Are the New Possibilities and Techniques in Donor Harvesting and Graft Availability?

### Split Cadaveric Donor Graft

OLT in small children has been limited by the shortage of suitable cadaveric donor (CD) organs. The number of new transplant candidates younger than 5 years of age has increased 5% annually since 1988, whereas the annual number of CD transplantations performed in this age group has fallen[33-35] (Fig. 74–8). In the adult recipient, the split is done using the extended right lobe of the CD graft, and in the pediatric recipient, the left lobe of the CD graft is used. The split CD graft was the obvious technical solution for this problem of pediatric graft availability, and has been used most frequently (Fig. 74–9). However, when emergency OLT was needed, and the technique of emergency living donor liver transplantation (LDLT) could not be applied or was not yet developed (before 1999),[36] split CD transplantation of two grafts was the only solution.

### Living Donor or Living Related Liver Transplantation

Initial reports on LDLT in the early 1990s established the technical feasibility of the procedure.[37,38] The donor hepatectomy can include left lobes, left lateral segments,[39,40] or an extended right lobe.[41] LDLT has some advantages for the pediatric recipient and the transplant population as a whole (Table 74–11), including increased graft availability and survival and decreased morbidity, mortality, rejections, and cost. Potential donor evaluation should include bedside ABO blood type compatibility with recipient (which is the only need in the CD graft). Also necessary is exclusion of acute, chronic, or viral illness, assessment of liver/biliary system function and anatomy, and psychological assessment (Table 74–12). Although the procedure is relatively safe for the donor, >10% of donors have presurgical complications.[39] Surgical experience and technical modifications have resulted in significant reduction of these complications. The mortality risk of hepatic resection in noncirrhotic people is extremely low when the operation is performed at an experienced center.[39,40,42,43] Emergency transplantation from living donors can increase OLT applicability from 10% to 37%, with high (85%) survival rates.[36] Thus, where cadaveric organ donation is scarce, emergency LDLT can be applied to high-urgency patients.

## What Should Be Known About Organ Preservation Techniques?

### Simple Hypothermia

Simple hypothermia is frequently used for preservation of the donor liver. It consists of irrigating the hepatic vascular

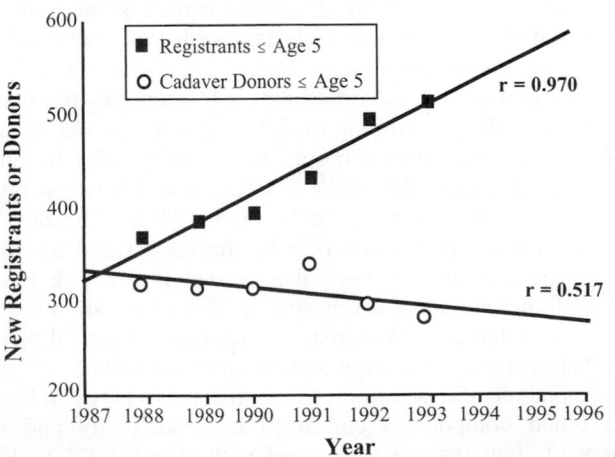

**FIGURE 74–8.** Trends in annual number of new liver transplant candidates 5 years of age or younger registered with the United Network for Organ Sharing, and the annual number of cadaver organ donors in this same age category. (From Jurim O, Shackleton CR, McDiarmid SV, et al. Living-donor liver transplantation at UCLA. *Am J Surg.* 1995;169:529.)

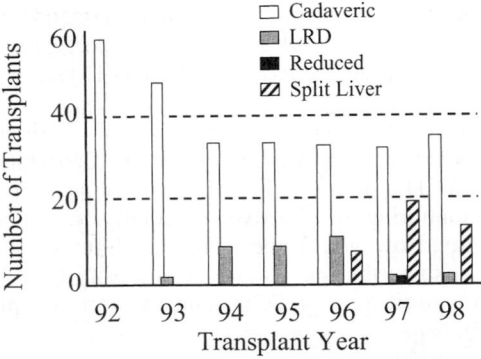

**FIGURE 74–9.** University of California, Los Angeles pediatric graft type (1992–1998). LRD, living related donor. (From Amersi F, Farmer DG, Busuttil RW. Fifteen-year experience with adult and pediatric liver transplantation at the University of California, Los Angeles. In: Ceckos JM, Teraski PI, eds. *Clinical Transplantation 1998.* Los Angeles, Calif: UCLA Tissue Typing Laboratory; 1998:257.)

**TABLE 74–8.** Intraoperative Blood and Blood Component Use (in Units) in the First 100 Liver Transplantations at the Mayo Clinic, Shown by Risk Category

| Type of Transfusion | High-Risk, Adult (n = 68) Mean | Median | Low-Risk, Adult (n = 27) Mean | Median | Child (n = 5) Mean | Median | P* |
|---|---|---|---|---|---|---|---|
| Erythrocytes | 19.2 | 14.8 | 19.0 | 8.4 | 5.2 | 4.7 | .02 |
| Fresh-frozen plasma | 15.3 | 12.0 | 11.9 | 7.0 | 4.6 | 3.0 | .03 |
| Cryoprecipitate | 19.6 | 17.0 | 13.4 | 10.0 | 9.0 | 10.0 | .11 |
| Platelets | 18.9 | 12.0 | 13.6 | 12.0 | 6.8 | 6.0 | .06 |

*Rank sum test, adult high-risk versus adult low-risk median use.

From Motschman TL, Taswell HF, Brecher ME, et al. Intraoperative blood loss and patient and graft survival in orthotopic liver transplantation: their relationship to clinical and laboratory data. *Mayo Clin Proc.* 1989;64:346. By permission.

tree and bathing the liver in iced preservation solution. Continuous perfusion is used rarely because complex equipment is required, vascular resistance may increase gradually, and the outcome is not superior to that with simple hypothermia.

## Preservation Solution

The preservation solution has an electrolyte composition similar to intracellular fluid (high potassium and low sodium concentrations). Collins' solution provides a clinically satisfactory cold ischemia time of 10 hours. The Wisconsin solution allows a cold ischemia time of 24 hours.[44] This long ischemia time permits the liver team to plan ahead for daytime surgery on a semiemergent basis. However, some reports[13] suggest a better outcome (related to biliary tract stenosis) if the total time from harvest to unclamping of the portal vein is <12 hours.

All preservation methods can affect recipient homeostasis. Rapid influx of acidic and metabolite-rich solution, flushed into the systemic circulation when the grafted liver is perfused, may cause hemodynamic instability, requiring therapy with epinephrine or phenylephrine (discussed later), especially if chlorpromazine is added in an attempt to maintain hepatocyte membrane integrity (Table 74–13).

## Timing

Most donors are declared brain-dead and eligible for organ donation during usual working hours. Additional time is needed for coordination of the different organ harvest teams,

traveling and harvesting, and selection and preparation of the OLT candidate. When the preservation time of the donor liver was short,[45] 85% of liver transplantations began outside usual working hours (Fig. 74–10). With roughly 5 to 6 hours required from the start of anesthesia to recirculation with the donor liver, timing must be considered. Time estimates reflect a 1- to 1½-hour anesthesia preparation time for induction and line placement before any surgical preparation.

## How Is the Preparation Phase Organized?

Use of resources is the prime consideration during preparation for OLT. The anesthesiologist should plan for an operating room time of 8 to 20 hours,[32] with an average total time of 8½ hours for anesthesia, of which 7 hours is devoted to surgery (Table 74–14).

The minimum anesthesia staff should comprise a 3:2 ratio of physicians to Certified Registered Nurse Anesthetists or technicians to deal with simultaneous administration of anesthesia and operation of the rapid-infusion device and the thromboelastograph (TEG). A courier, responsible solely for the transport of specimens and blood products, is indispensable.

## The Liver Team Approach

The liver team is a multidisciplinary team of administrators, hepatologists, surgeons, anesthesiologists, internists, technicians (including the perfusionist), and nurses. Among the administrators should be a central role coordinator who assembles the different services involved in the OLT and notifies

**TABLE 74–9.** Comparison of Intraoperative Blood Use (in Units) in Relationship to Prothrombin Time in the First 100 Liver Transplantations at the Mayo Clinic

| Type of Transfusion | PT > 15.0 (n = 28) Mean | Median | PT ≤ 15.0 (n = 72) Mean | Median | P* |
|---|---|---|---|---|---|
| Erythrocytes | 25.2 | 20.4 | 15.8 | 10.8 | .007 |
| Fresh-frozen plasma | 18.8 | 20.5 | 11.9 | 10.0 | .004 |
| Cryoprecipitate | 25.9 | 20.0 | 14.1 | 10.0 | .005 |
| Platelets | 22.1 | 19.0 | 14.8 | 12.0 | .001 |

*Rank sum test, comparison of median values.

PT, prothrombin time.

From Motschman TL, Taswell HF, Brecher ME, et al. Intraoperative blood loss and patient and graft survival in orthotopic liver transplantation: their relationship to clinical and laboratory data. *Mayo Clin Proc.* 1989;64:346. By permission.

**TABLE 74–10.** Comparison of Intraoperative Blood Use (in Units) in Relationship to Presence of Ascites in the First 100 Liver Transplantations at the Mayo Clinic

| Type of Transfusion | Ascites (n = 37) Mean | Median | No Ascites (n = 63) Mean | Median | P* |
|---|---|---|---|---|---|
| Erythrocytes | 26.4 | 22.3 | 13.7 | 9.7 | <.0001 |
| Fresh-frozen plasma | 19.2 | 18.0 | 10.7 | 8.0 | <.001 |
| Cryoprecipitate | 21.5 | 20.0 | 15.0 | 10.0 | .001 |
| Platelets | 20.9 | 18.0 | 14.5 | 12.0 | .001 |

*Rank sum test, adult high-risk versus adult low-risk median use.

**TABLE 74–11.** Living Donor Liver Transplantation (LDLT) Advantages

- Increases the number of organs available for the pediatric population
- Most LDLTs are elective, which should incur lower morbidity, mortality, and cost
- Minimal cold ischemia time and use of healthy donor contribute to graft survival
- Immunologic advantage of receiving LDL, supported by lower incidence of rejections

From Grewal HP, Thistlethwaite JR Jr, Loss GE, et al. Complications in 100 living-liver donors. *Ann Surg.* 1998;228:214.

laboratory and support personnel about expected candidates and donors.

Anesthesia personnel should see the patient, assemble medications and supplies, and set up the operating room. The liver team should meet for preoperative evaluations/discussions and postoperative analysis of complications or follow-up.

## What Should Be Accomplished During the Second-Stage Evaluation?

A brief second examination is performed immediately before surgery when a donor organ has been identified. Attention should be directed to evaluating any neurologic deterioration since the initial first-stage evaluation. Signs of progressive metabolic acidosis, infection, or sepsis should be sought. Cardiovascular instability, pulmonary infection, and severe coagulopathy should be corrected and treated.

The internist should ensure that a patient is in the best condition for surgery. Ideally, ascites should be controlled and nutrition improved, with PT showing a return toward normal. Parenteral vitamin K should have been given at least three days before surgery if possible; it corrects coagulation defects within 24 to 36 hours unless liver function is so poor that vitamin K-dependent proteins such as factor V and prothrombin cannot be synthesized. Albumin, FFP, and cryoprecipitate can be given immediately before surgery; platelets can be

**TABLE 74–12.** Presurgical Evaluation of Donors

1. ABO blood type compatibility with the recipient (including lymphocyte crossmatch)
2. Exclusion of acute and chronic medical illness (including history of physical examination, hematology, chemistry, electrolytes, kidney profile, chest radiograph, electrocardiogram, spirometry, arterial blood gases)
3. Screening for transmissible viral illness (serologic testing for hepatitis virus, herpes, cytomegalovirus, Epstein-Barr virus, human immunodeficiency virus)
4. Normal liver functions (liver profile, coagulation profile, protein, albumin)
5. Psychological assessment
6. Imaging for liver volume assessment and intraabdominal disease exclusion (abdominal ultrasound, computed tomography scan, and hepatic angiography)
7. Liver biopsy is not needed routinely, but may be considered in:
   a. Case of suspected steatosis
   b. Female donors because they have high probability of unsuspected steatosis
8. Endoscopic retrograde cholangiopancreatography to ensure adequacy of the biliary tract for parents of children with Alagille's syndrome

Data from Grewal HP, Thistlethwaite JR Jr, Loss GE, et al. Complications in 100 living-liver donors. *Ann Surg.* 1998;228:214; and Sterneck MR, Fischer L, Nischwitz U, et al. Selection of the living liver donor. *Transplantation.* 1995;60:667.

**TABLE 74–13.** Circulatory Effects of Preservation Solution During the Neohepatic Stage

| | Collins' Solution | Collins' Solution With Chlorpromazine | Wisconsin Solution |
|---|---|---|---|
| SBP (stage III + 5 min; mm Hg) | 102.5 ± 3.6 | 94.2 ± 7.9 | 95.0 ± 4.2 |
| SBP <100 (min) | 81.5 ± 16.9 | 127.0 ± 15.5* | 65.0 ± 11.4 |
| SBP <80 (min) | 6.5 ± 1.8 | 24.0 ± 5.1 | 10.5 ± 2.5* |
| Epinephrine (% of patients requiring) | 10.4 | 49.0* | 18.3 |
| Phenylephrine (% of patients requiring)† | 8.2 | 19.0* | 7.3 |

*Values are mean ± standard error of the mean.

†*P* < .05 compared with Collins' group. Retrospective study; endpoint to keep hemodynamic baseline level. No specific order.

SBP, systemic blood pressure.

From Kang YG, Freeman JA, Aggarwal S, et al. Hemodynamic instability during liver transplantation. *Transplant Proc.* 1989;21:3489.

infused (if the count is <50,000/mm³) immediately after induction or cannulation. Urine output and creatinine levels should be determined.

It is suggested that the preoperative (first-stage) evaluation report be available in the operating room chosen for the transplantation. During the second-stage evaluation, special attention should be directed to cytomegalovirus (CMV) status and coagulation (including fibrinogen and d-dimers). If the recipient is CMV immunoglobulin G negative, the status of the donor liver should be determined; if it is negative, the patient will need CMV-negative blood and prophylactic treatment.

### Premedication

Because preoperative coagulation may be abnormal, intramuscular premedication is ill advised. Hepatic encephalopathy is another contraindication. If coagulation and level of consciousness are normal, standard medications are not contraindicated. The dose is usually adjusted downward because of reduced hepatic function, including drug elimination. Premedication is frequently eliminated. Preoperative counseling often suffices for patient preparation and allows family inter-

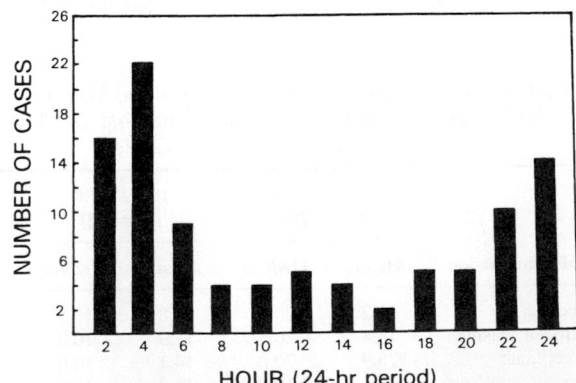

**FIGURE 74–10.** Comparison between time of day and number of liver transplantations begun (an analysis of the *first* 100 procedures at the Mayo Clinic). (By permission from Rettke SR, Chantigian RC, Janossy TA, et al. Anesthesia approach to hepatic transplantation. *Mayo Clin Proc.* 1989;64:224.)

**TABLE 74–14.** Mean Operating Room Times During Various Periods of Orthotopic Liver Transplantation at the Mayo Clinic

| | Total Time (min) | | |
|---|---|---|---|
| Group | Anesthesia | Surgical | Anhepatic |
| First 100 procedures | 510.1 ± 98.4 | 413.2 ± 87.5 | 130.4 ± 39.9 |
| By diagnosis: | | | |
| CAH (n = 24) | 541.0 ± 76.4 | 433.0 ± 76.5 | 145.1 ± 76.5 |
| PSC (n = 22) | 558.9 ± 75.7 | 459.2 ± 7 | 125.0 ± 75.7* |
| PBC (n = 20) | 444.0 ± 73.0† | 5.7357.1 ± 73.0† | 114.0 ± 73.0* |
| Retransplant (n = 17) | 471.8 ± 90.3 | 378.3 ± 77.4 | 134.3 ± 48.1 |

*Significantly lower than for CAH ($P < .05$).
†Significantly lower than for CAH and PSC ($P < .05$).
CAH, chronic active hepatitis; PBC, primary biliary cirrhosis; PSC, primary sclerosing cholangitis.
From Rettke SR, Chantigian RC, Janossy TA, et al. Anesthesia approach to hepatic transplantation. *Mayo Clin Proc.* 1989;64:224. By permission.

action with an alert patient before surgery. However, if a patient wishes premedication, short-acting benzodiazepines are often appropriate.

### Warming

During the final preoperative evaluation, an order should be written for the patient to be placed in a warm room and provided with abundant blankets. The operating room itself should be warmed before bringing the patient in. During catheter placement, the surgical team should be certain to have a heated humidifier operational, the room warmed appropriately, and covered forced air heating maintained as much as possible. In the transplantation room, we prepare disposable upper and lower body warmers, each one with its own heater unit. The lower body warmer goes under the foot of the table (Fig. 74–11), and the upper body warmer is often placed by the right arm of the patient.

### How Should the Operating Room Be Set Up?

The anesthesiologist should have access to the patient's head, neck (including insertion sites for left and right central catheters), and arms (including locations for a radial arterial catheter and the antecubital vein of the side opposite to the venovenous bypass [VVB]). Adequate space must be available at the anesthesia end/side of the room for the rapid-infusion system (RIS), TEG machine, monitors, infusion pumps, drug cart, and the anesthesia machine (see Fig. 74–11).

At the foot end of the operating room table and on both sides, space must be available for the VVB pump (reaching up to the patient's axilla), surgical instruments (including an area to work on the donor liver), blanket warmer, blood and blood product warmer, and fluid storage.

### What Equipment Is Needed by Anesthesia Personnel?

Equipment used by anesthesia personnel can be divided into three categories:

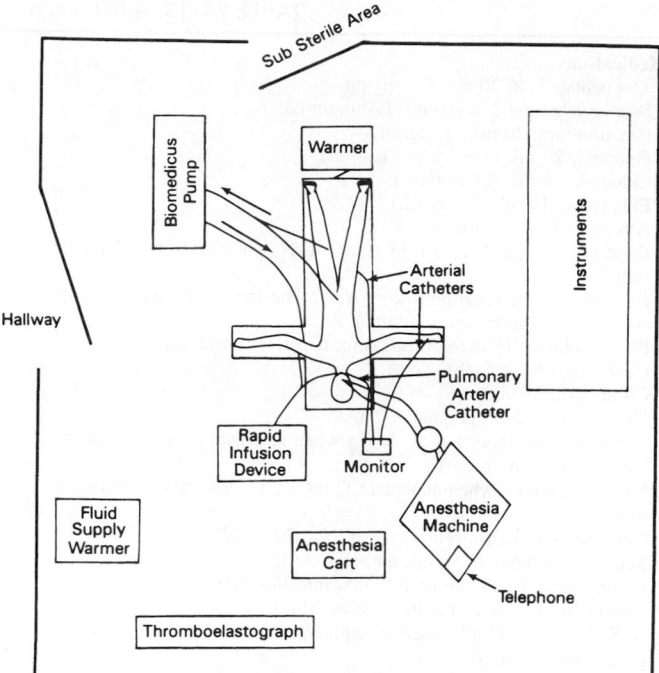

**FIGURE 74–11.** Suggested room layout for anesthesia and surgery in orthotopic liver transplantation.

1. That used for "regular" major abdominal surgery cases, including anesthesia gas machine, ventilator, positive end-expiratory pressure valves, humidifier, multiple-channel vital sign monitor, urinary catheter, automated record keeper (desirable, not routine), pulse oximeter, esophageal stethoscope, respiratory gas analyzer, nasogastric tube, warming blanket, medication infusion sets, supply cart, and telephone.

2. That used for a major vascular surgery case with the potential for significant blood or contractility loss: invasive blood pressure monitoring capabilities (radial *and* femoral, because of frequent blood sampling from a nonheparinized line in a vasoconstricted, cold patient), cardiac output monitor, on-line mixed venous oximetry, cardiac defibrillator, blood pump and blood warmer, nonautologous infusion system, and autotransfusion system. The latter device may be advantageous even with an RIS,[46] although most centers eliminate it if the RIS is present.

   Since 1995, we have routinely used two-dimensional surface ultrasound with the aid of a portable device to guide and facilitate central (internal jugular vein) venipuncture and avoid inadvertent carotid puncture, particularly in pediatric patients and those with significant clotting abnormalities.

3. That which is more specific to OLT: two invasive arterial pressure monitors, the RIS, TEG, and VVB devices.

Tables 74–15 and 74–16 outline the setups for adult and pediatric OLT.

### What Is the Recommendation for Venous Access?

#### Adults

Venous access entails a large, 10- to 12-gauge or 8 to 8.5 Fr catheter in the antecubital vein opposite to the VVB side

**TABLE 74–15.** Adult Setup for Orthotopic Liver Transplantation

**Medications**
- Thiopental: 3 × 20 mL (25 mg/mL)
- Succinylcholine: 2 × 10 mL (20 mg/mL)
- Pancuronium: 20 mL (1 mg/mL)
- Fentanyl: 20 mL or more (50 µg/mL)
- Lidocaine: 5 mL (20 mg/mL)
- Ephedrine: 10 mL (5 mg/mL)
- Atropine: 3 mL (0.4 mg/mL)
- Dopamine: 6 mg × kg wt, in 1000 mL NS → 10 mL/h = 1 µg/kg/min
  (Use to improve renal perfusion. *Note:* The larger volume allows more accurate administration in adults.)
- Phenylephrine: 10 mg/250 mL (mix if patient unstable)
- Cephazolin:* 1 g (q4h)
- Clindamycin:* 900 mg
- Gentamicin:* 2.5 mg/kg/dose q8h
- Methylprednisolone: 1 g × 2 (1 g when anhepatic; 2 mg/kg before leaving operating room)
- Imuran: 2 mg/kg when anhepatic; 2 mg/kg before leaving operating room
- Calcium chloride (injection): 10 mL × 20 vials
- Sodium bicarbonate: 50 mL ampules × 15
- Epinephrine: 3 or more of 1/10 000 injection (10 mL)
- Insulin (regular or Humulin U-100): 10 mL
- 50% Dextrose: 50 mL (used if required to lower potassium: 5 g glucose/unit insulin)

**Equipment**
- Positive end-expiratory pressure valves (5–20 cm)
- Blood infusion equipment
- Rapid-infusion device (~40 kg or more)
- Warming blanket and Bair Hugger for both lower and upper body (two heating plants required)
- Circuit humidifier/heater: mandatory! (*Note:* Be certain to get one that can reach a 45°C; not the type that reaches only 41°C)
- Oximetrix computer*
- TEG: Stored in an operating room dedicated for OLT. *Do not set up unless you are trained.*
- Reflective wraps (for heat and extremities), if available
- Blood collection tubes
- Two Alton-Dean high-pressure blood warmers

**Monitors**
- Electrocardiogram
- Invasive pressures:
  Arterial (radial, contralateral to VVB)
  Femoral or second radial (when setting up for two radials: arm board, arrow guidewire kit)
  Central venous pressure
  Pulmonary artery (If needed)
  *Note:*
  1. Do not use heparinized saline as flush; use NS.
  2. Be *very* careful that your lines are properly marked!
  3. Place blood pressure cuff on right arm (opposite VVB side)
- Esophageal stethoscope; nasogastric tube
- Temperature (esophageal and intravascular)
- Pulse oximeter
- Capnograph/gas monitor
- Twitch monitoring
- PA catheter (with oximeter*)
- TEG*
- Transesophageal echocardiogram two-dimensional probe, sterile gel, and two sets of 8½ size gloves

**Catheter Trays**
Prepare for the following lines:
1. VVB return line (venous line for return to the patient from the centrifugal pump): Use an 8.5 Fr (6.5 cm long) or 10 Fr (10 cm long) basilic catheter. If no antecubital line is possible, and the subclavian route is chosen, use the 10-cm length "femoral" catheter rather than the shorter basilic. *Note:* These catheters do not have diaphragms—you must connect a catheter to them. If a 9 Fr PA catheter introducer sidearm sheath is used, the port may leak at the pressures the VVB encounters; if you use the PA catheter, be certain to use the diaphragm cap. This line must be extremely reliable because the flow will be >1 L/min and typical pressures are >200 mm Hg.
2. RIJV line available for a PA catheter 9 Fr introducer: If a PA catheter is inserted, this line will not perform well as a volume infusion line. (Even with the 7 Fr PA catheter at 400 mL/min, the pressure rises well above the RIS limit of 300 mm Hg).
3. Additional volume line: Possibilities include a basilic on the opposite side as that for (1); or a second PA catheter introducer in the RIJV or subclavian. In some patients, (2) and (3) may be replaced by a double-lumen, 12 Fr catheter if there is no expected need for a PA catheter. The double-lumen, 12 Fr size cannot be used for VVB. One of its lumens alone is inadequate for the RIS. By comparison, one 9 Fr PA catheter introducer can easily handle the 400 mL/min bolus flow of the RIS.
4. Second arterial line: Usually a 4 Fr, 15-cm, single-lumen polyurethane femoral line, opposite side from the VVB. In very thin patients, the 8-cm, 3 Fr size may work. This requires a table/work area separate from that for the central lines in the neck.

*Optional.
NS, normal saline; PA, pulmonary artery; RIJV, right internal jugular vein; RIS, rapid-infusion system; TEG, thromboelastograph; VVB, venovenous bypass.

and a 9 Fr catheter in the left internal (IJV) or external jugular vein or subclavian vein. The right IJV is used for placement of a pulmonary artery (PA) catheter. Thus, we use three high-flow venous lines: typically either two 8.5-Fr basilic catheters and one 9-Fr IJV introducer; or one 8.5-Fr basilic catheter and two 9-Fr IJV introducers (same side, using double puncture and two wires in the IJV); or possibly some combination, including a 10- or 12-gauge intravenous line (see also Table 74–15). Impediment of cerebral venous return because of bilateral jugular cannulation has not been observed to be a problem, but we avoid it in all patients with suspected increased ICP. The large-bore access with infusion of warmed fluids may affect cardiac output measurement, making cardiac output readings falsely high. Since 1995, we have not used the oximetric PA catheter routinely because the typical patient with chronic liver disease has a high (>90%) venous satura-

tion, which declines significantly only after cardiac output and blood pressure change, and not before. Also, if the patient does not have cardiac or pulmonary involvement, we may consider using the 9-Fr PA introducer as a high-flow line, and float the PA line only if needed during the procedure.

### Children

For pediatric patients, smaller catheters are used for central venous pressure monitoring. A 5.5 or 4 Fr introducer for oximetric PA catheter placement is inserted. The oximeter catheter is placed just beyond the introducer tip because it does not have balloon flotation capabilities. Peripheral catheters are similar in number and location but smaller in dimension (14 to 20 gauge) according to the patient's size (see Table 74–16).

**TABLE 74–16.** Pediatric Setup for Orthotopic Liver Transplantation

**Medications**
- Atropine: adjust for weight
- Thiopental: adjust for weight
- Succinylcholine: adjust for weight
- Pancuronium: Adjust for weight
- Fentanyl
- Lidocaine: 5 mL (20 mg/mL)
- Ephedrine: 10 mL (5 mg/mL)
- Dopamine: 6 mg × kg wt, in 100 mL normal saline → 1 mL/h = 1 μg/kg/min (use to keep good renal perfusion)
- Phenylephrine 1/100 000(10 mL)
- Methylprednisolone (typical dose: 5 mg/kg)
  Mainstay of the acute immune suppression
  Calcium chloride injection: 10 mL × 20 vials
- Sodium bicarbonate: 15 ampules
- Epinephrine: 1/10 000 injection 10 mL
- Insulin (regular or Humulin U-100): 10 mL
- 50% Dextrose: 50 mL (Use if required to lower potassium: 5 g glucose/unit insulin)

**Equipment**
- Positive end-expiratory pressure valves: 5-20 cm
- Blood infusion equipment
  If less than 40 kg, venovenous bypass is not used
  Rapid-infusion system not used
  Consider Hot Line blood warmers (<20 kg) or Level One
  Access: multiple peripheral intravenous lines
  Right IJV 5 or 6 Fr introducer for oximetric catheter
  Left IJV introducer or central line
- Warming blanket: 2
- Circuit humidifier/heater: mandatory!
- Oximetrix computer*
- TEG
- Blood collection tubes: red top, blue top, purple top, and green top (ammonia)

**Monitors**
- Electrocardiogram
- Invasive pressures:
  Arterial (radial, contralateral to bypass)
  Femoral
  Central venous pressure
  PA (if older child, Swan-Ganz catheter is appropriate)
  *Note:* Be *very* careful that your lines are properly marked!
- Esophageal stethoscope
- Temperature (esophageal and intravascular)
- Pulse oximeter
- Capnograph/gas monitor
- Twitch monitor
- 5 Fr PA catheter for larger patients with severe cardiac risk; 4 Fr oximetric catheter for smaller patients with significant cardiac risk
- TEG

**Catheter Trays**
- Radial artery
- Peripheral intravenous line
- Femoral arterial line (most often 3 Fr, 8-cm polyurethane)
- Central line
- IJV (*Note:* requires minimum of two assembled, central line trays—one for head of bed, one for femoral)

*Optional.
IJV, internal jugular vein; PA, pulmonary artery; TEG, thromboelastograph.

## How Is Arterial Pressure Monitored?

Arterial pressure monitoring and blood sampling are carried out after insertion of a 20-gauge, 18-gauge, or 5 Fr cannula into the femoral artery (the side opposite the VVB), as well as a 20-gauge radial arterial catheter for backup. Since 1995, we have begun using two radial lines, avoiding a femoral puncture with great success. In pediatric patients, smaller catheters, 24 gauge or 3 Fr, are used for the femoral artery, and 22 or 24 gauge for the radial artery.

### Flush Solutions

Catheter flushing solutions are heparin free to avoid additional, unnecessary disturbances in the clotting mechanism. All arterial catheters should have continuous (3 mL/h), pressure-driven flush devices attached.

## What Are the Recommendations for Blood and Blood Product Availability?

### Adults

Preliminary reports of the 1981 to 1983 experience from the largest OLT center in the United States cited median and maximum intraoperative RBC use in adult patients of 28.5 and 251 units, respectively.[47] When the blood bank initiates an OLT program, it should plan for the extreme possibility of blood loss, even though later reports,[22,46] with and without autotransfusion (autologous) systems, claim lower median and maximum consumption of blood and blood products from 1985 to 1989.

Based on these data, we set aside blood products in two locations: the operating room (20 units of packed RBCs, 20 units of FFP, 20 units of cryoprecipitate) and the blood bank (200 units of packed RBCs).

### Children

For pediatric patients, we prepare half the amount of blood as for adults in the operating room (10 units of each), and one-fourth the amount (50 units) in the blood bank.

## How and When Is the Rapid-Infusion System Used?

### Adults

The RIS should be used in any adult OLT. Massive transfusion, up to 500 to 700 mL/min, is common. Even in cases that require <10 RBC units, rapid transfusion is necessary to maintain normovolemia[1] for short periods. The RIS is designed to deliver prewarmed (>35°C), premixed, air-free blood or fluid at low pressure (<300 mm Hg) through 170- and 40-μm filters at controlled, rapid rates up to 1500 mL/min. The RIS should be ready for use before the first stage of surgery (discussed later).

### Children

For pediatric patients, in whom total blood loss and rate of maximum transfusion are expected to be lower than in adults, the potential for RIS overtransfusion is higher, and catheter size is relatively small for the low pressure and adequate flow requirements of the RIS. Thus, I use two to four pneumatic pressure devices (Alton-Dean) instead. Regular pressure bags can also serve this function if they are attached to a tourniquet box. When the RIS system is not used, no air detector is in the system, and scrupulous care must be taken to avoid pressurized air infusion and embolization.

## Priming

Preparation of the RIS to deliver fluid, including loading of the reservoir and elimination of all air in the system, is called *priming*. Before this stage is complete, the system is not operable. The fluid used is saline or Plasma-Lyte A, which is compatible with blood administration. I usually do not prime with a blood product because debubbling is very difficult. Furthermore, not every patient needs blood or blood products as the first fluid dose at the initial stage of surgery.

## Plasma-Lyte A

Plasma-Lyte A (Table 74–17) is calcium and glucose free. It has a minimum amount of gluconate (23 mEq/L) without any lactate or citrate components. This feature is important because of a diseased liver's inability to handle acid metabolites.

## Red Blood Cells and Fresh-Frozen Plasma

When blood is added to the solutions, the resultant hematocrit should be 26% to 28% to reduce RBC loss and improve circulatory rheology. The low colloid oncotic pressure typical in these patients necessitates colloid or FFP. Fluid containing FFP, platelets, and cryoprecipitate is used to replace factors lost or reduced owing to bleeding or existing coagulopathies and to prevent dilution-induced coagulopathies.

These multiple goals are achieved by using a fixed ratio of RBCs, FFP, and Plasma-Lyte A. If the RIS is primed with blood, a combination of 300 mL (1 unit) of RBCs, 250 mL (1 unit) of FFP, and 250 mL of Plasma-Lyte A is used. The composition of the solution can be modified intraoperatively based on a patient's laboratory data (ie, hematocrit, platelet count, and coagulation profile).

# ANESTHETIC INDUCTION

## What Drugs Should Be Used?

Rapid-sequence induction is performed because many of these patients have ascites and, perhaps, the equivalent of a full stomach. Delayed gastric emptying often exists in patients taking cyclosporin orally. Thiopental, 4 mg/kg, ketamine, 1 to 2 mg/kg, or etomidate, 0.3 to 0.5 mg/kg, is used. Succinylcholine, 1 to 2 mg/kg, is added to facilitate tracheal intubation while cricoid pressure is maintained. The induction agents are protein bound, and the free drug fraction is increased in liver disease when serum albumin is low, leading to an enhanced effect. Thiopental and etomidate are metabolized in the liver, but their activity is terminated by redistribution. Hence, their

**TABLE 74–17.** Composition of Plasma-Lyte A

| | |
|---|---|
| Na$^+$ | 140 mEq/L |
| K | 5 mEq/L |
| Mg$^{2+}$ | 3 mEq/L |
| Acetate | 27 mEq/L |
| Gluconate | 23 mEq/L |
| Osmolality | 294 Osm |
| pH | 7.4 |

duration of action is normal unless the doses are large or repeated.

## Should Nasotracheal and Nasogastric Tubes Be Inserted?

Nasotracheal intubation, as a rule, is not performed because of the likelihood of preoperative as well as subsequent intraoperative abnormal coagulation function.

Similar concerns exist about insertion of nasogastric tubes. However, careful insertion after tracheal intubation and the application of topical vasoconstrictors provide the necessary gastric decompression during the procedure. If an incompletely corrected preoperative coagulopathy exists, an alternative approach is to place an orogastric tube, which can be converted to a nasogastric tube at a later time.

## How Is a Patient Positioned?

The recipient is placed on a gel pad-covered operating table with both arms abducted and resting on eggcrate foam-padded arm boards (see Fig. 74–11). The occiput and heels are also placed on eggcrate foam pads to prevent any pressure injury. Because the VVB involves axillary dissection, care should be taken to avoid extreme extension and brachial plexus injury.

The operating time is long, and the viscera are exposed. Thus, heat loss is significant, and the operating room table should have a warming blanket. After catheters are placed, the upper extremities and head are wrapped with vinyl covers to minimize heat loss. Other measures may be applicable (see Chapter 48).

## How Are Drugs Handled by Liver Transplant Recipients?

### Factors in Drug Tolerance/Intolerance

Patients with parenchymal liver disease represent a spectrum from mild to severe hepatic derangement (see Table 74–1). Although in early liver disease, particularly alcoholic disease, drug tolerance may be present, this is not the case in more severe forms. Drug tolerance/intolerance results from a multitude of factors:

1. Central nervous system changes. The blood-brain barrier in cirrhotic patients is abnormal, as are neural receptors.
2. Increased volume of distribution ($V_D$) suggests the need to increase the first dose of the drug.
3. Reduced synthesis of albumin reduces plasma-binding sites for the drug and increases the free active drug fraction (suggests the need to decrease the first drug dose).
4. Decreased hepatic blood flow.
5. Decreased biotransformation enzyme content and activity. Enzymes of phase 1 biotransformation (eg, oxidation) are impaired at an earlier stage than phase 2 (eg, conjugation).
6. Portacaval shunting may increase the bioavailability of orally administered drugs by reducing first-pass metabolism.
7. Coexisting impaired renal function decreases drug clearance.

Depending on which of these factors predominates, a drug may produce a more or less profound and prolonged or shortened effect than normal. The initial dose should be titrated against response. The effect of centrally acting agents may be particularly pronounced (eg, barbiturates, narcotics, and benzodiazepines).

Evidence shows that the benzodiazepine antagonist flumazenil can temporarily worsen hepatic encephalopathy. This observation may suggest a GABA-ergic (γ-aminobutyric acid) mechanism in the brains of patients with hepatic encephalopathy.[48] The effects of liver disease on some commonly used anesthetic agents are listed in Table 74–18.

## Biotransformation

Although the liver is the major site of drug biotransformation, the effects of hepatic dysfunction on drug handling are inconsistent. Such inconsistency may reflect the heterogeneous pathophysiologic process of liver disease with respect to hepatocellular function, protein binding, and hepatic blood flow.

For hepatic diseases with preserved hepatic blood flow but impaired hepatocellular function, the pharmacokinetic profile of a drug with high hepatic extraction dependency is relatively unaffected. On the other hand, a drug with a low extraction dependency has a pronounced alteration in its disposition and elimination.[49]

Some reports suggest that pharmacokinetic differences between children and adults in terms of anesthetic agents (eg, alfentanil) are a result of differences in the underlying pathophysiologic processes of cholestatic versus hepatocellular dysfunction; the latter is associated with lower clearance and longer elimination half-life.[50]

## Muscle Relaxants

The pharmacokinetics of muscle relaxants in adults with hepatic dysfunction has been studied extensively[51] (see Table 74–18). Vecuronium is less affected, although dose-dependent alterations have been observed. The pharmacokinetics of atracurium are unaffected by liver disease. However, the $V_D$ is larger for all relaxants; accordingly, the distribution half-lives are shorter in patients with severe hepatorenal dysfunction.

Any muscle relaxant can be used in patients with advanced liver disease; however, titration using nerve stimulation monitoring is recommended to avoid inadequate or prolonged effects. For OLT surgery that lasts 8 to 12 hours and with the significant time of postoperative intubation and ventilation, the clinical importance of prolonged relaxation usually is

**TABLE 74–18.** Anesthetic Drugs in Liver Disease

| Class of Drug | Drug | Effect of Decreased Serum Albumin | Effect of Decreased Hepatic Metabolism | Other Effects |
|---|---|---|---|---|
| Induction agents | Thiopental | Increased free drug | Increased elimination half-life | |
| | Ketamine | | Prolonged action, decreased clearance | Phase 1 metabolism affected |
| | Etomidate | Increased free drug | Increased elimination half-life | |
| Opioid analgesic agents | Meperidine | | Prolonged effect | Decreased first-pass metabolism |
| | Phenoperidine | | | |
| | Fentanyl | | | |
| | Sufentanil | Increased free drug | Prolonged effect | Decreased first-pass metabolism |
| | Morphine | | | Narcotic effect terminated by redistribution and extrahepatic glucuronidation |
| Benzodiazepines | Diazepam | Increased free drug | Prolonged action, decreased clearance | Phase 1 metabolism affected |
| | Chlordiazepoxide | | | |
| | Midazolam | | | |
| | Oxazepam | | Normal clearance and duration of action | Phase 2 metabolism spared |
| | Lorazepam | | | |
| β-Adrenergic blocking agents | Propranolol | Increased free drug | Increased oral bioavailability decreased clearance | Decreased first-pass metabolism, reduced dose for treatment of portal hypertension |
| Local anesthetic agents | Lidocaine | | Decreased clearance, increased elimination half-life | |
| Neuromuscular blocking agents | Succinylcholine | | | Decreased plasma cholinesterase Slightly prolonged apnea |
| Nondepolarizing muscle relaxants | Pancuronium | Bound to hemoglobin | Prolonged elimination half-life | Significantly metabolized Altered pharmacokinetics in patients with hepatic or biliary disease |
| | *d*-Tubocurarine | No effect | Prolonged elimination half-life | Significantly metabolized |
| | Vecuronium | No effect | Prolonged effect in large doses | Significantly metabolized Altered pharmacokinetics in patients with hepatic or biliary disease Metabolized to 3-acetyl derivative |
| | Rocuronium | Possibly bigger dose needed because of increased volume of distribution | Prolonged effect due to reduced clearance (less than vecuronium and pancuronium) | Minimal active metabolite formation |
| | Atracurium | No effect | Action unaffected by hepatic and renal disease | Significantly metabolized Elimination by Hoffman degradation and ester hydrolysis |

Modified from McEvedy BA, Shelley MP, Park GR. Anesthesia and liver disease. *Br J Hosp Med.* 1986;36:26.

minor. Even doxacurium, a long-acting relaxant, is satisfactory.[1] Finally, although the synthesis of pseudocholinesterase is reduced, the clinical effect on succinylcholine's duration of action is insignificant.

## ANESTHETIC MANAGEMENT

### Does It Differ From Typical Major Abdominal Cases?

#### Narcotics

Anesthetic maintenance is in many ways similar to that in other major abdominal surgery. A narcotic can be successfully used in patients with hepatic disease despite the pharmacologic consequences of decreased clearance and prolonged half-life (see Table 74–18). Fentanyl, sufentanil, and alfentanil are suitable opioid analgesic agents because they have short half-lives and inactive metabolites. Fentanyl does not decrease hepatic oxygen and blood supply or prevent increases in demand when used in moderate doses (50 µg/kg bolus and 0.5 µg/kg/min infusions).[52] Studies comparing fentanyl and morphine pharmacokinetics in adult patients with normal and abnormal liver function have not shown any differences with regard to disposition and elimination; similar findings have been reported for alfentanil in children.[50]

#### Inhalation Agents

Anesthesia can be maintained with an inhalation agent, as well as with tranquilizers or narcotics or any combination thereof. The effect of anesthetic drugs on hepatic function is as important as the effect of hepatic disease on the pharmacokinetics of the anesthetic agents. Halothane is avoided in favor of isoflurane for OLT.

Halothane, enflurane, and isoflurane all reduce liver blood flow, but halothane produces a proportionately larger decrement because it reduces hepatic arterial flow to a greater extent.[52]

Nitrous oxide has been used for many years without increased anesthesia-related postoperative hepatic complications. However, its sympathomimetic effect and accumulation in the intestinal lumen, with the potential for subsequent distention in protracted cases, make it counterproductive in many peoples' minds.

### Why Is Hourly Laboratory (Blood Sampling) Monitoring Recommended?

Tight control of physiologic parameters is essential to maintain homeostasis during OLT. Therefore, a system for rapid assessment of coagulation profile (hematocrit, PT, partial thromboplastin time [PTT], platelets), blood gas partial pressures (of oxygen and carbon dioxide), acid-base status (pH/bicarbonate/base excess), electrolytes (sodium, potassium, serum ionized calcium), blood glucose values, and lactate levels should be used at least hourly. In the operating room, TEG monitoring of the coagulation profile can be performed even more frequently. Perioperative fibrinogen or fibrin degradation product (FDP) measurements, serum osmolality, and urinary sodium determinations are desirable but are not essential hourly.

### What Are the Chances For Rejection?

Hyperacute rejection of the type seen after heart/kidney transplantation is not seen in liver transplant recipients, who seem to be protected from humoral rejection. Even livers with compatible blood groups but a cytotoxic crossmatch may be transplanted, although with increased risk. Histocompatibility testing to avoid rejection in OLT patients is less essential than determining blood type (ABO) compatibility, which is probably the only essential test.

### What Immunosuppressive Drugs Are Used?

Cyclosporin is the most commonly used maintenance immunosuppressive drug. Steroids are almost invariably added.[3] Azathioprine may be used as a third agent to reduce the dose of cyclosporin and, in some cases, may replace cyclosporin altogether when the latter is contraindicated or can no longer be used because of adverse side effects.

Antilymphocyte globulin preparations, including the monoclonal antibody OKT-3,[53] have been given prophylactically and for specific indications to prevent rejection. OKT-3 reacts against all mature T lymphocytes.

Other drugs have been developed and tested in multicenter trials in the 1990s.[54] The most prominent is tacrolimus (FK506), which has become an established immunosuppressant agent for primary and rescue therapy (when experiencing rejection or poor tolerance to cyclosporin) in patients with liver, kidney, and pancreatic transplants; it is also used to prevent graft-versus-host disease.[55] Although structurally unrelated, tacrolimus and cyclosporin have similar cellular actions that exert inhibitory effects on T-lymphocyte activation. Cyclosporin is given before surgery (orally or intravenously) as part of the premedication. It is not repeated during surgery because of the impracticality of controlling or monitoring effective or toxic blood levels, and is repeated after surgery only with dose adjustments on the basis of drug levels and creatinine clearance. Methylprednisolone, 500 mg, is given before surgery and repeated every 6 hours (before anastomosis, when anhepatic, and before leaving the operating room). Imuran (2 mg/kg) is normally given twice while anhepatic and during reperfusion.

## SURGICAL STAGES IN ORTHOTOPIC LIVER TRANSPLANTATION

### What Is the Preanhepatic Phase?

The first stage in OLT is the *preanhepatic phase*. It lasts from skin incision to the point at which the native liver is freed to its vascular pedicle. The skin incision is wide, bilateral, and subcostal, with cephalic extension to the xiphoid. The xiphoid process is removed without entering the thorax.

### What Is the Anhepatic Phase?

The second stage is referred to as the *anhepatic phase*. It begins with clamping of the suprahepatic and infrahepatic inferior vena cava (IVC), portal vein, and hepatic artery, after which the diseased liver is removed. This stage includes the hepatectomy and ends when vascular anastomosis of the IVC and portal vein is complete; the infrahepatic IVC anastomosis is prepared but not completed until late in this stage.

Three separate or combined techniques are used during this stage: (1) simple cross-clamping; (2) VVB (femoroaxillary) to avoid physiologic stress; and (3) either (1) or (2) combined with flushing of the donor liver with lactated Ringer's solution through the portal vein (100 mL in children, 200-300 mL in adults) to remove transport infusate and to clear the donor liver vasculature of air. The infrahepatic IVC and portal vein repairs are then completed.

## What Is the Neohepatic Phase?

The third stage is called the *neohepatic* or *postanhepatic phase*. Here, the donor liver is incorporated into the recipient's circulatory system by releasing, in sequence, clamps from the portal vein, the infrahepatic IVC, and the suprahepatic IVC. Subsequently, the portal artery anastomosis is performed, and after adequate hemostasis, the bile duct is reconstructed. If a patient has a normal extrahepatic bile duct system, duct-to-duct anastomosis is performed; if it is abnormal (biliary atresia, biliary cirrhosis, perisclerosing cholangitis), a Roux-en-Y choledochojejunostomy is performed. Finally, an intraoperative cholangiogram is obtained to assess patency of the biliary system and biliary drainage.

The average total surgical time (see Table 74–14) is >6 hours (range, 4-12 hours), and the average anhepatic phase is >2 hours (range, 1½-5 hours). The anhepatic time for patients with chronic active hepatitis is longer than for patients with primary biliary cirrhosis. This difference is attributable to more difficult surgical techniques and hemostatic conditions. Total surgical time for patients with primary biliary cirrhosis is significantly less than for those with chronic active hepatitis or perisclerosing cholangitis. Dissection to free the diseased liver is more difficult in the presence of portal hypertension, and hepaticojejunostomy with a Roux-en-Y loop takes longer than end-to-end choledochocholedochostomy.

## What Does the Anesthetist Need to Know About Venovenous Bypass?

### Indications

During the anhepatic phase, cross-clamping of the IVC and portal vein for hepatectomy reduces venous return to the heart and cardiac output by approximately 50%, creating congestion of the IVC and portal system. VVB is suggested for venous decompression, improved hemodynamic stability, and decreased intraoperative blood loss.[56] In addition, VVB has been reported to improve renal function, eliminate gastrointestinal hemorrhage, decrease operative mortality rates from 10% to 1%, and provide additional time for completion of the vascular anastomoses.

### Technique

Figure 74–12 illustrates the routine connection of the extracorporeal bypass circuit. Blood is pumped from the portal and

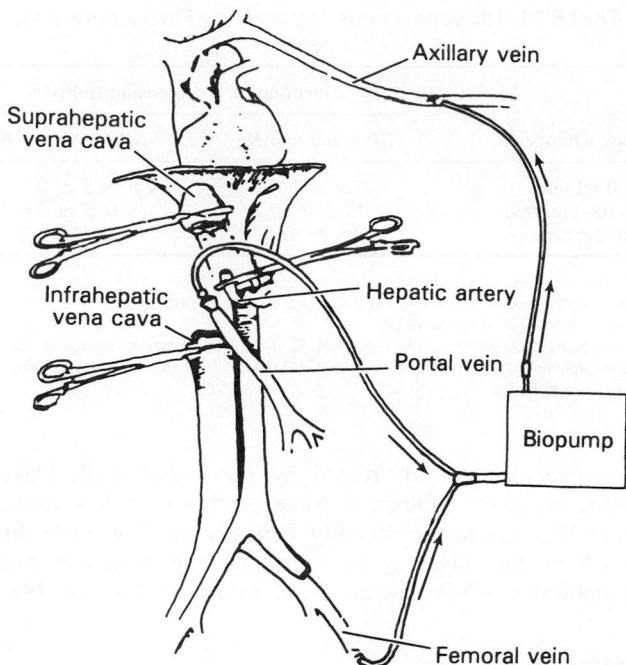

**FIGURE 74–12.** Diagram depicting the routine implementation of venovenous bypass in the adult patient. (From Paulsen AW, Whitten CW, Ramsay MAE, et al. Considerations for anesthetic management during veno-venous bypass in adult hepatic transplantation. *Anesth Analg.* 1989;58:489. © Williams & Wilkins, 1989.)

femoral veins by a centripetal pump without heparin, although the tubing may be heparin bonded. A small dose of heparin, 1000 to 2000 units, may be added to the bypass cannula. The VVB flow rate is up to 40% of cardiac output; hemodynamic changes usually do not occur if adequate flow is maintained.

Traditionally, VVB was accomplished through cannulas surgically placed into the femoral and portal veins for blood drainage and into the axillary vein for blood return.[56] In the last few years, reports of techniques for percutaneous placement of cannulas for VVB during OLT have been sparse.[57–59] The percutaneous modification is achieved by placing a large-bore catheter (7.5-21 Fr, depending on size and anatomy of the patient and the insertion site). The catheter is percutaneously inserted into the right internal jugular vein,[59] subclavian vein,[57] or basilic vein,[32] using the Seldinger technique. The cannula size should provide flow of at least 1.2 L/min (with 300 mm Hg pressure) by the VVB; this can be accomplished by using the minimum 8.5 Fr PA introducer or 15 to 21 Fr arterial inflow cannula originally designed for cardiopulmonary bypass. With the basilic approach, a short catheter should be used to avoid increased resistance. A Luer-lock port on the cannula allows use of the catheter for rapid volume infusion before and after VVB, or to connect to a centrifugal pump tubing (with ⅜-inch pump tubing). If the catheter is inserted centrally (internal jugular, subclavian vein), proper positioning of the cannula should be confirmed before its use with a chest radiograph to avoid an acute or slow-developing catastrophe due to iatrogenic tension hemothorax. If the catheter is inserted peripherally (basilic vein), frequent palpation is needed to check for problems or extravasation. The possibility of air emboli if the inflow lines are dislodged should be suspected.

During VVB, the patient's intravascular volume serves as a bypass reservoir. Bypass flow depends on inflow. It decreases

**TABLE 74–19.** Venovenous Bypass Flow Fluctuations and Hypotension

| Flow Changes* | Duration of Hypotension (min) | |
|---|---|---|
| | *SBP <100 mm Hg* | *SBP <80 mm Hg* |
| ≤500 mL/min | 27.5 ± 2.7 | 4.5 ± 0.7 |
| 500-1000 mL/min | 35 ± 3.1† | 14.5 ± 2.6† |
| >1000 mL/min | 49.5 ± 3.6† | 23.5 ± 3.2† |

*Values are mean ± standard error of the mean.
†$p < .05$ compared with minimum flow change group (<500 mL).
SBP, systemic blood pressure.
From Kang YG, Freeman JA, Aggarwal S, et al. Hemodynamic instability during liver transplantation. *Transplant Proc.* 1989;21:3489. © 1989. Reprinted by permission of Appleton & Lange.

when cannulas are obstructed by the vessel wall, kinked tubing, excessive centripetal force (suction), or low cardiac output. Hemodynamic stability depends on flow exceeding 2.5 L/min. Patients may have protracted hypotension when fluctuations in VVB flow are >500 mL/min (Table 74–19).

## Routine Use

Routine use of VVB during the anhepatic phase is somewhat controversial.[56] It is not recommended in younger patients or those who are in reasonably good physiologic condition and who are able to respond to the sudden loss of venous return with vasoconstriction and tachycardia. Vigorous volume infusion often results in some improvement, yet a penalty of fluid overload is paid when the liver is revascularized and venous return is restored. Some transplantation centers use VVB routinely, whereas others use various bypass techniques only for specific diagnoses or when suprahepatic IVC occlusion is not tolerated.[56] A few centers do not use it at all. Some centers use standard bypass in only 17% of cases and a variation of the technique (piggyback) in 68% of cases[23] (Fig. 74–13). Perhaps the most consistent approach for VVB use in OLT in the 1990s was its routine use only in patients with proven cardiovascular disease. Otherwise, in pediatric patients, young adults, and those with nonproven cardiac involvement, a trial of vena caval occlusion (suprahepatic and

infrahepatic) with fluid and catecholamine administration may be indicated.[32]

## Hypothermia

Hypothermia during VVB may pose another significant problem because it is potentiated by an extracorporeal circuit that does not contain a heat exchanger. A heat exchanger is avoided because of its large, potentially thrombogenic surface area. Heat loss from the bypass circuit can decrease core temperature three times more rapidly (0.9°C/h) during bypass than at any other time during OLT. It is directly related to VVB flow (Fig. 74–14).

## Miscellaneous Problems

Other complications of bypass include air emboli from the cannulation site, laceration of the portal vein, and pulmonary thromboembolism from migration of preexisting thrombi in the portal or deep venous systems through the low-resistance VVB circuit.[60] Plasma colloid oncotic pressure is decreased during VVB as a function of the flow (Fig. 74–15).

## *What Physiologic Changes Should Be Expected During the Preanhepatic Phase?*

Intraoperative changes in physiologic variables are listed in Table 74–20.

## Cardiovascular/Hemodynamic

At the beginning of surgery, high filling pressure due to fluid overload, ascites, pleural effusion, pulmonary hypertension, and a hyperdynamic cardiovascular state persists as long

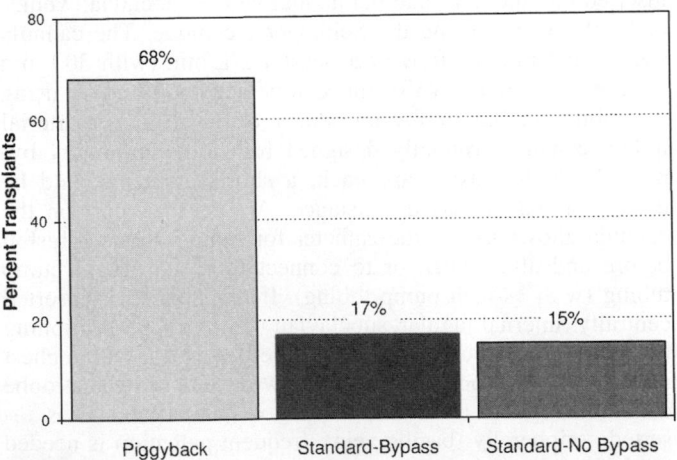

**FIGURE 74–13.** Mode of graft implantation (all transplants). (From Millan MT, Keeffe EB, Berquist WE, et al. Liver transplantation at Stanford University Medical Center. In: Ceckos JM, Teraski PI, eds. *Clinical Transplantation 1998.* Los Angeles, Calif: UCLA Tissue Typing Laboratory; 1998:293.)

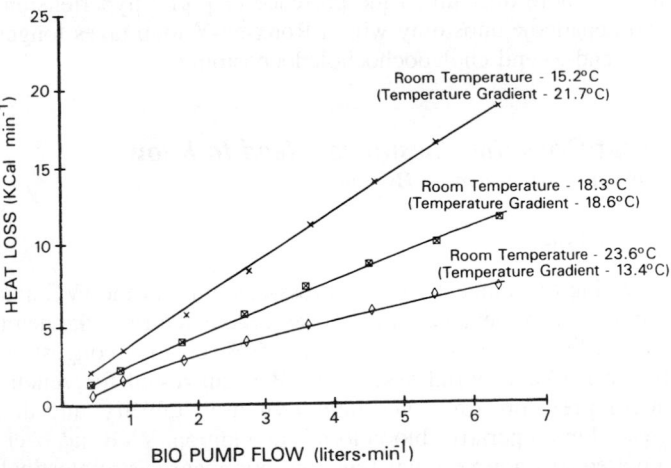

**FIGURE 74–14.** Calculated heat loss from the bypass circuit as a function of pump flow and room temperature, or temperature gradient between the circulating fluid and the room. Estimated heat loss for blood flowing through the bypass circuit was computed by substituting the specific gravity and specific heat of blood for those of distilled water. Because no consideration was given to the possibility that red blood cell motion may disturb the unstirred layer at the inner wall of the tubing, the heat loss may actually be underestimated. (From Paulsen AW, Whitten CW, Ramsay MAE, et al. Considerations for anesthetic management during veno-venous bypass in adult hepatic transplantation. *Anesth Analg.* 1989;58:489.)

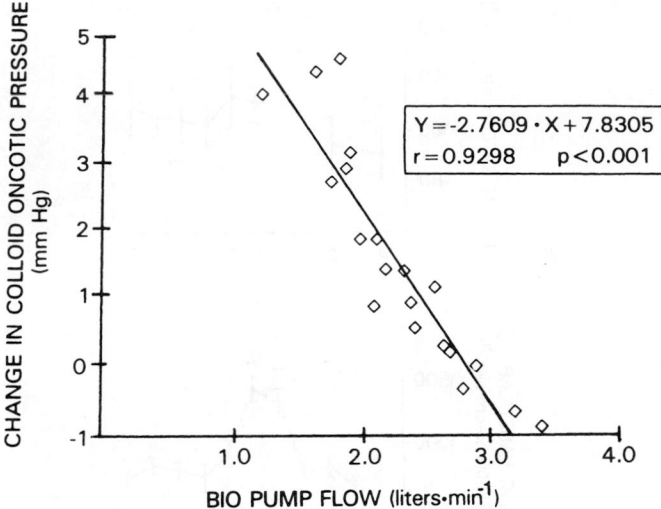

**FIGURE 74–15.** Changes in colloid oncotic pressure of the plasma as a function of the flow through the extracorporeal circuit. (From Paulsen AW, Whitten CW, Ramsay MAE, et al. Considerations for anesthetic management during veno-venous bypass in adult hepatic transplantation. *Anesth Analg.* 1989;58:489.)

as volume loss secondary to surgical bleeding and continuous formation of ascites is adequately replaced.

Surgical manipulation of major vessels reduces venous return, and prolonged hypotension may require adjustments of surgical technique. At the end of the preanhepatic phase, caudad traction on the liver to isolate the suprahepatic IVC may cause transient dysrhythmias and hypotension. Marginal cardiac performance necessitates a vasopressor (eg, dopamine, 2-5 μg/kg/min as a starting dose). End-stage liver disease may increase catecholamine resistance, necessitating a higher dose.

α-adrenergic agonists are of questionable value because they increase peripheral and coronary resistance. At the same time, they may decrease shunt fraction and improve tissue

**TABLE 74–20.** Characteristic Intraoperative Changes in Physiologic Variables

| Variable | Preanhepatic Stage | Anhepatic Stage | Neohepatic Stage | |
|---|---|---|---|---|
| | | | Early | Late |
| Cardiac output | High | Low | High | High |
| Heart rate | High | High | Low | High |
| Mean arterial pressure | Normal | Low | Very low | Normal |
| Filling pressure | Normal | Low | High | Normal |
| Vascular resistance | Low | High | Very low | Low |
| $Pao_2$ | Normal | Normal | Normal | Normal |
| $Pco_2$ | Normal | Low | Normal | Normal |
| Base deficit | Normal | High | Very high | Normal |
| Serum $Na^+$ | Low | Normal | Normal | Normal |
| Serum $K^+$ | Low | Normal | Very high | Low |
| Serum $Ca^{2+}$ | Normal | Very low | Low | Normal |
| Serum citrate | Normal | High | High | Low |

From Kang YG, Freeman JA, Aggarwal S, et al. Hemodynamic instability during liver transplantation. *Transplant Proc.* 1989;21:3489. © 1989. Reprinted by permission of Appleton & Lange.

perfusion. Continuous monitoring of mixed venous oxygen saturation ($S\bar{v}o_2$) helps to assess preload and cardiac output, assuming oxygen-carrying capacity, oxygen consumption, and myocardial contractility remain constant. Because of arteriovenous shunting, $S\bar{v}o_2$ and cardiac output are expected to be falsely high; thus, $S\bar{v}o_2$ serves more as a trend monitor. A more reliable sign of inadequate tissue perfusion is metabolic acidosis.

### Coagulation

During the preanhepatic phase, a dilutional coagulopathy is superimposed on the underlying disease-induced coagulopathy. FFP (given through the RIS) corrects low levels of coagulation factors, and platelet transfusion (not through the RIS) increases the platelet count (40 000-50 000 per 10-unit transfusion). Cryoprecipitate, which contains fibrinogen, factor VIII, and factor XIII, is rarely necessary during this period. Attempts should be made to correct coagulation problems during this stage.

### Temperature

Body temperature gradually decreases from the effects of anesthetics, muscle relaxants, cold environment, and insufficient energy production by the liver.

### Hypoglycemia

Hypoglycemia due to loss of liver gluconeogenic capacity may be a concern but has not been observed frequently. Transfusion of blood can maintain blood glucose at a normal level because each unit of whole blood contains 0.5 g of glucose before processing. When blood replacement is minimal, small intravenous doses of glucose avoid hypoglycemia.

### Hypocalcemia

Transient citrate-induced hypocalcemia from the banked blood may follow rapid transfusion. A 500-mL unit of whole blood contains 1.7 g of hydrated trisodium citrate. The amount of citrate in a unit of packed RBCs is variable. The volume and rate of transfusion correlate with a decrease in ionized calcium, but total calcium levels do not correlate with serum ionized calcium.

### *What Physiologic Changes Should Be Expected During the Anhepatic Phase?*

#### Cardiovascular/Hemodynamic

Cross-clamping of the IVC, which heralds the beginning of the anhepatic phase, causes significant hypotension because of reduced venous return. The loss of portal blood flow has little effect on total venous return, especially in patients with significant collateral flow. Reduced right- and left-sided filling pressures, systemic and pulmonary pressures, and cardiac index (Fig. 74–16) and increased heart rate, systemic resistance, and pulmonary resistance (Fig. 74–17) are all related to reduced venous return. Changes in systemic vascular resistance and afterload are less with venous inflow occlusion than with major arterial occlusion, in which reduced cardiac output is, in part, related to extreme afterload and hypertension.

Volume expansion and administration of inotropic agents can ameliorate the negative hemodynamic changes associated with IVC clamping. However, as noted earlier, with volume expansion comes the possibility of fluid overload during this stage (using the RIS) and later during stage 3 reperfusion. Vessel occlusion also promotes surgical bleeding, hematuria, and congestive ischemia of the bowel. All of these problems can be avoided by VVB.

### Venovenous Bypass

Initiation of VVB restores venous return but may produce transient bradycardia and peaked T waves, owing to rapid influx of room-temperature priming solution. Hypothermia due to heat loss and thromboembolism may be encountered, as also noted previously.

By the end of the anhepatic phase, portal vein anastomosis is completed. VVB then carries only systemic venous blood (partial bypass); the resulting hypovolemic state, lasting 10 to 15 minutes, may require additional fluids, with similar concerns about overloading.

### Coagulation

At the onset of VVB, a heparin effect may be detected by the TEG because a small dose of heparin may be added to

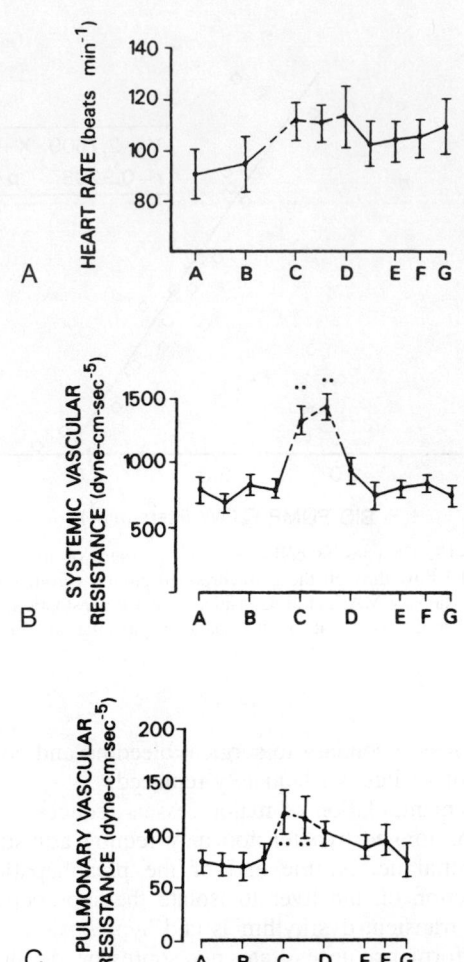

**FIGURE 74–17.** *A–C,* Changes in heart rate, systemic vascular resistance, and pulmonary vascular resistance during liver transplantation. Mean ± standard error of the mean for 9 patients. Phase: A, induction; B, dissection; C, anhepatic; D, partial anhepatic; E, gallbladder anastomosis; F, skin closure; G, end of procedure. **Different from preclamping values (*P* < .01). (From Carmichael FJ, Lindop MJ, Farman JV. Anesthesia for hepatic transplantation: cardiovascular and metabolic alterations and their management. *Anesth Analg.* 1985;64:108.)

the bypass cannula. This effect lasts only for 30 to 60 minutes. Dilutional coagulopathy may continue, although surgical bleeding is less severe owing to bypass decompression. Marked fibrinolysis related to progressively increased levels of plasminogen activators, which do not undergo hepatic clearance, can occur during the anhepatic phase. Administration of platelets and ε-aminocaproic acid (EACA) during this stage should be reserved for severe cases of bleeding due to thrombocytopenia or fibrinolysis to avoid thromboembolism in the unheparinized VVB system.

### Temperature

Further decreases in body temperature take place secondary to the absence of hepatic energy production, heat loss from the exposed viscera, and heat loss from the VVB.

### Hypoglycemia/Hypocalcemia

Hypoglycemia and hypocalcemia are most severe during VVB. Severe ionized hypocalcemia (<0.6 mmol/L) is some-

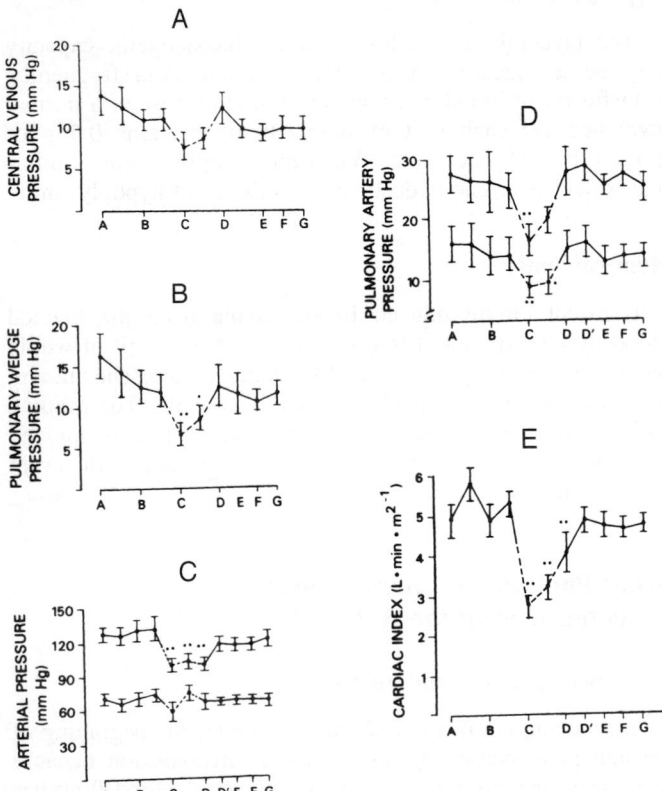

**FIGURE 74–16.** *A–E,* Changes in measured hemodynamic parameters during liver transplantation. Mean ± standard error of the mean for 9 patients. Phase: A, induction; B, dissection; C, anhepatic; D, partial anhepatic; E, gallbladder anastomosis; F, skin closure; G, end of procedure. *Different from preclamping values (*P* < .05); **different from preclamping values (*P* < .01). (From Carmichael FJ, Lindop MJ, Farman JV. Anesthesia for hepatic transplantation: cardiovascular and metabolic alterations and their management. *Anesth Analg.* 1985;64:108.)

times unavoidable during the anhepatic phase or during rapid blood transfusion. This change can produce myocardial depression if not corrected with exogenous calcium.

## Electrolytes

Preoperative hyponatremia and hypokalemia subside during surgery (see Table 74–20). Sodium and potassium are normalized by the large volume of FFP and Plasma-Lyte solution (5 mEq/L of potassium in Plasma-Lyte). Hypernatremia can emerge secondary to repeated sodium bicarbonate administration to correct metabolic acidosis. Progressive hyperkalemia may result from inadequate renal function and large volumes of transfused banked blood.

## Renal

Urine output should be maintained because hemolysis often occurs after massive transfusions; cyclosporin may damage renal function (usually after surgery); and IVC clamping can lead to renal venous congestion with hematuria. The latter usually resolves gradually at the end of surgery. Mannitol and low-dose dopamine (2-3 μg/kg/min) have been shown to improve postoperative renal function in this setting.[61]

## Acid-Base

Progressive metabolic acidosis (Fig. 74–18) and increased lactate levels during the anhepatic phase result from rapid transfusion of blood with acid metabolites, deficient hepatic clearance of acidic substances, and stagnation of blood flow below the diaphragm. Reduced perfusion leads to anaerobic metabolism. The acidosis becomes persistent in patients with unstable cardiovascular function, and further compromise of tissue perfusion follows.

Metabolic acidosis is treated with sodium bicarbonate to maintain a base excess no lower than −5 mEq/L, particularly at the end of the anhepatic phase and start of the neohepatic phase. Although this treatment may promote hypernatremia, hyperosmolarity, and postoperative alkalemia, these conditions are believed by many to be benign compared with the hemodynamic deterioration induced by severe metabolic acidosis. Severe myocardial depression and long-standing lactic acidosis, however, are thought by many investigators to be worsened by the administration of bicarbonate.

Complex changes in carbon dioxide ($CO_2$) homeostasis take place during OLT.[62] Patients may be hyperventilated to a mild degree of alkalemia to compensate partially for the metabolic acidosis. With hypothermia, the $CO_2$ production rate is expected to decrease; however, rapid transfusion of blood transiently increases the $CO_2$ load. A reduction of pulmonary gas exchange with arterial hypotension or reduced lung perfusion results in a progressive buildup of body stores of $CO_2$, an increase in arterial $CO_2$ partial pressure ($PaCO_2$), and a decrease in end-tidal $CO_2$ (Fig. 74–19).

## *What Physiologic Changes Should Be Expected in the Neohepatic Phase?*

### Cardiovascular/Hemodynamic

Before reperfusion of the new liver, preservative solution, air, and metabolites must be removed by flushing, or severe

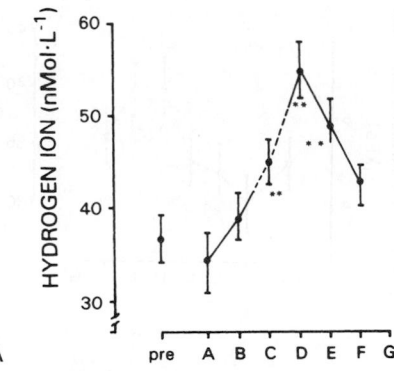

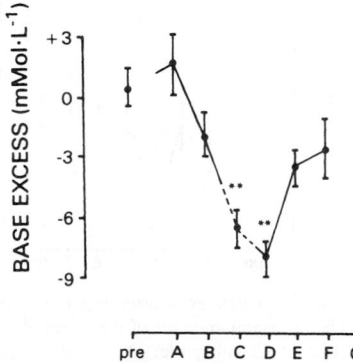

**FIGURE 74–18.** *A and B,* Changes in arterial plasma hydrogen ion concentrations and base deficit during liver transplantation. Mean ± standard error of the mean for 9 patients. Phase: A, induction; B, dissection; C, anhepatic; D, partial anhepatic; E, gallbladder anastomosis; F, skin closure; G, end of procedure. **Different from preclamping values ($P < .01$). (From Carmichael FJ, Lindop MJ, Farman JV. Anesthesia for hepatic transplantation: cardiovascular and metabolic alterations and their management. *Anesth Analg.* 1985;64:108.)

hyperkalemia may result (see also discussion of Acid-Base in this section). To ensure that a large amount of the preservation solution (0.5-1 L in adult) has been flushed through the liver, the surgeon may intentionally "lose" 0.5 to 1 L of blood through the anastomosis.

If a "split liver" is being transplanted, the practitioner should be aware of the potentially impressive blood loss that can occur on the cut surface (see previous section, What Are the New Possibilities and Techniques in Donor Harvesting and Graft Availability?).

Abrupt hemodynamic changes occur on reperfusion of a grafted liver. Subsequent unclamping of the portal vein and infrahepatic IVC decreases preload into the VVB. This decrease is followed by restoration of venous return on unclamping of the suprahepatic IVC. At this point (within a few minutes), the picture of *postperfusion syndrome* (similar to postacute arterial occlusion) appears. It consists of progressive bradycardia, hypotension, high filling pressures, and decreased systemic vascular resistance.

### Cardiac Output

During the early reperfusion period, thermodilution measurements of cardiac output are unreliable (falsely low) owing to rapid influx of cold preservation solution. In contrast, cardiac output studies using dye dilution technique show a real

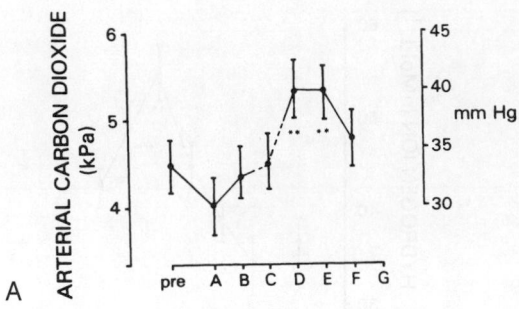

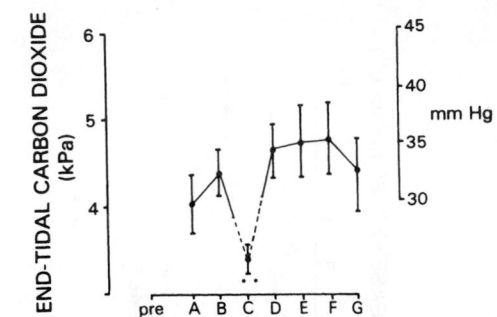

**FIGURE 74-19.** *A and B,* Changes in arterial and end-tidal $CO_2$ during liver transplantation. Mean ± standard error of the mean for 9 patients. Phase: A, induction; B, dissection; C, anhepatic; D, partial anhepatic; E, gallbladder anastomosis; F, skin closure; G, end of procedure. **Different from preclamping values ($P < .01$). (From Carmichael FJ, Lindop MJ, Farman JV. Anesthesia for hepatic transplantation: cardiovascular and metabolic alterations and their management. *Anesth Analg.* 1985;64:108.)

increase compared with the anhepatic phase, although output values remain lower than baseline levels.[62] In 30% of the cases in which extreme postperfusion hypotension (<70% of baseline) occurs, it is likely related to vasoactive substances released from the grafted liver. It does not correlate with the degree of hypokalemia, and symptoms persist even after core temperature returns to >34°C. The syndrome is treated with epinephrine (5- to 10-μg boluses) to restore heart rate and contractility.

Calcium chloride and bicarbonate are administered to treat hyperkalemia and acidosis. Calcium used prophylactically maintains cardiac output but does not prevent bradycardia and hypotension. Aggressive treatment of hyperkalemia usually is unnecessary because it disappears within minutes (Fig. 74-20A).

The acute reperfusion hemodynamic insult lasts 5 to 30 minutes; however, filling pressures stay high longer (30-120 minutes), whereas systemic vascular resistance remains low.

### Air Emboli

The high filling pressures are probably related to increased preload, myocardial depression, and air emboli. Air emboli originating from the donor liver can be detected immediately after reperfusion using echocardiography.

### Surgical Manipulation

The late neohepatic stage (see Table 74-20) is relatively uneventful as the hemodynamic profile returns to baseline.

However, surgical manipulation can still have a role: hepatic artery anastomosis to the aorta can cause acute or diffuse bleeding (eg, retroperitoneal dissection), hemodynamic instability (aortic clamping and unclamping), and bowel ischemia. Hypotension also can be caused suddenly by liver or major vessel manipulations. Hypertension at the end of surgery may result from fluid overload or cyclosporin (most typical in children). A final problem is that abdominal closure may interfere with the hemodynamic and respiratory status by decreasing filling pressures and thoracic compliance when the grafted liver is large in relation to the abdominal cavity size; secondary closure may be required.

### Coagulation

Reperfusion of the new liver often induces a severe coagulopathy for several reasons: (1) dilution by the preservation solution, (2) release of heparin or heparin-like substances from donor liver cells, (3) fibrinolysis due to release of plasminogen activator from the donor liver, and (4) inhibition of coagulation by unknown substances.[63]

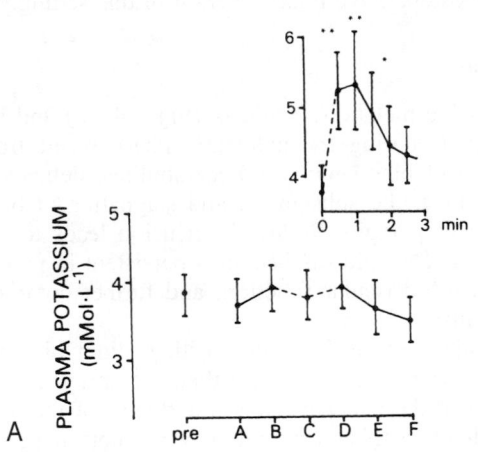

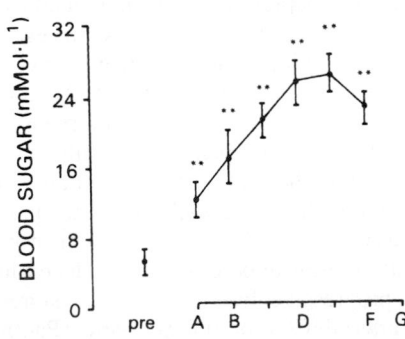

**FIGURE 74-20.** *A and B,* Changes in plasma potassium and blood sugar concentrations during liver transplantation. Mean ± standard error of the mean for 9 patients. Phase: A, induction; B, dissection; C, anhepatic; D, partial anhepatic; E, gallbladder anastomosis; F, skin closure; G, end of procedure. **Different from preclamping values ($P < .05$ or .01). *Inset,* Plasma potassium samples taken from the pulmonary artery catheter over 30-second periods after the release of clamps from the portal vein and suprahepatic artery in 8 patients. *Different from preclamping values ($P < .05$); **different from preclamping values ($P < .01$). (From Carmichael FJ, Lindop MJ, Farman JV. Anesthesia for hepatic transplantation: cardiovascular and metabolic alterations and their management. *Anesth Analg.* 1985;64:108.)

## Fibrinolysis

The fibrinolysis is probably primary, although it can be secondary to disseminated intravascular coagulation (DIC) because it is associated with high levels of fibrinogen, factors V and VIII, and plasminogen activator, and *not* coagulation factor consumption. Indeed, approximately 30% of patients before surgery have high levels of FDPs, which suggests the presence of DIC.[19]

The "explosive" nature of fibrinolysis in early stage 3, occurring within 5 minutes after reperfusion of the graft liver, makes sudden quantitative changes in coagulation factors and fibrinolytic proteins an unlikely cause. Qualitative changes probably account for the acute development of primary fibrinolysis. They may result from changes in cellular membrane permeability (even though the graft is preserved hypothermically in a solution with simulated intracellular composition).

**Diagnosis.** The differential diagnosis can be made by assessing the effect of different replacement therapies on the TEG. Protamine sulfate, 50 mg, reverses a persistent (>30 minutes postreperfusion) heparin effect. EACA, 1 g, treats severe fibrinolysis (<60 minutes TEG lysis time). Effectiveness of the latter agent without thrombotic complications also points to a primary fibrinolysis.

**Treatment.** Severe coagulopathy typically improves during the neohepatic phase unless the grafted liver does not function adequately or major surgical bleeding occurs. If bleeding is not severe, the coagulopathy should be treated aggressively, even if the TEG looks abnormal.

Perioperative graft failures due to technical complications occur in 10% of adults and 30% of children.[2] Iatrogenic problems, such as overzealous correction of clotting defects and polycythemia caused by overtransfusion, may contribute to hepatic artery or portal vein thrombosis. The risk in infants is inversely related to the patient's size, and complications are mainly attributed to vascular thrombosis.[64]

A hypercoagulable state sometimes occurs in patients with hepatic tumors or Budd-Chiari syndrome before surgery. With surgical bleeding, this situation probably will reverse. When surgical bleeding is minimal, low-dose heparin, 1000 to 2000 units, should be considered during VVB.

## Acid-Base

The acidosis and rise in $Paco_2$ at revascularization are the result of metabolites flushed out of the donor liver. Treatment of some patients with bicarbonate at this stage contributes to further $Paco_2$ elevation but also minimizes the fall in bicarbonate and pH levels. In any case, metabolic acidosis should be treated conservatively based on blood gas determinations; moderate to severe metabolic alkalosis is observed soon after OLT and may persist for days. This late alkalosis is a result of citrate metabolism and diuretic administration.

## Electrolytes

Acute hyperkalemia (potassium cardioplegia-like effect) with levels up to 11 mEq/L may be detected.[19] The early rise in potassium seen 1 minute after revascularization (see Fig. 74–20A) is probably the result of incomplete flushing of the liver preservation solution before revascularization. This solution is rich in potassium, which has been lost from cells during preservation (initially, the preservation solution has a low level of potassium). During the later neohepatic phase, potassium is taken up by the donor liver and by all cells of the body because of the alkalosis-induced intracellular shift. Supplemental potassium is usually required but may potentiate hyperkalemia in those cases of postoperative renal or liver donor dysfunction; its administration should be undertaken carefully.

## Hyperglycemia

On reperfusion, sudden, severe hyperglycemia may also occur, secondary to massive release of glucose from the donor liver. Glucose levels remain high during the third stage (see Fig. 74–20B) and slowly return to normal levels within 24 hours. Persistent hyperglycemia relates to impaired glucose reuptake and glycogenolysis by the new liver, low insulin levels during stages 2 and 3, and increased glucagon levels on reperfusion.

## When Does the New Liver Begin to Function?

Function of the grafted liver is detectable approximately 2 hours after reperfusion or occasionally at the end of the operation: citrate, lactate, and glucose levels decrease gradually; coagulopathy improves; bile is produced; and urine bilirubin is minimal. Liver enzymes, however, may still be very high, with serum levels of aspartate and alanine aminotransferases >100 IU/L owing to preservation injury. Persistent citrate intoxication, lactic acidosis, hyperglycemia, and coagulopathy are predictors of poor prognosis for new liver function.

## What Factors Cause Intraoperative Hypotension?

Intraoperative hypotension occurs because of one or more factors:

1. Inadequate replacement of the massive amounts of fluid and blood lost during the procedure
2. Cardiac dysfunction secondary to ionized hypocalcemia
3. Surgical manipulations that disturb preload (including IVC occlusion)
4. Dysrhythmias caused by metabolic disorders (ie, hypokalemia, hyperkalemia, and acidosis)
5. Preexisting myocardial disease
6. Emboli from the VVB or the donor liver
7. Myocardial ischemia secondary to hypotension, right ventricular overload due to overtransfusion, and paradoxical air emboli

## How Are the Metabolic Changes Treated?

### Hyperkalemia

Hyperkalemia may be treated by glucose and insulin: 1 to 2 g/kg glucose (2-4 mL/kg of 50% glucose) with 0.2 units of regular insulin per gram of glucose (5 g glucose per unit of insulin). Its effectiveness is unknown in patients with insulin resistance. Severe hyperkalemia (7-10 mEq/L), which can occur during reperfusion and lead to electrocardiographic and heart rate changes, is treated by intravenous calcium chloride ($CaCl_2$, adults 500 mg-1 g; children, 10-30 mg/kg) and bicarbonate, 1 to 2 mEq/kg, as symptomatic therapy in addition to glucose and insulin.

## Hypocalcemia

The treatment of hypocalcemia, which can produce myocardial ischemia, mandates frequent measurements and normalization of ionized calcium. Because calcium gluconate requires hepatic metabolism to liberate ionized calcium, the $CaCl_2$ preparation is preferred. However, equimolar doses of $CaCl_2$ and calcium gluconate have been shown to correct ionized hypocalcemia in patients undergoing OLT.[65] In any case, calcium is administered through a central catheter as a bolus dose of 15 mg/kg.

## Hyperglycemia

Hyperglycemia (glucose levels >250 mg/dL) should be treated with small insulin doses (5-10 units) after hourly blood glucose determination.

## Metabolic Acidosis

Progressive *acidosis* (base excess [BE] $> -7$ mEq/L) is treated with bicarbonate according to the following formula:

$$HCO_3^- \ (mEq) = (BE \times weight \ [kg] \times 0.3)/2$$

Aggressive treatment is not suggested if the donor liver is functional and urine formation is adequate.

## SPECIALIZED EQUIPMENT

Throughout this chapter, references have repeatedly been made to the RIS and TEG. A more detailed discussion of their function and use follows.

### How Does the Rapid-Infusion System Work?

The RIS is designed to deliver low-pressure, prewarmed, filtered, premixed, and air-free blood at a controlled and rapid rate. The Haemonetics RIS is a total fluid management system that can mix blood, FFP, Plasma-Lyte, saline, and other solutions with the same osmolality as blood in a 3-L reservoir. It offers a faster alternative to all conventional fluid and blood replacement techniques and is capable of fluid infusion in a controlled manner at a rate up to 1500 mL/min.

Avoidance of high pressure (>300 mm Hg), low temperature (<35°C), and infusion of aggregates or air during rapid fluid delivery is ensured through the use of infusate temperature monitoring, ultrasonic air detectors, and pressure sensors in the fluid line. The infusate is warmed by an in-line heat exchanger and filtered through high-capacity macroaggregate and microaggregate filters (Fig. 74-21).

Total fluid therapy can be managed by a single person. Simple, easy-to-use features give operators fingertip control (Fig. 74-22) of (1) flow rates as required (milliliters per minute or per hour); (2) continuous or bolus delivery of infusate; (3) fluid temperature, even when not in the infuse mode; and (4) uninterrupted fluid delivery during transport of patients or electrical failure by switchover to the battery mode.

The RIS has five modes of operation.

### Prime

This mode ensures that the disposable set is filled with fluid, thus getting rid of all the air in the system. The RIS

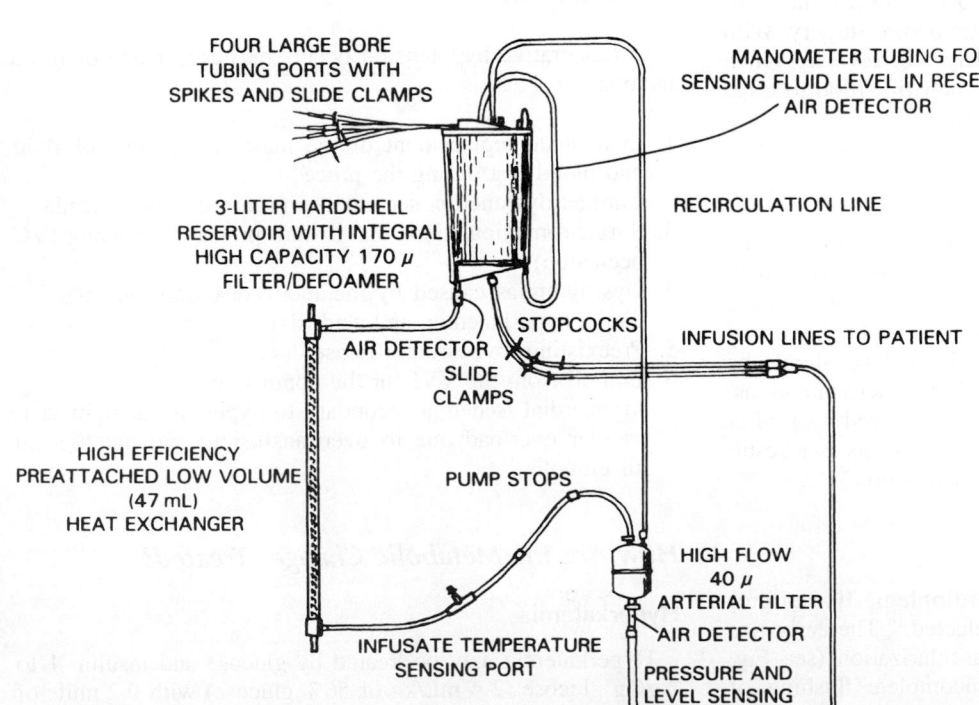

FOUR LARGE BORE TUBING PORTS WITH SPIKES AND SLIDE CLAMPS

MANOMETER TUBING FOR SENSING FLUID LEVEL IN RESERVOIR AIR DETECTOR

3-LITER HARDSHELL RESERVOIR WITH INTEGRAL HIGH CAPACITY 170 μ FILTER/DEFOAMER

RECIRCULATION LINE

STOPCOCKS

AIR DETECTOR SLIDE CLAMPS

INFUSION LINES TO PATIENT

HIGH EFFICIENCY PREATTACHED LOW VOLUME (47 mL) HEAT EXCHANGER

PUMP STOPS

INFUSATE TEMPERATURE SENSING PORT

HIGH FLOW 40 μ ARTERIAL FILTER AIR DETECTOR

PRESSURE AND LEVEL SENSING CHAMBER

FIGURE 74–21. The rapid-infusion system. (From *Directions for Use of RIS: Disposal Set List No. 400.* Mass: Haemonetics, Surgical Products Division.)

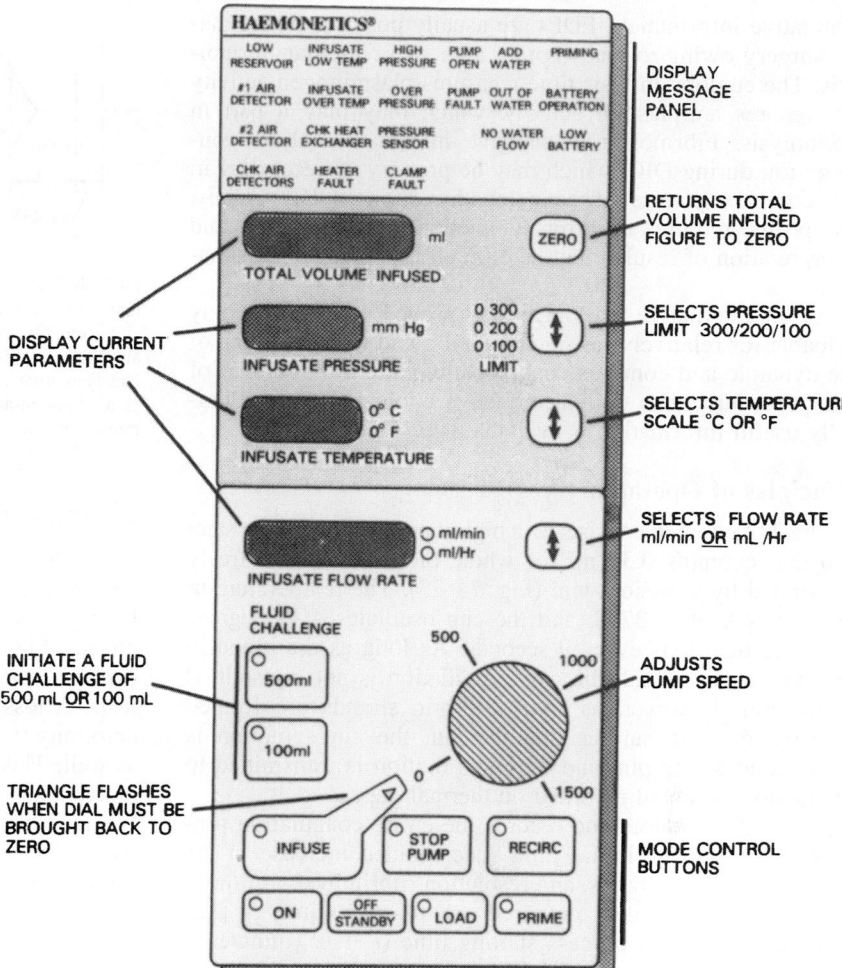

**FIGURE 74–22.** Rapid-infusion system, control panel. (From *Directions for Use of RIS.* Mass: Haemonetics, Surgical Products Division.)

operates in this mode only when power is on. "Load" opens the valves so that the disposable tubing may be installed. To prime the RIS, tubings should be connected as shown in Figure 74–21, not to the patient. Once priming is finished, the lower set of buttons in the bottom of the control panel should be shielded from further manipulation and covered, and infusion lines should be separated from the reservoir and connected to the patient.

## Infuse

This is the normal operating mode. Only after the infuse mode is set does the RIS infuse fluid automatically at the rate that is selected on the infuse dial.

## Stop

The machine may be placed in this mode before administering a fluid challenge or it will enter it automatically under certain circumstances, when the operation must be stopped. Whenever the system detects a condition requiring attention, such as low reservoir volume (200 mL), in-line air, high temperature (>41°C), or high pressure (>500 mm Hg), it stops the pump, sounds an alarm, and lights a display warning.

## Fluid Challenge

The fluid challenge mode initiates a fluid bolus of 100 mL or 1000 mL.

## Recirculate

This mode is used to warm fluid in the reservoir, to maintain the temperature >35°C, and to clear the filter of air bubbles by connecting it directly back to the reservoir.

## Safety Features

Safety features in the RIS include (1) temperature probe control of the heater power (below 34°C, the RIS pump is automatically slowed but not stopped); (2) pressure sensor slowing of the RIS pump at a chosen level (100, 200, 300 mm Hg), and stopping (540 mm Hg); and (3) system air detection by three ultrasonic air detectors: in the reservoir, in the fluid line as it leaves the reservoir, and in-line as fluid leaves the machine to be infused.

## *How Does the Thromboelastograph Work?*

Because of the possibility of severe coagulopathy, aggressive monitoring and proper treatment are essential. A simple coagulation profile (PT, PTT), platelet count, FDP, euglobulin lysis time, and fibrinogen level can be used, but they have drawbacks. The PT is already prolonged in many patients because it depends on hepatic function. The PTT may be clinically helpful, but heparin is not always a major cause of coagulopathy. Platelet counts provide quantitative but not qualitative information. FDPs are usually positive during major surgery owing to reabsorption after extravascular fibrinolysis. The euglobulin lysis time measures plasminogen activity but ignores antiplasmin activity, which may play a part in fibrinolysis. Fibrinogen levels give information about consumption during DIC, which may be primary or secondary in the complex picture of coagulopathy during OLT. Finally, this profile requires time for completion (>30 minutes), and interpretation of results may be difficult in this *dynamic* situation.

As an alternative, the TEG has proved to be extremely valuable for relatively fast interpretation and understanding of the dynamic and complex coagulopathy pattern that is part of this procedure, thus guiding effective clinical therapy. Clinically useful information is available *within* 30 minutes.[1]

## Principles of Operation

The TEG device consists of a highly polished stainless steel cup that contains 0.36 mL of whole blood and a pin freely suspended by a torsion wire (Fig. 74–23). The temperature in the cup is kept at 37°C, and the cup oscillates 4.45 degrees on its vertical axis every 9 seconds. As long as the blood in the cup remains fluid, the cup's oscillation is not transmitted to the pin. However, as soon as fibrin strands are formed between the cup surface and the pin, the cup's motion is transmitted to the pin, and the pin's motion is transmitted to the torsion wire and recorded on thermal paper.

The TEG monitors and records the entire coagulation process, including the initial fluid state, graded increase in the strength of fibrin strands, and resolution (fibrinolysis) of those strands. The variables measured are reaction time (r [minutes]); coagulation process starting time (r + k [minutes]); rate of clot formation (α [degrees]); maximum amplitude (MA [millimeters]); amplitude 60 minutes after MA ($\Lambda_{60}$ [millimeters]); and whole-blood clot lysis time (F [minutes]) (Fig. 74–24).

## Variations From Normal

The TEG output may be varied from normal (Fig. 74–25) to produce information on the following aspects of coagulation.

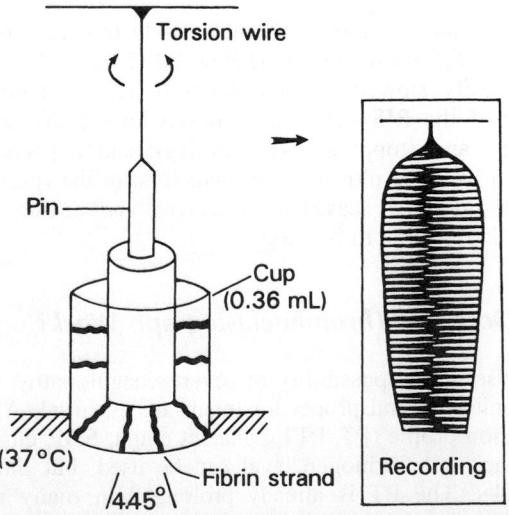

**FIGURE 74–23.** Schematic diagram of thromboelastography. (From Kang Y, Lewis JH, Navalgund A, et al. Epsilon-aminocaproic acid for treatment of fibrinolysis during liver transplantation. *Anesthesiology.* 1987;66:766.)

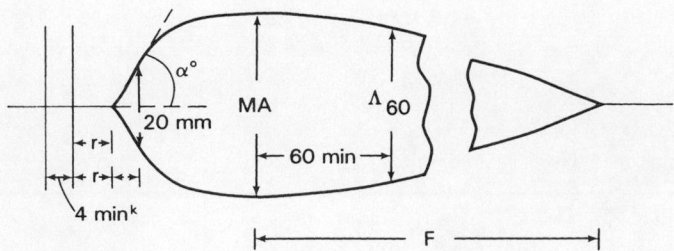

**FIGURE 74–24.** Variables measured by thromboelastography and their normal values. r, reaction time (minutes); r + k, coagulation time (minutes); α, clot formation rate (degrees); MA, maximum amplitude (millimeters); $\Lambda_{60}$, amplitude 60 minutes after maximum amplitude (millimeters); F, whole-blood clot lysis time (minutes). (Modified from Kang Y, Lewis JH, Navalgund A, et al. Epsilon-aminocaproic acid for treatment of fibrinolysis during liver transplantation. *Anesthesiology.* 1987;66:766.)

## Clotting Time

The onset of clotting on the TEG (r or r + k) correlates with whole-blood clotting time. A normal r is 6 to 8 minutes. In the presence of heparin, r + k is prolonged (see heparin profile, Fig. 74–25). This change suggests that protamine could be titrated to neutralize the heparin anticoagulant effects. A loss of clotting factors gives a similar TEG plotting deformity (r + k prolonged), but the MA angle α is decreased as well. This abnormality may be treated with FFP and cryoprecipitate.

Any clotting times shorter than these are hypercoagulable (see hypercoagulation, Fig. 74–25). This generalization, based on the onset of clotting and the MA angle α, is prone to error because clot structure and stability are not considered.

## Clot Strength

The strength of a clot determines its ability to perform hemostasis and can be determined from the MA of the TEG.

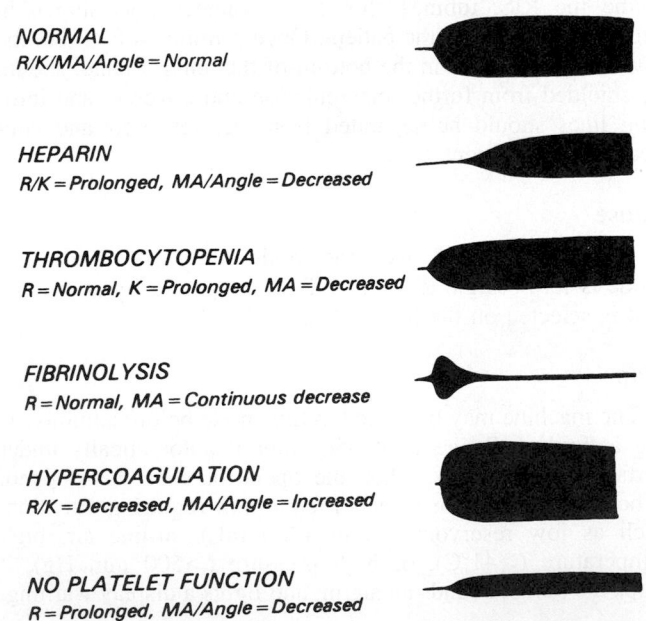

**NORMAL**
R/K/MA/Angle = Normal

**HEPARIN**
R/K = Prolonged, MA/Angle = Decreased

**THROMBOCYTOPENIA**
R = Normal, K = Prolonged, MA = Decreased

**FIBRINOLYSIS**
R = Normal, MA = Continuous decrease

**HYPERCOAGULATION**
R/K = Decreased, MA/Angle = Increased

**NO PLATELET FUNCTION**
R = Prolonged, MA/Angle = Decreased

**FIGURE 74–25.** Qualitative analysis from the thromboelastograph coagulation analyzer. (From Haemoscope Corporation. *Overview of Thromboelastograph Coagulation Analyzer: A Unique Analytical Device.* Morton Grove, Ill: Haemoscope Corporation; p 8.)

The strength is a direct result of platelet function and plasma factors (eg, fibrinogen) and their interaction. A normal MA is 50 to 70 mm. Thus, a clot with a low MA but normal r is missing platelet function (see thrombocytopenia, Fig. 74–25), and a clot with similar low MA but prolonged r is missing plasma factors *and* platelets.

Because platelets concentrate plasma factors and make clotting kinetics more effective, they should be the primary choice in therapy when MA is small (see no platelet function, Fig. 74–25). Hypercoagulable conditions can be identified as a result of either excess platelet function *or* elevated fibrinogen. The condition produces clots with MA >70 mm and usually with short reaction time. Such patients usually require anticoagulation. However, before any treatment is initiated, the clinician should determine if the clot is stable or unstable.

### Clot Stability

*Clot stability* refers to its potential to redissolve because of circulating fibrinolytic components that activate plasminogen within the clot. The TEG identifies this condition by showing early diminution of MA (see fibrinolysis profile, Fig. 74–25), with several low indices ($A_{60}$, F; see Fig. 74–24) showing the degree of dissolution over time. Patients with DIC or fibrinolytic conditions can be identified during early stages of this condition using TEG analysis even before clinical bleeding is evident. Possible correction of this condition can even be tested on the TEG by adding EACA to the specimen *in vitro* before it is given to a patient.[66]

### Clot Growth Kinetics

The TEG presents the rate of clot growth and formation as the angle $\alpha$ and K time (see Fig. 74–24). These parameters correlate with polymerization in clotting. Several aspects pertain to determining which factors are missing based on clot growth rate. In untreated people, this rate is a function of platelets and plasma components (complexes) residing on the platelet surface. Variation in growth rate results from decreased platelet function or plasma factors (eg, fibrinogen or specific enzyme complex proteins) or anticoagulants (eg, warfarin, heparin, FDP). Heparin gives the most characteristic shape, resembling a needle nose with angles of 5° to 15° (a normal $\alpha$ angle is >50°).

### Guidelines for Coagulation Therapy According to Thromboelastograph Monitoring

### Clot Formation

The most important consideration in TEG analysis is the fact that all aspects (clotting time, strength, stability, and kinetics) and the overall pattern of the TEG profile provide a more comprehensive clinical assessment of a patient's hemostasis than does any one variable of the TEG or coagulation test profile. A patient can have abnormal onset and growth kinetics but still form a normal, stable clot. Thus, although bleeding time can be prolonged, it may not represent a significant clinical problem. On the other hand, a short onset with rapid growth, good strength, and rapid lysis may predict or represent a dangerous clinical condition of consumption coagulopathy.

The clinical picture and evolution/resolution of the coagulation status also must be considered before treating coagulopathy according to TEG monitoring. This goal is accomplished hourly (or even half-hourly) during massive transfusion or early in the neohepatic phase.

### Fibrinolysis

Fibrinolysis occurring during OLT usually is primary in origin.[66] Although fibrinolysis is more dramatic on reperfusion of the graft liver, it may also occur during the preanhepatic and anhepatic phases. In these early stages, it may be caused by decreased clearance of plasminogen, release of plasminogen activator, and decreased synthesis of inhibitor. The previously discussed explosive fibrinolysis that occurs in the early neohepatic phase is probably caused by substances originating from the donor liver.

Although fibrinolysis increases progressively during OLT in >80% of patients, it is severe on reperfusion in only 34%.[66] A high incidence of hypercoagulable states and pulmonary emboli in OLT patients, both with and without EACA treatment, has led to the suggestion that because fibrinolysis during OLT is a self-limiting process, pharmacologic intervention is not necessary and might be harmful.[67]

### ε-Aminocaproic Acid Administration

The controversy surrounding EACA administration stems from evaluating unique patient populations (neoplasms with hypercoagulable state), overdose treatment (EACA up to 100 mg/kg), poor indications for treatment, and inadequate lysis monitoring. With the characteristic TEG tracing showing fibrinolysis, Kang and colleagues demonstrated the effectiveness of *in vitro* doses of EACA (0.03 mL of 1% EACA; Fig. 74–26). When this *in vitro* test showed effectiveness and reversed the TEG configuration to normal, 1 g of EACA (single intravenous dose) then was administered *in vivo* with

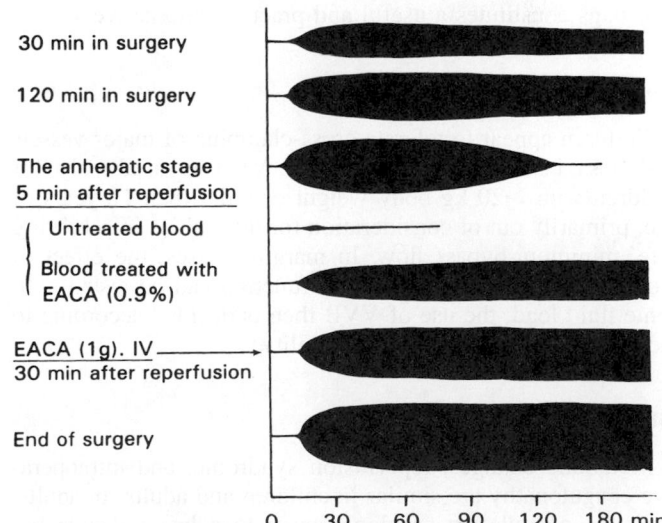

**FIGURE 74–26.** Thromboelastographic patterns in a patient undergoing liver transplantation. ε-aminocaproic acid (EACA, 1 g) was administered intravenously when severe fibrinolysis was observed on thromboelastography; generalized oozing occurred in a previously dry surgical field and EACA-treated fibrinolysis *in vitro*. (From Kang Y, Lewis JH, Navalgund A, et al. Epsilon-aminocaproic acid for treatment of fibrinolysis during liver transplantation. *Anesthesiology.* 1987;66:766.)

good results and no hemorrhagic or thrombotic complications.[66] Thus, for patients undergoing OLT, judicious use of small doses of EACA only after its effectiveness is confirmed *in vitro* is recommended. Our experience suggests that 0.25- to 0.5-g doses used judiciously with frequent TEG monitoring can ameliorate the brisk bleeding that results from fibrinolysis without causing portal vein/hepatic artery clot.

## PEDIATRIC ORTHOTOPIC LIVER TRANSPLANTATION

Some aspects of pediatric OLT have been discussed. More detailed information follows.

### How Does It Differ?

#### Type of Disease

Pediatric candidates for OLT most often have cholestatic disease or an inborn error of metabolism. This fact may be significant regarding the extent of hepatocellular damage, drug handling, bleeding tendencies, and survival.

#### Monitoring

PA catheterization does not appear to be necessary in many children because of their relatively healthy myocardium and difficult access. A central venous pressure oximeter catheter can be used to monitor the trend in cardiac output.

#### Blood and Fluid Management

Although blood transfusion requirements are proportional to those in adults (considering milliliters per kilogram consumption), the RIS may not be necessary because of the smaller total transfusion volumes. The use of pneumatic pressure bags constitutes a useful and practical alternative.

#### Hemodynamic Changes

Children appear to tolerate cross-clamping of major vessels with less hemodynamic instability. VVB is used only for children with >20 kg body weight or older than 12 years of age, primarily out of consideration for difficulties in achieving safe, minimum-bypass flow. In marginal cases, the effect of cross-clamping on hemodynamic function can be tested with some fluid load; the use of VVB then is decided according to the degree of hemodynamic instability.

#### Other Changes

Metabolic changes, reperfusion syndrome, and intraoperative coagulopathy are similar in children and adults. In adults, however, coagulation problems occur to a lesser degree because cholestatic disease is more prevalent in children.[68] The probability of postoperative hepatic vessel thrombosis is higher in children. This observation may influence the aggressiveness of treating coagulopathy in the neohepatic phase. In general, hypertension and metabolic alkalosis tend to develop earlier in children than in adults.

#### Donor Liver Size

Donor liver size may pose problems in pediatric patients in terms of dissection and surface bleeding of the liver, or decreased filling pressures and hemodynamic problems during abdominal closure, when it must adapt to the smaller abdominal cavity.

## RECOVERY AFTER ORTHOTOPIC LIVER TRANSPLANTATION

### How Long Is the Hospitalization Period?

The hospitalization period can vary between 2 weeks and 3 months (mean, 47 ± 25 days).[32] The average duration in the ICU is 1 to 2 weeks (mean, 5.9 ± 9 or 12.7 ± 12.6 days after OLT and 6.15 ± 7.0 days for readmission) according to several series.[32,69] A 10% death rate occurs in the ICU, and an additional 5% after OLT outside the ICU.[69] Considering the overall survival rate of 70% to 80%, the mortality rate in the ICU is relatively high.

### What Problems Occur in the Intensive Care Unit?

During the immediate postoperative period, hypothermia and hyperglycemia invariably occur. Later during the initial admission or on readmission, multiple problems are expected, but most significant are infections and renal insufficiency. Prompt diagnosis and treatment are also necessary for signs and symptoms of hypertension, hypokalemia, severe metabolic alkalosis (as citrate is metabolized), fever, altered mental status, oliguria, and signs of graft failure.

Repeated procedures, tests, and studies are needed to ensure graft function. These tests include liver biopsy, angiography, computed tomographic scan, and exploratory laparotomy. Selective bowel decontamination minimizes the occurrence of gram-negative and fungal sepsis, and the use of antihypertensive agents and correction of coagulopathies may decrease the risk of intracranial bleeding.

### Graft Survival

Graft survival depends primarily on donor and recipient factors (see also the section on Fulminant Hepatic Failure; see Figs. 74–6 and 74–7). Because hepatitis C is the most common cause of OLT, there is a concern that it will occur in the transplanted liver and inevitably lead to recurrent liver disease. However, the recurrence rate of hepatitis C was only 70% at 3 years, and graft loss attributable to it was infrequent.[70]

## ANESTHESIA FOR RETRANSPLANTATION

### How Does It Differ?

Retransplantation rates vary from center to center, but the overall incidence is <15% in adult patients.[1] The reasons for retransplantation are a poorly functioning donor liver, vascular complications (eg, hepatic arterial or portal venous thrombosis), and development of hyperacute rejection. These patients

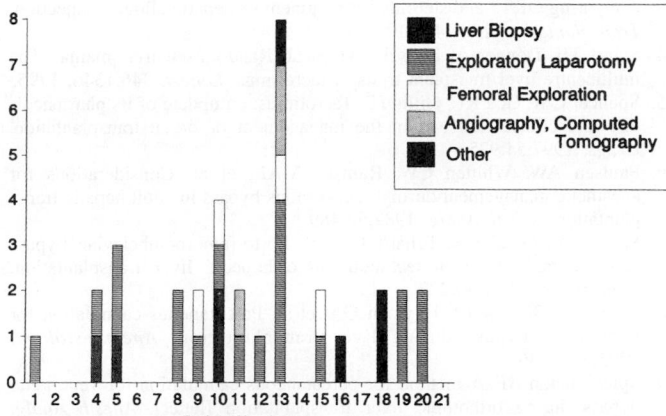

**FIGURE 74–27.** Additional procedures requiring general anesthesia (after orthotopic liver transplantation surgery) performed at the University of Florida in 1990 and 1991 in 21 patients during hospital stay.

may have other problems active at the same time (eg, adult respiratory distress syndrome, metabolic alkalosis) and require aggressive supportive therapy.

When severe liver necrosis develops, early removal of a dying graft minimizes its toxic effects. In these patients, retransplantation is relatively simple from a technical standpoint; all dissections have been performed, and all monitoring and infusion cannulas are *in situ*. Otherwise, anesthetic considerations are similar, but anesthetic and surgical times are expected to be significantly lower, and the physiologic effects (hemodynamic, blood loss) during the preanhepatic phase are less severe.

## ASSOCIATED PROCEDURES IMMEDIATELY AFTER ORTHOTOPIC LIVER TRANSPLANTATION

After surgery, patients are routinely kept intubated for the first 24 hours and are usually extubated on the second postoperative day.[19] However, because of the multiple physiologic (hemodynamic, metabolic) problems expected at this stage, a longer period of intubation may be necessary.

During the ICU stay, additional procedures may be needed to identify and treat sources of infection, bleeding, or graft failure, many of which require general anesthesia (Fig. 74–27). Such procedures are performed in up to 50% of post-OLT patients, and in half of these, more than one procedure may be required.[32] Because the procedures are relatively short and patients are already intubated or expected to stay that way, major issues concerning anesthesia are few. However, bleeding or hemodynamic stability is, as always, a concern.

### References

1. Kang Y. Anesthesia for liver transplantation. *Anesthesiol Clin North Am.* 1989;7:551.
2. Starzl TE, Demetris AJ, Van Thiel D. Liver transplantation (first of two parts). *N Engl J Med.* 1989;321:1014.
3. Starzl TE, Demetris AJ, Van Thiel D. Liver transplantation (second of two parts). *N Engl J Med.* 1989;321:1092.
4. Sidi A, Mahla ME. Noninvasive monitoring of cerebral perfusion by transcranial Doppler during fulminant hepatic failure and liver transplantation. *Anesth Analg.* 1995;80:194.
5. Pollard RJ, Sidi A, Gibby GL. Aortic stenosis with end-stage liver disease: prioritizing surgical and anesthetic therapies. Case Conference. *J Clin Anesth.* 1998;10:253.
6. Williams R, Gimson AES. Intensive liver care and management of acute hepatic failure. *Dig Dis Sci.* 1991;36:820.
7. Munoz SJ, Maddrey WC. Major complications of acute and chronic liver disease. *Gastroenterol Clin North Am.* 1988;17:265.
8. Lidofsky SD, Bass NM, Prager MC, et al. Intracranial pressure monitoring and liver transplantation for fulminant hepatic failure. *Hepatology.* 1992;16:1.
9. Morris JJ, Hellman CL, Gawey BJ, et al. Case 3-1995: three patients requiring both coronary artery bypass surgery and orthotopic liver transplantation. *J Cardiothorac Vasc Anesth.* 1995;9:322.
10. Figuera D, Ardaiz J, Martin-Judez V, et al. Combined transplantation of heart and liver from two different donors in a patient with familial type IIa hypercholesterolemia. *J Heart Transplant.* 1986;5:327.
11. Shaw BW Jr, Bahnson HT, Hardesty RL, et al. Combined transplantation of the heart and liver. *Ann Surg.* 1985;202:667.
12. Starzl TE, Bilheimer DW, Bahnson HT, et al. Heart-liver transplantation in a patient with familial hypercholesterolaemia. *Lancet.* 1984;1:1382.
13. Iwatsu S, Starzl TE, Todo S, et al. Experience in 1,000 liver transplants under cyclosporine-steroid therapy: a survival report. *Transplant Proc.* 1988;20:498.
14. Shaw BW Jr, Wood RP, Stratta RJ, et al. Stratifying the causes of death in liver transplant recipients. *Arch Surg.* 1989;124:895.
15. Trail KC, Stratta RJ, Larsen JL, et al. Orthotopic hepatic transplantation in patients with type I diabetes mellitus. *J Am Coll Surg.* 1994;178:337.
16. Trail KC, Stratta RJ, Larsen JL, et al. Results of liver transplantation in diabetic recipients. *Surgery.* 1993;114:650.
17. Starzl E, Iwatsuki S, Van Thiel DH, et al. Evolution of liver transplantation. *Hepatology.* 1982;2:614.
18. Borland LM, Martin DJ. Anesthesia considerations for orthotopic liver transplantation. *Contemp Anesth Pract.* 1987;10:157.
19. Samuel D, Benhamou JP, Bismuth H, et al. Criteria of selection for liver transplantation. *Transplant Proc.* 1987;19:2383.
20. Amersi F, Farmer DG, Busuttil RW. Fifteen-year experience with adult and pediatric liver transplantation at the University of California, Los Angeles. In: Ceckos JM, Teraski PI, eds. *Clinical Transplantation 1998.* Los Angeles, Calif: UCLA Tissue Typing Laboratory; 1998:255.
21. O'Grady JG, Alexander GJM, Hayllar KM, et al. Early indicators of prognosis in fulminant hepatic failure. *Gastroenterology.* 1989;97:439.
22. Motschman TL, Taswell HF, Brecher ME, et al. Intraoperative blood loss and patient and graft survival in orthotopic liver transplantation: their relationship to clinical and laboratory data. *Mayo Clin Proc.* 1989;64:346.
23. Millan MT, Keeffe EB, Berquist WE, et al. Liver transplantation at Stanford University Medical Center. In: Ceckos JM, Teraski PI, eds. *Clinical Transplantation 1998.* Los Angeles, Calif: UCLA Tissue Typing Laboratory; 1998:287.
24. Williams R, Gimson AES. Intensive liver care and management of acute hepatic failure. *Dig Dis Sci.* 1992;36:820.
25. Donovan JP, Shaw BW Jr, Langnas AN, et al. Brain water and acute liver failure: the emerging role of intracranial pressure monitoring [editorial]. *Hepatology.* 1992;16:267.
26. Keays R, Potter D, O'Grady J, et al. Intracranial and cerebral perfusion pressure changes before, during, and immediately after orthotopic liver transplantation for fulminant hepatic failure. *QJM.* 1991;79:425.
27. O'Grady JG, Alexander GJM, Thick M, et al. Outcome of orthotopic liver transplantation in the aetiological and clinical variants of acute liver failure. *QJM.* 1988;69:817.
28. O'Grady JG, Gimson AES, O'Brien CJ, et al. Controlled trials of charcoal hemoperfusion and prognostic factors in fulminant hepatic failure. *Gastroenterology.* 1988;94:1186.
29. Hanid MA, Davies M, Mellon PJ, et al. Clinical monitoring of intracranial pressure in fulminant hepatic failure. *Gut.* 1980;21:866.
30. Brajtbord D, Parks RI, Ramsay MA, et al. Management of acute elevation of intracranial pressure during hepatic transplantation. *Anesthesiology.* 1989;70:139.
31. Le Roux PD, Elliott JP, Perkins JD, et al. Intracranial pressure monitoring in fulminant hepatic failure and liver transplantation [abstract]. *Lancet.* 1990;335:1291.
32. Sidi A. Anesthesia for orthotopic liver transplantation (OLT): University of Florida data. In: *Refresher Course, 16th International Congress of the Israeli Society of Anesthesiologists.* 1992:233.
33. Jurim O, Shackleton CR, McDiarmid SV, et al. Living-donor liver transplantation at UCLA. *Am J Surg.* 1995;169:529.
34. 1993 Annual Report of the US Scientific Registry of Transplant Recipients and the Organ Procurement and Transplantation Network. *Transplant*

*Data: 1988–1991.* United Network for Organ Sharing (Richmond, Virginia) and the Division of Organ Transplantation; and Bureau of Health Resources Development, Health Resources and Services Administration, US Department of Health and Human Services Administration, US Department of Health and Human Services. Bethesda, Md: US Department of Health and Human Services; 1993.

35. United Network for Organ Sharing. Cadaveric and living donors recovered between 1988 and 1993 by age. *UNOS Update.* 1994;10:28.

36. Lo CM, Fan ST, Liu CL, et al. Applicability of living donor liver transplantation to high-urgency patients. *Transplantation.* 1999;67:73.

37. Raia S, Nery JR, Mies S. Liver transplantation from live donors. *Lancet.* 1989;21:497.

38. Strong RW, Lynch SV, Ong TN, et al. Successful liver transplantation from a living donor to her son. *N Engl J Med.* 1990;322:1505.

39. Grewal HP, Thistlethwaite JR Jr, Loss GE, et al. Complications in 100 living-liver donors. *Ann Surg.* 1998;228:214.

40. Tojimbara T, Fuchinque S, Nakajima I, et al. Analysis of postoperative liver function of donors in living-related liver transplantation. *Transplantation.* 1998;66:1035.

41. Lo CM, Fan ST, Liu CL, et al. Extending the limit on the size of adult recipient in living donor liver transplantation using extended right lobe graft. *Transplantation.* 1997;63:1524.

42. Iwatsuki S, Shaw BE Jr, Starzl TE. Experience with 150 liver resections. *Ann Surg.* 1983;197:247.

43. Sterneck MR, Fischer L, Nischwitz U, et al. Selection of the living liver donor. *Transplantation.* 1995;60:667.

44. Kalayoglu M, Sollinger HW, Stratta RJ, et al. Extended preservation of the liver for clinical transplantation. *Lancet.* 1988;1:617.

45. Rettke SR, Chantigian RC, Janossy TA, et al. Anesthesia approach to hepatic transplantation. *Mayo Clin Proc.* 1989;64:224.

46. Williamson KR, Taswell HF, Rettke SR, et al. Intraoperative autologous transfusion: its role in orthotopic liver transplantation. *Mayo Clin Proc.* 1989;64:340.

47. Butler P, Israel L, Jenkins DE, et al. Blood transfusion during liver transplantation [abstract]. *Transfusion.* 1983;23:433.

48. Brown BR. Anesthetizing the patient with abnormal liver function. In: *ASA 1990 Annual Refresher Course, Lecture 32.* Park Ridge, Ill: American Society of Anesthesiologists; 1990.

49. Williams R. Drug administration in hepatic disease. *N Engl J Med.* 1984;309:1616.

50. Davis PJ, Cook DR. Anesthetic problems in pediatric liver transplantation. *Transplant Proc.* 1989;21:3493.

51. McEvedy BA, Shelley MP, Park GR. Anesthesia and liver disease. *Br J Hosp Med.* 1986;36:26.

52. Gelman S. Anesthesia for the patient with liver disease. In: ASA 1990 Annual Refresher Course, Lecture 143. Park Ridge, Ill: American Society of Anesthesiologists; 1990.

53. Cosimi AB, Cho SI, Delmonico FL, et al. A randomized clinical trial comparing OKT3 and steroids for treatment of hepatic allograft rejection. *Transplantation.* 1987;43:91.

54. Starzl TE, Donner A, Eliasziw M, et al. Randomised trialomania? The multicentre liver transplant trials of tacrolimus. *Lancet.* 346:1346, 1995.

55. Spencer CM, Goa KL, Gillis JC. Tacrolimus: an update of its pharmacology and clinical efficacy in the management of organ transplantation. *Drugs.* 1997;54:925.

56. Paulsen AW, Whitten CW, Ramsay MAE, et al. Considerations for anesthetic management during veno-venous bypass in adult hepatic transplantation. *Anesth Analg.* 1989;58:489.

57. Scherer R, Giebler R, Erhard J, et al. Porto-femoro-subclavian bypass and the rapid infusion technique in orthopedic liver transplantation. *Anaesthetist.* 1991;40:222.

58. Smith MF, Klinck JR, Hayman GA, et al. Percutaneous cannulation for veno-veno bypass during liver transplantation. *Anesthesiology.* 1993;79:A486.

59. Spiekermann BF. A method for percutaneous cannulation for veno-veno bypass during orthotopic liver transplantation [letter]. *Anesth Analg.* 1995;80:432.

60. Kang Y, Aggarwal S, Freeman JA. Intraoperative mortality during liver transplantation. *Transplant Proc.* 1988;20(suppl 1):600.

61. Polson RJ, Parks GR, Lindop MJ, et al. The prevention of renal impairment in patients undergoing orthotopic liver transplantation by infusion of low dose of dopamine. *Anesthesiology.* 1987;42:15.

62. Carmichael FJ, Lindop MJ, Farman JV. Anesthesia for hepatic transplantation: cardiovascular and metabolic alterations and their management. *Anesth Analg.* 1985;64:108.

63. Groth CG, Pechet L, Starzl TE. Coagulation during and after orthotopic transplantation of the human liver. *Arch Surg.* 1969;98:31.

64. Esquivel CO, Koneru B, Karrer F, et al. Liver transplantation before 1 year of age. *J Pediatr.* 1987;110:545.

65. Martin T, Kang Y, Marquez JM, et al. Pharmacokinetics and hemodynamic effects of calcium chloride and calcium gluconate during liver transplantation. *Anesthesiology.* 1988;69:A451.

66. Kang Y, Lewis JH, Navalgund A, et al. Epsilon-aminocaproic acid for treatment of fibrinolysis during liver transplantation. *Anesthesiology.* 1987;66:766.

67. Von Kaulla KN, Kaye H, Von Kaulla E, et al. Changes in blood coagulation before and after hepatectomy or transplantation in dogs and man. *Arch Surg.* 1966;92:71.

68. Kang Y, Borland LM, Picone J, et al. Intraoperative changes in coagulation during liver transplantation in children. *Anesthesiology.* 1987;65:A525.

69. Plevak DJ, Southorn PA, Narr BJ, et al. Intensive-care unit experience in the Mayo liver transplantation program: the first 100 cases. *Mayo Clin Proc.* 1989;64:433.

70. Rosen HR, O'Reilly PM, Shackleton CR, et al. Graft loss following liver transplantation in patients with chronic hepatitis C. *Transplantation.* 1996;62:1773.

# Overview of Organ Transplantation

Ake Grenvik

Joseph M. Darby

Brian A. Broznick

Susan Stuart

Developments in organ transplantation have been spectacular. Almost 700 000 people worldwide have received organ transplants. The number of patients needing and wanting organ transplantation increases daily. By March 2001, 75 069 potential recipients were waiting for an organ in the United States alone.[1] This number almost quadrupled between 1990 and 2001. In comparison, the number of brain-dead donors increased by only 42% during these 11 years.

Because the number of patients awaiting transplantation has increased far more rapidly than the number of available donors, the shortage of donor organs has reached almost crisis proportions. Anesthesiologists may not be involved in the transplantation process until the patient is ready to come to the operating room, but they still will benefit by knowing the antecedent procedures and problems involving the acquisition and processing of donor organs.

## CURRENT TRANSPLANTATION ACTIVITIES

### What Is the Status of Solid Organ Transplantation?

#### Kidneys

Renal transplantation began more than 4 decades ago. Subsequently, over 150 000 patients have received renal allografts in the United States, and the current figure worldwide approximates 450 000. About 15 000 kidneys are transplanted each year in the United States, 20% from living donors (1-year graft survival is $\approx$95%) and 80% from brain-dead, heart-beating cadavers (1-year graft survival $\approx$85%). Patient 1-year survival is above 95% in prominent centers; almost 70% of kidney recipients are alive 10 years later, and more than 50% of their primary grafts are still functioning at that time.[2]

Approximately 22 000 Americans develop end-stage renal disease each year, and 30 000 transplantations could easily be performed annually if enough kidneys were available. The quality of life after transplantation is greatly improved, and long-term graft survival is achieved at a lower cost compared with that of chronic dialysis.

## Livers

In 1998, 4137 liver transplantations were performed in the United States and over 77 581 worldwide.[3] One-year graft survival exceeds 85% in prominent centers.

## Pancreata

The overall 1-year survival rate of pancreas recipients is approximately 80%, but graft *survival*, defined as lack of insulin dependence, approaches only 50%. Centers with the most experience report 90% patient survival and 80% graft survival at 1 year. The majority of successful procedures are performed in conjunction with renal transplantation.[4] Islet cell transplantation does not offer as high a success rate as that for solid or segmental pancreas grafts.

## Hearts

The first cardiac transplantation occurred in 1967.[5] Since then, heart transplantation has become a routine procedure and currently is performed in more than 170 medical centers in the United States. Results are excellent, with a 1-year graft survival rate of more than 80% in leading institutions. For comparison, the mortality rate at 1 year among candidates on the waiting list is significantly higher than 40%; our Pittsburgh experience indicates a death rate of approximately 80% in far sicker patients on our waiting list.

## Lungs

Single-lung and double-lung transplantations have increased in number over the past few years. Initially, only combined heart-lung procedures were carried out in numbers large enough to provide reliable data, but the heart is needed only in complex situations, with the disease process involving both organs. During 1997, almost 1300 lung transplantations were carried out worldwide; more than half of those were in the United States. Current 1-year survival rates exceed 70%.[6]

## Multiple Organs

Normally, double-organ transplantation is performed as two separate operations except for the combination of heart and lungs. The most common combination is the implantation of pancreas and a kidney in diabetic patients with renal failure.[7] Heart-liver,[8] heart-kidney,[9] and liver-kidney[10] transplantations are also done. In addition, multiple organs, which may include the liver, pancreas, stomach, small intestine, and colon, have been transplanted en bloc in recent years.

From the immunologic standpoint, transplantation of multiple organs from the same donor is advantageous. However, this approach is not always possible, as in the case of asynchronous transplantation of two organs. In multiple organ transplantation, rejection of one organ but not the other may occur even if the organs originate from a single donor.

## Who Are Potential Donors?

Of the more than 2 million individuals who die each year in the United States, 12 000 to 27 000 are considered suitable for organ donation, depending on age limits and medical criteria used. This number would meet the needs of the patients awaiting transplantation if a satisfactory method to bring all such cadavers into a pool of donors were available. However, this goal has not been achieved and probably never will be. The size of the potential brain-dead donor pool has not significantly increased in the United States since the 1990s. The increase in transplantations performed has resulted from the willingness of transplant surgeons to accept older donors and donors with a history of hypertension or diabetes. This change in philosophy has resulted in a 42% increase in the number of brain-dead donors during the past decade (Table 72–1).

The greatest obstacle in acquiring organs for transplantation remains the refusal of relatives to allow organ donation when the possibility exists. With increased efforts, however, nearly 10 000 brain-dead donors might be available for multiple organ procurement each year (ie, 70% of an estimated pool of 14 000 annual donors).[11]

## Which Are the Major Donor Categories?

Three major categories of organ donors can be identified:

- Living donors
- Brain-dead, heart-beating cadavers
- Non–heart-beating cadavers

**TABLE 75–1.** Brain-Dead Organ Donors in the United States, 1989–1998

| Year | Total No. of Donors | No. of Donors >50 Years of Age (%) | No. of Transplants | | | | |
|---|---|---|---|---|---|---|---|
| | | | Kidney | Liver | Heart | Lung | Pancreas |
| 1989 | 4018 | 565 (14) | 3815 | 2377 | 1781 | 191 | 799 |
| 1990 | 4513 | 702 (15) | 4311 | 2875 | 2169 | 276 | 950 |
| 1991 | 4530 | 796 (18) | 4271 | 3167 | 2198 | 395 | 1066 |
| 1992 | 4521 | 938 (21) | 4277 | 3335 | 2247 | 527 | 1004 |
| 1993 | 4860 | 998 (21) | 4608 | 3763 | 2443 | 790 | 1244 |
| 1994 | 5060 | 1151 (23) | 4738 | 3988 | 2497 | 838 | 1217 |
| 1995 | 5382 | 1211 (22.5) | 5002 | 4333 | 2505 | 583 | 1275 |
| 1996 | 5437 | 1333 (24.5) | 5038 | 4465 | 2483 | 763 | 1297 |
| 1997 | 5493 | 1363 (25) | 5082 | 4587 | 2433 | 839 | 1319 |
| 1998 | 5693 | 1429 (25) | 5314 | 4769 | 2436 | 748 | 1455 |
| Total | 49 507 | 10 486 (21.2) | 46 456 | 37 659 | 23 192 | 5950 | 11 626 |

125 000 organs from 50 000 brain-dead donors means 2.5 organs from each donor (average).

To enlarge the pool of organ donors, acceptable age limits have been expanded; particular organs with milder forms of disease or trauma have been less often excluded; and a segment of vital organs removed from living donors (eg, the tail of the pancreas or left lobe of the liver) have been used for transplantation from a parent to a child. Transplant surgeons even have removed a lobe of a lung of one family member to give to another.

## How Did the Brain Death Concept Evolve?

Herniation of a brain lethally injured by trauma or disease leads to death through respiratory and cardiac arrest. However, not until the implementation of intensive care and prolonged mechanical ventilation in the 1950s did brain death become a condition that could last for days and weeks rather than a few minutes. On the basis of criteria published by the Harvard Committee in 1968,[12] the Uniform Determination of Death Act was proposed jointly by the American Bar Association and the American Medical Association at the National Conference of Commissioners on Uniform State Laws in 1981. This Act, now accepted as law in all 50 of the United States, reads:

*An individual who has sustained either irreversible cessation of circulatory and respiratory functions, or irreversible cessation of all functions of the entire brain, including the brainstem, is dead.*

Debate is still ongoing concerning the relevance of the concept of brain death; in the future, certification of death may include not only conventional heart-beating cadavers who are brain-dead but also those with cerebral death (ie, patients in a permanent vegetative state[13,14] and those with an absent brain, or anencephalic infants[15]). A resolution in 1994 by the American Medical Association provided an ethical basis for the use of organs from anencephalic babies.[16] As long as these infants are considered alive, however, procurement of their organs remains illegal.

## What Are The Neurologic Criteria?

The neurologic criteria for certification of death include (1) documented cessation of cerebral function (cerebral death) and (2) unresponsiveness to stimulation of all cranial nerves (indicating death of the brainstem). Most important is verification that spontaneous breathing is absent when $Paco_2$ is greater than 60 mm Hg. Usually two neurologic examinations are required to avoid the possibility of misjudgment. However, the prescribed interval between the two examinations ranges from 2 to 24 hours. If confounding factors such as drug overdose, intoxication, administered muscle relaxants or anesthesia, hypothermia, shock, or metabolic coma are present, complete cessation of blood flow to the brain must be documented through four-vessel cerebral arteriography or another acceptable technique.

## How Is Consent Obtained?

After death has been certified, consent for organ donation must be obtained before procurement can take place. Even if consent in writing is available from the deceased, the practice in the United States has been to obtain consent from the next of kin as well. However, organ donor cards, including authorization on driver's licenses, are increasingly considered legal advance directives. Some states, such as Pennsylvania, have indicated that this prior decision by the deceased person cannot be overruled by relatives.

## What Is the Persistent Vegetative State?

Although irreversible cessation of all function of the entire brain is required for certification of brain death in the United States, demonstration of cessation of brainstem function is a satisfactory condition in the United Kingdom. Whereas the cerebral hemispheres cannot function independently if the whole brainstem is dead, the opposite is not true. In the persistent vegetative state (PVS), cerebral death is present but the brainstem is more or less intact.

Some ethicists are in favor of defining individuals with PVS as dead because (1) they have lost consciousness and cognition and (2) "personhood," as an indication of human life, is absent.[13,14] Because patients with PVS have the ability to breathe spontaneously, however, most people do not accept that life has ceased when the body is still breathing. Furthermore, variable degrees of cerebral death can be present in patients with PVS. Clinically, up to 3 months may be required to determine permanence in medical cases and up to 1 year in those cases caused by trauma.[17] This large group of patients ($\approx$10 000 annually in the United States) currently cannot be considered for organ donation unless treatment is withdrawn and death is certified based on cessation of cardiac function (so called non–heart-beating donors).

## Can Anencephalic Infants Be Considered?

Anencephaly refers to the absence of the cerebrum. If born alive, anencephalic infants rarely survive longer than 2 weeks without therapy. Because they have a brainstem with at least rudimentary function, they may be able to breathe spontaneously and cannot be certified dead unless they stop breathing or the heart ceases to function.

Although attempts to use organs from anencephalic donors have been made in various countries, no acceptable solution to the medicolegal and ethical problems involved in these procedures has resulted. However, a decreasing number of full-term anencephalic babies are born each year, making this potential donor category relatively unimportant.[18]

# PROCEDURAL CONSIDERATIONS

## How Are Donors Recognized?

Early recognition of potential donors who, depending on type of injury and clinical status, are likely to progress to brain death despite aggressive support, is crucial for ensuring a continuing supply, and it facilitates mobilization of personnel and resources essential to organ procurement. Anticipation, prevention, and aggressive treatment of physiologic instability and other complications associated with brain death result in enhanced organ function after transplantation. Most potential donors have been admitted to an intensive care unit (ICU) with severe blunt or penetrating head trauma or catastrophic intracranial hemorrhage that results in coma, marked impairment of brainstem reflexes, massive brain swelling with compression of basilar cisterns, and refractory intracranial hypertension.

### How Are Donors Assessed?

Medical eligibility criteria for organ donation continue to evolve. Physicians managing a potential donor in the ICU should involve the local organ procurement organization (OPO) in the determination of medical eligibility while focusing their efforts on maintaining vital organ function. A thorough patient history and physical examination as well as a general assessment of relevant organ function are the principal factors that determine medical eligibility of the potential donor.

The presence of the following main conditions exclude the potential organ donor from further consideration:

- Malignancy (except nonmetastasizing primary brain tumor or localized cutaneous or cervical cancer)
- Active viral infection
- Acquired immunodeficiency syndrome (AIDS)
- Tuberculosis
- Any other untreated or inadequately treated infectious disease

Although extremes of age were emphasized as a principal exclusionary factor in the past, more recent data indicate that age limits can be extended, [19-25] with physiologic function considered more important than chronologic age.

After general medical eligibility has been determined and consent for organ donation has been obtained, serologic testing and additional diagnostic examination directed at a more thorough evaluation of individual organ function and suitability are performed according to requirements of the local OPO. Details of individual organ assessment and suitability for organ donation can be found elsewhere.[26]

### How Is Death Certified?

In the United States, as was noted previously, brain death diagnostic criteria are based on the "whole brain" definition,[27] and brain death must be certified in accordance with local state laws. The diagnosis of brain death in pediatric patients less than 5 years of age is more complicated than in adults and requires special consideration of age, duration of observation after absent brain function is documented, and additional diagnostic tests, especially documentation of cessation of brain blood flow.[28]

### Confirmatory Tests

The diagnosis of brain death in most potential donors can be made on the basis of the clinical examination alone; however, adjunctive testing may be required in circumstances that might potentially mimic brain death (eg, high blood concentration of barbiturates or narcotics, pharmacologic neuromuscular blockade, hypothermia). In such circumstances, or if any ques-

tion regarding the validity of the clinical examination arises, brain death must be confirmed with studies that document absent cerebral blood flow.

Many diagnostic tests can be used.[29] Conventional bedside cranial radionuclide angiograms have the advantage of wide acceptance and simplicity. Another bedside technique increasingly used for confirmation of brain death employs the radionuclide tracer, technetium 99m hexamethylpropyleneamine oxime ($^{99m}$Tc-HM-PAO). This test evaluates brain perfusion rather than intracranial blood flow, and it can provide images of the posterior fossa.[30-32]

Physiologic deterioration of the potential donor may occur during brain death evaluation, particularly with prolonged apnea testing. Anesthesiologists not involved in critical care may be called in for this testing. Worsening hypotension[33] and hypoxemia are the most common problems encountered. Hypotension in conjunction with hypercarbia and acidosis during apneic oxygenation may be addressed by the administration of sodium bicarbonate or increased vasopressor infusion. Hypoxemia is minimized by preoxygenation before apnea testing and by tracheal insufflation of oxygen (eg, 4-6 L/min) during the apnea test. The date and time of death should be documented clearly in the patient's medical record after certification criteria are met. Physicians who declare brain death in potential donors may not be involved in either organ procurement or transplantation of the involved patient.

### Donor Management

The principal issues of concern after brain death has developed are hemodynamic instability and other complications that may have occurred as a consequence of brain death, associated injuries, or treatment directed at the primary brain insult. Commonly encountered complications include hypotension, hypothermia, diabetes mellitus, hypernatremia, hypokalemia, and metabolic acidosis. Because data are limited regarding donor management that optimizes subsequent allograft function, the goals of treatment in the ICU and operating room are similar to those for most critically ill patients. Support of organ perfusion and prevention of complications related to this management are the main objectives during organ donor maintenance.

### What Other Considerations Are Important?

#### General

Nasogastric suction minimizes the risk for large-volume pulmonary aspiration of gastric contents, and exposure to ambient temperature is minimized to prevent an excessive decrease in body temperature. All catheters placed under suboptimal conditions in the field should be removed and replaced, with aseptic technique used as indicated for further resuscitation and monitoring.

#### Monitoring

Hemodynamic instability and fluctuations in acid-base and electrolyte status necessitate invasive monitoring and frequent blood sampling in the prospective organ donor. Arterial pressure, central venous pressure (CVP), arterial blood oxygen saturation, and urine output are monitored. Pulmonary artery catheterization is occasionally needed if routine resuscitative efforts fail to restore adequate hemodynamic endpoints or in potential donors with cardiac tamponade, myocardial contusion, heart failure, or high positive end-expiratory pressure (PEEP) ventilation requirements. Arterial blood gas partial pressures, serum electrolytes, serum glucose, and hematocrit are measured as clinically indicated. Desirable physiologic endpoints are listed in Table 72–2.

## What Are the Critical Elements of Hemodynamic Support?

Hemodynamic instability should be expected in the brain-dead organ donor. Victims of multisystem trauma with ongoing blood loss and large fluid requirements are more likely to be unstable than donors who succumb to brain death as a result of isolated, unremitting intracranial hypertension. Hemodynamic instability in most brain-dead organ donors is manifested principally by hypotension.[34–37] The problem often is multifactorial, with loss of vascular tone compounded by fluid losses secondary to the use of osmotic or loop diuretics before brain death development and diabetes insipidus thereafter. Because ischemic organ injury is an important factor leading to allograft dysfunction,[38–41] donor hypotension must be aggressively treated, with titration of vasopressors and fluid administration as indicated.

### Fluids

Intravascular volume expansion with crystalloids, colloids, and blood is employed initially to treat established hypotension and to achieve indicated physiologic endpoints. Although crystalloids alone can be used, colloids may reduce the total fluid requirement, minimize body cooling, and reduce the potential risk of crystalloid-associated impairment in tissue oxygenation.[42] Excessive fluid administration is of particular concern for optimal function of donor lungs and heart. Fluid resuscitation in potential lung donors should be titrated to achieve a CVP of no more than 6 mm Hg (or a pulmonary artery occlusion pressure of 10 mm Hg) to minimize the adverse effects of pulmonary edema.[43] A high CVP and excessive fluid may also result in impaired heart function after brain death.[44,45]

### Vasopressors

Vasopressors should be titrated to their minimum effective doses to avoid end-organ damage caused by increased myocardial oxygen consumption or reduced splanchnic and renal blood flow. Dopamine usually is preferred because of potential beneficial effects on renal and mesenteric blood flow.[46] Donors in whom hemodynamic stability cannot be achieved or main-

tained should have a pulmonary artery catheter or transesophageal echocardiographic monitoring to better evaluate cardiac function and volume status and to guide therapy.

### Thyroid Hormones

Most anesthesiologists have little or no experience with thyroid hormone therapy. On the basis of experimental and uncontrolled clinical data, however, some investigators routinely administer triiodothyronine ($T_3$) or thyroxine ($T_4$) to improve hemodynamic stability and organ metabolism in the donor.[47–51] However, conflicting data regarding the value of thyroid hormone administration in organ donor management[52–58] have diminished the enthusiasm for the use of this novel therapy.

### Urine Output

Because of the frequent occurrence of polyuria caused by diabetes insipidus in brain death states, urine output cannot be relied on as an indication of the adequacy of fluid volume administration. Oliguria usually is not a problem in donors who receive early and vigorous volume resuscitation. However, because donor urine output appears to be an important determinant of renal graft function,[59] oliguria that is unresponsive to volume expansion should be treated with loop diuretics or mannitol to facilitate diuresis.

### Arrhythmias

Cardiac arrhythmias may complicate management, particularly during brain herniation and early after brain death.[26,60] Antiarrhythmic agents are occasionally required for ventricular or supraventricular tachyarrhythmias and bradyarrhythmias with associated hemodynamic instability. β-Blockers and calcium channel antagonists may cause untoward hypotension[61] and should be used with caution in the brain-dead patient. Atropine is ineffective in this condition; hence, isoproterenol and epinephrine should be used, if required, for treatment of bradyarrhythmias and in cardiac arrest situations.

### Cardiac Arrest

Cardiac arrest occurs in 4% to 28% of potential organ donors during the maintenance phase.[34,62] Shock, diabetes insipidus, and hypokalemia predispose the donor to unexpected cardiac arrest.[62] Sometimes organs can be recovered after successful cardiopulmonary resuscitation; therefore, vigorous resuscitative efforts should be instituted at the onset of cardiac arrest. If consent already has been obtained, the donor in cardiac arrest can be taken directly to the operating room for organ procurement after death certification, based on cessation of cardiac function.

### Ventilatory Support

Ventilatory support of the potential organ donor is adjusted to optimize oxygenation, carbon dioxide ($CO_2$) elimination, and hemodynamic function. Minimal lactic acidosis is commonly present in the potential organ donor[47–49,63,64] and can be managed simply with minor adjustments in minute ventilation. If severe acidosis is present, sodium bicarbonate or other buffers should be administered to minimize excessive ventila-

**TABLE 75–2.** Physiologic End Points in the Organ Donor

| | |
|---|---|
| Systolic blood pressure | 90–120 mm Hg |
| Central venous pressure | 5–10 mm Hg |
| Urine output | 100–250 mL/h |
| Core temperature | 35–38°C |
| Hematocrit | 25% |
| Oxygen saturation | >95% |
| pH | 7.4–7.45 |

tion. This strategy limits the adverse hemodynamic effects of both metabolic acidosis and excessive positive pressure ventilation.

If hypothermia is present, acid-base analysis and correction are probably best approached by the use of temperature-*uncorrected* blood gas values to adjust systemic pH. This approach results in higher in vivo pH values and may ultimately promote improved organ function.[65-67]

### Fluid and Electrolyte Management

Developing fluid and electrolyte disturbances must be addressed because they may be important contributors to instability and premature organ donor loss.[62,68] Hypokalemia and hypernatremia are the most common abnormalities and arise mainly as a result of polyuria and excessive solute diuresis associated with diabetes insipidus, hyperglycemia, hypothermia, mobilization of excess body fluids, or administration of mannitol.[26]

In the potential organ donor, polyuria in association with hypernatremia and hypotonic urine is sufficient to support the clinical diagnosis of diabetes insipidus. It often heralds clinical brain death.[69,70] Patients may be receiving intravenous (IV) desmopressin acetate (DDAVP), 1 to 2 µg every 8 to 12 hours, to minimize ongoing fluid and electrolyte losses after diabetes insipidus is recognized. Prophylactic administration of DDAVP is avoided because the polyuria of diabetes insipidus appears to protect against acute tubular necrosis after transplantation.[71]

Existing free water deficits and ongoing excess urinary losses should be replaced with hypotonic fluid and added electrolytes, as dictated by serum and urine electrolyte measurements. Additional supplements of potassium, phosphate, and magnesium are usually required to maintain normal electrolyte balance. Although excessive hyperglycemia should be avoided, glucose administration does appear to have a favorable effect on posttransplantation liver function.[72,73]

### Hypothermia

After brain death, the body becomes poikilothermic and at risk for hypothermia. Mean body temperatures range from 31.5° to 34°C.[74,75] Hypothermia may impair cardiac, renal, and hepatic function[76,77] and predisposes the donor to hemodynamic instability and unexpected cardiac arrest.[68] A reasonable therapeutic endpoint is the maintenance of core temperature at or above 35°C. Fluids and blood products should be warmed and heated. Humidified respiratory gases (37°-39°C) should be administered, and external warming devices should be used.

### Miscellaneous Problems

Brain trauma accompanied by disseminated intravascular coagulation (DIC), hypothermia, hemorrhage, and massive transfusion may predispose to coagulopathy. The frequency of DIC in one study was almost 30%, largely in those donors with penetrating brain injuries.[78] Specific therapy (eg, heparin) does not appear to be warranted. Donors with evidence of coagulopathy and ongoing hemorrhage should be treated with appropriate blood components to ensure adequate tissue oxygenation and to maintain hemodynamic stability. Antibiotic therapy should be administered to organ donors with documented or suspected infection.

## ORGAN PROCUREMENT AND PRESERVATION

### What Are Organ Procurement Organizations?

The responsibility for identification, procurement, and distribution of cadaveric organs for transplantation has been delegated to the nation's federally certified OPOs. Current OPOs include both independent and hospital-based agencies.[79] An independent agency is a freestanding, nonprofit organization that normally provides services to more than one transplant center; a hospital-based OPO usually is a subsidiary of a single transplant center.

### Responsibilities

One of the primary responsibilities of each OPO is professional public education. OPOs conduct more than 10 000 teaching programs per year across the United States. Many of these programs are presented to medical and nursing staffs, social services, and chaplaincy groups within area hospitals.[80] Most, however, are public-oriented programs that, if effectively delivered, result in increased referrals of potential donors, as has been demonstrated in the United Kingdom and Spain.

### Consent

The anesthesiologist must ensure that appropriate consent has been obtained before proceeding with operating room donor management. Obtaining consent is probably the most sensitive procedure in the donation process. Many health care professionals feel uncomfortable approaching families with the request for organ or tissue donation; however, organ procurement specialists are readily available 24 hours a day to provide this service. Whoever discusses donation with the family must be well versed in the entire process of donation and transplantation. One of the most unfortunate possible occurrences in the donation request process is for the family to be informed that their loved one is dead and then immediately to be approached about organ donation.[81]

Studies have shown that "coupling" of the notification of death with request for organ donation results in a consent rate of 30% or less, whereas 65% of families or more may consent if this information is provided separately (ie, "decoupled").[81]

After a donor has been identified, suitability determined, and family consent obtained, the next step is to secure permission from the coroner or medical examiner if required by law. Cooperation with these professionals is of utmost importance.[82,83] The anesthesiologist must ensure that this process has been completed before proceeding. On many occasions, the medical examiner or coroner may have specific requests that must be considered during the procurement process, such as preservation of evidence in homicide cases. One person should be responsible for coordinating the entire donation process to ensure that all aspects have been considered and that the procedure has been conducted accordingly.

### What Should the Anesthesiologist Know?

After all medical and legal aspects of the process have been completed, the donated organs are surgically removed. During the recovery of these organs, the process of preservation begins. Depending on which organs are procured, cannulas are introduced into the abdominal aorta, inferior vena cava, portal vein, aortic arch, or pulmonary artery. A hypothermic solution is infused through the cannulas to wash out the donor's blood and to cool the organs to a temperature of 4° to 7°C.

The most frequently used solution for preservation is commonly referred to as the University of Wisconsin, or UW, solution.[84] In some transplant centers, Euro-Collins solution,[85,86] a dextrose-based crystalloid, is used for lung preservation. Some surgeons also use a cardioplegic blood-based or plasma-based solution for heart preservation.

Hearts and lungs have the shortest hypothermic preservation tolerance; the maximum limit is 6 hours between the time of organ removal from the donor and restoration of circulation in the recipient. Pancreata and livers can be preserved safely for almost 24 hours, kidneys up to 72 hours. After the preservation process has begun and donated organs have been recovered, they are individually packaged in containers or sterilized plastic bags. The procured organs are then placed in a cooler that contains crushed ice and are shipped to the selected medical center for transplantation. This type of preservation is known as *simple static cold storage*.

Another method employed primarily for kidneys is known as *pulsatile perfusion preservation*. Instead of being packed in an ice cooler, the donated kidney is placed in a sterile environment with a cannula introduced into the renal artery. A cold solution is continually pumped through the organ. This process provides oxygen and nutrition to the organ and retains an organ temperature of 4° to 7°C. This method, although cumbersome and expensive, seems to result in better long-term preservation and initial organ function compared with the simple static cold storage technique.[87]

## TRANSPLANTATION ORGANIZATIONS AND ALLOCATION OF ORGANS

The list of candidates awaiting transplantation in the United States has grown from 10 000 to 60 000 in a little more than one decade. Because of this rapid growth, the government, the transplant community, and, most important, the public recognized early on the need to develop a formal organizational system to ensure high standards of care and equal access to transplantation.

### What Is the United Network for Organ Sharing?

In 1984, the federal government passed a law, commonly known as the National Organ Transplant Act, which mandated development of the National Organ and Transplantation System.[88] In 1986, the United Network for Organ Sharing (UNOS), located in Richmond, Virginia, was granted the responsibility for this function.

The purpose of UNOS is twofold: (1) to ensure equal access to organs for all patients awaiting transplantation and (2) to establish policies and procedures for standards of operation of all transplant-related organizations.

UNOS is governed by a board of directors of which no more than 50% may be physicians. The board also includes members of the transplant community and members of the general public, voluntary health organizations, donor families, patients awaiting transplantation, and transplant recipients. Membership requirements, organ procurement procedures, and histocompatibility standards are designed by UNOS committees and must be approved by the board of directors before implementation. All policy changes are published in the *Federal Register* for public comment. On the basis of public reaction, new policies may be altered before implementation.

### How Is Allocation Determined?

The single most difficult task facing UNOS has been the development of a fair and equitable system to allocate available organs for transplantation.[89] A sophisticated system exists today, but it continues to undergo further refinements.

#### Kidneys and Pancreata

Kidneys are allocated by matching ABO blood type, tissue type, percentage of reactive antibodies (PRA), and waiting time.[90] Other information regarding the donor is entered into the UNOS computer system, and patients are matched accordingly. Numeric values are assigned, and the eligible patient with the most points is offered the opportunity for transplantation first. A similar system is in place for allocation of pancreata.

#### Hearts, Lungs, and Livers

Tissue matching is impractical and is not deemed as important in the transplantation of the heart, the lung, and the liver. Lungs are allocated solely on the basis of waiting time and the recipient's distance from the donor site. Most transplantation surgeons agree that if a patient who is awaiting transplantation deteriorates to the point of ventilator dependency, transplantation is no longer an option. Therefore, medical criteria today are not used in allocating lungs.

With liver and heart transplantation, the patient's medical condition plays an important role in organ allocation. Numeric status codes are given to patients awaiting a transplant. A higher code value is assigned to a recipient who is maintained on mechanical support in an ICU, for example, than to one who is homebound and in fairly healthy condition. The total score is calculated for every waiting patient, and organs are distributed accordingly.

#### Local Primacy

Transplantation surgeons have some leeway to override the allocation system according to specific medical criteria, but they must provide a written explanation to UNOS in each such instance. This possibility was developed to allow individual physician judgment, which must be available in any area of medicine that involves patient selection.

With the exception of kidneys, which must be distributed on a national basis, the system always has recognized local primacy for organ distribution if a perfect match exists. One of the most important reasons for allocating organs on this basis is to stimulate donation. Local primacy allegedly stimulates organ donation from local patients. If all organs were placed into a national pool, health care workers and donor family members might be less eager to work compassionately toward obtaining or providing consent for organ donation.

Local primacy for organ distribution may not be in the best interests of recipients. Some experts question the appropriateness of giving a heart or liver to the sickest *local* recipient but not the sickest *national recipient* if the local patient is in a less critical condition. The current system of giving priority to local, then regional, and finally national allocation may result in an increased mortality rate for those patients awaiting organs other than kidneys.

## What Is the Role of Living Donors?

The first successful kidney transplantation was performed between identical twins and resulted in a 9-year recipient survival. However, when nontwin siblings or other close relatives were selected, the success rate was poor until the development of effective immunosuppression therapy. In addition to kidneys, the tail of the pancreas has been transplanted from living related donors, but the success rate of this procedure has been less than promising. The high frequency of complications in donors has also resulted in less enthusiasm for this procedure.

In recent years, the left liver lobe and even lung lobes have been transplanted from living related donors, usually from parents to children. Although these operations are not yet commonly performed, the results have been encouraging. Living nonrelated donors, usually spouses or other emotionally related donors, have been used. In the United States, organs cannot be sold or dealt with for profit. However, in developing countries, such as India, the selling of a kidney has provided a significant sum to a financially struggling family, sometimes as much as might be earned in a full decade.

## How Is Cardiac Arrest Managed During Evaluation for Brain Death?

If consent for organ donation already has been obtained, cardiopulmonary resuscitation may be initiated to maintain some perfusion of donated organs while the donor is brought to the operating room for emergent procurement of organs. Death must first be certified according to traditional cardiac criteria. Because cardiopulmonary resuscitation to save the patient's life in the presence of lethal head injury with evolving brain death is not indicated, cardiopulmonary resuscitation is interrupted in the operating room to permit certification of death after cessation of cardiac function is confirmed. Kidneys and livers have been transplanted from such donors with good results.

## How Are Withdrawal of Life Support and Organ Donation Managed After Death?

If life-sustaining therapy is to be withdrawn, the donor is taken to the operating room for terminal weaning from mechanical ventilation. After cardiac arrest has occurred, death is certified and organ procurement takes place immediately. A major ethical problem is that family members usually are not permitted to be present in the operating room during this terminal phase of life. This problem is solved if an adjacent room can be used for this purpose. Nonetheless, no time for prolonged grief and farewell after certification of death is possible, because warm ischemia rapidly reduces the success of graft transplantation. The University of Iowa and the University of Pittsburgh have reported successful transplantation of kidneys and livers in this setting.[90,91]

## References

1. United Network for Organ Sharing (UNOS). Critical Data. Available at: http://www.unos.org. Accessed, March 24, 2001.
2. Ellison M, Daily OP, Breen T, et al. *Annual Report of the U.S. Scientific Registry of Transplant Recipients and the Organ Procurement and Transplantation Network.* Richmond, Va: United Network for Organ Sharing; 1998.
3. Ceca JM, Terasaki PJ. Worldwide Transplant Center Directory. Liver Transplants. In: Terasaki PJ, Cecka JM, eds. *Clinical Transplants, 1998.* Los Angeles, Calif: UCLA Tissue Typing Lab; 1999:577.
4. Sutherland DER, Moudry-Munnis KC. International pancreas transplant registry report. In: Terasaki P, ed. *Clinical Transplants.* Los Angeles, Calif: UCLA Tissue Typing Laboratory; 1998.
5. Barnard CN. A human cardiac transplant: an interim report of a successful operation at Groote Schuur Hospital in Cape Town. *S Afr Med J.* 1967;41:1271.
6. Kawai A, Paradis IL, Keenan RJ, et al. Lung Transplantation at the University of Pittsburgh, 1982–1994. In: Terasaki PI, Cecka JM, eds. *Clinical Transplants, 1994.* Los Angeles, Calif: UCLA Tissue Typing Laboratory; 1995.
7. Kelly WD, Lillehei RC, Merkel FK, et al. Allotransplantation of the pancreas and duodenum along with the kidney in diabetic nephropathy. *Surgery.* 1967;61:827.
8. Shaw BW, Bahnson HT, Hardesty RL, et al. Combined transplantation of the heart and liver. *Ann Surg.* 1985;220:667.
9. Livesey SA, Rolles K, Calne RY, et al. Successful simultaneous heart and kidney transplantation using the same donor. *Clin Transpl.* 1988;2:1.
10. Margreiter R, Kramar R, Huber C, et al. Combined liver and kidney transplant. *Lancet.* 1984;1:1077.
11. Beasley CL. Maximizing donation. *Transplant Rev.* 1999;13:31.
12. Beecher H. A definition of irreversible coma: report of the Ad Hoc Committee of the Harvard Medical School to examine the definition of brain death. *JAMA.* 1968;205:337.
13. Veatch R. The whole-brain-oriented concept of death: an outmoded philosophical formulation. *J Thanatol.* 1975;13:3.
14. Youngner SJ, Bartlett ET. Human death and high technology: the failure of the whole brain formulations. *Ann Intern Med.* 1983;99:252.
15. Harrison MR. Fetal organ transplantation: organ procurement for children. The anencephalic fetus as a donor. *Lancet.* 1986;2:1383.
16. Warren J. AMA adopts resolution approving anencephalic as potential organ donor. *Transplant News.* 1994;4:5.
17. The Multisociety Task Force on Persistent Vegetative State: medical aspects of the persistent vegetative state. *N Engl J Med.* 1994;330:1572.
18. Peacock JL, Emery JR, Ashwal S. Experience with anencephalic infants as prospective organ donors. *N Engl J Med.* 1989;321:344.
19. Schuler S, Parnt R, Warnecke H, et al. Extended donor criteria for heart transplantation. *J Heart Transplant.* 1988;7:326.
20. Harjula A, Starnes VA, Oeyer PE, et al. Proper donor selection for heart-lung transplantation. *J Thorac Cardiovasc Surg.* 1987;94:874.
21. Szmidt J, Karolak T, Sablinski T, et al. Transplantation of kidneys harvested from donors over sixty years of age. *Transplant Proc.* 1988;20:772.
22. Klintmalm GB. The liver donor: special consideration. *Transplant Proc.* 1988;20(suppl 7):9.
23. Alexander JW, Vaughn WK. The use of marginal donor for organ transplantation: the influence of donor age on outcome. *Transplantation.* 1991;51:135.
24. Alexander JW, Bennett LE, Breen TJ. Effect of donor age on outcome of kidney transplantation: a two-year analysis of transplants reported to the United Network for Organ Sharing Registry. *Transplantation.* 1994;57:871.
25. Marino IR, Doyle HR, Doria C, et al. Outcome of liver transplantation using donors 60-79 years of age. *Transplant Proc.* 1995;27:1184.
26. Darby JNL, Stein K, Grenvik A, et al. Approach to the management of the heart-beating brain-dead organ donor. *JAMA.* 1989;261:2222.

27. Guidelines for the determination of death: report of the medical consultants on the diagnosis of death to the President's Commission for the Study of Ethical Problems in Medicine and Biomedical and Behavioral Research. *JAMA.* 1981;246:2184.

28. Task Force for the Determination of Brain Death in Children. Guidelines for the determination of brain death in children. *Ann Neurol.* 1987;21:616.

29. Powner DJ. The diagnosis of brain death in the adult patient. *J Intensive Care Med.* 1987;2:181.

30. De al Riva A, Gonzalez FM, Llamas-Elvira JM, et al. Diagnosis of brain death: superiority of perfusion studies with ⁹⁹ᵐTc-HMPAO over conventional radionuclide cerebral angiography. *Br J Radiol.* 1992;65:289.

31. Schlake H-P, Bottger IH, Groterneyer K-H, et al. Determination of cerebral perfusion by means of planar brain scintigraphy and ⁹⁹ᵐTc-HMPAO in brain death, persistent vegetative state and severe coma. *Intensive Care Med.* 1992;18:76.

32. Wilson K, Gordon L, Selby JB. The diagnosis of brain death with Tc-99m HMPAO. *Clin Nucl Med.* 1993;18:428.

33. Jeret JS, Benjamin JL. Risk of hypotension during apnea testing. *Arch Neurol.* 1994;51:595.

34. Emery RW, Cork RC, Levinson MM: The cardiac donor: a six-year experience. *Ann Thorac Surg.* 1986;41:356.

35. Robertson KM, Kramiak IM, Gelb AW, et al. Endocrine changes and hemodynamic stability after brain death. *Transplant Proc.* 1989;21:1197.

36. Powner DL, Jastremski K, Lagler RG, et al. Continuing care of multiorgan donor patients. *J Intensive Care Med.* 1989;4:75.

37. Fink MP. In vivo organ preservation in brain dead patients. *J Intensive Care.* 1989;4:53.

38. Gidepp RB, Stinson EB, Clark DA, et al. The cardiac donor. *Surg Gynecol Obstet.* 1971;133:792.

39. Flanigan WJ, Ardon LF, Brewer TE, et al. Etiology and diagnosis of early post-transplantation oliguria. *Am J Surg.* 1976;132:808.

40. Toledo-Pereyra LK, Simmons RL, Olson LC, et al. Cadaver kidney transplantation: effect of hypotension and donor pretreatment with methylprednisolone and phenoxybenzamine. *Minn Med.* 1979;62:159.

41. Starzl TE, Demetris AJ, Van Thiel D, et al. Liver transplantation. *N Engl J Med.* 1989;321:1014.

42. Randell T, Orko R, Hockerstedt K. Perioperative fluid management of the brain-dead multiorgan donor. *Acta Anaesthesiol Scand.* 1990;34:592.

43. Pennefather SH, Bullock RE, Dark JH. The effect of fluid therapy on alveolar arterial oxygen gradient in brain dead organ donors. *Transplantation.* 1993;56:1418.

44. Wicomb WN, Cooper DKC, Lanza RP, et al. The effects of brain death and 24 hours storage by hypothermic perfusion on donor heart function in the pig. *J Thorac Cardiovasc Surg.* 1986;91:896.

45. Mertes PM, el Abassi K, Jaboin Y. Changes in hemodynamic and metabolic parameters following induced brain death in the pig. *Transplantation.* 1994;59:414.

46. Goldberg LI. Cardiovascular and renal actions of dopamine: potential clinical applications. *Pharmacol Rev.* 1972;24:1.

47. Novitsky D, Cooper DKC, Morrell D, et al. Change from aerobic to anaerobic metabolism after brain death and reversal following triiodothyronine therapy. *Transplant.* 1988;45:32.

48. Novitsky D, Cooper DKC, Reichart B, et al. Hemodynamic and metabolic responses to hormonal therapy in brain dead potential organ donors. *Transplant.* 1987;43:852.

49. Novitsky D, Cooper DKC, Human PA, et al. Triiodothyronine therapy for heart donor and recipient. *J Heart Transplant.* 1988;7:370.

50. Orlowski JP, Spees EK. The use of thyroxine (T4) to promote hemodynamic stability in the vascular organ donor: a preliminary report on the Colorado experience. *J Transplant Coordination* 1991;1:19.

51. Orlowski JP, Spees EK. Eighteen-month graft and patient survival following liver transplantation with organs recovered from cadaveric donors managed with thyroxine: a retrospective study. *J Transplant Coordination.* 1991;1:144.

52. Howlett TA, Keogh AM, Perry L, et al. Anterior and posterior pituitary function in brain stem–dead donors. *Transplantation.* 1989;47:828.

53. Robertson KM, Hramiak IM, Gelb AW, et al. Endocrine changes and hemodynamic stability after brain death. *Transplant Proc.* 1989; 21:1197.

54. Macoviak JA, McDougall IR, Bayer MF, et al. Significance of thyroid dysfunction in human cardiac allograft procurement. *Transplantation.* 1987;43:24.

55. Wahlers T, Fieguth HG, Jurmann M, et al. Does hormone depletion of organ donors impair myocardial function after cardiac transplantation? *Transplant Proc.* 1988;20(suppl 1):792.

56. Gifford RRM, Weaver AS, Burg JE, et al. Thyroid hormone levels in heart and kidney cadaver donors. *J Heart Transplant.* 1986;5:49.

57. Koller J, Wieser C, Gottardis M, et al. Thyroid hormones and their impact on the hemodynamic and metabolic stability of organ donors and on kidney graft function after transplantation. *Transplant Proc.* 1990;22:355.

58. Garcia-Fages LC, Cabrer C, Valero R, et al. Hemodynamic and metabolic effects of substitute triiodothyronine therapy in organ donors. *Transplant Proc.* 1993;25:3038.

59. Lucas BA, Vaughn WK, Spees EK, et al. Identification of donor factors predisposing to high discard rates of cadaver kidneys and increased graft loss within one year post transplantation: SEOPF, 1977–1982. South-Eastern Organ Procurement Foundation. *Transplantation.* 1987; 43:253.

60. Nygaard CE, Townsend RN, Diamond DL. Organ donor management and organ outcome: a 6-year review from a level 1 trauma center. *J Trauma.* 1990;30:728.

61. Hayek DA, Veremakis C, O'Brien JA, et al. Enhanced vasomotor sensitivity to vasoactive agents during the evolution of brain death. *Chest.* 1990;98(suppl):633s.

62. Mallory DL, Nelson JE, Matuschak GM, et al. Risk factors for loss of donor organs in brain-dead ICU patients due to unexpected cardiac arrest. *Chest.* 1989;96(suppl 1):289s.

63. Nishimura N, Miyata Y. Cardiovascular changes in the terminal stage of disease. *Resuscitation.* 1984;12:175.

64. Powner DJ, Hendrich A, Lagler RG, et al. Hormonal changes in brain dead patients. *Crit Care Med.* 1990;18:70.

65. Kroncke GM, Nichols RD, Mendenhall JT, et al. Ectothermic philosophy of acid-base balance to prevent fibrillation during hypothermia. *Arch Surg.* 1986;121:303.

66. Swain JA. Hypothermia and blood pH: a review. *Arch Intern Med.* 1988;148:1643.

67. White FN. A comparative physiological approach to hypothermia. *J Thorac Cardiovasc Surg.* 1981;82:821.

68. Hayek DA, Veremakis C, O'Brien JA, et al. Time-dependent characteristics of hemodynamic instability in brain dead organ donors. *Crit Care Med.* 1990;18:S204.

69. Keren G, Schreiber K, Aladjem M, et al. Diabetes insipidus indicating a dying brain. *Crit Care Med.* 1982;10:798.

70. Outwater KM, Rockoff IMA. Diabetes insipidus accompanying brain death in children. *Neurology.* 1984;34:1243.

71. Rabanal JM, Teja JL, Quesada A, et al. Does diabetes insipidus in brain dead organ donors protect acute tubular necrosis in the renal grafts? *Transplant Proc.* 1993;25:3143.

72. Slapak M. The immediate care of potential donors for cadaveric organ transplantation. *Anesthesia.* 1978;33:700.

73. Palombo JD, Hirschberg Y, Pomposelli JJ, et al. Decreased loss of liver adenosine triphosphate during hypothermic preservation in rats pretreated with glucose: implications for organ donor management. *Gastroenterology.* 1988;95:1043.

74. Jastremski M, Powner D, Snyder J, et al. Problems in brain death. *Forensic Sci.* 1978;11:201.

75. Ouakinc GE: Bedside procedures in the diagnosis of brain death. *Resuscitation.* 1975;4:159.

76. Curley FJ, Irwin RS. Disorders of temperature control: hypothermia. Part III. *J Intensive Care Med.* 1986;1:270.

77. Wong KC. Physiology and pharmacology of hypothermia. *West J Med.* 1983;138:227.

78. Hefty TR, Cotterell LW, Fraser SC, et al. Disseminated intravascular coagulation in cadaveric organ donors: incidence and effect on renal transplantation. *Transplantation.* 1993;55:442.

79. Health Care and Finance Administration. Washington, DC: Certified Organ Procurement Organizations, 1990.

80. Association of Organ Procurement Organizations. www.aopo.org. Accessed, March 24, 2001.

81. Garrison RN, Bentley FR, Raque GH, et al. There is an answer to the shortage of organ donors. *Surg Gynecol Obstet.* 1991;173:391.

82. Miracle K, Broznick B, Stuart S. Coroner/medical examiner cooperation with the donation process: one OPO's experience. *J Transplant Coordination.* 1993;3:23.

83. Schafer T, Schkade LL, Warner HE, et al. Impact of medical examiner/coroner practices on organ recovery in the United States. *JAMA.* 1994;272:1607.

84. Wahlberg JA, Southard JH, Belzer FO. Development of a cold storage solution for pancreas preservation. *Cryobiology.* 1986;23:417.

85. Collins GM, Bravo-Sugarman M, Terasaki PL. Kidney preservation for

transportation: initial perfusion and 30 hours' ice storage. *Lancet.* 1969;2:1219.

86. Dreikorn K, Horsch R, Rohl L. 48- to 96-hour preservation of canine kidneys by initial perfusion and hypothermic storage using the Euro-Collins solution. *Eur Urol.* 1980;6:221.

87. Barber W, Laskaw D, Deiehoi M, et al. Comparison of simple hypothermic storage, pulsatile perfusion with Belzer's gluconate-albumin solution, and pulsatile perfusion with solution for renal allograft preservation. *Transplant Proc.* 1993;25:2394.

88. National Organ Transplant Act. Public Law 98-507, October 19, 1984.

89. Stratta R, Taylor R. Kidney allocation in the 1990s: progress and problems. *Transplant Proc.* 1993;25:3065.

90. D'Allessandro AM, Hoffman M, Knechtle SJ, et al. Controlled non–heart-beating donors: a potential source of extrarenal organs. *Transplant Proc.* 1995;27:707.

91. Casavilla A, Ramirez C, Shapiro R, et al. Liver and kidney transplantation from non–heart-beating donors: the Pittsburgh experience. *Transplant Proc.* 1995;27:710.

# 76

# Renal Transplantation

Avner Sidi

As with many other types of surgery, clinical experience and development of new techniques and drugs make the complex task of transplantation and, in particular, provision of anesthesia for renal transplantation more simple and successful. Today, the task seems fairly routine and has a low complication rate. During the 1980s and 1990s, well over 400 000 renal homografts were performed throughout the world; half of these patients were still alive with their grafted kidney in place.[1,2] About 12 000 renal transplantations are performed annually in the United States,[2,3] and a similar number are performed in foreign centers.[2] Advances in organ preservation, histocompatibility testing, and immunosuppression have enabled prolonged survival of both cadaveric allograft and living-related donor renal transplants. The actual technique of transplantation has changed little through the years (Fig. 76–1).

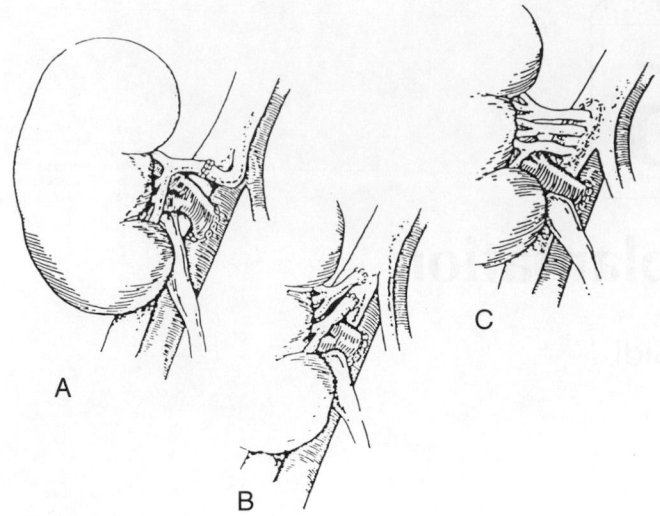

**FIGURE 76–1.** Techniques of reestablishing the allograft vascular supply. *A*, Renal artery to internal iliac artery. *B*, Anastomosis of multiple renal arteries to the external iliac artery. *C*, Carrel patch anastomosis to external iliac artery. (From Whelchel JD. Surgical aspects of renal transplantations. In: Graybar GB, Bready LL, eds. *Anesthesia for Renal Transplantation*. Boston, Mass: Martinus Nijhoff; 1987:90.)

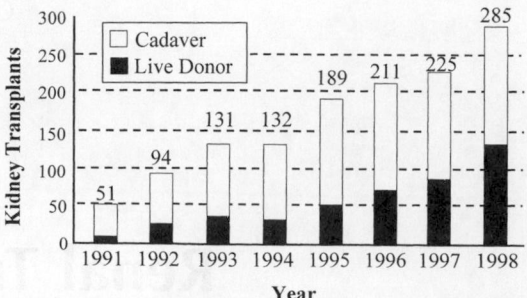

**FIGURE 76–2.** Annual number of cadaver and living donor kidney transplantations performed at the University of Maryland, Baltimore, since 1991. (From Bartlett ST, Farney AC, Jarrell BE, et al. Kidney transplantation at the University of Maryland. In: Cecka JM, Teraski PI, eds. *Clinical Transplants 1998*. Los Angeles, Calif: UCLA Tissue Typing Laboratory; 1999:178.)

## GENERAL CONSIDERATIONS

### How Long Can Donor Kidneys Be Preserved?

Kidney preservation allows time for transportation and evaluation of potential recipients for cytotoxic antibody tests. Preservation techniques include simple hypothermic storage, which preserves tissue for up to 48 hours. A more expensive and difficult option is pulsatile preservation, in which the organ's vascular system is flushed and supplied with preservation solutions delivered by a pulsatile pump. This method preserves tissue up to 60 hours. The preservation solution is cold (4°C), contains potassium, and is hyperosmolar.

### What Is Tissue Matching?

Tissue typing (HLA typing), or histocompatibility testing, consists of two main components: (1) antigen matching—with a match of six major histocompatibility antigens, outcome of cadaveric allograft is improved by 20%[4]; (2) detection of cytotoxic antibodies—cytotoxic antibodies in the potential recipient against donor antigen are predictive of a poor outcome; transplantation should be avoided in such patients.

### What Factors Are Major Determinants of Renal Allograft Function and Survival?

Many different factors affect the survival of renal allograft, such as those related to donor, recipient, donor-recipient, and external factors. The number of living-related donors and cadaveric grafts has increased since the 1990s (Fig. 76–2). Of these, donor-related factors appear to be more important.[5] A large collective study of 43 172 patients from the United Network for Organ Sharing (UNOS) Scientific Renal Trans-

plant Registry showed that graft survival is donor age–dependent, even when controlled for tissue typing; this cannot be overcome by improvement in immunosuppression.[6] The decreased survival rate associated with increases in donor age was attributed to the diminishing number of active nephrons with age. This study is disturbing in that it shows progressive diseases of graft survival in cases of donors older than 30 years of age.

### What Universal Immunosuppression Protocols Are Used?

Immunosuppression of the recipient often follows a different protocol in each transplantation center. Most centers include a protocol consisting of cyclosporine and steroid administration. In certain types of patients (eg, those undergoing retransplantation or those who cannot tolerate cyclosporine), the protocol may include azathioprine, antithymocyte, antilymphocyte globulin, monoclonal antibodies, or a combination of these (Table 76–1).

Other drugs have been developed and used for kidney transplantation recently. The most prominent of these is tacrolimus (FK-506), which has become an established immunosuppressant[7] (see Chapter 74).

## PREOPERATIVE CONCERNS

Kidney failure is associated with and induces systemic abnormalities, including behavioral, cardiovascular, pulmo-

**TABLE 76–1.** Intraoperative Drug Immunosuppression, Antibiotics, and Diuresis in a Protocol for Renal Transplantation

Cephazolin, 1 g IV, just after induction of anesthesia; gentamicin, 2 mg/kg, should be substituted if patient allergic to cephalosporins

Continue cyclosporine, 1.5 mg/kg in 120 mL of DW at 10 mL/h bid; cyclosporine is not compatible with other IV medications. Should be started preoperatively, if not already infusing at the time of arrival to the operating room, at 3 mg/kg

Methylprednisolone, 1 g IV (for children, use 20 mg/kg if weight is <50 kg), slow IV push; drip is continued

Azathioprine, 3 mg/kg (maximum, 250 mg) IV

Furosemide, 60 mg IV

Mannitol, 25 mg, at the start of anastomosis (with methylprednisolone sodium succinate [Solu-Medrol] bolus, azathioprine [Imuran], and furosemide [Lasix])

DW, dextrose in water; IV, intravenous.

nary, hematologic, metabolic, neurologic, endocrine, gastrointestinal, and immunologic changes (Table 76–2).

## What Abnormalities Are Likely?

### Cardiopulmonary

As the kidneys' ability to excrete water becomes impaired, peripheral and dependent edema, hypertension, and a hyperdynamic state often evolve.[8] Pulmonary edema and pericardial effusion may be present. Congestive heart failure, left ventricular hypertrophy, and cardiac tamponade are possible complications. A chest radiograph and electrocardiogram are obligatory.

The patient's usual blood pressure range and the medications that he or she is taking should be recorded, and antihypertensive drugs should be continued perioperatively. Hypertension may correlate with sodium and water loading or with renin levels; therefore, treatment should be directed toward controlling these factors. Blood volume should be normal or even slightly high before induction and maintenance of anesthesia if hypotension is to be avoided. At the end of the last preoperative dialysis or before induction, the patient's weight should be 1 to 2 kg above *dry* weight. Patients usually know their dry weight and how much fluid is taken off during each dialysis.

### Hematologic

Anemia of chronic renal disease is common, may be severe, and is often associated with a hematocrit that is less than half of normal. The cause is a decrease in the production and survival of red blood cells. The effects of anemia are compensated by increased cardiac output and a rightward shift of the oxyhemoglobin dissociation curve. Preoperative hemoglobin and hematocrit levels should be compared with the patient's usual values.

Anemia is usually well tolerated because of normovolemic or even hypervolemic compensation and because of its gradual onset and chronic nature. However, at some level, decompensation at rest or during stress occurs. This point varies and is a function of age, sympathetic activity, flow and volume in shunts and fistulas, and the presence of vascular disease.

A patient's ability to tolerate moderate activity without developing symptoms suggests that decompensation is not present and that a transfusion is unnecessary. Transfusion in these patients predisposes to fluid overload and congestive heart failure, along with the usual risk for disease transmission. However, in the presence of severe anemia (hemoglobin,

---

**TABLE 76–2.** Signs and Symptoms of Uremia

| Behavioral, Mental, or Neurologic | Hematologic |
|---|---|
| *Depressive* | *Anemia* |
| Fatigue, asthenia, malaise, shortening of concentration, memory defects, anorexia, drowsiness, suicidal thoughts, stupor, precoma, coma | Normochromic, normocytic |
| *Irritative* | *Bleeding Abnormalities* |
| Anxiety, fasciculations, twitching, headache, ataxia, asterixis, abnormal gait, vertigo, nausea, convulsions | Prolonged bleeding time, abnormal platelet aggregation<br>Lymphopenia, mild thrombocytopenia |
| *Psychiatric* | **Metabolic** |
| Personality change, bizarre behavior, phobias, organic psychosis, selective amnesia, denial, kleptomania | Hyperkalemia<br>Metabolic acidosis<br>Hypermagnesemia<br>Hyperphosphatemia |
| *Peripheral* | Hypocalcemia<br>Metastatic calcification |
| Pruritus, paresthesias, restless leg syndrome, monoplegia, paraplegia, sensory and motor defects, bladder atony, dysfunction | *Medium-sized* arteries: arterial insufficiency, ischemia, skin ulceration, gangrene |
| *Ophthalmic* | *Joints, Sites of Pressure* |
| Nystagmus, miosis, anisocoria, band keratopathy | Arthritis, decreased range of motion<br>Myocardium, skeletal muscle, lung |
| **Gastrointestinal** | Musculoskeletal muscle pain and weakness, proximal myopathy, bone pain, bone fractures |
| *Membrane Problems* | Aseptic necrosis of bone<br>Disturbances in multiple endocrine system |
| Glossitis, stomatitis, esophagitis, enteritis, pancreatitis, colitis, ileus | Carbohydrate intolerance<br>Hyperlipidemia |
| *Functional Problems* | Gout and pseudogout<br>Wasting and abnormalities in protein metabolism |
| Anorexia, dysgeusia, nausea, vomiting, hematemesis, constipation, diarrhea, abdominal distention | **Immunologic** |
| *Structural Problems* | Reduced T-cell–mediated immune function<br>Impaired phagocytosis and chemotaxis |
| Peptic and colonic ulceration | Atrophy of the lymphoid system, including the thymus<br>Reduced immune surveillance of neoplasia |
| **Cardiovascular and Pulmonary** | **Miscellaneous** |
| Pericarditis, acute and constrictive<br>Pleuritis<br>Congestive heart failure<br>Change in blood pressure<br>Dysrhythmias<br>Vascular calcification<br>Accelerated atherosclerosis<br>Cheyne-Stokes or Kussmaul's breathing, or both | Reduced wound healing<br>Hypothermia<br>Impaired response to pyrogen |

From Schreiner GE. Uremia. In: Massry SG, Glassock RJ, eds. *Textbook of Nephrology.* Baltimore, Md: Williams & Wilkins; 1983:452. © Williams & Wilkins, 1983.

<6 g/dL), hypovolemia, or signs and symptoms of myocardial or cerebral hypoxia, blood should be administered. Severe anemia may decrease the blood-gas partition coefficient for inhalation agents by as much as 25%, increasing the rates of induction and emergence.

## Coagulation

Platelet function may be abnormal as a consequence of decreased platelet factor 3, decreased adhesiveness, and decreased aggregation; bleeding times should be evaluated. The prothrombin time (PT) and partial thromboplastin time (PTT) are usually less affected. Platelet dysfunction can be treated and corrected by platelet transfusion or by the administration of desmopressin or even conjugated estrogens.[9,10] Although theoretic objection exists to perioperative blood transfusions, some clinicians transfuse preoperatively because of possible improvement in graft survival when a recipient shares at least one HLA-DR antigen with the donor.[9]

## Metabolic

Abnormalities of water balance, acid-base regulation, and electrolytes (sodium, potassium, chloride, phosphate, calcium, and magnesium) become more common as the degree of renal failure increases. Osteomalacia and osteosclerosis occur during renal failure and uremia. Glucose intolerance with insulin resistance is common. Hypoalbuminemia results from poor nutrition and urinary losses and leads to hypovolemia and extravascular edema.

## Neurologic

Encephalopathy, peripheral neuropathy, and autonomic dysfunction occur in uremic patients.[11] Patients with peripheral neuropathy often have autonomic neuropathy as well that is best detected by a tilt test. Such patients may respond abnormally to stress produced by surgery and anesthesia. Hypertensive encephalopathy may occur in these patients.

## Endocrine

Hyperparathyroidism due to hypocalcemia and adrenal insufficiency due to steroid use may be present and should be considered.

## Gastrointestinal

Hepatitis antigen status, PT, PTT, and fibrinogen levels should be checked in patients with renal failure or uremia. Parotitis, oral ulcers, delayed gastric emptying, hyperacidity, increased gastric volume, and gastroduodenal ulcers occur with increased frequency as renal function declines.[11] The most common gastrointestinal symptoms of uremia are anorexia, nausea, vomiting, bleeding, diarrhea, and hiccups. The last of these may be relieved by phenothiazines or may require mechanical stimulation of the nasopharynx with a soft rubber catheter (the tendency for bleeding should be borne in mind).

## Immunologic

Infections are common owing to defects in immunity and white blood cell function, specifically, reduced T-cell–mediated immune function caused by uremia, immunosuppressive therapy, and increased exposure to invasive procedures. Hepatitis, urinary tract infection, peritonitis with peritoneal dialysis, atrioventricular fistula infection, and pneumonia must all be considered. Strict sterile techniques should be adhered to for invasive procedures.

## What Are the Pertinent Laboratory Data?

Patients with end-stage renal disease (ESRD) often sustain metabolic acidosis, anemia, electrolyte abnormalities, cardiovascular disturbances, platelet dysfunction, residual heparin effect after dialysis, and a high incidence of serum hepatitis (40% of kidney recipients are positive for Australia antigen).[12]

Laboratory data that should be monitored in the preoperative and perioperative period are hemoglobin and hematocrit; concentrations of serum sodium, potassium, and calcium; platelets; bleeding time; and, less frequently, PT and PTT and bicarbonate or base excess.

## Hyperkalemia

Hyperkalemia is usually not a problem until late in the course of the disease; uremic patients tolerate moderate degrees of hyperkalemia well. The current practice of dialysis just before transplantation, together with better dialysis techniques, has almost eliminated this problem.

Little evidence supports the concept that patients with a serum potassium level that is more than 5.5 mEq/L should not be anesthetized; even higher levels are probably acceptable, provided that electrocardiogram changes are not present. In any case, when hyperkalemia is present, situations that elevate the serum potassium level further (eg, hypoventilation and succinylcholine administration) should be avoided.

The membrane effects of hyperkalemia can be reversed by calcium administration. Serum levels can also be reduced by hyperventilation or sodium bicarbonate administration or by producing "internal shifts" of potassium with glucose and insulin infusions.

## What Is the Role of Preoperative Dialysis?

All problems related to fluid and electrolyte disturbances can be reversed by adequate hemodialysis and ultrafiltration. Routine hemodialysis markedly decreases electrolyte abnormalities and the need for antihypertensive medications preoperatively. However, even in its absence, the metabolic and hemodynamic changes during induction and maintenance of anesthesia are manageable.

Problems related to uremia, for the most part, are partially, if not totally, reversible by adequate dialysis. Some abnormalities, however, are not significantly improved by dialysis. These include susceptibility to infection, refractory (renin-dependent) hypertension, and anemia.

Dialysis may also cause problems. Regionally administered heparin (ie, that within the dialysis machine) may *spill over* into the patient. Rebound heparinization may occur up to 2 hours after dialysis and present as a bleeding diathesis. It is reversible with protamine.

## What Abnormal Drug Responses Occur?

Patients with uremia may have unusual responses to drugs for several reasons (Table 76–3). Accordingly, narcotics and sedatives, including tranquilizers and antiemetic drugs, should be avoided or used carefully and in minimal doses.

### Narcotics

Morphine has a prolonged effect in anephric patients owing to longer-lasting plasma concentration and accumulation of its active metabolite (morphine-3-glucuronide).[13] The newer, synthetic narcotics (fentanyl, sufentanil, and alfentanil) also are reported to have a prolonged and more pronounced effect and to cause respiratory depression with elevated blood levels or increased unbound levels in renal failure.[14,15]

### Tranquilizers

Diazepam is metabolized by the liver, but the active metabolites are renally excreted, causing variable prolongation of the sedative effect in ESRD. Midazolam can delay emergence after induction.[16]

### Antiemetics

Metoclopramide kinetics correlate with creatinine clearance; its clearance is not improved by dialysis. Plasma concentrations of several histamine-2 blockers, including ranitidine, are reduced by dialysis.[15] Cimetidine should be of concern because of its significant clinical effect as an immunostimulating agent.[15]

### Diuretics

Pharmacokinetic studies with furosemide in ESRD reveal marked reduction in its clearance.[17] Furosemide has a direct depressant effect on the neuromuscular junction. However, when it is used in the treatment of congestive heart failure or for blood pressure control, it should be continued in the preoperative period.

### Antihypertensives

β-Blockers and clonidine are frequently used to treat hypertension in ESRD patients. They should be continued without interruption to prevent rebound hypertension, even though the usual dose of propranolol can result in higher peak blood concentrations because of reduced plasma clearance. Propranolol is not cleared by dialysis.[18] Verapamil and nifedipine enhance the neuromuscular blockade of nondepolarizing relaxants. Thus, when they are administered, careful neuromuscular junction monitoring is indicated.

### Antidysrhythmics

Dysrhythmias in ESRD compromise the cardiovascular system even further. Electrolyte and metabolic imbalance (eg, acidosis, alkalosis, hyperkalemia, hypokalemia) and untreated hypertension should be corrected as part of the antidysrhythmic regimen.

Lidocaine pharmacokinetics and metabolism are not significantly impaired in ESRD; however, active metabolites may accumulate. Procainamide urinary excretion is proportional to creatinine clearance. Quinidine, which undergoes hepatic oxidation, is 80% protein bound, but its therapeutic concentration does not exceed normal ranges in ESRD.[18]

## Does Immunosuppressive Treatment Influence Anesthesia?

Preoperative oral administration of cyclosporine creates "full-stomach" conditions. When it is used, induction is performed with thiopental and succinylcholine (unless the patient is hyperkalemic) and the Sellick maneuver.

Cyclosporine has been implicated as a cause of respiratory failure in anephric renal transplant recipients who received atracurium or vecuronium. This effect probably was caused by its solvent potentiating neuromuscular blockade.[19] Azathioprine may have similar effects on neuromuscular transmission.[20]

Antilymphocytic or antithymocytic globulin, which is administered for immunosuppression, may produce fever owing to an allergic (anaphylactic-type) reaction. High-dose steroid use may produce hyperglycemia as a side effect.

## ANESTHETIC INDUCTION

Hemodynamic control should be achieved by antihypertensive treatment before surgery or even during the preinduction period. The latter approach, however, prolongs induction. The combination of a short-acting β-blocker (eg, esmolol in 0.5 mg/kg increments) and a vasodilator (eg, hydralazine, 5-10 mg, or labetalol in 0.1-0.2 mg/kg increments) brings the blood pressure of most patients into a reasonable range. Invasive monitoring of blood pressure is helpful in patients who are labile or unusually sensitive to these drugs.

Sodium nitroprusside toxicity has been reported in renal transplant recipients; this is probably a result of the lack of detoxification, impaired excretion of cyanide, and use of the high doses necessary to control hypertension as well as other unclear causes of metabolic acidosis (eg, renal failure versus cyanide toxicity).

## What Drugs Should Be Used for Premedication?

Premedication, induction, and maintenance can vary according to the anesthesiologist's preference as long as the

---

**TABLE 76–3.** Reasons for Abnormal Drug Responses in Patients With Chronic Renal Failure

Protein binding is decreased; thus, highly protein-bound drugs may cause exaggerated responses (barbiturates, diazepam).

Pseudocholinesterase level is low (rarely significant clinically).

Electrolyte and acid-base abnormalities are present (acidosis prolongs effects of muscle relaxants).

Drug clearance reduced by decreased renal excretion; smaller than usual doses, increased interval between doses may be necessary. Use of drugs not dependent on renal excretion is preferable when possible (eg, vecuronium instead of pancuronium).

Total body water and volume of distribution are usually increased (however, they may be decreased in recently dialyzed patients).

appropriate doses and their redosing frequency are taken into account (see earlier section, What Abnormal Drug Responses Occur?). Patients can be premedicated with diazepam, midazolam, or promethazine (Phenergan) along with ranitidine, sodium citrate, or both.

## What Monitoring Is Advisable?

Monitors routinely used for renal transplantation (Table 76–4) are generally similar to those used for a typical abdominal surgery case. Invasive monitoring (if needed) and vascular access must be conducted with a sterile technique because of the immunosuppression related to the underlying disease and the treatment. The *relatively* healthy ESRD patient (one without major cardiovascular and respiratory complications) who has a short history of dialysis should not routinely require invasive monitoring.

## Central Venous Catheters

The renal transplant recipient who is medically compromised may need invasive perioperative monitoring. A central venous pressure catheter provides measurement of right-sided filling pressures, potentially large-bore venous access, a blood sampling site, and a route for administration of vasoactive drugs. Such monitoring, however, is not undertaken casually because of the possibility of bleeding abnormalities, the potential for infection, and the desire to preserve veins for dialysis access in these patients. It is indicated when fluid balance cannot be clarified, when the surgical procedure is complicated, or when the expected blood loss exceeds 20% of the blood volume. It provides valuable hemodynamic information when colloids, crystalloids, and osmotic diuretics are given as part of the renal transplantation protocol.

## Pulmonary Artery Catheters

Pulmonary artery pressure monitoring is performed even less routinely than central venous monitoring. The relationship among risk, benefit, and expense of this procedure is difficult to describe. However, the maintenance of a mean pulmonary artery pressure at more than 20 mm Hg is purported to prevent acute tubular necrosis and to improve postoperative function of cadaveric grafts.[21] In most transplantation centers, pulmonary artery catheters are not inserted unless left ventricular function is poor, fluid balance status cannot be clarified by other means, or disparity between left and right ventricular function is strongly suspected.[16]

## Arterial Catheters

Invasive blood pressure monitoring with a radial or other arterial catheter is not routine. In addition to the ordinary risks of arterial catheterization, radial artery damage can make this site unsuitable for vascular access later—a major consideration in these patients. The benefit of such monitoring is tighter hemodynamic control during volume infusion and regulation of hypertension and of autonomic insufficiency intraoperatively and postoperatively.

## Placement Sites

Placement of a 20- to 22-gauge radial artery catheter is associated with a low incidence of complications[22]; however, in the patient with ESRD, the placement site should be selected individually and carefully. When a vascular access for dialysis is present in one extremity, the radial artery of the opposite side should be cannulated. If both upper extremities have a vascular access, alternative sites in the lower extremities should be used. An arterial catheter placed at a location proximal or distal to an arteriovenous fistula underestimates central arterial pressure. If a lower extremity artery is cannulated, the limb contralateral to the transplantation site should be used because the ipsilateral iliac artery is occluded during vascular anastomosis.

Arterial or venous catheters should not be inserted electively into the limb containing an arteriovenous fistula because of the risk for thrombosis or infection. However, in acute situations in which large vessels are required for fluid resuscitation, this large, peripheral, easily identified venous access site should not be forgotten, denied, or contraindicated, especially in view of the fact that during each dialysis, larger-bore cannulas are inserted into it. In the case of a nonfunctioning arteriovenous fistula, retrograde flow from the ulnar artery may produce a palpable and usable radial artery. Catheterization is unlikely to succeed if the radial artery is permanently occluded above the pulse.

## Is Regional Anesthesia an Option?

A regional technique (spinal or epidural) may be considered. The pros and cons of this technique are listed in Table 76–5. With improved preoperative patient preparation, the use of newer anesthetic drugs that have reduced dependence on renal extraction, and improved monitoring, general anesthesia can be applied with great safety. Either regional or general anesthesia can be chosen to meet the individual needs of the patient, anesthesiologist, and surgeon. Because of the relative contraindications to regional anesthesia (see Table 76–5), we prefer general anesthesia for most transplant recipients.

If a regional technique is chosen, a bleeding time should be measured in addition to a platelet count, fibrinogen level, prothrombin time, and partial thromboplastin time. The amount of local anesthetic used and the frequency of its administration should be conservative; the anesthesiologist should take into account the increased potential for local anesthetic toxicity and the possibly higher regional anesthetic block level and its shorter duration in these patients.[23]

---

**TABLE 76–4.** Monitors Needed for Anesthesia in a "Routine" Renal Transplantation Case*

Stethoscope (precordial, esophageal, or both)
Electrocardiogram, preferably with printer
Arterial blood pressure monitor (indirect, direct, or both)
Monitor of inspired oxygen concentration
Anesthetic circuit pressure monitor
Pulse oximeter (to measure oxygen saturation)
Monitor of end-tidal carbon dioxide
Urinary catheter
Thermometer
Peripheral nerve stimulator (general anesthesia)

*Other monitors may be employed if indicated by patient's medical condition.
From Schreiner GE. Uremia. In: Massry SG, Glasscock RJ, eds. *Textbook of Nephrology.* Baltimore, Md: Williams & Wilkins; 1983:452. © Williams & Wilkins, 1983.

**TABLE 76–5.** Pros and Cons of Regional Anesthesia for Renal Transplantation

**Pros**

Avoids tracheal intubation
Avoids pharmacokinetic and pharmacodynamic problems of intravenous and inhalation agents
Induces peripheral vasodilation; decreases myocardial work, preload, and afterload

**Cons**

Coagulation problems may contraindicate
Peripheral neuropathies may be present
Intravascular volume estimates are difficult
Risk for infection (minimal)
Psychologic factors (needle intolerance, awareness during procedure)
Unpredictable duration of surgery
Hypotension because of dialysis- and anesthetic-induced hypovolemia
Volume overload as block recedes and central circulation becomes plethoric
Local anesthetic toxicity increased with acidosis (minimal)

## Which Muscle Relaxants Are Suitable?

### Succinylcholine

Succinylcholine is commonly used because it provides rapid-sequence anesthetic induction and is generally safe if serum potassium levels are less than 5.5 mEq/L. It will cause a predictable increase in potassium of about 0.5 mEq/L in patients with either normal renal function or renal failure. Cholinesterase levels are depressed by dialysis with cellophane membranes; this leads to a clinically increased but generally insignificantly longer duration of action when viewed in the context of the relatively lengthy operation time.

When succinylcholine is given after anticholinesterase administration to patients with ESRD, its duration of action is prolonged because of the prolonged duration of action of the anticholinesterase.[24] When infused for more than 2 hours, succinylcholine can produce a phase II (desensitization) block, even in patients with normal renal function. Many patients with chronic renal failure have decreased muscle mass; a reduced dose of muscle relaxant suffices in these patients.

### Atracurium

The volume of distribution, elimination half-life, and clearance of atracurium are not influenced by renal failure. Hence, its onset and duration of action are not different from that in patients with normal renal function. Metabolism produces levels of laudanosine (a central nervous system excitant) that are somewhat higher in patients with renal failure.[25]

### Vecuronium

The volume of distribution of vecuronium is also not affected by renal failure. About 20% is excreted unchanged in urine. Most of its excretion is biliary; hence, its clearance and elimination half-life may be slightly prolonged. Despite the pharmacokinetic changes, time to onset and duration of action of vecuronium are little different in ESRD than in other disease.[25] Although some accumulation has been reported, it has not been associated with major clinical problems.

In ESRD patients with normal liver function, atracurium or vecuronium is probably indicated. However, other relaxant use is also possible as long as one takes into consideration

(1) autonomic side effects, (2) duration of action (the dose should be decreased appropriately; eg, half the dose should be used with pancuronium), and (3) monitoring of neuromuscular function. The use of metocurine is not recommended because it is largely excreted by the kidney.

### Rocuronium

The relatively new aminosteroid neuromuscular blocking agent rocuronium has a major advantage over other currently used drugs of this kind (vecuronium and pancuronium)—fast onset of action. This advantage can make it the nondepolarizing muscle relaxant of choice for rapid facilitation of tracheal intubation, without causing hyperkalemia (unlike the depolarizing agent, succinylcholine). A further advantage of the new compound over vecuronium is less extensive formation of breakdown products, and thus, reduced contribution to neuromuscular blockade by active metabolites. The pharmacokinetics of vecuronium shows that hepatic and renal disease will prolong its effect because of reduced clearance.[26,27] However, this prolonged effect is less than that seen with its aminosteroid-blocking agent predecessors (vecuronium and pancuronium),[28] and it is suitable for clinical use in patients with chronic renal failure.[29] Also, one study showed that volume of distribution was greater for rocuronium in renal transplant recipients than in controls.[30]

### Curare

In renal failure, the clearance and half-life of curare are prolonged, but its biliary excretion increases fourfold. Protein binding is unchanged. Undesired drug effects include ganglionic blockade with hypotension and possible recurarization.[31]

### Pancuronium

The volume of distribution of pancuronium is probably not significantly changed in renal failure. Its half-life and clearance are prolonged, and its duration of action is increased.[32]

### Anticholinesterases

Neostigmine clearance is dependent on renal excretion for 50% of the dose; therefore, the duration of action is increased in patients with ESRD. Both relaxants and anticholinesterases appear to be similarly affected, providing some safety against recurarization.

## What Drugs Should Be Used for Induction?

Induction can be carried out with thiopental, fentanyl, and lidocaine. With thiopental, the volume of distribution is increased, the elimination half-life and clearance are only slightly prolonged, and the percentage of free drug state is increased. Nevertheless, it is generally considered the induction agent of choice.

## ANESTHETIC MAINTENANCE

The current choice for maintenance of general anesthesia is isoflurane with or without a supplemental narcotic (eg, fentanyl) and air/oxygen or nitrous oxide/oxygen. Although kidney recipients are anemic, they typically tolerate the cardiovascular effect of inhalation anesthetics as long as they are at least euvolemic.

## What Is the Role for Other Inhalation Agents?

Halothane is considered in some centers as a second-choice drug because it brings about more pronounced myocardial depression and has the potential for causing hepatitis.

At about the same time that renal transplantation became common, methoxyflurane was found to be nephrotoxic because of the fluoride ion metabolite that it produces. It never became popular for kidney transplantation.

Enflurane may also lead to slightly elevated fluoride levels (up to 20 mmol/L), even though in large series, it was reported to have been used without problem.[15]

## How Much Neuromuscular Blockade Is Needed?

Profound muscle relaxation is not a major consideration for this surgical procedure because the operative site is easily accessible. In adults, the lower abdominal extraperitoneal approach is used, and the donor kidney is placed in the iliac fossa. In children, the donor kidney is usually placed in the retroperitoneal space and only occasionally intraabdominally.

## How Should Volume and Pressure Be Managed During Revascularization?

### Fluids

The renal vein is anastomosed to the iliac vein or vena cava, and the renal artery is connected to the iliac artery, hypogastric artery, or aorta (see Fig. 76–1). Circulating blood volume and systemic pressure should be normal or slightly elevated at the time of revascularization to ensure adequate graft perfusion. Expansion of blood volume using crystalloids or colloids mandates careful assessment. For patients with marginal cardiac function, central venous pressure monitoring should be considered at a minimum. When in doubt, err on the side of excess volume replacement; if renal function is maintained, excess fluid can be removed by pharmacologic translocation (nitroglycerin) or diuresis as needed.

### Mannitol

Mannitol is used as both a blood volume expander and a diuretic; its diuretic effect is important after revascularization and during and after ureter reimplantation. Relatively large doses of mannitol (1.5-2.5 g/kg) are sometimes administered to patients in renal failure. A dilutional hyponatremia may result as water is drawn from the extracellular space.[33] I recommend moderate doses of mannitol (0.25-0.5 g/kg), depending on the patient's state of hydration. Mannitol usually decreases the serum potassium level. Occasionally, however, potassium increases as a result of water extraction and diuresis.[34]

### Pharmacologic Interventions

Various pharmacologic agents may also be infused during revascularization and immediately before unclamping. The routes of administration and the drugs used vary from direct papaverine injection into the renal artery to intravenous injection of hydrocortisone, procaine, furosemide, or dopamine (5-10 µg/kg/min). The common goal underlying the pharmacologic therapy at this stage is to maintain and promote graft vasodilation, kidney perfusion, and forced diuresis. The doses and timing of drug administration can differ according to the protocol used by the transplantation team (see Table 76–1).

## What Happens With Unclamping?

Unclamping increases the blood volume by up to 300 mL and releases various endogenous vasodilating agents. Significant myocardial depression is not associated with these substances. Hypotension can be treated with volume expanders, vasoactive agents, or both (eg, 10 µg/kg/min of dopamine). Vasoactive drugs with α-adrenergic effects constrict renal vessels and should be avoided. In rare cases of transplantation with an intact adrenal gland (cadaveric donor), a hypertensive crisis can result (including ventricular tachycardia or sinus bradycardia); this crisis should be treated with β-blockers.[35]

## How Are Fluids Managed?

Fluid replacement for patients with renal dysfunction is based on *conventional* principles. First, the preanesthetic deficit is determined (compare current weight to dry weight). Which fluids to administer intravenously is widely debated.[12] Lactated Ringer's solution probably should not be used in anuric patients. Dextrose, 5% and 0.2% saline, is the preferred maintenance fluid and should be used in amounts appropriate for the fluid requirements of anuric patients (400 mL/m²/d). Second, intraoperative fluid and blood losses and third space losses are determined, with the understanding that the patient's ability to compensate for fluid load by urine formation is gone. Deficits should be replaced preoperatively. If these are estimated to exceed 15% of blood volume, invasive monitoring should be considered. Anemia should be corrected only if the hemoglobin level is less than 6 g/dL.

### Preanesthetic Deficit

Fluid requirement is related to metabolic rate (protein and electrolyte intake): 1 mL of water is required for each kilocalorie consumed, and 0.7 mL/kcal is used for renal excretion of metabolites and electrolytes; the remainder, 0.3 mL/kcal, represents insensible loss.

Each 1 g of protein catabolized produces about 6 mOsm of urea; the daily production is about 6 mOsm/kg. Each milliequivalent of sodium or potassium administered is equivalent to about 2 mOsm (because of the accompanying anion); this amounts to about 6 mOsm/kg/d. Other metabolites account for an additional 2 to 3 mOsm/kg/d. The ideal time for dialysis is probably the day before anesthesia and surgery; this allows time for equilibration of dialysis-induced fluid and electrolyte shifts.

## Intraoperative Requirements

Intraoperative losses of more than 15% of blood volume should be replaced with colloid solution on a 1:1 or 1:2 ratio after red blood cell losses are corrected. Small losses can be replaced with the usual 3:1 ratio of crystalloid solution to blood loss. Crystalloid replacement of blood loss is usually with normal saline. Insufficient information is available to recommend 3% saline for volume replacement or expansion in ESRD. It may promote diuresis and decrease total water load. However, its clearance may be reduced, causing intravascular volume overload and electrolyte imbalance.

## Third Space Losses

I routinely have 2 units of red blood cells available perioperatively. Third space losses should be replaced initially by isotonic crystalloid solution *without* potassium and excess chloride or lactate. Bicarbonate salts can be used to decrease chloride concentration in fluid to about 100 mEq/L and to correct existing metabolic acidosis. Because the critical goal is to maintain blood volume, initial third space fluid replacement is 2 to 3 mL/kg/h; further titration is guided by monitored variables. The choice between crystalloid and colloid solutions can be guided by colloid oncotic pressure and hemoglobin and hematocrit monitoring. Generally speaking, if both values increase, crystalloid solutions are indicated, and if both fall, crystalloid solutions are probably in excess, and colloid solutions should be given. This interpretation also depends on an analysis of blood loss.

Urine output is usually monitored only after ureter anastomosis, which can be done by one of three different procedures: donor-to-recipient anastomosis, ureteral implant, or, rarely, urinary diversion. Urine output is the only real-time monitor of renal function. I sustain normal systemic pressure, intravascular volume, and renal perfusion to maintain and even to force diuresis.

## What Electrolyte and Acid-Base Changes Are Important?

### Hyperkalemia

Hyperkalemia may complicate intraoperative management of renal transplant recipients,[36] particularly those with diabetes. Numerous intraoperative events may cause an increase in serum potassium concentration (Table 76–6).

### Acidosis

Acidosis is a potential intraoperative complication (see Table 76–6). Treatment of metabolic acidosis with bicarbonate

**TABLE 76–6.** Causes of Intraoperative Hyperkalemia

Preexisting hyperkalemia not treated or corrected by dialysis
Succinylcholine administration (average increase, 0.5-0.7 mEq/L)
Metabolic acidosis due to renal insufficiency; lactic acid following hypotension or hypoperfusion; acid metabolites accumulating during vascular occlusion; ketoacidosis
Washout acidosis following declamping of grafted vessels
Red blood cell transfusion (a minor problem in most cases, but bank blood generally should be <3 day old[8])

should be started if the base excess exceeds −7 mEq/L. A functioning renal graft with appropriate diuresis should be sufficient to handle preexisting acidosis and hyperkalemia. Additional respiratory acidosis may be hazardous. A poorly prepared, acidotic patient may spontaneously hyperventilate preoperatively to compensate. Failure to maintain a similar degree of hyperventilation may result in a further decrease in pH with potentially significant increases in serum potassium and myocardial depression.

## How Is the Renal Transplant Recipient Positioned?

Handling and protection of an arteriovenous fistula in ESRD patients are important to avoid clotting, thrombosis, or infection. Continuous protection of the vascular access and periodic evaluation for a palpable thrill over the fistula are recommended. If the arm with vascular access is tucked at the patient's side, a cushioned rigid protector is helpful.

## POSTOPERATIVE CARE

### When Is Intensive Care Unit Admission Advisable?

Postoperatively, these patients should be observed in the postanesthesia care unit or special transplantation recovery unit. Special attention is directed to strict monitoring of fluid intake and output because massive, dilute urine output may be present immediately after transplantation and can lead to hypotension, electrolyte depletion, or both. Blood pressure monitoring should be done on the arm without the arteriovenous fistula. Fluid and electrolyte administration should be adjusted according to electrolyte and hemodynamic values because optimal hydration has been shown to improve the function of a new graft.[21]

This care can be provided in the postanesthesia care unit or in an intermediate care unit, even though hemodynamic, physiologic, and pharmacologic alterations make the recipient different from the routine postoperative patient. The prerequisite is that the patient be at *low risk* (ie, relatively young and otherwise healthy).

High-risk patients include those with other systemic diseases, such as diabetes, pancreatitis, hypertension, and uremia; a history of gastrointestinal bleeding; coronary artery disease; and age more than 50 years.[37] These patients are more likely to require and benefit from postoperative intensive care unit management.

## CADAVERIC DONOR HARVESTING

### What Factors Are Important?

#### General Criteria

Most transplanted kidneys are cadaveric in origin. Traditionally, the donors should be "heart-beating," with stable hemodynamic function and adequate respiratory support. Organs harvested after cardiopulmonary arrest and longer warm ischemia time are associated with a high incidence of graft

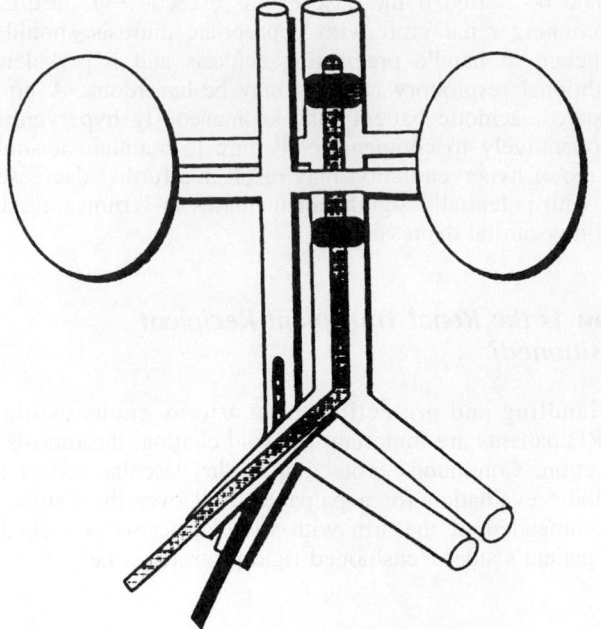

**FIGURE 76–3.** Scheme of in situ regional cooling using a triple-lumen double-balloon catheter and venous drainage tube. (From Hoshinaga K, Shiroki R, Fujita T, et al. The fate of 359 renal allografts harvested from non-heart beating cadaver donors at a single center. In: Cecka JM, Teraski PI, eds. *Clinical Transplants 1998*. Los Angeles, Calif: UCLA Tissue Typing Laboratory; 1999:213.)

failure. However, the technique of preservation of non–heart-beating donors has improved in recent years[38] (Figs. 76–3 and 76–4). Brain-dead donors must satisfy the additional requirements listed in Table 76–7.

### "Minimum Hundred Criteria"

I try to keep the donor normovolemic to hypervolemic before harvesting. Fluid infusion and blood pressure support mandate additional intravenous catheters for vascular access and possibly invasive monitoring. A guideline for care of the adult donor is satisfaction of the "minimum hundred criteria": maintenance of systolic blood pressure at more than 100 mm Hg; $PaO_2$ at more than 100 mm Hg; and urine output at more

**TABLE 76–7.** Additional Requirements for Brain-Dead Cadaveric Donors

| | |
|---|---|
| Age, <65 y | No insulin-dependent diabetes mellitus |
| Normal renal function | No active infection |
| No hypertension | No malignancy |

than 100 mL/h. Fluids may include crystalloids, colloids, and blood. Diuretics (mannitol, furosemide) can be used according to protocol. Blood pressure support and urine production can be achieved with dopamine (5-10 μg/kg/min). However, vasopressors with α-agonist effects may constrict renal vessels, compromise the graft, and adversely affect the function of a concurrently donated heart.

Respiratory support, mechanical ventilation, fraction of inspired oxygen, and positive end-expiratory pressure are provided to maintain normocarbia, normoxia, and normal pH. After heparin administration and removal of the organs, ventilation is discontinued, and anesthetic support ceases. Other organ tissues can still be harvested at this point (skin, bone, cornea). Although no anesthetic agents are used, muscle relaxation may be required.

## LIVING-RELATED DONOR HARVESTING

### How Is It Different From Cadaveric Renal Transplantation?

The number and percentage of living-related donors has been increasing[38] (see Fig. 76–2). The recipient survival rate in each age group is better for living-related donor transplants than for cadaveric donor transplants (Fig. 76–5). With living-related donor transplantation, anesthesia and surgery are scheduled electively, enabling complete preparation of both recipient and donor. The donor should be in good health and free of systemic and chronic disease, renal disease, or hypertension (Fig. 76–6). The exclusion criteria are similar to those described for the cadaveric donor.[39]

The allograft is a normal kidney with a minimal warm and cold ischemia time because it is removed under optimal conditions in a setting adjacent to the transplant recipient who is prepared simultaneously.

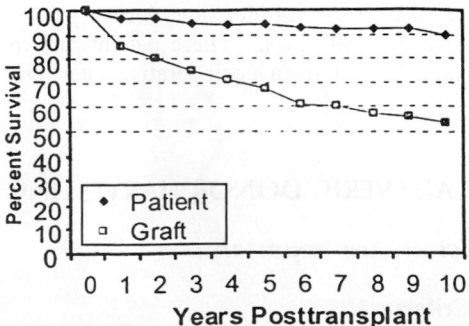

**FIGURE 76–4.** Patient and graft survival rates for 285 cadaveric renal transplantations using non–heart-beating donor grafts. (From Hoshinaga K, Shiroki R, Fujita T, et al. The fate of 359 renal allografts harvested from non-heart beating cadaver donors at a single center. In: Cecka JM, Teraski PI, eds. *Clinical Transplants 1998*. Los Angeles, Calif: UCLA Tissue Typing Laboratory; 1999:215.)

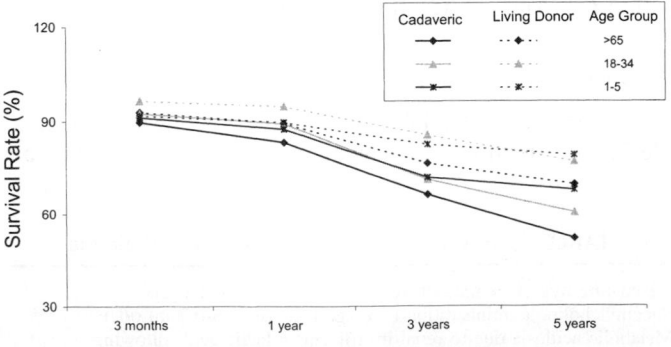

Time Post Transplantation

**FIGURE 76–5.** The survival (in months and years) of cadaveric kidney transplants and living-donor recipients, ages 1–5, 18–35, and >65 years. (Data from the *United Network of Organ Sharing (UNOS) 1998 Annual Report*, UNOS Scientific Registry Data, September 8, 1998.)

Chest X-Rays and
Pulmonary Function Tests*

Doppler U.S. FLOW Scan of
Epaiortic Vessels*

EKG and Echocardiography*

Abdominal U.S.

Doppler U.S. FLOW Scan of
Abdominal Aorta

Doppler U.S. FLOW Scan of
Femoral-Iliac Vessels*

**FIGURE 76–6.** Tests and studies performed for donor evaluation. (From Alfani D, Pretagostini R, Bruzzone P, et al. Kidney transplantation from living unrelated donors. In: Cecka JM, Teraski PI, eds. *Clinical Transplants 1998.* Los Angeles, Calif: UCLA Tissue Typing Laboratory; 1999:206.)

Urine Chemistry
BUN and Serum Creatinine
Creatinine Clearance
Renal Doppler Color FLOW/S Scan
    and U.S.
Renal Scan
Urography
Digital Angiography or Renal NMR

Blood Chemistry
Bacterial and Virological
Blood Tests

*If donor age > 50 years
U.S. = Ultrasound

## What Are the Effects of Positioning for a Flank Nephrectomy?

Donor nephrectomy is usually performed through a subcostal flank incision, with the patient positioned in a flank (nephrectomy, kidney) position or the prone position (Fig. 76–7). The flank position often impairs venous return. Several quick

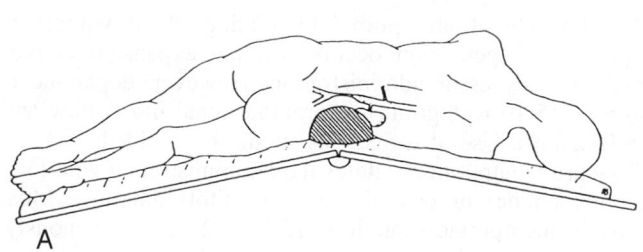

A

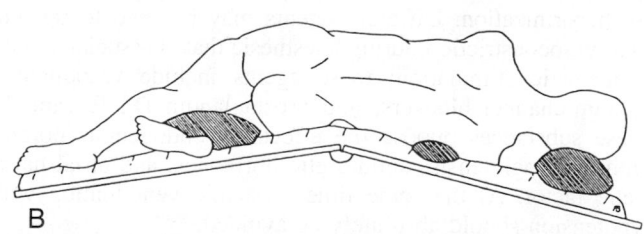

B

**FIGURE 76–7.** *A,* Incorrect lateral nephrectomy position. The top leg lies directly over the bottom leg, so that bone prominences are directly opposing each other, with inadequate padding between them. Inadequate support under the head permits excessive lateral flexion of the head. A lack of padding behind the rib cage leaves the head of the humerus directly under the thorax. Exaggerated kidney rest constricts the inferior vena cava. The brachial plexus is consequently compressed. *B,* Correct lateral nephrectomy position. The bottom leg is flexed more than the top leg, so that bone prominences are opposed by soft muscles. Padding between the legs is ample. A pillow prevents excessive lateral flexion of the head. Padding behind the lower rib cage permits slight posterior tilting of the upper part of the rib cage; as a result, the humeral head is anterior to the thorax, preventing compression of the brachial plexus. A small or no kidney rest ensures free flow of blood through the inferior vena cava. (From Britt BA, Joy N, Mackay MB. Positioning trauma. In: Orkin FK, Cooperman LH, eds. *Complications in Anesthesiology.* Philadelphia, Pa: JB Lippincott; 1983:646.)

blood pressure checks immediately after positioning identify position-related impairment of venous return. Wrapping the legs minimizes venous pooling. Extreme flexion should be avoided because it may injure the lower spine, compresses the abdominal aorta, and reduces cardiac output. Padding of the head, face, thorax, and bone prominences, as well as protection of the peripheral nerves, are essential to prevent compression injury, particularly in arthritic patients or in those with back problems. The flank position can produce adverse respiratory effects, which can lead to ventilation-perfusion mismatch. Decreased oxygenation may result from hyperperfusion and hypoventilation of the down-lung and hyperventilation and relative ischemia of the up-lung. Additionally, thoracic compliance is reduced by this position.

## How Should Anesthesia Be Administered?

### Agents

General anesthesia is preferred because of the awkwardness of the position and the length of the procedure. Induction and maintenance agents and muscle relaxants are titrated according to the patient's need and the anesthesiologist's preference. The main considerations are hemodynamic stability and maintenance of renal perfusion. Inhalation agents are widely used.[40] Potentially nephrotoxic inhalation agents (eg, methoxyflurane) obviously should not be used. High doses of drugs that are renally excreted should be avoided when possible because postnephrectomy renal reserve may decrease. Suggested simple, safe, and effective techniques include the use of nitrous oxide, oxygen, narcotics, and relaxants.

### Combined Techniques

A technique that combines epidural and general anesthesia has merit and allows an easy transition to postoperative pain management with peridural narcotics. This approach has been shown in a preliminary report to decrease the length of hospitalization when compared with conventional narcotic analgesic administration.[41]

Regardless of the agents chosen, mechanical ventilation should maintain normocapnia because hyperventilation or hypoventilation may cause renal artery constriction or venous pooling, respectively. The interaction between ventilation and renal function is complex. Mechanical ventilation has direct (renal) and indirect (cardiovascular, neural, humoral) effects, all of which decrease renal blood flow.

## How Should Ventilatory Support Be Provided?

### Direct Renal Effects

Direct renal effects of different modes of ventilatory support have been studied.[42] Intermittent positive pressure ventilation and continuous positive airway pressure may reduce renal blood flow, glomerular filtration rate, and urine output. Continuous positive pressure ventilation has the most adverse effects on these parameters and on urinary sodium excretion and osmolar clearance. Other coexisting variables, such as temperature, hematocrit, intravascular volume, and acid-base status, may also affect renal function, directly or indirectly, by modifying the cardiovascular response to ventilation. Thus, the renal effects of ventilation in an individual patient are impossible to predict.

### Hemodynamic Changes

Renal function is largely determined by hemodynamic alterations, which, in turn, may depend on the mode of ventilation, lung compliance, blood volume, and cardiac function. Mechanical ventilation, particularly continuous positive pressure ventilation, impairs renal function primarily by having an adverse effect on the effective intravascular volume and renal perfusion pressure rather than by directly decreasing cardiac output. The increase in intrathoracic pressure with continuous positive pressure ventilation results in an increase in inferior vena cava, hepatic, and renal venous pressures, all of which may further impede renal perfusion if systemic arterial pressure decreases. Careful fluid infusion often minimizes these changes.

### Baroreceptor and Humoral Changes

The relative importance of cardiac low-pressure receptors and renal high-pressure receptors in modulating renal function and intrarenal hemodynamics during mechanical ventilation is not yet established. Systemic baroreceptors (aortic arch, carotid sinus) may play a role in initiating renal dysfunction during continuous positive-pressure ventilation.[9] The primary role of antidiuretic hormone in the pathogenesis of reduced urine output is also not clear. However, plasma renin activity and aldosterone level may increase during continuous positive pressure ventilation[43]; this increase is probably related to reduction in renal perfusion pressure and glomerular filtration rate.

### Pharmacologic Support

Renal dysfunction during ventilation may resemble prerenal failure and should be treated as such. Adequate hydration to maintain filling pressures, cardiac output, and perfusion pressure is essential. A clinical dilemma may arise because what is therapeutically optimal for the kidney (ie, volume infusion) is not necessarily optimal for other organs (ie, the lungs and heart). Prophylaxis starts with choosing the ventilation mode that is least likely to depress cardiac performance. Also, pharmacologic agents (eg, dopamine) can be incorporated for prevention or treatment to improve renal function, cardiac performance, or both. The adverse effect of continuous positive pressure ventilation on renal function can be corrected by the administration of dopamine at a mean dose of 5 μg/kg/min.[44]

### Pneumothorax

Pneumothorax may develop during nephrectomy or in the immediate postoperative period. This is perhaps the most frequent serious acute perioperative complication after donor nephrectomy. Early recognition is critical. Hypotension after closure should provoke an examination to exclude pneumothorax. Nitrous oxide administration should be discontinued to avoid pneumothorax expansion; this should be followed by the institution of mechanical maneuvers (either tube drainage or needle aspiration) to ensure lung inflation. Regardless of whether a pneumothorax occurs or is suspected, a chest radiograph should be obtained immediately after nephrectomy.

## How Are the Kidneys Protected During Transplantation?

Maintenance of an optimal circulating blood volume is essential. If hypotension occurs, volume expansion is preferred to vasopressor administration. However, dopamine is also used (5-10 μg/kg/min) to promote renal blood flow and as a β-agonist. Use of α-agonists should be avoided.

Low urine output necessitates fluid administration with loop (eg, furosemide) or osmotic (eg, mannitol) diuretics. Most protocols incorporate mannitol, 12.5 to 25 g intravenously, when surgical manipulation of the kidney begins and if urine output decreases.

Local anesthetics may be applied to the renal vessels after dissection to minimize vascular spasm. Many protocols also use heparinization. Different agents may be used to prevent renal vasoconstriction during anesthesia that is associated with sympathetic stimulation; these agents include vasodilators, calcium-channel blockers, and prostaglandin $D_2$, $E_2$, and $I_2$. These substances oppose the effects of endogenous norepinephrine, angiotensin, antidiuretic hormones, and atrial natriuretic factor. At the same time, systemic venodilation with hypotension should absolutely be avoided.

## How Much Blood Loss Is Expected?

Imperfect hemostasis during nephrectomy can be associated with considerable blood loss. The use of two large-bore intravenous catheters is indicated because operative blood loss exceeds 500 mL in 25% of patients and transfusion is performed in 75%.[45] The need for transfusion may be less in the future as we continue to redefine and lower our "transfusion trigger"; however, this approach serves to increase other fluids and replace the blood loss.

# PANCREATIC TRANSPLANTATION (WITH OR WITHOUT KIDNEY)

## What Is the Indication for Pancreatic Transplantation?

Pancreatic transplantation is an alternative therapeutic option in the management of diabetes and its complications.[46,47] The purpose of pancreatic transplantation is twofold: (1) to establish normoglycemic insulin independence in a diabetic recipient; (2) to prevent recurrence of diabetic nephropathy in the transplanted kidney.[48] There are a relatively small number of medical centers performing this type of transplantation[2]: in 1998, 84 and 137 centers in the United States and worldwide, respectively, performed renal-pancreatic transplantation; 51 and 67 medical centers in the United States and worldwide, respectively, performed pancreatic transplantation only; and 232 and 578 centers in the United States and worldwide, respectively, performed renal transplantation only. In most centers, pancreatic transplantation is performed in patients who also require renal transplantation or in those who already have a functional renal allograft.[49]

## What Are the Expected Graft and Patient Survival Rates?

Unlike in liver or heart transplantation, in which the primary and immediate objective is to save life, the immediate objective of pancreatic transplantation is to improve the quality of life.[50] Thus, one must be selective in choosing patients in whom one can predict the severity of secondary complications (related to diabetes) that would exceed those of immunosuppression, with transplantation performed when the lesions are still at an early stage. Thus, the best candidates for solitary pancreatic transplantation are patients with poor quality of life, in whom chronic immunosuppression is justified to achieve insulin independence. Simultaneous transplantation of the pancreas and kidney had improved survival only in the post-cyclosporine era since 1980[51,52] (Fig. 76–8). In any case, 1- and 5-year pancreatic graft survival rates are significantly better with simultaneous (pancreas-kidney) transplantation

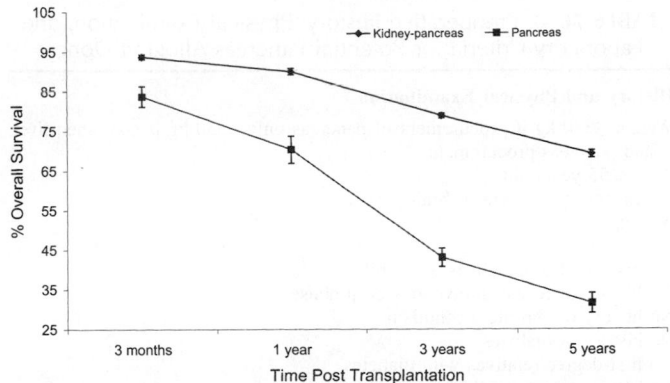

**FIGURE 76–9.** Survival rate and length of survival (in months and years) of grafts after solitary pancreas and simultaneous kidney-pancreas transplants. United Network of Organ Sharing (UNOS) 1998 Annual Report, UNOS Scientific Registry Data, September 8, 1998.

compared with single (pancreas only) transplantation (Fig. 76–9). The outcome after pancreatic transplantation is encouraging: a 1-year patient survival rate of more than 90% and a graft survival rate of more than 70% have been reported.[53] However, there is a consideration that increases morbidity (including infection), and side effects of immunosuppression associated with pancreatic transplantation may outweigh its potential benefits in the management (dialysis, insulin dependence) of anemic diabetic patients.[53,54] Infection is the major cause of morbidity and mortality among pancreas transplant recipients,[55] but not the primary cause of graft failure (Fig. 76–10). Risk factor analysis of graft survival after pancreatic transplantation reveal the following[56,57]: (1) older donors and those with cardiovascular disease should not be considered for any recipient category; (2) preservation time needs to be minimized; (3) strategies should be developed to decrease graft pancreatitis; and (4) surgically left-sided implantation, portal vein extension, and arterial reconstruction (other than Y graft) increase risk. Therefore, the renal transplant in type

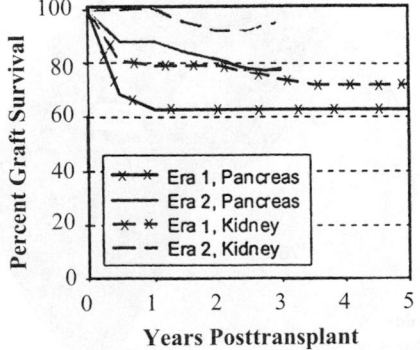

**FIGURE 76–8.** Death-censored pancreas and kidney graft survival rates for simultaneous pancreas-kidney (SPK) transplant recipients who underwent transplantation in Era 1 (1990–1995) compared with Era 2 (1995–1997). (From Stratta RJ, Gaber AO, Shokouh-Amiri MH, et al. Experience with portal-enteric pancreas transplant at the University of Tennessee-Memphis. In: Cecka JM, Teraski PI, eds. *Clinical Transplants 1998.* Los Angeles, Calif: UCLA Tissue Typing Laboratory; 1999:250.)

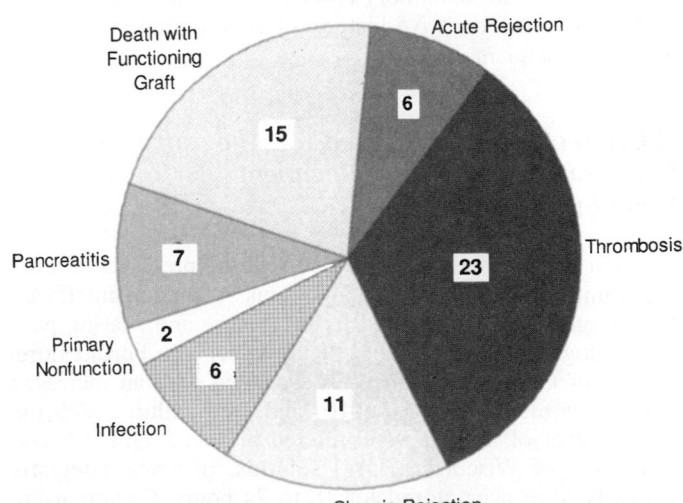

**FIGURE 76–10.** Causes of pancreas graft failure from 1989 to 1997. (From Stratta RJ, Gaber AO, Shokouh-Amiri MH, et al. Experience with portal-enteric pancreas transplant at the University of Tennessee-Memphis. In: Cecka JM, Teraski PI, eds. *Clinical Transplants 1998.* Los Angeles, Calif: UCLA Tissue Typing Laboratory; 1999:249.)

**TABLE 76–8.** Preoperative History, Physical Examination, and Laboratory Criteria for Potential Pancreas Allograft Donors

**History and Physical Examination**

Weight, ≥30 kg if procurement of pancreas only; ≥50 kg if combined liver and pancreas procurement
Age, ≤55 years old
No cancer except skin or brain
No sepsis
No hepatitis
No history of tuberculosis or syphilis
No history of recent intravenous drug abuse
No history of chronic alcoholism
No history of diabetes
No first-degree relatives with diabetes
No history of pancreatitis
No previous splenectomy
No severe chronic hypertension
Previous abdominal surgical procedure acceptable if in an area removed from the pancreas

**Laboratory Examination**

If blood glucose hemoglobin level must be normal, glycosylated hemoglobin level must be normal.
If serum amylase >3 times normal, measure isoenzymes; avoid if pancreatic fraction is increased.
Negative tests for hepatitis, syphilis, and human immunodeficiency virus

From Perkins JD, Fromme GA, Narr BJ, et al. Pancreas transplantation at Mayo, II: operative and perioperative management. *Mayo Clin Proc.* 1990;65:485.

I diabetic patients should always be placed on the left side, allowing right-side pancreatic graft placement.

## What Are the Contraindications to Pancreas Donation?

Contraindications to pancreas donation are diabetes mellitus (type I, II), chronic pancreatitis, and previous pancreatic surgical procedure or trauma. Relative contraindications include alcoholism and bouts of recurrent acute pancreatitis. Candidate (or potential pancreas allograft donors) screening and exclusion should be performed according to preoperative history, physical, and laboratory criteria described in Table 76–8. In donors with a negative history, graft condition is the most important factor in selection.

## What Techniques Are Used for Allograft Preservation and Donor-Recipient Combination?

When Collins preservation was used, the preservation time was limited to less than 6 hours. This restriction interfaced with surgery timing, detailed tissue typing, and sharing pancreas allografts between transplantation centers. Furthermore, the use of Collins solution was associated with an increased thrombosis rate (see Fig. 76–10) and graft failure. With the development of the silica gel-filtered plasma (SGFP-III) and University of Wisconsin (UW) solution, pancreas allografts routinely have been stored for 18 to 24 hours. Centers using those solutions reported a 0% graft thrombosis rate.[58]

For all donors, a lymphocytotoxic crossmatch to all ABO-compatible recipients is performed. When possible, the best HLA match is chosen. If possible, a cytomegalovirus-negative recipient is matched with a cytomegalovirus-negative donor.

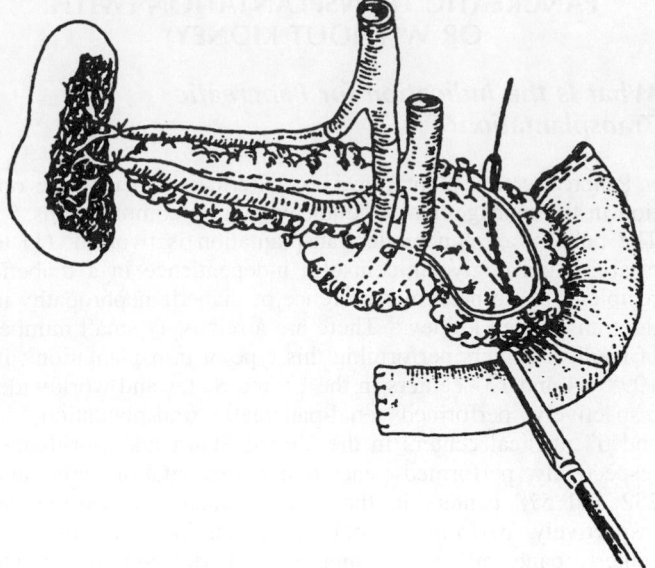

**FIGURE 76–11.** Bench reconstruction of pancreas allograft showing: (1) use of donor common iliac bifurcation Y graft to reconstruct the splenic and superior mesenteric arteries; (2) mobilization of the portal vein; (3) dissection in the splenic hilum with ligation of the splenic vessels in continuity; (4) oversewing, stapling, or individual suture ligation of the superior mesenteric vessels; and (5) tailoring of the duodenum with suture inversion of proximal duodenal staple line but preservation of the third and a variable part of the fourth portion of the duodenum for the portal-enteric procedure. (From Stratta RJ, Gaber AO, Shokouh-Amiri MH, et al. Experience with portal-enteric pancreas transplant at the University of Tennessee-Memphis. In: Cecka JM, Terasaki PI, eds. *Clinical Transplants 1998.* Los Angeles, Calif: UCLA Tissue Typing Laboratory; 1999:241.)

## What Is the Difference Between Pancreatic Transplantation and Other Solid Organ Transplantation That May Change Morbidity?

Underlying diabetes, resulting in abnormal neutrophilic and macrophagic function, and differences in surgical approach[52] (Fig. 76–11) may result in different types of morbidity and infectious complications.[56,58]

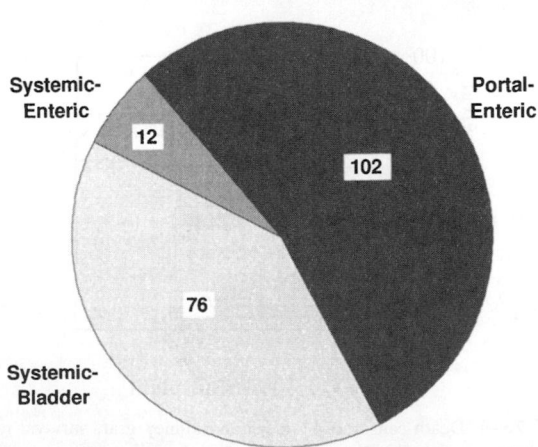

**FIGURE 76–12.** Total number of pancreas transplantations according to technique over the last 10 years. (From Kathaway DK, Winsett RP, Alloway RR, et al. Experience with portal-enteric pancreas transplant at the University of Tennessee-Memphis. In: Cecka JM, Terasaki PI, eds. *Clinical Transplants 1998.* Los Angeles, Calif: UCLA Tissue Typing Laboratory; 1999:240.)

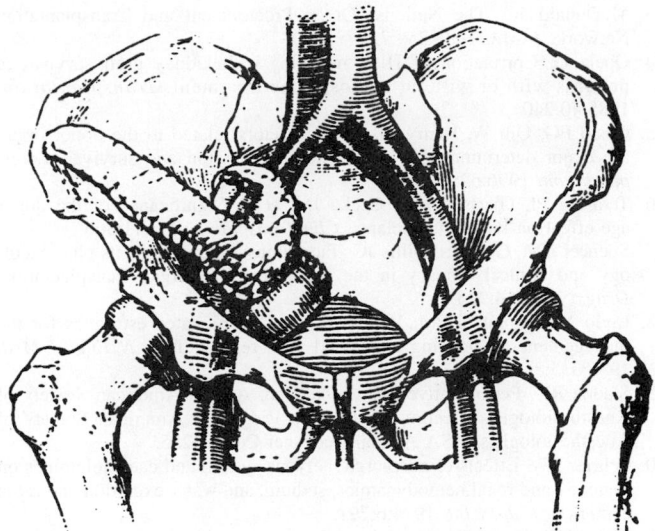

**FIGURE 76–13.** Diagram of pancreaticoduodenal transplant with duodenum anastomosed to posterolateral aspect of urinary bladder. (From Perkins JD, Fromme GA, Narr BJ, et al. Pancreas transplantation at Mayo, II: operative and perioperative management. *Mayo Clin Proc.* 1990;65:488.)

The specific areas of development include selection of donors, preservation procedures, engraftment (surgical) procedures, and anesthetic and intensive care management.[58]

## What Is the Surgical Technique Used in Pancreatic Transplantation?

The technique of pancreatic transplantation is a segmental transplantation with instantaneous or delayed duct occlusion using a portal-enteric procedure (Fig. 76–12) or a whole-organ pancreatic-duodenal transplant. Pancreatic transplantation is performed with portal venous drainage (of insulin) into the venous portal or systemic (ie, superior mesenteric) system and with enteric exocrine drainage into the bladder (Fig. 76–13) or into the gut (enteric or diverting Roux limb).[52,58]

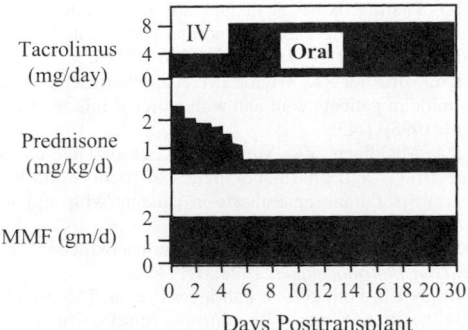

**FIGURE 76–14.** Methodology of triple immunosuppression with tacrolimus, mycophenolate mofetil (MMF), and steroids without antilymphocyte induction. (From Stratta RJ, Gaber AO, Shokouh-Amiri MH, et al. Experience with portal-enteric pancreas transplant at the University of Tennessee-Memphis. In: Cecka JM, Terasaki PI, eds. *Clinical Transplants 1998.* Los Angeles, Calif: UCLA Tissue Typing Laboratory; 1999:244.)

**TABLE 76–9.** Insulin Infusion Protocol for Pancreas Transplantation

| Blood glucose (mg/dL) | Insulin Infusion Rate (U/h) |
| --- | --- |
| ≥250 | 3.0 |
| 200–249 | 2.5 |
| 150–199 | 2.0 |
| 120–149 | 1.5 |
| 100–119 | 1.0 |
| 70–99 | 0.5 |
| <70 | 0.2 |

From Perkins JD, Fromme GA, Narr BJ, et al. Pancreas transplantation at Mayo, II: operative and perioperative management. *Mayo Clin Proc.* 1990;65:486.

## What Is the Typical Immunosuppressive Therapy Used in Pancreatic Transplantation?

Immunosuppressive therapy includes cyclosporine, azathioprine, corticosteroids (prednisone or methylprednisolone), and antilymphocytic globulin. Other new drugs used are tacrolimus[7] and mycophenolate mofetil.[52] A typical protocol for intraoperative and postoperative administration is presented in Figure 76–14.

## What Is Different in Pancreatic Transplantation for the Anesthesiologist?

The perioperative management of the diabetes in patients who undergo pancreatic transplantation is similar to the treatment of diabetes in patients who have undergone other major surgery: maintaining metabolic stability, avoiding hypoglycemia, and preventing excessive hyperglycemia and ketosis. The perioperative management of anesthesia should be focused on cardiovascular stability and viability of the transplanted organ.

During the evaluation phase for pancreatic transplantation, particular attention is paid to the cardiovascular status. After hospital admission, hourly glucose levels are obtained, and a continuous insulin infusion is commenced in accordance with

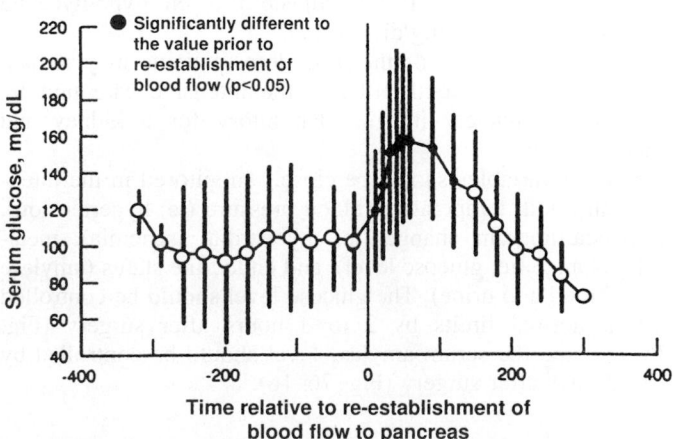

**FIGURE 76–15.** Serum glucose levels during pancreaticoduodenal transplantation. The *vertical* lines depict range of values. On *horizontal* axis, time is shown in minutes. (From Perkins JD, Fromme GA, Narr BJ, et al. Pancreas transplantation at Mayo, II: operative and perioperative management. *Mayo Clin Proc.* 1990;65:492.)

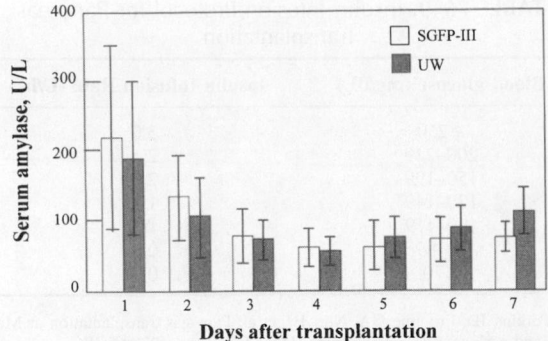

FIGURE 76–16. Serum amylase values after preservation of allograft in silica gel–filtered plasma (SGFP-III) or University of Wisconsin solution (UW). Data are shown as mean ± SE. (From Perkins JD, Fromme GA, Narr BJ, et al. Pancreas transplantation at Mayo, II: operative and perioperative management. *Mayo Clin Proc.* 1990;65:490).

a predetermined protocol (Table 76–9). This protocol can be continued in the operating room during surgery. A triple-lumen central venous catheter may be placed for intraoperative fluid management and postoperative hyperalimentation.

During anesthetic induction, regurgitation of gastric contents is prevented by using cricoid pressure. Otherwise, induction and maintenance of anesthesia is no different than that performed in any other abdominal case (with or without renal failure). The initial monitoring should include electrocardiogram lead V5, noninvasive blood pressure measurement, pulse oximetry, and central venous pressure (indicated in patients with potential cardiovascular instability). Patient temperature should be controlled during the procedure (eg, using a heating blanket or warm lines). Glucose levels should be determined at 30-minute intervals throughout the operation and at 10-minute intervals in the first hour after pancreas circulation is reestablished. Serum glucose values should be maintained at about 100 mg/dL by a continuous infusion of insulin (see Table 76–9). Arterial blood gases can be measured after induction (baseline) and before (10 minutes) and after (1 hour) pancreas circulation is reestablished. The patient should receive a dextrose-free solution with saline (combined kidney-pancreas transplantation) or lactated Ringer's solution (pancreas transplantation only). Dextrose-containing solutions are added (and insulin infusion adjusted) when hypoglycemia (glucose level, <50 mg/dL) occurs.

At the completion of the procedure, patients may remain intubated and are transported to the intensive care unit by way of the nuclear imaging laboratory for a kidney and pancreas scan.

Several variables should be closely monitored in the intensive care unit: temperature, blood pressure (ie, hypertension), electrocardiogram change (ie, myocardial ischemia), metabolic change (ie, glucose level), and endocrine status (amylase level blood and urine). The glucose level should be controlled within normal limits by 2 to 3 hours after surgery (Fig. 76–15), and the serum amylase level should be controlled by 2 to 3 days after surgery (Fig. 76–16).

## References

1. Terasaki PI, Perdue ST, Sasaki N, et al. Improving success rates of kidney transplantation. *JAMA.* 1983;250:1065.
2. Cecka JM, Terasaki PI, eds. *Clinical Transplants 1998.* Los Angeles, Calif: UCLA Tissue Typing Laboratory; 1999:1.
3. McDonald JC. The National Organ Procurement and Transplantation Network. *JAMA.* 1988;259:725.
4. Opelz G. Correlation of HLA matching with kidney graft survival in patients with or without cyclosporine treatment. *Transplantation.* 1985;40:240.
5. Cosio FG, Qiu W, Henry ML, et al. Factors related to the donor organ are major determinants of renal allograft function and survival. *Transplantation.* 1996;62:1571.
6. Terasaki PI, Gjertson DW, Cecka JM, et al. Significance of the donor age effect on kidney transplants. *Clin Transplant.* 1997;11:366.
7. Spencer CM, Goa KL, Gillis JC. Tacrolimus: an update of its pharmacology and clinical efficacy in the management of organ transplantation. *Drugs.* 1997;54:925.
8. Livio M, Mannucci PM, Vigano G, et al. Conjugated estrogens for the management of bleeding associated with renal failure. *N Engl J Med.* 1986;315:86.
9. Sladen RN. Perioperative renal protection. Annual American Society of Anesthesiologists Meeting; 1991; Park Ridge, Ill: American Society of Anesthesiologists. ASA Annual Refresher Course 255.
10. Schrier RW. Effects of adrenergic nervous system and catecholamines on systemic and renal hemodynamics, sodium, and water excretion and renin excretion. *Kidney Int.* 1974;6:291.
11. Weir PHC, Chung FF. Anaesthesia for patients with chronic renal disease. *Can Anaesth Soc J.* 1984;31:468.
12. Cook DR. Anesthetic considerations for organ transplantation. ASA Annual Refresher Course #255. 1989 Annual ASA meeting. Park Ridge, Ill: American Society of Anesthesiologists, 1991.
13. Don HF, Dieppa RA, Taylor P. Narcotic analgesics in anuric patients. *Anesthesiology.* 1975;42:745.
14. Wiggum DC, Cork RC, Weldon ST, et al. Postoperative respiratory depression and elevated sufentanil levels in a patient with chronic renal failure. *Anesthesiology.* 1985;63:708.
15. Smith BE. Renal failure, renal transplantation, and anesthesia. ASA Annual Refresher Course #241. 1990 Annual ASA meeting. Park Ridge, Ill: American Society of Anesthesiologists, 1990.
16. Bready LL. Kidney transplantation. *Anesth Clin North Am.* 1989;7:487.
17. Tilstone WJ, Fine A. Furosemide kinetics in renal failure. *Clin Pharmacol Ther.* 1978;23:644.
18. Lowenthal DT. Pharmacokinetics of propranolol, quinidine, procainamide, and lidocaine in chronic renal disease. *Am J Med.* 1977;62:532.
19. Sidi A, Kaplan RF, Davis RF. Prolonged neuromuscular blockade and ventilatory failure after renal transplantation and cyclosporine. *Can J Anaesth.* 1990;37:543.
20. Dretchen KL, Morgenroth VH, Standaert FG, et al. Azathioprine: effects on neuromuscular transmission. *Anesthesiology.* 1976;45:604.
21. Carlier M, Squifflet JP, Pirson Y, et al. Maximal hydration during anesthesia increases pulmonary artery pressures and improves early function of human renal transplant. *Transplantation.* 1982;34:201.
22. Slogoff S, Keats AS, Arlund C. On the safety of radial artery cannulation. *Anesthesiology.* 1983;59:42.
23. Orko R, Pitkanen M, Rosenberg PH. Subarachnoid anaesthesia with 0.75% bupivacaine in patients with chronic renal failure. *Br J Anaesth.* 1985;58:605.
24. Bishop MJ, Hornbein TF. Prolonged effect of succinylcholine after neostigmine and pyridostigmine administration in patients with renal failure. *Anesthesiology.* 1983;58:384.
25. Miller RD. Pharmacokinetics of atracurium and other nondepolarizing neuromuscular blocking agents in normal patients and those with renal or hepatic dysfunction. *Br J Anaesth.* 1986;58:11S.
26. Cooper RA, Mirakhur RK, Wierda JM, et al. Pharmacokinetics of rocuronium bromide in patients with and without renal failure. *Eur J Anaesthesiol Suppl.* 1995;11:43.
27. Cooper RA, Maddineni VR, Mirakhur RK, et al. Time course of neuromuscular effects and pharmacokinetics of rocuronium bromide (Org 9426) during isoflurane anaesthesia in patients with and without renal failure. *Br J Anaesth.* 1993;71:222.
28. Khuenl-Brady KS, Sparr N. Clinical pharmacokinetics of rocuronium bromide. *Clin Pharmacokinet.* 1996;31:174.
29. Khuenl-Brady KS, Pomaroli A, Puhringer F, et al. The use of rocuronium (ORG 9426) in patients with chronic renal failure. *Anaesthesia.* 1993;48:873.
30. Szenohradszky J, Fisher DM, Segredo V, et al. Pharmacokinetics of rocuronium bromide (ORG 9426) in patients with normal renal function or patients undergoing cadaver renal transplantation. *Anesthesiology.* 1992;77:899.
31. Miller RD, Cullen DJ. Renal failure and postoperative respiratory failure: recurarization? *Br J Anaesth.* 1976;48:253.

32. McLeod K, Watson MJ, Rawlings MD. Pharmacokinetics of pancuronium in patients with normal and impaired renal function. *Br J Anaesth.* 1976;48:341.

33. Borges HF, Hocks J, Kjellstrand CM. Mannitol intoxication in patients with renal failure. *Arch Intern Med.* 1982;142:63.

34. Charters P. Mannitol, osmolality and steroids during renal transplantation. *Anaesthesia.* 1983;38:327.

35. Freilich JD, Waterman PM, Rosenthal JT. Acute hemodynamic changes during renal transplantation. *Anesth Analg.* 1984;63:158.

36. Hirshman CA, Leon D, Edelstein G, et al. Risk of hyperkalemia in recipients of kidneys preserved with an intracellular electrolyte solution. *Anesth Analg.* 1980;59:283.

37. Ivey GL, Richie RE, Niblack GD, et al. Renal transplantation: a twenty-year experience in a Veterans Administration Medical Center. *Arch Surg.* 1985;120:1021.

38. Bartlett ST, Garney AC, Jarrell BE, et al. Kidney transplantation at the University of Maryland. In: In: Cecka JM, Terasaki PI, eds. *Clinical Transplants 1998.* Los Angeles, Calif: UCLA Tissue Typing Laboratory; 1999:177.

39. Phillips MG. Cadaver-donor nephrectomy. In: Glenn JF, ed. *Urologic Surgery.* Philadelphia, Pa: JB Lippincott; 1983:329.

40. Aldrete JA, Swanson JT, Penn I, et al. Anesthesia experience with living renal transplant donors. *Anesth Analg.* 1971;50:169.

41. Dixon C, Sefton W, Gravenstein N. Epidural analgesia after donor nephrectomy decreases duration of hospitalization [abstract]. *Reg Anesth.* 1992;17(3S):75.

42. Priebe HJ, Hedley-Whyte J. Respiratory support and renal function. *Int Anesth Clin.* 1984;22:203.

43. Annat G, Viale JP, Xuan BB, et al. Effect of PEEP ventilation on renal function, plasma renin, aldosterone, neurophysins and urinary ADH, and prostaglandins. *Anesthesiology.* 1983;58:136.

44. Lindner A, Cutler RE, Goodman G. Synergism of dopamine plus furosemide in preventing acute renal failure in the dog. *Kidney Int.* 1979;16:158.

45. Weiland D, Sutherland DER, Chavers B, et al. Information on 628 living-related kidney donors at a single institution, with long-term follow-up in 472 cases. *Transplant Proc.* 1984;16:5.

46. Sutherland DER, Dunn DL, Goetz FC, et al. A 10-year experience with 290 pancreas transplants at a single institution. *Ann Surg.* 1989;210:274.

47. Kennedy WR, Navarro X, Goetz FC, et al. Effects of pancreatic transplantation on diabetic neuropathy. *N Engl J Med.* 1990;322:1031.

48. Bilous RW, Mauer SM, Sutherland DER, et al. The effects of pancreas transplantation on the glomerular structure of renal allografts in patients with insulin-dependent diabetes. *N Engl J Med.* 1989;321:180.

49. Sutherland DE, Gruber SA. Pancreas transplantation. *Crit Care Clin.* 1990;6:947.

50. Milde FK, Hart LK, Zehr PS. Quality of life of pancreatic transplant recipients. *Diabetes Care.* 1992;15:1459.

51. Largiader F. Long-term results in pancreas transplantation in diabetes in the pre-cyclosporin era. *Schweiz Med Wochenschr.* 1996;126(ISS 34):1433.

52. Stratta RJ, Gaber AO, Shokouh-Amiri MH, et al. Experience with portal-enteric pancreas transplant at the University of Tennessee-Memphis. In: Cecka JM, Terasaki PI, eds. *Clinical Transplants 1998.* Los Angeles, Calif: UCLA Tissue Typing Laboratory; 1999:177.

53. Sutherland DE. Pancreatic transplantation: state of the art. *Transplant Proc.* 1992;24:762.

54. Remuzzi G, Ruggenenti P, Mauer SM. Pancreas and kidney/pancreas transplants: experimental medicine or real improvement? *Lancet.* 1994;343:27.

55. Cheung AHS, Sutherland DER, Gillingham KJ, et al. Simultaneous pancreas-kidney transplant versus kidney transplant alone in diabetic patients. *Kidney Int.* 1992;41:924.

56. Perkins JD, Frohnert PP, Service FJ, et al. Pancreas transplantation at Mayo, III: multidisciplinary management. *Mayo Clin Proc.* 1990;65:496.

57. Troppmann C, Gruessner AC, Benedetti E, et al. Vascular graft thrombosis after pancreatic transplantation: univariate and multivariate operative and nonoperative risk factor analysis [see comments]. *J Am Coll Surg.* 1996;182:285.

58. Perkins JD, Fromme GA, Narr BJ, et al. Pancreas transplantation at Mayo. II. Operative and perioperative management. *Mayo Clin Proc.* 1990;65:483.

# Index

Note: Page numbers followed by the letter f refer to figures; those followed by the letter t refer to tables.

A fibers, nerve, 664–665, 665t
A Severity Characterization of Trauma score, 718
a wave, of central venous pressure, 396, 396f
AARKs. *See* Automated anesthesia recordkeepers (AARKs).
ABCs of CPR, 892
Abdomen
  bleeding in, in trauma, 737
  blood flow in, carbon dioxide pneumoperitoneum effects on, 1523
  compression of, in circulation restoration, 896–897
  distention of
    hypoventilation in, 880
    radiography of, 224
  hypertension in. *See* Abdominal compartment syndrome/intraabdominal hypertension.
  injury of, 727–728
    thoracic injury with, 736
  insufflation of, with carbon dioxide, in laparoscopy, 1519–1523, 1521f–1523f, 1526–1528, 1527f, 1528f, 1528t
  motion of, monitoring of, 353
  pain in, in pediatric patients, 273
  position of, in supine to prone move, 550, 550f, 551f
  pressure in
    increased, larynx function in, 473–474, 474f
    measurement of, 1205
    versus functional residual capacity, 92
  radiography of, 224–230, 227f–230f
  surgery on. *See* Abdominal surgery.
  trauma to, in pregnancy, 1169
  visceral puncture in, during sympathetic blockade, 521
  wall of
    defects of, in neonates, 1075–1076, 1075f, 1076f
    hernia of, 1177–1178, 1203
    muscles of, tightness and relaxation of, 1177–1178
    surgery on, 1203
Abdominal compartment syndrome/intraabdominal hypertension, 737, 1203–1206
  causes of, 1204–1205
  diagnosis of, 1205
  pathophysiology of, 1204–1205, 1204f, 1205f
  pressure measurement in, 1205
  treatment of, 1205–1206
Abdominal surgery, 1176–1210
  anesthesia for
    biliary spasm in, 1185
    bowel distention in, 1184–1185, 1184f
    epidural, 269, 1182–1183, 1202–1203
    general, 1178
    in acute bleeding, 1190
    in liver resection, 1193–1194
    in portosystemic shunting, 1198
    spinal, 1182–1183

Abdominal surgery *(Continued)*
  bleeding in, 1190
  emergency, rapid-sequence induction in, 1185–1187, 1187f
  fluid management in, 1187–1190
    in acute pathology, 1189
    intraoperative deficit and, 1187
    losses and, 1189
    normovolemic oliguria and, 1188
    preoperative bowel preparation effects on, 1188–1189
    preoperative deficit and, 1187
    replacement in, 1188–1190
    third space losses and, 1188
  hypotension in, 1183–1184, 1183f, 1183t
  in ascites, 1194, 1195f
  in chronic obstructive lung disease, 1036, 1036t
  in obstructive jaundice, 1191
  in pediatric patients, epidural anesthesia for, 269
  induction in, rapid-sequence, 1185–1187, 1187f
  intestinal motility disorders after, 1202–1203
  intraabdominal hypertension in, 1203–1206, 1204f, 1205f
  laparoscopic. *See* Laparoscopy.
  liver resection as, 1191–1194, 1192f
  liver transplantation as. *See* Liver transplantation.
  lower, regional anesthesia for, 1182
  muscle relaxants/relaxation for, 1178–1182
    administration of, 1179
    bowel anastomosis and, 1181
    clinical criteria for, 1180
    duration of, 1179
    during peritoneal closure, 1181
    greatest need for, 1180
    hiccups and, 1180–1181
    nerve stimulator in, 1179–1180, 1180f
    reestablishment of, after reversal, 1181–1182
    selection of, 1179
  nasogastric tubes for, 1185–1187, 1186f
  pancreas transplantation as, 1605–1608, 1605f–1608f, 1607t
  peritoneovenous shunting as, 1195–1196, 1196f
  portosystemic shunting as, 1116f, 1196–1199, 1197f, 1198t
  pulmonary complications in, 164–165
  pulmonary effects of, 1199–1202, 1199f, 1200f, 1200t
  renal failure in, 1191
  splenectomy as, 1190–1191
  upper, regional anesthesia for, 1182
  wall, 1203
    tightness and relaxation in, 1177–1178
Abortion, spontaneous, in trace gas exposure, 952, 1165
Abruption, placental, in trauma, 1169
Abscess, pharyngeal, 1427
Abuse, drug. *See* Drug abuse.
Accelomyography, in neuromuscular block monitoring, 450, 450f